DRUG INFORMATION HANDBOOK for PSYCHIATRY

Including

Psychotropic, Nonpsychotropic, and Herbal Agents

Senior Editors:

Matthew A. Fuller, PharmD

Martha Sajatovic, MD

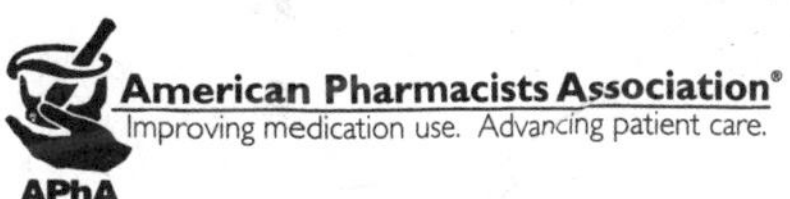

Lexi-Comp is the official drug reference for the American Pharmacists Association

7th Edition

DRUG INFORMATION HANDBOOK for PSYCHIATRY

Including

Psychotropic, Nonpsychotropic, and Herbal Agents

Matthew A. Fuller, PharmD, BCPS, BCPP, FASHP
Senior Editor
Clinical Pharmacy Specialist, Psychiatry
Cleveland Department of Veterans Affairs Medical Center
Brecksville, Ohio
Associate Clinical Professor of Psychiatry
Clinical Instructor of Psychology
Case Western Reserve University
Cleveland, Ohio
Adjunct Associate Professor of Clinical Pharmacy
University of Toledo
Toledo, Ohio

Martha Sajatovic, MD
Senior Editor
Professor of Psychiatry
Case Western Reserve University
Cleveland, Ohio
Department of Psychiatry
University Hospitals of Cleveland
Cleveland, Ohio

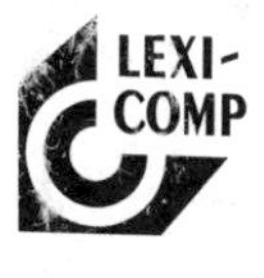

LEXI-COMP INC

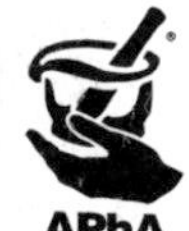

APhA

NOTICE

This data is intended to serve the user as a handy reference and not as a complete drug information resource. It does not include information on every therapeutic agent available. The publication covers over 1200 commonly used drugs and is specifically designed to present important aspects of drug data in a more concise format than is typically found in medical literature or product material supplied by manufacturers.

The nature of drug information is that it is constantly evolving because of ongoing research and clinical experience and is often subject to interpretation. While great care has been taken to ensure the accuracy of the information and recommendations presented, the reader is advised that the authors, editors, reviewers, contributors, and publishers cannot be responsible for the continued currency of the information or for any errors, omissions, or the application of this information, or for any consequences arising therefrom. Therefore, the author(s) and/or the publisher shall have no liability to any person or entity with regard to claims, loss, or damage caused, or alleged to be caused, directly or indirectly, by the use of information contained herein. Because of the dynamic nature of drug information, readers are advised that decisions regarding drug therapy must be based on the independent judgment of the clinician, changing information about a drug (eg, as reflected in the literature and manufacturer's most current product information), and changing medical practices. Therefore, this data is designed to be used in conjunction with other necessary information and is not designed to be solely relied upon by any user. The user of this data hereby and forever releases the authors and publishers of this data from any and all liability of any kind that might arise out of the use of this data. The editors are not responsible for any inaccuracy of quotation or for any false or misleading implication that may arise due to the text or formulas as used or due to the quotation of revisions no longer official.

Certain of the authors, editors, and contributors have written this book in their private capacities. No official support or endorsement by any federal or state agency or pharmaceutical company is intended or inferred.

The publishers have made every effort to trace any third party copyright holders, if any, for borrowed material. If they have inadvertently overlooked any, they will be pleased to make the necessary arrangements at the first opportunity.

If you have any suggestions or questions regarding any information presented in this data, please contact our drug information pharmacists at (330) 650-6506.

This manual was produced using Lexi-Comp's Information Management System™ (LIMS) — a complete publishing service of Lexi-Comp Inc.

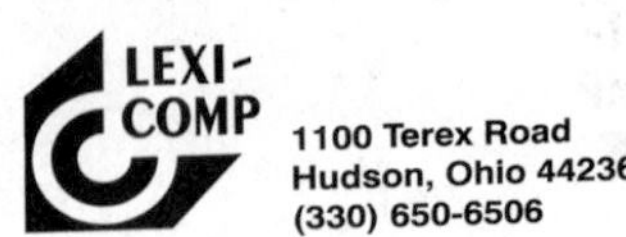

ISBN 978-1-59195-253-4

TABLE OF CONTENTS

About the Authors 2
Editorial Advisory Panel 4
Preface 11
Description of Fields and Sections in This Handbook 12
FDA Pregnancy Categories 16
FDA Name Differentiation Project The Use of Tall-Man Letters 17
Safe Writing 20

Alphabetical Listing of Drugs 21

Special Topics 1717
- Psychiatric Assessment 1718
- Diagnostic & Statistical Manual of Mental Disorders (DSM-IV) 1729

Appendix 1745
- Abbreviations and Measurements 1746
- Assessment of Renal Function 1749
- Comparative Drug Charts 1751
- Cytochrome P450 & Drug Interactions 1799
- Therapy Guidelines 1815
- Therapy Recommendations 1817
- Miscellaneous 1839

Alphabetical Index 1849

ABOUT THE AUTHORS

MATTHEW A. FULLER, PharmD

Dr Fuller received his Bachelor of Science in Pharmacy from Ohio Northern University and then earned a Doctor of Pharmacy degree from the University of Cincinnati. A residency in hospital pharmacy was completed at Bethesda hospital in Zanesville, Ohio. After completion of his training, Dr Fuller accepted a position at the Louis Stokes Department of Veterans Affairs Medical Center in Cleveland, Ohio

Dr Fuller has over 20 years of experience in psychiatric psychopharmacology in a variety of clinical settings including acute care and ambulatory care. Dr Fuller is currently a Clinical Pharmacy Specialist in Psychiatry at the Louis Stokes Cleveland Department of Veterans Affairs Medical Center in Cleveland, Ohio. He is also an Associate Clinical Professor of Psychiatry and Clinical Instructor of Psychology at Case Western Reserve University in Cleveland, Ohio and Adjunct Associate Professor of Clinical Pharmacy at the University of Toledo in Toledo, Ohio. In this position, Dr Fuller is responsible for providing service, education, and research. He is also the Director of an ASHP accredited Psychiatric Pharmacy Practice Residency Program.

Dr Fuller has received several awards including the Upjohn Excellence in Research Award and the OSHP Hospital Pharmacist of the Year Award in 1994. In 1996, he received the CSHP Evelyn Gray Scott Award (Pharmacist of the Year). In 2001, he received the OSHP Pharmacy Practice Research Award.

Dr Fuller is Board Certified by the Board of Pharmaceutical Specialties in both Pharmacotherapy and Psychiatric Pharmacy. He speaks regularly on the topic of psychotropic use and has published articles and abstracts on various issues in psychiatric psychopharmacology. His research interests include the psychopharmacologic treatment of schizophrenia and bipolar disorder.

Dr Fuller is a member of numerous professional organizations, including the College of Psychiatric and Neurologic Pharmacists (CPNP) where he recently completed his term is President. He is also a member of the American Society of Health-System Pharmacists (ASHP), where he is designated as a fellow. He completed his term as a member of the Commission on Therapeutics and is a member of the Clinical Specialist Section; Ohio Society of Health-System Pharmacists (OSHP) where he has served as an Educational Affairs Division member and a House of Delegates member; American College of Clinical Pharmacy (ACCP); Ohio College of Clinical Pharmacy where he served as secretary/treasurer; and Cleveland Society of Health-System Pharmacist (CSHP) where he has served as the education chair and treasurer. He is a member of the National Alliance for the Mentally Ill (NAMI) and also serves as a reviewer for pharmacy and psychiatric journals. He is also a member of the psychiatry editorial board for the *Annals of Pharmacotherapy*.

Special thanks from Dr Fuller to his parents, Raymond and Mary Fuller, who afforded him the opportunity to write this book; and to his wife and son, Jeanette and Samuel, who generously gave of their time and support.

MARTHA SAJATOVIC, MD

Dr Sajatovic is Professor of Psychiatry at Case Western Reserve University School of Medicine in Cleveland, Ohio. She is a researcher, educator, and clinician who has devoted herself to the study and treatment of traditionally hard-to-treat populations with serious mental illness. Dr Sajatovic is currently a clinical researcher and director of Geropsychiatry at University Hospitals of Cleveland.

Dr Sajatovic's research interests have focused on illness outcomes in serious mental illness such as bipolar disorder and schizophrenia. She also has research interests in the psychopharmacology of psychosis and serious mood disorders and in mental health rating scales. Over the last two decades, Dr Sajatovic has been the recipient of multiple research grants to study serious mental illness including support from the National Institute of Mental Health (NIMH), the Ohio Department of Mental Health (ODMH), the Veterans Health Administration (VHA), a variety of Mental Health Foundations, and Industry Sponsored clinical trials.

Dr Sajatovic has published widely on treatments and health services delivery among individuals with serious mental illness including geriatric and mixed-age individuals with bipolar disorder, schizophrenia, depression, and post-traumatic stress disorder as well as in the area of treatment adherence in bipolar disorder. She has authored or coauthored over 80 peer-reviewed publications and has published over 25 book chapters or books on serious mental illness topics.

Dr Sajatovic has been a guest lecturer at numerous academic and community settings, both on a national and international level, including speaking to consumer and family advocacy groups for individuals with psychiatric illness. Dr Sajatovic has been a recipient of the Exemplary Psychiatrist Award bestowed by the National Alliance for the Mentally Ill (NAMI) and was a Depression and Bipolar Support Alliance (DBSA) 2006 Gerald Klerman Young Investigator Award winner.

EDITORIAL ADVISORY PANEL

Harold L. Crossley, DDS, PhD
Associate Professor of Pharmacology
Baltimore College of Dental Surgery
Dental School
University of Maryland Baltimore
Baltimore, Maryland

Laura Cummings, PharmD, BCPS
Clinical Pharmacy Specialist, Pediatrics
The Children's Hospital at MetroHealth
Cleveland, Ohio

Andrew J. Donnelly, PharmD, MBA
Director of Pharmacy
and
Clinical Professor of Pharmacy Practice
University of Illinois Medical Center at Chicago
Chicago, Illinois

Julie A. Dopheide, PharmD, BCPP
Associate Professor of Clinical Pharmacy, Psychiatry and the Behavioral Sciences
University of Southern California
Schools of Pharmacy and Medicine
Los Angeles, California

Michael S. Edwards, PharmD, MBA
Chief, Oncology Pharmacy
Director, Oncology Pharmacy Residency Program
Walter Reed Army Medical Center
Washington, D.C.

Vicki L. Ellingrod, PharmD, BCPP
Associate Professor
University of Iowa
Iowa City, Iowa

Kelley K. Engle, BSPharm
Pharmacotherapy Specialist
Lexi-Comp, Inc
Hudson, Ohio

Erin Fabian, PharmD, RPh
Pharmacotherapy Specialist
Lexi-Comp, Inc
Hudson, Ohio

Margaret A. Fitzgerald, MS, APRN, BC, NP-C, FAANP
President
Fitzgerald Health Education Associates, Inc.
North Andover, Massachusetts
Family Nurse Practitioner
Greater Lawrence Family Health Center
Lawrence, Massachusetts

Lawrence A. Frazee, PharmD
Pharmacotherapy Specialist in Internal Medicine
Akron General Medical Center
Akron, Ohio

Matthew A. Fuller, PharmD, BCPS, BCPP, FASHP
Clinical Pharmacy Specialist, Psychiatry
Cleveland Department of Veterans Affairs Medical Center
Brecksville, Ohio
Associate Clinical Professor of Psychiatry
Clinical Instructor of Psychology
Case Western Reserve University
Cleveland, Ohio
Adjunct Associate Professor of Clinical Pharmacy
University of Toledo
Toledo, Ohio

Morton P. Goldman, RPh, PharmD, BCPS, FCCP
Director of Pharmacotherapy Services
The Cleveland Clinic Foundation
Cleveland, Ohio

Jill M. Kolesar, PharmD, FCCP, BCPS
Associate Professor
School of Pharmacy
Associate Professor
University of Wisconsin Paul P. Carbone Comprehensive Cancer Center
University of Wisconsin
Madison, Wisconsin

Donna M. Kraus, PharmD, FAPhA
Associate Professor of Pharmacy Practice
Departments of Pharmacy Practice and Pediatrics
Pediatric Clinical Pharmacist
University of Illinois
Chicago, Illinois

Kay Kyllonen, PharmD
Clinical Specialist
The Cleveland Clinic Children's Hospital
Cleveland, Ohio

Charles Lacy, MS, PharmD, FCSHP
Vice President for Executive Affairs
Professor, Pharmacy Practice
Professor, Business Leadership
University of Southern Nevada
Las Vegas, Nevada

Brenda R. Lance, RN, MSN
Program Development Director
Northcoast HealthCare Management Company
Northcoast Infusion Network
Beachwood, Ohio

Leonard L. Lance, RPh, BSPharm
Clinical Pharmacist
Lexi-Comp, Inc
Hudson, Ohio

Jerrold B. Leikin, MD, FACP, FACEP, FACMT, FAACT
Director, Medical Toxicology
Evanston Northwestern Healthcare-OMEGA
Glenbrook Hospital
Glenview, Illinois
Associate Director
Toxikon Consortium at Cook County Hospital
Chicago, Illinois
Professor of Medicine
Pharmacology and Health Systems Management
Rush Medical College
Chicago, Ilinois
Professor of Medicine
Feinberg School of Medicine
Northwestern University
Chicago, Ilinois

Jeffrey D. Lewis, PharmD
Pharmacotherapy Specialist
Lexi-Comp, Inc
Hudson, Ohio

Laurie S. Mauro, BS, PharmD
Professor of Clinical Pharmacy
College of Pharmacy
Adjunct Associate Professor of Medicine
College of Medicine
The University of Toledo
Toledo, Ohio

Vincent F. Mauro, BS, PharmD, FCCP
Professor of Clinical Pharmacy
College of Pharmacy
Adjunct Professor of Medicine
College of Medicine
The University of Toledo
Toledo, Ohio

Jennifer K. Sekeres, PharmD, BCPS
Infectious Diseases Clinical Specialist
The Cleveland Clinic Foundation
Cleveland, Ohio

Todd P. Semla, PharmD, BCPS, FCCP, AGSF
Clinical Pharmacy Specialist
Department of Veterans Affairs
Pharmacy Benefits Management Services
Associate Professor, Clinical
Department of Medicine and Psychiatry and Behavioral Health
Feinberg School of Medicine
Northwestern University
Chicago, Illinois

Joe Snoke, RPh, BCPS
Manager
Core Pharmacology Group
Lexi-Comp, Inc
Hudson, Ohio

Dominic A. Solimando, Jr, MA, FAPhA, FASHP, BCOP
Oncology Pharmacist
President, Oncology Pharmacy Services, Inc
Arlington, Virginia

Joni Lombardi Stahura, BS, PharmD, RPh
Pharmacotherapy Specialist
Lexi-Comp, Inc
Hudson, Ohio

Dan Streetman, PharmD, RPh
Pharmacotherapy Specialist
Lexi-Comp, Inc
Hudson, Ohio

Darcie-Ann Streetman, PharmD, RPh
Pharmacotherapy Specialist
Lexi-Comp, Inc
Hudson, Ohio

Carol K. Taketomo, PharmD
Pharmacy Manager
Children's Hospital Los Angeles
Los Angeles, California

Mary Temple, PharmD
Pediatric Clinical Research Specialist
Hillcrest Hospital
Mayfield Heights, Ohio

Elizabeth A. Tomsik, PharmD, BCPS
Manager
Adverse Drug Reactions Group
Lexi-Comp, Inc
Hudson, Ohio

Dana Travis, RPh
Pharmacotherapy Specialist
Lexi-Comp, Inc
Hudson, Ohio

Jennifer Trofe, PharmD
Clinical Transplant Pharmacist
Hospital of The University of Pennsylvania
Philadelphia, Pennsylvania

Beatrice B. Turkoski, RN, PhD
Associate Professor, Graduate Faculty,
Advanced Pharmacology
College of Nursing
Kent State University
Kent, Ohio

PREFACE

Our Seventh edition of the *Drug Information Handbook for Psychiatry* continues our efforts to provide an up-to-date, easy-to-use, portable source of drug information for mental healthcare professionals. To this aim, we have added new monographs and have updated our existing monographs with new indications, contraindications, warning/precautions, adverse effects, drug interactions, dosing information, and dosage forms that may have changed over the past year. The Effect on Mental Status and Effect on Psychiatric Treatment fields have been updated and included for new drugs. These fields were added in an effort to inform the mental health provider of potential psychiatric considerations. These considerations may require the practitioner to make adjustments to a patient's medication regimen. In addition, the Appendix, as well as the Psychiatric Special Topics/Issues section has been revised and updated. We have also added new drug comparison tables to the appendix.

We have condensed many monographs of infrequently-used compounds or ones not likely to be used by the mental healthcare practitioner. Therefore, all information fields are not included in all drug monographs. A Mental Health Comment field has been added to many psychotropic drug monographs. Our hope is that this information will provide useful clinical pearls for the practitioner. Herbal monographs have been included as in the past.

We hope this seventh edition proves to be a useful tool for the mental healthcare professional when evaluating clients' medication needs. More than ever, your comments are encouraged and appreciated, as we consider these suggestions for future editions, allowing us to better serve your needs.

— Matthew A. Fuller and Martha Sajatovic

DESCRIPTION OF FIELDS AND SECTIONS IN THIS HANDBOOK

Drug Information Handbook for Psychiatry is divided into five sections.

The first section is a compilation of introductory text pertinent to the use of this book.

The drug information section of the handbook, in which all drugs are listed alphabetically, includes comprehensive monographs for psychotropic medications and other drugs encountered frequently in psychiatric practice while a concise monograph is provided for nonpsychotropic agents. Extensive cross-referencing is provided by U.S. brand names and index terms.

The third section is comprised of general patient assessment and a description of rating scales used in patient evaluations. The text revision of the DSM-IV is also included.

The fourth section is an invaluable appendix with conversion information, charts, tables, nomograms, and management guidelines which can be helpful for patient care.

The last section of this handbook is an alphabetical index which includes generic names, U.S. brand names, Canadian brand names, Mexican brand names, and index terms.

The **Alphabetical Listing of Drugs** contains comprehensive monographs for psychotropic medications and other drugs or natural products encountered frequently in psychiatric practice while a concise monograph is provided for nonpsychotropic agents. Monographs may contain the following fields:

Drug Monographs

Generic Name	U.S. adopted name
Pronunciation	Phonetic pronunciation guide
Medication Safety Issues	In an effort to promote the safe use of medications, this field is intended to highlight possible sources of medication errors such as look-alike/sound-alike drugs or highly concentrated formulations which require vigilance on the part of healthcare professionals. In addition, medications which have been associated with severe consequences in the event of a medication error are also identified in this field.
Related Information	Cross-reference to other pertinent drug information found elsewhere in this handbook
U.S. Brand Names	U.S. trade names. The symbol [DSC] appears after trade names that have been recently discontinued (manufacturer-specific).
Canadian Brand Names	Trade names found in Canada
Mexican Brand Names	Trade names found in Mexico
Index Terms	Includes names or accepted abbreviations of the generic drug; may include common brand names no longer available; this field is used to create cross-references to monographs
Pharmacologic Category	Unique systematic classification of medications
Generic Available	Indicates if a generic form is available for medications
Use	Information pertaining to appropriate FDA-approved indications of the drug
Unlabeled/ Investigational Use	Information pertaining to non-FDA approved indications of the drug
Effect on Mental Status	Pertinent drug effects which may affect or alter a patient's mental status
Effect on Psychiatric Treatment	Information relative to the impact on psychiatric treatment
Mental Health Comment	Clinical pearls for the practitioner

Restrictions	The controlled substance classification from the Drug Enforcement Agency (DEA). U.S. schedules are I-V. Schedules vary by country and sometimes state (ie, Massachusetts uses I-VI)
Pregnancy Risk Factor	Five categories established by the FDA to indicate the potential of a systemically absorbed drug for causing risk to fetus.
Pregnancy Considerations	Information pertinent to or associated with the use of the drug as it relates to clinical effects on the fetus, newborn, and pregnant woman.
Lactation	Information describing characteristics of using the drug listed in the monograph while breast-feeding (where recommendation of American Academy of Pediatrics differs, notation is made).
Contraindications	Information pertaining to inappropriate use of the drug
Warnings/ Precautions	Precautionary considerations, hazardous conditions related to use of the drug, and disease states or patient populations in which the drug should be cautiously used. Boxed warnings, when present, are clearly identified and are adapted from the FDA approved labeling. Consult the product labeling for the exact black box warning through the manufacturer's or the FDA website.
Adverse Reactions	Side effects are grouped by percentage of incidence (if known) and/or body system; <1% of incidence are strung.
Metabolism/ Transport Effects	If a drug has demonstrated involvement with cytochrome P450 enzymes, or other metabolism or transport proteins, this field will identify the drug as an inhibitor, inducer, or substrate of the specific enzyme(s) (eg, CYP1A2 or UGT1A1). CYP450 isoenzymes are identified as substrates (minor or major), inhibitors (weak, moderate, or strong), and inducers (weak or strong).
Drug Interactions	This field presents a description of the interaction between the drug listed in the monograph and other drugs or drug classes. Following a description of the interaction for a drug class, any drugs from that class which are NOT likely to cause a similar interaction with the monograph drug are listed as exceptions. Lastly, the significance of the interaction is identified in the form of a risk rating. A brief description of the rating system is as follows (please note that the risk levels of A and B exist, reflecting no known interactions or clinically-insignificant interactions, respectively; however, for brevity, these interactions are not displayed in printed form: *Risk C: Monitor therapy* – data demonstrate that the specified agents may interact with each other in a clinically-significant manner, but the benefits of concomitant use usually outweigh any risks. An appropriate monitoring plan should be implemented to identify potential negative effects and dosage adjustments may be needed in a minority of patients. *Risk D: Consider therapy modification* - data demonstrate that the specified agents may interact with each other in a clinically-significant manner and patient-specific assessment must be conducted to determine whether the benefits of concomitant therapy outweigh the risks. Specific actions must be taken in order to realize the benefits and/or minimize toxicity of concomitant use. *Risk X: Avoid combination* - data demonstrate that the specified agents may interact with each other in a clinically-significant manner and the risk generally outweighs any potential benefit. Concurrent use of these agents is generally considered contraindicated.
Ethanol/Nutrition/ Herb Interactions	Information regarding potential interactions with food, nutritionals (including herbal products or vitamins), or ethanol.
Stability	Information regarding reconstitution, storage, and compatibility is supplied for the medications.
Mechanism of Action	How the drug works in the body to elicit a response
Pharmacodynamics/ Kinetics	The magnitude of a drug's effect depends on the drug concentration at the site of action. The pharmacodynamics are expressed in terms of onset of action and duration of action. Pharmacokinetics are expressed in terms of absorption, distribution (including appearance in breast milk and crossing of the placenta), protein binding, metabolism, bioavailability, half-life, time to peak serum concentration, and elimination.

Dosage	The amount of the drug to be typically given or taken during therapy for children and adults; also includes any dosing adjustment/comments for renal impairment or hepatic failure; **Note:** When **Dosage Summary** is listed, ranges separated by the word "or" may apply to differing indications.
Child/Adolescent Considerations	Information from clinical trials for children and adolescent patients
Dietary Considerations	Includes information on how the medication should be taken relative to meals or food
Administration	Information regarding the recommended final concentrations, rates of administration for parenteral drugs, or other guidelines when giving the medications
Monitoring Parameters	Laboratory tests and patient physical parameters that should be monitored for safety and efficacy of drug therapy
Reference Range	Therapeutic and toxic serum concentrations listed for psychotropic agents including peak and trough levels
Test Interactions	Listing of assay interferences when relevant; (B) = Blood; (S) = Serum; (U) = Urine
Additional Information	Information about sodium content and/or pertinent information about specific brands
Dosage Forms	Information with regard to form, strength, and availability of the drug. **Note:** Additional formulation information (eg, excipients, preservatives) is included when available. Please consult product labeling for further information.

Natural Product Monographs

Name	Common name with acronym or Latin binomial when appropriate
Pronunciation	Phonetic pronunciation guide
Natural Product Category	Identifies the natural product as an herb, nutraceutical, glandular, vitamin, mineral, or amino acid
Synonyms	Other names or accepted abbreviations
Plant Part	Most commonly used plant part with medicinal value
Dosage and Standardization (herbs only)	Standardized herbs are necessary to ensure consistent results. Dosages are based on currently accepted practice and clinical efficacy. As with all medicinal substances, dosages can be altered based on clinical presentation, including age, weight, health status, and other pertinent factors. Standardization numbers may also vary slightly, as more companies enter the market with clinical research. Ask the manufacturer for documented efficacy of its product.
Dosage (all products except herbs)	Amount of the natural product typically taken for common uses
Active Forms	Lists primary active chemical constituents of the commercially available natural products
Reported Uses	Reported uses are based on clinical efficacy in human and animal studies. These uses are not all-inclusive for each plant, but are the most widely recommended and currently accepted in the medical community.
Summary	A brief summary of the individual plant and its use as a therapeutic agent
Effect on Mental Status	Pertinent drug effects which may affect or alter a patient's mental status
Effect on Psychiatric Treatment	Information relative to the impact on psychiatric treatment
Pharmacology	Documented pharmacology based on reported studies. Some studies are reported on isolated chemical constituents in the herbs and extrapolated to the whole plant when standardized.
Warnings and Interactions (all products except herbs)	These warnings are categorized and based on (1) human clinical trials; (2) animal and/or *in vitro* studies; (3) case reports; (4) potential interaction based on pharmacology. Again, any individual taking pharmaceutical medications should use dietary supplements with caution.

Theoretical Cautions and Contraindications (herbs only)	See Warnings and Interactions
General Warnings (herbs only)	Warnings which apply to all herbal supplements, including general warnings about the potential for interactions with traditional medications and clinical situations in which herbal therapies must be approached with caution; occasionally, these warnings are superseded by information which may be listed in the Theoretical Cautions and Contraindications field and which is specific to the herb in question
Symptoms of Deficiency (all products except herbs)	List of symptoms caused by deficiency of the particular natural product
Theoretical Interactions Reported Interactions	List of potentially interacting medicines and/or nutrients based on either literature support, product pharmacology, or theoretical considerations
References	Sources used to verify included information

FDA PREGNANCY CATEGORIES

Throughout this book there is a field labeled Pregnancy Risk Factor (PRF) and the letter A, B, C, D, or X immediately following which signifies a category. The FDA has established these five categories to indicate the potential of a systemically absorbed drug for causing birth defects. The key differentiation among the categories rests upon the reliability of documentation and the risk:benefit ratio. Pregnancy Category X is particularly notable in that if any data exists that may implicate a drug as a teratogen and the risk:benefit ratio is clearly negative, the drug is contraindicated during pregnancy.

These categories are summarized as follows:

A — Controlled studies in pregnant women fail to demonstrate a risk to the fetus in the first trimester with no evidence of risk in later trimesters. The possibility of fetal harm appears remote.

B — Either animal-reproduction studies have not demonstrated a fetal risk but there are no controlled studies in pregnant women, or animal-reproduction studies have shown an adverse effect (other than a decrease in fertility) that was not confirmed in controlled studies in women in the first trimester and there is no evidence of a risk in later trimesters.

C — Either studies in animals have revealed adverse effects on the fetus (teratogenic or embryocidal effects or other) and there are no controlled studies in women, or studies in women and animals are not available. Drugs should be given only if the potential benefits justify the potential risk to the fetus.

D — There is positive evidence of human fetal risk, but the benefits from use in pregnant women may be acceptable despite the risk (eg, if the drug is needed in a life-threatening situation or for a serious disease for which safer drugs cannot be used or are ineffective).

X — Studies in animals or human beings have demonstrated fetal abnormalities or there is evidence of fetal risk based on human experience, or both, and the risk of the use of the drug in pregnant women clearly outweighs any possible benefit. The drug is contraindicated in women who are or may become pregnant.

FDA NAME DIFFERENTIATION PROJECT THE USE OF TALL-MAN LETTERS

Confusion between similar drug names is an important cause of medication errors. For years, The Institute For Safe Medication Practices (ISMP), has urged generic manufacturers to use a combination of large and small letters as well as bolding (ie, chlorpro**MAZINE** and chlorpro**PAMIDE**) to help distinguish drugs with look-alike names, especially when they share similar strengths. Recently the FDA's Division of Generic Drugs began to issue recommendation letters to manufacturers suggesting this novel way to label their products to help reduce this drug name confusion. Although this project has had marginal success, the method has successfully eliminated problems with products such as diphenhydr**AMINE** and dimenhy**DRINATE**. Hospitals should also follow suit by making similar changes in their own labels, preprinted order forms, computer screens and printouts, and drug storage location labels.

Lexi-Comp Medical Publishing will use "Tall-Man" letters for the drugs suggested by the FDA or recommended by ISMP.

The following is a list of generic product names and recommended revisions.

Drug Product	Recommended Revision
acetazolamide	aceta**ZOLAMIDE**
acetohexamide	aceto**HEXAMIDE**
alprazolam	**ALPRAZ**olam
amiloride	a**MIL**oride
amlodipine	am**LODIP**ine
azacitidine	aza**CITID**ine
azathioprine	aza**THIO**prine
bupropion	bu**PROP**ion
buspirone	bus**PIR**one
carbamazepine	car**BAM**azepine
carboplatin	**CARBO**platin
cefazolin	ce**FAZ**olin
ceftriaxone	cef**TRIAX**one
chlordiazepoxide	chlordiaze**POXIDE**
chlorpromazine	chlorpro**MAZINE**
chlorpropamide	chlorpro**PAMIDE**
cisplatin	**CIS**platin
clomiphene	clomi**PHENE**
clomipramine	clomi**PRAMINE**
clonazepam	clonaze**PAM**
clonidine	clo**NID**ine
cycloserine	cyclo**SERINE**
cyclosporine	cyclo**SPORINE**
dactinomycin	**DACTIN**omycin
daptomycin	**DAPTO**mycin
daunorubicin	**DAUNO**rubicin
dimenhydrinate	dimenhy**DRINATE**
diphenhydramine	diphenhydr**AMINE**
dobutamine	**DOBUT**amine
dopamine	**DOP**amine
doxorubicin	**DOXO**rubicin
duloxetine	**DUL**oxetine

Drug Product	Recommended Revision
ephedrine	e**PHED**rine
epinephrine	**EPINEPH**rine
fentanyl	fenta**NYL**
fluoxetine	**FLU**oxetine
glipizide	glipi**ZIDE**
glyburide	gly**BURIDE**
guaifenesin	guai**FEN**esin
guanfacine	guan**FACINE**
hydralazine	hydr**ALAZINE**
hydrocodone	**HYDRO**codone
hydromorphone	**HYDRO**morphone
hydroxyzine	hydr**OXY**zine
idarubicin	**IDA**rubicin
infliximab	in**FLIX**imab
lamivudine	lami**VUD**ine
lamotrigine	lamo**TRI**gine
lorazepam	**LOR**azepam
medroxyprogesterone	medroxy**PROGESTER**one
metformin	met**FORMIN**
methylprednisolone	methyl**PREDNIS**olone
methyltestosterone	methyl**TESTOSTER**one
metronidazole	metro**NIDAZOLE**
nicardipine	ni**CAR**dipine
nifedipine	**NIFE**dipine
nimodipine	ni**MOD**ipine
olanzapine	**OLANZ**apine
oxcarbazepine	**OX**carbazepine
oxycodone	oxy**CODONE**
paroxetine	**PAR**oxetine
pentobarbital	**PENT**obarbital
phenobarbital	**PHEN**obarbital
prednisolone	predniso**LONE**
prednisone	predni**SONE**
quetiapine	**QUE**tiapine
quinidine	qui**NID**ine
quinine	qui**NINE**
rituximab	ri**TUX**imab
sitagliptin	sita**GLIP**tin
sufentanil	**SUF**entanil
sulfadiazine	sulf**ADIAZINE**
sulfisoxazole	sulfi**SOXAZOLE**
sumatriptan	**SUMA**triptan
tiagabine	tia**GAB**ine
tizanidine	ti**ZAN**idine
tolazamide	**TOLAZ**amide
tolbutamide	**TOLBUT**amide
tramadol	tra**MAD**ol
trazodone	tra**ZOD**one

Drug Product	Recommended Revision
vinblastine	vin**BLAS**tine
vincristine	vin**CRIS**tine

Institute for Safe Medication Practices. "New Tall-Man Lettering Will Reduce Mix-Ups Due to Generic Drug Name Confusion," *ISMP Medication Safety Alert*, September 19, 2001. Available at: http://www.ismp.org.

Institute for Safe Medication Practices. "Prescription Mapping, Can Improve Efficiency While Minimizing Errors With Look-Alike Products," *ISMP Medication Safety Alert*, October 6, 1999. Available at: http://www.ismp.org.

Institute for Safe Medication Practices. "Use of Tall Man Letters Is Gaining Wide Acceptance," *ISMP Medication Safety Alert*, July 31, 2008. Available at: http://www.ismp.org.

U.S. Pharmacopeia, "USP Quality Review: Use Caution-Avoid Confusion," March 2001, No. 76. Available at: http://www.usp.org.

SAFE WRITING

Health professionals and their support personnel frequently produce handwritten copies of information they see in print; therefore, such information is subjected to even greater possibilities for error or misinterpretation on the part of others. Thus, particular care must be given to how drug names and strengths are expressed when creating written healthcare documents.

The following are a few examples of safe writing rules suggested by the Institute for Safe Medication Practices, Inc.[1]

1. There should be a space between a number and its units as it is easier to read. There should be no periods after the abbreviations mg or mL.

Correct	Incorrect
10 mg	10mg
100 mg	100mg

2. Never place a decimal and a zero after a whole number (2 mg is correct and 2.0 mg is **incorrect**). If the decimal point is not seen because it falls on a line or because individuals are working from copies where the decimal point is not seen, this causes a tenfold overdose.
3. Just the opposite is true for numbers less than one. Always place a zero before a naked decimal (0.5 mL is correct, .5 mL is **incorrect**).
4. Never abbreviate the word unit. The handwritten U or u, looks like a 0 (zero), and may cause a tenfold overdose error to be made.
5. IU is not a safe abbreviation for international units. The handwritten IU looks like IV. Write out international units or use int. units.
6. Q.D. is not a safe abbreviation for once daily, as when the Q is followed by a sloppy dot, it looks like QID which means four times daily.
7. O.D. is not a safe abbreviation for once daily, as it is properly interpreted as meaning "right eye" and has caused liquid medications such as saturated solution of potassium iodide and Lugol's solution to be administered incorrectly. There is no safe abbreviation for once daily. It must be written out in full.
8. Do not use chemical names such as 6-mercaptopurine or 6-thioguanine, as sixfold overdoses have been given when these were not recognized as chemical names. The proper names of these drugs are mercaptopurine or thioguanine.
9. Do not abbreviate drug names (5FC, 6MP, 5-ASA, MTX, HCTZ, CPZ, PBZ, etc) as they are misinterpreted and cause error.
10. Do not use the apothecary system or symbols.
11. Do not abbreviate microgram as µg; instead use mcg as there is less likelihood of misinterpretation.
12. When writing an outpatient prescription, write a complete prescription. A complete prescription can prevent the prescriber, the pharmacist, and/or the patient from making a mistake and can eliminate the need for further clarification. The legible prescriptions should contain:
    a. patient's full name
    b. for pediatric or geriatric patients: their age (or weight where applicable)
    c. drug name, dosage form and strength; if a drug is new or rarely prescribed, print this information
    d. number or amount to be dispensed
    e. complete instructions for the patient, including the purpose of the medication
    f. when there are recognized contraindications for a prescribed drug, indicate to the pharmacist that you are aware of this fact (ie, when prescribing a potassium salt for a patient receiving an ACE inhibitor, write "K serum level being monitored")

[1]From "Safe Writing" by Davis NM, PharmD and Cohen MR, MS, Lecturers and Consultants for Safe Medication Practices, 1143 Wright Drive, Huntington Valley, PA 19006. Phone: (215) 947-7566.

Alphabetical Listing of Drugs

Abacavir (a BAK a veer)

U.S. Brand Names Ziagen®
Canadian Brand Names Ziagen®
Mexican Brand Names Ampi-quim; Ziagenavir
Index Terms Abacavir Sulfate; ABC
Pharmacologic Category Antiretroviral Agent, Reverse Transcriptase Inhibitor (Nucleoside)
Use Treatment of HIV infections in combination with other antiretroviral agents
Effect on Mental Status May cause fatigue, lethargy, malaise, insomnia, and headache
Effect on Psychiatric Treatment Side effects mimic depressive symptoms; caution with benzodiazepines or other CNS depressants and antidepressants
Restrictions An FDA-approved medication guide and warning card (summarizing symptoms of hypersensitivity) must be distributed when dispensing an outpatient prescription (new or refill) where this medication is to be used without direct supervision of a healthcare provider. Medication guides are available at http://www.fda.gov/cder/Offices/ODS/medication_guides.htm.
Dosage Summary
Oral:
Children <3 months: Dosage not established
Children 3 months to 16 years: 8 mg/kg twice daily in combination with other antiretroviral agents (maximum: 300 mg twice daily)
Adults: 600 mg/day in 1-2 divided doses in combination with other antiretroviral agents (maximum: 600 mg/day)
Dosage Forms Excipient information presented when available (limited, particularly for generics); consult specific product labeling.
Solution, oral:
Ziagen®: 20 mg/mL (240 mL) [strawberry-banana flavor]
Tablet:
Ziagen®: 300 mg

Abacavir and Lamivudine (a BAK a veer & la MI vyoo deen)

U.S. Brand Names Epzicom®
Canadian Brand Names Kivexa™
Mexican Brand Names Kivexa
Index Terms Abacavir Sulfate and Lamivudine; Lamivudine and Abacavir
Pharmacologic Category Antiretroviral Agent, Reverse Transcriptase Inhibitor (Nucleoside)
Use Treatment of HIV infections in combination with other antiretroviral agents
Effect on Mental Status May cause anxiety, abnormal dreams, dizziness, depression, fatigue, lethargy, malaise, insomnia, and headache
Effect on Psychiatric Treatment Side effects mimic depressive symptoms; use caution with benzodiazepines, CNS depressants, or antidepressants. May rarely cause neutropenia; use caution with clozapine and carbamazepine.
Restrictions An FDA-approved medication guide and warning card (summarizing symptoms of hypersensitivity) must be distributed when dispensing an outpatient prescription (new or refill) where this medication is to be used without direct supervision of a healthcare provider. Medication guides are available at http://www.fda.gov/cder/Offices/ODS/medication_guides.htm.
Dosage Summary
Oral:
Children: Dosage not established
Adults: One tablet (abacavir 600 mg and lamivudine 300 mg) once daily
Dosage Forms Excipient information presented when available (limited, particularly for generics); consult specific product labeling.
Tablet:
Epzicom®: Abacavir 600 mg and lamivudine 300 mg

◆ **Abacavir Sulfate** *see* Abacavir *on page 22*
◆ **Abacavir Sulfate and Lamivudine** *see* Abacavir and Lamivudine *on page 22*

Abatacept (ab a TA sept)

Medication Safety Issues
Sound-alike/look-alike issues:
Orencia® may be confused with Oracea™
U.S. Brand Names Orencia®

Canadian Brand Names Orencia®
Index Terms CTLA-4Ig
Pharmacologic Category Antirheumatic, Disease Modifying
Use
Treatment of moderately- to severely-active adult rheumatoid arthritis (RA); may be used as monotherapy or in combination with other DMARDs
Treatment of moderately- to severely-active juvenile idiopathic arthritis (JIA); may be used as monotherapy or in combination with methotrexate
Note: Abatacept should **not** be used in combination with anakinra or TNF-blocking agents
Effect on Mental Status May cause dizziness
Effect on Psychiatric Treatment May cause nausea; concomitant use with SSRIs, lithium, valproic acid, and carbamazepine may produce additive effects
Dosage Summary
I.V.:
Children <6 years: Dosage not established
Children ≥6 years and <75 kg: 10 mg/kg, repeat dose at 2 and 4 weeks after initial infusion, and every 4 weeks thereafter; Maximum dose: 1000 mg
Children ≥6 years and >75 kg: **Note:** Dosage is according to body weight. Repeat dose at 2 weeks and 4 weeks after initial dose and every 4 weeks thereafter:
75-100 kg: 750 mg
>100 kg: 1000 mg
Adults: **Note:** Dosage is according to body weight. Repeat dose at 2 weeks and 4 weeks after initial dose and every 4 weeks thereafter:
<60 kg: 500 mg
60-100 kg: 750 mg
>100 kg: 1000 mg
Elderly: Use caution
Dosage Forms Excipient information presented when available (limited, particularly for generics); consult specific product labeling.
Injection, powder for reconstitution [preservative free]:
Orencia®: 250 mg [contains maltose]

- **Abbott-43818** *see* Leuprolide *on page 901*
- **ABC** *see* Abacavir *on page 22*
- **ABCD** *see* Amphotericin B Cholesteryl Sulfate Complex *on page 119*
- **Abelcet®** *see* Amphotericin B, Lipid Complex *on page 121*
- **ABI-007** *see* Paclitaxel (Protein Bound) *on page 1214*
- **Abilify®** *see* Aripiprazole *on page 133*
- **Abilify® Discmelt™** *see* Aripiprazole *on page 133*
- **ABLC** *see* Amphotericin B, Lipid Complex *on page 121*
- **Abraxane®** *see* Paclitaxel (Protein Bound) *on page 1214*
- **ABX-EGF** *see* Panitumumab *on page 1221*
- **9-AC** *see* Aminocamptothecin *on page 86*
- **AC 2993** *see* Exenatide *on page 609*
- **ACAM2000™** *see* Smallpox Vaccine *on page 1493*

Acamprosate (a kam PROE sate)

Related Information
Addiction Treatments *on page 1817*
U.S. Brand Names Campral®
Canadian Brand Names Campral®
Mexican Brand Names Campral
Index Terms Acamprosate Calcium; Calcium Acetylhomotaurinate
Pharmacologic Category GABA Agonist/Glutamate Antagonist
Generic Available No
Use Maintenance of alcohol abstinence
Pregnancy Risk Factor C
Pregnancy Considerations Teratogenic in animal studies. No adequate or well-controlled studies in pregnant women; use only if potential benefit outweighs possible risk to the fetus.
Lactation Excretion in breast milk unknown/use caution
Contraindications Hypersensitivity to acamprosate or any component of the formulation; severe renal impairment (Cl_{cr} <30 mL/minute)

Warnings/Precautions Should be used as part of a comprehensive program to treat alcohol dependence. Treatment should be initiated as soon as possible following the period of alcohol withdrawal, when the patient has achieved abstinence. Acamprosate does not eliminate or diminish the symptoms of alcohol withdrawal. Use caution in moderate renal impairment (Cl_{cr} 30-50 mL/minute). Suicidal ideation, attempted and completed suicides have occurred in acamprosate-treated patients; monitor for depression and/or suicidal thinking. Traces of sulfites may be present in the formulation. Safety and efficacy have not been established in pediatric patients.

Adverse Reactions

Note: Many adverse effects associated with treatment may be related to alcohol abstinence; reported frequency range may overlap with placebo.

>10%: Gastrointestinal: Diarrhea (10% to 17%)

1% to 10%:

Cardiovascular: Syncope, palpitation, edema (peripheral)

Central nervous system: Insomnia (6% to 9%), anxiety (5% to 8%), depression (4% to 8%), dizziness (3% to 4%), pain (2% to 4%), paresthesia (2% to 3%), headache, somnolence, amnesia, tremor, chills

Dermatologic: Pruritus (3% to 4%), rash

Endocrine & metabolic: Weight gain, libido decreased

Gastrointestinal: Anorexia (2% to 5%), flatulence (1% to 3%), nausea (3% to 4%), abdominal pain, dry mouth (1% to 3%), vomiting, dyspepsia, constipation, appetite increased, taste perversion

Genitourinary: Impotence

Neuromuscular & skeletal: Weakness (5% to 7%), back pain, myalgia, arthralgia

Ocular: Abnormal vision

Respiratory: Rhinitis, dyspnea, pharyngitis, bronchitis

Miscellaneous: Diaphoresis (2% to 3%), suicide attempt

<1%, postmarketing, and/or case reports (limited to important or life-threatening): Angina, asthma, exfoliative dermatitis, gastrointestinal hemorrhage, hallucinations, hypothyroidism, MI, ophthalmitis, pancreatitis, photosensitivity, psychosis, pulmonary embolus, renal calculus, renal failure, seizure, suicidal ideation, suicide attempts, suicide completion

Drug Interactions There are no known significant interactions.

Ethanol/Nutrition/Herb Interactions

Ethanol: Abstinence is required during treatment. Ethanol does not affect the pharmacokinetics of acamprosate; however, the continued use of ethanol will decrease desired efficacy of acamprosate.

Food: Food decreases absorption of acamprosate (not clinically significant).

Stability Store at 25°C (77°F); excursions permitted to 15°C to 30°C (59°F to 86°F).

Mechanism of Action Mechanism not fully defined. Structurally similar to gamma-amino butyric acid (GABA), acamprosate appears to increase the activity of the GABA-ergic system, and decreases activity of glutamate within the CNS, including a decrease in activity at N-methyl D-aspartate (NMDA) receptors; may also affect CNS calcium channels. Restores balance to GABA and glutamate activities which appear to be disrupted in alcohol dependence. During therapeutic use, reduces alcohol intake, but does not cause a disulfiram-like reaction following alcohol ingestion.

Pharmacodynamics/Kinetics

Distribution: V_d: 1 L/kg

Protein binding: Negligible

Metabolism: Not metabolized

Bioavailability: 11%

Half-life elimination: 20-33 hours

Excretion: Urine (as unchanged drug)

Dosage Oral: Adults: Alcohol abstinence: 666 mg 3 times/day (a lower dose may be effective in some patients)

Adjustment in patients with low body weight (unlabeled): A lower dose (4 tablets/day) may be considered in patients with low body weight (eg, <60 kg).

Note: Treatment should be initiated as soon as possible (following the period of alcohol withdrawal) when the patient has achieved abstinence.

Dosage adjustment in renal impairment:

Cl_{cr} 30-50 mL/minute: Initial dose should be reduced to 333 mg 3 times/day.

Cl_{cr} <30 mL/minute: Contraindicated in severe renal impairment.

Dietary Considerations May be taken without regard to meals. Each 333 mg tablet contains 33 mg of elemental calcium.

Administration May be administered without regard to meals. Tablet should be swallowed whole; do not crush or chew.

Dosage Forms Excipient information presented when available (limited, particularly for generics); consult specific product labeling.

Tablet, enteric coated, delayed release, as calcium:

Campral®: 333 mg [contains calcium 33 mg and sulfites]

◆ **Acamprosate Calcium** *see* Acamprosate *on page 23*

Acarbose (AY car bose)

Medication Safety Issues

Sound-alike/look-alike issues:

Precose® may be confused with PreCare®

International issues:

Precose® may be confused with Precosa® which is a brand name for *Saccharomyces boulardii* in Denmark, Finland, Norway, and Sweden

U.S. Brand Names Precose®

Canadian Brand Names Glucobay™

Mexican Brand Names Glucobay; Incardel; Sincrosa

Pharmacologic Category Antidiabetic Agent, Alpha-Glucosidase Inhibitor

Generic Available Yes

Use Adjunct to diet and exercise to lower blood glucose in patients with type 2 diabetes mellitus (noninsulin dependent, NIDDM)

Effect on Mental Status May cause drowsiness

Effect on Psychiatric Treatment Antipsychotics and tricyclic antidepressants may decrease the effects of acarbose. Monoamine oxidase inhibitors, SSRIs, and nefazodone may increase the effects of acarbose.

Pregnancy Risk Factor B

Pregnancy Considerations Adverse events have not been reported in animal reproduction studies; therefore, acarbose is classified as pregnancy category B. Low amounts of acarbose are absorbed systemically which should limit fetal exposure. Maternal hyperglycemia can be associated with adverse effects in the fetus, including macrosomia, neonatal hyperglycemia, and hyperbilirubinemia; the risk of congenital malformations is increased when the Hb A_{1c} is above the normal range. Diabetes can also be associated with adverse effects in the mother. Poorly-treated diabetes may cause end-organ damage that may in turn negatively affect obstetric outcomes. Physiologic glucose levels should be maintained prior to and during pregnancy to decrease the risk of adverse events in the mother and the fetus. Acarbose has been studied for its potential role in treating GDM; however, only limited information is available describing pregnancy outcomes. Until additional safety and efficacy data are obtained, the use of oral agents is generally not recommended as routine management of GDM or type 2 diabetes mellitus during pregnancy. Insulin is the drug of choice for the control of diabetes mellitus during pregnancy.

Lactation Excretion in breast milk unknown/not recommended

Contraindications Hypersensitivity to acarbose or any component of the formulation; patients with diabetic ketoacidosis or cirrhosis; patients with inflammatory bowel disease, colonic ulceration, partial intestinal obstruction, or in patients predisposed to intestinal obstruction; patients who have chronic intestinal diseases associated with marked disorders of digestion or absorption, and in patients who have conditions that may deteriorate as a result of increased gas formation in the intestine

Warnings/Precautions Acarbose given in combination with a sulfonylurea or insulin will cause a further lowering of blood glucose and may increase the hypoglycemic potential of the sulfonylurea or insulin. Treatment-emergent elevations of serum transaminases (AST and/or ALT) occurred in up to 14% of acarbose-treated patients in long-term studies. These serum transaminase elevations appear to be dose related and were asymptomatic, reversible, more common in females, and, in general, were not associated with other evidence of liver dysfunction. Fulminant hepatitis has been reported rarely. It may be necessary to discontinue acarbose and administer insulin if the patient is exposed to stress (ie, fever, trauma, infection, surgery). Use not recommended in patients with significant impairment (S_{cr} >2 mg/dL); use with caution in other patients with renal impairment. Safety and efficacy have not been established in children.

Adverse Reactions

>10%:

Gastrointestinal: Diarrhea (31%) and abdominal pain (19%) tend to return to pretreatment levels over time; frequency and intensity of flatulence (74%) tend to abate with time

Hepatic: Transaminases increased (≤4%)

Postmarketing and/or case reports: Edema, erythema, exanthema, hepatitis, ileus/subileus, jaundice, liver damage, rash, urticaria

Drug Interactions

Corticosteroids (Orally Inhaled): May diminish the hypoglycemic effect of Antidiabetic Agents. In some instances, corticosteroid-mediated HPA axis suppression has led to episodes of acute adrenal crisis, which may manifest as enhanced hypoglycemia, particularly in the setting of insulin or other antidiabetic agent use. *Risk C: Monitor therapy*

Corticosteroids (Systemic): May diminish the hypoglycemic effect of Antidiabetic Agents. In some instances, corticosteroid-mediated HPA axis suppression has led to episodes of acute adrenal crisis, which may manifest as enhanced hypoglycemia, particularly in the setting of insulin or other antidiabetic agent use. *Risk C: Monitor therapy*

Digoxin: Acarbose may decrease the serum concentration of Digoxin. *Risk C: Monitor therapy*

Herbs (Hypoglycemic Properties): May enhance the hypoglycemic effect of Hypoglycemic Agents. *Risk C: Monitor therapy*

Luteinizing Hormone-Releasing Hormone Analogs: May diminish the therapeutic effect of Antidiabetic Agents. *Risk C: Monitor therapy*

Pegvisomant: May enhance the hypoglycemic effect of Antidiabetic Agents. *Risk C: Monitor therapy*

Somatropin: May diminish the hypoglycemic effect of Antidiabetic Agents. *Risk D: Consider therapy modification*

Ethanol/Nutrition/Herb Interactions Ethanol: Limit ethanol.

Stability Store at <25°C (77°F). Protect from moisture.

Mechanism of Action Competitive inhibitor of pancreatic α-amylase and intestinal brush border α-glucosidases, resulting in delayed hydrolysis of ingested complex carbohydrates and disaccharides and absorption of glucose; dose-dependent reduction in postprandial serum insulin and glucose peaks; inhibits the metabolism of sucrose to glucose and fructose

Pharmacodynamics/Kinetics

Absorption: <2% as active drug; ~35% as metabolites

Metabolism: Exclusively via GI tract, principally by intestinal bacteria and digestive enzymes; 13 metabolites identified (major metabolites are sulfate, methyl, and glucuronide conjugates)

Bioavailability: Low systemic bioavailability of parent compound; acts locally in GI tract

Half-life elimination: ~2 hours

Time to peak: Active drug: ~1 hour

Excretion: Urine (~34% as inactive metabolites, <2% parent drug and active metabolite); feces (~51% as unabsorbed drug)

Dosage Oral:

Adults: Dosage must be individualized on the basis of effectiveness and tolerance while not exceeding the maximum recommended dose

Initial dose: 25 mg 3 times/day with the first bite of each main meal; to reduce GI effects, some patients may benefit from initiating at 25 mg once daily with gradual titration to 25 mg 3 times/day as tolerated

Maintenance dose: Should be adjusted at 4- to 8-week intervals based on 1-hour postprandial glucose levels and tolerance. Dosage may be increased from 25 mg 3 times/day to 50 mg 3 times/day. Some patients may benefit from increasing the dose to 100 mg 3 times/day.

Maintenance dose ranges: 50-100 mg 3 times/day.

Maximum dose:

≤60 kg: 50 mg 3 times/day

>60 kg: 100 mg 3 times/day

Patients receiving sulfonylureas or insulin: Acarbose given in combination with a sulfonylurea or insulin will cause a further lowering of blood glucose and may increase the hypoglycemic potential of the sulfonylurea or insulin. If hypoglycemia occurs, appropriate adjustments in the dosage of these agents should be made.

Dosing adjustment in renal impairment:

Cl_{cr} <25 mL/minute: Peak plasma concentrations were 5 times higher and AUCs were 6 times larger than in volunteers with normal renal function.

Significant renal dysfunction (S_{cr} >2 mg/dL): Use is not recommended.

Dietary Considerations Take with food (first bite of meal).

Administration Should be administered with the first bite of each main meal.

Monitoring Parameters Postprandial glucose, glycosylated hemoglobin levels, serum transaminase levels should be checked every 3 months during the first year of treatment and periodically thereafter, renal function (serum creatinine); blood pressure

Reference Range Recommendations for glycemic control in adults with diabetes:

Hb A_{1c}: <7%

Preprandial capillary plasma glucose: 70-130 mg/dL

Peak postprandial capillary blood glucose: <180 mg/dL

Dosage Forms Excipient information presented when available (limited, particularly for generics); consult specific product labeling.

Tablet: 25 mg, 50 mg, 100 mg

Precose®: 25 mg, 50 mg, 100 mg

- **Accolate®** *see* Zafirlukast *on page 1689*
- **AccuHist®** *see* Brompheniramine and Pseudoephedrine *on page 206*
- **AccuHist® PDX Drops** *see* Brompheniramine, Pseudoephedrine, and Dextromethorphan *on page 208*
- **AccuNeb®** *see* Albuterol *on page 54*
- **Accupril®** *see* Quinapril *on page 1386*
- **Accuretic®** *see* Quinapril and Hydrochlorothiazide *on page 1386*
- **Accutane®** *see* Isotretinoin *on page 871*
- **ACE** *see* Captopril *on page 264*

Acebutolol (a se BYOO toe lole)

Medication Safety Issues

Sound-alike/look-alike issues:

Sectral® may be confused with Factrel®, Seconal®, Septra®

Related Information

Beta-Blockers *on page 1776*

U.S. Brand Names Sectral®

Canadian Brand Names Apo-Acebutolol®; Gen-Acebutolol; Monitan®; Novo-Acebutolol; Nu-Acebutolol; Rhotral; Rhoxal-acebutolol; Sandoz-Acebutolol; Sectral®

Index Terms Acebutolol Hydrochloride

Pharmacologic Category Antiarrhythmic Agent, Class II; Beta Blocker With Intrinsic Sympathomimetic Activity

Generic Available Yes

Use Treatment of hypertension; management of ventricular arrhythmias

Unlabeled/Investigational Use Treatment of chronic stable angina

Effect on Mental Status Drowsiness/fatigue is common; may cause insomnia, depression, abnormal dreams, and polyuria

Effect on Psychiatric Treatment Additive hypotensive and/or sedative effects may be seen with concurrent use of antipsychotics, antidepressants, or benzodiazepines

Pregnancy Risk Factor B (manufacturer); D (2nd and 3rd trimesters - expert analysis)

Pregnancy Considerations Teratogenic effects were not observed in animal studies. Acebutolol and its metabolite cross the human placenta. The neonatal half-life of acebutolol is 6-14 hours and diacetolol is 24-30 hours. Decreased birth weight, blood pressure, and heart rate have been observed in neonates following maternal use of acebutolol during pregnancy. Neonatal hypoglycemia has also been reported. Available evidence suggests beta-blockers are generally safe during pregnancy (JNC 7). Monitoring of the newborn is recommended.

Lactation Enters breast milk/not recommended (AAP recommends "use with caution")

Contraindications Overt cardiac failure; cardiogenic shock; persistently-severe bradycardia or second- and third-degree heart block (except in patients with a functioning artificial pacemaker)

Warnings/Precautions Consider pre-existing conditions such as sick sinus syndrome before initiating. Beta-blocker therapy should not be withdrawn abruptly (particularly in patients with CAD), but gradually tapered to avoid acute tachycardia, hypertension, and/or ischemia. Use with caution in diabetic patients. Beta-blockers may impair glucose tolerance, potentiate hypoglycemia, and/or mask symptoms of hypoglycemia in a diabetic patient. Use with caution in bronchospastic lung disease, hepatic impairment, myasthenia gravis, psychiatric disease (may cause CNS depression), peripheral vascular disease or renal dysfunction. Use reduced doses in the elderly since metabolism and elimination are reduced. Beta-blockers with intrinsic sympathomimetic activity (eg, acebutolol) are likely to worsen survival in HF and should be avoided. Adequate $alpha_1$-receptor blockade is required prior to use of any beta-blocker for patients with untreated pheochromocytoma. Use caution in hyperthyroidism since beta-blockade may mask signs of thyrotoxicosis. Use caution with history of severe anaphylaxis to allergens; patients taking beta-blockers may become more sensitive to repeated challenges. Treatment of anaphylaxis (eg, epinephrine) in patients taking beta-blockers may be ineffective or promote undesirable effects. Safety and efficacy have not been established in children.

Adverse Reactions

>10%: Central nervous system: Fatigue (11%)

1% to 10%:

Cardiovascular: Chest pain (2%), edema (2%), bradycardia, hypotension, CHF

Central nervous system: Headache (6%), dizziness (6%), insomnia (3%), depression (2%), abnormal dreams (2%), anxiety, hyper-/hypoesthesia

Dermatologic: Rash (2%), pruritus

Gastrointestinal: Constipation (4%), diarrhea (4%), dyspepsia (4%), nausea (4%), flatulence (3%), abdominal pain, vomiting

Genitourinary: Micturition frequency (3%), dysuria, impotence, nocturia

Neuromuscular & skeletal: Myalgia (2%), back pain, joint pain

Ocular: Abnormal vision (2%), conjunctivitis, dry eyes, eye pain

Respiratory: Dyspnea (4%), rhinitis (2%), cough (1%), pharyngitis, wheezing

Postmarketing and/or case reports: Alkaline phosphatase increased, anorexia, AV block, bilirubin increased, cold extremities, drug-induced lupus-like syndrome, exacerbate pre-existing renal insufficiency, facial edema, hepatotoxic reaction, lichen planus, palpitation, pleurisy, pneumonitis, pulmonary granulomas, systemic lupus erythematosus, transaminases increased, urinary retention, ventricular arrhythmia, xerostomia

Potential adverse effects (based on experience with other beta-blocking agents) include agranulocytosis, allergic reactions, alopecia, catatonia, claudication, depression (reversible), disorientation, emotional lability, erythematous rash, ischemic colitis, laryngospasm, mesenteric artery thrombosis, Peyronie's disease, purpura, respiratory distress, short-term memory loss, slightly clouded sensorium, thrombocytopenia

Metabolism/Transport Effects Inhibits CYP2D6 (weak)

Drug Interactions

Acetylcholinesterase Inhibitors: May enhance the bradycardic effect of Beta-Blockers. *Risk C: Monitor therapy*

Alpha-/Beta-Agonists (Direct-Acting): Beta-Blockers may enhance the vasopressor effect of Alpha-/Beta-Agonists (Direct-Acting). Epinephrine used as a local anesthetic for dental procedures will not likely cause clinically relevant problems. **Exceptions:** Dipivefrin. *Risk D: Consider therapy modification*

Alpha$_1$-Blockers: Beta-Blockers may enhance the orthostatic effect of Alpha$_1$-Blockers. The risk associated with ophthalmic products is probably less than systemic products. *Risk D: Consider therapy modification*

Alpha$_2$-Agonists: Beta-Blockers may enhance the rebound hypertensive effect of Alpha$_2$-Agonists. This effect can occur when the alpha$_2$-agonist is abruptly withdrawn. **Exceptions:** Apraclonidine; Brimonidine. *Risk D: Consider therapy modification*

Aminoquinolines (Antimalarial): May decrease the metabolism of Beta-Blockers. *Risk C: Monitor therapy*

Amiodarone: May enhance the bradycardic effect of Beta-Blockers. Possibly to the point of cardiac arrest. Amiodarone may increase the serum concentration of Beta-Blockers. *Risk C: Monitor therapy*

Anilidopiperidine Opioids: May enhance the bradycardic effect of Beta-Blockers. Anilidopiperidine Opioids may enhance the hypotensive effect of Beta-Blockers. *Risk C: Monitor therapy*

Antipsychotic Agents (Phenothiazines): May enhance the hypotensive effect of Beta-Blockers. Beta-Blockers may decrease the metabolism of Antipsychotic Agents (Phenothiazines). Antipsychotic Agents (Phenothiazines) may decrease the metabolism of Beta-Blockers. *Risk C: Monitor therapy*

Barbiturates: May decrease the serum concentration of Beta-Blockers. *Risk C: Monitor therapy*

Beta$_2$-Agonists: Beta-Blockers (Beta$_1$ Selective) may diminish the bronchodilatory effect of Beta$_2$-Agonists. Of particular concern with nonselective beta-blockers or higher doses of the beta$_1$ selective beta-blockers. *Risk C: Monitor therapy*

Calcium Channel Blockers (Nondihydropyridine): May enhance the hypotensive effect of Beta-Blockers. Bradycardia and signs of heart failure have also been reported. Calcium Channel Blockers (Nondihydropyridine) may increase the serum concentration of Beta-Blockers. *Risk C: Monitor therapy*

Cardiac Glycosides: Beta-Blockers may enhance the bradycardic effect of Cardiac Glycosides. *Risk C: Monitor therapy*

Diazoxide: May enhance the hypotensive effect of Antihypertensives. *Risk C: Monitor therapy*

Dipyridamole: May enhance the bradycardic effect of Beta-Blockers. *Risk C: Monitor therapy*

Disopyramide: May enhance the bradycardic effect of Beta-Blockers. *Risk C: Monitor therapy*

Herbs (Hypertensive Properties): May diminish the antihypertensive effect of Antihypertensives. *Risk C: Monitor therapy*

Herbs (Hypotensive Properties): May enhance the hypotensive effect of Antihypertensives. *Risk C: Monitor therapy*

Insulin: Beta-Blockers may enhance the hypoglycemic effect of Insulin. *Risk C: Monitor therapy*

Lidocaine: Beta-Blockers may decrease the metabolism of Lidocaine. *Risk C: Monitor therapy*

Methacholine: Beta-Blockers may enhance the adverse/toxic effect of Methacholine. *Risk X: Avoid combination*

Methylphenidate: May diminish the antihypertensive effect of Antihypertensives. *Risk C: Monitor therapy*

Midodrine: Beta-Blockers may enhance the bradycardic effect of Midodrine. *Risk C: Monitor therapy*

Nonsteroidal Anti-Inflammatory Agents: May diminish the antihypertensive effect of Beta-Blockers. *Risk C: Monitor therapy*

Propafenone: May decrease the metabolism of Beta-Blockers. Propafenone possesses some independent beta blocking activity. *Risk C: Monitor therapy*

Propoxyphene: May decrease the metabolism of Beta-Blockers. *Risk C: Monitor therapy*

Prostacyclin Analogues: May enhance the hypotensive effect of Antihypertensives. *Risk C: Monitor therapy*

QuiNIDine: May decrease the metabolism of Beta-Blockers. *Risk C: Monitor therapy*

Reserpine: May enhance the hypotensive effect of Beta-Blockers. *Risk C: Monitor therapy*

Rifamycin Derivatives: May decrease the serum concentration of Beta-Blockers. **Exceptions:** Rifabutin. *Risk C: Monitor therapy*

RiTUXimab: Antihypertensives may enhance the hypotensive effect of RiTUXimab. *Risk D: Consider therapy modification*

Theophylline Derivatives: Beta-Blockers (Beta$_1$ Selective) may diminish the bronchodilatory effect of Theophylline Derivatives. This is true at higher beta-blockers doses where cardioselectivity is lost. *Risk C: Monitor therapy*

Ethanol/Nutrition/Herb Interactions

Food: Peak serum acebutolol levels may be slightly decreased if taken with food.

Herb/Nutraceutical: Avoid dong quai if using for hypertension (has estrogenic activity). Avoid yohimbe, ginseng (may worsen hypertension).

Stability Store at controlled room temperature of 20°C to 25°C (68°F to 77°F). Protect from light and dispense in a light-resistant, tight container.

Mechanism of Action Competitively blocks beta$_1$-adrenergic receptors with little or no effect on beta$_2$-receptors except at high doses; exhibits membrane stabilizing and intrinsic sympathomimetic activity

Pharmacodynamics/Kinetics

Onset of action: 1-2 hours

Duration: 12-24 hours

Absorption: Oral: 40%

Protein binding: ~26%

Metabolism: Extensive first-pass effect to equipotent and cardioselective diacetolol metabolite

Half-life elimination: Parent drug: 3-4 hours; Metabolite: 8-13 hours

Time to peak: 2-4 hours

Excretion: Feces (50% to 60%); urine (30% to 40%); diacetolol eliminated primarily in the urine

Dosage Oral:

Adults:

Hypertension: 400-800 mg/day (larger doses may be divided); maximum: 1200 mg/day; usual dose range (JNC 7): 200-800 mg/day in 2 divided doses

Ventricular arrhythmias: Initial: 400 mg/day in divided doses; maintenance: 600-1200 mg/day in divided doses

Elderly: Initial: 200-400 mg/day; dose reduction due to age-related decrease in Cl_{cr} will be necessary; do not exceed 800 mg/day

Dosing adjustment in renal impairment:

Cl_{cr} 25-49 mL/minute: Reduce dose by 50%.

Cl_{cr} <25 mL/minute: Reduce dose by 75%.

Dosing adjustment in hepatic impairment: Use with caution.

Dietary Considerations May be taken without regard to meals.

Administration To discontinue therapy, taper dose gradually over a period of 2 weeks. May be administered without regard to meals.

Monitoring Parameters Blood glucose; blood pressure, orthostatic hypotension, heart rate, CNS effects, ECG

Test Interactions Increased AST, ALT, alkaline phosphatase, bilirubin, cholesterol, glucose, LDH, potassium, thyroxine, triglycerides, uric acid; decreased HDL

Dosage Forms Excipient information presented when available (limited, particularly for generics); consult specific product labeling.

Capsule, as hydrochloride: 200 mg, 400 mg

Sectral®: 200 mg, 400 mg

◆ **Acebutolol Hydrochloride** *see* Acebutolol *on page 27*

◆ **Acenocoumarin** *see* Acenocoumarol *on page 30*

Acenocoumarol (a see no KOOM a rol)

Medication Safety Issues Interferes with hepatic synthesis of vitamin K-dependent coagulation factors (II, VII, IX, X)

High alert medication: The Institute for Safe Medication Practices (ISMP) includes this medication among its list of drug classes which have a heightened risk of causing significant patient harm when used in error.

Canadian Brand Names Sintrom®

Mexican Brand Names Sintrom

Index Terms Acenocoumarin; Nicoumalone

Pharmacologic Category Anticoagulant, Coumarin Derivative

Use Prophylaxis and treatment of venous thrombosis, pulmonary embolism, and thromboembolic disorders; atrial fibrillation with risk of embolism; adjunct in the prophylaxis of coronary occlusion and transient ischemic attacks

Effect on Mental Status None reported

Effect on Psychiatric Treatment Carbamazepine may decrease the effects of acenocoumarol; SSRIs may enhance the anticoagulant effects of acenocoumarol

Restrictions Not available in U.S.

Dosage Summary Note: Dosage must be individualized. The following information is based on the manufacturer's labeling in Canada.

Oral:

Children: Dosage not established

Adults: Initial: 8-12 mg on day 1, followed by 4-8 mg on day 2; Maintenance: 1-10 mg/day (based on PT/INR measurements)

Dosage Forms Excipient information presented when available (limited, particularly for generics); consult specific product labeling. [CAN] = Canadian brand name

Tablet:

Sintrom® [CAN]: 1 mg, 4 mg [not available in the U.S.]

◆ **Aceon®** *see* Perindopril Erbumine *on page 1254*

◆ **Acephen™ [OTC]** *see* Acetaminophen *on page 30*

◆ **Acerola [OTC]** *see* Ascorbic Acid *on page 141*

◆ **Acetadote®** *see* Acetylcysteine *on page 47*

◆ **Aceta-Gesic [OTC]** *see* Acetaminophen and Phenyltoloxamine *on page 36*

Acetaminophen (a seet a MIN oh fen)

Medication Safety Issues

Sound-alike/look-alike issues:

Acephen® may be confused with AcipHex®

FeverALL® may be confused with Fiberall®

Tylenol® may be confused with atenolol, timolol, Tuinal®, Tylox®

International issues:

Paralen® [Czech Republic] may be confused with Aralen® which is a brand name for chloroquine in the U.S.

Duorol® may be confused with Diuril® which is a brand name for chlorothiazide in the U.S.

Duplicate therapy issues: This product contains acetaminophen, which may be a component of combination products. Do not exceed the maximum recommended daily dose of acetaminophen.

U.S. Brand Names Acephen™ [OTC]; Apra Children's [OTC]; Aspirin Free Anacin® Maximum Strength [OTC]; Cetafen Extra® [OTC]; Cetafen® [OTC]; Comtrex® Sore Throat Maximum Strength [OTC]; FeverALL® [OTC]; Genapap™ Children [OTC]; Genapap™ Extra Strength [OTC]; Genapap™ Infant [OTC]; Genapap™ [OTC]; Genebs Extra Strength [OTC]; Genebs [OTC]; Infantaire [OTC]; Little Fevers™ [OTC]; Mapap Children's [OTC]; Mapap Extra Strength [OTC]; Mapap Infants [OTC]; Mapap [OTC]; Nortemp Children's [OTC]; Pain Eze [OTC]; Silapap® Children's [OTC]; Silapap® Infants [OTC]; Tycolene Maximum Strength [OTC]; Tycolene [OTC]; Tylenol® 8 Hour [OTC]; Tylenol® Arthritis Pain [OTC]; Tylenol® Children's with Flavor Creator [OTC]; Tylenol® Children's [OTC]; Tylenol® Extra Strength [OTC]; Tylenol® Infants [OTC]; Tylenol® Junior [OTC]; Tylenol® [OTC]; Valorin Extra [OTC]; Valorin [OTC]

Canadian Brand Names Abenol®; Apo-Acetaminophen®; Atasol®; Novo-Gesic; Pediatrix; Tempra®; Tylenol®

Mexican Brand Names Adinol; Analphen; Dismifen; Doluvital ; Dolviran; Filanc; Mejoralito Junior; Mejoralito Pediátrico; Nordinet Infantil; Pharmacen-M; Sedalito; Sinedol; Tempra; Tylenol; Tylex; XL-Dol Infantil

Index Terms APAP; N-Acetyl-P-Aminophenol; Paracetamol

Pharmacologic Category Analgesic, Miscellaneous

Generic Available Yes: Excludes extended release products

Use Treatment of mild-to-moderate pain and fever (antipyretic/analgesic); does not have antirheumatic or anti-inflammatory effects

Effect on Mental Status None reported

Effect on Psychiatric Treatment Barbiturates and carbamazepine may increase the hepatotoxic potential of acetaminophen

Pregnancy Risk Factor B

Pregnancy Considerations Acetaminophen crosses the placenta. It is generally considered to be safe for use during pregnancy when used at therapeutic doses for short periods of time.

Lactation Enters breast milk/compatible

Contraindications Hypersensitivity to acetaminophen or any component of the formulation

Warnings/Precautions Limit dose to <4 g/day. May cause severe hepatic toxicity on acute overdose; in addition, chronic daily dosing in adults has resulted in liver damage in some patients. Use with caution in patients with alcoholic liver disease; consuming ≥3 alcoholic drinks/day may increase the risk of liver damage. Use caution in patients with known G6PD deficiency.

OTC labeling: When used for self-medication, patients should be instructed to contact healthcare provider if used for fever lasting >3 days or for pain lasting >10 days in adults or >5 days in children.

Adverse Reactions Frequency not defined.

Dermatologic: Rash

Endocrine & metabolic: May increase chloride, uric acid, glucose; may decrease sodium, bicarbonate, calcium

Hematologic: Anemia, blood dyscrasias (neutropenia, pancytopenia, leukopenia)

Hepatic: Bilirubin increased, alkaline phosphatase increased

Renal: Ammonia increased, nephrotoxicity with chronic overdose, analgesic nephropathy

Miscellaneous: Hypersensitivity reactions (rare)

Metabolism/Transport Effects **Substrate** (minor) of CYP1A2, 2A6, 2C9, 2D6, 2E1, 3A4; **Inhibits** CYP3A4 (weak)

Drug Interactions

Anticonvulsants (Hydantoin): May increase the metabolism of Acetaminophen. This may 1) diminish the effect of acetaminophen; and 2) increase the risk of liver damage. *Risk C: Monitor therapy*

Barbiturates: May increase the metabolism of Acetaminophen. This may 1) diminish the effect of acetaminophen; and 2) increase the risk of liver damage. *Risk C: Monitor therapy*

CarBAMazepine: May increase the metabolism of Acetaminophen. This may 1) diminish the effect of acetaminophen; and 2) increase the risk of liver damage. *Risk C: Monitor therapy*

Cholestyramine Resin: May decrease the absorption of Acetaminophen. Effect is minimal if cholestyramine is administered 1 hour after acetaminophen. *Risk D: Consider therapy modification*

Imatinib: May increase the serum concentration of Acetaminophen. *Risk D: Consider therapy modification*

Isoniazid: May enhance the adverse/toxic effect of Acetaminophen. *Risk C: Monitor therapy*

Vitamin K Antagonists (eg, warfarin): Acetaminophen may enhance the anticoagulant effect of Vitamin K Antagonists. Most likely with daily acetaminophen doses >1.3 g for >1 week. *Risk C: Monitor therapy*

Ethanol/Nutrition/Herb Interactions

Ethanol: Excessive intake of ethanol may increase the risk of acetaminophen-induced hepatotoxicity. Avoid ethanol or limit to <3 drinks/day.

Food: Rate of absorption may be decreased when given with food.

Herb/Nutraceutical: St John's wort may decrease acetaminophen levels.

Stability Do not freeze suppositories.

Mechanism of Action Inhibits the synthesis of prostaglandins in the central nervous system and peripherally blocks pain impulse generation; produces antipyresis from inhibition of hypothalamic heat-regulating center

Pharmacodynamics/Kinetics

Onset of action: <1 hour

Duration: 4-6 hours

Absorption: Incomplete; varies by dosage form

Protein binding: 8% to 43% at toxic doses

Metabolism: At normal therapeutic dosages, hepatic to sulfate and glucuronide metabolites, while a small amount is metabolized by CYP to a highly reactive intermediate (acetylimidoquinone) which is conjugated with glutathione and inactivated; at toxic doses (as little as 4 g daily) glutathione conjugation becomes insufficient to meet the metabolic demand causing an increase in acetylimidoquinone concentration, which may cause hepatic cell necrosis

Half-life elimination: Prolonged following toxic doses

Neonates: 2-5 hours

Adults: 1-3 hours (may be increased in elderly; however, this should not affect dosing)

Time to peak, serum: Oral: 10-60 minutes; may be delayed in acute overdoses

Excretion: Urine (2% to 5% unchanged; 55% as glucuronide metabolites; 30% as sulphate metabolites)

Dosage Oral, rectal:

Children <12 years: 10-15 mg/kg/dose every 4-6 hours as needed; do **not** exceed 5 doses (2.6 g) in 24 hours; alternatively, the following age-based doses may be used; see table.

Acetaminophen Dosing

Age	Dosage (mg)	Age	Dosage (mg)
0-3 mo	40	4-5 y	240
4-11 mo	80	6-8 y	320
1-2 y	120	9-10 y	400
2-3 y	160	11 y	480

Note: Higher rectal doses have been studied for use in preoperative pain control in children. However, specific guidelines are not available and dosing may be product dependent. The safety and efficacy of alternating acetaminophen and ibuprofen dosing has not been established.

Adults: 325-650 mg every 4-6 hours or 1000 mg 3-4 times/day; do **not** exceed 4 g/day

Dosing interval in renal impairment:

Cl_{cr} 10-50 mL/minute: Administer every 6 hours

Cl_{cr} <10 mL/minute: Administer every 8 hours (metabolites accumulate)

Hemodialysis: Moderately dialyzable (20% to 50%)

Dosing adjustment/comments in hepatic impairment: Use with caution. Limited, low-dose therapy is usually well tolerated in hepatic disease/cirrhosis. However, cases of hepatotoxicity at daily acetaminophen dosages <4 g/day have been reported. Avoid chronic use in hepatic impairment.

Dietary Considerations Chewable tablets may contain phenylalanine (amount varies, ranges between 3-12 mg/tablet); consult individual product labeling.

Administration

Suppositories: Do not freeze.

Suspension, oral: Shake well before pouring a dose.

Monitoring Parameters Relief of pain or fever

Reference Range

Therapeutic concentration (analgesic/antipyretic): 10-30 mcg/mL

Toxic concentration (acute ingestion) with probable hepatotoxicity: >200 mcg/mL at 4 hours or 50 mcg/mL at 12 hours after ingestion

Test Interactions Increased chloride, bilirubin, uric acid, glucose, ammonia (B), chloride (S), uric acid (S), alkaline phosphatase (S), chloride (S); decreased sodium, bicarbonate, calcium (S)

Dosage Forms Excipient information presented when available (limited, particularly for generics); consult specific product labeling. [DSC] = Discontinued product

Caplet: 500 mg

Cetafen Extra® Strength, Genapap™ Extra Strength, Genebs Extra Strength, Mapap Extra Strength, Tycolene Maximum Strength, Tylenol® Extra Strength: 500 mg

Caplet, extended release:

Tylenol® 8 Hour, Tylenol® Arthritis Pain: 650 mg

Capsule: 500 mg

Elixir: 160 mg/5 mL (120 mL, 480 mL, 3780 mL [DSC])

Apra Children's: 160 mg/5 mL (120 mL, 480 mL, 3780 mL [DSC]) [alcohol free; contains benzoic acid; cherry and grape flavors]

Mapap Children's: 160 mg/5 mL (120 mL) [alcohol free; contains benzoic acid and sodium benzoate; cherry flavor]

Gelcap:

Mapap Extra Strength, Tylenol® Extra Strength: 500 mg

Geltab:

Tylenol® Extra Strength: 500 mg

Liquid, oral: 500 mg/15 mL (240 mL)

Comtrex® Sore Throat Maximum Strength: 500 mg/15 mL (240 mL) [contains sodium benzoate; honey lemon flavor]

Genapap™ Children: 160 mg/5 mL (120 mL) [contains sodium benzoate; cherry and grape flavors]

Silapap®: 160 mg/5 mL (120 mL, 240 mL, 480 mL) [sugar free; contains sodium benzoate; cherry flavor]

Tylenol® Extra Strength: 500 mg/15 mL (240 mL) [contains sodium benzoate; cherry flavor]

Solution, oral: 160 mg/5 mL (120 mL, 480 mL)

Solution, oral [drops]: 80 mg/0.8 mL (15 mL) [droppers are marked at 0.4 mL (40 mg) and at 0.8 mL (80 mg)]

Genapap™ Infant: 80 mg/0.8 mL (15 mL) [fruit flavor]

Infantaire: 80 mg/0.8mL (15 mL, 30 mL)

Little Fevers™: 80 mg/1 mL (30 mL) [alcohol free; contains propylene glycol, sodium benzoate; berry flavor; packaged with dropper and forehead thermometer]

Silapap® Infant's: 80 mg/0.8 mL (15 mL, 30 mL) [contains sodium benzoate; cherry flavor]

Suppository, rectal: 120 mg, 325 mg, 650 mg

Acephen™: 120 mg, 325 mg, 650 mg

FeverALL®: 80 mg, 120 mg, 325 mg, 650 mg

Mapap: 125 mg, 650 mg

Suspension, oral: 160 mg/5 mL (5 mL, 10 mL, 20 mL)

Mapap Children's: 160 mg/5 mL (120 mL) [contains sodium benzoate; cherry flavor]

Nortemp Children's: 160 mg/5 mL (120 mL) [alcohol free; contains sodium benzoate; cotton candy flavor]

Tylenol® Children's: 160 mg/5 mL (120 mL, 240 mL) [contains sodium benzoate; bubble gum yum, cherry blast, dye free cherry, grape splash, and very berry strawberry flavors]

Tylenol® Children's with Flavor Creator: 160 mg/5 mL (120 mL) [contains sodium 2 mg/5 mL and sodium benzoate; cherry blast flavor; packaged with apple (4), bubblegum (8), chocolate (4), & strawberry (4) sugar free flavor packets]

Suspension, oral [drops]:

Mapap Infants: 80 mg/0.8 mL (15 mL, 30 mL) [contains sodium benzoate; cherry flavor]

Tylenol® Infants: 80 mg/0.8 mL (15 mL, 30 mL) [contains sodium benzoate; cherry, dye free cherry, and grape flavors]

Tablet: 325 mg, 500 mg

Aspirin Free Anacin® Extra Strength, Genapap™ Extra Strength, Genebs Extra Strength, Mapap Extra Strength, Pain Eze, Tylenol® Extra Strength, Valorin Extra: 500 mg

Cetafen®, Genapap™, Genebs, Mapap, Tycolene, Tylenol®, Valorin: 325 mg

Tablet, chewable: 80 mg

Genapap™ Children: 80 mg [contains phenylalanine 6 mg/tablet; grape flavors] [DSC]

Mapap Children's: 80 mg [contains phenylalanine 3 mg/tablet; bubble gum, fruit, and grape flavors]
Mapap Junior Strength: 160 mg [contains phenylalanine 12 mg/tablet; grape flavor]
Tablet, orally disintegrating: 80 mg, 160 mg
Tylenol® Children's Meltaways: 80 mg [bubble gum, grape, and watermelon flavors]
Tylenol® Junior Meltaways: 160 mg [bubble gum and grape flavors]

- **Acetaminophen and Butalbital** *see* Butalbital and Acetaminophen *on page 236*
- **Acetaminophen and Chlorpheniramine** *see* Chlorpheniramine and Acetaminophen *on page 322*

Acetaminophen and Codeine (a seet a MIN oh fen & KOE deen)

Medication Safety Issues

Sound-alike/look-alike issues:
Capital® may be confused with Capitrol®
Tylenol® may be confused with atenolol, timolol, Tuinal®, Tylox®

T3 is an error-prone abbreviation (mistaken as liothyronine)

High alert medication: The Institute for Safe Medication Practices (ISMP) includes this medication among its list of drug classes which have a heightened risk of causing significant patient harm when used in error.

Duplicate therapy issues: This product contains acetaminophen, which may be a component of other combination products. Do not exceed the maximum recommended daily dose of acetaminophen.

U.S. Brand Names Capital® and Codeine; Tylenol® With Codeine

Canadian Brand Names ratio-Emtec; ratio-Lenoltec; Triatec-30; Triatec-8; Triatec-8 Strong; Tylenol Elixir with Codeine; Tylenol No. 1; Tylenol No. 1 Forte; Tylenol No. 2 with Codeine; Tylenol No. 3 with Codeine; Tylenol No. 4 with Codeine

Mexican Brand Names Tylex CD

Index Terms Codeine and Acetaminophen

Pharmacologic Category Analgesic, Opioid

Use Relief of mild-to-moderate pain

Effect on Mental Status Sedation is common; less commonly, codeine may produce euphoria or dysphoria

Effect on Psychiatric Treatment Codeine may produce physical and psychological dependence. Antipsychotics, TCAs, MAO inhibitors, barbiturates, benzodiazepines, and anticonvulsants may increase the toxicity of codeine. Barbiturates and carbamazepine may increase the hepatotoxic potential of acetaminophen. Diminution of pain relief may occur with the SSRIs.

Restrictions C-III; C-V

Note: In countries outside of the U.S., some formulations of Tylenol® with Codeine (eg, Tylenol® No. 3) include caffeine.

Dosage Summary

Oral:

Acetaminophen:
Children ≤12 years: 10-15 mg/kg/dose every 4-6 hours as needed (maximum: 2.6 g/day)
Children >12 years: 325-650 mg every 4-6 hours as needed (maximum: 4 g/day)
Adults: 325-650 mg every 4-6 hours as needed (maximum: 4 g/day)

Codeine:
Children: 0.5-1 mg/kg/dose every 4-6 hours (maximum: 60 mg/dose)
Adults: 15-60 mg/dose every 4-6 hours (maximum: 360 mg/day)

Dosage Forms Excipient information presented when available (limited, particularly for generics); consult specific product labeling. [DSC] = Discontinued product; [CAN] = Canadian brand name

Caplet:
ratio-Lenoltec No. 1 [CAN], Tylenol No. 1 [CAN]: Acetaminophen 300 mg, codeine phosphate 8 mg, and caffeine 15 mg [not available in the U.S.]
Tylenol No. 1 Forte [CAN]: Acetaminophen 500 mg, codeine phosphate 8 mg, and caffeine 15 mg [not available in the U.S.]

Elixir, oral [C-V]: Acetaminophen 120 mg and codeine phosphate 12 mg per 5 mL (5 mL, 10 mL, 12.5 mL, 15 mL, 120 mL, 480 mL) [contains alcohol 7%]
Tylenol® with Codeine [DSC]: Acetaminophen 120 mg and codeine phosphate 12 mg per 5 mL (480 mL) [contains alcohol 7%; cherry flavor]

Tylenol Elixir with Codeine [CAN]: Acetaminophen 160 mg and codeine phosphate 8 mg per 5 mL (500 mL) [contains alcohol 7%, sucrose 31%; cherry flavor; not available in the U.S.]

Suspension, oral [C-V] (Capital® and Codeine): Acetaminophen 120 mg and codeine phosphate 12 mg per 5 mL (480 mL) [alcohol free; fruit punch flavor]

Tablet [C-III]: Acetaminophen 300 mg and codeine phosphate 15 mg; acetaminophen 300 mg and codeine phosphate 30 mg; acetaminophen 300 mg and codeine phosphate 60 mg

ratio-Emtec [CAN], Triatec-30 [CAN]: Acetaminophen 300 mg and codeine phosphate 30 mg [not available in the U.S.]

ratio-Lenoltec No. 1 [CAN]: Acetaminophen 300 mg, codeine phosphate 8 mg, and caffeine 15 mg [not available in the U.S.]

ratio-Lenoltec No. 2 [CAN], Tylenol No. 2 with Codeine [CAN]: Acetaminophen 300 mg, codeine phosphate 15 mg, and caffeine 15 mg [not available in the U.S.]

ratio-Lenoltec No. 3 [CAN], Tylenol No. 3 with Codeine [CAN]: Acetaminophen 300 mg, codeine phosphate 30 mg, and caffeine 15 mg [not available in the U.S.]

ratio-Lenoltec No. 4 [CAN], Tylenol No. 4 with Codeine [CAN]: Acetaminophen 300 mg and codeine phosphate 60 mg [not available in the U.S.]

Triatec-8 [CAN]: Acetaminophen 325 mg, codeine phosphate 8 mg, and caffeine 30 mg [not available in the U.S.]

Triatec-8 Strong [CAN]: Acetaminophen 500 mg, codeine phosphate 8 mg, and caffeine 30 mg [not available in the U.S.]

Tylenol® with Codeine No. 3: Acetaminophen 300 mg and codeine phosphate 30 mg [contains sodium metabisulfite]

Tylenol® with Codeine No. 4: Acetaminophen 300 mg and codeine phosphate 60 mg [contains sodium metabisulfite]

Acetaminophen and Diphenhydramine

(a seet a MIN oh fen & dye fen HYE dra meen)

Medication Safety Issues

Sound-alike/look-alike issues:

Excedrin® may be confused with Dexatrim®, Dexedrine®

Percogesic® may be confused with paregoric, Percodan®

Tylenol® may be confused with atenolol, timolol, Tuinal®, Tylox®

Duplicate therapy issues: This product contains acetaminophen, which may be a component of other combination products. Do not exceed the maximum recommended daily dose of acetaminophen.

U.S. Brand Names Excedrin® P.M. [OTC]; Goody's PM® [OTC]; Legatrin PM® [OTC]; Percogesic® Extra Strength [OTC]; Tylenol® PM [OTC]; Tylenol® Severe Allergy [OTC]

Index Terms Diphenhydramine and Acetaminophen

Pharmacologic Category Analgesic, Miscellaneous

Use Aid in the relief of insomnia accompanied by minor pain

Effect on Mental Status Drowsiness is common

Effect on Psychiatric Treatment Concurrent use with CNS depressant may result in additive CNS depression. MAO inhibitor may cause additive anticholinergic effects.

Dosage Summary

Oral:

Children <12 years: Dosage not established

Children ≥12 years: 50 mg of diphenhydramine HCl (76 mg diphenhydramine citrate) at bedtime (maximum: Do not exceed recommended dosage)

Adults: 50 mg of diphenhydramine HCl (76 mg diphenhydramine citrate) at bedtime (maximum: Do not exceed recommended dosage)

Dosage Forms Excipient information presented when available (limited, particularly for generics); consult specific product labeling.

Caplet: Acetaminophen 500 mg and diphenhydramine hydrochloride 25 mg

Excedrin® P.M.: Acetaminophen 500 mg and diphenhydramine citrate 38 mg

Legatrin PM®: Acetaminophen 500 mg and diphenhydramine hydrochloride 50 mg

Percogesic® Extra Strength: Acetaminophen 500 mg and diphenhydramine hydrochloride 25 mg

Tylenol® PM: Acetaminophen 500 mg and diphenhydramine hydrochloride 25 mg [also available in vanilla caplets]

Tylenol® Severe Allergy: Acetaminophen 500 mg and diphenhydramine hydrochloride 12.5 mg

Gelcap:
Tylenol® PM: Acetaminophen 500 mg and diphenhydramine hydrochloride 25 mg
Geltab: Acetaminophen 500 mg and diphenhydramine hydrochloride 25 mg
Excedrin® P.M.: Acetaminophen 500 mg and diphenhydramine citrate 38 mg
Tylenol® PM: Acetaminophen 500 mg and diphenhydramine hydrochloride 25 mg
Liquid:
Tylenol® PM: Acetaminophen 500 mg and diphenhydramine hydrochloride 25 mg per 15 mL (240 mL) [contains sodium benzoate; vanilla flavor]
Powder for oral solution:
Goody's PM®: Acetaminophen 500 mg and diphenhydramine citrate 38 mg [contains potassium 41.9 mg and sodium 3.15 mg per powder]
Tablet: Acetaminophen 500 mg and diphenhydramine hydrochloride 25 mg
Excedrin® P.M.: Acetaminophen 500 mg and diphenhydramine citrate 38 mg

- **Acetaminophen and Hydrocodone** *see* Hydrocodone and Acetaminophen *on page 777*
- **Acetaminophen and Oxycodone** *see* Oxycodone and Acetaminophen *on page 1205*
- **Acetaminophen and Pentazocine** *see* Pentazocine and Acetaminophen *on page 1245*

Acetaminophen and Phenylephrine

(a seet a MIN oh fen & fen il EF rin)

Medication Safety Issues
Duplicate therapy issues: This product contains acetaminophen, which may be a component of combination products. Do not exceed the maximum recommended daily dose of acetaminophen.

U.S. Brand Names Alka-Seltzer Plus® Sinus Formula [OTC]; Contac® Cold + Flu Maximum Strength Non-Drowsy [OTC]; Mapap® Sinus Congestion and Pain Daytime [OTC]; Sinutab® Sinus [OTC]; Sudafed PE® Sinus Headache [OTC]; Tylenol® Sinus Congestion & Pain Daytime [OTC]

Index Terms Phenylephrine Hydrochloride and Acetaminophen

Pharmacologic Category Analgesic, Miscellaneous; Decongestant

Use Temporary relief of sinus/nasal congestion and pressure, headache, and minor aches and pains

Effect on Mental Status May cause anxiety and restlessness

Effect on Psychiatric Treatment Avoid concurrent use with MAO inhibitors; may result in hypertensive crisis and is contraindicated. Barbiturates and carbamazepine may increase the hepatotoxic potential of acetaminophen. Individuals consuming ≥3 alcoholic drinks/day may increase the risk of liver damage.

Dosage Forms Excipient information presented when available (limited, particularly for generics); consult specific product labeling.
Caplet, oral:
Contac® Cold + Flu Maximum Strength Non Drowsy: Acetaminophen 500 mg and phenylephrine hydrochloride 5 mg
Mapap® Sinus Congestion and Pain Daytime, Sinutab® Sinus, Sudafed PE® Sinus Headache: Acetaminophen 325 mg and phenylephrine hydrochloride 5 mg
Tylenol® Sinus Congestion & Pain Daytime: Acetaminophen 325 mg and phenylephrine hydrochloride 5 mg [Cool Burst™ flavor]
Gelcap, oral:
Tylenol® Sinus Congestion & Pain Daytime: Acetaminophen 325 mg and phenylephrine hydrochloride 5 mg
Gelcap, rapid release, oral:
Tylenol® Sinus Congestion & Pain Datyime: Acetaminophen 325 mg and phenylephrine hydrochloride 5 mg
Tablet for solution, oral [effervescent]:
Alka-Seltzer Plus® Sinus Formula: Acetaminophen 250 mg and phenylephrine hydrochloride 5 mg [contains sodium 477 mg/tablet and phenylalanine 4.2 mg/tablet; lemon zest flavor]

Acetaminophen and Phenyltoloxamine

(a seet a MIN oh fen & fen il to LOKS a meen)

Medication Safety Issues
Sound-alike/look-alike issues:
Percogesic® may be confused with paregoric, Percodan®

Duplicate therapy issues: This product contains acetaminophen, which may be a component of other combination products. Do not exceed the maximum recommended daily dose of acetaminophen.

U.S. Brand Names Aceta-Gesic [OTC]; Alpain; BeFlex; Dologesic®; Flextra 650; Flextra-DS; Genasec™ [OTC]; Hyflex-DS® [DSC]; Lagesic™; Percogesic® [OTC]; Phenagesic [OTC]; Phenylgesic [OTC]; RhinoFlex 650; RhinoFlex™; Staflex; Vistra 650; Zgesic

Index Terms Phenyltoloxamine Citrate and Acetaminophen

Pharmacologic Category Analgesic, Miscellaneous

Use Relief of mild-to-moderate pain

Effect on Mental Status None reported

Effect on Psychiatric Treatment Barbiturates and carbamazepine may increase the hepatotoxic potential of acetaminophen

Dosage Summary

Oral: Based on acetaminophen component:

Children <12 years: 10-15 mg/kg/dose every 4-6 hours as needed (maximum: 2.6 g/day)

Children ≥12 years: 325-650 mg every 4-6 hours as needed (maximum: 4 g/day)

Adults: 325-650 mg every 4-6 hours as needed (maximum: 4 g/day)

Dosage Forms Excipient information presented when available (limited, particularly for generics); consult specific product labeling. [DSC] = Discontinued product

Caplet:

Alpain: Acetaminophen 500 mg and phenyltoloxamine citrate 60 mg

BeFlex: Acetaminophen 500 mg and phenyltoloxamine citrate 55 mg

Dologesic®: Acetaminophen 500 mg and phenyltoloxamine citrate 30 mg

Staflex: Acetaminophen 500 mg and phenyltoloxamine citrate 55 mg

Caplet, extended release [scored]:

Lagesic™: Acetaminophen 600 mg and phenyltoloxamine citrate 66 mg

Capsule:

Dologesic®: Acetaminophen 500 mg and phenyltoloxamine citrate 30 mg

Liquid:

Dologesic®: Acetaminophen 500 mg and phenyltoloxamine citrate 30 mg per 15 mL (180 mL)

Tablet: Acetaminophen 325 mg and phenyltoloxamine citrate 30 mg

Aceta-Gesic, Genasec™, Percogesic®, Phenagesic, Phenylgesic: Acetaminophen 325 mg and phenyltoloxamine citrate 30 mg

Flextra-650, Vistra 650: Acetaminophen 650 mg and phenyltoloxamine citrate 60 mg

Flextra-DS, Hyflex-DS® [DSC], RhinoFlex™: Acetaminophen 500 mg and phenyltoloxamine citrate 50 mg

RhinoFlex™-650: Acetaminophen 650 mg and phenyltoloxamine citrate 50 mg

Tablet, prolonged release, oral:

Zgesic: Acetaminophen 600 mg and phenyltoloxamine citrate 66 mg

◆ **Acetaminophen and Propoxyphene** *see* Propoxyphene and Acetaminophen *on page 1354*

Acetaminophen and Pseudoephedrine

(a seet a MIN oh fen & soo doe e FED rin)

Medication Safety Issues

Sound-alike/look-alike issues:

Ornex® may be confused with Orexin®, Orinase®

Sudafed® may be confused with Sufenta®

Tylenol® may be confused with atenolol, timolol, Tuinal®, Tylox®

Duplicate therapy issues: This product contains acetaminophen, which may be a component of other combination products. Do not exceed the maximum recommended daily dose of acetaminophen.

U.S. Brand Names Allerest® Allergy and Sinus Relief [OTC]; Genapap™ Sinus Maximum Strength [OTC] [DSC]; Mapap Sinus Maximum Strength [OTC]; Medi-Synal [OTC]; Oranyl Plus [OTC]; Ornex® Maximum Strength [OTC]; Ornex® [OTC]; Sudafed® Multi-Symptom Sinus and Cold [OTC]; Tylenol® Cold Daytime, Children's [OTC]; Tylenol® Cold, Infants [OTC] [DSC]; Tylenol® Sinus Daytime [OTC]

Canadian Brand Names Contac® Cold and Sore Throat, Non Drowsy, Extra Strength; Dristan® N.D.; Dristan® N.D., Extra Strength; Sinutab® Non Drowsy; Sudafed® Head Cold and Sinus Extra Strength; Tylenol® Decongestant; Tylenol® Sinus

Index Terms Pseudoephedrine and Acetaminophen

Pharmacologic Category Alpha/Beta Agonist; Analgesic, Miscellaneous

Use Relief of mild-to-moderate pain; relief of congestion

Effect on Mental Status Anxiety, insomnia, excitability common; hallucination may be seen rarely

Effect on Psychiatric Treatment Hypertensive crisis may result with MAO inhibitor, effects of CNS depressants may be lessened

Dosage Summary

Oral:

Acetaminophen:

Children ≤12 years: 10-15 mg/kg/dose every 4-6 hours as needed (maximum: 2.6 g/day)

Children >12 years: 325-650 mg every 4-6 hours as needed (maximum: 4 g/day)

Adults: 325-650 mg every 4-6 hours as needed (maximum: 4 g/day)

Pseudoephedrine:

Children <2 years: Dosage not established

Children 2-6 years: 15 mg every 4 hours (maximum: 90 mg/day)

Children 6-12 years: 30 mg every 4 hours (maximum: 180 mg/day)

Children >12 years: 60 mg every 4 hours (maximum: 360 mg/day)

Dosage Forms Excipient information presented when available (limited, particularly for generics); consult specific product labeling. [DSC] = Discontinued product

Caplet:

Allerest® Allergy and Sinus Relief, Ornex®: Acetaminophen 325 mg and pseudoephedrine hydrochloride 30 mg

Genapap™ Sinus Maximum Strength [DSC], Mapap Sinus Maximum Strength, Ornex® Maximum Strength, Tylenol® Sinus Daytime: Acetaminophen 500 mg and pseudoephedrine hydrochloride 30 mg

Capsule, liquid:

Sudafed® Multi-Symptom Sinus and Cold: Acetaminophen 325 mg and pseudoephedrine hydrochloride 30 mg [contains sodium 16 mg]

Gelcap:

Tylenol® Sinus Daytime: Acetaminophen 500 mg and pseudoephedrine hydrochloride 30 mg

Liquid:

Childrens Tylenol® Cold Daytime: Acetaminophen 160 mg and pseudoephedrine hydrochloride 15 mg per 5 mL (120 mL) [contains sodium benzoate; fruit flavor]

Liquid, oral [drops]:

Infants Tylenol® Cold: Acetaminophen 80 mg and pseudoephedrine 7.5 mg per 0.8 mL [contains sodium benzoate; bubble gum flavor] [DSC]

Tablet:

Medi-Synal: Acetaminophen 325 mg and pseudoephedrine hydrochloride 30 mg

Oranyl Plus: Acetaminophen 500 mg and pseudoephedrine hydrochloride 30 mg

Acetaminophen and Tramadol (a seet a MIN oh fen & TRA ma dole)

Medication Safety Issues

Sound-alike/look-alike issues:

Ultracet® may be confused with Ultane®, Ultram®

Duplicate therapy issues: This product contains acetaminophen, which may be a component of other combination products. Do not exceed the maximum recommended daily dose of acetaminophen.

U.S. Brand Names Ultracet®

Canadian Brand Names Tramacet

Mexican Brand Names Tramacet; Zaldiar

Index Terms APAP and Tramadol; Tramadol Hydrochloride and Acetaminophen

Pharmacologic Category Analgesic, Miscellaneous; Analgesic, Opioid

Use Short-term (≤5 days) management of acute pain

Effect on Mental Status May cause sedation, dizziness, insomnia, anxiety, confusion, or euphoria; monitor with concurrent psychotropic use

Effect on Psychiatric Treatment Contraindicated with acute intoxication of psychotropic drugs. Use with extreme caution with MAO inhibitors. Seizure risk is increased with SSRIs, TCAs, antipsychotics, and MAO inhibitors. Carbamazepine may decrease the half-life of tramadol (concurrent use is not recommended). Fluoxetine and paroxetine may increase tramadol serum concentrations.

Dosage Summary

Oral:

Children: Dosage not established

Adults: Two tablets every 4-6 hours as needed (maximum: 8 tablets/day)

Dosage Forms Excipient information presented when available (limited, particularly for generics); consult specific product labeling.

Tablet: Acetaminophen 325 mg and tramadol hydrochloride 37.5 mg

Acetaminophen, Aspirin, and Caffeine

(a seet a MIN oh fen, AS pir in, & KAF een)

Medication Safety Issues

Sound-alike/look-alike issues:

Excedrin® may be confused with Dexatrim®, Dexedrine®

Duplicate therapy issues: This product contains acetaminophen, which may be a component of other combination products. Do not exceed the maximum recommended daily dose of acetaminophen.

U.S. Brand Names Excedrin® Extra Strength [OTC]; Excedrin® Migraine [OTC]; Fem-Prin® [OTC]; Genaced™ [OTC]; Goody's® Extra Strength Headache Powder [OTC]; Goody's® Extra Strength Pain Relief [OTC]; Pain-Off [OTC]; Vanquish® Extra Strength Pain Reliever [OTC]

Index Terms Aspirin, Acetaminophen, and Caffeine; Aspirin, Caffeine and Acetaminophen; Caffeine, Acetaminophen, and Aspirin; Caffeine, Aspirin, and Acetaminophen

Pharmacologic Category Analgesic, Miscellaneous

Use Relief of mild-to-moderate pain; mild-to-moderate pain associated with migraine headache

Effect on Mental Status May cause anxiety, insomnia, and excitability

Effect on Psychiatric Treatment Effects of CNS depressants may be lessened by caffeine component

Dosage Summary

Oral:

Children ≤12 years: Dosage not established

Children >12 years: 1-2 doses every 4-6 hours as needed (maximum: 4 g/day [based on acetaminophen and aspirin component])

Adults: 1-2 doses every 4-6 hours as needed (maximum: 4 g/day [based on acetaminophen and aspirin component])

Dosage Forms Excipient information presented when available (limited, particularly for generics); consult specific product labeling.

Caplet:

Excedrin® Extra Strength, Excedrin® Migraine: Acetaminophen 250 mg, aspirin 250 mg, and caffeine 65 mg

Vanquish® Extra Strength Pain Reliever: Acetaminophen 194 mg, aspirin 227 mg, and caffeine 33 mg

Geltab (Excedrin® Extra Strength, Excedrin® Migraine): Acetaminophen 250 mg, aspirin 250 mg, and caffeine 65 mg

Powder (Goody's® Extra Strength Headache Powder): Acetaminophen 260 mg, aspirin 520 mg, and caffeine 32.5 mg [contains lactose]

Tablet:

Excedrin® Extra Strength, Excedrin® Migraine, Genaced™, Pain-Off: Acetaminophen 250 mg, aspirin 250 mg, and caffeine 65 mg

Fem-Prin®: Acetaminophen 194.4 mg, aspirin 226.8 mg, and caffeine 32.4 mg

Goody's® Extra Strength Pain Relief: Acetaminophen 130 mg, aspirin 260 mg, and caffeine 16.25 mg

◆ **Acetaminophen, Butalbital, and Caffeine** *see* Butalbital, Acetaminophen, and Caffeine *on page 229*

Acetaminophen, Caffeine, and Dihydrocodeine

(a seet a MIN oh fen, KAF een, & dye hye droe KOE deen)

Medication Safety Issues

Sound-alike/look-alike issues:

Panlor® DC may be confused with Pamelor®

High alert medication: The Institute for Safe Medication Practices (ISMP) includes this medication among its list of drug classes which have a heightened risk of causing significant patient harm when used in error.

Duplicate therapy issues: This product contains acetaminophen, which may be a component of other combination products. Do not exceed the maximum recommended daily dose of acetaminophen.

U.S. Brand Names Panlor® DC; Panlor® SS; ZerLor™

Index Terms Caffeine, Dihydrocodeine, and Acetaminophen; Dihydrocodeine Bitartrate, Acetaminophen, and Caffeine

Pharmacologic Category Analgesic Combination (Opioid)

Use Relief of moderate to moderately-severe pain

Effect on Mental Status May cause dizziness or drowsiness

Effect on Psychiatric Treatment May cause nausea and vomiting; combined use with SSRIs, acetylcholinesterase inhibitors, aripiprazole, or ziprasidone may produce additive effects. The effects of benzodiazepines, mirtazapine, nefazodone, and venlafaxine may be enhanced by caffeine (CYP3A4 inhibitor). Use with chlorpromazine, fluoxetine, paroxetine, pergolide, or ropinirole may decrease the effects of dihydrocodeine. Fluvoxamine may increase the effects of caffeine. Reduce caffeine consumption by 50% or choose an alternative SSRI. Barbiturates, carbamazepine, and excessive intake of ethanol may decrease the effectiveness, as well as increase the hepatotoxic potential of acetaminophen. Combined use with psychotropics may produce additive sedative effects.

Restrictions C-III

Dosage Summary

Oral:

Children: Dosage not established

Adults: 1 tablet or 2 capsules every 4 hours as needed (maximum: 10 capsules/day or 5 tablets/day)

Dosage Forms Excipient information presented when available (limited, particularly for generics); consult specific product labeling.

Capsule:

Panlor® DC: Acetaminophen 356.4 mg, caffeine 30 mg, and dihydrocodeine bitartrate 16 mg

Tablet:

Panlor® SS, ZerLor™: Acetaminophen 712.8 mg, caffeine 60 mg, and dihydrocodeine bitartrate 32 mg

◆ **Acetaminophen, Caffeine, Codeine, and Butalbital** *see* Butalbital, Acetaminophen, Caffeine, and Codeine *on page 232*

Acetaminophen, Chlorpheniramine, and Pseudoephedrine

(a seet a MIN oh fen, klor fen IR a meen, & soo doe e FED rin)

Medication Safety Issues

Sound-alike/look-alike issues:

Thera-Flu® may be confused with Tamiflu®, Thera-Flur-N®

Tylenol® may be confused with atenolol, timolol, Tuinal®, Tylox®

Duplicate therapy issues: This product contains acetaminophen, which may be a component of other combination products. Do not exceed the maximum recommended daily dose of acetaminophen.

U.S. Brand Names Actifed® Cold and Sinus [OTC]; Comtrex® Flu Therapy Nighttime [OTC]; Drinex [OTC]; Kolephrin® [OTC]; Sinutab® Sinus Allergy Maximum Strength [OTC]; Tylenol® Children's Plus Cold Nighttime [OTC] [DSC]

Canadian Brand Names Sinutab® Sinus & Allergy; Tylenol® Allergy Sinus

Index Terms Acetaminophen, Pseudoephedrine, and Chlorpheniramine; Chlorpheniramine, Acetaminophen, and Pseudoephedrine; Chlorpheniramine, Pseudoephedrine, and Acetaminophen; Pseudoephedrine, Acetaminophen, and Chlorpheniramine; Pseudoephedrine, Chlorpheniramine, and Acetaminophen

Pharmacologic Category Alpha/Beta Agonist; Analgesic, Miscellaneous; Histamine H_1 Antagonist; Histamine H_1 Antagonist, First Generation

Use Temporary relief of sinus symptoms

Effect on Mental Status Sedation with chlorpheniramine is countered by the excitability associated with pseudoephedrine; one effect may predominate in any particular patient

Effect on Psychiatric Treatment Usually none; sedative effect of chlorpheniramine may be potentiated by other CNS depressants and MAO inhibitors

Dosage Summary

Oral:

Acetaminophen:

Children ≤12 years: 10-15 mg/kg/dose every 4-6 hours as needed (maximum: 2.6 g/day)

Children >12 years: 325-650 mg every 4-6 hours as needed (maximum: 4 g/day)

Adults: 325-650 mg every 4-6 hours as needed (maximum: 4 g/day)

Chlorpheniramine:

Children <2 years: Dosage not established

Children 2-6 years: 1 mg every 4-6 hours (maximum: 6 mg/day)

Children 6-12 years: 2 mg every 4-6 hours (maximum: 12 mg/day)

Children >12 years: 4 mg every 4-6 hours (maximum: 24 mg/day)

Adults: 4 mg every 4-6 hours (maximum: 24 mg/day)

Pseudoephedrine:

Children <2 years: Dosage not established

Children 2-6 years: 15 mg every 4 hours (maximum: 90 mg/day)

Children 6-12 years: 30 mg every 4 hours (maximum: 180 mg/day)

Children >12 years: 60 mg every 4 hours (maximum: 360 mg/day)

Adults: 60 mg every 4 hours (maximum: 360 mg/day)

Dosage Forms Excipient information presented when available (limited, particularly for generics); consult specific product labeling. [DSC] = Discontinued product

Caplet: Acetaminophen 325 mg, chlorpheniramine maleate 2 mg, and pseudoephedrine hydrochloride 30 mg

Actifed® Cold and Sinus, Sinutab® Sinus Allergy Maximum Strength: Acetaminophen 500 mg, chlorpheniramine maleate 2 mg, and pseudoephedrine hydrochloride 30 mg

Kolephrin®: Acetaminophen 325 mg, chlorpheniramine maleate 2 mg, and pseudoephedrine hydrochloride 30 mg

Liquid:

Comtrex® Flu Therapy Nighttime: Acetaminophen 100 mg, chlorpheniramine maleate 4 mg, and pseudoephedrine hydrochloride 60 mg per 30 mL (240 mL) [contains alcohol; cherry flavor]

Tylenol® Children's Plus Cold Nighttime: Acetaminophen 160 mg, chlorpheniramine maleate 1 mg, and pseudoephedrine hydrochloride 15 mg per 5 mL (120 mL) [contains sodium benzoate; grape flavor] [DSC]

Tablet:

Drinex: Acetaminophen 650 mg, chlorpheniramine maleate 4 mg, and pseudoephedrine hydrochloride 60 mg

Acetaminophen, Codeine, and Doxylamine

(a seet a MIN oh fen, KOE deen, & dox IL a meen)

Medication Safety Issues

High alert medication: The Institute for Safe Medication Practices (ISMP) includes this medication among its list of drug classes which have a heightened risk of causing significant patient harm when used in error.

Duplicate therapy issues: This product contains acetaminophen, which may be a component of other combination products. Do not exceed the maximum recommended daily dose of acetaminophen.

Canadian Brand Names Mersyndol® With Codeine

Index Terms Codeine, Doxylamine, and Acetaminophen; Doxylamine Succinate, Codeine Phosphate, and Acetaminophen

Pharmacologic Category Analgesic, Miscellaneous; Analgesic, Opioid; Antitussive; Histamine H_1 Antagonist; Histamine H_1 Antagonist, First Generation

Use Relief of headache, cold symptoms, neuralgia, and muscular aches/pain

Effect on Mental Status Drowsiness is common; may cause dizziness, disorientation, euphoria, confusion, insomnia, hallucinations, or depression

Effect on Psychiatric Treatment Concurrent use with psychotropics may produce additive sedation and anticholinergic effects; conversely, the effects of cholinergic agonists will be ameliorated. Concurrent use with fluoxetine or paroxetine may result in loss of codeine's analgesic effects.

Restrictions CDSA-1; Not available in U.S.

Dosage Summary

Oral:

Children ≤12 years: Dosage not established

Children >12 years: 1-2 tablets every 4 hours as needed (maximum: 12 tablets/day)

Adults: 1-2 tablets every 4 hours as needed (maximum: 12 tablets/day)

Dosage Forms Excipient information presented when available (limited, particularly for generics); consult specific product labeling. [CAN] = Canadian brand name

Tablet:

Mersyndol® With Codeine [CAN]: Acetaminophen 325 mg, codeine 8 mg, and doxylamine 5 mg [not available in the U.S.]

Acetaminophen, Dextromethorphan, and Phenylephrine

(a seet a MIN oh fen, deks troe meth OR fan, & fen il EF rin)

Medication Safety Issues

Duplicate therapy issues: This product contains acetaminophen, which may be a component of other combination products. Do not exceed the maximum recommended daily dose of acetaminophen.

U.S. Brand Names Alka-Seltzer Plus® Day Cold [OTC]; Little Colds® Multi-Symptom Cold Formula [OTC] [DSC]; Mapap® Multi-Symptom Cold [OTC]; Tylenol® Cold Head Congestion Daytime [OTC]; Tylenol® Cold Multi-Symptom Daytime [OTC]; Tylenol® Plus Infants Cold & Cough [OTC] [DSC]; Vicks® DayQuil® Cold/Flu Multi-Symptom Relief [OTC]

Index Terms Dextromethorphan Hydrobromide, Acetaminophen, and Phenylephrine Hydrochloride; Phenylephrine, Acetaminophen, and Dextromethorphan; Phenylephrine, Dextromethorphan, and Acetaminophen

Pharmacologic Category Analgesic, Miscellaneous; Antitussive; Decongestant

Use Temporary relief of common cold and flu symptoms (eg, pain, fever, cough, congestion)

Effect on Mental Status Sedation with dextromethorphan may be countered by the excitability associated with phenylephrine; one effect may predominate in any particular patient

Effect on Psychiatric Treatment Contraindicated with or within 14 days of MAO inhibitor treatment; avoid. Barbiturates and carbamazepine may increase the hepatotoxic potential of acetaminophen.

Dosage Summary

Oral:

Note: Dosage may vary considerably by product; ranges listed are representative. See specific product labeling.

Vicks® DayQuil® Cold/Flu Multi-Symptom Relief:

Children <6 years: Dosage not established

Children 6-11 years: 15 mL every 4 hours, up to 5 doses per day (maximum: 75 mL/24 hours)

Children ≥12 years: 2 doses every 4 hours or 30 mL every 4 hours (maximum: 6 doses/24 hours)

Adults: 2 doses every 4 hours or 30 mL every 4 hours (maximum: 6 doses/24 hours)

Dosage Forms Excipient information presented when available (limited, particularly for generics); consult specific product labeling. [DSC] = Discontinued product

Caplet:

Mapap® Multi-Symptom Cold: Acetaminophen 325 mg, dextromethorphan hydrobromide 10 mg, and phenylephrine hydrochloride 5 mg

Tylenol® Cold Head Congestion Daytime: Acetaminophen 325 mg, dextromethorphan hydrobromide 10 mg, and phenylephrine hydrochloride 5 mg [Cool Burst™ flavor]

Tylenol® Cold Multi-Symptom Daytime: Acetaminophen 325 mg, dextromethorphan hydrobromide 10 mg, and phenylephrine hydrochloride 5 mg [Cool Burst™ flavor]

Capsule, liquid gel:

Alka-Seltzer Plus® Day Cold: Acetaminophen 325 mg, dextromethorphan hydrobromide 10 mg, and phenylephrine hydrochloride 5 mg

Capsule, liquicap:

Vicks® DayQuil® Cold/Flu Multi-Symptom Relief: Acetaminophen 325 mg, dextromethorphan hydrobromide 10 mg, and phenylephrine hydrochloride 5 mg

Gelcap:

Tylenol® Cold Multi-Symptom Daytime: Acetaminophen 325 mg, dextromethorphan hydrobromide 10 mg, and phenylephrine hydrochloride 5 mg

Liquid:

Alka-Seltzer Plus® Day Cold: Acetaminophen 162.5 mg, dextromethorphan hydrobromide 5 mg, and phenylephrine hydrochloride 2.5 mg per 5 mL (180 mL) [alcohol free; contains sodium 3 mg/5 mL, propylene glycol, and sodium benzoate; berry flavor]

Tylenol® Cold Multi-Symptom Daytime: Acetaminophen 325 mg, dextromethorphan hydrobromide 10 mg, and phenylephrine hydrochloride 5 mg per 15 mL (240 mL) [contains sodium 5 mg/15 mL, sodium benzoate, and propylene glycol; Citrus Burst™ flavor]

Vicks® DayQuil® Cold/Flu Multi-Symptom Relief: Acetaminophen 325 mg, dextromethorphan hydrobromide 10 mg, and phenylephrine hydrochloride 5 mg per 15 mL (180 mL, 300 mL) [contains sodium 71 mg/15 mL and propylene glycol]

Liquid [drops]:

Little Colds® Multi-Symptom Cold Formula: Acetaminophen 80 mg, dextromethorphan hydrobromide 2.5 mg, and phenylephrine hydrochloride 1.25 mg per 1 mL (15 mL) [alcohol free, dye free; contains propylene glycol and sodium benzoate; berry flavor] [DSC]

Tylenol® Plus Infants Cold & Cough: Acetaminophen 80 mg, dextromethorphan hydrobromide 2.5 mg, and phenylephrine hydrochloride 1.25 mg per 0.8 mL (15 mL) [contains sodium benzoate; cherry flavor] [DSC]

Acetaminophen, Dextromethorphan, and Pseudoephedrine

(a seet a MIN oh fen, deks troe meth OR fan, & soo doe e FED rin)

Medication Safety Issues

Sound-alike/look-alike issues:

Sudafed® may be confused with Sufenta®

Thera-Flu® may be confused with Tamiflu®, Thera-Flur-N®

Tylenol® may be confused with atenolol, timolol, Tuinal®, Tylox®

Duplicate therapy issues: This product contains acetaminophen, which may be a component of other combination products. Do not exceed the maximum recommended daily dose of acetaminophen.

U.S. Brand Names Tylenol® Cold Day Non-Drowsy [OTC]; Tylenol® Flu Non-Drowsy Maximum Strength [OTC]

Canadian Brand Names Contac® Complete; Contac® Cough, Cold and Flu Day & Night™; Sudafed® Cold & Cough Extra Strength; Tylenol® Cold Daytime

Index Terms Dextromethorphan, Acetaminophen, and Pseudoephedrine; Pseudoephedrine, Acetaminophen, and Dextromethorphan; Pseudoephedrine, Dextromethorphan, and Acetaminophen

Pharmacologic Category Alpha/Beta Agonist; Analgesic, Miscellaneous; Antitussive

Use Treatment of mild-to-moderate pain and fever; symptomatic relief of cough and congestion

Effect on Mental Status Sedation with dextromethorphan tends to be countered by the excitability associated with pseudoephedrine; one effect may predominate in any particular patient

Effect on Psychiatric Treatment Increased toxicity and hypertensive crisis may be seen with concurrent use of MAO inhibitors and CNS depressants, effects of CNS depressants may be lessened

Dosage Summary

Oral:

Acetaminophen:

Children ≤12 years: 10-15 mg/kg/dose every 4-6 hours as needed (maximum: 2.6 g/day)

Children >12 years: 325-650 mg every 4-6 hours as needed (maximum: 4 g/day

Adults: 325-650 mg every 4-6 hours as needed (maximum: 4 g/day)

Dextromethorphan:

Children <6 years: Dosage not established

Children 6-12 years: 15 mg every 6-8 hours (maximum: 60 mg/day)

Children >12 years: 10-20 mg every 4-8 hours **or** 30 mg every 8 hours (maximum: 120 mg/day)

Adults: 10-20 mg every 4-8 hours **or** 30 mg every 8 hours (maximum: 120 mg/day)

Pseudoephedrine:

Children <2 years: Dosage not established

Children 2-6 years: 15 mg every 4 hours (maximum: 90 mg/day)

Children 6-12 years: 30 mg every 4 hours (maximum: 180 mg/day)

Children >12 years: 60 mg every 4 hours (maximum: 360 mg/day)

Adults: 60 mg every 4 hours (maximum: 360 mg/day)

Dosage Forms Excipient information presented when available (limited, particularly for generics); consult specific product labeling.

Caplet:

Tylenol® Cold Day Non-Drowsy: Acetaminophen 325 mg dextromethorphan hydrobromide 15 mg, and pseudoephedrine hydrochloride 30 mg

Gelcap:

Tylenol® Flu Non-Drowsy Maximum Strength: Acetaminophen 500 mg, dextromethorphan hydrobromide 15 mg, and pseudoephedrine hydrochloride 30 mg

◆ **Acetaminophen, Dichloralphenazone, and Isometheptene** *see* Acetaminophen, Isometheptene, and Dichloralphenazone *on page 45*

Acetaminophen, Diphenhydramine, and Phenylephrine

(a seet a MIN oh fen, dye fen HYE dra meen, & fen il EF rin)

Medication Safety Issues

Duplicate therapy issues: This product contains acetaminophen, which may be a component of combination products. Do not exceed the maximum recommended daily dose of acetaminophen.

U.S. Brand Names Benadryl® Allergy and Cold [OTC]; Benadryl® Allergy and Sinus Headache [OTC]; Children's Tylenol® Plus Cold and Allergy [OTC]; Sudafed PE® Nighttime Cold [OTC]; Sudafed PE® Severe Cold [OTC]; Tylenol® Allergy Multi-Symptom Nighttime [OTC]

Index Terms Acetaminophen, Phenylephrine, and Diphenhydramine; Diphenhydramine, Phenylephrine Hydrochloride, and Acetaminophen; Phenylephrine Hydrochloride, Acetaminophen, and Diphenhydramine

Pharmacologic Category Analgesic, Miscellaneous; Decongestant; Histamine H_1 Antagonist

Use Temporary relief of symptoms of hay fever and the common cold, including: sinus/nasal congestion and pain/pressure, headache, sneezing, runny nose, itchy/watery eyes, sore throat, cough, and minor aches and pains

Effect on Mental Status May cause drowsiness, anxiety, or restlessness

Effect on Psychiatric Treatment Contraindicated with or within 14 days of MAO inhibitor treatment. May cause CNS depression; concurrent use with psychotropics may produce additive effects. Barbiturates and carbamazepine may increase the hepatotoxic potential of acetaminophen. Individuals consuming ≥3 alcoholic drinks per day may increase the risk of liver damage.

Dosage Summary

Oral:

Caplet:

Children <6 years: Dosage not established

Children 6-11 years: One caplet every 4 hours as needed (maximum: 5 doses/caplets)

Children ≥12 years: Two caplets every 4 hours as needed (maximum: 12 caplets/24 hours)

Adults: Two caplets every 4 hours as needed (maximum: 12 caplets/24 hours)

Liquid:

Children <6 years and <48 lbs: Dosage not established

Children 6-11 years and 48-95 lbs: 10 mL every 4 hours as needed (maximum: 5 doses/24 hours)

Children ≥12 years and >95 lbs: Use alternative dosage form

Adults: Use alternative dosage form

Dosage Forms Excipient information presented when available (limited, particularly for generics); consult specific product labeling.

Caplet:

Benadryl® Allergy and Cold, Benadryl® Allergy and Sinus Headache, Sudafed PE® Severe Cold: Acetaminophen 325 mg, diphenhydramine hydrochloride 12.5 mg and phenylephrine hydrochloride 5 mg

Sudafed PE® Nighttime Cold: Acetaminophen 325 mg, diphenhydramine hydrochloride 25 mg and phenylephrine hydrochloride 5 mg

Tylenol® Allergy Multi-Symptom Nighttime: Acetaminophen 325 mg, diphenhydramine hydrochloride 25 mg and phenylephrine hydrochloride 5 mg [Cool Burst™ flavor]

Tablet:

Children's Tylenol® Plus Cold and Allergy: Acetaminophen 160 mg, Diphenhydramine 12.5 mg, and phenylephrine 2.5 mg per 5 mL (120 mL) [contains sodium benzoate; bubble gum flavor]

Acetaminophen, Isometheptene, and Dichloralphenazone

(a seet a MIN oh fen, eye soe me THEP teen, & dye KLOR al FEN a zone)

Medication Safety Issues

Sound-alike/look-alike issues:

Midrin® may be confused with Mydfrin®

Duplicate therapy issues: This product contains acetaminophen, which may be a component of other combination products. Do not exceed the maximum recommended daily dose of acetaminophen.

U.S. Brand Names Amidrine [DSC]; Duradrin® [DSC]; Midrin®; Migquin [DSC]; Migratine; Migrazone® [DSC]; Migrin-A [DSC]

Index Terms Acetaminophen, Dichloralphenazone, and Isometheptene; Dichloralphenazone, Acetaminophen, and Isometheptene; Dichloralphenazone, Isometheptene, and Acetaminophen; Isometheptene, Acetaminophen, and Dichloralphenazone; Isometheptene, Dichloralphenazone, and Acetaminophen

Pharmacologic Category Analgesic, Miscellaneous

Generic Available Yes

Use Relief of migraine and tension headache

Effect on Mental Status May cause drowsiness or dizziness

Effect on Psychiatric Treatment Contraindicated with MAO inhibitor

Restrictions C-IV

Lactation Excretion in breast milk unknown/use caution

Contraindications Hypersensitivity to acetaminophen, isometheptene, dichloralphenazone, or any component of the formulation; glaucoma; severe renal disease; hypertension; organic heart disease; hepatic disease; MAO inhibitor therapy

Adverse Reactions Frequency not defined.

Central nervous system: Transient dizziness

Dermatological: Rash

Metabolism/Transport Effects Acetaminophen: **Substrate** (minor) of CYP1A2, 2A6, 2C9, 2D6, 2E1, 3A4; **Inhibits** CYP3A4 (weak)

Drug Interactions

Antacids: May decrease the excretion of Alpha-/Beta-Agonists. **Exceptions:** Aluminum Hydroxide. *Risk C: Monitor therapy*

Anticonvulsants (Hydantoin): May increase the metabolism of Acetaminophen. This may 1) diminish the effect of acetaminophen; and 2) increase the risk of liver damage. *Risk C: Monitor therapy*

Barbiturates: May increase the metabolism of Acetaminophen. This may 1) diminish the effect of acetaminophen; and 2) increase the risk of liver damage. *Risk C: Monitor therapy*

Beta-Blockers: May enhance the vasopressor effect of Alpha-/Beta-Agonists (Direct-Acting). Epinephrine used as a local anesthetic for dental procedures will not likely cause clinically relevant problems. *Risk D: Consider therapy modification*

Bromocriptine: Alpha-/Beta-Agonists may enhance the adverse/toxic effect of Bromocriptine. Including increased blood pressure, ventricular arrhythmias, and seizure. *Risk C: Monitor therapy*

Cannabinoids: May enhance the tachycardic effect of Sympathomimetics. *Risk C: Monitor therapy*

CarBAMazepine: May increase the metabolism of Acetaminophen. This may 1) diminish the effect of acetaminophen; and 2) increase the risk of liver damage. *Risk C: Monitor therapy*

Carbonic Anhydrase Inhibitors: May decrease the excretion of Alpha-/Beta-Agonists. **Exceptions:** Brinzolamide; Dorzolamide. *Risk C: Monitor therapy*

Cholestyramine Resin: May decrease the absorption of Acetaminophen. Effect is minimal if cholestyramine is administered 1 hour after acetaminophen. *Risk D: Consider therapy modification*

Imatinib: May increase the serum concentration of Acetaminophen. *Risk D: Consider therapy modification*

Isoniazid: May enhance the adverse/toxic effect of Acetaminophen. *Risk C: Monitor therapy*

MAO Inhibitors: May enhance the vasopressor effect of Alpha-/Beta-Agonists (Direct-Acting). Primarily with oral administration of phenylephrine. *Risk D: Consider therapy modification*

Sympathomimetics: May enhance the adverse/toxic effect of other Sympathomimetics. *Risk C: Monitor therapy*

Tricyclic Antidepressants: May enhance the vasopressor effect of Alpha-/Beta-Agonists (Direct-Acting). *Risk D: Consider therapy modification*

Vitamin K Antagonists (eg, warfarin): Acetaminophen may enhance the anticoagulant effect of Vitamin K Antagonists. Most likely with daily acetaminophen doses >1.3 g for >1 week. *Risk C: Monitor therapy*

Ethanol/Nutrition/Herb Interactions Ethanol: Excessive intake of ethanol may increase the risk of acetaminophen-induced hepatotoxicity. Avoid ethanol or limit to <3 drinks/day.

Dosage Oral: Adults:

Migraine headache: 2 capsules to start, followed by 1 capsule every hour until relief is obtained (maximum: 5 capsules/12 hours)

Tension headache: 1-2 capsules every 4 hours (maximum: 8 capsules/24 hours)

Dosing adjustment in hepatic impairment: Use with caution. Limited, low-dose therapy is usually well tolerated in hepatic disease/cirrhosis; however, cases of hepatotoxicity at daily acetaminophen dosages <4 g/day have been reported. Avoid chronic use in hepatic impairment.

Dosage Forms Excipient information presented when available (limited, particularly for generics); consult specific product labeling. [DSC] = Discontinued product

Capsule: Acetaminophen 325 mg, isometheptene mucate 65 mg, dichloralphenazone 100 mg [DSC]

Amidrine [DSC], Duradrin® [DSC], Midrin®, Migquin [DSC], Migrazone® [DSC], Migratine, Migrin-A [DSC]: Acetaminophen 325 mg, isometheptene mucate 65 mg, and dichloralphenazone 100 mg

◆ **Acetaminophen, Phenylephrine, and Diphenhydramine** *see* Acetaminophen, Diphenhydramine, and Phenylephrine *on page 44*

◆ **Acetaminophen, Pseudoephedrine, and Chlorpheniramine** *see* Acetaminophen, Chlorpheniramine, and Pseudoephedrine *on page 40*

AcetaZOLAMIDE (a set a ZOLE a mide)

Medication Safety Issues

Sound-alike/look-alike issues:

AcetaZOLAMIDE may be confused with acetoHEXAMIDE

Diamox® Sequels® may be confused with Diabinese®, Dobutrex®, Trimox®

Related Information

Anticonvulsants By Seizure Type *on page 1759*

U.S. Brand Names Diamox® Sequels®

Canadian Brand Names Apo-Acetazolamide®; Diamox®

Mexican Brand Names Acetadiazol

Pharmacologic Category Anticonvulsant, Miscellaneous; Carbonic Anhydrase Inhibitor; Diuretic, Carbonic Anhydrase Inhibitor; Ophthalmic Agent, Antiglaucoma

Use Treatment of glaucoma (chronic simple open-angle, secondary glaucoma, preoperatively in acute angle-closure); drug-induced edema or edema due to congestive heart failure (adjunctive therapy); centrencephalic epilepsies (immediate release dosage form); prevention or amelioration of symptoms associated with acute mountain sickness

Unlabeled/Investigational Use Urine alkalinization; respiratory stimulant in COPD; metabolic alkalosis

Effect on Mental Status Drowsiness is common, may produce depression less commonly

Effect on Psychiatric Treatment Can rarely cause bone marrow suppression, therefore, use cautiously with clozapine and carbamazepine; may increase the excretion of lithium

Dosage Summary

I.V.:

Children: 20-40 mg/kg/day divided every 6 hours **or** 5 mg/kg (150 mg/m^2) once daily (maximum: 1 g/day)

Adults: 250-500 mg/day (may repeat in 2-4 hours for glaucoma) (maximum: 1 g/day)

Oral:

Immediate release:

Children: 5-30 mg/kg/day (150-900 mg/m^2/day) divided in 1-4 doses (maximum: 1 g/day)

Adults: 250-1000 mg/day in 1-4 divided doses (maximum: 1 g/day)

Elderly: Initial: 250 mg once or twice daily; use lowest effective dose possible.

Extended release:

Children: Dosage not established

Adults: 500 mg every 12-24 hours (maximum 1 g/day); **Note:** Extended release capsule not recommended for epilepsy.

Dosage Forms Excipient information presented when available (limited, particularly for generics); consult specific product labeling.

Capsule, extended release:

Diamox® Sequels®: 500 mg

Injection, powder for reconstitution: 500 mg

Tablet: 125 mg, 250 mg

◆ **Acetoxymethylprogesterone** *see* MedroxyPROGESTERone *on page 975*

Acetylcholine (a se teel KOE leen)

Medication Safety Issues

Sound-alike/look-alike issues:

Acetylcholine may be confused with acetylcysteine

U.S. Brand Names Miochol®-E

Canadian Brand Names Miochol®-E

Index Terms Acetylcholine Chloride

Pharmacologic Category Cholinergic Agonist; Ophthalmic Agent, Miotic

Use Produces complete miosis in cataract surgery, keratoplasty, iridectomy, and other anterior segment surgery where rapid miosis is required

Effect on Mental Status None reported

Effect on Psychiatric Treatment Intraocular product; should not impact psychiatric drug treatment

Dosage Summary

Intraocular:

Children: Dosage not established

Adults: Instill 0.5-2 mL of 1% injection (5-20 mg) before or after securing sutures

Dosage Forms Excipient information presented when available (limited, particularly for generics); consult specific product labeling.

Powder for solution, intraocular, as chloride:

Miochol®-E: 1:100 [20 mg; packaged with diluent (2 mL)]

◆ **Acetylcholine Chloride** *see* Acetylcholine *on page 47*

Acetylcysteine (a se teel SIS teen)

Medication Safety Issues

Sound-alike/look-alike issues:

Acetylcysteine may be confused with acetylcholine

Mucomyst® may be confused with Mucinex®

U.S. Brand Names Acetadote®

Canadian Brand Names Acetylcysteine Solution; Mucomyst®; Parvolex®

Mexican Brand Names ACC

Index Terms *N*-Acetyl-L-cysteine; *N*-Acetylcysteine; Acetylcysteine Sodium; Mercapturic Acid; Mucomyst; NAC

Pharmacologic Category Antidote; Mucolytic Agent

Use Adjunctive mucolytic therapy in patients with abnormal or viscid mucous secretions in acute and chronic bronchopulmonary diseases; pulmonary complications of surgery and cystic fibrosis; diagnostic bronchial studies; antidote for acute acetaminophen toxicity

Unlabeled/Investigational Use Prevention of radiocontrast-induced renal dysfunction (oral, I.V.); distal intestinal obstruction syndrome (DIOS, previously referred to as meconium ileus equivalent)

Effect on Mental Status May cause drowsiness

Effect on Psychiatric Treatment Sedative effects may be potentiated by psychotropic agents

Dosage Summary

Inhalation: Note: Patients should receive bronchodilator 10-15 minutes prior to dose

Nebulization:

Infants: 1-2 mL of 20% solution or 2-4 mL 10% solution 3-4 times/day

Children: 1-10 mL of 20% solution or 2-20 mL of 10% solution every 2-6 hours

Adults: 1-10 mL of 20% solution or 2-20 mL of 10% solution every 2-6 hours

Direct instillation:

Children: Dosage not established

Adults: 1-2 mL of 10% or 20% solution every 1-4 hours via tracheostomy **or** 1-2 mL of 20% or 2-4 mL of 10% solution every 1-4 hours via percutaneous intratracheal catheter

I.V.: Acetadote®:

Children: Loading dose: 150 mg/kg over 60 minutes; Maintenance: 50 mg/kg over 4 hours then 100 mg/kg over 16 hours (Total dose: 300 mg/kg over 21 hours)

Adults: Loading dose: 150 mg/kg over 60 minutes; Maintenance: 50 mg/kg over 4 hours then 100 mg/kg over 16 hours (Total dose: 300 mg/kg over 21 hours)

Oral:

Children Acetaminophen overdose: Loading dose: 140 mg/kg; Maintenance: 17 doses of 70 mg/kg every 4 hours

Adults

Acetaminophen overdose: Loading dose: 140 mg/kg; Maintenance: 17 doses of 70 mg/kg every 4 hours

Renal protectant for radiocontrast: 600-1200 mg twice daily for 2 days

Dosage Forms Excipient information presented when available (limited, particularly for generics); consult specific product labeling.

Injection, solution:

Acetadote®: 20% (30 mL) [200 mg/mL; contains disodium edetate]

Solution, inhalation/oral: 10% (4 mL, 10 mL, 30 mL) [100 mg/mL]; 20% (4 mL, 10 mL, 30 mL) [200 mg/mL]

◆ **Acetylcysteine Sodium** *see* Acetylcysteine *on page 47*

◆ **Acetylsalicylic Acid** *see* Aspirin *on page 143*

◆ **Achromycin** *see* Tetracycline *on page 1558*

◆ **Aciclovir** *see* Acyclovir *on page 49*

◆ **AcipHex®** *see* Rabeprazole *on page 1389*

◆ **Acitfed® Cold & Allergy [OTC]** ***[reformulation]*** *see* Chlorpheniramine and Phenylephrine *on page 323*

Acrivastine and Pseudoephedrine

(AK ri vas teen & soo doe e FED rin)

U.S. Brand Names Semprex®-D

Index Terms Pseudoephedrine Hydrochloride and Acrivastine

Pharmacologic Category Alpha/Beta Agonist; Histamine H_1 Antagonist; Histamine H_1 Antagonist, Second Generation

Use Temporary relief of nasal congestion, decongest sinus openings, running nose, itching of nose or throat, and itchy, watery eyes due to hay fever or other upper respiratory allergies

Effect on Mental Status Drowsiness is common; may produce anxiety and insomnia

Effect on Psychiatric Treatment Hypertensive crisis may result with MAO inhibitor; effects of CNS depressants may be lessened

Dosage Summary

Oral:

Children: Dosage not established

Adults: 1 capsule 3-4 times/day

Dosage Forms Excipient information presented when available (limited, particularly for generics); consult specific product labeling.

Capsule:

Semprex®-D: Acrivastine 8 mg and pseudoephedrine hydrochloride 60 mg

◆ **ACT** *see* DACTINomycin *on page 415*

◆ **Act-D** *see* DACTINomycin *on page 415*

◆ **ACTH** *see* Corticotropin *on page 401*

◆ **ActHIB®** *see Haemophilus* b Conjugate Vaccine *on page 753*

◆ **Actidose-Aqua® [OTC]** *see* Charcoal *on page 312*

◆ **Actidose® with Sorbitol [OTC]** *see* Charcoal *on page 312*

◆ **Actifed® Cold and Sinus [OTC]** *see* Acetaminophen, Chlorpheniramine, and Pseudoephedrine *on page 40*

◆ **Actigall®** *see* Ursodiol *on page 1639*

◆ **Actimmune®** *see* Interferon Gamma-1b *on page 849*

◆ **Actinomycin** *see* DACTINomycin *on page 415*

◆ **Actinomycin D** *see* DACTINomycin *on page 415*

◆ **Actinomycin CI** *see* DACTINomycin *on page 415*
◆ **Actiq®** *see* FentaNYL *on page 624*
◆ **Activated Carbon** *see* Charcoal *on page 312*
◆ **Activated Charcoal** *see* Charcoal *on page 312*
◆ **Activated Ergosterol** *see* Ergocalciferol *on page 550*
◆ **Activella®** *see* Estradiol and Norethindrone *on page 579*
◆ **Actonel®** *see* Risedronate *on page 1424*
◆ **Actonel® and Calcium** *see* Risedronate and Calcium *on page 1424*
◆ **Actoplus Met™** *see* Pioglitazone and Metformin *on page 1301*
◆ **Actos®** *see* Pioglitazone *on page 1297*
◆ **Acular®** *see* Ketorolac *on page 878*
◆ **Acular LS™** *see* Ketorolac *on page 878*
◆ **Acular® PF** *see* Ketorolac *on page 878*
◆ **ACV** *see* Acyclovir *on page 49*
◆ **Acycloguanosine** *see* Acyclovir *on page 49*

Acyclovir (ay SYE kloe veer)

Medication Safety Issues

Sound-alike/look-alike issues:

Zovirax® may be confused with Zostrix®, Zyvox®

International issues:

Opthavir® [Mexico] may be confused with Optivar® which is a brand name for azelastine in the U.S.

U.S. Brand Names Zovirax®

Canadian Brand Names Apo-Acyclovir®; Gen-Acyclovir; Nu-Acyclovir; ratio-Acyclovir; Zovirax®

Mexican Brand Names Acifur; Cicloferon; Clirbest; Clorixan; Clyvorax; Genovix; Hercivir; Ignis; Jersin; Laciken; Opthavir; Sophivir Ungena; Victoclir; Virestat; Zirconia; Ziverone; Zovirax

Index Terms Aciclovir; ACV; Acycloguanosine

Pharmacologic Category Antiviral Agent; Antiviral Agent, Topical

Use Treatment of genital herpes simplex virus (HSV), herpes labialis (cold sores), herpes zoster (shingles), HSV encephalitis, neonatal HSV, mucocutaneous HSV in immunocompromised patients, varicella-zoster (chickenpox)

Unlabeled/Investigational Use Prevention of HSV reactivation in HIV-positive patients; prevention of HSV reactivation in hematopoietic stem-cell transplant (HSCT); prevention of HSV reactivation during periods of neutropenia in patients with acute leukemia

Effect on Mental Status May see lethargy, confusion, or agitation; rarely may see depression or insomnia

Effect on Psychiatric Treatment Usually not a problem, may see additive sedation with sedating psychotropics

Dosage Summary Note: Obese patients should be dosed using ideal body weight

I.V.:

Neonates: Birth to 3 months: 10-20 mg/kg/dose every 8 hours (maximum: 60 mg/kg/day)

Children <12 years: 10-20 mg/kg/dose every 8 hours (maximum: 60 mg/kg/day)

Children ≥12 years: 5-10 mg/kg/dose **or** 500 mg/m^2/dose every 8 hours (maximum: 45 mg/kg/day)

Adults: 5-10 mg/kg/dose **or** 500 mg/m^2/dose every 8 hours (maximum: 45 mg/kg/day)

Oral:

Children <2 years: Dosage not established

Children ≥2 years and ≤40 kg: 20 mg/kg/dose 4 times/day (Maximum: 800 mg/dose)

Children >40 kg: 800 mg/dose 4 times a day

Adults: 200-800 mg/dose 3-5 times/day

Topical:

Children <12 years: Dosage not established

Children ≥12 years: Cream: Apply 5 times/day

Adults: Cream: Apply 5 times/day; Ointment: 1/2" ribbon of ointment for a 4" square surface area 6 times/day

Dosage Forms Excipient information presented when available (limited, particularly for generics); consult specific product labeling.

Capsule: 200 mg
Zovirax®: 200 mg
Cream, topical:
Zovirax®: 5% (2 g, 5 g)
Injection, powder for reconstitution, as sodium: 500 mg, 1000 mg
Injection, solution, as sodium [preservative free]: 50 mg/mL (10 mL, 20 mL)
Ointment, topical:
Zovirax®: 5% (15 g)
Suspension, oral: 200 mg/5 mL (480 mL)
Zovirax®: 200 mg/5 mL (480 mL) [banana flavor]
Tablet: 400 mg, 800 mg
Zovirax®: 400 mg, 800 mg

- **Aczone®** *see* Dapsone *on page 418*
- **AD3L** *see* Valrubicin *on page 1649*
- **Adalat® CC** *see* NIFEdipine *on page 1136*

Adalimumab (a da LIM yoo mab)

Medication Safety Issues
Sound-alike/look-alike issues:
Humira® may be confused with Humulin®, Humalog®
Humira® Pen may be confused with HumaPen® Memoir®

U.S. Brand Names Humira®

Canadian Brand Names Humira®

Mexican Brand Names Humira

Index Terms Antitumor Necrosis Factor Apha (Human); D2E7; Human Antitumor Necrosis Factor Alpha

Pharmacologic Category Antirheumatic, Disease Modifying; Gastrointestinal Agent, Miscellaneous; Monoclonal Antibody; Tumor Necrosis Factor (TNF) Blocking Agent

Use
Treatment of active rheumatoid arthritis (moderate-to-severe) and active psoriatic arthritis; may be used alone or in combination with disease-modifying antirheumatic drugs (DMARDs); treatment of ankylosing spondylitis
Treatment of moderately- to severely-active Crohn's disease in patients with inadequate response to conventional treatment, or patients who have lost response to or are intolerant of infliximab
Treatment of moderate-to-severe plaque psoriasis
Treatment of moderately- to severely-active juvenile idiopathic arthritis

Effect on Mental Status May cause confusion; may exacerbate pre-existing or recent-onset demyelinating CNS disorder

Effect on Psychiatric Treatment Rare reports of pancytopenia, including aplastic anemia, have been reported with TNF-α-blocking agents. Medically-significant thrombocytopenia and leukopenia have been infrequently reported; use with caution in patients receiving clozapine, carbamazepine, valproic acid, and mirtazapine.

Restrictions An FDA-approved medication guide must be distributed when dispensing an outpatient prescription (new or refill) where this medication is to be used without direct supervision of a healthcare provider. Medication guides are available at http://www.fda.gov/cder/Offices/ODS/medication_guides.htm.

Dosage Summary
SubQ:
Children <4 years or <15 kg: Dosage not established
Children ≥4 years: 15 kg to <30 kg: 20 mg every other week; ≥30 kg: 40 mg every other week
Adults: 40 mg every other week (maximum: 40 mg every week if not taking methotrexate in rheumatoid arthritis) **or** 160 mg (initially) given as 4 injections on day 1 or over 2 days, then 80 mg 2 weeks later (day 15); Maintenance: 40 mg every 2 weeks beginning day 29 **or** 80 mg (initially) as a single dose, followed by 40 mg every other week, beginning 1 week after initial dose

Dosage Forms Excipient information presented when available (limited, particularly for generics); consult specific product labeling.
Injection, solution [pediatric; preservative free]:
Humira®: 20 mg/0.4 mL (0.4 mL) [contains polysorbate 80]
Injection, solution [preservative free]:
Humira®: 40 mg/0.8 mL (0.8 mL) [contains polysorbate 80]

- **Adamantanamine Hydrochloride** *see* Amantadine *on page 79*

- **ADD 234037** *see* Lacosamide *on page 885*
- **Addaprin [OTC]** *see* Ibuprofen *on page 803*
- **Adderall®** *see* Dextroamphetamine and Amphetamine *on page 444*
- **Adderall XR®** *see* Dextroamphetamine and Amphetamine *on page 444*

Adefovir (a DEF o veer)

U.S. Brand Names Hepsera™

Canadian Brand Names Hepsera™

Index Terms Adefovir Dipivoxil; Bis-POM PMEA

Pharmacologic Category Antiretroviral Agent, Reverse Transcriptase Inhibitor (Nucleoside)

Use Treatment of chronic hepatitis B with evidence of active viral replication (based on persistent elevation of ALT/AST or histologic evidence), including patients with lamivudine-resistant hepatitis B

Effect on Mental Status None reported

Effect on Psychiatric Treatment Chronic administration may cause nephrotoxicity. In patients receiving lithium, gabapentin, or levetiracetam, a dosage adjustment may be needed; monitor.

Dosage Summary

Oral:

Children <12 years: Dosage not established

Children ≥12 years: 10 mg once daily

Adults: 10 mg once daily

Dosage Forms Excipient information presented when available (limited, particularly for generics); consult specific product labeling.

Tablet, as dipivoxil:

Hepsera®: 10 mg

- **Adefovir Dipivoxil** *see* Adefovir *on page 51*
- **Adenocard®** *see* Adenosine *on page 51*
- **Adenoscan®** *see* Adenosine *on page 51*

Adenosine (a DEN oh seen)

Medication Safety Issues

High alert medication: The Institute for Safe Medication Practices (ISMP) includes this medication among its list of drugs which have a heightened risk of causing significant patient harm when used in error.

U.S. Brand Names Adenocard®; Adenoscan®

Canadian Brand Names Adenocard®; Adenoscan®; Adenosine Injection, USP

Mexican Brand Names Krenosin

Index Terms 9-Beta-D-Ribofuranosyladenine

Pharmacologic Category Antiarrhythmic Agent, Class IV; Diagnostic Agent

Use

Adenocard®: Treatment of paroxysmal supraventricular tachycardia (PSVT) including that associated with accessory bypass tracts (Wolff-Parkinson-White syndrome); when clinically advisable, appropriate vagal maneuvers should be attempted prior to adenosine administration; **not effective in atrial flutter, atrial fibrillation, or ventricular tachycardia**

Adenoscan®: Pharmacologic stress agent used in myocardial perfusion thallium-201 scintigraphy

Unlabeled/Investigational Use Adenoscan®: Acute vasodilator testing in pulmonary artery hypertension

Effect on Mental Status Dizziness is common; may cause nervousness, anxiety, drowsiness, or emotional instability

Effect on Psychiatric Treatment Use caution with carbamazepine and tricyclic antidepressants, may increase heart block. Postmarking experience reports seizures as a potential adverse reaction. Psychotropics have the potential to lower seizure threshold. Monitor for seizure activity.

Dosage Summary

I.V.:

Children <50 kg: Initial: 0.05-0.1 mg/kg/dose; Repeat: 0.05-0.3 mg/kg/dose (maximum: 0.3 mg/kg/dose or 12 mg/dose)

Children ≥50 kg: Initial: 6 mg/dose; Repeat: 6-12 mg/dose (maximum: 12 mg/dose)

Adults: Initial: 6 mg/dose; Repeat: 6-12 mg/dose (maximum: 12 mg/dose); **Note:** May be administered via a central line at lower doses (ie, initial adult dose: 3 mg).

Dosage Forms Excipient information presented when available (limited, particularly for generics); consult specific product labeling.

Injection, solution [preservative free]: 3 mg/mL (2 mL, 4 mL)

Adenocard®: 3 mg/mL (2 mL, 4 mL)

Adenoscan®: 3 mg/mL (20 mL, 30 mL)

- ◆ **ADH** *see* Vasopressin *on page 1659*
- ◆ **Adipex-P®** *see* Phentermine *on page 1270*
- ◆ **AdoMet** *see* SAMe (S-adenosyl methionine) *on page 1460*
- ◆ **Adoxa®** *see* Doxycycline *on page 509*
- ◆ **Adrenalin®** *see* EPINEPHrine *on page 543*
- ◆ **Adrenaline** *see* EPINEPHrine *on page 543*
- ◆ **Adrenocorticotropic Hormone** *see* Corticotropin *on page 401*
- ◆ **ADR (error-prone abbreviation)** *see* DOXOrubicin *on page 507*
- ◆ **Adria** *see* DOXOrubicin *on page 507*
- ◆ **Adriamycin®** *see* DOXOrubicin *on page 507*
- ◆ **Adrucil®** *see* Fluorouracil *on page 649*
- ◆ **Adsorbent Charcoal** *see* Charcoal *on page 312*
- ◆ **Advair Diskus®** *see* Fluticasone and Salmeterol *on page 674*
- ◆ **Advair® HFA** *see* Fluticasone and Salmeterol *on page 674*
- ◆ **Advicor®** *see* Niacin and Lovastatin *on page 1127*
- ◆ **Advil® [OTC]** *see* Ibuprofen *on page 803*
- ◆ **Advil® Children's [OTC]** *see* Ibuprofen *on page 803*
- ◆ **Advil® Cold, Children's [OTC] [DSC]** *see* Pseudoephedrine and Ibuprofen *on page 1369*
- ◆ **Advil® Cold & Sinus [OTC]** *see* Pseudoephedrine and Ibuprofen *on page 1369*
- ◆ **Advil® Infants' [OTC]** *see* Ibuprofen *on page 803*
- ◆ **Advil® Junior [OTC] [DSC]** *see* Ibuprofen *on page 803*
- ◆ **Advil® Migraine [OTC]** *see* Ibuprofen *on page 803*
- ◆ **AeroBid®** *see* Flunisolide *on page 646*
- ◆ **AeroBid®-M** *see* Flunisolide *on page 646*
- ◆ **aerohist plus™** *see* Chlorpheniramine, Phenylephrine, and Methscopolamine *on page 329*
- ◆ **aeroKid™** *see* Chlorpheniramine, Phenylephrine, and Methscopolamine *on page 329*
- ◆ **Afeditab™ CR** *see* NIFEdipine *on page 1136*
- ◆ **Afluria®** *see* Influenza Virus Vaccine *on page 820*
- ◆ **Afrin® Extra Moisturizing [OTC]** *see* Oxymetazoline *on page 1208*
- ◆ **Afrin® Original [OTC]** *see* Oxymetazoline *on page 1208*
- ◆ **Afrin® Severe Congestion [OTC]** *see* Oxymetazoline *on page 1208*
- ◆ **Afrin® Sinus [OTC]** *see* Oxymetazoline *on page 1208*

Agalsidase Beta (aye GAL si days BAY ta)

Medication Safety Issues

Sound-alike/look-alike issues:

Agalsidase beta may be confused with agalsidase alfa, alglucerase, alglucosidase alfa

International issues:

Agalsidase beta may be confused with agalsidase alfa, which is available in international markets

U.S. Brand Names Fabrazyme®

Canadian Brand Names Fabrazyme®

Index Terms Alpha-Galactosidase-A (Recombinant); r-h α-GAL

Pharmacologic Category Enzyme

Use Replacement therapy for Fabry disease

Effect on Mental Status Anxiety and dizziness are common; may cause depression

Effect on Psychiatric Treatment None reported

Dosage Summary

I.V.:

Children <8 years of age: Dosage not established

Children ≥8 years of age: 1 mg/kg every 2 weeks

Adults: 1 mg/kg every 2 weeks

Dosage Forms Excipient information presented when available (limited, particularly for generics); consult specific product labeling.

Injection, powder for reconstitution:

Fabrazyme®: 5 mg [contains mannitol 33 mg; derived from Chinese hamster cells]; 35 mg [contains mannitol 222 mg; derived from Chinese hamster cells]

◆ **Agenerase® [DSC]** *see* Amprenavir *on page 123*

◆ **Aggrastat®** *see* Tirofiban *on page 1586*

◆ **Aggrenox®** *see* Aspirin and Dipyridamole *on page 145*

◆ **AGN 1135** *see* Rasagiline *on page 1403*

◆ **Agrylin®** *see* Anagrelide *on page 124*

◆ **AH-Chew®** *see* Chlorpheniramine, Phenylephrine, and Methscopolamine *on page 329*

◆ **AH-Chew™ Ultra** *see* Chlorpheniramine, Phenylephrine, and Methscopolamine *on page 329*

◆ **Ahist™** *see* Chlorpheniramine *on page 321*

◆ **A-hydroCort** *see* Hydrocortisone *on page 785*

◆ **AK-Con™** *see* Naphazoline *on page 1101*

◆ **AK-Dilate®** *see* Phenylephrine *on page 1273*

◆ **Akne-Mycin®** *see* Erythromycin *on page 557*

◆ **AK-Pentolate™** *see* Cyclopentolate *on page 407*

◆ **Akten™** *see* Lidocaine *on page 924*

◆ **AKTob®** *see* Tobramycin *on page 1590*

◆ **Akurza** *see* Salicylic Acid *on page 1454*

◆ **Alamag Plus [OTC]** *see* Aluminum Hydroxide, Magnesium Hydroxide, and Simethicone *on page 78*

◆ **Alavert™ [OTC]** *see* Loratadine *on page 946*

◆ **Alavert™ Allergy and Sinus [OTC]** *see* Loratadine and Pseudoephedrine *on page 948*

◆ **Alavert™ Allergy Relief 24-Hour [OTC]** *see* Loratadine *on page 946*

◆ **Alaway™ [OTC]** *see* Ketotifen *on page 879*

◆ **Albalon® [DSC]** *see* Naphazoline *on page 1101*

Albendazole (al BEN da zole)

Medication Safety Issues

International issues:

Albenza® may be confused with Avanza® which is a brand name for mirtazapine in Australia

U.S. Brand Names Albenza®

Mexican Brand Names Bruzol; Digezanol; Eskasole; Gascop; Lomsin; Lurdex; Vermin Plus; Zentel

Pharmacologic Category Anthelmintic

Use Treatment of parenchymal neurocysticercosis caused by *Taenia solium* and cystic hydatid disease of the liver, lung, and peritoneum caused by *Echinococcus granulosus*

Unlabeled/Investigational Use Albendazole has activity against *Ascaris lumbricoides* (roundworm); *Ancylostoma caninum*; *Ancylostoma duodenale* and *Necator americanus* (hookworms); cutaneous larva migrans; *Enterobius vermicularis* (pinworm); *Gnathostoma spinigerum*; *Gongylonema* sp; *Mansonella perstans* (filariasis); *Opisthorchis sinensis* (liver fluke); visceral larva migrans (toxocariasis); activity has also been shown against the liver fluke *Clonorchis sinensis*, *Giardia lamblia*, *Cysticercus cellulosae*, and *Echinococcus multilocularis*. Albendazole has also been used for the treatment of intestinal microsporidiosis (*Encephalitozoon intestinalis*), disseminated microsporidiosis (*E. hellem*, *E. cuniculi*, *E. intestinalis*, *Pleistophora* sp, *Trachipleistophora* sp, *Brachiola vesicularum*), and ocular microsporidiosis (*E. hellem*, *E. cuniculi*, *Vittaforma corneae*).

Effect on Mental Status None reported

Effect on Psychiatric Treatment May rarely cause bone marrow suppression; use caution with clozapine and carbamazepine. Carbamazepine may increase the metabolism of albendazole.

Dosage Summary

Oral:

Children <60 kg: 15 mg/kg/day in 2 divided doses (maximum: 800 mg/day; exceptions occur [indication specific])

Children ≥60 kg: 800 mg/day in 2 divided doses (maximum: 800 mg/day; exceptions occur [indication specific])

Adults <60 kg: 15 mg/kg/day in 2 divided doses (maximum: 800 mg/day; exceptions occur [indication specific])

Adults ≥60 kg: 800 mg/day in 2 divided doses (maximum: 800 mg/day; exceptions occur [indication specific])

Dosage Forms Excipient information presented when available (limited, particularly for generics); consult specific product labeling.

Tablet:

Albenza®: 200 mg

◆ **Albenza®** *see* Albendazole *on page 53*

◆ **Albumin-Bound Paclitaxel** *see* Paclitaxel (Protein Bound) *on page 1214*

Albuterol (al BYOO ter ole)

Medication Safety Issues

Sound-alike/look-alike issues:

Albuterol may be confused with Albutein®, atenolol

Proventil® may be confused with Bentyl®, Prilosec® Prinivil®

Salbutamol may be confused with salmeterol

Ventolin® may be confused with phentolamine, Benylin®, Vantin®

Volmax® may be confused with Flomax®

U.S. Brand Names AccuNeb®; ProAir™ HFA; Proventil® HFA; Proventil® [DSC]; Ventolin® HFA; VoSpire ER®

Canadian Brand Names Airomir; Alti-Salbutamol; Apo-Salvent®; Apo-Salvent® CFC Free; Apo-Salvent® Respirator Solution; Apo-Salvent® Sterules; Gen-Salbutamol; PMS-Salbutamol; ratio-Inspra-Sal; ratio-Salbutamol; Rhoxal-salbutamol; Salbu-2; Salbu-4; Ventolin®; Ventolin® Diskus; Ventolin® HFA; Ventolin® I.V. Infusion; Ventrodisk

Mexican Brand Names Assal; Avedox-FC; Brusal; Inbumed; Salbutalan; Unibron; Ventolin; Zibil

Index Terms Albuterol Sulfate; Salbutamol; Salbutamol Sulphate

Pharmacologic Category Beta$_2$-Adrenergic Agonist

Generic Available Yes

Use Bronchodilator in reversible airway obstruction due to asthma or COPD; prevention of exercise-induced bronchospasm

Unlabeled/Investigational Use As tocolytic agent (injectable form; not available in U.S.)

Effect on Mental Status May produce CNS stimulation resulting in anxiety, tremor, and insomnia

Effect on Psychiatric Treatment Effect of propranolol may be reduced; cardiovascular effects (tachycardia, palpitations) may be increased with MAO inhibitors, TCAs, and amphetamines

Pregnancy Risk Factor C

Pregnancy Considerations Albuterol crosses the placenta; tocolytic effects, fetal tachycardia, fetal hypoglycemia secondary to maternal hyperglycemia with oral or intravenous routes reported. Available evidence suggests safe use as an inhalation during pregnancy, and albuterol is the preferred short-acting beta agonist for use in asthma according to the NHLBI 2007 Guidelines for the Diagnosis and Management of Asthma.

Use of the parenteral formulation (not available in the U.S.) as a tocolytic agent has been associated with myocardial ischemia. Patients with a history of cardiac disease should be referred to a cardiologist for evaluation prior to initiating therapy in premature labor. If therapy is initiated, patients should be carefully monitored for ECG changes as well as for changes in fluid balance and cardiopulmonary function. Maternal pulse rate should not exceed 140 beats per minute during I.V. infusion of salbutamol. Consider discontinuing therapy with the development of signs of pulmonary edema or myocardial ischemia. Cautious use of parenteral salbutamol, as with other beta$_2$-agonists, is also warranted when used during labor and delivery for the relief of bronchospasm.

Lactation Excretion in breast milk unknown/use caution

Contraindications Hypersensitivity to albuterol, adrenergic amines, or any component of the formulation

Injection formulation (not available in U.S.): Patients with tachyarrhythmias; risk of abortion during first or second trimester

Warnings/Precautions Optimize anti-inflammatory treatment before initiating maintenance treatment with albuterol. Do not use as a component of chronic therapy without an anti-inflammatory agent. Only the mildest forms of asthma (Step 1 and/or exercise-induced) would not require concurrent use based upon asthma guidelines. Patient must be instructed to seek medical attention in cases where acute symptoms are not relieved or a previous level of response is diminished. The need to increase frequency of use may indicate deterioration of asthma, and treatment must not be delayed.

Use caution in patients with cardiovascular disease (arrhythmia or hypertension or HF), convulsive disorders, diabetes, glaucoma, hyperthyroidism, or hypokalemia. Beta-agonists may cause elevation in blood pressure, heart rate, and result in CNS stimulation/excitation. Beta$_2$-agonists may increase risk of arrhythmia, increase serum glucose, or decrease serum potassium.

Immediate hypersensitivity reactions (urticaria, angioedema, rash, bronchospasm) have been reported. Do not exceed recommended dose; serious adverse events, including fatalities, have been associated with excessive use of inhaled sympathomimetics. Rarely, paradoxical bronchospasm may occur with use of inhaled bronchodilating agents; this should be distinguished from inadequate response. All patients should utilize a spacer device or valved holding chamber when using a metered-dose inhaler; in addition, face masks should be used in children <4 years of age.

Patient response may vary between inhalers that contain chlorofluorocarbons and those which are chlorofluorocarbon-free.

Adverse Reactions Incidence of adverse effects is dependent upon age of patient, dose, and route of administration.

Cardiovascular: Angina, atrial fibrillation, arrhythmias, chest discomfort, chest pain, extrasystoles, flushing, hyper-/hypotension, palpitation, supraventricular tachycardia, tachycardia

Central nervous system: CNS stimulation, dizziness, drowsiness, headache, insomnia, irritability, lightheadedness, migraine, nervousness, nightmares, restlessness, seizure

Dermatologic: Angioedema, rash, urticaria

Endocrine & metabolic: Hyperglycemia, hypokalemia, lactic acidosis

Gastrointestinal: Diarrhea, dry mouth, dyspepsia, gastroenteritis, nausea, unusual taste, vomiting

Genitourinary: Micturition difficulty

Local: Injection: Pain, stinging

Neuromuscular & skeletal: Muscle cramps, musculoskeletal pain, tremor, weakness

Otic: Otitis media, vertigo

Respiratory: Asthma exacerbation, bronchospasm, cough, epistaxis, laryngitis, oropharyngeal drying/irritation, oropharyngeal edema, pharyngitis, rhinitis, upper respiratory inflammation, viral respiratory infection

Miscellaneous: Allergic reaction, anaphylaxis, diaphoresis, lymphadenopathy

Postmarketing and/or case reports: Anxiety, glossitis, hoarseness, myocardial ischemia, pulmonary edema, throat irritation, tongue ulceration

Drug Interactions

Alpha-/Beta-Blockers: May diminish the therapeutic effect of Beta$_2$-Agonists. *Risk D: Consider therapy modification*

Atomoxetine: May enhance the tachycardic effect of Beta$_2$-Agonists. *Risk C: Monitor therapy*

Beta-Blockers (Beta$_1$ Selective): May diminish the bronchodilatory effect of Beta$_2$-Agonists. Of particular concern with nonselective beta-blockers or higher doses of the beta$_1$ selective beta-blockers. *Risk C: Monitor therapy*

Beta-Blockers (Nonselective): May diminish the bronchodilatory effect of Beta$_2$-Agonists. *Risk D: Consider therapy modification*

Betahistine: May diminish the therapeutic effect of Beta$_2$-Agonists. *Risk C: Monitor therapy*

Cannabinoids: May enhance the tachycardic effect of Sympathomimetics. *Risk C: Monitor therapy*

MAO Inhibitors: May enhance the adverse/toxic effect of Beta$_2$-Agonists. *Risk C: Monitor therapy*

Sympathomimetics: May enhance the adverse/toxic effect of other Sympathomimetics. *Risk C: Monitor therapy*

Tricyclic Antidepressants: May enhance the adverse/toxic effect of $Beta_2$-Agonists. *Risk C: Monitor therapy*

Ethanol/Nutrition/Herb Interactions

Food: Avoid or limit caffeine (may cause CNS stimulation).

Herb/Nutraceutical: Avoid ephedra, yohimbe (may cause CNS stimulation). Avoid St John's wort (may decrease the levels/effects of albuterol).

Stability

HFA aerosols: Store at 15°C to 25°C (59°F to 77°F).

Ventolin® HFA: Discard after using 200 actuations or 3 months after removal from protective pouch, whichever comes first. Store with mouthpiece down.

Infusion solution (not available in U.S.): Ventolin® I.V.: Store at 15°C to 30°C (59°F to 86°F). Protect from light. After dilution, discard after 24 hours.

Inhalation solution:

Solution for nebulization (0.5%): Store at 2°C to 30°C (36°F to 86°F). To prepare a 2.5 mg dose, dilute 0.5 mL of solution to a total of 3 mL with normal saline; also compatible with cromolyn or ipratropium nebulizer solutions.

AccuNeb®: Store at 2°C to 25°C (36°F to 77°F). Do not use if solution changes color or becomes cloudy. Use within 1 week of opening foil pouch.

Syrup: Store at 2°C to 30°C (36°F to 86°F).

Tablet: Store at 2°C to 30°C (36°F to 86°F).

Tablet, extended release: Store at 20°C to 25°C (68°F to 77°F)

Mechanism of Action Relaxes bronchial smooth muscle by action on $beta_2$-receptors with little effect on heart rate

Pharmacodynamics/Kinetics

Onset of action: Peak effect:

Nebulization/oral inhalation: 0.5-2 hours

CFC-propelled albuterol: 10 minutes

Ventolin® HFA: 25 minutes

Oral: 2-3 hours

Duration: Nebulization/oral inhalation: 3-4 hours; Oral: 4-6 hours

Metabolism: Hepatic to an inactive sulfate

Half-life elimination: Inhalation: 3.8 hours; Oral: 3.7-5 hours

Excretion: Urine (30% as unchanged drug)

Dosage

Oral:

Children: Bronchospasm:

2-6 years: 0.1-0.2 mg/kg/dose 3 times/day; maximum dose not to exceed 12 mg/day (divided doses)

6-12 years: 2 mg/dose 3-4 times/day; maximum dose not to exceed 24 mg/day (divided doses)

Extended release: 4 mg every 12 hours; maximum dose not to exceed 24 mg/day (divided doses)

Children >12 years and Adults: Bronchospasm (treatment): 2-4 mg/dose 3-4 times/day; maximum dose not to exceed 32 mg/day (divided doses)

Extended release: 8 mg every 12 hours; maximum dose not to exceed 32 mg/day (divided doses). A 4 mg dose every 12 hours may be sufficient in some patients, such as adults of low body weight.

Elderly: Bronchospasm (treatment): 2 mg 3-4 times/day; maximum: 8 mg 4 times/day

Metered-dose inhaler (90 mcg/puff):

Children ≤4 years *(NIH Guidelines, 2007)*:

Quick relief: 1-2 puffs every 4-6 hours as needed

Exacerbation of asthma (acute, severe): 4-8 puffs every 20 minutes for 3 doses, then every 1-4 hours as needed

Exercise-induced bronchospasm (prevention): 1-2 puffs 5 minutes prior to exercise

Children 5-11 years *(NIH Guidelines, 2007)*:

Bronchospasm, quick relief: 2 puffs every 4-6 hours as needed

Exacerbation of asthma (acute, severe): 4-8 puffs every 20 minutes for 3 doses, then every 1-4 hours as needed

Exercise-induced bronchospasm (prevention): 2 puffs 5-30 minutes prior to exercise

Children ≥12 years and Adults:

Bronchospasm, quick relief *(NIH Guidelines, 2007)*: 2 puffs every 4-6 hours as needed

Exacerbation of asthma (acute, severe) *(NIH Guidelines, 2007)*: 4-8 puffs every 20 minutes for up to 4 hours, then every 1-4 hours as needed

Exercise-induced bronchospasm (prevention) *(NIH Guidelines, 2007)*: 2 puffs 5-30 minutes prior to exercise

Solution for nebulization:

Children 2-12 years (AccuNeb®): Bronchospasm: 0.63-1.25 mg every 4-6 hours as needed

Children ≤4 years *(NIH Guidelines, 2007)*:

Quick relief: 0.63-2.5 mg every 4-6 hours as needed

Exacerbation of asthma (acute, severe): 0.15 mg/kg (minimum: 2.5 mg) every 20 minutes for 3 doses, then 0.15-0.3 mg/kg (maximum: 10 mg) every 1-4 hours as needed **or** 0.5 mg/kg/hour by continuous nebulization

Children 5-11 years *(NIH Guidelines, 2007)*:

Quick relief: 1.25-5 mg every 4-8 hours as needed

Exacerbation of asthma (acute, severe): 0.15 mg/kg (minimum: 2.5 mg) every 20 minutes for 3 doses, then 0.15-0.3 mg/kg (maximum: 10 mg) every 1-4 hours as needed **or** 0.5 mg/kg/hour by continuous nebulization

Children ≥12 years and Adults:

Bronchospasm: 2.5 mg every 4-8 hours as needed

Quick relief *(NIH Guidelines, 2007)*: 1.25-5 mg every 4-8 hours as needed

Exacerbation of asthma (acute, severe) *(NIH Guidelines, 2007)*: 2.5-5 mg every 20 minutes for 3 doses then 2.5-10 mg every 1-4 hours as needed, **or** 10-15 mg/hour by continuous nebulization

I.V. continuous infusion: Adults (Ventolin® I.V. solution [not available in U.S.]): Severe bronchospasm and status asthmaticus: Initial: 5 mcg/minute; may increase up to 10-20 mcg/minute at 15- to 30-minute intervals if needed

Hemodialysis: Not removed

Peritoneal dialysis: Significant drug removal is unlikely based on physiochemical characteristics

Dietary Considerations Oral forms should be administered with water 1 hour before or 2 hours after meals.

Administration

Metered-dose inhaler: Shake well before use; prime prior to first use, and whenever inhaler has not been used for >2 weeks or when it has been dropped, by releasing 3-4 test sprays into the air (away from face). A spacer device or valved holding chamber is recommended for use with metered-dose inhalers.

Solution for nebulization: Concentrated solution should be diluted prior to use. Blow-by administration is not recommended, use a mask device if patient unable to hold mouthpiece in mouth for administration.

Infusion solution (Ventolin® I.V.): Do not inject undiluted. Reduce concentration by at least 50% before infusing. Administer as a continuous infusion via infusion pump. Discard unused portion of infusion within 24 hours of preparation.

Oral: Do not crush or chew extended release tablets.

Monitoring Parameters FEV_1, peak flow, and/or other pulmonary function tests; blood pressure, heart rate; CNS stimulation; serum glucose, serum potassium; asthma symptoms; arterial or capillary blood gases (if patients condition warrants)

Test Interactions Increased renin (S), increased aldosterone (S)

Additional Information The 2007 National Heart, Lung, and Blood Institute Guidelines for the Diagnosis and Management of Asthma do not recommend the use of oral systemic albuterol as a quick-relief medication and do not recommend regularly scheduled daily, chronic use of inhaled beta-agonists for long-term control of asthma.

Dosage Forms Excipient information presented when available (limited, particularly for generics); consult specific product labeling. [DSC] = Discontinued product; [CAN] = Canadian brand name

Aerosol, for oral inhalation: 90 mcg/metered inhalation (17 g) [200 metered inhalations; contains chlorofluorocarbons]

Proventil®: 90 mcg/metered inhalation (17 g) [200 metered inhalations; contains chlorofluorocarbons] [DSC]

Aerosol, for oral inhalation:

ProAir™ HFA: 90 mcg/metered inhalation (8.5 g) [200 metered inhalations; chlorofluorocarbon free]

Proventil® HFA: 90 mcg/metered inhalation (6.7 g) [200 metered inhalations; chlorofluorocarbon free]

Ventolin® HFA: 90 mcg/metered inhalation (8 g) [60 metered inhalation; chlorofluorocarbon free]; (18 g) [200 metered inhalations; chlorofluorocarbon free]

Injection, solution, as sulphate:

Ventolin® I.V. [CAN]: 1 mg/1mL (5 mL) [not available in U.S.]

Solution for nebulization: 0.042% (3 mL); 0.083% (3 mL); 0.5% (0.5 mL, 20 mL)

AccuNeb® [preservative free]: 0.63 mg/3 mL (3 mL) [0.021%]; 1.25 mg/3 mL (3 mL) [0.042%]

Proventil®: 0.083% (3 mL) [DSC] [preservative free]

Syrup, as sulfate: 2 mg/5 mL (480 mL)
Tablet: 2 mg, 4 mg
Tablet, extended release: 4 mg, 8 mg
VoSpire ER®: 4 mg, 8 mg

◆ **Albuterol and Ipratropium** *see* Ipratropium and Albuterol *on page 854*
◆ **Albuterol Sulfate** *see* Albuterol *on page 54*
◆ **Alcaine®** *see* Proparacaine *on page 1352*
◆ **Alcalak [OTC]** *see* Calcium Carbonate *on page 254*
◆ **Aldactazide®** *see* Hydrochlorothiazide and Spironolactone *on page 776*
◆ **Aldactone®** *see* Spironolactone *on page 1503*

Aldesleukin (al des LOO kin)

Medication Safety Issues
Sound-alike/look-alike issues:
Aldesleukin may be confused with oprelvekin
Proleukin® may be confused with oprelvekin

High alert medication: The Institute for Safe Medication Practices (ISMP) includes this medication among its list of drug classes which have a heightened risk of causing significant patient harm when used in error.

U.S. Brand Names Proleukin®
Canadian Brand Names Proleukin®
Index Terms Epidermal Thymocyte Activating Factor; IL-2; Interleukin-2; Lymphocyte Mitogenic Factor; NSC-373364; T-Cell Growth Factor; TCGF; Thymocyte Stimulating Factor
Pharmacologic Category Antineoplastic Agent, Miscellaneous; Biological Response Modulator
Use Treatment of metastatic renal cell cancer, metastatic melanoma
Unlabeled/Investigational Use HIV infection, and AIDS; non-Hodgkin's lymphoma
Effect on Mental Status Sedation, disorientation, delusions, and cognitive changes are common, reversible, and dose related
Effect on Psychiatric Treatment Propranolol potentiates hypotensive effects. Interaction may occur with other psychotropic given aldesleukin's effect on mental status.
Dosage Summary
I.V:
Children: Dosage not established
Adults: 600,000 int. units/kg every 8 hours (maximum: 14 doses); may repeat after 9 days for a total of 28 doses/course
Dosage Forms Excipient information presented when available (limited, particularly for generics); consult specific product labeling.
Injection, powder for reconstitution:
Proleukin®: 22 x 10^6 int. units [18 million int. units/mL = 1.1 mg/mL when reconstituted]

◆ **Aldex™** *see* Guaifenesin and Phenylephrine *on page 742*
◆ **Aldex® AN** *see* Doxylamine *on page 510*
◆ **Aldex® CT** *see* Diphenhydramine and Phenylephrine *on page 485*
◆ **Aldex®D** *see* Phenylephrine and Pyrilamine *on page 1275*
◆ **Aldex® DM** *see* Phenylephrine, Pyrilamine, and Dextromethorphan *on page 1278*
◆ **Aldomet** *see* Methyldopa *on page 1021*
◆ **Aldoril®** *see* Methyldopa and Hydrochlorothiazide *on page 1021*
◆ **Aldroxicon I [OTC]** *see* Aluminum Hydroxide, Magnesium Hydroxide, and Simethicone *on page 78*
◆ **Aldroxicon II [OTC]** *see* Aluminum Hydroxide, Magnesium Hydroxide, and Simethicone *on page 78*

Alefacept (a LE fa sept)

U.S. Brand Names Amevive®
Canadian Brand Names Amevive®
Index Terms B 9273; BG 9273; Human LFA-3/IgG(1) Fusion Protein; LFA-3/IgG (1) Fusion Protein, Human

Pharmacologic Category Monoclonal Antibody
Use Treatment of moderate to severe chronic plaque psoriasis in adults who are candidates for systemic therapy or phototherapy
Effect on Mental Status May cause dizziness
Effect on Psychiatric Treatment None reported
Restrictions Alefacept will be distributed directly to physician offices or to a specialty pharmacy; injections are intended to be administered in the physician's office
Dosage Summary
I.M.:
Children: Dosage not established
Adults: 15 mg once weekly for 12 weeks
Dosage Forms Excipient information presented when available (limited, particularly for generics); consult specific product labeling.
Injection, powder for reconstitution:
Amevive®: 15 mg [for I.M. administration; contains sucrose 12.5 mg; supplied with SWFI]

Alemtuzumab (ay lem TU zoo mab)

Medication Safety Issues
High alert medication: The Institute for Safe Medication Practices (ISMP) includes this medication among its list of drugs which have a heightened risk of causing significant patient harm when used in error.
U.S. Brand Names Campath®
Canadian Brand Names MabCampath®
Index Terms C1H; Campath-1H; Humanized IgG1 Anti-CD52 Monoclonal Antibody; NSC-715969
Pharmacologic Category Antineoplastic Agent, Monoclonal Antibody
Use Treatment of B-cell chronic lymphocytic leukemia (B-CLL)
Unlabeled/Investigational Use Treatment of refractory T-cell prolymphocytic leukemia (T-PLL); rheumatoid arthritis; graft-versus-host disease; multiple myeloma; preconditioning regimen for stem-cell transplantation and renal and liver transplantation; post-transplant rejection (renal); treatment of autoimmune cytopenias
Effect on Mental Status Fatigue is common; may cause dizziness, depression, insomnia
Effect on Psychiatric Treatment Hypotension is common; concurrent use with psychotropics may produce additive hypotensive effects; monitor. Nausea, vomiting, and diarrhea are common; may be additive when used with SSRIs; monitor. Neutropenia is common; use caution with clozapine and carbamazepine.
Dosage Summary Note: Dose escalation is required
I.V. (infusion):
Children: Dosage not established
Adults: Initial: 3 mg/day; Maintenance: 30 mg/day 3 times/week on alternate days; Maximum dose: 30 mg/day; 90 mg/week (cumulative)
Dosage Forms Excipient information presented when available (limited, particularly for generics); consult specific product labeling.
Injection, solution [preservative free]:
Campath®: 30 mg/mL (1 mL) [contains polysorbate 80; disodium edetate]

Alendronate (a LEN droe nate)

Medication Safety Issues
Sound-alike/look-alike issues:
Fosamax® may be confused with Flomax®

International issues:
Fosamax® may be confused with Fisamox® which is a brand name for amoxicillin in Australia
U.S. Brand Names Fosamax®
Canadian Brand Names Apo-Alendronate®; CO Alendronate; Dom-Alendronate; Fosamax®; Gen-Alendronate; Novo-Alendronate; PHL-Alendronate; PHL-Alendronate-FC; PMS-Alendronate; PMS-Alendronate-FC; ratio-Alendronate; Riva-Alendronate; Sandoz Alendronate
Mexican Brand Names Fosamax
Index Terms Alendronate Sodium
Pharmacologic Category Bisphosphonate Derivative

Generic Available Yes: Tablet

Use Treatment and prevention of osteoporosis in postmenopausal females; treatment of osteoporosis in males; Paget's disease of the bone in patients who are symptomatic, at risk for future complications, or with alkaline phosphatase ≥2 times the upper limit of normal; treatment of glucocorticoid-induced osteoporosis in males and females with low bone mineral density who are receiving a daily dosage ≥7.5 mg of prednisone (or equivalent)

Effect on Mental Status May rarely cause dizziness, weakness, and malaise

Effect on Psychiatric Treatment May produce GI side effects; concomitant use with SSRIs, carbamazepine, valproic acid, and lithium may produce additive effects

Pregnancy Risk Factor C

Pregnancy Considerations Safety and efficacy have not been established in pregnant women. Animal studies have shown delays in delivery and fetal/neonatal death (secondary to hypocalcemia). Bisphosphonates are incorporated into the bone matrix and gradually released over time. Theoretically, there may be a risk of fetal harm when pregnancy follows the completion of therapy. Based on limited case reports with pamidronate, serum calcium levels in the newborn may be altered if administered during pregnancy.

Lactation Excretion in breast milk unknown/use caution

Contraindications Hypersensitivity to alendronate, other bisphosphonates, or any component of the formulation; hypocalcemia; abnormalities of the esophagus which delay esophageal emptying such as stricture or achalasia; inability to stand or sit upright for at least 30 minutes; oral solution should not be used in patients at risk of aspiration

Warnings/Precautions Use caution in patients with renal impairment (not recommended for use in patients with Cl_{cr} <35 mL/minute); hypocalcemia must be corrected before therapy initiation; ensure adequate calcium and vitamin D intake. May cause irritation to upper gastrointestinal mucosa. Esophagitis, esophageal ulcers, esophageal erosions, and esophageal stricture (rare) have been reported; risk increases in patients unable to comply with dosing instructions. Use with caution in patients with dysphagia, esophageal disease, gastritis, duodenitis, or ulcers (may worsen underlying condition).

Bisphosphonate therapy has been associated with osteonecrosis, primarily of the jaw; this has been observed mostly in cancer patients, but also in patients with postmenopausal osteoporosis and other diagnoses. Dental exams and preventative dentistry should be performed prior to placing patients with risk factors on chronic bisphosphonate therapy. Invasive dental procedures should be avoided during treatment.

Severe (and occasionally debilitating) bone, joint, and/or muscle pain have been reported during bisphosphonate treatment. The onset of pain ranged from a single day to several months. Symptoms usually resolve upon discontinuation. Some patients experienced recurrence when rechallenged with same drug or another bisphosphonate; avoid use in patients with a history of these symptoms in association with bisphosphonate therapy. Discontinue use if severe symptoms occur.

Safety and efficacy in children have not been established.

Adverse Reactions Note: Incidence of adverse effects (mostly GI) increases significantly in patients treated for Paget's disease at 40 mg/day.

>10%: Endocrine & metabolic: Hypocalcemia (transient, mild, 18%); hypophosphatemia (transient, mild, 10%)

1% to 10%:

Cardiovascular: Atrial fibrillation (1% to 2%)

Central nervous system: Headache (up to 3%)

Gastrointestinal: Abdominal pain (1% to 7%), acid reflux (1% to 4%), dyspepsia (1% to 4%), nausea (1% to 4%), flatulence (up to 4%), diarrhea (1% to 3%), gastroesophageal reflux disease (1% to 3%), constipation (up to 3%), esophageal ulcer (up to 2%), abdominal distension (up to 1%), gastritis (up to 1%), vomiting (up to 1%), dysphagia (up to 1%), gastric ulcer (1%), melena (1%)

Neuromuscular & skeletal: Musculoskeletal pain (up to 6%), muscle cramps (up to 1%)

<1% (Limited to important or life-threatening): Alopecia, anastomotic ulcer, angioedema; bone, muscle, or joint pain (occasionally severe, considered incapacitating in rare cases); dizziness, duodenal ulcer, episcleritis, erythema, esophageal erosions, esophageal perforation, esophageal stricture, esophagitis, fever, flu-like syndrome, hypersensitivity reactions, hypocalcemia (symptomatic), joint swelling, lymphocytopenia, malaise, myalgia, oropharyngeal ulceration, osteonecrosis (jaw), peripheral edema,

photosensitivity (rare), pruritus, rash, scleritis (rare), Stevens-Johnson syndrome, taste perversion, toxic epidermal necrolysis, urticaria, uveitis (rare), vertigo, weakness

Drug Interactions

Aminoglycosides: May enhance the hypocalcemic effect of Bisphosphonate Derivatives. *Risk C: Monitor therapy*

Antacids: May decrease the absorption of Bisphosphonate Derivatives. Antacids containing aluminum, calcium, or magnesium are of specific concern. **Exceptions:** Magaldrate; Sodium Bicarbonate. *Risk D: Consider therapy modification*

Aspirin: May enhance the adverse/toxic effect of Alendronate. Specifically gastrointestinal adverse events. *Risk C: Monitor therapy*

Calcium Salts: May decrease the absorption of Bisphosphonate Derivatives. *Risk D: Consider therapy modification*

Iron Salts: May decrease the absorption of Bisphosphonate Derivatives. Only oral iron salts are of concern. **Exceptions:** Ferric Gluconate; Iron Dextran Complex; Iron Sucrose. *Risk D: Consider therapy modification*

Magnesium Salts: May decrease the absorption of Bisphosphonate Derivatives. Only oral magnesium salts are of concern. *Risk D: Consider therapy modification*

Nonsteroidal Anti-Inflammatory Agents: May enhance the adverse/toxic effect of Bisphosphonate Derivatives. Both an increased risk of gastrointestinal ulceration and an increased risk of nephrotoxicity are of concern. *Risk C: Monitor therapy*

Phosphate Supplements: Bisphosphonate Derivatives may enhance the hypocalcemic effect of Phosphate Supplements. *Risk C: Monitor therapy*

Ethanol/Nutrition/Herb Interactions

Ethanol: Avoid ethanol (may increase risk of osteoporosis and gastric irritation).

Food: All food and beverages interfere with absorption. Coadministration with caffeine may reduce alendronate efficacy. Coadministration with dairy products may decrease alendronate absorption. Beverages (especially orange juice and coffee) and food may reduce the absorption of alendronate as much as 60%.

Stability Store tablets and oral solution at room temperature of 15°C to 30°C (59°F to 86°F). Keep in well-closed container.

Mechanism of Action A bisphosphonate which inhibits bone resorption via actions on osteoclasts or on osteoclast precursors; decreases the rate of bone resorption, leading to an indirect increase in bone mineral density. In Paget's disease, characterized by disordered resorption and formation of bone, inhibition of resorption leads to an indirect decrease in bone formation; but the newly-formed bone has a more normal architecture.

Pharmacodynamics/Kinetics

Distribution: 28 L (exclusive of bone)

Protein binding: ~78%

Metabolism: None

Bioavailability: Fasting: 0.6%; reduced 60% with food or drink

Half-life elimination: Exceeds 10 years

Excretion: Urine; feces (as unabsorbed drug)

Dosage Oral: Adults: **Note:** Patients treated with glucocorticoids and those with Paget's disease should receive adequate amounts of calcium and vitamin D.

Osteoporosis in postmenopausal females:

Prophylaxis: 5 mg once daily **or** 35 mg once weekly

Treatment: 10 mg once daily **or** 70 mg once weekly

Osteoporosis in males: 10 mg once daily **or** 70 mg once weekly

Osteoporosis secondary to glucocorticoids in males and females: Treatment: 5 mg once daily; a dose of 10 mg once daily should be used in postmenopausal females who are not receiving estrogen.

Paget's disease of bone in males and females: 40 mg once daily for 6 months

Retreatment: Relapses during the 12 months following therapy occurred in 9% of patients who responded to treatment. Specific retreatment data are not available. Following a 6-month post-treatment evaluation period, retreatment with alendronate may be considered in patients who have relapsed based on increases in serum alkaline phosphatase, which should be measured periodically. Retreatment may also be considered in those who failed to normalize their serum alkaline phosphatase.

Elderly: No dosage adjustment is necessary

Dosage adjustment in renal impairment:

Cl_{cr} 35-60 mL/minute: None necessary

Cl_{cr} <35 mL/minute: Alendronate is not recommended due to lack of experience

Dosage adjustment in hepatic impairment: None necessary

Dietary Considerations Ensure adequate calcium and vitamin D intake; however, wait at least 30 minutes after taking alendronate before taking any supplement. Alendronate must be taken with plain water first thing in the morning and at least 30 minutes before the first food or beverage of the day.

Administration Alendronate must be taken with plain water (tablets 6-8 oz; oral solution follow with 2 oz) first thing in the morning and ≥30 minutes before the first food, beverage, or other medication of the day. Do not take with mineral water or with other beverages. Patients should be instructed to stay upright (not to lie down) for at least 30 minutes **and** until after first food of the day (to reduce esophageal irritation). Patients should receive supplemental calcium and vitamin D if dietary intake is inadequate.

Monitoring Parameters Alkaline phosphatase should be periodically measured; serum calcium and phosphorus; monitor pain and fracture rate; hormonal status (male and female) prior to therapy; bone mineral density (should be done prior to initiation of therapy and after 6-12 months of combined glucocorticoid and alendronate treatment)

Reference Range Calcium (total): Adults: 9.0-11.0 mg/dL (2.05-2.54 mmol/L), may slightly decrease with aging; phosphorus: 2.5-4.5 mg/dL (0.81-1.45 mmol/L)

Test Interactions Bisphosphonates may interfere with diagnostic imaging agents such as technetium-99m-diphosphonate in bone scans.

Dosage Forms Excipient information presented when available (limited, particularly for generics); consult specific product labeling.

Solution, oral:

Fosamax®: 70 mg/75 mL [contains parabens; raspberry flavor]

Tablet: 5 mg, 10 mg, 35 mg, 40 mg, 70 mg

Fosamax®: 5 mg, 10 mg, 35 mg, 40 mg, 70 mg

Alendronate and Cholecalciferol

(a LEN droe nate & kole e kal SI fer ole)

U.S. Brand Names Fosamax Plus D™

Canadian Brand Names Fosavance

Mexican Brand Names Fosamax Plus

Index Terms Alendronate Sodium and Cholecalciferol; Cholecalciferol and Alendronate; Vitamin D_3 and Alendronate

Pharmacologic Category Bisphosphonate Derivative; Vitamin D Analog

Generic Available No

Use Treatment of osteoporosis in postmenopausal females; increase bone mass in males with osteoporosis

Effect on Mental Status May cause irritability or sedation; rarely associated with psychosis

Effect on Psychiatric Treatment Symptoms of overdose are similar to those associated with lithium side effects/toxicity and psychogenic polydipsia.

Pregnancy Risk Factor C

Pregnancy Considerations Animal studies have shown delays in delivery and fetal/neonatal death (secondary to hypocalcemia). Bisphosphonates are incorporated into the bone matrix and gradually released over time. Theoretically, there may be a risk of fetal harm when pregnancy follows the completion of therapy. No animal data are available for the use of cholecalciferol in pregnancy; however, high-dose ergocalciferol has demonstrated abortifacient properties and aortic abnormalities in rabbits. There are no adequate and well-controlled studies in pregnant women.

Lactation Cholecalciferol enters breast milk; excretion of alendronate in breast milk unknown/use caution

Contraindications Hypersensitivity to alendronate, other bisphosphonates, vitamin D derivatives, or any component of the formulation; hypocalcemia; abnormalities of the esophagus which delay esophageal emptying such as stricture or achalasia; inability to stand or sit upright for at least 30 minutes

Warnings/Precautions Use caution in patients with renal impairment (not recommended for use in patients with Cl_{cr} <35 mL/minute). Hypocalcemia and/or vitamin D deficiency must be corrected before therapy initiation; ensure adequate calcium and vitamin D intake; do not use to treat vitamin D deficiency. May exacerbate hypercalcemia and/or hypercalciuria in certain disease states (eg, leukemia, lymphoma, sarcoidosis); monitor serum calcium levels. Increased doses of vitamin D supplementation may be required in patients with GI malabsorption syndrome; consider monitoring 25-hydroxyvitamin D levels. May cause irritation to upper gastrointestinal mucosa; ensure compliance with administration guidelines. Esophagitis, esophageal ulcers, esophageal erosions, and esophageal stricture (rare) have been reported; risk increases in patients unable to comply with dosing instructions. Use with caution in patients with dysphagia, esophageal disease, gastritis, duodenitis, or ulcers (may worsen underlying condition).

Bisphosphonate therapy has been associated with osteonecrosis, primarily of the jaw; this has been observed mostly in cancer patients, but also in patients with postmenopausal osteoporosis and other diagnoses. Risk factors include a diagnosis of cancer, with concomitant chemotherapy, radiotherapy, or corticosteroids; anemia, coagulopathy, infection or pre-existing dental disease. Symptoms included nonhealing extraction socket or an exposed jawbone. There are no data addressing whether discontinuation of therapy reduces the risk of developing osteonecrosis. Dental exams and preventative dentistry should be performed prior to placing patients with risk factors on chronic bisphosphonate therapy. Invasive dental procedures should be avoided during treatment.

Severe (and occasionally debilitating) bone, joint, and/or muscle pain have been reported during bisphosphonate treatment. The onset of pain ranged from a single day to several months. Symptoms usually resolve upon discontinuation. Some patients experienced recurrence when rechallenged with same drug or another bisphosphonate; avoid use in patients with a history of these symptoms in association with bisphosphonate therapy. Discontinue use if severe symptoms occur.

Safety and efficacy in pediatric patients have not been established.

Adverse Reactions See individual agents.

Drug Interactions

Aminoglycosides: May enhance the hypocalcemic effect of Bisphosphonate Derivatives. *Risk C: Monitor therapy*

Antacids: May decrease the absorption of Bisphosphonate Derivatives. Antacids containing aluminum, calcium, or magnesium are of specific concern. **Exceptions:** Magaldrate; Sodium Bicarbonate. *Risk D: Consider therapy modification*

Aspirin: May enhance the adverse/toxic effect of Alendronate. Specifically gastrointestinal adverse events. *Risk C: Monitor therapy*

Calcium Salts: May decrease the absorption of Bisphosphonate Derivatives. *Risk D: Consider therapy modification*

Iron Salts: May decrease the absorption of Bisphosphonate Derivatives. Only oral iron salts are of concern. **Exceptions:** Ferric Gluconate; Iron Dextran Complex; Iron Sucrose. *Risk D: Consider therapy modification*

Magnesium Salts: May decrease the absorption of Bisphosphonate Derivatives. Only oral magnesium salts are of concern. *Risk D: Consider therapy modification*

Nonsteroidal Anti-Inflammatory Agents: May enhance the adverse/toxic effect of Bisphosphonate Derivatives. Both an increased risk of gastrointestinal ulceration and an increased risk of nephrotoxicity are of concern. *Risk C: Monitor therapy*

Phosphate Supplements: Bisphosphonate Derivatives may enhance the hypocalcemic effect of Phosphate Supplements. *Risk C: Monitor therapy*

Ethanol/Nutrition/Herb Interactions See individual agents.

Stability Store at 20°C to 25°C (68°F to 77°F); excursions permitted to 15°C to 30°C (59°F to 86°F). Protect from moisture and light. Keep sealed in blister container or original bottle (with desiccant) until use.

Mechanism of Action See individual agents.

Dosage Oral: Adults: One tablet (alendronate 70 mg/cholecalciferol 2800 int. units **or** alendronate 70 mg/cholecalciferol 5600 int. units) once weekly. Appropriate dose in most osteoporotic women or men: Alendronate 70 mg/cholecalciferol 5600 int. units once weekly.

Dosage adjustment in renal impairment:

Cl_{cr} 35-60 mL/minute: No adjustment needed

Cl_{cr} <35 mL/minute: Not recommended

Dosage adjustment in hepatic impairment: Alendronate: None necessary. Cholecalciferol: May not be adequately absorbed in patients who have malabsorption due to inadequate bile production.

Dietary Considerations Ensure adequate calcium and vitamin D intake; supplemental calcium should be provided in patients whose dietary intake is inadequate. Recommended intake of vitamin D is 400-800 int. units daily. Certain patients may require additional vitamin D supplementation, particularly patients at risk for vitamin D deficiency (eg, malabsorption syndromes, chronically ill, >70 years of age). Consider monitoring 25-hydroxy vitamin D in patients with malabsorption syndromes. Wait at least 30 minutes after taking alendronate with cholecalciferol before taking any supplement. Must be taken with at least 6-8 oz. plain water first thing in the morning and at least 30 minutes before the first food or beverage of the day. Administer with plain water only; do not administer with mineral-enriched water.

Administration Alendronate must be taken with plain water (6-8 oz) first thing in the morning and ≥30 minutes before the first food, beverage, or other medication of the day. Patient should be instructed to stay upright (not to lie down) for at least 30 minutes and until after first food of the day (to reduce esophageal irritation).

Monitoring Parameters Alkaline phosphatase (measured periodically); urine and serum calcium, serum phosphorus, serum 25-hydroxy vitamin D; monitor pain and fracture rate; hormonal status (male and female) prior to therapy; bone mineral density (should be done prior to initiation of therapy and after 6-12 months of combined glucocorticoid and alendronate treatment)

Reference Range

Calcium (total): Adults: 9.0-11.0 mg/dL (2.05-2.54 mmol/L), may slightly decrease with aging

Phosphorus: 2.5-4.5 mg/dL (0.81-1.45 mmol/L)

25-hydroxyvitamin D: 10-80 ng/mL (higher during summer)

Test Interactions Bisphosphonates may interfere with diagnostic imaging agents such as technetium-99m-diphosphonate in bone scans.

Dosage Forms Excipient information presented when available (limited, particularly for generics); consult specific product labeling.

Tablet:

Fosamax Plus D™ 70/2800: Alendronate 70 mg and cholecalciferol 2800 int. units

Fosamax Plus D™ 70/5600: Alendronate 70 mg and cholecalciferol 5600 int. units

- **Alendronate Sodium** *see* Alendronate *on page 59*
- **Alendronate Sodium and Cholecalciferol** *see* Alendronate and Cholecalciferol *on page 62*
- **Aler-Cap [OTC]** *see* DiphenhydrAMINE *on page 481*
- **Aler-Dryl [OTC]** *see* DiphenhydrAMINE *on page 481*
- **Aler-Tab [OTC]** *see* DiphenhydrAMINE *on page 481*
- **Alesse®** *see* Ethinyl Estradiol and Levonorgestrel *on page 595*
- **Aleve® [OTC]** *see* Naproxen *on page 1102*
- **Aleve®-D Sinus & Cold [OTC]** *see* Naproxen and Pseudoephedrine *on page 1107*
- **Aleve®-D Sinus & Headache [OTC]** *see* Naproxen and Pseudoephedrine *on page 1107*
- **Aleve® Cold & Sinus [OTC] [DSC]** *see* Naproxen and Pseudoephedrine *on page 1107*
- **Aleve® Sinus & Headache [OTC] [DSC]** *see* Naproxen and Pseudoephedrine *on page 1107*
- **Alfenta®** *see* Alfentanil *on page 64*

Alfentanil (al FEN ta nil)

Medication Safety Issues

Sound-alike/look-alike issues:

Alfentanil may be confused with Anafranil®, fentanyl, remifentanil, sufentanil

Alfenta® may be confused with Sufenta®

High alert medication: The Institute for Safe Medication Practices (ISMP) includes this medication among its list of drug classes which have a heightened risk of causing significant patient harm when used in error.

Related Information

Narcotic / Opioid Analgesics *on page 1789*

U.S. Brand Names Alfenta®

Canadian Brand Names Alfentanil Injection, USP; Alfenta®

Index Terms Alfentanil Hydrochloride

Pharmacologic Category Analgesic, Opioid; Anilidopiperidine Opioid

Use Analgesic adjunct given by continuous infusion or in incremental doses in maintenance of anesthesia with barbiturate or N_2O or a primary anesthetic agent for the induction of anesthesia in patients undergoing general surgery in which endotracheal intubation and mechanical ventilation are required

Effect on Mental Status Sedation is common, may see depression or confusion, rarely may cause seizures or delirium

Effect on Psychiatric Treatment CNS depressant and beta-blockers may increase toxicity; phenothiazines may antagonize analgesic effect

Restrictions C-II

Dosage Summary Note: Dosage should be based on ideal body weight

I.V.:

Anesthetic Induction:

Children <12 years: Dosage not established

Children ≥12 years: Initial: 130-245 mcg/kg; Maintenance: 0.5-1.5 mcg/kg/minute

Adults: Initial: 130-245 mcg/kg; Maintenance: 0.5-1.5 mcg/kg/minute

Continuous infusion:

Children <12 years: Dosage not established

Children ≥12 years: Initial: 50-75 mcg/kg; Maintenance: 0.5-3 mcg/kg/minute

Adults: Initial: 50-75 mcg/kg; Maintenance: 0.5-3 mcg/kg/minute

Incremental injection:

Children <12 years: Dosage not established

Children ≥12 years:

≤30 minutes anesthesia: Initial: 8-20 mcg/kg; Maintenance: 3-5 mcg/kg **or** 0.5-1 mcg/kg/minute (maximum: 40 mcg/kg total dose)

≥30 minutes anesthesia: Initial: 20-50 mcg/kg; Maintenance: 5-15 mcg/kg (maximum: 75 mcg/kg total dose)

Adults:

≤30 minutes anesthesia: Initial: 8-20 mcg/kg; Maintenance: 3-5 mcg/kg **or** 0.5-1 mcg/kg/min (maximum: 40 mcg/kg total dose)

≥30 minutes anesthesia: Initial: 20-50 mcg/kg; Maintenance: 5-15 mcg/kg (maximum: 75 mcg/kg total dose)

Dosage Forms Excipient information presented when available (limited, particularly for generics); consult specific product labeling.

Injection, solution [preservative free]: 500 mcg/mL (2 mL, 5 mL)

Alfenta®: 500 mcg/mL (2 mL, 5 mL, 10 mL, 20 mL)

◆ **Alfentanil Hydrochloride** *see* Alfentanil *on page 64*

◆ **Alferon® N** *see* Interferon Alfa-n3 *on page 847*

Alfuzosin (al FYOO zoe sin)

U.S. Brand Names Uroxatral®

Canadian Brand Names Xatral

Mexican Brand Names Xatral OD

Index Terms Alfuzosin Hydrochloride

Pharmacologic Category $Alpha_1$ Blocker

Use Treatment of the functional symptoms of benign prostatic hyperplasia (BPH)

Effect on Mental Status May cause dizziness

Effect on Psychiatric Treatment Alfuzosin may cause orthostasis. Concomitant use with psychotropics may produce additive effects on blood pressure. Use caution with thioridazine and ziprasidone; may prolong QT interval. Use caution with nefazodone; may increase levels of alfuzosin resulting in toxicity.

Dosage Summary

Oral:

Children: Dosage not established

Adults: 10 mg once daily

Dosage Forms Excipient information presented when available (limited, particularly for generics); consult specific product labeling.

Tablet, extended release, as hydrochloride:

Uroxatral®: 10 mg

◆ **Alfuzosin Hydrochloride** *see* Alfuzosin *on page 65*

◆ **Aliclen™** *see* Salicylic Acid *on page 1454*

◆ **Alimta®** *see* Pemetrexed *on page 1238*

◆ **Alinia®** *see* Nitazoxanide *on page 1146*

Aliskiren (a lis KYE ren)

Medication Safety Issues

International issues:

Aliskiren may be confused with Aliseum which is a brand name for diazepam in Italy

Related Information

Angiotensin Agents *on page 1754*

U.S. Brand Names Tekturna®

Canadian Brand Names Rasilez®

Index Terms Aliskiren Hemifumarate; SPP100

Pharmacologic Category Renin Inhibitor

Use Treatment of hypertension, alone or in combination with other antihypertensive agents

Unlabeled/Investigational Use Treatment of persistent proteinuria in patients with type 2 diabetes mellitus, hypertension, and nephropathy despite administration of optimized recommended renoprotective therapy (eg, angiotensin II receptor blocker)

Effect on Mental Status May cause dizziness

Effect on Psychiatric Treatment Concomitant use with psychotropics (especially those with significant alpha-adrenergic blocking properties) may produce additive hypotensive effects.

Dosage Summary

Oral:

Children <18 years: Dosage not established

Adults: 150-300 mg once daily (maximum: 300 mg/day)

Dosage Forms Excipient information presented when available (limited, particularly for generics); consult specific product labeling.

Tablet:

Tekturna®: 150 mg, 300 mg

Aliskiren and Hydrochlorothiazide

(a lis KYE ren & hye droe klor oh THYE a zide)

U.S. Brand Names Tekturna HCT®

Index Terms Aliskiren Hemifumarate and Hydrochlorothiazide; Hydrochlorothiazide and Aliskiren

Pharmacologic Category Diuretic, Thiazide; Renin Inhibitor

Use Treatment of hypertension (not recommended for initial treatment)

Effect on Mental Status May cause dizziness

Effect on Psychiatric Treatment Concomitant use with psychotropics (especially those with significant alpha-adrenergic blocking properties) may produce additive hypotensive effects; monitor. Hydrochlorothiazide is used to treat lithium-induced diabetes insipidus; monitor for hypokalemia. May also decrease lithium clearance resulting in an increase in serum lithium levels and potential lithium toxicity; monitor serum lithium levels.

Dosage Summary

Oral:

Children: Dosage not established

Adults: Aliskiren 150-300 mg and hydrochlorothiazide 12.5-25 mg once daily (maximum: 300 mg/day [aliskiren]; 25 mg/day [hydrochlorothiazide])

Dosage Forms Excipient information presented when available (limited, particularly for generics); consult specific product labeling.

Tablet:

Tekturna HCT®:

150/12.5: Aliskiren 150 mg and hydrochlorothiazide 12.5 mg

150/25: Aliskiren 150 mg and hydrochlorothiazide 25 mg

300/12.5: Aliskiren 300 mg and hydrochlorothiazide 12.5 mg

300/25: Aliskiren 300 mg and hydrochlorothiazide 25 mg

◆ **Aliskiren Hemifumarate** *see* Aliskiren *on page 65*

◆ **Aliskiren Hemifumarate and Hydrochlorothiazide** *see* Aliskiren and Hydrochlorothiazide *on page 66*

Alitretinoin (a li TRET i noyn)

Medication Safety Issues

Sound-alike/look-alike issues:

Panretin® may be confused with pancreatin

High alert medication: The Institute for Safe Medication Practices (ISMP) includes this medication among its list of drugs which have a heightened risk of causing significant patient harm when used in error.

U.S. Brand Names Panretin®

Canadian Brand Names Panretin®

Pharmacologic Category Antineoplastic Agent, Miscellaneous; Retinoic Acid Derivative

Use Orphan drug: Topical treatment of cutaneous lesions in AIDS-related Kaposi's sarcoma

Unlabeled/Investigational Use Cutaneous T-cell lymphomas
Effect on Mental Status Pain is common
Effect on Psychiatric Treatment May be photosensitizing; caution with psychotropics
Dosage Summary
Topical:
Children: Dosage not established
Adults: Apply twice daily to cutaneous lesions
Dosage Forms Excipient information presented when available (limited, particularly for generics); consult specific product labeling.
Gel:
Panretin®: 0.1% (60 g)

- ◆ **Alka-Mints® [OTC]** *see* Calcium Carbonate *on page 254*
- ◆ **Alka-Seltzer Plus® Day Cold [OTC]** *see* Acetaminophen, Dextromethorphan, and Phenylephrine *on page 42*
- ◆ **Alka-Seltzer Plus® Sinus Formula [OTC]** *see* Acetaminophen and Phenylephrine *on page 36*
- ◆ **Alka-Seltzer® P.M. [OTC]** *see* Aspirin and Diphenhydramine *on page 145*
- ◆ **Alkeran®** *see* Melphalan *on page 983*
- ◆ **AllanHist PDX** *see* Brompheniramine, Pseudoephedrine, and Dextromethorphan *on page 208*
- ◆ **AllanTan Pediatric [DSC]** *see* Chlorpheniramine and Phenylephrine *on page 323*
- ◆ **AllanVan-DM** *see* Phenylephrine, Pyrilamine, and Dextromethorphan *on page 1278*
- ◆ **AllanVan-S [DSC]** *see* Phenylephrine and Pyrilamine *on page 1275*
- ◆ **Allegra®** *see* Fexofenadine *on page 629*
- ◆ **Allegra-D® 12 Hour** *see* Fexofenadine and Pseudoephedrine *on page 631*
- ◆ **Allegra-D® 24 Hour** *see* Fexofenadine and Pseudoephedrine *on page 631*
- ◆ **Allegra® ODT** *see* Fexofenadine *on page 629*
- ◆ **Aller-Chlor® [OTC]** *see* Chlorpheniramine *on page 321*
- ◆ **Allerest® Allergy and Sinus Relief [OTC]** *see* Acetaminophen and Pseudoephedrine *on page 37*
- ◆ **Allerest® Maximum Strength Allergy and Hay Fever [OTC]** *see* Chlorpheniramine and Pseudoephedrine *on page 325*
- ◆ **Allerfrim [OTC]** *see* Triprolidine and Pseudoephedrine *on page 1634*
- ◆ **Allergy Relief [OTC]** *see* Loratadine *on page 946*
- ◆ **AllerMax® [OTC]** *see* DiphenhydrAMINE *on page 481*
- ◆ **AllerTan™** *see* Chlorpheniramine, Pyrilamine, and Phenylephrine *on page 335*
- ◆ **AlleRx™-D** *see* Pseudoephedrine and Methscopolamine *on page 1370*
- ◆ **AlleRx™ Suspension** *see* Chlorpheniramine and Phenylephrine *on page 323*
- ◆ **Allfen-DM** *see* Guaifenesin and Dextromethorphan *on page 739*
- ◆ **Allfen Jr** *see* GuaiFENesin *on page 737*
- ◆ **Alli™ [OTC]** *see* Orlistat *on page 1184*

Allopurinol (al oh PURE i nole)

Medication Safety Issues
Sound-alike/look-alike issues:
Allopurinol may be confused with Apresoline
Zyloprim® may be confused with Xylo-Pfan®, ZORprin®
U.S. Brand Names Aloprim™; Zyloprim®
Canadian Brand Names Alloprin®; Apo-Allopurinol®; Novo-Purol; Zyloprim®
Mexican Brand Names Atisuril; Etindrax; Genozyl; Puribel 300; Unizuric 300; Zyloprim
Index Terms Allopurinol Sodium
Pharmacologic Category Xanthine Oxidase Inhibitor
Generic Available Yes
Use
Oral: Prevention of attack of gouty arthritis and nephropathy; treatment of secondary hyperuricemia which may occur during treatment of tumors or leukemia; prevention of recurrent calcium oxalate calculi

I.V.: Treatment of elevated serum and urinary uric acid levels when oral therapy is not tolerated in patients with leukemia, lymphoma, and solid tumor malignancies who are receiving cancer chemotherapy

Effect on Mental Status May cause drowsiness

Effect on Psychiatric Treatment Rarely may cause bone marrow suppression; use caution with clozapine and carbamazepine

Pregnancy Risk Factor C

Pregnancy Considerations There are few reports describing the use of allopurinol during pregnancy; no adverse fetal outcomes attributable to allopurinol have been reported in humans; use only if potential benefit outweighs the potential risk to the fetus.

Lactation Enters breast milk/use caution (AAP rates "compatible")

Contraindications Hypersensitivity to allopurinol or any component of the formulation

Warnings/Precautions Do not use to treat asymptomatic hyperuricemia. Has been associated with a number of hypersensitivity reactions, including severe reactions (vasculitis and Stevens-Johnson syndrome); discontinue at first sign of rash. Reversible hepatotoxicity has been reported; use with caution in patients with pre-existing hepatic impairment. Bone marrow suppression has been reported; use caution with other drugs causing myelosuppression. Caution in renal impairment, dosage adjustments needed. Use with caution in patients taking diuretics concurrently. Risk of skin rash may be increased in patients receiving amoxicillin or ampicillin. The risk of hypersensitivity may be increased in patients receiving thiazides, and possibly ACE inhibitors. Use caution with mercaptopurine or azathioprine; dosage adjustment necessary.

Adverse Reactions

>1%:

Dermatologic: Rash (increased with ampicillin or amoxicillin use, 1.5% per manufacturer, >10% in some reports)

Gastrointestinal: Nausea (1.3%), vomiting (1.2%)

Renal: Renal failure/impairment (1.2%)

<1% (Limited to important or life-threatening): Acute tubular necrosis, agranulocytosis, angioedema, aplastic anemia, bronchospasm, cataracts, exfoliative dermatitis, granuloma annulare, granulomatous hepatitis, hypersensitivity syndrome, interstitial nephritis, macular retinitis, nephrolithiasis, neuritis, pancreatitis, paresthesia, peripheral neuropathy, Stevens-Johnson syndrome, toxic epidermal necrolysis, toxic pustuloderma, vasculitis

Drug Interactions

ACE Inhibitors: May enhance the potential for allergic or hypersensitivity reactions to Allopurinol. *Risk D: Consider therapy modification*

Amoxicillin: Allopurinol may enhance the potential for allergic or hypersensitivity reactions to Amoxicillin. *Risk C: Monitor therapy*

Ampicillin: Allopurinol may enhance the potential for allergic or hypersensitivity reactions to Ampicillin. *Risk C: Monitor therapy*

Antacids: May decrease the absorption of Allopurinol. **Exceptions:** Sodium Bicarbonate. *Risk D: Consider therapy modification*

AzaTHIOprine: Allopurinol may decrease the metabolism of AzaTHIOprine. *Risk D: Consider therapy modification*

CarBAMazepine: Allopurinol may increase the serum concentration of CarBAMazepine. *Risk C: Monitor therapy*

ChlorproPAMIDE: Allopurinol may increase the serum concentration of ChlorproPAMIDE. *Risk C: Monitor therapy*

Cyclophosphamide: Allopurinol may enhance the adverse/toxic effect of Cyclophosphamide. Specifically, bone marrow suppression. *Risk C: Monitor therapy*

Didanosine: Allopurinol may decrease the metabolism of Didanosine. *Risk D: Consider therapy modification*

Loop Diuretics: May enhance the adverse/toxic effect of Allopurinol. Loop Diuretics may increase the serum concentration of Allopurinol. Specifically, Loop Diuretics may increase the concentration of Oxypurinolol, an active metabolite of Allopurinol. *Risk C: Monitor therapy*

Mercaptopurine: Allopurinol may decrease the metabolism of Mercaptopurine. *Risk D: Consider therapy modification*

Pivampicillin: Allopurinol may enhance the potential for allergic or hypersensitivity reactions to Pivampicillin. *Risk C: Monitor therapy*

Theophylline Derivatives: Allopurinol may increase the serum concentration of Theophylline Derivatives. **Exceptions:** Dyphylline. *Risk C: Monitor therapy*

Thiazide Diuretics: May enhance the potential for allergic or hypersensitivity reactions to Allopurinol. Thiazide Diuretics may increase the serum concentration of Allopurinol. Specifically, Thiazide Diuretics may increase the concentration of Oxypurinolol, an active metabolite of Allopurinol. *Risk C: Monitor therapy*

Vitamin K Antagonists (eg, warfarin): Allopurinol may enhance the anticoagulant effect of Vitamin K Antagonists. *Risk D: Consider therapy modification*

Ethanol/Nutrition/Herb Interactions

Ethanol: May decrease effectiveness.

Iron supplements: Hepatic iron uptake may be increased.

Vitamin C: Large amounts of vitamin C may acidify urine and increase kidney stone formation.

Stability

Powder for injection: Store at controlled room temperature of 15°C to 30°C (59°F to 86°F). Further dilution with NS or D_5W (50-100 mL) to ≤6 mg/mL is recommended. Following reconstitution, intravenous solutions should be stored at 20°C to 25°C (68°F to 77°F). Do not refrigerate reconstituted and/or diluted product. Must be administered within 10 hours of solution preparation.

Tablet: Store at controlled room temperature of 15°C to 25°C (59°F to 77°F).

Mechanism of Action Allopurinol inhibits xanthine oxidase, the enzyme responsible for the conversion of hypoxanthine to xanthine to uric acid. Allopurinol is metabolized to oxypurinol which is also an inhibitor of xanthine oxidase; allopurinol acts on purine catabolism, reducing the production of uric acid without disrupting the biosynthesis of vital purines.

Pharmacodynamics/Kinetics

Onset of action: Peak effect: 1-2 weeks

Absorption: Oral: ~80%; Rectal: Poor and erratic

Distribution: V_d: ~1.6 L/kg; V_{ss}: 0.84-0.87 L/kg; enters breast milk

Protein binding: <1%

Metabolism: ~75% to active metabolites, chiefly oxypurinol

Bioavailability: 49% to 53%

Half-life elimination:

Normal renal function: Parent drug: 1-3 hours; Oxypurinol: 18-30 hours

End-stage renal disease: Prolonged

Time to peak, plasma: Oral: 30-120 minutes

Excretion: Urine (76% as oxypurinol, 12% as unchanged drug)

Allopurinol and oxypurinol are dialyzable

Dosage

Oral: Doses >300 mg should be given in divided doses.

Children ≤10 years: Secondary hyperuricemia associated with chemotherapy: 10 mg/kg/day in 2-3 divided doses **or** 200-300 mg/m²/day in 2-4 divided doses, maximum: 800 mg/24 hours

Alternative (manufacturer labeling): <6 years: 150 mg/day in 3 divided doses; 6-10 years: 300 mg/day in 2-3 divided doses

Children >10 years and Adults:

Secondary hyperuricemia associated with chemotherapy: 600-800 mg/day in 2-3 divided doses for prevention of acute uric acid nephropathy for 2-3 days starting 1-2 days before chemotherapy

Gout: Mild: 200-300 mg/day; Severe: 400-600 mg/day; to reduce the possibility of acute gouty attacks, initiate dose at 100 mg/day and increase weekly to recommended dosage.

Recurrent calcium oxalate stones: 200-300 mg/day in single or divided doses

Elderly: Initial: 100 mg/day, increase until desired uric acid level is obtained

I.V.: Hyperuricemia secondary to chemotherapy: Intravenous daily dose can be given as a single infusion or in equally divided doses at 6-, 8-, or 12-hour intervals. A fluid intake sufficient to yield a daily urinary output of at least 2 L in adults and the maintenance of a neutral or, preferably, slightly alkaline urine are desirable.

Children ≤10 years: Starting dose: 200 mg/m²/day

Children >10 years and Adults: 200-400 mg/m²/day (maximum: 600 mg/day)

Dosing adjustment in renal impairment: Must be adjusted due to accumulation of allopurinol and metabolites:

Oral: Removed by hemodialysis; adult maintenance doses of allopurinol (mg) based on creatinine clearance (mL/minute): See table on next page.

Adult Maintenance Doses of Allopurinol[1]

Creatinine Clearance (mL/min)	Maintenance Dose of Allopurinol (mg)
140	400 daily
120	350 daily
100	300 daily
80	250 daily
60	200 daily
40	150 daily
20	100 daily
10	100 every 2 days
0	100 every 3 days

[1]This table is based on a standard maintenance dose of 300 mg of allopurinol per day for a patient with a creatinine clearance of 100 mL/min.

I.V.:

Cl_{cr} 10-20 mL/minute: 200 mg/day
Cl_{cr} 3-10 mL/minute: 100 mg/day
Cl_{cr} <3 mL/minute: 100 mg/day at extended intervals

Hemodialysis: Administer dose posthemodialysis or administer 50% supplemental dose

Dietary Considerations Should administer oral forms after meals with plenty of fluid. Fluid intake should be administered to yield neutral or slightly alkaline urine and an output of ~2 L (in adults).

Administration

Oral: Should administer oral forms after meals with plenty of fluid.

I.V.: Infuse over 15-60 minutes. The rate of infusion depends on the volume of the infusion. Whenever possible, therapy should be initiated at 24-48 hours before the start of chemotherapy known to cause tumor lysis (including adrenocorticosteroids). I.V. daily dose can be administered as a single infusion or in equally divided doses at 6-, 8-, or 12-hour interval.

Monitoring Parameters CBC, serum uric acid levels, I & O, hepatic and renal function, especially at start of therapy

Reference Range Uric acid, serum: An increase occurs during childhood

Adults:

Male: 3.4-7 mg/dL or slightly more
Female: 2.4-6 mg/dL or slightly more

Values >7 mg/dL are sometimes arbitrarily regarded as hyperuricemia, but there is no sharp line between normals on the one hand, and the serum uric acid of those with clinical gout. Normal ranges cannot be adjusted for purine ingestion, but high purine diet increases uric acid. Uric acid may be increased with body size, exercise, and stress.

Dosage Forms Excipient information presented when available (limited, particularly for generics); consult specific product labeling.

Injection, powder for reconstitution, as sodium: 500 mg
Aloprim™: 500 mg
Tablet: 100 mg, 300 mg
Zyloprim®: 100 mg, 300 mg

- **Allopurinol Sodium** *see* Allopurinol *on page 67*
- **All-*trans*-Retinoic Acid** *see* Tretinoin, Oral *on page 1617*
- **Almacone® [OTC]** *see* Aluminum Hydroxide, Magnesium Hydroxide, and Simethicone *on page 78*
- **Almacone Double Strength® [OTC]** *see* Aluminum Hydroxide, Magnesium Hydroxide, and Simethicone *on page 78*

Almotriptan (al moh TRIP tan)

Medication Safety Issues

Sound-alike/look-alike issues:

Axert™ may be confused with Antivert®

Related Information

Antimigraine Drugs: 5-HT_1 Receptor Agonists *on page 1766*

U.S. Brand Names Axert™

Canadian Brand Names Axert™

Index Terms Almotriptan Malate

Pharmacologic Category Antimigraine Agent; Serotonin 5-$HT_{1B,\ 1D}$ Receptor Agonist

Generic Available No

Use Acute treatment of migraine with or without aura

Pregnancy Risk Factor C

Pregnancy Considerations There are no adequate and well-controlled studies in pregnant women. Use in pregnancy should be limited to situations where benefit outweighs risk to fetus. In some (but not all) animal studies, administration was associated with embryolethality, fetal malformations, and decreased pup weight.

Lactation Excretion in breast milk unknown/use caution

Contraindications Hypersensitivity to almotriptan or any component of the formulation; use as prophylactic therapy for migraine; hemiplegic or basilar migraine; cluster headache; known or suspected ischemic heart disease (angina pectoris, MI, documented silent ischemia, coronary artery vasospasm, Prinzmetal's variant angina); peripheral vascular syndromes (including ischemic bowel disease); uncontrolled hypertension; use within 24 hours of another 5-HT_1 agonist; use within 24 hours of ergotamine derivative; concurrent administration or within 2 weeks of discontinuing an MAO inhibitor (specifically MAO type A inhibitors)

Warnings/Precautions Almotriptan is indicated only in patients ≥18 years of age with a clear diagnosis of migraine headache. If a patient does not respond to the first dose, the diagnosis of migraine should be reconsidered. Do not give to patients with risk factors for CAD until a cardiovascular evaluation has been performed; if evaluation is satisfactory, the healthcare provider should administer the first dose and cardiovascular status should be periodically re-evaluated. Cardiac events (coronary artery vasospasm, transient ischemia, myocardial infarction, ventricular tachycardia/fibrillation, cardiac arrest, and death), cerebral/subarachnoid hemorrhage, stroke, peripheral vascular ischemia, and colonic ischemia have been reported with 5-HT_1 agonist administration. Significant elevation in blood pressure, including hypertensive crisis, has also been reported on rare occasions in patients with and without a history of hypertension. Use with caution in liver or renal dysfunction. Symptoms of agitation, confusion, hallucinations, hyper-reflexia, myoclonus, shivering, and tachycardia (serotonin syndrome) may occur with concomitant proserotonergic drugs (ie, SSRIs/SNRIs or triptans) or agents which reduce almotriptan's metabolism. Safety and efficacy in pediatric patients have not been established.

Adverse Reactions

1% to 10%:

Central nervous system: Headache (>1%), dizziness (>1%), somnolence (>1%)

Gastrointestinal: Nausea (1% to 2%), xerostomia (1%)

Neuromuscular & skeletal: Paresthesia (1%)

<1% (Limited to important or life-threatening): Colitis, coronary artery vasospasm, hypertension, myocardial ischemia, MI, neuropathy, rash, syncope, tachycardia, ventricular fibrillation, ventricular tachycardia, vertigo

Metabolism/Transport Effects Substrate (minor) of CYP2D6, 3A4

Drug Interactions

Ergot Derivatives: May enhance the vasoconstricting effect of Serotonin 5-HT_{1D} Receptor Agonists. Serotonin 5-HT_{1D} Receptor Agonists may enhance the vasoconstricting effect of Ergot Derivatives. *Risk X: Avoid combination*

Ketoconazole: May increase the serum concentration of Almotriptan. *Risk C: Monitor therapy*

MAO Inhibitors: May decrease the metabolism of Serotonin 5-HT_{1D} Receptor Agonists. Management: If MAO inhibitor therapy is required, naratriptan, eletriptan or frovatriptan may be a suitable 5-HT_{1D} agonist to employ. *Risk X: Avoid combination*

Serotonin Modulators: May enhance the adverse/toxic effect of other Serotonin Modulators. The development of serotonin syndrome may occur. *Risk D: Consider therapy modification*

Sibutramine: May enhance the serotonergic effect of Serotonin Modulators. This may cause serotonin syndrome. *Risk X: Avoid combination*

Stability Store at 15°C to 30°C (59°F to 86°F).

Mechanism of Action Selective agonist for serotonin (5-HT_{1B}, 5-HT_{1D}, 5-HT_{1F} receptors) in cranial arteries; causes vasoconstriction and reduce sterile inflammation associated with antidromic neuronal transmission correlating with relief of migraine

Pharmacodynamics/Kinetics
Absorption: Well absorbed
Distribution: V_d: 180-200 L
Protein binding: ~35%
Metabolism: MAO type A oxidative deamination (~27% of dose); via CYP3A4 and 2D6 (~12% of dose) to inactive metabolites
Bioavailability: 70%
Half-life elimination: 3-4 hours
Time to peak: 1-3 hours
Excretion: Urine (40% as unchanged drug); feces (13% unchanged and metabolized)

Dosage Oral: Adults: Migraine: Initial: 6.25-12.5 mg in a single dose; if the headache returns, repeat the dose after 2 hours; no more than 2 doses in 24-hour period

Note: If the first dose is ineffective, diagnosis needs to be re-evaluated. Safety of treating more than 4 migraines/month has not been established.

Dosage adjustment in renal impairment: Initial: 6.25 mg in a single dose; maximum daily dose: ≤12.5 mg

Dosage adjustment in hepatic impairment: Initial: 6.25 mg in a single dose; maximum daily dose: ≤12.5 mg

Dietary Considerations May be taken without regard to meals

Dosage Forms Excipient information presented when available (limited, particularly for generics); consult specific product labeling.
Tablet, as malate:
Axert™: 6.25 mg, 12.5 mg

◆ **Almotriptan Malate** *see* Almotriptan *on page 70*
◆ **Alocril®** *see* Nedocromil *on page 1115*
◆ **Alomide®** *see* Lodoxamide *on page 942*
◆ **Aloprim™** *see* Allopurinol *on page 67*
◆ **Alora®** *see* Estradiol *on page 576*
◆ **Aloxi®** *see* Palonosetron *on page 1218*
◆ **Alpain** *see* Acetaminophen and Phenyltoloxamine *on page 36*
◆ **Alpha-Galactosidase-A (Recombinant)** *see* Agalsidase Beta *on page 52*
◆ **Alphagan® P** *see* Brimonidine *on page 199*
◆ **AlphaNine® SD** *see* Factor IX *on page 612*
◆ **Alph-E [OTC]** *see* Vitamin E *on page 1675*
◆ **Alph-E-Mixed [OTC]** *see* Vitamin E *on page 1675*

ALPRAZolam (al PRAY zoe lam)

Medication Safety Issues
Sound-alike/look-alike issues:
ALPRAZolam may be confused with alprostadil, LORazepam, triazolam
Xanax® may be confused with Lanoxin®, Tenex®, Tylox®, Xopenex®, Zantac®, Zyrtec®

Related Information

Benzodiazepines *on page 1774*
CMS: Long-Term Care Facility Thresholds *on page 1815*
Discontinuation of Psychotropic Drugs *on page 1839*

U.S. Brand Names Alprazolam Intensol®; Niravam™; Xanax XR®; Xanax®

Canadian Brand Names Alti-Alprazolam; Apo-Alpraz®; Apo-Alpraz® TS; Gen-Alprazolam; Novo-Alprazol; Nu-Alprax; Xanax TS™; Xanax®

Mexican Brand Names Alzam; Farmapram; Irizz.; Neupax; Tafil; Tazun

Pharmacologic Category Benzodiazepine

Generic Available Yes: Extended release tablet, immediate release tablet

Use Treatment of anxiety disorder (GAD); panic disorder, with or without agoraphobia; anxiety associated with depression

Unlabeled/Investigational Use Anxiety in children

Mental Health Comment In 2007, the FDA requested that all manufacturers of sedative-hypnotic drug products revise labeling to include a greater emphasis on the risks of adverse effects. These risks include severe allergic reactions (anaphylaxis, angioedema) and complex sleep-related behaviors, which may include sleep-driving (driving while not fully awake and with no memory of the event), making phone calls, and preparing and eating food while asleep.

There are two subtypes of GABA receptors (GABA-A and GABA-B) and three different benzodiazepine receptors (Bz_1, Bz_2, and Bz_3). Benzodiazepine receptors and effects appear to be linked to the GABA-A receptors. Benzodiazepines do not bind to GABA-B receptors. The role of GABA-B receptors is unclear. Benzodiazepines have no specificity for benzodiazepine receptor subtypes.

Alprazolam is a short half-life benzodiazepine. Duration of action after a single dose is determined by redistribution rather than metabolism. Tolerance develops to the sedative, hypnotic, and anticonvulsant effects. It does not develop to the anxiolytic or skeletal muscle-relaxing effects. Psychological and physical dependence may occur with prolonged use of benzodiazepines. The onset of withdrawal symptoms is usually seen on the first day without drug and lasts 5-7 days in patients receiving short half-life benzodiazepines, whereas, the onset occurs after 5 days with a duration of 10-14 days after abrupt discontinuance of long half-life benzodiazepines. Risk factors for abuse include personal or family history of substance abuse and personality disorder.

With the exception of a slower absorption rate, the extended release dosage form of alprazolam displays similar bioavailability and pharmacokinetics to the immediate release dosage form. The slower absorption rate results in a concentration that is maintained between 5-11 hours after dosing. The rate of absorption of benzodiazepines has been linked to abuse potential and side effect burden (sedation and cognitive impairment). The extended release dosage form may have less abuse potential and side effects relative to the immediate release dosage form.

Restrictions C-IV

Pregnancy Risk Factor D

Pregnancy Considerations Benzodiazepines have the potential to cause harm to the fetus, particularly when administered during the first trimester. In addition, withdrawal symptoms may occur in the neonate following *in utero* exposure. Use during pregnancy should be avoided.

Lactation Enters breast milk/not recommended (AAP rates "of concern")

Contraindications Hypersensitivity to alprazolam or any component of the formulation (cross-sensitivity with other benzodiazepines may exist); narrow-angle glaucoma; concurrent use with ketoconazole or itraconazole; pregnancy

Warnings/Precautions Rebound or withdrawal symptoms, including seizures, may occur 18 hours to 3 days following abrupt discontinuation or large decreases in dose (more common in patients receiving >4 mg/day or prolonged treatment). Breakthrough anxiety may occur at the end of dosing interval. Use with caution in patients receiving concurrent CYP3A4 inhibitors. Use with caution in renal impairment or predisposition to urate nephropathy. Use with caution in elderly or debilitated patients, patients with hepatic disease (including alcoholics), renal impairment, or obese patients.

Causes CNS depression (dose related) which may impair physical and mental capabilities. Patients must be cautioned about performing tasks that require mental alertness (eg, operating machinery or driving). Effects with other sedative drugs or ethanol may be potentiated. Benzodiazepines have been associated with falls and traumatic injury and should be used with extreme caution in patients who are at risk of these events (especially the elderly). Use with caution in patients with respiratory disease or impaired gag reflex.

Use caution in patients with depression, particularly if suicidal risk may be present. Episodes of mania or hypomania have occurred in depressed patients treated with alprazolam. May cause physical or psychological dependence. Acute withdrawal may be precipitated in patients after administration of flumazenil.

Benzodiazepines have been associated with anterograde amnesia. Paradoxical reactions have been reported with benzodiazepines, particularly in adolescent/pediatric or psychiatric patients. Does not have analgesic, antidepressant, or antipsychotic properties.

Adverse Reactions

>10%:

Central nervous system: Abnormal coordination, cognitive disorder, depression, drowsiness, fatigue, irritability, lightheadedness, memory impairment, sedation, somnolence

Gastrointestinal: Appetite increased/decreased, constipation, salivation decreased, weight gain/loss, xerostomia

Genitourinary: Micturition difficulty

Neuromuscular & skeletal: Dysarthria

1% to 10%:

Cardiovascular: Hypotension

Central nervous system: Agitation, attention disturbance, confusion, depersonalization, derealization, disorientation, disinhibition, dizziness, dream abnormalities, fear, hallucinations, hypersomnia, nightmares, seizure, talkativeness

Dermatologic: Dermatitis, pruritus, rash

Endocrine & metabolic: Libido decreased/increased, menstrual disorders

Gastrointestinal: Salivation increased

Genitourinary: Incontinence

Hepatic: Bilirubin increased, jaundice, liver enzymes increased

Neuromuscular & skeletal: Arthralgia, ataxia, myalgia, paresthesia

Ocular: Diplopia

Respiratory: Allergic rhinitis, dyspnea

<1% (Limited to important or life-threatening): Amnesia, falls, galactorrhea, gynecomastia, hepatic failure, hepatitis, hyperprolactinemia, Stevens-Johnson syndrome

Metabolism/Transport Effects Substrate of CYP3A4 (major)

Drug Interactions

Alcohol (Ethyl): CNS Depressants may enhance the CNS depressant effect of Alcohol (Ethyl). *Risk C: Monitor therapy*

Antifungal Agents (Azole Derivatives, Systemic): May decrease the metabolism of Benzodiazepines (metabolized by oxidation). *Risk D: Consider therapy modification*

Aprepitant: May increase the serum concentration of Benzodiazepines (metabolized by oxidation). *Risk C: Monitor therapy*

Calcium Channel Blockers (Nondihydropyridine): May decrease the metabolism of Benzodiazepines (metabolized by oxidation). *Risk D: Consider therapy modification*

CarBAMazepine: May increase the metabolism of Benzodiazepines (metabolized by oxidation). *Risk C: Monitor therapy*

Cimetidine: May decrease the metabolism of Benzodiazepines (metabolized by oxidation). *Risk C: Monitor therapy*

Clozapine: Benzodiazepines may enhance the adverse/toxic effect of Clozapine. *Risk D: Consider therapy modification*

CNS Depressants: May enhance the adverse/toxic effect of other CNS Depressants. *Risk C: Monitor therapy*

CYP3A4 Inducers (Strong): May increase the metabolism of CYP3A4 Substrates. *Risk C: Monitor therapy*

CYP3A4 Inhibitors (Moderate): May decrease the metabolism of CYP3A4 Substrates. *Risk C: Monitor therapy*

CYP3A4 Inhibitors (Strong): May decrease the metabolism of CYP3A4 Substrates. *Risk D: Consider therapy modification*

Dasatinib: May increase the serum concentration of CYP3A4 Substrates. *Risk C: Monitor therapy*

Deferasirox: May decrease the serum concentration of CYP3A4 Substrates. *Risk C: Monitor therapy*

Disulfiram: May decrease the metabolism of Benzodiazepines (metabolized by oxidation). *Risk C: Monitor therapy*

Fluconazole: May decrease the metabolism of Benzodiazepines (metabolized by oxidation). *Risk D: Consider therapy modification*

Fosaprepitant: May increase the serum concentration of Benzodiazepines (metabolized by oxidation). Specifically, the active metabolite aprepitant is likely responsible for this effect. *Risk C: Monitor therapy*

Grapefruit Juice: May decrease the metabolism of Benzodiazepines (metabolized by oxidation). *Risk D: Consider therapy modification*

Isoniazid: May decrease the metabolism of Benzodiazepines (metabolized by oxidation). *Risk C: Monitor therapy*

Macrolide Antibiotics: May decrease the metabolism of Benzodiazepines (metabolized by oxidation). **Exceptions:** Azithromycin; Dirithromycin [Off Market]; Spiramycin. *Risk D: Consider therapy modification*

Nefazodone: May decrease the metabolism of Benzodiazepines (metabolized by oxidation). *Risk D: Consider therapy modification*

Oral Contraceptive (Estrogens): May decrease the metabolism of Benzodiazepines (metabolized by oxidation). *Risk C: Monitor therapy*

Oral Contraceptive (Progestins): May decrease the metabolism of Benzodiazepines (metabolized by oxidation). *Risk C: Monitor therapy*

Protease Inhibitors: May decrease the metabolism of Benzodiazepines (metabolized by oxidation). Management: Amprenavir, atazanavir, darunavir, indinavir, nelfinavir, ritonavir, and tipranavir are contraindicated with midazolam and triazolam according to each protease inhibitor 's prescribing information. *Risk D: Consider therapy modification*

Proton Pump Inhibitors: May increase the serum concentration of Benzodiazepines (metabolized by oxidation). **Exceptions:** Lansoprazole; Pantoprazole; Rabeprazole. *Risk C: Monitor therapy*

Rifamycin Derivatives: May increase the metabolism of Benzodiazepines (metabolized by oxidation). *Risk D: Consider therapy modification*

Selective Serotonin Reuptake Inhibitors: May decrease the metabolism of Benzodiazepines (metabolized by oxidation). **Exceptions:** Citalopram; Escitalopram; PARoxetine; Sertraline. *Risk C: Monitor therapy*

St Johns Wort: May increase the metabolism of Benzodiazepines (metabolized by oxidation). *Risk C: Monitor therapy*

Theophylline Derivatives: May diminish the therapeutic effect of Benzodiazepines. *Risk D: Consider therapy modification*

Ethanol/Nutrition/Herb Interactions

Cigarette smoking: May decrease alprazolam concentrations up to 50%.

Ethanol: Avoid ethanol (may increase CNS depression).

Food: Alprazolam serum concentration is unlikely to be increased by grapefruit juice because of alprazolam's high oral bioavailability. The C_{max} of the extended release formulation is increased by 25% when a high-fat meal is given 2 hours before dosing. T_{max} is decreased 30% when food is given immediately prior to dose. T_{max} is increased by 30% when food is given ≥1 hour after dose.

Herb/Nutraceutical: St John's wort may decrease alprazolam levels. Avoid valerian, St John's wort, kava kava, gotu kola (may increase CNS depression).

Stability Orally-disintegrating tablet: Store at room temperature of 20°C to 25°C (68°F to 77°F). Protect from moisture. Seal bottle tightly and discard any cotton packaged inside bottle.

Mechanism of Action Binds to stereospecific benzodiazepine receptors on the postsynaptic GABA neuron at several sites within the central nervous system, including the limbic system, reticular formation. Enhancement of the inhibitory effect of GABA on neuronal excitability results by increased neuronal membrane permeability to chloride ions. This shift in chloride ions results in hyperpolarization (a less excitable state) and stabilization.

Pharmacodynamics/Kinetics

Onset of action: Immediate release and extended release formulations: 1 hour

Duration of action: Immediate release: 5.1 ± 1.7 hours; Extended release: 11.3 ± 4.2 hours

Absorption: Extended release: Slower relative to immediate release formulation resulting in a concentration that is maintained 5-11 hours after dosing

Distribution: V_d: 0.9-1.2 L/kg; enters breast milk

Protein binding: 80%; primarily to albumin

Metabolism: Hepatic via CYP3A4; forms two active metabolites (4-hydroxyalprazolam and α-hydroxyalprazolam)

Bioavailability: 90%

Half-life elimination:

Adults: 11.2 hours (immediate release range: 6.3-26.9; extended release range: 10.7-15.8)

Elderly: 16.3 hours (range: 9-26.9 hours)

Alcoholic liver disease: 19.7 hours (range: 5.8-65.3 hours)

Obesity: 21.8 hours (range: 9.9-40.4 hours)

Time to peak, serum: Immediate release: 1-2 hours; Extended release: ~9 hours; decreased by 1 hour following bedtime dosing compared to morning dosing

Excretion: Urine (as unchanged drug and metabolites)

Dosage Oral: **Note:** Treatment >4 months should be re-evaluated to determine the patient's continued need for the drug

Children: Anxiety (unlabeled use): Immediate release: Initial: 0.005 mg/kg/dose or 0.125 mg/dose 3 times/day; increase in increments of 0.125-0.25 mg, up to a maximum of 0.02 mg/kg/dose or 0.06 mg/kg/day (0.375-3 mg/day)

Adults:

Anxiety: Immediate release: Effective doses are 0.5-4 mg/day in divided doses; the manufacturer recommends starting at 0.25-0.5 mg 3 times/day; titrate dose upward; usual maximum: 4 mg/day. Patients requiring doses >4 mg/day should be increased cautiously. Periodic reassessment and consideration of dosage reduction is recommended.

Anxiety associated with depression: Immediate release: Average dose required: 2.5-3 mg/day in divided doses

Ethanol withdrawal (unlabeled use): Immediate release: Usual dose: 2-2.5 mg/day in divided doses

Panic disorder:

Immediate release: Initial: 0.5 mg 3 times/day; dose may be increased every 3-4 days in increments ≤1 mg/day. Mean effective dosage: 5-6 mg/day; many patients obtain relief at 2 mg/day, as much as 10 mg/day may be required

Extended release: 0.5-1 mg once daily; may increase dose every 3-4 days in increments ≤1 mg/day (range: 3-6 mg/day)

Switching from immediate release to extended release: Patients may be switched to extended release tablets by taking the total daily dose of the immediate release tablets and giving it once daily using the extended release preparation.

Preoperative sedation: 0.5 mg in evening at bedtime and 0.5 mg 1 hour before procedure

Dose reduction: Abrupt discontinuation should be avoided. Daily dose may be decreased by 0.5 mg every 3 days, however, some patients may require a slower reduction. If withdrawal symptoms occur, resume previous dose and discontinue on a less rapid schedule.

Elderly: Initial: 0.125-0.25 mg twice daily; increase by 0.125 mg/day as needed. The smallest effective dose should be used. **Note:** Elderly patients may be more sensitive to the effects of alprazolam including ataxia and oversedation. The elderly may also have impaired renal function leading to decreased clearance. Titrate gradually, if needed.

Immediate release: Initial: 0.25 mg 2-3 times/day

Extended release: Initial: 0.5 mg once daily

Dosing adjustment in renal impairment: No guidelines for adjustment; use caution

Dosing adjustment in hepatic impairment: Reduce dose by 50% to 60% or avoid in cirrhosis

Child/Adolescent Considerations Children <18 years: Anxiety: Dose not established; investigationally, in children 7-16 years of age (n=13), initial doses of 0.005 mg/kg or 0.125 mg/dose were given 3 times/day for situational anxiety; increments of 0.125-0.25 mg were used to increase doses to maximum of 0.02 mg/kg/dose or 0.06 mg/kg/day; a range of 0.375-3 mg/day was needed.

Note: A more recent study in 17 children (8-17 years of age) with overanxious disorder or avoidant disorders used initial daily doses of 0.25 mg for children <40 kg and 0.5 mg for those >40 kg. The dose was titrated at 2-day intervals to a maximum of 0.04 mg/kg/day. Required doses ranged from 0.5-3.5 mg/day (mean: 1.6 mg/day). Based on clinical global ratings, alprazolam appeared to be better than placebo, however, this difference was **not** statistically significant; further studies are needed (Simeon, 1992).

Simeon JG, Ferguson HB, Knott V, et al, "Clinical, Cognitive, and Neurophysiological Effects of Alprazolam in Children and Adolescents With Overanxious and Avoidant Disorders," *J Am Acad Child Adolesc Psychiatry*, 1992, 31(1):29-33.

Administration

Immediate release preparations: Can be administered sublingually with comparable onset and completeness of absorption.

Extended release tablet: Should be taken once daily in the morning; do not crush, break, or chew.

Orally-disintegrating tablets: Using dry hands, place tablet on top of tongue. If using one-half of tablet, immediately discard remaining half (may not remain stable). Administration with water is not necessary.

Monitoring Parameters Respiratory and cardiovascular status

Additional Information Not intended for management of anxieties and minor distresses associated with everyday life. Treatment longer than 4 months should be re-evaluated to determine the patient's need for the drug. Patients who become physically dependent on alprazolam tend to have a difficult time discontinuing it; withdrawal symptoms may be severe. To minimize withdrawal symptoms, taper dosage slowly; do not discontinue abruptly. Abrupt discontinuation after sustained use (generally >10 days) may cause withdrawal symptoms.

Dosage Forms Excipient information presented when available (limited, particularly for generics); consult specific product labeling.

Solution, oral [concentrate]:

Alprazolam Intensol®: 1 mg/mL (30 mL) [alcohol free, dye free, sugar free; contains propylene glycol]

Tablet: 0.25 mg, 0.5 mg, 1 mg, 2 mg

Xanax®: 0.25 mg, 0.5 mg, 1 mg, 2 mg

Tablet, extended release: 0.5 mg, 1 mg, 2 mg, 3 mg

Xanax XR®: 0.5 mg, 1 mg, 2 mg, 3 mg

Tablet, orally disintegrating [scored]:

Niravam™: 0.25 mg, 0.5 mg, 1 mg, 2 mg [orange flavor]

◆ **Alprazolam Intensol®** *see* ALPRAZolam *on page 72*

Alprostadil (al PROS ta dill)

Medication Safety Issues

Sound-alike/look-alike issues:

Alprostadil may be confused with alPRAZolam

U.S. Brand Names Caverject Impulse®; Caverject®; Edex®; Muse®; Prostin VR Pediatric®

Canadian Brand Names Caverject®; Muse® Pellet; Prostin® VR

Mexican Brand Names Caverject

Index Terms PGE_1; Prostaglandin E_1

Pharmacologic Category Prostaglandin; Vasodilator

Use

Prostin VR Pediatric®: Temporary maintenance of patency of ductus arteriosus in neonates with ductal-dependent congenital heart disease until surgery can be performed. These defects include cyanotic (eg, pulmonary atresia, pulmonary stenosis, tricuspid atresia, Fallot's tetralogy, transposition of the great vessels) and acyanotic (eg, interruption of aortic arch, coarctation of aorta, hypoplastic left ventricle) heart disease.

Caverject®: Treatment of erectile dysfunction of vasculogenic, psychogenic, or neurogenic etiology; adjunct in the diagnosis of erectile dysfunction

Edex®, Muse®: Treatment of erectile dysfunction of vasculogenic, psychogenic, or neurogenic etiology

Unlabeled/Investigational Use Investigational: Treatment of pulmonary hypertension in infants and children with congenital heart defects with left-to-right shunts

Effect on Mental Status May cause dizziness; rarely may produce irritability

Effect on Psychiatric Treatment May cause seizures; use caution with clozapine and bupropion

Dosage Summary

I.V.:

Neonates: Initial: 0.05-0.1 mcg/kg/minute; Maintenance: 0.01-0.4 mcg/kg/minute

Children: Dosage not established

Adults: Dosage not established

Intracavernous:

Children: Dosage not established

Adults: Initial: 1.25-2.5 mcg; increase by 2.5 mcg to 5 mcg then in increments of 5-10 mcg until suitable response; Maintenance: Effective dose no more than 3 times/week with at least 24 hours between doses (maximum: 40 mcg/dose [Edex®]; 60 mcg/dose [Caverject®])

Intraurethral:

Children: Dosage not established

Adults: Intial: 125-250 mcg; Maintenance: As needed (maximum: 2 doses/day)

Dosage Forms Excipient information presented when available (limited, particularly for generics); consult specific product labeling. [DSC] = Discontinued product

Injection, powder for reconstitution:

Caverject®: 20 mcg, 40 mcg [contains lactose; diluent contains benzyl alcohol]

Caverject Impulse®: 10 mcg, 20 mcg [prefilled injection system; contains lactose; diluent contains benzyl alcohol]

Edex®: 10 mcg, 20 mcg, 40 mcg [contains lactose; packaged in kits containing diluent, syringe, and alcohol swab]

Injection, solution: 500 mcg/mL (1 mL)

Prostin VR Pediatric®: 500 mcg/mL (1 mL) [contains dehydrated alcohol]

Pellet, urethral:

Muse®: 125 mcg (6s) [DSC], 250 mcg (6s), 500 mcg (6s), 1000 mcg (6s)

- **Altace®** *see* Ramipril *on page 1395*
- **Altafrin** *see* Phenylephrine *on page 1273*
- **Altamisa** *see* Feverfew *(Tanacetum parthenium) on page 628*
- **Altarussin DM [OTC]** *see* Guaifenesin and Dextromethorphan *on page 739*
- **Altaryl [OTC]** *see* DiphenhydrAMINE *on page 481*
- **ALternaGel® [OTC]** *see* Aluminum Hydroxide *on page 78*
- **Altoprev®** *see* Lovastatin *on page 956*

Altretamine (al TRET a meen)

Medication Safety Issues

High alert medication: The Institute for Safe Medication Practices (ISMP) includes this medication among its list of drugs which have a heightened risk of causing significant patient harm when used in error.

International issues:

Hexalen®: Brand name for hexetidine in Greece

U.S. Brand Names Hexalen®

Canadian Brand Names Hexalen®

Index Terms Hexamethylmelamine; HEXM; HMM; HXM; NSC-13875

Pharmacologic Category Antineoplastic Agent, Miscellaneous

Use Palliative treatment of persistent or recurrent ovarian cancer

Effect on Mental Status Neurotoxicity is common; rarely may produce depression

Effect on Psychiatric Treatment Bone marrow suppression may be seen; use caution with carbamazepine and clozapine; may produce seizures caution with bupropion and clozapine; may cause severe orthostatic hypotension when administered with MAO inhibitors

Dosage Summary

Oral:

Children: Dosage not established

Adults: 260 mg/m^2/day in 4 divided doses for 14 or 21 days of a 28-day cycle

Dosage Forms Excipient information presented when available (limited, particularly for generics); consult specific product labeling.

Gelcap:

Hexalen®: 50 mg

Aluminum Hydroxide (a LOO mi num hye DROKS ide)

U.S. Brand Names ALternaGel® [OTC]; Dermagran® [OTC]

Canadian Brand Names Amphojel®; Basaljel®

Pharmacologic Category Antacid; Antidote; Protectant, Topical

Use Treatment of hyperacidity; hyperphosphatemia; temporary protection of minor cuts, scrapes, and burns

Effect on Mental Status None reported

Effect on Psychiatric Treatment Constipation is common and may be additive when used with psychotropics; may decrease the absorption of benzodiazepines and phenothiazines

Dosage Summary

Oral:

Children: 50-150 mg/kg/day in divided doses every 4-6 hours

Adults: 300-1200 mg 3-4 times/day with meals

Topical:

Children: Apply to affected area as needed; reapply at least every 12 hours

Adults: Apply to affected area as needed; reapply at least every 12 hours

Dosage Forms Excipient information presented when available (limited, particularly for generics); consult specific product labeling.

Ointment:

Dermagran®: 0.275% (120 g)

Suspension, oral: 320 mg/5 mL (473 mL)

ALternaGel®: 600 mg/5 mL (360 mL)

Aluminum Hydroxide, Magnesium Hydroxide, and Simethicone

(a LOO mi num hye DROKS ide, mag NEE zhum hye DROKS ide, & sye METH i kone)

Medication Safety Issues

Sound-alike/look-alike issues:

Maalox® may be confused with Maox®, Monodox®

Mylanta® may be confused with Mynatal®

Maalox® is a different formulation than Maalox® Total Stomach Relief®

U.S. Brand Names Alamag Plus [OTC]; Aldroxicon I [OTC]; Aldroxicon II [OTC]; Almacone Double Strength® [OTC]; Almacone® [OTC]; Gelusil® [OTC]; Maalox® Max [OTC]; Maalox® [OTC]; Mi-Acid Maximum Strength [OTC]; Mi-Acid [OTC]; Mintox Extra Strength [OTC]; Mintox Plus [OTC]; Mylanta® Liquid [OTC]; Mylanta® Maximum Strength Liquid [OTC]

Canadian Brand Names Diovol Plus®; Gelusil®; Mylanta® Double Strength; Mylanta® Extra Strength; Mylanta® Regular Strength

Index Terms Magnesium Hydroxide, Aluminum Hydroxide, and Simethicone; Simethicone, Aluminum Hydroxide, and Magnesium Hydroxide

Pharmacologic Category Antacid; Antiflatulent

Use Temporary relief of hyperacidity associated with gas; may also be used for indications associated with other antacids

Effect on Mental Status None reported

Effect on Psychiatric Treatment Constipation is common; use with low potency antipsychotics and TCAs will likely result in additive effects

Dosage Summary

Oral:

Children: Dosage not established

Adults: 10-20 mL or 2-4 tablets 4-6 times/day between meals and at bedtime; **Note:** May be administered every hour for severe symptoms

Dosage Forms Excipient information presented when available (limited, particularly for generics); consult specific product labeling.

Liquid: Aluminum hydroxide 200 mg, magnesium hydroxide 200 mg, and simethicone 20 mg per 5 mL (360 mL); aluminum hydroxide 400 mg, magnesium hydroxide 400 mg, and simethicone 40 mg per 5 mL (360 mL)

Aldroxicon I: Aluminum hydroxide 200 mg, magnesium hydroxide 200 mg, and simethicone 20 mg per 5 mL (30 mL)

Aldroxicon II: Aluminum hydroxide 400 mg, magnesium hydroxide 400 mg, and simethicone 40 mg per 5 mL (30 mL)

Almacone®: Aluminum hydroxide 200 mg, magnesium hydroxide 200 mg, and simethicone 20 mg per 5 mL (360 mL)

Almacone Double Strength®: Aluminum hydroxide 400 mg, magnesium hydroxide 400 mg, and simethicone 40 mg per 5 mL (360 mL)

Maalox®: Aluminum hydroxide 200 mg, magnesium hydroxide 200 mg, and simethicone 20 mg per 5 mL (360 mL, 770 mL) [lemon and mint flavors]

Maalox® Max: Aluminum hydroxide 400 mg, magnesium hydroxide 400 mg, and simethicone 40 mg per 5 mL (360 mL, 770 mL) [cherry, vanilla creme, and wild berry flavors]

Mi-Acid: Aluminum hydroxide 200 mg, magnesium hydroxide 200 mg, and simethicone 20 mg per 5 mL (360 mL)

Mi-Acid Maximum Strength: Aluminum hydroxide 400 mg, magnesium hydroxide 400 mg, and simethicone 40 mg per 5 mL (360 mL)

Mintox Extra Strength: Aluminum hydroxide 500 mg, magnesium hydroxide 450 mg, and simethicone 40 mg per 5 mL (360 mL) [lemon creme flavor]

Mylanta®: Aluminum hydroxide 200 mg, magnesium hydroxide 200 mg, and simethicone 20 mg per 5 mL (180 mL, 360 mL, 720 mL) [original, cherry, and mint flavors]

Mylanta® Maximum Strength: Aluminum hydroxide 400 mg, magnesium hydroxide 400 mg, and simethicone 40 mg per 5 mL (180 mL, 360 mL, 720 mL) [original, cherry, orange creme, and mint flavors]

Suspension (Alamag Plus): Aluminum hydroxide 225 mg, magnesium hydroxide 200 mg, and simethicone 25 mg per 5 mL (360 mL)

Tablet, chewable: Aluminum hydroxide 200 mg, magnesium hydroxide 200 mg, and simethicone 25 mg

Alamag Plus: Aluminum hydroxide 200 mg, magnesium hydroxide 200 mg, and simethicone 25 mg [cherry flavor]

Almacone®: Aluminum hydroxide 200 mg, magnesium hydroxide 200 mg, and simethicone 20 mg [peppermint flavor]

Gelusil®: Aluminum hydroxide 200 mg, magnesium hydroxide 200 mg, and simethicone 25 mg [peppermint flavor]

Mintox Plus: Aluminum hydroxide 200 mg, magnesium hydroxide 200 mg, and simethicone 25 mg

◆ **Aluminum Sucrose Sulfate, Basic** *see* Sucralfate *on page 1514*

◆ **Alupent®** *see* Metaproterenol *on page 996*

◆ **Alvesco®** *see* Ciclesonide *on page 343*

Amantadine (a MAN ta deen)

Medication Safety Issues

Sound-alike/look-alike issues:

Amantadine may be confused with ranitidine, rimantadine

Symmetrel® may be confused with Synthroid®

International issues:

Symmetrel® may be confused with Somatrel® which is a brand name for somatorelin in Denmark

Related Information

Antiparkinsonian Agents *on page 1767*

Discontinuation of Psychotropic Drugs *on page 1839*

U.S. Brand Names Symmetrel®

Canadian Brand Names Endantadine®; PMS-Amantadine; Symmetrel®

Mexican Brand Names PK-Merz

Index Terms Adamantanamine Hydrochloride; Amantadine Hydrochloride

Pharmacologic Category Anti-Parkinson's Agent, Dopamine Agonist; Antiviral Agent, Adamantane

Generic Available Yes

Use Prophylaxis and treatment of influenza A viral infection (per manufacturer labeling; also refer to current ACIP guidelines for recommendations during current flu season); treatment of parkinsonism; treatment of drug-induced extrapyramidal symptoms

Note: In certain circumstances, the ACIP recommends use of amantadine in combination with oseltamivir for the treatment or prophylaxis of influenza A infection when resistance to oseltamivir is suspected.

Mental Health Comment This agent should not be used for an acute dystonic reaction. No injectable dosage form is available. Amantadine is generally considered to be less effective than anticholinergic antiparkinsonian agents and beta-blockers for the management of akathisia. It is effective for pseudoparkinsonism, but long-term efficacy has not been established. Given its high cost relative to anticholinergics, it is usually reserved for second-line therapy. Tolerance has also been reported to occur with long-term use (Zubenko, 1984). However, it does not impair cognition by adding anticholinergic load. Amantadine should not be abruptly discontinued; doing so may precipitate a parkinsonian crisis. Additionally, agitation, delirium, delusions, hallucinations, paranoia, stupor, anxiety, depression, and slurred speech may be seen if it is abruptly stopped.

Zubenko GS, Barreira P, and Lipinski JF Jr, "Development of Tolerance to the Therapeutic Effect of Amantadine on Akathisia," *J Clin Psychopharmacol*, 1984, 4(4):218-20.

Pregnancy Risk Factor C

Pregnancy Considerations Teratogenic effects were observed in animal studies; limited data in humans. Impaired fertility has also been reported during animal studies and during human *in vitro* fertilization.

Lactation Enters breast milk/not recommended

Contraindications Hypersensitivity to amantadine, rimantadine, or any component of the formulation

Warnings/Precautions May cause CNS depression, which may impair physical or mental abilities; patients must be cautioned about performing tasks which require mental alertness (eg, operating machinery or driving). There have been reports of suicidal ideation/attempt in patients with and without a history of psychiatric illness. Use with caution in patients with liver disease, a history of recurrent and eczematoid dermatitis, uncontrolled psychosis or severe psychoneurosis, seizures and in those receiving CNS stimulant drugs; reduce dose in renal disease; when treating Parkinson's disease, do not discontinue abruptly. In many patients, the therapeutic benefits of amantadine are limited to a few months. Elderly patients may be more susceptible to the CNS effects (using 2 divided daily doses may minimize this effect). Use with caution in patients with CHF, peripheral edema, or orthostatic hypotension. Avoid in untreated angle closure glaucoma.

Dopamine agonists have been associated with compulsive behaviors and/or loss of impulse control, which has manifested as pathological gambling, libido increases (hypersexuality), and/or binge eating. Causality has not been established, and controversy exists as to whether this phenomenon is related to the underlying disease, prior behaviors/addictions and/or drug therapy. Dose reduction or discontinuation of therapy has been reported to reverse these behaviors in some, but not all cases.

Due to increased resistance, the ACIP has recommended that rimantadine and amantadine no longer be used for the treatment or prophylaxis of influenza A in the United States until susceptibility has been re-established; consult current guidelines. Safety and efficacy have not been established in children <1 year of age.

Adverse Reactions

1% to 10%:

Cardiovascular: Orthostatic hypotension, peripheral edema

Central nervous system: Agitation, anxiety, ataxia, confusion, delirium, depression, dizziness, dream abnormality, fatigue, hallucinations, headache, insomnia, irritability, nervousness, somnolence

Dermatologic: Livedo reticularis

Gastrointestinal: Anorexia, constipation, diarrhea, nausea, xerostomia

Respiratory: Dry nose

<1% (Limited to important or life-threatening): Aggressive behavior, agranulocytosis, alkaline phosphatase increased, allergic reaction, ALT increased, AST increased, amnesia, anaphylaxis, arrhythmia, bilirubin increased, BUN increased, cardiac arrest, CHF, coma, CPK increased, creatinine increased, delirium, delusions, diaphoresis, dysphagia, dyspnea, eczematoid dermatitis, euphoria, GGT increased, hyperkinesis, LDH increased, leukopenia, mania, neutropenia, neuroleptic malignant syndrome (NMS; associated with dosage reduction or abrupt withdrawal of amantadine), oculogyric episodes, paresthesia, photosensitivity, psychosis, pulmonary edema, rash, respiratory failure (acute), seizures, suicidal ideation, suicide, urinary retention, withdrawal reactions (may include delirium, hallucinations, and psychosis), visual disturbances

Reported with dopamine agonists: Impulsive/compulsive behaviors (eg, pathological gambling, hypersexuality, binge eating)

Drug Interactions

Antipsychotics (Atypical): May diminish the therapeutic effect of Anti-Parkinson's Agents (Dopamine Agonist). *Risk D: Consider therapy modification*

Antipsychotics (Typical): May diminish the therapeutic effect of Anti-Parkinson's Agents (Dopamine Agonist). *Risk D: Consider therapy modification*

Influenza Virus Vaccine: Antiviral Agents (Influenza A and B) may diminish the therapeutic effect of Influenza Virus Vaccine. This only pertains to live, attentuated influenza virus vaccine. *Risk D: Consider therapy modification*

Metoclopramide: May diminish the therapeutic effect of Anti-Parkinson's Agents (Dopamine Agonist). *Risk C: Monitor therapy*

Ethanol/Nutrition/Herb Interactions Ethanol: Avoid ethanol (may increase CNS adverse effects).

Stability Store at 25°C (77°F).

Mechanism of Action As an antiviral, blocks the uncoating of influenza A virus preventing penetration of virus into host; antiparkinsonian activity may be due to its blocking the reuptake of dopamine into presynaptic neurons or by increasing dopamine release from presynaptic fibers

Pharmacodynamics/Kinetics

Onset of action: Antidyskinetic: Within 48 hours

Absorption: Well absorbed

Distribution: V_d: Normal: 1.5-6.1 L/kg; Renal failure: 5.1 ± 0.2 L/kg; in saliva, tear film, and nasal secretions; in animals, tissue (especially lung) concentrations higher than serum concentrations; crosses blood-brain barrier

Protein binding: Normal renal function: ~67%; Hemodialysis: ~59%

Metabolism: Not appreciable; small amounts of an acetyl metabolite identified

Bioavailability: 86% to 90%

Half-life elimination: Normal renal function: 16 ± 6 hours (9-31 hours); End-stage renal disease: 7-10 days

Excretion: Urine (80% to 90% unchanged) by glomerular filtration and tubular secretion

Total clearance: 2.5-10.5 L/hour

Dosage Oral:

Children:

Influenza A treatment:

1-9 years: 5 mg/kg/day in 2 divided doses (manufacturers range: 4.4-8.8 mg/kg/day); maximum dose: 150 mg/day

≥10 years and <40 kg: 5 mg/kg/day; maximum dose: 150 mg/day

≥10 years and ≥40 kg: 100 mg twice daily

Note: Initiate within 24-48 hours after onset of symptoms; discontinue as soon as possible based on clinical response (generally within 3-5 days or within 24-48 hours after symptoms disappear)

Influenza A prophylaxis: Refer to "Influenza A treatment" dosing

Note: Continue treatment throughout the peak influenza activity in the community or throughout the entire influenza season in patients who cannot be vaccinated. Development of immunity following vaccination takes ~2 weeks; amantadine therapy should be considered for high-risk patients from the time of vaccination until immunity has developed. For children <9 years receiving influenza vaccine for the first time, amantadine prophylaxis should continue for 6 weeks (4 weeks after the first dose and 2 weeks after the second dose).

Adults:

Drug-induced extrapyramidal symptoms: 100 mg twice daily; may increase to 300-400 mg/day, if needed

Parkinson's disease or Creutzfeldt-Jakob disease (unlabeled use): 100 mg twice daily as sole therapy; may increase to 400 mg/day if needed with close monitoring; initial dose: 100 mg/day if with other serious illness or with high doses of other anti-Parkinson drugs

Influenza A viral infection: 100 mg twice daily; initiate within 24-48 hours after onset of symptoms; discontinue as soon as possible based on clinical response (generally within 3-5 days or within 24-48 hours after symptoms disappear)

Influenza A prophylaxis: 100 mg twice daily

Note: Continue treatment throughout the peak influenza activity in the community or throughout the entire influenza season in patients who cannot be vaccinated. Development of immunity following vaccination takes ~2 weeks; amantadine therapy should be considered for high-risk patients from the time of vaccination until immunity has developed.

Elderly: Adjust dose based on renal function; some patients tolerate the drug better when it is given in 2 divided daily doses (to avoid adverse neurologic reactions).

Influenza A prophylaxis or treatment: ≤100 mg/day in patients ≥65 years

Dosing interval in renal impairment:

Cl_{cr} 30-50 mL/minute: Administer 200 mg on day 1, then 100 mg/day

Cl_{cr} 15-29 mL/minute: Administer 200 mg on day 1, then 100 mg on alternate days

Cl_{cr} <15 mL/minute: Administer 200 mg every 7 days

Hemodialysis: Administer 200 mg every 7 days

Peritoneal dialysis: No supplemental dose is needed

Continuous arteriovenous or venous-venous hemofiltration: No supplemental dose is needed

Monitoring Parameters Renal function, Parkinson's symptoms, mental status, influenza symptoms, blood pressure

Additional Information Patients with intolerable CNS side effects often do better with rimantadine.

Dosage Forms Excipient information presented when available (limited, particularly for generics); consult specific product labeling.

Capsule, as hydrochloride: 100 mg

Capsule, softgel, as hydrochloride: 100 mg

Solution, oral, as hydrochloride: 50 mg/5 mL (473 mL)

Syrup, oral, as hydrochloride: 50 mg/5 mL (10 mL, 480 mL)

Tablet, as hydrochloride: 100 mg

Symmetrel®: 100 mg

◆ **Amantadine Hydrochloride** *see* Amantadine *on page 79*

◆ **Amantilla** *see* Valerian *(Valeriana officinalis) on page 1641*

◆ **Amaryl®** *see* Glimepiride *on page 723*

Ambenonium (am be NOE nee um)

U.S. Brand Names Mytelase®

Canadian Brand Names Mytelase®

Index Terms Ambenonium Chloride

Pharmacologic Category Cholinergic Agonist

Use Treatment of myasthenia gravis

Effect on Mental Status May produce drowsiness

Effect on Psychiatric Treatment None reported; the cholinergic effects may counteract the anticholinergic effects of psychotropics

Dosage Summary

Oral:

Children: Dosage not established

Adults: 5-25 mg 3-4 times/day

Dosage Forms Excipient information presented when available (limited, particularly for generics); consult specific product labeling.

Caplet, as chloride [scored]:

Mytelase®: 10 mg

◆ **Ambenonium Chloride** *see* Ambenonium *on page 82*

◆ **Ambien®** *see* Zolpidem *on page 1705*

- **Ambien CR®** *see* Zolpidem *on page 1705*
- **Ambifed-G** *see* Guaifenesin and Pseudoephedrine *on page 744*
- **Ambifed-G DM** *see* Guaifenesin, Pseudoephedrine, and Dextromethorphan *on page 748*
- **AmBisome®** *see* Amphotericin B, Liposomal *on page 121*
- **Amdry-C** *see* Chlorpheniramine, Pseudoephedrine, and Methscopolamine *on page 334*
- **Amdry-D** *see* Pseudoephedrine and Methscopolamine *on page 1370*
- **Amerge®** *see* Naratriptan *on page 1107*
- **American coneflower** *see* Echinacea *(Echinacea purpurea, Echinacea angustifolia) on page 523*
- **A-Methapred** *see* MethylPREDNISolone *on page 1029*
- **Amethocaine Hydrochloride** *see* Tetracaine *on page 1557*
- **Amethopterin** *see* Methotrexate *on page 1014*
- **Amevive®** *see* Alefacept *on page 58*
- **Amfepramone** *see* Diethylpropion *on page 460*
- **AMG 073** *see* Cinacalcet *on page 345*
- **Amicar®** *see* Aminocaproic Acid *on page 87*
- **Amidrine [DSC]** *see* Acetaminophen, Isometheptene, and Dichloralphenazone *on page 45*

Amifostine (am i FOS teen)

Medication Safety Issues
Sound-alike/look-alike issues:
Ethyol® may be confused with ethanol

U.S. Brand Names Ethyol®

Canadian Brand Names Ethyol®

Mexican Brand Names Ethyol

Index Terms Ethiofos; Gammaphos; WR-2721; YM-08310

Pharmacologic Category Adjuvant, Chemoprotective Agent (Cytoprotective); Antidote

Use Reduce the incidence of moderate to severe xerostomia in patients undergoing postoperative radiation treatment for head and neck cancer, where the radiation port includes a substantial portion of the parotid glands; reduce the cumulative renal toxicity associated with repeated administration of cisplatin

Unlabeled/Investigational Use Prevention of radiation proctitis in patients with rectal cancer

Effect on Mental Status Drowsiness is common

Effect on Psychiatric Treatment Hypotension is common and may be additive with psychotropics

Dosage Summary Note: Antiemetic medication, including dexamethasone 20 mg I.V. and a serotonin 5-HT_3 receptor antagonist, is recommended prior to and in conjunction with amifostine.

I.V.:

Children: Dosage not established

Adults: 910 mg/m^2 once daily over 15 minutes 30 minutes prior to cytotoxic therapy **or** 200 mg/m^2/day over 3 minutes 15-30 minutes prior to radiation therapy

Dosage Forms Excipient information presented when available (limited, particularly for generics); consult specific product labeling.
Injection, powder for reconstitution: 500 mg
Ethyol®: 500 mg

- **Amigesic® [DSC]** *see* Salsalate *on page 1459*

Amikacin (am i KAY sin)

Medication Safety Issues
Sound-alike/look-alike issues:
Amikacin may be confused with Amicar®, anakinra
Amikin® may be confused with Amicar®

Canadian Brand Names Amikacin Sulfate Injection, USP; Amikin®

Mexican Brand Names Agnicin; Akacin; Amikafur; Amikayect; Amikin.; Biclin; Biokacin; Gamikal; Karmikin; Lisobac; Oprad; Yectamid

Index Terms Amikacin Sulfate

Pharmacologic Category Antibiotic, Aminoglycoside

Use Treatment of serious infections (bone infections, respiratory tract infections, endocarditis, and septicemia) due to organisms resistant to gentamicin and tobramycin, including *Pseudomonas*, *Proteus*, *Serratia*, and other gram-negative bacilli; documented infection of mycobacterial organisms susceptible to amikacin

Unlabeled/Investigational Use Bacterial endophthalmitis

Effect on Mental Status May cause drowsiness; case reports of delirium and psychosis

Effect on Psychiatric Treatment None reported

Dosage Summary Note: Use of ideal body weight (IBW) for determining the mg/kg/dose appears to be more accurate than dosing on the basis of total body weight (TBW); **Note:** Individualization of the dose is critical because of the low therapeutic index

I.M.:

Infants: 5-7.5 mg/kg/dose every 8 hours (maximum: 20 mg/kg/day)
Children: 5-7.5 mg/kg/dose every 8 hours (maximum: 20 mg/kg/day)
Adults: 5-7.5 mg/kg/dose every 8 hours (maximum: 20 mg/kg/day)

I.V:

Infants: 5-7.5 mg/kg/dose every 8 hours (maximum: 20 mg/kg/day)
Children: 5-7.5 mg/kg/dose every 8 hours (maximum: 20 mg/kg/day)
Adults: 5-7.5 mg/kg/dose every 8 hours **or** 15-20 mg/kg as a single daily dose (maximum: 20 mg/kg/day)

Dosage Forms Excipient information presented when available (limited, particularly for generics); consult specific product labeling.
Injection, solution, as sulfate: 50 mg/mL (2 mL); 250 mg/mL (2 mL, 4 mL)

◆ **Amikacin Sulfate** *see* Amikacin *on page 83*

AMILoride (a MIL oh ride)

Medication Safety Issues

Sound-alike/look-alike issues:

AMILoride may be confused with amiodarone, amLODIPine, amrinone

Canadian Brand Names Apo-Amiloride®

Mexican Brand Names Moduretic (Combinado con hidroclorotiazida)

Index Terms Amiloride Hydrochloride

Pharmacologic Category Diuretic, Potassium-Sparing

Generic Available Yes

Use Counteracts potassium loss induced by other diuretics in the treatment of hypertension or edematous conditions including CHF, hepatic cirrhosis, and hypoaldosteronism; usually used in conjunction with more potent diuretics such as thiazides or loop diuretics

Unlabeled/Investigational Use Investigational: Cystic fibrosis; reduction of lithium-induced polyuria; pediatric hypertension

Effect on Mental Status May cause drowsiness; rarely may cause insomnia and depression

Effect on Psychiatric Treatment May cause impotence and orthostatic hypotension which may be exacerbated by psychotropics; effective agent for the treatment of lithium-induced diabetes insipidus

Pregnancy Risk Factor B

Pregnancy Considerations Teratogenic effects were not observed in animal studies.

Lactation Excretion in breast milk unknown/not recommended

Contraindications Hypersensitivity to amiloride or any component of the formulation; presence of elevated serum potassium levels (>5.5 mEq/L); if patient is receiving other potassium-conserving agents (eg, spironolactone, triamterene) or potassium supplementation (medicine, potassium-containing salt substitutes, potassium-rich diet); anuria; acute or chronic renal insufficiency; evidence of diabetic nephropathy. Patients with evidence of renal impairment or diabetes mellitus should not receive this medicine without close, frequent monitoring of serum electrolytes and renal function.

Warnings/Precautions [U.S. Boxed Warning]: Hyperkalemia can occur; patients at risk include those with renal impairment, diabetes, the elderly, and the severely ill. Serum potassium levels must be monitored at frequent intervals especially when dosages are changed or with any illness that may cause renal dysfunction. Excess amounts can lead to profound diuresis with fluid and electrolyte loss; close medical supervision and dose evaluation are required. Watch for and correct electrolyte disturbances; adjust dose to avoid dehydration. In cirrhosis, avoid electrolyte and acid/base imbalances that might lead to hepatic encephalopathy. Use with extreme caution in patients with diabetes mellitus; monitor closely. Discontinue amiloride

3 days prior to glucose tolerance testing. Use with caution in patients who are at risk for metabolic or respiratory acidosis (eg, cardiopulmonary disease, uncontrolled diabetes). Safety and efficacy have not been established in children.

Adverse Reactions

1% to 10%:

Central nervous system: Headache, fatigue, dizziness

Endocrine & metabolic: Hyperkalemia (up to 10%; risk reduced in patients receiving kaliuretic diuretics), hyperchloremic metabolic acidosis, dehydration, hyponatremia, gynecomastia

Gastrointestinal: Nausea, diarrhea, vomiting, abdominal pain, gas pain, appetite changes, constipation

Genitourinary: Impotence

Neuromuscular & skeletal: Muscle cramps, weakness

Respiratory: Cough, dyspnea

<1% (Limited to important or life-threatening): Alopecia, arrhythmia, bladder spasms, chest pain, dyspnea, dysuria, GI bleeding, intraocular pressure increased, jaundice, orthostatic hypotension, palpitation, polyuria

Drug Interactions

ACE Inhibitors: Potassium-Sparing Diuretics may enhance the hyperkalemic effect of ACE Inhibitors. *Risk C: Monitor therapy*

Ammonium Chloride: Potassium-Sparing Diuretics may enhance the adverse/toxic effect of Ammonium Chloride. Specifically the risk of systemic acidosis. *Risk D: Consider therapy modification*

Angiotensin II Receptor Blockers: May enhance the hyperkalemic effect of Potassium-Sparing Diuretics. *Risk C: Monitor therapy*

Cardiac Glycosides: Potassium-Sparing Diuretics may diminish the therapeutic effect of Cardiac Glycosides. Specifically, the inotropic effects. *Risk C: Monitor therapy*

Diazoxide: May enhance the hypotensive effect of Antihypertensives. *Risk C: Monitor therapy*

Drospirenone: May enhance the hyperkalemic effect of Potassium-Sparing Diuretics. *Risk C: Monitor therapy*

Eplerenone: May enhance the hyperkalemic effect of Potassium-Sparing Diuretics. Management: This combination is contraindicated in patients receiving eplerenone for treatment of hypertension. *Risk D: Consider therapy modification*

Herbs (Hypertensive Properties): May diminish the antihypertensive effect of Antihypertensives. *Risk C: Monitor therapy*

Herbs (Hypotensive Properties): May enhance the hypotensive effect of Antihypertensives. *Risk C: Monitor therapy*

Methylphenidate: May diminish the antihypertensive effect of Antihypertensives. *Risk C: Monitor therapy*

Mitotane: Potassium-Sparing Diuretics may diminish the therapeutic effect of Mitotane. High dose diuretics (eg, Cushings syndrome) may present significantly higher risk than low doses (eg, CHF). *Risk D: Consider therapy modification*

Potassium Salts: May enhance the hyperkalemic effect of Potassium-Sparing Diuretics. *Risk D: Consider therapy modification*

Prostacyclin Analogues: May enhance the hypotensive effect of Antihypertensives. *Risk C: Monitor therapy*

QuiNIDine: Potassium-Sparing Diuretics may diminish the therapeutic effect of QuiNIDine. *Risk C: Monitor therapy*

RiTUXimab: Antihypertensives may enhance the hypotensive effect of RiTUXimab. *Risk D: Consider therapy modification*

Ethanol/Nutrition/Herb Interactions Food: Hyperkalemia may result if amiloride is taken with potassium-containing foods.

Mechanism of Action Inhibits sodium reabsorption in the distal tubule, cortical collecting tubule, and collecting duct subsequently reducing both potassium and hydrogen excretion resulting in weak natriuretic, diuretic, and antihypertensive activity; increases sodium loss; increases potassium retention; decreases calcium excretion; decreases magnesium loss

Pharmacodynamics/Kinetics

Onset of action: 2 hours

Duration: 24 hours

Absorption: ~15% to 25%

Distribution: V_d: 350-380 L

Protein binding: 23%

Metabolism: No active metabolites

Half-life elimination: Normal renal function: 6-9 hours; End-stage renal disease: 8-144 hours

Time to peak, serum: 6-10 hours

Excretion: Urine and feces (equal amounts as unchanged drug)

Dosage Oral:

Children 1-17 years: Hypertension (unlabeled use): 0.4-0.625 mg/kg/day (maximum: 20 mg/day)

Adults: 5-10 mg/day (up to 20 mg)

Hypertension (JNC 7): 5-10 mg/day in 1-2 divided doses

Elderly: Initial: 5 mg once daily or every other day

Dosing adjustment in renal impairment:

Cl_{cr} 10-50 mL/minute: Administer at 50% of normal dose.

Cl_{cr} <10 mL/minute: Avoid use.

Dietary Considerations Take with food or meals to avoid GI upset. Do not use salt substitutes or low salt milk without checking with your healthcare provider; too much potassium can be as harmful as too little.

Administration Administer with food or meals to avoid GI upset.

Monitoring Parameters I & O, daily weights, blood pressure, serum electrolytes, renal function

Test Interactions Increased potassium (S)

Additional Information Medication should be discontinued if potassium level exceeds 6.5 mEq/L. Combined with hydrochlorothiazide as Moduretic®. Amiloride is considered an alternative to triamterene or spironolactone.

Dosage Forms Excipient information presented when available (limited, particularly for generics); consult specific product labeling.

Tablet, as hydrochloride: 5 mg

Amiloride and Hydrochlorothiazide

(a MIL oh ride & hye droe klor oh THYE a zide)

Canadian Brand Names Apo-Amilzide®; Gen-Amilazide; Moduret; Novamilor; Nu-Amilzide

Mexican Brand Names Moduretic

Index Terms Hydrochlorothiazide and Amiloride

Pharmacologic Category Diuretic, Combination

Use Potassium-sparing diuretic; antihypertensive

Effect on Mental Status May cause drowsiness; rarely may cause insomnia and depression

Effect on Psychiatric Treatment May cause impotence and orthostatic hypotension which may be exacerbated by psychotropics; effective agent for the treatment of lithium-induced diabetes insipidus

Dosage Summary

Oral:

Children: Dosage not established

Adults: 1-2 tablets/day as a single dose (maximum: 2 tablets/day)

Elderly: Initial: 1/2 to 1 tablet/day (maximum: 2 tablets/day)

Dosage Forms Excipient information presented when available (limited, particularly for generics); consult specific product labeling.

Tablet: 5/50: Amiloride hydrochloride 5 mg and hydrochlorothiazide 50 mg

◆ **Amiloride Hydrochloride** *see* AMILoride *on page 84*

◆ **2-Amino-6-Mercaptopurine** *see* Thioguanine *on page 1569*

◆ **2-Amino-6-Methoxypurine Arabinoside** *see* Nelarabine *on page 1120*

◆ **2-Amino-6-Trifluoromethoxy-benzothiazole** *see* Riluzole *on page 1421*

◆ **Aminobenzylpenicillin** *see* Ampicillin *on page 122*

Aminocamptothecin (a min o camp to THE sin)

Index Terms 9-AC; 9-Aminocamptothecin; NSC-603071

Pharmacologic Category Antineoplastic Agent, DNA Binding Agent; Enzyme Inhibitor, Topoisomerase I Inhibitor

Unlabeled/Investigational Use Phase II trials: Relapsed lymphoma, refractory breast cancer, nonsmall cell lung cancer, untreated colorectal carcinoma

Effect on Mental Status May cause sedation

Effect on Psychiatric Treatment May cause GI side effects; concomitant use with SSRIs, lithium, or valproic acid may produce additive effects; monitor. May cause neutropenia and thrombocytopenia; monitor if using concomitantly with clozapine, valproic acid, and carbamazepine.

Restrictions Not available in U.S./Investigational

Dosage Forms Excipient information presented when available (limited, particularly for generics); consult specific product labeling.

Injection: 5 mg ampul

◆ **9-Aminocamptothecin** *see* Aminocamptothecin *on page 86*

Aminocaproic Acid (a mee noe ka PROE ik AS id)

Medication Safety Issues
Sound-alike/look-alike issues:
Amicar® may be confused with amikacin, Amikin®, Omacor®

U.S. Brand Names Amicar®

Index Terms EACA; Epsilon Aminocaproic Acid

Pharmacologic Category Antifibrinolytic Agent; Hemostatic Agent

Use To enhance hemostasis when fibrinolysis contributes to bleeding (causes may include cardiac surgery, hematologic disorders, neoplastic disorders, abruption placentae, hepatic cirrhosis, and urinary fibrinolysis)

Unlabeled/Investigational Use Treatment of traumatic hyphema; control bleeding in thrombocytopenia; control oral bleeding in congenital and acquired coagulation disorders; topical treatment (mouth rinse) of bleeding associated with dental procedures in patients on oral anticoagulant therapy; prevention of perioperative bleeding associated with cardiac surgery

Effect on Mental Status May cause drowsiness

Effect on Psychiatric Treatment May cause hypotension which may be exacerbated by psychotropics; rarely may cause seizures; use caution with clozapine and bupropion

Dosage Summary

I.V.:

Children (unlabeled use): Initial: Loading dose: 100-200 mg/kg for first hour; Maintenance: 100 mg/kg every 6 hours **or** 33.3 mg/kg/hour as a continuous infusion

Adults: Initial: Loading dose: 4-5 g for first hour; Maintenance: 1 g/hour for 8 hours or until bleeding controlled (maximum: 30 g/day) **or** 10 g prior to skin incision, followed by 1-2.5 g/hour (usual dose 2 g/hour) until the end of operation **or** 10 g prior to skin incision, followed by 10 g after heparin administration then 10 g at discontinuation of cardiopulmonary bypass prior to protamine reversal of heparin

Oral:

Children (unlabeled use): Initial: Loading dose: 100-200 mg/kg for first hour; Maintenance: 100 mg/kg every 6 hours

Adults: Initial: Loading dose: 4-5 g for first hour; Maintenance: 1 g/hour for 8 hours or until bleeding controlled (maximum: 30 g/day)

Dosage Forms Excipient information presented when available (limited, particularly for generics); consult specific product labeling.
Injection, solution: 250 mg/mL (20 mL)
Amicar®: 250 mg/mL (20 mL) [contains benzyl alcohol]
Solution, oral: 1.25 g/5 mL (240 mL, 480 mL)
Syrup:
Amicar®: 1.25 g/5 mL (480 mL) [raspberry flavor]
Tablet [scored]: 500 mg
Amicar®: 500 mg, 1000 mg

Aminoglutethimide (a mee noe gloo TETH i mide)

Medication Safety Issues
Sound-alike/look-alike issues:
Cytadren® may be confused with cytarabine

U.S. Brand Names Cytadren®

Index Terms BA-16038; Elipten

Pharmacologic Category Antineoplastic Agent, Aromatase Inhibitor; Enzyme Inhibitor; Hormone Antagonist, Anti-Adrenal; Nonsteroidal Aromatase Inhibitor

Use Suppression of adrenal function in selected patients with Cushing's syndrome

Unlabeled/Investigational Use Treatment of prostate cancer (androgen synthesis inhibitor)

Effect on Mental Status Drowsiness is common

Effect on Psychiatric Treatment May cause hypotension which may be exacerbated by psychotropics; may cause bone marrow suppression; use caution with clozapine and carbamazepine; propranolol may increase the risk of drowsiness

Dosage Summary

Oral:

Children: Dosage not established

Adults: 250-500 mg every 6 hours (maximum: 2 g/day); **Note:** Titration is recommended

Dosage Forms Excipient information presented when available (limited, particularly for generics); consult specific product labeling.

Tablet [scored]:

Cytadren®: 250 mg

Aminophylline (am in OFF i lin)

Medication Safety Issues

Sound-alike/look-alike issues:

Aminophylline may be confused with amitriptyline, ampicillin

Canadian Brand Names Phyllocontin®; Phyllocontin®-350

Mexican Brand Names Pharmafil

Index Terms Theophylline Ethylenediamine

Pharmacologic Category Theophylline Derivative

Use Bronchodilator in reversible airway obstruction due to asthma or COPD; increase diaphragmatic contractility

Unlabeled/Investigational Use Reversal of adenosine-, dipyridamole-, or regadenoson-induced adverse reactions (eg, angina, hypotension) during nuclear cardiac stress testing

Effect on Mental Status May cause nervousness or restlessness

Effect on Psychiatric Treatment Carbamazepine and barbiturates may decrease aminophylline levels; disulfiram and propranolol may increase aminophylline levels

Dosage Summary

I.V.:

Children <6 weeks: Dosage not established

Children 6 weeks to 6 months: Loading dose: 6 mg/kg over 20-30 minutes; Maintenance: 0.5 mg/kg/hour as a continuous infusion

Children 6 months to 1 year: Loading dose: 6 mg/kg over 20-30 minutes; Maintenance: 0.6-0.7 mg/kg/hour as a continuous infusion

Children 1-9 years: Loading dose: 6 mg/kg over 20-30 minutes; Maintenance: 1 mg/kg/hour as a continuous infusion

Children 9-16 years: Loading dose: 6 mg/kg over 20-30 minutes; Maintenance: 0.8 mg/kg/hour as a continuous infusion

Adults: Loading dose: 6 mg/kg over 20-30 minutes; Maintenance: 0.1-0.8 mg/kg/hour as a continuous infusion; **Note:** Dose dependent on age, smoker status, and heart/lung status.

Oral:

Children <45 kg: Dosage not established

Children ≥45 kg: Initial: 380 mg/day divided every 6-8 hours; Maintenance: 380-928 mg/day divided every 6-8 hours (maximum: 928 mg/day) **Note:** Titration is recommended

Adults: Initial: 380 mg/day divided every 6-8 hours; Maintenance: 380-928 mg/day divided every 6-8 hours (maximum: 928 mg/day) **Note:** Titration is recommended

Dosage Forms Excipient information presented when available (limited, particularly for generics); consult specific product labeling.

Injection, solution, as dihydrate: 25 mg/mL (10 mL, 20 mL)

Injection, solution, as dihydrate [preservative free]: 25 mg/mL (10 mL, 20 mL)

Tablet, as dihydrate: 100 mg

◆ **Aminosalicylate Sodium** *see* Aminosalicylic Acid *on page 88*

Aminosalicylic Acid (a mee noe sal i SIL ik AS id)

U.S. Brand Names Paser®

Index Terms 4-Aminosalicylic Acid; Aminosalicylate Sodium; Para-Aminosalicylate Sodium; PAS; Sodium PAS

Pharmacologic Category Salicylate

Use Adjunctive treatment of tuberculosis used in combination with other antitubercular agents

Unlabeled/Investigational Use Crohn's disease

Effect on Mental Status None reported

Effect on Psychiatric Treatment May cause bone marrow suppression; use caution with clozapine and carbamazepine

Dosage Summary

Oral:

Children: 200-300 mg/kg/day in 3-4 equally divided doses

Adults: 150 mg/kg/day in 2-3 equally divided doses

Dosage Forms Excipient information presented when available (limited, particularly for generics); consult specific product labeling.

Granules, delayed release:

Paser®: 4 g/packet (30s) [sugar free]

◆ **4-Aminosalicylic Acid** *see* Aminosalicylic Acid *on page 88*

◆ **5-Aminosalicylic Acid** *see* Mesalamine *on page 994*

◆ **Aminoxin [OTC]** *see* Pyridoxine *on page 1376*

Amiodarone (a MEE oh da rone)

Medication Safety Issues

Sound-alike/look-alike issues:

Amiodarone may be confused with aMILoride, amrinone

Cordarone® may be confused with Cardura®, Cordran®

High alert medication: The Institute for Safe Medication Practices (ISMP) includes this medication among its list of drugs which have a heightened risk of causing significant patient harm when used in error.

U.S. Brand Names Cordarone®; Pacerone®

Canadian Brand Names Alti-Amiodarone; Amiodarone Hydrochloride for Injection®; Apo-Amiodarone®; Cordarone®; Dom-Amiodarone; Gen-Amiodarone; Novo-Amiodarone; PHL-Amiodarone; PMS-Amiodarone; Ratio-Amiodarone; Ratio-Amiodarone I.V.; Sandoz-Amiodarone

Mexican Brand Names Braxan; Coedarone; Forken; Keritmon

Index Terms Amiodarone Hydrochloride

Pharmacologic Category Antiarrhythmic Agent, Class III

Use Management of life-threatening recurrent ventricular fibrillation (VF) or hemodynamically-unstable ventricular tachycardia (VT) refractory to other antiarrhythmic agents or in patients intolerant of other agents used for these conditions

Unlabeled/Investigational Use

Cardiac arrest with persistent ventricular tachycardia (VT) or ventricular fibrillation (VF) if defibrillation, CPR, and vasopressor administration have failed (ACLS/PALS guidelines)

Control of hemodynamically-stable VT, polymorphic VT with a normal QT interval, or wide-complex tachycardia of uncertain origin (ACLS/PALS guidelines)

Control of rapid ventricular rate due to accessory pathway conduction in pre-excited atrial arrhythmias (ACLS guidelines)

Heart rate control in patients with atrial fibrillation and heart failure [no accessory pathway] (ACC/AHA/ESC Practice Guidelines)

Paroxysmal supraventricular tachycardia (SVT)

Prevention of postoperative atrial fibrillation during cardiothoracic surgery

Pharmacologic adjunct to ICD therapy to suppress symptomatic ventricular tachyarrhythmias in otherwise optimally-treated patients with heart failure (ACC/AHA/ESC Practice Guidelines)

Pharmacologic conversion of atrial fibrillation to normal sinus rhythm; maintenance of normal sinus rhythm

Effect on Mental Status Insomnia, nightmares, and fatigue are common; postmarketing reports of confusion, delirium, disorientation, and hallucinations

Effect on Psychiatric Treatment Contraindicated with ziprasidone. May cause hypotension which may be exacerbated by psychotropics; may cause hypothyroidism; use caution with lithium. Postmarketing reports of agranulocytosis; use caution with clozapine and carbamazepine.

Restrictions An FDA-approved medication guide must be distributed when dispensing an outpatient prescription (new or refill) where this medication is to be used without direct supervision of a healthcare provider. Medication guides are available at http://www.fda.gov/cder/Offices/ODS/medication_guides.htm.

Dosage Summary

I.O.:

Children (PALS dosing): 5 mg/kg (maximum: 300 mg/day) rapid bolus or over 20-60 minutes; may repeat up to maximum dose of 15 mg/kg/day

Adults: Dosage not established

I.V.:

Children (PALS dosing): 5 mg/kg (maximum: 300 mg/day) rapid bolus or over 20-60 minutes; may repeat up to maximum dose of 15 mg/kg/day

Adults: Initial: 150-300 mg bolus **or** 5-7 mg/kg over 30-60 minutes; Maintenance: 1200-1800 mg/day continuous infusion until 10 g total

or 1 mg/minute infusion for 6 hours, then 0.5 mg/minute infusion (maximum: 2.1 g/day)

Oral:

Children <1 year (unlabeled use): Loading dose: 600-800 mg/1.73 m^2/day in 1-2 divided doses/day for 4-14 days; Maintenance: 200-400 mg/1.73 m^2/day as a single dose 5-7 days/week

Children ≥1 year (unlabeled use): Loading dose: 10-20 mg/kg/day in 1-2 doses for 4-14 days; Maintenance: 2.5-5 mg/kg/day as a single dose 5-7 days/week

Adults: Initial: 800-1600 mg/day in 1-2 doses for 1-3 weeks, then 600-800 mg/day in 1-2 doses for 1 month or 1200-1800 mg/day in divided doses until 10 g total; Maintenance: 100-400 mg/day

Dosage Forms Excipient information presented when available (limited, particularly for generics); consult specific product labeling.

Injection, solution, as hydrochloride: 50 mg/mL (3 mL, 9 mL, 18 mL) [contains benzyl alcohol and polysorbate 80]

Tablet, as hydrochloride [scored]: 200 mg, 400 mg

Cordarone®: 200 mg

Pacerone®: 100 mg [not scored], 200 mg, 400 mg

- **Amiodarone Hydrochloride** *see* Amiodarone *on page 89*
- **Amitiza®** *see* Lubiprostone *on page 963*

Amitriptyline (a mee TRIP ti leen)

Medication Safety Issues

Sound-alike/look-alike issues:

Amitriptyline may be confused with aminophylline, imipramine, nortriptyline

Elavil® may be confused with Aldoril®, Eldepryl®, enalapril, Equanil®, Mellaril®, Oruvail®, Plavix®

Related Information

Anticholinergic Effects of Common Psychotropics *on page 1758*

Antidepressant Agents *on page 1760*

Antidepressant Receptor Profile *on page 1764*

Discontinuation of Psychotropic Drugs *on page 1839*

Canadian Brand Names Apo-Amitriptyline®; Levate®; Novo-Triptyn; PMS-Amitriptyline

Mexican Brand Names Anapsique; Triptanol

Index Terms Amitriptyline Hydrochloride; Elavil

Pharmacologic Category Antidepressant, Tricyclic (Tertiary Amine)

Generic Available Yes

Use Relief of symptoms of depression

Unlabeled/Investigational Use Analgesic for certain chronic and neuropathic pain; prophylaxis against migraine headaches; treatment of depressive disorders in children

Mental Health Comment Tricyclic antidepressants may be classified as tertiary (amitriptyline, doxepin, clomipramine, imipramine, trimipramine) or secondary amines (nortriptyline, desipramine, protriptyline). The tertiary amines are not recommended to treat depression in the elderly. If a TCA is used in the elderly, it should be a secondary amine. The tertiary amines are commonly used in low dosages for various conditions associated with pain. Toxicity is generally dose dependent. Relatively small overdoses (1-week supply) can be potentially fatal.

Restrictions An FDA-approved medication guide concerning the use of antidepressants in children, adolescents, and young adults must be distributed when dispensing an outpatient prescription (new or refill) where this medication is to be used without direct supervision of a healthcare provider. Medication guides are available at http://www.fda.gov/cder/Offices/ODS/medication_guides.htm. Dispense to parents or guardians of children and adolescents receiving this medication.

Pregnancy Risk Factor C

Pregnancy Considerations Teratogenic effects have been observed in animal studies. Amitriptyline crosses the human placenta; CNS effects, limb deformities and developmental delay have been noted in case reports.

Lactation Enters breast milk/not recommended (AAP rates "of concern")

Contraindications Hypersensitivity to amitriptyline or any component of the formulation (cross-sensitivity with other tricyclics may occur); use of MAO inhibitors within past 14 days; acute recovery phase following myocardial infarction; concurrent use of cisapride

Warnings/Precautions **[U.S. Boxed Warning]: Antidepressants increase the risk of suicidal thinking and behavior in children, adolescents, and young adults (18-24 years of age) with major depressive disorder (MDD)**

and other psychiatric disorders; consider risk prior to prescribing. Short-term studies did not show an increased risk in patients >24 years of age and showed a decreased risk in patients ≥65 years. Closely monitor for clinical worsening, suicidality, or unusual changes in behavior; the patient's family or caregiver should be instructed to closely observe the patient and communicate condition with healthcare provider. Such observation would generally include at least weekly face-to-face contact with patients or their family members or caregivers during the first 4 weeks of treatment, then every other week visits for the next 4 weeks, then at 12 weeks, and as clinically indicated beyond 12 weeks. Additional contact by telephone may be appropriate between face-to-face visits. Adults treated with antidepressants should be observed similarly for clinical worsening and suicidality, especially during the initial few months of a course of drug therapy, or at times of dose changes, either increases or decreases. A medication guide should be dispensed with each prescription. **Amitriptyline is not FDA-approved for use in children <12 years of age.**

The possibility of a suicide attempt is inherent in major depression and may persist until remission occurs. Monitor for worsening of depression or suicidality, especially during initiation of therapy (generally first 1-2 months) or with dose increases or decreases. Worsening depression and severe abrupt suicidality that are not part of the presenting symptoms may require discontinuation or modification of drug therapy. The patient's family or caregiver should be alerted to monitor patients for the emergence of suicidality and associated behaviors (such as agitation, irritability, hostility, impulsivity, and hypomania) and notify healthcare provider.

May worsen psychosis in some patients or precipitate a shift to mania or hypomania in patients with bipolar disorder. Patients presenting with depressive symptoms should be screened for bipolar disorder. Monotherapy in patients with bipolar disorder should be avoided. **Amitriptyline is not FDA approved for bipolar depression.**

The degree of sedation, anticholinergic effects, orthostasis, and conduction abnormalities are high relative to other antidepressants. Amitriptyline often causes drowsiness/sedation, resulting in impaired performance of tasks requiring alertness (eg, operating machinery or driving). Sedative effects may be additive with other CNS depressants and/or ethanol. Use with caution in patients with a history of cardiovascular disease (including previous MI, stroke, tachycardia, or conduction abnormalities). Use with caution in patients with urinary retention, benign prostatic hyperplasia, narrow-angle glaucoma, xerostomia, visual problems, constipation, or a history of bowel obstruction.

TCAs may rarely cause bone marrow suppression; monitor for any signs of infection and obtain CBC if symptoms (eg, fever, sore throat) evident. May alter glucose control - use with caution in patients with diabetes. Consider discontinuing, when possible, prior to elective surgery. Therapy should not be abruptly discontinued in patients receiving high doses for prolonged periods. May lower seizure threshold - use caution in patients with a previous seizure disorder or condition predisposing to seizures such as brain damage, alcoholism, or concurrent therapy with other drugs which lower the seizure threshold. Hyperpyrexia has been observed with TCAs in combination with anticholinergics and/or neuroleptics, particularly during hot weather. May increase the risks associated with electroconvulsive therapy. Use with caution in hyperthyroid patients or those receiving thyroid supplementation. Use with caution in patients with hepatic or renal dysfunction and in elderly patients.

Adverse Reactions Anticholinergic effects may be pronounced; moderate to marked sedation can occur (tolerance to these effects usually occurs).

Frequency not defined.

Cardiovascular: Orthostatic hypotension, tachycardia, ECG changes (nonspecific), AV conduction changes, cardiomyopathy (rare), MI, stroke, heart block, arrhythmia, syncope, hypertension, palpitation

Central nervous system: Restlessness, dizziness, insomnia, sedation, fatigue, anxiety, cognitive function impaired, seizure, extrapyramidal symptoms, coma, hallucinations, confusion, disorientation, coordination impaired, ataxia, headache, nightmares, hyperpyrexia

Dermatologic: Allergic rash, urticaria, photosensitivity, alopecia

Endocrine & metabolic: Syndrome of inappropriate ADH secretion

Gastrointestinal: Weight gain, xerostomia, constipation, paralytic ileus, nausea, vomiting, anorexia, stomatitis, peculiar taste, diarrhea, black tongue

Genitourinary: Urinary retention

Hematologic: Bone marrow depression, purpura, eosinophilia

Neuromuscular & skeletal: Numbness, paresthesia, peripheral neuropathy, tremor, weakness

Ocular: Blurred vision, mydriasis, ocular pressure increased

Otic: Tinnitus

Miscellaneous: Diaphoresis, withdrawal reactions (nausea, headache, malaise)

Postmarketing and/or case reports: Neuroleptic malignant syndrome (rare), serotonin syndrome (rare)

Metabolism/Transport Effects Substrate of CYP1A2 (minor), 2B6 (minor), 2C9 (minor), 2C19 (minor), 2D6 (major), 3A4 (minor); **Inhibits** CYP1A2 (weak), 2C9 (weak), 2C19 (weak), 2D6 (weak), 2E1 (weak)

Drug Interactions

Acetylcholinesterase Inhibitors (Central): Anticholinergics may diminish the therapeutic effect of Acetylcholinesterase Inhibitors (Central). Acetylcholinesterase Inhibitors (Central) may diminish the therapeutic effect of Anticholinergics. If the anticholinergic action is a side effect of the agent, the result may be beneficial. *Risk C: Monitor therapy*

Alcohol (Ethyl): CNS Depressants may enhance the CNS depressant effect of Alcohol (Ethyl). *Risk C: Monitor therapy*

Alfuzosin: May enhance the QT_c-prolonging effect of QT_c-Prolonging Agents. *Risk C: Monitor therapy*

Alpha-/Beta-Agonists (Direct-Acting): Tricyclic Antidepressants may enhance the vasopressor effect of Alpha-/Beta-Agonists (Direct-Acting). **Exceptions:** Dipivefrin. *Risk D: Consider therapy modification*

Alpha$_1$-Agonists: Tricyclic Antidepressants may enhance the vasopressor effect of Alpha$_1$-Agonists. *Risk D: Consider therapy modification*

Alpha$_2$-Agonists: Tricyclic Antidepressants may diminish the antihypertensive effect of Alpha$_2$-Agonists. **Exceptions:** Apraclonidine; Brimonidine. *Risk D: Consider therapy modification*

Altretamine: May enhance the orthostatic effect of Tricyclic Antidepressants. *Risk C: Monitor therapy*

Amphetamines: Tricyclic Antidepressants may enhance the stimulatory effect of Amphetamines. Tricyclic Antidepressants may also potentiate the cardiovascular effects of Amphetamines. *Risk C: Monitor therapy*

Anticholinergics: May enhance the adverse/toxic effect of other Anticholinergics. **Exceptions:** Paliperidone. *Risk C: Monitor therapy*

Aspirin: Antidepressants (Tricyclic, Tertiary Amine) may enhance the antiplatelet effect of Aspirin. *Risk C: Monitor therapy*

Barbiturates: May increase the metabolism of Tricyclic Antidepressants. *Risk D: Consider therapy modification*

Beta$_2$-Agonists: Tricyclic Antidepressants may enhance the adverse/toxic effect of Beta$_2$-Agonists. *Risk C: Monitor therapy*

BuPROPion: May decrease the metabolism of Tricyclic Antidepressants. *Risk C: Monitor therapy*

CarBAMazepine: May increase the metabolism of Tricyclic Antidepressants. *Risk C: Monitor therapy*

Cimetidine: May decrease the metabolism of Tricyclic Antidepressants. *Risk C: Monitor therapy*

Cinacalcet: May increase the serum concentration of Tricyclic Antidepressants. *Risk C: Monitor therapy*

Ciprofloxacin: May enhance the QT_c-prolonging effect of QT_c-Prolonging Agents. *Risk C: Monitor therapy*

Cisapride: Amitriptyline may enhance the arrhythmogenic effect of Cisapride. *Risk X: Avoid combination*

CNS Depressants: May enhance the adverse/toxic effect of other CNS Depressants. *Risk C: Monitor therapy*

CYP2D6 Inhibitors (Moderate): May decrease the metabolism of CYP2D6 Substrates. *Risk C: Monitor therapy*

CYP2D6 Inhibitors (Strong): May decrease the metabolism of CYP2D6 Substrates. *Risk D: Consider therapy modification*

Darunavir: May increase the serum concentration of CYP2D6 Substrates. *Risk C: Monitor therapy*

Desmopressin: Tricyclic Antidepressants may enhance the adverse/toxic effect of Desmopressin. *Risk C: Monitor therapy*

Dexmethylphenidate: May decrease the metabolism of Tricyclic Antidepressants. *Risk C: Monitor therapy*

DULoxetine: May decrease the metabolism of Tricyclic Antidepressants. *Risk C: Monitor therapy*

Gadobutrol: May enhance the QT_c-prolonging effect of QT_c-Prolonging Agents. *Risk D: Consider therapy modification*

Lithium: May enhance the neurotoxic effect of Tricyclic Antidepressants. *Risk C: Monitor therapy*

MAO Inhibitors: May enhance the serotonergic effect of Tricyclic Antidepressants. This may cause serotonin syndrome. *Risk X: Avoid combination*

Methylphenidate: May decrease the metabolism of Tricyclic Antidepressants. *Risk C: Monitor therapy*

Nilotinib: May enhance the QT_c-prolonging effect of QT_c-Prolonging Agents. *Risk X: Avoid combination*

NSAID (COX-2 Inhibitor): Antidepressants (Tricyclic, Tertiary Amine) may enhance the antiplatelet effect of NSAID (COX-2 Inhibitor). *Risk C: Monitor therapy*

NSAID (Nonselective): Antidepressants (Tricyclic, Tertiary Amine) may enhance the antiplatelet effect of NSAID (Nonselective). *Risk C: Monitor therapy*

Pramlintide: May enhance the anticholinergic effect of Anticholinergics. These effects are specific to the GI tract. *Risk D: Consider therapy modification*

Propoxyphene: May enhance the CNS depressant effect of Tricyclic Antidepressants. *Risk C: Monitor therapy*

Protease Inhibitors: May increase the serum concentration of Tricyclic Antidepressants. *Risk C: Monitor therapy*

QT_c-Prolonging Agents: May enhance the adverse/toxic effect of other QT_c-Prolonging Agents. Their effects can be additive, causing life-threatening ventricular arrhythmias. *Risk D: Consider therapy modification*

QuiNIDine: Tricyclic Antidepressants may enhance the QT_c-prolonging effect of QuiNIDine. QuiNIDine may decrease the metabolism of Tricyclic Antidepressants. *Risk D: Consider therapy modification*

Selective Serotonin Reuptake Inhibitors: May decrease the metabolism of Tricyclic Antidepressants. *Risk D: Consider therapy modification*

Serotonin Modulators: May enhance the adverse/toxic effect of other Serotonin Modulators. The development of serotonin syndrome may occur. *Risk D: Consider therapy modification*

Sibutramine: May enhance the serotonergic effect of Serotonin Modulators. This may cause serotonin syndrome. *Risk X: Avoid combination*

St Johns Wort: May increase the metabolism of Tricyclic Antidepressants. The risk of serotonin syndrome may theoretically be increased. *Risk D: Consider therapy modification*

Sulfonylureas: Cyclic Antidepressants may enhance the hypoglycemic effect of Sulfonylureas. *Risk C: Monitor therapy*

Terbinafine: May decrease the metabolism of Tricyclic Antidepressants. *Risk D: Consider therapy modification*

Tetrabenazine: QT_c-Prolonging Agents may enhance the QT_c-prolonging effect of Tetrabenazine. *Risk X: Avoid combination*

Thioridazine: QT_c-Prolonging Agents may enhance the QT_c-prolonging effect of Thioridazine. *Risk X: Avoid combination*

TraMADol: Tricyclic Antidepressants may enhance the neuroexcitatory and/or seizure-potentiating effect of TraMADol. *Risk C: Monitor therapy*

Valproic Acid: May increase the serum concentration of Tricyclic Antidepressants. *Risk C: Monitor therapy*

Vitamin K Antagonists (eg, warfarin): Tricyclic Antidepressants may enhance the anticoagulant effect of Vitamin K Antagonists. *Risk C: Monitor therapy*

Ziprasidone: QT_c-Prolonging Agents may enhance the QT_c-prolonging effect of Ziprasidone. The risk of a severe arrhythmia may be increased. *Risk X: Avoid combination*

Ethanol/Nutrition/Herb Interactions

Ethanol: Avoid ethanol (may increase CNS depression).

Food: Grapefruit juice may inhibit the metabolism of some TCAs and clinical toxicity may result.

Herb/Nutraceutical: St John's wort may decrease amitriptyline levels. Avoid valerian, St John's wort, kava kava, gotu kola (may increase CNS depression).

Stability Protect Elavil® 10 mg tablets from light.

Mechanism of Action Increases the synaptic concentration of serotonin and/or norepinephrine in the central nervous system by inhibition of their reuptake by the presynaptic neuronal membrane

Pharmacodynamics/Kinetics

Onset of action: Migraine prophylaxis: 6 weeks, higher dosage may be required in heavy smokers because of increased metabolism; Depression: 4-6 weeks, reduce dosage to lowest effective level

Distribution: Crosses placenta; enters breast milk

Metabolism: Hepatic to nortriptyline (active), hydroxy and conjugated derivatives; may be impaired in the elderly

Half-life elimination: Adults: 9-27 hours (average: 15 hours)

Time to peak, serum: ~4 hours

Excretion: Urine (18% as unchanged drug); feces (small amounts)

Dosage

Children:

Chronic pain management (unlabeled use): Oral: Initial: 0.1 mg/kg at bedtime, may advance as tolerated over 2-3 weeks to 0.5-2 mg/kg at bedtime

Depressive disorders (unlabeled use): Oral: Initial doses of 1 mg/kg/day given in 3 divided doses with increases to 1.5 mg/kg/day have been reported in a small number of children (n=9) 9-12 years of age; clinically, doses up to 3 mg/kg/day (5 mg/kg/day if monitored closely) have been proposed

Migraine prophylaxis (unlabeled use): Oral: Initial: 0.25 mg/kg/day, given at bedtime; increase dose by 0.25 mg/kg/day to maximum 1 mg/kg/day. Reported dosing ranges: 0.1-2 mg/kg/day; maximum suggested dose: 10 mg.

Adolescents: Depressive disorders: Oral: Initial: 25-50 mg/day; may administer in divided doses; increase gradually to 100 mg/day in divided doses

Adults:

Depression:

Oral: 50-150 mg/day single dose at bedtime or in divided doses; dose may be gradually increased up to 300 mg/day

Migraine prophylaxis (unlabeled use): Oral: Initial: 10-25 mg at bedtime; usual dose: 150 mg; reported dosing ranges: 10-400 mg/day

Pain management (unlabeled use): Oral: Initial: 25 mg at bedtime; may increase as tolerated to 100 mg/day

Elderly: Depression: Oral: Initial: 10-25 mg at bedtime; dose should be increased in 10-25 mg increments every week if tolerated; dose range: 25-150 mg/day

Dosing interval in hepatic impairment: Use with caution and monitor plasma levels and patient response

Hemodialysis: Nondialyzable

Monitoring Parameters Monitor blood pressure and pulse rate prior to and during initial therapy; evaluate mental status, suicidal ideation (especially at the beginning of therapy or when doses are increased or decreased); monitor weight; ECG in older adults and patients with cardiac disease

Reference Range Therapeutic: Amitriptyline and nortriptyline 100-250 ng/mL (SI: 360-900 nmol/L); nortriptyline 50-150 ng/mL (SI: 190-570 nmol/L); Toxic: >0.5 mcg/mL; plasma levels do not always correlate with clinical effectiveness

Test Interactions May cause false-positive reaction to EMIT immunoassay for imipramine

Dosage Forms Excipient information presented when available (limited, particularly for generics); consult specific product labeling.

Tablet, as hydrochloride: 10 mg, 25 mg, 50 mg, 75 mg, 100 mg, 150 mg

Amitriptyline and Chlordiazepoxide

(a mee TRIP ti leen & klor dye az e POKS ide)

U.S. Brand Names Limbitrol®; Limbitrol® DS

Canadian Brand Names Limbitrol®

Index Terms Chlordiazepoxide and Amitriptyline Hydrochloride

Pharmacologic Category Antidepressant, Tricyclic (Tertiary Amine); Benzodiazepine

Generic Available Yes

Use Treatment of moderate to severe anxiety and/or agitation and depression

Mental Health Comment Tricyclic antidepressants may be classified as tertiary (amitriptyline, doxepin, clomipramine, imipramine, trimipramine) or secondary amines (nortriptyline, desipramine, protriptyline). The tertiary amines are not recommended to treat depression in the elderly. If a TCA is used in the elderly, it should be a secondary amine. The tertiary amines are commonly used in low dosages for various conditions associated with pain. Toxicity is generally dose dependent. Relatively small overdoses (1-week supply) can be potentially fatal.

In 2007, the FDA requested that all manufacturers of sedative-hypnotic drug products revise labeling to include a greater emphasis on the risks of adverse effects. These risks include severe allergic reactions (anaphylaxis, angioedema) and complex sleep-related behaviors, which may include sleep-driving (driving while not fully awake and with no memory of the event), making phone calls, and preparing and eating food while asleep.

Risk factors for abuse include personal or family history of substance abuse and personality disorder.

Restrictions C-IV

An FDA-approved medication guide concerning the use of antidepressants in children, adolescents, and young adults must be distributed when dispensing an outpatient prescription (new or refill) where this medication is to be used without direct supervision of a healthcare provider. Medication guides are available at http://www.fda.gov/cder/Offices/ODS/medication_guides.htm. Dispense to parents or guardians of children and adolescents receiving this medication.

Pregnancy Risk Factor D

Lactation Excretion in breast milk unknown/contraindicated

Contraindications Hypersensitivity to benzodiazepines, tricyclic antidepressants, or any component of the formulation; depression of CNS; MAO inhibitors; acute recovery phase following MI; angle-closure glaucoma; pregnancy

Warnings/Precautions See individual agents.

Adverse Reactions See individual agents.

Metabolism/Transport Effects

Amitriptyline: **Substrate** of CYP1A2 (minor), 2B6 (minor), 2C9 (minor), 2C19 (minor), 2D6 (major), 3A4 (minor); **Inhibits** CYP1A2 (weak), 2C9 (weak), 2C19 (weak), 2D6 (weak), 2E1 (weak)

Chlordiazepoxide: **Substrate** of CYP3A4 (major)

Drug Interactions

Acetylcholinesterase Inhibitors (Central): Anticholinergics may diminish the therapeutic effect of Acetylcholinesterase Inhibitors (Central). Acetylcholinesterase Inhibitors (Central) may diminish the therapeutic effect of Anticholinergics. If the anticholinergic action is a side effect of the agent, the result may be beneficial. *Risk C: Monitor therapy*

Alcohol (Ethyl): CNS Depressants may enhance the CNS depressant effect of Alcohol (Ethyl). *Risk C: Monitor therapy*

Alfuzosin: May enhance the QTc-prolonging effect of QTc-Prolonging Agents. *Risk C: Monitor therapy*

Alpha-/Beta-Agonists (Direct-Acting): Tricyclic Antidepressants may enhance the vasopressor effect of Alpha-/Beta-Agonists (Direct-Acting). **Exceptions:** Dipivefrin. *Risk D: Consider therapy modification*

Alpha1-Agonists: Tricyclic Antidepressants may enhance the vasopressor effect of Alpha1-Agonists. *Risk D: Consider therapy modification*

Alpha2-Agonists: Tricyclic Antidepressants may diminish the antihypertensive effect of Alpha2-Agonists. **Exceptions:** Apraclonidine; Brimonidine. *Risk D: Consider therapy modification*

Altretamine: May enhance the orthostatic effect of Tricyclic Antidepressants. *Risk C: Monitor therapy*

Amphetamines: Tricyclic Antidepressants may enhance the stimulatory effect of Amphetamines. Tricyclic Antidepressants may also potentiate the cardiovascular effects of Amphetamines. *Risk C: Monitor therapy*

Anticholinergics: May enhance the adverse/toxic effect of other Anticholinergics. **Exceptions:** Paliperidone. *Risk C: Monitor therapy*

Antifungal Agents (Azole Derivatives, Systemic): May decrease the metabolism of Benzodiazepines (metabolized by oxidation). *Risk D: Consider therapy modification*

Aprepitant: May increase the serum concentration of Benzodiazepines (metabolized by oxidation). *Risk C: Monitor therapy*

Aspirin: Antidepressants (Tricyclic, Tertiary Amine) may enhance the antiplatelet effect of Aspirin. *Risk C: Monitor therapy*

Barbiturates: May increase the metabolism of Tricyclic Antidepressants. *Risk D: Consider therapy modification*

Beta2-Agonists: Tricyclic Antidepressants may enhance the adverse/toxic effect of Beta2-Agonists. *Risk C: Monitor therapy*

BuPROPion: May decrease the metabolism of Tricyclic Antidepressants. *Risk C: Monitor therapy*

Calcium Channel Blockers (Nondihydropyridine): May decrease the metabolism of Benzodiazepines (metabolized by oxidation). *Risk D: Consider therapy modification*

CarBAMazepine: May increase the metabolism of Tricyclic Antidepressants. *Risk C: Monitor therapy*

CarBAMazepine: May increase the metabolism of Benzodiazepines (metabolized by oxidation). *Risk C: Monitor therapy*

Cimetidine: May decrease the metabolism of Tricyclic Antidepressants. *Risk C: Monitor therapy*

Cimetidine: May decrease the metabolism of Benzodiazepines (metabolized by oxidation). *Risk C: Monitor therapy*

Cinacalcet: May increase the serum concentration of Tricyclic Antidepressants. *Risk C: Monitor therapy*

Ciprofloxacin: May enhance the QTc-prolonging effect of QTc-Prolonging Agents. *Risk C: Monitor therapy*

Cisapride: Amitriptyline may enhance the arrhythmogenic effect of Cisapride. *Risk X: Avoid combination*

Clozapine: Benzodiazepines may enhance the adverse/toxic effect of Clozapine. *Risk D: Consider therapy modification*

CNS Depressants: May enhance the adverse/toxic effect of other CNS Depressants. *Risk C: Monitor therapy*

CYP2D6 Inhibitors (Moderate): May decrease the metabolism of CYP2D6 Substrates. *Risk C: Monitor therapy*

CYP2D6 Inhibitors (Strong): May decrease the metabolism of CYP2D6 Substrates. *Risk D: Consider therapy modification*

CYP3A4 Inducers (Strong): May increase the metabolism of CYP3A4 Substrates. *Risk C: Monitor therapy*

CYP3A4 Inhibitors (Moderate): May decrease the metabolism of CYP3A4 Substrates. *Risk C: Monitor therapy*

CYP3A4 Inhibitors (Strong): May decrease the metabolism of CYP3A4 Substrates. *Risk D: Consider therapy modification*

Darunavir: May increase the serum concentration of CYP2D6 Substrates. *Risk C: Monitor therapy*

Dasatinib: May increase the serum concentration of CYP3A4 Substrates. *Risk C: Monitor therapy*

Deferasirox: May decrease the serum concentration of CYP3A4 Substrates. *Risk C: Monitor therapy*

Desmopressin: Tricyclic Antidepressants may enhance the adverse/toxic effect of Desmopressin. *Risk C: Monitor therapy*

Dexmethylphenidate: May decrease the metabolism of Tricyclic Antidepressants. *Risk C: Monitor therapy*

Disulfiram: May decrease the metabolism of Benzodiazepines (metabolized by oxidation). *Risk C: Monitor therapy*

DULoxetine: May decrease the metabolism of Tricyclic Antidepressants. *Risk C: Monitor therapy*

Fluconazole: May decrease the metabolism of Benzodiazepines (metabolized by oxidation). *Risk D: Consider therapy modification*

Fosaprepitant: May increase the serum concentration of Benzodiazepines (metabolized by oxidation). Specifically, the active metabolite aprepitant is likely responsible for this effect. *Risk C: Monitor therapy*

Gadobutrol: May enhance the QTc-prolonging effect of QTc-Prolonging Agents. *Risk D: Consider therapy modification*

Grapefruit Juice: May decrease the metabolism of Benzodiazepines (metabolized by oxidation). *Risk D: Consider therapy modification*

Isoniazid: May decrease the metabolism of Benzodiazepines (metabolized by oxidation). *Risk C: Monitor therapy*

Lithium: May enhance the neurotoxic effect of Tricyclic Antidepressants. *Risk C: Monitor therapy*

Macrolide Antibiotics: May decrease the metabolism of Benzodiazepines (metabolized by oxidation). **Exceptions:** Azithromycin; Dirithromycin [Off Market]; Spiramycin. *Risk D: Consider therapy modification*

MAO Inhibitors: May enhance the serotonergic effect of Tricyclic Antidepressants. This may cause serotonin syndrome. *Risk X: Avoid combination*

Methylphenidate: May decrease the metabolism of Tricyclic Antidepressants. *Risk C: Monitor therapy*

Nefazodone: May decrease the metabolism of Benzodiazepines (metabolized by oxidation). *Risk D: Consider therapy modification*

Nilotinib: May enhance the QTc-prolonging effect of QTc-Prolonging Agents. *Risk X: Avoid combination*

NSAID (COX-2 Inhibitor): Antidepressants (Tricyclic, Tertiary Amine) may enhance the antiplatelet effect of NSAID (COX-2 Inhibitor). *Risk C: Monitor therapy*

NSAID (Nonselective): Antidepressants (Tricyclic, Tertiary Amine) may enhance the antiplatelet effect of NSAID (Nonselective). *Risk C: Monitor therapy*

Oral Contraceptive (Estrogens): May decrease the metabolism of Benzodiazepines (metabolized by oxidation). *Risk C: Monitor therapy*

Oral Contraceptive (Progestins): May decrease the metabolism of Benzodiazepines (metabolized by oxidation). *Risk C: Monitor therapy*

Phenytoin: Benzodiazepines may increase the serum concentration of Phenytoin. Short-term exposure to benzodiazepines may not present as much risk as chronic therapy. *Risk C: Monitor therapy*

Pramlintide: May enhance the anticholinergic effect of Anticholinergics. These effects are specific to the GI tract. *Risk D: Consider therapy modification*

Propoxyphene: May enhance the CNS depressant effect of Tricyclic Antidepressants. *Risk C: Monitor therapy*

Protease Inhibitors: May decrease the metabolism of Benzodiazepines (metabolized by oxidation). Management: Amprenavir, atazanavir, darunavir, indinavir, nelfinavir, ritonavir, and tipranavir are contraindicated with midazolam and triazolam according to each protease inhibitor's prescribing information. *Risk D: Consider therapy modification*

Protease Inhibitors: May increase the serum concentration of Tricyclic Antidepressants. *Risk C: Monitor therapy*

Proton Pump Inhibitors: May increase the serum concentration of Benzodiazepines (metabolized by oxidation). **Exceptions:** Lansoprazole; Pantoprazole; Rabeprazole. *Risk C: Monitor therapy*

QTc-Prolonging Agents: May enhance the adverse/toxic effect of other QTc-Prolonging Agents. Their effects can be additive, causing life-threatening ventricular arrhythmias. *Risk D: Consider therapy modification*

QuiNIDine: Tricyclic Antidepressants may enhance the QTc-prolonging effect of QuiNIDine. QuiNIDine may decrease the metabolism of Tricyclic Antidepressants. *Risk D: Consider therapy modification*

Rifamycin Derivatives: May increase the metabolism of Benzodiazepines (metabolized by oxidation). *Risk D: Consider therapy modification*

Selective Serotonin Reuptake Inhibitors: May decrease the metabolism of Tricyclic Antidepressants. *Risk D: Consider therapy modification*

Selective Serotonin Reuptake Inhibitors: May decrease the metabolism of Benzodiazepines (metabolized by oxidation). **Exceptions:** Citalopram; Escitalopram; PARoxetine; Sertraline. *Risk C: Monitor therapy*

Serotonin Modulators: May enhance the adverse/toxic effect of other Serotonin Modulators. The development of serotonin syndrome may occur. *Risk D: Consider therapy modification*

Sibutramine: May enhance the serotonergic effect of Serotonin Modulators. This may cause serotonin syndrome. *Risk X: Avoid combination*

St Johns Wort: May increase the metabolism of Tricyclic Antidepressants. The risk of serotonin syndrome may theoretically be increased. *Risk D: Consider therapy modification*

St Johns Wort: May increase the metabolism of Benzodiazepines (metabolized by oxidation). *Risk C: Monitor therapy*

Sulfonylureas: Cyclic Antidepressants may enhance the hypoglycemic effect of Sulfonylureas. *Risk C: Monitor therapy*

Terbinafine: May decrease the metabolism of Tricyclic Antidepressants. *Risk D: Consider therapy modification*

Tetrabenazine: QTc-Prolonging Agents may enhance the QTc-prolonging effect of Tetrabenazine. *Risk X: Avoid combination*

Theophylline Derivatives: May diminish the therapeutic effect of Benzodiazepines. *Risk D: Consider therapy modification*

Thioridazine: QTc-Prolonging Agents may enhance the QTc-prolonging effect of Thioridazine. *Risk X: Avoid combination*

TraMADol: Tricyclic Antidepressants may enhance the neuroexcitatory and/or seizure-potentiating effect of TraMADol. *Risk C: Monitor therapy*

Valproic Acid: May increase the serum concentration of Tricyclic Antidepressants. *Risk C: Monitor therapy*

Vitamin K Antagonists (eg, warfarin): Tricyclic Antidepressants may enhance the anticoagulant effect of Vitamin K Antagonists. *Risk C: Monitor therapy*

Ziprasidone: QTc-Prolonging Agents may enhance the QTc-prolonging effect of Ziprasidone. The risk of a severe arrhythmia may be increased. *Risk X: Avoid combination*

Mechanism of Action See individual agents.

Pharmacodynamics/Kinetics See individual agents.

Dosage Initial: 3-4 tablets in divided doses; this may be increased to 6 tablets/day as required; some patients respond to smaller doses and can be maintained on 2 tablets

Monitoring Parameters Suicidal ideation (especially at the beginning of therapy or when doses are increased or decreased)

Dosage Forms Excipient information presented when available (limited, particularly for generics); consult specific product labeling.

Tablet: 12.5/5: Amitriptyline hydrochloride 12.5 mg and chlordiazepoxide 5 mg; 25/10: Amitriptyline hydrochloride 25 mg and chlordiazepoxide 10 mg

Limbitrol®: 12.5/5: Amitriptyline hydrochloride 12.5 mg and chlordiazepoxide 5 mg

Limbitrol® DS: 25/10: Amitriptyline hydrochloride 25 mg and chlordiazepoxide 10 mg

Amitriptyline and Perphenazine

(a mee TRIP ti leen & per FEN a zeen)

Canadian Brand Names Etrafon®

Index Terms Perphenazine and Amitriptyline Hydrochloride

Pharmacologic Category Antidepressant, Tricyclic (Tertiary Amine); Antipsychotic Agent, Typical, Phenothiazine

Generic Available Yes

Use Treatment of patients with moderate to severe anxiety and depression

Unlabeled/Investigational Use Depression with psychotic features

Mental Health Comment Tricyclic antidepressants may be classified as tertiary (amitriptyline, doxepin, clomipramine, imipramine, trimipramine) or secondary amines (nortriptyline, desipramine, protriptyline). The tertiary amines are not recommended to treat depression in the elderly. If a TCA is used in the elderly, it should be a secondary amine. The tertiary amines are commonly used in low dosages for various conditions associated with pain. Toxicity is generally dose dependent. Relatively small overdoses (1-week supply) can be potentially fatal.

Not commonly used; use of individual drugs allows for more flexibility in dosing and discontinuation of unneeded agent.

Coadministration of two or more antipsychotics does not generally improve clinical response and may increase the potential for adverse effects. Long-term use of perphenazine, as is the case with any antipsychotic drug, may be associated with tardive dyskinesia (TD).

In 2008, the FDA issued a warning regarding increased mortality risk with typical **and** atypical antipsychotic drugs when used in elderly patients with dementia-related psychosis.

Restrictions An FDA-approved medication guide concerning the use of antidepressants in children, adolescents, and young adults must be distributed when dispensing an outpatient prescription (new or refill) where this medication is to be used without direct supervision of a healthcare provider. Medication guides are available at http://www.fda.gov/cder/Offices/ODS/medication_guides.htm. Dispense to parents or guardians of children and adolescents receiving this medication.

Pregnancy Risk Factor D

Lactation Enters breast milk/contraindicated

Contraindications Hypersensitivity to amitriptyline, perphenazine, or any component of the formulation (cross-sensitivity with other phenothiazines may exist); angle-closure glaucoma; bone marrow depression; severe liver or cardiac disease; pregnancy

Warnings/Precautions See individual agents. This combination is not FDA approved for use in children or for the treatment of bipolar depression.

Adverse Reactions See individual agents.

Metabolism/Transport Effects

Amitriptyline: **Substrate** of CYP1A2 (minor), 2B6 (minor), 2C9 (minor), 2C19 (minor), 2D6 (major), 3A4 (minor); **Inhibits** CYP1A2 (weak), 2C9 (weak), 2C19 (weak), 2D6 (weak), 2E1 (weak)

Perphenazine: **Substrate** of CYP1A2 (minor), 2C9 (minor), 2C19 (minor), 2D6 (major), 3A4 (minor); **Inhibits** CYP1A2 (weak), 2D6 (weak)

Drug Interactions

Acetylcholinesterase Inhibitors (Central): May enhance the neurotoxic (central) effect of Antipsychotics. Severe extrapyramidal symptoms have occurred in some patients. *Risk C: Monitor therapy*

Alcohol (Ethyl): CNS Depressants may enhance the CNS depressant effect of Alcohol (Ethyl). *Risk C: Monitor therapy*

Alfuzosin: May enhance the QTc-prolonging effect of QTc-Prolonging Agents. *Risk C: Monitor therapy*

Alpha-/Beta-Agonists (Direct-Acting): Tricyclic Antidepressants may enhance the vasopressor effect of Alpha-/Beta-Agonists (Direct-Acting). **Exceptions:** Dipivefrin. *Risk D: Consider therapy modification*

Alpha1-Agonists: Tricyclic Antidepressants may enhance the vasopressor effect of Alpha1-Agonists. *Risk D: Consider therapy modification*

Alpha2-Agonists: Tricyclic Antidepressants may diminish the antihypertensive effect of Alpha2-Agonists. **Exceptions:** Apraclonidine; Brimonidine. *Risk D: Consider therapy modification*

Altretamine: May enhance the orthostatic effect of Tricyclic Antidepressants. *Risk C: Monitor therapy*

Amphetamines: Tricyclic Antidepressants may enhance the stimulatory effect of Amphetamines. Tricyclic Antidepressants may also potentiate the cardiovascular effects of Amphetamines. *Risk C: Monitor therapy*

Amphetamines: Antipsychotics may diminish the stimulatory effect of Amphetamines. *Risk C: Monitor therapy*

Analgesics (Opioid): Antipsychotic Agents (Phenothiazines) may enhance the hypotensive effect of Analgesics (Opioid). *Risk C: Monitor therapy*

Antacids: May decrease the absorption of Antipsychotic Agents (Phenothiazines). *Risk C: Monitor therapy*

Anticholinergics: May enhance the adverse/toxic effect of other Anticholinergics. **Exceptions:** Paliperidone. *Risk C: Monitor therapy*

Antimalarial Agents: May increase the serum concentration of Antipsychotic Agents (Phenothiazines). *Risk C: Monitor therapy*

Anti-Parkinson's Agents (Dopamine Agonist): Antipsychotics (Typical) may diminish the therapeutic effect of Anti-Parkinson's Agents (Dopamine Agonist). *Risk D: Consider therapy modification*

Aspirin: Antidepressants (Tricyclic, Tertiary Amine) may enhance the antiplatelet effect of Aspirin. *Risk C: Monitor therapy*

Barbiturates: May increase the metabolism of Tricyclic Antidepressants. *Risk D: Consider therapy modification*

Beta2-Agonists: Tricyclic Antidepressants may enhance the adverse/toxic effect of Beta2-Agonists. *Risk C: Monitor therapy*

Beta-Blockers: Antipsychotic Agents (Phenothiazines) may enhance the hypotensive effect of Beta-Blockers. Beta-Blockers may decrease the metabolism of Antipsychotic Agents (Phenothiazines). Antipsychotic Agents (Phenothiazines) may decrease the metabolism of Beta-Blockers. **Exceptions:** Atenolol; Levobunolol; Metipranolol; Nadolol. *Risk C: Monitor therapy*

BuPROPion: May decrease the metabolism of Tricyclic Antidepressants. *Risk C: Monitor therapy*

CarBAMazepine: May increase the metabolism of Tricyclic Antidepressants. *Risk C: Monitor therapy*

Cimetidine: May decrease the metabolism of Tricyclic Antidepressants. *Risk C: Monitor therapy*

Cinacalcet: May increase the serum concentration of Tricyclic Antidepressants. *Risk C: Monitor therapy*

Ciprofloxacin: May enhance the QTc-prolonging effect of QTc-Prolonging Agents. *Risk C: Monitor therapy*

Cisapride: Amitriptyline may enhance the arrhythmogenic effect of Cisapride. *Risk X: Avoid combination*

CNS Depressants: May enhance the adverse/toxic effect of other CNS Depressants. *Risk C: Monitor therapy*

CYP2D6 Inhibitors (Moderate): May decrease the metabolism of CYP2D6 Substrates. *Risk C: Monitor therapy*

CYP2D6 Inhibitors (Strong): May decrease the metabolism of CYP2D6 Substrates. *Risk D: Consider therapy modification*

Darunavir: May increase the serum concentration of CYP2D6 Substrates. *Risk C: Monitor therapy*

Desmopressin: Tricyclic Antidepressants may enhance the adverse/toxic effect of Desmopressin. *Risk C: Monitor therapy*

Dexmethylphenidate: May decrease the metabolism of Tricyclic Antidepressants. *Risk C: Monitor therapy*

DULoxetine: May decrease the metabolism of Tricyclic Antidepressants. *Risk C: Monitor therapy*

Gadobutrol: May enhance the QTc-prolonging effect of QTc-Prolonging Agents. *Risk D: Consider therapy modification*

Lithium: May enhance the neurotoxic effect of Tricyclic Antidepressants. *Risk C: Monitor therapy*

Lithium formulations: May enhance the neurotoxic effect of Antipsychotics. Lithium formulations may decrease the serum concentration of Antipsychotics. Specifically noted with chlorpromazine. *Risk C: Monitor therapy*

MAO Inhibitors: May enhance the serotonergic effect of Tricyclic Antidepressants. This may cause serotonin syndrome. *Risk X: Avoid combination*

Methylphenidate: May decrease the metabolism of Tricyclic Antidepressants. *Risk C: Monitor therapy*

Nilotinib: May enhance the QTc-prolonging effect of QTc-Prolonging Agents. *Risk X: Avoid combination*

NSAID (COX-2 Inhibitor): Antidepressants (Tricyclic, Tertiary Amine) may enhance the antiplatelet effect of NSAID (COX-2 Inhibitor). *Risk C: Monitor therapy*

NSAID (Nonselective): Antidepressants (Tricyclic, Tertiary Amine) may enhance the antiplatelet effect of NSAID (Nonselective). *Risk C: Monitor therapy*

Pramlintide: May enhance the anticholinergic effect of Anticholinergics. These effects are specific to the GI tract. *Risk D: Consider therapy modification*

Propoxyphene: May enhance the CNS depressant effect of Tricyclic Antidepressants. *Risk C: Monitor therapy*

Protease Inhibitors: May increase the serum concentration of Tricyclic Antidepressants. *Risk C: Monitor therapy*

QTc-Prolonging Agents: May enhance the adverse/toxic effect of other QTc-Prolonging Agents. Their effects can be additive, causing life-threatening ventricular arrhythmias. *Risk D: Consider therapy modification*

QuiNIDine: Tricyclic Antidepressants may enhance the QTc-prolonging effect of QuiNIDine. QuiNIDine may decrease the metabolism of Tricyclic Antidepressants. *Risk D: Consider therapy modification*

Selective Serotonin Reuptake Inhibitors: May decrease the metabolism of Tricyclic Antidepressants. *Risk D: Consider therapy modification*

Serotonin Modulators: May enhance the adverse/toxic effect of other Serotonin Modulators. The development of serotonin syndrome may occur. *Risk D: Consider therapy modification*

Sibutramine: May enhance the serotonergic effect of Serotonin Modulators. This may cause serotonin syndrome. *Risk X: Avoid combination*

St Johns Wort: May increase the metabolism of Tricyclic Antidepressants. The risk of serotonin syndrome may theoretically be increased. *Risk D: Consider therapy modification*

Sulfonylureas: Cyclic Antidepressants may enhance the hypoglycemic effect of Sulfonylureas. *Risk C: Monitor therapy*

Terbinafine: May decrease the metabolism of Tricyclic Antidepressants. *Risk D: Consider therapy modification*

Tetrabenazine: May enhance the adverse/toxic effect of Antipsychotics. *Risk C: Monitor therapy*

Thioridazine: QTc-Prolonging Agents may enhance the QTc-prolonging effect of Thioridazine. *Risk X: Avoid combination*

TraMADol: Tricyclic Antidepressants may enhance the neuroexcitatory and/or seizure-potentiating effect of TraMADol. *Risk C: Monitor therapy*

Valproic Acid: May increase the serum concentration of Tricyclic Antidepressants. *Risk C: Monitor therapy*

Vitamin K Antagonists (eg, warfarin): Tricyclic Antidepressants may enhance the anticoagulant effect of Vitamin K Antagonists. *Risk C: Monitor therapy*

Ziprasidone: QTc-Prolonging Agents may enhance the QTc-prolonging effect of Ziprasidone. The risk of a severe arrhythmia may be increased. *Risk X: Avoid combination*

Ethanol/Nutrition/Herb Interactions Ethanol: Avoid ethanol (due to increased sedation).

Mechanism of Action

Amitriptyline increases the synaptic concentration of serotonin and/or norepinephrine in the central nervous system by inhibition of their reuptake by the presynaptic neuronal membrane.

Perphenazine is a piperazine phenothiazine antipsychotic which blocks postsynaptic mesolimbic dopaminergic receptors in the brain; exhibits alpha-adrenergic blocking effect and depresses the release of hypothalamic and hypophyseal hormones.

Pharmacodynamics/Kinetics See individual agents.

Dosage Oral: 1 tablet 2-4 times/day

Monitoring Parameters Vital signs; lipid profile, fasting blood glucose/Hb A_{1c}; BMI, weight; mental status, abnormal involuntary movement scale (AIMS), extrapyramidal symptoms (EPS), suicidal ideation (especially at the beginning of therapy or when doses are increased or decreased)

Dosage Forms Excipient information presented when available (limited, particularly for generics); consult specific product labeling.

Tablet:

2-10: Amitriptyline hydrochloride 10 mg and perphenazine 2 mg
2-25: Amitriptyline hydrochloride 25 mg and perphenazine 2 mg
4-10: Amitriptyline hydrochloride 10 mg and perphenazine 4 mg
4-25: Amitriptyline hydrochloride 25 mg and perphenazine 4 mg
4-50: Amitriptyline hydrochloride 50 mg and perphenazine 4 mg

◆ **Amitriptyline Hydrochloride** *see* Amitriptyline *on page 90*

◆ **AMJ 9701** *see* Palifermin *on page 1214*

AmLODIPine (am LOE di peen)

Medication Safety Issues

Sound-alike/look-alike issues:

AmLODIPine may be confused with aMILoride
Norvasc® may be confused with Navane®, Norvir®, Vascor®

Related Information

Calcium Channel Blockers *on page 1778*

U.S. Brand Names Norvasc®

Canadian Brand Names Norvasc®

Mexican Brand Names Avistar; Norvas; Sistopress

Index Terms Amlodipine Besylate

Pharmacologic Category Calcium Channel Blocker

Generic Available Yes

Use Treatment of hypertension; treatment of symptomatic chronic stable angina, vasospastic (Prinzmetal's) angina (confirmed or suspected); prevention of hospitalization due to angina with documented CAD (limited to patients without heart failure or ejection fraction <40%)

Effect on Mental Status May cause drowsiness; rarely may produce insomnia and nervousness

Effect on Psychiatric Treatment None reported

Pregnancy Risk Factor C

Pregnancy Considerations Embryotoxic effects have been demonstrated in small animals. No well-controlled studies have been conducted in pregnant women. Use in pregnancy only when clearly needed and when the benefits outweigh the potential hazard to the fetus.

Lactation Excretion in breast milk unknown/not recommended

Contraindications Hypersensitivity to amlodipine or any component of the formulation

Warnings/Precautions Increased angina and/or MI has occurred with initiation or dosage titration of calcium channel blockers. Symptomatic hypotension with or without syncope can rarely occur; blood pressure must be lowered at a rate appropriate for the patient's clinical condition. Use caution in severe aortic stenosis and/or hypertrophic cardiomyopathy. Use caution in patients with hepatic impairment. The most common side effect is peripheral edema; occurs within 2-3 weeks of starting therapy. Reflex tachycardia may occur with use. Dosage titration should occur after 7-14 days on a given dose. Initiate at a lower dose in the elderly. Safety and efficacy have not been established in children <6 years of age.

Adverse Reactions

>10%: Cardiovascular: Peripheral edema (2% to 15% dose related)

1% to 10%:

Cardiovascular: Flushing (1% to 3%), palpitation (1% to 4%)

Central nervous system: Headache (7%; similar to placebo 8%), dizziness (1% to 3%), fatigue (4%), somnolence (1% to 2%)

Dermatologic: Rash (1% to 2%), pruritus (1% to 2%)

Endocrine & metabolic: Male sexual dysfunction (1% to 2%)

Gastrointestinal: Nausea (3%), abdominal pain (1% to 2%), dyspepsia (1% to 2%), gingival hyperplasia

Neuromuscular & skeletal: Muscle cramps (1% to 2%), weakness (1% to 2%)

Respiratory: Dyspnea (1% to 2%), pulmonary edema (15% from PRAISE trial, CHF population)

<1% (Limited to important or life-threatening): Abnormal dreams, agitation alopecia, amnesia, anxiety, apathy, arrhythmia, ataxia, bradycardia, cardiac failure, cholestasis, depersonalization, depression, erythema multiforme, exfoliative dermatitis, extrapyramidal symptoms, gastritis, gynecomastia, hepatitis, hypotension, jaundice, leukocytoclastic vasculitis, migraine, non-thrombocytopenic purpura, paresthesia, peripheral ischemia, photosensitivity, postural hypotension, purpura, rash, skin discoloration, Stevens-Johnson syndrome, syncope, thrombocytopenia, tinnitus, transaminases increased, urticaria, weight loss, vertigo, xerophthalmia

Metabolism/Transport Effects **Substrate** of CYP3A4 (major); **Inhibits** CYP1A2 (moderate), 2A6 (weak), 2B6 (weak), 2C8 (weak), 2C9 (weak), 2D6 (weak), 3A4 (weak)

Drug Interactions

Alpha1-Blockers: May enhance the hypotensive effect of Calcium Channel Blockers. *Risk C: Monitor therapy*

Antifungal Agents (Azole Derivatives, Systemic): May decrease the metabolism of Calcium Channel Blockers. *Risk D: Consider therapy modification*

Barbiturates: May increase the metabolism of Calcium Channel Blockers. *Risk D: Consider therapy modification*

Calcium Channel Blockers (Nondihydropyridine): May enhance the hypotensive effect of Calcium Channel Blockers (Dihydropyridine). Calcium Channel Blockers (Nondihydropyridine) may decrease the metabolism of Calcium Channel Blockers (Dihydropyridine). *Risk C: Monitor therapy*

Calcium Salts: May diminish the therapeutic effect of Calcium Channel Blockers. *Risk C: Monitor therapy*

CarBAMazepine: May increase the metabolism of Calcium Channel Blockers (Dihydropyridine). *Risk C: Monitor therapy*

CycloSPORINE: May decrease the metabolism of Calcium Channel Blockers (Dihydropyridine). Nicardipine may likewise inhibit the metabolism of cyclosporine. Cyclosporine dosage adjustments might be needed. *Risk C: Monitor therapy*

CYP1A2 Substrates: CYP1A2 Inhibitors (Moderate) may decrease the metabolism of CYP1A2 Substrates. *Risk C: Monitor therapy*

CYP3A4 Inducers (Strong): May increase the metabolism of CYP3A4 Substrates. *Risk C: Monitor therapy*

CYP3A4 Inhibitors (Moderate): May decrease the metabolism of CYP3A4 Substrates. *Risk C: Monitor therapy*

CYP3A4 Inhibitors (Strong): May decrease the metabolism of CYP3A4 Substrates. *Risk D: Consider therapy modification*

Dasatinib: May increase the serum concentration of CYP3A4 Substrates. *Risk C: Monitor therapy*

Deferasirox: May decrease the serum concentration of CYP3A4 Substrates. *Risk C: Monitor therapy*

Diazoxide: May enhance the hypotensive effect of Antihypertensives. *Risk C: Monitor therapy*

Fluconazole: May decrease the metabolism of Calcium Channel Blockers. *Risk C: Monitor therapy*

Grapefruit Juice: May decrease the metabolism of Calcium Channel Blockers. *Risk C: Monitor therapy*

Herbs (CYP3A4 Inducers): May increase the metabolism of CYP3A4 Substrates. *Risk C: Monitor therapy*

Herbs (Hypertensive Properties): May diminish the antihypertensive effect of Antihypertensives. *Risk C: Monitor therapy*

Herbs (Hypotensive Properties): May enhance the hypotensive effect of Antihypertensives. *Risk C: Monitor therapy*

Macrolide Antibiotics: May decrease the metabolism of Calcium Channel Blockers. **Exceptions:** Azithromycin; Dirithromycin [Off Market]; Spiramycin. *Risk D: Consider therapy modification*

Magnesium Salts: Calcium Channel Blockers may enhance the adverse/toxic effect of Magnesium Salts. Magnesium Salts may enhance the hypotensive effect of Calcium Channel Blockers. *Risk C: Monitor therapy*

Methylphenidate: May diminish the antihypertensive effect of Antihypertensives. *Risk C: Monitor therapy*

Nafcillin: May increase the metabolism of Calcium Channel Blockers. *Risk D: Consider therapy modification*

Neuromuscular-Blocking Agents (Nondepolarizing): Calcium Channel Blockers may enhance the neuromuscular-blocking effect of Neuromuscular-Blocking Agents (Nondepolarizing). *Risk C: Monitor therapy*

Nitroprusside: Calcium Channel Blockers may enhance the hypotensive effect of Nitroprusside. *Risk C: Monitor therapy*

Phenytoin: Calcium Channel Blockers may decrease the metabolism of Phenytoin. *Risk D: Consider therapy modification*

Prostacyclin Analogues: May enhance the hypotensive effect of Antihypertensives. *Risk C: Monitor therapy*

Protease Inhibitors: May decrease the metabolism of Calcium Channel Blockers (Dihydropyridine). *Risk D: Consider therapy modification*

QuiNIDine: Calcium Channel Blockers (Dihydropyridine) may decrease the serum concentration of QuiNIDine. *Risk C: Monitor therapy*

Quinupristin: May decrease the metabolism of Calcium Channel Blockers. *Risk C: Monitor therapy*

Rifamycin Derivatives: May increase the metabolism of Calcium Channel Blockers. This primarily affects oral forms of calcium channel blockers. *Risk D: Consider therapy modification*

RiTUXimab: Antihypertensives may enhance the hypotensive effect of RiTUXimab. *Risk D: Consider therapy modification*

Tacrolimus: Calcium Channel Blockers (Dihydropyridine) may increase the serum concentration of Tacrolimus. *Risk C: Monitor therapy*

Ethanol/Nutrition/Herb Interactions

Food: Grapefruit juice may modestly increase amlodipine levels.

Herb/Nutraceutical: St John's wort may decrease amlodipine levels. Avoid dong quai if using for hypertension (has estrogenic activity). Avoid ephedra, yohimbe, ginseng (may worsen hypertension). Avoid garlic (may have increased antihypertensive effects).

Stability Store at room temperature of 15°C to 30°C (59°F to 86°F).

Mechanism of Action Inhibits calcium ion from entering the "slow channels" or select voltage-sensitive areas of vascular smooth muscle and myocardium during depolarization, producing a relaxation of coronary vascular smooth muscle and coronary vasodilation; increases myocardial oxygen delivery in patients with vasospastic angina

Pharmacodynamics/Kinetics

Onset of action: Antihypertensive: 30-50 minutes

Duration of antihypertensive effect: 24 hours

Absorption: Oral: Well absorbed

Distribution: V_d: 21 L/kg

Protein binding: 93% to 98%

Metabolism: Hepatic (>90%) to inactive metabolite

Bioavailability: 64% to 90%

Half-life elimination: 30-50 hours; increased with hepatic dysfunction

Time to peak, plasma: 6-12 hours

Excretion: Urine (10% as parent, 60% as metabolite)

Dosage Oral:

Children 6-17 years: Hypertension: 2.5-5 mg once daily

Adults:

Hypertension: Initial dose: 5 mg once daily; maximum dose: 10 mg once daily. In general, titrate in 2.5 mg increments over 7-14 days. Usual dosage range (JNC 7): 2.5-10 mg once daily.

Angina: Usual dose: 5-10 mg; lower dose suggested in elderly or hepatic impairment; most patients require 10 mg for adequate effect

Elderly: Dosing should start at the lower end of dosing range due to possible increased incidence of hepatic, renal, or cardiac impairment. Elderly patients also show decreased clearance of amlodipine.

Hypertension: 2.5 mg once daily

Angina: 5 mg once daily

Dialysis: Hemodialysis and peritoneal dialysis does not enhance elimination. Supplemental dose is not necessary.

Dosage adjustment in hepatic impairment:

Angina: Administer 5 mg once daily.

Hypertension: Administer 2.5 mg once daily.

Dietary Considerations May be taken without regard to meals.

Administration May be administered without regard to meals.

Monitoring Parameters Heart rate, blood pressure, peripheral edema

Dosage Forms Excipient information presented when available (limited, particularly for generics); consult specific product labeling.

Tablet: 2.5 mg, 5 mg, 10 mg

Norvasc®: 2.5 mg, 5 mg, 10 mg

Amlodipine and Atorvastatin (am LOW di peen & a TORE va sta tin)

U.S. Brand Names Caduet®

Canadian Brand Names Caduet®

Mexican Brand Names Caduet

Index Terms Atorvastatin Calcium and Amlodipine Besylate

Pharmacologic Category Antilipemic Agent, HMG-CoA Reductase Inhibitor; Calcium Channel Blocker

Use For use when treatment with both amlodipine and atorvastatin is appropriate:

Amlodipine: Treatment of hypertension; treatment of symptomatic chronic stable angina, vasospastic (Prinzmetal's) angina (confirmed or suspected); prevention of hospitalization due to angina with documented CAD (limited to patients without heart failure or ejection fraction <40%)

Atorvastatin: Treatment of dyslipidemias or primary prevention of cardiovascular disease (atherosclerotic) as detailed here:

Primary prevention of cardiovascular disease (high-risk for CVD): To reduce the risk of MI or stroke in patients without evidence of heart disease who have multiple CVD risk factors or type 2 diabetes. Treatment reduces the risk for angina or revascularization procedures in patients with multiple risk factors.

Treatment of dyslipidemias: To reduce elevations in total cholesterol, LDL-C, apolipoprotein B, and triglycerides in patients with elevations of one or more components, and/or to increase HDL-C as present in heterozygous hypercholesterolemia (Fredrickson type IIa hyperlipidemias); treatment of primary dysbetalipoproteinemia (Fredrickson type III), elevated serum TG levels (Fredrickson type IV), and homozygous familial hypercholesterolemia

Treatment of heterozygous familial hypercholesterolemia (HeFH) in adolescent patients (10-17 years of age, females >1 year postmenarche) having LDL-C ≥190 mg/dL or LDL-C ≥160 mg/dL with positive family history of premature cardiovascular disease (CVD) or with two or more CVD risk factors.

Effect on Mental Status May cause drowsiness; may rarely produce insomnia, nervousness, or euphoria
Effect on Psychiatric Treatment None reported
Dosage Summary
Oral:
Children <10 years: Dosage not established
Children 10-17 years (females >1 year postmenarche): 2.5-10 mg (amlodipine) and 10-80 mg (atorvastatin) once daily (maximum: amlodipine 10 mg/day; atorvastatin 80 mg/day)
Adults: 2.5-10 mg (amlodipine) and 10-80 mg (atorvastatin) once daily (maximum: amlodipine 10 mg/day; atorvastatin 80 mg/day)
Dosage Forms Excipient information presented when available (limited, particularly for generics); consult specific product labeling.
Tablet:
Caduet®
2.5/10: Amlodipine 2.5 mg and atorvastatin 10 mg
2.5/20: Amlodipine 2.5 mg and atorvastatin 20 mg
2.5/40: Amlodipine 2.5 mg and atorvastatin 40 mg
5/10: Amlodipine 5 mg and atorvastatin 10 mg
5/20: Amlodipine 5 mg and atorvastatin 20 mg
5/40: Amlodipine 5 mg and atorvastatin 40 mg
5/80: Amlodipine 5 mg and atorvastatin 80 mg
10/10: Amlodipine 10 mg and atorvastatin 10 mg
10/20: Amlodipine 10 mg and atorvastatin 20 mg
10/40: Amlodipine 10 mg and atorvastatin 40 mg
10/80: Amlodipine 10 mg and atorvastatin 80 mg

Amlodipine and Benazepril (am LOE di peen & ben AY ze pril)

U.S. Brand Names Lotrel®
Index Terms Benazepril Hydrochloride and Amlodipine Besylate
Pharmacologic Category Angiotensin-Converting Enzyme (ACE) Inhibitor; Calcium Channel Blocker
Use Treatment of hypertension
Effect on Mental Status May cause drowsiness; rarely may produce insomnia and nervousness
Effect on Psychiatric Treatment May decrease lithium clearance resulting in an increase in serum lithium levels and potential lithium toxicity; monitor serum lithium levels
Dosage Summary
Oral:
Children: Dosage not established
Adults: 2.5-10 mg (amlodipine) and 10-40 mg (benazepril) once daily (maximum: amlodipine 10 mg/day; benazepril 40 mg/day)
Elderly: Initial: 2.5 mg/day (based on amlodipine component)
Dosage Forms Excipient information presented when available (limited, particularly for generics); consult specific product labeling.
Capsule:
2.5/10: Amlodipine 2.5 mg and benazepril hydrochloride 10 mg
5/10: Amlodipine 5 mg and benazepril hydrochloride 10 mg
5/20: Amlodipine 5 mg and benazepril hydrochloride 20 mg
10/20: Amlodipine 10 mg and benazepril hydrochloride 20 mg
Lotrel® 2.5/10: Amlodipine 2.5 mg and benazepril hydrochloride 10 mg
Lotrel® 5/10: Amlodipine 5 mg and benazepril hydrochloride 10 mg
Lotrel® 5/20: Amlodipine 5 mg and benazepril hydrochloride 20 mg
Lotrel® 5/40: Amlodipine 5 mg and benazepril hydrochloride 40 mg
Lotrel® 10/20: Amlodipine 10 mg and benazepril hydrochloride 20 mg
Lotrel® 10/40: Amlodipine 10 mg and benazepril hydrochloride 40 mg

Amlodipine and Olmesartan (am LOE di peen & olme SAR tan)

U.S. Brand Names Azor™
Index Terms Amlodipine Besylate and Olmesartan Medoxomil; Olmesartan and Amlodipine
Pharmacologic Category Angiotensin II Receptor Blocker; Calcium Channel Blocker

Use Treatment of hypertension

Effect on Mental Status May cause drowsiness or dizziness; may rarely produce insomnia and nervousness

Effect on Psychiatric Treatment May cause hypotension, hyperglycemia, and hypertriglyceridemia; combined use with psychotropics (atypical antipsychotics and mirtazapine) may produce additive effects, May cause diarrhea, these effects may be additive with concurrent use of SSRIs, lithium, or valproate. May cause flu-like symptoms, take this into consideration if also concerned about SSRI discontinuation syndrome. Combined use with lithium may produce lithium toxicity; monitor lithium levels.

Dosage Summary

Oral:

Children: Dosage not established

Adults: Amlodipine 5-10 mg and olmesartan 20-40 mg once daily (maximum: 10 mg/day [amlodipine]; 40 mg/day [olmesartan]); **Note:** Titration is recommended

Dosage Forms Excipient information presented when available (limited, particularly for generics); consult specific product labeling.

Tablet:

Azor™:

5/20: Amlodipine besylate 5 mg and olmesartan medoxomil 20 mg
5/40: Amlodipine besylate 5 mg and olmesartan medoxomil 40 mg
10/20: Amlodipine besylate 10 mg and olmesartan medoxomil 20 mg
10/40: Amlodipine besylate 10 mg and olmesartan medoxomil 40 mg

Amlodipine and Valsartan (am LOE di peen & val SAR tan)

U.S. Brand Names Exforge®

Index Terms Amlodipine Besylate and Valsartan; Valsartan and Amlodipine

Pharmacologic Category Angiotensin II Receptor Blocker; Calcium Channel Blocker

Use Treatment of hypertension

Effect on Mental Status Headache is common; may cause anxiety, dizziness, or somnolence; may rarely cause insomnia and nervousness

Effect on Psychiatric Treatment May cause symptomatic hypotension; concomitant use with psychotropic agents may produce additive effects; monitor. Conversely, amphetamines may decrease the antihypertensive effects of valsartan. May increase the risk of lithium toxicity; monitor lithium levels.

Dosage Summary

Oral:

Children: Dosage not established

Adults: Amlodipine 5-10 mg and valsartan 160-320 mg once daily (maximum: 10 mg/day [amlodipine]; 320 mg/day [valsartan]. **Note:** Titration is recommended

Dosage Forms Excipient information presented when available (limited, particularly for generics); consult specific product labeling.

Tablet:

Exforge®:

5/160: Amlodipine 5 mg and valsartan 160 mg
5/320 mg: Amlodipine 5 mg and valsartan 320 mg
10/160: Amlodipine 10 mg and valsartan 160 mg
10/320: Amlodipine 10 mg and valsartan 320 mg

◆ **Amlodipine Besylate** *see* AmLODIPine *on page 100*

◆ **Amlodipine Besylate and Olmesartan Medoxomil** *see* Amlodipine and Olmesartan *on page 104*

◆ **Amlodipine Besylate and Valsartan** *see* Amlodipine and Valsartan *on page 105*

◆ **AMN107** *see* Nilotinib *on page 1140*

◆ **Amnesteem™** *see* Isotretinoin *on page 871*

Amobarbital (am oh BAR bi tal)

U.S. Brand Names Amytal®

Canadian Brand Names Amytal®

Index Terms Amobarbital Sodium; Amylobarbitone

Pharmacologic Category Barbiturate; General Anesthetic; Hypnotic; Sedative

Generic Available No

Use Hypnotic in short-term treatment of insomnia; reduce anxiety and provide sedation preoperatively

Unlabeled/Investigational Use Therapeutic or diagnostic "Amytal® Interviewing"; Wada test

Restrictions C-II

Pregnancy Risk Factor D

Pregnancy Considerations Barbiturates cross the placenta and distribute in fetal tissue. Teratogenic effects have been reported with 1st trimester exposure. Exposure during the 3rd trimester may lead to symptoms of acute withdrawal following delivery; symptoms may be delayed up to 14 days.

Lactation Excretion in breast milk unknown/use caution

Contraindications Hypersensitivity to barbiturates or any component of the formulation; marked hepatic impairment; dyspnea or airway obstruction; porphyria

Warnings/Precautions Tolerance to hypnotic effect can occur; do not use for >2 weeks to treat insomnia. Potential for drug dependency exists, abrupt cessation may precipitate withdrawal, including status epilepticus in epileptic patients. Do not administer to patients in acute or chronic pain. Use caution in elderly, debilitated, renally impaired, hepatic dysfunction, or pediatric patients. May cause paradoxical responses, including agitation and hyperactivity, particularly in acute pain and pediatric patients. An increased risk for hazardous sleep-related activities such as sleep-driving; cooking and eating food, and making phone calls while asleep has been noted with sedative-hypnotic medications. Discontinue treatment in patients who report a sleep-driving episode. Use with caution in patients with depression or suicidal tendencies, or in patients with a history of drug abuse. Tolerance, psychological and physical dependence may occur with prolonged use.

May cause CNS depression, which may impair physical or mental abilities. Patients must be cautioned about performing tasks which require mental alertness (eg, operating machinery or driving). Effects with other sedative drugs or ethanol may be potentiated. Use of this agent as a hypnotic in the elderly is not recommended.

May cause respiratory depression or hypotension, particularly when administered rapidly intravenously. Solution for injection is highly alkaline and extravasation may cause local tissue damage. Safety and efficacy have not been established in patients <6 years of age; use with caution in patients ≥6 years of age.

Adverse Reactions Frequency not defined and is reported as barbiturate use (not specifically amobarbital).

Cardiovascular: Bradycardia, hypotension, syncope

Central nervous system: Agitation, anxiety, ataxia, confusion, CNS depression, dizziness, fever, hallucinations, headache, insomnia, nightmares, nervousness, psychiatric disturbances, somnolence, thinking abnormal

Gastrointestinal: Constipation, nausea, vomiting

Hematologic: Megaloblastic anemia (following chronic phenobarbital use)

Hepatic: Liver damage

Local: Injection site reaction

Neuromuscular & skeletal: Hyperkinesia

Respiratory: Apnea, atelectasis (postoperative), hypoventilation

Miscellaneous: Hypersensitivity reaction (including angioedema, rash, and exfoliative dermatitis)

Metabolism/Transport Effects Induces CYP2A6 (strong)

Drug Interactions

Acetaminophen: Barbiturates may increase the metabolism of Acetaminophen. This may 1) diminish the effect of acetaminophen; and 2) increase the risk of liver damage. *Risk C: Monitor therapy*

Alcohol (Ethyl): CNS Depressants may enhance the CNS depressant effect of Alcohol (Ethyl). *Risk C: Monitor therapy*

Beta-Blockers: Barbiturates may decrease the serum concentration of Beta-Blockers. **Exceptions:** Atenolol; Levobunolol; Metipranolol; Nadolol. *Risk C: Monitor therapy*

Calcium Channel Blockers: Barbiturates may increase the metabolism of Calcium Channel Blockers. **Exceptions:** Clevidipine. *Risk D: Consider therapy modification*

Chloramphenicol: May decrease the metabolism of Barbiturates. Barbiturates may increase the metabolism of Chloramphenicol. *Risk D: Consider therapy modification*

CNS Depressants: May enhance the adverse/toxic effect of other CNS Depressants. *Risk C: Monitor therapy*

Contraceptive (Progestins): Barbiturates may diminish the therapeutic effect of Contraceptive (Progestins). Contraceptive failure is possible. *Risk D: Consider therapy modification*

Corticosteroids (Systemic): Barbiturates may increase the metabolism of Corticosteroids (Systemic). *Risk C: Monitor therapy*

CycloSPORINE: Barbiturates may increase the metabolism of CycloSPORINE. *Risk D: Consider therapy modification*

CYP2A6 Substrates: CYP2A6 Inducers (Strong) may increase the metabolism of CYP2A6 Substrates. *Risk C: Monitor therapy*

Disopyramide: Barbiturates may increase the metabolism of Disopyramide. *Risk D: Consider therapy modification*

Doxycycline: Barbiturates may decrease the serum concentration of Doxycycline. *Risk D: Consider therapy modification*

Etoposide: Barbiturates may increase the metabolism of Etoposide. *Risk C: Monitor therapy*

Etoposide Phosphate: Barbiturates may decrease the serum concentration of Etoposide Phosphate. Barbiturates may increase the metabolism, via CYP isoenzymes, of etoposide phosphate. *Risk C: Monitor therapy*

Felbamate: May increase the serum concentration of Barbiturates. *Risk C: Monitor therapy*

Griseofulvin: Barbiturates may decrease the absorption of Griseofulvin. *Risk D: Consider therapy modification*

LamoTRIgine: Barbiturates may increase the metabolism of LamoTRIgine. *Risk D: Consider therapy modification*

Meperidine: Barbiturates may enhance the CNS depressant effect of Meperidine. *Risk C: Monitor therapy*

Methadone: Barbiturates may increase the metabolism of Methadone. *Risk D: Consider therapy modification*

Oral Contraceptive (Estrogens): Barbiturates may diminish the therapeutic effect of Oral Contraceptive (Estrogens). Contraceptive failure is possible. *Risk D: Consider therapy modification*

Primidone: May enhance the adverse/toxic effect of Barbiturates. Primidone is converted to phenobarbital, and thus becomes additive with existing barbiturate therapy. *Risk C: Monitor therapy*

Propafenone: Barbiturates may increase the metabolism of Propafenone. *Risk D: Consider therapy modification*

Pyridoxine: May increase the metabolism of Barbiturates. Apparent in high pyridoxine doses (eg, 200 mg/day) *Risk C: Monitor therapy*

QuiNIDine: Barbiturates may increase the metabolism of QuiNIDine. *Risk D: Consider therapy modification*

Rifamycin Derivatives: May increase the metabolism of Barbiturates. *Risk C: Monitor therapy*

Teniposide: Barbiturates may increase the metabolism of Teniposide. *Risk C: Monitor therapy*

Theophylline Derivatives: Barbiturates may increase the metabolism of Theophylline Derivatives. **Exceptions:** Dyphylline. *Risk C: Monitor therapy*

Tricyclic Antidepressants: Barbiturates may increase the metabolism of Tricyclic Antidepressants. *Risk D: Consider therapy modification*

Valproic Acid: May decrease the metabolism of Barbiturates. Barbiturates may decrease the serum concentration of Valproic Acid. *Risk C: Monitor therapy*

Vitamin K Antagonists (eg, warfarin): Barbiturates may increase the metabolism of Vitamin K Antagonists. *Risk D: Consider therapy modification*

Voriconazole: Barbiturates may decrease the serum concentration of Voriconazole. *Risk X: Avoid combination*

Ethanol/Nutrition/Herb Interactions Ethanol: Avoid ethanol (may increase CNS depression).

Stability Powder should be stored at 15°C to 30°C (59°F to 86°F). Reconstitute with SWFI to make a 10% I.V. solution; a 20% solution may be made for I.M. use. Rotate vial to dissolve, do not shake. Do not use unless a clear solution forms within 5 minutes. Following reconstitution, solution should be used within 30 minutes.

Mechanism of Action Interferes with transmission of impulses from the thalamus to the cortex of the brain resulting in an imbalance in central inhibitory and facilitatory mechanisms

Pharmacodynamics/Kinetics

Onset of action: I.V.: Within 5 minutes

Distribution: Readily crosses placenta; small amounts enter breast milk

Metabolism: Primarily hepatic via microsomal enzymes

Half-life elimination: 15-40 hours (mean: 25 hours)

Excretion: Urine, feces

Dosage

Children:

Sedative: I.M., I.V.: 6-12 years: Manufacturer's dosing range: 65-500 mg

Hypnotic (unlabeled use): I.M.: 2-3 mg/kg (maximum: 500 mg)

Adults:

Hypnotic: I.M., I.V.: 65-200 mg at bedtime (maximum single dose: 1000 mg)

Sedative: I.M., I.V.: 30-50 mg 2-3 times/day (maximum single dose: 1000 mg)

"Amytal® interview" (unlabeled use): I.V.: 50-100 mg/minute for total dose of 200-1000 mg or until patient experiences drowsiness, impaired attention, slurred speech, or nystagmus

Wada test (unlabeled use): Intra-arterial: 100 mg over 4-5 seconds via percutaneous transfemoral catheter

Dosing adjustment in renal/hepatic impairment: Dosing should be reduced; specific recommendations not available.

Administration

I.M.: Administer deeply into a large muscle. Do not use more than 5 mL at any single site (may cause tissue damage). I.M. dosages should not exceed 500 mg. Use 20% solution to facilitate larger doses.

I.V.: Use only when I.M. administration is not feasible. Administer by slow I.V. injection (maximum: 50 mg/minute in adults).

Monitoring Parameters Vital signs should be monitored during injection and for several hours after administration.

Reference Range

Therapeutic: 1-5 mcg/mL (SI: 4-22 μmol/L)

Toxic: >10 mcg/mL (SI: >44 μmol/L)

Lethal: >50 mcg/mL

Dosage Forms Excipient information presented when available (limited, particularly for generics); consult specific product labeling.

Injection, powder for reconstitution, as sodium:

Amytal®: 500 mg

◆ **Amobarbital Sodium** *see* Amobarbital *on page 105*

◆ **Amoclan** *see* Amoxicillin and Clavulanate Potassium *on page 115*

Amonafide (a MON a fide)

Index Terms Amonafide Hydrochloride; Benzisoquinolinedione; BIDA; M-FA-142; Nafidimide; NSC-308847

Pharmacologic Category Antineoplastic Agent, DNA Binding Agent; Enzyme Inhibitor, Topoisomerase II Inhibitor

Unlabeled/Investigational Use Investigational: Breast, prostate, renal cell, ovarian, pancreatic, and nonsmall cell lung cancers

Effect on Mental Status May cause dizziness and sedation

Effect on Psychiatric Treatment Granulocytopenia is common; use caution with clozapine; monitor

Dosage Forms Excipient information presented when available (limited, particularly for generics); consult specific product labeling.

Powder for injection, lyophilized: 500 mg

◆ **Amonafide Hydrochloride** *see* Amonafide *on page 108*

Amoxapine (a MOKS a peen)

Medication Safety Issues

Sound-alike/look-alike issues:

Amoxapine may be confused with amoxicillin, Amoxil®

Asendin may be confused with aspirin

Related Information

Anticholinergic Effects of Common Psychotropics *on page 1758*

Antidepressant Agents *on page 1760*

Antidepressant Receptor Profile *on page 1764*

Discontinuation of Psychotropic Drugs *on page 1839*

Index Terms Asendin [DSC]

Pharmacologic Category Antidepressant, Tricyclic (Secondary Amine)

Generic Available Yes

Use Treatment of depression, psychotic depression, depression accompanied by anxiety or agitation

Mental Health Comment Amoxapine's metabolite (7-OH-amoxapine) blocks dopamine receptors. Therefore, extrapyramidal side effects noted with antipsychotic agents may also be seen with this antidepressant. May be useful as a third-line agent to treat depression with psychotic features. Generally not recommended for elderly patients.

Restrictions An FDA-approved medication guide concerning the use of antidepressants in children, adolescents, and young adults must be distributed when dispensing an outpatient prescription (new or refill) where this medication is to be used without direct supervision of a healthcare provider. Medication guides are available at http://www.fda.gov/cder/Offices/ODS/medication_guides.htm. Dispense to parents or guardians of children and adolescents receiving this medication.

Pregnancy Risk Factor C

Lactation Enters breast milk/contraindicated (AAP rates "of concern")

Contraindications Hypersensitivity to amoxapine or any component of the formulation; use of MAO inhibitors within past 14 days; acute recovery phase following myocardial infarction

Warnings/Precautions [U.S. Boxed Warning]: Antidepressants increase the risk of suicidal thinking and behavior in children, adolescents, and young adults (18-24 years of age) with major depressive disorder (MDD) and other psychiatric disorders; consider risk prior to prescribing. Short-term studies did not show an increased risk in patients >24 years of age and showed a decreased risk in patients ≥65 years. Closely monitor for clinical worsening, suicidality, or unusual changes in behavior; the patient's family or caregiver should be instructed to closely observe the patient and communicate condition with healthcare provider. A medication guide should be dispensed with each prescription. **Amoxapine is not FDA approved for use in patients <16 years of age.**

The possibility of a suicide attempt is inherent in major depression and may persist until remission occurs. Monitor for worsening of depression or suicidality, especially during initiation of therapy (generally first 1-2 months) or with dose increases or decreases. Use caution in high-risk patients. Worsening depression and severe abrupt suicidality that are not part of the presenting symptoms may require discontinuation or modification of drug therapy. The patient's family or caregiver should be alerted to monitor patients for the emergence of suicidality and associated behaviors (such as agitation, irritability, hostility, impulsivity, and hypomania) and notify the healthcare provider.

May worsen psychosis in some patients or precipitate a shift to mania or hypomania in patients with bipolar disorder. Patients presenting with depressive symptoms should be screened for bipolar disorder. Monotherapy in patients with bipolar disorder should be avoided. **Amoxapine is not FDA approved for bipolar depression.** May cause extrapyramidal symptoms, including pseudo-parkinsonism, acute dystonic reactions, akathisia, and tardive dyskinesia (risk of these reactions is low). May be associated with neuroleptic malignant syndrome.

The degree of sedation, anticholinergic effects, orthostasis, and conduction abnormalities are moderate relative to other antidepressants. May cause drowsiness/sedation, resulting in impaired performance of tasks requiring alertness (eg, operating machinery or driving). Sedative effects may be additive with other CNS depressants and/or ethanol. Use with caution in patients with a history of cardiovascular disease (including previous MI, stroke, tachycardia, or conduction abnormalities). Use with caution in patients with urinary retention, benign prostatic hyperplasia, narrow-angle glaucoma, xerostomia, visual problems, constipation, or a history of bowel obstruction.

Consider discontinuing, when possible, prior to elective surgery. Therapy should not be abruptly discontinued in patients receiving high doses for prolonged periods. May lower seizure threshold - use caution in patients with a previous seizure disorder or condition predisposing to seizures such as brain damage, alcoholism, or concurrent therapy with other drugs which lower the seizure threshold. May increase the risks associated with electroconvulsive therapy. Use with caution in hyperthyroid patients or those receiving thyroid supplementation. Use with caution in patients with hepatic or renal dysfunction and in elderly patients.

Adverse Reactions

>10%:

Central nervous system: Drowsiness

Gastrointestinal: Xerostomia, constipation

1% to 10%:

Central nervous system: Anxiety, ataxia, confusion, dizziness, excitement, headache, insomnia, nervousness, restlessness

Dermatologic: Edema, skin rash

Endocrine: Prolactin levels increased

Gastrointestinal: Nausea
Neuromuscular & skeletal: Tremor, weakness
Ocular: Blurred vision
Miscellaneous: Diaphoresis
<1% (Limited to important or life-threatening): Agranulocytosis, allergic reactions, diarrhea, extrapyramidal symptoms, galactorrhea, hypertension, impotence, incoordination, intraocular pressure increased, leukopenia, menstrual irregularity, mydriasis, neuroleptic malignant syndrome, numbness, painful ejaculation, paresthesia, photosensitivity, seizure, SIADH, syncope, tardive dyskinesia, testicular edema, tinnitus, urinary retention, vomiting

Metabolism/Transport Effects Substrate of CYP2D6 (major)

Drug Interactions

Acetylcholinesterase Inhibitors (Central): Anticholinergics may diminish the therapeutic effect of Acetylcholinesterase Inhibitors (Central). Acetylcholinesterase Inhibitors (Central) may diminish the therapeutic effect of Anticholinergics. If the anticholinergic action is a side effect of the agent, the result may be beneficial. *Risk C: Monitor therapy*

Alcohol (Ethyl): CNS Depressants may enhance the CNS depressant effect of Alcohol (Ethyl). *Risk C: Monitor therapy*

Alfuzosin: May enhance the QTc-prolonging effect of QTc-Prolonging Agents. *Risk C: Monitor therapy*

Alpha-/Beta-Agonists (Direct-Acting): Tricyclic Antidepressants may enhance the vasopressor effect of Alpha-/Beta-Agonists (Direct-Acting). **Exceptions:** Dipivefrin. *Risk D: Consider therapy modification*

Alpha1-Agonists: Tricyclic Antidepressants may enhance the vasopressor effect of Alpha1-Agonists. *Risk D: Consider therapy modification*

Alpha2-Agonists: Tricyclic Antidepressants may diminish the antihypertensive effect of Alpha2-Agonists. **Exceptions:** Apraclonidine; Brimonidine. *Risk D: Consider therapy modification*

Altretamine: May enhance the orthostatic effect of Tricyclic Antidepressants. *Risk C: Monitor therapy*

Amphetamines: Tricyclic Antidepressants may enhance the stimulatory effect of Amphetamines. Tricyclic Antidepressants may also potentiate the cardiovascular effects of Amphetamines. *Risk C: Monitor therapy*

Anticholinergics: May enhance the adverse/toxic effect of other Anticholinergics. **Exceptions:** Paliperidone. *Risk C: Monitor therapy*

Barbiturates: May increase the metabolism of Tricyclic Antidepressants. *Risk D: Consider therapy modification*

Beta2-Agonists: Tricyclic Antidepressants may enhance the adverse/toxic effect of Beta2-Agonists. *Risk C: Monitor therapy*

CarBAMazepine: May increase the metabolism of Tricyclic Antidepressants. *Risk C: Monitor therapy*

Cimetidine: May decrease the metabolism of Tricyclic Antidepressants. *Risk C: Monitor therapy*

Cinacalcet: May increase the serum concentration of Tricyclic Antidepressants. *Risk C: Monitor therapy*

Ciprofloxacin: May enhance the QTc-prolonging effect of QTc-Prolonging Agents. *Risk C: Monitor therapy*

CNS Depressants: May enhance the adverse/toxic effect of other CNS Depressants. *Risk C: Monitor therapy*

CYP2D6 Inhibitors (Moderate): May decrease the metabolism of CYP2D6 Substrates. *Risk C: Monitor therapy*

CYP2D6 Inhibitors (Strong): May decrease the metabolism of CYP2D6 Substrates. *Risk D: Consider therapy modification*

Darunavir: May increase the serum concentration of CYP2D6 Substrates. *Risk C: Monitor therapy*

Desmopressin: Tricyclic Antidepressants may enhance the adverse/toxic effect of Desmopressin. *Risk C: Monitor therapy*

Dexmethylphenidate: May decrease the metabolism of Tricyclic Antidepressants. *Risk C: Monitor therapy*

DULoxetine: May decrease the metabolism of Tricyclic Antidepressants. *Risk C: Monitor therapy*

Gadobutrol: May enhance the QTc-prolonging effect of QTc-Prolonging Agents. *Risk D: Consider therapy modification*

Lithium: May enhance the neurotoxic effect of Tricyclic Antidepressants. *Risk C: Monitor therapy*

MAO Inhibitors: May enhance the serotonergic effect of Tricyclic Antidepressants. This may cause serotonin syndrome. *Risk X: Avoid combination*

Methylphenidate: May decrease the metabolism of Tricyclic Antidepressants. *Risk C: Monitor therapy*

Nilotinib: May enhance the QTc-prolonging effect of QTc-Prolonging Agents. *Risk X: Avoid combination*

Pramlintide: May enhance the anticholinergic effect of Anticholinergics. These effects are specific to the GI tract. *Risk D: Consider therapy modification*

Propoxyphene: May enhance the CNS depressant effect of Tricyclic Antidepressants. *Risk C: Monitor therapy*

Protease Inhibitors: May increase the serum concentration of Tricyclic Antidepressants. *Risk C: Monitor therapy*

QTc-Prolonging Agents: May enhance the adverse/toxic effect of other QTc-Prolonging Agents. Their effects can be additive, causing life-threatening ventricular arrhythmias. *Risk D: Consider therapy modification*

QuiNIDine: Tricyclic Antidepressants may enhance the QTc-prolonging effect of QuiNIDine. QuiNIDine may decrease the metabolism of Tricyclic Antidepressants. *Risk D: Consider therapy modification*

Selective Serotonin Reuptake Inhibitors: May decrease the metabolism of Tricyclic Antidepressants. *Risk D: Consider therapy modification*

Serotonin Modulators: May enhance the adverse/toxic effect of other Serotonin Modulators. The development of serotonin syndrome may occur. *Risk D: Consider therapy modification*

Sibutramine: May enhance the serotonergic effect of Serotonin Modulators. This may cause serotonin syndrome. *Risk X: Avoid combination*

St Johns Wort: May increase the metabolism of Tricyclic Antidepressants. The risk of serotonin syndrome may theoretically be increased. *Risk D: Consider therapy modification*

Sulfonylureas: Cyclic Antidepressants may enhance the hypoglycemic effect of Sulfonylureas. *Risk C: Monitor therapy*

Terbinafine: May decrease the metabolism of Tricyclic Antidepressants. *Risk D: Consider therapy modification*

Tetrabenazine: QTc-Prolonging Agents may enhance the QTc-prolonging effect of Tetrabenazine. *Risk X: Avoid combination*

Thioridazine: QTc-Prolonging Agents may enhance the QTc-prolonging effect of Thioridazine. *Risk X: Avoid combination*

TraMADol: Tricyclic Antidepressants may enhance the neuroexcitatory and/or seizure-potentiating effect of TraMADol. *Risk C: Monitor therapy*

Valproic Acid: May increase the serum concentration of Tricyclic Antidepressants. *Risk C: Monitor therapy*

Vitamin K Antagonists (eg, warfarin): Tricyclic Antidepressants may enhance the anticoagulant effect of Vitamin K Antagonists. *Risk C: Monitor therapy*

Ziprasidone: QTc-Prolonging Agents may enhance the QTc-prolonging effect of Ziprasidone. The risk of a severe arrhythmia may be increased. *Risk X: Avoid combination*

Ethanol/Nutrition/Herb Interactions

Ethanol: Avoid ethanol (may increase CNS depression).

Food: Grapefruit juice may inhibit the metabolism of some TCAs and clinical toxicity may result.

Herb/Nutraceutical: Avoid valerian, St John's wort, SAMe, kava kava.

Mechanism of Action Reduces the reuptake of serotonin and norepinephrine. The metabolite, 7-OH-amoxapine has significant dopamine receptor blocking activity similar to haloperidol.

Pharmacodynamics/Kinetics

Onset of antidepressant effect: Usually occurs after 1-2 weeks, but may require 4-6 weeks

Absorption: Rapid and well absorbed

Distribution: V_d: 0.9-1.2 L/kg; enters breast milk

Protein binding: 80%

Metabolism: Primarily hepatic

Half-life elimination: Parent drug: 11-16 hours; Active metabolite (8-hydroxy): Adults: 30 hours

Time to peak, serum: 1-2 hours

Excretion: Urine (as unchanged drug and metabolites)

Dosage Oral:

Children: Not established in children <16 years of age.

Adolescents: Initial: 25-50 mg/day; increase gradually to 100 mg/day; may administer as divided doses or as a single dose at bedtime

Adults: Initial: 25 mg 2-3 times/day, if tolerated, dosage may be increased to 100 mg 2-3 times/day; may be given in a single bedtime dose when dosage <300 mg/day

Elderly: Initial: 25 mg at bedtime increased by 25 mg weekly for outpatients and every 3 days for inpatients if tolerated; usual dose: 50-150 mg/day, but doses up to 300 mg may be necessary

Maximum daily dose:

Inpatient: 600 mg

Outpatient: 400 mg

Administration May be administered with food to decrease GI distress.

Monitoring Parameters Monitor blood pressure and pulse rate prior to and during initial therapy evaluate mental status, suicidal ideation (especially at the beginning of therapy or when doses are increased or decreased); monitor weight; ECG in older adults

Reference Range Therapeutic: Amoxapine: 20-100 ng/mL (SI: 64-319 nmol/L); 8-OH amoxapine: 150-400 ng/mL (SI: 478-1275 nmol/L); both: 200-500 ng/mL (SI: 637-1594 nmol/L)

Test Interactions Increased glucose, liver function tests; decreased WBC

Additional Information Extrapyramidal reactions and tardive dyskinesia may occur.

Dosage Forms Excipient information presented when available (limited, particularly for generics); consult specific product labeling.

Tablet: 25 mg, 50 mg, 100 mg, 150 mg

Amoxicillin (a moks i SIL in)

Medication Safety Issues

Sound-alike/look-alike issues:

Amoxicillin may be confused with amoxapine, Amoxil®, Atarax®

Amoxil® may be confused with amoxapine, amoxicillin

International issues:

Fisamox® [Australia] may be confused with Fosamax® which is a brand name for alendronate in the U.S.

Fisamox® [Australia] may be confused with Vigamox™ which is a brand name for moxifloxacin in the U.S.

U.S. Brand Names Amoxil®

Canadian Brand Names Apo-Amoxi®; Gen-Amoxicillin; Lin-Amox; Novamoxin®; Nu-Amoxi; PHL-Amoxicillin; PMS-Amoxicillin

Mexican Brand Names Acimox; Amicil; Amobay; Amoxifur; Amoxil; Amoxinova; Amoxisol; Amoxivet; Bimxan; Dimopen; Gimalxina; Hidramox; Penamox; Polymox; Solciclina; Xalyn-Or

Index Terms *p*-Hydroxyampicillin; Amoxicillin Trihydrate; Amoxycillin

Pharmacologic Category Antibiotic, Penicillin

Generic Available Yes: Excludes drops

Use Treatment of otitis media, sinusitis, and infections caused by susceptible organisms involving the respiratory tract, skin, and urinary tract; prophylaxis of infective endocarditis in patients undergoing surgical or dental procedures; as part of a multidrug regimen for *H. pylori* eradication

Unlabeled/Investigational Use Postexposure prophylaxis for anthrax exposure with documented susceptible organisms

Effect on Mental Status Rarely large doses may produce confusion, hallucinations, and depression; penicillins have been reported to cause apprehension, illusions, agitation, insomnia, depersonalization, and encephalopathy

Effect on Psychiatric Treatment Disulfiram may increase amoxicillin levels

Pregnancy Risk Factor B

Pregnancy Considerations Adverse events have not been observed in animal studies; therefore, amoxicillin is classified as pregnancy category B. There is no documented increased risk of adverse pregnancy outcome or teratogenic affects caused by amoxicillin. It is the drug of choice for the treatment of chlamydial infections in pregnancy and for anthrax prophylaxis when penicillin susceptibility is documented.

Due to pregnancy-induced physiologic changes, amoxicillin clearance is increased during pregnancy resulting in lower concentrations and smaller AUCs. Oral ampicillin-class antibiotics are poorly-absorbed during labor.

Lactation Enters breast milk/compatible

Contraindications Hypersensitivity to amoxicillin, penicillin, or any component of the formulation

Warnings/Precautions In patients with renal impairment, doses and/or frequency of administration should be modified in response to the degree of renal impairment. A high percentage of patients with infectious mononucleosis have developed rash during therapy with amoxicillin; ampicillin-class antibiotics not recommended in these patients. Serious and occasionally severe or fatal hypersensitivity (anaphylactoid) reactions have been reported in patients on penicillin therapy, especially with a history of beta-lactam hypersensitivity history of sensitivity to multiple allergens, or previous IgE-mediated reactions (eg, anaphylaxis, angioedema, urticaria). Use with caution in asthmatic patients. Prolonged use may result in fungal or bacterial superinfection including *C. difficile*-associated diarrhea (CDAD) and pseudomembranous colitis; CDAD has been observed >2 months postantibiotic treatment. Chewable tablets contain phenylalanine.

Adverse Reactions Frequency not defined.

Central nervous system: Hyperactivity, agitation, anxiety, insomnia, confusion, convulsions, behavioral changes, dizziness

Dermatologic: Acute exanthematous pustulosis, erythematous maculopapular rash, erythema multiforme, mucocutaneous candidiasis, Stevens-Johnson syndrome, exfoliative dermatitis, toxic epidermal necrolysis, hypersensitivity vasculitis, urticaria

Gastrointestinal: Black hairy tongue, nausea, diarrhea, hemorrhagic colitis, pseudomembranous colitis, tooth discoloration (brown, yellow, or gray; rare), vomiting

Hematologic: Anemia, hemolytic anemia, thrombocytopenia, thrombocytopenia purpura, eosinophilia, leukopenia, agranulocytosis

Hepatic: AST and ALT increased, cholestatic jaundice, hepatic cholestasis, acute cytolytic hepatitis

Renal: Crystalluria

Drug Interactions

Allopurinol: May enhance the potential for allergic or hypersensitivity reactions to Amoxicillin. *Risk C: Monitor therapy*

Fusidic Acid: May diminish the therapeutic effect of Penicillins. *Risk D: Consider therapy modification*

Methotrexate: Penicillins may decrease the excretion of Methotrexate. *Risk C: Monitor therapy*

Tetracycline Derivatives: May diminish the therapeutic effect of Penicillins. *Risk D: Consider therapy modification*

Typhoid Vaccine: Antibiotics may diminish the therapeutic effect of Typhoid Vaccine. Only the live attenuated Ty21a strain is affected. *Risk D: Consider therapy modification*

Uricosuric Agents: May decrease the excretion of Penicillins. *Risk C: Monitor therapy*

Stability Amoxil®: Oral suspension remains stable for 14 days at room temperature or if refrigerated (refrigeration preferred). Unit-dose antibiotic oral syringes are stable for 48 hours.

Mechanism of Action Inhibits bacterial cell wall synthesis by binding to one or more of the penicillin-binding proteins (PBPs) which in turn inhibits the final transpeptidation step of peptidoglycan synthesis in bacterial cell walls, thus inhibiting cell wall biosynthesis. Bacteria eventually lyse due to ongoing activity of cell wall autolytic enzymes (autolysins and murein hydrolases) while cell wall assembly is arrested.

Pharmacodynamics/Kinetics

Absorption: Oral: Rapid and nearly complete; food does not interfere

Distribution: Widely to most body fluids and bone; poor penetration into cells, eyes, and across normal meninges

Pleural fluids, lungs, and peritoneal fluid; high urine concentrations are attained; also into synovial fluid, liver, prostate, muscle, and gallbladder; penetrates into middle ear effusions, maxillary sinus secretions, tonsils, sputum, and bronchial secretions

CSF:blood level ratio: Normal meninges: <1%; Inflamed meninges: 8% to 90%

Protein binding: 17% to 20%

Metabolism: Partially hepatic

Half-life elimination:

Neonates, full-term: 3.7 hours

Infants and Children: 1-2 hours

Adults: Normal renal function: 0.7-1.4 hours

Cl_{cr} <10 mL/minute: 7-21 hours

Time to peak: Capsule: 2 hours; Suspension: 1 hour

Excretion: Urine (80% as unchanged drug); lower in neonates

Dosage

Usual dosage range:

Children ≤3 months: Oral: 20-30 mg/kg/day divided every 12 hours

Children >3 months and <40 kg: Oral: 20-50 mg/kg/day in divided doses every 8-12 hours

Adults: Oral: 250-500 mg every 8 hours or 500-875 mg twice daily

Indication-specific dosing:

Children >3 months and <40 kg: Oral:

Acute otitis media: 80-90 mg/kg/day divided every 12 hours

Anthrax exposure (CDC guidelines): Note: Postexposure prophylaxis only with documented susceptible organisms: 80 mg/kg/day in divided doses every 8 hours (maximum: 500 mg/dose)

Community-acquired pneumonia:
4 months to <5 years: 80-100 mg/kg/day divided every 8 hours
5-15 years: 100 mg/kg/day divided every 8 hours; **Note:** Treatment with a macrolide or doxycycline (if age >8 years) is preferred due to higher prevalence of atypical pathogens in this age group

Ear, nose, throat, genitourinary tract, or skin/skin structure infections:
Mild to moderate: 25 mg/kg/day in divided doses every 12 hours **or** 20 mg/kg/day in divided doses every 8 hours
Severe: 45 mg/kg/day in divided doses every 12 hours **or** 40 mg/kg/day in divided doses every 8 hours

Lower respiratory tract infections: 45 mg/kg/day in divided doses every 12 hours **or** 40 mg/kg/day in divided doses every 8 hours

Lyme disease: 25-50 mg/kg/day divided every 8 hours (maximum: 500 mg)

Prophylaxis against infective endocarditis: 50 mg/kg 1 hour before procedure. **Note:** American Heart Association (AHA) guidelines now recommend prophylaxis only in patients undergoing invasive procedures and in whom underlying cardiac conditions may predispose to a higher risk of adverse outcomes should infection occur. As of April 2007, routine prophylaxis for GI/GU procedures is no longer recommended by the AHA.

Adults: Oral:

Anthrax exposure (CDC guidelines): Note: Postexposure prophylaxis in pregnant or nursing women only with documented susceptible organisms: 500 mg every 8 hours

Ear, nose, throat, genitourinary tract, or skin/skin structure infections:
Mild to moderate: 500 mg every 12 hours **or** 250 mg every 8 hours
Severe: 875 mg every 12 hours **or** 500 mg every 8 hours

***Helicobacter pylori* eradication:** 1000 mg twice daily; requires combination therapy with at least one other antibiotic and an acid-suppressing agent (proton pump inhibitor or H_2 blocker)

Lower respiratory tract infections: 875 mg every 12 hours **or** 500 mg every 8 hours

Lyme disease: 500 mg every 6-8 hours (depending on size of patient) for 21-30 days

Prophylaxis against infective endocarditis: 2 g 30-60 minutes before procedure. **Note:** American Heart Association (AHA) guidelines now recommend prophylaxis only in patients undergoing invasive procedures and in whom underlying cardiac conditions may predispose to a higher risk of adverse outcomes should infection occur. As of April 2007, routine prophylaxis for GI/GU procedures is no longer recommended by the AHA.

Prophylaxis in total joint replacement patients undergoing dental procedures which produce bacteremia: 2 g 1 hour prior to procedure

Dosing interval in renal impairment: The 875 mg tablet should not be used in patients with Cl_{cr} <30 mL/minute.
Cl_{cr} 10-30 mL/minute: 250-500 mg every 12 hours
Cl_{cr} <10 mL/minute: 250-500 mg every 24 hours

Dialysis: Moderately dialyzable (20% to 50%) by hemo- or peritoneal dialysis; approximately 50 mg of amoxicillin per liter of filtrate is removed by continuous arteriovenous or venovenous hemofiltration; dose as per Cl_{cr} <10 mL/minute guidelines

Dietary Considerations May be taken with food. Amoxil® chewable contains phenylalanine 1.82 mg per 200 mg tablet, phenylalanine 3.64 mg per 400 mg tablet.

Administration Administer around-the-clock to promote less variation in peak and trough serum levels. The appropriate amount of suspension may be mixed with formula, milk, fruit juice, water, ginger ale, or cold drinks; administer dose immediately after mixing.

Some penicillins (eg, carbenicillin, ticarcillin, and piperacillin) have been shown to inactivate aminoglycosides *in vitro*. This has been observed to a greater extent with tobramycin and gentamicin, while amikacin has shown greater stability against inactivation. Concurrent use of these agents may pose a risk of reduced antibacterial efficacy *in vivo*, particularly in the setting of profound renal impairment. However, definitive clinical evidence is lacking. If combination penicillin/aminoglycoside therapy is desired in a patient with renal dysfunction, separation of doses (if feasible), and routine monitoring of aminoglycoside levels, CBC, and clinical response should be considered.

Monitoring Parameters With prolonged therapy, monitor renal, hepatic, and hematologic function periodically; assess patient at beginning and throughout therapy for infection; monitor for signs of anaphylaxis during first dose

Test Interactions May interfere with urinary glucose tests using cupric sulfate (Benedict's solution, Clinitest®)

Some penicillin derivatives may accelerate the degradation of aminoglycosides *in vitro*, leading to a potential underestimation of aminoglycoside serum concentration.

Dosage Forms Excipient information presented when available (limited, particularly for generics); consult specific product labeling. [DSC] = Discontinued product

Capsule: 250 mg, 500 mg

Amoxil®: 500 mg

Powder for oral suspension: 125 mg/5 mL (80 mL, 100 mL, 150 mL); 200 mg/5 mL (50 mL, 75 mL, 100 mL); 250 mg/5 mL (80 mL, 100 mL, 150 mL); 400 mg/5 mL (50 mL, 75 mL, 100 mL)

Amoxil®: 200 mg/5 mL (50 mL, 75 mL, 100 mL) [contains sodium benzoate; bubble gum flavor] [DSC]; 250 mg/5 mL (100 mL, 150 mL) [contains sodium benzoate; bubble gum flavor]; 400 mg/5 mL (5 mL [DSC], 50 mL [DSC], 75 mL [DSC], 100 mL) [contains sodium benzoate; bubble gum flavor]

Powder for oral suspension [drops]:

Amoxil®: 50 mg/mL (30 mL) [contains sodium benzoate; bubble gum flavor]

Tablet: 500 mg, 875 mg

Amoxil®: 500 mg, 875 mg [DSC]

Tablet, chewable: 125 mg, 200 mg, 250 mg, 400 mg

Amoxil®: 200 mg [contains phenylalanine 1.82 mg/tablet; cherry banana peppermint flavor] [DSC]; 400 mg [contains phenylalanine 3.64 mg/tablet; cherry banana peppermint flavor] [DSC]

Amoxicillin and Clavulanate Potassium

(a moks i SIL in & klav yoo LAN ate poe TASS ee um)

Medication Safety Issues

Sound-alike/look-alike issues:

Augmentin® may be confused with Azulfidine®

U.S. Brand Names Amoclan; Augmentin ES-600®; Augmentin XR®; Augmentin®

Canadian Brand Names Alti-Amoxi-Clav; Apo-Amoxi-Clav®; Augmentin®; Clavulin®; Novo-Clavamoxin; ratio-Aclavulanate

Mexican Brand Names Acarbixin; Amobay Cl; Amoxiclav; Amoxiclav-BID; Augmentin; Clamoxin; Clavant; Clavipen; Clavucyd; Clavulin; Clavuser; Gimaclav; Moxlin; Riclasip; Servamox; Sinufin

Index Terms Amoxicillin and Clavulanic Acid; Clavulanic Acid and Amoxicillin

Pharmacologic Category Antibiotic, Penicillin

Generic Available Yes: Excludes extended release

Use Treatment of otitis media, sinusitis, and infections caused by susceptible organisms involving the lower respiratory tract, skin and skin structure, and urinary tract; spectrum same as amoxicillin with additional coverage of beta-lactamase producing *B. catarrhalis*, *H. influenzae*, *N. gonorrhoeae*, and *S. aureus* (not MRSA). The expanded coverage of this combination makes it a useful alternative when amoxicillin resistance is present and patients cannot tolerate alternative treatments.

Effect on Mental Status Penicillins have been reported to cause apprehension, illusions, agitation, insomnia, depersonalization, and encephalopathy

Effect on Psychiatric Treatment Disulfiram may increase amoxicillin levels

Pregnancy Risk Factor B

Pregnancy Considerations

Adverse events have not been observed in animal studies; therefore, amoxicillin/clavulanate is classified as pregnancy category B. Both amoxicillin and clavulanic acid cross the placenta. There is no documented increased risk of teratogenic affects caused by amoxicillin/clavulanate. A potential increased risk of necrotizing enterocolitis in the newborn has been noted after maternal use of amoxicillin/clavulanate for preterm labor or premature prolonged rupture of membranes. When used during pregnancy, pharmacokinetic changes have been observed with amoxicillin alone (refer to the Amoxicillin monograph for details).

Lactation Enters breast milk/use caution

Contraindications Hypersensitivity to amoxicillin, clavulanic acid, penicillin, or any component of the formulation; history of cholestatic jaundice or hepatic dysfunction with amoxicillin/clavulanate potassium therapy; Augmentin XR™: severe renal impairment (Cl_{cr} <30 mL/minute) and hemodialysis patients

Warnings/Precautions Hypersensitivity reactions, including anaphylaxis (some fatal), have been reported. Prolonged use may result in fungal or bacterial superinfection, including *C. difficile*-associated diarrhea (CDAD) and pseudomembranous colitis; CDAD has been observed >2 months postantibiotic treatment. In patients with renal impairment, doses and/or frequency of administration should be modified in response to the degree of renal impairment. High percentage of patients with infectious mononucleosis have developed rash during therapy; ampicillin-class antibiotics not recommended in these patients. Incidence of diarrhea is higher than with amoxicillin alone. Due to differing content of clavulanic acid, not all formulations are interchangeable. Low incidence of cross-allergy with cephalosporins exists. Some products contain phenylalanine.

Adverse Reactions

>10%: Gastrointestinal: Diarrhea (3% to 34%; incidence varies upon dose and regimen used)

1% to 10%:

Dermatologic: Diaper rash, skin rash, urticaria

Gastrointestinal: Abdominal discomfort, loose stools, nausea, vomiting

Genitourinary: Vaginitis, vaginal mycosis

Miscellaneous: Moniliasis

<1% (Limited to important or life-threatening): Cholestatic jaundice, flatulence, headache, hepatic dysfunction, prothrombin time increased, thrombocytosis

Additional adverse reactions seen with **ampicillin-class antibiotics:** Agitation, agranulocytosis, alkaline phosphatase increased, anaphylaxis, anemia, angioedema, anxiety, behavioral changes, bilirubin increased, black "hairy" tongue, confusion, convulsions, crystalluria, dizziness, enterocolitis, eosinophilia, erythema multiforme, exanthematous pustulosis, exfoliative dermatitis, gastritis, glossitis, hematuria, hemolytic anemia, hemorrhagic colitis, indigestion, insomnia, hyperactivity, interstitial nephritis, leukopenia, mucocutaneous candidiasis, pruritus, pseudomembranous colitis, serum sickness-like reaction, Stevens-Johnson syndrome, stomatitis, transaminases increased, thrombocytopenia, thrombocytopenic purpura, tooth discoloration, toxic epidermal necrolysis

Drug Interactions

Allopurinol: May enhance the potential for allergic or hypersensitivity reactions to Amoxicillin. *Risk C: Monitor therapy*

Fusidic Acid: May diminish the therapeutic effect of Penicillins. *Risk D: Consider therapy modification*

Methotrexate: Penicillins may decrease the excretion of Methotrexate. *Risk C: Monitor therapy*

Tetracycline Derivatives: May diminish the therapeutic effect of Penicillins. *Risk D: Consider therapy modification*

Typhoid Vaccine: Antibiotics may diminish the therapeutic effect of Typhoid Vaccine. Only the live attenuated Ty21a strain is affected. *Risk D: Consider therapy modification*

Uricosuric Agents: May decrease the excretion of Penicillins. *Risk C: Monitor therapy*

Stability

Powder for oral suspension: Store dry powder at room temperature of 25°C (77°F). Reconstitute powder for oral suspension with appropriate amount of water as specified on the bottle. Shake vigorously until suspended. Reconstituted oral suspension should be kept in refrigerator. Discard unused suspension after 10 days. Unit-dose antibiotic oral syringes are stable for 48 hours.

Tablet: Store at room temperature of 25°C (77°F).

Mechanism of Action Clavulanic acid binds and inhibits beta-lactamases that inactivate amoxicillin resulting in amoxicillin having an expanded spectrum of activity. Amoxicillin inhibits bacterial cell wall synthesis by binding to one or more of the penicillin-binding proteins (PBPs) which in turn inhibits the final transpeptidation step of peptidoglycan synthesis in bacterial cell walls, thus inhibiting cell wall biosynthesis. Bacteria eventually lyse due to ongoing activity of cell wall autolytic enzymes (autolysins and murein hydrolases) while cell wall assembly is arrested.

Pharmacodynamics/Kinetics Amoxicillin pharmacokinetics are not affected by clavulanic acid.

Amoxicillin: See Amoxicillin monograph.

Clavulanic acid:

Protein binding: ~25%

Metabolism: Hepatic

Half-life elimination: 1 hour

Time to peak: 1 hour

Excretion: Urine (30% to 40% as unchanged drug)

Dosage Note: Dose is based on the amoxicillin component; see "Augmentin® Product-Specific Considerations" table on page 118.

Usual dosage range:

Infants <3 months: Oral: 30 mg/kg/day divided every 12 hours using the 125 mg/5 mL suspension

Children ≥3 months and <40 kg: Oral: 20-90 mg/kg/day divided every 8-12 hours

Children >40 kg and Adults: Oral: 250-500 mg every 8 hours or 875 mg every 12 hours

Indication-specific dosing:

Children ≥3 months and <40 kg: Oral:

Lower respiratory tract infections, severe infections, sinusitis: 45 mg/kg/day divided every 12 hours **or** 40 mg/kg/day divided every 8 hours

Mild-to-moderate infections: 25 mg/kg/day divided every 12 hours or 20 mg/kg/day divided every 8 hours

Otitis media (Augmentin® ES-600): 90 mg/kg/day divided every 12 hours for 10 days in children with severe illness and when coverage for β-lactamase-positive *H. influenzae* and *M. catarrhalis* is needed.

Children ≥16 years and Adults: Oral:

Acute bacterial sinusitis: Extended release tablet: Two 1000 mg tablets every 12 hours for 10 days

Bite wounds (animal/human): 875 mg every 12 hours **or** 500 mg every 8 hours

Chronic obstructive pulmonary disease: 875 mg every 12 hours **or** 500 mg every 8 hours

Diabetic foot: Extended release tablet: Two 1000 mg tablets every 12 hours for 7-14 days

Diverticulitis, perirectal abscess: Extended release tablet: Two 1000 mg tablets every 12 hours for 7-10 days

Erysipelas: 875 mg every 12 hours **or** 500 mg every 8 hours

Febrile neutropenia: 875 mg every 12 hours

Pneumonia:

Aspiration: 875 mg every 12 hours

Community-acquired: Extended release tablet: Two 1000 mg tablets every 12 hours for 7-10 days

Pyelonephritis (acute, uncomplicated): 875 mg every 12 hours **or** 500 mg every 8 hours

Skin abscess: 875 mg every 12 hours

Dosing interval in renal impairment:

Cl_{cr} <30 mL/minute: Do not use 875 mg tablet or extended release tablets

Cl_{cr} 10-30 mL/minute: 250-500 mg every 12 hours

Cl_{cr} <10 mL/minute: 250-500 every 24 hours

Hemodialysis: Moderately dialyzable (20% to 50%)

250-500 mg every 24 hours; administer dose during and after dialysis. Do not use extended release tablets.

Peritoneal dialysis: Moderately dialyzable (20% to 50%)

Amoxicillin: Administer 250 mg every 12 hours

Clavulanic acid: Dose for Cl_{cr} <10 mL/minute

Continuous arteriovenous or venovenous hemofiltration effects:

Amoxicillin: ~50 mg of amoxicillin/L of filtrate is removed

Clavulanic acid: Dose for Cl_{cr} <10 mL/minute

Dietary Considerations May be taken with meals or on an empty stomach; take with meals to increase absorption and decrease GI intolerance; may mix with milk, formula, or juice. Extended release tablets should be taken with food. Some products contain phenylalanine. If you have phenylketonuria or PKU, avoid use. All dosage forms contain potassium.

Administration Administer around-the-clock to promote less variation in peak and trough serum levels. Administer with food to decrease stomach upset; shake suspension well before use. Extended release tablets should be administered with food.

Some penicillins (eg, carbenicillin, ticarcillin, and piperacillin) have been shown to inactivate aminoglycosides *in vitro*. This has been observed to a greater extent with tobramycin and gentamicin, while amikacin has shown greater stability against inactivation. Concurrent use of these agents may pose a risk of reduced antibacterial efficacy *in vivo*, particularly in the setting of profound renal impairment. However, definitive clinical evidence is lacking. If combination penicillin/aminoglycoside therapy is desired in a patient with renal dysfunction, separation of doses (if feasible), and routine monitoring of aminoglycoside levels, CBC, and clinical response should be considered.

Monitoring Parameters Assess patient at beginning and throughout therapy for infection; with prolonged therapy, monitor renal, hepatic, and hematologic function periodically; monitor for signs of anaphylaxis during first dose

Augmentin® Product-Specific Considerations

Strength	Form	Consideration
125 mg	CT, S	q8h dosing
	S	For adults having difficulty swallowing tablets, 125 mg/5 mL suspension may be substituted for 500 mg tablet.
200 mg	CT, S	q12h dosing
	CT	Contains phenylalanine
	S	For adults having difficulty swallowing tablets, 200 mg/5 mL suspension may be substituted for 875 mg tablet.
250 mg	CT, S, T	q8h dosing
	CT	Contains phenylalanine
	T	Not for use in patients <40 kg
	CT, T	Tablet and chewable tablet are not interchangeable due to differences in clavulanic acid.
	S	For adults having difficulty swallowing tablets, 250 mg/5 mL suspension may be substituted for 500 mg tablet.
400 mg	CT, S	q12h dosing
	CT	Contains phenylalanine
	S	For adults having difficulty swallowing tablets, 400 mg/5 mL suspension may be substituted for 875 mg tablet.
500 mg	T	q8h or q12h dosing
600 mg	S	q12h dosing
		Contains phenylalanine
		Not for use in adults or children ≥40 kg
		600 mg/5 mL suspension is not equivalent to or interchangeable with 200 mg/5 mL or 400 mg/5 mL due to differences in clavulanic acid.
875 mg	T	q12h dosing; not for use in Cl_{cr} <30 mL/minute
1000 mg	XR	q12h dosing
		Not for use in children <16 years of age
		Not interchangeable with two 500 mg tablets
		Not for use if Cl_{cr} <30 mL/minute or hemodialysis

Legend: CT = chewable tablet, S = suspension, T = tablet, XR = extended release.

Test Interactions May interfere with urinary glucose tests using cupric sulfate (Benedict's solution, Clinitest®, Fehling's solution); may inactivate aminoglycosides *in vitro*.

Some penicillin derivatives may accelerate the degradation of aminoglycosides *in vitro*, leading to a potential underestimation of aminoglycoside serum concentration.

Additional Information Two 250 mg tablets are not equivalent to a 500 mg tablet (both tablet sizes contain equivalent clavulanate). Two 500 mg tablets are not equivalent to a single 1000 mg extended release tablet.

Dosage Forms Excipient information presented when available (limited, particularly for generics); consult specific product labeling. [DSC] = Discontinued product

Powder for oral suspension: 200: Amoxicillin 200 mg and clavulanate potassium 28.5 mg per 5 mL (50 mL, 75 mL, 100 mL) [contains phenylalanine]; 400: Amoxicillin 400 mg and clavulanate potassium 57 mg per 5 mL (50 mL, 75 mL, 100 mL) [contains phenylalanine]; 600: Amoxicillin 600 mg and clavulanate potassium 42.9 mg per 5 mL (75 mL, 125 mL, 200 mL) [contains phenylalanine]

Amoclan:

200: Amoxicillin 200 mg and clavulanate potassium 28.5 mg per 5 mL (50 mL, 75 mL, 100 mL) [contains phenylalanine 7 mg/5 mL and potassium 0.14 mEq/5 mL; fruit flavor]

400: Amoxicillin 400 mg and clavulanate potassium 57 mg per 5 mL (50 mL, 75 mL, 100 mL) [contains phenylalanine 7 mg/5 mL and potassium 0.29 mEq/5 mL; fruit flavor]

Augmentin®:

125: Amoxicillin 125 mg and clavulanate potassium 31.25 mg per 5 mL (75 mL, 100 mL, 150 mL) [contains potassium 0.16 mEq/5 mL; banana flavor]

200: Amoxicillin 200 mg and clavulanate potassium 28.5 mg per 5 mL (50 mL, 75 mL, 100 mL) [contains phenylalanine 7 mg/5 mL and potassium 0.14 mEq/5 mL; orange flavor] [DSC]

250: Amoxicillin 250 mg and clavulanate potassium 62.5 mg per 5 mL (75 mL, 100 mL, 150 mL) [contains potassium 0.32 mEq/5 mL; orange flavor]
400: Amoxicillin 400 mg and clavulanate potassium 57 mg per 5 mL (50 mL [DSC], 75 mL [DSC], 100 mL) [contains phenylalanine 7 mg/5 mL and potassium 0.29 mEq/5 mL; orange flavor]
Augmentin ES-600®: Amoxicillin 600 mg and clavulanate potassium 42.9 mg per 5 mL (75 mL, 125 mL, 200 mL) [contains phenylalanine 7 mg/5 mL and potassium 0.23 mEq/5 mL; strawberry cream flavor]

Tablet: 250: Amoxicillin 250 mg and clavulanate potassium 125 mg; 500: Amoxicillin 500 mg and clavulanate potassium 125 mg; 875: Amoxicillin 875 mg and clavulanate potassium 125 mg
Augmentin®:
250: Amoxicillin 250 mg and clavulanate potassium 125 mg [contains potassium 0.63 mEq/tablet]
500: Amoxicillin 500 mg and clavulanate potassium 125 mg [contains potassium 0.63 mEq/tablet]
875: Amoxicillin 875 mg and clavulanate potassium 125 mg [contains potassium 0.63 mEq/tablet]

Tablet, chewable: 200: Amoxicillin 200 mg and clavulanate potassium 28.5 mg [contains phenylalanine]; 400: Amoxicillin 400 mg and clavulanate potassium 57 mg [contains phenylalanine]
Augmentin®:
125: Amoxicillin 125 mg and clavulanate potassium 31.25 mg [contains potassium 0.16 mEq/tablet; lemon-lime flavor] [DSC]
200: Amoxicillin 200 mg and clavulanate potassium 28.5 mg [contains phenylalanine 2.1 mg/tablet and potassium 0.14 mEq/tablet; cherry-banana flavor] [DSC]
250: Amoxicillin 250 mg and clavulanate potassium 62.5 mg [contains potassium 0.32 mEq/tablet; lemon-lime flavor]
400: Amoxicillin 400 mg and clavulanate potassium 57 mg [contains phenylalanine 4.2 mg/tablet and potassium 0.29 mEq/tablet; cherry-banana flavor] [DSC]

Tablet, extended release:
Augmentin XR®: Amoxicillin 1000 mg and clavulanate acid 62.5 mg [contains potassium 12.6 mg (0.32 mEq) and sodium 29.3 mg (1.27 mEq) per tablet; packaged in either a 7-day or 10-day package]

- ◆ **Amoxicillin and Clavulanic Acid** *see* Amoxicillin and Clavulanate Potassium *on page 115*
- ◆ **Amoxicillin, Lansoprazole, and Clarithromycin** *see* Lansoprazole, Amoxicillin, and Clarithromycin *on page 897*
- ◆ **Amoxicillin Trihydrate** *see* Amoxicillin *on page 112*
- ◆ **Amoxil®** *see* Amoxicillin *on page 112*
- ◆ **Amoxycillin** *see* Amoxicillin *on page 112*
- ◆ **Amphetamine and Dextroamphetamine** *see* Dextroamphetamine and Amphetamine *on page 444*
- ◆ **Amphocin® [DSC]** *see* Amphotericin B (Conventional) *on page 120*
- ◆ **Amphotec®** *see* Amphotericin B Cholesteryl Sulfate Complex *on page 119*

Amphotericin B Cholesteryl Sulfate Complex

(am foe TER i sin bee kole LES te ril SUL fate KOM plecks)

Medication Safety Issues

Safety issues:

Lipid-based amphotericin formulations (Amphotec®) may be confused with conventional formulations (Amphocin®, Fungizone®)

Large overdoses have occurred when conventional formulations were dispensed inadvertently for lipid-based products. Single daily doses of conventional amphotericin formulation never exceed 1.5 mg/kg.

High alert medication: The Institute for Safe Medication Practices (ISMP) includes this medication among its list of drugs which have a heightened risk of causing significant patient harm when used in error.

U.S. Brand Names Amphotec®

Canadian Brand Names Amphotec®

Mexican Brand Names Amphocil

Index Terms ABCD; Amphotericin B Colloidal Dispersion

Pharmacologic Category Antifungal Agent, Parenteral

Use Treatment of invasive aspergillosis in patients who have failed amphotericin B deoxycholate treatment, or who have renal impairment or experience unacceptable toxicity which precludes treatment with amphotericin B deoxycholate in effective doses.

Unlabeled/Investigational Use Effective in patients with serious *Candida* species infections

Effect on Mental Status None reported

Effect on Psychiatric Treatment May cause bone marrow suppression; use caution with clozapine and carbamazepine

Dosage Summary

I.V.:

Children: 3-4 mg/kg/day (maximum: 7.5 mg/kg/day)

Adults: 3-4 mg/kg/day (maximum: 7.5 mg/kg/day)

Dosage Forms Excipient information presented when available (limited, particularly for generics); consult specific product labeling.

Injection, powder for reconstitution:

Amphotec®: 50 mg, 100 mg

◆ **Amphotericin B Colloidal Dispersion** *see* Amphotericin B Cholesteryl Sulfate Complex *on page 119*

Amphotericin B (Conventional)

(am foe TER i sin bee con VEN sha nal)

Medication Safety Issues

Safety issues:

Conventional amphotericin formulations (Amphocin®, Fungizone®) may be confused with lipid-based formulations (AmBisome®, Abelcet®, Amphotec®).

Large overdoses have occurred when conventional formulations were dispensed inadvertently for lipid-based products. Single daily doses of conventional amphotericin formulation never exceed 1.5 mg/kg.

High alert medication: The Institute for Safe Medication Practices (ISMP) includes this medication (intrathecal administration) among its list of drugs which have a heightened risk of causing significant patient harm when used in error.

U.S. Brand Names Amphocin® [DSC]

Canadian Brand Names Fungizone®

Mexican Brand Names Amphocil; Terix

Index Terms Amphotericin B Desoxycholate

Pharmacologic Category Antifungal Agent, Parenteral

Use Treatment of severe systemic and central nervous system infections caused by susceptible fungi such as *Candida* species, *Histoplasma capsulatum*, *Cryptococcus neoformans*, *Aspergillus* species, *Blastomyces dermatitidis*, *Torulopsis glabrata*, and *Coccidioides immitis*; fungal peritonitis; irrigant for bladder fungal infections; used in fungal infection in patients with bone marrow transplantation, amebic meningoencephalitis, ocular aspergillosis (intraocular injection), candidal cystitis (bladder irrigation), chemoprophylaxis (low-dose I.V.), immunocompromised patients at risk of aspergillosis (intranasal/nebulized), refractory meningitis (intrathecal), coccidioidal arthritis (intra-articular/I.M.).

Low-dose amphotericin B has been administered after bone marrow transplantation to reduce the risk of invasive fungal disease.

Effect on Mental Status Sedation is common; may cause delirium

Effect on Psychiatric Treatment May cause bone marrow suppression; use caution with clozapine and carbamazepine

Dosage Summary

I.V.:

Infants: Test dose: 0.1 mg/kg/dose (maximum: 1 mg); Maintenance: 0.25-1 mg/kg/day given once daily; 1-1.5 mg/kg over 4-6 hours every other day may be given once therapy is established (maximum: 1.5-4 g cumulative dose).

Children: Test dose: 0.1 mg/kg/dose (maximum: 1 mg) infused over 30-60 minutes; Maintenance: 0.25-1 mg/kg/day given once daily; 1-1.5 mg/kg over 4-6 hours every other day may be given once therapy is established (maximum: 1.5-4 g cumulative dose).

Adults: Test dose: 1 mg infused over 20-30 minutes; Maintenance: 0.05-1.5 mg/kg/day given once daily; 1-1.5 mg/kg over 4-6 hours every other day may be given once therapy is established (maximum: 1.5 mg/kg/day)

Dosage Forms Excipient information presented when available (limited, particularly for generics); consult specific product labeling. [DSC] = Discontinued product

Injection, powder for reconstitution, as desoxycholate: 50 mg

Amphocin®: 50 mg [DSC]

◆ **Amphotericin B Desoxycholate** *see* Amphotericin B (Conventional) *on page 120*

Amphotericin B, Lipid Complex

(am foe TER i sin bee LIP id KOM pleks)

Medication Safety Issues

Safety issues:

Lipid-based amphotericin formulations (Abelcet®) may be confused with conventional formulations (Amphocin®, Fungizone®)

Large overdoses have occurred when conventional formulations were dispensed inadvertently for lipid-based products. Single daily doses of conventional amphotericin formulation never exceed 1.5 mg/kg.

High alert medication: The Institute for Safe Medication Practices (ISMP) includes this medication among its list of drugs which have a heightened risk of causing significant patient harm when used in error.

U.S. Brand Names Abelcet®

Canadian Brand Names Abelcet®; Amphotec®

Index Terms ABLC

Pharmacologic Category Antifungal Agent, Parenteral

Use Treatment of aspergillosis or any type of progressive fungal infection in patients who are refractory to or intolerant of conventional amphotericin B therapy

Unlabeled/Investigational Use Effective in patients with serious *Candida* species infections

Effect on Mental Status Sedation is common; may cause delirium

Effect on Psychiatric Treatment May cause bone marrow suppression; use caution with clozapine and carbamazepine

Dosage Summary

I.V.:

Children: 2.5-5 mg/kg/day as a single daily dose (maximum: 5 mg/kg/day)

Adults: 2.5-5 mg/kg/day as a single daily dose (maximum: 5 mg/kg/day)

Dosage Forms Excipient information presented when available (limited, particularly for generics); consult specific product labeling.

Injection, suspension [preservative free]:

Abelcet®: 5 mg/mL (20 mL)

Amphotericin B, Liposomal (am foe TER i sin bee lye po SO mal)

Medication Safety Issues

Safety issues:

Lipid-based amphotericin formulations (AmBisome®) may be confused with conventional formulations (Amphocin®, Fungizone®)

Large overdoses have occurred when conventional formulations were dispensed inadvertently for lipid-based products. Single daily doses of conventional amphotericin formulation never exceed 1.5 mg/kg.

High alert medication: The Institute for Safe Medication Practices (ISMP) includes this medication among its list of drugs which have a heightened risk of causing significant patient harm when used in error.

U.S. Brand Names AmBisome®

Canadian Brand Names AmBisome®

Index Terms L-AmB

Pharmacologic Category Antifungal Agent, Parenteral

Use Empirical therapy for presumed fungal infection in febrile, neutropenic patients; treatment of patients with *Aspergillus* species, *Candida* species, and/or *Cryptococcus* species infections refractory to amphotericin B desoxycholate, or in patients where renal impairment or unacceptable toxicity precludes the use of amphotericin B desoxycholate; treatment of cryptococcal meningitis in HIV-infected patients; treatment of visceral leishmaniasis

Unlabeled/Investigational Use Effective in patients with serious *Candida* species infections

Effect on Mental Status Sedation is common; may cause delirium

Effect on Psychiatric Treatment May cause bone marrow suppression; use caution with clozapine and carbamazepine

Dosage Summary

I.V.:

Children: 3-6 mg/kg/day as a single daily dose (maximum: 6 mg/kg/day)

Adults: 3-6 mg/kg/day as a single daily dose (maximum: 6 mg/kg/day)

Dosage Forms Excipient information presented when available (limited, particularly for generics); consult specific product labeling.

Injection, powder for reconstitution:

AmBisome®: 50 mg [contains soy and sucrose]

Ampicillin (am pi SIL in)

Medication Safety Issues

Sound-alike/look-alike issues:

Ampicillin may be confused with aminophylline

Canadian Brand Names Apo-Ampi®; Novo-Ampicillin; Nu-Ampi

Mexican Brand Names Alphapen; Amsapen; Binotal; Brupen; Dibacilina; Flamicina; Marovilina; Omnipen; Penbritin; Pentrexyl; Promecilina

Index Terms Aminobenzylpenicillin; Ampicillin Sodium; Ampicillin Trihydrate

Pharmacologic Category Antibiotic, Penicillin

Use Treatment of susceptible bacterial infections (nonbeta-lactamase-producing organisms); treatment or prophylaxis of infective endocarditis; susceptible bacterial infections caused by streptococci, pneumococci, nonpenicillinase-producing staphylococci, *Listeria*, meningococci; some strains of *H. influenzae*, *Salmonella*, *Shigella*, *E. coli*, *Enterobacter*, and *Klebsiella*

Effect on Mental Status Large I.V. doses may rarely produce encephalopathy; penicillins have been reported to cause apprehension, illusions, agitation, insomnia, depersonalization, and encephalopathy

Effect on Psychiatric Treatment Rarely may cause bone marrow suppression; use caution with clozapine and carbamazepine

Dosage Summary

I.M.:

Infants: 100-400 mg/kg/day divided every 6 hours (maximum: 12 g/day)

Children: 100-400 mg/kg/day divided every 6 hours (maximum: 12 g/day)

Adults: 250-500 mg every 6 hours or up to 150-250 mg/kg/day divided every 3-4 hours (maximum: 12 g/day)

I.V.:

Infants: 100-400 mg/kg/day divided every 6 hours (maximum: 12 g/day)

Children: 100-400 mg/kg/day divided every 6 hours (maximum: 12 g/day)

Adults: 250-500 mg every 6 hours or up to 150-250 mg/kg/day divided every 3-4 hours (maximum: 12 g/day)

Oral:

Infants: 50-100 mg/kg/day divided every 6 hours (maximum: 4 g/day)

Children: 50-100 mg/kg/day divided every 6 hours (maximum: 4 g/day)

Adults: 250-500 mg every 6 hours

Dosage Forms Excipient information presented when available (limited, particularly for generics); consult specific product labeling.

Capsule: 250 mg, 500 mg

Injection, powder for reconstitution, as sodium: 125 mg, 250 mg, 500 mg, 1 g, 2 g, 10 g

Powder for oral suspension: 125 mg/5 mL (100 mL, 200 mL); 250 mg/5 mL (100 mL, 200 mL)

Ampicillin and Sulbactam (am pi SIL in & SUL bak tam)

U.S. Brand Names Unasyn®

Canadian Brand Names Unasyn®

Index Terms Sulbactam and Ampicillin

Pharmacologic Category Antibiotic, Penicillin

Use Treatment of susceptible bacterial infections involved with skin and skin structure, intra-abdominal infections, gynecological infections; spectrum is that of ampicillin plus organisms producing beta-lactamases such as *S. aureus*, *H. influenzae*, *E. coli*, *Klebsiella*, *Acinetobacter*, *Enterobacter*, and anaerobes

Effect on Mental Status Large I.V. doses may rarely produce encephalopathy; penicillins have been reported to cause apprehension, illusions, agitation, insomnia, depersonalization, and encephalopathy

Effect on Psychiatric Treatment Rarely may cause bone marrow suppression; use caution with clozapine and carbamazepine

Dosage Summary Note: Dosage recommendations based on the ampicillin component

I.M.:

Children: Dosage not established

Adults: 1-2 g (1.5-3 g Unasyn®) ampicillin every 6 hours (maximum: 8 g ampicillin/day)

I.V.:

Children <1 year: Dosage not established

Children ≥1 year: 100-400 mg ampicillin/kg/day divided every 6 hours (maximum: 8 g ampicillin/day)

Adults: 1-2 g (1.5-3 g Unasyn®) ampicillin every 6 hours (maximum: 8 g ampicillin/day)

Dosage Forms Excipient information presented when available (limited, particularly for generics); consult specific product labeling.

Injection, powder for reconstitution: 1.5 g: Ampicillin 1 g and sulbactam 0.5 g [contains sodium 115 mg (5 mEq)/1.5 g)]; 3 g: Ampicillin 2 g and sulbactam 1 g [contains sodium 115 mg (5 mEq)/1.5 g)]; 15 g: Ampicillin 10 g and sulbactam 5 g [bulk package; contains sodium 115 mg (5 mEq)/1.5 g]

Unasyn®:

1.5 g: Ampicillin 1 g and sulbactam 0.5 g [contains sodium 115 mg (5 mEq)/1.5 g)]

3 g: Ampicillin 2 g and sulbactam 1 g [contains sodium 115 mg (5 mEq)/1.5 g)]

15 g: Ampicillin 10 g and sulbactam 5 g [bulk package; contains sodium 115 mg (5 mEq)/1.5 g)]

◆ **Ampicillin Sodium** *see* Ampicillin *on page 122*

◆ **Ampicillin Trihydrate** *see* Ampicillin *on page 122*

Amprenavir (am PREN a veer)

U.S. Brand Names Agenerase® [DSC]

Canadian Brand Names Agenerase®

Mexican Brand Names Agenerase

Pharmacologic Category Antiretroviral Agent, Protease Inhibitor

Use Treatment of HIV infections in combination with at least two other antiretroviral agents; oral solution should only be used when capsules or other protease inhibitors are not therapeutic options

Effect on Mental Status Depression is common; may cause headache and fatigue

Effect on Psychiatric Treatment Contraindicated with midazolam and triazolam. Concurrent use with vitamin E and sildenafil should be avoided. May increase concentrations of alprazolam, clorazepate, diazepam, flurazepam, sildenafil, carbamazepine, and pimozide. May increase adverse effects of TCAs (monitor serum levels). Concomitant use of amprenavir and St John's wort is not recommended. Coadministration of protease inhibitors (amprenavir) with St John's wort is expected to substantially decrease protease inhibitor serum concentrations leading to a loss of virologic response and possible resistance to amprenavir or to the class of protease inhibitors.

Dosage Summary Note: Capsule and oral solution are not interchangeable on a mg-per-mg basis.

Oral:

Children <4 years: Dosage not established

Children 4-12 years: Capsule: 20 mg/kg twice daily **or** 15 mg/kg 3 times daily (maximum: 2400 mg/day); Solution: 22.5 mg/kg twice daily **or** 17 mg/kg 3 times daily (maximum: 2800 mg/day)

Children 13-16 years and <50 kg: Capsule: 20 mg/kg twice daily **or** 15 mg/kg 3 times daily (maximum: 2400 mg/day); Solution: 22.5 mg/kg twice daily **or** 17 mg/kg 3 times daily (maximum: 2800 mg/day)

Children 13-16 years and ≥50 kg: Capsule: 1200 mg twice daily; Solution: 1400 mg twice daily

Adults <50 kg: Capsule: 20 mg/kg twice daily **or** 15 mg/kg 3 times daily (maximum: 2400 mg/day); Solution: 22.5 mg/kg twice daily **or** 17 mg/kg 3 times daily (maximum: 2800 mg/day)

Adults ≥50 kg: Capsule: 1200 mg twice daily; Solution: 1400 mg twice daily

Dosage Forms Excipient information presented when available (limited, particularly for generics); consult specific product labeling. [DSC] = Discontinued product

Capsule:

Agenerase®: 50 mg [contains vitamin E 36.3 int. units (as TPGS)] [DSC]

Solution, oral:
Agenerase®: 15 mg/mL (240 mL) [contains propylene glycol 550 mg/mL and vitamin E 46 int. units/mL; grape-bubble gum-peppermint flavor] [DSC]

- **AMPT** *see* Metyrosine *on page 1044*
- **Amrinone Lactate** *see* Inamrinone *on page 817*
- **Amrix®** *see* Cyclobenzaprine *on page 405*

Amyl Nitrite (AM il NYE trite)

Index Terms Isoamyl Nitrite
Pharmacologic Category Antidote; Vasodilator
Use Coronary vasodilator in angina pectoris; adjunct in treatment of cyanide poisoning; produce changes in the intensity of heart murmurs
Effect on Mental Status May cause headache
Effect on Psychiatric Treatment None reported
Dosage Summary
Nasal Inhalation:
Children: Dosage not established
Adults: 1-6 inhalations from 1 crushed ampul; may repeat in 3-5 minutes
Dosage Forms Excipient information presented when available (limited, particularly for generics); consult specific product labeling.
Vapor for inhalation [crushable covered glass capsules]: Amyl nitrite USP (0.3 mL)

- **Amylobarbitone** *see* Amobarbital *on page 105*
- **Amytal®** *see* Amobarbital *on page 105*
- **AN100226** *see* Natalizumab *on page 1109*
- **Anadrol®-50** *see* Oxymetholone *on page 1209*
- **Anafranil®** *see* ClomiPRAMINE *on page 368*

Anagrelide (an AG gre lide)

U.S. Brand Names Agrylin®
Canadian Brand Names Agrylin®; Dom-Anagrelide; Gen-Anagrelide; PHL-Anagrelide; PMS-Anagrelide; Sandoz-Anagrelide
Index Terms Anagrelide Hydrochloride; BL4162A; NSC-724577
Pharmacologic Category Phospholipase A_2 Inhibitor
Use Treatment of thrombocythemia associated with myeloproliferative disorders
Unlabeled/Investigational Use Treatment of essential thrombocythemia (ET)
Effect on Mental Status May impair ability to concentrate and produce bad dreams
Effect on Psychiatric Treatment May cause hypotension which may be exacerbated by psychotropics; may cause heart block; use caution with TCAs
Dosage Summary Note: Maintain for ≥1 week, then adjust to the lowest effective dose to reduce and maintain platelet count <600,000/µL ideally to the normal range; the dose must not be increased by >0.5 mg/day in any 1 week
Oral:
Children: Initial: 0.5 mg/day; Maintenance: 0.5 mg 1-4 times/day (maximum: 10 mg/day; 2.5 mg/dose)
Adults: 0.5 mg 4 times/day **or** 1 mg twice daily (maximum: 10 mg/day; 2.5 mg/dose)
Dosage Forms Excipient information presented when available (limited, particularly for generics); consult specific product labeling.
Capsule: 0.5 mg, 1 mg
Agrylin®: 0.5 mg

- **Anagrelide Hydrochloride** *see* Anagrelide *on page 124*

Anakinra (an a KIN ra)

Medication Safety Issues
Sound-alike/look-alike issues:
Anakinra may be confused with amikacin
U.S. Brand Names Kineret®
Canadian Brand Names Kineret®
Index Terms IL-1Ra; Interleukin-1 Receptor Antagonist

Pharmacologic Category Antirheumatic, Disease Modifying; Interleukin-1 Receptor Antagonist

Use Treatment of moderately- to severely-active rheumatoid arthritis in adult patients who have failed one or more disease-modifying antirheumatic drugs (DMARDs); may be used alone or in combination with DMARDs (other than tumor necrosis factor-blocking agents)

Effect on Mental Status None reported

Effect on Psychiatric Treatment May cause leukopenia and rarely neutropenia; use caution with clozapine and carbamazepine. May cause nausea and diarrhea; monitor with concurrent SSRI, lithium, or valproic acid use.

Dosage Summary

SubQ:

Children: Dosage not established

Adults: 100 mg once daily

Dosage Forms Excipient information presented when available (limited, particularly for generics); consult specific product labeling.

Injection, solution [preservative free]:

Kineret®: 100 mg/0.67 mL (1 mL) [prefilled syringe; needle cover contains latex]

◆ **Anaplex® DM** *see* Brompheniramine, Pseudoephedrine, and Dextromethorphan *on page 208*

◆ **Anaplex® DMX** *see* Brompheniramine, Pseudoephedrine, and Dextromethorphan *on page 208*

◆ **Anaprox®** *see* Naproxen *on page 1102*

◆ **Anaprox® DS** *see* Naproxen *on page 1102*

◆ **Anaspaz®** *see* Hyoscyamine *on page 799*

Anastrozole (an AS troe zole)

Medication Safety Issues

Sound-alike/look-alike issues:

Anastrozole may be confused with letrozole

U.S. Brand Names Arimidex®

Canadian Brand Names Arimidex®

Mexican Brand Names Arimidex

Index Terms ICI-D1033; NSC-719344; ZD1033

Pharmacologic Category Antineoplastic Agent, Aromatase Inhibitor

Use Treatment of locally-advanced or metastatic breast cancer (ER-positive or hormone receptor unknown) in postmenopausal women; treatment of advanced breast cancer in postmenopausal women with disease progression following tamoxifen therapy; adjuvant treatment of early ER-positive breast cancer in postmenopausal women

Effect on Mental Status Drowsiness, confusion, insomnia, and anxiety are common

Effect on Psychiatric Treatment None reported

Dosage Summary

Oral:

Children: Dosage not established

Adults: 1 mg once daily

Dosage Forms Excipient information presented when available (limited, particularly for generics); consult specific product labeling.

Tablet:

Arimidex®: 1 mg

◆ **Ancef** *see* CeFAZolin *on page 292*

◆ **Ancobon®** *see* Flucytosine *on page 640*

◆ **Andehist DM NR** *see* Brompheniramine, Pseudoephedrine, and Dextromethorphan *on page 208*

◆ **Andehist NR Drops [DSC]** *see* Carbinoxamine and Pseudoephedrine *on page 280*

◆ **Andehist NR Syrup** *see* Brompheniramine and Pseudoephedrine *on page 206*

◆ **Androderm®** *see* Testosterone *on page 1553*

◆ **AndroGel®** *see* Testosterone *on page 1553*

◆ **Android®** *see* MethylTESTOSTERone *on page 1030*

◆ **Androxy™** *see* Fluoxymesterone *on page 657*

- **Anectine®** *see* Succinylcholine *on page 1511*
- **Anestacon®** *see* Lidocaine *on page 924*
- **Anestafoam™ [OTC]** *see* Lidocaine *on page 924*
- **Aneurine Hydrochloride** *see* Thiamine *on page 1568*
- **Anextuss** *see* Guaifenesin, Dextromethorphan, and Phenylephrine *on page 746*
- **Angeliq®** *see* Drospirenone and Estradiol *on page 515*
- **Angiomax®** *see* Bivalirudin *on page 191*
- **Anolor 300** *see* Butalbital, Acetaminophen, and Caffeine *on page 229*
- **Ansamycin** *see* Rifabutin *on page 1418*
- **Antabuse®** *see* Disulfiram *on page 489*
- **Antara™** *see* Fenofibrate *on page 620*
- **Anti-4 Alpha Integrin** *see* Natalizumab *on page 1109*
- **131 I Anti-B1 Antibody** *see* Tositumomab and Iodine I 131 Tositumomab *on page 1603*
- **131 I-Anti-B1 Monoclonal Antibody** *see* Tositumomab and Iodine I 131 Tositumomab *on page 1603*
- **Anti-CD11a** *see* Efalizumab *on page 526*
- **Anti-CD20 Monoclonal Antibody** *see* RiTUXimab *on page 1434*
- **Anti-CD20-Murine Monoclonal Antibody I-131** *see* Tositumomab and Iodine I 131 Tositumomab *on page 1603*
- **Antidiuretic Hormone** *see* Vasopressin *on page 1659*

Antithymocyte Globulin (Equine)

(an te THY moe site GLOB yu lin, E kwine)

Medication Safety Issues
Sound-alike/look-alike issues:
Atgam® may be confused with Ativan®

U.S. Brand Names Atgam®

Canadian Brand Names Atgam®

Index Terms Antithymocyte Immunoglobulin; ATG; Horse Antihuman Thymocyte Gamma Globulin; Lymphocyte Immune Globulin

Pharmacologic Category Immune Globulin; Immunosuppressant Agent

Use Prevention and treatment of acute renal allograft rejection; treatment of moderate to severe aplastic anemia in patients not considered suitable candidates for bone marrow transplantation

Unlabeled/Investigational Use Prevention and treatment of other solid organ allograft rejection; prevention of graft-versus-host disease following bone marrow transplantation

Effect on Mental Status May cause malaise

Effect on Psychiatric Treatment Leukopenia is common; use caution with clozapine and carbamazepine

Dosage Summary Note: An intradermal skin test is recommended prior to administration of the initial dose of ATG; use 0.1 mL of a 1:1000 dilution of ATG in normal saline. **Note:** Premedication with diphenhydramine, hydrocortisone, and acetaminophen is recommended prior to first dose.

I.V.:

Children: Initial: 5-25 mg/kg/day administered daily for 8-14 days; may be followed by administration every other day (maximum: 21 doses in 28 days).

Adults: Initial: 10-20 mg/kg/day administered daily; may be followed by administraiton every other day (maximum: 21 doses in 28 days).

Dosage Forms Excipient information presented when available (limited, particularly for generics); consult specific product labeling.
Injection, solution:
Atgam®: 50 mg/mL (5 mL)

Antithymocyte Globulin (Rabbit)

(an te THY moe site GLOB yu lin RAB bit)

U.S. Brand Names Thymoglobulin®

Index Terms Antithymocyte Immunoglobulin; rATG

Pharmacologic Category Immune Globulin; Immunosuppressant Agent

Use Treatment of acute rejection of renal transplant; used in conjunction with concomitant immunosuppression

Unlabeled/Investigational Use Induction therapy in renal transplant

Effect on Mental Status None reported

Effect on Psychiatric Treatment Leukopenia and thrombocytopenia are common; use caution with clozapine, carbamazepine, and valproic acid

Dosage Summary

I.V.:

Children: 1.5 mg/kg/day as a single daily dose

Adults: 1.5 mg/kg/day as a single daily dose

Dosage Forms Excipient information presented when available (limited, particularly for generics); consult specific product labeling.

Injection, powder for reconstitution:

Thymoglobulin®: 25 mg

- ◆ **Antithymocyte Immunoglobulin** *see* Antithymocyte Globulin (Equine) *on page 126*
- ◆ **Antithymocyte Immunoglobulin** *see* Antithymocyte Globulin (Rabbit) *on page 126*
- ◆ **Antitumor Necrosis Factor Apha (Human)** *see* Adalimumab *on page 50*
- ◆ **Anti-VEGF Monoclonal Antibody** *see* Bevacizumab *on page 187*
- ◆ **Antivert®** *see* Meclizine *on page 974*
- ◆ **Antizol®** *see* Fomepizole *on page 685*
- ◆ **Anucort-HC®** *see* Hydrocortisone *on page 785*
- ◆ **Anu-Med [OTC]** *see* Phenylephrine *on page 1273*
- ◆ **Anusol-HC®** *see* Hydrocortisone *on page 785*
- ◆ **Anusol® HC-1 [OTC]** *see* Hydrocortisone *on page 785*
- ◆ **Anzemet®** *see* Dolasetron *on page 493*
- ◆ **APAP** *see* Acetaminophen *on page 30*
- ◆ **APAP and Tramadol** *see* Acetaminophen and Tramadol *on page 38*
- ◆ **Aphrodyne® [DSC]** *see* Yohimbine *on page 1688*
- ◆ **Apidra®** *see* Insulin Glulisine *on page 829*
- ◆ **Aplonidine** *see* Apraclonidine *on page 129*
- ◆ **Apokyn®** *see* Apomorphine *on page 127*

Apomorphine (a poe MOR feen)

Related Information

Antiparkinsonian Agents *on page 1767*

U.S. Brand Names Apokyn®

Index Terms Apomorphine Hydrochloride; Apomorphine Hydrochloride Hemihydrate

Pharmacologic Category Anti-Parkinson's Agent, Dopamine Agonist

Generic Available No

Use Treatment of hypomobility, "off" episodes with Parkinson's disease

Unlabeled/Investigational Use Treatment of erectile dysfunction

Pregnancy Risk Factor C

Pregnancy Considerations Reproduction studies have not been conducted; use only if clearly needed.

Lactation Excretion in breast milk unknown/contraindicated

Contraindications Hypersensitivity to apomorphine or any component of the formulation; **concomitant use with $5HT_3$ antagonists**; intravenous administration

Warnings/Precautions May cause orthostatic hypotension, especially during dosage escalation; use extreme caution, especially in patients on antihypertensives and/or vasodilators. If patient develops clinically-significant orthostatic hypotension with test dose then apomorphine should not be used. Ergot-derived dopamine agonists have also been associated with fibrotic complications (eg, retroperitoneal fibrosis, pleural thickening, and pulmonary infiltrates). **Pretreatment with antiemetic is necessary.** Monitor patients for drowsiness. May cause hallucinations. Use caution in patients with risk factors for torsade de pointes. Use caution in cardiovascular and cerebrovascular disease. Use caution in patients with hepatic or renal dysfunction. Use with caution in patients with pre-existing dyskinesias; may be exacerbated.

Dopamine agonists have been associated with compulsive behaviors and/or loss of impulse control, which has manifested as pathological gambling, libido increases (hypersexuality), and/or binge eating. Causality has not been established, and controversy exists as to whether this phenomenon is related to the underlying disease, prior behaviors/addictions and/or drug therapy. Dose reduction or discontinuation of therapy has been reported to reverse these behaviors in some, but not all cases. Dopaminergic agents have been associated with a syndrome resembling neuroleptic malignant syndrome on abrupt withdrawal or significant dosage reduction after long-term use. Retinal degeneration has been observed in animal studies when using dopamine agonists for prolonged periods. Rare cases of abuse have been reported. Contains metabisulfite. Safety and efficacy in pediatric patients have not been established.

Adverse Reactions

>10%:

Cardiovascular: Chest pain/pressure or angina (15%)

Central nervous system: Drowsiness or somnolence (35%), dizziness or orthostatic hypotension (20%)

Gastrointestinal: Nausea and/or vomiting (30%)

Neuromuscular & skeletal: Falls (30%), dyskinesias (24% to 35%)

Respiratory: Yawning (40%), rhinorrhea (20%)

1% to 10%:

Cardiovascular: Edema (10%), vasodilation (3%), hypotension (2%), syncope (2%), CHF

Central nervous system: Hallucinations or confusion (10%), anxiety, depression, fatigue, headache, insomnia, pain

Dermatologic: Bruising

Endocrine & metabolic: Dehydration

Gastrointestinal: Constipation, diarrhea

Local: Injection site reactions

Neuromuscular & skeletal: Arthralgias, weakness

Miscellaneous: Diaphoresis increased

<1% (Limited to important or life-threatening): Angina, cardiac arrest, focal panniculitis, libido increased, MI, priapism, psychosexual stimulation, skin nodules, sudden death

Reported with dopamine agonists: Impulsive/compulsive behaviors (eg, pathological gambling, hypersexuality, binge eating)

Metabolism/Transport Effects Substrate (minor) of CYP1A2, 3A4, 2C19; **Inhibits** CYP1A2 (weak), 3A (weak), 2C19 (weak)

Drug Interactions

Alfuzosin: May enhance the QTc-prolonging effect of QTc-Prolonging Agents. *Risk C: Monitor therapy*

Antiemetics (5HT3 Antagonists): May enhance the hypotensive effect of Apomorphine. *Risk X: Avoid combination*

Antipsychotics (Atypical): May diminish the therapeutic effect of Anti-Parkinson's Agents (Dopamine Agonist). *Risk D: Consider therapy modification*

Antipsychotics (Typical): May diminish the therapeutic effect of Anti-Parkinson's Agents (Dopamine Agonist). *Risk D: Consider therapy modification*

Ciprofloxacin: May enhance the QTc-prolonging effect of QTc-Prolonging Agents. *Risk C: Monitor therapy*

COMT Inhibitors: May decrease the metabolism of COMT Substrates. *Risk C: Monitor therapy*

Gadobutrol: May enhance the QTc-prolonging effect of QTc-Prolonging Agents. *Risk D: Consider therapy modification*

Metoclopramide: May diminish the therapeutic effect of Anti-Parkinson's Agents (Dopamine Agonist). *Risk C: Monitor therapy*

Nilotinib: May enhance the QTc-prolonging effect of QTc-Prolonging Agents. *Risk X: Avoid combination*

QTc-Prolonging Agents: May enhance the adverse/toxic effect of other QTc-Prolonging Agents. Their effects can be additive, causing life-threatening ventricular arrhythmias. *Risk D: Consider therapy modification*

Tetrabenazine: QTc-Prolonging Agents may enhance the QTc-prolonging effect of Tetrabenazine. *Risk X: Avoid combination*

Ethanol/Nutrition/Herb Interactions

Ethanol: Caution with ethanol consumption; may increase risk of hypotension.

Stability Store at 15°C to 30°C (59°F to 86°F).

Mechanism of Action Stimulates postsynaptic D2-type receptors within the caudate putamen in the brain.

Pharmacodynamics/Kinetics

Onset: SubQ: Rapid

Distribution: V_d: Mean: 218 L

Metabolism: Not established; potential routes of metabolism include sulfation, N-demethylation, glucuronidation, and oxidation; catechol-O methyltransferase and nonenzymatic oxidation. CYP isoenzymes do not appear to play a significant role.

Half-life elimination: Terminal: 40 minutes

Time to peak, plasma: Improved motor scores: 20 minutes
Excretion: Urine 93% (as metabolites); feces 16%

Dosage SubQ: Adults: Begin antiemetic therapy 3 days prior to initiation and continue for 2 months before reassessing need.

Parkinson's disease, "off" episode: Initial test dose 2 mg, **medical supervision required; see "Note"**. Subsequent dosing is based on both tolerance and response to initial test dose.

If patient tolerates test dose and responds: Starting dose: 2 mg as needed; may increase dose in 1 mg increments every few days; maximum dose: 6 mg

If patient tolerates but does not respond to 2 mg test dose: Second test dose: 4 mg

If patient tolerates and responds to 4 mg test dose: Starting dose: 3 mg, as needed for "off" episodes; may increase dose in 1 mg increments every few days; maximum dose 6 mg

If patient does not tolerate 4 mg test dose: Third test dose: 3 mg

If patient tolerates 3 mg test dose: Starting dose: 2 mg as needed for "off" episodes; may increase dose in 1 mg increments to a maximum of 3 mg

If therapy is interrupted for >1 week, restart at 2 mg and gradually titrate dose.

Note: Medical supervision is required for all test doses with standing and supine blood pressure monitoring predose and 20-, 40-, and 60 minutes postdose. If subsequent test doses are required, wait >2 hours before another test dose is given; next test dose should be timed with another "off" episode. If a single dose is ineffective for a particular "off" episode, then a second dose should not be given. The average dosing frequency was 3 times/day in the development program with limited experience in dosing >5 times/day and with total daily doses >20 mg. Apomorphine is intended to treat the "off" episodes associated with levodopa therapy of Parkinson's disease and has not been studied in levodopa-naive Parkinson's patients.

Dosage adjustment in renal impairment:

Mild-to-moderate impairment: Reduce test dose and starting dose: 1 mg
Severe impairment: Has not been studied

Dosage adjustment in hepatic impairment:

Mild-to-moderate impairment: Use caution
Severe impairment: Has not been studied

Dietary Considerations Avoid ethanol consumption.

Administration SubQ: Initiate antiemetic 3 days before test dose of apomorphine and continue for 2 months (if patient to be treated) before reassessment. Administer in abdomen, upper arm, or upper leg; change site with each injection. 3 mL cartridges are used with a manual, reusable, multidose injector pen. Injector pen can deliver doses up to 1 mL in 0.02 mL increments. Do not give intravenously; thrombus formation or pulmonary embolism may occur.

Monitoring Parameters Each test dose: Supine and standing blood pressure predose and 20, 40, and 60 minutes postdose; drowsiness

Dosage Forms Excipient information presented when available (limited, particularly for generics); consult specific product labeling.

Injection, solution, as hydrochloride:

Apokyn®: 10 mg/mL (2 mL) [ampul; contains sodium metabisulfite]; (3 mL) [multidose cartridge; contains sodium metabisulfite and benzyl alcohol]

- ◆ **Apomorphine Hydrochloride** *see* Apomorphine *on page 127*
- ◆ **Apomorphine Hydrochloride Hemihydrate** *see* Apomorphine *on page 127*
- ◆ **APPG** *see* Penicillin G Procaine *on page 1241*
- ◆ **Apra Children's [OTC]** *see* Acetaminophen *on page 30*

Apraclonidine (a pra KLOE ni deen)

Medication Safety Issues

Sound-alike/look-alike issues:

Iopidine® may be confused with indapamide, iodine, Lodine®

U.S. Brand Names Iopidine®

Canadian Brand Names Iopidine®

Index Terms Aplonidine; Apraclonidine Hydrochloride; p-Aminoclonidine

Pharmacologic Category $Alpha_2$ Agonist, Ophthalmic

Use Prevention and treatment of postsurgical intraocular pressure (IOP) elevation; short-term, adjunctive therapy in patients who require additional reduction of IOP

Effect on Mental Status May cause drowsiness

Effect on Psychiatric Treatment Dry mouth may be exacerbated by concurrent use of psychotropics

Dosage Summary

Ophthalmic:

Children: Dosage not established

Adults: 0.5%: Instill 1-2 drops in the affected eye(s) 3 times/day; 1%: Instill 1 drop in operative eye 1 hour prior to and upon completion of surgery

Dosage Forms Excipient information presented when available (limited, particularly for generics); consult specific product labeling.

Solution, ophthalmic:

Iopidine®: 0.5% (5 mL, 10 mL); 1% (0.1 mL) [contains benzalkonium chloride]

- **Apraclonidine Hydrochloride** *see* Apraclonidine *on page 129*

Aprepitant (ap RE pi tant)

Medication Safety Issues

Sound-alike/look-alike issues:

Aprepitant may be confused with fosaprepitant

Emend® (aprepitant) oral capsule formulation may be confused with Emend® for injection (fosaprepitant).

U.S. Brand Names Emend®

Canadian Brand Names Emend®

Mexican Brand Names Emend

Index Terms L 754030; MK 869

Pharmacologic Category Antiemetic; Substance P/Neurokinin 1 Receptor Antagonist

Use Prevention of acute and delayed nausea and vomiting associated with moderately- and highly-emetogenic chemotherapy (in combination with other antiemetics); prevention of postoperative nausea and vomiting (PONV)

Effect on Mental Status Fatigue and weakness are common; may cause dizziness

Effect on Psychiatric Treatment Contraindicated with pimozide. Nausea is common; may be additive when used with SSRIs; monitor. Nefazodone may inhibit aprepitant's metabolism, while carbamazepine may increase its metabolism. Plasma levels of alprazolam, midazolam, and triazolam may be increased when combined with aprepitant. Plasma levels of paroxetine may be decreased with combined use; monitor.

Dosage Summary

Oral:

Children: Dosage not established

Adults: 125 mg on day 1, followed by 80 mg on days 2 and 3 in combination with other antiemetics **or** 40 mg within 3 hours prior to induction with anesthesia

Dosage Forms Excipient information presented when available (limited, particularly for generics); consult specific product labeling.

Capsule:

Emend®: 40 mg, 80 mg, 125 mg

Combination package [each package contains]:

Emend®:

Capsule: 80 mg (2s)

Capsule: 125 mg (1s)

- **Aprepitant Injection** *see* Fosaprepitant *on page 690*
- **Apresazide [DSC]** *see* Hydralazine and Hydrochlorothiazide *on page 772*
- **Apresoline [DSC]** *see* HydrALAZINE *on page 772*
- **Apri®** *see* Ethinyl Estradiol and Desogestrel *on page 592*
- **Aprodine® [OTC]** *see* Triprolidine and Pseudoephedrine *on page 1634*

Aprotinin (a proe TYE nin)

U.S. Brand Names Trasylol®

Canadian Brand Names Trasylol®

Mexican Brand Names Trasylol

Pharmacologic Category Blood Product Derivative; Hemostatic Agent

Use Prevention of perioperative blood loss in patients who are at increased risk for blood loss and blood transfusions in association with cardiopulmonary bypass in coronary artery bypass graft surgery

Effect on Mental Status May cause confusion

Effect on Psychiatric Treatment May cause renal dysfunction; use caution with lithium and gabapentin; may rarely cause seizures; use caution with clozapine

Restrictions Available in U.S. under an investigational new drug (IND) process. The program will provide aprotinin for the treatment of adult patients undergoing coronary artery bypass graft (CABG) surgery requiring cardiopulmonary bypass (CPB) who are at increased risk of bleeding and transfusion during CABG surgery with no acceptable therapeutic alternative. Healthcare providers using aprotinin for this situation must also ensure that the benefits outweigh the risks for their patient. U.S. healthcare providers with patients who may qualify can access information and forms for enrollment at http://www.trasylol.com/main.-htm or contact Bayer Medical Communications at (888) 842-2937.

Dosage Summary

I.V.:

Children: Dosage not established

Adults: Test dose: 1 mL (1.4 mg) 10 minutes prior to loading dose; Loading dose: 1-2 million KIU (140-280 mg; 100-200 mL); Pump prime volume: 1-2 million KIU (140-280 mg, 100-200 mL); Infusion: 250,000-500,000 KIU/hour (35-70 mg/hour; 25-50 mL/hour)

Dosage Forms Excipient information presented when available (limited, particularly for generics); consult specific product labeling.

Injection, solution:

Trasylol®: 1.4 mg/mL [10,000 KIU/mL] (100 mL, 200 mL) [bovine derived]

- **Aptivus®** *see* Tipranavir *on page 1586*
- **Aquachloral® Supprettes® [DSC]** *see* Chloral Hydrate *on page 313*
- **Aquanil™ HC [OTC]** *see* Hydrocortisone *on page 785*
- **Aquasol E® [OTC]** *see* Vitamin E *on page 1675*
- **Aquavit-E [OTC]** *see* Vitamin E *on page 1675*
- **Aqueous Procaine Penicillin G** *see* Penicillin G Procaine *on page 1241*
- **Ara-C** *see* Cytarabine *on page 412*
- **Arabinosylcytosine** *see* Cytarabine *on page 412*
- **Aralen®** *see* Chloroquine Phosphate *on page 320*
- **Aranelle™** *see* Ethinyl Estradiol and Norethindrone *on page 597*
- **Aranesp®** *see* Darbepoetin Alfa *on page 419*
- **Arava®** *see* Leflunomide *on page 899*
- **Aredia®** *see* Pamidronate *on page 1220*

Arformoterol (ar for MOE ter ol)

U.S. Brand Names Brovana®

Index Terms (R,R)-Formoterol L-Tartrate; Arformoterol Tartrate

Pharmacologic Category Beta$_2$-Adrenergic Agonist

Generic Available No

Use Long-term maintenance treatment of bronchoconstriction in chronic obstructive pulmonary disease (COPD), including chronic bronchitis and emphysema

Effect on Mental Status May cause nervousness, restlessness, or anxiety with excessive use

Effect on Psychiatric Treatment Concurrent use with atomoxetine may enhance tachycardia

Restrictions An FDA-approved medication guide must be distributed when dispensing an outpatient prescription (new or refill) where this medication is to be used without direct supervision of a healthcare provider. Medication guides are available at http://www.fda.gov/cder/Offices/ODS/medication_guides.htm.

Pregnancy Risk Factor C

Pregnancy Considerations Teratogenic effects, decreased fetal weight and increased fetal loss were observed in animal studies. There are no adequate and well-controlled studies in pregnant women. Beta-agonists may interfere with uterine contractility if administered during labor. Use in pregnancy and/or during labor should be limited to situations where benefit outweighs risk to fetus.

Lactation Excretion in breast milk unknown/use caution

Contraindications Hypersensitivity to arformoterol, racemic formoterol, or any component of the formulation

Warnings/Precautions **[U.S. Boxed Warning]: Long-acting beta$_2$-agonists may increase the risk of asthma-related deaths.** In a large, randomized clinical trial (SMART, 2006), salmeterol was associated with a small, but statistically significant increase in asthma-related deaths (when added to usual asthma therapy); risk may be greater in African-American patients versus Caucasians. Data is not available to determine whether rate of death is increased with long-acting beta$_2$-agonists in COPD setting. Rarely, paradoxical bronchospasm may occur with use of inhaled bronchodilating agents; this should be distinguished from inadequate response. Immediate hypersensitivity reactions (urticaria, angioedema, rash, bronchospasm) have been reported. Do not exceed recommended dose; serious adverse events, including fatalities, have been associated with excessive use of inhaled sympathomimetics.

Use with caution in patients with cardiovascular disease (eg, arrhythmia, hypertension, HF); beta-agonists may cause elevation in blood pressure, heart rate and result in CNS stimulation/excitation. Beta$_2$-agonists may also increase risk of arrhythmias and prolong QT_c interval. Arformoterol should only be used for long-term maintenance treatment and should not be used as rescue therapy in treatment of acute episodes. It should not be initiated in patients with acutely deteriorating COPD or combined with other long-acting beta$_2$-agonists. Use with caution in patients with diabetes mellitus; beta$_2$-agonists may increase serum glucose. Use caution in hepatic impairment; systemic clearance prolonged in hepatic dysfunction. Use with caution in hyperthyroidism; may stimulate thyroid activity. Use with caution in patients with hypokalemia; beta$_2$-agonists may decrease serum potassium. Use with caution in patients with seizure disorders; beta$_2$-agonists may result in CNS stimulation/excitation.

Tolerance/tachyphylaxis to the bronchodilator effect, measured by FEV_1, has been observed in studies. Patients using inhaled, short-acting beta$_2$-agonists should be instructed to discontinue routine use of these medications prior to beginning treatment; short-acting agents should be reserved for symptomatic relief of acute symptoms. Patients must be instructed to seek medical attention in cases where acute symptoms are not relieved or a previous level of response is diminished. The need to increase frequency of use may indicate deterioration of COPD, and treatment must not be delayed. Safety and efficacy have not been established in children.

Adverse Reactions

2% to 10%:

Cardiovascular: Chest pain (7%), peripheral edema (3%)
Central nervous system: Pain (8%)
Dermatologic: Rash (4%)
Gastrointestinal: Diarrhea (6%)
Neuromuscular & skeletal: Back pain (6%), leg cramps (4%)
Respiratory: Dyspnea (4%), sinusitis (5%), congestive conditions (2%)
Miscellaneous: Flu-like syndrome (3%)

<2% (Limited to important or life-threatening): Abscess, agitation, allergic reaction, arteriosclerosis, arthralgia, arthritis, atrial flutter, AV block, bone disorder, calcium crystalluria, cystitis, cerebral infarct, CHF, circumoral paresthesia, constipation, dehydration, dry skin, ECG changes, edema, fever, gastritis, glaucoma, glucose tolerance decreased, glycosuria, gout, heart block, hematuria, hyper-/hypoglycemia, hyperlipemia, hypokalemia, hypokinesia, inverted T-wave, kidney calculus, lung carcinoma, melena, MI, neck rigidity, neoplasm, nocturia, oral moniliasis, paradoxical bronchospasm, paralysis, pelvic pain, periodontal abscess, PSA increased, pyuria, QT interval increased, rectal hemorrhage, retroperitoneal hemorrhage, rheumatoid arthritis, skin discoloration, skin hypertrophy, somnolence, supraventricular tachycardia, tendinous contracture, tremor, urinary tract disorder, urine abnormality, viral infection, vision abnormalities, voice alteration

Metabolism/Transport Effects Substrate of CY2D6 (minor) and CYP2C19 (minor)

Drug Interactions

Alpha-/Beta-Blockers: May diminish the therapeutic effect of Beta2-Agonists. *Risk D: Consider therapy modification*

Atomoxetine: May enhance the tachycardic effect of Beta2-Agonists. *Risk C: Monitor therapy*

Beta-Blockers (Beta1 Selective): May diminish the bronchodilatory effect of Beta2-Agonists. Of particular concern with nonselective beta-blockers or higher doses of the beta1 selective beta-blockers. *Risk C: Monitor therapy*

Beta-Blockers (Nonselective): May diminish the bronchodilatory effect of Beta2-Agonists. *Risk D: Consider therapy modification*

Betahistine: May diminish the therapeutic effect of Beta2-Agonists. *Risk C: Monitor therapy*

Cannabinoids: May enhance the tachycardic effect of Sympathomimetics. *Risk C: Monitor therapy*

MAO Inhibitors: May enhance the adverse/toxic effect of Beta2-Agonists. *Risk C: Monitor therapy*

Sympathomimetics: May enhance the adverse/toxic effect of other Sympathomimetics. *Risk C: Monitor therapy*

Tricyclic Antidepressants: May enhance the adverse/toxic effect of Beta2-Agonists. *Risk C: Monitor therapy*

Stability Prior to dispensing, store in protective foil pouch under refrigeration at 2°C to 8°C (36°F to 46°F). Protect from light and excessive heat. After dispensing, unopened foil pouches may be stored at room temperature at 20°C to 25°C (68°F to 77°F) for up to 6 weeks. Only remove vial from foil pouch immediately before use.

Mechanism of Action Arformoterol, the (R,R)-enantiomer of the racemic formoterol, is a long-acting beta$_2$-agonist that relaxes bronchial smooth muscle by selective action on beta$_2$-receptors with little effect on cardiovascular system.

Pharmacodynamics/Kinetics

Onset of action: 7-20 minutes

Peak effect: 1-3 hours

Absorption: A portion of inhaled dose is absorbed into systemic circulation

Protein binding: 52% to 65%

Metabolism: Hepatic via direct glucuronidation and secondarily via O-demethylation; CYP2D6 and CYP2C19 (to a lesser extent) involved in O-demethylation

Half-life elimination: 26 hours

Time to peak: 0.5-3 hours

Dosage Nebulization: Adults: COPD: 15 mcg twice daily; maximum: 30 mcg/day

Dosage adjustment in renal impairment: No adjustment required

Dosage adjustment in hepatic impairment: No dosage adjustment required, but use caution; systemic drug exposure prolonged (1.3- to 2.4-fold)

Administration Nebulization: Remove each vial from individually sealed foil pouch immediately before use. Use with standard jet nebulizer connected to an air compressor, administer with mouthpiece or face mask. Administer vial undiluted and do not mix with other medications in nebulizer.

Monitoring Parameters FEV$_1$, peak flow, and/or other pulmonary function tests; blood pressure, heart rate; CNS stimulation; serum glucose, serum potassium. Monitor for increased use of short-acting beta$_2$-agonist inhalers; may be marker of a deteriorating COPD condition.

Dosage Forms Excipient information presented when available (limited, particularly for generics); consult specific product labeling.

Solution for nebulization:

Brovana®: 15 mcg/2 mL (30s, 60s)

- **Arformoterol Tartrate** *see* Arformoterol *on page 131*
- **8-Arginine Vasopressin** *see* Vasopressin *on page 1659*
- **Aricept®** *see* Donepezil *on page 495*
- **Aricept® ODT** *see* Donepezil *on page 495*
- **Arimidex®** *see* Anastrozole *on page 125*

Aripiprazole (ay ri PIP ray zole)

Medication Safety Issues

Sound-alike/look-alike issues:

Aripiprazole may be confused with proton pump inhibitors (eg, rabeprazole)

Related Information

Agents Approved for Bipolar Disorder *on page 1752*

Antipsychotic Agents *on page 1769*

Antipsychotic Receptor Profile *on page 1772*

Atypical Antipsychotics *on page 1773*

CMS: Long-Term Care Facility Thresholds *on page 1815*

Liquid Compatibility of Antidepressants, Antipsychotics, and Mood Stabilizers *on page 1788*

U.S. Brand Names Abilify®; Abilify® Discmelt™

Mexican Brand Names Abilify

Index Terms BMS 337039; OPC-14597

Pharmacologic Category Antipsychotic Agent, Atypical

Generic Available No

Use

Oral: Acute and maintenance treatment of schizophrenia; stabilization, maintenance, and adjunctive therapy (to lithium or valproate) of bipolar disorder (with acute manic or mixed episodes); adjunctive treatment of major depressive disorder

Injection: Agitation associated with schizophrenia or bipolar mania

Unlabeled/Investigational Use Depression with psychotic features; aggression (children); conduct disorder (children); Tourette syndrome (children); psychosis/agitation related to Alzheimer's dementia

Mental Health Comment Aripiprazole is an antipsychotic agent of a class often referred to as atypical. Some have referred to this agent as a new generation agent since its pharmacology differs (partial dopamine agonist) from the other atypical agents. It should be noted that the definition of the term "atypical" is not universally agreed upon. Some prefer to describe antipsychotics based on their pharmacological properties. A common feature of all definitions used to describe "atypical" antipsychotics is the lack of significant acute or subacute EPS, at dosages generally associated with antipsychotic actions. Other experts have included definitions of atypicality that include a) failure to increase serum prolactin levels; b) superior efficacy for positive, negative, and cognitive symptoms; and c) lack of evidence of tardive dyskinesia or dystonia following chronic administration. Clinically, if a patient with schizophrenia is not doing well on a particular dose, it is not clear whether the dose should be increased or decreased (15 mg/day dose did not differ from 30 mg/day dose in schizophrenia clinical trials). It is helpful, however, for patients with significant GI side effects to lower the dose and wait for tolerance to develop before going to a higher dose. While the dose for individuals with bipolar is similar to those with schizophrenia (15-30 mg/day) when used as an adjunctive agent for the management of depression the dose is 2-15 mg/day.

The short-acting I.M. formulation appears to be as efficacious as other available agents for the management of acute agitation; however, comparative trials have not been conducted.

Tardive dyskinesia (TD) secondary to **typical** antipsychotics has an estimated incidence of 3% to 5% per year for the first 5 years of treatment. The incidence of TD associated with the atypical antipsychotics is estimated to be 0.5% to 1%. It is not clear if this estimate represents a risk associated with mental illness or to what extent drug therapy can be implicated. Atypical antipsychotics appear less likely to cause tardive dyskinesia than typical antipsychotics (fluphenazine, haloperidol).

Coadministration of two or more antipsychotics does not generally improve clinical response and may increase the potential for adverse effects.

In 2008, the FDA issued a warning regarding increased mortality risk with typical **and** atypical antipsychotic drugs when used in elderly patients with dementia-related psychosis.

Restrictions An FDA-approved medication guide concerning the use of antidepressants in children, adolescents, and young adults must be distributed when dispensing an outpatient prescription (new or refill) where this medication is to be used without direct supervision of a healthcare provider. Medication guides are available at http://www.fda.gov/cder/Offices/ODS/medication_guides.htm. Dispense to parents or guardians of children and adolescents receiving this medication.

Pregnancy Risk Factor C

Pregnancy Considerations Aripiprazole demonstrated developmental toxicity and teratogenic effects in animal models. There are no adequate and well-controlled trials in pregnant women. Should be used in pregnancy only when potential benefit to mother outweighs possible risk to the fetus.

Lactation Excretion in breast milk unknown/not recommended

Contraindications Hypersensitivity to aripiprazole or any component of the formulation

Warnings/Precautions **[U.S. Boxed Warning]: Elderly patients with dementia-related psychosis treated with atypical antipsychotics are at an increased risk of death compared to placebo.** An increased incidence of cerebrovascular adverse events (including fatalities) has been reported in elderly patients with dementia-related psychosis. Aripiprazole is not approved for this indication.

[U.S. Boxed Warning]: Antidepressants increase the risk of suicidal thinking and behavior in children, adolescents, and young adults (18-24 years of age) with major depressive disorder (MDD) and other psychiatric disorders; consider risk prior to prescribing. The possibility of a suicide attempt is inherent in major depression and may persist until remission occurs. Patients treated with antidepressants should be observed for clinical worsening and suicidality, especially during the initial few months of a course of drug therapy, or at times of dose changes, either increases or decreases. Prescriptions should be written for the smallest quantity consistent with good patient care. The patient's family or caregiver should be alerted to monitor patients for the emergence of suicidality and associated behaviors; patients should be instructed to notify their healthcare provider if any of these symptoms or worsening depression or psychosis occur.

A medication guide concerning the use of antidepressants should be dispensed with each prescription. **Aripiprazole is not FDA approved for adjunctive treatment of depression in children.**

May cause extrapyramidal symptoms (EPS), including pseudoparkinsonism, acute dystonic reactions, akathisia, and tardive dyskinesia (risk of these reactions is very low relative to typical/conventional antipsychotics, frequencies reported are similar to placebo). Risk of dystonia (and probably other EPS) may be greater with increased doses, use of conventional antipsychotics, males, and younger patients. May be associated with neuroleptic malignant syndrome (NMS).

May be sedating, use with caution in disorders where CNS depression is a feature. May cause orthostatic hypotension (although reported rates are similar to placebo); use caution in patients at risk of this effect or those who would not tolerate transient hypotensive episodes (cerebrovascular disease, cardiovascular disease, or other medications which may predispose).

Use caution in patients with Parkinson's disease; predisposition to seizures; and severe cardiac disease. May alter cardiac conduction; life-threatening arrhythmias have occurred with therapeutic doses of antipsychotics. Esophageal dysmotility and aspiration have been associated with antipsychotic use; use caution in patients at risk of pneumonia (eg, Alzheimer's disease). May alter temperature regulation. Significant weight gain has been observed with antipsychotic therapy; incidence varies with product. Monitor waist circumference and BMI.

Atypical antipsychotics have been associated with development of hyperglycemia; in some cases, may be extreme and associated with ketoacidosis, hyperosmolar coma, or death. Reports of hyperglycemia with aripiprazole therapy have been few and specific risk associated with this agent is not known. Use caution in patients with diabetes or other disorders of glucose regulation; monitor for worsening of glucose control.

Abilify® Discmelt™: Use caution in phenylketonuria; contains phenylalanine. Safety and efficacy in patients <10 years of age have not been established.

Adverse Reactions Unless otherwise noted, frequency of adverse reactions is shown as reported for adult patients receiving oral administration. Spectrum and incidence of adverse effects similar in children; exceptions noted when incidence much higher in children.

>10%:

Central nervous system: Headache (27%; children 16%; injection 12%), agitation (19%), insomnia (18%), anxiety (17%), akathisia (10% to 13%; injection 2%), lightheadedness (11%)

Gastrointestinal: Weight gain (8% to 30%; highest frequency in patients with BMI <23; children 3%), nausea (15%; injection 9%), dyspepsia (9% to 15%; injection 1%), constipation (11% to 13%), vomiting (11%; injection 3%)

1% to 10%:

Cardiovascular: Orthostatic hypotension (1% to 5%), tachycardia (injection 2%), chest pain, hypertension, peripheral edema

Central nervous system: Dizziness (10%; children 5%; injection 8%), sedation (dose-related 5% to 8%; children 20% to 23%; injection: 7%), EPS (5% to 6%; children 19% to 20%), restlessness (5% to 6%), fatigue (6%; children 7% to 11%), pain (3%), dystonia (children 2%), irritability, suicidal ideation

Dermatologic: Rash

Gastrointestinal: Salivation increased (children 4% to 8%), xerostomia (5%; children 2%; injection 1%), toothache (4%), abdominal discomfort (3%), diarrhea (children 3%), weight loss

Neuromuscular & skeletal: Tremor (5% to 9%), weakness (8%), arthralgia (5%; children 2%), extremity pain (4%), stiffness (4%), myalgia (2% to 4%), spasm (2%)

Ocular: Blurred vision (3%; children 5% to 8%)

Respiratory: Pharyngolaryngeal pain (3%), cough (3%), nasal congestion

<1% (Limited to important or life-threatening): Aggression, agitation, agranulocytosis, alopecia, akinesia, amenorrhea, anaphylactic reaction, anger, angina pectoris, angioedema, anorexia, anorgasmia, asphyxia, aspiration pneumonia, atrial fibrillation, atrial flutter, atrioventricular block, bilirubin increased, bradycardia, bradykinesia, breast pain, bundle branch block, cardiopulmonary failure, cardiorespiratory arrest, catatonia, cerebrovascular

accident, cholelithiasis, choreoathetosis, cogwheel rigidity, complete atrio-ventricular block, creatine phosphokinase increased, creatinine increased, deep vein thrombosis, delirium, diplopia, diabetes mellitus, DKA, dysphagia, dyspnea, edema (facial), erectile dysfunction, esophagitis, extrasystoles, galactorrhea, gastrointestinal hemorrhage, GGT increased, glycosylated hemoglobin increased, gynecomastia, heat stroke, hepatic enzyme increased, hepatitis, homicidal ideation, hostility, hyper-/hypoglycemia, hyperlipidemia, hypersensitivity, hyper-/hypotonia, hypotension, hypokalemia, hypokinesia, hyponatremia, hypothermia cholecystitis, idiopathic thrombocytopenic purpura, intentional self injury, jaundice, lactate dehydrogenase increased, leukopenia, libido changes, memory impairment, menstrual irregularities, MI, muscle rigidity, muscle spasms, myocardial ischemia, myoclonus, neutropenia, nocturia, oropharyngeal spasm, palpitation, pancreatitis, parkinsonism, phlebitis, photophobia, polydypsia, polyuria, priapism, prolactin increased, pruritus, psychomotor agitation, pulmonary embolism, QT_c prolonged, respiratory distress, rhabdomyolysis, seizure (grand mal), shock, speech disorder, suicide, suicide attempt, supraventricular tachycardia, swollen tongue, tardive dyskinesia, thrombocytopenia, thrombophlebitis, tic, ulcer, urea increased, urinary retention, urticaria, ventricular tachycardia

Metabolism/Transport Effects Substrate (major) of CYP2D6, 3A4

Drug Interactions

Acetylcholinesterase Inhibitors (Central): May enhance the neurotoxic (central) effect of Antipsychotics. Severe extrapyramidal symptoms have occurred in some patients. *Risk C: Monitor therapy*

Alcohol (Ethyl): CNS Depressants may enhance the CNS depressant effect of Alcohol (Ethyl). *Risk C: Monitor therapy*

Amphetamines: Antipsychotics may diminish the stimulatory effect of Amphetamines. *Risk C: Monitor therapy*

Anti-Parkinson's Agents (Dopamine Agonist): Antipsychotics (Atypical) may diminish the therapeutic effect of Anti-Parkinson's Agents (Dopamine Agonist). *Risk D: Consider therapy modification*

CarBAMazepine: May decrease the serum concentration of Aripiprazole. *Risk D: Consider therapy modification*

CNS Depressants: May enhance the adverse/toxic effect of other CNS Depressants. *Risk C: Monitor therapy*

CYP2D6 Inhibitors (Moderate): May decrease the metabolism of CYP2D6 Substrates. *Risk C: Monitor therapy*

CYP2D6 Inhibitors (Strong): May decrease the metabolism of CYP2D6 Substrates. *Risk D: Consider therapy modification*

CYP3A4 Inducers (Strong): May increase the metabolism of CYP3A4 Substrates. *Risk C: Monitor therapy*

CYP3A4 Inhibitors (Moderate): May decrease the metabolism of CYP3A4 Substrates. *Risk C: Monitor therapy*

CYP3A4 Inhibitors (Strong): May decrease the metabolism of CYP3A4 Substrates. *Risk D: Consider therapy modification*

Darunavir: May increase the serum concentration of CYP2D6 Substrates. *Risk C: Monitor therapy*

Dasatinib: May increase the serum concentration of CYP3A4 Substrates. *Risk C: Monitor therapy*

Deferasirox: May decrease the serum concentration of CYP3A4 Substrates. *Risk C: Monitor therapy*

Herbs (CYP3A4 Inducers): May increase the metabolism of CYP3A4 Substrates. *Risk C: Monitor therapy*

Lithium formulations: May enhance the neurotoxic effect of Antipsychotics. Lithium formulations may decrease the serum concentration of Antipsychotics. Specifically noted with chlorpromazine. *Risk C: Monitor therapy*

Tetrabenazine: May enhance the adverse/toxic effect of Antipsychotics. *Risk C: Monitor therapy*

Ethanol/Nutrition/Herb Interactions

Ethanol: Avoid ethanol (may increase CNS depression).

Food: Ingestion with a high-fat meal delays time to peak plasma level.

Herb/Nutraceutical: St John's wort may decrease aripiprazole levels. Avoid kava kava, gotu kola, valerian, St John's wort (may increase CNS depression).

Stability

Injection solution: Store at controlled room temperature of 25°C (77°F); excursions permitted to 15°C to 30°C (59°F to 86°F). Protect from light.

Oral solution: Store at controlled room temperature of 25°C (77°F); excursions permitted to 15°C to 30°C (59°F to 86°F). Use within 6 months after opening.

Tablet: Store at controlled room temperature of 25°C (77°F); excursions permitted to 15°C to 30°C (59°F to 86°F).

Mechanism of Action Aripiprazole is a quinolinone antipsychotic which exhibits high affinity for D_2, D_3, 5-HT_{1A}, and 5-HT_{2A} receptors; moderate affinity for D_4, 5-HT_{2C}, 5-HT_7, alpha$_1$ adrenergic, and H_1 receptors. It also possesses moderate affinity for the serotonin reuptake transporter; has no affinity for muscarinic (cholinergic) receptors. Aripiprazole functions as a partial agonist at the D_2 and 5-HT_{1A} receptors, and as an antagonist at the 5-HT_{2A} receptor.

Pharmacodynamics/Kinetics

Onset: Initial: 1-3 weeks

Absorption: Well absorbed

Distribution: V_d: 4.9 L/kg

Protein binding: ≥99%, primarily to albumin

Metabolism: Hepatic, via CYP2D6, CYP3A4 (dehydro-aripiprazole metabolite has affinity for D_2 receptors similar to the parent drug and represents 40% of the parent drug exposure in plasma)

Bioavailability: I.M.: 100%; Tablet: 87%

Half-life elimination: Aripiprazole: 75 hours; dehydro-aripiprazole: 94 hours

CYP2D6 poor metabolizers: Aripiprazole: 146 hours

Time to peak, plasma: I.M.: 1-3 hours; Tablet: 3-5 hours

With high-fat meal: Aripiprazole: Delayed by 3 hours; dehydro-aripiprazole: Delayed by 12 hours

Excretion: Feces (55%, ~18% unchanged drug); urine (25%, <1% unchanged drug)

Dosage Note: Oral solution may be substituted for the oral tablet on a mg-per-mg basis, up to 25 mg. Patients receiving 30 mg tablets should be given 25 mg oral solution. Orally disintegrating tablets (Abilify® Discmelt™) are bioequivalent to the immediate release tablets (Abilify®).

Children: Oral: Aggression, conduct disorder, Tourette syndrome (unlabeled uses): 5-20 mg/day

Children ≥10 years: Oral: Bipolar I disorder (acute manic or mixed episodes): Initial: 2 mg daily for 2 days, followed by 5 mg daily for 2 days with a further increase to target dose of 10 mg daily as monotherapy or adjunctive therapy; subsequent dose increases may be made in 5 mg increments, up to a maximum of 30 mg/day

Adolescents ≥13 years: Oral: Schizophrenia: Initial: 2 mg daily for 2 days, followed by 5 mg daily for 2 days with a further increase to target dose of 10 mg daily; subsequent dose increases may be made in 5 mg increments up to a maximum of 30 mg/day (30 mg/day not shown to be more efficacious than 10 mg/day)

Adults:

Acute agitation (schizophrenia/bipolar mania): I.M.: 9.75 mg as a single dose (range: 5.25-15 mg); repeated doses may be given at ≥2-hour intervals to a maximum of 30 mg/day. **Note:** If ongoing therapy with aripiprazole is necessary, transition to oral therapy as soon as possible.

Bipolar disorder (acute manic or mixed episodes): Oral:

Stabilization: Initial: 15 mg once daily as monotherapy or adjunctive to lithium or valproic acid. May increase to 30 mg once daily if clinically indicated; safety of doses >30 mg/day has not been evaluated.

Maintenance: Continue stabilization dose for up to 6 weeks; efficacy of continued treatment >6 weeks has not been established

Depression (adjunctive with antidepressants): Oral: Initial: 2-5 mg/day (range: 2-15 mg/day); dose adjustments of up to 5 mg/day may be made in intervals of ≥1 week. **Note:** Dosing based on patients already receiving antidepressant therapy.

Schizophrenia: Oral: 10-15 mg once daily; may be increased to a maximum of 30 mg once daily (efficacy at dosages above 10-15 mg has not been shown to be increased). Dosage titration should not be more frequent than every 2 weeks.

Dosage adjustment with concurrent CYP450 inducer or inhibitor therapy: Oral:

CYP3A4 inducers (eg, carbamazepine): Aripiprazole dose should be doubled (20-30 mg/day); dose should be subsequently reduced (10-15 mg/day) if concurrent inducer agent discontinued.

CYP3A4 inhibitors (eg, ketoconazole): Aripiprazole dose should be reduced to 1/2 of the usual dose, and proportionally increased upon discontinuation of the inhibitor agent.

CYP2D6 inhibitors (eg, fluoxetine, paroxetine): Aripiprazole dose should be reduced to 1/2 of the usual dose, and proportionally increased upon discontinuation of the inhibitor agent.

Dosage adjustment in renal impairment: No dosage adjustment required

Dosage adjustment in hepatic impairment: No dosage adjustment required

Dietary Considerations May be taken with or without food. Oral solution contains sucrose 400 mg/mL and fructose 200 mg/mL. Orally-disintegrating tablet contains phenylalanine; avoid use in phenylketonuria.

Administration

Injection: For I.M. use only; do not administer SubQ or I.V.; inject slowly into deep muscle mass

Oral: May be administered with or without food. Tablet and oral solution may be interchanged on a mg-per-mg basis, up to 25 mg. Doses using 30 mg tablets should be exchanged for 25 mg oral solution. Orally-disintegrating tablets (Abilify® Discmelt™) are bioequivalent to the immediate release tablets (Abilify®).

Orally-disintegrating tablet: Remove from foil blister by peeling back (do not push tablet through the foil). Place tablet in mouth immediately upon removal. Tablet dissolves rapidly in saliva and may be swallowed without liquid. If needed, can be taken with liquid. Do not split tablet.

Monitoring Parameters Vital signs; fasting lipid profile and fasting blood glucose/Hb A_{1c} (prior to treatment, at 3 months, then annually); BMI, personal/family history of diabetes, waist circumference, blood pressure, mental status, abnormal involuntary movement scale (AIMS), extrapyramidal symptoms (EPS). Weight should be assessed prior to treatment, at 4 weeks, 8 weeks, 12 weeks, and then at quarterly intervals. Consider titrating to a different antipsychotic agent for a weight gain ≥5% of the initial weight.

Dosage Forms Excipient information presented when available (limited, particularly for generics); consult specific product labeling.

Injection, solution:

Abilify®: 7.5 mg/mL (1.3 mL)

Solution, oral:

Abilify®: 1 mg/mL (150 mL) [contains propylene glycol, sucrose 400 mg/mL, and fructose 200 mg/mL; orange cream flavor]

Tablet:

Abilify®: 2 mg, 5 mg, 10 mg, 15 mg, 20 mg, 30 mg

Tablet, orally disintegrating:

Abilify® Discmelt™: 10 mg [contains phenylalanine 1.12 mg; creme de vanilla flavor]; 15 mg [contains phenylalanine 1.68 mg; creme de vanilla flavor]

◆ **Aristospan®** *see* Triamcinolone *on page 1617*

Armodafinil (ar moe DAF i nil)

U.S. Brand Names Nuvigil™

Index Terms R-modafinil

Pharmacologic Category Stimulant

Generic Available No

Use Improve wakefulness in patients with excessive daytime sleepiness associated with narcolepsy and shift work sleep disorder (SWSD); adjunctive therapy for obstructive sleep apnea/hypopnea syndrome (OSAHS)

Mental Health Comment Armodafinil is a stimulant and has been shown to worsen symptoms of psychosis (hallucinations), depression (suicidal thoughts), and mania in some vulnerable patients. Patients with bipolar disorder should not receive stimulant medication in the absence of treatment with a concomitant mood-stabilizing medication. Stimulants may also unmask tics in patients with Tourette's syndrome. Armodafinil has the potential to be abused and for individuals to become dependent. Assess patients' history of drug abuse. Monitor for life-threatening rashes including Stevens-Johnson syndrome. Armodafinil uses CYP3A4 as a major metabolic pathway. Evaluate medication regimen for potential drug-drug interactions.

Restrictions C-IV

Pregnancy Risk Factor C

Pregnancy Considerations There are no well-controlled studies of armodafinil in pregnant women. There have been reports of intrauterine growth retardation and spontaneous abortions in women using the both armodafinil and modafinil, but relationship to the drug is unknown.

Adverse events have been observed in animal studies. Armodafinil and modafinil have been studied in both rats and rabbits. Developmental toxicity (including visceral and skeletal abnormalities and decreased fetal weight) in rats (armodafinil and modafinil) and rabbits (modafinil) has been observed at doses correlating to those used clinically. Efficacy of steroidal contraceptives may be decreased; alternate means of contraception should be considered during therapy and for 1 month after modafinil is discontinued.

Lactation Excretion in breast milk unknown/use caution

Contraindications Hypersensitivity to armodafinil, modafinil, or any component of the formulation

Warnings/Precautions For use following complete evaluation of sleepiness and in conjunction with other standard treatments (eg, CPAP). The degree of sleepiness should be reassessed frequently; some patients may not return to a normal level of wakefulness. Use is not recommended with a history of angina, cardiac ischemia, recent history of myocardial infarction, left ventricular hypertrophy, or patients with mitral valve prolapse who have developed mitral valve prolapse syndrome with previous CNS stimulant use. Blood pressure monitoring may be required in patients on armodafinil. New or additional antihypertensive therapy may be needed.

Serious and life-threatening rashes including Stevens-Johnson syndrome, toxic epidermal necrolysis, and drug rash with eosinophilia and systemic symptoms have been reported with modafinil, the racemate of armodafinil. In clinical trials of modafinil, these rashes were more likely to occur in children; however, in the postmarketing period, serious reactions have occurred in both adults and children. Most cases have been reported within the first 5 weeks of initiating therapy; however, rare cases have occurred after prolonged therapy.

Caution should be exercised when modafinil is given to patients with a history of psychosis; may impair the ability to engage in potentially hazardous activities. Stimulants may unmask tics in individuals with coexisting Tourette's syndrome. Use caution with renal or hepatic impairment (dosage adjustment in hepatic dysfunction is recommended). Use reduced doses in elderly patients. Safety and efficacy in children <17 years of age have not been established.

Adverse Reactions

>10%: Central nervous system: Headache (14% to 23%; dose-related)

1% to 10%:

Cardiovascular: Palpitation (2%), increased heart rate (1%)

Central nervous system: Dizziness (5%), insomnia (4% to 6%; dose related), anxiety (4%), depression (1% to 3%; dose related), fatigue (2%), agitation (1%), attention disturbance (1%), depressed mood (1%), migraine (1%), nervousness (1%), pain (1%), pyrexia (1%), tremor (1%)

Dermatologic: Rash (1% to 4%; dose related), contact dermatitis (1%), hyperhidrosis (1%)

Gastrointestinal: Nausea (6% to 9%; dose related), xerostomia (2% to 7%; dose related), diarrhea (4%), abdominal pain (2%), dyspepsia (2%), anorexia (1%), appetite decreased (1%), constipation (1%), loose stools (1%), vomiting (1%)

Genitourinary: Polyuria (1%)

Hepatic: GGT increased (1%)

Neuromuscular & skeletal: Paresthesia (1%)

Respiratory: Dyspnea (1%)

Miscellaneous: Flu-like syndrome (1%), thirst (1%)

Postmarketing and/or case reports: Anaphylactoid reaction, angioedema, hypersensitivity, liver enzymes increased, pancytopenia, systolic blood pressure increased

Metabolism/Transport Effects

Substrate of CYP3A4 (major); **Inhibits** CYP2C19 (moderate); **Induces** CYP1A2 (weak), 3A4 (moderate)

Drug Interactions

Cannabinoids: May enhance the tachycardic effect of Sympathomimetics. *Risk C: Monitor therapy*

CYP2C19 Substrates: CYP2C19 Inhibitors (Moderate) may decrease the metabolism of CYP2C19 Substrates. *Risk C: Monitor therapy*

CYP3A4 Inducers (Strong): May increase the metabolism of CYP3A4 Substrates. *Risk C: Monitor therapy*

CYP3A4 Inhibitors (Moderate): May decrease the metabolism of CYP3A4 Substrates. *Risk C: Monitor therapy*

CYP3A4 Inhibitors (Strong): May decrease the metabolism of CYP3A4 Substrates. *Risk D: Consider therapy modification*

Dasatinib: May increase the serum concentration of CYP3A4 Substrates. *Risk C: Monitor therapy*

Deferasirox: May decrease the serum concentration of CYP3A4 Substrates. *Risk C: Monitor therapy*

Herbs (CYP3A4 Inducers): May increase the metabolism of CYP3A4 Substrates. *Risk C: Monitor therapy*

Maraviroc: CYP3A4 Inducers may decrease the serum concentration of Maraviroc. *Risk D: Consider therapy modification*

Oral Contraceptive (Estrogens): Armodafinil may decrease the serum concentration of Oral Contraceptive (Estrogens). *Risk D: Consider therapy modification*

Sympathomimetics: May enhance the adverse/toxic effect of other Sympathomimetics. *Risk C: Monitor therapy*

Ethanol/Nutrition/Herb Interactions

Ethanol: Avoid or limit ethanol.

Food: Delays absorption, but minimal effects on bioavailability. Food may affect the onset and time course of armodafinil.

Stability Store at 20°C to 25°C (68°F to 77°F).

Mechanism of Action The exact mechanism of action of armodafinil is unknown. It is the R-enantiomer of modafinil. Armodafinil binds to the dopamine transporter and inhibits dopamine reuptake, which may result in increased extracellular dopamine levels in the brain. However, it does not appear to be a dopamine receptor agonist and also does not appear to bind to or inhibit the most common receptors or enzymes that are relevant for sleep/wake regulation.

Pharmacodynamics/Kinetics

Absorption: Readily absorbed

Distribution: V_d: 42 L

Protein binding: ~60% (based on modafinil; primarily albumin)

Metabolism: Hepatic, multiple pathways, including CYP3A4/5; metabolites include R-modafinil acid and modafinil sulfone

Clearance: 33 mL/minute, mainly via hepatic metabolism

Half-life elimination: 15 hours; Steady state: ~7 days

Time to peak, plasma: 2 hours (fasted)

Excretion: Urine (80% predominantly as metabolites; <10% as unchanged drug)

Dosage Oral:

Adults:

Narcolepsy: 150-250 mg once daily in the morning

Obstructive sleep apnea/hypopnea syndrome (OSAHS): 150-250 mg once daily in the morning; 250 mg was not shown to have any increased benefit over 150 mg

Shift work sleep disorder (SWSD): 150 mg given once daily ~1 hour prior to work shift

Elderly: Consider lower initial dosage. Concentrations were almost doubled in clinical trials (based on modafinil)

Dosage adjustment in renal impairment: Inadequate data to determine safety and efficacy in severe renal impairment.

Dosage adjustment in hepatic impairment: Severe hepatic impairment (Child-Pugh classes B and C): Based on modafinil, dose should be reduced by half

Dietary Considerations Take with or without meals.

Administration May be administered without regard to food.

Monitoring Parameters Signs of hypersensitivity, rash, psychiatric symptoms, levels of sleepiness, blood pressure, and drug abuse

Dosage Forms Excipient information presented when available (limited, particularly for generics); consult specific product labeling.

Tablet:

Nuvigil™: 50 mg, 150 mg, 250 mg

◆ **Armour® Thyroid** *see* Thyroid, Desiccated *on page 1579*

◆ **Aromasin®** *see* Exemestane *on page 609*

◆ **Arranon®** *see* Nelarabine *on page 1120*

Arsenic Trioxide (AR se nik tri OKS id)

Medication Safety Issues

High alert medication: The Institute for Safe Medication Practices (ISMP) includes this medication among its list of drugs which have a heightened risk of causing significant patient harm when used in error.

U.S. Brand Names Trisenox®

Index Terms As_2O_3; NSC-706363

Pharmacologic Category Antineoplastic Agent, Miscellaneous

Use Induction of remission and consolidation in patients with relapsed or refractory acute promyelocytic leukemia (APL) which is specifically characterized by t(15;17) translocation or PML/RAR-alpha gene expression

Unlabeled/Investigational Use Treatment of myelodysplastic syndrome (MDS), multiple myeloma

Effect on Mental Status Fatigue, insomnia, anxiety, dizziness, and depression are common; may cause agitation and confusion

Effect on Psychiatric Treatment Contraindicated with ziprasidone. Gastrointestinal side effects are common; may produce additive GI side effects when used in combination with SSRIs. Hypotension is common and combined use with psychotropics may produce additive hypotension. May cause thrombocytopenia and neutropenia. Use caution with clozapine, carbamazepine, and valproic acid. Concurrent use with thioridazine may increase the risk of potentially fatal arrhythmias.

Dosage Summary

I.V.:

Children <5 years: Dosage not established

Children ≥5 years: Induction: 0.15 mg/kg/day (maximum: 60 doses); Consolidation: 0.15 mg/kg/day (maximum: 25 doses over 5 weeks)

Adults: Induction: 0.15 mg/kg/day (maximum: 60 doses); Consolidation: 0.15 mg/kg/day (maximum: 25 doses over 5 weeks)

Elderly ≥72 years: Dosage not established

Dosage Forms Excipient information presented when available (limited, particularly for generics); consult specific product labeling.

Injection, solution [preservative free]:

Trisenox®: 1 mg/mL (10 mL)

- **Artane** *see* Trihexyphenidyl *on page 1627*
- **Arthrotec®** *see* Diclofenac and Misoprostol *on page 458*
- **As_2O_3** *see* Arsenic Trioxide *on page 140*
- **ASA** *see* Aspirin *on page 143*
- **5-ASA** *see* Mesalamine *on page 994*
- **ASA and Diphenhydramine** *see* Aspirin and Diphenhydramine *on page 145*
- **Asacol®** *see* Mesalamine *on page 994*
- **Asco-Caps [OTC]** *see* Ascorbic Acid *on page 141*
- **Ascocid® [OTC]** *see* Ascorbic Acid *on page 141*
- **Ascomp® with Codeine** *see* Butalbital, Aspirin, Caffeine, and Codeine *on page 242*
- **Ascor L 500®** *see* Ascorbic Acid *on page 141*
- **Ascor L NC®** *see* Ascorbic Acid *on page 141*

Ascorbic Acid (a SKOR bik AS id)

Medication Safety Issues

International issues:

Rubex® [Ireland] may be confused with Revex® which is a brand name for nalmefene in the U.S.

Rubex® [Ireland]: Brand name for doxurbicin in the U.S.

U.S. Brand Names Acerola [OTC]; Asco-Caps [OTC]; Asco-Tabs [OTC]; Ascocid® [OTC]; Ascor L 500®; Ascor L NC®; C-Gel [OTC]; C-Gram [OTC]; C-Time [OTC]; Cecon® [OTC]; Cemill [OTC]; Cenolate®; Chew-C [OTC]; Dull-C® [OTC]; Mild-C® [OTC]; One Gram C [OTC]; Time-C [OTC]; Time-C-Bio [OTC]; Vicks® Vitamin C [OTC]; Vita-C® [OTC]

Canadian Brand Names Proflavanol C™; Revitalose C-1000®

Mexican Brand Names Cevalin; Femiprim; Ácido ascórbico

Index Terms Vitamin C

Pharmacologic Category Vitamin, Water Soluble

Use Prevention and treatment of scurvy; acidify the urine

Unlabeled/Investigational Use Investigational: In large doses, to decrease the severity of "colds"; dietary supplementation; a 20-year study was recently completed involving 730 individuals which indicates a possible decreased risk of death by stroke when ascorbic acid at doses ≥45 mg/day was administered

Effect on Mental Status Rare reports of drowsiness; usually well tolerated

Effect on Psychiatric Treatment May decrease fluphenazine levels; clinical significance unknown but likely not problematic

Dosage Summary

I.M.:

Children: 100-300 mg/day in divided doses

Adults: 100-250 mg 1-2 times/day

I.V.:

Children: 100-300 mg/day in divided doses (up to 500 mg every 6-8 hours for selected indications)

Adults: 100-250 mg 1-2 times/day (up to 4-12 g/day in 3-4 divided doses for selected indications)

Oral:

Children: 100-300 mg/day in divided doses (up to 500 mg every 6-8 hours for selected indications)

Adults: 100-250 mg 1-2 times/day (up to 4-12 g/day in 3-4 divided doses for selected indications)

SubQ:

Children: 100-300 mg/day in divided doses

Adults: 100-250 mg 1-2 times/day

Dosage Forms Excipient information presented when available (limited, particularly for generics); consult specific product labeling.

Caplet: 1000 mg

Caplet, timed release: 500 mg, 1000 mg

Capsule:
- Mild-C®: 500 mg

Capsule, softgel:
- C-Gel: 1000 mg

Capsule, sustained release:
- C-Time: 500 mg

Capsule, timed release: 500 mg
- Asco-Caps: 500 mg, 1000 mg [sugar free]
- Time-C®: 500 mg

Crystals for solution, oral: 4 g/teaspoonful (170 g, 1000 g)
- Mild-C®: 3600 mg/teaspoonful [contains calcium 400 mg/teaspoonful]
- Vita-C®: 4 g/teaspoonful (100 g, 454 g)

Injection, solution: 500 mg/mL (50 mL)
- Cenolate®: 500 mg/mL (1 mL, 2 mL) [contains aluminum, sodium hydrosulfite]

Injection, solution [preservative free]:
- Ascor L 500®: 500 mg/mL (50 mL) [contains edetate disodium]
- Ascor L NC®: 500 mg/mL (50 mL) [contains edetate disodium]

Liquid, oral: 500 mg/5 mL

Lozenge:
- Vicks® Vitamin C: 25 mg [contains sodium 5 mg; orange flavor]

Powder, for solution, oral:
- Ascocid®: 4000 mg/5 mL (227 g); 4300 mg/5 mL (227 g, 454 g); 5000 mg/5 mL (227 g, 454 g)
- Dull-C®: 4 g/teaspoonful

Solution, oral:
- Cecon®: 90 mg/mL

Tablet: 100 mg, 250 mg, 500 mg, 1000 mg
- Asco-Tabs: 1000 mg [sugar free]
- Ascocid®: 500 mg [sugar free]
- C-Gram, One Gram C: 1000 mg

Tablet, chewable: 250 mg, 500 mg
- Acerola: 500 mg [cherry flavor]
- Chew-C: 500 mg [orange flavor]
- Mild-C®: 250 mg

Tablet, timed release: 500 mg, 1000 mg
- Cemill: 500 mg, 1000 mg
- Mild-C®: 1000 mg
- Time-C-Bio: 500 mg

◆ **Ascorbic Acid and Ferrous Sulfate** *see* Ferrous Sulfate and Ascorbic Acid *on page 628*

◆ **Asco-Tabs [OTC]** *see* Ascorbic Acid *on page 141*

◆ **Ascriptin® [OTC]** *see* Aspirin *on page 143*

◆ **Ascriptin® Maximum Strength [OTC]** *see* Aspirin *on page 143*

◆ **Asendin [DSC]** *see* Amoxapine *on page 108*

◆ **Asian Ginseng** *see* Ginseng, Panax *(Panax ginseng) on page 718*

◆ **Asmanex® Twisthaler®** *see* Mometasone *on page 1071*

Asparaginase (a SPEAR a ji nase)

Medication Safety Issues

Sound-alike/look-alike issues:

Asparaginase may be confused with pegaspargase

Elspar® may be confused with Elaprase™

High alert medication: The Institute for Safe Medication Practices (ISMP) includes this medication among its list of classes of drugs which have a heightened risk of causing significant patient harm when used in error.

U.S. Brand Names Elspar®

Canadian Brand Names Elspar®; Kidrolase®

Mexican Brand Names Elspar

Index Terms *E. coli* Asparaginase; *Erwinia* Asparaginase; L-asparaginase; NSC-106977 (*Erwinia*); NSC-109229 (*E. coli*)

Pharmacologic Category Antineoplastic Agent, Miscellaneous

Use Treatment of acute lymphocytic leukemia (ALL)

Unlabeled/Investigational Use Treatment of lymphoma

Effect on Mental Status Rare reports of depression, disorientation, and hallucinations

Effect on Psychiatric Treatment May cause myelosuppression; use caution with clozapine and carbamazepine

Dosage Summary Note: Refer to individual protocols

I.M.:

Children: 6000 units/m^2/dose 3 times/week **or** 6000 units/m^2 every ~3 days for ~6-9 doses

Adults: 6000 units/m^2/dose 3 times/week for ~6-9 doses **or** 6000 units/m^2 every ~3 days for ~6-9 doses

I.V.:

Children: 6000 units/m^2/dose 3 times/week for ~6-9 doses **or** 6000 units/m^2 every ~3 days for ~6-9 doses **or** 1000 units/kg/day for 10 days

Adults: 6000 units/m^2/dose 3 times/week for ~6-9 doses **or** 6000 units/m^2 every ~3 days for ~6-9 doses **or** 1000 units/kg/day for 10 days **or** 200 units/kg/day (single agent therapy) for 28 days

Intradermal:

Children: Test dose: 0.1-0.2 mL of a 20-250 units/mL concentration

Adults: Test dose: 0.1-0.2 mL of a 20-250 units/mL concentration

Dosage Forms Excipient information presented when available (limited, particularly for generics); consult specific product labeling.

Injection, powder for reconstitution:

Elspar®: 10,000 units

◆ **Aspart Insulin** *see* Insulin Aspart *on page 822*

◆ **Aspercin [OTC]** *see* Aspirin *on page 143*

◆ **Aspergum® [OTC]** *see* Aspirin *on page 143*

Aspirin (AS pir in)

Medication Safety Issues

Sound-alike/look-alike issues:

Aspirin may be confused with Afrin®, Asendin®
Ascriptin® may be confused with Aricept®
Ecotrin® may be confused with Akineton®, Edecrin®, Epogen®
Halfprin® may be confused with Halfan®, Haltran®
ZORprin® may be confused with Zyloprim®

International issues:

Cartia® [multiple international markets] may be confused with Cartia XT™ which is a brand name for diltiazem in the U.S.

U.S. Brand Names Ascriptin® Maximum Strength [OTC]; Ascriptin® [OTC]; Aspercin [OTC]; Aspergum® [OTC]; Aspirtab [OTC]; Bayer® Aspirin Extra Strength [OTC]; Bayer® Aspirin Regimen Adult Low Dose [OTC]; Bayer® Aspirin Regimen Children's [OTC]; Bayer® Aspirin Regimen Regular Strength [OTC]; Bayer® Genuine Aspirin [OTC]; Bayer® Plus Extra Strength [OTC]; Bayer® with Heart Advantage [OTC]; Bayer® Women's Aspirin Plus Calcium [OTC]; Buffasal [OTC]; Bufferin® Extra Strength [OTC]; Bufferin® [OTC]; Buffinol [OTC]; Easprin®; Ecotrin® Low Strength [OTC]; Ecotrin® Maximum Strength [OTC]; Ecotrin® [OTC]; Genacote™ [OTC]; Halfprin® [OTC]; St. Joseph® Adult Aspirin [OTC]; ZORprin®

Canadian Brand Names Asaphen; Asaphen E.C.; Entrophen®; Novasen

Mexican Brand Names Adiro; Antacsal-E; Aspirina efervescente; Aspirina Junior; Ecotrin

Index Terms Acetylsalicylic Acid; ASA

Pharmacologic Category Salicylate

Use Treatment of mild-to-moderate pain, inflammation, and fever; may be used as prophylaxis of myocardial infarction; prophylaxis of stroke and/or transient ischemic episodes; management of rheumatoid arthritis, rheumatic fever, osteoarthritis, and gout (high dose); adjunctive therapy in revascularization procedures (coronary artery bypass graft [CABG], percutaneous transluminal coronary angioplasty [PTCA], carotid endarterectomy), stent implantation

Unlabeled/Investigational Use Low doses have been used in the prevention of pre-eclampsia, complications associated with autoimmune disorders such as lupus or antiphospholipid syndrome

Effect on Mental Status May cause drowsiness

Effect on Psychiatric Treatment May cause leukopenia; use caution with clozapine and carbamazepine; may displace valproic acid from binding sites resulting in an increase of unbound drug; monitor for toxicity

Dosage Summary

Oral:

Children: 10-15 mg/kg/dose every 4-6 hours (maximum: 4 g/day) **or** 60-100 mg/kg/day divided every 4-8 hours **or** 3-20 mg/kg/day as a single dose

Adults: 325-650 mg every 4-6 hours (maximum: 4 g/day) **or** 2.4-5.4 g/day in divided doses **or** 40-325 mg/day as a single dose

Rectal:

Children: 10-15 mg/kg/dose every 4-6 hours (maximum: 4 g/day)

Adults: 300-600 mg every 4-6 hours (maximum: 4 g/day)

Dosage Forms Excipient information presented when available (limited, particularly for generics); consult specific product labeling. [DSC] = Discontinued product

Caplet:
- Bayer® Aspirin Extra Strength: 500 mg
- Bayer® Aspirin Regimen Regular Strength: 325 mg
- Bayer® Genuine Aspirin: 325 mg
- Bayer® Plus Extra Strength: 500 mg [contains calcium carbonate]
- Bayer® with Heart Advantage: 81 mg [contains phytosterols, tartrazine]
- Bayer® Women's Aspirin Plus Calcium: 81 mg [contains elemental calcium 300 mg]

Caplet, buffered:
- Ascriptin® Maximum Strength: 500 mg [contains aluminum hydroxide, calcium carbonate, and magnesium hydroxide]

Gum:
- Aspergum®: 227 mg [cherry or orange flavor]

Suppository, rectal: 300 mg, 600 mg

Tablet: 325 mg
- Aspercin, Aspirtab: 325 mg
- Bayer® Genuine Aspirin: 325 mg

Tablet, buffered: 325 mg
- Ascriptin®: 325 mg [contains aluminum hydroxide, calcium carbonate, and magnesium hydroxide]
- Buffasal: 325 mg [contains magnesium oxide]
- Bufferin®: 325 mg [contains calcium carbonate, magnesium oxide, and magnesium carbonate; contains calcium 65 mg/tablet, magnesium 50 mg/tablet]
- Bufferin® Extra Strength: 500 mg [contains calcium carbonate, magnesium oxide, and magnesium carbonate; contains calcium 90 mg/tablet, magnesium 70 mg/tablet]
- Buffinol: 325 mg [contains magnesium oxide]

Tablet, chewable: 81 mg
- Bayer® Aspirin Regimen Children's: 81 mg [cherry or orange flavor]
- St. Joseph® Adult Aspirin: 81 mg [orange flavor]

Tablet, controlled release:
- ZORprin®: 800 mg

Tablet, delayed release, enteric coated:
- Easprin®: 975 mg

Tablet, enteric coated: 81 mg, 325 mg, 500 mg, 650 mg, 975 mg [DSC]
- Bayer® Aspirin Regimen Adult Low Dose, Ecotrin® Low Strength, St. Joseph Adult Aspirin: 81 mg
- Ecotrin®, Genacote™: 325 mg
- Ecotrin® Maximum Strength: 500 mg
- Halfprin®: 81 mg, 162 mg

◆ **Aspirin, Acetaminophen, and Caffeine** *see* Acetaminophen, Aspirin, and Caffeine *on page 39*

◆ **Aspirin and Carisoprodol** *see* Carisoprodol and Aspirin *on page 284*

Aspirin and Diphenhydramine (AS pir in & dye fen HYE dra meen)

U.S. Brand Names Alka-Seltzer® P.M. [OTC]; Bayer® PM [OTC]

Index Terms ASA and Diphenhydramine; Aspirin and Diphenhydramine Citrate; Diphenhydramine and ASA; Diphenhydramine and Aspirin; Diphenhydramine Citrate and Aspirin

Pharmacologic Category Analgesic, Miscellaneous

Use Aid in the relief of insomnia accompanied by minor pain or headache

Effect on Mental Status May cause confusion, dizziness, drowsiness, euphoria, excitation, fatigue, insomnia, irritability, nervousness, paradoxical excitement, and restlessness

Effect on Psychiatric Treatment May cause drowsiness and anticholinergic effects; concomitant use with psychotropic agents may produce additive effects. The anticholinergic effects of diphenhydramine may mitigate beneficial effects of acetylcholinesterase inhibitors. May cause leukopenia; use caution with clozapine and carbamazepine. Aspirin may displace valproic acid from binding sites resulting in an increase of unbound drug; monitor for toxicity. Diphenhydramine may diminish the therapeutic effect of tramadol via inhibition of CYP2D6 preventing the metabolic conversion of tramadol to its active metabolite that accounts for much of its opioid-like effects.

Dosage Summary

Oral:

Children <12 years: Dosage not established

Children ≥12 years: Two tablets (650 mg aspirin/76 mg diphenhydramine citrate) **or** 2 caplets (1000 mg aspirin/76 mg diphenhydramine citrate) at bedtime (maximum: Do not exceed recommended dosage)

Adults: Two tablets (650 mg aspirin/76 mg diphenhydramine citrate) **or** 2 caplets (1000 mg aspirin/76 mg diphenhydramine citrate) at bedtime (maximum: Do not exceed recommended dosage)

Dosage Forms Excipient information presented when available (limited, particularly for generics); consult specific product labeling.

Caplet:

Bayer® PM: Aspirin 500 mg and diphenhydramine citrate 38.3 mg

Tablet, effervescent:

Alka-Seltzer® PM: Aspirin 325 mg and diphenhydramine citrate 38 mg [contains phenylalanine 4 mg/tablet and sodium 504 mg/tablet]

◆ **Aspirin and Diphenhydramine Citrate** *see* Aspirin and Diphenhydramine *on page 145*

Aspirin and Dipyridamole (AS pir in & dye peer ID a mole)

Medication Safety Issues

Sound-alike/look-alike issues:

Aggrenox® may be confused with Aggrastat®

U.S. Brand Names Aggrenox®

Canadian Brand Names Aggrenox®

Index Terms Aspirin and Extended-Release Dipyridamole; Dipyridamole and Aspirin

Pharmacologic Category Antiplatelet Agent

Use Reduction in the risk of stroke in patients who have had transient ischemia of the brain or completed ischemic stroke due to thrombosis

Effect on Mental Status May cause amnesia, fatigue, and confusion

Effect on Psychiatric Treatment Effect of antidepressants may be blunted due to sedation and fatigue; rare reports of pancytopenia; use caution with clozapine and carbamazepine

Dosage Summary

Oral:

Children: Dosage not established

Adults: 1 capsule (200 mg dipyridamole, 25 mg aspirin) twice daily

Dosage Forms Excipient information presented when available (limited, particularly for generics); consult specific product labeling.

Capsule, variable release:

Aggrenox®: Aspirin 25 mg (immediate release) and dipyridamole 200 mg (extended release)

- **Aspirin and Extended-Release Dipyridamole** *see* Aspirin and Dipyridamole *on page 145*
- **Aspirin and Meprobamate** *see* Meprobamate and Aspirin *on page 992*
- **Aspirin and Oxycodone** *see* Oxycodone and Aspirin *on page 1208*

Aspirin and Pravastatin (AS pir in & PRA va stat in)

U.S. Brand Names Pravigard™ PAC [DSC]

Canadian Brand Names PravASA

Index Terms Buffered Aspirin and Pravastatin Sodium; Pravastatin and Aspirin

Pharmacologic Category Antilipemic Agent, HMG-CoA Reductase Inhibitor; Salicylate

Use Combination therapy in patients who need treatment with aspirin and pravastatin to reduce the incidence of cardiovascular events, including myocardial infarction, stroke, and death

Effect on Mental Status May cause drowsiness or dizziness

Effect on Psychiatric Treatment Aspirin may cause leukopenia; use caution with clozapine and carbamazepine; may also displace valproic acid from binding sites resulting in an increase of unbound drug; monitor for toxicity.

Dosage Summary

Oral:

Children: Dosage not established

Adults: Initial: Pravastatin 40 mg with aspirin 81 mg or 325 mg once daily; Maintenance: Pravastatin 20-80 mg with aspirin 81 mg or 325 mg once daily

Dosage Forms Excipient information presented when available (limited, particularly for generics); consult specific product labeling. [DSC] = Discontinued product

Combination package (Pravigard™ PAC) [each administration card contains] [DSC]:

81/20:

Tablet: Aspirin, buffered 81 mg (5/card) [contains calcium carbonate, and magnesium oxide, and magnesium carbonate]

Tablet (Pravachol®): Pravastatin sodium 20 mg (5/card) [contains lactose]

81/40:

Tablet: Aspirin, buffered 81 mg (5/card) [contains calcium carbonate, and magnesium oxide, and magnesium carbonate]

Tablet (Pravachol®): Pravastatin sodium 40 mg (5/card) [contains lactose]

81/80:

Tablet: Aspirin, buffered 81 mg (5/card) [contains calcium carbonate, and magnesium oxide, and magnesium carbonate]

Tablet (Pravachol®): Pravastatin sodium 80 mg (5/card) [contains lactose]

325/20:

Tablet: Aspirin, buffered 325 mg (5/card) [contains calcium carbonate, and magnesium oxide, and magnesium carbonate]

Tablet (Pravachol®): Pravastatin sodium 20 mg (5/card) [contains lactose]

325/40:

Tablet: Aspirin, buffered 325 mg (5/card) [contains calcium carbonate, and magnesium oxide, and magnesium carbonate]

Tablet (Pravachol®): Pravastatin sodium 40 mg (5/card) [contains lactose]

325/80:

Tablet: Aspirin, buffered 325 mg (5/card) [contains calcium carbonate, and magnesium oxide, and magnesium carbonate]

Tablet (Pravachol®): Pravastatin sodium 80 mg (5/card) [contains lactose]

- **Aspirin, Caffeine and Acetaminophen** *see* Acetaminophen, Aspirin, and Caffeine *on page 39*
- **Aspirin, Caffeine, and Butalbital** *see* Butalbital, Aspirin, and Caffeine *on page 239*
- **Aspirin, Caffeine, and Propoxyphene** *see* Propoxyphene, Aspirin, and Caffeine *on page 1355*
- **Aspirin, Caffeine, Codeine, and Butalbital** *see* Butalbital, Aspirin, Caffeine, and Codeine *on page 242*
- **Aspirin, Carisoprodol, and Codeine** *see* Carisoprodol, Aspirin, and Codeine *on page 284*
- **Aspirin Free Anacin® Maximum Strength [OTC]** *see* Acetaminophen *on page 30*
- **Aspirin, Orphenadrine, and Caffeine** *see* Orphenadrine, Aspirin, and Caffeine *on page 1187*

◆ **Aspirtab [OTC]** *see* Aspirin *on page 143*
◆ **Astelin®** *see* Azelastine *on page 162*
◆ **Astramorph/PF™** *see* Morphine Sulfate *on page 1077*
◆ **Atacand®** *see* Candesartan *on page 260*
◆ **Atacand HCT®** *see* Candesartan and Hydrochlorothiazide *on page 262*

Atazanavir (at a za NA veer)

U.S. Brand Names Reyataz®
Canadian Brand Names Reyataz®
Mexican Brand Names Reyataz
Index Terms Atazanavir Sulfate; BMS-232632
Pharmacologic Category Antiretroviral Agent, Protease Inhibitor
Use Treatment of HIV-1 infections in combination with at least two other antiretroviral agents
Note: In patients with prior virologic failure, coadministration with ritonavir is recommended.
Effect on Mental Status May cause depression, insomnia, dizziness, and fatigue
Effect on Psychiatric Treatment Contraindicated with midazolam, pimozide, St John's wort, triazolam, and ergot derivatives. Carbamazepine may decrease serum levels of atazanavir. TCA and sildenafil serum concentrations may be increased by atazanavir; monitor. Nausea, dizziness, hypotension, and syncope have been reported with concomitant use of trazodone and ritonavir.
Dosage Summary Note: Ritonavir unboosted regimen: Atazanavir without ritonavir is not recommended in antiretroviral-experienced patients with prior virologic failure.
Oral:
Children <6 years: Dosage not established
Children ≥6 years and Adolescents: Antiretroviral-naive patients:
15-24 kg: Atazanavir 150 mg once daily **plus** ritonavir 80 mg once daily
25-31 kg: Atazanavir 200 mg once daily **plus** ritonavir 100 mg once daily
32-38 kg: Atazanavir 250 mg once daily **plus** ritonavir 100 mg once daily
≥39 kg: Atazanavir 300 mg once daily **plus** 100 mg ritonavir once daily. **Note:** Treatment-naive patients ≥39 kg and ≥13 years of age who are unable to tolerate ritonavir, refer to adult dosing.
or
15-19 kg: Atazanavir 8.5 mg/kg/dose once daily (rounded to available capsule strengths) **plus** ritonavir 4 mg/kg once daily
≥20 kg: Atazanavir 7 mg/kg/dose once daily (round to available capsule strengths) (maximum 300 mg) **plus** ritonavir 4 mg/kg once daily
Children ≥13 years (≥39 kg): 400 mg once daily (antiretroviral-naive) **or** atazanavir 300 mg once daily **plus** ritonavir 100 mg once daily (antiretroviral-experienced)
25-31 kg: Atazanavir 200 mg once daily **plus** ritonavir 100 mg once daily
32-38 kg: Atazanavir 250 mg once daily **plus** ritonavir 100 mg once daily
≥39 kg: Atazanavir 300 mg once daily **plus** 100 mg ritonavir once daily
Adults: Atazanavir 300 mg once daily **plus** ritonavir 100 mg once daily **or** atazanavir 400 mg once daily (antiretroviral-naive unable to tolerate ritonavir)
Dosage Forms Excipient information presented when available (limited, particularly for generics); consult specific product labeling.
Capsule, as sulfate:
Reyataz®: 100 mg, 150 mg, 200 mg, 300 mg

◆ **Atazanavir Sulfate** *see* Atazanavir *on page 147*

Atenolol (a TEN oh lole)

Medication Safety Issues
Sound-alike/look-alike issues:
Atenolol may be confused with albuterol, Altenol®, timolol, Tylenol®
Tenormin® may be confused with Imuran®, Norpramin®, thiamine, Trovan®

International issues:
Betanol® [Bangladesh] may be confused with Patanol® which is a brand name for olopatadine in the U.S.
Related Information
Beta-Blockers *on page 1776*
Clozapine-Induced Side Effects *on page 1818*

U.S. Brand Names Tenormin®

Canadian Brand Names Apo-Atenol®; Gen-Atenolol; Novo-Atenol; Nu-Atenol; PMS-Atenolol; RAN™-Atenolol; Rhoxal-atenolol; Riva-Atenolol; Sandoz-Atenolol; Tenolin; Tenormin®

Mexican Brand Names Atoken; Biofilen; Blotex; Internol; Tenormin; Trebanol

Pharmacologic Category Beta Blocker, $Beta_1$ Selective

Generic Available Yes: Tablet

Use Treatment of hypertension, alone or in combination with other agents; management of angina pectoris, postmyocardial infarction patients

Unlabeled/Investigational Use Acute ethanol withdrawal, supraventricular and ventricular arrhythmias, and migraine headache prophylaxis

Effect on Mental Status May cause fatigue, insomnia, and confusion which can clinically look like depression

Effect on Psychiatric Treatment Concurrent use with other psychotropics may produce an additive hypotensive response (especially low-potency antipsychotics and TCAs)

Pregnancy Risk Factor D

Pregnancy Considerations Atenolol crosses the placenta; beta-blockers have been associated with persistent bradycardia, hypotension, and IUGR; IUGR is probably related to maternal hypertension. Available evidence suggests beta-blockers are generally safe during pregnancy (JNC 7). Cases of neonatal hypoglycemia have been reported following maternal use of beta-blockers at parturition or during breast-feeding. Monitor breast-fed infant for symptoms of beta-blockade.

Lactation Enters breast milk/use caution

Contraindications Hypersensitivity to atenolol or any component of the formulation; sinus bradycardia; sinus node dysfunction; heart block greater than first-degree (except in patients with a functioning artificial pacemaker); cardiogenic shock; uncompensated cardiac failure; pulmonary edema; pregnancy

Warnings/Precautions Consider pre-existing conditions such as sick sinus syndrome before initiating. Administer cautiously in compensated heart failure and monitor for a worsening of the condition (efficacy of atenolol in heart failure has not been established). **[U.S. Boxed Warning]: Beta-blocker therapy should not be withdrawn abruptly (particularly in patients with CAD), but gradually tapered to avoid acute tachycardia, hypertension, and/or ischemia.** Use caution with concurrent use of beta-blockers and either verapamil or diltiazem; bradycardia or heart block can occur. Avoid concurrent I.V. use of both agents. Beta-blockers should be avoided in patients with bronchospastic disease (asthma). Atenolol, with B_1 selectivity, has been used cautiously in bronchospastic disease with close monitoring. Use cautiously in peripheral arterial disease, especially if severe disease is present. Use cautiously in patients with diabetes - may mask hypoglycemic symptoms. Use cautiously in the renally impaired (dosage adjustment required). Use care with anesthetic agents which decrease myocardial function. Caution in myasthenia gravis or psychiatric disease (may cause CNS depression). Adequate alpha-blockade is required prior to use of any beta-blocker for patients with untreated pheochromocytoma. Use caution with history of severe anaphylaxis to allergens; patients taking beta-blockers may become more sensitive to repeated challenges. Treatment of anaphylaxis (eg, epinephrine) in patients taking beta-blockers may be ineffective or promote undesirable effects. Safety and efficacy have not been established in children.

Adverse Reactions

1% to 10%:

Cardiovascular: Persistent bradycardia, hypotension, chest pain, edema, heart failure, second- or third-degree AV block, Raynaud's phenomenon

Central nervous system: Dizziness, fatigue, insomnia, lethargy, confusion, mental impairment, depression, headache, nightmares

Gastrointestinal: Constipation, diarrhea, nausea

Genitourinary: Impotence

Miscellaneous: Cold extremities

<1% (Limited to important or life-threatening): Alopecia, dyspnea (especially with large doses), hallucinations, impotence, liver enzymes increased, lupus syndrome, Peyronie's disease, positive ANA, psoriasiform rash, psychosis, thrombocytopenia, wheezing

Drug Interactions

Acetylcholinesterase Inhibitors: May enhance the bradycardic effect of Beta-Blockers. *Risk C: Monitor therapy*

Alpha-/Beta-Agonists (Direct-Acting): Beta-Blockers may enhance the vasopressor effect of Alpha-/Beta-Agonists (Direct-Acting). Epinephrine used as a local anesthetic for dental procedures will not likely cause clinically relevant problems. **Exceptions:** Dipivefrin. *Risk D: Consider therapy modification*

Alpha1-Blockers: Beta-Blockers may enhance the orthostatic effect of Alpha1-Blockers. The risk associated with ophthalmic products is probably less than systemic products. *Risk D: Consider therapy modification*

Alpha2-Agonists: Beta-Blockers may enhance the rebound hypertensive effect of Alpha2-Agonists. This effect can occur when the alpha$_2$-agonist is abruptly withdrawn. **Exceptions:** Apraclonidine; Brimonidine. *Risk D: Consider therapy modification*

Amiodarone: May enhance the bradycardic effect of Beta-Blockers. Possibly to the point of cardiac arrest. Amiodarone may increase the serum concentration of Beta-Blockers. *Risk C: Monitor therapy*

Ampicillin: May decrease the bioavailability of Atenolol. *Risk C: Monitor therapy*

Anilidopiperidine Opioids: May enhance the bradycardic effect of Beta-Blockers. Anilidopiperidine Opioids may enhance the hypotensive effect of Beta-Blockers. *Risk C: Monitor therapy*

Beta2-Agonists: Beta-Blockers (Beta1 Selective) may diminish the bronchodilatory effect of Beta2-Agonists. Of particular concern with nonselective beta-blockers or higher doses of the beta1 selective beta-blockers. *Risk C: Monitor therapy*

Calcium Channel Blockers (Nondihydropyridine): May enhance the hypotensive effect of Beta-Blockers. Bradycardia and signs of heart failure have also been reported. Calcium Channel Blockers (Nondihydropyridine) may increase the serum concentration of Beta-Blockers. *Risk C: Monitor therapy*

Cardiac Glycosides: Beta-Blockers may enhance the bradycardic effect of Cardiac Glycosides. *Risk C: Monitor therapy*

Diazoxide: May enhance the hypotensive effect of Antihypertensives. *Risk C: Monitor therapy*

Dipyridamole: May enhance the bradycardic effect of Beta-Blockers. *Risk C: Monitor therapy*

Disopyramide: May enhance the bradycardic effect of Beta-Blockers. *Risk C: Monitor therapy*

Herbs (Hypertensive Properties): May diminish the antihypertensive effect of Antihypertensives. *Risk C: Monitor therapy*

Herbs (Hypotensive Properties): May enhance the hypotensive effect of Antihypertensives. *Risk C: Monitor therapy*

Insulin: Beta-Blockers may enhance the hypoglycemic effect of Insulin. *Risk C: Monitor therapy*

Lidocaine: Beta-Blockers may decrease the metabolism of Lidocaine. *Risk C: Monitor therapy*

Methacholine: Beta-Blockers may enhance the adverse/toxic effect of Methacholine. *Risk X: Avoid combination*

Methylphenidate: May diminish the antihypertensive effect of Antihypertensives. *Risk C: Monitor therapy*

Midodrine: Beta-Blockers may enhance the bradycardic effect of Midodrine. *Risk C: Monitor therapy*

Nonsteroidal Anti-Inflammatory Agents: May diminish the antihypertensive effect of Beta-Blockers. *Risk C: Monitor therapy*

Prostacyclin Analogues: May enhance the hypotensive effect of Antihypertensives. *Risk C: Monitor therapy*

Reserpine: May enhance the hypotensive effect of Beta-Blockers. *Risk C: Monitor therapy*

RiTUXimab: Antihypertensives may enhance the hypotensive effect of RiTUXimab. *Risk D: Consider therapy modification*

Theophylline Derivatives: Beta-Blockers (Beta1 Selective) may diminish the bronchodilatory effect of Theophylline Derivatives. This is true at higher beta-blockers doses where cardioselectivity is lost. *Risk C: Monitor therapy*

Ethanol/Nutrition/Herb Interactions

Food: Atenolol serum concentrations may be decreased if taken with food.

Herb/Nutraceutical: Avoid dong quai if using for hypertension (has estrogenic activity). Avoid ephedra, yohimbe, ginseng (may worsen hypertension). Avoid garlic (may have increased antihypertensive effect).

Stability Protect from light.

Mechanism of Action Competitively blocks response to beta-adrenergic stimulation, selectively blocks beta$_1$-receptors with little or no effect on beta$_2$-receptors except at high doses

Pharmacodynamics/Kinetics

Onset of action: Peak effect: Oral: 2-4 hours

Duration: Normal renal function: 12-24 hours

Absorption: Incomplete

Distribution: Low lipophilicity; does not cross blood-brain barrier

Protein binding: 3% to 15%

Metabolism: Limited hepatic
Half-life elimination: Beta:
Neonates: ≤35 hours; Mean: 16 hours
Children: 4.6 hours; children >10 years may have longer half-life (>5 hours) compared to children 5-10 years (<5 hours)
Adults: Normal renal function: 6-9 hours, prolonged with renal impairment; End-stage renal disease: 15-35 hours
Excretion: Feces (50%); urine (40% as unchanged drug)

Dosage
Oral:
Children: Hypertension: 0.5-1 mg/kg/dose given daily; range of 0.5-1.5 mg/kg/day; maximum dose: 2 mg/kg/day up to 100 mg/day
Adults:
Hypertension: 25-50 mg once daily, may increase to 100 mg/day. Doses >100 mg are unlikely to produce any further benefit.
Angina pectoris: 50 mg once daily, may increase to 100 mg/day. Some patients may require 200 mg/day.
Postmyocardial infarction: Follow I.V. dose with 100 mg/day or 50 mg twice daily for 6-9 days postmyocardial infarction.
I.V.:
Hypertension: Dosages of 1.25-5 mg every 6-12 hours have been used in short-term management of patients unable to take oral enteral beta-blockers
Postmyocardial infarction: Early treatment: 5 mg slow I.V. over 5 minutes; may repeat in 10 minutes. If both doses are tolerated, may start oral atenolol 50 mg every 12 hours or 100 mg/day for 6-9 days postmyocardial infarction.

Dosing interval for oral atenolol in renal impairment:
Cl_{cr} 15-35 mL/minute: Administer 50 mg/day maximum.
Cl_{cr} <15 mL/minute: Administer 50 mg every other day maximum.
Hemodialysis: Moderately dialyzable (20% to 50%) via hemodialysis; administer dose postdialysis or administer 25-50 mg supplemental dose.
Peritoneal dialysis: Elimination is not enhanced; supplemental dose is not necessary.

Dietary Considerations May be taken without regard to meals.

Administration When administered acutely for cardiac treatment, monitor ECG and blood pressure. The injection can be administered undiluted or diluted with a compatible I.V. solution. May administer by rapid infusion (I.V. push) at a rate of 1 mg/minute or by slow infusion over ~30 minutes. Necessary monitoring for surgical patients who are unable to take oral beta-blockers (prolonged ileus) has not been defined. Some institutions require monitoring of baseline and postinfusion heart rate and blood pressure when a patient's response to beta-blockade has not been characterized (ie, the patient's initial dose or following a change in dose). Consult individual institutional policies and procedures.

Monitoring Parameters Acute cardiac treatment: Monitor ECG and blood pressure with I.V. administration; heart rate and blood pressure with oral administration

Test Interactions Increased glucose; decreased HDL

Dosage Forms Excipient information presented when available (limited, particularly for generics); consult specific product labeling. [DSC] = Discontinued product
Injection, solution:
Tenormin®: 0.5 mg/mL (10 mL) [DSC]
Tablet: 25 mg, 50 mg, 100 mg
Tenormin®: 25 mg, 50 mg, 100 mg

Atenolol and Chlorthalidone (a TEN oh lole & klor THAL i done)

U.S. Brand Names Tenoretic®

Canadian Brand Names Apo-Atenidone®; Novo-Atenolthalidone; Tenoretic®

Mexican Brand Names Tenoretic

Index Terms Chlorthalidone and Atenolol

Pharmacologic Category Beta Blocker, $Beta_1$ Selective; Diuretic, Thiazide

Use Treatment of hypertension with a cardioselective beta-blocker and a diuretic

Effect on Mental Status May cause fatigue, insomnia, and confusion which can clinically look like depression

Effect on Psychiatric Treatment Concurrent use with other psychotropics may produce an additive hypotensive response (especially low-potency antipsychotics and TCAs)

Dosage Summary
Oral:
Children: Dosage not established
Adults: Initial: 50 mg (atenolol) and 25 mg (chlorthalidone) once daily; Maintenance: 50-100 mg (atenolol) and 25 mg (chlorthalidone) once daily (maximum: atenolol 100 mg/day; chlorthalidone 25 mg/day)

Dosage Forms Excipient information presented when available (limited, particularly for generics); consult specific product labeling.
Tablet:
50: Atenolol 50 mg and chlorthalidone 25 mg
100: Atenolol 100 mg and chlorthalidone 25 mg
Tenoretic®:
50: Atenolol 50 mg and chlorthalidone 25 mg
100: Atenolol 100 mg and chlorthalidone 25 mg

- **ATG** *see* Antithymocyte Globulin (Equine) *on page 126*
- **Atgam®** *see* Antithymocyte Globulin (Equine) *on page 126*
- **Ativan®** *see* LORazepam *on page 949*
- **ATNAA** *see* Atropine and Pralidoxime *on page 159*

Atomoxetine (AT oh mox e teen)

U.S. Brand Names Strattera®
Canadian Brand Names Strattera®
Mexican Brand Names Strattera
Index Terms Atomoxetine Hydrochloride; LY139603; Methylphenoxy-Benzene Propanamine; Tomoxetine
Pharmacologic Category Norepinephrine Reuptake Inhibitor, Selective
Generic Available No
Use Treatment of attention deficit/hyperactivity disorder (ADHD)
Restrictions An FDA-approved medication guide must be distributed when dispensing an outpatient prescription (new or refill) for this medication. Medication guides are available at http://www.fda.gov/cder/Offices/ODS/medication_guides.htm. Dispense to all patients or parents or guardians of children and teenagers receiving this medication.
Pregnancy Risk Factor C
Pregnancy Considerations Decreased pup weight and survival were observed in animal studies. There are no adequate and well-controlled studies in pregnant women. Use only if potential benefit to the mother outweighs possible risk to fetus.
Lactation Excretion in breast milk unknown/use caution
Contraindications Hypersensitivity to atomoxetine or any component of the formulation; use with or within 14 days of MAO inhibitors; narrow-angle glaucoma
Warnings/Precautions **[U.S. Boxed Warning]: Use caution in pediatric patients; may be an increased risk of suicidal ideation.** Closely monitor for clinical worsening, suicidality, or unusual changes in behavior; especially during the initial few months of a course of drug therapy, or at times of dose changes, either increases or decreases. The child's family or caregiver should be instructed to closely observe the patient and communicate condition with healthcare provider. New or worsening symptoms of hostility or aggressive behaviors have been associated with atomoxetine, particularly with the initiation of therapy. Use caution in patients with a history of psychotic illness or bipolar disorder; therapy may induce mixed/manic disorder or psychotic symptoms. Atomoxetine is not approved for major depressive disorder. Patients presenting with depressive symptoms should be screened for bipolar disorder. Recommended to be used as part of a comprehensive treatment program for attention deficit disorders. Atomoxetine does not worsen anxiety in patients with existing anxiety disorders or tics related to Tourette's disorder.

Use caution with hepatic (dosage adjustments necessary in hepatic impairment). Use may be associated with rare but severe hepatotoxicity; discontinue and do not restart if signs or symptoms of hepatotoxic reaction (eg, jaundice, pruritus, flu-like symptoms) are noted. Use caution in patients who are poor metabolizers of CYP2D6 metabolized drugs ("poor metabolizers"), bioavailability increases.

CNS stimulant use has been associated with serious cardiovascular events including sudden death in patients with pre-existing structural cardiac abnormalities or other serious heart problems (sudden death in children and adolescents; sudden death, stroke, and MI in adults). These products should be ▶

avoided in patients with known serious structural cardiac abnormalities, cardiomyopathy, serious heart rhythm abnormalities, or other serious cardiac problems that could increase the risk of sudden death that these conditions alone carry. Patients should be carefully evaluated for cardiac disease prior to initiation of therapy. May cause increased heart rate or blood pressure; use caution with hypertension or other cardiovascular disease. Use caution with renal impairment. May cause urinary retention/hesitancy; use caution in patients with history of urinary retention or bladder outlet obstruction. Priapism has been associated with use (rarely). Allergic reactions (including angioneurotic edema, urticaria, and rash) may occur (rare).

Growth should be monitored during treatment. Height and weight gain may be reduced during the first 9-12 months of treatment, but should recover by 3 years of therapy. Safety and efficacy have not been evaluated in pediatric patients <6 years of age.

Adverse Reactions Percentages as reported in children and adults; some adverse reactions may be increased in "poor metabolizers" (CYP2D6).

>10%:

Central nervous system: Headache (2% to 19%), insomnia (2% to 15%), somnolence (4% to 11%)

Gastrointestinal: Xerostomia (21%), nausea (7% to 21%), abdominal pain (7% to 18%), appetite decreased (11% to 16%), vomiting (3% to 11%)

1% to 10%:

Cardiovascular: Systolic blood pressure increased (4% to 5%), diastolic pressure increased (≤4%), palpitation (3%), flushing (≥2%), tachycardia (≤2%), orthostatic hypotension (<2%)

Central nervous system: Fatigue/lethargy (6% to 9%), dizziness (5% to 6%), irritability (≤6%), chills (3%), sleep disturbance (3%), mood swings (1% to 2%)

Dermatologic: Hyperhidrosis (4%), rash (2%)

Endocrine & metabolic: Hot flashes (8%), dysmenorrhea (6%), libido decreased (4%), menstruation disturbance (2%), orgasm abnormal (2%)

Gastrointestinal: Constipation (1% to 9%), dyspepsia (4%), anorexia (<3%), weight loss (2% to 3%)

Genitourinary: Erectile disturbance (9%), urinary hesitation/retention (7%), dysuria (3%), ejaculatory disturbance (3%), prostatitis (2%)

Neuromuscular & skeletal: Tremor (2%)

Ocular: Mydriasis (≥2%)

Respiratory: Sinus headache (3%)

Miscellaneous: Jittery feeling (2%)

Postmarketing and/or case reports: Allergic reactions, aggressiveness, agitation, akathisia, allergy, angioedema, anxiety, delusional thinking, growth suppression (children), hallucinations, hepatotoxicity, hostility, hypomania, impulsiveness, jaundice, mania, MI, panic attacks, pelvic pain, peripheral vascular instability, priapism, pruritus, QT prolongation, Raynaud's phenomenon, seizure (including patients with no prior history or known risk factors for seizure), stroke, suicidal ideation, syncope, urticaria

Metabolism/Transport Effects Substrate of CYP2C19 (minor), 2D6 (major)

Drug Interactions

Alcohol (Ethyl): CNS Depressants may enhance the CNS depressant effect of Alcohol (Ethyl). *Risk C: Monitor therapy*

Beta2-Agonists: Atomoxetine may enhance the tachycardic effect of Beta2-Agonists. *Risk C: Monitor therapy*

CNS Depressants: May enhance the adverse/toxic effect of other CNS Depressants. *Risk C: Monitor therapy*

CYP2D6 Inhibitors (Moderate): May decrease the metabolism of CYP2D6 Substrates. *Risk C: Monitor therapy*

CYP2D6 Inhibitors (Strong): May decrease the metabolism of CYP2D6 Substrates. *Risk D: Consider therapy modification*

Darunavir: May increase the serum concentration of CYP2D6 Substrates. *Risk C: Monitor therapy*

MAO Inhibitors: May enhance the neurotoxic (central) effect of Atomoxetine. *Risk X: Avoid combination*

PARoxetine: May decrease the metabolism of Atomoxetine. *Risk D: Consider therapy modification*

Ethanol/Nutrition/Herb Interactions Ethanol: Avoid ethanol (may increase CNS depression).

Stability Store at room temperature of 25°C (77°F).

Mechanism of Action Selectively inhibits the reuptake of norepinephrine (K 4.5nM) with little to no activity at the other neuronal reuptake pumps or receptor sites.

Pharmacodynamics/Kinetics

Absorption: Rapid

Distribution: V_d: I.V.: 0.85 L/kg

Protein binding: 98%, primarily albumin

Metabolism: Hepatic, via CYP2D6 and CYP2C19; forms metabolites (4-hydroxyatomoxetine, active, equipotent to atomoxetine; N-desmethylatomoxetine in poor metabolizers, limited activity)

Bioavailability: 63% in extensive metabolizers; 94% in poor metabolizers

Half-life elimination: Atomoxetine: 5 hours (up to 24 hours in poor metabolizers); Active metabolites: 4-hydroxyatomoxetine: 6-8 hours; N-desmethylatomoxetine: 6-8 hours (34-40 hours in poor metabolizers)

Time to peak, plasma: 1-2 hours

Excretion: Urine (80%, as conjugated 4-hydroxy metabolite); feces (17%)

Dosage Oral: **Note:** Atomoxetine may be discontinued without the need for tapering dose.

Children ≥6 years and ≤70 kg: ADHD: Initial: 0.5 mg/kg/day, increase after minimum of 3 days to ~1.2 mg/kg/day; may administer as either a single daily dose or 2 evenly divided doses in morning and late afternoon/early evening. Maximum daily dose: 1.4 mg/kg or 100 mg, whichever is less.

Dosage adjustment in patients receiving strong CYP2D6 inhibitors (eg, paroxetine, fluoxetine, quinidine) or patients known to be CYP2D6 poor metabolizers: Do not exceed 1.2 mg/kg/day; dose adjustments should occur only after 4 weeks.

Children ≥6 years and >70 kg and Adults: ADHD: Initial: 40 mg/day, increased after minimum of 3 days to ~80 mg/day; may administer as either a single daily dose or two evenly divided doses in morning and late afternoon/early evening. May increase to 100 mg/day in 2-4 additional weeks to achieve optimal response.

Dosage adjustment in patients receiving strong CYP2D6 inhibitors (eg, paroxetine, fluoxetine, quinidine) or patients known to be CYP2D6 poor metabolizers: Do not exceed 80 mg/day; dose adjustments should occur only after 4 weeks.

Elderly: Use has not been evaluated in the elderly

Dosage adjustment in renal impairment: No adjustment needed

Dosage adjustment in hepatic impairment:

Moderate hepatic insufficiency (Child-Pugh class B): All doses should be reduced to 50% of normal

Severe hepatic insufficiency (Child-Pugh class C): All doses should be reduced to 25% of normal

Dietary Considerations May be taken with or without food.

Administration May be administered with or without food. Swallow capsules whole; do not open capsules. Powder in capsules is an ocular irritant.

Monitoring Parameters Patient growth (weight/height gain in children); attention, hyperactivity, anxiety, worsening of aggressive behavior or hostility; blood pressure and pulse (baseline and following dose increases and periodically during treatment)

Family members and caregivers need to monitor patient daily for emergence of irritability, agitation, unusual changes in behavior, and suicidal ideation. Pediatric patients should be monitored closely for suicidality, clinical worsening, or unusual changes in behavior, especially during the initial for months of therapy or at times of dose changes. Appearance of symptoms needs to be immediately reported to healthcare provider. Weekly office visits from patient or caregiver are necessary for the first 4 weeks, then every other week for the next 4 weeks, then at 12 weeks, and as clinically indicated beyond 12 weeks. Additional contact may be required between office visits.

When used for the treatment of ADHD, thoroughly evaluate for cardiovascular risk. Monitor heart rate, blood pressure, and consider obtaining ECG prior to initiation (Vetter, 2008)

Dosage Forms Excipient information presented when available (limited, particularly for generics); consult specific product labeling.

Capsule:

Strattera®: 10 mg, 18 mg, 25 mg, 40 mg, 60 mg, 80 mg, 100 mg

◆ **Atomoxetine Hydrochloride** *see* Atomoxetine *on page 151*

Atorvastatin (a TORE va sta tin)

Medication Safety Issues

Sound-alike/look-alike issues:

Lipitor® may be confused with Levatol®

Related Information
Lipid-Lowering Agents *on page 1786*
U.S. Brand Names Lipitor®
Canadian Brand Names Lipitor®
Mexican Brand Names Lipitor
Pharmacologic Category Antilipemic Agent, HMG-CoA Reductase Inhibitor
Generic Available No
Use Treatment of dyslipidemias or primary prevention of cardiovascular disease (atherosclerotic) as detailed below:

Primary prevention of cardiovascular disease (high-risk for CVD): To reduce the risk of MI or stroke in patients without evidence of heart disease who have multiple CVD risk factors or type 2 diabetes. Treatment reduces the risk for angina or revascularization procedures in patients with multiple risk factors.
Secondary prevention of cardiovascular disease: To reduce the risk of MI, stroke, revascularization procedures, and angina in patients with evidence of heart disease. To reduce the risk of hospitalization for heart failure.
Treatment of dyslipidemias: To reduce elevations in total cholesterol, LDL-C, apolipoprotein B, and triglycerides in patients with elevations of one or more components, and/or to increase HDL-C as present in Fredrickson type IIa, IIb, III, and IV hyperlipidemias; treatment of primary dysbetalipoproteinemia, homozygous familial hypercholesterolemia
Treatment of heterozygous familial hypercholesterolemia (HeFH) in adolescent patients (10-17 years of age, females >1 year postmenarche) having LDL-C ≥190 mg/dL or LDL-C ≥160 mg/dL with positive family history of premature cardiovascular disease (CVD) or with two or more CVD risk factors.

Effect on Mental Status May cause fatigue; rare reports of euphoria
Effect on Psychiatric Treatment None reported
Pregnancy Risk Factor X
Pregnancy Considerations Cholesterol biosynthesis may be important in fetal development. Contraindicated in pregnancy. Administer to women of child-bearing potential only when conception is highly unlikely and patients have been informed of potential hazards.
Lactation Enters breast milk/contraindicated
Contraindications Hypersensitivity to atorvastatin or any component of the formulation; active liver disease; unexplained persistent elevations of serum transaminases; pregnancy
Warnings/Precautions Secondary causes of hyperlipidemia should be ruled out prior to therapy. Liver function must be monitored by periodic laboratory assessment. May cause hepatic dysfunction. Use with caution in patients who consume large amounts of ethanol or have a history of liver disease. Monitoring is recommended. Patients with a history of hemorrhagic stroke may be at increased risk for another with use.

Rhabdomyolysis with acute renal failure has occurred. Risk is dose related and is increased with concurrent use of lipid-lowering agents which may cause rhabdomyolysis (fibric acid derivatives or niacin at doses ≥1 g/day) or during concurrent use with potent CYP3A4 inhibitors (including amiodarone, clarithromycin, cyclosporine, erythromycin, itraconazole, ketoconazole, nefazodone, grapefruit juice in large quantities, verapamil, or protease inhibitors such as indinavir, nelfinavir, or ritonavir). Ensure patient is on the lowest effective atorvastatin dose. If concurrent use of clarithromycin or combination protease inhibitors (eg, lopinavir/ritonavir or ritonavir/saquinavir) is warranted consider dose adjustment of atorvastatin. Monitor closely if used with other drugs associated with myopathy. Weigh the risk versus benefit when combining any of these drugs with atorvastatin. Discontinue in any patient experiencing an acute or serious condition predisposing to renal failure secondary to rhabdomyolysis. Based upon current evidence, HMG-CoA reductase inhibitor therapy should be continued in the perioperative period unless risk outweighs cardioprotective benefit. Use with caution in patients with advanced age, these patients are predisposed to myopathy. Safety and efficacy have not been established in patients <10 years of age or in premenarcheal girls.

Adverse Reactions
>10%: Central nervous system: Headache (3% to 17%)
2% to 10%:
Cardiovascular: Chest pain, peripheral edema
Central nervous system: Insomnia, dizziness
Dermatologic: Rash (1% to 4%)
Gastrointestinal: Abdominal pain (up to 4%), constipation (up to 3%), diarrhea (up to 4%), dyspepsia (1% to 3%), flatulence (1% to 3%), nausea
Genitourinary: Urinary tract infection
Hepatic: Transaminases increased (2% to 3% with 80 mg/day dosing)

Neuromuscular & skeletal: Arthralgia (up to 5%), arthritis, back pain (up to 4%), myalgia (up to 6%), weakness (up to 4%)

Respiratory: Sinusitis (up to 6%), pharyngitis (up to 3%), bronchitis, rhinitis

Miscellaneous: Infection (3% to 10%), flu-like syndrome (up to 3%), allergic reaction (up to 3%)

<2% (Limited to important or life-threatening): Alopecia, anaphylaxis, angina, angioneurotic edema, arrhythmia, bullous rash, cholestatic jaundice, deafness, dyspnea, erythema multiforme, esophagitis, facial paralysis, fatigue, glaucoma, gout, hepatitis, hyperkinesias, impotence, migraine, myasthenia, myopathy, myositis, nephritis, pancreatitis, paresthesia, peripheral neuropathy, petechiae, photosensitivity, postural hypotension, pruritus, rectal hemorrhage, rhabdomyolysis, somnolence, Stevens-Johnson syndrome, syncope, tendinous contracture, tendon rupture, thrombocytopenia, tinnitus, torticollis, toxic epidermal necrolysis, urticaria, vaginal hemorrhage, vomiting

Metabolism/Transport Effects **Substrate** of CYP3A4 (major); **Inhibits** CYP3A4 (weak)

Drug Interactions

Aliskiren: Atorvastatin may increase the serum concentration of Aliskiren. *Risk C: Monitor therapy*

Amiodarone: May decrease the metabolism of HMG-CoA Reductase Inhibitors. Management: Dose of simvastatin should not exceed 20 mg/day during concurrent therapy. *Risk D: Consider therapy modification*

Antifungal Agents (Azole Derivatives, Systemic): May decrease the metabolism of HMG-CoA Reductase Inhibitors. *Risk D: Consider therapy modification*

Bosentan: May increase the metabolism of HMG-CoA Reductase Inhibitors. *Risk C: Monitor therapy*

Calcium Channel Blockers (Nondihydropyridine): May decrease the metabolism of HMG-CoA Reductase Inhibitors. *Risk D: Consider therapy modification*

Clopidogrel: Atorvastatin may diminish the therapeutic effect of Clopidogrel. *Risk C: Monitor therapy*

Colchicine: May enhance the myopathic (rhabdomyolysis) effect of HMG-CoA Reductase Inhibitors. Colchicine may increase the serum concentration of HMG-CoA Reductase Inhibitors. *Risk D: Consider therapy modification*

CycloSPORINE: May increase the serum concentration of HMG-CoA Reductase Inhibitors. *Risk D: Consider therapy modification*

CYP3A4 Inducers (Strong): May increase the metabolism of CYP3A4 Substrates. *Risk C: Monitor therapy*

CYP3A4 Inhibitors (Moderate): May decrease the metabolism of CYP3A4 Substrates. *Risk C: Monitor therapy*

CYP3A4 Inhibitors (Strong): May decrease the metabolism of CYP3A4 Substrates. *Risk D: Consider therapy modification*

Dabigatran Etexilate: Atorvastatin may decrease the serum concentration of Dabigatran Etexilate. *Risk C: Monitor therapy*

Danazol: May decrease the metabolism of HMG-CoA Reductase Inhibitors. *Risk C: Monitor therapy*

DAPTOmycin: HMG-CoA Reductase Inhibitors may enhance the adverse/toxic effect of DAPTOmycin. Specifically, the risk of skeletal muscle toxicity may be increased. Management: Consider temporarily stopping HMG-CoA reductase inhibitor therapy prior to daptomycin. If used together, regular (i.e., at least weekly) monitoring of CPK concentrations is recommended. *Risk D: Consider therapy modification*

Dasatinib: May increase the serum concentration of CYP3A4 Substrates. *Risk C: Monitor therapy*

Deferasirox: May decrease the serum concentration of CYP3A4 Substrates. *Risk C: Monitor therapy*

Digoxin: Atorvastatin may increase the serum concentration of Digoxin. *Risk C: Monitor therapy*

Etravirine: May decrease the serum concentration of HMG-CoA Reductase Inhibitors. This applies to atorvastatin, lovastatin and simvastatin. Conversely, levels of fluvastatin may be increased. Management: Dose adjustment of the HMG-CoA reductase inhibitor may be warranted. No interaction is expected with rosuvastatin or pravastatin. *Risk C: Monitor therapy*

Fenofibrate: May enhance the adverse/toxic effect of HMG-CoA Reductase Inhibitors. *Risk C: Monitor therapy*

Fluconazole: May decrease the metabolism of HMG-CoA Reductase Inhibitors. *Risk D: Consider therapy modification*

Gemfibrozil: May enhance the myopathic (rhabdomyolysis) effect of HMG-CoA Reductase Inhibitors. Gemfibrozil may increase the serum concentration of HMG-CoA Reductase Inhibitors. *Risk D: Consider therapy modification*

Grapefruit Juice: May decrease the metabolism of HMG-CoA Reductase Inhibitors. *Risk D: Consider therapy modification*

Macrolide Antibiotics: May decrease the metabolism of HMG-CoA Reductase Inhibitors. **Exceptions:** Azithromycin; Dirithromycin [Off Market]; Spiramycin. *Risk D: Consider therapy modification*

Midazolam: Atorvastatin may increase the serum concentration of Midazolam. *Risk C: Monitor therapy*

Nefazodone: May decrease the metabolism of HMG-CoA Reductase Inhibitors. *Risk D: Consider therapy modification*

Niacin: May enhance the adverse/toxic effect of HMG-CoA Reductase Inhibitors. *Risk C: Monitor therapy*

Niacinamide: May enhance the adverse/toxic effect of HMG-CoA Reductase Inhibitors. *Risk C: Monitor therapy*

P-Glycoprotein Inducers: May decrease the serum concentration of P-Glycoprotein Substrates. P-glycoprotein inducers may also further limit the distribution of p-glycoprotein substrates to specific cells/tissues/organs where p-glycoprotein is present in large amounts (e.g., brain, T-lymphocytes, testes, etc.). *Risk C: Monitor therapy*

P-Glycoprotein Inhibitors: May increase the serum concentration of P-Glycoprotein Substrates. P-glycoprotein inhibitors may also enhance the distribution of p-glycoprotein substrates to specific cells/tissues/organs where p-glycoprotein is present in large amounts (e.g., brain, T-lymphocytes, testes, etc.). *Risk C: Monitor therapy*

P-Glycoprotein Substrates: P-Glycoprotein Inhibitors may increase the serum concentration of P-Glycoprotein Substrates. P-glycoprotein inhibitors may also enhance the distribution of p-glycoprotein substrates to specific cells/tissues/organs where p-glycoprotein is present in large amounts (e.g., brain, T-lymphocytes, testes, etc.). *Risk C: Monitor therapy*

Phenytoin: May increase the metabolism of HMG-CoA Reductase Inhibitors. *Risk D: Consider therapy modification*

Protease Inhibitors: May increase the serum concentration of HMG-CoA Reductase Inhibitors. Limited data suggest pravastatin may slightly decrease protease inhibitor concentrations. Management: Lovastatin and simvastatin are contraindicated with many protease inhibitors; use lowest possible HMG-CoA reductase inhibitor dose and monitor for signs and symptoms of rhabdomyolysis if these agents are used concomitantly. *Risk D: Consider therapy modification*

Rifamycin Derivatives: May increase the metabolism of HMG-CoA Reductase Inhibitors. *Risk D: Consider therapy modification*

Rivaroxaban: P-Glycoprotein Inhibitors may increase the serum concentration of Rivaroxaban. *Risk X: Avoid combination*

Sildenafil: May decrease the metabolism of HMG-CoA Reductase Inhibitors. *Risk D: Consider therapy modification*

St Johns Wort: May increase the metabolism of HMG-CoA Reductase Inhibitors. *Risk C: Monitor therapy*

Topotecan: P-Glycoprotein Inhibitors may increase the serum concentration of Topotecan. *Risk X: Avoid combination*

Ethanol/Nutrition/Herb Interactions

Ethanol: Avoid excessive ethanol consumption (due to potential hepatic effects).

Food: Atorvastatin serum concentrations may be increased by grapefruit juice; avoid concurrent intake of large quantities (>1 quart/day). Red yeast rice contains an estimated 2.4 mg lovastatin per 600 mg rice.

Herb/Nutraceutical: St John's wort may decrease atorvastatin levels.

Mechanism of Action Inhibitor of 3-hydroxy-3-methylglutaryl coenzyme A (HMG-CoA) reductase, the rate-limiting enzyme in cholesterol synthesis (reduces the production of mevalonic acid from HMG-CoA); this then results in a compensatory increase in the expression of LDL receptors on hepatocyte membranes and a stimulation of LDL catabolism

Pharmacodynamics/Kinetics

Onset of action: Initial changes: 3-5 days; Maximal reduction in plasma cholesterol and triglycerides: 2 weeks

Absorption: Rapid

Distribution: V_d: 318 L

Protein binding: ≥98%

Metabolism: Hepatic; forms active ortho- and parahydroxylated derivates and an inactive beta-oxidation product

Bioavailability: ~14% (parent drug); ~30% (parent drug and equipotent metabolites)

Half-life elimination: Parent drug: 14 hours; Equipotent metabolites: 20-30 hours

Time to peak, serum: 1-2 hours

Excretion: Bile; urine (2% as unchanged drug)

Dosage Oral: **Note:** Doses should be individualized according to the baseline LDL-cholesterol levels, the recommended goal of therapy, and patient response; adjustments should be made at intervals of 2-4 weeks

Children 10-17 years (females >1 year postmenarche): Heterozygous familial hypercholesterolemia (HeFH): 10 mg once daily (maximum: 20 mg/day)

Adults:

Hypercholesterolemia (heterozygous familial and nonfamilial) and mixed hyperlipidemia (Fredrickson types IIa and IIb): Initial: 10-20 mg once daily; patients requiring >45% reduction in LDL-C may be started at 40 mg once daily; range: 10-80 mg once daily

Homozygous familial hypercholesterolemia: 10-80 mg once daily

Dosing adjustment in renal impairment: No dosage adjustment is necessary.

Dosing adjustment in hepatic impairment: Do not use in active liver disease.

Dietary Considerations May take with food if desired; may take without regard to time of day. Before initiation of therapy, patients should be placed on a standard cholesterol-lowering diet for 3-6 months and the diet should be continued during drug therapy. Red yeast rice contains an estimated 2.4 mg lovastatin per 600 mg rice.

Administration May be administered with food if desired; may take without regard to time of day.

Monitoring Parameters Lipid levels after 2-4 weeks; LFTs, CPK

It is recommended that liver function tests (LFTs) be performed prior to and at 12 weeks following both the initiation of therapy and any elevation in dose, and periodically (eg, semiannually) thereafter.

Dosage Forms Excipient information presented when available (limited, particularly for generics); consult specific product labeling.

Tablet:

Lipitor®: 10 mg, 20 mg, 40 mg, 80 mg

- **Atorvastatin Calcium and Amlodipine Besylate** *see* Amlodipine and Atorvastatin *on page 103*

Atovaquone (a TOE va kwone)

U.S. Brand Names Mepron®

Canadian Brand Names Mepron®

Pharmacologic Category Antiprotozoal

Use Acute oral treatment of mild-to-moderate *Pneumocystis jirovecii* pneumonia (PCP) in patients who are intolerant to co-trimoxazole; prophylaxis of PCP in patients who are intolerant to co-trimoxazole

Unlabeled/Investigational Use Treatment of babesiosis; treatment/suppression of *Toxoplasma gondii* encephalitis; primary prophylaxis of HIV-infected persons at high risk for developing *Toxoplasma gondii* encephalitis

Effect on Mental Status May cause anxiety

Effect on Psychiatric Treatment May cause anemia and neutropenia; use caution with clozapine and carbamazepine

Dosage Summary

Oral:

Children <1 month: Dosage not established

Children 1-3 months (unlabeled use): 30-40 mg/kg once daily

Children 3-24 months (unlabeled use): 45 mg/kg once daily

Children 2-13 years (unlabeled use): 30-40 mg/kg once daily

Children 13-16 years: 1500 mg/day in 1-2 divided doses

Adults: 1500 mg/day in 1-2 divided doses

Dosage Forms Excipient information presented when available (limited, particularly for generics); consult specific product labeling.

Suspension, oral:

Mepron®: 750 mg/5 mL (5 mL, 210 mL) [contains benzyl alcohol; citrus flavor]

Atovaquone and Proguanil (a TOE va kwone & pro GWA nil)

U.S. Brand Names Malarone®

Canadian Brand Names Malarone®; Malarone® Pediatric

Index Terms Atovaquone and Proguanil Hydrochloride; Proguanil and Atovaquone; Proguanil Hydrochloride and Atovaquone

Pharmacologic Category Antimalarial Agent

Use Prevention or treatment of acute, uncomplicated *P. falciparum* malaria

Effect on Mental Status May produce abnormal dreams; may rarely cause seizures and hallucinations

Effect on Psychiatric Treatment Significant adverse GI effects; use caution with SSRIs

Dosage Summary

Oral:

Children <5 kg: Dosage not established

Children 5-8 kg: 125 mg/50 mg as a single daily dose

Children 9-10 kg: 187.5 mg/75 mg as a single daily dose

Children 11-20 kg: Prophylaxis: 62.5 mg/25 mg; Treatment: 250 mg/100 mg as a single daily dose

Children 21-30 kg: Prophylaxis: 125 mg/50 mg; Treatment: 500 mg/200 mg as a single daily dose

Children 31-40 kg: Prophylaxis: 187.5 mg/75 mg; Treatment: 750 mg/300 mg as a single daily dose

Children >40 kg: Prophylaxis: 250 mg/100 mg; Treatment: 1 g/400 mg as a single daily dose

Adults: Prophylaxis: 250 mg/100 mg; Treatment: 1 g/400 mg as a single daily dose

Dosage Forms Excipient information presented when available (limited, particularly for generics); consult specific product labeling.

Tablet, oral:

Malarone®: Atovaquone 250 mg and proguanil hydrochloride 100 mg

Tablet, oral [pediatric]:

Malarone®: Atovaquone 62.5 mg and proguanil hydrochloride 25 mg

◆ **Atovaquone and Proguanil Hydrochloride** *see* Atovaquone and Proguanil *on page 157*

◆ **ATRA** *see* Tretinoin, Oral *on page 1617*

◆ **Atripla®** *see* Efavirenz, Emtricitabine, and Tenofovir *on page 527*

◆ **AtroPen®** *see* Atropine *on page 158*

Atropine (A troe peen)

Medication Safety Issues

International issues:

Genatropine® [France] may be confused with Genotropin®

U.S. Brand Names AtroPen®; Atropine-Care®; Isopto® Atropine; Sal-Tropine™

Canadian Brand Names Dioptic's Atropine Solution; Isopto® Atropine

Mexican Brand Names Redotex

Index Terms Atropine Sulfate

Pharmacologic Category Anticholinergic Agent; Anticholinergic Agent, Ophthalmic; Antidote; Antispasmodic Agent, Gastrointestinal; Ophthalmic Agent, Mydriatic

Use

Injection: Preoperative medication to inhibit salivation and secretions; treatment of symptomatic sinus bradycardia; AV block (nodal level); ventricular asystole; antidote for anticholinesterase inhibitor poisoning (carbamate insecticides, nerve agents, organophosphate insecticides)

Ophthalmic: Produce mydriasis and cycloplegia for examination of the retina and optic disc and accurate measurement of refractive errors; uveitis

Oral: Inhibit salivation and secretions

Unlabeled/Investigational Use Pulseless electric activity, asystole, neuromuscular blockade reversal

Effect on Mental Status Use of injectable dosage form may cause ataxia, hallucinations, dizziness, amnesia, difficulty concentrating, agitation, delirium, paranoia, anxiety, and mania

Effect on Psychiatric Treatment May decrease the effects of phenothiazines; concurrent use with psychotropics may result in additive anticholinergic side effects (dry mouth, blurred vision, constipation)

Restrictions The AtroPen® formulation is available for use primarily by the Department of Defense.

Dosage Summary Note: Doses <0.1 mg (children) and <0.5 mg (adults) have been associated with paradoxical bradycardia

I.M.:

Children ≤5 kg: 0.02 mg/kg/dose every 4-6 hours as needed

Children >5 kg: 0.01-0.2 mg/kg/dose every 4-6 hours as needed (maximum: 0.4 mg/dose; minimum: 0.1 mg/dose)

Adults: 0.4-0.6 mg every 4-6 hours as needed

AtroPen®:

Children <6.8 kg: Dosage not established

Children 6.8-18 kg: 0.5 mg/dose (maximum: 3 doses)
Children >41 kg: 2 mg/dose (maximum: 3 doses)
Adults: 2 mg/dose (maximum: 3 doses)

I.V.:

Children ≤5 kg: 0.02 mg/kg/dose every 4-6 hours as needed **or** 0.02 mg/kg repeated in 5-minute intervals to a maximum total dose of 1 mg (maximum: 0.5 mg/dose; 1 mg total dose) **or** 0.03-0.05 mg/kg every 10-20 minutes until atropine effect, then every 1-4 hours

Children >5 kg: 0.01-0.2 mg/kg/dose every 4-6 hours as needed (maximum: 0.4 mg/dose) **or** 0.02 mg/kg repeated in 5-minute intervals to a maximum total dose of 1 mg (maximum: 0.5 mg/dose; 1 mg total dose) **or** 0.03-0.05 mg/kg every 10-20 minutes until atropine effect, then every 1-4 hours

Adolescents: 0.01-0.2 mg/kg/dose every 4-6 hours as needed (maximum: 0.4 mg/dose) **or** 0.02 mg/kg repeated in 5-minute intervals to a maximum total dose of 1 mg (maximum: 0.5 mg/dose; 2 mg total dose) **or** 0.03-0.05 mg/kg every 10-20 minutes until atropine effect, then every 1-4 hours

Adults: 0.4-0.6 mg every 4-6 hours as needed **or** 0.5-1 mg every 3-5 minutes (maximum: 0.04 mg/kg total dose) **or** 2 mg every 15 minutes until adequate atropinization (maximum: 6 mg) **or** 10% to 20% of loading dose/hour

Intratracheal:

Children: 0.02 mg/kg repeated in 5-minute intervals to a maximum total dose of 1 mg (maximum: 0.5 mg/dose; 1 mg total dose)

Adolescents: 0.02 mg/kg repeated in 5-minute intervals to a maximum total dose of 1 mg (maximum: 0.5 mg/dose; 2 mg total dose)

Adults: Administer 2-2.5 times the recommended I.V. dose

Ophthalmic:

Children: Dosage not established

Adults: Ointment: Apply a small amount in the conjunctival sac up to 3 times/day; Solution (1%): Instill 1-2 drops 4 times/day

Oral:

Children ≤5 kg: 0.02 mg/kg/dose every 4-6 hours as needed

Children >5 kg: 0.01-0.2 mg/kg/dose every 4-6 hours as needed (maximum: 0.4 mg/dose)

Adults: 0.4 mg every 4-6 hours

SubQ:

Children ≤5 kg: 0.02 mg/kg/dose every 4-6 hours as needed

Children >5 kg: 0.01-0.2 mg/kg/dose every 4-6 hours as needed (maximum: 0.4 mg/dose)

Adults: 0.4-0.6 mg every 4-6 hours as needed

Dosage Forms Excipient information presented when available (limited, particularly for generics); consult specific product labeling.

Injection, solution, as sulfate: 0.05 mg/mL (5 mL); 0.1 mg/mL (5 mL, 10 mL); 0.4 mg/0.5 mL (0.5 mL); 0.4 mg/mL (0.5 mL, 1 mL, 20 mL); 1 mg/mL (1 mL)

AtroPen®: 0.25 mg/0.3 mL (0.3 mL); 0.5 mg/0.7 mL (0.7 mL); 1 mg/0.7 mL (0.7 mL); 2 mg/0.7 mL (0.7 mL) [prefilled autoinjector]

Ointment, ophthalmic, as sulfate: 1% (3.5 g)

Solution, ophthalmic, as sulfate: 1% (2 mL, 5 mL, 15 mL)

Atropine-Care®: 1% (2 mL) [contains benzalkonium chloride]

Isopto® Atropine: 1% (5 mL, 15 mL) [contains benzalkonium chloride]

Tablet, as sulfate:

Sal-Tropine™: 0.4 mg

◆ **Atropine and Difenoxin** *see* Difenoxin and Atropine *on page 462*

◆ **Atropine and Diphenoxylate** *see* Diphenoxylate and Atropine *on page 486*

Atropine and Pralidoxime (A troe peen & pra li DOKS eem)

U.S. Brand Names ATNAA; Duodote™

Index Terms Atropine and Pralidoxime Chloride; Mark 1™; NAAK; Nerve Agent Antidote Kit; Pralidoxime and Atropine

Pharmacologic Category Anticholinergic Agent; Antidote

Use

ATNAA: Treatment of poisoning by susceptible organophosphorous nerve agents having anticholinesterase activity for self or buddy-administration by military personnel

Duodote™: Treatment of poisoning by organophosphorous nerve agents (eg, tabun, sarin, soman) or organophosphorous insecticide for use by trained emergency medical services personnel

Effect on Mental Status May cause ataxia, hallucinations, dizziness, drowsiness, amnesia, difficulty concentrating, agitation, delirium, paranoia, anxiety, and mania

Effect on Psychiatric Treatment Atropine and pralidoxime may decrease the effects of acetylcholinesterase inhibitors. Concurrent use with psychotropics may result in additive anticholinergic side effects (eg, dry mouth, blurred vision, or constipation); avoid use with phenothiazines; effects of barbiturates may be increased by atropine and pralidoxime

Restrictions

ATNAA (**A**ntidote **T**reatment-**N**erve **A**gent **A**uto-Injector) is only available for use by U.S. Armed Forces military personnel. Information on distribution is available at Defense Services Supply Center-Philadelphia at https://dmmonline.dscp.dla.mil/pharm/nerve.asp.

Duodote™ is only available for use by trained emergency medical services personnel to treat civilians. Distribution is limited to directly from manufacturer (Meridian Medical Technologies, Inc.) to emergency medical service organizations or their suppliers.

Dosage Summary

I.M.:

Children <18 years: Dosage not established

Adults: 1-3 injections (maximum: 3 injections)

Dosage Forms Excipient information presented when available (limited, particularly for generics); consult specific product labeling.

Injection, solution:

ATNAA, Duodote™: Atropine 2.1 mg/0.7 mL and pralidoxime chloride 600 mg/2 mL [contains benzyl alcohol; prefilled autoinjector]

- **Atropine and Pralidoxime Chloride** *see* Atropine and Pralidoxime *on page 159*
- **Atropine-Care®** *see* Atropine *on page 158*
- **Atropine, Hyoscyamine, Scopolamine, and Phenobarbital** *see* Hyoscyamine, Atropine, Scopolamine, and Phenobarbital *on page 800*
- **Atropine Sulfate** *see* Atropine *on page 158*
- **Atropine Sulfate and Edrophonium Chloride** *see* Edrophonium and Atropine *on page 525*
- **Atrovent®** *see* Ipratropium *on page 852*
- **Atrovent® HFA** *see* Ipratropium *on page 852*
- **Atuss® HD [DSC]** *see* Pseudoephedrine, Hydrocodone, and Chlorpheniramine *on page 1372*
- **Atuss® HX [DSC]** *see* Hydrocodone and Guaifenesin *on page 779*
- **Augmentin®** *see* Amoxicillin and Clavulanate Potassium *on page 115*
- **Augmentin ES-600®** *see* Amoxicillin and Clavulanate Potassium *on page 115*
- **Augmentin XR®** *see* Amoxicillin and Clavulanate Potassium *on page 115*

Auranofin (au RANE oh fin)

Medication Safety Issues

Sound-alike/look-alike issues:

Ridaura® may be confused with Cardura®

U.S. Brand Names Ridaura®

Canadian Brand Names Ridaura®

Pharmacologic Category Gold Compound

Use Management of active stage of classic or definite rheumatoid arthritis in patients who do not respond to or tolerate other agents; psoriatic arthritis; adjunctive or alternative therapy for pemphigus

Effect on Mental Status None reported

Effect on Psychiatric Treatment May rarely produce agranulocytosis; use caution with clozapine and carbamazepine

Dosage Summary

Oral:

Children: Initial: 0.1 mg/kg/day; Maintenance: 0.15-0.2 mg/kg/day in 1-2 divided doses (maximum: 0.2 mg/kg/day)

Adults: Initial: 6 mg/day; Maintenance: 6-9 mg/day (maximum: 9 mg/day). **Note:** Titration may be recommended

Dosage Forms Excipient information presented when available (limited, particularly for generics); consult specific product labeling.

Capsule:

Ridaura®: 3 mg [29% gold]

- **Avage™** *see* Tazarotene *on page 1540*
- **Avalide®** *see* Irbesartan and Hydrochlorothiazide *on page 856*
- **Avandamet®** *see* Rosiglitazone and Metformin *on page 1449*
- **Avandaryl™** *see* Rosiglitazone and Glimepiride *on page 1448*
- **Avandia®** *see* Rosiglitazone *on page 1444*
- **Avapro®** *see* Irbesartan *on page 855*
- **Avapro® HCT** *see* Irbesartan and Hydrochlorothiazide *on page 856*
- **Avastin®** *see* Bevacizumab *on page 187*
- **Avelox®** *see* Moxifloxacin *on page 1084*
- **Avelox® I.V.** *see* Moxifloxacin *on page 1084*
- **Aviane™** *see* Ethinyl Estradiol and Levonorgestrel *on page 595*
- **Avian Influenza Virus Vaccine** *see* Influenza Virus Vaccine (H5N1) *on page 821*
- **Avinza®** *see* Morphine Sulfate *on page 1077*
- **Avodart®** *see* Dutasteride *on page 521*
- **Avonex®** *see* Interferon Beta-1a *on page 848*
- **Axert™** *see* Almotriptan *on page 70*
- **Axid®** *see* Nizatidine *on page 1149*
- **Axid® AR [OTC]** *see* Nizatidine *on page 1149*
- **AY-25650** *see* Triptorelin *on page 1635*
- **Aygestin®** *see* Norethindrone *on page 1150*
- **5-Aza-2'-deoxycytidine** *see* Decitabine *on page 422*
- **5-AzaC** *see* Decitabine *on page 422*

AzaCITIDine (ay za SYE ti deen)

Medication Safety Issues

Sound-alike/look-alike issues:

AzaCITIDine may be confused with azaTHIOprine

High alert medication: The Institute for Safe Medication Practices (ISMP) includes this medication among its list of drug classes which have a heightened risk of causing significant patient harm when used in error.

U.S. Brand Names Vidaza®

Index Terms 5-Azacytidine; 5-AZC; AZA-CR; Azacytidine; Ladakamycin; NSC-102816

Pharmacologic Category Antineoplastic Agent, DNA Methylation Inhibitor

Use Treatment of myelodysplastic syndrome (MDS)

Unlabeled/Investigational Use Treatment of acute myelogenous leukemia (AML)

Effect on Mental Status High doses may produce coma

Effect on Psychiatric Treatment Leukopenia is common; use caution with clozapine and carbamazepine

Dosage Summary

I.V.:

Children: Dosage not established

Adults: 75-100 mg/m^2/day for 7 days/28-day treatment cycle

SubQ:

Children: Dosage not established

Adults: 75-100 mg/m^2/day for 7 days/28-day treatment cycle

Dosage Forms Excipient information presented when available (limited, particularly for generics); consult specific product labeling.

Injection, powder for suspension [preservative free]:

Vidaza®: 100 mg [contains mannitol 100 mg]

- **AZA-CR** *see* AzaCITIDine *on page 161*
- **Azactam®** *see* Aztreonam *on page 168*
- **Azacytidine** *see* AzaCITIDine *on page 161*
- **5-Azacytidine** *see* AzaCITIDine *on page 161*
- **Azasan®** *see* AzaTHIOprine *on page 162*
- **AzaSite™** *see* Azithromycin *on page 163*

AzaTHIOprine (ay za THYE oh preen)

Medication Safety Issues

Sound-alike/look-alike issues:

AzaTHIOprine may be confused with azaCITIDine, azatadine, azidothymidine, azithromycin, Azulfidine®

Imuran® may be confused with Elmiron®, Enduron®, Imdur®, Inderal®, Tenormin®

Azathioprine is metabolized to mercaptopurine; concurrent use of these commercially-available products has resulted in profound myelosuppression.

U.S. Brand Names Azasan®; Imuran®

Canadian Brand Names Alti-Azathioprine; Apo-Azathioprine®; Gen-Azathioprine; Imuran®; Novo-Azathioprine

Mexican Brand Names Azatrilem; Imuran

Index Terms Azathioprine Sodium

Pharmacologic Category Immunosuppressant Agent

Use Adjunctive therapy in prevention of rejection of kidney transplants; management of active rheumatoid arthritis (RA)

Unlabeled/Investigational Use Adjunct in prevention of rejection of solid organ (nonrenal) transplants; steroid-sparing agent for corticosteroid-dependent Crohn's disease (CD) and ulcerative colitis (UC); maintenance of remission in CD; fistulizing Crohn's disease

Effect on Mental Status None reported

Effect on Psychiatric Treatment May produce pancytopenia; use caution with clozapine and carbamazepine

Dosage Summary

I.V.:

Children (unlabeled use): Transplant immunosuppression: Initial: 3-5 mg/kg/day as a single daily dose; Maintenance: 1-3 mg/kg/day as a single daily dose

Adults: Transplant immunosuppression: Initial: 3-5 mg/kg/day as a single daily dose; Maintenance: 1-3 mg/kg/day as a single daily dose

Oral:

Children (unlabeled use): Transplant immunosuppression: Initial: 3-5 mg/kg/day in 1-2 divided doses; Maintenance: 1-3 mg/kg/day in 1-2 divided doses

Adults:

Transplant immunosuppression: Initial: 3-5 mg/kg/day in 1-2 divided doses; Maintenance: 1-3 mg/kg/day in 1-2 divided doses

Rheumatoid arthritis: Initial: 1 mg/kg/day in 1-2 divided doses; Maintenance: 0.5-2.5 mg/kg/day in 1-2 divided doses

Dosage Forms Excipient information presented when available (limited, particularly for generics); consult specific product labeling.

Injection, powder for reconstitution: 100 mg

Tablet [scored]: 50 mg

Azasan®: 75 mg, 100 mg

Imuran®: 50 mg

◆ **Azathioprine Sodium** *see* AzaTHIOprine *on page 162*

◆ **5-AZC** *see* AzaCITIDine *on page 161*

Azelastine (a ZEL as teen)

Medication Safety Issues

Sound-alike/look-alike issues:

Optivar® may be confused with Optiray®, Optive™

International issues:

Optivar® may be confused with Opthavir® which is a brand name for acyclovir in Mexico

U.S. Brand Names Astelin®; Optivar®

Canadian Brand Names Astelin®

Mexican Brand Names Amsler; Astelin; Az Ofteno

Index Terms Azelastine Hydrochloride

Pharmacologic Category Histamine H_1 Antagonist; Histamine H_1 Antagonist, Second Generation

Use

Nasal spray: Treatment of the symptoms of seasonal allergic rhinitis such as rhinorrhea, sneezing, and nasal pruritus in children ≥5 years of age and adults; treatment of the symptoms of vasomotor rhinitis in children ≥12 years of age and adults

Ophthalmic: Treatment of itching of the eye associated with seasonal allergic conjunctivitis in children ≥3 years of age and adults

Effect on Mental Status Drowsiness is common; rare reports of anxiety and nervousness

Effect on Psychiatric Treatment Concurrent use with psychotropics may produce additive sedation

Dosage Summary

Intranasal:

Children <5 years: Dosage not established

Children 5-11 years: 1 spray in each nostril twice daily

Children ≥12 years: 1-2 sprays in each nostril twice daily

Adults: 1-2 sprays in each nostril twice daily

Ophthalmic:

Children <3 years: Dosage not established

Children ≥3 years: Instill 1 drop into affected eye(s) twice daily

Adults: Instill 1 drop into affected eye(s) twice daily

Dosage Forms Excipient information presented when available (limited, particularly for generics); consult specific product labeling.

Solution, intranasal, as hydrochloride [spray]:

Astelin®: 1 mg/mL (30 mL) [contains benzalkonium chloride; 137 mcg/spray; 200 metered sprays]

Solution, ophthalmic, as hydrochloride:

Optivar®: 0.05% (6 mL) [contains benzalkonium chloride]

◆ **Azelastine Hydrochloride** *see* Azelastine *on page 162*

◆ **Azidothymidine** *see* Zidovudine *on page 1695*

◆ **Azilect®** *see* Rasagiline *on page 1403*

Azithromycin (az ith roe MYE sin)

Medication Safety Issues

Sound-alike/look-alike issues:

Azithromycin may be confused with azathioprine, erythromycin

Zithromax® may be confused with Zinacef®

U.S. Brand Names AzaSite™; Zithromax®; Zmax™

Canadian Brand Names Apo-Azithromycin®; CO Azithromycin; Dom-Azithromycin; GMD-Azithromycin; Novo-Azithromycin; PHL-Azithromycin; PMS-Azithromycin; ratio-Azithromycin; Sandoz-Azithromycin; Zithromax®

Mexican Brand Names Azitrocin; Azitrohexal; Azo-Max; Koptin; Macrozit; Zithran

Index Terms Azithromycin Dihydrate; Azithromycin Hydrogencitrate; Azithromycin Monohydrate; Zithromax® TRI-PAK™; Zithromax® Z-PAK®

Pharmacologic Category Antibiotic, Macrolide; Antibiotic, Ophthalmic

Generic Available Yes: Injection, powder for oral suspension, tablet

Use

Oral, I.V.: Treatment of acute otitis media due to *H. influenzae*, *M. catarrhalis*, or *S. pneumoniae*; pharyngitis/tonsillitis due to *S. pyogenes*; treatment of mild-to-moderate upper and lower respiratory tract infections, infections of the skin and skin structure, community-acquired pneumonia, pelvic inflammatory disease (PID), sexually-transmitted diseases (urethritis/cervicitis), pharyngitis/tonsillitis (alternative to first-line therapy), and genital ulcer disease (chancroid) due to susceptible strains of *C. trachomatis*, *M. catarrhalis*, *H. influenzae*, *S. aureus*, *S. pneumoniae*, *Mycoplasma pneumoniae*, and *C. psittaci*; acute bacterial exacerbations of chronic obstructive pulmonary disease (COPD) due to *H. influenzae*, *M. catarrhalis*, or *S. pneumoniae*; acute bacterial sinusitis

Ophthalmic: Bacterial conjunctivitis

Unlabeled/Investigational Use Prevention of (or to delay onset of) or treatment of MAC in patients with advanced HIV infection; prophylaxis of infective endocarditis in patients who are allergic to penicillin and undergoing surgical or dental procedures; pertussis

Effect on Mental Status Macrolides have been reported to cause nightmares, confusion, anxiety, and mood lability; may rarely cause dizziness, agitation, nervousness, and insomnia

Effect on Psychiatric Treatment Contraindicated with pimozide; may increase concentration of bromocriptine, carbamazepine, and triazolam

Pregnancy Risk Factor B

Pregnancy Considerations Adverse events were not observed in animal studies; therefore, azithromycin is classified as pregnancy category B. Low levels of azithromycin have been shown to cross the placenta. Azithromycin ▶

may be used for the treatment of some infections during pregnancy. The CDC and IDSA provide recommendations for the treatment of chlamydial infections and MAC in pregnant patients. Since serum concentrations determine fetal exposure and azithromycin has much higher concentrations in tissue than serum, treatment results in the mother may be obtained with lower exposure to the fetus. Although no adverse reports in human or animal fetuses have been documented, information in pregnant women is limited.

Lactation Enters breast milk/use caution

Contraindications Hypersensitivity to azithromycin, other macrolide antibiotics, or any component of the formulation

Warnings/Precautions Use with caution in patients with pre-existing liver disease; hepatic impairment, including hepatocellular and/or cholestatic hepatitis, with or without jaundice, has been observed. Discontinue if symptoms of malaise, nausea, vomiting, abdominal colic, and fever. May mask or delay symptoms of incubating gonorrhea or syphilis, so appropriate culture and susceptibility tests should be performed prior to initiating azithromycin. Prolonged use may result in fungal or bacterial superinfection, including *C. difficile*-associated diarrhea (CDAD) and pseudomembranous colitis; CDAD has been observed >2 months postantibiotic treatment. Use caution with renal dysfunction. Prolongation of the QT_c interval has been reported with macrolide antibiotics; use caution in patients at risk of prolonged cardiac repolarization. Safety and efficacy of systemically-administered azithromycin (oral, intravenous) have not been established in children <6 months of age with acute otitis media, acute bacterial sinusitis, or community-acquired pneumonia, or in children <2 years of age with pharyngitis/tonsillitis. Safety and efficacy for ophthalmic use have not been established in children <1 year of age.

Ophthalmic solution should not be injected subconjunctivally or introduced directly into the anterior chamber of the eye. Ophthalmic solution contains benzalkonium chloride which may be absorbed by contact lenses; contact lens should not be worn during treatment of ophthalmic infections.

Oral suspensions (immediate release and extended release) are not interchangeable.

Adverse Reactions

>10%: Gastrointestinal: Diarrhea (4% to 9%; high single-dose regimens 14%), nausea (≤7%; high single-dose regimens 18%)

2% to 10%:

Dermatologic: Pruritus, rash

Gastrointestinal: Abdominal pain, anorexia, cramping, vomiting (especially with high single-dose regimens)

Genitourinary: Vaginitis

Local: (with I.V. administration): Injection site pain, inflammation

Ocular (with ophthalmic solution use): Eye irritation (1% to 2%)

≤1% (Limited to important or life-threatening): Systemic therapy: Agitation, allergic reaction, anemia, angioedema, bronchospasm, candidiasis, chest pain, cholestatic jaundice, conjunctivitis, constipation, cough increased, dermatitis (fungal), diaphoresis, dizziness, dyspepsia, eczema, enteritis, facial edema, fatigue, fever, flatulence, fungal infection, gastritis, headache, hyperkinesia, insomnia, jaundice, leukopenia, malaise, melena, mucositis, nephritis, nervousness, oral moniliasis, pain, palpitation, pharyngitis, photosensitivity, pleural effusion, rhinitis, somnolence, taste perversion, urticaria, vertigo, vesiculobullous rash

1%: Ophthalmic solution: Contact dermatitis, corneal erosion, dysgeusia, nasal congestion, ocular discharge, ocular dryness; ocular stinging, burning, and irritation upon instillation; punctate keratitis, sinusitis

Postmarketing and/or case reports (all formulations): Acute renal failure, aggressive behavior, anaphylaxis, anxiety, arrhythmia (including ventricular tachycardia), arthralgia, deafness, dehydration, edema, erythema multiforme (rare), hearing disturbance, hearing loss, hepatic failure (rare), hepatic necrosis (rare), hepatitis, hyperactivity, hypertrophic pyloric stenosis, hypotension, interstitial nephritis, loss of smell, loss of taste, LFTs increased, neutropenia (mild), oral candidiasis, pancreatitis, paresthesia, pseudomembranous colitis, QT_c prolongation (rare), seizure, smell perversion, somnolence, Stevens-Johnson syndrome (rare), syncope, thrombocytopenia, tinnitus, tongue discoloration (rare), torsade de pointes (rare), toxic epidermal necrolysis (rare), weakness

Metabolism/Transport Effects **Substrate** of CYP3A4 (minor); **Inhibits** CYP3A4 (weak)

Drug Interactions

Amiodarone: Azithromycin may enhance the QTc-prolonging effect of Amiodarone. *Risk D: Consider therapy modification*

Cardiac Glycosides: Macrolide Antibiotics may increase the serum concentration of Cardiac Glycosides. *Risk D: Consider therapy modification*

CycloSPORINE: Macrolide Antibiotics may decrease the metabolism of CycloSPORINE. *Risk C: Monitor therapy*

Nelfinavir: May decrease the excretion of Azithromycin. *Risk C: Monitor therapy*

Tacrolimus: Macrolide Antibiotics may increase the serum concentration of Tacrolimus. *Risk C: Monitor therapy*

Typhoid Vaccine: Antibiotics may diminish the therapeutic effect of Typhoid Vaccine. Only the live attenuated Ty21a strain is affected. *Risk D: Consider therapy modification*

Vitamin K Antagonists (eg, warfarin): Macrolide Antibiotics may decrease the metabolism of Vitamin K Antagonists. *Risk C: Monitor therapy*

Ethanol/Nutrition/Herb Interactions Food: Rate and extent of GI absorption may be altered depending upon the formulation. Azithromycin suspension, not tablet form, has significantly increased absorption (46%) with food.

Stability

Injection (Zithromax®): Store intact vials of injection at room temperature. Reconstitute the 500 mg vial with 4.8 mL of sterile water for injection and shake until all of the drug is dissolved. Each mL contains 100 mg azithromycin. Reconstituted solution is stable for 24 hours when stored below 30°C (86°F). Use of a standard syringe is recommended due to the vacuum in the vial (which may draw additional solution through an automated syringe).

The initial solution should be further diluted to a concentration of 1 mg/mL (500 mL) to 2 mg/mL (250 mL) in 0.9% sodium chloride, 5% dextrose in water, or lactated Ringer's. The diluted solution is stable for 24 hours at or below room temperature (30°C or 86°F) and for 7 days if stored under refrigeration (5°C or 41°F).

Ophthalmic solution: Prior to use, store unopened under refrigeration at 2°C to 8°C (36°F to 46°F). After opening, store at 2°C to 25°C (36°F to 77°F) for ≤14 days; discard any remaining solution after 14 days.

Suspension, immediate release (Zithromax®): Store dry powder below 30°C (86°F). Following reconstitution, store at 5°C to 30°C (41°F to 86°F).

Suspension, extended release (Zmax™): Store dry powder below 30°C (86°F). Following reconstitution, store at 15°C to 30°C (59°F to 86°F); do not freeze. Should be consumed within 12 hours following reconstitution.

Tablet (Zithromax®): Store between 15°C to 30°C (59°F to 86°F).

Mechanism of Action Inhibits RNA-dependent protein synthesis at the chain elongation step; binds to the 50S ribosomal subunit resulting in blockage of transpeptidation

Pharmacodynamics/Kinetics

Absorption: Oral: Rapid; Ophthalmic: Negligible

Distribution: Extensive tissue; distributes well into skin, lungs, sputum, tonsils, and cervix; penetration into CSF is poor; I.V.: 33.3 L/kg; Oral: 31.1 L/kg

Protein binding (concentration dependent): Oral, I.V.: 7% to 51%

Metabolism: Hepatic

Bioavailability: Oral: 38%, decreased by 17% with extended release suspension; variable effect with food (increased with immediate or delayed release oral suspension, unchanged with tablet)

Half-life elimination: Oral, I.V.: Terminal: Immediate release: 68-72 hours; Extended release: 59 hours

Time to peak, serum: Oral: Immediate release: 2-3 hours; Extended release: 5 hours

Excretion: Oral, I.V.: Biliary (major route); urine (6%)

Dosage Note: Extended release suspension (Zmax™) is not interchangeable with immediate release formulations. Use should be limited to approved indications. All doses are expressed as immediate release azithromycin unless otherwise specified.

Usual dosage range:

Children ≥6 months: Oral: 5-12 mg/kg given once daily (maximum: 500 mg/day) **or** 30 mg/kg as a single dose (maximum: 1500 mg)

Children ≥1 year and Adults: Ophthalmic: Instill 1 drop into affected eye(s) twice daily (8-12 hours apart) for 2 days, then 1 drop once daily for 5 days

Adolescents ≥16 years and Adults:

Oral: 250-600 mg once daily **or** 1-2 g as a single dose

I.V.: 250-500 mg once daily

Indication-specific dosing:

Children: Oral:

Bacterial sinusitis: 10 mg/kg once daily for 3 days (maximum: 500 mg/day)

Cat scratch disease (unlabeled use): <45.5 kg: 10 mg/kg as a single dose, then 5 mg/kg once daily for 4 days

Community-acquired pneumonia: 10 mg/kg on day 1 (maximum: 500 mg/day) followed by 5 mg/kg/day once daily on days 2-5 (maximum: 250 mg/day)

Disseminated *M. avium* (unlabeled use):

HIV-infected patients: 5 mg/kg/day once daily (maximum: 250 mg/day) or 20 mg/kg (maximum: 1200 mg) once weekly given alone or in combination with rifabutin

Treatment and secondary prevention in HIV-negative patients: 5 mg/kg/day once daily (maximum: 250 mg/day) in combination with ethambutol, with or without rifabutin

Prophylaxis against infective endocarditis (unlabeled use): 15 mg/kg 30-60 minutes before procedure (maximum: 500 mg). **Note:** American Heart Association (AHA) guidelines now recommend prophylaxis only in patients undergoing invasive procedures and in whom underlying cardiac conditions may predispose to a higher risk of adverse outcomes should infection occur. As of April 2007, routine prophylaxis for GI/GU procedures is no longer recommended by the AHA.

Otitis media:

1-day regimen: 30 mg/kg as a single dose (maximum: 1500 mg)

3-day regimen: 10 mg/kg once daily for 3 days (maximum: 500 mg/day)

5-day regimen: 10 mg/kg on day 1 (maximum: 500 mg/day) followed by 5 mg/kg/day once daily on days 2-5 (maximum: 250 mg/day)

Pharyngitis, tonsillitis: Children ≥2 years: 12 mg/kg/day once daily for 5 days (maximum: 500 mg/day)

Pertussis (CDC guidelines):

Children <6 months: 10 mg/kg/day for 5 days

Children ≥6 months: 10 mg/kg on day 1 (maximum: 500 mg/day) followed by 5 mg/kg/day once daily on days 2-5 (maximum: 250 mg/day)

Uncomplicated chlamydial urethritis or cervicitis (unlabeled use): Children ≥45 kg: 1 g as a single dose

Children ≥1 year and Adults: Ophthalmic:

Bacterial conjunctivitis: Instill 1 drop into affected eye(s) twice daily (8-12 hours apart) for 2 days, then 1 drop once daily for 5 days

Adolescents ≥16 years and Adults:

Bacterial sinusitis: Oral: 500 mg/day for a total of 3 days

Extended release suspension (Zmax™): 2 g as a single dose

Cat scratch disease (unlabeled use): Oral: >45.5 kg: 500 mg as a single dose, then 250 mg once daily for 4 days

Chancroid due to *H. ducreyi*: Oral: 1 g as a single dose

Community-acquired pneumonia:

Oral (Zmax™): 2 g as a single dose

I.V.: 500 mg as a single dose for at least 2 days, follow I.V. therapy by the oral route with a single daily dose of 500 mg to complete a 7- to 10-day course of therapy.

Disseminated *M. avium* complex disease in patients with advanced HIV infection (unlabeled use): Oral:

Prophylaxis: 1200 mg once weekly (may be combined with rifabutin)

Treatment: 600 mg daily (in combination with ethambutol 15 mg/kg)

Prophylaxis against infective endocarditis (unlabeled use): Oral: 500 mg 30-60 minutes prior to the procedure. **Note:** American Heart Association (AHA) guidelines now recommend prophylaxis only in patients undergoing invasive procedures and in whom underlying cardiac conditions may predispose to a higher risk of adverse outcomes should infection occur. As of April 2007, routine prophylaxis for GI/GU procedures is no longer recommended by the AHA.

Mild-to-moderate respiratory tract, skin, and soft tissue infections: Oral: 500 mg in a single loading dose on day 1 followed by 250 mg/day as a single dose on days 2-5

Alternative regimen: Bacterial exacerbation of COPD: 500 mg/day for a total of 3 days

Pelvic inflammatory disease (PID): I.V.: 500 mg as a single dose for 1-2 days, follow I.V. therapy by the oral route with a single daily dose of 250 mg to complete a 7-day course of therapy

Pertussis (CDC guidelines): Oral: 500 mg on day 1 followed by 250 mg/day on days 2-5 (maximum: 500 mg/day)

Urethritis/cervicitis: Oral:

Due to C. trachomatis: 1 g as a single dose

Due to N. gonorrhoeae: 2 g as a single dose

Dosage adjustment in renal impairment: Use caution in patients with Cl_{cr} <10 mL/minute

Dosage adjustment in hepatic impairment: Use with caution due to potential for hepatotoxicity (rare). Specific guidelines for dosing in hepatic impairment have not been established.

Dietary Considerations

Oral suspension, immediate release, may be administered with or without food.

Oral suspension, extended release, should be taken on an empty stomach (at least 1 hour before or 2 hours following a meal).

Tablet may be administered with food to decrease GI effects.

Sodium content:

Injection: 114 mg (4.96 mEq) per vial

Oral suspension, immediate release: 3.7 mg per 100 mg/5 mL of constituted suspension; 7.4 mg per 200 mg/5 mL of constituted suspension; 37 mg per 1 g single-dose packet

Oral suspension, extended release: 148 mg per 2 g constituted suspension

Tablet: 0.9 mg/250 mg tablet; 1.8 mg/500 mg tablet; 2.1 mg/600 mg tablet

Administration

I.V.: Infusate concentration and rate of infusion for azithromycin for injection should be either 1 mg/mL over 3 hours or 2 mg/mL over 1 hour. Other medications should not be infused simultaneously through the same I.V. line.

Ophthalmic: Shake bottle once prior to each administration. Wash hands before and after instillation.

Oral: Immediate release suspension and tablet may be taken without regard to food; extended release suspension should be taken on an empty stomach (at least 1 hour before or 2 hours following a meal), within 12 hours of reconstitution.

Monitoring Parameters Liver function tests, CBC with differential

Additional Information Zithromax® tablets and immediate release suspension may be interchanged (eg, two Zithromax® 250 mg tablets may be substituted for one Zithromax® 500 mg tablet or the tablets may be substituted with the immediate release suspension); however, the extended release suspension (Zmax™) is not bioequivalent with Zithromax® and therefore should not be interchanged.

Dosage Forms Excipient information presented when available (limited, particularly for generics); consult specific product labeling.

Note: Strength expressed as base

Injection, powder for reconstitution, as dihydrate: 500 mg

Zithromax®: 500 mg [contains sodium 114 mg (4.96 mEq) per vial]

Injection, powder for reconstitution, as hydrogencitrate: 500 mg

Injection, powder for reconstitution, as monohydrate: 500 mg

Microspheres for oral suspension, extended release, as dihydrate:

Zmax™: 2 g [single-dose bottle; contains sodium 148 mg per bottle; cherry and banana flavor]

Powder for oral suspension, as monohydrate: 100 mg/5 mL (15 mL); 200 mg/5 mL (15 mL, 22.5 mL, 30 mL)

Powder for oral suspension, immediate release, as dihydrate:

Zithromax®: 100 mg/5 mL (15 mL) [contains sodium 3.7 mg/ 5 mL; cherry creme de vanilla and banana flavor]; 200 mg/5 mL (15 mL, 22.5 mL, 30 mL) [contains sodium 7.4 mg/5 mL; cherry creme de vanilla and banana flavor]; 1 g/packet (3s, 10s) [single-dose packet; contains sodium 37 mg per packet; cherry creme de vanilla and banana flavor]

Solution, ophthalmic:

AzaSite™: 1% (2.5 mL) [contains benzalkonium chloride]

Tablet, as dihydrate:

Zithromax®: 250 mg [contains sodium 0.9 mg per tablet]; 500 mg [contains sodium 1.8 mg per tablet]; 600 mg [contains sodium 2.1 mg per tablet]

Zithromax® TRI-PAK™ [unit-dose pack]: 500 mg (3s) [contains sodium 1.8 mg per tablet]

Zithromax® Z-PAK® [unit-dose pack]: 250 mg (6s) [contains sodium 0.9 mg per tablet]

Tablet, as monohydrate: 250 mg, 500 mg, 600 mg

◆ **Azithromycin Dihydrate** *see* Azithromycin *on page 163*

◆ **Azithromycin Hydrogencitrate** *see* Azithromycin *on page 163*

◆ **Azithromycin Monohydrate** *see* Azithromycin *on page 163*

◆ **Azmacort®** *see* Triamcinolone *on page 1617*

◆ **AZO-Gesic® [OTC]** *see* Phenazopyridine *on page 1258*

◆ **Azopt®** *see* Brinzolamide *on page 199*

◆ **Azor™** *see* Amlodipine and Olmesartan *on page 104*

◆ **AZO-Standard® [OTC]** *see* Phenazopyridine *on page 1258*

◆ **AZO-Standard® Maximum Strength [OTC]** *see* Phenazopyridine *on page 1258*

◆ **AZT + 3TC (error-prone abbreviation)** *see* Zidovudine and Lamivudine *on page 1696*

◆ **AZT (error-prone abbreviation)** *see* Zidovudine *on page 1695*

◆ **Azthreonam** *see* Aztreonam *on page 168*

Aztreonam (AZ tree oh nam)

Medication Safety Issues

Sound-alike/look-alike issues:

Aztreonam may be confused with azidothymidine

U.S. Brand Names Azactam®

Canadian Brand Names Azactam®

Index Terms Azthreonam

Pharmacologic Category Antibiotic, Miscellaneous

Use Treatment of patients with urinary tract infections, lower respiratory tract infections, septicemia, skin/skin structure infections, intra-abdominal infections, and gynecological infections caused by susceptible gram-negative bacilli

Effect on Mental Status May rarely produce confusion

Effect on Psychiatric Treatment Rarely produces leukopenia and neutropenia; use caution with clozapine and carbamazepine

Dosage Summary

I.M.:

Children ≤1 month: Dosage not established

Children >1 month: 30-50 mg/kg/dose every 6-8 hours (maximum: 8 g/day)

Adults: 500 mg to 1 g every 8-12 hours

I.V.:

Children ≤1 month: Dosage not established

Children >1 month: 30-50 mg/kg/dose every 6-8 hours (maximum: 8 g/day)

Adults: 1-2 g every 6-12 hours (maximum: 8 g/day)

Dosage Forms Excipient information presented when available (limited, particularly for generics); consult specific product labeling. [DSC] = Discontinued product

Infusion premixed iso-osmotic solution:

Azactam®: 1 g (50 mL); 2 g (50 mL)

Injection, powder for reconstitution:

Azactam®: 500 mg [DSC], 1 g, 2 g

◆ **Azulfidine®** *see* Sulfasalazine *on page 1522*

◆ **Azulfidine® EN-tabs®** *see* Sulfasalazine *on page 1522*

◆ **B1** *see* Tositumomab and Iodine I 131 Tositumomab *on page 1603*

◆ **B1 Antibody** *see* Tositumomab and Iodine I 131 Tositumomab *on page 1603*

◆ **B2036-PEG** *see* Pegvisomant *on page 1237*

◆ **B 9273** *see* Alefacept *on page 58*

◆ **BA-16038** *see* Aminoglutethimide *on page 87*

◆ **Babee® Cof Syrup [OTC]** *see* Dextromethorphan *on page 448*

Baclofen (BAK loe fen)

Medication Safety Issues

Sound-alike/look-alike issues:

Baclofen may be confused with Bactroban®

Lioresal® may be confused with lisinopril, Lotensin®

High alert medication: The Institute for Safe Medication Practices (ISMP) includes this medication (intrathecal administration) among its list of drugs which have a heightened risk of causing significant patient harm when used in error.

U.S. Brand Names Lioresal®

Canadian Brand Names Apo-Baclofen®; Gen-Baclofen; Lioresal®; Liotec; Nu-Baclo; PMS-Baclofen

Pharmacologic Category Skeletal Muscle Relaxant

Generic Available Yes: Tablets only

Use Treatment of reversible spasticity associated with multiple sclerosis or spinal cord lesions

Orphan drug: Intrathecal: Treatment of intractable spasticity caused by spinal cord injury, multiple sclerosis, and other spinal disease (spinal ischemia or tumor, transverse myelitis, cervical spondylosis, degenerative myelopathy)

Unlabeled/Investigational Use Intractable hiccups, intractable pain relief, bladder spasticity, trigeminal neuralgia, cerebral palsy, Huntington's chorea

Effect on Mental Status Drowsiness and insomnia are common; rare reports of depression, euphoria, and hallucinations

Effect on Psychiatric Treatment Concurrent use with psychotropics may produce additive sedation; concurrent use with MAO inhibitors may potentiate their hypotensive effects

Pregnancy Risk Factor C

Lactation Enters breast milk (small amounts)/compatible

Contraindications Hypersensitivity to baclofen or any component of the formulation

Warnings/Precautions Use with caution in patients with seizure disorder or impaired renal function. **[U.S. Boxed Warning]: Avoid abrupt withdrawal of the drug; abrupt withdrawal of intrathecal baclofen has resulted in severe sequelae (hyperpyrexia, obtundation, rebound/exaggerated spasticity, muscle rigidity, and rhabdomyolysis), leading to organ failure and some fatalities.** Risk may be higher in patients with injuries at T-6 or above, history of baclofen withdrawal, or limited ability to communicate. May cause CNS depression, which may impair physical or mental abilities; patients must be cautioned about performing tasks which require mental alertness (eg, operating machinery or driving). Elderly are more sensitive to the effects of baclofen and are more likely to experience adverse CNS effects at higher doses.

Adverse Reactions

>10%:

- Central nervous system: Drowsiness, vertigo, dizziness, psychiatric disturbances, insomnia, slurred speech, ataxia, hypotonia
- Neuromuscular & skeletal: Weakness

1% to 10%:

- Cardiovascular: Hypotension
- Central nervous system: Fatigue, confusion, headache
- Dermatologic: Rash
- Gastrointestinal: Nausea, constipation
- Genitourinary: Polyuria

<1% (Limited to important or life-threatening): Chest pain, dyspnea, dysuria, enuresis, hematuria, impotence, inability to ejaculate, nocturia, palpitation, syncope, urinary retention; withdrawal reactions have occurred with abrupt discontinuation (particularly severe with intrathecal use).

Drug Interactions

Alcohol (Ethyl): CNS Depressants may enhance the CNS depressant effect of Alcohol (Ethyl). *Risk C: Monitor therapy*

CNS Depressants: May enhance the adverse/toxic effect of other CNS Depressants. *Risk C: Monitor therapy*

Ethanol/Nutrition/Herb Interactions

Ethanol: Avoid ethanol (may increase CNS depression).

Herb/Nutraceutical: Avoid valerian, St John's wort, kava kava, gotu kola.

Mechanism of Action Inhibits the transmission of both monosynaptic and polysynaptic reflexes at the spinal cord level, possibly by hyperpolarization of primary afferent fiber terminals, with resultant relief of muscle spasticity

Pharmacodynamics/Kinetics

Onset of action: 3-4 days

- Peak effect: 5-10 days

Absorption (dose dependent): Oral: Rapid

Protein binding: 30%

Metabolism: Hepatic (15% of dose)

Half-life elimination: 3.5 hours

Time to peak, serum: Oral: Within 2-3 hours

Excretion: Urine and feces (85% as unchanged drug)

Dosage

Oral (avoid abrupt withdrawal of drug):

Children (unlabeled use): Caution: Pediatric dosing expressed as a daily amount, and **NOT** in mg/kg. Limited published data in children; the following is a compilation of small prospective studies (Albright, 1996; Milla, 1977; Scheinberg, 2006) and one large retrospective study (Lubsch, 2006):

- <2 years: 10-20 mg daily divided every 8 hours; titrate dose every 3 days in increments of 5-15mg/day to a maximum of 40 mg daily
- 2-7 years: Initial: 20-30 mg daily divided every 8 hours; titrate dose every 3 days in increments of 5-15 mg/day to a maximum of 60 mg daily

≥8 years: 30-40 mg daily divided every 8 hours; titrate dose every 3 days in increments of 5-15 mg/day to a maximum of 120 mg daily

Note: Baclofen dose may need to be increased over time. One retrospective analysis (Lubsch, 2006) suggested that increased doses were needed as the time increased from spasticity onset, as age increased, and as the number of concomitant antispasticity medications increased. A small number of patients required daily doses exceeding 200 mg.

Adults: 5 mg 3 times/day, may increase 5 mg/dose every 3 days to a maximum of 80 mg/day

Hiccups (unlabeled use): Usual effective dose: 10-20 mg 2-3 times/day

Intrathecal: Children and Adults:

Test dose: 50-100 mcg, doses >50 mcg should be given in 25 mcg increments, separated by 24 hours. A screening dose of 25 mcg may be considered in very small patients. Patients not responding to screening dose of 100 mcg should not be considered for chronic infusion/implanted pump.

Maintenance: After positive response to test dose, a maintenance intrathecal infusion can be administered via an implanted intrathecal pump. Initial dose via pump: Infusion at a 24-hour rate dosed at twice the test dose. Avoid abrupt discontinuation.

Elderly: Oral (the lowest effective dose is recommended): Initial: 5 mg 2-3 times/day, increasing gradually as needed; if benefits are not seen, withdraw the drug slowly.

Dosing adjustment in renal impairment: May be necessary to reduce dosage in renal impairment, but there are no specific guidelines available

Hemodialysis: Poor water solubility allows for accumulation during chronic hemodialysis. Low-dose therapy is recommended. There have been several case reports of accumulation of baclofen resulting in toxicity symptoms (organic brain syndrome, myoclonia, deceleration and steep potentials in EEG) in patients with renal failure who have received normal doses of baclofen.

Administration Intrathecal: For screening dosages, dilute with preservative-free sodium chloride to a final concentration of 50 mcg/mL for bolus injection into the subarachnoid space. For maintenance infusions, concentrations of 500-2000 mcg/mL may be used.

Test Interactions Increased alkaline phosphatase, AST, glucose, ammonia (B); decreased bilirubin (S)

Dosage Forms Excipient information presented when available (limited, particularly for generics); consult specific product labeling.

Injection, solution, intrathecal [preservative free]:

Lioresal®: 50 mcg/mL (1 mL); 500 mcg/mL (20 mL); 2000 mcg/mL (5 mL, 20 mL)

Tablet: 10 mg, 20 mg

- ◆ **Bactrim™** *see* Sulfamethoxazole and Trimethoprim *on page 1517*
- ◆ **Bactrim™ DS** *see* Sulfamethoxazole and Trimethoprim *on page 1517*
- ◆ **Bactroban®** *see* Mupirocin *on page 1085*
- ◆ **Bactroban® Nasal** *see* Mupirocin *on page 1085*
- ◆ **Baking Soda** *see* Sodium Bicarbonate *on page 1494*
- ◆ **BAL** *see* Dimercaprol *on page 479*
- ◆ **Balacet 325™** *see* Propoxyphene and Acetaminophen *on page 1354*
- ◆ **BAL in Oil®** *see* Dimercaprol *on page 479*

Balsalazide (bal SAL a zide)

Medication Safety Issues

Sound-alike/look-alike issues:

Colazal® may be confused with Clozaril®

U.S. Brand Names Colazal®

Index Terms Balsalazide Disodium

Pharmacologic Category 5-Aminosalicylic Acid Derivative; Anti-inflammatory Agent

Use Treatment of mild-to-moderate active ulcerative colitis

Effect on Mental Status May cause insomnia, fatigue, and dizziness

Effect on Psychiatric Treatment None reported

Dosage Summary

Oral:

Children <5 years: Dosage not established

Children ≥5 years: 750 mg 3 times/day for up to 8 weeks **or** 2.25 g 3 times/day for 8 weeks
Adults: 2.25 g 3 times/day for 8-12 weeks

Dosage Forms Excipient information presented when available (limited, particularly for generics); consult specific product labeling.
Capsule, as disodium: 750 mg
Colazal®: 750 mg [contains sodium ~86 mg/capsule]

- **Balsalazide Disodium** *see* Balsalazide *on page 170*
- **Baltussin** *see* Dihydrocodeine, Chlorpheniramine, and Phenylephrine *on page 469*
- **Balziva™** *see* Ethinyl Estradiol and Norethindrone *on page 597*
- **Band-Aid® Hurt-Free™ Antiseptic Wash [OTC]** *see* Lidocaine *on page 924*
- **Banophen® [OTC]** *see* DiphenhydrAMINE *on page 481*
- **Banophen® Anti-Itch [OTC]** *see* DiphenhydrAMINE *on page 481*
- **Banzel™** *see* Rufinamide *on page 1452*
- **Baraclude®** *see* Entecavir *on page 540*
- **Baridium® [OTC]** *see* Phenazopyridine *on page 1258*

Basiliximab (ba si LIK si mab)

U.S. Brand Names Simulect®
Canadian Brand Names Simulect®
Mexican Brand Names Simulect
Pharmacologic Category Monoclonal Antibody
Use Prophylaxis of acute organ rejection in renal transplantation
Effect on Mental Status Dizziness, headache, and insomnia are common. May cause agitation, anxiety, depression, malaise, or fatigue.
Effect on Psychiatric Treatment Side effects mimic depressive symptoms; effects of benzodiazepines and antidepressants may be altered
Dosage Summary
I.V.:
Children <35 kg: 10 mg within 2 hours prior to transplant surgery, followed by a second 10 mg dose 4 days after transplantation
Children ≥35 kg: 20 mg within 2 hours prior to transplant surgery, followed by a second 20 mg dose 4 days after transplantation
Adults: 20 mg within 2 hours prior to transplant surgery, followed by a second 20 mg dose 4 days after transplantation

Dosage Forms Excipient information presented when available (limited, particularly for generics); consult specific product labeling.
Injection, powder for reconstitution [preservative free]:
Simulect®: 10 mg, 20 mg

- **BAY 43-9006** *see* Sorafenib *on page 1501*
- **Bayer® Aspirin Extra Strength [OTC]** *see* Aspirin *on page 143*
- **Bayer® Aspirin Regimen Adult Low Dose [OTC]** *see* Aspirin *on page 143*
- **Bayer® Aspirin Regimen Children's [OTC]** *see* Aspirin *on page 143*
- **Bayer® Aspirin Regimen Regular Strength [OTC]** *see* Aspirin *on page 143*
- **Bayer® Genuine Aspirin [OTC]** *see* Aspirin *on page 143*
- **Bayer® Plus Extra Strength [OTC]** *see* Aspirin *on page 143*
- **Bayer® PM [OTC]** *see* Aspirin and Diphenhydramine *on page 145*
- **Bayer® with Heart Advantage [OTC]** *see* Aspirin *on page 143*
- **Bayer® Women's Aspirin Plus Calcium [OTC]** *see* Aspirin *on page 143*
- **BCNU** *see* Carmustine *on page 284*
- **Bebulin® VH** *see* Factor IX Complex (Human) *on page 612*

Beclomethasone (be kloe METH a sone)

Medication Safety Issues
Sound-alike/look-alike issues:
Vanceril® may be confused with Vancenase®
U.S. Brand Names Beconase® AQ; QVAR®
Canadian Brand Names Apo-Beclomethasone®; Gen-Beclo; Nu-Beclomethasone; Propaderm®; QVAR®; Rivanase AQ; Vanceril® AEM
Mexican Brand Names Beclazone; Beconase; Becotide; Dobipro; Qvar
Index Terms Beclomethasone Dipropionate

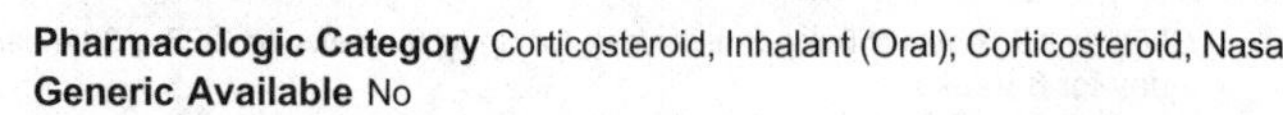

Pharmacologic Category Corticosteroid, Inhalant (Oral); Corticosteroid, Nasal

Generic Available No

Use

Oral inhalation: Maintenance and prophylactic treatment of asthma; includes those who require corticosteroids and those who may benefit from a dose reduction/elimination of systemically-administered corticosteroids. Not for relief of acute bronchospasm.

Nasal aerosol: Symptomatic treatment of seasonal or perennial rhinitis; prevent recurrence of nasal polyps following surgery.

Effect on Mental Status May cause agitation, depression, dizziness, euphoria, insomnia, mood swings, and personality changes; may cause exacerbation of pre-existing psychiatric conditions

Effect on Psychiatric Treatment None reported

Pregnancy Risk Factor C

Pregnancy Considerations Teratogenic effects were observed in animal studies. No human data on beclomethasone crossing the placenta or effects on the fetus. A decrease in fetal growth has not been observed with inhaled corticosteroid use during pregnancy. Inhaled corticosteroids are recommended for the treatment of asthma (most information available using budesonide) and allergic rhinitis during pregnancy.

Lactation Excretion in breast milk unknown/use caution

Contraindications Hypersensitivity to beclomethasone or any component of the formulation; status asthmaticus

Warnings/Precautions May cause hypercorticism or suppression of hypothalamic-pituitary-adrenal (HPA) axis, particularly in younger children or in patients receiving high doses for prolonged periods. HPA axis suppression may lead to adrenal crisis. Withdrawal and discontinuation of a corticosteroid should be done slowly and carefully. Particular care is required when patients are transferred from systemic corticosteroids to inhaled products due to possible adrenal insufficiency or withdrawal from steroids, including an increase in allergic symptoms. Patients receiving >20 mg per day of prednisone (or equivalent) may be most susceptible. Fatalities have occurred due to adrenal insufficiency in asthmatic patients during and after transfer from systemic corticosteroids to aerosol steroids; aerosol steroids do not provide the systemic steroid needed to treat patients having trauma, surgery, or infections.

Bronchospasm may occur with wheezing after inhalation; if this occurs stop steroid and treat with a fast-acting bronchodilator. Supplemental steroids (oral or parenteral) may be needed during stress or severe asthma attacks. Not to be used in status asthmaticus or for the relief of acute bronchospasm. Corticosteroid use may cause psychiatric disturbances, including depression, euphoria, insomnia, mood swings, and personality changes. Pre-existing psychiatric conditions may be exacerbated by corticosteroid use. Prolonged use of corticosteroids may also increase the incidence of secondary infection, mask acute infection (including fungal infections), prolong or exacerbate viral infections, or limit response to vaccines. Exposure to chickenpox should be avoided; corticosteroids should not be used to treat ocular herpes simplex. Corticosteroids should not be used for cerebral malaria. Close observation is required in patients with latent tuberculosis and/or TB reactivity; restrict use in active TB (only in conjunction with antituberculosis treatment). Prolonged treatment with corticosteroids has been associated with the development of Kaposi's sarcoma (case reports); if noted, discontinuation of therapy should be considered.

Use with caution in patients with thyroid disease, hepatic impairment, renal impairment, cardiovascular disease, diabetes, glaucoma, cataracts, myasthenia gravis, patients at risk for osteoporosis, patients at risk for seizures, or GI diseases (diverticulitis, peptic ulcer, ulcerative colitis) due to perforation risk. Use caution following acute MI (corticosteroids have been associated with myocardial rupture). Because of the risk of adverse effects, systemic corticosteroids should be used cautiously in the elderly in the smallest possible effective dose for the shortest duration. Avoid nasal corticosteroid use in patients with recent nasal septal ulcers, nasal surgery or nasal trauma until healing has occurred.

Orally-inhaled and intranasal corticosteroids may cause a reduction in growth velocity in pediatric patients (~1 centimeter per year [range: 0.3-1.8 cm per year] and related to dose and duration of exposure). To minimize the systemic effects of orally-inhaled and intranasal corticosteroids, each patient should be titrated to the lowest effective dose. Growth should be routinely monitored in pediatric patients. Safety and efficacy have not been established in children <5 years of age. There have been reports of systemic corticosteroid withdrawal symptoms (eg, joint/muscle pain, lassitude, depression) when withdrawing oral inhalation therapy.

Adverse Reactions Frequency not defined.

Central nervous system: Agitation, depression, dizziness, dysphonia, headache, lightheadedness, mental disturbances

Dermatologic: Acneiform lesions, angioedema, atrophy, bruising, pruritus, purpura, striae, rash, urticaria

Endocrine & metabolic: Cushingoid features, growth velocity reduction in children and adolescents, HPA function suppression

Gastrointestinal: Dry/irritated nose, throat and mouth, hoarseness, localized *Candida* or *Aspergillus* infection, loss of smell, loss of taste, nausea, unpleasant smell, unpleasant taste, vomiting, weight gain

Local: Nasal spray: Burning, epistaxis, localized *Candida* infection, nasal septum perforation (rare), nasal stuffiness, nosebleeds, rhinorrhea, sneezing, transient irritation, ulceration of nasal mucosa (rare)

Ocular: Cataracts, glaucoma, intraocular pressure increased

Respiratory: Cough, paradoxical bronchospasm, pharyngitis, sinusitis, wheezing

Miscellaneous: Anaphylactic/anaphylactoid reactions, death (due to adrenal insufficiency, reported during and after transfer from systemic corticosteroids to aerosol in asthmatic patients), immediate and delayed hypersensitivity reactions

Drug Interactions

Amphotericin B: Corticosteroids (Orally Inhaled) may enhance the hypokalemic effect of Amphotericin B. *Risk C: Monitor therapy*

Antidiabetic Agents: Corticosteroids (Orally Inhaled) may diminish the hypoglycemic effect of Antidiabetic Agents. In some instances, corticosteroid-mediated HPA axis suppression has led to episodes of acute adrenal crisis, which may manifest as enhanced hypoglycemia, particularly in the setting of insulin or other antidiabetic agent use. *Risk C: Monitor therapy*

Corticorelin: Corticosteroids may diminish the therapeutic effect of Corticorelin. Specifically, the plasma ACTH response to corticorelin may be blunted by recent or current corticosteroid therapy. *Risk C: Monitor therapy*

Loop Diuretics: Corticosteroids (Orally Inhaled) may enhance the hypokalemic effect of Loop Diuretics. *Risk C: Monitor therapy*

Thiazide Diuretics: Corticosteroids (Orally Inhaled) may enhance the hypokalemic effect of Thiazide Diuretics. *Risk C: Monitor therapy*

Stability Do not store near heat or open flame. Do not puncture canisters. Store at room temperature. Rest QVAR® on concave end of canister with actuator on top.

Mechanism of Action Controls the rate of protein synthesis; depresses the migration of polymorphonuclear leukocytes, fibroblasts; reverses capillary permeability and lysosomal stabilization at the cellular level to prevent or control inflammation

Pharmacodynamics/Kinetics

Onset of action: Therapeutic effect: 1-4 weeks

Absorption: Readily; quickly hydrolyzed by pulmonary esterases prior to absorption

Distribution: Beclomethasone: 20 L; active metabolite: 424 L

Protein binding: 87%

Metabolism: Hepatic via CYP3A4 to active metabolites

Bioavailability: Of active metabolite, 44% following nasal inhalation (43% from swallowed portion)

Half-life elimination: Initial: 3 hours

Excretion: Feces (60%); urine (12%)

Dosage Nasal inhalation and oral inhalation dosage forms are not to be used interchangeably

Inhalation, nasal: Rhinitis, nasal polyps (Beconase® AQ): Children ≥6 years and Adults: 1-2 inhalations each nostril twice daily; total dose 168-336 mcg/day

Inhalation, oral: Asthma (doses should be titrated to the lowest effective dose once asthma is controlled) (QVAR®):

- Children 5-11 years: Initial: 40 mcg twice daily; maximum dose: 80 mcg twice daily
- Children ≥12 years and Adults:
  - Patients previously on bronchodilators only: Initial dose 40-80 mcg twice daily; maximum dose: 320 mcg twice day
  - Patients previously on inhaled corticosteroids: Initial dose 40-160 mcg twice daily; maximum dose: 320 mcg twice daily

NIH Asthma Guidelines (NIH, 2007): HFA formulation (eg, QVAR®): Administer in divided doses:

Children 5-11 years:

"Low" dose: 80-160 mcg/day

"Medium" dose: >160-320 mcg/day

"High" dose: >320 mcg/day

Children ≥12 years and Adults:

"Low" dose: 80-240 mcg/day

"Medium" dose: >240-480 mcg/day

"High" dose: >480 mcg/day

Administration

Beconase AQ®: Shake well before use. Nasal applicator and dust cap may be washed in warm water and dry thoroughly.

QVAR®: Rinse mouth and throat after use to prevent *Candida* infection. Do not wash or put inhaler in water; mouth piece may be cleaned with a dry tissue or cloth. Prime canister before using.

Additional Information Effects of inhaled/intranasal steroids on growth have been observed in the absence of laboratory evidence of HPA axis suppression, suggesting that growth velocity is a more sensitive indicator of systemic corticosteroid exposure in pediatric patients than some commonly used tests of HPA axis function. The long-term effects of this reduction in growth velocity associated with orally-inhaled and intranasal corticosteroids, including the impact on final adult height, are unknown. The potential for "catch up" growth following discontinuation of treatment with inhaled corticosteroids has not been adequately studied.

Dosage Forms Excipient information presented when available (limited, particularly for generics); consult specific product labeling.

Aerosol for oral inhalation, as dipropionate:

QVAR®: 40 mcg/inhalation [100 metered actuations] (7.3 g); 80 mcg/inhalation [100 metered actuations] (7.3 g)

Suspension, intranasal, as dipropionate [aqueous spray]:

Beconase® AQ: 42 mcg/inhalation [180 metered sprays (25 g)

◆ **Beclomethasone Dipropionate** *see* Beclomethasone *on page 171*

◆ **Beconase® AQ** *see* Beclomethasone *on page 171*

◆ **BeFlex** *see* Acetaminophen and Phenyltoloxamine *on page 36*

◆ **Belladonna Alkaloids With Phenobarbital** *see* Hyoscyamine, Atropine, Scopolamine, and Phenobarbital *on page 800*

Belladonna and Opium (bel a DON a & OH pee um)

U.S. Brand Names B&O Supprettes® [DSC]

Index Terms Opium and Belladonna

Pharmacologic Category Analgesic Combination (Opioid); Antispasmodic Agent, Urinary

Use Relief of moderate-to-severe pain associated with ureteral spasms not responsive to nonopioid analgesics and to space intervals between injections of opiates

Effect on Mental Status None reported

Effect on Psychiatric Treatment Constipation and dry mouth are common; use with low potency antipsychotics and TCAs will likely result in additive effects

Restrictions C-II

Dosage Summary

Rectal:

Children >12 years: 1 suppository 1-2 times/day (maximum: 4 doses/day)

Adults: 1 suppository 1-2 times/day (maximum: 4 doses/day)

Dosage Forms Excipient information presented when available (limited, particularly for generics); consult specific product labeling. [DSC] = Discontinued product

Suppository: Belladonna extract 16.2 mg and opium 30 mg; belladonna extract 16.2 mg and opium 60 mg

B&O Supprettes® #15 A: Belladonna extract 16.2 mg and opium 30 mg [DSC]

B&O Supprettes® #16 A: Belladonna extract 16.2 mg and opium 60 mg [DSC]

Belladonna, Phenobarbital, and Ergotamine

(bel a DON a, fee noe BAR bi tal, & er GOT a meen)

U.S. Brand Names Bellamine S [DSC]; Eperbel-S [DSC]; Spastrin® [DSC]

Canadian Brand Names Bellergal® Spacetabs®

Index Terms Ergotamine Tartrate, Belladonna, and Phenobarbital; Phenobarbital, Belladonna, and Ergotamine Tartrate

Pharmacologic Category Ergot Derivative

Generic Available Yes

Use Management and treatment of menopausal disorders, GI disorders, and recurrent throbbing headache

Effect on Mental Status Drowsiness and dizziness are common

Effect on Psychiatric Treatment Combined use with TCAs and antipsychotics may potentiate the depressant actions

Pregnancy Risk Factor X

Pregnancy Considerations Potential uterotonic effects

Lactation Enters breast milk (ergotamine)/contraindicated

Contraindications Hypersensitivity to belladonna alkaloids, phenobarbital, ergotamine, or any component of the formulation; dopamine therapy; ergot alkaloids are contraindicated with potent inhibitors of CYP3A4 (includes protease inhibitors, azole antifungals, and some macrolide antibiotics); hypertension; glaucoma; coronary heart disease and peripheral vascular disease; impaired hepatic or renal function; sepsis; history of manifest or latent porphyria; pregnancy

Warnings/Precautions Ergot alkaloids have been associated with fibrotic valve thickening (eg, aortic, mitral, tricuspid); usually associated with long-term, chronic use; vasospasm or vasoconstriction can occur; ergot alkaloid use may result in ergotism (intense vasoconstriction) resulting in peripheral vascular ischemia and possible gangrene; rare cases of pleural and/or retroperitoneal fibrosis have been reported with prolonged daily use. Discontinuation after extended use may result in withdrawal symptoms (eg, rebound headache). Use with caution in patients with bronchial asthma or obstructive uropathy. Use with caution in the elderly. Safety and efficacy have not been established in children. Total weekly dosage of ergotamine should not exceed 10 mg. May be habit-forming. **[U.S. Boxed Warning]: Ergot alkaloids are contraindicated with potent inhibitors of CYP3A4 (includes protease inhibitors, azole antifungals, and some macrolide antibiotics); concomitant use associated with acute ergot toxicity (ergotism).**

Adverse Reactions

>10%:

- Cardiovascular: Peripheral vascular effects (numbness and tingling of fingers and toes)
- Central nervous system: Drowsiness, dizziness
- Dermatologic: Dry skin
- Gastrointestinal: Constipation, dry mouth and throat, diarrhea, nausea, vomiting
- Respiratory: Dry nose
- Miscellaneous: Diaphoresis decreased

1% to 10%:

- Cardiovascular: Precordial distress and pain, transient tachycardia or bradycardia
- Dermatologic: Photosensitivity
- Endocrine & metabolic: Breast milk flow decreased
- Gastrointestinal: Swallowing difficulty
- Neuromuscular & skeletal: Muscle pain in extremities, weakness in legs

<1% (Limited to important or life-threatening): Drowsiness, intraocular pain increased, memory loss, orthostatic hypotension, skin rash, tachycardia, ventricular fibrillation

Metabolism/Transport Effects

Phenobarbital: **Substrate** of CYP2C8/9 (minor), 2C19 (major), 2E1 (minor); **Induces** CYP1A2 (strong), 2A6 (strong), 2B6 (strong), 2C8/9 (strong), 3A4 (strong)

Ergotamine: **Substrate** of CYP3A4 (major); Inhibits 3A4 (weak)

Drug Interactions

Acetaminophen: Barbiturates may increase the metabolism of Acetaminophen. This may 1) diminish the effect of acetaminophen; and 2) increase the risk of liver damage. *Risk C: Monitor therapy*

Acetylcholinesterase Inhibitors (Central): Anticholinergics may diminish the therapeutic effect of Acetylcholinesterase Inhibitors (Central). Acetylcholinesterase Inhibitors (Central) may diminish the therapeutic effect of

Anticholinergics. If the anticholinergic action is a side effect of the agent, the result may be beneficial. *Risk C: Monitor therapy*

Alcohol (Ethyl): CNS Depressants may enhance the CNS depressant effect of Alcohol (Ethyl). *Risk C: Monitor therapy*

Aminocamptothecin: PHENobarbital may decrease the serum concentration of Aminocamptothecin. *Risk C: Monitor therapy*

Amphetamines: May decrease the serum concentration of PHENobarbital. *Risk C: Monitor therapy*

Anticholinergics: May enhance the adverse/toxic effect of other Anticholinergics. **Exceptions:** Paliperidone. *Risk C: Monitor therapy*

Bendamustine: CYP1A2 Inducers (Strong) may decrease the serum concentration of Bendamustine. Concentrations of active metabolites may be increased. *Risk C: Monitor therapy*

Beta-Blockers: Barbiturates may decrease the serum concentration of Beta-Blockers. **Exceptions:** Atenolol; Levobunolol; Metipranolol; Nadolol. *Risk C: Monitor therapy*

Calcium Channel Blockers: Barbiturates may increase the metabolism of Calcium Channel Blockers. **Exceptions:** Clevidipine. *Risk D: Consider therapy modification*

Cannabinoids: Anticholinergic Agents may enhance the tachycardic effect of Cannabinoids. *Risk C: Monitor therapy*

Carbonic Anhydrase Inhibitors: May enhance the adverse/toxic effect of Anticonvulsants (Barbiturate). Specifically, osteomalacia and rickets. **Exceptions:** Brinzolamide; Dorzolamide. *Risk C: Monitor therapy*

Chloramphenicol: May decrease the metabolism of Barbiturates. Barbiturates may increase the metabolism of Chloramphenicol. *Risk D: Consider therapy modification*

CNS Depressants: May enhance the adverse/toxic effect of other CNS Depressants. *Risk C: Monitor therapy*

Contraceptive (Progestins): Barbiturates may diminish the therapeutic effect of Contraceptive (Progestins). Contraceptive failure is possible. *Risk D: Consider therapy modification*

Corticosteroids (Systemic): Barbiturates may increase the metabolism of Corticosteroids (Systemic). *Risk C: Monitor therapy*

CycloSPORINE: Barbiturates may increase the metabolism of CycloSPORINE. *Risk D: Consider therapy modification*

CYP1A2 Substrates: CYP1A2 Inducers (Strong) may increase the metabolism of CYP1A2 Substrates. *Risk C: Monitor therapy*

CYP2A6 Substrates: CYP2A6 Inducers (Strong) may increase the metabolism of CYP2A6 Substrates. *Risk C: Monitor therapy*

CYP2B6 Substrates: CYP2B6 Inducers (Strong) may increase the metabolism of CYP2B6 Substrates. *Risk C: Monitor therapy*

CYP2C19 Inducers (Strong): May increase the metabolism of CYP2C19 Substrates. *Risk C: Monitor therapy*

CYP2C19 Inhibitors (Moderate): May decrease the metabolism of CYP2C19 Substrates. *Risk C: Monitor therapy*

CYP2C19 Inhibitors (Strong): May decrease the metabolism of CYP2C19 Substrates. *Risk D: Consider therapy modification*

CYP2C8 Substrates (High risk): CYP2C8 Inducers (Highly Effective) may increase the metabolism of CYP2C8 Substrates (High risk). *Risk C: Monitor therapy*

CYP2C9 Substrates (High risk): CYP2C9 Inducers (Highly Effective) may increase the metabolism of CYP2C9 Substrates (High risk). *Risk C: Monitor therapy*

CYP3A4 Inhibitors (Moderate): May decrease the metabolism of CYP3A4 Substrates. *Risk C: Monitor therapy*

CYP3A4 Inhibitors (Strong): May decrease the metabolism of CYP3A4 Substrates. *Risk D: Consider therapy modification*

CYP3A4 Substrates: CYP3A4 Inducers (Strong) may increase the metabolism of CYP3A4 Substrates. *Risk C: Monitor therapy*

Darunavir: PHENobarbital may decrease the serum concentration of Darunavir. *Risk X: Avoid combination*

Dasatinib: May increase the serum concentration of CYP3A4 Substrates. *Risk C: Monitor therapy*

Disopyramide: Barbiturates may increase the metabolism of Disopyramide. *Risk D: Consider therapy modification*

Doxycycline: Barbiturates may decrease the serum concentration of Doxycycline. *Risk D: Consider therapy modification*

Efavirenz: May enhance the adverse/toxic effect of Ergot Derivatives Specifically, the risk for peripheral vasospasm and ischemia may be increased. *Risk X: Avoid combination*

Etoposide: Barbiturates may increase the metabolism of Etoposide. *Risk C: Monitor therapy*

Etoposide Phosphate: Barbiturates may decrease the serum concentration of Etoposide Phosphate. Barbiturates may increase the metabolism, via CYP isoenzymes, of etoposide phosphate. *Risk C: Monitor therapy*

Etravirine: PHENobarbital may decrease the serum concentration of Etravirine. Management: The manufacturer of etravirine states these drugs should not be used in combination *Risk X: Avoid combination*

Felbamate: May increase the serum concentration of Barbiturates. *Risk C: Monitor therapy*

Folic Acid: May decrease the serum concentration of PHENobarbital. *Risk C: Monitor therapy*

Griseofulvin: Barbiturates may decrease the absorption of Griseofulvin. *Risk D: Consider therapy modification*

Ketorolac: May diminish the therapeutic effect of Anticonvulsants. *Risk C: Monitor therapy*

Lacosamide: PHENobarbital may decrease the serum concentration of Lacosamide. *Risk C: Monitor therapy*

LamoTRIgine: Barbiturates may increase the metabolism of LamoTRIgine. *Risk D: Consider therapy modification*

Leucovorin-Levoleucovorin: May decrease the serum concentration of PHENobarbital. *Risk C: Monitor therapy*

Macrolide Antibiotics: May enhance the adverse/toxic effect of Ergot Derivatives. Specifically leading the development of ergotism. **Exceptions:** Azithromycin; Dirithromycin [Off Market]; Spiramycin. *Risk D: Consider therapy modification*

Maraviroc: CYP3A4 Inducers may decrease the serum concentration of Maraviroc. *Risk D: Consider therapy modification*

Mefloquine: May diminish the therapeutic effect of Anticonvulsants. Mefloquine may decrease the serum concentration of Anticonvulsants. Management: Mefloquine is contraindicated in persons with a history of convulsions. If anticonvulsant is being used for another indication monitor response to treatment closely, as concurrent mefloquine may decrease response to treatment. *Risk D: Consider therapy modification*

Meperidine: Barbiturates may enhance the CNS depressant effect of Meperidine. *Risk C: Monitor therapy*

Methadone: Barbiturates may increase the metabolism of Methadone. *Risk D: Consider therapy modification*

Methylfolate: May decrease the serum concentration of PHENobarbital. *Risk C: Monitor therapy*

Nilotinib: CYP3A4 Inducers (Strong) may decrease the serum concentration of Nilotinib. *Risk X: Avoid combination*

Oral Contraceptive (Estrogens): Barbiturates may diminish the therapeutic effect of Oral Contraceptive (Estrogens). Contraceptive failure is possible. *Risk D: Consider therapy modification*

OXcarbazepine: PHENobarbital may decrease the serum concentration of OXcarbazepine. *Risk C: Monitor therapy*

Posaconazole: May increase the serum concentration of Ergot Derivatives. *Risk X: Avoid combination*

Potassium Chloride: Anticholinergic Agents may enhance the ulcerogenic effect of Potassium Chloride. *Risk D: Consider therapy modification*

Pramlintide: May enhance the anticholinergic effect of Anticholinergics. These effects are specific to the GI tract. *Risk D: Consider therapy modification*

Primidone: May enhance the adverse/toxic effect of Barbiturates. Primidone is converted to phenobarbital, and thus becomes additive with existing barbiturate therapy. *Risk C: Monitor therapy*

Propafenone: Barbiturates may increase the metabolism of Propafenone. *Risk D: Consider therapy modification*

Protease Inhibitors: May decrease the metabolism of Ergot Derivatives. *Risk X: Avoid combination*

Pyridoxine: May increase the metabolism of Barbiturates. Apparent in high pyridoxine doses (eg, 200 mg/day) *Risk C: Monitor therapy*

QuiNIDine: Barbiturates may increase the metabolism of QuiNIDine. *Risk D: Consider therapy modification*

Ranolazine: CYP3A4 Inducers (Strong) may decrease the serum concentration of Ranolazine. *Risk X: Avoid combination*

Rifamycin Derivatives: May increase the metabolism of Barbiturates. *Risk C: Monitor therapy*

Secretin: Anticholinergic Agents may diminish the stimulatory effect of Secretin. *Risk D: Consider therapy modification*

Serotonin 5-HT1D Receptor Agonists: Ergot Derivatives may enhance the vasoconstricting effect of Serotonin 5-HT1D Receptor Agonists. Serotonin

5-HT1D Receptor Agonists may enhance the vasoconstricting effect of Ergot Derivatives. *Risk X: Avoid combination*

Serotonin Modulators: May enhance the adverse/toxic effect of other Serotonin Modulators. The development of serotonin syndrome may occur. *Risk D: Consider therapy modification*

Sibutramine: May enhance the serotonergic effect of Ergot Derivatives. This may cause serotonin syndrome. *Risk X: Avoid combination*

Sorafenib: CYP3A4 Inducers (Strong) may decrease the serum concentration of Sorafenib. *Risk D: Consider therapy modification*

Teniposide: Barbiturates may increase the metabolism of Teniposide. *Risk C: Monitor therapy*

Theophylline Derivatives: Barbiturates may increase the metabolism of Theophylline Derivatives. **Exceptions:** Dyphylline. *Risk C: Monitor therapy*

Tipranavir: PHENobarbital may decrease the serum concentration of Tipranavir. Tipranavir may decrease the serum concentration of PHENobarbital. *Risk D: Consider therapy modification*

Tricyclic Antidepressants: Barbiturates may increase the metabolism of Tricyclic Antidepressants. *Risk D: Consider therapy modification*

Valproic Acid: May decrease the metabolism of Barbiturates. Barbiturates may decrease the serum concentration of Valproic Acid. *Risk C: Monitor therapy*

Vitamin K Antagonists (eg, warfarin): Barbiturates may increase the metabolism of Vitamin K Antagonists. *Risk D: Consider therapy modification*

Voriconazole: May increase the serum concentration of Ergot Derivatives. *Risk X: Avoid combination*

Voriconazole: Barbiturates may decrease the serum concentration of Voriconazole. *Risk X: Avoid combination*

Pharmacodynamics/Kinetics See individual agents.

Dosage Oral: Adults: 1 tablet each morning and evening

Dosage Forms Excipient information presented when available (limited, particularly for generics); consult specific product labeling. [DSC] = Discontinued product

Tablet:

Bellamie S [DSC], Eperbel-S [DSC], Spastrin® [DSC]: Belladonna alkaloids 0.2 mg, phenobarbital 40 mg, and ergotamine 0.6 mg

- **Bellamine S [DSC]** *see* Belladonna, Phenobarbital, and Ergotamine *on page 175*
- **Benadryl-D™ Allergy and Sinus Fastmelt™ [OTC]** *see* Diphenhydramine and Pseudoephedrine *on page 486*
- **Benadryl-D™ Children's Allergy and Sinus [OTC]** *see* Diphenhydramine and Pseudoephedrine *on page 486*
- **Benadryl® Allergy [OTC]** *see* DiphenhydrAMINE *on page 481*
- **Benadryl® Allergy and Cold [OTC]** *see* Acetaminophen, Diphenhydramine, and Phenylephrine *on page 44*
- **Benadryl® Allergy and Sinus Headache [OTC]** *see* Acetaminophen, Diphenhydramine, and Phenylephrine *on page 44*
- **Benadryl® Children's Allergy [OTC]** *see* DiphenhydrAMINE *on page 481*
- **Benadryl® Children's Allergy and Cold Fastmelt™ [OTC]** *see* Diphenhydramine and Pseudoephedrine *on page 486*
- **Benadryl® Children's Allergy Fastmelt® [OTC]** *see* DiphenhydrAMINE *on page 481*
- **Benadryl® Children's Dye-Free Allergy [OTC]** *see* DiphenhydrAMINE *on page 481*
- **Benadryl® Itch Stopping [OTC]** *see* DiphenhydrAMINE *on page 481*
- **Benadryl® Itch Stopping Extra Strength [OTC]** *see* DiphenhydrAMINE *on page 481*

Benazepril (ben AY ze pril)

Medication Safety Issues

Sound-alike/look-alike issues:

Benazepril may be confused with Benadryl®

Lotensin® may be confused with Lioresal®, lovastatin

International issues:

Lotensin® may be confused with Latensin® which is a brand name for bacillus cereus in Germany

Related Information

Angiotensin Agents *on page 1754*

U.S. Brand Names Lotensin®
Canadian Brand Names Apo-Benazepril®; Lotensin®
Mexican Brand Names Lotensin
Index Terms Benazepril Hydrochloride
Pharmacologic Category Angiotensin-Converting Enzyme (ACE) Inhibitor
Use Treatment of hypertension, either alone or in combination with other antihypertensive agents
Effect on Mental Status May cause drowsiness
Effect on Psychiatric Treatment May decrease lithium clearance resulting in an increase in serum lithium levels and potential lithium toxicity; monitor serum lithium levels
Dosage Summary
Oral:
Children <6 years: Dosage not established
Children ≥6 years: Initial: 0.2 mg/kg/day (up to 10 mg/day); Maintenance: 0.1-0.6 mg/kg/day (maximum: 40 mg/day)
Adults: Initial: 5-10 mg/day; Maintenance: 20-80 mg/day in 1-2 divided doses
Dosage Forms Excipient information presented when available (limited, particularly for generics); consult specific product labeling.
Tablet, as hydrochloride: 5 mg, 10 mg, 20 mg, 40 mg
Lotensin®: 5 mg, 10 mg, 20 mg, 40 mg

Benazepril and Hydrochlorothiazide

(ben AY ze pril & hye droe klor oh THYE a zide)

U.S. Brand Names Lotensin® HCT
Index Terms Hydrochlorothiazide and Benazepril
Pharmacologic Category Angiotensin-Converting Enzyme (ACE) Inhibitor; Diuretic, Thiazide
Use Treatment of hypertension
Effect on Mental Status May cause drowsiness
Effect on Psychiatric Treatment May decrease lithium clearance resulting in an increase in serum lithium levels and potential lithium toxicity; monitor serum lithium levels
Dosage Summary
Oral:
Children: Dosage not established
Adults: Benazepril 5-20 mg and hydrochlorothiazide 6.25-25 mg daily
Dosage Forms Excipient information presented when available (limited, particularly for generics); consult specific product labeling.
Tablet: 5/6.25: Benazepril hydrochloride 5 mg and hydrochlorothiazide 6.25 mg; 10/12.5: Benazepril hydrochloride 10 mg and hydrochlorothiazide 12.5 mg; 20/12.5: Benazepril hydrochloride 20 mg and hydrochlorothiazide 12.5 mg; 20/25: Benazepril hydrochloride 20 mg and hydrochlorothiazide 25 mg
Lotensin® HCT 5/6.25: Benazepril hydrochloride 5 mg and hydrochlorothiazide 6.25 mg
Lotensin® HCT 10/12.5: Benazepril hydrochloride 10 mg and hydrochlorothiazide 12.5 mg
Lotensin® HCT 20/12.5: Benazepril hydrochloride 20 mg and hydrochlorothiazide 12.5 mg
Lotensin® HCT 20/25: Benazepril hydrochloride 20 mg and hydrochlorothiazide 25 mg

◆ **Benazepril Hydrochloride** *see* Benazepril *on page 178*
◆ **Benazepril Hydrochloride and Amlodipine Besylate** *see* Amlodipine and Benazepril *on page 104*

Bendamustine (ben da MUS teen)

Medication Safety Issues
Sound-alike/look-alike issues:
Bendamustine may be confused with carmustine

High alert medication: The Institute for Safe Medication Practices (ISMP) includes this medication among its list of drug classes which have a heightened risk of causing significant patient harm when used in error.
U.S. Brand Names Treanda®
Index Terms Bendamustine Hydrochloride; Cytostasan; SDX-105
Pharmacologic Category Antineoplastic Agent, Alkylating Agent

Use Treatment of chronic lymphocytic leukemia (CLL); treatment of progressed indolent B-cell non-Hodgkin's lymphoma (NHL)

Unlabeled/Investigational Use Treatment of mantle cell lymphoma; salvage therapy for relapsed multiple myeloma

Effect on Mental Status May cause fatigue

Effect on Psychiatric Treatment Bone marrow suppression is common; use caution with clozapine, carbamazepine, and valproic acid. GI side effects are common; concomitant use with lithium, valproic acid, carbamazepine, and SSRIs may produce additive effects. Carbamazepine and phenobarbital may decease the levels/effects of bendamustine. Fluvoxamine may increase the levels/effects of bendamustine.

Dosage Summary

I.V.:

Children: Dosage not established

Adults: 100 mg/m^2 on days 1 and 2 of a 28-day treatment cycle for up to 6 cycles **or** 120 mg/m^2 on days 1 and 2 of a 21-day treatment cycle for up to 8 cycles

Dosage Forms Excipient information presented when available (limited, particularly for generics); consult specific product labeling.

Injection, powder for reconstitution:

Treanda®: 100 mg [contains mannitol 170 mg]

- **Bendamustine Hydrochloride** *see* Bendamustine *on page 179*
- **Bendroflumethiazide and Nadolol** *see* Nadolol and Bendroflumethiazide *on page 1092*
- **BeneFix®** *see* Factor IX *on page 612*
- **Benemid [DSC]** *see* Probenecid *on page 1338*
- **Benicar®** *see* Olmesartan *on page 1170*
- **Benicar HCT®** *see* Olmesartan and Hydrochlorothiazide *on page 1172*
- **Ben-Tann** *see* DiphenhydrAMINE *on page 481*
- **Bentyl®** *see* Dicyclomine *on page 459*
- **Benzathine Benzylpenicillin** *see* Penicillin G Benzathine *on page 1239*
- **Benzathine Penicillin G** *see* Penicillin G Benzathine *on page 1239*
- **Benzazoline Hydrochloride** *see* Tolazoline *on page 1592*
- **Benzene Hexachloride** *see* Lindane *on page 927*
- **Benzhexol Hydrochloride** *see* Trihexyphenidyl *on page 1627*
- **Benzisoquinolinedione** *see* Amonafide *on page 108*
- **Benzmethyzin** *see* Procarbazine *on page 1340*
- **Benzoic Acid, Methenamine, Methylene Blue, Phenyl Salicylate, and Hyoscyamine** *see* Methenamine, Phenyl Salicylate, Methylene Blue, Benzoic Acid, and Hyoscyamine *on page 1009*

Benzonatate (ben ZOE na tate)

U.S. Brand Names Tessalon®

Canadian Brand Names Tessalon®

Mexican Brand Names Tusitato

Pharmacologic Category Antitussive

Use Symptomatic relief of nonproductive cough

Effect on Mental Status May cause drowsiness

Effect on Psychiatric Treatment May potentiate sedative effects of sedating psychotropics

Dosage Summary

Oral:

Children ≤10 years: Dosage not established

Children >10 years: 100 mg 3 times/day **or** every 4 hours (maximum: 600 mg/day)

Adults: 100 mg 3 times/day **or** every 4 hours (maximum: 600 mg/day)

Dosage Forms Excipient information presented when available (limited, particularly for generics); consult specific product labeling.

Capsule, softgel: 100 mg, 200 mg

Tessalon®: 100 mg, 200 mg

Benzphetamine (benz FET a meen)

Medication Safety Issues

International issues:

Didrex® may be confused with Nitrex® which is a brand name for isosorbide mononitrate in Italy

U.S. Brand Names Didrex®

Canadian Brand Names Didrex®

Index Terms Benzphetamine Hydrochloride

Pharmacologic Category Anorexiant; Sympathomimetic

Generic Available Yes

Use Short-term (few weeks) adjunct in exogenous obesity

Restrictions C-III

Pharmacotherapy for weight loss is recommended only for obese patients with a body mass index ≥30 kg/m^2, or ≥27 kg/m^2 in the presence of other risk factors such as hypertension, diabetes, and/or dyslipidemia or a high waist circumference; therapy should be used in conjunction with a comprehensive weight management program. Rule out organic causes of obesity (eg, untreated hypothyroidism) prior to use.

Note: Benzphetamine is not approved for long-term use. The limited usefulness of medications in this class should be weighed against possible risks associated with their use. Consult weight loss guidelines for current pharmacotherapy recommendations.

Pregnancy Risk Factor X

Pregnancy Considerations Reproduction studies have not been conducted with benzphetamine. Amphetamines are teratogenic and embryotoxic in animal studies.

Lactation Enters breast milk/not recommended

Contraindications Hypersensitivity or idiosyncrasy to benzphetamine or other sympathomimetic amines; advanced arteriosclerosis, symptomatic cardiovascular disease, moderate-to-severe hypertension; pulmonary hypertension; hyperthyroidism; glaucoma; agitated states, history of drug abuse; during or within 14 days following MAO inhibitor therapy, concurrent use with other CNS stimulants; pregnancy

Warnings/Precautions The use of some anorexigens has been associated with the development of valvular heart disease. Avoid stimulants in patients with known serious structural cardiac abnormalities, cardiomyopathy, serious heart rhythm abnormalities, or other serious cardiac problems that could increase the risk of sudden death that these conditions alone carry. Caution should be used in patients with hypertension and other cardiovascular conditions that might be exacerbated by increases in blood pressure or heart rate.

Primary pulmonary hypertension (PPH), a rare and frequently fatal disease of the lungs, has been found to occur with increased frequency in patients receiving some anorexigens.

Use caution with diabetes; antidiabetic agent requirements may be altered with anorexigens and concomitant dietary restrictions. Stimulants may unmask tics in individuals with coexisting Tourette's syndrome. Use caution with seizure disorders. Benzphetamine is pharmacologically related to the amphetamines, which have a high abuse potential; prolonged use may lead to dependency. Prescriptions should be written for the smallest quantity consistent with good patient care to minimize possibility of overdose. Amphetamines may impair the ability to engage in potentially hazardous activities.

Not recommended for use in patients who have used other anorectic agents within the past year. Discontinue if satisfactory weight loss has not occurred within the first 4 weeks of treatment, or if tolerance develops. Safety and efficacy have not been established for use with other weight loss medications including over-the-counter or herbal products. Not recommended for children <12 years of age.

Adverse Reactions Frequency not defined.

Cardiovascular: Cardiomyopathy (with chronic amphetamine use), hypertension, palpitation, tachycardia

Central nervous system: Depression (with withdrawal), dizziness, headache, insomnia, nervousness, psychosis, restlessness

Dermatologic: Urticaria

Endocrine & metabolic: Libido changes

Gastrointestinal: Diarrhea, nausea, unpleasant taste, xerostomia

Neuromuscular & skeletal: Tremor

Ocular: Mydriasis

Miscellaneous: Diaphoresis, tachyphylaxis

Metabolism/Transport Effects Substrate of CYP2B6 (minor), 3A4 (major)

Drug Interactions

Alkalinizing Agents: May decrease the excretion of Amphetamines. *Risk D: Consider therapy modification*

Ammonium Chloride: May decrease the serum concentration of Amphetamines. This effect is likely due to an enhanced excretion of amphetamines in the urine. *Risk C: Monitor therapy*

Analgesics (Opioid): Amphetamines may enhance the analgesic effect of Analgesics (Opioid). *Risk C: Monitor therapy*

Antacids: May decrease the excretion of Amphetamines. *Risk C: Monitor therapy*

Antihistamines: Amphetamines may diminish the sedative effect of Antihistamines. *Risk C: Monitor therapy*

Antipsychotics: May diminish the stimulatory effect of Amphetamines. *Risk C: Monitor therapy*

Cannabinoids: May enhance the tachycardic effect of Sympathomimetics. *Risk C: Monitor therapy*

Carbonic Anhydrase Inhibitors: May decrease the excretion of Amphetamines. **Exceptions:** Brinzolamide; Dorzolamide. *Risk C: Monitor therapy*

CYP3A4 Inducers (Strong): May increase the metabolism of CYP3A4 Substrates. *Risk C: Monitor therapy*

CYP3A4 Inhibitors (Moderate): May decrease the metabolism of CYP3A4 Substrates. *Risk C: Monitor therapy*

CYP3A4 Inhibitors (Strong): May decrease the metabolism of CYP3A4 Substrates. *Risk D: Consider therapy modification*

Dasatinib: May increase the serum concentration of CYP3A4 Substrates. *Risk C: Monitor therapy*

Deferasirox: May decrease the serum concentration of CYP3A4 Substrates. *Risk C: Monitor therapy*

Ethosuximide: Amphetamines may diminish the therapeutic effect of Ethosuximide. Amphetamines may decrease the serum concentration of Ethosuximide. *Risk C: Monitor therapy*

Gastrointestinal Acidifying Agents: May decrease the serum concentration of Amphetamines. *Risk C: Monitor therapy*

Lithium: May diminish the stimulatory effect of Amphetamines. *Risk C: Monitor therapy*

MAO Inhibitors: May enhance the hypertensive effect of Amphetamines. *Risk X: Avoid combination*

Methenamine: May decrease the serum concentration of Amphetamines. This effect is likely due to an enhanced excretion of amphetamines in the urine. *Risk C: Monitor therapy*

PHENobarbital: Amphetamines may decrease the serum concentration of PHENobarbital. *Risk C: Monitor therapy*

Phenytoin: Amphetamines may decrease the serum concentration of Phenytoin. *Risk C: Monitor therapy*

Sympathomimetics: May enhance the adverse/toxic effect of other Sympathomimetics. *Risk C: Monitor therapy*

Tricyclic Antidepressants: May enhance the stimulatory effect of Amphetamines. Tricyclic Antidepressants may also potentiate the cardiovascular effects of Amphetamines. *Risk C: Monitor therapy*

Ethanol/Nutrition/Herb Interactions Herb/Nutraceutical: St John's wort may decrease benzphetamine levels.

Stability Store at room temperature of 20°C to 25°C (68°F to 77°F).

Mechanism of Action Benzphetamine is a sympathomimetic amine with pharmacologic properties similar to the amphetamines. The mechanism of action in reducing appetite appears to be secondary to CNS effects, including stimulation of the hypothalamus to release norepinephrine.

Dosage Children ≥12 years and Adults: Oral: Dose should be individualized based on patient response: Initial: 25-50 mg once daily; titrate to 25-50 mg 1-3 times/day; once-daily dosing should be administered midmorning or midafternoon; maximum dose: 50 mg 3 times/day

Dietary Considerations Most effective when combined with a low calorie diet and behavior modification counseling.

Monitoring Parameters Weight, waist circumference, blood pressure

Reference Range

Adult classification of weight by BMI (kg/m^2):

- Underweight: <18.5
- Normal: 18.5-24.9
- Overweight: 25-29.9
- Obese, class I: 30-34.9

Obese, class II: 35-39.9
Extreme obesity (class III): ≥40
Waist circumference: In adults with a BMI of 25-34.9 kg/m^2, high-risk waist circumference is defined as:
Men >102 cm (>40 in)
Women >88 cm (>35 in)

Dosage Forms Excipient information presented when available (limited, particularly for generics); consult specific product labeling.
Tablet, as hydrochloride: 50 mg
Didrex®: 50 mg

◆ **Benzphetamine Hydrochloride** *see* Benzphetamine *on page 181*

Benztropine (BENZ troe peen)

Medication Safety Issues
Sound-alike/look-alike issues:
Benztropine may be confused with bromocriptine

Related Information
Anticholinergic Effects of Common Psychotropics *on page 1758*
Antiparkinsonian Agents *on page 1767*
Clozapine-Induced Side Effects *on page 1818*
Discontinuation of Psychotropic Drugs *on page 1839*

U.S. Brand Names Cogentin®

Canadian Brand Names Apo-Benztropine®

Index Terms Benztropine Mesylate

Pharmacologic Category Anti-Parkinson's Agent, Anticholinergic; Anticholinergic Agent

Generic Available Yes: Tablet

Use Adjunctive treatment of Parkinson's disease; treatment of drug-induced extrapyramidal symptoms (except tardive dyskinesia)

Mental Health Comment Along with diphenhydramine, benztropine is considered the drug of choice for patients with acute dystonic reactions. The usual adult dosage is I.M. 2 mg. In an emergency situation (laryngeal spasm), it should be given intravenously. Benztropine has a long duration of action and may be given once daily, preferable at bedtime due to possible sedation when used to treat pseudoparkinsonism and akathisia.

Pregnancy Risk Factor C

Lactation Excretion in breast milk unknown/use caution

Contraindications Hypersensitivity to benztropine or any component of the formulation; pyloric or duodenal obstruction, stenosing peptic ulcers; bladder neck obstructions; achalasia; myasthenia gravis; children <3 years of age

Warnings/Precautions Use with caution in older children (dose has not been established). Use with caution in hot weather or during exercise. May cause anhydrosis and hyperthermia, which may be severe. The risk is increased in hot environments, particularly in the elderly, alcoholics, patients with CNS disease, and those with prolonged outdoor exposure.

Elderly patients frequently develop increased sensitivity and require strict dosage regulation - side effects may be more severe in elderly patients with atherosclerotic changes. Use with caution in patients with tachycardia, cardiac arrhythmias, hypertension, hypotension, glaucoma, prostatic hyperplasia (especially in the elderly), any tendency toward urinary retention, liver or kidney disorders, and obstructive disease of the GI or GU tract. When given in large doses or to susceptible patients, may cause weakness and inability to move particular muscle groups.

May be associated with confusion or hallucinations (generally at higher dosages). Intensification of symptoms or toxic psychosis may occur in patients with mental disorders. May cause CNS depression, which may impair physical or mental abilities; patients must be cautioned about performing tasks which require mental alertness (eg, operating machinery or driving). Benztropine does not relieve symptoms of tardive dyskinesia.

Adverse Reactions Frequency not defined.
Cardiovascular: Tachycardia
Central nervous system: Confusion, disorientation, memory impairment, toxic psychosis, visual hallucinations
Dermatologic: Rash
Endocrine & metabolic: Heat stroke, hyperthermia
Gastrointestinal: Constipation, dry throat, ileus, nasal dryness, nausea, vomiting, xerostomia
Genitourinary: Urinary retention, dysuria

Ocular: Blurred vision, mydriasis

Miscellaneous: Fever

Metabolism/Transport Effects Substrate of CYP2D6 (minor)

Drug Interactions

Acetylcholinesterase Inhibitors (Central): Anticholinergics may diminish the therapeutic effect of Acetylcholinesterase Inhibitors (Central). Acetylcholinesterase Inhibitors (Central) may diminish the therapeutic effect of Anticholinergics. If the anticholinergic action is a side effect of the agent, the result may be beneficial. *Risk C: Monitor therapy*

Anticholinergics: May enhance the adverse/toxic effect of other Anticholinergics. **Exceptions:** Paliperidone. *Risk C: Monitor therapy*

Cannabinoids: Anticholinergic Agents may enhance the tachycardic effect of Cannabinoids. *Risk C: Monitor therapy*

Potassium Chloride: Anticholinergic Agents may enhance the ulcerogenic effect of Potassium Chloride. *Risk D: Consider therapy modification*

Pramlintide: May enhance the anticholinergic effect of Anticholinergics. These effects are specific to the GI tract. *Risk D: Consider therapy modification*

Secretin: Anticholinergic Agents may diminish the stimulatory effect of Secretin. *Risk D: Consider therapy modification*

Ethanol/Nutrition/Herb Interactions Ethanol: Avoid ethanol (may increase CNS depression).

Mechanism of Action Possesses both anticholinergic and antihistaminic effects. *In vitro* anticholinergic activity approximates that of atropine; *in vivo* it is only about half as active as atropine. Animal data suggest its antihistaminic activity and duration of action approach that of pyrilamine maleate. May also inhibit the reuptake and storage of dopamine, thereby prolonging the action of dopamine.

Pharmacodynamics/Kinetics

Onset of action: Oral: Within 1 hour; Parenteral: Within 15 minutes

Duration: 6-48 hours

Metabolism: Hepatic (N-oxidation, N-dealkylation, and ring hydroxylation)

Bioavailability: 29%

Dosage Use in children ≤3 years of age should be reserved for life-threatening emergencies

Drug-induced extrapyramidal symptom: Oral, I.M., I.V.:

Children >3 years: 0.02-0.05 mg/kg/dose 1-2 times/day

Adults: 1-4 mg/dose 1-2 times/day

Acute dystonia: Adults: I.M., I.V.: 1-2 mg

Parkinsonism: Oral:

Adults: 0.5-6 mg/day in 1-2 divided doses; if one dose is greater, administer at bedtime; titrate dose in 0.5 mg increments at 5- to 6-day intervals

Elderly: Initial: 0.5 mg once or twice daily; increase by 0.5 mg as needed at 5-6 days; maximum: 4 mg/day

Monitoring Parameters Symptoms of EPS or Parkinson's, pulse, anticholinergic effects

Additional Information No significant difference in onset of I.M. or I.V. injection; therefore, there is usually no need to use the I.V. route. Improvement is sometimes noticeable a few minutes after injection.

Dosage Forms Excipient information presented when available (limited, particularly for generics); consult specific product labeling.

Injection, solution, as mesylate (Cogentin®): 1 mg/mL (2 mL)

Tablet, as mesylate: 0.5 mg, 1 mg, 2 mg

◆ **Benztropine Mesylate** *see* Benztropine *on page 183*

◆ **Benzylpenicillin Benzathine** *see* Penicillin G Benzathine *on page 1239*

◆ **Benzylpenicillin Potassium** *see* Penicillin G, Parenteral, Aqueous *on page 1241*

◆ **Benzylpenicillin Sodium** *see* Penicillin G, Parenteral, Aqueous *on page 1241*

◆ **9-Beta-D-Ribofuranosyladenine** *see* Adenosine *on page 51*

◆ **Betagan®** *see* Levobunolol *on page 907*

◆ **Beta-HC®** *see* Hydrocortisone *on page 785*

Betamethasone (bay ta METH a sone)

Medication Safety Issues

Sound-alike/look-alike issues:

Luxiq® may be confused with Lasix®

International issues:

Beta-Val® may be confused with Betanol® which is a brand name for metipranolol in Monaco

Related Information

Corticosteroids *on page 1780*

U.S. Brand Names Beta-Val®; Celestone®; Celestone® Soluspan®; Diprolene®; Diprolene® AF; Luxiq®

Canadian Brand Names Betaderm; Betaject™; Betnesol®; Betnovate®; Celestone® Soluspan®; Diprolene® Glycol; Diprosone®; Ectosone; Prevex® B; Taro-Sone®; Topilene®; Topisone®; Valisone® Scalp Lotion

Mexican Brand Names Betnovate; Celestone; Cronolevel; Diprofast; Dipronova; Diprosone; Diprospan; Erispan

Index Terms Betamethasone Dipropionate; Betamethasone Dipropionate, Augmented; Betamethasone Sodium Phosphate; Betamethasone Valerate; Flubenisolone

Pharmacologic Category Corticosteroid, Systemic; Corticosteroid, Topical

Use Inflammatory dermatoses such as seborrheic or atopic dermatitis, neurodermatitis, anogenital pruritus, psoriasis, inflammatory phase of xerosis

Unlabeled/Investigational Use Accelerate fetal lung maturation in patients with preterm labor

Effect on Mental Status May cause dizziness, insomnia, or nervousness

Effect on Psychiatric Treatment Enzyme inducers (barbiturates) may decrease the effects of corticosteroids

Dosage Summary

I.M.:

Children ≤12 years: 0.0175-0.125 mg base/kg/day **or** 0.5-7.5 mg base/m^2/day divided every 6-12 hours

Children ≥13 years: 0.6-9 mg/day (generally, 1/3 to 1/2 of oral dose) divided every 12-24 hours

Adults: 0.6-9 mg/day (generally, 1/3 to 1/2 of oral dose) divided every 12-24 hours

Intrabursal, intra-articular, intradermal:

Children: Dosage not established

Adults: 0.25-2 mL

Intralesional:

Children: Dosage not established

Adults: Very large joints: 1-2 mL; Large joints: 1 mL; Medium joints: 0.5-1 mL; Small joints: 0.25-0.5 mL

Oral:

Children ≤12 years: 0.0175-0.25 mg/kg/day **or** 0.5-7.5 mg/m^2/day divided every 6-8 hours

Children ≥13 years: 0.6-7.2 mg/day in 2-4 divided doses

Adults: 0.6-7.2 mg/day in 2-4 divided doses

Topical:

Children ≤12 years: Dosage not established

Children ≥13 years: Apply once or twice daily (maximum: 45-50 g/week; 50 mL/week; 2 weeks total therapy)

Adults: Apply once or twice daily (maximum: 45-50 g/week; 50 mL/week; 2 weeks total therapy)

Dosage Forms Excipient information presented when available (limited, particularly for generics); consult specific product labeling.

Note: Potency expressed as betamethasone base.

Aerosol, topical, as valerate [foam]:

Luxiq®: 0.12% (50 g, 100 g, 150 g) [strength expressed as salt; contains ethanol 60.4%]

Cream, topical, as dipropionate: 0.05% (15 g, 45 g)

Cream, topical, as dipropionate augmented: 0.05% (15 g, 50 g)

Diprolene® AF: 0.05% (15 g, 50 g)

Cream, topical, as valerate (Beta-Val®): 0.1% (15 g, 45 g)

Beta-Val®: 0.1% (15 g, 45 g)

Gel, topical, as dipropionate augmented: 0.05% (15 g, 50 g)

Injection, suspension:

Celestone® Soluspan®: Betamethasone sodium phosphate 3 mg and betamethasone acetate 3 mg per 1 mL (5 mL) [6 mg/mL]

Lotion, topical, as dipropionate: 0.05% (60 mL)

Lotion, topical, as dipropionate augmented:

Diprolene®: 0.05% (30 mL, 60 mL)

Lotion, topical, as valerate: 0.1% (60 mL)

Beta-Val®: 0.1% (60 mL)

Ointment, topical, as dipropionate: 0.05% (15 g, 45 g)

Ointment, topical, as dipropionate augmented: 0.05% (15 g, 50 g)

Diprolene®: 0.05% (15 g, 50 g)
Ointment, topical, as valerate: 0.1% (15 g, 45 g)
Solution, as base:
Celestone®: 0.6 mg/5 mL (118 mL) [contains alcohol and sodium benzoate; cherry-orange flavor]

- **Betamethasone Dipropionate** *see* Betamethasone *on page 184*
- **Betamethasone Dipropionate, Augmented** *see* Betamethasone *on page 184*
- **Betamethasone Sodium Phosphate** *see* Betamethasone *on page 184*
- **Betamethasone Valerate** *see* Betamethasone *on page 184*
- **Betapace®** *see* Sotalol *on page 1502*
- **Betapace AF®** *see* Sotalol *on page 1502*
- **Beta Sal® [OTC]** *see* Salicylic Acid *on page 1454*
- **Betaseron®** *see* Interferon Beta-1b *on page 848*
- **Beta-Val®** *see* Betamethasone *on page 184*

Betaxolol (be TAKS oh lol)

Medication Safety Issues
Sound-alike/look-alike issues:
Betaxolol may be confused with bethanechol, labetalol
Betoptic® S may be confused with Betagan®, Timoptic®
Related Information
Beta-Blockers *on page 1776*
U.S. Brand Names Betoptic® S; Kerlone®
Canadian Brand Names Betoptic® S; Sandoz-Betaxolol
Mexican Brand Names Betoptic S
Index Terms Betaxolol Hydrochloride
Pharmacologic Category Beta Blocker, $Beta_1$ Selective; Ophthalmic Agent, Antiglaucoma
Use
Ophthalmic: Treatment of chronic open-angle glaucoma or ocular hypertension
Oral: Management of hypertension
Effect on Mental Status May cause drowsiness; rare reports of depression and hallucinations
Effect on Psychiatric Treatment Has been used to treat akathisia; propranolol preferred
Dosage Summary
Ophthalmic:
Children:
Solution: Dosage not established
Suspension: Instill 1 drop twice daily
Adults:
Solution: Instill 1-2 drops twice daily
Suspension: Instill 1 drop twice daily
Oral:
Children: Dosage not established
Adults: 5-20 mg/day
Elderly: Initial dose: 5 mg/day; Range: 5-20 mg/day
Dosage Forms Excipient information presented when available (limited, particularly for generics); consult specific product labeling. [DSC] = Discontinued product
Solution, ophthalmic: 0.5% (5 mL, 10 mL, 15 mL) [contains benzalkonium chloride]
Suspension, ophthalmic:
Betoptic® S: 0.25% (5 mL [DSC], 10 mL, 15 mL) [contains benzalkonium chloride]
Tablet, as hydrochloride: 10 mg, 20 mg
Kerlone®: 10 mg, 20 mg

- **Betaxolol Hydrochloride** *see* Betaxolol *on page 186*

Bethanechol (be THAN e kole)

Medication Safety Issues
Sound-alike/look-alike issues:
Bethanechol may be confused with betaxolol
U.S. Brand Names Urecholine®
Canadian Brand Names Duvoid®; PMS-Bethanechol

Index Terms Bethanechol Chloride
Pharmacologic Category Cholinergic Agonist
Use Treatment of acute postoperative and postpartum nonobstructive (functional) urinary retention; treatment of neurogenic atony of the urinary bladder with retention
Unlabeled/Investigational Use Gastroesophageal reflux
Effect on Mental Status None reported
Effect on Psychiatric Treatment Contraindicated in Parkinson's disease
Dosage Summary
Oral:
Children (unlabeled use): 0.3-0.6 mg/kg/day in 3-4 divided doses
Adults: 10-100 mg 2-4 times/day; **Note:** Titration is recommended
Dosage Forms Excipient information presented when available (limited, particularly for generics); consult specific product labeling. [CAN] = Canadian brand name
Tablet, as chloride: 5 mg, 10 mg, 25 mg, 50 mg
Duvoid® [CAN]: 10 mg, 25 mg, 50 mg [not available in U.S.]
Urecholine®: 5 mg, 10 mg, 25 mg, 50 mg

- **Bethanechol Chloride** *see* Bethanechol *on page 186*
- **Betimol®** *see* Timolol *on page 1584*
- **Betoptic® S** *see* Betaxolol *on page 186*

Bevacizumab (be vuh SIZ uh mab)

Medication Safety Issues
Sound-alike/look-alike issues:
Bevacizumab may be confused with cetuximab

High alert medication: The Institute for Safe Medication Practices (ISMP) includes this medication among its list of drug classes which have a heightened risk of causing significant patient harm when used in error.
U.S. Brand Names Avastin®
Canadian Brand Names Avastin®
Mexican Brand Names Avastin
Index Terms Anti-VEGF Monoclonal Antibody; NSC-704865; rhuMAb-VEGF
Pharmacologic Category Antineoplastic Agent, Monoclonal Antibody; Vascular Endothelial Growth Factor (VEGF) Inhibitor
Use Treatment of metastatic colorectal cancer; treatment of nonsquamous, nonsmall cell lung cancer; treatment of breast cancer (metastatic, HER-2 negative)
Unlabeled/Investigational Use Treatment of ovarian cancer (early stage), renal cell cancer, age-related macular degeneration (AMD)
Effect on Mental Status Dizziness is common; may cause confusion
Effect on Psychiatric Treatment Gastrointestinal side effects are common; these effects may be additive with concurrent use of SSRIs, acetylcholinesterase inhibitors, aripiprazole, or ziprasidone. Hematologic adverse effects are common; use caution with clozapine, carbamazepine, valproate, mirtazapine. May cause hypokalemia; use caution with ziprasidone.
Dosage Summary
I.V.:
Children: Dosage not established
Adults: 5 or 10 mg/kg every 2 weeks **or** 15 mg/kg every 3 weeks
Dosage Forms Excipient information presented when available (limited, particularly for generics); consult specific product labeling.
Injection, solution [preservative free]:
Avastin®: 25 mg/mL (4 mL, 16 mL)

Bexarotene (beks AIR oh teen)

Medication Safety Issues
High alert medication: The Institute for Safe Medication Practices (ISMP) includes this medication among its list of drugs which have a heightened risk of causing significant patient harm when used in error.
U.S. Brand Names Targretin®
Canadian Brand Names Targretin®
Pharmacologic Category Antineoplastic Agent, Miscellaneous
Use
Oral: Treatment of cutaneous manifestations of cutaneous T-cell lymphoma in patients who are refractory to at least one prior systemic therapy

Topical: Treatment of cutaneous lesions in patients with refractory cutaneous T-cell lymphoma (stage 1A and 1B) or who have not tolerated other therapies

Effect on Mental Status May cause insomnia, agitation, confusion, and depression

Effect on Psychiatric Treatment Leukopenia is common; use caution with clozapine and carbamazepine; effects of psychotropics may be altered secondary to the insomnia, confusion, agitation, and depression seen with bexarotene

Dosage Summary

Oral:

Children: Dosage not established

Adults: 300-400 mg/m^2 once daily

Topical:

Children: Dosage not established

Adults: Apply once every other day for first week, then increase on a weekly basis to once daily, 2 times/day, 3 times/day, and finally 4 times/day, according to tolerance

Dosage Forms Excipient information presented when available (limited, particularly for generics); consult specific product labeling.

Capsule:

Targretin®: 75 mg

Gel: 1% (60 g)

Targretin®: 1% (60 g) [contains dehydrated alcohol]

◆ **Bexxar®** *see* Tositumomab and Iodine I 131 Tositumomab *on page 1603*
◆ **BG 9273** *see* Alefacept *on page 58*
◆ **Biaxin®** *see* Clarithromycin *on page 360*
◆ **Biaxin® XL** *see* Clarithromycin *on page 360*

Bicalutamide (bye ka LOO ta mide)

U.S. Brand Names Casodex®

Canadian Brand Names Casodex®; CO Bicalutamide; Gen-Bicalutamide; Novo-Bicalutamide; PHL-Bicalutamide; PMS-Bicalutamide; ratio-Bicalutamide; Sandoz-Bicalutamide

Mexican Brand Names Casodex

Index Terms CDX; ICI-176334; NC-722665

Pharmacologic Category Antineoplastic Agent, Antiandrogen

Use In combination therapy with LHRH agonist analogues in treatment of metastatic prostate cancer

Unlabeled/Investigational Use Monotherapy for locally-advanced prostate cancer

Effect on Mental Status May produce anxiety, depression, and confusion

Effect on Psychiatric Treatment None reported

Dosage Summary

Oral:

Children: Dosage not established

Adults: 50 mg once daily

Dosage Forms Excipient information presented when available (limited, particularly for generics); consult specific product labeling.

Tablet: 50 mg

◆ **Bicillin® L-A** *see* Penicillin G Benzathine *on page 1239*
◆ **Bicillin® C-R** *see* Penicillin G Benzathine and Penicillin G Procaine *on page 1240*
◆ **Bicillin® C-R 900/300** *see* Penicillin G Benzathine and Penicillin G Procaine *on page 1240*
◆ **BiCNU®** *see* Carmustine *on page 284*
◆ **BIDA** *see* Amonafide *on page 108*
◆ **Bidhist** *see* Brompheniramine *on page 205*
◆ **BiDil®** *see* Isosorbide Dinitrate and Hydralazine *on page 869*
◆ **Biltricide®** *see* Praziquantel *on page 1324*
◆ **Bird Flu Vaccine** *see* Influenza Virus Vaccine (H5N1) *on page 821*
◆ **bis-chloronitrosourea** *see* Carmustine *on page 284*
◆ **Bismatrol** *see* Bismuth *on page 189*
◆ **Bismatrol [OTC]** *see* Bismuth *on page 189*
◆ **Bismatrol Maximum Strength [OTC]** *see* Bismuth *on page 189*

Bismuth (BIZ muth)

Medication Safety Issues

Sound-alike/look-alike issues:

Kaopectate® may be confused with Kayexalate®

Maalox® Total Stomach Relief® is a different formulation than Maalox®

Note: Canadian formulation of Kaopectate® does not contain bismuth; the active ingredient in the Canadian formulation is attapulgite.

U.S. Brand Names Bismatrol Maximum Strength [OTC]; Bismatrol [OTC]; Diotame® [OTC]; Kao-Tin [OTC]; Kaopectate® Extra Strength [OTC]; Kaopectate® [OTC]; Kapectolin [OTC]; Maalox® Total Stomach Relief® [OTC]; Peptic Relief [OTC]; Pepto Relief [OTC]; Pepto-Bismol® Maximum Strength [OTC]; Pepto-Bismol® [OTC]

Mexican Brand Names A-Migdobis; Facidmol; Subsalicilato de Bismuto

Index Terms Bismatrol; Bismuth Subsalicylate; Pink Bismuth

Pharmacologic Category Antidiarrheal

Use Subsalicylate formulation: Symptomatic treatment of mild, nonspecific diarrhea; control of traveler's diarrhea (enterotoxigenic *Escherichia coli*); as part of a multidrug regimen for *H. pylori* eradication to reduce the risk of duodenal ulcer recurrence

Effect on Mental Status May rarely cause anxiety, confusion, or depression

Effect on Psychiatric Treatment None reported

Dosage Summary

Oral:

Subsalicylate based on 262 mg/5 mL liquid or 262 mg tablet (diarrhea):

Children <3 years: Dosage not established

Children 3-6 years: 1/3 tablet **or** 5 mL every 30 minutes to 1 hour as needed (maximum: 8 doses/day)

Children 6-9 years: 2/3 tablet **or** 10 mL every 30 minutes to 1 hour as needed (maximum: 8 doses/day)

Children 9-12 years: 1 tablet **or** 15 mL every 30 minutes to 1 hour as needed (maximum: 8 doses/day)

Subsalicylate based on 262 mg/15 mL liquid or 262 mg tablet:

Children >12 years: Diarrhea: 2 tablets **or** 30 mL every 30 minutes to 1 hour as needed (maximum: 8 doses/day)

Adults:

Diarrhea: 2 tablets **or** 30 mL every 30 minutes to 1 hour as needed (maximum: 8 doses/day)

H. pylori eradication: 524 mg 4 times/day

Dosage Forms Excipient information presented when available (limited, particularly for generics); consult specific product labeling.

Caplet, as subsalicylate:

Kaopectate®: 262 mg

Pepto-Bismol®: 262 mg [sugar free; contains sodium 2 mg/caplet]

Liquid, as subsalicylate: 262 mg/15 mL (240 mL)

Bismatrol: 262 mg/15 mL (240 mL)

Bismatrol Maximum Strength: 525 mg/15 mL (240 mL)

Diotame®: 262 mg/15 mL (30 mL) [sugar free]

Kaopectate®: 262 mg/15 mL (240 mL, 360 mL) [contains potassium 5 mg/15 mL, sodium 10 mg/15 mL; regular and peppermint flavors]

Kaopectate®: 262 mg/15 mL (180 mL) [contains sodium 10 mg/15 mL; cherry flavor]

Kaopectate® Extra Strength: 525 mg/15 mL (240 mL) [contains potassium 5 mg/15 mL, sodium 10 mg/15 mL; peppermint flavor]

Kao-Tin: 262 mg/15 mL (240 mL, 480 mL) [contains sodium benzoate]

Maalox® Total Stomach Relief®: 525 mg/15 mL (360 mL) [contains sodium 3.3 mg/15mL; strawberry and peppermint flavor]

Peptic Relief: 262 mg/15 mL (240 mL) [sugar free; mint flavor]

Pepto-Bismol®: 262 mg/15 mL (120 mL, 240 mL, 360 mL, 480 mL) [sugar free; contains sodium 6 mg/15 mL and benzoic acid; cherry and wintergreen flavors]

Pepto-Bismol® Maximum Strength: 525 mg/15 mL (120 mL, 240 mL, 360 mL) [sugar free; contains sodium 6 mg/15 mL and benzoic acid; wintergreen flavor]

Suspension, as subsalicylate:

Kapectolin: 262 mg/15 mL (480 mL) [mint flavor]

Tablet, chewable, as subsalicylate: 262 mg

Bismatrol: 262 mg

Diotame®: 262 mg [sugar free]

Peptic Relief, Pepto Relief: 262 mg

Pepto-Bismol®: 262 mg [sugar free; contains sodium <1 mg; cherry and wintergreen flavors]

Bismuth, Metronidazole, and Tetracycline

(BIZ muth, me troe NI da zole, & tet ra SYE kleen)

U.S. Brand Names Helidac®; Pylera™

Index Terms Bismuth Subcitrate Potassium, Tetracycline, and Metronidazole; Bismuth Subsalicylate, Tetracycline, and Metronidazole; Metronidazole, Bismuth Subcitrate Potassium, and Tetracycline; Metronidazole, Bismuth Subsalicylate, and Tetracycline; Tetracycline, Metronidazole, and Bismuth Subcitrate Potassium; Tetracycline, Metronidazole, and Bismuth Subsalicylate

Pharmacologic Category Antibiotic, Miscellaneous; Antibiotic, Tetracycline Derivative; Antidiarrheal

Use As part of a multidrug regimen for *H. pylori* eradication to reduce the risk of duodenal ulcer recurrence in combination with an H_2 agonist (Helidac®) or omeprazole (Pylera™)

Effect on Mental Status Dizziness common; metronidazole has been reported to cause depression, insomnia, confusion, panic, delusions, hallucinations, and exacerbation of schizophrenia; tetracycline has been reported to produce memory disturbances as well as mood stabilizing and antidepressant effects

Effect on Psychiatric Treatment Metronidazole and tetracycline may increase serum lithium levels and produce lithium toxicity; monitor serum lithium levels

Dosage Summary

Oral:

Children: Dosage not established

Adults:

Helidac®: Two bismuth subsalicylate 262.4 mg tablets, 1 metronidazole 250 mg tablet, and 1 tetracycline 500 mg capsule 4 times/day at meals and bedtime, plus an H_2 antagonist (at the appropriate dose) for 14 days; follow with 8 oz of water; the H_2 antagonist should be continued for a total of 28 days

Pylera™: Three capsules 4 times/day after meals and at bedtime, plus omeprazole 20 mg twice daily for 10 days; follow each dose with 8 oz of water (each capsule contains bismuth subcitrate potassium 140 mg, metronidazole 125 mg, and tetracycline 125 mg)

Dosage Forms Excipient information presented when available (limited, particularly for generics); consult specific product labeling.

Capsule:

Pylera™: Bismuth subcitrate potassium 140 mg, metronidazole 125 mg, and tetracycline hydrochloride 125 mg

Combination package:

Helidac® [each package contains 14 blister cards (2-week supply); each card contains the following]:

Capsule: Tetracycline hydrochloride: 500 mg (4)

Tablet, chewable: Bismuth subsalicylate: 262.4 mg (8)

Tablet: Metronidazole: 250 mg (4)

◆ **Bismuth Subcitrate Potassium, Tetracycline, and Metronidazole** *see* Bismuth, Metronidazole, and Tetracycline *on page 190*

◆ **Bismuth Subsalicylate** *see* Bismuth *on page 189*

◆ **Bismuth Subsalicylate, Tetracycline, and Metronidazole** *see* Bismuth, Metronidazole, and Tetracycline *on page 190*

Bisoprolol (bis OH proe lol)

Medication Safety Issues

Sound-alike/look-alike issues:

Zebeta® may be confused with DiaBeta®, Zetia®

Related Information

Beta-Blockers *on page 1776*

U.S. Brand Names Zebeta®

Canadian Brand Names Apo-Bisoprolol®; Monocor®; Novo-Bisoprolol; PMS-Bisoprolol; Sandoz-Bisoprolol; Zebeta®

Mexican Brand Names Concor

Index Terms Bisoprolol Fumarate

Pharmacologic Category Beta Blocker, $Beta_1$ Selective

Use Treatment of hypertension, alone or in combination with other agents

Unlabeled/Investigational Use Chronic stable angina, supraventricular arrhythmias, PVCs, heart failure (HF)

Effect on Mental Status Fatigue is common; may cause insomnia, confusion, depression, dizziness, headache, sleep disturbance, vivid dreams, anxiety, restlessness, and decreased concentration

Effect on Psychiatric Treatment Barbiturates may decrease the effects of beta-blockers

Dosage Summary

Oral:

Children: Dosage not established

Adults: Initial: 2.5-5 mg once daily; Maintenance: 2.5-20 mg once daily

Elderly: Initial: 2.5 mg/day, increase by 2.5-5 mg/day up to 20 mg/day

Dosage Forms Excipient information presented when available (limited, particularly for generics); consult specific product labeling.

Tablet, as fumarate: 5 mg, 10 mg

Bisoprolol and Hydrochlorothiazide

(bis OH proe lol & hye droe klor oh THYE a zide)

Medication Safety Issues

Sound-alike/look-alike issues:

Ziac® may be confused with Tiazac®, Zerit®

U.S. Brand Names Ziac®

Canadian Brand Names Ziac®

Mexican Brand Names Biconcor

Index Terms Hydrochlorothiazide and Bisoprolol

Pharmacologic Category Beta Blocker, $Beta_1$ Selective; Diuretic, Thiazide

Use Treatment of hypertension

Unlabeled/Investigational Use Pediatric hypertension

Effect on Mental Status Fatigue is common; may cause insomnia, confusion, depression, dizziness, headache, sleep disturbance, vivid dreams, anxiety, restlessness, and decreased concentration

Effect on Psychiatric Treatment Barbiturates may decrease the effects of beta-blockers; may decrease lithium clearance, resulting in elevated serum lithium levels and potential lithium toxicity; monitor serum lithium levels

Dosage Summary

Oral:

Children (unlabeled dose): Initial: Bisoprolol 2.5 mg/hydrochlorothiazide 6.25 mg once daily; up to a maximum of bisoprolol 10 mg/hydrochlorothiazide 6.25 mg daily

Adults: Bisoprolol 2.5-20 mg and hydrochlorothiazide 6.25-25 mg once daily

Dosage Forms Excipient information presented when available (limited, particularly for generics); consult specific product labeling.

Tablet:

2.5/6.25: Bisoprolol fumarate 2.5 mg and hydrochlorothiazide 6.25 mg

5/6.25: Bisoprolol fumarate 5 mg and hydrochlorothiazide 6.25 mg

10/6.25: Bisoprolol fumarate 10 mg and hydrochlorothiazide 6.25 mg

- ◆ **Bisoprolol Fumarate** *see* Bisoprolol *on page 190*
- ◆ **Bis-POM PMEA** *see* Adefovir *on page 51*
- ◆ **Bistropamide** *see* Tropicamide *on page 1636*

Bivalirudin (bye VAL i roo din)

Medication Safety Issues

High alert medication: The Institute for Safe Medication Practices (ISMP) includes this medication among its list of drugs which have a heightened risk of causing significant patient harm when used in error.

U.S. Brand Names Angiomax®

Canadian Brand Names Angiomax®

Index Terms Hirulog

Pharmacologic Category Anticoagulant, Thrombin Inhibitor

Use Anticoagulant used in conjunction with aspirin for patients with unstable angina undergoing percutaneous transluminal coronary angioplasty (PTCA) or percutaneous coronary intervention (PCI) with provisional glycoprotein IIb/IIIa inhibitor; anticoagulant used in patients undergoing PCI with (or at risk of) heparin-induced thrombocytopenia (HIT) / thrombosis syndrome (HITTS)

Unlabeled/Investigational Use Heparin-induced thrombocytopenia (HIT)

Effect on Mental Status May cause insomnia, anxiety, or nervousness

Effect on Psychiatric Treatment Nausea is common; this effect may be additive with concurrent use of SSRIs, lithium, or valproate. Do not administer bivalirudin in the same intravenous line with chlorpromazine, diazepam, or prochlorperazine; this results in haze formation, microparticulate formation, or gross precipitation.

Dosage Summary

I.V.:

Children: Dosage not established

Adults: Bolus: 0.75 mg/kg, may repeat at 0.3 mg/kg if necessary; Infusion: 1.75 mg/kg/hour for duration of procedure and up to 4 hours postprocedure if needed, after 4 hours may continue 0.2 mg/kg/minute for up to 20 hours if needed

Dosage Forms Excipient information presented when available (limited, particularly for generics); consult specific product labeling.

Injection, powder for reconstitution: 250 mg

- **BL4162A** *see* Anagrelide *on page 124*
- **Blenoxane® [DSC]** *see* Bleomycin *on page 192*
- **Bleo** *see* Bleomycin *on page 192*

Bleomycin (blee oh MYE sin)

Medication Safety Issues

Sound-alike/look-alike issues:

Bleomycin may be confused with Cleocin®

High alert medication: The Institute for Safe Medication Practices (ISMP) includes this medication among its list of drugs which have a heightened risk of causing significant patient harm when used in error.

U.S. Brand Names Blenoxane® [DSC]

Canadian Brand Names Blenoxane®; Bleomycin Injection, USP

Mexican Brand Names Bleolem; Bleomax

Index Terms Bleo; Bleomycin Sulfate; BLM; NSC-125066

Pharmacologic Category Antineoplastic Agent, Antibiotic

Use Treatment of squamous cell carcinomas, melanomas, sarcomas, testicular carcinoma, Hodgkin's lymphoma, and non-Hodgkin's lymphoma; sclerosing agent for malignant pleural effusion

Effect on Mental Status None reported

Effect on Psychiatric Treatment May rarely produce myelosuppression; use caution with clozapine and carbamazepine

Dosage Forms Excipient information presented when available (limited, particularly for generics); consult specific product labeling. [DSC] = Discontinued product

Injection, powder for reconstitution, as sulfate: 15 units, 30 units

Blenoxane®: 15 units [DSC], 30 units [DSC]

- **Bleomycin Sulfate** *see* Bleomycin *on page 192*
- **Blephamide®** *see* Sulfacetamide and Prednisolone *on page 1516*
- **BLM** *see* Bleomycin *on page 192*
- **BMS-232632** *see* Atazanavir *on page 147*
- **BMS 337039** *see* Aripiprazole *on page 133*
- **BMS-354825** *see* Dasatinib *on page 420*
- **Bonine® [OTC]** *see* Meclizine *on page 974*
- **Boniva®** *see* Ibandronate *on page 801*
- **Bontril PDM®** *see* Phendimetrazine *on page 1259*
- **Bontril® Slow-Release** *see* Phendimetrazine *on page 1259*

Bortezomib (bore TEZ oh mib)

Medication Safety Issues

High alert medication: The Institute for Safe Medication Practices (ISMP) includes this medication among its list of drug classes which have a heightened risk of causing significant patient harm when used in error.

U.S. Brand Names Velcade®

Canadian Brand Names Velcade®

Mexican Brand Names Velcade

Index Terms LDP-341; MLN341; NSC-681239; PS-341

Pharmacologic Category Antineoplastic Agent; Proteasome Inhibitor

Use Treatment of multiple myeloma; treatment of relapsed or refractory mantle cell lymphoma

Unlabeled/Investigational Use Treatment of non-Hodgkin's lymphomas (other than mantle cell lymphoma)

Effect on Mental Status Insomnia, dizziness, and anxiety are common; may cause agitation, confusion, psychosis, and suicidal ideation

Effect on Psychiatric Treatment Gastrointestinal side effects are common; use caution with SSRIs. May cause neutropenia and thrombocytopenia; use caution with clozapine, carbamazepine, and valproic acid. Fluoxetine, fluvoxamine, and nefazodone may increase bortezomib serum levels, while carbamazepine and barbiturates may decrease its serum levels.

Dosage Summary

I.V.:

Children: Dosage not established

Adults: 1.3 mg/m^2 days 1, 4, 8, 11, 22, 25, 29, and 32 of a 42-day treatment cycle for 4 cycles, followed by 1.3 mg/m^2 days 1, 8, 22 and 29 of a 42-day treatment cycle for 5 cycles **or** 1.3 mg/m^2 twice weekly for 2 weeks on days 1, 4, 8, and 11of a 21-day treatment regimen; therapy extending beyond 8 cycles may be given once weekly for 4 weeks (days 1, 8, 15, and 22)

Dosage Forms Excipient information presented when available (limited, particularly for generics); consult specific product labeling.

Injection, powder for reconstitution [preservative free]:

Velcade®: 3.5 mg [contains mannitol 35 mg]

◆ **B&O Supprettes® [DSC]** *see* Belladonna and Opium *on page 174*

◆ **Botox®** *see* Botulinum Toxin Type A *on page 193*

◆ **Botox® Cosmetic** *see* Botulinum Toxin Type A *on page 193*

Botulinum Toxin Type A (BOT yoo lin num TOKS in type aye)

U.S. Brand Names Botox®; Botox® Cosmetic

Canadian Brand Names Botox®; Botox® Cosmetic

Index Terms BTX-A

Pharmacologic Category Neuromuscular Blocker Agent, Toxin; Ophthalmic Agent, Toxin

Generic Available No

Use Treatment of strabismus and blepharospasm associated with dystonia (including benign essential blepharospasm or VII nerve disorders) in patients ≥12 years of age; cervical dystonia (spasmodic torticollis) in patients ≥16 years of age; temporary improvement in the appearance of lines/wrinkles of the face (moderate to severe glabellar lines associated with corrugator and/or procerus muscle activity) in adult patients ≤65 years of age; treatment of severe primary axillary hyperhidrosis in adults not adequately controlled with topical treatments

Canadian labeling: Additional use (not in U.S. labeling): Focal spasticity, including treatment of stroke related upper limb spasticity; dynamic equines foot deformity in pediatric cerebral palsy patients

Unlabeled/Investigational Use Treatment of oromandibular dystonia, spasmodic dysphonia (laryngeal dystonia) and other dystonias (ie, writer's cramp, focal task-specific dystonias); migraine treatment and prophylaxis; treatment of dynamic muscle contracture in pediatric cerebral palsy patients

Effect on Mental Status None reported

Effect on Psychiatric Treatment None reported

Pregnancy Risk Factor C

Pregnancy Considerations Decreased fetal body weight, delayed ossification, maternal toxicity, abortions, and fetal malformations were observed in animal studies. Human reproduction studies have not been conducted. Avoid use in pregnancy. Based on limited case reports, adverse fetal effects have not been observed with inadvertent administration during pregnancy. It is currently recommended to ensure adequate contraception in women of childbearing potential.

Lactation Excretion in breast milk unknown/use caution

Contraindications Hypersensitivity to albumin, botulinum toxin, or any component of the formulation; infection at the proposed injection site(s)

Canadian labeling: Additional contraindications (not in U.S. labeling): Myasthenia gravis or Eaton-Lambert syndrome

Warnings/Precautions Higher doses or more frequent administration may result in neutralizing antibody formation and loss of efficacy. Product contains albumin and may carry a remote risk of virus transmission. Use caution if there is excessive weakness or atrophy at the proposed injection site(s); use is contraindicated if infection is present at injection site. Have appropriate support in case of anaphylactic reaction. Use with caution in patients with neuromuscular diseases (such as myasthenia gravis), neuropathic disorders (such as amyotrophic lateral sclerosis), patients taking aminoglycosides, neuromuscular-blocking agents, or other drugs that interfere with neuromuscular transmission and patients with preexisting cardiovascular disease (rare reports of arrhythmia and MI). Long-term effects of chronic therapy unknown.

Cervical dystonia: Dysphagia is common. It may be severe requiring alternative feeding methods and may persist anywhere from 2 weeks up to 5 months after administration. Risk of upper respiratory infection may be increased. Risk factors include smaller neck muscle mass, bilateral injections into the sternocleidomastoid muscle, or injections into the levator scapulae.

Ocular disease: Blepharospasm: Reduced blinking from injection of the orbicularis muscle can lead to corneal exposure and ulceration. Strabismus: Retrobulbar hemorrhages may occur from needle penetration into orbit. Spatial disorientation, double vision, or past pointing may occur if one or more extraocular muscles are paralyzed. Covering the affected eye may help. Careful testing of corneal sensation, avoidance of lower lid injections, and treatment of epithelial defects are necessary. Use with caution in angle closure glaucoma.

Primary axillary hyperhidrosis: Evaluate for secondary causes prior to treatment (eg, hyperthyroidism). Safety and efficacy for treatment of hyperhidrosis in other areas of the body have not been established.

Temporary reduction in glabellar lines: Do not use more frequently than every 3 months. Patients with marked facial asymmetry, ptosis, excessive dermatochalasis, deep dermal scarring, thick sebaceous skin, or the inability to substantially lessen glabellar lines by physically spreading them apart were excluded from clinical trials. Reduced blinking from injection of the orbicularis muscle can lead to corneal exposure and ulceration. Spatial disorientation, double vision, or past pointing may occur if one or more extraocular muscles are paralyzed.

Adverse Reactions Adverse effects usually occur in 1 week and may last up to several months

>10%:

Cervical dystonia:

Central nervous system: Pain (32%), headache (up to 11%)
Gastrointestinal: Dysphagia (19%)
Neuromuscular & skeletal: Focal weakness (17%), neck pain (11%)
Respiratory: Upper respiratory infection (12%)

Other indications (blepharospasm, primary axillary hyperhidrosis, strabismus):

Neuromuscular & skeletal: Primary axillary hyperhidrosis (3% to 10%)
Ocular: Ptosis (blepharospasm 21%; strabismus 1% to 38%), vertical deviation (strabismus 17%)

2% to 10%:

Cervical dystonia:

Central nervous system: Dizziness, drowsiness, fever, malaise, speech disorder
Gastrointestinal: Nausea, xerostomia
Local: Injection site reaction: Soreness
Neuromuscular & skeletal: Back pain, hypertonia, weakness, stiffness
Respiratory: Cough, rhinitis
Miscellaneous: Flu-like syndrome

Cerebral palsy spasticity:

Central nervous system: Pain (1% to 2%), fever (1%), lethargy (1%)
Neuromuscular & skeletal: Falling, weakness

Focal spasticity:

Central nervous system: Arm pain (1% to 3%)
Dermatologic: Bruising (1% to 3%)
Local: Injection site reactions: burning, pain (1% to 3%)
Neuromuscular & skeletal: Hypertonia (1% to 3%), weakness (1% to 3%)

Other indications (blepharospasm, primary axillary hyperhidrosis, reduction of glabellar lines, strabismus):

Central nervous system: Anxiety, dizziness
Dermatologic: Pruritus
Gastrointestinal: Nausea
Local: Injection site reaction: Soreness
Neuromuscular & skeletal: Back pain, facial pain, weakness

Ocular: Irritation/tearing (includes dry eye, lagophthalmos, photophobia); ptosis, superficial punctate keratitis
Respiratory: Pharyngitis
Miscellaneous: Flu-like syndrome, infection, nonaxillary sweating

<2% (Limited to important or life-threatening): *Any indication:* Abdominal pain, acute angle closure glaucoma, allergic reactions, anaphylaxis, ankle pain, anterior segment eye ischemia, appetite decreased, arrhythmia, arthralgia, aspiration pneumonia, blurred vision, brachial plexopathy, bruising, ciliary ganglion damage, corneal perforation, dermatitis, diaphoresis, diarrhea, diplopia, dyspepsia, dysphonia, dyspnea, ectropion, entropion, erythema multiforme, eyelid edema, facial weakness, focal facial paralysis, glaucoma, hearing loss, hypoesthesia, hypertension, knee pain, leg cramps, lethargy, malaise, MI, myalgia, myasthenia gravis exacerbation, neutralizing antibody formation, numbness, pneumonia, pruritus, psoriasiform eruption, ptosis, rash, reduced blinking leading to corneal ulceration, retinal vein occlusion, retrobulbar hemorrhage, seizure, skin tightness, syncope, tooth disorder, urticaria, vertigo with nystagmus, vitreous hemorrhage, vomiting

Drug Interactions

Aminoglycosides: May enhance the neuromuscular-blocking effect of Botulinum Toxin Type A. *Risk C: Monitor therapy*

Botulinum Toxin Type B: Botulinum Toxin Type A may enhance the neuromuscular-blocking effect of Botulinum Toxin Type B. *Risk C: Monitor therapy*

Neuromuscular-Blocking Agents: May enhance the neuromuscular-blocking effect of Botulinum Toxin Type A. *Risk C: Monitor therapy*

Stability Store undiluted vials under refrigeration at 2°C to 8°C for up to 24 months (Botox® Cosmetic) or up to 36 months (Botox®). Reconstitute with sterile, preservative free 0.9% sodium chloride. Mix gently. After reconstitution, store in refrigerator (2°C to 8°C) and use within 4 hours (does not contain preservative).

Botox®: Reconstitute vials with 1 mL of diluent to obtain concentration of 10 units per 0.1 mL; 2 mL of diluent to obtain concentration of 5 units per 0.1 mL; 4 mL of diluent to obtain concentration of 2.5 units per 0.1 mL; 8 mL of diluent to obtain concentration of 1.25 units per 0.1 mL.

Botox® Cosmetic: Reconstitute vials with 2.5 mL of diluent to obtain concentration of 4 units per 0.1 mL (20 units per 0.5 mL).

Mechanism of Action Botulinum A toxin is a neurotoxin produced by *Clostridium botulinum,* spore-forming anaerobic bacillus, which appears to affect only the presynaptic membrane of the neuromuscular junction in humans, where it prevents calcium-dependent release of acetylcholine and produces a state of denervation. Muscle inactivation persists until new fibrils grow from the nerve and form junction plates on new areas of the muscle-cell walls. Intradermal injection results in temporary sweat gland denervation, reducing local sweating.

Pharmacodynamics/Kinetics

Onset of action (improvement):
- Blepharospasm: ~3 days
- Cervical dystonia: ~2 weeks
- Reduction of glabellar lines (Botox® Cosmetic): 1-2 days, increasing in intensity during first week
- Spasticity (focal and cerebral palsy related): <2 weeks
- Strabismus: ~1-2 days

Duration:
- Blepharospasm: ~3 months
- Cervical dystonia: <3 months
- Primary axillary hyperhidrosis: 201 days (mean)
- Reduction of glabellar lines (Botox® Cosmetic): ~3-4 months
- Spasticity (cerebral palsy related): ~3-3.5 months
- Strabismus: ~2-6 weeks

Absorption: Not expected to be present in peripheral blood at recommended doses following intramuscular (I.M.) injection

Time to peak:
- Blepharospasm: 1-2 weeks
- Cervical dystonia: ~6 weeks
- Spasticity (focal): 4-6 weeks
- Strabismus: Within first week

Dosage

Cervical dystonia: Children ≥16 years and Adults: I.M.: For dosing guidance, the mean dose is 236 units (25th to 75th percentile range 198-300 units) divided among the affected muscles in patients previously treated with botulinum toxin. Initial dose in previously untreated patients should be lower. Sequential dosing should be based on the patient's head and neck position, localization of pain, muscle hypertrophy, patient response, and previous adverse reactions. The total dose injected into the sternocleidomastoid muscles should be ≤100 units to decrease the occurrence of dysphagia.

Canadian labeling (not in U.S. labeling): Effective range of 200-360 units has been used in clinical practice; maximum dose: 6 units/kg every 2 months

Blepharospasm: Children ≥12 years and Adults: I.M.: Initial dose: 1.25-2.5 units injected into the medial and lateral pretarsal orbicularis oculi of the upper lid and lateral pretarsal orbicularis oculi of lower lid; dose may be increased up to twice the previous dose if the response from the initial dose lasted ≤2 months; maximum dose per site: 5 units. Tolerance may occur if treatments are given more often than every 3 months, but the effect is not usually permanent.

Cumulative dose:

U.S. labeling: ≤200 units in 30-day period

Canadian labeling (not in U.S. labeling): ≤200 units in 60-day period

Strabismus: Children ≥12 years and Adults: I.M.: **Note:** Several minutes prior to injection, administration of local anesthetic and ocular decongestant drops are recommended.

Initial dose:

Vertical muscles and for horizontal strabismus <20 prism diopters: 1.25-2.5 units in any one muscle

Horizontal strabismus of 20-50 prism diopters: 2.5-5 units in any one muscle

Persistent VI nerve palsy ≥1 month: 1.25-2.5 units in the medial rectus muscle

Re-examine patients 7-14 days after each injection to assess the effect of that dose. Subsequent doses for patients experiencing incomplete paralysis of the target may be increased up to twice the previous administered dose. The maximum recommended dose as a single injection for any one muscle is 25 units. Do not administer subsequent injections until the effects of the previous dose are gone.

Primary axillary hyperhidrosis: Adults ≥18 years: Intradermal: 50 units/axilla. Injection area should be defined by standard staining techniques. Injections should be evenly distributed into multiple sites (10-15), administered in 0.1-0.2 mL aliquots, ~1-2 cm apart. May repeat when clinical effect diminishes.

Reduction of glabellar lines: Adults ≤65 years: I.M.: An effective dose is determined by gross observation of the patient's ability to activate the superficial muscles injected. The location, size and use of muscles may vary markedly among individuals. Inject 0.1 mL (4 units) dose into each of five sites, two in each corrugator muscle and one in the procerus muscle for a total dose 0.5 mL (20 units) administered no more frequently than every 3-4 months.

Spasticity (cerebral palsy related; Canadian labeling [not approved in U.S. labeling]): Children ≥2 years: I.M.: 4 units/kg (total dose) divided into two injections into medial and lateral heads of the gastrocnemius of affected limb; if clinically indicated, may repeat every 2 months (maximum dose: 200 units)

Spasticity (focal; Canadian labeling [not approved in U.S. labeling]): Adults ≥18 years: I.M.: Individualize dose based on patient size, extent, and location of muscle involvement, degree of spasticity, local muscle weakness, and response to prior treatment. In clinical trials total doses up to 360 units were administered as separate injections typically divided among flexor muscles of the elbow, wrist, and fingers; may repeat therapy at 3-4 months with appropriate dosage based upon the clinical condition of patient at time of retreatment.

Suggested guidelines for the treatment of stroke-related upper limb spasticity:

Note: Dose listed is total dose administered as individual or separate intramuscular injection(s):

Biceps brachii: 100-200 units (up to 4 sites)

Flexor digitorum profundus: 15-50 units (1-2 sites)

Flexor digitorum sublimes: 15-50 units (1-2 sites)

Flexor carpi radialis: 15-60 units (1-2 sites)

Flexor carpi ulnaris: 10-50 units (1-2 sites)

Adductor pollicis: 20 units (1-2 sites)

Flexor pollicis longus: 20 units (1-2 sites)

Elderly: No specific adjustment recommended

Dosage adjustment in renal impairment: No specific adjustment recommended

Dosage adjustment in hepatic impairment: No specific adjustment recommended

Administration

Cervical dystonia: Use 25-, 27-, or 30-gauge needle for superficial muscles and a longer 22-gauge needle for deeper musculature; electromyography may help localize the involved muscles.

Blepharospasm: Use a 27- or 30-gauge needle without electromyography guidance. Avoid injecting near the levator palpebrae superioris (may decrease ptosis); avoid medial lower lid injections (may decrease diplopia). Apply pressure at the injection site to prevent ecchymosis in the soft eyelid tissues.

Spasticity (cerebral palsy related; Canadian labeling [not in U.S. labeling]): Use a 23 to 26-gauge needle for administration into the medial and lateral heads of the gastrocnemius muscle of the affected limb.

Spasticity (focal; Canadian labeling [not in U.S. labeling]): Use a 25, 27, or 30-gauge needle for superficial muscles and a longer 22-gauge needle for deeper musculature; electromyography or nerve stimulation may help localize the involved muscles.

Strabismus injections: Must use surgical exposure or electromyographic guidance; use the electrical activity recorded from the tip of the injections needle as a guide to placement within the target muscle. Local anesthetic and ocular decongestant should be given before injection. The volume of injection should be 0.05-0.15 mL per muscle. Many patients will require additional doses because of inadequate response to initial dose.

Primary axillary hyperhidrosis: Inject each dose intradermally to a depth of ~2 mm and at a 45° angle. Do not inject directly into areas marked in ink (to avoid permanent tattoo effect). Prior to administration, injection area should be defined by standard staining techniques such as Minor's Iodine-Starch Test.

Instructions for Minor's Iodine-Starch Test: Patient should shave underarms and refrain from using deodorants or antiperspirants for 24 hours prior to test. At 30 minutes prior to test, patient should be at rest, no exercise, and not consume hot beverages. Underarm area should be dried and immediately painted with iodine solution. After area dries, lightly sprinkle with starch powder. Gently blow off excess powder. A deep blue-black color will develop over the hyperhidrotic area in ~10 minutes.

Reduction of glabellar lines (Botox® Cosmetic): Use a 30-gauge needle. Ensure injected volume/dose is accurate and where feasible keep to a minimum. Avoid injection near the levator palpebrae superioris. Medial corrugator injections should be at least 1 cm above the bony supraorbital ridge. Do not inject toxin closer than 1 cm above the central eyebrow.

Additional Information Units of biological activity of Botox® cannot be compared with units of any other botulinum toxin.

Dosage Forms Excipient information presented when available (limited, particularly for generics); consult specific product labeling.

Injection, powder for reconstitution [preservative free]: *Clostridium botulinum* toxin type A 100 units [contains human albumin]

Botulinum Toxin Type B (BOT yoo lin num TOKS in type bee)

U.S. Brand Names Myobloc®

Pharmacologic Category Neuromuscular Blocker Agent, Toxin

Generic Available No

Use Treatment of cervical dystonia (spasmodic torticollis)

Unlabeled/Investigational Use Treatment of cervical dystonia in patients who have developed resistance to botulinum toxin type A

Effect on Mental Status May cause anxiety, dizziness, sedation, or confusion

Effect on Psychiatric Treatment May cause torticollis, use atypical antipsychotics with caution; may cause flu-like syndrome (take this into consideration if also concerned about SSRI discontinuation syndrome)

Pregnancy Risk Factor C (manufacturer)

Pregnancy Considerations Reproduction studies have not been conducted. Based on limited case reports using botulinum toxin A, adverse fetal effects have not been observed with inadvertent administration during pregnancy. It is currently recommended to ensure adequate contraception in women of childbearing years.

Lactation Excretion in breast milk unknown/use caution

Contraindications Hypersensitivity to albumin, botulinum toxin, or any component of the formulation; infection at the injection site(s). Relative contraindications include diseases of neuromuscular transmission; coagulopathy, including therapeutic anticoagulation; inability of patient to cooperate.

Warnings/Precautions Higher doses or more frequent administration may result in neutralizing antibody formation and loss of efficacy. Product contains albumin and may carry a remote risk of virus transmission. Use caution if there is inflammation, excessive weakness, or atrophy at the proposed injection site(s). Concurrent use of botulinum toxin type A or within <4 months of type B is not recommended. Have appropriate support in case of anaphylactic reaction. Use with caution in patients taking aminoglycosides or other drugs that interfere with neuromuscular transmission. Long-term effects of chronic therapy unknown. Increased risk of dysphagia and respiratory complications. Safety and efficacy in children have not been established.

Adverse Reactions

>10%:

Central nervous system: Headache (10% to 16%), pain (6% to 13%; placebo 10%)

Gastrointestinal: Dysphagia (10% to 25%), xerostomia (3% to 34%)

Local: Injection site pain (12% to 16%)

Neuromuscular & skeletal: Neck pain (up to 17%; placebo: 16%)

Miscellaneous: Infection (13% to 19%; placebo: 15%)

1% to 10%:

Cardiovascular: Chest pain, vasodilation, peripheral edema

Central nervous system: Dizziness (3% to 6%), fever, malaise, migraine, anxiety, tremor, hyperesthesia, somnolence, confusion, vertigo

Dermatologic: Pruritus, bruising

Gastrointestinal: Nausea (3% to 10%; placebo: 5%), dyspepsia (up to 10%; placebo: 5%), vomiting, stomatitis, taste perversion

Genitourinary: Urinary tract infection, cystitis, vaginal moniliasis

Hematologic: Serum neutralizing activity

Neuromuscular & skeletal: Torticollis (up to 8%; placebo: 7%), arthralgia (up to 7%; placebo: 5%), back pain (3% to 7%; placebo: 3%), myasthenia (3% to 6%; placebo: 3%), weakness (up to 6%; placebo: 4%), arthritis

Ocular: Amblyopia, abnormal vision

Otic: Otitis media, tinnitus

Respiratory: Cough (3% to 7%; placebo: 3%), rhinitis (1% to 5%; placebo: 6%), dyspnea, pneumonia

Miscellaneous: Flu-syndrome (6% to 9%), allergic reaction, viral infection, abscess, cyst

Drug Interactions

Aminoglycosides: May enhance the neuromuscular-blocking effect of Botulinum Toxin Type B. *Risk C: Monitor therapy*

Botulinum Toxin Type A: May enhance the neuromuscular-blocking effect of Botulinum Toxin Type B. *Risk C: Monitor therapy*

Neuromuscular-Blocking Agents: May enhance the neuromuscular-blocking effect of Botulinum Toxin Type B. *Risk C: Monitor therapy*

Stability Store vials under refrigeration at 2°C to 8°C (36°F to 46°F) for up to 21 months. May be diluted with normal saline; once diluted, use within 4 hours. Does not contain preservative. Single-use vial. Do not shake; do not freeze.

Mechanism of Action Botulinum B toxin is a neurotoxin produced by *Clostridium botulinum*, spore-forming anaerobic bacillus. It cleaves synaptic Vesicle Association Membrane Protein (VAMP; synaptobrevin) which is a component of the protein complex responsible for docking and fusion of the synaptic vesicle to the presynaptic membrane. By blocking neurotransmitter release, botulinum B toxin paralyzes the muscle.

Pharmacodynamics/Kinetics

Duration: 12-16 weeks

Absorption: Not expected to be present in peripheral blood at recommended doses

Dosage

Children: Not established in pediatric patients

Adults: Cervical dystonia: I.M.: Initial: 2500-5000 units divided among the affected muscles in patients **previously treated** with botulinum toxin; initial dose in **previously untreated** patients should be lower. Subsequent dosing should be optimized according to patient's response.

Elderly: No dosage adjustments required, but limited experience in patients ≥75 years old

Dosage adjustment in renal impairment: No specific adjustment recommended

Dosage adjustment in hepatic impairment: No specific adjustment recommended

Additional Information Units of biological activity of Myobloc® cannot be compared with units of any other botulinum toxin.

Dosage Forms Excipient information presented when available (limited, particularly for generics); consult specific product labeling.

Injection, solution [preservative free]:

Myobloc®: 5000 units/mL (0.5 mL, 1 mL, 2 mL) [contains albumin 0.05%]

◆ **Brethaire [DSC]** *see* Terbutaline *on page 1552*

◆ **Brevibloc®** *see* Esmolol *on page 569*

◆ **Brevicon®** *see* Ethinyl Estradiol and Norethindrone *on page 597*

◆ **Brevital® Sodium** *see* Methohexital *on page 1011*

◆ **Bricanyl [DSC]** *see* Terbutaline *on page 1552*

Brimonidine (bri MOE ni deen)

Medication Safety Issues
Sound-alike/look-alike issues:
Brimonidine may be confused with bromocriptine

U.S. Brand Names Alphagan® P

Canadian Brand Names Alphagan®; Apo-Brimonidine®; PMS-Brimonidine Tartrate; ratio-Brimonidine; Sandoz-Brimonidine

Mexican Brand Names Agglad Ofteno; Alphagan; Nor-Tenz

Index Terms Brimonidine Tartrate

Pharmacologic Category Alpha$_2$ Agonist, Ophthalmic; Ophthalmic Agent, Antiglaucoma

Use Lowering of intraocular pressure (IOP) in patients with open-angle glaucoma or ocular hypertension

Effect on Mental Status Drowsiness is common

Effect on Psychiatric Treatment Contraindicated with MAO inhibitors; concurrent use with psychotropics may produce additive sedation

Dosage Summary
Ophthalmic:
Children <2 years: Dosage not established
Children ≥2 years: Instill 1 drop in affected eye(s) 3 times/day
Adults: Instill 1 drop in affected eye(s) 3 times/day

Dosage Forms Excipient information presented when available (limited, particularly for generics); consult specific product labeling.
Solution, ophthalmic, as tartrate: 0.2% (5 mL, 10 mL, 15 mL) [may contain benzalkonium chloride]
Alphagan® P: 0.1% (5 mL, 10 mL, 15 mL) [contains Purite® as preservative]; 0.15% (5 mL, 10 mL, 15 mL) [contains Purite® as preservative]

◆ **Brimonidine Tartrate** *see* Brimonidine *on page 199*

Brinzolamide (brin ZOH la mide)

U.S. Brand Names Azopt®

Canadian Brand Names Azopt®

Mexican Brand Names Azopt

Pharmacologic Category Carbonic Anhydrase Inhibitor; Ophthalmic Agent, Antiglaucoma

Use Lowers intraocular pressure in patients with ocular hypertension or open-angle glaucoma

Effect on Mental Status May rarely cause dizziness

Effect on Psychiatric Treatment None reported

Dosage Summary
Ophthalmic:
Children: Dosage not established
Adults: Instill 1 drop in affected eye(s) 3 times/day

Dosage Forms Excipient information presented when available (limited, particularly for generics); consult specific product labeling. [DSC] = Discontinued product
Suspension, ophthalmic:
Azopt®: 1% (5 mL [DSC], 10 mL, 15 mL) [contains benzalkonium chloride]

◆ **Brioschi® [OTC]** *see* Sodium Bicarbonate *on page 1494*

◆ **British Anti-Lewisite** *see* Dimercaprol *on page 479*

◆ **BRL 43694** *see* Granisetron *on page 736*

◆ **Bromaline® [OTC]** *see* Brompheniramine and Pseudoephedrine *on page 206*

◆ **Bromaline® DM [OTC]** *see* Brompheniramine, Pseudoephedrine, and Dextromethorphan *on page 208*

◆ **Bromatane DX** *see* Brompheniramine, Pseudoephedrine, and Dextromethorphan *on page 208*

Bromazepam (broe MA ze pam)

Medication Safety Issues

International issues:

Lexotan® [multiple international markets] may be confused with Cefotan® which is a brand name for cefotetan in the U.S.

Lexotan® [multiple international markets] may be confused with Cefiton® which is a brand name for cefixime in Portugal

Lexotan® [multiple international markets] may be confused with Loxitane® which is a brand name for loxapine in the U.S.

Related Information

Discontinuation of Psychotropic Drugs *on page 1839*

Canadian Brand Names Apo-Bromazepam®; Gen-Bromazepam; Lectopam®; Novo-Bromazepam; Nu-Bromazepam; Pro Doc Limitee Bromazepam

Mexican Brand Names Lexotan; Otedram

Pharmacologic Category Benzodiazepine

Generic Available Yes

Use Short-term, symptomatic treatment of anxiety

Mental Health Comment In 2007, the FDA requested that all manufacturers of sedative-hypnotic drug products revise labeling to include a greater emphasis on the risks of adverse effects. These risks include severe allergic reactions (anaphylaxis, angioedema) and complex sleep-related behaviors, which may include sleep-driving (driving while not fully awake and with no memory of the event), making phone calls, and preparing and eating food while asleep.

Risk factors for abuse include personal or family history of substance abuse and personality disorder.

Restrictions CDSA IV; Not available in U.S.

Pregnancy Risk Factor D (based on other benzodiazepines)

Pregnancy Considerations Crosses the placenta. Oral clefts reported, however, more recent data does not support an association between drug and oral clefts; inguinal hernia, cardiac defects, spina bifida, dysmorphic facial features, skeletal defects, multiple other malformations reported; hypotonia and withdrawal symptoms reported following use near time of delivery.

Lactation Enters breast milk/contraindicated (AAP rates other benzodiazepines "of concern")

Contraindications Hypersensitivity to bromazepam or any component of the formulation (cross-sensitivity with other benzodiazepines may exist); myasthenia gravis; narrow-angle glaucoma; severe hepatic or respiratory disease; sleep apnea; pregnancy

Warnings/Precautions Rebound or withdrawal symptoms may occur following abrupt discontinuation or large decreases in dose. Use with caution in elderly or debilitated patients, patients with hepatic disease (including alcoholics), or renal impairment.

Causes CNS depression (dose related) resulting in sedation, dizziness, confusion, or ataxia which may impair physical and mental capabilities. Patients must be cautioned about performing tasks requiring alertness (eg operating machinery or driving). Use with caution in patients receiving other CNS depressants, psychoactive agents, sedative drugs or ethanol. Benzodiazepines have been associated with falls and traumatic injury and should be used with caution in patients who are at risk of these events (especially the elderly).

Use with caution in patients with respiratory disease or impaired gag reflex. Use caution in patients with depression, particularly if suicidal risk may be present. May cause physical or psychological dependence. Acute withdrawal, including seizures, may be precipitated by flumazenil in patients receiving long-term benzodiazepine therapy.

Benzodiazepines have been associated with anterograde amnesia. Paradoxical reactions have been reported with benzodiazepines, particularly in adolescent/pediatric or psychiatric patients. Does not have analgesic, antidepressant, or antipsychotic properties. Safety and efficacy not established in patients <18 years of age.

Adverse Reactions Frequency not defined.

Cardiovascular: Hypotension, palpitation, tachycardia

Central nervous system: Drowsiness, ataxia, dizziness, confusion, depression, euphoria, lethargy, slurred speech, stupor, headache, seizure, anterograde amnesia. In addition, paradoxical reactions (including excitation, agitation, hallucinations, and psychosis) are known to occur with benzodiazepines.

Dermatologic: Rash, pruritus

Endocrine & metabolic: Hyperglycemia, hypoglycemia
Gastrointestinal: Xerostomia, nausea, vomiting
Genitourinary: Incontinence, libido decreased
Hematologic: Hemoglobin decreased, hematocrit decreased, WBCs increased/ decreased
Hepatic: Transaminases increased, alkaline phosphatase increased, bilirubin increased
Neuromuscular & skeletal: Weakness, muscle spasm
Ocular: Blurred vision, depth perception decreased

Metabolism/Transport Effects **Substrate** of CYP3A4 (major); **Inhibits** CYP2E1 (weak)

Drug Interactions

Alcohol (Ethyl): CNS Depressants may enhance the CNS depressant effect of Alcohol (Ethyl). *Risk C: Monitor therapy*

Antifungal Agents (Azole Derivatives, Systemic): May decrease the metabolism of Benzodiazepines (metabolized by oxidation). *Risk D: Consider therapy modification*

Aprepitant: May increase the serum concentration of Benzodiazepines (metabolized by oxidation). *Risk C: Monitor therapy*

Calcium Channel Blockers (Nondihydropyridine): May decrease the metabolism of Benzodiazepines (metabolized by oxidation). *Risk D: Consider therapy modification*

CarBAMazepine: May increase the metabolism of Benzodiazepines (metabolized by oxidation). *Risk C: Monitor therapy*

Cimetidine: May decrease the metabolism of Benzodiazepines (metabolized by oxidation). *Risk C: Monitor therapy*

Clozapine: Benzodiazepines may enhance the adverse/toxic effect of Clozapine. *Risk D: Consider therapy modification*

CNS Depressants: May enhance the adverse/toxic effect of other CNS Depressants. *Risk C: Monitor therapy*

CYP3A4 Inducers (Strong): May increase the metabolism of CYP3A4 Substrates. *Risk C: Monitor therapy*

CYP3A4 Inhibitors (Moderate): May decrease the metabolism of CYP3A4 Substrates. *Risk C: Monitor therapy*

CYP3A4 Inhibitors (Strong): May decrease the metabolism of CYP3A4 Substrates. *Risk D: Consider therapy modification*

Dasatinib: May increase the serum concentration of CYP3A4 Substrates. *Risk C: Monitor therapy*

Deferasirox: May decrease the serum concentration of CYP3A4 Substrates. *Risk C: Monitor therapy*

Disulfiram: May decrease the metabolism of Benzodiazepines (metabolized by oxidation). *Risk C: Monitor therapy*

Fluconazole: May decrease the metabolism of Benzodiazepines (metabolized by oxidation). *Risk D: Consider therapy modification*

Fosaprepitant: May increase the serum concentration of Benzodiazepines (metabolized by oxidation). Specifically, the active metabolite aprepitant is likely responsible for this effect. *Risk C: Monitor therapy*

Grapefruit Juice: May decrease the metabolism of Benzodiazepines (metabolized by oxidation). *Risk D: Consider therapy modification*

Isoniazid: May decrease the metabolism of Benzodiazepines (metabolized by oxidation). *Risk C: Monitor therapy*

Macrolide Antibiotics: May decrease the metabolism of Benzodiazepines (metabolized by oxidation). **Exceptions:** Azithromycin; Dirithromycin [Off Market]; Spiramycin. *Risk D: Consider therapy modification*

Nefazodone: May decrease the metabolism of Benzodiazepines (metabolized by oxidation). *Risk D: Consider therapy modification*

Oral Contraceptive (Estrogens): May decrease the metabolism of Benzodiazepines (metabolized by oxidation). *Risk C: Monitor therapy*

Oral Contraceptive (Progestins): May decrease the metabolism of Benzodiazepines (metabolized by oxidation). *Risk C: Monitor therapy*

Phenytoin: Benzodiazepines may increase the serum concentration of Phenytoin. Short-term exposure to benzodiazepines may not present as much risk as chronic therapy. *Risk C: Monitor therapy*

Protease Inhibitors: May decrease the metabolism of Benzodiazepines (metabolized by oxidation). Management: Amprenavir, atazanavir, darunavir, indinavir, nelfinavir, ritonavir, and tipranavir are contraindicated with midazolam and triazolam according to each protease inhibitor 's prescribing information. *Risk D: Consider therapy modification*

Proton Pump Inhibitors: May increase the serum concentration of Benzodiazepines (metabolized by oxidation). **Exceptions:** Lansoprazole; Pantoprazole; Rabeprazole. *Risk C: Monitor therapy*

Rifamycin Derivatives: May increase the metabolism of Benzodiazepines (metabolized by oxidation). *Risk D: Consider therapy modification*

Selective Serotonin Reuptake Inhibitors: May decrease the metabolism of Benzodiazepines (metabolized by oxidation). **Exceptions:** Citalopram; Escitalopram; PARoxetine; Sertraline. *Risk C: Monitor therapy*

St Johns Wort: May increase the metabolism of Benzodiazepines (metabolized by oxidation). *Risk C: Monitor therapy*

Theophylline Derivatives: May diminish the therapeutic effect of Benzodiazepines. *Risk D: Consider therapy modification*

Ethanol/Nutrition/Herb Interactions

Ethanol: Avoid ethanol (may increase CNS depression).

Food: Serum concentration may be increased by grapefruit juice.

Herb/Nutraceutical: St John's wort may decrease bromazepam serum concentrations. Avoid valerian, St John's wort, kava kava, gotu kola (may increase CNS depression).

Stability Store at 20°C to 25°C (68°F to 77°F).

Mechanism of Action Binds to stereospecific benzodiazepine receptors on the postsynaptic GABA neuron at several sites within the central nervous system, including the limbic system, reticular formation. Enhancement of the inhibitory effect of GABA on neuronal excitability results by increased neuronal membrane permeability to chloride ions. This shift in chloride ions results in hyperpolarization (a less excitable state) and stabilization.

Pharmacodynamics/Kinetics

Protein binding: 70%

Metabolism: Hepatic

Bioavailability: 60%

Half-life elimination: 20 hours

Excretion: Urine (69%), as metabolites

Dosage Oral:

Adults: Initial: 6-18 mg/day in equally divided doses; initial course of treatment should not last longer than 1 week; optimal dosage range: 6-30 mg/day

Elderly/debilitated: Initial dose: 3 mg/day in divided doses

Dietary Considerations May be taken with or without food.

Administration May be administered with or without food.

Additional Information Not available in U.S.

Dosage Forms Excipient information presented when available (limited, particularly for generics); consult specific product labeling. [CAN] = Canadian brand name

Tablet: 1.5 mg, 3 mg, 6 mg [not available in the U.S.]

- **Brometane DX [DSC]** *see* Brompheniramine, Pseudoephedrine, and Dextromethorphan *on page 208*
- **Bromfenex® [DSC]** *see* Brompheniramine and Pseudoephedrine *on page 206*
- **Bromfenex® PD [DSC]** *see* Brompheniramine and Pseudoephedrine *on page 206*
- **Bromhist DM** *see* Brompheniramine, Pseudoephedrine, and Dextromethorphan *on page 208*
- **Bromhist-NR** *see* Brompheniramine and Pseudoephedrine *on page 206*
- **Bromhist PDX** *see* Brompheniramine, Pseudoephedrine, and Dextromethorphan *on page 208*
- **Bromhist Pediatric** *see* Brompheniramine and Pseudoephedrine *on page 206*

Bromocriptine (broe moe KRIP teen)

Medication Safety Issues

Sound-alike/look-alike issues:

Bromocriptine may be confused with benztropine, brimonidine

Parlodel® may be confused with pindolol, Provera®

Related Information

Antiparkinsonian Agents *on page 1767*

Discontinuation of Psychotropic Drugs *on page 1839*

U.S. Brand Names Parlodel®; Parlodel® SnapTabs®

Canadian Brand Names Apo-Bromocriptine®; Parlodel®; PMS-Bromocriptine

Mexican Brand Names Parlodel

Index Terms Bromocriptine Mesylate

Pharmacologic Category Anti-Parkinson's Agent, Dopamine Agonist; Ergot Derivative

Generic Available Yes

Use Treatment of hyperprolactinemia associated with amenorrhea with or without galactorrhea, infertility, or hypogonadism; treatment of prolactin-secreting adenomas; treatment of acromegaly; treatment of Parkinson's disease

Unlabeled/Investigational Use Neuroleptic malignant syndrome

Effect on Mental Status Drowsiness is common; may cause hallucinations

Effect on Psychiatric Treatment Used to treat neuroleptic malignant syndrome and cocaine abuse; fluvoxamine and nefazodone may increase bromocriptine concentrations; monitor for hypotension, headache, nausea

Pregnancy Risk Factor B

Pregnancy Considerations No evidence of teratogenicity or fetal toxicity in animal studies. Bromocriptine is used for ovulation induction in women with hyperprolactinemia. In general, therapy should be discontinued if pregnancy is confirmed unless needed for treatment of macroprolactinoma. Data collected from women taking bromocriptine during pregnancy suggest the incidence of birth defects is not increased with use. However, the majority of women discontinued use within 8 weeks of pregnancy. Women not seeking pregnancy should be advised to use appropriate contraception.

Lactation Enters breast milk/not recommended

Contraindications Hypersensitivity to bromocriptine, ergot alkaloids, or any component of the formulation; ergot alkaloids are contraindicated with potent inhibitors of CYP3A4 (includes protease inhibitors, azole antifungals, and some macrolide antibiotics); uncontrolled hypertension; severe ischemic heart disease or peripheral vascular disorders; pregnancy (risk to benefit evaluation must be performed in women who become pregnant during treatment for acromegaly, prolactinoma, or Parkinson's disease - hypertension during treatment should generally result in efforts to withdraw)

Warnings/Precautions Complete evaluation of pituitary function should be completed prior to initiation of treatment. Use caution in patients with a history of peptic ulcer disease, dementia, psychosis, or cardiovascular disease (myocardial infarction, arrhythmia). Symptomatic hypotension may occur in a significant number of patients. In addition, hypertension, seizures, MI, and stroke have been rarely associated with bromocriptine therapy. Severe headache or visual changes may precede events. The onset of reactions may be immediate or delayed (often may occur in the second week of therapy). Sudden sleep onset and somnolence have been reported with use, primarily in patients with Parkinson's disease. Patients must be cautioned about performing tasks which require mental alertness.

Concurrent antihypertensives or drugs which may alter blood pressure should be used with caution. Concurrent use with levodopa has been associated with an increased risk of hallucinations. Consider dosage reduction and/or discontinuation in patients with hallucinations. Hallucinations may require weeks to months before resolution.

Dopamine agonists have been associated with compulsive behaviors and/or loss of impulse control, which has manifested as pathological gambling, libido increases (hypersexuality), and/or binge eating. Causality has not been established, and controversy exists as to whether this phenomenon is related to the underlying disease, prior behaviors/addictions and/or drug therapy. Dose reduction or discontinuation of therapy has been reported to reverse these behaviors in some, but not all cases.

In the treatment of acromegaly, discontinuation is recommended if tumor expansion occurs during therapy. Digital vasospasm (cold sensitive) may occur in some patients with acromegaly; may require dosage reduction. Patients who receive bromocriptine during and immediately following pregnancy as a continuation of previous therapy (eg, acromegaly) should be closely monitored for cardiovascular effects. Should not be used postpartum in women with coronary artery disease or other cardiovascular disease. Use of bromocriptine to control or prevent lactation or in patients with uncontrolled hypertension is not recommended.

Monitoring and careful evaluation of visual changes during the treatment of hyperprolactinemia is recommended to differentiate between tumor shrinkage and traction on the optic chiasm; rapidly progressing visual field loss requires neurosurgical consultation. Discontinuation of bromocriptine in patients with macroadenomas has been associated with rapid regrowth of tumor and increased prolactin serum levels. Pleural and retroperitoneal fibrosis have been reported with prolonged daily use. Cardiac valvular fibrosis has also been associated with ergot alkaloids. Safety and efficacy have not been established in patients with hepatic or renal dysfunction. Safety and effectiveness in patients <11 years of age (for pituitary adenoma) have not been established. Safety has not been established for use >2 years in patients with Parkinson's disease.

Adverse Reactions Note: Frequency of adverse effects may vary by dose and/or indication.

>10%:

Central nervous system: Dizziness, headache

Gastrointestinal: Constipation, nausea

1% to 10%:

Cardiovascular: Hypotension (including postural/orthostatic), Raynaud's syndrome exacerbation, syncope

Central nervous system: Drowsiness, fatigue, lightheadedness

Gastrointestinal: Abdominal cramps, anorexia, diarrhea, dyspepsia, GI bleeding, vomiting, xerostomia

Neuromuscular & skeletal: Digital vasospasm

Respiratory: Nasal congestion

Frequency not defined, postmarketing, and/or case reports: Abdominal discomfort, alcohol potentiation, alopecia, anxiety, arrhythmia, ataxia, blepharospasm, blurred vision, bradycardia, cerebrospinal fluid rhinorrhea, cold tolerance decreased, confusion, constrictive pericarditis, delusional psychosis, depression, dyskinesia, dysphagia, dyspnea, ear tingling, epileptiform seizure, ergotism, erythromelalgia, facial pallor, faintness, hallucinations, heavy headedness, insomnia, involuntary movements, lassitude, lethargy, lightheadedness, mottling of skin, muscle cramps, nervousness, nightmares, "on-off" phenomenon, paranoia, paresthesia, pericardial effusion, peripheral edema, pleural effusion, pleural/pulmonary fibrosis, psychomotor agitation/excitation, rash, sleep requirement decreased, sluggishness, urinary frequency, urinary retention, vasovagal attack, ventricular tachycardia, vertigo, visual disturbance, weakness

Withdrawal reactions: Abrupt discontinuation has resulted in rare cases of a withdrawal reaction with symptoms similar to neuroleptic malignant syndrome.

Reported with dopamine agonists: Impulsive/compulsive behaviors (eg, pathological gambling, hypersexuality, binge eating)

Metabolism/Transport Effects **Substrate** of CYP3A4 (major); **Inhibits** CYP1A2 (weak), 3A4 (weak)

Drug Interactions

Alpha-/Beta-Agonists: May enhance the adverse/toxic effect of Bromocriptine. Including increased blood pressure, ventricular arrhythmias, and seizure. **Exceptions:** Dipivefrin. *Risk C: Monitor therapy*

Antipsychotics (Atypical): May diminish the therapeutic effect of Anti-Parkinson's Agents (Dopamine Agonist). *Risk D: Consider therapy modification*

Antipsychotics (Typical): May diminish the therapeutic effect of Anti-Parkinson's Agents (Dopamine Agonist) *Risk D: Consider therapy modification*

CycloSPORINE: Bromocriptine may increase the serum concentration of CycloSPORINE. *Risk C: Monitor therapy*

CYP3A4 Inhibitors (Moderate): May decrease the metabolism of CYP3A4 Substrates. *Risk C: Monitor therapy*

CYP3A4 Inhibitors (Strong): May decrease the metabolism of CYP3A4 Substrates. *Risk D: Consider therapy modification*

Dasatinib: May increase the serum concentration of CYP3A4 Substrates. *Risk C: Monitor therapy*

Efavirenz: May enhance the adverse/toxic effect of Ergot Derivatives. Specifically, the risk for peripheral vasospasm and ischemia may be increased. *Risk X: Avoid combination*

Macrolide Antibiotics: May enhance the adverse/toxic effect of Ergot Derivatives. Specifically leading the development of ergotism. **Exceptions:** Azithromycin; Dirithromycin [Off Market]; Spiramycin. *Risk D: Consider therapy modification*

Metoclopramide: May diminish the therapeutic effect of Anti-Parkinson's Agents (Dopamine Agonist). *Risk C: Monitor therapy*

Posaconazole: May increase the serum concentration of Ergot Derivatives. *Risk X: Avoid combination*

Protease Inhibitors: May decrease the metabolism of Ergot Derivatives. *Risk X: Avoid combination*

Serotonin 5-HT1D Receptor Agonists: Ergot Derivatives may enhance the vasoconstricting effect of Serotonin 5-HT1D Receptor Agonists. Serotonin 5-HT1D Receptor Agonists may enhance the vasoconstricting effect of Ergot Derivatives. *Risk X: Avoid combination*

Serotonin Modulators: May enhance the adverse/toxic effect of other Serotonin Modulators. The development of serotonin syndrome may occur. *Risk D: Consider therapy modification*

Sibutramine: May enhance the serotonergic effect of Ergot Derivatives. This may cause serotonin syndrome. *Risk X: Avoid combination*

Voriconazole: May increase the serum concentration of Ergot Derivatives. *Risk X: Avoid combination*

Ethanol/Nutrition/Herb Interactions

Ethanol: Avoid ethanol (may increase GI side effects or ethanol intolerance).

Herb/Nutraceutical: St John's wort may decrease bromocriptine levels.

Mechanism of Action Semisynthetic ergot alkaloid derivative and a dopamine receptor agonist which activates postsynaptic dopamine receptors in the tuberoinfundibular (inhibiting pituitary prolactin secretion) and nigrostriatal pathways (enhancing coordinated motor control).

Pharmacodynamics/Kinetics

Onset of action: Prolactin decreasing effect: 1-2 hours

Protein binding: 90% to 96%

Metabolism: Primarily hepatic via CYP3A; extensive first-pass biotransformation

Bioavailability: 28%

Half-life elimination: Biphasic: Terminal: 15 hours (range 8-20 hours)

Time to peak, serum: 1-3 hours

Excretion: Feces; urine (2% to 6% as unchanged drug and metabolites)

Dosage Oral:

Children: Hyperprolactinemia:

11-15 years (based on limited information): Initial: 1.25-2.5 mg daily; dosage may be increased as tolerated to achieve a therapeutic response (range: 2.5-10 mg daily).

≥16 years: Refer to adult dosing

Adults:

Parkinsonism: 1.25 mg twice daily, increased by 2.5 mg/day in 2- to 4-week intervals (usual dose range is 30-90 mg/day in 3 divided doses; maximum: 100 mg/day), though elderly patients can usually be managed on lower doses

Neuroleptic malignant syndrome (unlabeled use): 2.5-5 mg 3 times/day

Acromegaly: Initial: 1.25-2.5 mg daily increasing by 1.25-2.5 mg daily as necessary every 3-7 days; usual dose: 20-30 mg/day (maximum: 100 mg/day)

Hyperprolactinemia: Initial: 1.25-2.5 mg/day; may be increased by 2.5 mg/day as tolerated every 2-7 days until optimal response (range: 2.5-15 mg/day)

Dosing adjustment in hepatic impairment: No guidelines are available, however, may be necessary

Dietary Considerations May be taken with food to decrease GI distress.

Monitoring Parameters Monitor blood pressure closely as well as hepatic, hematopoietic, and cardiovascular function; visual field monitoring is recommended (prolactinoma); pregnancy test during amenorrheic period; growth hormone and prolactin levels.

Additional Information Usually used with levodopa or levodopa/carbidopa to treat Parkinson's disease. When adding bromocriptine, the dose of levodopa/carbidopa can usually be decreased.

Dosage Forms Excipient information presented when available (limited, particularly for generics); consult specific product labeling.

Capsule, as mesylate: 5 mg

Parlodel®: 5 mg

Tablet, as mesylate: 2.5 mg

Parlodel® SnapTabs®: 2.5 mg

◆ **Bromocriptine Mesylate** *see* Bromocriptine *on page 202*

◆ **Bromphenex DM** *see* Brompheniramine, Pseudoephedrine, and Dextromethorphan *on page 208*

Brompheniramine (brome fen IR a meen)

U.S. Brand Names B-Vex; Bidhist; BroveX™; BroveX™ CT; Lodrane® 12 Hour; Lodrane® 24; Lodrane® XR; LoHist-12; TanaCof-XR

Index Terms Brompheniramine Maleate; Brompheniramine Tannate

Pharmacologic Category Histamine H_1 Antagonist; Histamine H_1 Antagonist, First Generation

Use Symptomatic relief of perennial and seasonal allergic rhinitis, vasomotor rhinitis, and other respiratory allergies

Effect on Mental Status May cause agitation, confusion, dizziness, drowsiness, or fatigue. May cause paradoxical excitation in pediatric patients; may cause hallucinations in overdose.

Effect on Psychiatric Treatment Concurrent use with psychotropics may produce additive anticholinergic and/or sedative effects; monitor

Dosage Summary

Oral:

Children <1 year: Dosage not established

Children 1-2 years: B-Vex, BroveX™: 1.25 mL every 12 hours (maximum: 2.5 mL/day)

Children 2-6 years:

B-Vex, BroveX™: 2.5 mL every 12 hours (maximum: 5 mL/day)

BroveX™ CT: 1/2 tablet every 12 hours (maximum: 1 tablet/day)

Lodrane® XR, TanaCof-XR: 1.25 mL every 12 hours (maximum: 2.5 mL/day)

Children 6-12 years:

B-Vex, BroveX™: 5 mL every 12 hours (maximum: 10 mL/day)

BroveX™ CT: 1/2 to 1 tablet every 12 hours (maximum: 2 tablets/day)

Lodrane® 12 Hour, LoHist-12: One tablet every 12 hours (maximum: 2 tablets/day)

Lodrane® 24: One capsule once daily

Lodrane® XR, TanaCof-XR: 2.5 mL every 12 hours (maximum: 5 mL/day)

Children >12 years:

B-Vex, BroveX™: 5-10 mL every 12 hours (maximum: 20 mL/day)

BroveX™ CT: 1-2 tablets every 12 hours (maximum: 4 tablets/day)

Lodrane® 12 Hour, LoHist: 1-2 tablets every 12 hours (maximum: 4 tablets/day)

Lodrane® 24: 1-2 capsules once daily

Lodrane® XR, TanaCof-XR: 5 mL every 12 hours (maximum: 10 mL/day)

Adults:

B-Vex, BroveX™: 5-10 mL every 12 hours (maximum: 20 mL/day)

BroveX™ CT: 1-2 tablets every 12 hours (maximum: 4 tablets/day)

Lodrane® 12 Hour, LoHist: 1-2 tablets every 12 hours (maximum: 4 tablets/day)

Lodrane® 24: 1-2 capsules once daily

Lodrane® XR, TanaCof-XR: 5 mL every 12 hours (maximum: 10 mL/day)

Elderly (also refer to adult dosing): Initial:

B-Vex, BroveX™: 5 mL every 12 hours

BroveX™ CT, Lodrane® 12 Hour, LoHist: 1 tablet every 12 hours

Lodrane® 24: 1 capsule/24 hours

Lodrane® XR, TanaCof-XR: 2.5 mL every 12 hours

Dosage Forms Excipient information presented when available (limited, particularly for generics); consult specific product labeling.

Capsule, extended release:

Lodrane® 24: 12 mg [dye free]

Suspension, as tannate:

B-Vex, BroveX™: 12 mg/5 mL (120 mL) [contains sodium benzoate and tartrazine; banana flavor]

Lodrane® XR: 8 mg/5 mL (480 mL) [alcohol free, sugar free; strawberry flavor]

TanaCof-XR: 8 mg/5 mL (480 mL) [alcohol free, sugar free; contains phenylalanine; strawberry creme flavor]

Tablet, chewable, as tannate: 12 mg

BroveX™ CT: 12 mg [banana flavor]

Tablet, extended release, as maleate:

Bidhist: 6 mg

Tablet, extended release, as maleate [scored]:

Lodrane® 12 Hour, LoHist-12: 6 mg [dye free]

Tablet, timed release, as maleate: 6 mg

Brompheniramine and Pseudoephedrine

(brome fen IR a meen & soo doe e FED rin)

Medication Safety Issues

Sound-alike/look-alike issues:

Bromfed® may be confused with Bromphen®

U.S. Brand Names AccuHist®; Andehist NR Syrup; Bromaline® [OTC]; Bromfenex® PD [DSC]; Bromfenex® [DSC]; Bromhist Pediatric; Bromhist-NR; Brotapp; Brovex SR; Dimaphen [OTC]; Histex® SR; Lodrane® 12D; Lodrane® 24D; Lodrane® D; Lodrane® [DSC]; LoHist 12D; LoHist LQ; LoHist PD; Respahist®; Sildec Syrup; Touro® Allergy

Mexican Brand Names Dimetapp

Index Terms Brompheniramine Maleate and Pseudoephedrine Hydrochloride; Brompheniramine Maleate and Pseudoephedrine Sulfate; Pseudoephedrine and Brompheniramine

Pharmacologic Category Alpha/Beta Agonist; Histamine H_1 Antagonist; Histamine H_1 Antagonist, First Generation

Use Temporary relief of symptoms of seasonal and perennial allergic rhinitis, and vasomotor rhinitis, including nasal obstruction

Effect on Mental Status Drowsiness, nervousness, insomnia, and slight stimulation are common; may cause fatigue or dizziness; may rarely cause depression or hallucinations

Effect on Psychiatric Treatment Concurrent use with psychotropics and other CNS depressants may produce additive adverse effects; tachycardia is common; use caution with clozapine and TCAs

Dosage Forms Excipient information presented when available (limited, particularly for generics); consult specific product labeling. [DSC] = Discontinued product

Caplet, extended release:

Histex® SR: Brompheniramine maleate 10 mg and pseudoephedrine hydrochloride 120 mg

Capsule, extended release:

Bromfenex®: Brompheniramine maleate 12 mg and pseudoephedrine hydrochloride 120 mg [DSC]

Bromfenex® PD: Brompheniramine maleate 6 mg and pseudoephedrine hydrochloride 60 mg [DSC]

Lodrane® 24D: Brompheniramine maleate 12 mg and pseudoephedrine hydrochloride 90 mg

Capsule, sustained release:

Brovex SR: Brompheniramine maleate 9 mg and pseudoephedrine hydrochloride 90 mg

Respahist®: Brompheniramine maleate 6 mg and pseudoephedrine hydrochloride 60 mg

Touro® Allergy: Brompheniramine maleate 5.75 mg and pseudoephedrine hydrochloride 60 mg [DSC]

Elixir:

Dimaphen: Brompheniramine maleate 1 mg and pseudoephedrine hydrochloride 15 mg per 5 mL (120 mL, 480 mL)

Liquid: Brompheniramine maleate 4 mg and pseudoephedrine hydrochloride 60 mg per 5 mL (480 mL)

Brotapp: Brompheniramine maleate 1 mg and pseudoephedrine hydrochloride 15 mg per 5 mL (120 mL, 240 mL, 480 mL) [grape flavor]

Lodrane®: Brompheniramine maleate 4 mg and pseudoephedrine hydrochloride 60 mg per 5 mL (480 mL) [alcohol free, dye free, sugar free; cherry flavor] [DSC]

LoHist LQ: Brompheniramine maleate 4 mg and pseudoephedrine hydrochloride 60 mg per 5 mL (480 mL) [cherry flavor]

Liquid, oral [drops]:

AccuHist®: Brompheniramine maleate 1 mg and pseudoephedrine hydrochloride 12.5 mg per 1 mL (30 mL) [sugar free; cherry flavor]

Bromhist NR: Brompheniramine maleate 1 mg and pseudoephedrine hydrochloride 12.5 mg per 1 mL (30 mL) [cherry flavor]

Bromhist Pediatric: Brompheniramine maleate 1 mg and pseudoephedrine hydrochloride 15 mg per 1 mL (30 mL) [cherry flavor]

LoHist PD: Brompheniramine maleate 1 mg and pseudoephedrine hydrochloride 12.5 mg per 1 mL (30 mL) [cherry flavor]

Solution:

Bromaline®: Brompheniramine maleate 1 mg and pseudoephedrine hydrochloride 15 mg per 5 mL (120 mL, 480 mL) [alcohol free; contains sodium benzoate; grape flavor]

Suspension:

Lodrane® D: Brompheniramine tannate 8 mg and pseudoephedrine tannate 90 mg per 5 mL (480 mL) [alcohol free, sugar free; strawberry flavor]

Syrup:

Andehist NR: Brompheniramine maleate 4 mg and pseudoephedrine sulfate 45 mg per 5 mL (473 mL) [raspberry flavor]

Sildec: Brompheniramine maleate 4 mg and pseudoephedrine hydrochloride 45 mg per 5 mL (480 mL) [raspberry flavor]

Tablet, extended release:

Lodrane® 12D: Brompheniramine maleate 6 mg and pseudoephedrine hydrochloride 45 mg [dye free]

LoHist 12D: Brompheniramine maleate 6 mg and pseudoephedrine hydrochloride 45 mg

Tablet, prolonged release:
Touro® Allergy: Brompheniramine maleate 6 mg and pseudoephedrine hydrochloride 45 mg
Tablet, sustained release: Brompheniramine maleate 6 mg and pseudoephedrine hydrochloride 45 mg

- **Brompheniramine Maleate** *see* Brompheniramine *on page 205*
- **Brompheniramine Maleate and Pseudoephedrine Hydrochloride** *see* Brompheniramine and Pseudoephedrine *on page 206*
- **Brompheniramine Maleate and Pseudoephedrine Sulfate** *see* Brompheniramine and Pseudoephedrine *on page 206*

Brompheniramine, Pseudoephedrine, and Dextromethorphan

(brome fen IR a meen, soo doe e FED rin, & deks troe meth OR fan)

U.S. Brand Names AccuHist® PDX Drops; AllanHist PDX; Anaplex® DM; Anaplex® DMX; Andehist DM NR; Bromaline® DM [OTC]; Bromatane DX; Brometane DX [DSC]; Bromhist DM; Bromhist PDX; Bromphenex DM; Bromplex DX; Brotapp-DM; Carbofed DM; EndaCof-DM; EndaCof-PD; Histacol™ BD; Myphetane DX; PediaHist DM

Index Terms Dextromethorphan Hydrobromide, Brompheniramine Maleate, and Pseudoephedrine Hydrochloride; Pseudoephedrine Tannate, Dextromethorphan Tannate, and Brompheniramine Tannate

Pharmacologic Category Alpha/Beta Agonist; Antitussive; Histamine H_1 Antagonist; Histamine H_1 Antagonist, First Generation

Use Relief of cough and upper respiratory symptoms (including nasal congestion) associated with allergy or the common cold

Effect on Mental Status May cause CNS stimulation, insomnia, dizziness, hallucinations, irritability, nervousness, and drowsiness

Effect on Psychiatric Treatment Contraindicated with MAO inhibitors

Dosage Summary

Oral:

Children 1-3 months: AccuHist® PDX, EndaCof-PD: 0.25 mL 4 times/day
Children 3-6 months: AccuHist® PDX, EndaCof-PD: 0.5 mL 4 times/day
Children 6-12 months: AccuHist® PDX, EndaCof-PD: 0.75 mL 4 times/day
Children 12-24 months: AccuHist® PDX, EndaCof-PD:1 mL 4 times/day
Children 2-6 years:
Anaplex® DM, EndaCof-DM: 1.25 mL every 4-6 hours (maximum: 4 doses/day)
Anaplex® DMX: 1.25 mL every 12 hours (maximum: 2.5 mL/day)
Children 6-12 years:
Anaplex® DM, EndaCof-DM: 2.5 mL every 4-6 hours (maximum: 4 doses/day)
Anaplex® DMX: 2.5 mL every 12 hours (maximum: 5 mL/day)
Bromaline® DM, Dimaphen DM, Dimetapp® DM Children's Cough and Cold: 10 mL every 4-6 hours (maximum: 4 doses/day)
Children >12 years:
Anaplex® DM, EndaCof-DM: 5 mL every 4-6 hours (maximum: 4 doses/day)
Anaplex® DMX: 5 mL every 12 hours (maximum: 10 mL/day)
Bromaline® DM, Dimaphen DM, Dimetapp® DM Children's Cough and Cold: 20 mL every 4-6 hours (maximum: 4 doses/day)
Adults:
Anaplex® DM, EndaCof-DM: 5 mL every 4-6 hours (maximum: 4 doses/day)
Anaplex® DMX: 5 mL every 12 hours (maximum: 10 mL/day)
Bromaline® DM, Dimaphen DM, Dimetapp® DM Children's Cough and Cold: 20 mL every 4-6 hours (maximum: 4 doses/day)

Dosage Forms Excipient information presented when available (limited, particularly for generics); consult specific product labeling. [DSC] = Discontinued product

Elixir:
Bromaline® DM: Brompheniramine maleate 1 mg, pseudoephedrine hydrochloride 15 mg, and dextromethorphan hydrobromide 5 mg per 5 mL (12 mL, 480 mL) [alcohol free; contains sodium benzoate; grape flavor]

Liquid:
Bromplex DM: Brompheniramine maleate 4 mg, pseudoephedrine hydrochloride 60 mg, and dextromethorphan hydrobromide 30 mg per 5 mL (48 mL) [alcohol free, dye free, sugar free]

Brotapp-DM: Brompheniramine maleate 1 mg, pseudoephedrine hydrochloride 15 mg, and dextromethorphan hydrobromide 5 mg per 5 mL (120 mL, 240 mL) [grape flavor]

Solution, oral [drops]:

AccuHist® PDX, AllanHist PDX: Brompheniramine maleate 1 mg, pseudoephedrine hydrochloride 12.5 mg, and dextromethorphan hydrobromide 3 mg per 1 mL (30 mL) [alcohol free, sugar free; contains sodium benzoate; grape flavor]

Bromhist DM, PediaHist DM: Brompheniramine maleate 1 mg, pseudoephedrine hydrochloride 15 mg, and dextromethorphan hydrobromide 4 mg per 1 mL (30 mL) [grape flavor]

Bromhist PDX, EndaCof-PD: Brompheniramine maleate 1 mg, pseudoephedrine hydrochloride 12.5 mg, and dextromethorphan hydrobromide 3 mg per 1 mL (30 mL) [grape flavor]

Histacol™ BD: Brompheniramine maleate 1 mg, pseudoephedrine hydrochloride 12.5 mg, and dextromethorphan hydrobromide 3 mg per 1 mL (30 mL) [contains sodium benzoate; grape flavor]

Suspension: Brompheniramine tannate 8 mg, pseudoephedrine tannate 90 mg, and dextromethorphan tannate 60 mg per 5 mL (480 mL)

Anaplex® DMX: Brompheniramine tannate 8 mg, pseudoephedrine tannate 90 mg, and dextromethorphan tannate 60 mg per 5 mL (480 mL) [alcohol free, sugar free; grape flavor]

Syrup: Brompheniramine maleate 4 mg, pseudoephedrine hydrochloride 60 mg, and dextromethorphan hydrobromide 30 mg per 5 mL (480 mL)

Anaplex® DM: Brompheniramine maleate 4 mg, pseudoephedrine hydrochloride 60 mg, and dextromethorphan hydrobromide 30 mg per 5 mL (480 mL) [alcohol free, dye free, sugar free; fruit flavor]

Andehist DM NR: Brompheniramine maleate 4 mg, pseudoephedrine hydrochloride 45 mg, and dextromethorphan hydrobromide 15 mg per 5 mL (480 mL) [grape flavor]

Bromatane DX, Brometane DX [DSC]: Brompheniramine maleate 2 mg, pseudoephedrine hydrochloride 30 mg, and dextromethorphan hydrobromide 10 mg per 5 mL (480 mL)

Bromphenex DM: Brompheniramine maleate 4 mg, pseudoephedrine hydrochloride 60 mg, and dextromethorphan hydrobromide 30 mg per 5 mL (480 mL) [alcohol free, dye free, sugar free; fruit flavor]

Carbofed DM: Brompheniramine maleate 4 mg, pseudoephedrine hydrochloride 45 mg, and dextromethorphan hydrobromide 15 mg per 5 mL (480 mL) [alcohol free, sugar free; grape flavor]

EndaCof-DM: Brompheniramine maleate 4 mg, pseudoephedrine hydrochloride 60 mg, and dextromethorphan hydrobromide 30 mg per 5 mL (480 mL) [alcohol free, dye free, sugar free; fruit flavor]

Myphetane DX: Brompheniramine maleate 2 mg, pseudoephedrine hydrochloride 30 mg, and dextromethorphan hydrobromide 10 mg per 5 mL (480 mL) [contains alcohol <1%; butterscotch flavor]

Sildec-DM: Brompheniramine maleate 4 mg, pseudoephedrine hydrochloride 45 mg, and dextromethorphan hydrobromide 15 mg per 5 mL (480 mL) [grape flavor]

- ◆ **Brompheniramine Tannate** *see* Brompheniramine *on page 205*
- ◆ **Bromplex DX** *see* Brompheniramine, Pseudoephedrine, and Dextromethorphan *on page 208*
- ◆ **Brontex®** *see* Guaifenesin and Codeine *on page 738*
- ◆ **Brotapp** *see* Brompheniramine and Pseudoephedrine *on page 206*
- ◆ **Brotapp-DM** *see* Brompheniramine, Pseudoephedrine, and Dextromethorphan *on page 208*
- ◆ **Brovana®** *see* Arformoterol *on page 131*
- ◆ **BroveX™** *see* Brompheniramine *on page 205*
- ◆ **BroveX™ CT** *see* Brompheniramine *on page 205*
- ◆ **Brovex SR** *see* Brompheniramine and Pseudoephedrine *on page 206*
- ◆ **B-Tuss™** *see* Phenylephrine, Hydrocodone, and Chlorpheniramine *on page 1277*
- ◆ **BTX-A** *see* Botulinum Toxin Type A *on page 193*
- ◆ **B-type Natriuretic Peptide (Human)** *see* Nesiritide *on page 1123*
- ◆ **Budeprion XL®** *see* BuPROPion *on page 217*
- ◆ **Budeprion™ SR** *see* BuPROPion *on page 217*

Budesonide (byoo DES oh nide)

U.S. Brand Names Entocort® EC; Pulmicort Flexhaler™; Pulmicort Respules®; Rhinocort® Aqua®

Canadian Brand Names Entocort®; Gen-Budesonide AQ; Pulmicort®; Rhinocort® Aqua™; Rhinocort® Turbuhaler®

Mexican Brand Names Aerosial; Entocort; Miflonide; Numark; Pulmicort; Rhinocort

Pharmacologic Category Corticosteroid, Inhalant (Oral); Corticosteroid, Nasal; Corticosteroid, Systemic

Use

Intranasal: Management of symptoms of seasonal or perennial rhinitis

Canadian labeling: Additional use (not in U.S. labeling): Prevention and treatment of nasal polyps

Nebulization: Maintenance and prophylactic treatment of asthma

Oral capsule: Treatment of active Crohn's disease (mild-to-moderate) involving the ileum and/or ascending colon; maintenance of remission (for up to 3 months) of Crohn's disease (mild-to-moderate) involving the ileum and/or ascending colon

Oral inhalation: Maintenance and prophylactic treatment of asthma; includes patients who require oral corticosteroids and those who may benefit from systemic dose reduction/elimination

Effect on Mental Status May cause nervousness and insomnia

Effect on Psychiatric Treatment None reported

Dosage Summary

Inhalation:

Children <6 years: Dosage not established

Children ≥6 years: 180-360 mcg twice daily; Low dose: 180-400 mcg/day in 2 divided doses; Medium dose: >400-800 mcg/day in 2 divided doses; High dose: >800 mcg/day in 2 divided doses

Adults: 180-720 mcg twice daily, Low dose: 180-600 mcg/day in 2 divided doses; Medium dose: >600-1200 mcg/day in 2 divided doses; High dose: >1200 mcg/day in 2 divided doses

Intranasal:

Children <6 years: Dosage not established

Children ≥6 years: 64 mcg/day as a single 32 mcg spray in each nostril (maximum: 129 mcg/day [children <12 years])

Adults: 64 mcg/day as a single 32 mcg spray in each nostril (maximum: 256 mcg/day)

Nebulization:

Children <12 months: Dosage not established

Children 12 months to 8 years: 0.25-1 mg in 1-2 divided doses

Children >8 years: Dosage not established

Adults: Dosage not established

Oral:

Children: Dosage not established

Adults: Initial: 9 mg once daily; maintenance: 6 mg once daily

Dosage Forms Excipient information presented when available (limited, particularly for generics); consult specific product labeling. [CAN] = Canadian brand name; [DSC] = Discontinued product

Capsule, enteric coated:

Entocort® EC: 3 mg

Powder for nasal inhalation:

Rhinocort® Turbuhaler® [CAN]: 100 mcg/inhalation [delivers 200 metered actuations] [not available in the U.S.]

Powder for oral inhalation:

Pulmicort Flexhaler™: 90 mcg/inhalation (165 mg) [delivers ~80 mcg/inhalation; 60 actuations]

Pulmicort Flexhaler™: 180 mcg/inhalation (225 mg) [delivers ~160 mcg/inhalation; 120 actuations]

Pulmicort Turbuhaler® [CAN]: 100 mcg/inhalation [delivers 200 metered actuations]; 200 mcg/inhalation [delivers 200 metered actuations]; 400 mcg/inhalation [delivers 200 metered actuations] [not available in the U.S.]

Suspension, intranasal [spray]:

Rhinocort® Aqua®: 32 mcg/inhalation (8.6 g) [120 metered actuations]

Rhinocort® Aqua® [CAN]: 64 mcg/inhalation [120 metered actuations] [not available in the U.S.]

Suspension for nebulization:

Pulmicort Respules®: 0.25 mg/2 mL (2 mL); 0.5 mg/2 mL (2 mL); 1 mg/2 mL (2 mL)

- ◆ **Buffasal [OTC]** *see* Aspirin *on page 143*
- ◆ **Buffered Aspirin and Pravastatin Sodium** *see* Aspirin and Pravastatin *on page 146*
- ◆ **Bufferin® [OTC]** *see* Aspirin *on page 143*
- ◆ **Bufferin® Extra Strength [OTC]** *see* Aspirin *on page 143*
- ◆ **Buffinol [OTC]** *see* Aspirin *on page 143*

Bumetanide (byoo MET a nide)

Medication Safety Issues

Sound-alike/look-alike issues:

Bumetanide may be confused with Buminate®

Bumex® may be confused with Brevibloc®, Buprenex®, Permax®

U.S. Brand Names Bumex®

Canadian Brand Names Bumex®; Burinex®

Mexican Brand Names Drenural; Miccil

Pharmacologic Category Diuretic, Loop

Use Management of edema secondary to congestive heart failure or hepatic or renal disease including nephrotic syndrome; may be used alone or in combination with antihypertensives in the treatment of hypertension; can be used in furosemide-allergic patients

Effect on Mental Status May cause dizziness

Effect on Psychiatric Treatment Lithium excretion may be decreased; monitor serum lithium levels

Dosage Summary

I.M.:

Neonates: 0.01-0.05 mg/kg/dose every 24-48 hours

Infants and children: 0.015-0.1 mg/kg/dose every 6-24 hours (maximum: 10 mg/day)

Adults: 0.5-1 mg/dose, may repeat in 2-3 hours for up to 2 doses (maximum: 10 mg/day)

I.V.:

Neonates: 0.01-0.05 mg/kg/dose every 24-48 hours

Infants and children: 0.015-0.1 mg/kg/dose every 6-24 hours (maximum: 10 mg/day)

Adults: 0.5-1 mg/dose, may repeat in 2-3 hours for up to 2 doses (maximum: 10 mg/day) **or** 1 mg bolus followed by 0.5-2 mg/hour

Oral:

Neonates: 0.01-0.05 mg/kg/dose every 24-48 hours

Infants and children: 0.015-0.1 mg/kg/dose every 6-24 hours (maximum: 10 mg/day)

Adults: 0.5-2 mg 1-2 times/day (maximum: 5 mg/day [HTN]; 10 mg/day [edema])

Elderly: Initial: 0.5 mg once daily

Dosage Forms Excipient information presented when available (limited, particularly for generics); consult specific product labeling. [DSC] = Discontinued product

Injection, solution: 0.25 mg/mL (2 mL, 4 mL, 10 mL)

Tablet: 0.5 mg, 1 mg, 2 mg

Bumex®: 0.5 mg [DSC]; 1 mg; 2 mg [DSC]

- ◆ **Bumex®** *see* Bumetanide *on page 211*
- ◆ **Bupap** *see* Butalbital and Acetaminophen *on page 236*

Bupivacaine (byoo PIV a kane)

Medication Safety Issues

Sound-alike/look-alike issues:

Bupivacaine may be confused with mepivacaine, ropivacaine

Marcaine® may be confused with Narcan®

High alert medication: The Institute for Safe Medication Practices (ISMP) includes this medication (epidural administration) among its list of drug classes which have a heightened risk of causing significant patient harm when used in error.

U.S. Brand Names Marcaine®; Marcaine® Spinal; Sensorcaine®; Sensorcaine®-MPF; Sensorcaine®-MPF Spinal

Canadian Brand Names Marcaine®; Sensorcaine®

Index Terms Bupivacaine Hydrochloride

Pharmacologic Category Local Anesthetic

Use Local anesthetic (injectable) for peripheral nerve block, infiltration, sympathetic block, caudal or epidural block, retrobulbar block

Effect on Mental Status May cause anxiety and restlessness

Effect on Psychiatric Treatment Use with caution in patients receiving phenothiazines, MAO inhibitors, or TCAs; severe hypertension or hypotension may result

Dosage Summary Note: Dose varies with procedure, depth of anesthesia, vascularity of tissues, duration of anesthesia, and condition of patient. Do not use solutions containing preservatives for caudal or epidural block.

Caudal block:

Children ≤12 years: Dosage not established

Children >12 years: 15-30 mL of 0.25% or 0.5%

Adults: 15-30 mL of 0.25% or 0.5%

Epidural block:

Children ≤12 years: Dosage not established

Children >12 years: 10-20 mL of 0.25% or 0.5% in 3-5 mL increments **or** 10-20 mL of 0.75% if high degree of muscle relaxation and prolonged effects needed

Adults: 10-20 mL of 0.25% or 0.5% in 3-5 mL increments **or** 10-20 mL of 0.75% if high degree of muscle relaxation and prolonged effects needed

Infiltration (local):

Children ≤12 years: Dosage not established

Children >12 years: 0.25% (maximum: 175 mg)

Adults: 0.25% (maximum: 175 mg)

Nerve block:

Children ≤12 years: Dosage not established

Children >12 years: Peripheral: 5 mL of 0.25% or 0.5% (maximum: 400 mg/day); Sympathetic: 20-50 mL of 0.25%

Adults: Peripheral: 5 mL of 0.25% or 0.5% (maximum: 400 mg/day); Sympathetic: 20-50 mL of 0.25%

Retrobulbar anesthesia:

Children ≤12 years: Dosage not established

Children >12 years: 2-4 mL of 0.75%

Adults: 2-4 mL of 0.75%

Spinal:

Children: Dosage not established

Adults: Preservative free solution of 0.75% bupivacaine in 8.25% dextrose:

Cesarean section: 1-1.4 mL

Lower abdominal procedures: 1.6 mL

Lower extremity and perineal procedures: 1 mL

Normal vaginal delivery: 0.8 mL (higher doses may be required in some patients)

Dosage Forms Excipient information presented when available (limited, particularly for generics); consult specific product labeling.

Injection, solution, as hydrochloride [preservative free]: 0.25% (10 mL, 20 mL, 30 mL, 50 mL); 0.5% (10 mL, 20 mL, 30 mL); 0.75% (10 mL, 20 mL, 30 mL)

Marcaine®: 0.25% (10 mL, 30 mL); 0.5% (10 mL, 30 mL); 0.75% (10 mL, 30 mL)

Sensorcaine®-MPF: 0.25% (10 mL, 30 mL); 0.5% (10 mL, 30 mL); 0.75% (10 mL, 30 mL)

Injection, solution, as hydrochloride [preservative free]: 0.75% (2 mL) [in dextrose 8.25%]

Marcaine® Spinal: 0.75% (2 mL) [in dextrose 8.25%]

Sensorcaine®-MPF Spinal: 0.75% (2 mL) [in dextrose 8.25%]

Injection, solution, as hydrochloride:

Marcaine®, Sensorcaine®: 0.25% (50 mL); 0.5% (50 mL) [contains methylparaben]

◆ **Bupivacaine Hydrochloride** *see* Bupivacaine *on page 211*

◆ **Buprenex®** *see* Buprenorphine *on page 212*

Buprenorphine (byoo pre NOR feen)

Medication Safety Issues

Sound-alike/look-alike issues:

Buprenex® may be confused with Brevibloc®, Bumex®

High alert medication: The Institute for Safe Medication Practices (ISMP) includes this medication among its list of drug classes which have a heightened risk of causing significant patient harm when used in error.

Related Information

Addiction Treatments *on page 1817*

Narcotic / Opioid Analgesics *on page 1789*

U.S. Brand Names Buprenex®; Subutex®

Canadian Brand Names Buprenex®; Subutex®

Mexican Brand Names Brospina; Temgesic; Transtec

Index Terms Buprenorphine Hydrochloride

Pharmacologic Category Analgesic, Opioid

Generic Available Yes: Injection

Use

Injection: Management of moderate to severe pain

Tablet: Treatment of opioid dependence

Unlabeled/Investigational Use Injection: Heroin and opioid withdrawal

Effect on Mental Status Drowsiness is common; rare reports of euphoria

Effect on Psychiatric Treatment Concurrent use with benzodiazepines or barbiturates may result in CNS or respiratory depression

Restrictions Injection: C-V/C-III; Tablet: C-III

Prescribing of tablets for opioid dependence is limited to physicians who have met the qualification criteria and have received a DEA number specific to prescribing this product. Tablets will be available through pharmacies and wholesalers which normally provide controlled substances.

Pregnancy Risk Factor C

Pregnancy Considerations Withdrawal has been reported in infants of women receiving buprenorphine during pregnancy. Onset of symptoms ranged from day 1 to day 8 of life, most occurring on day 1.

Lactation Enters breast milk/not recommended

Contraindications Hypersensitivity to buprenorphine or any component of the formulation

Warnings/Precautions An opioid-containing analgesic regimen should be tailored to each patient's needs and based upon the type of pain being treated (acute versus chronic), the route of administration, degree of tolerance for opioids (naive versus chronic user), age, weight, and medical condition. The optimal analgesic dose varies widely among patients. Doses should be titrated to pain relief/prevention.

May cause CNS depression, which may impair physical or mental abilities. Effects with other sedative drugs or ethanol may be potentiated. Elderly may be more sensitive to CNS depressant and constipating effects. May cause respiratory depression - use caution in patients with respiratory disease or pre-existing respiratory depression. Potential for drug dependency exists, abrupt cessation may precipitate withdrawal. Use caution in elderly, debilitated, pediatric patients, depression or suicidal tendencies. Tolerance, psychological and physical dependence may occur with prolonged use. Partial antagonist activity may precipitate acute narcotic withdrawal in opioid-dependent individuals.

Use with caution in patients with hepatic, pulmonary, or renal function impairment. Also use caution in patients with head injury or increased ICP, biliary tract dysfunction, patients with history of hyperthyroidism, morbid obesity, adrenal insufficiency, prostatic hyperplasia, urinary stricture, CNS depression, toxic psychosis, pancreatitis, alcoholism, delirium tremens, or kyphoscoliosis. May cause hypotension; use with caution in patients with hypovolemia, cardiovascular disease (including acute MI), or drugs which may exaggerate hypotensive effects (including phenothiazines or general anesthetics). May obscure diagnosis or clinical course of patients with acute abdominal conditions.

Tablets, which are used for induction treatment of opioid dependence, should not be started until effects of withdrawal are evident. Safety and efficacy of the tablet formulation have not been established in children <16 years of age; safety and efficacy of the injection formulation have not been established in children <2 years of age.

Adverse Reactions

Injection:

>10%: Central nervous system: Sedation

1% to 10%:

Cardiovascular: Hypotension

Central nervous system: Respiratory depression, dizziness, headache

Gastrointestinal: Vomiting, nausea

Ocular: Miosis

Otic: Vertigo

Miscellaneous: Diaphoresis

<1% (Limited to important or life-threatening): Agitation, allergic reaction, apnea, appetite decreased, blurred vision, bradycardia, confusion,

constipation, convulsion, coma, cyanosis, depersonalization, depression, diplopia, dyspnea, dysphoria, euphoria, fatigue, flatulence, flushing, hallucinations, hypertension, injection site reaction, malaise, nervousness, pallor, paresthesia, pruritus, psychosis, rash, slurred speech, tachycardia, tinnitus, tremor, urinary retention, urticaria, weakness, Wenckebach block, xerostomia

Tablet:

>10%:

Central nervous system: Headache (30%), pain (24%), insomnia (21% to 25%), anxiety (12%), depression (11%)

Gastrointestinal: Nausea (10% to 14%), abdominal pain (12%), constipation (8% to 11%)

Neuromuscular & skeletal: Back pain (14%), weakness (14%)

Respiratory: Rhinitis (11%)

Miscellaneous: Withdrawal syndrome (19%; placebo 37%), infection (12% to 20%), diaphoresis (12% to 13%)

1% to 10%:

Central nervous system: Chills (6%), nervousness (6%), somnolence (5%), dizziness (4%), fever (3%)

Gastrointestinal: Vomiting (5% to 8%), diarrhea (5%), dyspepsia (3%)

Ocular: Lacrimation (5%)

Respiratory: Cough (4%), pharyngitis (4%)

Miscellaneous: Flu-like syndrome (6%)

Metabolism/Transport Effects Substrate of CYP3A4 (major); **Inhibits** CYP1A2 (weak), 2A6 (weak), 2C19 (weak), 2D6 (weak)

Drug Interactions

Alcohol (Ethyl): CNS Depressants may enhance the CNS depressant effect of Alcohol (Ethyl). *Risk C: Monitor therapy*

Alvimopan: Analgesics (Opioid) may enhance the adverse/toxic effect of Alvimopan. This is most notable for patients receiving long-term (i.e., more than 7 days) opiates prior to alvimopan initiation. Management: Alvimopan is contraindicated in patients receiving therapeutic doses of opioids for more than 7 consecutive days immediately prior to alvimopan initiation. *Risk D: Consider therapy modification*

Ammonium Chloride: May increase the excretion of Analgesics (Opioid). *Risk C: Monitor therapy*

Amphetamines: May enhance the analgesic effect of Analgesics (Opioid). *Risk C: Monitor therapy*

Antipsychotic Agents (Phenothiazines): May enhance the hypotensive effect of Analgesics (Opioid). *Risk C: Monitor therapy*

Atazanavir: May increase the serum concentration of Buprenorphine. *Risk C: Monitor therapy*

CNS Depressants: May enhance the adverse/toxic effect of other CNS Depressants. *Risk C: Monitor therapy*

CYP3A4 Inducers (Strong): May increase the metabolism of CYP3A4 Substrates. *Risk C: Monitor therapy*

CYP3A4 Inhibitors (Moderate): May decrease the metabolism of CYP3A4 Substrates. *Risk C: Monitor therapy*

CYP3A4 Inhibitors (Strong): May decrease the metabolism of CYP3A4 Substrates. *Risk D: Consider therapy modification*

Dasatinib: May increase the serum concentration of CYP3A4 Substrates. *Risk C: Monitor therapy*

Deferasirox: May decrease the serum concentration of CYP3A4 Substrates. *Risk C: Monitor therapy*

Desmopressin: Analgesics (Opioid) may enhance the adverse/toxic effect of Desmopressin. *Risk C: Monitor therapy*

Herbs (CYP3A4 Inducers): May increase the metabolism of CYP3A4 Substrates. *Risk C: Monitor therapy*

Pegvisomant: Analgesics (Opioid) may diminish the therapeutic effect of Pegvisomant. *Risk C: Monitor therapy*

Selective Serotonin Reuptake Inhibitors: Analgesics (Opioid) may enhance the serotonergic effect of Selective Serotonin Reuptake Inhibitors. This may cause serotonin syndrome. *Risk C: Monitor therapy*

Succinylcholine: May enhance the bradycardic effect of Analgesics (Opioid). *Risk C: Monitor therapy*

Ethanol/Nutrition/Herb Interactions

Ethanol: Avoid ethanol (may increase CNS depression).

Herb/Nutraceutical: Avoid valerian, St John's wort, kava kava, gotu kola (may increase CNS depression).

Stability

Injection: Protect from excessive heat >40°C (>104°F) and light.

Tablet: Store at room temperature of 25°C (77°F).

Mechanism of Action Buprenorphine exerts its analgesic effect via high affinity binding to μ opiate receptors in the CNS; displays both agonist and antagonist activity

Pharmacodynamics/Kinetics

Onset of action: Analgesic: 10-30 minutes
Duration: 6-8 hours
Absorption: I.M., SubQ: 30% to 40%
Distribution: V_d: 97-187 L/kg
Protein binding: High
Metabolism: Primarily hepatic; extensive first-pass effect
Half-life elimination: 2.2-3 hours
Excretion: Feces (70%); urine (20% as unchanged drug)

Dosage Long-term use is not recommended

Note: These are guidelines and do not represent the maximum doses that may be required in all patients. Doses should be titrated to pain relief/prevention. In high-risk patients (eg, elderly, debilitated, presence of respiratory disease) and/or concurrent CNS depressant use, reduce dose by one-half. Buprenorphine has an analgesic ceiling.

Acute pain (moderate to severe):

Children 2-12 years: I.M., slow I.V.: 2-6 mcg/kg every 4-6 hours

Children ≥13 years and Adults:

I.M.: Initial: Opiate-naive: 0.3 mg every 6-8 hours as needed; initial dose (up to 0.3 mg) may be repeated once in 30-60 minutes after the initial dose if needed; usual dosage range: 0.15-0.6 mg every 4-8 hours as needed

Slow I.V.: Initial: Opiate-naive: 0.3 mg every 6-8 hours as needed; initial dose (up to 0.3 mg) may be repeated once in 30-60 minutes after the initial dose if needed

Elderly: I.M., slow I.V.: 0.15 mg every 6 hours; elderly patients are more likely to suffer from confusion and drowsiness compared to younger patients

Heroin or opiate withdrawal (unlabeled use): Children ≥13 years and Adults: I.M., slow I.V.: Variable; 0.1-0.4 mg every 6 hours

Sublingual: Children ≥16 years and Adults: Opioid dependence:

Induction: Range: 12-16 mg/day (doses during an induction study used 8 mg on day 1, followed by 16 mg on day 2; induction continued over 3-4 days). Treatment should begin at least 4 hours after last use of heroin or short-acting opioid, preferably when first signs of withdrawal appear. Titrating dose to clinical effectiveness should be done as rapidly as possible to prevent undue withdrawal symptoms and patient drop-out during the induction period.

Maintenance: Target dose: 16 mg/day; range: 4-24 mg/day; patients should be switched to the buprenorphine/naloxone combination product for maintenance and unsupervised therapy

Administration

I.V.: Administer slowly, over at least 2 minutes.

Sublingual: Tablet should be placed under the tongue until dissolved; should not be swallowed. If two or more tablets are needed per dose, all may be placed under the tongue at once, or two at a time. To ensure consistent bioavailability, subsequent doses should always be taken the same way.

Monitoring Parameters Pain relief, respiratory and mental status, CNS depression, blood pressure; LFTs

Additional Information Subutex® (buprenorphine) should be limited to supervised use whenever possible; patients should be switched to Suboxone® (buprenorphine/naloxone) for maintenance and unsupervised therapy

Dosage Forms Excipient information presented when available (limited, particularly for generics); consult specific product labeling.

Injection, solution: 0.3 mg/mL (1 mL) [C-III]

Buprenex®: 0.3 mg/mL (1 mL) [C-V]

Tablet, sublingual:

Subutex®: 2 mg, 8 mg

Buprenorphine and Naloxone (byoo pre NOR feen & nal OKS one)

Medication Safety Issues

High alert medication: The Institute for Safe Medication Practices (ISMP) includes this medication among its list of drug classes which have a heightened risk of causing significant patient harm when used in error.

Related Information

Addiction Treatments *on page 1817*

U.S. Brand Names Suboxone®

Index Terms Buprenorphine Hydrochloride and Naloxone Hydrochloride Dihydrate; Naloxone and Buprenorphine; Naloxone Hydrochloride Dihydrate and Buprenorphine Hydrochloride

Pharmacologic Category Analgesic, Opioid

Generic Available No

Use Treatment of opioid dependence

Restrictions C-III; Prescribing of tablets for opioid dependence is limited to physicians who have met the qualification criteria and have received a DEA number specific to prescribing this product. Tablets will be available through pharmacies and wholesalers which normally provide controlled substances.

Pregnancy Risk Factor C

Pregnancy Considerations Withdrawal has been reported in infants of women receiving buprenorphine during pregnancy. Onset of symptoms ranged from day 1 to day 8 of life, most occurring on day 1.

Lactation Buprenorphine: Enters breast milk/not recommended

Contraindications Hypersensitivity to buprenorphine, naloxone, or any component of the formulation

Warnings/Precautions May cause respiratory depression - use caution in patients with respiratory disease or pre-existing respiratory depression. Potential for drug dependency exists, abrupt cessation may precipitate withdrawal. Use caution in elderly or debilitated patients. Use with caution in patients with hepatic, pulmonary, or renal function impairment. May cause CNS depression, which may impair physical or mental abilities. Patients must be cautioned about performing tasks which require mental alertness (eg, operating machinery or driving). Effects with other sedative drugs or ethanol may be potentiated. Elderly may be more sensitive to CNS depressant and constipating effects. Use with caution in patients with head injury or increased ICP, biliary tract dysfunction, pancreatitis, patients with history of ileus or bowel obstruction, glaucoma, hyperthyroidism, adrenal insufficiency, prostatic hyperplasia, urinary stricture, CNS depression, toxic psychosis, alcoholism, delirium tremens, kyphoscoliosis or morbidly obese patients. May obscure diagnosis or clinical course of patients with acute abdominal conditions. Partial antagonist activity of buprenorphine may precipitate acute narcotic withdrawal in opioid-dependent individuals upon rapid discontinuation. Naloxone may precipitate intense withdrawal symptoms in patients addicted to opiates when administered before the opioid effects have subsided, or misused parenterally in opioid-dependent individuals. Combination product is indicated for maintenance therapy and should not be used for induction. Oral buprenorphine is not approved for management of pain. Safety and efficacy in patients <16 years of age have not been established.

Adverse Reactions Also see individual agents.

>10%:

Central nervous system: Headache (36%), pain (22%)

Gastrointestinal: Nausea (15%), constipation (12%), abdominal pain (11%)

Miscellaneous: Withdrawal syndrome (25%; placebo 37%), diaphoresis (14%)

1% to 10%:

Cardiovascular: Vasodilation (9%)

Gastrointestinal: Vomiting (7%)

Drug Interactions

Alcohol (Ethyl): CNS Depressants may enhance the CNS depressant effect of Alcohol (Ethyl). *Risk C: Monitor therapy*

Alvimopan: Analgesics (Opioid) may enhance the adverse/toxic effect of Alvimopan. This is most notable for patients receiving long-term (i.e., more than 7 days) opiates prior to alvimopan initiation. Management: Alvimopan is contraindicated in patients receiving therapeutic doses of opioids for more than 7 consecutive days immediately prior to alvimopan initiation. *Risk D: Consider therapy modification*

Ammonium Chloride: May increase the excretion of Analgesics (Opioid). *Risk C: Monitor therapy*

Amphetamines: May enhance the analgesic effect of Analgesics (Opioid). *Risk C: Monitor therapy*

Antipsychotic Agents (Phenothiazines): May enhance the hypotensive effect of Analgesics (Opioid). *Risk C: Monitor therapy*

Atazanavir: May increase the serum concentration of Buprenorphine. *Risk C: Monitor therapy*

CNS Depressants: May enhance the adverse/toxic effect of other CNS Depressants. *Risk C: Monitor therapy*

CYP3A4 Inducers (Strong): May increase the metabolism of CYP3A4 Substrates. *Risk C: Monitor therapy*

CYP3A4 Inhibitors (Moderate): May decrease the metabolism of CYP3A4 Substrates. *Risk C: Monitor therapy*

CYP3A4 Inhibitors (Strong): May decrease the metabolism of CYP3A4 Substrates. *Risk D: Consider therapy modification*

Dasatinib: May increase the serum concentration of CYP3A4 Substrates. *Risk C: Monitor therapy*

Deferasirox: May decrease the serum concentration of CYP3A4 Substrates. *Risk C: Monitor therapy*

Desmopressin: Analgesics (Opioid) may enhance the adverse/toxic effect of Desmopressin. *Risk C: Monitor therapy*

Herbs (CYP3A4 Inducers): May increase the metabolism of CYP3A4 Substrates. *Risk C: Monitor therapy*

Pegvisomant: Analgesics (Opioid) may diminish the therapeutic effect of Pegvisomant. *Risk C: Monitor therapy*

Selective Serotonin Reuptake Inhibitors: Analgesics (Opioid) may enhance the serotonergic effect of Selective Serotonin Reuptake Inhibitors. This may cause serotonin syndrome. *Risk C: Monitor therapy*

Succinylcholine: May enhance the bradycardic effect of Analgesics (Opioid). *Risk C: Monitor therapy*

Stability Store at room temperature of 25°C (77°F).

Mechanism of Action See individual agents.

Pharmacodynamics/Kinetics See individual agents.

Absorption: Absorption of the combination product is variable among patients following sublingual use, but variability within each individual patient is low.

Dosage Sublingual: Children ≥16 years and Adults: Opioid dependence: **Note:** This combination product is not recommended for use during the induction period; initial treatment should begin using buprenorphine oral tablets. Patients should be switched to the combination product for maintenance and unsupervised therapy.

Maintenance: Target dose (based on buprenorphine content): 16 mg/day; range: 4-24 mg/day

Dietary Considerations

Ethanol: Avoid ethanol (may increase CNS depression).

Herb/Nutraceutical: Avoid valerian, St John's wort, kava kava, gotu kola (may increase CNS depression).

Administration Sublingual: Tablet should be placed under the tongue until dissolved; should not be swallowed. If two or more tablets are needed per dose, all may be placed under the tongue at once, or two at a time. To ensure consistent bioavailability, subsequent doses should always be taken the same way.

Monitoring Parameters Respiratory and mental status, CNS depression; symptoms of withdrawal

Dosage Forms Excipient information presented when available (limited, particularly for generics); consult specific product labeling.

Tablet, sublingual: Buprenorphine 2 mg and naloxone 0.5 mg; buprenorphine 8 mg and naloxone 2 mg [lemon-lime flavor]

◆ **Buprenorphine Hydrochloride** *see* Buprenorphine *on page 212*

◆ **Buprenorphine Hydrochloride and Naloxone Hydrochloride Dihydrate** *see* Buprenorphine and Naloxone *on page 215*

◆ **Buproban™** *see* BuPROPion *on page 217*

BuPROPion (byoo PROE pee on)

Medication Safety Issues

Sound-alike/look-alike issues:

BuPROPion may be confused with busPIRone

Wellbutrin SR® may be confused with Wellbutrin XL™

Wellbutrin XL™ may be confused with Wellbutrin SR®

Zyban® may be confused with Zagam®, Diovan®

Related Information

Addiction Treatments *on page 1817*

Antidepressant Agents *on page 1760*

Antidepressant Receptor Profile *on page 1764*

U.S. Brand Names Budeprion XL®; Budeprion™ SR; Buproban™; Wellbutrin SR®; Wellbutrin XL™; Wellbutrin®; Zyban®

Canadian Brand Names Novo-Bupropion SR; Wellbutrin XL™; Wellbutrin®; Zyban®

Mexican Brand Names Wellbutrin

Pharmacologic Category Antidepressant, Dopamine-Reuptake Inhibitor; Smoking Cessation Aid

Generic Available Yes

Use Treatment of major depressive disorder, including seasonal affective disorder (SAD); adjunct in smoking cessation

Unlabeled/Investigational Use Attention-deficit/hyperactivity disorder (ADHD); depression associated with bipolar disorder

Mental Health Comment Bupropion is an activating antidepressant that may be particularly useful for individuals whose depression is associated with fatigue and poor concentration. It is also used as an adjunct in smoking cessation and may benefit those with ADHD. While some evidence suggests that it is less likely to induce mania when used in individuals with bipolar disorder, the trials suggesting this are flawed. It is not associated with withdrawal symptoms so it can be stopped abruptly. Sexual dysfunction, seen commonly with the SSRI, is less problematic with bupropion.

Restrictions An FDA-approved medication guide concerning the use of antidepressants in children, adolescents, and young adults must be distributed when dispensing an outpatient prescription (new or refill) where this medication is to be used without direct supervision of a healthcare provider. Medication guides are available at http://www.fda.gov/cder/Offices/ODS/medication_guides.htm. Dispense to parents or guardians of children and adolescents receiving this medication.

Pregnancy Risk Factor C

Pregnancy Considerations Due to adverse events observed in some animal studies, bupropion is classified as pregnancy category C. A significant increase in major teratogenic effects has not been observed following exposure to bupropion during pregnancy; however, the risk of spontaneous abortions may be increased (additional studies are needed to confirm). The long-term effects on development and behavior have not been studied.

Pregnancy itself does not provide protection against depression. The ACOG recommends that therapy with antidepressants during pregnancy be individualized and should incorporate the clinical expertise of the mental health clinician, obstetrician, primary care provider, and pediatrician. If treatment is needed, consider gradually stopping antidepressants 10-14 days before the expected date of delivery to prevent potential withdrawal symptoms in the infant. If this is done and the woman is considered to be at risk of relapse from her major depressive disorder, the medication can be restarted following delivery, although the dose should be readjusted to that required before pregnancy. Bupropion has also been evaluated for smoking cessation during pregnancy; current recommendations suggest that pharmacologic treatments be considered only after other therapies have failed. A registry has been established for women exposed to bupropion during pregnancy (800-336-2176).

Lactation Enters breast milk/not recommended (AAP rates "of concern")

Contraindications Hypersensitivity to bupropion or any component of the formulation; seizure disorder; anorexia/bulimia; use of MAO inhibitors within 14 days; patients undergoing abrupt discontinuation of ethanol or sedatives (including benzodiazepines); patients receiving other dosage forms of bupropion

Warnings/Precautions **[U.S. Boxed Warning]: Antidepressants increase the risk of suicidal thinking and behavior in children, adolescents, and young adults (18-24 years of age) with major depressive disorder (MDD) and other psychiatric disorders;** consider risk prior to prescribing. Short-term studies did not show an increased risk in patients >24 years of age and showed a decreased risk in patients ≥65 years. All patients must be closely monitored for clinical worsening, suicidality, or unusual changes in behavior, especially during the initiation of therapy (generally first 1-2 months) or following an increase or decrease in dosage. The patient's family or caregiver should be instructed to closely observe the patient and communicate condition with healthcare provider. A medication guide should be dispensed with each prescription. **Bupropion is not FDA approved for use in children.**

The possibility of a suicide attempt is inherent in major depression and may persist until remission occurs. Use caution in high-risk patients. Worsening depression and severe abrupt suicidality that are not part of the presenting symptoms may require discontinuation or modification of drug therapy. The patient's family or caregiver should be alerted to monitor patients for the emergence of suicidality and associated behaviors (such as agitation, irritability hostility, impulsivity, and hypomania) and notify the healthcare provider.

May worsen psychosis in some patients or precipitate a shift to mania or hypomania in patients with bipolar disorder. Patients presenting with depressive symptoms should be screened for bipolar disorder. Monotherapy in patients with bipolar disorder should be avoided. **Bupropion is not FDA approved for bipolar depression.**

The risk of seizures is dose-dependent and increased in patients with a history of seizures, anorexia/bulimia, head trauma, CNS tumor, severe hepatic cirrhosis, abrupt discontinuation of sedative-hypnotics or ethanol, medications which lower seizure threshold (antipsychotics, antidepressants, theophyllines, systemic steroids), stimulants, or hypoglycemic agents. Discontinue and do not restart in patients experiencing a seizure. May cause CNS stimulation (restlessness, anxiety, insomnia) or anorexia. May increase the risks associated with electroconvulsive therapy. Consider discontinuing, when possible, prior to elective surgery. May cause weight loss; use caution in patients where weight loss is not desirable. The incidence of sexual dysfunction with bupropion is generally lower than with SSRIs.

Use caution in patients with cardiovascular disease, history of hypertension, or coronary artery disease; treatment-emergent hypertension (including some severe cases) has been reported, both with bupropion alone and in combination with nicotine transdermal systems. Use with caution in patients with hepatic or renal dysfunction and in elderly patients; reduced dose recommended. Elderly patients may be at greater risk of accumulation during chronic dosing. May cause motor or cognitive impairment in some patients; use with caution if tasks requiring alertness such as operating machinery or driving are undertaken. Arthralgia, myalgia, and fever with rash and other symptoms suggestive of delayed hypersensitivity resembling serum sickness have been reported.

Extended release tablet: Insoluble tablet shell may remain intact and be visible in the stool.

Adverse Reactions Frequencies, when reported, reflect highest incidence reported with sustained release product.

>10%:

Cardiovascular: Tachycardia (11%)

Central nervous system: Headache (25% to 34%), insomnia (11% to 20%), dizziness (6% to 11%)

Gastrointestinal: Xerostomia (17% to 26%), weight loss (14% to 23%), nausea (1% to 18%)

Respiratory: Pharyngitis (3% to 13%)

1% to 10%:

Cardiovascular: Palpitation (2% to 6%), arrhythmias (5%), chest pain (3% to 4%), hypertension (2% to 4%, may be severe), flushing (1% to 4%), hypotension (3%)

Central nervous system: Agitation (2% to 9%), confusion (8%), anxiety (5% to 7%), hostility (6%), nervousness (3% to 5%), sleep disturbance (4%), sensory disturbance (4%), migraine (1% to 4%), abnormal dreams (3%), irritability (2% to 3%), somnolence (2% to 3%), pain (2% to 3%), memory decreased (up to 3%), fever (1% to 2%), CNS stimulation (1% to 2%), depression

Dermatologic: Rash (1% to 5%), pruritus (2% to 4%), urticaria (1% to 2%)

Endocrine & metabolic: Menstrual complaints (2% to 5%), hot flashes (1% to 3%), libido decreased (3%)

Gastrointestinal: Constipation (5% to 10%), abdominal pain (2% to 9%), diarrhea (5% to 7%), flatulence (6%), anorexia (3% to 5%), appetite increased (4%), taste perversion (2% to 4%), vomiting (2% to 4%), dyspepsia (3%), dysphagia (up to 2%)

Genitourinary: Urinary frequency (2% to 5%), urinary urgency (up to 2%), vaginal hemorrhage (up to 2%), UTI (up to 1%)

Neuromuscular & skeletal: Tremor (3% to 6%), myalgia (2% to 6%), weakness (2% to 4%), arthralgia (1% to 4%), arthritis (2%), akathisia (2%), paresthesia (1% to 2%), twitching (1% to 2%), neck pain

Ocular: Amblyopia (2%), blurred vision (2% to 3%)

Otic: Tinnitus (3% to 6%), auditory disturbance (5%)

Respiratory: Upper respiratory infection (9%), cough increased (1% to 4%), sinusitis (1% to 5%)

Miscellaneous: Infection (8% to 9%), diaphoresis increased (5% to 6%), allergic reaction (including anaphylaxis, pruritus, urticaria)

Postmarketing and/or case reports: Accommodation abnormality, aggression, akinesia, alopecia, amnesia, anemia, angioedema, aphasia, ataxia, atrioventricular block, bronchospasm, bruxism, chills, colitis, coma, coordination abnormal, cystitis, deafness, delirium, delusions, depersonalization, derealization, diplopia, dry eye, dysarthria, dyskinesia, dyspareunia, dysphoria, dystonia, ecchymosis, EEG abnormality, ejaculation abnormality, emotional lability, esophagitis, euphoria, exfoliative dermatitis, extrapyramidal syndrome, extrasystoles, facial edema, fever with rash (and other symptoms suggestive of delayed hypersensitivity resembling serum sickness), gastric reflux, gastrointestinal hemorrhage, gingivitis, glossitis, glycosuria, gum hemorrhage, gynecomastia, hallucinations, hepatic damage, hepatitis, hirsutism, hostility, hyper-/hypokinesia, hypertonia, hypoesthesia, hyper-/hypoglycemia, hypomania, impotence, intestinal perforation, intraocular pressure increased, jaundice, leg cramps, leukocytosis, leukopenia, libido increased, liver function abnormal, lymphadenopathy, maculopapular rash, malaise, manic reaction, menopause, MI, mouth ulcers, muscle rigidity, muscle weakness, musculoskeletal chest pain, mydriasis, myoclonus, neuralgia, neuropathy, painful erection, pancreatitis, pancytopenia, paranoia, paranoid reaction, phlebitis, pneumonia, photosensitivity, postural hypotension, prostate disorder, pulmonary embolism, restlessness, rhabdomyolysis, salivation increased, salpingitis, sciatica, seizure, SIADH, stomach ulcer, stomatitis, stroke, suicidal ideation, syncope, tardive dyskinesia, thirst, thrombocytopenia, tongue edema, urinary incontinence, urinary retention, vaginitis, vasodilation, vertigo

Metabolism/Transport Effects Substrate of CYP1A2 (minor), 2A6 (minor), 2B6 (major), 2C9 (minor), 2D6 (minor), 2E1 (minor), 3A4 (minor); **Inhibits** CYP2D6 (weak)

Drug Interactions

Alcohol (Ethyl): CNS Depressants may enhance the CNS depressant effect of Alcohol (Ethyl). *Risk C: Monitor therapy*

CNS Depressants: May enhance the adverse/toxic effect of other CNS Depressants. *Risk C: Monitor therapy*

CYP2B6 Inducers (Strong): May increase the metabolism of CYP2B6 Substrates. *Risk C: Monitor therapy*

CYP2B6 Inhibitors (Moderate): May decrease the metabolism of CYP2B6 Substrates. *Risk C: Monitor therapy*

CYP2B6 Inhibitors (Strong): May decrease the metabolism of CYP2B6 Substrates. *Risk D: Consider therapy modification*

Lopinavir: May decrease the serum concentration of BuPROPion. Concentrations of the active metabolite, hydroxybupropion, may also be decreased. *Risk C: Monitor therapy*

MAO Inhibitors: May enhance the neurotoxic (central) effect of BuPROPion. *Risk X: Avoid combination*

Ritonavir: May decrease the serum concentration of BuPROPion. *Risk C: Monitor therapy*

Tricyclic Antidepressants: BuPROPion may decrease the metabolism of Tricyclic Antidepressants. **Exceptions:** Amoxapine; Protriptyline. *Risk C: Monitor therapy*

Ethanol/Nutrition/Herb Interactions

Ethanol: Avoid ethanol (may increase CNS depression).

Herb/Nutraceutical: Avoid valerian, St John's wort, SAMe, gotu kola, kava kava (may increase CNS depression).

Stability

Store at controlled room temperature of 20°C to 25°C (68°F to 77°F).

Wellbutrin XL™: Store at 15°C to 30°C (59°F to 86°F).

Mechanism of Action Aminoketone antidepressant structurally different from all other marketed antidepressants; like other antidepressants the mechanism of bupropion's activity is not fully understood. Bupropion is a relatively weak inhibitor of the neuronal uptake of norepinephrine and dopamine, and does not inhibit monoamine oxidase or the reuptake of serotonin. Metabolite inhibits the reuptake of norepinephrine. The primary mechanism of action is thought to be dopaminergic and/or noradrenergic.

Pharmacodynamics/Kinetics

Absorption: Rapid

Distribution: V_d: 19-21 L/kg

Protein binding: 82% to 88%

Metabolism: Extensively hepatic via CYP2B6 to hydroxybupropion; non-CYP-mediated metabolism to erythrohydrobupropion and threohydrobupropion. Metabolite activity ranges from 20% to 50% potency of bupropion.

Bioavailability: 5% to 20% in animals

Half-life:

Distribution: 3-4 hours

Elimination: 21 ± 9 hours; Metabolites: Hydroxybupropion: 20 ± 5 hours; Erythrohydrobupropion: 33 ± 10 hours; Threohydrobupropion: 37 ± 13 hours (metabolite accumulation has been noted in ESRD).

Time to peak, serum: Bupropion: ~3 hours; bupropion extended release: ~5 hours

Metabolites: Hydroxybupropion, erythrohydrobupropion, threohydrobupropion: 6 hours

Excretion: Urine (87%); feces (10%)

Dosage Oral:

Children and Adolescents: ADHD (unlabeled use): 1.4-6 mg/kg/day

Adults:

Depression:

Immediate release: 100 mg 3 times/day; begin at 100 mg twice daily; may increase to a maximum dose of 450 mg/day

Sustained release: Initial: 150 mg/day in the morning; may increase to 150 mg twice daily by day 4 if tolerated; target dose: 300 mg/day given as 150 mg twice daily; maximum dose: 400 mg/day given as 200 mg twice daily

Extended release: Initial: 150 mg/day in the morning; may increase as early as day 4 of dosing to 300 mg/day; maximum dose: 450 mg/day

SAD (Wellbutrin XL™): Initial: 150 mg/day in the morning; if tolerated, may increase after 1 week to 300 mg/day

Note: Prophylactic treatment should be reserved for those patients with frequent depressive episodes and/or significant impairment. Initiate treatment in the Autumn prior to symptom onset, and discontinue in early Spring with dose tapering to 150 mg/day for 2 weeks

Smoking cessation (Zyban®): Initiate with 150 mg once daily for 3 days; increase to 150 mg twice daily; treatment should continue for 7-12 weeks

Elderly: Depression: 50-100 mg/day, increase by 50-100 mg every 3-4 days as tolerated; there is evidence that the elderly respond at 150 mg/day in divided doses, but some may require a higher dose. **Note:** Patients with Alzheimer's dementia-related depression may require a lower starting dosage of 37.5 mg once or twice daily (100 mg/day sustained release), increased as needed up to 300 mg/day in divided doses (300 mg/day for sustained release)

Dosing conversion between immediate, sustained, and extended release products: Convert using same total daily dose (up to the maximum recommended dose for a given dosage form), but adjust frequency as indicated for sustained (twice daily) or extended (once daily) release products.

Dosing adjustment/comments in renal impairment: Per the manufacturer, the elimination of hydroxybupropion and threohydrobupropion are reduced in patients with end-stage renal failure. Other research has noted a reduction in bupropion clearance (Turpeinen, 2007). Consider a reduction in frequency and/or dosage in this patient population.

Dosing adjustment in hepatic impairment:

Note: The mean AUC increased by ~1.5-fold for hydroxybupropion and ~2.5-fold for erythro/threohydrobupropion; median T_{max} was observed 19 hours later for hydroxybupropion, 31 hours later for erythro/threohydrobupropion; mean half-life for hydroxybupropion increased fivefold, and increased twofold for erythro/threohydrobupropion in patients with severe hepatic cirrhosis compared to healthy volunteers.

Mild-to-moderate hepatic impairment: Use with caution and/or reduced dose/frequency

Severe hepatic cirrhosis: Use with extreme caution; maximum dose:

Wellbutrin®: 75 mg/day

Wellbutrin SR®: 100 mg/day or 150 mg every other day

Wellbutrin XL™: 150 mg every other day

Zyban®: 150 mg every other day

Child/Adolescent Considerations Attention-deficit/hyperactivity disorder (ADHD): 1.4-5.7 mg/kg/day (mean: 3.3 mg/kg/day) was utilized in 15 ADHD subjects 7-17 years of age (Barrickman, 1995); 72 children with ADHD (6-12 years of age) received 3-6 mg/kg/day (Conners, 1996); adolescents with conduct disorder and substance use disorder were titrated to a maximum fixed daily dose of 300 mg (Riggs, 1998). The immediate-release dosage form was studied in clinical trials for indications other than depression in 104 pediatric patients. This limited exposure does not allow for assessment of the safety of bupropion in pediatric patients. Bupropion 100–350 mg/day (mean: 3.5 ± 0.8 mg/kg/day) was given to 57 children and adolescents 9–18 years of age with ADHD in a randomized controlled trial to assess whether it prevented smoking in nonsmokers for ≤6.5 years (mean: 12 months). Bupropion was not found to be superior to placebo for smoking prevention in youth with ADHD. Adverse effects were similar in bupropion and placebo groups (Monuteaux, 2007).

A pharmacokinetic study of bupropion SR, showed the mean half-life and threohydrobupropion metabolite of bupropion were significantly shorter in children 11-17 years of age compared to adults. The AUC were 19% and 80%

higher for bupropion and its metabolite (respectively). This indicates it may be preferable to dose bupropion SR twice daily in children (Daviss, 2005).

Barrickman LL, Petty PJ, Allen AJ, et al, "Bupropion Versus Methylphenidate in the Treatment of Attention-Deficit Hyperactivity Disorder," *J Am Acad Child Adolesc Psychiatry*, 1995, 34(5):649-57.

Conners CK, Casat CD, Gualtieri CT, et al, "Bupropion Hydrochloride in Attention Deficit Disorder With Hyperactivity," *J Am Acad Child Adolesc Psychiatry*, 1996, 35(10):1314-21.

Daviss WB, Perel JM, Birmaher B, et al, "Steady-State Clinical Pharmacokinetics of Bupropion Extended-Release in Youths," *J Am Acad Child Adolesc Psychiatry*, 2006, 45(12):1503-9.

Monuteaux MC, Spencer TJ, Faraone SV, et al, "A Randomized, Placebo-Controlled Clinical Trial of Bupropion for the Prevention of Smoking in Children and Adolescents With Attention-Deficit/Hyperactivity Disorder," *J Clin Psychiatry*, 2007, 68(7):1094-101.

Riggs PD, Leon SL, Mikulich SK, et al, "An Open Trial of Bupropion for ADHD in Adolescents With Substance Use Disorders and Conduct Disorder," *J Am Acad Child Adolesc Psychiatry*, 1998, 37(12):1271-8.

Administration May be taken without regard to meals. Zyban® and extended release tablets should be swallowed whole; do not crush, chew, or divide. The insoluble shell of the extended-release tablet may remain intact during GI transit and is eliminated in the feces. Data from the manufacturer states that dividing Wellbutrin® SR tablets resulted in an increased rate of release at 15 minutes: "However, the divided tablet retained its sustained-release characteristics with similar increases of released bupropion at each sampling point beyond 15 minutes when compared to the intact Wellbutrin® SR tablet..." Bupropion is hydroscopic and therefore should be stored in a dry place. Splitting of large quantities in advance of administration is not advised since loss of potency may result. If necessary, splitting should be done cleanly without crushing.

Monitoring Parameters Body weight; mental status for depression, suicidal ideation (especially at the beginning of therapy or when doses are increased or decreased), anxiety, social functioning, mania, panic attacks

When used for the treatment of ADHD, thoroughly evaluate for cardiovascular risk. Monitor heart rate, blood pressure, and consider obtaining ECG prior to initiation (Vetter, 2008).

Reference Range Therapeutic levels (trough, 12 hours after last dose): 50-100 ng/mL

Additional Information Risk of seizures: When using immediate release tablets, seizure risk is increased at total daily dosage >450 mg, individual dosages >150 mg, or by sudden, large increments in dose. Data for the immediate-release formulation of bupropion revealed a seizure incidence of 0.4% in patients treated at doses in the 300-450 mg/day range. The estimated seizure incidence increases almost 10-fold between 450 mg and 600 mg per day. Data for the sustained release dosage form revealed a seizure incidence of 0.1% in patients treated at a dosage range of 100-300 mg/day, and increases to ~0.4% at the maximum recommended dose of 400 mg/day.

Dosage Forms Excipient information presented when available (limited, particularly for generics); consult specific product labeling.

Tablet, as hydrochloride: 75 mg [generic for Wellbutrin®], 100 mg [generic for Wellbutrin®]
- Wellbutrin®: 75 mg, 100 mg

Tablet, extended release, as hydrochloride: 100 mg [generic for Wellbutrin® SR], 150 mg [generic for Wellbutrin® SR], 150 mg [generic for Zyban®], 200 mg [generic for Wellbutrin® SR], 300 mg [generic for Wellbutrin XL™]
- Budeprion™ SR: 100 mg [generic for Wellbutrin® SR; contains tartrazine], 150 mg [generic for Wellbutrin® SR]
- Budeprion XL®: 150 mg [generic for Wellbutrin® XL], 300 mg [contains tartrazine; generic for Wellbutrin® XL]
- Buproban™: 150 mg [generic for Zyban®]
- Wellbutrin XL™: 150 mg, 300 mg

Tablet, sustained release, as hydrochloride: 100 mg [generic for Wellbutrin® SR], 150 mg [generic for Wellbutrin® SR], 150 mg [generic for Zyban®], 200 mg [generic for Wellbutrin® SR]
- Wellbutrin® SR: 100 mg, 150 mg, 200 mg
- Zyban®: 150 mg

◆ **Burnamycin [OTC]** *see* Lidocaine *on page 924*

◆ **Burn Jel® [OTC]** *see* Lidocaine *on page 924*

◆ **Burn-O-Jel [OTC]** *see* Lidocaine *on page 924*

◆ **BuSpar®** *see* BusPIRone *on page 223*

BusPIRone (byoo SPYE rone)

Medication Safety Issues

Sound-alike/look-alike issues:

BusPIRone may be confused with buPROPion

Related Information

Nonbenzodiazepine Anxiolytics and Hypnotics *on page 1791*

U.S. Brand Names BuSpar®

Canadian Brand Names Apo-Buspirone®; BuSpar®; Buspirex; Bustab®; CO Buspirone; Dom-Buspirone; Gen-Buspirone; Lin-Buspirone; Novo-Buspirone; Nu-Buspirone; PMS-Buspirone; ratio-Buspirone; Riva-Buspirone

Mexican Brand Names Buspar

Index Terms Buspirone Hydrochloride

Pharmacologic Category Antianxiety Agent, Miscellaneous

Generic Available Yes

Use Management of generalized anxiety disorder (GAD)

Unlabeled/Investigational Use Management of aggression in mental retardation and secondary mental disorders; major depression; potential augmenting agent for antidepressants; premenstrual syndrome

Mental Health Comment Buspirone is an azaspirodecanedione (nonbenzodiazepine) anxiolytic and is not GABA-ergic. It is extensively metabolized primarily by oxidation producing several hydroxylated derivatives and a pharmacologically-active metabolite, 1-pyrimidinyl piperazine (1-PP). 1-PP has about 20% the activity of buspirone. Buspirone decreases anxiety without causing sedation or having anticonvulsant or muscle relaxant properties. Initial therapeutic effect is usually seen as a decrease in irritability and worry. Buspirone may be as effective as the benzodiazepines in relieving anxiety, but has a slow onset of action. It is important to wait 3-4 weeks before assessing the response to buspirone.

The advantages of buspirone include a low abuse potential (no reinforcing value in substance abusers and tended to cause dysphoria at doses >40 mg/day), causes no impairment of psychomotor activity, is not associated with dependence and can be abruptly discontinued, produces minimal sedation, and does not potentiate the effects of alcohol. May be useful for those who become disinhibited on benzodiazepines, those with a history of benzodiazepines/substance abuse, and those with a medical history in whom the use of a benzodiazepines may be risky.

The disadvantages of buspirone include a lag time for onset of anxiolytic effect similar to antidepressants, the requirement for multiple daily dosing, an inability to use as a PRN medication, a lack of cross tolerance with benzodiazepines, an inability to prevent withdrawal from benzodiazepines or alcohol, the requirement for adherent patients, and the potential for patients with previous exposure to benzodiazepines to be less likely to respond. For these reasons, buspirone is uncommonly utilized as an anxiolytic in most clinical settings.

Pregnancy Risk Factor B

Pregnancy Considerations No impairment of fertility or fetotoxic effects were noted in animal studies with doses 30 times maximum recommended human dose. There are no adequate and well-controlled studies in pregnant women.

Lactation Excretion in breast milk unknown/not recommended

Contraindications Hypersensitivity to buspirone or any component of the formulation

Warnings/Precautions Use in severe hepatic or renal impairment is not recommended; does not prevent or treat withdrawal from benzodiazepines. Low potential for cognitive or motor impairment. Use with MAO inhibitors may result in hypertensive reactions. Restlessness syndrome has been reported in small number of patients; monitor for signs of any dopamine-related movement disorders. Buspirone does not exhibit cross-tolerance with benzodiazepines or other sedative/hypnotic agents. If substituting buspirone for any of these agents, gradually withdraw the drug(s) prior to initiating buspirone. Safety and efficacy of buspirone have not been established in children <6 years of age; no long-term safety/efficacy data available in children.

Adverse Reactions

>10%: Central nervous system: Dizziness (12%)

1% to 10%:

Cardiovascular: Chest pain (≥1%)

Central nervous system: Drowsiness (10%), headache (6%), nervousness (5%), lightheadedness (3%), anger/hostility (2%), confusion (2%), excitement (2%), dream disturbance (≥1%)

Dermatologic: Rash (1%)
Gastrointestinal: Nausea (8%), diarrhea (2%)
Neuromuscular & skeletal: Numbness (2%), weakness (2%), musculoskeletal pain (1%), paresthesia (1%), incoordination (1%), tremor (1%)
Ocular: Blurred vision (2%)
Otic: Tinnitus (≥1%)
Respiratory: Nasal congestion (≥1%), sore throat (≥1%)
Miscellaneous: Diaphoresis (1%)

<1% (Limited to important or life-threatening): Akathisia, allergic reaction, angioedema, anorexia, bradycardia, bruising, cardiomyopathy, cogwheel rigidity, conjunctivitis, CVA, dyskinesia, dyspnea, dystonia, edema, enuresis, eosinophilia, epistaxis, EPS, galactorrhea, hallucination, heart failure, hyper-/hypotension, hyperventilation, irritable colon, leukopenia, menstrual irregularity, MI, muscle spasms, parkinsonism, personality disorders, PID, psychosis, rectal bleeding, restless leg syndrome, seizure, serotonin syndrome, suicidal ideation, syncope, thrombocytopenia, thyroid abnormality, transaminase increases, visual disturbances (tunnel vision)

Metabolism/Transport Effects Substrate of CYP2D6 (minor), 3A4 (major)

Drug Interactions

Antidepressants (Serotonin Reuptake Inhibitor/Antagonist): BusPIRone may enhance the serotonergic effect of Antidepressants (Serotonin Reuptake Inhibitor/Antagonist). This may cause serotonin syndrome. *Risk C: Monitor therapy*

Antifungal Agents (Azole Derivatives, Systemic): May decrease the metabolism of BusPIRone. *Risk D: Consider therapy modification*

Calcium Channel Blockers (Nondihydropyridine): May decrease the metabolism of BusPIRone. *Risk D: Consider therapy modification*

CYP3A4 Inducers (Strong): May increase the metabolism of CYP3A4 Substrates. *Risk C: Monitor therapy*

CYP3A4 Inhibitors (Moderate): May decrease the metabolism of CYP3A4 Substrates. *Risk C: Monitor therapy*

CYP3A4 Inhibitors (Strong): May decrease the metabolism of CYP3A4 Substrates. *Risk D: Consider therapy modification*

Dasatinib: May increase the serum concentration of CYP3A4 Substrates. *Risk C: Monitor therapy*

Deferasirox: May decrease the serum concentration of CYP3A4 Substrates. *Risk C: Monitor therapy*

Grapefruit Juice: May decrease the metabolism of BusPIRone. *Risk D: Consider therapy modification*

Herbs (CYP3A4 Inducers): May increase the metabolism of CYP3A4 Substrates. *Risk C: Monitor therapy*

Macrolide Antibiotics: May decrease the metabolism of BusPIRone. **Exceptions:** Azithromycin; Dirithromycin [Off Market]; Spiramycin. *Risk D: Consider therapy modification*

MAO Inhibitors: BusPIRone may enhance the adverse/toxic effect of MAO Inhibitors. Elevated blood pressure has been reported. *Risk X: Avoid combination*

Rifamycin Derivatives: May increase the metabolism of BusPIRone. *Risk D: Consider therapy modification*

Selective Serotonin Reuptake Inhibitors: BusPIRone may enhance the serotonergic effect of Selective Serotonin Reuptake Inhibitors. This may cause serotonin syndrome. Selective Serotonin Reuptake Inhibitors may decrease the metabolism of BusPIRone. *Risk C: Monitor therapy*

Serotonin Modulators: May enhance the adverse/toxic effect of other Serotonin Modulators. The development of serotonin syndrome may occur. *Risk D: Consider therapy modification*

Sibutramine: May enhance the serotonergic effect of Serotonin Modulators. This may cause serotonin syndrome. *Risk X: Avoid combination*

Ethanol/Nutrition/Herb Interactions

Ethanol: Ethanol (may increase CNS depression).

Food: Food may decrease the absorption of buspirone, but it may also decrease the first-pass metabolism, thereby increasing the bioavailability of buspirone. Grapefruit juice may cause increased buspirone concentrations; avoid intake of large quantities of grapefruit juice.

Herb/Nutraceutical: St John's wort may decrease buspirone levels or increase CNS depression. Avoid valerian, gotu kola, kava kava (may increase CNS depression).

Stability Store at USP controlled room temperature of 25°C (77°F). Protect from light.

Mechanism of Action The mechanism of action of buspirone is unknown. Buspirone has a high affinity for serotonin 5-HT_{1A} and 5-HT_2 receptors, without affecting benzodiazepine-GABA receptors. Buspirone has moderate affinity for dopamine D_2 receptors.

Pharmacodynamics/Kinetics

Absorption: Rapid

Distribution: V_d: 5.3 L/kg

Protein binding: 86% to 95%

Metabolism: Hepatic oxidation, primarily via CYP3A4; extensive first-pass effect

Bioavailability: ~4%

Half-life elimination: 2-3 hours

Time to peak, serum: 40-90 minutes

Excretion: Urine: 29% to 63% (<0.1% dose excreted unchanged); feces: 18% to 38%

Dosage Oral:

Generalized anxiety disorder:

Children ≥6 years and Adolescents: Initial: 5 mg daily; increase in increments of 5 mg/day at weekly intervals as needed, to a maximum dose of 60 mg/day divided into 2-3 doses

Adults: 15 mg/day (7.5 mg twice daily); may increase in increments of 5 mg/day every 2-3 days to a maximum of 60 mg/day; target dose for most people is 20-30 mg/day (10-15 mg twice daily)

Elderly: Initial: 5 mg twice daily, increase by 5 mg/day every 2-3 days as needed up to 20-30 mg/day; maximum daily dose: 60 mg/day.

Dosing adjustment in renal impairment: Patients with impaired renal function demonstrated increased plasma levels and a prolonged half-life of buspirone. Use in patients with severe renal impairment not recommended.

Dosing adjustment in hepatic impairment: Patients with impaired hepatic function demonstrated increased plasma levels and a prolonged half-life of buspirone. Use in patients with severe hepatic impairment not recommended.

Child/Adolescent Considerations Anxiety disorders: One pilot study of 15 children, 6-14 years of age (mean: 10 years), with mixed anxiety disorders, used initial doses of 5 mg/day; doses were individualized with increases in increments of 5 mg/day weekly as needed, to a maximum dose of 20 mg/day divided into 2 doses (mean dose required: 18.6 mg/day). Some authors (Carrey, 1996 and Kutcher, 1992), based on their clinical experience, recommend higher doses. Open-label study in 25 prepubertal inpatients (mean age: 8 years) with anxiety symptoms and moderately-aggressive behavior utilized a mean optimal dose of 28 mg/day (Pfeffer, 1997). Dosages ranging from 15-45 mg/day were utilized in children 6-17 years of age with pervasive developmental disorders (Buitelaar, 1998). The safety and efficacy of buspirone were evaluated in two placebo-controlled 6-week trials involving a total of 559 pediatric patients (6-17 years of age) with generalized anxiety disorder (GAD). Doses studied were 7.5-30 mg twice daily (15-60 mg/day). There were no significant differences between buspirone and placebo with regard to the symptoms of GAD following doses recommended for the treatment of GAD in adults (Bristol-Myers Squibb, BuSpar® package labeling, July 2001).

An open-label pharmacokinetic study was conducted in children (n=13), adolescents (n=12) with anxiety disorders, and healthy adults (n=14) to measure blood levels and adverse effects over 3 weeks. Children had the highest blood levels, significantly higher than adults on all doses studied. The most frequently reported adverse events in children and adolescents were lightheadedness (68%), headache (48%), and dyspepsia (20%); two children withdrew from the study at the higher doses (15 mg and 30 mg twice daily) due to adverse effects (Salazar, 2001).

Buitelaar JK, van der Gaag RJ, and van der Hoeven J, "Buspirone in the Management of Anxiety and Irritability in Children With Pervasive Developmental Disorders: Results of an Open-Label Study," *J Clin Psychiatry*, 1998, 59(2):56-9.

Carrey NJ, Wiggins DM, and Milin RP, "Pharmacological Treatment of Psychiatric Disorders in Children and Adolescents," *Drugs*, 1996, 51 (5):750-9.

Kutcher SP, Reiter S, Gardner DM, et al, "The Pharmacotherapy of Anxiety Disorders in Children and Adolescents," *Psychiatr Clin North Am*, 1992, 15 (1):41-67.

Pfeffer CR, Jiang H, and Domeshek LJ, "Buspirone Treatment of Psychiatrically Hospitalized Prepubertal Children With Symptoms of Anxiety and Moderately Severe Aggression," *J Child Adolesc Psychopharmacol*, 1997, 7(3):145-55.

Salazar DE, Frackiewicz EJ, Dockens R, et al, "Pharmacokinetics and Tolerability of Buspirone During Oral Administration to Children and Adolescents With Anxiety Disorder and Normal Healthy Adults," *J Clin Pharmacol*, 2001, 41(12):1351-8.

Monitoring Parameters Mental status, symptoms of anxiety

Dosage Forms Excipient information presented when available (limited, particularly for generics); consult specific product labeling.

Tablet, as hydrochloride: 5 mg, 7.5 mg, 10 mg, 15 mg, 30 mg

BuSpar®: 5 mg, 10 mg, 15 mg, 30 mg

◆ **Buspirone Hydrochloride** *see* BusPIRone *on page 223*

Busulfan (byoo SUL fan)

Medication Safety Issues

Sound-alike/look-alike issues:

Busulfan may be confused with Butalan®

Myleran® may be confused with Alkeran®, Leukeran®, melphalan, Mylicon®

High alert medication: The Institute for Safe Medication Practices (ISMP) includes this medication among its list of drugs which have a heightened risk of causing significant patient harm when used in error.

U.S. Brand Names Busulfex®; Myleran®

Canadian Brand Names Busulfex®; Myleran®

Mexican Brand Names Myleran

Index Terms NSC-750

Pharmacologic Category Antineoplastic Agent, Alkylating Agent

Use

Oral: Chronic myelogenous leukemia (CML); conditioning regimens for bone marrow transplantation

I.V.: Combination therapy with cyclophosphamide as a conditioning regimen prior to allogeneic hematopoietic progenitor cell transplantation for chronic myelogenous leukemia

Unlabeled/Investigational Use Oral: Bone marrow disorders, such as polycythemia vera and myeloid metaplasia; thrombocytosis

Effect on Mental Status None reported

Effect on Psychiatric Treatment May cause severe pancytopenia; use caution with clozapine and carbamazepine

Dosage Summary

I.V.:

Children ≤12 kg: **BMT:** 1.1 mg/kg (ideal body weight) every 6 hours for 16 doses

Children >12 kg: **BMT:** 0.8 mg/kg (ideal body weight) every 6 hours for 16 doses

Adults: **BMT:** 0.8 mg/kg (ideal body weight or actual body weight, whichever is lower) every 6 hours for 16 doses

Oral:

Children: Induction: 0.06-0.12 mg/kg/day **or** 1.8-4.6 mg/m^2/day; Maintenance: Titrate to maintain leukocyte counts above 40,000/mm^3; **BMT:** 1 mg/kg (ideal body weight) every 6 hours for 16 doses

Adults: Induction: 60 mcg/kg/day or 1.8 mg/m^2/day; usual range: 4-12 mg/day; Maintenance: 1-4 mg/day to 2 mg/week; **BMT:** 1 mg/kg (ideal body weight) every 6 hours for 16 doses

Dosage Forms Excipient information presented when available (limited, particularly for generics); consult specific product labeling.

Injection, solution:

Busulfex®: 6 mg/mL (10 mL) [contains N,N-dimethylacetamide (DMA)]

Tablet:

Myleran®: 2 mg

◆ **Busulfex®** *see* Busulfan *on page 226*

Butabarbital (byoo ta BAR bi tal)

Medication Safety Issues

Sound-alike/look-alike issues:

Butabarbital may be confused with butalbital

U.S. Brand Names Butisol Sodium®

Pharmacologic Category Barbiturate

Generic Available No

Use Sedative; hypnotic

Effect on Mental Status Drowsiness is common

Effect on Psychiatric Treatment Rare reports of agranulocytosis; use caution with clozapine and carbamazepine; enzyme induction effects of barbiturates may decrease effects of psychotropics; CNS depressant effects of psychotropics may be enhanced by barbiturates

Mental Health Comment In 2007, the FDA requested that all manufacturers of sedative-hypnotic drug products revise labeling to include a greater emphasis on the risks of adverse effects. These risks include severe allergic reactions (anaphylaxis, angioedema) and complex sleep-related behaviors, which may include sleep-driving (driving while not fully awake and with no memory of the event), making phone calls, and preparing and eating food while asleep. Barbiturates are generally not utilized as first-line agents to manage anxiety or insomnia due to abuse potential and potential for drug interactions and adverse effects.

Restrictions C-III

Pregnancy Risk Factor D

Pregnancy Considerations Barbiturates cross the placenta and can be found in fetal tissues. Acute withdrawal symptoms may occur in the neonate following *in utero* exposure near term. Withdrawal symptoms may include seizures and hyperirritabilility and may be delayed for up to 14 days after birth.

Lactation Enters breast milk/use with caution

Contraindications Hypersensitivity to barbiturates or any component of the formulation; porphyria

Warnings/Precautions Symptomatic treatment of insomnia should be initiated only after careful evaluation of potential causes of sleep disturbance. Failure of sleep disturbance to resolve after 7-10 days may indicate psychiatric and/or medical illness. A worsening of insomnia or the emergence of new abnormalities of thought or behavior may represent unrecognized psychiatric or medical illness and requires immediate and careful evaluation. May cause CNS depression, which may impair physical or mental abilities. Patients must be cautioned about performing tasks which require mental alertness (eg, operating machinery or driving). Effects with other sedative drugs or ethanol may be potentiated. Postmarketing studies have indicated that the use of hypnotic/sedative agents for sleep has been associated with hypersensitivity reactions including anaphylaxis as well as angioedema. An increased risk for hazardous sleep-related activities such as sleep-driving; cooking and eating food, and making phone calls while asleep have also been noted.

May cause respiratory depression or hypotension. Use with caution in hemodynamically unstable patients or patients with respiratory disease. Use caution in elderly, debilitated, renal impairment, hepatic impairment, or pediatric patients. May cause paradoxical responses, including agitation and hyperactivity, particularly with pain, and pediatric patients. Potential for drug dependency exists; abrupt cessation may precipitate withdrawal, including status epilepticus in epileptic patients. Use with caution in patients with depression or suicidal tendencies, or in patients with a history of drug abuse. Tolerance, psychological and physical dependence may occur with prolonged use. Some products may contain tartrazine.

Adverse Reactions

1% to 3%: Central nervous system: Somnolence

<1% or frequency not defined (limited to important or life-threatening): Abnormal thinking, agitation, agranulocytosis, anaphylaxis, angioedema, anxiety, apnea, ataxia, bradycardia, complex sleep-related activities, confusion, constipation, dependence, depression, dizziness, exfoliative dermatitis, fever, hallucination, headache, hyperkinesias, hypersensitivity reactions, hypotension, hypoventilation, insomnia, liver damage, megaloblastic anemia, nausea, nervousness, nightmares, psychiatric disturbance, rash, respiratory depression, Stevens-Johnson syndrome, syncope, thrombocytopenia, thrombophlebitis, vomiting

Drug Interactions

Acetaminophen: Barbiturates may increase the metabolism of Acetaminophen. This may 1) diminish the effect of acetaminophen; and 2) increase the risk of liver damage. *Risk C: Monitor therapy*

Alcohol (Ethyl): CNS Depressants may enhance the CNS depressant effect of Alcohol (Ethyl). *Risk C: Monitor therapy*

Beta-Blockers: Barbiturates may decrease the serum concentration of Beta-Blockers. **Exceptions:** Atenolol; Levobunolol; Metipranolol; Nadolol. *Risk C: Monitor therapy*

Calcium Channel Blockers: Barbiturates may increase the metabolism of Calcium Channel Blockers. **Exceptions:** Clevidipine. *Risk D: Consider therapy modification*

Chloramphenicol: May decrease the metabolism of Barbiturates. Barbiturates may increase the metabolism of Chloramphenicol. *Risk D: Consider therapy modification*

CNS Depressants: May enhance the adverse/toxic effect of other CNS Depressants. *Risk C: Monitor therapy*

Contraceptive (Progestins): Barbiturates may diminish the therapeutic effect of Contraceptive (Progestins). Contraceptive failure is possible. *Risk D: Consider therapy modification*

Corticosteroids (Systemic): Barbiturates may increase the metabolism of Corticosteroids (Systemic). *Risk C: Monitor therapy*

CycloSPORINE: Barbiturates may increase the metabolism of CycloSPORINE. *Risk D: Consider therapy modification*

Disopyramide: Barbiturates may increase the metabolism of Disopyramide. *Risk D: Consider therapy modification*

Doxycycline: Barbiturates may decrease the serum concentration of Doxycycline. *Risk D: Consider therapy modification*

Etoposide: Barbiturates may increase the metabolism of Etoposide. *Risk C: Monitor therapy*

Etoposide Phosphate: Barbiturates may decrease the serum concentration of Etoposide Phosphate. Barbiturates may increase the metabolism, via CYP isoenzymes, of etoposide phosphate. *Risk C: Monitor therapy*

Felbamate: May increase the serum concentration of Barbiturates. *Risk C: Monitor therapy*

Griseofulvin: Barbiturates may decrease the absorption of Griseofulvin. *Risk D: Consider therapy modification*

LamoTRIgine: Barbiturates may increase the metabolism of LamoTRIgine. *Risk D: Consider therapy modification*

Meperidine: Barbiturates may enhance the CNS depressant effect of Meperidine. *Risk C: Monitor therapy*

Methadone: Barbiturates may increase the metabolism of Methadone. *Risk D: Consider therapy modification*

Oral Contraceptive (Estrogens): Barbiturates may diminish the therapeutic effect of Oral Contraceptive (Estrogens). Contraceptive failure is possible. *Risk D: Consider therapy modification*

Primidone: May enhance the adverse/toxic effect of Barbiturates. Primidone is converted to phenobarbital, and thus becomes additive with existing barbiturate therapy. *Risk C: Monitor therapy*

Propafenone: Barbiturates may increase the metabolism of Propafenone. *Risk D: Consider therapy modification*

Pyridoxine: May increase the metabolism of Barbiturates. Apparent in high pyridoxine doses (eg, 200 mg/day) *Risk C: Monitor therapy*

QuiNIDine: Barbiturates may increase the metabolism of QuiNIDine. *Risk D: Consider therapy modification*

Rifamycin Derivatives: May increase the metabolism of Barbiturates. *Risk C: Monitor therapy*

Teniposide: Barbiturates may increase the metabolism of Teniposide. *Risk C: Monitor therapy*

Theophylline Derivatives: Barbiturates may increase the metabolism of Theophylline Derivatives. **Exceptions:** Dyphylline. *Risk C: Monitor therapy*

Tricyclic Antidepressants: Barbiturates may increase the metabolism of Tricyclic Antidepressants. *Risk D: Consider therapy modification*

Valproic Acid: May decrease the metabolism of Barbiturates. Barbiturates may decrease the serum concentration of Valproic Acid. *Risk C: Monitor therapy*

Vitamin K Antagonists (eg, warfarin): Barbiturates may increase the metabolism of Vitamin K Antagonists. *Risk D: Consider therapy modification*

Voriconazole: Barbiturates may decrease the serum concentration of Voriconazole. *Risk X: Avoid combination*

Ethanol/Nutrition/Herb Interactions

Ethanol: Avoid ethanol (may increase CNS depression).

Food: Rate of absorption is increased if given as solution on an empty stomach.

Herb/Nutraceutical: Avoid valerian, St John's wort, kava kava, gotu kola (may increase CNS depression).

Mechanism of Action Interferes with transmission of impulses from the thalamus to the cortex of the brain resulting in an imbalance in central inhibitory and facilitatory mechanisms

Pharmacodynamics/Kinetics

Onset of action: 45-60 minutes

Duration: 6-8 hours

Absorption: Rapid

Metabolism: Hepatic

Half-life elimination: ~100 hours

Excretion: Urine (as metabolites)

Dosage Oral:

Children: Preoperative sedation: 2-6 mg/kg/dose (maximum: 100 mg)

Adults:
Sedative: 15-30 mg 3-4 times/day
Hypnotic: 50-100 mg at bedtime. When used for insomnia, treatment should be limited since barbiturates lose effectiveness for sleep induction and maintenance after 2 weeks.
Preop: 50-100 mg 1-1½ hours before surgery
Elderly: Use with caution; reduce dose if use is needed

Dosage adjustment in renal impairment: Reduce dose if use is needed
Dosage adjustment in hepatic impairment: Reduce dose if use is needed

Monitoring Parameters CBC, renal and hepatic function with prolonged therapy

Reference Range Serum plasma: Habitual/therapeutic: 1-15 mg/L; toxic: 10-20 mg/L; lethal 30 mg/L

Dosage Forms Excipient information presented when available (limited, particularly for generics); consult specific product labeling.
Elixir, as sodium:
Butisol Sodium®: 30 mg/5 mL (480 mL) [contains alcohol 7%, propylene glycol, sodium benzoate, and tartrazine]
Tablet, as sodium:
Butisol Sodium®: 30 mg [contains tartrazine], 50 mg [contains tartrazine]

Butalbital, Acetaminophen, and Caffeine

(byoo TAL bi tal, a seet a MIN oh fen, & KAF een)

Medication Safety Issues
Sound-alike/look-alike issues:
Fioricet® may be confused with Fiorinal®, Lorcet®
Repan® may be confused with Riopan®

Duplicate therapy issues: This product contains acetaminophen, which may be a component of other combination products. Do not exceed the maximum recommended daily dose of acetaminophen.

U.S. Brand Names Anolor 300; Dolgic® LQ; Dolgic® Plus; Esgic-Plus™; Esgic®; Fioricet®; Medigesic®; Repan®; Zebutal™

Index Terms Acetaminophen, Butalbital, and Caffeine

Pharmacologic Category Barbiturate

Generic Available Yes: Excludes solution

Use Relief of the symptomatic complex of tension or muscle contraction headache

Effect on Mental Status Drowsiness is common; may cause depression, nervousness, insomnia, and nightmares; rare reports of hallucinations

Effect on Psychiatric Treatment Rare reports of agranulocytosis; use caution with clozapine and carbamazepine; CNS depressant effects of psychotropics may be enhance by barbiturates; enzyme induction effects of barbiturates may decrease effects of psychotropics

Pregnancy Risk Factor C

Pregnancy Considerations Reproduction studies have not been conducted with this combination. The FDA pregnancy classification for most other barbiturates is Category D. Withdrawal seizures were reported in an infant 2 days after birth following maternal use of a butalbital product during the last 2 months of pregnancy; butalbital levels were measured in the infants serum. In general, barbiturates cross the placenta and distribute in fetal tissue. Teratogenic effects have been reported with 1st trimester exposure. Exposure during the third trimester may lead to symptoms of acute withdrawal following delivery; symptoms may be delayed up to 14 days. Refer to individual agents for specific information related to acetaminophen and caffeine.

Lactation Enters breast milk/not recommended

Contraindications Hypersensitivity to butalbital, acetaminophen, caffeine, or any component of the formulation; porphyria

Warnings/Precautions May cause CNS depression, which may impair physical or mental abilities; patients must be cautioned about performing tasks which require mental alertness (eg, operating machinery or driving). May cause severe hepatic toxicity on acute overdose; in addition, chronic daily dosing in adults has resulted in liver damage in some patients. Use with caution in patients with alcoholic liver disease; consuming ≥3 alcoholic drinks/day may increase the risk of liver damage. Effects may be potentiated when used with other sedative drugs or ethanol. Use caution in elderly and debilitated patients. Use with caution in patients with history of drug abuse, known G6PD deficiency, hepatic impairment, renal impairment, respiratory disease. Caffeine may cause CNS and cardiovascular stimulation, as well as GI irritation in high doses. Use with caution in patients with a history of peptic ulcer or GERD; avoid in patients with symptomatic cardiac arrhythmias. Limit acetaminophen to <4 g/day. Safety and efficacy in children <12 years of age have not been established.

Adverse Reactions Note: Specific percentages not reported.

Frequently observed:

Central nervous system: Dizziness, drowsiness, lightheadedness, sedation

Gastrointestinal: Abdominal pain, nausea, vomiting

Respiratory: Dyspnea

Miscellaneous: Intoxicated feeling

Infrequently observed:

Cardiovascular: Tachycardia

Central nervous system: Agitation, confusion, depression, euphoria, excitement, faintness, fever, headache, seizure

Dermatologic: Hyperhidrosis, pruritus

Endocrine & metabolic: Hot spells

Gastrointestinal: Constipation, dysphagia, heartburn, flatulence, xerostomia

Neuromuscular & skeletal: Leg pain, muscle fatigue, numbness, paresthesia

Ocular: Heavy eyelids

Otic: Earache, tinnitus

Renal: Diuresis

Respiratory: Nasal congestion

Miscellaneous: Allergic reaction, high energy, shaky feeling, sluggishness

Metabolism/Transport Effects

Acetaminophen: **Substrate** (minor) of CYP1A2, 2A6, 2C9, 2D6, 2E1, 3A4; **Inhibits** CYP3A4 (weak)

Caffeine: **Substrate** of CYP1A2 (major), 2C9 (minor), 2D6 (minor), 2E1 (minor), 3A4 (minor); **Inhibits** CYP1A2 (weak), 3A4 (moderate)

Drug Interactions

Acetaminophen: Barbiturates may increase the metabolism of Acetaminophen. This may 1) diminish the effect of acetaminophen; and 2) increase the risk of liver damage. *Risk C: Monitor therapy*

Alcohol (Ethyl): CNS Depressants may enhance the CNS depressant effect of Alcohol (Ethyl). *Risk C: Monitor therapy*

Anticonvulsants (Hydantoin): May increase the metabolism of Acetaminophen. This may 1) diminish the effect of acetaminophen; and 2) increase the risk of liver damage. *Risk C: Monitor therapy*

Barbiturates: May increase the metabolism of Acetaminophen. This may 1) diminish the effect of acetaminophen; and 2) increase the risk of liver damage. *Risk C: Monitor therapy*

Beta-Blockers: Barbiturates may decrease the serum concentration of Beta-Blockers. **Exceptions:** Atenolol; Levobunolol; Metipranolol; Nadolol. *Risk C: Monitor therapy*

Calcium Channel Blockers: Barbiturates may increase the metabolism of Calcium Channel Blockers. **Exceptions:** Clevidipine. *Risk D: Consider therapy modification*

Cannabinoids: May enhance the tachycardic effect of Sympathomimetics. *Risk C: Monitor therapy*

CarBAMazepine: May increase the metabolism of Acetaminophen. This may 1) diminish the effect of acetaminophen; and 2) increase the risk of liver damage. *Risk C: Monitor therapy*

Chloramphenicol: May decrease the metabolism of Barbiturates. Barbiturates may increase the metabolism of Chloramphenicol. *Risk D: Consider therapy modification*

Cholestyramine Resin: May decrease the absorption of Acetaminophen. Effect is minimal if cholestyramine is administered 1 hour after acetaminophen. *Risk D: Consider therapy modification*

CNS Depressants: May enhance the adverse/toxic effect of other CNS Depressants. *Risk C: Monitor therapy*

Contraceptive (Progestins): Barbiturates may diminish the therapeutic effect of Contraceptive (Progestins). Contraceptive failure is possible. *Risk D: Consider therapy modification*

Corticosteroids (Systemic): Barbiturates may increase the metabolism of Corticosteroids (Systemic). *Risk C: Monitor therapy*

CycloSPORINE: Barbiturates may increase the metabolism of CycloSPORINE. *Risk D: Consider therapy modification*

CYP1A2 Inhibitors (Moderate): May decrease the metabolism of CYP1A2 Substrates. *Risk C: Monitor therapy*

CYP1A2 Inhibitors (Strong): May decrease the metabolism of CYP1A2 Substrates. *Risk D: Consider therapy modification*

CYP3A4 Substrates: CYP3A4 Inhibitors (Moderate) may decrease the metabolism of CYP3A4 Substrates. *Risk C: Monitor therapy*

Disopyramide: Barbiturates may increase the metabolism of Disopyramide. *Risk D: Consider therapy modification*

Doxycycline: Barbiturates may decrease the serum concentration of Doxycycline. *Risk D: Consider therapy modification*

Eplerenone: CYP3A4 Inhibitors (Moderate) may increase the serum concentration of Eplerenone. Management: A lower starting dose of eplerenone (25 mg once daily) is recommended in patients with hypertension who are also taking drugs that are moderate inhibitors of CYP3A4. *Risk D: Consider therapy modification*

Etoposide: Barbiturates may increase the metabolism of Etoposide. *Risk C: Monitor therapy*

Etoposide Phosphate: Barbiturates may decrease the serum concentration of Etoposide Phosphate. Barbiturates may increase the metabolism, via CYP isoenzymes, of etoposide phosphate. *Risk C: Monitor therapy*

Felbamate: May increase the serum concentration of Barbiturates. *Risk C: Monitor therapy*

Griseofulvin: Barbiturates may decrease the absorption of Griseofulvin. *Risk D: Consider therapy modification*

Imatinib: May increase the serum concentration of Acetaminophen. *Risk D: Consider therapy modification*

Isoniazid: May enhance the adverse/toxic effect of Acetaminophen. *Risk C: Monitor therapy*

LamoTRIgine: Barbiturates may increase the metabolism of LamoTRIgine. *Risk D: Consider therapy modification*

Maraviroc: CYP3A4 Inhibitors may increase the serum concentration of Maraviroc. *Risk D: Consider therapy modification*

Meperidine: Barbiturates may enhance the CNS depressant effect of Meperidine. *Risk C: Monitor therapy*

Methadone: Barbiturates may increase the metabolism of Methadone. *Risk D: Consider therapy modification*

Oral Contraceptive (Estrogens): Barbiturates may diminish the therapeutic effect of Oral Contraceptive (Estrogens). Contraceptive failure is possible. *Risk D: Consider therapy modification*

Pimecrolimus: CYP3A4 Inhibitors (Moderate) may decrease the metabolism of Pimecrolimus. *Risk C: Monitor therapy*

Primidone: May enhance the adverse/toxic effect of Barbiturates. Primidone is converted to phenobarbital, and thus becomes additive with existing barbiturate therapy. *Risk C: Monitor therapy*

Propafenone: Barbiturates may increase the metabolism of Propafenone. *Risk D: Consider therapy modification*

Pyridoxine: May increase the metabolism of Barbiturates. Apparent in high pyridoxine doses (eg, 200 mg/day) *Risk C: Monitor therapy*

QuiNIDine: Barbiturates may increase the metabolism of QuiNIDine. *Risk D: Consider therapy modification*

Quinolone Antibiotics: May decrease the metabolism of Caffeine. **Exceptions:** Gatifloxacin; Gemifloxacin; Levofloxacin; Lomefloxacin; Moxifloxacin; Nalidixic Acid; Ofloxacin; Sparfloxacin; Trovafloxacin. *Risk C: Monitor therapy*

Ranolazine: CYP3A4 Inhibitors (Moderate) may increase the serum concentration of Ranolazine. Management: Limit the ranolazine dose to a maximum of 500mg twice daily in patients concurrently receiving moderate CYP3A4 inhibitors (e.g., diltiazem, verapamil, erythromycin, etc.). *Risk D: Consider therapy modification*

Regadenoson: Caffeine may diminish the vasodilatory effect of Regadenoson. *Risk D: Consider therapy modification*

Rifamycin Derivatives: May increase the metabolism of Barbiturates. *Risk C: Monitor therapy*

Salmeterol: CYP3A4 Inhibitors (Moderate) may increase the serum concentration of Salmeterol. *Risk C: Monitor therapy*

Sympathomimetics: May enhance the adverse/toxic effect of other Sympathomimetics. *Risk C: Monitor therapy*

Teniposide: Barbiturates may increase the metabolism of Teniposide. *Risk C: Monitor therapy*

Theophylline Derivatives: Barbiturates may increase the metabolism of Theophylline Derivatives. **Exceptions:** Dyphylline. *Risk C: Monitor therapy*

Tricyclic Antidepressants: Barbiturates may increase the metabolism of Tricyclic Antidepressants. *Risk D: Consider therapy modification*

Valproic Acid: May decrease the metabolism of Barbiturates. Barbiturates may decrease the serum concentration of Valproic Acid. *Risk C: Monitor therapy*

Vitamin K Antagonists (eg, warfarin): Barbiturates may increase the metabolism of Vitamin K Antagonists. *Risk D: Consider therapy modification*

Vitamin K Antagonists (eg, warfarin): Acetaminophen may enhance the anticoagulant effect of Vitamin K Antagonists. Most likely with daily acetaminophen doses >1.3 g for >1 week. *Risk C: Monitor therapy*

Voriconazole: Barbiturates may decrease the serum concentration of Voriconazole. *Risk X: Avoid combination*

Ethanol/Nutrition/Herb Interactions Ethanol: Avoid ethanol (may increase CNS depression).

Stability Store at room temperature below 30°C (86°F). Protect from moisture.

Mechanism of Action

Butalbital is a short- to intermediate-acting barbiturate. Barbiturates depress the sensory cortex, decrease motor activity, alter cerebellar function, and produce drowsiness, sedation, hypnosis, and dose-dependent respiratory depression.

Acetaminophen inhibits the synthesis of prostaglandins in the central nervous system and peripherally blocks pain impulse generation; produces antipyresis from inhibition of hypothalamic heat-regulating center

Caffeine increases levels of 3'5' cyclic AMP by inhibiting phosphodiesterase; CNS stimulant which increases medullary respiratory center sensitivity to carbon dioxide, stimulates central inspiratory drive, and improves skeletal muscle contraction (diaphragmatic contractility)

Pharmacodynamics/Kinetics

Absorption: Butalbital: Well absorbed

Protein binding: Butalbital: 45%

Half-life elimination: Butalbital: 35 hours

Excretion: Butalbital: Urine (59% to 88% as unchanged drug and metabolites)

Dosage

Adults: Oral: 1-2 tablets or capsules (or 15-30 mL solution) every 4 hours; not to exceed 6 tablets or capsules (or 180 mL solution) daily

Elderly: Not recommended for use in the elderly

Dosing interval in renal or hepatic impairment: Should be reduced

Test Interactions Acetaminophen may produce false-positive tests for urinary 5-hydroxyindoleacetic acid.

Dosage Forms Excipient information presented when available (limited, particularly for generics); consult specific product labeling.

Capsule:

Anolor 300, Esgic®, Medigesic®: Butalbital 50 mg, acetaminophen 325 mg, and caffeine 40 mg

Dolgic® Plus: Butalbital 50 mg, acetaminophen 750 mg, and caffeine 40 mg

Esgic-Plus™, Zebutal™: Butalbital 50 mg, acetaminophen 500 mg, and caffeine 40 mg

Solution:

Dolgic® LQ: Butalbital 50 mg, acetaminophen 325 mg, and caffeine 40 mg per 15 mL (480 mL) [contains alcohol 7%; tropical fruit punch flavor]

Tablet: Butalbital 50 mg, acetaminophen 325 mg, and caffeine 40 mg; butalbital 50 mg, acetaminophen 500 mg, and caffeine 40 mg

Esgic®, Fioricet®, Repan®: Butalbital 50 mg, acetaminophen 325 mg, and caffeine 40 mg

Esgic-Plus™: Butalbital 50 mg, acetaminophen 500 mg, and caffeine 40 mg

Butalbital, Acetaminophen, Caffeine, and Codeine

(byoo TAL bi tal, a seet a MIN oh fen, KAF een, & KOE deen)

Medication Safety Issues

Sound-alike/look-alike issues:

Fioricet® may be confused with Fiorinal®, Florinef®, Lorcet®, Percocet®

Phrenilin® may be confused with Phenergan®, Trinalin®

High alert medication: The Institute for Safe Medication Practices (ISMP) includes this medication among its list of drug classes which have a heightened risk of causing significant patient harm when used in error.

Duplicate therapy issues: This product contains acetaminophen, which may be a component of other combination products. Do not exceed the maximum recommended daily dose of acetaminophen.

U.S. Brand Names Fioricet® with Codeine; Phrenilin® with Caffeine and Codeine

Index Terms Acetaminophen, Caffeine, Codeine, and Butalbital; Caffeine, Acetaminophen, Butalbital, and Codeine; Codeine, Acetaminophen, Butalbital, and Caffeine

Pharmacologic Category Analgesic Combination (Opioid); Barbiturate

Generic Available Yes

Use Relief of symptoms of complex tension (muscle contraction) headache

Effect on Mental Status May cause confusion, disorientation, nervousness, hallucinations, euphoria, agitation, irritability, depression, or drowsiness

Effect on Psychiatric Treatment May cause severe hepatic toxicity in overdose, use caution in patients with alcoholic liver disease. May cause agranulocytosis, use caution with clozapine and carbamazepine. May cause thrombocytopenia, use caution with valproate.

Restrictions C-III

Pregnancy Risk Factor C (per manufacturer)

Pregnancy Considerations Reproduction studies have not been conducted with this combination. Refer to the acetaminophen, caffeine, and codeine monographs for additional information. Butalbital crosses the placenta; may cause withdrawal seizures when taken during pregnancy.

Lactation Enters breast milk/not recommended

Contraindications Hypersensitivity to butalbital, codeine, caffeine, acetaminophen, or any component of the formulation; porphyria

Warnings/Precautions May cause CNS depression, which may impair physical or mental abilities; patients must be cautioned about performing tasks which require mental alertness (eg, operating machinery or driving). Limit acetaminophen to <4 g/day. Use with caution in patients with alcoholic liver disease; consuming ≥3 alcoholic drinks/day may increase the risk of liver damage. Effects may be potentiated when used with other sedative drugs or ethanol. May cause severe hepatic toxicity in acute overdose. In addition, chronic daily dosing in adults has resulted in liver damage in some patients. Use with caution in patients with hypersensitivity reactions to other phenanthrene-derivative opioid agonists (eg, morphine, hydrocodone, oxycodone). Use caution with Addison's disease, known G6PD deficiency, severe renal or hepatic impairment. Use caution in patients with head injury or other intracranial lesions, acute abdominal conditions, urethral stricture of BPH, thyroid dysfunction, or in patients with respiratory diseases. Use caution in patients with two or more copies of the variant CYP2D6*2 allele; may have extensive conversion from codeine to morphine and thus increased opioid-mediated effects. Elderly (not recommended for use) and/or debilitated patients may be more susceptible to CNS depressants, as well as constipating effects of narcotics. Tolerance or drug dependence may result from extended use. Caffeine may cause CNS and cardiovascular stimulation, as well as GI irritation in high doses. Use with caution in patients with a history of peptic ulcer or GERD; avoid in patients with symptomatic cardiac arrhythmias. Safety and efficacy in pediatric patients have not been established.

Adverse Reactions Frequency not defined.

Cardiovascular: Syncope, tachycardia

Central nervous system: Agitation, depression, dizziness, drowsiness, euphoria, excitement, fatigue, fever, headache, high energy, intoxicated feeling, lightheadedness, mental confusion, sedation, seizure, sluggishness

Dermatologic: Hyperhidrosis, pruritus

Endocrine & metabolic: Hot flashes

Gastrointestinal: Abdominal pain, constipation, dysphagia, flatulence, heartburn, nausea, vomiting, xerostomia

Neuromuscular & skeletal: Leg pain, muscle fatigue, numbness, paresthesia, shaky feeling

Ocular: Heavy eyelids

Otic: Earache, tinnitus

Renal: Diuresis

Respiratory: Dyspnea, nasal congestion

Miscellaneous: Allergic reaction

Note: Potential reactions associated with components of Fioricet® with Codeine include agranulocytosis, cardiac stimulation, dependence, erythema multiforme, hyperglycemia, irritability, nephrotoxicity, rash, thrombocytopenia, toxic epidermal necrolysis, tremor

Metabolism/Transport Effects

Acetaminophen: **Substrate** (minor) of CYP1A2, 2A6, 2C9, 2D6, 2E1, 3A4; **Inhibits** CYP3A4 (weak)

Caffeine: **Substrate** of CYP1A2 (major), 2C9 (minor), 2D6 (minor), 2E1 (minor), 3A4 (minor); **Inhibits** CYP1A2 (weak), 3A4 (moderate)

Codeine: **Substrate** of CYP2D6 (major), 3A4 (minor); **Inhibits** CYP2D6 (weak)

Drug Interactions

Acetaminophen: Barbiturates may increase the metabolism of Acetaminophen. This may 1) diminish the effect of acetaminophen; and 2) increase the risk of liver damage. *Risk C: Monitor therapy*

Alcohol (Ethyl): CNS Depressants may enhance the CNS depressant effect of Alcohol (Ethyl). *Risk C: Monitor therapy*

Alvimopan: Analgesics (Opioid) may enhance the adverse/toxic effect of Alvimopan. This is most notable for patients receiving long-term (i.e., more than 7 days) opiates prior to alvimopan initiation. Management: Alvimopan is contraindicated in patients receiving therapeutic doses of opioids for more than 7 consecutive days immediately prior to alvimopan initiation. *Risk D: Consider therapy modification*

Ammonium Chloride: May increase the excretion of Analgesics (Opioid). *Risk C: Monitor therapy*

Amphetamines: May enhance the analgesic effect of Analgesics (Opioid). *Risk C: Monitor therapy*

Anticonvulsants (Hydantoin): May increase the metabolism of Acetaminophen. This may 1) diminish the effect of acetaminophen; and 2) increase the risk of liver damage. *Risk C: Monitor therapy*

Antipsychotic Agents (Phenothiazines): May enhance the hypotensive effect of Analgesics (Opioid). *Risk C: Monitor therapy*

Barbiturates: May increase the metabolism of Acetaminophen. This may 1) diminish the effect of acetaminophen; and 2) increase the risk of liver damage. *Risk C: Monitor therapy*

Beta-Blockers: Barbiturates may decrease the serum concentration of Beta-Blockers. **Exceptions:** Atenolol; Levobunolol; Metipranolol; Nadolol. *Risk C: Monitor therapy*

Calcium Channel Blockers: Barbiturates may increase the metabolism of Calcium Channel Blockers. **Exceptions:** Clevidipine. *Risk D: Consider therapy modification*

CarBAMazepine: May increase the metabolism of Acetaminophen. This may 1) diminish the effect of acetaminophen; and 2) increase the risk of liver damage. *Risk C: Monitor therapy*

Chloramphenicol: May decrease the metabolism of Barbiturates. Barbiturates may increase the metabolism of Chloramphenicol. *Risk D: Consider therapy modification*

Cholestyramine Resin: May decrease the absorption of Acetaminophen. Effect is minimal if cholestyramine is administered 1 hour after acetaminophen. *Risk D: Consider therapy modification*

CNS Depressants: May enhance the adverse/toxic effect of other CNS Depressants. *Risk C: Monitor therapy*

Contraceptive (Progestins): Barbiturates may diminish the therapeutic effect of Contraceptive (Progestins). Contraceptive failure is possible. *Risk D: Consider therapy modification*

Corticosteroids (Systemic): Barbiturates may increase the metabolism of Corticosteroids (Systemic). *Risk C: Monitor therapy*

CycloSPORINE: Barbiturates may increase the metabolism of CycloSPORINE. *Risk D: Consider therapy modification*

CYP1A2 Inhibitors (Moderate): May decrease the metabolism of CYP1A2 Substrates. *Risk C: Monitor therapy*

CYP1A2 Inhibitors (Strong): May decrease the metabolism of CYP1A2 Substrates. *Risk D: Consider therapy modification*

CYP2D6 Inhibitors (Moderate): May diminish the therapeutic effect of Codeine. These CYP2D6 inhibitors may prevent the metabolic conversion of codeine to its active metabolite morphine. *Risk C: Monitor therapy*

CYP2D6 Inhibitors (Strong): May diminish the therapeutic effect of Codeine. These CYP2D6 inhibitors may prevent the metabolic conversion of codeine to its active metabolite morphine. *Risk D: Consider therapy modification*

CYP3A4 Substrates: CYP3A4 Inhibitors (Moderate) may decrease the metabolism of CYP3A4 Substrates. *Risk C: Monitor therapy*

Desmopressin: Analgesics (Opioid) may enhance the adverse/toxic effect of Desmopressin. *Risk C: Monitor therapy*

Disopyramide: Barbiturates may increase the metabolism of Disopyramide. *Risk D: Consider therapy modification*

Doxycycline: Barbiturates may decrease the serum concentration of Doxycycline. *Risk D: Consider therapy modification*

Eplerenone: CYP3A4 Inhibitors (Moderate) may increase the serum concentration of Eplerenone. Management: A lower starting dose of eplerenone (25 mg once daily) is recommended in patients with hypertension who are also taking drugs that are moderate inhibitors of CYP3A4. *Risk D: Consider therapy modification*

Etoposide: Barbiturates may increase the metabolism of Etoposide. *Risk C: Monitor therapy*

Etoposide Phosphate: Barbiturates may decrease the serum concentration of Etoposide Phosphate. Barbiturates may increase the metabolism, via CYP isoenzymes, of etoposide phosphate. *Risk C: Monitor therapy*

Felbamate: May increase the serum concentration of Barbiturates. *Risk C: Monitor therapy*

Griseofulvin: Barbiturates may decrease the absorption of Griseofulvin. *Risk D: Consider therapy modification*

Imatinib: May increase the serum concentration of Acetaminophen. *Risk D: Consider therapy modification*

Isoniazid: May enhance the adverse/toxic effect of Acetaminophen. *Risk C: Monitor therapy*

LamoTRIgine: Barbiturates may increase the metabolism of LamoTRIgine. *Risk D: Consider therapy modification*

Maraviroc: CYP3A4 Inhibitors may increase the serum concentration of Maraviroc. *Risk D: Consider therapy modification*

Meperidine: Barbiturates may enhance the CNS depressant effect of Meperidine. *Risk C: Monitor therapy*

Methadone: Barbiturates may increase the metabolism of Methadone. *Risk D: Consider therapy modification*

Oral Contraceptive (Estrogens): Barbiturates may diminish the therapeutic effect of Oral Contraceptive (Estrogens). Contraceptive failure is possible. *Risk D: Consider therapy modification*

Pegvisomant: Analgesics (Opioid) may diminish the therapeutic effect of Pegvisomant. *Risk C: Monitor therapy*

Pimecrolimus: CYP3A4 Inhibitors (Moderate) may decrease the metabolism of Pimecrolimus. *Risk C: Monitor therapy*

Primidone: May enhance the adverse/toxic effect of Barbiturates. Primidone is converted to phenobarbital, and thus becomes additive with existing barbiturate therapy. *Risk C: Monitor therapy*

Propafenone: Barbiturates may increase the metabolism of Propafenone. *Risk D: Consider therapy modification*

Pyridoxine: May increase the metabolism of Barbiturates. Apparent in high pyridoxine doses (eg, 200 mg/day) *Risk C: Monitor therapy*

QuiNIDine: Barbiturates may increase the metabolism of QuiNIDine. *Risk D: Consider therapy modification*

Quinolone Antibiotics: May decrease the metabolism of Caffeine. **Exceptions:** Gatifloxacin; Gemifloxacin; Levofloxacin; Lomefloxacin; Moxifloxacin; Nalidixic Acid; Ofloxacin; Sparfloxacin; Trovafloxacin. *Risk C: Monitor therapy*

Ranolazine: CYP3A4 Inhibitors (Moderate) may increase the serum concentration of Ranolazine. Management: Limit the ranolazine dose to a maximum of 500mg twice daily in patients concurrently receiving moderate CYP3A4 inhibitors (e.g., diltiazem, verapamil, erythromycin, etc.). *Risk D: Consider therapy modification*

Regadenoson: Caffeine may diminish the vasodilatory effect of Regadenoson. *Risk D: Consider therapy modification*

Rifamycin Derivatives: May increase the metabolism of Barbiturates. *Risk C: Monitor therapy*

Salmeterol: CYP3A4 Inhibitors (Moderate) may increase the serum concentration of Salmeterol. *Risk C: Monitor therapy*

Selective Serotonin Reuptake Inhibitors: Analgesics (Opioid) may enhance the serotonergic effect of Selective Serotonin Reuptake Inhibitors. This may cause serotonin syndrome. *Risk C: Monitor therapy*

Somatostatin Analogs: May decrease the metabolism of Codeine. The formation of two major codeine metabolites (morphine and norcodeine) may be impaired by somatostatin analogs. *Risk C: Monitor therapy*

Succinylcholine: May enhance the bradycardic effect of Analgesics (Opioid). *Risk C: Monitor therapy*

Sympathomimetics: May enhance the adverse/toxic effect of other Sympathomimetics. *Risk C: Monitor therapy*

Teniposide: Barbiturates may increase the metabolism of Teniposide. *Risk C: Monitor therapy*

Theophylline Derivatives: Barbiturates may increase the metabolism of Theophylline Derivatives. **Exceptions:** Dyphylline. *Risk C: Monitor therapy*

Tricyclic Antidepressants: Barbiturates may increase the metabolism of Tricyclic Antidepressants. *Risk D: Consider therapy modification*

Valproic Acid: May decrease the metabolism of Barbiturates. Barbiturates may decrease the serum concentration of Valproic Acid. *Risk C: Monitor therapy*

Vitamin K Antagonists (eg, warfarin): Barbiturates may increase the metabolism of Vitamin K Antagonists. *Risk D: Consider therapy modification*

Vitamin K Antagonists (eg, warfarin): Acetaminophen may enhance the anticoagulant effect of Vitamin K Antagonists. Most likely with daily acetaminophen doses >1.3 g for >1 week. *Risk C: Monitor therapy*

Voriconazole: Barbiturates may decrease the serum concentration of Voriconazole. *Risk X: Avoid combination*

Ethanol/Nutrition/Herb Interactions Ethanol: Avoid ethanol (may increase CNS depression).

Stability Store below 30°C (86°F).

Mechanism of Action Combination product for the treatment of tension headache. Contains codeine (narcotic analgesic), butalbital (barbiturate), caffeine (CNS stimulant), and acetaminophen (nonopiate, nonsalicylate analgesic).

Dosage Oral: Adults: 1-2 capsules every 4 hours. Total daily dosage should not exceed 6 capsules.

Dosing adjustment/comments in hepatic impairment: Use with caution. Limited, low-dose therapy usually well tolerated in hepatic disease/cirrhosis. However, cases of hepatotoxicity at daily acetaminophen dosages <4 g/day have been reported. Avoid chronic use in hepatic impairment.

Monitoring Parameters Hepatic and renal function tests (in patients with impairment)

Test Interactions Acetaminophen may produce false-positive tests for urinary 5-hydroxyindoleacetic acid; codeine may increase serum amylase levels

Dosage Forms Excipient information presented when available (limited, particularly for generics); consult specific product labeling.

Capsule: Butalbital 50 mg, acetaminophen 325 mg, caffeine 40 mg, and codeine phosphate 30 mg

Fioricet® with Codeine: Butalbital 50 mg, acetaminophen 325 mg, caffeine 40 mg, and codeine phosphate 30 mg

Phrenilin® with Caffeine and Codeine: Butalbital 50 mg, acetaminophen 325 mg, caffeine 40 mg, and codeine phosphate 30 mg

Butalbital and Acetaminophen

(byoo TAL bi tal & a seet a MIN oh fen)

Medication Safety Issues

Duplicate therapy issues: This product contains acetaminophen, which may be a component of other combination products. Do not exceed the maximum recommended daily dose of acetaminophen.

U.S. Brand Names Bupap; Cephadyn; Phrenilin®; Phrenilin® Forte; Promacet; Sedapap®

Index Terms Acetaminophen and Butalbital

Pharmacologic Category Analgesic, Miscellaneous; Barbiturate

Generic Available Yes

Use Relief of the symptomatic complex of tension or muscle contraction headache

Effect on Mental Status Dizziness, drowsiness, and sedation are common; may cause agitation, confusion, euphoria, or excitement

Effect on Psychiatric Treatment Sedation is common; concomitant use with psychotropics may produce additive CNS depressant effects

Pregnancy Risk Factor C

Pregnancy Considerations Reproduction studies have not been conducted with this combination. The FDA pregnancy classification for most other barbiturates is Category D. Withdrawal seizures were reported in an infant 2 days after birth following maternal use of a butalbital product during the last 2 months of pregnancy; butalbital levels were measured in the infant's serum. In general, barbiturates cross the placenta and distribute in fetal tissue. Teratogenic effects have been reported with first trimester exposure. Exposure during the third trimester may lead to symptoms of acute withdrawal following delivery; symptoms may be delayed up to 14 days. Refer to Acetaminophen monograph for information specific to acetaminophen.

Lactation Enters breast milk/not recommended

Contraindications Hypersensitivity to butalbital, acetaminophen, or any component of the formulation; porphyria

Warnings/Precautions May cause CNS depression, which may impair physical or mental abilities; patients must be cautioned about performing tasks which require mental alertness (eg, operating machinery or driving). May cause severe hepatic toxicity on acute overdose; in addition, chronic daily dosing in adults has resulted in liver damage in some patients. Use with caution in patients with alcoholic liver disease; consuming ≥3 alcoholic drinks/day may increase the risk of liver damage. Effects may be potentiated when used with other sedative drugs or ethanol. Use caution in elderly and debilitated patients. Use with caution in patients with history of drug abuse, known G6PD deficiency, hepatic impairment, renal impairment, respiratory disease. Limit acetaminophen to <4 g/day. Safety and efficacy in children <12 years of age have not been established.

Adverse Reactions

Frequently observed:

Central nervous system: Dizziness, drowsiness, lightheadedness, sedation

Gastrointestinal: Abdominal pain, nausea, vomiting

Respiratory: Dyspnea

Miscellaneous: Intoxicated feeling

Infrequently observed:

Cardiovascular: Tachycardia

Central nervous system: Agitation, confusion, depression, euphoria, excitement, faintness, fever, headache, seizure

Dermatologic: Hyperhidrosis, pruritus

Endocrine & metabolic: Hot spells

Gastrointestinal: Constipation, dysphagia, heartburn, flatulence, xerostomia

Neuromuscular & skeletal: Leg pain, muscle fatigue, numbness, paresthesia

Ocular: Heavy eyelids

Otic: Earache, tinnitus

Renal: Diuresis

Respiratory: Nasal congestion

Miscellaneous: Allergic reaction, high energy, shaky feeling, sluggishness

Limited to important or life-threatening: Toxic epidermal necrolysis, erythema multiforme

Metabolism/Transport Effects

Acetaminophen: **Substrate** (minor) of CYP1A2, 2A6, 2C9, 2D6, 2E1, 3A4; **Inhibits** CYP3A4 (weak)

Butalbital: See Phenobarbital monograph

Drug Interactions

Acetaminophen: Barbiturates may increase the metabolism of Acetaminophen. This may 1) diminish the effect of acetaminophen; and 2) increase the risk of liver damage. *Risk C: Monitor therapy*

Alcohol (Ethyl): CNS Depressants may enhance the CNS depressant effect of Alcohol (Ethyl). *Risk C: Monitor therapy*

Anticonvulsants (Hydantoin): May increase the metabolism of Acetaminophen. This may 1) diminish the effect of acetaminophen; and 2) increase the risk of liver damage. *Risk C: Monitor therapy*

Barbiturates: May increase the metabolism of Acetaminophen. This may 1) diminish the effect of acetaminophen; and 2) increase the risk of liver damage. *Risk C: Monitor therapy*

Beta-Blockers: Barbiturates may decrease the serum concentration of Beta-Blockers. **Exceptions:** Atenolol; Levobunolol; Metipranolol; Nadolol. *Risk C: Monitor therapy*

Calcium Channel Blockers: Barbiturates may increase the metabolism of Calcium Channel Blockers. **Exceptions:** Clevidipine. *Risk D: Consider therapy modification*

CarBAMazepine: May increase the metabolism of Acetaminophen. This may 1) diminish the effect of acetaminophen; and 2) increase the risk of liver damage. *Risk C: Monitor therapy*

Chloramphenicol: May decrease the metabolism of Barbiturates. Barbiturates may increase the metabolism of Chloramphenicol. *Risk D: Consider therapy modification*

Cholestyramine Resin: May decrease the absorption of Acetaminophen. Effect is minimal if cholestyramine is administered 1 hour after acetaminophen. *Risk D: Consider therapy modification*

CNS Depressants: May enhance the adverse/toxic effect of other CNS Depressants. *Risk C: Monitor therapy*

Contraceptive (Progestins): Barbiturates may diminish the therapeutic effect of Contraceptive (Progestins). Contraceptive failure is possible. *Risk D: Consider therapy modification*

Corticosteroids (Systemic): Barbiturates may increase the metabolism of Corticosteroids (Systemic). *Risk C: Monitor therapy*

CycloSPORINE: Barbiturates may increase the metabolism of CycloSPORINE. *Risk D: Consider therapy modification*

Disopyramide: Barbiturates may increase the metabolism of Disopyramide. *Risk D: Consider therapy modification*

Doxycycline: Barbiturates may decrease the serum concentration of Doxycycline. *Risk D: Consider therapy modification*

Etoposide: Barbiturates may increase the metabolism of Etoposide. *Risk C: Monitor therapy*

Etoposide Phosphate: Barbiturates may decrease the serum concentration of Etoposide Phosphate. Barbiturates may increase the metabolism, via CYP isoenzymes, of etoposide phosphate. *Risk C: Monitor therapy*

Felbamate: May increase the serum concentration of Barbiturates. *Risk C: Monitor therapy*

Griseofulvin: Barbiturates may decrease the absorption of Griseofulvin. *Risk D: Consider therapy modification*

Imatinib: May increase the serum concentration of Acetaminophen. *Risk D: Consider therapy modification*

Isoniazid: May enhance the adverse/toxic effect of Acetaminophen. *Risk C: Monitor therapy*

LamoTRIgine: Barbiturates may increase the metabolism of LamoTRIgine. *Risk D: Consider therapy modification*

Meperidine: Barbiturates may enhance the CNS depressant effect of Meperidine. *Risk C: Monitor therapy*

Methadone: Barbiturates may increase the metabolism of Methadone. *Risk D: Consider therapy modification*

Oral Contraceptive (Estrogens): Barbiturates may diminish the therapeutic effect of Oral Contraceptive (Estrogens). Contraceptive failure is possible. *Risk D: Consider therapy modification*

Primidone: May enhance the adverse/toxic effect of Barbiturates. Primidone is converted to phenobarbital, and thus becomes additive with existing barbiturate therapy. *Risk C: Monitor therapy*

Propafenone: Barbiturates may increase the metabolism of Propafenone. *Risk D: Consider therapy modification*

Pyridoxine: May increase the metabolism of Barbiturates. Apparent in high pyridoxine doses (eg, 200 mg/day) *Risk C: Monitor therapy*

QuiNIDine: Barbiturates may increase the metabolism of QuiNIDine. *Risk D: Consider therapy modification*

Rifamycin Derivatives: May increase the metabolism of Barbiturates. *Risk C: Monitor therapy*

Teniposide: Barbiturates may increase the metabolism of Teniposide. *Risk C: Monitor therapy*

Theophylline Derivatives: Barbiturates may increase the metabolism of Theophylline Derivatives. **Exceptions:** Dyphylline. *Risk C: Monitor therapy*

Tricyclic Antidepressants: Barbiturates may increase the metabolism of Tricyclic Antidepressants. *Risk D: Consider therapy modification*

Valproic Acid: May decrease the metabolism of Barbiturates. Barbiturates may decrease the serum concentration of Valproic Acid. *Risk C: Monitor therapy*

Vitamin K Antagonists (eg, warfarin): Barbiturates may increase the metabolism of Vitamin K Antagonists. *Risk D: Consider therapy modification*

Vitamin K Antagonists (eg, warfarin): Acetaminophen may enhance the anticoagulant effect of Vitamin K Antagonists. Most likely with daily acetaminophen doses >1.3 g for >1 week. *Risk C: Monitor therapy*

Voriconazole: Barbiturates may decrease the serum concentration of Voriconazole. *Risk X: Avoid combination*

Ethanol/Nutrition/Herb Interactions Ethanol: Avoid ethanol (may increase CNS depression).

Stability Store at 15°C to 30°C (59°F to 86°F); protect from light

Mechanism of Action

Butalbital is a short- to intermediate-acting barbiturate. Barbiturates depress the sensory cortex, decrease motor activity, alter cerebellar function, and produce drowsiness, sedation, hypnosis, and dose-dependent respiratory depression.

Acetaminophen inhibits the synthesis of prostaglandins in the central nervous system and peripherally blocks pain impulse generation; produces antipyresis from inhibition of hypothalamic heat-regulating center.

Pharmacodynamics/Kinetics Also see Acetaminophen monograph.

Absorption: Butalbital: Well absorbed

Protein binding: Butalbital: 45%

Half-life elimination: Butalbital: 35 hours

Excretion: Butalbital: Urine (59% to 88% as unchanged drug or metabolites)

Dosage Oral: Adults: One tablet/capsule every 4 hours as needed (maximum dose: 6 tablets/day)

Phrenilin®: 1-2 tablets every 4 hours as needed (maximum: 6 tablets in 24 hours)

Elderly: Use with caution; see adult dosing

Dosage adjustment in renal impairment: Mild-to-moderate: Should decrease dose; in severe impairment, use with caution

Dosage adjustment in hepatic impairment: Mild-to-moderate: Should decrease dose; in severe impairment, use with caution

Test Interactions Acetaminophen may produce false-positive tests for urinary 5-hydroxyindoleacetic acid.

Dosage Forms Excipient information presented when available (limited, particularly for generics); consult specific product labeling.

Tablet:

Phrenilin®: Butalbital 50 mg and acetaminophen 325 mg

Bupap, Cephadyn, Promacet, Sedapap®: Butalbital 50 mg and acetaminophen 650 mg

Capsule:

Phrenilin® Forte: Butalbital 50 mg and acetaminophen 650 mg [may contain benzyl alcohol]

Butalbital, Aspirin, and Caffeine

(byoo TAL bi tal, AS pir in, & KAF een)

Medication Safety Issues

Sound-alike/look-alike issues:

Fiorinal® may be confused with Fioricet®, Florical®, Florinef®

U.S. Brand Names Fiorinal®

Canadian Brand Names Fiorinal®

Index Terms Aspirin, Caffeine, and Butalbital; Butalbital Compound

Pharmacologic Category Barbiturate

Generic Available Yes

Use Relief of the symptomatic complex of tension or muscle contraction headache

Effect on Mental Status Drowsiness is common; may cause depression, nervousness, insomnia, and nightmares; rare reports of hallucinations

Effect on Psychiatric Treatment Rare reports of agranulocytosis; use caution with clozapine and carbamazepine; CNS depressant effects of psychotropics may be enhance by barbiturates; enzyme induction effects of barbiturates may decrease effects of psychotropics

Restrictions C-III

Pregnancy Risk Factor C/D (prolonged use or high doses at term)

Lactation Enters breast milk/use caution due to aspirin content

Contraindications Hypersensitivity to butalbital or any component of the formulation; porphyria; pregnancy (prolonged use or high doses at term)

Warnings/Precautions May cause CNS depression, which may impair physical or mental abilities; patients must be cautioned about performing tasks which require mental alertness (eg, operating machinery or driving). Patients with sensitivity to tartrazine dyes, nasal polyps, and asthma may have an increased risk of salicylate sensitivity. Use cautions with patients on anticoagulant therapy. Effects may be potentiated when used with other sedative drugs or ethanol. Use caution in elderly. Use with caution in patients with abdominal conditions, bleeding disorders, history of drug abuse, gastrointestinal disease, hepatic impairment, renal impairment, respiratory disease. Caffeine may cause CNS and cardiovascular stimulation, as well as GI irritation in high doses. Use with caution in patients with a history of peptic ulcer or GERD; avoid in patients with symptomatic cardiac arrhythmias. Children and teenagers who have or are recovering from chickenpox or flu-like symptoms should not use this product. Changes in behavior (along with nausea and vomiting) may be an early sign of Reye's syndrome; patients should be instructed to contact their healthcare provider if these occur.

Adverse Reactions

>10%:

Central nervous system: Dizziness, lightheadedness, drowsiness, "hangover" effect

Gastrointestinal: Heartburn, stomach pain, dyspepsia, epigastric discomfort, nausea

1% to 10%:

Central nervous system: Confusion, mental depression, unusual excitement, nervousness, faint feeling, headache, insomnia, nightmares, fatigue

Dermatologic: Skin rash

Gastrointestinal: Constipation, vomiting, gastrointestinal ulceration

Hematologic: Hemolytic anemia

Neuromuscular & skeletal: Weakness

Respiratory: Troubled breathing

Miscellaneous: Anaphylactic shock

Metabolism/Transport Effects

Aspirin: **Substrate** of CYP2C9 (minor)

Caffeine: **Substrate** of CYP1A2 (major), 2C9 (minor), 2D6 (minor), 2E1 (minor), 3A4 (minor); **Inhibits** CYP1A2 (weak), 3A4 (moderate)

Drug Interactions

ACE Inhibitors: Salicylates may diminish the antihypertensive effect of ACE Inhibitors. They may also diminish other beneficial pharmacodynamic effects desired for the treatment of CHF. The effects are likely dose-related. 100 mg doses aspirin appear to cause no problems, whereas 300 mg doses appear to significantly affect ACE Inhibitor efficacy. *Risk C: Monitor therapy*

Acetaminophen: Barbiturates may increase the metabolism of Acetaminophen. This may 1) diminish the effect of acetaminophen; and 2) increase the risk of liver damage. *Risk C: Monitor therapy*

Alcohol (Ethyl): CNS Depressants may enhance the CNS depressant effect of Alcohol (Ethyl). *Risk C: Monitor therapy*

Alendronate: Aspirin may enhance the adverse/toxic effect of Alendronate. Specifically gastrointestinal adverse events. *Risk C: Monitor therapy*

Anticoagulants: Salicylates may enhance the anticoagulant effect of Anticoagulants. *Risk C: Monitor therapy*

Antidepressants (Serotonin/Norepinephrine Reuptake Inhibitor): May enhance the antiplatelet effect of Aspirin. *Risk C: Monitor therapy*

Antidepressants (Tricyclic, Tertiary Amine): May enhance the antiplatelet effect of Aspirin. *Risk C: Monitor therapy*

Antiplatelet Agents: May enhance the adverse/toxic effect of Salicylates. Increased risk of bleeding may result. *Risk C: Monitor therapy*

Beta-Blockers: Barbiturates may decrease the serum concentration of Beta-Blockers. **Exceptions:** Atenolol; Levobunolol; Metipranolol; Nadolol. *Risk C: Monitor therapy*

Calcium Channel Blockers: Barbiturates may increase the metabolism of Calcium Channel Blockers. **Exceptions:** Clevidipine. *Risk D: Consider therapy modification*

Calcium Channel Blockers (Nondihydropyridine): May enhance the anticoagulant effect of Salicylates. *Risk C: Monitor therapy*

Cannabinoids: May enhance the tachycardic effect of Sympathomimetics. *Risk C: Monitor therapy*

Carbonic Anhydrase Inhibitors: Salicylates may enhance the adverse/toxic effect of Carbonic Anhydrase Inhibitors. Salicylate toxicity might be enhanced by this same combination. *Risk D: Consider therapy modification*

Chloramphenicol: May decrease the metabolism of Barbiturates. Barbiturates may increase the metabolism of Chloramphenicol. *Risk D: Consider therapy modification*

CNS Depressants: May enhance the adverse/toxic effect of other CNS Depressants. *Risk C: Monitor therapy*

Contraceptive (Progestins): Barbiturates may diminish the therapeutic effect of Contraceptive (Progestins). Contraceptive failure is possible. *Risk D: Consider therapy modification*

Corticosteroids (Systemic): Salicylates may enhance the adverse/toxic effect of Corticosteroids (Systemic). These specifically include gastrointestinal ulceration and bleeding. Corticosteroids (Systemic) may decrease the serum concentration of Salicylates. Withdrawal of corticosteroids may result in salicylate toxicity. *Risk C: Monitor therapy*

Corticosteroids (Systemic): Barbiturates may increase the metabolism of Corticosteroids (Systemic). *Risk C: Monitor therapy*

CycloSPORINE: Barbiturates may increase the metabolism of CycloSPORINE. *Risk D: Consider therapy modification*

CYP1A2 Inhibitors (Moderate): May decrease the metabolism of CYP1A2 Substrates. *Risk C: Monitor therapy*

CYP1A2 Inhibitors (Strong): May decrease the metabolism of CYP1A2 Substrates. *Risk D: Consider therapy modification*

CYP3A4 Substrates: CYP3A4 Inhibitors (Moderate) may decrease the metabolism of CYP3A4 Substrates. *Risk C: Monitor therapy*

Dasatinib: May enhance the anticoagulant effect of Antiplatelet Agents. *Risk C: Monitor therapy*

Disopyramide: Barbiturates may increase the metabolism of Disopyramide. *Risk D: Consider therapy modification*

Doxycycline: Barbiturates may decrease the serum concentration of Doxycycline. *Risk D: Consider therapy modification*

Drotrecogin Alfa: Salicylates may enhance the adverse/toxic effect of Drotrecogin Alfa. Bleeding may occur. *Risk D: Consider therapy modification*

Eplerenone: CYP3A4 Inhibitors (Moderate) may increase the serum concentration of Eplerenone. Management: A lower starting dose of eplerenone (25 mg once daily) is recommended in patients with hypertension who are also taking drugs that are moderate inhibitors of CYP3A4. *Risk D: Consider therapy modification*

Etoposide: Barbiturates may increase the metabolism of Etoposide. *Risk C: Monitor therapy*

Etoposide Phosphate: Barbiturates may decrease the serum concentration of Etoposide Phosphate. Barbiturates may increase the metabolism, via CYP isoenzymes, of etoposide phosphate. *Risk C: Monitor therapy*

Felbamate: May increase the serum concentration of Barbiturates. *Risk C: Monitor therapy*

Ginkgo Biloba: May enhance the antiplatelet effect of Salicylates. *Risk D: Consider therapy modification*

Griseofulvin: Barbiturates may decrease the absorption of Griseofulvin. *Risk D: Consider therapy modification*

Heparin: Aspirin may enhance the anticoagulant effect of Heparin. *Risk C: Monitor therapy*

Herbs (Anticoagulant/Antiplatelet Properties) (eg, Alfalfa, Anise, Bilberry): May enhance the adverse/toxic effect of Salicylates. Bleeding may occur. *Risk D: Consider therapy modification*

Ibritumomab: Antiplatelet Agents may enhance the adverse/toxic effect of Ibritumomab. Both agents may contribute to impaired platelet function and an increased risk of bleeding. *Risk C: Monitor therapy*

Ketorolac: May enhance the adverse/toxic effect of Aspirin. *Risk X: Avoid combination*

LamoTRIgine: Barbiturates may increase the metabolism of LamoTRIgine. *Risk D: Consider therapy modification*

Maraviroc: CYP3A4 Inhibitors may increase the serum concentration of Maraviroc. *Risk D: Consider therapy modification*

Meperidine: Barbiturates may enhance the CNS depressant effect of Meperidine. *Risk C: Monitor therapy*

Methadone: Barbiturates may increase the metabolism of Methadone. *Risk D: Consider therapy modification*

Methotrexate: Salicylates may increase the serum concentration of Methotrexate. Salicylate doses used for prophylaxis of cardiovascular events are not likely to be of concern. *Risk D: Consider therapy modification*

Nonsteroidal Anti-Inflammatory Agents: May enhance the adverse/toxic effect of Antiplatelet Agents. An increased risk of bleeding may occur. *Risk C: Monitor therapy*

NSAID (Nonselective): May enhance the antiplatelet effect of Salicylates. NSAID (Nonselective) may diminish the cardioprotective effect of Salicylates. Salicylates may decrease the serum concentration of NSAID (Nonselective). **Exceptions:** Diclofenac. *Risk D: Consider therapy modification*

Omega-3-Acid Ethyl Esters: May enhance the antiplatelet effect of Antiplatelet Agents. *Risk C: Monitor therapy*

Oral Contraceptive (Estrogens): Barbiturates may diminish the therapeutic effect of Oral Contraceptive (Estrogens). Contraceptive failure is possible. *Risk D: Consider therapy modification*

Pentosan Polysulfate Sodium: May enhance the adverse/toxic effect of Antiplatelet Agents. Specifically, the risk of bleeding may be increased by concurrent use of these agents. *Risk C: Monitor therapy*

Pimecrolimus: CYP3A4 Inhibitors (Moderate) may decrease the metabolism of Pimecrolimus. *Risk C: Monitor therapy*

Primidone: May enhance the adverse/toxic effect of Barbiturates. Primidone is converted to phenobarbital, and thus becomes additive with existing barbiturate therapy. *Risk C: Monitor therapy*

Propafenone: Barbiturates may increase the metabolism of Propafenone. *Risk D: Consider therapy modification*

Prostacyclin Analogues: May enhance the antiplatelet effect of Antiplatelet Agents. *Risk C: Monitor therapy*

Pyridoxine: May increase the metabolism of Barbiturates. Apparent in high pyridoxine doses (eg, 200 mg/day) *Risk C: Monitor therapy*

QuiNIDine: Barbiturates may increase the metabolism of QuiNIDine. *Risk D: Consider therapy modification*

Quinolone Antibiotics: May decrease the metabolism of Caffeine. **Exceptions:** Gatifloxacin; Gemifloxacin; Levofloxacin; Lomefloxacin; Moxifloxacin; Nalidixic Acid; Ofloxacin; Sparfloxacin; Trovafloxacin. *Risk C: Monitor therapy*

Ranolazine: CYP3A4 Inhibitors (Moderate) may increase the serum concentration of Ranolazine. Management: Limit the ranolazine dose to a maximum of 500mg twice daily in patients concurrently receiving moderate CYP3A4 inhibitors (e.g., diltiazem, verapamil, erythromycin, etc.). *Risk D: Consider therapy modification*

Regadenoson: Caffeine may diminish the vasodilatory effect of Regadenoson. *Risk D: Consider therapy modification*

Rifamycin Derivatives: May increase the metabolism of Barbiturates. *Risk C: Monitor therapy*

Salicylates: May enhance the anticoagulant effect of other Salicylates. *Risk C: Monitor therapy*

Salmeterol: CYP3A4 Inhibitors (Moderate) may increase the serum concentration of Salmeterol. *Risk C: Monitor therapy*

Selective Serotonin Reuptake Inhibitors: May enhance the antiplatelet effect of Aspirin. *Risk C: Monitor therapy*

Sulfonylureas: Salicylates may enhance the hypoglycemic effect of Sulfonylureas. Of concern with regular, higher doses of salicylates, not sporadic, low doses. *Risk C: Monitor therapy*

Sympathomimetics: May enhance the adverse/toxic effect of other Sympathomimetics. *Risk C: Monitor therapy*

Teniposide: Barbiturates may increase the metabolism of Teniposide. *Risk C: Monitor therapy*

Theophylline Derivatives: Barbiturates may increase the metabolism of Theophylline Derivatives. **Exceptions:** Dyphylline. *Risk C: Monitor therapy*

Thrombolytic Agents: Salicylates may enhance the adverse/toxic effect of Thrombolytic Agents. An increased risk of bleeding may occur. *Risk C: Monitor therapy*

Tiludronate: Aspirin may decrease the serum concentration of Tiludronate. *Risk C: Monitor therapy*

Tositumomab and Iodine I 131 Tositumomab: Antiplatelet Agents may enhance the adverse/toxic effect of Tositumomab and Iodine I 131 Tositumomab. Specifically, the risk of bleeding-related adverse events may be increased. *Risk C: Monitor therapy*

Treprostinil: May enhance the adverse/toxic effect of Salicylates. Bleeding may occur. *Risk C: Monitor therapy*

Tricyclic Antidepressants: Barbiturates may increase the metabolism of Tricyclic Antidepressants. *Risk D: Consider therapy modification*

Uricosuric Agents: Salicylates may diminish the therapeutic effect of Uricosuric Agents. Specifically, uricosuria. *Risk C: Monitor therapy*

Valproic Acid: May decrease the metabolism of Barbiturates. Barbiturates may decrease the serum concentration of Valproic Acid. *Risk C: Monitor therapy*

Valproic Acid: Salicylates may increase the serum concentration of Valproic Acid. *Risk C: Monitor therapy*

Varicella Virus-Containing Vaccines: Salicylates may enhance the adverse/toxic effect of Varicella Virus-Containing Vaccines. Reye 's Syndrome may develop. *Risk D: Consider therapy modification*

Vitamin K Antagonists (eg, warfarin): Salicylates may enhance the anticoagulant effect of Vitamin K Antagonists. *Risk D: Consider therapy modification*

Vitamin K Antagonists (eg, warfarin): Barbiturates may increase the metabolism of Vitamin K Antagonists. *Risk D: Consider therapy modification*

Voriconazole: Barbiturates may decrease the serum concentration of Voriconazole. *Risk X: Avoid combination*

Ethanol/Nutrition/Herb Interactions Ethanol: Avoid ethanol (may increase CNS depression).

Stability Store below 25°C (77°F).

Dosage

Oral: Adults: 1-2 tablets or capsules every 4 hours; not to exceed 6/day

Elderly: Not recommended for use in the elderly

Dosing interval in renal or hepatic impairment: Should be reduced

Dosage Forms Excipient information presented when available (limited, particularly for generics); consult specific product labeling.

Capsule: Butalbital 50 mg, aspirin 325 mg, and caffeine 40 mg

Fiorinal®: Butalbital 50 mg, aspirin 325 mg, and caffeine 40 mg

Tablet: Butalbital 50 mg, aspirin 325 mg, and caffeine 40 mg

Butalbital, Aspirin, Caffeine, and Codeine

(byoo TAL bi tal, AS pir in, KAF een, & KOE deen)

Medication Safety Issues

Sound-alike/look-alike issues:

Fiorinal® may be confused with Fioricet®, Florical®, Florinef®

High alert medication: The Institute for Safe Medication Practices (ISMP) includes this medication among its list of drug classes which have a heightened risk of causing significant patient harm when used in error.

U.S. Brand Names Ascomp® with Codeine; Fiorinal® with Codeine

Canadian Brand Names Fiorinal®-C 1/2; Fiorinal®-C 1/4; Tecnal C 1/2; Tecnal C 1/4

Index Terms Aspirin, Caffeine, Codeine, and Butalbital; Butalbital Compound and Codeine; Codeine and Butalbital Compound; Codeine, Butalbital, Aspirin, and Caffeine

Pharmacologic Category Analgesic Combination (Opioid); Barbiturate

Generic Available Yes

Use Relief of symptoms of complex tension (muscle contraction) headache

Effect on Mental Status Drowsiness is common; may cause depression, nervousness, insomnia, and nightmares; rare reports of hallucinations

Effect on Psychiatric Treatment Rare reports of agranulocytosis; use caution with clozapine and carbamazepine; CNS depressant effects of psychotropics may be enhance by barbiturates; enzyme induction effects of barbiturates may decrease effects of psychotropics

Restrictions C-III

Pregnancy Risk Factor C (per manufacturer)

Pregnancy Considerations Reproduction studies have not been conducted with this combination. Refer to the individual monographs for Aspirin, Caffeine, and Codeine for additional information. Butalbital crosses the placenta; may cause withdrawal seizures when taken during pregnancy.

Lactation Enters breast milk/not recommended

Contraindications Hypersensitivity to butalbital, codeine, aspirin, caffeine, or any component of the formulation; opium derivatives; hemorrhagic diathesis (eg, hemophilia, hypoprothrombinemia, von Willebrand disease, the thrombocytopenias, thrombasthenia, and other ill-defined hereditary platelet dysfunctions, severe vitamin K deficiency, and severe liver damage); nasal polyp syndrome, angioedema, and bronchospastic reactivity to aspirin or other NSAIDs; peptic ulcer or other serious GI lesions; porphyria

Warnings/Precautions May cause CNS depression, which may impair physical or mental abilities; patients must be cautioned about performing tasks which require mental alertness (eg, operating machinery or driving). Use with caution in patients with hypersensitivity reactions to other phenanthrene-derivative opioid agonists (hydrocodone, hydromorphone, levorphanol, oxycodone, oxymorphone). Patients with sensitivity to tartrazine dyes, nasal polyps, and asthma may have an increased risk of salicylate sensitivity. Use cautions with patients on anticoagulant therapy. Effects may be potentiated when used with other sedative drugs or ethanol. Use caution in elderly and debilitated patients. Use with caution in patients with abdominal conditions, adrenal insufficiency, bleeding disorders, head trauma, history of drug abuse, gastrointestinal disease, hepatic impairment, prostatic hyperplasia, renal impairment, respiratory disease, thyroid dysfunction, or urinary stricture. Caffeine may cause CNS and cardiovascular stimulation, as well as GI irritation in high doses. Use with caution in patients with a history of peptic ulcer or GERD; avoid in patients with symptomatic cardiac arrhythmias. Use caution in patients with two or more copies of the variant CYP2D6*2 allele; may have extensive conversion from codeine to morphine and thus increased opioid-mediated effects. Children and teenagers who have or are recovering from chickenpox or flu-like symptoms should not use this product. Changes in behavior (along with nausea and vomiting) may be an early sign of Reye's syndrome; patients should be instructed to contact their healthcare provider if these occur.

Adverse Reactions

1% to 10%:

Central nervous system: Dizziness/lightheadedness (3%), drowsiness (2%), intoxicated feeling (1%)

Gastrointestinal: Abdominal pain/nausea (4%)

<1% (Limited to important or life-threatening): Agitation, allergic reaction, anaphylactic shock, anorexia, chest pain, cholangiocarcinoma, depression, disorientation, diuresis, dysphagia, dysuria, edema, epistaxis, erythema multiforme, esophagitis, exfoliative dermatitis, fainting, gastroenteritis, GI spasm, hallucinations, hives, hypotension, nervousness, neuropathy, numbness, palpitations, psychosis, pyloric ulcer, rash, renal impairment, slurred speech, syncope, tachycardia, tinnitus, toxic epidermal necrolysis, unconsciousness, vertigo, vomiting

Note: Potential reactions associated with components of Fiorinal® with Codeine include acute airway obstruction, anemia, bleeding time prolonged, cardiac stimulation, dependence, hemolytic anemia, hepatitis, hyperglycemia, irritability, nephrotoxicity, occult blood loss, peptic ulcer, pruritus, renal toxicity (high doses, prolonged therapy) thrombocytopenia, tremor, urate excretion impaired

Metabolism/Transport Effects

Aspirin: **Substrate** of CYP2C9 (minor)

Caffeine: **Substrate** of CYP1A2 (major), 2C9 (minor), 2D6 (minor), 2E1 (minor), 3A4 (minor); **Inhibits** CYP1A2 (weak), 3A4 (moderate)

Codeine: **Substrate** of CYP2D6 (major), 3A4 (minor); **Inhibits** CYP2D6 (weak)

Drug Interactions

ACE Inhibitors: Salicylates may diminish the antihypertensive effect of ACE Inhibitors. They may also diminish other beneficial pharmacodynamic effects desired for the treatment of CHF. The effects are likely dose-related. 100 mg doses aspirin appear to cause no problems, whereas 300 mg doses appear to significantly affect ACE Inhibitor efficacy. *Risk C: Monitor therapy*

Acetaminophen: Barbiturates may increase the metabolism of Acetaminophen. This may 1) diminish the effect of acetaminophen; and 2) increase the risk of liver damage. *Risk C: Monitor therapy*

Alcohol (Ethyl): CNS Depressants may enhance the CNS depressant effect of Alcohol (Ethyl). *Risk C: Monitor therapy*

Alendronate: Aspirin may enhance the adverse/toxic effect of Alendronate. Specifically gastrointestinal adverse events. *Risk C: Monitor therapy*

Alvimopan: Analgesics (Opioid) may enhance the adverse/toxic effect of Alvimopan. This is most notable for patients receiving long-term (i.e., more than 7 days) opiates prior to alvimopan initiation. Management: Alvimopan is contraindicated in patients receiving therapeutic doses of opioids for more than 7 consecutive days immediately prior to alvimopan initiation. *Risk D: Consider therapy modification*

Ammonium Chloride: May increase the excretion of Analgesics (Opioid). *Risk C: Monitor therapy*

Amphetamines: May enhance the analgesic effect of Analgesics (Opioid). *Risk C: Monitor therapy*

Anticoagulants: Salicylates may enhance the anticoagulant effect of Anticoagulants. *Risk C: Monitor therapy*

Antidepressants (Serotonin/Norepinephrine Reuptake Inhibitor): May enhance the antiplatelet effect of Aspirin. *Risk C: Monitor therapy*

Antidepressants (Tricyclic, Tertiary Amine): May enhance the antiplatelet effect of Aspirin. *Risk C: Monitor therapy*

Antiplatelet Agents: May enhance the adverse/toxic effect of Salicylates. Increased risk of bleeding may result. *Risk C: Monitor therapy*

Antipsychotic Agents (Phenothiazines): May enhance the hypotensive effect of Analgesics (Opioid). *Risk C: Monitor therapy*

Beta-Blockers: Barbiturates may decrease the serum concentration of Beta-Blockers. **Exceptions:** Atenolol; Levobunolol; Metipranolol; Nadolol. *Risk C: Monitor therapy*

Calcium Channel Blockers: Barbiturates may increase the metabolism of Calcium Channel Blockers. **Exceptions:** Clevidipine. *Risk D: Consider therapy modification*

Calcium Channel Blockers (Nondihydropyridine): May enhance the anticoagulant effect of Salicylates. *Risk C: Monitor therapy*

Carbonic Anhydrase Inhibitors: Salicylates may enhance the adverse/toxic effect of Carbonic Anhydrase Inhibitors. Salicylate toxicity might be enhanced by this same combination. *Risk D: Consider therapy modification*

Chloramphenicol: May decrease the metabolism of Barbiturates. Barbiturates may increase the metabolism of Chloramphenicol. *Risk D: Consider therapy modification*

CNS Depressants: May enhance the adverse/toxic effect of other CNS Depressants. *Risk C: Monitor therapy*

Contraceptive (Progestins): Barbiturates may diminish the therapeutic effect of Contraceptive (Progestins). Contraceptive failure is possible. *Risk D: Consider therapy modification*

Corticosteroids (Systemic): Salicylates may enhance the adverse/toxic effect of Corticosteroids (Systemic). These specifically include gastrointestinal ulceration and bleeding. Corticosteroids (Systemic) may decrease the serum concentration of Salicylates. Withdrawal of corticosteroids may result in salicylate toxicity. *Risk C: Monitor therapy*

Corticosteroids (Systemic): Barbiturates may increase the metabolism of Corticosteroids (Systemic). *Risk C: Monitor therapy*

CycloSPORINE: Barbiturates may increase the metabolism of CycloSPORINE. *Risk D: Consider therapy modification*

CYP1A2 Inhibitors (Moderate): May decrease the metabolism of CYP1A2 Substrates. *Risk C: Monitor therapy*

CYP1A2 Inhibitors (Strong): May decrease the metabolism of CYP1A2 Substrates. *Risk D: Consider therapy modification*

CYP2D6 Inhibitors (Moderate): May diminish the therapeutic effect of Codeine. These CYP2D6 inhibitors may prevent the metabolic conversion of codeine to its active metabolite morphine. *Risk C: Monitor therapy*

CYP2D6 Inhibitors (Strong): May diminish the therapeutic effect of Codeine. These CYP2D6 inhibitors may prevent the metabolic conversion of codeine to its active metabolite morphine. *Risk D: Consider therapy modification*

CYP3A4 Substrates: CYP3A4 Inhibitors (Moderate) may decrease the metabolism of CYP3A4 Substrates. *Risk C: Monitor therapy*

Dasatinib: May enhance the anticoagulant effect of Antiplatelet Agents. *Risk C: Monitor therapy*

Desmopressin: Analgesics (Opioid) may enhance the adverse/toxic effect of Desmopressin. *Risk C: Monitor therapy*

Disopyramide: Barbiturates may increase the metabolism of Disopyramide. *Risk D: Consider therapy modification*

Doxycycline: Barbiturates may decrease the serum concentration of Doxycycline. *Risk D: Consider therapy modification*

Drotrecogin Alfa: Salicylates may enhance the adverse/toxic effect of Drotrecogin Alfa. Bleeding may occur. *Risk D: Consider therapy modification*

Eplerenone: CYP3A4 Inhibitors (Moderate) may increase the serum concentration of Eplerenone. Management: A lower starting dose of eplerenone (25 mg once daily) is recommended in patients with hypertension who are also taking drugs that are moderate inhibitors of CYP3A4. *Risk D: Consider therapy modification*

Etoposide: Barbiturates may increase the metabolism of Etoposide. *Risk C: Monitor therapy*

Etoposide Phosphate: Barbiturates may decrease the serum concentration of Etoposide Phosphate. Barbiturates may increase the metabolism, via CYP isoenzymes, of etoposide phosphate. *Risk C: Monitor therapy*

Felbamate: May increase the serum concentration of Barbiturates. *Risk C: Monitor therapy*

Ginkgo Biloba: May enhance the antiplatelet effect of Salicylates. *Risk D: Consider therapy modification*

Griseofulvin: Barbiturates may decrease the absorption of Griseofulvin. *Risk D: Consider therapy modification*

Heparin: Aspirin may enhance the anticoagulant effect of Heparin. *Risk C: Monitor therapy*

Herbs (Anticoagulant/Antiplatelet Properties) (eg, Alfalfa, Anise, Bilberry): May enhance the adverse/toxic effect of Salicylates. Bleeding may occur. *Risk D: Consider therapy modification*

Ibritumomab: Antiplatelet Agents may enhance the adverse/toxic effect of Ibritumomab. Both agents may contribute to impaired platelet function and an increased risk of bleeding. *Risk C: Monitor therapy*

Ketorolac: May enhance the adverse/toxic effect of Aspirin. *Risk X: Avoid combination*

LamoTRIgine: Barbiturates may increase the metabolism of LamoTRIgine. *Risk D: Consider therapy modification*

Maraviroc: CYP3A4 Inhibitors may increase the serum concentration of Maraviroc. *Risk D: Consider therapy modification*

Meperidine: Barbiturates may enhance the CNS depressant effect of Meperidine. *Risk C: Monitor therapy*

Methadone: Barbiturates may increase the metabolism of Methadone. *Risk D: Consider therapy modification*

Methotrexate: Salicylates may increase the serum concentration of Methotrexate. Salicylate doses used for prophylaxis of cardiovascular events are not likely to be of concern. *Risk D: Consider therapy modification*

Nonsteroidal Anti-Inflammatory Agents: May enhance the adverse/toxic effect of Antiplatelet Agents. An increased risk of bleeding may occur. *Risk C: Monitor therapy*

NSAID (Nonselective): May enhance the antiplatelet effect of Salicylates. NSAID (Nonselective) may diminish the cardioprotective effect of Salicylates. Salicylates may decrease the serum concentration of NSAID (Nonselective). **Exceptions:** Diclofenac. *Risk D: Consider therapy modification*

Omega-3-Acid Ethyl Esters: May enhance the antiplatelet effect of Antiplatelet Agents. *Risk C: Monitor therapy*

Oral Contraceptive (Estrogens): Barbiturates may diminish the therapeutic effect of Oral Contraceptive (Estrogens). Contraceptive failure is possible. *Risk D: Consider therapy modification*

Pegvisomant: Analgesics (Opioid) may diminish the therapeutic effect of Pegvisomant. *Risk C: Monitor therapy*

Pentosan Polysulfate Sodium: May enhance the adverse/toxic effect of Antiplatelet Agents. Specifically, the risk of bleeding may be increased by concurrent use of these agents. *Risk C: Monitor therapy*

Pimecrolimus: CYP3A4 Inhibitors (Moderate) may decrease the metabolism of Pimecrolimus. *Risk C: Monitor therapy*

Primidone: May enhance the adverse/toxic effect of Barbiturates. Primidone is converted to phenobarbital, and thus becomes additive with existing barbiturate therapy. *Risk C: Monitor therapy*

Propafenone: Barbiturates may increase the metabolism of Propafenone. *Risk D: Consider therapy modification*

Prostacyclin Analogues: May enhance the antiplatelet effect of Antiplatelet Agents. *Risk C: Monitor therapy*

Pyridoxine: May increase the metabolism of Barbiturates. Apparent in high pyridoxine doses (eg, 200 mg/day) *Risk C: Monitor therapy*

QuiNIDine: Barbiturates may increase the metabolism of QuiNIDine. *Risk D: Consider therapy modification*

Quinolone Antibiotics: May decrease the metabolism of Caffeine. **Exceptions:** Gatifloxacin; Gemifloxacin; Levofloxacin; Lomefloxacin; Moxifloxacin; Nalidixic Acid; Ofloxacin; Sparfloxacin; Trovafloxacin. *Risk C: Monitor therapy*

Ranolazine: CYP3A4 Inhibitors (Moderate) may increase the serum concentration of Ranolazine. Management: Limit the ranolazine dose to a maximum of 500mg twice daily in patients concurrently receiving moderate CYP3A4 inhibitors (e.g., diltiazem, verapamil, erythromycin, etc.). *Risk D: Consider therapy modification*

Regadenoson: Caffeine may diminish the vasodilatory effect of Regadenoson. *Risk D: Consider therapy modification*

Rifamycin Derivatives: May increase the metabolism of Barbiturates. *Risk C: Monitor therapy*

Salicylates: May enhance the anticoagulant effect of other Salicylates. *Risk C: Monitor therapy*

Salmeterol: CYP3A4 Inhibitors (Moderate) may increase the serum concentration of Salmeterol. *Risk C: Monitor therapy*

Selective Serotonin Reuptake Inhibitors: Analgesics (Opioid) may enhance the serotonergic effect of Selective Serotonin Reuptake Inhibitors. This may cause serotonin syndrome. *Risk C: Monitor therapy*

Selective Serotonin Reuptake Inhibitors: May enhance the antiplatelet effect of Aspirin. *Risk C: Monitor therapy*

Somatostatin Analogs: May decrease the metabolism of Codeine. The formation of two major codeine metabolites (morphine and norcodeine) may be impaired by somatostatin analogs. *Risk C: Monitor therapy*

Succinylcholine: May enhance the bradycardic effect of Analgesics (Opioid). *Risk C: Monitor therapy*

Sulfonylureas: Salicylates may enhance the hypoglycemic effect of Sulfonylureas. Of concern with regular, higher doses of salicylates, not sporadic, low doses. *Risk C: Monitor therapy*

Sympathomimetics: May enhance the adverse/toxic effect of other Sympathomimetics. *Risk C: Monitor therapy*

Teniposide: Barbiturates may increase the metabolism of Teniposide. *Risk C: Monitor therapy*

Theophylline Derivatives: Barbiturates may increase the metabolism of Theophylline Derivatives. **Exceptions:** Dyphylline. *Risk C: Monitor therapy*

Thrombolytic Agents: Salicylates may enhance the adverse/toxic effect of Thrombolytic Agents. An increased risk of bleeding may occur. *Risk C: Monitor therapy*

Tiludronate: Aspirin may decrease the serum concentration of Tiludronate. *Risk C: Monitor therapy*

Tositumomab and Iodine I 131 Tositumomab: Antiplatelet Agents may enhance the adverse/toxic effect of Tositumomab and Iodine I 131 Tositumomab. Specifically, the risk of bleeding-related adverse events may be increased. *Risk C: Monitor therapy*

Treprostinil: May enhance the adverse/toxic effect of Salicylates. Bleeding may occur. *Risk C: Monitor therapy*

Tricyclic Antidepressants: Barbiturates may increase the metabolism of Tricyclic Antidepressants. *Risk D: Consider therapy modification*

Uricosuric Agents: Salicylates may diminish the therapeutic effect of Uricosuric Agents. Specifically, uricosuria. *Risk C: Monitor therapy*

Valproic Acid: May decrease the metabolism of Barbiturates. Barbiturates may decrease the serum concentration of Valproic Acid. *Risk C: Monitor therapy*

Valproic Acid: Salicylates may increase the serum concentration of Valproic Acid. *Risk C: Monitor therapy*

Varicella Virus-Containing Vaccines: Salicylates may enhance the adverse/toxic effect of Varicella Virus-Containing Vaccines. Reye 's Syndrome may develop. *Risk D: Consider therapy modification*

Vitamin K Antagonists (eg, warfarin): Salicylates may enhance the anticoagulant effect of Vitamin K Antagonists. *Risk D: Consider therapy modification*

Vitamin K Antagonists (eg, warfarin): Barbiturates may increase the metabolism of Vitamin K Antagonists. *Risk D: Consider therapy modification*

Voriconazole: Barbiturates may decrease the serum concentration of Voriconazole. *Risk X: Avoid combination*

Ethanol/Nutrition/Herb Interactions Ethanol: Avoid ethanol (may increase CNS depression).

Stability Store below 25°C (77°F). Protect from moisture.

Mechanism of Action Butalbital is a short-to-intermediate acting barbiturate; aspirin inhibits prostaglandin synthesis and has analgesic, antipyretic and anti-inflammatory actions; caffeine is a CNS stimulant; codeine is a narcotic analgesic and antitussive which produced generalized CNS depression. The combination product is for the treatment of tension headache; however, the role of each component in the relief of symptoms is not completely understood.

Pharmacodynamics/Kinetics See individual agents. Bioavailability of the combination is identical to their bioavailability when codeine is administered separately from butalbital, aspirin, and caffeine.

Dosage Oral:

Adults: 1-2 capsules every 4 hours as needed (maximum: 6 capsules/day)

Elderly: Use with caution; however, barbiturates (butalbital) are generally not recommended in the elderly.

Monitoring Parameters Serial hepatic and renal function tests (in patients with impairment)

Test Interactions Aspirin may interfere with amylase (S), fasting blood glucose (S), cholesterol (S), protein (S), glutamic-oxaloacetic transaminases (SGOT) (S), uric acid (S, U), prothrombin time (S), bleeding time (S), glucose, 5-hydroxy-indoleacetic acid (U), Gerhardt ketone (U), vanillylmandelic acid (U), diacetic acid (U), and spectrophotometric detection of barbiturates; codeine may increase amylase levels (S)

Dosage Forms Excipient information presented when available (limited, particularly for generics); consult specific product labeling.

Capsule: Butalbital 50 mg, aspirin 325 mg, caffeine 40 mg, and codeine phosphate 30 mg

Ascomp® with Codeine, Fiorinal® with Codeine: Butalbital 50 mg, aspirin 325 mg, caffeine 40 mg, and codeine phosphate 30 mg [may contain benzyl alcohol]

◆ **Butalbital Compound** *see* Butalbital, Aspirin, and Caffeine *on page 239*

◆ **Butalbital Compound and Codeine** *see* Butalbital, Aspirin, Caffeine, and Codeine *on page 242*

◆ **Butisol Sodium®** *see* Butabarbital *on page 226*

Butorphanol (byoo TOR fa nole)

Medication Safety Issues

Sound-alike/look-alike issues:

Stadol® may be confused with Haldol®, sotalol

High alert medication: The Institute for Safe Medication Practices (ISMP) includes this medication among its list of drug classes which have a heightened risk of causing significant patient harm when used in error.

Related Information

Narcotic / Opioid Analgesics *on page 1789*

U.S. Brand Names Stadol® [DSC]

Canadian Brand Names Apo-Butorphanol®; PMS-Butorphanol

Index Terms Butorphanol Tartrate

Pharmacologic Category Analgesic, Opioid

Use

Parenteral: Management of moderate-to-severe pain; preoperative medication; supplement to balanced anesthesia; management of pain during labor

Nasal spray: Management of moderate-to-severe pain, including migraine headache pain

Effect on Mental Status Drowsiness is common; may rarely produce CNS stimulation or depression, hallucinations, and confusion

Effect on Psychiatric Treatment Contraindicated in opiate dependent patients; may precipitate opiate withdrawal; concurrent use with psychotropic may produce additive sedation

Restrictions C-IV

Dosage Summary

I.M.:

Children: Dosage not established

Adults: Initial: 2 mg, may repeat every 3-4 hours as needed; Usual range: 1-4 mg every 3-4 hours as needed **or** 2 mg prior to surgery

Elderly: Initial: 1/2 of the recommended dose, repeated dosing generally should be at least 6 hours apart

I.V.:

Children: Dosage not established

Adults: Initial: 1 mg, may repeat every 3-4 hours as needed; Usual range: 0.5-2 mg every 3-4 hours as needed **or** 2 mg and/or an incremental dose of 0.5-1 mg (up to 0.06 mg/kg) as supplement to surgery

Elderly: Initial: 1/2 of the recommended dose, repeated dosing generally should be at least 6 hours apart

Intranasal:

Children: Dosage not established

Adults: Initial: 1 spray (~1 mg) in 1 nostril, may repeat in 60-90 minutes, then repeat initial dose sequence in 3-4 hours after last dose as needed; may use initial dose of 1 spray in each nostril (2 mg) in patients who will remain recumbent

Elderly: Initial: Should not exceed 1 mg, may repeat after 90-120 minutes

Dosage Forms Excipient information presented when available (limited, particularly for generics); consult specific product labeling.

Injection, solution, as tartrate [preservative free]: 1 mg/mL (1 mL); 2 mg/mL (1 mL, 2 mL)

Injection, solution, as tartrate [with preservative]: 2 mg/mL (10 mL)

Solution, intranasal, as tartrate [spray]: 10 mg/mL (2.5 mL) [14-15 doses]

- ◆ **Butorphanol Tartrate** *see* Butorphanol *on page 247*
- ◆ **B-Vex** *see* Brompheniramine *on page 205*
- ◆ **BW-430C** *see* LamoTRIgine *on page 889*
- ◆ **BW524W91** *see* Emtricitabine *on page 530*
- ◆ **Byetta®** *see* Exenatide *on page 609*
- ◆ **Bystolic™** *see* Nebivolol *on page 1115*
- ◆ **C1H** *see* Alemtuzumab *on page 59*
- ◆ **C2B8 Monoclonal Antibody** *see* RiTUXimab *on page 1434*
- ◆ **C8-CCK** *see* Sincalide *on page 1489*
- ◆ **311C90** *see* Zolmitriptan *on page 1703*
- ◆ **C225** *see* Cetuximab *on page 310*

Cabergoline (ca BER goe leen)

Related Information

Antiparkinsonian Agents *on page 1767*

U.S. Brand Names Dostinex® [DSC]

Canadian Brand Names CO Cabergoline; Dostinex®

Mexican Brand Names Dostinex

Pharmacologic Category Ergot Derivative

Generic Available Yes

Use Treatment of hyperprolactinemic disorders, either idiopathic or due to pituitary adenomas

Effect on Mental Status Dizziness is common; may cause depression

Effect on Psychiatric Treatment Antipsychotics may decrease the therapeutic effects of cabergoline; avoid combination

Pregnancy Risk Factor B

Pregnancy Considerations Teratogenic effects were not observed in most animal studies when administered in maternally nontoxic doses. Treatment of hyperprolactinemia may restore fertility in a previously infertile woman. Because information concerning the use of cabergoline in pregnancy is limited, bromocriptine is generally recommended to treat hyperprolactinemia in women who wish to conceive. Based on preliminary data, cabergoline has not been shown to increase the risk of congenital malformations or miscarriages when used early in pregnancy (treatment was generally stopped once pregnancy was diagnosed). Not recommended for use in patients with pregnancy-induced hypertension unless benefit outweighs potential risk.

Lactation Excretion in breast milk unknown/not recommended

Contraindications Hypersensitivity to ergot derivatives; uncontrolled hypertension; history of pulmonary, pericardial, cardiac valvular or retroperitoneal fibrotic disorders

Warnings/Precautions Initial doses >1 mg may cause orthostatic hypotension; concurrent use with antihypertensive agents may increase risk. Not indicated for the inhibition or suppression of physiologic lactation; other dopamine agonists are associated with cases of hypertension, stroke, and seizures. Use caution in patients with hepatic impairment; monitor LFTs. Should not be used in patients with pregnancy-induced hypertension unless benefit outweighs potential risk. In all patients, prolactin concentrations should be monitored monthly until normalized. Pleural effusion and pulmonary/retroperitoneal fibrosis have been reported with long-term use. Cardiac valvular disease (mitral, aortic, tricuspid regurgitation) has been associated with cabergoline (a potent 5-HT_{2B} agonist). Incidence may be higher for daily doses >2 mg and for duration of use ≥6 months. Following diagnosis of fibrosis/valvulopathy, discontinuation of cabergoline may result in improvement in condition. Safety and efficacy in children have not been established.

Adverse Reactions

>10%:

Central nervous system: Headache (26%), dizziness (15% to 17%)

Gastrointestinal: Nausea (27% to 29%)

1% to 10%:

Cardiovascular: Postural hypotension (4%), hypotension (1%), dependent edema (1%), edema (peripheral 1%), palpitation (1%), syncope (1%)

Central nervous system: Fatigue (5% to 7%), vertigo (1% to 4%), depression (3%), somnolence (2% to 5%), nervousness (1% to 2%), anxiety (1%), insomnia (1%), concentration impaired (1%), malaise (1%)

Dermatologic: Acne (1%), pruritus (1%)

Endocrine: Hot flashes (1% to 3%), breast pain (1% to 2%), dysmenorrhea (1%)

Gastrointestinal: Constipation (7% to 10%), abdominal pain (5%), dyspepsia (2% to 5%), vomiting (2% to 4%), xerostomia (2%), diarrhea (2%), flatulence (2%), anorexia (1%), throat irritation (1%), toothache (1%)

Neuromuscular & skeletal: Weakness (6% to 9%), pain (2%), paresthesia (1% to 2%), arthralgia (1%)

Ocular: Abnormal vision (1%), periorbital edema (1%)

Respiratory: Rhinitis (1%)

Miscellaneous: Flu-like syndrome (1%)

<1% (Limited to important or life-threatening): Aggression, alopecia, cardiac fibrosis, duodenal ulcer (in PD patients), gastric ulcer (in PD patients), pleural effusion, psychosis, pulmonary fibrosis, valvular regurgitation, valvulopathy

<1% (Limited to important or life-threatening): Aggression, alopecia, cardiac fibrosis, confusion (in patients with Parkinson's disease [PD]), constrictive pericarditis (in PD patients), duodenal ulcer (in PD patients), dyskinesia (in PD patients), epistaxis, facial edema, gastric ulcer (in PD patients), hallucinations (in PD patients), heart failure (in PD patients), hypersexuality, libido increased, pathological gambling, pleural effusion (in PD patients), psychosis, pulmonary fibrosis (in PD patients), valvulopathy, weight gain/loss

Drug Interactions

Efavirenz: May enhance the adverse/toxic effect of Ergot Derivatives. Specifically, the risk for peripheral vasospasm and ischemia may be increased. *Risk X: Avoid combination*

Posaconazole: May increase the serum concentration of Ergot Derivatives. *Risk X: Avoid combination*

Serotonin 5-HT1D Receptor Agonists: Ergot Derivatives may enhance the vasoconstricting effect of Serotonin 5-HT1D Receptor Agonists. Serotonin 5-HT1D Receptor Agonists may enhance the vasoconstricting effect of Ergot Derivatives. *Risk X: Avoid combination*

Serotonin Modulators: May enhance the adverse/toxic effect of other Serotonin Modulators. The development of serotonin syndrome may occur. *Risk D: Consider therapy modification*

Sibutramine: May enhance the serotonergic effect of Ergot Derivatives. This may cause serotonin syndrome. *Risk X: Avoid combination*

Voriconazole: May increase the serum concentration of Ergot Derivatives. *Risk X: Avoid combination*

Ethanol/Nutrition/Herb Interactions Herb/Nutraceutical: Avoid products that enhance serotonin activity (includes SAMe [S-adenosylmethionine] and St John's wort); may increase the risk of serotonin syndrome.

Stability Store at 20°C to 25°C (68°F to 77°F).

Mechanism of Action Cabergoline is a long acting dopamine receptor agonist with a high affinity for D_2 receptors; prolactin secretion by the anterior pituitary is predominantly under hypothalamic inhibitory control exerted through the release of dopamine. It is a potent $5\text{-}HT_{2B}$-receptor agonist, which may contribute to observed fibrotic/valvulopathic events.

Pharmacodynamics/Kinetics

Distribution: Extensive, particularly to the pituitary

Protein binding: 40% to 42%

Metabolism: Extensively hepatic via hydrolysis; minimal CYP mediated metabolism

Half-life elimination: 63-69 hours

Time to peak: 2-3 hours

Excretion: Primarily feces (~60%); urine (~22%, <4% as unchanged drug)

Dosage Initial dose: Oral: 0.25 mg twice weekly; the dose may be increased by 0.25 mg twice weekly up to a maximum of 1 mg twice weekly according to the patient's serum prolactin level. Dosage increases should not occur more rapidly than every 4 weeks. Once a normal serum prolactin level is maintained for 6 months, the dose may be discontinued and prolactin levels monitored to determine if cabergoline is still required. The durability of efficacy beyond 24 months of therapy has not been established.

Elderly: No dosage recommendations suggested, but start at the low end of the dosage range

Dosage adjustment in renal dysfunction: No adjustment required.

Dosage adjustment in hepatic dysfunction:

Mild-to-moderate dysfunction (Child-Pugh Class B): No adjustment required

Severe dysfunction (Child-Pugh Class C): Use caution; significant increase in AUC

Monitoring Parameters Blood pressure (both sitting/supine and standing); serum prolactin level, echocardiogram with long-term use (>6 months)

Additional Information Bromocriptine and cabergoline are the only drugs indicated for the treatment of hyperprolactinemia. In the largest comparative clinical trial, prolactin levels normalized in 77% of patients treated with cabergoline compared to 59% of patients treated with bromocriptine. In that trial, 3% of patients discontinued treatment due to adverse effects in the cabergoline group versus 12% of patients in the bromocriptine group. In addition to the improved safety and efficacy profile, cabergoline (administered twice weekly) is more convenient than bromocriptine (administered 1-3 times/day) for patients to take.

Dosage Forms Excipient information presented when available (limited, particularly for generics); consult specific product labeling. [DSC] = Discontinued product

Tablet: 0.5 mg

Dostinex®: 0.5 mg [DSC]

◆ **Caduet®** *see* Amlodipine and Atorvastatin *on page 103*

◆ **Cafcit®** *see* Caffeine *on page 250*

◆ **Cafergot®** *see* Ergotamine and Caffeine *on page 554*

Caffeine (KAF een)

U.S. Brand Names Cafcit®; Enerjets [OTC]; No Doz® Maximum Strength [OTC]; Vivarin® [OTC]

Index Terms Caffeine and Sodium Benzoate; Caffeine Citrate; Sodium Benzoate and Caffeine

Pharmacologic Category Stimulant

Generic Available Yes: Tablet, caffeine and sodium benzoate injection, injection, oral solution

Use

Caffeine citrate: Treatment of idiopathic apnea of prematurity

Caffeine and sodium benzoate: Treatment of acute respiratory depression (not a preferred agent)

Caffeine [OTC labeling]: Restore mental alertness or wakefulness when experiencing fatigue

Unlabeled/Investigational Use Caffeine and sodium benzoate: Treatment of spinal puncture headache; CNS stimulant; diuretic; augmentation of seizure induction during electroconvulsive therapy (ECT)

Effect on Mental Status May cause insomnia, nervousness, anxiety, and delirium.

Effect on Psychiatric Treatment May counteract sedative/hypnotics; may also lower seizure threshold and increase risk for epilepsy/convulsions

Pregnancy Risk Factor C

Pregnancy Considerations Caffeine crosses the placenta; serum levels in the fetus are similar to those in the mother. When large bolus doses are administered to animals, teratogenic effects have been reported. Similar doses are not probable following normal caffeine consumption and moderate consumption is not associated with congenital malformations, spontaneous abortions, preterm birth or low birth weight. According to one source, pregnant women who do not smoke or drink alcohol could consume ≤5 mg/kg of caffeine over the course of a day without reproductive risk. Another source recommends limiting caffeine intake to <150 mg/day. The half-life of caffeine is prolonged during the second and third trimesters of pregnancy.

Lactation Enters breast milk/use caution (AAP rates "compatible")

Contraindications Hypersensitivity to caffeine or any component of the formulation; sodium benzoate is not for use in neonates

Warnings/Precautions Use with caution in patients with a history of peptic ulcer, gastroesophageal reflux, impaired renal or hepatic function, seizure disorders, or cardiovascular disease. Avoid use in patients with symptomatic cardiac arrhythmias, agitation, anxiety, or tremor. Over-the-counter [OTC] products contain an amount of caffeine similar to one cup of coffee; limit the use of other caffeine-containing beverages or foods.

Caffeine citrate should not be interchanged with caffeine and sodium benzoate. Avoid use of products containing sodium benzoate in neonates; has been associated with a potentially fatal toxicity ("gasping syndrome"). Neonates receiving caffeine citrate should be closely monitored for the development of necrotizing enterocolitis. Caffeine serum levels should be closely monitored to optimize therapy and prevent serious toxicity.

Adverse Reactions Frequency not specified; primarily serum-concentration related.

Cardiovascular: Angina, arrhythmia (ventricular), chest pain, flushing, palpitation, sinus tachycardia, tachycardia (supraventricular), vasodilation

Central nervous system: Agitation, delirium, dizziness, hallucinations, headache, insomnia, irritability, psychosis, restlessness

Dermatologic: Urticaria

Gastrointestinal: Esophageal sphincter tone decreased, gastritis

Neuromuscular & skeletal: Fasciculations

Ocular: Intraocular pressure increased (>180 mg caffeine), miosis

Renal: Diuresis

Metabolism/Transport Effects Substrate of CYP1A2 (major), 2C9 (minor), 2D6 (minor), 2E1 (minor), 3A4 (minor); **Inhibits** CYP1A2 (weak), 3A4 (moderate)

Drug Interactions

Cannabinoids: May enhance the tachycardic effect of Sympathomimetics. *Risk C: Monitor therapy*

CYP1A2 Inhibitors (Moderate): May decrease the metabolism of CYP1A2 Substrates. *Risk C: Monitor therapy*

CYP1A2 Inhibitors (Strong): May decrease the metabolism of CYP1A2 Substrates. *Risk D: Consider therapy modification*

CYP3A4 Substrates: CYP3A4 Inhibitors (Moderate) may decrease the metabolism of CYP3A4 Substrates. *Risk C: Monitor therapy*

Eplerenone: CYP3A4 Inhibitors (Moderate) may increase the serum concentration of Eplerenone. Management: A lower starting dose of eplerenone (25 mg once daily) is recommended in patients with hypertension who are also taking drugs that are moderate inhibitors of CYP3A4. *Risk D: Consider therapy modification*

Maraviroc: CYP3A4 Inhibitors may increase the serum concentration of Maraviroc. *Risk D: Consider therapy modification*

Pimecrolimus: CYP3A4 Inhibitors (Moderate) may decrease the metabolism of Pimecrolimus. *Risk C: Monitor therapy*

Quinolone Antibiotics: May decrease the metabolism of Caffeine. **Exceptions:** Gatifloxacin; Gemifloxacin; Levofloxacin; Lomefloxacin; Moxifloxacin; Nalidixic Acid; Ofloxacin; Sparfloxacin; Trovafloxacin. *Risk C: Monitor therapy*

Ranolazine: CYP3A4 Inhibitors (Moderate) may increase the serum concentration of Ranolazine. Management: Limit the ranolazine dose to a maximum of 500mg twice daily in patients concurrently receiving moderate CYP3A4 inhibitors (e.g., diltiazem, verapamil, erythromycin, etc.). *Risk D: Consider therapy modification*

Regadenoson: Caffeine may diminish the vasodilatory effect of Regadenoson. *Risk D: Consider therapy modification*

Salmeterol: CYP3A4 Inhibitors (Moderate) may increase the serum concentration of Salmeterol. *Risk C: Monitor therapy*

Sympathomimetics: May enhance the adverse/toxic effect of other Sympathomimetics. *Risk C: Monitor therapy*

Stability Store at 20°C to 25°C (68°F to 77°F).

Caffeine citrate: Injection and oral solution contain no preservatives; injection is chemically stable for at least 24 hours at room temperature when diluted to 10 mg/mL (as caffeine citrate) with D_5W, $D_{50}W$, Intralipid® 20%, and Aminosyn® 8.5%; also compatible with dopamine (600 mcg/mL), calcium gluconate 10%, heparin (1 unit/mL), and fentanyl (10 mcg/mL) at room temperature for 24 hours.

Mechanism of Action Increases levels of 3'5' cyclic AMP by inhibiting phosphodiesterase; CNS stimulant which increases medullary respiratory center sensitivity to carbon dioxide, stimulates central inspiratory drive, and improves skeletal muscle contraction (diaphragmatic contractility); prevention of apnea may occur by competitive inhibition of adenosine

Pharmacodynamics/Kinetics

Distribution: V_d:

Neonates: 0.8-0.9 L/kg

Children >9 months to Adults: 0.6 L/kg

Protein binding: 17% (children) to 36% (adults)

Metabolism: Hepatic, via demethylation by CYP1A2. **Note:** In neonates, interconversion between caffeine and theophylline has been reported (caffeine levels are ~25% of measured theophylline after theophylline administration and ~3% to 8% of caffeine would be expected to be converted to theophylline)

Half-life elimination:

Neonates: 72-96 hours (range: 40-230 hours)

Children >9 months and Adults: 5 hours

Time to peak, serum: Oral: Within 30 minutes to 2 hours

Excretion:

Neonates ≤1 month: 86% excreted unchanged in urine

Infants >1 month and Adults: In urine, as metabolites

Dosage

Note: Caffeine citrate should not be interchanged with the caffeine sodium benzoate formulation.

Caffeine citrate: Neonates: Apnea of prematurity: Oral, I.V.:

Loading dose: 10-20 mg/kg as caffeine citrate (5-10 mg/kg as caffeine base). If theophylline has been administered to the patient within the previous 3 days, a full or modified loading dose (50% to 75% of a loading dose) may be given.

Maintenance dose: 5 mg/kg/day as caffeine citrate (2.5 mg/kg/day as caffeine base) once daily starting 24 hours after the loading dose. Maintenance dose is adjusted based on patient's response and serum caffeine concentrations.

Caffeine and sodium benzoate:

Children: Stimulant: I.M., I.V., SubQ: 8 mg/kg every 4 hours as needed

Children ≥12 years and Adults: OTC labeling (stimulant): Oral: 100-200 mg every 3-4 hours as needed

Adults:

Electroconvulsive therapy: I.V.: 300-2000 mg

Respiratory depression: I.M., I.V.: 250 mg as a single dose; may repeat as needed. Maximum single dose should be limited to 500 mg; maximum amount in any 24-hour period should generally be limited to 2500 mg.

Spinal puncture headache (unlabeled use):

I.V.: 500 mg in 1000 mL NS infused over 1 hour, followed by 1000 mL NS infused over 1 hour; a second course of caffeine can be given for unrelieved headache pain in 4 hours.

Oral: 300 mg as a single dose

Stimulant/diuretic (unlabeled use): I.M., I.V.: 500 mg, maximum single dose: 1 g

Dosage adjustment in renal impairment: No dosage adjustment required.

Administration

Oral: May be administered without regard to feedings or meals. May administer injectable formulation (caffeine citrate) orally.

Parenteral:

Caffeine citrate: Infuse loading dose over at least 30 minutes; maintenance dose may be infused over at least 10 minutes. May administer without dilution or diluted with D_5W to 10 mg caffeine citrate/mL.

Caffeine and sodium benzoate: I.V. as slow direct injection. For spinal headaches, dilute in 1000 mL NS and infuse over 1 hour. Follow with 1000 mL NS; infuse over 1 hour. May administer I.M. undiluted.

Reference Range

Therapeutic: Apnea of prematurity: 8-20 mcg/mL

Potentially toxic: >20 mcg/mL

Toxic: >50 mcg/mL

Dosage Forms Excipient information presented when available (limited, particularly for generics); consult specific product labeling. [DSC] = Discontinued product

Caplet:

NoDoz® Maximum Strength, Vivarin®: 200 mg

Injection, solution, as citrate [preservative free]: 20 mg/mL (3 mL) [equivalent to 10 mg/mL caffeine base]

Cafcit®: 20 mg/mL (3 mL) [equivalent to 10 mg/mL caffeine base]

Injection, solution [with sodium benzoate]: Caffeine 125 mg/mL and sodium benzoate 125 mg/mL (2 mL); caffeine 121 mg/mL and sodium benzoate 129 mg/mL (2 mL) [DSC]

Lozenge:

Enerjets®: 75 mg [classic coffee, hazelnut cream, or mochamint flavor]

Solution, oral, as citrate [preservative free]: 20 mg/mL (3 mL) [equivalent to 10 mg/mL caffeine base]

Cafcit®: 20 mg/mL (3 mL) [equivalent to 10 mg/mL caffeine base]

Tablet: 200 mg

Vivarin®: 200 mg

- **Caffeine, Acetaminophen, and Aspirin** *see* Acetaminophen, Aspirin, and Caffeine *on page 39*
- **Caffeine, Acetaminophen, Butalbital, and Codeine** *see* Butalbital, Acetaminophen, Caffeine, and Codeine *on page 232*
- **Caffeine and Ergotamine** *see* Ergotamine and Caffeine *on page 554*
- **Caffeine and Sodium Benzoate** *see* Caffeine *on page 250*
- **Caffeine, Aspirin, and Acetaminophen** *see* Acetaminophen, Aspirin, and Caffeine *on page 39*
- **Caffeine Citrate** *see* Caffeine *on page 250*
- **Caffeine, Dihydrocodeine, and Acetaminophen** *see* Acetaminophen, Caffeine, and Dihydrocodeine *on page 39*
- **Caffeine, Orphenadrine, and Aspirin** *see* Orphenadrine, Aspirin, and Caffeine *on page 1187*
- **Caffeine, Propoxyphene, and Aspirin** *see* Propoxyphene, Aspirin, and Caffeine *on page 1355*
- **Cal-C-Caps [OTC]** *see* Calcium Citrate *on page 257*
- **Calan®** *see* Verapamil *on page 1665*
- **Calan® SR** *see* Verapamil *on page 1665*
- **Calcarb 600 [OTC]** *see* Calcium Carbonate *on page 254*
- **Cal-Cee [OTC]** *see* Calcium Citrate *on page 257*
- **Calci-Chew® [OTC]** *see* Calcium Carbonate *on page 254*
- **Calci-Mix® [OTC]** *see* Calcium Carbonate *on page 254*
- **Calcionate [OTC]** *see* Calcium Glubionate *on page 258*

Calcitonin (kal si TOE nin)

Medication Safety Issues

Sound-alike/look-alike issues:

Calcitonin may be confused with calcitriol

Miacalcin® may be confused with Micatin®

Calcitonin nasal spray is administered as a single spray into **one** nostril daily, using alternate nostrils each day.

U.S. Brand Names Fortical®; Miacalcin®

Canadian Brand Names Apo-Calcitonin®; Calcimar®; Caltine®; Miacalcin® NS

Mexican Brand Names Miacalcic; Oseum

Index Terms Calcitonin (Salmon)

Pharmacologic Category Antidote; Hormone

Use Calcitonin (salmon): Treatment of Paget's disease of bone (osteitis deformans); adjunctive therapy for hypercalcemia; treatment of osteoporosis in women >5 years postmenopause

Effect on Mental Status May cause depression, dizziness, or fatigue. Rarely associated with agitation, anxiety, and insomnia.

Effect on Psychiatric Treatment May cause GI side effects; concomitant use with SSRIs, carbamazepine, valproic acid, and lithium may produce additive effects.

Dosage Summary

I.M.:

Children: Dosage not established

Adults: Paget's disease/osteoporosis: 50-100 units every 1-3 days; Hypercalcemia: 4-8 units/kg every 12 hours (maximum: 8 units/kg every 6 hours)

Intranasal:

Children: Dosage not established

Adults: 200 units (1 spray) in one nostril daily

SubQ:

Children: Dosage not established

Adults: Paget's disease/osteoporosis: 50-100 units every 1-3 days; Hypercalcemia: 4-8 units/kg every 12 hours (maximum: 8 units/kg every 6 hours)

Dosage Forms Excipient information presented when available (limited, particularly for generics); consult specific product labeling.

Injection, solution [calcitonin-salmon]:

Miacalcin®: 200 int. units/mL (2 mL)

Solution, intranasal [spray, calcitonin-salmon]:

Fortical®: 200 int. units/0.09 mL (3.7 mL) [rDNA origin; contains benzyl alcohol; delivers 30 doses, 200 units/actuation]

Miacalcin®: 200 int. units/0.09 mL (3.7 mL) [contains benzalkonium chloride; delivers 30 doses, 200 units/actuation]

◆ **Calcitonin (Salmon)** *see* Calcitonin *on page 253*

◆ **Cal-Citrate-225** *see* Calcium Citrate *on page 257*

◆ **Cal-Citrate® 250 [OTC] [DSC]** *see* Calcium Citrate *on page 257*

Calcium Acetate (KAL see um AS e tate)

Medication Safety Issues

Sound-alike/look-alike issues:

PhosLo® may be confused with Phos-Flur®, ProSom™

U.S. Brand Names PhosLo®

Canadian Brand Names PhosLo®

Mexican Brand Names Acid Mantle

Pharmacologic Category Antidote; Calcium Salt; Phosphate Binder

Use Control of hyperphosphatemia in end-stage renal failure; does not promote aluminum absorption

Effect on Mental Status May cause confusion and delirium (as a consequence of hypercalcemia)

Effect on Psychiatric Treatment None reported

Dosage Summary

Oral:

Children 0-6 months: RDA: 210 mg/day

Children 7-12 months: RDA: 270 mg/day

Children 1-3 years: RDA: 500 mg/day

Children 4-8 years: RDA: 800 mg/day

Children 9-18 years: RDA: 1300 mg/day

Adults: Initial: 1334 mg with each meal; Maintenance: 2001-2868 mg with each meal

Dosage Forms Excipient information presented when available (limited, particularly for generics); consult specific product labeling.

Gelcap: 667 mg

PhosLo®: 667 mg [equivalent to elemental calcium 169 mg (8.45 mEq)]

◆ **Calcium Acetylhomotaurinate** *see* Acamprosate *on page 23*

◆ **Calcium and Risedronate** *see* Risedronate and Calcium *on page 1424*

Calcium Carbonate (KAL see um KAR bun ate)

Medication Safety Issues

Sound-alike/look-alike issues:

Florical® may be confused with Fiorinal®

Mylanta® may be confused with Mynatal®

Nephro-Calci® may be confused with Nephrocaps®

Os-Cal® may be confused with Asacol®

International issues:

Remegel® [Great Britain, Ireland, Italy] may be confused with Renagel® which is a brand name for sevelamer in the U.S.

U.S. Brand Names Alcalak [OTC]; Alka-Mints® [OTC]; Cal-Gest [OTC]; Cal-Mint [OTC]; Calcarb 600 [OTC]; Calci-Chew® [OTC]; Calci-Mix® [OTC]; Caltrate® 600 [OTC]; Children's Pepto [OTC]; Chooz® [OTC]; Florical® [OTC]; Maalox® Regular Chewable [OTC]; Mylanta® Children's [OTC]; Nephro-Calci® [OTC]; Nutralox® [OTC]; Os-Cal® 500 [OTC] [DSC]; Oysco 500 [OTC]; Oyst-Cal 500 [OTC]; Rolaids® Softchews [OTC]; Titralac™ [OTC]; Tums® E-X [OTC]; Tums® Extra Strength Sugar Free [OTC]; Tums® Smoothies™ [OTC]; Tums® Ultra [OTC]; Tums® [OTC]

Canadian Brand Names Apo-Cal®; Calcite-500; Caltrate®; Caltrate® Select; Os-Cal®

Mexican Brand Names Calsan; Caltrate; Caltrón; Mubonet; Osteomin; Tums

Pharmacologic Category Antacid; Antidote; Calcium Salt; Electrolyte Supplement, Oral

Use As an antacid; treatment and prevention of calcium deficiency or hyperphosphatemia (eg, osteoporosis, osteomalacia, mild/moderate renal insufficiency, hypoparathyroidism, postmenopausal osteoporosis, rickets); has been used to bind phosphate

Effect on Mental Status May rarely produce irritability

Effect on Psychiatric Treatment None reported

Dosage Summary

Oral:

Neonates: 50-150 mg/kg/day in 4-6 divided doses (maximum: 1 g/day)

Children <2 years: 45-65 mg/kg/day in 4 divided doses

Children 2-5 years (24-47 lbs): Antacid: 161 mg (elemental calcium) as needed (maximum: 483 mg/day); Hypocalcemia: 45-65 mg/kg/day in 4 divided doses

Children 6-11 years (48-95 lbs): Antacid: 322 mg (elemental calcium) as needed (maximum: 966 mg/day); Hypocalcemia: 45-65 mg/kg/day in 4 divided doses

Children >11 years: 45-65 mg/kg/day in 4 divided doses

Adults ≤51 years: Antacid: 1-2 tablets or 5-10 mL every 2 hours (maximum: 7000 mg/day); Hypocalcemia/dietary: 500-2000 mg/day in 2-4 divided doses

Adults >51 years: Antacid: 1-2 tablets or 5-10 mL every 2 hours (maximum: 7000 mg/day); Hypocalcemia/dietary: 500-2000 mg/day in 2-4 divided doses; Osteoporosis: 1200 mg/day

Dosage Forms Excipient information presented when available (limited, particularly for generics); consult specific product labeling. [DSC] = Discontinued product

Capsule:

Calci-Mix®: 1250 mg [equivalent to elemental calcium 500 mg]

Florical®: 364 mg [equivalent to elemental calcium 145.6 mg; contains sodium fluoride 3.75 mg]

Gum, chewing: 250 mg (30s)

Chooz®: 500 mg [equivalent to elemental calcium 200 mg; mint flavor]

Powder: 4000 mg/teaspoonful (480 g) [equivalent to 1600 mg elemental calcium/teaspoonful]

Suspension, oral: 1250 mg/5 mL (5 mL, 500 mL) [equivalent to elemental calcium 500 mg/5 mL; mint flavor]

Tablet: 1250 mg [equivalent to elemental calcium 500 mg]; 1500 mg [equivalent to elemental calcium 600 mg]

Calcarb 600, Caltrate® 600, Nephro-Calci®: 1500 mg [equivalent to elemental calcium 600 mg]

Florical®: 364 mg [equivalent to elemental calcium 145.6 mg; contains sodium fluoride 8.3 mg]

Os-Cal® 500: 1250 mg [equivalent to elemental calcium 500 mg; contains tartrazine] [DSC]

Oysco 500, Oyst-Cal 500: 1250 mg [equivalent to elemental calcium 500 mg]

Tablet, chewable: 500 mg [equivalent to elemental calcium 200 mg]; 650 mg [equivalent to elemental calcium 260 mg]; 750 mg [equivalent to elemental calcium 300 mg]

Alcalak: 420 mg [equivalent to elemental calcium 168 mg; mint flavor]

Alka-Mints®: 850 mg [equivalent to elemental calcium 340 mg; spearmint flavor]

Cal-Gest: 500 mg [equivalent to elemental calcium 200 mg; assorted flavors]

Calci-Chew®: 1250 mg [equivalent to elemental calcium 500 mg; cherry, lemon, and orange flavors]

Cal-Mint: 650 mg [equivalent to elemental calcium 260 mg; mint flavor]

Children's Pepto: 400 mg [equivalent to elemental calcium 161 mg; bubble gum or watermelon flavors]

Maalox® Regular: 600 mg [equivalent to elemental calcium 222 mg; contains phenylalanine 0.5 mg/tablet; lemon flavor]

Mylanta® Children's: 400 mg [equivalent to elemental calcium 160 mg; bubble gum flavor]

Nutralox®: 420 mg [equivalent to elemental calcium 168 mg; sugar free; mint flavor]

Os-Cal® 500: 1250 mg [equivalent to elemental calcium 500 mg; Bavarian cream flavor] [DSC]

Titralac™: 420 mg [equivalent to elemental calcium 168 mg; sugar free; contains sodium 1.1 mg/tablet; spearmint flavor]

Tums®: 500 mg [equivalent to elemental calcium 200 mg; contains tartrazine; assorted fruit and peppermint flavors]

Tums® E-X: 750 mg [equivalent to elemental calcium 300 mg; contains tartrazine; assorted fruit, cool relief mint, fresh blend, tropical assorted fruit, wintergreen, and assorted berry flavors]

Tums® Extra Strength Sugar Free: 750 mg [equivalent to elemental calcium 300 mg; sugar free; contains phenylalanine <1 mg/tablet; orange cream flavor]

Tums® Smoothies™: 750 mg [equivalent to elemental calcium 300 mg; contains tartrazine; assorted fruit, assorted tropical fruit, peppermint flavors]

Tums® Ultra®: 1000 mg [equivalent to elemental calcium 400 mg; contains tartrazine; assorted berry, assorted fruit, assorted tropical fruit, peppermint, and spearmint flavors]

Tablet, softchew:

Rolaids®: 1177 mg [equivalent to elemental calcium 471 mg; contains coconut oil and soy lecithin; vanilla creme and wild cherry flavors]

♦ **Calcium Carbonate and Etidronate Disodium** *see* Etidronate and Calcium *on page 605*

Calcium Carbonate and Magnesium Hydroxide

(KAL see um KAR bun ate & mag NEE zhum hye DROKS ide)

Medication Safety Issues

Sound-alike/look-alike issues:

Mylanta® may be confused with Mynatal®

U.S. Brand Names Mi-Acid™ Double Strength [OTC]; Mylanta® Gelcaps® [OTC]; Mylanta® Supreme [OTC]; Mylanta® Ultra [OTC]; Rolaids® Extra Strength [OTC]; Rolaids® [OTC]

Index Terms Magnesium Hydroxide and Calcium Carbonate

Pharmacologic Category Antacid

Use Hyperacidity

Effect on Mental Status None reported

Effect on Psychiatric Treatment Antacids may decrease the excretion of amphetamines; monitor. Antacids may decrease the absorption of antipsychotics; monitor.

Dosage Summary

Oral:

Children: Dosage not established

Adults: 2-4 tablets between meals and at bedtime

Dosage Forms Excipient information presented when available (limited, particularly for generics); consult specific product labeling.

Gelcap (Mylanta® Gelcaps®): Calcium carbonate 550 mg and magnesium hydroxide 125 mg

Liquid (Mylanta® Supreme): Calcium carbonate 400 mg and magnesium hydroxide 135 mg per 5 mL (360 mL, 720 mL) [cherry flavor]

Tablet, chewable:

Mi-Acid™ Double Strength: Calcium carbonate 700 mg and magnesium hydroxide 300 mg

Mylanta® Ultra: Calcium carbonate 700 mg and magnesium hydroxide 300 mg [cherry créme and cool mint flavors]

Rolaids®: Calcium carbonate 550 mg and magnesium hydroxide 110 mg [sodium free; contains elemental calcium 220 mg and elemental magnesium 45 mg; original (peppermint), cherry, and spearmint flavors]

Rolaids® Extra Strength: Calcium carbonate 675 mg and magnesium hydroxide 135 mg [sodium free; contains elemental calcium 271 mg and elemental magnesium 56 mg, fruit flavor contains tartrazine; cool strawberry, fresh mint, fruit, and tropical fruit punch flavors]

♦ **Calcium Carbonate, Magnesium Hydroxide, and Famotidine** *see* Famotidine, Calcium Carbonate, and Magnesium Hydroxide *on page 614*

Calcium Chloride (KAL see um KLOR ide)

Medication Safety Issues

Dosing issues:

Calcium chloride may be confused with calcium gluconate

Confusion with the different intravenous salt forms of calcium has occurred. There is a threefold difference in the primary cation concentration between calcium chloride (in which 1g = 13.6 mEq [270 mg] of elemental Ca++) and calcium gluconate (in which 1g = 4.65 mEq [90 mg] of elemental Ca++).

Prescribers should specify which salt form is desired. Dosages should be expressed either as mEq, mg, or grams of the salt form.

Mexican Brand Names Solural

Pharmacologic Category Calcium Salt; Electrolyte Supplement, Parenteral

Use Treatment of acute symptomatic hypocalcemia; cardiac disturbances of hyperkalemia or hypocalcemia; emergent treatment of hypocalcemic tetany; treatment of severe hypermagnesemia

Unlabeled/Investigational Use Calcium channel blocker overdose; severe hyperkalemia (K+ >7 mEq/L with toxic ECG changes) [ACLS guidelines]; malignant arrhythmias associated with hypermagnesemia [ACLS guidelines]

Effect on Mental Status May cause drowsiness; rare reports of mania

Effect on Psychiatric Treatment None reported

Dosage Summary Note: One gram of calcium chloride is equal to 270 mg of elemental calcium. **Dosages are expressed in terms of the calcium chloride salt based on a solution concentration of 100 mg/mL (10%) containing 1.4 mEq (27.3 mg)/mL elemental calcium.**

I.V.:

Neonates:

Acute, symptomatic ionized hypocalcemia, hyperkalemia, or magnesium toxicity. **Note:** Routine use in cardiac arrest is not recommended due to the lack of improved survival [PALS 2005 Guidelines]: 20 mg/kg; may repeat as necessary

Calcium channel blocker overdose (unlabeled use) [PALS 2005 Guidelines]: 20 mg/kg (maximum: 1000 mg/dose) over 5-10 minutes; if favorable response obtained, consider I.V. infusion.

Hypocalcemia secondary to citrated blood transfusion: Give 32 mg (0.45 mEq elemental calcium) for each 100 mL citrated blood infused

Hypocalcemic tetany: 40-60 mg/kg/dose repeated every 6-8 hours

Infants and Children:

Acute, symptomatic ionized hypocalcemia, hyperkalemia, or magnesium toxicity. **Note:** Routine use in cardiac arrest is not recommended due to the lack of improved survival [PALS 2005 Guidelines]: 20 mg/kg, may repeat as necessary

Calcium channel blocker overdose (unlabeled use) [PALS 2005 Guidelines]: 20 mg/kg (maximum: 1000 mg per dose) over 5-10 minutes; if favorable response obtained, consider I.V. infusion.

Hypocalcemia secondary to citrated blood transfusion: Give 32 mg (0.45 mEq elemental calcium) for each 100 mL citrated blood infused

Hypocalcemic tetany: 10 mg/kg over 5-10 minutes, may repeat after 6-8 hours or follow with an infusion (maximum: 200 mg/kg/day) **or** 35-50 mg/kg every 6-8 hours

Adults:

Acute, symptomatic ionized hypocalcemia, hyperkalemia, or magnesium toxicity. **Note:** Routine use in cardiac arrest is not recommended due to the lack of improved survival [ACLS 2005 Guidelines]: 500-1000 mg, may repeat as necessary

Calcium channel blocker overdose (unlabeled use): 1000 mg every 10-20 minutes (total of 4 doses) **or** 1000 mg every 2-3 minutes until clinical effect is achieved; if favorable response obtained, consider I.V. infusion. I.V. infusion: 20-50 mg/kg/hour

Hypocalcemia secondary to citrated blood transfusion: 200-500 mg per 500 mL of citrated blood

Hypocalcemic tetany: 1000 mg, may repeat after 6 hours

Dosage Forms Excipient information presented when available (limited, particularly for generics); consult specific product labeling.

Injection, solution [preservative free]: 10% (10 mL) [present as calcium chloride 100 mg (1.36 mEq)/mL; provides elemental calcium 27.2 mg/mL (1.36 mEq)/mL]

Injection, solution: 10% (10 mL) [present as calcium chloride 100 mg (1.36 mEq)/mL; provides elemental calcium 27.2 mg (1.36 mEq)/mL]

Calcium Citrate (KAL see um SIT rate)

Medication Safety Issues

Sound-alike/look-alike issues:

Citracal® may be confused with Citrucel®

U.S. Brand Names Cal-C-Caps [OTC]; Cal-Cee [OTC]; Cal-Citrate-225; Cal-Citrate® 250 [OTC] [DSC]; Citracal® Kosher [OTC]

Canadian Brand Names Osteocit®

Mexican Brand Names Calcival

Pharmacologic Category Calcium Salt

Use Antacid; treatment and prevention of calcium deficiency or hyperphosphatemia (eg, osteoporosis, osteomalacia, mild/moderate renal insufficiency, hypoparathyroidism, postmenopausal osteoporosis, rickets)

Effect on Mental Status May cause confusion and delirium (as a consequence of hypercalcemia)

Effect on Psychiatric Treatment None reported

Dosage Summary

Oral:

Children 0-6 months: RDA: 210 mg/day
Children 7-12 months: RDA: 270 mg/day
Children 1-3 years: RDA: 500 mg/day
Children 4-8 years: RDA: 800 mg/day
Children 9-18 years: RDA: 1300 mg/day
Adults: 500-2000 mg 2-4 times/day

Dosage Forms Excipient information presented when available (limited, particularly for generics); consult specific product labeling. [DSC] = Discontinued product

Capsule:
Cal-C-Caps: Elemental calcium 180 mg
Cal-Citrate-225: Elemental calcium 225 mg
Granules: Elemental calcium 760 mg/teaspoonful (480 g)
Tablet: Elemental calcium 200 mg, 250 mg
Cal-Citrate®: Elemental calcium 250 mg [DSC]
Cal-Cee: Elemental calcium 250 mg
Citracal® Kosher: Elemental calcium 200 mg

Calcium Glubionate (KAL see um gloo BYE oh nate)

Medication Safety Issues

Sound-alike/look-alike issues:
Calcium glubionate may be confused with calcium gluconate

U.S. Brand Names Calcionate [OTC]

Pharmacologic Category Calcium Salt

Use Dietary supplement

Effect on Mental Status May cause confusion and delirium (as a consequence of hypercalcemia)

Effect on Psychiatric Treatment None reported

Dosage Summary

Oral:

Children 0-6 months: RDA: 210 mg/day
Children 7-12 months: RDA: 270 mg/day
Children 1-3 years: RDA: 500 mg/day
Children 4-8 years: RDA: 800 mg/day
Children 9-18 years: RDA: 1300 mg/day
Adults 19-50 years: RDA: 1000 mg/day
Adults ≥51 years: RDA: 1200 mg/day

Dosage Forms Excipient information presented when available (limited, particularly for generics); consult specific product labeling.

Syrup:
Calcionate: 1.8 g/5 mL (480 mL) [equivalent to elemental calcium 115 mg/5 mL; contains benzoic acid; caramel and orange flavor]

Calcium Gluconate (KAL see um GLOO koe nate)

Medication Safety Issues

Sound-alike/look-alike issues:
Calcium gluconate may be confused with calcium glubionate

U.S. Brand Names Cal-G [OTC]; Cal-GLU™

Pharmacologic Category Calcium Salt; Electrolyte Supplement, Oral; Electrolyte Supplement, Parenteral

Use Treatment and prevention of hypocalcemia; treatment of tetany, cardiac disturbances of hyperkalemia, cardiac resuscitation when epinephrine fails to improve myocardial contractions, hypocalcemia; calcium supplementation; hydrofluoric acid (HF) burns

Unlabeled/Investigational Use Calcium channel blocker overdose

Effect on Mental Status May cause drowsiness; may cause confusion and delirium (as a consequence of hypercalcemia)

Effect on Psychiatric Treatment None reported

Dosage Summary Note: 1 gram of calcium gluconate is equal to 90 mg of elemental calcium. The following dosages are expressed in terms of the calcium gluconate salt based on a solution concentration of 100 mg/mL (10%) containing 0.465 mEq (9.3 mg)/mL elemental calcium

I.V.:

Neonates:

Hypocalcemia: 200-800 mg/kg/day as a continuous infusion or in 4 divided doses (maximum: 1 g/dose)

Hypocalcemia secondary to citrated blood infusion: Give 98 mg (0.45 mEq elemental calcium) for each 100 mL citrated blood infused

Infants and Children:

Cardiac arrest or magnesium intoxication: 60-100 mg/kg/dose (maximum: 3 g/dose)

Hypocalcemia: 200-500 mg/kg/day as a continuous infusion or in 4 divided doses (maximum: 2-3 g/dose)

Hypocalcemia secondary to citrated blood infusion: Give 98 mg (0.45 mEq elemental calcium) for each 100 mL citrated blood infused

Hypocalcemic tetany: 100-200 mg/kg, may repeat every 6-8 hours or follow with an infusion of 500 mg/kg/day

Adults:

Cardiac arrest or magnesium intoxication: 500-800 mg/dose (maximum: 3 g/dose)

Hypocalcemia: 2-15 g/24 hours as a continuous infusion or in divided doses

Hypocalcemia secondary to citrated blood infusion: 500 mg to 1 g per 500 mL of citrated blood **or** up to 2 g as a single dose

Hypocalcemic tetany: 1-3 g/dose, may repeat until therapeutic response occurs

Maintenance electrolyte requirements for TPN: 1.7-3.4 g/1000 kcal/24 hours

Oral:

Children: Hypocalcemia: 200-500 mg/kg/day divided every 6 hours

Adults: Hypocalcemia: 500 mg to 2 g 2-4 times/day

Dosage Forms Excipient information presented when available (limited, particularly for generics); consult specific product labeling.

Capsule, oral:

Cal-G: 700 mg [gluten free, wheat free; equivalent to elemental calcium 65 mg]

Capsule, oral [preservative free]:

Cal-GLU™: 515 mg [dye free, sugar free; equivalent to elemental calcium 50 mg]

Injection, solution [preservative free]: 10% (10 mL, 50 mL, 100 mL, 200 mL) [100 mg/mL; equivalent to elemental calcium 9 mg/mL; calcium 0.46 mEq/mL]

Powder: 347 mg/tablespoonful (480 g)

Tablet: 500 mg [equivalent to elemental calcium 45 mg]; 650 mg [equivalent to elemental calcium 58.5 mg]; 975 mg [equivalent to elemental calcium 87.75 mg]

Calcium Lactate (KAL see um LAK tate)

Pharmacologic Category Calcium Salt

Use Adjunct in prevention of postmenopausal osteoporosis; treatment and prevention of calcium depletion

Effect on Mental Status May rarely cause confusion or dizziness

Effect on Psychiatric Treatment None reported

Dosage Summary

Oral:

Children 0-6 months: RDA: 210 mg/day

Children 7-12 months: RDA: 270 mg/day

Children 1-3 years: RDA: 500 mg/day

Children 4-8 years: RDA: 800 mg/day

Children 9-18 years: RDA: 1300 mg/day

Adults 19-50 years: RDA: 1000 mg/day

Adults ≥51 years: RDA: 1200 mg/day

Dosage Forms Excipient information presented when available (limited, particularly for generics); consult specific product labeling.

Tablet: 650 mg [equivalent to elemental calcium 84.5 mg]

◆ **Caldecort® [OTC]** *see* Hydrocortisone *on page 785*

◆ **Cal-G [OTC]** *see* Calcium Gluconate *on page 258*

◆ **Cal-Gest [OTC]** *see* Calcium Carbonate *on page 254*

◆ **Cal-GLU™** *see* Calcium Gluconate *on page 258*

◆ **Cal-Mint [OTC]** *see* Calcium Carbonate *on page 254*

◆ **CaloMist™** *see* Cyanocobalamin *on page 404*

- ◆ **Caltrate® 600 [OTC]** *see* Calcium Carbonate *on page 254*
- ◆ **Camila™** *see* Norethindrone *on page 1150*
- ◆ **Camomille Grande** *see* Feverfew *(Tanacetum parthenium) on page 628*
- ◆ **Campath®** *see* Alemtuzumab *on page 59*
- ◆ **Campath-1H** *see* Alemtuzumab *on page 59*
- ◆ **Camphorated Tincture of Opium (error-prone synonym)** *see* Paregoric *on page 1225*
- ◆ **Campral®** *see* Acamprosate *on page 23*
- ◆ **Camptosar®** *see* Irinotecan *on page 856*
- ◆ **Camptothecin-11** *see* Irinotecan *on page 856*
- ◆ **Canasa®** *see* Mesalamine *on page 994*
- ◆ **Cancidas®** *see* Caspofungin *on page 290*

Candesartan (kan de SAR tan)

Related Information
Angiotensin Agents *on page 1754*

U.S. Brand Names Atacand®

Canadian Brand Names Atacand®

Mexican Brand Names Atacand; Blopress

Index Terms Candesartan Cilexetil

Pharmacologic Category Angiotensin II Receptor Blocker

Generic Available No

Use Alone or in combination with other antihypertensive agents in treating essential hypertension; treatment of heart failure (NYHA class II-IV)

Effect on Mental Status May cause dizziness or drowsiness; may rarely cause anxiety or depression

Effect on Psychiatric Treatment None reported

Pregnancy Risk Factor C (1st trimester); D (2nd and 3rd trimesters)

Pregnancy Considerations Medications which act on the renin-angiotensin system are reported to have the following fetal/neonatal effects: Hypotension, neonatal skull hypoplasia, anuria, renal failure, and death; oligohydramnios is also reported. These effects are reported to occur with exposure during the second and third trimesters. There are no adequate and well-controlled studies in pregnant women. **[U.S. Boxed Warning]: Based on human data, drugs that act on the angiotensin system can cause injury and death to the developing fetus when used in the second and third trimesters. Angiotensin receptor blockers should be discontinued as soon as possible once pregnancy is detected.**

Lactation Enters breast milk/contraindicated

Contraindications Hypersensitivity to candesartan or any component of the formulation; severe hepatic impairment and/or cholestasis; pregnancy; breast-feeding

Warnings/Precautions [U.S. Boxed Warning]: Based on human data, drugs that act on the angiotensin system can cause injury and death to the developing fetus when used in the second and third trimesters. Angiotensin receptor blockers should be discontinued as soon as possible once pregnancy is detected. May cause hyperkalemia; avoid potassium supplementation unless specifically required by healthcare provider. Avoid use or use a smaller dose in patients who are volume depleted; correct depletion first. May be associated with deterioration of renal function and/or increases in serum creatinine, particularly in patients with low renal blood flow (eg, renal artery stenosis, heart failure) whose glomerular filtration rate (GFR) is dependent on efferent arteriolar vasoconstriction by angiotensin II. Use with caution in unstented unilateral/bilateral renal artery stenosis, pre-existing renal insufficiency, or significant aortic/mitral stenosis. Use with caution in patients with moderate hepatic impairment. Contraindicated with severe hepatic impairment and/or cholestasis. Use caution when initiating in heart failure; may need to adjust dose, and/or concurrent diuretic therapy, because of candesartan-induced hypotension. Hypotension may occur during major surgery and anesthesia; use cautiously before, during, and immediately after such interventions. Although some properties may be shared between these agents, concurrent therapy with ACE inhibitor may be rational in selected patients. Safety and efficacy have not been established in children.

Adverse Reactions
Cardiovascular: Angina, hypotension (CHF 19%), MI, palpitation, tachycardia
Central nervous system: Dizziness, lightheadedness, drowsiness, headache, vertigo, anxiety, depression, somnolence, fever

Dermatologic: Angioedema, rash
Endocrine & metabolic: Hyperglycemia, hyperkalemia (CHF <1% to 6%), hypertriglyceridemia, hyperuricemia
Gastrointestinal: Dyspepsia, gastroenteritis
Genitourinary: Hematuria
Neuromuscular & skeletal: Back pain, CPK increased, myalgia, paresthesia, weakness
Renal: Serum creatinine increased (up to 13% in patients with CHF with drug discontinuation required in 6%)
Respiratory: Dyspnea, epistaxis, pharyngitis, rhinitis, upper respiratory tract infection
Miscellaneous: Diaphoresis increased
<1%, postmarketing, and/or case reports: Abnormal hepatic function, agranulocytosis, anemia, hepatitis, hyponatremia, leukopenia, neutropenia, pruritus, renal failure, renal impairment, rhinitis, sinusitis, thrombocytopenia, urticaria; rhabdomyolysis has been reported (rarely) with angiotensin-receptor antagonists

Metabolism/Transport Effects **Substrate** of CYP2C9 (minor); **Inhibits** CYP2C8 (weak), 2C9 (weak)

Drug Interactions

ACE Inhibitors: Angiotensin II Receptor Blockers may enhance the adverse/toxic effect of ACE Inhibitors. *Risk C: Monitor therapy*
Diazoxide: May enhance the hypotensive effect of Antihypertensives. *Risk C: Monitor therapy*
Eplerenone: May enhance the hyperkalemic effect of Angiotensin II Receptor Blockers. *Risk C: Monitor therapy*
Herbs (Hypertensive Properties): May diminish the antihypertensive effect of Antihypertensives. *Risk C: Monitor therapy*
Herbs (Hypotensive Properties): May enhance the hypotensive effect of Antihypertensives. *Risk C: Monitor therapy*
Lithium: Angiotensin II Receptor Blockers may increase the serum concentration of Lithium. Management: Lithium dosage reductions will likely be needed following the addition of an angiotensin II receptor antagonist. *Risk D: Consider therapy modification*
Methylphenidate: May diminish the antihypertensive effect of Antihypertensives. *Risk C: Monitor therapy*
Nonsteroidal Anti-Inflammatory Agents: May diminish the therapeutic effect of Angiotensin II Receptor Blockers. The combination of these two agents may also significantly decrease glomerular filtration and renal function. *Risk C: Monitor therapy*
Potassium Salts: May enhance the hyperkalemic effect of Angiotensin II Receptor Blockers. *Risk C: Monitor therapy*
Potassium-Sparing Diuretics: Angiotensin II Receptor Blockers may enhance the hyperkalemic effect of Potassium-Sparing Diuretics. *Risk C: Monitor therapy*
Prostacyclin Analogues: May enhance the hypotensive effect of Antihypertensives. *Risk C: Monitor therapy*
RiTUXimab: Antihypertensives may enhance the hypotensive effect of RiTUXimab. *Risk D: Consider therapy modification*
Trimethoprim: May enhance the hyperkalemic effect of Angiotensin II Receptor Blockers. *Risk C: Monitor therapy*

Ethanol/Nutrition/Herb Interactions

Food: Food reduces the time to maximal concentration and increases the C_{max}.
Herb/Nutraceutical: Avoid dong quai if using for hypertension (has estrogenic activity). Avoid ephedra, yohimbe, ginseng (may worsen hypertension). Avoid garlic (may have increased antihypertensive effect).

Mechanism of Action Candesartan is an angiotensin receptor antagonist. Angiotensin II acts as a vasoconstrictor. In addition to causing direct vasoconstriction, angiotensin II also stimulates the release of aldosterone. Once aldosterone is released, sodium as well as water are reabsorbed. The end result is an elevation in blood pressure. Candesartan binds to the AT1 angiotensin II receptor. This binding prevents angiotensin II from binding to the receptor thereby blocking the vasoconstriction and the aldosterone secreting effects of angiotensin II.

Pharmacodynamics/Kinetics

Onset of action: 2-3 hours
  Peak effect: 6-8 hours
Duration: >24 hours
Distribution: V_d: 0.13 L/kg
Protein binding: 99%
Metabolism: To candesartan by the intestinal wall cells
Bioavailability: 15%

Half-life elimination (dose dependent): 5-9 hours
Time to peak: 3-4 hours
Excretion: Urine (26%)
Clearance: Total body: 0.37 mL/kg/minute; Renal: 0.19 mL/kg/minute

Dosage Adults: Oral:

Hypertension: Usual dose is 4-32 mg once daily; dosage must be individualized. Blood pressure response is dose related over the range of 2-32 mg. The usual recommended starting dose of 16 mg once daily when it is used as monotherapy in patients who are not volume depleted. It can be administered once or twice daily with total daily doses ranging from 8-32 mg. Larger doses do not appear to have a greater effect and there is relatively little experience with such doses.

Congestive heart failure: Initial: 4 mg once daily; double the dose at 2-week intervals, as tolerated; target dose: 32 mg

Note: In selected cases, concurrent therapy with an ACE inhibitor may provide additional benefit.

Elderly: No initial dosage adjustment is necessary for elderly patients (although higher concentrations (C_{max}) and AUC were observed in these populations), for patients with mildly impaired renal function, or for patients with mildly impaired hepatic function.

Dosage adjustment in hepatic impairment:

Mild hepatic impairment: No initial dosage adjustment required

Moderate hepatic impairment: Consider initiation at lower dosages (AUC increased by 145%).

Severe hepatic impairment and/or cholestasis: Contraindicated

Monitoring Parameters Supine blood pressure, electrolytes, serum creatinine, BUN, urinalysis, symptomatic hypotension, and tachycardia; in CHF, serum potassium during dose escalation and periodically thereafter

Additional Information May have an advantage over losartan due to minimal metabolism requirements and consequent use in mild-to-moderate hepatic impairment

Dosage Forms Excipient information presented when available (limited, particularly for generics); consult specific product labeling.

Tablet, as cilexetil:

Atacand®: 4 mg, 8 mg, 16 mg, 32 mg

Candesartan and Hydrochlorothiazide

(kan de SAR tan & hye droe klor oh THYE a zide)

U.S. Brand Names Atacand HCT®

Canadian Brand Names Atacand® Plus

Mexican Brand Names Atacand Plus

Index Terms Candesartan Cilexetil and Hydrochlorothiazide

Pharmacologic Category Angiotensin II Receptor Blocker; Diuretic, Thiazide

Use Treatment of hypertension; combination product should not be used for initial therapy

Effect on Mental Status May cause dizziness

Effect on Psychiatric Treatment May cause decreased renal lithium clearance; monitor serum lithium levels

Dosage Summary

Oral:

Children: Dosage not established

Adults: Candesartan 16-32 mg/day in 1-2 divided doses and hydrochlorothiazide 12.5-25 mg once daily

Dosage Forms Excipient information presented when available (limited, particularly for generics); consult specific product labeling.

Tablet:

Atacand HCT®:

16/12.5: Candesartan cilexetil 16 mg and hydrochlorothiazide 12.5 mg
32/12.5: Candesartan cilexetil 32 mg and hydrochlorothiazide 12.5 mg
32/25: Candesartan cilexetil 32 mg and hydrochlorothiazide 25 mg

◆ **Candesartan Cilexetil** *see* Candesartan *on page 260*

◆ **Candesartan Cilexetil and Hydrochlorothiazide** *see* Candesartan and Hydrochlorothiazide *on page 262*

◆ **Cannabidiol and Tetrahydrocannabinol** *see* Tetrahydrocannabinol and Cannabidiol *on page 1558*

Cantharidin (kan THAR e din)

Canadian Brand Names Canthacur®; Cantharone®

Pharmacologic Category Keratolytic Agent

Use Removal of ordinary and periungual warts

Effect on Mental Status May cause delirium

Effect on Psychiatric Treatment None reported

Dosage Summary

Topical:

Children: Apply directly to lesion, cover with nonporous tape, remove tape in 24 hours, reapply if necessary

Adults: Apply directly to lesion, cover with nonporous tape, remove tape in 24 hours, reapply if necessary

Dosage Forms Excipient information presented when available (limited, particularly for generics); consult specific product labeling.

- **Cantil® [DSC]** *see* Mepenzolate *on page 986*
- **Capastat® Sulfate** *see* Capreomycin *on page 263*

Capecitabine (ka pe SITE a been)

Medication Safety Issues

Sound-alike/look-alike issues:

Xeloda® may be confused with Xenical®

High alert medication: The Institute for Safe Medication Practices (ISMP) includes this medication among its list of drug classes which have a heightened risk of causing significant patient harm when used in error.

U.S. Brand Names Xeloda®

Canadian Brand Names Xeloda®

Mexican Brand Names Xeloda

Index Terms NSC-712807

Pharmacologic Category Antineoplastic Agent, Antimetabolite; Antineoplastic Agent, Antimetabolite (Pyrimidine Analog)

Use Treatment of metastatic colorectal cancer; adjuvant therapy of Dukes' C colon cancer; treatment of metastatic breast cancer

Unlabeled/Investigational Use Treatment of gastric cancer, pancreatic cancer, esophageal cancer, ovarian cancer, metastatic renal cell cancer, neuroendocrine tumors, metastatic CNS lesions

Effect on Mental Status Sedation is common; may cause dizziness or insomnia

Effect on Psychiatric Treatment Neutropenia is common; use caution with clozapine and carbamazepine

Dosage Summary

Oral:

Children: Dosage not established

Adults: 1250 mg/m^2 twice daily for 2 weeks, every 21 days

Dosage Forms Excipient information presented when available (limited, particularly for generics); consult specific product labeling.

Tablet:

Xeloda®: 150 mg, 500 mg

- **Capital® and Codeine** *see* Acetaminophen and Codeine *on page 34*
- **Capoten®** *see* Captopril *on page 264*
- **Capozide®** *see* Captopril and Hydrochlorothiazide *on page 265*

Capreomycin (kap ree oh MYE sin)

Medication Safety Issues

Sound-alike/look-alike issues:

Capastat® may be confused with Cepastat®

U.S. Brand Names Capastat® Sulfate

Index Terms Capreomycin Sulfate

Pharmacologic Category Antibiotic, Miscellaneous; Antitubercular Agent

Use Treatment of tuberculosis in conjunction with at least one other antituberculosis agent

Effect on Mental Status May cause dizziness

Effect on Psychiatric Treatment None reported

Dosage Summary

I.M.:

Infants and Children <15 years and ≤40 kg (unlabeled): 15-30 mg/kg/day (maximum: 1 g/day) for 2-4 months, followed by 15-30 mg/kg (maximum: 1 g/day) twice a week

Children ≥15 years or >40 kg (unlabeled): 15 mg/kg/day (maximum: 1 g/dose) for 2-4 months followed by 15 mg/kg (maximum: 1 g/dose) 2-3 times/week

Adults: 1 g/day (maximum: 20 mg/kg/day) for 60-120 days, followed by 1 g 2-3 times/week

I.V.:

Infants and Children <15 years and ≤40 kg (unlabeled): 15-30 mg/kg/day (maximum: 1 g/day) for 2-4 months, followed by 15-30 mg/kg (maximum: 1 g/day) twice a week

Children ≥15 years or >40 kg (unlabeled): 15 mg/kg/day (maximum: 1 g/dose) for 2-4 months followed by 15 mg/kg (maximum: 1 g/dose) 2-3 times/week

Adults: 1 g/day (maximum: 20 mg/kg/day) for 60-120 days, followed by 1 g 2-3 times/week

Dosage Forms Excipient information presented when available (limited, particularly for generics); consult specific product labeling.

Injection, powder for reconstitution, as sulfate:

Capastat® Sulfate: 1 g

◆ **Capreomycin Sulfate** *see* Capreomycin *on page 263*

Captopril (KAP toe pril)

Medication Safety Issues

Sound-alike/look-alike issues:

Captopril may be confused with Capitrol®, carvedilol

International issues:

Acepril® [Great Britain] may be confused with Accupril® which is a brand name for quinapril in the U.S.

Acepril®: Brand name for enalapril in Hungary and Switzerland; brand name for lisinopril in Denmark

Related Information

Angiotensin Agents *on page 1754*

Anticholinergic Effects of Common Psychotropics *on page 1758*

U.S. Brand Names Capoten®

Canadian Brand Names Alti-Captopril; Apo-Capto®; Capoten™; Gen-Captopril; Novo-Captopril; Nu-Capto; PMS-Captopril

Mexican Brand Names Capotena; Captral; Ecaten; Midrat

Index Terms ACE

Pharmacologic Category Angiotensin-Converting Enzyme (ACE) Inhibitor

Use Management of hypertension; treatment of heart failure, left ventricular dysfunction after myocardial infarction, diabetic nephropathy

Unlabeled/Investigational Use To delay the progression of nephropathy and reduce risks of cardiovascular events in hypertensive patients with type 1 or 2 diabetes mellitus; treatment of hypertensive crisis, rheumatoid arthritis; diagnosis of anatomic renal artery stenosis, hypertension secondary to scleroderma renal crisis; diagnosis of aldosteronism, idiopathic edema, Bartter's syndrome, postmyocardial infarction for prevention of ventricular failure; increase circulation in Raynaud's phenomenon, hypertension secondary to Takayasu's disease

Effect on Mental Status May cause drowsiness or insomnia

Effect on Psychiatric Treatment May rarely cause agranulocytosis; use caution with clozapine and carbamazepine; may decrease lithium clearance resulting in an increase in serum lithium levels and potential lithium toxicity; monitor serum lithium levels

Dosage Summary

Oral:

Infants: Initial: 0.15-0.3 mg/kg/dose; Maintenance: 2.5-6 mg/kg/day in 1-4 divided doses

Children: Initial: 0.5 mg/kg/dose; Maintenance: Up to 6 mg/kg/day in 2-4 divided doses

Older Children: Initial: 6.25-12.5 mg every 12-24 hours; Maintenance: Up to 6 mg/kg/day

Adolescents: Initial: 12.5-25 mg every 8-12 hours; Maintenance: Up tp 450 mg/day divided every 8-12 hours

Adults: Initial: 6.25-25 mg 2-3 times/day; Maintenance: 25-450 mg/day in 2-3 divided doses; CHF target dose: 50 mg 3 times/day; Usual dosage range (JNC 7): 25-100 mg in 2 divided doses

Dosage Forms Excipient information presented when available (limited, particularly for generics); consult specific product labeling.

Tablet: 12.5 mg, 25 mg, 50 mg, 100 mg

Captopril and Hydrochlorothiazide

(KAP toe pril & hye droe klor oh THYE a zide)

U.S. Brand Names Capozide®

Canadian Brand Names Capozide®

Mexican Brand Names Capozide

Index Terms Hydrochlorothiazide and Captopril

Pharmacologic Category Angiotensin-Converting Enzyme (ACE) Inhibitor; Diuretic, Thiazide

Use Management of hypertension

Effect on Mental Status May cause drowsiness or insomnia

Effect on Psychiatric Treatment May rarely cause agranulocytosis; use caution with clozapine and carbamazepine; may decrease lithium clearance resulting in an increase in serum lithium levels and potential lithium toxicity; monitor serum lithium levels

Dosage Summary

Oral:

Children: Dosage not established

Adults: Captopril 25-150 mg and hydrochlorothiazide 15-50 mg once daily

Dosage Forms Excipient information presented when available (limited, particularly for generics); consult specific product labeling.

Tablet:

25/15: Captopril 25 mg and hydrochlorothiazide 15 mg
25/25: Captopril 25 mg and hydrochlorothiazide 25 mg
50/15: Captopril 50 mg and hydrochlorothiazide 15 mg
50/25: Captopril 50 mg and hydrochlorothiazide 25 mg

◆ **Carac®** *see* Fluorouracil *on page 649*

◆ **Carafate®** *see* Sucralfate *on page 1514*

CarBAMazepine (kar ba MAZ e peen)

Medication Safety Issues

Sound-alike/look-alike issues:

CarBAMazepine may be confused with OXcarbazepine
Carbatrol® may be confused with Cartrol®
Epitol® may be confused with Epinal®
Tegretol®, Tegretol®-XR may be confused with Mebaral®, Tegrin®, Toprol-XL®, Toradol®, Trental®

Related Information

Adverse Effects of Approved Mood Stabilizers / Anticonvulsants *on page 1751*
Agents Approved for Bipolar Disorder *on page 1752*
Anticonvulsants By Seizure Type *on page 1759*
Liquid Compatibility of Antidepressants, Antipsychotics, and Mood Stabilizers *on page 1788*

U.S. Brand Names Carbatrol®; Epitol®; Equetro®; Tegretol®; Tegretol®-XR

Canadian Brand Names Apo-Carbamazepine®; Bio-Carbamazepine; Carbamazepine; Dom-Carbamazepine; Gen-Carbamazepine CR; Mapezine®; Novo-Carbamaz; Nu-Carbamazepine; PHL-Carbamazepine; PMS-Carbamazepine; Sandoz-Carbamazepine; Taro-Carbamazepine Chewable; Tegretol®

Mexican Brand Names Brucarcer; Carbazep; Carbazina; Carpin; Clostedal; Neugeron; Neurolep; Sepibest; Tegretol; Trepina

Index Terms CBZ; SPD417

Pharmacologic Category Anticonvulsant, Miscellaneous

Generic Available Yes: Excludes capsule (extended release), tablet (extended release)

Use

Carbatrol®, Tegretol®, Tegretol®-XR: Partial seizures with complex symptomatology (psychomotor, temporal lobe), generalized tonic-clonic seizures (grand mal), mixed seizure patterns, trigeminal neuralgia

Equetro®: Acute manic and mixed episodes associated with bipolar 1 disorder

Unlabeled/Investigational Use Treatment of resistant schizophrenia, ethanol withdrawal, restless leg syndrome, post-traumatic stress disorders

Mental Health Comment The extended-release capsule (Equetro®) is approved for acute manic and mixed episodes associated with bipolar I disorder. Like valproic acid and lithium, carbamazepine is considered a first-line agent. However, it is a significant inducer of hepatic enzymes. It is a heteroinducer and therefore, induces its own metabolism as well as metabolism of other drugs. Single-dose studies of carbamazepine show half-life ranges of 30-40 hours. After 3 weeks of continuous administration, the half-life decreases to ~20 hours. This reduction is caused by an increase in clearance resulting from autoinduction in metabolism. It is prudent to recheck serum carbamazepine levels after the first month of maintenance therapy. During chronic monotherapy, the half-life is ~12 hours and during polytherapy (with enzyme inducers; eg, phenytoin, phenobarbital), it is reduced to 8 hours. Maximal hepatic activation occurs within 2-4 weeks. Because of this, one has to be vigilant for drug-drug interactions. Studies have failed to document a correlation between plasma levels of carbamazepine and clinical response. However, correlation between CSF levels of carbamazepine's principle metabolite, the 10,11-epoxide, and clinical response in mania and depression have been observed. Therefore, this agent is best dosed clinically. Serum levels >12 mcg/mL do, however, correlate with toxicity. Carbamazepine is also used for a variety of other disorders such as aggressive behavior/episodic dyscontrol, eating disorders, alcohol withdrawal, anxiety disorders, behavioral disturbances in the developmentally disabled, and as an adjunctive agent to antipsychotic for the treatment of psychosis.

Pregnancy Risk Factor D

Pregnancy Considerations Crosses the placenta. Dysmorphic facial features, cranial defects, cardiac defects, spina bifida, IUGR, and multiple other malformations reported. Epilepsy itself, number of medications, genetic factors, or a combination of these probably influences the teratogenicity of anticonvulsant therapy. Benefit:risk ratio usually favors continued use during pregnancy and breast-feeding. Contraceptives may be rendered less effective by the coadministration of carbamazepine; alternative methods of contraception should be considered.

Lactation Enters breast milk/not recommended (AAP rates "compatible")

Contraindications Hypersensitivity to carbamazepine, tricyclic antidepressants, or any component of the formulation; bone marrow depression; with or within 14 days of MAO inhibitor use; concurrent use of nefazodone

Warnings/Precautions **[U.S. Boxed Warning]: Potentially fatal blood cell abnormalities have been reported.** Patients with a previous history of adverse hematologic reaction to any drug may be at increased risk. Administer carbamazepine with caution to patients with history of cardiac damage, ECG abnormalities (or at risk for ECG abnormalities), hepatic or renal disease. When used to treat bipolar disorder, the smallest effective dose is suggested to reduce the risk for overdose/suicide; high-risk patients should be monitored for suicidal ideations. Prescription should be written for the smallest quantity consistent with good patient care. May activate latent psychosis and/or cause confusion or agitation; elderly patients may be at an increased risk for psychiatric effects. Potentially serious, sometimes fatal multiorgan hypersensitivity reactions have been reported with some antiepileptic drugs; monitor for signs and symptoms of possible disparate manifestations associated with lymphatic, hepatic, renal, and/or hematologic organ systems; gradual discontinuation and conversion to alternate therapy may be required.

Carbamazepine is not effective in absence, myoclonic, or akinetic seizures; exacerbation of certain seizure types have been seen after initiation of carbamazepine therapy in children with mixed seizure disorders. Abrupt discontinuation is not recommended in patients being treated for seizures. Dizziness or drowsiness may occur; caution should be used when performing tasks which require alertness until the effects are known. Effects with other sedative drugs or ethanol may be potentiated. Carbamazepine has a high potential for drug interactions; use caution in patients taking strong CYP3A4 inducers or inhibitors or medications significantly metabolized via CYP1A2, 2B6, 2C9, 2C19, and 3A4. Coadministration of carbamazepine and nefazodone may lead to insufficient plasma levels of nefazodone; combination is contraindicated. Carbamazepine has mild anticholinergic activity; use with caution in patients with increased intraocular pressure, or sensitivity to anticholinergic effects. Severe dermatologic reactions, including toxic epidermal necrolysis and Stevens-Johnson syndrome, although rarely reported, have resulted in fatalities. **[U.S. Boxed Warning]: Use caution and screen for the genetic susceptibility genotype (*HLA-B*1502* allele) in Asian patients. Patients with a positive result should not be started on carbamazepine.** Discontinue if there are any signs of hypersensitivity. Elderly patients may have an increased risk of SIADH-like syndrome.

Administration of the suspension will yield higher peak and lower trough serum levels than an equal dose of the tablet form; consider a lower starting dose given more frequently (same total daily dose) when using the suspension.

Adverse Reactions Frequency not defined, unless otherwise specified.

Cardiovascular: Arrhythmias, AV block, bradycardia, chest pain (bipolar use), CHF, edema, hyper-/hypotension, lymphadenopathy, syncope, thromboembolism, thrombophlebitis

Central nervous system: Amnesia (bipolar use), anxiety (bipolar use), aseptic meningitis (case report), ataxia (bipolar use 15%), confusion, depression (bipolar use), dizziness (bipolar use 44%), fatigue, headache (bipolar use 22%), sedation, slurred speech, somnolence (bipolar use 32%)

Dermatologic: Alopecia, alterations in skin pigmentation, erythema multiforme, exfoliative dermatitis, photosensitivity reaction, pruritus (bipolar use 8%), purpura, rash, Stevens-Johnson syndrome, toxic epidermal necrolysis, urticaria

Endocrine & metabolic: Chills, fever, hyponatremia, syndrome of inappropriate ADH secretion (SIADH)

Gastrointestinal: Abdominal pain, anorexia, constipation, diarrhea, dyspepsia (bipolar use), gastric distress, nausea (bipolar use 29%), pancreatitis, vomiting (bipolar use 18%), xerostomia (bipolar use)

Genitourinary: Azotemia, impotence, renal failure, urinary frequency, urinary retention

Hematologic: Acute intermittent porphyria, agranulocytosis, aplastic anemia, bone marrow suppression, eosinophilia, leukocytosis, leukopenia, pancytopenia, thrombocytopenia

Hepatic: Abnormal liver function tests, hepatic failure, hepatitis, jaundice

Neuromuscular & skeletal: Back pain, pain (bipolar use 12%), peripheral neuritis, weakness

Ocular: Blurred vision, conjunctivitis, lens opacities, nystagmus

Otic: Hyperacusis, tinnitus

Miscellaneous: Diaphoresis, hypersensitivity (including multiorgan reactions, may include disorders mimicking lymphoma, eosinophilia, hepatosplenomegaly, vasculitis); infection (bipolar use 12%)

Postmarketing and/or case reports: Suicidal ideation

Metabolism/Transport Effects Substrate of CYP2C8 (minor), 3A4 (major); **Induces** CYP1A2 (strong), 2B6 (strong), 2C8 (strong), 2C9 (strong), 2C19 (strong), 3A4 (strong)

Drug Interactions

Acetaminophen: CarBAMazepine may increase the metabolism of Acetaminophen. This may 1) diminish the effect of acetaminophen; and 2) increase the risk of liver damage. *Risk C: Monitor therapy*

Alcohol (Ethyl): CNS Depressants may enhance the CNS depressant effect of Alcohol (Ethyl). *Risk C: Monitor therapy*

Allopurinol: May increase the serum concentration of CarBAMazepine. *Risk C: Monitor therapy*

Aminocamptothecin: CarBAMazepine may decrease the serum concentration of Aminocamptothecin. *Risk C: Monitor therapy*

Antifungal Agents (Azole Derivatives, Systemic): May decrease the metabolism of CarBAMazepine. *Risk C: Monitor therapy*

Aripiprazole: CarBAMazepine may decrease the serum concentration of Aripiprazole. *Risk D: Consider therapy modification*

Bendamustine: CYP1A2 Inducers (Strong) may decrease the serum concentration of Bendamustine. Concentrations of active metabolites may be increased. *Risk C: Monitor therapy*

Benzodiazepines (metabolized by oxidation): CarBAMazepine may increase the metabolism of Benzodiazepines (metabolized by oxidation). *Risk C: Monitor therapy*

Calcium Channel Blockers (Dihydropyridine): CarBAMazepine may increase the metabolism of Calcium Channel Blockers (Dihydropyridine). **Exceptions:** Clevidipine. *Risk C: Monitor therapy*

Calcium Channel Blockers (Nondihydropyridine): May decrease the metabolism of CarBAMazepine. CarBAMazepine may increase the metabolism of Calcium Channel Blockers (Nondihydropyridine). *Risk D: Consider therapy modification*

Carbonic Anhydrase Inhibitors: May increase the serum concentration of CarBAMazepine. **Exceptions:** Brinzolamide; Dorzolamide. *Risk C: Monitor therapy*

Caspofungin: Inducers of Drug Clearance may decrease the serum concentration of Caspofungin. Management: Consider using an increased caspofungin dose of 70 mg daily in adults (or 70 mg/m^2, up to a maximum of 70 mg, daily in pediatric patients) when coadministered with known inducers of drug clearance. *Risk D: Consider therapy modification*

Cimetidine: May increase the serum concentration of CarBAMazepine. The serum carbamazepine concentration might return to normal within one week of starting cimetidine. *Risk C: Monitor therapy*

ClomiPRAMINE: CarBAMazepine may increase the serum concentration of ClomiPRAMINE. *Risk C: Monitor therapy*

Clozapine: CarBAMazepine may increase the metabolism of Clozapine. *Risk D: Consider therapy modification*

CNS Depressants: May enhance the adverse/toxic effect of other CNS Depressants. *Risk C: Monitor therapy*

Contraceptive (Progestins): CarBAMazepine may diminish the therapeutic effect of Contraceptive (Progestins). Contraceptive failure is possible. *Risk D: Consider therapy modification*

CycloSPORINE: CarBAMazepine may decrease the serum concentration of CycloSPORINE. *Risk D: Consider therapy modification*

CYP1A2 Substrates: CYP1A2 Inducers (Strong) may increase the metabolism of CYP1A2 Substrates. *Risk C: Monitor therapy*

CYP2B6 Substrates: CYP2B6 Inducers (Strong) may increase the metabolism of CYP2B6 Substrates. *Risk C: Monitor therapy*

CYP2C19 Substrates: CYP2C19 Inducers (Strong) may increase the metabolism of CYP2C19 Substrates. *Risk C: Monitor therapy*

CYP2C8 Substrates (High risk): CYP2C8 Inducers (Highly Effective) may increase the metabolism of CYP2C8 Substrates (High risk). *Risk C: Monitor therapy*

CYP2C9 Substrates (High risk): CYP2C9 Inducers (Highly Effective) may increase the metabolism of CYP2C9 Substrates (High risk). *Risk C: Monitor therapy*

CYP3A4 Inducers (Strong): May increase the metabolism of CYP3A4 Substrates. *Risk C: Monitor therapy*

CYP3A4 Inhibitors (Moderate): May decrease the metabolism of CYP3A4 Substrates. *Risk C: Monitor therapy*

CYP3A4 Inhibitors (Strong): May decrease the metabolism of CYP3A4 Substrates. *Risk D: Consider therapy modification*

CYP3A4 Substrates: CYP3A4 Inducers (Strong) may increase the metabolism of CYP3A4 Substrates. *Risk C: Monitor therapy*

Dabigatran Etexilate: P-Glycoprotein Inducers may decrease the serum concentration of Dabigatran Etexilate. *Risk C: Monitor therapy*

Danazol: May decrease the metabolism of CarBAMazepine. *Risk D: Consider therapy modification*

Darunavir: CarBAMazepine may decrease the serum concentration of Darunavir. *Risk X: Avoid combination*

Dasatinib: May increase the serum concentration of CYP3A4 Substrates. *Risk C: Monitor therapy*

Deferasirox: May decrease the serum concentration of CYP3A4 Substrates. *Risk C: Monitor therapy*

Desmopressin: CarBAMazepine may enhance the adverse/toxic effect of Desmopressin. *Risk C: Monitor therapy*

Doxycycline: CarBAMazepine may decrease the serum concentration of Doxycycline. *Risk D: Consider therapy modification*

Etravirine: CarBAMazepine may decrease the serum concentration of Etravirine. Management: The manufacturer of etravirine states these drugs should not be used in combination. *Risk X: Avoid combination*

Fluconazole: May decrease the metabolism of CarBAMazepine. *Risk C: Monitor therapy*

Flunarizine: CarBAMazepine may decrease the serum concentration of Flunarizine. *Risk C: Monitor therapy*

Grapefruit Juice: May decrease the metabolism of CarBAMazepine. *Risk C: Monitor therapy*

Haloperidol: CarBAMazepine may increase the metabolism of Haloperidol. *Risk D: Consider therapy modification*

Herbs (CYP3A4 Inducers): May increase the metabolism of CYP3A4 Substrates. *Risk C: Monitor therapy*

Isoniazid: May decrease the metabolism of CarBAMazepine. *Risk D: Consider therapy modification*

Ketorolac: May diminish the therapeutic effect of Anticonvulsants. *Risk C: Monitor therapy*

Lacosamide: CarBAMazepine may decrease the serum concentration of Lacosamide. *Risk C: Monitor therapy*

LamoTRIgine: May enhance the adverse/toxic effect of CarBAMazepine. CarBAMazepine may increase the metabolism of LamoTRIgine. *Risk D: Consider therapy modification*

Lithium: CarBAMazepine may enhance the adverse/toxic effect of Lithium. *Risk C: Monitor therapy*

Macrolide Antibiotics: May decrease the metabolism of CarBAMazepine. **Exceptions:** Azithromycin; Dirithromycin [Off Market]; Spiramycin. *Risk D: Consider therapy modification*

Maraviroc: CYP3A4 Inducers may decrease the serum concentration of Maraviroc. *Risk D: Consider therapy modification*

Mebendazole: CarBAMazepine may decrease the serum concentration of Mebendazole. *Risk D: Consider therapy modification*

Mefloquine: May diminish the therapeutic effect of Anticonvulsants. Mefloquine may decrease the serum concentration of Anticonvulsants. Management: Mefloquine is contraindicated in persons with a history of convulsions. If anticonvulsant is being used for another indication monitor response to treatment closely, as concurrent mefloquine may decrease response to treatment. *Risk D: Consider therapy modification*

Methadone: CarBAMazepine may increase the metabolism of Methadone. *Risk D: Consider therapy modification*

Methylfolate: May decrease the serum concentration of CarBAMazepine. *Risk C: Monitor therapy*

Nilotinib: CYP3A4 Inducers (Strong) may decrease the serum concentration of Nilotinib. *Risk X: Avoid combination*

Oral Contraceptive (Estrogens): CarBAMazepine may diminish the therapeutic effect of Oral Contraceptive (Estrogens). Contraceptive failure is possible. *Risk D: Consider therapy modification*

Paliperidone: CarBAMazepine may decrease the serum concentration of Paliperidone. *Risk C: Monitor therapy*

P-Glycoprotein Substrates: P-Glycoprotein Inducers may decrease the serum concentration of P-Glycoprotein Substrates. P-glycoprotein inducers may also further limit the distribution of p-glycoprotein substrates to specific cells/tissues/organs where p-glycoprotein is present in large amounts (e.g., brain, T-lymphocytes, testes, etc.). *Risk C: Monitor therapy*

Phenytoin: CarBAMazepine may increase the metabolism of Phenytoin. Phenytoin may increase the metabolism of CarBAMazepine. CarBAMazepine may decrease the metabolism of Phenytoin. Possibly by competitive inhibition at sites of metabolism. *Risk D: Consider therapy modification*

Propoxyphene: May decrease the metabolism of CarBAMazepine. *Risk D: Consider therapy modification*

Protease Inhibitors: CarBAMazepine may increase the metabolism of Protease Inhibitors. Protease Inhibitors may decrease the metabolism of CarBAMazepine. *Risk D: Consider therapy modification*

Ranolazine: CYP3A4 Inducers (Strong) may decrease the serum concentration of Ranolazine. *Risk X: Avoid combination*

Risperidone: CarBAMazepine may decrease the serum concentration of Risperidone. *Risk C: Monitor therapy*

Selective Serotonin Reuptake Inhibitors: May decrease the metabolism of CarBAMazepine. Specifically those SSRIs that inhibit CYP3A4 isoenzymes. CarBAMazepine may increase the metabolism of Selective Serotonin Reuptake Inhibitors. Specifically those agents metabolized via CYP1A2, 2C, and/or 3A4 isoenzymes. *Risk D: Consider therapy modification*

Sorafenib: CYP3A4 Inducers (Strong) may decrease the serum concentration of Sorafenib. *Risk D: Consider therapy modification*

Temsirolimus: CarBAMazepine may decrease the serum concentration of Temsirolimus. Concentrations of the active metabolite, sirolimus, are also likely to be decreased (and maybe to an even greater degree). Management: Temsirolimus prescribing information recommends against coadministration with strong CYP3A4 inducers such as carbamazepine; however, if concurrent therapy is necessary, an increase in temsirolimus dose to 50 mg/week should be considered. *Risk D: Consider therapy modification*

Theophylline Derivatives: CarBAMazepine may increase the metabolism of Theophylline Derivatives. **Exceptions:** Dyphylline. *Risk C: Monitor therapy*

Thyroid Products: CarBAMazepine may decrease the serum concentration of Thyroid Products. *Risk C: Monitor therapy*

Topiramate: CarBAMazepine may decrease the serum concentration of Topiramate. *Risk D: Consider therapy modification*

Tricyclic Antidepressants: CarBAMazepine may increase the metabolism of Tricyclic Antidepressants. **Exceptions:** ClomiPRAMINE. *Risk C: Monitor therapy*

Valproic Acid: CarBAMazepine may increase the metabolism of Valproic Acid. Valproic Acid may decrease the serum concentration of CarBAMazepine. Carbamazepine-Epoxide concentrations might increase, offsetting the decreases in the parent compound. *Risk C: Monitor therapy*

Vecuronium: CarBAMazepine may decrease the serum concentration of Vecuronium. *Risk C: Monitor therapy*

Vitamin K Antagonists (eg, warfarin): CarBAMazepine may decrease the serum concentration of Vitamin K Antagonists. *Risk D: Consider therapy modification*

Voriconazole: CarBAMazepine may decrease the serum concentration of Voriconazole. *Risk X: Avoid combination*

Ziprasidone: CarBAMazepine may increase the metabolism of Ziprasidone. *Risk C: Monitor therapy*

Ethanol/Nutrition/Herb Interactions

Ethanol: Avoid ethanol (may increase CNS depression).

Food: Carbamazepine serum levels may be increased if taken with food. Carbamazepine serum concentration may be increased if taken with grapefruit juice; avoid concurrent use.

Herb/Nutraceutical: Avoid evening primrose (seizure threshold decreased). Avoid valerian, St John's wort, kava kava, gotu kola (may increase CNS depression).

Mechanism of Action In addition to anticonvulsant effects, carbamazepine has anticholinergic, antineuralgic, antidiuretic, muscle relaxant, antimanic, antidepressive, and antiarrhythmic properties; may depress activity in the nucleus ventralis of the thalamus or decrease synaptic transmission or decrease summation of temporal stimulation leading to neural discharge by limiting influx of sodium ions across cell membrane or other unknown mechanisms; stimulates the release of ADH and potentiates its action in promoting reabsorption of water; chemically related to tricyclic antidepressants

Pharmacodynamics/Kinetics

Absorption: Slow

Distribution: V_d: Neonates: 1.5 L/kg; Children: 1.9 L/kg; Adults: 0.59-2 L/kg

Protein binding: Carbamazepine: 75% to 90%, may be decreased in newborns; Epoxide metabolite: 50%

Metabolism: Hepatic via CYP3A4 to active epoxide metabolite; induces hepatic enzymes to increase metabolism

Bioavailability: 85%

Half-life elimination: **Note:** Half-life is variable because of autoinduction which is usually complete 3-5 weeks after initiation of a fixed carbamazepine regimen.

Carbamazepine: Initial: 25-65 hours; Extended release: 35-40 hours; Multiple doses: Children: 8-14 hours; Adults: 12-17 hours

Epoxide metabolite: Initial: 25-43 hours

Time to peak, serum: Unpredictable:

Immediate release: Suspension: 1.5 hour; tablet: 4-5 hours

Extended release: Carbatrol®, Equetro®: 12-26 hours (single dose), 4-8 hours (multiple doses); Tegretol®-XR: 3-12 hours

Excretion: Urine 72% (1% to 3% as unchanged drug); feces (28%)

Dosage Dosage must be adjusted according to patient's response and serum concentrations. Administer tablets (chewable or conventional) in 2-3 divided doses daily and suspension in 4 divided doses daily. Oral:

Epilepsy:

Children:

<6 years: Initial: 10-20 mg/kg/day divided twice or 3 times daily as tablets or 4 times/day as suspension; increase dose every week until optimal response and therapeutic levels are achieved

Maintenance dose: Divide into 3-4 doses daily (tablets or suspension); maximum recommended dose: 35 mg/kg/day

6-12 years: Initial: 200 mg/day in 2 divided doses (tablets or extended release tablets) or 4 divided doses (oral suspension); increase by up to 100 mg/day at weekly intervals using a twice daily regimen of extended release tablets or 3-4 times daily regimen of other formulations until optimal response and therapeutic levels are achieved

Maintenance: Usual: 400-800 mg/day; maximum recommended dose: 1000 mg/day

Note: Children <12 years who receive ≥400 mg/day of carbamazepine may be converted to extended release capsules (Carbatrol®) using the same total daily dosage divided twice daily

Children >12 years and Adults: Initial: 400 mg/day in 2 divided doses (tablets or extended release tablets) or 4 divided doses (oral suspension); increase by up to 200 mg/day at weekly intervals using a twice daily regimen of extended release tablets or capsules, or a 3-4 times/day regimen of other formulations until optimal response and therapeutic levels are achieved; usual dose: 800-1200 mg/day

Maximum recommended doses:

Children 12-15 years: 1000 mg/day

Children >15 years: 1200 mg/day

Adults: 1600 mg/day; however, some patients have required up to 1.6-2.4 g/day

Trigeminal or glossopharyngeal neuralgia: Adults: Initial: 200 mg/day in 2 divided doses (tablets, extended release tablets, or extended release capsules) or 4 divided doses (oral suspension) with food, gradually increasing in increments of 200 mg/day as needed

Maintenance: Usual: 400-800 mg daily in 2 divided doses (tablets, extended release tablets, or extended release capsules) or 4 divided doses (oral suspension); maximum dose: 1200 mg/day

Bipolar disorder: Adults: Initial: 400 mg/day in 2 divided doses (tablets, extended release tablets, or extended release capsules) or 4 divided doses (oral suspension), may adjust by 200 mg/day increments; maximum dose: 1600 mg/day.

Note: Equetro® is the only formulation specifically approved by the FDA for the management of bipolar disorder.

Dietary Considerations Drug may cause GI upset, take with large amount of water or food to decrease GI upset. May need to split doses to avoid GI upset.

Administration

Suspension: Must be given on a 3-4 times/day schedule versus tablets which can be given 2-4 times/day. Since a given dose of suspension will produce higher peak and lower trough levels than the same dose given as the tablet form, patients given the suspension should be started on lower doses given more frequently (same total daily dose) and increased slowly to avoid unwanted side effects. When carbamazepine suspension has been combined with chlorpromazine or thioridazine solutions, a precipitate forms which may result in loss of effect. Therefore, it is recommended that the carbamazepine suspension dosage form not be administered at the same time with other liquid medicinal agents or diluents. Should be administered with meals.

Extended release capsule (Carbatrol®, Equetro®): Consists of three different types of beads: Immediate release, extended-release, and enteric release. The bead types are combined in a ratio to allow twice daily dosing. May be opened and contents sprinkled over food such as a teaspoon of applesauce; may be administered with or without food; do not crush or chew.

Extended release tablet: Should be inspected for damage. Damaged extended release tablets (without release portal) should not be administered. Should be administered with meals; swallow whole, do not crush or chew.

Monitoring Parameters CBC with platelet count, reticulocytes, serum iron, lipid panel, liver function tests, urinalysis, BUN, serum carbamazepine levels, thyroid function tests, serum sodium; pregnancy test; ophthalmic exams (pupillary reflexes); observe patient for excessive sedation, especially when instituting or increasing therapy; signs of rash; *HLA-B*1502* genotype screening prior to therapy initiation in patients of Asian descent.

Reference Range

Timing of serum samples: Absorption is slow, peak levels occur 6-8 hours after ingestion of the first dose; the half-life ranges from 8-60 hours, therefore, steady-state is achieved in 2-5 days

Therapeutic levels: 4-12 mcg/mL (SI: 17-51 μmol/L)

Toxic concentration: >15 mcg/mL; patients who require higher levels of 8-12 mcg/mL (SI: 34-51 μmol/L) should be watched closely. Side effects including CNS effects occur commonly at higher dosage levels. If other anticonvulsants are given therapeutic range is 4-8 mcg/mL.

Test Interactions May interact with some pregnancy tests; increased BUN, AST, ALT, bilirubin, alkaline phosphatase (S); decreased calcium, T_3, T_4, sodium (S)

Dosage Forms Excipient information presented when available (limited, particularly for generics); consult specific product labeling.

Capsule, extended release:

Carbatrol®, Equetro®: 100 mg, 200 mg, 300 mg

Suspension, oral: 100 mg/5 mL (5 mL, 10 mL, 450 mL)

Tegretol®: 100 mg/5 mL (450 mL) [contains propylene glycol; citrus vanilla flavor]

Tablet: 200 mg

Epitol®, Tegretol®: 200 mg

Tablet, chewable: 100 mg

Tegretol®: 100 mg

Tablet, extended release:

Tegretol®-XR: 100 mg, 200 mg, 400 mg

◆ **Carbaphen 12®** *see* Carbetapentane, Phenylephrine, and Chlorpheniramine *on page 274*

- **Carbaphen 12 Ped®** *see* Carbetapentane, Phenylephrine, and Chlorpheniramine *on page 274*
- **Carbatrol®** *see* CarBAMazepine *on page 265*
- **Carbaxefed RF [DSC]** *see* Carbinoxamine and Pseudoephedrine *on page 280*

Carbenicillin (kar ben i SIL in)

U.S. Brand Names Geocillin® [DSC]

Index Terms Carbenicillin Indanyl Sodium; Carindacillin

Pharmacologic Category Antibiotic, Penicillin

Use Treatment of serious urinary tract infections and prostatitis caused by susceptible gram-negative aerobic bacilli

Effect on Mental Status Penicillins have been reported to cause apprehension, illusions, agitation, insomnia, depersonalization, and encephalopathy

Effect on Psychiatric Treatment Rare reports of leukopenia and neutropenia; use caution with clozapine and carbamazepine

Dosage Summary

Oral:

Children: 30-50 mg/kg/day divided every 6 hours (maximum: 3 g/day)

Adults: 1-2 tablets every 6 hours

Dosage Forms Excipient information presented when available (limited, particularly for generics); consult specific product labeling. [DSC] = Discontinued product

Tablet:

Geocillin®: 382 mg [contains sodium 23 mg/tablet] [DSC]

- **Carbenicillin Indanyl Sodium** *see* Carbenicillin *on page 272*

Carbetapentane and Chlorpheniramine

(kar bay ta PEN tane & klor fen IR a meen)

U.S. Brand Names C-Tanna 12; Tannate 12 S; Tannic-12 S; Tannic-12 [DSC]; Tannihist-12 RF [DSC]; Trionate® [DSC]; Tussi-12 S™; Tussi-12®; Tussizone-12 RF™; Tustan 12S™

Index Terms Carbetapentane Tannate and Chlorpheniramine Tannate; Chlorpheniramine and Carbetapentane

Pharmacologic Category Antitussive; Histamine H_1 Antagonist; Histamine H_1 Antagonist, First Generation

Use Symptomatic relief of cough associated with upper respiratory tract conditions, such as the common cold, bronchitis, bronchial asthma

Effect on Mental Status Sedation is common; combined use with psychotropics may produce additive sedation; monitor

Effect on Psychiatric Treatment Contraindicated with MAO inhibitors. Anticholinergic effects may be potentiated with combined psychotropic use.

Dosage Summary

Oral:

Children <2 years: Dosage not established

Children 2-6 years: Carbetapentane 15-30 mg and chlorpheniramine 2-4 mg every 12 hours

Children >6 years: Carbetapentane 30-60 mg and chlorpheniramine 4-8 mg every 12 hours

Adults: Carbetapentane 60-120 mg and chlorpheniramine 5-10 mg every 12 hours

Dosage Forms Excipient information presented when available (limited, particularly for generics); consult specific product labeling. [DSC] = Discontinued product

Suspension:

C-Tanna 12: Carbetapentane tannate 30 mg and chlorpheniramine tannate 4 mg per 5 mL (480 mL) [contains benzoic acid and tartrazine; strawberry currant flavor]

Tannate 12 S: Carbetapentane tannate 30 mg and chlorpheniramine tannate 4 mg per 5 mL (120 mL, 480 mL) [contains benzoic acid]

Tannic-12 S: Carbetapentane tannate 30 mg and chlorpheniramine tannate 4 mg per 5 mL (120 mL) [contains benzoic acid; strawberry flavor]

Tannihist-12 RF: Carbetapentane tannate 30 mg and chlorpheniramine tannate 4 mg per 5 mL (120 mL, 480 mL) [strawberry-black currant flavor] [DSC]

Tussi-12 S™: Carbetapentane tannate 30 mg and chlorpheniramine tannate 4 mg per 5 mL (120 mL) [contains benzoic acid and tartrazine; strawberry-currant flavor]

Tussizone-12 RF™: Carbetapentane tannate 30 mg and chlorpheniramine tannate 4 mg per 5 mL (120 mL, 480 mL) [contains benzoic acid and tartrazine; strawberry-black currant flavor] [DSC]

Tustan 12S™: Carbetapentane tannate 30 mg and chlorpheniramine tannate 4 mg per 5 mL (120 mL, 480 mL) [contains sodium benzoate; grape flavor]

Tablet:

Tannic-12 [DSC], Trionate® [DSC], Tussi-12®, Tussizone-12 RF™: Carbetapentane tannate 60 mg and chlorpheniramine tannate 5 mg

Carbetapentane and Phenylephrine

(kar bay ta PEN tane & fen il EF rin)

U.S. Brand Names L-All 12

Index Terms Phenylephrine Tannate and Carbetapentane Tannate

Pharmacologic Category Antitussive; Antitussive/Decongestant; Sympathomimetic

Use Symptomatic relief of upper respiratory tract conditions such as the common cold, bronchial asthma, and bronchitis (acute and chronic)

Effect on Mental Status May cause anxiety, restlessness, or sedation

Effect on Psychiatric Treatment Concurrent use with MAO inhibitors is contraindicated. May cause sedation and xerostomia; concomitant use with psychotropics may produce additive effects.

Dosage Summary

Oral:

Children <2 years: Dosage not established

Children 2-6 years: 2.5 mL every 12 hours (maximum: 5 mL/24 hours)

Children 6-12 years: 5 mL every 12 hours (maximum: 10 mL/24 hours)

Children >12 years: 5-10 mL every 12 hours (maximum: 20 mL/24 hours)

Adults: 5-10 mL every 12 hours (maximum: 20 mL/24 hours)

Dosage Forms Excipient information presented when available (limited, particularly for generics); consult specific product labeling.

Suspension:

L-All 12: Carbetapentane tannate 30 mg and phenylephrine tannate 30 mg per 5 mL (120 mL) [contains sodium benzoate and phenylalanine; strawberry flavor]

Carbetapentane and Pseudoephedrine

(kar bay ta PEN tane & soo doe e FED rin)

U.S. Brand Names Pseudacarb™; Respi-Tann™

Index Terms Carbetapentane Tannate and Pseudoephedrine Tannate; Pseudoephedrine and Carbetapentane

Pharmacologic Category Antitussive/Decongestant

Use Relief of cough and congestion due to the common cold, influenza, sinusitis, or bronchitis

Effect on Mental Status May cause anxiety, dizziness, insomnia, restlessness, hallucinations, or depression

Effect on Psychiatric Treatment Contraindicated with or within 14 days of MAO inhibitor treatment; may cause tremor which may be mistaken for EPS; may cause tachycardia; tachycardia is also common with clozapine; monitor vital signs

Dosage Summary

Oral:

Children <2 years: Dosage not established

Children 2-6 years: 1/2 tablet **or** 2.5 mL every 12 hours (maximum: 4 doses/day)

Children 6-12 years: 1 tablet **or** 5 mL every 12 hours (maximum: 4 doses/day)

Children >12 years: 2 tablets **or** 10 mL every 12 hours (maximum: 4 doses/day)

Adults: 2 tablets **or** 10 mL every 12 hours (maximum: 4 doses/day)

Dosage Forms Excipient information presented when available (limited, particularly for generics); consult specific product labeling.

Suspension: Carbetapentane tannate 25 mg and pseudoephedrine tannate 75 mg per 5 mL (480 mL)

Respi-Tann™: Carbetapentane tannate 25 mg and pseudoephedrine tannate 75 mg per 5 mL (480 mL) [dye free; contains sodium benzoate; cherry flavor]

Tablet, chewable:

Respi-Tann™: Carbetapentane tannate 25 mg and pseudoephedrine tannate 75 mg [dye free; cherry flavor]

Pseudacarb™: Carbetapentane tannate 25 mg and pseudoephedrine tannate 75 mg [dye free; grape flavor]

◆ **Carbetapentane, Ephedrine, Phenylephrine, and Chlorpheniramine** *see* Chlorpheniramine, Ephedrine, Phenylephrine, and Carbetapentane *on page 326*

Carbetapentane, Guaifenesin, and Phenylephrine

(kar bay ta PEN tane, gwye FEN e sin, & fen il EF rin)

U.S. Brand Names Carbetaplex; Extendryl® GCP; Gentex LQ; Levall™; Phencarb GG

Index Terms Guaifenesin, Carbetapentane Citrate, and Phenylephrine Hydrochloride; Phenylephrine Hydrochloride, Carbetapentane Citrate, and Guaifenesin

Pharmacologic Category Antitussive; Expectorant; Expectorant/Decongestant/Antitussive; Sympathomimetic

Use Relief of nonproductive cough accompanying respiratory tract congestion associated with the common cold, influenza, sinusitis, and bronchitis

Effect on Mental Status May cause dizziness, drowsiness, excitability, insomnia, nervousness, CNS stimulation, or restlessness

Effect on Psychiatric Treatment Contraindicated with MAO inhibitors or within 14 days of MAO inhibitor

Dosage Summary

Oral:

Children <2 years: Dosage not established

Children 2-6 years:

Gentex LQ: 2.5 mL every 4-6 hours

Levall™: 1.25 mL every 4-6 hours; maximum dose of phenylephrine: 15 mg/24 hours

Children 6-12 years:

Gentex LQ: 5 mL every 4-6 hours

Levall™: 2.5 mL every 4-6 hours; maximum dose of phenylephrine: 30 mg/24 hours

Children ≥12 years:

Gentex LQ: 5-10 mL every 4-6 hours

Levall™: 5 mL every 4-6 hours; maximum dose of phenylephrine: 60 mg/24 hours

Adults:

Gentex LQ: 5-10 mL every 4-6 hours

Levall™: 5 mL every 4-6 hours; maximum dose of phenylephrine: 60 mg/24 hours

Dosage Forms Excipient information presented when available (limited, particularly for generics); consult specific product labeling.

Liquid:

Carbetaplex: Carbetapentane citrate 20 mg, guaifenesin 100 mg, and phenylephrine hydrochloride 15 mg per 5 mL (480 mL) [alcohol free, sugar free, dye free; strawberry flavor]

Gentex LQ: Carbetapentane citrate 20 mg, guaifenesin 100 mg, and phenylephrine hydrochloride 10 mg per 5 mL [contains edetate disodium and benzoic acid; spearmint flavor]

Levall™: Carbetapentane citrate 15 mg, guaifenesin 100 mg, and phenylephrine hydrochloride 5 mg per 5 mL (480 mL) [alcohol free; strawberry flavor]

Phencarb GG: Carbetapentane citrate 20 mg, guaifenesin 100 mg, and phenylephrine hydrochloride 10 mg per 5 mL (480 mL) [spearmint flavor]

Solution, oral:

Extendryl® GCP: Carbetapentane citrate 15 mg, guaifenesin 100 mg, and phenylephrine hydrochloride 5 mg per 5 mL (473 mL) [alcohol free; contains propylene glycol; strawberry flavor]

Carbetapentane, Phenylephrine, and Chlorpheniramine

(kar bay ta PEN tane, fen il EF rin, & klor fen IR a meen)

U.S. Brand Names Carbaphen 12 Ped®; Carbaphen 12®; XiraTuss™ [DSC]

Index Terms Chlorpheniramine, Carbetapentane, and Phenylephrine; Phenylephrine, Chlorpheniramine, and Carbetapentane

Pharmacologic Category Alpha/Beta Agonist; Antitussive; Histamine H_1 Antagonist; Histamine H_1 Antagonist, First Generation

Use Symptomatic relief of cough, nasal congestion, and discharge associated with the common cold, bronchial asthma, acute and chronic bronchitis, and other respiratory tract conditions

Effect on Mental Status Sedation is common; concurrent use with psychotropic agents may produce additive sedative effects; monitor

Effect on Psychiatric Treatment Contraindicated with MAO inhibitors. Concurrent use with psychotropic agents may produce additive anticholinergic effects; monitor.

Dosage Summary

Oral:

Children <2 years: Dosage not established

Children 2-6 years:

Carbaphen 12 Ped®: 1-2 mL every 12 hours

XiraTuss: 2.5-5 mL every 12 hours

Children 6-12 years:

Carbaphen 12 Ped®: 2-4 mL every 12 hours

XiraTuss: 5-10 mL every 12 hours

Children >12 years:

Carbaphen 12®: 5-10 mL every 12 hours

XiraTuss: 1-2 tablets every 12 hours

Adults:

Carbaphen 12®: 5-10 mL every 12 hours

XiraTuss: 1-2 tablets every 12 hours

Dosage Forms Excipient information presented when available (limited, particularly for generics); consult specific product labeling. [DSC] = Discontinued product

Suspension:

Carbaphen 12®: Carbetapentane tannate 60 mg, phenylephrine tannate 20 mg, and chlorpheniramine tannate 8 mg per 5 mL (480 mL) [contains benzoic acid, phenylalanine 1 mg/5 mL; alcohol free, sugar free; blueberry-banana flavor]

Carbaphen 12 Ped®: Carbetapentane tannate 15 mg, phenylephrine tannate 2.5 mg, and chlorpheniramine tannate 2 mg per 1 mL (60 mL) [contains benzoic acid, phenylalanine 1.6 mg/mL; alcohol free, sugar free; blueberry-banana flavor]

XiraTuss™: Carbetapentane tannate 30 mg, phenylephrine tannate 12.5 mg, and chlorpheniramine tannate 4 mg per 5 mL (120 mL) [strawberry flavor] [DSC]

Tablet:

XiraTuss™: Carbetapentane tannate 60 mg, phenylephrine tannate 10 mg, and chlorpheniramine tannate 5 mg [DSC]

Carbetapentane, Phenylephrine, and Pyrilamine

(kar bay ta PEN tane, fen il EF rin, & peer II a meen)

U.S. Brand Names C-Tanna 12D; Tannihist-12 D [DSC]; Tussi-12® D; Tussi-12® DS

Index Terms Phenylephrine Tannate, Carbetapentane Tannate, and Pyrilamine Tannate; Pyrilamine, Phenylephrine, and Carbetapentane

Pharmacologic Category Alpha/Beta Agonist; Antitussive; Histamine H_1 Antagonist; Histamine H_1 Antagonist, First Generation

Use Symptomatic relief of cough associated with respiratory tract conditions such as the common cold, bronchial asthma, acute and chronic bronchitis

Effect on Mental Status Sedation is common; may cause paradoxical excitation in pediatric patients

Effect on Psychiatric Treatment Contraindicated with or within 14 days of MAO inhibitor treatment. Concurrent use with psychotropics may produce additive sedation and anticholinergic side effects; monitor.

Dosage Summary

Oral:

Children <2 years: Dosage not established

Children 2-6 years: Tussi-12® DS: 2.5-5 mL every 12 hours

Children 6-11 years:

Tussi-12® D: 1/2 to 1 tablet every 12 hours

Tussi-12® DS: 5-10 mL every 12 hours

Children ≥12 years: Tussi-12® D: 1-2 tablets every 12 hours

Adults: Tussi-12® D: 1-2 tablets every 12 hours

Dosage Forms Excipient information presented when available (limited, particularly for generics); consult specific product labeling. [DSC] = Discontinued product

Suspension:
- C-Tanna 12D: Carbetapentane tannate 30 mg, pyrilamine tannate 30 mg, and phenylephrine tannate 5 mg per 5 mL (120 mL) [contains benzoic acid and tartrazine; strawberry currant flavor]
- Tannihist-12 D: Carbetapentane tannate 30 mg, pyrilamine tannate 30 mg, and phenylephrine tannate 5 mg per 5 mL (120 mL) [alcohol free; contains sugar 15% and tartrazine; strawberry black currant flavor] [DSC]
- Tussi-12® DS: Carbetapentane tannate 30 mg, pyrilamine tannate 30 mg, and phenylephrine tannate 5 mg per 5 mL (120 mL) [contains benzoic acid and tartrazine; strawberry currant flavor; packaged with oral syringe]

Tablet:
- C-Tanna 12D, Tussi-12® D: Carbetapentane tannate 60 mg, pyrilamine tannate 40 mg, and phenylephrine tannate 10 mg

◆ **Carbetapentane Tannate and Chlorpheniramine Tannate** *see* Carbetapentane and Chlorpheniramine *on page 272*

◆ **Carbetapentane Tannate and Pseudoephedrine Tannate** *see* Carbetapentane and Pseudoephedrine *on page 273*

◆ **Carbetaplex** *see* Carbetapentane, Guaifenesin, and Phenylephrine *on page 274*

Carbidopa (kar bi DOE pa)

Medication Safety Issues

International issues:

Lodosyn® may be confused with Lidosen® which is a brand name for lidocaine in Italy

U.S. Brand Names Lodosyn®

Pharmacologic Category Anti-Parkinson's Agent, Dopamine Agonist

Generic Available No

Use Given with levodopa in the treatment of parkinsonism to enable a lower dosage of levodopa to be used and a more rapid response to be obtained and to decrease side effects; for details of administration and dosage, see Levodopa; has no effect without levodopa

Pregnancy Risk Factor C

Contraindications Hypersensitivity to carbidopa or levodopa, or any component of the formulation; use of nonselective MAO antagonists; narrow-angle glaucoma; history of melanoma or undiagnosed skin lesions

Adverse Reactions Adverse reactions are associated with concomitant administration with levodopa

>10%: Central nervous system: Anxiety, confusion, nervousness, mental depression

1% to 10%:
- Cardiovascular: Orthostatic hypotension, palpitation, cardiac arrhythmia
- Central nervous system: Memory loss, insomnia, fatigue, hallucinations, ataxia, dystonic movements
- Gastrointestinal: Nausea, vomiting, GI bleeding
- Ocular: Blurred vision

<1% (Limited to important or life-threatening): Duodenal ulcer, hemolytic anemia, hypertension

Drug Interactions

There are no known significant interactions.

Mechanism of Action Carbidopa is a peripheral decarboxylase inhibitor with little or no pharmacological activity when given alone in usual doses. It inhibits the peripheral decarboxylation of levodopa to dopamine; and as it does not cross the blood-brain barrier, unlike levodopa, effective brain concentrations of dopamine are produced with lower doses of levodopa. At the same time, reduced peripheral formation of dopamine reduces peripheral side-effects, notably nausea and vomiting, and cardiac arrhythmias, although the dyskinesias and adverse mental effects associated with levodopa therapy tend to develop earlier.

Pharmacodynamics/Kinetics

Absorption: 40% to 70%

Distribution: Does not cross the blood-brain barrier; in rats, reported to cross placenta and be excreted in milk

Protein binding: 36%

Half-life elimination: 1-2 hours

Excretion: Urine (as unchanged drug and metabolites)

Dosage Oral: Adults: 70-100 mg/day; maximum daily dose: 200 mg

Dietary Considerations May be taken with meals to decrease GI upset.

Administration Administer with meals to decrease GI upset.

Dosage Forms Excipient information presented when available (limited, particularly for generics); consult specific product labeling.

Tablet: 25 mg

Carbidopa and Levodopa (kar bi DOE pa & lee voe DOE pa)

Related Information

Antiparkinsonian Agents *on page 1767*

U.S. Brand Names Parcopa™; Sinemet®; Sinemet® CR

Canadian Brand Names Apo-Levocarb®; Apo-Levocarb® CR; Endo®-Levodopa/Carbidopa; Novo-Levocarbidopa; Nu-Levocarb; Sinemet®; Sinemet® CR

Mexican Brand Names Racovel; Sinemet

Index Terms Levodopa and Carbidopa

Pharmacologic Category Anti-Parkinson's Agent, Dopamine Agonist

Generic Available Yes

Use Idiopathic Parkinson's disease; postencephalitic parkinsonism; symptomatic parkinsonism

Unlabeled/Investigational Use Restless leg syndrome

Pregnancy Risk Factor C

Pregnancy Considerations Teratogenic effects were observed with levodopa and carbidopa in animal studies. There are case reports of levodopa crossing the placenta in humans.

Lactation Excretion in breast milk unknown/use caution

Contraindications Hypersensitivity to levodopa, carbidopa, or any component of the formulation; narrow-angle glaucoma; use of MAO inhibitors within prior 14 days (however, may be administered concomitantly with the manufacturer's recommended dose of an MAO inhibitor with selectivity for MAO type B); history of melanoma or undiagnosed skin lesions

Warnings/Precautions Use with caution in patients with history of cardiovascular disease (including myocardial infarction and arrhythmias), pulmonary dieases such as asthma, psychosis, wide-angle glaucoma, peptic ulcer disease, as well as in severe renal and hepatic dysfunction. Use with caution when interpreting plasma/urine catecholamine levels; falsely diagnosed pheochromocytoma has been rarely reported. Severe cases or rhabdomyolysis have been reported. Sudden discontinuation of levodopa may cause a worsening of Parkinson's disease. Elderly may be more sensitive to CNS effects of levodopa. May cause or exacerbate dyskinesias. Patients have reported falling asleep while engaging in activities of daily living; this has been reported to occur without significant warning signs. May cause orthostatic hypotension; Parkinson's disease patients appear to have an impaired capacity to respond to a postural challenge; use with caution in patients at risk of hypotension (such as those receiving antihypertensive drugs) or where transient hypotensive episodes would be poorly tolerated (cardiovascular disease or cerebrovascular disease). Observe patients closely for development of depression with concomitant suicidal tendencies.

Dopamine agonists have been associated with compulsive behaviors and/or loss of impulse control, which has manifested as pathological gambling, libido increases (hypersexuality), and/or binge eating. Causality has not been established, and controversy exists as to whether this phenomenon is related to the underlying disease, prior behaviors/addictions and/or drug therapy. Dose reduction or discontinuation of therapy has been reported to reverse these behaviors in some, but not all cases. Dopaminergic agents have been associated with a syndrome resembling neuroleptic malignant syndrome on abrupt withdrawal or significant dosage reduction after long-term use. Protein in the diet should be distributed throughout the day to avoid fluctuations in levodopa absorption. Safety and efficacy have not been established in children.

Adverse Reactions Frequency not defined.

Cardiovascular: Orthostatic hypotension, arrhythmia, chest pain, hypertension, syncope, palpitation, phlebitis

Central nervous system: Dizziness, anxiety, confusion, nightmares, headache, hallucinations, on-off phenomenon, decreased mental acuity, memory impairment, disorientation, delusions, euphoria, agitation, somnolence, insomnia, gait abnormalities, nervousness, ataxia, EPS, falling, psychosis, peripheral neuropathy, seizure (causal relationship not established)

Dermatologic: Rash, alopecia, malignant melanoma, hypersensitivity (angioedema, urticaria, pruritus, bullous lesions, Henoch-Schönlein purpura)

Endocrine & metabolic: Increased libido

Gastrointestinal: Anorexia, nausea, vomiting, constipation, GI bleeding, duodenal ulcer, diarrhea, dyspepsia, taste alterations, sialorrhea, heartburn

Genitourinary: Discoloration of urine, urinary frequency

Hematologic: Hemolytic anemia, agranulocytosis, thrombocytopenia, leukopenia; decreased hemoglobin and hematocrit; abnormalities in AST and ALT, LDH, bilirubin, BUN, Coombs' test

Neuromuscular & skeletal: Choreiform and involuntary movements, paresthesia, bone pain, shoulder pain, muscle cramps, weakness

Ocular: Blepharospasm, oculogyric crises (may be associated with acute dystonic reactions)

Renal: Difficult urination

Respiratory: Dyspnea, cough

Miscellaneous: Hiccups, discoloration of sweat, diaphoresis (increased)

Reported with dopamine agonists: Impulsive/compulsive behaviors (eg, pathological gambling, hypersexuality, binge eating)

Drug Interactions

Antipsychotics (Atypical): May diminish the therapeutic effect of Anti-Parkinson's Agents (Dopamine Agonist). *Risk D: Consider therapy modification*

Antipsychotics (Typical): May diminish the therapeutic effect of Anti-Parkinson's Agents (Dopamine Agonist). *Risk D: Consider therapy modification*

Iron Salts: May decrease the absorption of Levodopa. Only applies to oral iron preparations. **Exceptions:** Ferric Gluconate; Iron Dextran Complex; Iron Sucrose. *Risk D: Consider therapy modification*

MAO Inhibitors: Levodopa may enhance the adverse/toxic effect of MAO Inhibitors. Of particular concern is the development of hypertensive reactions when levodopa is used with nonselective MAOI. *Risk D: Consider therapy modification*

Methionine: May diminish the therapeutic effect of Levodopa. Probably only with large doses of methionine. Data was generated using 4.5gm daily. *Risk D: Consider therapy modification*

Metoclopramide: May diminish the therapeutic effect of Anti-Parkinson's Agents (Dopamine Agonist). *Risk C: Monitor therapy*

Phenytoin: May diminish the therapeutic effect of Levodopa. *Risk C: Monitor therapy*

Pyridoxine: May diminish the therapeutic effect of Levodopa. *Risk D: Consider therapy modification*

Sapropterin: May enhance the adverse/toxic effect of Levodopa. *Risk C: Monitor therapy*

Ethanol/Nutrition/Herb Interactions

Ethanol: Avoid ethanol (due to CNS depression).

Food: Avoid high protein diets and high intakes of vitamin B_6.

Herb/Nutraceutical: Avoid kava kava (may decrease effects). Pyridoxine in doses >10-25 mg (for levodopa alone) or higher doses >200 mg/day (for levodopa/carbidopa) may decrease efficacy.

Stability Store at 20°C to 25°C (68°F to 77°F); excursions permitted between 15°C to 30°C (59°F to 86°F). Protect from light and moisture.

Mechanism of Action Parkinson's symptoms are due to a lack of striatal dopamine; levodopa circulates in the plasma to the blood-brain-barrier (BBB), where it crosses, to be converted by striatal enzymes to dopamine; carbidopa inhibits the peripheral plasma breakdown of levodopa by inhibiting its decarboxylation, and thereby increases available levodopa at the BBB

Pharmacodynamics/Kinetics

Duration: Variable, 6-12 hours; longer with sustained release forms

See individual agents.

Dosage Oral: Adults:

Parkinson's disease:

Immediate release tablet:

Initial: Carbidopa 25 mg/levodopa 100 mg 3 times/day

Dosage adjustment: Alternate tablet strengths may be substituted according to individual carbidopa/levodopa requirements. Increase by 1 tablet every other day as necessary, except when using the carbidopa 25 mg/levodopa 250 mg tablets where increases should be made using 1/2-1 tablet every 1-2 days. Use of more than 1 dosage strength or dosing 4 times/day may be required (maximum: 8 tablets of any strength/day or 200 mg of carbidopa and 2000 mg of levodopa)

Sustained release tablet:

Initial: Carbidopa 50 mg/levodopa 200 mg 2 times/day, at intervals not <6 hours

Dosage adjustment: May adjust every 3 days; intervals should be between 4-8 hours during the waking day (maximum: 8 tablets/day)

Restless leg syndrome (unlabeled use): Carbidopa 25 mg/levodopa 100 mg given 30-60 minutes before bedtime; may repeat dose once

Elderly: Initial: Carbidopa 25 mg/levodopa 100 mg twice daily, increase as necessary

Dietary Considerations Levodopa peak serum concentrations may be decreased if taken with food. High protein diets (>2 g/kg) may decrease the efficacy of levodopa via competition with amino acids in crossing the blood-brain barrier.

Parcopa™: Contains phenylalanine 3.4 mg per 10/100 mg and 25/100 mg strengths; phenylalanine 8.4 mg in 25/250 mg strength

Administration Space doses evenly over the waking hours. Give with meals to decrease GI upset. Sustained release product should not be crushed. Orally-disintegrating tablets do not require water; the tablet should disintegrate on the tongue's surface before swallowing.

Monitoring Parameters Blood pressure, standing and sitting/supine; symptoms of parkinsonism, dyskinesias, mental status

Test Interactions False-positive reaction for urinary glucose with Clinitest®; false-negative reaction using Clinistix®; false-positive urine ketones with Acetest®, Ketostix®, Labstix®

Additional Information 50-100 mg/day of carbidopa is needed to block the peripheral conversion of levodopa to dopamine. "On-off" (a clinical syndrome characterized by sudden periods of drug activity/inactivity), can be managed by giving smaller, more frequent doses of Sinemet® or adding a dopamine agonist or selegiline; when adding a new agent, doses of Sinemet® can usually be decreased. Protein in the diet should be distributed throughout the day to avoid fluctuations in levodopa absorption. Levodopa is the drug of choice when rigidity is the predominant presenting symptom.

Conversion from levodopa to carbidopa/levodopa: **Note:** Levodopa must be discontinued at least 12 hours prior to initiation of levodopa/carbidopa:

Initial dose: Levodopa portion of carbidopa/levodopa should be at least 25% of previous levodopa therapy.

Levodopa <1500 mg/day: Sinemet® or Parcopa™ (levodopa 25 mg/carbidopa 100 mg) 3-4 times/day

Levodopa ≥1500 mg/day: Sinemet® or Parcopa™ (levodopa 25 mg/carbidopa 250 mg) 3-4 times/day

Conversion from immediate release carbidopa/levodopa (Sinemet® or Parcopa™) to Sinemet® CR (50/200):

Sinemet® or Parcopa™ [total daily dose of levodopa]/Sinemet® CR:

Sinemet® or Parcopa™ (levodopa 300-400 mg/day): Sinemet® CR (50/200) 1 tablet twice daily

Sinemet® or Parcopa™ (levodopa 500-600 mg/day): Sinemet® CR (50/200) 1 1/2 tablets twice daily or 1 tablet 3 times/day

Sinemet® or Parcopa™ (levodopa 700-800 mg/day): Sinemet® CR (50/200) 4 tablets in 3 or more divided doses

Sinemet® or Parcopa™ (levodopa 900-1000 mg/day): Sinemet® CR (50/200) 5 tablets in 3 or more divided doses

Intervals between doses of Sinemet® CR should be 4-8 hours while awake; when divided doses are not equal, smaller doses should be given toward the end of the day,

Dosage Forms Excipient information presented when available (limited, particularly for generics); consult specific product labeling.

Tablet: 10/100: Carbidopa 10 mg and levodopa 100 mg; 25/100: Carbidopa 25 mg and levodopa 100 mg; 25/250: Carbidopa 25 mg and levodopa 250 mg

Sinemet®:

10/100: Carbidopa 10 mg and levodopa 100 mg

25/100: Carbidopa 25 mg and levodopa 100 mg

25/250: Carbidopa 25 mg and levodopa 250 mg

Tablet, extended release: 25/100: Carbidopa 25 mg and levodopa 100 mg; 50/200: Carbidopa 50 mg and levodopa 200 mg

Tablet, orally disintegrating: 10/100: Carbidopa 10 mg and levodopa 100 mg; 25/100: Carbidopa 25 mg and levodopa 100 mg; 25/250: Carbidopa 25 mg and levodopa 250 mg

Parcopa™:

10/100: Carbidopa 10 mg and levodopa 100 mg [contains phenylalanine 3.4 mg/tablet; mint flavor]

25/100: Carbidopa 25 mg and levodopa 100 mg [contains phenylalanine 3.4 mg/tablet; mint flavor]

25/250: Carbidopa 25 mg and levodopa 250 mg [contains phenylalanine 8.4 mg/tablet; mint flavor]

Tablet, sustained release: 25/100: Carbidopa 25 mg and levodopa 100 mg; 50/200: Carbidopa 50 mg and levodopa 200 mg
Sinemet® CR:
25/100: Carbidopa 25 mg and levodopa 100 mg
50/200: Carbidopa 50 mg and levodopa 200 mg

◆ **Carbidopa, Levodopa, and Entacapone** *see* Levodopa, Carbidopa, and Entacapone *on page 911*

Carbinoxamine (kar bi NOKS a meen)

U.S. Brand Names Palgic®
Mexican Brand Names Prindex
Index Terms Carbinoxamine Maleate
Pharmacologic Category Histamine H_1 Antagonist; Histamine H_1 Antagonist, First Generation
Use Seasonal and perennial allergic rhinitis; vasomotor rhinitis; urticaria; decrease severity of other allergic reactions
Effect on Mental Status May cause dizziness, nervousness, or sedation; may cause excitability in children
Effect on Psychiatric Treatment Contraindicated with or within 14 days of MAO inhibitor treatment; concurrent use with psychotropics may produce additive sedation
Dosage Summary
Oral:
Children ≤3 years: Dosage not established
Children >3-6 years: Palgic®: 2-5 mg 3-4 times/day
Children >6 years: Palgic®: 4-6 mg 3-4 times/day
Adults: Palgic®: 4-8 mg 3-4 times/day
Dosage Forms Excipient information presented when available (limited, particularly for generics); consult specific product labeling.
Solution, as maleate:
Palgic®: 4 mg/5 mL (480 mL) [bubble gum flavor]
Tablet, as maleate [scored]:
Palgic®: 4 mg

Carbinoxamine and Pseudoephedrine
(kar bi NOKS a meen & soo doe e FED rin)

U.S. Brand Names Andehist NR Drops [DSC]; Carbaxefed RF [DSC]; Carboxine-PSE [DSC]; Cordron-D NR [DSC]; Hydro-Tussin™-CBX [DSC]; Palgic®-D [DSC]; Palgic®-DS [DSC]; Pediatex™-D [DSC]; Sildec [DSC]
Mexican Brand Names Prindex Pediátrico
Index Terms Pseudoephedrine and Carbinoxamine
Pharmacologic Category Alpha/Beta Agonist; Histamine H_1 Antagonist; Histamine H_1 Antagonist, First Generation
Use Seasonal and perennial allergic rhinitis; vasomotor rhinitis
Effect on Mental Status Drowsiness is common; may cause fatigue, nervousness, or dizziness; may rarely produce depression
Effect on Psychiatric Treatment Contraindicated with MAO inhibitors; concurrent use with sedating psychotropics or CNS depressants may produce additive adverse effects
Dosage Summary
Oral:
Children <1 month: Dosage not established
Children 1-3 months:
Andehist NR, Carbaxefed RF, Sildec: 0.25 mL 4 times/day
Hydro-Tussin™-CBX, Palgic®-DS, Pediatex™-D: 1.25 mL up to 4 times/day
Children 3-6 months:
Andehist NR, Carbaxefed RF, Sildec: 0.5 mL 4 times/day
Hydro-Tussin™-CBX, Palgic®-DS, Pediatex™-D: 2.5 mL up to 4 times/day
Children 6-9 months:
Andehist NR, Carbaxefed RF, Sildec: 0.75 mL 4 times/day
Hydro-Tussin™-CBX, Palgic®-DS, Pediatex™-D: 3.75 mL up to 4 times/day
Children 9-12 months:
Andehist NR, Carbaxefed RF, Sildec: 0.75 mL 4 times/day
Hydro-Tussin™-CBX, Palgic®-DS, Pediatex™-D: 3.75-5 mL up to 4 times/day

Children 12-18 months:
Andehist NR, Carbaxefed RF, Sildec: 1 mL 4 times/day
Hydro-Tussin™-CBX, Palgic®-DS, Pediatex™-D: 3.75-5 mL up to 4 times/day
Children 18-24 months:
Andehist NR, Carbaxefed RF, Sildec: 1 mL 4 times/day
Hydro-Tussin™-CBX, Palgic®-DS, Pediatex™-D: 5 mL 3-4 times/day
Children 2-6 years:
Hydro-Tussin™-CBX, Palgic®-DS, Pediatex™-D: 5 mL 3-4 times/day
Children 6-12 years:
Hydro-Tussin™-CBX, Palgic®-DS, Pediatex™-D: 10 mL 4 times/day
Palgic®-D: One-half tablet every 12 hours
Children >12 years:
Hydro-Tussin™-CBX, Palgic®-DS, Pediatex™-D: 10 mL 4 times/day
Palgic®-D: 1 tablet every 12 hours
Adults:
Hydro-Tussin™-CBX, Palgic®-DS, Pediatex™-D: 10 mL 4 times/day
Palgic®-D: 1 tablet every 12 hours

Dosage Forms Excipient information presented when available (limited, particularly for generics); consult specific product labeling. [DSC] = Discontinued product

Liquid:
Cordron-D NR: Carbinoxamine maleate 2 mg and pseudoephedrine hydrochloride 12.5 mg per 5 mL (480 mL) [cotton candy flavor] [DSC]
Pediatex™-D: Carbinoxamine maleate 2 mg and pseudoephedrine hydrochloride 20 mg per 5 mL (480 mL) [alcohol free, dye free, sugar free; cotton candy flavor] [DSC]

Solution: Carbinoxamine maleate 2 mg and pseudoephedrine hydrochloride 25 mg per 5 mL (480 mL) [DSC]
Carboxine-PSE: Carbinoxamine maleate 2 mg and pseudoephedrine hydrochloride 20 mg per 5 mL (480 mL) [peach flavor] [DSC]

Solution, oral drops:
Andehist NR: Carbinoxamine maleate 1 mg and pseudoephedrine hydrochloride 15 mg per mL (30 mL) [alcohol and sugar free; raspberry flavor] [DSC]
Carbaxefed RF: Carbinoxamine maleate 1 mg and pseudoephedrine hydrochloride 15 mg per mL (30 mL) [alcohol free; contains sodium benzoate; cherry flavor] [DSC]
Sildec: Carbinoxamine maleate 1 mg and pseudoephedrine hydrochloride 15 mg per mL (30 mL) [raspberry flavor] [DSC]

Syrup: Carbinoxamine maleate 2 mg and pseudoephedrine hydrochloride 25 mg per 5 mL (480 mL)
Hydro-Tussin™-CBX [DSC], Palgic®-DS [DSC]: Carbinoxamine maleate 2 mg and pseudoephedrine hydrochloride 25 mg per 5 mL (480 mL) [alcohol, dye, and sugar free; strawberry/pineapple flavor]

Tablet, timed release:
Palgic®-D: Carbinoxamine maleate 8 mg and pseudoephedrine hydrochloride 80 mg [dye free] [DSC]

- **Carbinoxamine Maleate** *see* Carbinoxamine *on page 280*
- **Carbinoxamine, Pseudoephedrine, and Hydrocodone** *see* Hydrocodone, Carbinoxamine, and Pseudoephedrine *on page 782*
- **Carbocaine®** *see* Mepivacaine *on page 990*
- **Carbofed DM** *see* Brompheniramine, Pseudoephedrine, and Dextromethorphan *on page 208*

CARBOplatin (KAR boe pla tin)

Medication Safety Issues

Sound-alike/look-alike issues:
CARBOplatin may be confused with CISplatin, oxaliplatin
Paraplatin® may be confused with Platinol®

High alert medication: The Institute for Safe Medication Practices (ISMP) includes this medication among its list of drugs which have a heightened risk of causing significant patient harm when used in error.

Canadian Brand Names Paraplatin-AQ

Mexican Brand Names Bagotanilo; Blastocarb RU; Carboplat; Carbotec

Index Terms CBDCA; NSC-241240

Pharmacologic Category Antineoplastic Agent, Alkylating Agent; Antineoplastic Agent, Platinum Analog

Use Treatment of ovarian cancer

Unlabeled/Investigational Use Lung cancer, head and neck cancer, endometrial cancer, esophageal cancer, bladder cancer, breast cancer, cervical cancer, CNS tumors, germ cell tumors, osteogenic sarcoma, and high-dose therapy with stem cell/bone marrow support

Effect on Mental Status None reported

Effect on Psychiatric Treatment May cause myelosuppression; use caution with clozapine and carbamazepine

Dosage Summary

I.V.:

Children (unlabeled):

Brain tumor: 175 mg/m^2 weekly for 4 weeks every 6 weeks, with a 2-week recovery period between courses

Solid tumor (unlabeled use): 300-600 mg/m^2 once every 4 weeks

Adults: 300-360 mg/m^2 every 4 weeks **or** AUC of 4-8 (using Calvert formula)

Elderly: The Calvert formula should be used to calculate dosing for elderly patients.

Intraperitoneal (unlabeled use):

Children: Dosage not established

Adults: 200-650 mg/m^2 in 2 L of dialysis fluid have been administered into the peritoneum of ovarian cancer patients **or** target AUC: 5-7

Dosage Forms Excipient information presented when available (limited, particularly for generics); consult specific product labeling. [DSC] = Discontinued product

Injection, powder for reconstitution: 50 mg, 150 mg, 450 mg

Injection, solution: 10 mg/mL (5 mL, 15 mL, 45 mL, 60 mL)

Injection, solution [preservative free]: 10 mg/mL (5 mL, 15 mL, 45 mL)

◆ **Carboprost** *see* Carboprost Tromethamine *on page 282*

Carboprost Tromethamine (KAR boe prost tro METH a meen)

U.S. Brand Names Hemabate®

Canadian Brand Names Hemabate®

Index Terms Carboprost; Prostaglandin F_2

Pharmacologic Category Abortifacient; Prostaglandin

Use Termination of pregnancy; treatment of refractory postpartum uterine bleeding

Unlabeled/Investigational Use Investigational: Hemorrhagic cystitis

Effect on Mental Status May cause drowsiness or nervousness; rare reports of dystonia

Effect on Psychiatric Treatment None reported

Dosage Summary

I.M.:

Children: Dosage not established

Adults (females):

Abortion: 250 mcg at 1.5- to 3.5-hour intervals, a 500 mcg dose may be given if uterine response is not adequate after several 250 mcg doses (maximum total dose: 12 mg)

Postpartum bleeding: 250 mcg; if needed, may repeat at 15- to 90-minute intervals; maximum total dose: 2 mg (8 doses)

Dosage Forms Excipient information presented when available (limited, particularly for generics); consult specific product labeling.

Injection, solution:

Hemabate®: Carboprost 250 mcg and tromethamine 83 mcg per mL (1 mL) [contains benzyl alcohol]

◆ **Carboxine-PSE [DSC]** *see* Carbinoxamine and Pseudoephedrine *on page 280*
◆ **Cardene®** *see* NiCARdipine *on page 1128*
◆ **Cardene® I.V.** *see* NiCARdipine *on page 1128*
◆ **Cardene® SR** *see* NiCARdipine *on page 1128*
◆ **Cardizem®** *see* Diltiazem *on page 473*
◆ **Cardizem® CD** *see* Diltiazem *on page 473*
◆ **Cardizem® LA** *see* Diltiazem *on page 473*
◆ **Cardura®** *see* Doxazosin *on page 500*
◆ **Cardura® XL** *see* Doxazosin *on page 500*
◆ **Carindacillin** *see* Carbenicillin *on page 272*
◆ **Carisoprodate** *see* Carisoprodol *on page 283*

Carisoprodol (kar eye soe PROE dole)

U.S. Brand Names Soma®

Canadian Brand Names Soma®

Index Terms Carisoprodate; Isobamate

Pharmacologic Category Skeletal Muscle Relaxant

Generic Available Yes

Use Short-term (2-3 weeks) relief of skeletal muscle pain

Effect on Mental Status Drowsiness is common; may produce depression or paradoxical CNS stimulation

Effect on Psychiatric Treatment Rarely may cause leukopenia or aplastic anemia; use caution with clozapine and carbamazepine; concurrent use with psychotropics may produce additive sedation

Pregnancy Risk Factor C

Pregnancy Considerations Animal data suggests that carisoprodol crosses placenta and adverse events have been observed in animal studies. Limited postmarketing data with meprobamate (the active metabolite) demonstrate a possible risk for congenital malformations. Use only if benefit outweighs the risk.

Lactation Enters breast milk/use caution

Contraindications Hypersensitivity to carisoprodol, meprobamate, or any component of the formulation; acute intermittent porphyria

Warnings/Precautions May cause CNS depression, which may impair physical or mental abilities. Effects with other sedative drugs or ethanol may be potentiated. Use with caution in patients with hepatic/renal dysfunction. Tolerance or drug dependence may result from extended use. Limit to 2-3 weeks; use caution in patients who may be prone to addiction. Idiosyncratic reactions and/or severe allergic reactions may occur. Idiosyncratic reactions occur following the initial dose and may include severe weakness, transient quadriplegia, euphoria, or vision loss (temporary). Has been associated (rarely) with seizures in patients with and without seizure history. Carisoprodol should be used with caution in patients who are poor metabolizers of CYP2C19; poor metabolizers have been shown to have a fourfold increase in exposure to carisoprodol and a 50% reduced exposure to the metabolite meprobamate compared to normal metabolizers. Safety and efficacy in children <16 years of age have not been established.

Adverse Reactions

>10%: Central nervous system: Drowsiness (13% to 17%)

1% to 10%: Central nervous system: Dizziness (7% to 8%), headache (3% to 5%)

Postmarketing and/or case reports: Agitation, anaphylaxis, angioedema, asthma exacerbation, ataxia, burning eyes, depression, dermatitis (allergic), dyspnea, epigastric pain, eosinophilia, erythema multiforme, fixed drug eruption, flushing of face, headache, hiccups, hypersensitivity reactions, hypotension (postural), idiosyncratic reaction (symptoms may include agitation, ataxia, confusion, diplopia, disorientation, dysarthria, euphoria, extreme weakness, mydriasis, temporary vision loss, and/or transient quadriplegia); insomnia, irritability, leukopenia, nausea, pancytopenia, paradoxical CNS stimulation, pruritus, rash, seizure, syncope, tachycardia, tremor, urticaria, vertigo, vomiting, weakness, withdrawal syndrome (abdominal cramps, headache, insomnia, nausea, seizure)

Metabolism/Transport Effects **Substrate** of CYP2C19 (major)

Drug Interactions

Alcohol (Ethyl): CNS Depressants may enhance the CNS depressant effect of Alcohol (Ethyl). *Risk C: Monitor therapy*

CNS Depressants: May enhance the adverse/toxic effect of other CNS Depressants. *Risk C: Monitor therapy*

CYP2C19 Inhibitors (Moderate): May decrease the metabolism of CYP2C19 Substrates. *Risk C: Monitor therapy*

CYP2C19 Inhibitors (Strong): May decrease the metabolism of CYP2C19 Substrates. *Risk D: Consider therapy modification*

Ethanol/Nutrition/Herb Interactions Ethanol: Avoid ethanol (may increase CNS depression).

Stability Store at controlled room temperature of 20°C to 25°C (68°F to 77°F).

Mechanism of Action Precise mechanism is not yet clear, but many effects have been ascribed to its central depressant actions. In animals, carisoprodol blocks interneuronal activity and depresses polysynaptic neuron transmission in the spinal cord and reticular formation of the brain. It is also metabolized to meprobamate, which has anxiolytic and sedative effects.

Pharmacodynamics/Kinetics
Onset of action: ~30 minutes
Duration: 4-6 hours
Metabolism: Hepatic, via CYP2C19 to active metabolite (meprobamate)
Half-life elimination: 2.4 hours; Meprobamate: 10 hours
Time to peak, plasma: 1.5-2 hours
Excretion: Urine, as metabolite

Dosage Note: Carisoprodol should only be used for short periods (2-3 weeks) due to lack of evidence of effectiveness with prolonged use.
Oral: Children ≥16 years and Adults: 250-350 mg 3 times/day and at bedtime

Dietary Considerations May give with or without food.

Administration Administer with or without food.

Monitoring Parameters Look for relief of pain and/or muscle spasm and avoid excessive drowsiness; signs of drug abuse in addiction-prone individuals

Dosage Forms Excipient information presented when available (limited, particularly for generics); consult specific product labeling.
Tablet: 350 mg
Soma®: 250 mg, 350 mg

Carisoprodol and Aspirin (kar eye soe PROE dole & AS pir in)

U.S. Brand Names Soma® Compound

Index Terms Aspirin and Carisoprodol

Pharmacologic Category Skeletal Muscle Relaxant

Use Skeletal muscle relaxant

Effect on Mental Status Drowsiness is common; may produce depression or paradoxical CNS stimulation

Effect on Psychiatric Treatment Rarely may cause leukopenia or aplastic anemia; use caution with clozapine and carbamazepine; concurrent use with psychotropics may produce additive sedation

Dosage Summary
Oral:
Children: Dosage not established
Adults: 1-2 tablets 4 times/day
Elderly: Use not recommended

Dosage Forms Excipient information presented when available (limited, particularly for generics); consult specific product labeling.
Tablet: Carisoprodol 200 mg and aspirin 325 mg

Carisoprodol, Aspirin, and Codeine
(kar eye soe PROE dole, AS pir in, and KOE deen)

U.S. Brand Names Soma® Compound w/Codeine [DSC]

Index Terms Aspirin, Carisoprodol, and Codeine; Codeine, Aspirin, and Carisoprodol

Pharmacologic Category Skeletal Muscle Relaxant

Use Skeletal muscle relaxant

Effect on Mental Status Drowsiness is common; may produce depression or paradoxical CNS stimulation

Effect on Psychiatric Treatment Rarely may cause leukopenia or aplastic anemia; use caution with clozapine and carbamazepine; concurrent use with psychotropics may produce additive sedation

Restrictions C-III

Dosage Summary
Oral:
Children: Dosage not established
Adults: 1-2 tablets 4 times/day (maximum: 8 tablets/day)

Dosage Forms Excipient information presented when available (limited, particularly for generics); consult specific product labeling. [DSC] = Discontinued product
Tablet: Carisoprodol 200 mg, aspirin 325 mg, and codeine phosphate 16 mg
Soma® Compound w/Codeine: Carisoprodol 200 mg, aspirin 325 mg, and codeine phosphate 16 mg [DSC]

Carmustine (kar MUS teen)

Medication Safety Issues
Sound-alike/look-alike issues:
Carmustine may be confused with bendamustine, lomustine

High alert medication: The Institute for Safe Medication Practices (ISMP) includes this medication among its list of drugs which have a heightened risk of causing significant patient harm when used in error.

U.S. Brand Names BiCNU®; Gliadel®

Canadian Brand Names BiCNU®; Gliadel Wafer®

Mexican Brand Names BiCNU

Index Terms BCNU; bis-chloronitrosourea; Carmustinum; NSC-409962; WR-139021

Pharmacologic Category Antineoplastic Agent; Antineoplastic Agent, Alkylating Agent (Nitrosourea); Antineoplastic Agent, DNA Adduct-Forming Agent; Antineoplastic Agent, DNA Binding Agent

Use

Injection: Treatment of brain tumors (glioblastoma, brainstem glioma, medulloblastoma, astrocytoma, ependymoma, and metastatic brain tumors), multiple myeloma, Hodgkin's disease (relapsed or refractory), non-Hodgkin's lymphomas (relapsed or refractory)

Wafer (implant): Adjunct to surgery in patients with recurrent glioblastoma multiforme; adjunct to surgery and radiation in patients with high-grade malignant glioma

Unlabeled/Investigational Use Melanoma

Effect on Mental Status Dizziness is common

Effect on Psychiatric Treatment May cause myelosuppression; use caution with clozapine and carbamazepine

Dosage Summary

I.V.:

Children (unlabeled): 200-250 mg/m^2 as a single dose every 4-6 weeks

Adults: 150-200 mg/m^2 every 6-8 weeks **or** 75-100 mg/m^2/day for 2 days every 6-8 weeks

Implantation:

Children: Dosage not established

Adults: Up to 8 wafers may be placed in the resection cavity (total dose 62.6 mg)

Dosage Forms Excipient information presented when available (limited, particularly for generics); consult specific product labeling.

Implant:

Gliadel®: 7.7 mg (8s)

Injection, powder for reconstitution:

BiCNU®: 100 mg [packaged with 3 mL of absolute alcohol as diluent]

◆ **Carmustinum** *see* Carmustine *on page 284*

Carteolol (KAR tee oh lole)

Medication Safety Issues

Sound-alike/look-alike issues:

Carteolol may be confused with carvedilol

Related Information

Beta-Blockers *on page 1776*

Canadian Brand Names Ocupress® Ophthalmic

Index Terms Carteolol Hydrochloride

Pharmacologic Category Ophthalmic Agent, Antiglaucoma

Use Treatment of chronic open-angle glaucoma and intraocular hypertension

Effect on Mental Status May cause fatigue, insomnia, confusion, and nightmares and clinically look like a major depression

Effect on Psychiatric Treatment Antipsychotics and MAO inhibitors may increase the effects of beta-blockers; conversely beta-blockers may increase the effects of antipsychotics and benzodiazepines

Dosage Summary

Ophthalmic:

Children: Dosage not established

Adults: Instill 1 drop in affected eye(s) twice daily

Dosage Forms Excipient information presented when available (limited, particularly for generics); consult specific product labeling.

Solution, ophthalmic, as hydrochloride: 1% (5 mL, 10 mL, 15 mL) [contains benzalkonium chloride]

◆ **Carteolol Hydrochloride** *see* Carteolol *on page 285*

◆ **Cartia XT™** *see* Diltiazem *on page 473*

Carvedilol (KAR ve dil ole)

Medication Safety Issues

Sound-alike/look-alike issues:

Carvedilol may be confused with atenolol, captopril, carbidopa, carteolol

Coreg® may be confused with Corgard®, Cortef®, Cozaar®

International issues:

Talliton® [Hungary] may be confused with Talacen® which is a brand name for pentazocine/acetaminophen combination in the U.S.

Related Information

Beta-Blockers *on page 1776*

U.S. Brand Names Coreg CR®; Coreg®

Canadian Brand Names Apo-Carvedilol®; Coreg®; Novo-Carvedilol; PMS-Carvedilol; RAN™-Carvedilol; ratio-Carvedilol

Mexican Brand Names Dilatrend

Pharmacologic Category Beta Blocker With Alpha-Blocking Activity

Generic Available Yes: Tablet

Use Mild-to-severe heart failure of ischemic or cardiomyopathic origin (usually in addition to standard therapy); left ventricular dysfunction following myocardial infarction (MI) (clinically stable with LVEF ≤40%); management of hypertension

Unlabeled/Investigational Use Angina pectoris

Effect on Mental Status May cause fatigue, insomnia, confusion, and nightmare and clinically look like a major depression

Effect on Psychiatric Treatment Fluoxetine and paroxetine may increase carvedilol's (a CYP2D6 substrate) serum levels

Pregnancy Risk Factor C (manufacturer); D (2nd and 3rd trimesters - expert analysis)

Pregnancy Considerations Postimplantation losses were observed in animal studies. No data available on whether carvedilol crosses the placenta. Beta-blockers have been associated with persistent bradycardia, hypotension, and IUGR; IUGR probably related to maternal hypertension. Cases of neonatal hypoglycemia have been reported following maternal use of beta-blockers at parturition or during breast-feeding.

Lactation Excretion in breast milk unknown/not recommended

Contraindications Serious hypersensitivity to carvedilol or any component of the formulation; decompensated cardiac failure requiring intravenous inotropic therapy; bronchial asthma or related bronchospastic conditions; second- or third-degree AV block, sick sinus syndrome, and severe bradycardia (except in patients with a functioning artificial pacemaker); cardiogenic shock; severe hepatic impairment

Warnings/Precautions Consider pre-existing conditions such as sick sinus syndrome before initiating. Heart failure patients may experience a worsening of renal function (rare); risk factors include ischemic heart disease, diffuse vascular disease, underlying renal dysfunction, and systolic BP <100 mm Hg. Initiate cautiously and monitor for possible deterioration in patient status (eg, symptoms of HF). Worsening heart failure or fluid retention may occur during upward titration; dose reduction or temporary discontinuation may be necessary. Adjustment of other medications (ACE inhibitors and/or diuretics) may also be required.

Symptomatic hypotension with or without syncope may occur with carvedilol (usually within the first 30 days of therapy); close monitoring of patient is required especially with initial dosing and dosing increases; blood pressure must be lowered at a rate appropriate for the patient's clinical condition. Initiation with a low dose, gradual up-titration, and administration with food may help to decrease the occurrence of hypotension or syncope. Patients should be advised to avoid driving or other hazardous tasks during initiation of therapy due to the risk of syncope. Beta-blocker therapy should not be withdrawn abruptly (particularly in patients with CAD), but gradually tapered to avoid acute tachycardia, hypertension, and/or ischemia.

In general, patients with bronchospastic disease should not receive beta-blockers; if used at all, should be used cautiously with close monitoring. May precipitate or aggravate symptoms of arterial insufficiency in patients with PVD and Raynaud's disease; use with caution and monitor for progression of arterial obstruction. Use caution with concurrent use of verapamil or diltiazem; bradycardia or heart block can occur. Use cautiously in patients with diabetes because it can mask prominent hypoglycemic symptoms. May mask signs of hyperthyroidism (eg, tachycardia); if hyperthyroidism is suspected, carefully manage and monitor; abrupt withdrawal may exacerbate symptoms of hyperthyroidism or precipitate thyroid storm. Use with caution in patients with myasthenia gravis or psychiatric disease (may cause CNS depression). Use with caution in patients with mild-to-moderate hepatic impairment; use is contraindicated in patients with severe impairment. Manufacturer recommends discontinuation of therapy if liver injury occurs (confirmed by laboratory testing). Adequate alpha-blockade is required prior to use of any beta-blocker for patients with untreated pheochromocytoma. Use caution with history of severe anaphylaxis to allergens; patients taking beta-blockers may become more sensitive to repeated challenges. Treatment of anaphylaxis (eg, epinephrine) in patients taking beta-blockers may be ineffective or promote undesirable effects. Use care with anesthetic agents that decrease myocardial function. Safety and efficacy in children <18 years of age have not been established.

Adverse Reactions Note: Frequency ranges include data from hypertension and heart failure trials. Higher rates of adverse reactions have generally been noted in patients with heart failure. However, the frequency of adverse effects associated with placebo is also increased in this population.

>10%:

Cardiovascular: Hypotension (9% to 20%)

Central nervous system: Dizziness (2% to 32%), fatigue (4% to 24%)

Endocrine & metabolic: Hyperglycemia (5% to 12%)

Gastrointestinal: Diarrhea (1% to 12%), weight gain (10% to 12%)

Neuromuscular & skeletal: Weakness (7% to 11%)

1% to 10%:

Cardiovascular: Bradycardia (2% to 10%), syncope (3% to 8%), peripheral edema (1% to 7%), generalized edema (5% to 6%), angina (1% to 6%), dependent edema (≤4%), AV block, cerebrovascular accident, hypertension, hyper-/hypovolemia, postural hypotension, palpitation

Central nervous system: Headache (5% to 8%), depression, fever, hypoesthesia, hypotonia, insomnia, malaise, somnolence, vertigo

Endocrine & metabolic: Hypercholesterolemia (1% to 4%), hypertriglyceridemia (1%), diabetes mellitus, gout, hyperkalemia, hyperuricemia, hypoglycemia, hyponatremia

Gastrointestinal: Nausea (2% to 9%), vomiting (1% to 6%), abdominal pain, melena, periodontitis, weight loss

Genitourinary: Impotence

Hematologic: Anemia, prothrombin decreased, purpura, thrombocytopenia

Hepatic: Alkaline phosphatase increased (1% to 3%), GGT increased, transaminases increased

Neuromuscular & skeletal: Back pain (2% to 7%), arthralgia (1% to 6%), arthritis, muscle cramps, paresthesia

Ocular: Blurred vision (1% to 5%)

Renal: BUN increased (≤6%), nonprotein nitrogen increased (6%), albuminuria, creatinine increased, glycosuria, hematuria, renal insufficiency

Respiratory: Cough (5% to 8%), nasopharyngitis (4%), rales (4%), dyspnea (>3%), pulmonary edema (>3%), rhinitis (2%), nasal congestion (1%), sinus congestion (1%)

Miscellaneous: Injury (3% to 6%), allergy, flu-like syndrome, sudden death

<1% (Limited to important or life-threatening): Anaphylactoid reaction, alopecia, aplastic anemia (rare, all events occurred in patients receiving other medications capable of causing this effect), amnesia, asthma, bronchospasm, bundle branch block, cholestatic jaundice, concentration decreased, diaphoresis, erythema multiforme, exfoliative dermatitis, GI hemorrhage, HDL decreased, hearing decreased, hyperbilirubinemia, hypokalemia, hypokinesia, interstitial pneumonitis, leukopenia, libido decreased, migraine, myocardial ischemia, nervousness, neuralgia, nightmares, pancytopenia, paresis, peripheral ischemia, photosensitivity, pruritus, rash (erythematous, maculopapular, and psoriaform), respiratory alkalosis, seizure, Stevens-Johnson syndrome, tachycardia, tinnitus, toxic epidermal necrolysis, urinary incontinence, xerostomia

Metabolism/Transport Effects Substrate of CYP1A2 (minor), 2C9 (major), 2D6 (major), 2E1 (minor), 3A4 (minor)

Drug Interactions

Acetylcholinesterase Inhibitors: May enhance the bradycardic effect of Beta-Blockers. *Risk C: Monitor therapy*

Alpha-/Beta-Agonists (Direct-Acting): Beta-Blockers may enhance the vasopressor effect of Alpha-/Beta-Agonists (Direct-Acting). Epinephrine used as a local anesthetic for dental procedures will not likely cause clinically relevant problems. **Exceptions:** Dipivefrin. *Risk D: Consider therapy modification*

Alpha1-Blockers: Beta-Blockers may enhance the orthostatic effect of Alpha1-Blockers. The risk associated with ophthalmic products is probably less than systemic products. *Risk D: Consider therapy modification*

Alpha2-Agonists: Beta-Blockers may enhance the rebound hypertensive effect of Alpha2-Agonists. This effect can occur when the alpha$_2$-agonist is abruptly withdrawn. **Exceptions:** Apraclonidine; Brimonidine. *Risk D: Consider therapy modification*

Aminoquinolines (Antimalarial): May decrease the metabolism of Beta-Blockers. *Risk C: Monitor therapy*

Amiodarone: May enhance the bradycardic effect of Beta-Blockers. Possibly to the point of cardiac arrest. Amiodarone may increase the serum concentration of Beta-Blockers. *Risk C: Monitor therapy*

Anilidopiperidine Opioids: May enhance the bradycardic effect of Beta-Blockers. Anilidopiperidine Opioids may enhance the hypotensive effect of Beta-Blockers. *Risk C: Monitor therapy*

Antipsychotic Agents (Phenothiazines): May enhance the hypotensive effect of Beta-Blockers. Beta-Blockers may decrease the metabolism of Antipsychotic Agents (Phenothiazines). Antipsychotic Agents (Phenothiazines) may decrease the metabolism of Beta-Blockers. *Risk C: Monitor therapy*

Barbiturates: May decrease the serum concentration of Beta-Blockers. *Risk C: Monitor therapy*

Beta2-Agonists: Beta-Blockers (Nonselective) may diminish the bronchodilatory effect of Beta2-Agonists. *Risk D: Consider therapy modification*

Beta2-Agonists: Alpha-/Beta-Blockers may diminish the therapeutic effect of Beta2-Agonists. *Risk D: Consider therapy modification*

Calcium Channel Blockers (Nondihydropyridine): May enhance the hypotensive effect of Beta-Blockers. Bradycardia and signs of heart failure have also been reported. Calcium Channel Blockers (Nondihydropyridine) may increase the serum concentration of Beta-Blockers. *Risk C: Monitor therapy*

Cardiac Glycosides: Beta-Blockers may enhance the bradycardic effect of Cardiac Glycosides. *Risk C: Monitor therapy*

Cimetidine: May decrease the metabolism of Carvedilol. *Risk C: Monitor therapy*

CycloSPORINE: Carvedilol may increase the serum concentration of CycloSPORINE. *Risk D: Consider therapy modification*

CYP2D6 Inhibitors (Moderate): May decrease the metabolism of CYP2D6 Substrates. *Risk C: Monitor therapy*

CYP2D6 Inhibitors (Strong): May decrease the metabolism of CYP2D6 Substrates. *Risk D: Consider therapy modification*

Dabigatran Etexilate: P-Glycoprotein Inhibitors may increase the serum concentration of Dabigatran Etexilate. *Risk X: Avoid combination*

Darunavir: May increase the serum concentration of CYP2D6 Substrates. *Risk C: Monitor therapy*

Diazoxide: May enhance the hypotensive effect of Antihypertensives. *Risk C: Monitor therapy*

Digoxin: Carvedilol may increase the serum concentration of Digoxin. *Risk C: Monitor therapy*

Dipyridamole: May enhance the bradycardic effect of Beta-Blockers. *Risk C: Monitor therapy*

Disopyramide: May enhance the bradycardic effect of Beta-Blockers. *Risk C: Monitor therapy*

Herbs (Hypertensive Properties): May diminish the antihypertensive effect of Antihypertensives. *Risk C: Monitor therapy*

Herbs (Hypotensive Properties): May enhance the hypotensive effect of Antihypertensives. *Risk C: Monitor therapy*

Insulin: Beta-Blockers may enhance the hypoglycemic effect of Insulin. *Risk C: Monitor therapy*

Lidocaine: Beta-Blockers may decrease the metabolism of Lidocaine. *Risk C: Monitor therapy*

Methacholine: Beta-Blockers may enhance the adverse/toxic effect of Methacholine. *Risk X: Avoid combination*

Methylphenidate: May diminish the antihypertensive effect of Antihypertensives. *Risk C: Monitor therapy*

Midodrine: Beta-Blockers may enhance the bradycardic effect of Midodrine. *Risk C: Monitor therapy*

Nonsteroidal Anti-Inflammatory Agents: May diminish the antihypertensive effect of Beta-Blockers. *Risk C: Monitor therapy*

P-Glycoprotein Inducers: May decrease the serum concentration of P-Glycoprotein Substrates. P-glycoprotein inducers may also further limit the distribution of p-glycoprotein substrates to specific cells/tissues/organs where p-glycoprotein is present in large amounts (e.g., brain, T-lymphocytes, testes, etc.). *Risk C: Monitor therapy*

P-Glycoprotein Inhibitors: May increase the serum concentration of P-Glycoprotein Substrates. P-glycoprotein inhibitors may also enhance the distribution of p-glycoprotein substrates to specific cells/tissues/organs where p-glycoprotein is present in large amounts (e.g., brain, T-lymphocytes, testes, etc.). *Risk C: Monitor therapy*

P-Glycoprotein Substrates: P-Glycoprotein Inhibitors may increase the serum concentration of P-Glycoprotein Substrates. P-glycoprotein inhibitors may also enhance the distribution of p-glycoprotein substrates to specific cells/tissues/organs where p-glycoprotein is present in large amounts (e.g., brain, T-lymphocytes, testes, etc.). *Risk C: Monitor therapy*

Propafenone: May decrease the metabolism of Beta-Blockers. Propafenone possesses some independent beta blocking activity. *Risk C: Monitor therapy*

Propoxyphene: May decrease the metabolism of Beta-Blockers. *Risk C: Monitor therapy*

Prostacyclin Analogues: May enhance the hypotensive effect of Antihypertensives. *Risk C: Monitor therapy*

QuiNIDine: May decrease the metabolism of Beta-Blockers. *Risk C: Monitor therapy*

Reserpine: May enhance the hypotensive effect of Beta-Blockers. *Risk C: Monitor therapy*

Rifamycin Derivatives: May decrease the serum concentration of Beta-Blockers. **Exceptions:** Rifabutin. *Risk C: Monitor therapy*

RiTUXimab: Antihypertensives may enhance the hypotensive effect of RiTUXimab. *Risk D: Consider therapy modification*

Rivaroxaban: P-Glycoprotein Inhibitors may increase the serum concentration of Rivaroxaban. *Risk X: Avoid combination*

Selective Serotonin Reuptake Inhibitors: May decrease the metabolism of Alpha-/Beta-Blockers. **Exceptions:** Fluvoxamine. *Risk C: Monitor therapy*

Selective Serotonin Reuptake Inhibitors: May enhance the bradycardic effect of Beta-Blockers. **Exceptions:** Fluvoxamine. *Risk C: Monitor therapy*

Theophylline Derivatives: Beta-Blockers (Nonselective) may diminish the bronchodilatory effect of Theophylline Derivatives. *Risk D: Consider therapy modification*

Topotecan: P-Glycoprotein Inhibitors may increase the serum concentration of Topotecan. *Risk X: Avoid combination*

Ethanol/Nutrition/Herb Interactions

Food: Food decreases rate but not extent of absorption. Administration with food minimizes risks of orthostatic hypotension.

Herb/Nutraceutical: Avoid herbs with hypertensive properties (bayberry, blue cohosh, cayenne, ephedra, ginger, ginseng [American], kola, licorice); may diminish the antihypertensive effect of carvedilol. Avoid herbs with hypotensive properties (black cohosh, California poppy, coleus, golden seal, hawthorn, mistletoe, periwinkle, quinine, shepherd's purse); may enhance the hypotensive effect of carvedilol.

Stability

Coreg®: Store at <30°C (<86°F). Protect from moisture.

Coreg CR®: Store at 25°C (77°F); excursions permitted to 15°C to 30°C (59°F to 86°F).

Mechanism of Action As a racemic mixture, carvedilol has nonselective beta-adrenoreceptor and alpha-adrenergic blocking activity. No intrinsic sympathomimetic activity has been documented. Associated effects in hypertensive patients include reduction of cardiac output, exercise- or beta-agonist-induced tachycardia, reduction of reflex orthostatic tachycardia, vasodilation, decreased peripheral vascular resistance (especially in standing position), decreased renal vascular resistance, reduced plasma renin activity, and increased levels of atrial natriuretic peptide. In CHF, associated effects include decreased pulmonary capillary wedge pressure, decreased pulmonary artery pressure, decreased heart rate, decreased systemic vascular resistance, increased stroke volume index, and decreased right arterial pressure (RAP).

Pharmacodynamics/Kinetics

Onset of action: 1-2 hours

Peak antihypertensive effect: ~1-2 hours

Absorption: Rapid and extensive

Distribution: V_d: 115 L

Protein binding: >98%, primarily to albumin

Metabolism: Extensively hepatic, via CYP2C9, 2D6, 3A4, and 2C19 (2% excreted unchanged); three active metabolites (4-hydroxyphenyl metabolite is 13 times more potent than parent drug for beta-blockade); first-pass effect; plasma concentrations in the elderly and those with cirrhotic liver disease are 50% and 4-7 times higher, respectively

Bioavailability: Immediate release: 25% to 35% (due to significant first-pass metabolism); Extended release: 85% of immediate release

Half-life elimination: 7-10 hours

Time to peak, plasma: Extended release: 5 hours

Excretion: Primarily feces

Dosage Oral: Adults: Reduce dosage if heart rate drops to <55 beats/minute.

Hypertension:

Immediate release: 6.25 mg twice daily; if tolerated, dose should be maintained for 1-2 weeks, then increased to 12.5 mg twice daily. If necessary, dosage may be increased to a maximum of 25 mg twice daily after 1-2 weeks.

Extended release: Initial: 20 mg once daily, if tolerated, dose should be maintained for 1-2 weeks then increased to 40 mg once daily if necessary; maximum dose: 80 mg once daily

Heart failure:

Immediate release: 3.125 mg twice daily for 2 weeks; if this dose is tolerated, may increase to 6.25 mg twice daily. Double the dose every 2 weeks to the highest dose tolerated by patient. (Prior to initiating therapy, other heart failure medications should be stabilized and fluid retention minimized.)

Maximum recommended dose:

Mild-to-moderate heart failure:

<85 kg: 25 mg twice daily

>85 kg: 50 mg twice daily

Severe heart failure: 25 mg twice daily

Extended release: Initial: 10 mg once daily for 2 weeks; if the dose is tolerated, increase dose to 20 mg, 40 mg, and 80 mg over successive intervals of at least 2 weeks. Maintain on lower dose if higher dose is not tolerated.

Left ventricular dysfunction following MI: **Note**: Should be initiated only after patient is hemodynamically stable and fluid retention has been minimized.

Immediate release: Initial 3.125-6.25 mg twice daily; increase dosage incrementally (ie, from 6.25-12.5 mg twice daily) at intervals of 3-10 days, based on tolerance, to a target dose of 25 mg twice daily.

Extended release: Initial: 10-20 mg once daily; increase dosage incrementally at intervals of 3-10 days, based on tolerance, to a target dose of 80 mg once daily.

Angina pectoris (unlabeled use): Immediate release: 25-50 mg twice daily

Conversion from immediate release to extended release (Coreg CR®):

Current dose immediate release tablets 3.125 mg twice daily: Convert to extended release capsules 10 mg once daily

Current dose immediate release tablets 6.25 mg twice daily: Convert to extended release capsules 20 mg once daily

Current dose immediate release tablets 12.5 mg twice daily: Convert to extended release capsules 40 mg once daily

Current dose immediate release tablets 25 mg twice daily: Convert to extended release capsules 80 mg once daily

Dosing adjustment in renal impairment: None necessary

Dosing adjustment in hepatic impairment: Use is contraindicated in severe liver dysfunction.

Dietary Considerations Should be taken with food to minimize the risk of orthostatic hypotension.

Administration Administer with food. Extended release capsules should not be crushed or chewed. Capsules may be opened and sprinkled on applesauce for immediate use.

Monitoring Parameters Heart rate, blood pressure (base need for dosage increase on trough blood pressure measurements and for tolerance on standing systolic pressure 1 hour after dosing); renal studies, BUN, liver function; in patient with increase risk for developing renal dysfunction, monitor during dosage titration.

Additional Information Fluid retention during therapy should be treated with an increase in diuretic dosage.

Dosage Forms Excipient information presented when available (limited, particularly for generics); consult specific product labeling.

Capsule, extended release; as phosphate:

Coreg CR®: 10 mg, 20 mg, 40 mg, 80 mg

Tablet: 3.125 mg, 6.25 mg, 12.5 mg, 25 mg

Coreg®: 3.125 mg, 6.25 mg, 12.5 mg, 25 mg

◆ **Casodex®** *see* Bicalutamide *on page 188*

Caspofungin (kas poe FUN jin)

U.S. Brand Names Cancidas®

Canadian Brand Names Cancidas®

Mexican Brand Names Cancidas

Index Terms Caspofungin Acetate

Pharmacologic Category Antifungal Agent, Parenteral; Echinocandin

Use Treatment of invasive *Aspergillus* infections in patients who are refractory or intolerant of other therapy; treatment of candidemia and other *Candida* infections (intra-abdominal abscesses, esophageal, peritonitis, pleural space); empirical treatment for presumed fungal infections in febrile neutropenic patient

Effect on Mental Status May cause dizziness and insomnia

Effect on Psychiatric Treatment Carbamazepine may decrease serum concentration of caspofungin

Dosage Summary

I.V.:

Children <3 months: Dosage not established

Children 3 months to 17 years: 70 mg/m^2 on day 1, subsequent dosing: 50 mg/m^2 once daily, if clinical response inadequate, may increase to 70 mg/m^2 once daily if tolerated, but increased efficacy not demonstrated (maximum dose: 70 mg/day)

Adults: Initial: 70 mg on day 1; Subsequent dose: 50 mg once daily; may increase to 70 mg once daily if clinical response inadequate or concomitant use with enzyme inducer

Dosage Forms Excipient information presented when available (limited, particularly for generics); consult specific product labeling.

Injection, powder for reconstitution, as acetate:

Cancidas®: 50 mg [contains sucrose 39 mg], 70 mg [contains sucrose 54 mg]

- ◆ **Caspofungin Acetate** *see* Caspofungin *on page 290*
- ◆ **Cataflam®** *see* Diclofenac *on page 457*
- ◆ **Catapres®** *see* CloNIDine *on page 377*
- ◆ **Catapres-TTS®** *see* CloNIDine *on page 377*
- ◆ **Caverject®** *see* Alprostadil *on page 77*
- ◆ **Caverject Impulse®** *see* Alprostadil *on page 77*
- ◆ **CB-1348** *see* Chlorambucil *on page 315*
- ◆ **CBDCA** *see* CARBOplatin *on page 281*
- ◆ **CBZ** *see* CarBAMazepine *on page 265*
- ◆ **CC-5013** *see* Lenalidomide *on page 899*
- ◆ **CCI-779** *see* Temsirolimus *on page 1547*
- ◆ **CCNU** *see* Lomustine *on page 943*
- ◆ **2-CdA** *see* Cladribine *on page 360*
- ◆ **CDDP** *see* CISplatin *on page 354*
- ◆ **CDP870** *see* Certolizumab Pegol *on page 307*
- ◆ **CDX** *see* Bicalutamide *on page 188*
- ◆ **CE** *see* Estrogens (Conjugated/Equine) *on page 582*
- ◆ **Cecon® [OTC]** *see* Ascorbic Acid *on page 141*
- ◆ **Cedax®** *see* Ceftibuten *on page 299*
- ◆ **CEE** *see* Estrogens (Conjugated/Equine) *on page 582*
- ◆ **CeeNU®** *see* Lomustine *on page 943*

Cefaclor (SEF a klor)

Medication Safety Issues

Sound-alike/look-alike issues:

Cefaclor may be confused with cephalexin

U.S. Brand Names Raniclor™

Canadian Brand Names Apo-Cefaclor®; Ceclor®; Novo-Cefaclor; Nu-Cefaclor; PMS-Cefaclor

Mexican Brand Names Cec; Ceclor; Ceflacid; Fasiclor; Ranclor; Serviclor

Pharmacologic Category Antibiotic, Cephalosporin (Second Generation)

Use Treatment of susceptible bacterial infections including otitis media, lower respiratory tract infections, acute exacerbations of chronic bronchitis, pharyngitis and tonsillitis, urinary tract infections, skin and skin structure infections

Effect on Mental Status May cause nervousness; case reports of euphoria, delusion, illusions, and depersonalization with cephalosporins

Effect on Psychiatric Treatment May rarely cause neutropenia; use caution with clozapine and carbamazepine

Dosage Summary

Oral:

Children ≤1 month: Dosage not established

Children >1 month: 20-40 mg/kg/day divided every 8-12 hours (maximum: 1 g/day)

Adults: 250-500 mg every 8 hours

Dosage Forms Excipient information presented when available (limited, particularly for generics); consult specific product labeling.

Capsule: 250 mg, 500 mg

Powder for oral suspension: 125 mg/5 mL (75 mL, 150 mL); 250 mg/5 mL (75 mL, 150 mL); 375 mg/5 mL (50 mL, 100 mL)

Tablet, chewable:

Raniclor™: 250 mg [contains phenylalanine 5.6 mg/tablet and tartrazine; fruity flavor]; 375 mg [contains phenylalanine 8.4 mg/tablet and tartrazine; fruity flavor]

Tablet, extended release: 500 mg

Cefadroxil (sef a DROKS il)

U.S. Brand Names Duricef® [DSC]

Canadian Brand Names Apo-Cefadroxil®; Duricef®; Novo-Cefadroxil

Mexican Brand Names Duracef

Index Terms Cefadroxil Monohydrate

Pharmacologic Category Antibiotic, Cephalosporin (First Generation)

Use Treatment of susceptible bacterial infections, including those caused by group A beta-hemolytic *Streptococcus*

Effect on Mental Status May cause nervousness; case reports of euphoria, delusion, illusions, and depersonalization with cephalosporins

Effect on Psychiatric Treatment May rarely cause neutropenia; use caution with clozapine and carbamazepine

Dosage Summary

Oral:

Children: 30 mg/kg/day in 2 divided doses (maximum: 2 g/day)

Adults: 1-2 g/day in 2 divided doses

Dosage Forms Excipient information presented when available (limited, particularly for generics); consult specific product labeling. [DSC] = Discontinued product

Note: Strength is expressed as base

Capsule, as hemihydrate: 500 mg

Capsule, as monohydrate: 500 mg

Powder for oral suspension, as monohydrate: 250 mg/5 mL (100 mL); 500 mg/5 mL (75 mL, 100 mL)

Duricef®: 250 mg/5 mL (50 mL, 100 mL) [DSC]; 500 mg/5 mL (75 mL, 100 mL) [contains sodium benzoate; orange-pineapple flavor] [DSC]

Tablet, as hemihydrate: 1 g

Tablet, as monohydrate: 1 g

◆ **Cefadroxil Monohydrate** *see* Cefadroxil *on page 292*

CeFAZolin (sef A zoe lin)

Medication Safety Issues

Sound-alike/look-alike issues:

CeFAZolin may be confused with cefprozil, cefTRIAXone, cephalexin, cephalothin

Kefzol® may be confused with Cefzil®

Index Terms Ancef; Cefazolin Sodium

Pharmacologic Category Antibiotic, Cephalosporin (First Generation)

Use Treatment of respiratory tract, skin and skin structure, genital, urinary tract, biliary tract, bone and joint infections, and septicemia due to susceptible gram-positive cocci (except enterococcus); some gram-negative bacilli including *E. coli*, *Proteus*, and *Klebsiella* may be susceptible; perioperative prophylaxis

Unlabeled/Investigational Use Prophylaxis against infective endocarditis

Effect on Mental Status May cause nervousness; case reports of euphoria, delusion, illusions, and depersonalization with cephalosporins

Effect on Psychiatric Treatment May rarely cause neutropenia; use caution with clozapine and carbamazepine

Dosage Summary

I.M.:

Children ≤1 month: Dosage not established

Children >1 month: 25-100 mg/kg/day divided every 6-8 hours (maximum: 6 g/day)
Adults: 250 mg to 2 g every 6-12 hours (maximum: 12 g/day)

I.V.:

Children ≤1 month: Dosage not established
Children >1 month: 25-100 mg/kg/day divided every 6-8 hours (maximum: 6 g/day)
Adults: 250 mg to 2 g every 6-12 hours (maximum: 12 g/day)

Dosage Forms Excipient information presented when available (limited, particularly for generics); consult specific product labeling.
Infusion [iso-osmotic dextrose solution]: 1 g (50 mL)
Injection, powder for reconstitution: 500 mg, 1 g, 10 g, 20 g

◆ **Cefazolin Sodium** *see* CeFAZolin *on page 292*

Cefdinir (SEF di ner)

U.S. Brand Names Omnicef®
Canadian Brand Names Omnicef®
Mexican Brand Names Omnicef R
Index Terms CFDN
Pharmacologic Category Antibiotic, Cephalosporin (Third Generation)
Use Treatment of community-acquired pneumonia, acute exacerbations of chronic bronchitis, acute bacterial otitis media, acute maxillary sinusitis, pharyngitis/tonsillitis, and uncomplicated skin and skin structure infections.
Effect on Mental Status May cause nervousness; case reports of euphoria, delusion, illusions, and depersonalization with cephalosporins
Effect on Psychiatric Treatment May rarely cause neutropenia; use caution with clozapine and carbamazepine
Dosage Summary

Oral:

Children <6 months: Dosage not established
Children 6 months to 12 years: 14 mg/kg/day in 1-2 divided doses (maximum: 600 mg/day)
Children >12 years: 600 mg/day in 1-2 divided doses
Adults: 600 mg/day in 1-2 divided doses

Dosage Forms Excipient information presented when available (limited, particularly for generics); consult specific product labeling.
Capsule: 300 mg
Omnicef®: 300 mg
Powder for oral suspension: 125 mg/5 mL (60 mL, 100 mL); 250 mg/5 mL (60 mL, 100 mL)
Omnicef®: 125 mg/5 mL (60 mL, 100 mL) [contains sodium benzoate and sucrose 2.86 g/5 mL; strawberry flavor]; 250 mg/5 mL (60 mL, 100 mL) [contains sodium benzoate and sucrose 2.86 g/5 mL; strawberry flavor]

Cefditoren (sef de TOR en)

Medication Safety Issues
International issues:
Spectracef® may be confused with Spectrocef® which is a brand name for cefotaxime in Italy
U.S. Brand Names Spectracef®
Index Terms Cefditoren Pivoxil
Pharmacologic Category Antibiotic, Cephalosporin (Third Generation)
Use Treatment of acute bacterial exacerbation of chronic bronchitis or community-acquired pneumonia (due to susceptible organisms including *Haemophilus influenzae*, *Haemophilus parainfluenzae*, *Streptococcus pneumoniae*-penicillin susceptible only, *Moraxella catarrhalis*); pharyngitis or tonsillitis (*Streptococcus pyogenes*); and uncomplicated skin and skin-structure infections (*Staphylococcus aureus* - not MRSA, *Streptococcus pyogenes*)
Effect on Mental Status May rarely cause abnormal dreams, insomnia, and dizziness
Effect on Psychiatric Treatment None reported
Dosage Summary

Oral:

Children <12 years: Dosage not established
Children ≥12 years: 200-400 mg twice daily
Adults: 200-400 mg twice daily

Dosage Forms Excipient information presented when available (limited, particularly for generics); consult specific product labeling.
Tablet:
Spectracef®: 200 mg [contains sodium caseinate]

◆ **Cefditoren Pivoxil** *see* Cefditoren *on page 293*

Cefepime (SEF e pim)

U.S. Brand Names Maxipime®
Canadian Brand Names Maxipime®
Mexican Brand Names Maxef; Maxipime
Index Terms Cefepime Hydrochloride
Pharmacologic Category Antibiotic, Cephalosporin (Fourth Generation)
Use Treatment of uncomplicated and complicated urinary tract infections, including pyelonephritis caused by typical urinary tract pathogens; monotherapy for febrile neutropenia; uncomplicated skin and skin structure infections caused by *Streptococcus pyogenes*; moderate-to-severe pneumonia caused by pneumococcus, *Pseudomonas aeruginosa*, and other gram-negative organisms; complicated intra-abdominal infections (in combination with metronidazole). Also active against methicillin-susceptible staphylococci, *Enterobacter* sp, and many other gram-negative bacilli.

Children 2 months to 16 years: Empiric therapy of febrile neutropenia patients, uncomplicated skin/soft tissue infections, pneumonia, and uncomplicated/complicated urinary tract infections.

Effect on Mental Status May cause nervousness; case reports of euphoria, delusion, illusions, and depersonalization with cephalosporins; has rarely been associated with encephalopathy (confusion, hallucinations, stupor, and coma); most cases occurred in patients with renal impairment who received doses that exceeded recommendations
Effect on Psychiatric Treatment May rarely cause neutropenia; use caution with clozapine and carbamazepine
Dosage Summary
I.M.:
Children <2 months: Dosage not established
Children ≥2 months: 50 mg/kg every 12 hours
Adults: 500-1000 mg every 12 hours
I.V.:
Children <2 months: Dosage not established
Children ≥2 months: 50 mg/kg every 8-12 hours
Adults: 1-2 g every 8-12 hours
Dosage Forms Excipient information presented when available (limited, particularly for generics); consult specific product labeling.
Injection, powder for reconstitution, as hydrochloride: 500 mg, 1 g, 2 g
Maxipime®: 500 mg, 1 g, 2 g

◆ **Cefepime Hydrochloride** *see* Cefepime *on page 294*

Cefixime (sef IKS eem)

Medication Safety Issues
Sound-alike/look-alike issues:
Suprax® may be confused with Sporanox®, Surbex®

International issues:
Cefiton® [Portugal] may be confused with Cefotan® which is a brand name for cefotetan in the U.S.
Cefiton® [Portugal] may be confused with Ceftim® which is a brand name for ceftazidime in Italy
Cefiton® [Portugal] may be confused with Ceftin® which is a brand name for cefuroxime in the U.S.
Cefiton® [Portugal] may be confused with Lexotan® which is a brand name for bromazepam in multiple international markets

U.S. Brand Names Suprax®
Canadian Brand Names Suprax®
Mexican Brand Names Denvar
Index Terms Cefixime Trihydrate
Pharmacologic Category Antibiotic, Cephalosporin (Third Generation)
Use Treatment of urinary tract infections, otitis media, respiratory infections due to susceptible organisms including *S. pneumoniae* and *S. pyogenes*, *H.*

influenzae, and many Enterobacteriaceae; uncomplicated cervical/urethral gonorrhea due to *N. gonorrhoeae*

Effect on Mental Status May cause nervousness; case reports of euphoria, delusion, illusions, and depersonalization with cephalosporins

Effect on Psychiatric Treatment May rarely cause neutropenia; use caution with clozapine and carbamazepine

Dosage Summary

Oral:

Children <6 months: Dosage not established

Children ≥6 months to 12 years and ≤50 kg: 8-20 mg/kg/day divided every 12-24 hours (maximum: 400 mg/day)

Children >12 years or >50 kg: 400 mg/day divided every 12-24 hours **or** 20-30 mg/kg/day in 2 divided doses

Adults: 400 mg/day divided every 12-24 hours **or** 20-30 mg/kg/day in 2 divided doses

Dosage Forms Excipient information presented when available (limited, particularly for generics); consult specific product labeling. [DSC] = Discontinued product

Powder for oral suspension, as trihydrate:

Suprax®: 100 mg/5 mL (50 mL, 75 mL [DSC], 100 mL) [contains sodium benzoate; strawberry flavor]; 200 mg/5 mL (50 mL, 75 mL) [contains sodium benzoate; strawberry flavor]

Tablet, oral, as trihydrate:

Suprax®: 400 mg

◆ **Cefixime Trihydrate** *see* Cefixime *on page 294*

◆ **Cefizox®** *see* Ceftizoxime *on page 299*

Cefotaxime (sef oh TAKS eem)

Medication Safety Issues

Sound-alike/look-alike issues:

Cefotaxime may be confused with cefoxitin, ceftizoxime, cefuroxime

International issues:

Spectrocef® [Italy] may be confused with Spectracef® which is a brand name for cefditoren in the U.S.

U.S. Brand Names Claforan®

Canadian Brand Names Claforan®

Mexican Brand Names Benaxima; Biosint; Fot-Amsa; Fotexina; Taporin; Tebruxim; Tirotax; Viken; Xedin

Index Terms Cefotaxime Sodium

Pharmacologic Category Antibiotic, Cephalosporin (Third Generation)

Use Treatment of susceptible infection in respiratory tract, skin and skin structure, bone and joint, urinary tract, gynecologic as well as septicemia, and documented or suspected meningitis. Active against most gram-negative bacilli (not *Pseudomonas*) and gram-positive cocci (not enterococcus). Active against many penicillin-resistant pneumococci.

Effect on Mental Status May cause nervousness; case reports of euphoria, delusion, illusions, and depersonalization with cephalosporins

Effect on Psychiatric Treatment May rarely cause neutropenia; use caution with clozapine and carbamazepine

Dosage Summary

I.M.:

Children <1 month: Dosage not established

Children 1 month to 12 years and <50 kg: 50-200 mg/kg/day in divided doses every 6-8 hours (maximum: 12 g/day)

Children >12 years and ≥50 kg: 1-2 g every 8-12 hours **or** as a single dose

Adults: 1-2 g every 8-12 hours **or** as a single dose

I.V.:

Children <1 month: Dosage not established

Children 1 month to 12 years and <50 kg: 50-200 mg/kg/day in divided doses every 6-8 hours (maximum: 12 g/day)

Children >12 years and ≥50 kg: 1-2 g every 4-12 hours

Adults: 1-2 g every 4-12 hours

Dosage Forms Excipient information presented when available (limited, particularly for generics); consult specific product labeling.

Infusion [premixed iso-osmotic solution]:

Claforan®: 1 g (50 mL); 2 g (50 mL) [contains sodium 50.5 mg (2.2 mEq) per cefotaxime 1 g]

Injection, powder for reconstitution: 500 mg, 1 g, 2 g, 10 g, 20 g
Claforan®: 500 mg, 1 g, 2 g, 10 g [contains sodium 50.5 mg (2.2 mEq) per cefotaxime 1 g]

◆ **Cefotaxime Sodium** *see* Cefotaxime *on page 295*

Cefotetan (SEF oh tee tan)

Medication Safety Issues

Sound-alike/look-alike issues:

Cefotetan may be confused with cefoxitin, Ceftin®

Cefotan® may be confused with Ceftin®

International issues:

Cefotan® may be confused with Lexotan® which is a brand name for bromazepam in multiple international markets

Cefotan® may be confused with Cefiton® which is a brand name for cefixime in Portugal

Index Terms Cefotetan Disodium

Pharmacologic Category Antibiotic, Cephalosporin (Second Generation)

Use Surgical prophylaxis; intra-abdominal infections and other mixed infections; respiratory tract, skin and skin structure, bone and joint, urinary tract and gynecologic as well as septicemia; active against gram-negative enteric bacilli including *E. coli*, *Klebsiella*, and *Proteus*; less active against staphylococci and streptococci than first generation cephalosporins, but active against anaerobes including *Bacteroides fragilis*

Effect on Mental Status May cause nervousness; case reports of euphoria, delusion, illusions, and depersonalization with cephalosporins

Effect on Psychiatric Treatment May rarely cause neutropenia; use caution with clozapine and carbamazepine

Dosage Summary

I.M.:

Children (unlabeled use): 20-40 mg/kg every 12 hours (maximum: 6 g/day) **or** 40 mg/kg prior to surgery

Adults: 1-6 g/day divided every 12 hours **or** 1-2 g every 24 hours **or** 1-2 g prior to surgery

I.V.:

Children (unlabeled use): 20-40 mg/kg every 12 hours (maximum: 6 g/day) **or** 40 mg/kg prior to surgery

Adolescents: PID: 2 g every 12 hours

Adults: 1-6 g/day divided every 12 hours **or** 1-2 g every 24 hours **or** 1-2 g prior to surgery

Dosage Forms Excipient information presented when available (limited, particularly for generics); consult specific product labeling.

Injection, powder for reconstitution: 1 g, 2 g [contains sodium 80 mg/g (3.5 mEq/g)]

◆ **Cefotetan Disodium** *see* Cefotetan *on page 296*

Cefoxitin (se FOKS i tin)

Medication Safety Issues

Sound-alike/look-alike issues:

Cefoxitin may be confused with cefotaxime, cefotetan, Cytoxan®

Mefoxin® may be confused with Lanoxin®

Canadian Brand Names Apo-Cefoxitin®

Index Terms Cefoxitin Sodium

Pharmacologic Category Antibiotic, Cephalosporin (Second Generation)

Use Less active against staphylococci and streptococci than first generation cephalosporins, but active against anaerobes including *Bacteroides fragilis*; active against gram-negative enteric bacilli including *E. coli*, *Klebsiella*, and *Proteus*; used predominantly for respiratory tract, skin and skin structure, bone and joint, urinary tract and gynecologic as well as septicemia; surgical prophylaxis; intra-abdominal infections and other mixed infections; indicated for bacterial *Eikenella corrodens* infections

Effect on Mental Status May cause nervousness; case reports of euphoria, delusion, illusions, and depersonalization with cephalosporins

Effect on Psychiatric Treatment May rarely cause neutropenia; use caution with clozapine and carbamazepine

Dosage Summary

I.M.:

Children ≤3 months: Dosage not established

Children >3 months: 80-160 mg/kg/day divided every 4-6 hours (maximum: 12 g/day)
Adolescents: 80-160 mg/kg/day divided every 4-6 hours (maximum: 12 g/day) **or** 1-2 g prior to surgery
Adults: 1-2 g every 4-8 hours (maximum: 12 g/day) **or** 1-2 g prior to surgery

I.V.:
Children ≤3 months: Dosage not established
Children >3 months: 80-160 mg/kg/day divided every 4-6 hours (maximum: 12 g/day) **or** 30-40 mg/kg prior to surgery
Adolescents: 80-160 mg/kg/day divided every 4-6 hours (maximum: 12 g/day) **or** 1-2 g prior to surgery
Adults: 1-2 g every 4-8 hours (maximum: 12 g/day) **or** 1-2 g prior to surgery

Dosage Forms Excipient information presented when available (limited, particularly for generics); consult specific product labeling.
Injection, powder for reconstitution: 1 g, 2 g, 10 g [contains sodium 53.8 mg/g (2.3 mEq/g)]
Powder for prescription compounding: 100 g

◆ **Cefoxitin Sodium** *see* Cefoxitin *on page 296*

Cefpodoxime (sef pode OKS eem)

Medication Safety Issues
Sound-alike/look-alike issues:
Vantin® may be confused with Ventolin®

U.S. Brand Names Vantin®

Canadian Brand Names Vantin®

Mexican Brand Names Orelox

Index Terms Cefpodoxime Proxetil

Pharmacologic Category Antibiotic, Cephalosporin (Third Generation)

Use Treatment of susceptible acute, community-acquired pneumonia caused by *S. pneumoniae* or nonbeta-lactamase producing *H. influenzae*; acute uncomplicated gonorrhea caused by *N. gonorrhoeae*; uncomplicated skin and skin structure infections caused by *S. aureus* or *S. pyogenes*; acute otitis media caused by *S. pneumoniae*, *H. influenzae*, or *M. catarrhalis*; pharyngitis or tonsillitis; and uncomplicated urinary tract infections caused by *E. coli*, *Klebsiella*, and *Proteus*

Effect on Mental Status May cause nervousness; case reports of euphoria, delusion, illusions, and depersonalization with cephalosporins

Effect on Psychiatric Treatment May rarely cause neutropenia; use caution with clozapine and carbamazepine

Dosage Summary

Oral:
Children <2 months: Dosage not established
Children 2 months to 12 years: 10 mg/kg/day divided every 12 hours (maximum: 400 mg/day)
Children ≥12 years: 100-400 mg every 12 hours **or** 200 mg as a single dose
Adults: 100-400 mg every 12 hours **or** 200 mg as a single dose

Dosage Forms Excipient information presented when available (limited, particularly for generics); consult specific product labeling. [DSC] = Discontinued product
Granules for oral suspension: 50 mg/5 mL (50 mL, 75 mL, 100 mL); 100 mg/5 mL (50 mL, 75 mL, 100 mL)
Vantin®: 50 mg/5 mL (100 mL) [contains sodium benzoate; lemon creme flavor] [DSC]; 100 mg/5 mL (100 mL) [contains sodium benzoate; lemon creme flavor] [DSC]
Tablet: 100 mg, 200 mg
Vantin®: 100 mg, 200 mg

◆ **Cefpodoxime Proxetil** *see* Cefpodoxime *on page 297*

Cefprozil (sef PROE zil)

Medication Safety Issues
Sound-alike/look-alike issues:
Cefprozil may be confused with ceFAZolin, cefuroxime
Cefzil® may be confused with Cefol®, Ceftin®, Kefzol®

Canadian Brand Names Apo-Cefprozil®; Cefzil®; Ran-Cefprozil; Sandoz-Cefprozil

Mexican Brand Names Procef

Pharmacologic Category Antibiotic, Cephalosporin (Second Generation)

Use Treatment of otitis media and infections involving the respiratory tract and skin and skin structure; active against methicillin-sensitive staphylococci, many streptococci, and various gram-negative bacilli including *E. coli*, some *Klebsiella*, *P. mirabilis*, *H. influenzae*, and *Moraxella*.

Effect on Mental Status May cause nervousness; case reports of euphoria, delusion, illusions, and depersonalization with cephalosporins

Effect on Psychiatric Treatment May rarely cause neutropenia; use caution with clozapine and carbamazepine

Dosage Summary

Oral:

Children ≤6 months: Dosage not established

Children 6 months to 2 years: 7.5-30 mg/kg/day divided every 12 hours

Children 2-12 years: 7.5-30 mg/kg/day divided every 12 hours **or** 20 mg/kg every 24 hours (maximum: 1 g/day)

Adolescents >12 years: 250-500 mg every 12 hours **or** 500 mg every 24 hours

Adults: 250-500 mg every 12 hours **or** 500 mg every 24 hours

Dosage Forms Excipient information presented when available (limited, particularly for generics); consult specific product labeling.

Powder for oral suspension, as anhydrous: 125 mg/5 mL (50 mL, 75 mL, 100 mL); 250 mg/5 mL (50 mL, 75 mL, 100 mL)

Tablet, as anhydrous: 250 mg, 500 mg

Ceftazidime (SEF tay zi deem)

Medication Safety Issues

Sound-alike/look-alike issues:

Ceftazidime may be confused with ceftizoxime

Ceptaz® may be confused with Septra®

Tazicef® may be confused with Tazidime®

Tazidime® may be confused with Tazicef®

International issues:

Ceftim® [Italy] may be confused with Ceftin® which is a brand name for cefuroxime in the U.S.

Ceftim® [Italy] may be confused with Cefiton® which is a brand name for cefixime in Portugal

Ceftim® [Italy] may be confused with Ceftina® which is a brand name for cefalotin in Mexico

U.S. Brand Names Fortaz®; Tazicef®

Canadian Brand Names Fortaz®

Mexican Brand Names Fortum; Tagal; Zadolina

Pharmacologic Category Antibiotic, Cephalosporin (Third Generation)

Use Treatment of documented susceptible *Pseudomonas aeruginosa* infection and infections due to other susceptible aerobic gram-negative organisms; empiric therapy of a febrile, granulocytopenic patient

Unlabeled/Investigational Use Bacterial endophthalmitis

Effect on Mental Status May cause nervousness; case reports of euphoria, delusion, illusions, and depersonalization with cephalosporins

Effect on Psychiatric Treatment May rarely cause neutropenia; use caution with clozapine and carbamazepine

Dosage Summary

I.M.:

Children: Dosage not established

Adults: 500 mg to 2 g every 8-12 hours

Elderly: Do not administer more frequently than every 12 hours

I.V.:

Children <1 month: Dosage not established

Children 1 month to 12 years: 30-50 mg/kg every 8 hours (maximum: 6 g/day)

Children ≥12 years: 500 mg to 2 g every 8-12 hours (maximum: 6 g/day)

Adults: 500 mg to 2 g every 8-12 hours (maximum: 6 g/day)

Elderly: Do not administer more frequently than every 12 hours

Dosage Forms Excipient information presented when available (limited, particularly for generics); consult specific product labeling.

Infusion [premixed iso-osmotic solution, frozen]:

Fortaz®: 1 g (50 mL) [contains sodium carbonate, sodium ~54 mg (2.3 mEq)/g]; 2 g (50 mL) [contains sodium ~54 mg (2.3 mEq)/g]

Injection, powder for reconstitution: 1 g, 2 g, 6 g

Fortaz®: 500 mg, 1 g, 2 g, 6 g [contains sodium ~54 mg (2.3 mEq)/g]

Tazicef®: 1 g, 2 g, 6 g [contains sodium ~54 mg (2.3 mEq)/g]

Ceftibuten (sef TYE byoo ten)

Medication Safety Issues

International issues:

Cedax® may be confused with Codex which is a brand name for *Saccharomyces boulardii* in Italy

U.S. Brand Names Cedax®

Mexican Brand Names Cedax

Pharmacologic Category Antibiotic, Cephalosporin (Third Generation)

Use Oral cephalosporin for treatment of bronchitis, otitis media, and pharyngitis/ tonsillitis due to *H. influenzae* and *M. catarrhalis*, both beta-lactamase-producing and nonproducing strains, as well as *S. pneumoniae* (weak) and *S. pyogenes*

Effect on Mental Status May cause nervousness; case reports of euphoria, delusion, illusions, and depersonalization with cephalosporins

Effect on Psychiatric Treatment May rarely cause neutropenia; use caution with clozapine and carbamazepine

Dosage Summary

Oral:

Children <12 years: 9 mg/kg/day (maximum: 400 mg/day)

Children ≥12 years: 400 mg once daily

Adults: 400 mg once daily

Dosage Forms Excipient information presented when available (limited, particularly for generics); consult specific product labeling.

Capsule:

Cedax®: 400 mg

Powder for oral suspension:

Cedax®: 90 mg/5 mL (30 mL, 60 mL, 90 mL, 120 mL) [contains sucrose 1g/5 mL and sodium benzoate; cherry flavor]

◆ **Ceftin®** *see* Cefuroxime *on page 300*

Ceftizoxime (sef ti ZOKS eem)

Medication Safety Issues

Sound-alike/look-alike issues:

Ceftizoxime may be confused with cefotaxime, ceftazidime, cefuroxime

U.S. Brand Names Cefizox®

Canadian Brand Names Cefizox®

Index Terms Ceftizoxime Sodium

Pharmacologic Category Antibiotic, Cephalosporin (Third Generation)

Use Treatment of susceptible bacterial infections, mainly respiratory tract, skin and skin structure, bone and joint, urinary tract and gynecologic, as well as septicemia; active against many gram-negative bacilli (not *Pseudomonas*), some gram-positive cocci (not *Enterococcus*), and some anaerobes

Effect on Mental Status May cause nervousness; case reports of euphoria, delusion, illusions, and depersonalization with cephalosporins

Effect on Psychiatric Treatment May rarely cause neutropenia; use caution with clozapine and carbamazepine

Dosage Summary

I.M.:

Children <6 months: Dosage not established

Children ≥6 months: 150-200 mg/kg/day divided every 6-8 hours (maximum: 12 g/day)

Adults: 1-2 g every 4-12 hours **or** 4 g every 8 hours (life-threatening infections) **or** 1 g as a single dose

I.V.:

Children <6 months: Dosage not established

Children ≥6 months: 150-200 mg/kg/day divided every 6-8 hours (maximum: 12 g/day)

Adults: 1-2 g every 4 hours **or** 1-4 g every 8-12 hours

Dosage Forms Excipient information presented when available (limited, particularly for generics); consult specific product labeling.

Infusion [premixed iso-osmotic solution]:

Cefizox®: 1 g (50 mL); 2 g (50 mL)

Injection, powder for reconstitution:

Cefizox®: 1 g, 2 g, 10 g [DSC]

◆ **Ceftizoxime Sodium** *see* Ceftizoxime *on page 299*

CefTRIAXone (sef trye AKS one)

Medication Safety Issues

Sound-alike/look-alike issues:

Rocephin® may be confused with Roferon®

U.S. Brand Names Rocephin®

Canadian Brand Names Rocephin®

Mexican Brand Names Amcef; Aurofox; Axtar; Benaxona; Cefaxona; Cefraden; Ceftrex; Ceftrianol; Ceftrilem; Megion; Rocephin; Tacex; Terbac; Triaken; Triox

Index Terms Ceftriaxone Sodium

Pharmacologic Category Antibiotic, Cephalosporin (Third Generation)

Use Treatment of lower respiratory tract infections, acute bacterial otitis media, skin and skin structure infections, bone and joint infections, intra-abdominal and urinary tract infections, pelvic inflammatory disease (PID), uncomplicated gonorrhea, bacterial septicemia, and meningitis; used in surgical prophylaxis

Unlabeled/Investigational Use Treatment of chancroid, epididymitis, complicated gonococcal infections; sexually-transmitted diseases (STD); periorbital or buccal cellulitis; salmonellosis or shigellosis; atypical community-acquired pneumonia; epiglottitis, Lyme disease; used in chemoprophylaxis for high-risk contacts and persons with invasive meningococcal disease; sexual assault; typhoid fever, Whipple's disease

Effect on Mental Status Case reports of euphoria, delusion, illusions, and depersonalization with cephalosporins

Effect on Psychiatric Treatment May rarely cause neutropenia; use caution with clozapine and carbamazepine

Dosage Summary

I.M.:

Children: 50-100 mg/kg/day divided every 12-24 hours (maximum: 4 g/day) **or** 125 mg or 50 mg/kg as a single dose

Adults: 1-2 g every 12-24 hours **or** 125-250 mg as a single dose

I.V.:

Children: 50-100 mg/kg/day divided every 12-24 hours (maximum: 4 g/day)

Adults: 1-2 g every 12-24 hours

Dosage Forms Excipient information presented when available (limited, particularly for generics); consult specific product labeling. [DSC] = Discontinued product

Infusion [premixed in dextrose]: 1 g (50 mL); 2 g (50 mL)

Injection, powder for reconstitution: 250 mg, 500 mg, 1 g, 2 g, 10 g

Rocephin®: 250 mg [DSC], 500 mg, 1 g, 2 g [DSC], 10 g [contains sodium ~83 mg (3.6 mEq) per ceftriaxone 1 g] [DSC]

◆ **Ceftriaxone Sodium** *see* CefTRIAXone *on page 300*

Cefuroxime (se fyoor OKS eem)

Medication Safety Issues

Sound-alike/look-alike issues:

Cefuroxime may be confused with cefotaxime, cefprozil, ceftizoxime, deferoxamine

Ceftin® may be confused with Cefzil®, Cipro®

Zinacef® may be confused with Zithromax®

International issues:

Ceftin® may be confused with Cefiton® which is a brand name for cefixime in Portugal

Ceftin® may be confused with Ceftina® which is a brand name for cefalotin in Mexico

Ceftin® may be confused with Ceftim® which is a brand name for ceftazidime in Italy

U.S. Brand Names Ceftin®; Zinacef®

Canadian Brand Names Apo-Cefuroxime®; Ceftin®; Cefuroxime For Injection ratio-Cefuroxime; Zinacef®

Mexican Brand Names Cefabiot; Cefuracet; Cetoxil; Furobioxin; Novador Xorufec; Zinnat

Index Terms Cefuroxime Axetil; Cefuroxime Sodium

Pharmacologic Category Antibiotic, Cephalosporin (Second Generation)

Use Treatment of infections caused by staphylococci, group B streptococci, *H. influenzae* (type A and B), *E. coli*, *Enterobacter*, *Salmonella*, and *Klebsiella*; treatment of susceptible infections of the upper and lower respiratory tract, otitis media, urinary tract, uncomplicated skin and soft tissue, bone and joint, sepsis uncomplicated gonorrhea, and early Lyme disease; preoperative prophylaxis of susceptible infections

Effect on Mental Status May cause nervousness; case reports of euphoria, delusion, illusions, and depersonalization with cephalosporins

Effect on Psychiatric Treatment May rarely cause neutropenia; use caution with clozapine and carbamazepine

Dosage Summary

I.M.:

Children 3 months to 12 years: 75-150 mg/kg/day divided every 8 hours (maximum: 6 g/day)

Adolescents >12 years: 750 mg to 1.5 g every 6-8 hours (maximum: 6 g/day) **or** 1.5 g as a single dose

Adults: 750 mg to 1.5 g every 6-8 hours (maximum: 6 g/day) **or** 1.5 g as a single dose

I.V.:

Children 3 months to 12 years: 75-150 mg/kg/day divided every 8 hours (maximum: 6 g/day)

Adolescents >12 years: 750 mg to 1.5 g every 6-8 hours (maximum: 6 g/day) **or** 1.5 g prior to surgery

Adults: 750 mg to 1.5 g every 6-8 hours (maximum: 6 g/day) **or** 1.5 g prior to surgery

Oral:

Children <3 months: Dosage not established

Children 3 months to 12 years: 20-30 mg/kg/day in 2 divided doses **or** 125-250 mg every 12 hours (maximum: 1 g/day)

Adolescents >12 years: 125-500 mg every 12 hours **or** 1 g as a single dose

Adults: 125-500 mg every 12 hours **or** 1 g as a single dose

Dosage Forms Excipient information presented when available (limited, particularly for generics); consult specific product labeling.

Note: Strength expressed as base

Infusion, as sodium [premixed]: 750 mg (50 mL); 1.5 g (50 mL)

Zinacef®: 750 mg (50 mL); 1.5 g (50 mL) [contains sodium 4.8 mEq (111 mg) per 750 mg]

Injection, powder for reconstitution, as sodium: 750 mg, 1.5 g, 7.5 g, 75 g, 225 g

Zinacef®: 750 mg, 1.5 g, 7.5 g [contains sodium 1.8 mEq (41 mg) per 750 mg]

Powder for suspension, oral, as axetil: 125 mg/5 mL (100 mL); 250 mg/5 mL (50 mL, 100 mL)

Ceftin®: 125 mg/5 mL (100 mL) [contains phenylalanine 11.8 mg/5 mL; tutti-frutti flavor]; 250 mg/5 mL (50 mL, 100 mL) [contains phenylalanine 25.2 mg/5 mL; tutti-frutti flavor]

Tablet, as axetil: 250 mg, 500 mg

Ceftin®: 250 mg, 500 mg

◆ **Cefuroxime Axetil** *see* Cefuroxime *on page 300*

◆ **Cefuroxime Sodium** *see* Cefuroxime *on page 300*

◆ **Celebrex®** *see* Celecoxib *on page 301*

Celecoxib (se le KOKS ib)

Medication Safety Issues

Sound-alike/look-alike issues:

Celebrex® may be confused with Celexa®, cerebra, Cerebyx®

Related Information

Nonsteroidal Anti-Inflammatory Agents *on page 1792*

U.S. Brand Names Celebrex®

Canadian Brand Names Celebrex®; GD-Celecoxib

Mexican Brand Names Celebrex

Pharmacologic Category Nonsteroidal Anti-inflammatory Drug (NSAID), COX-2 Selective

Generic Available No

Use Relief of the signs and symptoms of osteoarthritis, ankylosing spondylitis, juvenile rheumatoid arthritis (JRA), and rheumatoid arthritis; management of acute pain; treatment of primary dysmenorrhea; to reduce the number of intestinal polyps in familial adenomatous polyposis (FAP)

Canadian note: Celecoxib is only indicated for relief of symptoms of rheumatoid arthritis, osteoarthritis, and relief of acute pain in adults

Effect on Mental Status May cause dizziness and insomnia; may rarely, cause anxiety, depression, nervousness, or somnolence

Effect on Psychiatric Treatment Effects of benzodiazepines and antidepressants may be altered. Lithium concentrations may be increased by celecoxib via decreased renal lithium clearance; dose adjustment may be needed.

Restrictions An FDA-approved medication guide must be distributed when dispensing an oral outpatient prescription (new or refill) where this medication is to be used without direct supervision of a healthcare provider. Medication guides are available at http://www.fda.gov/cder/Offices/ODS/medication_guides.htm.

Pregnancy Risk Factor C/D (3rd trimester)

Pregnancy Considerations Teratogenic effects were observed in animal studies. Avoid use in the 3rd trimester of pregnancy, this drug may cause premature closure of the ductus arteriosus.

Lactation Enters breast milk/not recommended

Contraindications Hypersensitivity to celecoxib, sulfonamides, aspirin, other NSAIDs, or any component of the formulation; perioperative pain in the setting of coronary artery bypass surgery (CABG); pregnancy (3rd trimester)

Canadian labeling: Additional contraindications (not in U.S. labeling): Pregnancy (3rd trimester); women who are breast-feeding; severe, uncontrolled heart failure; active gastrointestinal ulcer (gastric, duodenal, peptic) or bleeding; inflammatory bowel disease; cerebrovascular bleeding; severe liver impairment or active hepatic disease; severe renal impairment (Cl_{cr} <30 mL/minute) or deteriorating renal disease; known hyperkalemia; use in children

Warnings/Precautions [U.S. Boxed Warning]: NSAIDs are associated with an increased risk of adverse cardiovascular thrombotic events, including MI, and new onset or worsening of pre-existing hypertension. Risk may be increased with duration of use or pre-existing cardiovascular risk factors or disease. Carefully evaluate individual cardiovascular risk profiles prior to prescribing. May cause sodium and fluid retention; use with caution in patients with CHF, edema, cerebrovascular disease, ischemic heart disease, or hypertension. Long-term cardiovascular risk in children has not been evaluated.

[U.S. Boxed Warning]: Celecoxib is contraindicated for treatment of perioperative pain in the setting of coronary artery bypass surgery (CABG). Risk of MI and stroke may be increased with use following CABG surgery.

[U.S. Boxed Warning]: NSAIDs may increase risk of gastrointestinal irritation, ulceration, bleeding, and perforation. These events may occur at any time during therapy and without warning. Use caution with a history of GI disease (bleeding or ulcers), concurrent therapy with aspirin, anticoagulants and/or corticosteroids, smoking, use of alcohol, the elderly or debilitated patients.

Use the lowest effective dose for the shortest duration of time, consistent with individual patient goals, to reduce risk of cardiovascular or GI adverse events. Alternate therapies should be considered for patients at high risk.

NSAIDs may cause serious skin adverse events including exfoliative dermatitis, Stevens-Johnson syndrome (SJS), and toxic epidermal necrolysis (TEN). Anaphylactoid reactions may occur, even without prior exposure; patients with "aspirin triad" (bronchial asthma, aspirin intolerance, rhinitis) may be at increased risk. Do not use in patients who experience bronchospasm, asthma, rhinitis, or urticaria with NSAID or aspirin therapy. Use caution in other forms of asthma.

Use with caution in patients with decreased hepatic (dosage adjustments are recommended for moderate hepatic impairment; not recommended for patients with severe hepatic impairment) or renal function. Closely monitor patients with any abnormal LFT. Severe hepatic reactions (eg, fulminant hepatitis, liver failure) have occurred with NSAID use, rarely; discontinue if signs or symptoms of liver disease develop, or if systemic manifestations occur. NSAID use may compromise existing renal function; dose-dependent decreases in prostaglandin synthesis may result from NSAID use, causing a reduction in renal blood flow which may cause renal decompensation. Patients with impaired renal function, dehydration, heart failure, liver dysfunction, those taking diuretics and ACEI, and the elderly are at greater risk for renal toxicity. Rehydrate patient before starting therapy; monitor renal function closely. Not recommended for use in patients with advanced renal disease. Long-term NSAID use may result in renal papillary necrosis.

Anaphylactoid reactions may occur, even with no prior exposure to celecoxib. Use with caution in patients with known or suspected deficiency of cytochrome

P450 isoenzyme 2C9; poor metabolizers may have higher plasma levels due to reduced metabolism.

When used for the treatment of FAP, routine monitoring and care should be continued. When used for JRA, celecoxib is not FDA-approved in children <2 years of age or in children <10 kg. Use caution with systemic onset JRA (may be at risk for disseminated intravascular coagulation). Safety and efficacy have not been established for use in children for indications other than JRA.

Adverse Reactions

>10%:

Cardiovascular: Hypertension (≤13%)

Central nervous system: Headache (10% to 16%)

Gastrointestinal: Diarrhea (4% to 11%)

2% to 10%:

Cardiovascular: Peripheral edema (2%)

Central nervous system: Fever (≤9%), insomnia (2%), dizziness (1% to 2%)

Dermatologic: Skin rash (2%)

Gastrointestinal: Dyspepsia (9%), nausea (4% to 7%), gastroesophageal reflux (≤5%), abdominal pain (4% to 8%), vomiting (≤6%), flatulence (2%)

Neuromuscular & skeletal: Arthralgia (≤7%), back pain (3%)

Respiratory: Upper respiratory tract infection (8%), cough (≤7%), nasopharyngitis (≤6%), sinusitis (5%), dyspnea (≤3%), pharyngitis (2%), rhinitis (2%)

Miscellaneous: Accidental injury (3%)

0.1% to 2%:

Cardiovascular: Angina, aortic valve incompetence, chest pain, coronary artery disorder, DVT, edema, facial edema, hypertension (aggravated), MI, palpitation, sinus bradycardia, tachycardia, ventricular hypertrophy

Central nervous system: Anxiety, cerebral infarction, depression, fatigue, hypoesthesia, migraine, nervousness, pain, somnolence, vertigo

Dermatologic: Alopecia, bruising, cellulitis, dermatitis, dry skin, nail disorder, photosensitivity, pruritus, rash (erythematous), rash (maculopapular), urticaria

Endocrine & metabolic: Breast fibroadenosis, breast neoplasm, breast pain, diabetes mellitus, dysmenorrhea, hot flashes, hypercholesterolemia, hyperglycemia, hyper-/hypokalemia, hypernatremia, menstrual disturbances, ovarian cyst, testosterone decreased

Gastrointestinal: Anorexia, appetite increased, constipation, diverticulitis, dysphagia, eructation, esophagitis, gastritis, gastroenteritis, gastrointestinal ulcer, hemorrhoids, hiatal hernia, melena, stomatitis, taste disturbance, tenesmus, tooth disorder, weight gain, xerostomia

Genitourinary: Cystitis, dysuria, incontinence, monilial vaginitis, prostate disorder, urinary frequency, urinary tract infection, vaginal bleeding, vaginitis

Hematologic: Anemia, thrombocytopenia

Hepatic: Alkaline phosphatase increased, transaminases increased

Neuromuscular & skeletal: Arthrosis, bone disorder, CPK increased, fracture, leg cramps, myalgia, neck stiffness, neuralgia, neuropathy, paresthesia, hypertonia, synovitis, tendon rupture, tendonitis, weakness

Ocular: Blurred vision, cataract, conjunctival hemorrhage, conjunctivitis, eye pain, glaucoma, vitreous floaters

Otic: Deafness, earache, labyrinthitis, otitis media, tinnitus

Renal: Albuminuria, BUN increased, creatinine increased, hematuria, nonprotein nitrogen increased, renal calculi

Respiratory: Bronchitis, bronchospasm, epistaxis, laryngitis, pneumonia

Miscellaneous: Allergic reactions, allergy aggravated, diaphoresis, flu-like syndrome, herpes infection, infection (bacterial, fungal, viral), moniliasis

<0.1% (Limited to important or life-threatening): Acute renal failure, agranulocytosis, anaphylactoid reactions, angioedema, aplastic anemia, aseptic meningitis, ataxia, cerebrovascular accident, CHF, cholelithiasis, colitis, erythema multiforme, esophageal perforation, exfoliative dermatitis, gangrene, gastrointestinal bleeding, hepatic failure, hepatic necrosis, hepatitis (including fulminant), hypoglycemia, hyponatremia, ileus, interstitial nephritis, intestinal obstruction, intestinal perforation, intracranial hemorrhage, jaundice, leukopenia, pancreatitis, pancytopenia, pulmonary embolism, renal papillary necrosis, sepsis, Stevens-Johnson syndrome, sudden death, suicide, syncope, thrombophlebitis, toxic epidermal necrolysis, vasculitis, ventricular fibrillation

Metabolism/Transport Effects **Substrate** of CYP2C9 (major), 3A4 (minor); **Inhibits** CYP2C8 (moderate), 2D6 (weak)

Drug Interactions

ACE Inhibitors: Nonsteroidal Anti-Inflammatory Agents may diminish the antihypertensive effect of ACE Inhibitors. *Risk C: Monitor therapy*

Aminoglycosides: Nonsteroidal Anti-Inflammatory Agents may decrease the excretion of Aminoglycosides. Data only in premature infants. *Risk C: Monitor therapy*

Angiotensin II Receptor Blockers: Nonsteroidal Anti-Inflammatory Agents may diminish the therapeutic effect of Angiotensin II Receptor Blockers. The combination of these two agents may also significantly decrease glomerular filtration and renal function. *Risk C: Monitor therapy*

Anticoagulants: Nonsteroidal Anti-Inflammatory Agents may enhance the anticoagulant effect of Anticoagulants. *Risk C: Monitor therapy*

Antidepressants (Tricyclic, Tertiary Amine): May enhance the antiplatelet effect of NSAID (COX-2 Inhibitor). *Risk C: Monitor therapy*

Antiplatelet Agents: Nonsteroidal Anti-Inflammatory Agents may enhance the adverse/toxic effect of Antiplatelet Agents. An increased risk of bleeding may occur. *Risk C: Monitor therapy*

Beta-Blockers: Nonsteroidal Anti-Inflammatory Agents may diminish the antihypertensive effect of Beta-Blockers. **Exceptions:** Levobunolol; Metipranolol. *Risk C: Monitor therapy*

Bile Acid Sequestrants: May decrease the absorption of Nonsteroidal Anti-Inflammatory Agents. *Risk D: Consider therapy modification*

Bisphosphonate Derivatives: Nonsteroidal Anti-Inflammatory Agents may enhance the adverse/toxic effect of Bisphosphonate Derivatives. Both an increased risk of gastrointestinal ulceration and an increased risk of nephrotoxicity are of concern. *Risk C: Monitor therapy*

Corticosteroids (Systemic): May enhance the adverse/toxic effect of NSAID (COX-2 Inhibitor). *Risk C: Monitor therapy*

CycloSPORINE: Nonsteroidal Anti-Inflammatory Agents may enhance the nephrotoxic effect of CycloSPORINE. Nonsteroidal Anti-Inflammatory Agents may increase the serum concentration of CycloSPORINE. *Risk D: Consider therapy modification*

CYP2C8 Substrates (High risk): CYP2C8 Inhibitors (Moderate) may decrease the metabolism of CYP2C8 Substrates (High risk). *Risk C: Monitor therapy*

CYP2C9 Inducers (Highly Effective): May increase the metabolism of CYP2C9 Substrates (High risk). *Risk C: Monitor therapy*

CYP2C9 Inhibitors (Moderate): May decrease the metabolism of CYP2C9 Substrates (High risk). *Risk C: Monitor therapy*

CYP2C9 Inhibitors (Strong): May decrease the metabolism of CYP2C9 Substrates (High risk). *Risk D: Consider therapy modification*

Desmopressin: Nonsteroidal Anti-Inflammatory Agents may enhance the adverse/toxic effect of Desmopressin. *Risk C: Monitor therapy*

Eplerenone: Nonsteroidal Anti-Inflammatory Agents may diminish the antihypertensive effect of Eplerenone. *Risk C: Monitor therapy*

Herbs (Anticoagulant/Antiplatelet Properties) (eg, Alfalfa, Anise, Bilberry): May enhance the adverse/toxic effect of Nonsteroidal Anti-Inflammatory Agents. Bleeding may occur. *Risk D: Consider therapy modification*

HydrALAZINE: Nonsteroidal Anti-Inflammatory Agents may diminish the antihypertensive effect of HydrALAZINE. *Risk C: Monitor therapy*

Ketorolac: May enhance the adverse/toxic effect of Nonsteroidal Anti-Inflammatory Agents. *Risk X: Avoid combination*

Lithium: Nonsteroidal Anti-Inflammatory Agents may increase the serum concentration of Lithium. *Risk D: Consider therapy modification*

Loop Diuretics: Nonsteroidal Anti-Inflammatory Agents may diminish the diuretic effect of Loop Diuretics. *Risk C: Monitor therapy*

Methotrexate: Nonsteroidal Anti-Inflammatory Agents may decrease the excretion of Methotrexate. *Risk D: Consider therapy modification*

Nonsteroidal Anti-Inflammatory Agents: May enhance the adverse/toxic effect of other Nonsteroidal Anti-Inflammatory Agents. *Risk C: Monitor therapy*

Probenecid: May increase the serum concentration of Nonsteroidal Anti-Inflammatory Agents. *Risk C: Monitor therapy*

Quinolone Antibiotics: Nonsteroidal Anti-Inflammatory Agents may enhance the neuroexcitatory and/or seizure-potentiating effect of Quinolone Antibiotics. *Risk C: Monitor therapy*

Selective Serotonin Reuptake Inhibitors: May enhance the antiplatelet effect of NSAID (COX-2 Inhibitor). *Risk D: Consider therapy modification*

Thiazide Diuretics: Nonsteroidal Anti-Inflammatory Agents may diminish the therapeutic effect of Thiazide Diuretics. *Risk C: Monitor therapy*

Thrombolytic Agents: Nonsteroidal Anti-Inflammatory Agents may enhance the adverse/toxic effect of Thrombolytic Agents. An increased risk of bleeding may occur. *Risk C: Monitor therapy*

Treprostinil: May enhance the adverse/toxic effect of Nonsteroidal Anti-Inflammatory Agents. Bleeding may occur. *Risk C: Monitor therapy*

Vancomycin: Nonsteroidal Anti-Inflammatory Agents may decrease the excretion of Vancomycin. *Risk C: Monitor therapy*

Vitamin K Antagonists (eg, warfarin): NSAID (COX-2 Inhibitor) may enhance the anticoagulant effect of Vitamin K Antagonists. *Risk C: Monitor therapy*

Ethanol/Nutrition/Herb Interactions

Ethanol: Avoid ethanol (increased GI irritation).

Food: Peak concentrations are delayed and AUC is increased by 10% to 20% when taken with a high-fat meal.

Herb/Nutraceutical: Avoid concomitant use with herbs possessing anticoagulation/antiplatelet properties, including alfalfa, anise, bilberry, bladderwrack, bromelain, cat's claw, celery, chamomile, coleus, cordyceps, dong quai, evening primrose, fenugreek, feverfew, garlic, ginger, ginkgo biloba, ginseng (American, Panax, Siberian), grapeseed, green tea, guggul, horse chestnuts, horseradish, licorice, prickly ash, red clover, reishi, SAMe (S-adenosylmethionine), sweet clover, turmeric, white willow.

Stability Store at controlled room temperature of 25°C (77°F); excursions permitted to 15°C to 30°C (59°F to 86°F).

Mechanism of Action Inhibits prostaglandin synthesis by decreasing the activity of the enzyme, cyclooxygenase-2 (COX-2), which results in decreased formation of prostaglandin precursors; has antipyretic, analgesic, and anti-inflammatory properties

Pharmacodynamics/Kinetics

Distribution: V_d (apparent): ~400 L

Protein binding: ~97% primarily to albumin

Metabolism: Hepatic via CYP2C9; forms inactive metabolites

Bioavailability: Absolute: Unknown

Half-life elimination: ~11 hours (fasted)

Time to peak: ~3 hours

Excretion: Feces (57% as metabolites, <3% as unchanged drug); urine (27% as metabolites, <3% as unchanged drug)

Dosage Note: Use the lowest effective dose for the shortest duration of time, consistent with individual patient goals. Oral:

Children ≥2 years: JRA:

- ≥10 kg to ≤25 kg: 50 mg twice daily
- >25 kg: 100 mg twice daily

Adults:

- Acute pain or primary dysmenorrhea: Initial dose: 400 mg, followed by an additional 200 mg if needed on day 1; maintenance dose: 200 mg twice daily as needed
- Ankylosing spondylitis: 200 mg/day as a single dose or in divided doses twice daily; if no effect after 6 weeks, may increase to 400 mg/day. If no response following 6 weeks of treatment with 400 mg/day, consider discontinuation and alternative treatment.
- Familial adenomatous polyposis: 400 mg twice daily
- Osteoarthritis: 200 mg/day as a single dose or in divided dose twice daily
- Rheumatoid arthritis: 100-200 mg twice daily

Elderly: No specific adjustment based on age is recommended. However, the AUC in elderly patients may be increased by 50% as compared to younger subjects. Initiate at the lowest recommended dose in patients weighing <50 kg.

Dosing adjustment in renal impairment: No specific dosage adjustment is recommended; not recommended in patients with severe renal dysfunction

Dosing adjustment in hepatic impairment: Reduced dosage is recommended (AUC may be increased by 40% to 180%); decrease dose by 50% in patients with moderate hepatic impairment (Child-Pugh class B). Not recommended for use with severe impairment.

Dietary Considerations Lower doses (200 mg twice daily) may be taken without regard to meals. Larger doses should be taken with food to improve absorption.

Administration Lower doses (200 mg twice daily) may be taken without regard to meals. Larger doses should be taken with food to improve absorption. Capsules may be swallowed whole or the entire contents emptied onto a teaspoon of cool or room temperature applesauce. The contents of the capsules sprinkled onto applesauce may be stored under refrigeration for up to 6 hours.

Monitoring Parameters CBC; blood chemistry profile; occult blood loss and periodic liver function tests; monitor renal function (urine output, serum BUN and creatinine; monitor response (pain, range of motion, grip strength, mobility, ADL function), inflammation; observe for weight gain, edema; observe for bleeding, bruising; evaluate gastrointestinal effects (abdominal pain, bleeding, dyspepsia); blood pressure

FAP: Continue routine endoscopic exams
JRA: Monitor for development of abnormal coagulation tests with systemic onset JRA

Additional Information Celecoxib does not inhibit cyclooxygenase-1 (COX-1) at therapeutic concentrations. Celecoxib does not affect platelet aggregation.

Dosage Forms Excipient information presented when available (limited, particularly for generics); consult specific product labeling.
Capsule:
Celebrex®: 50 mg, 100 mg, 200 mg, 400 mg

- ◆ **Celestone®** *see* Betamethasone *on page 184*
- ◆ **Celestone® Soluspan®** *see* Betamethasone *on page 184*
- ◆ **Celexa®** *see* Citalopram *on page 354*
- ◆ **CellCept®** *see* Mycophenolate *on page 1087*
- ◆ **Celontin®** *see* Methsuximide *on page 1019*
- ◆ **Cemill [OTC]** *see* Ascorbic Acid *on page 141*
- ◆ **Cenestin®** *see* Estrogens (Conjugated A/Synthetic) *on page 581*
- ◆ **Cenolate®** *see* Ascorbic Acid *on page 141*
- ◆ **Centany™ [DSC]** *see* Mupirocin *on page 1085*
- ◆ **Cephadyn** *see* Butalbital and Acetaminophen *on page 236*

Cephalexin (sef a LEKS in)

Medication Safety Issues
Sound-alike/look-alike issues:
Cephalexin may be confused with cefaclor, ceFAZolin, cephalothin, ciprofloxacin

U.S. Brand Names Keflex®

Canadian Brand Names Apo-Cephalex®; Keftab®; Novo-Lexin; Nu-Cephalex

Mexican Brand Names Cefalver; Ceporex; Keflex; Nafacil-S; Paferxin; Servicef

Index Terms Cephalexin Monohydrate

Pharmacologic Category Antibiotic, Cephalosporin (First Generation)

Use Treatment of susceptible bacterial infections including respiratory tract infections, otitis media, skin and skin structure infections, bone infections, and genitourinary tract infections, including acute prostatitis; alternative therapy for acute infective endocarditis prophylaxis

Effect on Mental Status May cause nervousness; case reports of euphoria, delusion, illusions, and depersonalization with cephalosporins

Effect on Psychiatric Treatment May rarely cause neutropenia; use caution with clozapine and carbamazepine

Dosage Summary

Oral:

Children ≤1 year: Dosage not established

Children >1-15 years: 25-100 mg/kg/day divided every 6-12 hours (maximum: 4 g/day) **or** 50 mg/kg prior to procedure (maximum: 2 g)

Adolescents >15 years: 25-100 mg/kg/day divided every 6-12 hours (maximum: 4 g/day) **or** 50 mg/kg prior to procedure (maximum: 2 g) **or** 500 mg every 12 hours (uncomplicated cystitis)

Adults: 250-1000 mg every 6 hours **or** 500 mg every 12 hours (maximum: 4 g/day) **or** 2 g prior to procedure

Dosage Forms Excipient information presented when available (limited, particularly for generics); consult specific product labeling.
Capsule: 250 mg, 500 mg
Keflex®: 250 mg, 500 mg, 750 mg
Powder for oral suspension: 125 mg/5 mL (100 mL, 200 mL); 250 mg/5 mL (100 mL, 200 mL)
Keflex®: 125 mg/5 mL (100 mL, 200 mL); 250 mg/5 mL (100 mL, 200 mL)
Tablet: 250 mg, 500 mg

- ◆ **Cephalexin Monohydrate** *see* Cephalexin *on page 306*
- ◆ **Cerebyx®** *see* Fosphenytoin *on page 692*
- ◆ **Cerezyme®** *see* Imiglucerase *on page 811*
- ◆ **Ceron** *see* Chlorpheniramine and Phenylephrine *on page 323*
- ◆ **Ceron-DM** *see* Chlorpheniramine, Phenylephrine, and Dextromethorphan *on page 327*

Certolizumab Pegol (cer to LIZ u mab PEG ol)

U.S. Brand Names Cimzia®

Index Terms CDP870

Pharmacologic Category Gastrointestinal Agent, Miscellaneous; Tumor Necrosis Factor (TNF) Blocking Agent

Use Treatment of moderately- to severely-active Crohn's disease in patients who have inadequate response to conventional therapy

Effect on Mental Status Headache is common; may cause dizziness

Effect on Psychiatric Treatment May cause neutropenia; use caution with clozapine, carbamazepine, and valproic acid. May cause GI side effects; concomitant use with SSRIs, lithium, carbamazepine, or valproic acid may produce additive effects.

Restrictions An FDA-approved medication guide is available, distribute to each patient to whom this medication is dispensed.

Dosage Summary

SubQ:

Children: Dosage not established

Adults: Initial: 400 mg, repeat dose 2 and 4 weeks after initial dose; Maintenance: 400 mg every 4 weeks

Dosage Forms Excipient information presented when available (limited, particularly for generics); consult specific product labeling.

Injection, powder for reconstitution:

Cimzia®: 200 mg [contains sterile water for reconstitution, syringes, and needles]

- **Certuss-D®** *see* Guaifenesin, Dextromethorphan, and Phenylephrine *on page 746*
- **Cerubidine®** *see* DAUNOrubicin Hydrochloride *on page 421*
- **Cervidil®** *see* Dinoprostone *on page 480*
- **C.E.S.** *see* Estrogens (Conjugated/Equine) *on page 582*
- **Cesamet®** *see* Nabilone *on page 1088*
- **Cesia™** *see* Ethinyl Estradiol and Desogestrel *on page 592*
- **Cetacort® [DSC]** *see* Hydrocortisone *on page 785*
- **Cetafen® [OTC]** *see* Acetaminophen *on page 30*
- **Cetafen Extra® [OTC]** *see* Acetaminophen *on page 30*

Cetirizine (se TI ra zeen)

Medication Safety Issues

Sound-alike/look-alike issues:

Zyrtec® may be confused with Serax®, Xanax®, Zantac®, Zyprexa®

U.S. Brand Names Zyrtec® Allergy [OTC]; Zyrtec® [OTC]; Zyrtec®, Children's Allergy [OTC]; Zyrtec®, Children's Hives Relief [OTC]

Canadian Brand Names Apo-Cetirizine®; Reactine™

Mexican Brand Names Cetitev; Reactine; Tradaxin

Index Terms Cetirizine Hydrochloride; P-071; UCB-P071

Pharmacologic Category Histamine H_1 Antagonist; Histamine H_1 Antagonist, Second Generation

Generic Available Yes

Use Perennial and seasonal allergic rhinitis and other allergic symptoms including urticaria; chronic idiopathic urticaria

Effect on Mental Status Drowsiness is common; may cause abnormal thinking, agitation, amnesia, anxiety, depersonalization, depression, emotional lability, euphoria, impaired concentration, insomnia, nervousness, paroniria, and sleep disturbances. May also cause aggressive reactions.

Effect on Psychiatric Treatment Concurrent use with psychotropics may produce additive sedation

Pregnancy Risk Factor B

Pregnancy Considerations Cetirizine was not shown to be teratogenic in animal studies; however, adequate studies have not been conducted in pregnant women. Use during pregnancy only if clearly needed.

Lactation Enters breast milk/not recommended

Contraindications Hypersensitivity to cetirizine, hydroxyzine, or any component of the formulation

Warnings/Precautions Cetirizine should be used cautiously in patients with hepatic or renal dysfunction; dosage adjustment recommended. Use with caution in the elderly; may be more sensitive to adverse effects. May cause drowsiness; use caution performing tasks which require alertness (eg, operating machinery or driving). Effects may be potentiated when used with other sedative drugs or ethanol. Safety and efficacy in pediatric patients <6 months of age have not been established.

Adverse Reactions

>10%: Central nervous system: Headache (children 11% to 14%, placebo 12%), somnolence (adults 14%, children 2% to 4%)

2% to 10%:

Central nervous system: Insomnia (children 9%, adults <2%), fatigue (adults 6%), malaise (4%), dizziness (adults 2%)

Gastrointestinal: Abdominal pain (children 4% to 6%), dry mouth (adults 5%), diarrhea (children 2% to 3%), nausea (children 2% to 3%, placebo 2%), vomiting (children 2% to 3%)

Respiratory: Epistaxis (children 2% to 4%, placebo 3%), pharyngitis (children 3% to 6%, placebo 3%), bronchospasm (children 2% to 3%, placebo 2%)

<2% (Limited to important or life-threatening; as reported in adults and/or children): Aggressive reaction, anaphylaxis, angioedema, ataxia, chest pain, confusion, convulsions, depersonalization, depression, edema, fussiness, hallucinations, hemolytic anemia, hepatitis, hypertension, hypotension (severe), irritability, liver function abnormal, nervousness, ototoxicity, palpitation, paralysis, paresthesia, photosensitivity, rash, suicidal ideation, suicide, taste perversion, tongue discoloration, tongue edema, tremor, visual field defect, weakness

Metabolism/Transport Effects Substrate of CYP3A4 (minor)

Drug Interactions

Acetylcholinesterase Inhibitors (Central): Anticholinergics may diminish the therapeutic effect of Acetylcholinesterase Inhibitors (Central). Acetylcholinesterase Inhibitors (Central) may diminish the therapeutic effect of Anticholinergics. If the anticholinergic action is a side effect of the agent, the result may be beneficial. *Risk C: Monitor therapy*

Alcohol (Ethyl): CNS Depressants may enhance the CNS depressant effect of Alcohol (Ethyl). *Risk C: Monitor therapy*

Amphetamines: May diminish the sedative effect of Antihistamines. *Risk C: Monitor therapy*

Anticholinergics: May enhance the adverse/toxic effect of other Anticholinergics. **Exceptions:** Paliperidone. *Risk C: Monitor therapy*

Betahistine: Antihistamines may diminish the therapeutic effect of Betahistine. *Risk C: Monitor therapy*

CNS Depressants: May enhance the adverse/toxic effect of other CNS Depressants. *Risk C: Monitor therapy*

P-Glycoprotein Inducers: May decrease the serum concentration of P-Glycoprotein Substrates. P-glycoprotein inducers may also further limit the distribution of p-glycoprotein substrates to specific cells/tissues/organs where p-glycoprotein is present in large amounts (e.g., brain, T-lymphocytes, testes, etc.). *Risk C: Monitor therapy*

P-Glycoprotein Inhibitors: May increase the serum concentration of P-Glycoprotein Substrates. P-glycoprotein inhibitors may also enhance the distribution of p-glycoprotein substrates to specific cells/tissues/organs where p-glycoprotein is present in large amounts (e.g., brain, T-lymphocytes, testes, etc.). *Risk C: Monitor therapy*

Pramlintide: May enhance the anticholinergic effect of Anticholinergics. These effects are specific to the GI tract. *Risk D: Consider therapy modification*

Ethanol/Nutrition/Herb Interactions Ethanol: Avoid ethanol (may increase CNS depression).

Stability

Syrup: Store at room temperature of 15°C to 30°C (59°F to 86°F), or under refrigeration at 2°C to 8°C (36°F to 46°F).

Tablet: Store at room temperature of 15°C to 30°C (59°F to 86°F).

Mechanism of Action Competes with histamine for H_1-receptor sites on effector cells in the gastrointestinal tract, blood vessels, and respiratory tract

Pharmacodynamics/Kinetics

Onset of action: 15-30 minutes

Absorption: Rapid

Protein binding, plasma: Mean: 93%

Metabolism: Limited hepatic

Half-life elimination: 8 hours

Time to peak, serum: 1 hour

Excretion: Urine (70%); feces (10%)

Dosage Oral:

Children:

6-12 months: Chronic urticaria, perennial allergic rhinitis: 2.5 mg once daily

12 months to <2 years: Chronic urticaria, perennial allergic rhinitis: 2.5 mg once daily; may increase to 2.5 mg every 12 hours if needed

2-5 years: Chronic urticaria, perennial or seasonal allergic rhinitis: Initial: 2.5 mg once daily; may be increased to 2.5 mg every 12 hours **or** 5 mg once daily

Children ≥6 years and Adults: Chronic urticaria, perennial or seasonal allergic rhinitis: 5-10 mg once daily, depending upon symptom severity

Elderly: Initial: 5 mg once daily; may increase to 10 mg/day. **Note:** Manufacturer recommends 5 mg/day in patients ≥77 years of age.

Dosage adjustment in renal/hepatic impairment:

Children <6 years: Cetirizine use not recommended

Children 6-11 years: <2.5 mg once daily

Children ≥12 and Adults:

Cl_{cr} 11-31 mL/minute, hemodialysis, or hepatic impairment: Administer 5 mg once daily

Cl_{cr} <11 mL/minute, not on dialysis: Cetirizine use not recommended

Dietary Considerations May be taken with or without food.

Administration May be administered with or without food.

Monitoring Parameters Relief of symptoms, sedation and anticholinergic effects

Dosage Forms Excipient information presented when available (limited, particularly for generics); consult specific product labeling. [DSC] = Discontinued product

Syrup, as hydrochloride: 5 mg/5 mL (120 mL, 473 mL)

Zyrtec®: 5 mg/5 mL (120 mL, 480 mL) [contains propylene glycol; banana-grape flavor]

Zyrtec®, Children's Allergy, Zyrtec®, Children's Hives Relief: 5 mg/5 mL (120 mL) [contains propylene glycol; grape flavor]

Tablet, as hydrochloride: 5 mg, 10 mg

Zyrtec®: 5 mg, 10 mg [DSC]

Zyrtec® Allergy: 10 mg

Tablet, chewable, as hydrochloride:

Zyrtec®: 5 mg, 10 mg [grape flavor] [DSC]

Zyrtec®, Children's Allergy: 5 mg, 10 mg [grape flavor]

Cetirizine and Pseudoephedrine

(se TI ra zeen & soo doe e FED rin)

Medication Safety Issues

Sound-alike/look-alike issues:

Zyrtec® may be confused with Serax®, Xanax®, Zantac®, Zyprexa®

U.S. Brand Names Zyrtec-D 12 Hour® [DSC]; Zytrec-D® Allergy & Congestion [OTC]

Canadian Brand Names Reactine® Allergy and Sinus

Mexican Brand Names Cipan; Virlix D; Zyrtec-D

Index Terms Cetirizine Hydrochloride and Pseudoephedrine Hydrochloride; Pseudoephedrine Hydrochloride and Cetirizine Hydrochloride

Pharmacologic Category Alpha/Beta Agonist; Histamine H_1 Antagonist; Histamine H_1 Antagonist, Second Generation

Use Treatment of symptoms of seasonal or perennial allergic rhinitis

Effect on Mental Status Drowsiness is common; may cause abnormal thinking, agitation, amnesia, anxiety, depersonalization, depression, emotional lability, euphoria, impaired concentration, insomnia, nervousness, paroniria, and sleep disturbances. May also cause aggressive reactions.

Effect on Psychiatric Treatment Contraindicated with MAO inhibitors or within 14 days of discontinuation of MAO inhibitors

Dosage Summary

Oral:

Children <12 years: Dosage not established

Children ≥12 years: 1 tablet twice daily

Adults: 1 tablet twice daily

Dosage Forms Excipient information presented when available (limited, particularly for generics); consult specific product labeling. [DSC] = Discontinued product

Tablet, extended release: Cetirizine hydrochloride 5 mg and pseudoephedrine hydrochloride 120 mg

Zyrtec-D 12 Hour® [DSC], Zytrec-D® Allergy & Congestion: Cetirizine hydrochloride 5 mg and pseudoephedrine hydrochloride 120 mg

◆ **Cetirizine Hydrochloride** *see* Cetirizine *on page 307*

- **Cetirizine Hydrochloride and Pseudoephedrine Hydrochloride** *see* Cetirizine and Pseudoephedrine *on page 309*

Cetuximab (se TUK see mab)

Medication Safety Issues
Sound-alike/look-alike issues:
Cetuximab may be confused with bevacizumab
U.S. Brand Names Erbitux®
Canadian Brand Names Erbitux®
Index Terms C225; IMC-C225; NSC-714692
Pharmacologic Category Antineoplastic Agent, Monoclonal Antibody; Epidermal Growth Factor Receptor (EGFR) Inhibitor
Use Treatment of metastatic colorectal cancer; treatment of squamous cell cancer of the head and neck
Unlabeled/Investigational Use Treatment of EGFR-expressing advanced nonsmall cell lung cancer (NSCLC)
Effect on Mental Status May cause malaise, insomnia, or depression
Effect on Psychiatric Treatment Gastrointestinal side effects are common; these effects may be additive with concurrent use of SSRIs, acetylcholinesterase inhibitors, aripiprazole, or ziprasidone. May cause anemia and leukopenia; use caution with clozapine and carbamazepine.
Dosage Summary
I.V.:
Children: Dosage not established
Adults: Loading dose: 400 mg/m^2; Maintenance: 250 mg/m^2 weekly
Dosage Forms Excipient information presented when available (limited, particularly for generics); consult specific product labeling.
Injection, solution [preservative free]:
Erbitux®: 2 mg/mL (50 mL, 100 mL)

Cevimeline (se vi ME leen)

Medication Safety Issues
Sound-alike/look-alike issues:
Evoxac® may be confused with Eurax®
U.S. Brand Names Evoxac®
Canadian Brand Names Evoxac®
Index Terms Cevimeline Hydrochloride
Pharmacologic Category Cholinergic Agonist
Use Treatment of symptoms of dry mouth in patients with Sjögren's syndrome
Effect on Mental Status May cause dizziness, insomnia, anxiety, and depression; rare reports of mania
Effect on Psychiatric Treatment Fluoxetine, nefazodone, and paroxetine may increase levels of cevimeline. TCAs, phenothiazine, clozapine, and olanzapine may antagonize the effects of cevimeline.
Dosage Summary
Oral:
Children: Dosage not established
Adults: 30 mg 3 times/day
Dosage Forms Excipient information presented when available (limited, particularly for generics); consult specific product labeling.
Capsule, as hydrochloride: 30 mg

- **Cevimeline Hydrochloride** *see* Cevimeline *on page 310*
- **CFDN** *see* Cefdinir *on page 293*
- **CG** *see* Chorionic Gonadotropin (Human) *on page 342*
- **C-Gel [OTC]** *see* Ascorbic Acid *on page 141*
- **CGP 33101** *see* Rufinamide *on page 1452*
- **CGP-42446** *see* Zoledronic Acid *on page 1702*
- **CGP-57148B** *see* Imatinib *on page 810*
- **C-Gram [OTC]** *see* Ascorbic Acid *on page 141*
- **CGS-20267** *see* Letrozole *on page 900*

Chamomile, German *(Matricaria chamomilla, Matricaria recutita)*

Natural Product Category Herb
Synonyms *Matricaria chamomilla, Matricaria recutita*

CHAMOMILE, GERMAN *(MATRICARIA CHAMOMILLA, MATRICARIA RECUTITA)*

Plant Part Flower

Dosage and Standardization

Oral: 400-1600 mg/day in divided doses, standardized to contain 1.2% apigenin and 0.5% essential oil per dose

Tea: 1 heaping teaspoonful of dried flowers in hot water; steep for 10 minutes, drink up to 3 times/day

Topical: Apply to affected area as needed

Reported Uses

Carminative, antispasmotic; insomnia (mild sedative); anxiolytic (Newall, 1996)
Colic (pharmacologic activity)
Common cold (Saller, 1990)
Diaper rash (pharmacologic activity)
Diarrhea (children); diarrhea (children, combination product) (Becker, 2006)
Indigestion (pharmacologic activity)
Minor injury (topical anti-inflammatory) (Bradley, 1992)
Nausea/vomiting (pharmacologic activity)
Oral health (as mouth rinse/gargle) (Bradley, 1992)
Stress/anxiety (pharmacologic activity)
Teething (pharmacologic activity)
Uterine tonic (Shipochiliev, 1981)
Vaginitis (Benetti, 1985)

Summary Chamomile has been used for centuries as a mild sedative and anxiolytic. In contrast to many anxiolytic agents, it does not generally cause drowsiness or motor impairment. Chamomile also has spasmolytic and anti-inflammatory properties which may contribute to its apparent value in relieving a number of gastrointestinal complaints.

Effect on Mental Status May cause sedation

Effect on Psychiatric Treatment Combined use with psychotropics may produce additive sedation

Pharmacology The sedative, spasmolytic, and anti-inflammatory activities of chamomile appear to be related to bisabolols, en-indicycloether, and flavonoids. In addition, azulene is claimed to inhibit histamine and serotonin release, which may decrease inflammation. Chamomile is considered a carminative (antiflatulent) agent. It has been used topically for a number of disorders, including acne, superficial infection, burns, and wounds. Chamomile also has been reported to have antibacterial activity against strains of *Staphylococcus, Streptococcus,* and *Candida* spp.

Theoretical Cautions and Contraindications Avoid use in individuals with allergies to members of the *Asteraceae/Compositae* family (chrysanthemum, daisy) or ragweed pollens (Subiza, 1989). Do not use in pregnancy and lactation (Bradley, 1992). Based on pharmacologic activity, may cause drowsiness in some individuals. Caution individuals to avoid hazardous tasks (eg, driving or operating machinery). Caution individuals taking sedative medications (eg, anxiolytics, benzodiazepines). Based on pharmacologic activity, this herb should be avoided in individuals with active bleeding (eg, peptic ulcer, intracranial bleeding). Use with caution in individuals with a history of bleeding, hemostatic disorders, or drug-related hemostatic problems. Use caution in individuals taking anticoagulant medications, including warfarin, aspirin or aspirin-containing products, NSAIDs, or antiplatelet agents (eg, ticlopidine, clopidogrel, dipyridamole). Discontinue use prior to dental or surgical procedures (generally at least 14 days before). Use with caution in individuals using cytochrome P450 metabolized agents.

General Warnings Use all herbal supplements with extreme caution in children <2 years of age and in pregnancy or lactation. Some herbs are contraindicated in pregnancy or lactation; make sure to observe warnings. Use with caution in individuals on medication and with pre-existing medical conditions. Always review for potential herb-drug interactions (HDIs) and other warnings. Large and prolonged doses may increase the potential for adverse effects. Herbs may cause transient adverse effects such as nausea, vomiting, and GI distress due to a variety of chemical constituents. Use caution in individuals having known allergies to plants.

Theoretical Interactions May increase effects of sedative medications (benzodiazepine, anxiolytics) and other herbs and natural products with this same effect.

In vitro data suggests this herb may inhibit the CYP3A4 isoenzyme. Theoretically, it may affect the disposition of the following medications: Protease inhibitors, cyclosporine, non-nucleoside reverse transcriptase inhibitors, certain benzodiazepines, calcium channel blockers, and other medications influenced by this enzyme system.

Anticoagulant medications (including warfarin), aspirin or asirin-containing products, NSAIDs, or antiplatelet agents (eg, ticlopidine, clopidogrel, dipyridamole)

References

Becker B, Kuhn U, and Hardewig-Budny B, "Double-Blind, Randomized Evaluation of Clinical Efficacy and Tolerability of an Apple Pectin-Chamomile Extract in Children With Unspecific Diarrhea," *Arzneimittelforschung*, 2006, 56(6):387-93.

Benetti C and Manganelli F, "Clinical Experiences in the Pharmacological Treatment of Vaginitis With a Camomile-Extract Vaginal Douche," *Minerva Ginecol*, 1985, 37 (12):799-801.

Bradley PR, ed, *British Herbal Compendium*, Vol 1, Bournemouth, England: British Herbal Medicine Association, 1992, 154-7.

Natural Standard Research Collaboration, Chief Editors: Ulbricht C, Basch E, *Natural Standard Herb and Supplement Reference - Evidence-Based Clinical Reviews*, USA: Elsevier/Mosby, 2005.

Newall CA, Anderson LA, and Phillipson JD, *Herbal Medicines: A Guide for Health Care Professionals*, London, England: The Pharmaceutical Press, 1996, 69-71.

Saller R, Beschomer M, Hellenbrecht D, et al, "Dose Dependency of Symptomatic Relief of Complaints by Chamomile Steam Inhalation in Patients With Common Cold," *Eur J Pharmacol*, 1990, 183:728-9.

Shipochiliev T, "Extracts From a Group of Medicinal Plants Enhancing Uterine Tonus," *Vet Med Nauk*, 1981, 18:94-8.

Subiza J, Subiza JL, Hinojosa M, et al, "Anaphylactic Reaction After Ingestion of Chamomile Tea: A Study of Cross-Reactivity With Other Composite Pollens," *Clin Immunol*, 1989, 84 (3):353-8.

◆ **Chantix®** *see* Varenicline *on page 1656*

◆ **Char-Caps [OTC]** *see* Charcoal *on page 312*

◆ **CharcoAid® G [OTC]** *see* Charcoal *on page 312*

Charcoal (CHAR kole AK tiv ay ted)

Medication Safety Issues

Sound-alike/look-alike issues:

Actidose® may be confused with Actos®

U.S. Brand Names Actidose-Aqua® [OTC]; Actidose® with Sorbitol [OTC]; Char-Caps [OTC]; CharcoAid® G [OTC]; Charcoal Plus® DS [OTC]; Charco-Caps® [OTC]; EZ-Char™ [OTC]; Kerr Insta-Char® [OTC]; Requa® Activated Charcoal [OTC]

Canadian Brand Names Charcadole®; Charcadole® TFS; Charcadole® Aqueous

Mexican Brand Names Carbotural

Index Terms Activated Carbon; Activated Charcoal; Adsorbent Charcoal; Liquid Antidote; Medicinal Carbon; Medicinal Charcoal

Pharmacologic Category Antidote

Use Emergency treatment in poisoning by drugs and chemicals; aids the elimination of certain drugs and improves decontamination of excessive ingestions of sustained-release products or in the presence of bezoars; repetitive doses have proven useful to enhance the elimination of certain drugs (eg, carbamazepine, dapsone, phenobarbital, quinine, or theophylline); repetitive doses for gastric dialysis in uremia to adsorb various waste products; dietary supplement (digestive aid)

Effect on Mental Status None reported

Effect on Psychiatric Treatment Does not effectively remove lithium

Dosage Summary Note: ~10 g of activated charcoal for each 1 g of toxin is considered adequate

Oral:

Children <1 year: 10-25 g **or** 0.5-1 g/kg as a single dose; additional doses can be given as 0.25 g/kg/hour or equivalent

Children 1-12 years: 25-50 g **or** 0.5-1 g/kg as a single dose; additional doses can be given as 0.25 g/kg/hour or equivalent

Children >12 years: 25-100 g **or** 1 g/kg as a single dose, additional doses can be given as 12.5 g/hour (0.25 g/kg/hour) or equivalent

Adults:

Acute poisoning: 25-100 mg as a single dose, additional doses can be given as 12.5 g/hour or equivalent

Dietary supplement: 500-520 mg after meals, may repeat in 2 hours (maximum: 10 g/day)

Dosage Forms Excipient information presented when available (limited, particularly for generics); consult specific product labeling.

Capsule:

Char-Caps, CharcoCaps®: 260 mg

Pellets, for suspension:
EZ-Char™: 25 g
Powder for suspension: 30 g, 240 g
CharcoAid® G: 15 g
Suspension:
Actidose-Aqua®: 15 g (72 mL); 25 g (120 mL); 50 g (240 mL)
Kerr Insta-Char®: 25 g (120 mL) [contains sodium benzoate; packaged with cherry flavor (cherry flavor contains propylene glycol and sodium benzoate)]; 50 g (240 mL) [contains sodium benzoate; unflavored or packaged with cherry flavor (cherry flavor contains propylene glycol and sodium benzoate)]
Suspension [with sorbitol]:
Actidose® with Sorbitol: 25 g (120 mL); 50 g (240 mL)
Kerr Insta-Char®: 25 g (120 mL) [contains sodium benzoate; packaged with cherry flavor (cherry flavor contains propylene glycol and sodium benzoate)]; 50 g (240 mL) [contains sodium benzoate; packaged with cherry flavor (cherry flavor contains propylene glycol and sodium benzoate)]
Tablet:
Requa® Activated Charcoal: 250 mg
Tablet, enteric coated:
Charcoal Plus® DS: 250 mg

- **Charcoal Plus® DS [OTC]** *see* Charcoal *on page 312*
- **CharcoCaps® [OTC]** *see* Charcoal *on page 312*
- **Chemet®** *see* Succimer *on page 1511*
- **Cheracol®** *see* Guaifenesin and Codeine *on page 738*
- **Cheracol® D [OTC]** *see* Guaifenesin and Dextromethorphan *on page 739*
- **Cheracol® Plus [OTC]** *see* Guaifenesin and Dextromethorphan *on page 739*
- **Chew-C [OTC]** *see* Ascorbic Acid *on page 141*
- **Children's Pepto [OTC]** *see* Calcium Carbonate *on page 254*
- **Children's Tylenol® Plus Cold and Allergy [OTC]** *see* Acetaminophen, Diphenhydramine, and Phenylephrine *on page 44*
- **Chinese Ephedra** *see* Ephedra *(Ephedra sinica) on page 541*
- **Chinese Joint Fir** *see* Ephedra *(Ephedra sinica) on page 541*
- **Chirocaine® [DSC]** *see* Levobupivacaine *on page 908*
- **Chloral** *see* Chloral Hydrate *on page 313*

Chloral Hydrate (KLOR al HYE drate)

Medication Safety Issues
High alert medication: The Institute for Safe Medication Practices (ISMP) includes this medication among its list of drugs which have a heightened risk of causing significant patient harm when used in error.

Related Information
CMS: Long-Term Care Facility Thresholds *on page 1815*
Nonbenzodiazepine Anxiolytics and Hypnotics *on page 1791*

U.S. Brand Names Aquachloral® Supprettes® [DSC]; Somnote®

Canadian Brand Names PMS-Chloral Hydrate

Index Terms Chloral; Hydrated Chloral; Trichloroacetaldehyde Monohydrate

Pharmacologic Category Hypnotic, Nonbenzodiazepine

Generic Available Yes: Syrup and suppositories

Use Short-term sedative and hypnotic (<2 weeks); sedative/hypnotic for diagnostic procedures; sedative prior to EEG evaluations

Restrictions C-IV

Pregnancy Risk Factor C

Lactation Enters breast milk/compatible

Contraindications Hypersensitivity to chloral hydrate or any component of the formulation; hepatic or renal impairment; gastritis or ulcers; severe cardiac disease

Warnings/Precautions Use with caution in patients with porphyria. Use with caution in neonates. Drug may accumulate with repeated use; prolonged use in neonates associated with hyperbilirubinemia. Tolerance to hypnotic effect develops, therefore, not recommended for use >2 weeks. Taper dosage to avoid withdrawal with prolonged use. Trichloroethanol (TCE), a metabolite of chloral hydrate, is a carcinogen in mice; there is no data in humans. Chloral hydrate is considered a second line hypnotic agent in the elderly. Recent interpretive guidelines from the Centers for Medicare and Medicaid Services

(CMS) discourage the use of chloral hydrate in residents of long-term care facilities.

Adverse Reactions Frequency not defined.

Central nervous system: Ataxia, disorientation, sedation, excitement (paradoxical), dizziness, fever, headache, confusion, lightheadedness, nightmares, hallucinations, drowsiness, "hangover" effect

Dermatologic: Rash, urticaria

Gastrointestinal: Gastric irritation, nausea, vomiting, diarrhea, flatulence

Hematologic: Leukopenia, eosinophilia, acute intermittent porphyria

Miscellaneous: Physical and psychological dependence may occur with prolonged use of large doses

Drug Interactions

Alcohol (Ethyl): CNS Depressants may enhance the CNS depressant effect of Alcohol (Ethyl). *Risk C: Monitor therapy*

CNS Depressants: May enhance the adverse/toxic effect of other CNS Depressants. *Risk C: Monitor therapy*

Flumazenil: May diminish the sedative effect of Hypnotics (Nonbenzodiazepine). *Risk C: Monitor therapy*

Ethanol/Nutrition/Herb Interactions

Ethanol: Avoid ethanol (may increase CNS depression).

Herb/Nutraceutical: Avoid valerian, St John's wort, kava kava, gotu kola (may increase CNS depression).

Stability Sensitive to light. Exposure to air causes volatilization. Store in light-resistant, airtight container.

Mechanism of Action Central nervous system depressant effects are due to its active metabolite trichloroethanol, mechanism unknown

Pharmacodynamics/Kinetics

Onset of action: Time to sleep: 0.5-1 hour

Duration: 4-8 hours

Absorption: Oral, rectal: Well absorbed

Distribution: Crosses placenta; negligible amounts enter breast milk

Metabolism: Rapidly hepatic to trichloroethanol (active metabolite); variable amounts hepatically and renally to trichloroacetic acid (inactive)

Half-life elimination: Active metabolite: 8-11 hours

Excretion: Urine (as metabolites); feces (small amounts)

Dosage

Children:

Sedation or anxiety: Oral, rectal: 5-15 mg/kg/dose every 8 hours (maximum: 500 mg/dose)

Prior to EEG: Oral, rectal: 20-25 mg/kg/dose, 30-60 minutes prior to EEG; may repeat in 30 minutes to maximum of 100 mg/kg or 2 g total

Hypnotic: Oral, rectal: 20-40 mg/kg/dose up to a maximum of 50 mg/kg/24 hours or 1 g/dose or 2 g/24 hours

Conscious sedation: Oral: 50-75 mg/kg/dose 30-60 minutes prior to procedure; may repeat 30 minutes after initial dose if needed, to a total maximum dose of 120 mg/kg or 1 g total

Adults: Oral, rectal:

Sedation, anxiety: 250 mg 3 times/day

Hypnotic: 500-1000 mg at bedtime or 30 minutes prior to procedure, not to exceed 2 g/24 hours

Discontinuation: Withdraw gradually over 2 weeks if patient has been maintained on high doses for prolonged period of time. Do not stop drug abruptly; sudden withdrawal may result in delirium.

Dosing adjustment/comments in renal impairment: Cl_{cr} <50 mL/minute: Avoid use

Hemodialysis: Dialyzable (50% to 100%); supplemental dose is not necessary

Dosing adjustment/comments in hepatic impairment: Avoid use in patients with severe hepatic impairment

Administration Chilling the syrup may help to mask unpleasant taste. Do not crush capsule (contains drug in liquid form). Gastric irritation may be minimized by diluting dose in water or other oral liquid.

Monitoring Parameters Vital signs, O_2 saturation and blood pressure with doses used for conscious sedation

Test Interactions False-positive urine glucose using Clinitest® method; may interfere with fluorometric urine catecholamine and urinary 17-hydroxycorticosteroid tests

Additional Information Not an analgesic

Dosage Forms Excipient information presented when available (limited, particularly for generics); consult specific product labeling. [DSC] = Discontinued product

Capsule:
Somnote®: 500 mg
Suppository, rectal: 500 mg
Aquachloral® Supprettes®: 325 mg [contains tartrazine] [DSC]
Syrup: 500 mg/5 mL (5 mL, 480 mL)

Chlorambucil (klor AM byoo sil)

Medication Safety Issues
Sound-alike/look-alike issues:
Chlorambucil may be confused with Chloromycetin®
Leukeran® may be confused with Alkeran®, leucovorin, Leukine®, Myleran®

High alert medication: The Institute for Safe Medication Practices (ISMP) includes this medication among its list of drugs which have a heightened risk of causing significant patient harm when used in error.

U.S. Brand Names Leukeran®

Canadian Brand Names Leukeran®

Mexican Brand Names Leukeran

Index Terms CB-1348; Chlorambucilum; Chloraminophene; Chlorbutinum; NSC-3088; WR-139013

Pharmacologic Category Antineoplastic Agent, Alkylating Agent

Use Management of chronic lymphocytic leukemia (CLL), Hodgkin's lymphoma, non-Hodgkin's lymphoma (NHL)

Unlabeled/Investigational Use Nephrotic syndrome, Waldenström's macroglobulinemia

Effect on Mental Status May rarely produce agitation, confusion, and hallucinations

Effect on Psychiatric Treatment Myelosuppression is common; use caution with clozapine and carbamazepine

Dosage Summary
Oral:
Children (unlabeled uses): 0.03-0.2 mg/kg/day **or** 0.4 mg/kg every 2 weeks, increasing by 0.1 mg/kg every 2 weeks until response **or** 0.4 mg/kg once a month, increasing by 0.1 mg/kg each month until response
Adults: 0.1-0.2 mg/kg/day for 3-6 weeks **or** 0.4 mg/kg biweekly or monthly (may increase by 0.1 mg/kg/dose) **or** 0.03-0.1 mg/kg/day
Elderly: Use lowest recommended dose; usual dose: 2-4 mg/day

Dosage Forms Excipient information presented when available (limited, particularly for generics); consult specific product labeling.
Tablet:
Leukeran®: 2 mg

◆ **Chlorambucilum** *see* Chlorambucil *on page 315*
◆ **Chloraminophene** *see* Chlorambucil *on page 315*

Chloramphenicol (klor am FEN i kole)

Medication Safety Issues
Sound-alike/look-alike issues:
Chloromycetin® may be confused with chlorambucil, Chlor-Trimeton®

Canadian Brand Names Chloromycetin®; Chloromycetin® Succinate; Diochloram®; Pentamycetin®

Mexican Brand Names Cloramfeni Ofteno; Cloran; Clordil; Exacol; Oftadil; Westenicol

Pharmacologic Category Antibiotic, Miscellaneous

Use Treatment of serious infections due to organisms resistant to other less toxic antibiotics or when its penetrability into the site of infection is clinically superior to other antibiotics to which the organism is sensitive; useful in infections caused by *Bacteroides*, *H. influenzae*, *Neisseria meningitidis*, *Salmonella*, and *Rickettsia*; active against many vancomycin-resistant enterococci

Effect on Mental Status May rarely cause nightmares

Effect on Psychiatric Treatment May cause bone marrow suppression; use caution with clozapine and carbamazepine

Dosage Summary
I.V.:
Neonates: Loading dose: 20 mg/kg, followed by maintenance dose based on postnatal age:
≤7 days: 25 mg/kg/day once every 24 hours
>7 days, ≤2000 g: 25 mg/kg/day once every 24 hours
>7 days, >2000 g: 50 mg/kg/day divided every 12 hours

Infants >30 days and Children: 50-100 mg/kg/day divided every 6 hours (maximum: 4 g/day)

Adults: 50-100 mg/kg/day divided every 6 hours (maximum: 4 g/day)

Dosage Forms Excipient information presented when available (limited, particularly for generics); consult specific product labeling.

Injection, powder for reconstitution: 1 g [contains sodium ~52 mg/g (2.25 mEq/g)]

◆ **Chlorbutinum** *see* Chlorambucil *on page 315*

◆ **Chlordex GP** *see* Dextromethorphan, Chlorpheniramine, Phenylephrine, and Guaifenesin *on page 450*

ChlordiazePOXIDE (klor dye az e POKS ide)

Medication Safety Issues

Sound-alike/look-alike issues:

ChlordiazePOXIDE may be confused with chlorproMAZINE

Librium® may be confused with Librax®

Related Information

Benzodiazepines *on page 1774*

CMS: Long-Term Care Facility Thresholds *on page 1815*

Discontinuation of Psychotropic Drugs *on page 1839*

U.S. Brand Names Librium®

Canadian Brand Names Apo-Chlordiazepoxide®

Index Terms Methaminodiazepoxide Hydrochloride

Pharmacologic Category Benzodiazepine

Generic Available Yes: Capsule

Use Management of anxiety disorder or for the short-term relief of symptoms of anxiety; withdrawal symptoms of acute alcoholism; preoperative apprehension and anxiety

Mental Health Comment In 2007, the FDA requested that all manufacturers of sedative-hypnotic drug products revise labeling to include a greater emphasis on the risks of adverse effects. These risks include severe allergic reactions (anaphylaxis, angioedema) and complex sleep-related behaviors, which may include sleep-driving (driving while not fully awake and with no memory of the event), making phone calls, and preparing and eating food while asleep.

There are two subtypes of GABA receptors (GABA-A and GABA-B) and three different benzodiazepine receptors (Bz_1, Bz_2, and Bz_3). Benzodiazepine receptors and effects appear to be linked to the GABA-A receptors. Benzodiazepines do not bind to GABA-B receptors. The role of GABA-B receptors is unclear. Benzodiazepines have no specificity for benzodiazepine receptor subtypes.

Chlordiazepoxide is poorly and erratically absorbed after I.M. administration; undergoes phase I metabolism. Chlordiazepoxide is a long half-life benzodiazepine. Duration of action after a single dose is determined by redistribution rather than metabolism. Tolerance develops to the sedative, hypnotic, and anticonvulsant effects. It does not develop to the anxiolytic or skeletal muscle-relaxing effects. Psychological and physical dependence may occur with prolonged use of benzodiazepines. The onset of withdrawal symptoms is usually seen on the first day without drug and lasts 5-7 days in patients receiving short half-life benzodiazepines, whereas, the onset occurs after 5 days with a duration of 10-14 days after abrupt discontinuance of long half-life benzodiazepines. Risk factors for abuse include personal or family history of substance abuse and personality disorder.

Restrictions C-IV

Pregnancy Risk Factor D

Lactation Enters breast milk/not recommended

Contraindications Hypersensitivity to chlordiazepoxide or any component of the formulation (cross-sensitivity with other benzodiazepines may also exist); narrow-angle glaucoma; pregnancy

Warnings/Precautions Active metabolites with extended half-lives may lead to delayed accumulation and adverse effects. Use with caution in elderly or debilitated patients, pediatric patients, patients with hepatic disease (including alcoholics) or renal impairment, patients with respiratory disease or impaired gag reflex, patients with porphyria.

Parenteral administration should be avoided in comatose patients or shock. Adequate resuscitative equipment/personnel should be available, and appropriate monitoring should be conducted at the time of injection and for several hours following administration. The parenteral formulation should be diluted for

I.M. administration with the supplied diluent only. This diluent should not be used when preparing the drug for intravenous administration.

Causes CNS depression (dose related) resulting in sedation, dizziness, confusion, or ataxia which may impair physical and mental capabilities. Patients must be cautioned about performing tasks which require mental alertness (eg, operating machinery or driving). Use with caution in patients receiving other CNS depressants or psychoactive agents (lithium, phenothiazines). Effects with other sedative drugs or ethanol may be potentiated. Benzodiazepines have been associated with falls and traumatic injury and should be used with extreme caution in patients who are at risk of these events (especially the elderly).

Use caution in patients with depression, particularly if suicidal risk may be present. Use with caution in patients with a history of drug dependence. Benzodiazepines have been associated with dependence and acute withdrawal symptoms on discontinuation or reduction in dose. Acute withdrawal, including seizures, may be precipitated in patients after administration of flumazenil to patients receiving long-term benzodiazepine therapy.

Benzodiazepines have been associated with anterograde amnesia. Paradoxical reactions, including hyperactive or aggressive behavior have been reported with benzodiazepines, particularly in adolescent/pediatric or psychiatric patients. Does not have analgesic, antidepressant, or antipsychotic properties.

Adverse Reactions

>10%:

Central nervous system: Drowsiness, fatigue, ataxia, lightheadedness, memory impairment, dysarthria, irritability

Dermatologic: Rash

Endocrine & metabolic: Libido decreased, menstrual disorders

Gastrointestinal: Xerostomia, salivation decreased, appetite increased or decreased, weight gain/loss

Genitourinary: Micturition difficulties

1% to 10%:

Cardiovascular: Hypotension

Central nervous system: Confusion, dizziness, disinhibition, akathisia

Dermatologic: Dermatitis

Endocrine & metabolic: Libido increased

Gastrointestinal: Salivation increased

Genitourinary: Sexual dysfunction, incontinence

Neuromuscular & skeletal: Rigidity, tremor, muscle cramps

Otic: Tinnitus

Respiratory: Nasal congestion

<1% (Limited to important or life-threatening): Photosensitivity

Metabolism/Transport Effects **Substrate** of CYP3A4 (major)

Drug Interactions

Alcohol (Ethyl): CNS Depressants may enhance the CNS depressant effect of Alcohol (Ethyl). *Risk C: Monitor therapy*

Antifungal Agents (Azole Derivatives, Systemic): May decrease the metabolism of Benzodiazepines (metabolized by oxidation). *Risk D: Consider therapy modification*

Aprepitant: May increase the serum concentration of Benzodiazepines (metabolized by oxidation). *Risk C: Monitor therapy*

Calcium Channel Blockers (Nondihydropyridine): May decrease the metabolism of Benzodiazepines (metabolized by oxidation). *Risk D: Consider therapy modification*

CarBAMazepine: May increase the metabolism of Benzodiazepines (metabolized by oxidation). *Risk C: Monitor therapy*

Cimetidine: May decrease the metabolism of Benzodiazepines (metabolized by oxidation). *Risk C: Monitor therapy*

Clozapine: Benzodiazepines may enhance the adverse/toxic effect of Clozapine. *Risk D: Consider therapy modification*

CNS Depressants: May enhance the adverse/toxic effect of other CNS Depressants. *Risk C: Monitor therapy*

CYP3A4 Inducers (Strong): May increase the metabolism of CYP3A4 Substrates. *Risk C: Monitor therapy*

CYP3A4 Inhibitors (Moderate): May decrease the metabolism of CYP3A4 Substrates. *Risk C: Monitor therapy*

CYP3A4 Inhibitors (Strong): May decrease the metabolism of CYP3A4 Substrates. *Risk D: Consider therapy modification*

Dasatinib: May increase the serum concentration of CYP3A4 Substrates. *Risk C: Monitor therapy*

Deferasirox: May decrease the serum concentration of CYP3A4 Substrates. *Risk C: Monitor therapy*

Disulfiram: May decrease the metabolism of Benzodiazepines (metabolized by oxidation). *Risk C: Monitor therapy*

Fluconazole: May decrease the metabolism of Benzodiazepines (metabolized by oxidation). *Risk D: Consider therapy modification*

Fosaprepitant: May increase the serum concentration of Benzodiazepines (metabolized by oxidation). Specifically, the active metabolite aprepitant is likely responsible for this effect. *Risk C: Monitor therapy*

Grapefruit Juice: May decrease the metabolism of Benzodiazepines (metabolized by oxidation). *Risk D: Consider therapy modification*

Isoniazid: May decrease the metabolism of Benzodiazepines (metabolized by oxidation). *Risk C: Monitor therapy*

Macrolide Antibiotics: May decrease the metabolism of Benzodiazepines (metabolized by oxidation). **Exceptions:** Azithromycin; Dirithromycin [Off Market]; Spiramycin. *Risk D: Consider therapy modification*

Nefazodone: May decrease the metabolism of Benzodiazepines (metabolized by oxidation). *Risk D: Consider therapy modification*

Oral Contraceptive (Estrogens): May decrease the metabolism of Benzodiazepines (metabolized by oxidation). *Risk C: Monitor therapy*

Oral Contraceptive (Progestins): May decrease the metabolism of Benzodiazepines (metabolized by oxidation). *Risk C: Monitor therapy*

Phenytoin: Benzodiazepines may increase the serum concentration of Phenytoin. Short-term exposure to benzodiazepines may not present as much risk as chronic therapy. *Risk C: Monitor therapy*

Protease Inhibitors: May decrease the metabolism of Benzodiazepines (metabolized by oxidation). Management: Amprenavir, atazanavir, darunavir, indinavir, nelfinavir, ritonavir, and tipranavir are contraindicated with midazolam and triazolam according to each protease inhibitor 's prescribing information. *Risk D: Consider therapy modification*

Proton Pump Inhibitors: May increase the serum concentration of Benzodiazepines (metabolized by oxidation). **Exceptions:** Lansoprazole; Pantoprazole; Rabeprazole. *Risk C: Monitor therapy*

Rifamycin Derivatives: May increase the metabolism of Benzodiazepines (metabolized by oxidation). *Risk D: Consider therapy modification*

Selective Serotonin Reuptake Inhibitors: May decrease the metabolism of Benzodiazepines (metabolized by oxidation). **Exceptions:** Citalopram; Escitalopram; PARoxetine; Sertraline. *Risk C: Monitor therapy*

St Johns Wort: May increase the metabolism of Benzodiazepines (metabolized by oxidation). *Risk C: Monitor therapy*

Theophylline Derivatives: May diminish the therapeutic effect of Benzodiazepines. *Risk D: Consider therapy modification*

Ethanol/Nutrition/Herb Interactions

Ethanol: Avoid ethanol (may increase CNS depression).

Food: Serum concentrations/effects may be increased with grapefruit juice, but unlikely because of high oral bioavailability of chlordiazepoxide.

Herb/Nutraceutical: Avoid valerian, St John's wort, kava kava, gotu kola (may increase CNS depression).

Stability Injection: Prior to reconstitution, store under refrigeration and protect from light. Solution should be used immediately following reconstitution.

I.M. use: Reconstitute by adding 2 mL of provided diluent; agitate gently until dissolved. Provided diluent is **not** for I.V. use.

I.V. use: Reconstitute by adding 5 mL NS or SWFI; agitate gently until dissolved; **do not administer this dilution I.M.**

Mechanism of Action Binds to stereospecific benzodiazepine receptors on the postsynaptic GABA neuron at several sites within the central nervous system, including the limbic system, reticular formation. Enhancement of the inhibitory effect of GABA on neuronal excitability results by increased neuronal membrane permeability to chloride ions. This shift in chloride ions results in hyperpolarization (a less excitable state) and stabilization.

Pharmacodynamics/Kinetics

Distribution: V_d: 3.3 L/kg; crosses placenta; enters breast milk

Protein binding: 90% to 98%

Metabolism: Extensively hepatic to desmethyldiazepam (active and long-acting)

Half-life elimination: 6.6-25 hours; End-stage renal disease: 5-30 hours; Cirrhosis: 30-63 hours

Time to peak, serum: Oral: Within 2 hours; I.M.: Results in lower peak plasma levels than oral

Excretion: Urine (minimal as unchanged drug)

Dosage

Children:

<6 years: Not recommended

>6 years: Anxiety: Oral, I.M.: 0.5 mg/kg/24 hours divided every 6-8 hours

Adults:

Anxiety:

Oral: 15-100 mg divided 3-4 times/day

I.M., I.V.: Initial: 50-100 mg followed by 25-50 mg 3-4 times/day as needed

Preoperative anxiety: I.M.: 50-100 mg prior to surgery

Ethanol withdrawal symptoms: Oral, I.V.: 50-100 mg to start, dose may be repeated in 2-4 hours as necessary to a maximum of 300 mg/24 hours

Note: Up to 300 mg may be given I.M. or I.V. during a 6-hour period, but not more than this in any 24-hour period.

Dosing adjustment in renal impairment: Cl_{cr} <10 mL/minute: Administer 50% of dose

Hemodialysis: Not dialyzable (0% to 5%)

Dosing adjustment/comments in hepatic impairment: Avoid use

Administration

I.M.: Administer by deep I.M. injection slowly into the upper outer quadrant of the gluteus muscle. Use only the diluent provided for I.M. use. Solutions made with SWFI or NS cause pain with I.M. administration.

I.V.: Administer slowly over at least 1 minute. Do not use the diluent provided for I.M. use. Air bubbles form during reconstitution.

Monitoring Parameters Respiratory and cardiovascular status, mental status, check for orthostasis

Reference Range Therapeutic: 0.1-3 mcg/mL (SI: 0-10 µmol/L); Toxic: >23 mcg/mL (SI: >77 µmol/L)

Additional Information Abrupt discontinuation after sustained use (generally >10 days) may cause withdrawal symptoms.

Dosage Forms Excipient information presented when available (limited, particularly for generics); consult specific product labeling.

Capsule, as hydrochloride: 5 mg, 10 mg, 25 mg

Injection, powder for reconstitution, as hydrochloride: 100 mg [diluent contains benzyl alcohol, polysorbate 80, and propylene glycol]

- **Chlordiazepoxide and Amitriptyline Hydrochloride** *see* Amitriptyline and Chlordiazepoxide *on page 94*
- **Chlordiazepoxide and Clidinium** *see* Clidinium and Chlordiazepoxide *on page 362*

Chlordiazepoxide and Methscopolamine

(klor dye az e POKS ide & meth skoe POL a meen)

Medication Safety Issues

Librax® formulation may be cause for confusion:

In November 2004, Valeant Pharmaceuticals licensed the Librax® trademark to Victory Pharmaceuticals. Subsequently, the product was reformulated to contain chlordiazepoxide and methscopolamine. In January 2006, Valeant Pharmaceuticals began redistributing the original formulation of Librax®, containing clidinium and chlordiazepoxide. Victory Pharmaceuticals has discontinued their product. **Note:** The formulation of Librax® distributed in Canada (Valeant Canada Ltd) always contained clidinium and chlordiazepoxide.

U.S. Brand Names Librax® *[reformulation]* [DSC]

Index Terms Methscopolamine Nitrate and Chlordiazepoxide Hydrochloride

Pharmacologic Category Anticholinergic Agent; Benzodiazepine

Use Adjunctive treatment of peptic ulcer; treatment of irritable bowel syndrome, acute enterocolitis

Effect on Mental Status Sedation is common; may cause dizziness, confusion, amnesia, and insomnia. May rarely be associated with paradoxical reactions that include hyperactive and aggressive behaviors.

Effect on Psychiatric Treatment Concomitant use with psychotropic agents may produce additive sedative and anticholinergic effects; enzyme inducers (carbamazepine) may decrease the therapeutic effects and inhibitors (nefazodone) may enhance therapeutic effects.

Mental Health Comment In 2007, the FDA requested that all manufacturers of sedative-hypnotic drug products revise labeling to include a greater emphasis on the risks of adverse effects. These risks include severe allergic reactions (anaphylaxis, angioedema) and complex sleep-related behaviors, which may include sleep-driving (driving while not fully awake and with no memory of the event), making phone calls, and preparing and eating food while asleep.

Risk factors for abuse include personal or family history of substance abuse and personality disorder.

Restrictions C-IV

Dosage Summary

Oral:

Children: Dosage not established

Adults: 1-2 capsules 3-4 times/day

Elderly: Initial: Do not exceed 2 capsules/day

Dosage Forms Excipient information presented when available (limited, particularly for generics); consult specific product labeling.

Capsule: Chlordiazepoxide hydrochloride 5 mg and methscopolamine nitrate 2.5 mg [DSC]

- **Chlorethazine** *see* Mechlorethamine *on page 974*
- **Chlorethazine Mustard** *see* Mechlorethamine *on page 974*
- **Chlorex-A** *see* Chlorpheniramine, Phenylephrine, and Phenyltoloxamine *on page 331*
- **Chlorex-A 12 [DSC]** *see* Chlorpheniramine, Pyrilamine, and Phenylephrine *on page 335*
- **Chlormeprazine** *see* Prochlorperazine *on page 1341*
- **Chlor-Mes** *see* Chlorpheniramine, Phenylephrine, and Methscopolamine *on page 329*
- **Chlor-Mes-D** *see* Chlorpheniramine, Phenylephrine, and Methscopolamine *on page 329*
- **2-Chlorodeoxyadenosine** *see* Cladribine *on page 360*
- **Chloromag®** *see* Magnesium Chloride *on page 965*

Chloroquine Phosphate (KLOR oh kwin FOS fate)

Medication Safety Issues

International issues:

Aralen® may be confused with Oralon® which is a brand name for povidone iodine in Japan

Aralen® may be confused with Paralen® which is a brand name fo acetaminophen in the Czech Republic

U.S. Brand Names Aralen®

Canadian Brand Names Aralen®; Novo-Chloroquine

Mexican Brand Names Aralen

Index Terms Chloroquine Phosphate

Pharmacologic Category Aminoquinoline (Antimalarial)

Use Suppression or chemoprophylaxis of malaria; treatment of uncomplicated c mild-to-moderate malaria; extraintestinal amebiasis

Unlabeled/Investigational Use Rheumatoid arthritis; discoid lupu erythematosus

Effect on Mental Status May cause psychosis, delirium, personality change and depression

Effect on Psychiatric Treatment May cause blood dyscrasias; use cautio with clozapine and carbamazepine. May cause seizures; use caution wi antipsychotics and antidepressants. May cause widening of QRS complex; us caution with ziprasidone.

Dosage Summary

Oral:

Children:

Extraintestinal amebiasis: 10 mg/kg (base) once daily (maximum: 300 m base/day)

Malaria prophylaxis:

No pretreatment: 10 mg/kg (base) in 2 divided doses given 6 hours apa followed by normal prophylactic regimen

Prior to exposure: 5 mg base/kg/week (maximum: 300 mg base/dose)

Malaria treatment: 10 mg/kg (base) on day 1, followed by 5 mg/kg (base) hours later and 5 mg/kg (base) on days 2 and 3

Adults:

Extraintestinal amebiasis: 1 g/day (600 mg base) for 2 days, then 500 m day (300 mg base)

Malaria prophylaxis:

No pretreatment: 1 g (600 mg base) in 2 divided doses given 6 hou apart, followed by normal prophylactic regimen

Prior to exposure: 500 mg/week (300 mg base)

Malaria treatment: 1 g (600 mg base) on day 1, followed by 500 mg (300 mg base) 6 hours later and 500 mg (300 mg base) on days 2 and 3

Dosage Forms Excipient information presented when available (limited, particularly for generics); consult specific product labeling.

Tablet, as phosphate: 250 mg [equivalent to 150 mg base]; 500 mg [equivalent to 300 mg base]

Aralen®: 500 mg [equivalent to 300 mg base]

◆ **Chloroquine Phosphate** *see* Chloroquine Phosphate *on page 320*

Chlorothiazide (klor oh THYE a zide)

Medication Safety Issues

International issues:

Diuril® may be confused with Duorol® which is a brand name for acetaminophen in Spain

U.S. Brand Names Diuril®; Sodium Diuril®

Canadian Brand Names Diuril®

Pharmacologic Category Diuretic, Thiazide

Use Management of mild-to-moderate hypertension; adjunctive treatment of edema

Effect on Mental Status May cause dizziness

Effect on Psychiatric Treatment Rare reports of agranulocytosis; use caution with clozapine and carbamazepine; thiazides decrease lithium clearance resulting in elevated serum lithium levels and potential toxicity; monitor serum lithium levels

Dosage Summary

I.V.:

Children <6 months (unlabeled): 2-8 mg/kg/day in 2 divided doses

Children ≥6 months (unlabeled): 4 mg/kg/day in 1-2 divided doses

Adults: 250-1000 mg once or twice daily (maximum: 1000 mg/day)

Oral:

Children <6 months: 10-30 mg/kg/day in 2 divided doses (maximum: 375 mg/day)

Children ≥6 months: 10-20 mg/kg/day in 1-2 divided doses (maximum: 375 mg/day)

Adults: 250-2000 mg/day in 1-2 divided doses (maximum: 1000 mg/day [CHF])

Dosage Forms Excipient information presented when available (limited, particularly for generics); consult specific product labeling.

Injection, powder for reconstitution, as sodium:

Sodium Diuril®: 500 mg

Suspension, oral:

Diuril®: 250 mg/5 mL (237 mL) [contains alcohol 0.5% and benzoic acid]

Tablet: 250 mg, 500 mg

◆ **Chlorphen [OTC]** *see* Chlorpheniramine *on page 321*

Chlorpheniramine (klor fen IR a meen)

Medication Safety Issues

Sound-alike/look-alike issues:

Chlor-Trimeton® may be confused with Chloromycetin®

U.S. Brand Names Ahist™; Aller-Chlor® [OTC]; Chlor-Trimeton® [OTC]; Chlorphen [OTC]; CPM-12; Diabetic Tussin® Allergy Relief [OTC]; PediaTan™; QDALL® AR; Teldrin® HBP [OTC]

Canadian Brand Names Chlor-Tripolon®; Novo-Pheniram

Mexican Brand Names Antadex-H; Bregamin; Cloro-Trimeton; Derimeton

Index Terms Chlorpheniramine Maleate; CTM

Pharmacologic Category Histamine H_1 Antagonist; Histamine H_1 Antagonist, First Generation

Use Perennial and seasonal allergic rhinitis and other allergic symptoms including urticaria

Effect on Mental Status Drowsiness is common; may cause excitability, nervousness, fatigue, or depression

Effect on Psychiatric Treatment Dry mouth and sedation may be exacerbated by concurrent psychotropic use

Dosage Summary

Oral:

Immediate release:

Children <2 years: 0.35 mg/kg/day divided every 4-6 hours

Children 2-6 years: 1 mg every 4-6 hours **or** 0.35 mg/kg/day divided every 4-6 hours (maximum: 6 mg/day)
Children 6-12 years: 2 mg every 4-6 hours or 0.35 mg/kg/day divided every 4-6 hours (maximum: 12 mg/day)
Children >12 years: 4 mg every 4-6 hours (maximum: 24 mg/day)
Adults: 4 mg every 4-6 hours (maximum: 24 mg/day)
Elderly: 4 mg once or twice daily

Sustained release:
Children <6 years: Dosage not established
Children 6-12 years: 8 mg at bedtime
Children >12 years: 8-12 mg every 8-12 hours (maximum: 24 mg/day)
Adults: 8-12 mg every 8-12 hours (maximum: 24 mg/day)
Elderly: 8 mg at bedtime

Dosage Forms Excipient information presented when available (limited, particularly for generics); consult specific product labeling.

Capsule, extended release:
CPM-12: Chlorpheniramine maleate 12 mg

Capsule, variable release, as maleate:
QDALL® AR: Chlorpheniramine 12 mg [immediate release and sustained release]

Suspension, as tannate:
PediaTan™: 8 mg/5 mL (480 mL) [sugar free; contains sodium benzoate; bubble gum flavor]

Syrup, as maleate:
Aller-Chlor®: 2 mg/5 mL (120 mL) [contains alcohol 5%]
Diabetic Tussin® Allergy Relief: 2 mg/5 mL (120 mL) [alcohol free, dye free, sugar free]

Tablet, as maleate: 4 mg
Aller-Chlor®, Chlor-Trimeton®, Chlorphen, Teldrin® HBP: 4 mg

Tablet, extended release, as maleate:
Chlor-Trimeton®: 12 mg

Tablet, long acting, as tannate [scored]:
Ahist™: 12 mg

◆ **Chlorpheniramine, Acetaminophen, and Pseudoephedrine** *see* Acetaminophen, Chlorpheniramine, and Pseudoephedrine *on page 40*

Chlorpheniramine and Acetaminophen

(klor fen IR a meen & a seet a MIN oh fen)

Medication Safety Issues

Duplicate therapy issues: This product contains acetaminophen, which may be a component of other combination products. Do not exceed the maximum recommended daily dose of acetaminophen.

U.S. Brand Names Coricidin HBP® Cold and Flu [OTC]

Index Terms Acetaminophen and Chlorpheniramine

Pharmacologic Category Analgesic, Miscellaneous; Histamine H_1 Antagonist; Histamine H_1 Antagonist, First Generation

Use Symptomatic relief of congestion, headache, aches and pains of colds and flu

Effect on Mental Status Drowsiness is common; may cause excitability, nervousness, fatigue, or depression

Effect on Psychiatric Treatment Dry mouth and sedation may be exacerbated by concurrent psychotropic use

Dosage Summary

Oral:
Children: Dosage not established
Adults: 2 tablets every 4 hours

Dosage Forms Excipient information presented when available (limited, particularly for generics); consult specific product labeling.

Tablet: Chlorpheniramine maleate 2 mg and acetaminophen 325 mg

◆ **Chlorpheniramine and Carbetapentane** *see* Carbetapentane and Chlorpheniramine *on page 272*

◆ **Chlorpheniramine and Dextromethorphan** *see* Dextromethorphan and Chlorpheniramine *on page 449*

Chlorpheniramine and Phenylephrine

(klor fen IR a meen & fen il EF rin)

Medication Safety Issues

Sound-alike/look-alike issues:

Rynatan® may be confused with Rynatuss®

U.S. Brand Names Actifed® Cold & Allergy [OTC] *[reformulation]*; AllanTan Pediatric [DSC]; AlleRx™ Suspension; C-Phen; Ceron; Dallergy Drops; Dallergy®-JR; Dec-Chlorphen; Ed A-Hist™; Ed ChlorPed D; NoHist; P-Tann D; PD-Hist-D; PediaTan™ D; Phenabid®; R-Tanna; R-Tanna Pediatric; Rescon-Jr®; Rinate™ Pediatric; Rondec® ; Rynatan®; Rynatan® Pediatric; Sildec PE [DSC]; Sudafed PE® Sinus & Allergy [OTC]; Tannate Pediatric; Triaminic® Cold and Allergy [OTC]

Index Terms Chlorpheniramine Maleate and Phenylephrine Hydrochloride; Chlorpheniramine Tannate and Phenylephrine Tannate; Phenylephrine and Chlorpheniramine

Pharmacologic Category Alpha/Beta Agonist; Histamine H_1 Antagonist; Histamine H_1 Antagonist, First Generation

Use Temporary relief of upper respiratory conditions such as nasal congestion, runny nose, and sneezing due to the common cold, hay fever, or allergic or vasomotor rhinitis

Effect on Mental Status Drowsiness is common; may cause excitability, nervousness, fatigue, or depression

Effect on Psychiatric Treatment Dry mouth and sedation may be exacerbated by concurrent psychotropic use

Dosage Summary

Oral:

Children <6 months: Dosage not established

Children 6-12 months: Rondec® Drops: 0.75 mL 4 times/day

Children 1-2 years: Rondec® Drops: 1 mL 4 times/day

Children 2-6 years:

AlleRx™: 1.25-2.5 mL every 12 hours1.25-2.5 mL every 12 hours

Rondec® Syrup: 1.25 mL every 4-6 hours (maximum 7.5 mL/day)

Rynatan®: Suspension: 2.5-5 mL every 12 hours

Children 6-12 years:

AlleRx™: 2.5-5 mL every 12 hours

Dallergy® Jr: One capsule every 12 hours (maximum: 2 capsules/day)

Ed A-Hist™: One-half caplet every 12 hours

Rondec®: 2.5 mL every 4-6 hours (maximum 15 mL/day)

Rynatan®: Suspension: 5-10 mL every 12 hours

Children ≥12 years:

AlleRx™: 15 mL every 12 hours

Dallergy® Jr: Two capsules every 12 hours (maximum: 4 capsules/day)

Ed A-Hist™: One caplet every 12 hours

R-Tanna: 1-2 tablets every 12 hours

Rondec®: 5 mL every 4-6 hours (maximum 30 mL/day)

Rynatan®: Tablet: 1-2 tablets every 12 hours

Adults:

AlleRx™: 15 mL every 12 hours

Dallergy® Jr: Two capsules every 12 hours (maximum: 4 capsules/day)

Ed A-Hist™: One caplet every 12 hours

R-Tanna: 1-2 tablets every 12 hours

Rondec®: 5 mL every 4-6 hours (maximum 30 mL/day)

Rynatan®: Tablet: 1-2 tablets every 12 hours

Dosage Forms Excipient information presented when available (limited, particularly for generics); consult specific product labeling. [DSC] = Discontinued product

Caplet, prolonged release:

Ed A-Hist™, NoHist: Chlorpheniramine maleate 8 mg and phenylephrine hydrochloride 20 mg

Capsule, extended release:

Dallergy®-JR: Chlorpheniramine maleate 4 mg and phenylephrine hydrochloride 20 mg

Liquid:

Ed A-Hist™: Chlorpheniramine maleate 4 mg and phenylephrine hydrochloride 10 mg per 5 mL (480 mL) [sugar free; contains alcohol 5%; grape flavor]

Triaminic® Cold and Allergy: Chlorpheniramine maleate 1 mg and phenylephrine hydrochloride 2.5 mg per 5 mL (120 mL) [contains sodium 5 mg/5 mL and benzoic acid; orange flavor]

Liquid, oral [drops]:
Dallergy: Chlorpheniramine maleate 1 mg and phenylephrine hydrochloride 2 mg per 1 mL (30 mL) [alcohol free, sugar free; contains propylene glycol; peach flavor]
Solution, oral [drops]:
C-Phen, PD-Hist-D: Chlorpheniramine maleate 1 mg and phenylephrine hydrochloride 3.5 mg per mL (30 mL) [alcohol free, sugar free; bubblegum flavor]
Ceron: Chlorpheniramine maleate 1 mg and phenylephrine hydrochloride 3.5 mg per mL (30 mL) [raspberry flavor]
Dec-Chlorphen: Chlorpheniramine maleate 1 mg and phenylephrine hydrochloride 3.5 mg per mL (30 mL) [alcohol free, dye free, sugar free; grape flavor]
Rondec®: Chlorpheniramine maleate 1 mg and phenylephrine hydrochloride 3.5 mg per mL (30 mL) [alcohol free, sugar free; contains propylene glycol; bubble gum flavor] [DSC]
Sildec PE: Chlorpheniramine maleate 1 mg and phenylephrine hydrochloride 3.5 mg per 1 mL (30 mL) [alcohol free, sugar free; raspberry flavor] [DSC]
Suspension, oral: Chlorpheniramine tannate 4 mg and phenylephrine tannate 20 mg per 5 mL (473 mL)
AllanTan Pediatric: Chlorpheniramine tannate 4.5 mg and phenylephrine tannate 5 mg per 5 mL (473 mL) [contains sodium benzoate; strawberry flavor] [DSC]
AlleRx™: Chlorpheniramine tannate 3 mg and phenylephrine tannate 7.5 per 5 mL (480 mL) [contains benzoic acid; raspberry flavor]
Dallergy®-JR: Chlorpheniramine tannate 4 mg and phenylephrine tannate 20 mg per 5 mL (480 mL) [contains sodium benzoate; peaches and cream flavor]
P-Tann D, PediaTan™ D: Chlorpheniramine tannate 8 mg and phenylephrine tannate 10 mg per 5 mL (480 mL) [sugar free; contains sodium benzoate bubblegum flavor]
R-Tanna Pediatric: Chlorpheniramine tannate 4.5 mg and phenylephrine tannate 5 mg per 5 mL (480 mL) [contains benzoic acid and tartrazine]
Rinate™ Pediatric: Chlorpheniramine tannate 4.5 mg and phenylephrine tannate 5 mg per 5 mL (120 mL, 480 mL) [contains sodium benzoate blueberry flavor]
Rynatan® Pediatric: Chlorpheniramine tannate 4.5 mg and phenylephrine tannate 5 mg per 5 mL (480 mL) [contains benzoic acid and tartrazine strawberry-currant flavor]
Tannate Pediatric: Chlorpheniramine tannate 4.5 mg and phenylephrine tannate 5 mg per 5 mL (480 mL) [contains sodium benzoate; raspberry flavor]
Suspension, oral [drops]:
Ed ChlorPed D: Chlorpheniramine tannate 2 mg and phenylephrine tannate 6 mg per 1 mL (60 mL) [apple sauce flavor]
Syrup:
C-Phen: Chlorpheniramine maleate 4 mg and phenylephrine hydrochloride 12. 5 mg per 5 mL (120 mL, 480 mL) [alcohol free, sugar free; contains sodium benzoate; bubble gum flavor]
Ceron, Sildec PE: Chlorpheniramine maleate 4 mg and phenylephrine hydrochloride 12. 5 mg per 5 mL (480 mL) [raspberry flavor]
PD-Hist-D: Chlorpheniramine maleate 4 mg and phenylephrine hydrochloride 12. 5 mg per 5 mL (480 mL)[alcohol free, sugar free; bubblegum flavor]
Rondec®: Chlorpheniramine maleate 4 mg and phenylephrine hydrochloride 12.5 mg per 5 mL (120 mL, 480 mL) [alcohol free, sugar free; contains propylene glycol; bubble gum flavor]
Tablet:
Actifed® Cold & Allergy, Sudafed PE® Sinus & Allergy: Chlorpheniramine maleate 4 mg and phenylephrine hydrochloride 10 mg
R-Tanna, Rynatan®: Chlorpheniramine tannate 9 mg and phenylephrine tannate 25 mg
Tablet, chewable:
Rynatan®: Chlorpheniramine tannate 4.5 mg and phenylephrine tannate 5 mg [grape flavor]
Tablet, sustained release:
Rescon-Jr®: Chlorpheniramine maleate 4 mg and phenylephrine hydrochloride 20 mg
Tablet, timed release:
Phenabid®: Chlorpheniramine maleate 8 mg and phenylephrine hydrochloride 20 mg [dye free, sugar free]

Chlorpheniramine and Pseudoephedrine

(klor fen IR a meen & soo doe e FED rin)

Medication Safety Issues

Sound-alike/look-alike issues:

Allerest® may be confused with Sinarest®

Chlor-Trimeton® may be confused with Chloromycetin®

Sudafed® may be confused with Sufenta®

U.S. Brand Names Allerest® Maximum Strength Allergy and Hay Fever [OTC]; Deconamine® SR; Dicel™; Duratuss® DA; Dynahist-ER Pediatric® [DSC]; Histade™ [DSC]; Histex™; LoHist-D; QDALL® [DSC]; Suclor™; Sudafed® Sinus & Allergy [OTC]; SudaHist®; Sudal® 12

Canadian Brand Names Triaminic® Cold & Allergy

Index Terms Chlorpheniramine Maleate and Pseudoephedrine Hydrochloride; Chlorpheniramine Tannate and Pseudoephedrine Tannate; Pseudoephedrine and Chlorpheniramine

Pharmacologic Category Alpha/Beta Agonist; Histamine H_1 Antagonist; Histamine H_1 Antagonist, First Generation

Use Relief of nasal congestion associated with the common cold, hay fever, and other allergies, sinusitis, eustachian tube blockage, and vasomotor and allergic rhinitis

Effect on Mental Status Drowsiness is common; may cause excitability, nervousness, fatigue, or depression

Effect on Psychiatric Treatment Dry mouth and sedation may be exacerbated by concurrent psychotropic use

Dosage Summary Note: General dosing guidelines; consult specific product labeling

Oral:

Immediate release:

Children <2 years: Dosage not established

Children 2-6 years: Chlorpheniramine maleate 1 mg and pseudoephedrine hydrochloride 15 mg every 4-6 hours **or** chlorpheniramine tannate 4.5 mg and pseudoephedrine tannate 75 mg: 2.5-5 mL every 12 hours (maximum: 10 mL/day)

Children 6-12 years: Chlorpheniramine maleate 2 mg and pseudoephedrine hydrochloride 30 mg every 4-6 hours

Children ≥12 years: Chlorpheniramine maleate 4 mg and pseudoephedrine hydrochloride 60 mg every 4-6 hours **or** chlorpheniramine tannate 4.5 mg and pseudoephedrine tannate 75 mg: 10-20 mL every 12 hours (maximum: 40 mL/day)

Adults: Chlorpheniramine maleate 4 mg and pseudoephedrine hydrochloride 60 mg every 4-6 hours **or** chlorpheniramine tannate 4.5 mg and pseudoephedrine tannate 75 mg: 10-20 mL every 12 hours (maximum: 40 mL/day)

Sustained release:

Children <12 years: Dosage not established

Children ≥12 years: Deconamine® SR: Chlorpheniramine maleate 8 mg and pseudoephedrine hydrochloride 120 mg every 12 hours

Adults: Deconamine® SR: Chlorpheniramine maleate 8 mg and pseudoephedrine hydrochloride 120 mg every 12 hours

Dosage Forms Excipient information presented when available (limited, particularly for generics); consult specific product labeling. [DSC] = Discontinued product

Capsule, extended release: Chlorpheniramine maleate 8 mg and pseudoephedrine hydrochloride 120 mg; chlorpheniramine maleate 12 mg and pseudoephedrine hydrochloride 100 mg

Duratuss® DA: Chlorpheniramine maleate 12 mg and pseudoephedrine hydrochloride 100 mg

Dynahist-ER Pediatric®: Chlorpheniramine maleate 4 mg and pseudoephedrine hydrochloride 60 mg [DSC]

Histade™: Chlorpheniramine maleate 12 mg and pseudoephedrine hydrochloride 120 mg [DSC]

QDALL®: Chlorpheniramine maleate 12 mg and pseudoephedrine hydrochloride 100 mg [DSC]

Suclor™: Chlorpheniramine maleate 8 mg and pseudoephedrine hydrochloride 120 mg

Capsule, sustained release: Chlorpheniramine maleate 8 mg and pseudoephedrine hydrochloride 120 mg

Deconamine® SR: Chlorpheniramine maleate 8 mg and pseudoephedrine hydrochloride 120 mg

Liquid:
Histex™: Chlorpheniramine maleate 2 mg and pseudoephedrine sulfate 30 mg per 5 mL (480 mL) [peach flavor]
LoHist-D: Chlorpheniramine maleate 2 mg and pseudoephedrine hydrochloride 30 mg per 5 mL (480 mL) [alcohol free, dye free; peach flavor]
Suspension:
Dicel™: Chlorpheniramine tannate 5 mg and pseudoephedrine tannate 75 mg per 5 mL (480 mL) [contains sodium benzoate; strawberry banana flavor]
Syrup: Chlorpheniramine maleate 2 mg and pseudoephedrine hydrochloride 30 mg per 5 mL (480 mL)
Tablet: Chlorpheniramine maleate 4 mg and pseudoephedrine hydrochloride 60 mg
Allerest® Maximum Strength Allergy and Hay Fever: Chlorpheniramine maleate 2 mg and pseudoephedrine hydrochloride 30 mg
Sudafed® Sinus & Allergy: Chlorpheniramine maleate 4 mg and pseudoephedrine hydrochloride 60 mg
Tablet, chewable:
Sudal® 12: Chlorpheniramine maleate 4 mg and pseudoephedrine hydrochloride 30 mg [contains phenylalanine 25 mg/tablet; grape flavor]
Tablet, sustained release:
SudaHist: Chlorpheniramine maleate 12 mg and pseudoephedrine hydrochloride 120 mg

◆ **Chlorpheniramine, Carbetapentane, and Phenylephrine** *see* Carbetapentane, Phenylephrine, and Chlorpheniramine *on page 274*

◆ **Chlorpheniramine, Dextromethorphan, Phenylephrine, and Guaifenesin** *see* Dextromethorphan, Chlorpheniramine, Phenylephrine, and Guaifenesin *on page 450*

Chlorpheniramine, Ephedrine, Phenylephrine, and Carbetapentane

(klor fen IR a meen, e FED rin, fen il EF rin, & kar bay ta PEN tane)

Medication Safety Issues
Sound-alike/look-alike issues:
Rynatuss® may be confused with Rynatan®

U.S. Brand Names Quad Tann®; Quad Tann® Pediatric; Rynatuss®; Tetra Tannate Pediatric

Index Terms Carbetapentane, Ephedrine, Phenylephrine, and Chlorpheniramine; Ephedrine, Chlorpheniramine, Phenylephrine, and Carbetapentane; Phenylephrine, Ephedrine, Chlorpheniramine, and Carbetapentane

Pharmacologic Category Alpha/Beta Agonist; Antitussive; Histamine H_1 Antagonist; Histamine H_1 Antagonist, First Generation

Use Symptomatic relief of cough with a decongestant and an antihistamine

Effect on Mental Status Drowsiness is common; may cause excitability, nervousness, fatigue, or depression

Effect on Psychiatric Treatment Dry mouth and sedation may be exacerbated by concurrent psychotropic use

Dosage Summary
Oral:
Children <2 years: Titrate dose individually
Children 2-6 years: 2.5-5 mL every 12 hours
Children >6 years: 5-10 mL every 12 hours
Adults: 1-2 tablets every 12 hours

Dosage Forms Excipient information presented when available (limited, particularly for generics); consult specific product labeling.
Suspension:
Quad Tann® Pediatric: Chlorpheniramine tannate 4 mg, ephedrine tannate 5 mg, phenylephrine tannate 5 mg, and carbetapentane tannate 30 mg per 5 mL (480 mL) [contains sodium benzoate; grape flavor]
Tetra Tannate Pediatric: Chlorpheniramine tannate 4 mg, ephedrine tannate 5 mg, phenylephrine tannate 5 mg, and carbetapentane tannate 30 mg per 5 mL (240 mL, 480 mL) [alcohol free; strawberry flavor]
Tablet:
Rynatuss®: Chlorpheniramine tannage 5 mg, ephedrine tannate 10 mg, phenylephrine tannate 10 mg, and carbetapentane tannate 60 mg
Tablet, long acting:
Quad Tann®: Chlorpheniramine tannage 5 mg, ephedrine tannate 10 mg, phenylephrine tannate 10 mg, and carbetapentane tannate 60 mg

- ◆ **Chlorpheniramine Maleate** *see* Chlorpheniramine *on page 321*
- ◆ **Chlorpheniramine Maleate and Dextromethorphan Hydrobromide** *see* Dextromethorphan and Chlorpheniramine *on page 449*
- ◆ **Chlorpheniramine Maleate and Hydrocodone Bitartrate** *see* Hydrocodone and Chlorpheniramine *on page 778*
- ◆ **Chlorpheniramine Maleate and Phenylephrine Hydrochloride** *see* Chlorpheniramine and Phenylephrine *on page 323*
- ◆ **Chlorpheniramine Maleate and Pseudoephedrine Hydrochloride** *see* Chlorpheniramine and Pseudoephedrine *on page 325*
- ◆ **Chlorpheniramine Maleate, Dihydrocodeine Bitartrate, and Phenylephrine Hydrochloride** *see* Dihydrocodeine, Chlorpheniramine, and Phenylephrine *on page 469*
- ◆ **Chlorpheniramine Maleate, Phenylephrine Hydrochloride, and Guaifenesin** *see* Chlorpheniramine, Phenylephrine, and Guaifenesin *on page 329*
- ◆ **Chlorpheniramine Maleate, Pseudoephedrine Hydrochloride, and Dextromethorphan Hydrobromide** *see* Chlorpheniramine, Pseudoephedrine, and Dextromethorphan *on page 333*

Chlorpheniramine, Phenylephrine, and Dextromethorphan

(klor fen IR a meen, fen il EF rin, & deks troe meth OR fan)

U.S. Brand Names C-Phen DM; Ceron-DM; Corfen DM; De-Chlor DM; De-Chlor DR; Dec-Chlorphen DM [DSC]; Dex PC; Donatussin DM [DSC]; Ed A-Hist DM; Father John's® Plus [OTC]; Mintuss DR; Neo DM; Norel DM™; PD-Cof; PE-Hist DM; Phenabid DM®; Poly Tussin DM; Robitussin® Cough and Allergy [OTC]; Robitussin® Cough and Cold Nighttime [OTC]; Robitussin® Pediatric Cough and Cold Nighttime [OTC]; Rondec®-DM; Sildec PE-DM; Statuss™ DM; Tri-Vent™ DPC [DSC]; Trital DM; Tussplex™ DM

Index Terms Dextromethorphan, Chlorpheniramine, and Phenylephrine; Phenylephrine, Chlorpheniramine, and Dextromethorphan

Pharmacologic Category Alpha/Beta Agonist; Antitussive; Histamine H_1 Antagonist; Histamine H_1 Antagonist, First Generation

Use Temporary relief of cough and upper respiratory symptoms associated with allergies or the common cold

Effect on Mental Status Drowsiness is common; may cause excitability, nervousness, fatigue, or depression

Effect on Psychiatric Treatment Dry mouth and sedation may be exacerbated by concurrent psychotropic use

Dosage Summary

Oral:

Children <6 months: Dosage not established

Children 6-12 months: Rondec®-DM Drops: 0.75 mL 4 times/day

Children 1-2 years: Rondec®-DM Drops: 1 mL 4 times/day

Children 2-6 years:

Rondec®-DM Syrup: 1.25 mL every 4-6 hours (maximum: 7.5 mL/day)
Tri-Vent™ DPC: 2.5 mL every 6 hours (maximum: 10 mL/day)

Children 6-12 years:

Rondec®-DM Syrup: 2.5 mL every 4-6 hours (maximum: 15 mL/day)
Tri-Vent™ DPC: 5 mL every 6 hours (maximum: 20 mL /day)

Children ≥12 years:

Rondec®-DM Syrup: 5 mL every 4-6 hours (maximum: 30 mL/day)
Tri-Vent™ DPC: 10 mL every 6 hours (maximum: 40 mL/day)

Adults:

Rondec®-DM Syrup: 5 mL every 4-6 hours (maximum: 30 mL/day)
Tri-Vent™ DPC: 10 mL every 6 hours (maximum: 40 mL/day)

Dosage Forms Excipient information presented when available (limited, particularly for generics); consult specific product labeling. [DSC] = Discontinued product

Liquid:

Corfen DM: Chlorpheniramine maleate 4 mg, phenylephrine hydrochloride 10 mg, and dextromethorphan hydrobromide 15 mg per 5 mL (480 mL) [grape flavor]

De-Chlor DM: Chlorpheniramine maleate 2 mg, phenylephrine hydrochloride 10 mg, and dextromethorphan hydrobromide 15 mg per 5 mL (480 mL) [strawberry flavor]

De-Chlor DR: Chlorpheniramine maleate 2 mg, phenylephrine hydrochloride 6 mg, and dextromethorphan hydrobromide 15 mg per 5 mL (480 mL) [strawberry flavor]

Father John's® Plus: Chlorpheniramine maleate 2 mg, phenylephrine hydrochloride 5 mg, and dextromethorphan hydrobromide 5 mg per 15 mL (118 mL) [alcohol free]

Norel DM™: Chlorpheniramine maleate 4 mg, phenylephrine hydrochloride 10 mg, and dextromethorphan hydrobromide 15 mg per 5 mL (480 mL) [alcohol free, dye free, sugar free; contains propylene glycol; grape flavor]

Trital DM: Chlorpheniramine maleate 4 mg, phenylephrine hydrochloride 10 mg, and dextromethorphan hydrobromide 15 mg per 5 mL (480 mL) [alcohol free, dye free, sugar free; contains sodium benzoate; grape flavor]

Liquid, oral [drops]:

Ceron DM: Chorpheniramine maleate 1 mg, phenylephrine hydrochloride 3.5 mg, and dextromethorphan hydrobromide 3 mg per 1 mL (30 mL) [alcohol free, sugar free; contains sodium benzoate; grape flavor] [DSC]

C-Phen DM: Chlorpheniramine maleate 1 mg, phenylephrine hydrochloride 3.5 mg, and dextromethorphan hydrobromide 3 mg per 1 mL (30 mL) [grape flavor]

Donatussin DM: Chlorpheniramine maleate 1 mg, phenylephrine hydrochloride 1.5 mg, and dextromethorphan hydrobromide 3 mg per 1 mL (30 mL) [alcohol free, sugar free; contains propylene glycol; bubblegum flavor] [DSC]

Neo DM: Chlorpheniramine maleate 0.75 mg, phenylephrine hydrochloride 1.75 mg, and dextromethorphan hydrobromide 2.75 mg per 1 mL (30 mL) [alcohol free, sugar free; contains propylene glycol; black cherry flavor]

PD-Cof: Chlorpheniramine maleate 1 mg, phenylephrine hydrochloride 3.5 mg, and dextromethorphan hydrobromide 3 mg per 1 mL (30 mL) [alcohol free, sugar free; grape flavor]

Rondec® DM, Sildec PE-DM [DSC]: Chlorpheniramine maleate 1 mg, phenylephrine hydrochloride 3.5 mg, and dextromethorphan hydrobromide 3 mg per 1 mL (30 mL) [alcohol free, sugar free; grape flavor]

Suspension:

Donatussin DM: Dexchlorpheniramine tannate 2 mg, phenylephrine tannate 20 mg, and dextromethorphan tannate 30 mg per 5 mL (480 mL) [alcohol free, sugar free; contains phenylalanine 7 mg/5 mL, propylene glycol; cotton candy strawberry flavor] [DSC]

Syrup:

Ceron-DM: Chlorpheniramine maleate 4 mg, phenylephrine hydrochloride 12.5 mg, and dextromethorphan hydrobromide 15 mg per 5 mL (480 mL) [alcohol free, sugar free; contains sodium benzoate; grape flavor]

C-Phen DM: Chlorpheniramine maleate 4 mg, phenylephrine hydrochloride 12.5 mg, and dextromethorphan hydrobromide 15 mg per 5 mL (120 mL, 480 mL) [grape flavor]

Dec-Chlorphen DM: Chlorpheniramine maleate 4 mg, phenylephrine hydrochloride 12.5 mg, and dextromethorphan hydrobromide 15 mg per 5 mL (120 mL, 480 mL) [alcohol free, dye free, sugar free; grape flavor] [DSC]

Dex PC: Chlorpheniramine maleate 2 mg, phenylephrine hydrochloride 6 mg, and dextromethorphan hydrobromide 15 mg per 5 mL (480 mL) [strawberry flavor]

Ed A-Hist DM: Chlorpheniramine maleate 4 mg, phenylephrine hydrochloride 10 mg, and dextromethorphan hydrobromide 15 mg per 5 mL (480 mL) [alcohol free, sugar free; contains propylene glycol; banana flavor]

Mintuss DR: Chlorpheniramine maleate 2 mg, phenylephrine hydrochloride 6 mg, and dextromethorphan hydrobromide 15 mg per 5 mL (480 mL) [alcohol free; strawberry flavor]

PD-Cof: Chlorpheniramine maleate 4 mg, phenylephrine hydrochloride 12.5 mg, and dextromethorphan hydrobromide 15 mg per 5 mL (480 mL) [alcohol free, sugar free; grape flavor]

PE-Hist DM: Chlorpheniramine maleate 2 mg, phenylephrine hydrochloride 5 mg, and dextromethorphan hydrobromide 15 mg per 5 mL (480 mL) [strawberry flavor]

Poly Tussin DM: Chlorpheniramine maleate 2 mg, phenylephrine hydrochloride 5 mg, and dextromethorphan hydrobromide 15 mg per 5 mL (480 mL) [alcohol free, sugar free]

Robitussion® Cough and Allergy: Chlorpheniramine maleate 2 mg, phenylephrine hydrochloride 5 mg, and dextromethorphan hydrobromide 10 mg per 5 mL (120 mL) [alcohol free; contains sodium 3 mg/5 mL, sodium benzoate, and propylene glycol] [DSC]

Robitussin® Cough and Cold Nighttime: Chlorpheniramine maleate 1 mg phenylephrine hydrochloride 2.5 mg, and dextromethorphan hydrobromide 5 mg per 5 mL (120 mL) [alcohol free; contains sodium 3 mg/5 mL, sodium benzoate, and propylene glycol]

Robitussin® Pediatric Cough and Cold Nighttime: Chlorpheniramine maleate 1 mg, phenylephrine hydrochloride 2.5 mg, and dextromethorphan hydrobromide 5 mg per 5 mL (120 mL) [alcohol free; contains sodium 3 mg/ 5 mL, sodium benzoate, and propylene glycol; fruit punch flavor]

Rondec®-DM: Chlorpheniramine maleate 4 mg, phenylephrine hydrochloride 12.5 mg, and dextromethorphan hydrobromide 15 mg per 5 mL (120 mL, 480 mL) [alcohol free, sugar free; contains propylene glycol; grape flavor]

Sildec PE-DM: Chlorpheniramine maleate 4 mg, phenylephrine hydrochloride 12.5 mg, and dextromethorphan hydrobromide 15 mg per 5 mL (480 mL) [grape flavor]

Statuss™: DM: Chlorpheniramine maleate 2 mg, phenylephrine hydrochloride 10 mg, and dextromethorphan hydrobromide 15 mg per 5 mL (480 mL) [alcohol free, sugar free; raspberry flavor]

Tri-Vent™ DPC: Chlorpheniramine maleate 2 mg, phenylephrine hydrochloride 6 mg, and dextromethorphan hydrobromide 15 mg per 5 mL (480 mL) [alcohol free; contains sodium benzoate, propylene glycol; strawberry flavor] [DSC]

Tussplex™ DM: Chlorpheniramine maleate 2 mg, phenylephrine hydrochloride 5 mg, and dextromethorphan hydrobromide 15 mg per 5 mL (480 mL) [alcohol free, sugar free; contains sodium benzoate; strawberry flavor]

Tablet, timed release:

Phenabid DM®: Chlorpheniramine maleate 8 mg, phenylephrine hydrochloride 20 mg, and dextromethorphan hydrobromide 30 mg [scored; dye free, sugar free]

Chlorpheniramine, Phenylephrine, and Guaifenesin

(klor fen IR a meen, fen il EF rin, & gwye FEN e sin)

U.S. Brand Names P Chlor GG

Index Terms Chlorpheniramine Maleate, Phenylephrine Hydrochloride, and Guaifenesin; Chlorpheniramine Tannate, Phenylephrine Tannate, and Guaifenesin; Guaifenesin, Phenylephrine, and Chlorpheniramine; Phenylephrine, Chlorpheniramine, and Guaifenesin

Pharmacologic Category Alpha/Beta Agonist; Expectorant; Histamine H_1 Antagonist; Histamine H_1 Antagonist, First Generation

Use Symptomatic relief of upper respiratory symptoms associated with infections such as the common cold or allergies

Effect on Mental Status May cause dizziness, drowsiness, insomnia, irritability, or nervousness

Effect on Psychiatric Treatment Contraindicated with MAO inhibitors or within 14 days of MAO inhibitor

Dosage Summary

Oral:

Children <3 months: 2-3 2-3 drops per month of age every 4-6 hours as needed (maximum: 4 doses/day)

Children 3-6 months: 0.3-0.6 mL every 4-6 hours as needed (maximum: 4 doses/day)

Children 6 months to 1 year: 0.6-1 mL every 4-6 hours as needed (maximum: 4 doses/day)

Children 1-2 years: 1-2 mL every 4-6 hours as needed (maximum: 4 doses/ day)

Dosage Forms Excipient information presented when available (limited, particularly for generics); consult specific product labeling.

Liquid:

P Chlor GG [drops]: Chlorpheniramine maleate 1 mg, phenylephrine hydrochloride 2 mg, and guaifenesin 20 mg per 1 mL (30 mL) [peach flavor]

◆ **Chlorpheniramine, Phenylephrine, and Hydrocodone** *see* Phenylephrine, Hydrocodone, and Chlorpheniramine *on page 1277*

Chlorpheniramine, Phenylephrine, and Methscopolamine

(klor fen IR a meen, fen il EF rin, & meth skoe POL a meen)

U.S. Brand Names aerohist plus™; aeroKid™; AH-Chew®; AH-Chew™ Ultra; Chlor-Mes; Chlor-Mes-D; Dallergy®; Dehistine; Duradryl®; Durahist™ PE; Extendryl®; Extendryl® JR; Extendryl® SR; Hista-Vent® DA [DSC]; Histatab PH; OMNIhist® II L.A.; PCM; PCM Allergy [DSC]; Phenylephrine CM; Ralix; Rescon®; Rescon® MX; Triall™

Index Terms Methscopolamine Nitrate, Chlorpheniramine Maleate, and Phenylephrine Hydrochloride; Phenylephrine Tannate, Chlorpheniramine Tannate, and Methscopolamine Nitrate

Pharmacologic Category Alpha/Beta Agonist; Anticholinergic Agent; Histamine H_1 Antagonist; Histamine H_1 Antagonist, First Generation

Use Treatment of upper respiratory symptoms such as respiratory congestion, allergic rhinitis, vasomotor rhinitis, sinusitis, and allergic skin reactions of urticaria and angioedema

Effect on Mental Status Drowsiness is common; may cause excitability, nervousness, fatigue, or depression

Effect on Psychiatric Treatment Dry mouth and sedation may be exacerbated by concurrent psychotropic use

Dosage Summary

Oral:

aeroKid™:
- *Children <6 years:* Dosage not established
- *Children 6-11 years:* 2.5-5 mL every 12 hours
- *Children ≥12 years:* 5-10 mL every 12 hours
- *Adults:* 5-10 mL every 12 hours

AH-Chew®:
- *Children <6 years:* Dosage not established
- *Children 6-11 years:* 2.5-5 mL every 4 hours
- *Children ≥12 years:* 5-10 mL every 3-4 hours
- *Adults:* 5-10 mL every 3-4 hours

Dallergy®:
- *Children <6 years:* Dosage not established
- *Children 6-11 years:* One-half caplet every 12 hours
- *Children ≥12 years:* 1 capsule every 12 hours
- *Adults:* 1 capsule every 12 hours

Extendryl® chewable tablet:
- *Children <6 years:* Dosage not established
- *Children 6-11 years:* One tablet every 4 hours (maximum: 4 doses/day)
- *Children ≥12 years:* 1-2 tablets every 4 hours
- *Adults:* 1-2 tablets every 4 hours

Extendryl® JR:
- *Children 6-11 years:* One tablet every 12 hours

Extendryl® SR:
- *Children ≥12 years:* 1 capsule every 12 hours
- *Adults:* 1 capsule every 12 hours

Extendryl® syrup:
- *Children 6-11 years:* 2.5-5 mL up to every 4 hours
- *Children ≥12 years:* 5-10 mL every 3-4 hours (4 times/day)
- *Adults:* 5-10 mL every 3-4 hours (4 times/day)

Dosage Forms Excipient information presented when available (limited, particularly for generics); consult specific product labeling. [DSC] = Discontinued product

Caplet, extended release:
- aerohist plus™: Chlorpheniramine maleate 8 mg, phenylephrine hydrochloride 20 mg, and methscopolamine nitrate 2.5 mg
- Chlor-Mes: Chlorpheniramine maleate 12 mg, phenylephrine hydrochloride 20 mg, and methscopolamine nitrate 2.5 mg [dye free, sugar free]
- Dallergy®: Chlorpheniramine maleate 12 mg, phenylephrine hydrochloride 20 mg, and methscopolamine nitrate 2.5 mg [scored]

Liquid:
- Chlor-Mes-D: Chlorpheniramine maleate 2 mg, phenylephrine hydrochloride 10 mg, and methscopolamine nitrate 0.625 mg per 5 mL (480 mL) [grape flavor]

Suspension:
- AH-Chew®: Chlorpheniramine tannate [equivalent to chlorpheniramine maleate 2 mg], phenylephrine tannate [equivalent to phenylephrine hydrochloride 10 mg], and methscopalamine nitrate 1.5 mg per 5 mL (120 mL) [grape flavor]

Syrup:
- aeroKid™: Chlorpheniramine maleate 4 mg, phenylephrine hydrochloride 10 mg, and methscopolamine nitrate 1.25 mg per 5 mL (120 mL, 480 mL) [contains propylene glycol; blue raspberry flavor]
- Dallergy: Chlorpheniramine maleate 2 mg, phenylephrine hydrochloride 8 mg, and methscopolamine nitrate 0.75 mg per 5 mL (480 mL) [contains propylene glycol; grape flavor]
- Dehistine: Chlorpheniramine maleate 2 mg, phenylephrine hydrochloride 10 mg, and methscopolamine nitrate 1.25 mg per 5 mL (480 mL) [root beer flavor]
- Duradryl®: Chlorpheniramine maleate 2 mg, phenylephrine hydrochloride 10 mg, and methscopolamine nitrate 1.25 mg per 5 mL (480 mL) [contains sodium benzoate; cherry flavor]

Extendryl®: Dexchlorpheniramine maleate 1 mg, phenylephrine hydrochloride 10 mg, and methscopolamine nitrate 1.25 mg per 5 mL (480 mL) [root beer flavor]

Triall™: Chlorpheniramine maleate 2 mg, phenylephrine hydrochloride 8 mg, and methscopolamine nitrate 0.75 mg per 5 mL (473 mL) [contains sodium benzoate; alcohol free; grape flavor]

Tablet [scored]:

Dallergy®: Chlorpheniramine maleate 4 mg, phenylephrine hydrochloride 10 mg, and methscopolamine nitrate 1.25 mg

Tablet, chewable:

AH-Chew™ Ultra: Chlorpheniramine tannate [equivalent to chlorpheniramine maleate 2 mg], phenylephrine tanneate [equivalent to phenylephrine hydrochloride 10 mg], and methscopolamine nitrate 1.5 mg [scored; grape flavor]

Extendryl: Chlorpheniramine maleate 2 mg, phenylephrine hydrochloride 10 mg, and methscopolamine nitrate 1.25 mg [root beer flavor]

PCM: Chlorpheniramine maleate 2 mg, phenylephrine hydrochloride 10 mg, and methscopolamine nitrate 1.25 mg [grape flavor]

Tablet, extended release: Chlorpheniramine maleate 8 mg, phenylephrine hydrochloride 20 mg, and methscopolamine nitrate 1.25 mg

Durahist™ PE: Chlorpheniramine maleate 8 mg, phenylephrine hydrochloride 20 mg, and methscopolamine nitrate 1.25 mg [scored]

Extendryl SR: Chlorpheniramine maleate 8 mg, phenylephrine hydrochloride 20 mg, and methscopolamine nitrate 2.5 mg [scored]

Extendryl® JR: Chlorpheniramine maleate 4 mg, phenylephrine hydrochloride 10 mg, and methscopolamine nitrate 1.25 mg [scored]

Hista-Vent® DA: Chlorpheniramine maleate 8 mg, phenylephrine hydrochloride 20 mg, and methscopolamine nitrate 2.5 mg [scored] [DSC]

PCM Allergy: Chlorpheniramine maleate 12 mg, phenylephrine hydrochloride 20 mg, and methscopolamine nitrate 2.5 mg [DSC]

Tablet, long acting [scored]:

OMNIhist® II L.A.: Chlorpheniramine maleate 8 mg, phenylephrine hydrochloride 25 mg, and methscopolamine nitrate 2.5 mg

Rescon® MX: Chlorpheniramine maleate 8 mg, phenylephrine hydrochloride 40 mg, and methscopolamine nitrate 2.5 mg

Tablet, sustained release:

Histatab PH: Chlorpheniramine maleate 8 mg, phenylephrine hydrochloride 20 mg, and methscopolamine nitrate 1.25 mg

Ralix: Chlorpheniramine maleate 8 mg, phenylephrine hydrochloride 40 mg, and methscopolamine nitrate 2 mg

Tablet, timed release:

Phenylephrine CM: Chlorpheniramine maleate 8 mg, phenylephrine hydrochloride 40 mg, and methscopolamine nitrate 2.5 mg

Tablet, variable release:

Rescon®: Chlorpheniramine maleate 12 mg and phenylephrine hydrochloride 40 mg [sustained release] and methscopolamine nitrate 2 mg [immediate release] [MaxRelent release]

Chlorpheniramine, Phenylephrine, and Phenyltoloxamine

(klor fen IR a meen, fen il EF rin, & fen il tole LOKS a meen)

U.S. Brand Names Chlorex-A; Comhist® [DSC]; Nalex®-A; NoHist-A; Rhinacon A

Index Terms Phenylephrine, Chlorpheniramine, and Phenyltoloxamine; Phenyltoloxamine, Chlorpheniramine, and Phenylephrine

Pharmacologic Category Alpha/Beta Agonist; Histamine H_1 Antagonist; Histamine H_1 Antagonist, First Generation

Use Symptomatic relief of rhinitis and nasal congestion due to colds or allergy

Effect on Mental Status Drowsiness is common; may cause excitability, nervousness, fatigue, or depression

Effect on Psychiatric Treatment Dry mouth and sedation may be exacerbated by concurrent psychotropic use

Dosage Forms Excipient information presented when available (limited, particularly for generics); consult specific product labeling. [DSC] = Discontinued product

Liquid: Chlorpheniramine maleate 2.5 mg, phenylephrine hydrochloride 5 mg, and phenyltoloxamine citrate 7.5 mg per 5 mL (480 mL)

Nalex®-A, NoHist-A, Rhinacon A: Chlorpheniramine maleate 2.5 mg, phenylephrine hydrochloride 5 mg, and phenyltoloxamine citrate 7.5 mg per 5 mL (480 mL) [alcohol free, sugar free; cotton candy flavor]

Tablet:
Comhist®: Chlorpheniramine maleate 2 mg, phenylephrine hydrochloride 10 mg, and phenyltoloxamine citrate 25 mg [DSC]
Tablet, extended release:
Rhinacon A: Chlorpheniramine maleate 4 mg, phenylephrine hydrochloride 20 mg, and phenyltoloxamine citrate 40 mg
Tablet, prolonged release:
Nalex®-A: Chlorpheniramine maleate 4 mg, phenylephrine hydrochloride 20 mg, and phenyltoloxamine citrate 40 mg
Tablet, sustained release:
Chlorex-A: Chlorpheniramine maleate 4 mg, phenylephrine hydrochloride 20 mg, and phenyltoloxamine citrate 40 mg

Chlorpheniramine, Phenylephrine, Codeine, and Potassium Iodide

(klor fen IR a meen, fen il EF rin, KOE deen, & poe TASS ee um EYE oh dide)

U.S. Brand Names Pediacof® [DSC]

Index Terms Codeine, Chlorpheniramine, Phenylephrine, and Potassium Iodide; Phenylephrine, Chlorpheniramine, Codeine, and Potassium Iodide; Potassium Iodide, Chlorpheniramine, Phenylephrine, and Codeine

Pharmacologic Category Alpha/Beta Agonist; Analgesic, Opioid; Antitussive; Expectorant; Histamine H_1 Antagonist; Histamine H_1 Antagonist, First Generation

Use Symptomatic relief of rhinitis, nasal congestion and cough due to colds or allergy

Effect on Mental Status Drowsiness is common; may cause excitability, nervousness, fatigue, or depression

Effect on Psychiatric Treatment Dry mouth and sedation may be exacerbated by concurrent psychotropic use

Restrictions C-V

Dosage Summary

Oral:

Children <6 months: Dosage not established
Children 6 months to 12 years: 1.25-10 mL every 4-6 hours
Children >12 years: Dosage not established
Adults: Dosage not established

Dosage Forms Excipient information presented when available (limited, particularly for generics); consult specific product labeling.

Syrup: Chlorpheniramine maleate 0.75 mg, phenylephrine hydrochloride 2.5 mg, codeine phosphate 5 mg, and potassium iodide 75 mg per 5 mL (480 mL) [contains alcohol 5% and sodium benzoate; raspberry flavor] [DSC]

◆ **Chlorpheniramine, Pseudoephedrine, and Acetaminophen** *see* Acetaminophen, Chlorpheniramine, and Pseudoephedrine *on page 40*

Chlorpheniramine, Pseudoephedrine, and Codeine

(klor fen IR a meen, soo doe e FED rin, & KOE deen)

U.S. Brand Names Dihistine® DH [DSC]

Index Terms Codeine, Chlorpheniramine, and Pseudoephedrine; Pseudoephedrine, Chlorpheniramine, and Codeine

Pharmacologic Category Alpha/Beta Agonist; Analgesic, Opioid; Antitussive; Histamine H_1 Antagonist; Histamine H_1 Antagonist, First Generation

Use Temporary relief of cough associated with minor throat or bronchial irritation or nasal congestion due to common cold, allergic rhinitis, or sinusitis

Effect on Mental Status Drowsiness is common; may cause excitability, nervousness, fatigue, or depression

Effect on Psychiatric Treatment Dry mouth and sedation may be exacerbated by concurrent psychotropic use

Restrictions C-V

Dosage Summary

Oral:

Children <25 lbs: Dosage not established
Children 25-50 lbs: 1.25-2.5 mL every 4-6 hours (maximum: 4 doses/day)
Children 50-90 lbs: 2.5-5 mL every 4-6 hours (maximum: 4 doses/day)
Adults: 10 mL every 4-6 hours (maximum: 4 doses/day)

Dosage Forms Excipient information presented when available (limited particularly for generics); consult specific product labeling. [DSC] = Discontinued product

Elixir:

Dihistine® DH: Chlorpheniramine maleate 2 mg, pseudoephedrine hydrochloride 30 mg, and codeine phosphate 10 mg per 5 mL (120 mL, 480 mL) [contains alcohol; grape flavor] [DSC]

Chlorpheniramine, Pseudoephedrine, and Dextromethorphan

(klor fen IR a meen, soo doe e FED rin, & deks troe meth OR fan)

U.S. Brand Names Dicel™ DM; DuraTan™ Forte; Kidkare Children's Cough and Cold [OTC]; Pedia Relief™ [OTC]; Rescon DM [OTC]; Tanafed DMX™; Tannate PD-DM

Index Terms Chlorpheniramine Maleate, Pseudoephedrine Hydrochloride, and Dextromethorphan Hydrobromide; Chlorpheniramine Tannate, Pseudoephedrine Tannate, and Dextromethorphan Tannate; Dexchlorpheniramine Tannate, Pseudoephedrine Tannate, and Dextromethorphan Tannate; Dextromethorphan, Chlorpheniramine, and Pseudoephedrine; Pseudoephedrine, Chlorpheniramine, and Dextromethorphan

Pharmacologic Category Alpha/Beta Agonist; Antitussive; Histamine H_1 Antagonist; Histamine H_1 Antagonist, First Generation

Use Temporarily relieves nasal congestion, runny nose, cough, and sneezing due to the common cold, hay fever, or allergic rhinitis

Effect on Mental Status May cause anxiety, dizziness, insomnia, restlessness, hallucinations, or depression

Effect on Psychiatric Treatment Contraindicated with or within 14 days of MAO inhibitor treatment; may cause tremor which may be mistaken for EPS; may cause tachycardia; tachycardia is also common with clozapine; monitor vital signs; may cause sedation (concurrent use with psychotropics may produce additive sedative effects)

Dosage Summary Note: General dosing guidelines; consult specific product labeling.

Oral:

Chlorpheniramine maleate 1 mg, pseudoephedrine 15 mg, and dextromethorphan hydrobromide 7.5 mg per 5 mL:

Children <6 years: Dosage not established

Children 6-12 years: 10 mL every 6 hours

Children >12 years: 20 mL every 6 hours

Chlorpheniramine maleate 1 mg, pseudoephedrine 15 mg, and dextromethorphan hydrobromide 5 mg per tablet or 5 mL:

Children <6 years: Dosage not established

Children 6-12 years: 2 tablets **or** 10 mL every 4-6 hours (maximum: 4 doses/day)

Chlorpheniramine maleate 2 mg, pseudoephedrine 30 mg, and dextromethorphan hydrobromide 10 mg per tablet or 5 mL (Rescon DM):

Children <6 years: Dosage not established

Children 6-12 years: 5 mL every 4-6 hours (maximum: 4 doses/day)

Children >12 years: 10 mL every 4-6 hours (maximum: 4 doses/day)

Adults: 10 mL every 4-6 hours (maximum: 4 doses/day)

Dexchlorpheniramine tannate 2.5 mg, pseudoephedrine tannate 75 mg, and dextromethorphan tannate 25 mg (Tanafed DMX™):

Children <2 years: Dosage not established

Children 2-6 years: 2.5-5 mL every 12 hours (maximum: 10 mL/day)

Children 6-12 years: 5-10 mL every 12 hours (maximum: 20 mL/day)

Children ≥12 years: 10-20 mL every 12 hours (maximum: 40 mL/day)

Adults: 10-20 mL every 12 hours (maximum: 40 mL/day)

Dosage Forms Excipient information presented when available (limited, particularly for generics); consult specific product labeling. [DSC] = Discontinued product

Liquid: Chlorpheniramine maleate 1 mg, pseudoephedrine hydrochloride 15 mg, and dextromethorphan hydrobromide 5 mg per 5 mL (120 mL)

Kidkare Children's Cough and Cold: Chlorpheniramine maleate 1 mg, pseudoephedrine hydrochloride 15 mg, and dextromethorphan hydrobromide 5 mg per 5 mL (120 mL) [alcohol free; contains propylene glycol and sodium benzoate; cherry flavor]

Pedia Relief™: Chlorpheniramine maleate 1 mg, pseudoephedrine hydrochloride 15 mg, and dextromethorphan hydrobromide 5 mg per 5 mL (120 mL) [alcohol free; contains propylene glycol and sodium benzoate; cherry flavor]

Rescon DM: Chlorpheniramine maleate 2 mg, pseudoephedrine hydrochloride 30 mg, and dextromethorphan hydrobromide 10 mg per 5 mL (120 mL, 480 mL) [dye free; contains propylene glycol; cherry flavor]

Suspension:

Dicel™ DM: Chlorpheniramine tannate 5 mg, pseudoephedrine tannate 75 mg, and dextromethorphan tannate 25 mg per 5 mL (480 mL) [contains sodium benzoate; cotton candy flavor]

DuraTan™ Forte: Dexchlorpheniramine tannate 3.5 mg, pseudoephedrine tannate 45 mg, and dextromethorphan tannate 30 mg per 5 mL (480 mL) [contains sodium benzoate; grape flavor]

Tanafed DMX™: Dexchlorpheniramine tannate 2.5 mg, pseudoephedrine tannate 75 mg, and dextromethorphan tannate 25 mg (120 mL, 480 mL) [contains sodium benzoate; cotton candy flavor]

Tannate PD-DM: Dexchlorpheniramine tannate 3 mg, pseudoephedrine tannate 50 mg, and dextromethorphan tannate 27.5 mg per 5 mL (473 mL) [contains sodium benzoate; grape flavor]

◆ **Chlorpheniramine, Pseudoephedrine, and Dihydrocodeine** *see* Pseudoephedrine, Dihydrocodeine, and Chlorpheniramine *on page 1371*

◆ **Chlorpheniramine, Pseudoephedrine, and Hydrocodone** *see* Pseudoephedrine, Hydrocodone, and Chlorpheniramine *on page 1372*

Chlorpheniramine, Pseudoephedrine, and Methscopolamine

(klor fen IR a meen, soo doe e FED rin, & meth skoe POL a meen)

U.S. Brand Names Amdry-C; Coldamine; Durahist™; Hista-Vent® PSE [DSC]

Index Terms Methscopolamine, Chlorpheniramine, and Pseudoephedrine; Methscopolamine, Pseudoephedrine, and Chlorpheniramine; Pseudoephedrine Hydrochloride, Methscopolamine Nitrate, and Chlorpheniramine Maleate; Pseudoephedrine, Methscopolamine, and Chlorpheniramine

Pharmacologic Category Alpha/Beta Agonist; Anticholinergic Agent; Histamine H_1 Antagonist; Histamine H_1 Antagonist, First Generation

Use Relief of symptoms of allergic rhinitis, vasomotor rhinitis, sinusitis, and the common cold

Effect on Mental Status May cause sedation, anxiety, dizziness, giddiness, hallucinations, insomnia, irritability, nervousness, restlessness, or tremor

Effect on Psychiatric Treatment Contraindicated with or within 2 weeks of discontinuing an MAO inhibitor. Sedating agent; concurrent use with CNS depressant or alcohol may produce additive effects. Contains an anticholinergic agent; concurrent use with anticholinergic psychotropics may produce additive effects.

Dosage Summary

Oral:

Children <6 years: Dosage not established

Children 6-11 years: Durahist™, Hista-Vent® PSE: One-half tablet every 12 hours (maximum: 1 tablet/day)

Children ≥12 years: Durahist™, Hista-Vent® PSE: One tablet every 12 hours (maximum: 2 tablets/day)

Adults: Durahist™, Hista-Vent® PSE: One tablet every 12 hours (maximum: 2 tablets/day)

Dosage Forms Excipient information presented when available (limited, particularly for generics); consult specific product labeling. [DSC] = Discontinued product

Tablet, extended release:

Coldamine: Chlorpheniramine maleate 8 mg, pseudoephedrine hydrochloride 90 mg, and methscopolamine nitrate 2.5 mg

Tablet, sustained release: Chlorpheniramine maleate 8 mg, pseudoephedrine hydrochloride 60 mg, and methscopolamine nitrate 1.25 mg; chlorpheniramine maleate 8 mg, pseudoephedrine hydrochloride 90 mg, and methscopolamine nitrate 2.5 mg

Amdry-C: Chlorpheniramine maleate 8 mg, pseudoephedrine hydrochloride 120 mg, and methscopolamine nitrate 2.5 mg [scored]

Durahist™: Chlorpheniramine maleate 8 mg, pseudoephedrine hydrochloride 60 mg, and methscopolamine nitrate 1.25 mg [scored]

Hista-Vent® PSE: Chlorpheniramine maleate 8 mg, pseudoephedrine hydrochloride 120 mg, and methscopolamine nitrate 2.5 mg [dye free; scored] [DSC]

Chlorpheniramine, Pyrilamine, and Phenylephrine

(klor fen IR a meen, pye RIL a meen, & fen il EF rin)

U.S. Brand Names AllerTan™; Chlor-Tan A 12 [DSC]; Chlorex-A 12 [DSC]; Conal; MyHist-PD; Nalex A 12; Poly Hist Forte®; Poly Hist PD; Ru-Hist Forte; Tri-Hist; Triplex™ AD

Pharmacologic Category Alpha/Beta Agonist; Histamine H_1 Antagonist; Histamine H_1 Antagonist, First Generation

Use Symptomatic relief of rhinitis and nasal congestion due to colds or allergy

Effect on Mental Status May cause dizziness, nervousness, sedation, or excitation (children).

Effect on Psychiatric Treatment Contraindicated with or within 14 days of MAO inhibitor treatment. May cause CNS depression; concomitant use with psychotropic agents may produce additive effects. May cause agranulocytosis; use with caution in patients receiving clozapine and carbamazepine. May cause anticholinergic side effects; concurrent use with psychotropic agents may produce additive effects. Use may mitigate effects of acetylcholinesterase inhibitors. Tricyclic antidepressants may enhance the vasopressor effect of phenylephrine.

Dosage Summary Oral:

Tablet:

Children <6 years: Dosage not established.
Children 6-12 years: 1/2 tablet 2-3 times/day
Children >12 years: 1 tablet 2-3 times/day
Adults: 1 tablet 2-3 times/day

Liquid (MyHist-PD, Poly Hist PD):

Children <6 years: Dosage not established.
Children 2-6 years: 2.5 mL every 4-6 hours (maximum: 10 mL/day)
Children 6-12 years: 5 mL every 4-6 hours (maximum: 20 mL/day)
Children >12 years: 5-10 mL every 4-6 hours (maximum: 40 mL/day)
Adults: 5-10 mL every 4-6 hours (maximum: 40 mL/day)

Liquid (Triplex™ AD):

Children <6 years: Dosage not established
Children 6-12 years: 5 mL every 4-6 hours (maximum: 20 mL/day)
Children >12: 5-10 mL every 4-6 hours (maximum: 40 mL/day)
Adults: 5-10 mL every 4-6 hours (maximum: 40 mL/day)

Suspension (AllerTan™, Conal):

Children 2-6 years: 2.5 mL every 12 hours (maximum: 5 mL/day)
Children 6-12 years: 5 mL every 12 hours (maximum: 10 mL/day)
Children >12 years and Adults: 5-10 mL every 12 hours (maximum: 20 mL/day)

Dosage Forms Excipient information presented when available (limited, particularly for generics); consult specific product labeling.

Liquid, oral:

MyHist-PD: Chlorpheniramine maleate 2 mg, pyrilamine maleate 12.5 mg, and phenylephrine hydrochloride 7.5 mg per 5 mL (473 mL) [dye free, ethanol free, sugar free; bubblegum flavor]

Poly Hist PD: Chlorpheniramine maleate 2 mg, pyrilamine maleate 12.5 mg, and phenylephrine hydrochloride 7.5 mg per 5 mL (480 mL) [dye free, ethanol free, sugar free; contains propylene glycol; bubblegum flavor]

Triplex™ AD: Chlorpheniramine maleate 2 mg, pyrilamine maleate 12.5 mg, and phenylephrine hydrochloride 7.5 mg per 5 mL (473 mL) [dye free, ethanol free, sugar free; contains sodium benzoate; bubblegum flavor]

Suspension, oral:

AllerTan™: Chlorpheniramine maleate 8 mg, pyrilamine maleate 12.5 mg, and phenylephrine hydrochloride 15 mg per 5 mL (473 mL) [contains sodium benzoate; grape flavor]

Chlor-Tan A 12: Chlorpheniramine maleate 2 mg, pyrilamine maleate 12.5 mg, and phenylephrine hydrochloride 5 mg per 5 mL (118 mL) [ethanol free, sugar free; raspberry flavor] [DSC]

Chlorex-A 12: Chlorpheniramine maleate 2 mg, pyrilamine maleate 12.5 mg, and phenylephrine hydrochloride 5 mg per 5 mL (120 mL) [raspberry flavor] [DSC]

Conal: Chlorpheniramine maleate 8 mg, pyrilamine maleate 12.5 mg, and phenylephrine hydrochloride 15 mg per 5 mL (473 mL) [contains phenylalanine 7 mg/5 mL, propylene glycol; raspberry flavor]

Nalex A 12: Chlorpheniramine tannate 2 mg, pyrilamine tannate 12.5 mg, and phenylephrine tannate 5 mg per 5 mL (120 mL) [contains benzoic acid; raspberry flavor]

Tri-Hist: Chlorpheniramine maleate 2 mg, pyrilamine maleate 12.5 mg, and phenylephrine hydrochloride 5 mg per 5 mL (120 mL)

Tablet, sustained release, oral:
Poly Hist Forte®: Chlorpheniramine maleate 4 mg, pyrilamine maleate 25 mg, and phenylephrine hydrochloride 10 mg
Tablet, time-released, oral: Chlorpheniramine maleate 4 mg, pyrilamine maleate 25 mg, and phenylephrine hydrochloride 10 mg
Ru-Hist Forte: Chlorpheniramine maleate 4 mg, pyrilamine maleate 25 mg, and phenylephrine hydrochloride 10 mg

◆ **Chlorpheniramine Tannate and Phenylephrine Tannate** *see* Chlorpheniramine and Phenylephrine *on page 323*

◆ **Chlorpheniramine Tannate and Pseudoephedrine Tannate** *see* Chlorpheniramine and Pseudoephedrine *on page 325*

◆ **Chlorpheniramine Tannate, Phenylephrine Tannate, and Guaifenesin** *see* Chlorpheniramine, Phenylephrine, and Guaifenesin *on page 329*

◆ **Chlorpheniramine Tannate, Pseudoephedrine Tannate, and Dextromethorphan Tannate** *see* Chlorpheniramine, Pseudoephedrine, and Dextromethorphan *on page 333*

ChlorproMAZINE (klor PROE ma zeen)

Medication Safety Issues
Sound-alike/look-alike issues:
ChlorproMAZINE may be confused with chlordiazePOXIDE, chlorproPAMIDE, clomiPRAMINE, prochlorperazine, promethazine
Thorazine® may be confused with thiamine, thioridazine

Related Information
Agents Approved for Bipolar Disorder *on page 1752*
Anticholinergic Effects of Common Psychotropics *on page 1758*
Antipsychotic Agents *on page 1769*
CMS: Long-Term Care Facility Thresholds *on page 1815*
Discontinuation of Psychotropic Drugs *on page 1839*
Liquid Compatibility of Antidepressants, Antipsychotics, and Mood Stabilizers *on page 1788*

Canadian Brand Names Largactil®; Novo-Chlorpromazine

Mexican Brand Names Largactil

Index Terms Chlorpromazine Hydrochloride; CPZ

Pharmacologic Category Antimanic Agent; Antipsychotic Agent, Typical, Phenothiazine

Generic Available Yes

Use Control of mania; treatment of schizophrenia; control of nausea and vomiting; relief of restlessness and apprehension before surgery; acute intermittent porphyria; adjunct in the treatment of tetanus; intractable hiccups; combativeness and/or explosive hyperexcitable behavior in children 1-12 years of age and in short-term treatment of hyperactive children

Unlabeled/Investigational Use Management of psychotic disorders; behavioral symptoms associated with dementia (elderly); psychosis/agitation related to Alzheimer's dementia

Mental Health Comment Chlorpromazine is a low-potency typical antipsychotic. Older antipsychotic medications (chlorpromazine, haloperidol), which do not meet specific criteria for "atypical" antipsychotics, are often referred to as typical antipsychotics. Compared to newer "atypical" antipsychotics, typical antipsychotics may have a greater propensity to cause extrapyramidal symptoms (EPS).

These drugs are thought to exert their antipsychotic activity by blocking dopamine D_2 receptors in the mesolimbic dopaminergic pathway. Side effects are often related to their ability to antagonize dopamine receptors in the nigrostriatal and tuberoinfundibular pathways.

Common side effects include sedation and neuroleptic effect (reduced initiative, interest in the environment, and display of emotion or affect). All **typical** antipsychotics are considered to be equally effective if given in equipotent doses. An inverse relationship exists between intrinsic antimuscarinic activity and propensity to cause extrapyramidal side effects. If dystonia or pseudoparkinsonism occurs, antiparkinsonian agents should be considered. If akathisia occurs, beta-blockers (eg, propranolol), benzodiazepines, or antiparkinsonian agents should be considered. Tardive dyskinesia (TD) secondary to typical antipsychotics has an estimated incidence of 3% to 5% per year for the first 5 years of treatment. After this time period, the incidence is estimated to be 2% to 3% per year. Prevalence rates are ~15% to 20%. Female gender and age constitute risk factors for TD. Indeed, prevalence rates have been reported to be as high as 70% in elderly females. No specific treatment exists for TD, however, patients are often initiated on/switched to an atypical antipsychotic because of their lower incidence to cause TD and hopes of suppression.

Typical antipsychotics are usually only indicated for schizophrenia, but are generally effective for mania and psychosis and/or behavioral syndromes secondary to other mental conditions. Nonpsychiatric uses include Tourette's syndrome, Huntington's disease, and occasionally, intractable hiccups, pruritus, nausea, and vomiting.

Coadministration of two or more antipsychotics does not generally improve clinical response and may increase the potential for adverse effects.

In 2008, the FDA issued a warning regarding increased mortality risk with typical **and** atypical antipsychotic drugs when used in elderly patients with dementia-related psychosis.

Pregnancy Risk Factor C

Lactation Enters breast milk/not recommended (AAP rates "of concern")

Contraindications Hypersensitivity to chlorpromazine or any component of the formulation (cross-reactivity between phenothiazines may occur); severe CNS depression; coma

Warnings/Precautions Highly sedating, use with caution in disorders where CNS depression is a feature and in patients with Parkinson's disease. Use with caution in patients with hemodynamic instability, bone marrow suppression, predisposition to seizures, subcortical brain damage, severe cardiac, hepatic, renal, or respiratory disease. Esophageal dysmotility and aspiration have been associated with antipsychotic use; use with caution in patients at risk of aspiration pneumonia (ie, Alzheimer's disease). Caution in breast cancer or other prolactin-dependent tumors (may elevate prolactin levels). May alter temperature regulation or mask toxicity of other drugs due to antiemetic effects. May alter cardiac conduction; life-threatening arrhythmias have occurred with therapeutic doses of neuroleptics.

Elderly patients with dementia-related psychosis treated with antipsychotics are at an increased risk of death compared to placebo. An increased incidence of cerebrovascular adverse events (including fatalities) has been reported in elderly patients with dementia-related psychosis. Chlorpromazine is not approved for this indication. Use with caution in patients at risk of hypotension (orthostasis is common) or those who would tolerate transient hypotensive episodes (cerebrovascular disease, cardiovascular disease, or other medications which may predispose). Significant hypotension may occur, particularly with parenteral administration. Injection contains sulfites.

Use with caution in patients with decreased gastrointestinal motility, urinary retention, BPH, xerostomia, or visual problems (ie, narrow-angle glaucoma - screening is recommended) and myasthenia gravis. Relative to other neuroleptics, chlorpromazine has a moderate potency of cholinergic blockade.

May cause extrapyramidal symptoms (EPS), including pseudoparkinsonism, acute dystonic reactions, akathisia, and tardive dyskinesia (risk of these reactions is low-moderate relative to other neuroleptics). Risk of dystonia (and possibly other EPS) may be greater with increased doses, use of conventional antipsychotics, males, and younger patients. May cause neuroleptic malignant syndrome (NMS) or pigmentary retinopathy.

Adverse Reactions Frequency not defined.

Cardiovascular: Postural hypotension, tachycardia, dizziness, nonspecific QT changes

Central nervous system: Drowsiness, dystonias, akathisia, pseudoparkinsonism, tardive dyskinesia, neuroleptic malignant syndrome, seizure

Dermatologic: Photosensitivity, dermatitis, skin pigmentation (slate gray)

Endocrine & metabolic: Lactation, breast engorgement, false-positive pregnancy test, amenorrhea, gynecomastia, hyper- or hypoglycemia

Gastrointestinal: Xerostomia, constipation, nausea

Genitourinary: Urinary retention, ejaculatory disorder, impotence

Hematologic: Agranulocytosis, eosinophilia, leukopenia, hemolytic anemia, aplastic anemia, thrombocytopenic purpura

Hepatic: Jaundice

Ocular: Blurred vision, corneal and lenticular changes, epithelial keratopathy, pigmentary retinopathy

Metabolism/Transport Effects **Substrate** of CYP1A2 (minor), 2D6 (major), 3A4 (minor); **Inhibits** CYP2D6 (strong), 2E1 (weak)

Drug Interactions

Acetylcholinesterase Inhibitors (Central): May enhance the neurotoxic (central) effect of Antipsychotics. Severe extrapyramidal symptoms have occurred in some patients. *Risk C: Monitor therapy*

Alcohol (Ethyl): CNS Depressants may enhance the CNS depressant effect of Alcohol (Ethyl). *Risk C: Monitor therapy*

Alfuzosin: May enhance the QTc-prolonging effect of QTc-Prolonging Agents. *Risk C: Monitor therapy*

Amphetamines: Antipsychotics may diminish the stimulatory effect of Amphetamines. *Risk C: Monitor therapy*

Analgesics (Opioid): Antipsychotic Agents (Phenothiazines) may enhance the hypotensive effect of Analgesics (Opioid). *Risk C: Monitor therapy*

Antacids: May decrease the absorption of Antipsychotic Agents (Phenothiazines). *Risk C: Monitor therapy*

Anticholinergics: May enhance the adverse/toxic effect of other Anticholinergics. **Exceptions:** Paliperidone. *Risk C: Monitor therapy*

Antimalarial Agents: May increase the serum concentration of Antipsychotic Agents (Phenothiazines). *Risk C: Monitor therapy*

Anti-Parkinson's Agents (Dopamine Agonist): Antipsychotics (Typical) may diminish the therapeutic effect of Anti-Parkinson's Agents (Dopamine Agonist). *Risk D: Consider therapy modification*

Beta-Blockers: Antipsychotic Agents (Phenothiazines) may enhance the hypotensive effect of Beta-Blockers. Beta-Blockers may decrease the metabolism of Antipsychotic Agents (Phenothiazines). Antipsychotic Agents (Phenothiazines) may decrease the metabolism of Beta-Blockers. **Exceptions:** Atenolol; Levobunolol; Metipranolol; Nadolol. *Risk C: Monitor therapy*

Ciprofloxacin: May enhance the QTc-prolonging effect of QTc-Prolonging Agents. *Risk C: Monitor therapy*

CNS Depressants: May enhance the adverse/toxic effect of other CNS Depressants. *Risk C: Monitor therapy*

CYP2D6 Inhibitors (Moderate): May decrease the metabolism of CYP2D6 Substrates. *Risk C: Monitor therapy*

CYP2D6 Inhibitors (Strong): May decrease the metabolism of CYP2D6 Substrates. *Risk D: Consider therapy modification*

CYP2D6 Substrates: CYP2D6 Inhibitors (Strong) may decrease the metabolism of CYP2D6 Substrates. **Exceptions:** Tamoxifen. *Risk D: Consider therapy modification*

Darunavir: May increase the serum concentration of CYP2D6 Substrates. *Risk C: Monitor therapy*

Desmopressin: ChlorproMAZINE may enhance the adverse/toxic effect of Desmopressin. *Risk C: Monitor therapy*

Gadobutrol: May enhance the QTc-prolonging effect of QTc-Prolonging Agents. *Risk D: Consider therapy modification*

Haloperidol: May enhance the QTc-prolonging effect of ChlorproMAZINE. ChlorproMAZINE may decrease the metabolism of Haloperidol. *Risk D: Consider therapy modification*

Lithium formulations: May enhance the neurotoxic effect of Antipsychotics. Lithium formulations may decrease the serum concentration of Antipsychotics. Specifically noted with chlorpromazine. *Risk C: Monitor therapy*

Nilotinib: May enhance the QTc-prolonging effect of QTc-Prolonging Agents. *Risk X: Avoid combination*

Pramlintide: May enhance the anticholinergic effect of Anticholinergics. These effects are specific to the GI tract. *Risk D: Consider therapy modification*

QTc-Prolonging Agents: May enhance the adverse/toxic effect of other QTc-Prolonging Agents. Their effects can be additive, causing life-threatening ventricular arrhythmias. *Risk D: Consider therapy modification*

Tamoxifen: CYP2D6 Inhibitors (Strong) may decrease the metabolism of Tamoxifen. Specifically, strong CYP2D6 inhibitors may decrease the formation of highly potent active metabolites. *Risk X: Avoid combination*

Tetrabenazine: May enhance the adverse/toxic effect of Antipsychotics. *Risk C: Monitor therapy*

Thioridazine: QTc-Prolonging Agents may enhance the QTc-prolonging effect of Thioridazine. *Risk X: Avoid combination*

Thioridazine: CYP2D6 Inhibitors may decrease the metabolism of Thioridazine. *Risk X: Avoid combination*

TraMADol: CYP2D6 Inhibitors (Strong) may diminish the therapeutic effect of TraMADol. These CYP2D6 inhibitors may prevent the metabolic conversion of tramadol to its active metabolite that accounts for much of its opioid-like effects. *Risk C: Monitor therapy*

Valproic Acid: ChlorproMAZINE may increase the serum concentration of Valproic Acid. *Risk C: Monitor therapy*

Ziprasidone: QTc-Prolonging Agents may enhance the QTc-prolonging effect of Ziprasidone. The risk of a severe arrhythmia may be increased. *Risk X: Avoid combination*

Ethanol/Nutrition/Herb Interactions

Ethanol: Avoid ethanol (may increase CNS depression).

Herb/Nutraceutical: Avoid St John's wort (may decrease chlorpromazine levels, increase photosensitization, or enhance sedative effect). Avoid dong quai (may enhance photosensitization). Avoid kava kava, gotu kola, valerian (may increase CNS depression).

Stability Injection: Protect from light. A slightly yellowed solution does not indicate potency loss, but a markedly discolored solution should be discarded. Diluted injection (1 mg/mL) with NS and stored in 5 mL vials remains stable for 30 days.

Mechanism of Action Chlorpromazine is an aliphatic phenothiazine antipsychotic which blocks postsynaptic mesolimbic dopaminergic receptors in the brain; exhibits a strong alpha-adrenergic blocking effect and depresses the release of hypothalamic and hypophyseal hormones; believed to depress the reticular activating system, thus affecting basal metabolism, body temperature, wakefulness, vasomotor tone, and emesis

Pharmacodynamics/Kinetics

Onset of action: I.M.: 15 minutes; Oral: 30-60 minutes

Absorption: Rapid

Distribution: V_d: 20 L/kg; crosses the placenta; enters breast milk

Protein binding: 92% to 97%

Metabolism: Extensively hepatic to active and inactive metabolites

Bioavailability: 20%

Half-life, biphasic: Initial: 2 hours; Terminal: 30 hours

Excretion: Urine (<1% as unchanged drug) within 24 hours

Dosage

Children ≥6 months:

Schizophrenia/psychoses:

Oral: 0.5-1 mg/kg/dose every 4-6 hours; older children may require 200 mg/day or higher

I.M., I.V.: 0.5-1 mg/kg/dose every 6-8 hours

<5 years (22.7 kg): Maximum: 40 mg/day

5-12 years (22.7-45.5 kg): Maximum: 75 mg/day

Nausea and vomiting:

Oral: 0.5-1 mg/kg/dose every 4-6 hours as needed

I.M., I.V.: 0.5-1 mg/kg/dose every 6-8 hours

<5 years (22.7 kg): Maximum: 40 mg/day

5-12 years (22.7-45.5 kg): Maximum: 75 mg/day

Adults:

Schizophrenia/psychoses:

Oral: Range: 30-2000 mg/day in 1-4 divided doses, initiate at lower doses and titrate as needed; usual dose: 400-600 mg/day; some patients may require 1-2 g/day

I.M., I.V.: Initial: 25 mg, may repeat (25-50 mg) in 1-4 hours, gradually increase to a maximum of 400 mg/dose every 4-6 hours until patient is controlled; usual dose: 300-800 mg/day

Intractable hiccups: Oral, I.M.: 25-50 mg 3-4 times/day

Nausea and vomiting:

Oral: 10-25 mg every 4-6 hours

I.M., I.V.: 25-50 mg every 4-6 hours

Elderly: Behavioral symptoms associated with dementia (unlabeled use): Initial: 10-25 mg 1-2 times/day; increase at 4- to 7-day intervals by 10-25 mg/day. Increase dose intervals (bid, tid, etc) as necessary to control behavior response or side effects; maximum daily dose: 800 mg; gradual increases (titration) may prevent some side effects or decrease their severity.

Dosing comments in renal impairment: Hemodialysis: Not dialyzable (0% to 5%)

Dosing adjustment/comments in hepatic impairment: Avoid use in severe hepatic dysfunction

Administration Note: Avoid skin contact with oral solution or injection solution; may cause contact dermatitis.

I.V.: Direct or intermittent infusion: Infuse 1 mg or portion thereof over 1 minute.

Monitoring Parameters Vital signs; lipid profile, fasting blood glucose/Hgb A_{1c}; BMI; mental status; abnormal involuntary movement scale (AIMS); extrapyramidal symptoms (EPS)

Reference Range

Therapeutic: 50-300 ng/mL (SI: 157-942 nmol/L)

Toxic: >750 ng/mL (SI: >2355 nmol/L); serum concentrations poorly correlate with expected response

Test Interactions False-positives for phenylketonuria, amylase, uroporphyrins, urobilinogen. May cause false-positive pregnancy test.

Dosage Forms Excipient information presented when available (limited, particularly for generics); consult specific product labeling.

Injection, solution, as hydrochloride: 25 mg/mL (1 mL, 2 mL)

Tablet, as hydrochloride: 10 mg, 25 mg, 50 mg, 100 mg, 200 mg

◆ **Chlorpromazine Hydrochloride** *see* ChlorproMAZINE *on page 336*

ChlorproPAMIDE (klor PROE pa mide)

Medication Safety Issues

Sound-alike/look-alike issues:

ChlorproPAMIDE may be confused with chlorproMAZINE

Diabinese® may be confused with DiaBeta®, Dialume®, Diamox®

High alert medication: The Institute for Safe Medication Practices (ISMP) includes this medication among its list of drugs which have a heightened risk of causing significant patient harm when used in error.

U.S. Brand Names Diabinese® [DSC]

Canadian Brand Names Apo-Chlorpropamide®; Novo-Propamide

Mexican Brand Names Diabenese; Insogen

Pharmacologic Category Antidiabetic Agent, Sulfonylurea

Use Management of blood sugar in type 2 diabetes mellitus (noninsulin dependent, NIDDM)

Unlabeled/Investigational Use Neurogenic diabetes insipidus

Effect on Mental Status Dizziness is common

Effect on Psychiatric Treatment Rare reports of agranulocytosis; use caution with clozapine and carbamazepine

Dosage Summary

Oral:

Children: Dosage not established

Adults: Initial: 250 mg/day; Maintenance: 100-500 mg/day (maximum: 750 mg/day); **Note:** Titration is recommended

Elderly: Initial: 100-125 mg/day

Dosage Forms Excipient information presented when available (limited, particularly for generics); consult specific product labeling. [DSC] = Discontinued product

Tablet: 100 mg, 250 mg

Diabinese®: 100 mg, 250 mg [DSC]

◆ **Chlor-Tan A 12 [DSC]** *see* Chlorpheniramine, Pyrilamine, and Phenylephrine *on page 335*

Chlorthalidone (klor THAL i done)

U.S. Brand Names Thalitone®

Canadian Brand Names Apo-Chlorthalidone®

Mexican Brand Names Higroton

Index Terms Hygroton

Pharmacologic Category Diuretic, Thiazide

Use Management of mild-to-moderate hypertension when used alone or in combination with other agents; treatment of edema associated with congestive heart failure or nephrotic syndrome. Recent studies have found chlorthalidone effective in the treatment of isolated systolic hypertension in the elderly.

Unlabeled/Investigational Use Pediatric hypertension

Effect on Mental Status None reported

Effect on Psychiatric Treatment Rare reports of blood dyscrasias; use caution with clozapine and carbamazepine; thiazides decrease lithium clearance resulting in elevated serum lithium levels and potential toxicity; monitor serum lithium levels

Dosage Summary

Oral:

Children (unlabeled use): 2 mg/kg 3 times/week **or** 0.3-2 mg/kg/day

Adults: 12.5-100 mg/day **or** 100 mg 3 times/week (maximum: 200 mg/day)

Elderly: Initial: 12.5-25 mg /day or every other day

Dosage Forms Excipient information presented when available (limited particularly for generics); consult specific product labeling.

Tablet: 25 mg, 50 mg, 100 mg

Thalitone®: 15 mg

- **Chlorthalidone and Atenolol** *see* Atenolol and Chlorthalidone *on page 150*
- **Chlorthalidone and Clonidine** *see* Clonidine and Chlorthalidone *on page 380*
- **Chlor-Trimeton® [OTC]** *see* Chlorpheniramine *on page 321*

Chlorzoxazone (klor ZOKS a zone)

Medication Safety Issues
Sound-alike/look-alike issues:
Parafon Forte® may be confused with Fam-Pren Forte
U.S. Brand Names Parafon Forte® DSC
Canadian Brand Names Parafon Forte®; Strifon Forte®
Mexican Brand Names Parafon Forte; Reumophan; Reumophan Alka; Reumophan Vit; Tafirol Flex
Pharmacologic Category Skeletal Muscle Relaxant
Use Symptomatic treatment of muscle spasm and pain associated with acute musculoskeletal conditions
Effect on Mental Status Drowsiness is common; may produce depression or paradoxical stimulation
Effect on Psychiatric Treatment May produce aplastic anemia and leukopenia; use caution with clozapine and carbamazepine
Dosage Summary
Oral:
Children: 20 mg/kg/day **or** 600 mg/m^2/day in 3-4 divided doses
Adults: 250-750 mg 3-4 times/day
Elderly: Initial: 250 mg 2-4 times/day, increase up to maximum of 750 mg 3-4 times/day
Dosage Forms Excipient information presented when available (limited, particularly for generics); consult specific product labeling.
Caplet (Parafon Forte® DSC): 500 mg
Tablet: 250 mg, 500 mg

Cholecalciferol (kole e kal SI fer ole)

U.S. Brand Names D-3 [OTC]; D3-50™ [OTC]; D3-5™ [OTC]; Delta-D® [OTC]; Maximum D3®; Vitamin D3 [OTC]
Canadian Brand Names D-Vi-Sol®
Index Terms D_3
Pharmacologic Category Vitamin D Analog
Use Dietary supplement, treatment of vitamin D deficiency, or prophylaxis of deficiency
Effect on Mental Status May cause irritability; rare reports of psychosis
Effect on Psychiatric Treatment None reported
Dosage Summary
Oral:
Children: Dosage not established
Adults: 400-1000 units/day
Dosage Forms Excipient information presented when available (limited, particularly for generics); consult specific product labeling.
Capsule, oral:
D-3: 1000 int. units
D3-5™: 5000 int. units
D3-50™: 50,000 int. units
Maximum D3®: 10,000 int. units [contains soybean lecithin]
Capsule, softgel, oral:
D-3: 2000 int. units
Tablet:
Delta-D®: 400 int. units

- **Cholecalciferol and Alendronate** *see* Alendronate and Cholecalciferol *on page 62*

Cholestyramine Resin (koe LES teer a meen REZ in)

Related Information
Lipid-Lowering Agents *on page 1786*
U.S. Brand Names Prevalite®; Questran®; Questran® Light
Canadian Brand Names Novo-Cholamine; Novo-Cholamine Light; PMS-Cholestyramine; Questran®; Questran® Light Sugar Free

Mexican Brand Names Questran

Pharmacologic Category Antilipemic Agent, Bile Acid Sequestrant

Use Adjunct in the management of primary hypercholesterolemia; pruritus associated with elevated levels of bile acids; diarrhea associated with excess fecal bile acids; binding toxicologic agents; pseudomembraneous colitis

Effect on Mental Status None reported

Effect on Psychiatric Treatment May decrease the absorption of psychotropics including TCAs, beta-blockers, valproic acid, barbiturates

Dosage Summary

Oral:

Children: 240 mg/kg/day in 3 divided doses

Adults: 4-24 g/day in 1-6 divided doses

Dosage Forms Excipient information presented when available (limited, particularly for generics); consult specific product labeling.

Powder for oral suspension: Cholestyramine resin 4 g/5 g packet (60s); cholestyramine resin 4 g/5 g of powder (210 g); cholestyramine resin 4 g/5.7 g packet (60s); cholestyramine resin 4 g/5.7 g of powder (240 g can); cholestyramine resin 4 g/9 g packet (60s); cholestyramine resin 4 g of resin/9 g of powder (378 g)

Prevalite®: Cholestyramine resin 4 g/5.5 g packet (42s, 60s) [contains phenylalanine 14.1 mg/5.5 g; orange flavor]; cholestyramine resin 4 g/5.5 g of powder (231 g) [contains phenylalanine 14.1 mg/5.5 g; orange flavor]

Questran®: Cholestyramine resin 4 g/9 g packet (60s); cholestyramine resin 4 g/9 g of powder (378 g)

Questran® Light: Cholestyramine resin 4 g/5 g packet (60s) [contains phenylalanine 14 mg/5 g]; cholestyramine resin 4 g/5 g of powder (210 g) [contains phenylalanine 14 mg/5 g]

Choline Magnesium Trisalicylate

(KOE leen mag NEE zhum trye sa LIS i late)

Index Terms Tricosal

Pharmacologic Category Salicylate

Use Management of osteoarthritis, rheumatoid arthritis, and other arthritis; acute painful shoulder

Effect on Mental Status May cause sedation; may rarely cause nervousness or insomnia

Effect on Psychiatric Treatment May rarely cause leukopenia; use caution with clozapine and carbamazepine

Dosage Summary

Oral:

Children <37 kg: 50 mg/kg/day in 2 divided doses

Children ≥37 kg: 2250 mg/day in divided doses

Adults: 500 mg to 1.5 g 2-3 times/day **or** 3 g at bedtime

Elderly: 750 mg 3 times/day

Dosage Forms Excipient information presented when available (limited, particularly for generics); consult specific product labeling.

Liquid: 500 mg/5 mL (240 mL) [choline salicylate 293 mg and magnesium salicylate 362 mg per 5 mL; cherry cordial flavor]

Tablet: 500 mg [choline salicylate 293 mg and magnesium salicylate 362 mg]; 750 mg [choline salicylate 440 mg and magnesium salicylate 544 mg]; 1000 mg [choline salicylate 587 mg and magnesium salicylate 725 mg]

◆ **Chooz® [OTC]** *see* Calcium Carbonate *on page 254*

◆ **Choriogonadotropin Alfa** *see* Chorionic Gonadotropin (Recombinant) *on page 343*

Chorionic Gonadotropin (Human)

(kor ee ON ik goe NAD oh troe pin, HYU man)

U.S. Brand Names Novarel®; Pregnyl®

Canadian Brand Names Humegon®; Pregnyl®; Profasi® HP

Mexican Brand Names Choragon; Choriomon; Pregnyl

Index Terms CG; hCG

Pharmacologic Category Gonadotropin; Ovulation Stimulator

Use Induces ovulation and pregnancy in anovulatory, infertile females; treatment of hypogonadotropic hypogonadism, prepubertal cryptorchidism; spermatogenesis induction with follitropin alfa

Effect on Mental Status May cause drowsiness or depression; rarely may cause restlessness or irritability

Effect on Psychiatric Treatment None reported

Dosage Summary

I.M.:

Children: 4000 units 3 times/week for 3 weeks **or** 5000 units every second day for 4 injections **or** 500 units 3 times/week for 4-6 weeks **or** 15 injections of 500-1000 units given over 6 weeks

Children (males): Hypogonadism: 500-1000 units 3 times/week for 3 weeks, followed by the same dose twice weekly for 3 weeks **or** 4000 units 3 times/week for 6-9 months, then reduce dosage to 2000 units 3 times/week for additional 3 months

Adults (females): 5000-10,000 units 1 day following last dose of menotropins

Adults (males): 1000-2000 units 2-3 times/week

Dosage Forms Excipient information presented when available (limited, particularly for generics); consult specific product labeling.

Injection, powder for reconstitution: 10,000 units [packaged with diluent; diluent contains benzyl alcohol and mannitol]

Novarel®: 10,000 units [packaged with diluent; diluent contains benzyl alcohol and mannitol]

Pregnyl®: 10,000 units [packaged with diluent; diluent contains benzyl alcohol]

Chorionic Gonadotropin (Recombinant)

(kor ee ON ik goe NAD oh troe pin ree KOM be nant)

U.S. Brand Names Ovidrel®

Canadian Brand Names Ovidrel®

Mexican Brand Names Ovidrel

Index Terms Choriogonadotropin Alfa; r-hCG

Pharmacologic Category Gonadotropin; Ovulation Stimulator

Use As part of an assisted reproductive technology (ART) program, induces ovulation in infertile females who have been pretreated with follicle stimulating hormones (FSH); induces ovulation and pregnancy in infertile females when the cause of infertility is functional

Effect on Mental Status May cause dizziness, emotional lability, and insomnia

Effect on Psychiatric Treatment None reported

Dosage Summary

SubQ:

Children: Dosage not established

Adults (female): 250 mcg given 1 day following last dose of follicle stimulating agent

Dosage Forms Excipient information presented when available (limited, particularly for generics); consult specific product labeling.

Injection, solution:

Ovidrel®: 257.5 mcg/0.515 mL (0.515 mL) [prefilled syringe; delivers 250 mcg r-hCG/0.5 mL]

◆ **CI-1008** *see* Pregabalin *on page 1332*

◆ **Cialis®** *see* Tadalafil *on page 1534*

Ciclesonide (sye KLES oh nide)

U.S. Brand Names Alvesco®; Omnaris™

Canadian Brand Names Alvesco®; Omnaris™

Mexican Brand Names Alvesco

Pharmacologic Category Corticosteroid, Inhalant (Oral); Corticosteroid, Nasal

Use

Intranasal: Management of seasonal and perennial allergic rhinitis

Oral inhalation: Prophylactic management of bronchial asthma

Effect on Mental Status None reported

Effect on Psychiatric Treatment Patients may experience symptoms of corticosteroid withdrawal (depression) when replacing a systemic agent with a topical corticosteroid.

Dosage Summary

Intranasal:

Children <6 years: Dosage not established

Children ≥6 years: 2 sprays (50 mcg/spray) per nostril once daily; maximum: 200 mcg/day

Adults: 2 sprays (50 mcg/spray) per nostril once daily; maximum: 200 mcg/day

Oral inhalation:

Children <12 years: Dosage not established

Children ≥12 years: 100-800 mcg/day (1-2 puffs once or twice daily); maximum: 640 mcg/day

Adults: 100-800 mcg/day (1-2 puffs once or twice daily); maximum 640 mcg/day

Dosage Forms Excipient information presented when available (limited, particularly for generics); consult specific product labeling. [CAN] = Canadian brand name

Aerosol for oral inhalation:

Alvesco® [U.S.]: 80 mcg/inhalation (6.1 g) [60 metered doses]; 160 mcg/inhalation (6.1 g) [60 metered doses]; 160 mcg/inhalation (9.6 g) [120 metered doses]

Alvesco® [CAN]: 50 mcg/inhalation [30-, 60-, and 120 metered doses] [not available in the U.S.]; 100 mcg/inhalation [30-, 60-, and 120 metered doses] [not available in the U.S.]; 200 mcg/inhalation [30-, 60-, and 120 metered doses] [not available in the U.S.]

Suspension, intranasal [spray]:

Omnaris™: 50 mcg/inhalation (12.5 g) [120 metered doses]

◆ **Cidecin** *see* DAPTOmycin *on page 418*

Cidofovir (si DOF o veer)

U.S. Brand Names Vistide®

Pharmacologic Category Antiviral Agent

Use Treatment of cytomegalovirus (CMV) retinitis in patients with acquired immunodeficiency syndrome (AIDS). **Note:** Should be administered with probenecid.

Effect on Mental Status Anxiety, confusion, amnesia, and insomnia are common; may cause depression or hallucinations

Effect on Psychiatric Treatment Anemia and neutropenia are common; use caution with clozapine and carbamazepine

Dosage Summary Note: Probenecid must be administered orally with each dose of cidofovir

I.V.:

Children: Dosage not established

Adults: Induction: 5 mg/kg once weekly for 2 consecutive weeks; Maintenance: 5 mg/kg once every 2 weeks

Dosage Forms Excipient information presented when available (limited, particularly for generics); consult specific product labeling.

Injection, solution [preservative free]: 75 mg/mL (5 mL)

Cilostazol (sil OH sta zol)

Medication Safety Issues

Sound-alike/look-alike issues:

Pletal® may be confused with Plendil®

U.S. Brand Names Pletal®

Canadian Brand Names Pletal®

Index Terms OPC-13013

Pharmacologic Category Antiplatelet Agent; Phosphodiesterase Enzyme Inhibitor

Use Symptomatic management of peripheral vascular disease, primarily intermittent claudication

Unlabeled/Investigational Use Adjunct with aspirin and clopidogrel for prevention of stent thrombosis and restenosis after coronary stent placement

Effect on Mental Status Headache and dizziness are common; may rarely cause anxiety or insomnia

Effect on Psychiatric Treatment CYP3A4 inhibitors (fluvoxamine, fluoxetine, nefazodone, sertraline) may increase the concentrations of cilostazol

Dosage Summary

Oral:

Children: Dosage not established

Adults: 100 mg twice daily; reduce to 50 mg twice daily during concurrent therapy with inhibitors of CYP3A4 or CYP2C19

Dosage Forms Excipient information presented when available (limited, particularly for generics); consult specific product labeling.

Tablet: 50 mg, 100 mg

Pletal®: 50 mg, 100 mg

◆ **Ciloxan®** *see* Ciprofloxacin *on page 346*

Cimetidine (sye MET i deen)

Medication Safety Issues
Sound-alike/look-alike issues:
Cimetidine may be confused with simethicone

Related Information
Anticholinergic Effects of Common Psychotropics *on page 1758*

U.S. Brand Names Tagamet® HB 200 [OTC]

Canadian Brand Names Apo-Cimetidine®; Gen-Cimetidine; Novo-Cimetidine; Nu-Cimet; PMS-Cimetidine; Tagamet® HB

Mexican Brand Names Cimetase; Tagamet

Pharmacologic Category Histamine H_2 Antagonist

Use Short-term treatment of active duodenal ulcers and benign gastric ulcers; long-term prophylaxis of duodenal ulcer; gastric hypersecretory states; gastroesophageal reflux; prevention of upper GI bleeding in critically-ill patients; labeled for OTC use for prevention or relief of heartburn, acid indigestion, or sour stomach

Unlabeled/Investigational Use Part of a multidrug regimen for *H. pylori* eradication to reduce the risk of duodenal ulcer recurrence

Effect on Mental Status May cause agitation or drowsiness; rare reports of confusion

Effect on Psychiatric Treatment Rare reports of agranulocytosis; use caution with clozapine and carbamazepine; may inhibit the metabolism of TCAs and benzodiazepines; monitor for adverse effects

Dosage Summary

I.M.:
Children: 20-40 mg/kg/day divided every 6 hours
Adults: 300-600 mg every 6 hours

I.V.:
Children: 20-40 mg/kg/day divided every 6 hours
Adults: 300-600 mg every 6 hours **or** 37.5-50 mg/hour continuous infusion

Oral:
Children <12 years: 20-40 mg/kg/day divided every 6 hours
Children ≥12 years: 20-40 mg/kg/day divided every 6 hours **or** 200 mg 1-2 times/day [OTC]
Adults: 300-600 mg 4 times/day **or** 400-800 mg 1-2 times/day **or** 200 mg 1-2 times/day [OTC]

Dosage Forms Excipient information presented when available (limited, particularly for generics); consult specific product labeling.
Note: Strength is expressed as base
Infusion [premixed in NS]: 300 mg (50 mL)
Injection, solution: 150 mg/mL (2 mL, 8 mL)
Solution, oral: 300 mg/5 mL (240 mL, 480 mL)
Tablet: 200 mg [OTC], 300 mg, 400 mg, 800 mg
Tagamet® HB 200: 200 mg

◆ **Cimzia®** *see* Certolizumab Pegol *on page 307*

Cinacalcet (sin a KAL cet)

U.S. Brand Names Sensipar®

Canadian Brand Names Sensipar®

Index Terms AMG 073; Cinacalcet Hydrochloride

Pharmacologic Category Calcimimetic

Use Treatment of secondary hyperparathyroidism in patients with chronic kidney disease (CKD) on dialysis; treatment of hypercalcemia in patients with parathyroid carcinoma
Note: In Canada, cinacalcet is approved only for the treatment of secondary hyperparathyroidism in patients with chronic kidney disease (CKD) on dialysis

Unlabeled/Investigational Use Primary hyperparathyroidism

Effect on Mental Status Dizziness is common

Effect on Psychiatric Treatment Gastrointestinal side effects are common; these effects may be additive with concurrent use of SSRIs, lithium, or valproate. Cinacalcet may increase levels of amitriptyline and nortriptyline; monitor for increased effects and/or serum levels.

Dosage Summary

Oral:
Children: Dosage not established

Adults:

Parathyroid carcinoma: Initial: 30 mg twice daily; Maintenance: Increase dose incrementally every 2-4 weeks to normalize calcium levels (maximum: 360 mg/day)

Secondary hyperparathyroidism: Initial: 30 mg once daily; Maintenance: Increase dose incrementally every 2-4 weeks to maintain iPTH level (maximum: 180 mg/day)

Dosage Forms Excipient information presented when available (limited, particularly for generics); consult specific product labeling.

Tablet:

Sensipar®: 30 mg, 60 mg, 90 mg

◆ **Cinacalcet Hydrochloride** *see* Cinacalcet *on page 345*

◆ **Cipro®** *see* Ciprofloxacin *on page 346*

Ciprofloxacin (sip roe FLOKS a sin)

Medication Safety Issues

Sound-alike/look-alike issues:

Ciprofloxacin may be confused with cephalexin

Ciloxan® may be confused with cinoxacin, Cytoxan®

Cipro® may be confused with Ceftin®

U.S. Brand Names Ciloxan®; Cipro®; Cipro® XR; Proquin® XR

Canadian Brand Names Apo-Ciproflox®; Ciloxan®; Cipro®; Cipro® XL; CO Ciprofloxacin; Dom-Ciprofloxacin; Gen-Ciprofloxacin; Novo-Ciprofloxacin; PHL-Ciprofloxacin; PMS-Ciprofloxacin; RAN™-Ciprofloxacin; ratio-Ciprofloxacin; Riva-Ciprofloxacin; Sandoz-Ciprofloxacin; Taro-Ciprofloxacin

Mexican Brand Names Ciloxan; Cimogal; Ciprobac; Ciproflox; Ciproxina; Eni; Floxager; Floxantina; Kenzoflex; Mitroken; Sophixin Ofteno; Zipra

Index Terms Ciprofloxacin Hydrochloride

Pharmacologic Category Antibiotic, Ophthalmic; Antibiotic, Quinolone

Generic Available Yes: Excludes ointment, suspension

Use

Children: Complicated urinary tract infections and pyelonephritis due to *E. coli*. **Note:** Although effective, ciprofloxacin is not the drug of first choice in children.

Children and Adults: To reduce incidence or progression of disease following exposure to aerolized *Bacillus anthracis*. Ophthalmologically, for superficial ocular infections (corneal ulcers, conjunctivitis) due to susceptible strains

Adults: Treatment of the following infections when caused by susceptible bacteria: Urinary tract infections; acute uncomplicated cystitis in females; chronic bacterial prostatitis; lower respiratory tract infections (including acute exacerbations of chronic bronchitis); acute sinusitis; skin and skin structure infections; bone and joint infections; complicated intra-abdominal infections (in combination with metronidazole); infectious diarrhea; typhoid fever due to *Salmonella typhi* (eradication of chronic typhoid carrier state has not been proven); uncomplicated cervical and urethra gonorrhea (due to *N. gonorrhoeae*); nosocomial pneumonia; empirical therapy for febrile neutropenic patients (in combination with piperacillin)

Note: As of April 2007, the CDC no longer recommends the use of fluoroquinolones for the treatment of gonococcal disease.

Unlabeled/Investigational Use Acute pulmonary exacerbations in cystic fibrosis (children); cutaneous/gastrointestinal/oropharyngeal anthrax (treatment, children and adults); disseminated gonococcal infection (adults); chancroid (adults); prophylaxis to *Neisseria meningitidis* following close contact with an infected person; empirical therapy (oral) for febrile neutropenia in low-risk cancer patients; HACEK group endocarditis; infectious diarrhea (children)

Effect on Mental Status Convulsions and toxic psychosis have been reported with quinolones. May cause dizziness, confusion, hallucinations, depression, and rarely suicidal ideation and attempts. These reactions may occur after the first dose. Discontinue drug and institute safety measures. Ciprofloxacin may also cause nervousness, agitation, insomnia, anxiety, nightmares or paranoia, phobia, depersonalization, manic reaction, ataxia, irritability, and drowsiness.

Effect on Psychiatric Treatment Inhibits CYP1A2 isoenzyme; use caution with clozapine; monitor for adverse effects. May rarely cause agranulocytosis; monitor with clozapine and carbamazepine. Use caution in patients with CNS disorders that may predispose them to seizures (epilepsy, alcohol/sedative hypnotic withdrawal).

Restrictions

An FDA-approved patient medication guide is available and must be distributed when dispensing an outpatient prescription (new or refill) where this medication is to be used without direct supervision of a healthcare provider. Medication guides are available at http://www.fda.gov/cder/Offices/ODS/medication_guides.htm.

Pregnancy Risk Factor C

Pregnancy Considerations Adverse events have been observed in some animal studies; therefore, the manufacturer classifies ciprofloxacin as pregnancy category C. Ciprofloxacin crosses the placenta and produces measurable concentrations in the amniotic fluid and cord serum. An increased risk of teratogenic effects has not been observed in animals or humans following ciprofloxacin use during pregnancy; however, because of concerns of cartilage damage in immature animals, ciprofloxacin should only be used during pregnancy if a safer option is not available. Ciprofloxacin is recommended for prophylaxis and treatment of pregnant women exposed to anthrax. Serum concentrations of ciprofloxacin may be lower during pregnancy than in nonpregnant patients.

Lactation Enters breast milk/not recommended (AAP rates "compatible")

Contraindications Hypersensitivity to ciprofloxacin, any component of the formulation, or other quinolones; concurrent administration of tizanidine

Warnings/Precautions [U.S. Boxed Warning]: There have been reports of tendon inflammation and/or rupture with quinolone antibiotics; risk may be increased with concurrent corticosteroids, organ transplant recipients, and in patients >60 years of age. Rupture of the Achilles tendon sometimes requiring surgical repair has been reported most frequently; but other tendon sites (eg, rotator cuff, biceps) have also been reported. Strenuous physical activity, rheumatoid arthritis, and renal impairment may be an independent risk factor for tendonitis. Discontinue at first sign of tendon inflammation or pain. May occur even after discontinuation of therapy. Use with caution in patients with rheumatoid arthritis; may increase risk of tendon rupture. CNS stimulation may occur (tremor, restlessness, confusion, and very rarely hallucinations or seizures). Use with caution in patients with known or suspected CNS disorder. Potential for seizures, although very rare, may be increased with concomitant NSAID therapy. Use with caution in individuals at risk of seizures. Fluoroquinolones may prolong QT_c interval; avoid use in patients with a history of QT_c prolongation, uncorrected hypokalemia, hypomagnesemia, or concurrent administration of other medications known to prolong the QT interval (including Class Ia and Class III antiarrhythmics, cisapride, erythromycin, antipsychotics, and tricyclic antidepressants). Prolonged use may result in fungal or bacterial superinfection, including *C. difficile*-associated diarrhea (CDAD) and pseudomembranous colitis; CDAD has been observed >2 months postantibiotic treatment. Rarely crystalluria has occurred; urine alkalinity may increase the risk. Ensure adequate hydration during therapy. Adverse effects, including those related to joints and/or surrounding tissues, are increased in pediatric patients and therefore, ciprofloxacin should not be considered as drug of choice in children (exception is anthrax treatment). Rare cases of peripheral neuropathy may occur.

Fluoroquinolones have been associated with the development of serious, and sometimes fatal, hypoglycemia, most often in elderly diabetics but also in patients without diabetes. This occurred most frequently with gatifloxicain (no longer available systemically), but may occur at a lower frequency with other quinolones.

Severe hypersensitivity reactions, including anaphylaxis, have occurred with quinolone therapy. Reactions may present as typical allergic symptoms after a single dose, or may manifest as severe idiosyncratic dermatologic, vascular, pulmonary, renal, hepatic, and/or hematologic events, usually after multiple doses. Prompt discontinuation of drug should occur if skin rash or other symptoms arise. Quinolones may exacerbate myasthenia gravis, use with caution (rare, potentially life-threatening weakness of respiratory muscles may occur). Use caution in renal impairment. Avoid excessive sunlight and take precautions to limit exposure (eg, loose fitting clothing, sunscreen); may cause moderate-to-severe phototoxicity reactions. Discontinue use if photosensitivity occurs. Since ciprofloxacin is ineffective in the treatment of syphilis and may mask symptoms, all patients should be tested for syphilis at the time of gonorrheal diagnosis and 3 months later. Hemolytic reactions may (rarely) occur with quinolone use in patients with latent or actual G6PD deficiency.

Ciprofloxacin is a potent inhibitor of CYP1A2. Coadministration of drugs which depend on this pathway may lead to substantial increases in serum concentrations and adverse effects.

Adverse Reactions

1% to 10%:

Central nervous system: Neurologic events (children 2%, includes dizziness, insomnia, nervousness, somnolence); fever (children 2%); headache (I.V. administration); restlessness (I.V. administration)

Dermatologic: Rash (children 2%, adults 1%)

Gastrointestinal: Nausea (children/adults 3%); diarrhea (children 5%, adults 2%); vomiting (children 5%, adults 1%); abdominal pain (children 3%, adults <1%); dyspepsia (children 3%)

Hepatic: ALT increased, AST increased (adults 1%)

Local: Injection site reactions (I.V. administration)

Respiratory: Rhinitis (children 3%)

<1% (Limited to important or life-threatening): Abnormal gait, acute renal failure, agitation, agranulocytosis, albuminuria, allergic reactions, anaphylactic shock, anaphylaxis, anemia, angina pectoris, angioedema, anorexia, anosmia, arthralgia, ataxia, atrial flutter, bone marrow depression (life-threatening), breast pain, bronchospasm, candidiasis, candiduria, cardiopulmonary arrest, cerebral thrombosis, chills, cholestatic jaundice, chromatopsia, confusion, constipation, crystalluria (particularly in alkaline urine), cylindruria, delirium, depersonalization, depression, dizziness, drowsiness, dyspepsia (adults), dysphagia, dyspnea, edema, eosinophilia, erythema multiforme, erythema nodosum, exfoliative dermatitis, fever (adults), fixed eruption, flatulence, gastrointestinal bleeding, hallucinations, headache (oral), hematuria, hemolytic anemia, hepatic failure (some fatal), hepatic necrosis, hyperesthesia, hyperglycemia, hyperpigmentation, hyper-/hypotension, hypertonia, insomnia, interstitial nephritis, intestinal perforation, irritability, jaundice, joint pain, laryngeal edema, lightheadedness, lymphadenopathy, malaise, manic reaction, methemoglobinemia, MI, migraine, moniliasis, myalgia, myasthenia gravis, myoclonus, nephritis, nightmares, nystagmus, orthostatic hypotension, palpitation, pancreatitis, pancytopenia (life-threatening or fatal), paranoia, paresthesia, peripheral neuropathy, petechia, photosensitivity, pneumonitis, prolongation of PT/INR, pseudomembranous colitis, psychosis, pulmonary edema, renal calculi, seizure; serum cholesterol, glucose, triglycerides increased; serum sickness-like reactions, Stevens-Johnson syndrome, syncope, tachycardia, taste loss, tendon rupture, tendonitis, thrombophlebitis, tinnitus, torsade de pointes, toxic epidermal necrolysis (Lyell's syndrome), tremor, twitching, urethral bleeding, vaginal candidiasis, vaginitis, vasculitis, ventricular ectopy, visual disturbance, weakness

Metabolism/Transport Effects Inhibits CYP1A2 (strong), 3A4 (weak)

Drug Interactions

Antacids: May decrease the absorption of Quinolone Antibiotics. Of concern only with oral administration of quinolones. **Exceptions:** Sodium Bicarbonate. *Risk D: Consider therapy modification*

Bendamustine: CYP1A2 Inhibitors (Strong) may increase the serum concentration of Bendamustine. Concentrations of the active metabolites of bendamustine may be decreased. *Risk C: Monitor therapy*

Caffeine: Quinolone Antibiotics may decrease the metabolism of Caffeine. *Risk C: Monitor therapy*

Calcium Salts: May decrease the absorption of Quinolone Antibiotics. Of concern only with oral administration of both agents. **Exceptions:** Calcium Chloride. *Risk D: Consider therapy modification*

Corticosteroids (Systemic): Quinolone Antibiotics may enhance the adverse/toxic effect of Corticosteroids (Systemic). Risk of tendon-related side effects, including tendonitis and rupture, may be enhanced. *Risk C: Monitor therapy*

CYP1A2 Substrates: CYP1A2 Inhibitors (Strong) may decrease the metabolism of CYP1A2 Substrates. *Risk D: Consider therapy modification*

Didanosine: May decrease the absorption of Quinolone Antibiotics. Of concern only with oral administration of both agents (excludes enteric coated formulation of didanosine). *Risk D: Consider therapy modification*

Insulin: May enhance the hyperglycemic effect of Quinolone Antibiotics. Insulin may enhance the hypoglycemic effect of Quinolone Antibiotics. *Risk C: Monitor therapy*

Iron Salts: May decrease the absorption of Quinolone Antibiotics. Of concern only with oral administration of both agents. **Exceptions:** Ferric Gluconate; Iron Dextran Complex; Iron Sucrose. *Risk D: Consider therapy modification*

Magnesium Salts: May decrease the absorption of Quinolone Antibiotics. Of concern only with oral administration of both agents. *Risk D: Consider therapy modification*

Methotrexate: Ciprofloxacin may increase the serum concentration of Methotrexate. *Risk C: Monitor therapy*

Mycophenolate: Quinolone Antibiotics may decrease the serum concentration of Mycophenolate. Specifically, quinolones may decrease concentrations of the active metabolite of mycophenolate. *Risk C: Monitor therapy*

Nonsteroidal Anti-Inflammatory Agents: May enhance the neuroexcitatory and/or seizure-potentiating effect of Quinolone Antibiotics. *Risk C: Monitor therapy*

Pentoxifylline: Ciprofloxacin may enhance the adverse/toxic effect of Pentoxifylline. *Risk C: Monitor therapy*

P-Glycoprotein Inducers: May decrease the serum concentration of P-Glycoprotein Substrates. P-glycoprotein inducers may also further limit the distribution of p-glycoprotein substrates to specific cells/tissues/organs where p-glycoprotein is present in large amounts (e.g., brain, T-lymphocytes, testes, etc.). *Risk C: Monitor therapy*

P-Glycoprotein Inhibitors: May increase the serum concentration of P-Glycoprotein Substrates. P-glycoprotein inhibitors may also enhance the distribution of p-glycoprotein substrates to specific cells/tissues/organs where p-glycoprotein is present in large amounts (e.g., brain, T-lymphocytes, testes, etc.). *Risk C: Monitor therapy*

Phenytoin: Ciprofloxacin may decrease the serum concentration of Phenytoin. *Risk C: Monitor therapy*

Probenecid: May increase the serum concentration of Quinolone Antibiotics. *Risk C: Monitor therapy*

QTc-Prolonging Agents: Ciprofloxacin may enhance the QTc-prolonging effect of QTc-Prolonging Agents. *Risk C: Monitor therapy*

Quinapril: May decrease the absorption of Quinolone Antibiotics. Of concern only with oral administration of quinolones. *Risk D: Consider therapy modification*

Ropinirole: Ciprofloxacin may decrease the metabolism of Ropinirole. *Risk C: Monitor therapy*

Ropivacaine: Ciprofloxacin may decrease the metabolism of Ropivacaine. *Risk C: Monitor therapy*

Sevelamer: May decrease the absorption of Quinolone Antibiotics. *Risk D: Consider therapy modification*

Sucralfate: May decrease the absorption of Quinolone Antibiotics. Of concern only with oral administration of quinolones. *Risk D: Consider therapy modification*

Sulfonylureas: Quinolone Antibiotics may enhance the hyperglycemic effect of Sulfonylureas. Quinolone Antibiotics may enhance the hypoglycemic effect of Sulfonylureas. *Risk C: Monitor therapy*

Theophylline Derivatives: Quinolone Antibiotics may decrease the metabolism of Theophylline Derivatives. Ciprofloxacin and enoxacin are of greatest concern. Theophylline/quinolone therapy might augment the seizure-producing potential of each of the individual agents. **Exceptions:** Dyphylline. *Risk D: Consider therapy modification*

TiZANidine: Ciprofloxacin may decrease the metabolism of TiZANidine. *Risk X: Avoid combination*

Typhoid Vaccine: Antibiotics may diminish the therapeutic effect of Typhoid Vaccine. Only the live attenuated Ty21a strain is affected. *Risk D: Consider therapy modification*

Vitamin K Antagonists (eg, warfarin): Quinolone Antibiotics may enhance the anticoagulant effect of Vitamin K Antagonists. *Risk C: Monitor therapy*

Zinc Salts: May decrease the absorption of Quinolone Antibiotics. Of concern only with oral administration of both agents. *Risk D: Consider therapy modification*

Ethanol/Nutrition/Herb Interactions

Food: Food decreases rate, but not extent, of absorption. Ciprofloxacin serum levels may be decreased if taken with dairy products or calcium-fortified juices. Ciprofloxacin may increase serum caffeine levels if taken with caffeine.

Enteral feedings may decrease plasma concentrations of ciprofloxacin probably by >30% inhibition of absorption. Ciprofloxacin should not be administered with enteral feedings. The feeding would need to be discontinued for 1-2 hours prior to and after ciprofloxacin administration. Nasogastric administration produces a greater loss of ciprofloxacin bioavailability than does nasoduodenal administration.

Herb/Nutraceutical: Avoid dong quai, St John's wort (may also cause photosensitization).

Stability

Injection:

Premixed infusion: Store between 5°C to 25°C (41°F to 77°F); avoid freezing. Protect from light.

Vial: Store between 5°C to 30°C (41°F to 86°F); avoid freezing. Protect from light. May be diluted with NS, D_5W, SWFI, $D_{10}W$, $D_5{}^1/_4NS$, $D_5{}^1/_2NS$, LR.

Diluted solutions of 0.5-2 mg/mL are stable for up to 14 days refrigerated or at room temperature.

Ophthalmic solution/ointment: Store at 36°F to 77°F (2°C to 25°C); protect from light.

Microcapsules for oral suspension: Prior to reconstitution, store below 25°C (77°F); protect from freezing. Following reconstitution, store below 30°C (86°F) for up to 14 days; protect from freezing.

Tablet:

Immediate release: Store below 30°C (86°F).

Extended release: Store at room temperature of 15°C to 30°C (59°F to 86°F).

Mechanism of Action Inhibits DNA-gyrase in susceptible organisms; inhibits relaxation of supercoiled DNA and promotes breakage of double-stranded DNA

Pharmacodynamics/Kinetics

Absorption: Oral: Immediate release tablet: Rapid (~50% to 85%)

Distribution: V_d: 2.1-2.7 L/kg; tissue concentrations often exceed serum concentrations especially in kidneys, gallbladder, liver, lungs, gynecological tissue, and prostatic tissue; CSF concentrations: 10% of serum concentrations (noninflamed meninges), 14% to 37% (inflamed meninges)

Protein binding: 20% to 40%

Metabolism: Partially hepatic; forms 4 metabolites (limited activity)

Half-life elimination: Children: 2.5 hours; Adults: Normal renal function: 3-5 hours

Time to peak: Oral:

Immediate release tablet: 0.5-2 hours

Extended release tablet: Cipro® XR: 1-2.5 hours, Proquin® XR: 3.5-8.7 hours

Excretion: Urine (30% to 50% as unchanged drug); feces (15% to 43%)

Dosage Note: Extended release tablets and immediate release formulations are not interchangeable. Unless otherwise specified, oral dosing reflects the use of immediate release formulations.

Usual dosage ranges:

Children (see Warnings/Precautions):

Oral: 20-30 mg/kg/day in 2 divided doses; maximum dose: 1.5 g/day

I.V.: 20-30 mg/kg/day divided every 12 hours; maximum dose: 800 mg/day

Adults:

Oral: 250-750 mg every 12 hours

I.V.: 200-400 mg every 12 hours

Indication-specific dosing:

Children:

Anthrax:

Inhalational (postexposure prophylaxis):

Oral: 15 mg/kg/dose every 12 hours for 60 days; maximum: 500 mg/dose

I.V.: 10 mg/kg/dose every 12 hours for 60 days; do **not** exceed 400 mg/dose (800 mg/day)

Cutaneous (treatment, CDC guidelines): Oral: 10-15 mg/kg every 12 hours for 60 days (maximum: 1 g/day); amoxicillin 80 mg/kg/day divided every 8 hours is an option for completion of treatment after clinical improvement. **Note:** In the presence of systemic involvement, extensive edema, lesions on head/neck, refer to I.V. dosing for treatment of inhalational/gastrointestinal/oropharyngeal anthrax.

Inhalational/gastrointestinal/oropharyngeal (treatment, CDC guidelines): I.V.: Initial: 10-15 mg/kg every 12 hours for 60 days (maximum: 500 mg/dose); switch to oral therapy when clinically appropriate; refer to adult dosing for notes on combined therapy and duration

Bacterial conjunctivitis: See adult dosing

Corneal ulcer: See adult dosing

Cystic fibrosis (unlabeled use):

Oral: 40 mg/kg/day divided every 12 hours administered following 1 week of I.V. therapy has been reported in a clinical trial; total duration of therapy: 10-21 days

I.V.: 30 mg/kg/day divided every 8 hours for 1 week, followed by oral therapy, has been reported in a clinical trial

Urinary tract infection (complicated) or pyelonephritis:

Oral: 20-30 mg/kg/day in 2 divided doses (every 12 hours) for 10-21 days; maximum: 1.5 g/day

I.V.: 6-10 mg/kg every 8 hours for 10-21 days (maximum: 400 mg/dose)

Adults:

Anthrax:

Inhalational (postexposure prophylaxis):

Oral: 500 mg every 12 hours for 60 days

I.V.: 400 mg every 12 hours for 60 days

Cutaneous (treatment, CDC guidelines): Oral: Immediate release formulation: 500 mg every 12 hours for 60 days. **Note:** In the presence of systemic involvement, extensive edema, lesions on head/neck, refer to I.V. dosing for treatment of inhalational/gastrointestinal/oropharyngeal anthrax

Inhalational/gastrointestinal/oropharyngeal (treatment, CDC guidelines): I.V.: 400 mg every 12 hours. **Note:** Initial treatment should include two or more agents predicted to be effective (per CDC recommendations). Continue combined therapy for 60 days.

Bacterial conjunctivitis:

Ophthalmic solution: Instill 1-2 drops in eye(s) every 2 hours while awake for 2 days and 1-2 drops every 4 hours while awake for the next 5 days

Ophthalmic ointment: Apply a 1/2" ribbon into the conjunctival sac 3 times/day for the first 2 days, followed by a 1/2" ribbon applied twice daily for the next 5 days

Bone/joint infections:

Oral: 500-750 mg twice daily for 4-6 weeks

I.V.: Mild to moderate: 400 mg every 12 hours for 4-6 weeks; Severe/complicated: 400 mg every 8 hours for 4-6 weeks

Chancroid (CDC guidelines): Oral: 500 mg twice daily for 3 days

Corneal ulcer: Ophthalmic solution: Instill 2 drops into affected eye every 15 minutes for the first 6 hours, then 2 drops into the affected eye every 30 minutes for the remainder of the first day. On day 2, instill 2 drops into the affected eye hourly. On days 3-14, instill 2 drops into affected eye every 4 hours. Treatment may continue after day 14 if re-epithelialization has not occurred.

Endocarditis due to HACEK organisms (AHA guidelines, unlabeled use): Note: Not first-line option; use only if intolerant of beta-lactam therapy:

Oral: 500 mg every 12 hours for 4 weeks

I.V.: 400 mg every 12 hours for 4 weeks

Febrile neutropenia*: I.V.: 400 mg every 8 hours for 7-14 days

Gonococcal infections:

Urethral/cervical gonococcal infections: Oral: 250-500 mg as a single dose (CDC recommends concomitant doxycycline or azithromycin due to possible coinfection with *Chlamydia*; **Note:** As of April 2007, the CDC no longer recommends the use of fluoroquinolones for the treatment of uncomplicated gonococcal disease.

Disseminated gonococcal infection (CDC guidelines): Oral: 500 mg twice daily to complete 7 days of therapy (initial treatment with ceftriaxone 1 g I.M./I.V. daily for 24-48 hours after improvement begins); **Note:** As of April 2007, the CDC no longer recommends the use of fluoroquinolones for the treatment of more serious gonococcal disease, unless no other options exist and susceptibility can be confirmed via culture.

Infectious diarrhea: Oral:

Salmonella: 500 mg twice daily for 5-7 days

Shigella: 500 mg twice daily for 3 days

Traveler's diarrhea: Mild: 750 mg for one dose; Severe: 500 mg twice daily for 3 days

Vibrio cholerae: 1 g for one dose

Intra-abdominal*:

Oral: 500 mg every 12 hours for 7-14 days

I.V.: 400 mg every 12 hours for 7-14 days

Lower respiratory tract, skin/skin structure infections:

Oral: 500-750 mg twice daily for 7-14 days

I.V.: Mild to moderate: 400 mg every 12 hours for 7-14 days; Severe/complicated: 400 mg every 8 hours for 7-14 days

Nosocomial pneumonia: I.V.: 400 mg every 8 hours for 10-14 days

Prostatitis (chronic, bacterial): Oral: 500 mg every 12 hours for 28 days

Sinusitis (acute): Oral: 500 mg every 12 hours for 10 days

Typhoid fever: Oral: 500 mg every 12 hours for 10 days

Urinary tract infection:

Acute uncomplicated, cystitis:

Oral:

Immediate release formulation: 250 mg every 12 hours for 3 days

Extended release formulation (Cipro® XR, Proquin® XR): 500 mg every 24 hours for 3 days

I.V.: 200 mg every 12 hours for 7-14 days

Complicated (including pyelonephritis):

Oral:

Immediate release formulation: 500 mg every 12 hours for 7-14 days

Extended release formulation (Cipro® XR): 1000 mg every 24 hours for 7-14 days

I.V.: 400 mg every 12 hours for 7-14 days

*Combination therapy generally recommended.

Elderly: No adjustment needed in patients with normal renal function

Dosing adjustment in renal impairment: Adults:

Cl_{cr} 30-50 mL/minute: Oral: 250-500 mg every 12 hours

Cl_{cr} <30 mL/minute: Acute uncomplicated pyelonephritis or complicated UTI: Oral: Extended release formulation: 500 mg every 24 hours

Cl_{cr} 5-29 mL/minute:

Oral: 250-500 mg every 18 hours

I.V.: 200-400 mg every 18-24 hours

Dialysis: Only small amounts of ciprofloxacin are removed by hemo- or peritoneal dialysis (<10%); usual dose: Oral: 250-500 mg every 24 hours following dialysis

Continuous renal replacement therapy (CRRT): I.V.:

CVVH: 200 mg every 12 hours

CVVHD or CVVHDF: 200-400 mg every 12 hours

Dietary Considerations

Food: Drug may cause GI upset; take without regard to meals (manufacturer prefers that immediate release tablet is taken 2 hours after meals). Extended release tablet may be taken with meals that contain dairy products (calcium content <800 mg), but not with dairy products alone.

Dairy products, calcium-fortified juices, oral multivitamins, and mineral supplements: Absorption of ciprofloxacin is decreased by divalent and trivalent cations. The manufacturer states that the usual dietary intake of calcium (including meals which include dairy products) has not been shown to interfere with ciprofloxacin absorption. Immediate release ciprofloxacin and Cipro® XR may be taken 2 hours before or 6 hours after, and Proquin® XR may be taken 4 hours before or 6 hours after, any of these products.

Caffeine: Patients consuming regular large quantities of caffeinated beverages may need to restrict caffeine intake if excessive cardiac or CNS stimulation occurs.

Administration

Oral: May administer with food to minimize GI upset; avoid antacid use; maintain proper hydration and urine output. Administer immediate release ciprofloxacin and Cipro® XR at least 2 hours before or 6 hours after, and Proquin® XR at least 4 hours before or 6 hours after antacids or other products containing calcium, iron, or zinc (including dairy products or calcium-fortified juices). Separate oral administration from drugs which may impair absorption (see Drug Interactions).

Oral suspension: Should not be administered through feeding tubes (suspension is oil-based and adheres to the feeding tube). Patients should avoid chewing on the microcapsules.

Nasogastric/orogastric tube: Crush immediate-release tablet and mix with water. Flush feeding tube before and after administration. Hold tube feedings at least 1 hour before and 2 hours after administration.

Tablet, extended release: Do not crush, split, or chew. May be administered with meals containing dairy products (calcium content <800 mg), but not with dairy products alone. Proquin® XR should be administered with a main meal of the day; evening meal is preferred.

Parenteral: Administer by slow I.V. infusion over 60 minutes to reduce the risk of venous irritation (burning, pain, erythema, and swelling); final concentration for administration should not exceed 2 mg/mL.

Monitoring Parameters Patients receiving concurrent ciprofloxacin, theophylline, or cyclosporine should have serum levels monitored; CBC, renal and hepatic function during prolonged therapy

Reference Range Therapeutic: 2.6-3 mcg/mL; Toxic: >5 mcg/mL

Test Interactions Some quinolones may produce a false-positive urine screening result for opiates using commercially-available immunoassay kits. This has been demonstrated most consistently for levofloxacin and ofloxacin, but other quinolones have shown cross-reactivity in certain assay kits. Confirmation of positive opiate screens by more specific methods should be considered.

Additional Information Although the systemic use of ciprofloxacin is only FDA approved in children for the treatment of complicated UTI and postexposure treatment of inhalation anthrax, use of the fluoroquinolones in pediatric patients is increasing. Current recommendations by the American Academy o Pediatrics note that the systemic use of these agents in children should be restricted to infections caused by multidrug resistant pathogens with no safe o effective alternative, and when parenteral therapy is not feasible or other oral agents are not available.

Dosage Forms Excipient information presented when available (limited, particularly for generics); consult specific product labeling.

Infusion [premixed in D_5W]: 200 mg (100 mL); 400 mg (200 mL)

Cipro®: 200 mg (100 mL); 400 mg (200 mL)

Injection, solution [concentrate]: 10 mg/mL (20 mL, 40 mL, 120 mL)

Cipro®: 10 mg/mL (20 mL, 40 mL)

Microcapsules for suspension, oral:

Cipro®: 250 mg/5 mL (100 mL); 500 mg/5 mL (100 mL) [strawberry flavor]

Ointment, ophthalmic, as hydrochloride:

Ciloxan®: 3.33 mg/g (3.5 g) [0.3% base]

Solution, ophthalmic, as hydrochloride: 3.5 mg/mL (2.5 mL, 5mL, 10 mL) [0.3% base]

Ciloxan®: 3.5 mg/mL (5 mL) [0.3% base; contains benzalkonium chloride]

Tablet, as hydrochloride: 100 mg [strength expressed as base], 250 mg [strength expressed as base], 500 mg [strength expressed as base], 750 mg [strength expressed as base]

Cipro®: 250 mg [strength expressed as base], 500 mg [strength expressed as base], 750 mg [strength expressed as base]

Tablet, extended release, as base and hydrochloride: 500 mg [strength expressed as base], 1000 mg [strength expressed as base]

Cipro® XR: 500 mg [strength expressed as base], 1000 mg [strength expressed as base]

Tablet, extended release, as hydrochloride:

Proquin® XR: 500 mg [strength expressed as base]

Tablet, extended release, as hydrochloride [dose pack]:

Proquin® XR: 500 mg (3s)

◆ **Ciprofloxacin Hydrochloride** *see* Ciprofloxacin *on page 346*

◆ **Cipro® XR** *see* Ciprofloxacin *on page 346*

Cisapride *U.S. - Available Via Limited-Access Protocol Only* (SIS a pride)

Medication Safety Issues

Sound-alike/look-alike issues:

Propulsid® may be confused with propranolol

U.S. Brand Names Propulsid®

Mexican Brand Names Enteropride; Kinestase; Lornakin; Presistin; Profercol; Tadasil; Unamol

Pharmacologic Category Gastrointestinal Agent, Prokinetic

Use Treatment of nocturnal symptoms of gastroesophageal reflux disease (GERD); has demonstrated effectiveness for gastroparesis, refractory constipation, and nonulcer dyspepsia

Effect on Mental Status May cause sedation, insomnia, anxiety, or extrapyramidal symptoms

Effect on Psychiatric Treatment Contraindicated with nefazodone and ziprasidone; may increase cisapride levels which have been associated with QT prolongation and torsade de pointes

Restrictions In U.S., available via limited-access protocol only (1-800-JANSSEN).

Dosage Summary

Oral:

Children: 0.15-0.3 mg/kg 3-4 times/day (maximum: 10 mg/dose)

Adults: Initial: 5-10 mg 4 times/day, may increase to 20 mg 4 times/day if needed

Cisatracurium (sis a tra KYOO ree um)

Medication Safety Issues

Sound-alike/look-alike issues:

Nimbex® may be confused with Revex®

High alert medication: The Institute for Safe Medication Practices (ISMP) includes this medication among its list of drugs which have a heightened risk of causing significant patient harm when used in error.

U.S. Brand Names Nimbex®

Canadian Brand Names Nimbex®

Mexican Brand Names Nimbex

Index Terms Cisatracurium Besylate

Pharmacologic Category Neuromuscular Blocker Agent, Nondepolarizing

Use Adjunct to general anesthesia to facilitate endotracheal intubation and to relax skeletal muscles during surgery; to facilitate mechanical ventilation in ICU patients; does not relieve pain or produce sedation

Effect on Mental Status None reported

Effect on Psychiatric Treatment Concurrent use with lithium may prolong neuromuscular blockade; conversely, neuromuscular blockade may be diminished if used with carbamazepine

Dosage Summary

I.V.:

Children <1 month: Dosage not established

Children 1-23 months: 0.15 mg/kg during either halothane or opioid anesthesia

Children 2-12 years: Intubating dose: 0.1-0.15 mg/kg over 5-15 seconds during either halothane or opioid anesthesia; Infusion: Initial: 3 mcg/kg/minute; Maintenance: 1-2 mcg/kg/minute (surgery) **or** 0.5-10 mcg/kg/minute (ICU)

Children >12 years: Infusion: Initial: 3 mcg/kg/minute; Maintenance: 1-2 mcg/kg/minute (surgery) **or** 0.5-10 mcg/kg/minute (ICU)

Adults: Intubating dose: 0.1-0.2 mg/kg; Infusion: Initial: 3 mcg/kg/minute; Maintenance: 1-2 mcg/kg/minute (surgery) **or** 0.5-10 mcg/kg/minute (ICU)

Dosage Forms Excipient information presented when available (limited, particularly for generics); consult specific product labeling.

Injection, solution: 2 mg/mL (5 mL); 10 mg/mL (20 mL)

Injection, solution: 2 mg/mL (10 mL) [contains benzyl alcohol]

◆ **Cisatracurium Besylate** *see* Cisatracurium *on page 353*

CISplatin (SIS pla tin)

Medication Safety Issues

Sound-alike/look-alike issues:

CISplatin may be confused with CARBOplatin

High alert medication: The Institute for Safe Medication Practices (ISMP) includes this medication among its list of drugs which have a heightened risk of causing significant patient harm when used in error.

Doses >100 mg/m^2 once every 3-4 weeks are rarely used and should be verified with the prescriber.

Mexican Brand Names Blastolem RU; Tecnoplatin

Index Terms CDDP

Pharmacologic Category Antineoplastic Agent, Alkylating Agent; Antineoplastic Agent, Platinum Analog

Use Treatment of bladder, testicular, and ovarian cancer

Unlabeled/Investigational Use Treatment of head and neck, breast, gastric, lung, esophageal, cervical, prostate and small cell lung cancer; Hodgkin's and non-Hodgkin's lymphoma; neuroblastoma; sarcomas, myeloma, melanoma, mesothelioma, and osteosarcoma

Effect on Mental Status None reported

Effect on Psychiatric Treatment May cause myelosuppression; use caution with clozapine and carbamazepine

Dosage Forms Excipient information presented when available (limited, particularly for generics); consult specific product labeling.

Injection, solution [preservative free]: 1 mg/mL (50 mL, 100 mL, 200 mL)

◆ **13-*cis*-Retinoic Acid** *see* Isotretinoin *on page 871*

Citalopram (sye TAL oh pram)

Medication Safety Issues

Sound-alike/look-alike issues:

Celexa® may be confused with Celebrex®, Cerebra®, Cerebyx®, Ranexa™, Zyprexa®

Related Information

Antidepressant Agents *on page 1760*

Antidepressant Receptor Profile *on page 1764*

Discontinuation of Psychotropic Drugs *on page 1839*

Liquid Compatibility of Antidepressants, Antipsychotics, and Mood Stabilizers *on page 1788*

Selective Serotonin Reuptake Inhibitors (SSRIs) CYP Profile *on page 1793*

Selective Serotonin Reuptake Inhibitors (SSRIs) FDA-Approved Indication(s) *on page 1794*

Selective Serotonin Reuptake Inhibitors (SSRIs) Pharmacokinetics *on page 1795*

Selective Serotonin Reuptake Inhibitors (SSRIs) Receptor Profile *on page 1796*

U.S. Brand Names Celexa®

Canadian Brand Names Apo-Citalopram®; Celexa®; Cipralex®; Citalopram-ODAN; CO Citalopram; CTP 30; Dom-Citalopram; Gen-Citalopram; IPG-Citalopram; JAMP-Citalopram; Mint-Citalopram; Novo-Citalopram; PHL-Citalopram; PMS-Citalopram; RAN™-Citalopram; ratio-Citalopram; Riva-Citalopram; Sandoz-Citalopram

Mexican Brand Names Citox; Seropram; Xylorane

Index Terms Citalopram Hydrobromide; Nitalapram

Pharmacologic Category Antidepressant, Selective Serotonin Reuptake Inhibitor

Generic Available Yes

Use Treatment of depression

Unlabeled/Investigational Use Treatment of mild dementia-associated agitation in nonpsychotic patients; smoking cessation; ethanol abuse; obsessive-compulsive disorder (OCD) in children; diabetic neuropathy

Mental Health Comment The SSRIs as a class are generally considered to be safe and equally effective. Allow sufficient dose-response time (6-12 weeks). Differences lie in approved indications, receptor profiles, pharmacokinetics, and cytochrome P450 activity profile. Subtle differences exist in adverse effect profiles. All SSRIs have the potential to cause sexual dysfunction. Among the SSRIs, citalopram possesses a mild effect on CYP isoenzymes.

Restrictions An FDA-approved medication guide concerning the use of antidepressants in children, adolescents, and young adults must be distributed when dispensing an outpatient prescription (new or refill) where this medication is to be used without direct supervision of a healthcare provider. Medication guides are available at http://www.fda.gov/cder/Offices/ODS/medication_guides.htm. Dispense to parents or guardians of children and adolescents receiving this medication.

Pregnancy Risk Factor C

Pregnancy Considerations Due to adverse effects observed in animal studies, citalopram is classified as pregnancy category C. Citalopram and its metabolites cross the human placenta. Nonteratogenic effects in the newborn following SSRI exposure late in the third trimester include respiratory distress, cyanosis, apnea, seizures, temperature instability, feeding difficulty, vomiting, hypoglycemia, hypo- or hypertonia, hyper-reflexia, jitteriness, irritability, constant crying, and tremor. An increased risk of low birth weight and lower APGAR scores have also been reported. Exposure to SSRIs after the twentieth week of gestation has been associated with persistent pulmonary hypertension of the newborn (PPHN). Adverse effects may be due to toxic effects of the SSRI or drug withdrawal without a taper. The long term effects of *in utero* SSRI exposure on infant development and behavior are not known.

Due to pregnancy-induced physiologic changes, women who are pregnant may require increased doses of citalopram to achieve euthymia. Women treated for major depression and who are euthymic prior to pregnancy are more likely to experience a relapse when medication is discontinued as compared to pregnant women who continue taking antidepressant medications. The ACOG recommends that therapy with SSRIs or SNRIs during pregnancy be individualized; treatment of depression during pregnancy should incorporate the clinical expertise of the mental health clinician, obstetrician, primary healthcare provider, and pediatrician (ACOG, 2007). If treatment during pregnancy is required, consider tapering therapy during the third trimester in order to prevent withdrawal symptoms in the infant. If this is done and the woman is considered to be at risk from her major depressive disorder, the medication can be restarted following delivery, although the dose should be readjusted to that required before pregnancy.

Lactation Enters breast milk/consider risk:benefit

Contraindications Hypersensitivity to citalopram or any component of the formulation; concomitant use with MAO inhibitors or within 2 weeks of discontinuing MAO inhibitors; concomitant use with pimozide

Warnings/Precautions **[U.S. Boxed Warning]: Antidepressants increase the risk of suicidal thinking and behavior in children, adolescents, and young adults (18-24 years of age) with major depressive disorder (MDD) and other psychiatric disorders;** consider risk prior to prescribing. Short-term studies did not show an increased risk in patients >24 years of age and showed a decreased risk in patients ≥65 years. Closely monitor patients for clinical worsening, suicidality, or unusual changes in behavior, particularly during the initial 1-2 months of therapy or during periods of dosage adjustments (increases or decreases); the patient's family or caregiver should be instructed to closely observe the patient and communicate condition with healthcare provider. A medication guide concerning the use of antidepressants should be dispensed with each prescription. **Citalopram is not FDA approved for use in children.**

The possibility of a suicide attempt is inherent in major depression and may persist until remission occurs. Use caution in high-risk patients. Worsening depression and severe abrupt suicidality that are not part of the presenting symptoms may require discontinuation or modification of drug therapy. The patient's family or caregiver should be alerted to monitor patients for the emergence of suicidality and associated behaviors (such as agitation, irritability, hostility, impulsivity, and hypomania) and call healthcare provider.

May worsen psychosis in some patients or precipitate a shift to mania or hypomania in patients with bipolar disorder. Patients presenting with depressive symptoms should be screened for bipolar disorder. Monotherapy in patients with bipolar disorder should be avoided. **Citalopram is not FDA approved for the treatment of bipolar depression.**

The potential for severe reaction exists when used with MAO inhibitors, SSRIs/SNRIs or triptans; serotonin syndrome (hyperthermia, muscular rigidity, mental status changes/agitation, and autonomic instability) may occur. Concurrent use with MAO inhibitors is contraindicated. May increase the risks associated with electroconvulsive therapy. Has a low potential to impair cognitive or motor performance; caution operating hazardous machinery or driving.

Use with caution in patients with hepatic or renal dysfunction, in elderly patients, concomitant CNS depressants, and pregnancy (high doses of citalopram have been associated with teratogenicity in animals). Use caution with concomitant use of aspirin, NSAIDs, warfarin, or other drugs that affect coagulation; the risk of bleeding may be potentiated. May cause hyponatremia/SIADH (elderly at increased risk); volume depletion and diuretics may increase risk. May cause or exacerbate sexual dysfunction. Upon discontinuation of citalopram therapy, gradually taper dose. If intolerable symptoms occur following a decrease in dosage or upon discontinuation of therapy, then resuming the previous dose with a more gradual taper should be considered.

Adverse Reactions

>10%:

- Central nervous system: Somnolence (18%; dose related), insomnia (15%; dose related)
- Gastrointestinal: Nausea (21%), xerostomia (20%)
- Miscellaneous: Diaphoresis (11%; dose related)

1% to 10%:

- Cardiovascular: Heart rate decreased, postural hypotension, tachycardia
- Central nervous system: Fatigue (5%; dose related), anorexia (4%), anxiety (4%), agitation (3%), fever (2%), yawning (2%; dose related), amnesia, apathy, concentration impaired, confusion, depression, migraine, suicide attempt
- Dermatologic: Rash, pruritus
- Endocrine & metabolic: Libido decreased (1% to 4%), dysmenorrhea (3%), amenorrhea, sexual dysfunction
- Gastrointestinal: Diarrhea (8%), dyspepsia (5%), vomiting (4%), abdominal pain (3%), flatulence, salivation increased, taste perversion, weight gain/loss
- Genitourinary: Ejaculation disorder (6%), impotence (3%; dose related), polyuria
- Neuromuscular & skeletal: Tremor (8%), arthralgia (2%), myalgia (2%), paresthesia
- Ocular: Abnormal accommodation
- Respiratory: Rhinitis (5%), upper respiratory tract infection (5%), sinusitis (3%), cough

<1% (Limited to important or life threatening): Acute renal failure, aggressiveness, akathisia, alkaline phosphatase increased, allergic reaction, alopecia, anaphylaxis, anemia, angina pectoris, angioedema, ataxia, cardiac failure, cerebral vascular accident, chest pain, choreoathetosis, delirium, dyskinesia, dyspnea, dystonia, ecchymosis, eczema, edema (extremities), epidermal necrolysis, epistaxis, erythema multiforme, extrapyramidal symptoms, extrasystoles, gastrointestinal hemorrhage, glaucoma, grand mal seizure, hallucinations, hemolytic anemia, hepatic necrosis, hypertension, hyponatremia, leukocytosis, leukopenia, liver enzymes increased, lymphadenopathy, muscle weakness, myocardial infarction, myoclonus, neuralgia, neuroleptic malignant syndrome, nystagmus, pancreatitis, photosensitivity, priapism, prolactinemia, prothrombin decreased, purpura, QT prolonged,

rhabdomyolysis, rigors, serotonin syndrome, SIADH, spontaneous abortion, thrombocytopenia, thrombosis, tinnitus, torsade de pointes, urinary incontinence, urinary retention, urticaria, ventricular arrhythmia, withdrawal syndrome

Metabolism/Transport Effects **Substrate** of CYP2C19 (major), 2D6 (minor), 3A4 (major); **Inhibits** CYP1A2 (weak), 2B6 (weak), 2C19 (weak), 2D6 (weak)

Drug Interactions

Alcohol (Ethyl): CNS Depressants may enhance the CNS depressant effect of Alcohol (Ethyl). *Risk C: Monitor therapy*

Alpha-/Beta-Blockers: Selective Serotonin Reuptake Inhibitors may decrease the metabolism of Alpha-/Beta-Blockers. *Risk C: Monitor therapy*

Analgesics (Opioid): May enhance the serotonergic effect of Selective Serotonin Reuptake Inhibitors. This may cause serotonin syndrome. *Risk C: Monitor therapy*

Anticoagulants: Antiplatelet Agents may enhance the anticoagulant effect of Anticoagulants. *Risk C: Monitor therapy*

Antidepressants (Serotonin Reuptake Inhibitor/Antagonist): Selective Serotonin Reuptake Inhibitors may enhance the serotonergic effect of Antidepressants (Serotonin Reuptake Inhibitor/Antagonist). This may cause serotonin syndrome. *Risk C: Monitor therapy*

Antiplatelet Agents: May enhance the anticoagulant effect of other Antiplatelet Agents. *Risk C: Monitor therapy*

Aspirin: Selective Serotonin Reuptake Inhibitors may enhance the antiplatelet effect of Aspirin. *Risk C: Monitor therapy*

Beta-Blockers: Selective Serotonin Reuptake Inhibitors may enhance the bradycardic effect of Beta-Blockers. **Exceptions:** Acebutolol; Atenolol; Carteolol; Esmolol; Levobunolol; Metipranolol; Nadolol; Penbutolol. *Risk C: Monitor therapy*

BusPIRone: May enhance the serotonergic effect of Selective Serotonin Reuptake Inhibitors. This may cause serotonin syndrome. Selective Serotonin Reuptake Inhibitors may decrease the metabolism of BusPIRone. *Risk C: Monitor therapy*

CarBAMazepine: Selective Serotonin Reuptake Inhibitors may decrease the metabolism of CarBAMazepine. Specifically those SSRIs that inhibit CYP3A4 isoenzymes. CarBAMazepine may increase the metabolism of Selective Serotonin Reuptake Inhibitors. Specifically those agents metabolized via CYP1A2, 2C, and/or 3A4 isoenzymes. *Risk D: Consider therapy modification*

Cimetidine: May decrease the metabolism of Selective Serotonin Reuptake Inhibitors. *Risk D: Consider therapy modification*

Clozapine: Selective Serotonin Reuptake Inhibitors may decrease the metabolism of Clozapine. *Risk D: Consider therapy modification*

CNS Depressants: May enhance the adverse/toxic effect of other CNS Depressants. *Risk C: Monitor therapy*

CYP2C19 Inducers (Strong): May increase the metabolism of CYP2C19 Substrates. *Risk C: Monitor therapy*

CYP2C19 Inhibitors (Moderate): May decrease the metabolism of CYP2C19 Substrates. *Risk C: Monitor therapy*

CYP2C19 Inhibitors (Strong): May decrease the metabolism of CYP2C19 Substrates. *Risk D: Consider therapy modification*

CYP3A4 Inducers (Strong): May increase the metabolism of CYP3A4 Substrates. *Risk C: Monitor therapy*

CYP3A4 Inhibitors (Moderate): May decrease the metabolism of CYP3A4 Substrates. *Risk C: Monitor therapy*

CYP3A4 Inhibitors (Strong): May decrease the metabolism of CYP3A4 Substrates. *Risk D: Consider therapy modification*

Cyproheptadine: May diminish the therapeutic effect of Selective Serotonin Reuptake Inhibitors. *Risk C: Monitor therapy*

Dasatinib: May enhance the anticoagulant effect of Antiplatelet Agents. *Risk C: Monitor therapy*

Dasatinib: May increase the serum concentration of CYP3A4 Substrates. *Risk C: Monitor therapy*

Deferasirox: May decrease the serum concentration of CYP3A4 Substrates. *Risk C: Monitor therapy*

Desmopressin: Selective Serotonin Reuptake Inhibitors may enhance the adverse/toxic effect of Desmopressin. *Risk C: Monitor therapy*

Dextromethorphan: Selective Serotonin Reuptake Inhibitors may enhance the adverse/toxic effect of Dextromethorphan. *Risk D: Consider therapy modification*

Drotrecogin Alfa: Antiplatelet Agents may enhance the adverse/toxic effect of Drotrecogin Alfa. Bleeding may occur. *Risk D: Consider therapy modification*

Haloperidol: Selective Serotonin Reuptake Inhibitors may decrease the metabolism of Haloperidol. *Risk C: Monitor therapy*

Herbs (Anticoagulant/Antiplatelet Properties) (eg, Alfalfa, Anise, Bilberry): May enhance the adverse/toxic effect of Antiplatelet Agents. Bleeding may occur. *Risk D: Consider therapy modification*

Herbs (CYP3A4 Inducers): May increase the metabolism of CYP3A4 Substrates. *Risk C: Monitor therapy*

Ibritumomab: Antiplatelet Agents may enhance the adverse/toxic effect of Ibritumomab. Both agents may contribute to impaired platelet function and an increased risk of bleeding. *Risk C: Monitor therapy*

Lithium: Selective Serotonin Reuptake Inhibitors may enhance the adverse/toxic effect of Lithium. *Risk C: Monitor therapy*

Macrolide Antibiotics: May decrease the metabolism of Selective Serotonin Reuptake Inhibitors. **Exceptions:** Azithromycin; Dirithromycin [Off Market]; Spiramycin. *Risk C: Monitor therapy*

MAO Inhibitors: May enhance the serotonergic effect of Selective Serotonin Reuptake Inhibitors. This may cause serotonin syndrome. *Risk X: Avoid combination*

Methadone: Selective Serotonin Reuptake Inhibitors may decrease the metabolism of Methadone. Fluvoxamine appears to be the only interacting SSRI. *Risk D: Consider therapy modification*

Mexiletine: Selective Serotonin Reuptake Inhibitors may decrease the metabolism of Mexiletine. *Risk D: Consider therapy modification*

NSAID (COX-2 Inhibitor): Selective Serotonin Reuptake Inhibitors may enhance the antiplatelet effect of NSAID (COX-2 Inhibitor). *Risk D: Consider therapy modification*

NSAID (Nonselective): Selective Serotonin Reuptake Inhibitors may enhance the antiplatelet effect of NSAID (Nonselective). *Risk D: Consider therapy modification*

Omega-3-Acid Ethyl Esters: May enhance the antiplatelet effect of Antiplatelet Agents. *Risk C: Monitor therapy*

Pentosan Polysulfate Sodium: May enhance the adverse/toxic effect of Antiplatelet Agents. Specifically, the risk of bleeding may be increased by concurrent use of these agents. *Risk C: Monitor therapy*

Phenytoin: Selective Serotonin Reuptake Inhibitors may decrease the metabolism of Phenytoin. *Risk D: Consider therapy modification*

Pimozide: Selective Serotonin Reuptake Inhibitors may enhance the adverse/toxic effect of Pimozide. *Risk X: Avoid combination*

Propafenone: Selective Serotonin Reuptake Inhibitors may decrease the metabolism of Propafenone. *Risk D: Consider therapy modification*

Prostacyclin Analogues: May enhance the antiplatelet effect of Antiplatelet Agents. *Risk C: Monitor therapy*

Risperidone: Selective Serotonin Reuptake Inhibitors may decrease the metabolism of Risperidone. *Risk C: Monitor therapy*

Salicylates: Antiplatelet Agents may enhance the adverse/toxic effect of Salicylates. Increased risk of bleeding may result. *Risk C: Monitor therapy*

Serotonin Modulators: May enhance the adverse/toxic effect of other Serotonin Modulators. The development of serotonin syndrome may occur. *Risk D: Consider therapy modification*

Sibutramine: May enhance the serotonergic effect of Serotonin Modulators. This may cause serotonin syndrome. *Risk X: Avoid combination*

Thrombolytic Agents: Antiplatelet Agents may enhance the anticoagulant effect of Thrombolytic Agents. *Risk C: Monitor therapy*

Tositumomab and Iodine I 131 Tositumomab: Antiplatelet Agents may enhance the adverse/toxic effect of Tositumomab and Iodine I 131 Tositumomab. Specifically, the risk of bleeding-related adverse events may be increased. *Risk C: Monitor therapy*

TraMADol: Selective Serotonin Reuptake Inhibitors may enhance the neuroexcitatory and/or seizure-potentiating effect of TraMADol. TraMADol may enhance the serotonergic effect of Selective Serotonin Reuptake Inhibitors. This may cause serotonin syndrome. *Risk D: Consider therapy modification*

Tricyclic Antidepressants: Selective Serotonin Reuptake Inhibitors may decrease the metabolism of Tricyclic Antidepressants. *Risk D: Consider therapy modification*

Tryptophan: May enhance the serotonergic effect of Selective Serotonin Reuptake Inhibitors. This may cause serotonin syndrome. *Risk D: Consider therapy modification*

Vitamin K Antagonists (eg, warfarin): Selective Serotonin Reuptake Inhibitors may enhance the anticoagulant effect of Vitamin K Antagonists. *Risk C: Monitor therapy*

Ethanol/Nutrition/Herb Interactions

Ethanol: Avoid ethanol (may increase CNS depression).

Herb/Nutraceutical: Avoid valerian, St John's wort, SAMe, kava kava, and gotu kola (may increase CNS depression).

Stability Store at 25°C (77°F); excursions permitted to 15°C to 30°C (59°F to 86°F).

Mechanism of Action A racemic bicyclic phthalane derivative, citalopram selectively inhibits serotonin reuptake in the presynaptic neurons and has minimal effects on norepinephrine or dopamine. Uptake inhibition of serotonin is primarily due to the *S*-enantiomer of citalopram. Displays little to no affinity for serotonin, dopamine, adrenergic, histamine, GABA, or muscarinic receptor subtypes.

Pharmacodynamics/Kinetics

Onset of action: Depression: The onset of action is within a week, however, individual response varies greatly and full response may not be seen until 8-12 weeks after initiation of treatment.

Distribution: V_d: 12 L/kg

Protein binding, plasma: ~80%

Metabolism: Extensively hepatic, via CYP3A4 and 2C19 (major pathways), and 2D6 (minor pathway); forms metabolites, N-demethylcitalopram (DCT) and didemethylcitalopram (DDCT) which are at least eight times less potent than citalopram

Bioavailability: 80%

Half-life elimination: 24-48 hours (average: 35 hours); doubled with hepatic impairment

Time to peak, serum: 1-6 hours, average within 4 hours

Excretion: Urine (Citalopram 10% and DCT 5%)

Note: Clearance was decreased, while AUC and half-life were significantly increased in elderly patients and in patients with hepatic impairment. Mild-to-moderate renal impairment may reduce clearance (17%) and prolong half-life of citalopram. No pharmacokinetic information is available concerning patients with severe renal impairment.

Dosage Oral:

Children and Adolescents: Obsessive-compulsive disorder (unlabeled use): 10-40 mg/day

Adults: Depression: Initial: 20 mg/day, generally with an increase to 40 mg/day; doses of more than 40 mg are not usually necessary. Should a dose increase be necessary, it should occur in 20 mg increments at intervals of no less than 1 week. Maximum dose: 60 mg/day; reduce dosage in elderly or those with hepatic impairment.

Elderly:

Depression: Initial: 20 mg once daily; increase dose to 40 mg/day in nonresponsive patients

Alzheimer's dementia-related depression (unlabeled use): Initial: 5-10 mg/day; may increase at multi-week intervals to maximum of 40 mg/day

Dosage adjustment in renal impairment:

Mild-to-moderate impairment: No dosage adjustment needed

Severe impairment: Cl_{cr} <20 mL/minute: Use with caution

Dosage adjustment in hepatic impairment: 20 mg once daily; increase dose to 40 mg/day in nonresponsive patients

Child/Adolescent Considerations Twenty-three patients with OCD (9-18 years of age) received 10-40 mg/day (40 mg modal) (Thomsen, 1997).

Thomsen PH, "Child and Adolescent Obsessive-Compulsive Disorder Treated With Citalopram: Findings From an Open Trial of 23 Cases," *J Child Adolesc Psychopharmacol*, 1997, 7(3):157-66.

Wagner KD, Robb AS, Findling RL, et al, "A Randomized, Placebo-Controlled Trial of Citalopram for the Treatment of Major Depression in Children and Adolescents," *Am J Psychiatry*, 2004, 161(6):1079-83.

Dietary Considerations May be taken without regard to food.

Monitoring Parameters Monitor patient periodically for symptom resolution; mental status for depression, suicidal ideation (especially at the beginning of therapy or when doses are increased or decreased), anxiety, social functioning, mania, panic attacks; akathisia

Dosage Forms Excipient information presented when available (limited, particularly for generics); consult specific product labeling.

Solution, oral: 10 mg/5 mL (240 mL)

Celexa®: 10 mg/5 mL (240 mL) [alcohol free, sugar free; contains propylene glycol; peppermint flavor]

Tablet: 10 mg, 20 mg, 40 mg

Celexa®: 10 mg, 20 mg, 40 mg

◆ **Citalopram Hydrobromide** *see* Citalopram *on page 354*

◆ **Citracal® Kosher [OTC]** *see* Calcium Citrate *on page 257*

◆ **CL-118,532** *see* Triptorelin *on page 1635*

- **CI-719** *see* Gemfibrozil *on page 711*
- **CL-184116** *see* Porfimer *on page 1314*
- **CL-232315** *see* Mitoxantrone *on page 1061*

Cladribine (KLA dri been)

Medication Safety Issues

Sound-alike/look-alike issues:

Cladribine may be confused with cleVIDipine, clofarabine

Leustatin® may be confused with lovastatin

High alert medication: The Institute for Safe Medication Practices (ISMP) includes this medication among its list of drugs which have a heightened risk of causing significant patient harm when used in error.

U.S. Brand Names Leustatin®

Canadian Brand Names Leustatin®

Index Terms 2-CdA; 2-Chlorodeoxyadenosine; NSC-105014

Pharmacologic Category Antineoplastic Agent, Antimetabolite; Antineoplastic Agent, Antimetabolite (Purine Antagonist)

Use Treatment of hairy cell leukemia

Unlabeled/Investigational Use Treatment of chronic lymphocytic leukemia (CLL), chronic myelogenous leukemia (CML), non-Hodgkin's lymphomas, progressive multiple sclerosis

Effect on Mental Status May cause drowsiness, dizziness, or insomnia

Effect on Psychiatric Treatment May cause bone marrow suppression; use caution with clozapine and carbamazepine

Dosage Summary

I.V.:

Children (unlabeled use): 6.2-7.5 mg/m^2/day continuous infusion for days 1-5 (maximum: 8.9 mg/m^2/day)

Adults: Continuous infusion: 0.09 mg/kg/day days 1-7 every 28-35 days

Dosage Forms Excipient information presented when available (limited, particularly for generics); consult specific product labeling.

Injection, solution [preservative free]: 1 mg/mL (10 mL)

- **Claforan®** *see* Cefotaxime *on page 295*
- **Claravis™** *see* Isotretinoin *on page 871*
- **Clarinex®** *see* Desloratadine *on page 430*
- **Clarinex-D® 12 Hour** *see* Desloratadine and Pseudoephedrine *on page 431*
- **Clarinex-D® 24 Hour** *see* Desloratadine and Pseudoephedrine *on page 431*

Clarithromycin (kla RITH roe mye sin)

Medication Safety Issues

Sound-alike/look-alike issues:

Clarithromycin may be confused with Claritin®, clindamycin, erythromycin

U.S. Brand Names Biaxin®; Biaxin® XL

Canadian Brand Names Apo-Clarithromycin; Biaxin®; Biaxin® XL; Gen-Clarithromycin; PMS-Clarithromycin; ratio-Clarithromycin

Mexican Brand Names Adel; Gervaken; Klaricid ; Klarmyn; Krobicin; Neo-Clarosip; Rolicytin

Pharmacologic Category Antibiotic, Macrolide

Use

Children:

Acute otitis media (*H. influenzae*, *M. catarrhalis*, or *S. pneumoniae*)

Community-acquired pneumonia due to susceptible *Mycoplasma pneumoniae*, *S. pneumoniae*, or *Chlamydia pneumoniae* (TWAR)

Pharyngitis/tonsillitis due to susceptible *S. pyogenes*, acute maxillary sinusitis due to susceptible *H. influenzae*, *S. pneumoniae*, or *Moraxella catarrhalis*, uncomplicated skin/skin structure infections due to susceptible *S. aureus*, *S. pyogenes*, and mycobacterial infections

Prevention of disseminated mycobacterial infections due to MAC disease in patients with advanced HIV infection

Adults:

Pharyngitis/tonsillitis due to susceptible *S. pyogenes*

Acute maxillary sinusitis and acute exacerbation of chronic bronchitis due to susceptible *H. influenzae*, *H. parainfluenzae*, *M. catarrhalis*, or *S. pneumoniae*

Community-acquired pneumonia due to susceptible *H. influenzae, H. parainfluenzae, Mycoplasma pneumoniae, S. pneumoniae,* or *Chlamydia pneumoniae* (TWAR), *Moraxella catarrhalis*

Uncomplicated skin/skin structure infections due to susceptible *S. aureus, S. pyogenes*

Disseminated mycobacterial infections due to *M. avium* or *M. intracellulare*

Prevention of disseminated mycobacterial infections due to *M. avium* complex (MAC) disease (eg, patients with advanced HIV infection)

Duodenal ulcer disease due to *H. pylori* in regimens with other drugs including amoxicillin and lansoprazole or omeprazole, ranitidine bismuth citrate, bismuth subsalicylate, tetracycline, and/or an H_2 antagonist

Unlabeled/Investigational Use Pertussis (CDC guidelines); alternate antibiotic for prophylaxis of infective endocarditis in patients who are allergic to penicillin and undergoing surgical or dental procedures (ACC/AHA guidelines)

Effect on Mental Status Macrolides have been reported to cause nightmares, confusion, anxiety, and mood lability

Effect on Psychiatric Treatment Contraindicated with pimozide; increases carbamazepine and triazolam levels; monitor for signs of toxicity

Dosage Summary

Oral:

Extended release:

Children: Dosage not established

Adults: 1000 mg once daily

Immediate release:

Children: 15 mg/kg/day divided every 12 hours (maximum: 1 g/day) **or** 15 mg/kg prior to procedure (maximum: 500 mg)

Adults: 250-500 mg every 8-12 hours **or** 500 mg prior to procedure

Dosage Forms Excipient information presented when available (limited, particularly for generics); consult specific product labeling.

Granules for oral suspension: 125 mg/5 mL (50 mL, 100 mL); 250 mg/5 mL (50 mL, 100 mL)

Biaxin®: 125 mg/5 mL (50 mL, 100 mL); 250 mg/5 mL (50 mL, 100 mL) [fruit punch flavor]

Tablet: 250 mg, 500 mg

Biaxin®: 250 mg, 500 mg

Tablet, extended release: 500 mg

Biaxin® XL: 500 mg

- **Clarithromycin, Lansoprazole, and Amoxicillin** *see* Lansoprazole, Amoxicillin, and Clarithromycin *on page 897*
- **Claritin® 24 Hour Allergy [OTC]** *see* Loratadine *on page 946*
- **Claritin-D® 12 Hour Allergy & Congestion [OTC]** *see* Loratadine and Pseudoephedrine *on page 948*
- **Claritin-D® 24 Hour Allergy & Congestion [OTC]** *see* Loratadine and Pseudoephedrine *on page 948*
- **Claritin® Children's [OTC]** *see* Loratadine *on page 946*
- **Claritin® Children's Allergy [OTC]** *see* Loratadine *on page 946*
- **Claritin® Hives Relief [OTC]** *see* Loratadine *on page 946*
- **Clavulanic Acid and Amoxicillin** *see* Amoxicillin and Clavulanate Potassium *on page 115*
- **Clear eyes® for Dry Eyes and ACR Relief [OTC]** *see* Naphazoline *on page 1101*
- **Clear eyes® for Dry Eyes and Redness Relief [OTC]** *see* Naphazoline *on page 1101*
- **Clear eyes® Redness Relief [OTC]** *see* Naphazoline *on page 1101*
- **Clear eyes® Seasonal Relief [OTC]** *see* Naphazoline *on page 1101*

Clemastine (KLEM as teen)

U.S. Brand Names Dayhist® Allergy [OTC]; Tavist® Allergy [OTC]

Index Terms Clemastine Fumarate

Pharmacologic Category Histamine H_1 Antagonist; Histamine H_1 Antagonist, First Generation

Use Perennial and seasonal allergic rhinitis and other allergic symptoms including urticaria

Effect on Mental Status Drowsiness is common; may cause nervousness; rare reports of depression

Effect on Psychiatric Treatment Concurrent use with psychotropics may result in additive sedation

Dosage Summary

Oral:

Children <6 years: 0.05 mg/kg/day (base) **or** 0.335-0.67 mg/day (fumarate) in 2-3 divided doses (maximum: 1.34 mg/day [fumarate] or 1 mg/day [base])

Children 6-12 years: 0.67-1.34 mg fumarate (0.5-1 mg base) twice daily (maximum: 4.02 mg/day [3 mg base])

Children ≥12 years: 1.34-2.68 mg fumarate (1-2 mg base) 2-3 times/day (maximum: 8.04 mg/day [6 mg base])

Adults: 1.34-2.68 mg fumarate (1-2 mg base) 2-3 times/day (maximum: 8.04 mg/day [6 mg base])

Dosage Forms Excipient information presented when available (limited, particularly for generics); consult specific product labeling.

Syrup, as fumarate: 0.67 mg/5 mL (120 mL, 480 mL) [prescription formulation; 0.5 mg base/5 mL]

Tablet, as fumarate: 1.34 mg [1 mg base; OTC], 2.68 mg [2 mg base; prescription formulation]

Dayhist® Allergy, Tavist® Allergy: 1.34 mg [1 mg base]

- **Clemastine Fumarate** *see* Clemastine *on page 361*
- **Cleocin®** *see* Clindamycin *on page 363*
- **Cleocin HCl®** *see* Clindamycin *on page 363*
- **Cleocin Pediatric®** *see* Clindamycin *on page 363*
- **Cleocin Phosphate®** *see* Clindamycin *on page 363*
- **Cleocin T®** *see* Clindamycin *on page 363*
- **Cleocin® Vaginal Ovule** *see* Clindamycin *on page 363*

Clidinium and Chlordiazepoxide

(kli DI nee um & klor dye az e POKS ide)

Medication Safety Issues

Sound-alike/look-alike issues:

Librax® may be confused with Librium®

Librax® formulation may be cause for confusion:

In November 2004, Valeant Pharmaceuticals licensed the Librax® trademark to Victory Pharmaceuticals. Subsequently, the product was reformulated to contain chlordiazepoxide and methscopolamine. In January 2006, Valeant Pharmaceuticals began redistributing the original formulation of Librax®, containing clidinium and chlordiazepoxide. Victory Pharmaceuticals has discontinued their product. **Note:** The formulation of Librax® distributed in Canada (Valeant Canada Ltd) always contained clidinium and chlordiazepoxide.

U.S. Brand Names Librax® *[original formulation]*

Canadian Brand Names Apo-Chlorax®; Librax®

Index Terms Chlordiazepoxide and Clidinium

Pharmacologic Category Antispasmodic Agent, Gastrointestinal; Benzodiazepine

Use Adjunct treatment of peptic ulcer; treatment of irritable bowel syndrome

Effect on Mental Status Drowsiness is common; may cause confusion

Effect on Psychiatric Treatment Concurrent use with psychotropics may result in additive sedation

Mental Health Comment In 2007, the FDA requested that all manufacturers of sedative-hypnotic drug products revise labeling to include a greater emphasis on the risks of adverse effects. These risks include severe allergic reactions (anaphylaxis, angioedema) and complex sleep-related behaviors, which may include sleep-driving (driving while not fully awake and with no memory of the event), making phone calls, and preparing and eating food while asleep.

Risk factors for abuse include personal or family history of substance abuse and personality disorder.

Dosage Summary

Oral:

Children: Dosage not established

Adults: 1-2 capsules 3-4 times/day

Dosage Forms Excipient information presented when available (limited, particularly for generics); consult specific product labeling.

Capsule: Clidinium bromide 2.5 mg and chlordiazepoxide hydrochloride 5 mg

Librax® [original formulation]: Clidinium bromide 2.5 mg and chlordiazepoxide hydrochloride 5 mg

◆ **Climara®** *see* Estradiol *on page 576*
◆ **Clindagel®** *see* Clindamycin *on page 363*
◆ **ClindaMax®** *see* Clindamycin *on page 363*

Clindamycin (klin da MYE sin)

Medication Safety Issues
Sound-alike/look-alike issues:
Cleocin® may be confused with bleomycin, Clinoril®, Cubicin®, Lincocin®
Clindamycin may be confused with clarithromycin, Claritin®, vancomycin

U.S. Brand Names Cleocin HCl®; Cleocin Pediatric®; Cleocin Phosphate®; Cleocin T®; Cleocin®; Cleocin® Vaginal Ovule; Clindagel®; ClindaMax®; ClindaReach™; Clindesse™; Evoclin®

Canadian Brand Names Alti-Clindamycin; Apo-Clindamycin®; Clindamycin Injection, USP; Clindoxyl®; Dalacin® C; Dalacin® T; Dalacin® Vaginal; Gen-Clindamycin; Novo-Clindamycin; PMS-Clindamycin; ratio-Clindamycin; Riva-Clindamycin; Taro-Clindamycin

Mexican Brand Names Biodaclin; Clidets; Clinamsa; Cutaclin 1%; Dalacin C; Galecin; Klamoxyl; Klin-Amsa; Lisiken; Trexen

Index Terms Clindamycin Hydrochloride; Clindamycin Palmitate; Clindamycin Phosphate

Pharmacologic Category Antibiotic, Lincosamide; Topical Skin Product, Acne

Use Treatment of susceptible bacterial infections, mainly those caused by anaerobes, streptococci, pneumococci, and staphylococci; bacterial vaginosis (vaginal cream, vaginal suppository); pelvic inflammatory disease (I.V.); topically in treatment of severe acne; vaginally for *Gardnerella vaginalis*

Unlabeled/Investigational Use May be useful in PCP; alternate treatment for toxoplasmosis

Effect on Mental Status None reported

Effect on Psychiatric Treatment May cause neutropenia; use caution with clozapine and carbamazepine

Dosage Summary

I.M.:
Children <1 month: 15-20 mg/kg/day in 3-4 divided doses
Children >1 month: 20-40 mg/kg/day in 3-4 divided doses
Adults: 1.2-2.7 g/day in 2-4 divided doses (maximum: 4.8 g/day)

I.V.:
Children <1 month: 15-20 mg/kg/day in 3-4 divided doses
Children >1 month: 20-40 mg/kg/day in 3-4 divided doses
Adults: 1.2-2.7 g/day in 2-4 divided doses (maximum: 4.8 g/day)

Intravaginal:
Children: Dosage not established
Adults: Insert one ovule or applicatorful once daily or one applicatorful as a single dose (Clindesse™)

Oral:
Children: 8-20 mg/kg/day as hydrochloride or 8-25 mg/kg/day as palmitate in 3-4 divided doses (minimum dose of palmitate: 37.5 mg 3 times/day)
Adults: 150-450 mg every 6-8 hours (maximum: 1.8 g/day)

Topical:
Children <12 years: Dosage not established
Children ≥12 years: Apply once or twice daily
Adults: Apply once or twice daily

Dosage Forms Excipient information presented when available (limited, particularly for generics); consult specific product labeling.
Note: Strength is expressed as base
Capsule, as hydrochloride: 75 mg, 150 mg, 300 mg
Cleocin HCl®: 75 mg [contains tartrazine], 150 mg [contains tartrazine], 300 mg
Cream, vaginal, as phosphate:
Cleocin®: 2% (40 g) [contains benzyl alcohol and mineral oil; packaged with 7 disposable applicators]
ClindaMax®: 2% (40 g) [contains benzyl alcohol and mineral oil; packaged with 7 disposable applicators]
Clindesse™: 2% (5 g) [contains mineral oil; prefilled single disposable applicator]
Foam, topical, as phosphate:
Evoclin®: 1% (50 g, 100 g) [contains ethanol 58%]
Gel, topical, as phosphate: 1% (30 g, 60 g)
Cleocin T®: 1% (30 g, 60 g)
Clindagel®: 1% (40 mL, 75 mL)
ClindaMax®: 1% (30 g, 60 g)

Granules for oral solution, as palmitate:
Cleocin Pediatric®: 75 mg/5 mL (100 mL) [cherry flavor]
Infusion, as phosphate [premixed in D_5W]:
Cleocin Phosphate®: 300 mg (50 mL); 600 mg (50 mL); 900 mg (50 mL) [contains benzyl alcohol and edetate disodium 0.5 mg/mL]
Injection, solution, as phosphate: 150 mg/mL (2 mL, 4 mL, 6 mL, 60 mL)
Cleocin Phosphate®: 150 mg/mL (2 mL, 4 mL, 6 mL, 60 mL) [contains benzyl alcohol and edetate disodium 0.5 mg/mL]
Lotion, as phosphate: 1% (60 mL)
Cleocin T®, ClindaMax®: 1% (60 mL)
Pledgets, topical: 1% (60s, 69s)
Cleocin T®: 1% (60s) [contains isopropyl alcohol 50%]
ClindaReach™: 1% (120s) [contains isopropyl alcohol 50%; packaged as a kit containing 1 collapsible applicator, 64 appliques, and 64 unmedicated pads]
Solution, topical, as phosphate: 1% (30 mL, 60 mL)
Cleocin T®: 1% (30 mL, 60 mL) [contains isopropyl alcohol 50%]
Suppository, vaginal, as phosphate:
Cleocin® Vaginal Ovule: 100 mg (3s) [contains oleaginous base; single reusable applicator]

Clindamycin and Tretinoin (klin da MYE sin & TRET i noyn)

U.S. Brand Names Ziana™
Index Terms Clindamycin Phosphate and Tretinoin; Tretinoin and Clindamycin
Pharmacologic Category Acne Products; Retinoic Acid Derivative; Topical Skin Product; Topical Skin Product, Acne
Use Treatment of acne vulgaris
Effect on Mental Status None reported
Effect on Psychiatric Treatment Diarrhea may occur with topical clindamycin. Concomitant use with SSRI, lithium, carbamazepine, or valproic acid and derivatives may produce additive effects. Tretinoin and psychotropics are associated with photosensitivity; monitor.
Dosage Summary
Topical:
Children <12 years: Dosage not established
Children ≥12 years: Apply pea-size amount to entire face once daily at bedtime
Adults: Apply pea-size amount to entire face once daily at bedtime
Dosage Forms Excipient information presented when available (limited, particularly for generics); consult specific product labeling.
Gel, topical:
Ziana™: Clindamycin phosphate 1.2% and tretinoin 0.025% (30 g, 60 g)

◆ **Clindamycin Hydrochloride** *see* Clindamycin *on page 363*
◆ **Clindamycin Palmitate** *see* Clindamycin *on page 363*
◆ **Clindamycin Phosphate** *see* Clindamycin *on page 363*
◆ **Clindamycin Phosphate and Tretinoin** *see* Clindamycin and Tretinoin *on page 364*
◆ **ClindaReach™** *see* Clindamycin *on page 363*
◆ **Clindesse™** *see* Clindamycin *on page 363*
◆ **Clinoril®** *see* Sulindac *on page 1523*

Clobazam (KLOE ba zam)

Related Information
Discontinuation of Psychotropic Drugs *on page 1839*
Canadian Brand Names Alti-Clobazam; Apo-Clobazam®; Clobazam-10; Dom-Clobazam; Frisium®; Novo-Clobazam; PMS-Clobazam; ratio-Clobazam
Pharmacologic Category Benzodiazepine
Generic Available Yes
Use Adjunctive treatment of epilepsy
Unlabeled/Investigational Use Monotherapy for epilepsy or intermittent seizures
Mental Health Comment In 2007, the FDA requested that all manufacturers of sedative-hypnotic drug products revise labeling to include a greater emphasis on the risks of adverse effects. These risks include severe allergic reactions (anaphylaxis, angioedema) and complex sleep-related behaviors, which may

include sleep-driving (driving while not fully awake and with no memory of the event), making phone calls, and preparing and eating food while asleep.

Risk factors for abuse include personal or family history of substance abuse and personality disorder.

Restrictions Not available in U.S.

Pregnancy Risk Factor Not assigned; similar agents rated D. Contraindicated in 1st trimester (per manufacturer).

Pregnancy Considerations Clobazam crosses the placenta. Oral clefts reported with benzodiazepines, however, more recent data does not support an association between drug and oral clefts. Inguinal hernia, cardiac defects, spina bifida, dysmorphic facial features, skeletal defects, multiple other malformations also reported. Hypotonia and withdrawal symptoms reported following use during 3rd trimester or near time of delivery.

Lactation Enters breast milk/contraindicated (AAP rates other benzodiazepines "of concern"); clinical effects on infant include sedation

Contraindications Hypersensitivity to clobazam or any component of the formulation (cross sensitivity with other benzodiazepines may exist); myasthenia gravis; narrow-angle glaucoma; severe hepatic or respiratory disease; sleep apnea; history of substance abuse; use in pregnancy (particularly 1st trimester); breast-feeding is contraindicated per manufacturer

Warnings/Precautions Rebound or withdrawal symptoms may occur following abrupt discontinuation or large decreases in dose (more common with prolonged treatment). Cautiously taper dose if drug discontinuation is required. Use with caution in elderly or debilitated patients, patients with hepatic disease (including alcoholics), or renal impairment.

Causes CNS depression (dose related) resulting in sedation, dizziness, confusion, or ataxia which may impair physical and mental capabilities. Patients must be cautioned about performing tasks which require mental alertness (eg, operating machinery or driving). Use with caution in patients receiving other CNS depressants or psychoactive agents. Effects with other sedative drugs or ethanol may be potentiated. Benzodiazepines have been associated with falls and traumatic injury and should be used with caution in patients who are at risk of these events (especially the elderly). Use with caution in patients with respiratory disease or impaired gag reflex.

Tolerance and loss of seizure control have been reported with chronic administration. Not recommended in patients with psychosis or depression (particularly if suicidal risk may be present). May cause physical or psychological dependence - avoid in patients with a history of drug dependence. Acute withdrawal, including seizures, may be precipitated in patients after administration of flumazenil to patients receiving long-term benzodiazepine therapy.

Benzodiazepines have been associated with anterograde amnesia. Paradoxical reactions, including hyperactive or aggressive behavior, have been reported with benzodiazepines, particularly in adolescent/pediatric or psychiatric patients. Does not have analgesic, antidepressant, or antipsychotic properties.

Adverse Reactions

Central nervous system: Drowsiness (17%), ataxia (4%), dizziness (2%), behavior disorder (1%), confusion, depression, lethargy, slurred speech, tremor, anterograde amnesia. In addition, paradoxical reactions (including excitation, agitation, hallucinations, and psychosis) are known to occur with benzodiazepines.

Dermatologic: Rash, pruritus, urticaria

Gastrointestinal: Weight gain (2%); dose related: Xerostomia, constipation, nausea

Hematologic: Decreased WBCs and other hematologic abnormalities have been rarely associated with benzodiazepines

Neuromuscular & skeletal: Muscle spasm

Ocular: Blurred vision (1%)

Metabolism/Transport Effects Substrate (major) of CYP2C19 and 3A4

Drug Interactions

Alcohol (Ethyl): CNS Depressants may enhance the CNS depressant effect of Alcohol (Ethyl). *Risk C: Monitor therapy*

Antifungal Agents (Azole Derivatives, Systemic): May decrease the metabolism of Benzodiazepines (metabolized by oxidation). *Risk D: Consider therapy modification*

Aprepitant: May increase the serum concentration of Benzodiazepines (metabolized by oxidation). *Risk C: Monitor therapy*

Calcium Channel Blockers (Nondihydropyridine): May decrease the metabolism of Benzodiazepines (metabolized by oxidation). *Risk D: Consider therapy modification*

CarBAMazepine: May increase the metabolism of Benzodiazepines (metabolized by oxidation). *Risk C: Monitor therapy*

Cimetidine: May decrease the metabolism of Benzodiazepines (metabolized by oxidation). *Risk C: Monitor therapy*

Clozapine: Benzodiazepines may enhance the adverse/toxic effect of Clozapine. *Risk D: Consider therapy modification*

CNS Depressants: May enhance the adverse/toxic effect of other CNS Depressants. *Risk C: Monitor therapy*

CYP2C19 Inducers (Strong): May increase the metabolism of CYP2C19 Substrates. *Risk C: Monitor therapy*

CYP2C19 Inhibitors (Moderate): May decrease the metabolism of CYP2C19 Substrates. *Risk C: Monitor therapy*

CYP2C19 Inhibitors (Strong): May decrease the metabolism of CYP2C19 Substrates. *Risk D: Consider therapy modification*

CYP3A4 Inducers (Strong): May increase the metabolism of CYP3A4 Substrates. *Risk C: Monitor therapy*

CYP3A4 Inhibitors (Moderate): May decrease the metabolism of CYP3A4 Substrates. *Risk C: Monitor therapy*

CYP3A4 Inhibitors (Strong): May decrease the metabolism of CYP3A4 Substrates. *Risk D: Consider therapy modification*

Dasatinib: May increase the serum concentration of CYP3A4 Substrates. *Risk C: Monitor therapy*

Deferasirox: May decrease the serum concentration of CYP3A4 Substrates. *Risk C: Monitor therapy*

Disulfiram: May decrease the metabolism of Benzodiazepines (metabolized by oxidation). *Risk C: Monitor therapy*

Fluconazole: May decrease the metabolism of Benzodiazepines (metabolized by oxidation). *Risk D: Consider therapy modification*

Fosaprepitant: May increase the serum concentration of Benzodiazepines (metabolized by oxidation). Specifically, the active metabolite aprepitant is likely responsible for this effect. *Risk C: Monitor therapy*

Grapefruit Juice: May decrease the metabolism of Benzodiazepines (metabolized by oxidation). *Risk D: Consider therapy modification*

Isoniazid: May decrease the metabolism of Benzodiazepines (metabolized by oxidation). *Risk C: Monitor therapy*

Macrolide Antibiotics: May decrease the metabolism of Benzodiazepines (metabolized by oxidation). **Exceptions:** Azithromycin; Dirithromycin [Off Market]; Spiramycin. *Risk D: Consider therapy modification*

Nefazodone: May decrease the metabolism of Benzodiazepines (metabolized by oxidation). *Risk D: Consider therapy modification*

Oral Contraceptive (Estrogens): May decrease the metabolism of Benzodiazepines (metabolized by oxidation). *Risk C: Monitor therapy*

Oral Contraceptive (Progestins): May decrease the metabolism of Benzodiazepines (metabolized by oxidation). *Risk C: Monitor therapy*

Phenytoin: Benzodiazepines may increase the serum concentration of Phenytoin. Short-term exposure to benzodiazepines may not present as much risk as chronic therapy. *Risk C: Monitor therapy*

Protease Inhibitors: May decrease the metabolism of Benzodiazepines (metabolized by oxidation). Management: Amprenavir, atazanavir, darunavir, indinavir, nelfinavir, ritonavir, and tipranavir are contraindicated with midazolam and triazolam according to each protease inhibitor's prescribing information. *Risk D: Consider therapy modification*

Proton Pump Inhibitors: May increase the serum concentration of Benzodiazepines (metabolized by oxidation). **Exceptions:** Lansoprazole; Pantoprazole; Rabeprazole. *Risk C: Monitor therapy*

Rifamycin Derivatives: May increase the metabolism of Benzodiazepines (metabolized by oxidation). *Risk D: Consider therapy modification*

Selective Serotonin Reuptake Inhibitors: May decrease the metabolism of Benzodiazepines (metabolized by oxidation). **Exceptions:** Citalopram; Escitalopram; PARoxetine; Sertraline. *Risk C: Monitor therapy*

St Johns Wort: May increase the metabolism of Benzodiazepines (metabolized by oxidation). *Risk C: Monitor therapy*

Theophylline Derivatives: May diminish the therapeutic effect of Benzodiazepines. *Risk D: Consider therapy modification*

Ethanol/Nutrition/Herb Interactions

Ethanol: Avoid ethanol (may increase CNS depression). Concomitant administration may increase bioavailability of clobazam by 50%.

Food: Serum concentrations may be increased by grapefruit juice.

Herb/Nutraceutical: St John's wort may decrease benzodiazepine levels. Avoid valerian, St John's wort, kava kava, gotu kola (may increase CNS depression).

Stability Store at 15°C to 30°C (59°F to 86°F).

Mechanism of Action Clobazam is a 1,5 benzodiazepine which binds to stereospecific benzodiazepine receptors on the postsynaptic GABA neuron at several sites within the central nervous system, including the limbic system, reticular formation. Enhancement of the inhibitory effect of GABA on neuronal excitability results by increased neuronal membrane permeability to chloride ions. This shift in chloride ions results in hyperpolarization (a less excitable state) and stabilization.

Pharmacodynamics/Kinetics

Absorption: Rapid

Protein binding: 85% to 91%

Metabolism: Hepatic via N-dealkylation (likely via CYP) to active metabolite (N-desmethyl), and glucuronidation

Bioavailability: 87%

Half-life elimination: 18 hours; N-desmethyl (active): 42 hours

Time to peak: 15 minutes to 4 hours

Excretion: Urine (90%), as metabolites

Dosage Oral:

Children:

<2 years: Initial 0.5-1 mg/kg/day

2-16 years: Initial: 5 mg/day; may be increased (no more frequently than every 5 days) to a maximum of 40 mg/day

Adults: Initial: 5-15 mg/day; dosage may be gradually adjusted (based on tolerance and seizure control) to a maximum of 80 mg/day

Note: Daily doses of up to 30 mg may be taken as a single dose at bedtime; higher doses should be divided.

Dosage adjustment in hepatic impairment: Avoid use in severe hepatic impairment. Use lower doses in mild-to-moderate impairment and monitor closely.

Dietary Considerations May be taken with or without food.

Administration May be administered with food.

Additional Information Not available in U.S.

Clobazam is a 1,5 benzodiazepine; other benzodiazepines are typically 1,4 substituted.

Dosage Forms Excipient information presented when available (limited, particularly for generics); consult specific product labeling. [CAN] = Canadian brand name

Tablet: 10 mg

Alti-Clobazam [CAN], Apo-Clobazam® [CAN], Clobazam-10 [CAN], Dom-Clobazam [CAN], Frisium® [CAN], Novo-Clobazam [CAN], PMS-Clobazam [CAN], ration-Clobazam [CAN]: 10 mg [not available in the U.S.]

Clofarabine (klo FARE a been)

Medication Safety Issues

Sound-alike/look-alike issues:

Clofarabine may be confused with cladribine, cleVIDipine

High alert medication: The Institute for Safe Medication Practices (ISMP) includes this medication among its list of drugs which have a heightened risk of causing significant patient harm when used in error.

U.S. Brand Names Clolar™

Index Terms Clofarex; NSC606869

Pharmacologic Category Antineoplastic Agent, Antimetabolite (Purine Antagonist)

Use Treatment of relapsed or refractory acute lymphoblastic leukemia

Unlabeled/Investigational Use Adults: Relapsed and refractory acute myeloid leukemia (AML), chronic myeloid leukemia (CML) in blast phase, acute lymphocytic leukemia (ALL), myelodysplastic syndrome

Effect on Mental Status May cause anxiety, dizziness, depression, irritability, and lethargy

Effect on Psychiatric Treatment GI side effects are common; concomitant use with SSRIs, lithium, valproic acid may produce additive effects.

Dosage Summary

I.V.:

Children <1 years: Dosage not established

Children >1 year: 52 mg/m²/day days 1 through 5; repeat every 2-6 weeks

Adults ≤21 years: 52 mg/m²/day days 1 through 5; repeat every 2-6 weeks

Adults >21 years: Dosage not established

Dosage Forms Excipient information presented when available (limited, particularly for generics); consult specific product labeling.
Injection, solution [preservative free]: 1 mg/mL (20 mL)

◆ **Clofarex** *see* Clofarabine *on page 367*

◆ **Clolar™** *see* Clofarabine *on page 367*

◆ **Clomid®** *see* ClomiPHENE *on page 368*

ClomiPHENE (KLOE mi feen)

Medication Safety Issues
Sound-alike/look-alike issues:
ClomiPHENE may be confused with clomiPRAMINE, clonidine
Clomid® may be confused with clonidine
Serophene® may be confused with Sarafem™

U.S. Brand Names Clomid®; Serophene®
Canadian Brand Names Clomid®; Milophene®; Serophene®
Mexican Brand Names Omifin; Serofene
Index Terms Clomiphene Citrate
Pharmacologic Category Ovulation Stimulator; Selective Estrogen Receptor Modulator (SERM)
Use Treatment of ovulatory failure in patients desiring pregnancy
Effect on Mental Status May cause insomnia, fatigue, or depression
Effect on Psychiatric Treatment None reported
Dosage Summary
Oral:
Children: Dosage not established
Adults (females): First course: 50 mg/day for 5 days; Second course (if needed): 100 mg/day for 5 days; **Note:** If ovulation does not occur after 3 courses, or if 3 ovulatory responses occur but pregnancy is not achieved, further treatment is not recommended.

Dosage Forms Excipient information presented when available (limited, particularly for generics); consult specific product labeling.
Tablet, as citrate [scored]: 50 mg
Clomid®, Serophene®: 50 mg

◆ **Clomiphene Citrate** *see* ClomiPHENE *on page 368*

ClomiPRAMINE (kloe MI pra meen)

Medication Safety Issues
Sound-alike/look-alike issues:
ClomiPRAMINE may be confused with chlorproMAZINE, cleVIDipine, clomiPHENE, desipramine, Norpramin®
Anafranil® may be confused with alfentanil, enalapril, nafarelin

Related Information
Antidepressant Agents *on page 1760*
Antidepressant Receptor Profile *on page 1764*
Discontinuation of Psychotropic Drugs *on page 1839*

U.S. Brand Names Anafranil®
Canadian Brand Names Anafranil®; Apo-Clomipramine®; CO Clomipramine; Gen-Clomipramine
Mexican Brand Names Anafranil
Index Terms Clomipramine Hydrochloride
Pharmacologic Category Antidepressant, Tricyclic (Tertiary Amine)
Generic Available Yes
Use Treatment of obsessive-compulsive disorder (OCD)
Unlabeled/Investigational Use Depression, panic attacks, chronic pain
Mental Health Comment Tricyclic antidepressants may be classified as tertiary (amitriptyline, doxepin, clomipramine, imipramine, trimipramine) or secondary amines (nortriptyline, desipramine, protriptyline). The tertiary amines are not recommended to treat depression in the elderly. If a TCA is used in the elderly, it should be a secondary amine. The tertiary amines are commonly used in low dosages for various conditions associated with pain. Toxicity is generally dose dependent. Relatively small overdoses (1-week supply) can be potentially fatal.

Seizures are dose dependent. The overall cumulative incidence is 0.7%. Doses ≤250 mg/day have an incidence of 0.5% and doses ≥300 mg/day have an incidence of 2.1%.

Restrictions An FDA-approved medication guide concerning the use of antidepressants in children, adolescents, and young adults must be distributed when dispensing an outpatient prescription (new or refill) where this medication is to be used without direct supervision of a healthcare provider. Medication guides are available at http://www.fda.gov/cder/Offices/ODS/medication_guides.htm. Dispense to parents or guardians of children and adolescents receiving this medication.

Pregnancy Risk Factor C

Pregnancy Considerations There are no adequate and well-controlled studies in pregnant women. Withdrawal symptoms (including dizziness, nausea, vomiting, headache, malaise, sleep disturbance, hyperthermia, and/or irritability) have been observed in neonates whose mothers took clomipramine up to delivery. Use in pregnancy only if the benefits to the mother outweigh the potential risks to the fetus.

Lactation Enters breast milk/not recommended (AAP rates "of concern")

Contraindications Hypersensitivity to clomipramine, other tricyclic agents, or any component of the formulation; use of MAO inhibitors within 14 days; use in a patient during the acute recovery phase of MI

Warnings/Precautions [U.S. Boxed Warning]: Antidepressants increase the risk of suicidal thinking and behavior in children, adolescents, and young adults (18-24 years of age) with major depressive disorder (MDD) and other psychiatric disorders; consider risk prior to prescribing. Short-term studies did not show an increased risk in patients >24 years of age and showed a decreased risk in patients ≥65 years. Closely monitor for clinical worsening, suicidality, or unusual changes in behavior; the patient's family or caregiver should be instructed to closely observe the patient and communicate condition with healthcare provider. A medication guide should be dispensed with each prescription. **Clomipramine is FDA approved for the treatment of OCD in children ≥10 years of age.**

The possibility of a suicide attempt is inherent in major depression and may persist until remission occurs. Monitor for worsening of depression or suicidality, especially during initiation of therapy (generally first 1-2 months) or with dose increases or decreases. Use caution in high-risk patients. Worsening depression and severe abrupt suicidality that are not part of the presenting symptoms may require discontinuation or modification of drug therapy. The patient's family or caregiver should be alerted to monitor patients for the emergence of suicidality and associated behaviors (such as agitation, irritability, hostility, impulsivity, and hypomania) and notify the healthcare provider.

May worsen psychosis in some patients or precipitate a shift to mania or hypomania in patients with bipolar disorder. Patients presenting with depressive symptoms should be screened for bipolar disorder. Monotherapy in patients with bipolar disorder should be avoided. **Clomipramine is not FDA approved for bipolar depression.**

TCAs may rarely cause bone marrow suppression; monitor for any signs of infection and obtain CBC if symptoms (eg, fever, sore throat) evident. May cause seizures (relationship to dose and/or duration of therapy) - do not exceed maximum doses. Use caution in patients with a previous seizure disorder or condition predisposing to seizures such as brain damage, alcoholism, or concurrent therapy with other drugs which lower the seizure threshold. May increase the risks associated with electroconvulsive therapy. Has been associated with a high incidence of sexual dysfunction. Weight gain may occur. Hyperpyrexia has been observed with TCAs in combination with anticholinergics and/or neuroleptics, particularly during hot weather.

The degree of sedation, anticholinergic effects, and conduction abnormalities are high relative to other antidepressants. Clomipramine often causes drowsiness/sedation, resulting in impaired performance of tasks requiring alertness (eg, operating machinery or driving). Sedative effects may be additive with other CNS depressants and/or ethanol. The risk of orthostasis is moderate to high relative to other antidepressants. Use with caution in patients with a history of cardiovascular disease (including previous MI, stroke, tachycardia, or conduction abnormalities). Use with caution in patients with urinary retention, benign prostatic hyperplasia, narrow-angle glaucoma, xerostomia, visual problems, constipation, or a history of bowel obstruction.

Consider discontinuing, when possible, prior to elective surgery. Therapy should not be abruptly discontinued in patients receiving high doses for prolonged periods. Use with caution in hyperthyroid patients or those receiving thyroid supplementation. Use with caution in patients with hepatic or renal dysfunction and in elderly patients.

Adverse Reactions Data shown for children reflects both children and adolescents studied in clinical trials.

>10%:

Central nervous system: Dizziness (54%), somnolence (54%), drowsiness, headache (52%; children 28%), fatigue (39%), insomnia (25%; children 11%), malaise, nervousness (18%; children 4%)

Endocrine & metabolic: Libido changes (21%), hot flushes (5%)

Gastrointestinal: Xerostomia (84%, children 63%) constipation (47%; children 22%), nausea (33%; children 9%), dyspepsia (22%; children 13%), weight gain (18%; children 2%), diarrhea (13%; children 7%), anorexia (12%; children 22%), abdominal pain (11%), appetite increased (11%)

Genitourinary: Ejaculation failure (42%), impotence (20%), micturition disorder (14%; children 4%)

Neuromuscular & skeletal: Tremor (54%), myoclonus (13%; children 2%), myalgia (13%)

Ocular: Abnormal vision (18%; children 7%)

Respiratory: Pharyngitis (14%), rhinitis (12%)

Miscellaneous: Diaphoresis increased (29%; children 9%)

1% to 10%:

Cardiovascular: Flushing (8%), postural hypotension (6%), palpitation (4%), tachycardia (4%; children 2%), chest pain (4%), edema (2%)

Central nervous system: Anxiety (9%), memory impairment (9%), twitching (7%), depression (5%), concentration impaired (5%), fever (4%), hypertonia (4%), abnormal dreaming (3%), agitation (3%), confusion (3%), migraine (3%), pain (3%), psychosomatic disorder (3%), speech disorder (3%), yawning (3%), aggressiveness (children 2%), chills (2%), depersonalization (2%), emotional lability (2%), irritability (2%), panic reaction (1%)

Dermatologic: Rash (8%), pruritus (6%), purpura (3%), dermatitis (2%), acne (2%), dry skin (2%), urticaria (1%)

Endocrine & metabolic: Amenorrhea (1%), breast enlargement (2%), breast pain (1%), hot flashes (5%), lactation (nonpuerperal) (4%)

Gastrointestinal: Taste disturbance (8%), vomiting (7%), flatulence (6%), tooth disorder (5%), dysphagia (2%), esophagitis (1%)

Genitourinary: UTI (2% to 6%), micturition frequency (5%), dysuria (2%), leucorrhea (2%), vaginitis (2%), urinary retention (2%)

Neuromuscular & skeletal: Paresthesia (9%), back pain (6%), arthralgia (3%), paresis (children 2%), weakness (1%)

Ocular: Lacrimation abnormal (3%), mydriasis (2%), conjunctivitis (1%)

Otic: Tinnitus (6%)

Respiratory: Sinusitis (6%), coughing (6%), bronchospasm (2%; children 7%), epistaxis (2%)

<1% (Limited to important or life-threatening): Accommodation abnormal, albuminuria, aneurysm, anticholinergic syndrome, aphasia, apraxia, arrhythmia, ataxia, atrial flutter, blepharitis, blood in stool, bradycardia, breast fibroadenosis, bronchitis, bundle branch block, cardiac arrest, cardiac failure, catalepsy, cellulitis, cerebral hemorrhage, cervical dysplasia, cheilitis, cholinergic syndrome, choreoathetosis, chromatopsia, chronic enteritis, coma, conjunctival hemorrhage, cyanosis, deafness, dehydration, delirium, delusion, diabetes mellitus, diplopia, dyskinesia, dysphonia, dystonia, EEG abnormal, encephalopathy, endometrial hyperplasia, endometriosis, epididymitis, erythematous rash, exophthalmos, extrapyramidal disorder, extrasystoles, gastric ulcer, generalized spasm, glaucoma, glycosuria, goiter, gynecomastia, hallucinations, heart block, hematuria, hemiparesis, hemoptysis, hepatitis, hostility, hyperacusis, hypercholesterolemia, hyper-/hypoesthesia, hyperglycemia, hyper-/hypokinesia, hyperreflexia, hyper-/hypothyroidism, hyperuricemia, hyper-/hypoventilation, hypnagogic hallucination, hypokalemia, ideation, intestinal obstruction, irritable bowel syndrome, keratitis, laryngismus, leukemoid reaction, lupus erythematosus rash, lymphadenopathy, lymphoma-like disorder, maculopapular rash, manic reaction, marrow depression, myocardial infarction, myocardial ischemia, myopathy, myositis, neuralgia, neuropathy, oculogyric crisis, oculomotor nerve paralysis, oral/pharyngeal edema, ovarian cyst, paralytic ileus, paranoia, parosmia, peptic ulcer, peripheral ischemia, phobic disorder, photophobia, photosensitivity reaction, pneumonia, polyarteritis nodosa, premature ejaculation, psychosis, pyelonephritis, pyuria, rectal hemorrhage, renal calculus, renal cyst, schizophrenic reaction, scleritis, seizure, sensory disturbance, skin ulceration, strabismus, stupor, suicidal ideation, suicide, suicide attempt, thrombophlebitis, tongue ulceration, tooth caries, torticollis, urinary incontinence, uterine hemorrhage, uterine inflammation, vaginal hemorrhage, vasospasm, ventricular tachycardia, visual field defect, withdrawal syndrome

Metabolism/Transport Effects Substrate of CYP1A2 (major), 2C19 (major), 2D6 (major), 3A4 (minor); **Inhibits** CYP2D6 (moderate)

Drug Interactions

Acetylcholinesterase Inhibitors (Central): Anticholinergics may diminish the therapeutic effect of Acetylcholinesterase Inhibitors (Central). Acetylcholinesterase Inhibitors (Central) may diminish the therapeutic effect of Anticholinergics. If the anticholinergic action is a side effect of the agent, the result may be beneficial. *Risk C: Monitor therapy*

Alcohol (Ethyl): CNS Depressants may enhance the CNS depressant effect of Alcohol (Ethyl). *Risk C: Monitor therapy*

Alfuzosin: May enhance the QTc-prolonging effect of QTc-Prolonging Agents. *Risk C: Monitor therapy*

Alpha-/Beta-Agonists (Direct-Acting): Tricyclic Antidepressants may enhance the vasopressor effect of Alpha-/Beta-Agonists (Direct-Acting). **Exceptions:** Dipivefrin. *Risk D: Consider therapy modification*

Alpha1-Agonists: Tricyclic Antidepressants may enhance the vasopressor effect of Alpha1-Agonists. *Risk D: Consider therapy modification*

Alpha2-Agonists: Tricyclic Antidepressants may diminish the antihypertensive effect of Alpha2-Agonists. **Exceptions:** Apraclonidine; Brimonidine. *Risk D: Consider therapy modification*

Altretamine: May enhance the orthostatic effect of Tricyclic Antidepressants. *Risk C: Monitor therapy*

Amphetamines: Tricyclic Antidepressants may enhance the stimulatory effect of Amphetamines. Tricyclic Antidepressants may also potentiate the cardiovascular effects of Amphetamines. *Risk C: Monitor therapy*

Anticholinergics: May enhance the adverse/toxic effect of other Anticholinergics. **Exceptions:** Paliperidone. *Risk C: Monitor therapy*

Aspirin: Antidepressants (Tricyclic, Tertiary Amine) may enhance the antiplatelet effect of Aspirin. *Risk C: Monitor therapy*

Barbiturates: May increase the metabolism of Tricyclic Antidepressants. *Risk D: Consider therapy modification*

Beta2-Agonists: Tricyclic Antidepressants may enhance the adverse/toxic effect of Beta2-Agonists. *Risk C: Monitor therapy*

BuPROPion: May decrease the metabolism of Tricyclic Antidepressants. *Risk C: Monitor therapy*

CarBAMazepine: May increase the serum concentration of ClomiPRAMINE. *Risk C: Monitor therapy*

Cimetidine: May decrease the metabolism of Tricyclic Antidepressants. *Risk C: Monitor therapy*

Cinacalcet: May increase the serum concentration of Tricyclic Antidepressants. *Risk C: Monitor therapy*

Ciprofloxacin: May enhance the QTc-prolonging effect of QTc-Prolonging Agents. *Risk C: Monitor therapy*

CNS Depressants: May enhance the adverse/toxic effect of other CNS Depressants. *Risk C: Monitor therapy*

Codeine: CYP2D6 Inhibitors (Moderate) may diminish the therapeutic effect of Codeine. These CYP2D6 inhibitors may prevent the metabolic conversion of codeine to its active metabolite morphine. *Risk C: Monitor therapy*

CYP1A2 Inducers (Strong): May increase the metabolism of CYP1A2 Substrates. *Risk C: Monitor therapy*

CYP1A2 Inhibitors (Moderate): May decrease the metabolism of CYP1A2 Substrates. *Risk C: Monitor therapy*

CYP1A2 Inhibitors (Strong): May decrease the metabolism of CYP1A2 Substrates. *Risk D: Consider therapy modification*

CYP2C19 Inducers (Strong): May increase the metabolism of CYP2C19 Substrates. *Risk C: Monitor therapy*

CYP2C19 Inhibitors (Moderate): May decrease the metabolism of CYP2C19 Substrates. *Risk C: Monitor therapy*

CYP2C19 Inhibitors (Strong): May decrease the metabolism of CYP2C19 Substrates. *Risk D: Consider therapy modification*

CYP2D6 Inhibitors (Moderate): May decrease the metabolism of CYP2D6 Substrates. *Risk C: Monitor therapy*

CYP2D6 Inhibitors (Strong): May decrease the metabolism of CYP2D6 Substrates. *Risk D: Consider therapy modification*

CYP2D6 Substrates: CYP2D6 Inhibitors (Moderate) may decrease the metabolism of CYP2D6 Substrates. **Exceptions:** Tamoxifen. *Risk C: Monitor therapy*

Darunavir: May increase the serum concentration of CYP2D6 Substrates. *Risk C: Monitor therapy*

Desmopressin: Tricyclic Antidepressants may enhance the adverse/toxic effect of Desmopressin. *Risk C: Monitor therapy*

Dexmethylphenidate: May decrease the metabolism of Tricyclic Antidepressants. *Risk C: Monitor therapy*

DULoxetine: May decrease the metabolism of Tricyclic Antidepressants. *Risk C: Monitor therapy*

Gadobutrol: May enhance the QTc-prolonging effect of QTc-Prolonging Agents. *Risk D: Consider therapy modification*

Lithium: May enhance the neurotoxic effect of Tricyclic Antidepressants. *Risk C: Monitor therapy*

MAO Inhibitors: May enhance the serotonergic effect of Tricyclic Antidepressants. This may cause serotonin syndrome. *Risk X: Avoid combination*

Methylphenidate: May decrease the metabolism of Tricyclic Antidepressants. *Risk C: Monitor therapy*

Nebivolol: CYP2D6 Inhibitors (Moderate) may increase the serum concentration of Nebivolol. *Risk C: Monitor therapy*

Nilotinib: May enhance the QTc-prolonging effect of QTc-Prolonging Agents. *Risk X: Avoid combination*

NSAID (COX-2 Inhibitor): Antidepressants (Tricyclic, Tertiary Amine) may enhance the antiplatelet effect of NSAID (COX-2 Inhibitor). *Risk C: Monitor therapy*

NSAID (Nonselective): Antidepressants (Tricyclic, Tertiary Amine) may enhance the antiplatelet effect of NSAID (Nonselective). *Risk C: Monitor therapy*

Pramlintide: May enhance the anticholinergic effect of Anticholinergics. These effects are specific to the GI tract. *Risk D: Consider therapy modification*

Propoxyphene: May enhance the CNS depressant effect of Tricyclic Antidepressants. *Risk C: Monitor therapy*

Protease Inhibitors: May increase the serum concentration of Tricyclic Antidepressants. *Risk C: Monitor therapy*

QTc-Prolonging Agents: May enhance the adverse/toxic effect of other QTc-Prolonging Agents. Their effects can be additive, causing life-threatening ventricular arrhythmias. *Risk D: Consider therapy modification*

QuiNIDine: Tricyclic Antidepressants may enhance the QTc-prolonging effect of QuiNIDine. QuiNIDine may decrease the metabolism of Tricyclic Antidepressants. *Risk D: Consider therapy modification*

Selective Serotonin Reuptake Inhibitors: May decrease the metabolism of Tricyclic Antidepressants. *Risk D: Consider therapy modification*

Serotonin Modulators: May enhance the adverse/toxic effect of other Serotonin Modulators. The development of serotonin syndrome may occur. *Risk D: Consider therapy modification*

Sibutramine: May enhance the serotonergic effect of Serotonin Modulators. This may cause serotonin syndrome. *Risk X: Avoid combination*

St Johns Wort: May increase the metabolism of Tricyclic Antidepressants. The risk of serotonin syndrome may theoretically be increased. *Risk D: Consider therapy modification*

Sulfonylureas: Cyclic Antidepressants may enhance the hypoglycemic effect of Sulfonylureas. *Risk C: Monitor therapy*

Tamoxifen: CYP2D6 Inhibitors (Moderate) may decrease the metabolism of Tamoxifen. Specifically, CYP2D6 inhibitors may decrease the formation of highly potent active metabolites. *Risk D: Consider therapy modification*

Terbinafine: May decrease the metabolism of Tricyclic Antidepressants. *Risk D: Consider therapy modification*

Tetrabenazine: QTc-Prolonging Agents may enhance the QTc-prolonging effect of Tetrabenazine. *Risk X: Avoid combination*

Thioridazine: QTc-Prolonging Agents may enhance the QTc-prolonging effect of Thioridazine. *Risk X: Avoid combination*

Thioridazine: CYP2D6 Inhibitors may decrease the metabolism of Thioridazine. *Risk X: Avoid combination*

TraMADol: Tricyclic Antidepressants may enhance the neuroexcitatory and/or seizure-potentiating effect of TraMADol. *Risk C: Monitor therapy*

Valproic Acid: May increase the serum concentration of Tricyclic Antidepressants. *Risk C: Monitor therapy*

Vitamin K Antagonists (eg, warfarin): Tricyclic Antidepressants may enhance the anticoagulant effect of Vitamin K Antagonists. *Risk C: Monitor therapy*

Ziprasidone: QTc-Prolonging Agents may enhance the QTc-prolonging effect of Ziprasidone. The risk of a severe arrhythmia may be increased. *Risk X: Avoid combination*

Ethanol/Nutrition/Herb Interactions

Ethanol: Avoid ethanol (may increase CNS depression).

Food: Serum concentrations/toxicity may be increased by grapefruit juice.

Herb/Nutraceutical: Avoid valerian, St John's wort, SAMe, kava kava.

Mechanism of Action Clomipramine appears to affect serotonin uptake while its active metabolite, desmethylclomipramine, affects norepinephrine uptake

Pharmacodynamics/Kinetics
Absorption: Rapid
Protein binding: 97%, primarily to albumin
Metabolism: Hepatic to desmethylclomipramine (DMI; active); extensive first-pass effect
Half-life elimination: Clomipramine: mean 32 hours (19-37 hours); DMI: mean 69 hours (range 54-77 hours)
Time to peak, plasma: 2-6 hours
Excretion: Urine and feces

Dosage Oral:
Children:
<10 years: Safety and efficacy have not been established.
≥10 years: OCD:
Initial: 25 mg/day; may gradually increase as tolerated over the first 2 weeks to 3 mg/kg/day or 100 mg/day (whichever is less) in divided doses
Maintenance: May further increase to recommended maximum of 3 mg/kg/day or 200 mg/day (whichever is less); may give as a single daily dose at bedtime once tolerated
Adults: OCD:
Initial: 25 mg/day; may gradually increase as tolerated over the first 2 weeks to 100 mg/day in divided doses
Maintenance: May further increase to recommended maximum of 250 mg/day; may give as a single daily dose at bedtime once tolerated

Administration During titration, may divide doses and administer with meals to decrease gastrointestinal side effects. After titration, may administer total daily dose at bedtime to decrease daytime sedation.

Monitoring Parameters Pulse rate and blood pressure prior to and during therapy; ECG/cardiac status in older adults and patients with cardiac disease; suicidal ideation (especially at the beginning of therapy or when doses are increased or decreased)

Test Interactions Increased glucose

Dosage Forms Excipient information presented when available (limited, particularly for generics); consult specific product labeling.
Capsule, as hydrochloride: 25 mg, 50 mg, 75 mg
Anafranil®: 25 mg, 50 mg, 75 mg

◆ **Clomipramine Hydrochloride** *see* ClomiPRAMINE *on page 368*

ClonazePAM (kloe NA ze pam)

Medication Safety Issues
Sound-alike/look-alike issues:
ClonazePAM may be confused with clofazimine, cloNIDine, clorazepate, clozapine, LORazepam
Klonopin® may be confused with clofazimine, clonNIDine, clorazepate, clozapine, LORazepam

Related Information
Anticonvulsants By Seizure Type *on page 1759*
Benzodiazepines *on page 1774*
CMS: Long-Term Care Facility Thresholds *on page 1815*
Discontinuation of Psychotropic Drugs *on page 1839*

U.S. Brand Names Klonopin®; Klonopin® Wafers

Canadian Brand Names Alti-Clonazepam; Apo-Clonazepam®; Clonapam; CO Clonazepam; Gen-Clonazepam; Klonopin®; Novo-Clonazepam; Nu-Clonazepam; PMS-Clonazepam; Rho®-Clonazepam; Rivotril®; Sandoz-Clonazepam

Mexican Brand Names Clonapilep; Clozer; Kenoket; Kriadex; Rivotril; Zymanta

Pharmacologic Category Benzodiazepine

Generic Available Yes

Use Alone or as an adjunct in the treatment of petit mal variant (Lennox-Gastaut), akinetic, and myoclonic seizures; petit mal (absence) seizures unresponsive to succimides; panic disorder with or without agoraphobia

Unlabeled/Investigational Use Restless legs syndrome; neuralgia; multifocal tic disorder; parkinsonian dysarthria; bipolar disorder; adjunct therapy for schizophrenia

Mental Health Comment In 2007, the FDA requested that all manufacturers of sedative-hypnotic drug products revise labeling to include a greater emphasis on the risks of adverse effects. These risks include severe allergic reactions (anaphylaxis, angioedema) and complex sleep-related behaviors, which may include sleep-driving (driving while not fully awake and with no memory of the event), making phone calls, and preparing and eating food while asleep.

There are two subtypes of GABA receptors (GABA-A and GABA-B) and three different benzodiazepine receptors (Bz_1, Bz_2, and Bz_3). Benzodiazepine receptors and effects appear to be linked to the GABA-A receptors. Benzodiazepines do not bind to GABA-B receptors. The role of GABA-B receptors is unclear. Benzodiazepines have no specificity for benzodiazepine receptor subtypes.

Clonazepam is a long half-life benzodiazepine. Duration of action after a single dose is determined by redistribution rather than metabolism. Tolerance develops to the sedative, hypnotic, and anticonvulsant effects. It does not develop to the anxiolytic or skeletal muscle relaxing effects. Psychological and physical dependence may occur with prolonged use of benzodiazepines. The onset of withdrawal symptoms is usually seen on the first day without drug and lasts 5-7 days in patients receiving short half-life benzodiazepines, whereas, the onset occurs after 5 days with a duration of 10-14 days after abrupt discontinuance of long half-life benzodiazepines. Risk factors for abuse include personal or family history of substance abuse and personality disorder.

Restrictions C-IV

Pregnancy Risk Factor D

Pregnancy Considerations Clonazepam was shown to be teratogenic in some animal studies. Clonazepam crosses the placenta. Benzodiazepine use during pregnancy is associated with increased risk of congenital malformations. Nonteratogenic effects (including neonatal flaccidity, respiratory and feeding problems, and withdrawal symptoms) during the postnatal period have also been reported with benzodiazepine use. Epilepsy itself, number of medications, genetic factors, or a combination of these probably influence the teratogenicity of anticonvulsant therapy.

Lactation Enters breast milk/not recommended

Contraindications Hypersensitivity to clonazepam or any component of the formulation (cross-sensitivity with other benzodiazepines may exist); significant liver disease; narrow-angle glaucoma; pregnancy

Warnings/Precautions Use with caution in elderly or debilitated patients, patients with hepatic disease (including alcoholics), or renal impairment. Use with caution in patients with respiratory disease or impaired gag reflex or ability to protect the airway from secretions (salivation may be increased). Worsening of seizures may occur when added to patients with multiple seizure types. Concurrent use with valproic acid may result in absence status. Monitoring of CBC and liver function tests has been recommended during prolonged therapy.

Causes CNS depression (dose related) resulting in sedation, dizziness, confusion, or ataxia which may impair physical and mental capabilities. Patients must be cautioned about performing tasks which require mental alertness (eg, operating machinery or driving). Use with caution in patients receiving other CNS depressants or psychoactive agents. Effects with other sedative drugs or ethanol may be potentiated. Benzodiazepines have been associated with falls and traumatic injury and should be used with extreme caution in patients who are at risk of these events (especially the elderly).

Use caution in patients with depression, particularly if suicidal risk may be present. Use with caution in patients with a history of drug dependence. Benzodiazepines have been associated with dependence and acute withdrawal symptoms, including seizures, on discontinuation or reduction in dose. Acute withdrawal, including seizures, may be precipitated in patients after administration of flumazenil to patients receiving long-term benzodiazepine therapy.

Benzodiazepines have been associated with anterograde amnesia. Paradoxical reactions, including hyperactive or aggressive behavior, have been reported with benzodiazepines, particularly in adolescent/pediatric or psychiatric patients. Does not have analgesic, antidepressant, or antipsychotic properties.

Adverse Reactions Reactions reported in patients with seizure and/or panic disorder. Frequency not defined.

Cardiovascular: Edema (ankle or facial), palpitation

Central nervous system: Amnesia, ataxia (seizure disorder ~30%; panic disorder 5%), behavior problems (seizure disorder ~25%), coma, confusion, depression, dizziness, drowsiness (seizure disorder ~50%), emotional lability, fatigue, fever, hallucinations, headache, hypotonia, hysteria, insomnia, intellectual ability reduced, memory disturbance, nervousness; paradoxical reactions (including aggressive behavior, agitation, anxiety, excitability, hostility, irritability, nervousness, nightmares, sleep disturbance, vivid dreams); psychosis, slurred speech, somnolence (panic disorder 37%), suicidal attempt, vertigo

Dermatologic: Hair loss, hirsutism, skin rash

Endocrine & metabolic: Dysmenorrhea, libido increased/decreased

Gastrointestinal: Abdominal pain, anorexia, appetite increased/decreased, coated tongue, constipation, dehydration, diarrhea, gastritis, gum soreness, nausea, weight changes (loss/gain), xerostomia

Genitourinary: Colpitis, dysuria, ejaculation delayed, enuresis, impotence, micturition frequency, nocturia, urinary retention, urinary tract infection

Hematologic: Anemia, eosinophilia, leukopenia, thrombocytopenia

Hepatic: Alkaline phosphatase increased (transient), hepatomegaly, transaminases increased (transient)

Neuromuscular & skeletal: Choreiform movements, coordination abnormal, dysarthria, muscle pain, muscle weakness, myalgia, tremor

Ocular: Blurred vision, eye movements abnormal, diplopia, nystagmus

Respiratory: Chest congestion, cough, bronchitis, hypersecretions, pharyngitis, respiratory depression, respiratory tract infection, rhinitis, rhinorrhea, shortness of breath, sinusitis

Miscellaneous: Allergic reaction, aphonia, dysdiadochokinesis, encopresis, "glassy-eyed" appearance, hemiparesis, lymphadenopathy

Metabolism/Transport Effects Substrate of CYP3A4 (major)

Drug Interactions

Alcohol (Ethyl): CNS Depressants may enhance the CNS depressant effect of Alcohol (Ethyl). *Risk C: Monitor therapy*

Antifungal Agents (Azole Derivatives, Systemic): May decrease the metabolism of Benzodiazepines (metabolized by oxidation). *Risk D: Consider therapy modification*

Aprepitant: May increase the serum concentration of Benzodiazepines (metabolized by oxidation). *Risk C: Monitor therapy*

Calcium Channel Blockers (Nondihydropyridine): May decrease the metabolism of Benzodiazepines (metabolized by oxidation). *Risk D: Consider therapy modification*

CarBAMazepine: May increase the metabolism of Benzodiazepines (metabolized by oxidation). *Risk C: Monitor therapy*

Cimetidine: May decrease the metabolism of Benzodiazepines (metabolized by oxidation). *Risk C: Monitor therapy*

Clozapine: Benzodiazepines may enhance the adverse/toxic effect of Clozapine. *Risk D: Consider therapy modification*

CNS Depressants: May enhance the adverse/toxic effect of other CNS Depressants. *Risk C: Monitor therapy*

CYP3A4 Inducers (Strong): May increase the metabolism of CYP3A4 Substrates. *Risk C: Monitor therapy*

CYP3A4 Inhibitors (Moderate): May decrease the metabolism of CYP3A4 Substrates. *Risk C: Monitor therapy*

CYP3A4 Inhibitors (Strong): May decrease the metabolism of CYP3A4 Substrates. *Risk D: Consider therapy modification*

Dasatinib: May increase the serum concentration of CYP3A4 Substrates. *Risk C: Monitor therapy*

Deferasirox: May decrease the serum concentration of CYP3A4 Substrates. *Risk C: Monitor therapy*

Disulfiram: May decrease the metabolism of Benzodiazepines (metabolized by oxidation). *Risk C: Monitor therapy*

Fluconazole: May decrease the metabolism of Benzodiazepines (metabolized by oxidation). *Risk D: Consider therapy modification*

Fosaprepitant: May increase the serum concentration of Benzodiazepines (metabolized by oxidation). Specifically, the active metabolite aprepitant is likely responsible for this effect. *Risk C: Monitor therapy*

Grapefruit Juice: May decrease the metabolism of Benzodiazepines (metabolized by oxidation). *Risk D: Consider therapy modification*

Isoniazid: May decrease the metabolism of Benzodiazepines (metabolized by oxidation). *Risk C: Monitor therapy*

Macrolide Antibiotics: May decrease the metabolism of Benzodiazepines (metabolized by oxidation). **Exceptions:** Azithromycin; Dirithromycin [Off Market]; Spiramycin. *Risk D: Consider therapy modification*

Nefazodone: May decrease the metabolism of Benzodiazepines (metabolized by oxidation). *Risk D: Consider therapy modification*

Oral Contraceptive (Estrogens): May decrease the metabolism of Benzodiazepines (metabolized by oxidation). *Risk C: Monitor therapy*

Oral Contraceptive (Progestins): May decrease the metabolism of Benzodiazepines (metabolized by oxidation). *Risk C: Monitor therapy*

Phenytoin: Benzodiazepines may increase the serum concentration of Phenytoin. Short-term exposure to benzodiazepines may not present as much risk as chronic therapy. *Risk C: Monitor therapy*

Protease Inhibitors: May decrease the metabolism of Benzodiazepines (metabolized by oxidation). Management: Amprenavir, atazanavir, darunavir, indinavir, nelfinavir, ritonavir, and tipranavir are contraindicated with midazolam and triazolam according to each protease inhibitor's prescribing information. *Risk D: Consider therapy modification*

Proton Pump Inhibitors: May increase the serum concentration of Benzodiazepines (metabolized by oxidation). **Exceptions:** Lansoprazole; Pantoprazole; Rabeprazole. *Risk C: Monitor therapy*

Rifamycin Derivatives: May increase the metabolism of Benzodiazepines (metabolized by oxidation). *Risk D: Consider therapy modification*

Selective Serotonin Reuptake Inhibitors: May decrease the metabolism of Benzodiazepines (metabolized by oxidation). **Exceptions:** Citalopram; Escitalopram; PARoxetine; Sertraline. *Risk C: Monitor therapy*

St Johns Wort: May increase the metabolism of Benzodiazepines (metabolized by oxidation). *Risk C: Monitor therapy*

Theophylline Derivatives: May diminish the therapeutic effect of Benzodiazepines. *Risk D: Consider therapy modification*

Ethanol/Nutrition/Herb Interactions

Ethanol: Avoid ethanol (may increase CNS depression).

Food: Clonazepam serum concentration is unlikely to be increased by grapefruit juice because of clonazepam's high oral bioavailability.

Herb/Nutraceutical: St John's wort may decrease clonazepam levels. Avoid valerian, St John's wort, kava kava, gotu kola (may increase CNS depression).

Mechanism of Action The exact mechanism is unknown, but believed to be related to its ability to enhance the activity of GABA; suppresses the spike-and-wave discharge in absence seizures by depressing nerve transmission in the motor cortex

Pharmacodynamics/Kinetics

Onset of action: 20-60 minutes

Duration: Infants and young children: 6-8 hours; Adults: ≤12 hours

Absorption: Well absorbed

Distribution: Adults: V_d: 1.5-4.4 L/kg

Protein binding: 85%

Metabolism: Extensively hepatic via glucuronide and sulfate conjugation

Half-life elimination: Children: 22-33 hours; Adults: 19-50 hours

Time to peak, serum: 1-3 hours; Steady-state: 5-7 days

Excretion: Urine (<2% as unchanged drug); metabolites excreted as glucuronide or sulfate conjugates

Dosage Oral:

Children <10 years or 30 kg: Seizure disorders:

Initial daily dose: 0.01-0.03 mg/kg/day (maximum: 0.05 mg/kg/day) given in 2-3 divided doses; increase by no more than 0.5 mg every third day until seizures are controlled or adverse effects seen

Usual maintenance dose: 0.1-0.2 mg/kg/day divided 3 times/day, not to exceed 0.2 mg/kg/day

Adults:

Burning mouth syndrome (dental use): 0.25-3 mg/day in 2 divided doses, in morning and evening

Seizure disorders:

Initial daily dose not to exceed 1.5 mg given in 3 divided doses; may increase by 0.5-1 mg every third day until seizures are controlled or adverse effects seen (maximum: 20 mg/day)

Usual maintenance dose: 0.05-0.2 mg/kg; do not exceed 20 mg/day

Panic disorder: 0.25 mg twice daily; increase in increments of 0.125-0.25 mg twice daily every 3 days; target dose: 1 mg/day (maximum: 4 mg/day)

Discontinuation of treatment: To discontinue, treatment should be withdrawn gradually. Decrease dose by 0.125 mg twice daily every 3 days until medication is completely withdrawn.

Elderly: Initiate with low doses and observe closely

Hemodialysis: Supplemental dose is not necessary

Administration Orally-disintegrating tablet: Open pouch and peel back foil on the blister; do not push tablet through foil. Use dry hands to remove tablet and place in mouth. May be swallowed with or without water. Use immediately after removing from package.

Monitoring Parameters CBC, liver function tests; observe patient for excess sedation, respiratory depression

Reference Range Relationship between serum concentration and seizure control is not well established

Timing of serum samples: Peak serum levels occur 1-3 hours after oral ingestion; the half-life is 20-40 hours; therefore, steady-state occurs in 5-7 days

Therapeutic levels: 20-80 ng/mL; Toxic concentration: >80 ng/mL

Additional Information Ethosuximide or valproic acid may be preferred for treatment of absence (petit mal) seizures. Clonazepam-induced behavioral disturbances may be more frequent in mentally handicapped patients. Abrupt discontinuation after sustained use (generally >10 days) may cause withdrawal symptoms. Flumazenil, a competitive benzodiazepine antagonist at the CNS receptor site, reverses benzodiazepine-induced CNS depression.

Dosage Forms Excipient information presented when available (limited, particularly for generics); consult specific product labeling.

Tablet: 0.5 mg, 1 mg, 2 mg

Klonopin®: 0.5 mg, 1 mg, 2 mg

Tablet, orally disintegrating: 0.125 mg, 0.25 mg, 0.5 mg, 1 mg, 2 mg

Klonopin® Wafers: 0.125 mg, 0.25 mg, 0.5 mg, 1 mg, 2 mg

CloNIDine (KLON i deen)

Medication Safety Issues

Sound-alike/look-alike issues:

CloNIDine may be confused with Clomid®, clomiPHENE, clonazePAM, clozapine, Klonopin®, quiNIDine

Catapres® may be confused with Cataflam®, Cetapred®, Combipres®

High alert medication: The Institute for Safe Medication Practices (ISMP) includes this medication (epidural administration) among its list of drug classes which have a heightened risk of causing significant patient harm when used in error.

Transdermal patch may contain conducting metal (eg, aluminum); remove patch prior to MRI.

Related Information

Addiction Treatments *on page 1817*

Clozapine-Induced Side Effects *on page 1818*

U.S. Brand Names Catapres-TTS®; Catapres®; Duraclon®

Canadian Brand Names Apo-Clonidine®; Carapres®; Dixarit®; Novo-Clonidine; Nu-Clonidine

Index Terms Clonidine Hydrochloride

Pharmacologic Category Alpha$_2$-Adrenergic Agonist

Generic Available Yes: Tablet

Use Management of mild-to-moderate hypertension; either used alone or in combination with other antihypertensives

Orphan drug: Duraclon®: For continuous epidural administration as adjunctive therapy with intraspinal opiates for treatment of cancer pain in patients tolerant to or unresponsive to intraspinal opiates

Unlabeled/Investigational Use Heroin or nicotine withdrawal; severe pain; dysmenorrhea; vasomotor symptoms associated with menopause; ethanol dependence; prophylaxis of migraines; glaucoma; diabetes-associated diarrhea; impulse control disorder, attention-deficit/hyperactivity disorder (ADHD), clozapine-induced sialorrhea

Effect on Mental Status Drowsiness is common

Effect on Psychiatric Treatment Dry mouth, orthostatic hypotension, and sedation may be increased with concurrent psychotropic use; used to treat clozapine-induced sialorrhea (unlabeled use); TCAs may antagonize clonidine's hypotensive effect

Pregnancy Risk Factor C

Pregnancy Considerations Clonidine crosses the placenta. Caution should be used with this drug due to the potential of rebound hypertension with abrupt discontinuation.

Lactation Enters breast milk/not recommended

Contraindications Hypersensitivity to clonidine hydrochloride or any component of the formulation

Warnings/Precautions Gradual withdrawal is needed (over 1 week for oral, 2-4 days with epidural) if drug needs to be stopped. Patients should be instructed about abrupt discontinuation (causes rapid increase in BP and symptoms of sympathetic overactivity). In patients on both a beta-blocker and clonidine where withdrawal of clonidine is necessary, withdraw the beta-blocker first and several days before clonidine. Then slowly decrease clonidine.

Use with caution in patients with severe coronary insufficiency; conduction disturbances; recent MI, CVA, or chronic renal insufficiency. Caution in sinus node dysfunction. Discontinue within 4 hours of surgery then restart as soon as possible after. Clonidine injection should be administered via a continuous epidural infusion device. **[U.S. Boxed Warning]: Epidural clonidine is not**

recommended for perioperative, obstetrical, or postpartum pain. It is not recommended for use in patients with severe cardiovascular disease or hemodynamic instability. In all cases, the epidural may lead to cardiovascular instability (hypotension, bradycardia). Transdermal patch may contain conducting metal (eg, aluminum); remove patch prior to MRI. Due to the potential for altered electrical conductivity, remove transdermal patch before cardioversion or defibrillation. Clonidine cause significant CNS depression and xerostomia. Caution in patients with pre-existing CNS disease or depression. Elderly may be at greater risk for CNS depressive effects, favoring other agents in this population.

Adverse Reactions Incidence of adverse events is not always reported.

>10%:

- Central nervous system: Drowsiness (35% oral, 12% transdermal), dizziness (16% oral, 2% transdermal)
- Dermatologic: Transient localized skin reactions characterized by pruritus, and erythema (15% to 50% transdermal)
- Gastrointestinal: Dry mouth (40% oral, 25% transdermal)
- Neuromuscular & skeletal: Weakness (10% transdermal)

1% to 10%:

- Cardiovascular: Orthostatic hypotension (3% oral)
- Central nervous system: Headache (1% oral, 5% transdermal), sedation (3% transdermal), fatigue (6% transdermal), lethargy (3% transdermal), insomnia (2% transdermal), nervousness (3% oral, 1% transdermal), mental depression (1% oral)
- Dermatologic: Rash (1% oral), allergic contact sensitivity (5% transdermal), localized vesiculation (7%), hyperpigmentation (5% at application site), edema (3%), excoriation (3%), burning (3%), throbbing, blanching (1%), papules (1%), and generalized macular rash (1%) has occurred in patients receiving transdermal clonidine.
- Endocrine & metabolic: Sodium and water retention, sexual dysfunction (3% oral, 2% transdermal), impotence (3% oral, 2% transdermal), weakness (10% transdermal)
- Gastrointestinal: Nausea (5% oral, 1% transdermal), vomiting (5% oral), anorexia and malaise (1% oral), constipation (10% oral, 1% transdermal), dry throat (2% transdermal), taste disturbance (1% transdermal), weight gain (1% oral)
- Genitourinary: Nocturia (1% oral)
- Hepatic: Liver function test (mild abnormalities, 1% oral)
- Miscellaneous: Withdrawal syndrome (1% oral)

<1% (Limited to important or life-threatening): Abdominal pain, agitation, alopecia, angioedema, AV block, behavioral changes, blurred vision, bradycardia, chest pain, CHF, contact dermatitis (transdermal), CVA, delirium, depression, dryness of eyes, ECG abnormalities, ethanol sensitivity increased, gynecomastia, hallucinations, hepatitis, localized hypo- or hyperpigmentation (transdermal), nightmares, orthostatic symptoms, pseudo-obstruction, rash, Raynaud's phenomenon, syncope, tachycardia, thrombocytopenia, urinary retention, urticaria, vomiting, withdrawal syndrome

Drug Interactions

- Antidepressants (Alpha2-Antagonist): May diminish the hypotensive effect of Alpha2-Agonists. *Risk D: Consider therapy modification*
- Beta-Blockers: May enhance the rebound hypertensive effect of Alpha2-Agonists. This effect can occur when the alpha$_2$-agonist is abruptly withdrawn. **Exceptions:** Levobunolol; Metipranolol. *Risk D: Consider therapy modification*
- Diazoxide: May enhance the hypotensive effect of Antihypertensives. *Risk C: Monitor therapy*
- Herbs (Hypertensive Properties): May diminish the antihypertensive effect of Antihypertensives. *Risk C: Monitor therapy*
- Herbs (Hypotensive Properties): May enhance the hypotensive effect of Antihypertensives. *Risk C: Monitor therapy*
- Methylphenidate: May enhance the adverse/toxic effect of CloNIDine. *Risk C: Monitor therapy*
- Prostacyclin Analogues: May enhance the hypotensive effect of Antihypertensives. *Risk C: Monitor therapy*
- RiTUXimab: Antihypertensives may enhance the hypotensive effect of RiTUXimab. *Risk D: Consider therapy modification*
- Tricyclic Antidepressants: May diminish the antihypertensive effect of Alpha2-Agonists. *Risk D: Consider therapy modification*

Ethanol/Nutrition/Herb Interactions

Ethanol: Avoid ethanol (may increase CNS depression).

Herb/Nutraceutical: Avoid dong quai if using for hypertension (has estrogenic activity). Avoid ephedra, yohimbe, ginseng (may worsen hypertension). Avoid valerian, St John's wort, kava kava, gotu kola (may increase CNS depression).

Mechanism of Action Stimulates alpha$_2$-adrenoceptors in the brain stem, thus activating an inhibitory neuron, resulting in reduced sympathetic outflow from the CNS, producing a decrease in peripheral resistance, renal vascular resistance, heart rate, and blood pressure; epidural clonidine may produce pain relief at spinal presynaptic and postjunctional alpha$_2$-adrenoceptors by preventing pain signal transmission; pain relief occurs only for the body regions innervated by the spinal segments where analgesic concentrations of clonidine exist

Pharmacodynamics/Kinetics

Onset of action: Oral: 0.5-1 hour; Transdermal: Initial application: 2-3 days

Duration: 6-10 hours

Distribution: V_d: Adults: 2.1 L/kg; highly lipid soluble; distributes readily into extravascular sites

Protein binding: 20% to 40%

Metabolism: Extensively hepatic to inactive metabolites; undergoes enterohepatic recirculation

Bioavailability: 75% to 95%

Half-life elimination: Adults: Normal renal function: 6-20 hours; Renal impairment: 18-41 hours

Time to peak: 2-4 hours

Excretion: Urine (65%, 32% as unchanged drug); feces (22%)

Dosage

Children:

Oral:

Hypertension: Children ≥12 years: Initial: 0.2 mg/day in 2 divided doses; increase gradually at 5- to 7-day intervals; maximum: 2.4 mg/day

Clonidine tolerance test (test of growth hormone release from pituitary): 0.15 mg/m^2 or 4 mcg/kg as single dose

ADHD (unlabeled use): Initial: 0.05 mg/day; increase every 3-7 days by 0.05 mg/day to 3-5 mcg/kg/day given in divided doses 3-4 times/day (maximum dose: 0.3-0.4 mg/day)

Epidural infusion: Pain management: Reserved for patients with severe intractable pain, unresponsive to other analgesics or epidural or spinal opiates: Initial: 0.5 mcg/kg/hour; adjust with caution, based on clinical effect

Adults:

Oral:

Acute hypertension (urgency): Initial 0.1-0.2 mg; may be followed by additional doses of 0.1 mg every hour, if necessary, to a maximum total dose of 0.6 mg.

Unlabeled route of administration: Sublingual clonidine 0.1-0.2 mg twice daily may be effective in patients unable to take oral medication

Hypertension: Initial dose: 0.1 mg twice daily (maximum recommended dose: 2.4 mg/day); usual dose range (JNC 7): 0.1-0.8 mg/day in 2 divided doses

Nicotine withdrawal symptoms: 0.1 mg twice daily to maximum of 0.4 mg/day for 3-4 weeks

Transdermal: Hypertension: Apply once every 7 days; for initial therapy start with 0.1 mg and increase by 0.1 mg at 1- to 2-week intervals (dosages >0.6 mg do not improve efficacy); usual dose range (JNC 7): 0.1-0.3 mg once weekly

Note: If transitioning from oral to transdermal therapy, overlap oral regimen for 1-2 days; transdermal route takes 2-3 days to achieve therapeutic effects.

Conversion from oral to transdermal:

Day 1: Place Catapres-TTS® 1; administer 100% of oral dose.

Day 2: Administer 50% of oral dose.

Day 3: Administer 25% of oral dose.

Day 4: Patch remains, no further oral supplement necessary.

Epidural infusion: Pain management: Starting dose: 30 mcg/hour; titrate as required for relief of pain or presence of side effects; minimal experience with doses >40 mcg/hour; should be considered an adjunct to intraspinal opiate therapy

Elderly: Initial: 0.1 mg once daily at bedtime, increase gradually as needed

Dosing adjustment in renal impairment: Cl_{cr} <10 mL/minute: Administer 50% to 75% of normal dose initially

Dialysis: Not dialyzable (0% to 5%) via hemo- or peritoneal dialysis; supplemental dose not necessary

Dietary Considerations Hypertensive patients may need to decrease sodium and calories in diet.

Administration

Oral: Do not discontinue clonidine abruptly. If needed, gradually reduce dose over 2-4 days to avoid rebound hypertension

Transdermal patch: Patches should be applied weekly at bedtime to a clean, hairless area of the upper outer arm or chest. Rotate patch sites weekly. Redness under patch may be reduced if a topical corticosteroid spray is applied to the area before placement of the patch.

Monitoring Parameters Blood pressure, standing and sitting/supine, mental status, heart rate

When used for the treatment of ADHD, thoroughly evaluate for cardiovascular risk. Monitor heart rate, blood pressure (when started and weaned), and consider obtaining ECG prior to initiation (Vetter, 2008).

Reference Range Therapeutic: 1-2 ng/mL (SI: 4.4-8.7 nmol/L)

Additional Information Transdermal clonidine should only be used in patients unable to take oral medication. The transdermal product is much more expensive than oral clonidine and produces no better therapeutic effects.

Dosage Forms Excipient information presented when available (limited, particularly for generics); consult specific product labeling.

Injection, solution, as hydrochloride [epidural; preservative free]:
- Duraclon®: 100 mcg/mL (10 mL); 500 mcg/mL (10 mL)

Tablet, as hydrochloride: 0.1 mg, 0.2 mg, 0.3 mg
- Catapres®: 0.1 mg, 0.2 mg, 0.3 mg

Transdermal system, topical [once-weekly patch]:
- Catapres-TTS®-1: 0.1 mg/24 hours (4s)
- Catapres-TTS®-2: 0.2 mg/24 hours (4s)
- Catapres-TTS®-3: 0.3 mg/24 hours (4s)

Clonidine and Chlorthalidone (KLON i deen & klor THAL i done)

Medication Safety Issues

Sound-alike/look-alike issues:
- Combipres® may be confused with Catapres®

U.S. Brand Names Clorpres®; Combipres® [DSC]

Index Terms Chlorthalidone and Clonidine

Pharmacologic Category Alpha$_2$-Adrenergic Agonist; Diuretic, Thiazide

Use Management of mild-to-moderate hypertension

Effect on Mental Status Drowsiness is common

Effect on Psychiatric Treatment Dry mouth, orthostatic hypotension, and sedation may be increased with concurrent psychotropic use; TCAs may antagonize clonidine's hypotensive effect; rare reports of blood dyscrasias; use caution with clozapine and carbamazepine; thiazides decrease lithium clearance resulting in elevated serum lithium levels and potential toxicity; monitor serum lithium levels

Dosage Summary

Oral:

Children: Dosage not established

Adults: 1 tablet 1-2 times/day (maximum: clonidine 0.6 mg; chlorthalidone 30 mg)

Dosage Forms Excipient information presented when available (limited, particularly for generics); consult specific product labeling.

Tablet:
- 0.1: Clonidine hydrochloride 0.1 mg and chlorthalidone 15 mg
- 0.2: Clonidine hydrochloride 0.2 mg and chlorthalidone 15 mg
- 0.3: Clonidine hydrochloride 0.3 mg and chlorthalidone 15 mg

◆ **Clonidine Hydrochloride** *see* CloNIDine *on page 377*

Clopidogrel (kloh PID oh grel)

Medication Safety Issues

Sound-alike/look-alike issues:
- Plavix® may be confused with Elavil®, Paxil®

U.S. Brand Names Plavix®

Canadian Brand Names Plavix®

Mexican Brand Names Plavix

Index Terms Clopidogrel Bisulfate

Pharmacologic Category Antiplatelet Agent

Generic Available No

Use Reduces rate of atherothrombotic events (myocardial infarction, stroke, vascular deaths) in patients with recent MI or stroke, or established peripheral arterial disease; reduces rate of atherothrombotic events in patients with unstable angina or non-ST-segment elevation acute coronary syndromes (unstable angina and non-ST-segment elevation MI) managed medically or through percutaneous coronary intervention (PCI) (with or without stent) or CABG; reduces rate of death and atherothrombotic events in patients with ST-segment elevation MI (STEMI) managed medically

Unlabeled/Investigational Use In aspirin-allergic patients, initial treatment of acute coronary syndromes (ACS) or prevention of coronary artery bypass graft closure (saphenous vein)

Effect on Mental Status May cause depression, dizziness, confusion, hallucinations, insomnia, or anxiety

Effect on Psychiatric Treatment GI side effects are common; concurrent use with SSRIs and/or valproic acid may produce additive effects. Flu-like syndrome may occur and present like SSRI-discontinuation symptoms. Hematologic side effects have rarely been reported; monitor with clozapine, carbamazepine, and valproate.

Pregnancy Risk Factor B

Pregnancy Considerations Teratogenic effects were not observed in animal studies. Use during pregnancy only if clearly needed.

Lactation Excretion in breast milk unknown/not recommended

Contraindications Hypersensitivity to clopidogrel or any component of the formulation; active pathological bleeding such as peptic ulcer disease (PUD) or intracranial hemorrhage; coagulation disorders

Warnings/Precautions Use with caution in patients who may be at risk of increased bleeding, including patients with PUD, trauma, or surgery. Consider discontinuing 5 days before elective surgery (except in patients with cardiac stents that have not completed their full course of dual antiplatelet therapy; patient-specific situations need to be discussed with cardiologist; AHA/ACC/SCAI/ACS/ADA Science Advisory provides recommendations). Use caution in concurrent treatment with anticoagulants (eg, heparin, warfarin) or other antiplatelet drugs; bleeding risk is increased. Use with caution in patients with severe liver or renal disease (experience is limited). Cases of thrombotic thrombocytopenic purpura (usually occurring within the first 2 weeks of therapy), resulting in some fatalities, have been reported; urgent plasmapheresis is required. Safety and efficacy have not been established in pediatric patients.

Adverse Reactions As with all drugs which may affect hemostasis, bleeding is associated with clopidogrel. Hemorrhage may occur at virtually any site. Risk is dependent on multiple variables, including the concurrent use of multiple agents which alter hemostasis and patient susceptibility.

>10%: Gastrointestinal: The overall incidence of gastrointestinal events (including abdominal pain, vomiting, dyspepsia, gastritis, and constipation) has been documented to be 27% compared to 30% in patients receiving aspirin.

3% to 10%:

- Cardiovascular: Chest pain (8%), edema (4%), hypertension (4%)
- Central nervous system: Headache (3% to 8%), dizziness (2% to 6%), depression (4%), fatigue (3%), general pain (6%)
- Dermatologic: Rash (4%), pruritus (3%)
- Endocrine & metabolic: Hypercholesterolemia (4%)
- Gastrointestinal: Abdominal pain (2% to 6%), dyspepsia (2% to 5%), diarrhea (2% to 5%), nausea (3%)
- Genitourinary: Urinary tract infection (3%)
- Hematologic: Bleeding (major 4%; minor 5%), purpura (5%), epistaxis (3%)
- Hepatic: Liver function test abnormalities (<3%; discontinued in 0.11%)
- Neuromuscular & skeletal: Arthralgia (6%), back pain (6%)
- Respiratory: Dyspnea (5%), rhinitis (4%), bronchitis (4%), cough (3%), upper respiratory infection (9%)
- Miscellaneous: Flu-like syndrome (8%)

1% to 3%:

- Cardiovascular: Atrial fibrillation, cardiac failure, palpitation, syncope
- Central nervous system: Fever, insomnia, vertigo, anxiety
- Dermatologic: Eczema
- Endocrine & metabolic: Gout, hyperuricemia
- Gastrointestinal: Constipation, GI hemorrhage, vomiting
- Genitourinary: Cystitis
- Hematologic: Hematoma, anemia

Neuromuscular & skeletal: Arthritis, leg cramps, neuralgia, paresthesia, weakness

Ocular: Cataract, conjunctivitis

<1% (Limited to important or life-threatening): Acute liver failure, agranulocytosis, allergic reaction, anaphylactoid reaction, angioedema, aplastic anemia, bilirubinemia, bronchospasm, bullous eruption, confusion, erythema multiforme, fatty liver, fever, granulocytopenia, hallucination, hematuria, hemoptysis, hemothorax, hepatitis, hypersensitivity, hypochromic anemia, interstitial pneumonitis, intracranial hemorrhage (0.4%), ischemic necrosis, leukopenia, lichen planus, maculopapular rash, menorrhagia, neutropenia (0.05%), ocular hemorrhage, pancreatitis, pancytopenia, pulmonary hemorrhage, purpura, retroperitoneal bleeding, serum sickness, Stevens-Johnson syndrome, stomatitis, taste disorder, thrombocytopenia, thrombotic thrombocytopenic purpura (TTP), toxic epidermal necrolysis, urticaria, vasculitis

Metabolism/Transport Effects **Substrate** (minor) of CYP1A2, 3A4; **Inhibits** CYP2C9 (weak)

Drug Interactions

Anticoagulants: Antiplatelet Agents may enhance the anticoagulant effect of Anticoagulants. *Risk C: Monitor therapy*

Antiplatelet Agents: May enhance the anticoagulant effect of other Antiplatelet Agents. *Risk C: Monitor therapy*

Atorvastatin: May diminish the therapeutic effect of Clopidogrel. *Risk C: Monitor therapy*

Dasatinib: May enhance the anticoagulant effect of Antiplatelet Agents. *Risk C: Monitor therapy*

Drotrecogin Alfa: Antiplatelet Agents may enhance the adverse/toxic effect of Drotrecogin Alfa. Bleeding may occur. *Risk D: Consider therapy modification*

Herbs (Anticoagulant/Antiplatelet Properties) (eg, Alfalfa, Anise, Bilberry): May enhance the adverse/toxic effect of Antiplatelet Agents. Bleeding may occur. *Risk D: Consider therapy modification*

Ibritumomab: Antiplatelet Agents may enhance the adverse/toxic effect of Ibritumomab. Both agents may contribute to impaired platelet function and an increased risk of bleeding. *Risk C: Monitor therapy*

Macrolide Antibiotics: May diminish the therapeutic effect of Clopidogrel. **Exceptions:** Azithromycin; Dirithromycin [Off Market]; Spiramycin. *Risk C: Monitor therapy*

Nonsteroidal Anti-Inflammatory Agents: May enhance the adverse/toxic effect of Antiplatelet Agents. An increased risk of bleeding may occur. *Risk C: Monitor therapy*

Omega-3-Acid Ethyl Esters: May enhance the antiplatelet effect of Antiplatelet Agents. *Risk C: Monitor therapy*

Pentosan Polysulfate Sodium: May enhance the adverse/toxic effect of Antiplatelet Agents. Specifically, the risk of bleeding may be increased by concurrent use of these agents. *Risk C: Monitor therapy*

Prostacyclin Analogues: May enhance the antiplatelet effect of Antiplatelet Agents. *Risk C: Monitor therapy*

Proton Pump Inhibitors: May diminish the therapeutic effect of Clopidogrel. This appears to be due to reduced formation of the active clopidogrel metabolite. *Risk C: Monitor therapy*

Rifamycin Derivatives: May enhance the therapeutic effect of Clopidogrel. *Risk C: Monitor therapy*

Salicylates: Antiplatelet Agents may enhance the adverse/toxic effect of Salicylates. Increased risk of bleeding may result. *Risk C: Monitor therapy*

Thrombolytic Agents: Antiplatelet Agents may enhance the anticoagulant effect of Thrombolytic Agents. *Risk C: Monitor therapy*

Tositumomab and Iodine I 131 Tositumomab: Antiplatelet Agents may enhance the adverse/toxic effect of Tositumomab and Iodine I 131 Tositumomab. Specifically, the risk of bleeding-related adverse events may be increased. *Risk C: Monitor therapy*

Warfarin: Clopidogrel may enhance the anticoagulant effect of Warfarin. *Risk D: Consider therapy modification*

Ethanol/Nutrition/Herb Interactions Herb/Nutraceutical: Avoid alfalfa, anise, bilberry, bladderwrack, bromelain, cat's claw, chamomile, coleus, cordyceps, dong quai, evening primrose oil, fenugreek, feverfew, garlic, ginger, ginkgo biloba, ginseng (American), ginseng (Panax), ginseng (Siberian), grape seed, green tea, guggul, horse chestnut seed, horseradish, licorice, prickly ash, red clover, reishi, SAMe (S-adenosylmethionine), sweet clover, turmeric, white willow (all have additional antiplatelet activity).

Stability Store at 25°C (77°F); excursions permitted to 15°C to 30°C (59°F to 86°F).

Mechanism of Action Clopidogrel requires *in vivo* biotransformation to an unidentified active metabolite. This active metabolite irreversibly blocks the

$P2Y_{12}$ component of ADP receptors on the platelet surface, which prevents activation of the GPIIb/IIIa receptor complex, thereby reducing platelet aggregation. Platelets blocked by clopidogrel are affected for the remainder of their lifespan.

Pharmacodynamics/Kinetics

Onset of action: Inhibition of platelet aggregation detected: 2 hours after 300 mg administered; after second day of treatment with 50-100 mg/day. At steady-state with 75 mg/day, the average inhibition level observed was 40% to 60%.

Peak effect: 50-100 mg/day: Bleeding time: 5-6 days; Platelet function: 3-7 days

Absorption: Well absorbed

Protein binding: Parent drug: 98%; metabolite: 94%

Metabolism: Extensively hepatic via hydrolysis; biotransformation primarily to carboxyl acid derivative (inactive). The active metabolite that inhibits platelet aggregation has not been isolated.

Half-life elimination: ~8 hours

Time to peak, serum: ~1 hour

Excretion: Urine (50%); feces (46%)

Dosage Oral: Adults:

Recent MI, recent stroke, or established arterial disease: 75 mg once daily

Acute coronary syndrome (ACS):

Unstable angina, non-ST-segment elevation myocardial infarction (UA/NSTEMI): Initial: 300 mg loading dose, followed by 75 mg once daily (in combination with aspirin 75-325 mg once daily). **Note:** A loading dose of 600 mg given at least 2 hours (or 24 hours in patients unable to take aspirin) prior to PCI followed by 75 mg once daily is recommended (*Chest* guidelines, 2008)

ST-segment elevation myocardial infarction (STEMI): 75 mg once daily (in combination with aspirin 75-162 mg/day). CLARITY used a 300 mg loading dose of clopidogrel (with thrombolysis). The duration of therapy was <28 days (usually until hospital discharge) (Sabatine, 2005).

The American College of Chest Physicians (Goodman, 2008) recommends:

Patients ≤75 years: Initial: 300 mg loading dose, followed by 75 mg once daily for up to 28 days (in combination with aspirin)

Patients >75 years: 75 mg once daily for up to 28 days (with or without thrombolysis)

Note: *Coronary artery stents:* Duration of clopidogrel (in combination with aspirin): According to the ACC/AHA/SCAI guidelines, ideally 12 months following drug-eluting stent (DES) placement in patients not at high risk for bleeding; at a minimum, 1, 3, and 6 months for bare metal (BMS), sirolimus eluting, and paclitaxel eluting stents, respectively, for uninterrupted therapy (Smith, 2005). The 2008 *Chest* guidelines recommend for patients who undergo PCI and receive a BMS (with ongoing ACS) or a DES (with or without ongoing ACS) that clopidogrel be continued for at least 12 months. In patients receiving a BMS without ongoing ACS, clopidogrel may be continued for at least 1 month. In patients receiving a DES, therapy with clopidogrel beyond 12 months may be considered in patients without bleeding or tolerability issues (Becker, 2008). Premature interruption of therapy may result in stent thrombosis with subsequent fatal and nonfatal myocardial infarction.

Prevention of coronary artery bypass graft closure (saphenous vein) [*Chest* guidelines, 2008]: Aspirin-allergic patients (unlabeled use): Loading dose: 300 mg 6 hours following procedure; maintenance: 75 mg/day

Dosing adjustment in renal impairment and elderly: None necessary

Dosing adjustment in hepatic impairment: No specific guidelines for patients with hepatic impairment; use with caution

Dietary Considerations May be taken without regard to meals.

Monitoring Parameters Signs of bleeding; hemoglobin and hematocrit periodically

Dosage Forms Excipient information presented when available (limited, particularly for generics); consult specific product labeling.

Tablet:

Plavix®: 75 mg, 300 mg

◆ **Clopidogrel Bisulfate** *see* Clopidogrel *on page 380*

Clorazepate (klor AZ e pate)

Medication Safety Issues

Sound-alike/look-alike issues:

Clorazepate may be confused with clofibrate, clonazepam

Related Information

Benzodiazepines *on page 1774*

CMS: Long-Term Care Facility Thresholds *on page 1815*

Discontinuation of Psychotropic Drugs *on page 1839*

U.S. Brand Names Tranxene® SD™; Tranxene® SD™-Half Strength; Tranxene® T-Tab®

Canadian Brand Names Apo-Clorazepate®; Novo-Clopate

Mexican Brand Names Tranxene

Index Terms Clorazepate Dipotassium; Tranxene T-Tab®

Pharmacologic Category Benzodiazepine

Generic Available Yes

Use Treatment of generalized anxiety disorder; management of ethanol withdrawal; adjunct anticonvulsant in management of partial seizures

Mental Health Comment In 2007, the FDA requested that all manufacturers of sedative-hypnotic drug products revise labeling to include a greater emphasis on the risks of adverse effects. These risks include severe allergic reactions (anaphylaxis, angioedema) and complex sleep-related behaviors, which may include sleep-driving (driving while not fully awake and with no memory of the event), making phone calls, and preparing and eating food while asleep.

There are two subtypes of GABA receptors (GABA-A and GABA-B) and three different benzodiazepine receptors (Bz_1, Bz_2, and Bz_3). Benzodiazepine receptors and effects appear to be linked to the GABA-A receptors. Benzodiazepines do not bind to GABA-B receptors. The role of GABA-B receptors is unclear. Benzodiazepines have no specificity for benzodiazepine receptor subtypes.

Clorazepate is a long half-life benzodiazepine. Duration of action after a single dose is determined by redistribution rather than metabolism. Tolerance develops to the sedative, hypnotic, and anticonvulsant effects. It does not develop to the anxiolytic or skeletal muscle relaxing effects. Psychological and physical dependence may occur with prolonged use of benzodiazepines. The onset of withdrawal symptoms is usually seen on the first day without drug and lasts 5-7 days in patients receiving short half-life benzodiazepines, whereas, the onset occurs after 5 days with a duration of 10-14 days after abrupt discontinuance of long half-life benzodiazepines. Risk factors for abuse include personal or family history of substance abuse and personality disorder.

Restrictions C-IV

Pregnancy Risk Factor D

Lactation Excretion in breast milk unknown/not recommended

Contraindications Hypersensitivity to clorazepate or any component of the formulation (cross-sensitivity with other benzodiazepines may exist); narrow-angle glaucoma; pregnancy

Warnings/Precautions Not recommended for use in patients <9 years of age or patients with depressive or psychotic disorders. Use with caution in elderly or debilitated patients, patients with hepatic disease (including alcoholics), or renal impairment. Active metabolites with extended half-lives may lead to delayed accumulation and adverse effects. Use with caution in patients with respiratory disease or impaired gag reflex. Avoid use in patients with sleep apnea.

Causes CNS depression (dose related) resulting in sedation, dizziness, confusion, or ataxia which may impair physical and mental capabilities. Patients must be cautioned about performing tasks which require mental alertness (eg, operating machinery or driving). Use with caution in patients receiving other CNS depressants or psychoactive agents. Effects with other sedative drugs or ethanol may be potentiated. Benzodiazepines have been associated with falls and traumatic injury and should be used with extreme caution in patients who are at risk of these events (especially the elderly).

Use caution in patients with depression, particularly if suicidal risk may be present. Use with caution in patients with a history of drug dependence. Benzodiazepines have been associated with dependence and acute withdrawal symptoms on discontinuation or reduction in dose. Acute withdrawal, including seizures, may be precipitated in patients after administration of flumazenil to patients receiving long-term benzodiazepine therapy.

Benzodiazepines have been associated with anterograde amnesia. Paradoxical reactions, including hyperactive or aggressive behavior, have been reported with benzodiazepines, particularly in adolescent/pediatric or psychiatric patients. Does not have analgesic, antidepressant, or antipsychotic properties.

Adverse Reactions Frequency not defined.

Cardiovascular: Hypotension

Central nervous system: Drowsiness, fatigue, ataxia, lightheadedness, memory impairment, insomnia, anxiety, headache, depression, slurred speech, confusion, nervousness, dizziness, irritability

Dermatologic: Rash

Endocrine & metabolic: Libido decreased

Gastrointestinal: Xerostomia, constipation, diarrhea, salivation decreased, nausea, vomiting, appetite increased or decreased

Neuromuscular & skeletal: Dysarthria, tremor

Ocular: Blurred vision, diplopia

Metabolism/Transport Effects Substrate of CYP3A4 (major)

Drug Interactions

Alcohol (Ethyl): CNS Depressants may enhance the CNS depressant effect of Alcohol (Ethyl). *Risk C: Monitor therapy*

Antifungal Agents (Azole Derivatives, Systemic): May decrease the metabolism of Benzodiazepines (metabolized by oxidation). *Risk D: Consider therapy modification*

Aprepitant: May increase the serum concentration of Benzodiazepines (metabolized by oxidation). *Risk C: Monitor therapy*

Calcium Channel Blockers (Nondihydropyridine): May decrease the metabolism of Benzodiazepines (metabolized by oxidation). *Risk D: Consider therapy modification*

CarBAMazepine: May increase the metabolism of Benzodiazepines (metabolized by oxidation). *Risk C: Monitor therapy*

Cimetidine: May decrease the metabolism of Benzodiazepines (metabolized by oxidation). *Risk C: Monitor therapy*

Clozapine: Benzodiazepines may enhance the adverse/toxic effect of Clozapine. *Risk D: Consider therapy modification*

CNS Depressants: May enhance the adverse/toxic effect of other CNS Depressants. *Risk C: Monitor therapy*

CYP3A4 Inducers (Strong): May increase the metabolism of CYP3A4 Substrates. *Risk C: Monitor therapy*

CYP3A4 Inhibitors (Moderate): May decrease the metabolism of CYP3A4 Substrates. *Risk C: Monitor therapy*

CYP3A4 Inhibitors (Strong): May decrease the metabolism of CYP3A4 Substrates. *Risk D: Consider therapy modification*

Dasatinib: May increase the serum concentration of CYP3A4 Substrates. *Risk C: Monitor therapy*

Deferasirox: May decrease the serum concentration of CYP3A4 Substrates. *Risk C: Monitor therapy*

Disulfiram: May decrease the metabolism of Benzodiazepines (metabolized by oxidation). *Risk C: Monitor therapy*

Fluconazole: May decrease the metabolism of Benzodiazepines (metabolized by oxidation). *Risk D: Consider therapy modification*

Fosaprepitant: May increase the serum concentration of Benzodiazepines (metabolized by oxidation). Specifically, the active metabolite aprepitant is likely responsible for this effect. *Risk C: Monitor therapy*

Grapefruit Juice: May decrease the metabolism of Benzodiazepines (metabolized by oxidation). *Risk D: Consider therapy modification*

Isoniazid: May decrease the metabolism of Benzodiazepines (metabolized by oxidation). *Risk C: Monitor therapy*

Macrolide Antibiotics: May decrease the metabolism of Benzodiazepines (metabolized by oxidation). **Exceptions:** Azithromycin; Dirithromycin [Off Market]; Spiramycin. *Risk D: Consider therapy modification*

Nefazodone: May decrease the metabolism of Benzodiazepines (metabolized by oxidation). *Risk D: Consider therapy modification*

Oral Contraceptive (Estrogens): May decrease the metabolism of Benzodiazepines (metabolized by oxidation). *Risk C: Monitor therapy*

Oral Contraceptive (Progestins): May decrease the metabolism of Benzodiazepines (metabolized by oxidation). *Risk C: Monitor therapy*

Phenytoin: Benzodiazepines may increase the serum concentration of Phenytoin. Short-term exposure to benzodiazepines may not present as much risk as chronic therapy. *Risk C: Monitor therapy*

Protease Inhibitors: May decrease the metabolism of Benzodiazepines (metabolized by oxidation). Management: Amprenavir, atazanavir, darunavir, indinavir, nelfinavir, ritonavir, and tipranavir are contraindicated with midazolam and triazolam according to each protease inhibitor's prescribing information. *Risk D: Consider therapy modification*

Proton Pump Inhibitors: May increase the serum concentration of Benzodiazepines (metabolized by oxidation). **Exceptions:** Lansoprazole; Pantoprazole; Rabeprazole. *Risk C: Monitor therapy*

Rifamycin Derivatives: May increase the metabolism of Benzodiazepines (metabolized by oxidation). *Risk D: Consider therapy modification*

Selective Serotonin Reuptake Inhibitors: May decrease the metabolism of Benzodiazepines (metabolized by oxidation). **Exceptions:** Citalopram; Escitalopram; PARoxetine; Sertraline. *Risk C: Monitor therapy*

St Johns Wort: May increase the metabolism of Benzodiazepines (metabolized by oxidation). *Risk C: Monitor therapy*

Theophylline Derivatives: May diminish the therapeutic effect of Benzodiazepines. *Risk D: Consider therapy modification*

Ethanol/Nutrition/Herb Interactions

Ethanol: Avoid ethanol (may increase CNS depression).

Food: Serum concentrations/toxicity may be increased by grapefruit juice.

Herb/Nutraceutical: Avoid valerian, St John's wort, kava kava, gotu kola (may increase CNS depression).

Mechanism of Action Binds to stereospecific benzodiazepine receptors on the postsynaptic GABA neuron at several sites within the central nervous system, including the limbic system, reticular formation. Enhancement of the inhibitory effect of GABA on neuronal excitability results by increased neuronal membrane permeability to chloride ions. This shift in chloride ions results in hyperpolarization (a less excitable state) and stabilization.

Pharmacodynamics/Kinetics

Onset of action: 1-2 hours

Duration: Variable, 8-24 hours

Distribution: Crosses placenta; appears in urine

Metabolism: Rapidly decarboxylated to desmethyldiazepam (active) in acidic stomach prior to absorption; hepatically to oxazepam (active)

Half-life elimination: Adults: Desmethyldiazepam: 48-96 hours; Oxazepam: 6-8 hours

Time to peak, serum: ~1 hour

Excretion: Primarily urine

Dosage Oral:

Children 9-12 years: Anticonvulsant: Initial: 3.75-7.5 mg/dose twice daily; increase dose by 3.75 mg at weekly intervals, not to exceed 60 mg/day in 2-3 divided doses

Children >12 years and Adults: Anticonvulsant: Initial: Up to 7.5 mg/dose 2-3 times/day; increase dose by 7.5 mg at weekly intervals, not to exceed 90 mg/day

Adults:

Anxiety:

Regular release tablets (Tranxene® T-Tab®): 7.5-15 mg 2-4 times/day

Sustained release (Tranxene® SD™): 11.25 or 22.5 mg once daily at bedtime

Ethanol withdrawal: Initial: 30 mg, then 15 mg 2-4 times/day on first day; maximum daily dose: 90 mg; gradually decrease dose over subsequent days

Monitoring Parameters Respiratory and cardiovascular status, excess CNS depression

Reference Range Therapeutic: 0.12-1 mcg/mL (SI: 0.36-3.01 μmol/L)

Test Interactions Decreased hematocrit; abnormal liver and renal function tests

Additional Information Abrupt discontinuation after sustained use (generally >10 days) may cause withdrawal symptoms.

Dosage Forms Excipient information presented when available (limited, particularly for generics); consult specific product labeling.

Tablet, as dipotassium: 3.75 mg, 7.5 mg, 15 mg

Tranxene® SD™: 22.5 mg [once daily]

Tranxene® SD™-Half Strength: 11.25 mg [once daily]

Tranxene® T-Tab®: 3.75 mg, 7.5 mg, 15 mg

◆ **Clorazepate Dipotassium** *see* Clorazepate *on page 384*

◆ **Clorpres®** *see* Clonidine and Chlorthalidone *on page 380*

Clozapine (KLOE za peen)

Medication Safety Issues

Sound-alike/look-alike issues:

Clozapine may be confused with clofazimine, clonidine, Klonopin®

Clozaril® may be confused with Clinoril®, Colazal®

Related Information

Anticholinergic Effects of Common Psychotropics *on page 1758*
Antipsychotic Agents *on page 1769*
Antipsychotic Receptor Profile *on page 1772*
Atypical Antipsychotics *on page 1773*
Clozapine-Induced Side Effects *on page 1818*
CMS: Long-Term Care Facility Thresholds *on page 1815*
Discontinuation of Psychotropic Drugs *on page 1839*

U.S. Brand Names Clozaril®; FazaClo®

Canadian Brand Names Apo-Clozapine®; Clozaril®; Gen-Clozapine

Mexican Brand Names Clopsine; Leponex

Pharmacologic Category Antipsychotic Agent, Atypical

Generic Available Yes

Use Treatment-refractory schizophrenia; to reduce risk of recurrent suicidal behavior in schizophrenia or schizoaffective disorder

Unlabeled/Investigational Use Schizoaffective disorder, bipolar disorder, childhood psychosis, severe obsessive-compulsive disorder; psychosis/agitation related to Alzheimer's dementia

Mental Health Comment Clozapine is the prototype drug from the antipsychotic class often referred to as atypical. It should be noted that the definition of the term "atypical" is not universally agreed upon. Some prefer to describe antipsychotics based on their pharmacological properties. A common feature of all definitions used to describe "atypical" antipsychotics is the lack of significant acute or subacute EPS, at dosages generally associated with antipsychotic actions. Other experts have included definitions of atypicality that include a) failure to increase serum prolactin levels; b) superior efficacy for positive, negative, and cognitive symptoms; and c) lack of evidence of tardive dyskinesia or dystonia following chronic administration. Clozapine meets all of these criteria and therefore is considered the standard by which other atypical antipsychotics should be compared.

Recently, questions have been raised about its ability (as well as other atypical antipsychotics) to differentiate itself on negative symptom improvement. However, clozapine is considered the drug of choice for treating refractory schizophrenia. Refractory illness is often defined by "Kane" criteria in which patients have failed to respond to at least two antipsychotics from different chemical classes at 1000 mg of chlorpromazine or its equivalent (Kane, 1988).

In a recent trial, clozapine therapy demonstrated superiority over olanzapine therapy in preventing suicide attempts in patients with schizophrenia and schizoaffective disorder at high risk for suicide (Meltzer, 2003). The authors concluded that the use of clozapine for 2 years in this population should lead to a significant reduction in suicidal behavior.

Tardive dyskinesia (TD) secondary to **typical** antipsychotics has an estimated incidence of 3% to 5% per year for the first 5 years of treatment. The incidence of TD associated with the atypical antipsychotics is estimated to be 0.5% to 1%. It is not clear if this estimate represents a risk associated with mental illness or to what extent drug therapy can be implicated. Clozapine appears less likely to cause tardive dyskinesia than typical antipsychotics (fluphenazine, haloperidol), but is generally associated with more weight gain and metabolic abnormalities such as diabetes.

Dose-dependent side effects associated with clozapine include seizures, tachycardia, and sedation.

Coadministration of two or more antipsychotics does not generally improve clinical response and may increase the potential for adverse effects.

In 2008, the FDA issued a warning regarding increased mortality risk with typical **and** atypical antipsychotic drugs when used in elderly patients with dementia-related psychosis.

Kane J, Honigfeld G, Singer J, et al, "Clozapine for the Treatment-Resistant Schizophrenic. A Double-Blind Comparison With Chlorpromazine," *Arch Gen Psychiatry*, 1988, 45(9):789-96.

Meltzer HY, Alphs L, Green AI, et al, "Clozapine Treatment for Suicidality in Schizophrenia: International Suicide Prevention Trial (InterSePT)," *Arch Gen Psychiatry*, 2003, 60(1):82-91.

Restrictions Patient-specific registration is required to dispense clozapine. Monitoring systems for individual clozapine manufacturers are independent. If a patient is switched from one brand/manufacturer of clozapine to another, the patient must be entered into a new registry (must be completed by the prescriber and delivered to the dispensing pharmacy). Healthcare providers, including pharmacists dispensing clozapine, should verify the patient's hematological status and qualification to receive clozapine with all existing registries. The manufacturer of Clozaril® requests that healthcare providers submit all WBC/ANC values following discontinuation of therapy to the Clozaril National Registry for all nonrechallengable patients until WBC is ≥3500/mm^3 and ANC is ≥2000/mm^3.

Pregnancy Risk Factor B

Pregnancy Considerations Teratogenic effects were not seen in animal studies; however, there are no adequate and well-controlled studies in pregnant women. Use during pregnancy only if clearly needed.

Lactation Enters breast milk/not recommended (AAP rates "of concern")

Contraindications Hypersensitivity to clozapine or any component of the formulation; history of agranulocytosis or granulocytopenia with clozapine; uncontrolled epilepsy, severe central nervous system depression or comatose state; paralytic ileus; myeloproliferative disorders or use with other agents which have a well-known risk of agranulocytosis or bone marrow suppression

Warnings/Precautions [U.S. Boxed Warning]: Elderly patients with dementia-related psychosis treated with atypical antipsychotics are at an increased risk of death compared to placebo. An increased incidence of cerebrovascular adverse events (including fatalities) has been reported in elderly patients with dementia-related psychosis. Clozapine is not approved for this indication.

[U.S. Boxed Warning]: Significant risk of agranulocytosis, potentially life-threatening. Therapy should not be initiated in patients with WBC <3500 cells/mm^3 or ANC <2000 cells/mm^3 or history of myeloproliferative disorder. WBC testing should occur periodically on an on-going basis (see prescribing information for monitoring details) to ensure that acceptable WBC/ANC counts are maintained. Initial episodes of moderate leukopenia or granulopoietic suppression confer up to a 12-fold increased risk for subsequent episodes of agranulocytosis. WBCs must be monitored weekly for at least 4 weeks after therapy discontinuation or until WBC is ≥3500/mm^3 and ANC is ≥2000/mm^3. Use with caution in patients receiving other marrow suppressive agents. Eosinophilia has been reported to occur with clozapine and may require temporary or permanent interruption of therapy. Due to the significant risk of agranulocytosis, it is strongly recommended that a patient must fail at least two trials of other primary medications for the treatment of schizophrenia (of adequate dose and duration) before initiating therapy with clozapine.

Cognitive and/or motor impairment (sedation) is common with clozapine, resulting in impaired performance of tasks requiring alertness (eg, operating machinery or driving); use caution in patients receiving general anesthesia. **[U.S. Boxed Warning]: Seizures have been associated with clozapine use in a dose-dependent manner;** use with caution in patients at risk of seizures, including those with a history of seizures, head trauma, brain damage, alcoholism, or concurrent therapy with medications which may lower seizure threshold. Has been associated with benign, self-limiting fever (<100.4°F, usually within first 3 weeks). However, clozapine may also be associated with severe febrile reactions, including neuroleptic malignant syndrome (NMS). Clozapine's potential for extrapyramidal symptoms (including tardive dyskinesia) appears to be extremely low. Risk of dystonia (and probably other EPS) may be greater with increased doses, use of conventional antipsychotics, males, and younger patients.

Deep vein thrombosis, myocarditis, pericarditis, pericardial effusion, cardiomyopathy, and HF have also been associated with clozapine. **[U.S. Boxed Warning]: Fatalities due to myocarditis have been reported; highest risk in the first month of therapy, however, later cases also reported.** Myocarditis or cardiomyopathy should be considered in patients who present with signs/symptoms of heart failure (dyspnea, fatigue, orthopnea, paroxysmal nocturnal dyspnea, peripheral edema), chest pain, palpitations, new electrocardiographic abnormalities (arrhythmias, ST-T wave abnormalities), or unexplained fever. Patients with tachycardia during the first month of therapy should be closely monitored for other signs of myocarditis. Discontinue clozapine if myocarditis is suspected; do not rechallenge in patients with clozapine-related myocarditis. The reported rate of myocarditis in clozapine-treated patients appears to be 17-322 times greater than in the general population. Clozapine should be discontinued in patients with confirmed cardiomyopathy unless benefit clearly outweighs risk. Rare cases of thromboembolism, including pulmonary embolism and stroke resulting in fatalities, have been associated with clozapine.

May cause anticholinergic effects; use with caution in patients with urinary retention, benign prostatic hyperplasia, narrow-angle glaucoma, xerostomia, visual problems, constipation, or history of bowel obstruction. May cause hyperglycemia; in some cases may be extreme and associated with ketoacidosis, hyperosmolar coma, or death. Use with caution in patients with diabetes or other disorders of glucose regulation; monitor for worsening of glucose control. Use with caution in patients with hepatic disease or impairment; hepatitis has been reported as a consequence of therapy.

Use caution with cardiovascular or renal disease. **[U.S. Boxed Warning]: May cause orthostatic hypotension (with or without syncope)** and tachycardia; use with caution in patients at risk of hypotension or in patients where transient hypotensive episodes would be poorly tolerated (cardiovascular disease or cerebrovascular disease). Concurrent use with benzodiazepines may increase the risk of severe cardiopulmonary reactions.

The possibility of a suicide attempt is inherent in psychotic illness or bipolar disorder; use caution in high-risk patients during initiation of therapy. Prescriptions should be written for the smallest quantity consistent with good patient care.

Medication should not be stopped abruptly; taper off over 1-2 weeks. If conditions warrant abrupt discontinuation (leukopenia, myocarditis, cardiomyopathy), monitor patient for psychosis and cholinergic rebound (headache, nausea, vomiting, diarrhea). Significant weight gain has been observed with antipsychotic therapy; incidence varies with product. Monitor waist circumference and BMI. Elderly patients are more susceptible to adverse effects (including agranulocytosis, cardiovascular, anticholinergic, and tardive dyskinesia). Safety and efficacy have not been established in children.

Adverse Reactions

>10%:

Cardiovascular: Tachycardia (25%)

Central nervous system: Drowsiness (39% to 46%), dizziness (19% to 27%), insomnia (2% to 20%)

Gastrointestinal: Constipation (14% to 25%), weight gain (4% to 31%), sialorrhea (31% to 48%), nausea/vomiting (3% to 17%)

1% to 10%:

Cardiovascular: Angina (1%), ECG changes (1%), hypertension (4%), hypotension (9%), syncope (6%)

Central nervous system: Akathisia (3%), seizure (3%), headache (7%), nightmares (4%), akinesia (4%), confusion (3%), myoclonic jerks (1%), restlessness (4%), agitation (4%), lethargy (1%), ataxia (1%), slurred speech (1%), depression (1%), anxiety (1%)

Dermatologic: Rash (2%)

Gastrointestinal: Abdominal discomfort/heartburn (4% to 14%), anorexia (1%), diarrhea (2%), xerostomia (6%), throat discomfort (1%)

Genitourinary: Urinary abnormalities (eg, abnormal ejaculation, retention, urgency, incontinence; 1% to 2%)

Hematologic: Eosinophilia (1%), leukopenia, leukocytosis, agranulocytosis (1%)

Hepatic: Liver function tests abnormal (1%)

Neuromuscular & skeletal: Tremor (6%), hypokinesia (4%), rigidity (3%), hyperkinesia (1%), weakness (1%), pain (1%), spasm (1%)

Ocular: Visual disturbances (5%)

Respiratory: Dyspnea (1%), nasal congestion (1%)

Miscellaneous: Diaphoresis increased, fever, tongue numbness (1%)

<1%, postmarketing, and/or case reports (limited to important or life-threatening): Amentia, amnesia, anemia, arrhythmia (atrial or ventricular), aspiration, blurred vision, bradycardia, bronchitis, cardiomyopathy (usually dilated), cataplexy, CHF, cholestasis, cyanosis, delusions, diabetes mellitus, difficult urination, edema, erythema multiforme, ESR increased, fecal impaction, gastroenteritis, granulocytopenia, hallucinations, hematemesis, hepatitis, hypercholesterolemia (rare), hyperglycemia, hypertriglyceridemia (rare), hyponatremia, hypothermia, impotence, interstitial nephritis (acute), intestinal obstruction, jaundice, loss of speech, MI, myasthenia syndrome, myocarditis, narrow-angle glaucoma, neuroleptic malignant syndrome, palpitations, pancreatitis (acute), paralytic ileus, Parkinsonism, pericardial effusion, pericarditis, phlebitis, pleural effusion, pneumonia, priapism, pulmonary embolism, rhabdomyolysis, rectal bleeding, salivary gland swelling, sepsis, status epilepticus, stroke, Stevens-Johnson syndrome, tardive dyskinesia, thrombocytopenia, thrombocytosis, thromboembolism, thrombophlebitis, vasculitis, wheezing

Metabolism/Transport Effects **Substrate** of CYP1A2 (major), 2A6 (minor), 2C9 (minor), 2C19 (minor), 2D6 (minor), 3A4 (minor); **Inhibits** CYP1A2 (weak), 2C9 (weak), 2C19 (weak), 2D6 (moderate), 2E1 (weak), 3A4 (weak)

Drug Interactions

Acetylcholinesterase Inhibitors (Central): May enhance the neurotoxic (central) effect of Antipsychotics. Severe extrapyramidal symptoms have occurred in some patients. *Risk C: Monitor therapy*

Alcohol (Ethyl): CNS Depressants may enhance the CNS depressant effect of Alcohol (Ethyl). *Risk C: Monitor therapy*

Amphetamines: Antipsychotics may diminish the stimulatory effect of Amphetamines. *Risk C: Monitor therapy*

Anticholinergics: May enhance the adverse/toxic effect of other Anticholinergics. **Exceptions:** Paliperidone. *Risk C: Monitor therapy*

Anti-Parkinson's Agents (Dopamine Agonist): Antipsychotics (Atypical) may diminish the therapeutic effect of Anti-Parkinson's Agents (Dopamine Agonist). *Risk D: Consider therapy modification*

Benzodiazepines: May enhance the adverse/toxic effect of Clozapine. *Risk D: Consider therapy modification*

CarBAMazepine: May increase the metabolism of Clozapine. *Risk D: Consider therapy modification*

Cimetidine: May decrease the metabolism of Clozapine. *Risk D: Consider therapy modification*

CNS Depressants: May enhance the adverse/toxic effect of other CNS Depressants. *Risk C: Monitor therapy*

Codeine: CYP2D6 Inhibitors (Moderate) may diminish the therapeutic effect of Codeine. These CYP2D6 inhibitors may prevent the metabolic conversion of codeine to its active metabolite morphine. *Risk C: Monitor therapy*

CYP1A2 Inducers (Strong): May increase the metabolism of CYP1A2 Substrates. *Risk C: Monitor therapy*

CYP1A2 Inhibitors (Moderate): May decrease the metabolism of CYP1A2 Substrates. *Risk C: Monitor therapy*

CYP1A2 Inhibitors (Strong): May decrease the metabolism of CYP1A2 Substrates. *Risk D: Consider therapy modification*

CYP2D6 Substrates: CYP2D6 Inhibitors (Moderate) may decrease the metabolism of CYP2D6 Substrates. **Exceptions:** Tamoxifen. *Risk C: Monitor therapy*

Lithium formulations: May enhance the neurotoxic effect of Antipsychotics. Lithium formulations may decrease the serum concentration of Antipsychotics. Specifically noted with chlorpromazine. *Risk C: Monitor therapy*

Macrolide Antibiotics: May decrease the metabolism of Clozapine. **Exceptions:** Azithromycin; Dirithromycin [Off Market]; Spiramycin. *Risk D: Consider therapy modification*

Nebivolol: CYP2D6 Inhibitors (Moderate) may increase the serum concentration of Nebivolol. *Risk C: Monitor therapy*

Nefazodone: May decrease the metabolism of Clozapine. *Risk C: Monitor therapy*

Omeprazole: May decrease the serum concentration of Clozapine. Omeprazole may increase the serum concentration of Clozapine. *Risk C: Monitor therapy*

Phenytoin: May increase the metabolism of Clozapine. *Risk C: Monitor therapy*

Pramlintide: May enhance the anticholinergic effect of Anticholinergics. These effects are specific to the GI tract. *Risk D: Consider therapy modification*

Selective Serotonin Reuptake Inhibitors: May decrease the metabolism of Clozapine. *Risk D: Consider therapy modification*

Tamoxifen: CYP2D6 Inhibitors (Moderate) may decrease the metabolism of Tamoxifen. Specifically, CYP2D6 inhibitors may decrease the formation of highly potent active metabolites. *Risk D: Consider therapy modification*

Tetrabenazine: May enhance the adverse/toxic effect of Antipsychotics. *Risk C: Monitor therapy*

Thioridazine: CYP2D6 Inhibitors may decrease the metabolism of Thioridazine. *Risk X: Avoid combination*

TraMADol: CYP2D6 Inhibitors (Moderate) may diminish the therapeutic effect of TraMADol. These CYP2D6 inhibitors may prevent the metabolic conversion of tramadol to its active metabolite that accounts for much of its opioid-like effects. *Risk C: Monitor therapy*

Ethanol/Nutrition/Herb Interactions

Ethanol: Avoid ethanol (may increase CNS depression).

Herb/Nutraceutical: St John's wort may decrease clozapine levels. Avoid kava kava, gotu kola, valerian, St John's wort (may increase CNS depression).

Stability Dispensed in "clozapine patient system" packaging. Store at controlled room temperature. FazaClo™: Protect from moisture; do not remove from package until ready to use.

Mechanism of Action Clozapine (dibenzodiazepine antipsychotic) exhibits weak antagonism of D_1, D_2, D_3, and D_5 dopamine receptor subtypes, but shows high affinity for D_4; in addition, it blocks the serotonin ($5HT_2$), alpha-adrenergic, histamine H_1, and cholinergic receptors

Pharmacodynamics/Kinetics

Protein binding: 97% to serum proteins

Metabolism: Extensively hepatic; forms metabolites with limited or no activity

Bioavailability: 12% to 81% (not affected by food)

Half-life elimination: Steady state: 12 hours (range: 4-66 hours)

Time to peak: 2.5 hours (range: 1-6 hours)

Excretion: Urine (~50%) and feces (30%) with trace amounts of unchanged drug

Dosage Oral:

Children and Adolescents: Childhood psychosis (unlabeled use): Initial: 25 mg/day; increase to a target dose of 25-400 mg/day

Adults:

Schizophrenia: Initial: 12.5 mg once or twice daily; increased, as tolerated, in increments of 25-50 mg/day to a target dose of 300-450 mg/day after 2-4 weeks; may require doses as high as 600-900 mg/day

Reduce risk of suicidal behavior: Initial: 12.5 mg once or twice daily; increased, as tolerated, in increments of 25-50 mg/day to a target dose of 300-450 mg/day after 2-4 weeks; median dose is ~300 mg/day (range: 12.5-900 mg)

Elderly:

Schizophrenia: Dose selection and titration should be cautious

Psychosis/agitation related to Alzheimer's dementia (unlabeled use): Initial: 12.5 mg/day; if necessary, gradually increase as tolerated not to exceed 75-100 mg/day

Termination of therapy: If dosing is interrupted for ≥48 hours, therapy must be reinitiated at 12.5-25 mg/day; may be increased more rapidly than with initial titration, unless cardiopulmonary arrest occurred during initial titration.

In the event of planned termination of clozapine, gradual reduction in dose over a 1- to 2-week period is recommended. If conditions warrant abrupt discontinuation (leukopenia), monitor patient for psychosis and cholinergic rebound (headache, nausea, vomiting, diarrhea).

Patients discontinued on clozapine therapy due to WBC <2000/mm^3 or ANC <1000/mm^3 should not be restarted on clozapine.

Dosage adjustment for toxicity:

Moderate leukopenia or granulocytopenia (WBC <3000/mm^3 and/or ANC <1500/mm^3): Discontinue therapy; may rechallenge patient when WBC is >3500/mm^3 and ANC is >2000/mm^3. **Note:** Patient is at greater risk for developing agranulocytosis.

Severe leukopenia or granulocytopenia (WBC <2000/mm^3 and/or ANC <1000/mm^3): Discontinue therapy and do not rechallenge patient.

Child/Adolescent Considerations Eleven adolescents with childhood-onset schizophrenia who failed a 6-week trial of haloperidol were treated with clozapine (mean 6-week daily dose: 370 mg) (Frazier, 1994). Twenty-one patients (mean age: 14 ± 2.3 years) with schizophrenia (DSM-III-R) who had been nonresponsive to typical antipsychotics received clozapine 176 ± 149 mg/day (final dose) (Kumra, 1996). Clozapine was evaluated in 11 neuroleptic-resistant children (<13 years of age) mean dosage: 227 mg/day (Turetz, 1997). A 15-year old boy with severe treatment-refractory bipolar disorder type I was treated successfully with clozapine 300 mg/day (Masi, 1998).

Frazier JA, Gordon CT, McKenna K, et al, "An Open Trial of Clozapine in 11 Adolescents With Childhood-Onset Schizophrenia," *J Am Acad Child Adolesc Psychiatry*, 1994, 33(5):658-63.

Kumra S, Frazier JA, Jacobsen LK, et al, "Childhood-Onset Schizophrenia. A Double-Blind Clozapine-Haloperidol Comparison," *Arch Gen Psychiatry*, 1996, 53(12):1090-7.

Kumra S, Oberstar JV, Sikich L, et al, "Efficacy and Tolerability of Second-Generation Antipsychotics in Children and Adolescents With Schizophrenia," *Schizophr Bull*, 2008, 34(1):60-71.

Masi G and Milone A, "Clozapine Treatment in an Adolescent With Bipolar Disorder," *Panminerva Med*, 1998, 40(3):254-7.

Turetz M, Mozes T, Toren P, et al, "An Open Trial of Clozapine in Neuroleptic-Resistant Childhood-Onset Schizophrenia," *Br J Psychiatry*, 1997, 170:507-10.

Dietary Considerations May be taken without regard to food. Fazaclo™ contains phenylalanine 0.87 mg per 12.5 mg tablet, phenylalanine 1.74 mg per 25 mg tablet, and phenylalanine 6.96 mg per 100 mg tablet.

Administration Orally-disintegrating tablet: Should be removed from foil blister by peeling apart (do not push tablet through the foil). Remove immediately prior to use. Place tablet in mouth and allow to dissolve; swallow with saliva. If dosing requires splitting tablet, throw unused portion away.

Monitoring Parameters Mental status, ECG, WBC (see below), vital signs, fasting lipid profile and fasting blood glucose/Hgb A_{1c} (prior to treatment, at 3 months, then annually; BMI, personal/family history of obesity; waist circumference (weight should be assessed prior to treatment, at 4 weeks, 8 weeks, 12 weeks, and then at quarterly intervals. Consider titrating to a different antipsychotic agent for a weight gain ≥5% of the initial weight); blood pressure; abnormal involuntary movement scale (AIMS).

WBC and ANC should be obtained at baseline and at least weekly for the first 6 months of continuous treatment. If counts remain acceptable (WBC ≥3500/mm^3, ANC ≥2000/mm^3) during this time period, then they may be monitored every other week for the next 6 months. If WBC/ANC continue to remain within these acceptable limits after the second 6 months of therapy, monitoring can be decreased to every 4 weeks. (**Note**: The decrease in monitoring to every 4 weeks is applicable in the United States. Blood monitoring requirements related to the use of clozapine have not changed in Canada). If clozapine is discontinued, a weekly WBC should be conducted for an additional 4 weeks or until WBC is ≥3500/mm^3 and ANC is ≥2000/mm^3. If clozapine therapy is interrupted due to moderate leukopenia, weekly WBC/ANC monitoring is required for 12 months in patients restarted on clozapine treatment. If therapy is interrupted for reasons other than leukopenia/granulocytopenia, the 6-month time period for initiation of biweekly WBCs may need to be reset. This determination depends upon the treatment duration, the length of the break in therapy, and whether or not an abnormal blood event occurred.

Consult full prescribing information for determination of appropriate WBC/ANC monitoring interval (http://www.clozaril.com/index.jsp).

Dosage Forms Excipient information presented when available (limited, particularly for generics); consult specific product labeling.

Tablet: 25 mg, 50 mg, 100 mg, 200 mg

Clozaril®: 25 mg [scored], 100 mg [scored]

Tablet, orally disintegrating:

FazaClo®: 12.5 mg [contains phenylalanine 0.87 mg/tablet; mint flavor], 25 mg [contains phenylalanine 1.74 mg/tablet; mint flavor], 100 mg [contains phenylalanine 6.96 mg/tablet; mint flavor]

- **Clozaril®** *see* Clozapine *on page 386*
- **CMA-676** *see* Gemtuzumab Ozogamicin *on page 713*
- **CNJ-016™** *see* Vaccinia Immune Globulin (Intravenous) *on page 1639*

Cocaine (koe KANE)

Related Information

Hallucinogenic Drugs *on page 1783*

Index Terms Cocaine Hydrochloride

Pharmacologic Category Local Anesthetic

Generic Available Yes

Use Topical anesthesia for mucous membranes

Effect on Mental Status CNS stimulation is common; may cause exacerbation of psychosis, nervousness, euphoria, restlessness, hallucinations, paranoia

Effect on Psychiatric Treatment Concurrent use with MAO inhibitors may result in hypertensive crisis

Restrictions C-II

Pregnancy Risk Factor C/X (nonmedicinal use)

Lactation Enters breast milk/contraindicated

Contraindications Hypersensitivity to cocaine or any component of the topical solution; ophthalmologic anesthesia (causing sloughing of the corneal epithelium); pregnancy (nonmedicinal use)

Warnings/Precautions For topical use only. Limit to office and surgical procedures only. Resuscitative equipment and drugs should be immediately available when any local anesthetic is used. Debilitated, elderly patients, acutely ill patients, and children should be given reduced doses consistent with their age and physical status. Use caution in patients with severely traumatized mucosa and sepsis in the region of the proposed application. Use with caution in patients with cardiovascular disease or a history of cocaine abuse. In patients being treated for cardiovascular complication of cocaine abuse, avoid beta-blockers for treatment.

Adverse Reactions

>10%:

Central nervous system: CNS stimulation

Gastrointestinal: Loss of taste perception

Respiratory: Rhinitis, nasal congestion
Miscellaneous: Loss of smell

1% to 10%:

Cardiovascular: Heart rate (decreased) with low doses, tachycardia with moderate doses, hypertension, cardiomyopathy, cardiac arrhythmia, myocarditis, QRS prolongation, Raynaud's phenomenon, cerebral vasculitis, thrombosis, fibrillation (atrial), flutter (atrial), sinus bradycardia, CHF, pulmonary hypertension, sinus tachycardia, tachycardia (supraventricular), arrhythmia (ventricular), vasoconstriction

Central nervous system: Fever, nervousness, restlessness, euphoria, excitation, headache, psychosis, hallucinations, agitation, seizure, slurred speech, hyperthermia, dystonic reactions, cerebral vascular accident, vasculitis, clonic-tonic reactions, paranoia, sympathetic storm

Dermatologic: Skin infarction, pruritus, madarosis

Gastrointestinal: Nausea, anorexia, colonic ischemia, spontaneous bowel perforation

Genitourinary: Priapism, uterine rupture

Hematologic: Thrombocytopenia

Neuromuscular & skeletal: Chorea (extrapyramidal), paresthesia, tremor, fasciculations

Ocular: Mydriasis (peak effect at 45 minutes; may last up to 12 hours), sloughing of the corneal epithelium, ulceration of the cornea, iritis, chemosis

Renal: Myoglobinuria, necrotizing vasculitis

Respiratory: Tachypnea, nasal mucosa damage (when snorting), hyposmia, bronchiolitis obliterans organizing pneumonia

Miscellaneous: "Washed-out" syndrome

Metabolism/Transport Effects **Substrate** of CYP3A4 (major); **Inhibits** CYP2D6 (strong), 3A4 (weak)

Drug Interactions

Cannabinoids: Cocaine may enhance the tachycardic effect of Cannabinoids. *Risk C: Monitor therapy*

Codeine: CYP2D6 Inhibitors (Strong) may diminish the therapeutic effect of Codeine. These CYP2D6 inhibitors may prevent the metabolic conversion of codeine to its active metabolite morphine. *Risk D: Consider therapy modification*

CYP2D6 Substrates: CYP2D6 Inhibitors (Strong) may decrease the metabolism of CYP2D6 Substrates. **Exceptions:** Tamoxifen. *Risk D: Consider therapy modification*

CYP3A4 Inhibitors (Moderate): May decrease the metabolism of CYP3A4 Substrates. *Risk C: Monitor therapy*

CYP3A4 Inhibitors (Strong): May decrease the metabolism of CYP3A4 Substrates. *Risk D: Consider therapy modification*

Dasatinib: May increase the serum concentration of CYP3A4 Substrates. *Risk C: Monitor therapy*

Nebivolol: CYP2D6 Inhibitors (Strong) may increase the serum concentration of Nebivolol. *Risk C: Monitor therapy*

Tamoxifen: CYP2D6 Inhibitors (Strong) may decrease the metabolism of Tamoxifen. Specifically, strong CYP2D6 inhibitors may decrease the formation of highly potent active metabolites. *Risk X: Avoid combination*

Tetrabenazine: CYP2D6 Inhibitors (Strong) may increase the serum concentration of Tetrabenazine. Specifically, concentrations of the active alpha- and beta-dihydrotetrabenazine metabolites may be increased. Management: Tetrabenazine dose should be reduced by 50% when starting a strong CYP2D6 inhibitor. Maximum tetrabenazine dose is 50mg/day when used with a strong CYP2D6 inhibitor. *Risk D: Consider therapy modification*

Thioridazine: CYP2D6 Inhibitors may decrease the metabolism of Thioridazine. *Risk X: Avoid combination*

TraMADol: CYP2D6 Inhibitors (Strong) may diminish the therapeutic effect of TraMADol. These CYP2D6 inhibitors may prevent the metabolic conversion of tramadol to its active metabolite that accounts for much of its opioid-like effects. *Risk C: Monitor therapy*

Stability Store in well closed, light-resistant containers.

Mechanism of Action Ester local anesthetic blocks both the initiation and conduction of nerve impulses by decreasing the neuronal membrane's permeability to sodium ions, which results in inhibition of depolarization with resultant blockade of conduction; interferes with the uptake of norepinephrine by adrenergic nerve terminals producing vasoconstriction

Pharmacodynamics/Kinetics Following topical administration to mucosa:

Onset of action: ~1 minute

Peak effect: ~5 minutes

Duration (dose dependent): ≥30 minutes; cocaine metabolites may appear in urine of neonates up to 5 days after birth due to maternal cocaine use shortly before birth

Absorption: Well absorbed through mucous membranes; limited by drug-induced vasoconstriction; enhanced by inflammation

Distribution: Enters breast milk

Metabolism: Hepatic; major metabolites are ecgonine methyl ester and benzoyl ecgonine

Half-life elimination: 75 minutes

Excretion: Primarily urine (<10% as unchanged drug and metabolites)

Dosage Topical application (ear, nose, throat, bronchoscopy): Dosage depends on the area to be anesthetized, tissue vascularity, technique of anesthesia, and individual patient tolerance; the lowest dose necessary to produce adequate anesthesia should be used; concentrations of 1% to 10% are used (not to exceed 1 mg/kg). Use reduced dosages for children, elderly, or debilitated patients.

Administration Topical: Use only on mucous membranes of the oral, laryngeal, and nasal cavities. Do not use on extensive areas of broken skin.

Monitoring Parameters Vital signs

Reference Range Therapeutic: 100-500 ng/mL (SI: 330 nmol/L); Toxic: >1000 ng/mL (SI: >3300 nmol/L)

Additional Information Cocaine intoxication of infants who are receiving breast milk from their mothers abusing cocaine has been reported.

Dosage Forms Excipient information presented when available (limited, particularly for generics); consult specific product labeling. [DSC] = Discontinued product

Powder, for prescription compounding, as hydrochloride: 1 g, 5 g, 25 g

Solution, topical, as hydrochloride: 4% (4 mL, 10 mL); 10% (4 mL, 10 mL) [DSC]

◆ **Cocaine Hydrochloride** *see* Cocaine *on page 392*

◆ **Codal-DM [OTC]** *see* Phenylephrine, Pyrilamine, and Dextromethorphan *on page 1278*

Codeine (KOE deen)

Medication Safety Issues

Sound-alike/look-alike issues:

Codeine may be confused with Cardene®, Cophene®, Cordran®, iodine, Lodine®

High alert medication: The Institute for Safe Medication Practices (ISMP) includes this medication among its list of drug classes which have a heightened risk of causing significant patient harm when used in error.

Related Information

Anticholinergic Effects of Common Psychotropics *on page 1758*

Narcotic / Opioid Analgesics *on page 1789*

Canadian Brand Names Codeine Contin®

Mexican Brand Names Coderit; Lertus CD; Tylex CD; Voltaren Forte

Index Terms Codeine Phosphate; Codeine Sulfate; Methylmorphine

Pharmacologic Category Analgesic, Opioid; Antitussive

Use Treatment of mild-to-moderate pain; antitussive in lower doses; dextromethorphan has equivalent antitussive activity but has much lower toxicity in accidental overdose

Effect on Mental Status Drowsiness is common; may cause euphoria, confusion, insomnia, hallucinations, or depression

Effect on Psychiatric Treatment Concurrent use with psychotropics may produce additive toxicity; concurrent use with fluoxetine or paroxetine may result in loss of pain control

Restrictions C-II

Dosage Summary

I.M.:

Children: 0.5-1 mg/kg every 4-6 hours as needed (maximum: 60 mg/dose; 1.5 mg/kg/dose)

Adults: Initial: 30 mg every 4-6 hours; Usual range: 15-120 mg every 4-6 hours as needed (maximum: 1.5 mg/kg/dose)

Oral:

Children:

Analgesic: 0.5-1 mg/kg every 4-6 hours as needed (maximum: 60 mg/dose; 1.5 mg/kg/dose)

Antitussive: 1-1.5 mg/kg/day divided every 4-6 hours as needed (maximum: 30 mg/day [2-6 years]; 60 mg/day [6-12 years])

Adults:

Analgesic: Initial: 30 mg every 4-6 hours as needed; Usual range: 15-120 mg every 4-6 hours as needed (maximum: 1.5 mg/kg/dose)

Antitussive: 10-20 mg every 4-6 hours as needed (maximum: 120 mg/day)

SubQ:

Children: 0.5-1 mg/kg every 4-6 hours as needed (maximum: 60 mg/dose; 1.5 mg/kg/dose)

Adults: Initial: 30 mg every 4-6 hours; Usual range: 15-120 mg every 4-6 hours as needed (maximum: 1.5 mg/kg/dose)

Dosage Forms Excipient information presented when available (limited, particularly for generics); consult specific product labeling. [CAN] = Canadian brand name

Injection, as phosphate: 15 mg/mL (2 mL); 30 mg/mL (2 mL) [contains sodium metabisulfite]

Powder, for prescription compounding: 10 g, 25 g

Tablet, as phosphate: 30 mg, 60 mg

Tablet, as sulfate: 15 mg, 30 mg, 60 mg

Tablet, controlled release (Codeine Contin®) [CAN]: 50 mg, 100 mg, 150 mg, 200 mg [not available in U.S.]

- ◆ **Codeine, Acetaminophen, Butalbital, and Caffeine** *see* Butalbital, Acetaminophen, Caffeine, and Codeine *on page 232*
- ◆ **Codeine and Acetaminophen** *see* Acetaminophen and Codeine *on page 34*
- ◆ **Codeine and Butalbital Compound** *see* Butalbital, Aspirin, Caffeine, and Codeine *on page 242*
- ◆ **Codeine and Guaifenesin** *see* Guaifenesin and Codeine *on page 738*
- ◆ **Codeine and Promethazine** *see* Promethazine and Codeine *on page 1349*
- ◆ **Codeine and Pseudoephedrine** *see* Pseudoephedrine and Codeine *on page 1368*
- ◆ **Codeine, Aspirin, and Carisoprodol** *see* Carisoprodol, Aspirin, and Codeine *on page 284*
- ◆ **Codeine, Butalbital, Aspirin, and Caffeine** *see* Butalbital, Aspirin, Caffeine, and Codeine *on page 242*
- ◆ **Codeine, Chlorpheniramine, and Pseudoephedrine** *see* Chlorpheniramine, Pseudoephedrine, and Codeine *on page 332*
- ◆ **Codeine, Chlorpheniramine, Phenylephrine, and Potassium Iodide** *see* Chlorpheniramine, Phenylephrine, Codeine, and Potassium Iodide *on page 332*
- ◆ **Codeine, Doxylamine, and Acetaminophen** *see* Acetaminophen, Codeine, and Doxylamine *on page 41*
- ◆ **Codeine, Guaifenesin, and Pseudoephedrine** *see* Guaifenesin, Pseudoephedrine, and Codeine *on page 747*
- ◆ **Codeine Phosphate** *see* Codeine *on page 394*
- ◆ **Codeine Phosphate and Pseudoephedrine Hydrochloride** *see* Pseudoephedrine and Codeine *on page 1368*
- ◆ **Codeine, Promethazine, and Phenylephrine** *see* Promethazine, Phenylephrine, and Codeine *on page 1350*
- ◆ **Codeine, Pseudoephedrine, and Triprolidine** *see* Triprolidine, Pseudoephedrine, and Codeine *on page 1635*
- ◆ **Codeine Sulfate** *see* Codeine *on page 394*
- ◆ **Codeine, Triprolidine, and Pseudoephedrine** *see* Triprolidine, Pseudoephedrine, and Codeine *on page 1635*
- ◆ **Codiclear® DH [DSC]** *see* Hydrocodone and Guaifenesin *on page 779*
- ◆ **codimal® DM [OTC]** *see* Phenylephrine, Pyrilamine, and Dextromethorphan *on page 1278*
- ◆ **Codituss DM [OTC]** *see* Phenylephrine, Pyrilamine, and Dextromethorphan *on page 1278*
- ◆ **Cogentin®** *see* Benztropine *on page 183*
- ◆ **Co-Gesic® [DSC]** *see* Hydrocodone and Acetaminophen *on page 777*
- ◆ **Cognex®** *see* Tacrine *on page 1531*
- ◆ **Colazal®** *see* Balsalazide *on page 170*
- ◆ **ColBenemid** *see* Colchicine and Probenecid *on page 398*

Colchicine (KOL chi seen)

Medication Safety Issues

Sound-alike/look-alike issues:

Colchicine may be confused with Cortrosyn®

High alert medication: The Institute for Safe Medication Practices (ISMP) includes this medication (I.V. formulation) among its list of drugs which have a heightened risk of causing significant patient harm when used in error.

Mexican Brand Names Colchiquim; Sixol

Pharmacologic Category Colchicine

Generic Available Yes

Use Treatment of acute gouty arthritis attacks and prevention of recurrences of such attacks

Unlabeled/Investigational Use Primary biliary cirrhosis; management of familial Mediterranean fever; pericarditis

Effect on Mental Status May cause drowsiness

Effect on Psychiatric Treatment Rare reports of agranulocytosis; use caution with clozapine and carbamazepine; CNS depressant effects may be enhanced

Pregnancy Risk Factor C (oral); D (parenteral)

Lactation Enters breast milk/use caution (AAP rates "compatible")

Contraindications Hypersensitivity to colchicine or any component of the formulation; severe renal, gastrointestinal, hepatic, or cardiac disorders; blood dyscrasias; pregnancy (parenteral)

Warnings/Precautions Use with caution in debilitated patients or elderly patients; use caution in patients with mild-to-moderate cardiac, GI, renal, or liver disease. Severe local irritation can occur following SubQ or I.M. administration. Dosage reduction is recommended in patients who develop weakness or gastrointestinal symptoms (anorexia, diarrhea, nausea, vomiting) related to drug therapy.

Intravenous: Use only with extreme caution; potential for serious, life-threatening complications. Should not be administered to patients with renal insufficiency, hepatobiliary obstruction, patients >70 years of age, or recent oral colchicine use. Should be reserved for hospitalized patients who are under the care of a physician experienced in the use of intravenous colchicine.

Adverse Reactions

>10%: Gastrointestinal: Nausea, vomiting, diarrhea, abdominal pain

1% to 10%:

Dermatologic: Alopecia

Gastrointestinal: Anorexia

<1% (Limited to important or life-threatening): Agranulocytosis, aplastic anemia, arrhythmia (with intravenous administration), azoospermia, bone marrow suppression, dermatosis, hepatotoxicity, hypersensitivity reaction, myopathy, peripheral neuritis, purpura, rash

Metabolism/Transport Effects Substrate of CYP3A4 (major); **Induces** CYP2C8 (weak), 2C9 (weak), 2E1 (weak), 3A4 (weak)

Drug Interactions

CycloSPORINE: May enhance the adverse/toxic effect of Colchicine. These include hepatotoxicity and myopathies. Colchicine may increase the serum concentration of CycloSPORINE. Nephrotoxicity and hepatotoxicity may also be increased. *Risk D: Consider therapy modification*

CYP3A4 Inhibitors (Moderate): May decrease the metabolism of CYP3A4 Substrates. *Risk C: Monitor therapy*

CYP3A4 Inhibitors (Strong): May decrease the metabolism of CYP3A4 Substrates. *Risk D: Consider therapy modification*

Dasatinib: May increase the serum concentration of CYP3A4 Substrates. *Risk C: Monitor therapy*

HMG-CoA Reductase Inhibitors: Colchicine may enhance the myopathic (rhabdomyolysis) effect of HMG-CoA Reductase Inhibitors. Colchicine may increase the serum concentration of HMG-CoA Reductase Inhibitors. *Risk D: Consider therapy modification*

Macrolide Antibiotics: May decrease the metabolism of Colchicine. **Exceptions:** Azithromycin; Dirithromycin [Off Market]; Spiramycin. *Risk D: Consider therapy modification*

Maraviroc: CYP3A4 Inducers may decrease the serum concentration of Maraviroc. *Risk D: Consider therapy modification*

P-Glycoprotein Inducers: May decrease the serum concentration of P-Glycoprotein Substrates. P-glycoprotein inducers may also further limit the distribution of p-glycoprotein substrates to specific cells/tissues/organs where p-glycoprotein is present in large amounts (e.g., brain, T-lymphocytes, testes, etc.). *Risk C: Monitor therapy*

P-Glycoprotein Inhibitors: May increase the serum concentration of P-Glycoprotein Substrates. P-glycoprotein inhibitors may also enhance the distribution of p-glycoprotein substrates to specific cells/tissues/organs where p-glycoprotein is present in large amounts (e.g., brain, T-lymphocytes, testes, etc.). *Risk C: Monitor therapy*

Verapamil: May enhance the nephrotoxic effect of Colchicine. Colchicine may increase the serum concentration of Verapamil. *Risk C: Monitor therapy*

Ethanol/Nutrition/Herb Interactions

Ethanol: Avoid ethanol.

Food: Cyanocobalamin (vitamin B_{12}): Malabsorption of the substrate. May result in macrocytic anemia or neurologic dysfunction.

Herb/Nutraceutical: Vitamin B_{12} absorption may be decreased by colchicine.

Stability Protect tablets from light.

Mechanism of Action Decreases leukocyte motility, decreases phagocytosis in joints and lactic acid production, thereby reducing the deposition of urate crystals that perpetuates the inflammatory response

Pharmacodynamics/Kinetics

Onset of action: Oral: Pain relief: ~12 hours if adequately dosed

Distribution: Concentrates in leukocytes, kidney, spleen, and liver; does not distribute in heart, skeletal muscle, and brain

Protein binding: 10% to 31%

Metabolism: Partially hepatic via deacetylation

Half-life elimination: 12-30 minutes; End-stage renal disease: 45 minutes

Time to peak, serum: Oral: 0.5-2 hours, declining for the next 2 hours before increasing again due to enterohepatic recycling

Excretion: Primarily feces; urine (10% to 20%)

Dosage

Familial Mediterranean fever (unlabeled use): Prophylaxis: Oral:

Children:

≤5 years: 0.5 mg/day

>5 years: 1-1.5 mg/day in 2-3 divided doses

Adults: 1-2 mg daily in divided doses (occasionally reduced to 0.6 mg/day in patients with GI intolerance)

Gouty arthritis: Adults:

Prophylaxis of acute attacks: Oral: 0.6 mg twice daily; initial and/or subsequent dosage may be decreased (ie, 0.6 mg once daily) in patients at risk of toxicity or in those who are intolerant (including weakness, loose stools, or diarrhea); range: 0.6 mg every other day to 0.6 mg 3 times/day

Acute attacks:

Oral: Initial: 0.6-1.2 mg, followed by 0.6 every 1-2 hours; some clinicians recommend a maximum of 3 doses; more aggressive approaches have recommended a maximum dose of up to 6 mg. Wait at least 3 days before initiating another course of therapy

I.V.: Initial: 1-2 mg, then 0.5 mg every 6 hours until response, not to exceed total dose of 4 mg. If pain recurs, it may be necessary to administer additional daily doses. The amount of colchicine administered intravenously in an acute treatment period (generally ~1 week) should not exceed a total dose of 4 mg. Do not administer more colchicine by any route for at least 7 days after a full course of I.V. therapy.

Note: Many experts would avoid use because of potential for serious, life-threatening complications. Should not be administered to patients with renal insufficiency, hepatobiliary obstruction, patients >70 years of age, or recent oral colchicine use. Should be reserved for hospitalized patients who are under the care of a physician experienced in the use of intravenous colchicine.

Surgery: Gouty arthritis, prophylaxis of recurrent attacks: Adults: Oral: 0.6 mg/day or every other day; patients who are to undergo surgical procedures may receive 0.6 mg 3 times/day for 3 days before and 3 days after surgery

Primary biliary cirrhosis (unlabeled use): Adults: Oral: 0.6 mg twice daily

Pericarditis (unlabeled use): Adults: Oral: 0.6 mg twice daily

Elderly: Reduce maintenance/prophylactic dose by 50% in individuals >70 years

Dosing adjustment in renal impairment: Gouty arthritis, acute attacks: Oral: Specific dosing recommendations not available from the manufacturer:

Prophylaxis:

Cl_{cr} 35-49 mL/minute: 0.6 mg once daily

Cl_{cr} 10-34 mL/minute: 0.6 mg every 2-3 days

Cl_{cr} <10 mL/minute: Avoid chronic use of colchicine. Use in serious renal impairment is contraindicated by the manufacturer.

Treatment: Cl_{cr} <10 mL/minute: Use in serious renal impairment is contraindicated by the manufacturer. If a decision is made to use colchicine, decrease dose by 75%.

Peritoneal dialysis: Supplemental dose is not necessary

Dosage adjustment in hepatic impairment: Avoid in hepatobiliary dysfunction and in patients with hepatic disease.

Dietary Considerations May need to supplement with vitamin B_{12}.

Administration

I.V.: Injection should be made over 2-5 minutes into tubing of free-flowing I.V. with compatible fluid. Do not administer I.M. or SubQ; severe local irritation can occur following SubQ or I.M. administration. Extravasation can cause tissue irritation.

Tablet: Administer orally with water and maintain adequate fluid intake.

Monitoring Parameters CBC and renal function test

Test Interactions May cause false-positive results in urine tests for erythrocytes or hemoglobin

Dosage Forms Excipient information presented when available (limited, particularly for generics); consult specific product labeling.

Injection, solution: 0.5 mg/mL (2 mL)

Tablet: 0.6 mg

Colchicine and Probenecid (KOL chi seen & proe BEN e sid)

Index Terms ColBenemid; Probenecid and Colchicine

Pharmacologic Category Anti-inflammatory Agent; Antigout Agent; Uricosuric Agent

Use Treatment of chronic gouty arthritis when complicated by frequent, recurrent acute attacks of gout

Effect on Mental Status May cause drowsiness or dizziness

Effect on Psychiatric Treatment Rare reports of agranulocytosis; use caution with clozapine and carbamazepine; CNS depressant effects may be enhanced

Dosage Summary

Oral:

Children: Dosage not established

Adults: Initial: 1 tablet daily for 1 week; Maintenance: 1 tablet twice daily

Dosage Forms Excipient information presented when available (limited, particularly for generics); consult specific product labeling.

Tablet: Colchicine 0.5 mg and probenecid 0.5 g

- **Coldamine** *see* Chlorpheniramine, Pseudoephedrine, and Methscopolamine *on page 334*
- **Coldcough** *see* Pseudoephedrine, Dihydrocodeine, and Chlorpheniramine *on page 1371*
- **Coldcough HC [DSC]** *see* Pseudoephedrine, Hydrocodone, and Chlorpheniramine *on page 1372*
- **Coldcough PD** *see* Dihydrocodeine, Chlorpheniramine, and Phenylephrine *on page 469*
- **Coldmist DM [DSC]** *see* Guaifenesin, Pseudoephedrine, and Dextromethorphan *on page 748*

Colesevelam (koh le SEV a lam)

Related Information

Lipid-Lowering Agents *on page 1786*

U.S. Brand Names WelChol®

Canadian Brand Names WelChol®

Pharmacologic Category Antilipemic Agent, Bile Acid Sequestrant

Use Management of elevated LDL in primary hypercholesterolemia (Fredrickson type IIa) when used alone or in combination with an HMG-CoA reductase inhibitor; improve control of type 2 diabetes mellitus (noninsulin dependent, NIDDM) in conjunction with insulin or oral antidiabetic agents

Effect on Mental Status None reported

Effect on Psychiatric Treatment Constipation is common, concurrent use with psychotropic agents may exacerbate this effect

Dosage Summary

Oral:

Children: Dosage not established

Adults: 6 tablets/day in 1-2 divided doses

Dosage Forms Excipient information presented when available (limited, particularly for generics); consult specific product labeling.
Tablet, as hydrochloride:
WelChol®: 625 mg

◆ **Colestid®** *see* Colestipol *on page 399*

Colestipol (koe LES ti pole)

Related Information
Lipid-Lowering Agents *on page 1786*
U.S. Brand Names Colestid®
Canadian Brand Names Colestid®
Index Terms Colestipol Hydrochloride
Pharmacologic Category Antilipemic Agent, Bile Acid Sequestrant
Use Adjunct in management of primary hypercholesterolemia; regression of arteriolosclerosis; relief of pruritus associated with elevated levels of bile acids; possibly used to decrease plasma half-life of digoxin in toxicity
Effect on Mental Status May cause drowsiness or anxiety
Effect on Psychiatric Treatment Constipation is common; may be exacerbated by concurrent psychotropic use; may decrease the absorption of TCAs
Dosage Summary
Oral:
Children: Dosage not established
Adults:
Granules: Initial: 5 g 1-2 times/day; Maintenance: 5-30 g/day in 1-4 divided doses; **Note:** Titration is recommended
Tablets: Initial: 2 g 1-2 times/day; Maintenance: 2-16 g/day; **Note:** Titration is recommended
Dosage Forms Excipient information presented when available (limited, particularly for generics); consult specific product labeling.
Granules for suspension, as hydrochloride, oral: 5 g/packet (30s, 90s); 5 g/scoopful (500 g)
Colestid®: 5 g/packet (30s, 90s); 5 g/teaspoon (300 g, 500 g) [unflavored]
Colestid®, flavored: 5 g/packet (60s) [contains phenylalanine (18.2 mg/packet); orange flavor]
Colestid®, flavored: 5 g/scoopful (450 g) [contains phenylalanine (18.2 mg/scoopful); orange flavor]
Tablet, as hydrochloride: 1 g
Tablet, as hydrochloride, oral [micronized]:
Colestid®: 1 g

◆ **Colestipol Hydrochloride** *see* Colestipol *on page 399*
◆ **Colocort®** *see* Hydrocortisone *on page 785*
◆ **Colyte®** *see* Polyethylene Glycol-Electrolyte Solution *on page 1310*
◆ **CombiPatch®** *see* Estradiol and Norethindrone *on page 579*
◆ **Combipres® [DSC]** *see* Clonidine and Chlorthalidone *on page 380*
◆ **Combivent®** *see* Ipratropium and Albuterol *on page 854*
◆ **Combivir®** *see* Zidovudine and Lamivudine *on page 1696*
◆ **Comhist® [DSC]** *see* Chlorpheniramine, Phenylephrine, and Phenyltoloxamine *on page 331*
◆ **Commit® [OTC]** *see* Nicotine *on page 1133*
◆ **Common Hops** *see* Hops *(Humulus lupulus) on page 770*
◆ **Compazine** *see* Prochlorperazine *on page 1341*
◆ **Compound E** *see* Cortisone *on page 401*
◆ **Compound F** *see* Hydrocortisone *on page 785*
◆ **Compound S** *see* Zidovudine *on page 1695*
◆ **Compound W® [OTC]** *see* Salicylic Acid *on page 1454*
◆ **Compound W® One-Step Wart Remover [OTC]** *see* Salicylic Acid *on page 1454*
◆ **Compound W® One-Step Wart Remover for Feet [OTC]** *see* Salicylic Acid *on page 1454*
◆ **Compound W® One-Step Wart Remover for Kids [OTC]** *see* Salicylic Acid *on page 1454*
◆ **Compoz® Nighttime Sleep Aid [OTC]** *see* DiphenhydrAMINE *on page 481*
◆ **Compro™** *see* Prochlorperazine *on page 1341*

- **Comtan®** *see* Entacapone *on page 538*
- **Comtrex® Flu Therapy Nighttime [OTC]** *see* Acetaminophen, Chlorpheniramine, and Pseudoephedrine *on page 40*
- **Comtrex® Sore Throat Maximum Strength [OTC]** *see* Acetaminophen *on page 30*
- **Comvax®** *see* *Haemophilus* b Conjugate and Hepatitis B Vaccine *on page 752*
- **Conal** *see* Chlorpheniramine, Pyrilamine, and Phenylephrine *on page 335*
- **Concerta®** *see* Methylphenidate *on page 1024*
- **Coneflower** *see* Echinacea *(Echinacea purpurea, Echinacea angustifolia) on page 523*
- **Congestac® [OTC]** *see* Guaifenesin and Pseudoephedrine *on page 744*

Conivaptan (koe NYE vap tan)

U.S. Brand Names Vaprisol®

Index Terms Conivaptan Hydrochloride; YM087

Pharmacologic Category Vasopressin Antagonist

Use Treatment of euvolemic and hypervolemic hyponatremia in hospitalized patients

Effect on Mental Status Headache is common; may cause insomnia or confusion

Effect on Psychiatric Treatment Adverse effects associated with this agent may mimic those of psychotropic agents (eg, headache with SSRIs or polyuria with lithium). Consider this when evaluating patients' side effect burden. Carbamazepine, phenytoin, and phenobarbital may decrease the effects of conivaptan. Conversely, nefazodone may increase conivaptan levels. Conivaptan may increase levels of benzodiazepines (midazolam and triazolam are contraindicated), mirtazapine, nefazodone, sildenafil, and venlafaxine.

Dosage Summary

I.V.:

Children: Dosage not established

Adults: Loading dose: 20 mg bolus, followed by 20 mg as continuous infusion over 24 hours; Maintenance: 20-40 mg/day as a continuous infusion over 24 hours (maximum therapy: 4 days)

Dosage Forms Excipient information presented when available (limited, particularly for generics); consult specific product labeling.

Injection, solution:

Vaprisol®: 5 mg/mL (4 mL) [single-use ampul; contains propylene glycol and ethanol]

- **Conivaptan Hydrochloride** *see* Conivaptan *on page 400*
- **Conjugated Estrogen** *see* Estrogens (Conjugated/Equine) *on page 582*
- **Conjugated Estrogen and Methyltestosterone** *see* Estrogens (Esterified) and Methyltestosterone *on page 587*
- **Constulose** *see* Lactulose *on page 886*
- **Contac® Cold + Flu Maximum Strength Non-Drowsy [OTC]** *see* Acetaminophen and Phenylephrine *on page 36*
- **Copaxone®** *see* Glatiramer Acetate *on page 722*
- **COPD** *see* Dyphylline and Guaifenesin *on page 522*
- **Copegus®** *see* Ribavirin *on page 1417*
- **Copolymer-1** *see* Glatiramer Acetate *on page 722*
- **Cordarone®** *see* Amiodarone *on page 89*
- **Cordron-D NR [DSC]** *see* Carbinoxamine and Pseudoephedrine *on page 280*
- **Coreg®** *see* Carvedilol *on page 286*
- **Coreg CR®** *see* Carvedilol *on page 286*
- **Corfen DM** *see* Chlorpheniramine, Phenylephrine, and Dextromethorphan *on page 327*
- **Corgard®** *see* Nadolol *on page 1090*
- **Coricidin HBP® Chest Congestion and Cough [OTC]** *see* Guaifenesin and Dextromethorphan *on page 739*
- **Coricidin HBP® Cold and Flu [OTC]** *see* Chlorpheniramine and Acetaminophen *on page 322*
- **Coricidin® HBP Cough & Cold [OTC]** *see* Dextromethorphan and Chlorpheniramine *on page 449*
- **Corlopam®** *see* Fenoldopam *on page 623*

- **Cortaid® Intensive Therapy [OTC]** *see* Hydrocortisone *on page 785*
- **Cortaid® Maximum Strength [OTC]** *see* Hydrocortisone *on page 785*
- **Cortaid® Sensitive Skin [OTC]** *see* Hydrocortisone *on page 785*
- **Cortef®** *see* Hydrocortisone *on page 785*
- **Cortenema®** *see* Hydrocortisone *on page 785*
- **Corticool® [OTC]** *see* Hydrocortisone *on page 785*

Corticotropin (kor ti koe TROE pin)

Medication Safety Issues

Sound-alike/look-alike issues:

Corticotropin may be confused with corticorelin

U.S. Brand Names H.P. Acthar® Gel

Index Terms ACTH; Adrenocorticotropic Hormone; Corticotropin, Repository

Pharmacologic Category Corticosteroid, Systemic

Use Acute exacerbations of multiple sclerosis; diagnostic aid in adrenocortical insufficiency, severe muscle weakness in myasthenia gravis

Cosyntropin is preferred over corticotropin for diagnostic test of adrenocortical insufficiency (cosyntropin is less allergenic and test is shorter in duration)

Effect on Mental Status Insomnia and nervousness are common; may cause euphoria or hallucinations

Effect on Psychiatric Treatment Barbiturates may decrease the levels of corticotropin

Dosage Summary

I.M.:

Children:

Anti-inflammatory/immunosuppressant: 0.8 units/kg/day or 25 units/m^2/day divided every 12-24 hours

Infantile spasms: Initial: 20 units/day for 2 weeks, if no response increase to 30 units/day for 4 weeks; Usual range: 5-160 units/day

Adults: 80-120 units/day for 2-3 weeks **or** 40-80 units every 24-72 hours

SubQ:

Children: Dosage not established

Adults: 40-80 units every 24-72 hours

Dosage Forms Excipient information presented when available (limited, particularly for generics); consult specific product labeling.

Injection, gelatin: 80 units/mL (5 mL)

- **Corticotropin, Repository** *see* Corticotropin *on page 401*
- **Cortifoam®** *see* Hydrocortisone *on page 785*
- **Cortisol** *see* Hydrocortisone *on page 785*

Cortisone (KOR ti sone)

Medication Safety Issues

Sound-alike/look-alike issues:

Cortisone may be confused with Cortizone®

Related Information

Corticosteroids *on page 1780*

Index Terms Compound E; Cortisone Acetate

Pharmacologic Category Corticosteroid, Systemic

Use Management of adrenocortical insufficiency

Effect on Mental Status Insomnia and nervousness are common; may cause euphoria or hallucinations

Effect on Psychiatric Treatment Barbiturates may decrease the levels of cortisone

Dosage Summary

Oral:

Children: 0.5-10 mg/kg/day **or** 20-300 mg/m^2/day divided every 6-8 hours

Adults: 25-300 mg /day divided every 12-24 hours

Dosage Forms Excipient information presented when available (limited, particularly for generics); consult specific product labeling.

Tablet, as acetate: 25 mg

- **Cortisone Acetate** *see* Cortisone *on page 401*
- **Cortizone®-10 Maximum Strength [OTC]** *see* Hydrocortisone *on page 785*
- **Cortizone®-10 Plus Maximum Strength [OTC]** *see* Hydrocortisone *on page 785*

- **Cortizone®-10 Quick Shot [OTC]** *see* Hydrocortisone *on page 785*
- **Cortrosyn®** *see* Cosyntropin *on page 402*
- **Corvert®** *see* Ibutilide *on page 808*
- **Corzide®** *see* Nadolol and Bendroflumethiazide *on page 1092*
- **Cosmegen®** *see* DACTINomycin *on page 415*
- **Cosopt®** *see* Dorzolamide and Timolol *on page 499*

Cosyntropin (koe sin TROE pin)

Medication Safety Issues
Sound-alike/look-alike issues:
Cortrosyn® may be confused with colchicine, Cotazym®

U.S. Brand Names Cortrosyn®

Canadian Brand Names Cortrosyn®

Index Terms Synacthen; Tetracosactide

Pharmacologic Category Diagnostic Agent

Use Diagnostic test to differentiate primary adrenal from secondary (pituitary) adrenocortical insufficiency

Effect on Mental Status None reported

Effect on Psychiatric Treatment Barbiturates may decrease the levels of cosyntropin

Dosage Forms Excipient information presented when available (limited, particularly for generics); consult specific product labeling.
Injection, powder for reconstitution: 0.25 mg

- **Co-Trimoxazole** *see* Sulfamethoxazole and Trimethoprim *on page 1517*
- **Coughcold HCM [DSC]** *see* Hydrocodone and Pseudoephedrine *on page 781*
- **Coughtuss** *see* Phenylephrine, Hydrocodone, and Chlorpheniramine *on page 1277*
- **Coumadin®** *see* Warfarin *on page 1679*
- **Covaryx™** *see* Estrogens (Esterified) and Methyltestosterone *on page 587*
- **Covaryx™ HS** *see* Estrogens (Esterified) and Methyltestosterone *on page 587*
- **Covera-HS®** *see* Verapamil *on page 1665*
- **Co-Vidarabine** *see* Pentostatin *on page 1250*
- **Coviracil** *see* Emtricitabine *on page 530*
- **Cozaar®** *see* Losartan *on page 952*
- **CP358774** *see* Erlotinib *on page 556*
- **C-Phen** *see* Chlorpheniramine and Phenylephrine *on page 323*
- **C-Phen DM** *see* Chlorpheniramine, Phenylephrine, and Dextromethorphan *on page 327*
- **CPM** *see* Cyclophosphamide *on page 408*
- **CPM-12** *see* Chlorpheniramine *on page 321*
- **CPT-11** *see* Irinotecan *on page 856*
- **CPZ** *see* ChlorproMAZINE *on page 336*
- **Crantex HC [DSC]** *see* Hydrocodone, Phenylephrine, and Guaifenesin *on page 783*
- **Crantex LA** *see* Guaifenesin and Phenylephrine *on page 742*
- ***Crataegus oxyacantha*** *see* Hawthorn *(Crataegus oxyacantha) on page 758*
- **Creomulsion® Cough [OTC]** *see* Dextromethorphan *on page 448*
- **Creomulsion® for Children [OTC]** *see* Dextromethorphan *on page 448*
- **Creo-Terpin® [OTC]** *see* Dextromethorphan *on page 448*
- **Crinone®** *see* Progesterone *on page 1345*
- **Crixivan®** *see* Indinavir *on page 818*
- **Crolom®** *see* Cromolyn *on page 402*
- **Cromoglycic Acid** *see* Cromolyn *on page 402*

Cromolyn (KROE moe lin)

Medication Safety Issues
Sound-alike/look-alike issues:
Intal® may be confused with Endal®
NasalCrom® may be confused with Nasacort®, Nasalide®

U.S. Brand Names Crolom®; Gastrocrom®; Intal®; NasalCrom® [OTC]

Canadian Brand Names Apo-Cromolyn®; Intal®; Nalcrom®; Nu-Cromolyn; Opticrom®

Mexican Brand Names Intal; Opticrom; Rynacrom

Index Terms Cromoglycic Acid; Cromolyn Sodium; Disodium Cromoglycate; DSCG

Pharmacologic Category Mast Cell Stabilizer

Use

Inhalation: May be used as an adjunct in the prophylaxis of allergic disorders, including asthma; prevention of exercise-induced bronchospasm

Nasal: Prevention and treatment of seasonal and perennial allergic rhinitis

Oral: Systemic mastocytosis

Ophthalmic: Treatment of vernal keratoconjunctivitis, vernal conjunctivitis, and vernal keratitis

Unlabeled/Investigational Use Oral: Food allergy, treatment of inflammatory bowel disease

Effect on Mental Status May cause dizziness

Effect on Psychiatric Treatment None reported

Dosage Summary

Inhalation:

Metered spray:

Children <5 years: Dosage not established

Children 5-12 years: Initial: 2 inhalations 4 times/day; Maintenance: 1-2 inhalations 3-4 times/day **or** 2 inhalations prior to exercise or allergen exposure

Children >12 years: Initial: 2 inhalations 4 times/day; Maintenance: 2-4 inhalations 3-4 times/day **or** 2 inhalations prior to exercise or allergen exposure

Adults: Initial: 2 inhalations 4 times/day; Maintenance: 2-4 inhalations 3-4 times/day **or** 2 inhalations prior to exercise or allergen exposure

Nebulization:

Children <2 years: Dosage not established

Children ≥2 years: Initial: 20 mg 4 times/day; Maintenance: 20 mg 3-4 times/day **or** 20 mg prior to exercise or allergen exposure

Adults: Initial: 20 mg 4 times/day; Maintenance: 20 mg 3-4 times/day **or** 20 mg prior to exercise or allergen exposure

Intranasal:

Children <2 years: Dosage not established

Children ≥2 years: Instill 1 spray in each nostril 3-4 times/day

Adults: Instill 1 spray in each nostril 3-4 times/day

Ophthalmic:

Children: Dosage not established

Adults: 1-2 drops in each eye 4-6 times/day

Oral:

Children <2 years: Dosage not established

Children 2-12 years: 100 mg 4 times/day; (maximum: 40 mg/kg/day)

Children >12 years: 200 mg 4 times/day (maximum: 40 mg/kg/day)

Adults: 200 mg 4 times/day (maximum: 40 mg/kg/day)

Dosage Forms Excipient information presented when available (limited, particularly for generics); consult specific product labeling.

Aerosol, for oral inhalation, as sodium:

Intal®: 800 mcg/inhalation (8.1 g) [112 metered inhalations; 56 doses], (14.2 g) [200 metered inhalations; 100 doses]

Solution for nebulization, as sodium: 20 mg/2 mL (60s, 120s)

Intal®: 20 mg/2 mL (60s, 120s)

Solution, intranasal, as sodium [spray]:

NasalCrom®: 40 mg/mL (13 mL, 26 mL) [5.2 mg/inhalation; contains benzalkonium chloride]

Solution, ophthalmic, as sodium: 4% (10 mL)

Crolom®: 4% (10 mL) [contains benzalkonium chloride]

Solution, oral, as sodium [concentrate]:

Gastrocrom®: 100 mg/5 mL (96s)

◆ **Cromolyn Sodium** *see* Cromolyn *on page 402*

◆ **Cryselle™** *see* Ethinyl Estradiol and Norgestrel *on page 601*

◆ **Crystalline Penicillin** *see* Penicillin G, Parenteral, Aqueous *on page 1241*

◆ **CsA** *see* CycloSPORINE *on page 409*

◆ **C-Tanna 12** *see* Carbetapentane and Chlorpheniramine *on page 272*

◆ **C-Tanna 12D** *see* Carbetapentane, Phenylephrine, and Pyrilamine *on page 275*

◆ **C-Time [OTC]** *see* Ascorbic Acid *on page 141*

◆ **CTLA-4Ig** *see* Abatacept *on page 22*

◆ **CTM** *see* Chlorpheniramine *on page 321*
◆ **CTX** *see* Cyclophosphamide *on page 408*
◆ **Cubicin®** *see* DAPTOmycin *on page 418*
◆ **Cuprimine®** *see* Penicillamine *on page 1239*
◆ **Cutivate®** *see* Fluticasone *on page 668*
◆ **CyA** *see* CycloSPORINE *on page 409*

Cyanocobalamin (sye an oh koe BAL a min)

U.S. Brand Names CaloMist™; Nascobal®; Twelve Resin-K

Mexican Brand Names Dolo-Neurobion Retard; Kiddi Pharmaton; Ledoxina; Tribedoce DX; Vitalen

Index Terms Vitamin B_{12}

Pharmacologic Category Vitamin, Water Soluble

Use Treatment of pernicious anemia; vitamin B_{12} deficiency due to dietary deficiencies or malabsorption diseases, inadequate secretion of intrinsic factor, and inadequate utilization of B_{12} (eg, during neoplastic treatment); increased B_{12} requirements due to pregnancy, thyrotoxicosis, hemorrhage, malignancy, liver or kidney disease

CaloMist™: Maintenance of vitamin B_{12} concentrations after initial correction in patients with B_{12} deficiency without CNS involvement

Effect on Mental Status None reported

Effect on Psychiatric Treatment Anticonvulsants may decrease the absorption of cyanocobalamin

Dosage Summary

I.M.:

Children:

B_{12} deficiency (dosage not well established): 0.2 mcg/kg for 2 days, followed by 1000 mcg/day for 2-7 days, followed by 100 mcg/week for one month, then 100 mcg monthly **or** 100 mcg/day for 10-15 days, then once or twice weekly for several months

Pernicious anemia: Initial: 30-50 mcg/day for 2 or more weeks (total dose: 1000-5000 mcg); Maintenance: 100 mcg/month

Adults:

B_{12} deficiency: Initial: 30 mcg/day for 5-10 days; Maintenance: 100-200 mcg/month

Pernicious anemia: Initial: 100 mcg/day for 6-7 days; if improvement, administer same dose on alternate days for 7 doses, then every 3-4 days for 2-3 weeks; Maintenance: 100-1000 mcg/month **or** 1000 mcg/day for 5 days, followed by 500-1000 mcg/month

Intranasal:

Children: Dosage not established

Adults: Nascobal®: 500 mcg in one nostril once weekly; CaloMist™: Maintenance therapy (following correction of vitamin B_{12} deficiency): 50-100 mcg/day

Oral:

Children: B_{12} deficiency: Dosage not established

Adults:

B_{12} deficiency: 250 mcg/day

Pernicious anemia: 1000-2000 mcg/day

SubQ:

Children:

B_{12} deficiency (dosage not well established): 0.2 mcg/kg for 2 days, followed by 1000 mcg/day for 2-7 days, followed by 100 mcg/week for one month, then 100 mcg monthly **or** 100 mcg/day for 10-15 days, then once or twice weekly for several months

Pernicious anemia: Initial: 30-50 mcg/day for 2 or more weeks (total dose: 1000-5000 mcg); Maintenance: 100 mcg/month

Adults:

B_{12} deficiency: Initial: 30 mcg/day for 5-10 days; Maintenance: 100-200 mcg/month

Pernicious anemia: Initial: 100 mcg/day for 6-7 days; if improvement, administer same dose on alternate days for 7 doses, then every 3-4 days for 2-3 weeks; Maintenance: 100-1000 mcg/month **or** 1000 mcg/day for 5 days, followed by 500-1000 mcg/month

Dosage Forms Excipient information presented when available (limited, particularly for generics); consult specific product labeling.

Injection, solution: 1000 mcg/mL (1 mL, 10 mL, 30 mL) [may contain benzyl alcohol]

Lozenge: 50 mcg, 100 mcg, 250 mcg, 500 mcg
Lozenge, sublingual: 500 mcg
Solution, intranasal [spray]:
CaloMist™: 25 mcg/0.1 mL actuation (18 mL) [contains benzyl alcohol, benzalkonium chloride; 60 metered sprays]
Nascobal®: 500 mcg/0.1 mL actuation (2.3 mL) [contains benzalkonium chloride; delivers 8 sprays]
Tablet: 50 mcg, 100 mcg, 250 mcg, 500 mcg, 1000 mcg
Twelve Resin-K: 1000 mcg [may be used as oral, sublingual, or buccal]
Tablet, timed release: 1000 mcg, 1500 mcg
Tablet, sublingual: 1000 mcg, 2500 mcg, 5000 mcg

◆ **Cyclessa®** *see* Ethinyl Estradiol and Desogestrel *on page 592*

Cyclizine (SYE kli zeen)

U.S. Brand Names Marezine® [OTC]
Index Terms Cyclizine Hydrochloride; Cyclizine Lactate
Pharmacologic Category Histamine H_1 Antagonist; Histamine H_1 Antagonist, First Generation
Use Prevention and treatment of nausea, vomiting, and vertigo associated with motion sickness; control of postoperative nausea and vomiting
Effect on Mental Status Drowsiness is common
Effect on Psychiatric Treatment Concurrent use with psychotropics may exacerbate the dry mouth and sedation commonly seen with cyclizine
Dosage Summary
Oral:
Children <6 years: Dosage not established
Children 6-12 years: 25 mg up to 3 times/day
Adults: 50 mg prior to departure, may repeat in 4-6 hours if needed (maximum: 200 mg/day)
Dosage Forms Excipient information presented when available (limited, particularly for generics); consult specific product labeling.
Tablet, as hydrochloride: 50 mg

◆ **Cyclizine Hydrochloride** *see* Cyclizine *on page 405*
◆ **Cyclizine Lactate** *see* Cyclizine *on page 405*

Cyclobenzaprine (sye kloe BEN za preen)

Medication Safety Issues
Sound-alike/look-alike issues:
Cyclobenzaprine may be confused with cycloSERINE, cyproheptadine
Flexeril® may be confused with Floxin®
U.S. Brand Names Amrix®; Fexmid™; Flexeril®
Canadian Brand Names Apo-Cyclobenzaprine®; Flexeril®; Flexitec; Gen-Cyclobenzaprine; Novo-Cycloprine; Nu-Cyclobenzaprine
Mexican Brand Names Yuredol
Index Terms Cyclobenzaprine Hydrochloride
Pharmacologic Category Skeletal Muscle Relaxant
Generic Available Yes: Excludes capsule
Use Treatment of muscle spasm associated with acute painful musculoskeletal conditions
Effect on Mental Status Drowsiness and dizziness are common; may cause nervousness or confusion
Effect on Psychiatric Treatment Contraindicated with MAO inhibitors or within 14 days of MAO inhibitor; concurrent use with psychotropics may exacerbate the dry mouth and sedation commonly seen with cyclobenzaprine
Pregnancy Risk Factor B
Pregnancy Considerations Teratogenic effects were not observed in animal studies. There are no adequate and well-controlled studies in pregnant women. Use during pregnancy only if clearly needed.
Lactation Excretion in breast milk unknown/use caution
Contraindications Hypersensitivity to cyclobenzaprine or any component of the formulation; do not use concomitantly or within 14 days of MAO inhibitors; hyperthyroidism; congestive heart failure, arrhythmias, heart block; acute recovery phase of MI
Warnings/Precautions May cause CNS depression, which may impair physical or mental abilities; patients must be cautioned about performing tasks which require mental alertness (eg, operating machinery or driving). ▶

Cyclobenzaprine shares the toxic potentials of the tricyclic antidepressants (including arrhythmias, tachycardia, and conduction time prolongation) and the usual precautions of tricyclic antidepressant therapy should be observed; use with caution in patients with urinary hesitancy or retention, angle-closure glaucoma or increased intraocular pressure, hepatic impairment, or in the elderly. Do not use concomitantly or within 14 days after MAO inhibitors; combination may cause hypertensive crisis, severe convulsions. Effects may be potentiated when used with other CNS depressants or ethanol. Safety and efficacy have not been established in patients <15 years of age.

Adverse Reactions

>10%:

Central nervous system: Drowsiness (29% to 39%), dizziness (1% to 11%)

Gastrointestinal: Xerostomia (21% to 32%)

1% to 10%:

Central nervous system: Fatigue (1% to 6%), confusion (1% to 3%), headache (1% to 3%), irritability (1% to 3%), mental acuity decreased (1% to 3%), nervousness (1% to 3%), somnolence (1% to 2%)

Gastrointestinal: Abdominal pain (1% to 3%), constipation (1% to 3%), diarrhea (1% to 3%), dyspepsia (≤4%), nausea (1% to 3%), unpleasant taste (1% to 3%)

Neuromuscular & skeletal: Weakness (1% to 3%)

Ocular: Blurred vision (1% to 3%)

Respiratory: Pharyngitis (1% to 3%), upper respiratory infection (1% to 3%)

<1% (Limited to important or life-threatening): Ageusia, agitation, anaphylaxis, angioedema, anorexia, anxiety, arrhythmia, ataxia, cholestasis, depression, diaphoresis, diplopia, disorientation, dysarthria, facial edema, flatulence, gastritis, hallucinations, hepatitis (rare), hypertonia, hypotension, insomnia, jaundice, liver function tests abnormal, malaise, muscle twitching, palpitation, paresthesia, pruritus, psychosis, rash, seizure, syncope, tachycardia, thirst, tinnitus, tongue edema, tremor, urinary retention, urticaria, vasodilation, vertigo, vomiting

Metabolism/Transport Effects Substrate of CYP1A2 (major), 2D6 (minor), 3A4 (minor)

Drug Interactions

Acetylcholinesterase Inhibitors (Central): Anticholinergics may diminish the therapeutic effect of Acetylcholinesterase Inhibitors (Central). Acetylcholinesterase Inhibitors (Central) may diminish the therapeutic effect of Anticholinergics. If the anticholinergic action is a side effect of the agent, the result may be beneficial. *Risk C: Monitor therapy*

Alcohol (Ethyl): CNS Depressants may enhance the CNS depressant effect of Alcohol (Ethyl). *Risk C: Monitor therapy*

Anticholinergics: May enhance the adverse/toxic effect of other Anticholinergics. **Exceptions:** Paliperidone. *Risk C: Monitor therapy*

CNS Depressants: May enhance the adverse/toxic effect of other CNS Depressants. *Risk C: Monitor therapy*

CYP1A2 Inhibitors (Moderate): May decrease the metabolism of CYP1A2 Substrates. *Risk C: Monitor therapy*

CYP1A2 Inhibitors (Strong): May decrease the metabolism of CYP1A2 Substrates. *Risk D: Consider therapy modification*

MAO Inhibitors: Cyclobenzaprine may enhance the serotonergic effect of MAO Inhibitors. This could result in serotonin syndrome. *Risk X: Avoid combination*

Pramlintide: May enhance the anticholinergic effect of Anticholinergics. These effects are specific to the GI tract. *Risk D: Consider therapy modification*

Ethanol/Nutrition/Herb Interactions

Food: Food increases bioavailability (peak plasma concentrations increased by 35% and area under the curve by 20%) of the extended release capsule.

Ethanol: Avoid ethanol (may increase CNS depression).

Herb/Nutraceutical: Avoid valerian, kava kava, gotu kola (may increase CNS depression).

Stability

Amrix®, Flexeril®: Store at room temperature of 15°C to 30°C (59°F to 86°F).

Fexmid™: Store at room temperature of 20°C to 25°C (68°F to 77°F).

Mechanism of Action Centrally-acting skeletal muscle relaxant pharmacologically related to tricyclic antidepressants; reduces tonic somatic motor activity influencing both alpha and gamma motor neurons

Pharmacodynamics/Kinetics

Onset of action: Immediate release tablet: ~1 hour

Duration: Immediate release tablet: 12-24 hours

Absorption: Complete

Metabolism: Hepatic via CYP3A4, 1A2, and 2D6; may undergo enterohepatic recirculation

Bioavailability: 33% to 55%

Half-life elimination: Range: 8-37 hours; Immediate release tablet: 18 hours; Extended release capsule: 32 hours

Time to peak, serum: Immediate release tablet: 3-8 hours; Extended release capsule: 7-8 hours

Excretion: Urine (as inactive metabolites); feces (as unchanged drug)

Dosage Oral: **Note:** Do not use longer than 2-3 weeks

Capsule, extended release:

Adults: Usual: 15 mg once daily; some patients may require up to 30 mg once daily

Elderly: Use not recommended

Tablet, immediate release:

Children ≥15 years and Adults: Initial: 5 mg 3 times/day; may increase to 7.5-10 mg 3 times/day if needed

Elderly: Initial: 5 mg; titrate dose slowly and consider less frequent dosing

Dosage adjustment in hepatic impairment:

Capsule, extended release: Mild-to-severe impairment: Use not recommended.

Tablet, immediate release:

Mild impairment: Initial: 5 mg; use with caution; titrate slowly and consider less frequent dosing

Moderate-to-severe impairment: Use not recommended

Administration Oral: Extended release capsules: Administer at the same time each day. Do not crush or chew.

Dosage Forms Excipient information presented when available (limited, particularly for generics); consult specific product labeling.

Capsule, extended release, as hydrochloride:

Amrix®: 15 mg, 30 mg

Tablet, as hydrochloride: 5 mg, 10 mg

Fexmid™: 7.5 mg

Flexeril®: 5 mg, 10 mg

◆ **Cyclobenzaprine Hydrochloride** *see* Cyclobenzaprine *on page 405*

◆ **Cyclogyl®** *see* Cyclopentolate *on page 407*

◆ **Cyclomydril®** *see* Cyclopentolate and Phenylephrine *on page 407*

Cyclopentolate (sye kloe PEN toe late)

U.S. Brand Names AK-Pentolate™; Cyclogyl®; Cylate™

Canadian Brand Names Cyclogyl®; Diopentolate®

Index Terms Cyclopentolate Hydrochloride

Pharmacologic Category Anticholinergic Agent, Ophthalmic

Use Diagnostic procedures requiring mydriasis and cycloplegia

Effect on Mental Status Cyclopentolate may cause restlessness, hallucinations, psychosis, hyperactivity, seizures, incoherent speech, or ataxia. The 2% solution may result in psychotic reactions and behavioral disturbances in children, usually occurring approximately 30-45 minutes after instillation.

Effect on Psychiatric Treatment None reported; may counteract the effects of antipsychotics, especially in children; monitor

Dosage Summary

Ophthalmic:

Neonates: Cyclopentolate and phenylephrine combination formulation is the preferred agent

Children: Instill 1 drop of 0.5%, 1%, or 2% in eye followed by 1 drop of 0.5% or 1% in 5 minutes, if necessary

Adults: Instill 1 drop of 1% followed by another drop in 5 minutes; 2% solution in heavily pigmented iris

Dosage Forms Excipient information presented when available (limited, particularly for generics); consult specific product labeling.

Solution, ophthalmic, as hydrochloride: 1% (2 mL, 15 mL)

AK-Pentolate™, Cylate™: 1% (2 mL, 15 mL) [contains benzalkonium chloride]

Cyclogyl®: 0.5% (15 mL); 1% (2 mL, 5 mL, 15 mL); 2% (2 mL, 5 mL, 15 mL) [contains benzalkonium chloride]

Cyclopentolate and Phenylephrine
(sye kloe PEN toe late & fen il EF rin)

U.S. Brand Names Cyclomydril®

Index Terms Phenylephrine and Cyclopentolate

Pharmacologic Category Ophthalmic Agent, Antiglaucoma

Use Induce mydriasis greater than that produced with cyclopentolate HCl alone

Effect on Mental Status Cyclopentolate may cause restlessness, hallucinations, psychosis, hyperactivity, seizures, incoherent speech, or ataxia. The 2% solution may result in psychotic reactions and behavioral disturbances in children, usually occurring approximately 30-45 minutes after instillation.

Effect on Psychiatric Treatment None reported; may counteract the effects of antipsychotics, especially in children; monitor

Dosage Summary

Ophthalmic:

Neonates: Instill 1 drop into eyes every 5-10 minutes, for up to 3 doses

Children: Instill 1 drop into eyes every 5-10 minutes, for up to 3 doses

Adults: Instill 1 drop into eyes every 5-10 minutes, for up to 3 doses

Dosage Forms Excipient information presented when available (limited, particularly for generics); consult specific product labeling.

Solution, ophthalmic: Cyclopentolate hydrochloride 0.2% and phenylephrine hydrochloride 1% (2 mL, 5 mL) [contains benzalkonium chloride]

◆ **Cyclopentolate Hydrochloride** *see* Cyclopentolate *on page 407*

Cyclophosphamide (sye kloe FOS fa mide)

Medication Safety Issues

Sound-alike/look-alike issues:

Cyclophosphamide may be confused with cycloSPORINE, ifosfamide

Cytoxan® may be confused with cefoxitin, Centoxin®, Ciloxan®, cytarabine, CytoGam®, Cytosar®, Cytosar-U®, Cytotec®

High alert medication: The Institute for Safe Medication Practices (ISMP) includes this medication among its list of drugs which have a heightened risk of causing significant patient harm when used in error.

U.S. Brand Names Cytoxan® [DSC]

Canadian Brand Names Cytoxan®; Procytox®

Mexican Brand Names Cryofaxol; Ledoxina

Index Terms CPM; CTX; CYT; Neosar; NSC-26271

Pharmacologic Category Antineoplastic Agent, Alkylating Agent

Use

Oncologic: Treatment of Hodgkin's and non-Hodgkin's lymphoma, Burkitt's lymphoma, chronic lymphocytic leukemia (CLL), chronic myelocytic leukemia (CML), acute myelocytic leukemia (AML), acute lymphocytic leukemia (ALL), mycosis fungoides, multiple myeloma, neuroblastoma, retinoblastoma, rhabdomyosarcoma, Ewing's sarcoma; breast, testicular, endometrial, ovarian, and lung cancers, and in conditioning regimens for bone marrow transplantation

Nononcologic: Prophylaxis of rejection for kidney, heart, liver, and bone marrow transplants, severe rheumatoid disorders, nephrotic syndrome, Wegener's granulomatosis, idiopathic pulmonary hemosideroses, myasthenia gravis, multiple sclerosis, systemic lupus erythematosus, lupus nephritis, autoimmune hemolytic anemia, idiopathic thrombocytic purpura (ITP), macroglobulinemia, and antibody-induced pure red cell aplasia

Effect on Mental Status May cause dizziness

Effect on Psychiatric Treatment May cause myelosuppression; use caution with clozapine and carbamazepine

Dosage Forms Excipient information presented when available (limited, particularly for generics); consult specific product labeling. [DSC] = Discontinued product

Injection, powder for reconstitution: 500 mg, 1 g, 2 g

Cytoxan®: 500 mg, 1 g, 2 g [DSC]

Tablet: 25 mg, 50 mg

Cytoxan®: 25 mg, 50 mg [DSC]

CycloSERINE (sye kloe SER een)

Medication Safety Issues

Sound-alike/look-alike issues:

CycloSERINE may be confused with cyclobenzaprine, cycloSPORINE

U.S. Brand Names Seromycin®

Pharmacologic Category Antibiotic, Miscellaneous; Antitubercular Agent

Use Adjunctive treatment in pulmonary or extrapulmonary tuberculosis

Unlabeled/Investigational Use Treatment of Gaucher's disease

Effect on Mental Status May cause drowsiness, confusion, depression, and psychosis

Effect on Psychiatric Treatment Low doses (50 mg) have been used to treat negative symptoms of schizophrenia

Dosage Summary

Oral:

Children: 10-20 mg/kg/day in 2 divided doses (maximum: 1000 mg/day)

Adults: Initial: 250 mg every 12 hours for 14 days; Maintenance: 500-1000 mg/day in 2 divided doses

Dosage Forms Excipient information presented when available (limited, particularly for generics); consult specific product labeling.

Capsule: 250 mg

◆ **Cyclosporin A** *see* CycloSPORINE *on page 409*

CycloSPORINE (SYE kloe spor een)

Medication Safety Issues

Sound-alike/look-alike issues:

CycloSPORINE may be confused with cyclophosphamide, Cyklokapron®, cycloSERINE

CycloSPORINE modified (Neoral®, Gengraf®) may be confused with cycloSPORINE non-modified (Sandimmne®)

Gengraf® may be confused with Prograf®

Neoral® may be confused with Neurontin®, Nizoral®

Sandimmune® may be confused with Sandostatin®

U.S. Brand Names Gengraf®; Neoral®; Restasis®; Sandimmune®

Canadian Brand Names Neoral®; Rhoxal-cyclosporine; Sandimmune® I.V.; Sandoz-Cyclosporine

Mexican Brand Names Modusik-A Ofteno; Neolem; Restasis; Sandimmun Neoral; Supremunn

Index Terms CsA; CyA; Cyclosporin A

Pharmacologic Category Immunosuppressant Agent

Use Prophylaxis of organ rejection in kidney, liver, and heart transplants, has been used with azathioprine and/or corticosteroids; severe, active rheumatoid arthritis (RA) not responsive to methotrexate alone; severe, recalcitrant plaque psoriasis in nonimmunocompromised adults unresponsive to or unable to tolerate other systemic therapy

Ophthalmic emulsion (Restasis®): Increase tear production when suppressed tear production is presumed to be due to keratoconjunctivitis sicca-associated ocular inflammation (in patients not already using topical anti-inflammatory drugs or punctal plugs)

Unlabeled/Investigational Use Short-term, high-dose cyclosporine as a modulator of multidrug resistance in cancer treatment; allogenic bone marrow transplants for prevention and treatment of graft-versus-host disease; also used in some cases of severe autoimmune disease (eg, SLE, myasthenia gravis, inflammatory bowel disease) that are resistant to corticosteroids and other therapy; focal segmental glomerulosclerosis

Effect on Mental Status None reported

Effect on Psychiatric Treatment Carbamazepine and phenobarbital may increase the clearance of cyclosporine resulting in decreased levels; nefazodone may inhibit the clearance of cyclosporine resulting in increased levels of cyclosporine. There have been reports of serious drug interactions between cyclosporine and St John's wort. This interaction produces a reduction in serum cyclosporine levels resulting in subtherapeutic levels, rejection of transplanted organs, and graft loss.

Dosage Summary Note: Modified (Neoral®/Genraf®) and non-modified (Sandimmune®) cyclosporine products are not bioequivalent and cannot be used interchangeably.

I.V. (non-modified):

Children: Initial dose: 5-6 mg/kg/day as a single dose (1/3 the oral dose); Maintenance: 3-7.5 mg/kg/day; **Note:** May divided into 2-3 doses for day or give as continuous infusion over 24 hours

Adults: Initial dose: 5-6 mg/kg/day as a single dose (1/3 the oral dose); Maintenance: 3-7.5 mg/kg/day; **Note:** May divided into 2-3 doses for day or give as continuous infusion over 24 hours

Ophthalmic (Restasis®):

Children <16 years: Dosage not established

Children >16 years: Instill 1 drop in each eye every 12 hours

Adults: Instill 1 drop in each eye every 12 hours

Oral:

Modified:

Children: Transplant: Heart: 7 ± 3 mg/kg/day in 2 divided doses; Liver: 8 ± 4 mg/kg/day in 2 divided doses; Renal: 9 ± 3 mg/kg/day in 2 divided doses

Adults:

Psoriasis: Initial: 2.5 mg/kg/day in 2 divided doses; Maintenance: May increase by 0.5 mg/kg/day after 4 weeks, if insufficient response; additional dosage increases may be made every 2 weeks if needed (maximum: 4 mg/kg/day; 1 year).

Rheumatoid arthritis: Initial: 2.5 mg/kg/day in 2 divided doses; Maintenance: May increase by 0.5-0.75 mg/kg/day after 8 weeks, if insufficient response; additional dosage increases may be made again at 12 weeks (maximum: 4 mg/kg/day)

Transplant: Heart: 7 ± 3 mg/kg/day in 2 divided doses; Liver: 8 ± 4 mg/kg/day in 2 divided doses; Renal: 9 ± 3 mg/kg/day in 2 divided doses

Non-modified:

Children: Initial: 10-18 mg/kg/day for 1-2 weeks; Maintenance: Taper by 5% per week to 3-10 mg/kg/day

Adults: Initial: 10-18 mg/kg/day for 1-2 weeks; Maintenance: Taper by 5% per week to 3-10 mg/kg/day

Dosage Forms Excipient information presented when available (limited, particularly for generics); consult specific product labeling.

Capsule [modified]:

Gengraf®: 25 mg [contains alcohol 12.8%]; 100 mg [contains alcohol 12.8%]

Capsule [non-modified]: 25 mg, 100 mg

Capsule, soft gel [modified]: 25 mg, 50 mg, 100 mg

Neoral®: 25 mg [contains alcohol 11.9% and corn oil]; 100 mg [contains alcohol 11.9% and corn oil]

Capsule, soft gel [non-modified]:

Sandimmune®: 25 mg [contains alcohol 12.7% and corn oil]; 100 mg [contains alcohol 12.7% and corn oil]

Emulsion, ophthalmic [preservative free]:

Restasis®: 0.05% (0.4 mL) [contains 30 single-use vials/box]

Injection, solution [non-modified]: 50 mg/mL (5 mL)

Sandimmune®: 50 mg/mL (5 mL) [contains Cremophor® EL (polyoxyethylated castor oil) and alcohol 32.9%]

Solution, oral [modified]: 100 mg/mL (50 mL)

Gengraf®: 100 mg/mL (50 mL) [contains propylene glycol]

Neoral®: 100 mg/mL (50 mL) [contains alcohol 11.9%, corn oil, and propylene glycol]

Solution, oral [non-modified]: 100 mg/mL (50 mL)

Sandimmune®: 100 mg/mL (50 mL) [contains alcohol 12.5%]

◆ **Cylate™** *see* Cyclopentolate *on page 407*

◆ **Cymbalta®** *see* DULoxetine *on page 516*

Cyproheptadine (si proe HEP ta deen)

Medication Safety Issues

Sound-alike/look-alike issues:

Cyproheptadine may be confused with cyclobenzaprine

Periactin may be confused with Perative®, Percodan®, Persantine®

Mexican Brand Names Pangavit Pediátrico

Index Terms Cyproheptadine Hydrochloride; Periactin

Pharmacologic Category Histamine H_1 Antagonist; Histamine H_1 Antagonist, First Generation

Generic Available Yes

Use Perennial and seasonal allergic rhinitis and other allergic symptoms including urticaria

Unlabeled/Investigational Use Appetite stimulation, blepharospasm, cluster headaches, migraine headaches, Nelson's syndrome, pruritus, schizophrenia, spinal cord damage associated spasticity, and tardive dyskinesia

Effect on Mental Status Drowsiness is common; may cause nervousness or depression

Effect on Psychiatric Treatment Contraindicated with MAO inhibitors; concurrent use with psychotropic may produce additive sedation

Pregnancy Risk Factor B

Lactation Excretion in breast milk unknown/contraindicated

Contraindications Hypersensitivity to cyproheptadine or any component of the formulation; narrow-angle glaucoma; bladder neck obstruction; symptomatic prostatic hyperplasia; acute asthmatic attack; stenosing peptic ulcer; GI tract obstruction; concurrent use of MAO inhibitors; avoid use in premature and term newborns due to potential association with SIDS

Warnings/Precautions May cause CNS depression, which may impair physical or mental abilities; patients must be cautioned about performing tasks which require mental alertness (eg, operating machinery or driving). Effects may be potentiated when used with other sedative drugs or ethanol. Use with caution in patients with cardiovascular disease; increased intraocular pressure; respiratory disease; or thyroid dysfunction. Use with caution in the elderly; may be more sensitive to adverse effects. In case reports, cyproheptadine has promoted weight gain in anorexic adults, though it has not been specifically studied in the elderly. All cases of weight loss or decreased appetite should be adequately assessed. Antihistamines may cause excitation in young children. Safety and efficacy have not been established in children <2 years of age.

Adverse Reactions

>10%:

Central nervous system: Slight to moderate drowsiness

Respiratory: Thickening of bronchial secretions

1% to 10%:

Central nervous system: Dizziness, fatigue, headache, nervousness

Gastrointestinal: Abdominal pain, appetitie stimulation, diarrhea, nausea, xerostomia

Neuromuscular & skeletal: Arthralgia

Respiratory: Pharyngitis

<1% (Limited to important or life-threatening): Bronchospasm, CNS stimulation, depression, epistaxis, hemolytic anemia, hepatitis, leukopenia, sedation, seizure, thrombocytopenia

Drug Interactions

Acetylcholinesterase Inhibitors (Central): Anticholinergics may diminish the therapeutic effect of Acetylcholinesterase Inhibitors (Central). Acetylcholinesterase Inhibitors (Central) may diminish the therapeutic effect of Anticholinergics. If the anticholinergic action is a side effect of the agent, the result may be beneficial. *Risk C: Monitor therapy*

Alcohol (Ethyl): CNS Depressants may enhance the CNS depressant effect of Alcohol (Ethyl). *Risk C: Monitor therapy*

Amphetamines: May diminish the sedative effect of Antihistamines. *Risk C: Monitor therapy*

Anticholinergics: May enhance the adverse/toxic effect of other Anticholinergics. **Exceptions:** Paliperidone. *Risk C: Monitor therapy*

Betahistine: Antihistamines may diminish the therapeutic effect of Betahistine. *Risk C: Monitor therapy*

CNS Depressants: May enhance the adverse/toxic effect of other CNS Depressants. *Risk C: Monitor therapy*

Pramlintide: May enhance the anticholinergic effect of Anticholinergics. These effects are specific to the GI tract. *Risk D: Consider therapy modification*

Selective Serotonin Reuptake Inhibitors: Cyproheptadine may diminish the therapeutic effect of Selective Serotonin Reuptake Inhibitors. *Risk C: Monitor therapy*

Ethanol/Nutrition/Herb Interactions Ethanol: Avoid ethanol (may increase CNS sedation).

Mechanism of Action A potent antihistamine and serotonin antagonist, competes with histamine for H_1-receptor sites on effector cells in the gastrointestinal tract, blood vessels, and respiratory tract

Pharmacodynamics/Kinetics

Absorption: Completely

Metabolism: Almost completely hepatic

Excretion: Urine (>50% primarily as metabolites); feces (~25%)

Dosage Oral:

Children:

Allergic conditions: 0.25 mg/kg/day or 8 mg/m^2/day in 2-3 divided doses **or**

2-6 years: 2 mg every 8-12 hours (not to exceed 12 mg/day)

7-14 years: 4 mg every 8-12 hours (not to exceed 16 mg/day)

Migraine headaches: 4 mg 2-3 times/day

Children ≥12 years and Adults: Spasticity associated with spinal cord damage: 4 mg at bedtime; increase by a 4 mg dose every 3-4 days; average daily dose: 16 mg in divided doses; not to exceed 36 mg/day

Children >13 years and Adults: Appetite stimulation (anorexia nervosa): 2 mg 4 times/day; may be increased gradually over a 3-week period to 8 mg 4 times/day

Adults:

Allergic conditions: 4-20 mg/day divided every 8 hours (not to exceed 0.5 mg/kg/day)

Cluster headaches: 4 mg 4 times/day

Migraine headaches: 4-8 mg 3 times/day

Dosage adjustment in hepatic impairment: Reduce dosage in patients with significant hepatic dysfunction

Test Interactions Diagnostic antigen skin test results may be suppressed; false positive serum TCA screen

Additional Information May stimulate appetite. In case reports, cyproheptadine has promoted weight gain in anorexic adults.

Dosage Forms Excipient information presented when available (limited, particularly for generics); consult specific product labeling.

Syrup, as hydrochloride: 2 mg/5 mL (473 mL) [contains alcohol 5%; mint flavor]

Tablet, as hydrochloride: 4 mg

◆ **Cyproheptadine Hydrochloride** *see* Cyproheptadine *on page 410*

◆ **Cystagon®** *see* Cysteamine *on page 412*

Cysteamine (sis TEE a meen)

U.S. Brand Names Cystagon®

Index Terms Cysteamine Bitartrate

Pharmacologic Category Anticystine Agent; Urinary Tract Product

Use Treatment of nephropathic cystinosis

Effect on Mental Status Sedation is common; may cause confusion, nervousness, impaired cognition, and hallucinations

Effect on Psychiatric Treatment Concurrent use with psychotropic may produce additive sedation

Dosage Summary Note: Initial dose should be 1/4 to 1/6 of maintenance dose

Oral:

Children <12 years: Maintenance: 1.3 g/m^2/day **or** 60 mg/kg/day in 4 divided doses (maximum dose: 1.95 g/m^2/day; 90 mg/kg/day)

Children ≥12 years and >110 lbs: Maintenance: 2 g/day in 4 divided doses (maximum: 1.95 g/m^2/day; 90 mg/kg/day)

Adults >110 lbs: Maintenance: 2 g/day in 4 divided doses (maximum: 1.95 g/m^2/day; 90 mg/kg/day)

Dosage Forms Excipient information presented when available (limited, particularly for generics); consult specific product labeling.

Capsule:

Cystagon®: 50 mg, 150 mg

◆ **Cysteamine Bitartrate** *see* Cysteamine *on page 412*

◆ **Cystospaz®** *see* Hyoscyamine *on page 799*

◆ **CYT** *see* Cyclophosphamide *on page 408*

◆ **Cytadren®** *see* Aminoglutethimide *on page 87*

Cytarabine (sye TARE a been)

Medication Safety Issues

Sound-alike/look-alike issues:

Cytarabine may be confused with Cytadren®, Cytosar®, Cytoxan®, vidarabine

Cytarabine (conventional) may be confused with cytarabine liposomal

Cytosar-U may be confused with cytarabine, Cytovene®, Cytoxan®, Neosar®

High alert medication: The Institute for Safe Medication Practices (ISMP) includes this medication among its list of drugs which have a heightened risk of causing significant patient harm when used in error.

Canadian Brand Names Cytosar®

Mexican Brand Names Laracit; Medsara

Index Terms Ara-C; Arabinosylcytosine; Cytarabine (Conventional); Cytarabine Hydrochloride; Cytosar-U; Cytosine Arabinosine Hydrochloride; NSC-63878

Pharmacologic Category Antineoplastic Agent, Antimetabolite; Antineoplastic Agent, Antimetabolite (Pyrimidine Analog)

Use Treatment of acute myeloid leukemia (AML), acute lymphocytic leukemia (ALL), chronic myelocytic leukemia (CML; blast phase), and lymphomas; prophylaxis and treatment of meningeal leukemia

Effect on Mental Status May cause sedation or confusion

Effect on Psychiatric Treatment May cause myelosuppression; use caution with clozapine and carbamazepine

Dosage Summary

I.M.:

Children: Dosage not established

Adults: 1-1.5 mg/kg at 1- to 4-week intervals

I.T.:

Children <1 year: 5-75 mg/m^2/dose **or** 15-20 mg per dose every 4 days until CNS findings normalize

Children 1-2 years: 5-75 mg/m^2/dose **or** 16-30 mg per dose every 4 days until CNS findings normalize

Children 2-3 years: 5-75 mg/m^2/dose **or** 20-50 mg per dose every 4 days until CNS findings normalize

Children >3 years: 5-75 mg/m^2/dose **or** 24-70 mg per dose every 4 days until CNS findings normalize

Adults: 5-75 mg/m^2/dose every 2-7 days until CNS findings normalize

I.V.:

Children: 75-200 mg/m^2/day for 5-10 days **or** every day until remission

Adults: Induction: 100-200 mg/m^2/day for 5-10-days, may repeat in 2-4 weeks if needed or 100 mg/m^2/day every 12 hours for 7 days; Maintenance: 70-200 mg/m^2/day for 2-5 days at monthly intervals; High dose: 1-3 g/m^2 every 12 hours for up to 12 doses (leukemia/lymphoma)

SubQ:

Children: Dosage not established

Adults: 1-1.5 mg/kg at 1- to 4-week intervals

Dosage Forms Excipient information presented when available (limited, particularly for generics); consult specific product labeling.

Injection, powder for reconstitution: 100 mg, 500 mg, 1 g, 2 g

Injection, solution: 20 mg/mL (5 mL, 25 mL, 50 mL); 100 mg/mL (20 mL)

◆ **Cytarabine (Conventional)** *see* Cytarabine *on page 412*

◆ **Cytarabine Hydrochloride** *see* Cytarabine *on page 412*

Cytarabine (Liposomal) (sye TARE a been lip po SOE mal)

Medication Safety Issues

Sound-alike/look-alike issues:

Cytarabine may be confused with Cytadren®, Cytosar®, Cytoxan®, vidarabine

Cytarabine liposomal may be confused with conventional cytarabine

DepoCyt® may be confused with Depoject®

High alert medication: The Institute for Safe Medication Practices (ISMP) includes this medication among its list of drugs which have a heightened risk of causing significant patient harm when used in error.

U.S. Brand Names DepoCyt®

Canadian Brand Names DepoCyt®

Pharmacologic Category Antineoplastic Agent, Antimetabolite (Pyrimidine Antagonist)

Use Treatment of lymphomatous meningitis

Effect on Mental Status Cerebellar syndrome is common; may cause dizziness, confusion, or sedation

Effect on Psychiatric Treatment Myelosuppression is common; use caution with clozapine and carbamazepine. GI side effects are common and dose related; use caution with SSRIs.

Dosage Summary

I.T.:

Children: Dosage not established

Adults: Induction: 50 mg every 14 days for a total of 2 doses (weeks 1 and 3); Consolidation: 50 mg every 14 days for 3 doses (weeks 5, 7, and 9), followed by 50 mg at week 13; Maintenance: 50 mg every 28 days for 4 doses (weeks 17, 21, 25, and 29)

Dosage Forms Excipient information presented when available (limited, particularly for generics); consult specific product labeling.

Injection, suspension, intrathecal [preservative free]:

Depocyt®: 10 mg/mL (5 mL)

◆ **Cytomel®** *see* Liothyronine *on page 928*

◆ **Cytosar-U** *see* Cytarabine *on page 412*

◆ **Cytosine Arabinosine Hydrochloride** *see* Cytarabine *on page 412*

◆ **Cytostasan** *see* Bendamustine *on page 179*

◆ **Cytovene®** *see* Ganciclovir *on page 708*

- **Cytoxan® [DSC]** *see* Cyclophosphamide *on page 408*
- **Cytuss HC** *see* Phenylephrine, Hydrocodone, and Chlorpheniramine *on page 1277*
- **D2E7** *see* Adalimumab *on page 50*
- **D_3** *see* Cholecalciferol *on page 341*
- **D-3 [OTC]** *see* Cholecalciferol *on page 341*
- **D3-5™ [OTC]** *see* Cholecalciferol *on page 341*
- **D3-50™ [OTC]** *see* Cholecalciferol *on page 341*
- **D-3-Mercaptovaline** *see* Penicillamine *on page 1239*
- **d4T** *see* Stavudine *on page 1505*
- **DAB_{389}IL-2** *see* Denileukin Diftitox *on page 425*
- **DAB389 Interleukin-2** *see* Denileukin Diftitox *on page 425*

Dacarbazine (da KAR ba zeen)

Medication Safety Issues
Sound-alike/look-alike issues:
Dacarbazine may be confused with Dicarbosil®, procarbazine

High alert medication: The Institute for Safe Medication Practices (ISMP) includes this medication among its list of drugs which have a heightened risk of causing significant patient harm when used in error.

Canadian Brand Names DTIC®

Mexican Brand Names Detilem

Index Terms DIC; Dimethyl Triazeno Imidazole Carboxamide; DTIC; Imidazole Carboxamide; Imidazole Carboxamide Dimethyltriazene; WR-139007

Pharmacologic Category Antineoplastic Agent, Alkylating Agent (Triazene)

Use Treatment of malignant melanoma, Hodgkin's disease, soft-tissue sarcomas, fibrosarcomas, rhabdomyosarcoma, islet cell carcinoma, medullary carcinoma of the thyroid, and neuroblastoma

Effect on Mental Status May cause headache

Effect on Psychiatric Treatment May cause myelosuppression; use caution with clozapine and carbamazepine

Dosage Forms Excipient information presented when available (limited, particularly for generics); consult specific product labeling.
Injection, powder for reconstitution: 100 mg, 200 mg

- **Dacex-DM** *see* Guaifenesin, Dextromethorphan, and Phenylephrine *on page 746*

Daclizumab (dac KLYE zue mab)

U.S. Brand Names Zenapax®

Canadian Brand Names Zenapax®

Mexican Brand Names Zenapax

Pharmacologic Category Immunosuppressant Agent

Use Part of an immunosuppressive regimen (including cyclosporine and corticosteroids) for the prophylaxis of acute organ rejection in patients receiving renal transplant

Unlabeled/Investigational Use Graft-versus-host disease; prevention of organ rejection after heart transplant

Effect on Mental Status May cause depression, anxiety, or insomnia

Effect on Psychiatric Treatment None reported

Dosage Summary
I.V.:
Children: 1 mg/kg within 24 hours before transplantation (day 0), then every 14 days for 4 additional doses
Adults: 1 mg/kg within 24 hours before transplantation (day 0), then every 14 days for 4 additional doses

Dosage Forms Excipient information presented when available (limited, particularly for generics); consult specific product labeling.
Injection, solution [concentrate; preservative free]:
Zenapax®: 5 mg/mL (5 mL) [contains polysorbate 80]

- **Dacogen™** *see* Decitabine *on page 422*
- **DACT** *see* DACTINomycin *on page 415*

DACTINomycin (dak ti noe MYE sin)

Medication Safety Issues

Sound-alike/look-alike issues:

DACTINomycin may be confused with DAPTOmycin, DAUNOrubicin

Actinomycin may be confused with achromycin

High alert medication: The Institute for Safe Medication Practices (ISMP) includes this medication among its list of drugs which have a heightened risk of causing significant patient harm when used in error.

U.S. Brand Names Cosmegen®

Canadian Brand Names Cosmegen®

Mexican Brand Names Ac-De

Index Terms ACT; Act-D; Actinomycin; Actinomycin Cl; Actinomycin D; DACT; NSC-3053

Pharmacologic Category Antineoplastic Agent, Antibiotic

Use Treatment of testicular tumors, melanoma, gestational trophoblastic neoplasm, Wilms' tumor, neuroblastoma, retinoblastoma, rhabdomyosarcoma, uterine sarcomas, Ewing's sarcoma, Kaposi's sarcoma, sarcoma botryoides, and soft tissue sarcoma

Effect on Mental Status Sedation is common

Effect on Psychiatric Treatment May cause myelosuppression; use caution with clozapine and carbamazepine

Dosage Summary

I.V.:

Children ≤6 months: Dosage not established

Children >6 months: 15 mcg/kg/day **or** 400-600 mcg/m^2/day for 5 days every 3-6 weeks

Adults: 2.5 mg/m^2 in divided doses over 1 week, repeated every 2 weeks **or** 12-15 mcg/kg/day for 5 days **or** 0.75-2 mg/m^2 every 1-4 weeks **or** 400-600 mcg/m^2/day for 2-5 days, repeated every 3-6 weeks

Dosage Forms Excipient information presented when available (limited, particularly for generics); consult specific product labeling.

Injection, powder for reconstitution:

Cosmegen®: 0.5 mg [contains mannitol 20 mg]

- **Dallergy®** *see* Chlorpheniramine, Phenylephrine, and Methscopolamine *on page 329*
- **Dallergy Drops** *see* Chlorpheniramine and Phenylephrine *on page 323*
- **Dallergy®-JR** *see* Chlorpheniramine and Phenylephrine *on page 323*
- **Dalmane®** *see* Flurazepam *on page 664*
- **d-Alpha-Gems™ [OTC]** *see* Vitamin E *on page 1675*
- ***d*-Alpha Tocopherol** *see* Vitamin E *on page 1675*

Danaparoid (da NAP a roid)

Medication Safety Issues

Sound-alike/look-alike issues:

Orgaran® may be confused with argatroban

Canadian Brand Names Orgaran®

Index Terms Danaparoid Sodium

Pharmacologic Category Anticoagulant

Use Prevention of postoperative deep vein thrombosis following elective hip replacement surgery

Unlabeled/Investigational Use Systemic anticoagulation for patients with heparin-induced thrombocytopenia: factor Xa inhibition is used to monitor degree of anticoagulation if necessary

Effect on Mental Status May cause insomnia

Effect on Psychiatric Treatment None reported

Restrictions Not available in U.S.

Dosage Summary

SubQ:

Children: Dosage not established

Adults: 750 anti-Xa units every 12 hours

Dosage Forms Excipient information presented when available (limited, particularly for generics); consult specific product labeling. [CAN] = Canadian brand name

Injection, solution:

Orgaran® [CAN]: 750 anti-Xa units/0.6 mL (0.6 mL) [not available in the U.S.]

◆ **Danaparoid Sodium** *see* Danaparoid *on page 415*

Danazol (DA na zole)

Medication Safety Issues

Sound-alike/look-alike issues:

Danazol may be confused with Dantrium®

Danocrine® may be confused with Dacriose®

U.S. Brand Names Danocrine® [DSC]

Canadian Brand Names Cyclomen®; Danocrine®

Mexican Brand Names Ladogal; Novaprin

Pharmacologic Category Androgen

Use Treatment of endometriosis, fibrocystic breast disease, and hereditary angioedema

Effect on Mental Status May cause dizziness

Effect on Psychiatric Treatment None reported

Dosage Summary

Oral:

Children: Dosage not established

Adults (females): 100-800 mg/day in 2 divided doses

Adults (females/males): Hereditary angioedema: Initial: 200 mg 2-3 times/day, after favorable response decrease dosage by 50% or less at intervals of 1-3 months

Dosage Forms Excipient information presented when available (limited, particularly for generics); consult specific product labeling. [DSC] = Discontinued product

Capsule: 50 mg, 100 mg, 200 mg

Danocrine®: 50 mg, 100 mg, 200 mg [DSC]

◆ **Danocrine® [DSC]** *see* Danazol *on page 416*

◆ **Dantrium®** *see* Dantrolene *on page 416*

Dantrolene (DAN troe leen)

Medication Safety Issues

Sound-alike/look-alike issues:

Dantrium® may be confused with danazol, Daraprim®

U.S. Brand Names Dantrium®

Canadian Brand Names Dantrium®

Index Terms Dantrolene Sodium

Pharmacologic Category Skeletal Muscle Relaxant

Generic Available Yes: Capsule

Use Treatment of spasticity associated with spinal cord injury, stroke, cerebral palsy, or multiple sclerosis; treatment of malignant hyperthermia

Unlabeled/Investigational Use Neuroleptic malignant syndrome (NMS)

Effect on Mental Status Drowsiness is common; may cause insomnia, nervousness, confusion, or depression

Effect on Psychiatric Treatment Concurrent use with psychotropic may result in additive sedation; use to treat neuroleptic malignant syndrome

Pregnancy Risk Factor C

Lactation Excretion in breast milk unknown/not recommended

Contraindications Active hepatic disease; should not be used where spasticity is used to maintain posture or balance

Warnings/Precautions Use with caution in patients with impaired cardiac function or impaired pulmonary function. **[U.S. Boxed Warning]: Has potential for hepatotoxicity.** Overt hepatitis has been most frequently observed between the third and twelfth month of therapy. Hepatic injury appears to be greater in females and in patients >35 years of age. Idiosyncratic and hypersensitivity reactions (sometimes fatal) of the liver have also occurred.

Adverse Reactions

>10%:

Central nervous system: Drowsiness, dizziness, lightheadedness, fatigue

Dermatologic: Rash

Gastrointestinal: Diarrhea (mild), vomiting

Neuromuscular & skeletal: Muscle weakness

1% to 10%:

Cardiovascular: Pleural effusion with pericarditis

Central nervous system: Chills, fever, headache, insomnia, nervousness, mental depression

Gastrointestinal: Diarrhea (severe), constipation, anorexia, stomach cramps

Ocular: Blurred vision

Respiratory: Respiratory depression

<1% (Limited to important or life-threatening): Confusion, hepatic necrosis, hepatitis, seizure

Metabolism/Transport Effects Substrate of CYP3A4 (major)

Drug Interactions

Alcohol (Ethyl): CNS Depressants may enhance the CNS depressant effect of Alcohol (Ethyl). *Risk C: Monitor therapy*

CNS Depressants: May enhance the adverse/toxic effect of other CNS Depressants. *Risk C: Monitor therapy*

CYP3A4 Inducers (Strong): May increase the metabolism of CYP3A4 Substrates. *Risk C: Monitor therapy*

CYP3A4 Inhibitors (Moderate): May decrease the metabolism of CYP3A4 Substrates. *Risk C: Monitor therapy*

CYP3A4 Inhibitors (Strong): May decrease the metabolism of CYP3A4 Substrates. *Risk D: Consider therapy modification*

Dasatinib: May increase the serum concentration of CYP3A4 Substrates. *Risk C: Monitor therapy*

Deferasirox: May decrease the serum concentration of CYP3A4 Substrates. *Risk C: Monitor therapy*

Herbs (CYP3A4 Inducers): May increase the metabolism of CYP3A4 Substrates. *Risk C: Monitor therapy*

Ethanol/Nutrition/Herb Interactions

Ethanol: Avoid ethanol (may increase CNS depression).

Herb/Nutraceutical: Avoid valerian, St John's wort, kava kava, gotu kola (may increase CNS depression).

Stability Reconstitute vial by adding 60 mL of sterile water for injection USP (**not bacteriostatic water for injection**). Protect from light. Use within 6 hours; avoid glass bottles for I.V. infusion.

Mechanism of Action Acts directly on skeletal muscle by interfering with release of calcium ion from the sarcoplasmic reticulum; prevents or reduces the increase in myoplasmic calcium ion concentration that activates the acute catabolic processes associated with malignant hyperthermia

Pharmacodynamics/Kinetics

Absorption: Oral: Slow and incomplete

Metabolism: Hepatic

Half-life elimination: 8.7 hours

Excretion: Feces (45% to 50%); urine (25% as unchanged drug and metabolites)

Dosage

Spasticity: Oral:

Children: Initial: 0.5 mg/kg/dose twice daily, increase frequency to 3-4 times/day at 4- to 7-day intervals, then increase dose by 0.5 mg/kg to a maximum of 3 mg/kg/dose 2-4 times/day up to 400 mg/day

Adults: 25 mg/day to start, increase frequency to 2-4 times/day, then increase dose by 25 mg every 4-7 days to a maximum of 100 mg 2-4 times/day or 400 mg/day

Malignant hyperthermia: Children and Adults:

Preoperative prophylaxis:

Oral: 4-8 mg/kg/day in 4 divided doses, begin 1-2 days prior to surgery with last dose 3-4 hours prior to surgery

I.V.: 2.5 mg/kg ~1¼ hours prior to anesthesia and infused over 1 hour with additional doses as needed and individualized

Crisis: I.V.: 2.5 mg/kg; may repeat dose up to cumulative dose of 10 mg/kg; if physiologic and metabolic abnormalities reappear, repeat regimen

Postcrisis follow-up: Oral: 4-8 mg/kg/day in 4 divided doses for 1-3 days; I.V. dantrolene may be used when oral therapy is not practical; individualize dosage beginning with 1 mg/kg or more as the clinical situation dictates

Neuroleptic malignant syndrome (unlabeled use): I.V.: 1 mg/kg; may repeat dose up to maximum cumulative dose of 10 mg/kg, then switch to oral dosage

Administration I.V.: Therapeutic or emergency dose can be administered with rapid continuous I.V. push. Follow-up doses should be administered over 2-3 minutes.

Monitoring Parameters Motor performance should be monitored for therapeutic outcomes; nausea, vomiting, and liver function tests should be monitored for potential hepatotoxicity; intravenous administration requires cardiac monitor and blood pressure monitor

Dosage Forms Excipient information presented when available (limited, particularly for generics); consult specific product labeling.

Capsule, as sodium: 25 mg, 50 mg, 100 mg

Dantrium®: 25 mg, 50 mg, 100 mg
Injection, powder for reconstitution, as sodium:
Dantrium®: 20 mg [contains mannitol 3 g]

◆ **Dantrolene Sodium** *see* Dantrolene *on page 416*

◆ **Dapcin** *see* DAPTOmycin *on page 418*

Dapsone (DAP sone)

Medication Safety Issues
Sound-alike/look-alike issues:
Dapsone may be confused with Diprosone®

U.S. Brand Names Aczone®

Mexican Brand Names Dapsoderm-X

Index Terms Diaminodiphenylsulfone

Pharmacologic Category Antibiotic, Miscellaneous; Topical Skin Product, Acne

Use Treatment of leprosy and dermatitis herpetiformis (infections caused by *Mycobacterium leprae*); topical treatment of acne vulgaris

Unlabeled/Investigational Use Prophylaxis of toxoplasmosis in severely-immunocompromised patients; alternative agent for *Pneumocystis carinii* pneumonia prophylaxis (monotherapy) and treatment (in combination with trimethoprim)

Effect on Mental Status May cause insomnia

Effect on Psychiatric Treatment None reported

Dosage Summary

Oral:
Children: 1-2 mg/kg once daily (maximum: 100 mg/day)
Adults: 50-300 mg once daily

Topical:
Children <12 years: Dosage not established
Children ≥12 years: Apply pea-sized amount (approximately) in thin layer to affected areas twice daily
Adults: Apply pea-sized amount (approximately) in thin layer to affected areas twice daily

Dosage Forms Excipient information presented when available (limited, particularly for generics); consult specific product labeling.
Gel, topical:
Aczone®: 5% (30 g)
Tablet: 25 mg, 100 mg

DAPTOmycin (DAP toe mye sin)

Medication Safety Issues
Sound-alike/look-alike issues:
Cubicin® may be confused with Cleocin®
DAPTOmycin may be confused with DACTINomycin

U.S. Brand Names Cubicin®

Canadian Brand Names Cubicin®

Index Terms Cidecin; Dapcin; LY146032

Pharmacologic Category Antibiotic, Cyclic Lipopeptide

Use Treatment of complicated skin and skin structure infections caused by susceptible aerobic gram-positive organisms; *Staphylococcus aureus* bacteremia, including right-sided infective endocarditis caused by MSSA or MRSA

Unlabeled/Investigational Use Treatment of severe infections caused by MRSA or VRE

Effect on Mental Status May cause insomnia or dizziness

Effect on Psychiatric Treatment May cause nausea, vomiting, and diarrhea; concurrent use with SSRIs may produce additive effects

Dosage Summary

I.V.:
Children: Dosage not established
Adults: 4-6 mg/kg once daily

Dosage Forms Excipient information presented when available (limited, particularly for generics); consult specific product labeling.
Injection, powder for reconstitution:
Cubicin®: 500 mg

◆ **Daranide®** *see* Dichlorphenamide *on page 457*

◆ **Daraprim®** *see* Pyrimethamine *on page 1377*

Darbepoetin Alfa (dar be POE e tin AL fa)

Medication Safety Issues

Sound-alike/look-alike issues:

Aranesp® may be confused with Aralast, Aricept®

Darbepoetin alfa may be confused with dalteparin, epoetin alfa, epoetin beta

U.S. Brand Names Aranesp®

Canadian Brand Names Aranesp®

Index Terms Erythropoiesis-Stimulating Agent (ESA); Erythropoiesis-Stimulating Protein; NSC-729969

Pharmacologic Category Colony Stimulating Factor; Growth Factor; Recombinant Human Erythropoietin

Use Treatment of anemia (elevate/maintain red blood cell level and decrease the need for transfusions) associated with chronic renal failure (including patients on dialysis and not on dialysis); treatment of anemia due to concurrent chemotherapy in patients with metastatic cancer (nonmyeloid malignancies)

Note: Darbepoetin is **not** indicated for use in cancer patients under the following conditions:

- receiving hormonal therapy, therapeutic biologic products, or radiation therapy unless also receiving concurrent myelosuppressive chemotherapy
- receiving myelosuppressive therapy when the expected outcome is curative

Unlabeled/Investigational Use Treatment of symptomatic anemia in myelodysplastic syndrome (MDS)

Effect on Mental Status May cause sedation or dizziness

Effect on Psychiatric Treatment Nausea, vomiting, and diarrhea are common; use caution with lithium, valproic acid, and SSRIs

Restrictions An FDA-approved medication guide is available; distribute to each patient to whom this medication is dispensed.

Dosage Summary

I.V.:

Children <1 year: Dosage not established

Children 1-18 years: 6.25-200 mcg/week

Adults: 0.45 mcg/kg once weekly **or** 0.75 mcg/kg once every 2 weeks (alternate dose for nondialysis patients); titrate to hemoglobin response

SubQ:

Children <1 year: Dosage not established

Children 1-18 years: 6.25-200 mcg/week

Adults: 0.45-4.5 mcg/kg/week **or** 0.75 mcg/kg once every 2 weeks (alternate dose for nondialysis patients) or 500 mcg once every 3 weeks; titrate to hemoglobin response

Dosage Forms Excipient information presented when available (limited, particularly for generics); consult specific product labeling.

Injection, solution [preservative free]:

Aranesp®: 25 mcg/0.42 mL (0.42 mL); 40 mcg/ 0.4 mL (0.4 mL); 60 mcg/0.3 mL (0.3 mL); 100 mcg/0.5 mL (0.5 mL); 150 mcg/0.3 mL (0.3 mL); 200 mcg/0.4 mL (0.4 mL); 300 mcg/0.6 mL (0.6 mL); 500 mcg/mL (1 mL) [contains polysorbate 80; prefilled syringe; needle cover contains latex]

Aranesp®: 25 mcg/mL (1 mL); 40 mcg/mL (1 mL); 60 mcg/mL (1 mL); 100 mcg/mL (1 mL); 150 mcg/0.75 mL (0.75 mL); 200 mcg/mL (1 mL); 300 mcg/mL (1 mL) [contains polysorbate 80; single-dose vial]

Darifenacin (dar i FEN a sin)

U.S. Brand Names Enablex®

Canadian Brand Names Enablex®

Index Terms Darifenacin Hydrobromide; UK-88,525

Pharmacologic Category Anticholinergic Agent

Use Management of symptoms of bladder overactivity (urge incontinence, urgency, and frequency)

Effect on Mental Status May cause dizziness

Effect on Psychiatric Treatment Concomitant use with acetylcholinesterase inhibitors will mitigate their clinical effects. Concomitant use with psychotropic agents may produce additive anticholinergic effects. Darifenacin may increase levels of fluoxetine, mirtazapine, nefazodone, paroxetine, risperidone, thioridazine, TCAs, and venlafaxine.

Dosage Summary

Oral:

Children: Dosage not established

Adults: Initial: 7.5 mg once daily, may increase to 15 mg once daily if response not adequate after 2 weeks

Note: Dosage should not exceed 7.5 mg/day with concurrent CYP3A4 inhibitors

Dosage Forms Excipient information presented when available (limited, particularly for generics); consult specific product labeling.

Tablet, extended release: 7.5 mg, 15 mg

◆ **Darifenacin Hydrobromide** *see* Darifenacin *on page 419*

Darunavir (dar OO na veer)

U.S. Brand Names Prezista®

Index Terms Darunavir Ethanolate; TMC-114

Pharmacologic Category Antiretroviral Agent, Protease Inhibitor

Use Treatment of HIV-1 infections in combination with ritonavir and other antiretroviral agents

Effect on Mental Status May cause headache

Effect on Psychiatric Treatment Contraindicated with midazolam, pimozide, and triazolam. Nausea is common; combined use with lithium, valproic acid, carbamazepine, and SSRIs may produce an additive risk. May cause neutropenia; use clozapine and carbamazepine with caution. Carbamazepine may decrease the levels of darunavir. St John's wort may decrease the plasma levels of darunavir. Concomitant use of darunavir and St John's wort is not recommended.

Dosage Summary

Oral:

Children: Dosage not established

Adults: 600 mg twice daily **or** 800 mg twice daily; **Note:** Coadministration with ritonavir (100 mg once or twice daily) is required

Dosage Forms Excipient information presented when available (limited, particularly for generics); consult specific product labeling.

Tablet:

Prezista®: 300 mg, 400 mg, 600 mg

◆ **Darunavir Ethanolate** *see* Darunavir *on page 420*

◆ **Darvocet A500®** *see* Propoxyphene and Acetaminophen *on page 1354*

◆ **Darvocet-N® 50** *see* Propoxyphene and Acetaminophen *on page 1354*

◆ **Darvocet-N® 100** *see* Propoxyphene and Acetaminophen *on page 1354*

◆ **Darvon®** *see* Propoxyphene *on page 1353*

◆ **Darvon® Compound [DSC]** *see* Propoxyphene, Aspirin, and Caffeine *on page 1355*

◆ **Darvon-N®** *see* Propoxyphene *on page 1353*

Dasatinib (da SA ti nib)

Medication Safety Issues

High alert medication: The Institute for Safe Medication Practices (ISMP) includes this medication among its list of drug classes which have a heightened risk of causing significant patient harm when used in error.

U.S. Brand Names Sprycel®

Canadian Brand Names Sprycel®

Index Terms BMS-354825; NSC-732517

Pharmacologic Category Antineoplastic Agent, Tyrosine Kinase Inhibitor

Use Treatment of chronic myelogenous leukemia (CML) in chronic, accelerated or blast (myeloid or lymphoid) phase resistant or intolerant to prior therapy (including imatinib); treatment of Philadelphia chromosome-positive (Ph+) acute lymphoblastic leukemia (ALL) resistant or intolerant to prior therapy

Effect on Mental Status Headache, fatigue, and dizziness are common; may cause anxiety, confusion, depression, insomnia, or sedation

Effect on Psychiatric Treatment Severe hemorrhage may occur due to thrombocytopenia; monitor valproic acid and derivatives closely. GI side effects are common; combined use with lithium, valproic acid, carbamazepine, and SSRIs may produce an additive risk. Hematologic side effects are common; use clozapine and carbamazepine with caution. Nefazodone may increase the levels of dasatinib. Concomitant use of dasatinib and nefazodone is not recommended.

Dosage Summary

Oral:

Children: Dosage not established

Adults: 70 mg twice daily or 100 mg once daily

Dosage Forms Excipient information presented when available (limited, particularly for generics); consult specific product labeling.

Tablet, oral:

Sprycel®: 20 mg, 50 mg, 70 mg, 100 mg

◆ **Daunomycin** *see* DAUNOrubicin Hydrochloride *on page 421*

DAUNOrubicin Citrate (Liposomal)

(daw noe ROO bi sin SI trate lip po SOE mal)

Medication Safety Issues

Sound-alike/look-alike issues:

DAUNOrubicin liposomal may be confused with DACTINomycin, DOXOrubicin, DOXOrubicin liposomal, epirubicin, IDArubicin

Liposomal formulation (DaunoXome®) may be confused with the conventional formulation (Cerubidine®, Rubex®)

High alert medication: The Institute for Safe Medication Practices (ISMP) includes this medication among its list of drug classes which have a heightened risk of causing significant patient harm when used in error.

U.S. Brand Names DaunoXome®

Index Terms DAUNOrubicin Liposomal; Liposomal DAUNOrubicin; NSC-697732

Pharmacologic Category Antineoplastic Agent, Anthracycline

Use First-line treatment of advanced HIV-associated Kaposi's sarcoma (KS)

Effect on Mental Status May produce myelosuppression; caution with clozapine and carbamazepine

Effect on Psychiatric Treatment None reported

Dosage Summary

I.V.:

Children: Dosage not established

Adults: 40 mg/m^2 every 2 weeks

Dosage Forms Excipient information presented when available (limited, particularly for generics); consult specific product labeling.

Injection, solution [preservative free]:

DaunoXome®: 2 mg/mL (25 mL) [contains sucrose 2125 mg/25 mL]

DAUNOrubicin Hydrochloride

(daw noe ROO bi sin hye droe KLOR ide)

Medication Safety Issues

Sound-alike/look-alike issues:

DAUNOrubicin may be confused with DACTINomycin, DOXOrubicin, DOXOrubicin liposomal, epirubicin, IDArubicin

Conventional formulation (Cerubidine®, DAUNOrubicin hydrochloride) may be confused with the liposomal formulation (DaunoXome®)

High alert medication: The Institute for Safe Medication Practices (ISMP) includes this medication among its list of drug classes which have a heightened risk of causing significant patient harm when used in error.

U.S. Brand Names Cerubidine®

Canadian Brand Names Cerubidine®

Mexican Brand Names Rubilem

Index Terms Daunomycin; NSC-82151; Rubidomycin Hydrochloride

Pharmacologic Category Antineoplastic Agent, Anthracycline

Use Treatment of acute lymphocytic (ALL) and nonlymphocytic (ANLL) leukemias

Effect on Mental Status None reported

Effect on Psychiatric Treatment May produce myelosuppression; use caution with clozapine and carbamazepine

Dosage Summary

I.V.:

Children <2 years or BSA <0.5 m^2: Dose should be based on weight, 1 mg/kg/dose per protocol with frequency dependent on regimen employed (maximum cumulative dose: 10 mg/kg)

Children ≥2 years and BSA ≥0.5 m²: on day 1 every week for 4 cycles **or** 30-60 mg/m²/day for 3 days (maximum cumulative dose: 300 mg/m²)

Adults <60 years: 30-60 mg/m²/day for 2-3 days (maximum cumulative dose: 550 mg/m²; 400 mg/m² with chest irradiation)

Adults ≥60 years: 30 mg/m²/day for 2-3 days (maximum cumulative dose: 550 mg/m²; 400 mg/m² with chest irradiation)

Dosage Forms Excipient information presented when available (limited, particularly for generics); consult specific product labeling. **Note: Strength expressed as base**

Injection, powder for reconstitution: 20 mg

Cerubidine®: 20 mg [contains mannitol 100 mg]

Injection, solution: 5 mg/mL (4 mL, 10 mL)

- **DAUNOrubicin Liposomal** *see* DAUNOrubicin Citrate (Liposomal) *on page 421*
- **DaunoXome®** *see* DAUNOrubicin Citrate (Liposomal) *on page 421*
- **Dayhist® Allergy [OTC]** *see* Clemastine *on page 361*
- **Daypro®** *see* Oxaprozin *on page 1193*
- **Daytrana™** *see* Methylphenidate *on page 1024*
- **dCF** *see* Pentostatin *on page 1250*
- **DDAVP®** *see* Desmopressin *on page 431*
- **ddC** *see* Zalcitabine *on page 1691*
- **ddI** *see* Didanosine *on page 460*
- **1-Deamino-8-D-Arginine Vasopressin** *see* Desmopressin *on page 431*
- **Dec-Chlorphen** *see* Chlorpheniramine and Phenylephrine *on page 323*
- **Dec-Chlorphen DM [DSC]** *see* Chlorpheniramine, Phenylephrine, and Dextromethorphan *on page 327*
- **De-Chlor DM** *see* Chlorpheniramine, Phenylephrine, and Dextromethorphan *on page 327*
- **De-Chlor DR** *see* Chlorpheniramine, Phenylephrine, and Dextromethorphan *on page 327*
- **De-Chlor G [DSC]** *see* Hydrocodone, Phenylephrine, and Guaifenesin *on page 783*
- **De-Chlor HC** *see* Phenylephrine, Hydrocodone, and Chlorpheniramine *on page 1277*

Decitabine (de SYE ta been)

Medication Safety Issues

High alert medication: The Institute for Safe Medication Practices (ISMP) includes this medication among its list of drug classes which have a heightened risk of causing significant patient harm when used in error.

U.S. Brand Names Dacogen™

Index Terms 5-Aza-2'-deoxycytidine; 5-AzaC; NSC-127716

Pharmacologic Category Antineoplastic Agent, DNA Methylation Inhibitor

Use Treatment of myelodysplastic syndrome (MDS)

Unlabeled/Investigational Use Treatment of acute myelogenous leukemia (AML), chronic myelogenous leukemia (CML), sickle cell anemia

Effect on Mental Status Insomnia, dizziness, confusion, lethargy, and anxiety are common

Effect on Psychiatric Treatment GI side effects are common; combined use with lithium, valproic acid, carbamazepine, and SSRIs may produce an additive risk. Neutropenia and thrombocytopenia are common; concomitant use with clozapine, carbamazepine, and valproic acid may produce additive risks.

Dosage Summary

I.V.:

Children: Dosage not established

Adults: MDS: 15 mg/m² over 3 hours every 8 hours for 3 days every 6 weeks

Dosage Forms Excipient information presented when available (limited, particularly for generics); consult specific product labeling.

Injection, powder for reconstitution:

Dacogen™: 50 mg

- **Declomycin®** *see* Demeclocycline *on page 424*
- **Deconamine® SR** *see* Chlorpheniramine and Pseudoephedrine *on page 325*
- **Deconsal® II** *see* Guaifenesin and Phenylephrine *on page 742*
- **Deconsal® CT** *see* Phenylephrine and Pyrilamine *on page 1275*

Deferasirox (de FER a sir ox)

Medication Safety Issues

Sound-alike/look-alike issues:

Deferasirox may be confused with deferoxamine

U.S. Brand Names Exjade®

Canadian Brand Names Exjade®

Mexican Brand Names Exjade

Index Terms ICL670

Pharmacologic Category Antidote; Chelating Agent

Use Treatment of chronic iron overload due to blood transfusions (transfusional hemosiderosis)

Effect on Mental Status May cause dizziness or fatigue; may rarely cause anxiety, hyperactivity, or insomnia

Effect on Psychiatric Treatment Associated with dose-related skin rash; monitor patients receiving anticonvulsants (especially lamotrigine). GI side effects are common; concomitant use with SSRIs, lithium, valproic acid, and carbamazepine may produce additive effects.

Dosage Summary

Oral:

Children <2 years: Dosage not established

Children ≥2 years: Initial: 20 mg/kg once daily; Maintenance: 20-30 mg/kg once daily; **Note:** Titration is recommended

Adults: Initial: 20 mg/kg once daily; Maintenance: 20-30 mg/kg once daily; **Note:** Titration is recommended

Dosage Forms Excipient information presented when available (limited, particularly for generics); consult specific product labeling.

Tablet, for oral suspension:

Exjade®: 125 mg, 250 mg, 500 mg

Deferoxamine (de fer OKS a meen)

Medication Safety Issues

Sound-alike/look-alike issues:

Deferoxamine may be confused with cefuroxime, deferasirox

Desferal® may be confused with desflurane, Dexferrum®, Disophrol®

International issues:

Desferal® may be confused with Deseril® which is a brand name for methysergide in multiple international markets

U.S. Brand Names Desferal®

Canadian Brand Names Desferal®; PMS-Deferoxamine

Mexican Brand Names Desferal

Index Terms Deferoxamine Mesylate; Desferrioxamine; NSC-644468

Pharmacologic Category Antidote; Chelating Agent

Use Acute iron intoxication or when clinical signs of significant iron toxicity exist; chronic iron overload secondary to multiple transfusions

Unlabeled/Investigational Use Removal of corneal rust rings following surgical removal of foreign bodies; diagnosis or treatment of aluminum induced toxicity associated with chronic kidney disease (CKD)

Effect on Mental Status None reported

Effect on Psychiatric Treatment Loss of consciousness has been reported with concurrent use of prochlorperazine

Dosage Summary

I.M.:

Children <3 years: Dosage not established

Children ≥3 years: 90 mg/kg/dose every 8 hours (maximum: 6 g/24 hours)

Adults: Initial: 1000 mg, followed by 500 mg every 4 hours for up to 2 doses; Maintenance: 500 mg every 4-12 hours or 500-1000 mg once daily (maximum: 6 g/day)

I.V.:

Children <3 years: Dosage not established

Children ≥3 years: 15 mg/kg/hour (maximum: 6-12 g/24 hours)

Adults: Initial: 1000 mg, followed by 500 mg every 4 hours for up to 2 doses; Maintenance: 500 mg every 4-12 hours or 2000 mg with each unit of blood (maximum: 1-6 g/day)

SubQ:

Children <3 years: Dosage not established

Children ≥3 years: 20-40 mg/kg/day over 8-12 hours (maximum: 2000 mg/day)

Adults: 1-2 g once daily over 8-24 hours

Dosage Forms Excipient information presented when available (limited, particularly for generics); consult specific product labeling.
Injection, powder for reconstitution, as mesylate: 500 mg, 2 g
Desferal®: 500 mg, 2 g

- ◆ **Deferoxamine Mesylate** *see* Deferoxamine *on page 423*
- ◆ **Dehistine** *see* Chlorpheniramine, Phenylephrine, and Methscopolamine *on page 329*
- ◆ **Dehydrobenzperidol** *see* Droperidol *on page 513*
- ◆ **Delatestryl®** *see* Testosterone *on page 1553*

Delavirdine (de la VIR deen)

U.S. Brand Names Rescriptor®
Canadian Brand Names Rescriptor®
Index Terms U-90152S
Pharmacologic Category Antiretroviral Agent, Reverse Transcriptase Inhibitor (Non-nucleoside)
Use Treatment of HIV-1 infection in combination with at least two additional antiretroviral agents
Effect on Mental Status May cause sedation
Effect on Psychiatric Treatment Fluoxetine may increase plasma concentrations of delavirdine; carbamazepine and phenobarbital may decrease plasma concentrations of delavirdine; delavirdine may increase concentrations of alprazolam, midazolam, and triazolam
Dosage Summary
Oral:
Children <16 years: Dosage not established
Children ≥16 years: 400 mg 3 times/day
Adults: 400 mg 3 times/day
Dosage Forms Excipient information presented when available (limited, particularly for generics); consult specific product labeling.
Tablet, as mesylate: 100 mg, 200 mg

- ◆ **Delestrogen®** *see* Estradiol *on page 576*
- ◆ **Delsym® [OTC]** *see* Dextromethorphan *on page 448*
- ◆ **Delta-9-tetrahydro-cannabinol** *see* Dronabinol *on page 512*
- ◆ **Delta-9-Tetrahydrocannabinol and Cannabinol** *see* Tetrahydrocannabinol and Cannabidiol *on page 1558*
- ◆ **Delta-9 THC** *see* Dronabinol *on page 512*
- ◆ **Delta-D® [OTC]** *see* Cholecalciferol *on page 341*
- ◆ **Deltacortisone** *see* PredniSONE *on page 1327*
- ◆ **Deltadehydrocortisone** *see* PredniSONE *on page 1327*
- ◆ **Deltahydrocortisone** *see* PrednisoLONE *on page 1326*
- ◆ **Demadex®** *see* Torsemide *on page 1603*

Demeclocycline (dem e kloe SYE kleen)

U.S. Brand Names Declomycin®
Canadian Brand Names Declomycin®
Index Terms Demeclocycline Hydrochloride; Demethylchlortetracycline
Pharmacologic Category Antibiotic, Tetracycline Derivative
Use Treatment of susceptible bacterial infections (acne, gonorrhea, pertussis, and urinary tract infections) caused by both gram-negative and gram-positive organisms
Unlabeled/Investigational Use Treatment of chronic syndrome of inappropriate secretion of antidiuretic hormone (SIADH)
Effect on Mental Status May cause dizziness
Effect on Psychiatric Treatment Barbiturates and carbamazepine may decrease the effects of demeclocycline. May cause photosensitivity and other dermatological reactions; consider this possibility when individuals are also taking psychotropics (eg, antipsychotics, carbamazepine, lamotrigine) since they may produce similar reactions.
Dosage Summary
Oral:
Children <8 years: Dosage not established

Children ≥8 years: 8-12 mg/kg/day divided every 6-12 hours
Adults: 600 mg/day in 2 or 4 divided doses

Dosage Forms Excipient information presented when available (limited, particularly for generics); consult specific product labeling.
Tablet, as hydrochloride: 150 mg, 300 mg
Declomycin®: 150 mg, 300 mg

- **Demeclocycline Hydrochloride** *see* Demeclocycline *on page 424*
- **Demerol®** *see* Meperidine *on page 986*
- **4-Demethoxydaunorubicin** *see* IDArubicin *on page 809*
- **Demethylchlortetracycline** *see* Demeclocycline *on page 424*
- **Demser®** *see* Metyrosine *on page 1044*

Denileukin Diftitox (de ni LOO kin DIF ti toks)

Medication Safety Issues
High alert medication: The Institute for Safe Medication Practices (ISMP) includes this medication among its list of drug classes which have a heightened risk of causing significant patient harm when used in error.

U.S. Brand Names ONTAK®

Index Terms DAB389 Interleukin-2; DAB_{389}IL-2; NSC-714744

Pharmacologic Category Antineoplastic Agent, Miscellaneous

Use Treatment of persistent or recurrent cutaneous (peripheral) T-cell lymphoma (CTCL) whose malignant cells express the CD25 component of the IL-2 receptor

Unlabeled/Investigational Use Treatment of CTCL types mycosis fungoides (MF) and Sézary syndrome (SS)

Effect on Mental Status Dizziness and nervousness are common; may cause insomnia or confusion

Effect on Psychiatric Treatment Hypotension and tachycardia are common; use caution with low potency antipsychotics and other psychotropics. Nausea and vomiting are common; use caution with SSRIs.

Dosage Summary
I.V.:
Children: Dosage not established
Adults: 9 or 18 mcg/kg/day days 1-5 every 21 days

Dosage Forms Excipient information presented when available (limited, particularly for generics); consult specific product labeling.
Injection, solution [frozen]:
ONTAK®: 150 mcg/mL (2 mL) [contains EDTA]

- **Deoxycoformycin** *see* Pentostatin *on page 1250*
- **2′-Deoxycoformycin** *see* Pentostatin *on page 1250*
- **Depacon®** *see* Valproic Acid and Derivatives *on page 1642*
- **Depade®** *see* Naltrexone *on page 1099*
- **Depakene®** *see* Valproic Acid and Derivatives *on page 1642*
- **Depakote®** *see* Valproic Acid and Derivatives *on page 1642*
- **Depakote® ER** *see* Valproic Acid and Derivatives *on page 1642*
- **Depakote® Sprinkle** *see* Valproic Acid and Derivatives *on page 1642*
- **Depen®** *see* Penicillamine *on page 1239*
- **Deplin™** *see* Methylfolate *on page 1022*
- **DepoCyt®** *see* Cytarabine (Liposomal) *on page 413*
- **DepoDur®** *see* Morphine Sulfate *on page 1077*
- **Depo®-Estradiol** *see* Estradiol *on page 576*
- **Depo-Medrol®** *see* MethylPREDNISolone *on page 1029*
- **Depo-Provera®** *see* MedroxyPROGESTERone *on page 975*
- **Depo-Provera® Contraceptive** *see* MedroxyPROGESTERone *on page 975*
- **depo-subQ provera 104™** *see* MedroxyPROGESTERone *on page 975*
- **Depo®-Testosterone** *see* Testosterone *on page 1553*
- **Deprenyl** *see* Selegiline *on page 1466*
- **Dermagran® [OTC]** *see* Aluminum Hydroxide *on page 78*
- **Dermamycin® [OTC]** *see* DiphenhydrAMINE *on page 481*
- **Dermarest Dricort® [OTC]** *see* Hydrocortisone *on page 785*

◆ **Dermarest® Psoriasis Medicated Moisturizer [OTC]** *see* Salicylic Acid *on page 1454*
◆ **Dermarest® Psoriasis Medicated Scalp Treatment [OTC]** *see* Salicylic Acid *on page 1454*
◆ **Dermarest® Psoriasis Medicated Shampoo/Conditioner [OTC]** *see* Salicylic Acid *on page 1454*
◆ **Dermarest® Psoriasis Medicated Skin Treatment [OTC]** *see* Salicylic Acid *on page 1454*
◆ **Dermarest® Psoriasis Overnight Treatment [OTC]** *see* Salicylic Acid *on page 1454*
◆ **Dermarest® Psoriasis Scalp Treatment Mousse [OTC] [DSC]** *see* Salicylic Acid *on page 1454*
◆ **Dermtex® HC [OTC]** *see* Hydrocortisone *on page 785*
◆ **Desferal®** *see* Deferoxamine *on page 423*
◆ **Desferrioxamine** *see* Deferoxamine *on page 423*
◆ **Desiccated Thyroid** *see* Thyroid, Desiccated *on page 1579*

Desipramine (des IP ra meen)

Medication Safety Issues

Sound-alike/look-alike issues:

Desipramine may be confused with clomiPRAMINE, deserpidine, diphenhydrAMINE, disopyramide, imipramine, nortriptyline

Norpramin® may be confused with clomiPRAMINE, imipramine, Norpace®, nortriptyline, Tenormin®

International issues:

Norpramin®: Brand name for omeprazole in Spain

Related Information

Anticholinergic Effects of Common Psychotropics *on page 1758*
Antidepressant Agents *on page 1760*
Antidepressant Receptor Profile *on page 1764*
Discontinuation of Psychotropic Drugs *on page 1839*

U.S. Brand Names Norpramin®

Canadian Brand Names Alti-Desipramine; Apo-Desipramine®; Norpramin®; Nu-Desipramine; PMS-Desipramine

Mexican Brand Names Norpramin

Index Terms Desipramine Hydrochloride; Desmethylimipramine Hydrochloride

Pharmacologic Category Antidepressant, Tricyclic (Secondary Amine)

Generic Available Yes

Use Treatment of depression

Unlabeled/Investigational Use Analgesic adjunct in chronic pain; peripheral neuropathies; substance-related disorders (eg, cocaine withdrawal); attention-deficit/hyperactivity disorder (ADHD); depression in children ≤12 years of age

Mental Health Comment Tricyclic antidepressants may be classified as tertiary (amitriptyline, doxepin, clomipramine, imipramine, trimipramine) or secondary amines (nortriptyline, desipramine, protriptyline). The tertiary amines are not recommended to treat depression in the elderly. If a TCA is used in the elderly, it should be a secondary amine. The tertiary amines are commonly used in low dosages for various conditions associated with pain. Plasma concentrations correlate with clinical response. A linear relationship appears to exist. Toxicity is generally dose dependent. Relatively small overdoses (1-week supply) can be potentially fatal.

Restrictions An FDA-approved medication guide concerning the use of antidepressants in children, adolescents, and young adults must be distributed when dispensing an outpatient prescription (new or refill) where this medication is to be used without direct supervision of a healthcare provider. Medication guides are available at http://www.fda.gov/cder/Offices/ODS/medication_guides.htm. Dispense to parents or guardians of children and adolescents receiving this medication.

Pregnancy Risk Factor C

Lactation Enters breast milk/not recommended (AAP rates "of concern")

Contraindications Hypersensitivity to desipramine, drugs of similar chemical class, or any component of the formulation; use of MAO inhibitors within 14 days; use in a patient during the acute recovery phase of MI; concurrent use of thioridazine

Warnings/Precautions **[U.S. Boxed Warning]: Antidepressants increase the risk of suicidal thinking and behavior in children, adolescents, and young adults (18-24 years of age) with major depressive disorder (MDD)**

and other psychiatric disorders; consider risk prior to prescribing. Short-term studies did not show an increased risk in patients >24 years of age and showed a decreased risk in patients ≥65 years. Closely monitor for clinical worsening, suicidality, or unusual changes in behavior; the patient's family or caregiver should be instructed to closely observe the patient and communicate condition with healthcare provider. A medication guide should be dispensed with each prescription. **Desipramine is FDA approved for the treatment of depression in adolescents.**

The possibility of a suicide attempt is inherent in major depression and may persist until remission occurs. Monitor for worsening of depression or suicidality, especially during initiation of therapy (generally first 1-2 months) or with dose increases or decreases. Use caution in high-risk patients. Worsening depression and severe abrupt suicidality that are not part of the presenting symptoms may require discontinuation or modification of drug therapy. The patient's family or caregiver should be alerted to monitor patients for the emergence of suicidality and associated behaviors (such as agitation, irritability, hostility, impulsivity, and hypomania) and notify healthcare provider.

May worsen psychosis in some patients or precipitate a shift to mania or hypomania in patients with bipolar disorder. Patients presenting with depressive symptoms should be screened for bipolar disorder. Monotherapy in patients with bipolar disorder should be avoided. **Desipramine is not FDA approved for the treatment of bipolar depression.**

TCAs may rarely cause bone marrow suppression; monitor for any signs of infection and obtain CBC if symptoms (eg, fever, sore throat) evident. The degree of anticholinergic blockade produced by this agent is low relative to other cyclic antidepressants - however, caution should be used in patients with urinary retention, benign prostatic hyperplasia, narrow-angle glaucoma, xerostomia, visual problems, constipation, or a history of bowel obstruction. The degree of sedation and conduction disturbances with desipramine are low relative to other antidepressants. However, desipramine may cause drowsiness/sedation, resulting in impaired performance of tasks requiring alertness (eg, operating machinery or driving). Sedative effects may be additive with other CNS depressants and/or ethanol. The risk of orthostasis is moderate relative to other antidepressants. Use with caution in patients with a history of cardiovascular disease (including previous MI, stroke, tachycardia, or conduction abnormalities). Use with caution in patients with diabetes mellitus; may alter glucose regulation.

Consider discontinuing, when possible, prior to elective surgery. Therapy should not be abruptly discontinued in patients receiving high doses for prolonged periods. May lower seizure threshold - use caution in patients with a previous seizure disorder or condition predisposing to seizures such as brain damage, alcoholism, or concurrent therapy with other drugs which lower the seizure threshold. May increase the risks associated with electroconvulsive therapy. Use with caution in hyperthyroid patients or those receiving thyroid supplementation. Use with caution in patients with hepatic or renal dysfunction and in elderly patients. Safety and efficacy have not been established in children.

Adverse Reactions Frequency not defined.

Cardiovascular: Arrhythmias, edema, flushing, heart block, hyper-/hypotension, MI, palpitation, stroke, tachycardia

Central nervous system: Agitation, anxiety, ataxia, confusion, delirium, disorientation, dizziness, drowsiness, drug fever, exacerbation of psychosis, extrapyramidal symptoms, fatigue, hallucinations, headache, hypomania, incoordination, insomnia, nervousness, parkinsonian syndrome, restlessness, seizure

Dermatologic: Alopecia, itching, petechiae, photosensitivity, skin rash, urticaria

Endocrine & metabolic: Breast enlargement, galactorrhea, hyper-/hypoglycemia, impotence, libido changes, SIADH

Gastrointestinal: Abdominal cramps, anorexia, black tongue, constipation, decreased lower esophageal sphincter tone may cause GE reflux, diarrhea, heartburn, nausea, paralytic ileus, stomatitis, unpleasant taste, vomiting, weight gain/loss, xerostomia

Genitourinary: Difficult urination, polyuria, sexual dysfunction, testicular edema, urinary retention

Hematologic: Agranulocytosis, eosinophilia, purpura, thrombocytopenia

Hepatic: Cholestatic jaundice, hepatitis, liver enzymes increased

Neuromuscular & skeletal: Fine muscle tremor, numbness, paresthesia of extremities, peripheral neuropathy, tingling, weakness

Ocular: Blurred vision, disturbances of accommodation, intraocular pressure increased, mydriasis

Otic: Tinnitus
Miscellaneous: Allergic reaction, diaphoresis (excessive)

Metabolism/Transport Effects Substrate of CYP1A2 (minor), 2D6 (major); **Inhibits** CYP2A6 (moderate), 2B6 (moderate), 2D6 (moderate), 2E1 (weak), 3A4 (moderate)

Drug Interactions

Acetylcholinesterase Inhibitors (Central): Anticholinergics may diminish the therapeutic effect of Acetylcholinesterase Inhibitors (Central). Acetylcholinesterase Inhibitors (Central) may diminish the therapeutic effect of Anticholinergics. If the anticholinergic action is a side effect of the agent, the result may be beneficial. *Risk C: Monitor therapy*

Alcohol (Ethyl): CNS Depressants may enhance the CNS depressant effect of Alcohol (Ethyl). *Risk C: Monitor therapy*

Alfuzosin: May enhance the QTc-prolonging effect of QTc-Prolonging Agents. *Risk C: Monitor therapy*

Alpha-/Beta-Agonists (Direct-Acting): Tricyclic Antidepressants may enhance the vasopressor effect of Alpha-/Beta-Agonists (Direct-Acting). **Exceptions:** Dipivefrin. *Risk D: Consider therapy modification*

Alpha1-Agonists: Tricyclic Antidepressants may enhance the vasopressor effect of Alpha1-Agonists. *Risk D: Consider therapy modification*

Alpha2-Agonists: Tricyclic Antidepressants may diminish the antihypertensive effect of Alpha2-Agonists. **Exceptions:** Apraclonidine; Brimonidine. *Risk D: Consider therapy modification*

Altretamine: May enhance the orthostatic effect of Tricyclic Antidepressants. *Risk C: Monitor therapy*

Amphetamines: Tricyclic Antidepressants may enhance the stimulatory effect of Amphetamines. Tricyclic Antidepressants may also potentiate the cardiovascular effects of Amphetamines. *Risk C: Monitor therapy*

Anticholinergics: May enhance the adverse/toxic effect of other Anticholinergics. **Exceptions:** Paliperidone. *Risk C: Monitor therapy*

Barbiturates: May increase the metabolism of Tricyclic Antidepressants. *Risk D: Consider therapy modification*

Beta2-Agonists: Tricyclic Antidepressants may enhance the adverse/toxic effect of Beta2-Agonists. *Risk C: Monitor therapy*

BuPROPion: May decrease the metabolism of Tricyclic Antidepressants. *Risk C: Monitor therapy*

CarBAMazepine: May increase the metabolism of Tricyclic Antidepressants. *Risk C: Monitor therapy*

Cimetidine: May decrease the metabolism of Tricyclic Antidepressants. *Risk C: Monitor therapy*

Cinacalcet: May increase the serum concentration of Tricyclic Antidepressants. *Risk C: Monitor therapy*

Ciprofloxacin: May enhance the QTc-prolonging effect of QTc-Prolonging Agents. *Risk C: Monitor therapy*

CNS Depressants: May enhance the adverse/toxic effect of other CNS Depressants. *Risk C: Monitor therapy*

Codeine: CYP2D6 Inhibitors (Moderate) may diminish the therapeutic effect of Codeine. These CYP2D6 inhibitors may prevent the metabolic conversion of codeine to its active metabolite morphine. *Risk C: Monitor therapy*

CYP2A6 Substrates: CYP2A6 Inhibitors (Moderate) may decrease the metabolism of CYP2A6 Substrates. *Risk C: Monitor therapy*

CYP2B6 Substrates: CYP2B6 Inhibitors (Moderate) may decrease the metabolism of CYP2B6 Substrates. *Risk C: Monitor therapy*

CYP2D6 Inhibitors (Moderate): May decrease the metabolism of CYP2D6 Substrates. *Risk C: Monitor therapy*

CYP2D6 Inhibitors (Strong): May decrease the metabolism of CYP2D6 Substrates. *Risk D: Consider therapy modification*

CYP2D6 Substrates: CYP2D6 Inhibitors (Moderate) may decrease the metabolism of CYP2D6 Substrates. **Exceptions:** Tamoxifen. *Risk C: Monitor therapy*

CYP3A4 Substrates: CYP3A4 Inhibitors (Moderate) may decrease the metabolism of CYP3A4 Substrates. *Risk C: Monitor therapy*

Darunavir: May increase the serum concentration of CYP2D6 Substrates. *Risk C: Monitor therapy*

Desmopressin: Tricyclic Antidepressants may enhance the adverse/toxic effect of Desmopressin. *Risk C: Monitor therapy*

Dexmethylphenidate: May decrease the metabolism of Tricyclic Antidepressants. *Risk C: Monitor therapy*

DULoxetine: May decrease the metabolism of Tricyclic Antidepressants. *Risk C: Monitor therapy*

Eplerenone: CYP3A4 Inhibitors (Moderate) may increase the serum concentration of Eplerenone. Management: A lower starting dose of eplerenone

(25 mg once daily) is recommended in patients with hypertension who are also taking drugs that are moderate inhibitors of CYP3A4. *Risk D: Consider therapy modification*

Gadobutrol: May enhance the QTc-prolonging effect of QTc-Prolonging Agents. *Risk D: Consider therapy modification*

Lithium: May enhance the neurotoxic effect of Tricyclic Antidepressants. *Risk C: Monitor therapy*

MAO Inhibitors: May enhance the serotonergic effect of Tricyclic Antidepressants. This may cause serotonin syndrome. *Risk X: Avoid combination*

Maraviroc: CYP3A4 Inhibitors may increase the serum concentration of Maraviroc. *Risk D: Consider therapy modification*

Methylphenidate: May decrease the metabolism of Tricyclic Antidepressants. *Risk C: Monitor therapy*

Nebivolol: CYP2D6 Inhibitors (Moderate) may increase the serum concentration of Nebivolol. *Risk C: Monitor therapy*

Nilotinib: May enhance the QTc-prolonging effect of QTc-Prolonging Agents. *Risk X: Avoid combination*

Pimecrolimus: CYP3A4 Inhibitors (Moderate) may decrease the metabolism of Pimecrolimus. *Risk C: Monitor therapy*

Pramlintide: May enhance the anticholinergic effect of Anticholinergics. These effects are specific to the GI tract. *Risk D: Consider therapy modification*

Propoxyphene: May enhance the CNS depressant effect of Tricyclic Antidepressants. *Risk C: Monitor therapy*

Protease Inhibitors: May increase the serum concentration of Tricyclic Antidepressants. *Risk C: Monitor therapy*

QTc-Prolonging Agents: May enhance the adverse/toxic effect of other QTc-Prolonging Agents. Their effects can be additive, causing life-threatening ventricular arrhythmias. *Risk D: Consider therapy modification*

QuiNIDine: Tricyclic Antidepressants may enhance the QTc-prolonging effect of QuiNIDine. QuiNIDine may decrease the metabolism of Tricyclic Antidepressants. *Risk D: Consider therapy modification*

Ranolazine: CYP3A4 Inhibitors (Moderate) may increase the serum concentration of Ranolazine. Management: Limit the ranolazine dose to a maximum of 500 mg twice daily in patients concurrently receiving moderate CYP3A4 inhibitors (e.g., diltiazem, verapamil, erythromycin, etc.). *Risk D: Consider therapy modification*

Selective Serotonin Reuptake Inhibitors: May decrease the metabolism of Tricyclic Antidepressants. *Risk D: Consider therapy modification*

Serotonin Modulators: May enhance the adverse/toxic effect of other Serotonin Modulators. The development of serotonin syndrome may occur. *Risk D: Consider therapy modification*

Sibutramine: May enhance the serotonergic effect of Serotonin Modulators. This may cause serotonin syndrome. *Risk X: Avoid combination*

St Johns Wort: May increase the metabolism of Tricyclic Antidepressants. The risk of serotonin syndrome may theoretically be increased. *Risk D: Consider therapy modification*

Sulfonylureas: Cyclic Antidepressants may enhance the hypoglycemic effect of Sulfonylureas. *Risk C: Monitor therapy*

Tamoxifen: CYP2D6 Inhibitors (Moderate) may decrease the metabolism of Tamoxifen. Specifically, CYP2D6 inhibitors may decrease the formation of highly potent active metabolites. *Risk D: Consider therapy modification*

Terbinafine: May decrease the metabolism of Tricyclic Antidepressants. *Risk D: Consider therapy modification*

Tetrabenazine: QTc-Prolonging Agents may enhance the QTc-prolonging effect of Tetrabenazine. *Risk X: Avoid combination*

Thioridazine: QTc-Prolonging Agents may enhance the QTc-prolonging effect of Thioridazine. *Risk X: Avoid combination*

Thioridazine: CYP2D6 Inhibitors may decrease the metabolism of Thioridazine. *Risk X: Avoid combination*

TraMADol: Tricyclic Antidepressants may enhance the neuroexcitatory and/or seizure-potentiating effect of TraMADol. *Risk C: Monitor therapy*

Valproic Acid: May increase the serum concentration of Tricyclic Antidepressants. *Risk C: Monitor therapy*

Vitamin K Antagonists (eg, warfarin): Tricyclic Antidepressants may enhance the anticoagulant effect of Vitamin K Antagonists. *Risk C: Monitor therapy*

Ziprasidone: QTc-Prolonging Agents may enhance the QTc-prolonging effect of Ziprasidone. The risk of a severe arrhythmia may be increased. *Risk X: Avoid combination*

Ethanol/Nutrition/Herb Interactions

Ethanol: Avoid ethanol (may increase CNS depression).

Food: Grapefruit juice may inhibit the metabolism of some TCAs and clinical toxicity may result.

Herb/Nutraceutical: Avoid valerian, St John's wort, SAMe, kava kava (may increase risk of serotonin syndrome and/or excessive sedation).

Mechanism of Action Traditionally believed to increase the synaptic concentration of norepinephrine (and to a lesser extent, serotonin) in the central nervous system by inhibition of its reuptake by the presynaptic neuronal membrane. However, additional receptor effects have been found including desensitization of adenyl cyclase, down regulation of beta-adrenergic receptors, and down regulation of serotonin receptors.

Pharmacodynamics/Kinetics

Onset of action: 1-3 weeks; Maximum antidepressant effect: >2 weeks

Absorption: Well absorbed

Metabolism: Hepatic

Half-life elimination: Adults: 7-60 hours

Time to peak, plasma: 4-6 hours

Excretion: Urine (70%)

Dosage Oral (dose is generally administered at bedtime):

Children 6-12 years: Depression (unlabeled use): 10-30 mg/day or 1-3 mg/kg/day in divided doses; do not exceed 5 mg/kg/day

Adolescents: Depression: Initial: 25-50 mg/day; gradually increase to 100 mg/day in single or divided doses (maximum: 150 mg/day)

Adults:

Depression: Initial: 75 mg/day in divided doses; increase gradually to 150-200 mg/day in divided or single dose (maximum: 300 mg/day)

Cocaine withdrawal (unlabeled use): 50-200 mg/day in divided or single dose

Elderly: Depression: Initial dose: 10-25 mg/day; increase by 10-25 mg every 3 days for inpatients and every week for outpatients if tolerated; usual maintenance dose: 75-100 mg/day, but doses up to 150 mg/day may be necessary

Hemodialysis/peritoneal dialysis: Supplemental dose is not necessary

Monitoring Parameters Monitor blood pressure and pulse rate prior to and during initial therapy; evaluate mental status, suicidal ideation (especially at the beginning of therapy or when doses are increased or decreased); monitor weight; ECG in older adults and those patients with cardiac disease; blood levels are useful for therapeutic monitoring

When used for the treatment of ADHD, thoroughly evaluate for cardiovascular risk. Monitor heart rate, blood pressure, and consider obtaining ECG prior to initiation (Vetter, 2008); ensure PR interval ≤200 ms, QRS duration ≤120 ms, and QT_c ≤460 ms.

Reference Range

Plasma levels do not always correlate with clinical effectiveness

Timing of serum samples: Draw trough just before next dose

Therapeutic: 50-300 ng/mL

In elderly patients the response rate is greatest with steady-state plasma concentrations >115 ng/mL

Possible toxicity: >300 ng/mL

Toxic: >1000 ng/mL

Additional Information Less sedation and anticholinergic effects than with amitriptyline or imipramine

Dosage Forms Excipient information presented when available (limited, particularly for generics); consult specific product labeling.

Tablet, as hydrochloride: 10 mg, 25 mg, 50 mg, 75 mg, 100 mg, 150 mg

Norpramin®: 10 mg, 25 mg, 50 mg, 75 mg, 100 mg, 150 mg [contains soy oil]

◆ **Desipramine Hydrochloride** *see* Desipramine *on page 426*

Desloratadine (des lor AT a deen)

U.S. Brand Names Clarinex®

Canadian Brand Names Aerius®

Mexican Brand Names Aviant; Azomyr

Pharmacologic Category Histamine H_1 Antagonist; Histamine H_1 Antagonist, Second Generation

Use Relief of nasal and non-nasal symptoms of seasonal allergic rhinitis (SAR) and perennial allergic rhinitis (PAR); treatment of chronic idiopathic urticaria (CIU)

Effect on Mental Status May cause sedation, fatigue, or dizziness

Effect on Psychiatric Treatment May cause nausea; concurrent use with SSRIs, lithium, and valproic acid may be additive

Dosage Summary

Oral:

Children <6 months: Dosage not established
Children 6-11 months: 1 mg once daily
Children 1-5 years: 1.25 mg once daily
Children 6-11 years: 2.5 mg once daily
Children ≥12 years: 5 mg once daily
Adults: 5 mg once daily

Dosage Forms Excipient information presented when available (limited, particularly for generics); consult specific product labeling.

Syrup:

Clarinex®: 0.5 mg/mL (480 mL) [contains propylene glycol, sodium benzoate; bubble gum flavor]

Tablet:

Clarinex®: 5 mg

Tablet, orally disintegrating:

Clarinex® RediTabs®: 2.5 mg [contains phenylalanine 1.4 mg/tablet; tutti-frutti flavor]; 5 mg [contains phenylalanine 2.9 mg/tablet; tutti-frutti flavor]

Desloratadine and Pseudoephedrine

(des lor AT a deen & soo doe e FED rin)

U.S. Brand Names Clarinex-D® 12 Hour; Clarinex-D® 24 Hour

Index Terms Pseudoephedrine and Desloratadine

Pharmacologic Category Alpha/Beta Agonist; Histamine H_1 Antagonist; Histamine H_1 Antagonist, Second Generation

Use Relief of symptoms of seasonal allergic rhinitis, in children ≥12 years of age and adults

Effect on Mental Status May cause dizziness, insomnia, restlessness, somnolence, or hyperactivity

Effect on Psychiatric Treatment Contraindicated with or within 14 days of MAO inhibitor therapy

Dosage Summary

Oral:

Children <12 years: Dosage not established
Children ≥12 years: 12 hour: 1 tablet twice daily; 24 hour: 1 tablet once daily
Adults: 12 hour: 1 tablet twice daily; 24 hour: 1 tablet once daily

Dosage Forms Excipient information presented when available (limited, particularly for generics); consult specific product labeling.

Tablet, variable release:

Clarinex-D® 12 Hour: Desloratadine 2.5 mg [immediate release] and pseudoephedrine 120 mg [extended release]

Clarinex-D® 24 Hour: Desloratadine 5 mg [immediate release] and pseudoephedrine 240 mg [extended release]

◆ **Desmethylimipramine Hydrochloride** *see* Desipramine *on page 426*

Desmopressin (des moe PRES in)

Related Information

Clozapine-Induced Side Effects *on page 1818*

U.S. Brand Names DDAVP®; Stimate®

Canadian Brand Names Apo-Desmopressin®; DDAVP®; DDAVP® Melt; Minirin®; Novo-Desmopressin; Octostim®; PMS-Desmopressin

Mexican Brand Names Nafiset; Octostim; Pizzard

Index Terms 1-Deamino-8-D-Arginine Vasopressin; Desmopressin Acetate

Pharmacologic Category Antihemophilic Agent; Hemostatic Agent; Vasopressin Analog, Synthetic

Use

Injection: Treatment of diabetes insipidus; maintenance of hemostasis and control of bleeding in hemophilia A with factor VIII coagulant activity levels >5% and mild-to-moderate classic von Willebrand's disease (type 1) with factor VIII coagulant activity levels >5%

Nasal solutions (DDAVP® Nasal Spray and DDAVP® Rhinal Tube): Treatment of central diabetes insipidus

Nasal spray (Stimate®): Maintenance of hemostasis and control of bleeding in hemophilia A with factor VIII coagulant activity levels >5% and mild to moderate classic von Willebrand's disease (type 1) with factor VIII coagulant activity levels >5%

Tablet: Treatment of central diabetes insipidus, temporary polyuria and polydipsia following pituitary surgery or head trauma, primary nocturnal enuresis

Unlabeled/Investigational Use Uremic bleeding associated with acute or chronic renal failure; prevention of surgical bleeding in patients with uremia

Effect on Mental Status May cause dizziness

Effect on Psychiatric Treatment May decrease lithium's effect on ADH, however, hydrochlorothiazide or amiloride are better choices

Dosage Summary

I.V.:

Children <3 months: Dosage not established

Children ≥3 months: 0.3 mcg/kg 30 minutes prior to procedure, may repeat dose if needed

Adults: 2-4 mcg/day in 2 divided doses **or** 1/10 of the intranasal maintenance dose **or** 0.3 mcg/kg 30 minutes prior to procedure

Intranasal:

Children <3 months: Dosage not established

Children 3-11 months: Initial: 5 mcg/day (0.05 mL/day) in 1-2 divided doses; Maintenance: 5-30 mcg/day (0.05-0.3 mL/day) in 1-2 divided doses

Children 12 months to 12 years: Initial: 5 mcg/day (0.05 mL/day) in 1-2 divided doses; Maintenance: 5-30 mcg/day (0.05-0.3 mL/day) in 1-2 divided doses **or** 150 mcg (1 spray of high concentration) 2 hours prior to surgery

Children >12 years and <50 kg: 10-40 mcg/day (0.1-0.4 mL) in 1-3 divided doses **or** 150 mcg (1 spray of high concentration spray) 2 hours prior to surgery

Children >12 years and ≥50 kg: 10-40 mcg/day in 1-3 divided doses **or** 300 mcg (1 spray each nostril of high concentration spray) 2 hours prior to surgery

Adults <50 kg: 10-40 mcg/day in 1-3 divided doses **or** 150 mcg (1 spray of high concentration spray) 2 hours prior to surgery

Adults ≥50 kg: 10-40 mcg/day in 1-3 divided doses **or** 300 mcg (1 spray each nostril of high concentration spray) 2 hours prior to surgery

Oral:

Children <4 years: Dosage not established

Children 4-5 years: Initial: 0.05 mg twice daily; Maintenance: 0.1-1.2 mg/day in 2-3 divided doses

Children ≥6 years: Initial: 0.05 mg twice daily **or** 0.2 mg at bedtime; Maintenance: 0.1-1.2 mg/day in 2-3 divided doses **or** 0.2-0.6 mg at bedtime

Adults: 0.2-0.6 mg at bedtime **or** 0.1-1.2 mg/day in 2-3 divided doses

SubQ:

Children: Dosage not established

Adults: 2-4 mcg/day in 2 divided doses **or** 1/10 of the intranasal maintenance dose

Dosage Forms Excipient information presented when available (limited, particularly for generics); consult specific product labeling. [CAN] = Canadian product

Injection, solution, as acetate: 4 mcg/mL (1 mL, 10 mL)

DDAVP®: 5 mcg/mL (1 mL, 10 mL)

Solution, intranasal, as acetate: 100 mcg/mL (2.5 mL)

DDAVP®: 100 mcg/mL (2.5 mL) [contains benzalkonium chloride; with rhinal tube]

Solution, as acetate, intranasal [spray]: 100 mcg/mL (5 mL)

DDAVP®: 100 mcg/mL (5 mL) [contains benzalkonium chloride; delivers 10 mcg/spray]

Stimate®: 1.5 mg/mL (2.5 mL) [delivers 150 mcg/spray]

Tablet, as acetate, oral: 0.1 mg, 0.2 mg

DDAVP®: 0.1 mg, 0.2 mg [scored]

Tablet, as acetate, sublingual:

DDAVP® Melt (CAN) [not available in U.S.]: 60 mcg, 120 mcg, 240 mcg

- **Desmopressin Acetate** *see* Desmopressin *on page 431*
- **Desogen®** *see* Ethinyl Estradiol and Desogestrel *on page 592*
- **Desogestrel and Ethinyl Estradiol** *see* Ethinyl Estradiol and Desogestrel *on page 592*
- **Desoxyephedrine Hydrochloride** *see* Methamphetamine *on page 1006*
- **Desoxyn®** *see* Methamphetamine *on page 1006*
- **Desoxyphenobarbital** *see* Primidone *on page 1336*

Desvenlafaxine (des ven la FAX een)

U.S. Brand Names Pristiq™

Index Terms O-desmethylvenlafaxine; ODV

Pharmacologic Category Antidepressant, Serotonin/Norepinephrine Reuptake Inhibitor

Generic Available No

Use Treatment of major depressive disorder

Mental Health Comment Desvenlafaxine is the active metabolite of venlafaxine (Effexor®). Both agents inhibit the reuptake of serotonin and norepinephrine and are referred to as serotonin/norepinephrine reuptake inhibitors (SNRIs). Both agents lack significant affinity for the muscarinic cholinergic, H_1-histaminergic, and alpha$_1$-adrenergic receptors. They also do not possess MAO inhibitory activity.

Parks et al, conducted a dose-finding study of desvenlafaxine in doses up to 750 mg and found that it was associated with less nausea than venlafaxine 150 mg extended release. Ahmed et al, conducted an open-label study in which patients were switched from venlafaxine extended release or placebo to desvenlafaxine. They found a low incidence of adverse reactions in the group switching from venlafaxine to desvenlafaxine, compared with the group switching from placebo to desvenlafaxine (nausea 4% vs 35%; $p<0.001$).

Overall, compared to venlafaxine, desvenlafaxine may be associated with an improved adverse effect profile and fewer drug-drug interactions, but head-to-head studies between these two agents are necessary to establish its place in therapy (Sproule, 2008).

Ahmed S, Zitek B, Ninan PT, et al, "Switch From Venlafaxine to Desvenlafaxine Succinate is Well Tolerated in Patients With Major Depressive Disorder," [abstract from the 160th Annual Meeting of the American Psychiatric Association, May 19-24, 2007, San Diego, CA] Available at: http://www.psych.org/edu/other_res/lib_archives/archives/meetings/AMS/2007saps.pdf.

Parks V, Patat A, Behrle J, et al, "Safety, Pharmacokinetics (PK) and Pharmacodynamics (PD) of Ascending Single Doses of Desvenlafaxine (DVS-233 SR) in Healthy Subjects," *Clin Pharmacol Ther*, 2005, 77:P28.

Sproule BA, Hazra M, and Pollock BG, "Desvenlafaxine Succinate for Major Depressive Disorder," *Drugs Today (Barc)*, 2008, 44(7):475-87.

Restrictions An FDA-approved medication guide concerning the use of antidepressants in children, adolescents, and young adults must be distributed when dispensing an outpatient prescription (new or refill) where this medication is to be used without direct supervision of a healthcare provider. Medication guides are available at http://www.wyeth.com/content/showlabeling.asp?id=498.

Pregnancy Risk Factor C

Pregnancy Considerations Desvenlafaxine is classified as pregnancy category C due to adverse effects observed in animal studies. Nonteratogenic effects in the newborn following SSRI/SNRI exposure late in the third trimester include respiratory distress, cyanosis, apnea, seizures, temperature instability, feeding difficulty, vomiting, hypoglycemia, hyper- or hypotonia, hyper-reflexia, jitteriness, irritability, constant crying, and tremor. The long-term effects on neurobehavior have not been studied.

Women treated for major depression and who are euthymic prior to pregnancy are more likely to experience a relapse when medication is discontinued as compared to pregnant women who continue taking antidepressant medications. The ACOG recommends that therapy with SSRIs or SNRIs during pregnancy be individualized; treatment of depression during pregnancy should incorporate the clinical expertise of the mental health clinician, obstetrician, primary healthcare provider, and pediatrician. If treatment during pregnancy is required, consider tapering therapy during the third trimester in order to prevent withdrawal symptoms in the infant. If this is done and the woman is considered to be at risk from her major depressive disorder, the medication can be restarted following delivery, although the dose should be readjusted to that required before pregnancy.

Desvenlafaxine is the major active metabolite of venlafaxine; also refer to the venlafaxine monograph.

Lactation Enters breast milk/not recommended

Contraindications Hypersensitivity to desvenlafaxine, venlafaxine or any component of the formulation; use of MAO inhibitors within 14 days; should not initiate MAO inhibitor within 7 days of discontinuing desvenlafaxine

Warnings/Precautions [U.S. Boxed Warning]: Antidepressants increase the risk of suicidal thinking and behavior in children, adolescents, and young adults (18-24 years of age) with major depressive disorder (MDD) and other psychiatric disorders; consider risk prior to prescribing. Short-term studies did not show an increased risk in patients >24 years of age and showed a decreased risk in patients ≥65 years. Closely monitor for clinical worsening, suicidality, or unusual changes in behavior; the patient's family or caregiver should be instructed to closely observe the patient and communicate condition with healthcare provider. A medication guide should be dispensed with each prescription. **Desvenlafaxine is not FDA approved for use in children.**

The possibility of a suicide attempt is inherent in major depression and may persist until remission occurs. Monitor for worsening of depression or suicidality, especially during initiation of therapy (generally first 1-2 months) or with dose increases or decreases. Use caution in high-risk patients. Worsening depression and severe abrupt suicidality that are not part of the presenting symptoms may require discontinuation or modification of drug therapy. The patient's family or caregiver should be alerted to monitor patients for the emergence of suicidality and associated behaviors (such as agitation, irritability, hostility, impulsivity, and hypomania) and call healthcare provider.

May worsen psychosis in some patients or precipitate a shift to mania or hypomania in patients with bipolar disorder. Patients presenting with depressive symptoms should be screened for bipolar disorder. Monotherapy in patients with bipolar disorder should be avoided. **Desvenlafaxine is not FDA approved for the treatment of bipolar depression.**

The potential for severe reactions exists when used with MAO inhibitors, proserotoneric drugs (myoclonus, diaphoresis, hyperthermia, NMS features, seizures, and death). May cause sustained increase in blood pressure or heart rate; dose related. Control pre-existing hypertension prior to initiation of desvenlafaxine. Use caution in patients with recent history of MI, unstable heart disease, or cerebrovascular disease; may cause increases in serum lipids (cholesterol, LDL, triglycerides). Use caution in patients with renal impairment; dose reduction required in severe renal impairment. Use caution in patients with hepatic impairment. May cause hyponatremia/SIADH (elderly at increased risk); volume depletion (diuretics may increase risk).

Interstitial lung disease and eosinophilic pneumonia have been rarely reported with venlafaxine (the parent drug of desvenlafaxine); may present as progressive dyspnea, cough, and/or chest pain. Prompt evaluation and possible discontinuation of therapy may be necessary. Use cautiously in patients with a history of seizures. The risks of cognitive or motor impairment are low. May cause or exacerbate sexual dysfunction. May impair platelet aggregation, resulting in bleeding.

Abrupt discontinuation or dosage reduction after extended (≥6 weeks) therapy may lead to agitation, dysphoria, nervousness, anxiety, and other symptoms. When discontinuing therapy, dosage should be tapered gradually over at least a 2-week period. If intolerable symptoms occur following a decrease in dosage or upon discontinuation of therapy, then resuming the previous dose with a more gradual taper should be considered. Use caution in patients with increased intraocular pressure or at risk of acute narrow-angle glaucoma.

Adverse Reactions Reported for 50-100 mg/day.

>10%:

Central nervous system: Dizziness (10% to 13%), insomnia (9% to 12%)

Gastrointestinal: Nausea (22% to 26%), xerostomia (11% to 17%), constipation (9% to 11%), diarrhea (9% to 11%)

Miscellaneous: Diaphoresis (10% to 14%)

1% to 10%:

Cardiovascular: Palpitation (≤3%), orthostatic hypotension (<2%), syncope (<2%), hypertension (dose related; ≤1% of patients taking 50-100 mg daily had sustained diastolic BP ≥90 mm Hg)

Central nervous system: Somnolence (≤9%), fatigue (7%), anxiety (3% to 5%), abnormal dreams (2% to 3%), irritability (2%), depersonalization (<2%), extrapyramidal symptoms (<2%), hypomania (<2%), seizures (<2%), concentration decreased (≤1%)

Dermatologic: Rash (1%)

Endocrine & metabolic: Libido decreased (males 4% to 5%), cholesterol increased (by ≥50 mg/dL and ≥261 mg/dL: 3% to 4%), anorgasmia (females 1%), low density lipoprotein cholesterol increased (by ≥50 mg/dL and ≥190 mg/dL: ≤1%), sexual dysfunction (males ≤1%)

Gastrointestinal: Anorexia (5% to 8%), vomiting (≤4%), weight loss (≤2%)

Genitourinary: Urinary hesitancy (≤1%)

Hepatic: Liver function tests abnormal (≤2%)
Neuromuscular & skeletal: Tremor (≤3%), paresthesia (≤2%), weakness (≤2%)
Ocular: Blurred vision (3% to 4%), mydriasis (2%)
Otic: Tinnitus (2%)
Renal: Proteinuria (6% to 8%)
Respiratory: Epistaxis (<2%)
Miscellaneous: Ejaculation retarded (1% to 5%), erectile dysfunction (3% to 6%), hypersensitivity reaction (<2%), ejaculation failure (≤1%)

<1% (Limited to important or life-threatening): Myocardial infarction, myocardial ischemia

Metabolism/Transport Effects **Substrate** of 3A4 (minor); **Inhibits** 3A4 (weak)

Drug Interactions

Alcohol (Ethyl): CNS Depressants may enhance the CNS depressant effect of Alcohol (Ethyl). *Risk C: Monitor therapy*

Aspirin: Antidepressants (Serotonin/Norepinephrine Reuptake Inhibitor) may enhance the antiplatelet effect of Aspirin. *Risk C: Monitor therapy*

CNS Depressants: May enhance the adverse/toxic effect of other CNS Depressants. *Risk C: Monitor therapy*

MAO Inhibitors: May enhance the serotonergic effect of Antidepressants (Serotonin/Norepinephrine Reuptake Inhibitor). This may cause serotonin syndrome. *Risk X: Avoid combination*

NSAID (Nonselective): Antidepressants (Serotonin/Norepinephrine Reuptake Inhibitor) may enhance the antiplatelet effect of NSAID (Nonselective). *Risk C: Monitor therapy*

Serotonin Modulators: May enhance the adverse/toxic effect of other Serotonin Modulators. The development of serotonin syndrome may occur. *Risk D: Consider therapy modification*

Sibutramine: May enhance the serotonergic effect of Serotonin Modulators. This may cause serotonin syndrome. *Risk X: Avoid combination*

Ethanol/Nutrition/Herb Interactions

Ethanol: Avoid ethanol (may increase CNS effects).

Herb/Nutraceutical: Avoid St John's wort (may increase risk of serotonin syndrome and/or excessive sedation).

Mechanism of Action Desvenlafaxine is a potent and selective serotonin and norepinephrine reuptake inhibitor.

Pharmacodynamics/Kinetics

Distribution: V_d: 3.4 L/kg
Protein binding: 30%
Metabolism: Hepatic via conjugation, and oxidation via CYP3A4 (minor pathway)
Bioavailability: 80%
Half-life elimination: 11 hours; prolonged in renal failure
Time to peak, serum: 7.5 hours
Excretion: Urine (45% as unchanged drug; ~24% as metabolites)

Dosage Oral: Adults: Depression: 50 mg once daily; up to 400 mg once daily have been studied; however, the manufacturer states there is no evidence that higher doses confer any additional benefit. A flat dose response curve for efficacy between 50-400 mg/day has been noted as well as an increase in adverse events.

Note: Gradually taper dose (by increasing dosing interval) if discontinuing.

Dosing adjustment in renal impairment:

Cl_{cr} ≥30 mL/minute: No dosage adjustment required
Cl_{cr} <30 mL/minute: 50 mg every other day (maximum).
Hemodialysis: 50 mg every other day (maximum). Supplemental doses not required after HD.

Dosing adjustment in hepatic impairment: Usual adult dose recommended; maximum dose: 100 mg/day

Dietary Considerations May be taken with or without food.

Administration May be taken with or without food. Swallow tablet whole; do not crush, chew, break, or dissolve. When discontinuing therapy, extend dosing interval to taper.

Monitoring Parameters Renal function for dosing purposes; blood pressure should be regularly monitored, especially in patients with a high baseline blood pressure; lipid panel (eg, total cholesterol, LDL, triglycerides); mental status for depression, suicidal ideation (especially at the beginning of therapy or when doses are increased or decreased). Intraocular pressure should be monitored in those with baseline elevations or a history of glaucoma.

Dosage Forms Excipient information presented when available (limited, particularly for generics); consult specific product labeling.

Tablet, extended release:
Pristiq™: 50 mg, 100 mg

◆ **Detemir Insulin** *see* Insulin Detemir *on page 825*

◆ **Detrol®** *see* Tolterodine *on page 1596*

◆ **Detrol® LA** *see* Tolterodine *on page 1596*

◆ **Detuss [DSC]** *see* Pseudoephedrine, Hydrocodone, and Chlorpheniramine *on page 1372*

◆ **Devil's Shrub** *see* Ginseng, Siberian *(Eleutherococcus senticosus)* *on page 720*

Dexamethasone (deks a METH a sone)

Medication Safety Issues

Sound-alike/look-alike issues:

Dexamethasone may be confused with desoximetasone, dextroamphetamine

Decadron® may be confused with Percodan®

Maxidex® may be confused with Maxzide®

Related Information

Corticosteroids *on page 1780*

U.S. Brand Names Dexamethasone Intensol™; DexPak® 10 Day TaperPak®; DexPak® TaperPak®; Maxidex®

Canadian Brand Names Apo-Dexamethasone®; Dexasone®; Diodex®; Maxidex®; PMS-Dexamethasone

Mexican Brand Names Alin; Brulin; Decadron; Decadronal; Decorex; Dexafrin Ofteno; Dibasona; Etacortilen; Examsa; Metax

Index Terms Dexamethasone Sodium Phosphate

Pharmacologic Category Anti-inflammatory Agent; Anti-inflammatory Agent, Ophthalmic; Antiemetic; Corticosteroid, Ophthalmic; Corticosteroid, Otic; Corticosteroid, Systemic

Use

Systemic: Primarily as an anti-inflammatory or immunosuppressant agent in the treatment of a variety of diseases including those of allergic, dermatologic, endocrine, hematologic, inflammatory, neoplastic, nervous system, renal, respiratory, rheumatic, and autoimmune origin; may be used in management of cerebral edema, septic shock, chronic swelling, as a diagnostic agent, diagnosis of Cushing's syndrome, antiemetic

Ophthalmic: Treatment of palpebral and bulbar conjunctivitis; corneal injury from chemical, radiation, thermal burns, or foreign body penetration

Otic: Treatment of inflammation of external auditory meatus; treatment of edema associated with infective otitis externa

Unlabeled/Investigational Use

Dexamethasone suppression test: General indicator consistent with depression and/or suicide

Accelerate fetal lung maturation in patients with preterm labor

Effect on Mental Status Insomnia and nervousness are common; may cause euphoria, confusion, or hallucinations

Effect on Psychiatric Treatment Barbiturates and carbamazepine may decrease dexamethasone effects

Dosage Summary Note: Dosage varies considerably by indication; ranges listed are representative

I.M.:

Children: 0.03-2 mg/kg/day **or** 0.6-10 mg/m^2/day divided every 6-12 hours

Adults: 0.75-9 mg/day **or** 0.03-2 mg/kg/day **or** 0.6-0.75 mg/m^2/day in divided doses every 6-12 hours **or** 4 mg every 4-6 hours

I.V.:

Children: 0.03-2 mg/kg/day **or** 0.6-10 mg/m^2/day divided every 6-12 hours **or** 5-20 mg prior to chemotherapy

Adults: 0.75-9 mg/day **or** 0.03-2 mg/kg/day **or** 0.6-0.75 mg/m^2/day in divided doses every 6-12 hours **or** 4 mg every 4-6 hours **or** 10-20 mg prior to chemotherapy **or** 10 mg every 12 hours **or** 40 mg **or** 1-6 mg/kg every 2-6 hours (shock)

Intra-articular, intralesional, or soft tissue:

Children: Dosage not established

Adults: 0.4-6 mg/day

Ophthalmic:

Solution:

Children: Dosage not established

Adults: Instill 1-2 drops into conjunctival sac every hour during the day and every other hour during the night; gradually reduce dose to every 3-4 hours, then to 3-4 times/day

Suspension:

Children: Dosage not established

Adults: Instill 1-2 drops up to 4-6 times/day or hourly in severe cases

Oral:

Children: 0.03-2 mg/kg/day **or** 0.6-10 mg/m^2/day divided every 6-12 hours

Adults: 0.75-9 mg/day **or** 0.03-2 mg/kg/day **or** 0.6-0.75 mg/m^2/day in divided doses every 6-12 hours **or** 10-20 mg prior to chemotherapy **or** 4-10 mg 1-2 times/day **or** 4 mg every 4-6 hours **or** 30 mg /day for 1 week, then 4-12 mg/day (MS) **or** 40 mg once daily (Multiple myeloma)

Otic:

Children: Dosage not established

Adults: Instill 3-4 drops 2-3 times/day

Dosage Forms Excipient information presented when available (limited, particularly for generics); consult specific product labeling.

Elixir, as base: 0.5 mg/5 mL (240 mL)

Injection, solution, as sodium phosphate: 4 mg/mL (1 mL, 5 mL, 30 mL); 10 mg/mL (10 mL)

Injection, solution, as sodium phosphate [preservative free]: 10 mg/mL (1 mL)

Solution, ophthalmic, as sodium phosphate [drops]: 0.1% (5 mL)

Solution, oral: 0.5 mg/5 mL (500 mL)

Solution, oral [concentrate]:

Dexamethasone Intensol™: 1 mg/mL (30 mL) [dye free, sugar free; contains alcohol 30% and propylene glycol]

Suspension, ophthalmic [drops]:

Maxidex®: 0.1% (5 mL) [contains benzalkonium chloride]

Tablet [scored]: 0.5 mg, 0.75 mg, 1 mg, 1.5 mg, 2 mg, 4 mg, 6 mg

DexPak® 10 Day TaperPak®: 1.5 mg [35 tablets on taper dose card]

DexPak® TaperPak®: 1.5 mg [51 tablets on taper dose card]

◆ **Dexamethasone Intensol™** *see* Dexamethasone *on page 436*

◆ **Dexamethasone Sodium Phosphate** *see* Dexamethasone *on page 436*

Dexbrompheniramine and Pseudoephedrine

(deks brom fen EER a meen & soo doe e FED rin)

U.S. Brand Names Drixoral® Cold & Allergy [OTC]

Canadian Brand Names Drixoral®

Index Terms Pseudoephedrine and Dexbrompheniramine

Pharmacologic Category Alpha/Beta Agonist; Histamine H_1 Antagonist; Histamine H_1 Antagonist, First Generation

Use Relief of symptoms of upper respiratory mucosal congestion in seasonal and perennial nasal allergies, acute rhinitis, rhinosinusitis, and eustachian tube blockage

Effect on Mental Status May cause drowsiness, anxiety, and nervousness

Effect on Psychiatric Treatment Dry mouth is common; this effect may be worsened by concurrent psychotropic use

Dosage Summary

Oral:

Children ≤12 years: Dosage not established

Children >12 years: 1 tablet every 8-12 hours

Adults: 1 tablet every 8-12 hours

Dosage Forms Excipient information presented when available (limited, particularly for generics); consult specific product labeling.

Tablet, sustained action: Dexbrompheniramine maleate 6 mg and pseudoephedrine sulfate 120 mg

Dexchlorpheniramine (deks klor fen EER a meen)

Mexican Brand Names Polaramine

Index Terms Dexchlorpheniramine Maleate

Pharmacologic Category Histamine H_1 Antagonist; Histamine H_1 Antagonist, First Generation

Use Perennial and seasonal allergic rhinitis and other allergic symptoms including urticaria

Effect on Mental Status Drowsiness is common; may cause nervousness and depression

Effect on Psychiatric Treatment Concurrent use with psychotropics may cause additive sedation

Dosage Summary

Oral:

Regular release:

Children <2 years: Dosage not established
Children 2-5 years: 0.5 mg every 4-6 hours
Children 6-11 years: 1 mg every 4-6 hours
Adults: 2 mg every 4-6 hours

Timed release:

Children <5 years: Dosage not established
Children 6-11 years: 4 mg at bedtime
Adults: 4-6 mg at bedtime **or** every 8-10 hours

Dosage Forms Excipient information presented when available (limited, particularly for generics); consult specific product labeling. [DSC] = Discontinued product

Syrup, as maleate: 2 mg/5 mL (480 mL) [contains alcohol 6%; orange flavor]
Tablet, sustained action, as maleate: 4 mg [DSC]

- **Dexchlorpheniramine Maleate** *see* Dexchlorpheniramine *on page 437*
- **Dexchlorpheniramine Tannate, Pseudoephedrine Tannate, and Dextromethorphan Tannate** *see* Chlorpheniramine, Pseudoephedrine, and Dextromethorphan *on page 333*
- **Dexcon-PE** *see* Guaifenesin, Dextromethorphan, and Phenylephrine *on page 746*
- **Dexedrine®** *see* Dextroamphetamine *on page 441*
- **Dexferrum®** *see* Iron Dextran Complex *on page 857*

Dexmedetomidine (deks MED e toe mi deen)

Medication Safety Issues

Sound-alike/look-alike issues:

Precedex™ may be confused with Peridex®

U.S. Brand Names Precedex™

Canadian Brand Names Precedex™

Mexican Brand Names Precedex

Index Terms Dexmedetomidine Hydrochloride

Pharmacologic Category $Alpha_2$-Adrenergic Agonist; Sedative

Use Sedation of initially intubated and mechanically ventilated patients during treatment in an intensive care setting; duration of infusion should not exceed 24 hours

Unlabeled/Investigational Use Unlabeled uses include premedication prior to anesthesia induction with thiopental; relief of pain and reduction of opioid dose following laparoscopic tubal ligation; as an adjunct anesthetic in ophthalmic surgery; treatment of shivering; premedication to attenuate the cardiostimulatory and postanesthetic delirium of ketamine

Effect on Mental Status Sedation is common

Effect on Psychiatric Treatment Hypotension and sedation are common; concurrent use with psychotropics may produce additive hypotension and sedation; monitor

Dosage Summary

I.V.:

Children: Dosage not established
Adults: Loading: 1 mcg/kg; Infusion: 0.2-0.7 mcg/kg/hour

Dosage Forms Excipient information presented when available (limited, particularly for generics); consult specific product labeling.

Injection, solution [preservative free]: 100 mcg/mL (2 mL)

- **Dexmedetomidine Hydrochloride** *see* Dexmedetomidine *on page 438*

Dexmethylphenidate (dex meth il FEN i date)

Medication Safety Issues

Sound-alike/look-alike issues:

Dexmethylphenidate may be confused with methadone

Related Information

Stimulant Agents Used for ADHD *on page 1797*

U.S. Brand Names Focalin®; Focalin® XR

Index Terms Dexmethylphenidate Hydrochloride

Pharmacologic Category Central Nervous System Stimulant

Generic Available Yes: Tablet

Use Treatment of attention-deficit/hyperactivity disorder (ADHD)

Restrictions C-II

An FDA-approved medication guide must be distributed when dispensing an outpatient prescription (new or refill) where this medication is to be used without direct supervision of a healthcare provider. Medication guides are available at http://www.fda.gov/cder/Offices/ODS/medication_guides.htm.

Pregnancy Risk Factor C

Pregnancy Considerations Teratogenic effects were noted in animal studies. There are no adequate and well-controlled studies in pregnant women. Use only if the potential benefit to the mother outweighs the possible risks to the fetus.

Lactation Excretion in breast milk unknown/use caution

Contraindications Hypersensitivity to dexmethylphenidate, methylphenidate, or any component of the formulation; marked anxiety, tension, and agitation; glaucoma, motor tics, family history or diagnosis of Tourette's syndrome; use with or within 14 days following MAO inhibitor therapy

Warnings/Precautions CNS stimulant use has been associated with serious cardiovascular events including sudden death in patients with pre-existing structural cardiac abnormalities or other serious heart problems (sudden death in children and adolescents; sudden death, stroke, and MI in adults). These products should be avoided in patients with known serious structural cardiac abnormalities, cardiomyopathy, serious heart rhythm abnormalities, or other serious cardiac problems that could increase the risk of sudden death that these conditions alone carry. Patients should be carefully evaluated for cardiac disease prior to initiation of therapy. Use of stimulants can cause an increase in blood pressure (average 2-4 mm Hg) and increases in heart rate (average 3-6 bpm), although some patients may have larger than average increases. Use caution with hypertension, hyperthyroidism, or other cardiovascular conditions that might be exacerbated by increases in blood pressure or heart rate.

Has demonstrated value as part of a comprehensive treatment program for ADHD. Use with caution in patients with bipolar disorder (may induce mixed/manic episode). May exacerbate symptoms of behavior and thought disorder in psychotic patients; new onset psychosis or mania may occur with stimulant use; observe for symptoms of aggression and/or hostility. Use caution with seizure disorders (may reduce seizure threshold). Use caution in patients with history of ethanol or drug abuse. May exacerbate symptoms of behavior and thought disorder in psychotic patients. **[U.S. Boxed Warning]: Potential for drug dependency exists - avoid abrupt discontinuation in patients who have received for prolonged periods.** Visual disturbances have been reported (rare). Stimulant use has been associated with growth suppression. Growth should be monitored during treatment. Safety and efficacy in children <6 years of age have not been established.

Adverse Reactions

>10%:

Central nervous system: Headache (25% to 26%), restlessness (12%)

Gastrointestinal: Appetite decreased (30%), abdominal pain (15%)

1% to 10%:

Cardiovascular: Tachycardia (3%)

Central nervous system: Dizziness (6%), anxiety (5% to 6%), fever (5%)

Gastrointestinal: Nausea (9%), dyspepsia (5% to 8%), xerostomia (7%), anorexia (6%), pharyngolaryngeal pain (4%)

Frequency not defined: Ocular: Accommodation difficulties, blurred vision

Also refer to Methylphenidate for adverse effects seen with other methylphenidate products.

Drug Interactions

Cannabinoids: May enhance the tachycardic effect of Sympathomimetics. *Risk C: Monitor therapy*

MAO Inhibitors: May enhance the hypertensive effect of Dexmethylphenidate. *Risk X: Avoid combination*

Phenytoin: Dexmethylphenidate may decrease the metabolism of Phenytoin. *Risk C: Monitor therapy*

Sympathomimetics: May enhance the adverse/toxic effect of other Sympathomimetics. *Risk C: Monitor therapy*

Tricyclic Antidepressants: Dexmethylphenidate may decrease the metabolism of Tricyclic Antidepressants. *Risk C: Monitor therapy*

Ethanol/Nutrition/Herb Interactions

Ethanol: Avoid ethanol (may cause CNS depression).

Food: High-fat meal may increase time to peak concentration.

Herb/Nutraceutical: Avoid ephedra (may cause hypertension or arrhythmias) and yohimbe (also has CNS stimulatory activity).

Stability Store at 15°C to 30°C (59°F to 86°F). Protect from light and moisture.

Mechanism of Action Dexmethylphenidate is the more active, *d-threo*-enantiomer, of racemic methylphenidate. It is a CNS stimulant; blocks the reuptake of norepinephrine and dopamine, and increases their release into the extraneuronal space.

Pharmacodynamics/Kinetics

Duration of action: Capsule: 12 hours

Absorption: Tablet: Rapid; Capsule: Bimodal

Distribution: V_d: 1.54-3.76 L/kg

Protein binding: 12% to 15%

Metabolism: Via de-esterification to inactive metabolite, *d*-α-phenyl-piperidine acetate (*d*-ritalinic acid)

Bioavailability: 22% to 25%

Half-life elimination: Immediate release: Adults: 2-4.5 hours; Children: 2-3 hours

Time to peak: Fasting:

Tablet: 1-1.5 hours

Capsule: First peak: 1.5 hours (range: 1-4 hours); Second peak: 6.5 hours (range: 4.5-7 hours)

Excretion: Urine (90%, primarily as inactive metabolite)

Dosage Treatment of ADHD: Oral:

Children ≥6 years: Patients not currently taking methylphenidate:

Tablet: Initial: 2.5 mg twice daily; dosage may be adjusted in increments of 2.5-5 mg at weekly intervals (maximum dose: 20 mg/day); doses should be taken at least 4 hours apart

Capsule: Initial: 5 mg/day; dosage may be adjusted in increments of 5 mg/day at weekly intervals (maximum dose: 20 mg/day)

Adults: Patients not currently taking methylphenidate:

Tablet: Initial: 2.5 mg twice daily; dosage may be adjusted in increments of 2.5-5 mg at weekly intervals (maximum dose: 20 mg/day); doses should be taken at least 4 hours apart

Capsule: Initial: 10 mg/day; dosage may be adjusted in increments of 10 mg/day at weekly intervals (maximum dose: 20 mg/day)

Conversion to dexmethylphenidate from methylphenidate: Tablet, capsule: Initial: Half the total daily dose of racemic methylphenidate (maximum dexmethylphenidate dose: 20 mg/day)

Conversion from dexmethylphenidate immediate release to dexmethylphenidate extended release: When changing from Focalin® tablets to Focalin® XR capsules, patients may be switched to the same daily dose using Focalin® XR (maximum dose: 20 mg/day)

Dose reductions and discontinuation: Reduce dose or discontinue in patients with paradoxical aggravation of symptoms. Discontinue if no improvement is seen after one month of treatment.

Dosage adjustment in renal impairment: No data available. However, considering extensive metabolism to inactive compounds, renal insufficiency expected to have minimal effect on kinetics of dexmethylphenidate.

Dosage adjustment in hepatic impairment: No data available.

Dietary Considerations May be taken with or without food. Food effects on Focalin® XR have not been studied and may need to be individually adjusted.

Administration

Capsule: Should be administered once daily in the morning; do not crush or chew. Capsules may be opened and contents sprinkled over a spoonful of applesauce; consume immediately; do not store for future use.

Tablet: Should be administered at least 4 hours apart; may be taken with or without food.

Monitoring Parameters Blood pressure and heart rate (especially in hypertensive patients), CBC with differential, platelet count; growth in children. Patients should be re-evaluated at appropriate intervals to assess continued need of the medication. Observe for signs/symptoms of aggression or hostility, or depression.

When used for the treatment of ADHD, thoroughly evaluate for cardiovascular risk. Monitor heart rate, blood pressure, and consider obtaining ECG prior to initiation (Vetter, 2008).

Additional Information Focalin® XR capsules use a bimodal release where 1/2 the dose is provided in immediate release beads and 1/2 the dose is in delayed release beads. A single, once-daily dose of a capsule provides the same amount of dexmethylphenidate as two tablets given 4 hours apart.

Dosage Forms Excipient information presented when available (limited, particularly for generics); consult specific product labeling.

Capsule, extended release:
Focalin® XR: 5 mg, 10 mg, 15 mg, 20 mg [bimodal release]
Tablet, as hydrochloride: 2.5 mg, 5 mg, 10 mg
Focalin®: 2.5 mg, 5 mg; 10 mg [dye free]

- **Dexmethylphenidate Hydrochloride** *see* Dexmethylphenidate *on page 438*
- **DexPak® 10 Day TaperPak®** *see* Dexamethasone *on page 436*
- **DexPak® TaperPak®** *see* Dexamethasone *on page 436*
- **Dex PC** *see* Chlorpheniramine, Phenylephrine, and Dextromethorphan *on page 327*

Dexrazoxane (deks ray ZOKS ane)

Medication Safety Issues
Sound-alike/look-alike issues:
Zinecard® may be confused with Gemzar®
U.S. Brand Names Totect™; Zinecard®
Canadian Brand Names Zinecard®
Mexican Brand Names Cardioxane
Index Terms ICRF-187; NSC-169780
Pharmacologic Category Antidote; Cardioprotectant
Use
Zinecard®: Reduction of the incidence and severity of cardiomyopathy associated with doxorubicin administration in women with metastatic breast cancer who have received a cumulative doxorubicin dose of 300 mg/m^2 and who would benefit from continuing therapy with doxorubicin. (Not recommended for use with initial doxorubicin therapy.)
Totect™: Treatment of anthracycline-induced extravasation.
Unlabeled/Investigational Use Reduction of the incidence and severity of cardiomyopathy associated with doxorubicin administration (cumulative doses >300 mg/m^2) in patients with malignancies other than metastatic breast cancer who would benefit from continuing therapy with doxorubicin; reduction of the incidence and severity of cardiomyopathy associated with continued epirubicin administration for advanced breast cancer
Effect on Mental Status None reported
Effect on Psychiatric Treatment May cause granulocytopenia; use caution with clozapine or carbamazepine
Dosage Summary
I.V.:
Children: Dosage not established
Adults:
Prevention of cardiomyopathy: A 10:1 ratio of dexrazoxane:doxorubicin (500 mg/m^2 dexrazoxane: 50 mg/m^2 doxorubicin)
Anthracycline-induced extravasation: 1000 mg/m^2 on days 1 and 2 (maximum dose: 2000 mg), followed by 500 mg/m^2 on day 3 (maximum dose: 1000 mg)
Dosage Forms Excipient information presented when available (limited, particularly for generics); consult specific product labeling.
Injection, powder for reconstitution: 250 mg, 500 mg
Totect™: 500 mg [provided with 0.167 Molar sodium lactate injection, USP]
Zinecard®: 250 mg, 500 mg [provided with 0.167 Molar sodium lactate injection, USP]

Dextroamphetamine (deks troe am FET a meen)

Medication Safety Issues
Sound-alike/look-alike issues:
Dexedrine® may be confused with dextran, Excedrin®
Dextroamphetamine may be confused with dexamethasone
Related Information
Stimulant Agents Used for ADHD *on page 1797*
U.S. Brand Names Dexedrine®; DextroStat®; Liquadd™
Canadian Brand Names Dexedrine®
Index Terms Dextroamphetamine Sulfate
Pharmacologic Category Stimulant
Generic Available Yes: Excludes oral suspension
Use Narcolepsy; attention-deficit/hyperactivity disorder (ADHD)
Unlabeled/Investigational Use Exogenous obesity; depression; abnormal behavioral syndrome in children (minimal brain dysfunction)

Restrictions C-II

An FDA-approved medication guide must be distributed when dispensing an outpatient prescription (new or refill) where this medication is to be used without direct supervision of a healthcare provider. Medication guides are available at http://www.fda.gov/cder/Offices/ODS/medication_guides.htm.

Pregnancy Risk Factor C

Pregnancy Considerations Teratogenic and embryocidal effects have been observed in animal studies. There are no adequate and well-controlled studies in pregnant women. Use only if potential benefit justifies the potential risk to the fetus.

Lactation Enters breast milk/not recommended

Contraindications Hypersensitivity or idiosyncrasy to dextroamphetamine, other sympathomimetic amines, or any component of the formulation; advanced arteriosclerosis, symptomatic cardiovascular disease, moderate-to-severe hypertension; hyperthyroidism; glaucoma; agitated states; patients with a history of drug abuse; during or within 14 days following MAO inhibitor therapy

Warnings/Precautions [U.S. Boxed Warning]: Use has been associated with serious cardiovascular events including sudden death in patients with pre-existing structural cardiac abnormalities or other serious heart problems (sudden death in children and adolescents; sudden death, stroke and MI in adults. These products should be avoided in the patients with known serious structural cardiac abnormalities, cardiomyopathy, serious heart rhythm abnormalities, or other serious cardiac problems that could increase the risk of sudden death that these conditions alone carry. Patients should be carefully evaluated for cardiac disease prior to initiation of therapy. Use with caution in patients with hypertension and other cardiovascular conditions that might be exacerbated by increases in blood pressure or heart rate. Amphetamines may impair the ability to engage in potentially hazardous activities. May cause visual disturbances.

Use with caution in patients with psychiatric or seizure disorders. May exacerbate symptoms of behavior and thought disorder in psychotic patients. Stimulants may unmask tics in individuals with coexisting Tourette's syndrome. **[U.S. Boxed Warning]: Potential for drug dependency exists; prolonged use may lead to drug dependency.** Use is contraindicated in patients with history of ethanol or drug abuse. Prescriptions should be written for the smallest quantity consistent with good patient care to minimize possibility of overdose. Abrupt discontinuation following high doses or for prolonged periods may result in symptoms for withdrawal. Products may contain tartrazine - use with caution in potentially sensitive individuals. Safety and efficacy have not been established in children <3 years of age; Dexedrine® is not recommended for use in children <6 years of age. Appetite suppression may occur; monitor weight during therapy, particularly in children. Use of stimulants has been associated with suppression of growth; monitor growth rate during treatment.

Adverse Reactions Frequency not defined.

Cardiovascular: Cardiomyopathy, hypertension, palpitation, tachycardia

Central nervous system: Aggression, dizziness, dyskinesia, dysphoria, euphoria, exacerbation of motor and phonic tics, headache, insomnia, mania, overstimulation, psychosis, restlessness, Tourette's syndrome

Dermatologic: Rash, urticaria

Endocrine & metabolic: Libido changes

Gastrointestinal: Anorexia, constipation, diarrhea, unpleasant taste, weight loss, xerostomia

Genitourinary: Impotence

Neuromuscular & skeletal: Tremor

Ocular: Accommodation abnormalities, blurred vision

Drug Interactions

Alkalinizing Agents: May decrease the excretion of Amphetamines. *Risk D: Consider therapy modification*

Ammonium Chloride: May decrease the serum concentration of Amphetamines. This effect is likely due to an enhanced excretion of amphetamines in the urine. *Risk C: Monitor therapy*

Analgesics (Opioid): Amphetamines may enhance the analgesic effect of Analgesics (Opioid). *Risk C: Monitor therapy*

Antacids: May decrease the excretion of Amphetamines. *Risk C: Monitor therapy*

Antihistamines: Amphetamines may diminish the sedative effect of Antihistamines. *Risk C: Monitor therapy*

Antipsychotics: May diminish the stimulatory effect of Amphetamines. *Risk C: Monitor therapy*

Cannabinoids: May enhance the tachycardic effect of Sympathomimetics. *Risk C: Monitor therapy*

Carbonic Anhydrase Inhibitors: May decrease the excretion of Amphetamines. **Exceptions:** Brinzolamide; Dorzolamide. *Risk C: Monitor therapy*

Ethosuximide: Amphetamines may diminish the therapeutic effect of Ethosuximide. Amphetamines may decrease the serum concentration of Ethosuximide. *Risk C: Monitor therapy*

Gastrointestinal Acidifying Agents: May decrease the serum concentration of Amphetamines. *Risk C: Monitor therapy*

Lithium: May diminish the stimulatory effect of Amphetamines. *Risk C: Monitor therapy*

MAO Inhibitors: May enhance the hypertensive effect of Amphetamines. *Risk X: Avoid combination*

Methenamine: May decrease the serum concentration of Amphetamines. This effect is likely due to an enhanced excretion of amphetamines in the urine. *Risk C: Monitor therapy*

PHENobarbital: Amphetamines may decrease the serum concentration of PHENobarbital. *Risk C: Monitor therapy*

Phenytoin: Amphetamines may decrease the serum concentration of Phenytoin. *Risk C: Monitor therapy*

Sympathomimetics: May enhance the adverse/toxic effect of other Sympathomimetics. *Risk C: Monitor therapy*

Tricyclic Antidepressants: May enhance the stimulatory effect of Amphetamines. Tricyclic Antidepressants may also potentiate the cardiovascular effects of Amphetamines. *Risk C: Monitor therapy*

Ethanol/Nutrition/Herb Interactions

Ethanol: Avoid ethanol (may increase CNS depression).

Food: Dextroamphetamine serum levels may be altered if taken with acidic food, juices, or vitamin C.

Herb/Nutraceutical: Avoid ephedra (may cause hypertension or arrhythmias).

Stability Store at controlled room temperature of 20°C to 25°C (68°F to 77°F). Protect from light.

Mechanism of Action Amphetamines are noncatecholamine, sympathomimetic amines. Blocks reuptake of dopamine and norepinephrine from the synapse, thus increases the amount of circulating dopamine and norepinephrine in cerebral cortex to reticular activating system; inhibits the action of monoamine oxidase and causes catecholamines to be released. Peripheral actions include elevated blood pressure, weak bronchodilator, and respiratory stimulant action.

Pharmacodynamics/Kinetics

Onset of action: 1-1.5 hours

Distribution: V_d: Adults: 3.5-4.6 L/kg; distributes into CNS; mean CSF concentrations are 80% of plasma; enters breast milk

Metabolism: Hepatic via CYP monooxygenase and glucuronidation

Half-life elimination: Adults: 10-13 hours

Time to peak, serum: T_{max}: Immediate release: ~3 hours; sustained release: ~8 hours

Excretion: Urine (as unchanged drug and inactive metabolites)

Dosage Oral:

Children:

Narcolepsy: 6-12 years: Initial: 5 mg/day; may increase at 5 mg increments in weekly intervals until side effects appear (maximum dose: 60 mg/day)

ADHD:

3-5 years: Initial: 2.5 mg/day given every morning; increase by 2.5 mg/day in weekly intervals until optimal response is obtained; usual range: 0.1-0.5 mg/kg/dose every morning with maximum of 40 mg/day

≥6 years: 5 mg once or twice daily; increase in increments of 5 mg/day at weekly intervals until optimal response is obtained; usual range: 0.1-0.5 mg/kg/dose every morning (5-20 mg/day) with maximum of 40 mg/day

Children >12 years and Adults:

Narcolepsy: Initial: 10 mg/day, may increase at 10 mg increments in weekly intervals until side effects appear; maximum: 60 mg/day

Exogenous obesity (unlabeled use): 5-30 mg/day in divided doses of 5-10 mg 30-60 minutes before meals

Dietary Considerations Should be taken 30 minutes before meals and at least 6 hours before bedtime.

Administration Do not crush sustained release drug product. Administer as single dose in morning or as divided doses with breakfast and lunch. Should be administered 30 minutes before meals and at least 6 hours before bedtime.

Monitoring Parameters Cardiac evaluation should be completed on any patient who develops chest pain, unexplained syncope, and any symptom of cardiac disease during treatment with stimulants; growth in children and CNS activity in all

When used for the treatment of ADHD, thoroughly evaluate for cardiovascular risk. Monitor heart rate, blood pressure, and consider obtaining ECG prior to initiation (Vetter, 2008).

Test Interactions Amphetamines may elevate plasma corticosteroid levels; may interfere with urinary steroid determinations.

Dosage Forms Excipient information presented when available (limited, particularly for generics); consult specific product labeling.

Capsule, extended release, as sulfate: 5 mg, 10 mg, 15 mg

Capsule, sustained release, as sulfate:

Dexedrine® Spansule®: 5 mg, 10 mg, 15 mg

Tablet, as sulfate: 5 mg, 10 mg

DextroStat®: 5 mg, 10 mg [contains tartrazine]

Solution, oral, as sulfate:

Liquadd™: 5 mg/5 mL (480 mL) [contains benzoic acid; bubblegum flavor]

Dextroamphetamine and Amphetamine

(deks troe am FET a meen & am FET a meen)

Medication Safety Issues

Sound-alike/look-alike issues:

Adderall® may be confused with Inderal®

Related Information

Stimulant Agents Used for ADHD *on page 1797*

U.S. Brand Names Adderall XR®; Adderall®

Canadian Brand Names Adderall XR®

Index Terms Amphetamine and Dextroamphetamine

Pharmacologic Category Stimulant

Generic Available Yes: Tablet

Use Attention-deficit/hyperactivity disorder (ADHD); narcolepsy

Restrictions C-II

An FDA-approved medication guide must be distributed when dispensing an outpatient prescription (new or refill) where this medication is to be used without direct supervision of a healthcare provider. Medication guides are available at http://www.fda.gov/cder/Offices/ODS/medication_guides.htm.

Pregnancy Risk Factor C

Pregnancy Considerations Use during pregnancy may lead to increased risk of premature delivery and low birth weight. Infants may experience symptoms of withdrawal. Teratogenic effects were reported when taken during the 1st trimester.

Lactation Enters breast milk/contraindicated

Contraindications Hypersensitivity to dextroamphetamine, amphetamine, or any component of the formulation; advanced arteriosclerosis; symptomatic cardiovascular disease; moderate to severe hypertension; hyperthyroidism; hypersensitivity or idiosyncrasy to the sympathomimetic amines; glaucoma; agitated states; patients with a history of drug abuse; with or within 14 days following MAO inhibitor (hypertensive crisis)

Warnings/Precautions **[U.S. Boxed Warning]: Use has been associated with serious cardiovascular events including sudden death in patients with pre-existing structural cardiac abnormalities or other serious heart problems (sudden death in children and adolescents; sudden death, stroke and MI in adults.** These products should be avoided in the patients with known serious structural cardiac abnormalities, cardiomyopathy, serious heart rhythm abnormalities, or other serious cardiac problems that could increase the risk of sudden death that these conditions alone carry. Patients should be carefully evaluated for cardiac disease prior to initiation of therapy. Use with caution in patients with hypertension and other cardiovascular conditions that might be exacerbated by increases in blood pressure or heart rate. Amphetamines may impair the ability to engage in potentially hazardous activities. May cause visual disturbances.

Use with caution in patients with psychiatric or seizure disorders. May exacerbate symptoms of behavior and thought disorder in psychotic patients. Stimulants may unmask tics in individuals with coexisting Tourette's syndrome. **[U.S. Boxed Warning]: Potential for drug dependency exists; prolonged use may lead to drug dependency.** Use is contraindicated in patients with history of ethanol or drug abuse. Prescriptions should be written for the smallest quantity consistent with good patient care to minimize possibility of overdose. Abrupt discontinuation following high doses or for prolonged periods may result in symptoms for withdrawal. Safety and efficacy have not been established in children <3 years of age. Appetite suppression may occur; monitor weight during therapy, particularly in children. Use of stimulants has been associated with suppression of growth; monitor growth rate during treatment.

Adverse Reactions

As reported with Adderall XR®:

>10%:

Central nervous system: Insomnia (12% to 27%), headache (up to 26% in adults)

Gastrointestinal: Appetite decreased (22% to 36%), abdominal pain (11% to 14%), dry mouth (2% to 35%), weight loss (4% to 11%)

1% to 10%:

Cardiovascular: Tachycardia (up to 6% in adults), palpitation (2% to 4%)

Central nervous system: Emotional lability (2% to 9%), agitation (up to 8% in adults), anxiety (8%), dizziness (2% to 7%), nervousness (6%), fever (5%), somnolence (2% to 4%)

Dermatologic: Photosensitization (2% to 4%)

Endocrine & metabolic: Dysmenorrhea (2% to 4%), impotence (2% to 4%), libido decreased (2% to 4%)

Gastrointestinal: Nausea (2% to 8%), vomiting (2% to 7%), diarrhea (2% to 6%), constipation (2% to 4%), dyspepsia (2% to 4%), tooth disorder (2% to 4%)

Genitourinary: Urinary tract infection (5%)

Neuromuscular & skeletal: Twitching (2% to 4%), weakness (2% to 6%)

Respiratory: Dyspnea (2% to 4%)

Miscellaneous: Diaphoresis (2% to 4%), infection (2% to 4%), speech disorder (2% to 4%)

<1% (Limited to important or life-threatening): MI, seizure, stroke, sudden death

Adverse reactions reported with other amphetamines include: Cardiomyopathy, dyskinesia, dysphoria, euphoria, exacerbation of motor and phonic tics, exacerbation of Tourette's syndrome, headache, hypertension, overstimulation, palpitation, psychosis, rash, restlessness, tachycardia, tremor, urticaria

Metabolism/Transport Effects Amphetamine: **Inhibits** CYP2D6 (weak)

Drug Interactions

Alkalinizing Agents: May decrease the excretion of Amphetamines. *Risk D: Consider therapy modification*

Ammonium Chloride: May decrease the serum concentration of Amphetamines. This effect is likely due to an enhanced excretion of amphetamines in the urine. *Risk C: Monitor therapy*

Analgesics (Opioid): Amphetamines may enhance the analgesic effect of Analgesics (Opioid). *Risk C: Monitor therapy*

Antacids: May decrease the excretion of Amphetamines. *Risk C: Monitor therapy*

Antihistamines: Amphetamines may diminish the sedative effect of Antihistamines. *Risk C: Monitor therapy*

Antipsychotics: May diminish the stimulatory effect of Amphetamines. *Risk C: Monitor therapy*

Cannabinoids: May enhance the tachycardic effect of Sympathomimetics. *Risk C: Monitor therapy*

Carbonic Anhydrase Inhibitors: May decrease the excretion of Amphetamines. **Exceptions:** Brinzolamide; Dorzolamide. *Risk C: Monitor therapy*

Ethosuximide: Amphetamines may diminish the therapeutic effect of Ethosuximide. Amphetamines may decrease the serum concentration of Ethosuximide. *Risk C: Monitor therapy*

Gastrointestinal Acidifying Agents: May decrease the serum concentration of Amphetamines. *Risk C: Monitor therapy*

Lithium: May diminish the stimulatory effect of Amphetamines. *Risk C: Monitor therapy*

MAO Inhibitors: May enhance the hypertensive effect of Amphetamines. *Risk X: Avoid combination*

Methenamine: May decrease the serum concentration of Amphetamines. This effect is likely due to an enhanced excretion of amphetamines in the urine. *Risk C: Monitor therapy*

PHENobarbital: Amphetamines may decrease the serum concentration of PHENobarbital. *Risk C: Monitor therapy*

Phenytoin: Amphetamines may decrease the serum concentration of Phenytoin. *Risk C: Monitor therapy*

Sympathomimetics: May enhance the adverse/toxic effect of other Sympathomimetics. *Risk C: Monitor therapy*

Tricyclic Antidepressants: May enhance the stimulatory effect of Amphetamines. Tricyclic Antidepressants may also potentiate the cardiovascular effects of Amphetamines. *Risk C: Monitor therapy*

Ethanol/Nutrition/Herb Interactions

Ethanol: Avoid ethanol (may increase CNS depression).

Food: Dextroamphetamine serum levels may be altered if taken with acidic food, juices, or vitamin C. Avoid caffeine.

Herb/Nutraceutical: Avoid ephedra (may cause hypertension or arrhythmias).

Stability Store at controlled room temperature of 15°C to 30°C (59°F to 86°F); protect from light

Mechanism of Action Blocks reuptake of dopamine and norepinephrine from the synapse, thus increases the amount of circulating dopamine and norepinephrine in cerebral cortex to reticular activating system; inhibits the action of monoamine oxidase and causes catecholamines to be released. Peripheral actions include elevation of blood pressure, weak bronchodilation, and respiratory stimulation.

Pharmacodynamics/Kinetics

Onset: 30-60 minutes

Duration: 4-6 hours

Absorption: Well-absorbed

Distribution: V_d: Adults: 3.5-4.6 L/kg; concentrates in breast milk (avoid breast-feeding); distributes into CNS, mean CSF concentrations are 80% of plasma

Half-life elimination:

Children 6-12 years: d-amphetamine: 9 hours; l-amphetamine: 11 hours

Adolescents 13-17 years: d-amphetamine: 11 hours; l-amphetamine: 13-14 hours

Adults: d-amphetamine: 10 hours; l-amphetamine: 13 hours

Metabolism: Hepatic via cytochrome P450 monooxygenase and glucuronidation

Time to peak: T_{max}: Adderall®: 3 hours; Adderall XR®: 7 hours

Excretion: Urine (highly dependent on urinary pH); 70% of a single dose is eliminated within 24 hours; excreted as unchanged amphetamine (30%, may range from ~1% in alkaline urine to ~75% in acidic urine), benzoic acid, hydroxyamphetamine, hippuric acid, norephedrine, and *p*-hydroxynorephedrine

Dosage Oral: **Note:** Use lowest effective individualized dose; administer first dose as soon as awake

ADHD:

Children: <3 years: Not recommended

Children: 3-5 years (Adderall®): Initial 2.5 mg/day given every morning; increase daily dose in 2.5 mg increments at weekly intervals until optimal response is obtained (maximum dose: 40 mg/day given in 1-3 divided doses); use intervals of 4-6 hours between additional doses

Children: ≥6 years:

Adderall®: Initial: 5 mg 1-2 times/day; increase daily dose in 5 mg increments at weekly intervals until optimal response is obtained (usual maximum dose: 40 mg/day given in 1-3 divided doses); use intervals of 4-6 hours between additional doses

Adderall XR®: 5-10 mg once daily in the morning; if needed, may increase daily dose in 5-10 mg increments at weekly intervals (maximum dose: 30 mg/day)

Adolescents 13-17 years (Adderall XR®): 10 mg once daily in the morning; maybe increased to 20 mg/day after 1 week if symptoms are not controlled; higher doses (up to 60 mg/day) have been evaluated; however, there is not adequate evidence that higher doses afford additional benefit.

Adults (Adderall XR®): Initial: 20 mg once daily in the morning; higher doses (up to 60 mg once daily) have been evaluated; however, there is not adequate evidence that higher doses afforded additional benefit

Narcolepsy (Adderall®):

Children: 6-12 years: Initial: 5 mg/day; increase daily dose in 5 mg at weekly intervals until optimal response is obtained (maximum dose: 60 mg/day given in 1-3 divided doses with intervals of 4-6 hours between doses)

Children >12 years and Adults: Initial: 10 mg/day; increase daily dose in 10 mg increments at weekly intervals until optimal response is obtained (maximum dose: 60 mg/day given in 1-3 divided doses with intervals of 4-6 hours between doses)

Administration

Adderall®: To avoid insomnia, last daily dose should be administered no less than 6 hours before retiring.

Adderall XR®: Should be given by noon. Capsule may be swallowed whole or it may be opened and the contents sprinkled on applesauce. Applesauce should be consumed immediately without chewing. Do not divide the contents of the capsule.

Monitoring Parameters CNS activity, blood pressure, pulse; height, weight, growth parameters; appetite; signs/symptoms of tolerance or dependence

When used for the treatment of ADHD, thoroughly evaluate for cardiovascular risk. Monitor heart rate, blood pressure, and consider obtaining ECG prior to initiation (Vetter, 2008).

Test Interactions May interfere with urinary steroid testing

Additional Information Treatment of ADHD may include "drug holidays" or periodic discontinuation of medication in order to assess the patient's requirements, decrease tolerance, and limit suppression of linear growth and weight; the combination of equal parts of *d*, *l*-amphetamine aspartate, *d*, *l*-amphetamine sulfate, dextroamphetamine saccharate and dextroamphetamine sulfate results in a 75:25 ratio of the dextro and levo isomers of amphetamine.

The duration of action of Adderall® is longer than methylphenidate; behavioral effects of a single morning dose of Adderall® may last throughout the school day; a single morning dose of Adderall® has been shown in several studies to be as effective as twice daily dosing of methylphenidate for the treatment of ADHD (see Pelham et al, *Pediatrics*, 1999, 104(6):1300-11; Manos, 1999; Pliszka, 2000).

Dosage Forms Excipient information presented when available (limited, particularly for generics); consult specific product labeling.

Capsule, extended release:

Adderall XR®:

5 mg [dextroamphetamine sulfate 1.25 mg, dextroamphetamine saccharate 1.25 mg, amphetamine aspartate monohydrate 1.25 mg, amphetamine sulfate 1.25 mg (equivalent to amphetamine base 3.1 mg)]

10 mg [dextroamphetamine sulfate 2.5 mg, dextroamphetamine saccharate 2.5 mg, amphetamine aspartate monohydrate 2.5 mg, amphetamine sulfate 2.5 mg (equivalent to amphetamine base 6.3 mg)]

15 mg [dextroamphetamine sulfate 3.75 mg, dextroamphetamine saccharate 3.75 mg, amphetamine aspartate monohydrate 3.75 mg, amphetamine sulfate 3.75 mg (equivalent to amphetamine base 9.4 mg)]

20 mg [dextroamphetamine sulfate 5 mg, dextroamphetamine saccharate 5 mg, amphetamine aspartate monohydrate 5 mg, amphetamine sulfate 5 mg (equivalent to amphetamine base 12.5 mg)]

25 mg [dextroamphetamine sulfate 6.25 mg, dextroamphetamine saccharate 6.25 mg, amphetamine aspartate monohydrate 6.25 mg, amphetamine sulfate 6.25 mg (equivalent to amphetamine base 15.6 mg)]

30 mg [dextroamphetamine sulfate 7.5 mg, dextroamphetamine saccharate 7.5 mg, amphetamine aspartate monohydrate 7.5 mg, amphetamine sulfate 7.5 mg (equivalent to amphetamine base 18.8 mg)]

Tablet:

5 mg [dextroamphetamine sulfate 1.25 mg, dextroamphetamine saccharate 1.25 mg, amphetamine aspartate monohydrate 1.25 mg, amphetamine sulfate 1.25 mg (equivalent to amphetamine base 3.13 mg)]

7.5 mg [dextroamphetamine 1.875 mg, dextroamphetamine saccharate 1.875 mg, amphetamine aspartate monohydrate 1.875 mg, amphetamine sulfate 1.875 mg (equivalent to amphetamine base 4.7 mg)]

10 mg [dextroamphetamine sulfate 2.5 mg, dextroamphetamine saccharate 2.5 mg, amphetamine aspartate monohydrate 2.5 mg, amphetamine sulfate 2.5 mg (equivalent to amphetamine base 6.3 mg)]

12.5 mg [dextroamphetamine sulfate 3.125 mg, dextroamphetamine saccharate 3.125 mg, amphetamine aspartate monohydrate 3.125 mg, amphetamine sulfate 3.125 mg (equivalent to amphetamine base 7.8 mg)]

15 mg [dextroamphetamine sulfate 3.75 mg, dextroamphetamine saccharate 3.75 mg, amphetamine aspartate monohydrate 3.75 mg, amphetamine sulfate 3.75 mg (equivalent to amphetamine base 9.4 mg)]

20 mg [dextroamphetamine sulfate 5 mg, dextroamphetamine saccharate 5 mg, amphetamine aspartate monohydrate 5 mg, amphetamine sulfate 5 mg (equivalent to amphetamine base 12.6 mg)]

30 mg [dextroamphetamine sulfate 7.5 mg, dextroamphetamine saccharate 7.5 mg, amphetamine aspartate monohydrate 7.5 mg, amphetamine sulfate 7.5 mg (equivalent to amphetamine base 18.8 mg)]

Adderall®:

5 mg [dextroamphetamine sulfate 1.25 mg, dextroamphetamine saccharate 1.25 mg, amphetamine aspartate monohydrate 1.25 mg, amphetamine sulfate 1.25 mg (equivalent to amphetamine base 3.13 mg)]

7.5 mg [dextroamphetamine 1.875 mg, dextroamphetamine saccharate 1.875 mg, amphetamine aspartate monohydrate 1.875 mg, amphetamine sulfate 1.875 mg (equivalent to amphetamine base 4.7 mg)]

10 mg [dextroamphetamine sulfate 2.5 mg, dextroamphetamine saccharate 2.5 mg, amphetamine aspartate monohydrate 2.5 mg, amphetamine sulfate 2.5 mg (equivalent to amphetamine base 6.3 mg)]
12.5 mg [dextroamphetamine sulfate 3.125 mg, dextroamphetamine saccharate 3.125 mg, amphetamine aspartate monohydrate 3.125 mg, amphetamine sulfate 3.125 mg (equivalent to amphetamine base 7.8 mg)]
15 mg [dextroamphetamine sulfate 3.75 mg, dextroamphetamine saccharate 3.75 mg, amphetamine aspartate monohydrate 3.75 mg, amphetamine sulfate 3.75 mg (equivalent to amphetamine base 9.4 mg)]
20 mg [dextroamphetamine sulfate 5 mg, dextroamphetamine saccharate 5 mg, amphetamine aspartate monohydrate 5 mg, amphetamine sulfate 5 mg (equivalent to amphetamine base 12.6 mg)]
30 mg [dextroamphetamine sulfate 7.5 mg, dextroamphetamine saccharate 7.5 mg, amphetamine aspartate monohydrate 7.5 mg, amphetamine sulfate 7.5 mg (equivalent to amphetamine base 18.8 mg)]

◆ **Dextroamphetamine Sulfate** *see* Dextroamphetamine *on page 441*

Dextromethorphan (deks troe meth OR fan)

Medication Safety Issues
Sound-alike/look-alike issues:
Benylin® may be confused with Benadryl®, Ventolin®
Delsym® may be confused with Delfen®, Desyrel®

U.S. Brand Names Babee® Cof Syrup [OTC]; Creo-Terpin® [OTC]; Creomulsion® Cough [OTC]; Creomulsion® for Children [OTC]; Delsym® [OTC]; ElixSure® Cough [OTC]; Hold® DM [OTC]; PediaCare® Infants' Long-Acting Cough [OTC] [DSC]; Robitussin® CoughGels™ [OTC]; Robitussin® Maximum Strength Cough [OTC]; Robitussin® Pediatric Cough [OTC]; Scot-Tussin DM® Cough Chasers [OTC] [DSC]; Silphen DM® [OTC]; Triaminic® Thin Strips™ Long Acting Cough [OTC]; Vicks® 44® Cough Relief [OTC]

Mexican Brand Names Athos; Brudex; Romilar; Tesafilm

Pharmacologic Category Antitussive

Use Symptomatic relief of coughs caused by minor viral upper respiratory tract infections or inhaled irritants; most effective for a chronic nonproductive cough

Unlabeled/Investigational Use *N*-methyl-D-aspartate (NMDA) antagonist in cerebral injury

Effect on Mental Status May cause drowsiness or depression

Effect on Psychiatric Treatment Use with MAO inhibitors may cause hypertensive crisis; avoid combination

Dosage Summary
Oral:
Extended release:
Children <2 years: Dosage not established
Children 2-6 years: 15 mg twice daily (maximum: 30 mg/day)
Children 6-12 years: 30 mg twice daily (maximum: 60 mg/day)
Children >12 years: 60 mg twice daily (maximum: 120 mg/day)
Adults: 60 mg twice daily (maximum: 120 mg/day)
Immediate release:
Children <2 years: Use only as directed by a physician
Children 2-6 years: 2.5-7.5 mg every 4-8 hours (maximum: 30 mg/day)
Children 6-12 years: 5-10 mg every 4 hours **or** 15 mg every 6-8 hours (maximum: 60 mg/day)
Children >12 years: 10-20 mg every 4 hours **or** 30 mg every 6-8 hours (maximum: 120 mg/day)
Adults: 10-20 mg every 4 hours **or** 30 mg every 6-8 hours (maximum: 120 mg/day)

Dosage Forms Excipient information presented when available (limited, particularly for generics); consult specific product labeling. [DSC] = Discontinued product
Gelcap, as hydrobromide:
Robitussin® CoughGels™: 15 mg [contains coconut oil]
Liquid, as hydrobromide:
Creo-Terpin®: 10 mg/15 mL (120 mL) [contains alcohol 25% and tartrazine]
Vicks® 44® Cough Relief: 10 mg/5 mL (120 mL) [contains alcohol, sodium 10 mg/5 mL, sodium benzoate]
Liquid, oral, as hydrobromide [drops]:
PediaCare® Infants' Long-Acting Cough: 7.5 mg/0.8 mL (15 mL) [alcohol free, dye free; contains sodium benzoate; grape flavor] [DSC]

Lozenge, as hydrobromide:
Hold® DM: 5 mg (10s) [cherry or original flavor]
Scot-Tussin DM® Cough Chasers: 5 mg (20s) [DSC]
Strips, oral, as hydrobromide:
Triaminic® Thin Strips™ Long Acting Cough: 7.5 mg [equivalent to dextromethorphan 5 mg; cherry flavor]
Suspension, extended release:
Delsym®: Dextromethorphan polistirex [equivalent to dextromethorphan hydrobromide 30 mg/5 mL] (78 mL, 148 mL) [contains sodium 6 mg/5 mL; orange flavor]
Syrup, as hydrobromide:
Babee® Cof Syrup: 7.5 mg/5 mL (120 mL) [alcohol free, dye free; cherry flavor]
Creomulsion® Cough: 20 mg/15 mL (120 mL) [alcohol free; contains sodium benzoate]
Creomulsion® for Children: 5 mg/5 mL (120 mL) [alcohol free; contains sodium benzoate; cherry flavor]
ElixSure® Cough: 7.5 mg/5 mL (120 mL) [cherry bubble gum flavor]
Robitussin® Maximum Strength Cough: 15 mg/5 mL (120 mL, 240 mL) [contains alcohol, sodium benzoate]
Robitussin® Pediatric Cough: 7.5 mg/5 mL (120 mL) [alcohol free; contains sodium benzoate; fruit punch flavor]
Silphen DM®: 10 mg/5 mL (120 mL) [strawberry flavor]

◆ **Dextromethorphan, Acetaminophen, and Pseudoephedrine** *see* Acetaminophen, Dextromethorphan, and Pseudoephedrine *on page 43*

Dextromethorphan and Chlorpheniramine

(deks troe meth OR fan & klor fen IR a meen)

U.S. Brand Names Coricidin® HBP Cough & Cold [OTC]; Dimetapp® Children's Long Acting Cough Plus Cold [OTC]; Robitussin® Children's Cough & Cold Long-Acting [OTC]; Robitussin® Cough & Cold Long-Acting [OTC]; Scot-Tussin® DM Maximum Strength [OTC]

Index Terms Chlorpheniramine and Dextromethorphan; Chlorpheniramine Maleate and Dextromethorphan Hydrobromide; Dextromethorphan Hydrobromide and Chlorpheniramine Maleate

Pharmacologic Category Antitussive; Histamine H_1 Antagonist; Histamine H_1 Antagonist, First Generation

Use Symptomatic relief of runny nose, sneezing, itchy/watery eyes, cough, and other upper respiratory symptoms associated with hay fever, common cold, or upper respiratory allergies

Effect on Mental Status May cause sedation, dizziness, excitability, nervousness

Effect on Psychiatric Treatment Contraindicated with or within 14 days of MAO inhibitor treatment. May cause sedation; concurrent use with psychotropics may produce additive effects. Combined use with serotoninergic agents may cause serotonin syndrome. The anticholinergic effects of chlorpheniramine may decrease the effects of acetylcholinesterase inhibitors. However, when combined with psychotropic agents, anticholinergic effects may be additive. Nefazodone may potentiate the effects of chlorpheniramine.

Dosage Summary

Oral:

Children <6 years: Dosage not established

Children 6-11 years: Dextromethorphan 15 mg and chlorpheniramine 2 mg every 6 hours as needed (maximum: 60 mg dextromethorphan and 8 mg chlorpheniramine/24 hours)

Children ≥12 years: Dextromethorphan 30 mg and chlorpheniramine 4 mg every 6 hours as needed (maximum: 120 mg dextromethorphan and 16 mg chlorpheniramine/24 hours)

Adults: Dextromethorphan 30 mg and chlorpheniramine 4 mg every 6 hours as needed (maximum: 120 mg dextromethorphan and 16 mg chlorpheniramine/24 hours)

Dosage Forms Excipient information presented when available (limited, particularly for generics); consult specific product labeling. [DSC] = Discontinued product

Syrup:
Dimetapp® Children's Long Acting Cough Plus Cold: Dextromethorphan hydrobromide 7.5 mg and chlorpheniramine maleate 1 mg per 5 mL (118 mL) [alcohol free, sugar free; contains sodium benzoate, propylene glycol; grape flavor]

Robitussin® Children's Cough and Cold Long-Acting: Dextromethorphan hydrobromide 15 mg and chlorpheniramine maleate 2 mg per 5 mL (118 mL) [alcohol free, sugar free; contains sodium benzoate, propylene glycol, fruit punch flavor]

Robitussin® Cough and Cold Long-Acting: Dextromethorphan hydrobromide 7.5 mg and chlorpheniramine maleate 1 mg per 5 mL (118 mL) [alcohol free, sugar free; contains sodium benzoate, propylene glycol]

Scot-Tussin® DM Maximum Strength: Dextromethorphan hydrobromide 15 mg and chlorpheniramine maleate 2 mg per 5 mL (118 mL) [alcohol free, sugar free, cherry-strawberry flavor]

Tablet:

Coricidin® HBP Cough and Cold: Dextromethorphan hydrobromide 30 mg and chlorpheniramine maleate 4 mg

◆ **Dextromethorphan and Guaifenesin** *see* Guaifenesin and Dextromethorphan *on page 739*

◆ **Dextromethorphan and Promethazine** *see* Promethazine and Dextromethorphan *on page 1350*

◆ **Dextromethorphan and Pseudoephedrine** *see* Pseudoephedrine and Dextromethorphan *on page 1369*

◆ **Dextromethorphan, Chlorpheniramine, and Phenylephrine** *see* Chlorpheniramine, Phenylephrine, and Dextromethorphan *on page 327*

◆ **Dextromethorphan, Chlorpheniramine, and Pseudoephedrine** *see* Chlorpheniramine, Pseudoephedrine, and Dextromethorphan *on page 333*

Dextromethorphan, Chlorpheniramine, Phenylephrine, and Guaifenesin

(deks troe meth OR fan, klor fen IR a meen, fen il EF rin, & gwye FEN e sin)

U.S. Brand Names Chlordex GP; Donatussin; Quartuss™

Index Terms Chlorpheniramine, Dextromethorphan, Phenylephrine, and Guaifenesin; Guaifenesin, Chlorpheniramine, Phenylephrine, and Dextromethorphan; Phenylephrine Hydrochloride, Chlorpheniramine maleate, Dextromethorphan Hydrobromide, and Guaifenesin

Pharmacologic Category Alpha/Beta Agonist; Antitussive; Expectorant; Histamine H_1 Antagonist; Histamine H_1 Antagonist, First Generation

Use Symptomatic relief of dry, nonproductive cough and upper respiratory symptoms associated with infections such as the common cold, bronchitis, or sinusitis

Effect on Mental Status May cause dizziness, drowsiness, insomnia, irritability, or nervousness

Effect on Psychiatric Treatment Contraindicated with MAO inhibitors or within 14 days of MAO inhibitor

Dosage Summary

Oral:

Children <2 year: Dosage not established

Children 2-6 years: 2.5 mL every 6 hours as needed (maximum: 10 mL/24 hours)

Children 6-12 years: 5 mL every 6 hours as needed (maximum: 20 mL/24 hours)

Children ≥12 years: 10 mL every 6 hours as needed (maximum: 40 mL/24 hours)

Adults: 10 mL every 6 hours as needed (maximum: 40 mL/24 hours)

Dosage Forms Excipient information presented when available (limited, particularly for generics); consult specific product labeling.

Syrup:

Chlordex GP®: Dextromethorphan hydrobromide 7.5 mg, chlorpheniramine maleate 2 mg, phenylephrine hydrochloride 10 mg, and guaifenesin 100 mg per 5 mL (480 mL) [grape flavor]

Donatussin: Dextromethorphan hydrobromide 15 mg, chlorpheniramine maleate 2 mg, phenylephrine hydrochloride 10 mg, and guaifenesin 100 mg per 5 mL (480 mL) [alcohol free; contains propylene glycol; cherry flavor]

Quartuss™: Dextromethorphan hydrobromide 15 mg, chlorpheniramine maleate 2 mg, phenylephrine hydrochloride 10 mg, and guaifenesin 100 mg per 5 mL (480 mL) [alcohol free, sugar free; contains sodium benzoate, propylene glycol; cherry flavor]

◆ **Dextromethorphan, Guaifenesin, and Pseudoephedrine** *see* Guaifenesin, Pseudoephedrine, and Dextromethorphan *on page 748*

- **Dextromethorphan Hydrobromide, Acetaminophen, and Phenylephrine Hydrochloride** *see* Acetaminophen, Dextromethorphan, and Phenylephrine *on page 42*
- **Dextromethorphan Hydrobromide and Chlorpheniramine Maleate** *see* Dextromethorphan and Chlorpheniramine *on page 449*
- **Dextromethorphan Hydrobromide, Brompheniramine Maleate, and Pseudoephedrine Hydrochloride** *see* Brompheniramine, Pseudoephedrine, and Dextromethorphan *on page 208*
- **Dextromethorphan Tannate, Pyrilamine Tannate, and Phenylephrine Tannate** *see* Phenylephrine, Pyrilamine, and Dextromethorphan *on page 1278*
- **Dextropropoxyphene** *see* Propoxyphene *on page 1353*
- **DextroStat®** *see* Dextroamphetamine *on page 441*
- **DFMO** *see* Eflornithine *on page 527*
- **DHAD** *see* Mitoxantrone *on page 1061*
- **DHAQ** *see* Mitoxantrone *on page 1061*
- **DHE** *see* Dihydroergotamine *on page 470*
- **D.H.E. 45®** *see* Dihydroergotamine *on page 470*
- **DHPG Sodium** *see* Ganciclovir *on page 708*
- **DHS™ Sal [OTC]** *see* Salicylic Acid *on page 1454*
- **DHT™ [DSC]** *see* Dihydrotachysterol *on page 472*
- **DHT™ Intensol™ [DSC]** *see* Dihydrotachysterol *on page 472*
- **Diabeta** *see* GlyBURIDE *on page 730*
- **Diabetic Tussin C®** *see* Guaifenesin and Codeine *on page 738*
- **Diabetic Tussin® Allergy Relief [OTC]** *see* Chlorpheniramine *on page 321*
- **Diabetic Tussin® DM [OTC]** *see* Guaifenesin and Dextromethorphan *on page 739*
- **Diabetic Tussin® DM Maximum Strength [OTC]** *see* Guaifenesin and Dextromethorphan *on page 739*
- **Diabetic Tussin® EX [OTC]** *see* GuaiFENesin *on page 737*
- **Diabinese® [DSC]** *see* ChlorproPAMIDE *on page 340*
- **Diaβeta®** *see* GlyBURIDE *on page 730*
- **Diaminocyclohexane Oxalatoplatinum** *see* Oxaliplatin *on page 1191*
- **Diaminodiphenylsulfone** *see* Dapsone *on page 418*
- **Diamode [OTC]** *see* Loperamide *on page 944*
- **Diamox® Sequels®** *see* AcetaZOLAMIDE *on page 46*
- **Diastat®** *see* Diazepam *on page 451*
- **Diastat® AcuDial™** *see* Diazepam *on page 451*

Diazepam (dye AZ e pam)

Medication Safety Issues

Sound-alike/look-alike issues:

Diazepam may be confused with diazoxide, Ditropan®, LORazepam

Valium® may be confused with Valcyte™

Related Information

Benzodiazepines *on page 1774*

CMS: Long-Term Care Facility Thresholds *on page 1815*

Discontinuation of Psychotropic Drugs *on page 1839*

U.S. Brand Names Diastat®; Diastat® AcuDial™; Diazepam Intensol®; Valium®

Canadian Brand Names Apo-Diazepam®; Diastat®; Diastat® Rectal Delivery System; Diazemuls®; Novo-Dipam; Valium®

Mexican Brand Names Ifa Fonal; Ortopsique; Sunzepam; Valium

Pharmacologic Category Benzodiazepine

Generic Available Yes: Injection, tablet, solution only

Use Management of anxiety disorders, ethanol withdrawal symptoms; skeletal muscle relaxant; status epilepticus; muscle spasm associated with tetanus

Rectal gel: Management of selected, refractory epilepsy patients on stable regimens of antiepileptic drugs (AEDs) requiring intermittent use of diazepam to control episodes of increased seizure activity

Unlabeled/Investigational Use Panic disorders; preoperative sedation, light anesthesia, amnesia

Mental Health Comment In 2007, the FDA requested that all manufacturers of sedative-hypnotic drug products revise labeling to include a greater emphasis on the risks of adverse effects. These risks include severe allergic reactions (anaphylaxis, angioedema) and complex sleep-related behaviors, which may include sleep-driving (driving while not fully awake and with no memory of the event), making phone calls, and preparing and eating food while asleep.

There are two subtypes of GABA receptors (GABA-A and GABA-B) and three different benzodiazepine receptors (Bz_1, Bz_2, and Bz_3). Benzodiazepine receptors and effects appear to be linked to the GABA-A receptors. Benzodiazepines do not bind to GABA-B receptors. The role of GABA-B receptors is unclear. Benzodiazepines have no specificity for benzodiazepine receptor subtypes.

Diazepam is a long half-life benzodiazepine. Duration of action after a single dose is determined by redistribution rather than metabolism. Tolerance develops to the sedative, hypnotic, and anticonvulsant effects. It does not develop to the anxiolytic or skeletal muscle relaxing effects. Psychological and physical dependence may occur with prolonged use of benzodiazepines. The onset of withdrawal symptoms is usually seen on the first day without drug and lasts 5-7 days in patients receiving short half-life benzodiazepines, whereas, the onset occurs after 5 days with a duration of 10-14 days after abrupt discontinuance of long half-life benzodiazepines. Risk factors for abuse include personal or family history of substance abuse and personality disorder.

Diazepam is the most rapidly absorbed benzodiazepine; poorly and erratically absorbed after I.M. administration; undergoes phase I metabolism; injection contains propylene glycol which may cause hypotension and bradycardia when injected rapidly. Therefore, maximum rate of infusion is 5 mg/minute.

Restrictions C-IV

Pregnancy Risk Factor D

Pregnancy Considerations Teratogenic effects have been reported in animal studies. In humans, diazepam crosses the placenta. An increased risk of congenital malformations and other developmental abnormalities have been associated with diazepam; epilepsy itself may also increase the risk. Hypotonia, hypothermia, withdrawal symptoms, respiratory and feeding difficulties have been reported in the infant following maternal use of benzodiazepines near time of delivery.

Lactation Enters breast milk/contraindicated (AAP rates "of concern")

Contraindications Hypersensitivity to diazepam or any component of the formulation (cross-sensitivity with other benzodiazepines may exist); myasthenia gravis; severe respiratory insufficiency; severe hepatic insufficiency; sleep apnea syndrome; acute narrow-angle glaucoma; not for use in children <6 months of age (oral)

Warnings/Precautions Withdrawal has also been associated with an increase in the seizure frequency. Use with caution with drugs which may decrease diazepam metabolism. Use with caution in elderly or debilitated patients, obese patients, patients with hepatic disease (including alcoholics), or renal impairment. Active metabolites with extended half-lives may lead to delayed accumulation and adverse effects. Use with caution in patients with respiratory disease or impaired gag reflex.

Acute hypotension, muscle weakness, apnea, and cardiac arrest have occurred with parenteral administration. Acute effects may be more prevalent in patients receiving concurrent barbiturates, narcotics, or ethanol. Appropriate resuscitative equipment and qualified personnel should be available during administration and monitoring. Avoid use of the injection in patients with shock, coma, or acute ethanol intoxication. Intra-arterial injection or extravasation of the parenteral formulation should be avoided. Parenteral formulation contains propylene glycol, which has been associated with toxicity when administered in high dosages. Administration of rectal gel should only be performed by individuals trained to recognize characteristic seizure activity and monitor response.

Causes CNS depression (dose-related) resulting in sedation, dizziness, confusion, or ataxia which may impair physical and mental capabilities. Patients must be cautioned about performing tasks which require mental alertness (eg, operating machinery or driving). Use with caution in patients receiving other CNS depressants or psychoactive agents. Effects with other sedative drugs or ethanol may be potentiated. The dosage of narcotics should be reduced by approximately 1/3 when diazepam is added. Benzodiazepines have been associated with falls and traumatic injury and should be used with extreme caution in patients who are at risk of these events (especially the elderly). Use with caution in patients taking strong CYP3A4 inhibitors, moderate or strong CYP3A4 and CYP2C19 inducers and major CYP3A4 substrates.

Use caution in patients with depression or anxiety associated with depression, particularly if suicidal risk may be present. Use with caution in patients with a history of drug dependence. Benzodiazepines have been associated with dependence and acute withdrawal symptoms on discontinuation or reduction in dose. Acute withdrawal, including seizures, may be precipitated in patients after administration of flumazenil to patients receiving long-term benzodiazepine therapy.

Diazepam has been associated with anterograde amnesia. Psychiatric and paradoxical reactions, including hyperactive or aggressive behavior, have been reported with benzodiazepines, particularly in adolescent/pediatric or elderly patients. Does not have analgesic, antidepressant, or antipsychotic properties.

Rectal gel: Safety and efficacy have not been established in children <2 years of age.

Oral: Safety and efficacy have not been established in children <6 months of age.

Injection: Safety and efficacy have not been established in children <30 days of age. Solution for injection may contain sodium benzoate, benzyl alcohol, or benzoic acid. Large amounts have been associated with "gasping syndrome" in neonates.

Adverse Reactions Frequency not defined. Adverse reactions may vary by route of administration.

Cardiovascular: Hypotension, vasodilatation

Central nervous system: Amnesia, ataxia, confusion, depression, drowsiness, fatigue, headache, slurred speech, paradoxical reactions (eg, aggressiveness, agitation, anxiety, delusions, hallucinations, inappropriate behavior, increased muscle spasms, insomnia, irritability, psychoses, rage, restlessness, sleep disturbances, stimulation), vertigo

Dermatologic: Rash

Endocrine & metabolic: Libido changes

Gastrointestinal: Constipation, diarrhea, nausea, salivation changes (dry mouth or hypersalivation)

Genitourinary: Incontinence, urinary retention

Hepatic: Jaundice

Local: Phlebitis, pain with injection

Neuromuscular & skeletal: Dysarthria, tremor, weakness

Ocular: Blurred vision, diplopia

Respiratory: Apnea, asthma, respiratory rate decreased

Metabolism/Transport Effects Substrate of CYP1A2 (minor), 2B6 (minor), 2C9 (minor), 2C19 (major), 3A4 (major); **Inhibits** CYP2C19 (weak), 3A4 (weak)

Drug Interactions

Alcohol (Ethyl): CNS Depressants may enhance the CNS depressant effect of Alcohol (Ethyl). *Risk C: Monitor therapy*

Antifungal Agents (Azole Derivatives, Systemic): May decrease the metabolism of Benzodiazepines (metabolized by oxidation). *Risk D: Consider therapy modification*

Aprepitant: May increase the serum concentration of Benzodiazepines (metabolized by oxidation). *Risk C: Monitor therapy*

Calcium Channel Blockers (Nondihydropyridine): May decrease the metabolism of Benzodiazepines (metabolized by oxidation). *Risk D: Consider therapy modification*

CarBAMazepine: May increase the metabolism of Benzodiazepines (metabolized by oxidation). *Risk C: Monitor therapy*

Cimetidine: May decrease the metabolism of Benzodiazepines (metabolized by oxidation). *Risk C: Monitor therapy*

Clozapine: Benzodiazepines may enhance the adverse/toxic effect of Clozapine. *Risk D: Consider therapy modification*

CNS Depressants: May enhance the adverse/toxic effect of other CNS Depressants. *Risk C: Monitor therapy*

CYP2C19 Inducers (Strong): May increase the metabolism of CYP2C19 Substrates. *Risk C: Monitor therapy*

CYP2C19 Inhibitors (Moderate): May decrease the metabolism of CYP2C19 Substrates. *Risk C: Monitor therapy*

CYP2C19 Inhibitors (Strong): May decrease the metabolism of CYP2C19 Substrates. *Risk D: Consider therapy modification*

CYP3A4 Inducers (Strong): May increase the metabolism of CYP3A4 Substrates. *Risk C: Monitor therapy*

CYP3A4 Inhibitors (Moderate): May decrease the metabolism of CYP3A4 Substrates. *Risk C: Monitor therapy*

CYP3A4 Inhibitors (Strong): May decrease the metabolism of CYP3A4 Substrates. *Risk D: Consider therapy modification*

Dasatinib: May increase the serum concentration of CYP3A4 Substrates. *Risk C: Monitor therapy*

Deferasirox: May decrease the serum concentration of CYP3A4 Substrates. *Risk C: Monitor therapy*

Disulfiram: May decrease the metabolism of Benzodiazepines (metabolized by oxidation). *Risk C: Monitor therapy*

Fluconazole: May decrease the metabolism of Benzodiazepines (metabolized by oxidation). *Risk D: Consider therapy modification*

Fosaprepitant: May increase the serum concentration of Benzodiazepines (metabolized by oxidation). Specifically, the active metabolite aprepitant is likely responsible for this effect. *Risk C: Monitor therapy*

Grapefruit Juice: May decrease the metabolism of Benzodiazepines (metabolized by oxidation). *Risk D: Consider therapy modification*

Isoniazid: May decrease the metabolism of Benzodiazepines (metabolized by oxidation). *Risk C: Monitor therapy*

Macrolide Antibiotics: May decrease the metabolism of Benzodiazepines (metabolized by oxidation). **Exceptions:** Azithromycin; Dirithromycin [Off Market]; Spiramycin. *Risk D: Consider therapy modification*

Nefazodone: May decrease the metabolism of Benzodiazepines (metabolized by oxidation). *Risk D: Consider therapy modification*

Oral Contraceptive (Estrogens): May decrease the metabolism of Benzodiazepines (metabolized by oxidation). *Risk C: Monitor therapy*

Oral Contraceptive (Progestins): May decrease the metabolism of Benzodiazepines (metabolized by oxidation). *Risk C: Monitor therapy*

Phenytoin: Benzodiazepines may increase the serum concentration of Phenytoin. Short-term exposure to benzodiazepines may not present as much risk as chronic therapy. *Risk C: Monitor therapy*

Protease Inhibitors: May decrease the metabolism of Benzodiazepines (metabolized by oxidation). Management: Amprenavir, atazanavir, darunavir, indinavir, nelfinavir, ritonavir, and tipranavir are contraindicated with midazolam and triazolam according to each protease inhibitor 's prescribing information. *Risk D: Consider therapy modification*

Proton Pump Inhibitors: May increase the serum concentration of Benzodiazepines (metabolized by oxidation). **Exceptions:** Lansoprazole; Pantoprazole; Rabeprazole. *Risk C: Monitor therapy*

Rifamycin Derivatives: May increase the metabolism of Benzodiazepines (metabolized by oxidation). *Risk D: Consider therapy modification*

Selective Serotonin Reuptake Inhibitors: May decrease the metabolism of Benzodiazepines (metabolized by oxidation). **Exceptions:** Citalopram; Escitalopram; PARoxetine; Sertraline. *Risk C: Monitor therapy*

St Johns Wort: May increase the metabolism of Benzodiazepines (metabolized by oxidation). *Risk C: Monitor therapy*

Theophylline Derivatives: May diminish the therapeutic effect of Benzodiazepines. *Risk D: Consider therapy modification*

Ethanol/Nutrition/Herb Interactions

Ethanol: Avoid ethanol (may increase CNS depression).

Food: Diazepam serum levels may be increased if taken with food. Diazepam effect/toxicity may be increased by grapefruit juice; avoid concurrent use.

Herb/Nutraceutical: St John's wort may decrease diazepam levels. Avoid valerian, St John's wort, kava kava, gotu kola (may increase CNS depression).

Stability

Injection: Store at 20° to 25°C (68° to 77°F); excursions permitted to 15°C to 30°C (59°F to 86°F). Protect from light. Potency is retained for up to 3 months when kept at room temperature. Most stable at pH 4-8; hydrolysis occurs at pH <3. Per manufacturer, do not mix I.V. product with other medications.

Rectal gel: Store at 25°C (77°F); excursion permitted to 15°C to 30°C (59°F to 86°F).

Tablet: Store at 15°C to 30°C (59°F to 86°F).

Mechanism of Action Binds to stereospecific benzodiazepine receptors on the postsynaptic GABA neuron at several sites within the central nervous system, including the limbic system, reticular formation. Enhancement of the inhibitory effect of GABA on neuronal excitability results by increased neuronal membrane permeability to chloride ions. This shift in chloride ions results in hyperpolarization (a less excitable state) and stabilization.

Pharmacodynamics/Kinetics

I.V.: Status epilepticus:

Onset of action: Almost immediate

Duration: 20-30 minutes

Absorption: Oral: 85% to 100%, more reliable than I.M.

Protein binding: 98%

Metabolism: Hepatic

Half-life elimination: Parent drug: Adults: 20-50 hours; increased half-life in neonates, elderly, and those with severe hepatic disorders; Active major metabolite (desmethyldiazepam): 50-100 hours; may be prolonged in neonates

Dosage Oral absorption is more reliable than I.M.

Children:

Conscious sedation for procedures: Oral: 0.2-0.3 mg/kg (maximum: 10 mg) 45-60 minutes prior to procedure

Muscle spasm associated with tetanus: I.V., I.M.:

Infants >30 days: 1-2 mg/dose every 3-4 hours as needed

Children ≥5 years: 5-10 mg/dose every 3-4 hours as needed

Sedation/muscle relaxant/anxiety:

Oral: 0.12-0.8 mg/kg/day in divided doses every 6-8 hours

I.M., I.V.: 0.04-0.3 mg/kg/dose every 2-4 hours to a maximum of 0.6 mg/kg within an 8-hour period if needed

Status epilepticus:

I.V.: Infants >30 days and Children: 0.1-0.3 mg/kg given over ≤5 mg/minute; may repeat dose after 5-10 minutes; maximum: 10 mg/dose (Hegenbarth, 2008)

Rectal gel: 0.5 mg/kg, then 0.25 mg/kg in 10 minutes if needed

Anticonvulsant (acute treatment): Rectal gel:

Children <2 years: Safety and efficacy have not been studied

Children 2-5 years: 0.5 mg/kg

Children 6-11 years: 0.3 mg/kg

Children ≥12 years: 0.2 mg/kg

Note: Dosage should be rounded upward to the next available dose, 2.5, 5, 7.5, 10, 12.5, 15, 17.5, and 20 mg/dose; dose may be repeated in 4-12 hours if needed; do not use for more than 5 episodes per month or more than one episode every 5 days

Adolescents: Conscious sedation for procedures:

Oral: 10 mg

I.V.: 5 mg, may repeat with 1/2 dose if needed

Adults:

Acute ethanol withdrawal: Oral: 10 mg 3-4 times during first 24 hours, then decrease to 5 mg 3-4 times/day as needed

Anticonvulsant (acute treatment): Rectal gel: 0.2 mg/kg

Note: Dosage should be rounded upward to the next available dose, 2.5, 5, 7.5, 10, 12.5, 15, 17.5, and 20 mg/dose; dose may be repeated in 4-12 hours if needed; do not use for more than 5 episodes per month or more than one episode every 5 days.

Anxiety (symptoms/disorders):

Oral: 2-10 mg 2-4 times/day

I.M., I.V.: 2-10 mg, may repeat in 3-4 hours if needed

Muscle spasm: I.V., I.M.: Initial: 5-10 mg; then 5-10 mg in 3-4 hours, if necessary. Larger doses may be required if associated with tetanus.

Sedation in the ICU patient: I.V.: 0.03-0.1 mg/kg every 30 minutes to 6 hours

Skeletal muscle relaxant (adjunct therapy): Oral: 2-10 mg 3-4 times/day

Status epilepticus:

I.V.: 5-10 mg every 5-10 minutes given over ≤5 mg/minute; maximum dose: 30 mg

Rectal gel: Premonitory/out-of-hospital treatment: 10 mg once; may repeat once if necessary

Rapid tranquilization of agitated patient (administer every 30-60 minutes): Oral: 5-10 mg; average total dose for tranquilization: 20-60 mg

Elderly/debilitated patients:

Oral: 2-2.5 mg 1-2 times/day initially; increase gradually as needed and tolerated

Rectal gel: Due to the increased half-life in elderly and debilitated patients, consider reducing dose.

Dosing adjustment in renal impairment: No dose adjustment recommended; decrease dose if administered for prolonged periods.

I.V.: Risk of propylene glycol toxicity; monitor closely if using for prolonged periods or at high doses

Hemodialysis: Not dialyzable (0% to 5%); supplemental dose is not necessary

Dosing adjustment in hepatic impairment: Use with caution

Administration Intensol® should be diluted before use.

In children, do not exceed 1-2 mg/minute IVP; adults 5 mg/minute.

Rectal gel: Prior to administration, confirm that prescribed dose is visible and correct, and that the green "ready" band is visible. Patient should be positioned on side (facing person responsible for monitoring), with top leg bent forward. Insert rectal tip (lubricated) into rectum and push in plunger gently over 3 seconds. Remove tip of rectal syringe after 3 additional seconds. Buttocks should be held together for 3 seconds after removal. Dispose of syringe appropriately.

Monitoring Parameters Respiratory, cardiovascular, and mental status; check for orthostasis

Reference Range Therapeutic: Diazepam: 0.2-1.5 mcg/mL (SI: 0.7-5.3 μmol/L); N-desmethyldiazepam (nordiazepam): 0.1-0.5 mcg/mL (SI: 0.35-1.8 μmol/L)

Test Interactions False-negative urinary glucose determinations when using Clinistix® or Diastix®

Additional Information Diazepam does not have any analgesic effects.

Diastat® AcuDial™: When dispensing, consult package information for directions on setting patient's dose; confirm green "ready" band is visible prior to dispensing product.

Dosage Forms Excipient information presented when available (limited, particularly for generics); consult specific product labeling.

Gel, rectal:

Diastat®: Pediatric rectal tip [4.4 cm]: 5 mg/mL (2.5 mg, 5 mg) [contains ethyl alcohol 10%, sodium benzoate, benzyl alcohol 1.5%; twin pack]

Diastat® AcuDial™ delivery system:

10 mg: Pediatric/adult rectal tip [4.4 cm]: 5 mg/mL (delivers set doses of 5 mg, 7.5 mg, and 10 mg) [contains ethyl alcohol 10%, sodium benzoate, benzyl alcohol 1.5%; twin pack]

20 mg: Adult rectal tip [6 cm]: 5 mg/mL (delivers set doses of 10 mg, 12.5 mg, 15 mg, 17.5 mg, and 20 mg) [contains ethyl alcohol 10%, sodium benzoate, benzyl alcohol 1.5%; twin pack]

Injection, solution: 5 mg/mL (2 mL, 10 mL)

Solution, oral: 5 mg/5 mL (5 mL, 500 mL)

Solution, oral concentrate:

Diazepam Intensol®: 5 mg/mL (30 mL)

Tablet: 2 mg, 5 mg, 10 mg

Valium®: 2 mg, 5 mg, 10 mg

◆ **Diazepam Intensol®** *see* Diazepam *on page 451*

Diazoxide (dye az OKS ide)

Medication Safety Issues

Sound-alike/look-alike issues:

Diazoxide may be confused with diazepam, Dyazide®

U.S. Brand Names Proglycem®

Canadian Brand Names Proglycem®

Pharmacologic Category Antihypoglycemic Agent; Vasodilator, Direct-Acting

Use Hypoglycemia related to islet cell adenoma, carcinoma, hyperplasia, or adenomatosis; nesidioblastosis; leucine sensitivity; extrapancreatic malignancy

Effect on Mental Status May cause dizziness; may rarely cause extrapyramidal symptoms

Effect on Psychiatric Treatment May cause leukopenia; use caution with clozapine and carbamazepine

Dosage Summary

Oral:

Infants: 8-15 mg/kg/day in divided doses every 8-12 hours

Children: 3-8 mg/kg/day in divided doses every 8-12 hours

Adults: 3-8 mg/kg/day in divided doses every 8-12 hours

Dosage Forms Excipient information presented when available (limited, particularly for generics); consult specific product labeling.

Capsule, oral:

Proglycem®: 50 mg [not available in the U.S.]

Suspension, oral:

Proglycem®: 50 mg/mL (30 mL) [contains ethanol 7.25%, sodium benzoate, propylene glycol; chocolate-mint flavor]

◆ **Dibenzyline®** *see* Phenoxybenzamine *on page 1270*

◆ **DIC** *see* Dacarbazine *on page 414*

◆ **Dicel™** *see* Chlorpheniramine and Pseudoephedrine *on page 325*

◆ **Dicel™ DM** *see* Chlorpheniramine, Pseudoephedrine, and Dextromethorphan *on page 333*

◆ **Dichloralphenazone, Acetaminophen, and Isometheptene** *see* Acetaminophen, Isometheptene, and Dichloralphenazone *on page 45*

◆ **Dichloralphenazone, Isometheptene, and Acetaminophen** *see* Acetaminophen, Isometheptene, and Dichloralphenazone *on page 45*

Dichlorphenamide (dye klor FEN a mide)

Medication Safety Issues

Sound-alike/look-alike issues:

Daranide® may be confused with Daraprim®

U.S. Brand Names Daranide®

Canadian Brand Names Daranide®

Index Terms Diclofenamide

Pharmacologic Category Carbonic Anhydrase Inhibitor; Diuretic, Carbonic Anhydrase Inhibitor; Ophthalmic Agent, Antiglaucoma

Use Adjunct in treatment of open-angle glaucoma and perioperative treatment for angle-closure glaucoma

Effect on Mental Status Sedation is common; may cause depression

Effect on Psychiatric Treatment May rarely cause bone marrow suppression; use caution with clozapine and carbamazepine; may increase the excretion of lithium but should not be used to treat lithium toxicity

Dosage Summary

Oral:

Children: Dosage not established

Adults: Initial: 100-200 mg, followed by 100 mg every 12 hours; Maintenance: 25-50 mg 1-3 times/day

Dosage Forms Excipient information presented when available (limited, particularly for generics); consult specific product labeling.

Tablet: 50 mg

◆ **Dichysterol** *see* Dihydrotachysterol *on page 472*

Diclofenac (dye KLOE fen ak)

Medication Safety Issues

Sound-alike/look-alike issues:

Diclofenac may be confused with Diflucan®, Duphalac®

Cataflam® may be confused with Catapres®

Voltaren® may be confused with traMADol, Ultram®, Verelan®

Related Information

Nonsteroidal Anti-Inflammatory Agents *on page 1792*

U.S. Brand Names Cataflam®; Flector®; Solaraze®; Voltaren Ophthalmic®; Voltaren®; Voltaren® Gel; Voltaren®-XR

Canadian Brand Names Apo-Diclo Rapide®; Apo-Diclo SR®; Apo-Diclo®; Cataflam®; Dom-Diclofenac; Dom-Diclofenac SR; Novo-Difenac; Novo-Difenac K; Novo-Difenac-SR; Nu-Diclo; Nu-Diclo-SR; Pennsaid®; PMS-Diclofenac; PMS-Diclofenac SR; Riva-Diclofenac; Riva-Diclofenac-K; Sab-Diclofenac; Sandoz-Diclofenac; Voltaren Ophtha®; Voltaren Rapide®; Voltaren®

Mexican Brand Names Cataflam; Deflox; Flankol

Index Terms Diclofenac Epolamine; Diclofenac Potassium; Diclofenac Sodium

Pharmacologic Category Nonsteroidal Anti-inflammatory Drug (NSAID); Nonsteroidal Anti-inflammatory Drug (NSAID), Ophthalmic; Nonsteroidal Anti-inflammatory Drug (NSAID), Oral; Nonsteroidal Anti-inflammatory Drug (NSAID), Topical

Use

Immediate release tablet: Ankylosing spondylitis; primary dysmenorrhea; acute and chronic treatment of rheumatoid arthritis, osteoarthritis

Delayed-release tablet: Acute and chronic treatment of rheumatoid arthritis, osteoarthritis, ankylosing spondylitis

Extended-release tablet: Chronic treatment of osteoarthritis, rheumatoid arthritis

Ophthalmic solution: Postoperative inflammation following cataract extraction; temporary relief of pain and photophobia in patients undergoing corneal refractive surgery

Topical gel 1%: Relief of osteoarthritis pain in joints amenable to topical therapy (eg, ankle, elbow, foot, hand, knee, wrist)

Topical gel 3%: Actinic keratosis (AK) in conjunction with sun avoidance

Topical patch: Acute pain due to minor strains, sprains, and contusions

Unlabeled/Investigational Use Juvenile rheumatoid arthritis

Effect on Mental Status May cause nervousness or dizziness; may rarely cause depression

Effect on Psychiatric Treatment May rarely cause agranulocytosis; use caution with clozapine and carbamazepine; may decrease the clearance of lithium resulting in elevated serum levels and potential toxicity; monitor serum lithium levels

Restrictions An FDA-approved medication guide must be distributed when dispensing an oral outpatient prescription (new or refill) where this medication is to be used without direct supervision of a healthcare provider. Medication guides are available at http://www.fda.gov/cder/Offices/ODS/medication_guides.htm.

Dosage Summary

Ophthalmic:

Children: Dosage not established

Adults: 1-2 drops into affected eye 4 times/day

Oral:

Immediate release:

Children: Dosage not established

Adults: 100-200 mg/day in 2-5 divided doses

Sustained release:

Children: Dosage not established

Adults: 100-200 mg/day

Topical:

Children: Dosage not established

Adults:

1% gel: Apply 2-4 g to affected joint 4 times daily (maximum: 16 g/day single joint of lower extremity, 8 g/day single joint of upper extremity); Maximum total body dose of 1% gel should not exceed 32 g per day.

3% gel: Apply to lesion area twice daily

Patch: Apply 1 patch twice daily

Dosage Forms Excipient information presented when available (limited, particularly for generics); consult specific product labeling. [DSC] = Discontinued product

Gel, as sodium:

Solaraze®: 3% (50 g, 100 g)

Voltaren® Gel: 1% (100 g)

Solution, ophthalmic, as sodium [drops]: 0.1% (2.5 mL, 5 mL)

Voltaren Ophthalmic®: 0.1% (2.5 mL, 5 mL)

Tablet, as potassium: 50 mg

Cataflam®: 50 mg

Tablet, delayed release, enteric coated, as sodium: 50 mg, 75 mg

Voltaren®: 25 mg [DSC], 50 mg [DSC], 75 mg

Tablet, extended release, as sodium: 100 mg

Voltaren®-XR: 100 mg

Transdermal system, topical, as epolamine:

Flector®: 1.3% (30s) [180 mg]

Diclofenac and Misoprostol (dye KLOE fen ak & mye soe PROST ole)

U.S. Brand Names Arthrotec®

Canadian Brand Names Arthrotec®

Mexican Brand Names Artrotec

Index Terms Misoprostol and Diclofenac

Pharmacologic Category Nonsteroidal Anti-inflammatory Drug (NSAID), Oral; Prostaglandin

Use The diclofenac component is indicated for the treatment of osteoarthritis and rheumatoid arthritis; the misoprostol component is indicated for the prophylaxis of NSAID-induced gastric and duodenal ulceration

Effect on Mental Status May cause nervousness or dizziness; may rarely cause depression

Effect on Psychiatric Treatment May rarely cause may agranulocytosis; use caution with clozapine and carbamazepine; may decrease the clearance of lithium resulting in elevated serum levels and potential toxicity; monitor serum lithium levels

Restrictions An FDA-approved medication guide must be distributed when dispensing an oral outpatient prescription (new or refill) where this medication is to be used without direct supervision of a healthcare provider. Medication guides are available at http://www.fda.gov/cder/Offices/ODS/medication_guides.htm.

Dosage Summary

Oral:

Children: Dosage not established

Adults: Arthrotec® 50: 1 tablet 2-4 times/day; Arthrotec® 75: 1 tablet twice daily if unable to tolerate 50 mg tablet

Dosage Forms Excipient information presented when available (limited, particularly for generics); consult specific product labeling.

Tablet: Diclofenac sodium 50 mg and misoprostol 200 mcg; diclofenac sodium 75 mg and misoprostol 200 mcg

- ◆ **Diclofenac Epolamine** *see* Diclofenac *on page 457*
- ◆ **Diclofenac Potassium** *see* Diclofenac *on page 457*
- ◆ **Diclofenac Sodium** *see* Diclofenac *on page 457*
- ◆ **Diclofenamide** *see* Dichlorphenamide *on page 457*

Dicloxacillin (dye kloks a SIL in)

Canadian Brand Names Dycill®; Pathocil®

Mexican Brand Names Brispen; Diamsalina; Ditterolina; Posipen

Index Terms Dicloxacillin Sodium

Pharmacologic Category Antibiotic, Penicillin

Use Treatment of systemic infections such as pneumonia, skin and soft tissue infections, and osteomyelitis caused by penicillinase-producing staphylococci

Effect on Mental Status Penicillins have been reported to cause apprehension, illusions, agitation, insomnia, depersonalization, and encephalopathy

Effect on Psychiatric Treatment Rarely may cause agranulocytosis; use caution with clozapine and carbamazepine

Dosage Summary

Oral:

Children <40 kg: 12.5-100 mg mg/kg/day divided every 6 hours

Children >40 kg: 125-250 mg every 6 hours

Adults: 125-1000 mg every 6-8 hours

Dosage Forms Excipient information presented when available (limited, particularly for generics); consult specific product labeling.

Capsule: 250 mg, 500 mg

- ◆ **Dicloxacillin Sodium** *see* Dicloxacillin *on page 459*

Dicyclomine (dye SYE kloe meen)

Medication Safety Issues

Sound-alike/look-alike issues:

Dicyclomine may be confused with diphenhydrAMINE, doxycycline, dyclonine

Bentyl® may be confused with Aventyl®, Benadryl®, Bontril®, Cantil®, Proventil®, Trental®

U.S. Brand Names Bentyl®

Canadian Brand Names Bentylol®; Formulex®; Lomine; Riva-Dicyclomine

Mexican Brand Names Bentyl

Index Terms Dicyclomine Hydrochloride; Dicycloverine Hydrochloride

Pharmacologic Category Anticholinergic Agent

Use Treatment of functional bowel/irritable bowel syndrome

Unlabeled/Investigational Use Urinary incontinence

Effect on Mental Status May cause nervousness, excitement, insomnia, confusion, drowsiness, dyskinesia

Effect on Psychiatric Treatment Concurrent use with psychotropics may produce additive sedation and dry mouth

Dosage Summary

I.M.:

Children: Dosage not established

Adults: 80 mg/day in 4 divided doses

Oral:

Children: Dosage not established

Adults: Initial: 20 mg 4 times/day; Maintenance: Up to 160 mg/day in 4 divided doses

Elderly: Initial: 10-20 mg 4 times/day; Maintenance: Up to 160 mg/day in 4 divided doses

Dosage Forms Excipient information presented when available (limited, particularly for generics); consult specific product labeling.

Capsule, as hydrochloride: 10 mg

Bentyl®: 10 mg

Injection, solution, as hydrochloride: 10 mg/mL (2 mL)

Bentyl®: 10 mg/mL (2 mL)

Syrup, as hydrochloride:
Bentyl®: 10 mg/5 mL (480 mL)
Tablet, as hydrochloride: 20 mg
Bentyl®: 20 mg

◆ **Dicyclomine Hydrochloride** *see* Dicyclomine *on page 459*
◆ **Dicycloverine Hydrochloride** *see* Dicyclomine *on page 459*

Didanosine (dye DAN oh seen)

Medication Safety Issues
Sound-alike/look-alike issues:
Videx® may be confused with Lidex®
U.S. Brand Names Videx®; Videx® EC
Canadian Brand Names Videx®; Videx® EC
Mexican Brand Names Didasten; Videx EC
Index Terms ddI; Dideoxyinosine
Pharmacologic Category Antiretroviral Agent, Reverse Transcriptase Inhibitor (Nucleoside)
Use Treatment of HIV infection; always to be used in combination with at least two other antiretroviral agents
Effect on Mental Status Anxiety; irritability and insomnia are common; may produce depression
Effect on Psychiatric Treatment May cause granulocytopenia; use caution with clozapine and carbamazepine
Dosage Summary
Oral:
Delayed release:
Children <20 kg: Dosage not established
Children 20 kg to <25 kg: 200 mg once daily
Children 25 kg to <60 kg: 250 mg once daily
Children ≥60 kg: 400 mg once daily
Adults <60 kg: 250 mg once daily
Adults ≥60 kg: 400 mg once daily
Pediatric powder for oral solution (Videx®):
Neonates <2 weeks: Dosage not established
Infants 2 weeks to 8 months: 100 mg/m^2 twice daily
Children >8 months to 12 years: 120 mg/m^2 twice daily
Adolescents <60 kg: 125 mg twice daily **or** 250 mg once daily
Adolescents ≥60 kg: 200 mg twice daily **or** 400 mg once daily
Adults <60 kg: 125 mg twice daily **or** 250 mg once daily
Adults ≥60 kg: 200 mg twice daily **or** 400 mg once daily
Dosage Forms Excipient information presented when available (limited, particularly for generics); consult specific product labeling.
Capsule, delayed release, enteric coated pellets: 200 mg, 250 mg, 400 mg
Capsule, delayed release, enteric coated beadlets:
Videx® EC: 125 mg, 200 mg, 250 mg, 400 mg
Powder for oral solution, pediatric:
Videx®: 2 g, 4 g [makes 10 mg/mL solution after final mixing]

◆ **Dideoxycytidine** *see* Zalcitabine *on page 1691*
◆ **Dideoxyinosine** *see* Didanosine *on page 460*
◆ **Didrex®** *see* Benzphetamine *on page 181*
◆ **Didronel®** *see* Etidronate Disodium *on page 605*

Diethylpropion (dye eth il PROE pee on)

Related Information
Phentermine *on page 1270*
Canadian Brand Names Tenuate®; Tenuate® Dospan®
Index Terms Amfepramone; Diethylpropion Hydrochloride
Pharmacologic Category Anorexiant; Sympathomimetic
Generic Available Yes
Use Short-term adjunct in a regimen of weight reduction based on exercise, behavioral modification, and caloric reduction in the management of exogenous obesity for patients with an initial body mass index ≥30 kg/m^2 or ≥27 kg/m^2 in the presence of other risk factors (diabetes, hypertension); see Body Mass Index on page 1746 in the Appendix
Effect on Mental Status Insomnia, nervousness, and euphoria are common; may cause confusion, depression, or psychosis

Effect on Psychiatric Treatment Concurrent use with MAO inhibitors may cause hypertensive crisis; avoid combination; antipsychotics may blunt effect of diethylpropion. May cause bone marrow depression; use caution with clozapine.

Restrictions C-IV

Pharmacotherapy for weight loss is recommended only for obese patients with a body mass index ≥30 kg/m^2, or ≥27 kg/m^2 in the presence of other risk factors such as hypertension, diabetes, and/or dyslipidemia or a high waist circumference; therapy should be used in conjunction with a comprehensive weight management program. Rule out organic causes of obesity (eg, untreated hypothyroidism) prior to use.

Note: Diethylpropion is not approved for long-term use. The limited usefulness of medications in this class should be weighed against possible risks associated with their use. Consult weight loss guidelines for current pharmacotherapy recommendations.

Pregnancy Risk Factor B

Pregnancy Considerations Teratogenic effects have not been observed in animal studies. Crosses the human placenta; spontaneous reports of congenital malformations have been reported, but an association with diethylpropion has not been established. Withdrawal symptoms may occur in the neonate following maternal use of diethylpropion.

Lactation Enters breast milk/use caution

Contraindications Hypersensitivity or idiosyncrasy to diethylpropion or other sympathomimetic amines; advanced arteriosclerosis, severe hypertension; pulmonary hypertension; hyperthyroidism; glaucoma; agitated states, history of drug abuse; during or within 14 days following MAO inhibitor therapy, concurrent use with other anorectic agents

Warnings/Precautions The use of some anorexigens, including diethylpropion, has been associated with the development of valvular heart disease. Avoid stimulants in patients with known serious structural cardiac abnormalities, cardiomyopathy, serious heart rhythm abnormalities, or other serious cardiac problems that could increase the risk of sudden death that these conditions alone carry. Caution should be used in patients with hypertension, symptomatic cardiovascular disease and other cardiovascular conditions that might be exacerbated by increases in blood pressure or heart rate.

Primary pulmonary hypertension (PPH), a rare and frequently fatal disease of the lungs, has been found to occur with increased frequency in patients receiving diethylpropion as well as other anorexigens.

Use caution with diabetes; antidiabetic agent requirements may be altered with anorexigens and concomitant dietary restrictions. Stimulants may unmask tics in individuals with coexisting Tourette's syndrome. Use caution with seizure disorders. Diethylpropion is pharmacologically related to the amphetamines, which have a high abuse potential; prolonged use may lead to dependency. Prescriptions should be written for the smallest quantity consistent with good patient care to minimize possibility of overdose. Amphetamines may impair the ability to engage in potentially hazardous activities.

Not recommended for use in patients who used other anorectic agents within the past year. Discontinue if satisfactory weight loss has not occurred within the first 4 weeks of treatment, or if tolerance develops. Safety and efficacy have not been established for use with other weight loss medications including over-the-counter or herbal products. Safety and efficacy have not been established in patients ≤16 years of age.

Adverse Reactions Frequency not defined.

Cardiovascular: Arrhythmia, ECG changes, hypertension, palpitation, precordial pain, pulmonary hypertension, tachycardia, valvulopathy

Central nervous system: Anxiety, CVA, depression, dizziness, drowsiness, dysphoria, euphoria, headache, insomnia, jitteriness, malaise, nervousness, overstimulation, psychosis, restlessness, seizure

Dermatologic: Alopecia, ecchymosis, erythema, rash, urticaria

Endocrine & metabolic: Libido changes, gynecomastia, menstrual irregularities

Gastrointestinal: Abdominal discomfort, constipation, diarrhea, nausea, unpleasant taste, vomiting, xerostomia

Genitourinary: Dysuria, impotence, polyuria

Hematologic: Bone marrow depression, agranulocytosis, leukopenia

Neuromuscular & skeletal: Dyskinesia, muscle pain, tremor

Ocular: Blurred vision, mydriasis

Respiratory: Dyspnea

Miscellaneous: Diaphoresis, tachyphylaxis

Drug Interactions
Cannabinoids: May enhance the tachycardic effect of Sympathomimetics. *Risk C: Monitor therapy*
Sympathomimetics: May enhance the adverse/toxic effect of other Sympathomimetics. *Risk C: Monitor therapy*

Ethanol/Nutrition/Herb Interactions Ethanol: Avoid ethanol (may increase CNS depression).

Stability Store at room temperature, below 30°C (86°F).

Mechanism of Action Diethylpropion s a sympathomimetic amine with pharmacologic properties similar to the amphetamines. It is also structurally similar to bupropion. The mechanism of action in reducing appetite appears to be secondary to CNS effects, including stimulation of the hypothalamus to release norepinephrine

Pharmacodynamics/Kinetics
Metabolism: Forms active metabolites via N-dealkylation and reduction
Half-life elimination: Aminoketone metabolites: ~4-6 hours
Excretion: Urine

Dosage Children >16 years and Adults: Oral:
Tablet: 25 mg 3 times/day before meals or food
Tablet, controlled release: 75 mg at midmorning

Dietary Considerations Most effective when combined with a low calorie diet and behavior modification counseling.

Administration Dose should not be administered in evening or at bedtime.
Tablet: Administer 1 hour before meals.
Tablet, controlled release: Do not crush tablet; administer at midmorning.

Monitoring Parameters Baseline cardiac evaluation (for preexisting valvular heart disease, pulmonary hypertension); echocardiogram during therapy; weight, waist circumference, blood pressure; renal function in elderly patients

Reference Range
Adult classification of weight by BMI (kg/m^2):
- Underweight: <18.5
- Normal: 18.5-24.9
- Overweight: 25-29.9
- Obese, class I: 30-34.9
- Obese, class II: 35-39.9
- Extreme obesity (class III): ≥40

Waist circumference: In adults with a BMI of 25-34.9 kg/m^2, high-risk waist circumference is defined as:
- Men >102 cm (>40 in)
- Women >88 cm (>35 in)

Dosage Forms Excipient information presented when available (limited, particularly for generics); consult specific product labeling.
Tablet, as hydrochloride: 25 mg
Tablet, controlled release, as hydrochloride: 75 mg

◆ **Diethylpropion Hydrochloride** *see* Diethylpropion *on page 460*

Difenoxin and Atropine (dye fen OKS in & A troe peen)

U.S. Brand Names Motofen® [DSC]
Index Terms Atropine and Difenoxin
Pharmacologic Category Antidiarrheal
Use Treatment of diarrhea
Effect on Mental Status May cause drowsiness; confusion
Effect on Psychiatric Treatment Concurrent use with psychotropic may cause additive sedation or dry mouth
Restrictions C-IV
Dosage Summary
Oral:
Children: Dosage not established
Adults: 2 tablets (each tablet contains difenoxin hydrochloride 1 mg and atropine sulfate 0.025 mg) initially, then 1 tablet after each loose stool (maximum: 8 tablets/day)

Dosage Forms Excipient information presented when available (limited, particularly for generics); consult specific product labeling. [DSC] = Discontinued product
Tablet, oral:
Motofen®: Difenoxin hydrochloride 1 mg and atropine sulfate 0.025 mg [DSC]

◆ **Difil-G** *see* Dyphylline and Guaifenesin *on page 522*

- **Difil®-G Forte** *see* Dyphylline and Guaifenesin *on page 522*
- **Diflucan®** *see* Fluconazole *on page 635*

Diflunisal (dye FLOO ni sal)

Medication Safety Issues

Sound-alike/look-alike issues:

Dolobid® (discontinued U.S. brand name [generics available]) may be confused with Slo-Bid®

International issues: Dolobid® (brand name product available in multiple international markets) may be confused with Slo-Bid®

Related Information

Nonsteroidal Anti-Inflammatory Agents *on page 1792*

Canadian Brand Names Apo-Diflunisal®; Novo-Diflunisal; Nu-Diflunisal

Mexican Brand Names Dolobid

Index Terms Dolobid

Pharmacologic Category Nonsteroidal Anti-inflammatory Drug (NSAID), Oral

Use Management of inflammatory disorders usually including rheumatoid arthritis and osteoarthritis; can be used as an analgesic for treatment of mild-to-moderate pain

Effect on Mental Status May cause dizziness; rarely may cause insomnia, nervousness, depression, and hallucinations

Effect on Psychiatric Treatment May rarely cause may agranulocytosis; use caution with clozapine and carbamazepine; may decrease the clearance of lithium resulting in elevated serum levels and potential toxicity; monitor serum lithium levels

Restrictions An FDA-approved medication guide must be distributed when dispensing an oral outpatient prescription (new or refill) where this medication is to be used without direct supervision of a healthcare provider. Medication guides are available at http://www.fda.gov/cder/Offices/ODS/medication_guides.htm.

Dosage Summary

Oral:

Children: Dosage not established

Adults: 250-500 mg every 8-12 hours (maximum: 1.5 g/day)

Dosage Forms Excipient information presented when available (limited, particularly for generics); consult specific product labeling.

Tablet: 500 mg

- **Digitek®** *see* Digoxin *on page 463*

Digoxin (di JOKS in)

Medication Safety Issues

Sound-alike/look-alike issues:

Digoxin may be confused with Desoxyn®, doxepin

Lanoxin® may be confused with Lasix®, Levoxyl®, Levsinex®, Lomotil®, Lonox®, Mefoxin®, Xanax®

High alert medication: The Institute for Safe Medication Practices (ISMP) includes this medication among its list of drugs which have a heightened risk of causing significant patient harm when used in error.

International issues:

Dilacor®: Brand name for diltiazem in the U.S.; brand name for verapamil in Brazil; brand name for barnidipine in Argentina

Lanoxin® may be confused with Lemoxin® which is a brand bane for cefuroxime in Mexico

Lanoxin® may be confused with Limoxin® which is a brand name for amoxicillin in Mexico

Related Information

Anticholinergic Effects of Common Psychotropics *on page 1758*

U.S. Brand Names Digitek®; Lanoxicaps® [DSC]; Lanoxin®

Canadian Brand Names Apo-Digoxin®; Digoxin CSD; Lanoxicaps®; Lanoxin®; Novo-Digoxin; Pediatric Digoxin CSD

Mexican Brand Names Lanoxin; Mapluxin; Vidaxil

Pharmacologic Category Antiarrhythmic Agent, Class IV; Cardiac Glycoside

Generic Available Yes: Excludes capsule

Use Treatment of congestive heart failure and to slow the ventricular rate in tachyarrhythmias such as atrial fibrillation, atrial flutter, and supraventricular tachycardia (paroxysmal atrial tachycardia); cardiogenic shock

Effect on Mental Status May cause sedation

Effect on Psychiatric Treatment Phenytoin may decrease levels of digoxin; monitor levels

Pregnancy Risk Factor C

Lactation Enters breast milk (small amounts)/compatible

Contraindications Hypersensitivity to digoxin or any component of the formulation; hypersensitivity to cardiac glycosides (another may be tried); history of toxicity; ventricular tachycardia or fibrillation; idiopathic hypertrophic subaortic stenosis; constrictive pericarditis; amyloid disease; second- or third-degree heart block (except in patients with a functioning artificial pacemaker); Wolff-Parkinson-White syndrome and atrial fibrillation concurrently

Warnings/Precautions Watch for proarrhythmic effects (especially with digoxin toxicity). Withdrawal in HF patients may lead to recurrence of HF symptoms. Use with caution in patients with hypoxia, myxedema, hypothyroidism, acute myocarditis; patients with incomplete AV block (Stokes-Adams attack) may progress to complete block with digitalis drug administration; use with caution in patients with acute myocardial infarction, severe pulmonary disease, advanced heart failure, idiopathic hypertrophic subaortic stenosis, Wolff-Parkinson-White syndrome, sick-sinus syndrome (bradyarrhythmias), amyloid heart disease, and constrictive cardiomyopathies; adjust dose with renal impairment and when verapamil, quinidine or amiodarone are added to a patient on digoxin; elderly and neonates may develop exaggerated serum/tissue concentrations due to age-related alterations in clearance and pharmacodynamic differences; exercise will reduce serum concentrations of digoxin due to increased skeletal muscle uptake; recent studies indicate photopsia, chromatopsia and decreased visual acuity may occur even with therapeutic serum drug levels; reduce or hold dose 1-2 days before elective electrical cardioversion. In the Cardiac Arrhythmia Suppression Trial (CAST), recent (>6 days but <2 years ago) myocardial infarction patients with asymptomatic, non-life-threatening ventricular arrhythmias did not benefit and may have been harmed by attempts to suppress the arrhythmia with flecainide or encainide. An increased mortality or nonfatal cardiac arrest rate (7.7%) was seen in the active treatment group compared with patients in the placebo group (3%). The applicability of the CAST results to other populations is unknown. Antiarrhythmic agents should be reserved for patients with life-threatening ventricular arrhythmias.

Adverse Reactions Incidence not always reported.

Cardiovascular: Heart block; first-, second- (Wenckebach), or third-degree heart block; asystole; atrial tachycardia with block; AV dissociation; accelerated junctional rhythm; ventricular tachycardia or ventricular fibrillation; PR prolongation; ST segment depression

Central nervous system: Visual disturbances (blurred or yellow vision), headache (3.2%), dizziness (4.9%), apathy, confusion, mental disturbances (4.1%), anxiety, depression, delirium, hallucinations, fever

Dermatologic: Maculopapular rash (1.6%); erythematous, scarlatiniform, papular, vesicular, or bullous rash; urticaria; pruritus; facial, angioneurotic, or laryngeal edema; shedding of fingernails or toenails; alopecia

Gastrointestinal: Nausea (3.2%), vomiting (1.6%), diarrhea (3.2%), abdominal pain

Neuromuscular & skeletal: Weakness

<1% (Limited to important or life-threatening): Abdominal pain, anorexia, eosinophilia, gynecomastia, hemorrhagic necrosis of the intestines, increased plasma estrogen and decreased serum luteinizing hormone in men and postmenopausal women and decreased plasma testosterone in men, intestinal ischemia, palpitation, sexual dysfunction, thrombocytopenia, unifocal or multiform ventricular premature contractions (especially bigeminy or trigeminy), vaginal cornification

Any arrhythmia seen in a child on digoxin should be considered as digoxin toxicity. The gastrointestinal and central nervous system symptoms are not frequently seen in children.

Metabolism/Transport Effects Substrate of CYP3A4 (minor)

Drug Interactions

5-ASA Derivatives: May decrease the absorption of Cardiac Glycosides. *Risk C: Monitor therapy*

Acarbose: May decrease the serum concentration of Digoxin. *Risk C: Monitor therapy*

Aminoglycosides: May decrease the absorption of Cardiac Glycosides. **Exceptions:** Amikacin; Gentamicin; Streptomycin; Tobramycin. *Risk C: Monitor therapy*

Aminoquinolines (Antimalarial): May increase the serum concentration of Cardiac Glycosides. *Risk D: Consider therapy modification*

Amiodarone: May increase the serum concentration of Cardiac Glycosides. *Risk D: Consider therapy modification*

Antifungal Agents (Azole Derivatives, Systemic): May increase the serum concentration of Cardiac Glycosides. **Exceptions:** Miconazole. *Risk D: Consider therapy modification*

Antineoplastic Agents: May decrease the absorption of Cardiac Glycosides. This may only affect digoxin tablets. **Exceptions:** Alitretinoin; Altretamine; Aminoglutethimide; Anastrozole; Asparaginase; AzaCITIDine; Busulfan; Capecitabine; CARBOplatin; Chlorambucil; CISplatin; Cladribine; Cytarabine (Liposomal); Dacarbazine; DACTINomycin; DAUNOrubicin Citrate (Liposomal); DAUNOrubicin Hydrochloride; Denileukin Diftitox; Docetaxel; Epirubicin; Estramustine; Etoposide; Etoposide Phosphate; Exemestane; Fludarabine; Fluorouracil; Gemcitabine; Goserelin; Hydroxyurea; IDArubicin; Ifosfamide; Irinotecan; Letrozole; Leuprolide; Lomustine; Mechlorethamine; Megestrol; Mercaptopurine; Mitomycin; Mitotane; Mitoxantrone; Nilutamide; Paclitaxel; Pegaspargase; Pentostatin; Polyestradiol; Porfimer; RiTUXimab; Streptozocin; Tamoxifen; Temozolomide; Teniposide; Thioguanine; Thiotepa; Topotecan; Toremifene; Tretinoin (Oral); Valrubicin; VinBLAStine; Vinorelbine. *Risk C: Monitor therapy*

Antineoplastic Agents (Anthracycline): Cardiac Glycosides may diminish the cardiotoxic effect of Antineoplastic Agents (Anthracycline). Antineoplastic Agents (Anthracycline) may decrease the serum concentration of Cardiac Glycosides. The effects of liposomal formulations may be unique from those of the free drug, as liposomal formulation have unique drug disposition and toxicity profiles, and liposomes themselves may alter digoxin absorption/distribution. *Risk C: Monitor therapy*

Atorvastatin: May increase the serum concentration of Digoxin. *Risk C: Monitor therapy*

Beta-Blockers: May enhance the bradycardic effect of Cardiac Glycosides. **Exceptions:** Levobunolol; Metipranolol. *Risk C: Monitor therapy*

Bile Acid Sequestrants: May decrease the absorption of Cardiac Glycosides. **Exceptions:** Colesevelam. *Risk C: Monitor therapy*

Calcitriol: May enhance the arrhythmogenic effect of Cardiac Glycosides. *Risk C: Monitor therapy*

Calcium Channel Blockers (Nondihydropyridine): May enhance the AV-blocking effect of Cardiac Glycosides. Calcium Channel Blockers (Nondihydropyridine) may decrease the metabolism of Cardiac Glycosides. *Risk D: Consider therapy modification*

Carvedilol: May increase the serum concentration of Digoxin. *Risk C: Monitor therapy*

Conivaptan: May increase the serum concentration of Digoxin. *Risk C: Monitor therapy*

CycloSPORINE: May decrease the metabolism of Cardiac Glycosides. *Risk D: Consider therapy modification*

Kaolin: May decrease the absorption of Cardiac Glycosides. *Risk C: Monitor therapy*

Macrolide Antibiotics: May increase the serum concentration of Cardiac Glycosides. *Risk D: Consider therapy modification*

Midodrine: Cardiac Glycosides may enhance the bradycardic effect of Midodrine. *Risk C: Monitor therapy*

Nefazodone: May increase the serum concentration of Cardiac Glycosides. *Risk C: Monitor therapy*

Neuromuscular-Blocking Agents: May enhance the arrhythmogenic effect of Cardiac Glycosides. *Risk C: Monitor therapy*

Penicillamine: May decrease the serum concentration of Digoxin. *Risk C: Monitor therapy*

P-Glycoprotein Inducers: May decrease the serum concentration of P-Glycoprotein Substrates. P-glycoprotein inducers may also further limit the distribution of p-glycoprotein substrates to specific cells/tissues/organs where p-glycoprotein is present in large amounts (e.g., brain, T-lymphocytes, testes, etc.). *Risk C: Monitor therapy*

P-Glycoprotein Inhibitors: May increase the serum concentration of P-Glycoprotein Substrates. P-glycoprotein inhibitors may also enhance the distribution of p-glycoprotein substrates to specific cells/tissues/organs where p-glycoprotein is present in large amounts (e.g., brain, T-lymphocytes, testes, etc.). *Risk C: Monitor therapy*

Potassium-Sparing Diuretics: May diminish the therapeutic effect of Cardiac Glycosides. Specifically, the inotropic effects. *Risk C: Monitor therapy*

Propafenone: May increase the serum concentration of Cardiac Glycosides. *Risk C: Monitor therapy*

Protease Inhibitors: May increase the serum concentration of Digoxin. Increased serum concentrations of digoxin may increase risk of AV nodal blockade. *Risk C: Monitor therapy*

QuiNIDine: May increase the serum concentration of Cardiac Glycosides. *Risk D: Consider therapy modification*

QuiNINE: May increase the serum concentration of Cardiac Glycosides. *Risk D: Consider therapy modification*

Ranolazine: May increase the serum concentration of Digoxin. *Risk C: Monitor therapy*

St Johns Wort: May decrease the serum concentration of Cardiac Glycosides. *Risk C: Monitor therapy*

Telmisartan: May increase the serum concentration of Cardiac Glycosides. *Risk C: Monitor therapy*

Ethanol/Nutrition/Herb Interactions

Food: Digoxin peak serum levels may be decreased if taken with food. Meals containing increased fiber (bran) or foods high in pectin may decrease oral absorption of digoxin.

Herb/Nutraceutical: Avoid ephedra (risk of cardiac stimulation). Avoid natural licorice (causes sodium and water retention and increases potassium loss).

Stability Protect elixir and injection from light.

Mechanism of Action

Congestive heart failure: Inhibition of the sodium/potassium ATPase pump which acts to increase the intracellular sodium-calcium exchange to increase intracellular calcium leading to increased contractility

Supraventricular arrhythmias: Direct suppression of the AV node conduction to increase effective refractory period and decrease conduction velocity - positive inotropic effect, enhanced vagal tone, and decreased ventricular rate to fast atrial arrhythmias. Atrial fibrillation may decrease sensitivity and increase tolerance to higher serum digoxin concentrations.

Pharmacodynamics/Kinetics

Onset of action: Oral: 1-2 hours; I.V.: 5-30 minutes

- Peak effect: Oral: 2-8 hours; I.V.: 1-4 hours

Duration: Adults: 3-4 days both forms

Absorption: By passive nonsaturable diffusion in the upper small intestine; food may delay, but does not affect extent of absorption

Distribution:

- Normal renal function: 6-7 L/kg
- V_d: Extensive to peripheral tissues, with a distinct distribution phase which lasts 6-8 hours; concentrates in heart, liver, kidney, skeletal muscle, and intestines. Heart/serum concentration is 70:1. Pharmacologic effects are delayed and do not correlate well with serum concentrations during distribution phase.
- Hyperthyroidism: Increased V_d
- Hyperkalemia, hyponatremia: Decreased digoxin distribution to heart and muscle
- Hypokalemia: Increased digoxin distribution to heart and muscles
- Concomitant quinidine therapy: Decreased V_d
- Chronic renal failure: 4-6 L/kg
- Decreased sodium/potassium ATPase activity - decreased tissue binding
- Neonates, full-term: 7.5-10 L/kg
- Children: 16 L/kg
- Adults: 7 L/kg, decreased with renal disease

Protein binding: 30%; in uremic patients, digoxin is displaced from plasma protein binding sites

Metabolism: Via sequential sugar hydrolysis in the stomach or by reduction of lactone ring by intestinal bacteria (in ~10% of population, gut bacteria may metabolize up to 40% of digoxin dose); metabolites may contribute to therapeutic and toxic effects of digoxin; metabolism is reduced with CHF

Bioavailability: Oral (formulation dependent): Elixir: 75% to 85%; Tablet: 70% to 80%

Half-life elimination (age, renal and cardiac function dependent):

- Neonates: Premature: 61-170 hours; Full-term: 35-45 hours
- Infants: 18-25 hours
- Children: 35 hours
- Adults: 38-48 hours
- Adults, anephric: 4-6 days

Half-life elimination: Parent drug: 38 hours; Metabolites: Digoxigenin: 4 hours; Monodigitoxoside: 3-12 hours

Time to peak, serum: Oral: ~1 hour

Excretion: Urine (50% to 70% as unchanged drug)

Dosage When changing from oral (tablets or liquid) or I.M. to I.V. therapy, dosage should be reduced by 20% to 25%. Refer to the following: See table on next page.

Dosage Recommendations for Digoxin

Age	Total Digitalizing Dose[2] (mcg/kg[1])		Daily Maintenance Dose[3] (mcg/kg[1])	
	P.O.	I.V. or I.M.	P.O.	I.V. or I.M.
Preterm infant[1]	20-30	15-25	5-7.5	4-6
Full-term infant[1]	25-35	20-30	6-10	5-8
1 mo - 2 y[1]	35-60	30-50	10-15	7.5-12
2-5 y[1]	30-40	25-35	7.5-10	6-9
5-10 y[1]	20-35	15-30	5-10	4-8
>10 y[1]	10-15	8-12	2.5-5	2-3
Adults	0.75-1.5 mg	0.5-1 mg	0.125-0.5 mg	0.1-0.4 mg

[1]Based on lean body weight and normal renal function for age. Decrease dose in patients with ↓ renal function; digitalizing dose often not recommended in infants and children.

[2]Give one-half of the total digitalizing dose (TDD) in the initial dose, then give one-quarter of the TDD in each of two subsequent doses at 6- to 8-hour intervals. Obtain ECG 6 hours after each dose to assess potential toxicity.

[3]Divided every 12 hours in infants and children <10 years of age. Given once daily to children >10 years of age and adults.

Dosing adjustment/interval in renal impairment:
Cl_{cr} 10-50 mL/minute: Administer 25% to 75% of dose or every 36 hours
Cl_{cr} <10 mL/minute: Administer 10% to 25% of dose or every 48 hours
Reduce loading dose by 50% in ESRD
Hemodialysis: Not dialyzable (0% to 5%)

Dietary Considerations Maintain adequate amounts of potassium in diet to decrease risk of hypokalemia (hypokalemia may increase risk of digoxin toxicity).

Administration

I.M.: Inject no more than 2 mL per injection site. May cause intense pain.

I.V.: May be administered undiluted or diluted fourfold in D_5W, NS, or SWFI for direct injection. Less than fourfold dilution may lead to drug precipitation. Inject slowly over ≥5 minutes.

Monitoring Parameters

When to draw serum digoxin concentrations: Digoxin serum concentrations are monitored because digoxin possesses a narrow therapeutic serum range; the therapeutic endpoint is difficult to quantify and digoxin toxicity may be life-threatening. Digoxin serum levels should be drawn **at least 4 hours after an intravenous dose** and **at least 6 hours after an oral dose (optimally 12-24 hours after a dose).**

Initiation of therapy:

If a loading dose is given: Digoxin serum concentration may be drawn within 12-24 hours after the initial loading dose administration. Levels drawn this early may confirm the relationship of digoxin plasma levels and response but are of little value in determining maintenance doses.

If a loading dose is not given: Digoxin serum concentration should be obtained after 3-5 days of therapy.

Maintenance therapy:

Trough concentrations should be followed just prior to the next dose or at a minimum of 4 hours after an I.V. dose and at least 6 hours after an oral dose.

Digoxin serum concentrations should be obtained within 5-7 days (approximate time to steady-state) after any dosage changes. Continue to obtain digoxin serum concentrations 7-14 days after any change in maintenance dose. **Note:** In patients with end-stage renal disease, it may take 15-20 days to reach steady-state.

Additionally, patients who are receiving potassium-depleting medications such as diuretics, should be monitored for potassium, magnesium, and calcium levels.

Digoxin serum concentrations should be obtained whenever any of the following conditions occur:

Questionable patient compliance or to evaluate clinical deterioration following an initial good response

Changing renal function

Suspected digoxin toxicity

Initiation or discontinuation of therapy with drugs (amiodarone, quinidine, verapamil) which potentially interact with digoxin; if quinidine therapy is started, the digoxin dose should be reduced by 25% to 50% and digoxin levels should be monitored closely. Any disease changes (hypothyroidism)

Any disease changes (hypothyroidism)

Heart rate and rhythm should be monitored along with periodic ECGs to assess both desired effects and signs of toxicity

Follow closely (especially in patients receiving diuretics or amphotericin) for decreased serum potassium and magnesium or increased calcium, all of which predispose to digoxin toxicity

Assess renal function

Be aware of drug interactions

Observe patients for noncardiac signs of toxicity, confusion, and depression

Reference Range

Digoxin therapeutic serum concentrations:

Congestive heart failure: 0.5-0.8 ng/mL

Arrhythmias: 0.8-2 ng/mL

Adults: <0.5 ng/mL; probably indicates underdigitalization unless there are special circumstances

Toxic: >2.5 ng/mL

Digoxin-like immunoreactive substance (DLIS) may cross-react with digoxin immunoassay. DLIS has been found in patients with renal and liver disease, congestive heart failure, neonates, and pregnant women (3rd trimester).

Dosage Forms Excipient information presented when available (limited, particularly for generics); consult specific product labeling. [CAN] = Canadian brand name; [DSC] = Discontinued product

Capsule:

Lanoxicaps®: 100 mcg [contains ethanol; DSC]; 200 mcg [contains ethanol; DSC]

Injection, solution: 250 mcg/mL (1 mL, 2 mL)

Lanoxin®: 250 mcg/mL (2 mL) [contains ethanol 10% and propylene glycol 40%]

Injection, solution [pediatric]: 100 mcg/mL (1 mL)

Solution, oral: 50 mcg/mL (2.5 mL, 5 mL, 60 mL)

Tablet: 125 mcg, 250 mcg

Digitek®, Lanoxin®: 125 mcg, 250 mcg

Apo-Digoxin® [CAN]: 62.5 mcg, 125 mcg, 250 mcg

◆ **Dihematoporphyrin Ether** *see* Porfimer *on page 1314*

◆ **Dihistine® DH [DSC]** *see* Chlorpheniramine, Pseudoephedrine, and Codeine *on page 332*

Dihydrocodeine, Aspirin, and Caffeine

(dye hye droe KOE deen, AS pir in, & KAF een)

Medication Safety Issues

Sound-alike/look-alike issues:

Synalgos®-DC may be confused with Synagis®

High alert medication: The Institute for Safe Medication Practices (ISMP) includes this medication among its list of drug classes which have a heightened risk of causing significant patient harm when used in error.

U.S. Brand Names Synalgos®-DC

Index Terms Dihydrocodeine Compound

Pharmacologic Category Analgesic, Opioid

Use Management of mild to moderate pain that requires relaxation

Effect on Mental Status Sedation is common

Effect on Psychiatric Treatment Concurrent use with MAO inhibitors may produce additive side effects

Restrictions C-III

Dosage Summary

Oral:

Children: Dosage not established

Adults: 1-2 capsules every 4-6 hours as needed

Dosage Forms Excipient information presented when available (limited, particularly for generics); consult specific product labeling.

Capsule: Dihydrocodeine bitartrate 16 mg, aspirin 356.4 mg, and caffeine 30 mg

◆ **Dihydrocodeine Bitartrate, Acetaminophen, and Caffeine** *see* Acetaminophen, Caffeine, and Dihydrocodeine *on page 39*

◆ **Dihydrocodeine Bitartrate, Phenylephrine Hydrochloride, and Chlorpheniramine Maleate** *see* Phenylephrine, Hydrocodone, and Chlorpheniramine *on page 1277*

◆ **Dihydrocodeine Bitartrate, Pseudoephedrine Hydrochloride, and Chlorpheniramine Maleate** *see* Pseudoephedrine, Dihydrocodeine, and Chlorpheniramine *on page 1371*

Dihydrocodeine, Chlorpheniramine, and Phenylephrine

(dye hye droe KOE deen, klor fen IR a meen, & fen il EF rin)

U.S. Brand Names Baltussin; Coldcough PD; Novahistine DH

Index Terms Chlorpheniramine Maleate, Dihydrocodeine Bitartrate, and Phenylephrine Hydrochloride; Phenylephrine, Chlorpheniramine, and Dihydrocodeine

Pharmacologic Category Alpha/Beta Agonist; Analgesic, Opioid; Antitussive; Histamine H_1 Antagonist; Histamine H_1 Antagonist, First Generation

Use Symptomatic relief of cough and congestion associated with the upper respiratory tract

Effect on Mental Status May cause paradoxical excitation in pediatric patients. Sedation is common; may cause anxiety, euphoria, confusion, insomnia, nervousness, fatigue, hallucinations, or depression.

Effect on Psychiatric Treatment Contraindicated with or within 14 days of MAO inhibitors. Concomitant use with psychotropics may produce additive sedation or hypotensive effects. May result in loss of pain control if used with fluoxetine or paroxetine.

Restrictions C-III/C-V

Dosage Summary

Oral:

Children <2 years: Dosage not established

Children 2-6 years: Novahistine DH: 1.25-2.5 mL every 4-6 hours as needed (maximum: 10 mL/day)

Children 6-12 years:

Baltussin: 2.5 mL every 4-6 hours as needed

Novahistine DH: 2.5-5 mL every 4-6 hours as needed (maximum: 20 mL/day)

Children >12 years:

Baltussin: 5 mL every 4-6 hours as needed

Novahistine DH: 5-10 mL every 4-6 hours as needed (maximum: 40 mL/day)

Adults:

Baltussin: 5 mL every 4-6 hours as needed

Novahistine DH: 5-10 mL every 4-6 hours as needed (maximum: 40 mL/day)

Dosage Forms Excipient information presented when available (limited, particularly for generics); consult specific product labeling.

Liquid:

Novahistine DH: Dihydrocodeine bitartrate 7.5 mg, chlorpheniramine maleate 2 mg and phenylephrine hydrochloride 5 mg per 5 mL (480 mL) [alcohol free, sugar free; contains propylene glycol; strawberry flavor; C-III]

Syrup:

Baltussin: Dihydrocodeine bitartrate 3 mg, chlorpheniramine maleate 5 mg, and phenylephrine hydrochloride 20 mg per 5 mL (480 mL) [alcohol free, sugar free; contains propylene glycol; fruit flavor; C-III]

Coldcough PD: Dihydrocodeine bitartrate 3 mg, chlorpheniramine maleate 2 mg, and phenylephrine hydrochloride 7.5 mg per 5 mL (120 mL) [alcohol free, sugar free; grape flavor; C-V]

◆ **Dihydrocodeine Compound** *see* Dihydrocodeine, Aspirin, and Caffeine *on page 468*

Dihydrocodeine, Pseudoephedrine, and Guaifenesin

(dye hye droe KOE deen, soo doe e FED rin, & gwye FEN e sin)

U.S. Brand Names DiHydro-GP; Hydro-Tussin™ EXP [DSC]; Pancof®-EXP

Index Terms Guaifenesin, Dihydrocodeine, and Pseudoephedrine; Pseudoephedrine Hydrochloride, Guaifenesin, and Dihydrocodeine Bitartrate

Pharmacologic Category Antitussive/Decongestant/Expectorant

Use Temporary relief of cough and congestion associated with upper respiratory tract infections and allergies

Effect on Mental Status Dizziness, nervousness, and insomnia are common; may cause CNS depression; concomitant use with psychotropic agents may produce additive effects; may rarely cause hallucinations

Effect on Psychiatric Treatment Contraindicated with or within 14 days of MAO inhibitor use

Dosage Summary

Oral:

Children <2 years: Dosage not established
Children 2-6 years: 1.25-2.5 mL every 4-6 hours as needed
Children 6-12 years: 2.5-5 mL every 4-6 hours as needed
Children ≥12 years: 5-10 mL every 4-6 hours as needed
Adults: 5-10 mL every 4-6 hours as needed

Dosage Forms Excipient information presented when available (limited, particularly for generics); consult specific product labeling. [DSC] = Discontinued product

Syrup:

DiHydro-GP: Dihydrocodeine bitartrate 7.5 mg, pseudoephedrine hydrochloride 15 mg, and guaifenesin 100 mg per 5 mL (480 mL) [vanilla flavor]

Hydro-Tussin™ EXP [DSC], Pancof®-EXP: Dihydrocodeine bitartrate 7.5 mg, pseudoephedrine hydrochloride 15 mg, and guaifenesin 100 mg per 5 mL (480 mL) [alcohol free, dye free, sugar free]

◆ **DiHydro-CP** *see* Pseudoephedrine, Dihydrocodeine, and Chlorpheniramine *on page 1371*

Dihydroergotamine (dye hye droe er GOT a meen)

U.S. Brand Names D.H.E. 45®; Migranal®

Canadian Brand Names Migranal®

Mexican Brand Names Parsel; Tonopan

Index Terms DHE; Dihydroergotamine Mesylate

Pharmacologic Category Antimigraine Agent; Ergot Derivative

Generic Available Yes: Injection

Use Treatment of migraine headache with or without aura; injection also indicated for treatment of cluster headaches

Unlabeled/Investigational Use Adjunct for DVT prophylaxis for hip surgery, for orthostatic hypotension, xerostomia secondary to antidepressant use, and pelvic congestion with pain

Effect on Mental Status Drowsiness is common

Effect on Psychiatric Treatment None reported

Pregnancy Risk Factor X

Pregnancy Considerations Dihydroergotamine is oxytocic and should not be used during pregnancy.

Lactation May be excreted in breast milk/contraindicated

Contraindications Hypersensitivity to dihydroergotamine or any component of the formulation; high-dose aspirin therapy; uncontrolled hypertension, ischemic heart disease, angina pectoris, history of MI, silent ischemia, or coronary artery vasospasm including Prinzmetal's angina; hemiplegic or basilar migraine; peripheral vascular disease; sepsis; severe hepatic or renal dysfunction; following vascular surgery; avoid use within 24 hours of sumatriptan, zolmitriptan, other serotonin agonists, or ergot-like agents; avoid during or within 2 weeks of discontinuing MAO inhibitors; ergot alkaloids are contraindicated with potent inhibitors of CYP3A4 (includes protease inhibitors, azole antifungals, and some macrolide antibiotics); pregnancy

Warnings/Precautions [U.S. Boxed Warning]: Ergot alkaloids are contraindicated with potent inhibitors of CYP3A4 (includes protease inhibitors, azole antifungals, and some macrolide antibiotics); concomitant use associated with acute ergot toxicity (ergotism). Do not give to patients with risk factors for CAD until a cardiovascular evaluation has been performed; if evaluation is satisfactory, the healthcare provider should administer the first dose and cardiovascular status should be periodically evaluated. May cause vasospastic reactions; persistent vasospasm may lead to gangrene or death in patients with compromised circulation. Discontinue if signs of vasoconstriction develop. Rare reports of increased blood pressure in patients without history of hypertension. Rare reports of adverse cardiac events (acute MI, life-threatening arrhythmias, death) have been reported following use of the injection. Cerebral hemorrhage, subarachnoid hemorrhage, and stroke have also occurred following use of the injection. Not for prolonged use. Pleural and peritoneal fibrosis have been reported with prolonged daily use. Cardiac valvular fibrosis has also been associated with ergot alkaloids. Use with caution in the elderly. Safety and efficacy in pediatric patients have not been established.

Migranal® Nasal Spray: Local irritation to nose and throat (usually transient and mild-moderate in severity) can occur; long-term consequences on nasal or respiratory mucosa have not been extensively evaluated.

Adverse Reactions

>10%: Nasal spray: Respiratory: Rhinitis (26%)

1% to 10%: Nasal spray:

Central nervous system: Dizziness (4%), somnolence (3%)

Endocrine & metabolic: Hot flashes (1%)

Gastrointestinal: Nausea (10%), taste disturbance (8%), vomiting (4%), diarrhea (2%)

Local: Application site reaction (6%)

Neuromuscular & skeletal: Weakness (1%), stiffness (1%)

Respiratory: Pharyngitis (3%)

<1% (Limited to important or life-threatening): Injection and nasal spray: Cerebral hemorrhage, coronary artery vasospasm, hypertension, MI, paresthesia, peripheral cyanosis, peripheral ischemia, rash, stroke, subarachnoid hemorrhage, ventricular fibrillation, ventricular tachycardia. Pleural and retroperitoneal fibrosis have been reported following prolonged use of the injection; cardiac valvular fibrosis has been associated with ergot alkaloids.

Metabolism/Transport Effects Substrate of CYP3A4 (major); **Inhibits** CYP3A4 (weak)

Drug Interactions

CYP3A4 Inhibitors (Moderate): May decrease the metabolism of CYP3A4 Substrates. *Risk C: Monitor therapy*

CYP3A4 Inhibitors (Strong): May decrease the metabolism of CYP3A4 Substrates. *Risk D: Consider therapy modification*

Dasatinib: May increase the serum concentration of CYP3A4 Substrates. *Risk C: Monitor therapy*

Efavirenz: May enhance the adverse/toxic effect of Ergot Derivatives. Specifically, the risk for peripheral vasospasm and ischemia may be increased. *Risk X: Avoid combination*

Macrolide Antibiotics: May enhance the adverse/toxic effect of Ergot Derivatives. Specifically leading the development of ergotism. **Exceptions:** Azithromycin; Dirithromycin [Off Market]; Spiramycin. *Risk D: Consider therapy modification*

Posaconazole: May increase the serum concentration of Ergot Derivatives. *Risk X: Avoid combination*

Protease Inhibitors: May decrease the metabolism of Ergot Derivatives. *Risk X: Avoid combination*

Serotonin 5-HT1D Receptor Agonists: Ergot Derivatives may enhance the vasoconstricting effect of Serotonin 5-HT1D Receptor Agonists. Serotonin 5-HT1D Receptor Agonists may enhance the vasoconstricting effect of Ergot Derivatives. *Risk X: Avoid combination*

Serotonin Modulators: May enhance the adverse/toxic effect of other Serotonin Modulators. The development of serotonin syndrome may occur. *Risk D: Consider therapy modification*

Sibutramine: May enhance the serotonergic effect of Ergot Derivatives. This may cause serotonin syndrome. *Risk X: Avoid combination*

Voriconazole: May increase the serum concentration of Ergot Derivatives. *Risk X: Avoid combination*

Stability

Injection: Store below 25°C (77°F); do not refrigerate or freeze. Protect from heat and light.

Nasal spray: Prior to use, store below 25°C (77°F); do not refrigerate or freeze. Once spray applicator has been prepared, use within 8 hours; discard any unused solution.

Mechanism of Action Ergot alkaloid alpha-adrenergic blocker directly stimulates vascular smooth muscle to vasoconstrict peripheral and cerebral vessels; also has effects on serotonin receptors

Pharmacodynamics/Kinetics

Onset of action: 15-30 minutes

Duration: 3-4 hours

Distribution: V_d: 14.5 L/kg

Protein binding: 93%

Metabolism: Extensively hepatic

Half-life elimination: 1.3-3.9 hours

Time to peak, serum: I.M.: 15-30 minutes

Excretion: Primarily feces; urine (10% mostly as metabolites)

Dosage Adults:

I.M., SubQ: 1 mg at first sign of headache; repeat hourly to a maximum dose of 3 mg total; maximum dose: 6 mg/week

I.V.: 1 mg at first sign of headache; repeat hourly up to a maximum dose of 2 mg total; maximum dose: 6 mg/week

Intranasal: 1 spray (0.5 mg) of nasal spray should be administered into each nostril; if needed, repeat after 15 minutes, up to a total of 4 sprays. **Note:** Do not exceed 3 mg (6 sprays) in a 24-hour period and no more than 8 sprays in a week.

Elderly: Patients >65 years of age were not included in controlled clinical studies

Dosing adjustment in renal impairment: Contraindicated in severe renal impairment

Dosing adjustment in hepatic impairment: Dosage reductions are probably necessary but specific guidelines are not available; contraindicated in severe hepatic dysfunction

Administration Prior to administration of nasal spray, the nasal spray applicator must be primed (pumped 4 times); in order to let the drug be absorbed through the skin in the nose, patients should not inhale deeply through the nose while spraying or immediately after spraying; for best results, treatment should be initiated at the first symptom or sign of an attack; however, nasal spray can be used at any stage of a migraine attack

Reference Range Minimum concentration for vasoconstriction is reportedly 0.06 ng/mL

Dosage Forms Excipient information presented when available (limited, particularly for generics); consult specific product labeling.

Injection, solution, as mesylate: 1 mg/mL (1 mL) [contains ethanol 6.2%]

D.H.E. 45®: 1 mg/mL (1 mL) [contains ethanol 6.2%]

Solution, intranasal spray, as mesylate (Migranal®): 4 mg/mL [0.5 mg/spray] (1 mL) [contains caffeine 10 mg/mL]

- **Dihydroergotamine Mesylate** *see* Dihydroergotamine *on page 470*
- **Dihydroergotoxine** *see* Ergoloid Mesylates *on page 551*
- **Dihydrogenated Ergot Alkaloids** *see* Ergoloid Mesylates *on page 551*
- **DiHydro-GP** *see* Dihydrocodeine, Pseudoephedrine, and Guaifenesin *on page 469*
- **Dihydrohydroxycodeinone** *see* OxyCODONE *on page 1201*
- **Dihydromorphinone** *see* HYDROmorphone *on page 791*

Dihydrotachysterol (dye hye droe tak ISS ter ole)

U.S. Brand Names DHT™ Intensol™ [DSC]; DHT™ [DSC]; Hytakerol® [DSC]

Canadian Brand Names Hytakerol®

Index Terms Dichysterol

Pharmacologic Category Vitamin D Analog

Use Treatment of hypocalcemia associated with hypoparathyroidism; prophylaxis of hypocalcemic tetany following thyroid surgery

Effect on Mental Status None reported

Effect on Psychiatric Treatment Concurrent use with phenytoin or phenobarbital may decrease effectiveness

Dosage Summary

Oral:

Infants and young children: Initial: 1-5 mg/day for 4 days; Maintenance: 0.1-0.5 mg/day

Older children: Initial: 0.8-2.4 mg/day for several days; Maintenance: 0.2-1 mg/day

Adults: Initial: 0.8-2.4 mg/day for several days; Maintenance: 0.2-1 mg/day **or** 13-50 mcg/day

Dosage Forms Excipient information presented when available (limited, particularly for generics); consult specific product labeling. [DSC] = Discontinued product

Capsule (Hytakerol®): 0.125 mg [contains sesame oil] [DSC]

Solution, oral concentrate (DHT™ Intensol™): 0.2 mg/mL (30 mL) [contains alcohol 20%] [DSC]

Tablet (DHT™): 0.125 mg, 0.2 mg, 0.4 mg [DSC]

- **Dihydroxyanthracenedione Dihydrochloride** *see* Mitoxantrone *on page 1061*
- **Dihydroxydeoxynorvinkaleukoblastine** *see* Vinorelbine *on page 1674*
- **Dihydroxypropyl Theophylline** *see* Dyphylline *on page 521*
- **Diiodohydroxyquin** *see* Iodoquinol *on page 851*
- **Dilacor® XR** *see* Diltiazem *on page 473*

- ◆ **Dilantin®** *see* Phenytoin *on page 1280*
- ◆ **Dilatrate®-SR** *see* Isosorbide Dinitrate *on page 866*
- ◆ **Dilaudid®** *see* HYDROmorphone *on page 791*
- ◆ **Dilaudid-HP®** *see* HYDROmorphone *on page 791*
- ◆ **Dilex-G** *see* Dyphylline and Guaifenesin *on page 522*
- ◆ **Dilor-G®** *see* Dyphylline and Guaifenesin *on page 522*
- ◆ **Dilt-CD** *see* Diltiazem *on page 473*

Diltiazem (dil TYE a zem)

Medication Safety Issues

Sound-alike/look-alike issues:

Cardizem® may be confused with Cardene®, Cardene SR®, Cardizem CD®, Cardizem SR®, cardiem

Cartia XT™ may be confused with Procardia XL®

Diltiazem may be confused with Dilantin®

Tiazac® may be confused with Tigan®, Tiazac® XC [CAN], Ziac®

High alert medication: The Institute for Safe Medication Practices (ISMP) includes this medication (I.V. formulation) among its list of drug classes which have a heightened risk of causing significant patient harm when used in error.

Significant differences exist between oral and I.V. dosing. Use caution when converting from one route of administration to another.

International issues:

Cardizem® may be confused with Cardem® which is a brand name for celiprolol in Spain

Cartia XT™ may be confused with Cartia® which is a brand name for aspirin in multiple international markets

Dilacor®: Brand name for digoxin in Serbia, a brand name for verapamil in Brazil, and a brand name for barnidipine in Argentina

Tiazac® may be confused with Tazac® which is a brand name for nizatidine in Australia

Tiazac® may be confused with Tiazac® XC which is a brand name for diltiazem available in Canada (not available in U.S.)

Related Information

Calcium Channel Blockers *on page 1778*

U.S. Brand Names Cardizem®; Cardizem® CD; Cardizem® LA; Cartia XT™; Dilacor® XR; Dilt-CD; Dilt-XR; Taztia XT™; Tiazac®

Canadian Brand Names Alti-Diltiazem CD; Apo-Diltiaz CD®; Apo-Diltiaz SR®; Apo-Diltiaz TZ®; Apo-Diltiaz®; Apo-Diltiaz® Injectable; Cardizem®; Cardizem® CD; Cardizem® SR; Diltiazem HCl ER®; Diltiazem Hydrochloride Injection; Gen-Diltiazem; Gen-Diltiazem CD; Med-Diltiazem; Novo-Diltazem; Novo-Diltazem-CD; Novo-Diltiazem HCl ER; Nu-Diltiaz; Nu-Diltiaz-CD; ratio-Diltiazem CD; Rhoxal-diltiazem CD; Rhoxal-diltiazem SR; Rhoxal-diltiazem T; Sandoz-Diltiazem CD; Sandoz-Diltiazem T; Syn-Diltiazem®; Tiazac® ; Tiazac® XC

Mexican Brand Names Angiotrofin; Angiotrofin Retard; Dasav; Tilazem

Index Terms Diltiazem Hydrochloride

Pharmacologic Category Calcium Channel Blocker

Generic Available Yes: Excludes extended release tablet

Use

Oral: Essential hypertension; chronic stable angina or angina from coronary artery spasm

Injection: Atrial fibrillation or atrial flutter; paroxysmal supraventricular tachycardia (PSVT)

Unlabeled/Investigational Use Investigational: Therapy of Duchenne muscular dystrophy

Effect on Mental Status May cause dizziness, insomnia, nervousness, or sedation

Effect on Psychiatric Treatment May produce leukopenia; use caution with clozapine and carbamazepine; lithium levels may be increased or decreased; monitor serum lithium levels; benzodiazepines (midazolam, triazolam), buspirone, and carbamazepine levels may be increased; monitor for increased side effects

Pregnancy Risk Factor C

Pregnancy Considerations Teratogenic and embryotoxic effects have been demonstrated in small animals. There are no adequate and well-controlled studies in pregnant women.

Lactation Enters breast milk/not recommended (AAP considers "compatible")

Contraindications

Oral: Hypersensitivity to diltiazem or any component of the formulation; sick sinus syndrome; second- or third-degree AV block (except in patients with a functioning artificial pacemaker); severe hypotension (systolic <90 mm Hg); acute MI and pulmonary congestion

Intravenous (I.V.): Hypersensitivity to diltiazem or any component of the formulation; sick sinus syndrome; second- or third-degree AV block (except in patients with a functioning artificial pacemaker); severe hypotension (systolic <90 mm Hg); acute MI and pulmonary congestion; administration concomitantly or within a few hours of the administration of I.V. beta-blockers; atrial fibrillation or flutter associated with accessory bypass tract (eg, Wolff-Parkinson-White syndrome); ventricular tachycardia (with wide-complex tachycardia, must determine whether origin is supraventricular or ventricular)

Canadian labeling: Additional contraindications (not in U.S. labeling): I.V. and oral: Pregnancy; use in women of childbearing potential

Warnings/Precautions Can cause first-, second-, and third-degree AV block or sinus bradycardia and risk increases with agents known to slow cardiac conduction. The most common side effect is peripheral edema; occurs within 2-3 weeks of starting therapy. Symptomatic hypotension with or without syncope can rarely occur; blood pressure must be lowered at a rate appropriate for the patient's clinical condition. Concomitant use with beta-blockers or digoxin can result in conduction disturbances. I.V. administration concomitantly or within a few hours of I.V. beta-blockers is contraindicated. Use caution in left ventricular dysfunction (may exacerbate condition). Use with caution with hypertrophic obstructive cardiomyopathy. Use with caution in hepatic or renal dysfunction.

Adverse Reactions Note: Frequencies represent ranges for various dosage forms. Patients with impaired ventricular function and/or conduction abnormalities may have higher incidence of adverse reactions.

>10%:

Cardiovascular: Edema (2% to 15%)

Central nervous system: Headache (5% to 12%)

2% to 10%:

Cardiovascular: AV block (first degree 2% to 8%), edema (lower limb, 2% to 8%), pain (6%), bradycardia (2% to 6%), hypotension (<2% to 4%), vasodilation (2% to 3%), extrasystoles (2%), flushing (1% to 2%), palpitation (1% to 2%)

Central nervous system: Dizziness (3% to 10%), nervousness (2%)

Dermatologic: Rash (1% to 4%)

Endocrine & metabolic: Gout (1% to 2%)

Gastrointestinal: Dyspepsia (1% to 6%), constipation (<2% to 4%), vomiting (2%), diarrhea (1% to 2%)

Local: Injection site reactions: Burning, itching (4%)

Neuromuscular & skeletal: Weakness (1% to 4%), myalgia (2%)

Respiratory: Rhinitis (<2% to 10%), pharyngitis (2% to 6%), dyspnea (1% to 6%), bronchitis (1% to 4%), sinus congestion (1% to 2%)

<2% (Limited to important or life-threatening): Alkaline phosphatase increased, allergic reaction, ALT increased, AST increased, amblyopia, amnesia, arrhythmia, AV block (second or third degree), bundle branch block, CHF, depression, dysgeusia, extrapyramidal symptoms, gingival hyperplasia, hemolytic anemia, petechiae, photosensitivity, Stevens-Johnson syndrome, syncope, tachycardia, thrombocytopenia, tremor, toxic epidermal necrolysis

Metabolism/Transport Effects Substrate of CYP2C9 (minor), 2D6 (minor), 3A4 (major); **Inhibits** CYP2C9 (weak), 2D6 (weak), 3A4 (moderate)

Drug Interactions

Alfentanil: Diltiazem may increase the serum concentration of Alfentanil. *Risk C: Monitor therapy*

Alpha1-Blockers: May enhance the hypotensive effect of Calcium Channel Blockers. *Risk C: Monitor therapy*

Amiodarone: Calcium Channel Blockers (Nondihydropyridine) may enhance the bradycardic effect of Amiodarone. Sinus arrest has been reported. *Risk D: Consider therapy modification*

Anilidopiperidine Opioids: May enhance the bradycardic effect of Calcium Channel Blockers (Nondihydropyridine). Anilidopiperidine Opioids may enhance the hypotensive effect of Calcium Channel Blockers (Nondihydropyridine). *Risk C: Monitor therapy*

Antifungal Agents (Azole Derivatives, Systemic): May decrease the metabolism of Calcium Channel Blockers. *Risk D: Consider therapy modification*

Aprepitant: May increase the serum concentration of Diltiazem. Diltiazem may increase the serum concentration of Aprepitant. *Risk C: Monitor therapy*

Barbiturates: May increase the metabolism of Calcium Channel Blockers. *Risk D: Consider therapy modification*

Benzodiazepines (metabolized by oxidation): Calcium Channel Blockers (Nondihydropyridine) may decrease the metabolism of Benzodiazepines (metabolized by oxidation). *Risk D: Consider therapy modification*

Beta-Blockers: Calcium Channel Blockers (Nondihydropyridine) may enhance the hypotensive effect of Beta-Blockers. Bradycardia and signs of heart failure have also been reported. Calcium Channel Blockers (Nondihydropyridine) may increase the serum concentration of Beta-Blockers. **Exceptions:** Levobunolol; Metipranolol. *Risk C: Monitor therapy*

BusPIRone: Calcium Channel Blockers (Nondihydropyridine) may decrease the metabolism of BusPIRone. *Risk D: Consider therapy modification*

Calcium Channel Blockers (Dihydropyridine): Calcium Channel Blockers (Nondihydropyridine) may enhance the hypotensive effect of Calcium Channel Blockers (Dihydropyridine). Calcium Channel Blockers (Nondihydropyridine) may decrease the metabolism of Calcium Channel Blockers (Dihydropyridine). **Exceptions:** Clevidipine. *Risk C: Monitor therapy*

Calcium Salts: May diminish the therapeutic effect of Calcium Channel Blockers. *Risk C: Monitor therapy*

CarBAMazepine: Calcium Channel Blockers (Nondihydropyridine) may decrease the metabolism of CarBAMazepine. CarBAMazepine may increase the metabolism of Calcium Channel Blockers (Nondihydropyridine). *Risk D: Consider therapy modification*

Cardiac Glycosides: Calcium Channel Blockers (Nondihydropyridine) may enhance the AV-blocking effect of Cardiac Glycosides. Calcium Channel Blockers (Nondihydropyridine) may decrease the metabolism of Cardiac Glycosides. *Risk D: Consider therapy modification*

Cimetidine: May decrease the metabolism of Calcium Channel Blockers. *Risk D: Consider therapy modification*

Colestipol: May decrease the absorption of Diltiazem. *Risk C: Monitor therapy*

Corticosteroids (Systemic): Calcium Channel Blockers (Nondihydropyridine) may decrease the metabolism of Corticosteroids (Systemic). *Risk C: Monitor therapy*

CycloSPORINE: Calcium Channel Blockers (Nondihydropyridine) may decrease the metabolism of CycloSPORINE. CycloSPORINE may decrease the metabolism of Calcium Channel Blockers (Nondihydropyridine). *Risk D: Consider therapy modification*

CYP3A4 Inducers (Strong): May increase the metabolism of CYP3A4 Substrates. *Risk C: Monitor therapy*

CYP3A4 Inhibitors (Moderate): May decrease the metabolism of CYP3A4 Substrates. *Risk C: Monitor therapy*

CYP3A4 Inhibitors (Strong): May decrease the metabolism of CYP3A4 Substrates. *Risk D: Consider therapy modification*

CYP3A4 Substrates: CYP3A4 Inhibitors (Moderate) may decrease the metabolism of CYP3A4 Substrates. *Risk C: Monitor therapy*

Dasatinib: May increase the serum concentration of CYP3A4 Substrates. *Risk C: Monitor therapy*

Deferasirox: May decrease the serum concentration of CYP3A4 Substrates. *Risk C: Monitor therapy*

Diazoxide: May enhance the hypotensive effect of Antihypertensives. *Risk C: Monitor therapy*

Eletriptan: Calcium Channel Blockers (Nondihydropyridine) may decrease the metabolism of Eletriptan. *Risk C: Monitor therapy*

Eplerenone: Calcium Channel Blockers (Nondihydropyridine) may decrease the metabolism of Eplerenone. *Risk C: Monitor therapy*

Fluconazole: May decrease the metabolism of Calcium Channel Blockers. *Risk C: Monitor therapy*

Fosaprepitant: May increase the serum concentration of Diltiazem. The active metabolite aprepitant is likely responsible for this effect. Diltiazem may increase the serum concentration of Fosaprepitant. Specifically, diltiazem may increase the concentration of the active metabolite aprepitant. *Risk C: Monitor therapy*

Grapefruit Juice: May decrease the metabolism of Calcium Channel Blockers. *Risk C: Monitor therapy*

Herbs (CYP3A4 Inducers): May increase the metabolism of CYP3A4 Substrates. *Risk C: Monitor therapy*

Herbs (Hypertensive Properties): May diminish the antihypertensive effect of Antihypertensives. *Risk C: Monitor therapy*

Herbs (Hypotensive Properties): May enhance the hypotensive effect of Antihypertensives. *Risk C: Monitor therapy*

HMG-CoA Reductase Inhibitors: Calcium Channel Blockers (Nondihydropyridine) may decrease the metabolism of HMG-CoA Reductase Inhibitors. ▶

Exceptions: Fluvastatin; Pravastatin; Rosuvastatin. *Risk D: Consider therapy modification*

Lithium: Calcium Channel Blockers (Nondihydropyridine) may enhance the neurotoxic effect of Lithium. Calcium Channel Blockers (Nondihydropyridine) may increase the serum concentration of Lithium. Decreased or unaltered lithium concentrations have also been reported with this combination. *Risk C: Monitor therapy*

Macrolide Antibiotics: May decrease the metabolism of Calcium Channel Blockers. **Exceptions:** Azithromycin; Dirithromycin [Off Market]; Spiramycin. *Risk D: Consider therapy modification*

Magnesium Salts: Calcium Channel Blockers may enhance the adverse/toxic effect of Magnesium Salts. Magnesium Salts may enhance the hypotensive effect of Calcium Channel Blockers. *Risk C: Monitor therapy*

Maraviroc: CYP3A4 Inhibitors may increase the serum concentration of Maraviroc. *Risk D: Consider therapy modification*

Methylphenidate: May diminish the antihypertensive effect of Antihypertensives. *Risk C: Monitor therapy*

Midodrine: Calcium Channel Blockers (Nondihydropyridine) may enhance the bradycardic effect of Midodrine. *Risk C: Monitor therapy*

Nafcillin: May increase the metabolism of Calcium Channel Blockers. *Risk D: Consider therapy modification*

Neuromuscular-Blocking Agents (Nondepolarizing): Calcium Channel Blockers may enhance the neuromuscular-blocking effect of Neuromuscular-Blocking Agents (Nondepolarizing). *Risk C: Monitor therapy*

Nitroprusside: Calcium Channel Blockers may enhance the hypotensive effect of Nitroprusside. *Risk C: Monitor therapy*

P-Glycoprotein Inducers: May decrease the serum concentration of P-Glycoprotein Substrates. P-glycoprotein inducers may also further limit the distribution of p-glycoprotein substrates to specific cells/tissues/organs where p-glycoprotein is present in large amounts (e.g., brain, T-lymphocytes, testes, etc.). *Risk C: Monitor therapy*

P-Glycoprotein Inhibitors: May increase the serum concentration of P-Glycoprotein Substrates. P-glycoprotein inhibitors may also enhance the distribution of p-glycoprotein substrates to specific cells/tissues/organs where p-glycoprotein is present in large amounts (e.g., brain, T-lymphocytes, testes, etc.). *Risk C: Monitor therapy*

Phenytoin: Calcium Channel Blockers may decrease the metabolism of Phenytoin. *Risk D: Consider therapy modification*

Pimecrolimus: CYP3A4 Inhibitors (Moderate) may decrease the metabolism of Pimecrolimus. *Risk C: Monitor therapy*

Prostacyclin Analogues: May enhance the hypotensive effect of Antihypertensives. *Risk C: Monitor therapy*

Protease Inhibitors: May decrease the metabolism of Calcium Channel Blockers (Nondihydropyridine). Increased serum concentrations of the calcium channel blocker may increase risk of AV nodal blockade. *Risk D: Consider therapy modification*

QuiNIDine: Calcium Channel Blockers (Nondihydropyridine) may increase the serum concentration of QuiNIDine. *Risk D: Consider therapy modification*

Quinupristin: May decrease the metabolism of Calcium Channel Blockers. *Risk C: Monitor therapy*

Ranolazine: Calcium Channel Blockers (Nondihydropyridine) may decrease the metabolism of Ranolazine. *Risk X: Avoid combination*

Rifamycin Derivatives: May increase the metabolism of Calcium Channel Blockers. This primarily affects oral forms of calcium channel blockers. *Risk D: Consider therapy modification*

RiTUXimab: Antihypertensives may enhance the hypotensive effect of RiTUXimab. *Risk D: Consider therapy modification*

Salicylates: Calcium Channel Blockers (Nondihydropyridine) may enhance the anticoagulant effect of Salicylates. *Risk C: Monitor therapy*

Salmeterol: CYP3A4 Inhibitors (Moderate) may increase the serum concentration of Salmeterol. *Risk C: Monitor therapy*

Tacrolimus: Calcium Channel Blockers (Nondihydropyridine) may decrease the metabolism of Tacrolimus. *Risk C: Monitor therapy*

Ethanol/Nutrition/Herb Interactions

Ethanol: Avoid ethanol (may increase risk of hypotension or vasodilation).

Food: Diltiazem serum levels may be elevated if taken with food. Serum concentrations were not altered by grapefruit juice in small clinical trials.

Herb/Nutraceutical: St John's wort may decrease diltiazem levels. Avoid bayberry, blue cohosh, cayenne, ephedra, ginger, ginseng (American), kola, licorice, yohimbe (may worsen hypertension). Avoid black cohosh, California poppy, coleus, garlic, golden seal, hawthorn, mistletoe, periwinkle, quinine, shepherd's purse (may have increased antihypertensive effect).

Stability

Capsule, tablet: Store at 15°C to 30°C (59°F to 86°F). Protect from light.

Solution for injection: Store in refrigerator at 2°C to 8°C (36°F to 46°F). May be stored at room temperature for up to 1 month; do not freeze. Following dilution with $D_5$1/2NS, D_5W, or NS, solution is stable for 24 hours at room temperature or under refrigeration.

Mechanism of Action Inhibits calcium ion from entering the "slow channels" or select voltage-sensitive areas of vascular smooth muscle and myocardium during depolarization, producing a relaxation of coronary vascular smooth muscle and coronary vasodilation; increases myocardial oxygen delivery in patients with vasospastic angina

Pharmacodynamics/Kinetics

Onset of action: Oral: Immediate release tablet: 30-60 minutes

Absorption: Immediate release tablet: >90%; Extended release capsule: ~93%

Distribution: V_d: 3-13 L/kg

Protein binding: 70% to 80%

Metabolism: Hepatic; extensive first-pass effect; following single I.V. injection, plasma concentrations of N-monodesmethyldiltiazem and desacetyldiltiazem are typically undetectable; however, these metabolites accumulate to detectable concentrations following 24-hour constant rate infusion. N-monodesmethyldiltiazem appears to have 20% of the potency of diltiazem; desacetyldiltiazem is about 25% to 50% as potent as the parent compound.

Bioavailability: Oral: ~40% (undergoes extensive first-pass metabolism)

Half-life elimination: Immediate release tablet: 3-4.5 hours, may be prolonged with renal impairment; Extended release tablet: 6-9 hours; Extended release capsules: 5-10 hours

Time to peak, serum: Immediate release tablet: 2-4 hours; Extended release tablet: 11-18 hours; Extended release capsule: 10-14 hours

Excretion: Urine (2% to 4% as unchanged drug; 6% to 7% as metabolites); feces

Dosage

Children (unlabeled use): Oral: Hypertension: Immediate release tablets: Initial: 1.5-2 mg/kg/day 3 times daily (maximum dose 6 mg/kg/day up to 360 mg/day)

Note: Doses up to 8 mg/kg/day given in 4 divided doses have been used for investigational therapy of Duchenne muscular dystrophy

Adults:

Oral:

Angina:

Capsule, extended release (Cardizem® CD, Cartia XT™, Dilacor® XR, Tiazac®): Initial: 120-180 mg once daily (maximum dose: 480 mg/day)

Tablet, extended release (Cardizem® LA), Tiazac® XC [CAN; not available in U.S.]): 180 mg once daily; may increase at 7- to 14-day intervals (maximum recommended dose: 360 mg/day)

Tablet, immediate release (Cardizem®): Usual starting dose: 30 mg 4 times/day; usual range: 180-360 mg/day

Hypertension:

Capsule, extended release (Cardizem® CD, Cartia XT™, Dilacor® XR, Tiazac®): Initial: 180-240 mg once daily; dose adjustment may be made after 14 days; usual dose range (JNC 7): 180-420 mg/day; Tiazac®: usual dose range: 120-540 mg/day

Capsule, sustained release: Initial: 60-120 mg twice daily; dose adjustment may be made after 14 days; usual range: 240-360 mg/day

Tablet, extended release (Cardizem® LA, Tiazac® XC [CAN; not available in U.S.]): Initial: 180-240 mg once daily; dose adjustment may be made after 14 days; usual dose range (JNC 7): 120-540 mg/day

Note: Elderly: Patients ≥60 years may respond to a lower initial dose (ie, 120 mg once daily using extended release capsule)

I.V.: Atrial fibrillation, atrial flutter, PSVT:

Initial bolus dose: 0.25 mg/kg actual body weight over 2 minutes (average adult dose: 20 mg)

Repeat bolus dose (may be administered after 15 minutes if the response is inadequate.): 0.35 mg/kg actual body weight over 2 minutes (average adult dose: 25 mg)

Continuous infusion (requires an infusion pump; infusions >24 hours or infusion rates >15 mg/hour are not recommended.): Initial infusion rate of 10 mg/hour; rate may be increased in 5 mg/hour increments up to 15 mg/hour as needed; some patients may respond to an initial rate of 5 mg/hour.

If diltiazem injection is administered by continuous infusion for >24 hours, the possibility of decreased diltiazem clearance, prolonged elimination half-life, and increased diltiazem and/or diltiazem metabolite plasma concentrations should be considered.

Conversion from I.V. diltiazem to oral diltiazem:

Oral dose (mg/day) is approximately equal to [rate (mg/hour) x 3 + 3] x 10.

3 mg/hour = 120 mg/day
5 mg/hour = 180 mg/day
7 mg/hour = 240 mg/day
11 mg/hour = 360 mg/day

Dosing comments in renal/hepatic impairment: Use with caution as extensively metabolized by the liver and excreted in the kidneys and bile.

Dialysis: Not removed by hemo- or peritoneal dialysis; supplemental dose is not necessary.

Administration

Oral: Do not crush long acting dosage forms.

Taztia XT™, Tiazac®: Capsules may be opened and sprinkled on a spoonful of applesauce. Applesauce should be swallowed without chewing, followed by drinking a glass of water.

Tiazac® XC [CAN; not available in U.S.]: Administer at bedtime

I.V.: Bolus doses given over 2 minutes with continuous ECG and blood pressure monitoring. Continuous infusion should be via infusion pump.

Monitoring Parameters Liver function tests, blood pressure, ECG

Dosage Forms Excipient information presented when available (limited, particularly for generics); consult specific product labeling. [CAN] = Canadian brand name

Capsule, extended release, as hydrochloride [once-daily dosing]: 120 mg, 180 mg, 240 mg, 300 mg, 360 mg, 420 mg
Cardizem® CD: 120 mg, 180 mg, 240 mg, 300 mg, 360 mg
Cartia XT™: 120 mg, 180 mg, 240 mg, 300 mg
Dilacor® XR, Dilt-XR: 120 mg, 180 mg, 240 mg
Dilt-CD: 120 mg, 180 mg, 240 mg, 300 mg
Taztia XT™: 120 mg, 180 mg, 240 mg, 300 mg, 360 mg
Tiazac®: 120 mg, 180 mg, 240 mg, 300 mg, 360 mg, 420 mg

Capsule, extended release, as hydrochloride [twice-daily dosing]: 60 mg, 90 mg, 120 mg

Injection, solution, as hydrochloride: 5 mg/mL (5 mL, 10 mL, 25 mL)

Injection, powder for reconstitution, as hydrochloride: 100 mg

Tablet, as hydrochloride: 30 mg, 60 mg, 90 mg, 120 mg
Cardizem®: 30 mg, 60 mg, 90 mg, 120 mg

Tablet, extended release, as hydrochloride:
Cardizem® LA: 120 mg, 180 mg, 240 mg, 300 mg, 360 mg, 420 mg
Tiazac® XC [CAN; not available in U.S.]: 120 mg, 180 mg, 240 mg, 300 mg, 360 mg

◆ **Diltiazem Hydrochloride** *see* Diltiazem *on page 473*
◆ **Dilt-XR** *see* Diltiazem *on page 473*
◆ **Dimaphen [OTC]** *see* Brompheniramine and Pseudoephedrine *on page 206*

DimenhyDRINATE (dye men HYE dri nate)

Medication Safety Issues

Sound-alike/look-alike issues:
DimenhyDRINATE may be confused with diphenhydrAMINE

U.S. Brand Names Dramamine® [OTC]; Driminate® [OTC]; TripTone® [OTC]

Canadian Brand Names Apo-Dimenhydrinate®; Children's Motion Sickness Liquid; Dinate®; Gravol®; Jamp® Travel Tablet; Nauseatol; Novo-Dimenate; SAB-Dimenhydrinate

Mexican Brand Names Dimenhidrinato; Dimicaps; Dramamine; Vomisin

Pharmacologic Category Histamine H_1 Antagonist; Histamine H_1 Antagonist, First Generation

Use Treatment and prevention of nausea, vertigo, and vomiting associated with motion sickness

Dosage forms available in Canada (not available in the U.S.), including parenteral formulations and suppositories, are also approved for the treatment of postoperative nausea and vomiting and treatment of radiation sickness.

Unlabeled/Investigational Use Treatment of Meniere's disease

Effect on Mental Status Drowsiness is common; may cause depression, nervousness, or paradoxical CNS stimulation

Effect on Psychiatric Treatment Concurrent use with psychotropic may result in additive sedation

Dosage Summary

Oral:

Children <2 years: Dosage not established

Children 2-5 years: 12.5-25 mg every 6-8 hours (maximum: 75 mg/day)

Children 6-12 years: 25-50 mg every 6-8 hours (maximum: 150 mg/day)

Adults: 50-100 mg every 4-6 hours (maximum: 400 mg/day)

Dosage Forms Excipient information presented when available (limited, particularly for generics); consult specific product labeling. [CAN] = Canadian brand name

Capsule, softgel (Gravol®) [CAN]: 50 mg [not available in the U.S.]

Capsule, long-acting (Gravol® L/A) [CAN]: 75 mg, 100 mg [not available in the U.S.]

Injection, solution: 50 mg/mL (1 mL)

Gravol® I.M. [CAN]: 50 mg/mL (1 mL, 5 mL) [not available in the U.S.]

Gravol® I.V. [CAN]: 10 mg/mL (5 mL) [not available in the U.S.]

Solution, oral (Gravol® [CAN], Children's Motion Sickness [CAN]): 3 mg/mL (75 mL) [not available in the U.S.]

Suppository, rectal (Gravol® [CAN], Sab-Dimenhydrinate [CAN]): 75 mg, 100 mg [not available in the U.S.]

Tablet:

Dinate® [CAN], Jamp® Travel Tablet [CAN], Nauseatol® [CAN]: 50 mg

Dramamine®: 50 mg

Driminate®: 50 mg [scored]

Gravol® Filmkote Jr [CAN]: 25 mg [not available in the U.S.]

Gravol® Filmkote [CAN]: 50 mg [not available in the U.S.]

TripTone®: 50 mg

Tablet, chewable:

Dramamine®: 50 mg [contains phenylalanine 1.5 mg/tablet and tartrazine; orange flavor]

Gravol® Chewable for Children [CAN]: 25 mg [not available in the U.S.]

Gravol® Chewable for Adults [CAN]: 50 mg [not available in the U.S.]

Dimercaprol (dye mer KAP role)

U.S. Brand Names BAL in Oil®

Index Terms BAL; British Anti-Lewisite; Dithioglycerol

Pharmacologic Category Antidote

Use Antidote to gold, arsenic (except arsine), or acute mercury poisoning (except nonalkyl mercury); adjunct to edetate CALCIUM disodium in lead poisoning

Effect on Mental Status May cause nervousness

Effect on Psychiatric Treatment May produce neutropenia; use caution with clozapine and carbamazepine

Dosage Summary

I.M.:

Children:

Arsenic or gold poisoning (mild): 2.5 mg/kg every 6 hours for 2 days, then every 12 hours for 1 day, followed by once daily for 10 days

Arsenic or gold poisoning (severe): 3 mg/kg every 4 hours for 2 days, then every 6 hours for 1 day, followed by every 12hours for 10 days

Lead encephalopathy: 4 mg/kg (75 mg/m^2) loading dose, followed by 4 mg/kg (75 mg/m^2) every 4 hours for 2-7 days

Symptomatic lead poisoning or blood lead levels ≥70 mcg/dL : 4 mg/kg/dose (75 mg/m^2) loading dose, followed by 3 mg/kg/dose (50 mg/m^2) every 4 hours for 2-7 days

Mercury poisoning: 5 mg/kg initially, followed by 2.5 mg/kg 1-2 times/day for 10 days

Adults:

Arsenic or gold poisoning (mild): 2.5 mg/kg every 6 hours for 2 days, then every 12 hours for 1 day, followed by once daily for 10 days

Arseni or gold poisoning (severe): 3 mg/kg every 4 hours for 2 days, then every 6 hours for 1 day, followed by every 12hours for 10 days

Lead encephalopathy: 4 mg/kg (75 mg/m^2) loading dose, followed by 4 mg/kg (75 mg/m^2) every 4 hours for 2-7 days

Symptomatic lead poisoning or blood lead levels ≥70 mcg/dL : 4 mg/kg/dose (75 mg/m^2) loading dose, followed by 3 mg/kg/dose (50 mg/m^2) every 4 hours for 2-7 days

Mercury poisoning: 5 mg/kg initially, followed by 2.5 mg/kg 1-2 times/day for 10 days

Dosage Forms Excipient information presented when available (limited, particularly for generics); consult specific product labeling.

Injection, oil:
BAL in Oil®: 100 mg/mL (3 mL) [contains benzyl benzoate and peanut oil]

- **Dimetapp® Children's Long Acting Cough Plus Cold [OTC]** *see* Dextromethorphan and Chlorpheniramine *on page 449*
- **Dimetapp® Children's Nighttime Cold & Congestion [OTC]** *see* Diphenhydramine and Phenylephrine *on page 485*
- **Dimetapp® ND Children's [OTC]** *see* Loratadine *on page 946*
- **Dimetapp® Toddler's [OTC]** *see* Phenylephrine *on page 1273*
- **β,β-Dimethylcysteine** *see* Penicillamine *on page 1239*

Dimethyl Sulfoxide (dye meth il sul FOKS ide)

U.S. Brand Names Rimso-50®
Canadian Brand Names Dimethyl Sulfoxide Irrigation, USP; Kemsol®; Rimso-50®
Index Terms DMSO
Pharmacologic Category Urinary Tract Product
Use Symptomatic relief of interstitial cystitis
Effect on Mental Status May cause sedation
Effect on Psychiatric Treatment None reported
Dosage Summary
Bladder instillation:
Children: Dosage not established
Adults: Instill 50 mL and allow to remain for 15 minutes, may repeat every 1-2 weeks
Dosage Forms Excipient information presented when available (limited, particularly for generics); consult specific product labeling.
Solution, intravesical:
Rimso-50®: 50% [500 mg/mL] (50 mL)

- **Dimethyl Triazeno Imidazole Carboxamide** *see* Dacarbazine *on page 414*

Dinoprostone (dye noe PROST one)

Medication Safety Issues
Sound-alike/look-alike issues:
Prepidil® may be confused with Bepridil®

International issues:
Cervidil®: Brand name for gemeprost in Italy
U.S. Brand Names Cervidil®; Prepidil®; Prostin E_2®
Canadian Brand Names Cervidil®; Prepidil®; Prostin E_2®
Index Terms PGE_2; Prostaglandin E_2
Pharmacologic Category Abortifacient; Prostaglandin
Use
Gel: Promote cervical ripening in patients at or near term in whom there is a medical or obstetrical indication for the induction of labor
Suppositories: Terminate pregnancy from 12th through 20th week of gestation; evacuate uterus in cases of missed abortion or intrauterine fetal death up to 28 weeks of gestation; manage benign hydatidiform mole (nonmetastatic gestational trophoblastic disease)
Vaginal insert: Initiation and/or continuation of cervical ripening in patients at or near term in whom there is a medical or obstetrical indication for the induction of labor
Effect on Mental Status May cause dizziness
Effect on Psychiatric Treatment None reported
Dosage Summary
Endocervical:
Children: Females of reproductive age: 0.5 mg; may repeat every 6 hours if needed. Maximum cumulative dose: 1.5 mg/24 hours
Adults (females): 0.5 mg; may repeat every 6 hours if needed. Maximum cumulative dose: 1.5 mg/24 hours
Intravaginal:
Children: Females of reproductive age: Insert: 10 mg; remove at onset of active labor or after 12 hours; Suppository: 20 mg every 3-5 hours until abortion occurs
Adults (females): Insert: 10 mg remove at onset of active labor or after 12 hours; Suppository: 20 mg every 3-5 hours until abortion occurs

Dosage Forms Excipient information presented when available (limited, particularly for generics); consult specific product labeling.
Gel, endocervical (Prepidil®): 0.5 mg/3 g syringe [each package contains a 10 mm and 20 mm shielded catheter]
Insert, vaginal (Cervidil®): 10 mg [releases 0.3 mg/hour]
Suppository, vaginal (Prostin E_2®): 20 mg

- **Diotame® [OTC]** *see* Bismuth *on page 189*
- **Diovan®** *see* Valsartan *on page 1650*
- **Diovan HCT®** *see* Valsartan and Hydrochlorothiazide *on page 1652*
- **Dipentum®** *see* Olsalazine *on page 1173*
- **Diphen® [OTC]** *see* DiphenhydrAMINE *on page 481*
- **Diphen® AF [OTC]** *see* DiphenhydrAMINE *on page 481*
- **Diphenhist [OTC]** *see* DiphenhydrAMINE *on page 481*

DiphenhydrAMINE (dye fen HYE dra meen)

Medication Safety Issues
Sound-alike/look-alike issues:
DiphenhydrAMINE may be confused with desipramine, dicyclomine, dimenhyDRINATE
Benadryl® may be confused with benazepril, Bentyl®, Benylin®, Caladryl®

Related Information
Anticholinergic Effects of Common Psychotropics *on page 1758*
Antiparkinsonian Agents *on page 1767*
CMS: Long-Term Care Facility Thresholds *on page 1815*
Discontinuation of Psychotropic Drugs *on page 1839*
Nonbenzodiazepine Anxiolytics and Hypnotics *on page 1791*

U.S. Brand Names Aler-Cap [OTC]; Aler-Dryl [OTC]; Aler-Tab [OTC]; AllerMax® [OTC]; Altaryl [OTC]; Banophen® Anti-Itch [OTC]; Banophen® [OTC]; Ben-Tann; Benadryl® Allergy [OTC]; Benadryl® Children's Allergy Fastmelt® [OTC]; Benadryl® Children's Allergy [OTC]; Benadryl® Children's Dye-Free Allergy [OTC]; Benadryl® Itch Stopping Extra Strength [OTC]; Benadryl® Itch Stopping [OTC]; Compoz® Nighttime Sleep Aid [OTC]; Dermamycin® [OTC]; Diphenhist [OTC]; Diphen® AF [OTC]; Diphen® [OTC]; Dytan™; Genahist® [OTC]; Hydramine® [OTC]; Nytol® Quick Caps [OTC]; Nytol® Quick Gels [OTC]; Siladryl® Allergy [OTC]; Silphen® [OTC]; Simply Sleep® [OTC]; Sleep-ettes D [OTC]; Sleepinal® [OTC]; Sominex® Maximum Strength [OTC]; Sominex® [OTC]; Triaminic® Thin Strips™ Cough and Runny Nose [OTC]; Twilite® [OTC]; Unisom® Maximum Strength SleepGels® [OTC]

Canadian Brand Names Allerdryl®; Allernix; Benadryl®; Nytol®; Nytol® Extra Strength; PMS-Diphenhydramine; Simply Sleep®

Mexican Brand Names Benadryl; Brudifen; Drafen; Indumir; Therafilm; Vicnite

Index Terms Diphenhydramine Citrate; Diphenhydramine Hydrochloride; Diphenhydramine Tannate

Pharmacologic Category Histamine H_1 Antagonist; Histamine H_1 Antagonist, First Generation

Generic Available Yes: Excludes chewable tablet, gel, orally-disintegrating tablet, stick, strip

Use Symptomatic relief of allergic symptoms caused by histamine release including nasal allergies and allergic dermatosis; adjunct to epinephrine in the treatment of anaphylaxis; nighttime sleep aid; prevention or treatment of motion sickness; antitussive; management of Parkinsonian syndrome including drug-induced extrapyramidal symptoms; topically for relief of pain and itching associated with insect bites, minor cuts and burns, or rashes due to poison ivy, poison oak, and poison sumac

Mental Health Comment Along with benztropine, considered the drug of choice for patients with acute dystonic reactions. The usual adult dosage is I.M. 50 mg. In an emergency situation (laryngeal spasm), it should be given intravenously. It is the most sedating antihistamine used to treat drug-induced EPS. Generally not a first-line agent for insomnia, but often utilized in individuals where benzodiazepines are contraindicated (eg, patients with a history of substance abuse).

Pregnancy Risk Factor B

Pregnancy Considerations Teratogenic effects were not observed in animal studies. Diphenhydramine crosses the human placenta. One retrospective study showed an increased risk of cleft palate formation following maternal use of diphenhydramine during the 1st trimester of pregnancy; however, later studies have not confirmed this finding. Signs of toxicity and symptoms of withdrawal have been reported in infants following high doses or chronic maternal use close to term. Diphenhydramine has been evaluated for the treatment of hyperemesis gravidarum. It is generally not considered the antihistamine of choice for treating allergic rhinitis or nausea and vomiting during pregnancy.

Lactation Enters breast milk/contraindicated

Contraindications Hypersensitivity to diphenhydramine or any component of the formulation; acute asthma; neonates or premature infants; breast-feeding; use as a local anesthetic (injection)

Warnings/Precautions Causes sedation, caution must be used in performing tasks which require alertness (eg, operating machinery or driving). Sedative effects of CNS depressants or ethanol are potentiated. Use with caution in the elderly; may be more sensitive to adverse effects. Antihistamines may cause excitation in young children. Use with caution in patients with angle-closure glaucoma, pyloroduodenal obstruction (including stenotic peptic ulcer), urinary tract obstruction (including bladder neck obstruction and symptomatic prostatic hyperplasia), asthma, hyperthyroidism, increased intraocular pressure, and cardiovascular disease (including hypertension and tachycardia). Some preparations contain soy protein; avoid use in patients with soy protein or peanut allergies. Some products may contain phenylalanine.

Self-medication (OTC use): Do not use with other products containing diphenhydramine, even ones used on the skin. Oral products are not for OTC use in children <6 years of age. Topical products should not be used on large areas of the body, or on chicken pox or measles. Healthcare provider should be contacted if topical use is needed for >7 days. Topical products are not for OTC use in children <2 years of age.

Adverse Reactions Frequency not defined.

Cardiovascular: Chest tightness, extrasystoles, hypotension, palpitation, tachycardia

Central nervous system: Chills, confusion, convulsion, disturbed coordination, dizziness, euphoria, excitation, fatigue, headache, insomnia, irritability, nervousness, paradoxical excitement, restlessness, sedation, sleepiness, vertigo

Dermatologic: Photosensitivity, rash, urticaria

Endocrine & metabolic: Menstrual irregularities (early menses)

Gastrointestinal: Anorexia, constipation, diarrhea, dry mucous membranes, epigastric distress, nausea, throat tightness, vomiting, xerostomia

Genitourinary: Difficult urination, urinary frequency, urinary retention

Hematologic: Agranulocytosis, hemolytic anemia, thrombocytopenia

Neuromuscular & skeletal: Neuritis, paresthesia, tremor

Ocular: Blurred vision, diplopia

Otic: Labyrinthitis (acute), tinnitus

Respiratory: Nasal stuffiness, thickening of bronchial secretions, wheezing

Miscellaneous: Anaphylactic shock, diaphoresis

Metabolism/Transport Effects Inhibits CYP2D6 (moderate)

Drug Interactions

Acetylcholinesterase Inhibitors (Central): Anticholinergics may diminish the therapeutic effect of Acetylcholinesterase Inhibitors (Central). Acetylcholinesterase Inhibitors (Central) may diminish the therapeutic effect of Anticholinergics. If the anticholinergic action is a side effect of the agent, the result may be beneficial. *Risk C: Monitor therapy*

Alcohol (Ethyl): CNS Depressants may enhance the CNS depressant effect of Alcohol (Ethyl). *Risk C: Monitor therapy*

Amphetamines: May diminish the sedative effect of Antihistamines. *Risk C: Monitor therapy*

Anticholinergics: May enhance the adverse/toxic effect of other Anticholinergics. **Exceptions:** Paliperidone. *Risk C: Monitor therapy*

Betahistine: Antihistamines may diminish the therapeutic effect of Betahistine. *Risk C: Monitor therapy*

CNS Depressants: May enhance the adverse/toxic effect of other CNS Depressants. *Risk C: Monitor therapy*

Codeine: CYP2D6 Inhibitors (Moderate) may diminish the therapeutic effect of Codeine. These CYP2D6 inhibitors may prevent the metabolic conversion of codeine to its active metabolite morphine. *Risk C: Monitor therapy*

CYP2D6 Substrates: CYP2D6 Inhibitors (Moderate) may decrease the metabolism of CYP2D6 Substrates. **Exceptions:** Tamoxifen. *Risk C: Monitor therapy*

Nebivolol: CYP2D6 Inhibitors (Moderate) may increase the serum concentration of Nebivolol. *Risk C: Monitor therapy*

Pramlintide: May enhance the anticholinergic effect of Anticholinergics. These effects are specific to the GI tract. *Risk D: Consider therapy modification*

Tamoxifen: CYP2D6 Inhibitors (Moderate) may decrease the metabolism of Tamoxifen. Specifically, CYP2D6 inhibitors may decrease the formation of highly potent active metabolites. *Risk D: Consider therapy modification*

TraMADol: CYP2D6 Inhibitors (Moderate) may diminish the therapeutic effect of TraMADol. These CYP2D6 inhibitors may prevent the metabolic conversion of tramadol to its active metabolite that accounts for much of its opioid-like effects. *Risk C: Monitor therapy*

Ethanol/Nutrition/Herb Interactions

Ethanol: Avoid ethanol (may increase CNS depression).

Herb/Nutraceutical: Avoid valerian, St John's wort, kava kava, gotu kola (may increase CNS depression).

Stability Injection: Store at room temperature of 15°C to 30°C (59°F to 86°F). Protect from light and freezing

Mechanism of Action Competes with histamine for H_1-receptor sites on effector cells in the gastrointestinal tract, blood vessels, and respiratory tract; anticholinergic and sedative effects are also seen

Pharmacodynamics/Kinetics

Onset of action: Maximum sedative effect: 1-3 hours

Duration: 4-7 hours

Distribution: V_d: 3-22 L/kg

Protein binding: 78%

Metabolism: Extensively hepatic n-demethylation via CYP2D6; minor demethylation via CYP1A2, 2C9 and 2C19; smaller degrees in pulmonary and renal systems; significant first-pass effect

Bioavailability: Oral: ~40% to 70%

Half-life elimination: 2-10 hours; Elderly: 13.5 hours

Time to peak, serum: 2-4 hours

Excretion: Urine (as unchanged drug)

Dosage Note: Dosages are expressed as the hydrochloride salt.

Children:

- Allergic reactions or motion sickness: Oral, I.M., I.V.: 5 mg/kg/day or 150 mg/m^2/day in divided doses every 6-8 hours, not to exceed 300 mg/day
  - Alternate dosing by age: Oral:
    - 2 to <6 years: 6.25 mg every 4-6 hours; maximum: 37.5 mg/day
    - 6 to <12 years: 12.5-25 mg every 4-6 hours; maximum: 150 mg/day
    - ≥12 years: 25-50 mg every 4-6 hours; maximum: 300 mg/day
- Night-time sleep aid: Oral: Children ≥12 years: 50 mg at bedtime
- Antitussive: Oral:
  - 2 to <6 years: 6.25 mg every 4 hours; maximum 37.5 mg/day
  - 6 to <12 years: 12.5 mg every 4 hours; maximum 75 mg/day
  - ≥12 years: 25 mg every 4 hours; maximum 150 mg/day
- Treatment of dystonic reactions: I.M., I.V.: 0.5-1 mg/kg/dose
- Relief of pain and itching: Topical: Children ≥2 years: Apply 1% or 2% to affected area up to 3-4 times/day

Adults:

- Allergic reactions or motion sickness: Oral: 25-50 mg every 6-8 hours
- Antitussive: Oral: 25 mg every 4 hours; maximum 150 mg/24 hours
- Nighttime sleep aid: Oral: 50 mg at bedtime
- Allergic reactions or motion sickness: I.M., I.V.: 10-50 mg per dose; single doses up to 100 mg may be used if needed; not to exceed 400 mg/day
- Dystonic reaction: I.M., I.V.: 50 mg in a single dose; may repeat in 20-30 minutes if necessary
- Relief of pain and itching: Topical: Apply 1% or 2% to affected area up to 3-4 times/day

Elderly: Initial: 25 mg 2-3 times/day increasing as needed

Dietary Considerations

Benadryl® Allergy strips contain sodium 4 mg per 25 mg strip.

Benadryl® Children's Allergy chewable tablets contain phenylalanine 4.2 mg, magnesium 15 mg, and sodium 2 mg per 12.5 mg tablet.

Benadryl® Children's Allergy Fastmelt® contains phenylalanine 4.5 mg/tablet and soy protein isolate (contraindicated in patients with soy protein allergies; use caution in peanut allergic individuals, ~10% are estimated to also have soy protein allergies).

Dytan™ chewable tablets contain phenylalanine.

Administration When used to prevent motion sickness, first dose should be given 30 minutes prior to exposure. Injection solution is for I.V. or I.M. administration only; local necrosis may result with SubQ or intradermal use. For I.V. administration, inject at a rate ≤25 mg/minute.

Monitoring Parameters Relief of symptoms, mental alertness

Reference Range

Antihistamine effects at levels >25 ng/mL

Drowsiness at levels 30-40 ng/mL
Mental impairment at levels >60 ng/mL
Therapeutic: Not established
Toxic: >0.1 mcg/mL

Test Interactions May suppress the wheal and flare reactions to skin test antigens

Additional Information Diphenhydramine citrate 19 mg is equivalent to diphenhydramine hydrochloride 12.5 mg

Dosage Forms Excipient information presented when available (limited, particularly for generics); consult specific product labeling. [DSC] = Discontinued product

Caplet, as hydrochloride: 25 mg, 50 mg
- Aler-Dryl, AllerMax®, Compoz® Nighttime Sleep Aid, Sleep-ettes D, Sominex® Maximum Strength, Twilite®: 50 mg
- Nytol® Quick Caps, Simply Sleep®: 25 mg

Capsule, as hydrochloride: 25 mg, 50 mg
- Aler-Cap, Banophen®, Benadryl® Allergy, Diphen®, Diphenhist, Genahist®: 25 mg
- Sleepinal®: 50 mg

Capsule, softgel, as hydrochloride: 50 mg
- Benadryl® Dye-Free Allergy: 25 mg [dye-free]
- Compoz® Nighttime Sleep Aid, Nytol® Quick Gels, Sleepinal®, Unisom® Maximum Strength SleepGels®: 50 mg

Captab, as hydrochloride:
- Diphenhist®: 25 mg

Cream, as hydrochloride: 2% (30 g)
- Banophen® Anti-Itch: 2% (30 g) [contains zinc acetate 0.1%]
- Benadryl® Itch Stopping: 1% (30 g) [contains zinc acetate 0.1%]
- Benadryl® Itch Stopping Extra Strength: 2% (30 g) [contains zinc acetate 0.1%]
- Diphenhist®: 2% (30 g) [contains zinc acetate 0.1%]

Elixir, as hydrochloride:
- Altaryl: 12.5 mg/5 mL (120 mL, 480 mL, 3840 mL) [cherry flavor]
- Banophen®: 12.5 mg/5 mL (120 mL)
- Diphen AF: 12.5 mg/5 mL (240 mL, 480 mL) [alcohol free; cherry flavor]

Gel, topical, as hydrochloride:
- Benadryl® Itch Stopping Extra Strength: 2% (120 mL)

Injection, solution, as hydrochloride: 50 mg/mL (1 mL, 10 mL)

Liquid, as hydrochloride:
- AllerMax®: 12.5 mg/5 mL (120 mL)
- Benadryl® Allergy: 12.5 mg/5 mL (120 mL, 240 mL) [alcohol free; contains sodium benzoate; cherry flavor]
- Benadryl® Children's Dye-Free Allergy: 12.5 mg/5 mL (120 mL) [alcohol free, dye free, sugar free; contains sodium benzoate; bubble gum flavor]
- Genahist®: 12.5 mg/5 mL (120 mL) [alcohol free, sugar free; contains sodium benzoate; cherry flavor]
- Hydramine®: 12.5 mg/5 mL (120 mL, 480 mL) [alcohol free]
- Siladryl® Allergy: 12.5 mg/5 mL (120 mL, 240 mL, 480 mL) [alcohol free, sugar free; black cherry flavor]

Liquid, topical, as hydrochloride [stick]:
- Benadryl® Itch Stopping Extra Strength: 2% (14 mL) [contains zinc acetate 0.1% and alcohol]

Solution, oral, as hydrochloride:
- Diphenhist: 12.5 mg/5 mL (120 mL, 480 mL) [alcohol free; contains sodium benzoate]

Solution, topical, as hydrochloride [spray]:
- Benadryl® Itch Stopping Extra Strength: 2% (60 mL) [contains zinc acetate 0.1% and alcohol]
- Dermamycin®: 2% (60 mL) [contains menthol 1%]

Strips, oral, as hydrochloride:
- Benadryl® Allergy: 25 mg (10s) [contains sodium 4 mg/strip; vanilla mint flavor]
- Benadryl® Children's Allergy: 12.5 mg (10s) [vanilla mint flavor]
- Triaminic® Thin Strips™ Cough and Runny Nose: 12. 5 mg (16s) [grape flavor]

Suspension, as tannate:
- Ben-Tann: 25 mg/5 mL (120 ml) [contains sodium benzoate; strawberry flavor]
- Dytan™: 25 mg/5 mL (120 mL) [strawberry flavor] [DSC]

Syrup, as hydrochloride:
- Silphen® Cough: 12.5 mg/5 mL (120 mL, 240 mL, 480 mL) [contains alcohol; 5%; strawberry flavor]

Tablet, as hydrochloride: 25 mg, 50 mg

Aler-Tab, Benadryl® Allergy, Genahist®, Sominex®: 25 mg

Tablet, chewable, as hydrochloride:

Benadryl® Children's Allergy: 12.5 mg [contains phenylalanine 4.2 mg, magnesium 15 mg, and sodium 2 mg per tablet; grape flavor]

Tablet, chewable, as tannate:

Dytan™: 25 mg [contains phenylalanine; strawberry flavor]

Tablet, orally disintegrating, as citrate:

Benadryl® Children's Allergy Fastmelt®: 19 mg [equivalent to diphenhydramine hydrochloride 12.5 mg; contains phenylalanine 4.5 mg/tablet and soy protein isolate; cherry flavor]

- **Diphenhydramine and Acetaminophen** *see* Acetaminophen and Diphenhydramine *on page 35*
- **Diphenhydramine and ASA** *see* Aspirin and Diphenhydramine *on page 145*
- **Diphenhydramine and Aspirin** *see* Aspirin and Diphenhydramine *on page 145*

Diphenhydramine and Phenylephrine

(dye fen HYE dra meen & fen il EF rin)

U.S. Brand Names Aldex® CT; D-Tann; Dimetapp® Children's Nighttime Cold & Congestion [OTC]; Robitussin® Night Time Cough & Cold [OTC]

Index Terms Diphenhydramine Hydrochloride and Phenylephrine Hydrochloride; Diphenhydramine Tannate and Phenylephrine Tannate; Phenylephrine and Diphenhydramine; Phenylephrine Hydrochloride and Diphenhydramine Hydrochloride; Phenylephrine Tannate and Diphenhydramine Tannate

Pharmacologic Category Alpha/Beta Agonist; Histamine H_1 Antagonist; Histamine H_1 Antagonist, First Generation

Use Temporary relief of symptoms of allergic rhinitis, sinusitis, and other upper respiratory conditions, including sinus/nasal congestion, sneezing, stuffy/runny nose, itchy/watery eyes, and cough

Effect on Mental Status May cause sedation, confusion, dizziness, euphoria, excitation, insomnia, irritability, nervousness, and restlessness

Effect on Psychiatric Treatment Contraindicated with or within 14 days of MAO inhibitor treatment. May cause sedation; concurrent use with psychotropics may produce additive effects

Dosage Summary

Oral:

Children <2 years: Dosage not established

Children 2-5 years: D-Tann: 1.25-2.5 mL every 12 hours

Children 6-11 years: Aldex® CT: One-half to 1 tablet every 6 hours; D-Tann: 2.5-5 mL **or** 1/2 to 1 tablet every 12 hours; OTC labeling: Dimetapp® Children's Nighttime Cold and Congestion: 10 mL every 4 hours as needed (maximum 6 doses/24 hours)

Children ≥12 years: Aldex® CT: 1-2 tablets every 6 hours; D-Tann: 5-10 mL **or** 1-2 tablets every 12 hours; OTC labeling: 20 mL every 4 hours as needed (maximum 6 doses/24 hours)

Adults: Aldex® CT: 1-2 tablets every 6 hours; D-Tann: 5-10 mL **or** 1-2 tablets every 12 hours; OTC labeling: 20 mL every 4 hours as needed (maximum 6 doses/24 hours)

Dosage Forms Excipient information presented when available (limited, particularly for generics); consult specific product labeling.

Suspension:

D-Tann: Diphenhydramine tannate 25 mg and phenylephrine tannate 7.5 mg per 5 mL [118 mL] [contains sodium benzoate, bubblegum flavor]

Syrup:

Dimetapp® Children's Nighttime Cold and Congestion: Diphenhydramine hydrochloride 6.25 mg and phenylephrine hydrochloride 2.5 mg per 5 mL [120 mL] [alcohol free, sugar free; grape flavor]

Robitussin® Night Time Cough and Cold: Diphenhydramine hydrochloride 6.25 mg and phenylephrine hydrochloride 2.5 mg per 5 mL [120 mL] [alcohol free, contains sodium benzoate]

Tablet, chewable:

Aldex® CT: Diphenhydramine hydrochloride 12.5 mg and phenylephrine hydrochloride 5 mg [strawberry flavor]

D-Tann: Diphenhydramine tannate 25 mg and phenylephrine tannate 10 mg [contains phenylalanine 5.7 mg/tablet, berry flavor]

Diphenhydramine and Pseudoephedrine

(dye fen HYE dra meen & soo doe e FED rin)

Medication Safety Issues

Sound-alike/look-alike issues:

Benadryl® may be confused with benazepril, Bentyl®, Benylin®, Caladryl®

U.S. Brand Names Benadryl-D™ Allergy and Sinus Fastmelt™ [OTC]; Benadryl-D™ Children's Allergy and Sinus [OTC]; Benadryl® Children's Allergy and Cold Fastmelt™ [OTC]

Index Terms Pseudoephedrine and Diphenhydramine

Pharmacologic Category Alpha/Beta Agonist; Histamine H_1 Antagonist; Histamine H_1 Antagonist, First Generation

Use Relief of symptoms of upper respiratory mucosal congestion in seasonal and perennial nasal allergies, acute rhinitis, rhinosinusitis, and eustachian tube blockage

Effect on Mental Status Diphenhydramine may cause paradoxical excitation in pediatric patients, and can result in hallucinations, coma, and death in overdose. May cause sedation, sleepiness, dizziness, disturbed coordination, headache, fatigue, nervousness, paradoxical excitement, insomnia, euphoria, or confusion. Pseudoephedrine may cause dizziness, drowsiness, nervousness, and insomnia; may rarely cause hallucinations.

Effect on Psychiatric Treatment Rare reports of agranulocytosis and thrombocytopenia; use caution with clozapine, carbamazepine, and valproic acid; may increase gastric degradation of levodopa and decrease the amount of levodopa absorbed by delaying gastric emptying. Therapeutic effects of cholinergic agents (tacrine, donepezil, rivastigmine, galantamine) and neuroleptics may be antagonized. Central and/or peripheral anticholinergic syndrome can occur when administered with amantadine, rimantadine, narcotic analgesics, phenothiazines, and other antipsychotics (especially with high anticholinergic activity), tricyclic antidepressants and antihistamines. Pseudoephedrine is contraindicated with MAO inhibitors.

Dosage Summary

Oral:

Children: Dosage not established

Adults: 60 mg (based on pseudoephedrine component) every 4-6 hours (maximum: 240 mg/day)

Dosage Forms Excipient information presented when available (limited, particularly for generics); consult specific product labeling.

Liquid:

Benadryl-D™ Children's Allergy and Sinus: Diphenhydramine hydrochloride 12.5 mg and pseudoephedrine hydrochloride 30 mg per 5 mL [alcohol free, sugar free; contains sodium 10 mg/5 mL and sodium benzoate; grape flavor]

Tablet, quick dissolving:

Benadryl® Children's Allergy and Cold Fastmelt™, Benadryl-D™ Allergy and Sinus Fastmelt™: Diphenhydramine citrate 19 mg [equivalent to diphenhydramine hydrochloride 12.5 mg] and pseudoephedrine 30 mg [contains phenylalanine 4.6 mg/tablet; cherry flavor]

◆ **Diphenhydramine Citrate** *see* DiphenhydrAMINE *on page 481*

◆ **Diphenhydramine Citrate and Aspirin** *see* Aspirin and Diphenhydramine *on page 145*

◆ **Diphenhydramine Hydrochloride** *see* DiphenhydrAMINE *on page 481*

◆ **Diphenhydramine Hydrochloride and Phenylephrine Hydrochloride** *see* Diphenhydramine and Phenylephrine *on page 485*

◆ **Diphenhydramine, Hydrocodone, and Phenylephrine** *see* Hydrocodone, Phenylephrine, and Diphenhydramine *on page 782*

◆ **Diphenhydramine, Phenylephrine Hydrochloride, and Acetaminophen** *see* Acetaminophen, Diphenhydramine, and Phenylephrine *on page 44*

◆ **Diphenhydramine Tannate** *see* DiphenhydrAMINE *on page 481*

◆ **Diphenhydramine Tannate and Phenylephrine Tannate** *see* Diphenhydramine and Phenylephrine *on page 485*

Diphenoxylate and Atropine (dye fen OKS i late & A troe peen)

Medication Safety Issues

Sound-alike/look-alike issues:

Lomotil® may be confused with Lamictal®, Lamisil®, lamotrigine, Lanoxin®, Lasix®, ludiomil

Lonox® may be confused with Lanoxin®, Loprox®

International issues:

Lomotil® may be confused with Lemesil® which is a brand name for nimesulide in Greece

Lonox® may be confused with Flomox® which is a brand of cefcapene in Japan

U.S. Brand Names Lomotil®; Lonox®

Canadian Brand Names Lomotil®

Index Terms Atropine and Diphenoxylate

Pharmacologic Category Antidiarrheal

Use Treatment of diarrhea

Effect on Mental Status May cause nervousness, restlessness, drowsiness, or insomnia; rarely may produce euphoria

Effect on Psychiatric Treatment Concurrent use with MAO inhibitors may result in hypertensive crisis; additive sedation and dry mouth with psychotropics; use with benztropine or other anticholinergic agents may result in ileus

Restrictions C-V

Dosage Summary

Oral:

Children <2 years: Dosage not established

Children 2-12 years: Initial: Diphenoxylate 0.3-0.4 mg/kg/day in 4 divided doses (maximum: 10 mg/day); Maintenance: Reduce as needed, may be as low as 25% of the initial daily dose

Adults: Initial: Diphenoxylate 5 mg 4 times/day (maximum: 20 mg/day); Maintenance: Reduce as needed, may be as low as 5 mg/day

Dosage Forms Excipient information presented when available (limited, particularly for generics); consult specific product labeling.

Solution, oral: Diphenoxylate hydrochloride 2.5 mg and atropine sulfate 0.025 mg per 5 mL (5 mL, 10 mL, 60 mL)

Lomotil®: Diphenoxylate hydrochloride 2.5 mg and atropine sulfate 0.025 mg per 5 mL (60 mL) [contains alcohol 15%; cherry flavor]

Tablet: Diphenoxylate hydrochloride 2.5 mg and atropine sulfate 0.025 mg

Lomotil®, Lonox®: Diphenoxylate hydrochloride 2.5 mg and atropine sulfate 0.025 mg

◆ **Diphenylhydantoin** *see* Phenytoin *on page 1280*

◆ **Diphtheria and Tetanus Toxoids and Acellular Pertussis Adsorbed, Hepatitis B (Recombinant) and Inactivated Poliovirus Vaccine Combined** *see* Diphtheria, Tetanus Toxoids, Acellular Pertussis, Hepatitis B (Recombinant), and Poliovirus (Inactivated) Vaccine *on page 487*

◆ **Diphtheria CRM_{197} Protein** *see* Pneumococcal Conjugate Vaccine, 7-Valent *on page 1308*

Diphtheria, Tetanus Toxoids, Acellular Pertussis, Hepatitis B (Recombinant), and Poliovirus (Inactivated) Vaccine

(dif THEER ee a, TET a nus TOKS oyds, ay CEL yoo lar per TUS sis, hep a TYE tis bee, & POE lee oh VYE rus, in ak ti VAY ted vak SEEN)

U.S. Brand Names Pediarix®

Canadian Brand Names Pediarix®

Index Terms Diphtheria and Tetanus Toxoids and Acellular Pertussis Adsorbed, Hepatitis B (Recombinant) and Inactivated Poliovirus Vaccine Combined; DTaP/IPV/HepB

Pharmacologic Category Vaccine, Inactivated (Bacterial); Vaccine, Inactivated (Viral)

Use Combination vaccine for the active immunization against diphtheria, tetanus, pertussis, hepatitis B virus (all known subtypes), and poliomyelitis (caused by poliovirus types 1, 2, and 3)

The Advisory Committee on Immunization Practices (ACIP) recommends Pediarix® for the following:

- Primary vaccination for DTaP, Hep B, and IPV in children at 2-, 4-, and 6 months of age.
- To complete the primary vaccination series in children who have received DTaP (Infanrix®) and who are scheduled to received the other components of the vaccine. Whenever feasible, the same manufacturer should be used to provide the pertussis component; however, vaccination should not be deferred if a specific brand is not known or is not available. HepB and IPV from different manufacturers are interchangeable.

Effect on Mental Status Sedation and restlessness are common

Effect on Psychiatric Treatment Contraindicated in patients with progressive neurologic disorders

Dosage Summary

I.M.:

Children <6 weeks: Dosage not established

Children 6 weeks to <7 years: 0.5 mL every 6-8 weeks for a total of 3 doses

Adults: Dosage not established

Dosage Forms Excipient information presented when available (limited, particularly for generics); consult specific product labeling.

Injection, suspension [preservative free]:

Pediarix®: Diphtheria toxoid 25 Lf, tetanus toxoid 10 Lf, acellular pertussis antigens [inactivated pertussis toxin 25 mcg, filamentous hemagglutin 25 mcg, pertactin 8 mcg, HBsAg 10 mcg, type 1 poliovirus 40 D antigen units, type 2 poliovirus 8 D antigen units and type 3 poliovirus 32 D antigen units] per 0.5 mL (0.5 mL) [contains aluminum, neomycin sulfate (trace amounts), polymyxin B (trace amounts), polysorbate 80, and yeast protein ≤5%; prefilled syringes contain natural rubber/natural latex]

- ◆ **Diphtheria Toxoid Conjugate** *see Haemophilus* b Conjugate Vaccine *on page 753*
- ◆ **Diprivan®** *see* Propofol *on page 1352*
- ◆ **Diprolene®** *see* Betamethasone *on page 184*
- ◆ **Diprolene® AF** *see* Betamethasone *on page 184*
- ◆ **Dipropylacetic Acid** *see* Valproic Acid and Derivatives *on page 1642*

Dipyridamole (dye peer ID a mole)

Medication Safety Issues

Sound-alike/look-alike issues:

Dipyridamole may be confused with disopyramide

Persantine® may be confused with Periactin®, Permitil®

Related Information

Anticholinergic Effects of Common Psychotropics *on page 1758*

U.S. Brand Names Persantine®

Canadian Brand Names Apo-Dipyridamole FC®; Dipyridamole For Injection; Persantine®

Mexican Brand Names Persantin

Pharmacologic Category Antiplatelet Agent; Vasodilator

Use

Oral: Used with warfarin to decrease thrombosis in patients after artificial heart valve replacement

I.V.: Diagnostic agent in CAD

Effect on Mental Status Dizziness is common

Effect on Psychiatric Treatment None reported

Dosage Summary

I.V.:

Children: Dosage not established

Adults: 0.14 mg/kg/minute for 4 minutes (maximum: 60 mg)

Oral:

Children ≥12 years: 75-100 mg 4 times/day

Adults: 75-100 mg 4 times/day

Dosage Forms Excipient information presented when available (limited, particularly for generics); consult specific product labeling.

Injection, solution: 5 mg/mL (2 mL, 10 mL)

Tablet: 25 mg, 50 mg, 75 mg

Persantine®: 25 mg, 50 mg, 75 mg

- ◆ **Dipyridamole and Aspirin** *see* Aspirin and Dipyridamole *on page 145*
- ◆ **Disalicylic Acid** *see* Salsalate *on page 1459*
- ◆ **Disodium Cromoglycate** *see* Cromolyn *on page 402*
- ◆ **Disodium Thiosulfate Pentahydrate** *see* Sodium Thiosulfate *on page 1497*
- ◆ ***d*-Isoephedrine Hydrochloride** *see* Pseudoephedrine *on page 1367*

Disopyramide (dye soe PEER a mide)

Medication Safety Issues

Sound-alike/look-alike issues:

Disopyramide may be confused with desipramine, dipyridamole

Norpace® may be confused with Norpramin®

U.S. Brand Names Norpace®; Norpace® CR

Canadian Brand Names Norpace®; Rythmodan®; Rythmodan®-LA

Mexican Brand Names Dimodan

Index Terms Disopyramide Phosphate

Pharmacologic Category Antiarrhythmic Agent, Class Ia

Use Suppression and prevention of unifocal and multifocal atrial and premature, ventricular premature complexes, coupled ventricular tachycardia; effective in the conversion of atrial fibrillation, atrial flutter, and paroxysmal atrial tachycardia to normal sinus rhythm and prevention of the recurrence of these arrhythmias after conversion by other methods

Unlabeled/Investigational Use Hypertrophic obstructive cardiomyopathy (HOCM)

Effect on Mental Status May cause drowsiness or nervousness; rare reports of depression and psychosis

Effect on Psychiatric Treatment Contraindicated with ziprasidone; use cautiously with TCAs; may cause AV block or QT prolongation; phenobarbital and carbamazepine may decrease the effects of disopyramide via enzyme induction

Dosage Summary

Oral:

Controlled release:

Children: Dosage not established

Adults <50 kg: 200 mg every 12 hours

Adults ≥50 kg: 300 mg every 12 hours

Immediate release:

Children <1 year: 10-30 mg/kg/day in 4 divided doses

Children 1-4 years: 10-20 mg/kg/day in 4 divided doses

Children 4-12 years: 10-15 mg/kg/day in 4 divided doses

Children 12-18 years: 6-15 mg/kg/day in 4 divided doses

Adults <50 kg: 100 mg every 6 hours

Adults ≥50 kg: Initial: 150 mg every 6 hours; Maintenance: 150-400 mg every 6 hours

Dosage Forms Excipient information presented when available (limited, particularly for generics); consult specific product labeling.

Capsule (Norpace®): 100 mg, 150 mg

Capsule, controlled release (Norpace® CR): 100 mg, 150 mg

◆ **Disopyramide Phosphate** *see* Disopyramide *on page 488*

Disulfiram (dye SUL fi ram)

Medication Safety Issues

Sound-alike/look-alike issues:

Disulfiram may be confused with Diflucan®

Antabuse® may be confused with Anturane®

Related Information

Addiction Treatments *on page 1817*

U.S. Brand Names Antabuse®

Mexican Brand Names Antabuse

Pharmacologic Category Aldehyde Dehydrogenase Inhibitor

Generic Available No

Use Management of chronic alcoholism

Effect on Mental Status Psychotic reactions have been noted

Pregnancy Risk Factor C

Lactation Excretion in breast milk unknown

Contraindications Hypersensitivity to disulfiram and related compounds or any component of the formulation; patients receiving or using ethanol, metronidazole, paraldehyde, or ethanol-containing preparations like cough syrup or tonics; psychosis; severe myocardial disease and coronary occlusion

Warnings/Precautions Use with caution in patients with diabetes, hypothyroidism, seizure disorders, nephritis (acute or chronic), hepatic cirrhosis or insufficiency. **[U.S. Boxed Warning]: Should never be administered to a patient when he/she is in a state of alcohol intoxication, or without his/her knowledge.** Patient must receive appropriate counseling, including information on "disguised" forms of alcohol (tonics, mouthwashes, etc) and the duration of the drug's activity (up to 14 days). Severe (sometimes fatal) hepatitis and/or hepatic failure have been associated with disulfiram. May occur in patients with or without prior history of abnormal hepatic function. Safety and efficacy have not been established in children.

Adverse Reactions Frequency not defined.

Central nervous system: Drowsiness, headache, fatigue, psychosis
Dermatologic: Rash, acneiform eruptions, allergic dermatitis
Gastrointestinal: Metallic or garlic-like aftertaste
Genitourinary: Impotence
Hepatic: Hepatitis
Neuromuscular & skeletal: Peripheral neuritis, polyneuritis, peripheral neuropathy
Ocular: Optic neuritis

Metabolism/Transport Effects Substrate (minor) of CYP1A2, 2A6, 2B6, 2D6, 2E1, 3A4; **Inhibits** CYP1A2 (weak), 2A6 (weak), 2B6 (weak), 2C9 (weak), 2D6 (weak), 2E1 (strong), 3A4 (weak)

Drug Interactions

Alcohol (Ethyl): Disulfiram may enhance the adverse/toxic effect of Alcohol (Ethyl). A disulfiram-like reaction may occur. *Risk X: Avoid combination*

Amprenavir: Disulfiram may enhance the adverse/toxic effect of Amprenavir. This is specifically related to the propylene glycol contained in amprenavir oral solution, not capsules. Management: Specifically, concurrent amprenavir oral solution and disulfiram is contraindicated due to the large amount of propylene glycol in the oral solution. *Risk X: Avoid combination*

Benzodiazepines (metabolized by oxidation): Disulfiram may decrease the metabolism of Benzodiazepines (metabolized by oxidation). *Risk C: Monitor therapy*

Chlorzoxazone: Disulfiram may decrease the metabolism of Chlorzoxazone. *Risk C: Monitor therapy*

CYP2E1 Substrates: CYP2E1 Inhibitors (Strong) may decrease the metabolism of CYP2E1 Substrates. *Risk D: Consider therapy modification*

MetroNIDAZOLE: Disulfiram may enhance the adverse/toxic effect of MetroNIDAZOLE. *Risk D: Consider therapy modification*

Phenytoin: Disulfiram may decrease the metabolism of Phenytoin. *Risk D: Consider therapy modification*

Ritonavir: Disulfiram may enhance the adverse/toxic effect of Ritonavir. This is specific for the lopinavir/ritonavir (Kaletra) oral solution due to its alcohol content (42%). Management: Concomitant use of Kaletra (lopinavir/ritonavir) oral solution and disulfiram should be avoided. Kaletra contains 42% alcohol. *Risk X: Avoid combination*

Sertraline: Disulfiram may enhance the adverse/toxic effect of Sertraline. This is specifically related to sertraline oral concentrate due to its alcohol content (12%). Management: Sertraline Oral Concentrate contains 12% alcohol, and its use should be avoided with disulfiram. *Risk X: Avoid combination*

Theophylline Derivatives: Disulfiram may increase the serum concentration of Theophylline Derivatives. **Exceptions:** Dyphylline. *Risk C: Monitor therapy*

Tipranavir: Disulfiram may enhance the adverse/toxic effect of Tipranavir. *Risk D: Consider therapy modification*

Vitamin K Antagonists (eg, warfarin): Disulfiram may increase the serum concentration of Vitamin K Antagonists. *Risk C: Monitor therapy*

Ethanol/Nutrition/Herb Interactions Ethanol: Disulfiram inhibits ethanol's usual metabolism. Avoid all ethanol. Patients can have a disulfiram reaction (headache, nausea, vomiting, chest, or abdominal pain) if they drink ethanol concurrently. Avoid cough syrups and elixirs containing ethanol. Avoid vinegars, cider, extracts, and foods containing ethanol.

Mechanism of Action Disulfiram is a thiuram derivative which interferes with aldehyde dehydrogenase. When taken concomitantly with alcohol, there is an increase in serum acetaldehyde levels. High acetaldehyde causes uncomfortable symptoms including flushing, nausea, thirst, palpitations, chest pain, vertigo, and hypotension. This reaction is the basis for disulfiram use in postwithdrawal long-term care of alcoholism.

Pharmacodynamics/Kinetics

Onset of action: Full effect: 12 hours
Duration: ~1-2 weeks after last dose
Absorption: Rapid
Metabolism: To diethylthiocarbamate
Excretion: Feces and exhaled gases (as metabolites)

Dosage Adults: Oral: Do not administer until the patient has abstained from ethanol for at least 12 hours

Initial: 500 mg/day as a single dose for 1-2 weeks; maximum daily dose is 500 mg

Average maintenance dose: 250 mg/day; range: 125-500 mg; duration of therapy is to continue until the patient is fully recovered socially and a basis for permanent self control has been established; maintenance therapy may be required for months or even years

Administration Administration of any medications containing alcohol, including topicals, is contraindicated. Do not administer disulfiram if ethanol has been consumed within the prior 12 hours.

Monitoring Parameters Hypokalemia; liver function tests at baseline and after 10-14 days of treatment; CBC, serum chemistries, liver function tests should be monitored during therapy

Dosage Forms Excipient information presented when available (limited, particularly for generics); consult specific product labeling.

Tablet:

Antabuse®: 250 mg, 500 mg

- **Dithioglycerol** *see* Dimercaprol *on page 479*
- **Ditropan®** *see* Oxybutynin *on page 1199*
- **Ditropan® XL** *see* Oxybutynin *on page 1199*
- **Diuril®** *see* Chlorothiazide *on page 321*
- **Divalproex Sodium** *see* Valproic Acid and Derivatives *on page 1642*
- **Divigel®** *see* Estradiol *on page 576*
- **5071-1DL(6)** *see* Megestrol *on page 977*
- ***dl*-Alpha Tocopherol** *see* Vitamin E *on page 1675*
- ***D*-Mannitol** *see* Mannitol *on page 968*
- **4-DMDR** *see* IDArubicin *on page 809*
- **DMSA** *see* Succimer *on page 1511*
- **DMSO** *see* Dimethyl Sulfoxide *on page 480*

Docetaxel (doe se TAKS el)

Medication Safety Issues

Sound-alike/look-alike issues:

Taxotere® may be confused with Taxol®

High alert medication: The Institute for Safe Medication Practices (ISMP) includes this medication among its list of drug classes which have a heightened risk of causing significant patient harm when used in error.

U.S. Brand Names Taxotere®

Canadian Brand Names Taxotere®

Mexican Brand Names Taxotere

Index Terms NSC-628503; RP-6976

Pharmacologic Category Antineoplastic Agent, Antimicrotubular; Antineoplastic Agent, Natural Source (Plant) Derivative; Antineoplastic Agent, Taxane Derivative

Use Treatment of breast cancer; locally-advanced or metastatic nonsmall cell lung cancer (NSCLC); hormone refractory, metastatic prostate cancer; advanced gastric adenocarcinoma; locally-advanced squamous cell head and neck cancer

Unlabeled/Investigational Use Treatment of bladder cancer, ovarian cancer, small cell lung cancer, and soft tissue sarcoma

Effect on Mental Status May cause confusion

Effect on Psychiatric Treatment May cause leukopenia; use caution with clozapine and carbamazepine

Dosage Summary

I.V.:

Children: Dosage not established

Adults: 60-100 mg/m^2 every 3 weeks

Dosage Forms Excipient information presented when available (limited, particularly for generics); consult specific product labeling.

Injection, solution [concentrate]:

Taxotere®: 20 mg/0.5 mL (0.5 mL, 2 mL) [contains Polysorbate 80®; diluent contains ethanol 13%]

Docusate and Senna (DOK yoo sate & SEN na)

Medication Safety Issues

Sound-alike/look-alike issues:

Senokot® may be confused with Depakote®

U.S. Brand Names Peri-Colace® [OTC]; Senokot-S® [OTC]; SenoSol™-SS [OTC]

Index Terms Senna and Docusate; Senna-S

Pharmacologic Category Laxative, Stimulant; Stool Softener

Use Short-term treatment of constipation

Unlabeled/Investigational Use Evacuate the colon for bowel or rectal examinations; management/prevention of opiate-induced constipation

Effect on Mental Status None reported

Effect on Psychiatric Treatment GI side effects are common; use caution with SSRIs

Dosage Summary

Oral:

Children <2 years: Dosage not established

Children 2-6 years: Initial: 4.3 mg sennosides plus 25 mg docusate (1/2 tablet) once daily (maximum: 1 tablet twice daily)

Children 6-12 years: Initial: 8.6 mg sennosides plus 50 mg docusate (1 tablet) once daily (maximum: 2 tablets twice daily)

Children ≥12 years: Initial: 2 tablets (17.2 mg sennosides plus 100 mg docusate) once daily (maximum: 4 tablets twice daily)

Adults: Initial: 2 tablets (17.2 mg sennosides plus 100 mg docusate) once daily (maximum: 4 tablets twice daily)

Dosage Forms Excipient information presented when available (limited, particularly for generics); consult specific product labeling.

Tablet: Docusate sodium 50 mg and sennosides 8.6 mg

Peri-Colace®: Docusate sodium 50 mg and sennosides 8.6 mg

Senokot-S®: Docusate sodium 50 mg and sennosides 8.6 mg [sugar free; contains sodium 4 mg/tablet]

SenoSol™-SS: Docusate sodium 50 mg and sennosides 8.6 mg [contains sodium 3 mg/tablet]

Dofetilide (doe FET il ide)

U.S. Brand Names Tikosyn®

Canadian Brand Names Tikosyn®

Pharmacologic Category Antiarrhythmic Agent, Class III

Use Maintenance of normal sinus rhythm in patients with chronic atrial fibrillation/atrial flutter of longer than 1-week duration who have been converted to normal sinus rhythm; conversion of atrial fibrillation and atrial flutter to normal sinus rhythm

Effect on Mental Status Insomnia is common

Effect on Psychiatric Treatment Contraindicated with drugs that prolong QT_c (phenothiazines, TCAs, ziprasidone)

Restrictions Tikosyn® is only available to prescribers and hospitals that have confirmed their participation in a designated Tikosyn® Education Program. The program provides comprehensive education about the importance of in-hospital treatment initiation and individualized dosing.

T.I.P.S. is the Tikosyn® In Pharmacy System designated to allow retail pharmacies to stock and dispense Tikosyn® once they have been enrolled. A participating pharmacy must confirm receipt of the T.I.P.S. program materials and educate its pharmacy staff about the procedures required to fill an outpatient prescription for Tikosyn®. The T.I.P.S. enrollment form is available at www.tikosyn.com. Tikosyn® is only available from a special mail order pharmacy, and enrolled retail pharmacies. Pharmacists must verify that the hospital/prescriber is a confirmed participant before Tikosyn® is provided. For participant verification, the pharmacist may call 1-800-788-7353 or use the web site located at www.tikosynlist.com. Further details and directions on the program are provided at www.tikosyn.com.

Dofetilide therapy must be initiated/adjusted in a hospital setting with proper monitoring under the guidance of experienced personnel.

Dosage Summary Note: QT_c must be determined prior to first dose. If QT_c >440 msec (>500 msec in patients with ventricular conduction abnormalities), dofetilide is contraindicated

Oral:

Children: Dosage not established

Adults: Initial: 500 mcg twice daily; Maintenance: 125-500 mcg twice daily **or** 125 mcg once daily

Dosage Forms Excipient information presented when available (limited, particularly for generics); consult specific product labeling.

Capsule: 125 mcg, 250 mcg, 500 mcg

Dolasetron (dol A se tron)

Medication Safety Issues
Sound-alike/look-alike issues:
Anzemet® may be confused with Aldomet® and Avandamet®
Dolasetron may be confused with granisetron, ondansetron, palonosetron
U.S. Brand Names Anzemet®
Canadian Brand Names Anzemet®
Mexican Brand Names Anzemet
Index Terms Dolasetron Mesylate; MDL 73,147EF
Pharmacologic Category Antiemetic; Selective 5-HT_3 Receptor Antagonist
Use Prevention of nausea and vomiting associated with emetogenic cancer chemotherapy; prevention of postoperative nausea and vomiting; treatment of postoperative nausea and vomiting (injectable form only).

Note: In Canada, the use of dolasetron is contraindicated for all uses in children <18 years of age or in the treatment of postoperative nausea and vomiting in adults. These are not labeled contraindications in the U.S.
Effect on Mental Status May cause drowsiness or dizziness
Effect on Psychiatric Treatment Contraindicated with ziprasidone
Dosage Summary
I.V.:
Children <2 years: Dosage not established
Children 2-16 years: 1.8 mg/kg prior to chemotherapy (maximum: 100 mg/dose) **or** 0.35 mg/kg as a single dose postoperatively (maximum: 12.5 mg)
Adults: 1.8 mg/kg or 100 mg prior to chemotherapy **or** 12.5 mg postoperatively
Oral:
Children <2 years: Dosage not established
Children 2-16 years: 1.8 mg/kg prior to chemotherapy **or** 1.2 mg/kg prior to surgery (maximum: 100 mg/dose)
Adults: 100 mg prior to chemotherapy or surgery

Note: In Canada, the use of dolasetron is contraindicated in the treatment of postoperative nausea and vomiting in adults. These are not labeled contraindications in the U.S.
Dosage Forms Excipient information presented when available (limited, particularly for generics); consult specific product labeling.
Injection, solution, as mesylate:
Anzemet®: 20 mg/mL (0.625 mL) [single-use Carpuject® or vial; contains mannitol 38.2 mg/mL]; 20 mg/mL (5 mL) [single-use vial; contains mannitol 38.2 mg/mL]; 20 mg/mL (25 mL) [multidose vial; contains mannitol 29 mg/mL]
Tablet, as mesylate:
Anzemet®: 50 mg, 100 mg

◆ **Dolasetron Mesylate** *see* Dolasetron *on page 493*
◆ **Dolgic® LQ** *see* Butalbital, Acetaminophen, and Caffeine *on page 229*
◆ **Dolgic® Plus** *see* Butalbital, Acetaminophen, and Caffeine *on page 229*
◆ **Dolobid** *see* Diflunisal *on page 463*
◆ **Dologesic®** *see* Acetaminophen and Phenyltoloxamine *on page 36*
◆ **Dolophine®** *see* Methadone *on page 1001*

Domperidone (dom PE ri done)

Canadian Brand Names Apo-Domperidone®; Dom-Domperidone; Novo-Domperidone; Nu-Domperidone; PHL-Domperidone; PMS-Domperidone; RAN™-Domperidone; ratio-Domperidone
Mexican Brand Names Motilium; Seronex
Index Terms Domperidone Maleate
Pharmacologic Category Dopamine Antagonist, Peripheral; Gastrointestinal Agent, Prokinetic
Generic Available Yes
Use Symptomatic management of upper GI motility disorders associated with chronic and subacute gastritis and diabetic gastroparesis; prevention of GI symptoms associated with use of dopamine-agonist anti-Parkinson agents
Restrictions Not available in U.S.
Pregnancy Risk Factor C
Pregnancy Considerations Animal studies have not shown drug-related teratogenic or primary embryotoxic effects on animal fetuses, however,

comparative studies have not been done in humans. Use only when benefit outweighs potential risk in a pregnant woman.

Lactation Enters breast milk/not recommended (AAP rates as "compatible")

Contraindications Hypersensitivity to domperidone or any component of the formulation; patients with GI hemorrhage, mechanical obstruction, or perforation; patients with prolactin-releasing pituitary tumor

Warnings/Precautions Domperidone may increase prolactin levels (dose-dependent response). Elevated prolactin may be asymptomatic (clinical consequence of chronically-elevated prolactin is unknown) or may present symptomatically as galactorrhea, gynecomastia, amenorrhea, or impotence (reversible upon decreasing dose or discontinuing drug).

QT_c prolongation, life-threatening tachyarrhythmias, and cardiac arrest have been reported after domperidone use; these adverse effects may be precipitated in hypokalemic patients. Use with caution in patients with hepatic impairment. Use caution when administering domperidone to patients with a personal or family history of breast cancer. Use with caution in patients on MAO inhibitors. Safety and efficacy have not been established in pediatric patients.

Adverse Reactions

1% to 10%:

Central nervous system: Headache/migraine (1%); does not cross blood-brain barrier; fewer CNS effects compared to metoclopramide

Gastrointestinal: Xerostomia (2%)

<1% (Limited to important or life-threatening): Dizziness, dysuria, edema, extrapyramidal symptoms (EPS) rarely, galactorrhea, gynecomastia, hot flashes, insomnia, irritability, nervousness, mastalgia, menstrual irregularities, pruritus, rash, serum prolactin increased

Metabolism/Transport Effects Substrate of CYP3A4 (minor)

Drug Interactions

Alfuzosin: May enhance the QTc-prolonging effect of QTc-Prolonging Agents. *Risk C: Monitor therapy*

Ciprofloxacin: May enhance the QTc-prolonging effect of QTc-Prolonging Agents. *Risk C: Monitor therapy*

Gadobutrol: May enhance the QTc-prolonging effect of QTc-Prolonging Agents. *Risk D: Consider therapy modification*

Nilotinib: May enhance the QTc-prolonging effect of QTc-Prolonging Agents. *Risk X: Avoid combination*

QTc-Prolonging Agents: May enhance the adverse/toxic effect of other QTc-Prolonging Agents. Their effects can be additive, causing life-threatening ventricular arrhythmias. *Risk D: Consider therapy modification*

Tetrabenazine: QTc-Prolonging Agents may enhance the QTc-prolonging effect of Tetrabenazine. *Risk X: Avoid combination*

Thioridazine: QTc-Prolonging Agents may enhance the QTc-prolonging effect of Thioridazine. *Risk X: Avoid combination*

Ziprasidone: QTc-Prolonging Agents may enhance the QTc-prolonging effect of Ziprasidone. The risk of a severe arrhythmia may be increased. *Risk X: Avoid combination*

Stability Store at room temperature of 15°C to 30°C (59°F to 86°F); protect from light and moisture.

Mechanism of Action Domperidone has peripheral dopamine receptor blocking properties. It increases esophageal peristalsis and increases lower esophageal sphincter pressure, increases gastric motility and peristalsis, and enhances gastroduodenal coordination, therefore, facilitating gastric emptying and decreasing small bowel transit time.

Pharmacodynamics/Kinetics

Protein binding: 93%

Metabolism: Hepatic via N-dealkylation (CYP3A4) and hydroxylation

Half-life elimination: 7 hours

Time to peak serum concentration: 30 minutes

Excretion: Feces (66%); urine (31%)

Dosage Oral: Adults:

GI motility disorders: 10 mg 3-4 times/day, 15-30 minutes before meals; severe/resistant cases: 20 mg 3-4 times/day, 15-30 minutes before meals

Nausea/vomiting associated with dopamine-agonist anti-Parkinson agents: 20 mg 3-4 times/day

Dosage adjustment in renal impairment: Decrease dose to 10-20 mg 1-2 times/day

Dietary Considerations In GI motility disorders, should be taken 15-30 minutes prior to meals.

Administration In GI motility disorders, administer 15-30 minutes prior to meals.

Monitoring Parameters Agitation, irritability, confusion, and rarely EPS

Additional Information Not available in U.S.

The Food and Drug Administration (FDA) has issued a warning concerning the off-label use of domperidone to increase milk production in breast-feeding women. Domperidone is not available for any use in the United States and does not have approval for this indication in other countries. However, the FDA is aware that women are obtaining domperidone from U.S. compounding pharmacies and foreign sources for this purpose. The FDA notes that there are health risks associated with the use of this product that is why it has been removed from marketing.

Dosage Forms Excipient information presented when available (limited, particularly for generics); consult specific product labeling. [CAN] = Canadian brand name

Tablet: 10 mg [domperidone maleate 12.72 mg; not available in the U.S.]

Alti-Domperidone [CAN], Apo-Domperidone® [CAN], Dom-Domperidone [CAN], Novo-Domperidone [CAN], Nu-Domperidone [CAN], PHL-Domperidone [CAN], PMS-Domperidone [CAN], ratio-Domperidone [CAN]: 10 mg [not available in the U.S.]

◆ **Domperidone Maleate** *see* Domperidone *on page 493*

◆ **Donatussin** *see* Dextromethorphan, Chlorpheniramine, Phenylephrine, and Guaifenesin *on page 450*

◆ **Donatussin DC [DSC]** *see* Hydrocodone, Phenylephrine, and Guaifenesin *on page 783*

◆ **Donatussin DM [DSC]** *see* Chlorpheniramine, Phenylephrine, and Dextromethorphan *on page 327*

◆ **Donatussin Drops** *see* Guaifenesin and Phenylephrine *on page 742*

Donepezil (doh NEP e zil)

Medication Safety Issues

Sound-alike/look-alike issues:

Aricept® may be confused with AcipHex®, Ascriptin®, and Azilect®

U.S. Brand Names Aricept®; Aricept® ODT

Canadian Brand Names Aricept®; Aricept® RDT

Mexican Brand Names Eranz

Index Terms E2020

Pharmacologic Category Acetylcholinesterase Inhibitor (Central)

Generic Available No

Use Treatment of mild, moderate, or severe dementia of the Alzheimer's type

Unlabeled/Investigational Use Attention-deficit/hyperactivity disorder (ADHD); behavioral syndromes in dementia; mild-to-moderate dementia associated with Parkinson's disease; Lewy body dementia

Mental Health Comment Be mindful of other medications (and their intrinsic anticholinergic activity) that an individual is receiving. The effects of donepezil may be completely mitigated. If tolerated, increase dosage from 5 mg/day to 10 mg/day after 4-6 weeks.

Pregnancy Risk Factor C

Pregnancy Considerations Teratogenic effects were not observed in animal studies. There are no adequate and well-controlled studies in pregnant women.

Lactation Excretion in breast milk unknown/not recommended

Contraindications Hypersensitivity to donepezil, piperidine derivatives, or any component of the formulation

Warnings/Precautions Cholinesterase inhibitors may have vagotonic effects which may cause bradycardia and/or heart block with or without a history of cardiac disease; syncopal episodes have been associated with donepezil. Alzheimer's treatment guidelines consider bradycardia to be a relative contraindication for use of centrally-active cholinesterase inhibitors. Use with caution with sick sinus syndrome or other supraventricular cardiac conduction abnormalities, with seizures, COPD, or asthma. Use with caution in patients at risk of ulcer disease (eg, previous history or NSAID use), or in patients with bladder outlet obstruction. May cause diarrhea, nausea, and/or vomiting, which may be dose-related. May exaggerate neuromuscular blockade effects of depolarizing neuromuscular-blocking agents like succinylcholine. Safety and efficacy in children have not been established.

Adverse Reactions

>10%:

Central nervous system: Insomnia (5% to 14%)

Gastrointestinal: Nausea (5% to 19%), diarrhea (8% to 15%)

Miscellaneous: Accident (7% to 13%), infection (11%)

1% to 10%:

Cardiovascular: Hypertension (3%), chest pain (2%), hemorrhage (2%), syncope (2%), hypotension, atrial fibrillation, bradycardia, ECG abnormal, edema, heart failure, hot flashes, peripheral edema, vasodilation

Central nervous system: Headache (4% to 10%), pain (3% to 9%), fatigue (3% to 8%), dizziness (2% to 8%), abnormal dreams (3%), depression (2% to 3%), hostility (3%), nervousness (3%), hallucinations (3%), confusion (2%), emotional lability (2%), personality disorder (2%), fever (2%), somnolence (2%), abnormal crying, aggression, agitation, anxiety, aphasia, delusions, irritability, restlessness, seizure

Dermatologic: Bruising (4% to 5%), eczema (3%), pruritus, rash, skin ulcer, urticaria

Endocrine & metabolic: Dehydration (2%), hyperlipemia (2%), libido increased

Gastrointestinal: Anorexia (3% to 8%), vomiting (3% to 8%), weight loss (3%), abdominal pain, constipation, dyspepsia, fecal incontinence, gastroenteritis, GI bleeding, bloating, epigastric pain, toothache

Genitourinary: Urinary frequency (2%), urinary incontinence (2%), hematuria, glycosuria, nocturia, UTI

Hematologic: Anemia

Hepatic: Alkaline phosphatase increased

Neuromuscular & skeletal: Muscle cramps (3% to 8%), back pain (3%), CPK increased (3%), arthritis (2%), ataxia, bone fracture, gait abnormal, lactate dehydrogenase increased, paresthesia, tremor, weakness

Ocular: Blurred vision, cataract, eye irritation

Respiratory: Cough increased, dyspnea, bronchitis, pharyngitis, pneumonia, sore throat

Miscellaneous: Diaphoresis, fungal infection, flu symptoms, wandering

<1%, postmarketing, and/or case reports (limited to important or life-threatening): Abscess, breast fibroadenosis, cellulitis, cerebrovascular accident, CHF, cholecystitis, conjunctival hemorrhage, conjunctivitis, deep vein thrombosis, diabetes mellitus, diverticulitis, ear pain, eosinophilia, fibrocystic breast, gastrointestinal ulcer, glaucoma, goiter, heart block, hemolytic anemia, hepatitis, hostility, hyperglycemia, hypertonia, hypokalemia, hypokinesia, hyponatremia, hypoxia, intracranial hemorrhage, jaundice, LFTs increased, MI, neuroleptic malignant syndrome, pancreatitis, pleurisy, pulmonary collapse, pulmonary congestion, pyelonephritis, renal failure, retinal hemorrhage, SVT, thrombocythemia, thrombocytopenia, tongue edema, transient ischemic attack, vision abnormal

Metabolism/Transport Effects Substrate (minor) of CYP2D6, 3A4

Drug Interactions

Anticholinergics: May diminish the therapeutic effect of Acetylcholinesterase Inhibitors (Central). Acetylcholinesterase Inhibitors (Central) may diminish the therapeutic effect of Anticholinergics. If the anticholinergic action is a side effect of the agent, the result may be beneficial. **Exceptions:** Paliperidone. *Risk C: Monitor therapy*

Antipsychotics: Acetylcholinesterase Inhibitors (Central) may enhance the neurotoxic (central) effect of Antipsychotics. Severe extrapyramidal symptoms have occurred in some patients. *Risk C: Monitor therapy*

Beta-Blockers: Acetylcholinesterase Inhibitors may enhance the bradycardic effect of Beta-Blockers. **Exceptions:** Levobunolol; Metipranolol. *Risk C: Monitor therapy*

Cholinergic Agonists: Acetylcholinesterase Inhibitors may enhance the adverse/toxic effect of Cholinergic Agonists. *Risk C: Monitor therapy*

Corticosteroids (Systemic): May enhance the adverse/toxic effect of Acetylcholinesterase Inhibitors. Increased muscular weakness may occur. *Risk C: Monitor therapy*

Ginkgo Biloba: May enhance the adverse/toxic effect of Acetylcholinesterase Inhibitors. *Risk C: Monitor therapy*

Neuromuscular-Blocking Agents (Nondepolarizing): Acetylcholinesterase Inhibitors may diminish the neuromuscular-blocking effect of Neuromuscular-Blocking Agents (Nondepolarizing). Acetylcholinesterase Inhibitors may decrease the metabolism of Neuromuscular-Blocking Agents (Nondepolarizing). This is only true for mivacurium in which case the neuromuscular blocking effects might be prolonged. *Risk C: Monitor therapy*

Succinylcholine: Acetylcholinesterase Inhibitors may enhance the neuromuscular-blocking effect of Succinylcholine. *Risk C: Monitor therapy*

Ethanol/Nutrition/Herb Interactions Herb/Nutraceutical: St John's wort may decrease donepezil levels. Gingko biloba may increase adverse effects/toxicity of acetylcholinesterase inhibitors.

Stability Store at 15°C to 30°C (59°F to 86°F).

Mechanism of Action Alzheimer's disease is characterized by cholinergic deficiency in the cortex and basal forebrain, which contributes to cognitive deficits. Donepezil reversibly and noncompetitively inhibits centrally-active acetylcholinesterase, the enzyme responsible for hydrolysis of acetylcholine. This appears to result in increased concentrations of acetylcholine available for synaptic transmission in the central nervous system.

Pharmacodynamics/Kinetics

Absorption: Well absorbed

Protein binding: 96%, primarily to albumin (75%) and α_1-acid glycoprotein (21%)

Metabolism: Extensively to four major metabolites (two are active) via CYP2D6 and 3A4; undergoes glucuronidation

Bioavailability: 100%

Half-life elimination: 70 hours; time to steady-state: 15 days

Time to peak, plasma: 3-4 hours

Excretion: Urine 57% (17% as unchanged drug); feces 15%

Dosage Oral:

Children: ADHD (unlabeled use): 5 mg/day

Adults: Dementia of Alzheimer's type: Initial: 5 mg/day at bedtime; may increase to 10 mg/day at bedtime after 4-6 weeks

Child/Adolescent Considerations Five children (8-17 years of age) with ADHD showed improvement when treated with donepezil (Wilens, 2000). Four of 8 patients with autism (mean age: 11 years of age; range: 7-19 years) showed significant improvement in behaviors in a retrospective pilot study (Hardan, 2002). A retrospective chart review case series of 8 individuals (10-17 years of age) with pervasive developmental disorder showed improvement in ADHD-like symptoms upon treatment with donepezil (Doyle, 2006). Mean treatment duration was 18 weeks and dosing ranged from 2.5-30 mg/day. However, a 12-week, open-label, adjunctive trial of donepezil (dose range: 2.5-10 mg/day) in 7 children and 6 adults with stimulant-stabilized ADHD showed no significant improvement in ADHD rating scale or Executive Function Checklist (Wilens, 2005).

An 18-week, prospective, open-label, dose-escalation study of donepezil (2.5 mg, 5 mg, 10 mg daily) in 20 patients 8-14 years of age with tics (including Tourette's syndrome) and comorbid ADHD showed significant improvement of tics at the 10 mg dose (Cubo, 2008). No improvement of ADHD was evident and a large number (65%) experienced adverse events, including a 50% study dropout rate.

Cubo E, Fern Ndez Jaén A, Moreno C, et al, "Donepezil Use in Children and Adolescents With Tics and Attention-Deficit/Hyperactivity Disorder: An 18-Week, Single-Center, Dose-Escalating, Prospective, Open-Label Study," *Clin Ther*, 2008, 30(1):182-9.

Doyle RL, Frazier J, Spencer TJ, et al, "Donepezil in the Treatment of ADHD-Like Symptoms in Youths With Pervasive Developmental Disorder: A Case Series," *J Atten Disord*, 2006, 9(3):543-9.

Hardan AY and Handen BL, "A Retrospective Open Trial of Adjunctive Donepezil in Children and Adolescents With Autistic Disorder," *J Child Adolesc Psychopharmacol*, 2002, 12(3): 237-41.

Wilens TE, Biederman J, Wong J, et al, "Adjunctive Donepezil in Attention Deficit Hyperactivity Disorder Youth: Case Series," *J Child Adolesc Psychopharmacol*, 2000, 10(3):217-22.

Wilens TE, Waxmonsky J, Scott M, et al, "An Open Trial of Adjunctive Donepezil in Attention-Deficit/Hyperactivity Disorder," *J Child Adolesc Psychopharmacol*, 2005, 15(6):947-55.

Dietary Considerations May take with or without food.

Administration Administer at bedtime without regard to food.

Aricept® ODT: Allow tablet to dissolve completely on tongue and follow with water.

Monitoring Parameters Behavior, mood, bowel function, cognitive function, general function (eg, activities of daily living)

Dosage Forms Excipient information presented when available (limited, particularly for generics); consult specific product labeling.

Tablet, as hydrochloride:

Aricept®: 5 mg, 10 mg

Tablet, orally disintegrating, as hydrochloride:

Aricept® ODT: 5 mg, 10 mg

◆ **Donnatal®** *see* Hyoscyamine, Atropine, Scopolamine, and Phenobarbital *on page 800*

- **Donnatal Extentabs®** *see* Hyoscyamine, Atropine, Scopolamine, and Phenobarbital *on page 800*

DOPamine (DOE pa meen)

Medication Safety Issues

Sound-alike/look-alike issues:

DOPamine may be confused with DOBUTamine, Dopram®

High alert medication: The Institute for Safe Medication Practices (ISMP) includes this medication among its list of drugs which have a heightened risk of causing significant patient harm when used in error.

Mexican Brand Names Drynalken

Index Terms Dopamine Hydrochloride; Intropin

Pharmacologic Category Adrenergic Agonist Agent

Use Adjunct in the treatment of shock (eg, MI, open heart surgery, renal failure, cardiac decompensation) which persists after adequate fluid volume replacement

Unlabeled/Investigational Use Symptomatic bradycardia or heart block unresponsive to atropine or pacing

Effect on Mental Status None reported

Effect on Psychiatric Treatment Dopamine's effects may be enhanced by MAO inhibitors

Dosage Summary

I.V.:

Neonates: 1-20 mcg/kg/minute

Children: 1-20 mcg/kg/minute (maximum: 50 mcg/kg/minute)

Adults: 1-50 mcg/kg/minute

Dosage Forms Excipient information presented when available (limited, particularly for generics); consult specific product labeling.

Infusion, as hydrochloride [premixed in D_5W]: 0.8 mg/mL (250 mL, 500 mL); 1.6 mg/mL (250 mL, 500 mL); 3.2 mg/mL (250 mL)

Injection, solution, as hydrochloride: 40 mg/mL (5 mL, 10 mL); 80 mg/mL (5 mL); 160 mg/mL (5 mL) [contains sodium metabisulfite]

- **Dopamine Hydrochloride** *see* DOPamine *on page 498*
- **Dopram®** *see* Doxapram *on page 499*
- **Doral®** *see* Quazepam *on page 1378*
- **Doribax™** *see* Doripenem *on page 498*

Doripenem (dore i PEN em)

U.S. Brand Names Doribax™

Index Terms S-4661

Pharmacologic Category Antibiotic, Carbapenem

Use Treatment of complicated intra-abdominal infections and complicated urinary tract infections (including pyelonephritis) due to susceptible gram-positive, gram-negative (including *Pseudomonas aeruginosa*), and anaerobic bacteria

Unlabeled/Investigational Use Treatment of nosocomial pneumonia

Effect on Mental Status None reported

Effect on Psychiatric Treatment GI side effects are common; concomitant use with SSRIs, carbamazepine, valproic acid, and lithium may produce additive effects. Doripenem may decrease valproic acid levels resulting in breakthrough seizures.

Dosage Summary

I.V.:

Children: Dosage not established

Adults: 500 mg every 8 hours

Dosage Forms Excipient information presented when available (limited, particularly for generics); consult specific product labeling.

Injection, powder for reconstitution:

Doribax™: 500 mg

- **Doryx®** *see* Doxycycline *on page 509*

Dorzolamide (dor ZOLE a mide)

U.S. Brand Names Trusopt®

Canadian Brand Names Trusopt®

Mexican Brand Names Trusopt

Index Terms Dorzolamide Hydrochloride

Pharmacologic Category Carbonic Anhydrase Inhibitor; Ophthalmic Agent, Antiglaucoma

Use Treatment of elevated intraocular pressure in patients with ocular hypertension or open-angle glaucoma

Effect on Mental Status May cause drowsiness

Effect on Psychiatric Treatment None reported

Dosage Summary

Ophthalmic:

Children: Instill 1 drop into affected eye(s) 3 times/day

Adults: Instill 1 drop into affected eye(s) 3 times/day

Dosage Forms Excipient information presented when available (limited, particularly for generics); consult specific product labeling.

Solution, ophthalmic: 2% (10 mL)

Trusopt®: 2% (10 mL) [contains benzalkonium chloride]

Dorzolamide and Timolol (dor ZOLE a mide & TYE moe lole)

U.S. Brand Names Cosopt®

Canadian Brand Names Cosopt®; Preservative-Free Cosopt®

Mexican Brand Names Cosopt

Index Terms Timolol and Dorzolamide

Pharmacologic Category Beta-Adrenergic Blocker, Nonselective; Carbonic Anhydrase Inhibitor; Ophthalmic Agent, Antiglaucoma

Use Treatment of elevated intraocular pressure in patients with ocular hypertension or open-angle glaucoma

Effect on Mental Status May cause drowsiness, dizziness, or fatigue; may rarely cause anxiety, depression, or hallucinations

Effect on Psychiatric Treatment Barbiturates and carbamazepine may decrease the effects of beta-blockers

Dosage Summary

Ophthalmic:

Children <2 years: Dosage not established

Children ≥2 years: Instill 1 drop into affected eye(s) twice daily

Adults: Instill 1 drop into affected eye(s) twice daily

Dosage Forms Excipient information presented when available (limited, particularly for generics); consult specific product labeling. [DSC] = Discontinued product

Solution, ophthalmic: Dorzolamide hydrochloride 2% (as base) and timolol maleate 0.5% (as base) (10 mL)

Cosopt®: Dorzolamide hydrochloride 2% (as base) and timolol maleate 0.5% (as base) (5 mL [DSC]; 10 mL) [contains benzalkonium chloride]

◆ **Dorzolamide Hydrochloride** *see* Dorzolamide *on page 498*

◆ **Dostinex® [DSC]** *see* Cabergoline *on page 248*

◆ **Double Tussin DM [OTC]** *see* Guaifenesin and Dextromethorphan *on page 739*

Doxapram (DOKS a pram)

Medication Safety Issues

Sound-alike/look-alike issues:

Doxapram may be confused with doxacurium, doxazosin, doxepin, Doxinate®, DOXOrubicin

Dopram® may be confused with DOPamine

U.S. Brand Names Dopram®

Index Terms Doxapram Hydrochloride

Pharmacologic Category Respiratory Stimulant; Stimulant

Use Respiratory and CNS stimulant for respiratory depression secondary to anesthesia, drug-induced CNS depression; acute hypercapnia secondary to COPD

Effect on Mental Status May cause CNS stimulation, restlessness, irritability, or hallucinations

Effect on Psychiatric Treatment May cause hypertensive crisis if used with MAO inhibitors

Dosage Summary

I.V.:

Children: Dosage not established

Adults: 0.5-1 mg/kg every 5 minutes until response (maximum total dose: 2 mg/kg) **or** 1-5 mg/minute until response, should not be continued >2 hours (maximum total dose: 4 mg/kg; 3 g/day)

Dosage Forms Excipient information presented when available (limited, particularly for generics); consult specific product labeling.

Injection, solution, as hydrochloride: 20 mg/mL (20 mL) [contains benzyl alcohol]

♦ **Doxapram Hydrochloride** *see* Doxapram *on page 499*

Doxazosin (doks AY zoe sin)

Medication Safety Issues

Sound-alike/look-alike issues:

Doxazosin may be confused with doxapram, doxepin, DOXOrubicin

Cardura® may be confused with Cardene®, Cordarone®, Cordran®, Coumadin®, K-Dur®, Ridaura®

U.S. Brand Names Cardura®; Cardura® XL

Canadian Brand Names Alti-Doxazosin; Apo-Doxazosin®; Cardura-1™; Cardura-2™; Cardura-4™; Gen-Doxazosin; Novo-Doxazosin

Mexican Brand Names Cardura

Index Terms Doxazosin Mesylate

Pharmacologic Category $Alpha_1$ Blocker

Generic Available Yes: Excludes extended release tablet

Use Treatment of hypertension alone or in conjunction with diuretics, ACE inhibitors, beta-blockers, or calcium antagonists; treatment of urinary outflow obstruction and/or obstructive and irritative symptoms associated with benign prostatic hyperplasia (BPH), particularly useful in patients with troublesome symptoms who are unable or unwilling to undergo invasive procedures, but who require rapid symptomatic relief; can be used in combination with finasteride

Unlabeled/Investigational Use Pediatric hypertension

Effect on Mental Status Dizziness is common.

Effect on Psychiatric Treatment Psychotropics may potentiate the hypotensive effects of doxazosin

Pregnancy Risk Factor C

Pregnancy Considerations Some studies demonstrated embryolethality resulting from doxazosin exposure during organogenesis. Delayed postnatal development was also noted. There are no adequate and well-controlled studies in pregnant women. Use only if benefit outweighs risk.

Lactation Excretion in breast milk unknown/not recommended

Contraindications Hypersensitivity to quinazolines (prazosin, terazosin), doxazosin, or any component of the formulation

Warnings/Precautions Can cause significant orthostatic hypotension and syncope, especially with first dose; anticipate a similar effect if therapy is interrupted for a few days, if dosage is rapidly increased, or if another antihypertensive drug (particularly vasodilators) or a PDE-5 inhibitor is introduced. Discontinue if symptoms of angina occur or worsen. Patients should be cautioned about performing hazardous tasks when starting new therapy or adjusting dosage upward. Prostate cancer should be ruled out before starting for BPH. Use with caution in mild to moderate hepatic impairment; not recommended in severe dysfunction. Intraoperative floppy iris syndrome has been observed in cataract surgery patients who were on or were previously treated with $alpha_1$-blockers. Causality has not been established and there appears to be no benefit in discontinuing alpha-blocker therapy prior to surgery. Safety and efficacy in children have not been established.

The extended release formulation consists of drug within a nondeformable matrix; following drug release/absorption, the matrix/shell is expelled in the stool. The use of nondeformable products in patients with known stricture/narrowing of the GI tract has been associated with symptoms of obstruction. Use caution in patients with increased GI retention (eg, chronic constipation) as doxazosin exposure may be increased. Extended release formulation is not approved for the treatment of hypertension.

Adverse Reactions Note: Type and frequency of adverse reactions reflect combined data from trials with immediate release and extended release products.

>10%: Central nervous system: Dizziness (5% to 19%), headache (5% to 14%)

1% to 10%:

Cardiovascular: Orthostatic hypotension (dose related; 0.3% up to 2%), edema (3% to 4%), hypotension (2%), palpitation (1% to 2%), chest pain (1% to 2%), arrhythmia (1%), syncope (2%), flushing (1%)

Central nervous system: Fatigue (8% to 12%), somnolence (1% to 5%), nervousness (2%), pain (2%), vertigo (2% to 4%), insomnia (1%), anxiety (1%), paresthesia (1%), movement disorder (1%), ataxia (1%), hypertonia (1%), depression (1%)

Dermatologic: Rash (1%), pruritus (1%)

Endocrine & metabolic: Sexual dysfunction (2%)

Gastrointestinal: Abdominal pain (2%), diarrhea (2%), dyspepsia (1% to 2%), nausea (1% to 3%), xerostomia (1% to 2%), constipation (1%), flatulence (1%)

Genitourinary: Urinary tract infection (1%), impotence (1%), polyuria (2%), incontinence (1%)

Neuromuscular & skeletal: Back pain (2% to 3%), weakness (1% to 7%), arthritis (1%), muscle weakness (1%), myalgia (≤1%), muscle cramps (1%)

Ocular: Abnormal vision (1% to 2%), conjunctivitis (1%)

Otic: Tinnitus (1%)

Respiratory: Respiratory tract infection (5%), rhinitis (3%), dyspnea (1% to 3%), respiratory disorder (1%), epistaxis (1%)

Miscellaneous: Diaphoresis increased (1%), flu-like syndrome (1%)

<1% (Limited to important or life-threatening): Abnormal thinking, agitation, allergic reaction, amnesia, angina, anorexia, bradycardia, breast pain, bronchospasm, cataplexy, cerebrovascular accident, cholestasis, confusion, depersonalization, emotional lability, enuresis, fecal incontinence, fever, gastroenteritis, gout, hematuria, hepatitis, hypoesthesia, hypokalemia, infection, intraoperative floppy iris syndrome (cataract surgery), jaundice, leukopenia, liver function tests increased, lymphadenopathy, MI, micturition abnormality, migraine, neutropenia, nocturia, pallor, paranoia, paresis, paresthesia, parosmia, peripheral ischemia, priapism, purpura, renal calculus, rigors stroke, syncope, systemic lupus erythematosus, tachycardia, thrombocytopenia, vomiting

Drug Interactions

Alfuzosin: Alpha1-Blockers may enhance the antihypertensive effect of Alfuzosin. Risk of orthostatic hypotension or syncope may be increased. Alfuzosin may enhance the antihypertensive effect of Alpha1-Blockers. *Risk X: Avoid combination*

Beta-Blockers: May enhance the orthostatic effect of Alpha1-Blockers. The risk associated with ophthalmic products is probably less than systemic products. **Exceptions:** Levobunolol; Metipranolol. *Risk D: Consider therapy modification*

Calcium Channel Blockers: Alpha1-Blockers may enhance the hypotensive effect of Calcium Channel Blockers. *Risk C: Monitor therapy*

Diazoxide: May enhance the hypotensive effect of Antihypertensives. *Risk C: Monitor therapy*

Herbs (Hypertensive Properties): May diminish the antihypertensive effect of Antihypertensives. *Risk C: Monitor therapy*

Herbs (Hypotensive Properties): May enhance the hypotensive effect of Antihypertensives. *Risk C: Monitor therapy*

Methylphenidate: May diminish the antihypertensive effect of Antihypertensives. *Risk C: Monitor therapy*

Phosphodiesterase 5 Inhibitors: May enhance the hypotensive effect of Alpha1-Blockers. *Risk D: Consider therapy modification*

Prostacyclin Analogues: May enhance the hypotensive effect of Antihypertensives. *Risk C: Monitor therapy*

RiTUXimab: Antihypertensives may enhance the hypotensive effect of RiTUXimab. *Risk D: Consider therapy modification*

Tamsulosin: Alpha1-Blockers may enhance the antihypertensive effect of Tamsulosin. Risk of orthostatic hypotension or syncope may be increased. Tamsulosin may enhance the antihypertensive effect of Alpha1-Blockers. *Risk X: Avoid combination*

Ethanol/Nutrition/Herb Interactions Herb/Nutraceutical: Avoid dong quai if using for hypertension (has estrogenic activity). Avoid ephedra, yohimbe, ginseng (may worsen hypertension). Avoid saw palmetto when used for BPH (due to limited experience with this combination). Avoid garlic (may have increased antihypertensive effect).

Mechanism of Action

Hypertension: Competitively inhibits postsynaptic alpha$_1$-adrenergic receptors which results in vasodilation of veins and arterioles and a decrease in total peripheral resistance and blood pressure; ~50% as potent on a weight by weight basis as prazosin.

BPH: Competitively inhibits postsynaptic alpha$_1$-adrenergic receptors in prostatic stromal and bladder neck tissues. This reduces the sympathetic tone-induced urethral stricture causing BPH symptoms.

Pharmacodynamics/Kinetics Not significantly affected by increased age

Duration: >24 hours

Protein binding: Extended release: 98%

Metabolism: Extensively hepatic to active metabolites; primarily via CYP3A4; secondary pathways involve CYP2D6 and 2C19

Bioavailability: Extended release relative to immediate release: 54% to 59%

Half-life elimination: 15-22 hours

Time to peak, serum: Immediate release: 2-3 hours; extended release: 8-9 hours

Excretion: Feces (63% primarily as metabolites); urine (9%)

Dosage Oral:

Children (unlabeled use): Hypertension: Immediate release: Initial: 1 mg once daily; maximum: 4 mg/day

Adults:

Immediate release: 1 mg once daily in morning or evening; may be increased to 2 mg once daily. Thereafter titrate upwards, if needed, over several weeks, balancing therapeutic benefit with doxazosin-induced postural hypotension. In the elderly, initiate at 0.5 mg once daily

Hypertension: Maximum dose: 16 mg/day

BPH: Goal: 4-8 mg/day; maximum dose: 8 mg/day

Extended release: BPH: 4 mg once daily with breakfast; titrate based on response and tolerability every 3-4 weeks to maximum recommended dose of 8 mg/day

Reinitiation of therapy: If therapy is discontinued for several days, restart at 4 mg dose and titrate as before.

Conversion to extended release from immediate release: Initiate with 4 mg once daily; omit final evening dose of immediate release prior to starting morning dosing with extended release product.

Dosing adjustment in hepatic impairment: Use with caution in mild-to-moderate hepatic dysfunction. Do not use with severe impairment.

Dietary Considerations Cardura® XL: Take with morning meal.

Administration Cardura® XL: Tablets should be swallowed whole; do not crush, chew, or divide.

Monitoring Parameters Blood pressure, standing and sitting/supine; syncope may occur usually within 90 minutes of the initial dose

Additional Information First-dose hypotension occurs less frequently with doxazosin as compared to prazosin; this may be due to its slower onset of action.

Dosage Forms Excipient information presented when available (limited, particularly for generics); consult specific product labeling.

Tablet: 1 mg, 2 mg, 4 mg, 8 mg

Cardura®: 1 mg, 2 mg, 4 mg, 8 mg

Tablet, extended release:

Cardura® XL: 4 mg, 8 mg

◆ **Doxazosin Mesylate** *see* Doxazosin *on page 500*

Doxepin (DOKS e pin)

Medication Safety Issues

Sound-alike/look-alike issues:

Doxepin may be confused with digoxin, doxapram, doxazosin, Doxidan®, doxycycline

Sinequan® may be confused with saquinavir, Serentil®, Seroquel®, Singulair®

Zonalon® may be confused with Zone-A Forte®

International issues:

Doxal® [Finland] may be confused with Doxil® which is a brand name for doxorubicin in the U.S.

Doxal® [Finland]: Brand name for doxycycline in Austria; brand name for pyridoxine/thiamine in Brazil

Related Information

Anticholinergic Effects of Common Psychotropics *on page 1758*

Antidepressant Agents *on page 1760*

Antidepressant Receptor Profile *on page 1764*

Discontinuation of Psychotropic Drugs *on page 1839*

Liquid Compatibility of Antidepressants, Antipsychotics, and Mood Stabilizers *on page 1788*

U.S. Brand Names Prudoxin™; Sinequan® [DSC]; Zonalon®

Canadian Brand Names Apo-Doxepin®; Novo-Doxepin; Sinequan®; Zonalon®

Mexican Brand Names Sinequan

Index Terms Doxepin Hydrochloride

Pharmacologic Category Antidepressant, Tricyclic (Tertiary Amine); Topical Skin Product

Generic Available Yes: Capsule, solution

Use

Oral: Depression

Topical: Short-term (<8 days) management of moderate pruritus in adults with atopic dermatitis or lichen simplex chronicus

Unlabeled/Investigational Use Analgesic for certain chronic and neuropathic pain; anxiety

Mental Health Comment Tricyclic antidepressants may be classified as tertiary (amitriptyline, doxepin, clomipramine, imipramine, trimipramine) or secondary amines (nortriptyline, desipramine, protriptyline). The tertiary amines are not recommended to treat depression in the elderly. If a TCA is used in the elderly, it should be a secondary amine. The tertiary amines are commonly used in low dosages for various conditions associated with pain. Toxicity is generally dose dependent. Relatively small overdoses (1-week supply) can be potentially fatal.

Restrictions An FDA-approved medication guide concerning the use of antidepressants in children, adolescents, and young adults must be distributed when dispensing an outpatient prescription (new or refill) where this medication is to be used without direct supervision of a healthcare provider. Medication guides are available at http://www.fda.gov/cder/Offices/ODS/medication_guides.htm. Dispense to parents or guardians of children and adolescents receiving this medication.

Pregnancy Risk Factor B (cream); C (all other forms)

Pregnancy Considerations Teratogenic effects were not observed in animal studies; however, there are no adequate and well-controlled studies in pregnant women. Use during pregnancy only if clearly needed.

Lactation Enters breast milk/not recommended (AAP rates "of concern")

Contraindications Hypersensitivity to doxepin, drugs from similar chemical class, or any component of the formulation; narrow-angle glaucoma; urinary retention; use of MAO inhibitors within 14 days; use in a patient during acute recovery phase of MI

Warnings/Precautions **[U.S. Boxed Warning]: Antidepressants increase the risk of suicidal thinking and behavior in children, adolescents, and young adults (18-24 years of age) with major depressive disorder (MDD) and other psychiatric disorders;** consider risk prior to prescribing. Short-term studies did not show an increased risk in patients >24 years of age and showed a decreased risk in patients ≥65 years. Closely monitor for clinical worsening, suicidality, or unusual changes in behavior; the patient's family or caregiver should be instructed to closely observe the patient and communicate condition with healthcare provider. A medication guide should be dispensed with each prescription. **Doxepin is approved for treatment of depression in adolescents.**

The possibility of a suicide attempt is inherent in major depression and may persist until remission occurs. Monitor for worsening of depression or suicidality, especially during initiation of therapy (generally first 1-2 months) or with dose increases or decreases. Use caution in high-risk patients. Worsening depression and severe abrupt suicidality that are not part of the presenting symptoms may require discontinuation or modification of drug therapy. The patient's family or caregiver should be alerted to monitor patients for the emergence of suicidality and associated behaviors (such as agitation, irritability, hostility, impulsivity, and hypomania) and call healthcare provider.

May worsen psychosis in some patients or precipitate a shift to mania or hypomania in patients with bipolar disorder. Patients presenting with depressive symptoms should be screened for bipolar disorder. Monotherapy in patients with bipolar disorder should be avoided. **Doxepin is not FDA approved for the treatment of bipolar depression.**

The risks of sedative and anticholinergic effects are high relative to other antidepressant agents. Doxepin frequently causes sedation, which may result in impaired performance of tasks requiring alertness (eg, operating machinery or driving). Sedative effects may be additive with other CNS depressants and/or ethanol. Also use caution in patients with benign prostatic hyperplasia, xerostomia, visual problems, constipation, or history of bowel obstruction.

May cause orthostatic hypotension or conduction disturbances (risks are moderate relative to other antidepressants). Use with caution in patients with a history of cardiovascular disease (including previous MI, stroke, tachycardia, or conduction abnormalities). Consider discontinuation, when possible, prior to elective surgery. Therapy should not be abruptly discontinued in patients receiving high doses for prolonged periods.

Use caution in patients with a previous seizure disorder or condition predisposing to seizures such as brain damage, alcoholism, or concurrent therapy with other drugs which lower the seizure threshold. Use with caution in hyperthyroid patients or those receiving thyroid supplementation. Use with caution in patients with hepatic or renal dysfunction and in elderly patients.

Cream formulation is for external use only (not for ophthalmic, vaginal, or oral use). Do not use occlusive dressings. Use for >8 days may increase risk of contact sensitization. Doxepin is significantly absorbed following topical administration; plasma levels may be similar to those achieved with oral administration.

Adverse Reactions

Oral: Frequency not defined.

Cardiovascular: Hyper-/hypotension, tachycardia

Central nervous system: Drowsiness, dizziness, headache, disorientation, ataxia, confusion, seizure

Dermatologic: Alopecia, photosensitivity, rash, pruritus

Endocrine & metabolic: Breast enlargement, galactorrhea, SIADH, blood sugar increased/decreased, libido increased/decreased

Gastrointestinal: Xerostomia, constipation, vomiting, indigestion, anorexia, aphthous stomatitis, nausea, unpleasant taste, weight gain, diarrhea, trouble with gums, lower esophageal sphincter tone decrease may cause GE reflux

Genitourinary: Urinary retention, testicular edema

Hematologic: Agranulocytosis, leukopenia, eosinophilia, thrombocytopenia, purpura

Neuromuscular & skeletal: Weakness, tremor, numbness, paresthesia, extrapyramidal symptoms, tardive dyskinesia

Ocular: Blurred vision

Otic: Tinnitus

Miscellaneous: Diaphoresis (excessive), allergic reactions

Topical:

>10%:

- Central nervous system: Drowsiness (22%)
- Dermatologic: Stinging/burning (23%)

1% to 10%:

- Cardiovascular: Edema: (1%)
- Central nervous system: Dizziness (2%), emotional changes (2%)
- Gastrointestinal: Xerostomia (10%), taste alteration (2%)

<1% (Limited to important or life-threatening): Contact dermatitis, tongue numbness, anxiety

Metabolism/Transport Effects Substrate (major) of CYP1A2, 2D6, 3A4

Drug Interactions

Acetylcholinesterase Inhibitors (Central): Anticholinergics may diminish the therapeutic effect of Acetylcholinesterase Inhibitors (Central). Acetylcholinesterase Inhibitors (Central) may diminish the therapeutic effect of Anticholinergics. If the anticholinergic action is a side effect of the agent, the result may be beneficial. *Risk C: Monitor therapy*

Alcohol (Ethyl): CNS Depressants may enhance the CNS depressant effect of Alcohol (Ethyl). *Risk C: Monitor therapy*

Alfuzosin: May enhance the QTc-prolonging effect of QTc-Prolonging Agents. *Risk C: Monitor therapy*

Alpha-/Beta-Agonists (Direct-Acting): Tricyclic Antidepressants may enhance the vasopressor effect of Alpha-/Beta-Agonists (Direct-Acting). **Exceptions:** Dipivefrin. *Risk D: Consider therapy modification*

Alpha1-Agonists: Tricyclic Antidepressants may enhance the vasopressor effect of Alpha1-Agonists. *Risk D: Consider therapy modification*

Alpha2-Agonists: Tricyclic Antidepressants may diminish the antihypertensive effect of Alpha2-Agonists. **Exceptions:** Apraclonidine; Brimonidine. *Risk D: Consider therapy modification*

Altretamine: May enhance the orthostatic effect of Tricyclic Antidepressants. *Risk C: Monitor therapy*

Amphetamines: Tricyclic Antidepressants may enhance the stimulatory effect of Amphetamines. Tricyclic Antidepressants may also potentiate the cardiovascular effects of Amphetamines. *Risk C: Monitor therapy*

Anticholinergics: May enhance the adverse/toxic effect of other Anticholinergics. **Exceptions:** Paliperidone. *Risk C: Monitor therapy*

Aspirin: Antidepressants (Tricyclic, Tertiary Amine) may enhance the antiplatelet effect of Aspirin. *Risk C: Monitor therapy*

Barbiturates: May increase the metabolism of Tricyclic Antidepressants. *Risk D: Consider therapy modification*

Beta2-Agonists: Tricyclic Antidepressants may enhance the adverse/toxic effect of Beta2-Agonists. *Risk C: Monitor therapy*

BuPROPion: May decrease the metabolism of Tricyclic Antidepressants. *Risk C: Monitor therapy*

CarBAMazepine: May increase the metabolism of Tricyclic Antidepressants. *Risk C: Monitor therapy*

Cimetidine: May decrease the metabolism of Tricyclic Antidepressants. *Risk C: Monitor therapy*

Cinacalcet: May increase the serum concentration of Tricyclic Antidepressants. *Risk C: Monitor therapy*

Ciprofloxacin: May enhance the QTc-prolonging effect of QTc-Prolonging Agents. *Risk C: Monitor therapy*

CNS Depressants: May enhance the adverse/toxic effect of other CNS Depressants. *Risk C: Monitor therapy*

CYP1A2 Inducers (Strong): May increase the metabolism of CYP1A2 Substrates. *Risk C: Monitor therapy*

CYP1A2 Inhibitors (Moderate): May decrease the metabolism of CYP1A2 Substrates. *Risk C: Monitor therapy*

CYP1A2 Inhibitors (Strong): May decrease the metabolism of CYP1A2 Substrates. *Risk D: Consider therapy modification*

CYP2D6 Inhibitors (Moderate): May decrease the metabolism of CYP2D6 Substrates. *Risk C: Monitor therapy*

CYP2D6 Inhibitors (Strong): May decrease the metabolism of CYP2D6 Substrates. *Risk D: Consider therapy modification*

CYP3A4 Inducers (Strong): May increase the metabolism of CYP3A4 Substrates. *Risk C: Monitor therapy*

CYP3A4 Inhibitors (Moderate): May decrease the metabolism of CYP3A4 Substrates. *Risk C: Monitor therapy*

CYP3A4 Inhibitors (Strong): May decrease the metabolism of CYP3A4 Substrates. *Risk D: Consider therapy modification*

Darunavir: May increase the serum concentration of CYP2D6 Substrates. *Risk C: Monitor therapy*

Dasatinib: May increase the serum concentration of CYP3A4 Substrates. *Risk C: Monitor therapy*

Deferasirox: May decrease the serum concentration of CYP3A4 Substrates. *Risk C: Monitor therapy*

Desmopressin: Tricyclic Antidepressants may enhance the adverse/toxic effect of Desmopressin. *Risk C: Monitor therapy*

Dexmethylphenidate: May decrease the metabolism of Tricyclic Antidepressants. *Risk C: Monitor therapy*

DULoxetine: May decrease the metabolism of Tricyclic Antidepressants. *Risk C: Monitor therapy*

Gadobutrol: May enhance the QTc-prolonging effect of QTc-Prolonging Agents. *Risk D: Consider therapy modification*

Lithium: May enhance the neurotoxic effect of Tricyclic Antidepressants. *Risk C: Monitor therapy*

MAO Inhibitors: May enhance the serotonergic effect of Tricyclic Antidepressants. This may cause serotonin syndrome. *Risk X: Avoid combination*

Methylphenidate: May decrease the metabolism of Tricyclic Antidepressants. *Risk C: Monitor therapy*

Nilotinib: May enhance the QTc-prolonging effect of QTc-Prolonging Agents. *Risk X: Avoid combination*

NSAID (COX-2 Inhibitor): Antidepressants (Tricyclic, Tertiary Amine) may enhance the antiplatelet effect of NSAID (COX-2 Inhibitor). *Risk C: Monitor therapy*

NSAID (Nonselective): Antidepressants (Tricyclic, Tertiary Amine) may enhance the antiplatelet effect of NSAID (Nonselective). *Risk C: Monitor therapy*

Pramlintide: May enhance the anticholinergic effect of Anticholinergics. These effects are specific to the GI tract. *Risk D: Consider therapy modification*

Propoxyphene: May enhance the CNS depressant effect of Tricyclic Antidepressants. *Risk C: Monitor therapy*

Protease Inhibitors: May increase the serum concentration of Tricyclic Antidepressants. *Risk C: Monitor therapy*

QTc-Prolonging Agents: May enhance the adverse/toxic effect of other QTc-Prolonging Agents. Their effects can be additive, causing life-threatening ventricular arrhythmias. *Risk D: Consider therapy modification*

QuiNIDine: Tricyclic Antidepressants may enhance the QTc-prolonging effect of QuiNIDine. QuiNIDine may decrease the metabolism of Tricyclic Antidepressants. *Risk D: Consider therapy modification*

Selective Serotonin Reuptake Inhibitors: May decrease the metabolism of Tricyclic Antidepressants. *Risk D: Consider therapy modification*

Serotonin Modulators: May enhance the adverse/toxic effect of other Serotonin Modulators. The development of serotonin syndrome may occur. *Risk D: Consider therapy modification*

Sibutramine: May enhance the serotonergic effect of Serotonin Modulators. This may cause serotonin syndrome. *Risk X: Avoid combination*

St Johns Wort: May increase the metabolism of Tricyclic Antidepressants. The risk of serotonin syndrome may theoretically be increased. *Risk D: Consider therapy modification*

Sulfonylureas: Cyclic Antidepressants may enhance the hypoglycemic effect of Sulfonylureas. *Risk C: Monitor therapy*

Terbinafine: May decrease the metabolism of Tricyclic Antidepressants. *Risk D: Consider therapy modification*

Tetrabenazine: QTc-Prolonging Agents may enhance the QTc-prolonging effect of Tetrabenazine. *Risk X: Avoid combination*

Thioridazine: QTc-Prolonging Agents may enhance the QTc-prolonging effect of Thioridazine. *Risk X: Avoid combination*

TraMADol: Tricyclic Antidepressants may enhance the neuroexcitatory and/or seizure-potentiating effect of TraMADol. *Risk C: Monitor therapy*

Valproic Acid: May increase the serum concentration of Tricyclic Antidepressants. *Risk C: Monitor therapy*

Vitamin K Antagonists (eg, warfarin): Tricyclic Antidepressants may enhance the anticoagulant effect of Vitamin K Antagonists. *Risk C: Monitor therapy*

Ziprasidone: QTc-Prolonging Agents may enhance the QTc-prolonging effect of Ziprasidone. The risk of a severe arrhythmia may be increased. *Risk X: Avoid combination*

Ethanol/Nutrition/Herb Interactions

Ethanol: Avoid ethanol (may increase CNS depression).

Food: Grapefruit juice may inhibit the metabolism of some TCAs and clinical toxicity may result.

Herb/Nutraceutical: Avoid valerian, St John's wort, SAMe, kava kava (may increase risk of serotonin syndrome and/or excessive sedation).

Stability Protect from light.

Mechanism of Action Increases the synaptic concentration of serotonin and norepinephrine in the central nervous system by inhibition of their reuptake by the presynaptic neuronal membrane

Pharmacodynamics/Kinetics

Onset of action: Peak effect: Antidepressant: Usually >2 weeks; Anxiolytic: may occur sooner

Absorption: Following topical application, plasma levels may be similar to those achieved with oral administration

Distribution: Crosses placenta; enters breast milk

Protein binding: 80% to 85%

Metabolism: Hepatic; metabolites include desmethyldoxepin (active)

Half-life elimination: Adults: 6-8 hours

Excretion: Urine

Dosage

Oral: Topical: Burning mouth syndrome (dental use): Cream: Apply 3-4 times daily

Oral (entire daily dose may be given at bedtime):

- Depression or anxiety:
  - Children (unlabeled use): 1-3 mg/kg/day in single or divided doses
  - Adolescents: Initial: 25-50 mg/day in single or divided doses; gradually increase to 100 mg/day
  - Adults: Initial: 25-150 mg/day at bedtime or in 2-3 divided doses; may gradually increase up to 300 mg/day; single dose should not exceed 150 mg; select patients may respond to 25-50 mg/day
  - Elderly: Use a lower dose and adjust gradually
- Chronic urticaria, angioedema, nocturnal pruritus: Adults and Elderly: 10-30 mg/day

Dosing adjustment in hepatic impairment: Use a lower dose and adjust gradually

Topical: Pruritus: Adults and Elderly: Apply a thin film 4 times/day with at least 3- to 4-hour interval between applications; not recommended for use >8 days. **Note:** Low-dose (25-50 mg) oral administration has also been used to treat pruritus, but systemic effects are increased.

Administration

Oral: Do not mix oral concentrate with carbonated beverages (physically incompatible).

Topical: Apply thin film to affected area; use of occlusive dressings is not recommended.

Monitoring Parameters Monitor blood pressure and pulse rate prior to and during initial therapy; monitor mental status, suicidal ideation (especially at the beginning of therapy or when doses are increased or decreased); weight; ECG in older adults; adverse effects may be increased if topical formulation is applied to >10% of body surface area

Reference Range Proposed therapeutic concentration (doxepin plus desmethyldoxepin): 110-250 ng/mL. Toxic concentration (doxepin plus desmethyldoxepin): >500 ng/mL. Utility of serum level monitoring is controversial.

Test Interactions Increased glucose

Dosage Forms Excipient information presented when available (limited, particularly for generics); consult specific product labeling. [DSC] = Discontinued product

Capsule, as hydrochloride: 10 mg, 25 mg, 50 mg, 75 mg, 100 mg, 150 mg
  Sinequan®: 10 mg, 25 mg, 50 mg, 75 mg, 100 mg, 150 mg [DSC]
Cream, as hydrochloride:
  Prudoxin™: 5% (45 g) [contains benzyl alcohol]
  Zonalon®: 5% (30 g, 45 g) [contains benzyl alcohol]
Solution, oral concentrate, as hydrochloride: 10 mg/mL (120 mL)
  Sinequan®: 10 mg/mL (120 mL) [DSC]

◆ **Doxepin Hydrochloride** *see* Doxepin *on page 502*

Doxercalciferol (doks er kal si fe FEER ole)

U.S. Brand Names Hectorol®

Canadian Brand Names Hectorol®

Index Terms 1α-Hydroxyergocalciferol

Pharmacologic Category Vitamin D Analog

Use Treatment of secondary hyperparathyroidism in patients with chronic kidney disease

Effect on Mental Status Dizziness and malaise are common; may cause confusion or sleep disorders

Effect on Psychiatric Treatment Nausea and vomiting are common; use caution with SSRIs

Dosage Summary

I.V.:

Children: Dosage not established

Adults: Initial: 4 mcg 3 times/week after dialysis; Titration: Dose can be increased by 1-2 mcg at 8-week intervals, as necessary (maximum: 18 mcg/week)

Oral:

Children: Dosage not established

Adults (dialysis patients): Initial: 10 mcg 3 times/week at dialysis; Titration: Dose can be increased by 2.5 mcg at 8-week intervals (maximum: 60 mcg/week)

Adults (predialysis patients): Initial: 1 mcg/day; Titration: Increase dose by 0.5 mcg at 2-week intervals (maximum: 3.5 mcg/day)

Dosage Forms Excipient information presented when available (limited, particularly for generics); consult specific product labeling.

Capsule, softgel:
  Hectorol®: 0.5 mcg, 2.5 mcg [contains coconut oil]
Injection, solution:
  Hectorol®: 2 mcg/mL (2 mL) [contains disodium edetate]

◆ **Doxil®** *see* DOXOrubicin (Liposomal) *on page 508*

DOXOrubicin (doks oh ROO bi sin)

Medication Safety Issues

Sound-alike/look-alike issues:

DOXOrubicin may be confused with DACTINomycin, DAUNOrubicin, DAUNOrubicin liposomal, doxacurium, doxapram, doxazosin, DOXOrubicin liposomal, epirubicin, IDArubicin

Adriamycin PFS® may be confused with achromycin, Aredia®, Idamycin®

Conventional formulation (Adriamycin PFS®, Adriamycin RDF®) may be confused with the liposomal formulation (Doxil®)

Use caution when selecting product for preparation and dispensing; indications, dosages and adverse event profiles differ between conventional DOXOrubicin hydrochloride solution and DOXOrubicin liposomal. Both formulations are the same concentration. As a result, serious errors have occurred.

High alert medication: The Institute for Safe Medication Practices (ISMP) includes this medication among its list of drug classes which have a heightened risk of causing significant patient harm when used in error.

ADR is an error-prone abbreviation

International issues:

Doxil® may be confused with Doxal® which is a brand name for doxepin in Finland, a brand name for doxycycline in Austria, and a brand name for pyridoxine/thiamine combination in Brazil

Rubex®: Brand name for ascorbic acid in Ireland

U.S. Brand Names Adriamycin®; Rubex® [DSC]

Canadian Brand Names Adriamycin®

Mexican Brand Names Adriblastina RD; Caelyx; Doxolem RU; Doxopeg; Doxotec; Doxtie

Index Terms ADR (error-prone abbreviation); Adria; Doxorubicin Hydrochloride; Hydroxydaunomycin Hydrochloride; Hydroxyldaunorubicin Hydrochloride; NSC-123127

Pharmacologic Category Antineoplastic Agent, Anthracycline

Use Treatment of leukemias, lymphomas, multiple myeloma, osseous and nonosseous sarcomas, mesotheliomas, germ cell tumors of the ovary or testis, and carcinomas of the head and neck, thyroid, lung, breast, stomach, pancreas, liver, ovary, bladder, prostate, uterus, neuroblastoma, and Wilms' tumor.

Effect on Mental Status None reported

Effect on Psychiatric Treatment Myelosuppression is common; use caution with clozapine and carbamazepine

Dosage Summary

I.V.:

Children: 35-75 mg/m^2/dose every 21 days **or** 20-30 mg/m^2/dose once weekly **or** 60-90 mg/m^2 infusion over 96 hours every 3-4 weeks

Adults: 60-75 mg/m^2/dose every 21 days **or** 60 mg/m^2/dose every 2 weeks **or** 40-60 mg/m^2/dose every 3-4 weeks **or** 20-30 mg/m^2/day for 2-3 days every 4 weeks **or** 20 mg/m^2/dose once weekly.

Dosage Forms Excipient information presented when available (limited, particularly for generics); consult specific product labeling.

Injection, powder for reconstitution, as hydrochloride: 10 mg, 50 mg

Adriamycin®: 10 mg, 20 mg, 50 mg, [contains lactose]

Rubex®: 50 mg, 100 mg [contains lactose] [DSC]

Injection, solution, as hydrochloride: 2 mg/mL (5 mL, 10 mL, 25 mL, 100 mL)

Adriamycin®: 2 mg/mL (5 mL, 10 mL, 25 mL, 100 mL)

◆ **Doxorubicin Hydrochloride** *see* DOXOrubicin *on page 507*

◆ **DOXOrubicin Hydrochloride (Liposomal)** *see* DOXOrubicin (Liposomal) *on page 508*

DOXOrubicin (Liposomal) (doks oh ROO bi sin lip pah SOW mal)

Medication Safety Issues

Sound-alike/look-alike issues:

DOXOrubicin liposomal may be confused with DACTINomycin, DAUNOrubicin, DAUNOrubicin liposomal, doxacurium, doxapram, doxazosin, DOXOrubicin, epirubicin, IDArubicin

DOXOrubicin liposomal may be confused with DAUNOrubicin liposomal

Doxil® may be confused with Doxy®, Paxil®

Liposomal formulation (Doxil®) may be confused with the conventional formulation (Adriamycin PFS®, Adriamycin RDF®)

High alert medication: The Institute for Safe Medication Practices (ISMP) includes this medication among its list of drug classes which have a heightened risk of causing significant patient harm when used in error.

Use caution when selecting product for preparation and dispensing; indications, dosages and adverse event profiles differ between conventional DOXOrubicin hydrochloride solution and DOXOrubicin liposomal. Both formulations are the same concentration. As a result, serious errors have occurred. Liposomal formulation of doxorubicin should NOT be substituted for doxorubicin hydrochloride on a mg-per-mg basis.

U.S. Brand Names Doxil®

Canadian Brand Names Caelyx®

Mexican Brand Names Caelyx; Doxolem

Index Terms DOXOrubicin Hydrochloride (Liposomal); Liposomal DOXOrubicin; NSC-712227; Pegylated Liposomal DOXOrubicin

Pharmacologic Category Antineoplastic Agent, Anthracycline

Use Treatment of ovarian cancer, multiple myeloma, and AIDS-related Kaposi's sarcoma

Unlabeled/Investigational Use Treatment of metastatic breast cancer

Effect on Mental Status None reported

Effect on Psychiatric Treatment Myelosuppression is common; use caution with clozapine and carbamazepine

Dosage Summary

I.V.:

Children: Dosage not established

Adults: 20-30 mg/m^2 every 3 weeks **or** 50 mg/m^2/dose every 4 weeks

Dosage Forms Excipient information presented when available (limited, particularly for generics); consult specific product labeling.

Injection, solution, as hydrochloride: 2 mg/mL (10 mL, 25 mL)

◆ **Doxy-100®** *see* Doxycycline *on page 509*

Doxycycline (doks i SYE kleen)

Medication Safety Issues

Sound-alike/look-alike issues:

Doxycycline may be confused with dicyclomine, doxepin, doxylamine

Doxy-100® may be confused with Doxil®

Monodox® may be confused with Maalox®

Oracea™ may be confused with Orencia®

Vibramycin® may be confused with vancomycin

U.S. Brand Names Adoxa®; Doryx®; Doxy-100®; Monodox®; Oracea™; Periostat®; Vibra-Tabs®; Vibramycin®

Canadian Brand Names Apo-Doxy Tabs®; Apo-Doxy®; Doxycin; Doxytec; Novo-Doxylin; Nu-Doxycycline; Periostat®; Vibra-Tabs®

Mexican Brand Names Biomixin; Ciclonal; Domiken; Genobiotic-Doxi; Vibramicina; Vivradoxil

Index Terms Doxycycline Calcium; Doxycycline Hyclate; Doxycycline Monohydrate

Pharmacologic Category Antibiotic, Tetracycline Derivative

Use Principally in the treatment of infections caused by susceptible *Rickettsia*, *Chlamydia*, and *Mycoplasma*; alternative to mefloquine for malaria prophylaxis; treatment for syphilis, uncomplicated *Neisseria gonorrhoeae*, *Listeria*, *Actinomyces israelii*, and *Clostridium* infections in penicillin-allergic patients; used for community-acquired pneumonia and other common infections due to susceptible organisms; anthrax due to *Bacillus anthracis*, including inhalational anthrax (postexposure); treatment of infections caused by uncommon susceptible gram-negative and gram-positive organisms including *Borrelia recurrentis*, *Ureaplasma urealyticum*, *Haemophilus ducreyi*, *Yersinia pestis*, *Francisella tularensis*, *Vibrio cholerae*, *Campylobacter fetus*, *Brucella* spp, *Bartonella bacilliformis*, and *Calymmatobacterium granulomatis*, Q fever, Lyme disease; treatment of inflammatory lesions associated with rosacea; intestinal amebiasis; severe acne

Unlabeled/Investigational Use Sclerosing agent for pleural effusion injection; vancomycin-resistant enterococci (VRE)

Effect on Mental Status Tetracyclines have been reported to cause memory disturbance, mood stabilizing and antidepressant effects

Effect on Psychiatric Treatment May cause neutropenia; use caution with clozapine and carbamazepine; barbiturates and carbamazepine increase the clearance of doxycycline

Dosage Summary

I.V.:

Children ≤8 years: Anthrax: 2.2 mg/kg every 12 hours

Children >8 years and ≤45 kg: 2-5 mg/kg/day in 1-2 divided doses (maximum: 200 mg/day)

Children >8 years and >45 kg: 100-200 mg/day in 1-2 divided doses

Adults: 100-200 mg/day in 1-2 divided doses

Oral:

Children ≤8 years: Anthrax: 2.2 mg/kg every 12 hours

Children >8 years and ≤45 kg: 2-5 mg/kg/day in 1-2 divided doses (maximum: 200 mg/day)

Children >8 years and >45 kg: 100-200 mg/day in 1-2 divided doses

Adults: 100-200 mg/day in 1-2 divided doses **or** 300 mg as a single dose (*Vibrio cholerae*) **or** 40 mg once daily (rosacea; Oracea™) **or** 20 mg twice daily (Periostat®)

Dosage Forms Excipient information presented when available (limited, particularly for generics); consult specific product labeling. [DSC] = Discontinued product

Note: Strength expressed as base.

Capsule, as hyclate: 50 mg, 100 mg
- Vibramycin®: 100 mg

Capsule, as monohydrate: 50 mg, 100 mg
- Monodox®: 50 mg, 75 mg, 100 mg

Capsule, variable release:
- Oracea™: 40 mg [30 mg (immediate-release) and 10 mg (delayed-release)]

Injection, powder for reconstitution, as hyclate: 100 mg
- Doxy-100®: 100 mg

Powder for oral suspension, as monohydrate: 25 mg/5 mL (60 mL)
- Vibramycin®: 25 mg/5 mL (60 mL) [raspberry flavor]

Syrup, as calcium:
- Vibramycin®: 50 mg/5 mL (480 mL) [contains sodium metabisulfite; raspberry-apple flavor]

Tablet, as hyclate: 20 mg, 100 mg
- Periostat®: 20 mg
- Vibra-Tabs®: 100 mg

Tablet, as monohydrate: 50 mg, 75 mg, 100 mg, 150 mg
- Adoxa®: 50 mg, 75 mg, 100 mg
- Adoxa® Pak™ 1/75 [unit-dose pack]: 75 mg (31s)
- Adoxa® Pak™ 1/100 [unit-dose pack]: 100 mg (31s)
- Adoxa® Pak™ 1/150 [unit-dose pack]: 150 mg (30s)
- Adoxa® Pak™ 2/100 [unit-dose pack]: 100 mg (60s)

Tablet, delayed-release coated pellets, as hyclate:
- Doryx®: 75 mg [contains sodium 4.5 mg (0.196 mEq); 100 mg [contains sodium 6 mg (0.261 mEq)]; 150 mg [contains sodium 9 mg (0.392 mEq)]

◆ **Doxycycline Calcium** *see* Doxycycline *on page 509*

◆ **Doxycycline Hyclate** *see* Doxycycline *on page 509*

◆ **Doxycycline Monohydrate** *see* Doxycycline *on page 509*

Doxylamine (dox IL a meen)

Medication Safety Issues

Sound-alike/look-alike issues:

Doxylamine may be confused with doxycycline

Related Information

Nonbenzodiazepine Anxiolytics and Hypnotics *on page 1791*

U.S. Brand Names Aldex® AN; Good Sense Sleep Aid [OTC]; Unisom® SleepTabs® [OTC]

Canadian Brand Names Unisom®-2

Index Terms Doxylamine Succinate

Pharmacologic Category Histamine H_1 Antagonist; Histamine H_1 Antagonist, First Generation

Generic Available Yes

Use Treatment of short-term insomnia

Effect on Mental Status May cause drowsiness, dizziness, disorientation, and paradoxical excitement

Effect on Psychiatric Treatment Concomitant use with psychotropic agents (including valerian, St John's wort, and kava kava) will produce additive sedative and anticholinergic effects. Conversely, the effects of cholinergic agonist will be ameliorated.

Pregnancy Risk Factor B

Pregnancy Considerations Doxylamine has been approved for used in pregnancy-associated nausea and vomiting.

Lactation Excretion in breast milk unknown

Contraindications Hypersensitivity to doxylamine or any component of the formulation

Warnings/Precautions May cause drowsiness; patient should avoid tasks requiring alertness (eg, driving, operating machinery) until effects are known. Sedative effects of CNS depressants or ethanol are potentiated. Use with caution in patients with angle-closure glaucoma, respiratory disease, urinary tract obstruction (including bladder neck obstruction and symptomatic prostatic hyperplasia), thyroid dysfunction, increased intraocular pressure, and cardiovascular disease (including hypertension and ischemic heart disease). If sleeplessness persists for >2 weeks, consult healthcare provider. Safety and efficacy not established in children <12 years of age.

Adverse Reactions Frequency not defined.

Cardiovascular: Palpitation, tachycardia

Central nervous system: Dizziness, disorientation, drowsiness, headache, paradoxical CNS stimulation, vertigo

Gastrointestinal: Anorexia, dry mucous membranes, diarrhea, constipation, epigastric pain, xerostomia

Genitourinary: Dysuria, urinary retention

Ocular: Blurred vision, diplopia

Drug Interactions

Acetylcholinesterase Inhibitors (Central): Anticholinergics may diminish the therapeutic effect of Acetylcholinesterase Inhibitors (Central). Acetylcholinesterase Inhibitors (Central) may diminish the therapeutic effect of Anticholinergics. If the anticholinergic action is a side effect of the agent, the result may be beneficial. *Risk C: Monitor therapy*

Alcohol (Ethyl): CNS Depressants may enhance the CNS depressant effect of Alcohol (Ethyl). *Risk C: Monitor therapy*

Amphetamines: May diminish the sedative effect of Antihistamines. *Risk C: Monitor therapy*

Anticholinergics: May enhance the adverse/toxic effect of other Anticholinergics. **Exceptions:** Paliperidone. *Risk C: Monitor therapy*

Betahistine: Antihistamines may diminish the therapeutic effect of Betahistine. *Risk C: Monitor therapy*

CNS Depressants: May enhance the adverse/toxic effect of other CNS Depressants. *Risk C: Monitor therapy*

Pramlintide: May enhance the anticholinergic effect of Anticholinergics. These effects are specific to the GI tract. *Risk D: Consider therapy modification*

Ethanol/Nutrition/Herb Interactions

Ethanol: Avoid ethanol (may increase CNS depression).

Herb/Nutraceutical: Avoid valerian, St John's wort, kava kava, gotu kola (may increase CNS depression).

Stability Store at 15°C to 30°C (59°F to 86°F).

Mechanism of Action Doxylamine competes with histamine for H_1-receptor sites on effector cells; blocks chemoreceptor trigger zone, diminishes vestibular stimulation, and depresses labyrinthine function through its central anticholinergic activity.

Pharmacodynamics/Kinetics

Absorption: Well absorbed

Distribution: V_d: 2.5 L/kg

Metabolism: Via multiple metabolic pathways including N-demethylation, oxidation, hydroxylation, N-acetylation to metabolites including nordoxylamine, dinordoxylamine

Half-life elimination: 10-12 hours

Excretion: Urine (primarily as metabolites)

Dosage Oral: Adults: One tablet 30 minutes before bedtime; once daily or as instructed by healthcare professional

Dosage adjustment in renal impairment: No dosage adjustment required

Administration Main dose should be taken at bedtime to provide relief in the early morning hours.

Dosage Forms Excipient information presented when available (limited, particularly for generics); consult specific product labeling.

Tablet, as succinate:

Good Sense Sleep Aid, Unisom® SleepTabs®: 25 mg

Tablet, chewable, as succinate:

Aldex® AN: 5 mg [orange flavor]

Doxylamine and Pyridoxine (dox IL a meen & peer i DOX een)

Medication Safety Issues

Sound-alike/look-alike issues:

Doxylamine may be confused with doxycycline

Canadian Brand Names Diclectin®

Index Terms Doxylamine Succinate and Pyridoxine Hydrochloride; Pyridoxine and Doxylamine

Pharmacologic Category Histamine H_1 Antagonist; Histamine H_1 Antagonist, First Generation; Vitamin, Water Soluble

Use Treatment of pregnancy-associated nausea and vomiting

Effect on Mental Status May cause drowsiness, dizziness, disorientation, and paradoxical excitement

Effect on Psychiatric Treatment Concomitant use with psychotropic agents (including valerian, St John's wort, and kava kava) will produce additive sedative and anticholinergic effects. Conversely, the effects of cholinergic agonist will be ameliorated.

Restrictions Not available in U.S.

Dosage Summary

Oral:

Children: Dosage not established

Adults: 2 tablets (a total of doxylamine 20 mg and pyridoxine 20 mg) at bedtime, may increase by 1 tablet in the morning and/or afternoon in severe cases

Dosage Forms Excipient information presented when available (limited, particularly for generics); consult specific product labeling. [CAN] = Canadian brand name

Tablet, delayed release:

Diclectin® [CAN]: Doxylamine 10 mg and pyridoxine 10 mg [not available in the U.S.]

- **Doxylamine Succinate** *see* Doxylamine *on page 510*
- **Doxylamine Succinate and Pyridoxine Hydrochloride** *see* Doxylamine and Pyridoxine *on page 511*
- **Doxylamine Succinate, Codeine Phosphate, and Acetaminophen** *see* Acetaminophen, Codeine, and Doxylamine *on page 41*
- **DPA** *see* Valproic Acid and Derivatives *on page 1642*
- **D-Penicillamine** *see* Penicillamine *on page 1239*
- **DPH** *see* Phenytoin *on page 1280*
- **D-Phen 1000** *see* Guaifenesin and Phenylephrine *on page 742*
- **Dramamine® [OTC]** *see* DimenhyDRINATE *on page 478*
- **Dramamine® Less Drowsy Formula [OTC]** *see* Meclizine *on page 974*
- **Dried Smallpox Vaccine** *see* Smallpox Vaccine *on page 1493*
- **Driminate® [OTC]** *see* DimenhyDRINATE *on page 478*
- **Drinex [OTC]** *see* Acetaminophen, Chlorpheniramine, and Pseudoephedrine *on page 40*
- **Drisdol®** *see* Ergocalciferol *on page 550*
- **Dristan™ 12-Hour [OTC]** *see* Oxymetazoline *on page 1208*
- **Drixoral® Cold & Allergy [OTC]** *see* Dexbrompheniramine and Pseudoephedrine *on page 437*

Dronabinol (droe NAB i nol)

Medication Safety Issues

Sound-alike/look-alike issues:

Dronabinol may be confused with droperidol

U.S. Brand Names Marinol®

Canadian Brand Names Marinol®

Index Terms Delta-9 THC; Delta-9-tetrahydro-cannabinol; Tetrahydrocannabinol; THC

Pharmacologic Category Antiemetic; Appetite Stimulant

Use Chemotherapy-associated nausea and vomiting refractory to other antiemetic(s); AIDS-related anorexia

Unlabeled/Investigational Use Cancer-related anorexia

Effect on Mental Status Drowsiness, anxiety, confusion, and mood changes are common; may cause depression or hallucinations

Effect on Psychiatric Treatment Concurrent use with barbiturates and benzodiazepines produce additive sedation

Restrictions C-III

Dosage Summary

Oral:

Children: Initial: 5 mg/m^2 before chemotherapy, then 5 mg/m^2/dose every 2-4 hours after chemotherapy for a total of 4-6 doses/day; Titration: Increase in increments of 2.5 mg/m^2 (maximum: 15 mg/m^2/dose)

Adults:

Antiemetic: Initial: 5 mg/m^2 before chemotherapy, then 5 mg/m^2/dose every 2-4 hours after chemotherapy for a total of 4-6 doses/day; Titration: Increase in increments of 2.5 mg/m^2 (maximum: 15 mg/m^2/dose)

Appetite stimulant: Initial: 2.5 mg twice daily; Maintenance: Titrate up to 20 mg/day in 2 divided doses

Dosage Forms Excipient information presented when available (limited, particularly for generics); consult specific product labeling.

Capsule, soft gelatin: 2.5 mg, 5 mg, 10 mg

Marinol®: 2.5 mg, 5 mg, 10 mg [contains sesame oil]

Droperidol (droe PER i dole)

Medication Safety Issues

Sound-alike/look-alike issues:

Droperidol may be confused with dronabinol

Inapsine® may be confused with Nebcin®

Related Information

Discontinuation of Psychotropic Drugs *on page 1839*

U.S. Brand Names Inapsine®

Canadian Brand Names Droperidol Injection, USP

Index Terms Dehydrobenzperidol

Pharmacologic Category Antiemetic; Antipsychotic Agent, Typical

Generic Available Yes

Use Antiemetic in surgical and diagnostic procedures; preoperative medication in patients when other treatments are ineffective or inappropriate

Effect on Psychiatric Treatment Contraindicated with ziprasidone

Mental Health Comment Primarily reserved as an agent in acute or intensive care setting for patients in whom rapid control of symptoms/behavior is needed.

In 2008, the FDA issued a warning regarding increased mortality risk with typical **and** atypical antipsychotic drugs when used in elderly patients with dementia-related psychosis.

Pregnancy Risk Factor C

Pregnancy Considerations Crosses the placenta

Lactation Excretion in breast milk unknown

Contraindications Hypersensitivity to droperidol or any component of the formulation; known or suspected QT prolongation, including congenital long QT syndrome (prolonged QT_c is defined as >440 msec in males or >450 msec in females)

Warnings/Precautions May alter cardiac conduction. **[U.S. Boxed Warning]: Cases of QT prolongation and torsade de pointes, including some fatal cases, have been reported.** Use extreme caution in patients with bradycardia (<50 bpm), cardiac disease, concurrent MAO inhibitor therapy, Class I and Class III antiarrhythmics or other drugs known to prolong QT interval, and electrolyte disturbances (hypokalemia or hypomagnesemia), including concomitant drugs which may alter electrolytes (diuretics).

Use with caution in patients with seizures or severe liver disease. May be sedating, use with caution in disorders where CNS depression is a feature. Caution in patients with hemodynamic instability, predisposition to seizures, subcortical brain damage, pheochromocytoma or renal disease. Esophageal dysmotility and aspiration have been associated with antipsychotic use - use with caution in patients at risk of pneumonia (ie, Alzheimer's disease). Caution in breast cancer or other prolactin-dependent tumors (may elevate prolactin levels). May alter temperature regulation or mask toxicity of other drugs due to antiemetic effects. May cause orthostatic hypotension - use with caution in patients at risk of this effect or those who would tolerate transient hypotensive episodes (cerebrovascular disease, cardiovascular disease, or other medications which may predispose). Significant hypotension may occur; injection contains benzyl alcohol; injection also contains sulfites which may cause allergic reaction.

May cause anticholinergic effects (confusion, agitation, constipation, xerostomia, blurred vision, urinary retention). Therefore, they should be used with caution in patients with decreased gastrointestinal motility, urinary retention, BPH, xerostomia, or visual problems. Conditions which also may be exacerbated by cholinergic blockade include narrow-angle glaucoma (screening is recommended) and worsening of myasthenia gravis. Relative to other neuroleptics, droperidol has a low potency of cholinergic blockade.

May cause extrapyramidal symptoms (EPS), including pseudoparkinsonism, acute dystonic reactions, akathisia, and tardive dyskinesia (risk of these reactions is high relative to other neuroleptics). Risk of dystonia (and possibly other EPS) may be greater with increased doses, use of conventional antipsychotics, males, and younger patients. May be associated with neuroleptic malignant syndrome (NMS) or pigmentary retinopathy. May mask toxicity of other drugs or conditions (eg, intestinal obstruction, Reye's syndrome, brain tumor) due to antiemetic effects. Use with caution in the elderly; reduce initial dose. Safety in children <2 years of age has not been established.

Adverse Reactions

>10%:

Cardiovascular: QT_c prolongation (dose dependent)

Central nervous system: Restlessness, anxiety, extrapyramidal symptoms, dystonic reactions, pseudoparkinsonian signs and symptoms, tardive dyskinesia, seizure, altered central temperature regulation, sedation, drowsiness

Endocrine & metabolic: Swelling of breasts

Gastrointestinal: Weight gain, constipation

1% to 10%:

Cardiovascular: Hypotension (especially orthostatic), tachycardia, abnormal T waves with prolonged ventricular repolarization, hypertension

Central nervous system: Hallucinations, persistent tardive dyskinesia, akathisia

Gastrointestinal: Nausea, vomiting

Genitourinary: Dysuria

<1% (Limited to important or life-threatening): Adynamic ileus, agranulocytosis, alopecia, arrhythmia, cholestatic jaundice, heat stroke, hyperpigmentation, laryngospasm, leukopenia, neuroleptic malignant syndrome (NMS), obstructive jaundice, photosensitivity (rare), priapism, rash, respiratory depression, retinal pigmentation, tardive dystonia, torsade de pointes, urinary retention, ventricular tachycardia, visual acuity decreased (may be irreversible)

Drug Interactions

Acetylcholinesterase Inhibitors (Central): May enhance the neurotoxic (central) effect of Antipsychotics. Severe extrapyramidal symptoms have occurred in some patients. *Risk C: Monitor therapy*

Alcohol (Ethyl): CNS Depressants may enhance the CNS depressant effect of Alcohol (Ethyl). *Risk C: Monitor therapy*

Alfuzosin: May enhance the QTc-prolonging effect of QTc-Prolonging Agents. *Risk C: Monitor therapy*

Amphetamines: Antipsychotics may diminish the stimulatory effect of Amphetamines. *Risk C: Monitor therapy*

Anticholinergics: May enhance the adverse/toxic effect of other Anticholinergics. **Exceptions:** Paliperidone. *Risk C: Monitor therapy*

Anti-Parkinson's Agents (Dopamine Agonist): Antipsychotics (Typical) may diminish the therapeutic effect of Anti-Parkinson's Agents (Dopamine Agonist). *Risk D: Consider therapy modification*

Ciprofloxacin: May enhance the QTc-prolonging effect of QTc-Prolonging Agents. *Risk C: Monitor therapy*

CNS Depressants: May enhance the adverse/toxic effect of other CNS Depressants. *Risk C: Monitor therapy*

Gadobutrol: May enhance the QTc-prolonging effect of QTc-Prolonging Agents. *Risk D: Consider therapy modification*

Lithium formulations: May enhance the neurotoxic effect of Antipsychotics. Lithium formulations may decrease the serum concentration of Antipsychotics. Specifically noted with chlorpromazine. *Risk C: Monitor therapy*

Nilotinib: May enhance the QTc-prolonging effect of QTc-Prolonging Agents. *Risk X: Avoid combination*

Pramlintide: May enhance the anticholinergic effect of Anticholinergics. These effects are specific to the GI tract. *Risk D: Consider therapy modification*

QTc-Prolonging Agents: May enhance the adverse/toxic effect of other QTc-Prolonging Agents. Their effects can be additive, causing life-threatening ventricular arrhythmias. *Risk D: Consider therapy modification*

Tetrabenazine: May enhance the adverse/toxic effect of Antipsychotics. *Risk C: Monitor therapy*

Thioridazine: QTc-Prolonging Agents may enhance the QTc-prolonging effect of Thioridazine. *Risk X: Avoid combination*

Ziprasidone: QTc-Prolonging Agents may enhance the QTc-prolonging effect of Ziprasidone. The risk of a severe arrhythmia may be increased. *Risk X: Avoid combination*

Stability Droperidol ampuls/vials should be stored at room temperature and protected from light. Solutions diluted in NS or D_5W are stable at room temperature for up to 7 days.

Mechanism of Action Droperidol is a butyrophenone antipsychotic; antiemetic effect is a result of blockade of dopamine stimulation of the chemoreceptor trigger zone. Other effects include alpha-adrenergic blockade, peripheral vascular dilation, and reduction of the pressor effect of epinephrine resulting in hypotension and decreased peripheral vascular resistance; may also reduce pulmonary artery pressure

Pharmacodynamics/Kinetics

Onset of action: Peak effect: Parenteral: ~30 minutes

Duration: Parenteral: 2-4 hours, may extend to 12 hours

Absorption: I.M.: Rapid

Distribution: Crosses blood-brain barrier and placenta

V_d: Children: ~0.25-0.9 L/kg; Adults: ~2 L/kg

Protein binding: Extensive

Metabolism: Hepatic, to *p*-fluorophenylacetic acid, benzimidazolone, *p*-hydroxypiperidine

Half-life elimination: Adults: 2.3 hours

Excretion: Urine (75%, <1% as unchanged drug); feces (22%, 11% to 50% as unchanged drug)

Dosage Titrate carefully to desired effect

Children 2-12 years: Nausea and vomiting: I.M., I.V.: 0.05-0.06 mg/kg (maximum initial dose: 0.1 mg/kg); additional doses may be repeated to achieve effect; administer additional doses with caution

Adults: Prevention of postoperative nausea and vomiting (PONV): I.M., I.V.: Initial: 0.625-2.5 mg; additional doses of 1.25 mg may be administered to achieve desired effect; administer additional doses with caution. Consensus guidelines recommend 0.625-1.25 mg I.V. administered after surgery (Gan, 2003).

Administration Administer I.M. or I.V.; according to the manufacturer, I.V. push administration should be slow (generally regarded as 2-5 minutes); however, many clinicians administer I.V. doses rapidly (over 30-60 seconds) in an effort to reduce the incidence of EPS. The effect, if any, of rapid administration on QT prolongation is unclear. For I.V. infusion, dilute in 50-100 mL NS or D_5W; ECG monitoring for 2-3 hours after administration is recommended regardless of rate of infusion.

Monitoring Parameters To identify QT prolongation, a 12-lead ECG prior to use is recommended; continued ECG monitoring for 2-3 hours following administration is recommended. Vital signs; lipid profile, fasting blood glucose/ Hgb A_{1c}, serum magnesium and potassium; BMI; mental status, abnormal involuntary movement scale (AIMS); observe for dystonias, extrapyramidal side effects, and temperature changes

Additional Information Does not possess analgesic effects; has little or no amnesic properties.

Dosage Forms Excipient information presented when available (limited, particularly for generics); consult specific product labeling.

Injection, solution [preservative free]: 2.5 mg/mL (1 mL, 2 mL)

Inapsine®: 2.5 mg/mL (1 mL, 2 mL)

Drospirenone and Estradiol (droh SPYE re none & es tra DYE ole)

U.S. Brand Names Angeliq®

Canadian Brand Names Angeliq®

Index Terms E2 and DRSP; Estradiol and Drospirenone

Pharmacologic Category Estrogen and Progestin Combination

Use Treatment of moderate-to-severe vasomotor symptoms associated with menopause; treatment of vulvar and vaginal atrophy associated with menopause

Effect on Mental Status May cause depression or other mood disturbances

Effect on Psychiatric Treatment Combined use with carbamazepine, felbamate, phenobarbital, phenytoin, or topiramate may increase the metabolism of ethinyl estradiol and/or some progestins, leading to possible decrease in contraceptive effectiveness. Estrogens may elevate triglycerides; combined use with clozapine, olanzapine, or quetiapine may produce additive risks; monitor lipid profile.

Mental Health Comment The role of hormone replacement therapy for postmenopausal women continues to evolve, given findings from a large-scale women's health initiative, which suggested a small but significant increased risk of dementia. Seizure frequency may also be increased in menopausal women with epilepsy.

Dosage Summary

Oral:

Children: Dosage not established

Adults (females): One tablet daily

Dosage Forms Excipient information presented when available (limited, particularly for generics); consult specific product labeling.

Tablet: Drospirenone 0.5 mg and estradiol 1 mg

- **Drospirenone and Ethinyl Estradiol** *see* Ethinyl Estradiol and Drospirenone *on page 593*
- **DroTuss-CP** *see* Phenylephrine, Hydrocodone, and Chlorpheniramine *on page 1277*
- **Droxia®** *see* Hydroxyurea *on page 796*
- **DSCG** *see* Cromolyn *on page 402*
- **D-Ser(Bu^{t})^{6},Azgly^{10}-LHRH** *see* Goserelin *on page 735*
- **D-Tann** *see* Diphenhydramine and Phenylephrine *on page 485*
- **D-Tann HC [DSC]** *see* Hydrocodone, Phenylephrine, and Diphenhydramine *on page 782*
- **DTaP/IPV/HepB** *see* Diphtheria, Tetanus Toxoids, Acellular Pertussis, Hepatitis B (Recombinant), and Poliovirus (Inactivated) Vaccine *on page 487*
- **DTIC** *see* Dacarbazine *on page 414*
- **DTO (error-prone abbreviation)** *see* Opium Tincture *on page 1183*
- **D-Trp(6)-LHRH** *see* Triptorelin *on page 1635*
- **Duetact™** *see* Pioglitazone and Glimepiride *on page 1300*
- **Dull-C® [OTC]** *see* Ascorbic Acid *on page 141*

DULoxetine (doo LOX e teen)

Medication Safety Issues

Sound-alike/look-alike issues:

DULoxetine may be confused with FLUoxetine

Related Information

Antidepressant Agents *on page 1760*

Antidepressant Receptor Profile *on page 1764*

U.S. Brand Names Cymbalta®

Canadian Brand Names Cymbalta®

Mexican Brand Names Cymbalta; Yentreve

Index Terms (+)-(*S*)-*N*-Methyl-γ-(1-naphthyloxy)-2-thiophenepropylamine Hydrochloride; Duloxetine Hydrochloride; LY248686

Pharmacologic Category Antidepressant, Serotonin/Norepinephrine Reuptake Inhibitor

Generic Available No

Use Acute and maintenance treatment of major depressive disorder (MDD); treatment of generalized anxiety disorder (GAD); management of pain associated with diabetic neuropathy; management of fibromyalgia

Unlabeled/Investigational Use Treatment of stress incontinence; management of chronic pain syndromes

Restrictions An FDA-approved medication guide concerning the use of antidepressants in children, adolescents, and young adults must be distributed when dispensing an outpatient prescription (new or refill) where this medication is to be used without direct supervision of a healthcare provider. Medication guides are available at http://www.fda.gov/cder/Offices/ODS/medication_guides.htm. Dispense to parents or guardians of children and adolescents receiving this medication.

Pregnancy Risk Factor C

Pregnancy Considerations Duloxetine is classified as pregnancy category C due to adverse effects observed in animal studies. Nonteratogenic effects in the newborn following SSRI/SNRI exposure late in the third trimester include respiratory distress, cyanosis, apnea, seizures, temperature instability, feeding difficulty, vomiting, hypoglycemia, hyper- or hypotonia, hyper-reflexia, jitteriness, irritability, constant crying, and tremor. The long-term effects on neurobehavior have not been studied.

Women treated for major depression and who are euthymic prior to pregnancy are more likely to experience a relapse when medication is discontinued as compared to pregnant women who continue taking antidepressant medications. The ACOG recommends that therapy with SSRIs or SNRIs during pregnancy be individualized; treatment of depression during pregnancy should incorporate the clinical expertise of the mental health clinician, obstetrician, primary healthcare provider, and pediatrician. If treatment during pregnancy is required, consider tapering therapy during the third trimester in order to prevent withdrawal symptoms in the infant. If this is done and the woman is considered to be at risk of relapse from her major depressive disorder, the medication can be restarted following delivery, although the dose should be readjusted to that required before pregnancy.

Lactation Enters breast milk/not recommended

Contraindications Concomitant use or within 2 weeks of MAO inhibitors; uncontrolled narrow-angle glaucoma

Canadian labeling: Additional contraindications (not in U.S. labeling): Hypersensitivity to duloxetine or any component of the formulation; hepatic impairment; severe renal impairment (eg, Cl_{cr} <30 mL/minute) or end-stage renal disease (ESRD); concomitant use with thioridazine or with CYP1A2 inhibitors

Warnings/Precautions [U.S. Boxed Warning]: Antidepressants increase the risk of suicidal thinking and behavior in children, adolescents, and young adults (18-24 years of age) with major depressive disorder (MDD) and other psychiatric disorders; consider risk prior to prescribing. Short-term studies did not show an increased risk in patients >24 years of age and showed a decreased risk in patients ≥65 years. Closely monitor for clinical worsening, suicidality, or unusual changes in behavior; the patient's family or caregiver should be instructed to closely observe the patient and communicate condition with healthcare provider. A medication guide concerning the use of antidepressants in children and teenagers should be dispensed with each prescription. **Duloxetine is not FDA approved for use in children.**

The possibility of a suicide attempt is inherent in major depression and may persist until remission occurs. Patients treated with antidepressants should be observed for clinical worsening and suicidality, especially during the initial (generally first 1-2 months) few months of a course of drug therapy, or at times of dose changes, either increases or decreases. Use caution in high-risk patients. Worsening depression and severe abrupt suicidality that are not part of the presenting symptoms may require discontinuation or modification of drug therapy. The patient's family or caregiver should be alerted to monitor patients for the emergence of suicidality and associated behaviors (such as agitation, irritability, hostility, impulsivity, and hypomania) and call healthcare provider.

May worsen psychosis in some patients or precipitate a shift to mania or hypomania in patients with bipolar disorder. Patients presenting with depressive symptoms should be screened for bipolar disorder. Monotherapy in patients with bipolar disorder should be avoided. **Duloxetine is not FDA approved for the treatment of bipolar depression.**

May cause orthostatic hypotension/syncope at therapeutic doses especially within the first week of therapy and after dose increases. Monitor blood pressure with initiation of therapy, dose increases (especially in patients receiving >60 mg/day), or with concomitant use of vasodilators or CYP1A2 inhibitors. Use caution in patients with hypertension. May increase blood pressure. Rare cases of hypertensive crisis have been reported in patients with pre-existing hypertension; evaluate blood pressure prior to initiating therapy and periodically thereafter; consider dose reduction or gradual discontinuation of therapy in individuals with sustained hypertension during therapy.

Modest increases in serum glucose and hemoglobin A_{1c} (Hb A_{1c}) levels have been observed in some diabetic patients receiving duloxetine therapy for diabetic peripheral neuropathy (DPN). Duloxetine may cause increased urinary resistance; advise patient to report symptoms of urinary hesitation/difficulty. Has a low potential to impair cognitive or motor performance. Use caution with a previous seizure disorder or condition predisposing to seizures such as brain damage or alcoholism. Avoid use in patients with substantial ethanol intake, evidence of chronic liver disease, or hepatic impairment (contraindicated in Canadian labeling). Rare cases of hepatic failure (including fatalities) have been reported with use. Hepatitis with abdominal pain, hepatomegaly, elevated transaminase levels >20 times the upper limit of normal (ULN) with and without jaundice have all been observed. Discontinue therapy with the presentation of jaundice or other signs of hepatic dysfunction and do not reinitiate therapy unless another source or cause is identified.

May cause hyponatremia/SIADH (elderly at increased risk); volume depletion (diuretics may increase risk). Use with caution in patients with controlled narrow angle glaucoma. May cause or exacerbate sexual dysfunction. Use caution with renal impairment (contraindicated in Canadian labeling for severe renal impairment or ESRD). Use caution with concomitant CNS depressants. May impair platelet aggregation; use caution with concomitant use of NSAIDs, ASA, or other drugs that affect coagulation; the risk of bleeding may be potentiated.

A potential exists for severe reactions when used with MAO inhibitors, SSRIs/SNRIs or triptans; serotonin syndrome (hyperthermia, muscular rigidity, mental status changes/agitation, autonomic instability) may occur. Use caution during concurrent therapy with other drugs which lower the seizure threshold. To discontinue therapy with duloxetine, gradually taper dose. If intolerable symptoms occur following a decrease in dosage or upon discontinuation of therapy, then resuming the previous dose with a more gradual taper should be considered. May increase the risks associated with electroconvulsive therapy. Consider discontinuing, when possible, prior to elective surgery. Formulation contains sucrose; patients with fructose intolerance, glucose-galactose malabsorption, or sucrose-isomaltase deficiency should avoid use. Safety and efficacy have not been established in patients <18 years of age.

Adverse Reactions

>10%:

Central nervous system: Fatigue (2% to 15%), somnolence (7% to 21%), dizziness (6% to 17%), headache (13% to 20%), insomnia (8% to 16%)

Gastrointestinal: Nausea (14% to 30%), xerostomia (5% to 18%), diarrhea (7% to 13%), constipation (5% to 15%), appetite decreased (3% to 11%)

1% to 10%:

Cardiovascular: Palpitation (1% to 2%)

Central nervous system: Agitation (5% to 6%), anxiety (3%), sleep disorder (3%), dreams abnormal (2% to 3%), fever (1% to 3%), yawning (1% to 2%), hypoesthesia (1%), lethargy (1%), nightmares (1%), vertigo (1%)

Dermatologic: Hyperhydrosis (6% to 8%), rash (4%), pruritus (3%)

Endocrine & metabolic: Libido decreased (2% to 4%), orgasm abnormality (3%), hot flushes (2% to 3%), anorgasmia (1%)

Gastrointestinal: Vomiting (5% to 6%), dyspepsia (4% to 5%), anorexia (3% to 5%), loose stools (2% to 3%), taste abnormal (1% to 3%), weight gain/loss (2%), flatulence (1%)

Genitourinary: Erectile dysfunction (1% to 5%), pollakiuria (1% to 5%), ejaculatory dysfunction (2% to 4%), ejaculation delayed (3%), penis disorder (2%)

Hepatic: ALT >3x ULN (1%)

Neuromuscular & skeletal: Weakness (2% to 8%), musculoskeletal pain (1% to 5%), muscle cramp (4% to 5%), muscle spasms (4%), tremor (3% to 4%), myalgia (1% to 4%), paresthesia (1%), rigors (1%)

Ocular: Blurred vision (1% to 3%)

Respiratory: Nasopharyngitis (7% to 9%), upper respiratory infection (7%), cough (3% to 6%), pharyngolaryngeal pain (1% to 6%)

Miscellaneous: Diaphoresis increased (6%), seasonal allergies (3%)

<1% (Limited to important or life-threatening): Abdominal pain, acne, agitation, aggression, alkaline phosphatase increased, alopecia, anaphylactic reaction, anger, anemia, angioneurotic edema, aphthous stomatitis, ataxia, atrial fibrillation, bloody stools, bundle branch block, CHF, colitis, CPK increased, dehydration, diastolic blood pressure increased, diplopia, disorientation, diverticulitis, dysarthria, dyskinesia, dyslipidemia, dysphagia, dysuria, ecchymosis, eczema, edema (peripheral), erythema, erythema multiforme, esophageal stenosis, EPS, facial edema, flu-like syndrome, flushing, gastric emptying impaired, gastric ulcer, gastritis, gastroenteritis, GI bleeding, gingivitis, glaucoma, hallucinations, Hb A_{1c} increased, hematochezia, hepatic failure, hepatic steatosis, hepatitis, hepatomegaly, hyperbilirubinemia, hypercholesterolemia, hyperglycemia, hyperlipidemia, hypersensitivity, hypertensive crisis, hyponatremia, hypothyroidism, irritability, irritable bowel syndrome, jaundice, keroconjunctivitis sicca, laryngitis, leukopenia, lymphadenopathy, macular degeneration, maculopathy, malaise, mania, melena, MI, micturition urgency, mood swings, muscle spasm, muscle tightness, muscle twitching, nephropathy, night sweats, nocturia, oropharyngeal edema, orthostatic hypotension, peripheral coldness, phlebitis, photosensitivity, polyuria, retinal detachment, seizure, serotonin syndrome, sexual dysfunction, SIADH, Stevens-Johnson syndrome, stomatitis, suicide, supraventricular arrhythmia, syncope, systolic blood pressure increased, tachycardia, thirst, throat tightness, thrombocytopenia, tinnitus, transaminases increased, trismus, urinary retention, urticaria, visual disturbance; withdrawal syndrome (including headache, dizziness, nightmares, irritability, paresthesia, and/or vomiting)

Metabolism/Transport Effects Substrate (major) of CYP1A2, 2D6; **inhibits** CYP2D6 (moderate)

Drug Interactions

Alcohol (Ethyl): CNS Depressants may enhance the CNS depressant effect of Alcohol (Ethyl). *Risk C: Monitor therapy*

Aspirin: Antidepressants (Serotonin/Norepinephrine Reuptake Inhibitor) may enhance the antiplatelet effect of Aspirin. *Risk C: Monitor therapy*

CNS Depressants: May enhance the adverse/toxic effect of other CNS Depressants. *Risk C: Monitor therapy*

Codeine: CYP2D6 Inhibitors (Moderate) may diminish the therapeutic effect of Codeine. These CYP2D6 inhibitors may prevent the metabolic conversion of codeine to its active metabolite morphine. *Risk C: Monitor therapy*

CYP1A2 Inducers (Strong): May increase the metabolism of CYP1A2 Substrates. *Risk C: Monitor therapy*

CYP1A2 Inhibitors (Moderate): May decrease the metabolism of CYP1A2 Substrates. *Risk C: Monitor therapy*

CYP1A2 Inhibitors (Strong): May decrease the metabolism of CYP1A2 Substrates. *Risk D: Consider therapy modification*

CYP2D6 Inhibitors (Moderate): May decrease the metabolism of CYP2D6 Substrates. *Risk C: Monitor therapy*

CYP2D6 Inhibitors (Strong): May decrease the metabolism of CYP2D6 Substrates. *Risk D: Consider therapy modification*

CYP2D6 Substrates: CYP2D6 Inhibitors (Moderate) may decrease the metabolism of CYP2D6 Substrates. **Exceptions:** Tamoxifen. *Risk C: Monitor therapy*

Darunavir: May increase the serum concentration of CYP2D6 Substrates. *Risk C: Monitor therapy*

Fluvoxamine: May decrease the metabolism of DULoxetine. *Risk C: Monitor therapy*

MAO Inhibitors: May enhance the serotonergic effect of Antidepressants (Serotonin/Norepinephrine Reuptake Inhibitor). This may cause serotonin syndrome. *Risk X: Avoid combination*

Nebivolol: CYP2D6 Inhibitors (Moderate) may increase the serum concentration of Nebivolol. *Risk C: Monitor therapy*

NSAID (Nonselective): Antidepressants (Serotonin/Norepinephrine Reuptake Inhibitor) may enhance the antiplatelet effect of NSAID (Nonselective). *Risk C: Monitor therapy*

PARoxetine: May decrease the metabolism of DULoxetine. *Risk C: Monitor therapy*

Serotonin Modulators: May enhance the adverse/toxic effect of other Serotonin Modulators. The development of serotonin syndrome may occur. *Risk D: Consider therapy modification*

Sibutramine: May enhance the serotonergic effect of Serotonin Modulators. This may cause serotonin syndrome. *Risk X: Avoid combination*

Tamoxifen: CYP2D6 Inhibitors (Moderate) may decrease the metabolism of Tamoxifen. Specifically, CYP2D6 inhibitors may decrease the formation of highly potent active metabolites. *Risk D: Consider therapy modification*

Thioridazine: CYP2D6 Inhibitors may decrease the metabolism of Thioridazine. *Risk X: Avoid combination*

TraMADol: CYP2D6 Inhibitors (Moderate) may diminish the therapeutic effect of TraMADol. These CYP2D6 inhibitors may prevent the metabolic conversion of tramadol to its active metabolite that accounts for much of its opioid-like effects. *Risk C: Monitor therapy*

Tricyclic Antidepressants: DULoxetine may decrease the metabolism of Tricyclic Antidepressants. *Risk C: Monitor therapy*

Ethanol/Nutrition/Herb Interactions

Ethanol: Avoid ethanol (may increase CNS depression and/or hepatotoxic potential of duloxetine).

Herb/Nutraceutical: Avoid valerian, St John's wort, SAMe, kava kava, and gotu kola (may increase CNS depression).

Stability Store at 25°C (77°F); excursions permitted to 15°C to 30°C (59°F to 86°F)

Mechanism of Action Duloxetine is a potent inhibitor of neuronal serotonin and norepinephrine reuptake and a weak inhibitor of dopamine reuptake. Duloxetine has no significant activity for muscarinic cholinergic, H_1-histaminergic, or alpha$_2$-adrenergic receptors. Duloxetine does not possess MAO-inhibitory activity.

Pharmacodynamics/Kinetics

Absorption: Well absorbed, 2-hour delay in absorption after ingestion; food decreases extent of absorption ~10% (no effect on C_{max})

Distribution: 1640 L (range: 701-3800 L)

Protein binding: >90%; primarily to albumin and α_1-acid glycoprotein

Metabolism: Hepatic, via CYP1A2 and CYP2D6; forms multiple metabolites (inactive)

Half-life elimination: 12 hours (range 8-17 hours)

Time to peak: 6 hours; 10 hours when ingested with food

Excretion: As metabolites; urine (72%), feces (19%)

Dosage Oral:

Adults:

Major depressive disorder: Initial: 40-60 mg/day; dose may be divided (ie, 20 or 30 mg twice daily) or given as a single daily dose of 60 mg; maintenance: 60 mg once daily; for doses >60 mg/day, titrate dose in increments of

30 mg/day over 1 week as tolerated to a maximum dose: 120 mg/day. **Note:** Doses >60 mg/day have not been demonstrated to be more effective.

Diabetic neuropathy: 60 mg once daily; lower initial doses may be considered in patients where tolerability is a concern and/or renal impairment is present. **Note:** Doses up to 120 mg/day administered in clinical trials offered no additional benefit and were less well tolerated than dose of 60 mg/day.

Fibromyalgia: Initial: 30 mg/day for 1 week, then increase to 60 mg/day as tolerated. **Note:** Doses up to 120 mg/day administered in clinical trials offered no additional benefit and were less well tolerated than dose of 60 mg/day.

Generalized anxiety disorder: Initial: 30-60 mg/day as a single daily dose; patients initiated at 30 mg/day should be titrated to 60 mg/day after 1 week; maximum dose: 120 mg/day. **Note:** Doses >60 mg/day have not been demonstrated to be more effective than 60 mg/day.

Chronic pain syndromes (unlabeled use): 60 mg once daily

Stress incontinence (unlabeled use): 40 mg twice daily

Elderly:

Major depressive disorder: Manufacturer does not recommend specific dosage adjustment. Conservatively, may initiate at a dose of 20 mg 1-2 times/day; increase to 40-60 mg/day as a single daily dose or in divided doses **or** initiate therapy at 30 mg/day for 1 week then increase to 60 mg/day as tolerated.

Other indications: Refer to adult dosing

Dosage adjustment in renal impairment: Not recommended for use in Cl_{cr} <30 mL/minute or ESRD (contraindicated in Canadian labeling); in mild-moderate impairment, lower initial doses may be considered with titration guided by response and tolerability

Dosage adjustment in hepatic impairment: Not recommended for use in hepatic impairment (contraindicated in Canadian labeling)

Dietary Considerations May be taken without regard to meals.

Administration Capsule should be swallowed whole; do not break open or crush.

Monitoring Parameters Blood pressure should be checked prior to initiating therapy and then regularly monitored, especially in patients with a high baseline blood pressure; mental status for depression, suicidal ideation (especially at the beginning of therapy or when doses are increased or decreased), anxiety, social functioning, mania, panic attacks; glucose levels and Hb A_{1c} levels in diabetic patients, creatinine, BUN, transaminases

Dosage Forms Excipient information presented when available (limited, particularly for generics); consult specific product labeling.

Capsule, delayed release, enteric coated pellets:

Cymbalta®: 20 mg, 30 mg, 60 mg

- **Duloxetine Hydrochloride** *see* DULoxetine *on page 516*
- **Duodote™** *see* Atropine and Pralidoxime *on page 159*
- **Duomax** *see* Guaifenesin and Phenylephrine *on page 742*
- **DuoNeb®** *see* Ipratropium and Albuterol *on page 854*
- **DuP 753** *see* Losartan *on page 952*
- **Duraclon®** *see* CloNIDine *on page 377*
- **Duradrin® [DSC]** *see* Acetaminophen, Isometheptene, and Dichloralphenazone *on page 45*
- **Duradryl®** *see* Chlorpheniramine, Phenylephrine, and Methscopolamine *on page 329*
- **Duragesic®** *see* FentaNYL *on page 624*
- **Durahist™** *see* Chlorpheniramine, Pseudoephedrine, and Methscopolamine *on page 334*
- **Durahist™ PE** *see* Chlorpheniramine, Phenylephrine, and Methscopolamine *on page 329*
- **Duramist® Plus [OTC]** *see* Oxymetazoline *on page 1208*
- **Duramorph®** *see* Morphine Sulfate *on page 1077*
- **Duraphen™ II DM** *see* Guaifenesin, Dextromethorphan, and Phenylephrine *on page 746*
- **Duraphen™ DM [DSC]** *see* Guaifenesin, Dextromethorphan, and Phenylephrine *on page 746*
- **Duraphen™ Forte** *see* Guaifenesin, Dextromethorphan, and Phenylephrine *on page 746*

- ◆ **DuraTan™ Forte** *see* Chlorpheniramine, Pseudoephedrine, and Dextromethorphan *on page 333*
- ◆ **Duration® [OTC] [DSC]** *see* Oxymetazoline *on page 1208*
- ◆ **Duratuss®** *see* Guaifenesin and Phenylephrine *on page 742*
- ◆ **Duratuss® DA** *see* Chlorpheniramine and Pseudoephedrine *on page 325*
- ◆ **Duratuss® DM** *see* Guaifenesin and Dextromethorphan *on page 739*
- ◆ **Duratuss GP®** *see* Guaifenesin and Phenylephrine *on page 742*
- ◆ **Duratuss® HD [DSC]** *see* Hydrocodone, Phenylephrine, and Guaifenesin *on page 783*
- ◆ **Duricef® [DSC]** *see* Cefadroxil *on page 292*

Dutasteride (doo TAS teer ide)

U.S. Brand Names Avodart®
Canadian Brand Names Avodart®
Mexican Brand Names Avodart
Pharmacologic Category 5 Alpha-Reductase Inhibitor
Use Treatment of symptomatic benign prostatic hyperplasia (BPH) as monotherapy or combination therapy with tamsulosin
Unlabeled/Investigational Use Treatment of male patterned baldness
Effect on Mental Status None reported
Effect on Psychiatric Treatment Nefazodone may increase dutasteride levels
Dosage Summary
Oral:
Children: Dosage not established
Adults (males): 0.5 mg once daily
Dosage Forms Excipient information presented when available (limited, particularly for generics); consult specific product labeling.
Capsule, softgel:
Avodart®: 0.5 mg

- ◆ **DW286** *see* Gemifloxacin *on page 712*
- ◆ **Dyazide®** *see* Hydrochlorothiazide and Triamterene *on page 776*
- ◆ **Dylix** *see* Dyphylline *on page 521*
- ◆ **Dynacin®** *see* Minocycline *on page 1056*
- ◆ **DynaCirc® CR** *see* Isradipine *on page 871*
- ◆ **Dynahist-ER Pediatric® [DSC]** *see* Chlorpheniramine and Pseudoephedrine *on page 325*
- ◆ **Dynatuss-EX** *see* Guaifenesin, Dextromethorphan, and Phenylephrine *on page 746*
- ◆ **Dynex [DSC]** *see* Guaifenesin and Pseudoephedrine *on page 744*

Dyphylline (DYE fi lin)

Medication Safety Issues
International issues:
Dilor® [Canada] may be confused with Dilar® which is a brand name for paramethasone in France and Mexico
U.S. Brand Names Dylix; Lufyllin®
Canadian Brand Names Dilor®; Lufyllin®
Index Terms Dihydroxypropyl Theophylline
Pharmacologic Category Theophylline Derivative
Use Bronchodilator in reversible airway obstruction due to asthma, chronic bronchitis, or emphysema
Effect on Mental Status May cause nervousness, restlessness, or insomnia
Effect on Psychiatric Treatment May decrease serum lithium levels; monitor; barbiturates and carbamazepine may decrease dyphylline levels; may antagonize effects of benzodiazepines
Dosage Summary
Oral:
Children: Dosage not established
Adults: Up to 15 mg/kg 4 times/day, individualize dosage
Dosage Forms Excipient information presented when available (limited, particularly for generics); consult specific product labeling.
Elixir:
Dylix: 100 mg/15 mL (473 mL) [contains alcohol 20%]

Tablet:
Lufyllin®: 200 mg, 400 mg

Dyphylline and Guaifenesin (DYE fi lin & gwye FEN e sin)

U.S. Brand Names COPD; Difil-G; Difil®-G Forte; Dilex-G; Dilor-G®; Lufyllin®-GG

Index Terms Guaifenesin and Dyphylline

Pharmacologic Category Expectorant; Theophylline Derivative

Use Treatment of bronchial asthma and reversible bronchospasm associated with chronic bronchitis and emphysema

Effect on Mental Status May cause agitation, dizziness, drowsiness, hyperexcitability, insomnia, irritability, nervousness, or restlessness

Effect on Psychiatric Treatment May decrease serum lithium levels, monitor; barbiturates and carbamazepine may decrease dyphylline levels; may antagonize effects of benzodiazepines

Dosage Summary

Oral:

Children <6 years: Dosage not established

Children 6-12 years:

Elixir: Lufyllin®-GG: 15-30 mL 3 or 4 times/day

Syrup: Dilex-G:

18-27 kg: 1.25-1.6 mL 4 times/day

27-36 kg: 2.5-3.3 mL 4 times/day

36.5-45 kg: 3.3-3.7 mL 4 times/day

Tablet: Lufyllin®-GG: 1/2 -1 tablet 3 or 4 times/day

Children >12 years:

Elixir: Lufyllin®-GG: 30 mL 4 times/day

Syrup:

Dilex-G: 5-10 mL 4 times/day

Difil®-G Forte: 5-10 mL 3 or 4 times/day; may double or triple (in severe cases) according to patient response

Tablet: Difil®-G, Dilex-G, Lufyllin®-GG: One tablet 3 or 4 times/day

Adults:

Elixir: Lufyllin®-GG: 30 mL 4 times/day

Syrup:

Dilex-G: 5-10 mL 4 times/day

Difil®-G Forte: 5-10 mL 3 or 4 times/day; may double or triple (in severe cases) according to patient response

Tablet: Difil®-G, Dilex-G, Lufyllin®-GG: One tablet 3 or 4 times/day

Dosage Forms Excipient information presented when available (limited, particularly for generics); consult specific product labeling.

Elixir: Dyphylline 100 mg and guaifenesin 100 mg per 15 mL (480 mL)

Lufyllin®-GG: Dyphylline 100 mg and guaifenesin 100 mg per 15 mL (480 mL) [contains alcohol 17%; wine-like flavor]

Liquid: Dyphylline 100 mg and guaifenesin 100 mg per 5 mL (480 mL)

Difil®-G Forte: Dyphylline 100 mg and guaifenesin 100 mg per 5 mL (240 mL) [menthol flavor]

Syrup:

Dilex-G: Dyphylline 100 mg and guaifenesin 200 mg per 5 mL (480 mL) [alcohol free, dye free, and sugar free]

Tablet: Dyphylline 200 mg and guaifenesin 200 mg

COPD, Lufyllin®-GG: Dyphylline 200 mg and guaifenesin 200 mg

Difil®-G: Dyphylline 200 mg and guaifenesin 300 mg

Dilex-G: Dyphylline 200 mg and guaifenesin 400 mg

- **Dyrenium®** *see* Triamterene *on page 1620*
- **Dytan™** *see* DiphenhydrAMINE *on page 481*
- **E2 and DRSP** *see* Drospirenone and Estradiol *on page 515*
- **E2020** *see* Donepezil *on page 495*
- **E 2080** *see* Rufinamide *on page 1452*
- **EACA** *see* Aminocaproic Acid *on page 87*
- **EarSol® HC** *see* Hydrocortisone *on page 785*
- **Easprin®** *see* Aspirin *on page 143*
- ***Echinacea angustifolia*** *see* Echinacea *(Echinacea purpurea, Echinacea angustifolia) on page 523*

Echinacea (*Echinacea purpurea, Echinacea angustifolia*)

Natural Product Category Herb

Synonyms *Echinacea angustifolia*; *Echinacea pallida*; *Echinacea purpurea*; American coneflower; Coneflower; Purple Coneflower

Plant Part Varies by species: *E. purpurea*: Flower, whole plant; *E. angustifolia*: Root

Dosage and Standardization Oral:

Capsule: 50-1000 mg 3 times/day on day 1, then 250 mg 4 times/day, standardized to contain 4% echinacosides (*E. angustifolia*) or 4% sesquiterpene esters (*E. purpurea*) per dose

NS has: Expressed juice: 6-9 mL daily in divided doses for 5-7 days

Plant juice: Freshly expressed (*E. purpurea*): 60 drops 3 times/day with food for 1 day, then 40 drops 3 times/day with food for up to 10 days, standardized to contain not less than 2.4% soluble beta-1,2 D-5 fructofuranosides per dose

Tea: 2 teaspoons (4 g *Echinacea*) of coarsely powdered herb simmered in 1 cup of boiling water for 10 minutes daily for 5-7 days; or 5-6 cups on the first day and titrated down by 1 cup daily for the next 5 days of *Echinacea* Plus® tea, manufactured by Traditional Medicinals (equivalent of 1.275 mg dried herb and root per tea bag)

Tincture: 0.75-1.5 mL, gargled then swallowed, 2-5 times/day for 5-7 days (daily dose equivalent to 900 mg dried *Echinacea* root

Topical: Apply to affected area as needed

Reported Uses

Antibacterial (topical: Boils, abscesses, tonsillitis, poison ivy) (Leung, 1996)
Antiviral (Orinda, 1973)
Arthritis (*E. augustifolia*) (Tubaro, 1987)
Genital herpes (Vonau, 2001)
Immune support (cold and other upper respiratory infections) (Bauer, 1996; Brinkeborn, 1999; Luettig, 1989)
Otitis media (pharmacologic activity)
Radiation-associated leucopenia (Bendel, 1989; Pohl, 1970; Sartor, 1972)
Upper respiratory infection (Taylor, 2003)
Uveitis (Neri, 2006)

Summary Echinacea is one of the most popular herbs and has been extensively studied for its effects on the immune system. It has been used as an immune stimulant for a variety of afflictions, including colds and flu. As opposed to its use during colds and flu, some published trials of this herb in the prevention of colds and upper respiratory infection have failed to demonstrate benefit (Grimm, 1999; Hoheisel, 1997), while others support its use. It has been promoted as a general health measure to improve resistance during seasonal outbreaks, but there is some concern related to the potential immunosuppressive effects of prolonged use; therefore, prolonged continuous use is not recommended.

Effect on Mental Status None reported

Effect on Psychiatric Treatment Contraindicated in patients with multiple sclerosis

Pharmacology Echinacea appears to have a variety of nonspecific stimulatory effects on the immune system. Echinacea is claimed to stimulate white blood cell function and cell-mediated immunity, including T lymphocytes, macrophages, and natural killer cells. As a consequence of macrophage stimulation, echinacea has been reported to increase the production of interferon, tumor necrosis factor, and interleukin-1. Echinacea activates white blood cells to scavenge for bacteria and cellular debris. In addition, echinacea inhibits hyaluronidase and stimulates fibroblast production of collagen. Echinacea is reported to have broad antimicrobial activity, including effects on bacteria, fungi, and viruses. It has been used externally for wound cleansing, eczema, burns, herpes, canker sores, and abscesses.

Theoretical Cautions and Contraindications Based on this agent's pharmacologic activity, use for more than 10 days in acute infections or in immunosuppressed individuals is not recommended (Bradley, 1992). When used as prophylaxis, ingestion should be cycled for 3 weeks on and 1 week off (Brown, 1999). Use with caution in individuals with renal disease or impairment; may cause electrolyte imbalance (Murray, 1995). Use with caution in individuals allergic to members of the *Asteraceae/Compositae* family (ragweed, daisy, aster, chrysanthemum) and other pollens; rare but severe reactions have been reported (Mullins, 1998). Use tinctures cautiously with alcoholic patients and in patients taking disulfiram or metronidazole; many tinctures contain significant concentrations of alcohol (range: 15% to 90%).

General Warnings Use all herbal supplements with extreme caution in children <2 years of age and in pregnancy or lactation. Some herbs are contraindicated in pregnancy or lactation; make sure to observe warnings. Use with caution in individuals on medication and with pre-existing medical conditions. Always review for potential herb-drug interactions (HDIs) and other warnings. Large and prolonged doses may increase the potential for adverse effects. Herbs may cause transient adverse effects such as nausea, vomiting, and GI distress due to a variety of chemical constituents. Caution should be used in individuals having known allergies to plants.

Theoretical Interactions Therapeutic immunosuppressants (cyclosporine, tacrolimus, sirolimus, methotrexate), corticosteroids

In vitro data suggests this herb may inhibit CYP3A4 isoenzyme. Theoretically, it may affect the following medications' disposition: Protease inhibitors, cyclosporine, non-nucleoside reverse transcriptase inhibitors, certain benzodiazepines, calcium channel blockers, grapefruit juice, and other medications influenced by this enzyme system.

Amoxicillin, disulfiram, metronidazole, econazole (topical)

References

Bauer R, "Echinacea Drugs - Effects and Active Ingredients," *Z Arztl Fortbild (Jena)*, 1996, 90(2):111-5.

Bendel R, Bendel V, Renner K, et al, "Additional Treatment With Esberitox N in Patients With Chemo-Radiotherapy Treatment of Advanced Breast Cancer," *Onkologie*, 1989, 12 Suppl 3:32-8.

Bradley PR, ed, *British Herbal Compendium*, Vol 1, Bournemouth, England: British Herbal Medicine Association, 1992, 81-3.

Brinkeborn RM, Shah DV, and Degenring FH, "Echinaforce and other Echinacea Fresh Plant Preparations in the Treatment of the Common Cold: A Randomized, Placebo Controlled, Double-Blind Clinical Trial," *Phytomedicine*, 1999, 6:1-5.

Brown D, "Echinacea Root Fails to Prevent Upper Respiratory Tract Infections," *HealthNotes Rev Complement Alternative Med*, 1999, 6(1):6-7.

Grimm W and Müller HH, "A Randomized Controlled Trial of the Effect of Fluid Extract of *Echinacea purpurea* on the Incidence and Severity of Colds and Respiratory Infections," *Am J Med*, 1999, 106(2):138-43.

Hoheisel O, Sandbers M, Bertram S, et al, "Echinacea Root Extracts for the Prevention of Upper Respiratory Tract Infections: A Double-Blind, Placebo Controlled Trial," *Eur J Clin Res*, 1997, 2:261-8.

Leung AY and Foster S, *Encyclopedia of Common Natural Ingredients Used in Foods, Drugs, and Cosmetics*, New York, NY: Wiley, 1996, 216-20.

Luettig B, Steinmuller C, Gifford GE, et al, "Macrophage Activation by the Polysaccharide Arabinogalactan Isolated From Plant Cell Cultures of *Echinacea purpurea*," *Natl Cancer Inst*, 1989, 81(9):669-75.

Mullins RJ, "Echinacea-Associated Anaphylaxis," *Med J Aust*, 1998, 168(4):170-1.

Murray MT, "Echinacea: Pharmacology and Clinical Applications," *Am J Natural Med*, 1995, 2:18-24.

Natural Standard Research Collaboration, Chief Editors: Ulbricht C, Basch E, *Natural Standard Herb and Supplement Reference - Evidence-Based Clinical Reviews*, USA: Elsevier/Mosby, 2005.

Neri PG, Stagni E, Filippello M, et al, "Oral *Echinacea purpurea* Extract in Low-Grade, Steroid-Dependent, Autoimmune Idiopathic Uveitis: A Pilot Study," *J Ocul Pharmacol Ther*, 2006, 22(6):431-6.

Orinda D, Diederich J, and Wacker A, "Antiviral Activity of Components of *Echinacea purpurea*," *Arzneimittelforschung*, 1973, 23(8):1119-20.

Pohl P, "Treatment of Radiation-Induced Leukopenia With Esberitox," *Ther Ggw*, 1970, 109 (6):902.

Sartor KJ, "Efficacy of Esberitox in the Treatment of Radiation-Induced Leukopenia," *Ther Ggw*, 1972, 111(8):1147-50.

Taylor JA, Weber W, Standish L, et al, "Efficacy and Safety of Echinacea in Treating Upper Respiratory Tract Infections in Children: A Randomized Controlled Trial," *JAMA*, 2003, 290 (21):2824-30.

Tubaro A, Tragni E, Del Negro P, et al, "Anti-inflammatory Activity of a Polysaccharidic Fraction of *Echinacea angustifolia*," *J Pharm Pharmacol*, 1987, 39(7):567-9.

Vonau B, Chard S, Mandalia S, et al, "Does the Extract of the Plant *Echinacea purpurea* Influence the Clinical Course of Recurrent Genital Herpes?" *Int J STD AIDS*, 2001, 12 (3):154-8.

- ***Echinacea pallida*** *see* Echinacea *(Echinacea purpurea, Echinacea angustifolia) on page 523*
- ***Echinacea purpurea*** *see* Echinacea *(Echinacea purpurea, Echinacea angustifolia) on page 523*
- **EC-Naprosyn®** *see* Naproxen *on page 1102*
- ***E. coli* Asparaginase** *see* Asparaginase *on page 142*
- **Econopred® Plus [DSC]** *see* PrednisoLONE *on page 1326*
- **Ecotrin® [OTC]** *see* Aspirin *on page 143*
- **Ecotrin® Low Strength [OTC]** *see* Aspirin *on page 143*
- **Ecotrin® Maximum Strength [OTC]** *see* Aspirin *on page 143*

- ◆ **Ed A-Hist™** *see* Chlorpheniramine and Phenylephrine *on page 323*
- ◆ **Ed A-Hist DM** *see* Chlorpheniramine, Phenylephrine, and Dextromethorphan *on page 327*
- ◆ **Ed ChlorPed D** *see* Chlorpheniramine and Phenylephrine *on page 323*
- ◆ **Edecrin®** *see* Ethacrynic Acid *on page 591*
- ◆ **Edex®** *see* Alprostadil *on page 77*

Edrophonium (ed roe FOE nee um)

U.S. Brand Names Enlon® [DSC]

Canadian Brand Names Enlon®; Tensilon®

Index Terms Edrophonium Chloride

Pharmacologic Category Antidote; Cholinergic Agonist; Diagnostic Agent

Use Diagnosis of myasthenia gravis; differentiation of cholinergic crises from myasthenia crises; reversal of nondepolarizing neuromuscular blockers; adjunct treatment of respiratory depression caused by curare overdose

Effect on Mental Status May cause drowsiness

Effect on Psychiatric Treatment None reported

Dosage Summary

I.M.:

Infants: 0.5-1 mg

Children ≤34 kg: 1 mg

Children >34 kg: 5 mg

Adults: 10 mg, if no cholinergic reactions administer 2 mg 30 minutes later

I.V.: Note: Following doses may be administered I.M. or SubQ if no I.V. access

Infants: 0.1 mg, followed by 0.4 mg if no response (maximum total dose: 0.5 mg)

Children ≤34 kg: 0.04 mg/kg, followed by 0.16 mg/kg if no response **or** 1 mg, followed by 1mg every 30-45 seconds if no response (maximum total dose: 5 mg) **or** 0.04 mg/kg as a single dose 1 hour after oral anticholinesterase therapy

Children >34 kg: 0.04 mg/kg, followed by 0.16 mg/kg if no response **or** 2 mg, followed by 1 mg every 30-45 seconds if no response (maximum total dose: 10 mg) **or** 0.04 mg/kg as a single dose 1 hour after oral anticholinesterase therapy

Adults: 2 mg test dose, followed by 8 mg after 30 minutes if no response **or** 1-2 mg as a single dose 1 hour after oral anticholinesterase therapy **or** 10 mg every 5-10 minutes up to 40 mg **or** 5-10 mg as a single dose **or** 1 mg, may repeat after 1 minute

Dosage Forms Excipient information presented when available (limited, particularly for generics); consult specific product labeling.

Injection, solution, as chloride:

Enlon®: 10 mg/mL (15 mL) [contains sodium sulfite]

Edrophonium and Atropine (ed roe FOE nee um & A troe peen)

U.S. Brand Names Enlon-Plus™ [DSC]

Index Terms Atropine Sulfate and Edrophonium Chloride; Edrophonium Chloride and Atropine Sulfate

Pharmacologic Category Anticholinergic Agent; Antidote; Cholinergic Agonist

Use Reversal of nondepolarizing neuromuscular blockers; adjunct treatment of respiratory depression caused by curare overdose

Effect on Mental Status None reported

Effect on Psychiatric Treatment Atropine is highly anticholinergic; concurrent use of atropine and other anticholinergics (eg, tricyclic antidepressants, antipsychotics, some antihistamines, antiparkinson drugs) may produce additive effects. Avoid use in myasthenia gravis; myasthenic weakness may be a symptom of anticholinesterase overdose. Concomitant use with propranolol may produce additive bradycardia.

Dosage Summary

I.V.:

Children: Dosage not established

Adults: 0.05 mL/kg (0.5-1 mg/kg of edrophonium and 0.007-0.015 mg/kg of atropine)

Dosage Forms Excipient information presented when available (limited, particularly for generics); consult specific product labeling. [DSC] = Discontinued product

Injection, solution:
Enlon-Plus™: Edrophonium chloride 10 mg/mL and atropine sulfate 0.14 mg/mL (5 mL, 15 mL) [contains sodium sulfite] [DSC]

- **Edrophonium Chloride** *see* Edrophonium *on page 525*
- **Edrophonium Chloride and Atropine Sulfate** *see* Edrophonium and Atropine *on page 525*
- **ED-TLC** *see* Phenylephrine, Hydrocodone, and Chlorpheniramine *on page 1277*
- **ED-Tuss HC** *see* Phenylephrine, Hydrocodone, and Chlorpheniramine *on page 1277*
- **E.E.M.T. D.S.** *see* Estrogens (Esterified) and Methyltestosterone *on page 587*
- **E.E.M.T. H.S.** *see* Estrogens (Esterified) and Methyltestosterone *on page 587*
- **E.E.S.®** *see* Erythromycin *on page 557*

Efalizumab (e fa li ZOO mab)

Medication Safety Issues
Sound-alike/look-alike issues:
Efalizumab may be confused with eculizumab
Raptiva® maybe confused with Rapaflo®

U.S. Brand Names Raptiva®

Mexican Brand Names Raptiva

Index Terms Anti-CD11a; hu1124

Pharmacologic Category Immunosuppressant Agent; Monoclonal Antibody

Use Treatment of chronic moderate-to-severe plaque psoriasis in patients who are candidates for systemic therapy or phototherapy

Effect on Mental Status May cause sedation

Effect on Psychiatric Treatment Nausea is common; concurrent use with SSRIs and/or valproic acid may produce additive effects. May cause acne or psoriasis; lithium may produce similar side effects; monitor. Flu-like syndrome has been reported and may present similarly to SSRI-discontinuation symptoms. May rarely cause thrombocytopenia; monitor with high-dose valproic acid use.

Dosage Summary
SubQ:
Children: Dosage not established
Adults: Initial: 0.7 mg/kg; Maintenance: 1 mg/kg once weekly (maximum: 200 mg/dose)

Dosage Forms Excipient information presented when available (limited, particularly for generics); consult specific product labeling.
Injection, powder for reconstitution:
Raptiva®: 150 mg [contains sucrose 123.2 mg/vial; delivers 125 mg/1.25 mL; packaged with prefilled syringe containing sterile water for injection]

Efavirenz (e FAV e renz)

U.S. Brand Names Sustiva®

Canadian Brand Names Sustiva®

Mexican Brand Names Stocrin

Pharmacologic Category Antiretroviral Agent, Reverse Transcriptase Inhibitor (Non-nucleoside)

Use Treatment of HIV-1 infections in combination with at least two other antiretroviral agents

Effect on Mental Status Serious psychiatric adverse effects have been reported. May cause severe depression, suicidal ideation, aggressive behavior, paranoia, and mania. Patients with a psychiatric history appear to be at a greater risk for these psychiatric effects. May cause difficulty in concentration, insomnia, abnormal dreams, sedation, nervousness, and fatigue. May rarely cause hallucinations, psychosis, anxiety, euphoria, emotional lability, agitation.

Effect on Psychiatric Treatment Should not be administered with other drugs known to be metabolized by the CYP3A4 system (midazolam, triazolam, ergot alkaloids) as combination may lead to life-threatening adverse effects. Coadministration with St John's wort is expected to substantially decrease NNRTI concentrations, and may result in suboptimal levels and lead to loss of virologic response and possible resistance to efavirenz or to the class of NNRTIs.

Dosage Summary
Oral:
Children <3 years: Dosage not established

Children ≥3 years and 10 kg to <15 kg: 200 mg once daily
Children ≥3 years and 15 kg to <20 kg: 250 mg once daily
Children ≥3 years and 20 kg to <25 kg: 300 mg once daily
Children ≥3 years and 25 kg to <32.5 kg: 350 mg once daily
Children ≥3 years and 32.5 kg to <40 kg: 400 mg once daily
Children ≥3 years and ≥40 kg: 600 mg once daily
Adults: 600 mg once daily

Dosage Forms Excipient information presented when available (limited, particularly for generics); consult specific product labeling. [DSC] = Discontinued product

Capsule:
Sustiva®: 50 mg; 100 mg [DSC]; 200 mg

Tablet:
Sustiva®: 600 mg

Efavirenz, Emtricitabine, and Tenofovir

(e FAV e renz, em trye SYE ta been, & te NOE fo veer)

U.S. Brand Names Atripla®

Canadian Brand Names Atripla®

Index Terms Emtricitabine, Efavirenz, and Tenofovir; FTC, TDF, and EFV; Tenofovir Disoproxil Fumarate, Efavirenz, and Emtricitabine

Pharmacologic Category Antiretroviral Agent, Reverse Transcriptase Inhibitor (Non-nucleoside); Antiretroviral Agent, Reverse Transcriptase Inhibitor (Nucleoside); Antiretroviral Agent, Reverse Transcriptase Inhibitor (Nucleotide)

Use Treatment of HIV infection

Effect on Mental Status May cause severe depression, suicidal ideation, paranoia, or mania. May also cause dizziness, drowsiness, and impaired concentration.

Effect on Psychiatric Treatment Contraindicated with midazolam, triazolam, and ergot alkaloids. Concurrent use with St John's wort is not recommended. Levels of citalopram, fluoxetine, and sertraline may be increased; monitor response.

Dosage Summary

Oral:

Children: Dosage not established
Adults: One tablet once daily

Dosage Forms Excipient information presented when available (limited, particularly for generics); consult specific product labeling.

Tablet:
Atripla™: Efavirenz 600 mg, emtricitabine 200 mg, and tenofovir disoproxil fumarate 300 mg

◆ **Effer-K™** *see* Potassium Bicarbonate and Potassium Citrate *on page 1315*

◆ **Effexor®** *see* Venlafaxine *on page 1659*

◆ **Effexor XR®** *see* Venlafaxine *on page 1659*

Eflornithine (ee FLOR ni theen)

Medication Safety Issues

Sound-alike/look-alike issues:
Vaniqa™ may be confused with Viagra®

U.S. Brand Names Vaniqa™

Canadian Brand Names Vaniqa™

Index Terms DFMO; Eflornithine Hydrochloride

Pharmacologic Category Antiprotozoal; Topical Skin Product

Use Cream: Females ≥12 years: Reduce unwanted hair from face and adjacent areas under the chin

Orphan status: Injection: Treatment of meningoencephalitic stage of *Trypanosoma brucei gambiense* infection (sleeping sickness)

Effect on Mental Status Dizziness is common

Effect on Psychiatric Treatment Leukopenia is common; use caution with clozapine and carbamazepine

Dosage Summary

I.V.:

Children: Dosage not established
Adults: 100 mg/kg/dose every 6 hours

Topical:

Children: Apply thin layer to affected areas twice daily (at least 8 hours apart)
Adults: Apply thin layer to affected areas twice daily (at least 8 hours apart) ▶

Dosage Forms Excipient information presented when available (limited, particularly for generics); consult specific product labeling.
Cream, topical, as hydrochloride: 13.9% (30 g)
Injection, solution, as hydrochloride: 200 mg/mL (100 mL) [orphan drug status]

- **Eflornithine Hydrochloride** *see* Eflornithine *on page 527*
- **Efudex®** *see* Fluorouracil *on page 649*
- **E-Gems® [OTC]** *see* Vitamin E *on page 1675*
- **E-Gems Elite® [OTC]** *see* Vitamin E *on page 1675*
- **E-Gems Plus® [OTC]** *see* Vitamin E *on page 1675*
- **EHDP** *see* Etidronate Disodium *on page 605*
- **Elavil** *see* Amitriptyline *on page 90*
- **Eldepryl®** *see* Selegiline *on page 1466*
- **Electrolyte Lavage Solution** *see* Polyethylene Glycol-Electrolyte Solution *on page 1310*
- **Elestrin™** *see* Estradiol *on page 576*

Eletriptan (el e TRIP tan)

Related Information
Antimigraine Drugs: 5-HT$_1$ Receptor Agonists *on page 1766*
U.S. Brand Names Relpax®
Canadian Brand Names Relpax®
Mexican Brand Names Relpax
Index Terms Eletriptan Hydrobromide
Pharmacologic Category Antimigraine Agent; Serotonin 5-HT$_{1B,\ 1D}$ Receptor Agonist
Generic Available No
Use Acute treatment of migraine, with or without aura
Pregnancy Risk Factor C
Pregnancy Considerations There are no adequate and well-controlled studies in pregnant women; use during pregnancy only if the potential benefit to the mother outweighs the possible risk to the fetus. Teratogenic effects were observed in animal studies.
Lactation Enters breast milk/use caution
Contraindications Hypersensitivity to eletriptan or any component of the formulation; ischemic heart disease or signs or symptoms of ischemic heart disease (including Prinzmetal's angina, angina pectoris, MI, silent myocardial ischemia); cerebrovascular syndromes (including strokes, transient ischemic attacks); peripheral vascular syndromes (including ischemic bowel disease); uncontrolled hypertension; use within 24 hours of ergotamine derivatives; use within 24 hours of another 5-HT$_1$ agonist; use within 72 hours of potent CYP3A4 inhibitors; management of hemiplegic or basilar migraine; prophylactic treatment of migraine; severe hepatic impairment
Warnings/Precautions Eletriptan is indicated only in patients ≥18 years of age with a clear diagnosis of migraine headache. If a patient does not respond to the first dose, the diagnosis of migraine should be reconsidered. Do not give to patients with risk factors for CAD until a cardiovascular evaluation has been performed; if evaluation is satisfactory, the healthcare provider should administer the first dose and cardiovascular status should be periodically evaluated. Cardiac events (coronary artery vasospasm, transient ischemia, MI, ventricular tachycardia/fibrillation, cardiac arrest, and death), cerebral/subarachnoid hemorrhage, stroke, peripheral vascular ischemia, and colonic ischemia have been reported with 5-HT$_1$ agonist administration. Significant elevation in blood pressure, including hypertensive crisis, has also been reported on rare occasions in patients with and without a history of hypertension. Use with caution with mild to moderate hepatic impairment. Symptoms of agitation, confusion, hallucinations, hyper-reflexia, myoclonus, shivering, and tachycardia (serotonin syndrome) may occur with concomitant proserotonergic drugs (ie, SSRIs/SNRIs or triptans) or agents which reduce eletriptan's metabolism. Concurrent use of serotonin precursors (eg, tryptophan) is not recommended. Safety and efficacy in pediatric patients have not been established.
Adverse Reactions
1% to 10%:
Cardiovascular: Chest pain/tightness (1% to 4%; placebo 1%), palpitation
Central nervous system: Dizziness (3% to 7%; placebo 3%), somnolence (3% to 7%; placebo 4%), headache (3% to 4%; placebo 3%), chills, pain, vertigo

Gastrointestinal: Nausea (4% to 8%; placebo 5%), xerostomia (2% to 4%, placebo 2%), dysphagia (1% to 2%), abdominal pain/discomfort (1% to 2%; placebo 1%), dyspepsia (1% to 2%; placebo 1%)

Neuromuscular & skeletal: Weakness (4% to 10%), paresthesia (3% to 4%), back pain, hypertonia, hypoesthesia

Respiratory: Pharyngitis

Miscellaneous: Diaphoresis

<1% (Limited to important or life-threatening): Agitation, allergic reaction, angina, arrhythmia, ataxia, confusion, constipation, CPK increased, depersonalization, depression, diarrhea, dreams (abnormal), dyspnea, edema, emotional lability, esophagitis, euphoria, hyperesthesia, hyperkinesia, hypertension, impotence, incoordination, insomnia, lacrimation disorder, liver function tests abnormal, myalgia, myasthenia, nervousness, peripheral vascular disorder, photophobia, polyuria, pruritus, rash, salivation increased, shock, speech disorder, stupor, tachycardia, taste perversion, thrombophlebitis, tinnitus, tongue edema, tremor, urinary frequency, vasospasm, vision abnormal

Metabolism/Transport Effects **Substrate** of CYP3A4 (major)

Drug Interactions

Antifungal Agents (Azole Derivatives, Systemic): May increase the serum concentration of Eletriptan. *Risk D: Consider therapy modification*

Calcium Channel Blockers (Nondihydropyridine): May decrease the metabolism of Eletriptan. *Risk C: Monitor therapy*

CYP3A4 Inhibitors (Moderate): May decrease the metabolism of CYP3A4 Substrates. *Risk C: Monitor therapy*

CYP3A4 Inhibitors (Strong): May decrease the metabolism of CYP3A4 Substrates. *Risk D: Consider therapy modification*

Dasatinib: May increase the serum concentration of CYP3A4 Substrates. *Risk C: Monitor therapy*

Ergot Derivatives: May enhance the vasoconstricting effect of Serotonin 5-HT1D Receptor Agonists. Serotonin 5-HT1D Receptor Agonists may enhance the vasoconstricting effect of Ergot Derivatives. *Risk X: Avoid combination*

Fluconazole: May decrease the metabolism of Eletriptan. *Risk C: Monitor therapy*

Macrolide Antibiotics: May decrease the metabolism of Eletriptan. **Exceptions:** Azithromycin; Dirithromycin [Off Market]; Spiramycin. *Risk D: Consider therapy modification*

Serotonin Modulators: May enhance the adverse/toxic effect of other Serotonin Modulators. The development of serotonin syndrome may occur. *Risk D: Consider therapy modification*

Sibutramine: May enhance the serotonergic effect of Serotonin Modulators. This may cause serotonin syndrome. *Risk X: Avoid combination*

Ethanol/Nutrition/Herb Interactions Food: High-fat meal increases bioavailability.

Stability Store at 25°C (77°F); excursions permitted to 15°C to 30°C (59°F to 86°F).

Mechanism of Action Selective agonist for serotonin (5-HT_{1B}, 5-HT_{1D}, 5-HT_{1F} receptors) in cranial arteries; causes vasoconstriction and reduce sterile inflammation associated with antidromic neuronal transmission correlating with relief of migraine

Pharmacodynamics/Kinetics

Absorption: Well absorbed

Distribution: V_d: 138 L

Protein binding: ~85%

Metabolism: Hepatic via CYP3A4; forms one metabolite (active)

Bioavailability: ~50%, increased with high-fat meal

Half-life elimination: 4 hours (Elderly: 4.4-5.7 hours); Metabolite: ~13 hours

Time to peak, plasma: 1.5-2 hours

Dosage Oral: Adults: Acute migraine: 20-40 mg; if the headache improves but returns, dose may be repeated after 2 hours have elapsed since first dose; maximum 80 mg/day.

Note: If the first dose is ineffective, diagnosis needs to be re-evaluated. Safety of treating >3 headaches/month has not been established.

Dosage adjustment in renal impairment: No dosing adjustment needed; monitor for increased blood pressure

Dosage adjustment in hepatic impairment:

Mild to moderate impairment: No adjustment necessary

Severe impairment: Use is contraindicated

Dosage Forms Excipient information presented when available (limited, particularly for generics); consult specific product labeling.

Tablet, as hydrobromide: 20 mg, 40 mg [as base]

- **Eletriptan Hydrobromide** *see* Eletriptan *on page 528*
- ***Eleutherococcus senticosus*** *see* Ginseng, Siberian *(Eleutherococcus senticosus) on page 720*
- **Eligard®** *see* Leuprolide *on page 901*
- **Elipten** *see* Aminoglutethimide *on page 87*
- **Elitek™** *see* Rasburicase *on page 1407*
- **Elixophyllin®** *see* Theophylline *on page 1562*
- **Elixophyllin-GG®** *see* Theophylline and Guaifenesin *on page 1567*
- **ElixSure® Cough [OTC]** *see* Dextromethorphan *on page 448*
- **Ellence®** *see* Epirubicin *on page 545*
- **Elmiron®** *see* Pentosan Polysulfate Sodium *on page 1250*
- **Elocon®** *see* Mometasone *on page 1071*
- **Eloxatin®** *see* Oxaliplatin *on page 1191*
- **Elspar®** *see* Asparaginase *on page 142*
- **Emcyt®** *see* Estramustine *on page 580*
- **Emend®** *see* Aprepitant *on page 130*
- **Emend® for Injection** *see* Fosaprepitant *on page 690*
- **Emsam®** *see* Selegiline *on page 1466*

Emtricitabine (em trye SYE ta been)

U.S. Brand Names Emtriva®

Canadian Brand Names Emtriva®

Mexican Brand Names Emtriva

Index Terms BW524W91; Coviracil; FTC

Pharmacologic Category Antiretroviral Agent, Reverse Transcriptase Inhibitor (Nucleoside)

Use Treatment of HIV infection in combination with at least two other antiretroviral agents

Unlabeled/Investigational Use Hepatitis B (with HIV coinfection)

Effect on Mental Status Insomnia and dizziness are common; may cause depression and abnormal dreams

Effect on Psychiatric Treatment GI side effects are common. Combined use with SSRIs may produce additive effects. May cause increases in serum triglycerides. Monitor in patients receiving concurrent psychotropic medication especially, clozapine, olanzapine, quetiapine, or mirtazapine. May cause glucose abnormalities; use caution with clozapine, olanzapine, and quetiapine, and risperidone.

Dosage Summary

Oral:

Capsule:

Children <3 months: Use solution

Children ≥3 months and ≤33 kg: Use solution

Children 3 months to 17 years and >33 kg: 200 mg once daily

Adults: 200 mg once daily

Solution:

Children <3 months: 3 mg/kg/day

Children 3 months to 17 years: 6 mg/kg once daily (maximum: 240 mg/day)

Adults: 240 mg once daily

Dosage Forms Excipient information presented when available (limited, particularly for generics); consult specific product labeling.

Capsule:

Emtriva®: 200 mg

Solution:

Emtriva®: 10 mg/mL (170 mL) [contains propylene glycol; cotton candy flavor]

Emtricitabine and Tenofovir (em trye SYE ta been & te NOE fo veer)

U.S. Brand Names Truvada®

Canadian Brand Names Truvada®

Mexican Brand Names Truvada

Index Terms Tenofovir and Emtricitabine

Pharmacologic Category Antiretroviral Agent, Reverse Transcriptase Inhibitor (Nucleoside); Antiretroviral Agent, Reverse Transcriptase Inhibitor (Nucleotide)

Use Treatment of HIV infection in combination with other antiretroviral agents

Effect on Mental Status Depression, insomnia, and dizziness are common; may cause abnormal dreams and anxiety

Effect on Psychiatric Treatment GI side effects are common; combined use with SSRIs (lithium or valproic acid) may produce additive effects. May cause increases in serum triglycerides; monitor in patients receiving concurrent psychotropic medication especially, clozapine, olanzapine, quetiapine, or mirtazapine. May cause glucose abnormalities; use caution with clozapine, olanzapine, quetiapine, and risperidone. May cause neutropenia; use caution with clozapine and carbamazepine.

Dosage Summary

Oral:

Children: Dosage not established

Adults: One tablet (emtricitabine 200 mg and tenofovir 300 mg) once daily

Dosage Forms Excipient information presented when available (limited, particularly for generics); consult specific product labeling.

Tablet: Emtricitabine 200 mg and tenofovir disoproxil fumarate 300 mg

- **Emtricitabine, Efavirenz, and Tenofovir** *see* Efavirenz, Emtricitabine, and Tenofovir *on page 527*
- **Emtriva®** *see* Emtricitabine *on page 530*
- **ENA 713** *see* Rivastigmine *on page 1435*
- **Enablex®** *see* Darifenacin *on page 419*

Enalapril (e NAL a pril)

Medication Safety Issues

Sound-alike/look-alike issues:

Enalapril may be confused with Anafranil®, Elavil®, Eldepryl®, nafarelin, ramipril

Significant differences exist between oral and I.V. dosing. Use caution when converting from one route of administration to another.

International issues:

Acepril® [Hungary, Switzerland] may be confused with Accupril® which is a brand name for quinapril in the U.S.

Acepril®: Brand name for lisinopril in Denmark; brand name for captopril in Great Britain

Nacor® [Spain] may be confused with Niacor® which is a brand name for niacin in the U.S.

Related Information

Angiotensin Agents *on page 1754*

U.S. Brand Names Vasotec®

Canadian Brand Names Apo-Enalapril®; CO Enalapril; Gen-Enalapril; Novo-Enalapril; PMS-Enalapril; ratio-Enalapril; Riva-Enalapril; Sandoz-Enalapril; Taro-Enalapril; Vasotec®; Vasotec® I.V.

Mexican Brand Names Ileveran

Index Terms Enalapril Maleate; Enalaprilat

Pharmacologic Category Angiotensin-Converting Enzyme (ACE) Inhibitor

Generic Available Yes

Use Treatment of hypertension; treatment of symptomatic heart failure; treatment of asymptomatic left ventricular dysfunction

Unlabeled/Investigational Use

Unlabeled: To delay the progression of nephropathy and reduce risks of cardiovascular events in hypertensive patients with type 1 or 2 diabetes mellitus; hypertensive crisis, diabetic nephropathy, hypertension secondary to scleroderma renal crisis, diagnosis of aldosteronism, idiopathic edema, Bartter's syndrome, postmyocardial infarction for prevention of ventricular failure

Investigational: Severe congestive heart failure in infants, neonatal hypertension, acute cardiogenic pulmonary edema (enalaprilat)

Effect on Mental Status May cause drowsiness and dizziness; rarely may cause insomnia, confusion, depression

Effect on Psychiatric Treatment May rarely cause agranulocytosis; use caution with clozapine and carbamazepine; may decrease lithium clearance resulting in an increase in serum lithium levels and potential lithium toxicity; monitor serum lithium levels

Pregnancy Risk Factor C (1st trimester); D (2nd and 3rd trimesters)

Pregnancy Considerations Due to adverse events observed in some animal studies, enalapril is considered pregnancy category C during the first trimester. Based on human data, enalapril is considered pregnancy category D if used during the second and third trimesters (per the manufacturer; however, one study suggests that fetal injury may occur at anytime during pregnancy). Enalaprilat, the active metabolite of enalapril, crosses the placenta. First trimester exposure to ACE inhibitors may cause major congenital malformations. An increased risk of cardiovascular and/or central nervous system malformations was observed in one study; however, an increased risk of teratogenic events was not observed in other studies. Second and third trimester use of an ACE inhibitor is associated with oligohydramnios. Oligohydramnios due to decreased fetal renal function may lead to fetal limb contractures, craniofacial deformation, and hypoplastic lung development. The use of ACE inhibitors during the second and third trimesters is also associated with anuria, hypotension, renal failure (reversible or irreversible), skull hypoplasia, and death in the fetus/neonate. Chronic maternal hypertension itself is also associated with adverse events in the fetus/infant. ACE inhibitors are not recommended during pregnancy to treat maternal hypertension or heart failure. Those who are planning a pregnancy should be considered for other medication options if an ACE inhibitor is currently prescribed or the ACE inhibitor should be discontinued as soon as possible once pregnancy is detected. The exposed fetus should be monitored for fetal growth, amniotic fluid volume, and organ formation. Infants exposed to an ACE inhibitor *in utero*, especially during the second and third trimester, should be monitored for hyperkalemia, hypotension, and oliguria.

[U.S. Boxed Warning]: Based on human data, ACE inhibitors can cause injury and death to the developing fetus when used in the second and third trimesters. ACE inhibitors should be discontinued as soon as possible once pregnancy is detected.

Lactation Enters breast milk/not recommended (AAP rates "compatible")

Contraindications Hypersensitivity to enalapril or enalaprilat; angioedema related to previous treatment with an ACE inhibitor; patients with idiopathic or hereditary angioedema

Warnings/Precautions Anaphylactic reactions may occur rarely with ACE inhibitors. At any time during treatment (especially following first dose) angioedema may occur rarely with ACE inhibitors; it may involve the head and neck (potentially compromising airway) or the intestine (presenting with abdominal pain). African-Americans may be at an increased risk. Prolonged frequent monitoring may be required especially if tongue, glottis, or larynx are involved as they are associated with airway obstruction. Patients with a history of airway surgery may have a higher risk of airway obstruction. Aggressive early and appropriate management is critical. Use in patients with idiopathic or hereditary angioedema or previous angioedema associated with ACE inhibitor therapy is contraindicated. Severe anaphylactoid reactions may be seen during hemodialysis (eg, CVVHD) with high-flux dialysis membranes (eg, AN69), and rarely, during low density lipoprotein apheresis with dextran sulfate cellulose. Rare cases of anaphylactoid reactions have been reported in patients undergoing sensitization treatment with hymenoptera (bee, wasp) venom while receiving ACE inhibitors.

Symptomatic hypotension with or without syncope can occur with ACE inhibitors (usually with the first several doses); effects are most often observed in volume depleted patients; correct volume depletion prior to initiation; close monitoring of patient is required especially with initial dosing and dosing increases; blood pressure must be lowered at a rate appropriate for the patient's clinical condition. Initiation of therapy in patients with ischemic heart disease or cerebrovascular disease warrants close observation due to the potential consequences posed by falling blood pressure (eg, MI, stroke). Use with caution in hypertrophic cardiomyopathy with outflow tract obstruction, severe aortic stenosis, or before, during, or immediately after major surgery. **[U.S. Boxed Warning]: Based on human data, ACEIs can cause injury and death to the developing fetus when used in the second and third trimesters. ACEIs should be discontinued as soon as possible once pregnancy is detected.**

Hyperkalemia may occur with ACE inhibitors; risk factors include renal dysfunction, diabetes mellitus, concomitant use of potassium-sparing diuretics, potassium supplements, and/or potassium-containing salts. Use cautiously, if at all, with these agents and monitor potassium closely. Cough may occur with ACE inhibitors. Other causes of cough should be considered (eg, pulmonary congestion in patients with heart failure) and excluded prior to discontinuation.

May be associated with deterioration of renal function and/or increases in serum creatinine, particularly in patients with low renal blood flow (eg, renal artery stenosis, heart failure) whose glomerular filtration rate (GFR) is dependent on efferent arteriolar vasoconstriction by angiotensin II; deterioration may result in oliguria, acute renal failure, and progressive azotemia. Small increases in serum creatinine may occur following initiation; consider discontinuation only in patients with progressive and/or significant deterioration in renal function. Use with caution in patients with unstented unilateral/bilateral renal artery stenosis. When unstented bilateral renal artery stenosis is present, use is generally avoided due to the elevated risk of deterioration in renal function unless possible benefits outweigh risks.

Rare toxicities associated with ACE inhibitors include cholestatic jaundice (which may progress to fulminant hepatic necrosis), agranulocytosis, neutropenia or leukopenia with myeloid hypoplasia. Patients with collagen vascular diseases (especially with concomitant renal impairment) or renal impairment alone may be at increased risk for hematologic toxicity; periodically monitor CBC with differential in these patients.

Adverse Reactions Note: Frequency ranges include data from hypertension and heart failure trials. Higher rates of adverse reactions have generally been noted in patients with CHF. However, the frequency of adverse effects associated with placebo is also increased in this population.

1% to 10%:

Cardiovascular: Hypotension (0.9% to 6.7%), chest pain (2%), syncope (0.5% to 2%), orthostasis (2%), orthostatic hypotension (2%)

Central nervous system: Headache (2% to 5%), dizziness (4% to 8%), fatigue (2% to 3%)

Dermatologic: Rash (1.5%)

Gastrointestinal: Abnormal taste, abdominal pain, vomiting, nausea, diarrhea, anorexia, constipation

Neuromuscular & skeletal: Weakness

Renal: Serum creatinine increased (0.2% to 20%), worsening of renal function (in patients with bilateral renal artery stenosis or hypovolemia)

Respiratory (1% to 2%): Bronchitis, cough, dyspnea

<1% (Limited to important or life-threatening): Agranulocytosis, alopecia, anaphylactoid reaction, angina pectoris, angioedema, ataxia, atrial fibrillation, atrial tachycardia, bone marrow suppression, bradycardia, bronchospasm, cardiac arrest, cerebral vascular accident, cholestatic jaundice, depression, eosinophilic pneumonitis, erythema multiforme, exfoliative dermatitis, flushing, giant cell arteritis, gynecomastia, hallucinations, hemolysis with G6PD, Henoch-Schönlein purpura, hepatitis, ileus, impotence, jaundice, lichen-form reaction, melena, MI, neutropenia, ototoxicity, pancreatitis, paresthesia, pemphigus, pemphigus foliaceus, peripheral neuropathy, photosensitivity, psychosis, pulmonary edema, pulmonary embolism, pulmonary infiltrates, Raynaud's phenomenon, sicca syndrome, somnolence, Stevens-Johnson syndrome, systemic lupus erythematosus, thrombocytopenia, toxic epidermal necrolysis, toxic pustuloderma, vertigo.

A syndrome which may include arthralgia, elevated ESR, eosinophilia and positive ANA, fever, interstitial nephritis, myalgia, rash, and vasculitis has been reported for enalapril and other ACE inhibitors.

Metabolism/Transport Effects Substrate of CYP3A4 (minor)

Drug Interactions

Allopurinol: ACE Inhibitors may enhance the potential for allergic or hypersensitivity reactions to Allopurinol. *Risk D: Consider therapy modification*

Angiotensin II Receptor Blockers: May enhance the adverse/toxic effect of ACE Inhibitors. *Risk C: Monitor therapy*

Antacids: May decrease the serum concentration of ACE Inhibitors. *Risk C: Monitor therapy*

Aprotinin: May diminish the antihypertensive effect of ACE Inhibitors. *Risk C: Monitor therapy*

AzaTHIOprine: ACE Inhibitors may enhance the neutropenic effect of AzaTHIOprine. *Risk C: Monitor therapy*

CycloSPORINE: ACE Inhibitors may enhance the nephrotoxic effect of CycloSPORINE. *Risk D: Consider therapy modification*

CYP3A4 Inducers (Strong): May increase the metabolism of CYP3A4 Substrates. *Risk C: Monitor therapy*

Deferasirox: May decrease the serum concentration of CYP3A4 Substrates. *Risk C: Monitor therapy*

Diazoxide: May enhance the hypotensive effect of Antihypertensives. *Risk C: Monitor therapy*

Eplerenone: May enhance the hyperkalemic effect of ACE Inhibitors. *Risk C: Monitor therapy*

Ferric Gluconate: ACE Inhibitors may enhance the adverse/toxic effect of Ferric Gluconate. *Risk C: Monitor therapy*

Gold Sodium Thiomalate: ACE Inhibitors may enhance the adverse/toxic effect of Gold Sodium Thiomalate. An increased risk of nitritoid reactions has been appreciated. *Risk C: Monitor therapy*

Herbs (CYP3A4 Inducers): May increase the metabolism of CYP3A4 Substrates. *Risk C: Monitor therapy*

Herbs (Hypertensive Properties): May diminish the antihypertensive effect of Antihypertensives. *Risk C: Monitor therapy*

Herbs (Hypotensive Properties): May enhance the hypotensive effect of Antihypertensives. *Risk C: Monitor therapy*

Lithium: ACE Inhibitors may increase the serum concentration of Lithium. *Risk D: Consider therapy modification*

Loop Diuretics: May enhance the hypotensive effect of ACE Inhibitors. Specifically, postural hypotension which can accompany ACE Inhibitor initiation. Loop Diuretics may enhance the nephrotoxic effect of ACE Inhibitors. *Risk C: Monitor therapy*

Methylphenidate: May diminish the antihypertensive effect of Antihypertensives. *Risk C: Monitor therapy*

Nonsteroidal Anti-Inflammatory Agents: May diminish the antihypertensive effect of ACE Inhibitors. *Risk C: Monitor therapy*

Potassium Salts: May enhance the hyperkalemic effect of ACE Inhibitors. *Risk C: Monitor therapy*

Potassium-Sparing Diuretics: May enhance the hyperkalemic effect of ACE Inhibitors. *Risk C: Monitor therapy*

Prostacyclin Analogues: May enhance the hypotensive effect of Antihypertensives. *Risk C: Monitor therapy*

RiTUXimab: Antihypertensives may enhance the hypotensive effect of RiTUXimab. *Risk D: Consider therapy modification*

Salicylates: May diminish the antihypertensive effect of ACE Inhibitors. They may also diminish other beneficial pharmacodynamic effects desired for the treatment of CHF. The effects are likely dose-related. 100 mg doses aspirin appear to cause no problems, whereas 300 mg doses appear to significantly affect ACE Inhibitor efficacy. *Risk C: Monitor therapy*

Sirolimus: May enhance the adverse/toxic effect of ACE Inhibitors. *Risk C: Monitor therapy*

Temsirolimus: May enhance the adverse/toxic effect of ACE Inhibitors. *Risk C: Monitor therapy*

Thiazide Diuretics: May enhance the hypotensive effect of ACE Inhibitors. Specifically, postural hypotension which can accompany ACE Inhibitor initiation. Thiazide Diuretics may enhance the nephrotoxic effect of ACE Inhibitors. *Risk C: Monitor therapy*

Trimethoprim: May enhance the hyperkalemic effect of ACE Inhibitors. *Risk C: Monitor therapy*

Ethanol/Nutrition/Herb Interactions Herb/Nutraceutical: Avoid bayberry, blue cohosh, cayenne, ephedra, ginger, ginseng (American), kola, licorice (may worsen hypertension). Avoid black cohosh, california poppy, coleus, golden seal, hawthorn, mistletoe, periwinkle, quinine, shepherd's purse (may have increased antihypertensive effect).

Stability Enalaprilat: Clear, colorless solution which should be stored at <30°C. I.V. is 24 hours at room temperature in D_5W or NS.

Mechanism of Action Competitive inhibitor of angiotensin-converting enzyme (ACE); prevents conversion of angiotensin I to angiotensin II, a potent vasoconstrictor; results in lower levels of angiotensin II which causes an increase in plasma renin activity and a reduction in aldosterone secretion

Pharmacodynamics/Kinetics

Onset of action: Oral: ~1 hour

Duration: Oral: 12-24 hours

Absorption: Oral: 55% to 75%

Protein binding: 50% to 60%

Metabolism: Prodrug, undergoes hepatic biotransformation to enalaprilat

Half-life elimination:

Enalapril: Adults: Healthy: 2 hours; Congestive heart failure: 3.4-5.8 hours

Enalaprilat: Infants 6 weeks to 8 months of age: 6-10 hours; Adults: 35-38 hours

Time to peak, serum: Oral: Enalapril: 0.5-1.5 hours; Enalaprilat (active): 3-4.5 hours

Excretion: Urine (60% to 80%); some feces

Dosage Use lower listed initial dose in patients with hyponatremia, hypovolemia, severe congestive heart failure, decreased renal function, or in those receiving diuretics.

Oral: **Enalapril**: Children 1 month to 17 years: Hypertension: Initial: 0.08 mg/kg/d (up to 5 mg) in 1-2 divided doses; adjust dosage based on patient response; doses >0.58 mg/kg (40 mg) have not been evaluated in pediatric patients

Investigational: Congestive heart failure: Initial oral doses of **enalapril**: 0.1 mg/kg/day increasing as needed over 2 weeks to 0.5 mg/kg/day have been used in infants

Investigational: Neonatal hypertension: I.V. doses of **enalaprilat**: 5-10 mcg/kg/dose administered every 8-24 hours have been used; monitor patients carefully; select patients may require higher doses

Adults:

Oral: **Enalapril:**

Hypertension: 2.5-5 mg/day then increase as required, usually at 1- to 2-week intervals; usual dose range (JNC 7): 2.5-40 mg/day in 1-2 divided doses. **Note:** Initiate with 2.5 mg if patient is taking a diuretic which cannot be discontinued. May add a diuretic if blood pressure cannot be controlled with enalapril alone.

Heart failure: Initial: 2.5 mg once or twice daily (usual range: 5-40 mg/day in 2 divided doses). Titrate slowly at 1- to 2-week intervals. Target dose: 10-20 mg twice daily (ACC/AHA 2005 Heart Failure Guidelines)

Asymptomatic left ventricular dysfunction: 2.5 mg twice daily, titrated as tolerated to 20 mg/day

I.V.: **Enalaprilat:**

Hypertension: 1.25 mg/dose, given over 5 minutes every 6 hours; doses as high as 5 mg/dose every 6 hours have been tolerated for up to 36 hours. **Note:** If patients are concomitantly receiving diuretic therapy, begin with 0.625 mg I.V. over 5 minutes; if the effect is not adequate after 1 hour, repeat the dose and administer 1.25 mg at 6-hour intervals thereafter; if adequate, administer 0.625 mg I.V. every 6 hours.

Heart failure: Avoid I.V. administration in patients with unstable heart failure or those suffering acute myocardial infarction.

Conversion from I.V. to oral therapy if not concurrently on diuretics: 5 mg once daily; subsequent titration as needed; if concurrently receiving diuretics and responding to 0.625 mg I.V. every 6 hours, initiate with 2.5 mg/day.

Dosing adjustment in renal impairment:

Oral: Enalapril:

Cl_{cr} 30-80 mL/minute: Administer 5 mg/day titrated upwards to maximum of 40 mg.

Cl_{cr} <30 mL/minute: Administer 2.5 mg day; titrated upward until blood pressure is controlled.

For heart failure patients with sodium <130 mEq/L or serum creatinine >1.6 mg/dL, initiate dosage with 2.5 mg/day, increasing to twice daily as needed. Increase further in increments of 2.5 mg/dose at >4-day intervals to a maximum daily dose of 40 mg.

I.V.: Enalaprilat:

Cl_{cr} >30 mL/minute: Initiate with 1.25 mg every 6 hours and increase dose based on response.

Cl_{cr} <30 mL/minute: Initiate with 0.625 mg every 6 hours and increase dose based on response.

Hemodialysis: Moderately dialyzable (20% to 50%); administer dose post-dialysis (eg, 0.625 mg I.V. every 6 hours) or administer 20% to 25% supplemental dose following dialysis; Clearance: 62 mL/minute.

Peritoneal dialysis: Supplemental dose is not necessary, although some removal of drug occurs.

Dosing adjustment in hepatic impairment: Hydrolysis of enalapril to enalaprilat may be delayed and/or impaired in patients with severe hepatic impairment, but the pharmacodynamic effects of the drug do not appear to be significantly altered; no dosage adjustment.

Dietary Considerations Limit salt substitutes or potassium-rich diet.

Administration Administer direct IVP over at least 5 minutes or dilute up to 50 mL and infuse; discontinue diuretic, if possible, for 2-3 days before beginning enalapril therapy

Monitoring Parameters Blood pressure; serum creatinine and potassium; if patient has collagen vascular disease and/or renal impairment, periodically monitor CBC with differential

Test Interactions Positive Coombs' [direct]; may cause false-positive results in urine acetone determinations using sodium nitroprusside reagent

Dosage Forms Excipient information presented when available (limited, particularly for generics); consult specific product labeling.

Injection, solution, as enalaprilat: 1.25 mg/mL (1 mL, 2 mL) [contains benzyl alcohol]

Tablet, as maleate (Vasotec®): 2.5 mg, 5 mg, 10 mg, 20 mg

Enalapril and Felodipine (e NAL a pril & fe LOE di peen)

U.S. Brand Names Lexxel® [DSC]

Canadian Brand Names Lexxel®

Index Terms Enalapril Maleate and Felodipine; Felodipine and Enalapril

Pharmacologic Category Angiotensin-Converting Enzyme (ACE) Inhibitor; Calcium Channel Blocker

Use Treatment of hypertension, however, not indicated for initial treatment of hypertension; replacement therapy in patients receiving separate dosage forms (for patient convenience); when monotherapy with one component fails to achieve desired antihypertensive effect, or when dose-limiting adverse effects limit upward titration of monotherapy

Effect on Mental Status May cause drowsiness and dizziness; rarely may cause nervousness, insomnia, confusion, or depression

Effect on Psychiatric Treatment May rarely cause agranulocytosis; use caution with clozapine and carbamazepine; may decrease lithium clearance resulting in an increase in serum lithium levels and potential lithium toxicity; monitor serum lithium levels; carbamazepine may decrease felodipine effect

Dosage Summary

Oral:

Children: Dosage not established

Adults: Enalapril 5-20 mg and felodipine 2.5-10 mg once daily

Elderly: Initial dose of felodipine is 2.5 mg daily

Dosage Forms Excipient information presented when available (limited, particularly for generics); consult specific product labeling. [DSC] = Discontinued product

Tablet, extended release:

Lexxel® 5/2.5: Enalapril maleate 5 mg and felodipine 2.5 mg [DSC]

Lexxel® 5/5: Enalapril maleate 5 mg and felodipine 5 mg [DSC]

Enalapril and Hydrochlorothiazide

(e NAL a pril & hye droe klor oh THYE a zide)

U.S. Brand Names Vaseretic®

Canadian Brand Names Vaseretic®

Mexican Brand Names Co-Renitec

Index Terms Enalapril Maleate and Hydrochlorothiazide; Hydrochlorothiazide and Enalapril

Pharmacologic Category Angiotensin-Converting Enzyme (ACE) Inhibitor; Diuretic, Thiazide

Use Treatment of hypertension

Effect on Mental Status May cause drowsiness and dizziness; rarely may cause insomnia, confusion, and depression

Effect on Psychiatric Treatment May rarely cause agranulocytosis; use caution with clozapine and carbamazepine; may decrease lithium clearance resulting in an increase in serum lithium levels and potential lithium toxicity; monitor serum lithium levels

Dosage Summary

Oral:

Children: Dosage not established

Adults: Enalapril 5-10 mg and hydrochlorothiazide 12.5-25 mg once daily (maximum: 40 mg/day [enalapril]; 50 mg/day [hydrochlorothiazide])

Dosage Forms Excipient information presented when available (limited, particularly for generics); consult specific product labeling.

Tablet:

5/12.5: Enalapril maleate 5 mg and hydrochlorothiazide 12.5 mg

10/25: Enalapril maleate 10 mg and hydrochlorothiazide 25 mg

Vaseretic®:

10/25: Enalapril maleate 10 mg and hydrochlorothiazide 25 mg

- ◆ **Enalaprilat** *see* Enalapril *on page 531*
- ◆ **Enalapril Maleate** *see* Enalapril *on page 531*
- ◆ **Enalapril Maleate and Felodipine** *see* Enalapril and Felodipine *on page 536*
- ◆ **Enalapril Maleate and Hydrochlorothiazide** *see* Enalapril and Hydrochlorothiazide *on page 536*
- ◆ **Enbrel®** *see* Etanercept *on page 591*
- ◆ **Encort™** *see* Hydrocortisone *on page 785*

- **EndaCof [DSC]** *see* Hydrocodone and Guaifenesin *on page 779*
- **EndaCof-DM** *see* Brompheniramine, Pseudoephedrine, and Dextromethorphan *on page 208*
- **EndaCof-PD** *see* Brompheniramine, Pseudoephedrine, and Dextromethorphan *on page 208*
- **EndaCof-XP [DSC]** *see* Hydrocodone and Guaifenesin *on page 779*
- **Endocet®** *see* Oxycodone and Acetaminophen *on page 1205*
- **Endodan®** *see* Oxycodone and Aspirin *on page 1208*
- **Endometrin®** *see* Progesterone *on page 1345*
- **Enduron® [DSC]** *see* Methyclothiazide *on page 1020*
- **Enerjets [OTC]** *see* Caffeine *on page 250*

Enfuvirtide (en FYOO vir tide)

U.S. Brand Names Fuzeon®

Canadian Brand Names Fuzeon®

Mexican Brand Names Fuzeon

Index Terms T-20

Pharmacologic Category Antiretroviral Agent, Fusion Protein Inhibitor

Use Treatment of HIV-1 infection in combination with other antiretroviral agents in treatment-experienced patients with evidence of HIV-1 replication despite ongoing antiretroviral therapy

Effect on Mental Status Insomnia is common; may cause depression and anxiety. Suicide attempts have been reported.

Effect on Psychiatric Treatment May cause an increase in triglycerides; use caution with clozapine, olanzapine, quetiapine, and mirtazapine. Smokers have an increased risk of pneumonia; monitor. May rarely cause neutropenia and thrombocytopenia; use caution with clozapine, carbamazepine, and valproic acid

Dosage Summary

SubQ:

Children <6 years: Dosage not established

Children 6-16 years: 2 mg/kg twice daily (maximum: 90 mg/dose)

Adolescents ≥16 years: 90 mg twice daily

Adults: 90 mg twice daily

Dosage Forms Excipient information presented when available (limited, particularly for generics); consult specific product labeling.

Injection, powder for reconstitution [preservative free]:

Fuzeon®: 108 mg [90 mg/mL following reconstitution; available in convenience kit of 60 vials, SWFI, syringes, alcohol wipes, patient instructions]

- **ENG** *see* Etonogestrel *on page 606*
- **Engerix-B®** *see* Hepatitis B Vaccine *on page 764*
- **Enjuvia™** *see* Estrogens (Conjugated B/Synthetic) *on page 581*
- **Enlon® [DSC]** *see* Edrophonium *on page 525*
- **Enlon-Plus™ [DSC]** *see* Edrophonium and Atropine *on page 525*

Enoxaparin (ee noks a PA rin)

Medication Safety Issues

Sound-alike/look-alike issues:

Lovenox® may be confused with Levaquin®, Lotronex®, Protonix®

High alert medication: The Institute for Safe Medication Practices (ISMP) includes this medication among its list of drugs which have a heightened risk of causing significant patient harm when used in error.

International issues:

Lovenox® may be confused with Lotanax® which is a brand name for terfenadine in the Czech Republic

2009 National Patient Safety Goals: The Joint Commission on Accreditation of Healthcare Organizations requires healthcare organizations that provide anticoagulant therapy to have a process in place to reduce the risk of anticoagulant-associated patient harm. Patients receiving anticoagulants should receive individualized care through a defined process that includes standardized ordering, dispensing, administration, monitoring and education. This does not apply to routine short-term use of anticoagulants for prevention of venous thromboembolism when the expectation is that the patient's laboratory values will remain within or close to normal values (NPSG.03.05.01).

U.S. Brand Names Lovenox®

Canadian Brand Names Enoxaparin Injection; Lovenox®; Lovenox® HP

Mexican Brand Names Clexane

Index Terms Enoxaparin Sodium

Pharmacologic Category Low Molecular Weight Heparin

Use

Acute coronary syndromes: Unstable angina (UA), non-ST-elevation (NSTEMI), and ST-elevation myocardial infarction (STEMI)

DVT prophylaxis: Following hip or knee replacement surgery, abdominal surgery, or in medical patients with severely-restricted mobility during acute illness who are at risk for thromboembolic complications

DVT treatment (acute): Inpatient treatment (patients with and without pulmonary embolism) and outpatient treatment (patients without pulmonary embolism)

Note: High-risk patients include those with one or more of the following risk factors: >40 years of age, obesity, general anesthesia lasting >30 minutes, malignancy, history of deep vein thrombosis or pulmonary embolism

Unlabeled/Investigational Use Prophylaxis and treatment of thromboembolism in children; anticoagulant bridge therapy during temporary interruption of vitamin K antagonist therapy in patients at high risk for thromboembolism; DVT prophylaxis following moderate-risk general surgery, major gynecologic surgery and following higher-risk general surgery for cancer; management of venous thromboembolism (VTE) during pregnancy (Hirsh, 2008)

Effect on Mental Status May cause confusion

Effect on Psychiatric Treatment None reported

Dosage Summary

SubQ:

Infants <2 months (unlabeled use): Prophylaxis: 0.75 mg/kg every 12 hours; Treatment: Initial: 1.5 mg/kg every 12 hours; Maintenance: Titrate dose based on antifactor Xa levels

Children ≥2 months to 18 years (unlabeled use): Prophylaxis: 0.5 mg/kg every 12 hours; Treatment: Initial: 1 mg/kg every 12 hours; Maintenance: Titrate dose based on antifactor Xa levels

Adults: Prophylaxis: 30 mg every 12 hours **or** 40 mg once daily; Treatment: 1 mg/kg every 12 hours **or** 1.5 mg/kg once daily

STEMI indication only:

<75 years: 30 mg I.V. bolus plus 1 mg/kg SubQ every 12 hours

≥75 years: 0.75 mg/kg SubQ every 12 hours; **Note:** I.V. bolus is omitted

Elderly: Refer to adult dosing.

Dosage Forms Excipient information presented when available (limited, particularly for generics); consult specific product labeling.

Injection, solution, as sodium [graduated prefilled syringe; preservative free]:

Lovenox®: 60 mg/0.6 mL (0.6 mL); 80 mg/0.8 mL (0.8 mL); 100 mg/mL (1 mL); 120 mg/0.8 mL (0.8 mL); 150 mg/mL (1 mL)

Injection, solution, as sodium [multidose vial]:

Lovenox®: 100 mg/mL (3 mL) [contains benzyl alcohol]

Injection, solution, as sodium [prefilled syringe; preservative free]:

Lovenox®: 30 mg/0.3 mL (0.3 mL); 40 mg/0.4 mL (0.4 mL)

◆ **Enoxaparin Sodium** *see* Enoxaparin *on page 537*

◆ **Enpresse™** *see* Ethinyl Estradiol and Levonorgestrel *on page 595*

Entacapone (en TA ka pone)

Related Information

Antiparkinsonian Agents *on page 1767*

U.S. Brand Names Comtan®

Canadian Brand Names Comtan®

Mexican Brand Names Comtan

Pharmacologic Category Anti-Parkinson's Agent, COMT Inhibitor

Generic Available No

Use Adjunct to levodopa/carbidopa therapy in patients with idiopathic Parkinson's disease who experience "wearing-off" symptoms at the end of a dosing interval

Pregnancy Risk Factor C

Pregnancy Considerations Not recommended

Lactation Excretion in breast milk unknown/use caution

Contraindications Hypersensitivity to entacapone or any of component of the formulation

Warnings/Precautions May cause orthostatic hypotension and syncope; Parkinson's disease patients appear to have an impaired capacity to respond to a postural challenge; use with caution in patients at risk of hypotension (such as those receiving antihypertensive drugs) or where transient hypotensive episodes would be poorly tolerated (cardiovascular disease or cerebrovascular disease). Parkinson's patients being treated with dopaminergic agonists ordinarily require careful monitoring for signs and symptoms of postural hypotension, especially during dose escalation, and should be informed of this risk. May cause hallucinations, which may improve with reduction in levodopa therapy. Use with caution in patients with pre-existing dyskinesias; exacerbation of pre-existing dyskinesia and severe rhabdomyolysis has been reported. Levodopa dosage reduction may be required, particularly in patients with levodopa dosages >600 mg daily or with moderate-to-severe dyskinesia prior to initiation. Entacapone, in conjunction with other drug therapy that alters brain biogenic amine concentrations (eg, MAO inhibitors, SSRIs), has been associated with a syndrome resembling neuroleptic malignant syndrome (hyperpyrexia and confusion - some fatal) on abrupt withdrawal or dosage reduction. Concomitant use of entacapone and nonselective MAO inhibitors should be avoided. Selegiline is a selective MAO type B inhibitor (when given orally at ≤10 mg/day) and can be taken with entacapone. Dopaminergic agents from the ergot class have also been associated with fibrotic complications, such as retroperitoneal fibrosis, pulmonary infiltrates or effusion and pleural thickening. It is unknown whether non-ergot, pro-dopaminergic agents like entacapone confer this risk. Use caution in patients with hepatic impairment or severe renal impairment. Do not withdraw therapy abruptly. Safety and efficacy in pediatric patients have not been established.

Adverse Reactions

>10%:

- Gastrointestinal: Nausea (14%)
- Neuromuscular & skeletal: Dyskinesia (25%), placebo (15%)

1% to 10%:

- Cardiovascular: Orthostatic hypotension (4.3%), syncope (1.2%)
- Central nervous system: Dizziness (8%), fatigue (6%), hallucinations (4%), anxiety (2%), somnolence (2%), agitation (1%)
- Dermatologic: Purpura (2%)
- Gastrointestinal: Diarrhea (10%), abdominal pain (8%), constipation (6%), vomiting (4%), dry mouth (3%), dyspepsia (2%), flatulence (2%), gastritis (1%), taste perversion (1%)
- Genitourinary: Brown-orange urine discoloration (10%)
- Neuromuscular & skeletal: Hyperkinesia (10%), hypokinesia (9%), back pain (4%), weakness (2%)
- Respiratory: Dyspnea (3%)
- Miscellaneous: Diaphoresis increased (2%), bacterial infection (1%)

<1% (Limited to important or life-threatening): Hyperpyrexia and confusion (resembling neuroleptic malignant syndrome), pulmonary fibrosis, retroperitoneal fibrosis, rhabdomyolysis

Metabolism/Transport Effects Inhibits CYP1A2 (weak), 2A6 (weak), 2C9 (weak), 2C19 (weak), 2D6 (weak), 2E1 (weak), 3A4 (weak)

Drug Interactions

Alcohol (Ethyl): CNS Depressants may enhance the CNS depressant effect of Alcohol (Ethyl). *Risk C: Monitor therapy*

CNS Depressants: May enhance the adverse/toxic effect of other CNS Depressants. *Risk C: Monitor therapy*

COMT Substrates: COMT Inhibitors may decrease the metabolism of COMT Substrates. *Risk C: Monitor therapy*

MAO Inhibitors: COMT Inhibitors may enhance the adverse/toxic effect of MAO Inhibitors. *Risk D: Consider therapy modification*

Ethanol/Nutrition/Herb Interactions

Ethanol: Avoid ethanol (may increase CNS adverse effects).

Food: Entacapone has been reported to chelate iron and decreasing serum iron levels were noted in clinical trials; however, clinically significant anemia has not been observed.

Mechanism of Action Entacapone is a reversible and selective inhibitor of catechol-O-methyltransferase (COMT). When entacapone is taken with levodopa, the pharmacokinetics are altered, resulting in more sustained levodopa serum levels compared to levodopa taken alone. The resulting levels of levodopa provide for increased concentrations available for absorption across the blood-brain barrier, thereby providing for increased CNS levels of dopamine, the active metabolite of levodopa.

Pharmacodynamics/Kinetics

Onset of action: Rapid

Peak effect: 1 hour

Absorption: Rapid

Distribution: I.V.: V_{dss}: 20 L

Protein binding: 98%, primarily to albumin

Metabolism: Isomerization to the *cis*-isomer, followed by direct glucuronidation of the parent and *cis*-isomer

Bioavailability: 35%

Half-life elimination: B phase: 0.4-0.7 hours; Y phase: 2.4 hours

Time to peak, serum: 1 hour

Excretion: Feces (90%); urine (10%)

Dosage Oral: Adults: 200 mg with each dose of levodopa/carbidopa, up to a maximum of 8 times/day (maximum daily dose: 1600 mg/day). To optimize therapy, the dosage of levodopa may need reduced or the dosing interval may need extended. Patients taking levodopa ≥800 mg/day or who had moderate-to-severe dyskinesias prior to therapy required an average decrease of 25% in the daily levodopa dose.

Dosage adjustment in hepatic impairment: Treat with caution and monitor carefully; AUC and C_{max} can be possibly doubled

Dietary Considerations May be taken with or without food.

Administration Always administer in association with levodopa/carbidopa; can be combined with both the immediate and sustained release formulations of levodopa/carbidopa. Can be taken with or without food. Should not be abruptly withdrawn from patient's therapy due to significant worsening of symptoms.

Monitoring Parameters Signs and symptoms of Parkinson's disease; liver function tests, blood pressure, patient's mental status; serum iron (if signs of anemia)

Dosage Forms Excipient information presented when available (limited, particularly for generics); consult specific product labeling.

Tablet: 200 mg

◆ **Entacapone, Carbidopa, and Levodopa** *see* Levodopa, Carbidopa, and Entacapone *on page 911*

Entecavir (en TE ka veer)

U.S. Brand Names Baraclude®

Canadian Brand Names Baraclude®

Pharmacologic Category Antiretroviral Agent, Reverse Transcriptase Inhibitor (Nucleoside)

Use Treatment of chronic hepatitis B infection in adults with evidence of active viral replication and either evidence of persistent transaminase elevations or histologically-active disease

Effect on Mental Status May cause sedation

Effect on Psychiatric Treatment None reported

Dosage Summary

Oral:

Children <16 years: Dosage not established

Adolescents ≥16 years: Nucleoside naive: 0.5 mg once daily; Lamivudine- or telbivudine-resistant: 1 mg once daily

Adults: Nucleoside naive: 0.5 mg once daily; Lamivudine- or telbivudine-resistant: 1 mg once daily

Dosage Forms Excipient information presented when available (limited, particularly for generics); consult specific product labeling.

Oral solution:

Baraclude®: 0.05 mg/mL (210 mL) [orange flavor]

Tablet:

Baraclude®: 0.5 mg, 1 mg

◆ **Entex® HC [DSC]** *see* Hydrocodone, Pseudoephedrine, and Guaifenesin *on page 784*

◆ **Entex® PSE** *see* Guaifenesin and Pseudoephedrine *on page 744*

◆ **Entocort® EC** *see* Budesonide *on page 210*

◆ **Enulose** *see* Lactulose *on page 886*

◆ **Eperbel-S [DSC]** *see* Belladonna, Phenobarbital, and Ergotamine *on page 175*

Ephedra *(Ephedra sinica)*

Natural Product Category Herb

Synonyms *Ephedra sinica*; Chinese Ephedra; Chinese Joint Fir; Ma Huang; Soma

Plant Part Stem

Dosage and Standardization No more than 8 mg total ephedra alkaloids per dose **or** no more than 24 mg total ephedra alkaloids per 24 hours

Oral: Weight loss: 8 mg every 6 hours for up to 7 days

Reported Uses

Allergies, sinusitis, hay fever (Langwinski, 1972)

Asthma (Redman, 1998)

Hypotension (Ducros, 2002; Furukawa, 1974; Kee, 2000; Lee, 2002; Ngan Kee, 2001; Powell, 1998; Saito, 1977; Saito, 1977; Ueda, 1995; Unger, 1968)

Sexual arousal (Meston, 1998)

Weight loss (monotherapy) (Betz, 1997; Pasquali, 1987)

Weight loss (combination therapy) (Astrup, 1992; Breum, 1994; Daly, 1993; Hackman, 2006; Mólnar, 2000)

Summary The Chinese have used ephedra medicinally for over 5000 years. It is listed as one of the original 365 herbs from the classical first century A.D. text on Chinese herbalism by Shen Nong. Ephedra's traditional medicinal uses include the alleviation of sweating, lung and bronchial constriction, and water retention. It was not until 1924 that the herb became popular with physicians in the United States for its bronchodilation and decongestant properties.

Effect on Mental Status Insomnia, nervousness, and restlessness are common; may cause anxiety, agitation, irritability, and psychosis

Effect on Psychiatric Treatment Contraindicated in anxiety disorders; avoid concurrent use with MAO inhibitors; may potentiate effects of CNS stimulants

Pharmacology Ephedra contains the alkaloids ephedrine and pseudoephedrine, which are routinely isolated and used in OTC products as decongestants. Ephedra is a potent sympathomimetic that stimulates alpha-, beta$_1$-, and beta$_2$-adrenergic receptors, and the release of norepinephrine (Langwinski, 1972). Its activity on the sympathetic nervous system causes vasoconstriction and cardiac stimulation. It is a sympathomimetic and produces a temporary rise in both systolic and diastolic blood pressure, causes mydriasis, produces bronchial muscle relaxation, and is a vasoconstrictor.

Warnings and Interactions Ephedra has been shown to cause hypertension, palpitations, arrhythmias, tachycardia, myocardial infarction, cardiac arrest, and sudden death. CNS events may include stroke, seizures, and transient ischemic attacks (Haller, 2000; Traub, 2001).

Theoretical Cautions and Contraindications Consult a physician before using in individuals with renal impairment (including nephrolithiasis) (Powell, 1998), hypertension, cardiovascular disease, thyroid disease, diabetes, prostate disorders, and glaucoma, as well as in individuals taking sympathomimetic medications and OTC stimulants (such as caffeine, phenylpropanolamine, and pseudoephedrine). Use is contraindicated in individuals taking MAO inhibitors (Dawson, 1995); use is contraindicated in pregnancy and lactation (Leung, 1996). Use with caution in individuals with diabetes or hypoglycemia and in those taking drugs, herbs, or supplements that affect blood sugar. In theory, ephedra may lower blood sugar levels. Ephedra may reduce the effects of steroids such as dexamethasone. Use with caution in individuals taking steroids. Some individuals may be sensitive to ephedra and may experience excitability and other complaints. If symptoms occur and continue for longer than 2 days, discontinue use. Ephedra has many reports of abuse. Use caution when considering this supplement.

Theoretical Interactions MAO inhibitors, sympathomimetic medications, OTC stimulants, thyroid medications, calcium channel blockers, antiarrhythmics, beta-blockers, angiotensin converting enzyme (ACE) inhibitors, cardiac glycosides, antidiabetic agents, ergot alkaloids, guanethidine, oxytocin, diuretics, morphine, anesthetic drugs, steroids

References

Astrup A, Breum L, Toubro S, et al, "The Effect and Safety of an Ephedrine/Caffeine Compound Compared to Ephedrine, Caffeine and Placebo in Obese Subjects on an Energy Restricted Diet. A Double Blind Trial," *Int J Obes Relat Metab Disord*, 1992, 16 (4):269-77.

Betz JM, Gay ML, Mossoba MM, et al, "Chiral Gas Chromatographic Determination of Ephedrine-Type Alkaloids in Dietary Supplements Containing Ma Huang," *J AOAC Int*, 1997, 80(2):303-15.

Breum L, Pedersen JK, Ahlstrøm F, et al, "Comparison of an Ephedrine/Caffeine Combination and Dexfenfluramine in the Treatment of Obesity. A Double-Blind Multi-Centre Trial in General Practice," *Int J Obes Relat Metab Disord*, 1994, 18(2):99-103.

Daly PA, Krieger DR, Dulloo AG, et al, "Ephedrine, Caffeine and Aspirin: Safety and Efficacy for Treatment of Human Obesity," *Int J Obes Relat Metab Disord*, 1993, 17 Suppl 1:S73-8.

Dawson JK, Earnshaw SM, and Graham CS, "Dangerous Monoamine Oxidase Inhibitor Interactions Are Still Occurring in the 1990s," *J Accid Emerg Med* 1995, 12(1):49-51.

Ducros L, Bonnin P, Cholley BP, et al, "Increasing Maternal Blood Pressure With Ephedrine Increases Uterine Artery Blood Flow Velocity During Uterine Contraction," *Anesthesiology*, 2002, 96(3):612-6.

Furukawa T and Kuroda M, "Effects of Ephedrine, Tyramine and Norepinephrine on the Blood Pressure Response to Dopamine," *Nippon Yakurigaku Zasshi*, 1974, 70(3):377-84.

Hackman RM, Havel PJ, Schwartz HJ, et al, "Multinutrient Supplement Containing Ephedra and Caffeine Causes Weight Loss and Improves Metabolic Risk Factors in Obese Women: A Randomized Controlled Trial," *Int J Obes (Lond)*, 2006, 30(10):1545-56.

Haller CA and Benowitz NL, "Adverse Cardiovascular and Central Nervous System Events Associated With Dietary Supplements Containing Ephedra Alkaloids," *N Engl J Med*, 2000, 343(25):1833-8.

Kee WD, Khaw KS, Lee BB, et al, "A Dose-Response Study of Prophylactic Intravenous Ephedrine for the Prevention of Hypotension During Spinal Anesthesia for Cesarean Delivery," *Anesth Analg*, 2000, 90(6):1390-5.

Langwinski R, "Central Effects of Ephedrine," *Pol Tyg Lek*, 1972, 27(31):1205-7.

Lee A, Ngan Kee WD, and Gin T, "A Quantitative, Systematic Review of Randomized Controlled Trials of Ephedrine Versus Phenylephrine for the Management of Hypotension During Spinal Anesthesia for Cesarean Delivery," *Anesth Analg*, 2002, 94(4):920-6.

Leung AY and Foster S, *Encyclopedia of Common Natural Ingredients Used in Foods, Drugs, and Cosmetics*, 2nd ed, New York, NY: John Wiley and Sons, Inc, 1996.

Meston CM and Heiman JR, "Ephedrine-Activated Physiological Sexual Arousal in Women," *Arch Gen Psychiatry*, 1998, 55(7):652-6.

Molnár D, Török K, Erhardt E, et al, "Safety and Efficacy of Treatment With an Ephedrine/Caffeine Mixture. The First Double-Blind Placebo-Controlled Pilot Study in Adolescents," *Int J Obes Relat Metab Disord*, 2000, 24(12):1573-8.

Natural Standard Research Collaboration, Chief Editors: Ulbricht C, Basch E, *Natural Standard Herb and Supplement Reference - Evidence-Based Clinical Reviews*, USA: Elsevier/Mosby, 2005.

Ngan Kee WD, Lau TK, Khaw KS, et al, "Comparison of Metaraminol and Ephedrine Infusions for Maintaining Arterial Pressure During Spinal Anesthesia for Elective Cesarean Section," *Anesthesiology*, 2001, 95(2):307-13.

Pasquali R, Cesari MP, Melchionda N, et al, "Does Ephedrine Promote Weight Loss in Low-Energy-Adapted Obese Women?" *Int J Obes*, 1987, 11(2):163-8.

Powell T, Hsu FF, Turk J, et al, "Ma-huang Strikes Again: Ephedrine Nephrolithiasis," *Am J Kidney Dis*, 1998, 32(1):153-9.

Redman CM and Druce HM, "Nonprescription Bronchodilator Use in Asthma," *Chest*, 1998, 11(4):657-8.

Saito H, "Mechanisms of Reversal of the Blood Pressure by Eephedrine (1)," *Nippon Yakurigaku Zasshi*, 1977, 73(1):73-82.

Saito H, "Mechanism of Reversal of the Blood Pressure by Ephedrine (2)," *Nippon Yakurigaku Zasshi*, 1977, 73(1):83-92.

Traub SJ, Hoyek W, and Hoffman RS, "Dietary Supplements Containing Ephedra Alkaloids," *N Engl J Med*, 2001, 344(14):1096.

Ueda W, Kataoka Y, Takimoto E, et al, "Ephedrine-Induced Increases in Arterial Blood Pressure Accelerate Regression of Epidural Block," *Anesth Analg*, 1995, 81(4):703-5.

Unger DL, "Blood Pressure and Pulse Rate Changes in Hypertensive Asthmatic Patients: Effects of an Ephedrine Compound," *Ann Allergy*, 1968, 26(12):637-8.

◆ ***Ephedra sinica*** *see* Ephedra *(Ephedra sinica) on page 541*

EPHEDrine (e FED rin)

Medication Safety Issues

Sound-alike/look-alike issues:

EPHEDrine may be confused with Epifrin®, EPINEPHrine

Related Information

Clozapine-Induced Side Effects *on page 1818*

U.S. Brand Names Pretz-D® [OTC]

Mexican Brand Names Coderit; Piralgina

Index Terms Ephedrine Sulfate

Pharmacologic Category Alpha/Beta Agonist

Use Treatment of bronchial asthma, nasal congestion, acute bronchospasm, idiopathic orthostatic hypotension, hypotension induced by spinal anesthesia

Effect on Mental Status Nervousness, anxiety, agitation, restlessness, and insomnia are common

Effect on Psychiatric Treatment Use with MAO inhibitors may produce hypertensive crisis; avoid combination

Dosage Summary

I.M.:

Children: 0.2-0.3 mg/kg/dose every 4-6 hours

Adults: 25-50 mg (maximum: 150 mg/day)

I.V.:

Children: 0.2-0.3 mg/kg/dose every 4-6 hours

Adults: 5-25 mg/dose, repeat after 5-10 minutes as needed, then every 3-4 hours (maximum: 150 mg/day)

Intranasal:

Children <6 years: Dosage not established

Children 6-12 years: 1-2 sprays into each nostril, not more frequently than every 4 hours

Children ≥12 years: 2-3 sprays into each nostril, not more frequently than every 4 hours

Adults: 2-3 sprays into each nostril, not more frequently than every 4 hours

Oral:

Children: 3 mg/kg/day **or** 25-100 mg/m^2/day in 4-6 divided doses (every 4-6 hours)

Adults: 25-50 mg every 3-4 hours as needed

SubQ:

Children: 3 mg/kg/day **or** 25-100 mg/m^2/day in 4-6 divided doses (every 4-6 hours)

Adults: 25-50 mg (maximum: 150 mg/day)

Dosage Forms Excipient information presented when available (limited, particularly for generics); consult specific product labeling.

Capsule, as sulfate: 25 mg

Injection, solution, as sulfate: 50 mg/mL (1 mL, 10 mL)

Solution, intranasal spray, as sulfate (Pretz-D®): 0.25% (50 mL)

- **Ephedrine, Chlorpheniramine, Phenylephrine, and Carbetapentane** *see* Chlorpheniramine, Ephedrine, Phenylephrine, and Carbetapentane *on page 326*
- **Ephedrine Sulfate** *see* EPHEDrine *on page 542*
- **Epidermal Thymocyte Activating Factor** *see* Aldesleukin *on page 58*

EPINEPHrine (ep i NEF rin)

Medication Safety Issues

Sound-alike/look-alike issues:

EPINEPHrine may be confused with ePHEDrine

Epifrin® may be confused with ephedrine, EpiPen®

EpiPen® may be confused with Epifrin®

High alert medication: The Institute for Safe Medication Practices (ISMP) includes this medication among its list of drugs which have a heightened risk of causing significant patient harm when used in error.

Medication errors have occurred due to confusion with epinephrine products expressed as ratio strengths (eg, 1:1000 vs 1:10,000).

Epinephrine 1:1000 = 1 mg/mL and is most commonly used I.M.

Epinephrine 1:10,000 = 0.1 mg/mL and is used I.V.

International issues:

EpiPen® may be confused with Epigen® which is a brand name for glycyrrhizinic acid in Mexico

EpiPen® may be confused with Epopen® which is a brand name for epoetin alfa in Spain

U.S. Brand Names Adrenalin®; EpiPen®; EpiPen® Jr; Primatene® Mist [OTC]; Raphon [OTC]; S2® [OTC]; Twinject™

Canadian Brand Names Adrenalin®; EpiPen®; EpiPen® Jr; Twinject™

Index Terms Adrenaline; Epinephrine Bitartrate; Epinephrine Hydrochloride; Racepinephrine

Pharmacologic Category Alpha/Beta Agonist; Antidote

Use Treatment of bronchospasms, bronchial asthma, nasal congestion, viral croup, anaphylactic reactions, cardiac arrest; added to local anesthetics to decrease systemic absorption of local anesthetics and increase duration of action; decrease superficial hemorrhage

Unlabeled/Investigational Use ACLS guidelines: Ventricular fibrillation (VF) or pulseless ventricular tachycardia (VT) unresponsive to initial defibrillatory shocks; pulseless electrical activity, asystole, hypotension unresponsive to volume resuscitation; symptomatic bradycardia or hypotension unresponsive to atropine or pacing; inotropic support

Effect on Mental Status Nervousness and restlessness are common; may cause insomnia

Effect on Psychiatric Treatment None reported; however, use cautiously with psychotropics that block alpha-receptors (phenothiazines); may produce paradoxical hypotension

Dosage Summary

I.M.:

Children: See specific products below

Adults: 0.3-0.5 mg (1:1000) every 15-20 minutes **or** see specific products below

EpiPen® Jr.:

Children <30 kg: 0.15 mg

EpiPen®:

Children ≥30 kg: 0.3 mg

Adults: 0.3 mg

Twinject™:

Children <15 kg: Dosage not established

Children 15-30 kg: 0.15 kg

Children >30 kg: 0.3 mg

Adults: 0.3 mg

I.O.:

Children: 0.01 mg/kg every 3-5 minutes as needed (maximum: 1 mg)

Adults: 1 mg every 3-5 minutes (up to 0.2 mg/kg may be needed for specific problems)

I.V. (1:10,000):

Neonates: 0.01-0.03 mg/kg every 3-5 minutes as needed

Children: 0.01 mg/kg every 3-5 minutes as needed (maximum: 1 mg) **or** 0.1-1 mcg/kg/minute as a continuous infusion **or** 0.01 mg/kg every 20 minutes (hypersensitivity reaction)

Adults: 1 mg every 3-5 minutes (up to 0.2 mg/kg may be needed for specific problems) **or** 1-10 mcg/minute as a continuous infusion

Inhalation:

Children <4 years: Dosage not established

Children ≥4 years: One inhalation, may repeat once after 1 minute, then do not use again for at least 3 hours

Adults: One inhalation, may repeat once after 1 minute, then do not use again for at least 3 hours

Intranasal:

Children <6 years: Dosage not established

Children ≥6 years: Apply 1:1000 locally as drops, spray or with sterile swab

Adults: Apply 1:1000 locally as drops, spray or with sterile swab

Intratracheal:

Neonates: 0.01-0.03 mg/kg every 3-5 minutes as needed

Children: 0.1 mg/kg every 3-5 minutes (maximum: 10 mg)

Adults: 2-2.5 mg diluted in 5-10 mL NS or distilled water

Nebulization:

Children: 1-3 inhalations up to every 3 hours (prepared with 10 drops of **1:100** solution for oral inhalation [Adrenalin®])

Adults: 1-3 inhalations up to every 3 hours (prepared with 10 drops of **1:100** solution for oral inhalation [Adrenalin®])

S2® (Racepinephrine, OTC):

Children <4 years: 0.05 mL/kg diluted in 3 mL NS up to every 2 hours (maximum: 0.5 mL/dose)

Adults: 0.5 mL up to every 3-4 hours as needed

SubQ:

Children: 0.01 mg/kg (1:1000) every 20 minutes for 3 doses or as condition requires (maximum: 0.5 mg/dose) **or** Twinject™, see below

Adults: 0.3-0.5 mg (1:1000) every 15-20 minutes for 3 doses or as condition requires **or** Twinject™, see below

Twinject™:

Children <15 kg: Dosage not established

Children 15-30 kg: 0.15 mg

Children >30 kg: 0.3 mg

Adults: 0.3 mg

Dosage Forms Excipient information presented when available (limited, particularly for generics); consult specific product labeling.

Aerosol for oral inhalation:

Primatene® Mist: 0.22 mg/inhalation (15 mL, 22.5 mL) [contains CFCs]

Injection, solution [prefilled auto injector]:

EpiPen®: 0.3 mg/0.3 mL (2 mL) [1:1000 solution; delivers 0.3 mg per injection; contains sodium metabisulfite; available as single unit or in double-unit pack with training unit]

EpiPen® Jr: 0.15 mg/0.3 mL (2 mL) [1:2000 solution; delivers 0.15 mg per injection; contains sodium metabisulfite; available as single unit or in double-unit pack with training unit]

Twinject™: 0.15 mg/0.15 mL (1.1 mL) [1:1000 solution; delivers 0.15 mg per injection; contains sodium bisulfite; two 0.15 mg doses per injector]; 0.3 mg/0.3 mL

(1.1 mL) [1:1000 solution; delivers 0.3 mg per injection; contains sodium bisulfite; two 0.3 mg doses per injector]

Injection, solution, as hydrochloride: 0.1 mg/mL (10 mL) [1:10,000 solution]; 1 mg/mL (1 mL) [1:1000 solution]

Adrenalin®: 1 mg/mL (1 mL) [1:1000 solution; contains sodium bisulfite]

Adrenalin®: 1 mg/mL (30 mL) [1:1000 solution; contains chlorobutanol, sodium bisulfite]

Solution for oral inhalation, as hydrochloride:

Adrenalin®: 1% (7.5 mL) [10 mg/mL, 1:100 solution; contains sodium bisulfite]

Solution for oral inhalation [racepinephrine; preservative free]:

S2®: 2.25% (0.5 mL) [as d-epinephrine 1.125% and l-epinephrine 1.125%]

Solution, intranasal, as hydrochloride [drops, spray]:

Adrenalin®: 1 mg/mL [1:1000 solution; contains sodium bisulfite]

Solution, topical [racepinephrine]:

Raphon: 2.25% (15 mL) [as d-epinephrine 1.125% and l-epinephrine 1.125%; contains benzoic acid, metabisulfites]

- **Epinephrine Bitartrate** *see* EPINEPHrine *on page 543*
- **Epinephrine Hydrochloride** *see* EPINEPHrine *on page 543*
- **EpiPen®** *see* EPINEPHrine *on page 543*
- **EpiPen® Jr** *see* EPINEPHrine *on page 543*
- **Epipodophyllotoxin** *see* Etoposide *on page 607*

Epirubicin (ep i ROO bi sin)

Medication Safety Issues

Sound-alike/look-alike issues:

Epirubicin may be confused with DOXOrubicin, DAUNOrubicin, idarubicin

Ellence® may be confused with Elase®

High alert medication: The Institute for Safe Medication Practices (ISMP) includes this medication among its list of drugs which have a heightened risk of causing significant patient harm when used in error.

U.S. Brand Names Ellence®

Canadian Brand Names Ellence®; Pharmorubicin®

Mexican Brand Names Binarin; Epilem; Farmorubicin; Farmorubicin RD

Index Terms Epirubicin Hydrochloride; NSC-256942; Pidorubicin; Pidorubicin Hydrochloride

Pharmacologic Category Antineoplastic Agent, Anthracycline

Use Adjuvant therapy for primary breast cancer

Effect on Mental Status Lethargy is common

Effect on Psychiatric Treatment Leukopenia is common; use caution with clozapine and carbamazepine

Dosage Summary

I.V.:

Children: Dosage not established

Adults: 100-120 mg/m^2 day 1 every 3-4 weeks **or** 50-60 mg/m^2 days 1 and 8 every 3-4 weeks

Dosage Forms Excipient information presented when available (limited, particularly for generics); consult specific product labeling.

Injection, powder for reconstitution, as hydrochloride, [preservative free]: 50 mg, 200 mg [contains lactose]

Injection, solution, as hydrochloride [preservative free]: 2 mg/mL (5 mL, 25 mL, 75 mL, 100 mL)

Ellence®: 2 mg/mL (25 mL, 100 mL)

- **Epirubicin Hydrochloride** *see* Epirubicin *on page 545*
- **Epitol®** *see* CarBAMazepine *on page 265*
- **Epivir®** *see* LamiVUDine *on page 888*
- **Epivir-HBV®** *see* LamiVUDine *on page 888*

Eplerenone (e PLER en one)

Medication Safety Issues

Sound-alike/look-alike issues:

Inspra™ may be confused with Spiriva®

U.S. Brand Names Inspra™

Mexican Brand Names Inspra IC

Pharmacologic Category Diuretic, Potassium-Sparing; Selective Aldosterone Blocker

Use Treatment of hypertension (may be used alone or in combination with other antihypertensive agents); treatment of heart failure (HF) following acute MI

Effect on Mental Status May cause dizziness

Effect on Psychiatric Treatment Hypertriglyceridemia is common; monitor when used with clozapine, olanzapine, quetiapine, and mirtazapine. Lithium levels should be monitored for possible effects on serum concentrations. Fluoxetine, fluvoxamine, and nefazodone may increase levels of eplerenone; initial dose should be 25 mg/day.

Dosage Summary

Oral:

Children: Dosage not established

Adults: Initial: 25-50 mg once daily; Maintenance: 50 mg once or twice daily (maximum: 100 mg/day); **Note:** Dosage may be adjusted according to serum potassium concentrations, see indication-specific dosing

Dosage Forms Excipient information presented when available (limited, particularly for generics); consult specific product labeling.

Tablet: 25 mg, 50 mg

Inspra™: 25 mg, 50 mg

◆ **EPO** *see* Epoetin Alfa *on page 546*

Epoetin Alfa (e POE e tin AL fa)

Medication Safety Issues

Sound-alike/look-alike issues:

Epoetin alfa may be confused with darbepoetin alfa, epoetin beta

Epogen® may be confused with Neupogen®

International issues:

Epopen® [Spain] may be confused with EpiPen® which is a brand name for epinephrine in the U.S.

U.S. Brand Names Epogen®; Procrit®

Canadian Brand Names Eprex®

Mexican Brand Names Eprex

Index Terms *r*HuEPO-α; EPO; Erythropoiesis-Stimulating Agent (ESA); Erythropoietin; NSC-724223

Pharmacologic Category Colony Stimulating Factor

Use Treatment of anemia (elevate/maintain red blood cell level and decrease the need for transfusions) associated with HIV (zidovudine) therapy, chronic renal failure (including patients on dialysis and not on dialysis); reduction of allogeneic blood transfusion for elective, noncardiac, nonvascular surgery; treatment of anemia due to concurrent chemotherapy in patients with metastatic cancer (nonmyeloid malignancies)

Note: Erythropoietin is **not** indicated for use in cancer patients under the following conditions:

- receiving hormonal therapy, therapeutic biologic products, or radiation therapy unless also receiving concurrent myelosuppressive chemotherapy
- receiving myelosuppressive therapy when the expected outcome is curative
- anemia due to other factors (eg, iron deficiency, folate deficiency, or gastrointestinal bleed)

Unlabeled/Investigational Use Treatment of anemia associated with critical illness; anemia of prematurity; symptomatic anemia in myelodysplastic syndrome (MDS)

Effect on Mental Status Sedation is common; may cause dizziness

Effect on Psychiatric Treatment None reported

Restrictions An FDA-approved medication guide is available; distribute to each patient to whom this medication is dispensed.

Dosage Summary

I.V.:

Children: Initial: 50 units/kg 3 times/week; Maintenance: 50-400 units/kg 1-3 times/week **or** 600 units/kg once weekly (maximum: 40,000 units)

Adults: Initial: 50-100 units/kg 3 times/week; Maintenance: 75-150 units/kg/week **or** 100-300 units/kg 3 times/week

SubQ:

Children: Initial: 50 units/kg 3 times/week; Maintenance: 50-400 units/kg 1-3 times/week

Adults: Initial: 50-100 units/kg 3 times/week; Maintenance: 75 units/kg 1-3 times/week **or** 75-150 units/kg/week **or** 100-300 units/kg 3 times/week **or** 10,000 units 3 times/week to 40,000-60,000 units once weekly (cancer patients) **or** 300 units/kg/day for 10 days before surgery, on the day of surgery, and for 4 days after surgery **or** 600 units/kg in once weekly doses (21, 14, and 7 days before surgery) plus a fourth dose on the day of surgery

Dosage Forms Excipient information presented when available (limited, particularly for generics); consult specific product labeling.

Injection, solution [preservative free]:

Epogen®, Procrit®: 2000 units/mL (1 mL); 3000 units/mL (1 mL); 4000 units/mL (1 mL); 10,000 units/mL (1 mL); 40,000 units/mL (1 mL) [contains human albumin]

Injection, solution [with preservative]:

Epogen®, Procrit®: 10,000 units/mL (2 mL); 20,000 units/mL (1 mL) [contains human albumin and benzyl alcohol]

◆ **Epogen®** *see* Epoetin Alfa *on page 546*

Epoprostenol (e poe PROST en ole)

Medication Safety Issues

High alert medication: The Institute for Safe Medication Practices (ISMP) includes this medication among its list of drugs which have a heightened risk of causing significant patient harm when used in error.

U.S. Brand Names Flolan®

Canadian Brand Names Flolan®

Index Terms Epoprostenol Sodium; PGI_2; PGX; Prostacyclin

Pharmacologic Category Prostacyclin; Prostaglandin; Vasodilator

Use Treatment of idiopathic pulmonary arterial hypertension (IPAH); pulmonary hypertension associated with the scleroderma spectrum of disease (SSD) in NYHA Class III and Class IV patients who do not respond adequately to conventional therapy

Effect on Mental Status Anxiety, nervousness are common; may cause confusion, insomnia, or depression

Effect on Psychiatric Treatment Hypotensive effects may be exacerbated by low potency antipsychotics (chlorpromazine) and TCAs

Restrictions Orders for epoprostenol are distributed by two sources in the United States. Information on orders or reimbursement assistance may be obtained from either Accredo Health, Inc (1-800-935-6526) or TheraCom, Inc (1-877-356-5264).

Dosage Summary

I.V.:

Children (unlabeled use): Initial: 1-2 ng/kg/minute, increase dose in increments of 1-2 ng/kg/minute every 15 minutes or longer until dose-limiting side effects are noted or tolerance limit to epoprostenol is observed

Adults: Initial: 1-2 ng/kg/minute, increase dose in increments of 1-2 ng/kg/minute every 15 minutes or longer until dose-limiting side effects are noted or tolerance limit to epoprostenol is observed

Dosage Forms Excipient information presented when available (limited, particularly for generics); consult specific product labeling.

Injection, powder for reconstitution: 0.5 mg, 1.5 mg [provided with 50 mL sterile diluent]

Flolan®: 0.5 mg, 1.5 mg

◆ **Epoprostenol Sodium** *see* Epoprostenol *on page 547*

Eprosartan (ep roe SAR tan)

Related Information

Angiotensin Agents *on page 1754*

U.S. Brand Names Teveten®

Canadian Brand Names Teveten®

Pharmacologic Category Angiotensin II Receptor Blocker

Generic Available No

Use Treatment of hypertension; may be used alone or in combination with other antihypertensives

Effect on Mental Status May cause fatigue or depression

Effect on Psychiatric Treatment Risk of lithium toxicity may be increased by eprosartan; monitor lithium levels

Pregnancy Risk Factor C (1st trimester); D (2nd and 3rd trimesters)

Pregnancy Considerations Medications which act on the renin-angiotensin system are reported to have the following fetal/neonatal effects: Hypotension, neonatal skull hypoplasia, anuria, renal failure, and death; oligohydramnios is also reported. These effects are reported to occur with exposure during the second and third trimesters. There are no adequate and well-controlled studies in pregnant women. **[U.S. Boxed Warning]: Based on human data, drugs that act on the angiotensin system can cause injury and death to the developing fetus when used in the second and third trimesters. Angiotensin receptor blockers should be discontinued as soon as possible once pregnancy is detected.**

Lactation Not recommended

Contraindications Hypersensitivity to eprosartan or any component of the formulation

Warnings/Precautions [U.S. Boxed Warning]: Based on human data, drugs that act on the angiotensin system can cause injury and death to the developing fetus when used in the second and third trimesters. Angiotensin receptor blockers should be discontinued as soon as possible once pregnancy is detected. May cause hyperkalemia; avoid potassium supplementation unless specifically required by healthcare provider. Avoid use or use a smaller dose in patients who are volume depleted; correct depletion first. May be associated with deterioration of renal function and/or increases in serum creatinine, particularly in patients with low renal blood flow (eg, renal artery stenosis, heart failure) whose glomerular filtration rate (GFR) is dependent on efferent arteriolar vasoconstriction by angiotensin II. Use with caution in unstented unilateral/bilateral renal artery stenosis. When unstented bilateral renal artery stenosis is present, use is generally avoided due to the elevated risk of deterioration in renal function unless possible benefits outweigh risks. Use with caution with pre-existing renal insufficiency; significant aortic/mitral stenosis. Safety and efficacy not established in pediatric patients.

Adverse Reactions

1% to 10%:

Central nervous system: Fatigue (2%), depression (1%)

Endocrine & metabolic: Hypertriglyceridemia (1%)

Gastrointestinal: Abdominal pain (2%)

Genitourinary: Urinary tract infection (1%)

Respiratory: Upper respiratory tract infection (8%), rhinitis (4%), pharyngitis (4%), cough (4%)

Miscellaneous: Viral infection (2%), injury (2%)

<1% (Limited to important or life-threatening): Abnormal ECG, angina, arthritis, asthma, ataxia, bradycardia, BUN increased, creatinine increased, eczema, edema, esophagitis, ethanol intolerance, gingivitis, gout, hypotension, influenza-like symptoms, leg cramps, leukopenia, maculopapular rash, migraine, neuritis, neutropenia, orthostasis, palpitation, paresthesia, peripheral ischemia, purpura, renal calculus, somnolence, tachycardia, tendonitis, thrombocytopenia, tinnitus, tremor, urinary incontinence, vertigo; rhabdomyolysis has been reported (rarely) with angiotensin-receptor antagonists.

Metabolism/Transport Effects Inhibits CYP2C9 (weak)

Drug Interactions

ACE Inhibitors: Angiotensin II Receptor Blockers may enhance the adverse/toxic effect of ACE Inhibitors. *Risk C: Monitor therapy*

Diazoxide: May enhance the hypotensive effect of Antihypertensives. *Risk C: Monitor therapy*

Eplerenone: May enhance the hyperkalemic effect of Angiotensin II Receptor Blockers. *Risk C: Monitor therapy*

Herbs (Hypertensive Properties): May diminish the antihypertensive effect of Antihypertensives. *Risk C: Monitor therapy*

Herbs (Hypotensive Properties): May enhance the hypotensive effect of Antihypertensives. *Risk C: Monitor therapy*

Lithium: Angiotensin II Receptor Blockers may increase the serum concentration of Lithium. Management: Lithium dosage reductions will likely be needed following the addition of an angiotensin II receptor antagonist. *Risk D: Consider therapy modification*

Methylphenidate: May diminish the antihypertensive effect of Antihypertensives. *Risk C: Monitor therapy*

Nonsteroidal Anti-Inflammatory Agents: May diminish the therapeutic effect of Angiotensin II Receptor Blockers. The combination of these two agents may also significantly decrease glomerular filtration and renal function. *Risk C: Monitor therapy*

Potassium Salts: May enhance the hyperkalemic effect of Angiotensin II Receptor Blockers. *Risk C: Monitor therapy*

Potassium-Sparing Diuretics: Angiotensin II Receptor Blockers may enhance the hyperkalemic effect of Potassium-Sparing Diuretics. *Risk C: Monitor therapy*

Prostacyclin Analogues: May enhance the hypotensive effect of Antihypertensives. *Risk C: Monitor therapy*

RiTUXimab: Antihypertensives may enhance the hypotensive effect of RiTUXimab. *Risk D: Consider therapy modification*

Trimethoprim: May enhance the hyperkalemic effect of Angiotensin II Receptor Blockers. *Risk C: Monitor therapy*

Ethanol/Nutrition/Herb Interactions Herb/Nutraceutical: Avoid dong quai if using for hypertension (has estrogenic activity). Avoid ephedra, yohimbe, ginseng (may worsen hypertension). Avoid garlic (may have increased antihypertensive effect).

Mechanism of Action Angiotensin II is formed from angiotensin I in a reaction catalyzed by angiotensin-converting enzyme (ACE, kininase II). Angiotensin II is the principal pressor agent of the renin-angiotensin system, with effects that include vasoconstriction, stimulation of synthesis and release of aldosterone, cardiac stimulation, and renal reabsorption of sodium. Eprosartan blocks the vasoconstrictor and aldosterone-secreting effects of angiotensin II by selectively blocking the binding of angiotensin II to the AT1 receptor in many tissues, such as vascular smooth muscle and the adrenal gland. Its action is therefore independent of the pathways for angiotensin II synthesis. Blockade of the renin-angiotensin system with ACE inhibitors, which inhibit the biosynthesis of angiotensin II from angiotensin I, is widely used in the treatment of hypertension. ACE inhibitors also inhibit the degradation of bradykinin, a reaction also catalyzed by ACE. Because eprosartan does not inhibit ACE (kininase II), it does not affect the response to bradykinin. Whether this difference has clinical relevance is not yet known. Eprosartan does not bind to or block other hormone receptors or ion channels known to be important in cardiovascular regulation.

Pharmacodynamics/Kinetics

Protein binding: 98%

Metabolism: Minimally hepatic

Bioavailability: 300 mg dose: 13%

Half-life elimination: Terminal: 5-9 hours

Time to peak, serum: Fasting: 1-2 hours

Excretion: Feces (90%); urine (7%, mostly as unchanged drug)

Clearance: 7.9 L/hour

Dosage Adults: Oral: Dosage must be individualized; can administer once or twice daily with total daily doses of 400-800 mg. Usual starting dose is 600 mg once daily as monotherapy in patients who are euvolemic. Limited clinical experience with doses >800 mg.

Dosage adjustment in renal impairment: No starting dosage adjustment is necessary; however, carefully monitor the patient

Dosage adjustment in hepatic impairment: No starting dosage adjustment is necessary; however, carefully monitor the patient

Elderly: No starting dosage adjustment is necessary; however, carefully monitor the patient

Dosage Forms Excipient information presented when available (limited, particularly for generics); consult specific product labeling.

Tablet: 400 mg, 600 mg

Eprosartan and Hydrochlorothiazide

(ep roe SAR tan & hye droe klor oh THYE a zide)

U.S. Brand Names Teveten® HCT

Canadian Brand Names Teveten® HCT; Teveten® Plus

Index Terms Eprosartan Mesylate and Hydrochlorothiazide; Hydrochlorothiazide and Eprosartan

Pharmacologic Category Angiotensin II Receptor Blocker; Diuretic, Thiazide

Use Treatment of hypertension (not indicated for initial treatment)

Effect on Mental Status May cause dizziness, fatigue, and depression

Effect on Psychiatric Treatment May decrease lithium clearance resulting in an increase in serum lithium levels and potential lithium toxicity; monitor serum lithium levels

Dosage Summary

Oral:

Children: Dosage not established

Adults: Eprosartan 600 mg and hydrochlorothiazide 12.5-25 mg once daily

Dosage Forms Excipient information presented when available (limited, particularly for generics); consult specific product labeling.

Tablet:

600 mg/12.5 mg: Eprosartan 600 mg and hydrochlorothiazide 12.5 mg

600 mg/25 mg: Eprosartan 600 mg and hydrochlorothiazide 25 mg

- **Eprosartan Mesylate and Hydrochlorothiazide** *see* Eprosartan and Hydrochlorothiazide *on page 549*
- **Epsilon Aminocaproic Acid** *see* Aminocaproic Acid *on page 87*
- **Epsom Salts** *see* Magnesium Sulfate *on page 966*
- **EPT** *see* Teniposide *on page 1549*

Eptifibatide (ep TIF i ba tide)

Medication Safety Issues

High alert medication: The Institute for Safe Medication Practices (ISMP) includes this medication among its list of drugs which have a heightened risk of causing significant patient harm when used in error.

U.S. Brand Names Integrilin®

Canadian Brand Names Integrilin®

Index Terms Intrifiban

Pharmacologic Category Antiplatelet Agent, Glycoprotein IIb/IIIa Inhibitor

Use Treatment of patients with acute coronary syndrome (unstable angina/non-Q wave myocardial infarction [UA/NQMI]), including patients who are to be managed medically and those undergoing percutaneous coronary intervention (PCI including angioplasty, intracoronary stenting)

Effect on Mental Status None reported

Effect on Psychiatric Treatment Contraindicated in patients with a recent stroke (within 30 days)

Dosage Summary

I.V.:

Children: Dosage not established

Adults: Bolus: 180 mcg/kg (maximum: 22.6 mg), repeat once for PCI; Infusion: 2 mcg/kg/minute (maximum: 15 mg/hour)

Dosage Forms Excipient information presented when available (limited, particularly for generics); consult specific product labeling.

Injection, solution: 0.75 mg/mL (100 mL); 2 mg/mL (10 mL, 100 mL)

- **Epzicom®** *see* Abacavir and Lamivudine *on page 22*
- **Equagesic®** *see* Meprobamate and Aspirin *on page 992*
- **Equanil** *see* Meprobamate *on page 991*
- **Equetro®** *see* CarBAMazepine *on page 265*
- **Erbitux®** *see* Cetuximab *on page 310*

Ergocalciferol (er goe kal SIF e role)

Medication Safety Issues

Sound-alike/look-alike issues:

Calciferol™ may be confused with calcitriol

Drisdol® may be confused with Drysol™

U.S. Brand Names Drisdol®

Canadian Brand Names Drisdol®; Ostoforte®

Mexican Brand Names Adekon; Aderowest; Aquasol AD; Axed; Pharmaton Complex

Index Terms Activated Ergosterol; Viosterol; Vitamin D_2

Pharmacologic Category Vitamin D Analog

Use Treatment of refractory rickets, hypophosphatemia, hypoparathyroidism; dietary supplement

Unlabeled/Investigational Use Prevention and treatment of vitamin D deficiency in patients with chronic kidney disease (CKD)

Effect on Mental Status May cause irritability or drowsiness; may rarely cause psychosis

Effect on Psychiatric Treatment None reported

Dosage Summary Note: Dosage varies considerably by indication; ranges listed are representative

Oral:

Children: 5-5000 mcg/day (200-200,000 int. units/day)

Adults 18-50 years: 5-7500 mcg/day (200-300,000 int. units/day)

Adults: 51-70 years: 10-7500 mcg/day (400-300,000 int. units/day)

Elderly >70 years: 15-7500 mcg/day (600-300,000 int. units/day)

Dosage Forms Excipient information presented when available (limited, particularly for generics); consult specific product labeling.

Capsule:

Drisdol®: 50,000 int. units [1.25 mg; contains tartrazine and soybean oil]

Liquid, oral [drops]:
Drisdol®: 8000 int. units/mL (60 mL) [200 mcg/mL; OTC]
Tablet: 400 int. units [10 mcg; OTC]

Ergoloid Mesylates (ER goe loid MES i lates)

Canadian Brand Names Hydergine®

Mexican Brand Names Hydergina

Index Terms Dihydroergotoxine; Dihydrogenated Ergot Alkaloids; Hydergine [DSC]

Pharmacologic Category Ergot Derivative

Generic Available Yes

Use Treatment of cerebrovascular insufficiency in primary progressive dementia, Alzheimer's dementia, and senile onset

Effect on Mental Status None reported

Effect on Psychiatric Treatment Contraindicated in individuals with psychosis

Pregnancy Risk Factor C

Contraindications Hypersensitivity to ergot or any component of the formulation; acute or chronic psychosis; ergot alkaloids are contraindicated with potent inhibitors of CYP3A4 (includes protease inhibitors, azole antifungals, and some macrolide antibiotics)

Warnings/Precautions Pleural and peritoneal fibrosis have been reported with prolonged daily use. Cardiac valvular fibrosis has also been associated with ergot alkaloids. Concomitant use with potent inhibitors of CYP3A4 (includes protease inhibitors, azole antifungals, and some macrolide antibiotics) and ergot alkaloids has been associated with acute ergot toxicity (ergotism); certain ergot alkaloids (eg, ergotamine and dihydroergotamine) are contraindicated by the manufacturer. Use with caution in the elderly. Safety and efficacy have not been established in children.

Adverse Reactions Adverse effects are minimal; most common include transient nausea, gastrointestinal disturbances and sublingual irritation with SL tablets; other common side effects include:

Cardiovascular: Orthostatic hypotension, bradycardia
Dermatologic: Skin rash, flushing
Ocular: Blurred vision
Respiratory: Nasal congestion

Metabolism/Transport Effects Substrate of CYP3A4 (major)

Drug Interactions

CYP3A4 Inhibitors (Moderate): May decrease the metabolism of CYP3A4 Substrates. *Risk C: Monitor therapy*

CYP3A4 Inhibitors (Strong): May decrease the metabolism of CYP3A4 Substrates. *Risk D: Consider therapy modification*

Dasatinib: May increase the serum concentration of CYP3A4 Substrates. *Risk C: Monitor therapy*

Efavirenz: May enhance the adverse/toxic effect of Ergot Derivatives. Specifically, the risk for peripheral vasospasm and ischemia may be increased. *Risk X: Avoid combination*

Macrolide Antibiotics: May enhance the adverse/toxic effect of Ergot Derivatives. Specifically leading the development of ergotism. **Exceptions:** Azithromycin; Dirithromycin [Off Market]; Spiramycin. *Risk D: Consider therapy modification*

Posaconazole: May increase the serum concentration of Ergot Derivatives. *Risk X: Avoid combination*

Protease Inhibitors: May decrease the metabolism of Ergot Derivatives. *Risk X: Avoid combination*

Serotonin 5-HT1D Receptor Agonists: Ergot Derivatives may enhance the vasoconstricting effect of Serotonin 5-HT1D Receptor Agonists. Serotonin 5-HT1D Receptor Agonists may enhance the vasoconstricting effect of Ergot Derivatives. *Risk X: Avoid combination*

Serotonin Modulators: May enhance the adverse/toxic effect of other Serotonin Modulators. The development of serotonin syndrome may occur. *Risk D: Consider therapy modification*

Sibutramine: May enhance the serotonergic effect of Ergot Derivatives. This may cause serotonin syndrome. *Risk X: Avoid combination*

Voriconazole: May increase the serum concentration of Ergot Derivatives. *Risk X: Avoid combination*

Mechanism of Action Ergoloid mesylates do not have the vasoconstrictor effects of the natural ergot alkaloids; exact mechanism in dementia is unknown; originally classed as peripheral and cerebral vasodilator, now considered a "metabolic enhancer"; there is no specific evidence which clearly establishes the mechanism by which ergoloid mesylate preparations produce mental effects, nor is there conclusive evidence that the drug particularly affects cerebral arteriosclerosis or cerebrovascular insufficiency

Pharmacodynamics/Kinetics

Absorption: Rapid yet incomplete

Half-life elimination, serum: 3.5 hours

Time to peak, serum: ~1 hour

Dosage Adults: Oral: 1 mg 3 times/day up to 4.5-12 mg/day; up to 6 months of therapy may be necessary

Dietary Considerations Should not eat or drink while tablet dissolves under tongue.

Dosage Forms Excipient information presented when available (limited, particularly for generics); consult specific product labeling.

Tablet: 1 mg

Tablet, sublingual: 1 mg

◆ **Ergomar®** *see* Ergotamine *on page 552*

◆ **Ergometrine Maleate** *see* Ergonovine *on page 552*

Ergonovine (er goe NOE veen)

U.S. Brand Names Ergotrate®

Mexican Brand Names Ergotrate

Index Terms Ergometrine Maleate; Ergonovine Maleate

Pharmacologic Category Ergot Derivative

Use Prevention and treatment of postpartum and postabortion hemorrhage caused by uterine atony or subinvolution

Unlabeled/Investigational Use Diagnostically to identify Prinzmetal's angina

Effect on Mental Status May cause dizziness

Effect on Psychiatric Treatment None reported

Dosage Summary

I.M.:

Children: Dosage not established

Adults: 0.2 mg, may repeat in 2-4 hours if needed

I.V.:

Children: Dosage not established

Adults: 0.2 mg, may repeat in 2-4 hours if needed

Oral:

Children: Dosage not established

Adults: 0.2-0.4 mg every 6-12 hours

SL:

Children: Dosage not established

Adults: 0.2-0.4 mg every 6-12 hours

Dosage Forms Excipient information presented when available (limited, particularly for generics); consult specific product labeling.

Injection, as maleate:

Ergotrate®: 0.2 mg/mL (1 mL)

Tablet, as maleate:

Ergotrate®: 0.2 mg

◆ **Ergonovine Maleate** *see* Ergonovine *on page 552*

Ergotamine (er GOT a meen)

U.S. Brand Names Ergomar®

Mexican Brand Names Cafergot; Caftar; Ergocaf; Sydolil; Trinergot

Index Terms Ergotamine Tartrate

Pharmacologic Category Antimigraine Agent; Ergot Derivative

Generic Available No

Use Abort or prevent vascular headaches, such as migraine, migraine variants, or so-called "histaminic cephalalgia"

Effect on Mental Status Drowsiness and dizziness are common

Effect on Psychiatric Treatment Use caution with propranolol; vasoconstriction has been reported; coadministration with strong CYP3A4 inhibitors has been associated with serious adverse events (some weaker inhibitors include nefazodone, fluoxetine and fluvoxamine)

Pregnancy Risk Factor X

Pregnancy Considerations May cause prolonged constriction of the uterine vessels and/or increased myometrial tone leading to reduced placental blood flow. This has contributed to fetal growth retardation in animals.

Lactation Enters breast milk/not recommended

Contraindications Hypersensitivity to ergotamine or any component of the formulation; peripheral vascular disease; hepatic or renal disease; coronary artery disease; hypertension; sepsis; ergot alkaloids are contraindicated with strong inhibitors of CYP3A4 (includes protease inhibitors, azole antifungals, and some macrolide antibiotics); pregnancy

Warnings/Precautions Ergot alkaloids have been associated with fibrotic valve thickening (eg, aortic, mitral, tricuspid); usually associated with long-term, chronic use; vasospasm or vasoconstriction can occur; ergot alkaloid use may result in ergotism (intense vasoconstriction) resulting in peripheral vascular ischemia and possible gangrene; rare cases of pleural and/or retroperitoneal fibrosis have been reported with prolonged daily use. Discontinuation after extended use may result in withdrawal symptoms (eg, rebound headache). Use with caution in the elderly. Safety and efficacy have not been established in children.

[U.S. Boxed Warning]: Ergot alkaloids are contraindicated with potent inhibitors of CYP3A4 (includes protease inhibitors, azole antifungals, and some macrolide antibiotics); concomitant use associated with acute ergot toxicity (ergotism).

Adverse Reactions Frequency not defined.

Cardiovascular: Absence of pulse, bradycardia, cardiac valvular fibrosis, cyanosis, edema, ECG changes, gangrene, hypertension, ischemia, precordial distress and pain, tachycardia, vasospasm

Central nervous system: Vertigo

Dermatologic: Itching

Gastrointestinal: Nausea, vomiting

Genitourinary: Retroperitoneal fibrosis

Neuromuscular & skeletal: Muscle pain, numbness, paresthesia, weakness

Respiratory: Pleuropulmonary fibrosis

Miscellaneous: Cold extremities

Metabolism/Transport Effects **Substrate** of CYP3A4 (major); Inhibits CYP3A4 (weak)

Drug Interactions

CYP3A4 Inhibitors (Moderate): May decrease the metabolism of CYP3A4 Substrates. *Risk C: Monitor therapy*

CYP3A4 Inhibitors (Strong): May decrease the metabolism of CYP3A4 Substrates. *Risk D: Consider therapy modification*

Dasatinib: May increase the serum concentration of CYP3A4 Substrates. *Risk C: Monitor therapy*

Efavirenz: May enhance the adverse/toxic effect of Ergot Derivatives. Specifically, the risk for peripheral vasospasm and ischemia may be increased. *Risk X: Avoid combination*

Macrolide Antibiotics: May enhance the adverse/toxic effect of Ergot Derivatives. Specifically leading the development of ergotism. **Exceptions:** Azithromycin; Dirithromycin [Off Market]; Spiramycin. *Risk D: Consider therapy modification*

Posaconazole: May increase the serum concentration of Ergot Derivatives. *Risk X: Avoid combination*

Protease Inhibitors: May decrease the metabolism of Ergot Derivatives. *Risk X: Avoid combination*

Serotonin 5-HT1D Receptor Agonists: Ergot Derivatives may enhance the vasoconstricting effect of Serotonin 5-HT1D Receptor Agonists. Serotonin 5-HT1D Receptor Agonists may enhance the vasoconstricting effect of Ergot Derivatives. *Risk X: Avoid combination*

Serotonin Modulators: May enhance the adverse/toxic effect of other Serotonin Modulators. The development of serotonin syndrome may occur. *Risk D: Consider therapy modification*

Sibutramine: May enhance the serotonergic effect of Ergot Derivatives. This may cause serotonin syndrome. *Risk X: Avoid combination*

Voriconazole: May increase the serum concentration of Ergot Derivatives. *Risk X: Avoid combination*

Ethanol/Nutrition/Herb Interactions Food: Avoid tea, cola, and coffee (caffeine may increase GI absorption of ergotamine). Grapefruit juice may cause increased blood levels of ergotamine, leading to increased toxicity.

Stability Store sublingual tablet at room temperature. Protect from light and heat.

Mechanism of Action Has partial agonist and/or antagonist activity against tryptaminergic, dopaminergic and alpha-adrenergic receptors depending upon their site; is a highly active uterine stimulant; it causes constriction of peripheral and cranial blood vessels and produces depression of central vasomotor centers

Pharmacodynamics/Kinetics

Absorption: Oral: Erratic; enhanced by caffeine coadministration

Metabolism: Extensively hepatic

Time to peak, serum: 0.5-3 hours

Half-life elimination: 2 hours

Excretion: Feces (90% as metabolites)

Dosage Sublingual: One tablet under tongue at first sign, then 1 tablet every 30 minutes if needed; maximum dose: 3 tablets/24 hours, 5 tablets/week

Administration Do not crush sublingual tablets.

Dosage Forms Excipient information presented when available (limited, particularly for generics); consult specific product labeling.

Tablet, sublingual, as tartrate:

Ergomar®: 2 mg [peppermint flavor]

Ergotamine and Caffeine (er GOT a meen & KAF een)

Medication Safety Issues

Sound-alike/look-alike issues:

Cafergot® may be confused with Carafate®

U.S. Brand Names Cafergot®; Migergot

Canadian Brand Names Cafergor®

Mexican Brand Names Cafergot; Sydolil; Trinergot

Index Terms Caffeine and Ergotamine; Ergotamine Tartrate and Caffeine

Pharmacologic Category Antimigraine Agent; Ergot Derivative; Stimulant

Generic Available Yes

Use Abort or prevent vascular headaches, such as migraine, migraine variants, or so-called "histaminic cephalalgia"

Effect on Mental Status Drowsiness and dizziness are common

Effect on Psychiatric Treatment Use caution with propranolol; vasoconstriction has been reported; coadministration with strong CYP3A4 inhibitors has been associated with serious adverse events (some weaker inhibitors include nefazodone, fluoxetine and fluvoxamine)

Pregnancy Risk Factor X

Pregnancy Considerations May cause prolonged constriction of the uterine vessels and/or increased myometrial tone leading to reduced placental blood flow. This has contributed to fetal growth retardation in animals.

Lactation Enters breast milk/not recommended

Contraindications Hypersensitivity to ergotamine, caffeine, or any component of the formulation; peripheral vascular disease; hepatic or renal disease; coronary artery disease; hypertension; sepsis; ergot alkaloids are contraindicated with strong inhibitors of CYP3A4 (includes protease inhibitors, azole antifungals, and some macrolide antibiotics); pregnancy

Warnings/Precautions Ergot alkaloids have been associated with fibrotic valve thickening (eg, aortic, mitral, tricuspid); usually associated with long-term, chronic use; vasospasm or vasoconstriction can occur; ergot alkaloid use may result in ergotism (intense vasoconstriction) resulting in peripheral vascular ischemia and possible gangrene; rare cases of pleural and/or retroperitoneal fibrosis have been reported with prolonged daily use. Discontinuation after extended use may result in withdrawal symptoms (eg, rebound headache). Use with caution in the elderly. Safety and efficacy have not been established in children.

[U.S. Boxed Warning]: Ergot alkaloids are contraindicated with potent inhibitors of CYP3A4 (includes protease inhibitors, azole antifungals, and some macrolide antibiotics); concomitant use associated with acute ergot toxicity (ergotism).

Adverse Reactions Frequency not defined.

Cardiovascular: Absence of pulse, bradycardia, cardiac valvular fibrosis, cyanosis, edema, ECG changes, gangrene, hypertension, ischemia, precordial distress and pain, tachycardia, vasospasm

Central nervous system: Vertigo

Dermatologic: Itching

Gastrointestinal: Anal or rectal ulcer (with overuse of suppository), nausea, vomiting

Genitourinary: Retroperitoneal fibrosis

Neuromuscular & skeletal: Muscle pain, numbness, paresthesia, weakness

Respiratory: Pleuropulmonary fibrosis
Miscellaneous: Cold extremities

Metabolism/Transport Effects

Ergotamine: **Substrate** of CYP3A4 (major); **Inhibits** CYP3A4 (weak)
Caffeine: **Substrate** of CYP1A2 (major), 2C9 (minor), 2D6 (minor), 2E1 (minor), 3A4 (minor); **Inhibits** CYP1A2 (weak), 3A4 (moderate)

Drug Interactions

Cannabinoids: May enhance the tachycardic effect of Sympathomimetics. *Risk C: Monitor therapy*

CYP1A2 Inhibitors (Moderate): May decrease the metabolism of CYP1A2 Substrates. *Risk C: Monitor therapy*

CYP1A2 Inhibitors (Strong): May decrease the metabolism of CYP1A2 Substrates. *Risk D: Consider therapy modification*

CYP3A4 Inhibitors (Moderate): May decrease the metabolism of CYP3A4 Substrates. *Risk C: Monitor therapy*

CYP3A4 Inhibitors (Strong): May decrease the metabolism of CYP3A4 Substrates. *Risk D: Consider therapy modification*

CYP3A4 Substrates: CYP3A4 Inhibitors (Moderate) may decrease the metabolism of CYP3A4 Substrates. *Risk C: Monitor therapy*

Dasatinib: May increase the serum concentration of CYP3A4 Substrates. *Risk C: Monitor therapy*

Efavirenz: May enhance the adverse/toxic effect of Ergot Derivatives. Specifically, the risk for peripheral vasospasm and ischemia may be increased. *Risk X: Avoid combination*

Eplerenone: CYP3A4 Inhibitors (Moderate) may increase the serum concentration of Eplerenone. Management: A lower starting dose of eplerenone (25 mg once daily) is recommended in patients with hypertension who are also taking drugs that are moderate inhibitors of CYP3A4. *Risk D: Consider therapy modification*

Macrolide Antibiotics: May enhance the adverse/toxic effect of Ergot Derivatives. Specifically leading the development of ergotism. **Exceptions:** Azithromycin; Dirithromycin [Off Market]; Spiramycin. *Risk D: Consider therapy modification*

Maraviroc: CYP3A4 Inhibitors may increase the serum concentration of Maraviroc. *Risk D: Consider therapy modification*

Pimecrolimus: CYP3A4 Inhibitors (Moderate) may decrease the metabolism of Pimecrolimus. *Risk C: Monitor therapy*

Posaconazole: May increase the serum concentration of Ergot Derivatives. *Risk X: Avoid combination*

Protease Inhibitors: May decrease the metabolism of Ergot Derivatives. *Risk X: Avoid combination*

Quinolone Antibiotics: May decrease the metabolism of Caffeine. **Exceptions:** Gatifloxacin; Gemifloxacin; Levofloxacin; Lomefloxacin; Moxifloxacin; Nalidixic Acid; Ofloxacin; Sparfloxacin; Trovafloxacin. *Risk C: Monitor therapy*

Ranolazine: CYP3A4 Inhibitors (Moderate) may increase the serum concentration of Ranolazine. Management: Limit the ranolazine dose to a maximum of 500 mg twice daily in patients concurrently receiving moderate CYP3A4 inhibitors (e.g., diltiazem, verapamil, erythromycin, etc.). *Risk D: Consider therapy modification*

Regadenoson: Caffeine may diminish the vasodilatory effect of Regadenoson. *Risk D: Consider therapy modification*

Salmeterol: CYP3A4 Inhibitors (Moderate) may increase the serum concentration of Salmeterol. *Risk C: Monitor therapy*

Serotonin 5-HT1D Receptor Agonists: Ergot Derivatives may enhance the vasoconstricting effect of Serotonin 5-HT1D Receptor Agonists. Serotonin 5-HT1D Receptor Agonists may enhance the vasoconstricting effect of Ergot Derivatives. *Risk X: Avoid combination*

Serotonin Modulators: May enhance the adverse/toxic effect of other Serotonin Modulators. The development of serotonin syndrome may occur. *Risk D: Consider therapy modification*

Sibutramine: May enhance the serotonergic effect of Ergot Derivatives. This may cause serotonin syndrome. *Risk X: Avoid combination*

Sympathomimetics: May enhance the adverse/toxic effect of other Sympathomimetics. *Risk C: Monitor therapy*

Voriconazole: May increase the serum concentration of Ergot Derivatives. *Risk X: Avoid combination*

Ethanol/Nutrition/Herb Interactions Food: Avoid tea, cola, and coffee (caffeine may increase GI absorption of ergotamine). Grapefruit juice may cause increased blood levels of ergotamine, leading to increased toxicity.

Stability

Suppositories: Store below 25°C (77°F) in sealed foil. Protect from moisture.
Tablet: Store at room temperature 15°C to 30°C (59°F to 86°F).

Mechanism of Action Has partial agonist and/or antagonist activity against tryptaminergic, dopaminergic and alpha-adrenergic receptors depending upon their site; is a highly active uterine stimulant; it causes constriction of peripheral and cranial blood vessels and produces depression of central vasomotor centers

Pharmacodynamics/Kinetics

Absorption: Ergotamine: Oral, rectal: Erratic; enhanced by caffeine coadministration

Metabolism: Extensively hepatic

Time to peak, serum: Ergotamine: 0.5-3 hours

Half-life elimination: 2 hours

Excretion: Feces (90% as metabolites)

Dosage Adults:

Oral: Two tablets at onset of attack; then 1 tablet every 30 minutes as needed; maximum: 6 tablets per attack; do not exceed 10 tablets/week.

Rectal: One suppository rectally at first sign of an attack; follow with second dose after 1 hour, if needed; maximum: 2 per attack; do not exceed 5/week.

Dosage Forms Excipient information presented when available (limited, particularly for generics); consult specific product labeling.

Suppository, rectal:

Migergot: Ergotamine tartrate 2 mg and caffeine 100 mg (12s)

Tablet: Ergotamine tartrate 1 mg and caffeine 100 mg

Cafergot®: Ergotamine tartrate 1 mg and caffeine 100 mg

- ◆ **Ergotamine Tartrate** *see* Ergotamine *on page 552*
- ◆ **Ergotamine Tartrate and Caffeine** *see* Ergotamine and Caffeine *on page 554*
- ◆ **Ergotamine Tartrate, Belladonna, and Phenobarbital** *see* Belladonna, Phenobarbital, and Ergotamine *on page 175*
- ◆ **Ergotrate®** *see* Ergonovine *on page 552*

Erlotinib (er LOE tye nib)

Medication Safety Issues

Sound-alike/look-alike issues:

Erlotinib may be confused with gefitinib

High alert medication: The Institute for Safe Medication Practices (ISMP) includes this medication among its list of drug classes which have a heightened risk of causing significant patient harm when used in error.

U.S. Brand Names Tarceva®

Canadian Brand Names Tarceva®

Mexican Brand Names Tarceva

Index Terms CP358774; Erlotinib Hydrochloride; NSC-718781; OSI-774; R 14-15

Pharmacologic Category Antineoplastic Agent, Tyrosine Kinase Inhibitor; Epidermal Growth Factor Receptor (EGFR) Inhibitor

Use Treatment of locally advanced or metastatic nonsmall cell lung cancer (NSCLC) as monotherapy; locally advanced, unresectable or metastatic pancreatic cancer (first-line therapy in combination with gemcitabine)

Effect on Mental Status Sedation is common

Effect on Psychiatric Treatment GI side effects and sedation are common. Concomitant use with lithium, SSRIs, or valproic acid may produce additive effects. Concomitant use with psychotropic agents may produce additive sedative effects; monitor. Carbamazepine, phenobarbital, phenytoin, and St John's wort may decrease the effects of erlotinib; monitor. Nefazodone may increase the effects of erlotinib secondary to enzyme inhibition; monitor.

Dosage Summary

Oral:

Children: Dosage not established

Adults: 150 mg/day **or** 100 mg/day with gemcitabine

Dosage Forms Excipient information presented when available (limited, particularly for generics); consult specific product labeling.

Tablet:

Tarceva®: 25 mg, 100 mg, 150 mg

- ◆ **Erlotinib Hydrochloride** *see* Erlotinib *on page 556*
- ◆ **Errin™** *see* Norethindrone *on page 1150*

Ertapenem (er ta PEN em)

Medication Safety Issues

Sound-alike/look-alike issues:

Ertapenem may be confused with imipenem, meropenem

Invanz® may be confused with Avinza™

U.S. Brand Names Invanz®

Canadian Brand Names Invanz®

Mexican Brand Names Invanz

Index Terms Ertapenem Sodium; L-749,345; MK0826

Pharmacologic Category Antibiotic, Carbapenem

Use Treatment of the following moderate-severe infections: Complicated intra-abdominal infections, complicated skin and skin structure infections (including diabetic foot infections without osteomyelitis), complicated UTI (including pyelonephritis), acute pelvic infections (including postpartum endomyometritis, septic abortion, post surgical gynecologic infections), and community-acquired pneumonia. Prophylaxis of surgical site infection following elective colorectal surgery. Antibacterial coverage includes aerobic gram-positive organisms, aerobic gram-negative organisms, anaerobic organisms.

Note: Methicillin-resistant *Staphylococcus*, *Enterococcus* spp, penicillin-resistant strains of *Streptococcus pneumoniae*, beta-lactamase-positive strains of *Haemophilus influenzae* are **resistant** to ertapenem, as are most *Pseudomonas aeruginosa*.

Effect on Mental Status May cause agitation, confusion, disorientation, decreased mental acuity, sedation, stupor, insomnia, dizziness, or anxiety

Effect on Psychiatric Treatment Nausea and diarrhea are common; use caution with lithium, valproic acid, and SSRIs. May increase hepatic enzymes; use caution with olanzapine and valproic acid.

Dosage Summary

I.M.:

Children <3 months: Dosage not established

Children 3 months to 12 years: 15 mg/kg twice daily (maximum: 1 g/day)

Adolescents ≥13 years: 1 g once daily

Adults: 1 g once daily

I.V.:

Children <3 months: Dosage not established

Children 3 months to 12 years: 15 mg/kg twice daily (maximum: 1 g/day)

Adolescents ≥13 years: 1 g once daily

Adults: 1 g once daily **or** 1 g given 1 hour prior to surgery

Dosage Forms Excipient information presented when available (limited, particularly for generics); consult specific product labeling.

Injection, powder for reconstitution:

Invanz®: 1 g [contains sodium 137 mg/g (~6 mEq/g)]

- **Ertapenem Sodium** *see* Ertapenem *on page 557*
- ***Erwinia* Asparaginase** *see* Asparaginase *on page 142*
- **Eryc® [DSC]** *see* Erythromycin *on page 557*
- **Eryderm® [DSC]** *see* Erythromycin *on page 557*
- **Erygel® [DSC]** *see* Erythromycin *on page 557*
- **EryPed®** *see* Erythromycin *on page 557*
- **Ery-Tab®** *see* Erythromycin *on page 557*
- **Erythrocin®** *see* Erythromycin *on page 557*

Erythromycin (er ith roe MYE sin)

Medication Safety Issues

Sound-alike/look-alike issues:

Erythromycin may be confused with azithromycin, clarithromycin, Ethmozine®

Akne-Mycin® may be confused with AK-Mycin®

E.E.S.® may be confused with DES®

Eryc® may be confused with Emcyt®, Ery-Tab®

Ery-Tab® may be confused with Eryc®

Erythrocin® may be confused with Ethmozine®

U.S. Brand Names Akne-Mycin®; E.E.S.®; Ery-Tab®; Eryc® [DSC]; Eryderm® [DSC]; Erygel® [DSC]; EryPed®; Erythro-RX; Erythrocin®; PCE®; Romycin®

Canadian Brand Names Apo-Erythro Base®; Apo-Erythro E-C®; Apo-Erythro-ES®; Apo-Erythro-S®; Diomycin®; EES®; Erybid™; Eryc®; Novo-Rythro

Estolate; Novo-Rythro Ethylsuccinate; Nu-Erythromycin-S; PCE®; PMS-Erythromycin; Sans Acne®

Mexican Brand Names Eritrocap; Eritropharma-S; Eryacnen 4; Ilosone; Iretron; Lauritran; Optomicin; Pantomicina; Sansacné; Stiemcyn; Tropharma

Index Terms Erythromycin Base; Erythromycin Ethylsuccinate; Erythromycin Lactobionate; Erythromycin Stearate

Pharmacologic Category Acne Products; Antibiotic, Macrolide; Antibiotic, Ophthalmic; Antibiotic, Topical; Topical Skin Product; Topical Skin Product, Acne

Generic Available Yes: Capsule, gel, ophthalmic ointment, topical solution, suspension (as ethylsuccinate), swab, tablet (as base, ethylsuccinate, and stearate)

Use

Systemic: Treatment of susceptible bacterial infections including *S. pyogenes*, some *S. pneumoniae*, some *S. aureus*, *M. pneumoniae*, *Legionella pneumophila*, diphtheria, pertussis, *Chlamydia*, erythrasma, *N. gonorrhoeae*, *E. histolytica*, syphilis and nongonococcal urethritis, and *Campylobacter* gastroenteritis; used in conjunction with neomycin for decontaminating the bowel

Ophthalmic: Treatment of superficial eye infections involving the conjunctiva or cornea; neonatal ophthalmia

Topical: Treatment of acne vulgaris

Unlabeled/Investigational Use Systemic: Treatment of gastroparesis, chancroid; preoperative gut sterilization

Effect on Mental Status Systemic: Macrolides have been reported to cause nightmares, confusion, anxiety, and mood lability

Effect on Psychiatric Treatment Systemic: Contraindicated with pimozide; may increase concentration of bromocriptine, carbamazepine, and triazolam

Pregnancy Risk Factor B

Pregnancy Considerations Adverse events were not observed in animal studies; therefore, erythromycin is classified as pregnancy category B. Low levels of erythromycin have been shown to cross the placenta and erythromycin is considered the drug of choice for certain illnesses in pregnant women. Most studies do not support a link between prenatal exposure to erythromycin and pyloric stenosis in the neonate. No increased risk for congenital abnormalities has been documented, with the exception of a possible slight increase in risk for cardiovascular anomalies. No adequate and well-controlled studies have been completed in pregnant women. The estolate form of erythromycin should not be used in pregnancy due to a potential increased risk for hepatic toxicity.

Lactation Enters breast milk/use caution (AAP considers "compatible")

Contraindications Hypersensitivity to erythromycin or any component of the formulation

Systemic: Concomitant use with pimozide or cisapride

Warnings/Precautions Systemic: Use caution with hepatic impairment with or without jaundice has occurred, it may be accompanied by malaise, nausea, vomiting, abdominal colic, and fever; discontinue use if these occur. Use caution with other medication relying on CYP3A4 metabolism; high potential for drug interactions exists. Prolonged use may result in fungal or bacterial superinfection, including *C. difficile*-associated diarrhea (CDAD) and pseudomembranous colitis; CDAD has been observed >2 months postantibiotic treatment. Use in infants has been associated with infantile hypertrophic pyloric stenosis (IHPS). Macrolides have been associated with rare QT_c prolongation and ventricular arrhythmias, including torsade de pointes. Use caution in elderly patients, as risk of adverse events may be increased. Use caution in myasthenia gravis patients; erythromycin may aggravate muscular weakness.

Adverse Reactions Frequency not defined. Incidence may vary with formulation.

Systemic:

Cardiovascular: QT_c prolongation, torsade de pointes, ventricular arrhythmia, ventricular tachycardia

Central nervous system: Seizure

Dermatitis: Pruritus, rash

Gastrointestinal: Abdominal pain, anorexia, diarrhea, infantile hypertrophic pyloric stenosis, nausea, oral candidiasis, pancreatitis, pseudomembranous colitis, vomiting

Hepatic: Cholestatic jaundice (most common with estolate), hepatitis, liver function tests abnormal

Local: Phlebitis at the injection site, thrombophlebitis

Neuromuscular & skeletal: Weakness

Otic: Hearing loss

Miscellaneous: Allergic reactions, anaphylaxis, hypersensitivity reactions, urticaria

Topical: 1% to 10%: Dermatologic: Erythema, desquamation, dryness, pruritus

Metabolism/Transport Effects Substrate of CYP2B6 (minor), 3A4 (major); **Inhibits** CYP1A2 (weak), 3A4 (moderate)

Drug Interactions

Alfentanil: Macrolide Antibiotics may decrease the metabolism of Alfentanil. *Risk D: Consider therapy modification*

Alfuzosin: May enhance the QTc-prolonging effect of QTc-Prolonging Agents. *Risk C: Monitor therapy*

Antifungal Agents (Azole Derivatives, Systemic): Macrolide Antibiotics may decrease the metabolism of Antifungal Agents (Azole Derivatives, Systemic). Antifungal Agents (Azole Derivatives, Systemic) may decrease the metabolism of Macrolide Antibiotics. *Risk D: Consider therapy modification*

Benzodiazepines (metabolized by oxidation): Macrolide Antibiotics may decrease the metabolism of Benzodiazepines (metabolized by oxidation). *Risk D: Consider therapy modification*

BusPIRone: Macrolide Antibiotics may decrease the metabolism of BusPIRone. *Risk D: Consider therapy modification*

Calcium Channel Blockers: Macrolide Antibiotics may decrease the metabolism of Calcium Channel Blockers. **Exceptions:** Clevidipine. *Risk D: Consider therapy modification*

CarBAMazepine: Macrolide Antibiotics may decrease the metabolism of CarBAMazepine. *Risk D: Consider therapy modification*

Cardiac Glycosides: Macrolide Antibiotics may increase the serum concentration of Cardiac Glycosides. *Risk D: Consider therapy modification*

Cilostazol: Macrolide Antibiotics may decrease the metabolism of Cilostazol. *Risk D: Consider therapy modification*

Ciprofloxacin: May enhance the QTc-prolonging effect of QTc-Prolonging Agents. *Risk C: Monitor therapy*

Cisapride: Macrolide Antibiotics may decrease the metabolism of Cisapride. *Risk X: Avoid combination*

Clopidogrel: Macrolide Antibiotics may diminish the therapeutic effect of Clopidogrel. *Risk C: Monitor therapy*

Clozapine: Macrolide Antibiotics may decrease the metabolism of Clozapine. *Risk D: Consider therapy modification*

Colchicine: Macrolide Antibiotics may decrease the metabolism of Colchicine. *Risk D: Consider therapy modification*

Corticosteroids (Systemic): Macrolide Antibiotics may decrease the metabolism of Corticosteroids (Systemic). *Risk D: Consider therapy modification*

CycloSPORINE: Macrolide Antibiotics may decrease the metabolism of CycloSPORINE. *Risk C: Monitor therapy*

CYP3A4 Inducers (Strong): May increase the metabolism of CYP3A4 Substrates. *Risk C: Monitor therapy*

CYP3A4 Inhibitors (Moderate): May decrease the metabolism of CYP3A4 Substrates. *Risk C: Monitor therapy*

CYP3A4 Inhibitors (Strong): May decrease the metabolism of CYP3A4 Substrates. *Risk D: Consider therapy modification*

CYP3A4 Substrates: CYP3A4 Inhibitors (Moderate) may decrease the metabolism of CYP3A4 Substrates. *Risk C: Monitor therapy*

Dabigatran Etexilate: P-Glycoprotein Inhibitors may increase the serum concentration of Dabigatran Etexilate. *Risk X: Avoid combination*

Dasatinib: May increase the serum concentration of CYP3A4 Substrates. *Risk C: Monitor therapy*

Deferasirox: May decrease the serum concentration of CYP3A4 Substrates. *Risk C: Monitor therapy*

Disopyramide: Macrolide Antibiotics may enhance the QTc-prolonging effect of Disopyramide. Macrolide Antibiotics may decrease the metabolism of Disopyramide. *Risk X: Avoid combination*

Eletriptan: Macrolide Antibiotics may decrease the metabolism of Eletriptan. *Risk D: Consider therapy modification*

Eplerenone: Macrolide Antibiotics may decrease the metabolism of Eplerenone. *Risk C: Monitor therapy*

Ergot Derivatives: Macrolide Antibiotics may enhance the adverse/toxic effect of Ergot Derivatives. Specifically leading the development of ergotism. **Exceptions:** Cabergoline. *Risk D: Consider therapy modification*

Etravirine: May decrease the serum concentration of Macrolide Antibiotics. Clarithromycin AUC is reduced and levels of the active metabolite (14-hydroxy-clarithromycin) are modestly increased. Management: For the treatment of *Mycobacterium avium* complex, consider changing to alternative agent, such as azithromycin. *Risk D: Consider therapy modification*

Fexofenadine: Erythromycin may increase the serum concentration of Fexofenadine. *Risk C: Monitor therapy*

Gadobutrol: May enhance the QTc-prolonging effect of QTc-Prolonging Agents. *Risk D: Consider therapy modification*

Herbs (CYP3A4 Inducers): May increase the metabolism of CYP3A4 Substrates. *Risk C: Monitor therapy*

HMG-CoA Reductase Inhibitors: Macrolide Antibiotics may decrease the metabolism of HMG-CoA Reductase Inhibitors. **Exceptions:** Fluvastatin; Pravastatin; Rosuvastatin. *Risk D: Consider therapy modification*

Lincosamide Antibiotics: May diminish the therapeutic effect of Erythromycin. *Risk X: Avoid combination*

Maraviroc: CYP3A4 Inhibitors may increase the serum concentration of Maraviroc. *Risk D: Consider therapy modification*

Nilotinib: May enhance the QTc-prolonging effect of QTc-Prolonging Agents. *Risk X: Avoid combination*

P-Glycoprotein Inducers: May decrease the serum concentration of P-Glycoprotein Substrates. P-glycoprotein inducers may also further limit the distribution of p-glycoprotein substrates to specific cells/tissues/organs where p-glycoprotein is present in large amounts (e.g., brain, T-lymphocytes, testes, etc.). *Risk C: Monitor therapy*

P-Glycoprotein Inhibitors: May increase the serum concentration of P-Glycoprotein Substrates. P-glycoprotein inhibitors may also enhance the distribution of p-glycoprotein substrates to specific cells/tissues/organs where p-glycoprotein is present in large amounts (e.g., brain, T-lymphocytes, testes, etc.). *Risk C: Monitor therapy*

P-Glycoprotein Substrates: P-Glycoprotein Inhibitors may increase the serum concentration of P-Glycoprotein Substrates. P-glycoprotein inhibitors may also enhance the distribution of p-glycoprotein substrates to specific cells/tissues/organs where p-glycoprotein is present in large amounts (e.g., brain, T-lymphocytes, testes, etc.). *Risk C: Monitor therapy*

Phosphodiesterase 5 Inhibitors: Macrolide Antibiotics may decrease the metabolism of Phosphodiesterase 5 Inhibitors. *Risk D: Consider therapy modification*

Pimecrolimus: CYP3A4 Inhibitors (Moderate) may decrease the metabolism of Pimecrolimus. *Risk C: Monitor therapy*

Pimozide: Macrolide Antibiotics may decrease the metabolism of Pimozide. QTc prolongation is a risk. *Risk X: Avoid combination*

QTc-Prolonging Agents: May enhance the adverse/toxic effect of other QTc-Prolonging Agents. Their effects can be additive, causing life-threatening ventricular arrhythmias. *Risk D: Consider therapy modification*

QuiNIDine: Macrolide Antibiotics may decrease the metabolism of QuiNIDine. *Risk D: Consider therapy modification*

Ranolazine: CYP3A4 Inhibitors (Moderate) may increase the serum concentration of Ranolazine. Management: Limit the ranolazine dose to a maximum of 500 mg twice daily in patients concurrently receiving moderate CYP3A4 inhibitors (e.g., diltiazem, verapamil, erythromycin, etc.). *Risk D: Consider therapy modification*

Repaglinide: Macrolide Antibiotics may increase the serum concentration of Repaglinide. *Risk C: Monitor therapy*

Rifamycin Derivatives: Macrolide Antibiotics may decrease the metabolism of Rifamycin Derivatives. **Exceptions:** Rifapentine. *Risk D: Consider therapy modification*

Rivaroxaban: Erythromycin may increase the serum concentration of Rivaroxaban. *Risk C: Monitor therapy*

Salmeterol: CYP3A4 Inhibitors (Moderate) may increase the serum concentration of Salmeterol. *Risk C: Monitor therapy*

Selective Serotonin Reuptake Inhibitors: Macrolide Antibiotics may decrease the metabolism of Selective Serotonin Reuptake Inhibitors. **Exceptions:** Fluvoxamine; PARoxetine. *Risk C: Monitor therapy*

Sirolimus: Macrolide Antibiotics may decrease the metabolism of Sirolimus. *Risk D: Consider therapy modification*

Tacrolimus: Macrolide Antibiotics may increase the serum concentration of Tacrolimus. *Risk C: Monitor therapy*

Temsirolimus: Macrolide Antibiotics may enhance the adverse/toxic effect of Temsirolimus. Levels of sirolimus, the active metabolite, may be increased, likely due to inhibition of CYP-mediated metabolism. *Risk D: Consider therapy modification*

Tetrabenazine: QTc-Prolonging Agents may enhance the QTc-prolonging effect of Tetrabenazine. *Risk X: Avoid combination*

Theophylline Derivatives: Macrolide Antibiotics may decrease the metabolism of Theophylline Derivatives. **Exceptions:** Dyphylline. *Risk D: Consider therapy modification*

Thioridazine: QTc-Prolonging Agents may enhance the QTc-prolonging effect of Thioridazine. *Risk X: Avoid combination*

Topotecan: P-Glycoprotein Inhibitors may increase the serum concentration of Topotecan. *Risk X: Avoid combination*

Typhoid Vaccine: Antibiotics may diminish the therapeutic effect of Typhoid Vaccine. Only the live attenuated Ty21a strain is affected. *Risk D: Consider therapy modification*

Vitamin K Antagonists (eg, warfarin): Macrolide Antibiotics may decrease the metabolism of Vitamin K Antagonists. *Risk C: Monitor therapy*

Zafirlukast: Erythromycin may decrease the serum concentration of Zafirlukast. *Risk C: Monitor therapy*

Ziprasidone: QTc-Prolonging Agents may enhance the QTc-prolonging effect of Ziprasidone. The risk of a severe arrhythmia may be increased. *Risk X: Avoid combination*

Zopiclone: Macrolide Antibiotics may increase the serum concentration of Zopiclone. *Risk D: Consider therapy modification*

Ethanol/Nutrition/Herb Interactions

Ethanol: Avoid ethanol (may decrease absorption of erythromycin or enhance ethanol effects).

Food: Erythromycin serum levels may be altered if taken with food (formulation-dependent).

Herb/Nutraceutical: St John's wort may decrease erythromycin levels.

Stability

Injection:

Store unreconstituted vials at 15°C to 30°C (59°F to 86°F). Erythromycin lactobionate should be reconstituted with sterile water for injection without preservatives to avoid gel formation. The reconstituted solution is stable for 2 weeks when refrigerated or for 8 hours at room temperature.

Erythromycin I.V. infusion solution is stable at pH 6-8. Stability of lactobionate is pH dependent. I.V. form has the longest stability in 0.9% sodium chloride (NS) and should be prepared in this base solution whenever possible. Do not use D_5W as a diluent unless sodium bicarbonate is added to solution. If I.V. must be prepared in D_5W, 0.5 mL of the 8.4% sodium bicarbonate solution should be added per each 100 mL of D_5W.

Stability of parenteral admixture at room temperature (25°C) and at refrigeration temperature (4°C) is 24 hours.

Standard diluent: 500 mg/250 mL D_5W/NS; 750 mg/250 mL D_5W/NS; 1 g/250 mL D_5W/NS.

Oral suspension:

Granules: Prior to mixing, store at <30°C (<86°F). After mixing, store under refrigeration and use within 10 days.

Powder: Refrigerate to preserve taste. Erythromycin ethylsuccinate may be stored at room temperature if used within 14 days. EryPed® drops should be used within 35 days following reconstitution. May store at room temperature or under refrigeration.

Tablet and capsule formulations: Store at <30°C (<86°F).

Topical and ophthalmic formulations: Store at room temperature.

Mechanism of Action Inhibits RNA-dependent protein synthesis at the chain elongation step; binds to the 50S ribosomal subunit resulting in blockage of transpeptidation

Pharmacodynamics/Kinetics

Absorption: Oral: Variable but better with salt forms than with base form; 18% to 45%; ethylsuccinate may be better absorbed with food

Distribution:

Relative diffusion from blood into CSF: Minimal even with inflammation

CSF:blood level ratio: Normal meninges: 2% to 13%; Inflamed meninges: 7% to 25%

Protein binding: Base: 73% to 81%

Metabolism: Demethylation primarily via hepatic CYP3A4

Half-life elimination: Peak: 1.5-2 hours; End-stage renal disease: 5-6 hours

Time to peak, serum: Base: 4 hours; Ethylsuccinate: 0.5-2.5 hours; delayed with food due to differences in absorption

Excretion: Primarily feces; urine (2% to 15% as unchanged drug)

Dosage Note: Due to differences in absorption, 400 mg erythromycin ethylsuccinate produces the same serum levels as 250 mg erythromycin base or stearate.

Usual dosage range:

Neonates: Ophthalmic: Prophylaxis of neonatal gonococcal or chlamydial conjunctivitis: 0.5-1 cm ribbon of ointment should be instilled into each conjunctival sac

Infants and Children:

Oral:

Base: 30-50 mg/kg/day in 2-4 divided doses; maximum: 2 g/day

Ethylsuccinate: 30-50 mg/kg/day in 2-4 divided doses; maximum: 3.2 g/day

Stearate: 30-50 mg/kg/day in 2-4 divided doses; maximum: 2 g/day

I.V.: Lactobionate: 15-50 mg/kg/day divided every 6 hours, not to exceed 4 g/day

Children and Adults:

Ophthalmic: Instill 1/2" (1.25 cm) 2-6 times/day depending on the severity of the infection

Topical: Acne: Apply over the affected area twice daily after the skin has been thoroughly washed and patted dry

Adults:

Oral:

Base: 250-500 mg every 6-12 hours; maximum 4 g/day

Ethylsuccinate: 400-800 mg every 6-12 hours; maximum: 4 g/day

I.V.: Lactobionate: 15-20 mg/kg/day divided every 6 hours or 500 mg to 1 g every 6 hours, or given as a continuous infusion over 24 hours; maximum: 4 g/24 hours

Indication-specific dosing:

Children:

***Bartonella sp* infections (bacillary angiomatosis [BA], peliosis hepatis [PH]) (unlabeled use):** Oral: 40 mg/kg/day (ethylsuccinate) in 4 divided doses (maximum: 2 g/day) for 3 months (BA) or 4 months (PH)

Conjunctivitis, neonatal *(C. trachomatis)*: Oral: 50 mg/kg/day (base or ethylsuccinate) in 4 divided doses for 14 days

Mild/moderate infection: Oral: 30-50 mg/kg/day in divided doses every 6-12 hours

Pertussis: Oral: 40-50 mg/kg/day in 4 divided doses for 14 days; maximum 2 g/day (not preferred agent for infants <1 month due to IHPS)

Pharyngitis, tonsillitis (streptococcal): Oral: 20 mg (base)/kg/day or 40 mg (ethylsuccinate)/kg/day in 2 divided doses for 10 days. **Note:** No longer preferred therapy due to increased organism resistance.

Pneumonia *(C. trachomatis)*: Oral: 50 mg/kg/day (base or ethylsuccinate) in 4 divided doses for 14-21 days

Preop bowel preparation: Oral: 20 mg (base)/kg at 1, 2, and 11 PM on the day before surgery combined with mechanical cleansing of the large intestine and oral neomycin

Severe infection: I.V.: 15-50 mg/kg/day; maximum: 4 g/day

Adults:

***Bartonella sp* infections (bacillary angiomatosis [BA], peliosis hepatis [PH]) (unlabeled use):** Oral: 500 mg (base) 4 times/day for 3 months (BA) or 4 months (PH)

Chancroid (unlabeled use): Oral: 500 mg (base) 3 times/day for 7 days; Note: Not a preferred agent; isolates with intermediate resistance have been documented

Gastrointestinal prokinetic (unlabeled use): I.V.: 200 mg initially followed by 250 mg (base) orally 3 times/day 30 minutes before meals. Lower dosages have been used in some trials.

Granuloma inguinale (*K. granulomatis*) (unlabeled use): Oral: 500 mg (base) 4 times/day for 21 days

Legionnaires' disease: Oral: 1.6-4 g (ethylsuccinate)/day or 1-4 g (base)/day in divided doses for 21 days. **Note:** No longer preferred therapy and only used in nonhospitalized patients.

Lymphogranuloma venereum: Oral: 500 mg (base) 4 times/day for 21 days

Nongonococcal urethritis (including coinfection with *C. trachomatis*): Oral: 500 mg (base) 4 times/day for 7 days or 800 mg (ethylsuccinate) 4 times/day for 7 days. **Note:** May use 250 mg (base) or 400 mg (ethylsuccinate) 4 times/day for 14 days if gastrointestinal intolerance.

Pelvic inflammatory disease: I.V.: 500 mg every 6 hours for 3 days, followed by 1000 mg (base)/day orally in 2-4 divided doses for 7 days. **Note:** Not recommended therapy per current treatment guidelines.

Pertussis: Oral: 500 mg (base) every 6 hours for 14 days

Preop bowel preparation (unlabeled use): Oral: 1 g erythromycin base at 1, 2, and 11 PM on the day before surgery combined with mechanical cleansing of the large intestine and oral neomycin

Syphilis, primary: Oral: 48-64 g (ethylsuccinate) or 30-40 g (base) in divided doses over 10-15 days. **Note:** Not recommended therapy per current treatment guidelines.

Dosage adjustment in renal impairment: Dialysis: Slightly dialyzable (5% to 20%); no supplemental dosage necessary in hemo- or peritoneal dialysis or in continuous arteriovenous or venovenous hemofiltration

Dietary Considerations

Systemic: Drug may cause GI upset; may take with food.

E.E.S.® granules for oral suspension contain sodium 25.9 mg (1.1 mEq)/5 mL

EryPed® powder for oral suspension contains sodium 117.5 mg (5.1 mEq)/5 mL; powder for oral suspension (drops) contains sodium 58.8 mg (2.6 mEq)/dropperful dose

Administration

Oral: Do not crush enteric coated drug product. GI upset, including diarrhea, is common. May be administered with food to decrease GI upset. Do not give with milk or acidic beverages.

I.V.: Infuse 1 g over 20-60 minutes. I.V. infusion may be very irritating to the vein. If phlebitis/pain occurs with used dilution, consider diluting further (eg, 1:5) if fluid status of the patient will tolerate, or consider administering in larger available vein. The addition of lidocaine or bicarbonate does not decrease the irritation of erythromycin infusions.

Ophthalmic: Avoid contact of tip of ophthalmic ointment tube with affected eye

Test Interactions False-positive urinary catecholamines

Dosage Forms Excipient information presented when available (limited, particularly for generics); consult specific product labeling. [DSC] = Discontinued product; [CAN] = Canadian brand name

Note: Strength expressed as base

Capsule, delayed release, enteric-coated pellets, as base: 250 mg
- Eryc®: 250 mg [DSC]

Gel, topical: 2% (30 g, 60 g)
- Erygel®: 2% (30 g, 60 g) [DSC] [contains alcohol 92%]

Granules for oral suspension, as ethylsuccinate:
- E.E.S.®: 200 mg/5 mL (100 mL, 200 mL) [contains sodium 25.9 mg (1.1 mEq)/5 mL; cherry flavor]

Injection, powder for reconstitution, as lactobionate:
- Erythrocin®: 500 mg, 1 g

Ointment, ophthalmic: 0.5% [5 mg/g] (1 g, 3.5 g)
- Romycin®: 0.5% [5 mg/g] (3.5 g)

Ointment, topical:
- Akne-Mycin®: 2% (25 g)

Powder for oral suspension, as ethylsuccinate:
- EryPed®: 200 mg/5 mL (100 mL, 200 mL [DSC]) [contains sodium 117.5 mg (5.1 mEq)/5 mL; fruit flavor]; 400 mg/5 mL (100 mL, 200 mL [DSC]) [contains sodium 117.5 mg (5.1 mEq)/5 mL; banana flavor]

Powder for oral suspension, as ethylsuccinate [drops]:
- EryPed®: 100 mg/2.5 mL (50 mL) [DSC] [contains sodium 58.8 mg (2.6 mEq)/dropperful; fruit flavor]

Powder, for prescription compounding:
- Erythro-RX: USP (50 g)

Solution, topical: 2% (60 mL)
- Eryderm®: 2% (60 mL) [contain alcohol] [DSC]
- Sans acne [CAN]: 2% (60 mL) [contains ethyl alcohol 44%; not available in U.S.]

Suspension, oral, as ethylsuccinate: 200 mg/5 mL (480 mL) [DSC]; 400 mg/5 mL (480 mL) [DSC]
- E.E.S.®: 200 mg/5 mL (100 mL, 480 mL) [fruit flavor] [DSC]; 400 mg/5 mL (100 mL, 480 mL) [orange flavor]

Tablet, as base: 250 mg, 500 mg

Tablet, as base [polymer-coated particles]:
- PCE®: 333 mg, 500 mg

Tablet, as ethylsuccinate: 400 mg
- E.E.S.®: 400 mg [DSC]

Tablet, as stearate: 250 mg, 500 mg
- Erythrocin®: 250 mg, 500 mg

Tablet, delayed release, enteric coated, as base:
- Ery-Tab®: 250 mg, 333 mg, 500 mg

Erythromycin and Sulfisoxazole

(er ith roe MYE sin & sul fi SOKS a zole)

Medication Safety Issues

Sound-alike/look-alike issues:
- Pediazole® may be confused with Pediapred®

U.S. Brand Names E.S.P.®

Canadian Brand Names Pediazole®

Mexican Brand Names Pediazole

Index Terms Sulfisoxazole and Erythromycin

Pharmacologic Category Antibiotic, Macrolide; Antibiotic, Macrolide Combination; Antibiotic, Sulfonamide Derivative

Use Treatment of susceptible bacterial infections of the upper and lower respiratory tract, otitis media in children caused by susceptible strains of *Haemophilus influenzae*, and many other infections in patients allergic to penicillin

Effect on Mental Status Macrolides have been reported to cause nightmares, confusion, anxiety, and mood lability; dizziness is common with sulfisoxazole; sulfonamides reported to cause restlessness, irritability, depression, euphoria, disorientation, panic, hallucinations, and delusions

Effect on Psychiatric Treatment Erythromycin is contraindicated with pimozide; may increase concentration of bromocriptine, carbamazepine, and triazolam; photosensitivity is common with sulfisoxazole; use caution with concurrent psychotropics; may cause leukopenia; caution with clozapine and carbamazepine

Dosage Summary

Oral:

Children <2 months: Dosage not established

Children ≥2 months: 50 mg/kg/day erythromycin and 150 mg/kg/day sulfisoxazole in divided doses every 6 hours

Adults: 400 mg erythromycin and 1200 mg sulfisoxazole every 6 hours

Elderly: Use not recommended

Dosage Forms Excipient information presented when available (limited, particularly for generics); consult specific product labeling.

Powder for oral suspension: Erythromycin ethylsuccinate 200 mg and sulfisoxazole acetyl 600 mg per 5 mL (100 mL, 150 mL, 200 mL)

E.S.P.®: Erythromycin ethylsuccinate 200 mg and sulfisoxazole acetyl 600 mg per 5 mL (100 mL, 150 mL, 200 mL) [cheri beri flavor]

◆ **Erythromycin Base** *see* Erythromycin *on page 557*
◆ **Erythromycin Ethylsuccinate** *see* Erythromycin *on page 557*
◆ **Erythromycin Lactobionate** *see* Erythromycin *on page 557*
◆ **Erythromycin Stearate** *see* Erythromycin *on page 557*
◆ **Erythropoiesis-Stimulating Agent (ESA)** *see* Darbepoetin Alfa *on page 419*
◆ **Erythropoiesis-Stimulating Agent (ESA)** *see* Epoetin Alfa *on page 546*
◆ **Erythropoiesis-Stimulating Protein** *see* Darbepoetin Alfa *on page 419*
◆ **Erythropoietin** *see* Epoetin Alfa *on page 546*
◆ **Erythro-RX** *see* Erythromycin *on page 557*

Escitalopram (es sye TAL oh pram)

Medication Safety Issues

Sound-alike/look-alike issues:

Lexapro® may be confused with Loxitane®

Related Information

Antidepressant Agents *on page 1760*
Antidepressant Receptor Profile *on page 1764*
Discontinuation of Psychotropic Drugs *on page 1839*
Liquid Compatibility of Antidepressants, Antipsychotics, and Mood Stabilizers *on page 1788*
Selective Serotonin Reuptake Inhibitors (SSRIs) CYP Profile *on page 1793*
Selective Serotonin Reuptake Inhibitors (SSRIs) FDA-Approved Indication(s) *on page 1794*
Selective Serotonin Reuptake Inhibitors (SSRIs) Pharmacokinetics *on page 1795*
Selective Serotonin Reuptake Inhibitors (SSRIs) Receptor Profile *on page 1796*

U.S. Brand Names Lexapro®

Canadian Brand Names Cipralex®

Index Terms Escitalopram Oxalate; Lu-26-054; S-Citalopram

Pharmacologic Category Antidepressant, Selective Serotonin Reuptake Inhibitor

Generic Available No

Use Treatment of major depressive disorder; generalized anxiety disorders (GAD)

Unlabeled/Investigational Use

Treatment of mild dementia-associated agitation in nonpsychotic patients

Mental Health Comment The SSRIs as a class are generally considered to be safe and equally effective. Allow sufficient dose-response time (6-12 weeks). Differences lie in approved indications, receptor profiles, pharmacokinetics, and cytochrome P450 activity profile. Subtle differences exist in adverse effect profiles. All SSRIs have the potential to cause sexual dysfunction. Escitalopram is the s-isomer of citalopram and therefore, similar to citalopram. Among the SSRIs, escitalopram possesses the lowest effects on CYP isoenzymes.

Restrictions An FDA-approved medication guide concerning the use of antidepressants in children, adolescents, and young adults must be distributed when dispensing an outpatient prescription (new or refill) where this medication is to be used without direct supervision of a healthcare provider. Medication guides are available at http://www.fda.gov/cder/Offices/ODS/medication_guides.htm. Dispense to parents or guardians of children and adolescents receiving this medication.

Pregnancy Risk Factor C

Pregnancy Considerations Due to adverse effects observed in animal studies, escitalopram is classified as pregnancy category C. Escitalopram is distributed into the amniotic fluid. Limited data is available concerning the use of escitalopram during pregnancy. Nonteratogenic effects in the newborn following SSRI exposure late in the third trimester include respiratory distress, cyanosis, apnea, seizures, temperature instability, feeding difficulty, vomiting, hypoglycemia, hypo- or hypertonia, hyper-reflexia, jitteriness, irritability, constant crying, and tremor. An increased risk of low birth weight and lower APGAR scores have also been reported. Exposure to SSRIs after the twentieth week of gestation has been associated with persistent pulmonary hypertension of the newborn (PPHN). Adverse effects may be due to toxic effects of the SSRI or drug withdrawal without a taper. The long-term effects of *in utero* SSRI exposure on infant development and behavior are not known. Escitalopram is the S-enantiomer of the racemic derivative citalopram; also refer to the Citalopram monograph.

Women treated for major depression and who are euthymic prior to pregnancy are more likely to experience a relapse when medication is discontinued as compared to pregnant women who continue taking antidepressant medications. The ACOG recommends that therapy with SSRIs or SNRIs during pregnancy be individualized; treatment of depression during pregnancy should incorporate the clinical expertise of the mental health clinician, obstetrician, primary healthcare provider, and pediatrician (ACOG, 2007). If treatment during pregnancy is required, consider tapering therapy during the third trimester in order to prevent withdrawal symptoms in the infant. If this is done and the woman is considered to be at risk from her major depressive disorder, the medication can be restarted following delivery, although the dose should be readjusted to that required before pregnancy.

Lactation Enters breast milk/consider risk:benefit

Contraindications Hypersensitivity to escitalopram, citalopram, or any component of the formulation; concomitant use with pimozide; concomitant use or within 2 weeks of MAO inhibitors

Warnings/Precautions **[U.S. Boxed Warning]: Antidepressants increase the risk of suicidal thinking and behavior in children, adolescents, and young adults (18-24 years of age) with major depressive disorder (MDD) and other psychiatric disorders;** consider risk prior to prescribing. Short-term studies did not show an increased risk in patients >24 years of age and showed a decreased risk in patients ≥65 years. Closely monitor patients for clinical worsening, suicidality, or unusual changes in behavior, particularly during the initial 1-2 months of therapy or during periods of dosage adjustments (increases or decreases); the patient's family or caregiver should be instructed to closely observe the patient and communicate condition with healthcare provider. A medication guide concerning the use of antidepressants should be dispensed with each prescription. **Escitalopram is not FDA approved for use in children.**

The possibility of a suicide attempt is inherent in major depression and may persist until remission occurs. Use caution in high-risk patients. Worsening depression and severe abrupt suicidality that are not part of the presenting symptoms may require discontinuation or modification of drug therapy. The patient's family or caregiver should be alerted to monitor patients for the emergence of suicidality and associated behaviors (such as agitation, irritability, hostility, impulsivity, and hypomania) and call healthcare provider.

May worsen psychosis in some patients or precipitate a shift to mania or hypomania in patients with bipolar disorder. Patients presenting with depressive symptoms should be screened for bipolar disorder. Monotherapy in patients with bipolar disorder should be avoided. Escitalopram is not FDA approved for the treatment of bipolar depression. Escitalopram is not FDA approved for the treatment of bipolar depression.

The potential for a severe reaction exists when used with MAO inhibitors, SSRIs/SNRIs or triptans; serotonin syndrome (hyperthermia, muscular rigidity, mental status changes/agitation, autonomic instability) may occur. Concurrent use with MAO inhibitors is contraindicated. May increase the risks associated with electroconvulsive therapy. Has a low potential to impair cognitive or motor performance; caution operating hazardous machinery or driving.

Use caution with a previous seizure disorder or condition predisposing to seizures such as brain damage, alcoholism, or concurrent therapy with other drugs which lower the seizure threshold. May cause hyponatremia/SIADH (elderly at increased risk); volume depletion (diuretics may increase risk) may occur. May cause or exacerbate sexual dysfunction. Use caution with renal or liver impairment; concomitant CNS depressants; pregnancy (high doses of citalopram have been associated with teratogenicity in animals). Use caution with concomitant use of aspirin, NSAIDs, warfarin, or other drugs that affect coagulation; the risk of bleeding may be potentiated.

Upon discontinuation of escitalopram therapy, gradually taper dose. If intolerable symptoms occur following a decrease in dosage or upon discontinuation of therapy, then resuming the previous dose with a more gradual taper should be considered.

Adverse Reactions

>10%:

- Central nervous system: Headache (24%), somnolence (6% to 13%), insomnia (9% to 12%)
- Gastrointestinal: Nausea (15% to 18%)
- Genitourinary: Ejaculation disorder (9% to 14%)

1% to 10%:

- Cardiovascular: Chest pain, hypertension, palpitation
- Central nervous system: Fatigue (5% to 8%), dizziness (5%), dreaming abnormal (3%), lethargy (1% to 3%), yawning (2%), concentration impaired, fever, irritability, lightheadedness, migraine
- Dermatologic: Rash
- Endocrine & metabolic: Libido decreased (3% to 7%), anorgasmia (2% to 6%), menstrual disorder (2%), hot flashes, menstrual cramps
- Gastrointestinal: Xerostomia (6% to 9%), diarrhea (8%), constipation (3% to 5%), appetite decreased (3%), indigestion (3%), vomiting (3%), abdominal pain (2%), flatulence (2%), toothache (2%), abdominal cramps, appetite increased, gastroenteritis, heartburn, weight gain
- Genitourinary: Impotence (2% to 3%), urinary tract infection, urinary frequency
- Neuromuscular & skeletal: Neck/shoulder pain (3%), paresthesia (2%), arthralgia, limb pain, muscle cramp, myalgia
- Ocular: Blurred vision
- Otic: Earache, tinnitus
- Respiratory: Rhinitis (5%), sinusitis (3%), bronchitis, cough, nasal or sinus congestion, sinus headache
- Miscellaneous: Diaphoresis (4% to 5%), flu-like syndrome (5%), allergy

<1% (Limited to important or life threatening): Abdominal discomfort, acute renal failure, aggression, agitation, akathisia, allergic reaction, amnesia, anaphylaxis, anemia, angioedema, anxiety attack, apathy, arthritis, arthropathy, asthma, atrial fibrillation, auditory hallucination, back discomfort, bilirubin increased, bradycardia, bruxism, carpal tunnel syndrome, chest tightness, chills, choreoathetosis, confusion, conjunctivitis, coordination abnormal, delirium, delusion, depersonalization, depression aggravated, depression, dermatitis, diplopia, disorientation, dyskinesia, dyspepsia, dyspnea, dystonia, dysuria, ecchymosis, ECG abnormal, eczema, edema, emotional lability, erythema multiforme, excitability, eye infection, flushing, folliculitis, furunculosis, gastritis, GERD, glaucoma, gout, grand mal seizure, hallucination, hematoma, hematuria, hemolytic anemia, hepatic necrosis, hepatitis, hypercholesterolemia, hyperglycemia, hyper-reflexia, INR increased, kidney stone, leg pain, lipoma, liver enzymes increased, liver failure, malaise, menorrhagia, muscle contractions (involuntary), muscle stiffness, muscle weakness, muscular tone increased, myocardial infarction, nervousness, neuroleptic malignant syndrome, nosebleed, nystagmus, pancreatitis, panic reaction, pneumonia, priapism, prolactinemia, prothrombin decreased, pruritus, pulmonary embolism, pupils dilated, QT prolonged, restless legs, restlessness aggravated, rhabdomyolysis, serotonin syndrome, shaking, SIADH, spontaneous abortion, spotting between menses, Stevens-Johnson syndrome, suicidal tendency, suicide attempt, syncope, tachycardia, taste alteration, thrombocytopenia, thrombosis, tics, torsade de pointes, toxic epidermal necrolysis, tracheitis, tremor, tremulousness nervous, twitching, urinary

urgency, varicose vein, ventricular arrhythmia, vertigo, vision abnormal, visual disturbance, weakness, weight loss, withdrawal syndrome

Metabolism/Transport Effects Substrate (major) of CYP2C19, 3A4; **Inhibits** CYP2D6 (weak)

Drug Interactions

Alcohol (Ethyl): CNS Depressants may enhance the CNS depressant effect of Alcohol (Ethyl). *Risk C: Monitor therapy*

Alpha-/Beta-Blockers: Selective Serotonin Reuptake Inhibitors may decrease the metabolism of Alpha-/Beta-Blockers. *Risk C: Monitor therapy*

Analgesics (Opioid): May enhance the serotonergic effect of Selective Serotonin Reuptake Inhibitors. This may cause serotonin syndrome. *Risk C: Monitor therapy*

Anticoagulants: Antiplatelet Agents may enhance the anticoagulant effect of Anticoagulants. *Risk C: Monitor therapy*

Antidepressants (Serotonin Reuptake Inhibitor/Antagonist): Selective Serotonin Reuptake Inhibitors may enhance the serotonergic effect of Antidepressants (Serotonin Reuptake Inhibitor/Antagonist). This may cause serotonin syndrome. *Risk C: Monitor therapy*

Antiplatelet Agents: May enhance the anticoagulant effect of other Antiplatelet Agents. *Risk C: Monitor therapy*

Aspirin: Selective Serotonin Reuptake Inhibitors may enhance the antiplatelet effect of Aspirin. *Risk C: Monitor therapy*

Beta-Blockers: Selective Serotonin Reuptake Inhibitors may enhance the bradycardic effect of Beta-Blockers. **Exceptions:** Acebutolol; Atenolol; Carteolol; Esmolol; Levobunolol; Metipranolol; Nadolol; Penbutolol. *Risk C: Monitor therapy*

BusPIRone: May enhance the serotonergic effect of Selective Serotonin Reuptake Inhibitors. This may cause serotonin syndrome. Selective Serotonin Reuptake Inhibitors may decrease the metabolism of BusPIRone. *Risk C: Monitor therapy*

CarBAMazepine: Selective Serotonin Reuptake Inhibitors may decrease the metabolism of CarBAMazepine. Specifically those SSRIs that inhibit CYP3A4 isoenzymes. CarBAMazepine may increase the metabolism of Selective Serotonin Reuptake Inhibitors. Specifically those agents metabolized via CYP1A2, 2C, and/or 3A4 isoenzymes. *Risk D: Consider therapy modification*

Cimetidine: May decrease the metabolism of Selective Serotonin Reuptake Inhibitors. *Risk D: Consider therapy modification*

Clozapine: Selective Serotonin Reuptake Inhibitors may decrease the metabolism of Clozapine. *Risk D: Consider therapy modification*

CNS Depressants: May enhance the adverse/toxic effect of other CNS Depressants. *Risk C: Monitor therapy*

CYP2C19 Inducers (Strong): May increase the metabolism of CYP2C19 Substrates. *Risk C: Monitor therapy*

CYP2C19 Inhibitors (Moderate): May decrease the metabolism of CYP2C19 Substrates. *Risk C: Monitor therapy*

CYP2C19 Inhibitors (Strong): May decrease the metabolism of CYP2C19 Substrates. *Risk D: Consider therapy modification*

CYP3A4 Inducers (Strong): May increase the metabolism of CYP3A4 Substrates. *Risk C: Monitor therapy*

CYP3A4 Inhibitors (Moderate): May decrease the metabolism of CYP3A4 Substrates. *Risk C: Monitor therapy*

CYP3A4 Inhibitors (Strong): May decrease the metabolism of CYP3A4 Substrates. *Risk D: Consider therapy modification*

Cyproheptadine: May diminish the therapeutic effect of Selective Serotonin Reuptake Inhibitors. *Risk C: Monitor therapy*

Dasatinib: May enhance the anticoagulant effect of Antiplatelet Agents. *Risk C: Monitor therapy*

Dasatinib: May increase the serum concentration of CYP3A4 Substrates. *Risk C: Monitor therapy*

Deferasirox: May decrease the serum concentration of CYP3A4 Substrates. *Risk C: Monitor therapy*

Desmopressin: Selective Serotonin Reuptake Inhibitors may enhance the adverse/toxic effect of Desmopressin. *Risk C: Monitor therapy*

Dextromethorphan: Selective Serotonin Reuptake Inhibitors may enhance the adverse/toxic effect of Dextromethorphan. *Risk D: Consider therapy modification*

Drotrecogin Alfa: Antiplatelet Agents may enhance the adverse/toxic effect of Drotrecogin Alfa. Bleeding may occur. *Risk D: Consider therapy modification*

Haloperidol: Selective Serotonin Reuptake Inhibitors may decrease the metabolism of Haloperidol. *Risk C: Monitor therapy*

Herbs (Anticoagulant/Antiplatelet Properties) (eg, Alfalfa, Anise, Bilberry): May enhance the adverse/toxic effect of Antiplatelet Agents. Bleeding may occur. *Risk D: Consider therapy modification*

Herbs (CYP3A4 Inducers): May increase the metabolism of CYP3A4 Substrates. *Risk C: Monitor therapy*

Ibritumomab: Antiplatelet Agents may enhance the adverse/toxic effect of Ibritumomab. Both agents may contribute to impaired platelet function and an increased risk of bleeding. *Risk C: Monitor therapy*

Lithium: Selective Serotonin Reuptake Inhibitors may enhance the adverse/toxic effect of Lithium. *Risk C: Monitor therapy*

Macrolide Antibiotics: May decrease the metabolism of Selective Serotonin Reuptake Inhibitors. **Exceptions:** Azithromycin; Dirithromycin [Off Market]; Spiramycin. *Risk C: Monitor therapy*

MAO Inhibitors: May enhance the serotonergic effect of Selective Serotonin Reuptake Inhibitors. This may cause serotonin syndrome. *Risk X: Avoid combination*

Methadone: Selective Serotonin Reuptake Inhibitors may decrease the metabolism of Methadone. Fluvoxamine appears to be the only interacting SSRI. *Risk D: Consider therapy modification*

Mexiletine: Selective Serotonin Reuptake Inhibitors may decrease the metabolism of Mexiletine. *Risk D: Consider therapy modification*

NSAID (COX-2 Inhibitor): Selective Serotonin Reuptake Inhibitors may enhance the antiplatelet effect of NSAID (COX-2 Inhibitor). *Risk D: Consider therapy modification*

NSAID (Nonselective): Selective Serotonin Reuptake Inhibitors may enhance the antiplatelet effect of NSAID (Nonselective). *Risk D: Consider therapy modification*

Omega-3-Acid Ethyl Esters: May enhance the antiplatelet effect of Antiplatelet Agents. *Risk C: Monitor therapy*

Pentosan Polysulfate Sodium: May enhance the adverse/toxic effect of Antiplatelet Agents. Specifically, the risk of bleeding may be increased by concurrent use of these agents. *Risk C: Monitor therapy*

Phenytoin: Selective Serotonin Reuptake Inhibitors may decrease the metabolism of Phenytoin. *Risk D: Consider therapy modification*

Pimozide: Selective Serotonin Reuptake Inhibitors may enhance the adverse/toxic effect of Pimozide. *Risk X: Avoid combination*

Propafenone: Selective Serotonin Reuptake Inhibitors may decrease the metabolism of Propafenone. *Risk D: Consider therapy modification*

Prostacyclin Analogues: May enhance the antiplatelet effect of Antiplatelet Agents. *Risk C: Monitor therapy*

Risperidone: Selective Serotonin Reuptake Inhibitors may decrease the metabolism of Risperidone. *Risk C: Monitor therapy*

Salicylates: Antiplatelet Agents may enhance the adverse/toxic effect of Salicylates. Increased risk of bleeding may result. *Risk C: Monitor therapy*

Serotonin Modulators: May enhance the adverse/toxic effect of other Serotonin Modulators. The development of serotonin syndrome may occur. *Risk D: Consider therapy modification*

Sibutramine: May enhance the serotonergic effect of Serotonin Modulators. This may cause serotonin syndrome. *Risk X: Avoid combination*

Thrombolytic Agents: Antiplatelet Agents may enhance the anticoagulant effect of Thrombolytic Agents. *Risk C: Monitor therapy*

Tositumomab and Iodine I 131 Tositumomab: Antiplatelet Agents may enhance the adverse/toxic effect of Tositumomab and Iodine I 131 Tositumomab. Specifically, the risk of bleeding-related adverse events may be increased. *Risk C: Monitor therapy*

TraMADol: Selective Serotonin Reuptake Inhibitors may enhance the neuroexcitatory and/or seizure-potentiating effect of TraMADol. TraMADol may enhance the serotonergic effect of Selective Serotonin Reuptake Inhibitors. This may cause serotonin syndrome. *Risk D: Consider therapy modification*

Tricyclic Antidepressants: Selective Serotonin Reuptake Inhibitors may decrease the metabolism of Tricyclic Antidepressants. *Risk D: Consider therapy modification*

Tryptophan: May enhance the serotonergic effect of Selective Serotonin Reuptake Inhibitors. This may cause serotonin syndrome. *Risk D: Consider therapy modification*

Vitamin K Antagonists (eg, warfarin): Selective Serotonin Reuptake Inhibitors may enhance the anticoagulant effect of Vitamin K Antagonists. *Risk C: Monitor therapy*

Ethanol/Nutrition/Herb Interactions

Ethanol: Avoid ethanol (may increase CNS depression).

Herb/Nutraceutical: Avoid valerian, St John's wort, SAMe, kava kava, and gotu kola (may increase CNS depression).

Stability Store at 25°C (77°F); excursions permitted to 15°C to 30°C (59°F to 86°F).

Mechanism of Action Escitalopram is the S-enantiomer of the racemic derivative citalopram, which selectively inhibits the reuptake of serotonin with little to no effect on norepinephrine or dopamine reuptake. It has no or very low affinity for 5-HT_{1-7}, alpha- and beta-adrenergic, D_{1-5}, H_{1-3}, M_{1-5}, and benzodiazepine receptors. Escitalopram does not bind to or has low affinity for Na^+, K^+, Cl^-, and Ca^{++} ion channels.

Pharmacodynamics/Kinetics

Onset of action: Depression: The onset of action is within a week, however, individual response varies greatly and full response may not be seen until 8-12 weeks after initiation of treatment.

Protein binding: 56% to plasma proteins

Metabolism: Hepatic via CYP2C19 and 3A4 to an active metabolite, S-desmethylcitalopram (S-DCT; 1/7 the activity); S-DCT is metabolized to S-didesmethylcitalopram (S-DDCT; active; 1/27 the activity) via CYP2D6

Half-life elimination: Escitalopram: 27-32 hours; S-desmethylcitalopram: 59 hours

Time to peak: Escitalopram: ~5 hours; S-desmethylcitalopram: 14 hours

Excretion: Urine (Escitalopram: 8%; S-DCT: 10%)

Clearance: Total body: 37-40 L/hour; Renal: Escitalopram: 2.7 L/hour; S-desmethylcitalopram: 6.9 L/hour

Dosage Oral:

Adults: Major depressive disorder, generalized anxiety disorder: Initial: 10 mg/day; dose may be increased to 20 mg/day after at least 1 week

Elderly: 10 mg once daily

Dosage adjustment in renal impairment:

Mild-to-moderate impairment: No dosage adjustment needed

Severe impairment: Cl_{cr} <20 mL/minute: Use with caution

Dosage adjustment in hepatic impairment: 10 mg/day

Dietary Considerations May be taken with or without food.

Administration Administer once daily (morning or evening), with or without food.

Monitoring Parameters Mental status for depression, suicidal ideation (especially at the beginning of therapy or when doses are increased or decreased), anxiety, social functioning, mania, panic attacks; akathisia

Additional Information The tablet and oral solution dosage forms are bioequivalent. Clinically, escitalopram 20 mg is equipotent to citalopram 40 mg. Do not coadminister with citalopram.

Dosage Forms Excipient information presented when available (limited, particularly for generics); consult specific product labeling.

Solution, oral:

Lexapro®: 1 mg/mL (240 mL) [contains propylene glycol; peppermint flavor]

Tablet:

Lexapro®: 5 mg, 10 mg, 20 mg

Note: Cipralex® [CAN] is available only in 10 mg and 20 mg strengths.

- **Escitalopram Oxalate** *see* Escitalopram *on page 564*
- **Esclim®** *see* Estradiol *on page 576*
- **Eserine Salicylate** *see* Physostigmine *on page 1288*
- **Esgic®** *see* Butalbital, Acetaminophen, and Caffeine *on page 229*
- **Esgic-Plus™** *see* Butalbital, Acetaminophen, and Caffeine *on page 229*
- **Eskalith® [DSC]** *see* Lithium *on page 938*
- **Eskalith CR® [DSC]** *see* Lithium *on page 938*

Esmolol (ES moe lol)

Medication Safety Issues

Sound-alike/look-alike issues:

Esmolol may be confused with Osmitrol®

Brevibloc® may be confused with bretylium, Brevital®, Bumex®, Buprenex®

High alert medication: The Institute for Safe Medication Practices (ISMP) includes this medication among its list of drugs which have a heightened risk of causing significant patient harm when used in error.

Related Information

Beta-Blockers *on page 1776*

U.S. Brand Names Brevibloc®

Canadian Brand Names Brevibloc®

Mexican Brand Names Brevibloc

Index Terms Esmolol Hydrochloride

Pharmacologic Category Antiarrhythmic Agent, Class II; Beta Blocker, $Beta_1$ Selective

Use Treatment of supraventricular tachycardia (SVT) and atrial fibrillation/flutter (control ventricular rate); treatment of tachycardia and/or hypertension (especially intraoperative or postoperative); treatment of noncompensatory sinus tachycardia

Unlabeled/Investigational Use In children, for SVT and postoperative hypertension

Effect on Mental Status May cause drowsiness, confusion, fatigue, or depression

Effect on Psychiatric Treatment Barbiturates may decease effects of esmolol

Dosage Summary

I.V.:

Children: Dosage not established

Adults: Bolus: 80 mg **or** 500 mcg/kg; Infusion: 50-200 mcg/kg/minute (maximum: 300 mcg/kg/minute)

Dosage Forms Excipient information presented when available (limited, particularly for generics); consult specific product labeling. [DSC] = Discontinued product

Infusion [premixed in sodium chloride; preservative free]:

Brevibloc®: 2000 mg (100 mL) [20 mg/mL; double strength]; 2500 mg (250 mL) [10 mg/mL]

Injection, solution, as hydrochloride: 10 mg/mL (10 mL)

Brevibloc®:

10 mg/mL (10 mL) [alcohol free; premixed in sodium chloride]

20 mg/mL (5 mL, 100 mL) [alcohol free; double strength; premixed in sodium chloride]

250 mg/mL (10 mL) [contains alcohol 25%, propylene glycol 25%; concentrate] [DSC]

◆ **Esmolol Hydrochloride** *see* Esmolol *on page 569*

Esomeprazole (es oh ME pray zol)

Medication Safety Issues

Sound-alike/look-alike issues:

Nexium® may be confused with Nexavar®

U.S. Brand Names Nexium®

Canadian Brand Names Nexium®

Mexican Brand Names Nexium IV; Nexium-MUPS

Index Terms Esomeprazole Magnesium; Esomeprazole Sodium

Pharmacologic Category Proton Pump Inhibitor; Substituted Benzimidazole

Generic Available No

Use

Oral: Short-term (4-8 weeks) treatment of erosive esophagitis; maintaining symptom resolution and healing of erosive esophagitis; treatment of symptomatic gastroesophageal reflux disease (GERD); as part of a multidrug regimen for *Helicobacter pylori* eradication in patients with duodenal ulcer disease (active or history of within the past 5 years); prevention of gastric ulcers in patients at risk (age ≥60 years and/or history of gastric ulcer) associated with continuous NSAID therapy; long-term treatment of pathological hypersecretory conditions including Zollinger-Ellison syndrome

Canadian labeling: Additional use (not in U.S. labeling): Oral: Treatment of nonerosive reflux disease (NERD)

I.V.: Short-term (≤10 days) treatment of gastroesophageal reflux disease (GERD) when oral therapy is not possible or appropriate

Effect on Mental Status May cause headache

Effect on Psychiatric Treatment The clearance of diazepam is decreased by 45% with concomitant use, resulting in increased diazepam levels and potential for toxicity; monitor

Pregnancy Risk Factor B

Pregnancy Considerations Teratogenic effects were not observed in animal studies. However, there are no adequate and well-controlled studies in pregnant women. Congenital abnormalities have been reported sporadically following omeprazole use during pregnancy.

Lactation Excretion in breast milk unknown/not recommended

Contraindications Hypersensitivity to esomeprazole, substituted benzimidazoles (ie, lansoprazole, omeprazole, pantoprazole, rabeprazole), or any component of the formulation

Warnings/Precautions Relief of symptoms does not preclude the presence of a gastric malignancy. Atrophic gastritis (by biopsy) has been noted with long-term omeprazole therapy; this may also occur with esomeprazole. No reports of enterochromaffin-like (ECL) cell carcinoids, dysplasia, or neoplasia have occurred. Severe liver dysfunction may require dosage reductions. Safety and efficacy of I.V. therapy >10 days have not been established; transition from I.V. to oral therapy as soon possible.

Adverse Reactions Unless otherwise specified, percentages represent adverse reactions identified in clinical trials evaluating the oral formulation.

>10%: Central nervous system: Headache (I.V. 11%; oral ≤8%)

1% to 10%:

Cardiovascular: Hypertension (≤3%), chest pain (>1%)

Central nervous system: Pain (4%), dizziness (oral >1%; I.V. 3%), anxiety (2%), insomnia (2%), pyrexia (2%), fatigue (>1%)

Dermatologic: Rash (>1%), pruritus (I.V. ≤1%)

Endocrine & metabolic: Hypercholesterolemia (2%)

Gastrointestinal: Flatulence (oral ≤5%; I.V. 10%), diarrhea (oral ≤7%; I.V. 4%), abdominal pain (oral ≤6%; I.V. 6%), nausea (oral 5%; I.V. 6%), dyspepsia (oral > 1%; I.V. 6%), gastritis (≤6%), constipation (oral 2%; I.V. 3%), vomiting (≤3%), benign GI neoplasm (>1%), dyspepsia (>1%), duodenitis (>1%), epigastric pain (>1%), esophageal disorder (>1%), gastroenteritis (>1%), GI mucosal discoloration (>1%), serum gastrin increased (>1%), tooth disorder (>1%), xerostomia (1%)

Genitourinary: Urinary tract infection (4%)

Hematologic: Anemia (>1%)

Hepatic: Transaminases increased (>1%)

Local: Local: Injection site reaction (I.V. 2%)

Neuromuscular & skeletal: Arthralgia (3%), back pain (>1%), fracture (>1%), arthropathy (1%), myalgia (1%)

Respiratory: Respiratory infection (oral ≤9%; I.V. 1%), bronchitis (4%), sinusitis (oral ≤4%; I.V. 2%), coughing (>1%), rhinitis (>1%), dyspnea (1%)

Miscellaneous: Accident/injury (≤8%), viral infection (4%), allergy (2%), ear infection (2%), hernia (>1%), flu-like syndrome (1%)

<1% (Limited to important or life-threatening): Abdominal rigidity, aggression, agitation, agranulocytosis, albuminuria, alkaline phosphatase increased, alopecia, anaphylactic reaction/shock, angioedema, anorexia, arthritis exacerbation, asthma exacerbation, benign polyps/nodules, bilirubinemia, blurred vision, bronchospasm, candidiasis (GI and genital), carcinoid tumor of stomach, cervical lymphadenopathy, conjunctivitis, cramps, creatinine increased, cystitis, dehydration, depression, dermatitis, dysmenorrhea, dysphagia, dysuria, edema (including facial, peripheral and tongue), epigastric pain, epistaxis, erythema multiforme, esophageal varices, fibromyalgia syndrome, flushing, fungal infection, gastric retention, GI dysplasia, glycosuria, goiter, gynecomastia, hallucinations, hematuria, hepatic encephalopathy, hepatic failure, hepatitis, hyperhidrosis, hyperparathyroidism, hypertonia, hyperuricemia, hypoesthesia, hypokalemia, hypomagnesemia, hyponatremia, impotence, interstitial nephritis, jaundice, larynx edema, leukocytosis, leukopenia, malaise, micturition increased, migraine, muscular weakness, nervousness, osteoporosis, otitis media, pancreatitis, pancytopenia, paresthesia, pharyngolaryngeal pain, pharyngitis, photosensitivity, polymyalgia rheumatica, polyuria, proteinuria, pruritus ani, rhinorrhea, rigors, sleep disorder, somnolence, Stevens-Johnson syndrome, stomatitis, tachycardia, taste disturbances, thrombocytopenia, thyroid-stimulating hormone increased, tinnitus, total bilirubin increased, toxic epidermal necrolysis, tremor, urticaria, vaginitis, vertigo, vitamin B_{12} deficiency, weight changes

Metabolism/Transport Effects Substrate of CYP2C19 (major), 3A4 (major); **Inhibits** CYP2C19 (moderate)

Drug Interactions

Antifungal Agents (Azole Derivatives, Systemic): Proton Pump Inhibitors may decrease the absorption of Antifungal Agents (Azole Derivatives, Systemic). **Exceptions:** Miconazole. *Risk D: Consider therapy modification*

Atazanavir: Proton Pump Inhibitors may decrease the absorption of Atazanavir. *Risk D: Consider therapy modification*

Benzodiazepines (metabolized by oxidation): Proton Pump Inhibitors may increase the serum concentration of Benzodiazepines (metabolized by oxidation). *Risk C: Monitor therapy*

Clopidogrel: Proton Pump Inhibitors may diminish the therapeutic effect of Clopidogrel. This appears to be due to reduced formation of the active clopidogrel metabolite. *Risk C: Monitor therapy*

CYP2C19 Inducers (Strong): May increase the metabolism of CYP2C19 Substrates. *Risk C: Monitor therapy*

CYP2C19 Substrates: CYP2C19 Inhibitors (Moderate) may decrease the metabolism of CYP2C19 Substrates. *Risk C: Monitor therapy*

Dabigatran Etexilate: Proton Pump Inhibitors may decrease the serum concentration of Dabigatran Etexilate. *Risk C: Monitor therapy*

Dasatinib: Proton Pump Inhibitors may decrease the absorption of Dasatinib. *Risk D: Consider therapy modification*

Erlotinib: Proton Pump Inhibitors may decrease the serum concentration of Erlotinib. *Risk X: Avoid combination*

Indinavir: Proton Pump Inhibitors may decrease the absorption of Indinavir. *Risk C: Monitor therapy*

Iron Salts: Proton Pump Inhibitors may decrease the absorption of Iron Salts. **Exceptions:** Ferric Gluconate; Iron Dextran Complex; Iron Sucrose. *Risk C: Monitor therapy*

Methotrexate: Proton Pump Inhibitors may decrease the excretion of Methotrexate. Antirheumatic doses of methotrexate probably hold minimal risk. *Risk C: Monitor therapy*

Mycophenolate: Proton Pump Inhibitors may decrease the serum concentration of Mycophenolate. Specifically, concentrations of the active mycophenolic acid may be reduced. *Risk C: Monitor therapy*

Saquinavir: Proton Pump Inhibitors may increase the serum concentration of Saquinavir. *Risk C: Monitor therapy*

Tipranavir: May decrease the serum concentration of Proton Pump Inhibitors. These data are derived from studies with Ritonavir-boosted Tipranavir. *Risk C: Monitor therapy*

Ethanol/Nutrition/Herb Interactions Food: Absorption is decreased by 43% to 53% when taken with food.

Stability

Capsule, granules: Store at 15°C to 30°C (59°F to 86°F). Keep container tightly closed.

Powder for injection: Store at 15°C to 30°C (59°F to 86°F). Protect from light.

For I.V. injection: Reconstitute powder with 5 mL NS.

For I.V. infusion: Initially reconstitute powder with 5 mL of NS, LR, or D_5W, then further dilute to a final volume of 50 mL.

Following reconstitution, solution for injection prepared in NS, and solution for infusion prepared in NS or LR should be used within 12 hours. Following reconstitution, solution for infusion prepared in D_5W should be used within 6 hours. Refrigeration is not required following reconstitution.

Mechanism of Action Proton pump inhibitor suppresses gastric acid secretion by inhibition of the H^+/K^+-ATPase in the gastric parietal cell

Pharmacodynamics/Kinetics

Distribution: V_{dss}: 16 L

Protein binding: 97%

Metabolism: Hepatic via CYP2C19 and 3A4 enzymes to hydroxy, desmethyl, and sulfone metabolites (all inactive)

Bioavailability: Oral: 90% with repeat dosing

Half-life elimination: ~1-1.5 hours

Time to peak: Oral: 1.5-2 hours

Excretion: Urine (80%, primarily as inactive metabolites; <1% as active drug); feces (20%)

Dosage

Children 1-11 years: Oral: **Note:** Safety and efficacy of doses >1 mg/kg/day and/or therapy beyond 8 weeks have not been established.

Symptomatic GERD: 10 mg once daily for up to 8 weeks

Erosive esophagitis (healing):

<20 kg: 10 mg once daily for 8 weeks

≥20 kg: 10-20 mg once daily for 8 weeks

Nonerosive reflux disease (NERD) (Canadian labeling): 10 mg once daily for up to 8 weeks

Adolescents 12-17 years: Oral:

GERD: 20-40 mg once daily for up to 8 weeks

NERD (Canadian labeling): 20 mg once daily for 2-4 weeks; lack of symptom control after 4 weeks warrants further evaluation

Adults:

Oral:

Erosive esophagitis (healing): Initial: 20-40 mg once daily for 4-8 weeks; if incomplete healing, may continue for an additional 4-8 weeks; maintenance: 20 mg once daily (controlled studies did not extend beyond 6 months)

Symptomatic GERD: 20 mg once daily for 4 weeks; may continue an additional 4 weeks if symptoms persist

NERD (Canadian labeling): Initial: 20 mg once daily for 2-4 weeks; lack of symptom control after 4 weeks warrants further evaluation; maintenance (in patients with successful initial therapy): 20 mg once daily as needed

Helicobacter pylori eradication: 40 mg once daily for 10 days; requires combination therapy **Note:** Various regimens available.

Canadian labeling: 20 mg twice daily for 7 days; requires combination therapy

Prevention of NSAID-induced gastric ulcers: 20-40 mg once daily for up to 6 months

Treatment of NSAID-induced gastric ulcers (Canadian labeling): 20 mg once daily for 4-8 weeks.

Pathological hypersecretory conditions (Zollinger-Ellison syndrome): 40 mg twice daily; adjust regimen to individual patient needs; doses up to 240 mg/day have been administered

I.V.: GERD: 20 mg or 40 mg once daily for ≤10 days; change to oral therapy as soon as appropriate

Elderly: No dosage adjustment needed.

Dosage adjustment in renal impairment: No dosage adjustment needed

Dosage adjustment in hepatic impairment:

Safety and efficacy not established in children with hepatic impairment.

Mild-to-moderate hepatic impairment (Child-Pugh class A or B): No dosage adjustment needed

Severe hepatic impairment (Child-Pugh class C): Dose should not exceed 20 mg/day

Dietary Considerations Take at least 1 hour before meals; best if taken before breakfast. The contents of the capsule may be mixed in applesauce or water; pellets also remain intact when exposed to orange juice, apple juice, and yogurt.

Administration

Oral:

Capsule: Should be swallowed whole and taken at least 1 hour before eating (best if taken before breakfast). Capsule can be opened and contents mixed with 1 tablespoon of applesauce. Swallow immediately; mixture should not be chewed or warmed. For patients with difficulty swallowing, use of granules may be easiest.

Granules: Empty into container with 1 tablespoon of water and stir; leave 2-3 minutes to thicken. Stir and drink within 30 minutes. If any medicine remains after drinking, add more water, stir and drink immediately.

Tablet (Canadian formulation, not available in U.S.): Swallow whole or may be dispersed in a half a glass of noncarbonated water. Stir until tablets disintegrate, leaving a liquid containing pellets. Drink contents within 30 minutes. Do not chew or crush pellets. After drinking, rinse glass with water and drink.

I.V.: May be administered by injection (≥3 minutes) or infusion (10-30 minutes). Flush line prior to and after administration with NS, LR, or D_5W.

Nasogastric tube:

Capsule: Open capsule and place intact granules into a 60 mL syringe; mix with 50 mL of water. Replace plunger and shake vigorously for 15 seconds. Ensure that no granules remain in syringe tip. Do not administer if pellets dissolve or disintegrate. Use immediately after preparation. After administration, flush nasogastric tube with additional water.

Granules: Delayed release oral suspension granules can also be given by nasogastric or gastric tube. Add 15 mL of water to a syringe, add granules from packet. Shake the syringe, leave 2-3 minutes to thicken. Shake the syringe and administer through nasogastric or gastric tube (French size 6 or greater) within 30 minutes. Refill the syringe with 15 mL of water, shake and flush nasogastric/gastric tube.

Tablet (Canadian formulation, not available in U.S.): Disperse tablets in 50 mL of noncarbonated water. Stir until tablets disintegrate leaving a liquid containing pellets. After administration, flush with additional 25-50 mL of water to clear the syringe and tube.

Monitoring Parameters Susceptibility testing recommended in patients who fail *H. pylori* eradication regimen (esomeprazole, clarithromycin, and amoxicillin)

Additional Information Esomeprazole is the S-isomer of omeprazole.

Dosage Forms Excipient information presented when available (limited, particularly for generics); consult specific product labeling. [CAN] = Canadian availability

Note: Strength expressed as base

Capsule, delayed release, as magnesium:

Nexium®: 20 mg, 40 mg

Granules, for oral suspension, delayed release, as magnesium:
  Nexium®: 10 mg/packet (30s); 20 mg/packet (30s); 40 mg/packet (30s)
  Nexium® [CAN]: 10 mg/packet (28s)
Injection, powder for reconstitution, as sodium:
  Nexium®: 20 mg, 40 mg [contains edetate sodium]
Tablet, extended release, as magnesium:
  Nexium® [CAN]: 20 mg, 40 mg [not available in U.S.]

- **Esomeprazole Magnesium** *see* Esomeprazole *on page 570*
- **Esomeprazole Sodium** *see* Esomeprazole *on page 570*
- **E.S.P.®** *see* Erythromycin and Sulfisoxazole *on page 563*

Estazolam (es TA zoe lam)

Medication Safety Issues
Sound-alike/look-alike issues:
ProSom® may be confused with PhosLo®, Proscar®, Pro-Sof® Plus, Prozac®, Psorcon®

Related Information
Benzodiazepines *on page 1774*
CMS: Long-Term Care Facility Thresholds *on page 1815*
Discontinuation of Psychotropic Drugs *on page 1839*

U.S. Brand Names ProSom® [DSC]

Mexican Brand Names Tasedan

Pharmacologic Category Benzodiazepine

Generic Available Yes

Use Short-term management of insomnia

Mental Health Comment In 2007, the FDA requested that all manufacturers of sedative-hypnotic drug products revise labeling to include a greater emphasis on the risks of adverse effects. These risks include severe allergic reactions (anaphylaxis, angioedema) and complex sleep-related behaviors, which may include sleep-driving (driving while not fully awake and with no memory of the event), making phone calls, and preparing and eating food while asleep.

There are two subtypes of GABA receptors (GABA-A and GABA-B) and three different benzodiazepine receptors (Bz_1, Bz_2, and Bz_3). Benzodiazepine receptors and effects appear to be linked to the GABA-A receptors. Benzodiazepines do not bind to GABA-B receptors. The role of GABA-B receptors is unclear. Benzodiazepines have no specificity for benzodiazepine receptor subtypes.

Estazolam is a short half-life benzodiazepine. Duration of action after a single dose is determined by redistribution rather than metabolism. Tolerance develops to the sedative, hypnotic, and anticonvulsant effects. It does not develop to the anxiolytic or skeletal muscle relaxing effects. Psychological and physical dependence may occur with prolonged use of benzodiazepines. The onset of withdrawal symptoms is usually seen on the first day without drug and lasts 5-7 days in patients receiving short half-life benzodiazepines, whereas, the onset occurs after 5 days with a duration of 10-14 days after abrupt discontinuance of long half-life benzodiazepines. Risk factors for abuse include personal or family history of substance abuse and personality disorder.

Restrictions C-IV

Pregnancy Risk Factor X

Lactation Enters breast milk/contraindicated

Contraindications Hypersensitivity to estazolam or any component of the formulation (cross-sensitivity with other benzodiazepines may exist); pregnancy

Note: Manufacturer states concurrent therapy with itraconazole or ketoconazole is contraindicated.

Warnings/Precautions As a hypnotic, should be used only after evaluation of potential causes of sleep disturbance. Failure of sleep disturbance to resolve after 7-10 days may indicate psychiatric or medical illness. Use is not recommended in patients with depressive disorders or psychoses. Avoid use in patients with sleep apnea. Postmarketing studies have indicated that the use of hypnotic/sedative agents for sleep has been associated with hypersensitivity reactions including anaphylaxis as well as angioedema. An increased risk for hazardous sleep-related activities such as sleep-driving; cooking and eating food, and making phone calls while asleep have also been noted. Use with caution in patients receiving concurrent CYP3A4 inhibitors, particularly when these agents are added to therapy. Use with caution in elderly or debilitated patients, patients with hepatic disease (including alcoholics), renal impairment, respiratory disease, impaired gag reflex, or obese patients. Rebound or withdrawal symptoms may occur following abrupt discontinuation or large decreases in dose. Use caution when reducing dose or withdrawing therapy; decrease slowly and monitor for withdrawal symptoms.

Causes CNS depression (dose related) which may impair physical and mental capabilities. Use with caution in patients receiving other CNS depressants or psychoactive agents. Benzodiazepines have been associated with falls and traumatic injury and should be used with extreme caution in patients who are at risk of these events (especially the elderly). May cause physical or psychological dependence - use with caution in patients with a history of drug dependence.

Benzodiazepines have been associated with anterograde amnesia. Paradoxical reactions, including hyperactive or aggressive behavior, have been reported with benzodiazepines, particularly in adolescent/pediatric or psychiatric patients. Does not have analgesic, antidepressant, or antipsychotic properties.

Adverse Reactions

>10%:

Central nervous system: Somnolence
Neuromuscular & skeletal: Weakness

1% to 10%:

Cardiovascular: Flushing, palpitation
Central nervous system: Anxiety, confusion, dizziness, hypokinesia, abnormal coordination, hangover effect, agitation, amnesia, apathy, emotional lability, euphoria, hostility, seizure, sleep disorder, stupor, twitch
Dermatologic: Dermatitis, pruritus, rash, urticaria
Gastrointestinal: Xerostomia, constipation, appetite increased/decreased, flatulence, gastritis, perverse taste
Genitourinary: Frequent urination, menstrual cramps, urinary hesitancy, urinary frequency, vaginal discharge/itching
Neuromuscular & skeletal: Paresthesia
Ocular: Photophobia, eye pain, eye swelling
Respiratory: Cough, dyspnea, asthma, rhinitis, sinusitis
Miscellaneous: Diaphoresis

<1% (Limited to important or life-threatening): Allergic reactions, anaphylaxis, angioedema, chills, complex sleep-related behavior (sleep-driving, cooking or eating food, making phone calls), drug dependence, fever, muscle spasm, myalgia, neck pain

Metabolism/Transport Effects **Substrate** of CYP3A4 (minor)

Drug Interactions

Alcohol (Ethyl): CNS Depressants may enhance the CNS depressant effect of Alcohol (Ethyl). *Risk C: Monitor therapy*

Antifungal Agents (Azole Derivatives, Systemic): May decrease the metabolism of Benzodiazepines (metabolized by oxidation). *Risk D: Consider therapy modification*

Aprepitant: May increase the serum concentration of Benzodiazepines (metabolized by oxidation). *Risk C: Monitor therapy*

Calcium Channel Blockers (Nondihydropyridine): May decrease the metabolism of Benzodiazepines (metabolized by oxidation). *Risk D: Consider therapy modification*

CarBAMazepine: May increase the metabolism of Benzodiazepines (metabolized by oxidation). *Risk C: Monitor therapy*

Cimetidine: May decrease the metabolism of Benzodiazepines (metabolized by oxidation). *Risk C: Monitor therapy*

Clozapine: Benzodiazepines may enhance the adverse/toxic effect of Clozapine. *Risk D: Consider therapy modification*

CNS Depressants: May enhance the adverse/toxic effect of other CNS Depressants. *Risk C: Monitor therapy*

Disulfiram: May decrease the metabolism of Benzodiazepines (metabolized by oxidation). *Risk C: Monitor therapy*

Fluconazole: May decrease the metabolism of Benzodiazepines (metabolized by oxidation). *Risk D: Consider therapy modification*

Fosaprepitant: May increase the serum concentration of Benzodiazepines (metabolized by oxidation). Specifically, the active metabolite aprepitant is likely responsible for this effect. *Risk C: Monitor therapy*

Grapefruit Juice: May decrease the metabolism of Benzodiazepines (metabolized by oxidation). *Risk D: Consider therapy modification*

Isoniazid: May decrease the metabolism of Benzodiazepines (metabolized by oxidation). *Risk C: Monitor therapy*

Macrolide Antibiotics: May decrease the metabolism of Benzodiazepines (metabolized by oxidation). **Exceptions:** Azithromycin; Dirithromycin [Off Market]; Spiramycin. *Risk D: Consider therapy modification*

Nefazodone: May decrease the metabolism of Benzodiazepines (metabolized by oxidation). *Risk D: Consider therapy modification*
Oral Contraceptive (Estrogens): May decrease the metabolism of Benzodiazepines (metabolized by oxidation). *Risk C: Monitor therapy*
Oral Contraceptive (Progestins): May decrease the metabolism of Benzodiazepines (metabolized by oxidation). *Risk C: Monitor therapy*
Phenytoin: Benzodiazepines may increase the serum concentration of Phenytoin. Short-term exposure to benzodiazepines may not present as much risk as chronic therapy. *Risk C: Monitor therapy*
Protease Inhibitors: May decrease the metabolism of Benzodiazepines (metabolized by oxidation). Management: Amprenavir, atazanavir, darunavir, indinavir, nelfinavir, ritonavir, and tipranavir are contraindicated with midazolam and triazolam according to each protease inhibitor 's prescribing information. *Risk D: Consider therapy modification*
Proton Pump Inhibitors: May increase the serum concentration of Benzodiazepines (metabolized by oxidation). **Exceptions:** Lansoprazole; Pantoprazole; Rabeprazole. *Risk C: Monitor therapy*
Rifamycin Derivatives: May increase the metabolism of Benzodiazepines (metabolized by oxidation). *Risk D: Consider therapy modification*
Selective Serotonin Reuptake Inhibitors: May decrease the metabolism of Benzodiazepines (metabolized by oxidation). **Exceptions:** Citalopram; Escitalopram; PARoxetine; Sertraline. *Risk C: Monitor therapy*
St Johns Wort: May increase the metabolism of Benzodiazepines (metabolized by oxidation). *Risk C: Monitor therapy*
Theophylline Derivatives: May diminish the therapeutic effect of Benzodiazepines. *Risk D: Consider therapy modification*

Ethanol/Nutrition/Herb Interactions
Ethanol: Avoid ethanol (may increase CNS depression).
Food: Serum levels and/or toxicity may be increased by grapefruit juice.

Mechanism of Action Binds to stereospecific benzodiazepine receptors on the postsynaptic GABA neuron at several sites within the central nervous system, including the limbic system, reticular formation. Enhancement of the inhibitory effect of GABA on neuronal excitability results by increased neuronal membrane permeability to chloride ions. This shift in chloride ions results in hyperpolarization (a less excitable state) and stabilization.

Pharmacodynamics/Kinetics
Onset of action: ~1 hour
Duration: Variable
Metabolism: Extensively hepatic
Half-life elimination: 10-24 hours (no significant changes in elderly)
Time to peak, serum: 0.5-1.6 hours
Excretion: Urine (<5% as unchanged drug)

Dosage Adults: Oral: 1 mg at bedtime, some patients may require 2 mg; start at doses of 0.5 mg in debilitated or small elderly patients
Dosing adjustment in hepatic impairment: May be necessary

Monitoring Parameters Respiratory and cardiovascular status

Additional Information Abrupt discontinuation after sustained use (generally >10 days) may cause withdrawal symptoms.

Dosage Forms Excipient information presented when available (limited, particularly for generics); consult specific product labeling. [DSC] = Discontinued product
Tablet: 1 mg, 2 mg
ProSom®: 1 mg, 2 mg [DSC]

- **Ester-E™ [OTC]** *see* Vitamin E *on page 1675*
- **Esterified Estrogen and Methyltestosterone** *see* Estrogens (Esterified) and Methyltestosterone *on page 587*
- **Esterified Estrogens** *see* Estrogens, Esterified *on page 587*
- **Estrace®** *see* Estradiol *on page 576*
- **Estraderm®** *see* Estradiol *on page 576*

Estradiol (es tra DYE ole)

Medication Safety Issues
Sound-alike/look-alike issues:
Alora® may be confused with Aldara®
Elestrin™ may be confused with alosetron
Estraderm® may be confused with Testoderm®

International issues:
Vivelle®: Brand name for ethinyl estradiol and norgestimate in Austria

Estring® may be confused with Estrena® [Finland]
Estrena® [Finland] may be confused with estrone in the U.S.

Transdermal patch may contain conducting metal (eg, aluminum); remove patch prior to MRI.

U.S. Brand Names Alora®; Climara®; Delestrogen®; Depo®-Estradiol; Divigel®; Elestrin™; Esclim®; Estrace®; Estraderm®; Estrasorb™; Estring®; EstroGel®; Evamist™; Femring®; Femtrace®; Gynodiol® [DSC]; Menostar®; Vagifem®; Vivelle-Dot®; Vivelle® [DSC]

Canadian Brand Names Climara®; Depo®-Estradiol; Estrace®; Estraderm®; Estradot®; Estring®; EstroGel®; Menostar®; Oesclim®; Sandoz-Estradiol Derm 100; Sandoz-Estradiol Derm 50; Sandoz-Estradiol Derm 75; Vagifem®

Mexican Brand Names Climaderm; Evorel; Ginedisc; Oestrogel; Sandrena; Systen

Index Terms Estradiol Acetate; Estradiol Cypionate; Estradiol Hemihydrate; Estradiol Transdermal; Estradiol Valerate

Pharmacologic Category Estrogen Derivative

Use Treatment of moderate-to-severe vasomotor symptoms associated with menopause; treatment of vulvar and vaginal atrophy; hypoestrogenism (due to hypogonadism, castration, or primary ovarian failure); prostatic cancer (palliation), breast cancer (palliation), osteoporosis (prophylaxis); abnormal uterine bleeding due to hormonal imbalance; postmenopausal urogenital symptoms of the lower urinary tract (urinary urgency, dysuria)

Effect on Mental Status May cause dizziness, headache, depression, insomnia, nervousness, irritability, and mood disturbances

Effect on Psychiatric Treatment The Women's Health Initiative (WHI) Memory Study reported an increased risk of developing dementia in postmenopausal women ≥65 years of age during 4 years of treatment with oral conjugated equine estrogens and medroxyprogesterone acetate relative to placebo (1.8% vs 0.9%). Relative risk was 2.05 (95% CI 1.21-3.48). Therefore, estrogens and progestins should not be used for the prevention of dementia. The WHI also reported an increased risk of stroke (29 vs 21 per 10,000 women-years) compared to women receiving placebo. The increase in risk was observed after the first year and persisted. May cause hypertriglyceridemia; monitor in patients receiving antipsychotics especially clozapine, olanzapine, and quetiapine.

Dosage Summary

I.M.:

Cypionate:

Females (hypogonadism): 1.5-2 mg monthly

Adults (females): Menopause: 1-5 mg every 3-4 weeks

Valerate:

*Females (hypogonadism):*10-20 mg every 4 weeks

Adults (females): Menopause: 10-20 mg every 4 weeks

Adults (males): Prostate cancer: ≥30 mg or more every 1-2 weeks

Oral:

Females (hypogonadism): 1-2 mg/day cyclically (3 weeks on, 1 week off)

Adults (females):

Breast cancer: 10 mg 3 times/day

Other indications: 0.5-2 mg/day cyclically (3 weeks on, 1 week off)

Adults (males): Prostate cancer: 10 mg 3 times/day

Intravaginal:

Children: Dosage not established

Adults (females):

Cream: Initial: 2-4 g/day for 2 weeks, then 1/2 the initial dose for 2 weeks; Maintenance: 1 g 1-3 times/week

Ring: Insert 2 mg (Estring®) **or** 0.05-0.1 mg (Femring®), leave in place for 3 months

Tablet: Initial: Insert 1 tablet once daily for 2 weeks; Maintenance: Insert 1 tablet twice weekly

Topical:

Children: Dosage not established

Adults (females):

Emulsion: 3.84 g applied once daily in the morning

Gel: 1.25 g/day (EstroGel®) or 0.87 g/day (Elestrin™) or 0.25-1 g/day (Divigel®) applied at the same time each day

Spray: One spray (1.53 mg) per day; dosing range: 1-3 sprays/day

Transdermal:

Children: Dosage not established

Adults (females):

Alora®, Esclim®, Estraderm®, Vivelle®, Vivelle-Dot®: Apply twice weekly continuously or cyclically (3 weeks on, 1 week off)

Climara®, Menostar®: Apply once weekly continuously or cyclically (3 weeks on, 1 week off)

Dosage Forms Excipient information presented when available (limited, particularly for generics); consult specific product labeling. [DSC] = Discontinued product

Cream, vaginal:
Estrace®: 0.1 mg/g (12 g) [refill]; 0.1 mg/g (42.5 g) [packaged with applicator]

Emulsion, topical, as hemihydrate:
Estrasorb™: 2.5 mg/g (56s) [each pouch contains 4.35 mg estradiol hemihydrate; contents of two pouches delivers estradiol 0.05 mg/day]

Gel, topical:
Divigel®: 0.1% (0.25 g) [foil packet; delivers estradiol 0.25 mg/packet]; (0.5 g) [foil packet; delivers 0.5 mg estradiol/packet]; (1 g) [foil packet; delivers estradiol 1 mg/packet]
Elestrin™: 0.06% (144 g) [pump; delivers estradiol 0.52 mg/0.87 g; 100 actuations]
EstroGel®:
0.06% (50 g) [pump; delivers estradiol 0.75 mg/1.25 g; 32 actuations]
0.06% (93 g) [pump; delivers estradiol 0.75 mg/1.25 g; 64 actuations] [DSC]

Injection, oil, as cypionate:
Depo®-Estradiol: 5 mg/mL (5 mL) [contains chlorobutanol; in cottonseed oil]

Injection, oil, as valerate: 10 mg/mL (5 mL); 20 mg/mL (5 mL); 40 mg/mL (5 mL)
Delestrogen®:
10 mg/mL (5 mL) [contains chlorobutanol; in sesame oil]
20 mg/mL (5 mL) [contains benzyl alcohol; in castor oil]
40 mg/mL (5 mL) [contains benzyl alcohol; in castor oil]

Ring, vaginal, as base:
Estring®: 2 mg (1s) [total estradiol 2 mg; releases 7.5 mcg/day over 90 days]

Ring, vaginal, as acetate:
Femring®: 0.05 mg (1s) [total estradiol 12.4 mg; releases 0.05 mg/day over 3 months]; 0.1 mg (1s) [total estradiol 24.8 mg; releases 0.1 mg/day over 3 months]

Solution, topical [spray]:
Evamist™: 1.53 mg/spray (8.1 mL) [contains 56 sprays after priming; contains alcohol]

Tablet, oral, as acetate:
Femtrace®: 0.45 mg, 0.9 mg, 1.8 mg

Tablet, oral, micronized: 0.5 mg, 1 mg, 2 mg
Estrace®: 0.5 mg, 1 mg, 2 mg [2 mg tablets contain tartrazine]
Gynodiol®: 0.5 mg [DSC], 1 mg [DSC], 1.5 mg [DSC], 2 mg [DSC]

Tablet, vaginal, as base:
Vagifem®: 25 mcg [contains lactose]

Transdermal system: 0.025 mg/24 hours (4s) [once-weekly patch]; 0.0375 mg/24 hours (4s) [once-weekly patch]; 0.05 mg/24 hours (4s) [once-weekly patch]; 0.06 mg/24 hours (4s) [once-weekly patch]; 0.075 mg/24 hours [once-weekly patch]; 0.1 mg/24 hours (4s) [once-weekly patch]

Alora® [twice-weekly patch]:
0.025 mg/24 hours (8s) [9 cm^2, total estradiol 0.77 mg]
0.05 mg/24 hours (8s, 24s) [18 cm^2, total estradiol 1.5 mg]
0.075 mg/24 hours (8s) [27 cm^2, total estradiol 2.3 mg]
0.1 mg/24 hours (8s) [36 cm^2, total estradiol 3.1 mg]

Climara® [once-weekly patch]:
0.025 mg/24 hours (4s) [6.5 cm^2, total estradiol 2.04 mg]
0.0375 mg/24 hours (4s) [9.375 cm^2, total estradiol 2.85 mg]
0.05 mg/24 hours (4s) [12.5 cm^2, total estradiol 3.8 mg]
0.06 mg/24 hours (4s) [15 cm^2, total estradiol 4.55 mg]
0.075 mg/24 hours (4s) [18.75 cm^2, total estradiol 5.7 mg]
0.1 mg/24 hours (4s) [25 cm^2, total estradiol 7.6 mg]

Esclim® [twice-weekly patch]:
0.025 mg/day (8s) [11 cm^2, total estradiol 5 mg]
0.0375 mg/day (8s) [16.5 cm^2, total estradiol 7.5 mg]
0.05 mg/day (8s) [22 cm^2, total estradiol 10 mg]
0.075 mg/day (8s) [33 cm^2, total estradiol 15 mg]
0.1 mg/day (8s) [44 cm^2, total estradiol 20 mg]

Estraderm® [twice-weekly patch]:
0.05 mg/24 hours (8s) [10 cm^2, total estradiol 4 mg]
0.1 mg/24 hours (8s) [20 cm^2, total estradiol 8 mg]

Menostar® [once-weekly patch]: 0.014 mg/24 hours (4s) [3.25 cm^2, total estradiol 1 mg]

Vivelle® [twice-weekly patch]:
0.05 mg/24 hours (8s) [14.5 cm^2, total estradiol 4.33 mg] [DSC]
0.1 mg/24 hours (8s) [29 cm^2, total estradiol 8.66 mg] [DSC]

Vivelle-Dot® [twice-weekly patch]:
- 0.025 mg/day (8s) [2.5 cm^2, total estradiol 0.39 mg]
- 0.0375 mg/day (8s) [3.75 cm^2, total estradiol 0.585 mg]
- 0.05 mg/day (8s) [5 cm^2, total estradiol 0.78 mg]
- 0.075 mg/day (8s) [7.5 cm^2, total estradiol 1.17 mg]
- 0.1 mg/day (8s) [10 cm^2, total estradiol 1.56 mg]

◆ **Estradiol Acetate** *see* Estradiol *on page 576*

◆ **Estradiol and Drospirenone** *see* Drospirenone and Estradiol *on page 515*

◆ **Estradiol and NGM** *see* Estradiol and Norgestimate *on page 580*

Estradiol and Norethindrone (es tra DYE ole & nor eth IN drone)

Medication Safety Issues
Transdermal patch may contain conducting metal (eg, aluminum); remove patch prior to MRI.

U.S. Brand Names Activella®; CombiPatch®

Canadian Brand Names Estalis-Sequi®; Estalis®

Index Terms Norethindrone and Estradiol

Pharmacologic Category Estrogen and Progestin Combination

Use Women with an intact uterus:

Tablet: Treatment of moderate-to-severe vasomotor symptoms associated with menopause; treatment of vulvar and vaginal atrophy; prophylaxis for postmenopausal osteoporosis

Transdermal patch: Treatment of moderate-to-severe vasomotor symptoms associated with menopause; treatment of vulvar and vaginal atrophy; treatment of hypoestrogenism due to hypogonadism, castration, or primary ovarian failure

Effect on Mental Status May cause dizziness, headache, depression, insomnia, nervousness, irritability, and mood disturbances

Effect on Psychiatric Treatment The Women's Health Initiative (WHI) Memory Study reported an increased risk of developing dementia in postmenopausal women ≥65 years of age during 4 years of treatment with oral conjugated equine estrogens and medroxyprogesterone acetate relative to placebo (1.8% vs 0.9%). Relative risk was 2.05 (95% CI 1.21-3.48). Therefore, estrogens and progestins should not be used for the prevention of dementia. The WHI also reported an increased risk of stroke (29 vs 21 per 10,000 women-years) compared to women receiving placebo. The increase in risk was observed after the first year and persisted. May cause hypertriglyceridemia; monitor in patients receiving antipsychotics especially clozapine, olanzapine, and quetiapine.

Dosage Summary

Oral:

Children: Dosage not established

Adults (females): POne tablet daily

Transdermal:

Children: Dosage not established

Adults (females): Apply 1 patch twice weekly

Dosage Forms Excipient information presented when available (limited, particularly for generics); consult specific product labeling.

Combination pack:

Estalis-Sequi® 140/50 [CAN; not available in U.S.]:
- Transdermal system (Vivelle®): Estradiol 50 mcg per day (4s) [14.5 sq cm; total estradiol 4.33 mg]
- Transdermal system (Estalis®): Norethindrone acetate 140 mcg and estradiol 50 mcg per day (4s) [9 sq cm; total norethindrone acetate 2.7 mg, total estradiol 0.62 mg; not available in U.S.]

Estalis-Sequi® 250/50 [CAN; not available in U.S.]:
- Transdermal system (Vivelle®): Estradiol 50 mcg per day (4s) [14.5 sq cm; total estradiol 4.33 mg]
- Transdermal system (Estalis®): Norethindrone acetate 250 mcg and estradiol 50 mcg per day (4s) [16 sq cm; total norethindrone acetate 4.8 mg, total estradiol 0.51 mg; not available in U.S.]

Tablet:
- Activella® 0.5/0.1: Estradiol 0.5 mg and norethindrone acetate 0.1mg (28s)
- Activella® 1/0.5: Estradiol 1 mg and norethindrone acetate 0.5 mg (28s)

Transdermal system:

CombiPatch®:
- 0.05/0.14: Estradiol 0.05 mg and norethindrone acetate 0.14 mg per day (8s) [9 sq cm]

0.05/0.25: Estradiol 0.05 mg and norethindrone acetate 0.25 mg per day (8s) [16 sq cm]

Estalis® [CAN]:

140/50: Norethindrone acetate 140 mcg and estradiol 50 mcg per day (8s) [9 sq cm; total norethindrone acetate 2.7 mg, total estradiol 0.62 mg; not available in U.S.]

250/50 Norethindrone acetate 250 mcg and estradiol 50 mcg per day (8s) [16 sq cm; total norethindrone acetate 4.8 mg, total estradiol 0.51 mg; not available in U.S.]

Estradiol and Norgestimate (es tra DYE ole & nor JES ti mate)

U.S. Brand Names Prefest™

Index Terms Estradiol and NGM; Norgestimate and Estradiol; Ortho Prefest

Pharmacologic Category Estrogen and Progestin Combination

Use Women with an intact uterus: Treatment of moderate to severe vasomotor symptoms associated with menopause; treatment of atrophic vaginitis; prevention of osteoporosis

Effect on Mental Status May cause dizziness, headache, depression, insomnia, nervousness, irritability, and mood disturbances

Effect on Psychiatric Treatment May cause flu-like symptoms, take this into consideration if also concerned about SSRI discontinuation syndrome. Carbamazepine and topiramate may increase the metabolism of estradiol, leading to a decrease in serum concentrations. Estrogens may inhibit the metabolism of some benzodiazepines (alprazolam, chlordiazepoxide, diazepam), TCAs, and selegiline. Estrogens may increase the clearance of lorazepam, oxazepam, and temazepam.

The Women's Health Initiative (WHI) Memory Study reported an increased risk of developing dementia in postmenopausal women ≥65 years of age during 4 years of treatment with oral conjugated equine estrogens and medroxyprogesterone acetate relative to placebo (1.8% vs 0.9%). Relative risk was 2.05 (95% CI 1.21-3.48). Therefore, estrogens and progestins should not be used for the prevention of dementia. The WHI also reported an increased risk of stroke (29 vs 21 per 10,000 women-years) compared to women receiving placebo. The increase in risk was observed after the first year and persisted. May cause hypertriglyceridemia; monitor in patients receiving antipsychotics especially clozapine, olanzapine, and quetiapine.

Dosage Summary

Oral:

Children: Dosage not established

Adults (females): One tablet of estradiol 1 mg once daily for 3 days, followed by 1 tablet of estradiol 1 mg and norgestimate 0.09 mg once daily for 3 days; repeat sequence continuously

Dosage Forms Excipient information presented when available (limited, particularly for generics); consult specific product labeling.

Tablet: Estradiol 1 mg [15 pink tablets] and estradiol 1 mg and norgestimate 0.09 mg [15 white tablets] (supplied in blister card of 30)

◆ **Estradiol Cypionate** *see* Estradiol *on page 576*
◆ **Estradiol Hemihydrate** *see* Estradiol *on page 576*
◆ **Estradiol Transdermal** *see* Estradiol *on page 576*
◆ **Estradiol Valerate** *see* Estradiol *on page 576*

Estramustine (es tra MUS teen)

Medication Safety Issues

Sound-alike/look-alike issues:

Emcyt® may be confused with Eryc®

Estramustine may be confused with exemestane.

High alert medication: The Institute for Safe Medication Practices (ISMP) includes this medication among its list of drugs which have a heightened risk of causing significant patient harm when used in error.

U.S. Brand Names Emcyt®

Canadian Brand Names Emcyt®

Mexican Brand Names Emcyt

Index Terms Estramustine Phosphate; Estramustine Phosphate Sodium; NSC-89199

Pharmacologic Category Antineoplastic Agent, Alkylating Agent; Antineoplastic Agent, Hormone; Antineoplastic Agent, Hormone (Estrogen/Nitrogen Mustard)

Use Palliative treatment of prostatic carcinoma (progressive or metastatic)

Effect on Mental Status May cause sedation or insomnia; rarely may cause depression

Effect on Psychiatric Treatment None reported

Dosage Summary

Oral:

Children: Dosage not established

Adults (males): 14 mg/kg/day (range: 10-16 mg/kg/day) in 3 or 4 divided doses

Dosage Forms Excipient information presented when available (limited, particularly for generics); consult specific product labeling.

Capsule, as phosphate sodium:

Emcyt®: 140 mg

- ◆ **Estramustine Phosphate** *see* Estramustine *on page 580*
- ◆ **Estramustine Phosphate Sodium** *see* Estramustine *on page 580*
- ◆ **Estrasorb™** *see* Estradiol *on page 576*
- ◆ **Estratest®** *see* Estrogens (Esterified) and Methyltestosterone *on page 587*
- ◆ **Estratest® H.S.** *see* Estrogens (Esterified) and Methyltestosterone *on page 587*
- ◆ **Estring®** *see* Estradiol *on page 576*
- ◆ **EstroGel®** *see* Estradiol *on page 576*
- ◆ **Estrogenic Substances, Conjugated** *see* Estrogens (Conjugated/Equine) *on page 582*

Estrogens (Conjugated A/Synthetic)

(ES troe jenz, KON joo gate ed, aye, sin THET ik)

Medication Safety Issues

Sound-alike/look-alike issues:

Cenestin® may be confused with Senexon®

International issues:

Cenestin® may be confused with Canesten® which is a brand name for clotrimazole in multiple international markets and a brand name for fluconazole in Great Britain

U.S. Brand Names Cenestin®

Canadian Brand Names Cenestin

Pharmacologic Category Estrogen Derivative

Use Treatment of moderate-to-severe vasomotor symptoms of menopause; treatment of vulvar and vaginal atrophy

Effect on Mental Status May cause dizziness, headache, depression, insomnia, nervousness, irritability, and mood disturbances

Effect on Psychiatric Treatment The Women's Health Initiative (WHI) Memory Study reported an increased risk of developing dementia in postmenopausal women ≥65 years of age during 4 years of treatment with oral conjugated equine estrogens and medroxyprogesterone acetate relative to placebo (1.8% vs 0.9%). Relative risk was 2.05 (95% CI 1.21-3.48). Therefore, estrogens and progestins should not be used for the prevention of dementia. The WHI also reported an increased risk of stroke (29 vs 21 per 10,000 women-years) compared to women receiving placebo. The increase in risk was observed after the first year and persisted. May cause hypertriglyceridemia; monitor in patients receiving antipsychotics especially clozapine, olanzapine, and quetiapine.

Dosage Summary

Oral:

Children: Dosage not established

Adults (females): 0.3-1.25 mg once daily; **Note:** Titration is recommended

Dosage Forms Excipient information presented when available (limited, particularly for generics); consult specific product labeling.

Tablet: 0.3 mg, 0.45 mg, 0.625 mg, 0.9 mg, 1.25 mg

Estrogens (Conjugated B/Synthetic)

(ES troe jenz, KON joo gate ed, bee, sin THET ik)

U.S. Brand Names Enjuvia™

Pharmacologic Category Estrogen Derivative

Use Treatment of moderate-to-severe vasomotor symptoms of menopause; treatment of vulvar and vaginal atrophy associated with menopause; treatment of moderate-to-severe vaginal dryness and pain with intercourse associated with menopause

Effect on Mental Status May cause dizziness, irritability, depression, mood disturbances, and nervousness

Effect on Psychiatric Treatment The risk of dementia may be increased in postmenopausal women. Increased incidence of dementia was observed in women ≥65 years of age who were taking conjugated equine estrogens alone or in combination with medroxyprogesterone acetate. May increase triglycerides; combined use with clozapine, olanzapine, and quetiapine may produce an additive risk. Nausea is common; combined use with lithium, valproic acid, carbamazepine, and SSRIs may produce an additive risk. Carbamazepine and St John's wort may reduce the effectiveness or estrogens.

Dosage Summary

Oral:

Children: Dosage not established

Adults (females): 0.3-1.25 mg once daily; **Note:** Titration is recommended

Dosage Forms Excipient information presented when available (limited, particularly for generics); consult specific product labeling.

Tablet:

Enjuvia™: 0.3 mg, 0.45 mg, 0.625 mg, 0.9 mg, 1.25 mg

Estrogens (Conjugated/Equine)

(ES troe jenz KON joo gate ed, EE kwine)

Medication Safety Issues

Sound-alike/look-alike issues:

Premarin® may be confused with Primaxin®, Provera®, Remeron®

U.S. Brand Names Premarin®

Canadian Brand Names C.E.S.®; Premarin®

Mexican Brand Names C.E.S; Premarin

Index Terms C.E.S.; CE; CEE; Conjugated Estrogen; Estrogenic Substances, Conjugated

Pharmacologic Category Estrogen Derivative

Use Treatment of moderate-to-severe vasomotor symptoms associated with menopause; treatment of vulvar and vaginal atrophy; hypoestrogenism (due to hypogonadism, castration, or primary ovarian failure); prostatic cancer (palliation); breast cancer (palliation); osteoporosis (prophylaxis, postmenopausal women at significant risk only); abnormal uterine bleeding; moderate-to-severe dyspareunia (pain during intercourse) due to vaginal/vulvar atrophy of menopause

Unlabeled/Investigational Use Uremic bleeding

Effect on Mental Status May cause dizziness, headache, depression, insomnia, nervousness, irritability, and mood disturbances

Effect on Psychiatric Treatment Barbiturates and carbamazepine may decrease estrogen levels. The Women's Health Initiative (WHI) Memory Study reported an increased risk of developing dementia in postmenopausal women ≥65 years of age during 4 years of treatment with oral conjugated equine estrogens and medroxyprogesterone acetate relative to placebo (1.8% vs 0.9%). Relative risk was 2.05 (95% CI 1.21-3.48). Therefore, estrogens and progestins should not be used for the prevention of dementia. The WHI also reported an increased risk of stroke (29 vs 21 per 10,000 women-years) compared to women receiving placebo. The increase in risk was observed after the first year and persisted. May cause hypertriglyceridemia; monitor in patients receiving antipsychotics especially clozapine, olanzapine, and quetiapine.

Dosage Summary Note: Cyclic administration: Either 3 weeks on, 1 week off **or** 25 days on, 5 days off

I.M.:

Children (premenarche): Dosage not established

Children (postmenarche): Abnormal uterine bleeding: 25 mg, may repeat in 6-12 hours if needed

Adults (females): Abnormal uterine bleeding: 25 mg, may repeat in 6-12 hours if needed

I.V.:

Children (premenarche): Dosage not established

Children (postmenarche): Abnormal uterine bleeding: 25 mg, may repeat in 6-12 hours if needed

Adults (females): Abnormal uterine bleeding: 25 mg, may repeat in 6-12 hours if needed

Intravaginal:

Children: Dosage not established

Adults (females): Vaginal atrophy: 0.5-2 g/day given cyclically; Moderate-to-severe dyspareunia: 0.5 g twice weekly (eg, Monday and Thursday) or once daily cyclically*

Oral:

Females (hypogonadism): 0.3-0.625 mg/day given cyclically

Adults (females):

Breast cancer: 10 mg 3 times/day

Other indications: 0.3-1.25 mg daily or cyclically; **Note:** Titration is recommended

Adults (males):

Breast cancer: 10 mg 3 times/day

Prostate cancer: 1.25-2.5 mg 3 times/day

Dosage Forms Excipient information presented when available (limited, particularly for generics); consult specific product labeling.

Cream, vaginal:

Premarin®: 0.625 mg/g (42.5 g)

Injection, powder for reconstitution:

Premarin®: 25 mg [contains benzyl alcohol (in diluent), lactose 200 mg]

Tablet:

Premarin®: 0.3 mg, 0.45 mg, 0.625 mg, 0.9 mg, 1.25 mg

Estrogens (Conjugated/Equine) and Medroxyprogesterone

(ES troe jenz KON joo gate ed/EE kwine & me DROKS ee proe JES te rone)

Medication Safety Issues

Sound-alike/look-alike issues:

Premphase® may be confused with Prempro™

Prempro™ may be confused with Premphase®

U.S. Brand Names Premphase®; Prempro™

Canadian Brand Names Premphase®; Premplus®; Prempro™

Mexican Brand Names Premelle

Index Terms Medroxyprogesterone and Estrogens (Conjugated); MPA and Estrogens (Conjugated)

Pharmacologic Category Estrogen and Progestin Combination

Generic Available No

Use Women with an intact uterus: Treatment of moderate-to-severe vasomotor symptoms associated with menopause; treatment of atrophic vaginitis; osteoporosis (prophylaxis)

Effect on Mental Status May cause dizziness, headache, depression, insomnia, nervousness, irritability, and mood disturbances

Effect on Psychiatric Treatment Barbiturates and carbamazepine may decrease the effects of estrogens; estrogens may affect metabolism of benzodiazepines; monitor for clinical effect. The Women's Health Initiative (WHI) Memory Study reported an increased risk of developing dementia in postmenopausal women ≥65 years of age during 4 years of treatment with oral conjugated equine estrogens and medroxyprogesterone acetate relative to placebo (1.8% vs 0.9%). Relative risk was 2.05 (95% CI 1.21-3.48). Therefore, estrogens and progestins should not be used for the prevention of dementia. The WHI also reported an increased risk of stroke (29 vs 21 per 10,000 women-years) compared to women receiving placebo. The increase in risk was observed after the first year and persisted. May cause hypertriglyceridemia; monitor in patients receiving antipsychotics especially clozapine, olanzapine, and quetiapine.

Pregnancy Considerations See individual agents; use of this combination is contraindicated during pregnancy

Lactation Enters breast milk/use caution

Contraindications Hypersensitivity to conjugated estrogens, medroxyprogesterone (MPA), or any component of the formulation; undiagnosed abnormal vaginal bleeding; history of or current thrombophlebitis or venous thromboembolic disorders (including DVT, PE); active or recent (within 1 year) arterial thromboembolic disease (eg, stroke, MI); carcinoma of the breast; estrogen-dependent tumor; hepatic dysfunction or disease; pregnancy

Warnings/Precautions

Cardiovascular-related considerations: **[U.S. Boxed Warning]: Estrogens with or without progestin should not be used to prevent coronary heart disease.** Use caution with cardiovascular disease or dysfunction. May increase the risks of hypertension, myocardial infarction (MI), stroke, pulmonary emboli (PE), and deep vein thrombosis; incidence of these effects was shown to be significantly increased in postmenopausal women using conjugated equine estrogens (CEE) in combination with medroxyprogesterone acetate (MPA). Nonfatal MI, PE, and thrombophlebitis have also been reported in males taking high doses of CEE (eg, for prostate cancer). Estrogen compounds are generally associated with lipid effects such as increased HDL-cholesterol and decreased LDL-cholesterol. Triglycerides may also be increased; use with caution in patients with familial defects of lipoprotein metabolism. Whenever possible, estrogens should be discontinued at least 4 weeks prior to and for 2 weeks following elective surgery associated with an increased risk of thromboembolism or during periods of prolonged immobilization.

Neurological considerations: **[U.S. Boxed Warning]: The risk of dementia may be increased in postmenopausal women;** increased incidence was observed in women ≥65 years of age taking CEE alone or in combination with MPA.

Cancer-related considerations: Unopposed estrogens may increase the risk of endometrial carcinoma in postmenopausal women. Estrogens may exacerbate endometriosis. Malignant transformation of residual endometrial implants has been reported posthysterectomy with estrogen only therapy. Estrogens may increase the risk of breast cancer. An increased risk of invasive breast cancer was observed in postmenopausal women using CEE in combination with MPA; a smaller increase in risk was seen with estrogen therapy alone in observational studies. An increase in abnormal mammograms has also been reported with estrogen and progestin therapy. Estrogen use may lead to severe hypercalcemia in patients with breast cancer and bone metastases; discontinue estrogen if hypercalcemia occurs.

Estrogens may cause retinal vascular thrombosis; discontinue permanently if papilledema or retinal vascular lesions are observed on examination. Use with caution in patients with diseases which may be exacerbated by fluid retention, including asthma, epilepsy, migraine, diabetes, or renal dysfunction. Use with caution in patients with a history of severe hypocalcemia, SLE, hepatic hemangiomas, porphyria, endometriosis, and gallbladder disease. Use caution with history of cholestatic jaundice associated with past estrogen use or pregnancy. Safety and efficacy in pediatric patients have not been established. Prior to puberty, estrogens may cause premature closure of the epiphyses, premature breast development in girls, or gynecomastia in boys. Vaginal bleeding and vaginal cornification may also be induced in girls.

Before prescribing estrogen therapy to postmenopausal women, the risks and benefits must be weighed for each patient. Women should be informed of these risks and benefits, as well as possible effects of progestin when added to estrogen therapy. Estrogens with or without progestin should be used for shortest duration possible consistent with treatment goals. Conduct periodic risk:benefit assessments.

When used solely for prevention of osteoporosis in women at significant risk, nonestrogen treatment options should be considered. When used solely for the treatment of vulvar and vaginal atrophy, topical vaginal products should be considered.

Adverse Reactions

>10%:

- Central nervous system: Headache (28% to 37%), pain (11% to 13%), depression (6% to 11%)
- Endocrine & metabolic: Breast pain (32% to 38%), dysmenorrhea (8% to 13%)
- Gastrointestinal: Abdominal pain (16% to 23%), nausea (9% to 11%)
- Neuromuscular & skeletal: Back pain (13% to 16%)
- Respiratory: Pharyngitis (11% to 13%)
- Miscellaneous: Infection (16% to 18%), flu-like syndrome (10% to 13%)

1% to 10%:

- Cardiovascular: Peripheral edema (3% to 4%)
- Central nervous system: Dizziness (3% to 5%)
- Dermatologic: Pruritus (5% to 10%), rash (4% to 6%)
- Endocrine & metabolic: Leukorrhea (5% to 9%)
- Gastrointestinal: Flatulence (8% to 9%), diarrhea (5% to 6%), dyspepsia (5% to 6%)
- Genitourinary: Vaginitis (5% to 7%), cervical changes (4% to 5%), vaginal hemorrhage (1% to 3%)
- Neuromuscular & skeletal: Weakness (6% to 10%), arthralgia (7% to 9%), leg cramps (3% to 5%), hypertonia (3% to 4%)
- Respiratory: Sinusitis (7% to 8%), rhinitis (6% to 8%)

Additional adverse effects reported with conjugated estrogens and/or progestins (limited): Abnormal vaginal bleeding, amenorrhea, anaphylactoid reactions, anaphylaxis, breast enlargement/tenderness, cerebral embolism/thrombosis, cholecystitis, cholelithiasis, cholestatic jaundice, chorea, coagulation factor changes, contact lens intolerance, decreased carbohydrate tolerance, endometrial hyperplasia, erythema multiforme, erythema nodosum, HDL-cholesterol increased, hirsutism, hypertension, increase in size of uterine leiomyomata, gallbladder disease, libido changes, LDL-cholesterol decreased, migraine, optic neuritis, pancreatitis, pulmonary embolism, retinal thrombosis, thrombophlebitis, triglycerides increased, urticaria

Metabolism/Transport Effects

Based on estradiol and estrone: **Substrate** of CYP1A2 (major), 2A6 (minor), 2B6 (minor), 2C9 (minor), 2C19 (minor), 2D6 (minor), 2E1 (minor), 3A4 (major); **Inhibits** CYP1A2 (weak), 2C8 (weak); **Induces** CYP3A4 (weak)

Medroxyprogesterone: **Substrate** of CYP3A4 (major); **Induces** CYP3A4 (weak)

Drug Interactions

Acitretin: May diminish the therapeutic effect of Contraceptive (Progestins). Contraceptive failure is possible. *Risk X: Avoid combination*

Aminoglutethimide: May increase the metabolism of Progestins. *Risk D: Consider therapy modification*

Aprepitant: May decrease the serum concentration of Contraceptive (Progestins). *Risk D: Consider therapy modification*

Barbiturates: May diminish the therapeutic effect of Contraceptive (Progestins). Contraceptive failure is possible. *Risk D: Consider therapy modification*

CarBAMazepine: May diminish the therapeutic effect of Contraceptive (Progestins). Contraceptive failure is possible. *Risk D: Consider therapy modification*

Corticosteroids (Systemic): Estrogen Derivatives may increase the serum concentration of Corticosteroids (Systemic). *Risk C: Monitor therapy*

CYP1A2 Inducers (Strong): May increase the metabolism of CYP1A2 Substrates. *Risk C: Monitor therapy*

CYP3A4 Inducers (Strong): May increase the metabolism of CYP3A4 Substrates. *Risk C: Monitor therapy*

Deferasirox: May decrease the serum concentration of CYP3A4 Substrates. *Risk C: Monitor therapy*

Fosaprepitant: May decrease the serum concentration of Contraceptive (Progestins). The active metabolite aprepitant is likely responsible for this effect. *Risk D: Consider therapy modification*

Griseofulvin: May diminish the therapeutic effect of Contraceptive (Progestins). Contraceptive failure is possible. *Risk X: Avoid combination*

Herbs (Estrogenic Properties): May enhance the adverse/toxic effect of Estrogen Derivatives. *Risk C: Monitor therapy*

Herbs (Progestogenic Properties) (eg, Bloodroot, Yucca): May enhance the adverse/toxic effect of Progestins. *Risk C: Monitor therapy*

Maraviroc: CYP3A4 Inducers may decrease the serum concentration of Maraviroc. *Risk D: Consider therapy modification*

Phenytoin: May diminish the therapeutic effect of Contraceptive (Progestins). Contraceptive failure is possible. *Risk D: Consider therapy modification*

Rifamycin Derivatives: May decrease the serum concentration of Contraceptive (Progestins). Contraceptive failure is possible. *Risk D: Consider therapy modification*

Ropinirole: Estrogen Derivatives may increase the serum concentration of Ropinirole. *Risk C: Monitor therapy*

Somatropin: Estrogen Derivatives may diminish the therapeutic effect of Somatropin. Shown to be a concern with oral hormone replacement therapy in postmenopausal women. *Risk D: Consider therapy modification*

St Johns Wort: May diminish the therapeutic effect of Contraceptive (Progestins). Contraceptive failure is possible. *Risk D: Consider therapy modification*

Thyroid Products: Estrogen Derivatives may diminish the therapeutic effect of Thyroid Products. *Risk C: Monitor therapy*

Tipranavir: Estrogen Derivatives may enhance the dermatologic adverse effect of Tipranavir. The combination of tipranavir/ritonavir and ethinyl estradiol/norethindrone was associated with a high incidence of skin rash. Tipranavir may decrease the serum concentration of Estrogen Derivatives. *Risk D: Consider therapy modification*

Vitamin K Antagonists (eg, warfarin): Contraceptive (Progestins) may diminish the anticoagulant effect of Vitamin K Antagonists. In contrast, enhanced anticoagulant effects have also been noted with some products. *Risk D: Consider therapy modification*

Ethanol/Nutrition/Herb Interactions

Ethanol: Avoid ethanol (routine use increases estrogen level and risk of breast cancer). Ethanol may also increase the risk of osteoporosis.

Food: Folic acid absorption may be decreased.

Herb/Nutraceutical: St John's wort may decrease levels. Avoid black cohosh, dong quai (has estrogenic activity). Avoid red clover, saw palmetto, ginseng (due to potential hormonal effects).

Stability Store at room temperature 20°C to 25°C (68°F to 77°F).

Mechanism of Action

Conjugated estrogens contain a mixture of estrone sulfate, equilin sulfate, 17 alpha-dihydroequilin, 17 alpha-estradiol, and 17 beta-dihydroequilin. Estrogens are responsible for the development and maintenance of the female reproductive system and secondary sexual characteristics. Estradiol is the principle intracellular human estrogen and is more potent than estrone and estriol at the receptor level; it is the primary estrogen secreted prior to menopause. Following menopause, estrone and estrone sulfate are more highly produced. Estrogens modulate the pituitary secretion of gonadotropins, luteinizing hormone, and follicle-stimulating hormone through a negative feedback system; estrogen replacement reduces elevated levels of these hormones in postmenopausal women.

MPA inhibits gonadotropin production which then prevents follicular maturation and ovulation. In women with adequate estrogen, MPA transforms a proliferative endometrium into a secretory endometrium; when administered with conjugated estrogens, reduces the incidence of endometrial hyperplasia and risk of adenocarcinoma.

Pharmacodynamics/Kinetics See individual agents.

Dosage Oral: Adults:

Treatment of moderate-to-severe vasomotor symptoms associated with menopause or treatment of atrophic vaginitis in females with an intact uterus. (The lowest dose that will control symptoms should be used; medication should be discontinued as soon as possible):

Premphase®: One maroon conjugated estrogen 0.625 mg tablet daily on days 1 through 14 and one light blue conjugated estrogen 0.625 mg/MPA 5 mg tablet daily on days 15 through 28; re-evaluate patients at 3- and 6-month intervals to determine if treatment is still necessary; monitor patients for signs of endometrial cancer; rule out malignancy if unexplained vaginal bleeding occurs

Prempro™: One conjugated estrogen 0.3 mg/MPA 1.5 mg tablet daily; re-evaluate at 3-and 6-month intervals to determine if therapy is still needed; dose may be increased to a maximum of one conjugated estrogen 0.625 mg/MPA 5 mg tablet daily in patients with bleeding or spotting, once malignancy has been ruled out

Osteoporosis prophylaxis in females with an intact uterus:

Premphase®: One maroon conjugated estrogen 0.625 tablet daily on days 1 through 14 and one light blue conjugated estrogen 0.625 mg/MPA 5 mg tablet daily on days 15 through 28; monitor patients for signs of endometrial cancer; rule out malignancy if unexplained vaginal bleeding occurs

Prempro™: One conjugated estrogen 0.3 mg/MPA 1.5 mg tablet daily; dose may be increased to one conjugated estrogen 0.625 mg/MPA 5 mg tablet daily; in patients with bleeding or spotting, once malignancy has been ruled out

Elderly: Refer to adult dosing; a higher incidence of stroke and invasive breast cancer was observed in women >75 years in a WHI substudy.

Dietary Considerations Administration with food decreases nausea, administer with food. Ensure adequate calcium and vitamin D intake when used for the prevention of osteoporosis.

Monitoring Parameters Yearly physical examination that includes blood pressure and Papanicolaou smear, breast exam, mammogram. Monitor for signs of endometrial cancer. Adequate diagnostic measures, including endometrial sampling, if indicated, should be performed to rule out malignancy in all cases of undiagnosed abnormal vaginal bleeding. Monitor for loss of vision, sudden onset of proptosis, diplopia, migraine; signs and symptoms of thromboembolic disorders; glycemic control in patients with diabetes; lipid profiles in patients being treated for hyperlipidemias; thyroid function in patients on thyroid hormone replacement therapy.

Menopausal symptoms: Assess need for therapy at 3- to 6-month intervals

Prevention of osteoporosis: Bone density measurement

Test Interactions Pathologist should be advised of estrogen/progesterone therapy when specimens are submitted. Reduced response to metyrapone test.

Dosage Forms Excipient information presented when available (limited, particularly for generics); consult specific product labeling.

Tablet:
Premphase® [therapy pack contains 2 separate tablet formulations]: Conjugated estrogens 0.625 mg [14 maroon tablets] and conjugated estrogen 0.625 mg/medroxyprogesterone acetate 5 mg [14 light blue tablets] (28s)
Prempro™:
0.3/1.5: Conjugated estrogens 0.3 mg and medroxyprogesterone acetate 1.5 mg (28s)
0.45/1.5: Conjugated estrogens 0.45 mg and medroxyprogesterone acetate 1.5 mg (28s)
0.625/2.5: Conjugated estrogens 0.625 mg and medroxyprogesterone acetate 2.5 mg (28s)
0.625/5: Conjugated estrogens 0.625 mg and medroxyprogesterone acetate 5 mg (28s)

Estrogens, Esterified (ES troe jenz, es TER i fied)

Medication Safety Issues
Sound-alike/look-alike issues:
Estratab® may be confused with Estratest®, Estratest® H.S.

U.S. Brand Names Menest®

Canadian Brand Names Estratab®; Menest®

Index Terms Esterified Estrogens

Pharmacologic Category Estrogen Derivative

Use Treatment of moderate to severe vasomotor symptoms associated with menopause; treatment of vulvar and vaginal atrophy; hypoestrogenism (due to hypogonadism, castration, or primary ovarian failure); prostatic cancer (palliation); breast cancer (palliation); osteoporosis (prophylaxis, in women at significant risk only)

Effect on Mental Status May cause dizziness, headache, depression, insomnia, nervousness, irritability, and mood disturbances

Effect on Psychiatric Treatment The Women's Health Initiative (WHI) Memory Study reported an increased risk of developing dementia in postmenopausal women ≥65 years of age during 4 years of treatment with oral conjugated equine estrogens and medroxyprogesterone acetate relative to placebo (1.8% vs 0.9%). Relative risk was 2.05 (95% CI 1.21-3.48). Therefore, estrogens and progestins should not be used for the prevention of dementia. The WHI also reported an increased risk of stroke (29 vs 21 per 10,000 women-years) compared to women receiving placebo. The increase in risk was observed after the first year and persisted. May cause hypertriglyceridemia; monitor in patients receiving antipsychotics especially clozapine, olanzapine, and quetiapine.

Dosage Summary

Oral:

Females (hypogonadism): 2.5-7.5 mg daily for 20 days followed by a 10-day rest, repeat until response

Adults (females):
Breast cancer: 10 mg 3 times/day
Other indications: 0.3-1.25 mg daily or cyclically (3 weeks on and 1 week off)

Adults (males):
Breast cancer: 10 mg 3 times/day
Prostate cancer: 1.25-2.5 mg 3 times/day

Dosage Forms Tablet: 0.3 mg, 0.625 mg, 1.25 mg, 2.5 mg

Estrogens (Esterified) and Methyltestosterone
(ES troe jenz es TER i fied & meth il tes TOS te rone)

Medication Safety Issues
Sound-alike/look-alike issues:
Estratest® may be confused with Eskalith®, Estratab®, Estratest® H.S.
Estratest® H.S. may be confused with Eskalith®, Estratab®, Estratest®

U.S. Brand Names Covaryx™; Covaryx™ HS; E.E.M.T. D.S.; E.E.M.T. H.S.; Estratest®; Estratest® H.S.; Syntest D.S. [DSC]; Syntest H.S. [DSC]

Canadian Brand Names Estratest®

Index Terms Conjugated Estrogen and Methyltestosterone; Esterified Estrogen and Methyltestosterone

Pharmacologic Category Estrogen and Progestin Combination

Use Vasomotor symptoms of menopause

Effect on Mental Status May cause dizziness, headache, depression, insomnia, nervousness, irritability, and mood disturbances

Effect on Psychiatric Treatment Barbiturates and carbamazepine may decrease the effects of estrogens; estrogens may affect metabolism of benzodiazepines; monitor for clinical effect. The Women's Health Initiative (WHI) Memory Study reported an increased risk of developing dementia in postmenopausal women ≥65 years of age during 4 years of treatment with oral conjugated equine estrogens and medroxyprogesterone acetate relative to placebo (1.8% vs 0.9%). Relative risk was 2.05 (95% CI 1.21-3.48). Therefore, estrogens and progestins should not be used for the prevention of dementia. The WHI also reported an increased risk of stroke (29 vs 21 per 10,000 women-years) compared to women receiving placebo. The increase in risk was observed after the first year and persisted. May cause hypertriglyceridemia; monitor in patients receiving antipsychotics especially clozapine, olanzapine, and quetiapine.

Dosage Summary

Oral:

Children: Dosage not established

Adults (females): Lowest dose that will control symptoms should be chosen, normally given 3 weeks on and 1 week off

Dosage Forms Excipient information presented when available (limited, particularly for generics); consult specific product labeling. [DSC] = Discontinued product

Tablet: Esterified estrogens 1.25 mg and methyltestosterone 2.5 mg [contains tartrazine]; esterified estrogen 0.625 mg and methyltestosterone 1.25 mg

Covaryx™: Esterified estrogens 1.25 mg and methyltestosterone 2.5 mg [contains tartrazine]

Covaryx™ H.S.: Esterified estrogens 1.25 mg and methyltestosterone 2.5 mg [contains tartrazine]

Estratest®: Esterified estrogen 1.25 mg and methyltestosterone 2.5 mg

Estratest® H.S.: Esterified estrogen 0.625 mg and methyltestosterone 1.25 mg

E.E.M.T. D.S., Syntest D.S. [DSC]: Esterified estrogen 1.25 mg and methyltestosterone 2.5 mg

E.E.M.T. H.S., Syntest H.S. [DSC]: Esterified estrogen 0.625 mg and methyltestosterone 1.25 mg

Estropipate (ES troe pih pate)

U.S. Brand Names Ogen®; Ortho-Est®

Canadian Brand Names Ogen®

Index Terms Ortho Est; Piperazine Estrone Sulfate

Pharmacologic Category Estrogen Derivative

Use Treatment of moderate to severe vasomotor symptoms associated with menopause; treatment of vulvar and vaginal atrophy; hypoestrogenism (due to hypogonadism, castration, or primary ovarian failure); osteoporosis (prophylaxis, in women at significant risk only)

Effect on Mental Status May cause dizziness, headache, depression, insomnia, nervousness, irritability, and mood disturbances

Effect on Psychiatric Treatment The Women's Health Initiative (WHI) Memory Study reported an increased risk of developing dementia in postmenopausal women ≥65 years of age during 4 years of treatment with oral conjugated equine estrogens and medroxyprogesterone acetate relative to placebo (1.8% vs 0.9%). Relative risk was 2.05 (95% CI 1.21-3.48). Therefore, estrogens and progestins should not be used for the prevention of dementia. The WHI also reported an increased risk of stroke (29 vs 21 per 10,000 women-years) compared to women receiving placebo. The increase in risk was observed after the first year and persisted. May cause hypertriglyceridemia; monitor in patients receiving antipsychotics especially clozapine, olanzapine, and quetiapine.

Dosage Summary

Oral:

Children: Dosage not established

Adults (females): 0.75-6 mg once daily or cyclically [menopause] **or** 1.5-9 mg for the first 3 weeks, followed by a rest period of 8-10 days [hypoestrogenism] **or** 0.75 mg for 25 days of a 31 day cycle [osteoporosis]

Dosage Forms Excipient information presented when available (limited, particularly for generics); consult specific product labeling.

Tablet: 0.625 mg [estropipate 0.75 mg]; 1.25 mg [estropipate 1.5 mg]; 2.5 mg [estropipate 3 mg]

Ogen®: 0.625 mg [estropipate 0.75 mg]; 1.25 mg [estropipate 1.5 mg]; 2.5 mg [estropipate 3 mg]

Ortho-Est®: 0.625 mg [estropipate 0.75 mg]; 1.25 mg [estropipate 1.5 mg]

◆ **Estrostep® Fe** *see* Ethinyl Estradiol and Norethindrone *on page 597*

Eszopiclone (es zoe PIK lone)

Medication Safety Issues

Sound-alike/look-alike issues:

Lunesta® may be confused with Neulasta®

Related Information

CMS: Long-Term Care Facility Thresholds *on page 1815*

Nonbenzodiazepine Anxiolytics and Hypnotics *on page 1791*

U.S. Brand Names Lunesta®

Pharmacologic Category Hypnotic, Nonbenzodiazepine

Generic Available No

Use Treatment of insomnia

Mental Health Comment In 2007, the FDA requested that all manufacturers of sedative-hypnotic drug products revise labeling to include a greater emphasis on the risks of adverse effects. These risks include severe allergic reactions (anaphylaxis, angioedema) and complex sleep-related behaviors, which may include sleep-driving (driving while not fully awake and with no memory of the event), making phone calls, and preparing and eating food while asleep. Eszopiclone may be associated with a lower potential for abuse compared to benzodiazepines.

Restrictions C-IV

An FDA-approved patient medication guide is available and must be distributed when dispensing an outpatient prescription (new or refill) where this medication is to be used without direct supervision of a healthcare provider. Medication guides are available at http://www.fda.gov/cder/Offices/ODS/medication_guides.htm.

Pregnancy Risk Factor C

Pregnancy Considerations No evidence of teratogenicity in animal models (high dose). There are no adequate or well-controlled studies in pregnant women; use only if clearly needed.

Lactation Excretion in breast milk unknown/use caution

Contraindications There are no contraindications listed within the manufacturer's labeling.

Warnings/Precautions Symptomatic treatment of insomnia should be initiated only after careful evaluation of potential causes of sleep disturbance. Tolerance did not develop over 6 months of use. Use with caution in patients with depression or a history of drug dependence. Abrupt discontinuance may lead to withdrawal symptoms. Use with caution in patients receiving other CNS depressants or psychoactive medications. Hypnotics/sedatives have been associated with abnormal thinking and behavior changes including decreased inhibition, aggression, bizarre behavior, agitation, hallucinations, and depersonalization. These changes may occur unpredictably and may indicate previously unrecognized psychiatric disorders; evaluate appropriately. Amnesia may occur. May impair physical and mental capabilities. Postmarketing studies have indicated that the use of hypnotic/sedative agents for sleep has been associated with hypersensitivity reactions including anaphylaxis as well as angioedema. An increased risk for hazardous sleep-related activities such as sleep-driving; cooking and eating food, and making phone calls while asleep have also been noted. Use caution in patients with respiratory compromise, hepatic dysfunction, elderly or those taking strong CYP3A4 inhibitors. Because of the rapid onset of action, administer immediately prior to bedtime or after the patient has gone to bed and is having difficulty falling asleep. Safety and efficacy in children have not been established.

Adverse Reactions

>10%:

Central nervous system: Headache (15% to 21%)

Gastrointestinal: Unpleasant taste (8% to 34%)

1% to 10%:

Cardiovascular: Chest pain, peripheral edema

Central nervous system: Somnolence (8% to 10%), dizziness (5% to 7%), pain (4% to 5%), nervousness (up to 5%), depression (1% to 4%), confusion (up to 3%), hallucinations (1% to 3%), anxiety (1% to 3%), abnormal dreams (1% to 3%), migraine

Dermatologic: Rash (3% to 4%), pruritus (1% to 4%)

Endocrine & metabolic: Libido decreased (up to 3%), dysmenorrhea (up to 3%), gynecomastia (males up to 3%)

Gastrointestinal: Xerostomia (3% to 7%), dyspepsia (2% to 6%), nausea (4% to 5%), diarrhea (2% to 4%), vomiting (up to 3%)

Genitourinary: Urinary tract infection (up to 3%)
Neuromuscular & skeletal: Neuralgia (up to 3%)
Miscellaneous: Infection (5% to 10%), viral infection (3%), accidental injury (up to 3%)

<1% (Limited to important or life-threatening): Abnormal gait, agitation, alopecia, allergic reaction, amenorrhea, anaphylaxis, angioedema, anorexia, asthma, ataxia, breast enlargement, breast neoplasm, bronchitis, cholelithiasis, colitis; complex sleep-related behavior (sleep-driving, cooking or eating food, making phone calls); conjunctivitis, contact dermatitis, cystitis, dehydration, diaphoresis, dry eyes, dyspnea, dysphagia, dysuria, eczema, emotional lability, epistaxis, erythema multiforme, euphoria, facial edema, fever, gout, heat stroke, hematuria, hepatitis, hepatomegaly, herpes zoster, hostility, hypercholesterolemia, hypertension, hypokalemia, kidney calculus, kidney pain, liver damage, maculopapular rash, malaise, mastitis, melena, memory impairment, menorrhagia, myasthenia, mydriasis, myopathy, neck rigidity, neuritis, neuropathy, neurosis, nystagmus, oliguria, paresthesia, photophobia, photosensitivity, pyelonephritis, rectal hemorrhage, reflexes decreased, stomach ulcer, swelling, thrombophlebitis, tinnitus, tongue edema, tremor, twitching, ulcerative stomatitis, urinary frequency, urinary incontinence, urticaria, urethritis, vaginal hemorrhage, vaginitis, vestibular disorder, vertigo, vesiculobullous rash

Metabolism/Transport Effects Substrate of CYP2E1 (minor), 3A4 (major)

Drug Interactions

Alcohol (Ethyl): CNS Depressants may enhance the CNS depressant effect of Alcohol (Ethyl). *Risk C: Monitor therapy*

Antifungal Agents (Azole Derivatives, Systemic): May decrease the metabolism of Eszopiclone. *Risk C: Monitor therapy*

CNS Depressants: May enhance the adverse/toxic effect of other CNS Depressants. *Risk C: Monitor therapy*

CYP3A4 Inducers (Strong): May increase the metabolism of CYP3A4 Substrates. *Risk C: Monitor therapy*

CYP3A4 Inhibitors (Moderate): May decrease the metabolism of CYP3A4 Substrates. *Risk C: Monitor therapy*

CYP3A4 Inhibitors (Strong): May decrease the metabolism of CYP3A4 Substrates. *Risk D: Consider therapy modification*

Dasatinib: May increase the serum concentration of CYP3A4 Substrates. *Risk C: Monitor therapy*

Deferasirox: May decrease the serum concentration of CYP3A4 Substrates. *Risk C: Monitor therapy*

Flumazenil: May diminish the sedative effect of Hypnotics (Nonbenzodiazepine). *Risk C: Monitor therapy*

Herbs (CYP3A4 Inducers): May increase the metabolism of CYP3A4 Substrates. *Risk C: Monitor therapy*

Ethanol/Nutrition/Herb Interactions

Ethanol: Use caution with concurrent use. Effects are additive and may decrease psychomotor function.

Food: Onset of action may be reduced if taken with or immediately after a heavy meal.

Herb/Nutraceutical: Avoid valerian, St John's wort, kava kava, gotu kola (may increase CNS depression).

Stability Store at controlled room temperature of 25°C (77°F).

Mechanism of Action May interact with GABA-receptor complexes at binding domains located close to or allosterically coupled to benzodiazepine receptors.

Pharmacodynamics/Kinetics

Absorption: Rapid; high-fat/heavy meal may delay absorption

Protein binding: 52% to 59%

Metabolism: Hepatic via oxidation and demethylation (CYP2E1, 3A4); 2 primary metabolites; one with activity less than parent.

Half-life elimination: ~6 hours; Elderly (≥65 years): ~9 hours

Time to peak, plasma: ~1 hour

Excretion: Urine (up to 75%, primarily as metabolites; <10% as parent drug)

Dosage Oral:

Adults: Insomnia: Initial: 2 mg immediately before bedtime (maximum dose: 3 mg)

Concurrent use with strong CYP3A4 inhibitor: 1 mg immediately before bedtime; if needed, dose may be increased to 2 mg

Elderly:

Difficulty **falling** asleep: Initial: 1 mg immediately before bedtime; maximum dose: 2 mg

Difficulty **staying** asleep: 2 mg immediately before bedtime

Dosage adjustment in renal impairment: None required

Dosage adjustment in hepatic impairment:

Mild-to-moderate: Use with caution; dosage adjustment unnecessary

Severe: Initial dose: 1 mg; maximum dose: 2 mg

Dietary Considerations Avoid taking after a heavy meal; may delay onset.

Administration Because of the rapid onset of action, eszopiclone should be administered immediately prior to bedtime or after the patient has gone to bed and is having difficulty falling asleep. Do not take with, or immediately following, a high-fat meal; do not crush or break tablet.

Dosage Forms Excipient information presented when available (limited, particularly for generics); consult specific product labeling.

Tablet: 1 mg, 2 mg, 3 mg

Etanercept (et a NER sept)

U.S. Brand Names Enbrel®

Canadian Brand Names Enbrel®

Mexican Brand Names Enbrel

Pharmacologic Category Antirheumatic, Disease Modifying; Tumor Necrosis Factor (TNF) Blocking Agent

Use Treatment of moderately- to severely-active rheumatoid arthritis (RA); moderately- to severely-active polyarticular juvenile idiopathic arthritis (JIA); psoriatic arthritis; active ankylosing spondylitis (AS); moderate-to-severe chronic plaque psoriasis

Effect on Mental Status Dizziness is common; may cause depression

Effect on Psychiatric Treatment None reported

Restrictions

An FDA-approved patient medication guide is available and must be distributed when dispensing an outpatient prescription (new or refill) where this medication is to be used without direct supervision of a healthcare provider. Medication guides are available at http://www.fda.gov/cder/Offices/ODS/medication_guides.htm.

Dosage Summary

SubQ:

Children <2 years: Dosage not established

Children 2-17 years: 0.8 mg/kg (maximum: 50 mg) once weekly **or** 0.4 mg/kg (maximum: 25 mg) twice weekly

Adults: 50 mg once weekly **or** 25-50 mg twice weekly

Dosage Forms Excipient information presented when available (limited, particularly for generics); consult specific product labeling.

Injection, powder for reconstitution:

Enbrel®: 25 mg [contains sucrose 10 mg; diluent contains benzyl alcohol]

Injection, solution [preservative free]:

Enbrel®: 50 mg/mL (0.51 mL, 0.98 mL) [contains sucrose 1%; natural rubber/natural latex in packaging]

◆ **Ethacrynate Sodium** *see* Ethacrynic Acid *on page 591*

Ethacrynic Acid (eth a KRIN ik AS id)

Medication Safety Issues

Sound-alike/look-alike issues:

Edecrin® may be confused with Eulexin®, Ecotrin®

U.S. Brand Names Edecrin®

Canadian Brand Names Edecrin®

Index Terms Ethacrynate Sodium

Pharmacologic Category Diuretic, Loop

Use Management of edema associated with congestive heart failure; hepatic cirrhosis or renal disease; short-term management of ascites due to malignancy, idiopathic edema, and lymphedema

Effect on Mental Status May cause dizziness; may rarely cause drowsiness, nervousness, or confusion

Effect on Psychiatric Treatment Rare reports of agranulocytosis; use caution with clozapine and carbamazepine; may increase serum lithium levels, however, more likely with thiazide diuretic

Dosage Summary

I.V.:

Children: Dosage not established

Adults: 0.5-1 mg/kg/dose (maximum: 100 mg/dose)

Oral:

Children: 1-3 mg/kg/day

Adults: 50-400 mg/day in 1-2 divided doses
Elderly: Initial: 25-50 mg/day

Dosage Forms Excipient information presented when available (limited, particularly for generics); consult specific product labeling.
Injection, powder for reconstitution, as ethacrynate sodium: 50 mg
Tablet: 25 mg

Ethambutol (e THAM byoo tole)

Medication Safety Issues
Sound-alike/look-alike issues:
Myambutol® may be confused with Nembutal®

U.S. Brand Names Myambutol®

Canadian Brand Names Etibi®

Mexican Brand Names Manzida

Index Terms Ethambutol Hydrochloride

Pharmacologic Category Antitubercular Agent

Use Treatment of tuberculosis and other mycobacterial diseases in conjunction with other antituberculosis agents

Effect on Mental Status May cause confusion and disorientation

Effect on Psychiatric Treatment None reported

Dosage Summary

Oral:

Children: 15-20 mg/kg/day (maximum: 1 g/day) **or** 50 mg/kg twice weekly (maximum: 4 g/dose)

Adults:
Daily therapy: 15-25 mg/kg/day (maximum 1600 mg)
Three times/week DOT: 25-30 mg/kg/dose (maximum: 2.4 g/dose)
Twice weekly DOT: 50 mg/kg/dose (maximum: 4 g/dose)

Dosage Forms Excipient information presented when available (limited, particularly for generics); consult specific product labeling.
Tablet, as hydrochloride: 100 mg, 400 mg

◆ **Ethambutol Hydrochloride** *see* Ethambutol *on page 592*

Ethinyl Estradiol and Desogestrel
(ETH in il es tra DYE ole & des oh JES trel)

Medication Safety Issues
Sound-alike/look-alike issues:
Apri® may be confused with Apriso™
Ortho-Cept® may be confused with Ortho-Cyclen®

U.S. Brand Names Apri®; Cesia™; Cyclessa®; Desogen®; Kariva™; Mircette®; Ortho-Cept®; Reclipsen™; Solia™; Velivet™

Canadian Brand Names Cyclessa®; Linessa®; Marvelon®; Ortho-Cept®

Mexican Brand Names Marvelon

Index Terms Desogestrel and Ethinyl Estradiol; Ortho Cept

Pharmacologic Category Contraceptive; Estrogen and Progestin Combination

Use Prevention of pregnancy

Unlabeled/Investigational Use Treatment of hypermenorrhea (menorrhagia); pain associated with endometriosis; dysmenorrhea; dysfunctional uterine bleeding

Effect on Mental Status May cause dizziness, headache, depression, insomnia, nervousness, irritability, and mood disturbances

Effect on Psychiatric Treatment Barbiturates decrease the effects of oral contraceptives; may increase the toxicity of the benzodiazepines and TCAs. The Women's Health Initiative (WHI) Memory Study reported an increased risk of developing dementia in postmenopausal women ≥65 years of age during 4 years of treatment with oral conjugated equine estrogens and medroxyprogesterone acetate relative to placebo (1.8% vs 0.9%). Relative risk was 2.05 (95% CI 1.21-3.48). Therefore, estrogens and progestins should not be used for the prevention of dementia. The WHI also reported an increased risk of stroke (29 vs 21 per 10,000 women-years) compared to women receiving placebo. The increase in risk was observed after the first year and persisted. May cause hypertriglyceridemia; monitor in patients receiving antipsychotics especially clozapine, olanzapine, and quetiapine.

Dosage Summary

Oral:

Children (premenarche): Dosage not established

Children (postmenarche): 21-tablet package: 1 tablet daily for 21 days, followed by 7 days off; 28-tablet package: 1 tablet daily

Adults (females): 21-tablet package: 1 tablet daily for 21 days, followed by 7 days off; 28-tablet package: 1 tablet daily

Dosage Forms Excipient information presented when available (limited, particularly for generics); consult specific product labeling.

Tablet, low-dose formulations:

Kariva™:

Day 1-21: Ethinyl estradiol 0.02 mg and desogestrel 0.15 mg [21 white tablets]

Day 22-23: 2 inactive light green tablets

Day 24-28: Ethinyl estradiol 0.01 mg [5 light blue tablets] (28s)

Mircette®:

Day 1-21: Ethinyl estradiol 0.02 mg and desogestrel 0.15 mg [21 white tablets]

Day 22-23: 2 inactive green tablets

Day 24-28: Ethinyl estradiol 0.01 mg [5 yellow tablets] (28s)

Tablet, monophasic formulations:

Apri® 28: Ethinyl estradiol 0.03 mg and desogestrel 0.15 mg (28s) [21 rose tablets and 7 white inactive tablets]

Desogen®, Reclipsen™, Solia™: Ethinyl estradiol 0.03 mg and desogestrel 0.15 mg (28s) [21 white tablets and 7 green inactive tablets]

Ortho-Cept® 28: Ethinyl estradiol 0.03 mg and desogestrel 0.15 mg (28s) [21 orange tablets and 7 green inactive tablets]

Tablet, triphasic formulations:

Cesia™, Cyclessa®:

Day 1-7: Ethinyl estradiol 0.025 mg and desogestrel 0.1 mg [7 light yellow tablets]

Day 8-14: Ethinyl estradiol 0.025 mg and desogestrel 0.125 mg [7 orange tablets]

Day 14-21: Ethinyl estradiol 0.025 mg and desogestrel 0.15 mg [7 red tablets]

Day 21-28: 7 green inactive tablets (28s)

Velivet™:

Day 1-7: Ethinyl estradiol 0.025 mg and desogestrel 0.1 mg [7 beige tablets]

Day 8-14: Ethinyl estradiol 0.025 mg and desogestrel 0.125 mg [7 orange tablets]

Day 14-21: Ethinyl estradiol 0.025 mg and desogestrel 0.15 mg [7 pink tablets]

Day 21-28: 7 white inactive tablets (28s)

Ethinyl Estradiol and Drospirenone

(ETH in il es tra DYE ole & droh SPYE re none)

U.S. Brand Names Ocella™; Yasmin®; Yaz®

Canadian Brand Names Yasmin®

Mexican Brand Names Yasmin

Index Terms Drospirenone and Ethinyl Estradiol

Pharmacologic Category Contraceptive; Estrogen and Progestin Combination

Use Females: Prevention of pregnancy; treatment of premenstrual dysphoric disorder (PMDD); treatment of acne

Unlabeled/Investigational Use Treatment of hypermenorrhea (menorrhagia); pain associated with endometriosis; dysmenorrhea; dysfunctional uterine bleeding

Effect on Mental Status May cause dizziness, headache, depression, insomnia, nervousness, irritability, and mood disturbances

Effect on Psychiatric Treatment May cause flu-like symptoms, take this into consideration if also concerned about SSRI discontinuation syndrome. Carbamazepine and topiramate may increase the metabolism of estradiol, leading to a decrease in serum concentrations. Estrogens may inhibit the metabolism of some benzodiazepines (alprazolam, chlordiazepoxide, diazepam), TCAs, and selegiline. Estrogens may increase the clearance of lorazepam, oxazepam, and temazepam. The Women's Health Initiative (WHI) Memory Study reported an increased risk of developing dementia in postmenopausal women ≥65 years of age during 4 years of treatment with oral conjugated equine estrogens and medroxyprogesterone acetate relative to placebo (1.8% vs 0.9%). Relative risk was 2.05 (95% CI 1.21-3.48). Therefore, estrogens and progestins should not be used for the prevention of dementia.

The WHI also reported an increased risk of stroke (29 vs 21 per 10,000 women-years) compared to women receiving placebo. The increase in risk was observed after the first year and persisted. May cause hypertriglyceridemia; monitor in patients receiving antipsychotics especially clozapine, olanzapine, and quetiapine.

Dosage Summary

Oral:

Children (premenarche): Use not indicated
Children (females, postmenarche): One tablet daily
Adults (females): One tablet daily

Dosage Forms Excipient information presented when available (limited, particularly for generics); consult specific product labeling.

Tablet:

Ocella™: Ethinyl estradiol 0.03 mg and drospirenone 3 mg (28s) [21 yellow active tablets and 7 white inactive tablets]

Yasmin®: Ethinyl estradiol 0.03 mg and drospirenone 3 mg (28s) [21 yellow active tablets and 7 white inactive tablets]

Yaz®: Ethinyl estradiol 0.02 mg and drospirenone 3 mg (28s) [24 light pink tablets and 4 white inactive tablets]

Ethinyl Estradiol and Ethynodiol Diacetate

(ETH in il es tra DYE ole & e thye noe DYE ole dye AS e tate)

Medication Safety Issues

Sound-alike/look-alike issues:

Demulen® may be confused with Dalmane®, Demerol®

U.S. Brand Names Kelnor™; Zovia®

Canadian Brand Names Demulen® 30

Index Terms Ethynodiol Diacetate and Ethinyl Estradiol

Pharmacologic Category Contraceptive; Estrogen and Progestin Combination

Use Prevention of pregnancy

Unlabeled/Investigational Use Treatment of hypermenorrhea (menorrhagia); pain associated with endometriosis; dysmenorrhea; dysfunctional uterine bleeding

Effect on Mental Status May cause dizziness, headache, depression, insomnia, nervousness, irritability, and mood disturbances

Effect on Psychiatric Treatment The Women's Health Initiative (WHI) Memory Study reported an increased risk of developing dementia in postmenopausal women ≥65 years of age during 4 years of treatment with oral conjugated equine estrogens and medroxyprogesterone acetate relative to placebo (1.8% vs 0.9%). Relative risk was 2.05 (95% CI 1.21-3.48). Therefore, estrogens and progestins should not be used for the prevention of dementia. The WHI also reported an increased risk of stroke (29 vs 21 per 10,000 women-years) compared to women receiving placebo. The increase in risk was observed after the first year and persisted. May cause hypertriglyceridemia; monitor in patients receiving antipsychotics especially clozapine, olanzapine, and quetiapine.

Dosage Summary

Oral:

Children (premenarche): Dosage not established
Children (postmenarche): 21-tablet package: 1 tablet daily for 21 days, followed by 7 days off; 28-tablet package: 1 tablet daily
Adults (females): 21-tablet package: 1 tablet daily for 21 days, followed by 7 days off; 28-tablet package: 1 tablet daily

Dosage Forms Excipient information presented when available (limited, particularly for generics); consult specific product labeling.

Tablet, monophasic formulations:

Kelnor™ 1/35: Ethinyl estradiol 0.035 mg and ethynodiol diacetate 1 mg [21 light yellow tablets and 7 white inactive tablets] (28s)

Zovia® 1/35-28: Ethinyl estradiol 0.035 mg and ethynodiol diacetate 1 mg [21 light pink tablets and 7 white inactive tablets] (28s)

Zovia® 1/50-28: Ethinyl estradiol 0.05 mg and ethynodiol diacetate 1 mg [21 pink tablets and 7 white inactive tablets] (28s)

Ethinyl Estradiol and Etonogestrel

(ETH in il es tra DYE ole & et oh noe JES trel)

U.S. Brand Names NuvaRing®

Canadian Brand Names NuvaRing®

Mexican Brand Names NuvaRing

Index Terms Etonogestrel and Ethinyl Estradiol

Pharmacologic Category Contraceptive; Estrogen and Progestin Combination

Use Prevention of pregnancy

Unlabeled/Investigational Use Treatment of hypermenorrhea (menorrhagia); pain associated with endometriosis; dysmenorrhea; dysfunctional uterine bleeding

Effect on Mental Status May cause dizziness, headache, depression, insomnia, nervousness, irritability, and mood disturbances

Effect on Psychiatric Treatment May cause flu-like symptoms, take this into consideration if also concerned about SSRI discontinuation syndrome. Carbamazepine and topiramate may increase the metabolism of estradiol, leading to a decrease in serum concentrations. Estrogens may inhibit the metabolism of some benzodiazepines (alprazolam, chlordiazepoxide, diazepam), TCAs, and selegiline. Estrogens may increase the clearance of lorazepam, oxazepam, and temazepam. The Women's Health Initiative (WHI) Memory Study reported an increased risk of developing dementia in postmenopausal women ≥65 years of age during 4 years of treatment with oral conjugated equine estrogens and medroxyprogesterone acetate relative to placebo (1.8% vs 0.9%). Relative risk was 2.05 (95% CI 1.21-3.48). Therefore, estrogens and progestins should not be used for the prevention of dementia. The WHI also reported an increased risk of stroke (29 vs 21 per 10,000 women-years) compared to women receiving placebo. The increase in risk was observed after the first year and persisted. May cause hypertriglyceridemia; monitor in patients receiving antipsychotics especially clozapine, olanzapine, and quetiapine.

Dosage Summary

Vaginal:

Children (females, premenarche): Dosage not established

Children (females, postmenarche): Insert one ring and leave in place for 3 consecutive weeks, then remove for 1 week

Adults (females): Insert one ring and leave in place for 3 consecutive weeks, then remove for 1 week

Dosage Forms Excipient information presented when available (limited, particularly for generics); consult specific product labeling.

Ring, vaginal:

NuvaRing®: Ethinyl estradiol 0.015 mg/day and etonogestrel 0.12 mg/day (1s) [3-week duration]

Ethinyl Estradiol and Levonorgestrel

(ETH in il es tra DYE ole & LEE voe nor jes trel)

Medication Safety Issues

Sound-alike/look-alike issues:

Alesse® may be confused with Aleve®
Nordette® may be confused with Nicorette®
PREVEN® may be confused with Prevnar®
Seasonale® may be confused with Seasonique™
Seasonique™ may be confused with Seasonale®
Tri-Levlen® may be confused with Trilafon®
Triphasil® may be confused with Tri-Norinyl®

U.S. Brand Names Alesse®; Aviane™; Enpresse™; Jolessa™; Lessina™; Levlen®; Levlite™; Levora®; Lutera™; Lybrel™; Nordette®; Portia™; Quasense™; Seasonale®; Seasonique™; Sronyx™; Triphasil®; Trivora®

Canadian Brand Names Alesse®; Aviane®; Min-Ovral®; Seasonale®; Triphasil®; Triquilar®

Mexican Brand Names Microgynon; Microgynon CD; Nordet; Trinordiol; Triquilar

Index Terms Levonorgestrel and Ethinyl Estradiol

Pharmacologic Category Contraceptive; Estrogen and Progestin Combination

Use Prevention of pregnancy; postcoital contraception

Unlabeled/Investigational Use Treatment of hypermenorrhea (menorrhagia); pain associated with endometriosis; dysmenorrhea; dysfunctional uterine bleeding

Effect on Mental Status May cause dizziness, headache, depression, insomnia, nervousness, irritability, and mood disturbances

Effect on Psychiatric Treatment Barbiturates decrease the effects of oral contraceptives; may increase the toxicity of the benzodiazepines and TCAs. The Women's Health Initiative (WHI) Memory Study reported an increased risk of developing dementia in postmenopausal women ≥65 years of age during

4 years of treatment with oral conjugated equine estrogens and medroxyprogesterone acetate relative to placebo (1.8% vs 0.9%). Relative risk was 2.05 (95% CI 1.21-3.48). Therefore, estrogens and progestins should not be used for the prevention of dementia. The WHI also reported an increased risk of stroke (29 vs 21 per 10,000 women-years) compared to women receiving placebo. The increase in risk was observed after the first year and persisted. May cause hypertriglyceridemia; monitor in patients receiving antipsychotics especially clozapine, olanzapine, and quetiapine.

Dosage Summary

Oral:

Children (premenarche): Use not indicated

Children (postmenarche):

Contraception: 21-tablet package: 1 tablet daily for 21 days, followed by 7 days off; 28-tablet package: 1 tablet daily

Emergency contraception: 2 tablets as soon as possible (but within 72 hours of unprotected intercourse), followed by 2 tablets 12 hours later

Adults (females):

Contraception: 21-tablet package: 1 tablet daily for 21 days, followed by 7 days off; 28-tablet package: 1 tablet daily

Emergency contraception: 2 tablets as soon as possible (but within 72 hours of unprotected intercourse), followed by 2 tablets 12 hours later

Dosage Forms Excipient information presented when available (limited, particularly for generics); consult specific product labeling. [DSC] = Discontinued product

Tablet, low-dose formulations:

Alesse® 28: Ethinyl estradiol 0.02 mg and levonorgestrel 0.1 mg (28s) [21 pink tablets and 7 light green inactive tablets]

Aviane™ 28: Ethinyl estradiol 0.02 mg and levonorgestrel 0.1 mg (28s) [21 orange tablets and 7 light green inactive tablets]

Lessina™ 28, Levlite™ 28: Ethinyl estradiol 0.02 mg and levonorgestrel 0.1 mg (28s) [21 pink tablets and 7 white inactive tablets]

Lutera™, Sronyx™: Ethinyl estradiol 0.02 mg and levonorgestrel 0.1 mg (28s) [21 white tablets and 7 peach inactive tablets]

Lybrel™: Ethinyl estradiol 0.02 mg and levonorgestrel 0.09 mg (28s) [28 yellow tablets]

Tablet, monophasic formulations:

Levlen® 28: Ethinyl estradiol 0.03 mg and levonorgestrel 0.15 mg (28s) [21 light orange tablets and 7 pink inactive tablets]

Levora® 28: Ethinyl estradiol 0.03 mg and levonorgestrel 0.15 mg (28s) [21 white tablets and 7 peach inactive tablets]

Nordette® 28: Ethinyl estradiol 0.03 mg and levonorgestrel 0.15 mg (28s) [21 light orange tablets and 7 pink inactive tablets]

Portia™ 28: Ethinyl estradiol 0.03 mg and levonorgestrel 0.15 mg (28s) [21 pink tablets and 7 white inactive tablets]

Tablet, monophasic formulations [extended cycle regimen]:

Jolessa™, Seasonale®: Ethinyl estradiol 0.03 mg and levonorgestrel 0.15 mg (91s) [84 pink tablets and 7 white inactive tablets]

Quasense™: Ethinyl estradiol 0.03 mg and levonorgestrel 0.15 mg (91s) [84 white tablets and 7 peach inactive tablets]

Seasonique™: Ethinyl estradiol 0.03 mg and levonorgestrel 0.15 mg (91s) [84 light blue-green tablets] and ethinyl estradiol 0.01 mg [7 yellow tablets]

Tablet, triphasic formulations:

Enpresse™:

Day 1-6: Ethinyl estradiol 0.03 mg and levonorgestrel 0.05 mg [6 pink tablets]

Day 7-11: Ethinyl estradiol 0.04 mg and levonorgestrel 0.075 mg [5 white tablets]

Day 12-21: Ethinyl estradiol 0.03 mg and levonorgestrel 0.125 mg [10 orange tablets]

Day 22-28: 7 light green inactive tablets (28s)

Triphasil® 28:

Day 1-6: Ethinyl estradiol 0.03 mg and levonorgestrel 0.05 mg [6 brown tablets]

Day 7-11: Ethinyl estradiol 0.04 mg and levonorgestrel 0.075 mg [5 white tablets]

Day 12-21: Ethinyl estradiol 0.03 mg and levonorgestrel 0.125 mg [10 light yellow tablets]

Day 22-28: 7 light green inactive tablets (28s)

Trivora® 28:

Day 1-6: Ethinyl estradiol 0.03 mg and levonorgestrel 0.05 mg [6 blue tablets]

Day 7-11: Ethinyl estradiol 0.04 mg and levonorgestrel 0.075 mg [5 white tablets]

Day 12-21: Ethinyl estradiol 0.03 mg and levonorgestrel 0.125 mg [10 pink tablets]

Day 22-28: 7 peach inactive tablets (28s)

◆ **Ethinyl Estradiol and NGM** *see* Ethinyl Estradiol and Norgestimate *on page 600*

Ethinyl Estradiol and Norelgestromin

(ETH in il es tra DYE ole & nor el JES troe min)

Medication Safety Issues

Transdermal patch may contain conducting metal (eg, aluminum); remove patch prior to MRI.

U.S. Brand Names Ortho Evra®

Canadian Brand Names Evra®

Index Terms Norelgestromin and Ethinyl Estradiol; Ortho-Evra

Pharmacologic Category Contraceptive; Estrogen and Progestin Combination

Use Prevention of pregnancy

Effect on Mental Status May cause dizziness, headache, depression, insomnia, nervousness, irritability, and mood disturbances

Effect on Psychiatric Treatment May cause flu-like symptoms, take this into consideration if also concerned about SSRI discontinuation syndrome. Carbamazepine and topiramate may increase the metabolism of estradiol, leading to a decrease in serum concentrations. Estrogens may inhibit the metabolism of some benzodiazepines (alprazolam, chlordiazepoxide, diazepam), TCAs, and selegiline. Estrogens may increase the clearance of lorazepam, oxazepam, and temazepam. The Women's Health Initiative (WHI) Memory Study reported an increased risk of developing dementia in postmenopausal women ≥65 years of age during 4 years of treatment with oral conjugated equine estrogens and medroxyprogesterone acetate relative to placebo (1.8% vs 0.9%). Relative risk was 2.05 (95% CI 1.21-3.48). Therefore, estrogens and progestins should not be used for the prevention of dementia. The WHI also reported an increased risk of stroke (29 vs 21 per 10,000 women-years) compared to women receiving placebo. The increase in risk was observed after the first year and persisted. May cause hypertriglyceridemia; monitor in patients receiving antipsychotics especially clozapine, olanzapine, and quetiapine.

Dosage Summary

Topical:

Children (premenarche): Dosage not established

Children (postmenarche): Apply one patch weekly for 3 weeks, followed by one week that is patch-free

Adults (females): Apply one patch weekly for 3 weeks, followed by one week that is patch-free

Dosage Forms Excipient information presented when available (limited, particularly for generics); consult specific product labeling. [CAN] = Canadian brand name

Note: The formulation available in Canada differs from the U.S. product in both composition and the manufacturing process (although delivery rates appear similar).

Patch, transdermal:

Ortho Evra®: Ethinyl estradiol 0.75 mg and norelgestromin 6 mg [releases ethinyl estradiol 20 mcg and norelgestromin 150 mcg per day] (1s, 3s)

Evra® [CAN]: Ethinyl estradiol 0.6 mg and norelgestromin 6 mg [releases ethinyl estradiol 20 mcg and norelgestromin 150 mcg per day] (1s, 3s) [Not available in U.S.]

Ethinyl Estradiol and Norethindrone

(ETH in il es tra DYE ole & nor eth IN drone)

Medication Safety Issues

Sound-alike/look-alike issues:

femhrt® may be confused with Femara®

Modicon® may be confused with Mylicon®

Norinyl® may be confused with Nardil®

Tri-Norinyl® may be confused with Triphasil®

International issues:

Notrel™ may be confused with Nostril® which is a brand name for chlorhexidine and cetrimonium in France

U.S. Brand Names Aranelle™; Balziva™; Brevicon®; Estrostep® Fe; Femcon™ Fe; femhrt®; Junel™; Junel™ Fe; Leena™; Loestrin®; Loestrin® 24 Fe; Loestrin® Fe; Microgestin™; Microgestin™ Fe; Modicon®; Necon® 0.5/35; Necon® 1/35; Necon® 10/11; Necon® 7/7/7; Norinyl® 1+35; Nortrel™; Nortrel™ 7/7/7; Ortho-Novum®; Ovcon®; Tilia™ Fe; Tri-Norinyl®; Zenchent™

Canadian Brand Names Brevicon® 0.5/35; Brevicon® 1/35; FemHRT®; Loestrin™ 1.5/30; Minestrin™ 1/20; Ortho® 0.5/35; Ortho® 1/35; Ortho® 7/7/7; Select™ 1/35; Synphasic®

Mexican Brand Names Evorelconti

Index Terms Norethindrone Acetate and Ethinyl Estradiol; Ortho Novum

Pharmacologic Category Contraceptive; Estrogen and Progestin Combination

Use Prevention of pregnancy; treatment of acne; moderate-to-severe vasomotor symptoms associated with menopause; prevention of osteoporosis (in women at significant risk only)

Unlabeled/Investigational Use Treatment of hypermenorrhea (menorrhagia); pain associated with endometriosis, dysmenorrhea; dysfunctional uterine bleeding

Effect on Mental Status May cause dizziness, headache, depression, insomnia, nervousness, irritability, and mood disturbances

Effect on Psychiatric Treatment Barbiturates decrease the effects of oral contraceptives; may increase the toxicity of the benzodiazepines and TCAs. The Women's Health Initiative (WHI) Memory Study reported an increased risk of developing dementia in postmenopausal women ≥65 years of age during 4 years of treatment with oral conjugated equine estrogens and medroxyprogesterone acetate relative to placebo (1.8% vs 0.9%). Relative risk was 2.05 (95% CI 1.21-3.48). Therefore, estrogens and progestins should not be used for the prevention of dementia. The WHI also reported an increased risk of stroke (29 vs 21 per 10,000 women-years) compared to women receiving placebo. The increase in risk was observed after the first year and persisted. May cause hypertriglyceridemia; monitor in patients receiving antipsychotics especially clozapine, olanzapine, and quetiapine.

Dosage Summary

Oral:

Children (premenarche): Dosage not established

Children (postmenarche): 21-tablet package: 1 tablet daily for 21 days, followed by 7 days off; 28-tablet package: 1 tablet daily

Adults (females): 21-tablet package: 1 tablet daily for 21 days, followed by 7 days off; 28-tablet package: 1 tablet daily

Dosage Forms Excipient information presented when available (limited, particularly for generics); consult specific product labeling.

Tablet:

femhrt® 1/5: Ethinyl estradiol 5 mcg and norethindrone acetate 1 mg [white tablets]

femhrt® 0.5/2.5: Ethinyl estradiol 2.5 mcg and norethindrone acetate 0.5 mg [white tablets]

Tablet, monophasic formulations:

Balziva™: Ethinyl estradiol 0.035 mg and norethindrone 0.4 mg (28s) [21 light peach tablets and 7 white inactive tablets]

Brevicon®: Ethinyl estradiol 0.035 mg and norethindrone 0.5 mg (28s) [21 blue tablets and 7 orange inactive tablets]

Junel™ 21 1/20: Ethinyl estradiol 0.02 mg and norethindrone acetate 1 mg (21s) [yellow tablets]

Junel™ 21 1.5/30: Ethinyl estradiol 0.03 mg and norethindrone acetate 1.5 mg (21s) [pink tablets]

Junel™ Fe 1/20: Ethinyl estradiol 0.02 mg and norethindrone acetate 1 mg (28s) [21 yellow tablets] and ferrous fumarate 75 mg [7 brown tablets]

Junel™ Fe 1.5/30: Ethinyl estradiol 0.03 mg and norethindrone acetate 1.5 mg (28s) [21 pink tablets] and ferrous fumarate 75 mg [7 brown tablets]

Loestrin® 21 1/20, Microgestin™ 1/20: Ethinyl estradiol 0.02 mg and norethindrone acetate 1 mg (21s) [white tablets]

Loestrin® 21 1.5/30, Microgestin™ 1.5/30: Ethinyl estradiol 0.03 mg and norethindrone acetate 1.5 mg (21s) [green tablets]

Loestrin® 24 Fe: 1/20: Ethinyl estradiol 0.02 mg and norethindrone acetate 1 mg (28s) [24 white tablets] and ferrous fumarate 75 mg [4 brown tablets]

Loestrin® Fe 1/20, Microgestin™ Fe 1/20: Ethinyl estradiol 0.02 mg and norethindrone acetate 1 mg (28s) [21 white tablets] and ferrous fumarate 75 mg [7 brown tablets]
Loestrin® Fe 1.5/30, Microgestin™ Fe 1.5/30: Ethinyl estradiol 0.03 mg and norethindrone acetate 1.5 mg (28s) [21 green tablets] and ferrous fumarate 75 mg [7 brown tablets]
Modicon® 28: Ethinyl estradiol 0.035 mg and norethindrone 0.5 mg (28s) [21 white tablets and 7 green inactive tablets]
Necon® 0.5/35-28: Ethinyl estradiol 0.035 mg and norethindrone 0.5 mg (28s) [21 light yellow tablets and 7 white inactive tablets]
Necon® 1/35-28: Ethinyl estradiol 0.035 mg and norethindrone 1 mg (28s) [21 dark yellow tablets and 7 white inactive tablets]
Norinyl® 1+35: Ethinyl estradiol 0.035 mg and norethindrone 1 mg (28s) [21 yellow-green tablets and 7 orange inactive tablets]
Nortrel™ 0.5/35 mg:
Ethinyl estradiol 0.035 mg and norethindrone 0.5 mg (21s) [light yellow tablets]
Ethinyl estradiol 0.035 mg and norethindrone 0.5 mg (28s) [21 light yellow tablets and 7 white inactive tablets]
Nortrel™ 1/35 mg:
Ethinyl estradiol 0.035 mg and norethindrone 1 mg (21s) [yellow tablets]
Ethinyl estradiol 0.035 mg and norethindrone 1 mg (28s) [21 yellow tablets and 7 white inactive tablets]
Ortho-Novum® 1/35 28: Ethinyl estradiol 0.035 mg and norethindrone 1 mg (28s) [21 peach tablets and 7 green inactive tablets]
Ovcon® 35 21-day: Ethinyl estradiol 0.035 mg and norethindrone 0.4 mg (21s) [peach tablets]
Ovcon® 35 28-day: Ethinyl estradiol 0.035 mg and norethindrone 0.4 mg (28s) [21 peach tablets and 7 green inactive tablets]
Ovcon® 50: Ethinyl estradiol 0.05 mg and norethindrone 1 mg (28s) [21 yellow tablets and 7 green inactive tablets]
Zenchent™: Ethinyl estradiol 0.035 mg and norethindrone 0.4 mg (28s) [21 light peach tablets and 7 white inactive tablets]

Tablet, chewable, monophasic formulations:
Femcon™ Fe: Ethinyl estradiol 0.035 mg and norethindrone 0.4 mg (28s) [21 white tablets and 7 brown inactive tablets] [spearmint flavor]

Tablet, biphasic formulations:
Necon® 10/11-28:
Day 1-10: Ethinyl estradiol 0.035 mg and norethindrone 0.5 mg [10 light yellow tablets]
Day 11-21: Ethinyl estradiol 0.035 mg and norethindrone 1 mg [11 dark yellow tablets]
Day 22-28: 7 white inactive tablets (28s)
Ortho-Novum® 10/11-28:
Day 1-10: Ethinyl estradiol 0.035 mg and norethindrone 0.5 mg [10 white tablets]
Day 11-21: Ethinyl estradiol 0.035 mg and norethindrone 1 mg [11 peach tablets]
Day 22-28: 7 green inactive tablets (28s)

Tablet, triphasic formulations:
Aranelle™:
Day 1-7: Ethinyl estradiol 0.035 mg and norethindrone 0.5 mg [7 light yellow tablets]
Day 8-16: Ethinyl estradiol 0.035 mg and norethindrone 1 mg [9 white tablets]
Day 17-21: Ethinyl estradiol 0.035 mg and norethindrone 0.5 mg [5 light yellow tablets]
Day 22-28: 7 peach inactive tablets (28s)
Estrostep® Fe:
Day 1-5: Ethinyl estradiol 0.02 mg and norethindrone acetate 1 mg [5 white triangular tablets]
Day 6-12: Ethinyl estradiol 0.03 mg and norethindrone acetate 1 mg [7 white square tablets]
Day 13-21: Ethinyl estradiol 0.035 mg and norethindrone acetate 1 mg [9 white round tablets]
Day 22-28: Ferrous fumarate 75 mg [7 brown tablets] (28s)
Leena™:
Day 1-7: Ethinyl estradiol 0.035 mg and norethindrone 0.5 mg [7 light blue tablets]

Day 8-16: Ethinyl estradiol 0.035 mg and norethindrone 1 mg [9 light yellow-green tablets]
Day 17-21: Ethinyl estradiol 0.035 mg and norethindrone 0.5 mg [5 light blue tablets]
Day 22-28: 7 orange inactive tablets (28s)

Necon® 7/7/7, Ortho-Novum® 7/7/7 28:
Day 1-7: Ethinyl estradiol 0.035 mg and norethindrone 0.5 mg [7 white tablets]
Day 8-14: Ethinyl estradiol 0.035 mg and norethindrone 0.75 mg [7 light peach tablets]
Day 15-21: Ethinyl estradiol 0.035 mg and norethindrone 1 mg [7 peach tablets]
Day 22-28: 7 green inactive tablets (28s)

Nortrel™ 7/7/7 28:
Day 1-7: Ethinyl estradiol 0.035 mg and norethindrone 0.5 mg [7 light yellow tablets]
Day 8-14: Ethinyl estradiol 0.035 mg and norethindrone 0.75 mg [7 blue tablets]
Day 15-21: Ethinyl estradiol 0.035 mg and norethindrone 1 mg [7 peach tablets]
Day 22-28: 7 white inactive tablets (28s)

Ortho-Novum® 7/7/7 28:
Day 1-7: Ethinyl estradiol 0.035 mg and norethindrone 0.5 mg [7 white tablets]
Day 8-14: Ethinyl estradiol 0.035 mg and norethindrone 0.75 mg [7 light peach tablets]
Day 15-21: Ethinyl estradiol 0.035 mg and norethindrone 1 mg [7 peach tablets]
Day 22-28: 7 green inactive tablets (28s)

Tilia™ Fe:
Day 1-5: Ethinyl estradiol 0.02 mg and norethindrone acetate 1 mg [5 white triangular tablets]
Day 6-12: Ethinyl estradiol 0.03 mg and norethindrone acetate 1 mg [7 white square tablets]
Day 13-21: Ethinyl estradiol 0.035 mg and norethindrone acetate 1 mg [9 white round tablets]
Day 22-28: Ferrous fumarate 75 mg [7 brown tablets] (28s)

Tri-Norinyl® 28:
Day 1-7: Ethinyl estradiol 0.035 mg and norethindrone 0.5 mg [7 blue tablets]
Day 8-16: Ethinyl estradiol 0.035 mg and norethindrone 1 mg [9 yellow-green tablets]
Day 17-21: Ethinyl estradiol 0.035 mg and norethindrone 0.5 mg [5 blue tablets]
Day 22-28: 7 orange inactive tablets (28s)

Ethinyl Estradiol and Norgestimate

(ETH in il es tra DYE ole & nor JES ti mate)

Medication Safety Issues

Sound-alike/look-alike issues:

Ortho-Cyclen® may be confused with Ortho-Cept®

U.S. Brand Names MonoNessa™; Ortho Tri-Cyclen®; Ortho Tri-Cyclen® Lo; Ortho-Cyclen®; Previfem™; Sprintec™; Tri-Previfem™; Tri-Sprintec™; TriNessa™

Canadian Brand Names Cyclen®; Tri-Cyclen® ; Tri-Cyclen® Lo

Mexican Brand Names Cilest

Index Terms Ethinyl Estradiol and NGM; Norgestimate and Ethinyl Estradiol; Ortho Cyclen; Ortho Tri Cyclen

Pharmacologic Category Contraceptive; Estrogen and Progestin Combination

Use Prevention of pregnancy; treatment of acne

Unlabeled/Investigational Use Treatment of hypermenorrhea (menorrhagia); pain associated with endometriosis; dysmenorrhea; dysfunctional uterine bleeding

Effect on Mental Status May cause dizziness, headache, depression, insomnia, nervousness, irritability, and mood disturbances

Effect on Psychiatric Treatment Barbiturates decrease the effects of oral contraceptives; may increase the toxicity of the benzodiazepines and TCAs. The Women's Health Initiative (WHI) Memory Study reported an increased risk of developing dementia in postmenopausal women ≥65 years of age during

4 years of treatment with oral conjugated equine estrogens and medroxyprogesterone acetate relative to placebo (1.8% vs 0.9%). Relative risk was 2.05 (95% CI 1.21-3.48). Therefore, estrogens and progestins should not be used for the prevention of dementia. The WHI also reported an increased risk of stroke (29 vs 21 per 10,000 women-years) compared to women receiving placebo. The increase in risk was observed after the first year and persisted. May cause hypertriglyceridemia; monitor in patients receiving antipsychotics especially clozapine, olanzapine, and quetiapine.

Dosage Summary

Oral:

Children (premenarche): Dosage not established

Children (postmenarche): 21-tablet package: 1 tablet daily for 21 days, followed by 7 days off; 28-tablet package: 1 tablet daily

Adults (females): 21-tablet package: 1 tablet daily for 21 days, followed by 7 days off; 28-tablet package: 1 tablet daily

Dosage Forms Excipient information presented when available (limited, particularly for generics); consult specific product labeling.

Tablet, monophasic formulations:

MonoNessa™, Ortho-Cyclen®: Ethinyl estradiol 0.035 mg and norgestimate 0.25 mg (28s) [21 blue tablets and 7 green inactive tablets]

Previfem™: Ethinyl estradiol 0.035 mg and norgestimate 0.25 mg (28s) [21 blue tablets and 7 teal inactive tablets]

Sprintec™: Ethinyl estradiol 0.035 mg and norgestimate 0.25 mg (28s) [21 blue tablets and 7 white inactive tablets]

Tablet, triphasic formulations:

Ortho Tri-Cyclen®, TriNessa™:

Day 1-7: Ethinyl estradiol 0.035 mg and norgestimate 0.18 mg [7 white tablets]

Day 8-14: Ethinyl estradiol 0.035 mg and norgestimate 0.215 mg [7 light blue tablets]

Day 15-21: Ethinyl estradiol 0.035 mg and norgestimate 0.25 mg [7 blue tablets]

Day 22-28: 7 green inactive tablets (28s)

Tri-Previfem™:

Day 1-7: Ethinyl estradiol 0.035 mg and norgestimate 0.18 mg [7 white tablets]

Day 8-14: Ethinyl estradiol 0.035 mg and norgestimate 0.215 mg [7 light blue tablets]

Day 15-21: Ethinyl estradiol 0.035 mg and norgestimate 0.25 mg [7 blue tablets]

Day 22-28: 7 teal inactive tablets (28s)

Tri-Sprintec™:

Day 1-7: Ethinyl estradiol 0.035 mg and norgestimate 0.18 mg [7 gray tablets]

Day 8-14: Ethinyl estradiol 0.035 mg and norgestimate 0.215 mg [7 light blue tablets]

Day 15-21: Ethinyl estradiol 0.035 mg and norgestimate 0.25 mg [7 blue tablets]

Day 22-28: 7 white inactive tablets (28s)

Ortho Tri-Cyclen® Lo:

Day 1-7: Ethinyl estradiol 0.025 mg and norgestimate 0.18 mg [7 white tablets]

Day 8-14: Ethinyl estradiol 0.025 mg and norgestimate 0.215 mg [7 light blue tablets]

Day 15-21: Ethinyl estradiol 0.025 mg and norgestimate 0.25 mg [7 dark blue tablets]

Day 22-28: 7 green inactive tablets (28s)

Ethinyl Estradiol and Norgestrel

(ETH in il es tra DYE ole & nor JES trel)

U.S. Brand Names Cryselle™; Lo/Ovral®; Low-Ogestrel®; Ogestrel®

Canadian Brand Names Ovral®

Mexican Brand Names Ovral

Index Terms Morning After Pill; Norgestrel and Ethinyl Estradiol

Pharmacologic Category Contraceptive; Estrogen and Progestin Combination

Use Prevention of pregnancy; postcoital contraceptive or "morning after" pill

Unlabeled/Investigational Use Treatment of hypermenorrhea (menorrhagia); pain associated with endometriosis; dysmenorrhea; dysfunctional uterine bleeding

Effect on Mental Status May cause dizziness, headache, depression, insomnia, nervousness, irritability, and mood disturbances

Effect on Psychiatric Treatment Barbiturates decrease the effects of oral contraceptives; may increase the toxicity of the benzodiazepines and TCAs. The Women's Health Initiative (WHI) Memory Study reported an increased risk of developing dementia in postmenopausal women ≥65 years of age during 4 years of treatment with oral conjugated equine estrogens and medroxyprogesterone acetate relative to placebo (1.8% vs 0.9%). Relative risk was 2.05 (95% CI 1.21-3.48). Therefore, estrogens and progestins should not be used for the prevention of dementia. The WHI also reported an increased risk of stroke (29 vs 21 per 10,000 women-years) compared to women receiving placebo. The increase in risk was observed after the first year and persisted. May cause hypertriglyceridemia; monitor in patients receiving antipsychotics especially clozapine, olanzapine, and quetiapine.

Dosage Summary

Oral:

Children (premenarche): Dosage not established

Children (females, postmenarche):

Contraception: 21-tablet package: 1 tablet daily for 21 days, followed by 7 days off; 28-tablet package: 1 tablet daily

Postcoital contraception: Ethinyl estradiol 0.03 mg and norgestrel 0.3 mg formulation: 4 tablets within 72 hours of unprotected intercourse and 4 tablets 12 hours after first dose **or** ethinyl estradiol 0.05 mg and norgestrel 0.5 mg formulation: 2 tablets within 72 hours of unprotected intercourse and 2 tablets 12 hours after first dose

Adults (females):

Contraception: 21-tablet package: 1 tablet daily for 21 days, followed by 7 days off; 28-tablet package: 1 tablet daily

Postcoital contraception: Ethinyl estradiol 0.03 mg and norgestrel 0.3 mg formulation: 4 tablets within 72 hours of unprotected intercourse and 4 tablets 12 hours after first dose **or** ethinyl estradiol 0.05 mg and norgestrel 0.5 mg formulation: 2 tablets within 72 hours of unprotected intercourse and 2 tablets 12 hours after first dose

Dosage Forms Excipient information presented when available (limited, particularly for generics); consult specific product labeling.

Tablet, monophasic formulations:

Cryselle™: Ethinyl estradiol 0.03 mg and norgestrel 0.3 mg [21 white tablets and 7 light green inactive tablets] (28s)

Low-Ogestrel® 28: Ethinyl estradiol 0.03 mg and norgestrel 0.3 mg [21 white tablets and 7 peach inactive tablets] (28s)

Lo/Ovral® 28: Ethinyl estradiol 0.03 mg and norgestrel 0.3 mg [21 white tablets and 7 pink inactive tablets] (28s)

Ogestrel® 28: Ethinyl estradiol 0.05 mg and norgestrel 0.5 mg [21 white tablets and 7 peach inactive tablets] (28s)

◆ **Ethiofos** *see* Amifostine *on page 83*

Ethionamide (e thye on AM ide)

U.S. Brand Names Trecator®

Canadian Brand Names Trecator®

Pharmacologic Category Antitubercular Agent

Use Treatment of tuberculosis and other mycobacterial diseases, in conjunction with other antituberculosis agents, when first-line agents have failed or resistance has been demonstrated

Effect on Mental Status May cause drowsiness or dizziness; case reports of depression and psychosis

Effect on Psychiatric Treatment None reported

Dosage Summary

Oral:

Children: 15-20 mg/kg/day in 2-3 divided doses (maximum: 1 g/day)

Adults: 250-750 mg/day in 1-4 divided doses (maximum: 1 g/day)

Dosage Forms Excipient information presented when available (limited, particularly for generics); consult specific product labeling.

Tablet: 250 mg

◆ **Ethmozine® [DSC]** *see* Moricizine *on page 1077*

Ethosuximide (eth oh SUKS i mide)

Medication Safety Issues

Sound-alike/look-alike issues:

Ethosuximide may be confused with methsuximide

Zarontin® may be confused with Xalatan®, Zantac®, Zaroxolyn®

Related Information

Anticonvulsants By Seizure Type *on page 1759*

U.S. Brand Names Zarontin®

Canadian Brand Names Zarontin®

Mexican Brand Names Fluozoid

Pharmacologic Category Anticonvulsant, Succinimide

Generic Available Yes

Use Management of absence (petit mal) seizures

Effect on Mental Status May cause sedation, euphoria, insomnia, or hallucinations; may rarely cause depression

Effect on Psychiatric Treatment Barbiturates and carbamazepine may decrease the clinical effects of ethosuximide

Pregnancy Considerations

Ethosuximide crosses the placenta. Cases of birth defects have been reported in infants. Epilepsy itself, the number of medications, genetic factors, or a combination of these probably influence the teratogenicity of anticonvulsant therapy. Health professionals and patients are encouraged to contact the North American Antiepileptic Drug Pregnancy registry to monitor outcomes of pregnant women exposed to ethosuximide and other antiepileptic drugs (888-233-2334).

Lactation Enters breast milk/use caution (AAP rates "compatible")

Contraindications Hypersensitivity to ethosuximide, other succinimides, or any component of the formulation

Warnings/Precautions Use with caution in patients with hepatic or renal disease; abrupt withdrawal of the drug may precipitate absence status; ethosuximide may increase tonic-clonic seizures in patients with mixed seizure disorders; ethosuximide must be used in combination with other anticonvulsants in patients with both absence and tonic-clonic seizures. Succinimides have been associated with severe blood dyscrasias and cases of systemic lupus erythematosus. Consider evaluation of blood counts in patients with signs/symptoms of infection. Effects with other sedative drugs or ethanol may be potentiated. Safety and efficacy in patients <3 years of age have not been established.

Adverse Reactions Frequency not defined.

Central nervous system: Aggressiveness, ataxia, disturbance in sleep, dizziness, drowsiness, euphoria, fatigue, headache, hyperactivity, inability to concentrate, irritability, lethargy, mental depression (with cases of overt suicidal intentions), night terrors, paranoid psychosis

Dermatologic: Hirsutism, pruritus, rash, Stevens-Johnson syndrome, urticaria

Endocrine & metabolic: Libido increased

Gastrointestinal: Abdominal pain, anorexia, cramps, diarrhea, epigastric pain, gastric upset, gum hypertrophy, nausea, tongue swelling, vomiting, weight loss

Genitourinary: Hematuria (microscopic), vaginal bleeding

Hematologic: Agranulocytosis, eosinophilia, leukopenia, pancytopenia

Ocular: Myopia

Miscellaneous: Hiccups, systemic lupus erythematosus

Metabolism/Transport Effects Substrate of CYP3A4 (major)

Drug Interactions

Alcohol (Ethyl): CNS Depressants may enhance the CNS depressant effect of Alcohol (Ethyl). *Risk C: Monitor therapy*

Amphetamines: May diminish the therapeutic effect of Ethosuximide. Amphetamines may decrease the serum concentration of Ethosuximide. *Risk C: Monitor therapy*

CNS Depressants: May enhance the adverse/toxic effect of other CNS Depressants. *Risk C: Monitor therapy*

CYP3A4 Inducers (Strong): May increase the metabolism of CYP3A4 Substrates. *Risk C: Monitor therapy*

CYP3A4 Inhibitors (Moderate): May decrease the metabolism of CYP3A4 Substrates. *Risk C: Monitor therapy*

CYP3A4 Inhibitors (Strong): May decrease the metabolism of CYP3A4 Substrates. *Risk D: Consider therapy modification*

Dasatinib: May increase the serum concentration of CYP3A4 Substrates. *Risk C: Monitor therapy*

Deferasirox: May decrease the serum concentration of CYP3A4 Substrates. *Risk C: Monitor therapy*
Herbs (CYP3A4 Inducers): May increase the metabolism of CYP3A4 Substrates. *Risk C: Monitor therapy*
Ketorolac: May diminish the therapeutic effect of Anticonvulsants. *Risk C: Monitor therapy*
Mefloquine: May diminish the therapeutic effect of Anticonvulsants. Mefloquine may decrease the serum concentration of Anticonvulsants. Management: Mefloquine is contraindicated in persons with a history of convulsions. If anticonvulsant is being used for another indication monitor response to treatment closely, as concurrent mefloquine may decrease response to treatment. *Risk D: Consider therapy modification*
Valproic Acid: Ethosuximide may decrease the serum concentration of Valproic Acid. Valproic Acid may increase the serum concentration of Ethosuximide. *Risk C: Monitor therapy*

Ethanol/Nutrition/Herb Interactions
Ethanol: Avoid ethanol (may increase CNS depression).
Herb/Nutraceutical: St John's wort may decrease ethosuximide levels.

Mechanism of Action Increases the seizure threshold and suppresses paroxysmal spike-and-wave pattern in absence seizures; depresses nerve transmission in the motor cortex

Pharmacodynamics/Kinetics
Distribution: Adults: V_d: 0.62-0.72 L/kg
Metabolism: Hepatic (~80% to 3 inactive metabolites)
Half-life elimination, serum: Children: 30 hours; Adults: 50-60 hours
Time to peak, serum: Capsule: ~2-4 hours; Syrup: <2-4 hours
Excretion: Urine, slowly (50% as metabolites, 10% to 20% as unchanged drug); feces (small amounts)

Dosage Oral:
Children 3-6 years: Initial: 250 mg/day; increase every 4-7 days; usual maintenance dose: 20 mg/kg/day; maximum dose: 1.5 g/day in divided doses
Children >6 years and Adults: Initial: 500 mg/day; increase by 250 mg as needed every 4-7 days, up to 1.5 g/day in divided doses; usual maintenance dose for most pediatric patients is 20 mg/kg/day.
Dosing comment in renal/hepatic dysfunction: Use with caution.

Dietary Considerations Increase dietary intake of folate; may be administered with food or milk.

Administration Administer with food or milk to avoid GI upset

Monitoring Parameters Seizure frequency, trough serum concentrations; CBC, platelets, liver enzymes, urinalysis

Reference Range Therapeutic: 40-100 mcg/mL

Dosage Forms Excipient information presented when available (limited, particularly for generics); consult specific product labeling.
Capsule: 250 mg
Zarontin®: 250 mg
Syrup: 250 mg/5 mL (473 mL)
Zarontin®: 250 mg/5 mL [contains sodium benzoate; raspberry flavor]

Ethotoin (ETH oh toyn)

U.S. Brand Names Peganone®
Canadian Brand Names Peganone®
Index Terms Ethylphenylhydantoin
Pharmacologic Category Anticonvulsant, Hydantoin
Use Generalized tonic-clonic or complex-partial seizures
Effect on Mental Status Drowsiness and dizziness are common; may cause insomnia or confusion
Effect on Psychiatric Treatment None reported
Dosage Summary
Oral:
Children <1 year: Dosage not established
Children ≥1 year: Maximum initial dose: 750 mg/day; usual maintenance dose: 0.5-1 g/day; maximum dose: 3 g/day
Adults: Initial dose: ≤1 g/day; usual maintenance dose: 2-3 g/day

Dosage Forms Excipient information presented when available (limited, particularly for generics); consult specific product labeling.
Tablet:
Peganone®: 250 mg

◆ **ETH-Oxydose™** *see* OxyCODONE *on page 1201*

- **Ethoxynaphthamido Penicillin Sodium** *see* Nafcillin *on page 1093*
- **Ethyl Esters of Omega-3 Fatty Acids** *see* Omega-3-Acid Ethyl Esters *on page 1175*
- **Ethylphenylhydantoin** *see* Ethotoin *on page 604*
- **Ethynodiol Diacetate and Ethinyl Estradiol** *see* Ethinyl Estradiol and Ethynodiol Diacetate *on page 594*
- **Ethyol®** *see* Amifostine *on page 83*

Etidronate and Calcium (e ti DROE nate & KAL see um)

Canadian Brand Names Didrocal™

Index Terms Calcium Carbonate and Etidronate Disodium

Pharmacologic Category Bisphosphonate Derivative; Calcium Salt

Use Treatment and prevention of postmenopausal osteoporosis; prevention of corticosteroid-induced osteoporosis

Effect on Mental Status May cause dizziness

Effect on Psychiatric Treatment Bisphosphonates have been associated with renal toxicity manifested as deterioration of renal function and potential renal failure. use caution in patients receiving lithium. GI side effects are common, concurrent use with SSRIs, lithium, valproic acid, or carbamazepine may produce additive effects.

Restrictions Not available in U.S.

Dosage Summary

Oral:

Children: Dosage not established

Adults: Etidronate disodium 400 mg once daily for 14 days, followed by calcium carbonate 1250 mg (500 mg elemental calcium) once daily for 76 days

Dosage Forms Excipient information presented when available (limited, particularly for generics); consult specific product labeling. [CAN] = Canadian brand name

Combination package [each package contains five blister cards (90-day supply)]:

Didrocal™ [CAN; not available in the U.S.]

Tablet, etidronate disodium 400 mg (14s) [first card (white tablets)]

Tablet, calcium carbonate: 1250 mg (76s) [equivalent to elemental calcium 500 mg; remaining cards (blue tablets)]

Etidronate Disodium (e ti DROE nate dye SOW dee um)

Medication Safety Issues

Sound-alike/look-alike issues:

Etidronate may be confused with etidocaine, etomidate, etretinate

U.S. Brand Names Didronel®

Canadian Brand Names Didronel®; Gen-Etidronate

Index Terms EHDP; Sodium Etidronate

Pharmacologic Category Bisphosphonate Derivative

Use Symptomatic treatment of Paget's disease; prevention and treatment of heterotopic ossification due to spinal cord injury or after total hip replacement

Unlabeled/Investigational Use Postmenopausal osteoporosis

Effect on Mental Status None reported

Effect on Psychiatric Treatment Bisphosphonates have been associated with renal toxicity manifested as deterioration of renal function and potential renal failure. Use caution in patients receiving lithium.

Dosage Summary

Oral:

Children: Dosage not established

Adults:

Heterotopic ossification:

Caused by spinal cord injury: 20 mg/kg/day for 2 weeks, then 10 mg/kg/day for 10 weeks (total treatment period: 12 weeks)

Complicating total hip replacement: 20 mg/kg/day for 1 month preoperatively then 20 mg/kg/day for 3 months postoperatively (total treatment period: 4 months)

Paget's disease: 5-10 mg/kg/day for up to 6 months or 11-20 mg/kg/day for up to 3 months; may retreat after etidronate-free period ≥90 days

Dosage Forms Excipient information presented when available (limited, particularly for generics); consult specific product labeling.

Tablet: 200 mg, 400 mg

Etodolac (ee toe DOE lak)

Medication Safety Issues

Sound-alike/look-alike issues:

Lodine® may be confused with codeine, iodine, Iopidine®, Lopid®

Related Information

Nonsteroidal Anti-Inflammatory Agents *on page 1792*

Canadian Brand Names Apo-Etodolac®; Utradol™

Mexican Brand Names Lodine; Lodine Retard

Index Terms Etodolic Acid

Pharmacologic Category Nonsteroidal Anti-inflammatory Drug (NSAID), Oral

Use Acute and long-term use in the management of signs and symptoms of osteoarthritis; rheumatoid arthritis and juvenile rheumatoid arthritis; management of acute pain

Effect on Mental Status Dizziness is common; may cause nervousness; rarely produces confusion, depression, insomnia, or hallucinations

Effect on Psychiatric Treatment May rarely cause agranulocytosis; use caution with clozapine and carbamazepine; may decrease the clearance of lithium resulting in elevated serum levels and potential toxicity; monitor serum lithium levels

Restrictions An FDA-approved medication guide must be distributed when dispensing an oral outpatient prescription (new or refill) where this medication is to be used without direct supervision of a healthcare provider. Medication guides are available at http://www.fda.gov/cder/Offices/ODS/medication_guides.htm.

Dosage Summary

Oral:

Extended release:

Children <6 years: Dosage not established

Children 6-16 years and 20-30 kg: 400 mg once daily

Children 6-16 years and 31-45 kg: 600 mg once daily

Children 6-16 years and 46-60 kg: 800 mg once daily

Children 6-16 years and >60 kg: 1000 mg once daily

Adults: 400-1000 mg once daily

Regular release:

Children: Dosage not established

Adults: 200-400 mg every 6-12 hours as needed **or** 500 mg 2 times/day (maximum: 1 g/day)

Dosage Forms Excipient information presented when available (limited, particularly for generics); consult specific product labeling.

Capsule: 200 mg, 300 mg

Tablet: 400 mg, 500 mg

Tablet, extended release: 400 mg, 500 mg, 600 mg

◆ **Etodolic Acid** *see* Etodolac *on page 606*

Etonogestrel (e toe noe JES trel)

U.S. Brand Names Implanon™

Mexican Brand Names Implanon

Index Terms 3-Keto-desogestrel; ENG

Pharmacologic Category Contraceptive; Progestin

Use Prevention of pregnancy; for use in women who request long-acting (up to 3 years) contraception

Effect on Mental Status Headache is common; may cause dizziness, depression, nervousness, or mood lability

Effect on Psychiatric Treatment Etonogestrel is not recommended for patients receiving potent enzyme inducers (eg, phenobarbital, carbamazepine, St John's wort). Weight gain is common; concomitant use with psychotropics may produce additive effects.

Restrictions Only healthcare providers who have undergone training in the insertion and removal procedures will be able to order Implanon™.

Dosage Summary

Subdermal:

Children: Not for use prior to menarche

Adults: Implant 1 rod for up to 3 years

Elderly: Not for use after menopause

Dosage Forms Excipient information presented when available (limited, particularly for generics); consult specific product labeling.

Rod, subdermal:
Implanon™: 68 mg [latex free]

- **Etonogestrel and Ethinyl Estradiol** *see* Ethinyl Estradiol and Etonogestrel *on page 594*
- **Etopophos®** *see* Etoposide Phosphate *on page 607*

Etoposide (e toe POE side)

Medication Safety Issues
Sound-alike/look-alike issues:
Etoposide may be confused with teniposide
VePesid® may be confused with Versed

High alert medication: The Institute for Safe Medication Practices (ISMP) includes this medication among its list of drugs which have a heightened risk of causing significant patient harm when used in error.

U.S. Brand Names Toposar®; VePesid® [DSC]
Canadian Brand Names VePesid®
Mexican Brand Names Cryosid; Etonco; Etopos; VP-TEC
Index Terms Epipodophyllotoxin; VP-16; VP-16-213
Pharmacologic Category Antineoplastic Agent, Podophyllotoxin Derivative
Use Treatment of refractory testicular tumors; treatment of small cell lung cancer
Unlabeled/Investigational Use Treatment of lymphomas, acute nonlymphocytic leukemia (ANLL); lung, bladder, and prostate carcinoma; hepatoma, rhabdomyosarcoma, uterine carcinoma, neuroblastoma, mycosis fungoides, Kaposi's sarcoma, histiocytosis, gestational trophoblastic disease, Ewing's sarcoma, Wilms' tumor, brain tumors
Effect on Mental Status May cause sedation
Effect on Psychiatric Treatment May cause myelosuppression; use caution with clozapine and carbamazepine
Dosage Summary
I.V.:
Children (unlabeled use): 60-120 mg/m²/day for 3-5 days every 3-6 weeks **or** 150 mg/m²/day for 2-3 days for 2-3 cycles **or** 250 mg/m²/day for 3 days, courses 2-5 **or** 150 mg/m²/day on days 2 and 3 of treatment course **or** 100 mg/m²/day on days 1-5 of cycle, repeat cycle every 4 weeks; **BMT:** 160 mg/m²/day as continuous infusion for 4 days **or** 60 mg/kg/dose as a single dose
Adults: 35 mg/m²/day for 4 days every 3-4 weeks **or** 50-100 mg/m²/day for 5 days every 3-4 weeks **or** 60-100 mg/m²/day for 3 days **or** 500 mg/m² over 24 hours every 3 weeks **or** 100 mg/m² every other day for 3 doses repeated every 3-4 weeks
Oral:
Children: Dosage not established
Adults: Doses should be twice the I.V. dose (rounded to the nearest 50 mg) given once daily
Dosage Forms Excipient information presented when available (limited, particularly for generics); consult specific product labeling. [DSC] = Discontinued product
Capsule, softgel: 50 mg
VePesid®: 50 mg [DSC]
Injection, solution: 20 mg/mL (5 mL, 25 mL, 50 mL)
Toposar®: 20 mg/mL (5 mL, 25 mL, 50 mL) [contains alcohol 33% and polysorbate 80]

Etoposide Phosphate (e toe POE side FOS fate)

Medication Safety Issues
Sound-alike/look-alike issues:
Etoposide may be confused with teniposide
Etoposide phosphate is a prodrug of etoposide and is rapidly converted in the plasma to etoposide. To avoid confusion or dosing errors, **dosage should be expressed as the desired etoposide dose,** not as the etoposide phosphate dose (eg, etoposide phosphate equivalent to ____ mg etoposide).

High alert medication: The Institute for Safe Medication Practices (ISMP) includes this medication among its list of drugs which have a heightened risk of causing significant patient harm when used in error.

U.S. Brand Names Etopophos®

Mexican Brand Names Etopos
Pharmacologic Category Antineoplastic Agent, Podophyllotoxin Derivative
Use Treatment of refractory testicular tumors; treatment of small cell lung cancer
Effect on Mental Status May cause sedation
Effect on Psychiatric Treatment May cause myelosuppression; use caution with clozapine and carbamazepine
Dosage Summary Note: Etoposide phosphate is a prodrug of etoposide, doses should be expressed as the desired ETOPOSIDE dose; not as the etoposide phosphate dose.

I.V.:

Children: Dosage not established

Adults: 35 mg/m²/day for 4 days to 50-100 mg/m²/day for 5 days every 3-4 weeks **or** 100 mg/m²/day on days 1, 3, and 5 every 3-4 weeks

Dosage Forms Excipient information presented when available (limited, particularly for generics); consult specific product labeling.

Injection, powder for reconstitution:

Etopophos®: 100 mg

Etravirine (et ra VIR een)

U.S. Brand Names Intelence™
Canadian Brand Names Intelence™
Index Terms TMC125
Pharmacologic Category Antiretroviral Agent, Reverse Transcriptase Inhibitor (Non-nucleoside)
Use Treatment of HIV-1 infection in combination with at least two additional antiretroviral agents in treatment-experienced patients exhibiting viral replication with documented non-nucleoside reverse transcriptase inhibitor (NNRTI) resistance
Effect on Mental Status May rarely cause amnesia, confusion, insomnia, and hypersomnia
Effect on Psychiatric Treatment Etravirine is associated with Stevens-Johnson syndrome; monitor patients also receiving lamotrigine. May cause elevations in lipid panel; concomitant use with atypical antipsychotics may produce additive effects. GI side effects are common; concomitant use with lithium, SSRIs, valproic acid, and carbamazepine may produce additive effects. Associated with a high potential for drug-drug interactions; monitor. Carbamazepine, phenobarbital, and St John's wort may decrease the levels/effects of etravirine; do not coadminister. Etravirine may increase the levels/effects of citalopram, diazepam, fluoxetine, propranolol, and sertraline. Etravirine may decrease the levels/effects of benzodiazepines, methadone, mirtazapine, nefazodone, and venlafaxine.

Dosage Summary

Oral:

Children: Dosage not established

Adults: 200 mg twice daily after meals

Dosage Forms Excipient information presented when available (limited, particularly for generics); consult specific product labeling.

Tablet:

Intelence™: 100 mg

- **Eudal®-SR** *see* Guaifenesin and Pseudoephedrine *on page 744*
- **Eulexin®** *see* Flutamide *on page 667*
- **Eun-haeng** *see* Ginkgo *(Ginkgo biloba) on page 715*
- **Evamist™** *see* Estradiol *on page 576*
- **Evista®** *see* Raloxifene *on page 1391*
- **Evoclin®** *see* Clindamycin *on page 363*
- **Evoxac®** *see* Cevimeline *on page 310*
- **Excedrin® Extra Strength [OTC]** *see* Acetaminophen, Aspirin, and Caffeine *on page 39*
- **Excedrin® Migraine [OTC]** *see* Acetaminophen, Aspirin, and Caffeine *on page 39*
- **Excedrin® P.M. [OTC]** *see* Acetaminophen and Diphenhydramine *on page 35*
- **ExeClear [DSC]** *see* Hydrocodone and Guaifenesin *on page 779*
- **ExeCof** *see* Guaifenesin, Dextromethorphan, and Phenylephrine *on page 746*
- **ExeCof-XP [DSC]** *see* Hydrocodone and Guaifenesin *on page 779*
- **ExeFen** *see* Guaifenesin and Pseudoephedrine *on page 744*

- ◆ **ExeFen-DMX** *see* Guaifenesin, Pseudoephedrine, and Dextromethorphan *on page 748*
- ◆ **ExeFen-PD** *see* Guaifenesin and Phenylephrine *on page 742*
- ◆ **Exelon®** *see* Rivastigmine *on page 1435*

Exemestane (ex e MES tane)

Medication Safety Issues
Sound-alike/look-alike issues:
Exemestane may be confused with estramustine.
U.S. Brand Names Aromasin®
Canadian Brand Names Aromasin®
Pharmacologic Category Antineoplastic Agent, Aromatase Inactivator
Use Treatment of advanced breast cancer in postmenopausal women whose disease has progressed following tamoxifen therapy; adjuvant treatment of postmenopausal estrogen receptor-positive early breast cancer following 2-3 years of tamoxifen (for a total of 5 years of adjuvant therapy)
Effect on Mental Status Drowsiness, depression, insomnia, and anxiety are common; may cause confusion
Effect on Psychiatric Treatment None reported
Dosage Summary
Oral:
Children: Dosage not established
Adults (postmenopausal females): 25 mg once daily (50 mg once daily with CYP3A4 inducers)
Dosage Forms Excipient information presented when available (limited, particularly for generics); consult specific product labeling.
Tablet: 25 mg

Exenatide (ex EN a tide)

U.S. Brand Names Byetta®
Index Terms AC 2993; AC002993; Exendin-4 ; LY2148568
Pharmacologic Category Antidiabetic Agent, Incretin Mimetic
Use Management (adjunctive) of type 2 diabetes mellitus (noninsulin dependent, NIDDM) in patients receiving a sulfonylurea, thiazolidinedione, or metformin (or a combination of these agents)
Effect on Mental Status May cause dizziness
Effect on Psychiatric Treatment
GI side effects are common; use caution with SSRIs, lithium, and valproic acid
Dosage Summary
SubQ:
Children: Dosage not established
Adults: Initial: 5 mcg twice daily for 1 month; Maintenance: 5-10 mcg twice daily
Dosage Forms Excipient information presented when available (limited, particularly for generics); consult specific product labeling.
Injection, solution:
Byetta®: 250 mcg/mL (1.2 mL [5 mcg/0.02 mL; 60-dose pen]); (2.4 mL [10 mcg/0.04 mL; 60-dose pen])

- ◆ **Exendin-4** *see* Exenatide *on page 609*
- ◆ **ExeTuss [DSC]** *see* Guaifenesin and Phenylephrine *on page 742*
- ◆ **ExeTuss-DM** *see* Guaifenesin, Dextromethorphan, and Phenylephrine *on page 746*
- ◆ **ExeTuss-GP** *see* Guaifenesin and Phenylephrine *on page 742*
- ◆ **ExeTuss HC [DSC]** *see* Hydrocodone, Phenylephrine, and Guaifenesin *on page 783*
- ◆ **Exforge®** *see* Amlodipine and Valsartan *on page 105*
- ◆ **Exjade®** *see* Deferasirox *on page 423*
- ◆ **Extendryl®** *see* Chlorpheniramine, Phenylephrine, and Methscopolamine *on page 329*
- ◆ **Extendryl® GCP** *see* Carbetapentane, Guaifenesin, and Phenylephrine *on page 274*
- ◆ **Extendryl® HC [DSC]** *see* Hydrocodone and Guaifenesin *on page 779*
- ◆ **Extendryl® JR** *see* Chlorpheniramine, Phenylephrine, and Methscopolamine *on page 329*

- ◆ **Extendryl PSE** *see* Pseudoephedrine and Methscopolamine *on page 1370*
- ◆ **Extendryl® SR** *see* Chlorpheniramine, Phenylephrine, and Methscopolamine *on page 329*
- ◆ **Extina®** *see* Ketoconazole *on page 876*
- ◆ **Exubera® [DSC]** *see* Insulin Inhalation *on page 830*
- ◆ **EYE001** *see* Pegaptanib *on page 1235*
- ◆ **Eye-Sine™ [OTC] [DSC]** *see* Tetrahydrozoline *on page 1560*
- ◆ **EZ-Char™ [OTC]** *see* Charcoal *on page 312*

Ezetimibe (ez ET i mibe)

Medication Safety Issues
Sound-alike/look-alike issues:
Zetia® may be confused with Zebeta®, Zestril®

U.S. Brand Names Zetia®

Canadian Brand Names Ezetrol®

Mexican Brand Names Ezetrol; Zient

Pharmacologic Category Antilipemic Agent, 2-Azetidinone

Generic Available No

Use Use in combination with dietary therapy for the treatment of primary hypercholesterolemia (as monotherapy or in combination with HMG-CoA reductase inhibitors); homozygous sitosterolemia; homozygous familial hypercholesterolemia (in combination with atorvastatin or simvastatin); mixed hyperlipidemia (in combination with fenofibrate)

Effect on Mental Status May cause dizziness and fatigue

Effect on Psychiatric Treatment None reported

Pregnancy Risk Factor C

Pregnancy Considerations Safety and efficacy have not been established; use during pregnancy only if the potential benefit to the mother outweighs the possible risk to the fetus.

Lactation Excretion in breast milk unknown/not recommended

Contraindications Hypersensitivity to ezetimibe or any component of the formulation; concomitant use with an HMG-CoA reductase inhibitor in patients with active hepatic disease, unexplained persistent elevations in serum transaminases; pregnancy; breast-feeding

Warnings/Precautions Secondary causes of hyperlipidemia should be ruled out prior to therapy. Use caution with severe renal (Cl_{cr} <30 mL/minute) or mild hepatic impairment (Child-Pugh class A); not recommended for use with moderate or severe hepatic impairment (Child-Pugh classes B and C). Concurrent use of ezetimibe and fibric acid derivatives may increase the risk of cholelithiasis. Safety and efficacy have not been established in patients <10 years of age.

Adverse Reactions
1% to 10%:
Central nervous system: Fatigue (2%)
Gastrointestinal: Diarrhea (4%)
Hepatic: Transaminases increased (with HMG-CoA reductase inhibitors) (≥3 x ULN, 1%)
Neuromuscular & skeletal: Arthralgia (3%), pain in extremity (3%)
Respiratory: Upper respiratory tract infection (4%), sinusitis (3%)
Miscellaneous: Influenza (2%)

Postmarketing and/or case reports: Anaphylaxis, angioedema, autoimmune hepatitis (Stolk, 2006), cholecystitis, cholelithiasis, cholestatic hepatitis (Stolk, 2006), CPK increased, depression, dizziness, hepatitis, hypersensitivity reactions, myalgia, myopathy, nausea, pancreatitis, paresthesia, rash, rhabdomyolysis, thrombocytopenia, urticaria

Drug Interactions
Bile Acid Sequestrants: May decrease the absorption of Ezetimibe. *Risk C: Monitor therapy*
CycloSPORINE: May increase the serum concentration of Ezetimibe. Ezetimibe may increase the serum concentration of CycloSPORINE. *Risk D: Consider therapy modification*
Fibric Acid Derivatives: May increase the serum concentration of Ezetimibe. *Risk C: Monitor therapy*

Ethanol/Nutrition/Herb Interactions Food: Ezetimibe did not cause meaningful reductions in fat-soluble vitamin concentrations during a 2-week clinical trial. Effects of long-term therapy have not been evaluated.

Stability Store at controlled room temperature of 25°C (77°F). Protect from moisture.

Mechanism of Action Inhibits absorption of cholesterol at the brush border of the small intestine via the sterol transporter, Niemann-Pick C1-Like1 (NPC1L1). This leads to a decreased delivery of cholesterol to the liver, reduction of hepatic cholesterol stores and an increased clearance of cholesterol from the blood; decreases total C, LDL-cholesterol (LDL-C), ApoB, and triglycerides (TG) while increasing HDL-cholesterol (HDL-C).

Pharmacodynamics/Kinetics

Protein binding: >90% to plasma proteins

Metabolism: Undergoes glucuronide conjugation in the small intestine and liver; forms metabolite (active); may undergo enterohepatic recycling

Bioavailability: Variable

Half-life elimination: 22 hours (ezetimibe and metabolite)

Time to peak, plasma: 4-12 hours

Excretion: Feces (78%, 69% as ezetimibe); urine (11%, 9% as metabolite)

Dosage Oral:

Children ≥10 years and Adults: 10 mg/day

Elderly: Refer to adult dosing

Dosage adjustment in renal impairment: AUC increased with severe impairment (Cl_{cr} <30 mL/minute); no dosing adjustment recommended

Dosage adjustment in hepatic impairment: AUC increased with hepatic impairment

Mild impairment (Child-Pugh class A): No dosing adjustment necessary

Moderate-to-severe impairment (Child-Pugh classes B and C): Use of ezetimibe not recommended

Dietary Considerations May be taken without regard to meals. Before initiation of therapy, patients should be placed on a standard cholesterol-lowering diet for 6 weeks and the diet should be continued during drug therapy.

Administration May be administered without regard to meals. May be taken at the same time as HMG-CoA reductase inhibitors. Administer ≥2 hours before or ≥4 hours after bile acid sequestrants.

Monitoring Parameters Total cholesterol profile prior to therapy, and when clinically indicated and/or periodically thereafter. When used in combination with fenofibrate, monitor LFTs and signs and symptoms of cholelithiasis.

Additional Information When studied in combination with fenofibrate for mixed hyperlipidemia, the dose of fenofibrate was 160 mg daily.

Dosage Forms Excipient information presented when available (limited, particularly for generics); consult specific product labeling.

Tablet:

Zetia®: 10 mg

Ezetimibe and Simvastatin (ez ET i mibe & SIM va stat in)

Medication Safety Issues

Sound-alike/look-alike issues:

Vytorin® may be confused with Vyvanse™

U.S. Brand Names Vytorin®

Mexican Brand Names Vytorin; Zintrepid

Index Terms Simvastatin and Ezetimibe

Pharmacologic Category Antilipemic Agent, 2-Azetidinone; Antilipemic Agent, HMG-CoA Reductase Inhibitor

Use Used in combination with dietary modification for the treatment of primary hypercholesterolemia and homozygous familial hypercholesterolemia

Effect on Mental Status May cause dizziness or fatigue; may rarely cause anxiety, depression, insomnia, or memory loss

Effect on Psychiatric Treatment Rhabdomyolysis with acute renal failure has occurred; risk increased with concurrent use of fluvoxamine, nefazodone, and verapamil

Dosage Summary

Oral:

Children: Dosage not established

Adults: Ezetimibe 10 mg and simvastatin 10-80 mg once daily

Dosage Forms Excipient information presented when available (limited, particularly for generics); consult specific product labeling.

Tablet:

10/10: Ezetimibe 10 mg and simvastatin 10 mg

10/20: Ezetimibe 10 mg and simvastatin 20 mg

10/40: Ezetimibe 10 mg and simvastatin 40 mg

10/80: Ezetimibe 10 mg and simvastatin 80 mg

◆ **Fabrazyme®** *see* Agalsidase Beta *on page 52*

- **Factive®** *see* Gemifloxacin *on page 712*
- **Factor IX Concentrate** *see* Factor IX *on page 612*

Factor IX (FAK ter nyne)

U.S. Brand Names AlphaNine® SD; BeneFix®; Mononine®
Canadian Brand Names BeneFix®; Immunine® VH; Mononine®
Mexican Brand Names Berinin P; Octanine F
Index Terms Factor IX Concentrate
Pharmacologic Category Antihemophilic Agent; Blood Product Derivative
Use Control bleeding in patients with factor IX deficiency (hemophilia B or Christmas disease)
Effect on Mental Status May rarely cause sedation
Effect on Psychiatric Treatment None reported
Dosage Summary Note: Dosage is expressed in int. units of factor IX activity and must be individualized

I.V.:

AlphaNine® SD, Mononine®:

Children: Number of factor IX int. units required = body weight (in kg) x desired factor IX level increase (int. units/dL or % of normal) x 1 int. unit/kg every 12-24 hours or every 18-30 hours

Adults: Number of factor IX int. units required = body weight (in kg) x desired factor IX level increase (int. units/dL or % of normal) x 1 int. unit/kg every 12-24 hours or every 18-30 hours

BeneFix®:

Children <15 years: Number of factor IX int. units required = body weight (in kg) x desired factor IX level increase (int. units/dL or % of normal) x 1.4 int. units/kg every 12-24 hours

Children ≥15 years: Number of factor IX int. units required = body weight (in kg) x desired factor IX level increase (int. units/dL or % of normal) x 1.3 int. units/kg every 12-24 hours

Adults: Number of factor IX int. units required = body weight (in kg) x desired factor IX level increase (int. units/dL or % of normal) x 1.3 int. units/kg every 12-24 hours

Dosage Forms Excipient information presented when available (limited, particularly for generics); consult specific product labeling.

Injection, powder for reconstitution (**Note:** Exact potency labeled on each vial):

BeneFix® [contains polysorbate 80; sucrose 0.8%; recombinant formulation; supplied with diluent]

Injection, powder for reconstitution [human derived] (**Note:** Exact potency labeled on each vial):

AlphaNine® SD [contains polysorbate 80; solvent detergent treated; virus filtered; contains nondetectable levels of factors II, VII, X; supplied with diluent]

Mononine® [contains polysorbate 80; monoclonal antibody purified; contains nondetectable levels of factors II, VII, X; supplied with diluent]

Factor IX Complex (Human) (FAK ter nyne KOM pleks HYU man)

U.S. Brand Names Bebulin® VH; Profilnine® SD; Proplex® T [DSC]
Mexican Brand Names Replenine-VF
Index Terms Prothrombin Complex Concentrate
Pharmacologic Category Antihemophilic Agent; Blood Product Derivative; Prothrombin Complex Concentrate (PCC)
Use Control bleeding in patients with factor IX deficiency (hemophilia B or Christmas disease) **Note:** Factor IX concentrate containing **only** factor IX is also available and preferable for this indication.
Unlabeled/Investigational Use Emergency correction of the coagulopathy of warfarin excess in critical situations. **Note:** Products contain low or non-therapeutic levels of factor VII component.
Effect on Mental Status May rarely cause sedation
Effect on Psychiatric Treatment None reported
Dosage Summary Note: Dosage is expressed in units of factor IX activity and must be individualized

I.V.:

Children: Number of units = desired level increase [desired level - actual level] x plasma volume (in mL) given once and repeated in 24 hours if necessary or given every 18-30 hours **or** 75 units/kg/dose every 6-12 hours **or** 15 units/kg as a single dose

Adults: Number of units = desired level increase [desired level - actual level] x plasma volume (in mL) given once and repeated in 24 hours if necessary or given every 18-30 hours **or** 75 units/kg/dose every 6-12 hours **or** 15 units/kg as a single dose

Dosage Forms Excipient information presented when available (limited, particularly for generics); consult specific product labeling. [DSC] = Discontinued product

Injection, powder for reconstitution (**Note:** Exact potency labeled on each vial):

Bebulin® VH [single-dose vial; vapor heated; supplied with sterile water for injection]

Profilnine® SD [single-dose vial; solvent detergent treated]

Proplex® T [single-dose vial; heat treated; supplied with sterile water for injection] [DSC]

◆ **Factrel®** *see* Gonadorelin *on page 734*

Famciclovir (fam SYE kloe veer)

Medication Safety Issues

Sound-alike/look-alike issues:

Famvir® may be confused with Femara®

U.S. Brand Names Famvir®

Canadian Brand Names Apo-Famciclovir; Famvir®; PMS-Famciclovir; Sandoz-Famciclovir

Pharmacologic Category Antiviral Agent

Use Treatment of acute herpes zoster (shingles); treatment and suppression of recurrent episodes of genital herpes in immunocompetent patients; treatment of herpes labialis (cold sores) in immunocompetent patients; treatment of recurrent mucocutaneous/genital herpes simplex in HIV-infected patients

Effect on Mental Status May cause sedation

Effect on Psychiatric Treatment None reported

Dosage Summary

Oral:

Children: Dosage not established

Adults: 125-500 mg twice daily **or** 500 mg every 8 hours

Dosage Forms Excipient information presented when available (limited, particularly for generics); consult specific product labeling.

Tablet: 125 mg, 250 mg, 500 mg

Famvir®: 125 mg, 250 mg, 500 mg

Famotidine (fa MOE ti deen)

U.S. Brand Names Pepcid®; Pepcid® AC Maximum Strength [OTC]; Pepcid® AC [OTC]

Canadian Brand Names Apo-Famotidine®; Apo-Famotidine® Injectable; Famotidine Omega; Gen-Famotidine; Novo-Famotidine; Nu-Famotidine; Pepcid®; Pepcid® AC; Pepcid® I.V.; ratio-Famotidine; Riva-Famotidine; Ulcidine

Mexican Brand Names Androtin; Durater; Facidex; Ludex; Pepcidine

Pharmacologic Category Histamine H_2 Antagonist

Use Maintenance therapy and treatment of duodenal ulcer; treatment of gastroesophageal reflux, active benign gastric ulcer, and pathological hypersecretory conditions

OTC labeling: Relief of heartburn, acid indigestion, and sour stomach

Unlabeled/Investigational Use Part of a multidrug regimen for *H. pylori* eradication to reduce the risk of duodenal ulcer recurrence; stress ulcer prophylaxis in critically-ill patients; symptomatic relief in gastritis

Effect on Mental Status May cause dizziness or drowsiness; may rarely cause insomnia

Effect on Psychiatric Treatment May cause agranulocytosis; use caution with clozapine and carbamazepine

Dosage Summary

I.V.:

Children <1 year: Dosage not established

Children 1-16 years: 0.25 mg/kg every 12 hours (maximum: 40 mg/day)

Adults: 20 mg every 12 hours

Oral:

Children <3 months: 0.5 mg/kg once daily

Children 3-12 months: 0.5 mg/kg twice daily

Children 1-11 years: 0.5-1 mg/kg/day in 1-2 divided doses (maximum: 80 mg/day; Exceptions occur - Indication specific)

Children 12-16 years: 0.5-1 mg/kg/day in 1-2 divided doses (maximum: 80 mg/day; Exceptions occur - Indication specific)
OTC dosing: 10-20 mg every 12 hours (OTC dosing)
Adults: 20-40 mg/day in 1-2 divided doses
OTC dosing: 10-20 mg every 12 hours
Hypersecretory conditions: 20 mg every 6 hours, may increase in increments up to 160 mg every 6 hours

Dosage Forms Excipient information presented when available (limited, particularly for generics); consult specific product labeling.
Gelcap:
Pepcid® AC: 10 mg
Infusion [premixed in NS]: 20 mg (50 mL)
Pepcid®: 20 mg (50 mL)
Injection, solution: 10 mg/mL (4 mL, 20 mL, 50 mL)
Pepcid®: 10 mg/mL (20 mL) [contains benzyl alcohol]
Injection, solution [preservative free]: 10 mg/mL (2 mL)
Pepcid®: 10 mg/mL (2 mL)
Powder for oral suspension:
Pepcid®: 40 mg/5 mL (50 mL) [contains sodium benzoate; cherry-banana-mint flavor]
Tablet: 10 mg [OTC], 20 mg, 40 mg
Pepcid®: 20 mg, 40 mg
Pepcid® AC: 10 mg, 20 mg
Pepcid® AC Maximum Strength: 20 mg

Famotidine, Calcium Carbonate, and Magnesium Hydroxide

(fa MOE ti deen, KAL see um KAR bun ate, & mag NEE zhum hye DROKS ide)

U.S. Brand Names Pepcid® Complete [OTC]
Canadian Brand Names Pepcid® Complete [OTC]
Index Terms Calcium Carbonate, Magnesium Hydroxide, and Famotidine; Magnesium Hydroxide, Famotidine, and Calcium Carbonate
Pharmacologic Category Antacid; Histamine H_2 Antagonist
Use Relief of heartburn due to acid indigestion
Effect on Mental Status May cause dizziness or drowsiness; may rarely cause insomnia
Effect on Psychiatric Treatment May cause agranulocytosis; use caution with clozapine and carbamazepine
Dosage Summary
Oral:
Children <12 years: Dosage not established
Children ≥12 years: 1 tablet as needed (maximum: 2 tablets/day)
Adults: 1 tablet as needed (maximum: 2 tablets/day)
Dosage Forms Excipient information presented when available (limited, particularly for generics); consult specific product labeling.
Tablet, chewable: Famotidine 10 mg, calcium carbonate 800 mg, and magnesium hydroxide 165 mg [berry blend and mint flavors]

- **Famvir®** *see* Famciclovir *on page 613*
- **Fansidar®** *see* Sulfadoxine and Pyrimethamine *on page 1517*
- **Fareston®** *see* Toremifene *on page 1603*
- **Faslodex®** *see* Fulvestrant *on page 698*
- **Father John's® Plus [OTC]** *see* Chlorpheniramine, Phenylephrine, and Dextromethorphan *on page 327*
- **FazaClo®** *see* Clozapine *on page 386*
- **5-FC** *see* Flucytosine *on page 640*
- **FC1157a** *see* Toremifene *on page 1603*
- **Featherfew** *see* Feverfew *(Tanacetum parthenium) on page 628*
- **Featherfoil** *see* Feverfew *(Tanacetum parthenium) on page 628*
- **Febrifuge Plant** *see* Feverfew *(Tanacetum parthenium) on page 628*

Felbamate (FEL ba mate)

U.S. Brand Names Felbatol®
Pharmacologic Category Anticonvulsant, Miscellaneous

Generic Available No

Use Not as a first-line antiepileptic treatment; only in those patients who respond inadequately to alternative treatments and whose epilepsy is so severe that a substantial risk of aplastic anemia and/or liver failure is deemed acceptable in light of the benefits conferred by its use. Patient must be fully advised of risk and provide signed written informed consent. Felbamate can be used as either monotherapy or adjunctive therapy in the treatment of partial seizures (with and without generalization) and in adults with epilepsy. Used as adjunctive therapy in the treatment of partial and generalized seizures associated with Lennox-Gastaut syndrome in children.

Effect on Mental Status Anxiety and dizziness are common; may cause drowsiness, insomnia, or depression

Effect on Psychiatric Treatment Carbamazepine may decrease effects of felbamate; may increase effects of valproic acid

Restrictions A patient "informed consent" form should be completed and signed by the patient and physician. Copies are available from Wallace Pharmaceuticals by calling 800-526-3840 or 609-655-6147.

Pregnancy Risk Factor C

Pregnancy Considerations There are no adequate and well-controlled studies in pregnant women. Postmarketing case reports in humans include fetal death, genital malformation, anencephaly, encephalocele, and placental disorder.

Lactation Enters breast milk/not recommended

Contraindications Hypersensitivity to felbamate any component of the formulation; or known sensitivity to other carbamates; history of any blood dyscrasia; hepatic dysfunction

Warnings/Precautions Use with caution in patients allergic to other carbamates (eg, meprobamate); antiepileptic drugs should not be suddenly discontinued because of the possibility of increasing seizure frequency. **[U.S. Boxed Warning]: Felbamate is associated with an increased risk of aplastic anemia. [U.S. Boxed Warning]: Felbamate has been associated with rare cases of hepatic failure (estimated >6 cases per 75,000 patients per year).** Do not initiate treatment in patients with pre-existing hepatic dysfunction. Use caution in renal impairment (dose adjustment recommended). "Informed consent" (concerning hematological/hepatic risks) should be documented prior to initiation of therapy. Effects with other sedative drugs or ethanol may be potentiated.

Adverse Reactions

>10%:

Central nervous system: Somnolence (children 48%; adults 19%), headache (children 7%; adults 7% to 37%), fever (children 23%; adults 3%), dizziness (18%), insomnia (9% to 18%), fatigue (7% to 17%), nervousness (7% to 16%)

Dermatologic: Purpura (children 13%)

Gastrointestinal: Anorexia (children 55%; adults 19%), vomiting (children 39%; adults 9% to 17%), nausea (children 7%; adults 34%), constipation (7% to 13%), dyspepsia (7% to 12%)

Respiratory: Upper respiratory infection (children 45%; adults 5% to 9%)

1% to 10%:

Cardiovascular: Chest pain (3%), facial edema (3%), palpitation (≥1%), tachycardia (≥1%)

Central nervous system: Nervousness (7% to 16%), abnormal thinking (7%), emotional lability (children 7%), ataxia (4% to 7%), depression (5%), anxiety (5%), stupor (3%), malaise ≥1%), agitation (≥1%) psychological disturbances (≥1%), aggressive reaction (≥1%), euphoria (≤1%), hallucination (≤1%), migraine (≤1%), suicide attempt (≤1%)

Dermatologic: Skin rash (children 10%; adults 3% to 4%), acne (3%), pruritus (≥1%), bullous eruption (≤1%), urticaria (≤1%)

Endocrine and metabolic: Hypophosphatemia (≤1% to 3%), intramenstrual bleeding (3%), hypokalemia (≤1%), hyponatremia (≤1%)

Gastrointestinal: Hiccup (children 10%), weight loss (3% to 7%), taste perversion (6%), diarrhea (5%), abdominal pain (5%), xerostomia (3%), weight gain (≥1%), appetite increased (≤1%), esophagitis (≤1%)

Genitourinary: Urinary tract infection (3%)

Hematologic: Leukopenia (1% to 7%), granulocytopenia (≤1%), lymphadenopathy (≤1%), leukocytosis (≤1%), thrombocytopenia (≤1%)

Hepatic: Liver function tests increased (1% to 4%), alkaline phosphatase increased (≤1%)

Neuromuscular & skeletal: Abnormal gait (children 10%; adults 5%), pain (children 7%), tremor (6%), paresthesia (4%), myalgia (3%), weakness (≥1%), dystonia (≤1%)

Ocular: Miosis (7%), diplopia (3% to 6%), abnormal vision (5%)
Otic: Otitis media (children 10%; adults 3%)
Respiratory: Pharyngitis (children 10%; adults 3%), cough (children 7%), rhinitis (7%), sinusitis (4%)
Miscellaneous: Flu-like syndrome (≥1%), lymphadenopathy (≥1%)
<1% (Limited to important or life-threatening): Acute renal failure, agranulocytosis, allergic reaction, alopecia, anaphylactoid reaction, anemia, aplastic anemia, atrial arrhythmia, atrial fibrillation, bradycardia, cardiac arrest, cardiac failure, cerebrovascular disorder, cerebral edema, choreoathetosis, coagulation disorder, coma, concentration impaired, confusion, CPK increased, delusion, diaphoresis, DIC, dysphagia, dyspnea, dysarthria, dyskinesia, dysuria, embolism, encephalopathy, enteritis, eosinophilia, epistaxis, extrapyramidal disorder, flushing, gastric ulcer, gastritis, gastroesophageal reflux, GI hemorrhage, gingival bleeding, glossitis, hematemesis, hematuria, hemolytic anemia, Henoch-Schönlein vasculitis, hepatic failure, hepatitis, hepatorenal syndrome, hyperammonemia, hyper-/hypoglycemia, hyper-/hypotension, hypernatremia, hypocalcemia, hypomagnesemia, hypoxia, ileus, ischemic necrosis, jaundice, manic reaction, mononeuritis, nephrosis, nystagmus, pancreatitis, pancytopenia, paralysis, paranoid reaction, peripheral ischemia, photosensitivity, platelet disorder, pleural effusion, pneumonitis, psychosis, pulmonary hemorrhage, rectal hemorrhage, renal function abnormal, respiratory depression, rhabdomyolysis, SIADH, Stevens-Johnson syndrome, sudden death, suicidal behavior/ideation, SVT, thrombophlebitis, torsade de pointes, toxic epidermal necrolysis, ulcerative stomatitis, urinary retention, urticaria

Metabolism/Transport Effects Substrate of CYP2E1 (minor), 3A4 (major); **Inhibits** CYP2C19 (weak); **Induces** CYP3A4 (weak)

Drug Interactions

Alcohol (Ethyl): CNS Depressants may enhance the CNS depressant effect of Alcohol (Ethyl). *Risk C: Monitor therapy*

Barbiturates: Felbamate may increase the serum concentration of Barbiturates. *Risk C: Monitor therapy*

CNS Depressants: May enhance the adverse/toxic effect of other CNS Depressants. *Risk C: Monitor therapy*

CYP3A4 Inducers (Strong): May increase the metabolism of CYP3A4 Substrates. *Risk C: Monitor therapy*

CYP3A4 Inhibitors (Moderate): May decrease the metabolism of CYP3A4 Substrates. *Risk C: Monitor therapy*

CYP3A4 Inhibitors (Strong): May decrease the metabolism of CYP3A4 Substrates. *Risk D: Consider therapy modification*

Dasatinib: May increase the serum concentration of CYP3A4 Substrates. *Risk C: Monitor therapy*

Deferasirox: May decrease the serum concentration of CYP3A4 Substrates. *Risk C: Monitor therapy*

Herbs (CYP3A4 Inducers): May increase the metabolism of CYP3A4 Substrates. *Risk C: Monitor therapy*

Ketorolac: May diminish the therapeutic effect of Anticonvulsants. *Risk C: Monitor therapy*

Maraviroc: CYP3A4 Inducers may decrease the serum concentration of Maraviroc. *Risk D: Consider therapy modification*

Mefloquine: May diminish the therapeutic effect of Anticonvulsants. Mefloquine may decrease the serum concentration of Anticonvulsants. Management: Mefloquine is contraindicated in persons with a history of convulsions. If anticonvulsant is being used for another indication monitor response to treatment closely, as concurrent mefloquine may decrease response to treatment. *Risk D: Consider therapy modification*

Oral Contraceptive (Estrogens): Felbamate may decrease the serum concentration of Oral Contraceptive (Estrogens). Contraceptive failure is possible. *Risk D: Consider therapy modification*

Oral Contraceptive (Progestins): Felbamate may decrease the serum concentration of Oral Contraceptive (Progestins). Contraceptive failure is possible. *Risk D: Consider therapy modification*

Phenytoin: May increase the metabolism of Felbamate. Felbamate may increase the serum concentration of Phenytoin. *Risk D: Consider therapy modification*

Primidone: Felbamate may increase the serum concentration of Primidone. Specifically, the concentration of its metabolite, phenobarbital. *Risk C: Monitor therapy*

Valproic Acid: Felbamate may increase the serum concentration of Valproic Acid. *Risk D: Consider therapy modification*

Ethanol/Nutrition/Herb Interactions

Ethanol: Avoid ethanol (may increase CNS depression).

Food: Food does not affect absorption.
Herb/Nutraceutical: Avoid evening primrose (seizure threshold decreased).

Stability Store in tightly closed container at controlled room temperature of 20°C to 25°C (68°F to 77°F).

Mechanism of Action Mechanism of action is unknown but has properties in common with other marketed anticonvulsants; has weak inhibitory effects on GABA-receptor binding, benzodiazepine receptor binding, and is devoid of activity at the MK-801 receptor binding site of the NMDA receptor-ionophore complex.

Pharmacodynamics/Kinetics

Absorption: Rapid and almost complete; food has no effect upon the tablet's absorption
Distribution: V_d: 0.7-0.8 L/kg
Protein binding: 22% to 25%, primarily to albumin
Half-life elimination: 20-23 hours (average); prolonged in renal dysfunction
Time to peak, serum: 3-5 hours
Excretion: Urine (40% to 50% as unchanged drug, 40% as inactive metabolites)

Dosage Anticonvulsant:

Monotherapy: Children >14 years and Adults:

Initial: 1200 mg/day in divided doses 3 or 4 times/day; titrate previously untreated patients under close clinical supervision, increasing the dosage in 600 mg increments every 2 weeks to 2400 mg/day based on clinical response and thereafter to 3600 mg/day as clinically indicated

Conversion to monotherapy: Initiate at 1200 mg/day in divided doses 3 or 4 times/day, reduce the dosage of the concomitant anticonvulsant(s) by 20% to 33% at the initiation of felbamate therapy; at week 2, increase the felbamate dosage to 2400 mg/day while reducing the dosage of the other anticonvulsant(s) up to an additional 33% of their original dosage; at week 3, increase the felbamate dosage up to 3600 mg/day and continue to reduce the dosage of the other anticonvulsant(s) as clinically indicated

Adjunctive therapy: **Note:** Dose of concomitant carbamazepine, phenobarbital, phenytoin, or valproic acid should be decreased by 20% to 33% when initiating felbamate therapy. Further dosage reductions may be necessary as dose of felbamate is increased.

Children 2-14 years with Lennox-Gastaut syndrome: Initial: 15 mg/kg/day in divided doses 3 or 4 times/day; may increase once per week by 15 mg/kg/day increments up to 45 mg/kg/day in divided doses 3 or 4 times/day.

Children >14 years and Adults: Initial: 1200 mg/day in divided doses 3 or 4 times/day; may increase once per week by 1200 mg/day increments up to 3600 mg/day in divided doses 3 or 4 times/day.

Dosage adjustment in renal impairment: Use caution; reduce initial and maintenance doses by 50% (half-life prolonged by 9-15 hours)

Dietary Considerations May be taken without regard to meals.

Administration Administer on an empty stomach for best absorption.

Monitoring Parameters Monitor serum levels of concomitant anticonvulsant therapy; obtain transaminases (AST, ALT) levels before initiation of therapy and periodically thereafter and bilirubin weekly. Hematologic evaluations before therapy begins, frequently during therapy, and for a significant period after discontinuation.

Reference Range Not necessary to routinely monitor serum drug levels, since dose should be titrated to clinical response

Additional Information Monotherapy has not been associated with gingival hyperplasia, impaired concentration, weight gain, or abnormal thinking. Because felbamate is the only drug shown effective in Lennox-Gastaut syndrome, it is considered an orphan drug for this indication.

Dosage Forms Excipient information presented when available (limited, particularly for generics); consult specific product labeling.

Suspension, oral:
Felbatol®: 600 mg/5 mL (240 mL, 960 mL)

Tablet:
Felbatol®: 400 mg; 600 mg

◆ **Felbatol®** *see* Felbamate *on page 614*
◆ **Feldene®** *see* Piroxicam *on page 1307*

Felodipine (fe LOE di peen)

Medication Safety Issues

Sound-alike/look-alike issues:
Plendil® may be confused with Isordil®, pindolol, Pletal®, Prilosec®, Prinivil®

Related Information
Calcium Channel Blockers *on page 1778*

U.S. Brand Names Plendil®

Canadian Brand Names Plendil®; Renedil®

Mexican Brand Names Munobal; Plendil

Pharmacologic Category Calcium Channel Blocker

Generic Available Yes

Use Treatment of hypertension

Unlabeled/Investigational Use Pediatric hypertension

Effect on Mental Status May cause dizziness; rarely may cause nervousness, insomnia, or depression

Effect on Psychiatric Treatment Carbamazepine may decrease felodipine effect

Pregnancy Risk Factor C

Pregnancy Considerations Potentially, calcium channel blockers may prolong labor. There are no adequate or well-controlled studies in pregnant women.

Lactation Excretion in breast milk unknown/not recommended

Contraindications Hypersensitivity to felodipine, any component of the formulation, or other calcium channel blocker

Warnings/Precautions Increased angina and/or MI has occurred with initiation or dosage titration of dihydropyridine calcium channel blockers, reflex tachycardia may occur resulting in angina and/or MI in patients with obstructive coronary disease especially in the absence of concurrent beta-blockade. Use with extreme caution in patients with severe aortic stenosis. Use caution in patients with heart failure and/or hypertrophic cardiomyopathy with outflow tract obstruction. Elderly patients and patients with hepatic impairment should start off with a lower dose. Peripheral edema (dose dependent) is the most common side effect (occurs within 2-3 weeks of starting therapy). Symptomatic hypotension with or without syncope can rarely occur; blood pressure must be lowered at a rate appropriate for the patient's clinical condition. Safety and efficacy in children have not been established. Dosage titration should occur after 14 days on a given dose.

Adverse Reactions

>10%: Central nervous system: Headache (11% to 15%)

2% to 10%: Cardiovascular: Peripheral edema (2% to 17%), tachycardia (0.4% to 2.5%), flushing (4% to 7%)

<1% (Limited to important or life-threatening): Angina, angioedema, anxiety, arrhythmia, CHF, CVA, libido decreased, depression, dizziness, gingival hyperplasia, dyspnea, dysuria, gynecomastia, hypotension, impotence, insomnia, irritability, leukocytoclastic vasculitis, MI, nervousness, paresthesia, somnolence, syncope, urticaria, vomiting

Metabolism/Transport Effects Substrate of CYP3A4 (major); **Inhibits** CYP2C8 (moderate), 2C9 (weak), 2D6 (weak), 3A4 (weak)

Drug Interactions

Alpha1-Blockers: May enhance the hypotensive effect of Calcium Channel Blockers. *Risk C: Monitor therapy*

Antifungal Agents (Azole Derivatives, Systemic): May decrease the metabolism of Calcium Channel Blockers. *Risk D: Consider therapy modification*

Barbiturates: May increase the metabolism of Calcium Channel Blockers. *Risk D: Consider therapy modification*

Calcium Channel Blockers (Nondihydropyridine): May enhance the hypotensive effect of Calcium Channel Blockers (Dihydropyridine). Calcium Channel Blockers (Nondihydropyridine) may decrease the metabolism of Calcium Channel Blockers (Dihydropyridine). *Risk C: Monitor therapy*

Calcium Salts: May diminish the therapeutic effect of Calcium Channel Blockers. *Risk C: Monitor therapy*

CarBAMazepine: May increase the metabolism of Calcium Channel Blockers (Dihydropyridine). *Risk C: Monitor therapy*

Cimetidine: May decrease the metabolism of Calcium Channel Blockers. *Risk D: Consider therapy modification*

CycloSPORINE: May decrease the metabolism of Calcium Channel Blockers (Dihydropyridine). Nicardipine may likewise inhibit the metabolism of cyclosporine. Cyclosporine dosage adjustments might be needed. *Risk C: Monitor therapy*

CYP2C8 Substrates (High risk): CYP2C8 Inhibitors (Moderate) may decrease the metabolism of CYP2C8 Substrates (High risk). *Risk C: Monitor therapy*

CYP3A4 Inducers (Strong): May increase the metabolism of CYP3A4 Substrates. *Risk C: Monitor therapy*

CYP3A4 Inhibitors (Moderate): May decrease the metabolism of CYP3A4 Substrates. *Risk C: Monitor therapy*

CYP3A4 Inhibitors (Strong): May decrease the metabolism of CYP3A4 Substrates. *Risk D: Consider therapy modification*

Dasatinib: May increase the serum concentration of CYP3A4 Substrates. *Risk C: Monitor therapy*

Deferasirox: May decrease the serum concentration of CYP3A4 Substrates. *Risk C: Monitor therapy*

Diazoxide: May enhance the hypotensive effect of Antihypertensives. *Risk C: Monitor therapy*

Fluconazole: May decrease the metabolism of Calcium Channel Blockers. *Risk C: Monitor therapy*

Grapefruit Juice: May decrease the metabolism of Calcium Channel Blockers. *Risk C: Monitor therapy*

Herbs (CYP3A4 Inducers): May increase the metabolism of CYP3A4 Substrates. *Risk C: Monitor therapy*

Herbs (Hypertensive Properties): May diminish the antihypertensive effect of Antihypertensives. *Risk C: Monitor therapy*

Herbs (Hypotensive Properties): May enhance the hypotensive effect of Antihypertensives. *Risk C: Monitor therapy*

Macrolide Antibiotics: May decrease the metabolism of Calcium Channel Blockers. **Exceptions:** Azithromycin; Dirithromycin [Off Market]; Spiramycin. *Risk D: Consider therapy modification*

Magnesium Salts: Calcium Channel Blockers may enhance the adverse/toxic effect of Magnesium Salts. Magnesium Salts may enhance the hypotensive effect of Calcium Channel Blockers. *Risk C: Monitor therapy*

Methylphenidate: May diminish the antihypertensive effect of Antihypertensives. *Risk C: Monitor therapy*

Nafcillin: May increase the metabolism of Calcium Channel Blockers. *Risk D: Consider therapy modification*

Neuromuscular-Blocking Agents (Nondepolarizing): Calcium Channel Blockers may enhance the neuromuscular-blocking effect of Neuromuscular-Blocking Agents (Nondepolarizing). *Risk C: Monitor therapy*

Nitroprusside: Calcium Channel Blockers may enhance the hypotensive effect of Nitroprusside. *Risk C: Monitor therapy*

Phenytoin: Calcium Channel Blockers may decrease the metabolism of Phenytoin. *Risk D: Consider therapy modification*

Prostacyclin Analogues: May enhance the hypotensive effect of Antihypertensives. *Risk C: Monitor therapy*

Protease Inhibitors: May decrease the metabolism of Calcium Channel Blockers (Dihydropyridine). *Risk D: Consider therapy modification*

Quinupristin: May decrease the metabolism of Calcium Channel Blockers. *Risk C: Monitor therapy*

Rifamycin Derivatives: May increase the metabolism of Calcium Channel Blockers. This primarily affects oral forms of calcium channel blockers. *Risk D: Consider therapy modification*

RiTUXimab: Antihypertensives may enhance the hypotensive effect of RiTUXimab. *Risk D: Consider therapy modification*

Tacrolimus: Calcium Channel Blockers (Dihydropyridine) may increase the serum concentration of Tacrolimus. *Risk C: Monitor therapy*

Ethanol/Nutrition/Herb Interactions

Ethanol: Increases felodipine's absorption; watch for a greater hypotensive effect.

Food: Increased therapeutic and vasodilator side effects, including severe hypotension and myocardial ischemia, may occur if felodipine is taken with grapefruit juice; avoid concurrent use. High-fat/carbohydrate meals will increase C_{max} by 60%; grapefruit juice will increase C_{max} by twofold.

Herb/Nutraceutical: St John's wort may decrease felodipine levels. Avoid dong quai if using for hypertension (has estrogenic activity). Avoid ephedra, yohimbe, ginseng (may worsen hypertension). Avoid garlic (may have increased antihypertensive effect).

Mechanism of Action Inhibits calcium ions from entering the "slow channels" or select voltage-sensitive areas of vascular smooth muscle and myocardium during depolarization, producing a relaxation of coronary vascular smooth muscle and coronary vasodilation; increases myocardial oxygen delivery in patients with vasospastic angina

Pharmacodynamics/Kinetics

Onset of action: Antihypertensive: 2-5 hours

Duration of antihypertensive effect: 24 hours

Absorption: 100%; Absolute: 20% due to first-pass effect

Protein binding: >99%

Metabolism: Hepatic; CYP3A4 substrate (major); extensive first-pass effect

Half-life elimination: Immediate release: 11-16 hours

Excretion: Urine (70% as metabolites); feces 10%

Dosage Oral: Hypertension:
Children (unlabeled use): Initial: 2.5 mg once daily; maximum: 10 mg/day
Adults: Oral: 2.5-10 mg once daily; usual initial dose: 5 mg; increase by 5 mg at 2-week intervals, as needed, to a maximum of 20 mg/day
Usual dose range (JNC 7) for hypertension: 2.5-20 mg once daily
Elderly: Begin with 2.5 mg/day
Dosing adjustment/comments in hepatic impairment: Initial: 2.5 mg/day; monitor blood pressure

Dietary Considerations Should be taken without food.

Administration Do not crush or chew extended release tablets; swallow whole.

Additional Information Felodipine maintains renal and mesenteric blood flow during hemorrhagic shock in animals.

Dosage Forms Excipient information presented when available (limited, particularly for generics); consult specific product labeling.
Tablet, extended release: 2.5 mg, 5 mg, 10 mg
Plendil®: 2.5 mg, 5 mg, 10 mg

- **Felodipine and Enalapril** *see* Enalapril and Felodipine *on page 536*
- **Femara®** *see* Letrozole *on page 900*
- **Femcon™ Fe** *see* Ethinyl Estradiol and Norethindrone *on page 597*
- **femhrt®** *see* Ethinyl Estradiol and Norethindrone *on page 597*
- **Femiron® [OTC]** *see* Ferrous Fumarate *on page 626*
- **Fem-Prin® [OTC]** *see* Acetaminophen, Aspirin, and Caffeine *on page 39*
- **Femring®** *see* Estradiol *on page 576*
- **Femtrace®** *see* Estradiol *on page 576*
- **Fenesin DM IR** *see* Guaifenesin and Dextromethorphan *on page 739*
- **Fenesin IR** *see* GuaiFENesin *on page 737*
- **Fenesin PE IR** *see* Guaifenesin and Phenylephrine *on page 742*

Fenofibrate (fen oh FYE brate)

Medication Safety Issues
Sound-alike/look-alike issues:
TriCor® may be confused with Tracleer®

Related Information
Lipid-Lowering Agents *on page 1786*

U.S. Brand Names Antara™; Fenoglide™; Lipofen™; Lofibra®; TriCor®; Triglide™

Canadian Brand Names Apo-Feno-Micro®; Apo-Fenofibrate®; Dom-Fenofibrate Supra; Gen-Fenofibrate Micro; Lipidil EZ®; Lipidil Micro®; Lipidil Supra®; Novo-Fenofibrate; Novo-Fenofibrate-S; Nu-Fenofibrate; PHL-Fenofibrate Supra; PMS-Fenofibrate Micro; PMS-Fenofibrate Supra; ratio-Fenofibrate MC; Sandoz Fenofibrate S; TriCor®

Mexican Brand Names Controlip

Index Terms Procetofene; Proctofene

Pharmacologic Category Antilipemic Agent, Fibric Acid

Generic Available Yes: Micronized capsule and tablet

Use Adjunct to dietary therapy for the treatment of adults with elevations of serum triglyceride levels (types IV and V hyperlipidemia); adjunct to dietary therapy for the reduction of low density lipoprotein cholesterol (LDL-C), total cholesterol (total-C), triglycerides, and apolipoprotein B (apo B) in adult patients with primary hypercholesterolemia or mixed dyslipidemia (Fredrickson types IIa and IIb)

Effect on Mental Status May rarely cause drowsiness or insomnia

Effect on Psychiatric Treatment None reported

Pregnancy Risk Factor C

Pregnancy Considerations Animal studies have shown embryocidal and teratogenic effect. There are no adequate and well-controlled studies in pregnant women. Use should be avoided, if possible, in pregnant women since the neonatal glucuronide conjugation pathways are immature.

Lactation Excretion in breast milk unknown/not recommended

Contraindications Hypersensitivity to fenofibrate or any component of the formulation; hepatic dysfunction including primary biliary cirrhosis and unexplained persistent liver function abnormalities; severe renal dysfunction; pre-existing gallbladder disease; breast-feeding (only Fenoglide™)

Warnings/Precautions Secondary causes of hyperlipidemia should be ruled out prior to therapy. Hepatic transaminases can become significantly elevated (dose-related); hepatocellular, chronic active, and cholestatic hepatitis have been reported. Regular monitoring of liver function tests is required. May cause cholelithiasis. Use caution with warfarin; adjustments in warfarin therapy may be required. Use caution with HMG-CoA reductase inhibitors (may lead to myopathy, rhabdomyolysis). In combination with HMG-CoA reductase inhibitors, fenofibrate is generally regarded as safer than gemfibrozil due to limited pharmacokinetic interaction with statins. Therapy should be withdrawn if an adequate response is not obtained after 2 months of therapy at the maximal daily dose. The occurrence of pancreatitis may represent a failure of efficacy in patients with severely elevated triglycerides. May cause mild-to-moderate decreases in hemoglobin, hematocrit, and WBC upon initiation of therapy which usually stabilizes with long-term therapy. Rare hypersensitivity reactions may occur. Use has been associated with pulmonary embolism (PE) and deep vein thrombosis (DVT). Use with caution in patients with risk factors for VTE. Dose adjustment is required for renal impairment and elderly patients. Safety and efficacy in children have not been established.

Adverse Reactions

>10%: Hepatic: ALT increased (dose related; 3% to 13%), AST increased (dose related; 3% to 13%)

1% to 10%:

Central nervous system: Headache (3%)
Gastrointestinal: Abdominal pain (5%), constipation (2%)
Neuromuscular & skeletal: Back pain (3%)
Respiratory: Respiratory disorder (6%), rhinitis (2%)

Postmarketing and/or case reports (limited to important or life-threatening): Abnormal vision, acne, agranulocytosis, allergic reaction, alopecia, amblyopia, anemia, angina pectoris, anorexia, anxiety, appetite increased, arrhythmia, arthralgia, arthritis, arthrosis, asthma, atrial fibrillation, bruising, bursitis, cataract, chest pain, cholecystitis, cholelithiasis, cholestatic hepatitis, cirrhosis, colitis, conjunctivitis, contact dermatitis, cough increased, creatine phosphokinase increased, creatinine increased, cyst, cystitis, deep venous thrombosis, depression, diabetes mellitus, diaphoresis, diarrhea, dizziness, dry mouth, duodenal ulcer, dyspepsia, dyspnea, dysuria, ear pain, eczema, edema, electrocardiogram abnormality, eosinophilia, eructation, esophagitis, extrasystoles, eye disorder, fatty liver deposits, fever, flatulence, fungal dermatitis, gastritis, gastroenteritis, gastrointestinal disorder, gout, gynecomastia, hepatitis, hernia, herpes simplex, herpes zoster, hyper-/hypotension, hypersensitivity reaction, hypertonia, hyperuricemia, hypoglycemia, infection, insomnia, joint disorder, kidney function abnormality, laryngitis, leg cramps, leukopenia, libido decreased, lymphadenopathy, maculopapular rash, malaise, MI, myalgia, myasthenia, myopathy, myositis, nail disorder, nausea, nervousness, neuralgia, otitis media, pain, palpitation, pancreatitis, paresthesia, peptic ulcer, peripheral edema, peripheral vascular disorder, pharyngitis, phlebitis, photosensitivity reaction, pneumonia, prostatic disorder, pruritus, pulmonary embolus, rectal disorder, rectal hemorrhage, refraction disorder, rhabdomyolysis, skin ulcer, somnolence, Stevens-Johnson syndrome, tachycardia, tenosynovitis, thrombocytopenia, tooth disorder, toxic epidermal necrolysis, urinary frequency, urolithiasis, urticaria, vaginal moniliasis, varicose veins, vasodilatation, vertigo, vomiting, weakness, weight gain/loss

Metabolism/Transport Effects **Substrate** of CYP3A4 (minor); **Inhibits** CYP2A6 (weak), 2C8 (weak), 2C9 (weak), 2C19 (weak)

Drug Interactions

Bile Acid Sequestrants: May decrease the absorption of Fibric Acid Derivatives. **Exceptions:** Colesevelam. *Risk D: Consider therapy modification*

Ezetimibe: Fibric Acid Derivatives may increase the serum concentration of Ezetimibe. *Risk C: Monitor therapy*

HMG-CoA Reductase Inhibitors: Fenofibrate may enhance the adverse/toxic effect of HMG-CoA Reductase Inhibitors. *Risk C: Monitor therapy*

Sulfonylureas: Fibric Acid Derivatives may enhance the hypoglycemic effect of Sulfonylureas. *Risk C: Monitor therapy*

Vitamin K Antagonists (eg, warfarin): Fibric Acid Derivatives may enhance the anticoagulant effect of Vitamin K Antagonists. *Risk D: Consider therapy modification*

Warfarin: Fenofibrate may enhance the anticoagulant effect of Warfarin. Fenofibrate may increase the serum concentration of Warfarin. *Risk D: Consider therapy modification*

Stability Store at 15°C to 30°C (59°F to 86°F). Protect from light and moisture. Store tablets in moisture-protective container.

Mechanism of Action Fenofibric acid, an agonist for the nuclear transcription factor peroxisome proliferator-activated receptor-alpha (PPAR-alpha), down-regulates apoprotein C-III (an inhibitor of lipoprotein lipase) and upregulates the synthesis of apolipoprotein A-I, fatty acid transport protein, and lipoprotein lipase resulting in an increase in VLDL catabolism, fatty acid oxidation, and elimination of triglyceride-rich particles; as a result of a decrease in VLDL levels, total plasma triglycerides are reduced by 30% to 60%; modest increase in HDL occurs in some hypertriglyceridemic patients.

Pharmacodynamics/Kinetics

Absorption: Increased when taken with meals

Distribution: Widely to most tissues

Protein binding: >99%

Metabolism: Tissue and plasma via esterases to active form, fenofibric acid; undergoes inactivation by glucuronidation hepatically or renally

Half-life elimination: Fenofibric acid: Mean: 20 hours (range: 10-35 hours)

Time to peak: 3-8 hours

Excretion: Urine (60% as metabolites); feces (25%); hemodialysis has no effect on removal of fenofibric acid from plasma

Dosage Oral:

Adults:

Hypertriglyceridemia: Initial:

Antara™ (micronized): 43-130 mg/day; maximum dose: 130 mg/day

Fenoglide™: 40-120 mg/day; maximum dose: 120 mg/day

Lipofen™: 50-150 mg/day; maximum dose: 150 mg/day

Lofibra® (micronized): 67-200 mg/day with meals; maximum dose: 200 mg/day

Lofibra® (tablets): 54-160 mg/day; maximum dose: 160 mg/day

TriCor®: 48-145 mg/day; maximum dose: 145 mg/day

Triglide™: 50-160 mg/day; maximum dose: 160 mg/day

Hypercholesterolemia or mixed hyperlipidemia:

Antara™ (micronized): 130 mg/day

Fenoglide™: 120 mg/day

Lipofen™: 150 mg/day

Lofibra® (micronized): 200 mg/day

Lofibra® (tablets): 160 mg/day

TriCor®: 145 mg/day

Triglide™: 160 mg/day

Elderly: Initial:

Antara™ (micronized): 43 mg/day

Fenoglide™: Adjust dosage based on creatinine clearance

Lipofen™: 50 mg/day

Lofibra® (micronized): 67 mg/day

Lofibra® (tablets): 54 mg/day

TriCor®: Adjust dosage based on creatinine clearance

Triglide™: 50 mg/day

Dosage adjustment/interval in renal impairment: Monitor renal function and lipid panel before adjusting. Decrease dose or increase dosing interval for patients with renal failure: Initial:

Antara™ (micronized): 43 mg/day

Fenoglide™:

Cl_{cr} 31-80 mL/minute: 40 mg/day

Cl_{cr} ≤30 mL/minute: **Contraindicated**

Lipofen™: 50 mg/day

Lofibra® (micronized): 67 mg/day

Lofibra® (tablets): 54 mg/day

TriCor®:

Cl_{cr} 31-80 mL/minute: 48 mg/day

Cl_{cr} ≤30 mL/minute: **Contraindicated**

Triglide™: 50 mg/day

Dietary Considerations

Fenoglide™, Lofibra® (capsules [micronized] and tablets), Lipofen™: Take with meals.

Antara™, TriCor®, Triglide™: May be taken with or without food.

Administration 6-8 weeks of therapy is required to determine efficacy.

Fenoglide™, Lofibra® (capsules [micronized] and tablets), Lipofen™: Administer with meals.

Antara™, TriCor®: May be administered with or without food.

Triglide™: Do not consume chipped or broken tablets. May be administered with or without food.

Monitoring Parameters Periodic blood counts during first year of therapy. Total cholesterol, LDL-C, triglycerides, and HDL-C should be measured periodically; If only marginal changes are noted in 6-8 weeks, the drug should be discontinued. Monitor LFTs regularly and discontinue therapy if levels remain >3 times normal limits.

Dosage Forms Excipient information presented when available (limited, particularly for generics); consult specific product labeling. [DSC] = Discontinued product

Capsule:

Lipofen™: 50 mg; 100 mg [DSC]; 150 mg

Capsule [micronized]: 67 mg, 134 mg, 200 mg

Antara™: 43 mg, 130 mg

Lofibra®: 67 mg, 134 mg, 200 mg

Tablet: 54 mg, 160 mg

Fenoglide™: 40 mg, 120 mg

Lofibra®: 54 mg, 160 mg

TriCor®: 48 mg, 145 mg

Triglide™: 50 mg, 160 mg

◆ **Fenoglide™** *see* Fenofibrate *on page 620*

Fenoldopam (fe NOL doe pam)

U.S. Brand Names Corlopam®

Canadian Brand Names Corlopam®

Index Terms Fenoldopam Mesylate

Pharmacologic Category Dopamine Agonist

Use Treatment of severe hypertension (up to 48 hours in adults), including in patients with renal compromise; short-term (up to 4 hours) blood pressure reduction in pediatric patients

Effect on Mental Status May cause dizziness

Effect on Psychiatric Treatment Causes hypotension; caution with low potency antipsychotics and TCAs

Dosage Summary

I.V.:

Children: Initial: 0.2 mcg/kg/minute, may increase to 0.3-0.5 mcg/kg/minute every 20-30 minutes (maximum: 0.8 mcg/kg/minute)

Adults: Initial: 0.1-0.3 mcg/kg/minute, may increase in increments of 0.05-0.1 mcg/kg/minute every 15 minutes (maximum: 1.6 mcg/kg/minute)

Dosage Forms Excipient information presented when available (limited, particularly for generics); consult specific product labeling.

Injection, solution: 10 mg/mL (1 mL, 2 mL) [contains sodium metabisulfite and propylene glycol]

◆ **Fenoldopam Mesylate** *see* Fenoldopam *on page 623*

Fenoprofen (fen oh PROE fen)

Medication Safety Issues

Sound-alike/look-alike issues:

Fenoprofen may be confused with flurbiprofen

Nalfon® may be confused with Naldecon®

Related Information

Nonsteroidal Anti-Inflammatory Agents *on page 1792*

U.S. Brand Names Nalfon®

Canadian Brand Names Nalfon®

Mexican Brand Names Nalfon

Index Terms Fenoprofen Calcium

Pharmacologic Category Nonsteroidal Anti-inflammatory Drug (NSAID), Oral

Use Symptomatic treatment of acute and chronic rheumatoid arthritis and osteoarthritis; relief of mild to moderate pain

Effect on Mental Status Dizziness is common; may cause nervousness; rarely may cause insomnia, confusion, depression, or hallucinations

Effect on Psychiatric Treatment May rarely cause may agranulocytosis; use caution with clozapine and carbamazepine; may decrease the clearance of lithium resulting in elevated serum levels and potential toxicity; monitor serum lithium levels; use acetaminophen, if possible, for pain

Restrictions An FDA-approved medication guide must be distributed when dispensing an oral outpatient prescription (new or refill) where this medication is to be used without direct supervision of a healthcare provider. Medication guides are available at http://www.fda.gov/cder/Offices/ODS/medication_guides.htm.

Dosage Summary

Oral:

Children: Dosage not established

Adults: 200 mg every 4-6 hours as needed **or** 300-600 mg 3-4 times/day (maximum: 3.2 g/day)

Dosage Forms Excipient information presented when available (limited, particularly for generics); consult specific product labeling.

Capsule, as calcium:

Nalfon®: 200 mg

Tablet, as calcium: 600 mg

◆ **Fenoprofen Calcium** *see* Fenoprofen *on page 623*

FentaNYL (FEN ta nil)

Medication Safety Issues

Sound-alike/look-alike issues:

FentaNYL may be confused with alfentanil, SUFentanil

Dosing of transdermal fentanyl patches may be confusing. Transdermal fentanyl patches should always be prescribed in mcg/hour, not size. Patch dosage form of Duragesic®-12 actually delivers 12.5 mcg/hour of fentanyl. Use caution, as orders may be written as "Duragesic 12.5" which can be erroneously interpreted as a 125 mcg dose.

Fentora® and Actiq® are not interchangeable; do not substitute doses on a mcg-per-mcg basis.

High alert medication: The Institute for Safe Medication Practices (ISMP) includes this medication among its list of drug classes which have a heightened risk of causing significant patient harm when used in error.

Fentanyl transdermal system patches: Leakage of fentanyl gel from the patch has been reported; patch may be less effective; do not use. Thoroughly wash any skin surfaces coming into direct contact with gel with water (do not use soap).

Transdermal patch (eg, Duragesic®) does not contain any metal-based compounds; however, the printed ink used to indicate strength on the outer surface of the patch does contain titanium dioxide, but the amount is minimal.

Related Information

Narcotic / Opioid Analgesics *on page 1789*

U.S. Brand Names Actiq®; Duragesic®; Fentora®; Sublimaze®

Canadian Brand Names Actiq®; Duragesic®; Fentanyl Citrate Injection, USP; RAN™-Fentanyl Transdermal System; ratio-Fentanyl

Mexican Brand Names Durogesic; Fentanest

Index Terms Fentanyl Citrate; Fentanyl Hydrochloride; OTFC (Oral Transmucosal Fentanyl Citrate)

Pharmacologic Category Analgesic, Opioid; Anilidopiperidine Opioid; General Anesthetic

Use

Injection: Sedation, relief of pain, preoperative medication, adjunct to general or regional anesthesia

Transdermal patch (eg, Duragesic®): Management of persistent moderate-to-severe chronic pain

Transmucosal lozenge (eg, Actiq®), buccal tablet (Fentora®): Management of breakthrough cancer pain in opioid-tolerant patients

Effect on Mental Status Drowsiness, sedation, and depression are common; may rarely cause paradoxical CNS excitement or delirium

Effect on Psychiatric Treatment Concurrent use with low potency antipsychotics and TCAs may produce additive hypotension

Restrictions C-II

An FDA-approved medication guide for buccal tablet (Fentora®), transmucosal lozenge (eg, Actiq®), and transdermal patch (eg, Duragesic®) must be distributed when dispensing an outpatient prescription (new or refill) where this medication is to be used without direct supervision of a healthcare provider. Medication guides are available at http://www.fda.gov/cder/Offices/ODS/medication_guides.htm.

Dosage Summary Note: These are guidelines and do not represent the maximum doses that may be required in all patients. Doses should be titrated to pain relief/prevention.

I.M.:

Children: Dosage not established

Adults: 50-100 mcg/dose every 1-2 hours as needed (unlabeled) **or** 50-100 mcg/dose prior to surgery

I.V.:

Children <2 year: Dosage not established

Children 2-12 years: 2-3 mcg/kg/dose every 1-2 hours as adjunct to anesthesia **or** 0.5-2 mcg/kg/dose given every 1-2 hours as needed (unlabeled)

Children >12 years: 50-100 mcg given 30-60 minutes prior to surgery or 25-100 mcg over 1-2 minutes as adjunct to general anesthesia **or** 25-50 mcg every 1-2 hours as needed (unlabeled)

Adults: 50-100 mcg given 30-60 minutes prior to surgery or 25-100 mcg over 1-2 minutes as adjunct to general anesthesia **or** 50-100 mcg every 1-2 hours as needed (unlabeled)

Adults: Mechanically-ventilated patients (based on 70 kg patient) (unlabeled): 0.35-1.5 mcg/kg every 30-60 minutes as needed; Infusion: 0.7-10 mcg/kg/hour

PCA (unlabeled):

Children: Dosage not established

Adults: Usual concentration: 10 mcg/mL; Basal rate ≤50 mcg/hour; Demand dose: 10-50 mcg; Lockout interval: 5-8 minutes

Transmucosal buccal tablet (Fentora®):

Children <18 years: Dosage not established

Adults: Initial: 100 mcg; a second dose, if needed, may be started 30 minutes after the start of the first dose (maximum: 2 doses per breakthrough pain episode every 4 hours)

Transmucosal lozenge (Actiq®):

Children <16 years: Dosage not established

Children ≥16 years: Initial: 200 mcg; the second dose may be started 15 minutes after completion of the first dose (maximum: 4 units/day)

Adults: Initial: 200 mcg; the second dose may be started 15 minutes after completion of the first dose (maximum: 4 units/day)

Elderly: In clinical trials, patients who were >65 years of age were titrated to a mean dose that was 200 mcg less than that of younger patients.

Transdermal:

Patch:

Children <2 years: Dosage not established

Children ≥2 years: Initial: Opioid-tolerant: Convert 24-hour analgesic requirements to patch using tables; Fentanyl infusion: Dose at rate equivalent to the I.V. rate; Patches range from 12.5-300 mcg/hour applied every 72 hours; **Note:** Titration is recommended

Adults: Initial: Opioid-tolerant: Convert 24-hour analgesic requirements to patch using tables; Fentanyl infusion: Dose at rate equivalent to the I.V. rate; Patches range from 12.5-300 mcg/hour applied every 72 hours; **Note:** Titration is recommended

Dosage Forms Excipient information presented when available (limited, particularly for generics); consult specific product labeling.

Note: Strengths expressed as base.

Injection, solution, as citrate [preservative free]: 0.05 mg/mL (2 mL, 5 mL, 10 mL, 20 mL; 30 mL [DSC]; 50 mL)

Sublimaze®: 0.05 mg/mL (2 mL, 5 mL, 10 mL [DSC], 20 mL)

Lozenge, oral, as citrate [transmucosal]: 200 mcg, 400 mcg, 600 mcg, 800 mcg, 1200 mcg, 1600 mcg

Actiq®: 200 mcg, 400 mcg, 600 mcg, 800 mcg, 1200 mcg, 1600 mcg [contains sugar 2 g/lozenge; berry flavor]

Powder, for prescription compounding, as citrate: USP (1 g)

Tablet, for buccal application, as citrate:

Fentora®: 100 mcg, 200 mcg, 300 mcg, 400 mcg, 600 mcg, 800 mcg

Transdermal system, topical, as base: 12 (5s) [delivers 12.5 mcg/hour; 3.13 cm^2]; 12 (5s) [delivers 12.5 mcg/hour; 5 cm^2]; 25 (5s) [delivers 25 mcg/hour; 10 cm^2]; 25 (5s) [delivers 25 mcg/hour; 6.25 cm^2]; 50 (5s) [delivers 50 mcg/hour; 12.5 cm^2]; 50 (5s) [delivers 50 mcg/hour; 20 cm^2]; 75 (5s) [delivers 75 mcg/hour; 18.75 cm^2]; 75 (5s) [delivers 75 mcg/hour; 30 cm^2]; 100 (5s) [delivers 100 mcg/hour; 25 cm^2]; 100 (5s) [delivers 100 mcg/hour; 40 cm^2]

Duragesic®: 12 (5s) [delivers 12.5 mcg/hour; 5 cm^2; contains ethanol 0.1 mL/10 cm^2]; 25 (5s) [delivers 25 mcg/hour; 10 cm^2; contains ethanol 0.1 mL/10 cm^2]; 50 (5s) [delivers 50 mcg/hour; 20 cm^2; contains ethanol 0.1 mL/10 cm^2]; 75 (5s) [delivers 75 mcg/hour; 30 cm^2; contains ethanol 0.1 mL/10 cm^2]; 100 (5s) [delivers 100 mcg/hour; 40 cm^2; contains ethanol 0.1 mL/10 cm^2]

◆ **Fentanyl Citrate** *see* FentaNYL *on page 624*

◆ **Fentanyl Hydrochloride** *see* FentaNYL *on page 624*

◆ **Fentora®** *see* FentaNYL *on page 624*

◆ **Feosol® [OTC]** *see* Ferrous Sulfate *on page 627*
◆ **Feostat® [OTC] [DSC]** *see* Ferrous Fumarate *on page 626*
◆ **Feratab® [OTC]** *see* Ferrous Sulfate *on page 627*
◆ **Fer-Gen-Sol [OTC]** *see* Ferrous Sulfate *on page 627*
◆ **Fergon® [OTC]** *see* Ferrous Gluconate *on page 627*
◆ **Fer-In-Sol® [OTC]** *see* Ferrous Sulfate *on page 627*
◆ **Fer-Iron® [OTC]** *see* Ferrous Sulfate *on page 627*
◆ **Fero-Grad 500® [OTC]** *see* Ferrous Sulfate and Ascorbic Acid *on page 628*
◆ **Ferretts [OTC]** *see* Ferrous Fumarate *on page 626*
◆ **Ferrex 150 [OTC]** *see* Polysaccharide-Iron Complex *on page 1313*

Ferric Gluconate (FER ik GLOO koe nate)

Medication Safety Issues
Sound-alike/look-alike issues:
Ferrlecit® may be confused with Ferralet®
U.S. Brand Names Ferrlecit®
Canadian Brand Names Ferrlecit®
Index Terms Sodium Ferric Gluconate
Pharmacologic Category Iron Salt
Use Repletion of total body iron content in patients with iron-deficiency anemia who are undergoing hemodialysis in conjunction with erythropoietin therapy
Effect on Mental Status May cause drowsiness, dizziness, insomnia, agitation
Effect on Psychiatric Treatment May cause hypotension; caution with low potency antipsychotics
Dosage Summary
I.V.:
Children <6 years: Dosage not established
Children ≥6 years: 1.5 mg/kg of elemental iron at 8 sequential dialysis sessions (maximum: 125 mg/dose)
Adults: 125 mg of elemental iron at ~8 sequential dialysis treatments to make a cumulative dose of 1 g
Dosage Forms Excipient information presented when available (limited, particularly for generics); consult specific product labeling.
Injection, solution:
Ferrlecit®: Elemental iron 12.5 mg/mL (5 mL) [contains benzyl alcohol and sucrose 20%]

◆ **Ferrlecit®** *see* Ferric Gluconate *on page 626*
◆ **Ferro-Sequels® [OTC]** *see* Ferrous Fumarate *on page 626*

Ferrous Fumarate (FER us FYOO ma rate)

Medication Safety Issues
Sound-alike/look-alike issues:
Feostat® may be confused with Feosol®
U.S. Brand Names Femiron® [OTC]; Feostat® [OTC] [DSC]; Ferretts [OTC]; Ferro-Sequels® [OTC]; Hemocyte® [OTC]; Ircon® [OTC]; Nephro-Fer® [OTC]
Canadian Brand Names Palafer®
Mexican Brand Names Ferval
Index Terms Iron Fumarate
Pharmacologic Category Iron Salt
Use Prevention and treatment of iron-deficiency anemias
Effect on Mental Status None reported
Effect on Psychiatric Treatment Constipation is common; concurrent use with psychotropic agents may increase the risk
Dosage Summary Doses expressed in terms of elemental iron.
Oral:
Children: 1-6 mg elemental iron/kg/day in 1-3 divided doses
Adults: 60 mg elemental iron 2-4 times/day
Elderly: 200 mg elemental iron 3-4 times/day
Dosage Forms Excipient information presented when available (limited, particularly for generics); consult specific product labeling. [DSC] = Discontinued product
Tablet: 324 mg [elemental iron 106 mg]
Femiron®: 63 mg [elemental iron 20 mg]
Ferretts: 325 mg [elemental iron 106 mg]
Hemocyte®: 324 mg [elemental iron 106 mg]

Ircon®: 200 mg [elemental iron 66 mg]
Nephro-Fer®: 350 mg [elemental iron 115 mg; contains tartrazine]
Tablet, chewable (Feostat®): 100 mg [elemental iron 33 mg; chocolate flavor] [DSC]
Tablet, timed release (Ferro-Sequels®): 150 mg [elemental iron 50 mg; contains docusate sodium and sodium benzoate]

Ferrous Gluconate (FER us GLOO koe nate)

U.S. Brand Names Fergon® [OTC]
Canadian Brand Names Apo-Ferrous Gluconate®; Novo-Ferrogluc
Index Terms Iron Gluconate
Pharmacologic Category Iron Salt
Use Prevention and treatment of iron-deficiency anemias
Effect on Mental Status None reported
Effect on Psychiatric Treatment Constipation is common; concurrent use with psychotropic agents may increase the risk
Dosage Summary
Oral:
Children: 1-6 mg Fe/kg/day in 1-3 divided doses
Adults: 60 mg 1-4 times/day
Dosage Forms Excipient information presented when available (limited, particularly for generics); consult specific product labeling. [DSC] = Discontinued product
Tablet: 246 mg [elemental iron 28 mg]; 300 mg [elemental iron 34 mg] [DSC]; 325 mg [elemental iron 36 mg]
Fergon®: 240 mg [elemental iron 27 mg]

Ferrous Sulfate (FER us SUL fate)

Medication Safety Issues
Sound-alike/look-alike issues:
Feosol® may be confused with Feostat®, Fer-In-Sol®
Fer-In-Sol® may be confused with Feosol®
Slow FE® may be confused with Slow-K®
U.S. Brand Names Feosol® [OTC]; Fer-Gen-Sol [OTC]; Fer-In-Sol® [OTC]; Fer-Iron® [OTC]; Feratab® [OTC]; MyKidz Iron 10™; Slow FE® [OTC]
Canadian Brand Names Apo-Ferrous Sulfate®; Fer-In-Sol®; Ferodan™
Mexican Brand Names Hemobion
Index Terms $FeSO_4$; Iron Sulfate
Pharmacologic Category Iron Salt
Use Prevention and treatment of iron-deficiency anemias
Effect on Mental Status None reported
Effect on Psychiatric Treatment GI side effects are common; concomitant use with SSRIs, carbamazepine, valproic acid, and lithium may produce additive effects
Dosage Summary
Oral:
Extended release:
Children: Dosage not established
Adults: 250 mg 1-2 times/day
Immediate release:
Children: 1-6 mg Fe/kg/day in 1-3 divided doses (maximum: 15 mg/day [prophylaxis dosing])
Adults: 300 mg 1-4 times/day
Dosage Forms Excipient information presented when available (limited, particularly for generics); consult specific product labeling.
Elixir: 220 mg/5 mL (480 mL) [elemental iron 44 mg/5 mL; contains alcohol]
Liquid, oral drops: 75 mg/0.6 mL (50 mL) [elemental iron 15 mg/0.6 mL]
Fer-Gen-Sol: 75 mg/0.6 mL (50 mL) [elemental iron 15 mg/0.6 mL]
Fer-In-Sol®: 75 mg/1 mL (50 mL) [elemental iron 15 mg/1 mL; contains alcohol 0.2% and sodium bisulfite]
Fer-Iron®: 75 mg/0.6 mL (50 mL) [elemental iron 15 mg/0.6 mL]
Suspension, oral [drops]:
MyKidz Iron 10™: 75 mg/1.5 mL [elemental iron 15 mg/1.5 mL] (118 mL) [contains propylene glycol; ethanol free, dye free; strawberry-banana flavor]
Tablet: 324 mg [elemental iron 65 mg]; 325 mg [elemental iron 65 mg]
Feratab®: 300 mg [elemental iron 60 mg]
Tablet, exsiccated (Feosol®): 200 mg [elemental iron 65 mg]
Tablet, exsiccated, timed release (Slow FE®): 160 mg [elemental iron 50 mg]

Ferrous Sulfate and Ascorbic Acid

(FER us SUL fate & a SKOR bik AS id)

U.S. Brand Names Fero-Grad 500® [OTC]; Vitelle™ Irospan® [OTC] [DSC]

Index Terms Ascorbic Acid and Ferrous Sulfate; Iron Sulfate and Vitamin C

Pharmacologic Category Iron Salt; Vitamin

Use Treatment of iron deficiency in nonpregnant adults; treatment and prevention of iron deficiency in pregnant adults

Effect on Mental Status None reported

Effect on Psychiatric Treatment Constipation is common; concurrent use with psychotropic agents may increase the risk

Dosage Summary

Oral:

Children: Dosage not established

Adults: 1 tablet daily

Dosage Forms Excipient information presented when available (limited, particularly for generics); consult specific product labeling. [DSC] = Discontinued product

Capsule, extended release (Vitelle™ Irospan®): Ferrous sulfate [elemental iron 65 mg] and ascorbic acid 150 mg [DSC]

Tablet, controlled release (Fero-Grad 500®): Ferrous sulfate 525 mg [elemental iron 105 mg] and ascorbic acid 500 mg

Tablet, extended release (Vitelle™ Irospan®): Ferrous sulfate [elemental iron 65 mg] and ascorbic acid 150 mg [DSC]

◆ **$FeSO_4$** *see* Ferrous Sulfate *on page 627*

◆ **FeverALL® [OTC]** *see* Acetaminophen *on page 30*

Feverfew *(Tanacetum parthenium)*

Natural Product Category Herb

Synonyms *Tanacetum parthenium*; Altamisa; Camomille Grande; Featherfew; Featherfoil; Febrifuge Plant; Midsummer Daisy; Mutterkraut; Wild Chamomile; Wild Quinine

Plant Part Leaf

Dosage and Standardization Oral:

Migraine prevention:100-250 mg, standardized to contain 0.2% parthenolide

Anti-inflammatory and rheumatoid arthritis: 250 mg 3 times/day

NS has a different dose for rheumatoid arthritis: 70-86 dried chopped feverfew leaves daily or 76 mg dried feverfew leaf, corresponding to 2-3 µmol parthenolide, in capsules

Reported Uses

Anti-inflammatory, rheumatoid arthritis (Pattrick, 1989)

Migraine headache (preventive) (Diener, 2005; Johnson, 1985)

Muscle soreness (pharmacologic activity)

Summary Feverfew contains a number of compounds with anti-inflammatory and smooth muscle relaxant activities. It has increased in popularity in recent years, particularly for migraines. Since the effects of this herb may take several weeks of continuous use, individuals should be encouraged to use the herb for a minimum of 1 month before determining whether it has been effective.

Effect on Mental Status May cause insomnia and nervousness

Effect on Psychiatric Treatment Feverfew blocks 5-HT_{2B} and 5-HT_{2A} receptors. Clinical effects of serotonergic antipsychotics and antidepressants may be antagonized; monitor.

Pharmacology Feverfew reportedly inhibits the synthesis of leukotrienes, prostaglandins, and thromboxanes which mediate inflammation. In addition, feverfew is claimed to inhibit platelet aggregation and induce smooth muscle relaxation. It has been used most commonly for migraine headaches. Feverfew has been claimed to relax uterine smooth muscle and should be avoided in pregnancy. It also may inhibit platelet aggregation and blood coagulation.

Theoretical Cautions and Contraindications Use of feverfew is contraindicated in pregnancy (animal data suggests emmenagogue activity) (Bradley, 1992) or in individuals with allergies to members of the *Asteraceae/Compositae* family (chrysanthemum, daisy). The onset of feverfew's effects may be delayed for several weeks. Abrupt discontinuation may increase migraine frequency, rebound headaches, and anxiety. A "post-feverfew syndrome" has been described, including nervousness, insomnia, joint stiffness, and pain which may occur following discontinuation in some individuals.

Pharmacologic activity may include inhibition of platelet aggregation (Makheja, 1982). Based on pharmacologic activity, this herb may be contraindicated in individuals with active bleeding (eg, peptic ulcer, intracranial bleeding). Use with caution in individuals with a history of bleeding, hemostatic disorders, or drug-related hemostatic problems. Use with caution in individuals taking anticoagulant medications, including warfarin, aspirin, aspirin-containing products, NSAIDs, or antiplatelet agents (eg, ticlopidine, clopidogrel, dipyridamole). Discontinue use prior to dental or surgical procedures (generally at least 14 days before).

This herb may also cause gastrointestinal upset and irritation of oral mucosa/tongue.

Feverfew may increase the risk of photosensitivity. Use caution in individuals taking photosensitizing agents.

General Warnings Use all herbal supplements with extreme caution in children <2 years of age and in pregnancy or lactation. Some herbs are contraindicated in pregnancy or lactation; make sure to observe warnings. Use with caution in individuals on medication and with pre-existing medical conditions. Always review for potential herb-drug interactions (HDIs) and other warnings. Large and prolonged doses may increase the potential for adverse effects. Herbs may cause transient adverse effects such as nausea, vomiting, and GI distress due to a variety of chemical constituents. Use caution in individuals having known allergies to plants.

Theoretical Interactions Anticoagulant medications (including warfarin), aspirin or aspirin-containing products, NSAIDs, antiplatelet agents (eg, ticlopidine, clopidogrel, dipyridamole), photosensitizers

References

Bradley PR, ed, *British Herbal Compendium*, Vol 1, Bournemouth, England: British Herbal Medicine Association, 1992, 96-8.

Diener HC, Pfaffenrath V, Schnitker J, et al, "Efficacy and Safety of 6.25 mg t.i.d. Feverfew CO2-Extract (MIG-99) in Migraine Prevention - A Randomized, Double-Blind, Multicentre, Placebo-Controlled Study," *Cephalalgia*, 2005, 25(11):1031-41.

Johnson ES, Kadam NP, Hylands DM, et al, "Efficacy of Feverfew as Prophylactic Treatment of Migraine," *Br Med J (Clin Res Ed)*, 1985, 291(6495):569-73.

Makheja AN and Bailey JM, "A Platelet Phospholipase Inhibitor From the Medicinal Herb Feverfew (*Tanacetum parthenium*)," *Prostaglandins Leukot Med*, 1982, 8(6):653-60.

Natural Standard Research Collaboration, Chief Editors: Ulbricht C, Basch E, *Natural Standard Herb and Supplement Reference - Evidence-Based Clinical Reviews*, USA: Elsevier/Mosby, 2005.

Newall CA, Anderson LA, and Phillipson JD, *Herbal Medicines: A Guide for Health Care Professionals*, London, England: The Pharmaceutical Press, 1996, 119-21.

Pattrick M, Heptinstall S, and Doherty M, "Feverfew in Rheumatoid Arthritis: A Double-Blind Placebo Controlled Study," *Ann Rheum Dis*, 1989, 48(7):547-49.

◆ **Fexmid™** *see* Cyclobenzaprine *on page 405*

Fexofenadine (feks oh FEN a deen)

Medication Safety Issues

Sound-alike/look-alike issues:

Fexofenadine may be confused with fesoterodine

Allegra® may be confused with Viagra®

International issues:

Allegra® may be confused with Allegro® which is a brand name for frovatriptan in Germany; a brand name for fluticasone in Israel

U.S. Brand Names Allegra®; Allegra® ODT

Canadian Brand Names Allegra®

Mexican Brand Names Allegra

Index Terms Fexofenadine Hydrochloride

Pharmacologic Category Histamine H_1 Antagonist; Histamine H_1 Antagonist, Second Generation

Generic Available Yes: Excludes orally disintegrating tablet and suspension

Use Relief of symptoms associated with seasonal allergic rhinitis; treatment of chronic idiopathic urticaria

Effect on Mental Status May cause drowsiness or dizziness

Effect on Psychiatric Treatment None reported

Pregnancy Risk Factor C

Pregnancy Considerations Decreased fetal weight gain and survival were observed in animal studies. There are no adequate and well-controlled studies in pregnant women; use during pregnancy only if potential benefit to mother outweighs possible risk to fetus.

Lactation Excretion in breast milk unknown/use caution (AAP rates "compatible")

Contraindications Hypersensitivity to fexofenadine or any component of the formulation

Warnings/Precautions Use with caution in patients with renal impairment; dosage adjustment recommended. Safety and efficacy in children <6 months of age have not been established; orally disintegrating tablet not recommended for use in children <6 years of age. Orally disintegrating tablet contains phenylalanine.

Adverse Reactions

>10%:

Central nervous system: Headache (5% to 11%)

Gastrointestinal: Vomiting (children 6 months to 5 years: 4% to 12%)

1% to 10%:

Central nervous system: Fatigue (1% to 3%), somnolence (1% to 3%), dizziness (2%), fever (2%), pain (2%), drowsiness (1%)

Endocrine & metabolic: Dysmenorrhea (2%)

Gastrointestinal: Dyspepsia (1% to 2%), diarrhea (3% to 4%), nausea (2%)

Neuromuscular & skeletal: Myalgia (3%), back pain (2% to 3%), pain in extremities (2%)

Otic: Otitis media (2% to 4%)

Respiratory: Upper respiratory tract infection (3% to 4%), cough (2% to 4%), rhinorrhea (1% to 2%)

Miscellaneous: Viral infection (3%)

<1% (Limited to important or life-threatening): Hypersensitivity reactions (anaphylaxis, angioedema, chest tightness, dyspnea, flushing, pruritus, rash, urticaria); insomnia, nervousness, sleep disorders, paroniria

Metabolism/Transport Effects Substrate of CYP3A4 (minor); **Inhibits** CYP2D6 (weak)

Drug Interactions

Acetylcholinesterase Inhibitors (Central): Anticholinergics may diminish the therapeutic effect of Acetylcholinesterase Inhibitors (Central). Acetylcholinesterase Inhibitors (Central) may diminish the therapeutic effect of Anticholinergics. If the anticholinergic action is a side effect of the agent, the result may be beneficial. *Risk C: Monitor therapy*

Alcohol (Ethyl): CNS Depressants may enhance the CNS depressant effect of Alcohol (Ethyl). *Risk C: Monitor therapy*

Amphetamines: May diminish the sedative effect of Antihistamines. *Risk C: Monitor therapy*

Antacids: May decrease the serum concentration of Fexofenadine. Management: No specific recommendations concerning the time required between their administration are provided. Separate administration of each agent by as much time as possible to decrease the risk of an interaction. **Exceptions:** Calcium Carbonate; Magaldrate; Sodium Bicarbonate. *Risk D: Consider therapy modification*

Anticholinergics: May enhance the adverse/toxic effect of other Anticholinergics. **Exceptions:** Paliperidone. *Risk C: Monitor therapy*

Betahistine: Antihistamines may diminish the therapeutic effect of Betahistine. *Risk C: Monitor therapy*

CNS Depressants: May enhance the adverse/toxic effect of other CNS Depressants. *Risk C: Monitor therapy*

Erythromycin: May increase the serum concentration of Fexofenadine. *Risk C: Monitor therapy*

Grapefruit Juice: May decrease the serum concentration of Fexofenadine. *Risk C: Monitor therapy*

Ketoconazole: May increase the serum concentration of Fexofenadine. *Risk C: Monitor therapy*

P-Glycoprotein Inducers: May decrease the serum concentration of P-Glycoprotein Substrates. P-glycoprotein inducers may also further limit the distribution of p-glycoprotein substrates to specific cells/tissues/organs where p-glycoprotein is present in large amounts (e.g., brain, T-lymphocytes, testes, etc.). *Risk C: Monitor therapy*

P-Glycoprotein Inhibitors: May increase the serum concentration of P-Glycoprotein Substrates. P-glycoprotein inhibitors may also enhance the distribution of p-glycoprotein substrates to specific cells/tissues/organs where p-glycoprotein is present in large amounts (e.g., brain, T-lymphocytes, testes, etc.). *Risk C: Monitor therapy*

Pramlintide: May enhance the anticholinergic effect of Anticholinergics. These effects are specific to the GI tract. *Risk D: Consider therapy modification*

Rifampin: May decrease the serum concentration of Fexofenadine. *Risk C: Monitor therapy*

Verapamil: May increase the bioavailability of Fexofenadine. *Risk C: Monitor therapy*

Ethanol/Nutrition/Herb Interactions

Ethanol: Avoid ethanol (although limited with fexofenadine, may increase risk of sedation).

Food: Fruit juice (apple, grapefruit, orange) may decrease bioavailability of fexofenadine by ~36%.

Herb/Nutraceutical: St John's wort may decrease fexofenadine levels.

Stability Store at controlled room temperature of 20°C to 25°C (68°F to 77°F). Protect from excessive moisture.

Mechanism of Action Fexofenadine is an active metabolite of terfenadine and like terfenadine it competes with histamine for H_1-receptor sites on effector cells in the gastrointestinal tract, blood vessels and respiratory tract; it appears that fexofenadine does not cross the blood brain barrier to any appreciable degree, resulting in a reduced potential for sedation

Pharmacodynamics/Kinetics

Onset of action: 60 minutes

Duration: Antihistaminic effect: ≥12 hours

Protein binding: 60% to 70%, primarily albumin and $alpha_1$-acid glycoprotein

Metabolism: Minimal (~5%)

Half-life elimination: 14.4 hours (31% to 72% longer in renal impairment)

Time to peak, serum: ODT: 2 hours (4 hours with high-fat meal); Tablet: ~2.6 hours; Suspension: ~1 hour

Excretion: Feces (~80%) and urine (~11%) as unchanged drug

Dosage Oral:

Chronic idiopathic urticaria: Children 6 months to <2 years: 15 mg twice daily

Chronic idiopathic urticaria, seasonal allergic rhinitis:

Children 2-11 years: 30 mg twice daily

Children ≥12 years and Adults: 60 mg twice daily **or** 180 mg once daily

Elderly: Starting dose: 60 mg once daily; adjust for renal impairment

Dosing adjustment in renal impairment: Cl_{cr} <80 mL/minute:

Children 6 months to <2 years: Initial: 15 mg once daily

Children 2-11 years: Initial: 30 mg once daily

Children ≥12 years and Adults: Initial: 60 mg once daily

Dietary Considerations Allegra® ODT 30 mg contains phenylalanine 5.3 mg/tablet.

Administration

Suspension, tablet: Administer with water only; do not administer with fruit juices. Shake suspension well before use.

Orally disintegrating tablet: Take on an empty stomach. Do not remove from blister pack until administered. Using dry hands, place immediately on tongue. Tablet will dissolve within seconds, and may be swallowed with or without liquid. Do not split or chew.

Monitoring Parameters Relief of symptoms

Dosage Forms Excipient information presented when available (limited, particularly for generics); consult specific product labeling. [DSC] = Discontinued product

Suspension, oral, as hydrochloride:

Allegra®: 6 mg/mL (30 mL [DSC], 300 mL) [contains propylene glycol; raspberry cream]

Tablet, oral, as hydrochloride: 30 mg, 60 mg, 180 mg

Allegra®: 30 mg [DSC], 60 mg, 180 mg

Tablet, orally disintegrating, oral, as hydrochloride:

Allegra® ODT: 30 mg [contains phenylalanine 5.3 mg/tablet; orange cream flavor]

Fexofenadine and Pseudoephedrine

(feks oh FEN a deen & soo doe e FED rin)

Medication Safety Issues

Sound-alike/look-alike issues:

Allegra-D® may be confused with Viagra®

U.S. Brand Names Allegra-D® 12 Hour; Allegra-D® 24 Hour

Canadian Brand Names Allegra-D®

Mexican Brand Names Allegra-D

Index Terms Pseudoephedrine and Fexofenadine

Pharmacologic Category Alpha/Beta Agonist; Histamine H_1 Antagonist; Histamine H_1 Antagonist, Second Generation

Use Relief of symptoms associated with seasonal allergic rhinitis in adults and children ≥12 years of age

Effect on Mental Status May cause drowsiness or dizziness, nervousness, and insomnia; may rarely cause hallucinations

Effect on Psychiatric Treatment Contraindicated with MAO inhibitors

Dosage Summary

Oral:

Children <12 years: Dosage not established

Children ≥12 years:

Allegra-D® 12 Hour: One tablet twice daily

Allegra-D® 24 Hour: One tablet once daily

Adults:

Allegra-D® 12 Hour: One tablet twice daily

Allegra-D® 24 Hour: One tablet once daily

Dosage Forms Excipient information presented when available (limited, particularly for generics); consult specific product labeling.

Tablet, extended release:

Allegra-D® 12 Hour: Fexofenadine hydrochloride 60 mg [immediate release] and pseudoephedrine hydrochloride 120 mg [extended release]

Allegra-D® 24 Hour: Fexofenadine hydrochloride 180 mg [immediate release] and pseudoephedrine hydrochloride 240 mg [extended release]

◆ **Fexofenadine Hydrochloride** *see* Fexofenadine *on page 629*

Filgrastim (fil GRA stim)

Medication Safety Issues

Sound-alike/look-alike issues:

Neupogen® may be confused with Epogen®, Neumega®, Neupro®, Nutramigen®

Related Information

Clozapine-Induced Side Effects *on page 1818*

U.S. Brand Names Neupogen®

Canadian Brand Names Neupogen®

Mexican Brand Names Biocilin; Biofilgran; Filatil; Inmunef; Neupogen

Index Terms G-CSF; Granulocyte Colony Stimulating Factor; NSC-614629

Pharmacologic Category Colony Stimulating Factor

Use Stimulation of granulocyte production in chemotherapy-induced neutropenia (nonmyeloid malignancies, acute myeloid leukemia, and bone marrow transplantation); severe chronic neutropenia (SCN); patients undergoing peripheral blood progenitor cell (PBPC) collection

Unlabeled/Investigational Use Treatment of anemia in myelodysplastic syndrome; treatment of drug-induced (nonchemotherapy) agranulocytosis in the elderly

Effect on Mental Status None reported

Effect on Psychiatric Treatment May be used to treat clozapine-induced agranulocytosis; lithium may potentiate the release of neutrophils; use with caution

Dosage Summary Note: Dosing should be based on actual body weight (even in morbidly obese patients).

I.V.:

Children: 5-10 mcg/kg/day

Adults: 5-10 mcg/kg/day

SubQ:

Children: 5-10 mcg/kg/day **or** 6 mcg/kg twice daily

Adults: 5-10 mcg/kg/day **or** 6 mcg/kg twice daily

Dosage Forms Excipient information presented when available (limited, particularly for generics); consult specific product labeling.

Injection, solution [preservative free]:

Neupogen®: 300 mcg/mL (1 mL, 1.6 mL) [vial; contains sodium 0.035 mg/mL and sorbitol]

Injection, solution [preservative free]:

Neupogen®: 600 mcg/mL (0.5 mL, 0.8 mL) [prefilled Singleject® syringe; contains sodium 0.035 mg/mL and sorbitol; needle cover contains latex]

◆ **Fioricet®** *see* Butalbital, Acetaminophen, and Caffeine *on page 229*

◆ **Fioricet® with Codeine** *see* Butalbital, Acetaminophen, Caffeine, and Codeine *on page 232*

◆ **Fiorinal®** *see* Butalbital, Aspirin, and Caffeine *on page 239*

◆ **Fiorinal® with Codeine** *see* Butalbital, Aspirin, Caffeine, and Codeine *on page 242*

◆ **First™-Progesterone VGS** *see* Progesterone *on page 1345*

- **First®-Testosterone** *see* Testosterone *on page 1553*
- **First®-Testosterone MC** *see* Testosterone *on page 1553*
- **Fisalamine** *see* Mesalamine *on page 994*
- **Fish Oil** *see* Omega-3-Acid Ethyl Esters *on page 1175*
- **FK506** *see* Tacrolimus *on page 1533*
- **Flagyl®** *see* MetroNIDAZOLE *on page 1040*
- **Flagyl ER®** *see* MetroNIDAZOLE *on page 1040*
- **Flavan** *see* Flavocoxid *on page 633*

Flavocoxid (fla vo KOKS id)

U.S. Brand Names Limbrel™

Index Terms Flavan; Flavonoid

Pharmacologic Category Anti-inflammatory Agent

Use Clinical dietary management of osteoarthritis, including associated inflammation

Effect on Mental Status May cause dizziness

Effect on Psychiatric Treatment Lithium concentrations may be increased with flavocoxid via decreased renal lithium clearance; dose adjustment may be needed

Dosage Summary

Oral:

Children: Dosage not established

Adults: 250 mg every 8-12 hours

Dosage Forms Excipient information presented when available (limited, particularly for generics); consult specific product labeling.

Capsule:

Limbrel™: 250 mg, 500 mg [gluten free]

- **Flavonoid** *see* Flavocoxid *on page 633*

Flavoxate (fla VOKS ate)

Medication Safety Issues

Sound-alike/look-alike issues:

Flavoxate may be confused with fluvoxamine

Urispas® may be confused with Urised®

U.S. Brand Names Urispas®

Canadian Brand Names Apo-Flavoxate®; Urispas®

Index Terms Flavoxate Hydrochloride

Pharmacologic Category Antispasmodic Agent, Urinary

Use Antispasmodic to provide symptomatic relief of dysuria, nocturia, suprapubic pain, urgency, and incontinence due to detrusor instability and hyper-reflexia in elderly with cystitis, urethritis, urethrocystitis, urethrotrigonitis, and prostatitis

Effect on Mental Status Drowsiness is common; may cause nervousness

Effect on Psychiatric Treatment None reported

Dosage Summary

Oral:

Children ≤12 years: Dosage not established

Children >12 years: 100-200 mg 3-4 times/day

Adults: 100-200 mg 3-4 times/day

Dosage Forms Excipient information presented when available (limited, particularly for generics); consult specific product labeling.

Tablet, as hydrochloride: 100 mg

- **Flavoxate Hydrochloride** *see* Flavoxate *on page 633*

Flecainide (fle KAY nide)

Medication Safety Issues

Sound-alike/look-alike issues:

Flecainide may be confused with fluconazole

Tambocor™ may be confused with tamoxifen

U.S. Brand Names Tambocor™

Canadian Brand Names Apo-Flecainide®; Tambocor™

Mexican Brand Names Tambocor

Index Terms Flecainide Acetate

Pharmacologic Category Antiarrhythmic Agent, Class Ic

Use Prevention and suppression of documented life-threatening ventricular arrhythmias (eg, sustained ventricular tachycardia); controlling symptomatic, disabling supraventricular tachycardias in patients without structural heart disease in whom other agents fail

Effect on Mental Status Dizziness is common; may cause sedation; may rarely cause nervousness

Effect on Psychiatric Treatment Use beta-blockers with caution; may produce additive negative inotropic effect; use caution with TCAs; may affect cardiac conduction; CYP2D6 substrate; use caution with the SSRIs

Dosage Summary

Oral:

Children: Initial: 3 mg/kg/day **or** 50-100 mg/m^2/day in 3 divided doses; Maintenance: 3-6 mg/kg/day **or** 100-150 mg/m^2/day in 3 divided doses (maximum: 11 mg/kg/day; 200 mg/m^2/day)

Adults: Initial: 50-100 mg every 12 hours; Maintenance: 100-400 mg/day in 2 divided doses (maximum: 400 mg/day-Exceptions occur-Indication specific); **Note:** Titration is recommended

Dosage Forms Excipient information presented when available (limited, particularly for generics); consult specific product labeling.

Tablet, as acetate: 50 mg, 100 mg, 150 mg

- ◆ **Flecainide Acetate** *see* Flecainide *on page 633*
- ◆ **Flector®** *see* Diclofenac *on page 457*
- ◆ **Fleet® Mineral Oil Enema [OTC]** *see* Mineral Oil *on page 1055*
- ◆ **Flexeril®** *see* Cyclobenzaprine *on page 405*
- ◆ **Flextra 650** *see* Acetaminophen and Phenyltoloxamine *on page 36*
- ◆ **Flextra-DS** *see* Acetaminophen and Phenyltoloxamine *on page 36*
- ◆ **Flolan®** *see* Epoprostenol *on page 547*
- ◆ **Flomax®** *see* Tamsulosin *on page 1537*
- ◆ **Flonase®** *see* Fluticasone *on page 668*
- ◆ **Florical® [OTC]** *see* Calcium Carbonate *on page 254*
- ◆ **Florinef® [DSC]** *see* Fludrocortisone *on page 641*
- ◆ **Flovent® Diskus®** *see* Fluticasone *on page 668*
- ◆ **Flovent® HFA** *see* Fluticasone *on page 668*
- ◆ **Floxin®** *see* Ofloxacin *on page 1159*
- ◆ **Floxin Otic Singles** *see* Ofloxacin *on page 1159*

Floxuridine (floks YOOR i deen)

Medication Safety Issues

Sound-alike/look-alike issues:

Floxuridine may be confused with Fludara®, fludarabine

FUDR® may be confused with Fludara®

High alert medication: The Institute for Safe Medication Practices (ISMP) includes this medication among its list of drugs which have a heightened risk of causing significant patient harm when used in error.

U.S. Brand Names FUDR®

Canadian Brand Names FUDR®

Index Terms 5-FUDR; Fluorodeoxyuridine; FUDR; NSC-27640

Pharmacologic Category Antineoplastic Agent, Antimetabolite (Pyrimidine Analog)

Use Management of hepatic metastases of colorectal and gastric cancers

Effect on Mental Status May cause drowsiness

Effect on Psychiatric Treatment May rarely cause agranulocytosis; use caution with clozapine and carbamazepine

Dosage Summary

Intra-arterial:

Children: Dosage not established

Adults: 0.1-0.6 mg/kg/day

Dosage Forms Excipient information presented when available (limited, particularly for generics); consult specific product labeling.

Injection, powder for reconstitution: 500 mg

- ◆ **Fluarix®** *see* Influenza Virus Vaccine *on page 820*
- ◆ **Flubenisolone** *see* Betamethasone *on page 184*

Fluconazole (floo KOE na zole)

Medication Safety Issues

Sound-alike/look-alike issues:

Fluconazole may be confused with flecainide

Diflucan® may be confused with diclofenac, Diprivan®, disulfiram

International issues:

Canesten® [Great Britain]: Brand name for clotrimazole in multiple international markets

U.S. Brand Names Diflucan®

Canadian Brand Names Apo-Fluconazole®; Co-Fluconazole; Diflucan®; Dom-Fluconazole; Fluconazole Injection; Fluconazole Omega; Gen-Fluconazole; GMD-Fluconazole; Novo-Fluconazole; PHL-Fluconazole; PMS-Fluconazole; Riva-Fluconazole; Taro-Fluconazole; Zym-Fluconazole

Mexican Brand Names Afungil; Diflucan; Flucoxan; Oxifungol; Zoldicam

Pharmacologic Category Antifungal Agent, Oral; Antifungal Agent, Parenteral

Generic Available Yes

Use Treatment of candidiasis (vaginal, oropharyngeal, esophageal, urinary tract infections, peritonitis, pneumonia, and systemic infections); cryptococcal meningitis; antifungal prophylaxis in allogeneic bone marrow transplant recipients

Effect on Mental Status May cause dizziness and seizures

Effect on Psychiatric Treatment None reported; CYP3A4 inhibitor; use caution with triazolam, alprazolam, and midazolam

Pregnancy Risk Factor C

Pregnancy Considerations When used in high doses, fluconazole is teratogenic in animal studies. Following exposure during the first trimester, case reports have noted similar malformations in humans when used in higher doses (400 mg/day) over extended periods of time. Use of lower doses (150 mg as a single dose or 200 mg/day) may have less risk; however, additional data is needed. Use during pregnancy only if the potential benefit to the mother outweighs any potential risk to the fetus.

Lactation Enters breast/not recommended (AAP rates "compatible")

Contraindications Hypersensitivity to fluconazole, other azoles, or any component of the formulation; concomitant administration with cisapride

Warnings/Precautions Should be used with caution in patients with renal and hepatic dysfunction or previous hepatotoxicity from other azole derivatives. Patients who develop abnormal liver function tests during fluconazole therapy should be monitored closely and discontinued if symptoms consistent with liver disease develop. Rare exfoliative skin disorders have been observed; monitor closely if rash develops. The manufacturer reports rare cases of QT_c prolongation and TdP associated with fluconazole use and advises caution in patients with concomitant medications or conditions which are arrhythmogenic. However, given the limited number of cases and the presence of multiple confounding variables, the likelihood that fluconazole causes conduction abnormalities appears remote.

Adverse Reactions Frequency not always defined.

Cardiovascular: Angioedema, pallor, QT prolongation (rare, case reports), torsade de pointes(rare, case reports)

Central nervous system: Headache (2% to 13%), seizure, dizziness

Dermatologic: Rash (2%), alopecia, toxic epidermal necrolysis, Stevens-Johnson syndrome

Endocrine & metabolic: Hypercholesterolemia, hypertriglyceridemia, hypokalemia

Gastrointestinal: Nausea (4% to 7%), vomiting (2%), abdominal pain (2% to 6%), diarrhea (2% to 3%), taste perversion, dyspepsia

Hematologic: Agranulocytosis, leukopenia, neutropenia, thrombocytopenia

Hepatic: Alkaline phosphatase increased, ALT increased, AST increased, cholestasis, hepatic failure (rare), hepatitis, jaundice

Respiratory: Dyspnea

Miscellaneous: Anaphylactic reactions (rare)

Metabolism/Transport Effects Inhibits CYP1A2 (weak), 2C9 (strong), 2C19 (strong), 3A4 (moderate)

Drug Interactions

Alfentanil: Antifungal Agents (Azole Derivatives, Systemic) may decrease the metabolism of Alfentanil. *Risk D: Consider therapy modification*

Alfentanil: Fluconazole may decrease the metabolism of Alfentanil. *Risk D: Consider therapy modification*

Alfuzosin: May enhance the QTc-prolonging effect of QTc-Prolonging Agents. *Risk C: Monitor therapy*

Antacids: May decrease the absorption of Antifungal Agents (Azole Derivatives, Systemic). *Risk D: Consider therapy modification*

Aprepitant: Antifungal Agents (Azole Derivatives, Systemic) may decrease the metabolism of Aprepitant. *Risk C: Monitor therapy*

Benzodiazepines (metabolized by oxidation): Antifungal Agents (Azole Derivatives, Systemic) may decrease the metabolism of Benzodiazepines (metabolized by oxidation). **Exceptions:** Quazepam. *Risk D: Consider therapy modification*

Benzodiazepines (metabolized by oxidation): Fluconazole may decrease the metabolism of Benzodiazepines (metabolized by oxidation). *Risk D: Consider therapy modification*

Bosentan: Antifungal Agents (Azole Derivatives, Systemic) may decrease the metabolism of Bosentan. *Risk C: Monitor therapy*

BusPIRone: Antifungal Agents (Azole Derivatives, Systemic) may decrease the metabolism of BusPIRone. *Risk D: Consider therapy modification*

Busulfan: Antifungal Agents (Azole Derivatives, Systemic) may decrease the metabolism of Busulfan. *Risk C: Monitor therapy*

Calcium Channel Blockers: Antifungal Agents (Azole Derivatives, Systemic) may decrease the metabolism of Calcium Channel Blockers. **Exceptions:** Clevidipine. *Risk D: Consider therapy modification*

Calcium Channel Blockers: Fluconazole may decrease the metabolism of Calcium Channel Blockers. **Exceptions:** Clevidipine. *Risk C: Monitor therapy*

CarBAMazepine: Antifungal Agents (Azole Derivatives, Systemic) may decrease the metabolism of CarBAMazepine. *Risk C: Monitor therapy*

CarBAMazepine: Fluconazole may decrease the metabolism of CarBAMazepine. *Risk C: Monitor therapy*

Cardiac Glycosides: Antifungal Agents (Azole Derivatives, Systemic) may increase the serum concentration of Cardiac Glycosides. *Risk D: Consider therapy modification*

Cilostazol: Antifungal Agents (Azole Derivatives, Systemic) may decrease the metabolism of Cilostazol. *Risk D: Consider therapy modification*

Cinacalcet: Antifungal Agents (Azole Derivatives, Systemic) may decrease the metabolism of Cinacalcet. *Risk C: Monitor therapy*

Ciprofloxacin: May enhance the QTc-prolonging effect of QTc-Prolonging Agents. *Risk C: Monitor therapy*

Cisapride: Antifungal Agents (Azole Derivatives, Systemic) may increase the serum concentration of Cisapride. *Risk X: Avoid combination*

Conivaptan: Antifungal Agents (Azole Derivatives, Systemic) may decrease the metabolism of Conivaptan. *Risk X: Avoid combination*

Corticosteroids (Orally Inhaled): Antifungal Agents (Azole Derivatives, Systemic) may decrease the metabolism of Corticosteroids (Orally Inhaled). **Exceptions:** Beclomethasone; Flunisolide; Triamcinolone. *Risk C: Monitor therapy*

Corticosteroids (Systemic): Antifungal Agents (Azole Derivatives, Systemic) may decrease the metabolism of Corticosteroids (Systemic). *Risk C: Monitor therapy*

Corticosteroids (Systemic): Fluconazole may decrease the metabolism of Corticosteroids (Systemic). *Risk C: Monitor therapy*

CycloSPORINE: Antifungal Agents (Azole Derivatives, Systemic) may decrease the metabolism of CycloSPORINE. *Risk D: Consider therapy modification*

CycloSPORINE: Fluconazole may decrease the metabolism of CycloSPORINE. *Risk D: Consider therapy modification*

CYP2C19 Substrates: CYP2C19 Inhibitors (Strong) may decrease the metabolism of CYP2C19 Substrates. *Risk D: Consider therapy modification*

CYP2C9 Substrates (High risk): CYP2C9 Inhibitors (Strong) may decrease the metabolism of CYP2C9 Substrates (High risk). *Risk D: Consider therapy modification*

CYP3A4 Substrates: CYP3A4 Inhibitors (Moderate) may decrease the metabolism of CYP3A4 Substrates. *Risk C: Monitor therapy*

Didanosine: May decrease the absorption of Antifungal Agents (Azole Derivatives, Systemic). Enteric coated didanosine capsules are not expected to affect these antifungals. *Risk D: Consider therapy modification*

Docetaxel: Antifungal Agents (Azole Derivatives, Systemic) may decrease the metabolism of Docetaxel. *Risk D: Consider therapy modification*

Dofetilide: Antifungal Agents (Azole Derivatives, Systemic) may decrease the metabolism of Dofetilide. *Risk X: Avoid combination*

Eletriptan: Antifungal Agents (Azole Derivatives, Systemic) may increase the serum concentration of Eletriptan. *Risk D: Consider therapy modification*

Eletriptan: Fluconazole may decrease the metabolism of Eletriptan. *Risk C: Monitor therapy*

Eplerenone: Antifungal Agents (Azole Derivatives, Systemic) may decrease the metabolism of Eplerenone. *Risk D: Consider therapy modification*

Eplerenone: Fluconazole may decrease the metabolism of Eplerenone. *Risk C: Monitor therapy*

Erlotinib: Antifungal Agents (Azole Derivatives, Systemic) may decrease the metabolism of Erlotinib. *Risk C: Monitor therapy*

Eszopiclone: Antifungal Agents (Azole Derivatives, Systemic) may decrease the metabolism of Eszopiclone. *Risk C: Monitor therapy*

Fosaprepitant: Antifungal Agents (Azole Derivatives, Systemic) may increase the serum concentration of Fosaprepitant. Specifically, concentrations of aprepitant are likely to be increased. *Risk C: Monitor therapy*

Gadobutrol: May enhance the QTc-prolonging effect of QTc-Prolonging Agents. *Risk D: Consider therapy modification*

Gefitinib: Antifungal Agents (Azole Derivatives, Systemic) may decrease the metabolism of Gefitinib. *Risk C: Monitor therapy*

Grapefruit Juice: May increase the metabolism of Antifungal Agents (Azole Derivatives, Systemic). This specifically applies to oral antifungal administration. *Risk D: Consider therapy modification*

H2-Antagonists: May decrease the absorption of Antifungal Agents (Azole Derivatives, Systemic). *Risk D: Consider therapy modification*

HMG-CoA Reductase Inhibitors: Antifungal Agents (Azole Derivatives, Systemic) may decrease the metabolism of HMG-CoA Reductase Inhibitors. **Exceptions:** Fluvastatin; Rosuvastatin. *Risk D: Consider therapy modification*

HMG-CoA Reductase Inhibitors: Fluconazole may decrease the metabolism of HMG-CoA Reductase Inhibitors. **Exceptions:** Pravastatin; Rosuvastatin. *Risk D: Consider therapy modification*

Imatinib: Antifungal Agents (Azole Derivatives, Systemic) may decrease the metabolism of Imatinib. *Risk C: Monitor therapy*

Irbesartan: Fluconazole may decrease the metabolism of Irbesartan. *Risk C: Monitor therapy*

Irinotecan: Antifungal Agents (Azole Derivatives, Systemic) may enhance the adverse/toxic effect of Irinotecan. *Risk D: Consider therapy modification*

Losartan: Antifungal Agents (Azole Derivatives, Systemic) may decrease the metabolism of Losartan. *Risk C: Monitor therapy*

Losartan: Fluconazole may decrease the metabolism of Losartan. *Risk C: Monitor therapy*

Macrolide Antibiotics: May decrease the metabolism of Antifungal Agents (Azole Derivatives, Systemic). Antifungal Agents (Azole Derivatives, Systemic) may decrease the metabolism of Macrolide Antibiotics. **Exceptions:** Azithromycin; Dirithromycin [Off Market]; Spiramycin. *Risk D: Consider therapy modification*

Maraviroc: CYP3A4 Inhibitors may increase the serum concentration of Maraviroc. *Risk D: Consider therapy modification*

Methadone: Antifungal Agents (Azole Derivatives, Systemic) may increase the serum concentration of Methadone. *Risk C: Monitor therapy*

Nilotinib: May enhance the QTc-prolonging effect of QTc-Prolonging Agents. *Risk X: Avoid combination*

Phenytoin: Antifungal Agents (Azole Derivatives, Systemic) may increase the serum concentration of Phenytoin. Phenytoin may decrease the serum concentration of Antifungal Agents (Azole Derivatives, Systemic). *Risk D: Consider therapy modification*

Phenytoin: Fluconazole may decrease the metabolism of Phenytoin. *Risk D: Consider therapy modification*

Phosphodiesterase 5 Inhibitors: Antifungal Agents (Azole Derivatives, Systemic) may decrease the metabolism of Phosphodiesterase 5 Inhibitors. *Risk D: Consider therapy modification*

Pimecrolimus: CYP3A4 Inhibitors (Moderate) may decrease the metabolism of Pimecrolimus. *Risk C: Monitor therapy*

Pimozide: Antifungal Agents (Azole Derivatives, Systemic) may decrease the metabolism of Pimozide. *Risk X: Avoid combination*

Protease Inhibitors: Antifungal Agents (Azole Derivatives, Systemic) may increase the serum concentration of Protease Inhibitors. Protease Inhibitors may increase the serum concentration of Antifungal Agents (Azole Derivatives, Systemic). Management: Limit indinavir to 600 mg every 8 hours with itraconazole or ketoconazole. When used with ritonavir, limit ketoconazole to 200 mg/day. Tipranavir labeling recommends limiting fluconazole, itraconazole, and ketoconazole to 200 mg with tipranavir/ritonavir. *Risk D: Consider therapy modification*

Proton Pump Inhibitors: May decrease the absorption of Antifungal Agents (Azole Derivatives, Systemic). *Risk D: Consider therapy modification*

QTc-Prolonging Agents: May enhance the adverse/toxic effect of other QTc-Prolonging Agents. Their effects can be additive, causing life-threatening ventricular arrhythmias. *Risk D: Consider therapy modification*

QuiNIDine: Antifungal Agents (Azole Derivatives, Systemic) may decrease the metabolism of QuiNIDine. Management: Itraconazole, voriconazole, and posaconazole are specifically contraindicated with quinidine. Use of quinidine with any azole antifungal may require quinidine dose adjustment and should be done with caution and close monitoring. *Risk X: Avoid combination*

QuiNIDine: Fluconazole may decrease the metabolism of QuiNIDine. *Risk C: Monitor therapy*

Ramelteon: Antifungal Agents (Azole Derivatives, Systemic) may decrease the metabolism of Ramelteon. *Risk C: Monitor therapy*

Ramelteon: Fluconazole may decrease the metabolism of Ramelteon. *Risk C: Monitor therapy*

Ranolazine: Antifungal Agents (Azole Derivatives, Systemic) may decrease the metabolism of Ranolazine. *Risk X: Avoid combination*

Repaglinide: Antifungal Agents (Azole Derivatives, Systemic) may increase the serum concentration of Repaglinide. Management: Concurrent use of an azole antifungal with both repaglinide and gemfibrozil should be avoided. *Risk C: Monitor therapy*

Rifamycin Derivatives: Antifungal Agents (Azole Derivatives, Systemic) may increase the serum concentration of Rifamycin Derivatives. Only rifabutin appears to be affected. Rifamycin Derivatives may decrease the serum concentration of Antifungal Agents (Azole Derivatives, Systemic). *Risk D: Consider therapy modification*

Rifamycin Derivatives: Fluconazole may decrease the metabolism of Rifamycin Derivatives. This appears only affect rifabutin. Rifamycin Derivatives may increase the metabolism of Fluconazole. *Risk C: Monitor therapy*

Saccharomyces boulardii: Antifungal Agents may diminish the therapeutic effect of Saccharomyces boulardii. *Risk D: Consider therapy modification*

Salmeterol: CYP3A4 Inhibitors (Moderate) may increase the serum concentration of Salmeterol. *Risk C: Monitor therapy*

Sirolimus: Antifungal Agents (Azole Derivatives, Systemic) may increase the serum concentration of Sirolimus. Management: Sirolimus dose reductions of up to 50-90% may be necessary when starting an azole antifungal. Use of sirolimus with the azole antifungals voriconazole and posaconazole is contraindicated. *Risk D: Consider therapy modification*

Solifenacin: Antifungal Agents (Azole Derivatives, Systemic) may decrease the metabolism of Solifenacin. *Risk D: Consider therapy modification*

Sucralfate: May decrease the absorption of Antifungal Agents (Azole Derivatives, Systemic). *Risk C: Monitor therapy*

Sulfonylureas: Fluconazole may increase the serum concentration of Sulfonylureas. *Risk C: Monitor therapy*

Sunitinib: Antifungal Agents (Azole Derivatives, Systemic) may decrease the metabolism of Sunitinib. *Risk D: Consider therapy modification*

Tacrolimus: Antifungal Agents (Azole Derivatives, Systemic) may decrease the metabolism of Tacrolimus. *Risk D: Consider therapy modification*

Tacrolimus: Fluconazole may decrease the metabolism of Tacrolimus. *Risk D: Consider therapy modification*

Temsirolimus: Antifungal Agents (Azole Derivatives, Systemic) may increase the serum concentration of Temsirolimus. Concentrations of the active metabolite, sirolimus, are likely to be increased more substantially than those of the parent temsirolimus. *Risk D: Consider therapy modification*

Tetrabenazine: QTc-Prolonging Agents may enhance the QTc-prolonging effect of Tetrabenazine. *Risk X: Avoid combination*

Thioridazine: QTc-Prolonging Agents may enhance the QTc-prolonging effect of Thioridazine. *Risk X: Avoid combination*

Tolterodine: Antifungal Agents (Azole Derivatives, Systemic) may decrease the metabolism of Tolterodine. This is likely only of concern in CYP2D6-deficient patients (ie, "poor metabolizers") *Risk D: Consider therapy modification*

Tolterodine: Fluconazole may decrease the metabolism of Tolterodine. This is likely only of concern in CYP2D6-deficient patients (ie, "poor metabolizers") *Risk C: Monitor therapy*

VinCRIStine: Antifungal Agents (Azole Derivatives, Systemic) may decrease the metabolism of VinCRIStine. *Risk D: Consider therapy modification*

Vitamin K Antagonists (eg, warfarin): Antifungal Agents (Azole Derivatives, Systemic) may decrease the metabolism of Vitamin K Antagonists. *Risk D: Consider therapy modification*

Vitamin K Antagonists (eg, warfarin): Fluconazole may decrease the metabolism of Vitamin K Antagonists. *Risk D: Consider therapy modification*

Zidovudine: Fluconazole may decrease the metabolism of Zidovudine. *Risk C: Monitor therapy*

Ziprasidone: Antifungal Agents (Azole Derivatives, Systemic) may decrease the metabolism of Ziprasidone. *Risk C: Monitor therapy*

Zolpidem: Antifungal Agents (Azole Derivatives, Systemic) may decrease the metabolism of Zolpidem. *Risk D: Consider therapy modification*

Stability

Powder for oral suspension: Store dry powder at ≤30°C (86°F). Following reconstitution, store at 5°C to 30°C (41°F to 86°F). Discard unused portion after 2 weeks. Do not freeze.

Injection: Store injection in glass at 5°C to 30°C (41°F to 86°F). Store injection in Viaflex® at 5°C to 25°C (41°F to 77°F). Do not freeze. Do not unwrap unit until ready for use.

Mechanism of Action Interferes with fungal cytochrome P450 activity (lanosterol 14-α-demethylase), decreasing ergosterol synthesis (principal sterol in fungal cell membrane) and inhibiting cell membrane formation

Pharmacodynamics/Kinetics

Distribution: Widely throughout body with good penetration into CSF, eye, peritoneal fluid, sputum, skin, and urine

Relative diffusion blood into CSF: Adequate with or without inflammation (exceeds usual MICs)

CSF:blood level ratio: Normal meninges: 70% to 80%; Inflamed meninges: >70% to 80%

Protein binding, plasma: 11% to 12%

Bioavailability: Oral: >90%

Half-life elimination: Normal renal function: ~30 hours

Time to peak, serum: Oral: 1-2 hours

Excretion: Urine (80% as unchanged drug)

Dosage The daily dose of fluconazole is the same for oral and I.V. administration

Usual dosage ranges:

Neonates: First 2 weeks of life, especially premature neonates: Same dose as older children every 72 hours

Children: Loading dose: 6-12 mg/kg; maintenance: 3-12 mg/kg/day; duration and dosage depends on severity of infection

Adults: 200-800 mg/day; duration and dosage depends on severity of infection

Indication-specific dosing:

Children:

Candidiasis:

Oropharyngeal: Loading dose: 6 mg/kg; maintenance: 3 mg/kg/day for 2 weeks

Esophageal: Loading dose: 6 mg/kg; maintenance: 3-12 mg/kg/day for 21 days and at least 2 weeks following resolution of symptoms

Systemic infection: 6 mg/kg every 12 hours for 28 days

Meningitis, cryptococcal: Loading dose: 12 mg/kg; maintenance: 6-12 mg/kg/day for 10-12 weeks following negative CSF culture; relapse suppression (HIV-positive): 6 mg/kg/day

Adults:

Candidiasis:

Candidemia (neutropenic and non-neutropenic): 400-800 mg/day for 14 days after last positive blood culture and resolution of signs/symptoms

Chronic, disseminated: 400-800 mg/day for 3-6 months

Oropharyngeal (long-term suppression): 200 mg/day; chronic therapy is recommended in immunocompromised patients with history of oropharyngeal candidiasis (OPC)

Osteomyelitis: 400-800 mg/day for 6-12 months

Esophageal: 200 mg on day 1, then 100-200 mg/day for 2-3 weeks after clinical improvement

Prophylaxis in bone marrow transplant: 400 mg/day; begin 3 days before onset of neutropenia and continue for 7 days after neutrophils >1000 cells/mm^3

Urinary: 200 mg/day for 1-2 weeks

Vaginal: 150 mg as a single dose

Coccidiomycosis (unlabeled use, IDSA guideline): 400 mg/day; doses of 800-1000 mg/day have been used for meningeal disease; usual duration of therapy ranges from 3-6 months for primary uncomplicated infections and up to 1 year for pulmonary (chronic and diffuse) infection

Endocarditis, prosthetic valve, early (unlabeled use, IDSA guideline): 400-800 mg/day for 6 weeks after valve replacement; long-term suppression in absence of valve replacement: 200-400 mg/day

Endophthalmitis: 400-800 mg/day for 6-12 weeks after surgical intervention.

Meningitis, cryptococcal: Amphotericin 0.7-1 mg/kg +/- 5-FC for 2 weeks then fluconazole 400 mg/day for at least 10 weeks (consider life-long in HIV-positive); maintenance (HIV-positive): 200-400 mg/day life-long

Pneumonia, cryptococcal (mild-to-moderate) (unlabeled use, IDSA guideline): 200-400 mg/day for 6-12 months (consider life-long in HIV-positive patients)

Dosing adjustment/interval in renal impairment:

No adjustment for vaginal candidiasis single-dose therapy

For multiple dosing, administer usual load then adjust daily doses as follows:

Cl_{cr} ≤50 mL/minute (no dialysis): Administer 50% of recommended dose or administer every 48 hours.

Hemodialysis: 50% is removed by hemodialysis; administer 100% of daily dose (according to indication) after each dialysis treatment.

Continuous renal replacement therapy (CRRT): Drug clearance is highly dependent on the method of renal replacement, filter type, and flow rate. Appropriate dosing requires close monitoring of pharmacologic response, signs of adverse reactions due to drug accumulation, as well as drug levels in relation to target trough (if appropriate). The following are general recommendations only (based on dialysate flow/ultrafiltration rates of 1 L/hour) and should not supersede clinical judgment:

CVVH: 200-400 mg every 24 hours

CVVHD/CVVHDF: 400-800 mg every 24 hours

Note: Higher daily doses of 400 mg (CVVH) and 800 mg (CVVHD/CVVHDF) should be considered when treating resistant organisms and/or when employing combined ultrafiltration and dialysis flow rates of ≥2 L/hour for CVVHD/CVVHDF (Trotman, 2005).

Dietary Considerations Take with or without regard to food.

Administration

I.V.: Infuse over approximately 1-2 hours; do not exceed 200 mg/hour

Oral: May be administered with or without food

Monitoring Parameters Periodic liver function tests (AST, ALT, alkaline phosphatase) and renal function tests, potassium

Dosage Forms Excipient information presented when available (limited, particularly for generics); consult specific product labeling.

Infusion [premixed in sodium chloride or dextrose]: 200 mg (100 mL); 400 mg (200 mL)

Diflucan® [premixed in sodium chloride or dextrose]: 200 mg (100 mL); 400 mg (200 mL)

Powder for oral suspension: 10 mg/mL (35 mL); 40 mg/mL (35 mL)

Diflucan®: 10 mg/mL (35 mL); 40 mg/mL (35 mL) [contains sodium benzoate; orange flavor]

Tablet: 50 mg, 100 mg, 150 mg, 200 mg

Diflucan®: 50 mg, 100 mg, 150 mg, 200 mg

Flucytosine (floo SYE toe seen)

Medication Safety Issues

Sound-alike/look-alike issues:

Flucytosine may be confused with fluorouracil

Ancobon® may be confused with Oncovin®

High alert medication: The Institute for Safe Medication Practices (ISMP) includes this medication among its list of drugs which have a heightened risk of causing significant patient harm when used in error.

U.S. Brand Names Ancobon®

Canadian Brand Names Ancobon®

Index Terms 5-FC; 5-Fluorocytosine; 5-Flurocytosine

Pharmacologic Category Antifungal Agent, Oral

Use Adjunctive treatment of systemic fungal infections (eg, septicemia, endocarditis, UTI, meningitis, or pulmonary) caused by susceptible strains of *Candida* or *Cryptococcus*

Effect on Mental Status May rarely cause drowsiness, confusion, or hallucinations

Effect on Psychiatric Treatment May cause bone marrow suppression; use caution with clozapine and carbamazepine

Dosage Summary

Oral:

Children (unlabeled): 50-150 mg/kg/day in divided doses every 6 hours

Adults: 50-150 mg/kg/day in divided doses every 6 hours

Dosage Forms Excipient information presented when available (limited, particularly for generics); consult specific product labeling.

Capsule: 250 mg, 500 mg

◆ **Fludara®** *see* Fludarabine *on page 641*

Fludarabine (floo DARE a been)

Medication Safety Issues

Sound-alike/look-alike issues:

Fludarabine may be confused with floxuridine, Flumadine®

Fludara® may be confused with FUDR®

High alert medication: The Institute for Safe Medication Practices (ISMP) includes this medication among its list of drug classes which have a heightened risk of causing significant patient harm when used in error.

U.S. Brand Names Fludara®

Canadian Brand Names Beneflur®; Fludara®

Mexican Brand Names Beneflur

Index Terms Fludarabine Phosphate; NSC-312887

Pharmacologic Category Antineoplastic Agent, Antimetabolite (Purine Antagonist)

Use

U.S. labeling: I.V.: Treatment of chronic lymphocytic leukemia (CLL) (including refractory CLL)

Canadian labeling:

I.V.: Treatment of chronic lymphocytic leukemia (CLL) (including refractory CLL); treatment of low-grade, refractory non-Hodgkin's lymphoma (NHL)

Oral (formulation not available in U.S.): Treatment of CLL

Unlabeled/Investigational Use Treatment of non-Hodgkin's lymphoma (NHL); refractory acute leukemias and solid tumors (in pediatric patients); Waldenström's macroglobulinemia (WM); reduced-intensity conditioning regimens prior to allogeneic hematopoietic stem cell transplantation (generally administered in combination with busulfan and antithymocyte globulin or lymphocyte immune globulin, or in combination with melphalan and alemtuzumab)

Effect on Mental Status Sedation is common; may cause agitation, confusion, coma

Effect on Psychiatric Treatment Myelosuppression is common; use caution with clozapine and carbamazepine; concurrent use with low potency antipsychotics and TCAs may produce additive sedation. May cause nausea, vomiting, diarrhea, and GI bleeding; concomitant use with SSRIs may produce additive risk (use caution).

Dosage Summary

I.V.:

Children (unlabeled use): 10 mg/m^2 bolus followed by 30.5 mg/m^2/day for 5 days **or** 10.5 mg/m^2 bolus followed by 30.5 mg/m^2/day for 48 hours **or** 7 mg/m^2 bolus followed by 20 mg/m^2/day for 5 days

Adults: 25 mg/m^2/day for 5 days every 28 days

Dosage Forms Excipient information presented when available (limited, particularly for generics); consult specific product labeling. [CAN] = Canadian brand name

Injection, powder for reconstitution, as phosphate: 50 mg

Fludara®: 50 mg [contains mannitol 50 mg/vial]

Tablet, as phosphate:

Fludara® [CAN]: 10 mg [not available in U.S.]

◆ **Fludarabine Phosphate** *see* Fludarabine *on page 641*

Fludrocortisone (floo droe KOR ti sone)

Medication Safety Issues

Sound-alike/look-alike issues:

Florinef® may be confused with Fioricet®, Fiorinal®

Related Information

Corticosteroids *on page 1780*

U.S. Brand Names Florinef® [DSC]

Canadian Brand Names Florinef®

Index Terms 9α-Fluorohydrocortisone Acetate; Fludrocortisone Acetate; Fluohydrisone Acetate; Fluohydrocortisone Acetate

Pharmacologic Category Corticosteroid, Systemic

Generic Available Yes

Use Partial replacement therapy for primary and secondary adrenocortical insufficiency in Addison's disease; treatment of salt-losing adrenogenital syndrome

Effect on Mental Status May cause dizziness

Effect on Psychiatric Treatment Barbiturates and carbamazepine may decrease corticosteroid effects; useful in the management of psychotropic-induced hypotension

Pregnancy Risk Factor C

Pregnancy Considerations Animal reproduction studies have not been conducted with fludrocortisone; adverse events have been observed with corticosteroids in animal reproduction studies. Some studies have shown an association between first trimester systemic corticosteroid use and oral clefts; adverse events in the fetus/neonate have been noted in case reports following large doses of systemic corticosteroids during pregnancy.

Lactation Excretion in breast milk unknown/use caution

Contraindications Hypersensitivity to fludrocortisone or any component of the formulation; systemic fungal infections

Warnings/Precautions May cause hypercorticism or suppression of hypothalamic-pituitary-adrenal (HPA) axis, particularly in younger children or in patients receiving high doses for prolonged periods. HPA axis suppression may lead to adrenal crisis. Withdrawal and discontinuation of a corticosteroid should be done slowly and carefully. Fludrocortisone is primarily a mineralocorticoid agonist, but may also inhibit the HPA axis. May increase risk of infection and/or limit response to vaccinations; close observation is required in patients with latent tuberculosis and/or TB reactivity. Restrict use in active TB (only in conjunction with antituberculosis treatment). Use with caution in patients with sodium retention and potassium loss, hepatic impairment, myocardial infarction, osteoporosis, and/or renal impairment. Use with caution in the elderly. Withdraw therapy with gradual tapering of dose. Safety and efficacy have not been established in children.

Adverse Reactions Frequency not defined.

Cardiovascular: Hypertension, edema, CHF

Central nervous system: Convulsions, headache, dizziness

Dermatologic: Acne, rash, bruising

Endocrine & metabolic: Hypokalemic alkalosis, suppression of growth, hyperglycemia, HPA suppression

Gastrointestinal: Peptic ulcer

Neuromuscular & skeletal: Muscle weakness

Ocular: Cataracts

Miscellaneous: Diaphoresis, anaphylaxis (generalized)

Drug Interactions

Acetylcholinesterase Inhibitors: Corticosteroids (Systemic) may enhance the adverse/toxic effect of Acetylcholinesterase Inhibitors. Increased muscular weakness may occur. *Risk C: Monitor therapy*

Aminoglutethimide: May increase the metabolism of Corticosteroids (Systemic). *Risk C: Monitor therapy*

Amphotericin B: Corticosteroids (Systemic) may enhance the hypokalemic effect of Amphotericin B. *Risk C: Monitor therapy*

Antacids: May decrease the bioavailability of Corticosteroids (Oral). *Risk D: Consider therapy modification*

Antidiabetic Agents: Corticosteroids (Systemic) may diminish the hypoglycemic effect of Antidiabetic Agents. In some instances, corticosteroid-mediated HPA axis suppression has led to episodes of acute adrenal crisis, which may manifest as enhanced hypoglycemia, particularly in the setting of insulin or other antidiabetic agent use. *Risk C: Monitor therapy*

Antifungal Agents (Azole Derivatives, Systemic): May decrease the metabolism of Corticosteroids (Systemic). *Risk C: Monitor therapy*

Aprepitant: May increase the serum concentration of Corticosteroids (Systemic). *Risk D: Consider therapy modification*

Barbiturates: May increase the metabolism of Corticosteroids (Systemic). *Risk C: Monitor therapy*

Bile Acid Sequestrants: May decrease the absorption of Corticosteroids (Oral). *Risk C: Monitor therapy*

Calcitriol: Corticosteroids (Systemic) may diminish the therapeutic effect of Calcitriol. *Risk C: Monitor therapy*

Calcium Channel Blockers (Nondihydropyridine): May decrease the metabolism of Corticosteroids (Systemic). *Risk C: Monitor therapy*

Corticorelin: Corticosteroids may diminish the therapeutic effect of Corticorelin. Specifically, the plasma ACTH response to corticorelin may be blunted by recent or current corticosteroid therapy. *Risk C: Monitor therapy*

CycloSPORINE: Corticosteroids (Systemic) may increase the serum concentration of CycloSPORINE. CycloSPORINE may increase the serum concentration of Corticosteroids (Systemic). *Risk C: Monitor therapy*

Echinacea: May diminish the therapeutic effect of Immunosuppressants. *Risk D: Consider therapy modification*

Estrogen Derivatives: May increase the serum concentration of Corticosteroids (Systemic). *Risk C: Monitor therapy*

Fluconazole: May decrease the metabolism of Corticosteroids (Systemic). *Risk C: Monitor therapy*

Fosaprepitant: May increase the serum concentration of Corticosteroids (Systemic). The active metabolite aprepitant is likely responsible for this effect. *Risk D: Consider therapy modification*

Isoniazid: Corticosteroids (Systemic) may decrease the serum concentration of Isoniazid. *Risk C: Monitor therapy*

Loop Diuretics: Corticosteroids (Systemic) may enhance the hypokalemic effect of Loop Diuretics. *Risk C: Monitor therapy*

Macrolide Antibiotics: May decrease the metabolism of Corticosteroids (Systemic). **Exceptions:** Azithromycin; Dirithromycin [Off Market]; Spiramycin. *Risk D: Consider therapy modification*

Natalizumab: Immunosuppressants may enhance the adverse/toxic effect of Natalizumab. Specifically, the risk of concurrent infection may be increased. *Risk X: Avoid combination*

Neuromuscular-Blocking Agents (Nondepolarizing): May enhance the adverse neuromuscular effect of Corticosteroids (Systemic). Increased muscle weakness, possibly progressing to polyneuropathies and myopathies, may occur. *Risk D: Consider therapy modification*

NSAID (COX-2 Inhibitor): Corticosteroids (Systemic) may enhance the adverse/toxic effect of NSAID (COX-2 Inhibitor). *Risk C: Monitor therapy*

NSAID (Nonselective): Corticosteroids (Systemic) may enhance the adverse/toxic effect of NSAID (Nonselective). *Risk C: Monitor therapy*

Primidone: May increase the metabolism of Corticosteroids (Systemic). *Risk C: Monitor therapy*

Quinolone Antibiotics: May enhance the adverse/toxic effect of Corticosteroids (Systemic). Risk of tendon-related side effects, including tendonitis and rupture, may be enhanced. *Risk C: Monitor therapy*

Rifamycin Derivatives: May increase the metabolism of Corticosteroids (Systemic). *Risk C: Monitor therapy*

Salicylates: May enhance the adverse/toxic effect of Corticosteroids (Systemic). These specifically include gastrointestinal ulceration and bleeding. Corticosteroids (Systemic) may decrease the serum concentration of Salicylates. Withdrawal of corticosteroids may result in salicylate toxicity. *Risk C: Monitor therapy*

Thiazide Diuretics: Corticosteroids (Systemic) may enhance the hypokalemic effect of Thiazide Diuretics. *Risk C: Monitor therapy*

Trastuzumab: May enhance the neutropenic effect of Immunosuppressants. *Risk C: Monitor therapy*

Vaccines (Inactivated): Immunosuppressants may diminish the therapeutic effect of Vaccines (Inactivated). *Risk C: Monitor therapy*

Vaccines (Live): Immunosuppressants may enhance the adverse/toxic effect of Vaccines (Live). Vaccinal infections may develop. Immunosuppressants may also decrease therapeutic response to vaccines. *Risk X: Avoid combination*

Warfarin: Corticosteroids (Systemic) may enhance the anticoagulant effect of Warfarin. *Risk C: Monitor therapy*

Mechanism of Action Promotes increased reabsorption of sodium and loss of potassium from renal distal tubules

Pharmacodynamics/Kinetics

Absorption: Rapid and complete

Protein binding: 42%

Metabolism: Hepatic

Half-life elimination, plasma: 30-35 minutes; Biological: 18-36 hours

Time to peak, serum: ~1.7 hours

Dosage Oral:

Infants and Children: 0.05-0.1 mg/day

Adults: 0.1-0.2 mg/day with ranges of 0.1 mg 3 times/week to 0.2 mg/day

Addison's disease: Initial: 0.1 mg/day; if transient hypertension develops, reduce the dose to 0.05 mg/day. Preferred administration with cortisone (10-37.5 mg/day) or hydrocortisone (10-30 mg/day).

Salt-losing adrenogenital syndrome: 0.1-0.2 mg/day

Dietary Considerations Systemic use of mineralocorticoids/corticosteroids may require a diet with increased potassium, vitamins A, B_6, C, D, folate, calcium, zinc, and phosphorus, and decreased sodium. With fludrocortisone, a decrease in dietary sodium is often not required as the increased retention of sodium is usually the desired therapeutic effect.

Administration Administration in conjunction with a glucocorticoid is preferable

Monitoring Parameters Monitor blood pressure and signs of edema when patient is on chronic therapy; very potent mineralocorticoid with high glucocorticoid activity; monitor serum electrolytes, serum renin activity, and blood pressure; monitor for evidence of infection; stop treatment if a significant increase in weight or blood pressure, edema, or cardiac enlargement occurs

Additional Information In patients with salt-losing forms of congenital adrenogenital syndrome, use along with cortisone or hydrocortisone. Fludrocortisone 0.1 mg has sodium retention activity equal to DOCA® 1 mg.

Dosage Forms Excipient information presented when available (limited, particularly for generics); consult specific product labeling. [DSC] = Discontinued product

Tablet, as acetate: 0.1 mg
  Florinef®: 0.1 mg [DSC]

◆ **Fludrocortisone Acetate** *see* Fludrocortisone *on page 641*

◆ **FluLaval™** *see* Influenza Virus Vaccine *on page 820*

◆ **Flumadine®** *see* Rimantadine *on page 1422*

Flumazenil (FLOO may ze nil)

U.S. Brand Names Romazicon®

Canadian Brand Names Anexate®; Flumazenil Injection; Flumazenil Injection, USP; Romazicon®

Mexican Brand Names Lanexat

Pharmacologic Category Antidote

Generic Available Yes

Use Benzodiazepine antagonist; reverses sedative effects of benzodiazepines used in conscious sedation and general anesthesia; treatment of benzodiazepine overdose

Pregnancy Risk Factor C

Pregnancy Considerations Teratogenic effects were not seen in animal studies. Embryocidal effects were seen at large doses. There are no adequate or well-controlled studies in pregnant women. Use only if clearly needed.

Lactation Excretion in breast milk unknown/use caution

Contraindications Hypersensitivity to flumazenil, benzodiazepines, or any component of the formulation; patients given benzodiazepines for control of potentially life-threatening conditions (eg, control of intracranial pressure or status epilepticus); patients who are showing signs of serious cyclic-antidepressant overdosage

Warnings/Precautions **[U.S. Boxed Warning]: Benzodiazepine reversal may result in seizures in some patients.** Patients who may develop seizures include patients on benzodiazepines for long-term sedation, tricyclic antidepressant overdose patients, concurrent major sedative-hypnotic drug withdrawal, recent therapy with repeated doses of parenteral benzodiazepines, myoclonic jerking or seizure activity prior to flumazenil administration. Flumazenil may not reliably reverse respiratory depression/hypoventilation. Flumazenil is not a substitute for evaluation of oxygenation; establishing an airway and assisting ventilation, as necessary, is always the initial step in overdose management. Resedation occurs more frequently in patients where a large single dose or cumulative dose of a benzodiazepine is administered along with a neuromuscular-blocking agent and multiple anesthetic agents. Flumazenil should be used with caution in the intensive care unit because of increased risk of unrecognized benzodiazepine dependence in such settings. Should not be used to diagnose benzodiazepine-induced sedation. Reverse neuromuscular blockade before considering use. Flumazenil does not antagonize the CNS effects of other GABA agonists (such as ethanol, barbiturates, or general anesthetics); nor does it reverse narcotics. Flumazenil does not consistently reverse amnesia; patient may not recall verbal instructions after procedure.

Use with caution in patients with a history of panic disorder; may provoke panic attacks. Use caution in drug and ethanol-dependent patients; these patients may also be dependent on benzodiazepines. Not recommended for treatment of benzodiazepine dependence. Use with caution in head injury patients. Use caution in patients with mixed drug overdoses; toxic effects of other drugs taken may emerge once benzodiazepine effects are reversed. Use caution in hepatic dysfunction and in patients relying on a benzodiazepine for seizure control. Safety and efficacy have not been established in children <1 year of age.

Adverse Reactions

>10%: Gastrointestinal: Vomiting, nausea

1% to 10%:

Cardiovascular: Vasodilation (1% to 3%), palpitation

Central nervous system: Headache (1% to 3%), agitation (3% to 9%), dizziness (10%), emotional lability (1% to 3%), fatigue (1% to 3%)

Gastrointestinal: Xerostomia

Local: Pain at injection site (3% to 9%)

Neuromuscular & skeletal: Tremor, weakness, paresthesia (1% to 3%)

Ocular: Abnormal vision, blurred vision (3% to 9%)

Respiratory: Dyspnea, hyperventilation (3% to 9%)

Miscellaneous: Diaphoresis

<1%: Abnormal hearing, altered blood pressure (increases and decreases), confusion, sensation of coldness, bradycardia, chest pain, generalized seizure, hiccups, hypertension, junctional tachycardia, shivering, somnolence, tachycardia, thick tongue, ventricular tachycardia, withdrawal syndrome

Drug Interactions

Hypnotics (Nonbenzodiazepine): Flumazenil may diminish the sedative effect of Hypnotics (Nonbenzodiazepine). **Exceptions:** Ramelteon. *Risk C: Monitor therapy*

Stability Store at 15°C to 30°C (59°F to 86°F). For I.V. use only. Once drawn up in the syringe or mixed with solution use within 24 hours. Discard any unused solution after 24 hours.

Mechanism of Action Competitively inhibits the activity at the benzodiazepine receptor site on the GABA/benzodiazepine receptor complex. Flumazenil does not antagonize the CNS effect of drugs affecting GABA-ergic neurons by means other than the benzodiazepine receptor (ethanol, barbiturates, general anesthetics) and does not reverse the effects of opioids

Pharmacodynamics/Kinetics

Onset of action: 1-3 minutes; 80% response within 3 minutes

Peak effect: 6-10 minutes

Duration: Resedation: ~1 hour; duration related to dose given and benzodiazepine plasma concentrations; reversal effects of flumazenil may wear off before effects of benzodiazepine

Distribution: Initial V_d: 0.5 L/kg; V_{dss} 0.77-1.6 L/kg

Protein binding: 40% to 50%

Metabolism: Hepatic; dependent upon hepatic blood flow

Half-life elimination: Adults: Alpha: 7-15 minutes; Terminal: 41-79 minutes; Moderate hepatic dysfunction: 1.3 hours; severe hepatic impairment: 2.4 hours

Excretion: Feces; urine (0.2% as unchanged drug)

Dosage

Children and Adults: I.V.: See table on next page.

Resedation: Repeated doses may be given at 20-minute intervals as needed; repeat treatment doses of 1 mg (at a rate of 0.5 mg/minute) should be given at any time and no more than 3 mg should be given in any hour. After intoxication with high doses of benzodiazepines, the duration of a single dose of flumazenil is not expected to exceed 1 hour; if desired, the period of wakefulness may be prolonged with repeated low intravenous doses of flumazenil, or by an infusion of 0.1-0.4 mg/hour. Most patients with benzodiazepine overdose will respond to a cumulative dose of 1-3 mg and doses >3 mg do not reliably produce additional effects. Rarely, patients with a partial response at 3 mg may require additional titration up to a total dose of 5 mg. **If a patient has not responded 5 minutes after receiving a cumulative dose of 5 mg, the major cause of sedation is not likely to be due to benzodiazepines.**

Elderly: No differences in safety or efficacy have been reported. However, increased sensitivity may occur in some elderly patients.

Dosing in renal impairment: Not significantly affected by renal failure (Cl_{cr} <10 mL/minute) or hemodialysis beginning 1 hour after drug administration

Dosing in hepatic impairment: Use caution with initial and/or repeat doses in patients with liver disease

Flumazenil

Pediatric Dosage	
Pediatric dosage for **reversal of conscious sedation and general anesthesia:**	
Initial dose	0.01 mg/kg over 15 seconds (maximum: 0.2 mg)
Repeat doses (maximum: 4 doses)	0.005-0.01 mg/kg (maximum: 0.2 mg) repeated at 1-minute intervals
Maximum total cumulative dose	1 mg or 0.05 mg/kg (whichever is lower)
Adult Dosage	
Adult dosage for **reversal of conscious sedation and general anesthesia:**	
Initial dose	0.2 mg intravenously over 15 seconds
Repeat doses (maximum: 4 doses)	If desired level of consciousness is not obtained, 0.2 mg may be repeated at 1-minute intervals.
Maximum total cumulative dose	1 mg (usual dose: 0.6-1 mg) **In the event of resedation:** Repeat doses may be given at 20-minute intervals with maximum of 1 mg/dose and 3 mg/hour.
Adult dosage for **suspected benzodiazepine overdose:**	
Initial dose	0.2 mg intravenously over 30 seconds; if the desired level of consciousness is not obtained, 0.3 mg can be given over 30 seconds
Repeat doses	0.5 mg over 30 seconds repeated at 1-minute intervals
Maximum total cumulative dose	3 mg (usual dose 1-3 mg) Patients with a partial response at 3 mg may require additional titration up to a total dose of 5 mg. If a patient has not responded 5 minutes after cumulative dose of 5 mg, the major cause of sedation is not likely due to benzodiazepines. **In the event of resedation:** May repeat doses at 20-minute intervals with maximum of 1 mg/dose and 3 mg/hour.

Administration I.V.: Administer in freely-running I.V. into large vein. Inject over 15 seconds for conscious sedation and general anesthesia and over 30 seconds for overdose.

Monitoring Parameters Monitor patients for return of sedation or respiratory depression

Dosage Forms Excipient information presented when available (limited, particularly for generics); consult specific product labeling.

Injection, solution: 0.1 mg/mL (5 mL, 10 mL)

Romazicon®: 0.1 mg/mL (5 mL, 10 mL) [contains edetate disodium]

◆ **FluMist®** *see* Influenza Virus Vaccine *on page 820*

Flunisolide (floo NISS oh lide)

Medication Safety Issues

Sound-alike/look-alike issues:

Flunisolide may be confused with Flumadine®, fluocinonide

Nasarel® may be confused with Nizoral®

U.S. Brand Names AeroBid®; AeroBid®-M; Nasarel®

Canadian Brand Names Alti-Flunisolide; Apo-Flunisolide®; Nasalide®; PMS-Flunisolide; Rhinalar®

Pharmacologic Category Corticosteroid, Inhalant (Oral); Corticosteroid, Nasal

Generic Available Yes: Nasal spray

Use Steroid-dependent asthma; nasal solution is used for seasonal or perennial rhinitis

Effect on Mental Status Dizziness and nervousness are common; may cause insomnia

Effect on Psychiatric Treatment None reported

Pregnancy Risk Factor C

Pregnancy Considerations No data on crossing the placenta or effects on the fetus.

Lactation Excretion in breast milk unknown/use caution

Contraindications Hypersensitivity to flunisolide or any component of the formulation; acute status asthmaticus; viral, tuberculosis, fungal, or bacterial respiratory infections; infections of the nasal mucosa

Warnings/Precautions May cause hypercorticism or suppression of hypothalamic-pituitary-adrenal (HPA) axis, particularly in younger children or in patients receiving high doses for prolonged periods. HPA axis suppression may lead to adrenal crisis. Withdrawal and discontinuation of a corticosteroid should be done slowly and carefully. Particular care is required when patients are transferred from systemic corticosteroids to inhaled products due to possible adrenal insufficiency or withdrawal from steroids, including an increase in allergic symptoms. Patients receiving >20 mg per day of prednisone (or equivalent) may be most susceptible. Fatalities have occurred due to adrenal insufficiency in asthmatic patients during and after transfer from systemic corticosteroids to aerosol steroids; aerosol steroids do **not** provide the systemic steroid needed to treat patients having trauma, surgery, or infections. Do not use this product to transfer patients from oral corticosteroid therapy.

Bronchospasm may occur with wheezing after inhalation; if this occurs stop steroid and treat with a fast-acting bronchodilator. Supplemental steroids (oral or parenteral) may be needed during stress or severe asthma attacks. Not to be used in status asthmaticus or for the relief of acute bronchospasm. Corticosteroid use may cause psychiatric disturbances, including depression, euphoria, insomnia, mood swings, and personality changes. Pre-existing psychiatric conditions may be exacerbated by corticosteroid use. Prolonged use of corticosteroids may also increase the incidence of secondary infection, mask acute infection (including fungal infections), prolong or exacerbate viral infections, or limit response to vaccines. Exposure to chickenpox should be avoided; corticosteroids should not be used to treat ocular herpes simplex. Corticosteroids should not be used for cerebral malaria. Close observation is required in patients with latent tuberculosis and/or TB reactivity; restrict use in active TB (only in conjunction with antituberculosis treatment). Prolonged treatment with corticosteroids has been associated with the development of Kaposi's sarcoma (case reports); if noted, discontinuation of therapy should be considered.

Use with caution in patients with thyroid disease, hepatic impairment, renal impairment, cardiovascular disease, diabetes, glaucoma, cataracts, myasthenia gravis, patients at risk for osteoporosis, patients at risk for seizures, or GI diseases (diverticulitis, peptic ulcer, ulcerative colitis) due to perforation risk. Use caution following acute MI (corticosteroids have been associated with myocardial rupture). Because of the risk of adverse effects, systemic corticosteroids should be used cautiously in the elderly in the smallest possible effective dose for the shortest duration. Avoid nasal corticosteroid use in patients with recent nasal septal ulcers, nasal surgery or nasal trauma until healing has occurred.

Orally-inhaled and intranasal corticosteroids may cause a reduction in growth velocity in pediatric patients (~1 centimeter per year [range 0.3-1.8 cm per year] and related to dose and duration of exposure). To minimize the systemic effects of orally-inhaled and intranasal corticosteroids, each patient should be titrated to the lowest effective dose. Growth should be routinely monitored in pediatric patients. There have been reports of systemic corticosteroid withdrawal symptoms (eg, joint/muscle pain, lassitude, depression) when withdrawing oral inhalation therapy.

Adverse Reactions

>10%:

Central nervous system: Headache (intranasal <5%; oral 9% to 25%)

Gastrointestinal: Aftertaste (10% to 17%)

Respiratory: Nasal burning (intranasal 45%), pharyngitis (14% to 20%), rhinitis (<15%), nasal irritation (>1% to 13%)

1% to 10%:

Cardiovascular: Chest pain (1% to 3%), edema (1% to 3%), chest tightness, hypertension, palpitation, tachycardia

Central nervous system: Fever (1% to 9%), dizziness (1% to 3%), insomnia (1% to 3%), migraine (1% to 3%), chills, malaise, irritability, shakiness, anxiety, depression, faintness, fatigue, moodiness, vertigo

Dermatologic: Erythema multiform (1% to 3%), acne, eczema, pruritus, urticaria

Endocrine & metabolic: Dysmenorrhea (1% to 3%)

Gastrointestinal: Dyspepsia (2% to 4%), abdominal pain (1% to 3%), diarrhea (1% to 10%), gastroenteritis (1% to 3%), nausea (Aerospan™: 1% to 3%), oral candidiasis (1% to 3%), taste perversion (1% to 3%), abdominal fullness, constipation, gas, heartburn, sore throat, dry throat, mouth discomfort, throat irritation

Genitourinary: Vaginitis (1% to 3%), urinary tract infection (1% to 4%)

Neuromuscular & skeletal: Myalgia (1% to 3%), neck pain (1% to 3%), numbness, weakness
Ocular: Conjunctivitis (1% to 3%), blurred vision
Renal: Laryngitis (1% to 3%)
Respiratory: Sinusitis (<9%), epistaxia (<3%), bronchospasm, cough increased, dyspnea, hoarseness, nasal ulcer, sneezing, wheezing
Miscellaneous: Allergy (4% to 5%), infection (3% to 9%), loss of smell, voice alteration (1% to 3%), flu-like syndrome, diaphoresis
<1% (Limited to important or life-threatening): Adrenal suppression

Metabolism/Transport Effects
Substrate of CYP3A4 (major)

Drug Interactions
Amphotericin B: Corticosteroids (Orally Inhaled) may enhance the hypokalemic effect of Amphotericin B. *Risk C: Monitor therapy*
Antidiabetic Agents: Corticosteroids (Orally Inhaled) may diminish the hypoglycemic effect of Antidiabetic Agents. In some instances, corticosteroid-mediated HPA axis suppression has led to episodes of acute adrenal crisis, which may manifest as enhanced hypoglycemia, particularly in the setting of insulin or other antidiabetic agent use. *Risk C: Monitor therapy*
Corticorelin: Corticosteroids may diminish the therapeutic effect of Corticorelin. Specifically, the plasma ACTH response to corticorelin may be blunted by recent or current corticosteroid therapy. *Risk C: Monitor therapy*
CYP3A4 Inhibitors (Moderate): May decrease the metabolism of CYP3A4 Substrates. *Risk C: Monitor therapy*
CYP3A4 Inhibitors (Strong): May decrease the metabolism of CYP3A4 Substrates. *Risk D: Consider therapy modification*
Dasatinib: May increase the serum concentration of CYP3A4 Substrates. *Risk C: Monitor therapy*
Loop Diuretics: Corticosteroids (Orally Inhaled) may enhance the hypokalemic effect of Loop Diuretics. *Risk C: Monitor therapy*
Thiazide Diuretics: Corticosteroids (Orally Inhaled) may enhance the hypokalemic effect of Thiazide Diuretics. *Risk C: Monitor therapy*

Stability
Aerospan™: Store at 15°C to 30°C (59°F to 86°F). Do not store near heat or flame. Protect from freezing and sunlight.
AeroBid®: Store below 49°C (below 120°F).

Mechanism of Action Decreases inflammation by suppression of migration of polymorphonuclear leukocytes and reversal of increased capillary permeability; does not depress hypothalamus

Pharmacodynamics/Kinetics
Absorption: Nasal inhalation: ~50%
Metabolism: Rapidly hepatic to active metabolites
Bioavailability: 40% to 50%
Half-life elimination: 1.8 hours
Excretion: Urine and feces (equal amounts)

Dosage Note: AeroBid® and Aerospan™ are not interchangeable; dosing changes when switching from one to the other.
Oral inhalation: Asthma:
AeroBid®:
Children 6-15 years: 2 inhalations twice daily (morning and evening); up to 4 inhalations/day
Children ≥16 years and Adults: 2 inhalations twice daily (morning and evening); up to 8 inhalations/day maximum
NIH Asthma Guidelines (NIH, 2007) (administer in divided doses twice daily):
Children 5-11 years:
"Low" dose: 500-750 mcg/day
"Medium" dose: 1000-1250 mcg/day
"High" dose: >1250 mcg/day
Children ≥12 years and Adults:
"Low" dose: 500-1000 mcg/day
"Medium" dose: >1000-2000 mcg/day
"High" dose: >2000 mcg/day
Aerospan™:
Children 6-11 years: 1 inhalation twice daily; up to 4 inhalations/day
Children ≥12 years and Adults: 2 inhalations twice daily; up to 8 inhalations/day
NIH Asthma Guidelines (NIH, 2007) (administer in divided doses twice daily):
Children 5-11 years:
"Low" dose: 160 mcg/day
"Medium" dose: 320 mcg/day

"High" dose: ≥640 mcg/day
Children ≥12 years and Adults:
"Low" dose: 320 mcg/day
"Medium" dose: >320-640 mcg/day
"High" dose: >640 mcg/day

Intranasal: Rhinitis:

Children 6-14 years: 1 spray each nostril 3 times daily **or** 2 sprays in each nostril twice daily; not to exceed 4 sprays/day in each nostril (200 mcg/day)

Children ≥15 years and Adults: 2 sprays each nostril twice daily (morning and evening); may increase to 2 sprays 3 times daily; maximum dose: 8 sprays/day in each nostril (400 mcg/day)

Administration Inhalation: Shake well before using. Rinse mouth following use of oral inhalers.

Aerospan™: Has a self-contained spacer; do not use with another spacer. Prime inhaler prior to first use. Begin inhalation immediately prior to actuation; a delay may reduce dose by ≥75%.

Additional Information Aerospan™and AeroBid® doses are not interchangeable because of differences in delivery characteristics.

Effects of inhaled/intranasal steroids on growth have been observed in the absence of laboratory evidence of HPA axis suppression, suggesting that growth velocity is a more sensitive indicator of systemic corticosteroid exposure in pediatric patients than some commonly used tests of HPA axis function. The long-term effects of this reduction in growth velocity associated with orally-inhaled and intranasal corticosteroids, including the impact on final adult height, are unknown. The potential for "catch up" growth following discontinuation of treatment with inhaled corticosteroids has not been adequately studied.

Dosage Forms Excipient information presented when available (limited, particularly for generics); consult specific product labeling.

Aerosol for oral inhalation:

AeroBid®: 250 mcg/actuation (7 g) [100 metered inhalations; contains chlorofluorocarbon]

AeroBid®-M: 250 mcg/actuation (7 g) [100 metered inhalations; contains chlorofluorocarbon; menthol flavor]

Solution, intranasal [spray]: 25 mcg/actuation (25 mL); 29 mcg/actuation (25 mL) [200 sprays]

Nasarel®: 29 mcg/actuation (25 mL) [200 sprays; contains benzalkonium chloride]

- **Fluohydrisone Acetate** *see* Fludrocortisone *on page 641*
- **Fluohydrocortisone Acetate** *see* Fludrocortisone *on page 641*
- **5-Fluorocytosine** *see* Flucytosine *on page 640*
- **Fluorodeoxyuridine** *see* Floxuridine *on page 634*
- **9α-Fluorohydrocortisone Acetate** *see* Fludrocortisone *on page 641*
- **Fluoroplex®** *see* Fluorouracil *on page 649*

Fluorouracil (flure oh YOOR a sil)

Medication Safety Issues

Sound-alike/look-alike issues:

Carac® may be confused with Kuric™
Fluorouracil may be confused with flucytosine
Efudex® may be confused with Efidac (Efidac 24®), Eurax®

High alert medication: The Institute for Safe Medication Practices (ISMP) includes this medication among its list of drugs which have a heightened risk of causing significant patient harm when used in error.

International issues:

Carac® may be confused with Carace® which is a brand name for lisinopril in Ireland and Great Britain

U.S. Brand Names Adrucil®; Carac®; Efudex®; Fluoroplex®; Fluorouracil®

Canadian Brand Names Efudex®

Mexican Brand Names Efudix; Tecflu

Index Terms 5-Fluorouracil; 5-FU; FU

Pharmacologic Category Antineoplastic Agent, Antimetabolite (Pyrimidine Analog)

Use Treatment of carcinomas of the breast, colon, head and neck, pancreas, rectum, or stomach; topically for the management of actinic or solar keratoses and superficial basal cell carcinomas

Effect on Mental Status May cause drowsiness

Effect on Psychiatric Treatment Myelosuppression is common; use caution with clozapine and carbamazepine

Dosage Forms Excipient information presented when available (limited, particularly for generics); consult specific product labeling.

Cream, topical:
 Carac™: 0.5% (30 g)
 Efudex®: 5% (40 g)
 Fluoroplex®: 1% (30 g) [contains benzyl alcohol]
Injection, solution: 50 mg/mL (10 mL, 20 mL, 50 mL, 100 mL)
 Adrucil®: 50 mg/mL (10 mL, 50 mL, 100 mL)
Solution, topical: 2% (10 mL); 5% (10 mL)
 Efudex®: 2% (10 mL); 5% (10 mL)
 Fluorouracil®: 5% (10 mL)

◆ **Fluorouracil®** *see* Fluorouracil *on page 649*

◆ **5-Fluorouracil** *see* Fluorouracil *on page 649*

FLUoxetine (floo OKS e teen)

Medication Safety Issues

Sound-alike/look-alike issues:
 FLUoxetine may be confused with DULoxetine, fluvastatin, fluvoxamine, PARoxetine
 Prozac® may be confused with Prilosec®, Prograf®, Proscar®, ProSom®, ProStep®
 Sarafem® may be confused with Serophene®

International issues:
 Fluoxin® [Czech Republic and Romania] may be confused with Floxin® which is a brand name for ofloxacin in the U.S.
 Prozac® may be confused with Prazac® a brand of prazosin in Denmark
 Reneuron® [Spain] may be confused with Remeron® a brand of mirtazapine in the U.S.

Related Information

Anticholinergic Effects of Common Psychotropics *on page 1758*
Antidepressant Agents *on page 1760*
Antidepressant Receptor Profile *on page 1764*
Discontinuation of Psychotropic Drugs *on page 1839*
Liquid Compatibility of Antidepressants, Antipsychotics, and Mood Stabilizers *on page 1788*
Selective Serotonin Reuptake Inhibitors (SSRIs) CYP Profile *on page 1793*
Selective Serotonin Reuptake Inhibitors (SSRIs) FDA-Approved Indication(s) *on page 1794*
Selective Serotonin Reuptake Inhibitors (SSRIs) Pharmacokinetics *on page 1795*
Selective Serotonin Reuptake Inhibitors (SSRIs) Receptor Profile *on page 1796*

U.S. Brand Names Prozac®; Prozac® Weekly™; Sarafem®; Selfemra™

Canadian Brand Names Apo-Fluoxetine®; BCI-Fluoxetine; CO Fluoxetine; Dom-Fluoxetine; Fluoxetine; FXT; Gen-Fluoxetine; Novo-Fluoxetine; Nu-Fluoxetine; PHL-Fluoxetine; PMS-Fluoxetine; Prozac®; ratio-Fluoxetine; Rhoxal-Fluoxetine; Riva-Fluoxetine; Sandoz-Fluoxetine

Mexican Brand Names Symbyax

Index Terms Fluoxetine Hydrochloride

Pharmacologic Category Antidepressant, Selective Serotonin Reuptake Inhibitor

Generic Available Yes: Excludes delayed release capsule

Use Treatment of major depressive disorder (MDD); treatment of binge-eating and vomiting in patients with moderate-to-severe bulimia nervosa; obsessive-compulsive disorder (OCD); premenstrual dysphoric disorder (PMDD); panic disorder with or without agoraphobia

Unlabeled/Investigational Use Selective mutism; treatment of mild dementia-associated agitation in nonpsychotic patients

Mental Health Comment The SSRIs as a class are generally considered to be safe and equally effective. Allow sufficient dose-response time (6-12 weeks). Differences lie in approved indications, receptor profiles, pharmacokinetics, and cytochrome P450 activity profile. Subtle differences exist in adverse effect profiles. All SSRIs have the potential to cause sexual dysfunction. Among the SSRIs, fluoxetine is felt to be the most activating. The once-weekly dosing formulation may be appropriate for psychiatric populations that are non-compliant with daily administration.

Restrictions An FDA-approved medication guide concerning the use of antidepressants in children, adolescents, and young adults must be distributed when dispensing an outpatient prescription (new or refill) where this medication is to be used without direct supervision of a healthcare provider. Medication guides are available at http://www.fda.gov/cder/Offices/ODS/medication_guides.htm. Dispense to parents or guardians of children and adolescents receiving this medication.

Pregnancy Risk Factor C

Pregnancy Considerations Due to adverse effects observed in animal studies, fluoxetine is classified as pregnancy category C. Fluoxetine and its metabolite cross the human placenta. Nonteratogenic effects in the newborn following SSRIs exposure late in the third trimester include respiratory distress, cyanosis, apnea, seizures, temperature instability, feeding difficulty, vomiting, hypoglycemia, hypo- or hypertonia, hyper-reflexia, jitteriness, irritability, constant crying, and tremor. An increased risk of low birth weight, lower APGAR scores, and blunted behavioral response to pain for a prolonged period after delivery have also been reported. Exposure to SSRIs after the twentieth week of gestation has been associated with persistent pulmonary hypertension of the newborn (PPHN). Adverse effects may be due to toxic effects of the SSRI or drug withdrawal without a taper. The long term effects of *in utero* SSRI exposure on infant development and behavior are not known.

Due to pregnancy-induced physiologic changes, women who are pregnant may require increased doses of fluoxetine to achieve euthymia. Women treated for major depression and who are euthymic prior to pregnancy are more likely to experience a relapse when medication is discontinued as compared to pregnant women who continue taking antidepressant medications. The ACOG recommends that therapy with SSRIs or SNRIs during pregnancy be individualized; treatment of depression during pregnancy should incorporate the clinical expertise of the mental health clinician, obstetrician, primary healthcare provider, and pediatrician (ACOG, 2007). If treatment during pregnancy is required, consider tapering therapy during the third trimester in order to prevent withdrawal symptoms in the infant. If this is done and the woman is considered to be at risk from her major depressive disorder, the medication can be restarted following delivery, although the dose should be readjusted to that required before pregnancy.

Lactation Enters breast milk/not recommended (AAP rates "of concern")

Contraindications Hypersensitivity to fluoxetine or any component of the formulation; patients currently receiving MAO inhibitors, pimozide, or thioridazine

Note: MAO inhibitor therapy must be stopped for 14 days before fluoxetine is initiated. Treatment with MAO inhibitors, thioridazine, or mesoridazine should not be initiated until 5 weeks after the discontinuation of fluoxetine.

Warnings/Precautions **[U.S. Boxed Warning]: Antidepressants increase the risk of suicidal thinking and behavior in children, adolescents, and young adults (18-24 years of age) with major depressive disorder (MDD) and other psychiatric disorders;** consider risk prior to prescribing. Short-term studies did not show an increased risk in patients >24 years of age and showed a decreased risk in patients ≥65 years. Closely monitor patients for clinical worsening, suicidality, or unusual changes in behavior, particularly during the initial 1-2 months of therapy or during periods of dosage adjustments (increases or decreases); the patient's family or caregiver should be instructed to closely observe the patient and communicate condition with healthcare provider. A medication guide concerning the use of antidepressants should be dispensed with each prescription. **Fluoxetine is FDA approved for the treatment of OCD in children ≥7 years of age and MDD in children ≥8 years of age.**

The possibility of a suicide attempt is inherent in major depression and may persist until remission occurs. Use caution in high-risk patients. Worsening depression and severe abrupt suicidality that are not part of the presenting symptoms may require discontinuation or modification of drug therapy. The patient's family or caregiver should be alerted to monitor patients for the emergence of suicidality and associated behaviors (such as agitation, irritability, hostility, impulsivity, and hypomania) and call healthcare provider.

May worsen psychosis in some patients or precipitate a shift to mania or hypomania in patients with bipolar disorder. Patients presenting with depressive symptoms should be screened for bipolar disorder. Monotherapy in patients with bipolar disorder should be avoided. **Fluoxetine is not FDA approved for the treatment of bipolar depression.** May cause insomnia, anxiety, nervousness, or anorexia. Use with caution in patients where weight loss is undesirable. May impair cognitive or motor performance; caution operating hazardous machinery or driving.

The potential for severe reactions exists when used with MAO inhibitors, SSRIs/SNRIs or triptans; serotonin syndrome (hyperthermia, muscular rigidity, mental status changes/agitation, autonomic instability) may occur. Concurrent use with MAO inhibitors is contraindicated. Fluoxetine may elevate plasma levels of thioridazine and increase the risk of QT_c interval prolongation. This may lead to serious ventricular arrhythmias, such as torsade de pointes-type arrhythmias, and sudden death. Fluoxetine use has been associated with occurrences of significant rash and allergic events, including vasculitis, lupus-like syndrome, laryngospasm, anaphylactoid reactions, and pulmonary inflammatory disease. Discontinue if underlying cause of rash cannot be identified.

Use caution in patients with a previous seizure disorder or condition predisposing to seizures such as brain damage, alcoholism, or concurrent therapy with other drugs which lower the seizure threshold. Use with caution in patients with hepatic or renal dysfunction and in elderly patients. May cause hyponatremia/SIADH (elderly at increased risk); volume depletion (diuretics may increase risk). May increase the risks associated with electroconvulsive treatment. Use caution with concomitant use of NSAIDs, ASA, or other drugs that affect coagulation; the risk of bleeding may be potentiated.Use caution with history of MI or unstable heart disease; use in these patients is limited. May alter glycemic control in patients with diabetes. Due to the long half-life of fluoxetine and its metabolites, the effects and interactions noted may persist for prolonged periods following discontinuation. May cause or exacerbate sexual dysfunction. Discontinuation symptoms (eg, dysphoric mood, irritability, agitation, confusion, anxiety, insomnia, hypomania) may occur upon abrupt discontinuation. Taper dose when discontinuing therapy.

Adverse Reactions Percentages listed for adverse effects as reported in placebo-controlled trials and were generally similar in adults and children; actual frequency may be dependent upon diagnosis and in some cases the range presented may be lower than or equal to placebo for a particular disorder.

>10%:

Central nervous system: Insomnia (10% to 33%), headache (21%), anxiety (6% to 15%), nervousness (8% to 14%), somnolence (5% to 17%)

Endocrine & metabolic: Libido decreased (1% to 11%)

Gastrointestinal: Nausea (12% to 29%), diarrhea (8% to 18%), anorexia (4% to 11%), xerostomia (4% to 12%)

Neuromuscular & skeletal: Weakness (7% to 21%), tremor (3% to 13%)

Respiratory: Pharyngitis (3% to 11%), yawn (<1% to 11%)

1% to 10%:

Cardiovascular: Vasodilation (1% to 5%), fever (2%), chest pain, hemorrhage, hypertension, palpitation

Central nervous system: Dizziness (9%), dream abnormality (1% to 5%), thinking abnormality (2%), agitation, amnesia, chills, confusion, emotional lability, sleep disorder

Dermatologic: Rash (2% to 6%), pruritus (4%)

Endocrine & metabolic: Ejaculation abnormal (<1% to 7%), impotence (<1% to 7%)

Gastrointestinal: Dyspepsia (6% to 10%), constipation (5%), flatulence (3%), vomiting (3%), weight loss (2%), appetite increased, taste perversion, weight gain

Genitourinary: Urinary frequency

Ocular: Vision abnormal (2%)

Otic: Ear pain, tinnitus

Respiratory: Sinusitis (1% to 6%)

Miscellaneous: Flu-like syndrome (3% to 10%), diaphoresis (2% to 8%)

<1% (Limited to important or life-threatening): Allergies, alopecia, anaphylactoid reactions, angina, arrhythmia, asthma, cataract, CHF, cholelithiasis, cholestatic jaundice, colitis, dyskinesia, dysphagia, eosinophilic pneumonia, erythema nodosum, esophagitis, euphoria, exfoliative dermatitis, extrapyramidal symptoms (rare), gout, hallucinations, hepatic failure/necrosis, hemorrhage, hyperprolactinemia, hyponatremia (possibly in association with SIADH), immune-related hemolytic anemia, laryngospasm, lupus-like syndrome, MI, neuroleptic malignant syndrome (NMS), optic neuritis, pancreatitis, pancytopenia, photosensitivity reaction, postural hypotension, priapism, pulmonary embolism, pulmonary fibrosis, pulmonary hypertension, QT prolongation, renal failure, serotonin syndrome, Stevens-Johnson syndrome, syncope, thrombocytopenia, thrombocytopenic purpura, vasculitis, ventricular tachycardia (including torsade de pointes)

Metabolism/Transport Effects **Substrate** of CYP1A2 (minor), 2B6 (minor), 2C9 (major), 2C19 (minor), 2D6 (major), 2E1 (minor), 3A4 (minor); **Inhibits**

CYP1A2 (moderate), 2B6 (weak), 2C9 (weak), 2C19 (moderate), 2D6 (strong), 3A4 (weak)

Drug Interactions

Alcohol (Ethyl): CNS Depressants may enhance the CNS depressant effect of Alcohol (Ethyl). *Risk C: Monitor therapy*

Alfuzosin: May enhance the QTc-prolonging effect of QTc-Prolonging Agents. *Risk C: Monitor therapy*

Alpha-/Beta-Blockers: Selective Serotonin Reuptake Inhibitors may decrease the metabolism of Alpha-/Beta-Blockers. *Risk C: Monitor therapy*

Analgesics (Opioid): May enhance the serotonergic effect of Selective Serotonin Reuptake Inhibitors. This may cause serotonin syndrome. *Risk C: Monitor therapy*

Anticoagulants: Antiplatelet Agents may enhance the anticoagulant effect of Anticoagulants. *Risk C: Monitor therapy*

Antidepressants (Serotonin Reuptake Inhibitor/Antagonist): Selective Serotonin Reuptake Inhibitors may enhance the serotonergic effect of Antidepressants (Serotonin Reuptake Inhibitor/Antagonist). This may cause serotonin syndrome. *Risk C: Monitor therapy*

Antiplatelet Agents: May enhance the anticoagulant effect of other Antiplatelet Agents. *Risk C: Monitor therapy*

Aspirin: Selective Serotonin Reuptake Inhibitors may enhance the antiplatelet effect of Aspirin. *Risk C: Monitor therapy*

Benzodiazepines (metabolized by oxidation): Selective Serotonin Reuptake Inhibitors may decrease the metabolism of Benzodiazepines (metabolized by oxidation). *Risk C: Monitor therapy*

Beta-Blockers: Selective Serotonin Reuptake Inhibitors may enhance the bradycardic effect of Beta-Blockers. **Exceptions:** Acebutolol; Atenolol; Carteolol; Esmolol; Levobunolol; Metipranolol; Nadolol; Penbutolol. *Risk C: Monitor therapy*

BusPIRone: May enhance the serotonergic effect of Selective Serotonin Reuptake Inhibitors. This may cause serotonin syndrome. Selective Serotonin Reuptake Inhibitors may decrease the metabolism of BusPIRone. *Risk C: Monitor therapy*

CarBAMazepine: Selective Serotonin Reuptake Inhibitors may decrease the metabolism of CarBAMazepine. Specifically those SSRIs that inhibit CYP3A4 isoenzymes. CarBAMazepine may increase the metabolism of Selective Serotonin Reuptake Inhibitors. Specifically those agents metabolized via CYP1A2, 2C, and/or 3A4 isoenzymes. *Risk D: Consider therapy modification*

Cimetidine: May decrease the metabolism of Selective Serotonin Reuptake Inhibitors. *Risk D: Consider therapy modification*

Ciprofloxacin: May enhance the QTc-prolonging effect of QTc-Prolonging Agents. *Risk C: Monitor therapy*

Clozapine: Selective Serotonin Reuptake Inhibitors may decrease the metabolism of Clozapine. *Risk D: Consider therapy modification*

CNS Depressants: May enhance the adverse/toxic effect of other CNS Depressants. *Risk C: Monitor therapy*

CYP1A2 Substrates: CYP1A2 Inhibitors (Moderate) may decrease the metabolism of CYP1A2 Substrates. *Risk C: Monitor therapy*

CYP2C19 Substrates: CYP2C19 Inhibitors (Moderate) may decrease the metabolism of CYP2C19 Substrates. *Risk C: Monitor therapy*

CYP2C9 Inducers (Highly Effective): May increase the metabolism of CYP2C9 Substrates (High risk). *Risk C: Monitor therapy*

CYP2C9 Inhibitors (Moderate): May decrease the metabolism of CYP2C9 Substrates (High risk). *Risk C: Monitor therapy*

CYP2C9 Inhibitors (Strong): May decrease the metabolism of CYP2C9 Substrates (High risk). *Risk D: Consider therapy modification*

CYP2D6 Inhibitors (Moderate): May decrease the metabolism of CYP2D6 Substrates. *Risk C: Monitor therapy*

CYP2D6 Inhibitors (Strong): May decrease the metabolism of CYP2D6 Substrates. *Risk D: Consider therapy modification*

CYP2D6 Substrates: CYP2D6 Inhibitors (Strong) may decrease the metabolism of CYP2D6 Substrates. **Exceptions:** Tamoxifen. *Risk D: Consider therapy modification*

Cyproheptadine: May diminish the therapeutic effect of Selective Serotonin Reuptake Inhibitors. *Risk C: Monitor therapy*

Darunavir: May increase the serum concentration of CYP2D6 Substrates. *Risk C: Monitor therapy*

Dasatinib: May enhance the anticoagulant effect of Antiplatelet Agents. *Risk C: Monitor therapy*

Desmopressin: Selective Serotonin Reuptake Inhibitors may enhance the adverse/toxic effect of Desmopressin. *Risk C: Monitor therapy*

Dextromethorphan: Selective Serotonin Reuptake Inhibitors may enhance the adverse/toxic effect of Dextromethorphan. *Risk D: Consider therapy modification*

Drotrecogin Alfa: Antiplatelet Agents may enhance the adverse/toxic effect of Drotrecogin Alfa. Bleeding may occur. *Risk D: Consider therapy modification*

Gadobutrol: May enhance the QTc-prolonging effect of QTc-Prolonging Agents. *Risk D: Consider therapy modification*

Galantamine: Selective Serotonin Reuptake Inhibitors may decrease the metabolism of Galantamine. *Risk C: Monitor therapy*

Haloperidol: Selective Serotonin Reuptake Inhibitors may decrease the metabolism of Haloperidol. *Risk C: Monitor therapy*

Herbs (Anticoagulant/Antiplatelet Properties) (eg, Alfalfa, Anise, Bilberry): May enhance the adverse/toxic effect of Antiplatelet Agents. Bleeding may occur. *Risk D: Consider therapy modification*

Ibritumomab: Antiplatelet Agents may enhance the adverse/toxic effect of Ibritumomab. Both agents may contribute to impaired platelet function and an increased risk of bleeding. *Risk C: Monitor therapy*

Lithium: Selective Serotonin Reuptake Inhibitors may enhance the adverse/toxic effect of Lithium. *Risk C: Monitor therapy*

Macrolide Antibiotics: May decrease the metabolism of Selective Serotonin Reuptake Inhibitors. **Exceptions:** Azithromycin; Dirithromycin [Off Market]; Spiramycin. *Risk C: Monitor therapy*

MAO Inhibitors: May enhance the serotonergic effect of Selective Serotonin Reuptake Inhibitors. This may cause serotonin syndrome. *Risk X: Avoid combination*

Methadone: Selective Serotonin Reuptake Inhibitors may decrease the metabolism of Methadone. Fluvoxamine appears to be the only interacting SSRI. *Risk D: Consider therapy modification*

Mexiletine: Selective Serotonin Reuptake Inhibitors may decrease the metabolism of Mexiletine. *Risk D: Consider therapy modification*

Nilotinib: May enhance the QTc-prolonging effect of QTc-Prolonging Agents. *Risk X: Avoid combination*

NSAID (COX-2 Inhibitor): Selective Serotonin Reuptake Inhibitors may enhance the antiplatelet effect of NSAID (COX-2 Inhibitor). *Risk D: Consider therapy modification*

NSAID (Nonselective): Selective Serotonin Reuptake Inhibitors may enhance the antiplatelet effect of NSAID (Nonselective). *Risk D: Consider therapy modification*

Omega-3-Acid Ethyl Esters: May enhance the antiplatelet effect of Antiplatelet Agents. *Risk C: Monitor therapy*

Pentosan Polysulfate Sodium: May enhance the adverse/toxic effect of Antiplatelet Agents. Specifically, the risk of bleeding may be increased by concurrent use of these agents. *Risk C: Monitor therapy*

Phenytoin: Selective Serotonin Reuptake Inhibitors may decrease the metabolism of Phenytoin. *Risk D: Consider therapy modification*

Pimozide: Selective Serotonin Reuptake Inhibitors may enhance the adverse/toxic effect of Pimozide. *Risk X: Avoid combination*

Propafenone: Selective Serotonin Reuptake Inhibitors may decrease the metabolism of Propafenone. *Risk D: Consider therapy modification*

Prostacyclin Analogues: May enhance the antiplatelet effect of Antiplatelet Agents. *Risk C: Monitor therapy*

QTc-Prolonging Agents: May enhance the adverse/toxic effect of other QTc-Prolonging Agents. Their effects can be additive, causing life-threatening ventricular arrhythmias. *Risk D: Consider therapy modification*

QuiNIDine: Selective Serotonin Reuptake Inhibitors may decrease the metabolism of QuiNIDine. Fluvoxamine appears to be the only SSRI of concern. *Risk D: Consider therapy modification*

Risperidone: Selective Serotonin Reuptake Inhibitors may decrease the metabolism of Risperidone. *Risk C: Monitor therapy*

Salicylates: Antiplatelet Agents may enhance the adverse/toxic effect of Salicylates. Increased risk of bleeding may result. *Risk C: Monitor therapy*

Serotonin Modulators: May enhance the adverse/toxic effect of other Serotonin Modulators. The development of serotonin syndrome may occur. *Risk D: Consider therapy modification*

Sibutramine: May enhance the serotonergic effect of Serotonin Modulators. This may cause serotonin syndrome. *Risk X: Avoid combination*

Tamoxifen: CYP2D6 Inhibitors (Strong) may decrease the metabolism of Tamoxifen. Specifically, strong CYP2D6 inhibitors may decrease the formation of highly potent active metabolites. *Risk X: Avoid combination*

Tetrabenazine: QTc-Prolonging Agents may enhance the QTc-prolonging effect of Tetrabenazine. *Risk X: Avoid combination*

Tetrabenazine: CYP2D6 Inhibitors (Strong) may increase the serum concentration of Tetrabenazine. Specifically, concentrations of the active alpha- and beta-dihydrotetrabenazine metabolites may be increased. Management: Tetrabenazine dose should be reduced by 50% when starting a strong CYP2D6 inhibitor. Maximum tetrabenazine dose is 50 mg/day when used with a strong CYP2D6 inhibitor. *Risk D: Consider therapy modification*

Thioridazine: QTc-Prolonging Agents may enhance the QTc-prolonging effect of Thioridazine. *Risk X: Avoid combination*

Thioridazine: CYP2D6 Inhibitors may decrease the metabolism of Thioridazine. *Risk X: Avoid combination*

Thrombolytic Agents: Antiplatelet Agents may enhance the anticoagulant effect of Thrombolytic Agents. *Risk C: Monitor therapy*

Tositumomab and Iodine I 131 Tositumomab: Antiplatelet Agents may enhance the adverse/toxic effect of Tositumomab and Iodine I 131 Tositumomab. Specifically, the risk of bleeding-related adverse events may be increased. *Risk C: Monitor therapy*

TraMADol: Selective Serotonin Reuptake Inhibitors may enhance the neuroexcitatory and/or seizure-potentiating effect of TraMADol. TraMADol may enhance the serotonergic effect of Selective Serotonin Reuptake Inhibitors. This may cause serotonin syndrome. *Risk D: Consider therapy modification*

Tricyclic Antidepressants: Selective Serotonin Reuptake Inhibitors may decrease the metabolism of Tricyclic Antidepressants. *Risk D: Consider therapy modification*

Tryptophan: May enhance the serotonergic effect of Selective Serotonin Reuptake Inhibitors. This may cause serotonin syndrome. *Risk D: Consider therapy modification*

Vitamin K Antagonists (eg, warfarin): Selective Serotonin Reuptake Inhibitors may enhance the anticoagulant effect of Vitamin K Antagonists. *Risk C: Monitor therapy*

Ziprasidone: QTc-Prolonging Agents may enhance the QTc-prolonging effect of Ziprasidone. The risk of a severe arrhythmia may be increased. *Risk X: Avoid combination*

Ethanol/Nutrition/Herb Interactions

Ethanol: Avoid ethanol (may increase CNS depression). Depressed patients should avoid/limit intake.

Herb/Nutraceutical: Avoid valerian, St John's wort, kava kava, gotu kola (may increase CNS depression).

Stability All dosage forms should be stored at controlled room temperature of 15°C to 30°C (50°F to 86°F). Oral liquid should be dispensed in a light-resistant container.

Mechanism of Action Inhibits CNS neuron serotonin reuptake; minimal or no effect on reuptake of norepinephrine or dopamine; does not significantly bind to alpha-adrenergic, histamine, or cholinergic receptors

Pharmacodynamics/Kinetics

Onset of action: Depression: The onset of action is within a week, however, individual response varies greatly and full response may not be seen until 8-12 weeks after initiation of treatment.

Absorption: Well absorbed; delayed 1-2 hours with weekly formulation

Distribution: V_d: 12-43 L/kg

Protein binding: 95% to albumin and $alpha_1$ glycoprotein

Metabolism: Hepatic, via CYP2C19 and 2D6, to norfluoxetine (activity equal to fluoxetine)

Half-life elimination: Adults:

Parent drug: 1-3 days (acute), 4-6 days (chronic), 7.6 days (cirrhosis)

Metabolite (norfluoxetine): 9.3 days (range: 4-16 days), 12 days (cirrhosis)

Time to peak, serum: 6-8 hours

Excretion: Urine (10% as norfluoxetine, 2.5% to 5% as fluoxetine)

Note: Weekly formulation results in greater fluctuations between peak and trough concentrations of fluoxetine and norfluoxetine compared to once-daily dosing (24% daily/164% weekly; 17% daily/43% weekly, respectively). Trough concentrations are 76% lower for fluoxetine and 47% lower for norfluoxetine than the concentrations maintained by 20 mg once-daily dosing. Steady-state fluoxetine concentrations are ~50% lower following the once-weekly regimen compared to 20 mg once daily. Average steady-state concentrations of once-daily dosing were highest in children ages 6 to <13 (fluoxetine 171 ng/mL; norfluoxetine 195 ng/mL), followed by adolescents ages 13 to <18 (fluoxetine 86 ng/mL; norfluoxetine 113 ng/mL); concentrations were considered to be within the ranges reported in adults (fluoxetine 91-302 ng/mL; norfluoxetine 72-258 ng/mL).

Dosage Oral: **Note:** Upon discontinuation of fluoxetine therapy, gradually taper dose. If intolerable symptoms occur following a dose reduction, consider resuming the previously prescribed dose and/or decrease dose at a more gradual rate.

Children:

Depression: 8-18 years: 10-20 mg/day; lower-weight children can be started at 10 mg/day, may increase to 20 mg/day after 1 week if needed

Obsessive-compulsive disorder: 7-18 years: Initial: 10 mg/day; in adolescents and higher-weight children, dose may be increased to 20 mg/day after 2 weeks. Range: 10-60 mg/day.

Selective mutism (unlabeled use):

<5 years: No dosing information available

5-18 years: Initial: 5-10 mg/day; titrate upwards as needed (usual maximum dose: 60 mg/day)

Adults: 20 mg/day in the morning; may increase after several weeks by 20 mg/day increments; maximum: 80 mg/day; doses >20 mg may be given once daily or divided twice daily. **Note:** Lower doses of 5-10 mg/day have been used for initial treatment.

Usual dosage range:

Bulimia nervosa: 60-80 mg/day

Depression: 20-40 mg/day; patients maintained on Prozac® 20 mg/day may be changed to Prozac® Weekly™ 90 mg/week, starting dose 7 days after the last 20 mg/day dose

Obsessive-compulsive disorder: 40-80 mg/day

Panic disorder: Initial: 10 mg/day; after 1 week, increase to 20 mg/day; may increase after several weeks; doses >60 mg/day have not been evaluated

Premenstrual dysphoric disorder (Sarafem™): 20 mg/day continuously, **or** 20 mg/day starting 14 days prior to menstruation and through first full day of menses (repeat with each cycle)

Elderly: Depression: Some patients may require an initial dose of 10 mg/day with dosage increases of 10 and 20 mg every several weeks as tolerated; should not be taken at night unless patient experiences sedation

Dosing adjustment in renal impairment:

Single dose studies: Pharmacokinetics of fluoxetine and norfluoxetine were similar among subjects with all levels of impaired renal function, including anephric patients on chronic hemodialysis

Chronic administration: Additional accumulation of fluoxetine or norfluoxetine may occur in patients with severely impaired renal function

Hemodialysis: Not removed by hemodialysis; use of lower dose or less frequent dosing is not usually necessary.

Dosing adjustment in hepatic impairment: Elimination half-life of fluoxetine is prolonged in patients with hepatic impairment; a lower or less frequent dose of fluoxetine should be used in these patients

Cirrhosis patients: Administer a lower dose or less frequent dosing interval

Compensated cirrhosis without ascites: Administer 50% of normal dose

Child/Adolescent Considerations A study in children 8-15 years of age with obsessive compulsive disorder (n=14) used a fixed dose of 20 mg/day (Riddle, 1992). A study of children 10-18 years of age with obsessive compulsive symptoms and Tourette's syndrome (n=5) used 20-40 mg/day (Kurlan, 1993). Six children 6-12 years of age with selective mutism were treated with initial doses of 0.2 mg/kg/day for 1 week, then 0.4 mg/kg/day for 1 week, then 0.6 mg/kg/day for 10 weeks (Black, 1994). Twenty-one children (mean age: 8.2 years) with selective mutism received a mean end dose of 28.1 mg (10-60 mg) in a 9 week open trial (Dummit, 1996). Ninety-six outpatients 7-17 years of age with nonpsychotic major depression received 20 mg/day (Emslie, 1997); further studies are needed.

Numerous studies show a modest effect, at best, for selective serotonin reuptake inhibitors in the treatment of pediatric depression. However, data from these studies has suggested that fluoxetine may be more effective than other SSRIs, particularly in adolescents (Hetrick, 2007; Tsapakis, 2008; Usala, 2008). However, concerns remain for the risk of increased suicidal thinking/behaviors in children and adolescents.

Black B and Uhde TW, "Treatment of Elective Mutism With Fluoxetine: A Double Blind, Placebo-Controlled Study," *J Am Acad Child Adolesc Psychiatry*, 1994, 33(7):1000-6.

Bridge JA, Iyengar S, Salary CB, et al, "Clinical Response and Risk for Reported Suicidal Ideation and Suicide Attempts in Pediatric Antidepressant Treatment: A Meta-Analysis of Randomized Controlled Trials," *JAMA*, 2007, 297(15):1683-96.

Dummit ES 3rd, Klein RG, Tancer NK, et al, "Fluoxetine Treatment of Children With Selective Mutism: An Open Trial," *J Am Acad Child Adolesc Psychiatry*, 1996, 35(5):615-21.

Emslie GJ, Rush AJ, Weinberg WA, et al, "A Double-Blind, Randomized, Placebo-Controlled Trial of Fluoxetine in Children and Adolescents With Depression," *Arch Gen Psychiatry*, 1997, 54(11):1031-7.

Hetrick S, Merry S, McKenzie J, et al, "Selective Serotonin Reuptake Inhibitors (SSRIs) for Depressive Disorders in Children and Adolescents," *Cochrane Database Syst Rev*, 2007, 3:CD004851.

Kurlan R, Como PG, Deeley C, et al, "A Pilot Controlled Study of Fluoxetine for Obsessive-Compulsive Symptoms in Children With Tourette's Syndrome," *Clin Neuropharmacol*, 1993, 16(2):167-72.

Riddle MA, Scahill L, King RA, et al, "Double-Blind, Crossover Trial of Fluoxetine and Placebo in Children and Adolescents With Obsessive-Compulsive Disorder," *J Am Acad Child Adolesc Psychiatry*, 1992, 31 (6):1062-9.

Tsapakis EM, Soldani F, Tondo L, et al, "Efficacy of Antidepressants in Juvenile Depression: Meta-Analysis," *Br J Psychiatry*, 2008, 193(1):10-7.

Usala T, Clavenna A, Zuddas A, et al, "Randomised Controlled Trials of Selective Serotonin Reuptake Inhibitors in Treating Depression in Children and Adolescents: A Systematic Review and Meta-Analysis," *Eur Neuropsychopharmacol*, 2008, 18(1):62-73.

Dietary Considerations May be taken with or without food.

Monitoring Parameters Mental status for depression, suicidal ideation (especially at the beginning of therapy or when doses are increased or decreased), anxiety, social functioning, mania, panic attacks; akathisia, sleep

Reference Range Therapeutic levels have not been well established

Therapeutic: Fluoxetine: 100-800 ng/mL (SI: 289-2314 nmol/L); Norfluoxetine: 100-600 ng/mL (SI: 289-1735 nmol/L)

Toxic: Fluoxetine plus norfluoxetine: >2000 ng/mL

Additional Information ECG may reveal S-T segment depression. Not shown to be teratogenic in rodents; 15-60 mg/day, buspirone and cyproheptadine, may be useful in treatment of sexual dysfunction during treatment with a selective serotonin reuptake inhibitor.

Weekly capsules are a delayed release formulation containing enteric-coated pellets of fluoxetine hydrochloride, equivalent to 90 mg fluoxetine. Therapeutic equivalence of weekly formulation with daily formulation for delaying time to relapse has not been established.

Dosage Forms Excipient information presented when available (limited, particularly for generics); consult specific product labeling. **Note:** Strength expressed as base unless otherwise noted. [DSC] = Discontinued product

Capsule: 10 mg, 20 mg, 40 mg
- Prozac®: 10 mg, 20 mg, 40 mg
- Sarafem®: 10 mg, 20 mg [DSC]
- Selfemra™: 10 mg, 20 mg [contains soya lecithin]

Capsule, delayed release, enteric coated pellets:
- Prozac® Weekly™: 90 mg

Solution, oral: 20 mg/5 mL (5 mL, 120 mL) [contains ethanol 0.23% and benzoic acid; mint flavor]
- Prozac®: 20 mg/5 mL (120 mL) [contains ethanol 0.23% and benzoic acid; mint flavor]

Tablet: 10 mg, 20 mg
- Prozac® [scored]: 10 mg [DSC]
- Sarafem®: 10 mg, 20 mg

◆ **Fluoxetine and Olanzapine** *see* Olanzapine and Fluoxetine *on page 1165*

◆ **Fluoxetine Hydrochloride** *see* FLUoxetine *on page 650*

Fluoxymesterone (floo oks i MES te rone)

Medication Safety Issues

Sound-alike/look-alike issues:

Halotestin® may be confused with Haldol®, haloperidol, halothane

U.S. Brand Names Androxy™

Mexican Brand Names Stenox

Pharmacologic Category Androgen

Use Replacement of endogenous testicular hormone; in females, palliative treatment of breast cancer

Unlabeled/Investigational Use Stimulation of erythropoiesis, angioneurotic edema

Effect on Mental Status None reported

Effect on Psychiatric Treatment May cause leukopenia; use caution with clozapine and carbamazepine

Restrictions C-III

Dosage Summary

Oral:

Children: Dosage not established

Adults (females): 10-40 mg/day in divided doses

Adults (males): 2.5-20 mg/day

Dosage Forms Excipient information presented when available (limited, particularly for generics); consult specific product labeling.

Tablet: 10 mg

Androxy™: 10 mg

Flupenthixol (floo pen THIKS ol)

Related Information

Discontinuation of Psychotropic Drugs *on page 1839*

Canadian Brand Names Fluanxol®

Index Terms Flupenthixol Decanoate; Flupenthixol Dihydrochloride

Pharmacologic Category Antipsychotic Agent, Typical

Generic Available No

Use Maintenance therapy of chronic schizophrenic patients whose main manifestations do **not** include excitement, agitation, or hyperactivity

Mental Health Comment Primarily used as a long-acting injectable antipsychotic for patients who are nonadherent to oral medication treatment.

Coadministration of two or more antipsychotics does not generally improve clinical response and may increase the potential for adverse effects.

In 2008, the FDA issued a warning regarding increased mortality risk with typical **and** atypical antipsychotic drugs when used in elderly patients with dementia-related psychosis.

Restrictions Not available in U.S.

Pregnancy Risk Factor C (based on similar agents)

Lactation Enters breast milk/not recommended

Contraindications Hypersensitivity to flupenthixol, phenothiazines, thioxanthenes, or any component of the formulation; acute intoxication (ethanol, barbiturate, or opioid); severe CNS depression; coma; severely-agitated patients; suspected or established subcortical brain damage; cerebrovascular or renal insufficiency; severe cardiovascular disease/circulatory collapse; blood dyscrasias; pheochromocytoma

Warnings/Precautions May alter cardiac conduction; life-threatening arrhythmias have occurred with therapeutic doses of antipsychotics. Avoid use in patients with underlying QT prolongation, in those taking medicines that prolong the QT interval, or cause polymorphic ventricular tachycardia; monitor ECG closely for dose-related QT effects. Adverse effects of decanoate may be prolonged. Myelosuppression (eg, leukopenia, agranulocytosis) has been observed with antipsychotic use; check blood counts periodically and discontinue at first signs of blood dyscrasias; use is contraindicated in patients with bone marrow suppression. Antipsychotic use has been associated with esophageal dysmotility and aspiration; use with caution in patients at risk of pneumonia (ie, Alzheimer's disease). May cause extrapyramidal symptoms (EPS), including pseudoparkinsonism, acute dystonic reactions, akathisia, and tardive dyskinesia (risk of these reactions is high relative to other neuroleptics). Risk of dystonia (and possibly other EPS) may be greater with increased doses, use of conventional antipsychotics, males, and younger patients. Use may be associated with NMS; monitor for mental status changes, fever, muscle rigidity, and/or autonomic instability (risk may be increased in patients with Parkinson's disease or Lewy body dementia). May cause orthostatic hypotension; use with caution in patients at risk of this effect or in those who would not tolerate transient hypotensive episodes (cerebrovascular disease, cardiovascular disease, hypovolemia, or concurrent medication use which may predispose to hypotension/bradycardia). May be associated with pigmentary retinopathy. May be sedating, use with caution in disorders where CNS depression is a feature; patients must be cautioned about performing tasks which require mental alertness (eg, operating machinery or driving). Impaired core body temperature regulation may occur; caution with strenuous exercise, heat exposure, dehydration, and concomitant medication possessing anticholinergic effects.

Elderly patients with dementia-related psychosis treated with antipsychotics are at an increased risk of death compared to placebo. An increased incidence of cerebrovascular adverse events (including fatalities) has been reported in elderly patients with dementia-related psychosis. Flupenthixol is not approved for this indication.

May be sedating, use with caution in disorders where CNS depression is a feature; patients must be cautioned about performing tasks which require mental alertness (eg, operating machinery or driving). May cause anticholinergic effects (constipation, xerostomia, blurred vision, urinary retention); use with caution in patients with decreased gastrointestinal motility, paralytic ileus, urinary retention, BPH, xerostomia, or visual problems. Relative to other neuroleptics, flupenthixol has a low potency of cholinergic blockade. May mask toxicity of other drugs or conditions (eg, intestinal obstruction, Reye's syndrome, brain tumor) due to antiemetic effects.

Use with caution in patients with severe cardiovascular disease, narrow-angle glaucoma, hepatic impairment, myasthenia gravis, Parkinson's disease, breast cancer or other prolactin-dependent tumors, renal impairment, respiratory disease, or seizure disorder. Safety and efficacy have not been established in children.

Adverse Reactions Frequency not defined.

Central nervous system: Extrapyramidal effects (up to 30%; including akathisia, dystonia, pseudoparkinsonism, tardive dyskinesia), anxiety/nervousness, insomnia, headache, dizziness, depression, fatigue

Dermatologic: Contact dermatitis, exfoliative dermatitis, pruritus, rash

Endocrine & metabolic: Galactorrhea, glycosuria, gynecomastia, hyperglycemia, libido decreased, weight gain

Gastrointestinal: Nausea, salivation increased, vomiting, xerostomia

Genitourinary: Micturition disorder

Neuromuscular & skeletal: Hypertonia, tremor, weakness

Ocular: Abnormal accommodation, abnormal vision

Miscellaneous: Diaphoresis increased

Additional adverse events associated with antipsychotics include arrhythmias, angioedema, hematologic adverse effects (agranulocytosis, hemolytic anemia, pancytopenia, thrombocytopenia), neuroleptic malignant syndrome (NMS), photosensitivity, seizure

Drug Interactions

Acetylcholinesterase Inhibitors (Central): May enhance the neurotoxic (central) effect of Antipsychotics. Severe extrapyramidal symptoms have occurred in some patients. *Risk C: Monitor therapy*

Alcohol (Ethyl): CNS Depressants may enhance the CNS depressant effect of Alcohol (Ethyl). *Risk C: Monitor therapy*

Alfuzosin: May enhance the QTc-prolonging effect of QTc-Prolonging Agents. *Risk C: Monitor therapy*

Amphetamines: Antipsychotics may diminish the stimulatory effect of Amphetamines. *Risk C: Monitor therapy*

Anticholinergics: May enhance the adverse/toxic effect of other Anticholinergics. **Exceptions:** Paliperidone. *Risk C: Monitor therapy*

Anti-Parkinson's Agents (Dopamine Agonist): Antipsychotics (Typical) may diminish the therapeutic effect of Anti-Parkinson's Agents (Dopamine Agonist). *Risk D: Consider therapy modification*

Ciprofloxacin: May enhance the QTc-prolonging effect of QTc-Prolonging Agents. *Risk C: Monitor therapy*

CNS Depressants: May enhance the adverse/toxic effect of other CNS Depressants. *Risk C: Monitor therapy*

Gadobutrol: May enhance the QTc-prolonging effect of QTc-Prolonging Agents. *Risk D: Consider therapy modification*

Lithium formulations: May enhance the neurotoxic effect of Antipsychotics. Lithium formulations may decrease the serum concentration of Antipsychotics. Specifically noted with chlorpromazine. *Risk C: Monitor therapy*

Nilotinib: May enhance the QTc-prolonging effect of QTc-Prolonging Agents. *Risk X: Avoid combination*

Pramlintide: May enhance the anticholinergic effect of Anticholinergics. These effects are specific to the GI tract. *Risk D: Consider therapy modification*

QTc-Prolonging Agents: May enhance the adverse/toxic effect of other QTc-Prolonging Agents. Their effects can be additive, causing life-threatening ventricular arrhythmias. *Risk D: Consider therapy modification*

Tetrabenazine: May enhance the adverse/toxic effect of Antipsychotics. *Risk C: Monitor therapy*

Thioridazine: QTc-Prolonging Agents may enhance the QTc-prolonging effect of Thioridazine. *Risk X: Avoid combination*

Ziprasidone: QTc-Prolonging Agents may enhance the QTc-prolonging effect of Ziprasidone. The risk of a severe arrhythmia may be increased. *Risk X: Avoid combination*

Stability Solution: Store at room temperature. Protect from light.

Mechanism of Action Flupenthixol is a thioxanthene antipsychotic which blocks postsynaptic dopamine receptors in the CNS, resulting in inhibition of dopamine-mediated effects.

Pharmacodynamics/Kinetics

Onset: I.M. depot: 24-72 hours following injection

Duration: I.M. depot: 2-4 weeks

Metabolism: Hepatic

Time to peak:

- I.M. depot: 4-7 days
- Oral: 3-8 hours

Excretion: Feces (as metabolites); urine (small amounts)

Dosage

I.M. (depot): Flupenthixol is administered by deep I.M. injection, preferably in the gluteus maximus, **NOT for I.V. use**; maintenance dosages are given at 2- to 3-week intervals

Patients not previously treated with long-acting depot neuroleptics should be given an initial test dose of 5-20 mg. An initial dose of 20 mg is usually well tolerated; however, a 5 mg test dose is recommended in elderly, frail, and cachectic patients, and in patients whose individual or family history suggests a predisposition to extrapyramidal reactions. In the subsequent 5-10 days, the therapeutic response and the appearance of extrapyramidal symptoms should be carefully monitored. Oral neuroleptic drugs may be continued, but dosage should be reduced during this overlapping period and eventually discontinued.

Oral: Initial: 1 mg 3 times/day; dose must be individualized. May be increased by 1 mg every 2-3 days based on tolerance and control of symptoms. Usual maintenance dosage: 3-6 mg/day in divided doses (doses ≥12 mg/day used in some patients).

Administration Administer by deep I.M. injection, preferably in the gluteus maximum; **not for I.V. use**

Monitoring Parameters Vital signs; lipid profile, fasting blood glucose/Hgb A_{1c}; BMI; mental status, abnormal involuntary movement scale (AIMS), extrapyramidal symptoms (EPS)

Additional Information Not available in U.S.

Dosage Forms Excipient information presented when available (limited, particularly for generics); consult specific product labeling.

Injection, solution, as decanoate [depot]: 20 mg/mL (10 mL); 100 mg/mL (2 mL)

Tablet, as dihydrochloride: 0.5 mg, 3 mg

◆ **Flupenthixol Decanoate** *see* Flupenthixol *on page 658*

◆ **Flupenthixol Dihydrochloride** *see* Flupenthixol *on page 658*

Fluphenazine (floo FEN a zeen)

Medication Safety Issues

Sound-alike/look-alike issues:

Prolixin® may be confused with Proloprim®

International issues:

Prolixin® may be confused with Prolixan® which is a brand name for azapropazone in multiple international markets

Related Information

Anticholinergic Effects of Common Psychotropics *on page 1758*

Antipsychotic Agents *on page 1769*

CMS: Long-Term Care Facility Thresholds *on page 1815*

Discontinuation of Psychotropic Drugs *on page 1839*

Liquid Compatibility of Antidepressants, Antipsychotics, and Mood Stabilizers *on page 1788*

Canadian Brand Names Apo-Fluphenazine Decanoate®; Apo-Fluphenazine®; Modecate®; Modecate® Concentrate; PMS-Fluphenazine Decanoate

Index Terms Fluphenazine Decanoate

Pharmacologic Category Antipsychotic Agent, Typical, Phenothiazine

Generic Available Yes

Use Management of manifestations of psychotic disorders and schizophrenia; depot formulation may offer improved outcome in individuals with psychosis who are nonadherent with oral antipsychotics

Unlabeled/Investigational Use Pervasive developmental disorder; nonpsychotic patient, dementia behavior in the elderly; psychosis/agitation related to Alzheimer's dementia

Mental Health Comment Fluphenazine is a high-potency antipsychotic. Older antipsychotic medications (chlorpromazine, haloperidol), which do not meet specific criteria for "atypical" antipsychotics, are often referred to as typical antipsychotics. They are associated with the troubling side effect, EPS. However, it is commonly believed that in order for a drug to treat psychosis, it must block dopamine is some manner.

Common side effects include sedation and neuroleptic effect (reduced initiative, interest in the environment, and display of emotion or affect). All **typical** antipsychotics are considered to be equally effective if given in equipotent doses. An inverse relationship exists between intrinsic antimuscarinic activity and propensity to cause extrapyramidal side effects. If dystonia or pseudoparkinsonism occurs, antiparkinsonian agents should be considered. If akathisia occurs, beta-blockers (eg, propranolol), benzodiazepines, or antiparkinsonian agents should be considered. Tardive dyskinesia (TD) secondary to typical antipsychotics has an estimated incidence of 3% to 5% per year for the first 5 years of treatment. After this time period, the incidence is estimated to be 2% to 3% per year. Prevalence rates are ~15% to 20%. Female gender and age constitute risk factors for TD. Indeed, prevalence rates have been reported to be as high as 70% in elderly females. No specific treatment exists for TD, however, patients are often initiated on/switched to an atypical antipsychotic because of their lower incidence to cause TD and hopes of suppression.

Typical antipsychotics are usually only indicated for schizophrenia, but are generally effective for mania and psychosis and/or behavioral syndromes secondary to other mental conditions. Nonpsychiatric uses include Tourette's syndrome, Huntington's disease, and occasionally, intractable hiccups, pruritus, nausea, and vomiting.

These drugs are thought to exert their antipsychotic activity by blocking dopamine D_2 receptors in the mesolimbic dopaminergic pathway. Side effects are often related to their ability to antagonize dopamine receptors in the nigrostriatal and tuberoinfundibular pathways.

Long-acting dosage form is useful in patients nonadherent to treatment.

Coadministration of two or more antipsychotics does not generally improve clinical response and may increase the potential for adverse effects.

In 2008, the FDA issued a warning regarding increased mortality risk with typical **and** atypical antipsychotic drugs when used in elderly patients with dementia-related psychosis.

Pregnancy Risk Factor C

Lactation Enters breast milk/not recommended

Contraindications Hypersensitivity to fluphenazine or any component of the formulation (cross-reactivity between phenothiazines may occur); severe CNS depression; coma; subcortical brain damage; blood dyscrasias; hepatic disease

Warnings/Precautions May be sedating; use with caution in disorders where CNS depression is a feature. Use with caution in Parkinson's disease. Caution in patients with hemodynamic instability; predisposition to seizures; or severe cardiac, renal, or respiratory disease. Esophageal dysmotility and aspiration have been associated with antipsychotic use - use with caution in patients at risk of pneumonia (ie, Alzheimer's disease). Caution in breast cancer or other prolactin-dependent tumors (may elevate prolactin levels). May alter temperature regulation or mask toxicity of other drugs due to antiemetic effects. May alter cardiac conduction; life-threatening arrhythmias have occurred with therapeutic doses of phenothiazines. Hypotension may occur, particularly with I.M. administration. May cause orthostatic hypotension - use with caution in patients at risk of this effect or those who would tolerate transient hypotensive episodes (cerebrovascular disease, cardiovascular disease, or other medications which may predispose). Adverse effects of depot injections may be prolonged. Check blood counts periodically and discontinue at first signs of blood dyscrasias; use is contraindicated in patients with bone marrow suppression.

Due to anticholinergic effects, use caution in patients with decreased gastrointestinal motility, urinary retention, BPH, xerostomia, visual problems, narrow-angle glaucoma (screening is recommended), and myasthenia gravis. Relative to other antipsychotics, fluphenazine has a low potency of cholinergic blockade.

May cause extrapyramidal symptoms, including pseudoparkinsonism, acute dystonic reactions, akathisia, and tardive dyskinesia (risk of these reactions is high relative to other antipsychotics). Use caution in the elderly. May be associated with neuroleptic malignant syndrome (NMS) or pigmentary retinopathy.

Adverse Reactions Frequency not defined.

Cardiovascular: Tachycardia, fluctuations in blood pressure, hyper-/hypotension, arrhythmia, edema

Central nervous system: Parkinsonian symptoms, akathisia, dystonias, tardive dyskinesia, dizziness, hyper-reflexia, headache, cerebral edema, drowsiness, lethargy, restlessness, excitement, bizarre dreams, EEG changes, depression, seizure, NMS, altered central temperature regulation

Dermatologic: Dermatitis, eczema, erythema, itching, photosensitivity, rash, seborrhea, skin pigmentation, urticaria

Endocrine & metabolic: Menstrual cycle changes, breast pain, amenorrhea, galactorrhea, gynecomastia, libido changes, prolactin increased, SIADH

Gastrointestinal: Weight gain, appetite loss, salivation, xerostomia, constipation, paralytic ileus, laryngeal edema

Genitourinary: Ejaculatory disturbances, impotence, polyuria, bladder paralysis, enuresis

Hematologic: Agranulocytosis, leukopenia, thrombocytopenia, nonthrombocytopenic purpura, eosinophilia, pancytopenia

Hepatic: Cholestatic jaundice, hepatotoxicity

Neuromuscular & skeletal: Trembling of fingers, SLE, facial hemispasm

Ocular: Pigmentary retinopathy, cornea and lens changes, blurred vision, glaucoma

Respiratory: Nasal congestion, asthma

Metabolism/Transport Effects **Substrate** of CYP2D6 (major); **Inhibits** CYP1A2 (weak), 2C9 (weak), 2D6 (weak), 2E1 (weak)

Drug Interactions

Acetylcholinesterase Inhibitors (Central): May enhance the neurotoxic (central) effect of Antipsychotics. Severe extrapyramidal symptoms have occurred in some patients. *Risk C: Monitor therapy*

Alcohol (Ethyl): CNS Depressants may enhance the CNS depressant effect of Alcohol (Ethyl). *Risk C: Monitor therapy*

Amphetamines: Antipsychotics may diminish the stimulatory effect of Amphetamines. *Risk C: Monitor therapy*

Analgesics (Opioid): Antipsychotic Agents (Phenothiazines) may enhance the hypotensive effect of Analgesics (Opioid). *Risk C: Monitor therapy*

Antacids: May decrease the absorption of Antipsychotic Agents (Phenothiazines). *Risk C: Monitor therapy*

Anticholinergics: May enhance the adverse/toxic effect of other Anticholinergics. **Exceptions:** Paliperidone. *Risk C: Monitor therapy*

Antimalarial Agents: May increase the serum concentration of Antipsychotic Agents (Phenothiazines). *Risk C: Monitor therapy*

Anti-Parkinson's Agents (Dopamine Agonist): Antipsychotics (Typical) may diminish the therapeutic effect of Anti-Parkinson's Agents (Dopamine Agonist). *Risk D: Consider therapy modification*

Beta-Blockers: Antipsychotic Agents (Phenothiazines) may enhance the hypotensive effect of Beta-Blockers. Beta-Blockers may decrease the metabolism of Antipsychotic Agents (Phenothiazines). Antipsychotic Agents (Phenothiazines) may decrease the metabolism of Beta-Blockers. **Exceptions:** Atenolol; Levobunolol; Metipranolol; Nadolol. *Risk C: Monitor therapy*

CNS Depressants: May enhance the adverse/toxic effect of other CNS Depressants. *Risk C: Monitor therapy*

CYP2D6 Inhibitors (Moderate): May decrease the metabolism of CYP2D6 Substrates. *Risk C: Monitor therapy*

CYP2D6 Inhibitors (Strong): May decrease the metabolism of CYP2D6 Substrates. *Risk D: Consider therapy modification*

Darunavir: May increase the serum concentration of CYP2D6 Substrates. *Risk C: Monitor therapy*

Lithium formulations: May enhance the neurotoxic effect of Antipsychotics. Lithium formulations may decrease the serum concentration of Antipsychotics. Specifically noted with chlorpromazine. *Risk C: Monitor therapy*

Pramlintide: May enhance the anticholinergic effect of Anticholinergics. These effects are specific to the GI tract. *Risk D: Consider therapy modification*

Tetrabenazine: May enhance the adverse/toxic effect of Antipsychotics. *Risk C: Monitor therapy*

Ethanol/Nutrition/Herb Interactions

Ethanol: Avoid ethanol (may increase CNS depression).

Herb/Nutraceutical: Avoid dong quai, St John's wort (may also cause photosensitization). Avoid kava kava, gotu kola, valerian, St John's wort (may increase CNS depression).

Stability Avoid freezing. Protect all dosage forms from light. Clear or slightly yellow solutions may be used. Should be dispensed in amber or opaque vials/

bottles. Solutions may be diluted or mixed with fruit juices or other liquids, but must be administered immediately after mixing. Do not prepare bulk dilutions or store bulk dilutions.

Mechanism of Action Fluphenazine is a piperazine phenothiazine antipsychotic which blocks postsynaptic mesolimbic dopaminergic D_1 and D_2 receptors in the brain; depresses the release of hypothalamic and hypophyseal hormones; believed to depress the reticular activating system, thus affecting basal metabolism, body temperature, wakefulness, vasomotor tone, and emesis

Pharmacodynamics/Kinetics

Onset of action: I.M., SubQ (derivative dependent): Hydrochloride salt: ~1 hour
Peak effect: Neuroleptic: Decanoate: 48-96 hours

Duration: Hydrochloride salt: 6-8 hours; Decanoate: 24-72 hours

Absorption: Oral: Erratic and variable

Distribution: Crosses placenta; enters breast milk

Protein binding: 91% and 99%

Metabolism: Hepatic

Half-life elimination (derivative dependent): Hydrochloride: 33 hours; Decanoate: 163-232 hours

Excretion: Urine (as metabolites)

Dosage

Children: Oral: Childhood-onset pervasive developmental disorder (unlabeled use): 0.04 mg/kg/day

Adults: Psychoses:

Oral: 0.5-10 mg/day in divided doses at 6- to 8-hour intervals; some patients may require up to 40 mg/day

I.M.: 2.5-10 mg/day in divided doses at 6- to 8-hour intervals (parenteral dose is 1/3 to 1/2 the oral dose for the hydrochloride salts)

I.M. (decanoate): 12.5-37.5 mg every 2 weeks

Conversion from hydrochloride to decanoate I.M. 0.5 mL (12.5 mg) decanoate every 3 weeks is approximately equivalent to 10 mg hydrochloride/day; **Note:** Clinically, an every-2-week interval is frequently utilized

Elderly: Nonpsychotic patient, dementia behavior (unlabeled use): Oral: 1-2.5 mg/day; increase dose at 4- to 7-day intervals by 1-2.5 mg/day. Increase dosing intervals (bid, tid) as necessary to control response or side effects. Maximum daily dose: 20 mg; gradual increases (titration) may prevent some side effects or decrease their severity.

Hemodialysis: Not dialyzable (0% to 5%)

Child/Adolescent Considerations Twelve hospitalized children 7-11 years of age with childhood-onset pervasive developmental disorder received haloperidol or fluphenazine at an average dose of 0.04 mg/kg/day (Joshi, 1988).

Joshi PT, Capozzoli JA, and Coyle JT, "Low-Dose Neuroleptic Therapy for Children With Childhood-Onset Pervasive Developmental Disorder," *Am J Psychiatry*, 1988, 145(3):335-8.

Administration Avoid contact of oral solution or injection with skin (contact dermatitis). Oral liquid should be diluted in the following **only**: Water, saline, homogenized milk, carbonated orange beverages, pineapple, apricot, prune, orange, tomato, and grapefruit juices. Do **not** dilute in beverages containing caffeine, tannics, or pectinate. Watch for hypotension when administering I.M.

Monitoring Parameters Vital signs; lipid profile, fasting blood glucose/Hgb A_{1c}; BMI; mental status, abnormal involuntary movement scale (AIMS), extrapyramidal symptoms (EPS)

Reference Range Therapeutic: 0.3-3 ng/mL (SI: 0.6-6.0 nmol/L); correlation of serum concentrations and efficacy is controversial; most often dosed to best response

Additional Information Less sedative and hypotensive effects than chlorpromazine.

Dosage Forms Excipient information presented when available (limited, particularly for generics); consult specific product labeling. [DSC] = Discontinued product

Elixir, as hydrochloride: 2.5 mg/5 mL (60 mL) [contains alcohol 14% and sodium benzoate] [DSC]

Injection, oil, as decanoate: 25 mg/mL (5 mL) [may contain benzyl alcohol, sesame oil]

Injection, solution, as hydrochloride: 2.5 mg/mL (10 mL)

Solution, oral concentrate, as hydrochloride: 5 mg/mL (120 mL) [contains alcohol 14%]

Tablet, as hydrochloride: 1 mg, 2.5 mg, 5 mg, 10 mg

◆ **Fluphenazine Decanoate** *see* Fluphenazine *on page 660*

Flurazepam (flure AZ e pam)

Medication Safety Issues

Sound-alike/look-alike issues:

Flurazepam may be confused with temazepam

Dalmane® may be confused with Demulen®, Dialume®

Related Information

Benzodiazepines *on page 1774*

CMS: Long-Term Care Facility Thresholds *on page 1815*

Discontinuation of Psychotropic Drugs *on page 1839*

U.S. Brand Names Dalmane®

Canadian Brand Names Apo-Flurazepam®; Dalmane®; Som Pam

Index Terms Flurazepam Hydrochloride

Pharmacologic Category Hypnotic, Benzodiazepine

Generic Available Yes

Use Short-term treatment of insomnia

Mental Health Comment In 2007, the FDA requested that all manufacturers of sedative-hypnotic drug products revise labeling to include a greater emphasis on the risks of adverse effects. These risks include severe allergic reactions (anaphylaxis, angioedema) and complex sleep-related behaviors, which may include sleep-driving (driving while not fully awake and with no memory of the event), making phone calls, and preparing and eating food while asleep.

There are two subtypes of GABA receptors (GABA-A and GABA-B) and three different benzodiazepine receptors (Bz_1, Bz_2, and Bz_3). Benzodiazepine receptors and effects appear to be linked to the GABA-A receptors. Benzodiazepines do not bind to GABA-B receptors. The role of GABA-B receptors is unclear. Benzodiazepines have no specificity for benzodiazepine receptor subtypes.

Flurazepam is a long half-life benzodiazepine. Duration of action after a single dose is determined by redistribution rather than metabolism. Tolerance develops to the sedative, hypnotic, and anticonvulsant effects. It does not develop to the anxiolytic or skeletal muscle-relaxing effects. Psychological and physical dependence may occur with prolonged use of benzodiazepines. The onset of withdrawal symptoms is usually seen on the first day without drug and lasts 5-7 days in patients receiving short half-life benzodiazepines, whereas, the onset occurs after 5 days with a duration of 10-14 days after abrupt discontinuance of long half-life benzodiazepines. Risk factors for abuse include personal or family history of substance abuse and personality disorder.

Restrictions C-IV

Pregnancy Risk Factor X

Pregnancy Considerations An increased risk of fetal malformations has been associated with maternal use of other benzodiazepines during the 1st trimester of pregnancy. Neonatal depression has been observed, specifically following exposure to flurazepam when used maternally for 10 consecutive days prior to delivery. Serum levels of N-desalkylflurazepam were measurable in the infant during the first 4 days of life. Use of flurazepam during pregnancy is contraindicated.

Lactation Excretion in breast milk unknown/not recommended

Contraindications Hypersensitivity to flurazepam or any component of the formulation (cross-sensitivity with other benzodiazepines may exist); narrow-angle glaucoma; pregnancy

Warnings/Precautions Use with caution in elderly or debilitated patients, patients with hepatic disease (including alcoholics), or renal impairment. Use with caution in patients with respiratory disease or impaired gag reflex. Avoid use in patients with sleep apnea.

Causes CNS depression (dose related); patients must be cautioned about performing tasks which require mental alertness (eg, operating machinery or driving). Use with caution in patients receiving other CNS depressants or psychoactive agents. Benzodiazepines have been associated with falls and traumatic injury and should be used with extreme caution in patients who are at risk of these events (especially the elderly).

Use caution in patients with depression, particularly if suicidal risk may be present. Use with caution in patients with a history of drug dependence. Benzodiazepines have been associated with dependence and acute withdrawal symptoms on discontinuation or reduction in dose (may occur after as little as 10 days of use).

As a hypnotic, should be used only after evaluation of potential causes of sleep disturbance. Failure of sleep disturbance to resolve after 7-10 days may indicate psychiatric or medical illness. A worsening of insomnia or the emergence of new abnormalities of thought or behavior may represent unrecognized psychiatric or medical illness and requires immediate and careful evaluation. Postmarketing studies have indicated that the use of hypnotic/sedative agents for sleep has been associated with hypersensitivity reactions including anaphylaxis as well as angioedema. An increased risk for hazardous sleep-related activities such as sleep-driving; cooking and eating food, and making phone calls while asleep have also been noted.

Benzodiazepines have been associated with anterograde amnesia. Paradoxical reactions have been reported, particularly in adolescent/pediatric or psychiatric patients. Does not have analgesic, antidepressant, or antipsychotic properties.

Safety and efficacy have not been established in children <15 years of age.

Adverse Reactions Frequency not defined.

Cardiovascular: Chest pain, flushing, hypotension, palpitation

Central nervous system: Apprehension, ataxia, confusion, depression, dizziness, drowsiness, euphoria, faintness, falling, hallucinations, hangover effect, headache, irritability, lightheadedness, memory impairment, nervousness, paradoxical reactions, restlessness, slurred speech, staggering, talkativeness

Dermatologic: Pruritus, rash

Gastrointestinal: Appetite increased/decreased, bitter taste, constipation, diarrhea, GI pain, heartburn, nausea, salivation increased/excessive, upset stomach, vomiting, weight gain/loss, xerostomia

Hematologic: Granulocytopenia, leukopenia

Hepatic: Alkaline phosphatase increased, ALT increased, AST increased, cholestatic jaundice, total bilirubin increased

Neuromuscular & skeletal: Body/joint pain, dysarthria, reflex slowing, weakness

Ocular: Blurred vision, burning eyes, difficulty focusing

Respiratory: Apnea, dyspnea

Miscellaneous: Diaphoresis, drug dependence

Metabolism/Transport Effects **Substrate** of CYP3A4 (major); **Inhibits** CYP2E1 (weak)

Drug Interactions

Alcohol (Ethyl): CNS Depressants may enhance the CNS depressant effect of Alcohol (Ethyl). *Risk C: Monitor therapy*

Antifungal Agents (Azole Derivatives, Systemic): May decrease the metabolism of Benzodiazepines (metabolized by oxidation). *Risk D: Consider therapy modification*

Aprepitant: May increase the serum concentration of Benzodiazepines (metabolized by oxidation). *Risk C: Monitor therapy*

Calcium Channel Blockers (Nondihydropyridine): May decrease the metabolism of Benzodiazepines (metabolized by oxidation). *Risk D: Consider therapy modification*

CarBAMazepine: May increase the metabolism of Benzodiazepines (metabolized by oxidation). *Risk C: Monitor therapy*

Cimetidine: May decrease the metabolism of Benzodiazepines (metabolized by oxidation). *Risk C: Monitor therapy*

Clozapine: Benzodiazepines may enhance the adverse/toxic effect of Clozapine. *Risk D: Consider therapy modification*

CNS Depressants: May enhance the adverse/toxic effect of other CNS Depressants. *Risk C: Monitor therapy*

CYP3A4 Inducers (Strong): May increase the metabolism of CYP3A4 Substrates. *Risk C: Monitor therapy*

CYP3A4 Inhibitors (Moderate): May decrease the metabolism of CYP3A4 Substrates. *Risk C: Monitor therapy*

CYP3A4 Inhibitors (Strong): May decrease the metabolism of CYP3A4 Substrates. *Risk D: Consider therapy modification*

Dasatinib: May increase the serum concentration of CYP3A4 Substrates. *Risk C: Monitor therapy*

Deferasirox: May decrease the serum concentration of CYP3A4 Substrates. *Risk C: Monitor therapy*

Disulfiram: May decrease the metabolism of Benzodiazepines (metabolized by oxidation). *Risk C: Monitor therapy*

Fluconazole: May decrease the metabolism of Benzodiazepines (metabolized by oxidation). *Risk D: Consider therapy modification*

Fosaprepitant: May increase the serum concentration of Benzodiazepines (metabolized by oxidation). Specifically, the active metabolite aprepitant is likely responsible for this effect. *Risk C: Monitor therapy*

Grapefruit Juice: May decrease the metabolism of Benzodiazepines (metabolized by oxidation). *Risk D: Consider therapy modification*

Isoniazid: May decrease the metabolism of Benzodiazepines (metabolized by oxidation). *Risk C: Monitor therapy*

Macrolide Antibiotics: May decrease the metabolism of Benzodiazepines (metabolized by oxidation). **Exceptions:** Azithromycin; Dirithromycin [Off Market]; Spiramycin. *Risk D: Consider therapy modification*

Nefazodone: May decrease the metabolism of Benzodiazepines (metabolized by oxidation). *Risk D: Consider therapy modification*

Oral Contraceptive (Estrogens): May decrease the metabolism of Benzodiazepines (metabolized by oxidation). *Risk C: Monitor therapy*

Oral Contraceptive (Progestins): May decrease the metabolism of Benzodiazepines (metabolized by oxidation). *Risk C: Monitor therapy*

Phenytoin: Benzodiazepines may increase the serum concentration of Phenytoin. Short-term exposure to benzodiazepines may not present as much risk as chronic therapy. *Risk C: Monitor therapy*

Protease Inhibitors: May decrease the metabolism of Benzodiazepines (metabolized by oxidation). Management: Amprenavir, atazanavir, darunavir, indinavir, nelfinavir, ritonavir, and tipranavir are contraindicated with midazolam and triazolam according to each protease inhibitor 's prescribing information. *Risk D: Consider therapy modification*

Proton Pump Inhibitors: May increase the serum concentration of Benzodiazepines (metabolized by oxidation). **Exceptions:** Lansoprazole; Pantoprazole; Rabeprazole. *Risk C: Monitor therapy*

Rifamycin Derivatives: May increase the metabolism of Benzodiazepines (metabolized by oxidation). *Risk D: Consider therapy modification*

Selective Serotonin Reuptake Inhibitors: May decrease the metabolism of Benzodiazepines (metabolized by oxidation). **Exceptions:** Citalopram; Escitalopram; PARoxetine; Sertraline. *Risk C: Monitor therapy*

St Johns Wort: May increase the metabolism of Benzodiazepines (metabolized by oxidation). *Risk C: Monitor therapy*

Theophylline Derivatives: May diminish the therapeutic effect of Benzodiazepines. *Risk D: Consider therapy modification*

Ethanol/Nutrition/Herb Interactions

Ethanol: Avoid ethanol (may increase CNS depression).

Food: Serum levels and response to flurazepam may be increased by grapefruit juice, but unlikely because of flurazepam's high oral bioavailability.

Herb/Nutraceutical: Avoid valerian, St John's wort, kava kava, gotu kola (may increase CNS depression).

Stability Store at 15°C to 30°C (59°F to 86°F).

Mechanism of Action Binds to stereospecific benzodiazepine receptors on the postsynaptic GABA neuron at several sites within the central nervous system, including the limbic system, reticular formation. Enhancement of the inhibitory effect of GABA on neuronal excitability results by increased neuronal membrane permeability to chloride ions. This shift in chloride ions results in hyperpolarization (a less excitable state) and stabilization.

Pharmacodynamics/Kinetics

Onset of action: Hypnotic: 15-20 minutes

Peak effect: 3-6 hours

Duration: 7-8 hours

Metabolism: Hepatic to N-desalkylflurazepam (active) and N-hydroxyethylflurazepam

Half-life elimination:

Flurazepam: 2.3 hours

N-desalkylflurazepam:

Adults: Single dose: 74-90 hours; Multiple doses: 111-113 hours

Elderly (61-85 years): Single dose: 120-160 hours; Multiple doses: 126-158 hours

Excretion: Urine: N-hydroxyethylflurazepam (22% to 55%); N-desalkylflurazepam (<1%)

Dosage Oral:

Children: Insomnia:

<15 years: Dose not established

≥15 years: 15 mg at bedtime

Adults: Insomnia: 15-30 mg at bedtime

Elderly: Insomnia: Oral: 15 mg at bedtime; avoid use if possible

Administration Give 30 minutes to 1 hour before bedtime on an empty stomach with full glass of water. May be taken with food if GI distress occurs.

Monitoring Parameters Respiratory and cardiovascular status

Reference Range Therapeutic: 0-4 ng/mL (SI: 0-9 nmol/L); Metabolite N-desalkylflurazepam: 20-110 ng/mL (SI: 43-240 nmol/L); Toxic: >0.12 mcg/mL

Dosage Forms Excipient information presented when available (limited, particularly for generics); consult specific product labeling.
Capsule, as hydrochloride: 15 mg, 30 mg
Dalmane®: 15 mg, 30 mg

◆ **Flurazepam Hydrochloride** *see* Flurazepam *on page 664*

Flurbiprofen (flure BI proe fen)

Medication Safety Issues
Sound-alike/look-alike issues:
Flurbiprofen may be confused with fenoprofen
Ansaid® may be confused with Asacol®, Axid®
Ocufen® may be confused with Ocuflox®, Ocupress®

Related Information
Nonsteroidal Anti-Inflammatory Agents *on page 1792*

U.S. Brand Names Ocufen®

Canadian Brand Names Alti-Flurbiprofen; Ansaid®; Apo-Flurbiprofen®; Froben-SR®; Froben®; Novo-Flurprofen; Nu-Flurprofen; Ocufen®

Mexican Brand Names Ansaid; Ocufen

Index Terms Flurbiprofen Sodium

Pharmacologic Category Nonsteroidal Anti-inflammatory Drug (NSAID), Ophthalmic; Nonsteroidal Anti-inflammatory Drug (NSAID), Oral

Use
Oral: Treatment of rheumatoid arthritis and osteoarthritis
Ophthalmic: Inhibition of intraoperative miosis

Effect on Mental Status Dizziness is common; may cause nervousness; may rarely cause drowsiness, confusion, depression, or hallucinations

Effect on Psychiatric Treatment May rarely cause agranulocytosis; use caution with clozapine and carbamazepine; may decrease the clearance of lithium resulting in elevated serum levels and potential toxicity; monitor serum lithium levels

Restrictions An FDA-approved medication guide must be distributed when dispensing an oral outpatient prescription (new or refill) where this medication is to be used without direct supervision of a healthcare provider. Medication guides are available at http://www.fda.gov/cder/Offices/ODS/medication_guides.htm.

Dosage Summary
Ophthalmic:
Children: Dosage not established
Adults: Instill 1 drop to each eye every 30 minutes, beginning 2 hours prior to surgery (maximum: 4 doses)
Oral:
Children: Dosage not established
Adults: 200-300 mg/day in 2-4 divided doses (maximum: 100 mg/dose; 300 mg/day)

Dosage Forms Excipient information presented when available (limited, particularly for generics); consult specific product labeling.
Solution, ophthalmic, as sodium: 0.03% (2.5 mL)
Ocufen®: 0.03% (2.5 mL)
Tablet: 50 mg, 100 mg

◆ **Flurbiprofen Sodium** *see* Flurbiprofen *on page 667*
◆ **5-Flurocytosine** *see* Flucytosine *on page 640*

Flutamide (FLOO ta mide)

Medication Safety Issues
Sound-alike/look-alike issues:
Flutamide may be confused with Flumadine®, thalidomide
Eulexin® may be confused with Edecrin®, Eurax®

U.S. Brand Names Eulexin®

Canadian Brand Names Apo-Flutamide®; Euflex®; Eulexin®; Novo-Flutamide

Mexican Brand Names Eulexin; Fluken; Flulem; Tafenil

Index Terms 4'-Nitro-3'-Trifluoromethylisobutyrantide; Niftolid; NSC-147834; SCH 13521

Pharmacologic Category Antineoplastic Agent, Antiandrogen

Use Treatment of metastatic prostatic carcinoma in combination therapy with LHRH agonist analogues

Unlabeled/Investigational Use Female hirsutism

Effect on Mental Status May rarely cause nervousness or confusion

Effect on Psychiatric Treatment None reported

Dosage Summary

Oral:

Children: Dosage not established

Adults: 250 mg 3 times/day

Dosage Forms Excipient information presented when available (limited, particularly for generics); consult specific product labeling.

Capsule: 125 mg

Fluticasone (floo TIK a sone)

Medication Safety Issues

Sound-alike/look-alike issues:

Cutivate® may be confused with Ultravate®

International issues:

Allegro® [Israel] may be confused with Allegra® which is a brand name for fexofenadine in the U.S.

Allegro®: Brand name for frovatriptan in Germany

Flovent® may be confused with Flogen® which is a brand name for naproxen in Mexico

Related Information

Corticosteroids *on page 1780*

U.S. Brand Names Cutivate®; Flonase®; Flovent® Diskus®; Flovent® HFA; Veramyst™

Canadian Brand Names Apo-Fluticasone; Avamys™; Cutivate™; Flonase®; Flovent® Diskus®; Flovent® HFA; ratio-Fluticasone

Mexican Brand Names Cutivate; Flixonase; Flixotide

Index Terms Fluticasone Furoate; Fluticasone Propionate

Pharmacologic Category Corticosteroid, Inhalant (Oral); Corticosteroid, Nasal; Corticosteroid, Topical

Generic Available Yes: Cream, nasal spray, ointment

Use

Oral inhalation: Maintenance treatment of asthma as prophylactic therapy; also indicated for patients requiring oral corticosteroid therapy for asthma to assist in total discontinuation or reduction of total oral dose

Intranasal:

Flonase®: Management of seasonal and perennial allergic rhinitis and nonallergic rhinitis

Veramyst™: Management of seasonal and perennial allergic rhinitis

Avamys™ [CAN]: Management of seasonal allergic rhinitis

Topical: Relief of inflammation and pruritus associated with corticosteroid-responsive dermatoses; atopic dermatitis

Effect on Mental Status May cause agitation, aggression, anxiety, depression, hyperactivity, irritability, and restlessness

Effect on Psychiatric Treatment None reported

Pregnancy Risk Factor C

Pregnancy Considerations Teratogenic events have been observed in some, but not all, animal studies. There are no adequate and well-controlled studies using inhaled fluticasone in pregnant women. Oral corticosteroid use has shown animals to be more prone to teratogenic effects than humans. Due to the natural increase in corticosteroid production during pregnancy, most women may require a lower steroid dose; use with caution.

Lactation Excretion in breast milk unknown/use caution

Contraindications Hypersensitivity to fluticasone or any component of the formulation; primary treatment of status asthmaticus or acute bronchospasm

Topical: Do not use if infection is present at treatment site, in the presence of skin atrophy, or for the treatment of rosacea or perioral dermatitis

Warnings/Precautions May cause hypercorticism or suppression of hypothalamic-pituitary-adrenal (HPA) axis, particularly in younger children or in patients receiving high doses for prolonged periods. HPA axis suppression may lead to adrenal crisis. Withdrawal and discontinuation of a corticosteroid should be done slowly and carefully. Particular care is required when patients are transferred from systemic corticosteroids to inhaled products due to possible adrenal insufficiency or withdrawal from steroids, including an increase in allergic symptoms. Patients receiving ≥20 mg per day of prednisone (or equivalent) may be most susceptible. Concurrent use of ritonavir (and potentially other strong inhibitors of CYP3A4) may increase fluticasone levels and effects on HPA suppression. Fatalities have occurred due to adrenal insufficiency in asthmatic patients during and after transfer from systemic corticosteroids to aerosol steroids; aerosol steroids do **not** provide the systemic steroid needed to treat patients having trauma, surgery, or infections.

Bronchospasm may occur with wheezing after inhalation; if this occurs, stop steroid and treat with a fast-acting bronchodilator. Supplemental steroids (oral or parenteral) may be needed during stress or severe asthma attacks. Corticosteroid use may cause psychiatric disturbances, including depression, euphoria, insomnia, mood swings, and personality changes. Pre-existing psychiatric conditions may be exacerbated by corticosteroid use. Prolonged use of corticosteroids may also increase the incidence of secondary infection, mask acute infection (including fungal infections), prolong or exacerbate viral infections, or limit response to vaccines. Exposure to chickenpox should be avoided; corticosteroids should not be used to treat ocular herpes simplex. Corticosteroids should not be used for cerebral malaria. Close observation is required in patients with latent tuberculosis and/or TB reactivity; restrict use in active TB (only in conjunction with antituberculosis treatment). Rare cases of vasculitis (Churg-Strauss syndrome) or other eosinophilic conditions can occur. Prolonged treatment with corticosteroids has been associated with the development of Kaposi's sarcoma (case reports); if noted, discontinuation of therapy should be considered.

Use with caution in patients with thyroid disease, hepatic impairment, renal impairment, cardiovascular disease, diabetes, glaucoma, cataracts, myasthenia gravis, patients at risk for osteoporosis, patients at risk for seizures, or GI diseases (diverticulitis, peptic ulcer, ulcerative colitis) due to perforation risk. Use caution following acute MI (corticosteroids have been associated with myocardial rupture). Because of the risk of adverse effects, systemic corticosteroids should be used cautiously in the elderly in the smallest possible effective dose for the shortest duration. Avoid nasal corticosteroid use in patients with recent nasal septal ulcers, nasal surgery, or nasal trauma until healing has occurred.

Orally-inhaled and intranasal corticosteroids may cause a reduction in growth velocity in pediatric patients (~1 centimeter per year [range 0.3-1.8 cm per year] and related to dose and duration of exposure). To minimize the systemic effects of orally-inhaled and intranasal corticosteroids, each patient should be titrated to the lowest effective dose. Growth should be routinely monitored in pediatric patients. Safety and efficacy have not been established in children <4 years of age.

Inhalation: Not to be used in status asthmaticus or for the relief of acute bronchospasm. Flovent® Diskus® contains lactose; very rare anaphylactic reactions have been reported in patients with severe milk protein allergy. There have been reports of systemic corticosteroid withdrawal symptoms (eg, joint/muscle pain, lassitude, depression) when withdrawing oral inhalation therapy. Local yeast infections (eg, oral pharyngeal candidiasis) may occur. Lower respiratory tract infections, including pneumonia, have been reported in patients with COPD with an even higher incidence in the elderly.

Topical: May also cause suppression of HPA axis, especially when used on large areas of the body, denuded areas, for prolonged periods of time, or with an occlusive dressing. Pediatric patients may be more susceptible to systemic toxicity.

Adverse Reactions

Oral inhalation (includes reactions from Flovent® HFA and Flovent® Diskus® trials):

>10%:

- Central nervous system: Headache (2% to 14%)
- Respiratory: Upper respiratory tract infection (14% to 21%), throat irritation (3% to 22%)

3% to 10%:

- Central nervous system: Fever (1% to 7%)
- Gastrointestinal: Oral candidiasis (≤9%), nausea/vomiting (1% to 8%), gastrointestinal infection (including viral; 1% to 5%), gastrointestinal discomfort/pain (1% to 4%)
- Neuromuscular & skeletal: Musculoskeletal pain (2% to 5%), muscle injury (1% to 5%)
- Respiratory: Sinusitis/sinus infection (4% to 10%), lower respiratory tract infections/pneumonia (1% to 7%; COPD diagnosis and age >65 years increase risk), cough (1% to 6%), bronchitis (≤8%), hoarseness/dysphonia (2% to 6%), upper respiratory tract inflammation (≤5%), viral respiratory infection (1% to 5%), rhinitis (1% to 4%)
- Miscellaneous: Viral infection (≤5%)

1% to 3%:

Cardiovascular: Chest symptoms, edema, palpitation

Central nervous system: Cranial nerve paralysis, dizziness, fatigue, malaise, migraine, mood disorders, pain, sleep disorder

Dermatologic: Acne, dermatitis/dermatosis, eczema, folliculitis, photodermatitis, infection (fungal, viral), pruritus, rash, urticaria

Endocrine metabolic: Fluid disturbance, goiter, uric acid metabolism disturbance

Gastrointestinal: Abdominal discomfort/pain, appetite changes, dental discomfort/pain, diarrhea, dyspepsia, gastroenteritis, hyposalivation, oral discomfort/pain, oral erythema/rash, oral ulcerations, oropharyngeal plaques, tooth decay, weight gain

Genitourinary: Reproductive organ infections (bacterial), urinary tract infection

Hematologic: Hematoma

Hepatic: Cholecystitis

Neuromuscular & skeletal: Arthralgia, articular rheumatism, muscle cramps/spasms, muscle pain, muscle stiffness/tightness/rigidity, musculoskeletal inflammation

Ocular: Blepharoconjunctivitis, conjunctivitis, keratitis

Otic: Otitis

Respiratory: Epistaxis, hoarseness/dysphonia, laryngitis, nasal sinus disorder, pharyngitis/throat infection, rhinorrhea/postnasal drip, throat constriction

Miscellaneous: Infection (bacterial, fungal); injuries (including muscle, soft tissue); polyps (ear, nose, throat); tonsillitis

Postmarketing and/or case reports: Aggression, agitation, anaphylactic reaction (rare; Diskus®: some patients with severe milk allergy), angioedema, anxiety, aphonia, asthma exacerbation, behavioral changes (eg, hyperactivity and irritability in children; rare), bronchospasm (immediate and delayed), cataracts, chest tightness, Churg-Strauss syndrome, contusion, Cushingoid features, cutaneous hypersensitivity, depression, dyspnea, ecchymoses, eosinophilia, facial edema, growth velocity reduction in children/adolescents, HPA axis suppression, hyperglycemia, hypersensitivity reactions (immediate and delayed), oropharyngeal edema, osteoporosis, paradoxical bronchospasm, restlessness, throat soreness, vasculitis, wheeze

Nasal inhalation (includes reactions from Flonase®, Veramyst™, and Avamys™ [CAN] trials):

>10%: Central nervous system: Headache (7% to 16%)

1% to 10%:

Central nervous system: Dizziness (1% to 3%), fever (1% to 5%)

Gastrointestinal: Nausea/vomiting (3% to 5%), abdominal pain (1% to 3%), diarrhea (1% to 3%)

Neuromuscular & skeletal: Back pain (1%)

Respiratory: Pharyngitis (6% to 8%), epistaxis (4% to 7%), asthma symptoms (3% to 7%), cough (3% to 4%), pharyngolaryngeal pain (2% to 4%), blood in nasal mucous (1% to 3%), bronchitis (1% to 3%), runny nose (1% to 3%), nasal ulcer (1%)

Miscellaneous: Aches and pains (1% to 3%), flu-like syndrome (1% to 3%)

<1% (Limited to important or life-threatening): Alteration or loss of sense of taste and/or smell, anaphylaxis/anaphylactoid reactions, angioedema, AST increased, AV block (second degree), blurred vision, bronchospasm, cataracts, conjunctivitis, dry/irritated eyes, dry throat, dyspnea, edema (face and tongue), glaucoma, hoarseness, hypersensitivity reactions, increased intraocular pressure, nasal candidiasis, nasal septal perforation (rare), palpitations, pruritus, psychomotor hyperactivity, sinus congestion, skin rash, sore throat, throat irritation, tremor, urticaria, vaginal candidiasis, voice changes, wheezing

Topical: Pruritus (3%), skin irritation (3%), exacerbation of eczema (2%), dryness (1%), numbness of fingers (1%)

Reported with other topical corticosteroids (in decreasing order of occurrence): Irritation, folliculitis, acneiform eruptions, hypopigmentation, perioral dermatitis, allergic contact dermatitis, secondary infection, skin atrophy, striae, miliaria, pustular psoriasis from chronic plaque psoriasis

Metabolism/Transport Effects Substrate of CYP3A4 (major)

Drug Interactions

Amphotericin B: Corticosteroids (Orally Inhaled) may enhance the hypokalemic effect of Amphotericin B. *Risk C: Monitor therapy*

Antidiabetic Agents: Corticosteroids (Orally Inhaled) may diminish the hypoglycemic effect of Antidiabetic Agents. In some instances, corticosteroid-mediated HPA axis suppression has led to episodes of acute adrenal crisis, which may manifest as enhanced hypoglycemia, particularly in the setting of insulin or other antidiabetic agent use. *Risk C: Monitor therapy*

Antifungal Agents (Azole Derivatives, Systemic): May decrease the metabolism of Corticosteroids (Orally Inhaled). *Risk C: Monitor therapy*

Corticorelin: Corticosteroids may diminish the therapeutic effect of Corticorelin. Specifically, the plasma ACTH response to corticorelin may be blunted by recent or current corticosteroid therapy. *Risk C: Monitor therapy*

CYP3A4 Inhibitors (Moderate): May decrease the metabolism of CYP3A4 Substrates. *Risk C: Monitor therapy*

CYP3A4 Inhibitors (Strong): May decrease the metabolism of CYP3A4 Substrates. *Risk D: Consider therapy modification*

Dasatinib: May increase the serum concentration of CYP3A4 Substrates. *Risk C: Monitor therapy*

Loop Diuretics: Corticosteroids (Orally Inhaled) may enhance the hypokalemic effect of Loop Diuretics. *Risk C: Monitor therapy*

Protease Inhibitors: May decrease the metabolism of Corticosteroids (Orally Inhaled). *Risk D: Consider therapy modification*

Thiazide Diuretics: Corticosteroids (Orally Inhaled) may enhance the hypokalemic effect of Thiazide Diuretics. *Risk C: Monitor therapy*

Ethanol/Nutrition/Herb Interactions Herb/Nutraceutical: In theory, St John's wort may decrease serum levels of fluticasone by inducing CYP3A4 isoenzymes.

Stability

Nasal spray:

Flonase®: Store between 4°C to 30°C (39°F to 86°F).

Veramyst™: Store between 15°C to 30°C (59°F to 86°F); do not refrigerate or freeze. Store in upright position with cap on.

Avamys™ [CAN]: Store between 4°C to 30°C (39°F to 86°F); do not refrigerate or freeze. Store in upright position with cap on.

Oral inhalation:

Flovent® HFA: Store at 15°C to 30°C (59°F to 86°F). Discard device when the dose counter reads "000". Store with mouthpiece down.

Flovent® Diskus®: Store at 20°C to 25°C (68°F to 77°F) in a dry place away from direct heat or sunlight. Discard after 6 weeks from removal from protective foil pouch or when the dose counter reads "0" (whichever comes first); device is not reusable.

Topical, cream: Store at 15°C to 30°C (59°F to 86°F).

Cutivate® lotion: Store at 15°C to 30°C (59°F to 86°F); do not refrigerate.

Cutivate® cream, ointment: Store at 2°C to 30°C (36°F to 86°F).

Mechanism of Action Fluticasone belongs to a group of corticosteroids which utilizes a fluorocarbothioate ester linkage at the 17 carbon position; extremely potent vasoconstrictive and anti-inflammatory activity; has a weak HPA inhibitory potency when applied topically, which gives the drug a high therapeutic index. The effectiveness of inhaled fluticasone is due to its direct local effect. The mechanism of action for all topical corticosteroids is believed to be a combination of three important properties: anti-inflammatory activity, immunosuppressive properties, and antiproliferative actions.

Pharmacodynamics/Kinetics

Onset of action: Intranasal: Maximal benefit may take several days

Flovent® HFA, Flovent® Diskus®: Maximal benefit may take 1-2 weeks or longer

Absorption:

Topical cream: 5% (increased with inflammation)

Oral inhalation: Absorbed systemically (Flovent® Diskus®: ~18%) primarily via lungs, minimal GI absorption (<1%) due to presystemic metabolism

Distribution: Propionate: 4.2 L/kg

Protein binding: 91% to 99%

Metabolism: Hepatic via CYP3A4 to 17β-carboxylic acid (negligible activity)

Bioavailability: Nasal: ≤2%; Oral inhalation: (~18% to 21%)

Excretion: Feces (as parent drug and metabolites); urine (<5% as metabolites)

Dosage

Children:

Asthma: Inhalation, oral:

Flovent® HFA:

Children 4-11 years: 88 mcg twice daily

Children ≥12 years: Refer to adult dosing.

NIH Asthma Guidelines (NIH, 2007) (administer in divided doses twice daily):

"Low" dose:

0-4 years: 176 mcg/day

5-11 years: 88-176 mcg/day

≥12 years: 88-264 mcg/day

"Medium" dose:
0-4 years: >176-352 mcg/day
5-11 years: >176-352 mcg/day
≥12 years: >264-440 mcg/day
"High" dose:
0-4 years: >352 mcg/day
5-11 years: >352 mcg/day
≥12 years: >440 mcg/day

Flovent® Diskus® *(U.S. labeling)*:
Children 4-11 years: Usual starting dose: 50 mcg twice daily; may increase to 100 mcg twice daily in patients not adequately controlled after 2 weeks of therapy. Higher starting doses may be considered in patients with poorer asthma control or those requiring high ranges of inhaled corticosteroids. Titrate to the lowest effective dose once asthma stability is achieved (maximum dose: 100 mcg twice daily)
Children >11 years: Refer to adult dosing.

Flovent® Diskus® *(Canadian labeling)*:
Children 4-16 years: Usual starting dose: 50-100 mcg twice daily; may increase to 200 mcg twice daily in patients not adequately controlled; titrate to the lowest effective dose once asthma stability is achieved
Children ≥16 years: Refer to adult dosing.

Corticosteroid-responsive dermatoses: Topical: Children ≥3 months: Cream: Apply sparingly to affected area twice daily. If no improvement is seen within 2 weeks, reassessment of diagnosis may be necessary. **Note:** Safety and efficacy of treatment >4 weeks duration have not been established.

Atopic dermatitis: Topical:
Children ≥3 months: Cream: Apply sparingly to affected area 1-2 times/day. If no improvement is seen within 2 weeks, reassessment of diagnosis may be necessary.
Children ≥1 year: Lotion: Apply sparingly to affected area once daily
Note: Safety and efficacy of treatment >4 weeks duration have not been established.

Rhinitis: Intranasal:
Flonase® (fluticasone propionate): Children ≥4 years and Adolescents: Initial: 1 spray (50 mcg/spray) per nostril once daily; patients not adequately responding or patients with more severe symptoms may use 2 sprays (100 mcg) per nostril. Depending on response, dosage may be reduced to 100 mcg daily. Total daily dosage should not exceed 2 sprays in each nostril (200 mcg)/day. Dosing should be at regular intervals.

Veramyst™ (fluticasone furoate):
Children 2-11 years: Initial: 1 spray (27.5 mcg/spray) per nostril once daily (55 mcg/day); patients not adequately responding may use 2 sprays per nostril once daily (110 mcg/day). Once symptoms are controlled, dosage may be reduced to 55 mcg once daily. Total daily dosage should not exceed 2 sprays in each nostril (110 mcg)/day.
Children ≥12 years and Adolescents: Initial: 2 sprays (27.5 mcg/spray) per nostril once daily (110 mcg/day). Once symptoms are controlled, dosage may be reduced to 1 spray per nostril once daily (55 mcg/day). Total daily dosage should not exceed 2 sprays in each nostril (110 mcg)/day.

Avamys™ [CAN] (fluticasone furoate): Children ≥12 years: 2 sprays (27.5 mcg/spray) in each nostril once daily (110 mcg/day). Total daily dosage should not exceed 2 sprays in each nostril (110 mcg)/day.

Adults:
Asthma: Inhalation, oral: **Note:** Titrate to the lowest effective dose once asthma stability is achieved
Flovent® HFA: Manufacturers labeling: Dosing based on previous therapy
Bronchodilator alone: Recommended starting dose: 88 mcg twice daily; highest recommended dose: 440 mcg twice daily
Inhaled corticosteroids: Recommended starting dose: 88-220 mcg twice daily; highest recommended dose: 440 mcg twice daily; a higher starting dose may be considered in patients previously requiring higher doses of inhaled corticosteroids
Oral corticosteroids: Recommended starting dose: 440 mcg twice daily
Highest recommended dose: 880 mcg twice daily; starting dose is patient dependent. In patients on chronic oral corticosteroids therapy, reduce prednisone dose no faster than 2.5-5 mg/day on a weekly basis; begin taper after 1 week of fluticasone therapy.

NIH Asthma Guidelines (NIH, 2007) (administer in divided doses twice daily):
"Low" dose: 88-264 mcg/day
"Medium" dose: >264-440 mcg/day

"High" dose: >440 mcg/day

Flovent® Diskus® *(U.S. labeling)*: **Note:** May increase dose after 2 weeks of therapy in patients not adequately controlled. Higher starting doses may be considered in patients with poorer asthma control or those requiring high ranges of inhaled corticosteroids. Titrate to the lowest effective dose once asthma stability is achieved.

Bronchodilator alone: Recommended starting dose: 100 mcg twice daily; maximum recommended dose: 500 mcg twice daily

Inhaled corticosteroids: Recommended starting dose: 100-250 mcg twice daily; maximum recommended dose: 500 mcg twice daily

Oral corticosteroids: Recommended starting dose: 500-1000 mcg twice daily; maximum recommended dose: 1000 mcg twice daily. Starting dose is patient dependent. In patients on chronic oral corticosteroids therapy, reduce prednisone dose no faster than 2.5 mg/day on a weekly basis; begin taper after 1 week of fluticasone therapy.

Flovent® Diskus® *(Canadian labeling)*:

Mild asthma: 100-250 mcg twice daily

Moderate asthma: 250-500 mcg twice daily

Severe asthma: 500 mcg twice daily; may increase to 1000 mcg twice daily in very severe patients requiring high doses of corticosteroids

Corticosteroid-responsive dermatoses: Topical: Cream, lotion, ointment: Apply sparingly to affected area twice daily. If no improvement is seen within 2 weeks, reassessment of diagnosis may be necessary.

Atopic dermatitis: Topical: Cream, lotion: Apply sparingly to affected area once or twice daily. If no improvement is seen within 2 weeks, reassessment of diagnosis may be necessary.

Rhinitis: Intranasal:

Flonase® (fluticasone propionate): Initial: 2 sprays (50 mcg/spray) per nostril once daily; may also be divided into 100 mcg twice a day. After the first few days, dosage may be reduced to 1 spray per nostril once daily for maintenance therapy.

Veramyst™ (fluticasone furoate): Initial: 2 sprays (27.5 mcg/spray) per nostril once daily (110 mcg/day). Once symptoms are controlled, may reduce dosage to 1 spray per nostril once daily (55 mcg/day) for maintenance therapy.

Avamys™ [CAN] (fluticasone furoate): 2 sprays (27.5 mcg/spray) in each nostril once daily (110 mcg/day). Total daily dosage should not exceed 2 sprays in each nostril (110 mcg)/day.

Elderly: No differences in safety have been observed in the elderly when compared to younger patients. Based on current data, no dosage adjustment is needed based on age.

Dosage adjustment in hepatic impairment: Fluticasone is primarily cleared in the liver. Fluticasone plasma levels may be increased in patients with hepatic impairment, use with caution; monitor.

Dietary Considerations Flovent® Diskus® contains lactose; very rare anaphylactic reactions have been reported in patients with severe milk protein allergy.

Administration

Aerosol inhalation: Flovent® HFA: Shake container thoroughly before using. Take 3-5 deep breaths. Use inhaler on inspiration. Allow 1 full minute between inhalations. Rinse mouth with water after use to reduce aftertaste and incidence of candidiasis; do not swallow. Inhaler must be primed before first use, when not used for 7 days, or if dropped. To prime the first time, release 4 sprays into air; shake well before each spray and spray away from face. If dropped or not used for 7 days, prime by releasing a single test spray. Patient should contact pharmacy for refill when the dose counter reads "020". Discard device when the dose counter reads "000". Do not use "float" test to determine contents.

Nasal spray: Administer at regular intervals. Shake bottle gently before using. Blow nose to clear nostrils. Insert applicator into nostril, keeping bottle upright, and close off the other nostril. Breathe in through nose. While inhaling, press pump to release spray. Discard after labeled number of doses has been used, even if bottle is not completely empty.

Flonase®: Prime pump (press 6 times until fine spray appears) prior to first use or if spray unused for ≥7 days. Once weekly, nasal applicator may be removed and rinsed with warm water to clean.

Veramyst™, Avamys™ [CAN]: Prime pump (press 6 times until fine spray appears) prior to first use, if spray unused for ≥30 days, or if cap left off bottle for ≥5 days. After each use, nozzle should be wiped with a clean, dry tissue. Once weekly, inside of cap should be cleaned with a clean, dry tissue.

Powder for oral inhalation: Flovent® Diskus®: Do not use with a spacer device. Do not exhale into Diskus®. Do not wash or take apart. Use in horizontal position. Mouth should be rinsed with water after use (do not swallow). Discard after 6 weeks once removed from protective pouch or when the dose counter reads "0", whichever comes first (device is not reusable).

Topical cream, lotion, ointment: Apply sparingly in a thin film. Rub in lightly. Unless otherwise directed by healthcare professional, do not use with occlusive dressing; do not use on children's skin covered by diapers or plastic pants.

Monitoring Parameters Growth (adolescents and children); signs/symptoms of HPA axis suppression/adrenal insufficiency; possible eosinophilic conditions (including Churg-Strauss syndrome); FEV_1, peak flow, and/or other pulmonary function tests; asthma symptoms

Additional Information Effects of inhaled/intranasal steroids on growth have been observed in the absence of laboratory evidence of HPA axis suppression, suggesting that growth velocity is a more sensitive indicator of systemic corticosteroid exposure in pediatric patients than some commonly used tests of HPA axis function. The long-term effects of this reduction in growth velocity associated with orally-inhaled and intranasal corticosteroids, including the impact on final adult height, are unknown. The potential for "catch up" growth following discontinuation of treatment with inhaled corticosteroids has not been adequately studied. The product labeling notes that intranasal administration was not associated with a statistically-significant reduction in growth velocity (based on a small study conducted over 1 year).

In the United States, dosage for the metered dose inhaler (Flovent® HFA) is expressed as the amount of drug which leaves the actuater and is delivered to the patient. This differs from other countries, which express the dosage as the amount of drug which leaves the valve.

Dosage Forms Excipient information presented when available (limited, particularly for generics); consult specific product labeling. [CAN] = Canadian brand name

Aerosol for oral inhalation, as propionate [CFC free]:
- Flovent® HFA: 44 mcg/inhalation (10.6 g) [120 metered actuations]
- Flovent® HFA: 110 mcg/inhalation (12 g) [120 metered actuations]
- Flovent® HFA: 220 mcg/inhalation (12 g) [120 metered actuations]

Cream, as propionate: 0.05% (15 g, 30 g, 60 g)
- Cutivate®: 0.05% (30 g, 60 g)

Lotion, as propionate:
- Cutivate®: 0.05% (120 mL)

Ointment, as propionate: 0.005% (15 g, 30 g, 60 g)
- Cutivate®: 0.005% (30 g, 60 g)

Powder for oral inhalation, as propionate:
- Flovent® Diskus® [U.S.]: 50 mcg (60s) [contains lactose; prefilled blister pack]
- Flovent® Diskus® [CAN]: 50 mcg (28s, 60s) [contains lactose; prefilled blister pack] [not available in the U.S.]
- Flovent® Diskus® [CAN]: 100 mcg (28s, 60s) [contains lactose; prefilled blister pack] [not available in the U.S.]
- Flovent® Diskus® [CAN]: 250 mcg (28s, 60s) [contains lactose; prefilled blister pack] [not available in the U.S.]
- Flovent® Diskus® [CAN]: 500 mcg (28s, 60s) [contains lactose; prefilled blister pack] [not available in the U.S.]

Suspension, intranasal, as furoate [spray]:
- Avamys™ [CAN]: 27.5 mcg/inhalation (4.5 g) [30 metered actuations; contains benzalkonium chloride]; (10 g) [120 metered actuations; contains benzalkonium chloride] [not available in the U.S.]
- Veramyst™: 27.5 mcg/inhalation (10 g) [120 metered actuations; contains benzalkonium chloride]

Suspension, intranasal, as propionate [spray]: 50 mcg/inhalation (16 g) [120 metered actuations]
- Flonase®: 50 mcg/inhalation (16 g) [120 metered actuations; contains benzalkonium chloride]

Fluticasone and Salmeterol (floo TIK a sone & sal ME te role)

Medication Safety Issues

Sound-alike/look-alike issues:

Advair may be confused with Advicor®

U.S. Brand Names Advair Diskus®; Advair® HFA

Canadian Brand Names Advair Diskus®; Advair®

Mexican Brand Names Seretide

Index Terms Fluticasone Propionate and Salmeterol Xinafoate; Salmeterol and Fluticasone

Pharmacologic Category Beta2-Adrenergic Agonist, Long-Acting; $Beta_2$-Adrenergic Agonist; Corticosteroid, Inhalant (Oral)

Use Maintenance treatment of asthma; maintenance treatment of COPD

Effect on Mental Status May cause headache, nervousness, dizziness, fatigue, or sleep disorders

Effect on Psychiatric Treatment Propranolol may decrease the effects of salmeterol and cause bronchospasm in asthmatics. Combined use with MAO inhibitors and TCAs may increase the risk of cardiovascular toxicity (avoid concurrent use and within 14 days after discontinuing this agents).

Restrictions An FDA-approved medication guide must be distributed when dispensing an outpatient prescription (new or refill) where this medication is to be used without direct supervision of a healthcare provider. Medication guides are available at http://www.fda.gov/cder/Offices/ODS/medication_guides.htm.

Dosage Summary

Oral inhalation:

Children <4 years: Advair Diskus®: Dosage not established

Children 4-11 years: Advair Diskus®: Fluticasone 100 mcg/salmeterol 50 mcg/inhalation: One inhalation twice daily (maximum dose)

Children <12 years: Advair® HFA: Dosage not established

Children ≥12 years: Asthma:

Advair Diskus®: Fluticasone 100-500 mcg/salmeterol 50 mcg/inhalation: One inhalation twice daily. Maximum: Fluticasone 500 mcg/salmeterol 50 mcg/inhalation twice daily

Advair® HFA: Fluticasone 45-230 mcg/salmeterol 21 mcg/inhalation: Two inhalations twice daily

Advair® 125 or Advair® 250 [Canadian labeling; not in approved U.S. labeling]: Fluticasone 125-250 mcg/salmeterol 25 mcg/inhalation: Two inhalations twice daily

Adults:

COPD:

Advair Diskus®: Initial, maximum: Fluticasone 250 mcg/salmeterol 50 mcg twice daily

Advair Diskus® [Canadian labeling; not in approved U.S. labeling]: Fluticasone 250-500 mcg/salmeterol 50 mcg: One inhalation twice daily

Asthma:

Advair Diskus®: Maximum dose: Fluticasone 500 mcg/salmeterol 50 mcg/inhalation: One inhalation twice daily

Advair® HFA: Fluticasone 45-230 mcg/salmeterol 50 mcg/inhalation: Two inhalations twice daily

Advair® 125 or Advair® 250 [Canadian labeling; not in approved U.S. labeling]: Fluticasone 125-250 mcg/salmeterol 25 mcg/inhalation: Two inhalations twice daily

Dosage Forms Excipient information presented when available (limited, particularly for generics); consult specific product labeling. [DSC] = Discontinued product; [CAN] = Canadian brand name/formulation

Aerosol, for oral inhalation:

Advair® HFA:

45/21: Fluticasone propionate 45 mcg and salmeterol 21 mcg (12 g) [120 metered inhalations]

115/21: Fluticasone propionate 115 mcg and salmeterol 21 mcg (12 g) [120 metered inhalations]

230/21: Fluticasone propionate 230 mcg and salmeterol 21 mcg (12 g) [120 metered inhalations]

Advair® [CAN]:

125/25: Fluticasone propionate 125 mcg and salmeterol 25 mcg (12 g) [120 metered inhalations] [not available in the U.S.]

250/25: Fluticasone propionate 250 mcg and salmeterol 25 mcg (12 g) [120 metered inhalations] [not available in the U.S.]

Powder, for oral inhalation:

Advair Diskus®:

100/50: Fluticasone propionate 100 mcg and salmeterol 50 mcg (14s, 28s [DSC], 60s) [contains lactose; chlorofluorocarbon free]

250/50: Fluticasone propionate 250 mcg and salmeterol 50 mcg (14s [DSC], 60s) [contains lactose; chlorofluorocarbon free]

500/50: Fluticasone propionate 500 mcg and salmeterol 50 mcg (14s [DSC], 60s) [contains lactose; chlorofluorocarbon free]

◆ **Fluticasone Furoate** *see* Fluticasone *on page 668*

◆ **Fluticasone Propionate** *see* Fluticasone *on page 668*

◆ **Fluticasone Propionate and Salmeterol Xinafoate** *see* Fluticasone and Salmeterol *on page 674*

Fluvastatin (FLOO va sta tin)

Medication Safety Issues
Sound-alike/look-alike issues:
Fluvastatin may be confused with fluoxetine

Related Information
Lipid-Lowering Agents *on page 1786*

U.S. Brand Names Lescol®; Lescol® XL

Canadian Brand Names Lescol®; Lescol® XL

Mexican Brand Names Lescol; Lescol XL

Pharmacologic Category Antilipemic Agent, HMG-CoA Reductase Inhibitor

Generic Available No

Use To be used as a component of multiple risk factor intervention in patients at risk for atherosclerosis vascular disease due to hypercholesterolemia

Adjunct to dietary therapy to reduce elevated total cholesterol (total-C), LDL-C, triglyceride, and apolipoprotein B (apo-B) levels and to increase HDL-C in primary hypercholesterolemia and mixed dyslipidemia (Fredrickson types IIa and IIb); to slow the progression of coronary atherosclerosis in patients with coronary heart disease; reduce risk of coronary revascularization procedures in patients with coronary heart disease

Effect on Mental Status May cause dizziness, insomnia, or drowsiness

Effect on Psychiatric Treatment None reported

Pregnancy Risk Factor X

Pregnancy Considerations Cholesterol biosynthesis may be important in fetal development. Contraindicated in pregnancy. Administer to women of child-bearing potential only when conception is highly unlikely and patients have been informed of potential hazards.

Lactation Enters breast milk/contraindicated

Contraindications Hypersensitivity to fluvastatin or any component of the formulation; active liver disease; unexplained persistent elevations of serum transaminases; pregnancy; breast-feeding

Warnings/Precautions Secondary causes of hyperlipidemia should be ruled out prior to therapy. Liver function must be monitored by periodic laboratory assessment. Rhabdomyolysis with acute renal failure has occurred with fluvastatin and other HMG-CoA reductase inhibitors. Risk may be increased with concurrent use of other drugs which may cause rhabdomyolysis (including colchicine, gemfibrozil, fibric acid derivatives, or niacin at doses ≥1 g/day). Temporarily discontinue in any patient experiencing markedly elevated CPK levels, myopathy, or an acute/serious condition predisposing to renal failure secondary to rhabdomyolysis. Based upon current evidence, HMG-CoA reductase inhibitor therapy should be continued in the perioperative period unless risk outweighs cardioprotective benefit. Use with caution in patients with advanced age; these patients are predisposed to myopathy. Use caution in patients with previous liver disease or heavy ethanol use. Use caution in patients with concurrent medications or conditions which reduce steroidogenesis. Safety and efficacy in children <10 years of age have not been established.

Adverse Reactions As reported with fluvastatin capsules; in general, adverse reactions reported with fluvastatin extended release tablet were similar, but the incidence was less.

1% to 10%:
- Central nervous system: Headache (9%), fatigue (3%), insomnia (3%)
- Gastrointestinal: Dyspepsia (8%), diarrhea (5%), abdominal pain (5%), nausea (3%)
- Genitourinary: Urinary tract infection (2%)
- Neuromuscular & skeletal: Myalgia (5%)
- Respiratory: Sinusitis (3%), bronchitis (2%)

<1% (Limited to important or life-threatening) including additional class-related events (not necessarily reported with fluvastatin therapy): Alopecia, anaphylaxis, angioedema, arthralgia, arthritis, cataracts, cholestatic jaundice, cirrhosis, CPK increased (>10x normal), depression, dermatomyositis, dyspnea, eosinophilia, erectile dysfunction, erythema multiforme, ESR increased, facial paresis, fatty liver, fever, fulminant hepatic necrosis, gynecomastia, hemolytic anemia, hepatitis, hepatoma, hypersensitivity reaction, impotence, leukopenia, memory loss, muscle cramps, myopathy, nodules, ophthalmoplegia, pancreatitis, paresthesia, peripheral nerve palsy, peripheral neuropathy, photosensitivity, polymyalgia rheumatica, positive

ANA, pruritus, psychic disturbance, purpura, rash, renal failure (secondary to rhabdomyolysis), rhabdomyolysis, skin discoloration, Stevens-Johnson syndrome, systemic lupus erythematosus-like syndrome, taste alteration, thrombocytopenia, thyroid dysfunction, toxic epidermal necrolysis, transaminases increased, tremor, urticaria, vasculitis, vertigo

Metabolism/Transport Effects Substrate of CYP2C9 (major), 2C8 (minor), 2D6 (minor), 3A4 (minor); **Inhibits** CYP1A2 (weak), 2C8 (weak), 2C9 (moderate), 2D6 (weak), 3A4 (weak)

Drug Interactions

Amiodarone: May decrease the metabolism of HMG-CoA Reductase Inhibitors. Management: Dose of simvastatin should not exceed 20 mg/day during concurrent therapy. *Risk D: Consider therapy modification*

Colchicine: May enhance the myopathic (rhabdomyolysis) effect of HMG-CoA Reductase Inhibitors. Colchicine may increase the serum concentration of HMG-CoA Reductase Inhibitors. *Risk D: Consider therapy modification*

CYP2C9 Substrates (High risk): CYP2C9 Inhibitors (Moderate) may decrease the metabolism of CYP2C9 Substrates (High risk). *Risk C: Monitor therapy*

DAPTOmycin: HMG-CoA Reductase Inhibitors may enhance the adverse/toxic effect of DAPTOmycin. Specifically, the risk of skeletal muscle toxicity may be increased. Management: Consider temporarily stopping HMG-CoA reductase inhibitor therapy prior to daptomycin. If used together, regular (i.e., at least weekly) monitoring of CPK concentrations is recommended. *Risk D: Consider therapy modification*

Etravirine: May decrease the serum concentration of HMG-CoA Reductase Inhibitors. This applies to atorvastatin, lovastatin and simvastatin. Conversely, levels of fluvastatin may be increased. Management: Dose adjustment of the HMG-CoA reductase inhibitor may be warranted. No interaction is expected with rosuvastatin or pravastatin. *Risk C: Monitor therapy*

Fenofibrate: May enhance the adverse/toxic effect of HMG-CoA Reductase Inhibitors. *Risk C: Monitor therapy*

Fluconazole: May decrease the metabolism of HMG-CoA Reductase Inhibitors. *Risk D: Consider therapy modification*

Niacin: May enhance the adverse/toxic effect of HMG-CoA Reductase Inhibitors. *Risk C: Monitor therapy*

Niacinamide: May enhance the adverse/toxic effect of HMG-CoA Reductase Inhibitors. *Risk C: Monitor therapy*

Phenytoin: May increase the metabolism of HMG-CoA Reductase Inhibitors. *Risk D: Consider therapy modification*

Rifamycin Derivatives: May increase the metabolism of HMG-CoA Reductase Inhibitors. *Risk D: Consider therapy modification*

Vitamin K Antagonists (eg, warfarin): HMG-CoA Reductase Inhibitors may enhance the anticoagulant effect of Vitamin K Antagonists. *Risk C: Monitor therapy*

Ethanol/Nutrition/Herb Interactions

Ethanol: Avoid excessive ethanol consumption (due to potential hepatic effects).

Food: Reduces rate but not the extent of absorption. Red yeast rice contains an estimated 2.4 mg lovastatin per 600 mg rice.

Stability Store at 15°C to 30°C (59°F to 86°F). Protect from light.

Mechanism of Action Acts by competitively inhibiting 3-hydroxyl-3-methylglutaryl-coenzyme A (HMG-CoA) reductase, the enzyme that catalyzes the reduction of HMG-CoA to mevalonate; this is an early rate-limiting step in cholesterol biosynthesis. HDL is increased while total, LDL, and VLDL cholesterols; apolipoprotein B; and plasma triglycerides are decreased.

Pharmacodynamics/Kinetics

Onset of action: Peak effect: Maximal LDL-C reductions achieved within 4 weeks

Distribution: V_d: 0.35 L/kg

Protein binding: >98%

Metabolism: To inactive and active metabolites (oxidative metabolism via CYP2C9 [75%], 2C8 [~5%], and 3A4 [~20%] isoenzymes); active forms do not circulate systemically; extensive (saturable) first-pass hepatic extraction

Bioavailability: Absolute: Capsule: 24%; Extended release tablet: 29%

Half-life elimination: Capsule: <3 hours; Extended release tablet: 9 hours

Time to peak: Capsule: 1 hour; Extended release tablet: 3 hours

Excretion: Feces (90%): urine (5%)

Dosage

Adolescents 10-16 years: Oral: Heterozygous familial hypercholesterolemia: Initial: 20 mg once daily; may increase every 6 weeks based on tolerability and response to a maximum recommended dose of 80 mg/day, given in 2 divided doses (immediate release capsule) or as a single daily dose (extended release tablet)

Note: Indicated only for adjunctive therapy when diet alone cannot reduce LDL-C below 190 mg/dL, or 160 mg/dL (with cardiovascular risk factors). Female patients must be 1 year postmenarche.

Adults: Oral:

Patients requiring ≥25% decrease in LDL-C: 40 mg capsule once daily in the evening, 80 mg extended release tablet once daily (anytime), or 40 mg capsule twice daily

Patients requiring <25% decrease in LDL-C: Initial: 20 mg capsule once daily in the evening; may increase based on tolerability and response to a maximum recommended dose of 80 mg/day, given in 2 divided doses (immediate release capsule) or as a single daily dose (extended release tablet)

Dosage adjustment in renal impairment: Less than 6% excreted renally; no dosage adjustment needed with mild-to-moderate renal impairment; use with caution in severe impairment

Dosage adjustment in hepatic impairment: Levels may accumulate in patients with liver disease (increased AUC and C_{max}); use caution with severe hepatic impairment or heavy ethanol ingestion; contraindicated in active liver disease or unexplained transaminase elevations; decrease dose and monitor effects carefully in patients with hepatic insufficiency

Elderly: No dosage adjustment necessary based on age

Dietary Considerations Generally, patients should be placed on a standard cholesterol-lowering diet and other lifestyle modifications for 3-6 months prior to the initiation of drug therapy. The diet should be continued during drug therapy. However, for patients with advanced risk factors (eg, known coronary heart disease), drug therapy may be initiated concurrently with diet modification. May be taken without regard to meals. Red yeast rice contains an estimated 2.4 mg lovastatin per 600 mg rice.

Administration Patient should be placed on a standard cholesterol-lowering diet before and during treatment. Fluvastatin may be taken without regard to meals. Adjust dosage as needed in response to periodic lipid determinations during the first 4 weeks after a dosage change; lipid-lowering effects are additive when fluvastatin is combined with a bile-acid binding resin or niacin, however, it must be administered at least 2 hours following these drugs. Do not break, chew, or crush extended release tablets; do not open capsules.

Monitoring Parameters Obtain baseline LFTs and total cholesterol profile; repeat tests at 12 weeks after initiation of therapy or elevation in dose, and periodically thereafter. Monitor LDL-C at intervals no less than 4 weeks.

Dosage Forms Excipient information presented when available (limited, particularly for generics); consult specific product labeling.

Capsule (Lescol®): 20 mg, 40 mg

Tablet, extended release (Lescol® XL): 80 mg

◆ **Fluvirin®** *see* Influenza Virus Vaccine *on page 820*

Fluvoxamine (floo VOKS a meen)

Medication Safety Issues

Sound-alike/look-alike issues:

Fluvoxamine may be confused with flavoxate, fluoxetine

Luvox may be confused with Lasix®, Levoxyl®, Lovenox®

Related Information

Antidepressant Agents *on page 1760*

Antidepressant Receptor Profile *on page 1764*

Discontinuation of Psychotropic Drugs *on page 1839*

Selective Serotonin Reuptake Inhibitors (SSRIs) CYP Profile *on page 1793*

Selective Serotonin Reuptake Inhibitors (SSRIs) FDA-Approved Indication(s) *on page 1794*

Selective Serotonin Reuptake Inhibitors (SSRIs) Pharmacokinetics *on page 1795*

Selective Serotonin Reuptake Inhibitors (SSRIs) Receptor Profile *on page 1796*

U.S. Brand Names Luvox® CR

Canadian Brand Names Alti-Fluvoxamine; Apo-Fluvoxamine®; Luvox®; Novo-Fluvoxamine; Nu-Fluvoxamine; PMS-Fluvoxamine; Rhoxal-fluvoxamine; Sandoz-Fluvoxamine

Mexican Brand Names Luvox; Vuminix

Index Terms Luvox

Pharmacologic Category Antidepressant, Selective Serotonin Reuptake Inhibitor

Generic Available Yes: Excludes extended release capsule

Use Treatment of obsessive-compulsive disorder (OCD); treatment of social anxiety disorder

Unlabeled/Investigational Use Treatment of major depression; panic disorder; anxiety disorders in children; treatment of mild dementia-associated agitation in nonpsychotic patients

Mental Health Comment The SSRIs as a class are generally considered to be safe and equally effective. Allow sufficient dose-response time (6-12 weeks). Differences lie in approved indications, receptor profiles, pharmacokinetics, and cytochrome P450 activity profile. Subtle differences exist in adverse effect profiles. All SSRIs have the potential to cause sexual dysfunction. Fluvoxamine is only approved in U.S. for obsessive-compulsive disorder (OCD), offers no advantage over other SSRIs, and is associated with significant CYP inhibitory properties.

Restrictions An FDA-approved medication guide concerning the use of antidepressants in children, adolescents, and young adults must be distributed when dispensing an outpatient prescription (new or refill) where this medication is to be used without direct supervision of a healthcare provider. Medication guides are available at http://www.fda.gov/cder/Offices/ODS/medication_guides.htm. Dispense to parents or guardians of children and adolescents receiving this medication.

Pregnancy Risk Factor C

Pregnancy Considerations Due to adverse effects observed in animal studies, fluvoxamine is classified as pregnancy category C. Fluvoxamine crosses the human placenta. Nonteratogenic effects in the newborn following SSRI exposure late in the third trimester include respiratory distress, cyanosis, apnea, seizures, temperature instability, feeding difficulty, vomiting, hypoglycemia, hypo- or hypertonia, hyper-reflexia, jitteriness, irritability, constant crying, and tremor. An increased risk of low birth weight and low APGAR scores has also been reported. Exposure to SSRIs after the twentieth week of gestation has been associated with persistent pulmonary hypertension of the newborn (PPHN). Adverse effects may be due to toxic effects of the SSRI or drug withdrawal due to discontinuation. The long-term effects of *in utero* SSRI exposure on infant development and behavior are not known.

Women treated for major depression and who are euthymic prior to pregnancy are more likely to experience a relapse when medication is discontinued as compared to pregnant women who continue taking antidepressant medications. The ACOG recommends that therapy with SSRIs or SNRIs during pregnancy be individualized; treatment of depression during pregnancy should incorporate the clinical expertise of the mental health clinician, obstetrician, primary healthcare provider, and pediatrician (ACOG, 2007). If treatment during pregnancy is required, consider tapering therapy during the third trimester in order to prevent withdrawal symptoms in the infant. If this is done and the woman is considered to be at risk from her major depressive disorder, the medication can be restarted following delivery, although the dose should be readjusted to that required before pregnancy.

Lactation Enters breast milk/consider risk:benefit (AAP rates "of concern")

Contraindications Hypersensitivity to fluvoxamine or any component of the formulation; concurrent use with alosetron, pimozide, thioridazine, or tizanidine; use with or within 14 days of MAO inhibitors

Warnings/Precautions **[U.S. Boxed Warning]: Antidepressants increase the risk of suicidal thinking and behavior in children, adolescents, and young adults (18-24 years of age) with major depressive disorder (MDD) and other psychiatric disorders;** consider risk prior to prescribing. Short-term studies did not show an increased risk in patients >24 years of age and showed a decreased risk in patients ≥65 years. Closely monitor patients for clinical worsening, suicidality, or unusual changes in behavior, particularly during the initial 1-2 months of therapy or during periods of dosage adjustments (increases or decreases); the patient's family or caregiver should be instructed to closely observe the patient and communicate condition with healthcare provider. A medication guide concerning the use of antidepressants should be dispensed with each prescription. **Fluvoxamine is FDA approved for the treatment of OCD in children ≥8 years of age; extended release capsules are not FDA approved for use in children.**

The possibility of a suicide attempt is inherent in major depression and may persist until remission occurs. Use caution in high-risk patients. Worsening depression and severe abrupt suicidality that are not part of the presenting symptoms may require discontinuation or modification of drug therapy. The patient's family or caregiver should be alerted to monitor patients for the emergence of suicidality and associated behaviors (such as agitation, irritability, hostility, impulsivity, and hypomania) and call healthcare provider.

May worsen psychosis in some patients or precipitate a shift to mania or hypomania in patients with bipolar disorder. Patients presenting with depressive symptoms should be screened for bipolar disorder. Monotherapy in patients with bipolar disorder should be avoided. **Fluvoxamine is not FDA approved for the treatment of bipolar depression.**

The potential for severe reaction exits when used with MAO inhibitors, SSRIs/SNRIs, or triptans; serotonin syndrome (hyperthermia, muscular rigidity, mental status changes/agitation, autonomic instability) may occur. Concurrent use with MAO inhibitors is contraindicated. Fluvoxamine has a low potential to impair cognitive or motor performance; caution operating hazardous machinery or driving. Use caution in patients with a previous seizure disorder or condition predisposing to seizures such as brain damage, alcoholism, or concurrent therapy with other drugs which lower the seizure threshold. Fluvoxamine may significantly increase alosetron concentrations; concurrent use **contraindicated.** Potential for QT_C prolongation and arrhythmia with thioridazine and pimozide; concurrent use of fluvoxamine with either of these agents is **contraindicated.** Concomitant use with tizanidine may cause a significant decrease in blood pressure and increase in drowsiness; concurrent use is **contraindicated.** Fluvoxamine levels may be lower in patients who smoke.

May increase the risks associated with electroconvulsive therapy. Use with caution in patients with hepatic dysfunction and in elderly patients. May cause hyponatremia/SIADH (elderly at increased risk); volume depletion (diuretics may increase risk). Use with caution in patients at risk of bleeding or receiving concurrent anticoagulant therapy, although not consistently noted, fluvoxamine may cause impairment in platelet function. May cause or exacerbate sexual dysfunction.

Adverse Reactions Frequency varies by dosage form and indication. Adverse reactions reported as a composite of all indications.

>10%:

Central nervous system: Headache (22% to 35%), insomnia (21% to 35%), somnolence (22% to 27%), dizziness (11% to 15%), nervousness (10% to 12%)

Gastrointestinal: Nausea (34% to 40%), diarrhea (11% to 18%), xerostomia (10% to 14%), anorexia (6% to 14%)

Genitourinary: Ejaculation abnormal (8% to 11%)

Neuromuscular & skeletal: Weakness (14% to 26%)

1% to 10%:

Cardiovascular: Chest pain (3%), palpitation (3%), vasodilation (2% to 3%), hypertension (1% to 2%), edema (≤1%), hypotension (≤1%), syncope (≤1%), tachycardia (≤1%)

Central nervous system: Pain (10%), anxiety (5% to 8%), abnormal dreams (3%), abnormal thinking (3%), agitation (2% to 3%), apathy (≥1% to 3%), chills (2%), CNS stimulation (2%), depression (2%), neurosis (2%), amnesia, malaise, manic reaction, psychotic reaction

Dermatologic: Bruising (4%), acne (2%)

Endocrine & metabolic: Libido decreased (2% to 10%; incidence higher in males), anorgasmia (2% to 5%), sexual function abnormal (2% to 4%), menorrhagia (3%)

Gastrointestinal: Dyspepsia (8% to 10%), constipation (4% to 10%), vomiting (4% to 6%), abdominal pain (5%), flatulence (4%), taste perversion (2% to 3%), tooth disorder (2% to 3%), dysphagia (2%), gingivitis (2%), weight loss (≤1% to 2%), weight gain

Genitourinary: Polyuria (2% to 3%), impotence (2%), urinary tract infection (2%), urinary retention (1%)

Hepatic: Liver function tests abnormal (≥1% to 2%)

Neuromuscular & skeletal: Tremor (5% to 8%), myalgia (5%), paresthesia (3%), hypertonia (2%), twitching (2%), hyper-/hypokinesia, myoclonus

Ocular: Amblyopia (2% to 3%)

Respiratory: Upper respiratory infection (9%), pharyngitis (6%), yawn (2% to 5%), laryngitis (3%), bronchitis (2%), dyspnea (2%), epistaxis (2%), cough increased, sinusitis

Miscellaneous: Diaphoresis (6% to 7%), flu-like syndrome (3%), viral infection (2%)

<1% (Limited to important or life-threatening): Acute renal failure, agranulocytosis, akinesia, allergic reaction, anaphylactic reaction, anemia, angina, angioedema, anuria, aplastic anemia, apnea, asthma, ataxia, AV block, bradycardia, bullous eruption, cardiomyopathy, cerebrovascular accident, cholecystitis, cholelithiasis, colitis, conduction delay, coronary artery disease,

diplopia, dyskinesia, dystonia, extrapyramidal syndrome, embolus, GI bleeding, goiter, hallucinations, heart failure, hematemesis, hematuria, Henoch-Schönlein purpura, hepatitis, hemoptysis, hypercholesterolemia, hyper-/hypoglycemia, hypokalemia, hyponatremia, hypothyroidism, ileus, intestinal obstruction, jaundice, leukopenia, leukocytosis, lymphadenopathy, MI, myasthenia, myopathy, neuralgia, neuroleptic malignant syndrome, neuropathy, pancreatitis, paralysis, pericarditis, porphyria, purpura, retinal detachment, serotonin syndrome, ST segment changes, seizure, Stevens-Johnson syndrome, suicidal tendencies, supraventricular extrasystoles, tardive dyskinesia, thrombocytopenia, toxic epidermal necrolysis, vasculitis, ventricular tachycardia (including torsade de pointes)

Metabolism/Transport Effects **Substrate** (major) of CYP1A2, 2D6; **Inhibits** CYP1A2 (strong), 2B6 (weak), 2C9 (weak), 2C19 (strong), 2D6 (weak), 3A4 (weak)

Drug Interactions

Alcohol (Ethyl): CNS Depressants may enhance the CNS depressant effect of Alcohol (Ethyl). *Risk C: Monitor therapy*

Alosetron: Fluvoxamine may decrease the metabolism of Alosetron. *Risk X: Avoid combination*

Analgesics (Opioid): May enhance the serotonergic effect of Selective Serotonin Reuptake Inhibitors. This may cause serotonin syndrome. *Risk C: Monitor therapy*

Anticoagulants: Antiplatelet Agents may enhance the anticoagulant effect of Anticoagulants. *Risk C: Monitor therapy*

Antidepressants (Serotonin Reuptake Inhibitor/Antagonist): Selective Serotonin Reuptake Inhibitors may enhance the serotonergic effect of Antidepressants (Serotonin Reuptake Inhibitor/Antagonist). This may cause serotonin syndrome. *Risk C: Monitor therapy*

Antiplatelet Agents: May enhance the anticoagulant effect of other Antiplatelet Agents. *Risk C: Monitor therapy*

Aspirin: Selective Serotonin Reuptake Inhibitors may enhance the antiplatelet effect of Aspirin. *Risk C: Monitor therapy*

Bendamustine: CYP1A2 Inhibitors (Strong) may increase the serum concentration of Bendamustine. Concentrations of the active metabolites of bendamustine may be decreased. *Risk C: Monitor therapy*

Benzodiazepines (metabolized by oxidation): Selective Serotonin Reuptake Inhibitors may decrease the metabolism of Benzodiazepines (metabolized by oxidation). *Risk C: Monitor therapy*

BusPIRone: May enhance the serotonergic effect of Selective Serotonin Reuptake Inhibitors. This may cause serotonin syndrome. Selective Serotonin Reuptake Inhibitors may decrease the metabolism of BusPIRone. *Risk C: Monitor therapy*

CarBAMazepine: Selective Serotonin Reuptake Inhibitors may decrease the metabolism of CarBAMazepine. Specifically those SSRIs that inhibit CYP3A4 isoenzymes. CarBAMazepine may increase the metabolism of Selective Serotonin Reuptake Inhibitors. Specifically those agents metabolized via CYP1A2, 2C, and/or 3A4 isoenzymes. *Risk D: Consider therapy modification*

Cimetidine: May decrease the metabolism of Selective Serotonin Reuptake Inhibitors. *Risk D: Consider therapy modification*

Clozapine: Selective Serotonin Reuptake Inhibitors may decrease the metabolism of Clozapine. *Risk D: Consider therapy modification*

CNS Depressants: May enhance the adverse/toxic effect of other CNS Depressants. *Risk C: Monitor therapy*

CYP1A2 Inducers (Strong): May increase the metabolism of CYP1A2 Substrates. *Risk C: Monitor therapy*

CYP1A2 Inhibitors (Moderate): May decrease the metabolism of CYP1A2 Substrates. *Risk C: Monitor therapy*

CYP1A2 Inhibitors (Strong): May decrease the metabolism of CYP1A2 Substrates. *Risk D: Consider therapy modification*

CYP1A2 Substrates: CYP1A2 Inhibitors (Strong) may decrease the metabolism of CYP1A2 Substrates. *Risk D: Consider therapy modification*

CYP2C19 Substrates: CYP2C19 Inhibitors (Strong) may decrease the metabolism of CYP2C19 Substrates. *Risk D: Consider therapy modification*

CYP2D6 Inhibitors (Moderate): May decrease the metabolism of CYP2D6 Substrates. *Risk C: Monitor therapy*

CYP2D6 Inhibitors (Strong): May decrease the metabolism of CYP2D6 Substrates. *Risk D: Consider therapy modification*

Cyproheptadine: May diminish the therapeutic effect of Selective Serotonin Reuptake Inhibitors. *Risk C: Monitor therapy*

Darunavir: May increase the serum concentration of CYP2D6 Substrates. *Risk C: Monitor therapy*

Dasatinib: May enhance the anticoagulant effect of Antiplatelet Agents. *Risk C: Monitor therapy*

Desmopressin: Selective Serotonin Reuptake Inhibitors may enhance the adverse/toxic effect of Desmopressin. *Risk C: Monitor therapy*

Drotrecogin Alfa: Antiplatelet Agents may enhance the adverse/toxic effect of Drotrecogin Alfa. Bleeding may occur. *Risk D: Consider therapy modification*

DULoxetine: Fluvoxamine may decrease the metabolism of DULoxetine. *Risk C: Monitor therapy*

Haloperidol: Selective Serotonin Reuptake Inhibitors may decrease the metabolism of Haloperidol. *Risk C: Monitor therapy*

Herbs (Anticoagulant/Antiplatelet Properties) (eg, Alfalfa, Anise, Bilberry): May enhance the adverse/toxic effect of Antiplatelet Agents. Bleeding may occur. *Risk D: Consider therapy modification*

Ibritumomab: Antiplatelet Agents may enhance the adverse/toxic effect of Ibritumomab. Both agents may contribute to impaired platelet function and an increased risk of bleeding. *Risk C: Monitor therapy*

Lithium: Selective Serotonin Reuptake Inhibitors may enhance the adverse/toxic effect of Lithium. *Risk C: Monitor therapy*

MAO Inhibitors: May enhance the serotonergic effect of Selective Serotonin Reuptake Inhibitors. This may cause serotonin syndrome. *Risk X: Avoid combination*

Methadone: Selective Serotonin Reuptake Inhibitors may decrease the metabolism of Methadone. Fluvoxamine appears to be the only interacting SSRI. *Risk D: Consider therapy modification*

Mexiletine: Selective Serotonin Reuptake Inhibitors may decrease the metabolism of Mexiletine. *Risk D: Consider therapy modification*

NSAID (COX-2 Inhibitor): Selective Serotonin Reuptake Inhibitors may enhance the antiplatelet effect of NSAID (COX-2 Inhibitor). *Risk D: Consider therapy modification*

NSAID (Nonselective): Selective Serotonin Reuptake Inhibitors may enhance the antiplatelet effect of NSAID (Nonselective). *Risk D: Consider therapy modification*

OLANZapine: Fluvoxamine may decrease the metabolism of OLANZapine. *Risk D: Consider therapy modification*

Omega-3-Acid Ethyl Esters: May enhance the antiplatelet effect of Antiplatelet Agents. *Risk C: Monitor therapy*

Pentosan Polysulfate Sodium: May enhance the adverse/toxic effect of Antiplatelet Agents. Specifically, the risk of bleeding may be increased by concurrent use of these agents. *Risk C: Monitor therapy*

Phenytoin: Selective Serotonin Reuptake Inhibitors may decrease the metabolism of Phenytoin. *Risk D: Consider therapy modification*

Pimozide: Selective Serotonin Reuptake Inhibitors may enhance the adverse/toxic effect of Pimozide. *Risk X: Avoid combination*

Propranolol: Fluvoxamine may increase the serum concentration of Propranolol. Management: Use a lower initial propranolol dose and be cautious with propranolol dose titration. *Risk D: Consider therapy modification*

Prostacyclin Analogues: May enhance the antiplatelet effect of Antiplatelet Agents. *Risk C: Monitor therapy*

QuiNIDine: Selective Serotonin Reuptake Inhibitors may decrease the metabolism of QuiNIDine. Fluvoxamine appears to be the only SSRI of concern. *Risk D: Consider therapy modification*

Ramelteon: Fluvoxamine may decrease the metabolism of Ramelteon. *Risk X: Avoid combination*

Ropivacaine: Fluvoxamine may decrease the metabolism of Ropivacaine. *Risk C: Monitor therapy*

Salicylates: Antiplatelet Agents may enhance the adverse/toxic effect of Salicylates. Increased risk of bleeding may result. *Risk C: Monitor therapy*

Serotonin Modulators: May enhance the adverse/toxic effect of other Serotonin Modulators. The development of serotonin syndrome may occur. *Risk D: Consider therapy modification*

Sibutramine: May enhance the serotonergic effect of Serotonin Modulators. This may cause serotonin syndrome. *Risk X: Avoid combination*

Tacrine: Fluvoxamine may decrease the metabolism of Tacrine. *Risk D: Consider therapy modification*

Theophylline Derivatives: Fluvoxamine may decrease the metabolism of Theophylline Derivatives. **Exceptions:** Dyphylline. *Risk D: Consider therapy modification*

Thioridazine: Fluvoxamine may increase the serum concentration of Thioridazine. *Risk X: Avoid combination*

Thrombolytic Agents: Antiplatelet Agents may enhance the anticoagulant effect of Thrombolytic Agents. *Risk C: Monitor therapy*

TiZANidine: Fluvoxamine may decrease the metabolism of TiZANidine. *Risk X: Avoid combination*

Tositumomab and Iodine I 131 Tositumomab: Antiplatelet Agents may enhance the adverse/toxic effect of Tositumomab and Iodine I 131 Tositumomab. Specifically, the risk of bleeding-related adverse events may be increased. *Risk C: Monitor therapy*

TraMADol: Selective Serotonin Reuptake Inhibitors may enhance the neuroexcitatory and/or seizure-potentiating effect of TraMADol. TraMADol may enhance the serotonergic effect of Selective Serotonin Reuptake Inhibitors. This may cause serotonin syndrome. *Risk D: Consider therapy modification*

Tricyclic Antidepressants: Selective Serotonin Reuptake Inhibitors may decrease the metabolism of Tricyclic Antidepressants. *Risk D: Consider therapy modification*

Tryptophan: May enhance the serotonergic effect of Selective Serotonin Reuptake Inhibitors. This may cause serotonin syndrome. *Risk D: Consider therapy modification*

Vitamin K Antagonists (eg, warfarin): Selective Serotonin Reuptake Inhibitors may enhance the anticoagulant effect of Vitamin K Antagonists. *Risk C: Monitor therapy*

Ethanol/Nutrition/Herb Interactions

Ethanol: Avoid ethanol. Patients with depression should avoid/limit intake.

Food: The bioavailability of melatonin has been reported to be increased by fluvoxamine.

Herb/Nutraceutical: Avoid valerian, St John's wort, SAMe, kava kava (may increase risk of serotonin syndrome and/or excessive sedation). Avoid alfalfa, anise, bilberry, bladderwrack, bromelain, cat's claw, celery, chamomile, coleus, cordyceps, dong quai, evening primrose, fenugreek, feverfew, garlic, ginger, ginkgo biloba, ginseng (American), ginseng (Panax), ginseng (Siberian), grape seed, green tea, guggul, horse chestnuts, horseradish, licorice, prickly ash, red clover, reishi, SAMe (S-adenosylmethionine), sweet clover, turmeric, white willow (all have additional antiplatelet activity).

Stability Protect from high humidity and store at controlled room temperature 25°C (77°F).

Mechanism of Action Inhibits CNS neuron serotonin uptake; minimal or no effect on reuptake of norepinephrine or dopamine; does not significantly bind to alpha-adrenergic, histamine or cholinergic receptors

Pharmacodynamics/Kinetics

Onset of action: Depression: The onset of action is within a week; however, individual response varies greatly and full response may not be seen until 8-12 weeks after initiation of treatment.

Absorption: Steady-state plasma concentrations have been noted to be 2-3 times higher in children than those in adolescents; female children demonstrated a significantly higher AUC than males

Distribution: V_d: ~25 L/kg

Protein binding: ~80%, primarily to albumin

Metabolism: Extensively hepatic via oxidative demethylation and deamination

Bioavailability: Immediate release: 53%; not significantly affected by food

Half-life elimination: 15-16 hours; 17-26 hours in the elderly

Time to peak, plasma: 3-8 hours

Excretion: Urine (~85% as metabolites; ~2% as unchanged drug)

Dosage Oral:

Obsessive-compulsive disorder:

Children 8-17 years: Immediate release: Initial: 25 mg once daily at bedtime; may be increased in 25 mg increments at 4- to 7-day intervals, as tolerated, to maximum therapeutic benefit; usual dose range: 50-200 mg/day. **Note:** When total daily dose exceeds 50 mg, the dose should be given in 2 divided doses with larger portion administered at bedtime.

Maximum: Children: 8-11 years: 200 mg/day, adolescents: 300 mg/day; lower doses may be effective in female versus male patients

Adults:

Immediate release: Initial: 50 mg once daily at bedtime; may be increased in 50 mg increments at 4- to 7-day intervals, as tolerated; usual dose range: 100-300 mg/day; maximum dose: 300 mg/day. **Note:** When total daily dose exceeds 100 mg, the dose should be given in 2 divided doses with larger portion administered at bedtime.

Extended release: Initial: 100 mg once daily at bedtime; may be increased in 50 mg increments at intervals of at least 1 week; usual dosage range: 100-300 mg/day; maximum dose: 300 mg/day

Social anxiety disorder: Adults: Extended release: Initial: 100 mg once daily at bedtime; may be increased in 50 mg increments at intervals of at least 1 week; usual dosage range: 100-300 mg/day; maximum dose: 300 mg/day

Elderly: Reduce dose, titrate slowly

Dosage adjustment in hepatic impairment: Reduce dose, titrate slowly

Child/Adolescent Considerations Children 8-17 years of age with obsessive-compulsive disorder (OCD) received 50-200 mg/day for 10 weeks (Riddle, 2001). One hundred twenty-eight children 6-17 years of age with social phobia, separation anxiety disorder, or generalized anxiety disorder, who had received psychological treatment for 3 weeks without improvement, received fluvoxamine up to 300 mg/day for 8 weeks (Research Unit, 2001).

"Fluvoxamine for the Treatment of Anxiety Disorders in Children and Adolescents. The Research Unit on Pediatric Psychopharmacology Anxiety Study Group," *N Engl J Med*, 2001, 344(17):1279-85.

Riddle MA, Reeve EA, Yaryura-Tobias JA, et al, "Fluvoxamine for Children and Adolescents With Obsessive-Compulsive Disorder: A Randomized, Controlled, Multicenter Trial," *J Am Acad Child Adolesc Psychiatry*, 2001, 40 (2):222-9.

Dietary Considerations May be taken with or without food.

Administration May be administered with or without food. Do not crush, open, or chew extended release capsules.

Monitoring Parameters Mental status for depression, suicidal ideation (especially at the beginning of therapy or when doses are increased or decreased), anxiety, social functioning, mania, panic attacks; akathisia, weight gain or loss, nutritional intake, sleep; liver function assessment prior to beginning drug therapy

Dosage Forms Excipient information presented when available (limited, particularly for generics); consult specific product labeling.

Tablet, as maleate: 25 mg, 50 mg, 100 mg

Capsule, extended release, as maleate:

Luvox® CR: 100 mg, 150 mg [gluten free]

◆ **Fluzone®** *see* Influenza Virus Vaccine *on page 820*

◆ **Focalin®** *see* Dexmethylphenidate *on page 438*

◆ **Focalin® XR** *see* Dexmethylphenidate *on page 438*

◆ **Folacin** *see* Folic Acid *on page 684*

◆ **Folacin-800 [OTC]** *see* Folic Acid *on page 684*

◆ **Folate** *see* Folic Acid *on page 684*

Folic Acid (FOE lik AS id)

Medication Safety Issues

Sound-alike/look-alike issues:

Folic acid may be confused with folinic acid

U.S. Brand Names Folacin-800 [OTC]

Canadian Brand Names Apo-Folic®

Mexican Brand Names A.F. Valdecasas; Folivital; Prinac AC

Index Terms Folacin; Folate; Pteroylglutamic Acid

Pharmacologic Category Vitamin, Water Soluble

Generic Available Yes

Use Treatment of megaloblastic and macrocytic anemias due to folate deficiency; dietary supplement to prevent neural tube defects

Unlabeled/Investigational Use Adjunctive cofactor therapy in methanol toxicity (alternative to leucovorin)

Effect on Mental Status May cause drowsiness

Effect on Psychiatric Treatment None reported

Pregnancy Risk Factor A

Pregnancy Considerations Folic acid requirements are increased during pregnancy; a deficiency may result in fetal harm.

Lactation Enters breast milk/compatible

Contraindications Hypersensitivity to folic acid or any component of the formulation

Warnings/Precautions Not appropriate for monotherapy with pernicious, aplastic, or normocytic anemias when anemia is present with vitamin B_{12} deficiency. Doses >0.1 mg/day may obscure pernicious anemia with continuing irreversible nerve damage progression. Resistance to treatment may occur with depressed hematopoiesis, alcoholism, and deficiencies of other vitamins. Injection contains benzyl alcohol (1.5%) as preservative (use care in administration to neonates).

Adverse Reactions Frequency not defined.

Allergic reaction, bronchospasm, flushing (slight), malaise (general), pruritus, rash

Drug Interactions

PHENobarbital: Folic Acid may decrease the serum concentration of PHENobarbital. *Risk C: Monitor therapy*

Phenytoin: Folic Acid may decrease the serum concentration of Phenytoin. *Risk C: Monitor therapy*

Primidone: Folic Acid may decrease the serum concentration of Primidone. Additionally, folic acid may decrease concentrations of active metabolites of primidone (e.g., phenobarbital). *Risk C: Monitor therapy*

Raltitrexed: Folic Acid may diminish the therapeutic effect of Raltitrexed. *Risk X: Avoid combination*

Stability Do not use with oxidizing and reducing agents or heavy metal ions.

Mechanism of Action Folic acid is necessary for formation of a number of coenzymes in many metabolic systems, particularly for purine and pyrimidine synthesis; required for nucleoprotein synthesis and maintenance in erythropoiesis; stimulates WBC and platelet production in folate deficiency anemia. Folic acid enhances the elimination of formic acid, the toxic metabolite of methanol (unlabeled use).

Pharmacodynamics/Kinetics

Onset of action: Peak effect: Oral: 0.5-1 hour

Absorption: Proximal part of small intestine

Dosage

Oral, I.M., I.V., SubQ: Anemia:

- Infants: 0.1 mg/day
- Children <4 years: Up to 0.3 mg/day
- Children >4 years and Adults: 0.4 mg/day
- Pregnant and lactating women: 0.8 mg/day

Oral:

- RDA: Expressed as dietary folate equivalents:
  - Children:
    - 1-3 years: 150 mcg/day
    - 4-8 years: 200 mcg/day
    - 9-13 years: 300 mcg/day
  - Children ≥14 years and Adults: 400 mcg/day
  - Elderly: Vitamin B_{12} deficiency must be ruled out before initiating folate therapy due to frequency of combined nutritional deficiencies: RDA requirements (1999): 400 mcg/day (0.4 mg) minimum
- Prevention of neural tube defects:
  - Females of childbearing potential: 400 mcg/day
  - Females at high risk or with family history of neural tube defects: 4 mg/day

Dietary Considerations As of January 1998, the FDA has required manufacturers of enriched flour, bread, corn meal, pasta, rice, and other grain products to add folic acid to their products. The intent is to help decrease the risk of neural tube defects by increasing folic acid intake. Other foods which contain folic acid include dark green leafy vegetables, citrus fruits and juices, and lentils.

Administration Oral preferred, but may also be administered by deep I.M., SubQ, or I.V. injection.

Reference Range Therapeutic: 0.005-0.015 mcg/mL

Test Interactions Falsely low serum concentrations may occur with the *Lactobacillus casei* assay method in patients on anti-infectives (eg, tetracycline)

Additional Information The RDA for folic acid is presented as dietary folate equivalents (DFE). DFE adjusts for the difference in bioavailability of folic acid from food as compared to dietary supplements.

Dosage Forms Excipient information presented when available (limited, particularly for generics); consult specific product labeling.

Injection, solution, as sodium folate: 5 mg/mL (10 mL) [contains benzyl alcohol, edetate disodium]

Tablet: 0.4 mg, 0.8 mg, 1 mg

- Folacin-800: 0.8 mg

Fomepizole (foe ME pi zole)

U.S. Brand Names Antizol®

Index Terms 4-Methylpyrazole; 4-MP

Pharmacologic Category Antidote

Use Treatment of methanol or ethylene glycol poisoning alone or in combination with hemodialysis

Unlabeled/Investigational Use Treatment of propylene glycol toxicity
Effect on Mental Status Dizziness is common; may cause drowsiness
Effect on Psychiatric Treatment None reported
Dosage Summary
I.V.:
Children: Dosage not established
Adults: Loading dose of 15 mg/kg, followed by 10 mg/kg every 12 hours for 4 doses, then 15 mg/kg every 12 hours until levels have been reduced <20 mg/dL and patient is asymptomatic
Dosage Forms Excipient information presented when available (limited, particularly for generics); consult specific product labeling.
Injection, solution [preservative free]: 1 g/mL (1.5 mL)
Antizol®: 1 g/mL (1.5 mL)

◆ **Foradil® Aerolizer®** *see* Formoterol *on page 686*

Formoterol (for MOH te rol)

Medication Safety Issues
Sound-alike/look-alike issues:
Foradil® may be confused with Toradol®
Foradil® capsules for inhalation are for administration via Aerolizer™ inhaler and are **not** for oral use.

International issues:
Foradil® may be confused with Theradol® which is a brand name for tramadol in the Netherlands.
U.S. Brand Names Foradil® Aerolizer®; Perforomist™
Canadian Brand Names Foradil®; Oxeze® Turbuhaler®
Mexican Brand Names Foradil; Oxis Turbuhaler
Index Terms Formoterol Fumarate; Formoterol Fumarate Dihydrate
Pharmacologic Category Beta$_2$-Adrenergic Agonist
Generic Available No
Use Maintenance treatment of asthma and prevention of bronchospasm in patients ≥5 years of age with reversible obstructive airway disease, including patients with symptoms of nocturnal asthma, who require regular treatment with inhaled, short-acting beta$_2$-agonists; maintenance treatment of bronchoconstriction in patients with COPD; prevention of exercise-induced bronchospasm in patients ≥5 years of age

Note:
Oxeze® is also approved in Canada for acute relief of symptoms ("on demand" treatment) in patients ≥6 years of age.
Perforomist™ is only indicated for maintenance treatment of bronchoconstriction in patients with COPD.
Effect on Mental Status May cause dizziness or insomnia
Effect on Psychiatric Treatment Concurrent use with MAO inhibitors, TCAs, thioridazine, or mesoridazine may potentiate cardiovascular effects
Restrictions An FDA-approved medication guide must be distributed when dispensing an outpatient prescription (new or refill) where this medication is to be used without direct supervision of a healthcare provider. Medication guides are available at http://www.fda.gov/cder/Offices/ODS/medication_guides.htm.
Pregnancy Risk Factor C
Pregnancy Considerations When given orally to rats throughout organogenesis, formoterol caused delayed ossification and decreased fetal weight, but no malformations. There were no adverse events when given to pregnant rats in late pregnancy. Doses used were ≥70 times the recommended daily inhalation dose in humans. There are no adequate and well-controlled studies in pregnant women. Use only if benefit outweighs risk to the fetus. Beta-agonists interfere with uterine contractility so use during labor only if benefit outweighs risk to the fetus.
Lactation Excretion in breast milk unknown/use caution
Contraindications
Foradil®: Hypersensitivity to formoterol, or any component of the formulation
Oxeze®: Hypersensitivity to formoterol, inhaled lactose, or any component of the formulation; presence of tachyarrhythmias
Perforomist™: No contraindications listed in the product labeling
Warnings/Precautions [U.S. Boxed Warning]: Long-acting beta$_2$-agonists may increase the risk of asthma-related deaths. Foradil® should only be used as adjuvant therapy in patients not adequately controlled on other asthma medications (eg, low-to-medium dose inhaled corticosteroids) or whose

disease warrants initiation of two maintenance therapies. Optimize anti-inflammatory treatment before initiating maintenance treatment with formoterol. Do not use as a component of chronic therapy without an anti-inflammatory agent. Corticosteroids should not be stopped or reduced at formoterol initiation. Patients using inhaled, short-acting beta$_2$-agonists should be instructed to discontinue routine use of these medications prior to beginning treatment; short-acting agents should still be provided to patients; however, use should be reserved for symptomatic relief of acute symptoms. Patient must be instructed to seek medical attention in cases where acute symptoms are not relieved by a rapid-onset beta-agonist or when a previous level of response is diminished. Treatment must not be delayed. Rarely, paradoxical bronchospasm may occur with use of inhaled bronchodilating agents; this should be distinguished from inadequate response. The safety and efficacy of Perforomist™ in the treatment of asthma have not been established.

Acute episodes should be treated with a rapid-onset beta$_2$-agonist. Oxeze® is a formulation of formoterol (available outside the U.S. [eg, Canada]) approved for acute treatment of asthmatic symptoms. The labelings for U.S. approved formulations (Foradil®, Perforomist™) state that formoterol is not meant to relieve acute asthmatic symptoms.

Formoterol should not be used for the treatment of rapidly deteriorating COPD or for acute symptomatic COPD. Increased use and/or ineffectiveness of short-acting beta$_2$-agonists may indicate rapidly deteriorating disease and should prompt re-evaluation of the patient's condition.

Immediate hypersensitivity reactions (urticaria, angioedema, rash, bronchospasm) have been reported. Do not exceed recommended dose or frequency; serious adverse events (including serious asthma exacerbations and fatalities) have been associated with excessive use of inhaled sympathomimetics. Beta$_2$-agonists may increase risk of arrhythmias, decrease serum potassium, prolong QT_c interval, or increase serum glucose. These effects may be exacerbated in hypoxemia. Use caution in patients with cardiovascular disease (arrhythmia, coronary insufficiency, hypertension, or HF), seizures, diabetes, glaucoma, hyperthyroidism, or hypokalemia. Beta-agonists may cause elevation in blood pressure and heart rate, and result in CNS stimulation/excitation.

Powder for oral inhalation contains lactose; very rare anaphylactic reactions have been reported in patients with severe milk protein allergy. The contents of the Foradil® capsules are for inhalation via the Aerolizer™ device. There have been reports of incorrect administration (swallowing of the capsules).Safety and efficacy of Foradil® have not been established in children <5 years of age; safety and efficacy of Perforomist™ have not been established in children <18 years of age.

Adverse Reactions

1% to 10%:

Cardiovascular: Chest pain (2%), palpitation

Central nervous system: Anxiety (2%), dizziness (2%), fever (2%), insomnia (2%), dysphonia (1%), headache

Dermatologic: Rash (1%)

Gastrointestinal: Diarrhea (5%), nausea (5%), xerostomia (1% to 3%), vomiting (2%), abdominal pain, dyspepsia, gastroenteritis

Neuromuscular & skeletal: Tremor

Respiratory: Asthma exacerbation (age 5-12 years: 5% to 6%; age >12 years: <4%), bronchitis (5%), infection (3% to 7%), pharyngitis (3% to 4%), sinusitis (3%), dyspnea (2%), tonsillitis (1%)

<1% (Limited to important or life-threatening): Acute asthma deterioration, anaphylactic reactions (severe hypotension/angioedema), agitation, angina, arrhythmia, bronchospasm (paradoxical), fatigue, hyperglycemia, hypertension, hypokalemia, glucose intolerance, malaise, metabolic acidosis, muscle cramps, nervousness, tachycardia

Metabolism/Transport Effects **Substrate** (minor) of CYP2A6, 2C9, 2C19, 2D6

Drug Interactions

Alpha-/Beta-Blockers: May diminish the therapeutic effect of Beta2-Agonists. *Risk D: Consider therapy modification*

Atomoxetine: May enhance the tachycardic effect of Beta2-Agonists. *Risk C: Monitor therapy*

Beta-Blockers (Beta1 Selective): May diminish the bronchodilatory effect of Beta2-Agonists. Of particular concern with nonselective beta-blockers or higher doses of the beta1 selective beta-blockers. *Risk C: Monitor therapy*

Beta-Blockers (Nonselective): May diminish the bronchodilatory effect of Beta2-Agonists. *Risk D: Consider therapy modification*

Betahistine: May diminish the therapeutic effect of Beta2-Agonists. *Risk C: Monitor therapy*

Cannabinoids: May enhance the tachycardic effect of Sympathomimetics. *Risk C: Monitor therapy*

MAO Inhibitors: May enhance the adverse/toxic effect of Beta2-Agonists. *Risk C: Monitor therapy*

Sympathomimetics: May enhance the adverse/toxic effect of other Sympathomimetics. *Risk C: Monitor therapy*

Tricyclic Antidepressants: May enhance the adverse/toxic effect of Beta2-Agonists. *Risk C: Monitor therapy*

Stability

Foradil®: Prior to dispensing, store in refrigerator at 2°C to 8°C (36°F to 46°F). After dispensing, store at room temperature at 20°C to 25°C (68°F to 77°F). Protect from heat and moisture. Capsules should always be stored in the blister and only removed immediately before use. Always check expiration date. Use within 4 months of purchase date or product expiration date, whichever comes first.

Perforomist™: Prior to dispensing, store in refrigerator at 2°C to 8°C (36°F to 46°F). After dispensing, store at 2°C to 25°C (36°F to 77°F) for up to 3 months. Protect from heat. Unit-dose vials should always be stored in the foil pouch and only removed immediately before use.

Mechanism of Action Relaxes bronchial smooth muscle by selective action on $beta_2$ receptors with little effect on heart rate. Formoterol has a long-acting effect.

Pharmacodynamics/Kinetics

Onset: Within 3 minutes

Peak effect: 80% of peak effect within 15 minutes

Duration: Improvement in FEV_1 observed for 12 hours in most patients

Absorption: Rapidly into plasma

Protein binding: 61% to 64% *in vitro* at higher concentrations than achieved with usual dosing

Metabolism: Hepatic via direct glucuronidation and O-demethylation; CYP2D6, CYP2C8/9, CYP2C19, CYP2A6 involved in O-demethylation

Half-life elimination: Powder: ~10-14 hours; Nebulized solution: ~7 hours

Time to peak: Maximum improvement in FEV_1 in 1-3 hours

Excretion:

Children 5-12 years: Urine (7% to 9% as direct glucuronide metabolites, 6% as unchanged drug)

Adults: Urine (15% to 18% as direct glucuronide metabolites, 2% to 10% as unchanged drug)

Dosage

Asthma maintenance treatment: Children ≥5 years and Adults: Inhalation:

Foradil®: 12 mcg capsule inhaled every 12 hours via Aerolizer™ device

Oxeze® (CAN): **Note:** Not labeled for use in the U.S.: Children ≥6 years and Adults: Inhalation: 6 mcg or 12 mcg every 12 hours. Maximum dose: Children: 24 mcg/day; Adults: 48 mcg/day

Prevention of exercise-induced bronchospasm: Children ≥5 years and Adults: Inhalation:

Foradil®:12 mcg capsule inhaled via Aerolizer™ device at least 15 minutes before exercise on an "as needed" basis; additional doses should not be used for another 12 hours. **Note:** If already using for asthma maintenance, then should not use additional doses for exercise-induced bronchospasm.

Oxeze® (CAN): **Note:** Not labeled for use in the U.S.: Children ≥6 years and Adults: Inhalation: 6 mcg or 12 mcg at least 15 minutes before exercise.

COPD maintenance treatment: Adults: Inhalation:

Foradil®: 12 mcg capsule inhaled every 12 hours via Aerolizer™ device

Perforomist™: 20 mcg unit-dose vial twice daily (maximum dose: 40 mcg/day)

Additional indication for Oxeze® (approved in Canada): Acute ("on demand") relief of bronchoconstriction: Children ≥12 years and Adults: 6 mcg or 12 mcg as a single dose (maximum dose: 72 mcg in any 24-hour period). The prolonged use of high dosages (48 mcg/day for ≥3 consecutive days) may be a sign of suboptimal control, and should prompt the re-evaluation of therapy.

Administration

Foradil®: Remove capsule from foil blister **immediately** before use. Place capsule in the capsule-chamber in the base of the Aerolizer™ Inhaler. Must only use the Aerolizer™ Inhaler. Press both buttons **once only** and then release. Keep inhaler in a level, horizontal position. Exhale fully. Do not exhale into inhaler. Tilt head slightly back and inhale (rapidly, steadily, and deeply). Hold breath as long as possible. If any powder remains in capsule, exhale and inhale again. Repeat until capsule is empty. Throw away empty capsule; do not leave in inhaler. Do not use a spacer with the Aerolizer™ Inhaler. Always keep capsules and inhaler dry.

Perforomist™: Remove unit-dose vial from foil pouch **immediately** before use. Solution does not require dilution prior to administration; do not mix other medications with formoterol solution. Place contents of unit-dose vial into the reservoir of a standard jet nebulizer connected to an air compressor; assemble nebulizer based on the manufacturer's instructions and turn nebulizer on; breathe deeply and evenly until all of the medication has been inhaled. Discard any unused medication immediately; do not ingest contents of vial. Clean nebulizer after use.

Monitoring Parameters FEV_1, peak flow, and/or other pulmonary function tests; blood pressure, heart rate; CNS stimulation; serum glucose, serum potassium

Dosage Forms Excipient information presented when available (limited, particularly for generics); consult specific product labeling. [CAN] = Canadian brand name

Powder for oral inhalation, as fumarate:

Foradil® Aerolizer™ [capsule]: 12 mcg (12s, 60s) [contains lactose 25 mg]

Oxeze® Turbuhaler® [CAN]: 6 mcg/inhalation [delivers 60 metered doses; contains lactose 600 mcg/dose]; 12 mcg/inhalation [delivers 60 metered doses; contains lactose 600 mcg/dose] [not available in the U.S.]

Solution for nebulization, as fumarate dihydrate:

Perforomist™: 20 mcg/2 mL (2 mL)

◆ **Formoterol Fumarate** *see* Formoterol *on page 686*

◆ **Formoterol Fumarate Dihydrate** *see* Formoterol *on page 686*

◆ **Formulation R™ [OTC]** *see* Phenylephrine *on page 1273*

◆ **Fortamet®** *see* MetFORMIN *on page 997*

◆ **Fortaz®** *see* Ceftazidime *on page 298*

◆ **Forteo®** *see* Teriparatide *on page 1553*

◆ **Fortical®** *see* Calcitonin *on page 253*

◆ **Fosamax®** *see* Alendronate *on page 59*

◆ **Fosamax Plus D™** *see* Alendronate and Cholecalciferol *on page 62*

Fosamprenavir (FOS am pren a veer)

Medication Safety Issues

Sound-alike/look-alike issues:

Lexiva® may be confused with Levitra®

U.S. Brand Names Lexiva®

Canadian Brand Names Telzir®

Mexican Brand Names Telzer

Index Terms Fosamprenavir Calcium; GW433908G

Pharmacologic Category Antiretroviral Agent, Protease Inhibitor

Use Treatment of HIV infections in combination with at least two other antiretroviral agents

Effect on Mental Status Fatigue is common; may cause depression

Effect on Psychiatric Treatment Contraindicated in patients receiving midazolam, pimozide, and triazolam; concurrent use with other benzodiazepines may produce additive effects. Oral solution contraindicated with disulfiram. Do not use fosamprenavir with St John's wort; may lead to loss of response. Rash is common; consider in differential in patients receiving lamotrigine. GI side effects are common; concurrent use with SSRIs may produce additive GI effects. May produce hypertriglyceridemia; monitor with atypical antipsychotics. May produce neutropenia; use caution with clozapine and carbamazepine. Effects of methadone may be diminished with maintenance therapy; consider an alternative antiretroviral. Amprenavir may increase serum concentration/toxicity of sildenafil, tricyclic antidepressants, and vardenafil.

Dosage Summary Notes: The adult regimen of 1400 mg twice daily may be used for pediatric patients who weigh ≥47 kg. When combined with ritonavir, fosamprenavir tablets may be administered to children who weigh ≥39 kg while ritonavir capsules may be used for pediatric patients who weigh ≥33 kg.

Oral:

Children <2 years: Dosage not established

Children 2-5 years: 30 mg/kg twice daily (maximum: 1400 mg twice daily) ▶

Children ≥6 years:
Unboosted regimen: 30 mg/kg twice daily (maximum: 1400 mg twice daily)
Ritonavir-boosted regimen: 18 mg/kg twice daily (maximum: 700 mg twice daily)
Adults:
Unboosted regimen: 1400 mg twice daily
Ritonavir-boosted regimen: 700 mg twice daily **or** 1400 mg once daily

Dosage Forms Excipient information presented when available (limited, particularly for generics); consult specific product labeling. [CAN] = Canadian brand name
Tablet, as calcium:
Lexiva®: 700 mg [equivalent to amprenavir ~600 mg)
Telzir® [CAN]: 700 mg [not available in the U.S.]
Suspension, oral, as calcium:
Lexiva®: 50 mg/mL (225 mL) [equivalent to amprenavir ~43 mg/mL; contains propylene glycol; grape-bubblegum-peppermint flavored]
Telzir® [CAN]: 50 mg/mL (225 mL) [not available in the U.S.]

◆ **Fosamprenavir Calcium** *see* Fosamprenavir *on page 689*

Fosaprepitant (fos a PRE pi tant)

Medication Safety Issues
Sound-alike/look-alike issues:
Fosaprepitant may be confused with aprepitant, fosamprenavir
Emend® for injection (fosaprepitant) may be confused with Emend® (aprepitant) which is an oral capsule formulation.

U.S. Brand Names Emend® for Injection

Index Terms Aprepitant Injection; Fosaprepitant Dimeglumine; L-758,298; MK 0517

Pharmacologic Category Antiemetic; Substance P/Neurokinin 1 Receptor Antagonist

Use Prevention of acute and delayed nausea and vomiting associated with moderately- and highly-emetogenic chemotherapy (in combination with other antiemetics)

Effect on Mental Status Fatigue is common; may cause dizziness

Effect on Psychiatric Treatment Concurrent use with pimozide is contraindicated; avoid combination. GI side effects are common; concurrent use with SSRIs, carbamazepine, lithium, and valproic acid may produce additive effects. May produce neutropenia; use caution with clozapine and carbamazepine. A potential for numerous drug-drug interactions exists. Aprepitant may increase the serum concentration of benzodiazepines including alprazolam, chlordiazepoxide, clonazepam, clorazepate, diazepam, estazolam, flurazepam, midazolam, quazepam, and triazolam (metabolized by oxidation). CYP3A4 inducers (eg, carbamazepine, phenobarbital, and phenytoin) may decrease levels/effects of aprepitant. CYP3A4 inhibitors (eg, nefazodone and verapamil) may increase levels/effects of aprepitant. Aprepitant may increase the levels/effects of CYP3A4 substrates (eg, benzodiazepines, calcium channel blockers, ergot derivatives, mirtazapine, nefazodone, and venlafaxine. Avoid St John's wort (may decrease aprepitant levels).

Dosage Summary
I.V.:
Children: Dosage not established
Adults: 115 mg 30 minutes prior to chemotherapy on day 1

Dosage Forms Excipient information presented when available (limited, particularly for generics); consult specific product labeling.
Injection, powder for reconstitution:
Emend® for Injection: 115 mg [contains edetate disodium; lactose; polysorbate 80]

◆ **Fosaprepitant Dimeglumine** *see* Fosaprepitant *on page 690*

Foscarnet (fos KAR net)

U.S. Brand Names Foscavir®

Canadian Brand Names Foscavir®

Index Terms PFA; Phosphonoformate; Phosphonoformic Acid

Pharmacologic Category Antiviral Agent

Use Treatment of acyclovir-resistant mucocutaneous herpes simplex virus (HSV) infections in immunocompromised persons (eg, with advanced AIDS); treatment of CMV retinitis in persons with HIV

Unlabeled/Investigational Use Other CMV infections (eg, colitis, esophagitis, neurological disease); CMV prophylaxis for cancer patients receiving alemtuzumab therapy or allogeneic stem cell transplant

Effect on Mental Status Dizziness, anxiety, confusion, and depression are common; may rarely produce abnormal crying

Effect on Psychiatric Treatment Leukopenia is common; use caution with clozapine and carbamazepine

Dosage Summary

I.V.:

Children ≤12 years: Dosage not established

Adolescents: Induction: CMV: 60 mg/kg every 8 hours **or** 90 mg/kg every 12 hours for 14-21 day; HSV: 40 mg/kg/dose every 8-12 hours for 14-21 days; Maintenance: CMV: 90-120 mg/kg once daily

Adults: Induction: CMV: 60 mg/kg every 8 hours **or** 90 mg/kg every 12 hours for 14-21 day; HSV: 40 mg/kg/dose every 8-12 hours for 14-21 days; Maintenance: CMV: 90-120 mg/kg once daily

Dosage Forms Excipient information presented when available (limited, particularly for generics); consult specific product labeling.

Injection, solution, as sodium [preservative-free]: 24 mg/mL (250 mL, 500 mL)

Foscavir®: 24 mg/mL (500 mL)

◆ **Foscavir®** *see* Foscarnet *on page 690*

Fosfomycin (fos foe MYE sin)

Medication Safety Issues

Sound-alike/look-alike issues:

Monurol® may be confused with Monopril®

U.S. Brand Names Monurol®

Canadian Brand Names Monurol®

Mexican Brand Names Monurol

Index Terms Fosfomycin Tromethamine

Pharmacologic Category Antibiotic, Miscellaneous

Use Single oral dose in the treatment of uncomplicated urinary tract infections in women due to susceptible strains of *E. coli* and *Enterococcus faecalis*

Unlabeled/Investigational Use Multiple doses have been investigated for complicated urinary tract infections in men

Effect on Mental Status May cause drowsiness

Effect on Psychiatric Treatment None reported

Dosage Summary

Oral:

Children: Dosage not established

Adults (females): Single dose of 3 g in 3-4 oz (90-120 mL) of water

Adults males (unlabeled use): 3 g every 2-3 days

Dosage Forms Excipient information presented when available (limited, particularly for generics); consult specific product labeling.

Powder for solution:

Monurol®: 3 g/sachet (3s) [orange flavor]

◆ **Fosfomycin Tromethamine** *see* Fosfomycin *on page 691*

Fosinopril (foe SIN oh pril)

Medication Safety Issues

Sound-alike/look-alike issues:

Fosinopril may be confused with lisinopril

Monopril® may be confused with Accupril®, minoxidil, moexipril, Monoket®, Monurol™, ramipril

Related Information

Angiotensin Agents *on page 1754*

U.S. Brand Names Monopril®

Canadian Brand Names Apo-Fosinopril®; Gen-Fosinopril; Lin-Fosinopril; Monopril®; Novo-Fosinopril; PMS-Fosinopril; RAN-Fosinopril; ratio-Fosinopril; Riva-Fosinopril

Mexican Brand Names Monopril

Index Terms Fosinopril Sodium

Pharmacologic Category Angiotensin-Converting Enzyme (ACE) Inhibitor

Use Treatment of hypertension, either alone or in combination with other antihypertensive agents; treatment of heart failure (HF)

Effect on Mental Status May cause drowsiness or dizziness; may rarely cause insomnia

Effect on Psychiatric Treatment May rarely cause agranulocytosis; use caution with clozapine and carbamazepine; may decrease lithium clearance resulting in an increase in serum lithium levels and potential lithium toxicity; monitor serum lithium levels

Dosage Summary

Oral:

Children ≤50 kg: Dosage not established

Children ≥6 years and >50 kg: Initial: 5-10 mg once daily (maximum: 40 mg/day)

Adults: Initial: 10 mg once daily; Maintenance: 10-40 mg/day in 1-2 divided doses (maximum: 80 mg/day)

Dosage Forms Excipient information presented when available (limited, particularly for generics); consult specific product labeling.

Tablet, as sodium: 10 mg, 20 mg, 40 mg

Monopril®: 10 mg, 20 mg, 40 mg

Fosinopril and Hydrochlorothiazide

(foe SIN oh pril & hye droe klor oh THYE a zide)

Medication Safety Issues

Sound-alike/look-alike issues:

Monopril® may be confused with Accupril®, minoxidil, moexipril, Monoket®, Monurol™, ramipril

U.S. Brand Names Monopril-HCT®

Canadian Brand Names Monopril-HCT®

Index Terms Hydrochlorothiazide and Fosinopril

Pharmacologic Category Angiotensin-Converting Enzyme (ACE) Inhibitor; Diuretic, Thiazide

Use Treatment of hypertension; not indicated for first-line treatment

Effect on Mental Status May cause drowsiness or dizziness; may rarely cause depression

Effect on Psychiatric Treatment Neutropenia and agranulocytosis may rarely occur; use caution with clozapine and carbamazepine. Thiazide diuretics may decrease the renal clearance of lithium increasing the risk for toxicity; monitor. May cause photosensitivity; concomitant use with psychotropics may further the risk. Use sunscreen, wear protective clothing and eyewear, and avoid direct sunlight.

Dosage Summary

Oral:

Children: Dosage not established

Adults: Fosinopril 10-80 mg and hydrochlorothiazide 12.5-50 mg once daily; **Note:** JNC 7 recommends fosinopril 10-40 mg/day

Dosage Forms Excipient information presented when available (limited, particularly for generics); consult specific product labeling.

Tablet: 10/12.5: Fosinopril sodium 10 mg and hydrochlorothiazide 12.5 mg; 20/12.5: Fosinopril sodium 20 mg and hydrochlorothiazide 12.5 mg

Monopril-HCT® 10/12.5: Fosinopril sodium 10 mg and hydrochlorothiazide 12.5 mg

Monopril-HCT® 20/12.5: Fosinopril sodium 20 mg and hydrochlorothiazide 12.5 mg

◆ **Fosinopril Sodium** *see* Fosinopril *on page 691*

Fosphenytoin (FOS fen i toyn)

Medication Safety Issues

Sound-alike/look-alike issues:

Cerebyx® may be confused with Celebrex®, Celexa™, Cerezyme®

Overdoses have occurred due to confusion between the **mg per mL concentration** of fosphenytoin (50 mg PE/mL) and **total drug content per vial** (either 100 mg PE/2 mL vial or 500 mg PE/10 mL vial). ISMP recommends that the total drug content per container is identified instead of the concentration in mg per mL to avoid confusion and potential overdosages. Additionally, since most errors have occurred with overdoses in children, they recommend that pediatric hospitals should consider stocking only the 2 mL vial.

Related Information

Phenytoin *on page 1280*

U.S. Brand Names Cerebyx®

Canadian Brand Names Cerebyx®

Index Terms Fosphenytoin Sodium

Pharmacologic Category Anticonvulsant, Hydantoin

Generic Available Yes

Use Used for the control of generalized convulsive status epilepticus and prevention and treatment of seizures occurring during neurosurgery; indicated for short-term parenteral administration when other means of phenytoin administration are unavailable, inappropriate, or deemed less advantageous (the safety and effectiveness of fosphenytoin in this use has not been systematically evaluated for more than 5 days)

Effect on Mental Status May cause dizziness, drowsiness, or visual hallucinations

Effect on Psychiatric Treatment May cause neutropenia; use caution with clozapine and carbamazepine

Pregnancy Risk Factor D

Pregnancy Considerations Fosphenytoin is the prodrug of phenytoin. Refer to Phenytoin on page 1280 for additional information.

Lactation Excretion in breast milk unknown/not recommended

Contraindications Hypersensitivity to phenytoin, other hydantoins, or any component of the formulation; patients with sinus bradycardia, sinoatrial block, second- and third-degree AV block, or Adams-Stokes syndrome; occurrence of rash during treatment (should not be resumed if rash is exfoliative, purpuric, or bullous); treatment of absence seizures

Warnings/Precautions Doses of fosphenytoin are expressed as their phenytoin sodium equivalent (PE). Antiepileptic drugs should not be abruptly discontinued. Hypotension may occur, especially after I.V. administration at high doses and high rates of administration. Administration of phenytoin has been associated with atrial and ventricular conduction depression and ventricular fibrillation. Careful cardiac monitoring is needed when administering I.V. loading doses of fosphenytoin. Acute hepatotoxicity associated with a hypersensitivity syndrome characterized by fever, skin eruptions, and lymphadenopathy has been reported to occur within the first 2 months of treatment. Discontinue if skin rash or lymphadenopathy occurs. A spectrum of hematologic effects have been reported with use (eg, neutropenia, leukopenia, thrombocytopenia, pancytopenia, and anemias). Use with caution in patients with hypotension, severe myocardial insufficiency, diabetes mellitus, porphyria, hypoalbuminemia, hypothyroidism, fever, or hepatic or renal dysfunction. Effects with other sedative drugs or ethanol may be potentiated. Safety and efficacy have not been established in children. Severe reactions, including toxic epidermal necrolysis and Stevens-Johnson syndromes, although rarely reported, have resulted in fatalities; drug should be discontinued if there are any signs of rash. Patients of Asian descent with the variant *HLA-B*1502* may be at an increased risk of developing Stevens-Johnson syndrome and/or toxic epidermal necrolysis.

Adverse Reactions The more important adverse clinical events caused by the I.V. use of fosphenytoin or phenytoin are cardiovascular collapse and/or central nervous system depression. Hypotension can occur when either drug is administered rapidly by the I.V. route. Do not exceed a rate of 150 mg phenytoin equivalent/minute when administering fosphenytoin.

The adverse clinical events most commonly observed with the use of fosphenytoin in clinical trials were nystagmus, dizziness, pruritus, paresthesia, headache, somnolence, and ataxia. Paresthesia and pruritus were seen more often following fosphenytoin (versus phenytoin) administration and occurred more often with I.V. fosphenytoin than with I.M. administration. These events were dose and rate related (doses ≥15 mg/kg at a rate of 150 mg/minute). These sensations, generally described as itching, burning, or tingling are usually not at the infusion site. The location of the discomfort varied with the groin mentioned most frequently. The paresthesia and pruritus were transient events that occurred within several minutes of the start of infusion and generally resolved within 10 minutes after completion of infusion.

Transient pruritus, tinnitus, nystagmus, somnolence, and ataxia occurred 2-3 times more often at doses ≥15 mg/kg and rates ≥150 mg/minute.

I.V. administration (maximum dose/rate):

>10%:

Central nervous system: Nystagmus, dizziness, somnolence, ataxia

Dermatologic: Pruritus

1% to 10%:

Cardiovascular: Hypotension, vasodilation, tachycardia

Central nervous system: Stupor, incoordination, paresthesia, extrapyramidal syndrome, tremor, agitation, hypoesthesia, dysarthria, vertigo, brain edema, headache
Gastrointestinal: Nausea, tongue disorder, dry mouth, vomiting
Neuromuscular & skeletal: Pelvic pain, muscle weakness, back pain
Ocular: Diplopia, amblyopia
Otic: Tinnitus, deafness
Miscellaneous: Taste perversion

I.M. administration (substitute for oral phenytoin):

1% to 10%:

Central nervous system: Nystagmus, tremor, ataxia, headache, incoordination, somnolence, dizziness, paresthesia, reflexes decreased
Dermatologic: Pruritus
Gastrointestinal: Nausea, vomiting
Hematologic/lymphatic: Ecchymosis
Neuromuscular & skeletal: Muscle weakness

<1% (Limited to important or life-threatening): Acidosis, acute hepatic failure, acute hepatotoxicity, alkalosis, anemia, atrial flutter, bundle branch block, cardiac arrest, cardiomegaly, cerebral hemorrhage, cerebral infarct, CHF, cyanosis, dehydration, hyperglycemia, hyperkalemia, hypertension, hypochromic anemia, hypokalemia, hypophosphatemia, ketosis, leukocytosis, leukopenia, lymphadenopathy, palpitation, postural hypotension, pulmonary embolus, QT interval prolongation, sinus bradycardia, syncope, Stevens-Johnson syndrome, thrombocytopenia, thrombophlebitis, toxic epidermal necrolysis, ventricular extrasystoles

Metabolism/Transport Effects As phenytoin: **Substrate** of CYP2C9 (major), 2C19 (major), 3A4 (minor); **Induces** CYP2B6 (strong), 2C8 (strong), 2C9 (strong), 2C19 (strong), 3A4 (strong)

Drug Interactions

Acetaminophen: Anticonvulsants (Hydantoin) may increase the metabolism of Acetaminophen. This may 1) diminish the effect of acetaminophen; and 2) increase the risk of liver damage. *Risk C: Monitor therapy*

Alcohol (Ethyl): CNS Depressants may enhance the CNS depressant effect of Alcohol (Ethyl). *Risk C: Monitor therapy*

Antacids: May decrease the serum concentration of Anticonvulsants (Hydantoin). *Risk C: Monitor therapy*

Carbonic Anhydrase Inhibitors: May enhance the adverse/toxic effect of Anticonvulsants (Hydantoin). Specifically, osteomalacia and rickets. **Exceptions:** Brinzolamide; Dorzolamide. *Risk C: Monitor therapy*

Chloramphenicol: May decrease the metabolism of Anticonvulsants (Hydantoin). Anticonvulsants (Hydantoin) may decrease the serum concentration of Chloramphenicol. Increased chloramphenicol concentrations have also been seen. *Risk D: Consider therapy modification*

Cimetidine: May decrease the metabolism of Anticonvulsants (Hydantoin). *Risk D: Consider therapy modification*

CNS Depressants: May enhance the adverse/toxic effect of other CNS Depressants. *Risk C: Monitor therapy*

CYP2B6 Substrates: CYP2B6 Inducers (Strong) may increase the metabolism of CYP2B6 Substrates. *Risk C: Monitor therapy*

CYP2C19 Inducers (Strong): May increase the metabolism of CYP2C19 Substrates. *Risk C: Monitor therapy*

CYP2C19 Inhibitors (Moderate): May decrease the metabolism of CYP2C19 Substrates. *Risk C: Monitor therapy*

CYP2C19 Inhibitors (Strong): May decrease the metabolism of CYP2C19 Substrates. *Risk D: Consider therapy modification*

CYP2C19 Substrates: CYP2C19 Inducers (Strong) may increase the metabolism of CYP2C19 Substrates. *Risk C: Monitor therapy*

CYP2C8 Substrates (High risk): CYP2C8 Inducers (Highly Effective) may increase the metabolism of CYP2C8 Substrates (High risk). *Risk C: Monitor therapy*

CYP2C9 Inducers (Highly Effective): May increase the metabolism of CYP2C9 Substrates (High risk). *Risk C: Monitor therapy*

CYP2C9 Inhibitors (Moderate): May decrease the metabolism of CYP2C9 Substrates (High risk). *Risk C: Monitor therapy*

CYP2C9 Inhibitors (Strong): May decrease the metabolism of CYP2C9 Substrates (High risk). *Risk D: Consider therapy modification*

CYP2C9 Substrates (High risk): CYP2C9 Inducers (Highly Effective) may increase the metabolism of CYP2C9 Substrates (High risk). *Risk C: Monitor therapy*

CYP3A4 Substrates: CYP3A4 Inducers (Strong) may increase the metabolism of CYP3A4 Substrates. *Risk C: Monitor therapy*

Ketorolac: May diminish the therapeutic effect of Anticonvulsants. *Risk C: Monitor therapy*

Maraviroc: CYP3A4 Inducers may decrease the serum concentration of Maraviroc. *Risk D: Consider therapy modification*

Mefloquine: May diminish the therapeutic effect of Anticonvulsants. Mefloquine may decrease the serum concentration of Anticonvulsants. Management: Mefloquine is contraindicated in persons with a history of convulsions. If anticonvulsant is being used for another indication monitor response to treatment closely, as concurrent mefloquine may decrease response to treatment. *Risk D: Consider therapy modification*

Nilotinib: CYP3A4 Inducers (Strong) may decrease the serum concentration of Nilotinib. *Risk X: Avoid combination*

Nisoldipine: CYP3A4 Inducers (Strong) may decrease the serum concentration of Nisoldipine. *Risk X: Avoid combination*

Ranolazine: CYP3A4 Inducers (Strong) may decrease the serum concentration of Ranolazine. *Risk X: Avoid combination*

Sorafenib: CYP3A4 Inducers (Strong) may decrease the serum concentration of Sorafenib. *Risk D: Consider therapy modification*

Ethanol/Nutrition/Herb Interactions

Ethanol:

Acute use: Avoid or limit ethanol (inhibits metabolism of phenytoin); watch for sedation.

Chronic use: Avoid or limit ethanol (stimulates metabolism of phenytoin).

Stability Refrigerate at 2°C to 8°C (36°F to 46°F). Do not store at room temperature for more than 48 hours. Do not use vials that develop particulate matter. Must be diluted to concentrations of 1.5-25 mg PE/mL, in normal saline or D_5W, for I.V. infusion.

Mechanism of Action Diphosphate ester salt of phenytoin which acts as a water soluble prodrug of phenytoin; after administration, plasma esterases convert fosphenytoin to phosphate, formaldehyde, and phenytoin as the active moiety; phenytoin works by stabilizing neuronal membranes and decreasing seizure activity by increasing efflux or decreasing influx of sodium ions across cell membranes in the motor cortex during generation of nerve impulses

Pharmacodynamics/Kinetics Also refer to Phenytoin monograph for additional information.

Protein binding: Fosphenytoin: 95% to 99% to albumin; can displace phenytoin and increase free fraction (up to 30% unbound) during the period required for conversion of fosphenytoin to phenytoin

Metabolism: Fosphenytoin is rapidly converted via hydrolysis to phenytoin; phenytoin is metabolized in the liver and forms metabolites

Bioavailability: I.M.: Fosphenytoin: 100%

Half-life elimination:

Fosphenytoin: 15 minutes

Phenytoin: Variable (mean: 12-29 hours); kinetics of phenytoin are saturable

Time to peak: Conversion to phenytoin: Following I.V. administration (maximum rate of administration): 15 minutes; following I.M. administration, peak phenytoin levels are reached in 3 hours

Excretion: Phenytoin: Urine (as inactive metabolites)

Dosage The dose, concentration in solutions, and infusion rates for fosphenytoin are expressed as phenytoin sodium equivalents (PE); fosphenytoin should always be prescribed and dispensed in phenytoin sodium equivalents (PE)

Infants and Children (unlabeled use): I.V.:

Loading dose: 10-20 mg PE/kg for the treatment of generalized convulsive status epilepticus

Maintenance dosing: Phenytoin dosing guidelines in pediatric patients are used when dosing fosphenytoin using doses in PE equal to the phenytoin doses (ie, phenytoin 1 mg = fosphenytoin 1 PE); maintenance doses may be started 8-12 hours after a loading dose

Adults:

Status epilepticus: I.V.: Loading dose: 15-20 mg PE/kg I.V. administered at 100-150 mg PE/minute

Nonemergent loading and maintenance dosing: I.V. or I.M.:

Loading dose: 10-20 mg PE/kg I.V. or I.M. (maximum I.V. rate: 150 mg PE/minute)

Initial daily maintenance dose: 4-6 mg PE/kg/day I.V. or I.M.

I.M. or I.V. substitution for oral phenytoin therapy: May be substituted for oral phenytoin sodium at the same total daily dose; however, Dilantin® capsules are ~90% bioavailable by the oral route; phenytoin, supplied as fosphenytoin, is 100% bioavailable by both the I.M. and I.V. routes; for this reason, plasma phenytoin concentrations may increase when I.M. or I.V. fosphenytoin is substituted for oral phenytoin sodium therapy; in clinical trials, I.M. fosphenytoin was administered as a single daily dose utilizing either 1 or 2 injection sites; some patients may require more frequent dosing

Dosing adjustments in renal/hepatic impairment: Phenytoin clearance may be substantially reduced in cirrhosis and plasma level monitoring with dose adjustment advisable; free phenytoin levels should be monitored closely in patients with renal or hepatic disease or in those with hypoalbuminemia; furthermore, fosphenytoin clearance to phenytoin may be increased without a similar increase in phenytoin in these patients leading to increased frequency and severity of adverse events

Dietary Considerations Provides phosphate 0.0037 mmol/mg PE fosphenytoin

Administration

I.M.: May be administered as a single daily dose using either 1 or 2 injection sites.

I.V.: Rates of infusion:

Children: 1-3 mg PE/kg/minute

Adults: Should not exceed 150 mg PE/minute

Monitoring Parameters Continuous blood pressure, ECG, and respiratory function monitoring with loading dose and for 10-20 minutes following infusion; vital signs, CBC, liver function tests, plasma level monitoring (plasma levels should not be measured until conversion to phenytoin is complete, ~2 hours after an I.V. infusion or ~4 hours after an I.M. injection)

Reference Range

Therapeutic: 10-20 mcg/mL (SI: 40-79 µmol/L); toxicity is measured clinically, and some patients require levels outside the suggested therapeutic range

Toxic: 30-50 mcg/mL (SI: 120-200 µmol/L)

Lethal: >100 mcg/mL (SI: >400 µmol/L)

Manifestations of toxicity:

Nystagmus: 20 mcg/mL (SI: 79 µmol/L)

Ataxia: 30 mcg/mL (SI: 118.9 µmol/L)

Decreased mental status: 40 mcg/mL (SI: 159 µmol/L)

Coma: 50 mcg/mL (SI: 200 µmol/L)

Peak serum phenytoin level after a 375 mg I.M. fosphenytoin dose in healthy males: 5.7 mcg/mL

Peak serum fosphenytoin levels and phenytoin levels after a 1.2 g infusion (I.V.) in healthy subjects over 30 minutes were 129 mcg/mL and 17.2 mcg/mL, respectively

Test Interactions Increased glucose, alkaline phosphatase (S); decreased thyroxine (S), calcium (S); serum sodium increased in overdose setting

Additional Information 1.5 mg fosphenytoin is approximately equivalent to 1 mg phenytoin. Equimolar fosphenytoin dose is 375 mg (75 mg/mL solution) to phenytoin 250 mg (50 mg/mL).

Dosage Forms Excipient information presented when available (limited, particularly for generics); consult specific product labeling.

Injection, solution, as sodium: 75 mg/mL (2 mL, 10 mL) [equivalent to phenytoin sodium 50 mg/mL]

Cerebyx®: 75 mg/mL (2 mL, 10 mL) [equivalent to phenytoin sodium 50 mg/mL]

- **Fosphenytoin Sodium** *see* Fosphenytoin *on page 692*
- **Fosrenol®** *see* Lanthanum *on page 898*
- **Fossil Tree** *see* Ginkgo *(Ginkgo biloba) on page 715*
- **Freezone® [OTC]** *see* Salicylic Acid *on page 1454*
- **Frova®** *see* Frovatriptan *on page 696*

Frovatriptan (froe va TRIP tan)

Medication Safety Issues

International issues:

Allegro® [Germany] may be confused with Allegra® which is a brand name for fexofenadine in the U.S.

Allegro®: Brand name for fluticasone in Israel

Related Information

Antimigraine Drugs: 5-HT_1 Receptor Agonists *on page 1766*

U.S. Brand Names Frova®

Canadian Brand Names Frova®

Index Terms Frovatriptan Succinate

Pharmacologic Category Antimigraine Agent; Serotonin 5-$HT_{1B,\ 1D}$ Receptor Agonist

Generic Available No

Use Acute treatment of migraine with or without aura in adults

Pregnancy Risk Factor C

Pregnancy Considerations There are no adequate and well-controlled studies using frovatriptan in pregnant women. Use only if potential benefit to the mother outweighs the potential risk to the fetus.

Lactation Excretion in breast milk unknown/use caution

Contraindications Hypersensitivity to frovatriptan or any component of the formulation; patients with ischemic heart disease or signs or symptoms of ischemic heart disease (including Prinzmetal's angina, angina pectoris, myocardial infarction, silent myocardial ischemia); cerebrovascular syndromes (including strokes, transient ischemic attacks); peripheral vascular syndromes (including ischemic bowel disease); uncontrolled hypertension; use within 24 hours of ergotamine derivatives; use within 24 hours of another 5-HT_1 agonist; management of hemiplegic or basilar migraine; prophylactic treatment of migraine

Canadian labeling: Additional contraindications (not in U.S. labeling): Cardiac arrhythmias, valvular heart disease, congenital heart disease, atherosclerotic disease; management of ophthalmoplegic migraine; severe hepatic impairment

Warnings/Precautions Not intended for migraine prophylaxis, or treatment of cluster headaches, hemiplegic or basilar migraines. Rule out underlying neurologic disease in patients with atypical headache, migraine (with no prior history of migraine) or inadequate clinical response to initial dosing. Cardiac events (coronary artery vasospasm, transient ischemia, MI, ventricular tachycardia/fibrillation, cardiac arrest, and death), cerebral/subarachnoid hemorrhage, stroke, peripheral vascular ischemia, and colonic ischemia have been reported with 5-HT_1 agonist administration. May cause vasospastic reactions resulting in colonic, peripheral, or coronary ischemia. Do not give to patients with risk factors for CAD until a cardiovascular evaluation has been performed; if evaluation is satisfactory, the healthcare provider should administer the first dose and cardiovascular status should be periodically evaluated. Significant elevation in blood pressure, including hypertensive crisis, has also been reported on rare occasions in patients using other 5-HT_{1D} agonists with and without a history of hypertension. May lower seizure threshold, use caution in epilepsy or structural brain lesions. Symptoms of agitation, confusion, hallucinations, hyper-reflexia, myoclonus, shivering, and tachycardia (serotonin syndrome) may occur with concomitant proserotonergic drugs (ie, SSRIs/SNRIs or triptans) or agents which reduce frovatriptan's metabolism. Safety and efficacy in pediatric patients have not been established.

Adverse Reactions

1% to 10%:

Cardiovascular: Chest pain (2%), flushing (4%), palpitation (1%)

Central nervous system: Dizziness (8%), fatigue (5%), headache (4%), hot or cold sensation (3%), anxiety (1%), dysesthesia (1%), hypoesthesia (1%), insomnia (1%), pain (1%)

Gastrointestinal: Xerostomia (3%), dyspepsia (2%), abdominal pain (1%), diarrhea (1%), vomiting (1%)

Neuromuscular & skeletal: Paresthesia (4%), skeletal pain (3%)

Ocular: Vision abnormal (1%)

Otic: Tinnitus (1%)

Respiratory: Rhinitis (1%), sinusitis (1%)

Miscellaneous: Diaphoresis (1%)

<1% (Limited to important or life-threatening): Abnormal dreaming, abnormal gait, abnormal lacrimation, abnormal reflexes, abnormal urine, agitation, amnesia, arthralgia, arthrosis, ataxia, back pain, bradycardia, bullous eruption, cheilitis, concentration impaired, confusion, conjunctivitis, constipation, dehydration, depersonalization, depression, dysphagia, dyspnea, earache, ECG changes, emotional lability, epistaxis, eructation, esophagospasm, euphoria, eye pain, fever, gastroesophageal reflux, hiccup, hot flushes, hyperacusis, hyperesthesia, hypertonia, hyperventilation, hypocalcemia, hypoglycemia, hypotonia, involuntary muscle contractions, laryngitis, leg cramps, malaise, micturition, muscle weakness, myalgia, nervousness, nocturia, peptic ulcer, personality disorder, pharyngitis, polyuria, pruritus, purpura, renal pain, rigors, saliva increased, salivary gland pain, seizure, speech disorder, stomatitis, syncope, tachycardia, taste perversion, thirst, tongue paralysis, toothache, tremor, unspecified pain, urinary frequency, vertigo, weakness

Metabolism/Transport Effects Substrate of CYP1A2 (minor)

Drug Interactions

Ergot Derivatives: May enhance the vasoconstricting effect of Serotonin 5-HT1D Receptor Agonists. Serotonin 5-HT1D Receptor Agonists may enhance the vasoconstricting effect of Ergot Derivatives. *Risk X: Avoid combination*

Serotonin Modulators: May enhance the adverse/toxic effect of other Serotonin Modulators. The development of serotonin syndrome may occur. *Risk D: Consider therapy modification*

Sibutramine: May enhance the serotonergic effect of Serotonin Modulators. This may cause serotonin syndrome. *Risk X: Avoid combination*

Ethanol/Nutrition/Herb Interactions Food: Food does not affect frovatriptan bioavailability.

Stability Store at room temperature of 25°C (77°F); excursions permitted to 15°C to 30°C (59°F to 86°F). Protect from moisture and light.

Mechanism of Action Selective agonist for serotonin (5-HT_{1B} and 5-HT_{1D} receptor) in cranial arteries to cause vasoconstriction and reduces sterile inflammation associated with antidromic neuronal transmission correlating with relief of migraine.

Pharmacodynamics/Kinetics

Distribution: Male: 4.2 L/kg; Female: 3.0 L/kg

Protein binding: 15%

Metabolism: Primarily hepatic via CYP1A2

Bioavailability: 20% to 30%

Half-life elimination: 26 hours

Time to peak: 2-4 hours

Excretion: Feces (62%); urine (32%)

Dosage Oral: Adults: Migraine:

U.S. labeling: 2.5 mg; if headache recurs, a second dose may be given if first dose provided relief and at least 2 hours have elapsed since the first dose (maximum daily dose: 7.5 mg)

Canadian labeling: 2.5 mg; if headache recurs, a second dose may be given if first dose provided relief and at least 4 hours have elapsed since the first dose (maximum daily dose: 5 mg)

Dosage adjustment in renal impairment: No adjustment necessary

Dosage adjustment in hepatic impairment: No adjustment necessary in mild-to-moderate hepatic impairment; use with caution in severe impairment (has not been studied in severe impairment).

Canadian labeling (not in U.S. labeling): Use is contraindicated in severe hepatic impairment.

Administration Administer with fluids.

Dosage Forms Excipient information presented when available (limited, particularly for generics); consult specific product labeling.

Tablet, as base: 2.5 mg

- **Frovatriptan Succinate** *see* Frovatriptan *on page 696*
- **Frusemide** *see* Furosemide *on page 699*
- **FTC** *see* Emtricitabine *on page 530*
- **FTC, TDF, and EFV** *see* Efavirenz, Emtricitabine, and Tenofovir *on page 527*
- **FU** *see* Fluorouracil *on page 649*
- **5-FU** *see* Fluorouracil *on page 649*
- **FUDR** *see* Floxuridine *on page 634*
- **FUDR®** *see* Floxuridine *on page 634*
- **5-FUDR** *see* Floxuridine *on page 634*

Fulvestrant (fool VES trant)

U.S. Brand Names Faslodex®

Mexican Brand Names Faslodex

Index Terms ICI-182,780; Zeneca 182,780; ZM-182,780

Pharmacologic Category Antineoplastic Agent, Estrogen Receptor Antagonist

Use Treatment of hormone receptor positive metastatic breast cancer in postmenopausal women with disease progression following antiestrogen therapy

Unlabeled/Investigational Use Endometriosis; uterine bleeding

Effect on Mental Status May cause depression, anxiety, insomnia, or dizziness

Effect on Psychiatric Treatment Gastrointestinal side effects are common, these effects may be additive with concurrent use of SSRIs, lithium, or valproate; rare reports of leukopenia; use caution with clozapine and carbamazepine; fluoxetine, fluvoxamine, and nefazodone may increase the serum levels and/or toxicity of fulvestrant; barbiturates and carbamazepine may decrease the therapeutic effect via increased metabolism

Dosage Summary

I.M.:

Children: Dosage not established

Adults: 250 mg at 1-month intervals

Dosage Forms Excipient information presented when available (limited, particularly for generics); consult specific product labeling.

Injection, solution:

Faslodex®: 50 mg/mL (2.5 mL, 5 mL) [contains alcohol, benzyl alcohol, benzyl stearate, castor oil]

◆ **Fung-O® [OTC]** *see* Salicylic Acid *on page 1454*

◆ **Furadantin®** *see* Nitrofurantoin *on page 1147*

◆ **Furazosin** *see* Prazosin *on page 1325*

Furosemide (fyoor OH se mide)

Medication Safety Issues

Sound-alike/look-alike issues:

Furosemide may be confused with torsemide

Lasix® may be confused with Esidrix®, Lanoxin®, Lidex®, Lomotil®, Luvox®, Luxiq®

International issues:

Urex® [Australia] may be confused with Eurax® which is a brand name for crotamiton in the U.S.

Urex® [Australia]: Brand name for methenamine in the U.S.

Related Information

Anticholinergic Effects of Common Psychotropics *on page 1758*

U.S. Brand Names Lasix®

Canadian Brand Names Apo-Furosemide®; Dom-Furosemide; Furosemide Injection, USP; Furosemide Special; Lasix®; Lasix® Special; Novo-Semide; Nu-Furosemide; PMS-Furosemide

Mexican Brand Names Lasix

Index Terms Frusemide

Pharmacologic Category Diuretic, Loop

Generic Available Yes

Use Management of edema associated with congestive heart failure and hepatic or renal disease; alone or in combination with antihypertensives in treatment of hypertension

Effect on Mental Status Dizziness is common

Effect on Psychiatric Treatment Orthostatic hypotension is common; use caution with low potency antipsychotics and TCAs; may rarely cause agranulocytosis; caution with clozapine and carbamazepine; may decrease renal clearance of lithium resulting in elevated serum levels and risk for toxicity; more common with thiazide diuretics; monitor lithium levels

Pregnancy Risk Factor C

Pregnancy Considerations Crosses the placenta. Increased fetal urine production, electrolyte disturbances reported. Generally, use of diuretics during pregnancy is avoided due to risk of decreased placental perfusion.

Lactation Enters breast milk/use caution

Contraindications Hypersensitivity to furosemide, any component, or sulfonylureas; anuria; patients with hepatic coma or in states of severe electrolyte depletion until the condition improves or is corrected

Warnings/Precautions Loop diuretics are potent diuretics; excess amounts can lead to profound diuresis with fluid and electrolyte loss; close medical supervision and dose evaluation are required. Watch for and correct electrolyte disturbances; adjust dose to avoid dehydration. In cirrhosis, avoid electrolyte and acid/base imbalances that might lead to hepatic encephalopathy. Coadministration of antihypertensives may increase the risk of hypotension.

Monitor fluid status and renal function in an attempt to prevent oliguria, azotemia, and reversible increases in BUN and creatinine; close medical supervision of aggressive diuresis is required. Rapid I.V. administration, renal impairment, excessive doses, and concurrent use of other ototoxins is associated with ototoxicity. Asymptomatic hyperuricemia has been reported with use.

Chemical similarities are present among sulfonamides, sulfonylureas, carbonic anhydrase inhibitors, thiazides, and loop diuretics (except ethacrynic acid). Use in patients with sulfonylurea allergy is specifically contraindicated in product labeling, however, a risk of cross-reaction exists in patients with allergy to any of these compounds; avoid use when previous reaction has been severe. Discontinue if signs of hypersensitivity are noted.

Adverse Reactions Frequency not defined.

Cardiovascular: Acute hypotension, chronic aortitis, necrotizing angiitis, orthostatic hypotension, thrombophlebitis, sudden death from cardiac arrest (with I.V. or I.M. administration)

Central nervous system: Blurred vision, dizziness, fever, headache, lightheadedness, restlessness, vertigo, xanthopsia

Dermatologic: Cutaneous vasculitis, erythema multiforme, exfoliative dermatitis, photosensitivity, pruritus, purpura, rash, urticaria

Endocrine & metabolic: Gout, hyperglycemia, hyperuricemia, hypocalcemia, hypochloremia, hypokalemia, hypomagnesemia, hyponatremia, metabolic alkalosis

Gastrointestinal: Anorexia, constipation, cramping, diarrhea, intrahepatic cholestatic jaundice, ischemia hepatitis, nausea, oral and gastric irritation, pancreatitis, vomiting

Genitourinary: Urinary bladder spasm, urinary frequency

Hematological: Agranulocytosis (rare), anemia, aplastic anemia (rare), hemolytic anemia, leukopenia, purpura, thrombocytopenia

Neuromuscular & skeletal: Muscle spasm, paresthesia, weakness

Otic: Hearing impairment (reversible or permanent with rapid I.V. or I.M. administration), reversible deafness (with rapid I.V. or I.M. administration), tinnitus

Renal: Allergic interstitial nephritis, fall in glomerular filtration rate and renal blood flow (due to overdiuresis), glycosuria, transient rise in BUN, vasculitis

Miscellaneous: Anaphylaxis (rare), exacerbate or activate systemic lupus erythematosus

Drug Interactions

ACE Inhibitors: Loop Diuretics may enhance the hypotensive effect of ACE Inhibitors. Specifically, postural hypotension which can accompany ACE Inhibitor initiation. Loop Diuretics may enhance the nephrotoxic effect of ACE Inhibitors. *Risk C: Monitor therapy*

Aliskiren: May decrease the serum concentration of Furosemide. *Risk C: Monitor therapy*

Allopurinol: Loop Diuretics may enhance the adverse/toxic effect of Allopurinol. Loop Diuretics may increase the serum concentration of Allopurinol. Specifically, Loop Diuretics may increase the concentration of Oxypurinolol, an active metabolite of Allopurinol. *Risk C: Monitor therapy*

Aminoglycosides: Loop Diuretics may enhance the adverse/toxic effect of Aminoglycosides. Specifically, nephrotoxicity and ototoxicity. *Risk C: Monitor therapy*

Bile Acid Sequestrants: May decrease the absorption of Loop Diuretics. *Risk D: Consider therapy modification*

Corticosteroids (Orally Inhaled): May enhance the hypokalemic effect of Loop Diuretics. *Risk C: Monitor therapy*

Corticosteroids (Systemic): May enhance the hypokalemic effect of Loop Diuretics. *Risk C: Monitor therapy*

Diazoxide: May enhance the hypotensive effect of Antihypertensives. *Risk C: Monitor therapy*

Dofetilide: Loop Diuretics may enhance the QTc-prolonging effect of Dofetilide. *Risk C: Monitor therapy*

Herbs (Hypertensive Properties): May diminish the antihypertensive effect of Antihypertensives. *Risk C: Monitor therapy*

Herbs (Hypotensive Properties): May enhance the hypotensive effect of Antihypertensives. *Risk C: Monitor therapy*

Methylphenidate: May diminish the antihypertensive effect of Antihypertensives. *Risk C: Monitor therapy*

Neuromuscular-Blocking Agents: Loop Diuretics may diminish the neuromuscular-blocking effect of Neuromuscular-Blocking Agents. Loop Diuretics may enhance the neuromuscular-blocking effect of Neuromuscular-Blocking Agents. *Risk C: Monitor therapy*

Nonsteroidal Anti-Inflammatory Agents: May diminish the diuretic effect of Loop Diuretics. *Risk C: Monitor therapy*

Phenytoin: May diminish the diuretic effect of Loop Diuretics. *Risk C: Monitor therapy*

Prostacyclin Analogues: May enhance the hypotensive effect of Antihypertensives. *Risk C: Monitor therapy*

RiTUXimab: Antihypertensives may enhance the hypotensive effect of RiTUXimab. *Risk D: Consider therapy modification*

Ethanol/Nutrition/Herb Interactions

Food: Furosemide serum levels may be decreased if taken with food.

Herb/Nutraceutical: Avoid dong quai if using for hypertension (has estrogenic activity). Avoid ephedra, yohimbe, and ginseng (may worsen hypertension). Limit intake of natural licorice. Avoid garlic (may have increased antihypertensive effect).

Stability Furosemide injection should be stored at controlled room temperature and protected from light. Exposure to light may cause discoloration; do not use furosemide solutions if they have a yellow color. Furosemide solutions are unstable in acidic media, but very stable in basic media Refrigeration may result in precipitation or crystallization, however, resolubilization at room temperature or warming may be performed without affecting the drug's stability.

I.V. infusion solution mixed in NS or D_5W solution is stable for 24 hours at room temperature. May also be diluted for infusion 1-2 mg/mL (maximum: 10 mg/mL) over 10-15 minutes (following infusion rate parameters).

Mechanism of Action Inhibits reabsorption of sodium and chloride in the ascending loop of Henle and distal renal tubule, interfering with the chloride-binding cotransport system, thus causing increased excretion of water, sodium, chloride, magnesium, and calcium

Pharmacodynamics/Kinetics

Onset of action: Diuresis: Oral: 30-60 minutes; I.M.: 30 minutes; I.V.: ~5 minutes
Peak effect: Oral: 1-2 hours

Duration: Oral: 6-8 hours; I.V.: 2 hours

Absorption: Oral: 60% to 67%

Protein binding: >98%

Metabolism: Minimally hepatic

Half-life elimination: Normal renal function: 0.5-1.1 hours; End-stage renal disease: 9 hours

Excretion: Urine (Oral: 50%, I.V.: 80%) within 24 hours; feces (as unchanged drug); nonrenal clearance prolonged in renal impairment

Dosage

Infants and Children:

Oral: 0.5-2 mg/kg/dose increased in increments of 1 mg/kg/dose with each succeeding dose until a satisfactory effect is achieved to a maximum of 6 mg/kg/dose no more frequently than 6 hours.

I.M., I.V.: 1 mg/kg/dose, increasing by each succeeding dose at 1 mg/kg/dose at intervals of 6-12 hours until a satisfactory response up to 6 mg/kg/dose.

Adults:

Oral: 20-80 mg/dose initially increased in increments of 20-40 mg/dose at intervals of 6-8 hours; usual maintenance dose interval is twice daily or every day; may be titrated up to 600 mg/day with severe edematous states. Hypertension (JNC 7): 20-80 mg/day in 2 divided doses

I.M., I.V.: 20-40 mg/dose, may be repeated in 1-2 hours as needed and increased by 20 mg/dose until the desired effect has been obtained. Usual dosing interval: 6-12 hours; for acute pulmonary edema, the usual dose is 40 mg I.V. over 1-2 minutes. If not adequate, may increase dose to 80 mg. **Note:** ACC/AHA 2005 guidelines for chronic congestive heart failure recommend a maximum single dose of 160-200 mg.

Continuous I.V. infusion: Initial I.V. bolus dose 20-40 mg, followed by continuous I.V. infusion doses of 10-40 mg/hour. If urine output is <1 mL/kg/hour, double as necessary to a maximum of 80-160 mg/hour. The risk associated with higher infusion rates (80-160 mg/hour) must be weighed against alternative strategies. **Note:** ACC/AHA 2005 guidelines for chronic congestive heart failure recommend 40 mg I.V. load, then 10-40 mg/hour infusion.

Refractory heart failure: Oral, I.V.: Doses up to 8 g/day have been used.

Elderly: Oral, I.M., I.V.: Initial: 20 mg/day; increase slowly to desired response.

Dosing adjustment/comments in renal impairment: Acute renal failure: High doses (up to 1-3 g/day - oral/I.V.) have been used to initiate desired response; avoid use in oliguric states.

Dialysis: Not removed by hemo- or peritoneal dialysis; supplemental dose is not necessary.

Dosing adjustment/comments in hepatic disease: Diminished natriuretic effect with increased sensitivity to hypokalemia and volume depletion in cirrhosis; monitor effects, particularly with high doses.

Dietary Considerations May cause a potassium loss; potassium supplement or dietary changes may be required. Administer on an empty stomach. May be administered with food or milk if GI distress occurs. Do not mix with acidic solutions.

Administration

I.V.: I.V. injections should be given slowly. In adults, undiluted direct I.V. injections may be administered at a rate of 40 mg over 1-2 minutes; maximum rate of administration for IVPB or continuous infusion: 4 mg/minute. In children, a maximum rate of 0.5 mg/kg/minute has been recommended.

Oral: May be taken with or without food.

Monitoring Parameters Monitor weight and I & O daily; blood pressure, orthostasis, serum electrolytes, renal function; in high doses, monitor hearing

Dosage Forms Excipient information presented when available (limited, particularly for generics); consult specific product labeling.

Injection, solution: 10 mg/mL (2 mL, 4 mL, 10 mL)

Injection, solution [preservative free]: 10 mg/mL (2 mL, 4 mL, 10 mL)

Solution, oral: 10 mg/mL (60 mL, 120 mL) [orange flavor]; 40 mg/5 mL (5 mL, 500 mL) [pineapple-peach flavor]

Tablet: 20 mg, 40 mg, 80 mg

Lasix®: 20 mg

Lasix®: 40 mg, 80 mg [scored]

◆ **Fuzeon®** *see* Enfuvirtide *on page 537*

Gabapentin (GA ba pen tin)

Medication Safety Issues

Sound-alike/look-alike issues:

Neurontin® may be confused with Neoral®, Noroxin®

Related Information

Anticonvulsants By Seizure Type *on page 1759*

U.S. Brand Names Neurontin®

Canadian Brand Names Apo-Gabapentin®; BCI-Gabapentin; Gen-Gabapentin; Neurontin®; Novo-Gabapentin; Nu-Gabapentin; PMS-Gabapentin

Mexican Brand Names Bapex; Blugat; Gabantin; Gapridol; Neurontin; Nopatic

Pharmacologic Category Anticonvulsant, Miscellaneous

Generic Available Yes: Capsule, tablet

Use Adjunct for treatment of partial seizures with and without secondary generalized seizures in patients >12 years of age with epilepsy; adjunct for treatment of partial seizures in pediatric patients 3-12 years of age; management of postherpetic neuralgia (PHN) in adults

Unlabeled/Investigational Use Social phobia; chronic pain

Mental Health Comment Double-blind studies have failed to differentiate this drug from placebo when used as an adjunctive treatment for bipolar disorder. Gabapentin may be useful for some of the anxiety disorders.

Pregnancy Risk Factor C

Pregnancy Considerations Animal studies have documented teratogenic effects. There are no adequate and well-controlled studies in pregnant women. Use during pregnancy only if the potential benefit to the mother outweighs the potential risk to the fetus.

Lactation Enters breast milk/use caution

Contraindications Hypersensitivity to gabapentin or any component of the formulation

Warnings/Precautions Avoid abrupt withdrawal, may precipitate seizures; use cautiously in patients with severe renal dysfunction; male rat studies demonstrated an association with pancreatic adenocarcinoma (clinical implication unknown). May cause CNS depression, which may impair physical or mental abilities. Patients must be cautioned about performing tasks which require mental alertness (eg, operating machinery or driving). Effects with other sedative drugs or ethanol may be potentiated. Pediatric patients (3-12 years of age) have shown increased incidence of CNS-related adverse effects, including emotional lability, hostility, thought disorder, and hyperkinesia. Safety and efficacy in children <3 years of age have not been established.

Adverse Reactions As reported in patients >12 years of age, unless otherwise noted in children (3-12 years)

>10%:

Central nervous system: Somnolence (20%; children 8%), dizziness (17% to 28%; children 3%), ataxia (13%), fatigue (11%)

Miscellaneous: Viral infection (children 11%)

1% to 10%:

Cardiovascular: Peripheral edema (2% to 8%), vasodilatation (1%)

Central nervous system: Fever (children 10%), hostility (children 8%), emotional lability (children 4%), fatigue (children 3%), headache (3%), ataxia (3%), abnormal thinking (2% to 3%; children 2%), amnesia (2%), depression (2%), dysarthria (2%), nervousness (2%), abnormal coordination (1% to 2%), twitching (1%), hyperesthesia (1%)
Dermatologic: Pruritus (1%), rash (1%)
Endocrine & metabolic: Hyperglycemia (1%)
Gastrointestinal: Diarrhea (6%), nausea/vomiting (3% to 4%; children 8%), abdominal pain (3%), weight gain (adults and children 2% to 3%), dyspepsia (2%), flatulence (2%), dry throat (2%), xerostomia (2% to 5%), constipation (2% to 4%), dental abnormalities (2%), appetite stimulation (1%)
Genitourinary: Impotence (2%)
Hematologic: Leukopenia (1%), decreased WBC (1%)
Neuromuscular & skeletal: Tremor (7%), weakness (6%), hyperkinesia (children 3%), abnormal gait (2%), back pain (2%), myalgia (2%), fracture (1%)
Ocular: Nystagmus (8%), diplopia (1% to 6%), blurred vision (3% to 4%), conjunctivitis (1%)
Otic: Otitis media (1%)
Respiratory: Rhinitis (4%), bronchitis (children 3%), respiratory infection (children 3%), pharyngitis (1% to 3%), cough (2%)
Miscellaneous: Infection (5%)

Postmarketing and additional clinical reports (limited to important or life-threatening): Acute renal failure, anemia, angina, angioedema, aphasia, arrhythmias (various), aspiration pneumonia, blindness, bradycardia, bronchospasm, cerebrovascular accident, CNS tumors, coagulation defect, colitis, Cushingoid appearance, dyspnea, encephalopathy, facial paralysis, fecal incontinence, glaucoma, glycosuria, heart block, hearing loss, hematemesis, hematuria, hemiplegia, hemorrhage, hepatitis, hepatomegaly, hyper-/hypotension, hyperlipidemia, hyper-/hypothyroidism, hyper-/hypoventilation, gastroenteritis, heart failure, leukocytosis, liver function tests increased, local myoclonus, lymphadenopathy, lymphocytosis, meningismus, MI, migraine, nephrosis, nerve palsy, non-Hodgkin's lymphoma, ovarian failure, pulmonary thrombosis, pericardial rub, pulmonary embolus, pericardial effusion, pericarditis, pancreatitis, peptic ulcer, purpura, paresthesia, palpitation, peripheral vascular disorder, pneumonia, psychosis, renal stone, retinopathy, skin necrosis, status epilepticus, subdural hematoma, suicidal behavior/ideation, syncope, tachycardia, thrombocytopenia, thrombophlebitis

Drug Interactions

Alcohol (Ethyl): CNS Depressants may enhance the CNS depressant effect of Alcohol (Ethyl). *Risk C: Monitor therapy*
CNS Depressants: May enhance the adverse/toxic effect of other CNS Depressants. *Risk C: Monitor therapy*
Ketorolac: May diminish the therapeutic effect of Anticonvulsants. *Risk C: Monitor therapy*
Mefloquine: May diminish the therapeutic effect of Anticonvulsants. Mefloquine may decrease the serum concentration of Anticonvulsants. Management: Mefloquine is contraindicated in persons with a history of convulsions. If anticonvulsant is being used for another indication monitor response to treatment closely, as concurrent mefloquine may decrease response to treatment. *Risk D: Consider therapy modification*

Ethanol/Nutrition/Herb Interactions

Ethanol: Avoid ethanol (may increase CNS depression).
Food: Does not change rate or extent of absorption.
Herb/Nutraceutical: Avoid evening primrose (seizure threshold decreased). Avoid valerian, St John's wort, kava kava, gotu kola (may increase CNS depression).

Stability Store at 25°C (77°F); excursions permitted to 15°C to 30°C (59°F to 86°F).

Mechanism of Action Gabapentin is structurally related to GABA. However, it does not bind to $GABA_A$ or $GABA_B$ receptors, and it does not appear to influence synthesis or uptake of GABA. High affinity gabapentin binding sites have been located throughout the brain; these sites correspond to the presence of voltage-gated calcium channels specifically possessing the alpha-2-delta-1 subunit. This channel appears to be located presynaptically, and may modulate the release of excitatory neurotransmitters which participate in epileptogenesis and nociception.

Pharmacodynamics/Kinetics

Absorption: 50% to 60% from proximal small bowel by L-amino transport system
Distribution: V_d: 0.6-0.8 L/kg

Protein binding: <3%
Bioavailability: Inversely proportional to dose due to saturable absorption:
900 mg/day: 60%
1200 mg/day: 47%
2400 mg/day: 34%
3600 mg/day: 33%
4800 mg/day: 27%
Half-life elimination: 5-7 hours; anuria 132 hours; during dialysis 3.8 hours
Excretion: Proportional to renal function; urine (as unchanged drug)

Dosage Oral:
Children: Anticonvulsant:
3-12 years: Initial: 10-15 mg/kg/day in 3 divided doses; titrate to effective dose over ~3 days; dosages of up to 50 mg/kg/day have been tolerated in clinical studies
3-4 years: Effective dose: 40 mg/kg/day in 3 divided doses
≥5-12 years: Effective dose: 25-35 mg/kg/day in 3 divided doses
See "Note" in adult dosing.
Children >12 years and Adults:
Anticonvulsant: Initial: 300 mg 3 times/day; if necessary the dose may be increased up to 1800 mg/day. Doses of up to 2400 mg/day have been tolerated in long-term clinical studies; up to 3600 mg/day has been tolerated in short-term studies.
Note: If gabapentin is discontinued or if another anticonvulsant is added to therapy, it should be done slowly over a minimum of 1 week
Pain (unlabeled use): 300-1800 mg/day given in 3 divided doses has been the most common dosage range
Adults: Postherpetic neuralgia or neuropathic pain: Day 1: 300 mg, Day 2: 300 mg twice daily, Day 3: 300 mg 3 times/day; dose may be titrated as needed for pain relief (range: 1800-3600 mg/day, daily doses >1800 mg do not generally show greater benefit)
Elderly: Studies in elderly patients have shown a decrease in clearance as age increases. This is most likely due to age-related decreases in renal function; dose reductions may be needed.

Dosing adjustment in renal impairment: Children ≥12 years and Adults: See table.
Hemodialysis: Dialyzable

Gabapentin Dosing Adjustments in Renal Impairment

Creatinine Clearance (mL/min)	Daily Dose Range
≥60	300-1200 mg tid
>30-59	200-700 mg bid
>15-29	200-700 mg daily
15[1]	100-300 mg daily
Hemodialysis[2]	125-350 mg

[1]Cl_{cr}<15 mL/minute: Reduce daily dose in proportion to creatinine clearance.

[2]Single supplemental dose administered after each 4 hours of hemodialysis.

Dietary Considerations May be taken without regard to meals.

Administration Administer first dose on first day at bedtime to avoid somnolence and dizziness. Dosage must be adjusted for renal function; when given 3 times daily, the maximum time between doses should not exceed 12 hours.

Monitoring Parameters Monitor serum levels of concomitant anticonvulsant therapy

Test Interactions False positives have been reported with the Ames N-Multistix SG® dipstick test for urine protein

Dosage Forms Excipient information presented when available (limited, particularly for generics); consult specific product labeling.
Capsule: 100 mg, 300 mg, 400 mg
Neurontin®: 100 mg, 300 mg, 400 mg
Solution, oral:
Neurontin®: 250 mg/5 mL (480 mL) [cool strawberry anise flavor]
Tablet: 100 mg, 300 mg, 400 mg, 600 mg, 800 mg
Neurontin®: 600 mg, 800 mg

◆ **Gabitril®** *see* TiaGABine *on page 1580*

◆ **Gadolinium-DTPA** *see* Gadopentetate Dimeglumine *on page 705*

Gadopentetate Dimeglumine

(gad oh PEN te tate dye MEG loo meen)

Medication Safety Issues

High alert medication: The Institute for Safe Medication Practices (ISMP) includes this medication among its list of drugs which have a heightened risk of causing significant patient harm when used in error.

U.S. Brand Names Magnevist®

Canadian Brand Names Magnevist®

Index Terms Gadolinium-DTPA; Gd-DTPA

Pharmacologic Category Gadolinium-Containing Contrast Agent; Radiological/Contrast Media, Ionic (High Osmolality); Radiological/Contrast Media, Paramagnetic Agent

Use Contrast medium for magnetic resonance imaging (MRI) to visualize lesions with abnormal vascularity in the brain, spine and associated tissues, head and neck, and body (excluding the heart)

Effect on Mental Status May cause dizziness; may rarely cause agitation, anxiety, or sedation

Effect on Psychiatric Treatment None reported

Dosage Summary Note: Dosing for patients >130 kg (286 pounds) has not been studied.

I.V.:

Children <2 years: Dosage not established

Children ≥2 years: 0.1 mmol/kg (0.2 mL/kg)

Adults: 0.1 mmol/kg (0.2 mL/kg)

Dosage Forms Excipient information presented when available (limited, particularly for generics); consult specific product labeling.

Injection, solution [preservative free]:

Magnevist®: Gadopentetate dimeglumine 469.01 mg/mL (5 mL, 10 mL, 15 mL, 20 mL, 50 mL, 100 mL)

Galantamine (ga LAN ta meen)

Medication Safety Issues

Sound-alike/look-alike issues:

Razedyne™ may be confused with Rozerem™

Reminyl® may be confused with Amaryl®

Due to patient safety concerns regarding prescribing and dispensing errors between Reminyl® and Amaryl®, Reminyl® (galantamine) is being renamed to Razadyne™ (immediate-release) and Razadyne™ ER (extended-release). The brand name Reminyl® was discontinued with the July, 2005 distribution of Razadyne™.

U.S. Brand Names Razadyne™; Razadyne™ ER; Reminyl® [DSC]

Canadian Brand Names Reminyl®; Reminyl® ER

Mexican Brand Names Reminyl

Index Terms Galantamine Hydrobromide

Pharmacologic Category Acetylcholinesterase Inhibitor (Central)

Generic Available Yes: Tablet

Use Treatment of mild-to-moderate dementia of Alzheimer's disease

Unlabeled/Investigational Use Severe dementia associated with Alzheimer's disease; mild-to-moderate dementia associated with Parkinson's disease; Lewy body dementia

Pregnancy Risk Factor B

Pregnancy Considerations In animal studies, there was a slight increased in the incident of skeletal variations when given during organogenesis. Adequate, well-controlled studies in pregnant women do not exist. Should be used in pregnancy only if benefit outweighs potential risk to the fetus.

Lactation Excretion in breast milk unknown/not recommended

Contraindications Hypersensitivity to galantamine or any component of the formulation; severe liver dysfunction (Child-Pugh score 10-15); severe renal dysfunction (Cl_{cr} <9 mL/minute)

Warnings/Precautions Use caution in patients with supraventricular conduction delays (without a functional pacemaker in place); Alzheimer's treatment guidelines consider bradycardia to be a relative contraindication for use of centrally-active cholinesterase inhibitors. Use caution in patients taking medicines that slow conduction through SA or AV node. Use caution in peptic ulcer disease (or in patients at risk); seizure disorder; asthma; COPD; mild-to-moderate liver dysfunction; moderate renal dysfunction. May cause bladder outflow obstruction. May exaggerate neuromuscular blockade effects of succinylcholine and like agents. May cause nausea, vomiting, diarrhea, weight loss, and anorexia. Safety and efficacy in children have not been established.

Adverse Reactions

>10%: Gastrointestinal: Nausea (6% to 24%), vomiting (4% to 13%), diarrhea (6% to 12%)

1% to 10%:

Cardiovascular: Bradycardia (2% to 3%), syncope (0.4% to 2.2%: dose related), chest pain (≥1%)

Central nervous system: Dizziness (9%), headache (8%), depression (7%), fatigue (5%), insomnia (5%), somnolence (4%)

Gastrointestinal: Anorexia (7% to 9%), weight loss (5% to 7%), abdominal pain (5%), dyspepsia (5%), flatulence (≥1%)

Genitourinary: Urinary tract infection (8%), hematuria (<1% to 3%), incontinence (≥1%)

Hematologic: Anemia (3%)

Neuromuscular & skeletal: Tremor (3%)

Respiratory: Rhinitis (4%)

<1% (Limited to important or life-threatening): Aggression, alkaline phosphatase increased, aphasia, apraxia, ataxia, atrial fibrillation, AV block, bundle branch block, convulsions, dehydration, delirium, diverticulitis, dysphagia, epistaxis, esophageal perforation, fever, gastrointestinal bleeding, heart failure, hyper-/hypokinesia, hypokalemia, hypotension, malaise, melena, MI, palpitation, paranoid reaction, paresthesia, paroniria, postural hypotension, purpura, QT prolongation, rectal hemorrhage, renal calculi, renal failure (due to dehydration), stroke, suicide, supraventricular tachycardia, T-wave inversion, thrombocytopenia, TIA, ventricular tachycardia, vertigo, weakness

Metabolism/Transport Effects Substrate (minor) of CYP2D6, 3A4

Drug Interactions

Anticholinergics: May diminish the therapeutic effect of Acetylcholinesterase Inhibitors (Central). Acetylcholinesterase Inhibitors (Central) may diminish the therapeutic effect of Anticholinergics. If the anticholinergic action is a side effect of the agent, the result may be beneficial. **Exceptions:** Paliperidone. *Risk C: Monitor therapy*

Antipsychotics: Acetylcholinesterase Inhibitors (Central) may enhance the neurotoxic (central) effect of Antipsychotics. Severe extrapyramidal symptoms have occurred in some patients. *Risk C: Monitor therapy*

Beta-Blockers: Acetylcholinesterase Inhibitors may enhance the bradycardic effect of Beta-Blockers. **Exceptions:** Levobunolol; Metipranolol. *Risk C: Monitor therapy*

Cholinergic Agonists: Acetylcholinesterase Inhibitors may enhance the adverse/toxic effect of Cholinergic Agonists. *Risk C: Monitor therapy*

Corticosteroids (Systemic): May enhance the adverse/toxic effect of Acetylcholinesterase Inhibitors. Increased muscular weakness may occur. *Risk C: Monitor therapy*

Ginkgo Biloba: May enhance the adverse/toxic effect of Acetylcholinesterase Inhibitors. *Risk C: Monitor therapy*

Neuromuscular-Blocking Agents (Nondepolarizing): Acetylcholinesterase Inhibitors may diminish the neuromuscular-blocking effect of Neuromuscular-Blocking Agents (Nondepolarizing). Acetylcholinesterase Inhibitors may decrease the metabolism of Neuromuscular-Blocking Agents (Nondepolarizing). This is only true for mivacurium in which case the neuromuscular blocking effects might be prolonged. *Risk C: Monitor therapy*

Selective Serotonin Reuptake Inhibitors: May decrease the metabolism of Galantamine. **Exceptions:** Citalopram; Escitalopram; Fluvoxamine. *Risk C: Monitor therapy*

Succinylcholine: Acetylcholinesterase Inhibitors may enhance the neuromuscular-blocking effect of Succinylcholine. *Risk C: Monitor therapy*

Ethanol/Nutrition/Herb Interactions

Ethanol: Avoid ethanol (may increase CNS adverse events).

Herb/Nutraceutical: St John's wort may decrease galantamine serum levels; avoid concurrent use.

Stability Store at 15°C to 30°C (59°F to 86°F). Do not freeze oral solution; protect from light.

Mechanism of Action Centrally-acting cholinesterase inhibitor (competitive and reversible). It elevates acetylcholine in cerebral cortex by slowing the degradation of acetylcholine. Modulates nicotinic acetylcholine receptor to increase acetylcholine from surviving presynaptic nerve terminals. May increase glutamate and serotonin levels.

Pharmacodynamics/Kinetics

Duration: 3 hours; maximum inhibition of erythrocyte acetylcholinesterase ~40% at 1 hour post 8 mg oral dose; levels return to baseline at 30 hours

Absorption: Rapid and complete
Distribution: 175 L; levels in the brain are 2-3 times higher than in plasma
Protein binding: 18%
Metabolism: Hepatic; linear, CYP2D6 and 3A4; metabolized to epigalanthaminone and galanthaminone both of which have acetylcholinesterase inhibitory activity 130 times less than galantamine
Bioavailability: ~90%
Half-life elimination: 7 hours
Time to peak: Immediate release: 1 hour (2.5 hours with food); extended release: 4.5-5 hours
Excretion: Urine (25%)

Dosage Oral: Adults:

Note: Oral solution and tablet should be taken with breakfast and dinner; capsule should be taken with breakfast. If therapy is interrupted for ≥3 days, restart at the lowest dose and increase to current dose.

Immediate release tablet or solution: Mild-to-moderate dementia of Alzheimer's:
Initial: 4 mg twice a day for 4 weeks; if tolerated, increase to 8 mg twice daily for ≥4 weeks; if tolerated, increase to 12 mg twice daily
Range: 16-24 mg/day in 2 divided doses

Extended-release capsule: Initial: 8 mg once daily for 4 weeks; if tolerated, increase to 16 mg once daily for ≥4 weeks; if tolerated, increase to 24 mg once daily
Range: 16-24 mg once daily

Conversion to galantamine from other cholinesterase inhibitors: Patients experiencing poor tolerability with donepezil or rivastigmine should wait until side effects subside or allow a 7-day washout period prior to beginning galantamine. Patients not experiencing side effects with donepezil or rivastigmine may begin galantamine therapy the day immediately following discontinuation of previous therapy (Morris, 2001).

Elderly: No dosage adjustment needed

Dosage adjustment in renal impairment:
Moderate renal impairment: Maximum dose: 16 mg/day.
Severe renal dysfunction (Cl_{cr} <9 mL/minute): Use is not recommended

Dosage adjustment in hepatic impairment:
Moderate liver dysfunction (Child-Pugh score 7-9): Maximum dose: 16 mg/day
Severe liver dysfunction (Child-Pugh score 10-15): Use is not recommended

Dietary Considerations
Administration with food is preferred, but not required; should be taken with breakfast and dinner (tablet or solution) or with breakfast (capsule).

Administration Oral: Administer solution or tablet with breakfast and dinner; administer extended release capsule with breakfast. If therapy is interrupted for ≥3 days, restart at the lowest dose and increase to current dose. If using oral solution, mix dose with 3-4 ounces of any nonalcoholic beverage; mix well and drink immediately.

Monitoring Parameters Mental status

Dosage Forms Excipient information presented when available (limited, particularly for generics); consult specific product labeling.
Capsule, extended release, oral, as hydrobromide:
Razadyne™ ER: 8 mg, 16 mg, 24 mg [contains gelatin]
Solution, oral, as hydrobromide:
Razadyne™: 4 mg/mL (100 mL) [with calibrated pipette]
Tablet, as hydrobromide: 4 mg, 8 mg, 12 mg
Razadyne™: 4 mg, 8 mg, 12 mg

◆ **Galantamine Hydrobromide** *see* Galantamine *on page 705*

Gallium Nitrate (GAL ee um NYE trate)

U.S. Brand Names Ganite™
Index Terms NSC-15200
Pharmacologic Category Calcium-Lowering Agent
Use Treatment of symptomatic cancer-related hypercalcemia
Effect on Mental Status None reported
Effect on Psychiatric Treatment Nausea is common; risk may be increased with concomitant SSRI use
Dosage Summary
I.V.:
Children: Dosage not established
Adults: 100-200 mg/m^2/day

Dosage Forms Excipient information presented when available (limited, particularly for generics); consult specific product labeling.
Injection, solution [preservative free]:
Ganite™: 25 mg/mL (20 mL)

Galsulfase (gal SUL fase)

U.S. Brand Names Naglazyme™
Index Terms Recombinant N-Acetylgalactosamine 4-Sulfatase; rhASB
Pharmacologic Category Enzyme
Use Replacement therapy in mucopolysaccharidosis VI (MPS VI; Maroteaux-Lamy Syndrome) for improvement of walking and stair-climbing capacity
Effect on Mental Status May cause sedation
Effect on Psychiatric Treatment Concomitant administration with psychotropic agents may produce additive sedation; monitor
Dosage Summary Note: Premedicate with antihistamines with/without antipyretics 30-60 minutes prior to infusion.
I.V.:
Children <5 years: Dosage not established
Children >5 years: 1 mg/kg once weekly
Adults: 1 mg/kg once weekly
Dosage Forms Excipient information presented when available (limited, particularly for generics); consult specific product labeling.
Injection, solution [preservative free]:
Naglazyme™: 5 mg/5 mL (5 mL) [contains polysorbate 80]

◆ **Gamma Benzene Hexachloride** *see* Lindane *on page 927*
◆ **Gamma E-Gems® [OTC]** *see* Vitamin E *on page 1675*
◆ **Gamma-E Plus [OTC]** *see* Vitamin E *on page 1675*
◆ **Gamma Hydroxybutyric Acid** *see* Sodium Oxybate *on page 1495*
◆ **Gammaphos** *see* Amifostine *on page 83*

Ganciclovir (gan SYE kloe veer)

Medication Safety Issues
Sound-alike/look-alike issues:
Cytovene® may be confused with Cytosar®, Cytosar-U®
U.S. Brand Names Cytovene®; Vitrasert®
Canadian Brand Names Cytovene®; Vitrasert®
Mexican Brand Names Cymevene
Index Terms DHPG Sodium; GCV Sodium; Nordeoxyguanosine
Pharmacologic Category Antiviral Agent
Use
Parenteral: Treatment of CMV retinitis in immunocompromised individuals, including patients with acquired immunodeficiency syndrome; prophylaxis of CMV infection in transplant patients
Oral: Alternative to the I.V. formulation for maintenance treatment of CMV retinitis in immunocompromised patients, including patients with AIDS, in whom retinitis is stable following appropriate induction therapy and for whom the risk of more rapid progression is balanced by the benefit associated with avoiding daily I.V. infusions.
Implant: Treatment of CMV retinitis
Unlabeled/Investigational Use May be given in combination with foscarnet in patients who relapse after monotherapy with either drug
Effect on Mental Status May cause confusion; may rarely cause nervousness, psychosis, hallucinations, or disorientation
Effect on Psychiatric Treatment Leukopenia is common; use caution with clozapine and carbamazepine
Dosage Summary Note: Dosing is based on total body weight
I.V.:
Children ≤3 months: Dosage not established
Children >3 months: Induction: 5 mg/kg every 12 hours for 14-21 days; Maintenance: 30-35 mg/kg/week, given as once daily dose for 5-7 days per week
Adults: Induction: 5 mg/kg every 12 hours for 14-21 days; Maintenance: 30-35 mg/kg/week, given as once daily dose for 5-7 days per week
Ocular Implant:
Children <9 years: Dosage not established
Children ≥9 years: One implant every 5-8 months

Adults: One implant for 5- to 8-month period

Oral:

Children <3 months: Dosage not established

Children ≥3 months: 3 g/day given in 3 or 6 divided doses

Adults: 3 g/day given in 3 or 6 divided doses

Dosage Forms Excipient information presented when available (limited, particularly for generics); consult specific product labeling.

Capsule: 250 mg, 500 mg

Implant, intravitreal:

Vitrasert®: 4.5 mg [released gradually over 5-8 months]

Injection, powder for reconstitution, as sodium:

Cytovene®: 500 mg

- ◆ **Ganidin NR** *see* GuaiFENesin *on page 737*
- ◆ **Ganite™** *see* Gallium Nitrate *on page 707*
- ◆ **Gani-Tuss DM NR** *see* Guaifenesin and Dextromethorphan *on page 739*
- ◆ **Gani-Tuss® NR** *see* Guaifenesin and Codeine *on page 738*
- ◆ **Gantrisin®** *see* SulfiSOXAZOLE *on page 1523*
- ◆ **GAR-936** *see* Tigecycline *on page 1583*
- ◆ **Gastrocrom®** *see* Cromolyn *on page 402*

Gatifloxacin (gat i FLOKS a sin)

U.S. Brand Names Zymar®

Canadian Brand Names Zymar®

Mexican Brand Names Tequin

Pharmacologic Category Antibiotic, Ophthalmic; Antibiotic, Quinolone

Use Treatment of bacterial conjunctivitis

Effect on Mental Status Gatifloxacin may cause dizziness, insomnia; may rarely produce abnormal thinking, agitation, anorexia, anxiety, asthenia, ataxia, confusion, depersonalization, depression, euphoria, hallucination, hostility, nervousness, panic attacks, paranoia, psychosis, somnolence, or stress

Effect on Psychiatric Treatment May have potential to prolong QT interval; should avoid in patients with uncorrected hypokalemia, or concurrent administration of other medications known to prolong the QT interval (antipsychotics, tricyclic antidepressants, ziprasidone)

Dosage Summary

Ophthalmic:

Children <1 year: Dosage not established

Children ≥1 year: Days 1 and 2: 1 drop into affected eye(s) every 2 hours while awake (maximum: 8 times/day); Days 3-7: 1 drop into affected eye(s) up to 4 times/day

Adults: Days 1 and 2: 1 drop into affected eye(s) every 2 hours while awake (maximum: 8 times/day); Days 3-7: 1 drop into affected eye(s) up to 4 times/day

Dosage Forms Excipient information presented when available (limited, particularly for generics); consult specific product labeling.

Solution, ophthalmic:

Zymar®: 0.3% (5 mL) [contains benzalkonium chloride]

- ◆ **G-CSF** *see* Filgrastim *on page 632*
- ◆ **G-CSF (PEG Conjugate)** *see* Pegfilgrastim *on page 1236*
- ◆ **GCV Sodium** *see* Ganciclovir *on page 708*
- ◆ **Gd-DTPA** *see* Gadopentetate Dimeglumine *on page 705*

Gefitinib (ge FI tye nib)

Medication Safety Issues

Sound-alike/look-alike issues:

Gefitinib may be confused with erlotinib

High alert medication: The Institute for Safe Medication Practices (ISMP) includes this medication among its list of drugs which have a heightened risk of causing significant patient harm when used in error.

U.S. Brand Names IRESSA®

Index Terms NSC-715055; ZD1839

Pharmacologic Category Antineoplastic Agent, Tyrosine Kinase Inhibitor

Use

U.S. labeling: Treatment of locally advanced or metastatic nonsmall cell lung cancer after failure of platinum-based and docetaxel therapies. Treatment is limited to patients who are benefiting or have benefited from treatment with gefitinib.

Note: Due to the lack of improved survival data from clinical trials of gefitinib, and in response to positive survival data with another EGFR inhibitor, physicians are advised to use other treatment options in advanced nonsmall cell lung cancer patients following one or two prior chemotherapy regimens when they are refractory/intolerant to their most recent regimen.

Canada labeling: Approved indication is limited to NSCLC patients with epidermal growth factor receptor (EGFR) expression status positive or unknown.

Effect on Mental Status None reported

Effect on Psychiatric Treatment GI side effects are common; use caution with SSRIs. Carbamazepine may decrease gefitinib concentrations, while nefazodone and fluvoxamine may increase its concentrations.

Restrictions As of September 15, 2005, distribution will be limited to patients enrolled in the Iressa Access Program. Under this program, access to gefitinib will be limited to the following groups:

Patients who are currently receiving and benefitting from gefitinib (IRESSA®)

Patients who have previously received and benefited from gefitinib (IRESSA®)

Previously-enrolled patients or new patients in non-Investigational New Drug (IND) clinical trials involving gefitinib (IRESSA®) if these protocols were approved by an IRB prior to June 17, 2005

New patients may also receive Iressa if the manufacturer (AstraZeneca) decides to make it available under IND, and the patients meet the criteria for enrollment under the IND

Additional information on the IRESSA® Access Program, including enrollment forms, may be obtained by calling AstraZeneca at 1-800-601-8933 or via the web at www.Iressa-access.com

Dosage Summary

Oral:

Children: Dosage not established

Adults: 250 mg once daily; **Note:** May need 500 mg/day in patients receiving effective CYP3A4 inducers

Dosage Forms Excipient information presented when available (limited, particularly for generics); consult specific product labeling.

Tablet: 250 mg

◆ **Gelusil® [OTC]** *see* Aluminum Hydroxide, Magnesium Hydroxide, and Simethicone *on page 78*

Gemcitabine (jem SITE a been)

Medication Safety Issues

Sound-alike/look-alike issues:

Gemcitabine may be confused with gemtuzumab

Gemzar® may be confused with Zinecard®

High alert medication: The Institute for Safe Medication Practices (ISMP) includes this medication among its list of drugs which have a heightened risk of causing significant patient harm when used in error.

U.S. Brand Names Gemzar®

Canadian Brand Names Gemzar®

Mexican Brand Names Gemzar

Index Terms Gemcitabine Hydrochloride; NSC-613327

Pharmacologic Category Antineoplastic Agent, Antimetabolite (Pyrimidine Analog)

Use Treatment of metastatic breast cancer; locally-advanced or metastatic nonsmall cell lung cancer (NSCLC) or pancreatic cancer; advanced, relapsed ovarian cancer

Unlabeled/Investigational Use Treatment of bladder cancer, acute leukemia

Effect on Mental Status None reported

Effect on Psychiatric Treatment Leukopenia is common; use caution with clozapine and carbamazepine

Dosage Summary

I.V.:

Children: Dosage not established

Adults: Initial: 1000 mg/m^2 once weekly for up to 7 weeks; 21-day cycle: 1250 mg/m^2 days 1and 8; repeat cycle every 21 days; 28-day cycle: 1000 mg/m^2 days 1, 8, and 15; repeat cycle every 28 days

Dosage Forms Excipient information presented when available (limited, particularly for generics); consult specific product labeling.

Injection, powder for reconstitution:

Gemzar®: 200 mg, 1 g

◆ **Gemcitabine Hydrochloride** *see* Gemcitabine *on page 710*

Gemfibrozil (jem FI broe zil)

Medication Safety Issues

Sound-alike/look-alike issues:

Lopid® may be confused with Levbid®, Lodine®, Lorabid®, Slo-bid™

Related Information

Lipid-Lowering Agents *on page 1786*

U.S. Brand Names Lopid®

Canadian Brand Names Apo-Gemfibrozil®; Gen-Gemfibrozil; GMD-Gemfibrozil; Lopid®; Novo-Gemfibrozil; Nu-Gemfibrozil; PMS-Gemfibrozil

Mexican Brand Names Lopid

Index Terms CI-719

Pharmacologic Category Antilipemic Agent, Fibric Acid

Generic Available Yes

Use Treatment of hypertriglyceridemia in types IV and V hyperlipidemia for patients who are at greater risk for pancreatitis and who have not responded to dietary intervention

Effect on Mental Status May rarely cause sedation or depression

Effect on Psychiatric Treatment None reported

Pregnancy Risk Factor C

Lactation Excretion in breast milk unknown/contraindicated

Contraindications Hypersensitivity to gemfibrozil or any component of the formulation; significant hepatic or renal dysfunction; primary biliary cirrhosis; pre-existing gallbladder disease

Warnings/Precautions Secondary causes of hyperlipidemia should be ruled out prior to therapy. Possible increased risk of malignancy and cholelithiasis. No evidence of cardiovascular mortality benefit. Anemia and leukopenia have been reported. Elevations in serum transaminases can be seen. Discontinue if lipid response not seen. Be careful in patient selection; this is not a first- or second-line choice. Other agents may be more suitable. Adjustments in warfarin therapy may be required with concurrent use. Has been associated with rare myositis or rhabdomyolysis; patients should be monitored closely. Patients should be instructed to report unexplained muscle pain, tenderness, weakness, or brown urine. Use caution when combining gemfibrozil with HMG-CoA reductase inhibitors (may lead to myopathy, rhabdomyolysis). Renal function deterioration has been seen when used in patients with a serum creatinine >2.0 mg/dL. Safety and efficacy in pediatric patients have not been established.

Adverse Reactions

>10%: Gastrointestinal: Dyspepsia (20%)

1% to 10%:

Central nervous system: Fatigue (4%), vertigo (2%), headache (1%)

Dermatologic: Eczema (2%), rash (2%)

Gastrointestinal: Abdominal pain (10%), diarrhea (7%), nausea/vomiting (3%), constipation (1%)

<1% (Limited to important or life-threatening): Alopecia, anaphylaxis, angioedema, bone marrow hypoplasia, cataracts, cholelithiasis, cholecystitis, depression, dermatomyositis/polymyositis, drug-induced lupus-like syndrome, eosinophilia, exfoliative dermatitis, hypokalemia, impotence, intracranial hemorrhage, jaundice, laryngeal edema, leukopenia, myasthenia, myopathy, nephrotoxicity, pancreatitis, paresthesia, peripheral neuritis, photosensitivity, positive ANA, rash, Raynaud's phenomenon, retinal edema, rhabdomyolysis, seizure, syncope, thrombocytopenia, urticaria, vasculitis

Metabolism/Transport Effects **Substrate** of CYP3A4 (minor); **Inhibits** CYP1A2 (moderate), 2C8 (strong), 2C9 (strong), 2C19 (strong)

Drug Interactions

Antidiabetic Agents (Thiazolidinedione): Gemfibrozil may decrease the metabolism of Antidiabetic Agents (Thiazolidinedione). *Risk C: Monitor therapy*

Bile Acid Sequestrants: May decrease the absorption of Fibric Acid Derivatives. **Exceptions:** Colesevelam. *Risk D: Consider therapy modification*

CYP1A2 Substrates: CYP1A2 Inhibitors (Moderate) may decrease the metabolism of CYP1A2 Substrates. *Risk C: Monitor therapy*

CYP2C19 Substrates: CYP2C19 Inhibitors (Strong) may decrease the metabolism of CYP2C19 Substrates. *Risk D: Consider therapy modification*

CYP2C8 Substrates (High risk): CYP2C8 Inhibitors (Strong) may decrease the metabolism of CYP2C8 Substrates (High risk). *Risk D: Consider therapy modification*

CYP2C9 Substrates (High risk): CYP2C9 Inhibitors (Strong) may decrease the metabolism of CYP2C9 Substrates (High risk). *Risk D: Consider therapy modification*

Ezetimibe: Fibric Acid Derivatives may increase the serum concentration of Ezetimibe. *Risk C: Monitor therapy*

HMG-CoA Reductase Inhibitors: Gemfibrozil may enhance the myopathic (rhabdomyolysis) effect of HMG-CoA Reductase Inhibitors. Gemfibrozil may increase the serum concentration of HMG-CoA Reductase Inhibitors. **Exceptions:** Fluvastatin. *Risk D: Consider therapy modification*

Repaglinide: Gemfibrozil may increase the serum concentration of Repaglinide. The addition of itraconazole may augment the effect of gemfibrozil on repaglinide. Management: Consider alternative therapy combinations to avoid this potentially significant interaction. Avoid concurrent use when also used with a CYP3A4 inhibitor. *Risk D: Consider therapy modification*

Sulfonylureas: Fibric Acid Derivatives may enhance the hypoglycemic effect of Sulfonylureas. *Risk C: Monitor therapy*

Vitamin K Antagonists (eg, warfarin): Fibric Acid Derivatives may enhance the anticoagulant effect of Vitamin K Antagonists. *Risk D: Consider therapy modification*

Ethanol/Nutrition/Herb Interactions Ethanol: Avoid ethanol to decrease triglycerides.

Mechanism of Action The exact mechanism of action of gemfibrozil is unknown, however, several theories exist regarding the VLDL effect; it can inhibit lipolysis and decrease subsequent hepatic fatty acid uptake as well as inhibit hepatic secretion of VLDL; together these actions decrease serum VLDL levels; increases HDL-cholesterol; the mechanism behind HDL elevation is currently unknown

Pharmacodynamics/Kinetics

Onset of action: May require several days

Absorption: Well absorbed

Protein binding: 99%

Metabolism: Hepatic via oxidation to two inactive metabolites; undergoes enterohepatic recycling

Half-life elimination: 1.4 hours

Time to peak, serum: 1-2 hours

Excretion: Urine (70% primarily as conjugated drug); feces (6%)

Dosage Adults: Oral: 1200 mg/day in 2 divided doses, 30 minutes before breakfast and dinner

Hemodialysis: Not removed by hemodialysis; supplemental dose is not necessary

Dietary Considerations Before initiation of therapy, patients should be placed on a standard cholesterol-lowering diet for 3-6 months and the diet should be continued during drug therapy.

Monitoring Parameters Serum cholesterol, LFTs

Dosage Forms Excipient information presented when available (limited, particularly for generics); consult specific product labeling.

Tablet, oral: 600 mg

Lopid®: 600 mg [scored]

Gemifloxacin (je mi FLOKS a sin)

U.S. Brand Names Factive®

Canadian Brand Names Factive®

Index Terms DW286; Gemifloxacin Mesylate; LA 20304a; SB-265805

Pharmacologic Category Antibiotic, Quinolone; Respiratory Fluoroquinolone

Use Treatment of acute exacerbation of chronic bronchitis; treatment of community-acquired pneumonia (CAP), including pneumonia caused by multidrug-resistant strains of *S. pneumoniae* (MDRSP)

Unlabeled/Investigational Use Acute sinusitis

Effect on Mental Status May cause dizziness, hallucinations, and suicidal ideation

Effect on Psychiatric Treatment Contraindicated with ziprasidone. May lower seizure threshold; use caution with clozapine. Gemifloxacin may prolong QT interval; avoid use with antipsychotics and TCAs.

Restrictions An FDA-approved patient medication guide is available and must be distributed when dispensing an outpatient prescription (new or refill) where this medication is to be used without direct supervision of a healthcare provider. Medication guides are available at http://www.fda.gov/cder/Offices/ODS/medication_guides.htm.

Dosage Summary

Oral:

Children: Dosage not established

Adults: 320 mg once daily

Dosage Forms Excipient information presented when available (limited, particularly for generics); consult specific product labeling.

Tablet:

Factive®: 320 mg

- **Gemifloxacin Mesylate** *see* Gemifloxacin *on page 712*

Gemtuzumab Ozogamicin (gem TOO zoo mab oh zog a MY sin)

Medication Safety Issues

Sound-alike/look-alike issues:

Gemtuzumab may be confused with gemcitabine

High alert medication: The Institute for Safe Medication Practices (ISMP) includes this medication among its list of drug classes which have a heightened risk of causing significant patient harm when used in error.

U.S. Brand Names Mylotarg®

Canadian Brand Names Mylotarg®

Index Terms CMA-676; NSC-720568

Pharmacologic Category Antineoplastic Agent, Monoclonal Antibody

Use Treatment of relapsed CD33 positive acute myeloid leukemia (AML) in patients ≥60 years of age who are not candidates for cytotoxic chemotherapy

Unlabeled/Investigational Use Salvage therapy for acute promyelocytic leukemia (APL), relapsed/ refractory CD33 positive acute myeloid leukemia in children and adults <60 years

Effect on Mental Status Dizziness, insomnia, and depression are common

Effect on Psychiatric Treatment Hypotension is common; caution with low potency antipsychotics and TCAs; nausea and vomiting are common, use caution with the SSRIs. Neutropenia is common, use caution with carbamazepine and clozapine.

Dosage Summary

I.V.:

Children <3 years (unlabeled use): 0.2 mg/kg every 2 weeks for 2 doses **or** 4-9 mg/m^2 every 2 weeks for 1-3 doses

Children ≥3 years (unlabeled use): 6 mg/m^2 every 2 weeks for 2 doses **or** 4-9 mg/m^2 every 2 weeks for a total of 1-3 doses per treatment course

Adults <60 years (unlabeled use): 9 mg/m^2 every 2 weeks for a total of 2 doses per treatment course

Adults ≥60 years: 9 mg/m^2 every 2 weeks for a total of 2 doses per treatment course

Dosage Forms Excipient information presented when available (limited, particularly for generics); consult specific product labeling.

Injection, powder for reconstitution [preservative free]:

Mylotarg®: 5 mg

- **Gemzar®** *see* Gemcitabine *on page 710*
- **Genac® [OTC]** *see* Triprolidine and Pseudoephedrine *on page 1634*
- **Genaced™ [OTC]** *see* Acetaminophen, Aspirin, and Caffeine *on page 39*
- **Genacote™ [OTC]** *see* Aspirin *on page 143*
- **Genahist® [OTC]** *see* DiphenhydrAMINE *on page 481*
- **Genapap™ [OTC]** *see* Acetaminophen *on page 30*
- **Genapap™ Children [OTC]** *see* Acetaminophen *on page 30*
- **Genapap™ Extra Strength [OTC]** *see* Acetaminophen *on page 30*
- **Genapap™ Infant [OTC]** *see* Acetaminophen *on page 30*
- **Genapap™ Sinus Maximum Strength [OTC] [DSC]** *see* Acetaminophen and Pseudoephedrine *on page 37*
- **Genaphed® [OTC]** *see* Pseudoephedrine *on page 1367*
- **Genasal [OTC]** *see* Oxymetazoline *on page 1208*
- **Genasec™ [OTC]** *see* Acetaminophen and Phenyltoloxamine *on page 36*
- **Genatuss DM® [OTC]** *see* Guaifenesin and Dextromethorphan *on page 739*

- ◆ **Genebs [OTC]** *see* Acetaminophen *on page 30*
- ◆ **Genebs Extra Strength [OTC]** *see* Acetaminophen *on page 30*
- ◆ **Generlac** *see* Lactulose *on page 886*
- ◆ **Genexa™ LA [DSC]** *see* Guaifenesin and Phenylephrine *on page 742*
- ◆ **Geneye [OTC]** *see* Tetrahydrozoline *on page 1560*
- ◆ **Gengraf®** *see* CycloSPORINE *on page 409*
- ◆ **Genotropin®** *see* Somatropin *on page 1499*
- ◆ **Genotropin Miniquick®** *see* Somatropin *on page 1499*
- ◆ **Genpril® [OTC] [DSC]** *see* Ibuprofen *on page 803*
- ◆ **Gentak®** *see* Gentamicin *on page 714*

Gentamicin (jen ta MYE sin)

Medication Safety Issues

Sound-alike/look-alike issues:

Garamycin® may be confused with kanamycin, Terramycin®

Gentamicin may be confused with gentian violet, kanamycin, vancomycin

High alert medication: The Institute for Safe Medication Practices (ISMP) includes this medication (intrathecal administration) among its list of drug classes which have a heightened risk of causing significant patient harm when used in error.

U.S. Brand Names Gentak®; Gentasol™

Canadian Brand Names Alcomicin®; Diogent®; Garamycin®; Gentamicin Injection, USP; SAB-Gentamicin

Mexican Brand Names Garamicina; Garamsa; Genkova; Genrex; Gentamil; Gentazol; Misinex; Servigenta; Tondex; Yectamicina

Index Terms Gentamicin Sulfate

Pharmacologic Category Antibiotic, Aminoglycoside; Antibiotic, Ophthalmic; Antibiotic, Topical

Use Treatment of susceptible bacterial infections, normally gram-negative organisms including *Pseudomonas*, *Proteus*, *Serratia*, and gram-positive *Staphylococcus*; treatment of bone infections, respiratory tract infections, skin and soft tissue infections, as well as abdominal and urinary tract infections, and septicemia; treatment of infective endocarditis; used topically to treat superficial infections of the skin or ophthalmic infections caused by susceptible bacteria

Effect on Mental Status Dizziness is common; may cause drowsiness

Effect on Psychiatric Treatment May rarely cause agranulocytosis; use caution with clozapine and carbamazepine

Dosage Summary Note: Use of ideal body weight (IBW) for determining the mg/kg/dose appears to be more accurate than dosing on the basis of total body weight (TBW). In morbid obesity, dosage requirement may best be estimated using a dosing weight of IBW + 0.4 (TBW - IBW).

I.M.:

Children <5 years: 2.5 mg/kg/dose every 8 hours; **Note:** Higher individual doses and/or more frequent intervals (eg, every 6 hours) may be required in selected clinical situations (cystic fibrosis) or if serum levels document the need

Children ≥5 years: 2-2.5 mg/kg/dose every 8 hours; **Note:** Higher individual doses and/or more frequent intervals (eg, every 6 hours) may be required in selected clinical situations (cystic fibrosis) or if serum levels document the need hours

Adults: 1-2.5 mg/kg/dose every 8-12 hours **or** 4-7 mg/kg once daily

I.V.:

Neonates 0-7 days and <2000 g: 2.5 mg/kg every 18-24 hours

Neonates 0-7 days and >2000 g: 2.5 mg/kg every 12 hours

Neonates 8-28 days and <2000 g: 2.5 mg/kg every 8-12 hours

Neonates 8-28 days and >2000 g: 2.5 mg/kg every 8 hours

Children <5 years: 2.5 mg/kg/dose every 8 hours; **Note:** Higher individual doses and/or more frequent intervals (eg, every 6 hours) may be required in selected clinical situations (cystic fibrosis) or if serum levels document the need

Children ≥5 years: 2-2.5 mg/kg/dose every 8 hours; **Note:** Higher individual doses and/or more frequent intervals (eg, every 6 hours) may be required in selected clinical situations (cystic fibrosis) or if serum levels document the need hours

Adults: 1-2.5 mg/kg/dose every 8-12 hours **or** 4-7 mg/kg once daily

Intrathecal:

Children: Dosage not established

Adults: 4-8 mg/day

Ophthalmic:

Ointment:

Children: Instill 1/2" (1.25 cm) 2-3 times/day to every 3-4 hours

Adults: Instill 1/2" (1.25 cm) 2-3 times/day to every 3-4 hours

Solution:

Children: Instill 1-2 drops every 2-4 hours, up to 2 drops every hour for severe infections

Adults: Instill 1-2 drops every 2-4 hours, up to 2 drops every hour for severe infections

Topical:

Children: Apply 3-4 times/day to affected area

Adults: Apply 3-4 times/day to affected area

Dosage Forms Excipient information presented when available (limited, particularly for generics); consult specific product labeling. [DSC] = Discontinued product

Cream, topical, as sulfate: 0.1% (15 g, 30 g)

Infusion, as sulfate [premixed in NS]: 40 mg (50 mL); 60 mg (50 mL, 100 mL); 70 mg (50 mL); 80 mg (50 mL, 100 mL); 90 mg (100 mL); 100 mg (50 mL, 100 mL); 120 mg (100 mL)

Injection, solution, as sulfate: 10 mg/mL (6 mL, 8 mL, 10 mL)

Injection, solution, as sulfate: 40 mg/mL (2 mL, 20 mL)

Injection, solution [pediatric], as sulfate: 10 mg/mL (2 mL)

Injection, solution [pediatric], as sulfate [preservative free]: 10 mg/mL (2 mL)

Ointment, ophthalmic, as sulfate (Gentak®): 0.3% [3 mg/g] (3.5 g)

Ointment, topical, as sulfate: 0.1% (15 g, 30 g)

Solution, ophthalmic, as sulfate: 0.3% (5 mL, 15 mL) [contains benzalkonium chloride]

Gentak®: 0.3% (5 mL; 15 mL [DSC]) [contains benzalkonium chloride]

Gentasol™: 0.3% (5 mL) [contains benzalkonium chloride]

- **Gentamicin Sulfate** *see* Gentamicin *on page 714*
- **Gentasol™** *see* Gentamicin *on page 714*
- **Gentex HC [DSC]** *see* Hydrocodone, Phenylephrine, and Guaifenesin *on page 783*
- **Gentex LA [DSC]** *see* Guaifenesin and Phenylephrine *on page 742*
- **Gentex LQ** *see* Carbetapentane, Guaifenesin, and Phenylephrine *on page 274*
- **Gentuss-HC** *see* Hydrocodone, Phenylephrine, and Diphenhydramine *on page 782*
- **Geocillin® [DSC]** *see* Carbenicillin *on page 272*
- **Geodon®** *see* Ziprasidone *on page 1698*
- **GF196960** *see* Tadalafil *on page 1534*
- **GG** *see* GuaiFENesin *on page 737*
- **GHB** *see* Sodium Oxybate *on page 1495*
- **GI87084B** *see* Remifentanil *on page 1408*
- **Gilphex TR®** *see* Guaifenesin and Phenylephrine *on page 742*
- **Giltuss®** *see* Guaifenesin, Dextromethorphan, and Phenylephrine *on page 746*
- **Giltuss HC® [DSC]** *see* Hydrocodone, Phenylephrine, and Guaifenesin *on page 783*
- **Giltuss Pediatric®** *see* Guaifenesin, Dextromethorphan, and Phenylephrine *on page 746*
- **Giltuss TR®** *see* Guaifenesin, Dextromethorphan, and Phenylephrine *on page 746*
- ***Ginkgo biloba*** *see* Ginkgo *(Ginkgo biloba) on page 715*

Ginkgo *(Ginkgo biloba)*

Natural Product Category Herb

Synonyms *Ginkgo biloba*; Eun-haeng; Fossil Tree; Kew Tree; Silver Apricot

Plant Part Leaf

Dosage and Standardization Oral: 40-80 mg 3 times/day, standardized to contain 24% to 27% ginkgo flavone glycosides and 6% to 7% triterpenes per dose

Reported Uses

Acute ischemic stroke (Garg, 1995)

Alzheimer's disease, dementia (Ernst, 1999; Itil, 1998; Le Bars, 1997; Napryeyenko, 2007; Oken, 1998)

Contradictory study (Schneider, 2005)

Anxiety (Woelk, 2007)
Asthma (Braquet, 1987)
Chemotherapy (adjunct) (Hauns, 1999)
Chronic cochleovestibular disorders (Hahn, 2000)
Cognitive function (Carlson, 2007)
Depression (pharmacologic activity)
Epilepsy (pharmacologic activity)
Functional measures (in patients with multiple sclerosis) (Johnson, 2006)
Gastric cancer (Xu, 2003)
Glaucoma (Quaranta, 2003)
Headache (pharmacologic activity)
Intermittent claudication (Ernst, 1996; Peters, 1998; Pittler, 2000)
Macular degeneration (Lebuisson, 1986)
Memory enhancement (Allain, 1993; Kleijnen, 1992)
Mountain sickness (Roncin, 1996)
Multiple sclerosis (Brochet, 1992; Brochet, 1995; Lovera, 2007)
Ocular blood flow (contradictory study) (Wimpissinger, 2007)
Parkinson's disease (pharmacologic activity)
Peripheral blood flow: Cerebral vascular disease, peripheral vascular insufficiency, impotence, tinnitus, and depression (Kleijnen, 1992)
Premenstrual syndrome (PMS) (Tamborini, 1993)
Quality of life (Cockle, 2000; Trick, 2004)
Raynaud's phenomenon (Muir, 2002)
Retinopathy (Huang, 2004)
Seasonal affective disorder (SAD) (Lingaerde, 1999)
Seizures (pharmacologic activity)
Sexual dysfunction (antidepressant-induced) (Cohen, 1998)
Tinnitus (Drew, 2001; Holgers, 1994; Meyer, 1986; Morgenstern, 2002; Rejali, 2004)
Vertigo (Haguenauer, 1986)
Vitiligo (Parsad, 2003)

Summary Ginkgo has been used in China for thousands of years and is one of the most frequently prescribed medicinal herbs in Europe. Most uses of ginkgo have centered on improvement in regional (ie, CNS) or peripheral blood flow and oxygen delivery. Claims of benefit range from improved cognitive function in Alzheimer's disease to decreased symptoms of peripheral vascular disease. Other neurologic uses include tinnitus and vertigo. It has also become popular among students who hope to enhance memory during their academic studies.

Effect on Mental Status May cause restlessness and dizziness

Effect on Psychiatric Treatment Effects of acetylcholinesterase inhibitors and MAO inhibitors may be increased by ginkgo biloba

Pharmacology The primary activity of ginkgo appears to be derived from flavoglycosides. These compounds are potent-free radical scavengers and demonstrate a variety of pharmacologic activities. Ginkgo has also been reported to inhibit platelet-activating factor (PAF). It may stimulate endothelial releasing factor and prostacyclin and may augment venous tone and improve the clearance of toxins during periods of ischemia. In addition, ginkgo may improve cholinergic neurotransmission. The effect of ginkgo may be to increase cerebral blood flow and, therefore, improve oxygen and nutrient delivery while enhancing the elimination of metabolic end products. Ginkgo may reduce capillary fragility and function as an antioxidant. Ginkgo has been reported to improve circulation in the elderly and has been proposed to enhance memory, potentially delaying the onset of senile dementia and Alzheimer's.

Warnings and Interactions May cause abdominal problems, nausea, and dyspepsia (Pittler, 2000).

Theoretical Cautions and Contraindications Ginkgo demonstrates *in vitro* inhibition of platelet aggregation and has been associated with case reports of bleeding (Matthews, 1998; Odawara, 1997; Rosenblatt, 1997; Skogh, 1998; Vale, 1998). Based on pharmacologic activity, this herb may be contraindicated in individuals with active bleeding (eg, peptic ulcer, intracranial bleeding). Use with caution in individuals with a history of bleeding, hemostatic disorders, or drug-related hemostatic problems, and in individuals taking anticoagulant medications, including warfarin, aspirin, aspirin-containing products, NSAIDs, or antiplatelet agents (eg, ticlopidine, clopidogrel, dipyridamole). Discontinue use prior to dental or surgical procedures (generally at least 14 days before).

Based on pharmacologic activity, may increase effect or toxicity of monoamine oxidase inhibitors (MAOIs) (White, 1966; Wu 1999).

General Warnings Use all herbal supplements with extreme caution in children <2 years of age and in pregnancy or lactation. Some herbs are contraindicated in pregnancy or lactation; make sure to observe warnings. Use with caution in individuals on medication and with pre-existing medical conditions. Always review for potential herb-drug interactions (HDIs) and other warnings. Large and prolonged doses may increase the potential for adverse effects. Herbs may cause transient adverse effects such as nausea, vomiting, and GI distress due to a variety of chemical constituents. Use caution in individuals having known allergies to plants.

Theoretical Interactions Anticoagulant medications (including warfarin), aspirin or aspirin-containing products, NSAIDs, antiplatelet agents (eg, ticlopidine, clopidogrel, dipyridamole), MAO inhibitors, acetylcholinesterase inhibitors, 5-fluorouracil, anticonvulsants, antihypertensives, antipsychotics, colchicine, antidiabetic medications, insulin, erectile dysfunction agents, SSRIs, thiazide diuretics

Data from one case report suggests this herb may induce the CYP3A4 isoenzyme. Theoretically, it may affect the following medications' disposition: Trazodone, protease inhibitors, cyclosporine, non-nucleoside reverse transcriptase inhibitors, certain benzodiazepines, calcium channel blockers, grapefruit juice, and other medications influenced by this enzyme system.

Reported interaction with trazodone; after 3 days of concomitant therapy with ginkgo and trazodone, an 80-year old female was found to have instability, drowsiness, and unresponsiveness. The patient regained consciousness quickly with discontinuation of both products. Mechanism for interaction unknown.

References

Allain H, Raoul P, Lieury A, et al, "Effect of Two Doses of *Ginkgo biloba* Extract (EGb 761) on the Dual-Coding Test in Elderly Subjects," *Clin Ther*, 1993, 15(3):549-58.

Balon R, "*Ginkgo biloba* for Antidepressant-Induced Sexual Dysfunction," *J Sex Marital Ther*, 1999, 25(1):1-2.

Braquet P, "The Ginkgolides: Potent Platelet-Activating Factor Antagonists Isolated from *Ginkgo biloba* L.: Chemistry, Pharmacology, and Clinical Applications," *Drugs of the Future*, 1987, 12:643-99.

Brochet B, Guinot P, Orgogozo JM, et al, "Double Blind Placebo Controlled Multicentre Study of Ginkgolide B in Treatment of Acute Exacerbations of Multiple Sclerosis. The Ginkgolide Study Group in Multiple Sclerosis," *J Neurol Neurosurg Psychiatry*, 1995, 58(3):360-2.

Brochet B, Orgogozo JM, Guinot P, et al, "Pilot Study of Ginkgolide B, a PAF-acether Specific Inhibitor in the Treatment of Acute Outbreaks of Multiple Sclerosis," *Rev Neurol (Paris)*, 1992, 148(4):299-301.

Carlson JJ, Farquhar JW, DiNucci E, et al, "Safety and Efficacy of a *Ginkgo biloba*-Containing Dietary Supplement on Cognitive Function, Quality of Life, and Platelet Function in Healthy, Cognitively Intact Older Adults," *J Am Diet Assoc*, 2007, 107 (3):422-32.

Cockle SM, Kimber S, and Hindmarch I, "The Effects of *Ginkgo biloba* Extract (LI 1370) Supplementation on Activities of Daily Living in Free Living Older Volunteers: A Questionnaire Survey," *Hum Psychopharmacol*, 2000, 15(4):227-35.

Cohen AJ and Bartlik B, "*Ginkgo biloba* for Antidepressant-Induced Sexual Dysfunction," *J Sex Marital Ther*, 1998, 24(2):139-43.

Drew S and Davies E, "Effectiveness of *Ginkgo biloba* in Treating Tinnitus: Double Blind, Placebo Controlled Trial," *BMJ*, 2001, 322(7278):73.

Ernst E, "*Ginkgo biloba* in Treatment of Intermittent Claudication. A Systematic Research Based on Controlled Studies in the Literature," *Fortschr Med*, 1996, 114(8):85-7.

Ernst E and Pittler MH, "*Ginkgo biloba* for Dementia: A Systematic Review of Double-Blind, Placebo-Controlled Trials," *Clin Drug Invest*, 1999, 17(4):301-8.

Galluzzi S, Zanetti O, Binetti G, et al, "Coma in a Patient With Alzheimer's Disease Taking Low Dose Trazodone and Gingko Biloba," *J Neurol Neurosurg Psychiatry*, 2000, 68 (5):679-80.

Garg RK, Nag D, and Agrawal A, "A Double Blind Placebo Controlled Trial of *Ginkgo biloba* Extract in Acute Cerebral Ischaemia," *J Assoc Physicians India*, 1995, 43(11):760-3.

Haguenauer JP, Cantenot F, Koskas H, et al, "Treatment of Equilibrium Disorders With *Ginkgo biloba* Extract. A Multicenter Double-Blind Drug Vs. Placebo Study," *Presse Med*, 1986, 15(31):1569-72.

Hahn A and Stolbova K, "*Ginkgo biloba*: Local Experiences," *Int Tinnitus J*, 2000, 6(1):54-5.

Hauns B, Haring B, Kohler S, et al, "Phase II Study With 5-Fluorouracil and *Ginkgo biloba* Extract (GBE 761 ONC) in Patients With Pancreatic Cancer," *Arzneimittelforschung*, 1999, 49(12):1030-4.

Holgers KM, Axelsson A, and Pringle I, "*Ginkgo biloba* Extract for the Treatment of Tinnitus," *Audiology*, 1994, 33(2):85-92.

Huang SY, Jeng C, Kao SC, et al, "Improved Haemorrheological Properties by *Ginkgo biloba* Extract (Egb 761) in Type 2 Diabetes Mellitus Complicated With Retinopathy," *Clin Nutr*, 2004, 23(4):615-21.

Itil TM, Erlap E, Ahmed I, et al, "The Pharmacological Effects of *Ginkgo biloba*, a Plant Extract, on the Brain of Dementia Patients in Comparison With Tacrine," *Psychopharmacol Bull*, 1998, 34(3):391-7.

Johnson SK, Diamond BJ, Rausch S, et al, "The Effect of *Ginkgo biloba* on Functional Measures in Multiple Sclerosis: A Pilot Randomized Controlled Trial," *Explore (NY)*, 2006, 2(1):19-24.

Kleijnen J and Knipschild P, "*Ginkgo biloba*," *Lancet*, 1992, 340(8828):1136-9.

Le Bars PL, Katz MM, Berman N, et al, "A Placebo-Controlled, Double-Blind, Randomized Trial of an Extract of *Ginkgo biloba* for Dementia. North American EGb Study Group," *JAMA*, 1997, 278(16):1327-32.

Lebuissen DA, Leroy L, and Rigal G, "Treatment of Senile Macular Degeneration With *Ginkgo biloba* Extract. A Preliminary Double-Blind Drug vs Placebo Study," *Presse Med*, 1986, 15(31):1556-8.

Lingaerde O, Foreland AR, and Magnusson A, "Can Winter Depression Be Prevented by *Ginkgo biloba* Extract? A Placebo-Controlled Trial," *Acta Psychiatr Scand*, 1999, 100 (1):62-6.

Lovera J, Bagert B, Smoot K, et al, "*Ginkgo biloba* for the Improvement of Cognitive Performance in Multiple Sclerosis: A Randomized, Placebo-Controlled Trial," *Mult Scler*, 2007, 13(3):376-85.

Matthews MK Jr, "Association of *Ginkgo biloba* With Intracerebral Hemorrhage," *Neurology*, 1998, 50(6):1933-4.

Meyer B, "Multicenter Randomized Double-Blind Drug vs Placebo Study of the Treatment of Tinnitus With *Ginkgo biloba* Extract," *Presse Med*, 1986, 15(31):1562-4.

Morgenstern C and Biermann E, "The Efficacy of Ginkgo Special Extract EGb 761 in Patients With Tinnitus," *Int J Clin Pharmacol Ther*, 2002, 40(5):188-97.

Muir AH, Robb R, McLaren M, et al, "The Use of *Ginkgo biloba* in Raynaud's Disease: A Double-Blind Placebo-Controlled Trial," *Vasc Med*, 2002, 7(4):265-7.

Napryeyenko O, Borzenko I, and GINDEM-NP Study Group, "*Ginkgo biloba* Special Extract in Dementia With Neuropsychiatric Features. A Randomised, Placebo-Controlled, Double-Blind Clinical Trial," *Arzneimittelforschung*, 2007, 57(1):4-11.

Natural Standard Research Collaboration, Chief Editors: Ulbricht C, Basch E, *Natural Standard Herb and Supplement Reference - Evidence-Based Clinical Reviews*, USA: Elsevier/Mosby, 2005.

Odawara M, Tamaoka A, and Yamashita K, "*Ginkgo biloba*," *Neurology*, 1997, 48(3):789-90.

Oken BS, Storzbach DM, and Kaye JA, "The Efficacy of *Ginkgo biloba* on Cognitive Function in Alzheimer Disease," *Arch Neurol*, 1998, 55(11):1409-15.

Parsad D, Pandhi R, and Juneja A, "Effectiveness of Oral *Ginkgo biloba* in Treating Limited, Slowly Spreading Vitiligo," *Clin Exp Dermatol*, 2003, 28(3):285-7.

Peters H, Kieser M, and Holscher U, "Demonstration of the Efficacy of *Ginkgo biloba* Special Extract EGb 761 on Intermittent Claudication - A Placebo-Controlled, Double-Blind Multicenter Trial," *Vasa*, 1998, 27(2):106-10.

Pittler MH and Ernst E, "*Ginkgo biloba* Extract for the Treatment of Intermittent Claudication: A Meta-analysis of Randomized Trials," *Am J Med*, 2000, 108(4):276-81.

Quaranta L, Bettelli S, Uva MG, et al, "Effect of Ginkgo Biloba Extract on Preexisting Visual Field Damage in Normal Tension Glaucoma," *Ophthalmology*, 2003, 110(2):359-62.

Rejali D, Sivakumar A, and Balaji N, "*Ginkgo biloba* Does Not Benefit Patients With Tinnitus: A Randomized Placebo-Controlled Double-Blind Trial and Meta-Analysis of Randomized Trials," *Clin Otolaryngol Allied Sci*, 2004, 29(3):226-31.

Roncin JP, Schwartz F, and D'Arbigny P, "EGb 761 in Control of Acute Mountain Sickness and Vascular Reactivity to Cold Exposure," *Aviat Space Environ Med*, 1996, 67(5):445-52.

Rosenblatt M and Mindel J, "Spontaneous Hyphema Associated With Ingestion of *Ginko biloba* Extract," *N Engl J Med*, 1997, 336(15):1108.

Sasaki K, Hatta S, Haga M, et al, "Effects of Bilobalide on Gamma-Aminobutyric Acid Levels and Glutamic Acid Decarboxylase in Mouse Brain," *Eur J Pharmacol*, 1999, 367 (2-3):165-73.

Schneider LS, DeKosky ST, Farlow MR, et al, "A Randomized, Double-Blind, Placebo-Controlled Trial of Two Doses of *Ginkgo biloba* Extract in Dementia of the Alzheimer's Type," *Curr Alzheimer Res*, 2005, 2(5):541-51.

Skogh M, "Extracts of *Ginkgo biloba*, and Bleeding or Haemorrhage," *Lancet*, 1998, 352 (9134):1145-6.

Tamborini A and Taurelle R, "Value of Standardized *Ginkgo biloba* Extract (EGb 761) in the Management of Congestive Symptoms of Premenstrual Syndrome," *Rev Fr Gynecol Obstet*, 1993, 88(7-9):447-57.

Trick L, Boyle J, and Hindmarch I, "The Effects of *Ginkgo biloba* Extract (LI 1370) Supplementation and Discontinuation on Activities of Daily Living and Mood in Free Living Older Volunteers," *Phytother Res*, 2004, 18(7):531-7.

Vale S, "Subarachnoid Haemorrhage Associated With *Ginkgo biloba*," *Lancet*, 1998, 352 (9121):36.

White HL, Scates PW, and Cooper BR, "Extracts of *Ginkgo biloba* Leaves Inhibit Monoamine Oxidase," *Life Sci*, 1966, 58(16):1315-21.

Wimpissinger B, Berisha F, Garhoefer G, et al, "Influence of *Ginkgo biloba* on Ocular Blood Flow," *Acta Ophthalmol Scand*, 2007, 85(4):445-9.

Woelk H, Arnoldt KH, Kieser M, et al, "*Ginkgo biloba* Special Extract EGB 761 in Generalized Anxiety Disorder and Adjustment Disorder With Anxious Mood: A Randomized, Double-Blind, Placebo-Controlled Trial," *J Psychiatr Res*, 2007, 41(6):472-80.

Wu WR and Zhu XZ, "Involvement of Monoamine Oxidase Inhibition in Neuroprotective and Neurorestorative Effects of *Ginkgo biloba* Extract Against MPTP-Induced Nigrostriatal Dopaminergic Toxicity in C57 Mice," *Life Sci*, 1999, 65(2):157-64.

Xu AH, Chen HS, Sun BC, et al, "Therapeutic Mechanism of *Ginkgo biloba* Exocarp Polysaccharides on Gastric Cancer," *World J Gastroenterol*, 2003, 9(11):2424-7.

Ginseng, Panax *(Panax ginseng)*

Natural Product Category Herb

Synonyms *Panax ginseng*; Asian Ginseng; Ninjin

Plant Part Root

Dosage and Standardization Oral: 100-600 mg/day in divided doses, standardized to contain a minimum of 5% ginsenosides per dose. A regimen of 4 weeks on, followed by 2 weeks off, is recommended for maximum benefit.

Reported Uses

Adrenal tonic (Hiai, 1979)

Diabetes (Ng, 1985; Reay, 2006; Vuksan, 2000)

Immune support (Kim, 1990)

Physical and mental performance; energy enhancement; chemotherapy and radiation (adjunct) (Chong, 1988)

Summary Historically, *Panax ginseng* has been used primarily for its reported ability to help people during fatigue or stress (adaptogenic properties). It is promoted to enhance wellness by increasing the ability to cope with physiologic, emotional, and environmental stressors, reducing susceptibility to illness. In addition, it may assist in physiologic adaptation to the stress of illness, including chemotherapeutic regimens or radiation therapy.

Effect on Mental Status May cause agitation, insomnia, mania, or nervousness

Effect on Psychiatric Treatment Avoid concurrent use with MAO inhibitors. Avoid use in patients with psychosis or bipolar disorder. Effects of barbiturates and CNS stimulants may be increased; use caution. May produce hypotension; concurrent use with psychotropic agents may produce additive effects.

Pharmacology The primary active constituents of ginseng are believed to be the ginsenosides, which include more than 20 saponin triterpenes similar in structure to steroid hormones. These are believed to act via hormone receptors in the hypothalamus, pituitary glands, and other tissues. Ginsenosides stimulate secretion of adrenocorticotropic hormone (ACTH), leading to production of increased release of adrenal hormones, including cortisol. Ginsenosides reportedly stimulate RNA transcription, protein synthesis, and hepatic cholesterol production. In addition, they may stimulate synthesis of adrenal hormone precursors. Evidence suggests that *Panax ginseng* lowers cortisol levels in individuals with diabetes, while increasing cortisol levels in nondiabetic individuals.

Specific triterpenoid saponins (diols) are claimed to cause improvements in endurance and learning. These compounds are also believed to contribute to sedative and antihypertensive properties. A second group (triols) reportedly increase blood pressure and function as central nervous system stimulants. Ginsenosides have carbohydrate-sparing actions and may increase muscle stamina.

The effects of *Panax ginseng* have been reported to be dose-dependent. Low doses increase blood pressure, while high doses exhibit a hypotensive effect. Additionally, *Panax ginseng* is reported to have immunostimulating effects on the reticuloendothelial system. *Panax ginseng* has been postulated to decrease weight loss and stabilize white blood cell counts during chemotherapy and may also accelerate postsurgical recovery. *Panax ginseng* helps the body adapt to stresses caused by chemotherapy and radiation (Chong, 1988; Kim, 1990).

Theoretical Cautions and Contraindications Use of *Panax ginseng* is contraindicated in renal failure and acute infection. Avoid in pregnancy and lactation (Bradley, 1992). Use with caution in individuals receiving MAO inhibitors (based on pharmacologic activity and case reports). Use caution with stimulant medications, including decongestants, caffeine, and caffeine-containing beverages (based on pharmacologic activity). May be associated with a syndrome of diarrhea, hypertension, nervousness, dermatologic eruptions, and insomnia (Ginseng Abuse Syndrome) after prolonged use or high dosages (Chen, 1981). May also cause mastalgia in prolonged, high-dose use (case reports, Dukes, 1978). May cause vaginal breakthrough bleeding (case reports, Hopkins, 1988). Due to pharmacologic activity, may interfere with hormonal therapy.

May cause palpitations and tachycardia in sensitive individuals or in high doses. Based on pharmacologic activity, use with caution in individuals with hypertension or in those receiving antihypertensives (Siegel, 1980). Also use caution in individuals at risk of hypotension (including those taking antihypertensive medication or agents that predispose to orthostasis), elderly individuals, or those who would not tolerate transient hyper- or hypotensive episodes (ie, cerebrovascular or cardiovascular disease). May increase the QT_c interval (Caron, 2002).

May alter glucose regulation. Use with caution in individuals with diabetes or in those who may be predisposed to hypoglycemia. Effects of drugs with hypoglycemic activity may be potentiated (including insulin and oral hypoglycemics). Blood sugar should be closely monitored, and the dosage of hypoglycemic medications may require adjustment. This should be carefully coordinated among the individual's healthcare providers.

Based on pharmacologic activity and case reports, may alter hemostasis (Janetsky, 1997; Teng, 1989) and may be contraindicated in individuals with active bleeding (eg, peptic ulcer, intracranial bleeding). Use with caution in individuals with a history of bleeding, hemostatic disorders, or drug-related hemostatic problems; and in individuals taking anticoagulant medications, including warfarin, aspirin, aspirin-containing products, NSAIDs, antiplatelet agents (eg, ticlopidine, clopidogrel, dipyridamole). Discontinue use prior to dental or surgical procedures (generally at least 14 days before).

General Warnings Use with caution in pregnancy (based on a study in rat embryos and the effects of ginsenoside Rb1, a chemical found in many commercially available products).

Use all herbal supplements with extreme caution in children <2 years of age and in pregnancy or lactation. Some herbs are contraindicated in pregnancy or lactation; make sure to observe warnings. Use with caution in individuals on medication and with pre-existing medical conditions. Always review for potential herb-drug interactions (HDIs) and other warnings. Large and prolonged doses may increase the potential for adverse effects. Herbs may cause transient adverse effects such as nausea, vomiting, and GI distress due to a variety of chemical constituents. Use caution in individuals having known allergies to plants.

Theoretical Interactions Antihypertensives, anticoagulant medications (including warfarin), aspirin or aspirin-containing products, NSAIDs, antiplatelet agents (eg, ticlopidine, clopidogrel, dipyridamole), central nervous stimulants (caffeine), sympathomimetics, and hormonal therapies

References

Caron MF, Hotsko AL, Robertson S, et al, "Electrocardiographic and Hemodynamic Effects of *Panax Ginseng*," *Ann Pharmacother*, 2002, 36(5):758-63.

Chan LY, Chiu PY, and Lau TK, "An *In vitro* Study of Ginsenoside Rb1-Induced Teratogenicity Using a Whole Rat Embryo Culture Model," *Hum Reprod*, 2003, 18(10):2166-8.

Chen KJ, "The Effect and Abuse Syndrome of Ginseng," *J Tradit Chin Med*, 1981, 1 (1):69-72.

Chong SK and Oberholzer VG, "Ginseng - Is There a Use in Clinical Medicine?" *Postgrad Med J*, 1988, 64(757):841-6.

Dukes MN, "Ginseng and Mastalgia," *Br Med J*, 1978, 1(6127):1621.

Hiai S, et al, "Stimulation of Pituitary-Adrenocortical System by Ginseng Saponin," *J Endocrinol Jpn*, 1979, 26(6):661-5.

Hopkins MP, Androff L, and Benninghoff AS, "Ginseng Face Cream and Unexplained Vaginal Bleeding," *Am J Obstet Gynecol*, 1988, 159(5):1121-2

Janetzky K and Morreale AP, "Probable Interaction Between Warfarin and Ginseng," *Am J Health Syst Pharm*, 1997, 54(6):692-3.

Jones BD and Runikis AM, "Interaction of Ginseng With Phenelzine," *J Clin Psychopharmacol*, 1987, 7(3):201-2.

Kim JY, Germolec DR, and Luster MI, "*Panax ginseng* as a Potential Immunomodulator: Studies in Mice," *Immunopharmacol Immunotoxicol*, 1990, 12(2):257-76.

Natural Standard Research Collaboration, Chief Editors: Ulbricht C, Basch E, *Natural Standard Herb and Supplement Reference - Evidence-Based Clinical Reviews*, USA: Elsevier/Mosby, 2005.

Ng TB and Yeung HW, "Hypoglycemic Constituents of *Panax ginseng*," *Gen Pharmacol*, 1985, 16(6):549-52.

Palop-Larrea V, González-Perales JL, Catálan-Oliver C, et al, "Metrorrhagia and Ginseng," *Ann Pharmacother*, 2000, 34(11):1347-8.

Reay JL, Kennedy DO, and Scholey AB, "The Glycaemic Effects of Single Doses of *Panax ginseng* in Young Healthy Volunteers," *Br J Nutr*, 2006, 96(4):639-42.

Siegel RK, "Ginseng and High Blood Pressure," *JAMA*, 1980, 243(1):32.

Teng CM, Kuo SC, Kof N, et al, "Antiplatelet Actions of Panaxynol and Ginsenosides Isolated From Ginseng," *Biochim Biophys Acta*, 1989, 990(3):315-20.

Vuksan V, Sievenpiper JL, Koo VY, et al, "American Ginseng (*Panax quinquefolius* L) Reduces Postprandial Glycemia in Nondiabetic Subjects and Subjects With Type 2 Diabetes Mellitus," *Arch Intern Med*, 2000, 160(7):1009-13.

Vuksan V, Stavro MP, Sievenpiper JL, et al, "Similar Postprandial Glycemic Reductions With Escalation of Dose and Administration Time of American Ginseng in Type 2 Diabetes," *Diabetes Care*, 2000, 23(9):1221-6.

Ginseng, Siberian *(Eleutherococcus senticosus)*

Natural Product Category Herb

Synonyms *Eleutherococcus senticosus*; Devil's Shrub; Siberian Ginseng

Plant Part Root

Dosage and Standardization Oral: 100-200 mg twice daily, standardized to contain 0.8% eleutherosides B and E per dose. A regimen of 4 weeks on, 2 weeks off is recommended for maximum benefit.

Reported Uses

Adaptogen/tonic (promote wellness) (Brekhman, 1965; Brekhman, 1969)

Athletic performance (enhancement); stress (decrease fatigue); immune support (Hikino, 1986)

Summary Although Siberian ginseng is a member of the ginseng family, it is of a different genus than the *Panax* or Asian varieties. It has been used for thousands of years in traditional Chinese medicine and in Russia and has been shown to improve energy and vitality. Siberian ginseng has been reported to increase stamina and endurance and to protect the body systems against stress-induced illness. It is believed to increase the body's ability to adapt to chemical, physical, psychological, and biological stressors (adaptogen). As an aid to general health, it has been used in chronic illnesses such as atherosclerosis, diabetes mellitus, and hypertension.

Effect on Mental Status May cause agitation, insomnia, mania, or nervousness

Effect on Psychiatric Treatment Avoid concurrent use with MAO inhibitors. Avoid use in patients with psychosis or bipolar disorder. Effects of barbiturates and CNS stimulants may be increased; use caution. May produce hypotension; concurrent use with psychotropic agents may produce additive effects.

Pharmacology The eleutheroside content of Siberian ginseng is believed to be responsible for its ability to facilitate adaptation to stress. In addition, polysaccharides in Siberian ginseng appear to act as immune stimulants. Siberian ginseng has been demonstrated to improve adaptation to reduced cellular oxygen levels, thermal changes, and radiation and toxic exposures (chemotherapy, alcohol, and environmental). It enhances immunity, leading to resistance against viral and microbial infections. Reported benefits include increased physical endurance, mental alertness, increased amount and quality of work performed, decreased sick days, and enhanced athletic performance.

Theoretical Cautions and Contraindications Based on pharmacologic activity, use with caution with stimulant products, including decongestants, caffeine, and caffeine-containing beverages.

Based on pharmacologic activity, use with caution in individuals with hypertension or in individuals receiving antihypertensive medications; and in individuals at risk of hypotension (including those taking antihypertensive medication or agents that predispose to orthostasis), elderly individuals, or those who would not tolerate transient hyper- or hypotensive episodes (ie, cerebrovascular or cardiovascular disease). May potentiate effects of antihypertensives.

Use with caution in individuals taking barbiturates (based on *in vitro* or animal studies) (McRae, 1996; Medon, 1984).

Use with caution in individuals with diabetes or in those who may be predisposed to hypoglycemia; may alter glucose regulation. Effects of drugs with hypoglycemic activity may be potentiated (including insulin and oral hypoglycemics). Blood sugar should be closely monitored and the dosage of hypoglycemic medications may require adjustment. This should be carefully coordinated among the individual's healthcare providers.

Based on pharmacologic activity and case reports, hemostasis may be affected. Based on pharmacologic activity, this herb may be contraindicated in individuals with active bleeding (eg, peptic ulcer, intracranial bleeding). Use with caution in individuals with a history of bleeding, hemostatic disorders, or drug-related hemostatic problems; and in individuals taking anticoagulant medications, including warfarin, aspirin, aspirin-containing products, NSAIDs, or antiplatelet agents (eg, ticlopidine, clopidogrel, dipyridamole). Discontinue use prior to dental or surgical procedures (generally at least 14 days before).

Extensive or prolonged use may heighten estrogenic activity (based on pharmacologic activity).

General Warnings Use with caution in pregnancy (based on a study in rat embryos and the effects of ginsenoside Rb1, a chemical found in many commercially available products).

Use all herbal supplements with extreme caution in children <2 years of age and in pregnancy or lactation. Some herbs are contraindicated in pregnancy or lactation; make sure to observe warnings. Use with caution in individuals on medication and with pre-existing medical conditions. Always review for potential herb-drug interactions (HDIs) and other warnings. Large and prolonged doses may increase the potential for adverse effects. Herbs may cause transient adverse effects such as nausea, vomiting, and GI distress due to a variety of chemical constituents. Use caution in individuals having known allergies to plants.

Theoretical Interactions Barbiturates, antihypertensives, anticoagulant medications (including warfarin), aspirin or aspirin-containing products, NSAIDs, antiplatelet agents (eg, ticlopidine, clopidogrel, dipyridamole), insulin, oral hypoglycemics, digoxin, stimulants (including OTC stimulants)

References

Brekhman II and Kirillov OI, "Effect of *Eleutherococcus* on Alarm-Phase of Stress," *Life Sci*, 1969, 8(3):113-21.

Brekhman II and Maianskii GM, "*Eleutherococcus* - a Means of Increasing the Nonspecific Resistance of the Organism," *Izv Akad Nauk SSSR Biol*, 1965, 5:762-5.

Chan LY, Chiu PY, and Lau TK, "An *In-Vitro* Study of Ginsenoside Rb1-Induced Teratogenicity Using a Whole Rat Embryo Culture Model," *Hum Reprod*, 2003, 18 (10):2166-8.

Hikino H, Takahashi M, Otakek, et al, "Isolation and Hypoglycemic Activity of Eleutherans A, B, C, D, E, F and G: Glycans of *Eleutherococcus senticosus* Roots," *J Nat Prod*, 1986, 49 (2):293-7.

McRae S, "Elevated Serum Digoxin Levels in a Patient Taking Digoxin and Siberian Ginseng," *CMAJ*, 1996, 155(3):293-5.

Medon PJ, Ferguson PW, and Watson CF, "Effects of *Eleutherococcus senticosus* Extracts on Hexobarbital Metabolism *In Vivo* and *In Vitro*," *J Ethnopharmacol*, 1984, 10(2):235-41.

Natural Standard Research Collaboration, Chief Editors: Ulbricht C, Basch E, *Natural Standard Herb and Supplement Reference - Evidence-Based Clinical Reviews*, USA: Elsevier/Mosby, 2005.

◆ **Glargine Insulin** *see* Insulin Glargine *on page 827*

Glatiramer Acetate (gla TIR a mer AS e tate)

Medication Safety Issues

Sound-alike/look-alike issues:

Copaxone® may be confused with Compazine®

U.S. Brand Names Copaxone®

Canadian Brand Names Copaxone®

Index Terms Copolymer-1

Pharmacologic Category Biological, Miscellaneous

Generic Available No

Use Management of relapsing-remitting type multiple sclerosis

Effect on Mental Status May cause anxiety or depression

Effect on Psychiatric Treatment None reported

Pregnancy Risk Factor B

Pregnancy Considerations Adverse events were not observed in animal studies. There are no adequate and well-controlled studies in pregnant women. Use in pregnancy only if clearly necessary.

Lactation Excretion in breast milk unknown/use caution

Contraindications Hypersensitivity to glatiramer acetate, mannitol, or any component of the formulation

Warnings/Precautions For SubQ use only, **not for I.V. administration**. Glatiramer acetate is antigenic, and may possibly lead to the induction of untoward host responses. Immediate postinjection systemic reactions occur in a substantial percentage of patients (~10% in premarketing studies); symptoms may begin within minutes of injection and usually spontaneously resolve within 30 minutes. Most patients only have one reaction despite repeated administration. Safety and efficacy has not been established in patients with renal impairment, in the elderly, or in patients <18 years of age.

Adverse Reactions

>10%:

Cardiovascular: Vasodilation (27%), chest pain (21%), palpitation (17%)

Central nervous system: Pain (28%), anxiety (23%)

Dermatologic: Pruritus (18%), rash (18%)

Gastrointestinal: Nausea (22%), diarrhea (12%)

Local: Injection site reactions: Pain (73%), erythema (66%), inflammation (49%), pruritus (40%), mass (27%), induration (13%), welt (11%)

Neuromuscular & skeletal: Weakness (41%), arthralgia (24%), hypertonia (22%), back pain (16%)

Respiratory: Dyspnea (19%), rhinitis (14%)

Miscellaneous: Infection (50%), flu-like syndrome (19%), diaphoresis (15%), lymphadenopathy (12%)

1% to 10%:

Cardiovascular: Peripheral edema (7%), facial edema (6%), syncope (5%), tachycardia (5%), edema (3%), hypertension (1%)

Central nervous system: Fever (8%), vertigo (6%), migraine (5%), agitation (4%), chills (4%), confusion (2%), nervousness (2%), speech disorder (2%)

Dermatologic: Bruising (8%), erythema (4%), urticaria (4%), skin nodule (2%), eczema (1%), pustular rash (1%), skin atrophy (1%)

Endocrine & metabolic: Dysmenorrhea (6%)

Gastrointestinal: Anorexia (8%), vomiting (6%), gastrointestinal disorder (5%), gastroenteritis (3%), weight gain (3%), oral moniliasis (1%), salivary gland enlargement (1%), ulcerative stomatitis (1%)

Genitourinary: Urinary urgency (10%), vaginal moniliasis (8%), hematuria (1%)
Local: Injection site reactions: Hemorrhage (5%), urticaria (5%), edema (1%), atrophy (1%), abscess (1%), hypersensitivity (1%)
Neuromuscular & skeletal: Neck pain (8%), tremor (7%), foot drop (3%)
Ocular: Eye disorder (4%), nystagmus (2%)
Otic: Ear pain (7%)
Respiratory: Bronchitis (9%), laryngismus (5%)
Miscellaneous: Bacterial infection (5%), herpes simplex (4%), cyst (2%), herpes zoster (1%)

<1% (Limited to important or life-threatening): Allergic reaction, anaphylactoid reaction, angina, angioedema, aphasia, arrhythmia, atrial fibrillation, blindness; carcinoma (breast, bladder, lung); cardiomyopathy, CHF, cholecystitis, cholelithiasis, cirrhosis, CNS neoplasm, coma, corneal ulcer, effusion, esophageal ulcer, esophagitis, ethanol intolerance, gastrointestinal hemorrhage, GI carcinoma, glaucoma, gout, hallucination, hematemesis, hepatitis, hepatomegaly, hypotension, injection site abscess, injection site fibrosis, leukopenia, lupus erythematosus, manic reaction, meningitis, MI, neuralgia, optic neuritis, pancreatitis, pancytopenia, paraplegia, pericardial, photosensitivity reaction, postural hypotension, priapism, pulmonary embolism, rash, renal failure, rheumatoid arthritis, seizure, sepsis, serum sickness, splenomegaly, stomatitis, stroke, thrombocytopenia, thrombosis

Drug Interactions

There are no known significant interactions.

Stability Store in refrigerator at 2°C to 8°C (36°F to 46°F); excursions to room temperature for up to 1 month do not have a negative impact on potency. Avoid heat; protect from intense light.

Mechanism of Action Glatiramer is a mixture of random polymers of four amino acids; L-alanine, L-glutamic acid, L-lysine and L-tyrosine, the resulting mixture is antigenically similar to myelin basic protein, which is an important component of the myelin sheath of nerves; glatiramer is thought to induce and activate T-lymphocyte suppressor cells specific for a myelin antigen, it is also proposed that glatiramer interferes with the antigen-presenting function of certain immune cells opposing pathogenic T-cell function

Pharmacodynamics/Kinetics

Distribution: Small amounts of intact and partial hydrolyzed drug enter lymphatic circulation
Metabolism: SubQ: Large percentage hydrolyzed locally

Dosage Adults: SubQ: 20 mg daily

Administration For SubQ administration in the arms, abdomen, hips, or thighs; rotate injection sites to prevent lipoatrophy. Bring to room temperature prior to use. Visually inspect the solution; discard if solution is cloudy or contains any particulate matter.

Dosage Forms Excipient information presented when available (limited, particularly for generics); consult specific product labeling.

Injection, solution [preservative free]:
Copaxone®: 20 mg/mL (1 mL) [prefilled syringe; contains mannitol; packaged with alcohol pads]

◆ **Gleevec®** *see* Imatinib *on page 810*
◆ **Gliadel®** *see* Carmustine *on page 284*
◆ **Glibenclamide** *see* GlyBURIDE *on page 730*

Glimepiride (GLYE me pye ride)

Medication Safety Issues

Sound-alike/look-alike issues:
Glimepiride may be confused with glipiZIDE
Amaryl® may be confused with Altace®, Amerge®, Reminyl®

High alert medication: The Institute for Safe Medication Practices (ISMP) includes this medication among its list of drugs which have a heightened risk of causing significant patient harm when used in error.

U.S. Brand Names Amaryl®

Canadian Brand Names Amaryl®; Apo-Glimepiride; CO Glimepiride; Novo-Glimepiride; PMS-Glimepiride; ratio-Glimepiride; Rhoxal-glimepiride; Sandoz-Glimepiride

Mexican Brand Names Amaryl

Pharmacologic Category Antidiabetic Agent, Sulfonylurea

Generic Available Yes

Use Management of type 2 diabetes mellitus (noninsulin dependent, NIDDM) as an adjunct to diet and exercise to lower blood glucose; may be used in combination with metformin or insulin in patients whose hyperglycemia cannot be controlled by diet and exercise in conjunction with a single oral hypoglycemic agent

Effect on Mental Status None reported

Effect on Psychiatric Treatment May rarely cause agranulocytosis; use caution with clozapine and carbamazepine; phenothiazines and TCAs may antagonize glimepiride hypoglycemic effects; MAO inhibitors and TCAs may enhance hypoglycemic effects

Pregnancy Risk Factor C

Pregnancy Considerations

Adverse events have been observed in animal studies; therefore, glimepiride is classified as pregnancy category C. Severe hypoglycemia lasting 4-10 days has been noted in infants born to mothers taking a sulfonylurea at the time of delivery. The manufacturer recommends that patients be switched to insulin during pregnancy. Maternal hyperglycemia can be associated with adverse effects in the fetus, including macrosomia, neonatal hyperglycemia, and hyperbilirubinemia; the risk of congenital malformations is increased when the Hb A_{1c} is above the normal range. Diabetes can also be associated with adverse effects in the mother. Poorly-treated diabetes may cause end-organ damage that may in turn negatively affect obstetric outcomes. Physiologic glucose levels should be maintained prior to and during pregnancy to decrease the risk of adverse events in the mother and the fetus. Until additional safety and efficacy data are obtained, the use of oral agents is generally not recommended as routine management of GDM or type 2 diabetes mellitus during pregnancy. Insulin is the drug of choice for the control of diabetes mellitus during pregnancy.

Lactation Excretion in breast milk unknown/not recommended

Contraindications Hypersensitivity to glimepiride, any component of the formulation, or sulfonamides; diabetic ketoacidosis (with or without coma)

Warnings/Precautions All sulfonylurea drugs are capable of producing severe hypoglycemia. Hypoglycemia is more likely to occur when caloric intake is deficient, after severe or prolonged exercise, when ethanol is ingested, or when more than one glucose-lowering drug is used. It is also more likely in elderly patients, malnourished patients and in patients with impaired renal or hepatic function; use with caution.

Chemical similarities are present among sulfonamides, sulfonylureas, carbonic anhydrase inhibitors, thiazides, and loop diuretics (except ethacrynic acid). Use in patients with sulfonamide allergy is specifically contraindicated in product labeling, however, a risk of cross-reaction exists in patients with allergy to any of these compounds; avoid use when previous reaction has been severe.

Product labeling states oral hypoglycemic drugs may be associated with an increased cardiovascular mortality as compared to treatment with diet alone or diet plus insulin. Data to support this association are limited, and several studies, including a large prospective trial (UKPDS) have not supported an association.

It may be necessary to discontinue therapy and administer insulin if the patient is exposed to stress (fever, trauma, infection, surgery). Safety and efficacy have not been established in children.

Adverse Reactions

1% to 10%:

- Central nervous system: Dizziness (2%), headache (2%)
- Endocrine & metabolic: Hypoglycemia (1% to 2%)
- Gastrointestinal: Nausea (1%)
- Neuromuscular & skeletal: Weakness (2%)

<1% or frequency not defined: Agranulocytosis, anorexia, aplastic anemia, cholestatic jaundice, constipation, diarrhea, disulfiram-like reaction, diuretic effect, edema, epigastric fullness, gastrointestinal pain, erythema, heartburn, hemolytic anemia, hepatitis, hypoglycemia, hyponatremia, leukopenia, liver function tests abnormal, nausea, pancytopenia, photosensitivity, porphyria cutanea tarda, pruritus, rash (morbilliform or maculopapular), SIADH, thrombocytopenia, urticaria, vasculitis (allergic), visual accommodation changes (early treatment), vomiting

Metabolism/Transport Effects Substrate of CYP2C9 (major)

Drug Interactions

Alcohol (Ethyl): Sulfonylureas may enhance the adverse/toxic effect of Alcohol (Ethyl). A flushing reaction may occur. *Risk C: Monitor therapy*

Chloramphenicol: May decrease the metabolism of Sulfonylureas. *Risk C: Monitor therapy*

Cimetidine: May decrease the metabolism of Sulfonylureas. *Risk C: Monitor therapy*

Corticosteroids (Orally Inhaled): May diminish the hypoglycemic effect of Antidiabetic Agents. In some instances, corticosteroid-mediated HPA axis suppression has led to episodes of acute adrenal crisis, which may manifest as enhanced hypoglycemia, particularly in the setting of insulin or other antidiabetic agent use. *Risk C: Monitor therapy*

Corticosteroids (Systemic): May diminish the hypoglycemic effect of Antidiabetic Agents. In some instances, corticosteroid-mediated HPA axis suppression has led to episodes of acute adrenal crisis, which may manifest as enhanced hypoglycemia, particularly in the setting of insulin or other antidiabetic agent use. *Risk C: Monitor therapy*

Cyclic Antidepressants: May enhance the hypoglycemic effect of Sulfonylureas. *Risk C: Monitor therapy*

CycloSPORINE: Sulfonylureas may increase the serum concentration of CycloSPORINE. *Risk C: Monitor therapy*

CYP2C9 Inducers (Highly Effective): May increase the metabolism of CYP2C9 Substrates (High risk). *Risk C: Monitor therapy*

CYP2C9 Inhibitors (Moderate): May decrease the metabolism of CYP2C9 Substrates (High risk). *Risk C: Monitor therapy*

CYP2C9 Inhibitors (Strong): May decrease the metabolism of CYP2C9 Substrates (High risk). *Risk D: Consider therapy modification*

Fibric Acid Derivatives: May enhance the hypoglycemic effect of Sulfonylureas. *Risk C: Monitor therapy*

Fluconazole: May increase the serum concentration of Sulfonylureas. *Risk C: Monitor therapy*

Herbs (Hypoglycemic Properties): May enhance the hypoglycemic effect of Hypoglycemic Agents. *Risk C: Monitor therapy*

Luteinizing Hormone-Releasing Hormone Analogs: May diminish the therapeutic effect of Antidiabetic Agents. *Risk C: Monitor therapy*

Pegvisomant: May enhance the hypoglycemic effect of Antidiabetic Agents. *Risk C: Monitor therapy*

Quinolone Antibiotics: May enhance the hyperglycemic effect of Sulfonylureas. Quinolone Antibiotics may enhance the hypoglycemic effect of Sulfonylureas. *Risk C: Monitor therapy*

Rifampin: May increase the metabolism of Sulfonylureas. *Risk C: Monitor therapy*

Salicylates: May enhance the hypoglycemic effect of Sulfonylureas. Of concern with regular, higher doses of salicylates, not sporadic, low doses. *Risk C: Monitor therapy*

Somatropin: May diminish the hypoglycemic effect of Antidiabetic Agents. *Risk D: Consider therapy modification*

Sulfonamide Derivatives: May enhance the hypoglycemic effect of Sulfonylureas. **Exceptions:** Sulfacetamide. *Risk C: Monitor therapy*

Ethanol/Nutrition/Herb Interactions

Ethanol: Caution with ethanol (may cause hypoglycemia).

Herb/Nutraceutical: Caution with chromium, garlic, gymnema (may cause hypoglycemia).

Mechanism of Action Stimulates insulin release from the pancreatic beta cells; reduces glucose output from the liver; insulin sensitivity is increased at peripheral target sites

Pharmacodynamics/Kinetics

Onset of action: Peak effect: Blood glucose reductions: 2-3 hours

Duration: 24 hours

Absorption: 100%; delayed when given with food

Distribution: V_d: 8.8 L

Protein binding: >99.5%

Metabolism: Hepatic oxidation via CYP2C9 to M1 metabolite (~33% activity of parent compound); further oxidative metabolism to inactive M2 metabolite

Half-life elimination: 5-9 hours

Time to peak, plasma: 2-3 hours

Excretion: Urine (60%, 80% to 90% as M1 and M2); feces (40%, 70% as M1 and M2)

Dosage Oral:

Children 10-18 years (unlabeled use): Initial: 1 mg once daily; maintenance: 1-4 mg once daily

Adults: Initial: 1-2 mg once daily, administered with breakfast or the first main meal; usual maintenance dose: 1-4 mg once daily; after a dose of 2 mg once daily, increase in increments of 2 mg at 1- to 2-week intervals based upon the patient's blood glucose response to a maximum of 8 mg once daily. If inadequate response to maximal dose, combination therapy with metformin may be considered.

Combination with insulin therapy (fasting glucose level for instituting combination therapy is in the range of >150 mg/dL in plasma or serum depending on the patient): initial recommended dose: 8 mg once daily with the first main meal

After starting with low-dose insulin, upward adjustments of insulin can be done approximately weekly as guided by frequent measurements of fasting blood glucose. Once stable, combination-therapy patients should monitor their capillary blood glucose on an ongoing basis, preferably daily.

Conversion from therapy with long half-life agents: Observe patient carefully for 1-2 weeks when converting from a longer half-life agent (eg, chlorpropamide) to glimepiride due to overlapping hypoglycemic effects.

Dosing adjustment/comments in renal impairment: Cl_{cr} <22 mL/minute: Initial starting dose should be 1 mg and dosage increments should be based on fasting blood glucose levels

Dosing adjustment in hepatic impairment: No data available

Elderly: Initial: 1 mg/day; dose titration and maintenance dosing should be conservative to avoid hypoglycemia

Dietary Considerations Administer with breakfast or the first main meal of the day. Dietary modification based on ADA recommendations is a part of therapy. Decreases blood glucose concentration. Hypoglycemia may occur. Must be able to recognize symptoms of hypoglycemia (palpitations, sweaty palms, lightheadedness).

Administration Administer once daily with breakfast or first main meal of the day. Patients who are NPO may need to have their dose held to avoid hypoglycemia.

Monitoring Parameters Urine for glucose and ketones; monitor for signs and symptoms of hypoglycemia (fatigue, excessive hunger, profuse sweating, numbness of extremities), fasting blood glucose, hemoglobin A_{1c}, fructosamine

Reference Range Recommendations for glycemic control in adults with diabetes:

Hb A_{1c}: <7%

Preprandial capillary plasma glucose: 70-130 mg/dL

Peak postprandial capillary blood glucose: <180 mg/dL

Blood pressure: <130/80 mm Hg

Dosage Forms Excipient information presented when available (limited, particularly for generics); consult specific product labeling.

Tablet: 1 mg, 2 mg, 4 mg

Amaryl®: 1 mg, 2 mg, 4 mg

◆ **Glimepiride and Pioglitazone** *see* Pioglitazone and Glimepiride *on page 1300*

◆ **Glimepiride and Pioglitazone Hydrochloride** *see* Pioglitazone and Glimepiride *on page 1300*

◆ **Glimepiride and Rosiglitazone Maleate** *see* Rosiglitazone and Glimepiride *on page 1448*

GlipiZIDE (GLIP i zide)

Medication Safety Issues

Sound-alike/look-alike issues:

GlipiZIDE may be confused with glimepiride, glyBURIDE

Glucotrol® may be confused with Glucophage®, Glucotrol® XL, glyBURIDE

Glucotrol® XL may be confused with Glucotrol®

High alert medication: The Institute for Safe Medication Practices (ISMP) includes this medication among its list of drugs which have a heightened risk of causing significant patient harm when used in error.

U.S. Brand Names Glucotrol XL®; Glucotrol®

Mexican Brand Names Flumedil; Gabaz; Luditec; Minodiab; Singloben

Index Terms Glydiazinamide

Pharmacologic Category Antidiabetic Agent, Sulfonylurea

Generic Available Yes

Use Management of type 2 diabetes mellitus (noninsulin dependent, NIDDM)

Effect on Mental Status None reported

Effect on Psychiatric Treatment May rarely cause agranulocytosis; use caution with clozapine and carbamazepine; phenothiazines and TCAs may antagonize glipizide hypoglycemic effects; MAO inhibitors and TCAs may enhance hypoglycemic effects

Pregnancy Risk Factor C

Pregnancy Considerations Adverse events have been observed in animal studies; therefore, glipizide is classified as pregnancy category C. Glipizide crosses the placenta. Severe hypoglycemia lasting 4-10 days has been noted in infants born to mothers taking a sulfonylurea at the time of delivery. Maternal hyperglycemia can be associated with adverse effects in the fetus, including macrosomia, neonatal hyperglycemia, and hyperbilirubinemia; the risk of congenital malformations is increased when the Hb A_{1c} is above the normal range. Diabetes can also be associated with adverse effects in the mother. Poorly-treated diabetes may cause end-organ damage that may in turn negatively affect obstetric outcomes. Physiologic glucose levels should be maintained prior to and during pregnancy to decrease the risk of adverse events in the mother and the fetus. Until additional safety and efficacy data are obtained, the use of oral agents is generally not recommended as routine management of GDM or type 2 diabetes mellitus during pregnancy. The manufacturer recommends if glipizide is used during pregnancy it should be discontinued at least 1 month before the expected delivery date. Insulin is the drug of choice for the control of diabetes mellitus during pregnancy.

Lactation Excretion in breast milk unknown/not recommended

Contraindications Hypersensitivity to glipizide or any component of the formulation, other sulfonamides; type 1 diabetes mellitus (insulin dependent, IDDM); diabetic ketoacidosis

Warnings/Precautions All sulfonylurea drugs are capable of producing severe hypoglycemia. Hypoglycemia is more likely to occur when caloric intake is deficient, after severe or prolonged exercise, when ethanol is ingested, or when more than one glucose-lowering drug is used. It is also more likely in elderly patients, malnourished patients and in patients with impaired renal or hepatic function; use with caution.

Chemical similarities are present among sulfonamides, sulfonylureas, carbonic anhydrase inhibitors, thiazides, and loop diuretics (except ethacrynic acid). Use in patients with sulfonamide allergy is specifically contraindicated in product labeling, however, a risk of cross-reaction exists in patients with allergy to any of these compounds; avoid use when previous reaction has been severe.

Product labeling states oral hypoglycemic drugs may be associated with an increased cardiovascular mortality as compared to treatment with diet alone or diet plus insulin. Data to support this association are limited, and several studies, including a large prospective trial (UKPDS) have not supported an association.

Use with caution in patients with severe hepatic disease. It may be necessary to discontinue therapy and administer insulin if the patient is exposed to stress (fever, trauma, infection, surgery). Safety and efficacy have not been established in children.

Avoid use of extended release tablets (Glucotrol® XL) in patients with known stricture/narrowing of the GI tract.

Adverse Reactions Frequency not defined.

Cardiovascular: Edema, syncope

Central nervous system: Anxiety, depression, dizziness, drowsiness, headache, hypoesthesia, insomnia, nervousness, pain

Dermatologic: Eczema, erythema, maculopapular eruptions, morbilliform eruptions, photosensitivity, pruritus, rash, urticaria

Endocrine & metabolic: Disulfiram-like reaction, hypoglycemia, hyponatremia, SIADH (rare)

Gastrointestinal: Anorexia, constipation, diarrhea, epigastric fullness, flatulence, gastralgia, heartburn, nausea, vomiting

Hematologic: Agranulocytopenia, aplastic anemia, blood dyscrasias, hemolytic anemia, leukopenia, pancytopenia, porphyria cutanea tarda, thrombocytopenia

Hepatic: Cholestatic jaundice, hepatic porphyria

Neuromuscular & skeletal: Arthralgia, leg cramps, myalgia, paresthesia, tremor

Ocular: Blurred vision

Renal: Diuretic effect (minor)

Respiratory: Rhinitis

Miscellaneous: Diaphoresis

Postmarketing and/or case reports: Abdominal pain

Metabolism/Transport Effects Substrate of 2C9 (major)

Drug Interactions

Alcohol (Ethyl): Sulfonylureas may enhance the adverse/toxic effect of Alcohol (Ethyl). A flushing reaction may occur. *Risk C: Monitor therapy*

Chloramphenicol: May decrease the metabolism of Sulfonylureas. *Risk C: Monitor therapy*

Cimetidine: May decrease the metabolism of Sulfonylureas. *Risk C: Monitor therapy*

Corticosteroids (Orally Inhaled): May diminish the hypoglycemic effect of Antidiabetic Agents. In some instances, corticosteroid-mediated HPA axis suppression has led to episodes of acute adrenal crisis, which may manifest as enhanced hypoglycemia, particularly in the setting of insulin or other antidiabetic agent use. *Risk C: Monitor therapy*

Corticosteroids (Systemic): May diminish the hypoglycemic effect of Antidiabetic Agents. In some instances, corticosteroid-mediated HPA axis suppression has led to episodes of acute adrenal crisis, which may manifest as enhanced hypoglycemia, particularly in the setting of insulin or other antidiabetic agent use. *Risk C: Monitor therapy*

Cyclic Antidepressants: May enhance the hypoglycemic effect of Sulfonylureas. *Risk C: Monitor therapy*

CycloSPORINE: Sulfonylureas may increase the serum concentration of CycloSPORINE. *Risk C: Monitor therapy*

CYP2C9 Inducers (Highly Effective): May increase the metabolism of CYP2C9 Substrates (High risk). *Risk C: Monitor therapy*

CYP2C9 Inhibitors (Moderate): May decrease the metabolism of CYP2C9 Substrates (High risk). *Risk C: Monitor therapy*

CYP2C9 Inhibitors (Strong): May decrease the metabolism of CYP2C9 Substrates (High risk). *Risk D: Consider therapy modification*

Fibric Acid Derivatives: May enhance the hypoglycemic effect of Sulfonylureas. *Risk C: Monitor therapy*

Fluconazole: May increase the serum concentration of Sulfonylureas. *Risk C: Monitor therapy*

Herbs (Hypoglycemic Properties): May enhance the hypoglycemic effect of Hypoglycemic Agents. *Risk C: Monitor therapy*

Luteinizing Hormone-Releasing Hormone Analogs: May diminish the therapeutic effect of Antidiabetic Agents. *Risk C: Monitor therapy*

Pegvisomant: May enhance the hypoglycemic effect of Antidiabetic Agents. *Risk C: Monitor therapy*

Quinolone Antibiotics: May enhance the hyperglycemic effect of Sulfonylureas. Quinolone Antibiotics may enhance the hypoglycemic effect of Sulfonylureas. *Risk C: Monitor therapy*

Rifampin: May increase the metabolism of Sulfonylureas. *Risk C: Monitor therapy*

Salicylates: May enhance the hypoglycemic effect of Sulfonylureas. Of concern with regular, higher doses of salicylates, not sporadic, low doses. *Risk C: Monitor therapy*

Somatropin: May diminish the hypoglycemic effect of Antidiabetic Agents. *Risk D: Consider therapy modification*

Sulfonamide Derivatives: May enhance the hypoglycemic effect of Sulfonylureas. **Exceptions:** Sulfacetamide. *Risk C: Monitor therapy*

Ethanol/Nutrition/Herb Interactions

Ethanol: Caution with ethanol (may cause hypoglycemia or rare disulfiram reaction).

Food: A delayed release of insulin may occur if glipizide is taken with food. Immediate release tablets should be administered 30 minutes before meals to avoid erratic absorption.

Herb/Nutraceutical: Herbs with hypoglycemic properties may enhance the hypoglycemic effect of glipizide. This includes alfalfa, aloe, bilberry, bitter melon, burdock, celery, damiana, fenugreek, garcinia, garlic, ginger, ginseng (American), gymnema, marshmallow, stinging nettle

Mechanism of Action Stimulates insulin release from the pancreatic beta cells; reduces glucose output from the liver; insulin sensitivity is increased at peripheral target sites

Pharmacodynamics/Kinetics

Duration: 12-24 hours

Absorption: Rapid and complete; delayed with food

Distribution: 10-11 L

Protein binding: 98% to 99%; primarily to albumin

Bioavailability: 90% to 100%

Metabolism: Hepatic via CYP2C9; forms metabolites (inactive)

Half-life elimination: 2-5 hours

Time to peak: 1-3 hours; extended release tablets: 6-12 hours

Excretion: Urine (60% to 80%, 91% to 97% as metabolites); feces (11%)

Dosage Oral (allow several days between dose titrations): Adults: Initial: 5 mg/day; adjust dosage at 2.5-5 mg daily increments as determined by blood glucose response at intervals of several days.

Immediate release tablet: Maximum recommended once-daily dose: 15 mg; maximum recommended total daily dose: 40 mg. Doses >15 mg/day should be administered in divided doses.

Extended release tablet (Glucotrol XL®): Maximum recommended dose: 20 mg

When transferring from insulin to glipizide:

Current insulin requirement ≤20 units: Discontinue insulin and initiate glipizide at usual dose

Current insulin requirement >20 units: Decrease insulin by 50% and initiate glipizide at usual dose; gradually decrease insulin dose based on patient response. Several days should elapse between dosage changes.

Elderly: Initial: 2.5 mg/day; increase by 2.5-5 mg/day at 1- to 2-week intervals

Dosing adjustment/comments in renal impairment: Cl_{cr} <10 mL/minute: Some investigators recommend not using

Dosing adjustment in hepatic impairment: Initial dosage should be 2.5 mg/day

Dietary Considerations Take immediate release tablets 30 minutes before meals; extended release tablets should be taken with breakfast. Dietary modification based on ADA recommendations is a part of therapy. Decreases blood glucose concentration. Hypoglycemia may occur. Must be able to recognize symptoms of hypoglycemia (palpitations, sweaty palms, lightheadedness).

Administration Administer immediate release tablets 30 minutes before a meal to achieve greatest reduction in postprandial hyperglycemia. Extended release tablets should be given with breakfast. Patients who are NPO may need to have their dose held to avoid hypoglycemia.

Monitoring Parameters Signs and symptoms of hypoglycemia (fatigue, excessive hunger, profuse sweating, numbness of extremities), blood glucose, hemoglobin A_{1c}

Reference Range Recommendations for glycemic control in adults with diabetes:

Hb A_{1c}: <7%

Preprandial capillary plasma glucose: 70-130 mg/dL

Peak postprandial capillary blood glucose: <180 mg/dL

Blood pressure: <130/80 mm Hg

Dosage Forms Excipient information presented when available (limited, particularly for generics); consult specific product labeling.

Tablet: 5 mg, 10 mg

Glucotrol®: 5 mg, 10 mg

Tablet, extended release: 2.5 mg, 5 mg, 10 mg

Glucotrol XL®: 2.5 mg, 5 mg, 10 mg

Glipizide and Metformin (GLIP i zide & met FOR min)

Medication Safety Issues

High alert medication: The Institute for Safe Medication Practices (ISMP) includes this medication among its list of drugs which have a heightened risk of causing significant patient harm when used in error.

U.S. Brand Names Metaglip™

Index Terms Glipizide and Metformin Hydrochloride; Metformin and Glipizide

Pharmacologic Category Antidiabetic Agent, Biguanide; Antidiabetic Agent, Sulfonylurea

Use Indicated as an adjunct to diet and exercise to improve glycemic control in adults with type 2 diabetes mellitus (noninsulin dependent, NIDDM)

Effect on Mental Status May cause dizziness

Effect on Psychiatric Treatment Diarrhea is common; use caution with SSRIs. May rarely cause agranulocytosis; use caution with clozapine and carbamazepine. Phenothiazines and TCAs may antagonize glipizide hypoglycemic effects; MAO inhibitors and TCAs may enhance hypoglycemic effects.

Dosage Summary

Oral:

Children: Dosage not established

Adults: Initial: Glipizide 2.5 mg and metformin 250 mg once daily; Maintenance: Increase dose by 1 tablet/day every 2 weeks up to a maximum of glipizide 20 mg/day and metformin 2000 mg/day in divided doses

Elderly ≥80 years: Do not use unless renal function verified as normal

Dosage Forms Excipient information presented when available (limited, particularly for generics); consult specific product labeling.

Tablet: 2.5/250: Glipizide 2.5 mg and metformin hydrochloride 250 mg; 2.5/500: Glipizide 2.5 mg and metformin hydrochloride 500 mg; 5/500: Glipizide 5 mg and metformin hydrochloride 500 mg
Metaglip™ 2.5/250: Glipizide 2.5 mg and metformin hydrochloride 250 mg
Metaglip™ 2.5/500: Glipizide 2.5 mg and metformin hydrochloride 500 mg
Metaglip™ 5/500: Glipizide 5 mg and metformin hydrochloride 500 mg

- **Glipizide and Metformin Hydrochloride** *see* Glipizide and Metformin *on page 729*
- **Glivec** *see* Imatinib *on page 810*
- **Glucophage®** *see* MetFORMIN *on page 997*
- **Glucophage® XR** *see* MetFORMIN *on page 997*
- **Glucotrol®** *see* GlipiZIDE *on page 726*
- **Glucotrol XL®** *see* GlipiZIDE *on page 726*
- **Glucovance®** *see* Glyburide and Metformin *on page 733*
- **Glulisine Insulin** *see* Insulin Glulisine *on page 829*
- **Glumetza™** *see* MetFORMIN *on page 997*
- **Glybenclamide** *see* GlyBURIDE *on page 730*
- **Glybenzcyclamide** *see* GlyBURIDE *on page 730*

GlyBURIDE (GLYE byoor ide)

Medication Safety Issues

Sound-alike/look-alike issues:

GlyBURIDE may be confused with glipiZIDE, Glucotrol®
Diaβeta® may be confused with Diabinese®, Zebeta®
Micronase® may be confused with microK®, miconazole, Micronor®, Microzide™

High alert medication: The Institute for Safe Medication Practices (ISMP) includes this medication among its list of drugs which have a heightened risk of causing significant patient harm when used in error.

U.S. Brand Names Diaβeta®; Glynase® PresTab®; Micronase®

Canadian Brand Names Albert® Glyburide; Apo-Glyburide®; Diaβeta®; Euglucon®; Gen-Glybe; Novo-Glyburide; Nu-Glyburide; PMS-Glyburide; ratio-Glyburide; Sandoz-Glyburide

Mexican Brand Names Daonil; Euglucon; Glucal; Norboral

Index Terms Diabeta; Glibenclamide; Glybenclamide; Glybenzcyclamide

Pharmacologic Category Antidiabetic Agent, Sulfonylurea

Generic Available Yes

Use Management of type 2 diabetes mellitus (noninsulin dependent, NIDDM)

Unlabeled/Investigational Use Alternative to insulin in women for the treatment of gestational diabetes mellitus (GDM) (11-33 weeks gestation)

Effect on Mental Status Dizziness is common

Effect on Psychiatric Treatment May rarely cause agranulocytosis; use caution with clozapine and carbamazepine; phenothiazines and TCAs may antagonize glimepiride hypoglycemic effects; MAO inhibitors and TCAs may enhance hypoglycemic effects

Pregnancy Risk Factor B/C (manufacturer dependent)

Pregnancy Considerations Reproduction studies differ by manufacturer labeling. Because adverse events were not observed in animal reproduction studies, one manufacturer classifies glyburide as pregnancy category B. Because adverse events were noted in animal studies during the period of lactation, another manufacturer classifies glyburide as pregnancy category C.

Glyburide was not found to significantly cross the placenta *in vitro* and was not found in the cord serum infants of mothers taking glyburide for gestational diabetes mellitus (GDM). Nonteratogenic effects such as hypoglycemia in the neonate have been associated with maternal glyburide use. Maternal hyperglycemia can be associated with adverse effects in the fetus, including macrosomia, neonatal hyperglycemia, and hyperbilirubinemia; the risk of congenital malformations is increased when the Hb A_{1c} is above the normal range. Diabetes can also be associated with adverse effects in the mother. Poorly-treated diabetes may cause end-organ damage that may in turn negatively affect obstetric outcomes. Physiologic glucose levels should be maintained prior to and during pregnancy to decrease the risk of adverse events in the mother and the fetus. The manufacturer recommends that if glyburide is used during pregnancy, it should be discontinued at least 2 weeks before the expected delivery date. Although studies have shown positive outcomes using glyburide for the treatment of GDM, use may not be appropriate for all women. Until additional safety and efficacy data are obtained, the use of oral agents is generally not recommended as routine management of type 2 diabetes mellitus during pregnancy. Insulin is considered the drug of choice for the control of diabetes mellitus during pregnancy.

Lactation Does not enter breast milk/use caution

Contraindications Hypersensitivity to glyburide, any component of the formulation, or other sulfonamides; type 1 diabetes mellitus (insulin dependent, IDDM), diabetic ketoacidosis; concurrent use with bosentan

Warnings/Precautions All sulfonylurea drugs are capable of producing severe hypoglycemia. Hypoglycemia is more likely to occur when caloric intake is deficient, after severe or prolonged exercise, when ethanol is ingested, or when more than one glucose-lowering drug is used. It is also more likely in elderly patients, malnourished patients and in patients with impaired renal or hepatic function; use with caution.

Elderly: Rapid and prolonged hypoglycemia (>12 hours) despite hypertonic glucose injections have been reported; age and hepatic and renal impairment are independent risk factors for hypoglycemia; dosage titration should be made at weekly intervals.

Chemical similarities are present among sulfonamides, sulfonylureas, carbonic anhydrase inhibitors, thiazides, and loop diuretics (except ethacrynic acid). Use in patients with sulfonamide allergy is specifically contraindicated in product labeling, however, a risk of cross-reaction exists in patients with allergy to any of these compounds; avoid use when previous reaction has been severe.

Product labeling states oral hypoglycemic drugs may be associated with an increased cardiovascular mortality as compared to treatment with diet alone or diet plus insulin. Data to support this association are limited, and several studies, including a large prospective trial (UKPDS) have not supported an association.

It may be necessary to discontinue therapy and administer insulin if the patient is exposed to stress (fever, trauma, infection, surgery). Safety and efficacy have not been established in children.

Adverse Reactions Frequency not defined.

Cardiovascular: Vasculitis

Central nervous system: Headache, dizziness

Dermatologic: Erythema, maculopapular eruptions, morbilliform eruptions, pruritus, purpura, rash, urticaria, photosensitivity reaction

Endocrine & metabolic: Disulfiram-like reaction, hypoglycemia, hyponatremia (SIADH reported with other sulfonylureas)

Gastrointestinal: Nausea, epigastric fullness, heartburn, constipation, diarrhea, anorexia

Genitourinary: Nocturia

Hematologic: Leukopenia, thrombocytopenia, hemolytic anemia, agranulocytosis, aplastic anemia, pancytopenia, porphyria cutanea tarda

Hepatic: Cholestatic jaundice, hepatitis, transaminase increased

Neuromuscular & skeletal: Arthralgia, myalgia, paresthesia

Ocular: Blurred vision

Renal: Diuretic effect (minor)

Miscellaneous: Allergic reaction

Metabolism/Transport Effects Inhibits CYP2C8 (weak), 3A4 (weak)

Drug Interactions

Alcohol (Ethyl): Sulfonylureas may enhance the adverse/toxic effect of Alcohol (Ethyl). A flushing reaction may occur. *Risk C: Monitor therapy*

Bosentan: GlyBURIDE may enhance the hepatotoxic effect of Bosentan. GlyBURIDE may increase the metabolism of Bosentan. Bosentan may increase the metabolism of GlyBURIDE. *Risk X: Avoid combination*

Chloramphenicol: May decrease the metabolism of Sulfonylureas. *Risk C: Monitor therapy*

Cimetidine: May decrease the metabolism of Sulfonylureas. *Risk C: Monitor therapy*

Colesevelam: May decrease the serum concentration of GlyBURIDE. *Risk D: Consider therapy modification*

Corticosteroids (Orally Inhaled): May diminish the hypoglycemic effect of Antidiabetic Agents. In some instances, corticosteroid-mediated HPA axis suppression has led to episodes of acute adrenal crisis, which may manifest as enhanced hypoglycemia, particularly in the setting of insulin or other antidiabetic agent use. *Risk C: Monitor therapy*

Corticosteroids (Systemic): May diminish the hypoglycemic effect of Antidiabetic Agents. In some instances, corticosteroid-mediated HPA axis suppression has led to episodes of acute adrenal crisis, which may manifest as enhanced hypoglycemia, particularly in the setting of insulin or other antidiabetic agent use. *Risk C: Monitor therapy*

Cyclic Antidepressants: May enhance the hypoglycemic effect of Sulfonylureas. *Risk C: Monitor therapy*

CycloSPORINE: Sulfonylureas may increase the serum concentration of CycloSPORINE. *Risk C: Monitor therapy*

Fibric Acid Derivatives: May enhance the hypoglycemic effect of Sulfonylureas. *Risk C: Monitor therapy*

Fluconazole: May increase the serum concentration of Sulfonylureas. *Risk C: Monitor therapy*

Herbs (Hypoglycemic Properties): May enhance the hypoglycemic effect of Hypoglycemic Agents. *Risk C: Monitor therapy*

Luteinizing Hormone-Releasing Hormone Analogs: May diminish the therapeutic effect of Antidiabetic Agents. *Risk C: Monitor therapy*

Pegvisomant: May enhance the hypoglycemic effect of Antidiabetic Agents. *Risk C: Monitor therapy*

Quinolone Antibiotics: May enhance the hyperglycemic effect of Sulfonylureas. Quinolone Antibiotics may enhance the hypoglycemic effect of Sulfonylureas. *Risk C: Monitor therapy*

Rifampin: May increase the metabolism of Sulfonylureas. *Risk C: Monitor therapy*

Salicylates: May enhance the hypoglycemic effect of Sulfonylureas. Of concern with regular, higher doses of salicylates, not sporadic, low doses. *Risk C: Monitor therapy*

Somatropin: May diminish the hypoglycemic effect of Antidiabetic Agents. *Risk D: Consider therapy modification*

Sulfonamide Derivatives: May enhance the hypoglycemic effect of Sulfonylureas. **Exceptions:** Sulfacetamide. *Risk C: Monitor therapy*

Ethanol/Nutrition/Herb Interactions

Ethanol: Caution with ethanol (may cause hypoglycemia).

Herb/Nutraceutical: Herbs with hypoglycemic properties may enhance the hypoglycemic effect of glyburide. This includes alfalfa, aloe, bilberry, bitter melon, burdock, celery, damiana, fenugreek, garcinia, garlic, ginger, ginseng (American), gymnema, marshmallow, stinging nettle

Mechanism of Action Stimulates insulin release from the pancreatic beta cells; reduces glucose output from the liver; insulin sensitivity is increased at peripheral target sites

Pharmacodynamics/Kinetics

Onset of action: Serum insulin levels begin to increase 15-60 minutes after a single dose

Duration: ≤24 hours

Absorption: Significant within 1 hour

Distribution: 9-10 L

Protein binding, plasma: >99% primarily to albumin

Metabolism: Hepatic; forms metabolites (weakly active)

Half-life elimination: Diabeta®, Micronase®: 10 hours; Glynase® PresTab®: ~4 hours; may be prolonged with renal or hepatic impairment

Time to peak, serum: Adults: 2-4 hours

Excretion: Feces (50%) and urine (50%) as metabolites

Dosage Oral: Adults:

DiaBeta®, Micronase®:

Initial: 2.5-5 mg/day, administered with breakfast or the first main meal of the day. In patients who are more sensitive to hypoglycemic drugs, start at 1.25 mg/day.

Increase in increments of no more than 2.5 mg/day at weekly intervals based on the patient's blood glucose response

Maintenance: 1.25-20 mg/day given as single or divided doses; maximum: 20 mg/day

Elderly: Initial: 1.25-2.5 mg/day, increase by 1.25-2.5 mg/day every 1-3 weeks

Micronized tablets (Glynase® PresTab®): Adults:

Initial: 1.5-3 mg/day, administered with breakfast or the first main meal of the day in patients who are more sensitive to hypoglycemic drugs, start at 0.75 mg/day. Increase in increments of no more than 1.5 mg/day in weekly intervals based on the patient's blood glucose response.

Maintenance: 0.75-12 mg/day given as a single dose or in divided doses. Some patients (especially those receiving >6 mg/day) may have a more satisfactory response with twice-daily dosing. Maximum: 12 mg/day

Dosing adjustment/comments in renal impairment: Cl_{cr} <50 mL/minute: **Not recommended**

Dosing adjustment in hepatic impairment: Use conservative initial and maintenance doses and avoid use in severe disease

Dietary Considerations Should be taken with meals at the same time each day. Dietary modification based on ADA recommendations is a part of therapy. Decreases blood glucose concentration. Hypoglycemia may occur. Must be able to recognize symptoms of hypoglycemia (palpitations, sweaty palms, lightheadedness).

Administration Administer with meals at the same time each day. Patients who are anorexic or NPO may need to have their dose held to avoid hypoglycemia.

Monitoring Parameters Signs and symptoms of hypoglycemia, fasting blood glucose, hemoglobin A_{1c}

Reference Range Recommendations for glycemic control in adults with diabetes:

Hb A_{1c}: <7%

Preprandial capillary plasma glucose: 70-130 mg/dL

Peak postprandial capillary blood glucose: <180 mg/dL

Blood pressure: <130/80 mm Hg

Dosage Forms Excipient information presented when available (limited, particularly for generics); consult specific product labeling. [DSC] = Discontinued product

Tablet: 1.25 mg, 2.5 mg, 5 mg

DiaβetaⓇ: 1.25 mg, 2.5 mg, 5 mg

MicronaseⓇ: 1.25 mg, 2.5 mg [DSC], 5 mg

Tablet, micronized: 1.5 mg, 3 mg, 6 mg

GlynaseⓇ PresTabⓇ: 1.5 mg, 3 mg, 6 mg

Glyburide and Metformin (GLYE byoor ide & met FOR min)

Medication Safety Issues

Sound-alike/look-alike issues:

Glucovance may be confused with Vyvanse™

High alert medication: The Institute for Safe Medication Practices (ISMP) includes this medication among its list of drugs which have a heightened risk of causing significant patient harm when used in error.

U.S. Brand Names GlucovanceⓇ

Mexican Brand Names Bi-Euglucon M "5"

Index Terms Glyburide and Metformin Hydrochloride; Metformin and Glyburide

Pharmacologic Category Antidiabetic Agent, Biguanide; Antidiabetic Agent, Sulfonylurea

Use Adjunct to diet and exercise for the management of type 2 diabetes mellitus (noninsulin dependent, NIDDM)

Effect on Mental Status Dizziness is common; may cause sedation

Effect on Psychiatric Treatment May rarely cause agranulocytosis; use caution with clozapine and carbamazepine; phenothiazines and TCAs may antagonize glyburide's hypoglycemic effects; MAO inhibitors and TCAs may enhance hypoglycemic effects; concurrent use with psychotropics may produce additive sedation

Dosage Summary

Oral:

Children: Dosage not established

Adults: Initial: Glyburide 1.25-5 mg and metformin 250-500 mg once or twice daily; Maintenance: Up to glyburide 20 mg/day and /metformin 2000 mg/day

Elderly ≥80 years: Do not use unless renal function verified as normal

Dosage Forms Excipient information presented when available (limited, particularly for generics); consult specific product labeling.

Tablet: 1.25 mg/250 mg: Glyburide 1.25 mg and metformin hydrochloride 250 mg; 2.5 mg/500 mg: Glyburide 2.5 mg and metformin hydrochloride 500 mg; 5 mg/500 mg: Glyburide 5 mg and metformin hydrochloride 500 mg

GlucovanceⓇ: 1.25 mg/250 mg: Glyburide 1.25 mg and metformin hydrochloride 250 mg

GlucovanceⓇ: 2.5 mg/500 mg: Glyburide 2.5 mg and metformin hydrochloride 500 mg

GlucovanceⓇ: 5 mg/500 mg: Glyburide 5 mg and metformin hydrochloride 500 mg

◆ **Glyburide and Metformin Hydrochloride** *see* Glyburide and Metformin *on page 733*

◆ **Glycerol Guaiacolate** *see* GuaiFENesin *on page 737*

◆ **Glyceryl Trinitrate** *see* Nitroglycerin *on page 1147*

Glycopyrrolate (glye koe PYE roe late)

U.S. Brand Names Robinul®; Robinul® Forte
Canadian Brand Names Glycopyrrolate Injection, USP
Index Terms Glycopyrronium Bromide
Pharmacologic Category Anticholinergic Agent
Use Inhibit salivation and excessive secretions of the respiratory tract preoperatively; reversal of neuromuscular blockade; control of upper airway secretions; adjunct in treatment of peptic ulcer
Effect on Mental Status May rarely cause drowsiness, confusion, amnesia
Effect on Psychiatric Treatment Concurrent use with other psychotropics may produce additive sedation and dry mouth
Dosage Forms Excipient information presented when available (limited, particularly for generics); consult specific product labeling. [DSC] = Discontinued product

Injection, solution: 0.2 mg/mL (1 mL, 2 mL, 5 mL, 20 mL)
Robinul®: 0.2 mg/mL (1 mL, 2 mL, 5 mL; 20 mL [DSC]) [contains benzyl alcohol]
Tablet: 1 mg, 2 mg
Robinul®: 1 mg
Robinul® Forte: 2 mg

◆ **Glycopyrronium Bromide** *see* Glycopyrrolate *on page 734*
◆ **Glydiazinamide** *see* GlipiZIDE *on page 726*
◆ **Glynase® PresTab®** *see* GlyBURIDE *on page 730*
◆ **Glyset®** *see* Miglitol *on page 1052*
◆ **GM-CSF** *see* Sargramostim *on page 1462*
◆ **GnRH** *see* Gonadorelin *on page 734*
◆ **GnRH Agonist** *see* Histrelin *on page 769*

Gold Sodium Thiomalate (gold SOW dee um thye oh MAL ate)

U.S. Brand Names Myochrysine®
Canadian Brand Names Myochrysine®
Index Terms Sodium Aurothiomalate
Pharmacologic Category Gold Compound
Use Treatment of progressive rheumatoid arthritis
Effect on Mental Status None reported
Effect on Psychiatric Treatment May rarely cause agranulocytosis; use caution with clozapine and carbamazepine
Dosage Summary

I.M.:

Children: Test dose (recommended): 10 mg first week; Initial dosing: 1 mg/kg/week for 20 weeks; Maintenance: 1 mg/kg every 2-4 weeks

Adults: Test dose: 10 mg first week; Initial dosing: 25 mg second week, then 25-50 mg/week until 1 g cumulative dose has been given; Maintenance: 25-50 mg every 2-3 weeks for 2-20 weeks, then every 3-4 weeks

Dosage Forms Excipient information presented when available (limited, particularly for generics); consult specific product labeling.

Injection, solution:
Myochrysine®: 50 mg/mL (1 mL, 10 mL)

◆ **GoLYTELY®** *see* Polyethylene Glycol-Electrolyte Solution *on page 1310*

Gonadorelin (goe nad oh RELL in)

Medication Safety Issues

Sound-alike/look-alike issues:
Gonadorelin may be confused with gonadotropin, guanadrel
Factrel® may be confused with Sectral®
Gonadotropin may be confused with gonadorelin

U.S. Brand Names Factrel®
Canadian Brand Names Lutrepulse™
Index Terms GnRH; Gonadorelin Acetate; Gonadorelin Hydrochloride; Gonadotropin Releasing Hormone; LHRH; LRH; Luteinizing Hormone Releasing Hormone
Pharmacologic Category Diagnostic Agent; Gonadotropin

Use Evaluation of functional capacity and response of gonadotrophic hormones; evaluate abnormal gonadotropin regulation as in precocious puberty and delayed puberty.

Orphan drug: Lutrepulse®: Induction of ovulation in females with hypothalamic amenorrhea

Effect on Mental Status None reported

Effect on Psychiatric Treatment Antipsychotics may decrease the effects of gonadorelin

Dosage Summary

I.V.:

Acetate:

Children: Dosage not established

Adults: 5 mcg every 90 minutes via Lutrepulse® pump kit at treatment intervals of 21 days (pump will pulsate every 90 minutes for 7 days)

Hydrochloride:

Children <12 years: Use not indicated

Children ≥12 years: 100 mcg administered in women during early phase of menstrual cycle (day 1-7)

Adults: 100 mcg administered in women during early phase of menstrual cycle (day 1-7)

SubQ:

Children <12 years: Dosage not established

Children ≥12 years: 100 mcg administered in women during early phase of menstrual cycle (day 1-7)

Adults: 100 mcg administered in women during early phase of menstrual cycle (day 1-7)

Dosage Forms Excipient information presented when available (limited, particularly for generics); consult specific product labeling.

Injection, powder for reconstitution, as hydrochloride: 100 mcg [diluent contains benzyl alcohol]

◆ **Gonadorelin Acetate** *see* Gonadorelin *on page 734*

◆ **Gonadorelin Hydrochloride** *see* Gonadorelin *on page 734*

◆ **Gonadotropin Releasing Hormone** *see* Gonadorelin *on page 734*

◆ **Good Sense Sleep Aid [OTC]** *see* Doxylamine *on page 510*

◆ **Goody's® Extra Strength Headache Powder [OTC]** *see* Acetaminophen, Aspirin, and Caffeine *on page 39*

◆ **Goody's® Extra Strength Pain Relief [OTC]** *see* Acetaminophen, Aspirin, and Caffeine *on page 39*

◆ **Goody's PM® [OTC]** *see* Acetaminophen and Diphenhydramine *on page 35*

◆ **Gordofilm® [OTC]** *see* Salicylic Acid *on page 1454*

Goserelin (GOE se rel in)

U.S. Brand Names Zoladex®

Canadian Brand Names Zoladex®; Zoladex® LA

Index Terms D-Ser(Bu^t)^6,Azgly^{10}-LHRH; Goserelin Acetate; ICI-118630; NSC-606864

Pharmacologic Category Antineoplastic Agent, Gonadotropin-Releasing Hormone Agonist; Gonadotropin Releasing Hormone Agonist

Use Palliative treatment of advanced breast cancer and carcinoma of the prostate; treatment of endometriosis, including pain relief and reduction of endometriotic lesions; endometrial thinning agent as part of treatment for dysfunctional uterine bleeding

Effect on Mental Status May cause sedation or insomnia

Effect on Psychiatric Treatment Sexual dysfunction is common; concurrent use with SSRIs may produce additive dysfunction

Dosage Summary

SubQ:

Children: Dosage not established

Adults: 3.6 mg every 28 days **or** 10.8 mg every 12 weeks

Dosage Forms Excipient information presented when available (limited, particularly for generics); consult specific product labeling.

Implant, subcutaneous:

Zoladex®:

3.6 mg [1-month implant packaged with 16-gauge hypodermic needle]

10.8 mg [3-month implant packaged with 14-gauge hypodermic needle]

◆ **Goserelin Acetate** *see* Goserelin *on page 735*

◆ **GP 47680** *see* OXcarbazepine *on page 1195*

◆ **GR38032R** *see* Ondansetron *on page 1180*

Granisetron (gra NI se tron)

Medication Safety Issues

Sound-alike/look-alike issues:

Granisetron may be confused with dolasetron, ondansetron, palonosetron

U.S. Brand Names Granisol™; Kytril®; Sancuso®

Canadian Brand Names Kytril®

Mexican Brand Names Kytril

Index Terms BRL 43694

Pharmacologic Category Antiemetic; Selective 5-HT_3 Receptor Antagonist

Use Prophylaxis of nausea and vomiting associated with emetogenic chemotherapy and radiation therapy, (including total body irradiation and fractionated abdominal radiation); prophylaxis and treatment of postoperative nausea and vomiting (PONV)

Transdermal patch: Prophylaxis of nausea and vomiting associated with moderate-to-high emetogenic chemotherapy regimens ≤5 days consecutive duration

Generally **not** recommended for treatment of existing chemotherapy-induced emesis (CIE) or for prophylaxis of nausea from agents with a low emetogenic potential.

Effect on Mental Status May cause anxiety or insomnia

Effect on Psychiatric Treatment None reported

Dosage Summary

I.V.:

Children <2 years: Dosage not established

Children ≥2 years: 10 mcg/kg/dose (maximum: 1 mg/dose) prior to chemotherapy **or** every 12 hours

Adults: 10 mcg/kg/dose (maximum: 1 mg/dose) prior to chemotherapy **or** every 12 hours or 1 mg as a single dose [PONV]

Oral:

Children: Dosage not established

Adults: 2 mg/day in 1-2 divided dose

Transdermal:

Children: Dosage not established

Adults: One patch applied ≥24 hours to ≤48 hours prior to chemotherapy regimen. Maximum duration: Patch may be worn up to 7 days

Dosage Forms Excipient information presented when available (limited, particularly for generics); consult specific product labeling. [DSC] = Discontinued product

Injection, solution: 1 mg/mL (1 mL, 4 mL)

Kytril®: 1 mg/mL (1 mL, 4 mL) [contains benzyl alcohol]

Injection, solution [preservative free]: 0.1 mg/mL (1 mL); 1 mg/mL (1 mL)

Kytril®: 0.1 mg/mL (1 mL)

Solution, oral:

Granisol™: 2 mg/10 mL (30 mL) [contains sodium benzoate; orange flavor]

Kytril®: 2 mg/10 mL (30 mL) [contains sodium benzoate; orange flavor] [DSC]

Tablet: 1 mg

Kytril®: 1 mg

Transdermal system, topical:

Sancuso®: 3.1 mg/24 hours (1s) [52 cm^2, total granisetron 34.3 mg]

◆ **Granisol™** *see* Granisetron *on page 736*

◆ **Granulocyte Colony Stimulating Factor** *see* Filgrastim *on page 632*

◆ **Granulocyte Colony Stimulating Factor (PEG Conjugate)** *see* Pegfilgrastim *on page 1236*

◆ **Granulocyte-Macrophage Colony Stimulating Factor** *see* Sargramostim *on page 1462*

◆ **Grifulvin® V** *see* Griseofulvin *on page 736*

Griseofulvin (gri see oh FUL vin)

Medication Safety Issues

Sound-alike/look-alike issues:

International issues: Fulvicin® (brand name used in international markets) may be confused with Furacin®

U.S. Brand Names Grifulvin® V; Gris-PEG®

Mexican Brand Names Fulcin Forte; Grisovin

Index Terms Griseofulvin Microsize; Griseofulvin Ultramicrosize

Pharmacologic Category Antifungal Agent, Oral

Use Treatment of susceptible tinea infections of the skin, hair, and nails

Effect on Mental Status May cause dizziness, confusion, or insomnia

Effect on Psychiatric Treatment May rarely cause leukopenia; use caution with clozapine and carbamazepine; barbiturates may decrease levels of griseofulvin

Dosage Summary

Oral:

Microsize:

Children ≤2 years: Dosage not established

Children >2 years: 10-15 mg/kg/day in single or divided doses

Adults: 500-1000 mg/day in single or divided doses

Ultramicrosize:

Children ≤2 years: Dosage not established

Children >2 years: 5-15 mg/kg/day in single dose or 2 divided doses (maximum: 750 mg/day)

Adults: 375-750 mg/day in single or divided doses

Dosage Forms Excipient information presented when available (limited, particularly for generics); consult specific product labeling.

Suspension, oral [microsize]: 125 mg/5mL (120 mL)

Grifulvin® V: 125 mg/5 mL (120 mL) [contains alcohol 0.2%]

Tablet, oral [microsize]:

Grifulvin® V: 500 mg

Tablet, oral [ultramicrosize]:

Gris-PEG®: 125 mg, 250 mg

◆ **Griseofulvin Microsize** *see* Griseofulvin *on page 736*

◆ **Griseofulvin Ultramicrosize** *see* Griseofulvin *on page 736*

◆ **Gris-PEG®** *see* Griseofulvin *on page 736*

◆ **Guaicon DM [OTC]** *see* Guaifenesin and Dextromethorphan *on page 739*

◆ **Guaicon DMS [OTC]** *see* Guaifenesin and Dextromethorphan *on page 739*

◆ **Guaifed®** *see* Guaifenesin and Phenylephrine *on page 742*

◆ **Guaifed-PD®** *see* Guaifenesin and Phenylephrine *on page 742*

◆ **Guaifen™ DM [DSC]** *see* Guaifenesin, Dextromethorphan, and Phenylephrine *on page 746*

GuaiFENesin (gwye FEN e sin)

Medication Safety Issues

Sound-alike/look-alike issues:

GuaiFENesin may be confused with guanFACINE

Mucinex® may be confused with Mucomyst®

Naldecon® may be confused with Nalfon®

International issues:

Mucolex® [Hong Kong] may be confused with Mycelex® which is a brand name for clotrimazole in the U.S.

U.S. Brand Names Allfen Jr; Diabetic Tussin® EX [OTC]; Fenesin IR; Ganidin NR; Guiatuss™ [OTC]; Mucinex® Maximum Strength [OTC]; Mucinex® [OTC]; Mucinex®, Children's Mini-Melts™ [OTC]; Mucinex®, Children's [OTC]; Mucinex®, Junior Mini-Melts™ [OTC]; Organidin® NR; Phanasin® Diabetic Choice [OTC]; Phanasin® [OTC]; Refenesen™ 400 [OTC]; Refenesen™ [OTC]; Robitussin® [OTC]; Scot-Tussin® Expectorant [OTC]; Siltussin DAS [OTC]; Siltussin SA [OTC]; Vicks® Casero™ Chest Congestion Relief [OTC]; XPECT™ [OTC]

Canadian Brand Names Balminil Expectorant; Benylin® E Extra Strength; Koffex Expectorant; Robitussin®

Mexican Brand Names Deflenol; Robitussin

Index Terms GG; Glycerol Guaiacolate

Pharmacologic Category Expectorant

Use Help loosen phlegm and thin bronchial secretions to make coughs more productive

Effect on Mental Status May cause drowsiness
Effect on Psychiatric Treatment None reported
Dosage Summary
Oral:
Extended release:
Children <12 years: Dosage not established
Children ≥12 years: 600-1200 mg every 12 hours (maximum: 2.4 g/day)
Adults: 600-1200 mg every 12 hours (maximum: 2.4 g/day)
Immediate release:
Children <6 months: Dosage not established
Children 6 months to 2 years: 25-50 mg every 4 hours (maximum: 300 mg/day)
Children 2-5 years: 50-100 mg every 4 hours (maximum: 600 mg/day)
Children 6-11 years: 100-200 mg every 4 hours (maximum: 1.2 g/day)
Children ≥12 years: 200-400 mg every 4 hours (maximum: 2.4 g/day)
Adults: 200-400 mg every 4 hours (maximum: 2.4 g/day)

Dosage Forms Excipient information presented when available (limited, particularly for generics); consult specific product labeling.
Caplet:
Fenesin IR, Refenesen™ 400: 400 mg
Granules, oral:
Mucinex® Children's Mini-Melts™: 50 mg/packet (12s) [contains phenylalanine 0.6 mg/packet and magnesium 6 mg/packet; grape flavor]
Mucinex® Junior Mini-Melts™: 100 mg/packet (12s) [contains phenylalanine 1 mg/packet and magnesium 10 mg/packet; bubble gum flavor]
Liquid: 100 mg/5 mL (120 mL, 480 mL)
Diabetic Tussin EX®: 100 mg/5 mL (120 mL) [alcohol free, sugar free, dye free; contains phenylalanine 8.4 mg/5 mL]
Ganidin NR: 100 mg/5 mL (480 mL) [raspberry flavor]
Mucinex® Children's: 100 mg/5 mL (120 mL) [alcohol free; grape flavor]
Organidin® NR: 100 mg/5 mL (480 mL) [contains sodium benzoate; raspberry flavor]
Siltussin DAS: 100 mg/5 mL (120 mL) [alcohol free, dye free, sugar free; strawberry flavor]
Syrup: 100 mg/5 mL (120 mL, 480 mL)
Guiatuss™: 100 mg/5 mL (120 mL, 480 mL) [alcohol free; fruit-mint flavor]
Phanasin®: 100 mg/5 mL (120 mL, 240 mL) [alcohol free, sugar free; mint flavor]
Phanasin® Diabetic Choice: 100 mg/5 mL (120 mL) [alcohol free, sugar free; mint flavor]
Robitussin®: 100 mg/5 mL (5 mL, 10 mL, 15 mL, 30 mL, 120 mL, 240 mL, 480 mL) [alcohol free; contains sodium benzoate]
Scot-Tussin® Expectorant: 100 mg/5 mL (120 mL) [alcohol free, dye free, sugar free; contains benzoic acid; grape flavor]
Siltussin SA: 100 mg/5 mL (120 mL, 240 mL, 480 mL) [alcohol free, sugar free; strawberry flavor]
Vicks® Casero™ Chest Congestion Relief: 100 mg/6.25 mL (120 mL, 240 mL) [contains phenylalanine 5.5 mg/12.5 mL, sodium 32 mg/12.5 mL, and sodium benzoate; honey menthol flavor]
Tablet: 200 mg
Allfen Jr: 400 mg [dye free]
Organidin® NR: 200 mg
Refenesen™: 200 mg
XPECT™: 400 mg
Tablet, extended release:
Mucinex®: 600 mg
Mucinex® Maximum Strength: 1200 mg

◆ **Guaifenesin AC** *see* Guaifenesin and Codeine *on page 738*

Guaifenesin and Codeine (gwye FEN e sin & KOE deen)

U.S. Brand Names Brontex®; Cheracol®; Diabetic Tussin C®; Gani-Tuss® NR; Guaifenesin AC; Guaituss AC; Kolephrin® #1; Mytussin® AC; Robafen® AC; Romilar® AC; Tussi-Organidin® NR; Tussi-Organidin® S-NR; Tusso-C™
Index Terms Codeine and Guaifenesin
Pharmacologic Category Antitussive; Cough Preparation; Expectorant
Use Temporary control of cough due to minor throat and bronchial irritation
Effect on Mental Status Drowsiness is common; may cause confusion, headache, dizziness, lightheadedness, false feeling of well being, restlessness,

paradoxical CNS stimulation, or malaise; may rarely cause hallucinations, mental depression, nightmares, or insomnia

Effect on Psychiatric Treatment Constipation and drowsiness are common, this effect may be additive when used concurrently with psychotropics

Restrictions C-V

Dosage Summary

Oral: Also refer to specific product labeling; not all products indicated for each age group

Children <2 years: Dosage not established

Children 2-6 years: Dose based on codeine 1 mg/kg/day in 4 divided doses

Children 6-12 years: 5 mL every 4 hours; maximum 30 mL/day

Children ≥12 years: 1 tablet or 10 mL every 4 hours; maximum 6 tablets or 60 mL per day

Adults: 1 tablet or 10 mL every 4 hours; maximum 6 tablets or 60 mL per day

Dosage Forms Excipient information presented when available (limited, particularly for generics); consult specific product labeling.

Liquid: Guaifenesin 300 mg and codeine phosphate 10 mg per 5 mL (120 mL, 480 mL)

Brontex®: Guaifenesin 75 mg and codeine phosphate 2.5 mg per 5 mL (480 mL) [alcohol free; strawberry mint flavor]

Diabetic Tussin C®: Guaifenesin 200 mg and codeine phosphate 10 mg per 5 mL (480 mL) [contains phenylalanine 0.03 mcg/5 mL; cherry vanilla flavor]

Gani-Tuss® NR: Guaifenesin 100 mg and codeine phosphate 10 mg per 5 mL (480 mL) [raspberry flavor]

Guaifenesin AC: Guaifenesin 100 mg and codeine phosphate 10 mg per 5 mL (120 mL, 480 mL) [alcohol free, sugar free; raspberry flavor]

Kolephrin® #1: Guaifenesin 100 mg and codeine phosphate 10 mg per 5 mL (120 mL) [contains sodium 1.1 mg/5 mL and sodium benzoate]

Tussi-Organidin® NR: Guaifenesin 300 mg and codeine phosphate 10 mg per 5 mL (480 mL) [alcohol free, sugar free; contains sodium benzoate; raspberry flavor]

Tussi-Organidin® S-NR: Guaifenesin 300 mg and codeine phosphate 10 mg per 5 mL (120 mL) [alcohol free, sugar free; contains sodium benzoate; raspberry flavor]

Syrup:

Cheracol®: Guaifenesin 100 mg and codeine phosphate 10 mg per 5 mL (120 mL) [contains alcohol 4.75% and benzoic acid]

Guaituss AC: Guaifenesin 100 mg and codeine phosphate 10 mg per 5 mL (120 mL, 480 mL) [contains alcohol; sugar free; fruit-mint flavor]

Mytussin® AC: Guaifenesin 100 mg and codeine phosphate 10 mg per 5 mL (120 mL, 480 mL) [contains alcohol; sugar free; fruit flavor]

Robafen® AC: Guaifenesin 100 mg and codeine phosphate 10 mg per 5 mL (120 mL, 480 mL)

Romilar® AC: Guaifenesin 100 mg and codeine phosphate 10 mg per 5 mL (480 mL) [alcohol free, sugar free, dye free; contains benzoic acid and phenylalanine; grape flavor]

Tusso-C™: Guaifenesin 200 mg and codeine phosphate 10 mg per 5 mL (480 mL) [alcohol free, dye free, sugar free; contains phenylalanine 0.03 mcg/5 mL; cherry vanilla flavor]

Tablet: Guaifenesin 300 mg and codeine phosphate 10 mg

Brontex®: Guaifenesin 300 mg and codeine phosphate 10 mg

Guaifenesin and Dextromethorphan

(gwye FEN e sin & deks troe meth OR fan)

Medication Safety Issues

Sound-alike/look-alike issues:

Benylin® may be confused with Benadryl®, Ventolin®

U.S. Brand Names Allfen-DM; Altarussin DM [OTC]; Cheracol® D [OTC]; Cheracol® Plus [OTC]; Coricidin HBP® Chest Congestion and Cough [OTC]; Diabetic Tussin® DM Maximum Strength [OTC]; Diabetic Tussin® DM [OTC]; Double Tussin DM [OTC]; Duratuss® DM; Fenesin DM IR; Gani-Tuss DM NR; Genatuss DM® [OTC]; Guaicon DM [OTC]; Guaicon DMS [OTC]; Guaifenex® DM [DSC]; Guia-D; Guiatuss-DM® [OTC]; Hydro-Tussin™ DM [DSC]; Kolephrin® GG/DM [OTC]; Mintab DM; Mucinex® Children's Cough [OTC]; Mucinex® DM Maximum Strength [OTC]; Mucinex® DM [OTC]; Phanatuss® DM [OTC]; Phlemex; Refenesen™ DM [OTC]; Respa-DM®; Robafen DM Clear [OTC]; Robafen DM [OTC]; Robitussin® Cough and Congestion [OTC]; Robitussin® DM Infant [OTC] [DSC]; Robitussin® DM [OTC]; Robitussin® Sugar Free Cough [OTC]; Safe Tussin® DM [OTC]; Scot-Tussin® Senior [OTC]; Silexin [OTC]; Siltussin DM DAS [OTC]; Siltussin DM [OTC]; Simuc-DM;

Su-Tuss DM; Touro® DM; Tussi-Organidin® DM NR; Tussi-Organidin® DM-S NR; Vicks® 44E [OTC]; Vicks® Pediatric Formula 44E [OTC]; Z-Cof LA™

Canadian Brand Names Balminil DM E; Benylin® DM-E; Koffex DM-Expectorant; Robitussin® DM

Mexican Brand Names Bre-A-Col; Cheracol D; Debequin C; Dequin; Dexometorfano-Guaifenesina; Dimacol; Exiadol; Megal; Robitussin DM; Tukol D

Index Terms Dextromethorphan and Guaifenesin

Pharmacologic Category Antitussive; Cough Preparation; Expectorant

Use Temporary control of cough due to minor throat and bronchial irritation

Effect on Mental Status May cause drowsiness

Effect on Psychiatric Treatment Concurrent use with psychotropics may produce additive sedation

Dosage Summary

Oral:

Children <2 years: Dosage not established

Children 2-6 years: Guaifenesin 50-100 mg and dextromethorphan 2.5-5 mg every 4 hours (maximum: Guaifenesin 600 mg/day; Dextromethorphan 30 mg/day)

Children 6-12 years: Guaifenesin 100-200 mg and dextromethorphan 5-10 mg every 4 hours (maximum: Guaifenesin 1200 mg/day; Dextromethorphan 60 mg/day)

Children ≥12 years: Guaifenesin 200-400 mg and dextromethorphan 10-20 mg every 4 hours (maximum: Guaifenesin 2400 mg/day; Dextromethorphan 120 mg/day)

Adults: Guaifenesin 200-400 mg and dextromethorphan 10-20 mg every 4 hours (maximum: Guaifenesin 2400 mg/day; Dextromethorphan 120 mg/day)

Dosage Forms Excipient information presented when available (limited, particularly for generics); consult specific product labeling. [DSC] = Discontinued product

Caplet:

Fenesin DM IR: Guaifenesin 400 mg and dextromethorphan hydrobromide 15 mg

Refenesen™ DM: Guaifenesin 400 mg and dextromethorphan hydrobromide 20 mg

Capsule, softgel:

Coricidin HBP® Chest Congestion and Cough: Guaifenesin 200 mg and dextromethorphan hydrobromide 10 mg

Elixir:

Duratuss DM®: Guaifenesin 225 mg and dextromethorphan hydrobromide 25 mg per 5 mL (480 mL) [contains sodium benzoate; grape flavor]

Simuc-DM: Guaifenesin 225 mg and dextromethorphan hydrobromide 25 mg per 5 mL (480 mL) [grape flavor]

Su-Tuss DM: Guaifenesin 200 mg and dextromethorphan hydrobromide 20 mg per 5 mL (480 mL) [fruit flavor]

Liquid: Guaifenesin 100 mg and dextromethorphan hydrobromide 10 mg per 5 mL (480 mL); guaifenesin 300 mg and dextromethorphan hydrobromide 10 mg per 5 mL (120 mL, 480 mL)

Diabetic Tussin® DM: Guaifenesin 100 mg and dextromethorphan hydrobromide 10 mg per 5 mL (120 mL) [alcohol free, sugar free, dye free; contains phenylalanine 8.4 mg/5 mL]

Diabetic Tussin® DM Maximum Strength: Guaifenesin 200 mg and dextromethorphan hydrobromide 10 mg per 5 mL (120 mL) [alcohol free, sugar free, dye free; contains phenylalanine 8.4 mg/5 mL]

Double Tussin DM: Guaifenesin 300 mg and dextromethorphan hydrobromide 200 mg per 5 mL (120 mL, 480 mL) [alcohol free, dye free, sugar free]

Gani-Tuss® DM NR: Guaifenesin 100 mg and dextromethorphan hydrobromide 10 mg per 5 mL (480 mL) [raspberry flavor]

Hydro-Tussin™ DM: Guaifenesin 200 mg and dextromethorphan hydrobromide 20 mg per 5 mL (480 mL) [alcohol free, sugar free; contains sodium benzoate] [DSC]

Kolephrin® GG/DM: Guaifenesin 150 mg and dextromethorphan hydrobromide 10 mg per 5 mL (120 mL) [alcohol free; cherry flavor]

Mucinex® Children's Cough: Guaifenesin 100 mg and dextromethorphan hydrobromide 5 mg per 5 mL (120 mL) [contains sodium 3 mg/5 mL; cherry flavor]

Safe Tussin® DM: Guaifenesin 100 mg and dextromethorphan hydrobromide 15 mg per 5 mL (120 mL) [contains phenylalanine 4.2 mg/5 mL, benzoic acid, and propylene glycol; orange and mint flavors]

Scot-Tussin® Senior: Guaifenesin 200 mg and dextromethorphan hydrobromide 15 mg per 5 mL (120 mL) [alcohol free, sodium free, sugar free]

Tussi-Organidin® DM NR: Guaifenesin 300 mg and dextromethorphan hydrobromide 10 mg per 5 mL (480 mL) [alcohol free, sugar free; contains sodium benzoate; grape flavor]

Tussi-Organidin® DM-S NR: Guaifenesin 300 mg and dextromethorphan hydrobromide 10 mg per 5 mL (120 mL) [alcohol free, sugar free; contains sodium benzoate; grape flavor]

Vicks® 44E: Guaifenesin 200 mg and dextromethorphan hydrobromide 20 mg per 15 mL (120 mL, 235 mL) [contains sodium 31 mg/15 mL, alcohol, sodium benzoate]

Vicks® Pediatric Formula 44E: Guaifenesin 100 mg and dextromethorphan hydrobromide 10 mg per 15 mL (120 mL) [alcohol free; contains sodium 30 mg/15 mL, sodium benzoate; cherry flavor]

Liquid, oral [drops]:

Robitussin® DM Infant: Guaifenesin 100 mg and dextromethorphan hydrobromide 5 mg per 2.5 mL (30 mL) [alcohol free; contains sodium benzoate; fruit punch flavor] [DSC]

Syrup: Guaifenesin 100 mg and dextromethorphan hydrobromide 10 mg per 5 mL (120 mL, 480 mL)

Altarussin DM: Guaifenesin 100 mg and dextromethorphan hydrobromide 10 mg per 5 mL (120 mL, 240 mL, 480 mL, 3840 mL)

Cheracol® D: Guaifenesin 100 mg and dextromethorphan hydrobromide 10 mg per 5 mL (120 mL, 180 mL) [contains alcohol 4.75%, benzoic acid]

Cheracol® Plus: Guaifenesin 100 mg and dextromethorphan hydrobromide 10 mg per 5 mL (120 mL) [contains alcohol 4.75%, benzoic acid]

Genatuss DM®: Guaifenesin 100 mg and dextromethorphan hydrobromide 10 mg per 5 mL (120 mL)

Guiatuss® DM: Guaifenesin 100 mg and dextromethorphan hydrobromide 10 mg per 5 mL (120 mL, 480 mL, 3840 mL) [alcohol free; contains sodium benzoate]

Guaicon DM®: Guaifenesin 100 mg and dextromethorphan hydrobromide 10 mg per 5 mL (10 mL) [alcohol free]

Guaicon DMS®: Guaifenesin 100 mg and dextromethorphan hydrobromide 10 mg per 5 mL (10 mL) [alcohol free, sugar free]

Mintab DM: Guaifenesin 200 mg and dextromethorphan hydrobromide 10 mg per 5 mL (480 mL) [alcohol free, dye free; cherry vanilla flavor]

Phanatuss® DM: Guaifenesin 100 mg and dextromethorphan hydrobromide 10 mg per 5 mL (120 mL) [alcohol free, sugar free]

Robafen® DM: Guaifenesin 100 mg and dextromethorphan hydrobromide 10 mg per 5 mL (120 mL, 240 mL, 480 mL) [cherry flavor]

Robafen® DM Clear: Guaifenesin 100 mg and dextromethorphan hydrobromide 10 mg per 5 mL (120 mL)

Robitussin® Cough and Congestion: Guaifenesin 100 mg and dextromethorphan hydrobromide 10 mg per 5 mL (120 mL) [alcohol free; contains sodium benzoate]

Robitussin®-DM: Guaifenesin 100 mg and dextromethorphan hydrobromide 10 mg per 5 mL (5 mL, 120 mL, 340 mL, 360 mL) [alcohol free; contains sodium benzoate]

Robitussin® Sugar Free Cough: Guaifenesin 100 mg and dextromethorphan hydrobromide 10 mg per 5 mL (120 mL) [alcohol free, sugar free; contains sodium benzoate]

Silexin: Guaifenesin 100 mg and dextromethorphan hydrobromide 10 mg per 5 mL (45 mL) [alcohol free, sugar free)]

Siltussin DM: Guaifenesin 100 mg and dextromethorphan hydrobromide 10 mg per 5 mL (120 mL, 240 mL, 480 mL) [strawberry flavor]

Siltussin DM DAS: Guaifenesin 100 mg and dextromethorphan hydrobromide 10 mg per 5 mL (120 mL) [alcohol free, dye free, sugar free; strawberry flavor]

Tablet: Guaifenesin 1000 mg and dextromethorphan hydrobromide 60 mg; guaifenesin 1200 mg and dextromethorphan hydrobromide 60 mg

Silexin: Guaifenesin 100 mg and dextromethorphan hydrobromide 10 mg

Tablet, extended release: 800/30: Guaifenesin 800 mg and dextromethorphan hydrobromide 30 mg; 1200/20: Guaifenesin 1200 mg and dextromethorphan hydrobromide 20 mg

Guaifenex® DM: Guaifenesin 600 mg and dextromethorphan hydrobromide 30 mg [DSC]

Mucinex® DM, Respa-DM®: Guaifenesin 600 mg and dextromethorphan hydrobromide 30 mg

Mucophen® DM: Guaifenesin 1000 mg and dextromethorphan hydrobromide 60 mg

Mucinex® DM Maximum Strength: Guaifenesin 1200 mg and dextromethorphan hydrobromide 60 mg

Phlemex: Guaifenesin 1200 mg and dextromethorphan hydrobromide 20 mg

Touro® DM: Guaifenesin 575 mg and dextromethorphan hydrobromide 30 mg

Tablet, long-acting: Guaifenesin 1000 mg and dextromethorphan hydrobromide 60 mg

Z-Cof LA [scored]: Guaifenesin 650 mg and dextromethorphan hydrobromide 30 mg

Tablet, sustained release:

Allfen-DM: Guaifenesin 1000 mg and dextromethorphan hydrobromide 55 mg

Relacon LAX: Guaifenesin 835 mg and dextromethorphan hydrobromide 30 mg

Tussi-Bid®: Guaifenesin 1200 mg and dextromethorphan hydrobromide 60 mg

Tablet, timed release [scored]: Guaifenesin 1200 mg and dextromethorphan hydrobromide 60 mg

Guia-D: Guaifenesin 1000 mg and dextromethorphan hydrobromide 60 mg [dye free]

◆ **Guaifenesin and Dyphylline** *see* Dyphylline and Guaifenesin *on page 522*

◆ **Guaifenesin and Hydrocodone** *see* Hydrocodone and Guaifenesin *on page 779*

Guaifenesin and Phenylephrine (gwye FEN e sin & fen il EF rin)

Medication Safety Issues

Sound-alike/look-alike issues:

Endal® may be confused with Depen®, Intal®

Entex® may be confused with Tenex®

Entex® LA brand name represents a different product in the U.S. than it does in Canada. In the U.S., Entex® LA contains guaifenesin and phenylephrine, while in Canada the product bearing this brand name contains guaifenesin and pseudoephedrine.

U.S. Brand Names Aldex™; Crantex LA; D-Phen 1000; Deconsal® II; Donatussin Drops; Duomax; Duratuss GP®; Duratuss®; ExeFen-PD; ExeTuss [DSC]; ExeTuss-GP; Fenesin PE IR; Genexa™ LA [DSC]; Gentex LA [DSC]; Gilphex TR®; Guaifed-PD®; Guaifed®; Guaiphen-D; Guaiphen-D 1200; Guaiphen-PD; Liquibid-D®; MyDex; Nasex-G; Nexphen PD; norel® EX; Pendex; PhenaVent™ D [DSC]; PhenaVent™ LA [DSC]; PhenaVent™ Ped [DSC]; PhenaVent™ [DSC]; Prolex®-D [DSC]; Prolex®-PD [DSC]; Refenesen™ PE [OTC]; Rescon GG [OTC]; Respa® PE [DSC]; Sil-Tex; Simuc [DSC]; Sina-12X; SINUvent® PE; XPECT-PE™ [DSC]

Index Terms Guaifenesin and Phenylephrine Tannate; Phenylephrine Hydrochloride and Guaifenesin

Pharmacologic Category Decongestant; Expectorant

Use Temporary relief of nasal congestion, sinusitis, rhinitis, and hay fever; temporary relief of cough associated with upper respiratory tract conditions, especially when associated with dry, nonproductive cough

Effect on Mental Status Guaifenesin may cause drowsiness; phenylephrine may cause anxiety or restlessness

Effect on Psychiatric Treatment Concurrent use with psychotropics may produce additive sedation or lessen the effects of anxiolytics depending on whether the effects of guaifenesin or phenylephrine predominate; concurrent use with MAO inhibitors may result in hypertensive crisis; avoid combination

Dosage Summary Note: Dosage varies considerably by product, ranges listed are representative. See specific product labeling.

Oral:

Children 3-6 months: 0.3-0.6 mL; may repeat every 4-6 hours as needed (maximum 4 doses/24 hours) [Donatussin liquid drops]

Children 6 months to 1 year: 0.6-1 mL; may repeat every 4-6 hours as needed (maximum 4 doses/24 hours) [Donatussin liquid drops]

Children 1-2 years: 1-2 mL; may repeat every 4-6 hours as needed (maximum 4 doses/24 hours) [Donatussin liquid drops]

Children 2-6 years: 2.5 mL every 4-6 hours (maximum: 10 mL/day) [Rescon GG] **or** 2.5-5 mL every 12 hours [Sina-12X suspension]

Children 6-12 years: One-half to 1 tablet every 12 hours [Liquibid-D®] **or** 1 capsule every 12 hours [Deconsal® II] **or** 5 mL every 4-6 hours (maximum: 20 mL/day) [Rescon GG] **or** 5-10 mL every 12 hours [Sina-12X suspension]

Children ≥12 years: 1-2 capsules/tablets every 12 hours [Prolex®-PD] **or** 5-10 mL every 4-6 hours (maximum: 40 mL/day) **or** 5-10 mL every 12 hours [Sina-12X suspension]

Adults: 1-2 capsules/tablets every 12 hours [Prolex®-PD] **or** 5-10 mL every 4-6 hours (maximum: 40 mL/day) **or** 5-10 mL every 12 hours [Sina-12X suspension]

Dosage Forms Excipient information presented when available (limited, particularly for generics); consult specific product labeling. [DSC] = Discontinued product

Caplet:
- Fenesin PE IR, Refenesen™ PE: Guaifenesin 400 mg and phenylephrine hydrochloride 10 mg

Capsule:
- Nexphen PD: Guaifenesin 200 mg and phenylephrine hydrochloride 7 mg

Capsule, variable release:
- Deconsal® II: Guaifenesin 375 mg [immediate release] and phenylephrine hydrochloride 20 mg [extended release] [contains tartrazine]
- Genexa™ LA [DSC], PhenaVent™ LA [DSC]: Guaifenesin 400 mg [immediate release] and phenylephrine hydrochloride 30 mg [extended release]
- Guaifed®, PhenaVent™ [DSC]: Guaifenesin 400 mg [immediate release] and phenylephrine hydrochloride 15 mg [extended release]
- Guaifed-PD®, PhenaVent™ Ped [DSC]: Guaifenesin 200 mg [immediate release] and phenylephrine hydrochloride 7.5 mg [extended release]

Liquid: Guaifenesin 100 mg and phenylephrine hydrochloride 7.5 mg per 5 mL (480 mL)
- Sil-Tex: Guaifenesin 100 mg and phenylephrine hydrochloride 7.5 mg per 5 mL (480 mL) [alcohol free, dye-free, sugar free; punch flavor]
- Rescon GG: Guaifenesin 100 mg and phenylephrine hydrochloride 5 mg per 5 mL (120 mL, 480 mL) [cherry orange-pineapple flavor]

Liquid [drops]:
- Donatussin: Guaifenesin 20 mg and phenylephrine hydrochloride 1.5 mg (30 mL) [raspberry flavor]

Suspension:
- Sina-12X: Guaifenesin 100 mg and phenylephrine tannate 5 mg per 5 mL (120 mL) [contains benzoic acid; grape flavor]

Tablet: Guaifenesin 900 mg and phenylephrine hydrochloride 30 mg
- Sina-12X: Guaifenesin 200 mg and phenylephrine tannate 25 mg

Tablet, extended release: Guaifenesin 600 mg and phenylephrine hydrochloride 20 mg; guaifenesin 600 mg and phenylephrine hydrochloride 40 mg; guaifenesin 1200 mg and phenylephrine hydrochloride 40 mg
- Aldex™: Guaifenesin 650 mg and phenylephrine hydrochloride 25 mg
- D-Phen: Guaifenesin 1000 mg and phenylephrine hydrochloride 30 mg
- Duomax: Guaifenesin 1200 mg and phenylephrine hydrochloride 40 mg [Duomatrix release]
- ExeFen-PD: Guaifenesin 600 mg and phenylephrine hydrochloride 10 mg
- Gentex LA: Guaifenesin 650 mg and phenylephrine hydrochloride 23.75 mg [DSC]
- PhenaVent™ D: Guaifenesin 1200 mg and phenylephrine hydrochloride 40 mg [DSC]
- Simuc: Guaifenesin 900 mg and phenylephrine hydrochloride 25 mg [DSC]
- SINUvent® PE: Guaifenesin 600 mg and phenylephrine hydrochloride 15 mg

Tablet, long acting: Guaifenesin 900 mg and phenylephrine hydrochloride 25 mg; guaifenesin 1200 mg and phenylephrine hydrochloride 25 mg

Tablet, prolonged release: Guaifenesin 600 mg and phenylephrine hydrochloride 15 mg
- Respa® PE: Guaifenesin 600 mg and phenylephrine hydrochloride 18 mg [DSC]

Tablet, sustained release: Guaifenesin 600 mg and phenylephrine hydrochloride 30 mg; guaifenesin 1200 mg and phenylephrine hydrochloride 30 mg
- Crantex LA: Guaifenesin 600 mg and phenylephrine hydrochloride 30 mg [dye-free]
- Duratuss®, ExeTuss [DSC]: Guaifenesin 900 mg and phenylephrine hydrochloride 25 mg
- Duratuss GP®, ExeTuss-GP: Guaifenesin 1200 mg and phenylephrine hydrochloride 25 mg
- MyDex: Guaifenesin 900 mg and phenylephrine hydrochloride 30 mg
- Nasex-G: Guaifenesin 835 mg and phenylephrine hydrochloride 25 mg
- Pendex, Prolex®-PD: Guaifenesin 600 mg and phenylephrine hydrochloride 10 mg
- Prolex™-D: Guaifenesin 600 mg and phenylephrine hydrochloride 20 mg [dye-free] [DSC]

XPECT-PE™: Guaifenesin 1200 mg and phenylephrine hydrochloride 25 mg [DSC]

Tablet, timed release:

Gilphex TR®: Guaifenesin 600 mg and phenylephrine hydrochloride 25 mg [sugar free, dye free; scored]

Guaiphen-D: Guaifenesin 600 mg and phenylephrine hydrochloride 40 mg

Guaiphen-D 1200: Guaifenesin 1200 mg and phenylephrine hydrochloride 40 mg

Guaiphen-PD: Guaifenesin 275 mg and phenylephrine hydrochloride 25 mg

Tablet, variable release:

Liquibid-D®: Guaifenesin 400 mg and phenylephrine 10 mg [immediate release] and guaifenesin 800 mg and phenylephrine hydrochloride 30 mg [sustained release]

norel® EX: Guaifenesin 400 mg [immediate release] and guaifenesin 400 mg and phenylephrine hydrochloride 40 mg [extended release]

◆ **Guaifenesin and Phenylephrine Tannate** *see* Guaifenesin and Phenylephrine *on page 742*

Guaifenesin and Pseudoephedrine

(gwye FEN e sin & soo doe e FED rin)

Medication Safety Issues

Sound-alike/look-alike issues:

Entex® may be confused with Tenex®

Entex® LA brand name represents a different product in the U.S. than it does in Canada. In the U.S., Entex® LA contains guaifenesin and phenylephrine, while in Canada the product bearing this brand name contains guaifenesin and pseudoephedrine.

Profen II® may be confused with Profen II DM®, Profen Forte®, Profen Forte™ DM

Profen Forte® may be confused with Profen II®, Profen II DM®, Profen Forte™ DM

U.S. Brand Names Ambifed-G; Congestac® [OTC]; Dynex [DSC]; Entex® PSE; Eudal®-SR; ExeFen; Guaifenex® GP [DSC]; Guaifenex® PSE [DSC]; Guaimax-D®; Levall G; Maxifed-G®; Maxifed®; Medent LD; Mucinex® D Maximum Strength [OTC]; Mucinex®-D [OTC]; Nasatab® LA; Profen II® [DSC]; Pseudo GG TR; Pseudo Max; Pseudovent™ 400 [DSC]; Pseudovent™ [DSC]; Pseudovent™-Ped [DSC]; Refenesen Plus [OTC]; Respaire®-120 SR [DSC]; Respaire®-60 SR [DSC]; Respa®-1st; Rutuss Jr; Sinutab® Non-Drying [OTC]; SudaTex-G; Touro LA®

Canadian Brand Names Contac® Cold-Chest Congestion, Non Drowsy, Regular Strength; Entex® LA; Novahistex® Expectorant with Decongestant

Index Terms Pseudoephedrine and Guaifenesin

Pharmacologic Category Alpha/Beta Agonist; Expectorant

Use Temporary relief of nasal congestion and to help loosen phlegm and thin bronchial secretions in the treatment of cough

Effect on Mental Status Guaifenesin may cause drowsiness; pseudoephedrine may cause anxiety or restlessness

Effect on Psychiatric Treatment Concurrent use with psychotropics may produce additive sedation or lessen the effects of anxiolytics depending on whether the effects of guaifenesin or pseudoephedrine predominate; concurrent use with MAO inhibitors may result in hypertensive crisis; avoid combination

Dosage Summary Note: Dosage varies considerably by product, ranges listed are representative. See specific product labeling.

Oral:

Children <2 years: Dosage not established

Children 2-6 years: One-third to 1/2 tablet every 12 hours (maximum: 1 tablet/12 hours) **or** 2.5 mg every 4-6 hours (maximum: 4 dose/day)

Children 6-12 years: One-half to 1 caplet/tablet every 12-24 hours (maximum: 1-2 caplets/tablets per day) **or** One-half caplet/tablet every 4-6 hours (maximum: 2 caplets/tablets per day) **or** 5 mL every 4-6 hours (maximum: 4 doses/day)

Children >12 years: 1-2 tablets or capsules every 12 hours **or** 1-2 capsules/tablets every 4-6 hours (maximum: 4 doses/day) **or** 10 mL every 4-6 hours (maximum: 4 doses/24 hours)

Adults: 1-2 tablets or capsules every 12 hours **or** 1-2 capsules/tablets every 4-6 hours (maximum: 4 doses/day) **or** 10 mL every 4-6 hours (maximum: 4 doses/24 hours)

Dosage Forms Excipient information presented when available (limited, particularly for generics); consult specific product labeling. [DSC] = Discontinued product

Caplet:
- Congestac®, Refenesen Plus: Guaifenesin 400 mg and pseudoephedrine hydrochloride 60 mg

Caplet, long acting:
- Touro LA®: Guaifenesin 500 mg and pseudoephedrine hydrochloride 120 mg

Caplet, prolonged release:
- Ambifed-G: Guaifenesin 1000 mg and pseudoephedrine hydrochloride 60 mg

Capsule, extended release:
- Respaire®-60 SR: Guaifenesin 200 mg and pseudoephedrine hydrochloride 60 mg [DSC]
- Respaire®-120 SR: Guaifenesin 250 mg and pseudoephedrine hydrochloride 120 mg [DSC]

Capsule, liquicap:
- Sinutab® Non-Drying: Guaifenesin 200 mg and pseudoephedrine hydrochloride 30 mg

Capsule, variable release:
- Entex® PSE: Guaifenesin 400 mg [immediate release] and pseudoephedrine hydrochloride 120 mg [extended release]
- Levall G: Guaifenesin 400 mg [immediate release] and pseudoephedrine hydrochloride 90 mg [extended release]
- Pseudovent™: Guaifenesin 250 mg [immediate release] and pseudoephedrine hydrochloride 120 mg [prolonged release] [DSC]
- Pseudovent™-Ped: Guaifenesin 300 mg [immediate release] and pseudoephedrine hydrochloride 60 mg [prolonged release] [DSC]
- Pseudovent™ 400: Guaifenesin 400 mg [immediate release] and pseudoephedrine hydrochloride 120 mg [extended release] [DSC]

Syrup: Guaifenesin 200 mg and pseudoephedrine hydrochloride 40 mg per 5 mL (480 mL)

Tablet:
- ExeFen: Guaifenesin 780 mg and pseudoephedrine hydrochloride 80 mg
- Rutuss Jr: 600/45: Guaifenesin 600 mg and pseudoephedrine hydrochloride 45 mg

Tablet, extended release:
- Guaifenesin 550 mg and pseudoephedrine hydrochloride 60 mg
- Guaifenesin 595 mg and pseudoephedrine hydrochloride 48 mg
- Guaifenesin 600 mg and pseudoephedrine hydrochloride 120 mg
- Guaifenesin 1200 mg and pseudoephedrine hydrochloride 50 mg
- Guaifenesin 1200 mg and pseudoephedrine hydrochloride 75 mg
- Guaifenesin 1200 mg and pseudoephedrine hydrochloride 120 mg
- Guaifenex® GP: Guaifenesin 1200 mg and pseudoephedrine hydrochloride 120 mg [dye free] [DSC]
- Guaifenex® PSE 60: Guaifenesin 600 mg and pseudoephedrine hydrochloride 60 mg [DSC]
- Guaifenex® PSE 80: Guaifenesin 800 mg and pseudoephedrine hydrochloride 80 mg [DSC]
- Guaifenex® PSE 85: Guaifenesin 795 mg and pseudoephedrine hydrochloride 85 mg [DSC]
- Guaifenex® PSE 120: Guaifenesin 600 mg and pseudoephedrine hydrochloride 120 mg [dye free] [DSC]
- Guaimax-D®: Guaifenesin 600 mg and pseudoephedrine hydrochloride 120 mg
- Maxifed®: Guaifenesin 780 mg and pseudoephedrine hydrochloride 80 mg
- Maxifed-G®: Guaifenesin 580 mg and pseudoephedrine hydrochloride 60 mg
- Mucinex®-D 600/60: Guaifenesin 600 mg and pseudoephedrine hydrochloride 60 mg
- Mucinex® D Maximum Strength [OTC]: Guaifenesin 1200 mg and pseudoephedrine hydrochloride 120 mg
- Profen II®: Guaifenesin 800 mg and pseudoephedrine hydrochloride 45 mg [DSC]
- Pseudo Max: Guaifenesin 700 mg and pseudoephedrine hydrochloride 80 mg

Tablet, long acting:
- Dynex: Guaifenesin 1200 mg and pseudoephedrine hydrochloride 90 mg [DSC]
- Medent LD: Guaifenesin 800 mg and pseudoephedrine hydrochloride 60 mg [dye free; scored]

Tablet, sustained release:
Nasatab® LA: Guaifenesin 500 mg and pseudoephedrine hydrochloride 120 mg
Respa®-1st: Guaifenesin 600 mg and pseudoephedrine hydrochloride 58 mg
SudaTex-G: Guaifenesin 580 mg and pseudoephedrine hydrochloride 60 mg [dye free; scored]

- **Guaifenesin and Theophylline** *see* Theophylline and Guaifenesin *on page 1567*
- **Guaifenesin, Carbetapentane Citrate, and Phenylephrine Hydrochloride** *see* Carbetapentane, Guaifenesin, and Phenylephrine *on page 274*
- **Guaifenesin, Chlorpheniramine, Phenylephrine, and Dextromethorphan** *see* Dextromethorphan, Chlorpheniramine, Phenylephrine, and Guaifenesin *on page 450*

Guaifenesin, Dextromethorphan, and Phenylephrine

(gwye FEN e sin, deks troe meth OR fan, & fen il EF rin)

U.S. Brand Names Anextuss; Certuss-D®; Dacex-DM; Dexcon-PE; Duraphen™ DM [DSC]; Duraphen™ Forte; Duraphen™ II DM; Dynatuss-EX; ExeCof; ExeTuss-DM; Giltuss Pediatric®; Giltuss TR®; Giltuss®; Guaifen™ DM [DSC]; Maxiphen DM; Robitussin® Cold and Cough CF [OTC]; Robitussin® Pediatric Cold and Cough CF [OTC]; SINUtuss® DM; TriTuss®; TriTuss® ER; Tusso™-DMR

Index Terms Guaifenesin, Dextromethorphan Hydrobromide, and Phenylephrine Hydrochloride; Phenylephrine Hydrochloride, Guaifenesin, and Dextromethorphan Hydrobromide

Pharmacologic Category Antitussive; Decongestant

Use Symptomatic relief of dry nonproductive coughs and upper respiratory symptoms associated with hay fever, colds, or the flu

Effect on Mental Status May cause anxiety, dizziness, drowsiness, hallucinations, insomnia, irritability, or nervousness

Effect on Psychiatric Treatment Contraindicated with or within 14 days of MAO inhibitor treatment. Concurrent use with psychotropic agents may produce additive CNS depression.

Dosage Summary

Oral:

Children <6 years: Dosage not established

Children 6-12 years: Certuss-D®, Duraphen™ DM, Duraphen™ Forte, Duraphen™ II DM, Maxiphen DM: One-half tablet every 12 hours (maximum: 1 tablet/day)

Children ≥12 years:

Certuss-D®, Duraphen™ DM, Duraphen™ Forte, Maxiphen DM: One tablet every 12 hours (maximum: 2 tablets/day)

Duraphen™ II DM: 1-1½ tablets twice daily (maximum: 3 tablets/day)

Adults:

Certuss-D, Duraphen™ DM, Duraphen™ Forte, Maxiphen DM: One tablet every 12 hours (maximum: 2 tablets/day)

Duraphen™ II DM: 1-1½ tablets twice daily (maximum: 3 tablets/day)

Dosage Forms Excipient information presented when available (limited, particularly for generics); consult specific product labeling. [DSC] = Discontinued product

Caplet:
Dexcon-PE: Guaifenesin 550 mg, dextromethorphan hydrobromide 25 mg, and phenylephrine hydrochloride 20 mg

Caplet, extended release:
TriTuss®-ER: Guaifenesin 600 mg, dextromethorphan hydrobromide 30 mg, and phenylephrine hydrochloride 10 mg

Capsule:
Tusso™-DMR: Guaifenesin 288 mg, dextromethorphan hydrobromide 14 mg, and phenylephrine hydrochloride 7 mg [gluten free, sodium free, sugar free]

Liquid:
Giltuss®: Guaifenesin 300 mg, dextromethorphan hydrobromide 15 mg, and phenylephrine hydrochloride 10 mg per 5 mL (237 mL) [alcohol free, sugar free; contains phenylalanine 3.75 mg per 5 mL; natural grape flavor]
Giltuss Pediatric®: Guaifenesin 50 mg, dextromethorphan hydrobromide 5 mg, and phenylephrine hydrochloride 2.5 mg per mL (60 mL) [alcohol free, dye free, sugar free; grape flavor]

Liquid, oral [drops]: Guaifenesin 50 mg, dextromethorphan hydrobromide 5 mg, and phenylephrine 2.5 mg per mL (30 mL) [alcohol free; cherry flavor]

Robitussin® Pediatric Cold and Cough CF: Guaifenesin 100 mg, dextromethorphan hydrobromide 5 mg, and phenylephrine hydrochloride 2.5 mg per 2.5 mL (30 mL) [alcohol free; contains propylene glycol and sodium benzoate; fruit punch flavor]

Syrup: Guaifenesin 200 mg, dextromethorphan hydrobromide 30 mg, and phenylephrine hydrochloride 10 mg (473 mL) [cherry flavor]

Dacex-DM: Guaifenesin 175 mg, dextromethorphan hydrobromide 25 mg, and phenylephrine hydrochloride 12.5 mg per 5 mL (480 mL) [strawberry flavor]

Dynatuss-Ex: Guaifenesin 200 mg, dextromethorphan hydrobromide 30 mg, and phenylephrine hydrochloride 10 mg (473 mL) [alcohol free; cherry vanilla flavor]

Robitussin® Cold and Cough CF: Guaifenesin 100 mg, dextromethorphan hydrobromide 10 mg, and phenylephrine hydrochloride 5 mg per 5 mL (120 mL, 240 mL, 355 mL) [alcohol free; contains sodium benzoate and propylene glycol]

TriTuss®: Guaifenesin 175 mg, dextromethorphan hydrobromide 25 mg, and phenylephrine hydrochloride 12.5 mg per 5 mL (480 mL) [alcohol free, sugar free]

Tablet [scored]:

SINUtuss™ DM: Guaifenesin 600 mg, dextromethorphan hydrobromide 30 mg, and phenylephrine hydrochloride 15 mg

Tablet, extended release [scored]:

Duraphen™ II DM: Guaifenesin 800 mg, dextromethorphan hydrobromide 20 mg, and phenylephrine hydrochloride 20 mg [dye free]

Duraphen™ Forte: Guaifenesin 1200 mg, dextromethorphan hydrobromide 30 mg, and phenylephrine hydrochloride 30 mg [dye free, sugar free]

Tablet, prolonged release [scored]:

Maxiphen DM: Guaifenesin 1000 mg, dextromethorphan hydrobromide 60 mg, and phenylephrine hydrochloride 40 mg [dye free]

Tablet, sustained release: Guaifenesin 600 mg, dextromethorphan hydrobromide 60 mg, and phenylephrine hydrochloride 40 mg

Anextuss: Guaifenesin 600 mg, dextromethorphan hydrobromide 60 mg, and phenylephrine hydrochloride 40 mg

Certuss-D® [scored]: Guaifenesin 600 mg, dextromethorphan hydrobromide 60 mg, and phenylephrine hydrochloride 40 mg

Duraphen™ DM [scored]: Guaifenesin 1200 mg, dextromethorphan hydrobromide 20 mg, and phenylephrine hydrochloride 40 mg [dye free] [DSC]

ExeCof: Guaifenesin 100 mg, dextromethorphan hydrobromide 60 mg, and phenylephrine hydrochloride 40 mg [dye free; scored]

ExeTuss-DM: Guaifenesin 600 mg, dextromethorphan hydrobromide 25 mg, and phenylephrine hydrochloride 20 mg

Guaifen™ DM [scored]: Guaifenesin 1200 mg, dextromethorphan hydrobromide 20 mg, and phenylephrine hydrochloride 40 mg [dye free] [DSC]

Tablet, timed release [scored]:

Giltuss TR®: Guaifenesin 600 mg, dextromethorphan hydrobromide 30 mg, and phenylephrine hydrochloride 20 mg [dye free, sugar free]

◆ **Guaifenesin, Dextromethorphan Hydrobromide, and Phenylephrine Hydrochloride** *see* Guaifenesin, Dextromethorphan, and Phenylephrine *on page 746*

◆ **Guaifenesin, Dihydrocodeine, and Pseudoephedrine** *see* Dihydrocodeine, Pseudoephedrine, and Guaifenesin *on page 469*

◆ **Guaifenesin, Hydrocodone, and Pseudoephedrine** *see* Hydrocodone, Pseudoephedrine, and Guaifenesin *on page 784*

◆ **Guaifenesin, Hydrocodone Bitartrate, and Phenylephrine Hydrochloride** *see* Hydrocodone, Phenylephrine, and Guaifenesin *on page 783*

◆ **Guaifenesin, Phenylephrine, and Chlorpheniramine** *see* Chlorpheniramine, Phenylephrine, and Guaifenesin *on page 329*

Guaifenesin, Pseudoephedrine, and Codeine

(gwye FEN e sin, soo doe e FED rin, & KOE deen)

U.S. Brand Names Guiatuss DAC; Mytussin® DAC; Nucofed® Expectorant [DSC]; Nucofed® Pediatric Expectorant [DSC]

Canadian Brand Names Benylin® 3.3 mg-D-E; Calmylin with Codeine

Index Terms Codeine, Guaifenesin, and Pseudoephedrine; Pseudoephedrine, Guaifenesin, and Codeine

Pharmacologic Category Antitussive/Decongestant/Expectorant

Use Temporarily relieves nasal congestion and controls cough associated with upper respiratory infections and related conditions (common cold, sinusitis, bronchitis, influenza)

Effect on Mental Status Guaifenesin may cause drowsiness or dizziness; pseudoephedrine may cause anxiety or restlessness; codeine may cause drowsiness; may cause euphoria, confusion, insomnia, hallucinations, or depression

Effect on Psychiatric Treatment Concurrent use with psychotropics may produce additive sedation or lessen the effects of anxiolytics depending on whether the effects of guaifenesin/codeine or pseudoephedrine predominate; concurrent use with MAO inhibitors may result in hypertensive crisis; avoid combination

Restrictions C-III; C-V

Dosage Summary

Oral:

Children 2-6 years:

Nucofed® Pediatric: 2.5 mL every 6 hours (maximum 10 mL/24 hours)

Nucofed®: 1.25 mL every 6 hours (maximum 5 mL/24 hours)

Children 6-12 years:

Guaituss DAC: 5 mL every 4 hours (maximum 20 mL/24 hours)

Nucofed® Pediatric: 5 mL every 6 hours (maximum 20 mL/24 hours)

Nucofed®: 2.5 mL every 6 hours (maximum 10 mL/24hours)

Children >12 years:

Guaituss DAC: 10 mL every 4 hours (maximum 40 mL/24 hours)

Nucofed® Pediatric: 10 mL every 6 hours (maximum 40 mL/24 hours)

Nucofed®: 5 mL every 6 hours (maximum 20 mL/24 hours)

Adults:

Guaituss DAC: 10 mL every 4 hours (maximum 40 mL/24 hours)

Nucofed® Pediatric: 10 mL every 6 hours (maximum 40 mL/24 hours)

Nucofed®: 5 mL every 6 hours (maximum 20 mL/24 hours)

Dosage Forms Excipient information presented when available (limited, particularly for generics); consult specific product labeling. [DSC] = Discontinued product

Syrup:

Guiatuss DAC: Guaifenesin 100 mg, pseudoephedrine hydrochloride 30 mg, and codeine phosphate 10 mg per 5 mL (480 mL)

Mytussin® DAC: Guaifenesin 100 mg, pseudoephedrine hydrochloride 30 mg, and codeine phosphate 10 mg per 5 mL (120 mL, 480 mL) [sugar free; contains alcohol 1.7%; strawberry-raspberry flavor]

Nucofed® Expectorant: Guaifenesin 200 mg, pseudoephedrine hydrochloride 60 mg, and codeine phosphate 20 mg per 5 mL (480 mL) [contains alcohol 12.5%; cherry flavor] [DSC]

Nucofed® Pediatric Expectorant: Guaifenesin 100 mg, pseudoephedrine hydrochloride 30 mg, and codeine phosphate 10 mg per 5 mL (480 mL) [contains alcohol 6%; strawberry flavor] [DSC]

Guaifenesin, Pseudoephedrine, and Dextromethorphan

(gwye FEN e sin, soo doe e FED rin, & deks troe meth OR fan)

Medication Safety Issues

Sound-alike/look-alike issues:

Profen II DM® may be confused with Profen II®, Profen Forte®, Profen Forte™ DM

Profen Forte™ DM may be confused with Profen II®, Profen II DM®, Profen Forte®

U.S. Brand Names Ambifed-G DM; Coldmist DM [DSC]; ExeFen-DMX; Maxifed DM; Maxifed DMX; Medent-DM; Profen Forte™ DM; Profen II DM®; Pseudo Max DMX; Pseudovent™ DM [DSC]; Relacon-DM NR; Robitussin® Cough and Cold CF [OTC]; Robitussin® Cough and Cold Infant CF [OTC]; Robitussin® Cough and Cold [OTC]; Ru-Tuss DM; SudaTex-DM; Touro® CC; Touro® CC-LD; Tri-Vent™ DM [DSC]; Trikof-D® [DSC]; Tusnel Liquid®; Tusnel Pediatric®; Tusnel-DM Pediatric®; Z-Cof™ 12DM

Canadian Brand Names Balminil DM + Decongestant + Expectorant; Benylin® DM-D-E; Koffex DM + Decongestant + Expectorant; Novahistex® DM Decongestant Expectorant; Novahistine® DM Decongestant Expectorant; Robitussin® Cough & Cold®

Index Terms Dextromethorphan, Guaifenesin, and Pseudoephedrine; Pseudoephedrine, Dextromethorphan, and Guaifenesin

Pharmacologic Category Antitussive/Decongestant/Expectorant

Use Temporarily relieves nasal congestion and controls cough due to minor throat and bronchial irritation; helps loosen phlegm and thin bronchial secretions to make coughs more productive

Effect on Mental Status Guaifenesin may cause drowsiness or dizziness; pseudoephedrine may cause anxiety or restlessness; dextromethorphan may cause drowsiness

Effect on Psychiatric Treatment Concurrent use with psychotropics may produce additive sedation or lessen the effects of anxiolytics depending on whether the effects of guaifenesin/dextromethorphan or pseudoephedrine predominate; concurrent use with MAO inhibitors may result in hypertensive crisis; avoid combination

Dosage Forms Excipient information presented when available (limited, particularly for generics); consult specific product labeling. [DSC] = Discontinued product

Caplet, prolonged release:

Ambifed-G DM: Guaifenesin 1000 mg, pseudoephedrine hydrochloride 60 mg, and dextromethorphan hydrobromide 30 mg

Caplet, sustained release [scored]:

Touro® CC: Guaifenesin 575 mg, pseudoephedrine hydrochloride 60 mg, and dextromethorphan hydrobromide 30 mg [dye free]

Touro® CC-LD: Guaifenesin 575 mg, pseudoephedrine hydrochloride 25 mg, and dextromethorphan hydrobromide 30 mg

Capsule, softgel:

Robitussin® Cough and Cold: Guaifenesin 200 mg, pseudoephedrine hydrochloride 30 mg, and dextromethorphan hydrobromide 10 mg

Liquid: Guaifenesin 100 mg, pseudoephedrine hydrochloride 30 mg, and dextromethorphan hydrobromide 10 mg per 5 mL (120 mL)

Profen II DM®: Guaifenesin 200 mg, pseudoephedrine hydrochloride 15 mg, and dextromethorphan hydrobromide 10 mg per 5 mL (480 mL) [alcohol free, dye free, sugar free; cherry flavor]

Relacon-DM NR: Guaifenesin 200 mg, pseudoephedrine hydrochloride 32 mg, and dextromethorphan hydrobromide 15 mg (480 mL) [alcohol free, sugar free; grape flavor]

Tusnel Liquid®: Guaifenesin 200 mg, pseudoephedrine hydrochloride 30 mg, and dextromethorphan hydrobromide 15 mg per 5 mL (180 mL) [alcohol free, dye free, sugar free]

Tusnel Pediatric®: Guaifenesin 50 mg, pseudoephedrine hydrochloride 15 mg, and dextromethorphan hydrobromide 5 mg per 5 mL (120 mL) [alcohol free]

Liquid, oral [drops]:

Robitussin® Cough and Cold Infant CF: Guaifenesin 100 mg, pseudoephedrine hydrochloride 15 mg, and dextromethorphan hydrobromide 5 mg per 2.5 mL (30 mL) [alcohol free; contains sodium benzoate]

Tusnel-DM Pediatric®: Guaifenesin 25 mg, pseudoephedrine hydrochloride 5 mg, and dextromethorphan hydrobromide 5 mg per 1 mL (60 mL)

Suspension:

Z-Cof™ 12DM: Guaifenesin 175 mg, pseudoephedrine tannate (equivalent to pseudoephedrine hydrochloride 30 mg), and dextromethorphan tannate (equivalent to dextromethorphan hydrobromide 15 mg) per 5 mL (480 mL) [alcohol free; contains phenylalanine 25.26 mg/5 mL and sodium benzoate; grape flavor]

Syrup: Guaifenesin 100 mg, pseudoephedrine hydrochloride 45 mg, and dextromethorphan hydrobromide 15 mg per 5 mL (480 mL)

Robitussin® Cough and Cold CF: Guaifenesin 100 mg, pseudoephedrine hydrochloride 30 mg, and dextromethorphan hydrobromide 10 mg per 5 mL (120 mL, 240 mL, 360 mL) [alcohol free; contains sodium benzoate]

Ru-Tuss DM: Guaifenesin 100 mg, pseudoephedrine hydrochloride 45 mg, and dextromethorphan hydrobromide 15 mg per 5 mL (480 mL) [alcohol free, dye free, sugar free; strawberry flavor]

Tri-Vent™ DM: Guaifenesin 100 mg, pseudoephedrine hydrochloride 40 mg, and dextromethorphan hydrobromide 15 mg per 5 mL (480 mL) [alcohol free, dye free, sugar free; strawberry flavor] [DSC]

Tablet, extended release: Guaifenesin 100 mg, pseudoephedrine hydrochloride 30 mg, and dextromethorphan hydrobromide 10 mg; guaifenesin 800 mg, pseudoephedrine hydrochloride 60 mg, and dextromethorphan hydrobromide 30 mg; guaifenesin 1200 mg, pseudoephedrine hydrochloride 60 mg, and dextromethorphan hydrobromide 60 mg; guaifenesin 1200 mg, pseudoephedrine hydrochloride 120 mg, and dextromethorphan hydrobromide 60 mg; guaifenesin 800 mg, pseudoephedrine hydrochloride 90 mg, and dextromethorphan hydrobromide 60 mg; guaifenesin 550 mg, pseudoephedrine hydrochloride 60 mg, and dextromethorphan hydrobromide 30 mg; guaifenesin 595 mg, pseudoephedrine hydrochloride 48 mg, and dextromethorphan hydrobromide 32 mg; guaifenesin 600 mg, pseudoephedrine hydrochloride 60 mg, and dextromethorphan hydrobromide 30 mg

Coldmist DM: Guaifenesin 595 mg, pseudoephedrine hydrochloride 48 mg, and dextromethorphan hydrobromide 32 mg [DSC]

Profen Forte™ DM: Guaifenesin 800 mg, pseudoephedrine hydrochloride 90 mg, and dextromethorphan hydrobromide 60 mg

Profen II DM®: Guaifenesin 800 mg, pseudoephedrine hydrochloride 45 mg, and dextromethorphan hydrobromide 30 mg

Pseudovent™ DM: Guaifenesin 595 mg, pseudoephedrine hydrochloride 48 mg, and dextromethorphan hydrobromide 32 mg [DSC]

Tablet, long acting [scored]: Guaifenesin 800 mg, pseudoephedrine hydrochloride 60 mg, and dextromethorphan hydrobromide 30 mg

Medent-DM: Guaifenesin 800 mg, pseudoephedrine hydrochloride 60 mg, and dextromethorphan hydrobromide 30 mg [dye free]

Tablet, sustained release:

ExeFen-DMX: Guaifenesin 780 mg, pseudoephedrine hydrochloride 80 mg, and dextromethorphan hydrobromide 40 mg [dye free]

Maxifed DM, SudaTex-DM: Guaifenesin 580 mg, pseudoephedrine hydrochloride 60 mg, and dextromethorphan hydrobromide 30 mg [dye free; scored]

Maxifed DM: Guaifenesin 780 mg, pseudoephedrine hydrochloride 80 mg, and dextromethorphan hydrobromide 40 mg [dye free; scored]

Pseudo Max DMX: Guaifenesin 700 mg, pseudoephedrine hydrochloride 80 mg, and dextromethorphan hydrobromide 40 mg

Trikof-D®: Guaifenesin 600 mg, pseudoephedrine hydrochloride 50 mg, and dextromethorphan hydrobromide 30 mg [DSC]

- ◆ **Guaifenesin, Pyrilamine Tannate, and Phenylephrine Tannate** *see* Phenylephrine, Pyrilamine, and Guaifenesin *on page 1279*
- ◆ **Guaifenex® DM [DSC]** *see* Guaifenesin and Dextromethorphan *on page 739*
- ◆ **Guaifenex® GP [DSC]** *see* Guaifenesin and Pseudoephedrine *on page 744*
- ◆ **Guaifenex® PSE [DSC]** *see* Guaifenesin and Pseudoephedrine *on page 744*
- ◆ **Guaimax-D®** *see* Guaifenesin and Pseudoephedrine *on page 744*
- ◆ **Guaiphen-D** *see* Guaifenesin and Phenylephrine *on page 742*
- ◆ **Guaiphen-D 1200** *see* Guaifenesin and Phenylephrine *on page 742*
- ◆ **Guaiphen-PD** *see* Guaifenesin and Phenylephrine *on page 742*
- ◆ **Guaituss AC** *see* Guaifenesin and Codeine *on page 738*

Guanabenz (GWAHN a benz)

Medication Safety Issues

Sound-alike/look-alike issues:

Guanabenz may be confused with guanadrel, guanfacine

Canadian Brand Names Wytensin®

Index Terms Guanabenz Acetate

Pharmacologic Category Alpha$_2$-Adrenergic Agonist

Use Management of hypertension

Effect on Mental Status Drowsiness and dizziness are common; may cause anxiety or depression

Effect on Psychiatric Treatment Has been used to treat ADHD; concurrent use with psychotropics may produce additive sedation and dry mouth; TCAs may decrease the hypotensive effect of guanabenz

Dosage Summary

Oral:

Children: Dosage not established

Adults: Initial: 4 mg twice daily; Maintenance: 4-32 mg twice daily; **Note:** Titration is recommended

Elderly: Initial: 4 mg once daily, increase every 1-2 weeks

Dosage Forms Excipient information presented when available (limited, particularly for generics); consult specific product labeling.

Tablet: 4 mg, 8 mg

◆ **Guanabenz Acetate** *see* Guanabenz *on page 750*

GuanFACINE (GWAHN fa seen)

Medication Safety Issues

Sound-alike/look-alike issues:

GuanFACINE may be confused with guaiFENesin, guanabenz, guanidine

Tenex® may be confused with Entex®, Ten-K®, Xanax®

International issues:

Tenex® may be confused with Kinex® which is a brand name for biperiden in Mexico

U.S. Brand Names Tenex®

Canadian Brand Names Tenex®

Index Terms Guanfacine Hydrochloride

Pharmacologic Category $Alpha_2$-Adrenergic Agonist

Generic Available Yes

Use Management of hypertension

Unlabeled/Investigational Use ADHD, tic disorder, aggression

Effect on Mental Status Drowsiness is common; may cause insomnia or dizziness, may rarely cause confusion or depression

Effect on Psychiatric Treatment Has been used to treat ADHD; concurrent use with psychotropics may produce additive sedation and dry mouth; TCAs may decrease the hypotensive effect of guanfacine

Pregnancy Risk Factor B

Contraindications Hypersensitivity to guanfacine or any component of the formulation

Warnings/Precautions Use caution with severe coronary insufficiency, recent MI, cerebrovascular disease, or chronic renal or hepatic disease. Abrupt discontinuation can result in nervousness, anxiety and rarely, rebound hypertension (occurs 2-4 days after withdrawal). Avoid use in CNS disease, elderly, or with other CNS depressants (can cause sedation and drowsiness alone). Caution in diabetes; may mask signs of hypoglycemia. Safety and efficacy in children <12 years of age have not been demonstrated. May cause orthostasis.

Adverse Reactions

>10%:

Central nervous system: Somnolence (5% to 40%), headache (3% to 13%), dizziness (2% to 15%)

Gastrointestinal: Xerostomia (10% to 54%), constipation (2% to 15%)

1% to 10%:

Central nervous system: Fatigue (2% to 10%)

Endocrine & metabolic: Impotence (up to 7%)

<1% (Limited to important or life-threatening): Agitation, alopecia, amnesia, blurred vision, bradycardia, chest pain, confusion, depression, dermatitis, diaphoresis, dysphagia, dyspnea, edema, exfoliative dermatitis, hypokinesia, hypotension, insomnia, leg cramps, malaise, nervousness, orthostasis, palpitation, paresthesia, pruritus, rash, rebound hypertension, syncope, tinnitus, urinary incontinence, vertigo; **Note:** Mania and aggressive behavior have been reported in pediatric patients with ADHD who received guanfacine.

Drug Interactions

Antidepressants (Alpha2-Antagonist): May diminish the hypotensive effect of Alpha2-Agonists. *Risk D: Consider therapy modification*

Beta-Blockers: May enhance the rebound hypertensive effect of Alpha2-Agonists. This effect can occur when the $alpha_2$-agonist is abruptly withdrawn. **Exceptions:** Levobunolol; Metipranolol. *Risk D: Consider therapy modification*

Diazoxide: May enhance the hypotensive effect of Antihypertensives. *Risk C: Monitor therapy*

Herbs (Hypertensive Properties): May diminish the antihypertensive effect of Antihypertensives. *Risk C: Monitor therapy*

Herbs (Hypotensive Properties): May enhance the hypotensive effect of Antihypertensives. *Risk C: Monitor therapy*

Methylphenidate: May diminish the antihypertensive effect of Antihypertensives. *Risk C: Monitor therapy*

Prostacyclin Analogues: May enhance the hypotensive effect of Antihypertensives. *Risk C: Monitor therapy*

RiTUXimab: Antihypertensives may enhance the hypotensive effect of RiTUXimab. *Risk D: Consider therapy modification*

Tricyclic Antidepressants: May diminish the antihypertensive effect of Alpha2-Agonists. *Risk D: Consider therapy modification*

Mechanism of Action Stimulates $alpha_2$-adrenoreceptors in the brain stem, thus activating an inhibitory neuron, resulting in reduced sympathetic outflow, producing a decrease in vasomotor tone and heart rate

Pharmacodynamics/Kinetics

Onset of action: Peak effect: 8-11 hours

Duration: 24 hours following single dose

Half-life elimination, serum: 17 hours

Time to peak, serum: 1-4 hours

Dosage Oral: Adults:

Hypertension: 1 mg usually at bedtime, may increase if needed at 3- to 4-week intervals; usual dose range (JNC 7): 0.5-2 mg once daily

ADHD, tic disorder, aggression (unlabeled uses): Initial: 0.5 mg at bedtime; increase as tolerated (every 3-14 days) to usual dose range (1.5-3 mg/day) given in 3 divided doses (maximum: 4 mg/day)

Monitoring Parameters Heart rate, blood pressure

When used for the treatment of ADHD, thoroughly evaluate for cardiovascular risk. Monitor heart rate, blood pressure (when started and weaned), and consider obtaining ECG prior to initiation (Vetter, 2008).

Additional Information More selective $alpha_2$ agonist than clonidine; withdrawal effects rarely occur due to its long half-life.

Dosage Forms Excipient information presented when available (limited, particularly for generics); consult specific product labeling.

Tablet: 1 mg, 2 mg

Tenex®: 1 mg, 2 mg

- **Guanfacine Hydrochloride** *see* GuanFACINE *on page 750*
- **Guia-D** *see* Guaifenesin and Dextromethorphan *on page 739*
- **Guiaplex™ HC [DSC]** *see* Hydrocodone, Phenylephrine, and Guaifenesin *on page 783*
- **Guiatuss™ [OTC]** *see* GuaiFENesin *on page 737*
- **Guiatuss DAC** *see* Guaifenesin, Pseudoephedrine, and Codeine *on page 747*
- **Guiatuss-DM® [OTC]** *see* Guaifenesin and Dextromethorphan *on page 739*
- **GW506U78** *see* Nelarabine *on page 1120*
- **GW-1000-02** *see* Tetrahydrocannabinol and Cannabidiol *on page 1558*
- **GW433908G** *see* Fosamprenavir *on page 689*
- **GW572016** *see* Lapatinib *on page 898*
- **Gynodiol® [DSC]** *see* Estradiol *on page 576*
- **H5N1 Influenza Vaccine** *see* Influenza Virus Vaccine (H5N1) *on page 821*
- **Habitrol** *see* Nicotine *on page 1133*

Haemophilus b Conjugate and Hepatitis B Vaccine

(he MOF i lus bee KON joo gate & hep a TYE tis bee vak SEEN)

Medication Safety Issues

Sound-alike/look-alike issues:

Comvax® may be confused with Recombivax [Recombivax HB®]

U.S. Brand Names Comvax®

Mexican Brand Names Comvax

Index Terms *Haemophilus* b (meningococcal protein conjugate) Conjugate Vaccine; Hepatitis B Vaccine (Recombinant); Hib Conjugate Vaccine

Pharmacologic Category Vaccine, Inactivated (Bacterial); Vaccine, Inactivated (Viral)

Use

Immunization against invasive disease caused by *H. influenzae* type b and against infection caused by all known subtypes of hepatitis B virus in infants 6 weeks to 15 months of age born of hepatitis B surface antigen (HB_sAg) negative mothers

Infants born of HB_sAg-positive mothers or mothers of unknown HB_sAg status should receive hepatitis B immune globulin and hepatitis B vaccine (recombinant) at birth and should complete the hepatitis B vaccination series given according to a particular schedule

Effect on Mental Status May cause irritability or lethargy

Effect on Psychiatric Treatment May lessen or potentiate the effects of anxiolytics or mood stabilizers

Dosage Summary

I.M.

Infants <6 weeks: Dosage not established

Infants ≥6 weeks: 0.5 mL at 2, 4, and 12-15 months of age (total of 3 doses); Modified schedule: Children who receive one dose of hepatitis B vaccine at or shortly after birth may receive Comvax® on a schedule of 2, 4, and 12-15 months of age

Dosage Forms Excipient information presented when available (limited, particularly for generics); consult specific product labeling.

Injection, suspension [preservative free]:

Comvax®: *Haemophilus* b capsular polysaccharide 7.5 mcg (bound to *Neisseria meningitides* OMPC 125 mcg) and hepatitis B surface antigen 5 mcg per 0.5 mL (0.5 mL) [contains aluminum; contains natural rubber/natural latex in packaging]

Haemophilus b Conjugate Vaccine

(he MOF fi lus bee KON joo gate vak SEEN)

Medication Safety Issues

Sound-alike/look-alike issues:

International issues:

Hiberix is also a brand name for influenza virus vaccine in multiple international markets

U.S. Brand Names ActHIB®; PedvaxHIB®

Canadian Brand Names ActHIB®; PedvaxHIB®

Index Terms *Haemophilus* b Oligosaccharide Conjugate Vaccine; *Haemophilus* b Polysaccharide Vaccine; Diphtheria Toxoid Conjugate; HbCV; Hib Conjugate Vaccine; Hib Polysaccharide Conjugate; PRP-OMP; PRP-T

Pharmacologic Category Vaccine, Inactivated (Bacterial)

Use Routine immunization of children against invasive disease caused by *H. influenzae* type b

The Advisory Committee on Immunization Practices (ACIP) recommends routine vaccination of all children through age 59 months. Efficacy data is not available for use in older children and adults with chronic conditions associated with an increased risk of Hib disease. However, a single dose may also be considered for older children, adolescents, and adults who did not receive the childhood series and who have had splenectomies or who have sickle cell disease, leukemia or HIV infection.

Effect on Mental Status May cause irritability or lethargy

Effect on Psychiatric Treatment May lessen or potentiate the effects of anxiolytics or mood stabilizers

Dosage Summary

I.M.

Children: 0.5 mL as a single dose administered according to one of the "brand-specific" schedules

ActHIB®: Age at first dose:

2 months of age: Immunization consists of 3 doses (0.5 mL/dose) administered at 2-, 4- and 6 months of age (may reconstitute with provided diluent or DTP vaccine). A booster dose is given at 15-18 months of age (may reconstitute with provided diluent or Tripedia® vaccine).

7-11 months of age: Two doses (0.5 mL/dose) administered 8 months apart, with a booster dose at 15-18 months of age

12-14 months of age: One dose (0.5 mL) followed by a booster dose 2 months later

PedvaxHIB®: Age at first dose:

2-10 months of age: Two doses (0.5 mL/dose) administered 2 months apart; booster dose at 12-15 months of age

11-14 months of age: Two doses (0.5 mL/dose) administered 1 months apart

15-71 months of age: One 0.5 mL dose

Dosage Forms Excipient information presented when available (limited, particularly for generics); consult specific product labeling.

Injection, powder for reconstitution [preservative free]:

ActHIB® *Haemophilus* b capsular polysaccharide 10 mcg (bound to tetanus toxoid 24 mcg) per 0.5 mL [contains sucrose; may be reconstituted with provided diluent (forms solution; contains natural rubber/natural latex in packaging) or Tripedia® (forms suspension)]

Injection, suspension:

PedvaxHIB®: *Haemophilus* b capsular polysaccharide 7.5 mcg [bound to *Neisseria meningitidis* OMPC 125 mcg] per 0.5 mL (0.5 mL) [contains aluminum]

◆ ***Haemophilus* b (meningococcal protein conjugate) Conjugate Vaccine** *see* *Haemophilus* b Conjugate and Hepatitis B Vaccine *on page 752*

◆ ***Haemophilus* b Oligosaccharide Conjugate Vaccine** *see* *Haemophilus* b Conjugate Vaccine *on page 753*

◆ ***Haemophilus* b Polysaccharide Vaccine** *see* *Haemophilus* b Conjugate Vaccine *on page 753*

◆ **Halcion®** *see* Triazolam *on page 1620*
◆ **Haldol®** *see* Haloperidol *on page 754*
◆ **Haldol® Decanoate** *see* Haloperidol *on page 754*
◆ **Halfprin® [OTC]** *see* Aspirin *on page 143*

Haloperidol (ha loe PER i dole)

Medication Safety Issues

Sound-alike/look-alike issues:

Haloperidol may be confused Halotestin®

Haldol® may be confused with Halcion®, Halenol®, Halog®, Halotestin®, Stadol®

Related Information

Anticholinergic Effects of Common Psychotropics *on page 1758*
Antipsychotic Agents *on page 1769*
Antipsychotic Receptor Profile *on page 1772*
CMS: Long-Term Care Facility Thresholds *on page 1815*
Discontinuation of Psychotropic Drugs *on page 1839*
Liquid Compatibility of Antidepressants, Antipsychotics, and Mood Stabilizers *on page 1788*

U.S. Brand Names Haldol®; Haldol® Decanoate

Canadian Brand Names Apo-Haloperidol LA®; Apo-Haloperidol®; Haloperidol Injection, USP; Haloperidol Long Acting; Haloperidol-LA; Haloperidol-LA Omega; Novo-Peridol; Peridol; PMS-Haloperidol LA

Mexican Brand Names Haldol; Haloperil

Index Terms Haloperidol Decanoate; Haloperidol Lactate

Pharmacologic Category Antipsychotic Agent, Typical

Generic Available Yes

Use Management of schizophrenia; control of tics and vocal utterances of Tourette's disorder in children and adults; severe behavioral problems in children

Unlabeled/Investigational Use Treatment of non-schizophrenia psychosis; may be used for the emergency sedation of severely-agitated or delirious patients; adjunctive treatment of ethanol dependence; antiemetic; psychosis/agitation related to Alzheimer's dementia

Mental Health Comment Haloperidol is a high-potency antipsychotic. Older antipsychotic medications (chlorpromazine, haloperidol), which do not meet specific criteria for "atypical" antipsychotics, are often referred to as typical antipsychotics. They are associated with the troubling side effect, EPS. However, it is commonly believed that in order for a drug to treat psychosis, it must block dopamine is some manner.

Common side effects include sedation and neuroleptic effect (reduced initiative, interest in the environment, and display of emotion or affect). All **typical** antipsychotics are considered to be equally effective if given in equipotent doses. An inverse relationship exists between intrinsic antimuscarinic activity and propensity to cause extrapyramidal side effects. If dystonia or pseudo-parkinsonism occurs, antiparkinsonian agents should be considered. If akathisia occurs, beta-blockers (eg, propranolol), benzodiazepines, or anti-parkinsonian agents should be considered. Tardive dyskinesia (TD) secondary to typical antipsychotics has an estimated incidence of 3% to 5% per year for the first 5 years of treatment. After this time period, the incidence is estimated to be 2% to 3% per year. Prevalence rates are ~15% to 20%. Female gender and age constitute risk factors for TD. Indeed, prevalence rates have been reported to be as high as 70% in elderly females. No specific treatment exists for TD, however, patients are often initiated on/switched to an atypical antipsychotic because of their lower incidence to cause TD and hopes of suppression.

Typical antipsychotics are usually only indicated for schizophrenia, but are generally effective for mania and psychosis and/or behavioral syndromes secondary to other mental conditions. Nonpsychiatric uses include Tourette's syndrome, Huntington's disease, and occasionally, intractable hiccups, pruritus, nausea, and vomiting.

These drugs are thought to exert their antipsychotic activity by blocking dopamine D_2 receptors in the mesolimbic dopaminergic pathway. Side effects are often related to their ability to antagonize dopamine receptors in the nigrostriatal and tuberoinfundibular pathways.

Long-acting dosage form is useful in patients nonadherent to treatment.

Coadministration of two or more antipsychotics does not generally improve clinical response and may increase the potential for adverse effects.

In 2008, the FDA issued a warning regarding increased mortality risk with typical **and** atypical antipsychotic drugs when used in elderly patients with dementia-related psychosis.

Pregnancy Risk Factor C

Lactation Enters breast milk/not recommended (AAP rates "of concern")

Contraindications Hypersensitivity to haloperidol or any component of the formulation; Parkinson's disease; severe CNS depression; bone marrow suppression; severe cardiac or hepatic disease; coma

Warnings/Precautions **[U.S. Boxed Warning]: Elderly patients with dementia-related psychosis treated with antipsychotics are at an increased risk of death compared to placebo.** An increased incidence of cerebrovascular adverse events (including fatalities) has been reported in elderly patients with dementia-related psychosis. Haloperidol is not approved for this indication. Hypotension may occur, particularly with parenteral administration. Although the short-acting form (lactate) is used clinically, the I.V. use of the injection is not an FDA-approved route of administration; the decanoate form should never be administered intravenously.

May alter cardiac conduction and prolong QT interval; life-threatening arrhythmias have occurred with therapeutic doses of antipsychotics but risk may be increased with doses exceeding recommendations and/or intravenous administration (unlabeled route). Use caution or avoid use in patients with electrolyte abnormalities (eg, hypokalemia, hypomagnesemia), hypothyroidism, familial long QT syndrome, concomitant medications which may augment QT prolongation, or any underlying cardiac abnormality which may also potentiate risk. Monitor ECG closely for dose-related QT effects. Adverse effects of decanoate may be prolonged. Avoid in thyrotoxicosis. Myelosuppression (eg, leukopenia, agranulocytosis) has been observed with antipsychotic use; check blood counts periodically and discontinue at first signs of blood dyscrasias; use is contraindicated in patients with bone marrow suppression. May be sedating, use with caution in disorders where CNS depression is a feature. Caution in patients with severe cardiovascular disease, predisposition to seizures, subcortical brain damage, renal or respiratory disease. Esophageal dysmotility and aspiration have been associated with antipsychotic use - use with caution in patients at risk of pneumonia (eg, Alzheimer's disease). Caution in breast cancer or other prolactin-dependent tumors (may elevate prolactin levels). May alter temperature regulation or mask toxicity of other drugs due to antiemetic effects. May cause orthostatic hypotension; use with caution in patients at risk of this effect or those who would tolerate transient hypotensive episodes (cerebrovascular disease, cardiovascular disease, or other medications which may predispose). Some tablets contain tartrazine.

May cause anticholinergic effects (confusion, agitation, constipation, xerostomia, blurred vision, urinary retention). Therefore, they should be used with caution in patients with decreased gastrointestinal motility, urinary retention, BPH, xerostomia, or visual problems. Conditions which also may be exacerbated by cholinergic blockade include narrow-angle glaucoma (screening is recommended) and worsening of myasthenia gravis. Relative to other neuroleptics, haloperidol has a low potency of cholinergic blockade.

May cause extrapyramidal symptoms (EPS), including pseudoparkinsonism, acute dystonic reactions, akathisia, and tardive dyskinesia (risk of these reactions is high relative to other neuroleptics). Risk of dystonia (and possibly other EPS) may be greater with increased doses, use of conventional antipsychotics, males, and younger patients. May be associated with neuroleptic malignant syndrome (NMS) or pigmentary retinopathy.

Adverse Reactions Frequency not defined.

Cardiovascular: Abnormal T waves with prolonged ventricular repolarization, arrhythmia, hyper-/hypotension, QT prolongation, sudden death, tachycardia, torsade de pointes

Central nervous system: Agitation, akathisia, altered central temperature regulation, anxiety, confusion, depression, drowsiness, dystonic reactions, euphoria, extrapyramidal reactions, headache, insomnia, lethargy, neuroleptic malignant syndrome (NMS), pseudoparkinsonian signs and symptoms, restlessness, seizure, tardive dyskinesia, tardive dystonia, vertigo

Dermatologic: Alopecia, contact dermatitis, hyperpigmentation, photosensitivity (rare), pruritus, rash

Endocrine & metabolic: Amenorrhea, breast engorgement, galactorrhea, gynecomastia, hyper-/hypoglycemia, hyponatremia, lactation, mastalgia, menstrual irregularities, sexual dysfunction

Gastrointestinal: Anorexia, constipation, diarrhea, dyspepsia, hypersalivation, nausea, vomiting, xerostomia

Genitourinary: Priapism, urinary retention

Hematologic: Cholestatic jaundice, obstructive jaundice
Ocular: Blurred vision
Respiratory: Bronchospasm, laryngospasm
Miscellaneous: Diaphoresis, heat stroke

Metabolism/Transport Effects Substrate of CYP1A2 (minor), 2D6 (major), 3A4 (major); **Inhibits** CYP2D6 (moderate), 3A4 (moderate)

Drug Interactions

Acetylcholinesterase Inhibitors (Central): May enhance the neurotoxic (central) effect of Antipsychotics. Severe extrapyramidal symptoms have occurred in some patients. *Risk C: Monitor therapy*

Alcohol (Ethyl): CNS Depressants may enhance the CNS depressant effect of Alcohol (Ethyl). *Risk C: Monitor therapy*

Alfuzosin: May enhance the QTc-prolonging effect of QTc-Prolonging Agents. *Risk C: Monitor therapy*

Amphetamines: Antipsychotics may diminish the stimulatory effect of Amphetamines. *Risk C: Monitor therapy*

Anticholinergics: May enhance the adverse/toxic effect of other Anticholinergics. **Exceptions:** Paliperidone. *Risk C: Monitor therapy*

Anti-Parkinson's Agents (Dopamine Agonist): Antipsychotics (Typical) may diminish the therapeutic effect of Anti-Parkinson's Agents (Dopamine Agonist). *Risk D: Consider therapy modification*

CarBAMazepine: May increase the metabolism of Haloperidol. *Risk D: Consider therapy modification*

ChlorproMAZINE: Haloperidol may enhance the QTc-prolonging effect of ChlorproMAZINE. ChlorproMAZINE may decrease the metabolism of Haloperidol. *Risk D: Consider therapy modification*

Ciprofloxacin: May enhance the QTc-prolonging effect of QTc-Prolonging Agents. *Risk C: Monitor therapy*

CNS Depressants: May enhance the adverse/toxic effect of other CNS Depressants. *Risk C: Monitor therapy*

Codeine: CYP2D6 Inhibitors (Moderate) may diminish the therapeutic effect of Codeine. These CYP2D6 inhibitors may prevent the metabolic conversion of codeine to its active metabolite morphine. *Risk C: Monitor therapy*

CYP2D6 Inhibitors (Moderate): May decrease the metabolism of CYP2D6 Substrates. *Risk C: Monitor therapy*

CYP2D6 Inhibitors (Strong): May decrease the metabolism of CYP2D6 Substrates. *Risk D: Consider therapy modification*

CYP2D6 Substrates: CYP2D6 Inhibitors (Moderate) may decrease the metabolism of CYP2D6 Substrates. **Exceptions:** Tamoxifen. *Risk C: Monitor therapy*

CYP3A4 Inducers (Strong): May increase the metabolism of CYP3A4 Substrates. *Risk C: Monitor therapy*

CYP3A4 Inhibitors (Moderate): May decrease the metabolism of CYP3A4 Substrates. *Risk C: Monitor therapy*

CYP3A4 Inhibitors (Strong): May decrease the metabolism of CYP3A4 Substrates. *Risk D: Consider therapy modification*

CYP3A4 Substrates: CYP3A4 Inhibitors (Moderate) may decrease the metabolism of CYP3A4 Substrates. *Risk C: Monitor therapy*

Darunavir: May increase the serum concentration of CYP2D6 Substrates. *Risk C: Monitor therapy*

Dasatinib: May increase the serum concentration of CYP3A4 Substrates. *Risk C: Monitor therapy*

Deferasirox: May decrease the serum concentration of CYP3A4 Substrates. *Risk C: Monitor therapy*

Eplerenone: CYP3A4 Inhibitors (Moderate) may increase the serum concentration of Eplerenone. Management: A lower starting dose of eplerenone (25 mg once daily) is recommended in patients with hypertension who are also taking drugs that are moderate inhibitors of CYP3A4. *Risk D: Consider therapy modification*

Gadobutrol: May enhance the QTc-prolonging effect of QTc-Prolonging Agents. *Risk D: Consider therapy modification*

Herbs (CYP3A4 Inducers): May increase the metabolism of CYP3A4 Substrates. *Risk C: Monitor therapy*

Lithium formulations: May enhance the neurotoxic effect of Antipsychotics. Lithium formulations may decrease the serum concentration of Antipsychotics. Specifically noted with chlorpromazine. *Risk C: Monitor therapy*

Maraviroc: CYP3A4 Inhibitors may increase the serum concentration of Maraviroc. *Risk D: Consider therapy modification*

Nebivolol: CYP2D6 Inhibitors (Moderate) may increase the serum concentration of Nebivolol. *Risk C: Monitor therapy*

Nilotinib: May enhance the QTc-prolonging effect of QTc-Prolonging Agents. *Risk X: Avoid combination*

Pimecrolimus: CYP3A4 Inhibitors (Moderate) may decrease the metabolism of Pimecrolimus. *Risk C: Monitor therapy*

Pramlintide: May enhance the anticholinergic effect of Anticholinergics. These effects are specific to the GI tract. *Risk D: Consider therapy modification*

QTc-Prolonging Agents: May enhance the adverse/toxic effect of other QTc-Prolonging Agents. Their effects can be additive, causing life-threatening ventricular arrhythmias. *Risk D: Consider therapy modification*

QuiNIDine: May increase the serum concentration of Haloperidol. *Risk C: Monitor therapy*

Ranolazine: CYP3A4 Inhibitors (Moderate) may increase the serum concentration of Ranolazine. Management: Limit the ranolazine dose to a maximum of 500 mg twice daily in patients concurrently receiving moderate CYP3A4 inhibitors (e.g., diltiazem, verapamil, erythromycin, etc.). *Risk D: Consider therapy modification*

Salmeterol: CYP3A4 Inhibitors (Moderate) may increase the serum concentration of Salmeterol. *Risk C: Monitor therapy*

Selective Serotonin Reuptake Inhibitors: May decrease the metabolism of Haloperidol. *Risk C: Monitor therapy*

Tamoxifen: CYP2D6 Inhibitors (Moderate) may decrease the metabolism of Tamoxifen. Specifically, CYP2D6 inhibitors may decrease the formation of highly potent active metabolites. *Risk D: Consider therapy modification*

Tetrabenazine: May enhance the adverse/toxic effect of Antipsychotics. *Risk C: Monitor therapy*

Thioridazine: QTc-Prolonging Agents may enhance the QTc-prolonging effect of Thioridazine. *Risk X: Avoid combination*

Thioridazine: CYP2D6 Inhibitors may decrease the metabolism of Thioridazine. *Risk X: Avoid combination*

TraMADol: CYP2D6 Inhibitors (Moderate) may diminish the therapeutic effect of TraMADol. These CYP2D6 inhibitors may prevent the metabolic conversion of tramadol to its active metabolite that accounts for much of its opioid-like effects. *Risk C: Monitor therapy*

Ziprasidone: QTc-Prolonging Agents may enhance the QTc-prolonging effect of Ziprasidone. The risk of a severe arrhythmia may be increased. *Risk X: Avoid combination*

Ethanol/Nutrition/Herb Interactions

Ethanol: Avoid ethanol (may increase CNS depression).

Herb/Nutraceutical: Avoid valerian, St John's wort, kava kava, gotu kola (may increase CNS depression).

Stability

Protect oral dosage forms from light.

Haloperidol lactate injection should be stored at controlled room temperature; do not freeze or expose to temperatures >40°C. Protect from light; exposure to light may cause discoloration and the development of a grayish-red precipitate over several weeks.

Haloperidol lactate may be administered IVPB or I.V. infusion in D_5W solutions. NS solutions should not be used due to reports of decreased stability and incompatibility.

Standardized dose: 0.5-100 mg/50-100 mL D_5W.

Stability of standardized solutions is 38 days at room temperature (24°C).

Mechanism of Action Haloperidol is a butyrophenone antipsychotic which blocks postsynaptic mesolimbic dopaminergic D_1 and D_2 receptors in the brain; depresses the release of hypothalamic and hypophyseal hormones; believed to depress the reticular activating system thus affecting basal metabolism, body temperature, wakefulness, vasomotor tone, and emesis

Pharmacodynamics/Kinetics

Onset of action: Sedation: I.M., I.V.: 30-60 minutes

Duration: Decanoate: 2-4 weeks

Distribution: V_d: 8-18 L/kg; crosses placenta; enters breast milk

Protein binding: 90%

Metabolism: Hepatic to inactive compounds

Bioavailability: Oral: 60%

Half-life elimination: 18 hours; Decanoate: ~1 day

Time to peak, serum: Oral: 2-6 hours; I.M.: 20 minutes; Decanoate: 7 days

Excretion: Urine (33% to 40% as metabolites) within 5 days; feces (15%)

Clearance: 550 ± 133 mL/minute

Dosage

Children: 3-12 years (15-40 kg): Oral:

Initial: 0.05 mg/kg/day or 0.25-0.5 mg/day given in 2-3 divided doses; increase by 0.25-0.5 mg every 5-7 days; maximum: 0.15 mg/kg/day

Usual maintenance:

Agitation or hyperkinesia: 0.01-0.03 mg/kg/day once daily

Nonpsychotic disorders: 0.05-0.075 mg/kg/day in 2-3 divided doses

Psychotic disorders: 0.05-0.15 mg/kg/day in 2-3 divided doses

Children 6-12 years: Sedation/psychotic disorders: I.M. (as lactate): 1-3 mg/dose every 4-8 hours to a maximum of 0.15 mg/kg/day; change over to oral therapy as soon as able

Adults:

Psychosis:

Oral: 0.5-5 mg 2-3 times/day; usual maximum: 30 mg/day

I.M. (as lactate): 2-5 mg every 4-8 hours as needed

I.M. (as decanoate): Initial: 10-20 times the daily oral dose administered at 4-week intervals

Maintenance dose: 10-15 times initial oral dose; used to stabilize psychiatric symptoms

Delirium in the intensive care unit (unlabeled use, unlabeled route):

I.V.: 2-10 mg; may repeat bolus doses every 20-30 minutes until calm achieved then administer 25% of the maximum dose every 6 hours; monitor ECG and QT_c interval

Intermittent I.V.: 0.03-0.15 mg/kg every 30 minutes to 6 hours

Oral: Agitation: 5-10 mg

Continuous intravenous infusion (100 mg/100 mL D_5W): Rates of 3-25 mg/hour have been used

Rapid tranquilization of severely-agitated patient (unlabeled use): Administer every 30-60 minutes:

Oral: 5-10 mg

I.M. (as lactate): 5 mg

Average total dose (oral or I.M.) for tranquilization: 10-20 mg

Elderly: Nonpsychotic patient, dementia behavior (unlabeled use): Initial: Oral: 0.25-0.5 mg 1-2 times/day; increase dose at 4- to 7-day intervals by 0.25-0.5 mg/day; increase dosing intervals (twice daily, 3 times/day, etc) as necessary to control response or side effects

Hemodialysis/peritoneal dialysis: Supplemental dose is not necessary

Administration The decanoate injectable formulation should be administered I.M. only, **do not administer decanoate I.V.** Dilute the oral concentrate with water or juice before administration. Avoid skin contact with oral suspension or solution; may cause contact dermatitis.

Monitoring Parameters Vital signs; lipid profile, fasting blood glucose/Hgb A_{1c}; BMI; mental status, abnormal involuntary movement scale (AIMS), extrapyramidal symptoms (EPS); ECG (with off-label intravenous administration)

Reference Range

Therapeutic: 5-20 ng/mL (SI: 10-40 nmol/L) (psychotic disorders - less for Tourette's and mania)

Toxic: >42 ng/mL (SI: >84 nmol/L)

Dosage Forms Excipient information presented when available (limited, particularly for generics); consult specific product labeling. [DSC] = Discontinued product

Note: Strength expressed as base.

Injection, oil, as decanoate: 50 mg/mL (1 mL, 5 mL); 100 mg/mL (1 mL, 5 mL)

Haldol® Decanoate: 50 mg/mL (1 mL; 5 mL [DSC]); 100 mg/mL (1 mL; 5 mL [DSC]) [contains benzyl alcohol, sesame oil]

Injection, solution, as lactate: 5 mg/mL (1 mL, 10 mL)

Haldol®: 5 mg/mL (1 mL)

Solution, oral concentrate, as lactate: 2 mg/mL (15 mL, 120 mL)

Tablet: 0.5 mg, 1 mg, 2 mg, 5 mg, 10 mg, 20 mg

◆ **Haloperidol Decanoate** *see* Haloperidol *on page 754*

◆ **Haloperidol Lactate** *see* Haloperidol *on page 754*

◆ **Harkoseride** *see* Lacosamide *on page 885*

◆ **HAVRIX®** *see* Hepatitis A Vaccine *on page 760*

Hawthorn *(Crataegus oxyacantha)*

Natural Product Category Herb

Synonyms *Crataegus oxyacantha*; Maybush; Shanzha Rou; Whitethorn

Plant Part Flower, leaf, berry

Dosage and Standardization Oral: 250 mg 1-3 times/day, standardized to contain at least 2% vitexin and/or 20% procyanidins per dose, **or** 160-900 mg hawthorn extract/day in 2-3 divided doses (corresponding to 3.5-19.8 mg flavonoids or 30-168.8 mg oligomeric procyanidines)

Reported Uses
Angina, hypotension, hypertension, peripheral vascular disease, tachycardia; cardiotonic; congestive heart failure (Schussler, 1995; Walker, 2006; Weihmayr, 1996)
Heart failure (Pittler, 2003)

Summary Hawthorn is a vasodilator and cardiotonic with a variety of applications in the support of cardiovascular function. It has been used in both hypertension and hypotension, and is used in mild heart failure, angina, and peripheral vascular disorders. In traditional Chinese medicine, hawthorn berries (shanzha) were used for gastrointestinal complaints.

Effect on Mental Status May cause sedation, fatigue, and depression

Effect on Psychiatric Treatment None reported

Pharmacology The effect of hawthorn as an antihypertensive may be mediated by several mechanisms. Hawthorn bioflavonoids reportedly cause dilation of both peripheral and coronary vessels. Hawthorn is also believed to inhibit angiotensin-converting enzyme and demonstrates a modest diuretic effect. In addition, hawthorn-derived glycosides reportedly increase vagal tone.

The vasodilating properties have been noted to improve the symptoms of angina and peripheral vascular disease. Proanthocyanidins of hawthorn are claimed to have spasmolytic effects and have been reported to reverse atherosclerotic processes in laboratory studies.

Hawthorn has been reported to improve cardiac performance without affecting coronary blood flow. Flavonoid compounds in hawthorn are reported to have a variety of positive effects on collagen structure in blood vessels.

Theoretical Cautions and Contraindications Contraindicated in pregnancy (based on animal studies and human case reports) (Ammon, 1981). Due to pharmacologic activity, use with caution in individuals receiving antihypertensive medications, including vasodilators and angiotensin converting enzyme inhibitors (Ammon, 1981), and in individuals receiving cardiac glycosides. It has been used in Europe to decrease the need for digoxin. May cause dizziness, headache, or hypotension. Use caution in individuals at risk of hypotension including those taking antihypertensive medication or agents that predispose to orthostasis, elderly individuals, or those who would not tolerate transient hypotensive episodes (ie, cerebrovascular or cardiovascular disease).

Theoretically, based on its proposed pharmacologic activity, hawthorn has the potential to share some effects associated with ACE inhibitors. Cough is frequently associated with ACE inhibition and serious, rare reactions (including angioedema and renal impairment) have been attributed to these agents; however, these have not been reported with hawthorn despite broad experience.

General Warnings Use all herbal supplements with extreme caution in children <2 years of age and in pregnancy or lactation. Some herbs are contraindicated in pregnancy or lactation; make sure to observe warnings. Use with caution in individuals on medication and with pre-existing medical conditions. Always review for potential herb-drug interactions (HDIs) and other warnings. Large and prolonged doses may increase the potential for adverse effects. Herbs may cause transient adverse effects such as nausea, vomiting, and GI distress due to a variety of chemical constituents. Use caution in individuals having known allergies to plants.

Theoretical Interactions Antiarrhythmics, antihypertensives (vasodilators, ACE inhibitors, angiotensin receptor blockers), cardiac glycosides (digoxin), vasodilators, antilipemic agents

References

Ammon HP and Handel M, "Crataegus, Toxicology and Pharmacology, Part I: Toxicity," *Plant Med*, 1981, 43(2):105-20.

McGuffin M, et al, eds, *American Herbal Products Association's Botanical Safety Handbook*, Boca Raton, FL: CRC Press, 1997, 37.

Natural Standard Research Collaboration, Chief Editors: Ulbricht C, Basch E, *Natural Standard Herb and Supplement Reference - Evidence-Based Clinical Reviews*, USA: Elsevier/Mosby, 2005.

Pittler MH, Schmidt K, and Ernst E, "Hawthorn Extract for Treating Chronic Heart Failure: Meta-Analysis of Randomized Trials," *Am J Med*, 2003, 114(8):665-74.

Schussler M, Holzl J, and Fricke U, "Myocardial Effects of Flavonoids From *Crataegus* Species," *Arzneimittelforschung*, 1995, 45(8):842-5.

Walker AF, Marakis G, Simpson F, et al, "Hypotensive Effects of Hawthorn for Patients With Diabetes Taking Prescription Drugs: A Randomised Controlled Trial," *BR J Gen Pract*, 2006, 56(527):437-43.

Weihmayr T and Ernst E, "Therapeutic Effectiveness of *Crataegus*," *Fortschr Med*, 1996, 114 (1-2):27-9.

◆ **HbCV** *see Haemophilus* b Conjugate Vaccine *on page 753*

◆ **HBIG** *see* Hepatitis B Immune Globulin *on page 762*

◆ **hBNP** *see* Nesiritide *on page 1123*
◆ **hCG** *see* Chorionic Gonadotropin (Human) *on page 342*
◆ **HCTZ (error-prone abbreviation)** *see* Hydrochlorothiazide *on page 773*
◆ **Heavy Mineral Oil** *see* Mineral Oil *on page 1055*
◆ **Hectorol®** *see* Doxercalciferol *on page 507*
◆ **Helidac®** *see* Bismuth, Metronidazole, and Tetracycline *on page 190*
◆ **Hemabate®** *see* Carboprost Tromethamine *on page 282*
◆ **Hematin** *see* Hemin *on page 760*

Hemin (HEE min)

U.S. Brand Names Panhematin®
Index Terms Hematin
Pharmacologic Category Blood Modifiers
Use Treatment of recurrent attacks of acute intermittent porphyria (AIP)
Effect on Mental Status None reported
Effect on Psychiatric Treatment Avoid concurrent use with barbiturates
Dosage Summary
I.V.:
Children <16 years: Dosage not established
Children ≥16 years: 1-4 mg/kg/day repeated no earlier than every 12 hours (maximum: 6 mg/kg in any 24-hour period)
Adults: 1-4 mg/kg/day repeated no earlier than every 12 hours; (maximum: 6 mg/kg/24-hour period)
Dosage Forms Excipient information presented when available (limited, particularly for generics); consult specific product labeling.
Injection, powder for reconstitution [preservative free]:
Panhematin®: 313 mg [provides 7 mg/mL when reconstituted]

◆ **Hemocyte® [OTC]** *see* Ferrous Fumarate *on page 626*
◆ **Hemorrhoidal HC** *see* Hydrocortisone *on page 785*
◆ **Hemril®-30** *see* Hydrocortisone *on page 785*
◆ **HepaGam B™** *see* Hepatitis B Immune Globulin *on page 762*

Hepatitis A Vaccine (hep a TYE tis aye vak SEEN)

U.S. Brand Names HAVRIX®; VAQTA®
Canadian Brand Names Avaxim®; Avaxim®-Pediatric; HAVRIX®; VAQTA®
Mexican Brand Names Havrix 1440; Havrix Junior; Vaqta
Pharmacologic Category Vaccine, Inactivated (Viral)
Generic Available No
Use
Active immunization against disease caused by hepatitis A virus (HAV)
The Advisory Committee on Immunization Practices (ACIP) recommends routine vaccination for:
- All children ≥12 months of age
- Travelers to countries with intermediate to high endemicity of HAV (a list of countries is available at http://wwwn.cdc.gov/travel/contentdiseases.aspx)
- Men who have sex with men
- Illegal drug users
- Patients with chronic liver disease
- Patients who receive clotting-factor concentrates
- Persons who work with HAV-infected primates or with HAV in a research laboratory setting

Effect on Mental Status Irritability and drowsiness are common; may cause weakness and fatigue
Effect on Psychiatric Treatment None reported
Pregnancy Risk Factor C
Pregnancy Considerations Reproduction studies have not been conducted. The safety of vaccination during pregnancy has not been determined, however, the theoretical risk to the infant is expected to be low.
Lactation Excretion in breast milk unknown/use caution
Contraindications Hypersensitivity to hepatitis A vaccine or any component of the formulation
Warnings/Precautions Use caution in patients on anticoagulants, with thrombocytopenia, or bleeding disorders (bleeding may occur following intramuscular injection). Treatment for anaphylactic reactions should be immediately available. Postpone vaccination with acute infection or febrile

illness. May not prevent infection if adequate antibody titers are not achieved (including immunosuppressed patients, patients on immunosuppressant therapy). Packaging may contain natural latex rubber; some products may contain neomycin. In order to maximize vaccination rates, the ACIP recommends simultaneous administration of all age-appropriate vaccines (live or inactivated) for which a person is eligible at a single clinic visit, unless contraindications exist. Safety and efficacy have not been established in children <12 months of age.

Adverse Reactions All serious adverse reactions must be reported to the U.S. Department of Health and Human Services (DHHS) Vaccine Adverse Event Reporting System (VAERS)) at 1-800-822-7967 or online at https://secure.vaers.org.

Frequency dependent upon age, product used, and concomitant vaccine administration. In general, injection site reactions were less common in younger children.

>10%:

Central nervous system: Irritability (11% to 36%), drowsiness (15% to 17%), headache (≤1% to 16%), fever ≥100.4°F (9% to 11%)

Gastrointestinal: Anorexia (1% to 19%)

Local: Injection site: Pain, soreness, tenderness (3% to 56%), erythema (1% to 22%), warmth (<1% to 17%), swelling (1% to 14%)

1% to 10%:

Central nervous system: Fever ≥102°F (3%)

Dermatologic: Rash (≤1% to 5%)

Endocrine & metabolic: Menstrual disorder (1%)

Gastrointestinal: Diarrhea (<1% to 6%), vomiting (<1% to 4%), nausea (2%), abdominal pain (<1% to 2%), anorexia (1%)

Local: Injection site bruising (1% to 2%)

Neuromuscular & skeletal: Weakness/fatigue (4%), myalgia (<1% to 2%), arm pain (1%), back pain (1%), stiffness (1%)

Ocular: Conjunctivitis (1%)

Otic: Otitis media (8%), otitis (2%)

Respiratory: Upper respiratory tract infection (<1% to 10%), rhinorrhea (6%), cough (1% to 5%), pharyngitis (<1% to 3%), respiratory congestion (2%), nasal congestion (1%), laryngotracheobronchitis (1%)

Miscellaneous: Crying (2%), viral exanthema (1%)

<1% (Limited to important or life threatening): Allergic reaction, anaphylaxis, angioedema, arthralgia, asthma, bronchial constriction, bronchiolitis, cerebellar ataxia, CK increased, dehydration, dermatitis, diabetes mellitus, dizziness, dyspnea, encephalitis, erythema multiforme, eosinophilia, eye irritation, gastroenteritis, Guillain-Barré syndrome, hepatitis, hyperhidrosis, hypertonic episode, injection site hematoma, injection site itching, injection site rash, insomnia, jaundice, Kawasaki's disease, liver function tests increased, lymphadenopathy, multiple sclerosis, myelitis, neuropathy, paresthesia, photophobia, pneumonia, pruritus, seizure, somnolence, syncope, taste disturbance, thrombocytopenia, urine protein increased, urticaria, vertigo, wheezing

Drug Interactions

Immunosuppressants: May diminish the therapeutic effect of Vaccines (Inactivated). *Risk C: Monitor therapy*

Stability Store under refrigeration at 2°C to 8°C (36°F to 46°F); do not freeze.

Mechanism of Action As an inactivated virus vaccine, hepatitis A vaccine offers active immunization against hepatitis A virus infection at an effective immune response rate in up to 99% of subjects

Pharmacodynamics/Kinetics

Onset of action (protection): 2-4 weeks after a single dose; 2 weeks after vaccine administration, 54% to 62% of patients develop neutralizing antibodies; this percentage increases to 94% to 100% at 1 month postvaccination (CDC, 2006)

Duration: Neutralizing antibodies have persisted for up to 8 years; based on kinetic models, antibodies may be present ≥14-20 years in children and ≥25 years in adults who receive the complete vaccination series (CDC, 2006; Van Damme, 2003).

Dosage I.M.: **Note:** When used for primary immunization, the vaccine should be given at least 2 weeks prior to expected HAV exposure. When used for post-exposure prophylaxis, the vaccine should be given as soon as possible.

HAVRIX®:

Children 12 months to 18 years: 720 ELISA units (0.5 mL) with a booster dose of 720 ELISA units to be given 6-12 months following primary immunization

Adults: 1440 ELISA units (1 mL) with a booster dose of 1440 ELISA units to be given 6-12 months following primary immunization

VAQTA®:

Children 12 months to 18 years: 25 units (0.5 mL) with 25 units (0.5 mL) booster dose of 25 units to be given 6-18 months after primary immunization (6-12 months if initial dose was with HAVRIX®)

Adults: 50 units (1 mL) with 50 units (1 mL) booster dose of 50 units to be given 6-18 months after primary immunization (6-12 months if initial dose was with HAVRIX®)

Administration The deltoid muscle is the preferred site for injection; gluteal administration may decrease efficacy. Do not administer intravenously, intradermally, or subcutaneously. Shake well prior to use; discard if the suspension is discolored or does not appear homogenous after shaking. When used for primary immunization, the vaccine should be given at least 2 weeks prior to expected HAV exposure. When used for post-exposure prophylaxis, the vaccine should be given as soon as possible. For patients at risk of hemorrhage following intramuscular injection, the ACIP recommends "it should be administered intramuscularly if, in the opinion of the physician familiar with the patients bleeding risk, the vaccine can be administered with reasonable safety by this route. If the patient receives antihemophilia or other similar therapy, intramuscular vaccination can be scheduled shortly after such therapy is administered. A fine needle (23 gauge or smaller) can be used for the vaccination and firm pressure applied to the site (without rubbing) for at least 2 minutes. The patient should be instructed concerning the risk of hematoma from the injection."

Administration with other vaccines:

Hepatitis A vaccine with live vaccines: May be given simultaneously or at any interval between doses.

Hepatitis A vaccine with other inactivated vaccines: May be given simultaneously or at any interval between doses.

Vaccine administration with antibody-containing products: Hepatitis A vaccine may be given simultaneously at different sites or at any interval between doses. Examples of antibody-containing products include I.M. and I.V. immune globulin, hepatitis B immune globulin, tetanus immune globulin, varicella zoster immune globulin, rabies immune globulin, whole blood, packed red cells, plasma, and platelet products.

Monitoring Parameters Liver function tests

Additional Information The ACIP currently recommends that older adults, the immunocompormised, or persons with underlying medical conditions (including chronic liver disease) that are vaccinated <2 weeks from departure to an area with a high risk of hepatitis A infection also receive immune globulin.

Federal law requires that the date of administration, the vaccine manufacturer, lot number of vaccine, and the administering person's name, title and address be entered into the patient's permanent medical record.

Dosage Forms Excipient information presented when available (limited, particularly for generics); consult specific product labeling.

Injection, suspension [adult formulation; preservative free]:

HAVRIX®: Hepatitis A virus antigen 1440 ELISA units/mL (1 mL) [contains aluminum, trace amounts of neomycin; prefilled syringe contains natural rubber/natural latex]

VAQTA®: Hepatitis A virus antigen 50 units/mL (1 mL) [contains aluminum, natural rubber/natural latex in packaging]

Injection, suspension [pediatric formulation; preservative free]:

HAVRIX®: Hepatitis A virus antigen 720 ELISA units/0.5 mL (0.5 mL) [contains aluminum, trace amounts of neomycin; prefilled syringe contains natural rubber/natural latex]

Injection, suspension [pediatric/adolescent formulation; preservative free]:

VAQTA®: Hepatitis A virus antigen 25 units/0.5 mL (0.5 mL) [contains aluminum, natural rubber/natural latex in packaging]

Hepatitis B Immune Globulin

(hep a TYE tis bee i MYUN GLOB yoo lin YU man)

Medication Safety Issues

Sound-alike/look-alike issues:

HBIG may be confused with BabyBIG

U.S. Brand Names HepaGam B™; HyperHEP B™ S/D; Nabi-HB®

Canadian Brand Names HepaGam B™; HyperHep B®

Index Terms HBIG

Pharmacologic Category Immune Globulin

Generic Available No

Use

Passive prophylactic immunity to hepatitis B following: Acute exposure to blood containing hepatitis B surface antigen (HBsAg); perinatal exposure of infants born to HBsAg-positive mothers; sexual exposure to HBsAg-positive persons; household exposure to persons with acute HBV infection

Prevention of hepatitis B virus recurrence after liver transplantation in HBsAg-positive transplant patients

Note: Hepatitis B immune globulin is not indicated for treatment of active hepatitis B infection and is ineffective in the treatment of chronic active hepatitis B infection.

Effect on Mental Status May cause dizziness or drowsiness

Effect on Psychiatric Treatment Sedative effects may be additive with concurrent psychotropic use

Pregnancy Risk Factor C

Pregnancy Considerations Reproduction studies have not been conducted.

Lactation Excretion in breast milk unknown/use caution

Contraindications Hypersensitivity to hepatitis B immune globulin or any component of the formulation; severe allergy to gamma globulin or anti-immunoglobulin therapies

Warnings/Precautions Hypersensitivity and anaphylactic reactions can occur; immediate treatment (including epinephrine 1:1000) should be available. Use with caution in patients with previous systemic hypersensitivity to human immunoglobulins. Use with caution in patients with thrombocytopenia or coagulation disorders; I.M. injections may be contraindicated. Use with caution in patients with IgA deficiency. Product of human plasma; may potentially contain infectious agents which could transmit disease. Screening of donors, as well as testing and/or inactivation or removal of certain viruses, reduces the risk. Infections thought to be transmitted by this product should be reported to the manufacturer. Some products may contain maltose, which may result in falsely-elevated blood glucose readings.

Adverse Reactions Reported with postexposure prophylaxis. Adverse events reported in liver transplant patients included tremor and hypotension, were associated with a single infusion during the first week of treatment, and did not recur with additional infusions.

Central nervous system: Fainting, headache, lightheadedness, malaise

Dermatologic: Angioedema, bruising, urticaria

Gastrointestinal: Nausea, vomiting

Hematologic: WBC decreased

Hepatic: Alkaline phosphatase increased, AST increased

Local: Ache, erythema, pain, and/or tenderness at injection site

Neuromuscular & skeletal: Arthralgia, joint stiffness, myalgia

Renal: Creatinine increased

Respiratory: Cold symptoms

Miscellaneous: Anaphylaxis, flu-like syndrome

Drug Interactions

Vaccines (Live): Immune Globulins may diminish the therapeutic effect of Vaccines (Live). **Exceptions:** Influenza Virus Vaccine; Yellow Fever Vaccine. *Risk D: Consider therapy modification*

Stability Refrigerate at 2°C to 8°C (36°F to 46°F); do not freeze. Use within 6 hours of entering vial. Do not shake vial; avoid foaming.

Mechanism of Action Hepatitis B immune globulin (HBIG) is a nonpyrogenic sterile solution containing immunoglobulin G (IgG) specific to hepatitis B surface antigen (HB_sAg). HBIG differs from immune globulin in the amount of anti-HB_s. Immune globulin is prepared from plasma that is not preselected for anti-HB_s content. HBIG is prepared from plasma preselected for high titer anti-HB_s. In the U.S., HBIG has an anti-HB_s high titer >1:100,000 by IRA.

Pharmacodynamics/Kinetics

Duration of action: Postexposure prophylaxis: 3-6 months

Absorption: I.M.: Slow

Half-life: 17-25 days

Distribution: V_d: 7-15 L

Time to peak, serum: I.M.: 2-10 days

Dosage

I.M.:

Newborns: Perinatal exposure of infants born to HBsAg-positive mothers: 0.5 mL as soon after birth as possible (within 12 hours); active vaccination with hepatitis B vaccine may begin at the same time in a different site (if not contraindicated). If first dose of hepatitis B vaccine is delayed for as long as 3 months, dose may be repeated. If hepatitis B vaccine is refused, dose may be repeated at 3 and 6 months.

Infants <12 months: Household exposure prophylaxis: 0.5 mL (to be administered if mother or primary caregiver has acute HBV infection)

Children ≥12 months and Adults: Postexposure prophylaxis: 0.06 mL/kg as soon as possible after exposure (ie, within 24 hours of needlestick, ocular, or mucosal exposure or within 14 days of sexual exposure); usual dose: 3-5 mL; repeat at 28-30 days after exposure in nonresponders to hepatitis B vaccine or in patients who refuse vaccination

Note: HBIG may be administered at the same time (but at a different site) or up to 1 month preceding hepatitis B vaccination without impairing the active immune response

I.V.: Adults: Prevention of hepatitis B virus recurrence after liver transplantation (HepaGam B™): 20,000 int. units/dose according to the following schedule:

Anhepatic phase (Initial dose): One dose given with the liver transplant

Week 1 postop: One dose daily for 7 days (days 1-7)

Weeks 2-12 postop: One dose every 2 weeks starting day 14

Month 4 onward: One dose monthly starting on month 4

Dose adjustment: Adjust dose to reach anti-HBs levels of 500 int. units/L within the first week after transplantation. In patients with surgical bleeding, abdominal fluid drainage >500 mL or those undergoing plasmapheresis, administer 10,000 int. units/dose every 6 hours until target anti-HBs levels are reached.

Administration

I.M.: Postexposure prophylaxis: I.M. injection only in anterolateral aspect of upper thigh and deltoid muscle of upper arm; to prevent injury from injection, care should be taken when giving to patients with thrombocytopenia or bleeding disorders

I.V.:

HepaGam B™: Liver transplant: Administer at 2 mL/minute. Decrease infusion to ≤1 mL/minute for patient discomfort or infusion-related adverse events. Actual volume of infusion is dependant upon potency labeled on each individual vial.

Nabi-HB®: Although not an FDA-approved for this purpose, Nabi-HB® has been administered intravenously in hepatitis B-positive liver transplant patients

Monitoring Parameters Liver transplant: Serum HBsAg; infusion-related adverse events

Test Interactions

Glucose testing: HepaGam B™ contains maltose. Falsely-elevated blood glucose levels may occur when glucose monitoring devices and test strips utilizing the glucose dehydrogenase pyrroloquinolinequinone (GDH-PQQ) based methods are used.

Serological testing: Antibodies transferred following administration of immune globulins may provide misleading positive test results (eg, Coombs' test)

Additional Information Each vial contains anti-HB_s antibody equivalent to or exceeding the potency of anti-HB_s in a U.S. reference standard hepatitis B immune globulin (FDA). The U.S. reference standard has been tested against the WHO standard hepatitis B immune globulin with listed values between 207 int. units/mL and 220 int. units/mL (included in individual product information).

Dosage Forms Excipient information presented when available (limited, particularly for generics); consult specific product labeling.

Note: Potency expressed in international units (as compared to the WHO standard) is noted by individual lot on the vial label.

Injection, solution [preservative free]:

HyperHEP B™ S/D: Anti-HBs ≥220 int. units/mL (0.5 mL, 1 mL, 5 mL)

Nabi-HB®: Anti-HBs >312 int. units/mL (1 mL, 5 mL) [contains polysorbate 80]

HepaGam B™: Anti-HBs 312 int. units/mL (1 mL, 5 mL) [contains maltose and polysorbate 80]

◆ **Hepatitis B Inactivated Virus Vaccine (recombinant DNA)** *see* Hepatitis B Vaccine *on page 764*

Hepatitis B Vaccine (hep a TYE tis bee vak SEEN ree KOM be nant)

Medication Safety Issues

Sound-alike/look-alike issues:

Recombivax HB® may be confused with Comvax®

U.S. Brand Names Engerix-B®; Recombivax HB®

Canadian Brand Names Engerix-B®; Recombivax HB®

Mexican Brand Names Engerix-B

Index Terms Hepatitis B Inactivated Virus Vaccine (recombinant DNA)

Pharmacologic Category Vaccine, Inactivated (Viral)

Generic Available No

Use Immunization against infection caused by all known subtypes of hepatitis B virus (HBV), in individuals seeking protection from HBV infection and/or in the following individuals considered at high risk of potential exposure to hepatitis B virus or HBsAg-positive materials:

Workplace Exposure:

- Healthcare workers[1] (including students, custodial staff, lab personnel, etc)
- Police and fire personnel
- Military personnel
- Morticians and embalmers
- Clients/staff of institutions for the developmentally disabled

Lifestyle Factors:

- Homosexual men
- Heterosexually-active persons with multiple partners in a 6-month period or those with recently acquired sexually-transmitted disease
- Intravenous drug users

Specific Patient Groups:

- Those on hemodialysis[2], receiving transfusions[3], or in hematology/oncology units
- Adolescents
- Infants born of HBsAG-positive mothers
- Individuals with chronic liver disease
- Individual with HIV infection

Others:

- Prison inmates and staff of correctional facilities
- Household and sexual contacts of HBV carriers
- Residents, immigrants, adoptees, and refugees from areas with endemic HBV infection (eg, Alaskan Eskimos, Pacific Islanders, Indochinese, and Haitian descent)
- International travelers to areas of endemic HBV
- Children born after 11/21/1991

[1]The risk of hepatitis B virus (HBV) infection for healthcare workers varies both between hospitals and within hospitals. Hepatitis B vaccination is recommended for all healthcare workers with blood exposure.

[2]Hemodialysis patients often respond poorly to hepatitis B vaccination; higher vaccine doses or increased number of doses are required. A special formulation of one vaccine is now available for such persons (Recombivax HB®, 40 mcg/mL). The anti-HB_s (antibody to hepatitis B surface antigen) response of such persons should be tested after they are vaccinated, and those who have not responded should be revaccinated with 1-3 additional doses. Patients with chronic renal disease should be vaccinated as early as possible, ideally before they require hemodialysis. In addition, their anti-HB^s levels should be monitored at 6- to 12-month intervals to assess the need for revaccination.

[3]Patients with hemophilia should be immunized subcutaneously, not intramuscularly.

In addition, the Advisory Committee on Immunization Practices (ACIP) recommends vaccination for any persons who are wounded in bombings or similar mass casualty events who have penetrating injuries or nonintact skin exposure, or who have contact with mucous membranes (exception - superficial contact with intact skin), and who cannot confirm receipt of a hepatitis B vaccination.

Effect on Mental Status Malaise and fatigue are common; may rarely cause lightheadedness, somnolence, insomnia, irritability, agitation, anorexia

Effect on Psychiatric Treatment Sedative effects may be additive with concurrent psychotropic use

Pregnancy Risk Factor C

Pregnancy Considerations Reproduction studies have not been conducted. The ACIP recommends HBsAg testing for all pregnant women. Based on limited data, there is no apparent risk to the fetus when the hepatitis B vaccine is administered during pregnancy. Pregnancy itself is not a contraindication to vaccination; vaccination should be considered if otherwise indicated.

Lactation Excretion in breast milk unknown/use caution

Contraindications Hypersensitivity to yeast, hepatitis B vaccine, or any component of the formulation

Warnings/Precautions Immediate treatment for anaphylactic/anaphylactoid reaction should be available during vaccine use. Consider delaying vaccination during acute, moderate-to-severe febrile illness. Use caution with decreased cardiopulmonary function Unrecognized hepatitis B infection may be present, immunization may not prevent infection in these patients. Patients >65 years may have lower response rates. Consider delaying vaccination for ≥3 months after receiving immunosuppressive therapy. Use caution in multiple sclerosis patients; rare exacerbations of symptoms have been observed. Some dosage forms contain dry natural latex rubber. In order to maximize vaccination rates, the ACIP recommends simultaneous administration of all age-appropriate vaccines (live or inactivated) for which a person is eligible at a single clinic visit, unless contraindications exist.

Adverse Reactions All serious adverse reactions must be reported to the U.S. Department of Health and Human Services (DHHS) Vaccine Adverse Event Reporting System (VAERS) 1-800-822-7967.

Frequency not defined. The most common adverse effects reported with both products included injection site reactions (>10%).

Cardiovascular: Flushing, hypotension

Central nervous system: Agitation, chills, dizziness, fatigue, fever (≥37.5°C / 100°F), headache, insomnia, irritability, lightheadedness, malaise, somnolence, vertigo

Dermatologic: Angioedema, petechiae, pruritus, rash, urticaria

Gastrointestinal: Abdominal pain, appetite decreased, constipation, cramps, diarrhea, dyspepsia, nausea, vomiting

Genitourinary: Dysuria

Local: Injection site reactions: Ecchymosis, erythema, induration, pain, nodule formation, soreness, swelling, tenderness, warmth

Neuromuscular & skeletal: Achiness, arthralgia, back pain, myalgia, neck pain, neck stiffness, paresthesia, shoulder pain, tingling, weakness

Otic: Earache

Respiratory: Cough, pharyngitis, rhinitis, upper respiratory tract infection

Miscellaneous: Diaphoresis, lymphadenopathy, flu-like syndrome

Postmarketing and/or case reports: Alopecia, anaphylaxis, arthritis, Bell's palsy, bronchospasm, conjunctivitis, eczema, encephalitis, erythema nodosum, erythema multiforme, erythrocyte sedimentation rate increased, febrile seizure, Guillain-Barré syndrome, herpes zoster, hypoesthesia, keratitis, liver enzymes increased, lupus-like syndrome, migraine, multiple sclerosis, muscle weakness, neuropathy, optic neuritis, palpitation, paresis, paresthesia, polyarteritis nodosa, purpura, seizure, serum-sickness like syndrome (may be delayed days to weeks), Stevens-Johnson syndrome, SLE, syncope, tachycardia, thrombocytopenia, tinnitus, transverse myelitis, vasculitis, visual disturbances, vertigo

Drug Interactions

Immunosuppressants: May diminish the therapeutic effect of Vaccines (Inactivated). *Risk C: Monitor therapy*

Stability Refrigerate at 2°C to 8°C (36°F to 46°F); do not freeze.

Mechanism of Action Recombinant hepatitis B vaccine is a noninfectious subunit viral vaccine, which confers active immunity via formation of antihepatitis B antibodies. The vaccine is derived from hepatitis B surface antigen (HBsAg) produced through recombinant DNA techniques from yeast cells. The portion of the hepatitis B gene which codes for HBsAg is cloned into yeast which is then cultured to produce hepatitis B vaccine.

Pharmacodynamics/Kinetics Duration of action: Following a 3-dose series in children, up to 50% of patients will have low or undetectable anti-HB antibody 5-15 years postvaccination. However, anamnestic increases in anti-HB have been shown up to 23 years later suggesting a lifelong immune memory response.

Dosage I.M.:

Immunization regimen: Regimen consists of 3 doses (0, 1, and 6 months): First dose given on the elected date, second dose given 1 month later, third dose given 6 months after the first dose; see table.

When used for immediate prophylactic intervention (eg, administration to persons who are wounded in bombings or similar mass casualty events), vaccination should begin within 24 hours and no later than 7 days following the event.

Note: Infants born to mothers whose HBsAg status is unknown should follow the regimen for HBsAg-positive mothers, omitting the dose of HBIG.

Note: Preterm infants <2000 g and born to HBsAg-negative mothers should have the first dose delayed until 1 month after birth or hospital discharge due to decreased immune response in underweight infants.

Routine Immunization Regimen of Three I.M. Hepatitis B Vaccine Doses

Age	Initial		1 mo		2 mo	6 mo[1]	
	Recombivax HB® (mL)	Engerix-B® (mL)	Recombivax HB® (mL)	Engerix-B® (mL)	Engerix-B® (mL)	Recombivax HB® (mL)	Engerix-B® (mL)
Birth[2] to 19 y	0.5[3]	0.5[4]	0.5[3]	0.5[4]	–	0.5[3]	0.5[4]
≥20 y[5]	1[6]	1[7]	1[6]	1[7]	–	1[6]	1[7]
Dialysis or immunocompromised patients[8]	1[9]	2[10]	1[9]	2[10]	2[10]	1[9]	2[10]

[1]Final dose in series should not be administered before age of 24 weeks.

[2]Infants born of HBsAg **negative** mothers.

[3]5 mcg/0.5 mL pediatric/adolescent formulation.

[4]10 mcg/0.5 mL formulation.

[5]Alternately, doses may be administered at 0, 1, and 4 months **or** at 0, 2, and 4 months.

[6]10 mcg/mL adult formulation.

[7]20 mcg/mL formulation.

[8]Revaccinate if anti-HB_s <10 mIU/mL ≥1-2 months after third dose.

[9]40 mcg/mL dialysis formulation.

[10]Two 1 mL doses given at different sites using the 20 mcg/mL formulation.

Alternative dosing schedule for **Recombivax HB®**:

Children 11-15 years (10 mcg/mL adult formulation): First dose of 1 mL given on the elected date, second dose given 4-6 months later

Adults ≥20 years: Doses may be administered at 0, 1, and 4 months **or** at 0, 2, and 4 months

Alternative dosing schedules for **Engerix-B®**:

Children ≤10 years (10 mcg/0.5 mL formulation): High-risk children: 0.5 mL at 0, 1, 2, and 12 months; lower-risk children ages 5-10 who are candidates for an extended administration schedule may receive an alternative regimen of 0.5 mL at 0, 12, and 24 months. If booster dose is needed, revaccinate with 0.5 mL.

Adolescents 11-19 years (20 mcg/mL formulation): 1 mL at 0, 1, and 6 months. High-risk adolescents: 1 mL at 0, 1, 2, and 12 months; lower-risk adolescents 11-16 years who are candidates for an extended administration schedule may receive an alternative regimen of 0.5 mL (using the 10 mcg/0.5 mL) formulation at 0, 12, and 24 months. If booster dose is needed, revaccinate with 20 mcg.

Adults ≥20 years:

Doses may be administered at 0, 1, and 4 months **or** at 0, 2, and 4 months

High-risk adults (20 mcg/mL formulation): 1 mL at 0, 1, 2, and 12 months. If booster dose is needed, revaccinate with 1 mL.

Postexposure prophylaxis: **Note:** High-risk individuals may include children born of hepatitis B-infected mothers, those who have been or might be exposed or those who have traveled to high-risk areas. See table.

Postexposure Prophylaxis Recommended Dosage for Infants Born to HBsAg-Positive Mothers

Treatment	Birth ≤12 h	1 mo	6 mo
Engerix-B® (pediatric formulation 10 mcg/0.5 mL)[1]	0.5 mL[2]	0.5 mL	0.5 mL
Recombivax HB® (pediatric/adolescent formulation 5 mcg/0.5 mL)	0.5 mL[2]	0.5 mL	0.5 mL
Hepatitis B immune globulin	0.5 mL[2]	—	—

[1]An alternate regimen is administration of the vaccine at birth, and 1, 2, and 12 months later.

[2]The first dose of vaccine may be given at birth at the same time as HBIG, but give in the opposite anterolateral thigh. This may better ensure vaccine absorption. HBIG should be given immediately if mother is determined to be HBsAg-positive within 7 days of birth.

Administration It is possible to interchange the vaccines for completion of a series or for booster doses; the antibody produced in response to each type of vaccine is comparable, however, the quantity of the vaccine will vary

I.M. injection only; in adults, the deltoid muscle is the preferred site; the anterolateral thigh is the recommended site in infants and young children. Not for gluteal administration. Shake well prior to withdrawal and use.

For patients at risk of hemorrhage following intramuscular injection, hepatitis B vaccine may be administered subcutaneously although lower titers and/or increased incidence of local reactions may result. The ACIP recommends "it should be administered intramuscularly if, in the opinion of the physician familiar with the patients bleeding risk, the vaccine can be administered with reasonable safety by this route. If the patient receives antihemophilia or other similar therapy, intramuscular vaccination can be scheduled shortly after such therapy is administered. A fine needle (23 gauge or smaller) can be used for the vaccination and firm pressure applied to the site (without rubbing) for at least 2 minutes. The patient should be instructed concerning the risk of hematoma from the injection."

Administration with other vaccines:

Hepatitis B vaccine with live vaccines: May be given simultaneously or at any interval between doses.

Hepatitis B vaccine with other inactivated vaccines: May be given simultaneously or at any interval between doses.

Vaccine administration with antibody-containing products: Hepatitis B vaccine may be given simultaneously at different sites or at any interval between doses. Examples of antibody containing products include I.M. and I.V. immune globulin, hepatitis B immune globulin, tetanus immune globulin, varicella zoster immune globulin, rabies immune globulin, whole blood, packed red cells, plasma, and platelet products

Vaccination at the time of HBsAg testing: For persons in whom vaccination is recommended, the first dose of hepatitis B vaccine can be given after blood is drawn to test for HBsAg.

Additional Information Federal law requires that the date of administration, the vaccine manufacturer, lot number of vaccine, and the administering person's name, title, and address be entered into the patient's permanent medical record.

Dosage Forms Excipient information presented when available (limited, particularly for generics); consult specific product labeling.

Injection, suspension [adult; preservative free]:

Engerix-B®: Hepatitis B surface antigen 20 mcg/mL (1 mL) [contains aluminum, trace amounts of thimerosal; prefilled syringes contain natural rubber/natural latex]

Recombivax HB®: Hepatitis B surface antigen 10 mcg/mL (1 mL, 3 mL) [contains aluminum and yeast protein]

Injection, suspension [pediatric/adolescent]; preservative free]:

Engerix-B®: Hepatitis B surface antigen 10 mcg/0.5 mL (0.5 mL) [contains aluminum, trace amounts of thimerosal; prefilled syringes contain natural rubber/natural latex]

Recombivax HB®: Hepatitis B surface antigen 5 mcg/0.5 mL (0.5 mL) [contains aluminum and yeast protein]

Injection, suspension [dialysis formulation; preservative free]:

Recombivax HB®: Hepatitis B surface antigen 40 mcg/mL (1 mL) [contains aluminum and yeast protein]

- **Hepatitis B Vaccine (Recombinant)** *see Haemophilus* b Conjugate and Hepatitis B Vaccine *on page 752*
- **Hepsera™** *see* Adefovir *on page 51*
- **Herceptin®** *see* Trastuzumab *on page 1613*
- **Hexachlorocyclohexane** *see* Lindane *on page 927*
- **Hexalen®** *see* Altretamine *on page 78*
- **Hexamethylmelamine** *see* Altretamine *on page 78*
- **HEXM** *see* Altretamine *on page 78*
- **hGH** *see* Somatropin *on page 1499*
- **Hib Conjugate Vaccine** *see Haemophilus* b Conjugate and Hepatitis B Vaccine *on page 752*
- **Hib Conjugate Vaccine** *see Haemophilus* b Conjugate Vaccine *on page 753*
- **Hib Polysaccharide Conjugate** *see Haemophilus* b Conjugate Vaccine *on page 753*

◆ **High Gamma Vitamin E Complete™ [OTC]** *see* Vitamin E *on page 1675*

◆ **High-Molecular-Weight Iron Dextran (DexFerrum®)** *see* Iron Dextran Complex *on page 857*

◆ **Hirulog** *see* Bivalirudin *on page 191*

◆ **Histacol™ BD** *see* Brompheniramine, Pseudoephedrine, and Dextromethorphan *on page 208*

◆ **Histade™ [DSC]** *see* Chlorpheniramine and Pseudoephedrine *on page 325*

◆ **Histatab PH** *see* Chlorpheniramine, Phenylephrine, and Methscopolamine *on page 329*

◆ **Hista-Vent® DA [DSC]** *see* Chlorpheniramine, Phenylephrine, and Methscopolamine *on page 329*

◆ **Hista-Vent® PSE [DSC]** *see* Chlorpheniramine, Pseudoephedrine, and Methscopolamine *on page 334*

◆ **Histex™** *see* Chlorpheniramine and Pseudoephedrine *on page 325*

◆ **Histex® SR** *see* Brompheniramine and Pseudoephedrine *on page 206*

◆ **Histinex® HC** *see* Phenylephrine, Hydrocodone, and Chlorpheniramine *on page 1277*

Histrelin (his TREL in)

U.S. Brand Names Supprelin® LA; Vantas™

Canadian Brand Names Vantas™

Index Terms GnRH Agonist; Histrelin Acetate; LH-RH Agonist

Pharmacologic Category Gonadotropin Releasing Hormone Agonist

Use Palliative treatment of advanced prostate cancer; treatment of children with central precocious puberty (CPP)

Effect on Mental Status May cause fatigue and insomnia; may rarely cause depression, dizziness, irritability, lethargy, or malaise

Effect on Psychiatric Treatment May cause sexual dysfunction; concomitant use with psychotropic agents (especially SSRIs) may produce additive effects. May cause renal dysfunction; monitor serum levels in patients receiving lithium.

Dosage Summary

SubQ:

Children <2 years: Dosage not established

Children ≥2 years: 50 mg implant, inserted every 12 months [Supprelin® LA]

Adults: 50 mg implant, inserted every 12 months [Vantas™]

Dosage Forms Excipient information presented when available (limited, particularly for generics); consult specific product labeling.

Implant, subcutaneous:

Supprelin® LA: 50 mg (1) [releases ~65 mcg/day over 12 months; packaged with implantation kit]

Vantas™: 50 mg (1) [releases 50-60 mcg/day over 12 months; packaged with implantation kit]

◆ **Histrelin Acetate** *see* Histrelin *on page 769*

◆ **Hivid® [DSC]** *see* Zalcitabine *on page 1691*

◆ **HMM** *see* Altretamine *on page 78*

◆ **HMR 3647** *see* Telithromycin *on page 1542*

◆ **HN_2** *see* Mechlorethamine *on page 974*

◆ **Hold® DM [OTC]** *see* Dextromethorphan *on page 448*

Homatropine (hoe MA troe peen)

U.S. Brand Names Isopto® Homatropine

Index Terms Homatropine Hydrobromide

Pharmacologic Category Anticholinergic Agent, Ophthalmic; Ophthalmic Agent, Mydriatic

Use Producing cycloplegia and mydriasis for refraction; treatment of acute inflammatory conditions of the uveal tract; optical aid in axial lens opacities

Effect on Mental Status May cause drowsiness

Effect on Psychiatric Treatment None reported

Dosage Summary

Ophthalmic:

Children: Instill 1 drop (2% solution) 2-3 times/day **or** immediately prior to procedure, repeat every 10 minutes intervals as needed

Adults: Instill 1-2 drops (2% or 5% solution) 2-3 times/day, up to every 3-4 hours as needed **or** 1-2 drops (2% solution) or 1 drop (5% solution) prior to procedure, repeat every 5-10 minutes as needed up to 3 doses

Dosage Forms Excipient information presented when available (limited, particularly for generics); consult specific product labeling.

Solution, ophthalmic, as hydrobromide:

Isopto® Homatropine: 2% (5 mL); 5% (5 mL, 15 mL) [contains benzalkonium chloride]

◆ **Homatropine and Hydrocodone** *see* Hydrocodone and Homatropine *on page 780*

◆ **Homatropine Hydrobromide** *see* Homatropine *on page 769*

Hops *(Humulus lupulus)*

Natural Product Category Herb

Synonyms *Humulus lupulus*; Common Hops; Lupulus; Small Wolf

Plant Part Strobiles

Dosage and Standardization Oral: 100 mg twice daily as needed, standardized to contain 5.2% bitter acids and 4% flavonoids per dose

Reported Uses

Sedative/hypnotic (mild) (Hansel, 1980; Wohlfart, 1983)

Summary Hops have been used for centuries in brewing and as a traditional nerve and sedative tonic. Hops are thought to possess sedative and hypnotic properties. Traditional uses of hops include neuralgia, insomnia, excitability, and for the restlessness associated with nervous tension.

Effect on Mental Status May cause sedation

Effect on Psychiatric Treatment Combined use with psychotropics may produce additive CNS depression

Pharmacology The sedative effect of hops is not fully understood. Hops is reported to improve sleep disturbances when given in combination with other sedative herbs such as valerian root and passion flower. The constituent 2-methyl-3-buten-2-ol may have central nervous system depressant activity. It is usually formed *in vivo* through metabolism of the α-bitter acids, humulone and lupulone; may explain part of the sedative action of hops.

Theoretical Cautions and Contraindications Use with caution in individuals on the following medications (action may be potentiated): Antianxiety agents, antidepressants, antipsychotics, ethanol, hypnotics, sedatives (reported to increase sleeping time induced by pentobarbital) (Hansel, 1980). Use with caution when driving an automobile or operating heavy machinery and in individuals with hormone-sensitive conditions, such as breast, uterine, cervical, or prostate cancer, or endometriosis, due to the presence of phytoestrogens in hops which may exert estrogen receptor agonist or antagonist properties.

General Warnings Use all herbal supplements with extreme caution in children <2 years of age and in pregnancy or lactation. Some herbs are contraindicated in pregnancy or lactation; make sure to observe warnings. Use with caution in individuals on medication and with pre-existing medical conditions. Always review for potential herb-drug interactions (HDIs) and other warnings. Large and prolonged doses may increase the potential for adverse effects. Herbs may cause transient adverse effects such as nausea, vomiting, and GI distress due to a variety of chemical constituents. Use caution in individuals having known allergies to plants.

Theoretical Interactions Antianxiety agents, antidepressants, antipsychotics, ethanol, hypnotics, pentobarbital, sedatives, oral contraceptives, hormone replacement therapy, tamoxifen, raloxifene, cytochrome P450 metabolized agents, antidiabetic agents, disulfiram, metronidazole

References

Hansel R, Wohlfart R, and Coper H, "Sedative-Hypnotic Compounds in the Exhalation of Hops, II," *Z Naturforsch [C]*, 1980, 35(11-12):1096-7.

Lee KM, et al, "Effects of *Humulus lupulus* Extract on the Central Nervous System in Mice," *Planta Med*, 1993, 59(Supp):A691.

Natural Standard Research Collaboration, Chief Editors: Ulbricht C, Basch E, *Natural Standard Herb and Supplement Reference - Evidence-Based Clinical Reviews*, USA: Elsevier/Mosby, 2005.

Wohlfart R, Wurm G, Hansel R, et al, "Detection of Sedative-Hypnotic Active Ingredients in Hops. 5. Degradation of Bitter Acids to 2-Methyl-3-Buten-2-Ol, a Hop Constituent With Sedative-Hypnotic Activity," *Arch Pharm (Weinheim)*, 1983, 316(2):132-7.

◆ **Horse Antihuman Thymocyte Gamma Globulin** *see* Antithymocyte Globulin (Equine) *on page 126*

◆ **H.P. Acthar® Gel** *see* Corticotropin *on page 401*

◆ **HTF919** *see* Tegaserod *on page 1541*

- **hu1124** *see* Efalizumab *on page 526*
- **Humalog®** *see* Insulin Lispro *on page 832*
- **Humalog® Mix 50/50™** *see* Insulin Lispro Protamine and Insulin Lispro *on page 834*
- **Humalog® Mix 75/25™** *see* Insulin Lispro Protamine and Insulin Lispro *on page 834*
- **Human Antitumor Necrosis Factor Alpha** *see* Adalimumab *on page 50*
- **Human Growth Hormone** *see* Somatropin *on page 1499*
- **Humanized IgG1 Anti-CD52 Monoclonal Antibody** *see* Alemtuzumab *on page 59*
- **Human LFA-3/IgG(1) Fusion Protein** *see* Alefacept *on page 58*
- **Humatin® [DSC]** *see* Paromomycin *on page 1226*
- **Humatrope®** *see* Somatropin *on page 1499*
- **Humira®** *see* Adalimumab *on page 50*
- **Humulin® 50/50** *see* Insulin NPH and Insulin Regular *on page 836*
- **Humulin® 70/30** *see* Insulin NPH and Insulin Regular *on page 836*
- **Humulin® N** *see* Insulin NPH *on page 835*
- **Humulin® R** *see* Insulin Regular *on page 838*
- **Humulin® R U-500** *see* Insulin Regular *on page 838*
- ***Humulus lupulus*** *see* Hops *(Humulus lupulus) on page 770*
- ***Huperzia serrata*** *see* HuperzineA *(Huperzia serrata) on page 771*

HuperzineA *(Huperzia serrata)*

Natural Product Category Herb

Synonyms *Huperzia serrata*

Plant Part Isolated from *Huperzia serrata* (Chinese club moss)

Dosage and Standardization Oral: 50 mcg 1-3 times/day

Reported Uses

Myasthenia gravis (Cheng, 1986)

Senile dementia and Alzheimer's disease (Wang, 1998)

Summary Huperzia (Chinese club moss) has been used for centuries for various problems including memory and alertness. The isolated constituent is currently used as an acetylcholinesterase (ACE) inhibitor in senile dementia and Alzheimer's disease.

Effect on Mental Status None reported

Effect on Psychiatric Treatment Purported acetylcholinesterase activity may be diminished by anticholinergic effects of psychotropic agents. Side effects may be enhanced if used in combination with other acetylcholinesterase inhibitors.

Pharmacology In the 1980s, scientists demonstrated that purified huperzineA kept ACE from breaking down into acetylcholine.

Theoretical Cautions and Contraindications Based on pharmacologic activity, use with caution in individuals taking other acetylcholinesterase inhibitors.

General Warnings Use all herbal supplements with extreme caution in children <2 years of age and in pregnancy or lactation. Some herbs are contraindicated in pregnancy or lactation; make sure to observe warnings. Use with caution in individuals on medication and with pre-existing medical conditions. Always review for potential herb-drug interactions (HDIs) and other warnings. Large and prolonged doses may increase the potential for adverse effects. Herbs may cause transient adverse effects such as nausea, vomiting, and GI distress due to a variety of chemical constituents. Use caution in individuals having known allergies to plants.

Theoretical Interactions Acetylcholinesterase inhibitors (tacrine, donepezil), anticholinergic drugs, memantine, beta agonists

References

Cheng YS, Lu CZ, Ying ZL, et al, "128 Cases of Myasthenia Gravis Treated With Huperzine A," *New Drugs Clin Rem*, 1986, 5:260-2.

Natural Standard Research Collaboration, Chief Editors: Ulbricht C, Basch E, *Natural Standard Herb and Supplement Reference - Evidence-Based Clinical Reviews*, USA: Elsevier/Mosby, 2005.

Wang H and Tang XC, "Anticholinesterase Effects of HuperzineA, E2020, and Tacrine in Rats," *Chung Kuo Yao Li Hsueh Pao*, 1998, 19(1):27-30.

- **HXM** *see* Altretamine *on page 78*
- **Hycamptamine** *see* Topotecan *on page 1602*

- **Hycamtin®** *see* Topotecan *on page 1602*
- **hycet™** *see* Hydrocodone and Acetaminophen *on page 777*
- **Hycodan® [DSC]** *see* Hydrocodone and Homatropine *on page 780*
- **Hycotuss® [DSC]** *see* Hydrocodone and Guaifenesin *on page 779*
- **Hydergine [DSC]** *see* Ergoloid Mesylates *on page 551*

HydrALAZINE (hye DRAL a zeen)

Medication Safety Issues

Sound-alike/look-alike issues:

HydrALAZINE may be confused with hydrOXYzine

Canadian Brand Names Apo-Hydralazine®; Apresoline®; Novo-Hylazin; Nu-Hydral

Mexican Brand Names Apresolina

Index Terms Apresoline [DSC]; Hydralazine Hydrochloride

Pharmacologic Category Vasodilator

Use Management of moderate to severe hypertension, congestive heart failure, hypertension secondary to pre-eclampsia/eclampsia; treatment of primary pulmonary hypertension

Effect on Mental Status May cause drowsiness

Effect on Psychiatric Treatment Concurrent use with MAO inhibitors may result in significant decrease in blood pressure; use cautiously

Dosage Summary

I.M.:

Children: 0.1-0.2 mg/kg/dose (not to exceed 20 mg) every 4-6 hours as needed (maximum: 3.5 mg/kg/day in 4-6 divided doses)

Adults: Initial: 10-20 mg/dose every 4-6 hours as needed; Maintenance: Up to 40 mg/dose every 4-6 hours **or** Eclampsia/Pre-eclampsia: 5 mg/dose then 5-10 mg every 20-30 minutes as needed

I.V.:

Children: 0.1-0.2 mg/kg/dose (not to exceed 20 mg) every 4-6 hours as needed (maximum: 3.5 mg/kg/day in 4-6 divided doses)

Adults: Initial: 10-20 mg/dose every 4-6 hours as needed; Maintenance: Up to 40 mg/dose every 4-6 hours **or** Eclampsia/Pre-eclampsia: 5 mg/dose then 5-10 mg every 20-30 minutes as needed

Oral:

Children: Initial: 0.75-1 mg/kg/day in 2-4 divided doses; Maintenance: Up to 7.5 mg/kg/day in 2-4 divided doses (maximum: 200 mg/day)

Adults: Initial: 10-25 mg 3-4 times/day; Maintenance: 25-300 mg/day (Target dose: 225-300 mg/day for CHF) in 2-4 divided doses (maximum: 300 mg/day)

Elderly: Initial: 10 mg 2-3 times/day, increase by 10-25 mg/day every 2-5 days; Target dose: 225-300 mg/day for CHF

Dosage Forms Excipient information presented when available (limited, particularly for generics); consult specific product labeling.

Injection, solution, as hydrochloride: 20 mg/mL (1 mL)

Tablet, as hydrochloride: 10 mg, 25 mg, 50 mg, 100 mg

Hydralazine and Hydrochlorothiazide

(hye DRAL a zeen & hye droe klor oh THYE a zide)

Index Terms Apresazide [DSC]; Hydrochlorothiazide and Hydralazine

Pharmacologic Category Diuretic, Thiazide; Vasodilator, Direct-Acting

Use Management of moderate to severe hypertension and treatment of congestive heart failure

Effect on Mental Status May cause drowsiness or depression

Effect on Psychiatric Treatment Concurrent use with MAO inhibitors may result in significant decrease in blood pressure, use cautiously; may decrease lithium clearance resulting in an increase in serum lithium levels and potential lithium toxicity; monitor serum lithium levels

Dosage Summary

Oral:

Children: Dosage not established

Adults: Hydralazine 25-100 mg/day and hydrochlorothiazide 25-50 mg/day in 2 divided doses (maximum: Hydrochlorothiazide: 50 mg/day)

Dosage Forms Excipient information presented when available (limited, particularly for generics); consult specific product labeling.

Capsule:

25/25: Hydralazine hydrochloride 25 mg and hydrochlorothiazide 25 mg

50/50: Hydralazine hydrochloride 50 mg and hydrochlorothiazide 50 mg
100/50: Hydralazine hydrochloride 100 mg and hydrochlorothiazide 50 mg

- **Hydralazine and Isosorbide Dinitrate** *see* Isosorbide Dinitrate and Hydralazine *on page 869*
- **Hydralazine Hydrochloride** *see* HydrALAZINE *on page 772*
- **Hydramine® [OTC]** *see* DiphenhydrAMINE *on page 481*
- **Hydrated Chloral** *see* Chloral Hydrate *on page 313*
- **Hydrea®** *see* Hydroxyurea *on page 796*
- **Hydrisalic™ [OTC]** *see* Salicylic Acid *on page 1454*

Hydrochlorothiazide (hye droe klor oh THYE a zide)

Medication Safety Issues

Sound-alike/look-alike issues:

Esidrix may be confused with Lasix®

HCTZ is an error-prone abbreviation (mistaken as hydrocortisone)

Hydrochlorothiazide may be confused with hydrocortisone, hydroflumethiazide

Microzide™ may be confused with Maxzide®, Micronase®

International issues:

Microzide™ may be confused with Nitrobide® which is a brand name for isosorbide dinitrate in Japan

Microzide™ may be confused with Mikrozid® which is a brand name for ethanol/propanol combination in Great Britain

U.S. Brand Names Microzide®

Canadian Brand Names Apo-Hydro®; Novo-Hydrazide; PMS-Hydrochlorothiazide

Mexican Brand Names Acortiz; Rofucal

Index Terms HCTZ (error-prone abbreviation)

Pharmacologic Category Diuretic, Thiazide

Generic Available Yes

Use Management of mild to moderate hypertension; treatment of edema in congestive heart failure and nephrotic syndrome

Unlabeled/Investigational Use Treatment of lithium-induced diabetes insipidus

Effect on Mental Status None reported

Effect on Psychiatric Treatment Used to treat lithium-induced diabetes insipidus; monitor for hypokalemia; may decrease lithium clearance resulting in an increase in serum lithium levels and potential lithium toxicity; monitor serum lithium levels

Pregnancy Risk Factor B (manufacturer); D (expert analysis)

Pregnancy Considerations Although there are no adequate and well-controlled studies using hydrochlorothiazide in pregnancy, thiazide diuretics may cause an increased risk of congenital defects. Hypoglycemia, hypokalemia, hyponatremia, jaundice, and thrombocytopenia are also reported as possible complications to the fetus or newborn.

Lactation Enters breast milk/use caution (AAP rates "compatible")

Contraindications Hypersensitivity to hydrochlorothiazide or any component of the formulation, thiazides, or sulfonamide-derived drugs; anuria; renal decompensation; pregnancy

Warnings/Precautions Avoid in severe renal disease (ineffective as a diuretic). Electrolyte disturbances (hypokalemia, hypochloremic alkalosis, hyponatremia) can occur. Use with caution in severe hepatic dysfunction; hepatic encephalopathy can be caused by electrolyte disturbances. Gout may be precipitated in certain patients with a history of gout, a familial predisposition to gout, or chronic renal failure. Use with caution in patients with prediabetes and diabetes; may alter glucose control. May cause SLE exacerbation or activation. Use with caution in patients with moderate or high cholesterol concentrations. Photosensitization may occur. Correct hypokalemia before initiating therapy.

Chemical similarities are present among sulfonamides, sulfonylureas, carbonic anhydrase inhibitors, thiazides, and loop diuretics (except ethacrynic acid). Use in patients with sulfonamide allergy is specifically contraindicated in product labeling, however, a risk of cross-reaction exists in patients with allergy to any of these compounds; avoid use when previous reaction has been severe. Discontinue if signs of hypersensitivity are noted.

Adverse Reactions

1% to 10%:

Cardiovascular: Orthostatic hypotension, hypotension

Dermatologic: Photosensitivity

Endocrine & metabolic: Hypokalemia

Gastrointestinal: Anorexia, epigastric distress

<1% (Limited to important or life-threatening): Agranulocytosis, allergic myocarditis, allergic reactions (possibly with life-threatening anaphylactic shock), alopecia, aplastic anemia, eosinophilic pneumonitis, erythema multiforme, exfoliative dermatitis, hemolytic anemia, hepatic function impairment, hypercalcemia, interstitial nephritis, leukopenia, pancreatitis, renal failure, respiratory distress, Stevens-Johnson syndrome, thrombocytopenia, toxic epidermal necrolysis

Drug Interactions

ACE Inhibitors: Thiazide Diuretics may enhance the hypotensive effect of ACE Inhibitors. Specifically, postural hypotension which can accompany ACE Inhibitor initiation. Thiazide Diuretics may enhance the nephrotoxic effect of ACE Inhibitors. *Risk C: Monitor therapy*

Allopurinol: Thiazide Diuretics may enhance the potential for allergic or hypersensitivity reactions to Allopurinol. Thiazide Diuretics may increase the serum concentration of Allopurinol. Specifically, Thiazide Diuretics may increase the concentration of Oxypurinolol, an active metabolite of Allopurinol. *Risk C: Monitor therapy*

Bile Acid Sequestrants: May decrease the absorption of Thiazide Diuretics. The diuretic response is likewise decreased. *Risk D: Consider therapy modification*

Calcitriol: Thiazide Diuretics may enhance the hypercalcemic effect of Calcitriol. *Risk C: Monitor therapy*

Calcium Salts: Thiazide Diuretics may decrease the excretion of Calcium Salts. Continued concomitant use can also result in metabolic alkalosis. *Risk C: Monitor therapy*

Corticosteroids (Orally Inhaled): May enhance the hypokalemic effect of Thiazide Diuretics. *Risk C: Monitor therapy*

Corticosteroids (Systemic): May enhance the hypokalemic effect of Thiazide Diuretics. *Risk C: Monitor therapy*

Dofetilide: Thiazide Diuretics may enhance the QTc-prolonging effect of Dofetilide. Thiazide Diuretics may increase the serum concentration of Dofetilide. *Risk D: Consider therapy modification*

Herbs (Hypertensive Properties): May diminish the antihypertensive effect of Antihypertensives. *Risk C: Monitor therapy*

Herbs (Hypotensive Properties): May enhance the hypotensive effect of Antihypertensives. *Risk C: Monitor therapy*

Lithium: Thiazide Diuretics may decrease the excretion of Lithium. *Risk D: Consider therapy modification*

Methylphenidate: May diminish the antihypertensive effect of Antihypertensives. *Risk C: Monitor therapy*

Nonsteroidal Anti-Inflammatory Agents: May diminish the therapeutic effect of Thiazide Diuretics. *Risk C: Monitor therapy*

Prostacyclin Analogues: May enhance the hypotensive effect of Antihypertensives. *Risk C: Monitor therapy*

RiTUXimab: Antihypertensives may enhance the hypotensive effect of RiTUXimab. *Risk D: Consider therapy modification*

Ethanol/Nutrition/Herb Interactions

Food: Hydrochlorothiazide peak serum levels may be decreased if taken with food. This product may deplete potassium, sodium, and magnesium.

Herb/Nutraceutical: Avoid dong quai if using for hypertension (has estrogenic activity). Dong quai may also cause photosensitization. Avoid ephedra, ginseng, yohimbe (may worsen hypertension). Avoid garlic (may have increased antihypertensive effect).

Mechanism of Action Inhibits sodium reabsorption in the distal tubules causing increased excretion of sodium and water as well as potassium and hydrogen ions

Pharmacodynamics/Kinetics

Onset of action: Diuresis: ~2 hours

Peak effect: 4-6 hours

Duration: 6-12 hours

Absorption: ~50% to 80%

Distribution: 3.6-7.8 L/kg

Protein binding: 68%

Metabolism: Not metabolized

Bioavailability: 50% to 80%

Half-life elimination: 5.6-14.8 hours

Time to peak: 1-2.5 hours
Excretion: Urine (as unchanged drug)

Dosage Oral (effect of drug may be decreased when used every day):

Children (in pediatric patients, chlorothiazide may be preferred over hydrochlorothiazide as there are more dosage formulations [eg, suspension] available): Edema, hypertension:

<6 months: 1-3 mg/kg/day in 2 divided doses
>6 months to 2 years: 1-3 mg/kg/day in 2 divided doses; maximum: 37.5 mg/day
>2-17 years: Initial: 1 mg/kg/day; maximum: 3 mg/kg/day (50 mg/day)

Adults:

Edema: 25-100 mg/day in 1-2 doses; maximum: 200 mg/day
Hypertension: 12.5-50 mg/day; minimal increase in response and more electrolyte disturbances are seen with doses >50 mg/day

Elderly: 12.5-25 mg once daily

Dosing adjustment/comments in renal impairment: Cl_{cr} <10 mL/minute: Avoid use. Usually ineffective with GFR <30 mL/minute. Effective at lower GFR in combination with a loop diuretic.

Administration May be taken with food or milk. Take early in day to avoid nocturia. Take the last dose of multiple doses no later than 6 PM unless instructed otherwise.

Monitoring Parameters Assess weight, I & O reports daily to determine fluid loss; blood pressure, serum electrolytes, BUN, creatinine

Test Interactions Increased creatine phosphokinase [CPK] (S), ammonia (B), amylase (S), calcium (S), chloride (S), cholesterol (S), glucose, increased acid (S), decreased chloride (S), magnesium, potassium (S), sodium (S); Tyramine and phentolamine tests, histamine tests for pheochromocytoma

Additional Information If given the morning of surgery it may render the patient volume depleted and blood pressure may be labile during general anesthesia. Effect of drug may be decreased when used every day.

Dosage Forms Excipient information presented when available (limited, particularly for generics); consult specific product labeling.

Capsule: 12.5 mg
Microzide®: 12.5 mg
Tablet: 25 mg, 50 mg

- **Hydrochlorothiazide and Aliskiren** *see* Aliskiren and Hydrochlorothiazide *on page 66*
- **Hydrochlorothiazide and Amiloride** *see* Amiloride and Hydrochlorothiazide *on page 86*
- **Hydrochlorothiazide and Benazepril** *see* Benazepril and Hydrochlorothiazide *on page 179*
- **Hydrochlorothiazide and Bisoprolol** *see* Bisoprolol and Hydrochlorothiazide *on page 191*
- **Hydrochlorothiazide and Captopril** *see* Captopril and Hydrochlorothiazide *on page 265*
- **Hydrochlorothiazide and Enalapril** *see* Enalapril and Hydrochlorothiazide *on page 536*
- **Hydrochlorothiazide and Eprosartan** *see* Eprosartan and Hydrochlorothiazide *on page 549*
- **Hydrochlorothiazide and Fosinopril** *see* Fosinopril and Hydrochlorothiazide *on page 692*
- **Hydrochlorothiazide and Hydralazine** *see* Hydralazine and Hydrochlorothiazide *on page 772*
- **Hydrochlorothiazide and Irbesartan** *see* Irbesartan and Hydrochlorothiazide *on page 856*
- **Hydrochlorothiazide and Lisinopril** *see* Lisinopril and Hydrochlorothiazide *on page 938*
- **Hydrochlorothiazide and Losartan** *see* Losartan and Hydrochlorothiazide *on page 956*
- **Hydrochlorothiazide and Methyldopa** *see* Methyldopa and Hydrochlorothiazide *on page 1021*
- **Hydrochlorothiazide and Metoprolol** *see* Metoprolol and Hydrochlorothiazide *on page 1040*
- **Hydrochlorothiazide and Metoprolol Tartrate** *see* Metoprolol and Hydrochlorothiazide *on page 1040*

◆ **Hydrochlorothiazide and Moexipril** *see* Moexipril and Hydrochlorothiazide *on page 1068*

◆ **Hydrochlorothiazide and Olmesartan Medoxomil** *see* Olmesartan and Hydrochlorothiazide *on page 1172*

◆ **Hydrochlorothiazide and Propranolol** *see* Propranolol and Hydrochlorothiazide *on page 1361*

◆ **Hydrochlorothiazide and Quinapril** *see* Quinapril and Hydrochlorothiazide *on page 1386*

Hydrochlorothiazide and Spironolactone

(hye droe klor oh THYE a zide & speer on oh LAK tone)

Medication Safety Issues

Sound-alike/look-alike issues:

Aldactazide® may be confused with Aldactone®

U.S. Brand Names Aldactazide®

Canadian Brand Names Aldactazide 25®; Aldactazide 50®; Novo-Spirozine

Index Terms Spironolactone and Hydrochlorothiazide

Pharmacologic Category Diuretic, Thiazide; Selective Aldosterone Blocker

Use Management of mild-to-moderate hypertension; treatment of edema in congestive heart failure and nephrotic syndrome, and cirrhosis of the liver accompanied by edema and/or ascites

Effect on Mental Status May cause lethargy or anorexia

Effect on Psychiatric Treatment May decrease lithium clearance resulting in an increase in serum lithium levels and potential lithium toxicity; monitor serum lithium levels

Dosage Summary

Oral:

Children: 1.5-3 mg/kg/day in 2-4 divided doses (maximum: 200 mg/day)

Adults: 12.5-50 mg hydrochlorothiazide and 12.5-50 mg spironolactone/day in 1-2 divided doses

Dosage Forms Excipient information presented when available (limited, particularly for generics); consult specific product labeling.

Tablet: Hydrochlorothiazide 25 mg and spironolactone 25 mg

Aldactazide®:

25/25: Hydrochlorothiazide 25 mg and spironolactone 25 mg

50/50: Hydrochlorothiazide 50 mg and spironolactone 50 mg

◆ **Hydrochlorothiazide and Telmisartan** *see* Telmisartan and Hydrochlorothiazide *on page 1544*

Hydrochlorothiazide and Triamterene

(hye droe klor oh THYE a zide & trye AM ter een)

Medication Safety Issues

Sound-alike/look-alike issues:

Dyazide® may be confused with diazoxide, Dynacin®

Maxzide® may be confused with Maxidex®, Microzide®

U.S. Brand Names Dyazide®; Maxzide®; Maxzide®-25

Canadian Brand Names Apo-Triazide®; Novo-Triamzide; Nu-Triazide; Penta-Triamterene HCTZ; Riva-Zide

Mexican Brand Names Dyazide

Index Terms Triamterene and Hydrochlorothiazide

Pharmacologic Category Diuretic, Potassium-Sparing; Diuretic, Thiazide

Use Treatment of hypertension or edema (not recommended for initial treatment) when hypokalemia has developed on hydrochlorothiazide alone or when the development of hypokalemia must be avoided

Effect on Mental Status May cause lethargy or anorexia

Effect on Psychiatric Treatment May decrease lithium clearance resulting in an increase in serum lithium levels and potential lithium toxicity; monitor serum lithium levels

Dosage Summary

Oral:

Children: Dosage not established

Adults: 25-50 mg hydrochlorothiazide and 37.5-75 mg triamterene once daily

Dosage Forms Excipient information presented when available (limited, particularly for generics); consult specific product labeling.

Capsule, oral: Hydrochlorothiazide 25 mg and triamterene 37.5 mg; hydrochlorothiazide 25 mg and triamterene 50 mg

Dyazide®: Hydrochlorothiazide 25 mg and triamterene 37.5 mg

Tablet: Hydrochlorothiazide 25 mg and triamterene 37.5 mg; hydrochlorothiazide 50 mg and triamterene 75 mg
Maxzide®: Hydrochlorothiazide 50 mg and triamterene 75 mg [scored]
Maxzide®-25: Hydrochlorothiazide 25 mg and triamterene 37.5 mg [scored]

◆ **Hydrochlorothiazide and Valsartan** *see* Valsartan and Hydrochlorothiazide *on page 1652*

Hydrocodone and Acetaminophen

(hye droe KOE done & a seet a MIN oh fen)

Medication Safety Issues

Sound-alike/look-alike issues:
Lorcet® may be confused with Fioricet®
Lortab® may be confused with Cortef®, Lorabid®, Luride®
Vicodin® may be confused with Hycodan®, Hycomine®, Indocin®, Uridon®
Zydone® may be confused with Vytone®

High alert medication: The Institute for Safe Medication Practices (ISMP) includes this medication among its list of drug classes which have a heightened risk of causing significant patient harm when used in error.

Duplicate therapy issues: This product contains acetaminophen, which may be a component of other combination products. Do not exceed the maximum recommended daily dose of acetaminophen.

U.S. Brand Names Co-Gesic® [DSC]; hycet™; Lorcet® 10/650; Lorcet® Plus; Lortab®; Margesic® H; Maxidone®; Norco®; Stagesic™; Vicodin®; Vicodin® ES; Vicodin® HP; Xodol® 10/300; Xodol® 5/300; Xodol® 7.5/300; Zamicet®; Zydone®

Index Terms Acetaminophen and Hydrocodone

Pharmacologic Category Analgesic Combination (Opioid)

Use Relief of moderate to severe pain

Effect on Mental Status Sedation is common; may cause confusion; may rarely cause hallucinations

Effect on Psychiatric Treatment May result in loss of pain control when used in combination with SSRIs (especially paroxetine and fluoxetine); concurrent use with psychotropics may produce additive sedation

Restrictions C-III

Dosage Summary

Oral:

Children <2 years: Dosage not established
Children 2-13 years or <50 kg: Hydrocodone 0.135 mg/kg/dose every 4-6 hours (maximum: 6 doses/day or maximum recommended dose of acetaminophen for age/weight)
Children ≥50 kg: Hydrocodone 2.5-10 mg every 4-6 hours (maximum: 4 g/day [acetaminophen]; 60 mg/day [hydrocodone])
Adults: Hydrocodone 2.5-10 mg every 4-6 hours (maximum: 4 g/day [acetaminophen]; 60 mg/day [hydrocodone])
Elderly: Hydrocodone 2.5-5 mg every 4-6 hours

Dosage Forms Excipient information presented when available (limited, particularly for generics); consult specific product labeling. [DSC] = Discontinued product

Capsule:
Margesic® H, Stagesic™: Hydrocodone bitartrate 5 mg and acetaminophen 500 mg

Elixir: Hydrocodone bitartrate 7.5 mg and acetaminophen 500 mg per 15 mL (480 mL)
Lortab®: Hydrocodone bitartrate 7.5 mg and acetaminophen 500 mg per 15 mL (480 mL) [contains ethanol 7%, propylene glycol; tropical fruit punch flavor]

Solution, oral: Hydrocodone bitartrate 7.5 mg and acetaminophen 500 mg per 15 mL (5 mL, 10 mL, 15 mL, 118 mL, 473 mL)
hycet™: Hydrocodone bitartrate 7.5 mg and acetaminophen 325 mg per 15 mL (473 mL) [contains ethanol 6.7%, propylene glycol; fruit flavor]
Zamicet™: Hydrocodone bitartrate 10 mg and acetaminophen 325 mg per 15 mL (473 mL) [contains ethanol 6.7%, propylene glycol; fruit flavor]

Tablet:
Hydrocodone bitartrate 2.5 mg and acetaminophen 500 mg
Hydrocodone bitartrate 5 mg and acetaminophen 325 mg
Hydrocodone bitartrate 5 mg and acetaminophen 500 mg
Hydrocodone bitartrate 7.5 mg and acetaminophen 325 mg
Hydrocodone bitartrate 7.5 mg and acetaminophen 500 mg

Hydrocodone bitartrate 7.5 mg and acetaminophen 650 mg
Hydrocodone bitartrate 7.5 mg and acetaminophen 750 mg
Hydrocodone bitartrate 10 mg and acetaminophen 325 mg
Hydrocodone bitartrate 10 mg and acetaminophen 500 mg
Hydrocodone bitartrate 10 mg and acetaminophen 650 mg
Hydrocodone bitartrate 10 mg and acetaminophen 660 mg
Hydrocodone bitartrate 10 mg and acetaminophen 750 mg
Co-Gesic® 5/500: Hydrocodone bitartrate 5 mg and acetaminophen 500 mg
Lorcet® 10/650: Hydrocodone bitartrate 10 mg and acetaminophen 650 mg
Lorcet® Plus: Hydrocodone bitartrate 7.5 mg and acetaminophen 650 mg
Lortab®:
- 5/500: Hydrocodone bitartrate 5 mg and acetaminophen 500 mg
- 7.5/500: Hydrocodone bitartrate 7.5 mg and acetaminophen 500 mg
- 10/500: Hydrocodone bitartrate 10 mg and acetaminophen 500 mg

Maxidone™: Hydrocodone bitartrate 10 mg and acetaminophen 750 mg
Norco®:
- Hydrocodone bitartrate 5 mg and acetaminophen 325 mg
- Hydrocodone bitartrate 7.5 mg and acetaminophen 325 mg
- Hydrocodone bitartrate 10 mg and acetaminophen 325 mg

Vicodin®: Hydrocodone bitartrate 5 mg and acetaminophen 500 mg
Vicodin® ES: Hydrocodone bitartrate 7.5 mg and acetaminophen 750 mg
Vicodin® HP: Hydrocodone bitartrate 10 mg and acetaminophen 660 mg
Xodol®:
- 10/300: Hydrocodone bitartrate 10 mg and acetaminophen 300 mg
- 5/300: Hydrocodone bitartrate 5 mg and acetaminophen 300 mg
- 7/300: Hydrocodone bitartrate 7 mg and acetaminophen 300 mg

Zydone®:
- Hydrocodone bitartrate 5 mg and acetaminophen 400 mg
- Hydrocodone bitartrate 7.5 mg and acetaminophen 400 mg
- Hydrocodone bitartrate 10 mg and acetaminophen 400 mg

Hydrocodone and Chlorpheniramine

(hye droe KOE done & klor fen IR a meen)

U.S. Brand Names TussiCaps™; Tussionex®

Index Terms Chlorpheniramine Maleate and Hydrocodone Bitartrate ; Hydrocodone Polistirex and Chlorpheniramine Polistirex

Pharmacologic Category Alpha/Beta Agonist; Antitussive; Histamine H_1 Antagonist; Histamine H_1 Antagonist, First Generation

Use Symptomatic relief of cough and upper respiratory symptoms associated with cold and allergy

Effect on Mental Status Sedation is common; may cause confusion, dizziness, excitability, nervousness, fatigue, or depression; may rarely cause hallucinations

Effect on Psychiatric Treatment May result in loss of pain control when used in combination with SSRIs (especially paroxetine and fluoxetine); concurrent use with psychotropics may produce additive sedation or dry mouth

Restrictions C-III

Dosage Summary

Oral:

Children <6 years: Dosage not established

Children 6-12 years: TussiCaps™ 5 mg/4 mg: One capsule every 12 hours (maximum: 2 capsules/24 hours); Tussionex®: 2.5 mL every 12 hours (maximum: 5 mL/24 hours)

Children >12 years: TussiCaps™ 10 mg/8 mg: One capsule every 12 hours (maximum: 2 capsules/24 hours); Tussionex®: 5 mL every 12 hours (maximum: 10 mL/24 hours)

Adults: TussiCaps™ 10 mg/8 mg: One capsule every 12 hours (maximum: 2 capsules/24 hours); Tussionex®: 5 mL every 12 hours (maximum: 10 mL/24 hours)

Dosage Forms Excipient information presented when available (limited, particularly for generics); consult specific product labeling.

Capsule, extended release:

TussiCaps™ 5 mg/4 mg: Hydrocodone polistirex [equivalent to hydrocodone bitartrate 5 mg] and chlorpheniramine polistirex [equivalent to chlorpheniramine maleate 4 mg]

TussiCaps™ 10 mg/8 mg: Hydrocodone polistirex [equivalent to hydrocodone bitartrate 10 mg] and chlorpheniramine polistirex [equivalent to chlorpheniramine maleate 8 mg]

Suspension, extended release:

Tussionex®: Hydrocodone polistirex [equivalent to hydrocodone bitartrate 10 mg] and chlorpheniramine polistirex [equivalent to chlorpheniramine maleate 8 mg] per 5 mL (480 mL)

Hydrocodone and Guaifenesin

(hye droe KOE done & gwye FEN e sin)

U.S. Brand Names Atuss® HX [DSC]; Codiclear® DH [DSC]; EndaCof [DSC]; EndaCof-XP [DSC]; ExeClear [DSC]; ExeCof-XP [DSC]; Extendryl® HC [DSC]; Hycotuss® [DSC]; Kwelcof® [DSC]; Maxi-Tuss HCG [DSC]; Pancof-XP [DSC]; Phanatuss® HC [DSC]; Pneumotussin® [DSC]; Touro® HC [DSC]; Tusso-DF® [DSC]; Vitussin [DSC]; Xpect-HC™ [DSC]; Ztuss™ ZT [DSC]

Index Terms Guaifenesin and Hydrocodone

Pharmacologic Category Antitussive/Expectorant

Use Symptomatic relief of nonproductive coughs associated with upper and lower respiratory tract congestion

Effect on Mental Status May cause drowsiness, sedation, mental clouding, mental impairment, anxiety, fear, dysphoria, dizziness, psychotic dependence, mood changes

Effect on Psychiatric Treatment Concurrent use with psychotropics may produce additive sedation

Restrictions C-III

Dosage Summary

Oral:

Children <6 years (unlabeled use): Hydrocodone 0.3 mg/kg/day in 4 divided doses

Children 6-12 years:

Atuss® HX: One capsule every 8 hours

Codiclear® DH, Hycotuss®, Kwelcof®, Maxi-Tuss HCG: 2.5-5 mL every 4 hours

Pneumotussin®: One tablet **or** 5 mL every 4-6 hours (maximum: 4 doses/24 hours)

Children >12 years:

Codiclear® DH, Hycotuss®, Kwelcof®, Maxi-Tuss HCG: 5-10 mL every 4 hours

Pneumotussin®: 1-2 tablets **or** 10 mL every 4-6 hours (maximum: 4 doses/24 hours)

Children ≥12 years: Atuss® HX: 1-2 capsules every 8 hours

Adults:

Atuss® HX: 1-2 capsules every 8 hours

Codiclear® DH, Kwelcof®, Hycotuss®: 5-15 mL every 4 hours (maximum: 30 mL/24 hours)

Maxi-Tuss HCG: 5-10 mL every 4 hours

Pneumotussin®: 1-2 tablets **or** 10 mL every 4-6 hours (maximum: 4 doses/24 hours)

Dosage Forms Excipient information presented when available (limited, particularly for generics); consult specific product labeling. [DSC] = Discontinued product

Caplet:

Ztuss™ ZT: Hydrocodone bitartrate 5 mg and guaifenesin 300 mg [DSC]

Capsule, variable release:

Atuss® HX: Hydrocodone bitartrate 5 mg [immediate release] and guaifenesin 100 mg [sustained release] [DSC]

Liquid: Hydrocodone bitartrate 5 mg and guaifenesin 100 mg per 5 mL (480 mL, 960 mL) [DSC]

ExeCof-XP: Hydrocodone bitartrate 3 mg and guaifenesin 90 mg per 5 mL (3840 mL) [contains benzoic acid] [DSC]

Kwelcof®: Hydrocodone bitartrate 5 mg and guaifenesin 100 mg per 5 mL (480 mL) [alcohol free, dye free, sugar free; contains benzoic acid; apricot-pineapple flavor] [DSC]

Pancof-XP: Hydrocodone bitartrate 3 mg and guaifenesin 90 mg per 5 mL (3840 mL) [contains benzoic acid] [DSC]

Phanatuss® HC: Hydrocodone bitartrate 5 mg and guaifenesin 100 mg per 5 mL (480 mL) [alcohol free, sugar free; mint flavor] [DSC]

Vitussin: Hydrocodone bitartrate 5 mg and guaifenesin 100 mg per 5 mL (480 mL) [alcohol free, sugar free, dye free; cherry flavor] [DSC]

Syrup: Hydrocodone bitartrate 3.5 mg and guaifenesin 100 mg per 5 mL (120 mL, 480 mL); hydrocodone bitartrate 3.5 mg and guaifenesin 300 mg per 5 mL (120 mL, 480 mL); hydrocodone bitartrate 5 mg and guaifenesin 100 mg per 5 mL (480 mL) [DSC]

Codiclear® DH: Hydrocodone bitartrate 3.5 mg and guaifenesin 300 mg per 5 mL (120 mL, 480 mL) [alcohol free, dye free, sugar free; contains sodium benzoate; grape flavor] [DSC]

EndaCof-XP: Hydrocodone bitartrate 2.5 mg and guaifenesin 200 mg per 5 mL (480 mL) [alcohol free, dye free, sugar free; contains phenylalanine; cherry punch flavor] [DSC]

ExeClear: Hydrocodone bitartrate 3.5 mg and guaifenesin 100 mg per 5 mL (480 mL) [DSC]

Hycotuss®: Hydrocodone bitartrate 5 mg and guaifenesin 100 mg per 5 mL (480 mL) [contains alcohol 10%; butterscotch flavor] [DSC]

Maxi-Tuss HCG: Hydrocodone bitartrate 6 mg and guaifenesin 200 mg per 5 mL (480 mL) [alcohol free, sugar free; contains aspartame; butterscotch flavor] [DSC]

Pneumotussin®: Hydrocodone bitartrate 2.5 mg and guaifenesin 200 mg per 5 mL (480 mL) [alcohol free, dye free, sugar free; cherry punch flavor] [DSC]

Tusso-DF®: Hydrocodone bitartrate 2.5 mg and guaifenesin 100 mg per 5 mL (480 mL) [cherry flavor] [DSC]

Tablet:

EndaCof: Hydrocodone bitartrate 2.5 mg and guaifenesin 300 mg [DSC]

Touro® HC: Hydrocodone bitartrate 5 mg and guaifenesin 575 mg [DSC]

Tablet, sustained release:

Extendryl® HC: Hydrocodone bitartrate 10 mg and guaifenesin 1000 mg [DSC]

Xpect-HC™: Hydrocodone bitartrate 5 mg and guaifenesin 600 mg [DSC]

Hydrocodone and Homatropine

(hye droe KOE done & hoe MA troe peen)

Medication Safety Issues

Sound-alike/look-alike issues:

Hycodan® may be confused with Hycomine®, Vicodin®

U.S. Brand Names Hycodan® [DSC]; Hydromet®; Tussigon®

Mexican Brand Names Hydromet

Index Terms Homatropine and Hydrocodone

Pharmacologic Category Antitussive

Use Symptomatic relief of cough

Effect on Mental Status Lightheadedness, dizziness, sedation, drowsiness, and fatigue are common; may cause confusion; may rarely cause hallucinations

Effect on Psychiatric Treatment Concurrent use with psychotropics may produce additive sedation

Restrictions C-III

Dosage Summary

Oral:

Children <6 years: Dosage not established

Children 6-12 years: 1/2 tablet or 2.5 mL every 4-6 hours as needed (maximum: 3 tablets or 15 mL/24 hours)

Children ≥12 years: 1 tablet or 5 mL every 4-6 hours as needed (maximum: 6 tablets/24 hours or 30 mL/24 hours)

Adults: 1 tablet or 5 mL every 4-6 hours as needed (maximum: 6 tablets/24 hours or 30 mL/24 hours)

Dosage Forms Excipient information presented when available (limited, particularly for generics); consult specific product labeling.

Syrup:

Hycodan® [DSC], Hydromet®: Hydrocodone bitartrate 5 mg and homatropine methylbromide 1.5 mg per 5 mL (480 mL) [cherry flavor]

Tablet: Hydrocodone bitartrate 5 mg and homatropine methylbromide 1.5 mg [DSC]

Hycodan® [DSC], Tussigon®: Hydrocodone bitartrate 5 mg and homatropine methylbromide 1.5 mg

Hydrocodone and Ibuprofen

(hye droe KOE done & eye byoo PROE fen)

Medication Safety Issues

High alert medication: The Institute for Safe Medication Practices (ISMP) includes this medication among its list of drug classes which have a heightened risk of causing significant patient harm when used in error.

U.S. Brand Names Ibudone™; Reprexain®; Vicoprofen®

Canadian Brand Names Vicoprofen®

Index Terms Hydrocodone Bitartrate and Ibuprofen; Ibuprofen and Hydrocodone

Pharmacologic Category Analgesic, Opioid; Nonsteroidal Anti-inflammatory Drug (NSAID), Oral

Use Short-term (generally <10 days) management of moderate to severe acute pain; is not indicated for treatment of such conditions as osteoarthritis or rheumatoid arthritis

Effect on Mental Status Sedation, drowsiness, and fatigue are common; may cause nervousness or confusion; may rarely cause hallucinations, depression, or insomnia

Effect on Psychiatric Treatment Hypotension is common and may be potentiated by low potency antipsychotics and other psychotropics. May rarely cause agranulocytosis, caution with clozapine and carbamazepine. Sedation may be additive with psychotropics. Ibuprofen may inhibit the clearance of lithium resulting in elevated serum lithium levels; may need to adjust dosage downward.

Restrictions C-III; An FDA-approved medication guide for NSAIDs must be distributed when dispensing an oral outpatient prescription (new or refill) where this medication is to be used without direct supervision of a healthcare provider. Medication guides are available at http://www.fda.gov/cder/Offices/ODS/medication_guides.htm.

Dosage Summary

Oral:

Children: Dosage not established

Adults: 1 tablet every 4-6 hours (maximum: 5 tablets/day; <10 days total therapy)

Dosage Forms Excipient information presented when available (limited, particularly for generics); consult specific product labeling.

Tablet: Hydrocodone bitartrate 5 mg and ibuprofen 200 mg; hydrocodone bitartrate 7.5 mg and ibuprofen 200 mg

Ibudone™:

5/200: Hydrocodone bitartrate 5 mg and ibuprofen 200 mg

10/200: Hydrocodone bitartrate 10 mg and ibuprofen 200 mg

Reprexain®: Hydrocodone bitartrate 5 mg and ibuprofen 200 mg; hydrocodone bitartrate 7.5 mg and ibuprofen 200 mg

Vicoprofen®: Hydrocodone bitartrate 7.5 mg and ibuprofen 200 mg

Hydrocodone and Pseudoephedrine

(hye droe KOE done & soo doe e FED rin)

U.S. Brand Names Coughcold HCM [DSC]; P-V Tussin Tablet [DSC]; SymTan™ [DSC]

Index Terms Hydrocodone Tannate and Pseudoephedrine Tannate; Pseudoephedrine Hydrochloride and Hydrocodone Bitartrate

Pharmacologic Category Antitussive/Decongestant

Use Symptomatic relief of cough and nasal congestion

Effect on Mental Status May cause sedation, drowsiness, mental clouding, lethargy, impairment of mental performance, anxiety, fear, dysphoria, dizziness, psychic dependence, mood changes

Effect on Psychiatric Treatment Contraindicated with MAO inhibitors

Restrictions C-III

Dosage Summary

Oral:

Children 2-6 years: Coldcough HCM: 1.25-2.5 mL 4 times/day as needed

Children 6-12 years: Coldcough HCM: 2.5-5 mL 4 times/day as needed **or** SymTan™: 2.5 mL every 12 hours

Children >12 years: Coldcough HCM: 5-10 mL 4 times/day as needed **or** SymTan™: 5 mL every 12 hours

Adults: Coldcough HCM 5-10 mL 4 times/day as needed **or** SymTan™: 5 mL every 12 hours

Dosage Forms Excipient information presented when available (limited, particularly for generics); consult specific product labeling. [DSC] = Discontinued product

Solution:

SymTan™: Hydrocodone tannate 10 mg and pseudoephedrine tannate 45 mg per 5 mL (480 mL) [contains aspartame, propylene glycol; cherry mint flavor] [DSC]

Syrup:

Coldcough HCM: Hydrocodone bitartrate 3 mg and pseudoephedrine hydrochloride 15 mg per 5 mL (480 mL) [alcohol, dye and sugar free; contains propylene glycol; grape flavor] [DSC]

Tablet:
P-V Tussin: Hydrocodone bitartrate 5 mg and pseudoephedrine hydrochloride 60 mg [DSC]

◆ **Hydrocodone Bitartrate and Ibuprofen** *see* Hydrocodone and Ibuprofen *on page 780*

◆ **Hydrocodone Bitartrate, Carbinoxamine Maleate, and Pseudoephedrine Hydrochloride** *see* Hydrocodone, Carbinoxamine, and Pseudoephedrine *on page 782*

◆ **Hydrocodone Bitartrate, Phenylephrine Hydrochloride, and Diphenhydramine Hydrochloride** *see* Hydrocodone, Phenylephrine, and Diphenhydramine *on page 782*

Hydrocodone, Carbinoxamine, and Pseudoephedrine

(hye droe KOE done, kar bi NOKS a meen, & soo doe e FED rin)

U.S. Brand Names Tri-Vent™ HC [DSC]

Index Terms Carbinoxamine, Pseudoephedrine, and Hydrocodone; Hydrocodone Bitartrate, Carbinoxamine Maleate, and Pseudoephedrine Hydrochloride; Pseudoephedrine, Hydrocodone, and Carbinoxamine

Pharmacologic Category Alpha/Beta Agonist; Analgesic, Opioid; Antitussive; Histamine H_1 Antagonist; Histamine H_1 Antagonist, First Generation

Use Symptomatic relief of cough, congestion, and rhinorrhea associated with the common cold, influenza, bronchitis, or sinusitis

Effect on Mental Status May cause anxiety, dizziness, insomnia, restlessness, hallucinations, or depression

Effect on Psychiatric Treatment Contraindicated with or within 14 days of MAO inhibitor treatment; may cause tremor which may be mistaken for EPS; may cause tachycardia; tachycardia is also common with clozapine; monitor vital signs; may cause sedation (concurrent use with psychotropics may produce additive sedative effects)

Restrictions C-III

Dosage Summary

Oral:

Children <2 years: Dosage not established

Children 2-4 years: 1.25 mL every 4-6 hours (maximum: 7.5 mL/day)

Children 4-10 years: 2.5 mL every 4-6 hours (maximum: 15 mL/day)

Children >10 years: 5-10 mL every 4-6 hours (maximum: 30 mL/day)

Adults: 5-10 mL every 4-6 hours (maximum: 30 mL/day)

Dosage Forms Excipient information presented when available (limited, particularly for generics); consult specific product labeling. [DSC] = Discontinued product

Liquid:

Tri-Vent™ HC: Hydrocodone bitartrate 5 mg, carbinoxamine maleate 2 mg, and pseudoephedrine hydrochloride 30 mg per 5 mL (480 mL) [alcohol free, sugar free; peach flavor] [DSC]

◆ **Hydrocodone, Chlorpheniramine, and Pseudoephedrine** *see* Pseudoephedrine, Hydrocodone, and Chlorpheniramine *on page 1372*

◆ **Hydrocodone, Phenylephrine, and Chlorpheniramine** *see* Phenylephrine, Hydrocodone, and Chlorpheniramine *on page 1277*

Hydrocodone, Phenylephrine, and Diphenhydramine

(hye droe KOE done, fen il EF rin, & dye fen HYE dra meen)

Medication Safety Issues

Sound-alike/look-alike issues:

Endal® may be confused with Depen®, Intal®

U.S. Brand Names D-Tann HC [DSC]; Gentuss-HC; Hydro DP; Rindal HPD [DSC]; TussiNate™ [DSC]

Index Terms Diphenhydramine, Hydrocodone, and Phenylephrine; Hydrocodone Bitartrate, Phenylephrine Hydrochloride, and Diphenhydramine Hydrochloride; Hydrocodone Tannate, Phenylephrine Tannate, and Diphenhydramine Tannate; Phenylephrine, Diphenhydramine, and Hydrocodone

Pharmacologic Category Alpha/Beta Agonist; Analgesic, Opioid; Antitussive; Histamine H_1 Antagonist; Histamine H_1 Antagonist, First Generation

Use Symptomatic relief of cough and congestion associated with the common cold, sinusitis, or acute upper respiratory tract infections

Effect on Mental Status Diphenhydramine may cause paradoxical excitation in pediatric patients and can result in hallucinations, coma, and death in overdose.

Sedation is common; may cause dizziness, fatigue, nervousness, insomnia, euphoria, or confusion; may rarely cause hallucinations.

Effect on Psychiatric Treatment Contraindicated with MAO inhibitors. Rare reports of agranulocytosis and thrombocytopenia; use caution with clozapine, carbamazepine, valproic acid, and mirtazapine. Therapeutic effects of cholinergic agents (donepezil, rivastigmine, and galantamine) may be antagonized. Concurrent use with psychotropic agents may result in additive sedative and anticholinergic effects; monitor.

Restrictions C-III

Dosage Summary

Oral:

Children <6 years: Dosage not established

Children 6-12 years: 5 mL every 4 hours (maximum: 20 mL/day) [Rindal HPD, TussiNate™]

Children >12 years: 10 mL every 4 hours (maximum: 40 mL/day) [Rindal HPD, TussiNate™]

Adults: 10 mL every 4 hours (maximum: 40 mL/day) [Rindal HPD, TussiNate™]

Dosage Forms Excipient information presented when available (limited, particularly for generics); consult specific product labeling. [DSC] = Discontinued product

Suspension:

D-Tann HC: Hydrocodone tannate 3.5 mg, phenylephrine tannate 7.5 mg, and diphenhydramine tannate 25 mg per 5 mL (120 mL) [alcohol free, sugar free; contains phenylalanine; grape flavor] [DSC]

Syrup:

Gestuss-HC: Hydrocodone bitartrate 3 mg, phenylephrine hydrochloride 5 mg, and diphenhydramine hydrochloride 12.5 mg per 5 mL (480 mL) [black raspberry flavor]

Hydro DP: Hydrocodone bitartrate 2 mg, phenylephrine hydrochloride 7.5 mg, and diphenhydramine hydrochloride 12.5 mg per 5 mL (480 mL) [cherry flavor]

Rindal HPD: Hydrocodone bitartrate 2 mg, phenylephrine hydrochloride 7.5 mg, and diphenhydramine hydrochloride 12.5 mg per 5 mL (480 mL) [alcohol free, sugar free; black raspberry flavor] [DSC]

TussiNate™: Hydrocodone bitartrate 3.5 mg, phenylephrine hydrochloride 5 mg, and diphenhydramine hydrochloride 12.5 mg per 5 mL (480 mL) [alcohol free; contains sodium benzoate; black raspberry flavor] [DSC]

Hydrocodone, Phenylephrine, and Guaifenesin

(hye droe KOE done, fen il EF rin, & gwye FEN e sin)

U.S. Brand Names Crantex HC [DSC]; De-Chlor G [DSC]; Donatussin DC [DSC]; Duratuss® HD [DSC]; ExeTuss HC [DSC]; Gentex HC [DSC]; Giltuss HC® [DSC]; Guiaplex™ HC [DSC]; Hydro-GP [DSC]; HydroFed [DSC]; Levall 5.0 [DSC]; Mintuss G [DSC]; Tussafed® HC [DSC]; Tussafed® HCG [DSC]

Index Terms Guaifenesin, Hydrocodone Bitartrate, and Phenylephrine Hydrochloride; Phenylephrine, Guaifenesin, and Hydrocodone

Pharmacologic Category Antitussive/Decongestant/Expectorant

Use Temporary relief of cough, congestion, and other symptoms associated with colds or allergies

Effect on Mental Status Drowsiness and giddiness are common; may cause CNS depression; concomitant use with psychotropic agents may produce additive effects

Effect on Psychiatric Treatment Contraindicated with or within 14 days of MAO inhibitor use; CNS depressants, MAO inhibitors, and tricyclic antidepressants may potentiate the effects of opiate agonists. Dextroamphetamine may enhance the analgesic effect of opiate agonists. Chlorpromazine, fluoxetine, paroxetine, pergolide, and ropinirole may decrease the effects of hydrocodone.

Restrictions C-III

Dosage Summary

Oral:

Children <2 years: Dosage not established

Children 2-6 years: Crantex HC: 2.5 mL every 4-6 hours (maximum: 10 mL/day)

Children 3-6 years:

Giltuss HC®: 1.25 mL every 6 hours (maximum: 6 doses/day)

Tussafed® HC: 2.5 mL every 4-6 hours as needed (maximum: 6 doses/day)

Children 6-12 years:

Crantex HC: 5 mL every 4-6 hours (maximum: 4 doses/day)

Giltuss HC®: 2.5 mL every 6 hours (maximum: 6 doses/day)

Tussafed® HC: 2.5 mL every 4-6 hours as needed (maximum: 6 doses/day)

Children ≥12 years:

Crantex HC: 5-10 mL every 4-6 hours (maximum: 40 mL/day)

Giltuss HC®: 5 mL every 6 hours (maximum: 6 doses/day)

Tussafed® HC: 10 mL every 4-6 hours as needed (maximum: 6 doses/day)

Adults:

Crantex HC: 5-10 mL every 4-6 hours (maximum: 40 mL/day)

Giltuss HC®: 5 mL every 6 hours (maximum: 6 doses/day)

Tussafed® HC: 10 mL every 4-6 hours as needed (maximum: 6 doses/day)

Dosage Forms Excipient information presented when available (limited, particularly for generics); consult specific product labeling. [DSC] = Discontinued product

Elixir:

Duratuss® HD: Hydrocodone bitartrate 2.5 mg, phenylephrine hydrochloride 10 mg, and guaifenesin 225 mg per 5 mL (480 mL) [contains sodium benzoate; cherry flavor] [DSC]

Liquid:

Crantex HC: Hydrocodone bitartrate 5 mg, phenylephrine hydrochloride 7.5 mg, and guaifenesin 100 mg per 5 mL (480 mL) [alcohol free, dye free, sugar free; black cherry flavor] [DSC]

De-Chlor G: Hydrocodone bitartrate 2 mg, phenylephrine hydrochloride 10 mg, and guaifenesin 100 mg per 5 mL (480 mL) [grape-menthol mint flavor] [DSC]

ExeTuss HC: Hydrocodone bitartrate 2.5 mg, phenylephrine hydrochloride 10 mg, and guaifenesin 225 mg per 5 mL (480 mL) [alcohol free, sugar free; cherry flavor] [DSC]

Gentex HC: Hydrocodone bitartrate 2.5 mg, phenylephrine hydrochloride 7.5 mg, and guaifenesin 100 mg per 5 mL (480 mL) [cherry flavor] [DSC]

Giltuss HC®: Hydrocodone bitartrate 5 mg, phenylephrine hydrochloride 10 mg, and guaifenesin 300 mg per 5 mL (480 mL) [alcohol free, dye free, sugar free; strawberry banana flavor] [DSC]

Guiaplex™ HC: Hydrocodone bitartrate 5 mg, phenylephrine hydrochloride 15 mg, and guaifenesin 100 mg per 5 mL (480 mL) [alcohol free, sugar free; contains sodium benzoate; grape flavor] [DSC]

Hydro-GP: Hydrocodone bitartrate 2.5 mg, phenylephrine hydrochloride 7.5 mg, and guaifenesin 50 mg per 5 mL (480 mL) [cherry flavor] [DSC]

Levall 5.0: Hydrocodone bitartrate 5 mg, phenylephrine hydrochloride 15 mg, and guaifenesin 100 mg per 5 mL (480 mL) [grape flavor] [DSC]

Mintuss G: Hydrocodone bitartrate 2 mg, phenylephrine hydrochloride 10 mg, and guaifenesin 100 mg per 5 mL (480 mL) [alcohol free; contains sodium benzoate; grape flavor] [DSC]

Syrup:

Donatussin DC: Hydrocodone bitartrate 2.5 mg, phenylephrine hydrochloride 6 mg, and guaifenesin 120 mg per 5 mL (480 mL) [cherry flavor] [DSC]

HydroFed: Hydrocodone bitartrate 2.5 mg, phenylephrine hydrochloride 6 mg, and guaifenesin 150 mg per 5 mL (480 mL) [alcohol free, sugar free; contains propylene glycol; cherry flavor] [DSC]

Tussafed® HC: Hydrocodone bitartrate 2.5 mg, phenylephrine hydrochloride 7.5 mg, and guaifenesin 50 mg per 5 mL (480 mL) [alcohol free] [DSC]

Tussafed® HCG: Hydrocodone bitartrate 2.5 mg, phenylephrine hydrochloride 6 mg, and guaifenesin 150 mg per 5 mL (480 mL) [alcohol free, sugar free; cherry flavor] [DSC]

◆ **Hydrocodone Polistirex and Chlorpheniramine Polistirex** *see* Hydrocodone and Chlorpheniramine *on page 778*

Hydrocodone, Pseudoephedrine, and Guaifenesin

(hye droe KOE done, soo doe e FED rin & gwye FEN e sin)

U.S. Brand Names Entex® HC [DSC]; Hydro-Tussin™ HD [DSC]; Hydro-Tussin™ XP [DSC]; Su-Tuss®-HD [DSC]; Ztuss™ Tablet [DSC]

Index Terms Guaifenesin, Hydrocodone, and Pseudoephedrine; Pseudoephedrine, Hydrocodone, and Guaifenesin

Pharmacologic Category Antitussive/Decongestant/Expectorant

Use Symptomatic relief of irritating, nonproductive cough associated with upper respiratory conditions and allergies

Effect on Mental Status May cause drowsiness, fear, anxiety, tenseness, restlessness, insomnia, hallucinations, CNS depression

Effect on Psychiatric Treatment Contraindicated with MAO inhibitors

Restrictions C-III

Dosage Summary

Oral:

Children <2 years: Dosage not established

Children 2-6 years: Hydro-Tussin™ XP: 1.25-2.5 mL 4 times/day as needed

Children 6-12 years:

Hydro-Tussin™ XP: 2.5-5 mL 4 times/day as needed

Hydro-Tussin™ HD: 5 mL every 4-6 hours as needed

Ztuss™: One-half to 1 tablet every 4-6 hours (maximum: 6 tablets/day)

Children ≥12 years:

Hydro-Tussin™ XP: 5-10 mL 4 times/day as needed

Hydro-Tussin™ HD: 10 mL every 4-6 hours as needed

Ztuss™: 1-1½ tablets every 4-6 hours (maximum: 8 tablets/day)

Adults:

Hydro-Tussin™ XP: 5-10 mL 4 times/day as needed

Hydro-Tussin™ HD: 10 mL every 4-6 hours as needed

Ztuss™: 1-1½ tablets every 4-6 hours (maximum: 8 tablets/day)

Dosage Forms Excipient information presented when available (limited, particularly for generics); consult specific product labeling.

Elixir:

Su-Tuss®-HD: Hydrocodone bitartrate 2.5 mg, pseudoephedrine hydrochloride 30 mg, and guaifenesin 100 mg per 5 mL (480 mL) [contains alcohol; fruit punch flavor] [DSC]

Liquid:

Entex® HC: Hydrocodone bitartrate 3.75 mg, pseudoephedrine hydrochloride 22.5 mg, and guaifenesin 50 mg per 5 mL (480 mL) [alcohol free, sugar free; contains propylene glycol; tropical fruit punch flavor] [DSC]

Hydro-Tussin™ HD: Hydrocodone bitartrate 2.5 mg, pseudoephedrine hydrochloride 30 mg, and guaifenesin 100 mg per 5 mL (480 mL) [alcohol free; contains sodium benzoate] [DSC]

Hydro-Tussin® XP: Hydrocodone bitartrate 3 mg, pseudoephedrine hydrochloride 15 mg, and guaifenesin 100 mg per 5 mL (480 mL) [alcohol free, dye free] [DSC]

Tablet:

Ztuss™: Hydrocodone bitartrate 5 mg, pseudoephedrine hydrochloride 30 mg, and guaifenesin 300 mg [sugar free] [DSC]

◆ **Hydrocodone Tannate and Pseudoephedrine Tannate** *see* Hydrocodone and Pseudoephedrine *on page 781*

◆ **Hydrocodone Tannate, Phenylephrine Tannate, and Diphenhydramine Tannate** *see* Hydrocodone, Phenylephrine, and Diphenhydramine *on page 782*

Hydrocortisone (hye droe KOR ti sone)

Medication Safety Issues

Sound-alike/look-alike issues:

Hydrocortisone may be confused with hydrocodone, hydroxychloroquine, hydrochlorothiazide

Anusol® may be confused with Anusol-HC®, Aplisol®, Aquasol®

Anusol-HC® may be confused with Anusol®

Cortef® may be confused with Coreg®, Lortab®

Cortizone® may be confused with cortisone

HCT (occasional abbreviation for hydrocortisone) is an error-prone abbreviation (mistaken as hydrochlorothiazide)

Hytone® may be confused with Vytone®

Proctocort® may be confused with ProctoCream®

ProctoCream® may be confused with Proctocort®

Solu-Cortef® may be confused with Solu-Medrol®

International issues:

Hytone® may be confused with Hysone® [Australia]

Nutracort® may be confused with Nitrocor® which is a brand name of nitroglycerin in Chile and Italy

Related Information

Corticosteroids *on page 1780*

U.S. Brand Names Anucort-HC®; Anusol-HC®; Anusol® HC-1 [OTC]; Aquanil™ HC [OTC]; Beta-HC®; Caldecort® [OTC]; Cetacort® [DSC]; Colocort®; Cortaid® Intensive Therapy [OTC]; Cortaid® Maximum Strength [OTC]; Cortaid® Sensitive Skin [OTC]; Cortef®; Cortenema®; Corticool® [OTC]; Cortifoam®; Cortizone®-10 Maximum Strength [OTC]; Cortizone®-10

Plus Maximum Strength [OTC]; Cortizone®-10 Quick Shot [OTC]; Dermarest Dricort® [OTC]; Dermtex® HC [OTC]; EarSol® HC; Encort™; Hemril®-30; Hydro-Rx; HydroZone Plus [OTC]; Hytone®; IvySoothe® [OTC]; Locoid Lipocream®; Locoid®; Nupercainal® Hydrocortisone Cream [OTC]; Nutracort®; Pandel®; Post Peel Healing Balm [OTC]; Preparation H® Hydrocortisone [OTC]; Procto-Kit™; Procto-Pak™; Proctocort®; ProctoCream® HC; Proctosert; Proctosol-HC®; Proctozone-HC™; Sarnol®-HC [OTC]; Solu-Cortef®; Summer's Eve® SpecialCare™ Medicated Anti-Itch Cream [OTC] [DSC]; Texacort®; Tucks® Anti-Itch [OTC]; Westcort®

Canadian Brand Names Aquacort®; Cortamed®; Cortef®; Cortenema®; Cortifoam™; Emo-Cort®; Hycort™; Hyderm; HydroVal®; Locoid®; Prevex® HC; Sarna® HC; Solu-Cortef®; Westcort®

Mexican Brand Names Aquanil HC; Efficort Lipo; Flebocortid; Flkeboconadrol; Microsona; Nositrol; Nutracort; Paxosit; Solhidrol

Index Terms A-hydroCort; Compound F; Cortisol; Hemorrhoidal HC; Hydrocortisone Acetate; Hydrocortisone Butyrate; Hydrocortisone Probutate; Hydrocortisone Sodium Succinate; Hydrocortisone Valerate

Pharmacologic Category Corticosteroid, Rectal; Corticosteroid, Systemic; Corticosteroid, Topical

Generic Available Yes: Excludes acetate foam, butyrate cream and ointment, gel as base, otic drops as base, probutate cream, sodium succinate injection

Use Management of adrenocortical insufficiency; relief of inflammation of corticosteroid-responsive dermatoses (low and medium potency topical corticosteroid); adjunctive treatment of ulcerative colitis

Unlabeled/Investigational Use Management of septic shock when blood pressure is poorly responsive to fluid resuscitation and vasopressor therapy

Effect on Mental Status Insomnia and nervousness are common; rare reports of delirium, euphoria, hallucinations, and mood swings

Effect on Psychiatric Treatment Barbiturates may increase the metabolism of hydrocortisone; lithium has been used to treat mood swings associated with hydrocortisone

Pregnancy Risk Factor C

Pregnancy Considerations Adverse events have been observed with corticosteroids in animal reproduction studies. Hydrocortisone crosses the placenta. Some studies have shown an association between first trimester systemic corticosteroid use and oral clefts; adverse events in the fetus/neonate have been noted in case reports following large doses of systemic corticosteroids during pregnancy. Topical products are not recommended for extensive use, in large quantities, or for long periods of time in pregnant women.

Lactation Enters breast milk/use caution

Contraindications Hypersensitivity to hydrocortisone or any component of the formulation; serious infections, except septic shock or tuberculous meningitis; viral, fungal, or tubercular skin lesions; I.M. administration contraindicated in idiopathic thrombocytopenia purpura

Rectal suspension: Systemic fungal infections; ileocolostomy during the immediate or early postoperative period

Warnings/Precautions Use with caution in patients with thyroid disease, hepatic impairment, renal impairment, heart failure, hypertension, diabetes, glaucoma, cataracts, myasthenia gravis, patients at risk for osteoporosis, patients at risk for seizures, or GI diseases (diverticulitis, peptic ulcer, ulcerative colitis) due to perforation risk. Use caution following acute MI (corticosteroids have been associated with myocardial rupture). Because of the risk of adverse effects, systemic corticosteroids should be used cautiously in the elderly in the smallest possible effective dose for the shortest duration. May affect growth velocity; growth should be routinely monitored in pediatric patients. Withdraw therapy with gradual tapering of dose.

May cause hypercorticism or suppression of hypothalamic-pituitary-adrenal (HPA) axis, particularly in younger children or in patients receiving high doses for prolonged periods. HPA axis suppression may lead to adrenal crisis. Withdrawal and discontinuation of a corticosteroid should be done slowly and carefully. Particular care is required when patients are transferred from systemic corticosteroids to inhaled products due to possible adrenal insufficiency or withdrawal from steroids, including an increase in allergic symptoms. Patients receiving >20 mg per day of prednisone (or equivalent) may be most susceptible. Fatalities have occurred due to adrenal insufficiency in asthmatic patients during and after transfer from systemic corticosteroids to aerosol steroids; aerosol steroids do not provide the systemic steroid needed to treat patients having trauma, surgery, or infections. Avoid use of topical preparations with occlusive dressings or on weeping or exudative lesions.

Acute myopathy has been reported with high dose corticosteroids, usually in patients with neuromuscular transmission disorders; may involve ocular and/or respiratory muscles; monitor creatine kinase; recovery may be delayed. Corticosteroid use may cause psychiatric disturbances, including depression, euphoria, insomnia, mood swings, and personality changes. Pre-existing psychiatric conditions may be exacerbated by corticosteroid use. Prolonged use of corticosteroids may also increase the incidence of secondary infection, mask acute infection (including fungal infections), prolong or exacerbate viral infections, or limit response to vaccines. Exposure to chickenpox should be avoided; corticosteroids should not be used to treat ocular herpes simplex. Corticosteroids should not be used for cerebral malaria or viral hepatitis. Close observation is required in patients with latent tuberculosis and/or TB reactivity; restrict use in active TB (only in conjunction with antituberculosis treatment). Prolonged treatment with corticosteroids has been associated with the development of Kaposi's sarcoma (case reports); if noted, discontinuation of therapy should be considered. High-dose corticosteroids should not be used to manage acute head injury.

Adverse Reactions

Systemic:

Frequency not defined:

Cardiovascular: Edema, hypertension

Central nervous system: Delirium, euphoria, hallucinations, headache, insomnia, nervousness, pseudotumor cerebri, psychoses, seizure, vertigo

Dermatologic: Bruising, hyperpigmentation, skin atrophy

Endocrine & metabolic: Adrenal suppression, alkalosis, amenorrhea, Cushing's syndrome, diabetes mellitus, glucose intolerance, growth suppression, hyperglycemia, hyperlipidemia, hypokalemia, pituitary-adrenal axis suppression, sodium and water retention

Gastrointestinal: Abdominal distention, appetite increased, indigestion, nausea, pancreatitis, peptic ulcer, ulcerative esophagitis, vomiting

Hematologic: Leukocytosis (transient)

Neuromuscular & skeletal: Arthralgia, fractures, muscle weakness, osteoporosis

Ocular: Cataracts, glaucoma

Miscellaneous: Avascular necrosis, hypersensitivity reactions, infection, secondary malignancy

Topical:

>10%: Dermatologic: Eczema (12.5%)

1% to 10%: Dermatologic: Pruritus (6%), stinging (2%), dry skin (2%)

<1% (Limited to important or life-threatening): Allergic contact dermatitis, burning, dermal atrophy, folliculitis, HPA axis suppression, hypopigmentation; metabolic effects (hyperglycemia, hypokalemia); striae

Metabolism/Transport Effects **Substrate** of CYP3A4 (minor); **Induces** CYP3A4 (weak)

Drug Interactions

Acetylcholinesterase Inhibitors: Corticosteroids (Systemic) may enhance the adverse/toxic effect of Acetylcholinesterase Inhibitors. Increased muscular weakness may occur. *Risk C: Monitor therapy*

Aminoglutethimide: May increase the metabolism of Corticosteroids (Systemic). *Risk C: Monitor therapy*

Amphotericin B: Corticosteroids (Systemic) may enhance the hypokalemic effect of Amphotericin B. *Risk C: Monitor therapy*

Antacids: May decrease the bioavailability of Corticosteroids (Oral). *Risk D: Consider therapy modification*

Antidiabetic Agents: Corticosteroids (Systemic) may diminish the hypoglycemic effect of Antidiabetic Agents. In some instances, corticosteroid-mediated HPA axis suppression has led to episodes of acute adrenal crisis, which may manifest as enhanced hypoglycemia, particularly in the setting of insulin or other antidiabetic agent use. *Risk C: Monitor therapy*

Antifungal Agents (Azole Derivatives, Systemic): May decrease the metabolism of Corticosteroids (Systemic). *Risk C: Monitor therapy*

Aprepitant: May increase the serum concentration of Corticosteroids (Systemic). *Risk D: Consider therapy modification*

Barbiturates: May increase the metabolism of Corticosteroids (Systemic). *Risk C: Monitor therapy*

Bile Acid Sequestrants: May decrease the absorption of Corticosteroids (Oral). *Risk C: Monitor therapy*

Calcitriol: Corticosteroids (Systemic) may diminish the therapeutic effect of Calcitriol. *Risk C: Monitor therapy*

Calcium Channel Blockers (Nondihydropyridine): May decrease the metabolism of Corticosteroids (Systemic). *Risk C: Monitor therapy*

Corticorelin: Corticosteroids may diminish the therapeutic effect of Corticorelin. Specifically, the plasma ACTH response to corticorelin may be blunted by recent or current corticosteroid therapy. *Risk C: Monitor therapy*

CycloSPORINE: Corticosteroids (Systemic) may increase the serum concentration of CycloSPORINE. CycloSPORINE may increase the serum concentration of Corticosteroids (Systemic). *Risk C: Monitor therapy*

Echinacea: May diminish the therapeutic effect of Immunosuppressants. *Risk D: Consider therapy modification*

Estrogen Derivatives: May increase the serum concentration of Corticosteroids (Systemic). *Risk C: Monitor therapy*

Fluconazole: May decrease the metabolism of Corticosteroids (Systemic). *Risk C: Monitor therapy*

Fosaprepitant: May increase the serum concentration of Corticosteroids (Systemic). The active metabolite aprepitant is likely responsible for this effect. *Risk D: Consider therapy modification*

Isoniazid: Corticosteroids (Systemic) may decrease the serum concentration of Isoniazid. *Risk C: Monitor therapy*

Loop Diuretics: Corticosteroids (Systemic) may enhance the hypokalemic effect of Loop Diuretics. *Risk C: Monitor therapy*

Macrolide Antibiotics: May decrease the metabolism of Corticosteroids (Systemic). **Exceptions:** Azithromycin; Dirithromycin [Off Market]; Spiramycin. *Risk D: Consider therapy modification*

Maraviroc: CYP3A4 Inducers may decrease the serum concentration of Maraviroc. *Risk D: Consider therapy modification*

Natalizumab: Immunosuppressants may enhance the adverse/toxic effect of Natalizumab. Specifically, the risk of concurrent infection may be increased. *Risk X: Avoid combination*

Neuromuscular-Blocking Agents (Nondepolarizing): May enhance the adverse neuromuscular effect of Corticosteroids (Systemic). Increased muscle weakness, possibly progressing to polyneuropathies and myopathies, may occur. *Risk D: Consider therapy modification*

NSAID (COX-2 Inhibitor): Corticosteroids (Systemic) may enhance the adverse/toxic effect of NSAID (COX-2 Inhibitor). *Risk C: Monitor therapy*

NSAID (Nonselective): Corticosteroids (Systemic) may enhance the adverse/toxic effect of NSAID (Nonselective). *Risk C: Monitor therapy*

P-Glycoprotein Inducers: May decrease the serum concentration of P-Glycoprotein Substrates. P-glycoprotein inducers may also further limit the distribution of p-glycoprotein substrates to specific cells/tissues/organs where p-glycoprotein is present in large amounts (e.g., brain, T-lymphocytes, testes, etc.). *Risk C: Monitor therapy*

P-Glycoprotein Inhibitors: May increase the serum concentration of P-Glycoprotein Substrates. P-glycoprotein inhibitors may also enhance the distribution of p-glycoprotein substrates to specific cells/tissues/organs where p-glycoprotein is present in large amounts (e.g., brain, T-lymphocytes, testes, etc.). *Risk C: Monitor therapy*

Primidone: May increase the metabolism of Corticosteroids (Systemic). *Risk C: Monitor therapy*

Quinolone Antibiotics: May enhance the adverse/toxic effect of Corticosteroids (Systemic). Risk of tendon-related side effects, including tendonitis and rupture, may be enhanced. *Risk C: Monitor therapy*

Rifamycin Derivatives: May increase the metabolism of Corticosteroids (Systemic). *Risk C: Monitor therapy*

Salicylates: May enhance the adverse/toxic effect of Corticosteroids (Systemic). These specifically include gastrointestinal ulceration and bleeding. Corticosteroids (Systemic) may decrease the serum concentration of Salicylates. Withdrawal of corticosteroids may result in salicylate toxicity. *Risk C: Monitor therapy*

Thiazide Diuretics: Corticosteroids (Systemic) may enhance the hypokalemic effect of Thiazide Diuretics. *Risk C: Monitor therapy*

Trastuzumab: May enhance the neutropenic effect of Immunosuppressants. *Risk C: Monitor therapy*

Vaccines (Inactivated): Immunosuppressants may diminish the therapeutic effect of Vaccines (Inactivated). *Risk C: Monitor therapy*

Vaccines (Live): Immunosuppressants may enhance the adverse/toxic effect of Vaccines (Live). Vaccinal infections may develop. Immunosuppressants may also decrease therapeutic response to vaccines. *Risk X: Avoid combination*

Warfarin: Corticosteroids (Systemic) may enhance the anticoagulant effect of Warfarin. *Risk C: Monitor therapy*

Ethanol/Nutrition/Herb Interactions

Ethanol: Avoid ethanol (may enhance gastric mucosal irritation).

Food: Hydrocortisone interferes with calcium absorption.

Herb/Nutraceutical: St John's wort may decrease hydrocortisone levels. Avoid cat's claw, echinacea (have immunostimulant properties).

Stability Store at controlled room temperature 20°C to 25°C (68°F to 77°F). Protect from light. Hydrocortisone sodium phosphate and hydrocortisone sodium succinate are clear, light yellow solutions which are heat labile.

Sodium succinate: Reconstitute 100 mg vials with bacteriostatic water (not >2 mL). Act-O-Vial (self-contained powder for injection plus diluent) may be reconstituted by pressing the activator to force diluent into the powder compartment. Following gentle agitation, solution may be withdrawn via syringe through a needle inserted into the center of the stopper. May be administered (I.V. or I.M.) without further dilution. After initial reconstitution, hydrocortisone sodium succinate solutions are stable for 3 days at room temperature or under refrigeration when protected from light. Stability of parenteral admixture (Solu-Cortef®) at room temperature (25°C) and at refrigeration temperature (4°C) is concentration-dependent:

Stability of concentration 1 mg/mL: 24 hours.

Stability of concentration 2 mg/mL to 60 mg/mL: At least 4 hours.

Solutions for I.V. infusion: Reconstituted solutions may be added to an appropriate volume of compatible solution for infusion. Concentration should generally not exceed 1 mg/mL. However, in cases where administration of a small volume of fluid is desirable, 100-3000 mg may be added to 50 mL of D_5W or NS (stability limited to 4 hours).

Mechanism of Action Decreases inflammation by suppression of migration of polymorphonuclear leukocytes and reversal of increased capillary permeability

Pharmacodynamics/Kinetics

Onset of action:

Hydrocortisone acetate: Slow

Hydrocortisone sodium succinate (water soluble): Rapid

Duration: Hydrocortisone acetate: Long

Absorption: Rapid by all routes, except rectally

Metabolism: Hepatic

Half-life elimination: Biologic: 8-12 hours

Excretion: Urine (primarily as 17-hydroxysteroids and 17-ketosteroids)

Dosage Dose should be based on severity of disease and patient response

Adrenal hyperplasia (congenital): Children: Oral: Initial: 10-20 mg/m^2/day in 3 divided doses; a variety of dosing schedules have been used. **Note:** Inconsistencies have occurred with liquid formulations; tablets may provide more reliable levels. Doses must be individualized by monitoring growth, bone age, and hormonal levels. Mineralocorticoid and sodium supplementation may be required based upon electrolyte regulation and plasma renin activity.

Adrenal insufficiency (acute): I.M., I.V.:

Infants and young Children: Succinate: 1-2 mg/kg/dose bolus, then 25-150 mg/day in divided doses every 6-8 hours

Older Children: Succinate: 1-2 mg/kg bolus then 150-250 mg/day in divided doses every 6-8 hours

Adults: Succinate: 100 mg I.V. bolus, then 300 mg/day in divided doses every 8 hours or as a continuous infusion for 48 hours; once patient is stable change to oral, 50 mg every 8 hours for 6 doses, then taper to 30-50 mg/day in divided doses

Adrenal insufficiency (chronic): Adults: Oral: 20-30 mg/day

Anti-inflammatory or immunosuppressive:

Infants and Children:

Oral: 2.5-10 mg/kg/day **or** 75-300 mg/m^2/day every 6-8 hours

I.M., I.V.: Succinate: 1-5 mg/kg/day **or** 30-150 mg/m^2/day divided every 12-24 hours

Adolescents and Adults: Oral, I.M., I.V.: Succinate: 15-240 mg every 12 hours

Physiologic replacement: Children:

Oral: 0.5-0.75 mg/kg/day **or** 20-25 mg/m^2/day every 8 hours

I.M.: Succinate: 0.25-0.35 mg/kg/day **or** 12-15 mg/m^2/day once daily

Rheumatic diseases: Adults:

Intralesional, intra-articular, soft tissue injection: Acetate:

Large joints: 25 mg (up to 37.5 mg)

Small joints: 10-25 mg

Tendon sheaths: 5-12.5 mg

Soft tissue infiltration: 25-50 mg (up to 75 mg)

Bursae: 25-37.5 mg

Ganglia: 12.5-25 mg

Septic shock (unlabeled; Dellinger, 2008): I.V.: 50 mg every 6 hours. Wean once vasopressors are no longer required. **Note:** Fludrocortisone 50 mcg orally once daily is optional with hydrocortisone.

Shock: I.M., I.V.: Succinate:
Children: Initial: 50 mg/kg, then repeated in 4 hours and/or every 24 hours as needed
Adolescents and Adults: 500 mg to 2 g every 2-6 hours
Status asthmaticus: Children and Adults: I.V.: Succinate: 1-2 mg/kg/dose every 6 hours for 24 hours, then maintenance of 0.5-1 mg/kg every 6 hours
Stress dosing (surgery) in patients known to be adrenally-suppressed or on chronic systemic steroids: I.V.: Adults:
Minor stress (ie, inguinal herniorrhaphy): 25 mg/day for 1 day
Moderate stress (ie, joint replacement, cholecystectomy): 50-75 mg/day (25 mg every 8-12 hours) for 1-2 days
Major stress (pancreatoduodenectomy, esophagogastrectomy, cardiac surgery): 100-150 mg/day (50 mg every 8-12 hours) for 2-3 days
Dermatosis: Children >2 years and Adults: Topical: Apply to affected area 2-4 times/day (Buteprate: Apply once or twice daily). Therapy should be discontinued when control is achieved; if no improvement is seen, reassessment of diagnosis may be necessary.
Ulcerative colitis: Adults: Rectal: 10-100 mg 1-2 times/day for 2-3 weeks

Dietary Considerations Systemic use of corticosteroids may require a diet with increased potassium, vitamins A, B_6, C, D, folate, calcium, zinc, phosphorus, and decreased sodium. Sodium content of 1 g (sodium succinate injection): 47.5 mg (2.07 mEq)

Administration
Oral: Administer with food or milk to decrease GI upset
Parenteral: Hydrocortisone sodium succinate may be administered by I.M. or I.V. routes
I.V. bolus: Dilute to 50 mg/mL and administer over 30 seconds or over 10 minutes for doses ≥500 mg
I.V. intermittent infusion: Dilute to 1 mg/mL and administer over 20-30 minutes
Topical: Apply a thin film to clean, dry skin and rub in gently

Monitoring Parameters Blood pressure, weight, serum glucose, and electrolytes

Reference Range Therapeutic: AM: 5-25 mcg/dL (SI: 138-690 nmol/L), PM: 2-9 mcg/dL (SI: 55-248 nmol/L) depending on test, assay

Additional Information Hydrocortisone base topical cream, lotion, and ointments in concentrations of 0.25%, 0.5%, and 1% may be OTC or prescription depending on the product labeling.

Dosage Forms Excipient information presented when available (limited, particularly for generics); consult specific product labeling. [DSC] = Discontinued product
Aerosol, rectal, as acetate (Cortifoam®): 10% (15 g) [90 mg/applicator]
Cream, rectal, as acetate (Nupercainal® Hydrocortisone Cream): 1% (30 g) [strength expressed as base]
Cream, rectal, as base:
Cortizone®-10: 1% (30 g) [contains aloe]
Preparation H® Hydrocortisone: 1% (27 g)
Cream, topical, as acetate: 0.5% (9 g, 30 g, 60 g) [available with aloe]; 1% (30 g, 454 g) [available with aloe]
Cream, topical, as base: 0.5% (30 g); 1% (1.5 g, 30 g, 114 g, 454 g); 2.5% (20 g, 30 g, 454 g)
Anusol-HC®: 2.5% (30 g) [contains benzyl alcohol]
Caldecort®: 1% (30 g) [contains aloe vera gel]
Cortaid® Intensive Therapy: 1% (60 g)
Cortaid® Maximum Strength: 1% (15 g, 30 g, 40 g, 60 g) [contains aloe vera gel and benzyl alcohol]
Cortaid® Sensitive Skin: 0.5% (15 g) [contains aloe vera gel]
Cortizone®-10 Maximum Strength: 1% (15 g, 30 g, 60 g) [contains aloe]
Cortizone®-10 Plus Maximum Strength: 1% (30 g, 60 g) [contains vitamins A, D, E and aloe]
Dermarest® Dricort®: 1% (15 g, 30 g)
HydroZone Plus, Proctocort®, Procto-Pak™: 1% (30 g)
Hytone®: 2.5% (30 g, 60 g)
IvySoothe®: 1% (30 g) [contains aloe]
Post Peel Healing Balm: 1% (23 g)
ProctoCream® HC: 2.5% (30 g) [contains benzyl alcohol]
Procto-Kit™: 1% (30 g) [packaged with applicator tips and finger cots]; 2.5% (30 g) [packaged with applicator tips and finger cots]
Proctosol-HC®, Proctozone-HC™: 2.5% (30 g)
Summer's Eve® SpecialCare™ Medicated Anti-Itch Cream: 1% (30 g) [DSC]
Cream, topical, as butyrate (Locoid®, Locoid Lipocream®): 0.1% (15 g, 45 g)
Cream, topical, as probutate (Pandel®): 0.1% (15 g, 45 g, 80 g)
Cream, topical, as valerate (Westcort®): 0.2% (15 g, 45 g, 60 g)

Gel, topical, as base (Corticool®): 1% (45 g)
Injection, powder for reconstitution, as sodium succinate:
A-Hydrocort®: 100 mg [contains monobasic sodium phosphate 0.8 mg, anhydrous dibasic sodium phosphate 8.73 mg; strength expressed as base]
Solu-Cortef®: 100 mg, 250 mg, 500 mg, 1 g [diluent contains benzyl alcohol; strength expressed as base]
Lotion, topical, as base: 1% (120 mL); 2.5% (60 mL)
Aquanil™ HC: 1% (120 mL)
Beta-HC®, Cetacort® [DSC], Sarnol®-HC: 1% (60 mL)
HydroZone Plus: 1% (120 mL)
Hytone®: 2.5% (60 mL)
Nutracort®: 1% (60 mL, 120 mL); 2.5% (60 mL, 120 mL)
Lotion, topical, as butyrate:
Locoid®: 0.1% (60 mL)
Ointment, topical, as acetate: 1% (30 g) [strength expressed as base; available with aloe]
Anusol® HC-1: 1% (21 g) [strength expressed as base]
Cortaid® Maximum Strength: 1% (15 g, 30 g) [strength expressed as base]
Ointment, topical, as base: 0.5% (30 g); 1% (30 g, 454 g); 2.5% (20 g, 30 g, 454 g)
Cortizone®-10 Maximum Strength: 1% (30 g, 60 g)
Hytone®: 2.5% (30 g) [DSC]
Ointment, topical, as butyrate (Locoid®): 0.1% (15 g, 45 g)
Ointment, topical, as valerate (Westcort®): 0.2% (15 g, 45 g, 60 g)
Powder, for prescription compounding [micronized]:
Hydro-Rx: USP (10 g, 25 g, 50 g, 100 g)
Powder, for prescription compounding, as acetate [micronized]: USP (10 g, 25 g, 50 g)
Solution, otic, as base (EarSol® HC): 1% (30 mL) [contains alcohol 44%, benzyl benzoate, yerba santa]
Solution, topical, as base (Texacort®): 2.5% (30 mL) [contains ethanol 48%]
Solution, topical, as butyrate (Locoid®): 0.1% (20 mL, 60 mL) [contains alcohol 50%]
Solution, topical spray, as base:
Cortaid® Intensive Therapy: 1% (60 mL) [contains alcohol]
Cortizone®-10 Quick Shot: 1% (44 mL) [contains benzyl alcohol]
Dermtex® HC: 1% (52 mL) [contains menthol 1%]
Suppository, rectal, as acetate: 25 mg (12s, 24s, 100s)
Anucort-HC®, Tucks® Anti-Itch: 25 mg (12s, 24s, 100s) [strength expressed as base; Anucort-HC® *renamed* Tucks® Anti-Itch]
Anusol-HC®, Proctosol-HC®: 25 mg (12s, 24s)
Encort™, Proctocort®: 30 mg (12s)
Hemril®-30, Proctosert: 30 mg (12s, 24s)
Suspension, rectal, as base: 100 mg/60 mL (7s)
Colocort®, Cortenema®: 100 mg/60 mL (1s, 7s)
Tablet, as base: 20 mg
Cortef®: 5 mg, 10 mg, 20 mg

◆ **Hydrocortisone Acetate** *see* Hydrocortisone *on page 785*

◆ **Hydrocortisone Butyrate** *see* Hydrocortisone *on page 785*

◆ **Hydrocortisone Probutate** *see* Hydrocortisone *on page 785*

◆ **Hydrocortisone Sodium Succinate** *see* Hydrocortisone *on page 785*

◆ **Hydrocortisone Valerate** *see* Hydrocortisone *on page 785*

◆ **Hydro DP** *see* Hydrocodone, Phenylephrine, and Diphenhydramine *on page 782*

◆ **HydroFed [DSC]** *see* Hydrocodone, Phenylephrine, and Guaifenesin *on page 783*

◆ **Hydro-GP [DSC]** *see* Hydrocodone, Phenylephrine, and Guaifenesin *on page 783*

◆ **Hydromet®** *see* Hydrocodone and Homatropine *on page 780*

HYDROmorphone (hye droe MOR fone)

Medication Safety Issues

Sound-alike/look-alike issues:
Dilaudid® may be confused with Demerol®, Dilantin®
HYDROmorphone may be confused with morphine; significant overdoses have occurred when hydromorphone products have been inadvertently administered instead of morphine sulfate. Commercially available prefilled

syringes of both products looks similar and are often stored in close proximity to each other. **Note:** Hydromorphone 1 mg oral is approximately equal to morphine 4 mg oral; hydromorphone 1 mg I.V. is approximately equal to morphine 5 mg I.V.

High alert medication: The Institute for Safe Medication Practices (ISMP) includes this medication among its list of drug classes which have a heightened risk of causing significant patient harm when used in error.

Dilaudid®, Dilaudid-HP®: Extreme caution should be taken to avoid confusing the highly-concentrated (Dilaudid-HP®) injection with the less-concentrated (Dilaudid®) injectable product.

Significant differences exist between oral and I.V. dosing. Use caution when converting from one route of administration to another.

Related Information

Narcotic / Opioid Analgesics *on page 1789*

U.S. Brand Names Dilaudid-HP®; Dilaudid®

Canadian Brand Names Dilaudid-HP-Plus®; Dilaudid-HP®; Dilaudid-XP®; Dilaudid®; Dilaudid® Sterile Powder; Hydromorph Contin®; Hydromorph-IR®; Hydromorphone HP; Hydromorphone HP® 10; Hydromorphone HP® 20; Hydromorphone HP® 50; Hydromorphone HP® Forte; Hydromorphone Hydrochloride Injection, USP; PMS-Hydromorphone

Mexican Brand Names Liberaxim

Index Terms Dihydromorphinone; Hydromorphone Hydrochloride

Pharmacologic Category Analgesic, Opioid

Generic Available Yes: Excludes capsule, liquid, powder for injection

Use Management of moderate-to-severe pain

Unlabeled/Investigational Use Antitussive

Effect on Mental Status Drowsiness and dizziness are common; may cause nervousness or restlessness; may rarely cause hallucinations or depression

Effect on Psychiatric Treatment Concurrent use with psychotropics may produce additive sedation

Restrictions C-II

Pregnancy Risk Factor C/D (prolonged use or high doses at term)

Pregnancy Considerations Hydromorphone was teratogenic in some, but not all, animal studies; however, maternal toxicity was also reported. Hydromorphone crosses the placenta. Chronic opioid use during pregnancy may lead to a withdrawal syndrome in the neonate. Symptoms include irritability, hyperactivity, loss of sleep pattern, abnormal crying, tremor, vomiting, diarrhea, weight loss, or failure to gain weight.

Lactation Excretion in breast milk unknown/not recommended

Contraindications Hypersensitivity to hydromorphone, any component of the formulation; acute or severe asthma, severe respiratory depression (in absence of resuscitative equipment or ventilatory support); severe CNS depression; pregnancy (prolonged use or high doses at term); obstetrical analgesia

Warnings/Precautions Use with caution in patients with hypersensitivity reactions to other phenanthrene derivative opioid agonists (codeine, hydrocodone, levorphanol, oxycodone, oxymorphone). Hydromorphone shares toxic potential of opiate agonists, including CNS depression and respiratory depression. Precautions associated with opiate agonist therapy should be observed. May cause CNS depression, which may impair physical or mental abilities; patients must be cautioned about performing tasks which require mental alertness (eg, operating machinery or driving). Myoclonus and seizures have been reported with high doses. Critical respiratory depression may occur, even at therapeutic dosages, particularly in elderly or debilitated patients or in patients with pre-existing respiratory compromise (hypoxia and/or hypercapnia). Use caution in COPD or other obstructive pulmonary disease. Use with caution in patients with hypersensitivity to other phenanthrene opiates, kyphoscoliosis, biliary tract disease, acute pancreatitis, morbid obesity, adrenocortical insufficiency, hypothyroidism, acute alcoholism, toxic psychoses, prostatic hyperplasia and/or urinary stricture, or severe liver or renal failure. Use extreme caution in patients with head injury, intracranial lesions, or elevated intracranial pressure; exaggerated elevation of ICP may occur (in addition, hydromorphone may complicate neurologic evaluation due to pupillary dilation and CNS depressant effects). Use with caution in patients with depleted blood volume or drugs which may exaggerate hypotensive effects (including phenothiazines or general anesthetics). May obscure diagnosis or clinical course of patients with acute abdominal conditions.

[U.S. Boxed Warning]: Hydromorphone has a high potential for abuse. Those at risk for opioid abuse include patients with a history of substance abuse or mental illness. Tolerance or drug dependence may result from extended use; however, concerns for abuse should not prevent effective management of pain. In general, abrupt discontinuation of therapy in dependent patients should be avoided.

An opioid-containing analgesic regimen should be tailored to each patient's needs and based upon the type of pain being treated (acute versus chronic), the route of administration, degree of tolerance for opioids (naive versus chronic user), age, weight, and medical condition. The optimal analgesic dose varies widely among patients. Doses should be titrated to pain relief/prevention. I.M. use may result in variable absorption and a lag time to peak effect.

Dosage form specific warnings:

[U.S. Boxed Warning]: Dilaudid-HP®: Extreme caution should be taken to avoid confusing the highly-concentrated (Dilaudid-HP®) injection with the less-concentrated (Dilaudid®) injectable product. Dilaudid-HP® should only be used in patients who are opioid-tolerant.

Controlled release: Capsules should only be used when continuous analgesia is required over an extended period of time. Controlled release products are not to be used on an "as needed" (PRN) basis.

Some dosage forms contain trace amounts of sodium metabisulfite which may cause allergic reactions in susceptible individuals.

Adverse Reactions Frequency not defined.

Cardiovascular: Bradycardia, flushing of face, hyper-/hypotension, palpitation, peripheral vasodilation, syncope, tachycardia

Central nervous system: Agitation, chills, CNS depression, dizziness, drowsiness, dysphoria, euphoria, fatigue, hallucinations, headache, increased intracranial pressure, insomnia, lightheadedness, mental depression, nervousness, restlessness, sedation, seizure

Dermatologic: Pruritus, rash, urticaria

Endocrine & metabolic: Antidiuretic hormone release

Gastrointestinal: Anorexia, biliary tract spasm, constipation, diarrhea, nausea, paralytic ileus, stomach cramps, taste perversion, vomiting, xerostomia

Genitourinary: Ureteral spasm, urinary retention, urinary tract spasm, urination decreased

Hepatic: AST/ALT increased, LFTs increased

Local: Pain at injection site (I.M.), wheal/flare over vein (I.V.)

Neuromuscular & skeletal: Myoclonus, paresthesia, trembling, tremor, weakness

Ocular: Blurred vision, diplopia, miosis, nystagmus

Respiratory: Apnea, bronchospasm, dyspnea, laryngospasm, respiratory depression

Miscellaneous: Diaphoresis, histamine release, physical and psychological dependence

Drug Interactions

Alcohol (Ethyl): CNS Depressants may enhance the CNS depressant effect of Alcohol (Ethyl). *Risk C: Monitor therapy*

Alvimopan: Analgesics (Opioid) may enhance the adverse/toxic effect of Alvimopan. This is most notable for patients receiving long-term (i.e., more than 7 days) opiates prior to alvimopan initiation. Management: Alvimopan is contraindicated in patients receiving therapeutic doses of opioids for more than 7 consecutive days immediately prior to alvimopan initiation. *Risk D: Consider therapy modification*

Ammonium Chloride: May increase the excretion of Analgesics (Opioid). *Risk C: Monitor therapy*

Amphetamines: May enhance the analgesic effect of Analgesics (Opioid). *Risk C: Monitor therapy*

Antipsychotic Agents (Phenothiazines): May enhance the hypotensive effect of Analgesics (Opioid). *Risk C: Monitor therapy*

CNS Depressants: May enhance the adverse/toxic effect of other CNS Depressants. *Risk C: Monitor therapy*

Desmopressin: Analgesics (Opioid) may enhance the adverse/toxic effect of Desmopressin. *Risk C: Monitor therapy*

Pegvisomant: Analgesics (Opioid) may diminish the therapeutic effect of Pegvisomant. *Risk C: Monitor therapy*

Selective Serotonin Reuptake Inhibitors: Analgesics (Opioid) may enhance the serotonergic effect of Selective Serotonin Reuptake Inhibitors. This may cause serotonin syndrome. *Risk C: Monitor therapy*

Succinylcholine: May enhance the bradycardic effect of Analgesics (Opioid). *Risk C: Monitor therapy*

Ethanol/Nutrition/Herb Interactions

Ethanol: Avoid ethanol (may increase CNS depression).

Herb/Nutraceutical: Avoid valerian, St John's wort, kava kava, gotu kola (may increase CNS depression).

Stability Store injection and oral dosage forms at 15°C to 30°C (59°F to 86°F). Protect tablets from light. A slightly yellowish discoloration has not been associated with a loss of potency.

Mechanism of Action Binds to opiate receptors in the CNS, causing inhibition of ascending pain pathways, altering the perception of and response to pain; causes cough supression by direct central action in the medulla; produces generalized CNS depression

Pharmacodynamics/Kinetics

Onset of action: Analgesic: Immediate release formulations:
- Oral: 15-30 minutes
- Peak effect: Oral: 30-60 minutes

Duration: Immediate release formulations: 4-5 hours
Absorption: I.M.: Variable and delayed
Distribution: V_d: 4 L/kg
Protein binding: ~8% to 19%
Metabolism: Hepatic via glucuronidation; to inactive metabolites
Bioavailability: 62%
Half-life elimination: Immediate release formulations: 1-3 hours
Excretion: Urine (primarily as glucuronide conjugates)

Dosage

Acute pain (moderate to severe): **Note:** These are guidelines and do not represent the maximum doses that may be required in all patients. Doses should be titrated to pain relief/prevention.

Children ≥6 months and <50 kg:
- Oral: 0.03-0.08 mg/kg/dose every 3-4 hours as needed
- I.V.: 0.015 mg/kg/dose every 3-6 hours as needed

Children >50 kg and Adults:
- Oral: Initial: Opiate-naive: 2-4 mg every 3-6 hours as needed; elderly/debilitated patients may require lower doses; patients with prior opiate exposure may require higher initial doses; usual dosage range: 2-8 mg every 3-4 hours as needed
- I.V.: Initial: Opiate-naive: 0.2-0.6 mg every 2-3 hours as needed; patients with prior opiate exposure may tolerate higher initial doses
  - Critically-ill patients (unlabeled dose): 0.7-2 mg (based on 70 kg patient) every 1-2 hours as needed. **Note:** More frequent dosing may be needed (eg, mechanically-ventilated patients).
    - Continuous infusion: Usual dosage range: 0.5-1 mg/hour (based on 70 kg patient) or 7-15 mcg/kg/hour
- Patient-controlled analgesia (PCA): (Opiate-naive: Consider lower end of dosing range)
  - Usual concentration: 0.2 mg/mL
  - Demand dose: Usual: 0.1-0.2 mg; range: 0.05-0.5 mg
  - Lockout interval: 5-15 minutes
  - 4-hour limit: 4-6 mg
- Epidural:
  - Bolus dose: 1-1.5 mg
  - Infusion concentration: 0.05-0.075 mg/mL
  - Infusion rate: 0.04-0.4 mg/hour
  - Demand dose: 0.15 mg
  - Lockout interval: 30 minutes
- I.M., SubQ: **Note:** I.M. use may result in variable absorption and a lag time to peak effect.
  - Initial: Opiate-naive: 0.8-1 mg every 4-6 hours as needed; patients with prior opiate exposure may require higher initial doses; usual dosage range: 1-2 mg every 3-6 hours as needed
- Rectal: 3 mg every 4-8 hours as needed

Chronic pain: Adults: Oral: **Note:** Patients taking opioids chronically may become tolerant and require doses higher than the usual dosage range to maintain the desired effect. Tolerance can be managed by appropriate dose titration. There is no optimal or maximal dose for hydromorphone in chronic pain. The appropriate dose is one that relieves pain throughout its dosing interval without causing unmanageable side effects.

Controlled release formulation (Hydromorph Contin®, not available in U.S.): 3-30 mg every 12 hours. **Note:** A patient's hydromorphone requirement should be established using prompt release formulations; conversion to long acting products may be considered when chronic, continuous treatment is required. Higher dosages should be reserved for use only in opioid-tolerant patients.

Antitussive (unlabeled use): Oral:
- Children 6-12 years: 0.5 mg every 3-4 hours as needed
- Children >12 years and Adults: 1 mg every 3-4 hours as needed

Dosing adjustment in hepatic impairment: Should be considered

Administration

Parenteral: May be given SubQ or I.M.; vial stopper contains latex

I.V.: For IVP, must be given slowly over 2-3 minutes (rapid IVP has been associated with an increase in side effects, especially respiratory depression and hypotension)

Oral: Hydromorph Contin®: Capsule should be swallowed whole; do not crush or chew; contents may be sprinkled on soft food and swallowed

Monitoring Parameters Pain relief, respiratory and mental status, blood pressure

Test Interactions Some quinolones may produce a false-positive urine screening result for opiates using commercially-available immunoassay kits. This has been demonstrated most consistently for levofloxacin and ofloxacin, but other quinolones have shown cross-reactivity in certain assay kits. Confirmation of positive opiate screens by more specific methods should be considered.

Additional Information Equianalgesic doses: Morphine 10 mg I.M. = hydromorphone 1.5 mg I.M.

Dosage Forms Excipient information presented when available (limited, particularly for generics); consult specific product labeling. [CAN] = Canadian brand name

Capsule, controlled release:

Hydromorph Contin® [CAN]: 3 mg, 6 mg, 12 mg, 18 mg, 24 mg, 30 mg [not available in U.S.]

Injection, powder for reconstitution, as hydrochloride:

Dilaudid-HP®: 250 mg [may contain trace amounts of sodium bisulfite]

Injection, solution, as hydrochloride: 1 mg/mL (1 mL); 2 mg/mL (1 mL, 20 mL); 4 mg/mL (1 mL)

Dilaudid®: 1 mg/mL (1 mL); 2 mg/mL (1 mL, 20 mL) [20 mL size contains edetate sodium; vial stopper contains latex]; 4 mg/mL (1 mL)

Injection, solution, as hydrochloride [preservative free]: 10 mg/mL (1 mL, 5 mL, 50 mL)

Dilaudid-HP®: 10 mg/mL (1 mL, 5 mL) [contains sodium metabisulfate]

Dilaudid-HP®: 10 mg/mL (50 mL) [contains natural rubber/natural latex in packaging, sodium metabisulfate]

Liquid, oral, as hydrochloride:

Dilaudid®: 1 mg/mL (480 mL) [may contain trace amounts of sodium bisulfite]

Powder, for prescription compounding: 100% (15 grain)

Suppository, rectal, as hydrochloride: 3 mg

Dilaudid®: 3 mg (6s)

Tablet, as hydrochloride: 2 mg, 4 mg, 8 mg

Dilaudid®: 2 mg, 4 mg, 8 mg (8 mg tablets may contain trace amounts of sodium bisulfite)

- ◆ **Hydromorphone Hydrochloride** *see* HYDROmorphone *on page 791*
- ◆ **Hydron CP** *see* Phenylephrine, Hydrocodone, and Chlorpheniramine *on page 1277*
- ◆ **Hydron PSC [DSC]** *see* Pseudoephedrine, Hydrocodone, and Chlorpheniramine *on page 1372*
- ◆ **Hydro-PC II** *see* Phenylephrine, Hydrocodone, and Chlorpheniramine *on page 1277*
- ◆ **Hydro PC II Plus** *see* Phenylephrine, Hydrocodone, and Chlorpheniramine *on page 1277*
- ◆ **Hydro-Rx** *see* Hydrocortisone *on page 785*
- ◆ **Hydro-Tussin™-CBX [DSC]** *see* Carbinoxamine and Pseudoephedrine *on page 280*
- ◆ **Hydro-Tussin™ DHC [DSC]** *see* Pseudoephedrine, Dihydrocodeine, and Chlorpheniramine *on page 1371*
- ◆ **Hydro-Tussin™ DM [DSC]** *see* Guaifenesin and Dextromethorphan *on page 739*
- ◆ **Hydro-Tussin™ EXP [DSC]** *see* Dihydrocodeine, Pseudoephedrine, and Guaifenesin *on page 469*
- ◆ **Hydro-Tussin™ HD [DSC]** *see* Hydrocodone, Pseudoephedrine, and Guaifenesin *on page 784*
- ◆ **Hydro-Tussin™ XP [DSC]** *see* Hydrocodone, Pseudoephedrine, and Guaifenesin *on page 784*
- ◆ **4-Hydroxybutyrate** *see* Sodium Oxybate *on page 1495*
- ◆ **Hydroxycarbamide** *see* Hydroxyurea *on page 796*

Hydroxychloroquine (hye droks ee KLOR oh kwin)

Medication Safety Issues
Sound-alike/look-alike issues:
Hydroxychloroquine may be confused with hydrocortisone
Plaquenil® may be confused with Platinol®

U.S. Brand Names Plaquenil®

Canadian Brand Names Apo-Hydroxyquine®; Gen-Hydroxychloroquine; Plaquenil®

Mexican Brand Names Plaquenil

Index Terms Hydroxychloroquine Sulfate

Pharmacologic Category Aminoquinoline (Antimalarial)

Use Suppression and treatment of acute attacks of malaria; treatment of systemic lupus erythematosus (SLE) and rheumatoid arthritis

Unlabeled/Investigational Use Porphyria cutanea tarda, polymorphous light eruptions

Effect on Mental Status May cause dizziness or nervousness

Effect on Psychiatric Treatment May rarely cause agranulocytosis; use caution with clozapine and carbamazepine

Dosage Summary Note: Hydroxychloroquine sulfate 200 mg is equivalent to 155 mg hydroxychloroquine base and 250 mg chloroquine phosphate.

Oral:

Children:
SLE (unlabeled use): 3-5 mg/kg/day (base) divided 1-2 times/day (maximum: 7 mg/kg/day)
Malaria prophylaxis:
No pretreatment: 10 mg/kg (base) in 2 divided doses 6 hours apart, followed by normal prophylactic regimen
Prior to exposure: 5 mg/kg (base) once weekly
Malaria treatment: 10 mg/kg (base) initially, followed by 5 mg/kg at 6, 24, and 48 hours
Rheumatoid arthritis: 3-5 mg/kg/day (base) divided 1-2 times/day (maximum: 7 mg/kg/day)

Adults:
SLE: Initial: 310-620 mg/day (base) divided 1-2 times/day; Maintenance: 155-310 mg/day (base)
Malaria prophylaxis:
No pretreatment: 620 mg (base) in 2 divided doses 6 hours apart, followed by normal prophylactic regimen
Prior to exposure: 310 mg (base) once weekly
Malaria treatment: 620 mg (base) initially, followed by 310 mg (base) at 6, 24, and 48 hours
Rheumatoid arthritis: Initial: 310-465 mg/day (base); Maintenance: 155-310 mg/day (base)

Dosage Forms Excipient information presented when available (limited, particularly for generics); consult specific product labeling.
Tablet, as sulfate: 200 mg [equivalent to 155 mg base]

- **Hydroxychloroquine Sulfate** *see* Hydroxychloroquine *on page 796*
- **Hydroxydaunomycin Hydrochloride** *see* DOXOrubicin *on page 507*
- **1α-Hydroxyergocalciferol** *see* Doxercalciferol *on page 507*
- **Hydroxyldaunorubicin Hydrochloride** *see* DOXOrubicin *on page 507*
- **9-hydroxy-risperidone** *see* Paliperidone *on page 1215*

Hydroxyurea (hye droks ee yoor EE a)

Medication Safety Issues
Sound-alike/look-alike issues:
Hydroxyurea may be confused with hydrOXYzine

High alert medication: The Institute for Safe Medication Practices (ISMP) includes this medication among its list of drugs which have a heightened risk of causing significant patient harm when used in error.

International issues:
Hydrea® may be confused with Hydra® which is a brand name for isoniazid in Japan

U.S. Brand Names Droxia®; Hydrea®; Mylocel™

Canadian Brand Names Apo-Hydroxyurea®; Gen-Hydroxyurea; Hydrea®

Mexican Brand Names Hydrea

Index Terms Hydroxycarbamide

Pharmacologic Category Antineoplastic Agent, Antimetabolite

Use Treatment of melanoma, refractory chronic myelocytic leukemia (CML), relapsed and refractory metastatic ovarian cancer; radiosensitizing agent in the treatment of squamous cell head and neck cancer (excluding lip cancer); adjunct in the management of sickle cell patients who have had at least three painful crises in the previous 12 months (to reduce frequency of these crises and the need for blood transfusions)

Unlabeled/Investigational Use Treatment of HIV; treatment of psoriasis, treatment of hematologic conditions such as essential thrombocythemia, polycythemia vera, hypereosinophilia, and hyperleukocytosis due to acute leukemia; treatment of uterine, cervix and nonsmall cell lung cancers; radiosensitizing agent in the treatment of primary brain tumors; has shown activity against renal cell cancer and prostate cancer

Effect on Mental Status Drowsiness is common; may rarely cause disorientation and hallucinations

Effect on Psychiatric Treatment Myelosuppression is common; use caution with clozapine and carbamazepine

Dosage Summary

Oral:

Children: Dosage not established

Adults: 10-35 mg/kg/day **or** 500-3000 mg/day as single or divided dose **or** 80 mg/kg as a single dose every third day

Dosage Forms Excipient information presented when available (limited, particularly for generics); consult specific product labeling.

Capsule: 500 mg

Droxia®: 200 mg, 300 mg, 400 mg

Hydrea®: 500 mg

Tablet:

Mylocel™: 1000 mg

HydrOXYzine (hye DROKS i zeen)

Medication Safety Issues

Sound-alike/look-alike issues:

HydrOXYzine may be confused with hydrALAZINE, hydroxyurea

Atarax® may be confused with amoxicillin, Ativan®

Vistaril® may be confused with Restoril®, Versed, Zestril®

International issues:

Vistaril® may be confused with Vastarel® which is a brand name for trimetazidine in multiple international markets

Related Information

CMS: Long-Term Care Facility Thresholds *on page 1815*

Nonbenzodiazepine Anxiolytics and Hypnotics *on page 1791*

U.S. Brand Names Vistaril®

Canadian Brand Names Apo-Hydroxyzine®; Atarax®; Hydroxyzine Hydrochloride Injection, USP; Novo-Hydroxyzin; PMS-Hydroxyzine; Vistaril®

Mexican Brand Names Atarax

Index Terms Hydroxyzine Hydrochloride; Hydroxyzine Pamoate

Pharmacologic Category Antiemetic; Histamine H_1 Antagonist; Histamine H_1 Antagonist, First Generation

Generic Available Yes

Use Treatment of anxiety; preoperative sedative; antipruritic

Unlabeled/Investigational Use Antiemetic; ethanol withdrawal symptoms

Mental Health Comment Commonly used as an anxiolytic, especially in individuals with a history of or active substance use. Postmarketing experience revealed cases of headache and hallucinations.

Pregnancy Risk Factor C

Pregnancy Considerations Hydroxyzine-induced fetal abnormalities at high dosages in animal studies. Neonatal withdrawal symptoms have been reported following long-term maternal use or the use of large doses near term. Use in early pregnancy is contraindicated by the manufacturer.

Lactation Excretion in breast milk unknown/not recommended

Contraindications Hypersensitivity to hydroxyzine or any component of the formulation; early pregnancy; SubQ, intra-arterial, or I.V. administration of injection

Warnings/Precautions Causes sedation, caution must be used in performing tasks which require alertness (eg, operating machinery or driving). Sedative effects of CNS depressants or ethanol are potentiated. SubQ, I.V., and intra-arterial administration are contraindicated since tissue damage, intravascular hemolysis, thrombosis, and digital gangrene can occur. Use with caution with narrow-angle glaucoma, prostatic hyperplasia, bladder neck obstruction, asthma, or COPD.

Anticholinergic effects are not well tolerated in the elderly. Hydroxyzine may be useful as a short-term antipruritic, but it is not recommended for use as a sedative or anxiolytic in the elderly.

Adverse Reactions Frequency not defined.

Central nervous system: Dizziness, drowsiness, fatigue, hallucination, headache, nervousness, seizure

Dermatologic: Pruritus, rash, urticaria

Gastrointestinal: Xerostomia

Neuromuscular & skeletal: Involuntary movements, paresthesia, tremor

Ocular: Blurred vision

Respiratory: Thickening of bronchial secretions

Miscellaneous: Allergic reaction

Metabolism/Transport Effects Inhibits CYP2D6 (weak)

Drug Interactions

Acetylcholinesterase Inhibitors (Central): Anticholinergics may diminish the therapeutic effect of Acetylcholinesterase Inhibitors (Central). Acetylcholinesterase Inhibitors (Central) may diminish the therapeutic effect of Anticholinergics. If the anticholinergic action is a side effect of the agent, the result may be beneficial. *Risk C: Monitor therapy*

Alcohol (Ethyl): CNS Depressants may enhance the CNS depressant effect of Alcohol (Ethyl). *Risk C: Monitor therapy*

Amphetamines: May diminish the sedative effect of Antihistamines. *Risk C: Monitor therapy*

Anticholinergics: May enhance the adverse/toxic effect of other Anticholinergics. **Exceptions:** Paliperidone. *Risk C: Monitor therapy*

Betahistine: Antihistamines may diminish the therapeutic effect of Betahistine. *Risk C: Monitor therapy*

CNS Depressants: May enhance the adverse/toxic effect of other CNS Depressants. *Risk C: Monitor therapy*

Pramlintide: May enhance the anticholinergic effect of Anticholinergics. These effects are specific to the GI tract. *Risk D: Consider therapy modification*

Ethanol/Nutrition/Herb Interactions

Ethanol: Avoid ethanol (may increase CNS depression).

Herb/Nutraceutical: Avoid valerian, St John's wort, kava kava, gotu kola (may increase CNS depression).

Stability Injection: Store at 15°C to 30°C. Protect from light.

Mechanism of Action Competes with histamine for H_1-receptor sites on effector cells in the gastrointestinal tract, blood vessels, and respiratory tract. Possesses skeletal muscle relaxing, bronchodilator, antihistamine, antiemetic, and analgesic properties.

Pharmacodynamics/Kinetics

Onset of action: Oral: 15-30 minutes

Duration: 4-6 hours

Absorption: Oral: Rapid

Metabolism: Forms metabolites

Half-life elimination: 3-7 hours

Time to peak: ~2 hours

Excretion: Urine

Dosage

Children:

- Preoperative sedation:
  - Oral: 0.6 mg/kg/dose
  - I.M.: 0.5-1 mg/kg/dose
- Pruritus, anxiety: Oral:
  - <6 years: 50 mg daily in divided doses
  - ≥6 years: 50-100 mg daily in divided doses

Adults:

- Antiemetic (unlabeled use): I.M.: 25-100 mg/dose every 4-6 hours as needed
- Anxiety: Oral, I.M.: 50-100 mg 4 times/day
- Preoperative sedation:
  - Oral: 50-100 mg
  - I.M.: 25-100 mg
- Pruritus: Oral, I.M.: 25 mg 3-4 times/day

Dosing interval in hepatic impairment: Change dosing interval to every 24 hours in patients with primary biliary cirrhosis

Administration Do not administer SubQ or intra-arterially. Administer I.M. deep in large muscle. With I.V. administration, extravasation can result in sterile abscess and marked tissue induration.

Monitoring Parameters Relief of symptoms, mental status, blood pressure

Dosage Forms Excipient information presented when available (limited, particularly for generics); consult specific product labeling. [DSC] = Discontinued product

Capsule, as pamoate: 25 mg, 50 mg, 100 mg
 Vistaril®: 25 mg, 50 mg

Injection, solution, as hydrochloride: 25 mg/mL (1 mL); 50 mg/mL (1 mL, 2 mL, 10 mL)

Suspension, oral, as pamoate:
 Vistaril®: 25 mg/5 mL (120 mL, 480 mL) [lemon flavor] [DSC]

Syrup, as hydrochloride: 10 mg/5 mL (120 mL, 480 mL)

Tablet, as hydrochloride: 10 mg, 25 mg, 50 mg

- **Hydroxyzine Hydrochloride** *see* HydrOXYzine *on page 797*
- **Hydroxyzine Pamoate** *see* HydrOXYzine *on page 797*
- **HydroZone Plus [OTC]** *see* Hydrocortisone *on page 785*
- **Hyflex-DS® [DSC]** *see* Acetaminophen and Phenyltoloxamine *on page 36*
- **Hygroton** *see* Chlorthalidone *on page 340*
- **Hyoscine Butylbromide** *see* Scopolamine Derivatives *on page 1463*
- **Hyoscine Hydrobromide** *see* Scopolamine Derivatives *on page 1463*

Hyoscyamine (hye oh SYE a meen)

Medication Safety Issues

Sound-alike/look-alike issues:
 Anaspaz® may be confused with Anaprox®, Antispas®
 Levbid® may be confused with Lithobid®, Lopid®, Lorabid®
 Levsinex® may be confused with Lanoxin®
 Levsin/SL® maybe confused with Levaquin®

U.S. Brand Names Anaspaz®; Cystospaz®; Hyosyne; Levbid®; Levsin®; Levsin®/SL; NuLev™ [DSC]; Spacol T/S [DSC]; Spacol [DSC]; Symax SL; Symax SR

Canadian Brand Names Cystospaz®; Levsin®

Index Terms *l*-Hyoscyamine Sulfate; Hyoscyamine Sulfate

Pharmacologic Category Anticholinergic Agent

Use

Oral: Adjunctive therapy for peptic ulcers, irritable bowel, neurogenic bladder/bowel; treatment of infant colic, GI tract disorders caused by spasm; to reduce rigidity, tremors, sialorrhea, and hyperhidrosis associated with parkinsonism; as a drying agent in acute rhinitis

Injection: Preoperative antimuscarinic to reduce secretions and block cardiac vagal inhibitory reflexes; to improve radiologic visibility of the kidneys; symptomatic relief of biliary and renal colic; reduce GI motility to facilitate diagnostic procedures (ie, endoscopy, hypotonic duodenography); reduce pain and hypersecretion in pancreatitis, certain cases of partial heart block associated with vagal activity; reversal of neuromuscular blockade

Effect on Mental Status May cause drowsiness; may rarely cause restlessness, amnesia, or delirium

Effect on Psychiatric Treatment Concurrent use with psychotropics may produce additive sedation and dry mouth

Dosage Summary

I.M.:

Children: Dosage not established

Adults: 0.25-0.5 mg 4 times/day as needed

I.V.:

Children <2 years: Dosage not established

Children ≥2 years: 5 mcg/kg given 30-60 minutes prior to induction of anesthesia

Adults: 0.125-0.5 mg 4 times/day as needed **or** 0.25-0.5 mg 5-10 minutes prior to procedure **or** 5 mcg/kg given 30-60 minutes prior to induction of anesthesia **or** 0.2 mg for every 1 mg neostigmine

Oral:

Regular release:

Children <2 years and 3.4 kg: 4 drops every 4 hours as needed (maximum: 24 drops/day)

Children <2 years and 5 kg: 5 drops every 4 hours as needed (maximum: 30 drops/day)
Children <2 years and 7 kg: 6 drops every 4 hours as needed (maximum: 36 drops/day)
Children <2 years and 10 kg: 8 drops every 4 hours as needed (maximum: 48 drops/day)
Children ≥2 years and 10 kg: 0.031-0.033 mg every 4 hours as needed (maximum: 0.75 mg/day)
Children ≥2 years and 20 kg: 0.0625 mg every 4 hours as needed (maximum: 0.75 mg/day)
Children ≥2 years and 40 kg: 0.0938 mg every 4 hours as needed (maximum: 0.75 mg/day)
Children ≥2 years and 50 kg: 0.125 mg every 4 hours as needed (maximum: 0.75 mg/day)
Adults: 0.125-0.25 mg every 4 hours or as needed **or** 0.15-0.3 mg (Cystospaz®) up to 4 times/day (maximum: 1.5 mg/day)

Timed release:
Children: Dosage not established
Adults: 0.375-0.75 mg every 12 hours (maximum: 1.5 mg/day)

S.L.:
Children <2 years: Dosage not established
Children ≥2 years and 10 kg: 0.031-0.033 mg every 4 hours as needed (maximum: 0.75 mg/day)
Children ≥2 years and 20 kg: 0.0625 mg every 4 hours as needed (maximum: 0.75 mg/day)
Children ≥2 years and 40 kg: 0.0938 mg every 4 hours as needed (maximum: 0.75 mg/day)
Children ≥2 years and 50 kg: 0.125 mg every 4 hours as needed (maximum: 0.75 mg/day)
Adults: 0.125-0.25 mg every 4 hours or as needed **or** 0.15-0.3 mg (Cystospaz®) up to 4 times/day (maximum: 1.5 mg/day)

SubQ:
Children: Dosage not established
Adults: 0.25-0.5 mg 4 times/day as needed

Dosage Forms Excipient information presented when available (limited, particularly for generics); consult specific product labeling. [DSC] = Discontinued product

Capsule, timed release, as sulfate: 0.375 mg
Elixir, as sulfate: 0.125 mg/5 mL (480 mL)
Hyosyne: 0.125 mg/5 mL (480 mL) [contains ethanol 20% and sodium benzoate; orange flavor]
Levsin®: 0.125 mg/5 mL (480 mL) [contains ethanol 20%; orange flavor]
Injection, solution, as sulfate: 0.5 mg/mL (1 mL)
Levsin®: 0.5 mg/mL (1 mL)
Solution, oral, as sulfate [drops]: 0.125 mg/mL (15 mL)
Hyosyne: 0.125 mg/mL (15 mL) [contains ethanol 5% and sodium benzoate; orange flavor]
Levsin®: 0.125 mg/mL (15 mL) [contains ethanol 5%; orange flavor]
Tablet:
Cystospaz®: 0.15 mg [DSC]
Tablet, as sulfate: 0.125 mg
Anaspaz®: 0.125 mg
Levsin®: 0.125 mg
Tablet, extended release, as sulfate: 0.375 mg
Levbid®: 0.375 mg
Symax SR: 0.375 mg
Tablet, orally disintegrating, as sulfate: 0.125 mg
NuLev™: 0.125 mg [contains phenylalanine 1.7 mg/tablet, mint flavor] [DSC]
Tablet, sublingual, as sulfate: 0.125 mg
Levsin®/SL: 0.125 mg
Symax SL: 0.125 mg

Hyoscyamine, Atropine, Scopolamine, and Phenobarbital

(hye oh SYE a meen, A troe peen, skoe POL a meen, & fee noe BAR bi tal)

Medication Safety Issues
Sound-alike/look-alike issues:
Donnatal® may be confused with Donnagel®

U.S. Brand Names Donnatal Extentabs®; Donnatal®

Index Terms Atropine, Hyoscyamine, Scopolamine, and Phenobarbital; Belladonna Alkaloids With Phenobarbital; Phenobarbital, Hyoscyamine, Atropine, and Scopolamine; Scopolamine, Hyoscyamine, Atropine, and Phenobarbital

Pharmacologic Category Anticholinergic Agent; Antispasmodic Agent, Gastrointestinal

Use Adjunct in treatment of irritable bowel syndrome, acute enterocolitis, duodenal ulcer

Effect on Mental Status May rarely cause confusion, drowsiness, headache, loss of memory, fatigue, ataxia

Effect on Psychiatric Treatment Anticholinergic effects are common and may be increased with concurrent psychotropic use

Dosage Summary

Oral:

Extended release:

Children: Dosage not established

Adults: 1 tablet every 12 hours, may increase to every 8 hours

Regular release:

Children 4.5 kg: 0.5 mL every 4 hours **or** 0.75 mL every 6 hours

Children 10 kg: 1 mL every 4 hours **or** 1.5 mL every 6 hours

Children 14 kg: 1.5 mL every 4 hours **or** 2 mL every 6 hours

Children 23 kg: 2.5 mL every 4 hours **or** 3.8 mL every 6 hours

Children 34 kg: 3.8 mL every 4 hours **or** 5 mL every 6 hours

Children ≥45 kg: 5 mL every 4 hours **or** 7.5 mL every 6 hours

Adults: 1-2 tablets **or** 5-10 mL of elixir 3-4 times/day

Dosage Forms Excipient information presented when available (limited, particularly for generics); consult specific product labeling.

Elixir:

Donnatal®: Hyoscyamine sulfate 0.1037 mg, atropine sulfate 0.0194 mg, scopolamine hydrobromide 0.0065 mg, and phenobarbital 16.2 mg per 5 mL (120 mL, 480 mL) [contains alcohol 95%; grape flavor]

Tablet: Hyoscyamine sulfate 0.1037 mg, atropine sulfate 0.0194 mg, scopolamine hydrobromide 0.0065 mg, and phenobarbital 16.2 mg

Donnatal®: Hyoscyamine sulfate 0.1037 mg, atropine sulfate 0.0194 mg, scopolamine hydrobromide 0.0065 mg, and phenobarbital 16.2 mg

Tablet, extended release:

Donnatal Extentabs®: Hyoscyamine sulfate 0.3111 mg, atropine sulfate 0.0582 mg, scopolamine hydrobromide 0.0195 mg, and phenobarbital 48.6 mg

- ◆ **Hyoscyamine, Methenamine, Benzoic Acid, Phenyl Salicylate, and Methylene Blue** *see* Methenamine, Phenyl Salicylate, Methylene Blue, Benzoic Acid, and Hyoscyamine *on page 1009*
- ◆ **Hyoscyamine, Methenamine, Sodium Biphosphate, Phenyl Salicylate, and Methylene Blue** *see* Methenamine, Sodium Biphosphate, Phenyl Salicylate, Methylene Blue, and Hyoscyamine *on page 1010*
- ◆ **Hyoscyamine Sulfate** *see* Hyoscyamine *on page 799*
- ◆ **Hyosyne** *see* Hyoscyamine *on page 799*
- ◆ **Hyperforin** *see* St John's Wort *(Hypericum perforatum) on page 1506*
- ◆ **HyperHEP B™ S/D** *see* Hepatitis B Immune Globulin *on page 762*
- ◆ **Hypericum** *see* St John's Wort *(Hypericum perforatum) on page 1506*
- ◆ ***Hypericum perforatum*** *see* St John's Wort *(Hypericum perforatum) on page 1506*
- ◆ **HyperRHO™ S/D Full Dose** *see* Rh_o(D) Immune Globulin *on page 1415*
- ◆ **HyperRHO™ S/D Mini Dose** *see* Rh_o(D) Immune Globulin *on page 1415*
- ◆ **Hyphed [DSC]** *see* Pseudoephedrine, Hydrocodone, and Chlorpheniramine *on page 1372*
- ◆ **Hytakerol® [DSC]** *see* Dihydrotachysterol *on page 472*
- ◆ **Hytone®** *see* Hydrocortisone *on page 785*
- ◆ **Hyzaar®** *see* Losartan and Hydrochlorothiazide *on page 956*
- ◆ **I^{123} Iobenguane** *see* Iobenguane I 123 *on page 849*
- ◆ **I-123 MIBG** *see* Iobenguane I 123 *on page 849*

Ibandronate (eye BAN droh nate)

U.S. Brand Names Boniva®

Canadian Brand Names Bondronat®

Mexican Brand Names Bondronat; Bonviva
Index Terms Ibandronate Sodium; Ibandronic Acid; NSC-722623
Pharmacologic Category Bisphosphonate Derivative
Use Treatment and prevention of osteoporosis in postmenopausal females
Unlabeled/Investigational Use Hypercalcemia of malignancy; corticosteroid-induced osteoporosis; Paget's disease; reduce bone pain and skeletal complications from metastatic bone disease
Effect on Mental Status May cause dizziness
Effect on Psychiatric Treatment None reported
Dosage Summary
I.V.:
Children: Dosage not established
Adults: 3 mg every 3 months
Oral:
Children: Dosage not established
Adults: 2.5 mg/day **or** 150 mg once a month
Dosage Forms Excipient information presented when available (limited, particularly for generics); consult specific product labeling.
Injection, solution: 1 mg/mL (3 mL) [prefilled syringe]
Tablet: 2.5 mg [once-daily formulation]; 150 mg [once-monthly formulation]

◆ **Ibandronate Sodium** *see* Ibandronate *on page 801*
◆ **Ibandronic Acid** *see* Ibandronate *on page 801*
◆ **Ibidomide Hydrochloride** *see* Labetalol *on page 881*

Ibritumomab (ib ri TYOO mo mab)

Medication Safety Issues
High alert medication: The Institute for Safe Medication Practices (ISMP) includes this medication among its list of drug classes which have a heightened risk of causing significant patient harm when used in error.
Dosage maximum: Do not exceed the Y-90 Ibritumomab maximum allowable dose of 32 mCi, regardless of the patient's body weight.
U.S. Brand Names Zevalin®
Canadian Brand Names Zevalin®
Index Terms Ibritumomab Tiuxetan; IDEC-Y2B8; In-111 Ibritumomab; In-111 Zevalin; Y-90 Ibritumomab; Y-90 Zevalin
Pharmacologic Category Antineoplastic Agent, Monoclonal Antibody; Radiopharmaceutical
Use Treatment of relapsed or refractory low-grade or follicular B-cell non-Hodgkin's lymphoma
Effect on Mental Status May cause dizziness, insomnia, or anxiety
Effect on Psychiatric Treatment Gastrointestinal side effects are common; use caution with SSRIs, lithium, and valproic acid. Hematologic side effects are common; use caution with clozapine, carbamazepine, and valproic acid.
Dosage Summary
I.V.:
Children: Dosage not established
Adults:
Day 1: In-111: Within 4 hours of the completion of rituximab, inject 5 mCi (1.6 mg total antibody dose)
Day 7, 8, or 9: Y-90: Within 4 hours of the completion of rituximab infusion, inject 0.3 mCi/kg (11.1 MBq/kg actual body weight) if platelet count 100,000-149,000 cell/mm^3 **or** 0.4 mCi/kg (14.8 MBq/kg actual body weight) if platelet count ≥150,000 cell/mm^3 (maximum: 32 mCi [1184 MBq])
Dosage Forms Excipient information presented when available (limited, particularly for generics); consult specific product labeling.
Each kit contains 4 vials for preparation of either In-111 or Y-90 conjugate (as indicated on container label)
Injection, solution:
Zevalin®: 1.6 mg/mL (2 mL) [supplied with sodium acetate solution, formulation buffer vial (includes albumin 750 mg), and an empty reaction vial]

◆ **Ibritumomab Tiuxetan** *see* Ibritumomab *on page 802*
◆ **Ibu®** *see* Ibuprofen *on page 803*
◆ **Ibu-200 [OTC]** *see* Ibuprofen *on page 803*
◆ **Ibudone™** *see* Hydrocodone and Ibuprofen *on page 780*

Ibuprofen (eye byoo PROE fen)

Medication Safety Issues

Sound-alike/look-alike issues:

Haltran® may be confused with Halfprin®

Related Information

Nonsteroidal Anti-Inflammatory Agents *on page 1792*

U.S. Brand Names Addaprin [OTC]; Advil® Children's [OTC]; Advil® Infants' [OTC]; Advil® Junior [OTC] [DSC]; Advil® Migraine [OTC]; Advil® [OTC]; Genpril® [OTC] [DSC]; I-Prin [OTC]; Ibu-200 [OTC]; Ibu®; Midol® Cramp and Body Aches [OTC]; Motrin® Children's [OTC]; Motrin® IB [OTC]; Motrin® Infants' [OTC]; Motrin® Junior [OTC]; Motrin® [DSC]; NeoProfen®; Proprinal [OTC]; Ultraprin [OTC]

Canadian Brand Names Advil®; Apo-Ibuprofen®; Motrin® (Children's); Motrin® IB; Novo-Profen; Nu-Ibuprofen

Mexican Brand Names Advil; Bestafen; Febratic; Ibuflam; Motrin; Quadrax; Tabalon 400

Index Terms *p*-Isobutylhydratropic Acid; Ibuprofen Lysine

Pharmacologic Category Nonsteroidal Anti-inflammatory Drug (NSAID), Oral; Nonsteroidal Anti-inflammatory Drug (NSAID), Parenteral

Generic Available Yes: Caplet, suspension, tablet

Use

Oral: Inflammatory diseases and rheumatoid disorders including juvenile rheumatoid arthritis, mild-to-moderate pain, fever, dysmenorrhea

Injection: Ibuprofen lysine is for use in premature infants weighing between 500-1500 g and who are ≤32 weeks gestational age (GA) to induce closure of a clinically-significant patent ductus arteriosus (PDA) when usual treatments are ineffective

Unlabeled/Investigational Use Cystic fibrosis, gout, ankylosing spondylitis, acute migraine headache

Effect on Mental Status Drowsiness and dizziness are common; may cause nervousness; may rarely cause insomnia, confusion, hallucinations, or depression

Effect on Psychiatric Treatment May rarely cause agranulocytosis; use caution with clozapine and carbamazepine; may decrease lithium clearance resulting in an increase in serum lithium levels and potential lithium toxicity; monitor serum lithium levels

Restrictions An FDA-approved medication guide must be distributed when dispensing an oral outpatient prescription (new or refill) where this medication is to be used without direct supervision of a healthcare provider. Medication guides are available at http://www.fda.gov/cder/Offices/ODS/medication_guides.htm.

Pregnancy Risk Factor C/D (3rd trimester)

Lactation Enters breast milk/use caution (AAP rates "compatible")

Contraindications Hypersensitivity to ibuprofen, aspirin, other NSAIDs, or any component of the formulation; perioperative pain in the setting of coronary artery bypass graft (CABG) surgery

Ibuprofen lysine is contraindicated in preterm infants with untreated proven or suspected infection; congenital heart disease where patency of the PDA is necessary for pulmonary or systemic blood flow; bleeding (especially with active intracranial hemorrhage or GI bleed); thrombocytopenia; coagulation defects; proven or suspected necrotizing enterocolitis (NEC); significant renal dysfunction

Warnings/Precautions **[U.S. Boxed Warning]: NSAIDs are associated with an increased risk of adverse cardiovascular thrombotic events, including MI, stroke, and new onset or worsening of pre-existing hypertension.** Risk may be increased with duration of use or pre-existing cardiovascular risk factors or disease. Carefully evaluate individual cardiovascular risk profiles prior to prescribing. Use caution with fluid retention, heart failure, or hypertension. Concurrent administration of ibuprofen, and potentially other nonselective NSAIDs, may interfere with aspirin's cardioprotective effect. **[U.S. Boxed Warning]: Use is contraindicated for treatment of perioperative pain in the setting of coronary artery bypass graft (CABG) surgery.** Risk of MI and stroke may be increased with use following CABG surgery.

May increase the risk of aseptic meningitis, especially in patients with systemic lupus erythematosus (SLE) and mixed connective tissue disorders. Platelet adhesion and aggregation may be decreased; may prolong bleeding time; patients with coagulation disorders or who are receiving anticoagulants should be monitored closely. Anemia may occur; patients on long-term NSAID therapy should be monitored for anemia. NSAID use may compromise existing renal function; dose-dependent decreases in prostaglandin synthesis may result from NSAID use, reducing renal blood flow which may cause renal decompensation. Patients with impaired renal function, dehydration, heart failure, liver dysfunction, those taking diuretics, and ACE inhibitors, and the elderly are at greater risk of renal toxicity. Rehydrate patient before starting therapy; monitor renal function closely. Not recommended for use in patients with advanced renal disease. Long-term NSAID use may result in renal papillary necrosis.

NSAIDs may increase risk of gastrointestinal irritation, inflammation, ulceration, bleeding, and perforation. These events may occur at any time during therapy and without warning. Use caution with a history of GI disease (bleeding or ulcers), concurrent therapy with aspirin, anticoagulants and/or corticosteroids, smoking, use of alcohol, the elderly or debilitated patients.

Use the lowest effective dose for the shortest duration of time, consistent with individual patient goals, to reduce risk of cardiovascular or GI adverse events. Alternate therapies should be considered for patients at high risk.

NSAIDs may cause serious skin adverse events including exfoliative dermatitis, Stevens-Johnson Syndrome (SJS) and toxic epidermal necrolysis (TEN); discontinue use at first sign of skin rash or hypersensitivity. Anaphylactoid reactions may occur, even without prior exposure; patients with "aspirin triad" (bronchial asthma, aspirin intolerance, rhinitis) may be at increased risk. Do not use in patients who experience bronchospasm, asthma, rhinitis, or urticaria with NSAID or aspirin therapy. Use caution in other forms of asthma.

Use with caution in patients with decreased hepatic function. Closely monitor patients with any abnormal LFT. Severe hepatic reactions (eg, fulminant hepatitis, liver failure) have occurred with NSAID use, rarely; discontinue if signs or symptoms of liver disease develop, or if systemic manifestations occur.

The elderly are at increased risk for adverse effects (especially peptic ulceration, CNS effects, renal toxicity) from NSAIDs even at low doses.

Withhold for at least 4-6 half-lives prior to surgical or dental procedures. Some products may contain phenylalanine.

Injection: Hold second or third doses if urinary output is <0.6 mL/kg/hour. May alter signs of infection. May inhibit platelet aggregation; monitor for signs of bleeding. May displace bilirubin; use caution when total bilirubin is elevated. Long-term evaluations of neurodevelopment, growth, or diseases associated with prematurity following treatment have not been conducted. A second course of treatment, alternative pharmacologic therapy or surgery may be needed if the ductus arteriosus fails to close or reopens following the initial course of therapy.

Self medication (OTC use): Prior to self-medication, patients should contact healthcare provider if they have had recurring stomach pain or upset, ulcers, bleeding problems, high blood pressure, heart or kidney disease, other serious medical problems, are currently taking a diuretic, aspirin, anticoagulant, or are ≥60 years of age. If patients are using for migraines, they should also contact healthcare provider if they have not had a migraine diagnosis by healthcare provider, a headache that is different from usual migraine, worst headache of life, fever and neck stiffness, headache from head injury or coughing, first headache at ≥50 years of age, daily headache, or migraine requiring bed rest. Recommended dosages should not be exceeded, due to an increased risk of GI bleeding. Stop use and consult a healthcare provider if symptoms get worse, newly appear, fever lasts for >3 days or pain lasts >3 days (children) and >10 days (adults). Do not give for >10 days unless instructed by healthcare provider. Consuming ≥3 alcoholic beverages/day or taking longer than recommended may increase the risk of GI bleeding.

Adverse Reactions

Oral:

1% to 10%:

Cardiovascular: Edema (1% to 3%)

Central nervous system: Dizziness (3% to 9%), headache (1% to 3%), nervousness (1% to 3%)

Dermatologic: Rash (3% to 9%), itching (1% to 3%)

Endocrine & metabolic: Fluid retention (1% to 3%)

Gastrointestinal: Epigastric pain (3% to 9%), heartburn (3% to 9%), nausea (3% to 9%), abdominal pain/cramps/distress (1% to 3%), appetite decreased (1% to 3%), constipation (1% to 3%), diarrhea (1% to 3%), dyspepsia (1% to 3%), flatulence (1% to 3%), vomiting (1% to 3%)

Otic: Tinnitus (3% to 9%)

<1% (Limited to important or life-threatening): Acute renal failure, agranulocytosis, anaphylaxis, aplastic anemia, azotemia, blurred vision, bone marrow suppression, confusion, creatinine clearance decreased, duodenal ulcer,

edema, eosinophilia, epistaxis, erythema multiforme, gastric ulcer, GI bleed, GI hemorrhage, GI ulceration, hallucinations, hearing decreased, hematuria, hematocrit decreased, hemoglobin decreased, hemolytic anemia, hepatitis, hypertension, inhibition of platelet aggregation, jaundice, liver function tests abnormal, leukopenia, melena, neutropenia, pancreatitis, photosensitivity, Stevens-Johnson syndrome, thrombocytopenia, toxic amblyopia, toxic epidermal necrolysis, urticaria, vesiculobullous eruptions, vision changes

Injection:

>10%:

Cardiovascular: Intraventricular hemorrhage (29%; grade 3/4: 15%)

Dermatologic: Skin irritation (16%)

Endocrine & metabolic: Hypocalcemia (12%), hypoglycemia (12%)

Gastrointestinal: GI disorders, non NEC (22%)

Hematologic: Anemia (32%)

Respiratory: Apnea (28%), respiratory infection (19%)

Miscellaneous: Sepsis (43%)

1% to 10%:

Cardiovascular: Edema (4%)

Endocrine & metabolic: Adrenal insufficiency (7%), hypernatremia (7%)

Genitourinary: Urinary tract infection (9%)

Renal: Urea increased (7%), renal impairment (6%), creatinine increased (3%), urine output decreased (3%; small decrease reported on days 2-6 with compensatory increase in output on day 9), renal failure (1%)

Respiratory: Respiratory failure (10%), atelectasis (4%)

Frequency not defined: Abdominal distension, cholestasis, feeding problems, gastritis, GI reflux, heart failure, hyperglycemia, hypotension, ileus, infection, inguinal hernia, injection site reaction, jaundice, neutropenia, seizure, tachycardia, thrombocytopenia

Postmarketing and/or case reports: GI perforation, necrotizing enterocolitis

Metabolism/Transport Effects Substrate (minor) of CYP2C9, 2C19; **Inhibits** CYP2C9 (strong)

Drug Interactions

ACE Inhibitors: Nonsteroidal Anti-Inflammatory Agents may diminish the antihypertensive effect of ACE Inhibitors. *Risk C: Monitor therapy*

Aminoglycosides: Nonsteroidal Anti-Inflammatory Agents may decrease the excretion of Aminoglycosides. Data only in premature infants. *Risk C: Monitor therapy*

Angiotensin II Receptor Blockers: Nonsteroidal Anti-Inflammatory Agents may diminish the therapeutic effect of Angiotensin II Receptor Blockers. The combination of these two agents may also significantly decrease glomerular filtration and renal function. *Risk C: Monitor therapy*

Anticoagulants: Nonsteroidal Anti-Inflammatory Agents may enhance the anticoagulant effect of Anticoagulants. *Risk C: Monitor therapy*

Antidepressants (Serotonin/Norepinephrine Reuptake Inhibitor): May enhance the antiplatelet effect of NSAID (Nonselective). *Risk C: Monitor therapy*

Antidepressants (Tricyclic, Tertiary Amine): May enhance the antiplatelet effect of NSAID (Nonselective). *Risk C: Monitor therapy*

Antiplatelet Agents: Nonsteroidal Anti-Inflammatory Agents may enhance the adverse/toxic effect of Antiplatelet Agents. An increased risk of bleeding may occur. *Risk C: Monitor therapy*

Beta-Blockers: Nonsteroidal Anti-Inflammatory Agents may diminish the antihypertensive effect of Beta-Blockers. **Exceptions:** Levobunolol; Metipranolol. *Risk C: Monitor therapy*

Bile Acid Sequestrants: May decrease the absorption of Nonsteroidal Anti-Inflammatory Agents. *Risk D: Consider therapy modification*

Bisphosphonate Derivatives: Nonsteroidal Anti-Inflammatory Agents may enhance the adverse/toxic effect of Bisphosphonate Derivatives. Both an increased risk of gastrointestinal ulceration and an increased risk of nephrotoxicity are of concern. *Risk C: Monitor therapy*

Corticosteroids (Systemic): May enhance the adverse/toxic effect of NSAID (Nonselective). *Risk C: Monitor therapy*

CycloSPORINE: Nonsteroidal Anti-Inflammatory Agents may enhance the nephrotoxic effect of CycloSPORINE. Nonsteroidal Anti-Inflammatory Agents may increase the serum concentration of CycloSPORINE. *Risk D: Consider therapy modification*

CYP2C9 Substrates (High risk): CYP2C9 Inhibitors (Strong) may decrease the metabolism of CYP2C9 Substrates (High risk). *Risk D: Consider therapy modification*

Desmopressin: Nonsteroidal Anti-Inflammatory Agents may enhance the adverse/toxic effect of Desmopressin. *Risk C: Monitor therapy*

Eplerenone: Nonsteroidal Anti-Inflammatory Agents may diminish the antihypertensive effect of Eplerenone. *Risk C: Monitor therapy*

Herbs (Anticoagulant/Antiplatelet Properties) (eg, Alfalfa, Anise, Bilberry): May enhance the adverse/toxic effect of Nonsteroidal Anti-Inflammatory Agents. Bleeding may occur. *Risk D: Consider therapy modification*

HydrALAZINE: Nonsteroidal Anti-Inflammatory Agents may diminish the antihypertensive effect of HydrALAZINE. *Risk C: Monitor therapy*

Ketorolac: May enhance the adverse/toxic effect of Nonsteroidal Anti-Inflammatory Agents. *Risk X: Avoid combination*

Lithium: Nonsteroidal Anti-Inflammatory Agents may increase the serum concentration of Lithium. *Risk D: Consider therapy modification*

Loop Diuretics: Nonsteroidal Anti-Inflammatory Agents may diminish the diuretic effect of Loop Diuretics. *Risk C: Monitor therapy*

Methotrexate: Nonsteroidal Anti-Inflammatory Agents may decrease the excretion of Methotrexate. *Risk D: Consider therapy modification*

Nonsteroidal Anti-Inflammatory Agents: May enhance the adverse/toxic effect of other Nonsteroidal Anti-Inflammatory Agents. *Risk C: Monitor therapy*

Pemetrexed: NSAID (Nonselective) may decrease the excretion of Pemetrexed. *Risk D: Consider therapy modification*

Probenecid: May increase the serum concentration of Nonsteroidal Anti-Inflammatory Agents. *Risk C: Monitor therapy*

Quinolone Antibiotics: Nonsteroidal Anti-Inflammatory Agents may enhance the neuroexcitatory and/or seizure-potentiating effect of Quinolone Antibiotics. *Risk C: Monitor therapy*

Salicylates: NSAID (Nonselective) may enhance the antiplatelet effect of Salicylates. NSAID (Nonselective) may diminish the cardioprotective effect of Salicylates. Salicylates may decrease the serum concentration of NSAID (Nonselective). **Exceptions:** Choline Magnesium Trisalicylate. *Risk D: Consider therapy modification*

Selective Serotonin Reuptake Inhibitors: May enhance the antiplatelet effect of NSAID (Nonselective). *Risk D: Consider therapy modification*

Thiazide Diuretics: Nonsteroidal Anti-Inflammatory Agents may diminish the therapeutic effect of Thiazide Diuretics. *Risk C: Monitor therapy*

Thrombolytic Agents: Nonsteroidal Anti-Inflammatory Agents may enhance the adverse/toxic effect of Thrombolytic Agents. An increased risk of bleeding may occur. *Risk C: Monitor therapy*

Treprostinil: May enhance the adverse/toxic effect of Nonsteroidal Anti-Inflammatory Agents. Bleeding may occur. *Risk C: Monitor therapy*

Vancomycin: Nonsteroidal Anti-Inflammatory Agents may decrease the excretion of Vancomycin. *Risk C: Monitor therapy*

Vitamin K Antagonists (eg, warfarin): NSAID (Nonselective) may enhance the anticoagulant effect of Vitamin K Antagonists. *Risk D: Consider therapy modification*

Ethanol/Nutrition/Herb Interactions

Ethanol: Avoid ethanol (may enhance gastric mucosal irritation).

Food: Ibuprofen peak serum levels may be decreased if taken with food.

Herb/Nutraceutical: Avoid alfalfa, anise, bilberry, bladderwrack, bromelain, cat's claw, celery, chamomile, coleus, cordyceps, dong quai, evening primrose, fenugreek, feverfew, garlic, ginger, ginkgo biloba, ginseng (American, Panax, Siberian), grapeseed, green tea, guggul, horse chestnut seed, horseradish, licorice, prickly ash, red clover, reishi, SAMe (S-adenosylmethionine), sweet clover, turmeric, white willow (all have additional antiplatelet activity).

Stability

Injection: Store at room temperature of 20°C to 25°C (68°F to 77°F). Protect from light. Dilute with dextrose or saline to an appropriate volume. Following dilution, administer within 30 minutes of preparation.

Suspension, tablet: Store at room temperature of 20°C to 25°C (68°F to 77°F).

Mechanism of Action Reversibly inhibits cyclooxygenase-1 and 2 (COX-1 and 2) enzymes, which result in decreased formation of prostaglandin precursors; has antipyretic, analgesic, and anti-inflammatory properties

Pharmacodynamics/Kinetics

Onset of action: Analgesic: 30-60 minutes; Anti-inflammatory: ≤7 days

Peak effect: 1-2 weeks

Duration: 4-6 hours

Absorption: Oral: Rapid (85%)

Distribution: Premature infants with ductal closure (highly variable between studies):

Day 3: 145-349 mL/kg

Day 5: 72-222 mL/kg

Protein binding: 90% to 99%

Metabolism: Hepatic via oxidation

Half-life elimination:
- Premature infants (highly variable between studies):
  - Day 3: 35-51 hours
  - Day 5: 20-33 hours
- Children 3 months to 10 years: 1.6 ± 0.7 hours
- Adults: 2-4 hours; End-stage renal disease: Unchanged

Time to peak: ~1-2 hours

Excretion: Urine (80% as metabolites; 1% as unchanged drug); some feces

Dosage

I.V.: Infants between 500-1500 g and ≤32 weeks GA: Patent ductus arteriosus: Initial dose: Ibuprofen 10 mg/kg, followed by two doses of 5 mg/kg at 24 and 48 hours. Dose should be based on birth weight.

Oral:

Children:
- Antipyretic: 6 months to 12 years: Temperature <102.5°F (39°C): 5 mg/kg/dose; temperature >102.5°F: 10 mg/kg/dose given every 6-8 hours (maximum daily dose: 40 mg/kg/day)
- Juvenile rheumatoid arthritis: 30-50 mg/kg/24 hours divided every 8 hours; start at lower end of dosing range and titrate upward (maximum: 2.4 g/day)
- Analgesic: 4-10 mg/kg/dose every 6-8 hours
- Cystic fibrosis (unlabeled use): Chronic (>4 years) twice daily dosing adjusted to maintain serum levels of 50-100 mcg/mL has been associated with slowing of disease progression in younger patients with mild lung disease
- OTC labeling (analgesic, antipyretic): **Note:** Treatment for >10 days is not recommended unless directed by healthcare provider.
  - Children 6 months to 11 years: See table; use of weight to select dose is preferred; doses may be repeated every 6-8 hours (maximum: 4 doses/day)
  - Children ≥12 years: 200 mg every 4-6 hours as needed (maximum: 1200 mg/24 hours)

Ibuprofen Dosing

Weight (lb)	Age	Dosage (mg)
12-17	6-11 mo	50
18-23	12-23 mo	75
24-35	2-3 y	100
36-47	4-5 y	150
48-59	6-8 y	200
60-71	9-10 y	250
72-95	11 y	300

Adults:
- Inflammatory disease: 400-800 mg/dose 3-4 times/day (maximum dose: 3.2 g/day)
- Analgesia/pain/fever/dysmenorrhea: 200-400 mg/dose every 4-6 hours (maximum daily dose: 1.2 g, unless directed by physician; under physician supervision daily doses ≤2.4 g may be used)
- OTC labeling (analgesic, antipyretic): 200 mg every 4-6 hours as needed (maximum: 1200 mg/24 hours); treatment for >10 days is not recommended unless directed by healthcare provider.
  - Migraine: 2 capsules at onset of symptoms (maximum: 400 mg/24 hours unless directed by healthcare provider)

Dosing adjustment/comments in renal impairment: If anuria or oliguria evident, hold dose until renal function returns to normal

Dosing adjustment/comments in severe hepatic impairment: Avoid use

Dietary Considerations Should be taken with food. Chewable tablets may contain phenylalanine; amount varies by product, consult manufacturers labeling.

Administration

Oral: Administer with food

I.V.: For I.V. administration only; administration via umbilical arterial line has not been evaluated. Infuse over 15 minutes through port closest to insertion site. Avoid extravasation. Do not administer simultaneously via same line with TPN. If needed, interrupt TPN for 15 minutes prior to and after ibuprofen administration, keeping line open with dextrose or saline.

Monitoring Parameters CBC; occult blood loss and periodic liver function tests; monitor response (pain, range of motion, grip strength, mobility, ADL function), inflammation; observe for weight gain, edema; monitor renal function (urine output, serum BUN and creatinine); observe for bleeding, bruising; evaluate gastrointestinal effects (abdominal pain, bleeding, dyspepsia); mental confusion, disorientation; with long-term therapy, periodic ophthalmic exams

Injection: Renal function, signs of infection or bleeding, ECG

Reference Range Plasma concentrations >200 mcg/mL may be associated with severe toxicity

PDA: Minimum effective level: 10-12 mg/L

Dosage Forms Excipient information presented when available (limited, particularly for generics); consult specific product labeling. [DSC] = Discontinued product

Caplet: 200 mg [OTC]

Advil®: 200 mg [contains sodium benzoate]

Ibu-200, Motrin® IB: 200 mg

Motrin® Junior: 100 mg [scored]

Capsule, liquid-filled:

Advil®: 200 mg [solubilized ibuprofen; contains potassium 20 mg]

Advil® Migraine: 200 mg [solubilized ibuprofen; contains potassium 20 mg]

Gelcap:

Advil®: 200 mg [contains coconut oil]

Injection, solution, as lysine [preservative free]:

NeoProfen®: 17.1 mg/mL (2 mL) [equivalent to ibuprofen 10 mg/mL]

Suspension, oral: 100 mg/5 mL (5 mL, 10 mL, 120 mL, 240 mL, 480 mL)

Advil® Children's: 100 mg/5 mL (120 mL) [contains sodium benzoate, sodium, propylene glycol; blue raspberry, fruit, and grape flavors]

Motrin® Children's: 100 mg/5 mL (60 mL, 120 mL) [contains sodium benzoate; berry, dye free berry, bubble gum, and grape flavors]

Suspension, oral [concentrate, drops]: 40 mg/mL (15 mL)

Advil® Infants': 40 mg/mL (15 mL) [contains sodium benzoate; fruit, grape, and white grape flavors]

Motrin® Infants': 40 mg/mL (15 mL) [contains sodium benzoate; ethanol free; berry and dye-free berry flavors]

Tablet: 200 mg [OTC], 400 mg, 600 mg, 800 mg

Addaprin: 200 mg

Advil®: 200 mg [contains sodium benzoate]

Advil® Junior: 100 mg [contains sodium benzoate; coated tablets] [DSC]

Genpril® [DSC], I-Prin, Midol® Cramp and Body Aches, Motrin® IB, Proprinal, Ultraprin: 200 mg

Ibu®: 400 mg, 600 mg, 800 mg

Ibu-200: 200 mg

Motrin®: 400 mg, 600 mg, 800 mg [DSC]

Proprinal: 200 mg [contains sodium benzoate]

Ultraprin: 200 mg [sugar free]

Tablet, chewable:

Advil® Children's: 50 mg [contains phenylalanine 2.1 mg; grape flavors]

Advil® Junior: 100 mg [contains phenylalanine 4.2 mg; grape flavors] [DSC]

Motrin® Junior: 100 mg [contains phenylalanine 2.1 mg; grape and orange flavors]

◆ **Ibuprofen and Hydrocodone** *see* Hydrocodone and Ibuprofen *on page 780*

◆ **Ibuprofen and Pseudoephedrine** *see* Pseudoephedrine and Ibuprofen *on page 1369*

◆ **Ibuprofen Lysine** *see* Ibuprofen *on page 803*

Ibutilide (i BYOO ti lide)

Medication Safety Issues

High alert medication: The Institute for Safe Medication Practices (ISMP) includes this medication among its list of drugs which have a heightened risk of causing significant patient harm when used in error.

U.S. Brand Names Corvert®

Index Terms Ibutilide Fumarate

Pharmacologic Category Antiarrhythmic Agent, Class III

Use Acute termination of atrial fibrillation or flutter of recent onset; the effectiveness of ibutilide has not been determined in patients with arrhythmias >90 days in duration

Effect on Mental Status None reported

Effect on Psychiatric Treatment Concurrent use with phenothiazine and antidepressants may produce prolongation of the QT interval; use combination with caution; consider a nonphenothiazine antipsychotic

Dosage Summary

I.V.:

Children: Dosage not established

Adults <60 kg: 0.01 mg/kg, may repeat once

Adults ≥60 kg: 1 mg, may repeat once

Dosage Forms Excipient information presented when available (limited, particularly for generics); consult specific product labeling.

Injection, solution, as fumarate: 0.1 mg/mL (10 mL)

- **Ibutilide Fumarate** *see* Ibutilide *on page 808*
- **ICI-182,780** *see* Fulvestrant *on page 698*
- **ICI-204,219** *see* Zafirlukast *on page 1689*
- **ICI-46474** *see* Tamoxifen *on page 1537*
- **ICI-118630** *see* Goserelin *on page 735*
- **ICI-176334** *see* Bicalutamide *on page 188*
- **ICI-D1033** *see* Anastrozole *on page 125*
- **ICL670** *see* Deferasirox *on page 423*
- **ICRF-187** *see* Dexrazoxane *on page 441*
- **Idamycin PFS®** *see* IDArubicin *on page 809*

IDArubicin (eye da ROO bi sin)

Medication Safety Issues

Sound-alike/look-alike issues:

IDArubicin may be confused with DOXOrubicin, DAUNOrubicin, epirubicin

Idamycin PFS® may be confused with Adriamycin

High alert medication: The Institute for Safe Medication Practices (ISMP) includes this medication among its list of drugs which have a heightened risk of causing significant patient harm when used in error.

U.S. Brand Names Idamycin PFS®

Canadian Brand Names Idamycin®

Mexican Brand Names Idamycin

Index Terms 4-Demethoxydaunorubicin; 4-DMDR; Idarubicin Hydrochloride; IDR; IMI 30; NSC-256439; SC 33428

Pharmacologic Category Antineoplastic Agent, Anthracycline; Antineoplastic Agent, Antibiotic

Use Treatment of acute leukemias (AML, ANLL, ALL), accelerated phase or blast crisis of chronic myelogenous leukemia (CML), breast cancer

Unlabeled/Investigational Use Autologous hematopoietic stem cell transplantation

Effect on Mental Status None reported

Effect on Psychiatric Treatment Leukopenia is common; use caution with clozapine and carbamazepine

Dosage Summary

I.V.:

Children: 5 mg/m^2 **or** 10-12 mg/m^2 once daily for 3 days every 3 weeks

Adults: Induction: 12 mg/m^2/day for 3 days; Consolidation: 10-12 mg/m^2/day for 2 days

Dosage Forms Excipient information presented when available (limited, particularly for generics); consult specific product labeling.

Injection, solution, as hydrochloride [preservative free] (Idamycin PFS®): 1 mg/mL (5 mL, 10 mL, 20 mL)

- **Idarubicin Hydrochloride** *see* IDArubicin *on page 809*
- **IDEC-C2B8** *see* RiTUXimab *on page 1434*
- **IDEC-Y2B8** *see* Ibritumomab *on page 802*
- **IDR** *see* IDArubicin *on page 809*
- **Ifex®** *see* Ifosfamide *on page 809*
- **IFLrA** *see* Interferon Alfa-2a *on page 844*

Ifosfamide (eye FOSS fa mide)

Medication Safety Issues

Sound-alike/look-alike issues:

Ifosfamide may be confused with cyclophosphamide

High alert medication: The Institute for Safe Medication Practices (ISMP) includes this medication among its list of drugs which have a heightened risk of causing significant patient harm when used in error.

U.S. Brand Names Ifex®

Canadian Brand Names Ifex®

Mexican Brand Names Ifadex; Ifolem; Ifomida

Index Terms Isophosphamide; NSC-109724; Z4942

Pharmacologic Category Antineoplastic Agent, Alkylating Agent; Antineoplastic Agent, Alkylating Agent (Nitrogen Mustard)

Use Treatment of testicular cancer

Unlabeled/Investigational Use Treatment of bladder, breast, cervical, ovarian, pancreatic, and lung cancers; Hodgkin's and non-Hodgkin's lymphoma; acute lymphocytic leukemia; Ewing's sarcoma, osteosarcoma, and soft tissue sarcomas

Effect on Mental Status Sedation, confusion, and hallucinations are common

Effect on Psychiatric Treatment May cause myelosuppression; use caution with clozapine and carbamazepine; barbiturates and chloral hydrate may increase the metabolism of ifosfamide

Dosage Summary

I.V.:

Children (unlabeled use): 1200-1800 mg/m²/day for 3-5 days every 21-28 days **or** 5 g/m² once every 21-28 days **or** 3 g/m²/day for 2 days every 21-28 days

Adults: 4000-5000 mg/m²/day for 1 day every 14-28 days **or** 1000-3000 mg/m²/day for 2-5 days every 21-28 days

Dosage Forms Excipient information presented when available (limited, particularly for generics); consult specific product labeling.

Injection, powder for reconstitution: 1 g

Ifex®: 1 g, 3 g

Injection, solution: 50 mg/mL (20 mL, 60 mL)

◆ **IgG4-Kappa Monoclonal Antibody** *see* Natalizumab *on page 1109*

◆ **IL-1Ra** *see* Anakinra *on page 124*

◆ **IL-2** *see* Aldesleukin *on page 58*

◆ **IL-11** *see* Oprelvekin *on page 1184*

Iloprost (EYE loe prost)

U.S. Brand Names Ventavis®

Index Terms Iloprost Tromethamine; Prostacyclin PGI_2

Pharmacologic Category Prostacyclin; Prostaglandin; Vasodilator

Use Treatment of idiopathic pulmonary arterial hypertension in patients with NYHA Class III or IV symptoms

Effect on Mental Status May cause insomnia

Effect on Psychiatric Treatment None reported

Dosage Summary

Inhalation:

Children: Dosage not established

Adults: Initial: 2.5 mcg/dose; Maintenance: 2.5-5 mcg/dose 6-9 times/day (maximum: 45 mcg/day)

Dosage Forms Excipient information presented when available (limited, particularly for generics); consult specific product labeling.

Solution for oral inhalation [preservative-free]:

Ventavis®: 10 mcg/mL (1 mL, 2 mL) [ampul]

◆ **Iloprost Tromethamine** *see* Iloprost *on page 810*

Imatinib (eye MAT eh nib)

Medication Safety Issues

High alert medication: The Institute for Safe Medication Practices (ISMP) includes this medication among its list of drug classes which have a heightened risk of causing significant patient harm when used in error.

U.S. Brand Names Gleevec®

Canadian Brand Names Gleevec®

Mexican Brand Names Glivec

Index Terms CGP-57148B; Glivec; Imatinib Mesylate; NSC-716051; STI-571

Pharmacologic Category Antineoplastic Agent, Tyrosine Kinase Inhibitor

Use Treatment of:

Gastrointestinal stromal tumors (GIST) kit-positive (CD117) unresectable and/or metastatic malignant

Philadelphia chromosome-positive (Ph+) chronic myeloid leukemia (CML) in chronic phase (newly-diagnosed)

Ph+ CML in chronic phase in pediatric patients recurring following stem cell transplant or who are resistant to interferon-alpha therapy (**not** an approved use in Canada)

Ph+ CML in blast crisis, accelerated phase, or chronic phase after failure of interferon therapy

Ph+ acute lymphoblastic leukemia (ALL) (relapsed or refractory)

Aggressive systemic mastocytosis (ASM) without D816V c-Kit mutation (or c-Kit mutation status unknown)

Dermatofibrosarcoma protuberans (DFSP) (unresectable, recurrent and/or metastatic)

Hypereosinophilic syndrome (HES) and/or chronic eosinophilic leukemia (CEL)

Myelodysplastic/myeloproliferative disease (MDS/MPD) associated with platelet-derived growth factor receptor (PDGFR) gene rearrangements

Note: The following use is approved in Canada (not an approved indication in the U.S.):

Ph+ ALL induction therapy (newly diagnosed)

Unlabeled/Investigational Use Treatment of desmoid tumors (soft tissue sarcoma)

Effect on Mental Status Sedation is common; may infrequently cause depression, anxiety, insomnia, somnolence, migraine, and memory impairment; may rarely cause confusion and convulsions

Effect on Psychiatric Treatment Gastrointestinal irritation is common; use caution with lithium, valproic acid, and SSRIs. May cause hepatotoxicity; use caution with valproic acid and olanzapine. May cause neutropenia or thrombocytopenia; use caution with clozapine, carbamazepine, and valproic acid. Imatinib may inhibit the metabolism of alprazolam, carbamazepine, clozapine, diazepam, fluoxetine, haloperidol, nefazodone, phenothiazines (avoid thioridazine and mesoridazine), sertraline, TCAs, trazodone, and triazolam resulting in elevated serum levels. Fluoxetine and nefazodone may inhibit the metabolism of imatinib. Carbamazepine, St John's wort, and phenobarbital may increase the metabolism of imatinib.

Dosage Summary

Oral:

Children <2 years: Dosage not established

Children ≥2 years: 260-340 mg/m^2/day in 1-2 divided doses (maximum 600 mg/day)

Adults: 100-800 mg/day in 1-2 divided doses

Dosage Forms Excipient information presented when available (limited, particularly for generics); consult specific product labeling.

Tablet:

Gleevec®: 100 mg; 400 mg

- ◆ **Imatinib Mesylate** *see* Imatinib *on page 810*
- ◆ **IMC-C225** *see* Cetuximab *on page 310*
- ◆ **Imdur®** *see* Isosorbide Mononitrate *on page 869*
- ◆ **123I-Metaiodobenzylguanidine (MIBG)** *see* Iobenguane I 123 *on page 849*
- ◆ **Imferon** *see* Iron Dextran Complex *on page 857*
- ◆ **IMI 30** *see* IDArubicin *on page 809*
- ◆ **IMid-3** *see* Lenalidomide *on page 899*
- ◆ **Imidazole Carboxamide** *see* Dacarbazine *on page 414*
- ◆ **Imidazole Carboxamide Dimethyltriazene** *see* Dacarbazine *on page 414*

Imiglucerase (i mi GLOO ser ace)

Medication Safety Issues

Sound-alike/look-alike issues:

Cerezyme® may be confused with Cerebyx®, Ceredase®

U.S. Brand Names Cerezyme®

Canadian Brand Names Cerezyme®

Pharmacologic Category Enzyme

Use Long-term enzyme replacement therapy for patients with Type 1 Gaucher's disease

Effect on Mental Status May cause dizziness

Effect on Psychiatric Treatment None reported

Dosage Summary

I.V.:

Children <2 years: Dosage not established

Children ≥2 years: Initial: 30-60 units/kg every 2 weeks; Range: 2.5 units/kg 3 times/week to 60 units/kg once weekly; Average dose: 60 units/kg every 2 weeks

Adults: Initial: 30-60 units/kg every 2 weeks; Range: 2.5 units/kg 3 times/week to 60 units/kg once weekly; Average dose: 60 units/kg every 2 weeks

Dosage Forms Excipient information presented when available (limited, particularly for generics); consult specific product labeling.

Injection, powder for reconstitution:

Cerezyme®: 200 units, 400 units [derived from Chinese hamster cells; contains mannitol and polysorbate 80]

◆ **Imipemide** *see* Imipenem and Cilastatin *on page 812*

Imipenem and Cilastatin (i mi PEN em & sye la STAT in)

Medication Safety Issues

Sound-alike/look-alike issues:

Imipenem may be confused with ertapenem, meropenem

Primaxin® may be confused with Premarin®, Primacor®

U.S. Brand Names Primaxin®

Canadian Brand Names Primaxin®; Primaxin® I.V.

Mexican Brand Names Arzobema; Iminen; Tienam

Index Terms Imipemide

Pharmacologic Category Antibiotic, Carbapenem

Use Treatment of lower respiratory tract, urinary tract, intra-abdominal, gynecologic, bone and joint, skin and skin structure, and polymicrobic infections as well as bacterial septicemia and endocarditis. Antibacterial activity includes resistant gram-negative bacilli (*Pseudomonas aeruginosa* and *Enterobacter* sp), gram-positive bacteria (methicillin-sensitive *Staphylococcus aureus* and *Streptococcus* sp) and anaerobes.

Unlabeled/Investigational Use Hepatic abscess; neutropenic fever; melioidosis

Effect on Mental Status Reports of encephalopathy

Effect on Psychiatric Treatment May rarely cause neutropenia; use caution with clozapine and carbamazepine

Dosage Summary

I.M.:

Children: Dosage not established

Adults: 500-750 mg every 12 hours

I.V.:

Neonates <1 week and ≥1500 g: 25 mg/kg every 12 hours

Neonates 1-4 weeks and ≥1500 g: 25 mg/kg every 8 hours

Neonates 4 weeks to 3 months and ≥1500 g: 25 mg/kg every 6 hours

Children >3 months: 15-25 mg/kg every 6 hours (maximum: 4 g/day)

Adults 30 to <70 kg: 125 mg every 12 hours up to 1000 mg every 8 hours (weight dependent)

Adults ≥70 kg: 250-1000 mg every 6-8 hours (maximum: 50 mg/kg/day; 4 g/day)

Dosage Forms Excipient information presented when available (limited, particularly for generics); consult specific product labeling.

Injection, powder for reconstitution [I.M.]:

Primaxin®: Imipenem 500 mg and cilastatin 500 mg [contains sodium 32 mg (1.4 mEq)]

Injection, powder for reconstitution [I.V.]:

Primaxin®: Imipenem 250 mg and cilastatin 250 mg [contains sodium 18.8 mg (0.8 mEq)]; imipenem 500 mg and cilastatin 500 mg [contains sodium 37.5 mg (1.6 mEq)]

Imipramine (im IP ra meen)

Medication Safety Issues

Sound-alike/look-alike issues:

Imipramine may be confused with amitriptyline, desipramine, Norpramin®

Related Information

Anticholinergic Effects of Common Psychotropics *on page 1758*

Antidepressant Agents *on page 1760*
Antidepressant Receptor Profile *on page 1764*
Discontinuation of Psychotropic Drugs *on page 1839*

U.S. Brand Names Tofranil-PM®; Tofranil®

Canadian Brand Names Apo-Imipramine®; Novo-Pramine; Tofranil®

Mexican Brand Names Talpramin; Tofranil

Index Terms Imipramine Hydrochloride; Imipramine Pamoate

Pharmacologic Category Antidepressant, Tricyclic (Tertiary Amine)

Generic Available Yes

Use Treatment of depression; treatment of nocturnal enuresis in children

Unlabeled/Investigational Use Analgesic for certain chronic and neuropathic pain; panic disorder; attention-deficit/hyperactivity disorder (ADHD)

Mental Health Comment Tricyclic antidepressants may be classified as tertiary (amitriptyline, doxepin, clomipramine, imipramine, trimipramine) or secondary amines (nortriptyline, desipramine, protriptyline). The tertiary amines are not recommended to treat depression in the elderly. If a TCA is used in the elderly, it should be a secondary amine. The tertiary amines are commonly used in low dosages for various conditions associated with pain. Toxicity is generally dose dependent. Relatively small overdoses (1-week supply) can be potentially fatal.

Plasma concentrations correlate with clinical response. A linear relationship exists.

Restrictions An FDA-approved medication guide concerning the use of antidepressants in children, adolescents, and young adults must be distributed when dispensing an outpatient prescription (new or refill) where this medication is to be used without direct supervision of a healthcare provider. Medication guides are available at http://www.fda.gov/cder/Offices/ODS/medication_guides.htm. Dispense to parents or guardians of children and adolescents receiving this medication.

Pregnancy Risk Factor D

Lactation Enters breast milk/not recommended (AAP rates "of concern")

Contraindications Hypersensitivity to imipramine (cross-reactivity with other dibenzodiazepines may occur) or any component of the formulation; concurrent use of MAO inhibitors (within 14 days); in a patient during acute recovery phase of MI; pregnancy

Warnings/Precautions **[U.S. Boxed Warning]: Antidepressants increase the risk of suicidal thinking and behavior in children, adolescents, and young adults (18-24 years of age) with major depressive disorder (MDD) and other psychiatric disorders;** consider risk prior to prescribing. Short-term studies did not show an increased risk in patients >24 years of age and showed a decreased risk in patients ≥65 years. Closely monitor for clinical worsening, suicidality, or unusual changes in behavior; the patient's family or caregiver should be instructed to closely observe the patient and communicate condition with healthcare provider. A medication guide should be dispensed with each prescription. **Imipramine is FDA approved for the treatment of nocturnal enuresis in children ≥6 years of age.**

The possibility of a suicide attempt is inherent in major depression and may persist until remission occurs. Monitor for worsening of depression or suicidality, especially during initiation of therapy (generally first 1-2 months) or with dose increases or decreases. Use caution in high-risk patients. Worsening depression and severe abrupt suicidality that are not part of the presenting symptoms may require discontinuation or modification of drug therapy. The patient's family or caregiver should be alerted to monitor patients for the emergence of suicidality and associated behaviors (such as agitation, irritability, hostility, impulsivity, and hypomania) and notify healthcare provider.

May worsen psychosis in some patients or precipitate a shift to mania or hypomania in patients with bipolar disorder. Patients presenting with depressive symptoms should be screened for bipolar disorder. Monotherapy in patients with bipolar disorder should be avoided. **Imipramine is not FDA approved for the treatment of bipolar depression.**

TCAs may rarely cause bone marrow suppression; monitor for any signs of infection and obtain CBC if symptoms (eg, fever, sore throat) evident. The degree of sedation, anticholinergic effects, orthostasis, and conduction abnormalities are high relative to other antidepressants. Imipramine often causes drowsiness/sedation, resulting in impaired performance of tasks requiring alertness (eg, operating machinery or driving). Sedative effects may be additive with other CNS depressants and/or ethanol. Use with caution in patients with a history of cardiovascular disease (including previous MI, stroke, tachycardia, or conduction abnormalities). Use with caution in patients with urinary retention, benign prostatic hyperplasia, narrow-angle glaucoma, xerostomia, visual problems, constipation, or a history of bowel obstruction.

Consider discontinuing, when possible, prior to elective surgery. Therapy should not be abruptly discontinued in patients receiving high doses for prolonged periods. May lower seizure threshold - use caution in patients with a previous seizure disorder or condition predisposing to seizures such as brain damage, alcoholism, or concurrent therapy with other drugs which lower the seizure threshold. May increase the risks associated with electroconvulsive therapy. Use with caution in hyperthyroid patients or those receiving thyroid supplementation. Use with caution in patients with diabetes mellitus; may alter glucose regulation. Use with caution in patients with hepatic or renal dysfunction and in elderly patients. Has been associated with photosensitization.

Adverse Reactions Reported for tricyclic antidepressants in general. Frequency not defined.

Cardiovascular: Arrhythmia, CHF, ECG changes, heart block, hypertension, MI, orthostatic hypotension, palpitation, stroke, tachycardia

Central nervous system: Agitation, anxiety, confusion, delusions, disorientation, dizziness, drowsiness, fatigue, hallucination, headache, hypomania, insomnia, nightmares, psychosis, restlessness, seizure

Dermatologic: Alopecia, itching, petechiae, photosensitivity, purpura, rash, urticaria

Endocrine & metabolic: Breast enlargement, galactorrhea, gynecomastia, increase or decrease in blood sugar, increase or decrease in libido, SIADH

Gastrointestinal: Abdominal cramps, anorexia, black tongue, constipation, diarrhea, epigastric disorders, ileus, nausea, stomatitis, taste disturbance, vomiting, weight gain/loss, xerostomia

Genitourinary: Impotence, testicular swelling, urinary retention

Hematologic: Agranulocytosis, eosinophilia, thrombocytopenia

Hepatic: Cholestatic jaundice, transaminases increased

Neuromuscular & skeletal: Ataxia, extrapyramidal symptoms, incoordination, numbness, paresthesia, peripheral neuropathy, tingling, tremor, weakness

Ocular: Blurred vision, disturbances of accommodation, mydriasis

Otic: Tinnitus

Miscellaneous: Diaphoresis, falling, hypersensitivity (eg, drug fever, edema)

Metabolism/Transport Effects Substrate of CYP1A2 (minor), 2B6 (minor), 2C19 (major), 2D6 (major), 3A4 (minor); **Inhibits** CYP1A2 (weak), 2C19 (weak), 2D6 (moderate), 2E1 (weak)

Drug Interactions

Acetylcholinesterase Inhibitors (Central): Anticholinergics may diminish the therapeutic effect of Acetylcholinesterase Inhibitors (Central). Acetylcholinesterase Inhibitors (Central) may diminish the therapeutic effect of Anticholinergics. If the anticholinergic action is a side effect of the agent, the result may be beneficial. *Risk C: Monitor therapy*

Alcohol (Ethyl): CNS Depressants may enhance the CNS depressant effect of Alcohol (Ethyl). *Risk C: Monitor therapy*

Alfuzosin: May enhance the QTc-prolonging effect of QTc-Prolonging Agents. *Risk C: Monitor therapy*

Alpha-/Beta-Agonists (Direct-Acting): Tricyclic Antidepressants may enhance the vasopressor effect of Alpha-/Beta-Agonists (Direct-Acting). **Exceptions:** Dipivefrin. *Risk D: Consider therapy modification*

Alpha1-Agonists: Tricyclic Antidepressants may enhance the vasopressor effect of Alpha1-Agonists. *Risk D: Consider therapy modification*

Alpha2-Agonists: Tricyclic Antidepressants may diminish the antihypertensive effect of Alpha2-Agonists. **Exceptions:** Apraclonidine; Brimonidine. *Risk D: Consider therapy modification*

Altretamine: May enhance the orthostatic effect of Tricyclic Antidepressants. *Risk C: Monitor therapy*

Amphetamines: Tricyclic Antidepressants may enhance the stimulatory effect of Amphetamines. Tricyclic Antidepressants may also potentiate the cardiovascular effects of Amphetamines. *Risk C: Monitor therapy*

Anticholinergics: May enhance the adverse/toxic effect of other Anticholinergics. **Exceptions:** Paliperidone. *Risk C: Monitor therapy*

Aspirin: Antidepressants (Tricyclic, Tertiary Amine) may enhance the antiplatelet effect of Aspirin. *Risk C: Monitor therapy*

Barbiturates: May increase the metabolism of Tricyclic Antidepressants. *Risk D: Consider therapy modification*

Beta2-Agonists: Tricyclic Antidepressants may enhance the adverse/toxic effect of Beta2-Agonists. *Risk C: Monitor therapy*

BuPROPion: May decrease the metabolism of Tricyclic Antidepressants. *Risk C: Monitor therapy*

CarBAMazepine: May increase the metabolism of Tricyclic Antidepressants. *Risk C: Monitor therapy*

Cimetidine: May decrease the metabolism of Tricyclic Antidepressants. *Risk C: Monitor therapy*

Cinacalcet: May increase the serum concentration of Tricyclic Antidepressants. *Risk C: Monitor therapy*

Ciprofloxacin: May enhance the QTc-prolonging effect of QTc-Prolonging Agents. *Risk C: Monitor therapy*

CNS Depressants: May enhance the adverse/toxic effect of other CNS Depressants. *Risk C: Monitor therapy*

Codeine: CYP2D6 Inhibitors (Moderate) may diminish the therapeutic effect of Codeine. These CYP2D6 inhibitors may prevent the metabolic conversion of codeine to its active metabolite morphine. *Risk C: Monitor therapy*

CYP2C19 Inducers (Strong): May increase the metabolism of CYP2C19 Substrates. *Risk C: Monitor therapy*

CYP2C19 Inhibitors (Moderate): May decrease the metabolism of CYP2C19 Substrates. *Risk C: Monitor therapy*

CYP2C19 Inhibitors (Strong): May decrease the metabolism of CYP2C19 Substrates. *Risk D: Consider therapy modification*

CYP2D6 Inhibitors (Moderate): May decrease the metabolism of CYP2D6 Substrates. *Risk C: Monitor therapy*

CYP2D6 Inhibitors (Strong): May decrease the metabolism of CYP2D6 Substrates. *Risk D: Consider therapy modification*

CYP2D6 Substrates: CYP2D6 Inhibitors (Moderate) may decrease the metabolism of CYP2D6 Substrates. **Exceptions:** Tamoxifen. *Risk C: Monitor therapy*

Darunavir: May increase the serum concentration of CYP2D6 Substrates. *Risk C: Monitor therapy*

Desmopressin: Tricyclic Antidepressants may enhance the adverse/toxic effect of Desmopressin. *Risk C: Monitor therapy*

Dexmethylphenidate: May decrease the metabolism of Tricyclic Antidepressants. *Risk C: Monitor therapy*

DULoxetine: May decrease the metabolism of Tricyclic Antidepressants. *Risk C: Monitor therapy*

Gadobutrol: May enhance the QTc-prolonging effect of QTc-Prolonging Agents. *Risk D: Consider therapy modification*

Lithium: May enhance the neurotoxic effect of Tricyclic Antidepressants. *Risk C: Monitor therapy*

MAO Inhibitors: May enhance the serotonergic effect of Tricyclic Antidepressants. This may cause serotonin syndrome. *Risk X: Avoid combination*

Methylphenidate: May decrease the metabolism of Tricyclic Antidepressants. *Risk C: Monitor therapy*

Nebivolol: CYP2D6 Inhibitors (Moderate) may increase the serum concentration of Nebivolol. *Risk C: Monitor therapy*

Nilotinib: May enhance the QTc-prolonging effect of QTc-Prolonging Agents. *Risk X: Avoid combination*

NSAID (COX-2 Inhibitor): Antidepressants (Tricyclic, Tertiary Amine) may enhance the antiplatelet effect of NSAID (COX-2 Inhibitor). *Risk C: Monitor therapy*

NSAID (Nonselective): Antidepressants (Tricyclic, Tertiary Amine) may enhance the antiplatelet effect of NSAID (Nonselective). *Risk C: Monitor therapy*

Pramlintide: May enhance the anticholinergic effect of Anticholinergics. These effects are specific to the GI tract. *Risk D: Consider therapy modification*

Propoxyphene: May enhance the CNS depressant effect of Tricyclic Antidepressants. *Risk C: Monitor therapy*

Protease Inhibitors: May increase the serum concentration of Tricyclic Antidepressants. *Risk C: Monitor therapy*

QTc-Prolonging Agents: May enhance the adverse/toxic effect of other QTc-Prolonging Agents. Their effects can be additive, causing life-threatening ventricular arrhythmias. *Risk D: Consider therapy modification*

QuiNIDine: Tricyclic Antidepressants may enhance the QTc-prolonging effect of QuiNIDine. QuiNIDine may decrease the metabolism of Tricyclic Antidepressants. *Risk D: Consider therapy modification*

Selective Serotonin Reuptake Inhibitors: May decrease the metabolism of Tricyclic Antidepressants. *Risk D: Consider therapy modification*

Serotonin Modulators: May enhance the adverse/toxic effect of other Serotonin Modulators. The development of serotonin syndrome may occur. *Risk D: Consider therapy modification*

Sibutramine: May enhance the serotonergic effect of Serotonin Modulators. This may cause serotonin syndrome. *Risk X: Avoid combination*

St Johns Wort: May increase the metabolism of Tricyclic Antidepressants. The risk of serotonin syndrome may theoretically be increased. *Risk D: Consider therapy modification*

Sulfonylureas: Cyclic Antidepressants may enhance the hypoglycemic effect of Sulfonylureas. *Risk C: Monitor therapy*

Tamoxifen: CYP2D6 Inhibitors (Moderate) may decrease the metabolism of Tamoxifen. Specifically, CYP2D6 inhibitors may decrease the formation of highly potent active metabolites. *Risk D: Consider therapy modification*

Terbinafine: May decrease the metabolism of Tricyclic Antidepressants. *Risk D: Consider therapy modification*

Tetrabenazine: QTc-Prolonging Agents may enhance the QTc-prolonging effect of Tetrabenazine. *Risk X: Avoid combination*

Thioridazine: QTc-Prolonging Agents may enhance the QTc-prolonging effect of Thioridazine. *Risk X: Avoid combination*

Thioridazine: CYP2D6 Inhibitors may decrease the metabolism of Thioridazine. *Risk X: Avoid combination*

TraMADol: Tricyclic Antidepressants may enhance the neuroexcitatory and/or seizure-potentiating effect of TraMADol. *Risk C: Monitor therapy*

Valproic Acid: May increase the serum concentration of Tricyclic Antidepressants. *Risk C: Monitor therapy*

Vitamin K Antagonists (eg, warfarin): Tricyclic Antidepressants may enhance the anticoagulant effect of Vitamin K Antagonists. *Risk C: Monitor therapy*

Ziprasidone: QTc-Prolonging Agents may enhance the QTc-prolonging effect of Ziprasidone. The risk of a severe arrhythmia may be increased. *Risk X: Avoid combination*

Ethanol/Nutrition/Herb Interactions

Ethanol: Avoid ethanol (may increase CNS depression).

Herb/Nutraceutical: St John's wort may decrease imipramine levels. Avoid valerian, St John's wort, SAMe, kava kava (may increase risk of serotonin syndrome and/or excessive sedation).

Mechanism of Action Traditionally believed to increase the synaptic concentration of serotonin and/or norepinephrine in the central nervous system by inhibition of their reuptake by the presynaptic neuronal membrane. However, additional receptor effects have been found including desensitization of adenyl cyclase, down regulation of beta-adrenergic receptors, and down regulation of serotonin receptors.

Pharmacodynamics/Kinetics

Onset of action: Peak antidepressant effect: Usually after ≥2 weeks

Absorption: Well absorbed

Distribution: Crosses placenta

Metabolism: Hepatic, primarily via CYP2D6 to desipramine (active) and other metabolites; significant first-pass effect

Half-life elimination: 6-18 hours

Excretion: Urine (as metabolites)

Dosage Oral:

Children:

Depression (unlabeled use): 1.5 mg/kg/day with dosage increments of 1 mg/kg every 3-4 days to a maximum dose of 5 mg/kg/day in 1-4 divided doses; monitor carefully especially with doses ≥3.5 mg/kg/day

Enuresis: ≥6 years: Initial: 25 mg at bedtime, if inadequate response still seen after 1 week of therapy, increase by 25 mg/day; dose should not exceed 2.5 mg/kg/day or 50 mg at bedtime if 6-12 years of age or 75 mg at bedtime if ≥12 years of age

Adjunct in the treatment of cancer pain (unlabeled use): Initial: 0.2-0.4 mg/kg at bedtime; dose may be increased by 50% every 2-3 days up to 1-3 mg/kg/dose at bedtime

Adolescents: Depression: Initial: 25-50 mg/day; increase gradually; maximum: 100 mg/day in single or divided doses

Adults: Depression:

Outpatients: Initial: 75 mg/day; may increase gradually to 150 mg/day. May be given in divided doses or as a single bedtime dose; maximum: 200 mg/day

Inpatients: Initial: 100-150 mg/day; may increase gradually to 200 mg/day; if no response after 2 weeks, may further increase to 250-300 mg/day. May be given in divided doses or as a single bedtime dose; maximum: 300 mg/day.

Elderly: Depression: Initial: 25-50 mg at bedtime; may increase every 3 days for inpatients and weekly for outpatients if tolerated to a recommended maximum of 100 mg/day.

Monitoring Parameters Monitor blood pressure and pulse rate prior to and during initial therapy; ECG in older adults, with high doses, and/or in patients with pre-existing cardiovascular disease; evaluate mental status, suicidal ideation (especially at the beginning of therapy or when doses are increased or decreased); blood levels are useful for therapeutic monitoring

When used for the treatment of ADHD, thoroughly evaluate for cardiovascular risk. Monitor heart rate, blood pressure, and consider obtaining ECG prior to initiation (Vetter, 2008); ensure PR interval ≤200 ms, QRS duration ≤120 ms, and QT_c ≤460 ms.

Reference Range Therapeutic: Imipramine and desipramine: 150-250 ng/mL (SI: 530-890 nmol/L); desipramine: 150-300 ng/mL (SI: 560-1125 nmol/L); Toxic: >500 ng/mL (SI: 446-893 nmol/L); utility of serum level monitoring controversial

Dosage Forms Excipient information presented when available (limited, particularly for generics); consult specific product labeling.

Capsule, as pamoate: 75 mg, 100 mg, 125 mg, 150 mg

Tofranil-PM®: 75 mg, 100 mg, 125 mg, 150 mg

Tablet, as hydrochloride: 10 mg, 25 mg, 50 mg

Tofranil®): 10 mg, 25 mg, 50 mg

- **Imipramine Hydrochloride** *see* Imipramine *on page 812*
- **Imipramine Pamoate** *see* Imipramine *on page 812*
- **Imitrex®** *see* SUMAtriptan *on page 1527*
- **Imodium® A-D [OTC]** *see* Loperamide *on page 944*
- **Imodium® Advanced** *see* Loperamide and Simethicone *on page 944*
- **Implanon™** *see* Etonogestrel *on page 606*
- **Imuran®** *see* AzaTHIOprine *on page 162*
- **In-111 Ibritumomab** *see* Ibritumomab *on page 802*
- **In-111 Zevalin** *see* Ibritumomab *on page 802*

Inamrinone (eye NAM ri none)

Medication Safety Issues

Sound-alike/look-alike issues:

Amrinone may be confused with aMILoride, amiodarone

High alert medication: The Institute for Safe Medication Practices (ISMP) includes this medication among its list of drug classes which have a heightened risk of causing significant patient harm when used in error.

Index Terms Amrinone Lactate

Pharmacologic Category Phosphodiesterase Enzyme Inhibitor

Use Short-term therapy in patients with intractable heart failure

Effect on Mental Status None reported

Effect on Psychiatric Treatment May cause hypotension which may be exacerbated by psychotropics

Dosage Summary

I.V.:

Children (unlabeled population): Bolus: 0.75 mg/kg, may repeat; Infusion: 5-10 mcg/kg/minute

Adults: Bolus: 0.75 mg/kg, may repeat; Infusion: 5-10 mcg/kg/minute

Dosage Forms Excipient information presented when available (limited, particularly for generics); consult specific product labeling.

Injection, solution, as lactate: 5 mg/mL (20 mL) [contains sodium metabisulfite]

- **Inapsine®** *see* Droperidol *on page 513*
- **Increlex™** *see* Mecasermin *on page 973*

Indapamide (in DAP a mide)

Medication Safety Issues

Sound-alike/look-alike issues:

Indapamide may be confused with Iopidine®

International issues:

Pretanix® [Hungary] may be confused with Protonix® which is a brand name for pantoprazole in the U.S.

Canadian Brand Names Apo-Indapamide®; Gen-Indapamide; Lozide®; Lozol®; Novo-Indapamide; Nu-Indapamide; PMS-Indapamide

Pharmacologic Category Diuretic, Thiazide-Related

Use Management of mild to moderate hypertension; treatment of edema in congestive heart failure and nephrotic syndrome

Effect on Mental Status May rarely cause mood changes

Effect on Psychiatric Treatment May decrease lithium clearance resulting in an increase in serum lithium levels and potential lithium toxicity; monitor serum lithium levels

Dosage Summary

Oral:

Children: Dosage not established

Adults: 1.25-5 mg once daily

Dosage Forms Excipient information presented when available (limited, particularly for generics); consult specific product labeling.

Tablet: 1.25 mg, 2.5 mg

◆ **Inderal®** *see* Propranolol *on page 1355*

◆ **Inderal® LA** *see* Propranolol *on page 1355*

◆ **Inderide®** *see* Propranolol and Hydrochlorothiazide *on page 1361*

Indinavir (in DIN a veer)

Medication Safety Issues

Sound-alike/look-alike issues:

Indinavir may be confused with Denavir™

U.S. Brand Names Crixivan®

Canadian Brand Names Crixivan®

Mexican Brand Names Aviran; Crixivan; Indilan

Index Terms Indinavir Sulfate

Pharmacologic Category Antiretroviral Agent, Protease Inhibitor

Use Treatment of HIV infection; should always be used as part of a multidrug regimen (at least three antiretroviral agents)

Effect on Mental Status May cause insomnia; may rarely cause dizziness or drowsiness

Effect on Psychiatric Treatment Contraindicated with midazolam and triazolam; use caution with other benzodiazepines; may produce additive sedation and respiratory depression. Concomitant use of indinavir and St John's wort is not recommended. Coadministration of protease inhibitors (indinavir) with St John's wort is expected to substantially decrease protease inhibitor serum concentrations leading to a loss of virologic response and possible resistance to indinavir or to the class of protease inhibitors.

Dosage Summary

Oral:

Children: Dosage not established

Adults: 800 mg every 8 hours; Boosted regimen: 400-800 mg every 12 hours

Dosage Forms Excipient information presented when available (limited, particularly for generics); consult specific product labeling.

Capsule:

Crixivan®: 100 mg, 200 mg, 333 mg, 400 mg

◆ **Indinavir Sulfate** *see* Indinavir *on page 818*

◆ **Indocin®** *see* Indomethacin *on page 818*

◆ **Indocin® I.V.** *see* Indomethacin *on page 818*

◆ **Indometacin** *see* Indomethacin *on page 818*

Indomethacin (in doe METH a sin)

Medication Safety Issues

Sound-alike/look-alike issues:

Indocin® may be confused with Imodium®, Lincocin®, Minocin®, Vicodin®

International issues:

Flexin® [Great Britain] may be confused with Floxin® which is a brand name for ofloxacin in the U.S.

Flexin® [Great Britain]: Brand name for orphenadrine in Israel

Related Information

Nonsteroidal Anti-Inflammatory Agents *on page 1792*

U.S. Brand Names Indocin®; Indocin® I.V.

Canadian Brand Names Apo-Indomethacin®; Indo-Lemmon; Indocid® P.D.A.; Indocin®; Indotec; Novo-Methacin; Nu-Indo; Rhodacine®

Mexican Brand Names Antalgin; Indaflex; Indanet; Indocid; Malival; Stratasin

Index Terms Indometacin; Indomethacin Sodium Trihydrate

Pharmacologic Category Nonsteroidal Anti-inflammatory Drug (NSAID), Oral; Nonsteroidal Anti-inflammatory Drug (NSAID), Parenteral

Use Acute gouty arthritis, acute bursitis/tendonitis, moderate to severe osteoarthritis, rheumatoid arthritis, ankylosing spondylitis; I.V. form used as alternative to surgery for closure of patent ductus arteriosus in neonates

Effect on Mental Status Dizziness is common; may cause nervousness; may rarely cause sedation, confusion, depression, and hallucinations

Effect on Psychiatric Treatment May cause bone marrow suppression; use caution with clozapine and carbamazepine; may decrease lithium clearance resulting in an increase in serum lithium levels and potential lithium toxicity; monitor serum lithium levels

Restrictions An FDA-approved medication guide must be distributed when dispensing an oral outpatient prescription (new or refill) where this medication is to be used without direct supervision of a healthcare provider. Medication guides are available at http://www.fda.gov/cder/Offices/ODS/medication_guides.htm.

Dosage Summary

I.V.:

Neonates <48 hours old at time of first dose: Initial: 0.2 mg/kg, followed by 2 doses of 0.1 mg/kg at 12- to 24- hour intervals

Neonates 2-7 days old at time of first dose: Initial: 0.2 mg/kg, followed by 2 doses of 0.2 mg/kg at 12- to 24-hour intervals

Neonates >7 days old at time of first dose: Initial: 0.2 mg/kg, followed by 0.25 mg/kg at 12- to 24-hour intervals

Children: Dosage not established

Adults: Dosage not established

Oral:

Extended release:

Children ≤14 years: Dosage not established

Children >14 years: 75-150 mg/day in 1-2 divided doses (maximum: 150 mg/day)

Adults: 75-150 mg/day in 1-2 divided doses (maximum: 150 mg/day)

Immediate release:

Children ≥2 years: 1-2 mg/kg/day in 2-4 divided doses (maximum: 4 mg/kg/day; 200 mg/day)

Adults: 50-150 mg/day in 2-4 divided doses (maximum: 200 mg/day)

Dosage Forms Excipient information presented when available (limited, particularly for generics); consult specific product labeling.

Capsule: 25 mg, 50 mg

Capsule, extended release, oral: 75 mg

Injection, powder for reconstitution:

Indocin® I.V: 1 mg

Suppository, rectal: 50 mg (30s)

Suspension, oral:

Indocin®: 25 mg/5 mL (237 mL) [contains alcohol 1%; pineapple-coconut-mint flavor]

◆ **Indomethacin Sodium Trihydrate** *see* Indomethacin *on page 818*
◆ **INF-alpha 2** *see* Interferon Alfa-2b *on page 844*
◆ **Infantaire [OTC]** *see* Acetaminophen *on page 30*
◆ **INFeD®** *see* Iron Dextran Complex *on page 857*
◆ **Infergen®** *see* Interferon Alfacon-1 *on page 847*

InFLIXimab (in FLIKS e mab)

Medication Safety Issues

Sound-alike/look-alike issues:

Remicade® may be confused with Renacidin®, Rituxan®

InFLIXimab may be confused with riTUXimab

U.S. Brand Names Remicade®

Canadian Brand Names Remicade®

Mexican Brand Names Remicade

Index Terms Infliximab, Recombinant; NSC-728729

Pharmacologic Category Antirheumatic, Disease Modifying; Gastrointestinal Agent, Miscellaneous; Monoclonal Antibody; Tumor Necrosis Factor (TNF) Blocking Agent

Use Treatment of rheumatoid arthritis (moderate-to-severe, with methotrexate); treatment of Crohn's disease (moderate-to-severe with inadequate response to conventional therapy) for induction and maintenance of remission, and/or to reduce the number of draining enterocutaneous and rectovaginal fistulas, and to maintain fistula closure; treatment of psoriatic arthritis; treatment of plaque psoriasis (chronic severe); treatment of ankylosing spondylitis; treatment of and maintenance of healing of ulcerative colitis (moderately- to severely-active with inadequate response to conventional therapy)

Unlabeled/Investigational Use Acute graft-versus-host disease (GVHD), juvenile rheumatoid arthritis (JRA)

Effect on Mental Status Fatigue is common; may cause dizziness

Effect on Psychiatric Treatment None reported

Restrictions An FDA-approved medication guide is available at www.fda.gov/cder/Offices/ODS/labeling.htm; distribute to each patient to whom this medication is dispensed.

Dosage Summary

I.V.:

Children: U.S. labeling <6 years, Canadian labeling <9 years: Dosage not established

Children: U.S. labeling ≥6 years, Canadian labeling ≥9 years: Initial: 5 mg/kg at 0, 2, and 6 weeks; Maintenance: 5 mg/kg every 8 weeks (Crohn's disease)

Adults: Initial: 3-10 mg/kg (specific dose varies by indication) at 0, 2, and 6 weeks; Maintenance: 3-10 mg/kg every 8 weeks **or** 5 mg/kg every 6 weeks

Dosage Forms Excipient information presented when available (limited, particularly for generics); consult specific product labeling.

Injection, powder for reconstitution [preservative free]:

Remicade®: 100 mg [contains sucrose 500 mg and polysorbate 80]

◆ **Infliximab, Recombinant** *see* InFLIXimab *on page 819*

Influenza Virus Vaccine (in floo EN za VYE rus vak SEEN)

Medication Safety Issues

Sound-alike/look-alike issues:

Fluarix® may be confused with Flarex®

Influenza virus vaccine may be confused with tetanus toxoid and tuberculin products. Medication errors have occurred when tuberculin skin tests (PPD) have been inadvertently administered instead of tetanus toxoid products and influenza virus vaccine. These products are refrigerated and often stored in close proximity to each other.

Influenza virus vaccine (human strain) may be confused with the avian strain (H5N1) of influenza virus vaccine

International issues:

Hiberix is also a brand name for *Haemophilus* b conjugate vaccine in Slovenia

U.S. Brand Names Afluria®; Fluarix®; FluLaval™; FluMist®; Fluvirin®; Fluzone®

Canadian Brand Names Fluviral S/F®; Vaxigrip®

Mexican Brand Names Fluarix; Fluzone

Index Terms Influenza Virus Vaccine (Purified Surface Antigen); Influenza Virus Vaccine (Split-Virus); Influenza Virus Vaccine (Trivalent, Live); Live Attenuated Influenza Vaccine (LAIV); Trivalent Inactivated Influenza Vaccine (TIV)

Pharmacologic Category Vaccine, Inactivated (Viral); Vaccine, Live (Viral)

Use Provide active immunity to influenza virus strains contained in the vaccine

Advisory Committee on Immunization Practices (ACIP) recommends annual vaccination for all children (6 months to 18 years) and adults. Target groups for vaccination (those at higher risk of complications from influenza infection and their close contacts) include the following:

- Persons ≥50 years of age
- Residents of nursing homes and other chronic-care facilities that house persons of any age with chronic medical conditions
- Adults and children with chronic disorders of the pulmonary or cardiovascular systems (except hypertension), including asthma
- Adults and children who have chronic metabolic diseases (including diabetes mellitus), hepatic disease, renal dysfunction, hematologic disorders, hemoglobinopathies, or immunosuppression (including immunosuppression caused by medications or HIV)
- Adults and children with conditions which may compromise respiratory function, the handling of respiratory secretions, or that can increase the risk of aspiration (eg, cognitive dysfunction, spinal; cord injuries, seizure disorders, other neuromuscular disorders)
- Children and adolescents (6 months to 18 years of age) who are receiving long-term aspirin therapy and therefore, may be at risk for developing Reye's syndrome after influenza
- Women who will be pregnant during the influenza season

- Children 6-59 months of age
- Healthcare personnel
- Household contacts and caregivers of children <5 years (particularly children <6 months) and adults ≥50 years
- Household contacts and caregivers of persons with medical conditions which put them at high risk of complications from influenza infection

Effect on Mental Status May cause fatigue, irritability, insomnia, and malaise

Effect on Psychiatric Treatment None reported

Dosage Summary Note: Children <9 years who are not previously vaccinated or who received only 1 dose of vaccine during the previous season should receive 2 doses, in order to achieve satisfactory antibody response.

I.M.:

Children <6 months: Dosage not established

Children 6-35 months: Fluzone®: 0.25 mL/dose (1 or 2 doses per season; see **Note**)

Children 3-4 years: Fluzone®: 0.5 mL/dose (1 or 2 doses per season; see **Note**)

Children 4-8 years: Fluvirin®, Fluzone®: 0.5 mL/dose (1 or 2 doses per season; see **Note**)

Children ≥9 years: Fluvirin®, Fluzone®: 0.5 mL/dose (1 dose per season)

Adults: Afluria®, Fluarix®, FluLaval™, Fluvirin®, Fluzone®: 0.5 mL/dose (1 dose per season)

Intranasal:

Children <2 years: Dosage not established

Children 2-8 years: Previously not vaccinated: Initial season: Two 0.2 mL doses separated by at least 4 weeks; Previously vaccinated: 0.2 mL/dose (1 or 2 doses separated by at least 4 weeks; see **Note**)

Children ≥9 years: 0.2 mL/dose (1 dose per season)

Adults ≤49 years: 0.2 mL/dose (1 dose per season)

Dosage Forms Excipient information presented when available (limited, particularly for generics); consult specific product labeling.

Injection, suspension [purified split-virus]:

Afluria®: 5 mL [TIV; contains chicken egg protein, thimerosal, neomycin (trace amounts), and polymyxin (trace amounts)]

FluLaval™: 5 mL [TIV; contains chicken egg protein and thimerosal]

Fluvirin®: 5 mL [TIV; contains chicken egg protein, thimerosal, neomycin (trace amounts), and polymyxin (trace amounts)]

Fluzone®: 5 mL [TIV; contains chicken egg protein and thimerosal]

Injection, suspension [purified split-virus; preservative free]:

Afluria®: 0.5 mL [TIV; contains chicken egg protein, neomycin (trace amounts), and polymyxin (trace amounts)]

Fluarix®: 0.5 mL [TIV; contains chicken egg protein, gentamicin (trace amounts), natural rubber/natural latex in packaging, polysorbate 80, and thimerosal (trace amounts)]

Fluvirin®: 0.5 mL [TIV; contains chicken egg protein, thimerosal (trace amounts), neomycin (trace amounts), and polymyxin (trace amounts)]

Fluzone®: 0.25 mL, 0.5 mL [TIV; contains chicken egg protein]

Solution, intranasal [preservative free; spray]:

FluMist®: 0.2 mL [trivalent, LAIV; contains arginine, chicken egg protein, gelatin, and gentamicin]

Influenza Virus Vaccine (H5N1)

(in floo EN za VYE rus vak SEEN H5N1)

Medication Safety Issues

Sound-alike/look-alike issues:

Influenza virus vaccine (H5N1) may be confused with the nonavian strain of influenza virus vaccine

Index Terms Avian Influenza Virus Vaccine; Bird Flu Vaccine; H5N1 Influenza Vaccine; Influenza Virus Vaccine (Monovalent)

Pharmacologic Category Vaccine

Use Active immunization of adults at increased risk of exposure to the H5N1 viral subtype of influenza

Effect on Mental Status Malaise is common

Effect on Psychiatric Treatment None reported

Restrictions Commercial distribution is not planned. The vaccine will be included as part of the U.S. Strategic National Stockpile. It will be distributed by public health officials if needed.

Dosage Summary

I.M.:

Children: Dosage not established

Adults 18-64 years: 1 mL, followed by second 1 mL dose given 28 days later

Dosage Forms Injection, suspension [monovalent]: Hemagglutinin (H5N1 strain) 90 mcg/1 mL (5 mL) [contains thimerosal, and chicken, porcine, and egg proteins]

◆ **Influenza Virus Vaccine (Monovalent)** *see* Influenza Virus Vaccine (H5N1) *on page 821*

◆ **Influenza Virus Vaccine (Purified Surface Antigen)** *see* Influenza Virus Vaccine *on page 820*

◆ **Influenza Virus Vaccine (Split-Virus)** *see* Influenza Virus Vaccine *on page 820*

◆ **Influenza Virus Vaccine (Trivalent, Live)** *see* Influenza Virus Vaccine *on page 820*

◆ **Infumorph®** *see* Morphine Sulfate *on page 1077*

◆ **Infuvite® Adult** *see* Vitamins (Multiple/Injectable) *on page 1677*

◆ **Infuvite® Pediatric** *see* Vitamins (Multiple/Injectable) *on page 1677*

◆ **INH** *see* Isoniazid *on page 862*

◆ **Inhaled Insulin** *see* Insulin Inhalation *on page 830*

◆ **Innohep®** *see* Tinzaparin *on page 1585*

◆ **InnoPran XL™** *see* Propranolol *on page 1355*

◆ **Inspra™** *see* Eplerenone *on page 545*

Insulin Aspart

(IN soo lin AS part)

Medication Safety Issues

Sound-alike/look-alike issues:

NovoLog® may be confused with Novolin®

NovoLog® Mix 70/30 may be confused with NovoLog®

High alert medication: The Institute for Safe Medication Practices (ISMP) includes this medication among its list of drugs which have a heightened risk of causing significant patient harm when used in error. ***Due to the number of insulin preparations, it is essential to identify/clarify the type of insulin to be used.***

Cross-contamination may occur if insulin pens are shared among multiple patients. Steps should be taken to prohibit sharing of insulin pens.

Related Information

Insulin Regular *on page 838*

U.S. Brand Names NovoLog®

Canadian Brand Names NovoRapid®

Mexican Brand Names Novomix 30

Index Terms Aspart Insulin

Pharmacologic Category Antidiabetic Agent, Insulin

Generic Available No

Use Treatment of type 1 diabetes mellitus (insulin dependent, IDDM) and type 2 diabetes mellitus (noninsulin dependent, NIDDM) to improve glycemic control

Effect on Mental Status May cause drowsiness or confusion

Effect on Psychiatric Treatment MAO inhibitors may enhance the hypoglycemic effects of insulin; TCAs may antagonize the effects of insulin

Pregnancy Risk Factor B

Pregnancy Considerations Adverse events have generally not been observed in animal reproduction studies; therefore, the manufacturer classifies insulin aspart as pregnancy category B. When compared to regular insulin, the use of insulin aspart during pregnancy has not been found to increase the risk of adverse events to the fetus. Maternal hyperglycemia can be associated with adverse effects in the fetus, including macrosomia, neonatal hyperglycemia, and hyperbilirubinemia; the risk of congenital malformations is increased when the Hb A_{1c} is above the normal range.

Insulin requirements tend to fall during the first trimester of pregnancy and increase in the later trimesters, peaking at 28-32 weeks of gestation. Following delivery, insulin requirements decrease rapidly. Diabetes can be associated with adverse effects in the mother. Poorly-treated diabetes may cause end-organ damage that may in turn negatively affect obstetric outcomes. Physiologic glucose levels should be maintained prior to and during pregnancy to decrease the risk of adverse events in the fetus and the mother. Insulin is the drug of choice for the control of diabetes mellitus during pregnancy. Insulin aspart has been demonstrated to be as safe and effective as regular human insulin when used during pregnancy and may have advantages over regular insulin during pregnancy.

Lactation Excretion in breast milk unknown/compatible

Contraindications Hypersensitivity to insulin aspart or any component of the formulation; during episodes of hypoglycemia

Warnings/Precautions Refer to Insulin Regular on page 838.

Due to short duration of action, a longer acting insulin or continuous basal administration of insulin via a SubQ infusion pump is needed to maintain adequate glucose control in type 1 diabetes mellitus (insulin dependent, IDDM). In type 2 diabetes mellitus (noninsulin dependent, NIDDM), insulin aspart may be used without a long-acting insulin or continuous basal administration of insulin via a SubQ infusion pump when used in combination with a sulfonylurea. Preprandial administration should be immediately followed by a meal within 5-10 minutes. Insulin aspart may be administered I.V. in selected clinical situations to control hyperglycemia.

Adverse Reactions Refer to Insulin Regular on page 838.

Drug Interactions Refer to Insulin Regular on page 838.

Ethanol/Nutrition/Herb Interactions Refer to Insulin Regular on page 838.

Stability Insulin aspart (NovoLog®): Store unopened vials, cartridges, and syringes in refrigerator between 2°C and 8°C (36°F to 46°F); do not use if frozen. If stored at room temperature of <30°C (<86°F), use within 28 days and protect from heat and light. Once punctured (in use), vials may be stored for up to 28 days at temperatures of <30°C (<86°F); do not freeze. Cartridges that are punctured (in use) should be stored at temperatures <30°C (<86°F) and used within 28 days; do not freeze or refrigerate. For insulin pumps, the insulin aspart in the reservoir should be replaced every 48 hours. Discard if exposed to temperatures ≥37°C (98.6°F).

For SubQ administration: May be diluted with insulin-diluting medium to a concentration of 10 units/mL (U-10) or 50 units/mL (U-50). Should be stored at temperatures <30°C (<86°F) and used within 28 days; do not freeze or refrigerate.

For I.V. infusion; May be diluted in NS, D_5W, or $D_{10}W$ with 40 mEq/L potassium chloride at concentrations from 0.05 units/mL to 1 unit/mL using polypropylene infusion bags. Stable for 24 hours at room temperature of <30°C (<86°F).

Mechanism of Action Refer to Insulin Regular on page 838. Insulin aspart is a rapid-acting insulin analog.

Pharmacodynamics/Kinetics Note: Rate of absorption, onset, and duration of activity may be affected by site of injection, exercise, presence of lipodystrophy, local blood supply, and/or temperature.

Onset of action: 0.2-0.5 hours

Peak effect: 1-3 hours

Duration: 3-5 hours

Protein binding: <10%

Half-life elimination: 81 minutes

Time to peak, plasma: 40-50 minutes

Excretion: Urine

Dosage Refer to Insulin Regular on page 838. Insulin aspart is a rapid-acting insulin analog which is normally administered as a a premeal component of the insulin regimen. It is normally used along with a long-acting (basal) form of insulin.

Dosing adjustment in renal impairment: Insulin requirements are reduced due to changes in insulin clearance or metabolism.

Dietary Considerations Dietary modification based on ADA recommendations is a key component of therapy.

Administration Do not use if solution is viscous or cloudy; use only if clear and colorless.

SubQ: Should be administered immediately before a meal (within 5-10 minutes of the start of a meal). Cold injections should be avoided. SubQ administration is usually made into the thighs, arms, buttocks, or abdomen, with sites rotated. If mixed with human NPH insulin, insulin aspart should be drawn into syringe first. Can be infused SubQ by external insulin pump; however, when used in an external pump, should not be diluted with other insulins. **Do not administer insulin mixtures intravenously.**

SubQ infusion pump: When used in an external SubQ infusion pump, insulin aspart should not be diluted or mixed with other insulins. The reservoir, infusion sets, and infusion set insertion site must be changed at least every 48 hours.

I.V.: Insulin aspart may be administered I.V. in selected clinical situations to control hyperglycemia. Appropriate medical supervision is required. **Do not administer insulin mixtures intravenously.**

Because of adsorption, the actual amount of insulin aspart being administered via I.V. infusion could be substantially less than the apparent amount. Therefore, adjustment of the insulin aspart I.V. infusion rate should be based on effect and not solely on the apparent insulin aspart dose. The apparent dose may be used as a starting point for determining the subsequent SubQ dosing regimen (Schmeltz, 2006); however, frequent monitoring of blood glucose and adjustment of therapy is required. Infusion requires continuous medical supervision.

Monitoring Parameters Serum glucose, electrolytes, Hb A_{1c}

Reference Range Refer to Insulin Regular on page 838.

Dosage Forms Excipient information presented when available (limited, particularly for generics); consult specific product labeling.

Injection, solution:

NovoLog®: 100 units/mL (3 mL) [FlexPen® prefilled syringe or PenFill® prefilled cartridge]; (10 mL) [vial]

◆ **Insulin Aspart and Insulin Aspart Protamine** *see* Insulin Aspart Protamine and Insulin Aspart *on page 824*

Insulin Aspart Protamine and Insulin Aspart

(IN soo lin AS part PROE ta meen & IN soo lin AS part)

Medication Safety Issues

Sound-alike/look-alike issues:

NovoLog® Mix 70/30 may be confused with Novolin® 70/30

High alert medication: The Institute for Safe Medication Practices (ISMP) includes this medication among its list of drugs which have a heightened risk of causing significant patient harm when used in error. ***Due to the number of insulin preparations, it is essential to identify/clarify the type of insulin to be used.***

Cross-contamination may occur if insulin pens are shared among multiple patients. Steps should be taken to prohibit sharing of insulin pens.

Related Information

Insulin Regular *on page 838*

U.S. Brand Names NovoLog® Mix 70/30

Canadian Brand Names NovoMix® 30

Index Terms Insulin Aspart and Insulin Aspart Protamine

Pharmacologic Category Antidiabetic Agent, Insulin

Generic Available No

Use Treatment of type 1 diabetes mellitus (insulin dependent, IDDM) and type 2 diabetes mellitus (noninsulin dependent, NIDDM) to improve glycemic control

Effect on Mental Status May cause drowsiness or confusion

Effect on Psychiatric Treatment MAO inhibitors may enhance the hypoglycemic effects of insulin; TCAs may antagonize the effects of insulin

Pregnancy Risk Factor C

Pregnancy Considerations Reproduction studies have not been conducted with this combination; see Insulin Aspart monograph

Lactation See Insulin Aspart monograph.

Contraindications Hypersensitivity to any component of the formulation; during episodes of hypoglycemia

Warnings/Precautions Refer to Insulin Regular on page 838. Safety and efficacy of this insulin product have not been established in pediatric patients.

Adverse Reactions Refer to Insulin Regular on page 838.

Drug Interactions

Antidiabetic Agents (Thiazolidinedione): Insulin may enhance the fluid-retaining effect of Antidiabetic Agents (Thiazolidinedione). *Risk C: Monitor therapy*

Beta-Blockers: May enhance the hypoglycemic effect of Insulin. **Exceptions:** Levobunolol; Metipranolol. *Risk C: Monitor therapy*

Corticosteroids (Orally Inhaled): May diminish the hypoglycemic effect of Antidiabetic Agents. In some instances, corticosteroid-mediated HPA axis suppression has led to episodes of acute adrenal crisis, which may manifest as enhanced hypoglycemia, particularly in the setting of insulin or other antidiabetic agent use. *Risk C: Monitor therapy*

Corticosteroids (Systemic): May diminish the hypoglycemic effect of Antidiabetic Agents. In some instances, corticosteroid-mediated HPA axis suppression has led to episodes of acute adrenal crisis, which may manifest as enhanced hypoglycemia, particularly in the setting of insulin or other antidiabetic agent use. *Risk C: Monitor therapy*

Edetate CALCIUM Disodium: May enhance the hypoglycemic effect of Insulin. *Risk C: Monitor therapy*

Edetate Disodium: May enhance the hypoglycemic effect of Insulin. *Risk C: Monitor therapy*

Herbs (Hypoglycemic Properties): May enhance the hypoglycemic effect of Hypoglycemic Agents. *Risk C: Monitor therapy*

Luteinizing Hormone-Releasing Hormone Analogs: May diminish the therapeutic effect of Antidiabetic Agents. *Risk C: Monitor therapy*

Pegvisomant: May enhance the hypoglycemic effect of Antidiabetic Agents. *Risk C: Monitor therapy*

Quinolone Antibiotics: Insulin may enhance the hyperglycemic effect of Quinolone Antibiotics. Insulin may enhance the hypoglycemic effect of Quinolone Antibiotics. *Risk C: Monitor therapy*

Somatropin: May diminish the hypoglycemic effect of Antidiabetic Agents. *Risk D: Consider therapy modification*

Stability NovoLog® Mix 70/30: Store unopened container in refrigerator. Do not use if frozen. If refrigeration is not possible, vial (in use) may be stored at room temperature for up to 28 days. The pen in use should **not** be refrigerated, store below 30°C (86°F) away from direct heat or light; discard after 14 days. If refrigeration is not available, opened vials may be stored unrefrigerated in cool place away from heat and sunlight.

Mechanism of Action Refer to Insulin Regular on page 838. Insulin aspart protamine and insulin aspart is a combination insulin product with intermediate-acting characteristics. Normally administered twice daily.

Pharmacodynamics/Kinetics Note: Rate of absorption, onset, and duration of activity may be affected by site of injection, exercise, presence of lipodystrophy, local blood supply, and/or temperature.

Onset of action: 0.2 hours

Peak effect: 1-4 hours

Duration: 18-24 hours

Half-life: 8-9 hours

Time to peak, plasma: 1-1.5 hours

Excretion: Urine

Dosage Refer to Insulin Regular on page 838. Fixed ratio insulins (such as insulin aspart protamine and insulin aspart combination) are normally administered in 2 daily doses.

Dosing adjustment in renal impairment: Insulin requirements are reduced due to changes in insulin clearance or metabolism.

Administration Aspart protamine human suspension and aspart human solution (NovoLog® Mix 70/30): SubQ administration only. Cold injections should be avoided. Should be administered within 15 minutes before a meal. Normally administered twice daily (before breakfast and supper). SubQ administration is usually made into the thighs, arms, buttocks, or abdomen, with sites rotated. Resuspend immediately prior to use. Gently roll vial or pen in the palms of the hands to resuspend before using. Do not mix or dilute with other insulins.

Additional Information Refer to Insulin Regular on page 838 for additional details on adverse effects, drug interactions, warnings, and dosing of insulin products.

Dosage Forms Excipient information presented when available (limited, particularly for generics); consult specific product labeling.

Injection, suspension:

NovoLog® Mix 70/30: Insulin aspart protamine suspension 70% [intermediate acting] and insulin aspart solution 30% [rapid acting]: 100 units/mL (3 mL) [FlexPen® prefilled syringe]; (10 mL) [vial]

Insulin Detemir (IN soo lin DE te mir)

Medication Safety Issues

High alert medication: The Institute for Safe Medication Practices (ISMP) includes this medication among its list of drugs which have a heightened risk of causing significant patient harm when used in error. ***Due to the number of insulin preparations, it is essential to identify/clarify the type of insulin to be used.***

Note: Insulin detemir is a clear solution, but it is NOT intended for I.V. or I.M. administration.

Cross-contamination may occur if insulin pens are shared among multiple patients. Steps should be taken to prohibit sharing of insulin pens.

Related Information

Insulin Regular *on page 838*

U.S. Brand Names Levemir®

Canadian Brand Names Levemir®

Mexican Brand Names Levemir

Index Terms Detemir Insulin

Pharmacologic Category Antidiabetic Agent, Insulin

Generic Available No

Use Treatment of type 1 diabetes mellitus (insulin dependent, IDDM) and type 2 diabetes mellitus (noninsulin dependent, NIDDM) to improve glycemic control

Effect on Mental Status May cause drowsiness or confusion

Effect on Psychiatric Treatment MAO inhibitors may enhance the hypoglycemic effects of insulin; TCAs may antagonize the effects of insulin

Pregnancy Risk Factor C

Pregnancy Considerations Adverse events were observed in animal reproduction studies; therefore, the manufacturer classifies insulin detemir as pregnancy category C. Maternal hyperglycemia can be associated with adverse effects in the fetus, including macrosomia, neonatal hyperglycemia, and hyperbilirubinemia; the risk of congenital malformations is increased when the Hb A_{1c} is above the normal range. Insulin requirements tend to fall during the first trimester of pregnancy and increase in the later trimesters, peaking at 28-32 weeks of gestation. Following delivery, insulin requirements decrease rapidly. Diabetes can be associated with adverse effects in the mother. Poorly-treated diabetes may cause end-organ damage that may in turn negatively affect obstetric outcomes. Physiologic glucose levels should be maintained prior to and during pregnancy to decrease the risk of adverse events in the fetus and the mother. Insulin is the drug of choice for the control of diabetes mellitus during pregnancy. Pregnant women using insulin detemir should be switched to NPH insulin pending additional safety information with this agent.

Lactation Excretion in breast milk unknown/compatible

Contraindications Hypersensitivity to any component of the formulation

Warnings/Precautions Refer to Insulin Regular on page 838. Safety and efficacy not established in children <6 years of age.

Careful adjustment of dosage and timing is required to achieve glycemic targets. Adjustment of other antidiabetic therapy (short-acting or oral antidiabetic agents) may be required. The duration of of action of insulin detemir is dose-dependent and this factor must be considered during dosage adjustment and titration. Insulin detemir is a clear solution, but it is not for intravenous administration.

Adverse Reactions Refer to Insulin Regular on page 838.

Metabolism/Transport Effects Refer to Insulin Regular on page 838.

Drug Interactions Refer to Insulin Regular on page 838.

Ethanol/Nutrition/Herb Interactions Refer to Insulin Regular on page 838.

Stability Insulin detemir (Levemir®): Store unopened container in refrigerator; do not use if it has been frozen. Once opened (in use), vials may be stored in refrigerator or for up to 42 days at room temperature (below 30°C). Cartridges and prefilled syringes that are in use should be stored at room temperature and used within 42 days; do not refrigerate. Do not store with needle in place. All opened (in-use) vials should be stored away from direct heat and sunlight.

Mechanism of Action Refer to Insulin Regular on page 838. The product labeling identifies this product as a long-acting insulin analog; however, at lower dosages (<0.6 units/kg) its pharmacodynamic characteristics and dosing are consistent with intermediate insulin forms. In some patients, or at higher dosages, it may have a duration of action approaching 24 hours, which is consistent with a long-acting insulin.

Pharmacodynamics/Kinetics Note: Rate of absorption, onset, and duration of activity may be affected by site of injection, exercise, presence of lipodystrophy, local blood supply, and/or temperature.

Onset of action: 3-4 hours

Peak effect: 3-14 hours

Duration: Dose dependent: 6-23 hours; **Note:** Duration is dose-dependent. At lower dosages (0.1-0.2 units/kg), mean duration is variable (5.7-12.1 hours). At 0.6 units/kg, the mean duration was 19.9 hours. At high dosages (>0.6 units/kg) the duration is longer and less variable (mean of 22-23 hours).

Bioavailability: 60%

Half-life: 5-7 hours (dose dependent)

Protein binding: >98% (albumin)

Distribution: V_d: 0.1 L/kg

Time to peak, plasma: 6-8 hours

Excretion: Urine

Dosage Also refer to Insulin Regular on page 838.

Notes: Duration is dose-dependent. Dosage must be carefully titrated (adjustment of dose and timing. Adjustment of concomitant antidiabetic treatment (short-acting insulins or oral antidiabetic agents) may be required. In Canada, insulin detemir is not approved for use in children.

SubQ: Children ≥6 years and Adults: Type 1 or type 2 diabetes:

Basal insulin or basal-bolus: May be substituted on a unit-per-unit basis. Adjust dose to achieve glycemic targets.

Insulin-naive patients (type 2 diabetes only): 0.1-0.2 units/kg once daily in the evening or 10 units once or twice daily. Adjust dose to achieve glycemic targets. **Note:** Canadian labeling recommends 10 units once daily (twice daily dosing is not included).

Dosage adjustment in renal impairment: Insulin requirements are reduced due to changes in insulin clearance or metabolism.

Dietary Considerations Dietary modification based on ADA recommendations is a key component of therapy.

Administration Insulin detemir is a clear solution but it is NOT intended for I.V. or I.M. administration.

Insulin detemir (Levemir®): SubQ administration: Cold injections should be avoided. SubQ administration is usually made into the thighs, arms, buttocks, or abdomen, with sites rotated. Not for infusion pumps. Cannot be diluted or mixed with other insulins.

Once daily: Administer with evening meal or at bedtime.

Twice daily: Administer evening dose with evening meal, at bedtime, or 12 hours following morning dose.

Monitoring Parameters Urine sugar and acetone, serum glucose, electrolytes, Hb A_{1c}, lipid profile

Reference Range Refer to Insulin Regular on page 838.

Additional Information The product labeling identifies this product as a long-acting form of insulin; however, at lower dosages (≤0.6 units/kg) its pharmacodynamic characteristics and dosing are consistent with intermediate insulin forms such as NPH.

Dosage Forms Excipient information presented when available (limited, particularly for generics); consult specific product labeling.

Injection, solution:

Levemir®: 100 units/mL (3 mL) [FlexPen® prefilled syringe]; (10 mL) [vial]

Insulin Glargine (IN soo lin GLAR jeen)

Medication Safety Issues

Sound-alike/look-alike issues:

Insulin glargine may be confused with insulin glulisine

Lantus® may be confused with Lente®

Lente® may be confused with Lantus®

High alert medication: The Institute for Safe Medication Practices (ISMP) includes this medication among its list of drugs which have a heightened risk of causing significant patient harm when used in error. ***Due to the number of insulin preparations, it is essential to identify/clarify the type of insulin to be used.***

Related Information

Insulin Regular *on page 838*

U.S. Brand Names Lantus®

Canadian Brand Names Lantus®; Lantus® OptiSet®

Mexican Brand Names Lantus

Index Terms Glargine Insulin

Pharmacologic Category Antidiabetic Agent, Insulin

Generic Available No

Use Treatment of type 1 diabetes mellitus (insulin dependent, IDDM) and type 2 diabetes mellitus (noninsulin dependent, NIDDM) requiring basal (long-acting) insulin to improve glycemic control

Effect on Mental Status May cause drowsiness or confusion

Effect on Psychiatric Treatment MAO inhibitors may enhance the hypoglycemic effects of insulin; TCAs may antagonize the effects of insulin

Pregnancy Risk Factor C

Pregnancy Considerations Adverse events have been shown in some animal studies; therefore, the manufacturer classifies insulin glargine as pregnancy category C. Maternal hyperglycemia can be associated with adverse effects in the fetus, including macrosomia, neonatal hyperglycemia, and hyperbilirubinemia; the risk of congenital malformations is increased when Hb A_{1c} is above the normal range.

Insulin requirements tend to fall during the first trimester of pregnancy and increase in the later trimesters, peaking at 28-32 weeks of gestation. Following delivery, insulin requirements decrease rapidly. Diabetes can be associated with adverse effects in the mother. Poorly-treated diabetes may cause end-organ damage that may in turn negatively affect obstetric outcomes. Physiologic glucose levels should be maintained prior to and during pregnancy to decrease the risk of adverse events in the fetus and the mother. Insulin is the drug of choice for the control of diabetes mellitus during pregnancy. Pregnancy outcome information following the use of insulin glargine is available from case reports and small studies. Current reports indicate that insulin glargine is effective when used during pregnancy and may be an option for pregnant women with significantly uncontrolled diabetes; however, pregnant women using insulin glargine should be switched to NPH insulin pending additional safety information with this agent.

Lactation Excretion in breast milk unknown/compatible

Contraindications Hypersensitivity to insulin glargine or any component of the formulation

Warnings/Precautions Refer to Insulin Regular on page 838. Safety and efficacy not established in children <6 years of age. Insulin glargine is a clear solution, but it is **NOT** intended for I.V. or I.M. administration.

Adverse Reactions Refer to Insulin Regular on page 838.

Metabolism/Transport Effects Refer to Insulin Regular on page 838.

Drug Interactions Refer to Insulin Regular on page 838.

Ethanol/Nutrition/Herb Interactions Refer to Insulin Regular on page 838.

Stability Insulin glargine (Lantus®): Store unopened vials, cartridges, and disposable insulin devices in refrigerator; do not use if it has been frozen. If not refrigerated, use within 28 days and protect from heat and light. Once opened (in use), vials may be stored in refrigerator or for up to 28 days at room temperature. Opened cartridge systems (OptiClik®) and disposable insulin devices (SoloStar®) (in use) should be stored at room temperature and used within 28 days; do not refrigerate.

Mechanism of Action Refer to Insulin Regular on page 838. Insulin glargine is a long-acting insulin analog.

Pharmacodynamics/Kinetics Note: Rate of absorption, onset, and duration of activity may be affected by site of injection, exercise, presence of lipodystrophy, local blood supply, and/or temperature.

Onset of action: 3-4 hours

Peak effect: No pronounced peak

Duration: Generally 24 hours or longer; reported range: 10.8 to >24 hours (up to 32 hours documented in some studies)

Absorption: Slow; upon injection into the subcutaneous tissue, microprecipitates form which allow small amounts of insulin glargine to release over time

Metabolism: Partially metabolized in the skin to form two active metabolites

Time to peak, plasma: No pronounced peak

Excretion: Urine

Dosage SubQ: Adults:

Type 1 diabetes: Refer to Insulin Regular on page 838.

Type 2 diabetes:

Patient not already on insulin: 10 units once daily, adjusted according to patient response (range in clinical study: 2-100 units/day)

Patient already receiving insulin: In clinical studies, when changing to insulin glargine from once-daily NPH or Ultralente® insulin, the initial dose was not changed; when changing from twice-daily NPH to once-daily insulin glargine, the total daily dose was reduced by 20% and adjusted according to patient response

Dosage adjustment in renal impairment: Insulin requirements are reduced due to changes in insulin clearance or metabolism.

Administration Insulin glargine (Lantus®): SubQ administration: Should be administered once daily, at any time of day, but should be administered at the same time each day. Cold injections should be avoided. SubQ administration is usually made into the thighs, arms, buttocks, or abdomen, with sites rotated. Cannot be diluted or mixed with any other insulin or solution. Solution should be clear and colorless with no visible particles; inspect solution prior to administration.

Monitoring Parameters Urine sugar and acetone, serum glucose, electrolytes, Hb A_{1c}

Reference Range Refer to Insulin Regular on page 838.

Additional Information The duration of action of insulin glargine is generally 24 hours or longer with a relatively flat action profile throughout this interval. Many pharmacokinetic and pharmacodynamic studies were terminated at 24 hours despite the fact that insulin glargine continued to exhibit hypoglycemic activity beyond 24 hours; therefore, it is difficult to determine the absolute duration of action.

Clinicians should be aware that, in rare cases, patients may exhibit hypoglycemic activity beyond 24 hours and that accumulation of insulin glargine is possible. Adequate monitoring and subsequent dosage adjustments should be made in patients who are requiring less insulin to maintain euglycemia after several days of therapy.

On the other hand, insulin glargine has a reported duration of action that ranges from 10.8 to >24 hours. On rare occasions, patients may require twice-daily injections of insulin glargine to deliver adequate basal insulin coverage over 24 hours. Some clinicians may also switch to twice-daily dosing in patients who require >100 units of insulin glargine per day to allow for complete absorption. Dosing insulin glargine 3 times daily is not recommended.

Dosage Forms Excipient information presented when available (limited, particularly for generics); consult specific product labeling.

Injection, solution:

Lantus®: 100 units/mL (3 mL) [OptiClik® prefilled cartridge or SoloStar® disposable insulin device]; (10 mL) [vial]

Insulin Glulisine (IN soo lin gloo LIS een)

Medication Safety Issues

Sound-alike/look-alike issues:

Insulin glulisine may be confused with insulin glargine

High alert medication: The Institute for Safe Medication Practices (ISMP) includes this medication among its list of drugs which have a heightened risk of causing significant patient harm when used in error. ***Due to the number of insulin preparations, it is essential to identify/clarify the type of insulin to be used.***

Related Information

Insulin Regular *on page 838*

U.S. Brand Names Apidra®

Canadian Brand Names Apidra®

Index Terms Glulisine Insulin

Pharmacologic Category Antidiabetic Agent, Insulin

Generic Available No

Use Treatment of type 1 diabetes mellitus (insulin dependent, IDDM) and type 2 diabetes mellitus (noninsulin dependent, NIDDM) to improve glycemic control

Effect on Mental Status May cause drowsiness or confusion

Effect on Psychiatric Treatment MAO inhibitors may enhance the hypoglycemic effects of insulin; TCAs may antagonize the effects of insulin

Pregnancy Risk Factor C

Pregnancy Considerations Adverse events were observed in some animal reproduction studies; therefore, the manufacturer classifies insulin glulisine as pregnancy category C. Maternal hyperglycemia can be associated with adverse effects in the fetus, including macrosomia, neonatal hyperglycemia, and hyperbilirubinemia; the risk of congenital malformations is increased when the Hb A_{1c} is above the normal range.

Insulin requirements tend to fall during the first trimester of pregnancy and increase in the later trimesters, peaking at 28-32 weeks of gestation. Following delivery, insulin requirements decrease rapidly. Diabetes can be associated with adverse effects in the mother. Poorly-treated diabetes may cause end-organ damage that may in turn negatively affect obstetric outcomes. Physiologic glucose levels should be maintained prior to and during pregnancy to decrease the risk of adverse events in the fetus and mother. Insulin is the drug of choice for the control of diabetes mellitus during pregnancy. Due to lack of clinical studies with insulin glulisine in pregnant women, the manufacturer recommends use during pregnancy only if the potential benefit to the mother justifies any potential risk to the fetus.

Lactation Excretion in breast milk unknown/compatible

Contraindications Hypersensitivity to insulin glulisine or any component of the formulation; during episodes of hypoglycemia

Warnings/Precautions Refer to Insulin Regular on page 838.

Due to short duration of action, a longer acting insulin or continuous basal administration of insulin via a SubQ infusion pump is needed to maintain adequate glucose control in type 1 diabetes mellitus (insulin dependent, IDDM). In type 2 diabetes mellitus (noninsulin dependent, NIDDM), insulin glulisine may be used without a long-acting insulin or continuous basal administration of insulin via a SubQ infusion pump when used in combination with a sulfonylurea. Preprandial administration should be immediately followed by a meal within

5-10 minutes. Insulin glulisine may be administered I.V. in selected clinical situations to control hyperglycemia.

Adverse Reactions Refer to Insulin Regular on page 838.

Drug Interactions Refer to Insulin Regular on page 838.

Ethanol/Nutrition/Herb Interactions Refer to Insulin Regular on page 838.

Stability Insulin glulisine (Apidra®): Store unopened vials in refrigerator at 2°C to 8°C (36°F to 46°F); do not freeze. Protect from light. Once opened, may store under refrigeration or at room temperature ≤25°C (77°F); use within 28 days. Stable in infusion pump for up to 48 hours. Discard if exposed to temperatures >37°C (98.6°F). Open, in-use cartridges inserted in the Opti-Clik® system should not be refrigerated; keep at room temperature ≤25°C (77°F); use within 28 days.

For I.V. infusion in a controlled clinical setting: The recommended infusion concentration is 0.05-1 unit/mL in NS using PVC bags; store at room temperature. Stable for 48 hours.

Mechanism of Action Refer to Insulin Regular on page 838. Insulin glulisine is a rapid-acting insulin analog.

Pharmacodynamics/Kinetics Note: Rate of absorption, onset, and duration of activity may be affected by site of injection, exercise, presence of lipodystrophy, local blood supply, and/or temperature.

Onset of action: 0.2-0.5 hours

Peak effect: 1.6-2.8 hours

Duration: 3-4 hours

Distribution: I.V.: 13 L

Bioavailability: SubQ: ~70%

Half-life

I.V.: 13 minutes

SubQ: 42 minutes

Time to peak, plasma: 0.6-2 hours

Excretion: Urine

Dosage Refer to Insulin Regular on page 838.

Dosing adjustment in renal impairment: Insulin requirements are reduced due to changes in insulin clearance or metabolism.

Administration Insulin glulisine (Apidra®): SubQ administration: Cold injections should be avoided. SubQ administration is usually made into the thighs, arms, buttocks, or abdomen, with sites rotated. Insulin glulisine should be administered within 15 minutes before or within 20 minutes after start of a meal. Can be infused SubQ into the abdominal wall by external insulin pump; however, when used in an external pump, should not be diluted or mixed with other insulins. Rotate infusion site.

Insulin glulisine may be administered by the I.V. route only in a carefully controlled clinical setting with medical supervision and close monitoring of blood glucose as well as serum potassium. A dedicated infusion line should be used. **Do not administer insulin mixtures intravenously.** The recommended infusion concentration is 0.05-1 unit/mL in NS using PVC bags.

Monitoring Parameters Urine sugar and acetone, serum glucose, electrolytes, Hb A_{1c}, lipid profile

Blood glucose and serum potassium should be closely monitored during I.V. infusion.

Reference Range Refer to Insulin Regular on page 838.

Dosage Forms Excipient information presented when available (limited, particularly for generics); consult specific product labeling.

Injection, solution:

Apidra®: 100 units/mL (3 mL [cartridge], 10 mL [vial])

Insulin Inhalation (IN soo lin in ha LAY shun)

Medication Safety Issues

High alert medication: The Institute for Safe Medication Practices (ISMP) includes this medication among its list of drugs which have a heightened risk of causing significant patient harm when used in error. **Due to the number of insulin preparations, it is essential to identify/clarify the type of insulin to be used. The inhalation form of insulin is expressed in milligrams rather than units, potentially leading to confusion. Absolute conversion between doses of inhalation and injection insulin is not possible.**

Related Information

Insulin Regular *on page 838*

U.S. Brand Names Exubera® [DSC]

Canadian Brand Names Exubera® [DSC]

Mexican Brand Names Exubera

Index Terms Inhaled Insulin

Pharmacologic Category Antidiabetic Agent, Insulin

Generic Available No

Use Treatment of type 1 diabetes mellitus (insulin dependent, IDDM); type 2 diabetes mellitus (noninsulin dependent, NIDDM)

Effect on Mental Status May cause drowsiness or confusion

Effect on Psychiatric Treatment MAO inhibitors may enhance the hypoglycemic effects of insulin; TCAs may antagonize the effects of insulin

Restrictions Product is available only through the Extended Transition Program (ETP) by Pfizer for certain patients meeting inclusion/exclusion requirements unable to transition off inhaled insulin to other agents following the product market withdrawal in October 2007. The ETP allows for continued limited availability through September 2008 to provide additional transition time for these patients. Information on the ETP program is available by calling AmeriPharm (program administrator) at 1-866-376-6500 or at http://www.-exubera.com.

Pregnancy Risk Factor C

Pregnancy Considerations Animal reproduction studies have not been conducted with this dosage form. Absorption of insulin inhalation (Exubera®) in women with gestational and pregestational type 2 diabetes is similar to nonpregnant women with type 2 diabetes. Does not cross the placenta. Insulin is the drug of choice for control of diabetes mellitus during pregnancy.

Lactation Excretion in breast milk unknown/compatible

Contraindications Hypersensitivity to any component of the formulation; smokers or patients who have discontinued smoking for <6 months; poorly-controlled or unstable lung disease

Warnings/Precautions Also refer to Insulin Regular on page 838.

Due to increased systemic absorption, the risk of hypoglycemia is greatly increased in patients who smoke or who have stopped smoking for less than 6 months. The effect of passive exposure to smoke has not been fully evaluated but may result in alteration in absorption and/or hypoglycemia. Insulin inhalation should be immediately discontinued in any patient who resumes smoking.

Decreases in pulmonary function have been associated with use. Due the potential impact on pulmonary function, testing should be performed prior to the initiation of inhaled insulin therapy. Not recommended for use in patients with lung disease (asthma, COPD). Monitor closely during periods of intercurrent respiratory illness. Newly diagnosed cases of primary lung malignancy have been observed rarely in clinical trials and postmarketing. Due to the low incidence, it is unclear if these cases are related to use of inhaled insulin. Patients diagnosed with lung cancer had a prior history of cigarette smoking.

In type 1 diabetes mellitus (insulin dependent, IDDM), rapid-acting insulins including insulin inhalation should be used in combination with a long-acting insulin. However, in type 2 diabetes mellitus (noninsulin dependent, NIDDM), rapid-acting agents may be used without a long-acting insulin when used as monotherapy or combined with an oral antidiabetic agent.

Use caution in renal and/or hepatic impairment.

Adverse Reactions Also refer to Insulin Regular on page 838.

Cardiovascular: Chest pain (5%; usually mild to moderate)

Dermatologic: Rash (rare)

Endocrine & metabolic: Hypoglycemia

Gastrointestinal: Xerostomia (2%)

Otic: Otitis media (pediatric patients 7%), ear pain (4%), ear disorder (1%)

Respiratory: Respiratory infection (30% to 43%), cough increased (22% to 30%), pharyngitis (10% to 18%), rhinitis (9% to 15%), sinusitis (5% to 10%), dyspnea (4%), sputum increased (3% to 4%), bronchitis (3% to 5%), epistaxis (1%), laryngitis (1%), voice alteration (1%), bronchospasm (rare)

Note: Decreases in pulmonary function (reduced FEV1, DLco) have been associated with use, usually noted in the initial weeks of therapy; declines from baseline of 20% in, respectively, FEV1 and DLco, were reported in 5.1% and 1.5% of patients as compared to 3.6% and 1.3% in comparator-treated patients.

Miscellaneous: Allergic reactions, anaphylaxis (including tachycardia and hypotension), diaphoresis increased

Metabolism/Transport Effects Refer to Insulin Regular on page 838.

Drug Interactions Refer to Insulin Regular on page 838.

Ethanol/Nutrition/Herb Interactions Refer to Insulin Regular on page 838.

Stability Insulin inhalation (Exubera®): Store unopened blisters, in-use blisters, and inhaler at controlled room temperature (25°C); excursions permitted to 15°C to 30°C (59°F to 86°F); do not freeze or refrigerate. Once foil overwrap is opened, blisters should be used within 3 months. Avoid exposure to excess humidity.

Mechanism of Action Refer to Insulin Regular on page 838. Insulin inhalation is a rapid-acting form of human insulin.

Pharmacodynamics/Kinetics

Onset of action: 0.2-0.4 hours

Duration: 6-8 hours

Absorption: Rapid

Bioavailability: Absolute bioavailability not defined (depends on inspiratory flow characteristics); systemic exposure may be up to 2-5 times higher in smokers

Time to peak, plasma: 30-90 minutes

Excretion: Urine

Dosage Inhalation: Children ≥6 years and Adults:

Initial: 0.05 mg/kg (rounded down to nearest whole milligram) 3 times/daily administered within 10 minutes of a meal

Adjustment: Dosage may be increased or decreased based on serum glucose monitoring, meal size, nutrient composition, time of day, and exercise patterns.

Note: A 1 mg blister is approximately equivalent to 3 units of regular insulin, while a 3 mg blister is approximately equivalent to 8 units of regular insulin administered subcutaneously. Patients should combine 1 mg and 3 mg blisters so that the fewest blisters are required to achieve the prescribed dose. Consecutive inhalation of three 1 mg blisters results in significantly higher insulin levels as compared to inhalation of a single 3 mg blister (do not substitute). In a patient stabilized on a dosage which uses 3 mg blisters, if 3 mg blister is temporarily unavailable, inhalation of two 1 mg blisters may be substituted.

Dosing adjustment in renal impairment: Insulin requirements are reduced due to changes in insulin clearance or metabolism.

Dietary Considerations Dietary modification based on ADA recommendations is a key component of therapy.

Administration Insulin inhalation (Exubera®): Administer no more than 10 minutes before a meal using the Exubera® inhalation device. The Exubera® Release Unit in the inhaler should be changed every 2 weeks; the Exubera® inhaler may be used for 1 year.

Monitoring Parameters Pulmonary function testing at baseline and periodically during therapy; blood glucose, urine sugar and acetone, serum glucose, electrolytes, Hb A_{1c}, lipid profile

Reference Range Refer to Insulin Regular on page 838.

Dosage Forms Excipient information presented when available (limited, particularly for generics); consult specific product labeling. [DSC] = Discontinued product

Combination package:

- Exubera® Kit [packaged with inhaler, chamber and release unit]:
  - Powder for oral inhalation [prefilled blister pack]: 1 mg/blister (180s) [DSC]
  - Powder for oral inhalation [prefilled blister pack]: 3 mg/blister (90s) [DSC]
- Exubera® Combination Pack 15 [packaged with 2 release units]:
  - Powder for oral inhalation [prefilled blister pack]: 1 mg/blister (180s) [DSC]
  - Powder for oral inhalation [prefilled blister pack]: 3 mg/blister (90s) [DSC]
- Exubera® Combination Pack 12 [packaged with 2 release units]:
  - Powder for oral inhalation [prefilled blister pack]: 1 mg/blister (90s) [DSC]
  - Powder for oral inhalation [prefilled blister pack]: 3 mg/blister (90s) [DSC]

Insulin Lispro (IN soo lin LYE sproe)

Medication Safety Issues

Sound-alike/look-alike issues:

Humalog® may be confused with Humulin®, Humira®

High alert medication: The Institute for Safe Medication Practices (ISMP) includes this medication among its list of drugs which have a heightened risk of causing significant patient harm when used in error. ***Due to the number of insulin preparations, it is essential to identify/clarify the type of insulin to be used.***

Cross-contamination may occur if insulin pens are shared among multiple patients. Steps should be taken to prohibit sharing of insulin pens.

Related Information

Insulin Regular *on page 838*

U.S. Brand Names Humalog®

Canadian Brand Names Humalog®

Mexican Brand Names Humalog

Index Terms Lispro Insulin

Pharmacologic Category Antidiabetic Agent, Insulin

Generic Available No

Use Treatment of type 1 diabetes mellitus (insulin dependent, IDDM) and type 2 diabetes mellitus (noninsulin dependent, NIDDM) to improve glycemic control

Effect on Mental Status May cause drowsiness or confusion

Effect on Psychiatric Treatment MAO inhibitors may enhance the hypoglycemic effects of insulin; TCAs may antagonize the effects of insulin

Pregnancy Risk Factor B

Pregnancy Considerations Adverse events have not been observed in animal reproduction studies; therefore, the manufacturer classifies insulin lispro as pregnancy category B. Insulin lispro has not been shown to cross the placenta at standard clinical doses. Although congenital anomalies have been noted in case reports, when compared to regular insulin, insulin lispro has not been found to increase the risk of adverse events to the fetus in larger studies. Maternal hyperglycemia can be associated with adverse effects in the fetus, including macrosomia, neonatal hyperglycemia, and hyperbilirubinemia; the risk of congenital malformations is increased when Hb A_{1c} is above the normal range.

Insulin requirements tend to fall during the first trimester of pregnancy and increase in the later trimesters, peaking at 28-32 weeks of gestation. Following delivery, insulin requirements decrease rapidly. Diabetes can be associated with adverse effects in the mother. Poorly-treated diabetes may cause end-organ damage that may in turn negatively affect obstetric outcomes. Physiologic glucose levels should be maintained prior to and during pregnancy to decrease the risk of adverse events in the fetus and mother. Insulin is the drug of choice for the control of diabetes mellitus during pregnancy. The use of insulin lispro has been shown to be as effective as regular insulin to treat diabetes in pregnancy and may have advantages over regular insulin during pregnancy.

Lactation Excretion in breast milk unknown/compatible

Contraindications Hypersensitivity to any component of the formulation

Warnings/Precautions Refer to Insulin Regular on page 838 .

Due to short duration of action, a longer acting insulin or continuous basal administration of insulin via a SubQ infusion pump is needed to maintain adequate glucose control in type 1 diabetes mellitus (insulin dependent, IDDM). In type 2 diabetes mellitus (noninsulin dependent, NIDDM), insulin lispro may be used without a long-acting insulin or continuous basal administration of insulin via a SubQ infusion pump when used in combination with a sulfonylurea. Preprandial administration should be immediately followed by a meal within 5-10 minutes. Insulin lispro may be administered I.V. in selected clinical situations to control hyperglycemia.

Adverse Reactions Refer to Insulin Regular on page 838.

Metabolism/Transport Effects Refer to Insulin Regular on page 838.

Drug Interactions Refer to Insulin Regular on page 838.

Ethanol/Nutrition/Herb Interactions Refer to Insulin Regular on page 838.

Stability Insulin lispro (Humalog®): Store unopened container in refrigerator; do not use if it has been frozen. If not refrigerated, use within 28 days and protect from heat and light. Once opened (in use), vials may be stored in refrigerator or for up to 28 days at room temperature. Cartridges/pens should be stored at room temperature and used within 28 days. When used in an external pump, replace insulin in reservoir within 48 hours and cartridges within 7 days; do not expose to temperatures >37°C (98.6°F). If diluted with sterile diluent (available from manufacturer), 1:10 dilutions are stable for 28 days stored at 5°C (41°F) or 14 days stored at 30°C (86°F).

Mechanism of Action Refer to Insulin Regular on page 838. Insulin lispro is a rapid-acting form of insulin.

Pharmacodynamics/Kinetics Note: Rate of absorption, onset, and duration of activity may be affected by site of injection, exercise, presence of lipodystrophy, local blood supply, and/or temperature.

Onset of action: 0.2-0.5 hours

  Peak effect: 1.5-2.5 hours

Duration: 3-4 hours

Distribution: 0.26-0.36 L/kg

Bioavailability: 55% to 77%

Time to peak, plasma: 0.5-1.5 hours

Excretion: Urine

Dosage Refer to Insulin Regular on page 838. Insulin lispro is equipotent to insulin regular, but has a more rapid onset.

Dosing adjustment in renal impairment: Insulin requirements are reduced due to changes in insulin clearance or metabolism.

Dietary Considerations Dietary modification based on ADA recommendations is a key component of therapy.

Administration Insulin lispro (Humalog®): SubQ administration: May be administered within 15 minutes before or immediately after a meal. Cold injections should be avoided. SubQ administration is usually made into the thighs, arms, buttocks, or abdomen, with sites rotated. Can be infused SubQ by external insulin pump; however, when used in an external pump, should not be diluted or mixed with other insulins.

Note: May be mixed in the same syringe as Humulin® N or Humulin® U, but Humalog® should be drawn into the syringe first.

Monitoring Parameters Urine sugar and acetone, serum glucose, electrolytes, Hb A_{1c}, lipid profile

Reference Range Refer to Insulin Regular on page 838.

Dosage Forms Excipient information presented when available (limited, particularly for generics); consult specific product labeling.

Injection, solution:

Humalog®: 100 units/mL (3 mL) [prefilled cartridge or prefilled disposable pen]; (10 mL) [vial]

◆ **Insulin Lispro and Insulin Lispro Protamine** *see* Insulin Lispro Protamine and Insulin Lispro *on page 834*

Insulin Lispro Protamine and Insulin Lispro

(IN soo lin LYE sproe PROE ta meen & IN soo lin LYE sproe)

Medication Safety Issues

Sound-alike/look-alike issues:

Humalog® Mix 75/25™ may be confused with Humulin® 70/30.

High alert medication: The Institute for Safe Medication Practices (ISMP) includes this medication among its list of drugs which have a heightened risk of causing significant patient harm when used in error. ***Due to the number of insulin preparations, it is essential to identify/clarify the type of insulin to be used.***

Cross-contamination may occur if insulin pens are shared among multiple patients. Steps should be taken to prohibit sharing of insulin pens.

Related Information

Insulin Regular *on page 838*

U.S. Brand Names Humalog® Mix 50/50™; Humalog® Mix 75/25™

Canadian Brand Names Humalog® Mix 25

Mexican Brand Names Humalog Mix 25

Index Terms Insulin Lispro and Insulin Lispro Protamine

Pharmacologic Category Antidiabetic Agent, Insulin

Generic Available No

Use Treatment of type 1 diabetes mellitus (insulin dependent, IDDM) and type 2 diabetes mellitus (noninsulin dependent, NIDDM) to improve glycemic control

Effect on Mental Status May cause drowsiness or confusion

Effect on Psychiatric Treatment MAO inhibitors may enhance the hypoglycemic effects of insulin; TCAs may antagonize the effects of insulin

Pregnancy Risk Factor B

Pregnancy Considerations See Insulin Lispro monograph.

Lactation See Insulin Lispro monograph.

Contraindications Hypersensitivity to any component of the formulation; during episodes of hypoglycemia

Warnings/Precautions Refer to Insulin Regular on page 838. Safety and efficacy in children <18 years of age have not been established.

Adverse Reactions Refer to Insulin Regular on page 838.

Drug Interactions Refer to Insulin Regular on page 838.

Ethanol/Nutrition/Herb Interactions Refer to Insulin Regular on page 838.

Stability Insulin lispro protamine and insulin lispro (Humalog® Mix): Store unopened container in refrigerator; do not use if it has been frozen. Once opened (in use), vials may be stored in refrigerator or for up to 28 days at room temperature. Pens should be stored at room temperature and used within 10 days. Do not expose to temperatures >37°C (98.6°F).

Mechanism of Action Refer to Insulin Regular on page 838. Insulin lispro protamine and insulin lispro is a combination product with a rapid onset, and a duration of action which is similar to intermediate-acting insulin products.

Pharmacodynamics/Kinetics Note: Rate of absorption, onset, and duration of activity may be affected by site of injection, exercise, presence of lipodystrophy, local blood supply, and/or temperature.

Onset of action: 0.2-0.5 hours

Peak effect: 2-4 hours

Duration: 18-24 hours

Time to peak, plasma: 0.5-4 hours

Excretion: Urine

Dosage Refer to Insulin Regular on page 838. Fixed ratio insulins (such as insulin lispro protamine and insulin lispro) are normally administered in 2 daily doses.

Dosage adjustment in renal impairment: Insulin requirements are reduced due to changes in insulin clearance or metabolism.

Dietary Considerations Dietary modification based on ADA recommendations is a key component of therapy.

Administration Insulin lispro protamine and insulin lispro (Humalog® Mix 75/25™): SubQ administration only. Should be administered within 15 minutes before or after a meal. Normally administered twice daily (breakfast and supper). Cold injections should be avoided. SubQ administration is usually made into the thighs, arms, buttocks, or abdomen, with sites rotated. Resuspend immediately prior to use. Gently roll vial or pen in the palms of the hands to resuspend before using. Do not mix or dilute with other insulins.

Reference Range Refer to Insulin Regular on page 838.

Additional Information Refer to Insulin Regular on page 838 for additional details on adverse effects, drug interactions, warnings, and dosing of insulin products.

Dosage Forms Excipient information presented when available (limited, particularly for generics); consult specific product labeling.

Injection, suspension:

Humalog® Mix 50/50™: Insulin lispro protamine suspension 50% [intermediate acting] and insulin lispro solution 50% [rapid acting]: 100 units/mL (3 mL) [disposable pen]

Humalog® Mix 75/25™: Insulin lispro protamine suspension 75% [intermediate acting] and insulin lispro solution 25% [rapid acting]: 100 units/mL (3 mL) [disposable pen]; (10 mL) [vial]

Insulin NPH (IN soo lin N P H)

Medication Safety Issues

Sound-alike/look-alike issues:

Humulin® may be confused with Humalog®, Humira®

Novolin® may be confused with NovoLog®

High alert medication: The Institute for Safe Medication Practices (ISMP) includes this medication among its list of drugs which have a heightened risk of causing significant patient harm when used in error. ***Due to the number of insulin preparations, it is essential to identify/clarify the type of insulin to be used.***

Cross-contamination may occur if insulin pens are shared among multiple patients. Steps should be taken to prohibit sharing of insulin pens.

Related Information

Insulin Regular *on page 838*

U.S. Brand Names Humulin® N; Novolin® N

Canadian Brand Names Humulin® N; Novolin® ge NPH

Mexican Brand Names Humulin N; Novolin N

Index Terms Isophane Insulin; NPH Insulin

Pharmacologic Category Antidiabetic Agent, Insulin

Generic Available No

Use Treatment of type 1 diabetes mellitus (insulin dependent, IDDM) and type 2 diabetes mellitus (noninsulin dependent, NIDDM) to improve glycemic control

Effect on Mental Status May cause drowsiness or confusion

Effect on Psychiatric Treatment MAO inhibitors may enhance the hypoglycemic effects of insulin; TCAs may antagonize the effects of insulin

Pregnancy Considerations Maternal hyperglycemia can be associated with adverse effects in the fetus, including macrosomia, neonatal hyperglycemia, and hyperbilirubinemia; the risk of congenital malformations is increased when the Hb A_{1c} is above the normal range. Insulin requirements tend to fall during the first trimester of pregnancy and increase in the later trimesters, peaking at 28-32 weeks of gestation. Following delivery, insulin requirements decrease rapidly. Diabetes can be associated with adverse effects in the mother. Poorly-treated diabetes may cause end-organ damage that may in turn negatively affect obstetric outcomes. Physiologic glucose levels should be maintained prior to and during pregnancy to decrease the risk of adverse events in the fetus and the mother. Insulin is the drug of choice for the control of diabetes mellitus during pregnancy. NPH insulin is preferred over other intermediate-acting insulin products during pregnancy.

Lactation Excretion in breast milk unknown/compatible

Contraindications Hypersensitivity to any component of the formulation

Warnings/Precautions Refer to Insulin Regular on page 838.

Adverse Reactions Refer to Insulin Regular on page 838.

Metabolism/Transport Effects Refer to Insulin Regular on page 838.

Drug Interactions Refer to Insulin Regular on page 838.

Ethanol/Nutrition/Herb Interactions Refer to Insulin Regular on page 838.

Stability Insulin NPH (Humulin® N, Novolin® N): Store unopened container in refrigerator at 2°C to 8°C (36°F to 46°F); do not freeze. Vial in use may be stored under refrigeration or at room temperature. Humulin® N Pen in use should not be refrigerated; store below 30°C (86°F) away from direct heat or light; discard after 2 weeks.

Mechanism of Action Refer to Insulin Regular on page 838. Insulin NPH is an intermediate-acting form of insulin.

Pharmacodynamics/Kinetics Note: Rate of absorption, onset, and duration of activity may be affected by site of injection, exercise, presence of lipodystrophy, local blood supply, and/or temperature.

Onset of action: 1-2 hours

Peak effect: 4-12 hours

Duration: 18-24 hours

Time to peak, plasma: 6-12 hours

Excretion: Urine

Dosage Refer to Insulin Regular on page 838. Insulin NPH is usually administered 1-2 times daily.

Dosing adjustment in renal impairment: Insulin requirements are reduced due to changes in insulin clearance or metabolism.

Dietary Considerations Dietary modification based on ADA recommendations is a key component of therapy.

Administration Insulin NPH (intermediate-acting insulin): SubQ administration: May be administered 1-2 times/day. Cold injections should be avoided. SubQ administration is usually made into the thighs, arms, buttocks, or abdomen, with sites rotated. When mixing regular insulin with other preparations of insulin, regular insulin should be drawn into syringe first. Gently roll vial or pen in the palms of the hands to resuspend before using. Insulin lispro (Humalog®) may be mixed in the same syringe as Humulin® N, but Humalog® should be drawn into the syringe first.

Monitoring Parameters Urine sugar and acetone, serum glucose, electrolytes, Hb A_{1c}, lipid profile

Reference Range Refer to Insulin Regular on page 838.

Dosage Forms Excipient information presented when available (limited, particularly for generics); consult specific product labeling. [CAN] = Canadian brand name

Injection, suspension:

Humulin® N: 100 units/mL (3 mL) [disposable pen]; (10 mL) [vial]

Novolin® ge NPH [CAN]: 100 units/mL (3 mL) [NovolinSet® prefilled syringe or PenFill® prefilled cartridge]; 10 mL [vial]

Novolin® N: 100 units/mL (3 mL) [InnoLet® prefilled syringe or PenFill® prefilled cartridge]; (10 mL) [vial]

Insulin NPH and Insulin Regular

(IN soo lin N P H & IN soo lin REG yoo ler)

Medication Safety Issues

Sound-alike/look-alike issues:

Humulin® 70/30 may be confused with Humalog® Mix 75/25

Novolin® 70/30 may be confused with NovoLog® Mix 70/30

High alert medication: The Institute for Safe Medication Practices (ISMP) includes this medication among its list of drugs which have a heightened risk of causing significant patient harm when used in error. ***Due to the number of insulin preparations, it is essential to identify/clarify the type of insulin to be used.***

Cross-contamination may occur if insulin pens are shared among multiple patients. Steps should be taken to prohibit sharing of insulin pens.

Related Information

Insulin Regular *on page 838*

U.S. Brand Names Humulin® 50/50; Humulin® 70/30; Novolin® 70/30

Canadian Brand Names Humulin® 20/80; Humulin® 70/30; Novolin® ge 30/70; Novolin® ge 40/60; Novolin® ge 50/50

Mexican Brand Names Humulin 30 70; Novolin 70/30

Index Terms Insulin Regular and Insulin NPH; Isophane Insulin and Regular Insulin; NPH Insulin and Regular Insulin

Pharmacologic Category Antidiabetic Agent, Insulin

Generic Available No

Use Treatment of type 1 diabetes mellitus (insulin dependent, IDDM) and type 2 diabetes mellitus (noninsulin dependent, NIDDM) to improve glycemic control

Effect on Mental Status May cause drowsiness or confusion

Effect on Psychiatric Treatment MAO inhibitors may enhance the hypoglycemic effects of insulin; TCAs may antagonize the effects of insulin

Pregnancy Considerations See individual agents.

Contraindications Hypersensitivity to any component of the formulation; during episodes of hypoglycemia

Warnings/Precautions Refer to Insulin Regular on page 838.

Drug Interactions

Antidiabetic Agents (Thiazolidinedione): Insulin may enhance the fluid-retaining effect of Antidiabetic Agents (Thiazolidinedione). *Risk C: Monitor therapy*

Beta-Blockers: May enhance the hypoglycemic effect of Insulin. **Exceptions:** Levobunolol; Metipranolol. *Risk C: Monitor therapy*

Corticosteroids (Orally Inhaled): May diminish the hypoglycemic effect of Antidiabetic Agents. In some instances, corticosteroid-mediated HPA axis suppression has led to episodes of acute adrenal crisis, which may manifest as enhanced hypoglycemia, particularly in the setting of insulin or other antidiabetic agent use. *Risk C: Monitor therapy*

Corticosteroids (Systemic): May diminish the hypoglycemic effect of Antidiabetic Agents. In some instances, corticosteroid-mediated HPA axis suppression has led to episodes of acute adrenal crisis, which may manifest as enhanced hypoglycemia, particularly in the setting of insulin or other antidiabetic agent use. *Risk C: Monitor therapy*

Edetate CALCIUM Disodium: May enhance the hypoglycemic effect of Insulin. *Risk C: Monitor therapy*

Edetate Disodium: May enhance the hypoglycemic effect of Insulin. *Risk C: Monitor therapy*

Herbs (Hypoglycemic Properties): May enhance the hypoglycemic effect of Hypoglycemic Agents. *Risk C: Monitor therapy*

Luteinizing Hormone-Releasing Hormone Analogs: May diminish the therapeutic effect of Antidiabetic Agents. *Risk C: Monitor therapy*

Pegvisomant: May enhance the hypoglycemic effect of Antidiabetic Agents. *Risk C: Monitor therapy*

Quinolone Antibiotics: Insulin may enhance the hyperglycemic effect of Quinolone Antibiotics. Insulin may enhance the hypoglycemic effect of Quinolone Antibiotics. *Risk C: Monitor therapy*

Somatropin: May diminish the hypoglycemic effect of Antidiabetic Agents. *Risk D: Consider therapy modification*

Stability Store unopened container in refrigerator. Do not use if it has been frozen. The pen in use should not be refrigerated; store below 30°C (86°F) away from direct heat or light; discard after 10 days. If refrigeration is not available, opened vials may be stored unrefrigerated in cool place away from heat and sunlight.

Mechanism of Action Refer to Insulin Regular on page 838. Insulin NPH and insulin regular is a combination insulin product with intermediate-acting characteristics. It may be administered once or twice daily.

Pharmacodynamics/Kinetics Note: Rate of absorption, onset, and duration of activity may be affected by site of injection, exercise, presence of lipodystrophy, local blood supply, and/or temperature.

Onset of action: 0.5 hours

Peak effect: 2-12 hours

Duration: 18-24 hours

Time to peak, plasma: 0.8-2 hours

Excretion: Urine

Dosage Refer to Insulin Regular on page 838. Fixed ratio insulins are normally administered in 1-2 daily doses.

Administration SubQ administration only. Should be administered ~30 minutes before a meal. Normally administered once or twice daily (before breakfast and supper). Cold injections should be avoided. SubQ administration is usually made into the thighs, arms, buttocks, or abdomen, with sites rotated. Resuspend immediately prior to use. Gently roll vial or pen in the palms of the hands to resuspend before using.

Reference Range Refer to Insulin Regular on page 838.

Additional Information Refer to Insulin Regular on page 838 for additional details on adverse effects, drug interactions, warnings, and dosing of insulin products.

Dosage Forms Excipient information presented when available (limited, particularly for generics); consult specific product labeling.

Injection, suspension:

Humulin® 50/50: Insulin NPH suspension 50% [intermediate acting] and insulin regular solution 50% [short acting]: 100 units/mL (10 mL) [vial]

Humulin® 70/30: Insulin NPH suspension 70% [intermediate acting] and insulin regular solution 30% [short acting]: 100 units/mL (3 mL) [disposable pen]; (10 mL) [vial]

Novolin® 70/30: Insulin NPH suspension 70% [intermediate acting] and insulin regular solution 30% [short acting]: 100 units/mL (3 mL) [InnoLet® prefilled syringe or PenFill® prefilled cartridge]; (10 mL) [vial]

Additional formulations available in Canada: Injection, suspension:

Humulin® 20/80: Insulin regular solution 20% [short acting] and insulin NPH suspension 80% [intermediate acting]: 100 units/mL (3 mL) [PenFill® prefilled cartridge]

Novolin® ge 30/70: Insulin regular solution 30% [short acting] and insulin NPH suspension 70% [intermediate acting]: 100 units/mL (3 mL) [prefilled syringe or PenFill® prefilled cartridge]; (10 mL) [vial]

Novolin® ge 40/60: Insulin regular solution 40% [short acting] and insulin NPH suspension 60% [intermediate acting]: 100 units/mL (3 mL) [PenFill® prefilled cartridge]

Novolin® ge 50/50: Insulin regular solution 50% [short acting] and insulin NPH suspension 50% [intermediate acting]: 100 units/mL (3 mL) [PenFill® prefilled cartridge]

Insulin Regular (IN soo lin REG yoo ler)

Medication Safety Issues

Sound-alike/look-alike issues:

Humulin® may be confused with Humalog®, Humira®

Novolin® may be confused with NovoLog®

High alert medication: The Institute for Safe Medication Practices (ISMP) includes this medication among its list of drugs which have a heightened risk of causing significant patient harm when used in error. ***Due to the number of insulin preparations, it is essential to identify/clarify the type of insulin to be used.***

Concentrated solutions (eg, U-500) should not be available in patient care areas.

Cross-contamination may occur if insulin pens are shared among multiple patients. Steps should be taken to prohibit sharing of insulin pens.

Related Information

Insulin Aspart *on page 822*
Insulin Aspart Protamine and Insulin Aspart *on page 824*
Insulin Detemir *on page 825*
Insulin Glargine *on page 827*
Insulin Glulisine *on page 829*
Insulin Lispro *on page 832*
Insulin Lispro Protamine and Insulin Lispro *on page 834*
Insulin NPH *on page 835*
Insulin NPH and Insulin Regular *on page 836*

U.S. Brand Names Humulin® R; Humulin® R U-500; Novolin® R

Canadian Brand Names Humulin® R; Novolin® ge Toronto

Index Terms Regular Insulin

Pharmacologic Category Antidiabetic Agent, Insulin; Antidote

Generic Available No

Use Treatment of type 1 diabetes mellitus (insulin dependent, IDDM); type 2 diabetes mellitus (noninsulin dependent, NIDDM) unresponsive to treatment with diet and/or oral hypoglycemics, to improve glycemic control; adjunct to parenteral nutrition; diabetic ketoacidosis (DKA)

Unlabeled/Investigational Use Hyperkalemia (regular insulin only; use with glucose to shift potassium into cells to lower serum potassium levels)

Effect on Mental Status May cause drowsiness or confusion

Effect on Psychiatric Treatment MAO inhibitors may enhance the hypoglycemic effects of insulin; TCAs may antagonize the effects of insulin

Pregnancy Risk Factor B

Pregnancy Considerations Insulin has not been found to cross the placenta, but insulin bound to anti-insulin antibodies has been detected in cord blood. Maternal hyperglycemia can be associated with adverse effects in the fetus, including macrosomia, neonatal hyperglycemia, and hyperbilirubinemia; the risk of congenital malformations is increased when the Hb A_{1c} is above the normal range. Insulin requirements tend to fall during the first trimester of pregnancy and increase in the later trimesters, peaking at 28-32 weeks of gestation. Following delivery, insulin requirements decrease rapidly. Diabetes can be associated with adverse effects in the mother. Poorly-treated diabetes may cause end-organ damage that may in turn negatively affect obstetric outcomes. Physiologic glucose levels should be maintained prior to and during pregnancy to decrease the risk of adverse events in the fetus and the mother. Insulin is the drug of choice for the control of diabetes mellitus during pregnancy.

Lactation Excretion in breast milk unknown/compatible

Contraindications Hypersensitivity to any component of the formulation

Warnings/Precautions Hypoglycemia is the most common adverse effect of insulin. The timing of hypoglycemia differs among various insulin formulations. Hypoglycemia may result from increased work or exercise without eating; use of long-acting insulin preparations (insulin detemir, insulin glargine) may delay recovery from hypoglycemia. Profound and prolonged episodes of hypoglycemia may result in convulsions, unconsciousness, temporary or permanent brain damage or even death. Insulin requirements may be altered during illness, emotional disturbances or other stresses. Insulin may produce hypokalemia which, if left untreated, may result in respiratory paralysis, ventricular arrhythmia and even death. Use with caution in patients at risk for hypokalemia (eg, I.V. insulin use). Use with caution in renal or hepatic impairment.

Human insulin differs from animal-source insulin. Any change of insulin should be made cautiously; changing manufacturers, type, and/or method of manufacture may result in the need for a change of dosage.

Regular insulin is the only insulin to be used intravenously. Insulin aspart may also be administered I.V. in selected clinical situations to control hyperglycemia; close medical supervision is required.

The general objective of exogenous insulin therapy is to approximate the physiologic pattern of insulin secretion which is characterized by two distinct phases. Phase 1 insulin secretion suppresses hepatic glucose production and phase 2 insulin secretion occurs in response to carbohydrate ingestion; therefore, exogenous insulin therapy may consist of basal insulin (eg, intermediate- or long-acting insulin or continuous insulin infusion administered via an external SubQ insulin infusion pump) and/or preprandial insulin (eg, short- or rapid-acting insulin). Patients with type 1 diabetes do not produce endogenous insulin; therefore, these patients require both basal and preprandial insulin administration. Patients with type 2 diabetes retain some beta-cell function in the early stages of their disease; however, as the disease progresses, phase 1 insulin secretion may become completely impaired and phase 2 insulin secretion becomes delayed and/or inadequate in response to meals. Therefore, patients with type 2 diabetes may be treated with oral antidiabetic agents, basal insulin, and/or preprandial insulin depending on the stage of disease and current glycemic control. Since treatment regimens often consist of multiple agents, dosage adjustments must address the specific phase of insulin release that is primarily contributing to the patient's impaired glycemic control. Treatment and monitoring regimens must be individualized.

Adverse Reactions Frequency not defined.

Cardiovascular: Palpitation, pallor, tachycardia

Central nervous system: Fatigue, headache, hypothermia, loss of consciousness, mental confusion

Dermatologic: Urticaria, redness

Endocrine & metabolic: Hypoglycemia, hypokalemia

Gastrointestinal: Hunger, nausea, numbness of mouth, weight gain

Local: Atrophy or hypertrophy of SubQ fat tissue; edema, itching, pain or warmth at injection site; stinging

Neuromuscular & skeletal: Muscle weakness, paresthesia, tremor

Ocular: Transient presbyopia or blurred vision

Miscellaneous: Anaphylaxis, antibodies to insulin (no change in efficacy), diaphoresis, local allergy, systemic allergic symptoms

Metabolism/Transport Effects Induces CYP1A2 (weak)

Drug Interactions

Antidiabetic Agents (Thiazolidinedione): Insulin may enhance the fluid-retaining effect of Antidiabetic Agents (Thiazolidinedione). *Risk C: Monitor therapy*

Beta-Blockers: May enhance the hypoglycemic effect of Insulin. **Exceptions:** Levobunolol; Metipranolol. *Risk C: Monitor therapy*

Corticosteroids (Orally Inhaled): May diminish the hypoglycemic effect of Antidiabetic Agents. In some instances, corticosteroid-mediated HPA axis suppression has led to episodes of acute adrenal crisis, which may manifest as enhanced hypoglycemia, particularly in the setting of insulin or other antidiabetic agent use. *Risk C: Monitor therapy*

Corticosteroids (Systemic): May diminish the hypoglycemic effect of Antidiabetic Agents. In some instances, corticosteroid-mediated HPA axis suppression has led to episodes of acute adrenal crisis, which may manifest as enhanced hypoglycemia, particularly in the setting of insulin or other antidiabetic agent use. *Risk C: Monitor therapy*

Edetate CALCIUM Disodium: May enhance the hypoglycemic effect of Insulin. *Risk C: Monitor therapy*

Edetate Disodium: May enhance the hypoglycemic effect of Insulin. *Risk C: Monitor therapy*

Herbs (Hypoglycemic Properties): May enhance the hypoglycemic effect of Hypoglycemic Agents. *Risk C: Monitor therapy*

Luteinizing Hormone-Releasing Hormone Analogs: May diminish the therapeutic effect of Antidiabetic Agents. *Risk C: Monitor therapy*

Pegvisomant: May enhance the hypoglycemic effect of Antidiabetic Agents. *Risk C: Monitor therapy*

Quinolone Antibiotics: Insulin may enhance the hyperglycemic effect of Quinolone Antibiotics. Insulin may enhance the hypoglycemic effect of Quinolone Antibiotics. *Risk C: Monitor therapy*

Somatropin: May diminish the hypoglycemic effect of Antidiabetic Agents. *Risk D: Consider therapy modification*

Ethanol/Nutrition/Herb Interactions

Ethanol: Caution with ethanol (may increase hypoglycemia).

Food: Insulin shifts potassium from extracellular to intracellular space. Decreases potassium serum concentration.

Herb/Nutraceutical: Use caution with chromium, garlic, gymnema (may increase hypoglycemia).

Stability Insulin, regular (Humulin® R, Novolin® R): Store unopened containers in refrigerator at 2°C to 8°C (36°F to 46°F); do not freeze. Vial in use may be stored under refrigeration or at room temperature; store below 30°C (86°F) away from direct heat or light. Regular insulin should only be used if clear.

Note: Standard diluent for regular insulin: 100 units/100 mL NS; all bags should be prepared fresh; tubing should be flushed 30 minutes prior to administration to allow adsorption as time permits. Can be given as a more diluted solution (eg, 100 units/250 mL 0.45% NS).

Mechanism of Action Insulin acts via specific membrane-bound receptors on target tissues to regulate metabolism of carbohydrate, protein, and fats. Insulin facilitates entry of glucose into muscle, adipose, and other tissues via hexose transporters, including GLUT4. Insulin stimulates the cellular uptake of amino acids and increases cellular permeability to several ions, including potassium, magnesium, and phosphate. By activating sodium-potassium ATPases, insulin promotes the intracellular movement of potassium.

Target organs for insulin include the liver, skeletal muscle, and adipose tissue. Within the liver, insulin stimulates hepatic glycogen synthesis through the activation of the enzymes hexokinase, phosphofructokinase, and glycogen synthase as well as the inhibition of glucose-6 phosphatase. Insulin promotes hepatic synthesis of fatty acids, which are released into the circulation as lipoproteins. Skeletal muscle effects of insulin include increased protein synthesis and increased glycogen synthesis. Within adipose tissue, insulin stimulates the processing of circulating lipoproteins to provide free fatty acids, facilitating triglyceride synthesis and storage by adipocytes. Insulin also directly inhibits the hydrolysis of triglycerides.

Normally secreted by the pancreas, insulin products are manufactured for pharmacologic use through recombinant DNA technology using either *E. coli* or *Saccharomyces cerevisiae*. Insulins are categorized based on promptness and duration of effect, including rapid-, short-, intermediate-, and long-acting insulins.

Pharmacodynamics/Kinetics Note: Rate of absorption, onset, and duration of activity may be affected by site of injection, exercise, presence of lipodystrophy, local blood supply, and/or temperature.

Onset of action: 0.5 hours

Peak effect: 2.5-5 hours

Duration: 4-12 hours (may increase with dose)

Time to peak, plasma: 0.8-2 hours

Excretion: Urine

Dosage SubQ (regular insulin may also be administered I.V.): The number and size of daily doses, time of administration, and diet and exercise require continuous medical supervision. In addition, specific formulations may require distinct administration procedures.

Type 1 Diabetes Mellitus: Children and Adults: **Note:** Multiple daily doses guided by blood glucose monitoring are the standard of diabetes care. Combinations of insulin are commonly used.

Initial dose: 0.2-0.6 units/kg/day in divided doses. Conservative initial doses of 0.2-0.4 units/kg/day are often recommended to avoid the potential for hypoglycemia.

Division of daily insulin requirement: Generally, 50% to 75% of the daily insulin dose is given as an intermediate- or long-acting form of insulin (in 1-2 daily injections). The remaining portion of the 24-hour insulin requirement is divided and administered as a rapid-acting or short-acting form of insulin. These may be given with meals (before or at the time of meals depending on the form of insulin) or at the same time as injections of intermediate forms (some premixed combinations are intended for this purpose).

Adjustment of dose: Dosage must be titrated to achieve glucose control and avoid hypoglycemia. Adjust dose to maintain premeal and bedtime glucose of 80-140 mg/dL (children <5 years: 100-200 mg/dL). Since combinations of agents are frequently used, dosage adjustment must address the individual component of the insulin regimen which most directly influences the blood glucose value in question, based on the known onset and duration of the insulin component. Also see Additional Information.

Usual maintenance range: 0.5-1.2 units/kg/day in divided doses. An estimate of anticipated needs may be based on body weight and/or activity factors as follows:

Adolescents: May require ≤1.5 units/kg/day during growth spurts

Nonobese: 0.4-0.6 units/kg/day

Obese: 0.8-1.2 units/kg/day

Renal failure: Due to alterations in pharmacokinetics of insulin, may require <0.2 units/kg/day

Type 2 Diabetes Mellitus:

Augmentation therapy: Dosage must be carefully adjusted.

Insulins other than glargine: Initial dosage of 0.15-0.2 units/kg/day have been recommended

Insulin glargine: Initial dose: 10 units/day

Note: Administered when residual beta-cell function is present, as a supplemental agent when oral hypoglycemics have not achieved goal glucose control. Twice daily NPH, or an evening dose of NPH, lente, or glargine insulin may be added to oral therapy with metformin or a sulfonylurea. Augmentation to control postprandial glucose may be accomplished with regular, glulisine, aspart, or lispro insulin.

Monotherapy: Initial dose: Highly variable: See Augmentation therapy dosing.

Note: An empirically-defined scheme for dosage estimation based on fasting plasma glucose and degree of obesity has been published with recommended doses ranging from 6-77 units/day (Holman, 1995). In the setting of glucose toxicity (loss of beta-cell sensitivity to glucose concentrations), insulin therapy may be used for short-term management to restore sensitivity of beta-cells; in these cases, the dose may need to be rapidly reduced/withdrawn when sensitivity is re-established.

Diabetic ketoacidosis:

Children <20 years:

I.V.: Regular insulin infused at 0.1 units/kg/hour; continue until acidosis clears, then decrease to 0.05 units/kg/hour until SubQ replacement dosing can be initiated

SubQ, I.M.: If no I.V. infusion access, regular insulin 0.1 units/kg I.M. bolus followed by 0.1 units/kg/hour SubQ or I.M.; continue until acidosis clears, then decrease to 0.05 units/kg/hour until SubQ replacement dosing can be initiated

Adults:

I.V.: Regular insulin 0.15 units/kg initially followed by an infusion of 0.1 units/kg/hour

SubQ, I.M.: Regular insulin 0.4 units/kg given half as I.V. bolus and half as SubQ or I.M., followed by 0.1 units/kg/hour SubQ or I.M.

If serum glucose does not fall by 50-70 mg/dL in the first hour, double insulin dose hourly until glucose falls at an hourly rate of 50-70 mg/dL. Decrease dose to 0.05-0.1 units/kg/hour once serum glucose reaches 250 mg/dL.

Note: Newly-diagnosed patients with IDDM presenting in DKA and patients with blood sugars <800 mg/dL may be relatively "sensitive" to insulin and should receive loading and initial maintenance doses ~50% of those indicated.

Infusion should continue until reversal of acid-base derangement/ketonemia. Serum glucose is not a direct indicator of these abnormalities, and may decrease more rapidly than correction of the range of metabolic abnormalities.

Hyperkalemia (unlabeled use): Children and Adults: I.V.: Administer dextrose at 0.5-1 mL/kg and regular insulin 1 unit for every 4-5 g dextrose given

Dosing adjustment in renal impairment (regular): Insulin requirements are reduced due to changes in insulin clearance or metabolism. Close monitoring of blood glucose and adjustment of therapy is required in renal impairment.

Cl_{cr} 10-50 mL/minute: Administer at 75% of normal dose

Cl_{cr} <10 mL/minute: Administer at 25% to 50% of normal dose and monitor glucose closely

Hemodialysis: Because of a large molecular weight (6000 daltons), insulin is not significantly removed by either peritoneal or hemodialysis

Supplemental dose is not necessary

Peritoneal dialysis: Supplemental dose is not necessary

Continuous arteriovenous or venovenous hemofiltration effects: Supplemental dose is not necessary

Dietary Considerations Dietary modification based on ADA recommendations is a part of therapy.

Administration

SubQ administration: Cold injections should be avoided. SubQ administration is usually made into the thighs, arms, buttocks, or abdomen, with sites rotated. When mixing regular insulin with other preparations of insulin, regular insulin should be drawn into syringe first. Except for rapid-acting, short-acting, or insulin detemir or glargine, gently roll vial or pen in the palms of the hands to resuspend before using. When rapid-acting insulin is mixed with an intermediate- or long-acting insulin, it should be administered within 15 minutes before a meal.

Human regular insulin: Should be administered within 30-60 minutes before a meal; may be administered by SubQ, I.M., or I.V. routes.

I.V. administration (requires use of an infusion pump): May be administered I.V. with close monitoring of blood glucose and serum potassium.

I.V. infusions: To minimize adsorption problems to I.V. solution bag:

If new tubing is **not** needed: Wait a minimum of 30 minutes between the preparation of the solution and the initiation of the infusion.

If new tubing is needed: After receiving the insulin drip solution, the administration set should be attached to the I.V. container and the line should be flushed with the insulin solution. The nurse should wait 30 minutes, then flush the line again with the insulin solution prior to initiating the infusion.

If insulin is required prior to the availability of the insulin drip, regular insulin should be administered by I.V. push injection.

Because of adsorption, the actual amount of insulin being administered could be substantially less than the apparent amount. Therefore, adjustment of the insulin drip rate should be based on effect and not solely on the apparent insulin dose. Furthermore, the apparent dose should not be used as the basis for determining the subsequent insulin dose upon discontinuing the insulin drip. Dose requires continuous medical supervision.

Monitoring Parameters Urine sugar and acetone, serum glucose, electrolytes, Hb A_{1c}, lipid profile

DKA: Arterial blood gases, CBC with differential, urinalysis, serum glucose (baseline and every hour until reaches 250 mg/dL), BUN, creatinine, electrolytes, anion gap

Hyperkalemia: Serum potassium and glucose must be closely monitored to avoid hypoglycemia and/or hypokalemia.

Reference Range

Therapeutic, serum insulin (fasting): 5-20 µIU/mL (SI: 35-145 pmol/L)

Glucose, fasting:

Newborns: 60-110 mg/dL

Adults: 60-110 mg/dL

Elderly: 100-180 mg/dL

Recommendations for glycemic control, adults with type 1 diabetes:

Hb A_{1c}: <7%

Preprandial capillary plasma glucose: 70-130 mg/dL

Peak postprandial capillary blood glucose: <180 mg/dL

Blood pressure: <130/80 mm Hg

Criteria for diagnosis of DKA:

Serum glucose: >250 mg/dL

Arterial pH: <7.3
Bicarbonate: <15 mEq/L
Moderate ketonuria or ketonemia

Additional Information

Split-mixed or basal-bolus regimens: Combination regimens which exploit differences in the onset and duration of different insulin products are commonly used to approximate physiologic secretion. In split-mixed regimens, an intermediate-acting insulin (such as NPH insulin) is administered once or twice daily and supplemented by short-acting (regular) or rapid-acting (lispro, aspart, or glulisine) insulin. Blood glucose measurements are completed several times daily. Dosages are adjusted emphasizing the individual component of the regimen which most directly influences the blood sugar in question (either the intermediate-acting component or the shorter-acting component). Fixed-ratio formulations (eg, 70/30 mix) may be used as twice daily injections in this scenario; however, the ability to titrate the dosage of an individual component is limited. A example of a "split-mixed" regimen would be 21 units of NPH plus 9 units of regular insulin in the morning and an evening meal dose consisting of 14 units of NPH plus 6 units of regular insulin.

Basal-bolus regimens are designed to more closely mimic physiologic secretion. These employ a long-acting insulin (eg, glargine) to simulate basal insulin secretion. The basal component is frequently administered at bedtime or in the early morning. This is supplemented by multiple daily injections of very rapid-acting products (lispro or aspart) immediately prior to a meal, which provides insulin at the time when nutrients are absorbed. An example of a basal-bolus regimen would be 30 units of glargine at bedtime and 12 units of lispro insulin prior to each meal.

Estimation of the effect per unit: A "Rule of 1500" has been frequently used as a means to estimate the change in blood sugar relative to each unit of insulin administered. In fact, the recommended values used in these calculations may vary from 1500-2200 (a value of 1500 is generally recommended for regular insulin while 1800 is recommended for "rapid-acting insulins"). The higher values lead to more conservative estimates of the effect per unit of insulin, and therefore lead to more cautious adjustments. The effect per unit of insulin is approximated by dividing the selected numerical value (eg, 1500-2200) by the number of units/day received by the patient. This may be used as a crude approximation of the patient's insulin sensitivity as adjustments to individual components of the regimen are made. Each additional unit of insulin added to the corresponding insulin dose may be expected to lower the blood glucose by this amount.

To illustrate, in the "basal-bolus" regimen example presented above, the rule of 1800 would indicate an expected change of 27 mg/dL per unit of lispro insulin (the total daily insulin dose is 66 units; using the formula: 1800/66 = 27). A patient may be instructed to add additional insulin if the preprandial glucose is >125 mg/dL. For a prelunch glucose of 195 mg/dL, this would mean the patient would administer the scheduled 12 units of lispro along with an additional "correctional" 3 units for a total of 15 units prior to the meal. If correctional doses are required on a consistent basis, an adjustment of the patients diet and/or scheduled insulin dose may be necessary.

Dosage Forms Excipient information presented when available (limited, particularly for generics); consult specific product labeling.

Injection, solution:
- Humulin® R: 100 units/mL (10 mL)
- Novolin® R: 100 units/mL (3 mL) [InnoLet® prefilled syringe or PenFill® prefilled cartridge]; (10 mL) [vial]

Injection, solution [concentrate]:
- Humulin® R U-500: 500 units/mL (20 mL vial)

- ◆ **Insulin Regular and Insulin NPH** *see* Insulin NPH and Insulin Regular *on page 836*
- ◆ **Intal®** *see* Cromolyn *on page 402*
- ◆ **Integrilin®** *see* Eptifibatide *on page 550*
- ◆ **Intelence™** *see* Etravirine *on page 608*
- ◆ **α-2-interferon** *see* Interferon Alfa-2b *on page 844*
- ◆ **Interferon Alfa-2a (PEG Conjugate)** *see* Peginterferon Alfa-2a *on page 1236*
- ◆ **Interferon Alfa-2b and Ribavirin Combination Pack** *see* Interferon Alfa-2b and Ribavirin *on page 846*
- ◆ **Interferon Alfa-2b (PEG Conjugate)** *see* Peginterferon Alfa-2b *on page 1237*

Interferon Alfa-2a (in ter FEER on AL fa too aye)

Medication Safety Issues

Sound-alike/look-alike issues:

Interferon alfa-2a may be confused with interferon alfa-2b, interferon alfa-n3, pegylated interferon alfa-2b

Roferon-A® may be confused with Rocephin®

International issues:

Interferon alfa-2a may be confused with interferon alpha multi-subtype which is available in international markets

U.S. Brand Names Roferon®-A [DSC]

Canadian Brand Names Roferon®-A

Mexican Brand Names Multiferon; Roferon-A; Roquiferon

Index Terms IFLrA; Interferon Alpha-2a; NSC-367982; rIFN-A

Pharmacologic Category Interferon

Use

Patients >18 years of age: Treatment of hairy cell leukemia, chronic hepatitis C

Children and Adults: Treatment of Philadelphia chromosome-positive (Ph+) chronic myelogenous leukemia (CML) in chronic phase, within 1 year of diagnosis (limited experience in children)

Unlabeled/Investigational Use Adjuvant therapy for malignant melanoma; treatment of AIDS-related Kaposi's sarcoma, carcinoid tumors; bladder, cervical, and ovarian cancers; hemangioma; chronic hepatitis D; low-grade non-Hodgkin's lymphoma; multiple myeloma; renal cell carcinoma; basal and squamous cell skin cancer; cutaneous T-cell lymphoma

Effect on Mental Status Severe psychiatric disorders including depression, suicidal behavior, ideation, attempts, and suicides have been reported with alfa interferons in patients with and without a previous psychiatric history. Extreme caution should be used in individuals who report a history of depression and patients should be informed of these potential side effects and how to respond if they occur. Careful neuropsychiatric monitoring for depressive symptoms is recommended. Dizziness and drowsiness are common. May cause memory impairment, agitation, manic behavior, and psychotic reactions; may rarely cause delirium.

Effect on Psychiatric Treatment May cause leukopenia; use caution with clozapine and carbamazepine; concurrent use with psychotropics may produce additive sedation and dry mouth

Restrictions An FDA-approved medication guide must be distributed when dispensing an outpatient prescription (new or refill) where this medication is to be used without direct supervision of a healthcare provider. Medication guides are available at http://www.fda.gov/cder/Offices/ODS/medication_guides.htm.

Dosage Summary

I.M.:

Children: 2.5-5 million units/m^2/day

Adults: Dosage not established

SubQ:

Children: Dosage not established

Adults: 3, 6, or 9 million units/day **or** 3 million units 3 times/week

Dosage Forms Excipient information presented when available (limited, particularly for generics); consult specific product labeling. [DSC] = Discontinued product

Injection, solution:

Roferon®-A: 3 million units/0.5 mL (0.5 mL) [contains benzyl alcohol and polysorbate 80] [DSC]; 6 million units/0.5 mL (0.5 mL) [contains benzyl alcohol and polysorbate 80] [DSC]; 9 million units/0.5 mL (0.5 mL) [contains benzyl alcohol and polysorbate 80] [DSC]

Interferon Alfa-2b (in ter FEER on AL fa too bee)

Medication Safety Issues

Sound-alike/look-alike issues:

Interferon alfa-2b may be confused with interferon alfa-2a, interferon alfa-n3, pegylated interferon alfa-2b

Intron® A may be confused with PEG-Intron®

International issues:

Interferon alfa-2b may be confused with interferon alpha multi-subtype which is available in international markets

U.S. Brand Names Intron® A

Canadian Brand Names Intron® A

Mexican Brand Names FNI 2B

Index Terms INF-alpha 2; Interferon Alpha-2b; NSC-377523; rLFN-α2; α-2-interferon

Pharmacologic Category Interferon

Use

Patients ≥1 year of age: Chronic hepatitis B

Patients ≥3 years of age: Chronic hepatitis C (in combination with ribavirin)

Patients ≥18 years of age: Condyloma acuminata, chronic hepatitis B, chronic hepatitis C, hairy cell leukemia, malignant melanoma, AIDS-related Kaposi's sarcoma, follicular non-Hodgkin's lymphoma

Unlabeled/Investigational Use AIDS-related thrombocytopenia, cutaneous ulcerations of Behçet's disease, neuroendocrine tumors (including carcinoid syndrome and islet cell tumor), cutaneous T-cell lymphoma, desmoid tumor, lymphomatoid granulomatosis, hepatitis D, chronic myelogenous leukemia (CML), non-Hodgkin's lymphomas (other than follicular lymphoma, see approved use), multiple myeloma, renal cell carcinoma, basal and squamous cell skin cancers, West Nile virus

Effect on Mental Status Dizziness and drowsiness are common; may rarely cause delirium. Severe psychiatric disorders, including depression and suicidal behavior, have been associated with some interferons. Careful neuropsychiatric monitoring is recommended.

Effect on Psychiatric Treatment May cause leukopenia; use caution with clozapine and carbamazepine; concurrent use with psychotropics may produce additive sedation and dry mouth

Restrictions An FDA-approved medication guide is available at http://www.fda.gov/cder/Offices/ODS/labeling.htm; distribute to each patient to whom this medication is dispensed.

Dosage Summary

I.M.:

Children: Dosage not established

Adults:

AIDS-related Kaposi's sarcoma: 30 million units/m^2 3 times/week

Chronic hepatitis B: 5 million units/day or 10 million units 3 times/week

Chronic hepatitis C: 3 million units 3 times/week

Hairy cell leukemia: 2 million units/m^2 3 times/week

I.V.:

Children: Dosage not established

Adults: 20 million units/m^2 for 5 consecutive days per week for 4 weeks

Intralesionally:

Children: Dosage not established

Adults: 1 million units/lesion 3 times/week, on alternate days (maximum: 5 lesions/treatment)

SubQ:

Children <1 year: Dosage not established

Children 1-17 years: Initial: 3 million units/m^2 3 times/week for 1 week; Maintenance: 6 million units/m^2 3 times/week (maximum: 10 million units 3 times/week)

Children 3-17 years: Initial: 3 million units/m^2 3 times/week (combination therapy) for up to 48 weeks

Adults:

AIDS-related Kaposi's sarcoma: 30 million units/m^2 3 times/week

Chronic hepatitis B: 5 million units/day or 10 million units 3 times/week

Chronic hepatitis C: 3 million units 3 times/week

Hairy cell leukemia: 2 million units/m^2 3 times/week

Lymphoma (follicular): 5 million units 3 times/week

Malignant melanoma: 10 million units/m^2 3 times/week

Dosage Forms Excipient information presented when available (limited, particularly for generics); consult specific product labeling. [DSC] = Discontinued product

Injection, powder for reconstitution [preservative free]:

Intron® A: 10 million units; 18 million units; 50 million units [contains human albumin]

Injection, solution [multidose prefilled pen]:

Intron® A:

Delivers 3 million units/0.2 mL (1.5 mL) [delivers 6 doses; 18 million units; contains polysorbate 80; edetate disodium]

Delivers 5 million units/0.2 mL (1.5 mL) [delivers 6 doses; 30 million units; contains polysorbate 80; edetate disodium]

Delivers 10 million units/0.2 mL (1.5 mL) [delivers 6 doses; 60 million units; contains polysorbate 80; edetate disodium]

Injection, solution [multidose vial]:
Intron® A: 6 million units/mL (3 mL); 10 million units/mL (2.5 mL) [contains polysorbate 80; edetate disodium]
Injection, solution [single-dose vial]:
Intron® A: 10 million units/ mL (1 mL) [DSC] [contains polysorbate 80; edetate disodium]

See also Interferon Alfa-2b and Ribavirin Combination Pack monograph.

Interferon Alfa-2b and Ribavirin

(in ter FEER on AL fa too bee & rye ba VYE rin)

U.S. Brand Names Rebetron®

Mexican Brand Names Hepatron C

Index Terms Interferon Alfa-2b and Ribavirin Combination Pack; Ribavirin and Interferon Alfa-2b Combination Pack

Pharmacologic Category Antiviral Agent; Interferon

Use Combination therapy for the treatment of chronic hepatitis C in patients with compensated liver disease previously untreated with alpha interferon or who have relapsed after alpha interferon therapy

Effect on Mental Status Severe psychiatric disorders, including depression and suicidal behavior, have been associated with interferon use. Careful neuropsychiatric monitoring is recommended.

Effect on Psychiatric Treatment None reported

Restrictions An FDA-approved medication guide must be distributed when dispensing an outpatient prescription (new or refill) for treatment of hepatitis C where this medication is to be used without direct supervision of a healthcare provider. Medication guides are available at http://www.fda.gov/cder/Offices/ODS/medication_guides.htm.

Dosage Summary

Oral (Rebetol®):

Children <3 years: Dosage not established
Children 3-5 years or ≤25 kg: 15 mg/kg/day in 2 divided doses
Children >5 years and 26-36 kg: 200 mg twice daily
Children >5 years and 37-49 kg: 200 mg in the morning and 400 mg in the evening
Children >5 years and 50-61 kg: 400 mg twice daily
Children >5 years and >61-75 kg: 400 mg in the morning and 600 mg in the evening
Children >5 years and >75 kg: 600 mg twice daily
Adults ≤75 kg: 400 mg in the morning and 600 mg in the evening
Adults >75 kg: 600 mg twice daily

SubQ (Intron® A):

Children <3 years: Dosage not established
Children ≥3 years and 25-61 kg: 3 million int. units/m^2 3 times/week
Children ≥3 years and >61 kg: 3 million int. units 3 times/week
Adults: 3 million int. units 3 times/week

Dosage Forms Excipient information presented when available (limited, particularly for generics); consult specific product labeling.

Combination package:

For patients ≤75 kg [contains single-dose vials]:
Injection, solution: Interferon alfa-2b (Intron® A): 3 million int. units/0.5 mL (0.5 mL) [6 vials (3 million int. units/vial), 6 syringes, and alcohol swabs]
Capsule: Ribavirin (Rebetol®): 200 mg (70s)

For patients ≤75 kg [contains multidose vials]:
Injection, solution: Interferon alfa-2b (Intron® A): 3 million int. units/0.5 mL (3.8 mL) [1 multidose vial (18 million int. units/vial), 6 syringes, and alcohol swabs]
Capsule: Ribavirin (Rebetol®): 200 mg (70s)

For patients ≤75 kg [contains multidose pen]:
Injection, solution: Interferon alfa-2b (Intron® A): 3 million int. units/0.2 mL (1.5 mL) [1 multidose pen (18 million int. units/pen), 6 needles, and alcohol swabs]
Capsule: Ribavirin (Rebetol®): 200 mg (70s)

For patients >75 kg [contains single-dose vials]:
Injection, solution: Interferon alfa-2b (Intron® A): 3 million int. units/0.5 mL (0.5 mL) [6 vials (3 million int. units/vial), 6 syringes, and alcohol swabs]
Capsule: Ribavirin (Rebetol®): 200 mg (84s)

For patients >75 kg [contains multidose vials]:
Injection, solution: Interferon alfa-2b (Intron® A): 3 million int. units/0.5 mL (3.8 mL) [1 multidose vial (18 million int. units/vial), 6 syringes, and alcohol swabs]

Capsule: Ribavirin (Rebetol®): 200 mg (84s)

For patients >75 kg [contains multidose pen]:

Injection, solution: Interferon alfa-2b (Intron® A): 3 million int. units/0.2 mL (1.5 mL) [1 multidose pen (18 million int. units/pen), 6 needles, and alcohol swabs]

Capsule: Ribavirin (Rebetol®): 200 mg (84s)

For Rebetol® dose reduction [contains single-dose vials]:

Injection, solution: Interferon alfa-2b (Intron® A): 3 million int. units/0.5 mL (0.5 mL) [6 vials (3 million int. units/vial), 6 syringes, and alcohol swabs]

Capsule: Ribavirin (Rebetol®): 200 mg (42s)

For Rebetol® dose reduction [contains multidose vials]:

Injection, solution: Interferon alfa-2b (Intron® A): 3 million int. units/0.5 mL (3.8 mL) [1 multidose vial (18 million int. units/vial), 6 syringes, and alcohol swabs]

Capsule: Ribavirin (Rebetol®): 200 mg (42s)

For Rebetol® dose reduction [contains multidose pen]:

Injection, solution: Interferon alfa-2b (Intron® A): 3 million int. units/0.2 mL (1.5 mL) [1 multidose pen (18 million int. units/pen), 6 needles, and alcohol swabs]

Capsule: Ribavirin (Rebetol®): 200 mg (42s)

Interferon Alfacon-1 (in ter FEER on AL fa con one)

Medication Safety Issues

Sound-alike/look-alike issues:

Interferon alfacon-1 may be confused with interferon alfa-2a, interferon alfa-2b, interferon alfa-n3, peginterferon alfa-2b

International issues:

Interferon alfacon-1 may be confused with interferon alpha multi-subtype which is available in international markets

U.S. Brand Names Infergen®

Pharmacologic Category Interferon

Use Treatment of chronic hepatitis C virus (HCV) infection in patients ≥18 years of age with compensated liver disease and anti-HCV serum antibodies or HCV RNA.

Effect on Mental Status Use caution in those patients with depressive disorders. Severe psychiatric adverse effects, including depression, suicidal ideation, and suicide attempt may occur. Fatigue, insomnia, nervousness, depression, anxiety, and emotional lability are common.

Effect on Psychiatric Treatment Granulocytopenia, thrombocytopenia, and leukopenia are common. Use caution with clozapine, carbamazepine, and valproate.

Restrictions An FDA-approved medication guide must be distributed when dispensing an outpatient prescription (new or refill) where this medication is to be used without direct supervision of a healthcare provider. Medication guides are available at http://www.fda.gov/cder/Offices/ODS/medication_guides.htm.

Dosage Summary

SubQ:

Children: Dosage not established

Adults: 9 mcg 3 times/week. Patients who do not respond or relapse after tolerating initial therapy may be increased to 15 mcg 3 times/week.

Dosage Forms Excipient information presented when available (limited, particularly for generics); consult specific product labeling.

Injection, solution [preservative free]:

Infergen®: 30 mcg/mL (0.3 mL, 0.5 mL)

Interferon Alfa-n3 (in ter FEER on AL fa en three)

Medication Safety Issues

Sound-alike/look-alike issues:

Alferon® may be confused with Alkeran®

U.S. Brand Names Alferon® N

Canadian Brand Names Alferon® N

Pharmacologic Category Interferon

Use Patients ≥18 years of age: Intralesional treatment of refractory or recurring genital or venereal warts (condylomata acuminata)

Effect on Mental Status Dizziness and drowsiness are common; may cause delirium or neurotoxicity. Severe psychiatric disorders, including depression and suicidal behavior, have been associated with some interferons. Careful neuropsychiatric monitoring is recommended.

Effect on Psychiatric Treatment May cause leukopenia; use caution with clozapine and carbamazepine; concurrent use with psychotropics may produce additive sedation and dry mouth

Dosage Summary

Intralesional:

Children: Dosage not established

Adults: Inject 250,000 units (0.05 mL) in each wart twice weekly (maximum: 8 weeks)

Dosage Forms Excipient information presented when available (limited, particularly for generics); consult specific product labeling.

Injection, solution: 5 million int. units (1 mL) [contains albumin]

◆ **Interferon Alpha-2a** *see* Interferon Alfa-2a *on page 844*

◆ **Interferon Alpha-2b** *see* Interferon Alfa-2b *on page 844*

Interferon Beta-1a (in ter FEER on BAY ta won aye)

Medication Safety Issues

Sound-alike/look-alike issues:

Avonex® may be confused with Avelox®

U.S. Brand Names Avonex®; Rebif®

Canadian Brand Names Avonex®; Rebif®

Mexican Brand Names Rebif

Index Terms rIFN beta-1a

Pharmacologic Category Interferon

Use Treatment of relapsing forms of multiple sclerosis (MS)

Effect on Mental Status May cause sedation, anxiety, agitation, or confusion. Severe psychiatric disorders, including depression and suicidal behavior, have been associated with the use of some interferons. Careful neuropsychiatric monitoring is recommended.

Effect on Psychiatric Treatment May cause leukopenia; use caution with clozapine and carbamazepine; concurrent use with psychotropics may produce additive sedation

Restrictions An FDA-approved medication guide must be distributed when dispensing an outpatient prescription (new or refill) where this medication is to be used without direct supervision of a healthcare provider. Medication guides are available at http://www.fda.gov/cder/Offices/ODS/medication_guides.htm.

Dosage Summary

I.M.:

Children: Dosage not established

Adults: 30 mcg once weekly

SubQ:

Children: Dosage not established

Adults: Initial: 4.4 or 8.8 mcg 3 times/week for 2 weeks; Titration: 11 or 22 mcg 3 times/week for 2 weeks; Maintenance: 22 or 44 mcg 3 times/week

Dosage Forms Excipient information presented when available (limited, particularly for generics); consult specific product labeling.

Combination package [preservative free] (Rebif® Titration Pack):

Injection, solution: 8.8 mcg/0.2 mL (0.2 mL) [6 prefilled syringes; contains albumin]

Injection, solution: 22 mcg/0.5 mL (0.5 mL) [6 prefilled syringes; contains albumin]

Injection, powder for reconstitution (Avonex®): 33 mcg [6.6 million units; provides 30 mcg/mL following reconstitution] [contains albumin; packaged with SWFI, alcohol wipes, and access pin and needle]

Injection, solution (Avonex®): 30 mcg/0.5 mL (0.5 mL) [albumin free; prefilled syringe; syringe cap contains latex; packaged with alcohol wipes, gauze pad, and adhesive bandages]

Injection, solution [preservative free] (Rebif®): 22 mcg/0.5 mL (0.5 mL) [prefilled syringe; contains albumin]; 44 mcg/0.5 mL (0.5 mL) [prefilled syringe; contains albumin]

Interferon Beta-1b (in ter FEER on BAY ta won bee)

U.S. Brand Names Betaseron®

Canadian Brand Names Betaseron®

Mexican Brand Names Betaferon

Index Terms rIFN beta-1b

Pharmacologic Category Interferon

Use Treatment of relapsing forms of multiple sclerosis (MS); treatment of first clinical episode with MRI features consistent with MS

Effect on Mental Status May cause sedation, anxiety, agitation, or confusion. Severe psychiatric disorders, including depression and suicidal behavior, have been associated with use of some interferons. Careful neuropsychiatric monitoring is recommended.

Effect on Psychiatric Treatment May cause leukopenia; use caution with clozapine and carbamazepine; concurrent use with psychotropics may produce additive sedation

Restrictions An FDA-approved medication guide must be distributed when dispensing an outpatient prescription (new or refill) where this medication is to be used without direct supervision of a healthcare provider. Medication guide is available at http://www.berlex.com/html/products/pi/Betaseron_Medication_Guide.pdf.

Dosage Summary

SubQ:

Children: Use not recommended

Adults: 0.25 mg (8 million units) every other day

Dosage Forms Excipient information presented when available (limited, particularly for generics); consult specific product labeling.

Injection, powder for reconstitution [preservative free]:

Betaseron®: 0.3 mg [9.6 million units] [contains albumin; packaged with prefilled syringe containing diluent]

Interferon Gamma-1b (in ter FEER on GAM ah won bee)

U.S. Brand Names Actimmune®

Canadian Brand Names Actimmune®

Pharmacologic Category Interferon

Use Reduce frequency and severity of serious infections associated with chronic granulomatous disease; delay time to disease progression in patients with severe, malignant osteopetrosis

Effect on Mental Status Sedation is common; may rarely cause depression

Effect on Psychiatric Treatment May cause leukopenia; use caution with clozapine and carbamazepine; concurrent use with psychotropics may produce additive sedation

Dosage Summary

SubQ:

Children:

BSA ≤0.5 m^2: 1.5 mcg/kg/dose 3 times/week

BSA >0.5 m^2: 50 mcg/m^2 (1 million int. $units/m^2$) 3 times/week

Adults:

BSA ≤0.5 m^2: 1.5 mcg/kg/dose 3 times/week

BSA >0.5 m^2: 50 mcg/m^2 (1 million int. $units/m^2$) 3 times/week

Dosage Forms Excipient information presented when available (limited, particularly for generics); consult specific product labeling.

Injection, solution [preservative free]:

Actimmune®: 100 mcg [2 million int. units] (0.5 mL)

- **Interleukin-1 Receptor Antagonist** *see* Anakinra *on page 124*
- **Interleukin-2** *see* Aldesleukin *on page 58*
- **Interleukin-11** *see* Oprelvekin *on page 1184*
- **Intrifiban** *see* Eptifibatide *on page 550*
- **Intron® A** *see* Interferon Alfa-2b *on page 844*
- **Intropin** *see* DOPamine *on page 498*
- **Invanz®** *see* Ertapenem *on page 557*
- **Invega®** *see* Paliperidone *on page 1215*
- **Inversine®** *see* Mecamylamine *on page 973*
- **Invirase®** *see* Saquinavir *on page 1461*

Iobenguane I 123 (eye oh BEN gwane eye one TWEN tee three)

Index Terms 123 Meta-Iodobenzlyguanidine Sulfate; 123I-Metaiodobenzylguanidine (MIBG); I-123 MIBG; I^{123} Iobenguane; Iobenguane Sulfate I 123

Pharmacologic Category Radiopharmaceutical

Use As an adjunct to other diagnostic tests, in the detection of primary or metastatic pheochromocytoma or neuroblastoma

Effect on Mental Status May cause dizziness

Effect on Psychiatric Treatment Norepinephrine reuptake inhibitors (most antidepressants and ziprasidone) may interfere with the uptake of iobenguane I 123 in neuroendocrine tumors leading to false-negative results. If possible taper/discontinue norepinephrine reuptake inhibitor and allow 5 half-lives to elapse prior to administration of iobenguane.

Dosage Summary

Infants <1 month: Dosage not established
Children <16 years and 3 kg: 1 mCi (37 MBq)
Children <16 years and 4 kg: 1.4 mCi (52 MBq)
Children <16 years and 6 kg: 1.9 mCi (70 MBq)
Children <16 years and 8 kg: 2.3 mCi (85.1 MBq)
Children <16 years and 10 kg: 2.7 mCi (99.9 MBq)
Children <16 years and 12 kg: 3.2 mCi (118.4 MBq)
Children <16 years and 14 kg: 3.6 mCi (133.2 MBq)
Children <16 years and 16 kg: 4 mCi (148 MBq)
Children <16 years and 18 kg: 4.4 mCi (162.8 MBq)
Children <16 years and 20 kg: 4.6 mCi (170.2 MBq)
Children <16 years and 22 kg: 5 mCi (185 MBq)
Children <16 years and 24 kg: 5.3 mCi (196.1 MBq)
Children <16 years and 26 kg: 5.6 mCi (207.2 MBq)
Children <16 years and 28 kg: 5.8 mCi (214.6 MBq)
Children <16 years and 30 kg: 6.2 mCi (229.4 MBq)
Children <16 years and 32 kg: 6.5 mCi (240.5 MBq)
Children <16 years and 34 kg: 6.8 mCi (251.6 MBq)
Children <16 years and 36 kg: 7.1 mCi (262.7 MBq)
Children <16 years and 38 kg: 7.3 mCi (270.1 MBq)
Children <16 years and 40 kg: 7.6 mCi (281.2 MBq)
Children <16 years and 42 kg: 7.8 mCi (288.6 MBq)
Children <16 years and 44 kg: 8 mCi (296 MBq)
Children <16 years and 46 kg: 8.2 mCi (303.4 MBq)
Children <16 years and 48 kg: 8.5 mCi (314.5 MBq)
Children <16 years and 50 kg: 8.8 mCi (325.6 MBq)
Children <16 years and 52-54 kg: 9 mCi (333 MBq)
Children <16 years and 56-58 kg: 9.2 mCi (340.4 MBq)
Children <16 years and 60-62 kg: 9.6 mCi (355.2 MBq)
Children <16 years and 64-66 kg: 9.8 mCi (362.6 MBq)
Children <16 years and 68 kg: 9.9 mCi (366.3 MBq)
Children <16 years and ≥70 kg: 10 mCi (370 MBq)
Children ≥16 years: 10 mCi (370 MBq)
Adults: 10 mCi (370 MBq)

Dosage Forms Excipient information presented when available (limited, particularly for generics); consult specific product labeling.

Injection, solution:
AdreView®: Iobenguane sulfate 0.08 mg and I 123 74 MBq (2 mCi) per mL (5 mL) [contains benzyl alcohol]

◆ **Iobenguane Sulfate I 123** *see* Iobenguane I 123 *on page 849*

◆ **Iodine I 131 Tositumomab and Tositumomab** *see* Tositumomab and Iodine I 131 Tositumomab *on page 1603*

Iodixanol (EYE oh dix an ole)

Medication Safety Issues

Not for intrathecal use

High alert medication: The Institute for Safe Medication Practices (ISMP) includes this medication among its list of drugs which have a heightened risk of causing significant patient harm when used in error.

U.S. Brand Names Visipaque™

Pharmacologic Category Iodinated Contrast Media; Radiological/Contrast Media, Nonionic (Iso-Osmolality)

Use

Intra-arterial: Digital subtraction angiography, angiocardiography, peripheral arteriography, visceral arteriography, cerebral arteriography

Intravenous: Contrast enhanced computed tomography imaging, excretory urography, and peripheral venography

Effect on Mental Status May cause serious thromboembolic events including stroke

Effect on Psychiatric Treatment None reported

Dosage Summary

I.V.:

Children ≤1 year: Dosage not established

Children >1-12 years: Iodixanol 270 mg iodine/mL: 1-2 mL/kg (maximum: 2 mL/kg)

Children >12 years: Iodixanol 270 mg and 320 mg iodine /mL: concentration and dose vary based on study type; refer to product labeling (maximum total dose: 80 g iodine)

Adults: Iodixanol 270 mg and 320 mg iodine /mL: concentration and dose vary based on study type; refer to product labeling (maximum total dose: 80 g iodine)

Intra-arterial:

Children ≤1 year: Dosage not established

Children >1-12 years: Iodixanol 320 mg iodine/mL: 1-2 mL/kg (maximum: 4 mL/kg)

Children >12 years: Iodixanol 320 mg iodine/mL: Dose individualized based on injection site and study type; refer to product labeling (maximum total dose: 80 g iodine)

Adults: Iodixanol 320 mg iodine/mL: Dose individualized based on injection site and study type; refer to product labeling (maximum total dose: 80 g iodine)

Dosage Forms Excipient information presented when available (limited, particularly for generics); consult specific product labeling.

Injection, solution [preservative free]:

Visipaque™ 270: 550 mg/mL (50 mL, 100 mL, 125 mL, 150 mL, 200 mL) [provides organically-bound iodine 270 mg/mL; contains tromethamine 1.2 mg/mL, edetate calcium disodium]

Visipaque™ 320: 652 mg/mL (50 mL, 100 mL, 125 mL, 150 mL, 200 mL) [provides organically-bound iodine 320 mg/mL; contains tromethamine 1.2 mg/mL, edetate calcium disodium]

Iodoquinol (eye oh doe KWIN ole)

U.S. Brand Names Yodoxin®

Canadian Brand Names Diodoquin®

Mexican Brand Names Depofin

Index Terms Diiodohydroxyquin

Pharmacologic Category Amebicide

Use Treatment of acute and chronic intestinal amebiasis; asymptomatic cyst passers; *Blastocystis hominis* infections; ineffective for amebic hepatitis or hepatic abscess

Effect on Mental Status May cause agitation or amnesia

Effect on Psychiatric Treatment None reported

Dosage Summary

Oral:

Children: 30-40 mg/kg/day in 3 divided doses (maximum: 1.95 g/day)

Adults: 650 mg 3 times/day (maximum: 1.95 g/day)

Elderly: Only use if other therapy contraindicated or has failed; due to optic nerve damage use cautiously

Dosage Forms Excipient information presented when available (limited, particularly for generics); consult specific product labeling.

Tablet: 210 mg, 650 mg

- **Ionamin®** *see* Phentermine *on page 1270*
- **Ionil® [OTC]** *see* Salicylic Acid *on page 1454*
- **Ionil Plus® [OTC]** *see* Salicylic Acid *on page 1454*
- **Iopidine®** *see* Apraclonidine *on page 129*
- **Iosat™ [OTC]** *see* Potassium Iodide *on page 1317*

Ipecac Syrup (IP e kak SIR up)

Index Terms Syrup of Ipecac

Pharmacologic Category Antidote

Use Treatment of acute oral drug overdosage and in certain poisonings

Effect on Mental Status May cause sedation

Effect on Psychiatric Treatment Combination with chlorpromazine has been associated with dystonic reactions

Dosage Summary

Oral:

Children <6 months: Dosage not established

Children 6-12 months: 5-10 mL followed by 10-20 mL/kg of water, may repeat if vomiting does not occur within 20 minutes

Children 1-12 years: 15 mL followed by 10-20 mL/kg of water, may repeat if vomiting does not occur within 20 minutes

Adults: 15-30 mL followed by 200-300 mL of water; may repeat if vomiting does not occur within 20 minutes

Dosage Forms Excipient information presented when available (limited, particularly for generics); consult specific product labeling.

Syrup: 70 mg/mL (30 mL) [contains alcohol]

◆ **Iplex™ [DSC]** *see* Mecasermin *on page 973*

Ipratropium (i pra TROE pee um)

Medication Safety Issues

Sound-alike/look-alike issues:

Atrovent® may be confused with Alupent®

U.S. Brand Names Atrovent®; Atrovent® HFA

Canadian Brand Names Alti-Ipratropium; Apo-Ipravent®; Atrovent®; Atrovent® HFA; Gen-Ipratropium; Novo-Ipramide; Nu-Ipratropium; PMS-Ipratropium

Mexican Brand Names Atrovent

Index Terms Ipratropium Bromide

Pharmacologic Category Anticholinergic Agent

Generic Available Yes: Excludes solution for oral inhalation, aerosol for oral inhalation

Use

Oral inhalation: Anticholinergic bronchodilator used in bronchospasm associated with COPD, bronchitis, and emphysema

Nasal spray: Symptomatic relief of rhinorrhea associated with the common cold and allergic and nonallergic rhinitis

Unlabeled/Investigational Use Oral inhalation: Adjunct to short-acting beta-adrenergic agonists therapy in moderate-to-severe exacerbations of acute asthma in the emergency room

Effect on Mental Status Nervousness, dizziness, and fatigue are common; may cause insomnia

Effect on Psychiatric Treatment Concurrent use with psychotropics may produce additive anticholinergic effects

Pregnancy Risk Factor B

Pregnancy Considerations Teratogenic effects were not observed in animal studies.

Lactation Excretion in breast milk unknown/use caution

Contraindications Hypersensitivity to ipratropium, atropine (and its derivatives), or any component of the formulation

Warnings/Precautions Immediate hypersensitivity reactions (urticaria, angioedema, rash, bronchospasm) have been reported. Rarely, paradoxical bronchospasm may occur with use of inhaled bronchodilating agents; this should be distinguished from inadequate response. Not indicated for the initial treatment of acute episodes of bronchospasm where rescue therapy is required for rapid response. Should only be used in acute exacerbations of asthma in conjunction with short-acting beta-adrenergic agonists for acute episodes. Use with caution in patients with myasthenia gravis, narrow-angle glaucoma, benign prostatic hyperplasia (BPH), or bladder neck obstruction

Adverse Reactions

Inhalation aerosol and inhalation solution:

>10%: Respiratory: Upper respiratory tract infection (9% to 34%), bronchitis (10% to 23%), sinusitis (1% to 11%)

1% to 10%:

Cardiovascular: Chest pain (3%), palpitation

Central nervous system: Headache (6% to 7%), dizziness (2% to 3%)

Gastrointestinal: Dyspepsia (1% to 5%), nausea (4%), xerostomia (2% to 4%)

Genitourinary: Urinary tract infection (2% to 10%)

Neuromuscular & skeletal: Back pain (2% to 7%)

Respiratory: Dyspnea (7% to 10%), rhinitis (2% to 6%), cough (3% to 5%), pharyngitis (4%), bronchospasm (2%), sputum increased (1%)

Miscellaneous: Flu-like syndrome (4% to 8%)

<1% (Limited to important or life-threatening): Anaphylactic reaction, angioedema, arthritis, atrial fibrillation, bitter taste, constipation, diarrhea, eye pain

(acute), glaucoma, hypersensitivity reactions, hypotension, insomnia, laryngospasm, mydriasis, nervousness, pruritus, rash, tachycardia (including supraventricular), tremor, urinary retention, urticaria

Nasal spray:

1% to 10%:Central nervous system: Headache (4% to 10%)

Gastrointestinal: Taste perversion (≤4%), xerostomia (1% to 4%), diarrhea (2%), nausea (2%)

Respiratory: Epistaxis (6% to 9%), pharyngitis (≤8%), upper respiratory tract infection (5% to 10%), nasal dryness (<1% to 5%), nasal irritation (2%), nasal congestion (1%)

<2% (Limited to important or life-threatening): Anaphylactic reaction, angioedema, blurred vision, conjunctivitis, cough, dizziness, hoarseness, laryngospasm, nasal burning, ocular irritation, palpitation, rash, tachycardia, thirst, tinnitus, urticaria, xerostomia

Drug Interactions

Acetylcholinesterase Inhibitors (Central): Anticholinergics may diminish the therapeutic effect of Acetylcholinesterase Inhibitors (Central). Acetylcholinesterase Inhibitors (Central) may diminish the therapeutic effect of Anticholinergics. If the anticholinergic action is a side effect of the agent, the result may be beneficial. *Risk C: Monitor therapy*

Anticholinergics: May enhance the adverse/toxic effect of other Anticholinergics. **Exceptions:** Paliperidone. *Risk C: Monitor therapy*

Cannabinoids: Anticholinergic Agents may enhance the tachycardic effect of Cannabinoids. *Risk C: Monitor therapy*

Potassium Chloride: Anticholinergic Agents may enhance the ulcerogenic effect of Potassium Chloride. *Risk D: Consider therapy modification*

Pramlintide: May enhance the anticholinergic effect of Anticholinergics. These effects are specific to the GI tract. *Risk D: Consider therapy modification*

Secretin: Anticholinergic Agents may diminish the stimulatory effect of Secretin. *Risk D: Consider therapy modification*

Stability

Oral inhalation aerosol and nasal spray: Store at controlled room temperature of 25°C (77°F). Do not store near heat or open flame.

Oral inhalation solution: Store at 15°C to 30°C (59°F to 86°F). Protect from light.

Mechanism of Action Blocks the action of acetylcholine at parasympathetic sites in bronchial smooth muscle causing bronchodilation; local application to nasal mucosa inhibits serous and seromucous gland secretions.

Pharmacodynamics/Kinetics

Onset of action: Bronchodilation: Within 15 minutes

Peak effect: 1-2 hours

Duration: 2-5 hours

Absorption: Negligible

Distribution: Inhalation: 15% of dose reaches lower airways

Protein Binding: ≤9%

Half-life elimination: 2 hours

Excretion: Urine

Dosage

Nebulization:

Children ≤12 years: Asthma exacerbation, acute (*NIH Asthma Guidelines, 2007*): 250-500 mcg every 20 minutes for 3 doses, then as needed. **Note:** Should be given in combination with a short-acting beta-adrenergic agonist.

Children >12 years and Adults:

Bronchodilator for COPD: 500 mcg (one unit-dose vial) 3-4 times/day with doses 6-8 hours apart

Asthma exacerbation, acute (*NIH Asthma Guidelines, 2007*): 500 mcg every 20 minutes for 3 doses, then as needed. **Note:** Should be given in combination with a short-acting beta-adrenergic agonist.

Oral inhalation: MDI:

Children ≤12 years: Asthma exacerbation, acute (*NIH Asthma Guidelines, 2007*): 4-8 inhalations every 20 minutes as needed for up to 3 hours. **Note:** Should be given in combination with a short-acting beta-adrenergic agonist.

Children >12 years and Adults:

Bronchodilator for COPD: 2 inhalations 4 times/day, up to 12 inhalations/24 hours

Asthma exacerbation, acute (*NIH Asthma Guidelines, 2007*): 8 inhalations every 20 minutes as needed for up to 3 hours. **Note:** Should be given in combination with a short-acting beta-adrenergic agonist.

Intranasal: Nasal spray:

Symptomatic relief of rhinorrhea associated with the common cold (safety and efficacy of use beyond 4 days in patients with the common cold have not been established):

Children 5-11 years: 0.06%: 2 sprays in each nostril 3 times/day

Children ≥12 years and Adults: 0.06%: 2 sprays in each nostril 3-4 times/day

Symptomatic relief of rhinorrhea associated with allergic/nonallergic rhinitis: Children ≥6 years and Adults: 0.03%: 2 sprays in each nostril 2-3 times/day

Symptomatic relief of rhinorrhea associated with seasonal allergic rhinitis (safety and efficacy of use beyond 3 weeks in patients with seasonal allergic rhinitis has not been established): Children ≥5 years and Adults: 0.06%: 2 sprays in each nostril 4 times/day

Administration Avoid spraying into the eyes.

Atrovent® HFA: Prior to initial use, prime inhaler by releasing 2 test sprays into the air. If the inhaler has not been used for >3 days, reprime.

Nasal spray: Prior to initial use, prime inhaler by releasing 7 test sprays into the air. If the inhaler has not been used for >24 hours, reprime by releasing 2 test sprays into the air.

Dosage Forms Excipient information presented when available (limited, particularly for generics); consult specific product labeling.

Aerosol for oral inhalation, as bromide:

Atrovent® HFA: 17 mcg/actuation (12.9 g)

Solution for nebulization, as bromide: 0.02% (2.5 mL)

Solution, intranasal, as bromide [spray]:

Atrovent®: 0.03% (30 mL); 0.06% (15 mL)

Ipratropium and Albuterol (i pra TROE pee um & al BYOO ter ole)

Medication Safety Issues

Sound-alike/look-alike issues:

Combivent® may be confused with Combivir®

International issues:

DuoNeb® may be confused with DuoTrav™ which is a brand name for travoprost/timolol combination product in Canada

U.S. Brand Names Combivent®; DuoNeb®

Canadian Brand Names CO Ipra-Sal; Combivent®; Gen-Combo Sterinebs; ratio-Ipra Sal UDV

Mexican Brand Names Combivent

Index Terms Albuterol and Ipratropium; Salbutamol and Ipratropium

Pharmacologic Category Bronchodilator

Generic Available Yes: Solution for nebulization

Use Treatment of COPD in those patients who are currently on a regular bronchodilator who continue to have bronchospasms and require a second bronchodilator

Effect on Mental Status Nervousness, dizziness, fatigue, headache are common; may cause insomnia or anxiety

Effect on Psychiatric Treatment May produce additive anticholinergic effects if used concurrently with psychotropics; effect of propranolol may be reduced; cardiovascular effects (tachycardia, palpitations) may be increased with MAO inhibitors, TCAs, and amphetamines

Pregnancy Risk Factor C

Pregnancy Considerations Reproduction studies have not been conducted with this combination. See individual agents.

Contraindications Hypersensitivity to ipratropium, albuterol, atropine (and its derivatives) or any component of the formulation

Warnings/Precautions See individual agents. Some dosage forms of this combination contain soya lecithin; may cause allergic reactions in patients with allergy to soya lecithin or related food products (eg, soybean and peanut)

Adverse Reactions See individual agents.

Metabolism/Transport Effects Albuterol: **Substrate** of CYP3A4 (major)

Drug Interactions

Acetylcholinesterase Inhibitors (Central): Anticholinergics may diminish the therapeutic effect of Acetylcholinesterase Inhibitors (Central). Acetylcholinesterase Inhibitors (Central) may diminish the therapeutic effect of Anticholinergics. If the anticholinergic action is a side effect of the agent, the result may be beneficial. *Risk C: Monitor therapy*

Alpha-/Beta-Blockers: May diminish the therapeutic effect of Beta2-Agonists. *Risk D: Consider therapy modification*

Anticholinergics: May enhance the adverse/toxic effect of other Anticholinergics. **Exceptions:** Paliperidone. *Risk C: Monitor therapy*

Atomoxetine: May enhance the tachycardic effect of Beta2-Agonists. *Risk C: Monitor therapy*

Beta-Blockers (Beta1 Selective): May diminish the bronchodilatory effect of Beta2-Agonists. Of particular concern with nonselective beta-blockers or higher doses of the beta1 selective beta-blockers. *Risk C: Monitor therapy*

Beta-Blockers (Nonselective): May diminish the bronchodilatory effect of Beta2-Agonists. *Risk D: Consider therapy modification*

Betahistine: May diminish the therapeutic effect of Beta2-Agonists. *Risk C: Monitor therapy*

Cannabinoids: Anticholinergic Agents may enhance the tachycardic effect of Cannabinoids. *Risk C: Monitor therapy*

MAO Inhibitors: May enhance the adverse/toxic effect of Beta2-Agonists. *Risk C: Monitor therapy*

Potassium Chloride: Anticholinergic Agents may enhance the ulcerogenic effect of Potassium Chloride. *Risk D: Consider therapy modification*

Pramlintide: May enhance the anticholinergic effect of Anticholinergics. These effects are specific to the GI tract. *Risk D: Consider therapy modification*

Secretin: Anticholinergic Agents may diminish the stimulatory effect of Secretin. *Risk D: Consider therapy modification*

Sympathomimetics: May enhance the adverse/toxic effect of other Sympathomimetics. *Risk C: Monitor therapy*

Tricyclic Antidepressants: May enhance the adverse/toxic effect of Beta2-Agonists. *Risk C: Monitor therapy*

Stability

DuoNeb®: Store at 2°C to 30°C (36°F to 86°F). Protect from light.

Combivent®: Store at 15°C to 30°C (59°F to 86°F). Avoid excessive humidity. Do not store near heat or open flame.

Mechanism of Action See individual agents.

Pharmacodynamics/Kinetics See individual agents.

Dosage Adults:

Aerosol for inhalation: 2 inhalations 4 times/day (maximum: 12 inhalations/24 hours)

Solution for nebulization: Initial: 3 mL every 6 hours (maximum: 3 mL every 4 hours)

Dietary Considerations Some dosage forms may contain soya lecithin. Do not use in patients allergic to soya lecithin or related food products such as soybean and peanut.

Administration Nebulization: Administer via jet nebulizer to an air compressor with an adequate air flow, equipped with a mouthpiece or face mask. MDI: Shake canister vigorously for ≥10 seconds. Prior to first use (or if not used for >24 hours) a test spray of 3 sprays is recommended. Avoid spraying into eyes.

Monitoring Parameters Spirometry (FEV, FVC); weight

Dosage Forms Excipient information presented when available (limited, particularly for generics); consult specific product labeling.

Aerosol for oral inhalation:

Combivent®: Ipratropium bromide 18 mcg and albuterol sulfate 103 mcg per actuation (14.7 g) [contains chlorofluorocarbon, soya lecithin; 200 metered actuations]

Solution for nebulization: Ipratropium bromide 0.5 mg and albuterol base 2.5 mg per 3 mL (30s, 60s)

DuoNeb®: Ipratropium bromide 0.5 mg and albuterol base 2.5 mg per 3 mL (30s, 60s)

◆ **Ipratropium Bromide** *see* Ipratropium *on page 852*

◆ **I-Prin [OTC]** *see* Ibuprofen *on page 803*

◆ **Iproveratril Hydrochloride** *see* Verapamil *on page 1665*

◆ **Iquix®** *see* Levofloxacin *on page 913*

Irbesartan (ir be SAR tan)

Medication Safety Issues

Sound-alike/look-alike issues:

Avapro® may be confused with Anaprox®

Related Information

Angiotensin Agents *on page 1754*

U.S. Brand Names Avapro®

Canadian Brand Names Avapro®

Mexican Brand Names Aprovel; Avapro

Pharmacologic Category Angiotensin II Receptor Blocker

Use Treatment of hypertension alone or in combination with other antihypertensives; treatment of diabetic nephropathy in patients with type 2 diabetes mellitus (noninsulin dependent, NIDDM) and hypertension

Unlabeled/Investigational Use To slow the rate of progression of aortic-root dilation in pediatric patients with Marfan's syndrome

Effect on Mental Status May cause anxiety, dizziness, nervousness

Effect on Psychiatric Treatment None reported

Dosage Summary

Oral:

Children <6 years: Dosage not established

Children 6-12 years: Initial: 75 mg once daily; Maintenance: May be titrated up to 150 mg once daily

Children ≥13 years: Initial: 75-150 mg once daily; Maintenance: May be titrated up to 300 mg once daily

Adults: Initial: 75-150 mg once daily; Maintenance: May be titrated up to 300 mg once daily

Dosage Forms Excipient information presented when available (limited, particularly for generics); consult specific product labeling.

Tablet: 75 mg, 150 mg, 300 mg

Irbesartan and Hydrochlorothiazide

(ir be SAR tan & hye droe klor oh THYE a zide)

Medication Safety Issues

Sound-alike/look-alike issues:

Avalide® may be confused with Avandia®

U.S. Brand Names Avalide®

Canadian Brand Names Avalide®

Mexican Brand Names Co-Aprovel

Index Terms Avapro® HCT; Hydrochlorothiazide and Irbesartan

Pharmacologic Category Angiotensin II Receptor Blocker; Diuretic, Thiazide

Use Combination therapy for the management of hypertension; may be used as initial therapy in patients likely to need multiple drugs to achieve blood pressure goals

Note: In Canada, this combination product is approved for initial therapy in severe, essential hypertension (sitting diastolic blood pressure [DBP] ≥110 mm Hg).

Effect on Mental Status May cause anxiety, dizziness, nervousness

Effect on Psychiatric Treatment May decrease lithium clearance resulting in an increase in serum lithium levels and potential lithium toxicity; monitor serum lithium levels

Dosage Summary

Oral:

Children: Dosage not established

Adults: Irbesartan 150-300 mg and hydrochlorothiazide 12.5-25 mg once daily

Dosage Forms Excipient information presented when available (limited, particularly for generics); consult specific product labeling.

Tablet:

Irbesartan 150 mg and hydrochlorothiazide 12.5 mg

Irbesartan 300 mg and hydrochlorothiazide 12.5 mg

Irbesartan 300 mg and hydrochlorothiazide 25 mg

◆ **Ircon® [OTC]** *see* Ferrous Fumarate *on page 626*

◆ **IRESSA®** *see* Gefitinib *on page 709*

Irinotecan (eye rye no TEE kan)

Medication Safety Issues

High alert medication: The Institute for Safe Medication Practices (ISMP) includes this medication among its list of drug classes which have a heightened risk of causing significant patient harm when used in error.

U.S. Brand Names Camptosar®

Canadian Brand Names Camptosar®; Irinotecan Hydrochloride Trihydrate

Mexican Brand Names Camptosar; Terican

Index Terms Camptothecin-11; CPT-11; NSC-616348

Pharmacologic Category Antineoplastic Agent, Camptothecin; Antineoplastic Agent, Natural Source (Plant) Derivative

Use Treatment of metastatic carcinoma of the colon or rectum

Unlabeled/Investigational Use Lung cancer (small cell and nonsmall cell), cervical cancer, gastric cancer, pancreatic cancer, leukemia, lymphoma, breast cancer, brain tumors

Effect on Mental Status Dizziness and insomnia are common

Effect on Psychiatric Treatment May cause myelosuppression; use caution with clozapine and carbamazepine; concurrent use with prochlorperazine has produced akathisia. Two severe (life-threatening) forms of diarrhea may occur; these effects may be additive with concurrent use of SSRIs, lithium, or valproate; use caution.

Dosage Summary

Note: A reduction in the starting dose by one dose level should be considered for patients ≥65 years of age, prior pelvic/abdominal radiotherapy, performance status of 2, homozygosity for UGT1A1*28 allele, or increased bilirubin (dosing for patients with a bilirubin >2 mg/dL cannot be recommended based on lack of data per manufacturer); **Note:** For combination therapy refer to individual protocols

I.V.:

Children: Dosage not established

Adults:

Once weekly regimen: 125 mg/m^2 on days 1, 8, 15, and 22, every 42 days; Adjusted dose level-1: 100 mg/m^2; Adjusted dose level-2: 75 mg/m^2

Once-every-3 week regimen: 350 mg/m^2; Adjusted dose level-1: 300 mg/m^2; Adjusted dose level-2: 250 mg/m^2

Dosage Forms Excipient information presented when available (limited, particularly for generics); consult specific product labeling.

Injection, solution, as hydrochloride: 20 mg/mL (2 mL, 5 mL)

Camptosar®: 20 mg/mL (2 mL, 5 mL) [contains sorbitol 45 mg/mL]

◆ **Iron Dextran** *see* Iron Dextran Complex *on page 857*

Iron Dextran Complex (EYE ern DEKS tran KOM pleks)

Medication Safety Issues

Sound-alike/look-alike issues:

Dexferrum® may be confused with Desferal®

U.S. Brand Names Dexferrum®; INFeD®

Canadian Brand Names Dexiron™; Infufer®

Mexican Brand Names Driken

Index Terms High-Molecular-Weight Iron Dextran (DexFerrum®); Imferon; Iron Dextran; Low-Molecular-Weight Iron Dextran (INFeD®)

Pharmacologic Category Iron Salt

Use Treatment of iron deficiency in patients in whom oral administration is infeasible or ineffective

Effect on Mental Status May cause dizziness

Effect on Psychiatric Treatment None reported

Dosage Summary Note: A 0.5 mL test dose (0.25 mL in infants) should be given prior to starting iron dextran therapy.

I.M.:

Children <4 months: Use not recommended

Children <5 kg: (INFeD®): Replacement iron (mg) = blood loss (mL) x Hct; **Note:** Total dose should be divided daily at not more than 25 mg/day

Children 5-15 kg: (INFeD®): Total Dose (mL) = 0.0442 (desired Hgb [usually 12 g/dL] - observed Hgb) x W (in kg) + (0.26 x W [in kg]) **or** replacement iron (mg) = blood loss (mL) x hematocrit; **Note:** Total dose should be divided daily at not more than 50 mg/day [5-10 kg] or 100 mg/day [10-15 kg]

Children >15 kg: (INFeD®): Total Dose (mL) = 0.0442 (desired Hgb [usually 14.8 g/dL] - observed Hgb) x LBW + (0.26 x LBW) **or** replacement iron (mg) = blood loss (mL) x Hct; **Note:** Total dose should be divided daily at not more than 100 mg/day

Adults: (INFeD®): Total Dose (mL) = 0.0442 (desired Hgb [usually 14.8 g/dL] - observed Hgb) x LBW + (0.26 x LBW) **or** replacement iron (mg) = blood loss (mL) x Hct; **Note:** Total dose should be divided daily at not more than 100 mg/day

I.V.:

Children <4 months: Use not recommended

Children <5 kg: Replacement iron (mg) = blood loss (mL) x Hct; **Note:** Total dose should be divided daily at not more than 100 mg/day

Children 5-15 kg: Total Dose (mL) = 0.0442 (desired Hgb [usually 12 g/dL] - observed Hgb) x W (in kg) + (0.26 x W [in kg]) **or** replacement iron (mg) = blood loss (mL) x hematocrit; **Note:** Total dose should be divided daily at not more than 100 mg/day

Children >15 kg: Total Dose (mL) = 0.0442 (desired Hgb [usually 14.8 g/dL] - observed Hgb) x LBW + (0.26 x LBW) **or** replacement iron (mg) = blood loss (mL) x Hct (maximum: 100 mg/day); **Note:** Total dose should be divided daily at not more than 100 mg/day

Adults: Total Dose (mL) = 0.0442 (desired Hgb [usually 14.8 g/dL] - observed Hgb) x LBW + (0.26 x LBW) **or** replacement iron (mg) = blood loss (mL) x Hct (maximum: 100 mg/day); **Note:** Total dose should be divided daily at not more than 100 mg/day

Dosage Forms Excipient information presented when available (limited, particularly for generics); consult specific product labeling.

Note: Strength expressed as elemental iron

Injection, solution:

Dexferrum®: 50 mg/mL (1 mL, 2 mL) [high-molecular-weight iron dextran]

INFeD®: 50 mg/mL (2 mL) [low-molecular-weight iron dextran]

- **Iron Fumarate** *see* Ferrous Fumarate *on page 626*
- **Iron Gluconate** *see* Ferrous Gluconate *on page 627*
- **Iron-Polysaccharide Complex** *see* Polysaccharide-Iron Complex *on page 1313*

Iron Sucrose (EYE ern SOO krose)

U.S. Brand Names Venofer®

Canadian Brand Names Venofer®

Pharmacologic Category Iron Salt

Use Treatment of iron-deficiency anemia in chronic renal failure, including nondialysis-dependent patients (with or without erythropoietin therapy) and dialysis-dependent patients receiving erythropoietin therapy

Effect on Mental Status May cause dizziness and malaise

Effect on Psychiatric Treatment Hypotension is common; concurrent use with psychotropic medications may produce additive hypotensive effects; use caution. Nausea and vomiting are common; concurrent use with SSRIs, valproic acid, and lithium may produce additive effects; monitor.

Dosage Summary

I.V.:

Children: Dosage not established

Adults: 100 mg (5 mL) 1-3 times/week during dialysis **or** 200 mg on 5 different occasions within a 14-day period **or** two 300 mg infusion 14 days apart, followed by a single 400 mg infusion 14 days later (maximum: 1000 mg cumulative total)

Dosage Forms Excipient information presented when available (limited, particularly for generics); consult specific product labeling.

Injection, solution [preservative free]:

Venofer®: 20 mg of elemental iron/mL (5 mL, 10 mL)

- **Iron Sulfate** *see* Ferrous Sulfate *on page 627*
- **Iron Sulfate and Vitamin C** *see* Ferrous Sulfate and Ascorbic Acid *on page 628*
- **ISD** *see* Isosorbide Dinitrate *on page 866*
- **ISDN** *see* Isosorbide Dinitrate *on page 866*
- **Isentress™** *see* Raltegravir *on page 1393*
- **ISMN** *see* Isosorbide Mononitrate *on page 869*
- **Ismo®** *see* Isosorbide Mononitrate *on page 869*
- **Isoamyl Nitrite** *see* Amyl Nitrite *on page 124*
- **Isobamate** *see* Carisoprodol *on page 283*

Isocarboxazid (eye soe kar BOKS a zid)

Related Information

Antidepressant Agents *on page 1760*

U.S. Brand Names Marplan®

Pharmacologic Category Antidepressant, Monoamine Oxidase Inhibitor

Generic Available No

Use Treatment of depression

Mental Health Comment Not commonly used due to a required low tyramine diet and drug-drug interactions. It is estimated that 20 mg of tranylcypromine = 40 mg of isocarboxazid = 45 mg phenelzine. Phenelzine and isocarboxazid are hydrazine MAO inhibitors and tranylcypromine is a nonhydrazine. These drugs produce irreversible inhibition of MAO inhibitors. The half-life for regeneration is 2-3 days. Therefore, a 2-week period is required when switching from an MAO inhibitor to another antidepressant.

While hypertension and hypertensive crisis are risks associated with MAO inhibitor therapy, orthostatic hypotension may also occur. Orthostasis associated with MAO inhibitor therapy is not related to alpha$_1$-adrenergic receptor blockade. The "false transmitter" concept is used to explain this side effect. This concept states that MAO inhibitors promote gradual accumulation in sympathetic nerve ending of amines lacking direct sympathomimetic activity (octopamine) at the expense of the normal synaptic transmitter, norepinephrine. Since octopamine has little ability to activate either alpha- or beta-adrenergic receptors, a functional impairment of sympathetic neurotransmission occurs.

The MAO inhibitors are usually reserved for patients who do not tolerate or respond to other antidepressants. The brain activity of monoamine oxidase increases with age and even more so in patients with Alzheimer's disease. Therefore, the MAO inhibitors may have an increased role in patients with Alzheimer's disease who are depressed. Phenelzine is less stimulating than tranylcypromine.

Restrictions An FDA-approved medication guide concerning the use of antidepressants in children, adolescents, and young adults must be distributed when dispensing an outpatient prescription (new or refill) where this medication is to be used without direct supervision of a healthcare provider. Medication guides are available at http://www.fda.gov/cder/Offices/ODS/medication_guides.htm. Dispense to parents or guardians of children and adolescents receiving this medication.

Pregnancy Risk Factor C

Lactation Excretion in breast milk unknown/not recommended

Contraindications

Hypersensitivity to isocarboxazid or any component of the formulation; cardiovascular disease (including CHF, or HTN); cerebrovascular disease; history of hepatic disease or abnormal liver function tests; pheochromocytoma; renal disease or severe renal impairment

Concurrent use of sympathomimetics (including amphetamines, cocaine, dopamine, epinephrine, methylphenidate, norepinephrine, or phenylephrine) and related compounds (methyldopa, levodopa, phenylalanine, tryptophan, or tyrosine), as well as ophthalmic alpha$_2$-agonists (apraclonidine, brimonidine); may result in behavioral and neurologic symptoms

CNS depressants, cyclobenzaprine, dextromethorphan, ethanol, meperidine, bupropion, buspirone; may result in delirium, excitation, hyper-/hypotension, hyperpyrexia, seizures, and coma

Isocarboxazid **initiation**: At least 2 weeks should elapse between the discontinuation of serotoninergic agents (including SSRIs and tricyclics) and the initiation of isocarboxazid; at least 5 weeks should elapse between the discontinuation of fluoxetine and the initiation of isocarboxazid; at least 1 week should elapse between the discontinuation of other monoamine oxidase (MAO) inhibitors and the initiation of isocarboxazid (using half the normal starting dose). In all cases, a sufficient amount of time must be allowed for the clearance of the serotoninergic agent and any active metabolites prior to the initiation of isocarboxazid.

Isocarboxazid **discontinuation**: At least 2 weeks should elapse between the discontinuation of isocarboxazid and the initiation of the following agents: Serotoninergic agents (including SSRIs, fluoxetine, and tricyclics), bupropion, and other antidepressants. Two to 3 weeks should elapse between the discontinuation of isocarboxazid and the initiation of meperidine. At least 10 days should elapse between the discontinuation of isocarboxazid and initiation of buspirone. At least 1 week should elapse between the discontinuation of isocarboxazid and the initiation of other MAO inhibitors (see specific agent for details).

Antihypertensive agents (including thiazide diuretics): may result in potentiation of antihypertensive effects.

General anesthesia, spinal anesthesia (hypotension may be exaggerated). Use caution with local anesthetics containing sympathomimetic agents. Discontinue drug 10 days prior to elective surgery.

Foods high in tyramine or dopamine content; foods and/or supplements containing tyrosine, phenylalanine, tryptophan, or caffeine; may result in hypertensive reactions.

Warnings/Precautions [U.S. Boxed Warning]: Antidepressants increase the risk of suicidal thinking and behavior in children, adolescents, and young adults (18-24 years of age) with major depressive disorder (MDD) and other psychiatric disorders; consider risk prior to prescribing. Short-term studies did not show an increased risk in patients >24 years of age and showed a decreased risk in patients ≥65 years. Closely monitor for clinical worsening, suicidality, or unusual changes in behavior; the patient's family or caregiver should be instructed to closely observe the patient and communicate condition with healthcare provider. A medication guide should be dispensed with each prescription. **Isocarboxazid is FDA approved for the treatment of depression in children ≥16 years of age.**

The possibility of a suicide attempt is inherent in major depression and may persist until remission occurs. Monitor for worsening of depression or suicidality, especially during initiation of therapy (generally first 1-2 months) or with dose increases or decreases. Use caution in high-risk patients. Worsening depression and severe abrupt suicidality that are not part of the presenting symptoms may require discontinuation or modification of drug therapy. The patient's family or caregiver should be alerted to monitor patients for the emergence of suicidality and associated behaviors (such as agitation, irritability, hostility, impulsivity, and hypomania) and notify healthcare provider.

May worsen psychosis in some patients or precipitate a shift to mania or hypomania in patients with bipolar disorder. Patients presenting with depressive symptoms should be screened for bipolar disorder. Monotherapy in patients with bipolar disorder should be avoided. Isocarboxazid is not FDA approved for the treatment of bipolar depression. Isocarboxazid should not be used for initial therapy but reserved for patients who have not responded to other antidepressants.

Use with caution in patients who are hyperactive, hyperexcitable, have a seizure disorder, or who have glaucoma, hyperthyroidism, or diabetes, or renal impairment; avoid use in hepatic impairment or severe renal impairment. High potential for interactions; do not use with other MAO inhibitors or antidepressants. Avoid products containing sympathomimetic stimulants, dextromethorphan, disulfiram, and meperidine. Concurrent use with antihypertensive agents may lead to exaggeration of hypotensive effects. May cause orthostatic hypotension (especially at dosages >30 mg/day). Use with caution in patients with hypotension or patients who would not tolerate transient hypotensive episodes; effects may be additive when used with other agents known to cause orthostasis (phenothiazines). Hypertensive crisis may occur with foods/supplements high in tyramine, tryptophan, phenylalanine, or tyrosine content.

Discontinue at least 48 hours prior to myelography. May increase the risks associated with electroconvulsive therapy. Consider discontinuing, when possible, prior to elective surgery. Use with caution in patients receiving disulfiram.

Adverse Reactions

>10%: Central nervous system: Dizziness (29%), headache (15%)

1% to 10%:

- Cardiovascular: Orthostatic hypotension (4%), syncope (2%), palpitation (2%)
- Central nervous system: Sleep disturbance (5%), drowsiness (4%), anxiety (2%), chills (2%), forgetfulness (2%), hyperactivity (2%), lethargy (2%), sedation (2%)
- Gastrointestinal: Xerostomia (9%), constipation (7%), nausea (6%), diarrhea (2%)
- Genitourinary: Urinary frequency (2%), impotence (2%), urinary hesitancy (1%)
- Neuromuscular & skeletal: Tremor (4%), myoclonus (2%), paresthesia (2%)
- Miscellaneous: Diaphoresis (2%), heavy feeling (2%)

<1% (Limited to important or life-threatening): Ataxia, black tongue, coma, hallucination, hematologic changes, hepatitis, SIADH, Parkinsonian syndrome, sexual disturbances, toxic amblyopia

Drug Interactions

Acetylcholinesterase Inhibitors (Central): Anticholinergics may diminish the therapeutic effect of Acetylcholinesterase Inhibitors (Central). Acetylcholinesterase Inhibitors (Central) may diminish the therapeutic effect of Anticholinergics. If the anticholinergic action is a side effect of the agent, the result may be beneficial. *Risk C: Monitor therapy*

Alcohol (Ethyl): CNS Depressants may enhance the CNS depressant effect of Alcohol (Ethyl). *Risk C: Monitor therapy*

Alpha-/Beta-Agonists (Direct-Acting): MAO Inhibitors may enhance the vasopressor effect of Alpha-/Beta-Agonists (Direct-Acting). Primarily with oral administration of phenylephrine. **Exceptions:** Dipivefrin. *Risk D: Consider therapy modification*

Alpha-/Beta-Agonists (Indirect-Acting): MAO Inhibitors may enhance the hypertensive effect of Alpha-/Beta-Agonists (Indirect-Acting). *Risk X: Avoid combination*

Alpha1-Agonists: MAO Inhibitors may enhance the hypertensive effect of Alpha1-Agonists. *Risk X: Avoid combination*

Alpha2-Agonists (Ophthalmic): MAO Inhibitors may enhance the hypertensive effect of Alpha2-Agonists (Ophthalmic). *Risk X: Avoid combination*

Altretamine: May enhance the orthostatic effect of MAO Inhibitors. *Risk C: Monitor therapy*

Amphetamines: MAO Inhibitors may enhance the hypertensive effect of Amphetamines. *Risk X: Avoid combination*

Anilidopiperidine Opioids: May enhance the serotonergic effect of MAO Inhibitors. This could result in serotonin syndrome. Management: Avoid use of fentanyl (and other anilidopiperidine opioids when possible) in patients who have used a monoamine oxidase inhibitor within the past 14 days due to reports of unpredictable but severe adverse effects. *Risk D: Consider therapy modification*

Anticholinergics: May enhance the adverse/toxic effect of other Anticholinergics. **Exceptions:** Paliperidone. *Risk C: Monitor therapy*

Antidepressants (Serotonin/Norepinephrine Reuptake Inhibitor): MAO Inhibitors may enhance the serotonergic effect of Antidepressants (Serotonin/Norepinephrine Reuptake Inhibitor). This may cause serotonin syndrome. *Risk X: Avoid combination*

Atomoxetine: MAO Inhibitors may enhance the neurotoxic (central) effect of Atomoxetine. *Risk X: Avoid combination*

Beta2-Agonists: MAO Inhibitors may enhance the adverse/toxic effect of Beta2-Agonists. *Risk C: Monitor therapy*

BuPROPion: MAO Inhibitors may enhance the neurotoxic (central) effect of BuPROPion. *Risk X: Avoid combination*

BusPIRone: May enhance the adverse/toxic effect of MAO Inhibitors. Elevated blood pressure has been reported. *Risk X: Avoid combination*

CNS Depressants: May enhance the adverse/toxic effect of other CNS Depressants. *Risk C: Monitor therapy*

COMT Inhibitors: May enhance the adverse/toxic effect of MAO Inhibitors. *Risk D: Consider therapy modification*

Cyclobenzaprine: May enhance the serotonergic effect of MAO Inhibitors. This could result in serotonin syndrome. *Risk X: Avoid combination*

Dexmethylphenidate: MAO Inhibitors may enhance the hypertensive effect of Dexmethylphenidate. *Risk X: Avoid combination*

Dextromethorphan: MAO Inhibitors may enhance the serotonergic effect of Dextromethorphan. This may cause serotonin syndrome. *Risk X: Avoid combination*

Levodopa: May enhance the adverse/toxic effect of MAO Inhibitors. Of particular concern is the development of hypertensive reactions when levodopa is used with nonselective MAOI. *Risk D: Consider therapy modification*

Linezolid: MAO Inhibitors may enhance the adverse/toxic effect of Linezolid. *Risk X: Avoid combination*

Lithium: MAO Inhibitors may enhance the adverse/toxic effect of Lithium. *Risk C: Monitor therapy*

Maprotiline: May enhance the adverse/toxic effect of MAO Inhibitors. *Risk X: Avoid combination*

Meperidine: MAO Inhibitors may enhance the serotonergic effect of Meperidine. This may cause serotonin syndrome. *Risk X: Avoid combination*

Methyldopa: MAO Inhibitors may enhance the adverse/toxic effect of Methyldopa. *Risk X: Avoid combination*

Methylphenidate: MAO Inhibitors may enhance the hypertensive effect of Methylphenidate. *Risk X: Avoid combination*

Mirtazapine: MAO Inhibitors may enhance the neurotoxic (central) effect of Mirtazapine. *Risk X: Avoid combination*

Pramlintide: May enhance the anticholinergic effect of Anticholinergics. These effects are specific to the GI tract. *Risk D: Consider therapy modification*

Propoxyphene: May enhance the adverse/toxic effect of MAO Inhibitors. Specifically, the risk of serotonin syndrome or other serotonergic adverse events may be increased. *Risk X: Avoid combination*

Rauwolfia Alkaloids: MAO Inhibitors may enhance the adverse/toxic effect of Rauwolfia Alkaloids. Existing MAOI therapy can result in paradoxical effects of added rauwolfia alkaloids (eg, excitation, hypertension). *Risk D: Consider therapy modification*

Selective Serotonin Reuptake Inhibitors: MAO Inhibitors may enhance the serotonergic effect of Selective Serotonin Reuptake Inhibitors. This may cause serotonin syndrome. *Risk X: Avoid combination*

Serotonin 5-HT1D Receptor Agonists: MAO Inhibitors may decrease the metabolism of Serotonin 5-HT1D Receptor Agonists. Management: If MAO inhibitor therapy is required, naratriptan, eletriptan or frovatriptan may be a suitable 5-HT1D agonist to employ. **Exceptions:** Eletriptan; Frovatriptan; Naratriptan. *Risk X: Avoid combination*

Serotonin Modulators: May enhance the adverse/toxic effect of other Serotonin Modulators. The development of serotonin syndrome may occur. *Risk D: Consider therapy modification*

Sibutramine: May enhance the serotonergic effect of Serotonin Modulators. This may cause serotonin syndrome. *Risk X: Avoid combination*

Tetrabenazine: May enhance the adverse/toxic effect of MAO Inhibitors. *Risk X: Avoid combination*

TraMADol: May enhance the neuroexcitatory and/or seizure-potentiating effect of MAO Inhibitors. *Risk D: Consider therapy modification*

Tricyclic Antidepressants: MAO Inhibitors may enhance the serotonergic effect of Tricyclic Antidepressants. This may cause serotonin syndrome. *Risk X: Avoid combination*

Ethanol/Nutrition/Herb Interactions

Ethanol: Avoid ethanol (based on CNS depressant effects and potential tyramine content)

Food: Concurrent ingestion of foods rich in tyramine may cause sudden and severe high blood pressure (hypertensive crisis). Avoid tyramine-containing foods with MAO inhibitors. Food's freshness is also an important concern; improperly stored or spoiled food can create an environment where tyramine concentrations may increase.

Herb/Nutraceuticals: Avoid supplements containing caffeine, tyrosine, tryptophan or phenylalanine. Ingestion of large quantities may increase the risk of severe side effects (eg, hypertensive reactions, serotonin syndrome).

Mechanism of Action Thought to act by increasing endogenous concentrations of epinephrine, norepinephrine, dopamine, and serotonin through inhibition of the enzyme (monoamine oxidase) responsible for the breakdown of these neurotransmitters

Dosage Oral: Adults: Initial: 10 mg 2-4 times/day; may increase by 10 mg/day every 2-4 days to 40 mg/day by the end of the first week (divided into 2-4 doses). After first week, may increase by up to 20 mg/week to a maximum of 60 mg/day. May take 3-6 weeks to see effects. Dose should be reduced once maximum clinical effect is seen. If no response obtained within 6 weeks, additional titration is unlikely to be beneficial. **Note:** Use caution in patients on >40 mg/day; experience is limited.

Dietary Considerations Avoid tyramine-containing foods/beverages. Some examples include aged or matured cheese, air-dried or cured meats (including sausages and salamis), fava or broad bean pods, tap/draft beers, Marmite concentrate, sauerkraut, soy sauce and other soybean condiments.

Monitoring Parameters

Blood pressure, heart rate; mood, suicidal ideation (especially at the beginning of therapy or when doses are increased or decreased)

Dosage Forms Excipient information presented when available (limited, particularly for generics); consult specific product labeling.

Tablet: 10 mg

- **Isochron™** *see* Isosorbide Dinitrate *on page 866*
- **Isometheptene, Acetaminophen, and Dichloralphenazone** *see* Acetaminophen, Isometheptene, and Dichloralphenazone *on page 45*
- **Isometheptene, Dichloralphenazone, and Acetaminophen** *see* Acetaminophen, Isometheptene, and Dichloralphenazone *on page 45*
- **IsonaRif™** *see* Rifampin and Isoniazid *on page 1419*

Isoniazid (eye soe NYE a zid)

Medication Safety Issues

International issues:

Hydra® [Japan] may be confused with Hydrea®

Canadian Brand Names Isotamine®; PMS-Isoniazid

Mexican Brand Names Valifol

Index Terms INH; Isonicotinic Acid Hydrazide

Pharmacologic Category Antitubercular Agent

Generic Available Yes

Use Treatment of susceptible tuberculosis infections; treatment of latent tuberculosis infection (LTBI)

Effect on Mental Status May cause drowsiness or dizziness; may rarely cause depression or psychosis; reports of insomnia, restlessness, disorientation, hallucinations, delusions, obsessive-compulsive symptoms, and exacerbation of schizophrenia

Effect on Psychiatric Treatment Isoniazid may impair the metabolism of carbamazepine and oxidatively metabolized benzodiazepines; monitor for adverse effects

Pregnancy Risk Factor C

Pregnancy Considerations Isoniazid was found to be embryocidal in animal studies; teratogenic effects were not noted. Isoniazid crosses the human placenta. Due to the risk of tuberculosis to the fetus, treatment is recommended when the probability of maternal disease is moderate to high. The CDC recommends isoniazid as part of the initial treatment regimen (CDC, 2003). Pyridoxine supplementation is recommended (25 mg/day).

Lactation Enters breast milk/compatible

Contraindications Hypersensitivity to isoniazid or any component of the formulation; acute liver disease; previous history of hepatic damage during isoniazid therapy; previous severe adverse reaction (drug fever, chills, arthritis) to isoniazid

Warnings/Precautions Use with caution in patients with severe renal impairment and liver disease. **[U.S. Boxed Warning]: Severe and sometimes fatal hepatitis may occur; usually occurs within the first 3 months of treatment, although may develop even after many months of treatment.** The risk of developing hepatitis is age-related; daily ethanol consumption may also increase the risk. Patients must report any prodromal symptoms of hepatitis, such as fatigue, weakness, malaise, anorexia, nausea, or vomiting. Treatment with isoniazid for latent tuberculosis infection should be deferred in patients with acute hepatic diseases. Periodic ophthalmic examinations are recommended even when usual symptoms do not occur. Pyridoxine (10-50 mg/day) is recommended in individuals at risk for development of peripheral neuropathies (eg, HIV infection, nutritional deficiency, diabetes, pregnancy). Children with low milk and low meat intake should receive concomitant pyridoxine therapy. Multidrug regimens should be utilized for the treatment of active tuberculosis to prevent the emergence of drug resistance.

Adverse Reactions Frequency not defined.

Cardiovascular: Hypertension, palpitation, tachycardia, vasculitis

Central nervous system: Depression, dizziness, encephalopathy, fever, lethargy, memory impairment, psychosis, seizure, slurred speech

Dermatologic: Flushing, rash (morbilliform, maculopapular, pruritic, or exfoliative)

Endocrine & metabolic: Gynecomastia, hyperglycemia, metabolic acidosis, pellagra, pyridoxine deficiency

Gastrointestinal: Anorexia, nausea, vomiting, stomach pain

Hematologic: Agranulocytosis, anemia (sideroblastic, hemolytic, or aplastic), eosinophilia, thrombocytopenia

Hepatic: LFTs mildly increased (10% to 20%); hyperbilirubinemia, bilirubinuria, jaundice, hepatitis (may involve progressive liver damage; risk increases with age; 2.3% in patients >50 years), hepatic dysfunction

Neuromuscular & skeletal: Arthralgia, hyper-reflexia, peripheral neuropathy (dose-related incidence, 10% to 20% incidence with 10 mg/kg/day), weakness

Ocular: Blurred vision, loss of vision, optic neuritis and atrophy

Miscellaneous: Lupus-like syndrome, lymphadenopathy, rheumatic syndrome

Metabolism/Transport Effects Substrate of CYP2E1 (major); **Inhibits** CYP1A2 (weak), 2A6 (moderate), 2C9 (weak), 2C19 (strong), 2D6 (moderate), 2E1 (moderate), 3A4 (strong); **Induces** CYP2E1 (after discontinuation) (weak)

Drug Interactions

Acetaminophen: Isoniazid may enhance the adverse/toxic effect of Acetaminophen. *Risk C: Monitor therapy*

Alfuzosin: CYP3A4 Inhibitors (Strong) may increase the serum concentration of Alfuzosin. *Risk X: Avoid combination*

Alosetron: CYP3A4 Inhibitors (Strong) may increase the serum concentration of Alosetron. *Risk C: Monitor therapy*

Antacids: May decrease the absorption of Isoniazid. *Risk D: Consider therapy modification*

Benzodiazepines (metabolized by oxidation): Isoniazid may decrease the metabolism of Benzodiazepines (metabolized by oxidation). *Risk C: Monitor therapy*

CarBAMazepine: Isoniazid may decrease the metabolism of CarBAMazepine. *Risk D: Consider therapy modification*

Chlorzoxazone: Isoniazid may decrease the metabolism of Chlorzoxazone. *Risk C: Monitor therapy*

Ciclesonide: CYP3A4 Inhibitors (Strong) may increase the serum concentration of Ciclesonide. Specifically, concentrations of the active des-ciclesonide metabolite may be increased. *Risk C: Monitor therapy*

Codeine: CYP2D6 Inhibitors (Moderate) may diminish the therapeutic effect of Codeine. These CYP2D6 inhibitors may prevent the metabolic conversion of codeine to its active metabolite morphine. *Risk C: Monitor therapy*

Corticosteroids (Systemic): May decrease the serum concentration of Isoniazid. *Risk C: Monitor therapy*

CycloSERINE: May enhance the CNS depressant effect of Isoniazid. *Risk D: Consider therapy modification*

CYP2A6 Substrates: CYP2A6 Inhibitors (Moderate) may decrease the metabolism of CYP2A6 Substrates. *Risk C: Monitor therapy*

CYP2C19 Substrates: CYP2C19 Inhibitors (Strong) may decrease the metabolism of CYP2C19 Substrates. *Risk D: Consider therapy modification*

CYP2D6 Substrates: CYP2D6 Inhibitors (Moderate) may decrease the metabolism of CYP2D6 Substrates. **Exceptions:** Tamoxifen. *Risk C: Monitor therapy*

CYP2E1 Substrates: CYP2E1 Inhibitors (Moderate) may decrease the metabolism of CYP2E1 Substrates. *Risk C: Monitor therapy*

CYP3A4 Substrates: CYP3A4 Inhibitors (Strong) may decrease the metabolism of CYP3A4 Substrates. *Risk D: Consider therapy modification*

Eplerenone: CYP3A4 Inhibitors (Strong) may increase the serum concentration of Eplerenone. *Risk X: Avoid combination*

Ixabepilone: CYP3A4 Inhibitors (Strong) may increase the serum concentration of Ixabepilone. *Risk D: Consider therapy modification*

Maraviroc: CYP3A4 Inhibitors may increase the serum concentration of Maraviroc. *Risk D: Consider therapy modification*

Nebivolol: CYP2D6 Inhibitors (Moderate) may increase the serum concentration of Nebivolol. *Risk C: Monitor therapy*

Nilotinib: CYP3A4 Inhibitors (Strong) may increase the serum concentration of Nilotinib. *Risk X: Avoid combination*

Nisoldipine: CYP3A4 Inhibitors (Strong) may increase the serum concentration of Nisoldipine. *Risk X: Avoid combination*

Phenytoin: Isoniazid may decrease the metabolism of Phenytoin. *Risk D: Consider therapy modification*

Pimecrolimus: CYP3A4 Inhibitors (Strong) may decrease the metabolism of Pimecrolimus. *Risk C: Monitor therapy*

Ranolazine: CYP3A4 Inhibitors (Strong) may increase the serum concentration of Ranolazine. *Risk X: Avoid combination*

Rifamycin Derivatives: May enhance the hepatotoxic effect of Isoniazid. Even so, this is a frequently employed combination regimen. *Risk C: Monitor therapy*

Rivaroxaban: CYP3A4 Inhibitors (Strong) may increase the serum concentration of Rivaroxaban. *Risk X: Avoid combination*

Salmeterol: CYP3A4 Inhibitors (Strong) may increase the serum concentration of Salmeterol. *Risk X: Avoid combination*

Sorafenib: CYP3A4 Inhibitors (Strong) may increase the serum concentration of Sorafenib. *Risk C: Monitor therapy*

Tamoxifen: CYP2D6 Inhibitors (Moderate) may decrease the metabolism of Tamoxifen. Specifically, CYP2D6 inhibitors may decrease the formation of highly potent active metabolites. *Risk D: Consider therapy modification*

Theophylline Derivatives: Isoniazid may decrease the metabolism of Theophylline Derivatives. **Exceptions:** Dyphylline. *Risk D: Consider therapy modification*

Thioridazine: CYP2D6 Inhibitors may decrease the metabolism of Thioridazine. *Risk X: Avoid combination*

TraMADol: CYP2D6 Inhibitors (Moderate) may diminish the therapeutic effect of TraMADol. These CYP2D6 inhibitors may prevent the metabolic conversion of tramadol to its active metabolite that accounts for much of its opioid-like effects. *Risk C: Monitor therapy*

Ethanol/Nutrition/Herb Interactions

Ethanol: Avoid ethanol (increases the risk of hepatitis).

Food: Isoniazid should not be taken with food; serum levels may be decreased if taken with food. Has some ability to inhibit tyramine metabolism; several case reports of mild reactions (flushing, palpitations) after ingestion of cheese (with or without wine). Reactions resembling allergic symptoms following ingestion of fish high in histamine content have been reported. Isoniazid decreases folic acid absorption. Isoniazid alters pyridoxine metabolism.

Stability

Tablet: Store at 20°C to 25°C (68°F to 77°F). Protect from light.

Oral solution: Store at 15°C to 30°C (59°F to 86°F). Protect from light.

Mechanism of Action Unknown, but may include the inhibition of mycolic acid synthesis resulting in disruption of the bacterial cell wall

Pharmacodynamics/Kinetics

Absorption: Rapid and complete; rate can be slowed with food

Distribution: All body tissues and fluids including CSF; crosses placenta; enters breast milk

Protein binding: 10% to 15%

Metabolism: Hepatic with decay rate determined genetically by acetylation phenotype

Half-life elimination: Fast acetylators: 30-100 minutes; Slow acetylators: 2-5 hours; may be prolonged with hepatic or severe renal impairment

Time to peak, serum: 1-2 hours

Excretion: Urine (75% to 95%); feces; saliva

Dosage

Usual dosage ranges: Oral, I.M.:

Infants and Children: 10-15 mg/kg/day in 1-2 divided doses (maximum: 300 mg/day) or 20-40 mg/kg given 2-3 times per week (maximum: 900 mg/dose)

Adults: 5 mg/kg/day (usual: 300 mg/day) as a single daily dose or 15 mg/kg (maximum: 900 mg/dose) given 2-3 times per week

Indication-specific dosing: Oral, I.M.: Recommendations often change due to resistant strains and newly-developed information; consult *MMWR* for current CDC recommendations. Intramuscular injection is available for patients who are unable to either take or absorb oral therapy.

Infants and Children:

Tuberculosis, active:

Daily therapy: 10-15 mg/kg/day in 1-2 divided doses (maximum: 300 mg/day)

Twice weekly or 3 times/week directly observed therapy (DOT): 20-40 mg/kg (maximum: 900 mg)

Tuberculosis, latent infection (LTBI): 10 mg/kg/day as a single dose (maximum: 300 mg/day) **or** 20-30 mg/kg (maximum: 900 mg/dose) twice weekly for 9 months

Adults: **Note:** Concomitant administration of 10-50 mg/day pyridoxine is recommended in malnourished patients or those prone to neuropathy (eg, alcoholics, patients with diabetes).

Nontuberculous mycobacterium (*M. kansasii*) (unlabeled use): 5 mg/kg/day (maximum: 300 mg/day) for duration to include 12 months of culture-negative sputum; typically used in combination with ethambutol and rifampin

Tuberculosis, active:

Daily therapy: 5 mg/kg/day given daily (usual dose: 300 mg/day)

Twice weekly or 3 times/week directly observed therapy (DOT): 15 mg/kg (maximum: 900 mg). **Note:** CDC guidelines state that once-weekly therapy (15 mg/kg/dose) may be considered, but only after the first 2 months of initial therapy in HIV-negative patients, and only in combination with rifapentine.

Note: Treatment may be defined by the number of doses administered (eg, "six-month" therapy involves 182 doses of INH and rifampin, and 56 doses of pyrazinamide). Six months is the shortest interval of time over which these doses may be administered, assuming no interruption of therapy.

Tuberculosis, latent infection (LTBI): 300 mg/day or 900 mg twice weekly for 6-9 months in patients who do not have HIV infection (9 months is optimal, 6 months may be considered to reduce costs of therapy) and 9 months in patients who have HIV infection. Extend to 12 months of therapy if interruptions in treatment occur.

Dosing adjustment in renal impairment: No adjustment necessary

Hemodialysis: Dialyzable (50% to 100%); administer dose post dialysis

Dosing adjustment in hepatic impairment: No adjustment required, however, use with caution; may accumulate and additional liver damage may occur in patients with pre-existing liver disease. For ALT or AST >3 times the ULN: discontinue or temporarily withhold treatment. Treatment with isoniazid for latent tuberculosis infection should be deferred in patients with acute hepatic diseases.

Dietary Considerations Should be taken 1 hour before or 2 hours after meals on an empty stomach; increase dietary intake of folate, niacin, magnesium. Avoid tyramine-containing foods. Avoid histamine-containing foods.

Administration Should be administered 1 hour before or 2 hours after meals on an empty stomach.

Monitoring Parameters Baseline and periodic (more frequently in patients with higher risk for hepatitis) liver function tests (ALT and AST); sputum cultures monthly (until 2 consecutive negative cultures reported); monitoring for prodromal signs of hepatitis

Reference Range Therapeutic: 1-7 mcg/mL (SI: 7-51 µmol/L); Toxic: 20-710 mcg/mL (SI: 146-5176 µmol/L)

Test Interactions False-positive urinary glucose with Clinitest®

Additional Information The AAP recommends that pyridoxine supplementation (1-2 mg/kg/day) should be administered to malnourished patients, children or adolescents on meat or milk-deficient diets, breast-feeding infants, and those predisposed to neuritis to prevent peripheral neuropathy; administration of isoniazid syrup has been associated with diarrhea

Dosage Forms Excipient information presented when available (limited, particularly for generics); consult specific product labeling.
Injection, solution: 100 mg/mL (10 mL)
Oral solution: 50 mg/5 mL (473 mL) [orange flavor]
Tablet: 100 mg, 300 mg

- ◆ **Isoniazid and Rifampin** *see* Rifampin and Isoniazid *on page 1419*
- ◆ **Isoniazid, Rifampin, and Pyrazinamide** *see* Rifampin, Isoniazid, and Pyrazinamide *on page 1419*
- ◆ **Isonicotinic Acid Hydrazide** *see* Isoniazid *on page 862*
- ◆ **Isonipecaine Hydrochloride** *see* Meperidine *on page 986*
- ◆ **Isophane Insulin** *see* Insulin NPH *on page 835*
- ◆ **Isophane Insulin and Regular Insulin** *see* Insulin NPH and Insulin Regular *on page 836*
- ◆ **Isophosphamide** *see* Ifosfamide *on page 809*

Isoproterenol (eye soe proe TER e nole)

Medication Safety Issues
Sound-alike/look-alike issues:
Isuprel® may be confused with Disophrol®, Ismelin®, Isordil®

U.S. Brand Names Isuprel®

Index Terms Isoproterenol Hydrochloride

Pharmacologic Category Beta$_1$- & Beta$_2$-Adrenergic Agonist Agent

Use Ventricular arrhythmias due to AV nodal block; hemodynamically compromised bradyarrhythmias or atropine- and dopamine-resistant bradyarrhythmias (when transcutaneous/venous pacing is not available); temporary use in third-degree AV block until pacemaker insertion

Unlabeled/Investigational Use Pharmacologic overdrive pacing for torsade de pointes; diagnostic aid (vasovagal syncope)

Effect on Mental Status Insomnia and restlessness are common

Effect on Psychiatric Treatment None reported

Dosage Summary
I.V.:
Children: Initial: 0.1 mcg/kg/minute; Maintenance: 0.2-2 mcg/kg/minute
Adults: Initial: 2 mcg/minute; Maintenance: 2-10 mcg/minute

Dosage Forms Excipient information presented when available (limited, particularly for generics); consult specific product labeling.
Injection, solution, as hydrochloride:
Isuprel®: 0.2 mg/mL (1:5000) (1 mL, 5 mL) [contains sodium metabisulfite]

- ◆ **Isoproterenol Hydrochloride** *see* Isoproterenol *on page 866*
- ◆ **Isoptin® SR** *see* Verapamil *on page 1665*
- ◆ **Isopto® Atropine** *see* Atropine *on page 158*
- ◆ **Isopto® Carpine** *see* Pilocarpine *on page 1290*
- ◆ **Isopto® Homatropine** *see* Homatropine *on page 769*
- ◆ **Isopto® Hyoscine** *see* Scopolamine Derivatives *on page 1463*
- ◆ **Isordil®** *see* Isosorbide Dinitrate *on page 866*

Isosorbide Dinitrate (eye soe SOR bide dye NYE trate)

Medication Safety Issues
Sound-alike/look-alike issues:
Isordil® may be confused with Inderal®, Isuprel®

International issues:
Nitrobide® [Japan] may be confused with Microzide® which is a brand name for hydrochlorothiazide in the U.S.

Related Information
Anticholinergic Effects of Common Psychotropics *on page 1758*

U.S. Brand Names Dilatrate®-SR; Isochron™; Isordil®

Canadian Brand Names Apo-ISDN®; Cedocard®-SR; Coronex®; Novo-Sorbide; PMS-Isosorbide

Mexican Brand Names Isorbid

Index Terms ISD; ISDN

Pharmacologic Category Vasodilator

Generic Available Yes: Tablet, sublingual tablet

Use Prevention and treatment of angina pectoris; for congestive heart failure; to relieve pain, dysphagia, and spasm in esophageal spasm with GE reflux

Unlabeled/Investigational Use Esophageal spastic disorders

Effect on Mental Status May cause dizziness

Effect on Psychiatric Treatment None reported

Pregnancy Risk Factor C

Lactation Excretion in breast milk unknown

Contraindications Hypersensitivity to isosorbide dinitrate or any component of the formulation; hypersensitivity to organic nitrates; concurrent use with phosphodiesterase-5 (PDE-5) inhibitors (sildenafil, tadalafil, or vardenafil); angle-closure glaucoma (intraocular pressure may be increased); head trauma or cerebral hemorrhage (increase intracranial pressure); severe anemia

Warnings/Precautions Use with caution in patients with increased intracranial pressure, hypotension, hypovolemia, right ventricular infarctions, and glaucoma. Paradoxical bradycardia and increased angina pectoris can accompany hypotension. Postural hypotension may also occur; ethanol may potentiate this effect. Tolerance does develop to nitrates and appropriate dosing is needed to minimize this. Nitrates may aggravate angina caused by hypertrophic cardiomyopathy. Avoid concurrent use with PDE-5 inhibitors (eg, sildenafil, tadalafil, vardenafil). Safety and efficacy have not been established in children.Sustained release products may be absorbed erratically in patients with GI hypermotility or malabsorption syndrome; do not crush or chew sublingual dosage form.

Adverse Reactions Frequency not defined.

Cardiovascular: Hypotension (infrequent), postural hypotension, crescendo angina (uncommon), rebound hypertension (uncommon), pallor, cardiovascular collapse, tachycardia, shock, flushing, peripheral edema, syncope (uncommon)

Central nervous system: Headache (most common), lightheadedness (related to blood pressure changes), dizziness, restlessness

Gastrointestinal: Nausea, vomiting, bowel incontinence, xerostomia

Genitourinary: Urinary incontinence

Hematologic: Methemoglobinemia (rare, overdose)

Neuromuscular & skeletal: Weakness

Ocular: Blurred vision

Miscellaneous: Cold sweat

The incidence of hypotension and adverse cardiovascular events may be increased when used in combination with sildenafil (Viagra®).

Metabolism/Transport Effects Substrate of CYP3A4 (major)

Drug Interactions

CYP3A4 Inducers (Strong): May increase the metabolism of CYP3A4 Substrates. *Risk C: Monitor therapy*

CYP3A4 Inhibitors (Moderate): May decrease the metabolism of CYP3A4 Substrates. *Risk C: Monitor therapy*

CYP3A4 Inhibitors (Strong): May decrease the metabolism of CYP3A4 Substrates. *Risk D: Consider therapy modification*

Dasatinib: May increase the serum concentration of CYP3A4 Substrates. *Risk C: Monitor therapy*

Deferasirox: May decrease the serum concentration of CYP3A4 Substrates. *Risk C: Monitor therapy*

Diazoxide: May enhance the hypotensive effect of Antihypertensives. *Risk C: Monitor therapy*

Herbs (CYP3A4 Inducers): May increase the metabolism of CYP3A4 Substrates. *Risk C: Monitor therapy*

Herbs (Hypertensive Properties): May diminish the antihypertensive effect of Antihypertensives. *Risk C: Monitor therapy*

Herbs (Hypotensive Properties): May enhance the hypotensive effect of Antihypertensives. *Risk C: Monitor therapy*

Methylphenidate: May diminish the antihypertensive effect of Antihypertensives. *Risk C: Monitor therapy*

Phosphodiesterase 5 Inhibitors: May enhance the vasodilatory effect of Vasodilators (Organic Nitrates). *Risk X: Avoid combination*

Prostacyclin Analogues: May enhance the hypotensive effect of Antihypertensives. *Risk C: Monitor therapy*

RiTUXimab: Antihypertensives may enhance the hypotensive effect of RiTUXimab. *Risk D: Consider therapy modification*

Rosiglitazone: Vasodilators (Organic Nitrates) may enhance the adverse/toxic effect of Rosiglitazone. Specifically, a greater risk of myocardial ischemia was reported for users of this combination in a meta-analysis. Management: Consider alternatives to this combination when possible. Rosiglitazone prescribing information states that the combination of rosiglitazone and a nitrate is not recommended. *Risk D: Consider therapy modification*

Ethanol/Nutrition/Herb Interactions Ethanol: Caution with ethanol (may increase risk of hypotension).

Mechanism of Action Stimulation of intracellular cyclic-GMP results in vascular smooth muscle relaxation of both arterial and venous vasculature. Increased venous pooling decreases left ventricular pressure (preload) and arterial dilatation decreases arterial resistance (afterload). Therefore, this reduces cardiac oxygen demand by decreasing left ventricular pressure and systemic vascular resistance by dilating arteries. Additionally, coronary artery dilation improves collateral flow to ischemic regions; esophageal smooth muscle is relaxed via the same mechanism.

Pharmacodynamics/Kinetics

Onset of action: Sublingual tablet: 2-10 minutes; Chewable tablet: 3 minutes; Oral tablet: 45-60 minutes

Duration: Sublingual tablet: 1-2 hours; Chewable tablet: 0.5-2 hours; Oral tablet: 4-6 hours

Metabolism: Extensively hepatic to conjugated metabolites, including isosorbide 5-mononitrate (active) and 2-mononitrate (active)

Half-life elimination: Parent drug: 1-4 hours; Metabolite (5-mononitrate): 4 hours

Excretion: Urine and feces

Dosage Adults (elderly should be given lowest recommended daily doses initially and titrate upward): Oral:

Angina: 5-40 mg 4 times/day or 40 mg every 8-12 hours in sustained-release dosage form

Sublingual: 2.5-5 mg every 5-10 minutes for maximum of 3 doses in 15-30 minutes; may also use prophylactically 15 minutes prior to activities which may provoke an attack

Congestive heart failure:

Initial dose: 20 mg 3-4 times per day

Target dose: 120-160 mg/day in divided doses; use in combination with hydralazine

Esophageal spastic disorders (unlabeled use):

Oral: 5-10 mg before meals

Sublingual: 2.5 mg after meals

Tolerance to nitrate effects develops with chronic exposure: Dose escalation does not overcome this effect. Tolerance can only be overcome by short periods of nitrate absence from the body. Short periods (10-12 hours) of nitrate withdrawal help minimize tolerance. General recommendations are to take the last dose of short-acting agents no later than 7 PM; administer 2-3 times/day rather than 4 times/day. Sustained release preparations could be administered at times to allow a 15- to 17-hour interval between first and last daily dose. Example: Administer sustained release at 8 AM and 2 PM for a twice daily regimen.

Hemodialysis: During hemodialysis, administer dose postdialysis or administer supplemental 10-20 mg dose

Peritoneal dialysis: Supplemental dose is not necessary

Administration Do not administer around-the-clock; the first dose of nitrates should be administered in a physician's office to observe for maximal cardiovascular dynamic effects and adverse effects (orthostatic blood pressure drop, headache); when immediate release products are prescribed twice daily (recommend 7 AM and noon); for 3 times/day dosing (recommend 7 AM, noon, and 5 PM); when sustained-release products are indicated, suggest once a day in morning or via twice daily dosing at 8 AM and 2 PM. Do not crush sublingual tablets.

Monitoring Parameters Monitor for orthostasis

Test Interactions Decreased cholesterol (S)

Dosage Forms Excipient information presented when available (limited, particularly for generics); consult specific product labeling. [DSC] = Discontinued product

Capsule, sustained release (Dilatrate®-SR): 40 mg

Tablet: 5 mg, 10 mg, 20 mg, 30 mg

Isordil®: 5 mg, 10 mg [DSC], 20 mg [DSC], 30 mg [DSC], 40 mg

Tablet, extended release (Isochron™): 40 mg
Tablet, sublingual: 2.5 mg, 5 mg
Isordil®: 2.5 mg, 5 mg, 10 mg [DSC]

Isosorbide Dinitrate and Hydralazine

(eye soe SOR bide dye NYE trate & hye DRAL a zeen)

U.S. Brand Names BiDil®

Index Terms Hydralazine and Isosorbide Dinitrate

Pharmacologic Category Vasodilator

Use Treatment of heart failure, adjunct to standard therapy, in self-identified African-Americans

Effect on Mental Status May cause drowsiness or dizziness

Effect on Psychiatric Treatment Concomitant use with MAO inhibitors may result in large decreases in blood pressure; monitor

Dosage Summary

Oral:

Children: Dosage not established

Adults: 1-2 tablets 3 times/day

Dosage Forms Excipient information presented when available (limited, particularly for generics); consult specific product labeling.

Tablet: Isosorbide dinitrate 20 mg and hydralazine 37.5 mg

Isosorbide Mononitrate (eye soe SOR bide mon oh NYE trate)

Medication Safety Issues

Sound-alike/look-alike issues:

Imdur® may be confused with Imuran®, Inderal LA®, K-Dur®

Monoket® may be confused with Monopril®

International issues:

Nitrex® [Italy] may be confused with Imitrex® which is a brand name for sumatriptan in the U.S.

U.S. Brand Names Imdur®; Ismo®; Monoket®

Canadian Brand Names Apo-ISMN®; Imdur®; PMS-ISMN

Mexican Brand Names Elantan; Imdur 60; Mono Mack

Index Terms ISMN

Pharmacologic Category Vasodilator

Generic Available Yes

Use Long-acting metabolite of the vasodilator isosorbide dinitrate used for the prophylactic treatment of angina pectoris

Effect on Mental Status May cause dizziness; may rarely cause drowsiness, agitation, anxiety, confusion, nervousness, or insomnia

Effect on Psychiatric Treatment None reported

Pregnancy Risk Factor C

Lactation Excretion in breast milk unknown

Contraindications Hypersensitivity to isosorbide or any component of the formulation; hypersensitivity to organic nitrates; concurrent use with phosphodiesterase-5 (PDE-5) inhibitors (sildenafil, tadalafil, or vardenafil); angle-closure glaucoma (intraocular pressure may be increased); head trauma or cerebral hemorrhage (increase intracranial pressure); severe anemia

Warnings/Precautions Use with caution in volume depletion, hypotension, and right ventricular infarctions. Postural hypotension, transient episodes of weakness, dizziness, or syncope may occur even with small doses; ethanol accentuates these effects; tolerance and cross-tolerance to nitrate antianginal and hemodynamic effects may occur during prolonged isosorbide mononitrate therapy; (minimized by using the smallest effective dose, by alternating coronary vasodilators or offering drug-free intervals of as little as 12 hours). Excessive doses may result in severe headache, blurred vision, or xerostomia; increased anginal symptoms may be a result of dosage increases. Nitrates may aggravate angina caused by hypertrophic cardiomyopathy. Avoid concurrent use with PDE-5 inhibitors (eg, sildenafil, tadalafil, vardenafil). Safety and efficacy have not been established in children.

Adverse Reactions

>10%: Central nervous system: Headache (19% to 38%)

1% to 10%:

Central nervous system: Dizziness (3% to 5%)

Gastrointestinal: Nausea/vomiting (2% to 4%)

<1% (Limited to important or life-threatening): Angina pectoris, arrhythmia, atrial fibrillation, impotence, methemoglobinemia (rare), pruritus, rash, supraventricular tachycardia, syncope, vomiting

The incidence of hypotension and adverse cardiovascular events may be increased when used in combination with sildenafil (Viagra®).

Metabolism/Transport Effects Substrate of CYP3A4 (major)

Drug Interactions

CYP3A4 Inducers (Strong): May increase the metabolism of CYP3A4 Substrates. *Risk C: Monitor therapy*

CYP3A4 Inhibitors (Moderate): May decrease the metabolism of CYP3A4 Substrates. *Risk C: Monitor therapy*

CYP3A4 Inhibitors (Strong): May decrease the metabolism of CYP3A4 Substrates. *Risk D: Consider therapy modification*

Dasatinib: May increase the serum concentration of CYP3A4 Substrates. *Risk C: Monitor therapy*

Deferasirox: May decrease the serum concentration of CYP3A4 Substrates. *Risk C: Monitor therapy*

Diazoxide: May enhance the hypotensive effect of Antihypertensives. *Risk C: Monitor therapy*

Herbs (CYP3A4 Inducers): May increase the metabolism of CYP3A4 Substrates. *Risk C: Monitor therapy*

Herbs (Hypertensive Properties): May diminish the antihypertensive effect of Antihypertensives. *Risk C: Monitor therapy*

Herbs (Hypotensive Properties): May enhance the hypotensive effect of Antihypertensives. *Risk C: Monitor therapy*

Methylphenidate: May diminish the antihypertensive effect of Antihypertensives. *Risk C: Monitor therapy*

Phosphodiesterase 5 Inhibitors: May enhance the vasodilatory effect of Vasodilators (Organic Nitrates). *Risk X: Avoid combination*

Prostacyclin Analogues: May enhance the hypotensive effect of Antihypertensives. *Risk C: Monitor therapy*

RiTUXimab: Antihypertensives may enhance the hypotensive effect of RiTUXimab. *Risk D: Consider therapy modification*

Rosiglitazone: Vasodilators (Organic Nitrates) may enhance the adverse/toxic effect of Rosiglitazone. Specifically, a greater risk of myocardial ischemia was reported for users of this combination in a meta-analysis. Management: Consider alternatives to this combination when possible. Rosiglitazone prescribing information states that the combination of rosiglitazone and a nitrate is not recommended. *Risk D: Consider therapy modification*

Ethanol/Nutrition/Herb Interactions Ethanol: Caution with ethanol (may increase risk of hypotension).

Stability Tablets should be stored in a tight container at room temperature of 15°C to 30°C (59°F to 86°F).

Mechanism of Action Prevailing mechanism of action for nitroglycerin (and other nitrates) is systemic venodilation, decreasing preload as measured by pulmonary capillary wedge pressure and left ventricular end diastolic volume and pressure; the average reduction in left ventricular end diastolic volume is 25% at rest, with a corresponding increase in ejection fractions of 50% to 60%. This effect improves congestive symptoms in heart failure and improves the myocardial perfusion gradient in patients with coronary artery disease.

Pharmacodynamics/Kinetics

Onset of action: 30-60 minutes

Absorption: Nearly complete and low intersubject variability in its pharmacokinetic parameters and plasma concentrations

Metabolism: Hepatic

Half-life elimination: Mononitrate: ~4 hours

Excretion: Urine and feces

Dosage Adults and Geriatrics (start with lowest recommended dose): Oral:

Regular tablet: 5-20 mg twice daily with the two doses given 7 hours apart (eg, 8 AM and 3 PM) to decrease tolerance development; then titrate to 10 mg twice daily in first 2-3 days.

Extended release tablet: Initial: 30-60 mg given in morning as a single dose; titrate upward as needed, giving at least 3 days between increases; maximum daily single dose: 240 mg

Dosing adjustment in renal impairment: Not necessary for elderly or patients with altered renal or hepatic function.

Tolerance to nitrate effects develops with chronic exposure. Dose escalation does not overcome this effect. Tolerance can only be overcome by short periods of nitrate absence from the body. Short periods (10-12 hours) of nitrate withdrawal help minimize tolerance. Recommended dosage regimens incorporate this interval. General recommendations are to take the last dose of short-acting agents no later than 7 PM; administer 2 times/day rather than 4 times/day. Administer sustained release tablet once daily in the morning.

Administration Do not administer around-the-clock; Monoket® and Ismo® should be scheduled twice daily with doses 7 hours apart (8 AM and 3 PM); Imdur® may be administered once daily. Extended release tablets should not be chewed or crushed. Should be swallowed with a half-glassful of fluid.

Monitoring Parameters Monitor for orthostasis, increased hypotension

Dosage Forms Excipient information presented when available (limited, particularly for generics); consult specific product labeling.

Tablet: 10 mg, 20 mg
  Ismo®: 20 mg
  Monoket®: 10 mg, 20 mg
Tablet, extended release: 30 mg, 60 mg, 120 mg
  Imdur®: 30 mg, 60 mg, 120 mg

Isotretinoin (eye soe TRET i noyn)

Medication Safety Issues

Sound-alike/look-alike issues:
  Accutane® may be confused with Accolate®, Accupril®
  Claravis™ may be confused with Cleviprex™
  Isotretinoin may be confused with tretinoin

U.S. Brand Names Accutane®; Amnesteem™; Claravis™; Sotret®

Canadian Brand Names Accutane®; Clarus™; Isotrex®

Mexican Brand Names Isoface; Isotrex; Neotrex; Roaccutan; Sotrexe

Index Terms 13-*cis*-Retinoic Acid

Pharmacologic Category Acne Products; Retinoic Acid Derivative

Use Treatment of severe recalcitrant nodular acne unresponsive to conventional therapy

Unlabeled/Investigational Use Investigational: Treatment of children with metastatic neuroblastoma or leukemia that does not respond to conventional therapy

Effect on Mental Status May cause depression, psychosis; may rarely cause suicidal ideation, suicide attempts, suicide, and aggressive and/or violent behaviors

Effect on Psychiatric Treatment May increase the clearance of carbamazepine, leading to decreased levels; monitor. Avoid dong quai and St John's wort (may cause photosensitization).

Restrictions All patients (male and female), prescribers, wholesalers, and dispensing pharmacists must register and be active in the iPLEDGE™ risk management program, designed to eliminate fetal exposures to isotretinoin. This program covers all isotretinoin products (brand and generic). The iPLEDGE™ program requires that all patients meet qualification criteria and monthly program requirements. Registration, activation, and additional information are provided at www.ipledgeprogram.com or by calling 866-495-0654.

An FDA-approved medication guide must be distributed when dispensing an outpatient prescription (new or refill) where this medication is to be used without direct supervision of a healthcare provider. Medication guides are available at http://www.fda.gov/cder/Offices/ODS/medication_guides.htm.

Dosage Summary

Oral:

Children <12 years: Dosage not established

Children 12-17 years: 0.5-1 mg/kg/day in 2 divided doses; doses as low as 0.05 mg/kg/day have been reported to be beneficial

Adults: 0.5-2 mg/kg/day in 2 divided doses; doses as low as 0.05 mg/kg/day have been reported to be beneficial

Dosage Forms Excipient information presented when available (limited, particularly for generics); consult specific product labeling.

Capsule:
  Accutane®: 10 mg, 20 mg, 40 mg [contains soybean oil and parabens]
  Amnesteem™: 10 mg, 20 mg, 40 mg [contains soybean oil]
  Claravis™: 10 mg, 20 mg, 40 mg
  Sotret®: 10 mg, 20 mg, 30 mg, 40 mg [contains soybean oil]

Isradipine (iz RA di peen)

Medication Safety Issues

Sound-alike/look-alike issues:
  DynaCirc® may be confused with Dynabac®, Dynacin®

Related Information

Calcium Channel Blockers *on page 1778*

U.S. Brand Names DynaCirc® CR

Canadian Brand Names DynaCirc®
Mexican Brand Names Dynacirc; Dynacirc SRO
Pharmacologic Category Calcium Channel Blocker
Use Treatment of hypertension
Unlabeled/Investigational Use Pediatric hypertension
Effect on Mental Status May cause dizziness or drowsiness
Effect on Psychiatric Treatment None reported
Dosage Summary

Oral:

Children (unlabeled use): Capsule: Initial: 0.15-0.2 mg/kg/day in 2-3 divided doses; maximum 0.8 mg/kg/day, up to 20 mg/day; controlled release formulation is administered once daily or in 2 divided doses

Adults:

Capsule: Initial: 2.5 mg twice daily; titrate dose in 2- to 4-week intervals; usual range: 2.5-10 mg/day

Controlled release tablet: Initial: 5 mg once daily; Maintenance: 5-20 mg once daily (maximum: 20 mg/day)

Dosage Forms Excipient information presented when available (limited, particularly for generics); consult specific product labeling.

Capsule: 2.5 mg, 5 mg

Tablet, controlled release:

DynaCirc® CR: 5 mg, 10 mg

◆ **Istalol®** *see* Timolol *on page 1584*

◆ **Isuprel®** *see* Isoproterenol *on page 866*

Itraconazole (i tra KOE na zole)

Medication Safety Issues

Sound-alike/look-alike issues:

Sporanox® may be confused with Suprax®

U.S. Brand Names Sporanox®
Canadian Brand Names Sporanox®
Mexican Brand Names Isox; Itranax; Sinozol; Sporanox
Pharmacologic Category Antifungal Agent, Oral
Use Treatment of susceptible fungal infections in immunocompromised and immunocompetent patients including blastomycosis and histoplasmosis; indicated for aspergillosis, and onychomycosis of the toenail; treatment of onychomycosis of the fingernail without concomitant toenail infection via a pulse-type dosing regimen; has activity against *Aspergillus*, *Candida*, *Coccidioides*, *Cryptococcus*, *Sporothrix*, tinea unguium

Oral: Useful in superficial mycoses including dermatophytoses (eg, tinea capitis), pityriasis versicolor, sebopsoriasis, vaginal and chronic mucocutaneous candidiases; systemic mycoses including candidiasis, meningeal and disseminated cryptococcal infections, paracoccidioidomycosis, coccidioidomycoses; miscellaneous mycoses such as sporotrichosis, chromomycosis, leishmaniasis, fungal keratitis, alternariosis, zygomycosis

Oral solution: Treatment of oral and esophageal candidiasis

Intravenous solution: Indicated in the treatment of blastomycosis, histoplasmosis (nonmeningeal), and aspergillosis (in patients intolerant or refractory to amphotericin B therapy); empiric therapy of febrile neutropenic fever

Effect on Mental Status May cause sedation
Effect on Psychiatric Treatment Contraindicated with oral midazolam, pimozide, and triazolam
Dosage Summary

I.V.:

Children: Dosage not established

Adults: 100-400 mg/day; doses >200 mg/day are given in 2 divided doses

Oral:

Children: Dosage not established

Adults: 100-800 mg/day; doses >200 mg/day are given in 2-3 divided doses

Dosage Forms Excipient information presented when available (limited, particularly for generics); consult specific product labeling. [DSC] = Discontinued product

Capsule: 100 mg

Sporanox®: 100 mg

Injection, solution:

Sporanox®: 10 mg/mL (25 mL) [packaged in a kit containing sodium chloride 0.9% (50 mL); filtered infusion set (1)] [DSC]

Solution, oral:
Sporanox®: 100 mg/10 mL (150 mL) [cherry flavor]

Ivermectin (eye ver MEK tin)

U.S. Brand Names Stromectol®
Mexican Brand Names Ivexterm
Pharmacologic Category Anthelmintic
Use Treatment of the following infections: Strongyloidiasis of the intestinal tract due to the nematode parasite *Strongyloides stercoralis*. Onchocerciasis due to the nematode parasite *Onchocerca volvulus*. Ivermectin is only active against the immature form of *Onchocerca volvulus*, and the intestinal forms of *Strongyloides stercoralis*.
Unlabeled/Investigational Use Has been used for other parasitic infections including *Ascaris lumbricoides*, Bancroftian filariasis, *Brugia malayi*, scabies, *Enterobius vermicularis*, *Mansonella ozzardi*, *Gnathostomia spingerum*, *Mansonella ozzardi*, *Mansonella streptocera*, pediculosis pubis, *Trichuris trichiura*.
Effect on Mental Status May cause dizziness, drowsiness, or insomnia
Effect on Psychiatric Treatment May cause leukopenia; use caution with clozapine and carbamazepine
Dosage Summary
Oral:
Children <15 kg: Dosage not established
Children ≥15 kg: 150-200 mcg/kg as a single dose
Adults: 150-200 mcg/kg as a single dose
Dosage Forms Excipient information presented when available (limited, particularly for generics); consult specific product labeling.
Tablet [scored]:
Stromectol®: 3 mg

- **IvySoothe® [OTC]** *see* Hydrocortisone *on page 785*
- **Jantoven®** *see* Warfarin *on page 1679*
- **Janumet™** *see* Sitagliptin and Metformin *on page 1492*
- **Januvia™** *see* SitaGLIPtin *on page 1491*
- **Jolessa™** *see* Ethinyl Estradiol and Levonorgestrel *on page 595*
- **Jolivette™** *see* Norethindrone *on page 1150*
- **Junel™** *see* Ethinyl Estradiol and Norethindrone *on page 597*
- **Junel™ Fe** *see* Ethinyl Estradiol and Norethindrone *on page 597*
- **Kadian®** *see* Morphine Sulfate *on page 1077*
- **Kaletra®** *see* Lopinavir and Ritonavir *on page 945*

Kanamycin (kan a MYE sin)

Medication Safety Issues
Sound-alike/look-alike issues:
Kanamycin may be confused with Garamycin®, gentamicin
U.S. Brand Names Kantrex®
Canadian Brand Names Kantrex®
Mexican Brand Names Kantrex
Index Terms Kanamycin Sulfate
Pharmacologic Category Antibiotic, Aminoglycoside
Use Treatment of serious infections caused by susceptible strains of *E. coli*, *Proteus* species, *Enterobacter aerogenes*, *Klebsiella pneumoniae*, *Serratia marcescens*, and *Acinetobacter* species; second-line treatment of *Mycobacterium tuberculosis*
Effect on Mental Status May cause drowsiness or dizziness; case reports of delirium and psychosis with aminoglycosides
Effect on Psychiatric Treatment May cause agranulocytosis; use caution with clozapine and carbamazepine
Dosage Summary Note: Dosing should be based on ideal body weight
I.M.:
Children: 15 mg/kg/day divided every 8-12 hours
Adults: 5-7.5 mg/kg every 8-12 hours
Elderly: 5-7.5 mg/kg every 12-24 hours
I.V.:
Children: 15 mg/kg/day divided every 8-12 hours
Adults: 5-7.5 mg/kg every 8-12 hours
Elderly: 5-7.5 mg/kg every 12-24 hours

Inhalation: Aerosol:
Children: Dosage not established
Adults: 250 mg 2-4 times/day
Intraperitoneal:
Children: Dosage not established
Adults: 500 mg
Irrigation:
Children: Dosage not established
Adults: 0.25% (maximum: 1.5 g/day)

Dosage Forms Excipient information presented when available (limited, particularly for generics); consult specific product labeling.
Injection, solution, as sulfate: 1 g/3 mL (3 mL) [contains sodium bisulfate]

- **Kanamycin Sulfate** *see* Kanamycin *on page 873*
- **Kantrex®** *see* Kanamycin *on page 873*
- **Kaon-Cl-10®** *see* Potassium Chloride *on page 1315*
- **Kao-Paverin® [OTC]** *see* Loperamide *on page 944*
- **Kaopectate® [OTC]** *see* Bismuth *on page 189*
- **Kaopectate® Extra Strength [OTC]** *see* Bismuth *on page 189*
- **Kao-Tin [OTC]** *see* Bismuth *on page 189*
- **Kapectolin [OTC]** *see* Bismuth *on page 189*
- **Kariva™** *see* Ethinyl Estradiol and Desogestrel *on page 592*

Kava Kava *(Piper methysticum)*

Natural Product Category Herb
Synonyms *Piper methysticum*; Kawa; Kew; Yagona
Plant Part Root, rhizome
Dosage and Standardization Oral:
Children: Attention deficit disorder/attention deficit hyperactivity disorder: Liquid extract (1:1 w/v fresh plant or 1:4 w/v dry plant): 5-15 drops diluted in favorite beverage 2-3 times/day
Adult:
Anxiety: 100-250 mg 1-3 times/day as needed, standardized to contain 30% kavalactones per dose
Sedation: 250-500 mg at bedtime, standardized to contain 30% kavalactones per dose

Reported Uses
Fibromyalgia (pharmacologic activity)
Insomnia; anxiety/stress, skeletal muscle relaxation, postischemic episodes (Davies, 1992; Kinzler, 1991; Lehmann, 1996; Malsch, 2001; Pittler, 2000; Singh, 1992; Warnecke, 1991)
Muscle soreness (pharmacologic activity)

Summary Kava kava is a unique plant native to the South Pacific. It has gained popularity as an anxiolytic and sleep aid and appears to act through a unique mechanism and is claimed to induce relaxation without impairment in memory or motor function. In fact, cognitive function improvement and sharpened awareness have been claimed to accompany relaxation induced by this product. It is available as capsules or in teas. Individuals should be warned against overindulgence in tea consumption, in particular.

Effect on Mental Status May cause depression, euphoria, and sedation

Effect on Psychiatric Treatment Contraindicated in patients with depression. Avoid use with benzodiazepines; combined use with psychotropics may produce addictive CNS depression.

Pharmacology Kava kava appears to act on the amygdala complex in the limbic system, which moderates many emotional processes. In contrast to benzodiazepines and barbiturates, it is not believed to exhibit significant binding or influence on gamma-aminobutyric acid (GABA). Kava kava is claimed to protect against CNS ischemia. Tolerance to the effects of kava kava has not been described. The whole plant extract appears to exhibit more activity than the isolated kavalactones.

Warnings and Interactions The U.S. Food and Drug Administration (FDA) is attempting to determine whether dietary supplements containing the herbal extract kava (*Piper methysticum*) are directly responsible for causing certain types of hepatotoxicity. Recently, more than 20 cases of hepatitis, cirrhosis, and liver failure have been reported in Europe, with at least one individual requiring a liver transplant. Healthcare providers are urged to query their patients about the use of kava and to evaluate closely these individuals for potential liver complications. In addition, physicians are urged to review all their cases of liver toxicity to determine if kava-containing products may be involved. Kava is marketed for a variety of uses, including stress relief, tension, anxiety, insomnia, and postmenstrual syndrome (PMS).

The "Dear Healthcare Professional" letter is viewable at http://www.fda.gov/medwatch/safety/2001/kava.htm, last accessed January 10, 2002.

For additional information, contact Steven Gitterman, MD, PhD, at the FDA at (301) 436-2371.

Theoretical Cautions and Contraindications Use of kava kava is contraindicated in pregnancy and lactation (based on case reports) (Meyer). Due to the potential for dopamine antagonism, use is also contraindicated in Parkinson's disease (Schelosky, 1995). Use with caution in individuals receiving antianxiety agents (ie, alprazolam), antidepressants, antipsychotics, or other agents which cause CNS depression such as sedative/hypnotics (based on pharmacologic activity and case reports) (Almeida, 1996). May potentiate the effects of concurrent ethanol (Jamieson, 1990). Some conflicting evidence concerning effects with ethanol have been published (Herberg, 1993). May cause drowsiness or sedation in higher doses; use caution when performing tasks which require alertness (driving or operating heavy machinery). Long-term use of high doses may cause rash.

General Warnings Use all herbal supplements with extreme caution in children <2 years of age and in pregnancy or lactation. Some herbs are contraindicated in pregnancy or lactation; make sure to observe warnings. Use with caution in individuals on medication and with pre-existing medical conditions. Always review for potential herb-drug interactions (HDIs) and other warnings. Large and prolonged doses may increase the potential for adverse effects. Herbs may cause transient adverse effects such as nausea, vomiting, and GI distress due to a variety of chemical constituents. Use caution in individuals having known allergies to plants.

Theoretical Interactions Ethanol, CNS depressants (including alprazolam and other benzodiazepines, antidepressants, and sedative-hypnotics), antipsychotics, levodopa, dopamine, dopamine antagonists, dopamine agonists, MAOIs, anesthetics, antiplatelet medications, hepatotoxic agents, cytochrome P450 metabolized agents

References

Almeida JC and Grimsley EW, "Coma From the Health Food Store: Interaction Between Kava and Alprazolam," *Ann Intern Med*, 1996, 125(11):940-1.

Davies LP, Drew CA, Duffield P, et al, "Kava Pyrones and Resin: Studies on GABAA, GABAB and Benzodiazepine Binding Sites in Rodent Brain," *Pharmacol Toxicol*, 1992, 71 (2):120-6.

Herberg KW, "Effect of Kava-Special Extract WS 1490 Combined With Ethyl Alcohol on Safety-Relevant Performance Parameters," *Blutalkohol*, 1993, 30(2):96-105.

Jamieson DD and Duffield PH, "Positive Interaction of Ethanol and Kava Resin in Mice," *Clin Exp Pharmacol Physiol*, 1990, 17(7):509-14.

Kinzler E, Krömer J, and Lehmann E, "Effect of a Special Kava Extract in Patients With Anxiety-, Tension-, and Excitation States of Non-Psychotic Genesis. Double Blind Study With Placebos Over 4 Weeks," *Arzneimittelforschung*, 1991, 41(6):584-8.

Lehmann E, Kinzler E, and Friedemann J, "Efficacy of a Special Kava Extract (*Piper methysticum*) in Patients With States of Anxiety, Tension and Excitedness of Non-Mental Origin - A Double-Blind Placebo-Controlled Study of Four Weeks Treatment," *Phytomedicine*, 1996, 3(2):113-9.

Malsch U and Kieser M, "Efficacy of Kava-Kava in the Treatment of Non-Psychotic Anxiety, Following Pretreatment With Benzodiazepines," *Psychopharmacology (Berl)*, 2001, 157 (3):277-83.

Meyer JJ, "Pharmacology of Kava," Ethnopharmacologic Search for Psychoactive Drugs, U.S. Dept Health, Education, and Welfare, Pub No 1645, Washington, DC: Government Printing Office, 133-40.

Natural Standard Research Collaboration, Chief Editors: Ulbricht C, Basch E, *Natural Standard Herb and Supplement Reference - Evidence-Based Clinical Reviews*, USA: Elsevier/Mosby, 2005.

Pittler MH and Ernst E, "Efficacy of Kava Extract for Treating Anxiety: Systematic Review and Meta-Analysis," *J Clin Psychopharmacol*, 2000, 20(1):84-9.

Schelosky L, Raffauf C, Jendroska K, et al, "Kava and Dopamine Antagonism," *J Neurol Neurosurg Psychiatry*, 1995, 58(5):639-40.

Singh YN, "Kava: An Overview," *J Ethnopharmacol*, 1992, 37(1):13-45.

Warnecke G, "Psychosomatic Dysfunctions in the Female Climacteric. Clinical Effectiveness and Tolerance of Kava Extract WS 1490," *Fortschr Med*, 1991, 109(4):119-22.

- **Kawa** *see* Kava Kava *(Piper methysticum) on page 874*
- **Kay Ciel® [DSC]** *see* Potassium Chloride *on page 1315*
- **KCl** *see* Potassium Chloride *on page 1315*
- **Keflex®** *see* Cephalexin *on page 306*
- **Kelnor™** *see* Ethinyl Estradiol and Ethynodiol Diacetate *on page 594*
- **Kemadrin® [DSC]** *see* Procyclidine *on page 1344*

- **Kenalog®** *see* Triamcinolone *on page 1617*
- **Kenalog-10®** *see* Triamcinolone *on page 1617*
- **Kenalog-40®** *see* Triamcinolone *on page 1617*
- **Keoxifene Hydrochloride** *see* Raloxifene *on page 1391*
- **Kepivance™** *see* Palifermin *on page 1214*
- **Keppra®** *see* Levetiracetam *on page 905*
- **Keppra XR™** *see* Levetiracetam *on page 905*
- **Keralyt® [OTC]** *see* Salicylic Acid *on page 1454*
- **Kerlone®** *see* Betaxolol *on page 186*
- **Kerr Insta-Char® [OTC]** *see* Charcoal *on page 312*
- **Ketalar®** *see* Ketamine *on page 876*

Ketamine (KEET a meen)

Medication Safety Issues

Sound-alike/look-alike issues:

Ketalar® may be confused with Kenalog®, ketorolac

High alert medication: The Institute for Safe Medication Practices (ISMP) includes this medication among its list of drugs which have a heightened risk of causing significant patient harm when used in error.

U.S. Brand Names Ketalar®

Canadian Brand Names Ketalar®; Ketamine Hydrochloride Injection, USP

Mexican Brand Names Ketalin

Index Terms Ketamine Hydrochloride

Pharmacologic Category General Anesthetic

Use Induction and maintenance of general anesthesia

Unlabeled/Investigational Use Analgesia, sedation

Effect on Mental Status Vivid dreams and hallucinations common

Effect on Psychiatric Treatment Contraindicated in patients with psychotic disorders; barbiturates and hydroxyzine may increase the effects of ketamine; avoid combination

Restrictions C-III

Dosage Summary

I.M.:

Children: 4-5 mg/kg

Adults: 6.5-13 mg/kg

I.V.:

Children: 1-2 mg/kg **or** 5-20 mcg/kg/minute as a continuous infusion

Adults: 1-4.5 mg/kg **or** 1-2 mg/kg infused over 0.5 mg/kg/minute

Oral:

Children: 6-10 mg/kg for 1 dose given 30 minutes before the procedure

Adults: Dosage not established

Dosage Forms Excipient information presented when available (limited, particularly for generics); consult specific product labeling.

Injection, solution: 50 mg/mL (10 mL); 100 mg/mL (5 mL)

Ketalar®: 10 mg/mL (20 mL); 50 mg/mL (10 mL); 100 mg/mL (5 mL)

- **Ketamine Hydrochloride** *see* Ketamine *on page 876*
- **Ketek®** *see* Telithromycin *on page 1542*

Ketoconazole (kee toe KOE na zole)

Medication Safety Issues

Sound-alike/look-alike issues:

Kuric™ may be confused with Carac®

Nizoral® may be confused with Nasarel®, Neoral®, Nitrol®

U.S. Brand Names Extina®; Kuric™; Nizoral®; Nizoral® A-D [OTC]; Xolegel™

Canadian Brand Names Apo-Ketoconazole®; Ketoderm®; Novo-Ketoconazole; Xolegel™

Mexican Brand Names Akorazol; Conazol; Fungoral; Konaturil; Nastil; Nizoral; Tiniazol

Pharmacologic Category Antifungal Agent, Oral; Antifungal Agent, Topical

Use

Systemic: Treatment of susceptible fungal infections, including candidiasis, oral thrush, blastomycosis, histoplasmosis, paracoccidioidomycosis, coccidioidomycosis, chromomycosis, candiduria, chronic mucocutaneous candidiasis, as well as certain recalcitrant cutaneous dermatophytoses

Topical:

Cream: Treatment of tinea corporis, tinea cruris, tinea versicolor, cutaneous candidiasis, seborrheic dermatitis

Foam, gel: Treatment of seborrheic dermatitis

Shampoo: Treatment of dandruff, seborrheic dermatitis, tinea versicolor

Unlabeled/Investigational Use Tablet: Treatment of prostate cancer (androgen synthesis inhibitor)

Effect on Mental Status May cause drowsiness, dizziness, or depression

Effect on Psychiatric Treatment May cause leukopenia; use caution with clozapine and carbamazepine

Dosage Summary

Oral:

Children <2 years: Dosage not established

Children ≥2 years: 3.3-6.6 mg/kg/day as a single daily dose

Adults: 200-400 mg/day as a single daily dose

Topical:

Cream:

Children <12 years: Dosage not established

Children ≥12 years: Rub gently into the affected area 1-2 times daily

Adults: Rub gently into the affected area 1-2 times daily

Foam:

Children <12 years: Dosage not established

Children ≥12 years: Apply to affected area twice daily for 4 weeks

Adults: Apply to affected area twice daily for 4 weeks

Gel:

Children <12 years: Dosage not established

Children ≥12 years: Apply gently to affected area once daily

Adults: Apply gently to affected area once daily

Shampoo:

Children <12 years: Dosage not established

Children ≥12 years: Apply twice weekly with at least 3 days between each shampoo

Adults: Apply twice weekly with at least 3 days between each shampoo

Dosage Forms Excipient information presented when available (limited, particularly for generics); consult specific product labeling.

Aerosol, topical [foam]:

Extina®: 2% (50 g, 100 g)

Cream, topical: 2% (15 g, 30 g, 60 g)

Kuric™: 2%: (75 g)

Gel, topical:

Xolegel™: 2% (15 g) [contains dehydrated alcohol 34%]

Shampoo, topical: 1% (120 mL), 2% (120 mL)

Nizoral®: 2% (120 mL)

Nizoral® A-D: 1% (120 mL, 210 mL)

Tablet: 200 mg

◆ **3-Keto-desogestrel** *see* Etonogestrel *on page 606*

Ketoprofen (kee toe PROE fen)

Medication Safety Issues

Sound-alike/look-alike issues:

Ketoprofen may be confused with ketotifen

Oruvail® may be confused with Clinoril®, Elavil®

Related Information

Nonsteroidal Anti-Inflammatory Agents *on page 1792*

Canadian Brand Names Apo-Keto SR®; Apo-Keto-E®; Apo-Keto®; Novo-Keto; Novo-Keto-EC; Nu-Ketoprofen; Nu-Ketoprofen-E; Oruvail®; Rhodis SR™; Rhodis-EC™; Rhodis™

Mexican Brand Names Profenid

Pharmacologic Category Nonsteroidal Anti-inflammatory Drug (NSAID), Oral

Use Acute and long-term treatment of rheumatoid arthritis and osteoarthritis; primary dysmenorrhea; mild-to-moderate pain

Effect on Mental Status Dizziness is common; may cause nervousness; may rarely cause insomnia, confusion, depression, or hallucinations

Effect on Psychiatric Treatment May rarely cause agranulocytosis; use caution with clozapine and carbamazepine; may decrease lithium clearance resulting in an increase in serum lithium levels and potential lithium toxicity; monitor serum lithium levels

Restrictions An FDA-approved medication guide must be distributed when dispensing an oral outpatient prescription (new or refill) where this medication is to be used without direct supervision of a healthcare provider. Medication guides are available at http://www.fda.gov/cder/Offices/ODS/medication_guides.htm.

Dosage Summary

Oral:

Extended release:

Children: Dosage not established

Adults: 200 mg once daily

Regular release:

Children: Dosage not established

Adults: 25-50 mg 4 times/day or 75 mg 3 times a day (maximum: 300 mg/day)

Elderly: Initial: 25-50 mg 3-4 times/day; Maintenance: 150-300 mg/day (maximum: 300 mg/day)

Dosage Forms Excipient information presented when available (limited, particularly for generics); consult specific product labeling.

Capsule, regular release: 50 mg, 75 mg

Capsule, extended release: 200 mg

Ketorolac (KEE toe role ak)

Medication Safety Issues

Sound-alike/look-alike issues:

Acular® may be confused with Acthar®, Ocular®

Ketorolac may be confused with Ketalar®

Toradol® may be confused with Foradil®, Inderal®, Tegretol®, Torecan®, traMADol, tromethamine

International issues:

Toradol® may be confused with Theradol® which is a brand name for tramadol in the Netherlands

Related Information

Nonsteroidal Anti-Inflammatory Agents *on page 1792*

U.S. Brand Names Acular LS™; Acular®; Acular® PF

Canadian Brand Names Acular LS™; Acular®; Apo-Ketorolac Injectable®; Apo-Ketorolac®; Ketorolac Tromethamine Injection, USP; Novo-Ketorolac; ratio-Ketorolac; Toradol®; Toradol® IM

Mexican Brand Names Alidol; Dolac; Estopein; Supradol; Toloran; Toral; Torkol

Index Terms Ketorolac Tromethamine

Pharmacologic Category Nonsteroidal Anti-inflammatory Drug (NSAID), Ophthalmic; Nonsteroidal Anti-inflammatory Drug (NSAID), Oral; Nonsteroidal Anti-inflammatory Drug (NSAID), Parenteral

Use

Oral, injection: Short-term (≤5 days) management of moderate-to-severe acute pain requiring analgesia at the opioid level

Ophthalmic: Temporary relief of ocular itching due to seasonal allergic conjunctivitis; postoperative inflammation following cataract extraction; reduction of ocular pain and photophobia following incisional refractive surgery; reduction of ocular pain, burning, and stinging following corneal refractive surgery

Effect on Mental Status May cause drowsiness or dizziness; may rarely produce depression

Effect on Psychiatric Treatment May decrease lithium clearance resulting in an increase in serum lithium levels and potential lithium toxicity; monitor serum lithium levels

Restrictions An FDA-approved medication guide must be distributed when dispensing an oral outpatient prescription (new or refill) where this medication is to be used without direct supervision of a healthcare provider. Medication guides are available at http://www.fda.gov/cder/Offices/ODS/medication_guides.htm.

Dosage Summary Note: The maximum combined duration of treatment (for parenteral and oral) is 5 days

I.M.:

Children <16 years: Dosage not established

Children ≥16 years and <50 kg: 30 mg as a single dose **or** 15 mg every 6 hours (maximum: 60 mg/day)

Children ≥16 years and ≥50 kg: 60 mg as a single dose **or** 30 mg every 6 hours (maximum: 120 mg/day)

Adults <50 kg: 30 mg as a single dose **or** 15 mg every 6 hours (maximum: 60 mg/day)

Adults ≥50 kg: 60 mg as a single dose **or** 30 mg every 6 hours (maximum: 120 mg/day)

Elderly ≥65 years: 30 mg as a single dose **or** 15 mg every 6 hours (maximum: 60 mg/day)

I.V.:

Children <16 years: Dosage not established

Children ≥16 years and <50 kg: 15 mg as a single dose **or** 15 mg every 6 hours (maximum: 60 mg/day)

Children ≥16 years and ≥50 kg: 30 mg as a single dose **or** 30 mg every 6 hours (maximum: 120 mg/day)

Adults <50 kg: 15 mg as a single dose **or** 15 mg every 6 hours (maximum: 60 mg/day)

Adults ≥50 kg: 30 mg as a single dose **or** 30 mg every 6 hours (maximum: 120 mg/day)

Elderly ≥65 years: 15 mg as a single dose **or** 15 mg every 6 hours (maximum: 60 mg/day)

Ophthalmic:

Children <3 years: Dosage not established

Children ≥3 years: Instill 1 drop (0.25 mg) 4 times/day to eye(s)

Adults: Instill 1 drop (0.25 mg) 4 times/day to eye(s)

Oral:

Children <17 years: Dosage not established

Children ≥17 years and <50 kg: 10 mg every 4-6 hours (maximum: 40 mg/day)

Children ≥17 years and ≥50 kg: 20 mg, followed by 10 mg every 4-6 hours (maximum: 40 mg/day)

Adults <50 kg: 10 mg every 4-6 hours (maximum: 40 mg/day)

Adults ≥50 kg: 20 mg, followed by 10 mg every 4-6 hours (maximum: 40 mg/day)

Elderly ≥65 years: 10 mg every 4-6 hours (maximum: 40 mg/day)

Dosage Forms Excipient information presented when available (limited, particularly for generics); consult specific product labeling.

Injection, solution, as tromethamine: 15 mg/mL (1 mL); 30 mg/mL (1 mL, 2 mL, 10 mL) [contains ethanol]

Solution, ophthalmic, as tromethamine:

Acular®: 0.5% (3 mL, 5 mL, 10 mL) [contains benzalkonium chloride]

Acular LS™: 0.4% (5 mL) [contains benzalkonium chloride]

Solution, ophthalmic, as tromethamine [preservative free]:

Acular® P.F.: 0.5% (0.4 mL)

Tablet, as tromethamine: 10 mg

◆ **Ketorolac Tromethamine** *see* Ketorolac *on page 878*

Ketotifen (kee toe TYE fen)

Medication Safety Issues

Sound-alike/look-alike issues:

Ketotifen may be confused with ketoprofen

U.S. Brand Names Alaway™ [OTC]; Zaditor® [OTC]

Canadian Brand Names Novo-Ketotifen®; Nu-Ketotifen®; Zaditen®; Zaditor®

Mexican Brand Names Butifeno; Hyalcrom NF; Kedrop; Ketaxal; Zaditen

Index Terms Ketotifen Fumarate

Pharmacologic Category Histamine H_1 Antagonist; Histamine H_1 Antagonist, Second Generation; Mast Cell Stabilizer

Use

Ophthalmic: Temporary prevention of eye itching due to allergic conjunctivitis

Oral (Canadian use; not approved in U.S.): Adjunctive therapy in the chronic treatment of pediatric patients ≥6 months of age with mild, atopic asthma

Effect on Mental Status None reported

Effect on Psychiatric Treatment May cause dry eyes which can be exacerbated by anticholinergic agents or psychotropics with significant anticholinergic activity

Restrictions Oral formulation not available in U.S.

Dosage Summary

Ophthalmic:

Children <3 years: Dosage not established

Children ≥3 years: Instill 1 drop into the affected eye(s) twice daily, every 8-12 hours

Adults: Instill 1 drop into the affected eye(s) twice daily, every 8-12 hours

Oral (not approved in U.S.):

Children 6 months to 3 years: Initial: 0.025 mg/kg once daily or in 2 divided doses for 5 days; Maintenance: 0.05 mg/kg twice daily

Children >3 years: Initial: 0.5 mg once daily or in 2 divided doses for 5 days; Maintenance: 1 mg twice daily

Adults: Dosage not established

Dosage Forms Excipient information presented when available (limited, particularly for generics); consult specific product labeling. [CAN] = Canadian brand name

Solution, ophthalmic [drops]: 0.025% (5 mL)

Alaway™: 0.025% (10 mL) [contains benzalkonium chloride]

Zaditor®: 0.025% (5 mL) [contains benzalkonium chloride]

Syrup: 1 mg/5 mL (250 mL) [not available in U.S.]

Novo-Ketotifen® [CAN]: 1 mg/5 mL (250 mL) [not available in U.S.; contains alcohol, benzoate compounds; strawberry flavor]

Nu-Ketotifen® [CAN]: 1 mg/5 mL (250 mL) [not available in U.S.]

Zaditen® [CAN]: 1 mg/5 mL (250 mL) [not available in U.S.]

Tablet: 1 mg [not available in U.S.]

Novo-Ketotifen® [CAN]: 1 mg [not available in U.S.]

Zaditen® [CAN]: 1 mg [not available in U.S.]

- **Ketotifen Fumarate** *see* Ketotifen *on page 879*
- **Kew** *see* Kava Kava *(Piper methysticum) on page 874*
- **Kew Tree** *see* Ginkgo *(Ginkgo biloba) on page 715*
- **Key-E® [OTC]** *see* Vitamin E *on page 1675*
- **Key-E® Kaps [OTC]** *see* Vitamin E *on page 1675*
- **KI** *see* Potassium Iodide *on page 1317*
- **Kidkare Children's Cough and Cold [OTC]** *see* Chlorpheniramine, Pseudoephedrine, and Dextromethorphan *on page 333*
- **Kidkare Decongestant [OTC]** *see* Pseudoephedrine *on page 1367*
- **Kineret®** *see* Anakinra *on page 124*
- **Kinevac®** *see* Sincalide *on page 1489*
- **Klonopin®** *see* ClonazePAM *on page 373*
- **Klonopin® Wafers** *see* ClonazePAM *on page 373*
- **K-Lor®** *see* Potassium Chloride *on page 1315*
- **Klor-Con®** *see* Potassium Chloride *on page 1315*
- **Klor-Con® 8** *see* Potassium Chloride *on page 1315*
- **Klor-Con® 10** *see* Potassium Chloride *on page 1315*
- **Klor-Con®/25** *see* Potassium Chloride *on page 1315*
- **Klor-Con® M** *see* Potassium Chloride *on page 1315*
- **Klor-Con®/EF** *see* Potassium Bicarbonate and Potassium Citrate *on page 1315*
- **K-Lyte®** *see* Potassium Bicarbonate and Potassium Citrate *on page 1315*
- **K-Lyte® DS** *see* Potassium Bicarbonate and Potassium Citrate *on page 1315*
- **Kolephrin® [OTC]** *see* Acetaminophen, Chlorpheniramine, and Pseudoephedrine *on page 40*
- **Kolephrin® #1** *see* Guaifenesin and Codeine *on page 738*
- **Kolephrin® GG/DM [OTC]** *see* Guaifenesin and Dextromethorphan *on page 739*
- **Kondremul® [OTC]** *see* Mineral Oil *on page 1055*
- **K-Pek II [OTC]** *see* Loperamide *on page 944*
- **Kristalose®** *see* Lactulose *on page 886*
- **K-Tab®** *see* Potassium Chloride *on page 1315*
- **K-Tan [DSC]** *see* Phenylephrine and Pyrilamine *on page 1275*
- **K-Tan 4 [DSC]** *see* Phenylephrine and Pyrilamine *on page 1275*
- **Kuric™** *see* Ketoconazole *on page 876*
- **Kwelcof® [DSC]** *see* Hydrocodone and Guaifenesin *on page 779*
- **Kytril®** *see* Granisetron *on page 736*
- **L-749,345** *see* Ertapenem *on page 557*
- **L-758,298** *see* Fosaprepitant *on page 690*
- **L-M-X™ 4 [OTC]** *see* Lidocaine *on page 924*
- **L-M-X™ 5 [OTC]** *see* Lidocaine *on page 924*
- **L 754030** *see* Aprepitant *on page 130*

◆ **LA 20304a** *see* Gemifloxacin *on page 712*

Labetalol (la BET a lole)

Medication Safety Issues

Sound-alike/look-alike issues:

Labetalol may be confused with betaxolol, Hexadrol®, lamoTRIgine

Trandate® may be confused with traMADol, Trendar®, Trental®, Tridrate®

High alert medication: The Institute for Safe Medication Practices (ISMP) includes this medication among its list of drugs which have a heightened risk of causing significant patient harm when used in error.

Significant differences exist between oral and I.V. dosing. Use caution when converting from one route of administration to another.

Related Information

Beta-Blockers *on page 1776*

U.S. Brand Names Trandate®

Canadian Brand Names Apo-Labetalol®; Labetalol Hydrochloride Injection, USP; Normodyne®; Trandate®

Index Terms Ibidomide Hydrochloride; Labetalol Hydrochloride

Pharmacologic Category Beta Blocker With Alpha-Blocking Activity

Generic Available Yes

Use Treatment of mild-to-severe hypertension; I.V. for severe hypertension (eg, hypertensive emergencies)

Unlabeled/Investigational Use Pediatric hypertension

Effect on Mental Status Dizziness is common; may cause sedation

Effect on Psychiatric Treatment Barbiturates may decrease effects of beta-blockers; low potency antipsychotic and TCAs may potentiate the hypotensive effects of beta-blockers

Pregnancy Risk Factor C (manufacturer); D (2nd and 3rd trimesters - expert analysis)

Pregnancy Considerations Labetalol crosses the placenta. Beta-blockers have been associated with persistent bradycardia, hypotension, and IUGR; IUGR is probably related to maternal hypertension. Available evidence suggests beta-blockers are generally safe during pregnancy (JNC 7). Cases of neonatal hypoglycemia have been reported following maternal use of beta-blockers at parturition or during breast-feeding. Monitor breast-fed infant for symptoms of beta-blockade.

Lactation Enters breast milk/use caution (AAP rates "compatible")

Contraindications Hypersensitivity to labetalol or any component of the formulation; severe bradycardia; heart block greater than first degree (except in patients with a functioning artificial pacemaker); cardiogenic shock; bronchial asthma; uncompensated cardiac failure; conditions associated with severe and prolonged hypotension

Warnings/Precautions Consider pre-existing conditions such as sick sinus syndrome before initiating. Symptomatic hypotension with or without syncope may occur with labetalol; close monitoring of patient is required especially with initial dosing and dosing increases; blood pressure must be lowered at a rate appropriate for the patient's clinical condition. Initiation with a low dose and gradual up-titration may help to decrease the occurrence of hypotension or syncope. Patients should be advised to avoid driving or other hazardous tasks during initiation of therapy due to the risk of syncope. Orthostatic hypotension may occur with I.V. administration; patient should remain supine during and for up to 3 hours after I.V. administration. Use with caution in impaired hepatic function; bioavailability is increased due to decreased first-pass metabolism. Severe hepatic injury including some fatalities have also been rarely reported with use: periodically monitor LFTs with prolonged use. Use with caution in patients with diabetes mellitus; may potentiate hypoglycemia and/or mask signs and symptoms. May also reduce release of insulin in response to hyperglycemia; dosage of antidiabetic agents may need to be adjusted. Elimination of labetalol is reduced in elderly patients; lower maintenance doses may be required.

Use only with extreme caution in compensated heart failure and monitor for a worsening of the condition. Beta-blocker therapy should not be withdrawn abruptly (particularly in patients with CAD), but gradually tapered to avoid acute tachycardia, hypertension, and/or ischemia. Use caution with concurrent use of beta-blockers and either verapamil or diltiazem; bradycardia or heart block can occur. Patients with bronchospastic disease should not receive beta-blockers; if used at all, should be used cautiously with close monitoring. Use with caution in patients with myasthenia gravis, psychiatric disease (may cause or exacerbate ▶

CNS depression), or peripheral vascular disease. If possible, obtain diagnostic tests for pheochromocytoma prior to use. Labetalol has been shown to be effective in lowering blood pressure and relieving symptoms in patients with pheochromocytoma. However, some patients have experienced paradoxical hypertensive responses; use with caution in patients with pheochromocytoma. Additional alpha-blockade may be required during use of labetalol. Use caution with history of severe anaphylaxis to allergens; patients taking beta-blockers may become more sensitive to repeated challenges. Treatment of anaphylaxis (eg, epinephrine) in patients taking beta-blockers may be ineffective or promote undesirable effects. Use with caution in patients receiving anesthetic agents which decrease myocardial function.

Adverse Reactions

>10%:

- Cardiovascular: Postural hypotension (I.V. use; ≤58%)
- Central nervous system: Dizziness (1% to 20%), fatigue (1% to 11%)
- Gastrointestinal: Nausea (≤19%)

1% to 10%:

- Cardiovascular: Hypotension (1% to 5%), edema (≤2%), flushing (1%), ventricular arrhythmia (I.V. use; 1%)
- Central nervous system: Somnolence (3%), headache (2%), vertigo (1% to 2%)
- Dermatologic: Scalp tingling (≤7%), pruritus (1%), rash (1%)
- Gastrointestinal: Dyspepsia (≤4%), vomiting (≤3%), taste disturbance (1%)
- Genitourinary: Ejaculatory failure (≤5%), impotence (1% to 4%)
- Hepatic: Transaminases increased (4%)
- Neuromuscular & skeletal: Paresthesia (≤5%), weakness (1%)
- Ocular: Vision abnormal (1%)
- Renal: BUN increased (≤8%)
- Respiratory: Nasal congestion (1% to 6%), dyspnea (2%)
- Miscellaneous: Diaphoresis (≤4%)

<1% (Limited to important or life-threatening): Alopecia (reversible), anaphylactoid reaction, ANA positive, angioedema, bradycardia, bronchospasm, cholestatic jaundice, CHF, diabetes insipidus, heart block, hepatic necrosis, hepatitis, hypersensitivity, Peyronie's disease, Raynaud's syndrome, syncope, systemic lupus erythematosus, toxic myopathy, urinary retention, urticaria

Other adverse reactions noted with beta-adrenergic blocking agents include mental depression, catatonia, disorientation, short-term memory loss, emotional lability, clouded sensorium, intensification of pre-existing AV block, laryngospasm, respiratory distress, agranulocytosis, thrombocytopenic purpura, nonthrombocytopenic purpura, mesenteric artery thrombosis, and ischemic colitis.

Drug Interactions

Acetylcholinesterase Inhibitors: May enhance the bradycardic effect of Beta-Blockers. *Risk C: Monitor therapy*

Alpha-/Beta-Agonists (Direct-Acting): Beta-Blockers may enhance the vasopressor effect of Alpha-/Beta-Agonists (Direct-Acting). Epinephrine used as a local anesthetic for dental procedures will not likely cause clinically relevant problems. **Exceptions:** Dipivefrin. *Risk D: Consider therapy modification*

Alpha1-Blockers: Beta-Blockers may enhance the orthostatic effect of Alpha1-Blockers. The risk associated with ophthalmic products is probably less than systemic products. *Risk D: Consider therapy modification*

Alpha2-Agonists: Beta-Blockers may enhance the rebound hypertensive effect of Alpha2-Agonists. This effect can occur when the alpha$_2$-agonist is abruptly withdrawn. **Exceptions:** Apraclonidine; Brimonidine. *Risk D: Consider therapy modification*

Aminoquinolines (Antimalarial): May decrease the metabolism of Beta-Blockers. *Risk C: Monitor therapy*

Amiodarone: May enhance the bradycardic effect of Beta-Blockers. Possibly to the point of cardiac arrest. Amiodarone may increase the serum concentration of Beta-Blockers. *Risk C: Monitor therapy*

Anilidopiperidine Opioids: May enhance the bradycardic effect of Beta-Blockers. Anilidopiperidine Opioids may enhance the hypotensive effect of Beta-Blockers. *Risk C: Monitor therapy*

Antipsychotic Agents (Phenothiazines): May enhance the hypotensive effect of Beta-Blockers. Beta-Blockers may decrease the metabolism of Antipsychotic Agents (Phenothiazines). Antipsychotic Agents (Phenothiazines) may decrease the metabolism of Beta-Blockers. *Risk C: Monitor therapy*

Barbiturates: May decrease the serum concentration of Beta-Blockers. *Risk C: Monitor therapy*

Beta2-Agonists: Beta-Blockers (Nonselective) may diminish the bronchodilatory effect of Beta2-Agonists. *Risk D: Consider therapy modification*

Beta2-Agonists: Alpha-/Beta-Blockers may diminish the therapeutic effect of Beta2-Agonists. *Risk D: Consider therapy modification*

Calcium Channel Blockers (Nondihydropyridine): May enhance the hypotensive effect of Beta-Blockers. Bradycardia and signs of heart failure have also been reported. Calcium Channel Blockers (Nondihydropyridine) may increase the serum concentration of Beta-Blockers. *Risk C: Monitor therapy*

Cardiac Glycosides: Beta-Blockers may enhance the bradycardic effect of Cardiac Glycosides. *Risk C: Monitor therapy*

Diazoxide: May enhance the hypotensive effect of Antihypertensives. *Risk C: Monitor therapy*

Dipyridamole: May enhance the bradycardic effect of Beta-Blockers. *Risk C: Monitor therapy*

Disopyramide: May enhance the bradycardic effect of Beta-Blockers. *Risk C: Monitor therapy*

Herbs (Hypertensive Properties): May diminish the antihypertensive effect of Antihypertensives. *Risk C: Monitor therapy*

Herbs (Hypotensive Properties): May enhance the hypotensive effect of Antihypertensives. *Risk C: Monitor therapy*

Insulin: Beta-Blockers may enhance the hypoglycemic effect of Insulin. *Risk C: Monitor therapy*

Lidocaine: Beta-Blockers may decrease the metabolism of Lidocaine. *Risk C: Monitor therapy*

Methacholine: Beta-Blockers may enhance the adverse/toxic effect of Methacholine. *Risk X: Avoid combination*

Methylphenidate: May diminish the antihypertensive effect of Antihypertensives. *Risk C: Monitor therapy*

Midodrine: Beta-Blockers may enhance the bradycardic effect of Midodrine. *Risk C: Monitor therapy*

Nonsteroidal Anti-Inflammatory Agents: May diminish the antihypertensive effect of Beta-Blockers. *Risk C: Monitor therapy*

Propafenone: May decrease the metabolism of Beta-Blockers. Propafenone possesses some independent beta blocking activity. *Risk C: Monitor therapy*

Propoxyphene: May decrease the metabolism of Beta-Blockers. *Risk C: Monitor therapy*

Prostacyclin Analogues: May enhance the hypotensive effect of Antihypertensives. *Risk C: Monitor therapy*

QuiNIDine: May decrease the metabolism of Beta-Blockers. *Risk C: Monitor therapy*

Reserpine: May enhance the hypotensive effect of Beta-Blockers. *Risk C: Monitor therapy*

Rifamycin Derivatives: May decrease the serum concentration of Beta-Blockers. **Exceptions:** Rifabutin. *Risk C: Monitor therapy*

RiTUXimab: Antihypertensives may enhance the hypotensive effect of RiTUXimab. *Risk D: Consider therapy modification*

Selective Serotonin Reuptake Inhibitors: May decrease the metabolism of Alpha-/Beta-Blockers. **Exceptions:** Fluvoxamine. *Risk C: Monitor therapy*

Selective Serotonin Reuptake Inhibitors: May enhance the bradycardic effect of Beta-Blockers. **Exceptions:** Fluvoxamine. *Risk C: Monitor therapy*

Theophylline Derivatives: Beta-Blockers (Nonselective) may diminish the bronchodilatory effect of Theophylline Derivatives. *Risk D: Consider therapy modification*

Ethanol/Nutrition/Herb Interactions

Food: Labetalol serum concentrations may be increased if taken with food.

Herb/Nutraceutical: Avoid dong quai if using for hypertension (has estrogenic activity). Avoid ephedra, yohimbe, ginseng (may worsen hypertension). Avoid natural licorice (causes sodium and water retention and increases potassium loss). Avoid garlic (may have increased antihypertensive effect).

Stability

Tablets: Store tablets at 2°C to 30°C (36°F to 86°F). Protect from light and excessive moisture.

Vials: Store unopened injectable vials at 20°C to 25°C (68°F to 77°F); do not freeze. Protect from light. The solution is clear to slightly yellow.

Parenteral admixture: Stability of parenteral admixture at room temperature (25°C) and refrigeration temperature (4°C): 3 days.

Standard concentration: 500 mg/250 mL D_5W.

Minimum volume: 250 mL D_5W.

Mechanism of Action Blocks alpha-, $beta_1$-, and $beta_2$-adrenergic receptor sites; elevated renins are reduced. The ratios of alpha- to beta-blockade differ depending on the route of administration: 1:3 (oral) and 1:7 (I.V.).

Pharmacodynamics/Kinetics

Onset of action: Oral: 20 minutes to 2 hours; I.V.: 2-5 minutes

Peak effect: Oral: 1-4 hours; I.V.: 5-15 minutes

Duration: Blood pressure response:
Oral: 8-12 hours (dose dependent)
I.V.: 2-18 hours (dose dependent; based on single and multiple sequential doses of 0.25-0.5 mg/kg with cumulative dosing up to 3.25 mg/kg)
Distribution: V_d: Adults: 3-16 L/kg; mean: <9.4 L/kg; moderately lipid soluble, therefore, can enter CNS; crosses placenta; small amounts enter breast milk
Protein binding: 50%
Metabolism: Hepatic, primarily via glucuronide conjugation; extensive first-pass effect
Bioavailability: Oral: 25%; increased with liver disease, elderly, and concurrent cimetidine
Half-life elimination: Oral: 6-8 hours; I.V.: ~5.5 hours
Excretion: Urine (55% to 60% as glucuronide conjugates, <5% as unchanged drug)
Clearance: Possibly decreased in neonates/infants

Dosage

Children: Due to limited documentation of its use, labetalol should be initiated cautiously in pediatric patients with careful dosage adjustment and blood pressure monitoring.
Oral: Hypertension (unlabeled use): Initial: 1-3 mg/kg/day, in 2 divided doses; maximum: 10-12 mg/kg/day, up to 1200 mg/day
I.V., intermittent bolus doses of 0.3-1 mg/kg/dose have been reported.
For treatment of pediatric hypertensive emergencies, initial continuous infusions of 0.4-1 mg/kg/hour with a maximum of 3 mg/kg/hour have been used. Administration requires the use of an infusion pump.

Adults:
Oral: Initial: 100 mg twice daily, may increase as needed every 2-3 days by 100 mg twice daily (titration increments not to exceed 200 mg twice daily) until desired response is obtained; usual dose: 200-400 mg twice daily; may require up to 2.4 g/day.
Usual dose range (JNC 7): 200-800 mg/day in 2 divided doses
I.V.: 20 mg (0.25 mg/kg for an 80 kg patient) I.V. push over 2 minutes; may administer 40-80 mg at 10-minute intervals, up to 300 mg total dose.
I.V. infusion (acute loading): Initial: 2 mg/minute; titrate to response up to 300 mg total dose, if needed. Administration requires the use of an infusion pump.
I.V. infusion (500 mg/250 mL D_5W) rates:
1 mg/minute: 30 mL/hour
2 mg/minute: 60 mL/hour
3 mg/minute: 90 mL/hour
4 mg/minute: 120 mL/hour
5 mg/minute: 150 mL/hour
6 mg/minute: 180 mL/hour

Note: Although loading infusions are well described in the product labeling, the labeling is silent in specific clinical situations, such as in the patient who has an initial response to labetalol infusions but cannot be converted to an oral route for subsequent dosing. There is limited documentation of prolonged continuous infusions. In rare clinical situations, higher continuous infusion dosages (up to 6 mg/minute) have been used in the critical care setting (eg, aortic dissection). At the other extreme, continuous infusions at relatively low doses (0.03-0.1 mg/minute) have been used in some settings (following loading infusion in patients who are unable to be converted to oral regimens or in some cases as a continuation of outpatient oral regimens). These prolonged infusions should not be confused with loading infusions. Because of wide variation in the use of infusions, an awareness of institutional policies and practices is extremely important. Careful clarification of orders and specific infusion rates/units is required to avoid confusion. Due to the prolonged duration of action, careful monitoring should be extended for the duration of the infusion and for several hours after the infusion. Excessive administration may result in prolonged hypotension and/or bradycardia.

Elderly: Initial dose: Refer to adult dosing. Usual maintenance: 100-200 mg twice daily

Dosage adjustment in renal impairment: Dialysis: Not removed by hemo- or peritoneal dialysis; supplemental dose is not necessary.

Dosage adjustment in hepatic impairment: Dosage reduction may be necessary.

Administration Bolus dose may be administered I.V. push at a rate of 10 mg/minute; may follow with continuous I.V. infusion

Monitoring Parameters Blood pressure, standing and sitting/supine, pulse, cardiac monitor and blood pressure monitor required for I.V. administration

Test Interactions False-positive urine catecholamines, vanillylmandelic acid (VMA) if measured by fluorometric or photometric methods; use HPLC or specific catecholamine radioenzymatic technique; false-positive amphetamine if measured by thin-layer chromatography or radioenzymatic assay (gas chromatographic-mass spectrometer technique should be used)

Dosage Forms Excipient information presented when available (limited, particularly for generics); consult specific product labeling.

Injection, solution, as hydrochloride: 5 mg/mL (4 mL, 8 mL, 20 mL, 40 mL)

Trandate®: 5 mg/mL (20 mL, 40 mL) [contains edetate disodium]

Tablet, as hydrochloride: 100 mg, 200 mg, 300 mg

Trandate®: 100 mg, 200 mg [contains sodium benzoate], 300 mg

◆ **Labetalol Hydrochloride** *see* Labetalol *on page 881*

Lacosamide (la KOE sa mide)

Medication Safety Issues

Sound-alike/look-alike issues:

Lacosamide may be confused with zonisamide

U.S. Brand Names Vimpat®

Index Terms ADD 234037; Harkoseride; LCM; SPM 927

Pharmacologic Category Anticonvulsant, Miscellaneous

Generic Available No

Use Adjunctive therapy in the treatment of partial-onset seizures

Effect on Mental Status May cause suicidal behavior or ideation, dizziness, fatigue, somnolence, memory impairment, and depression

Effect on Psychiatric Treatment May cause GI side effects; concomitant use with lithium, carbamazepine, valproic acid, and SSRIs may produce additive effects

Restrictions An FDA-approved medication guide is available. Distribute to each patient to whom this medication is dispensed.

Pregnancy Risk Factor C

Pregnancy Considerations Developmental toxicities were observed in animal studies. There are no adequate and well-controlled studies in pregnant women; only use during pregnancy if potential benefit justifies the potential risk to the fetus. Two registries are available for women exposed to lacosamide during pregnancy:

Antiepileptic Drug Pregnancy Registry (888-233-2334 or http://www.-aedpregnancyregistry.org)

Vimpat® pregnancy registry (888-537-7734)

Lactation Excretion in breast milk unknown/use caution

Contraindications There are no contraindications listed in manufacturer's labeling.

Warnings/Precautions Suicidal ideation may occur; monitor patients for change in mood or emergence of depression/suicidal thoughts. CNS effects may occur; patients should be cautioned about performing tasks which require alertness (eg, operating machinery or driving). Use caution in patients with cardiovascular disease. Use caution with renal or hepatic impairment; dosage adjustment may be necessary. Multiorgan hypersensitivity reactions can occur (rare); monitor patient and discontinue therapy if necessary. Withdraw therapy gradually (≥1 week) to minimize the potential of increased seizure frequency. Effects with ethanol may be potentiated. Safety and efficacy in children <17 years of age have not been established.

Adverse Reactions

>10%:

Central nervous system: Dizziness (31%), headache (13%)

Gastrointestinal: Nausea (11%)

Ocular: Diplopia (11%)

1% to 10%:

Cardiovascular: Syncope (1%; dose-related: >400 mg/day)

Central nervous system: Fatigue (9%), ataxia (8%), somnolence (7%), coordination impaired (4%), vertigo (4%), depression (2%), memory impairment (2%)

Dermatologic: Pruritus (2%)

Gastrointestinal: Vomiting (9%), diarrhea (4%)

Local: Contusion (3%), skin laceration (3%), injection site pain/discomfort (2.5%), irritation (1%)

Neuromuscular & skeletal: Tremor (7%), weakness (2%)

Ocular: Blurred vision (8%), nystagmus (5%)

<1% (Limited to important or life-threatening): ALT increased, anemia, atrial fibrillation/flutter, atrioventricular block, concentration (decreased in),

bradycardia, cerebellar syndrome, cognitive dysfunction, confusion, constipation, depression, dysarthria, dyspepsia, erythema (injection site), falling, fever, hepatitis, hypoesthesia (including oral), inebriation-like feeling, irritability, mood changes, multiorgan hypersensitivity, muscle spasm, nephritis, neutropenia, palpitation, paresthesia, tinnitus, xerostomia

Drug Interactions

CarBAMazepine: May decrease the serum concentration of Lacosamide. *Risk C: Monitor therapy*

PHENobarbital: May decrease the serum concentration of Lacosamide. *Risk C: Monitor therapy*

Phenytoin: May decrease the serum concentration of Lacosamide. *Risk C: Monitor therapy*

Ethanol/Nutrition/Herb Interactions Ethanol: Avoid ethanol (may increase CNS depression).

Stability

Injection: Store at 20°C to 25°C (68°F to 77°F); excursions permitted between 15°C to 30°C (59°F to 86°F). Can be administered without further dilution or may be mixed with compatible diluents (NS, LR, D_5W). Reconstituted solution is stable for ≤24 hours in glass or PVC at room temperature of 15°C to 30°C (59°F to 86°F). Any unused portion should be discarded.

Tablets: Store at 20°C to 25°C (68°F to 77°F); excursions permitted between 15°C to 30°C (59°F to 86°F).

Mechanism of Action *In vitro* studies have shown that lacosamide stabilizes hyperexcitable neuronal membranes and inhibits repetitive neuronal firing by enhancing the slow inactivation of sodium channels (with no effects on fast inactivation of sodium channels).

Pharmacodynamics/Kinetics

Absorption: Oral: Completely

Distribution: V_d: ~0.6 L/kg

Protein binding: <15%

Metabolism: Hepatic; forms metabolite, O-desmethyl-lacosamide (inactive)

Bioavailability: ~100%

Half-life elimination: 13 hours

Time to peak, plasma: Oral: 1-4 hours postdose

Excretion: Urine (95%; 40% as unchanged drug, 30% as inactive metabolite, 20% as uncharacterized metabolite); feces (<0.5%)

Dosage Oral, I.V.: Adolescents ≥17 years and Adults: Partial onset seizure:

Initial: 50 mg twice daily; may be increased at weekly intervals by 100 mg/day

Maintenance dose: 200-400 mg/day

Note: When switching from oral to I.V. formulations, the total daily dose and frequency should be the same; I.V. therapy should only be used temporarily.

Dosing adjustment in renal impairment:

Mild-to-moderate renal impairment: No dose adjustment necessary

Severe renal impairment (Cl_{cr} ≤30 mL/minute): Maximum dose: 300 mg/day

Hemodialysis: Removed by hemodialysis; after 4-hour HD treatment, a supplemental dose of up to 50% should be considered.

Dosing adjustment in hepatic impairment:

Mild-to-moderate hepatic impairment: Maximum dose: 300 mg/day

Severe hepatic impairment: Use is not recommended

Dietary Considerations Tablets may be taken with or without food.

Administration

Injection: Administer over 30-60 minutes. Twice daily I.V. infusions have been used for up to 5 days.

Tablet: May be administered with or without food.

Monitoring Parameters Patients with conduction problems or severe cardiac disease should have ECG tracing prior to start of therapy and when at steady-state

Dosage Forms Excipient information presented when available (limited, particularly for generics); consult specific product labeling.

Injection, solution:

Vimpat®: 200 mg/20 mL

Tablet:

Vimpat®: 50 mg, 100 mg, 150 mg, 200 mg

Lactulose (LAK tyoo lose)

Medication Safety Issues

Sound-alike/look-alike issues:

Lactulose may be confused with lactose

Related Information

Laxatives, Classification and Properties *on page 1785*

U.S. Brand Names Constulose; Enulose; Generlac; Kristalose®

Canadian Brand Names Acilac; Apo-Lactulose®; Laxilose; PMS-Lactulose

Mexican Brand Names Lactulax; Regulact

Pharmacologic Category Ammonium Detoxicant; Laxative, Osmotic

Generic Available Yes

Use Adjunct in the prevention and treatment of portal-systemic encephalopathy; treatment of chronic constipation

Effect on Mental Status None reported

Effect on Psychiatric Treatment The therapeutic GI effect of laxation is desired; however, concomitant use with SSRIs, carbamazepine, valproic acid, and lithium may produce additive GI side effects

Pregnancy Risk Factor B

Lactation Excretion in breast milk unknown

Contraindications Hypersensitivity to lactulose or any component of the formulation; galactosemia (or patients requiring a low galactose diet)

Warnings/Precautions Use with caution in patients with diabetes mellitus; solution contains galactose and lactose; monitor periodically for electrolyte imbalance when lactulose is used >6 months or in patients predisposed to electrolyte abnormalities (eg, elderly); patients receiving lactulose and an oral anti-infective agent should be monitored for possible inadequate response to lactulose

Adverse Reactions Frequency not defined: Gastrointestinal: Flatulence, diarrhea (excessive dose), abdominal discomfort, nausea, vomiting, cramping

Drug Interactions

There are no known significant interactions.

Stability Keep solution at room temperature to reduce viscosity. Discard solution if cloudy or very dark.

Mechanism of Action The bacterial degradation of lactulose resulting in an acidic pH inhibits the diffusion of NH_3 into the blood by causing the conversion of NH_3 to NH_4+; also enhances the diffusion of NH_3 from the blood into the gut where conversion to NH_4+ occurs; produces an osmotic effect in the colon with resultant distention promoting peristalsis

Pharmacodynamics/Kinetics

Absorption: Not appreciable

Metabolism: Via colonic flora to lactic acid and acetic acid; requires colonic flora for drug activation

Excretion: Primarily feces and urine (~3%)

Dosage Diarrhea may indicate overdosage and responds to dose reduction

Prevention of portal systemic encephalopathy (PSE): Oral:

- Infants: 2.5-10 mL/day divided 3-4 times/day; adjust dosage to produce 2-3 stools/day
- Older Children: Daily dose of 40-90 mL divided 3-4 times/day; if initial dose causes diarrhea, then reduce it immediately; adjust dosage to produce 2-3 stools/day

Constipation: Oral:

- Children: 5 g/day (7.5 mL) after breakfast
- Adults: 15-30 mL/day increased to 60 mL/day in 1-2 divided doses if necessary

Acute PSE: Adults:

- Oral: 20-30 g (30-45 mL) every 1-2 hours to induce rapid laxation; adjust dosage daily to produce 2-3 soft stools; doses of 30-45 mL may be given hourly to cause rapid laxation, then reduce to recommended dose; usual daily dose: 60-100 g (90-150 mL) daily
- Rectal administration: 200 g (300 mL) diluted with 700 mL of H_2O or NS; administer rectally via rectal balloon catheter and retain 30-60 minutes every 4-6 hours

Dietary Considerations Contraindicated in patients on galactose-restricted diet; may be mixed with fruit juice, milk, water, or citrus-flavored carbonated beverages.

Administration Dilute lactulose in water, usually 60-120 mL, prior to administering through a gastric or feeding tube. Syrup formulation has been used in preparation of rectal solution.

Monitoring Parameters Blood pressure, standing/supine; serum potassium, bowel movement patterns, fluid status, serum ammonia

Dosage Forms Excipient information presented when available (limited, particularly for generics); consult specific product labeling.

Crystals for solution, oral:

Kristalose®: 10 g/packet (30s), 20 g/packet (30s)

Solution, oral: 10 g/15 mL (15 mL, 30 mL, 237 mL, 473 mL, 946 mL, 1890 mL)
  Constulose: 10 g/15 mL (240 mL, 960 mL)
  Enulose: 10 g/15 mL (480 mL)
  Generlac: 10 g/15 mL (480 mL, 1920 mL)
Solution, oral/rectal: 10 g/15 mL (473 mL)

- **Ladakamycin** *see* AzaCITIDine *on page 161*
- **Lagesic™** *see* Acetaminophen and Phenyltoloxamine *on page 36*
- **L-All 12** *see* Carbetapentane and Phenylephrine *on page 273*
- **L-AmB** *see* Amphotericin B, Liposomal *on page 121*
- **Lamictal®** *see* LamoTRIgine *on page 889*
- **Lamisil®** *see* Terbinafine *on page 1551*
- **Lamisil AT® [OTC]** *see* Terbinafine *on page 1551*

LamiVUDine (la MI vyoo deen)

Medication Safety Issues
Sound-alike/look-alike issues:
  LamiVUDine may be confused with lamoTRIgine
  Epivir® may be confused with Combivir®

U.S. Brand Names Epivir-HBV®; Epivir®

Canadian Brand Names 3TC®; Heptovir®

Mexican Brand Names 3TC

Index Terms 3TC

Pharmacologic Category Antiretroviral Agent, Reverse Transcriptase Inhibitor (Nucleoside)

Use
Epivir®: Treatment of HIV infection when antiretroviral therapy is warranted; should always be used as part of a multidrug regimen (at least three antiretroviral agents)
Epivir-HBV®: Treatment of chronic hepatitis B associated with evidence of hepatitis B viral replication and active liver inflammation

Unlabeled/Investigational Use Postexposure prophylaxis for HIV exposure as part of a multidrug regimen

Effect on Mental Status Fatigue and insomnia are common; may cause dizziness or depression

Effect on Psychiatric Treatment May rarely cause neutropenia; use caution with clozapine and carbamazepine

Dosage Summary
Oral:
Neonates <30 days: HIV (AIDSinfo guidelines): 2 mg/kg/dose twice daily
Infants 1-3 months: HIV (AIDSinfo guidelines): 4 mg/kg/dose twice daily
Children 3 months to 2 years: HIV: 4 mg/kg/dose twice daily (maximum: 150 mg/dose twice daily)
Children 2-16 years:
  Hepatitis B: 3 mg/kg/dose once daily (maximum: 100 mg/day)
  HIV: 4 mg/kg/dose twice daily (maximum: 150 mg/dose twice daily)
Children >16 years and <50 kg:
  Hepatitis B: 3 mg/kg/dose once daily (maximum: 100 mg/day)
  HIV (AIDSinfo guidelines): 4 mg/kg/dose twice daily (maximum: 150 mg/dose twice daily)
Children >16 years and ≥50 kg:
  Hepatitis B: 3 mg/kg/dose once daily (maximum: 100 mg/day)
  HIV: 150 mg twice daily **or** 300 mg once daily
Adults <50 kg:
  Hepatitis B: 100 mg/day
  HIV (AIDSinfo guidelines): 4 mg/kg/dose twice daily (maximum: 150 mg/dose twice daily)
Adults ≥50 kg:
  Hepatitis B: 100 mg/day
  HIV: 150 mg twice daily **or** 300 mg once daily

Dosage Forms Excipient information presented when available (limited, particularly for generics); consult specific product labeling.
Solution, oral:
  Epivir®: 10 mg/mL (240 mL) [strawberry-banana flavor]
  Epivir-HBV®: 5 mg/mL (240 mL) [strawberry-banana flavor]
Tablet:
  Epivir®: 150 mg [scored], 300 mg
  Epivir-HBV®: 100 mg

- **Lamivudine and Abacavir** *see* Abacavir and Lamivudine *on page 22*

◆ **Lamivudine and Zidovudine** *see* Zidovudine and Lamivudine *on page 1696*

LamoTRIgine (la MOE tri jeen)

Medication Safety Issues

Sound-alike/look-alike issues:

LamoTRIgine may be confused with labetalol, Lamisil®, lamiVUDine, Lomotil®, ludiomil

Lamictal® may be confused with Lamisil®, Lomotil®, ludiomil

Related Information

Adverse Effects of Approved Mood Stabilizers / Anticonvulsants *on page 1751*
Agents Approved for Bipolar Disorder *on page 1752*
Anticonvulsants By Seizure Type *on page 1759*

U.S. Brand Names Lamictal®

Canadian Brand Names Apo-Lamotrigine®; Gen-Lamotrigine; Lamictal®; Novo-Lamotrigine; PMS-Lamotrigine; ratio-Lamotrigine

Mexican Brand Names Lamdra SBK; Lamictal; Protalgine

Index Terms BW-430C; LTG

Pharmacologic Category Anticonvulsant, Miscellaneous

Generic Available Yes

Use Adjunctive therapy in the treatment of generalized seizures of Lennox-Gastaut syndrome, primary generalized tonic-clonic seizures, and partial seizures in adults and children ≥2 years of age; conversion to monotherapy in adults with partial seizures who are receiving treatment with valproic acid or a single enzyme-inducing antiepileptic drug (specifically carbamazepine, phenytoin, phenobarbital or primidone); maintenance treatment of bipolar I disorder

Effect on Mental Status May cause sedation

Effect on Psychiatric Treatment Valproic acid decreases clearance of lamotrigine; carbamazepine may decrease effects of lamotrigine

Mental Health Comment Lamotrigine is useful for the maintenance treatment of bipolar disorder. Best efficacy appears to be in the prophylaxis of depressive episodes. This medication requires a slow titration process. If patient is receiving valproic acid and/or carbamazepine, a dosage adjustment is necessary (see Dosage).

Potentially life-threatening skin rashes have been reported. These appear to be more frequent in pediatric patients and is associated with high serum levels, use of higher than recommended starting dose, and rapid dose titration. The majority of cases occur within the first 8 weeks of treatment. The combination use with valproate may increase this risk. Discontinue if rash develops.

Pregnancy Risk Factor C

Pregnancy Considerations Lamotrigine has been found to decrease folate concentrations in animal studies. Teratogenic effects in animals were not observed. Lamotrigine crosses the human placenta and can be measured in the plasma of exposed newborns. Preliminary data from the North American Antiepileptic Drug Pregnancy Registry (NAAED) suggest an increased incidence of cleft lip and/or cleft palate following first trimester exposure. Healthcare providers may enroll patients in the Lamotrigine Pregnancy Registry by calling (800) 336-2176. Patients may enroll themselves in the NAAED registry by calling (888) 233-2334. Dose of lamotrigine may need adjustment during pregnancy to maintain clinical response; lamotrigine serum levels may decrease during pregnancy and return to prepartum levels following delivery. Monitor frequently during pregnancy, following delivery, and when adding or discontinuing combination hormonal contraceptives.

Lactation Enters breast milk/not recommended (AAP rates "of concern")

Contraindications Hypersensitivity to lamotrigine or any component of the formulation

Warnings/Precautions [U.S. Boxed Warning]: Severe and potentially life-threatening skin rashes requiring hospitalization have been reported; risk may be increased by coadministration with valproic acid, higher than recommended starting doses, and rapid dose titration. The majority of cases occur in the first 8 weeks; however, isolated cases may occur after prolonged treatment. Discontinue at first sign of rash unless rash is clearly not drug related. Acute multiorgan failure has also been reported. A spectrum of hematologic effects have been reported with use (eg, neutropenia, leukopenia, thrombocytopenia, pancytopenia, and anemias); patients with a previous history of adverse hematologic reaction to any drug may be at increased risk. Early detection of hematologic change is important; advise patients of early signs and symptoms including fever, sore throat, mouth ulcers, infections, easy bruising, petechial or purpuric hemorrhage. May be associated with hypersensitivity syndrome. Use caution in patients with impaired renal, hepatic, or ▶

cardiac function. Avoid abrupt cessation, taper over at least 2 weeks if possible. May cause CNS depression, which may impair physical or mental abilities. Patients must be cautioned about performing tasks which require mental alertness (eg, operating machinery or driving). Effects with other sedative drugs or ethanol may be potentiated. Binds to melanin and may accumulate in the eye and other melanin-rich tissues; the clinical significance of this is not known. Safety and efficacy have not been established for use as initial monotherapy, conversion to monotherapy from antiepileptic drugs (AED) other than carbamazepine, phenytoin, phenobarbital, primidone or valproic acid or conversion to monotherapy from two or more AEDs. Patients treated for bipolar disorder should be monitored closely for clinical worsening or suicidality; prescriptions should be written for the smallest quantity consistent with good patient care. Hormonal contraceptives may cause a decrease in lamotrigine levels requiring dose adjustment.

Adverse Reactions Percentages reported in adults on monotherapy for epilepsy or bipolar disorder.

>10%: Gastrointestinal: Nausea (7% to 14%)

1% to 10%:

Cardiovascular: Chest pain (5%), peripheral edema (2% to 5%), edema (1% to 5%)

Central nervous system: Somnolence (9%), fatigue (8%), dizziness (7%), anxiety (5%), insomnia (5% to 10%), pain (5%), ataxia (2% to 5%), irritability (2% to 5%), suicidal ideation (2% to 5%), agitation (1% to 5%), amnesia (1% to 5%), depression (1% to 5%), dream abnormality (1% to 5%), emotional lability (1% to 5%), fever (1% to 5%), hypoesthesia (1% to 5%), migraine (1% to 5%), thought abnormality (1% to 5%), confusion (1%)

Dermatologic: Rash (nonserious: 7%), dermatitis (2% to 5%), dry skin (2% to 5%)

Endocrine & metabolic: Dysmenorrhea (5%), libido increased (2% to 5%)

Gastrointestinal: Vomiting (5% to 9%), dyspepsia (7%), abdominal pain (6%), xerostomia (2% to 6%), constipation (5%), weight loss (5%), anorexia (2% to 5%), peptic ulcer (2% to 5%), rectal hemorrhage (2% to 5%), flatulence (1% to 5%), weight gain (1% to 5%)

Genitourinary: Urinary frequency (1% to 5%)

Neuromuscular & skeletal: Back pain (8%), coordination abnormal (7%), weakness (2% to 5%), arthralgia (1% to 5%), myalgia (1% to 5%), neck pain (1% to 5%), paresthesia (1%)

Ocular: Nystagmus (2% to 5%), vision abnormal (2% to 5%), amblyopia (1%)

Respiratory: Rhinitis (7%), cough (5%), pharyngitis (5%), bronchitis (2% to 5%), dyspnea (2% to 5%), epistaxis (2% to 5%), sinusitis (1% to 5%)

Miscellaneous: Infection (5%), diaphoresis (2% to 5%), reflexes increased/decreased (2% to 5%), dyspraxia (1% to 5%)

<1%: Any indication (limited to important or life-threatening): Accommodation abnormality, acne, agranulocytosis, alcohol intolerance, allergic reaction, alopecia, anemia, angina, angioedema, aphasia, aplastic anemia, apnea, appetite increased, arthritis, atrial fibrillation, breast pain, bruising, cerebellar syndrome, cerebral sinus thrombosis, cerebrovascular accident, chills, choreoathetosis, CNS depression/stimulation, conjunctivitis, deafness, deep thrombophlebitis, delirium, delusions, dermatitis (exfoliative, fungal), disseminated intravascular coagulation, dry eyes, dysphagia, dysphoria, dystonia, ear pain, ECG abnormality, ejaculation abnormal, eructation, esophagitis, euphoria, extrapyramidal syndrome, faintness, flushing, gastritis, gingivitis, goiter, halitosis, hallucinations, hematuria, hemiplegia, hemolytic anemia, hemorrhage, hiccup, hirsutism, hot flashes, hyperalgesia, hyperglycemia, hypersensitivity reactions, hypertension, hyperventilation, hypokinesia, hypothyroidism, hypotonia, impotence, kidney failure (acute), leg cramps, leukopenia, liver function tests abnormal, lupus-like reaction, maculopapular rash, malaise, menorrhagia, MI, mouth ulceration, movement disorder, multiorgan failure, muscle spasm, myasthenia, neuralgia, neurosis, neutropenia, palpitation, pancreatitis, pancytopenia, paralysis, parkinsonian exacerbation, peripheral neuritis, photophobia, polyuria, postural hypotension, progressive immunosuppression, red cell aplasia, rhabdomyolysis, salivation increased, skin discoloration, Stevens-Johnson syndrome, suicide, syncope, tachycardia, taste loss/perversion, thrombocytopenia, tic, tinnitus, tongue edema, toxic epidermal necrolysis, twitching, urinary incontinence, urticaria, vasculitis, vasodilation, yawn

Also observed: Rash requiring hospitalization: Children <16 years 0.8% (epilepsy adjunctive therapy); Adults 0.3% (epilepsy adjunctive therapy), 0.13% (epilepsy monotherapy), 0.8% (bipolar disorder, monotherapy)

Drug Interactions

Alcohol (Ethyl): CNS Depressants may enhance the CNS depressant effect of Alcohol (Ethyl). *Risk C: Monitor therapy*

Barbiturates: May increase the metabolism of LamoTRIgine. *Risk D: Consider therapy modification*

CarBAMazepine: LamoTRIgine may enhance the adverse/toxic effect of CarBAMazepine. CarBAMazepine may increase the metabolism of LamoTRIgine. *Risk D: Consider therapy modification*

CNS Depressants: May enhance the adverse/toxic effect of other CNS Depressants. *Risk C: Monitor therapy*

Desmopressin: LamoTRIgine may enhance the adverse/toxic effect of Desmopressin. LamoTRIgine may enhance the therapeutic effect of Desmopressin. *Risk C: Monitor therapy*

Ketorolac: May diminish the therapeutic effect of Anticonvulsants. *Risk C: Monitor therapy*

Mefloquine: May diminish the therapeutic effect of Anticonvulsants. Mefloquine may decrease the serum concentration of Anticonvulsants. Management: Mefloquine is contraindicated in persons with a history of convulsions. If anticonvulsant is being used for another indication monitor response to treatment closely, as concurrent mefloquine may decrease response to treatment. *Risk D: Consider therapy modification*

OLANZapine: LamoTRIgine may enhance the sedative effect of OLANZapine. *Risk C: Monitor therapy*

Oral Contraceptive (Estrogens): May decrease the serum concentration of LamoTRIgine. *Risk D: Consider therapy modification*

Phenytoin: May increase the metabolism of LamoTRIgine. *Risk D: Consider therapy modification*

Primidone: May increase the metabolism of LamoTRIgine. *Risk D: Consider therapy modification*

Rifampin: May increase the metabolism of LamoTRIgine. *Risk C: Monitor therapy*

Ritonavir: May decrease the serum concentration of LamoTRIgine. *Risk D: Consider therapy modification*

Valproic Acid: May enhance the adverse/toxic effect of LamoTRIgine. Valproic Acid may increase the serum concentration of LamoTRIgine. *Risk D: Consider therapy modification*

Ethanol/Nutrition/Herb Interactions

Ethanol: Avoid ethanol (may increase CNS depression).

Food: Has no effect on absorption.

Herb/Nutraceutical: Avoid evening primrose (seizure threshold decreased).

Stability Store at 25°C (77°F); excursions permitted to 15°C to 30°C (59°F to 86°F). Protect from light.

Mechanism of Action A triazine derivative which inhibits release of glutamate (an excitatory amino acid) and inhibits voltage-sensitive sodium channels, which stabilizes neuronal membranes. Lamotrigine has weak inhibitory effect on the 5-HT_3 receptor; *in vitro* inhibits dihydrofolate reductase.

Pharmacodynamics/Kinetics

Absorption: Rapid and complete

Distribution: V_d: ~1 L/kg

Protein binding: 55%

Metabolism: Hepatic and renal; metabolized by glucuronic acid conjugation to inactive metabolites

Bioavailability: 98%

Half-life elimination: Adults: 25-33 hours

- Concomitant valproic acid therapy: 59-70 hours
- Concomitant phenytoin or carbamazepine therapy: 13-14 hours
- Chronic renal failure: 43 hours
- Hemodialysis: 13 hours during dialysis; 57 hours between dialysis
- Hepatic impairment: 26-148 hours

Time to peak, plasma: 1-5 hours

Excretion: Urine (94%, ~90% as glucuronide conjugates and ~10% unchanged); feces (2%)

Dosage Note: Only whole tablets should be used for dosing, round calculated dose down to the nearest whole tablet. Enzyme-inducing regimens specifically refer to those containing carbamazepine, phenytoin, phenobarbital, or primidone. Oral:

Children 2-12 years: Lennox-Gastaut (adjunctive), primary generalized tonic-clonic seizures (adjunctive), or partial seizures (adjunctive): **Note:** Children <30 kg will likely require maintenance doses to be increased as much as 50% based on clinical response regardless of regimen below:

Initial: 0.3 mg/kg/day in 1-2 divided doses for weeks 1 and 2, then increase to 0.6 mg/kg/day in 1-2 divided doses for weeks 3 and 4. Maintenance: Titrate dose to effect; after week 4, increase daily dose every 1-2 weeks by

0.6 mg/kg/day; usual maintenance: 4.5-7.5 mg/kg/day in 2 divided doses; maximum: 300 mg/day in 2 divided doses

Adjustment for AED regimens **containing** valproic acid (see "Note"): Initial: 0.15 mg/kg/day in 1-2 divided doses for weeks 1 and 2, then increase to 0.3 mg/kg/day in 1-2 divided doses for weeks 3 and 4. Maintenance: Titrate dose to effect; after week 4, increase daily dose every 1-2 weeks by 0.3 mg/kg/day; usual maintenance: 1-5 mg/kg/day in 2 divided doses; maximum: 200 mg/day in 1-2 divided doses

Note: For patients >6.7 kg and <14 kg, initial dosing should be 2 mg every other day for first 2 weeks, then increased to 2 mg daily for weeks 3-4. For patients taking lamotrigine with valproic acid alone, the usual maintenance dose is 1-3 mg/kg/day in 2 divided doses

Adjustment for **enzyme-inducing** AED regimens **without** valproic acid: Initial: 0.6 mg/kg/day in 2 divided doses for weeks 1 and 2, then increase to 1.2 mg/kg/day in 2 divided doses for weeks 3 and 4. Maintenance: Titrate dose to effect; after week 4, increase daily dose every 1-2 weeks by 1.2 mg/kg/day; usual maintenance: 5-15 mg/kg/day in 2 divided doses; maximum: 400 mg/day in 2 divided doses

Children >12 years: Lennox-Gastaut (adjunctive), primary generalized tonic-clonic seizures (adjunctive), or partial seizures (adjunctive): Refer to adult dosing.

Children ≥16 years: Conversion from adjunctive therapy with valproic acid or a single enzyme-inducing AED regimen to monotherapy with lamotrigine: Refer to adult dosing.

Adults:

Lennox-Gastaut (adjunctive), primary generalized tonic-clonic seizures (adjunctive) or partial seizures (adjunctive): Initial: 25 mg/day for weeks 1 and 2, then increase to 50 mg/day for weeks 3 and 4. Maintenance: Titrate dose to effect; after week 4 increase daily dose every 1-2 weeks by 50 mg/day; usual maintenance: 225-375 mg/day in 2 divided doses

Adjustment for AED regimens **containing** valproic acid (see "Note"): Initial: 25 mg every other day for weeks 1 and 2, then increase to 25 mg every day for weeks 3 and 4. Maintenance: Titrate dose to effect; after week 4 increase daily dose every 1-2 weeks by 25-50 mg/day; usual maintenance: 100-400 mg/day in 1 or 2 divided doses

Note: For patients taking lamotrigine with valproic acid alone, the usual maintenance dose is 100-200 mg/day

Adjustment for **enzyme-inducing** AED regimens **without** valproic acid: Initial: 50 mg/day for weeks 1 and 2, then increase to 100 mg/day in 2 divided doses for weeks 3 and 4. Maintenance: titrate dose to effect; after week 4 increase daily dose every 1-2 weeks by 100 mg/day; usual maintenance: 300-500 mg/day in 2 divided doses. Doses as high as 700 mg/day have been used, though additional benefit has not been established.

Conversion to monotherapy with lamotrigine:

Conversion from adjunctive therapy with valproic acid: Initiate and titrate as per recommendations to a lamotrigine dose of 200 mg/day. Then taper valproic acid dose in decrements of not >500 mg/day at intervals of 1 week (or longer) to a valproic acid dosage of 500 mg/day; this dosage should be maintained for 1 week. The lamotrigine dosage should then be increased to 300 mg/day while valproic acid is decreased to 250 mg/day; this dosage should be maintained for 1 week. Valproic acid may then be discontinued, while the lamotrigine dose is increased by 100 mg/day at weekly intervals to achieve a lamotrigine maintenance dose of 500 mg/day.

Conversion from adjunctive therapy with carbamazepine, phenytoin, phenobarbital, or primidone: Initiate and titrate as per recommendations to a lamotrigine dose of 500 mg/day. Concomitant enzyme-inducing AED should then be withdrawn by 20% decrements each week over a 4-week period. Patients should be monitored for rash.

Conversion from adjunctive therapy with AED other than carbamazepine, phenytoin, phenobarbital, primidone or valproic acid: No specific guidelines available

Bipolar disorder:

Initial: 25 mg/day for weeks 1 and 2, then increase to 50 mg/day for weeks 3 and 4, then increase to 100 mg/day for week 5; maintenance: increase dose to 200 mg/day beginning week 6

Adjustment for regimens **containing** valproic acid: Initial: 25 mg every other day for weeks 1 and 2, then increase to 25 mg every day for weeks 3 and 4, then increase to 50 mg/day for week 5; maintenance: 100 mg/day beginning week 6

Adjustment for **enzyme-inducing** regimens **without** valproic acid: Initial: 50 mg/day for weeks 1 and 2, then increase to 100 mg/day in divided doses for weeks 3 and 4, then increase to 200 mg/day in divided doses for week 5, then increase to 300 mg/day in divided dose for week 6; maintenance: 400 mg/day in divided doses beginning week 7

Adjustment following discontinuation of psychotropic medication:

Discontinuing valproic acid with current dose of lamotrigine 100 mg/day: 150 mg/day for week 1, then increase to 200 mg/day beginning week 2

Discontinuing carbamazepine, phenytoin, phenobarbital, primidone, or rifampin with current dose of lamotrigine 400 mg/day: 400 mg/day for week 1, then decrease to 300 mg/day for week 2, then decrease to 200 mg/day beginning week 3

Discontinuing therapy: Children and Adults: Decrease dose by ~50% per week, over at least 2 weeks unless safety concerns require a more rapid withdrawal. Discontinuing carbamazepine, phenytoin, phenobarbital, or primidone should prolong the half-life of lamotrigine; discontinuing valproic acid should shorten the half-life of lamotrigine

Restarting therapy after discontinuation: If lamotrigine has been withheld for >5 half-lives, consider restarting according to initial dosing recommendations.

Dosage adjustment with combination hormonal contraceptives: Follow initial dosing guidelines, maintenance dose should be adjusted as follows:

Patients taking carbamazepine, phenytoin, phenobarbital, primidone or rifampin: No dosing adjustment required

Patients **not** taking carbamazepine, phenytoin, phenobarbital, primidone or rifampin: Maintenance dose may need increased by twofold over target dose. If already taking a stable dose of lamotrigine and starting contraceptive, maintenance dose may need increased by twofold. Dose increases should start when contraceptive is started and titrated to clinical response increasing no more rapidly than 50-100 mg/day every week. Gradual increases of lamotrigine plasma levels may occur during the inactive "pill-free" week and will be greater when dose increases are made the week before. If increased adverse events consistently occur during "pill-free" week, overall dose adjustments may be required. When discontinuing combination hormonal contraceptive, dose of lamotrigine may need decreased by as much as 50%; do not decrease by more than 25% of total daily dose over a 2-week period unless clinical response or plasma levels indicate otherwise. Dose adjustments during "pill-free" week are not recommended.

Dosage adjustment in renal impairment: Decreased dosage may be effective in patients with significant renal impairment; use with caution

Dosage adjustment in hepatic impairment:

Moderate-to-severe impairment without ascites: Decrease initial, escalation, and maintenance doses by ~25%

Moderate-to-severe impairment with ascites: Decrease initial, escalation, and maintenance doses by ~50%

Dietary Considerations Take without regard to meals; drug may cause GI upset.

Administration Doses should be rounded down to the nearest whole tablet. Dispersible tablets may be chewed, dispersed in water or diluted fruit juice, or swallowed whole. To disperse tablets, add to a small amount of liquid (just enough to cover tablet); let sit ~1 minute until dispersed; swirl solution and consume immediately. Do not administer partial amounts of liquid. If tablets are chewed, a small amount of water or diluted fruit juice should be used to aid in swallowing.

Monitoring Parameters Seizure, frequency and duration, serum levels of concurrent anticonvulsants, hypersensitivity reactions, especially rash

Reference Range A therapeutic serum concentration range has not been established for lamotrigine. Dosing should be based on therapeutic response. Lamotrigine plasma concentrations of 0.25-29.1 mcg/mL have been reported in the literature.

Dosage Forms Excipient information presented when available (limited, particularly for generics); consult specific product labeling.

Tablet: 25 mg, 100 mg, 150 mg, 200 mg

Lamictal®: 25 mg, 100 mg, 150 mg, 200 mg

Tablet, combination package [each unit-dose starter kit contains]:

Lamictal® (blue kit; for patients taking valproic acid):

Tablet: Lamotrigine 25 mg (35s)

Lamictal® (green kit; for patients taking carbamazepine, phenytoin, phenobarbital, primidone, or rifampin and **not** taking valproic acid):

Tablet: Lamotrigine 25 mg (84s)

Tablet: Lamotrigine 100 mg (14s)

Lamictal® (orange kit; for patients **not** taking carbamazepine, phenytoin, phenobarbital, primidone, rifampin, or valproic acid):
Tablet: Lamotrigine 25 mg (42s)
Tablet: Lamotrigine 100 mg (7s)
Tablet, dispersible/chewable: 5 mg, 25 mg
Lamictal®: 2 mg, 5 mg, 25 mg [black currant flavor]

◆ **Lanoxicaps® [DSC]** *see* Digoxin *on page 463*

◆ **Lanoxin®** *see* Digoxin *on page 463*

Lansoprazole (lan SOE pra zole)

Medication Safety Issues
Sound-alike/look-alike issues:
Prevacid® may be confused with Pravachol®, Prevpac®, Prilosec®, Prinivil®

U.S. Brand Names Prevacid®; Prevacid® SoluTab™

Canadian Brand Names Prevacid®

Mexican Brand Names Imidex; Lanodizol; Ogastro; Olan; Palatrin; Prilosan; Safemar; Sorifran; Uldapril; Ulpax

Pharmacologic Category Proton Pump Inhibitor; Substituted Benzimidazole

Generic Available No

Use Short-term treatment of active duodenal ulcers; maintenance treatment of healed duodenal ulcers; as part of a multidrug regimen for *H. pylori* eradication to reduce the risk of duodenal ulcer recurrence; short-term treatment of active benign gastric ulcer; treatment of NSAID-associated gastric ulcer; to reduce the risk of NSAID-associated gastric ulcer in patients with a history of gastric ulcer who require an NSAID; short-term treatment of symptomatic GERD; short-term treatment for all grades of erosive esophagitis; to maintain healing of erosive esophagitis; long-term treatment of pathological hypersecretory conditions, including Zollinger-Ellison syndrome

Effect on Mental Status May cause drowsiness or dizziness

Effect on Psychiatric Treatment None reported

Pregnancy Risk Factor B

Pregnancy Considerations Animal studies have not shown teratogenic effects to the fetus. However, there are no adequate and well-controlled studies in pregnant women; use during pregnancy only if clearly needed.

Lactation Excretion in breast milk unknown/not recommended

Contraindications Hypersensitivity to lansoprazole, substituted benzimidazoles (ie, esomeprazole, omeprazole, pantoprazole, rabeprazole), or any component of the formulation

Warnings/Precautions Relief of symptoms does not preclude the presence of a gastric malignancy. Atrophic gastritis (by biopsy) has been noted with long-term omeprazole therapy; this may also occur with lansoprazole. No reports of enterochromaffin-like (ECL) cell carcinoids, dysplasia, or neoplasia have occurred. Severe liver dysfunction may require dosage reductions. Safety and efficacy have not been established in children <1 year of age.

Adverse Reactions
1% to 10%:
Central nervous system: Headache (children 1-11 years 3%, 12-17 years 7%)
Gastrointestinal: Abdominal pain (children 12-17 years 5%; adults 2%), constipation (children 1-11 years 5%; adults 1%), diarrhea (60 mg/day; adults 7%), nausea (children 12-17 years 3%; adults 1%)

<1% (Limited to important or life-threatening): Abnormal vision, agitation, allergic reaction, ALT increased, anaphylactoid reaction, anemia, angina, anxiety, aplastic anemia, arrhythmia, AST increased, chest pain, convulsion, depression, dizziness, dry eyes, dry mouth, erythema multiforme, esophagitis, gastrin levels increased, glucocorticoids increased, globulins increased, hemolysis, hemolytic anemia, hepatotoxicity, hyperglycemia, interstitial nephritis, LDH increased, maculopapular rash, myositis, pancreatitis, photophobia, rash, RBC abnormal, taste perversion, Stevens-Johnson syndrome, thrombocytopenia, tinnitus, toxic epidermal necrolysis, tremor, vertigo, visual field defect, vomiting, WBC abnormal

Metabolism/Transport Effects Substrate of CYP2C9 (minor), 2C19 (major), 3A4 (major); **Inhibits** CYP2C9 (weak), 2C19 (moderate), 2D6 (weak), 3A4 (weak); **Induces** CYP1A2 (weak)

Drug Interactions
Antifungal Agents (Azole Derivatives, Systemic): Proton Pump Inhibitors may decrease the absorption of Antifungal Agents (Azole Derivatives, Systemic). **Exceptions:** Miconazole. *Risk D: Consider therapy modification*

Atazanavir: Proton Pump Inhibitors may decrease the absorption of Atazanavir. *Risk D: Consider therapy modification*

Clopidogrel: Proton Pump Inhibitors may diminish the therapeutic effect of Clopidogrel. This appears to be due to reduced formation of the active clopidogrel metabolite. *Risk C: Monitor therapy*

CYP2C19 Inducers (Strong): May increase the metabolism of CYP2C19 Substrates. *Risk C: Monitor therapy*

CYP2C19 Substrates: CYP2C19 Inhibitors (Moderate) may decrease the metabolism of CYP2C19 Substrates. *Risk C: Monitor therapy*

CYP3A4 Inducers (Strong): May increase the metabolism of CYP3A4 Substrates. *Risk C: Monitor therapy*

Dabigatran Etexilate: Proton Pump Inhibitors may decrease the serum concentration of Dabigatran Etexilate. *Risk C: Monitor therapy*

Dasatinib: Proton Pump Inhibitors may decrease the absorption of Dasatinib. *Risk D: Consider therapy modification*

Deferasirox: May decrease the serum concentration of CYP3A4 Substrates. *Risk C: Monitor therapy*

Erlotinib: Proton Pump Inhibitors may decrease the serum concentration of Erlotinib. *Risk X: Avoid combination*

Herbs (CYP3A4 Inducers): May increase the metabolism of CYP3A4 Substrates. *Risk C: Monitor therapy*

Imatinib: Lansoprazole may enhance the dermatologic adverse effect of Imatinib. *Risk C: Monitor therapy*

Indinavir: Proton Pump Inhibitors may decrease the absorption of Indinavir. *Risk C: Monitor therapy*

Iron Salts: Proton Pump Inhibitors may decrease the absorption of Iron Salts. **Exceptions:** Ferric Gluconate; Iron Dextran Complex; Iron Sucrose. *Risk C: Monitor therapy*

Methotrexate: Proton Pump Inhibitors may decrease the excretion of Methotrexate. Antirheumatic doses of methotrexate probably hold minimal risk. *Risk C: Monitor therapy*

Mycophenolate: Proton Pump Inhibitors may decrease the serum concentration of Mycophenolate. Specifically, concentrations of the active mycophenolic acid may be reduced. *Risk C: Monitor therapy*

Saquinavir: Proton Pump Inhibitors may increase the serum concentration of Saquinavir. *Risk C: Monitor therapy*

Tipranavir: May decrease the serum concentration of Proton Pump Inhibitors. These data are derived from studies with Ritonavir-boosted Tipranavir. *Risk C: Monitor therapy*

Ethanol/Nutrition/Herb Interactions

Ethanol: Avoid ethanol (may cause gastric mucosal irritation).

Food: Lansoprazole serum concentrations may be decreased if taken with food.

Herb/Nutraceutical: Avoid St John's wort (may decrease the levels/effect of lansoprazole).

Stability Store at 25°C (77°F); excursions permitted to 15°C to 30°C (59°F to 86°F).

Mechanism of Action Decreases acid secretion in gastric parietal cells through inhibition of (H+, K+)-ATPase enzyme system, blocking the final step in gastric acid production.

Pharmacodynamics/Kinetics

Duration: >1 day

Absorption: Rapid

Distribution: V_d: 14-18 L

Protein binding: 97%

Metabolism: Hepatic via CYP2C19 and 3A4, and in parietal cells to two active metabolites that are not present in systemic circulation

Bioavailability: 80%; decreased 50% to 70% if given 30 minutes after food

Half-life elimination: 1-2 hours; Elderly: 2-3 hours; Hepatic impairment: ≤7 hours

Time to peak, plasma: 1.7 hours

Excretion: Feces (67%); urine (33%)

Dosage Oral:

Children 1-11 years: GERD, erosive esophagitis:

- ≤30 kg: 15 mg once daily
- >30 kg: 30 mg once daily
- **Note:** Doses were increased in some pediatric patients if still symptomatic after 2 or more weeks of treatment (maximum dose: 30 mg twice daily)

Children 12-17 years:

- Nonerosive GERD: 15 mg once daily for up to 8 weeks
- Erosive esophagitis: 30 mg once daily for up to 8 weeks

Adults:

- Duodenal ulcer: Short-term treatment: 15 mg once daily for 4 weeks; maintenance therapy: 15 mg once daily

Gastric ulcer: Short-term treatment: 30 mg once daily for up to 8 weeks

NSAID-associated gastric ulcer (healing): 30 mg once daily for 8 weeks; controlled studies did not extend past 8 weeks of therapy

NSAID-associated gastric ulcer (to reduce risk): 15 mg once daily for up to 12 weeks; controlled studies did not extend past 12 weeks of therapy

Symptomatic GERD: Short-term treatment: 15 mg once daily for up to 8 weeks

Erosive esophagitis: Short-term treatment: 30 mg once daily for up to 8 weeks; continued treatment for an additional 8 weeks may be considered for recurrence or for patients who do not heal after the first 8 weeks of therapy; maintenance therapy: 15 mg once daily

Hypersecretory conditions: Initial: 60 mg once daily; adjust dose based upon patient response and to reduce acid secretion to <10 mEq/hour (5 mEq/hour in patients with prior gastric surgery); doses of 90 mg twice daily have been used; administer doses >120 mg/day in divided doses

Helicobacter pylori eradication: Currently accepted recommendations (may differ from product labeling): Dose varies with regimen: 30 mg once daily or 60 mg/day in 2 divided doses; requires combination therapy with antibiotics

Elderly: No dosage adjustment is needed in elderly patients with normal hepatic function

Dosage adjustment in renal impairment: No dosage adjustment is needed

Dosing adjustment in hepatic impairment: Dose reduction is necessary for severe hepatic impairment

Dietary Considerations Should be taken before eating; best if taken before breakfast. Prevacid® SoluTab™ contains phenylalanine 2.5 mg per 15 mg tablet; phenylalanine 5.1 mg per 30 mg tablet.

Administration

Oral: Administer before food; best if taken before breakfast. The intact granules should not be chewed or crushed; however, several options are available for those patients unable to swallow capsules:

Capsules may be opened and the intact granules sprinkled on 1 tablespoon of applesauce, Ensure® pudding, cottage cheese, yogurt, or strained pears. The granules should then be swallowed immediately.

Capsules may be opened and emptied into ~60 mL orange juice, apple juice, or tomato juice; mix and swallow immediately. Rinse the glass with additional juice and swallow to assure complete delivery of the dose.

Orally-disintegrating tablets: Should not be swallowed whole or chewed. Place tablet on tongue; allow to dissolve (with or without water) until particles can be swallowed. Orally-disintegrating tablets may also be administered via an oral syringe: Place the 15 mg tablet in an oral syringe and draw up ~4 mL water, or place the 30 mg tablet in an oral syringe and draw up ~10 mL water. After tablet has dispersed, administer within 15 minutes. Refill the syringe with water (2 mL for the 15 mg tablet; 4 mL for the 30 mg tablet), shake gently, then administer any remaining contents.

Nasogastric tube administration:

Capsule: Capsule can be opened, the granules mixed (not crushed) with 40 mL of apple juice and then injected through the NG tube into the stomach, then flush tube with additional apple juice. Do not mix with other liquids.

Orally-disintegrating tablet: Nasogastric tube ≥8 French: Place a 15 mg tablet in a syringe and draw up ~4 mL water, or place the 30 mg tablet in a syringe and draw up ~10 mL water. After tablet has dispersed, administer within 15 minutes. Refill the syringe with ~5 mL water, shake gently, and then flush the nasogastric tube.

Monitoring Parameters Patients with Zollinger-Ellison syndrome should be monitored for gastric acid output, which should be maintained at ≤10 mEq/hour during the last hour before the next lansoprazole dose; lab monitoring should include CBC, liver function, renal function, and serum gastrin levels

Dosage Forms Excipient information presented when available (limited, particularly for generics); consult specific product labeling. [DSC] = Discontinued product

Capsule, delayed release:

Prevacid®: 15 mg, 30 mg

Tablet, delayed release, orally disintegrating:

Prevacid® SoluTab™: 15 mg [contains phenylalanine 2.5 mg; strawberry flavor]; 30 mg [contains phenylalanine 5.1 mg; strawberry flavor]

Lansoprazole, Amoxicillin, and Clarithromycin
(lan SOE pra zole, a moks i SIL in, & kla RITH roe mye sin)

Medication Safety Issues
Sound-alike/look-alike issues:
Prevpac® may be confused with Prevacid®

U.S. Brand Names Prevpac®

Canadian Brand Names Hp-PAC®; Prevpac®

Index Terms Amoxicillin, Lansoprazole, and Clarithromycin; Clarithromycin, Lansoprazole, and Amoxicillin

Pharmacologic Category Antibiotic, Macrolide Combination; Antibiotic, Penicillin; Gastrointestinal Agent, Miscellaneous

Use Eradication of *H. pylori* to reduce the risk of recurrent duodenal ulcer

Effect on Mental Status May cause drowsiness or dizziness; rarely large doses may produce confusion, hallucinations, and depression; penicillins have been reported to cause apprehension, illusions, agitation, insomnia, depersonalization, and encephalopathy; macrolides have been reported to cause nightmares, confusion, anxiety, and mood lability

Effect on Psychiatric Treatment Disulfiram may increase amoxicillin levels; macrolides are contraindicated with pimozide and increase carbamazepine and triazolam levels; monitor for signs of toxicity

Dosage Summary

Oral:

Children: Dosage not established

Adults: Lansoprazole 30 mg, amoxicillin 1 g, and clarithromycin 500 mg taken together twice daily

Dosage Forms Excipient information presented when available (limited, particularly for generics); consult specific product labeling.

Combination package [each administration card contains]:

Prevpac®:

Capsule: Amoxicillin 500 mg (4 capsules/day)

Capsule, delayed release (Prevacid®): Lansoprazole 30 mg (2 capsules/day)

Tablet (Biaxin®): Clarithromycin 500 mg (2 tablets/day)

Lansoprazole and Naproxen (lan SOE pra zole & na PROKS en)

Medication Safety Issues
Sound-alike/look-alike issues:
Prevacid® may be confused with Pravachol®, Prevpac®, Prilosec®, Prinivil®

U.S. Brand Names Prevacid® NapraPAC™

Index Terms NapraPAC™; Naproxen and Lansoprazole

Pharmacologic Category Nonsteroidal Anti-inflammatory Drug (NSAID), Oral; Proton Pump Inhibitor

Use Reduction of the risk of NSAID-associated gastric ulcers in patients with history of gastric ulcer who require an NSAID for the treatment of rheumatoid arthritis, osteoarthritis, and ankylosing spondylitis

Effect on Mental Status Dizziness is common; may cause nervousness or sedation; may rarely cause confusion, insomnia, depression, or hallucinations

Effect on Psychiatric Treatment May rarely cause agranulocytosis; use caution with clozapine, carbamazepine, and mirtazapine. May decrease lithium clearance resulting in an increase in serum lithium levels and potential lithium toxicity; monitor serum lithium levels. Combined use with SSRIs may increase bleeding risk.

Restrictions An FDA-approved medication guide must be distributed when dispensing an oral outpatient prescription (new or refill) where this medication is to be used without direct supervision of a healthcare provider. Medication guides are available at http://www.fda.gov/cder/Offices/ODS/medication_guides.htm.

Dosage Summary

Oral:

Children: Dosage not established

Adults: 15 mg once daily of lansoprazole and 500 mg twice daily of naproxen

Elderly: Naproxen dosing adjustment should be considered

Dosage Forms Excipient information presented when available (limited, particularly for generics); consult specific product labeling. [DSC] = Discontinued product

Combination package:
Prevacid® NapraPAC™ 375 [each administration card contains] [DSC]:
Capsule, delayed release (Prevacid®): Lansoprazole 15 mg (7 capsules per card)
Tablet (Naprosyn®): Naproxen 375 mg (14 tablets per card)
Prevacid® NapraPAC™ 500 [each administration card contains]:
Capsule, delayed release (Prevacid®): Lansoprazole 15 mg (7 capsules per card)
Tablet (Naprosyn®): Naproxen 500 mg (14 tablets per card)

Lanthanum (LAN tha num)

U.S. Brand Names Fosrenol®
Canadian Brand Names Fosrenol®
Index Terms Lanthanum Carbonate
Pharmacologic Category Phosphate Binder
Use Reduction of serum phosphate in patients with stage 5 chronic kidney disease (kidney failure: GFR <15 mL/minute/1.73 m^2 or dialysis)
Effect on Mental Status None reported
Effect on Psychiatric Treatment GI side effects are common; concurrent use with SSRIs, lithium, or valproic acid may produce additive GI effects; may bind with gabapentin; separate administration by at least 2 hours
Dosage Summary
Oral:
Children: Dosage not established
Adults: Initial: 750-1500 mg/day in divided doses with meals; Usual range: 1500-3000 mg/day. **Note:** Titration is recommended
Dosage Forms Excipient information presented when available (limited, particularly for generics); consult specific product labeling. [DSC] = Discontinued product
Tablet, chewable:
Fosrenol®: 250 mg [DSC], 500 mg, 750 mg, 1000 mg

◆ **Lanthanum Carbonate** *see* Lanthanum *on page 898*
◆ **Lantus®** *see* Insulin Glargine *on page 827*

Lapatinib (la PA ti nib)

Medication Safety Issues
Sound-alike/look-alike issues:
Lapatinib may be confused with dasatinib, erlotinib, imatinib
High alert medication: The Institute for Safe Medication Practices (ISMP) includes this medication among its list of drug classes which have a heightened risk of causing significant patient harm when used in error.
U.S. Brand Names Tykerb®
Index Terms GW572016; Lapatinib Ditosylate; NSC-727989
Pharmacologic Category Antineoplastic Agent, Tyrosine Kinase Inhibitor; Epidermal Growth Factor Receptor (EGFR) Inhibitor
Use Treatment (in combination with capecitabine) of HER2/neu overexpressing advanced or metastatic breast cancer, in patients who have received prior therapy (with an anthracycline, a taxane, and trastuzumab)
Unlabeled/Investigational Use Treatment of head and neck cancers
Effect on Mental Status Fatigue is common; may cause insomnia
Effect on Psychiatric Treatment Diarrhea is common; concurrent use with SSRIs or lithium may produce additive effects. May prolong QT_c interval; concurrent use with ziprasidone, paliperidone, and thioridazine is not recommended. Hematologic side effects are common; use caution with clozapine, carbamazepine, and valproic acid. Lapatinib is a CYP3A4 substrate and inhibitor. CYP3A4 inducers (St John's wort, carbamazepine, barbiturates) may decrease the levels/effects of lapatinib. The effects/levels of CYP3A4 substrates (benzodiazepines, mirtazapine, venlafaxine, and nefazodone) may be increased by lapatinib. Selected benzodiazepines (midazolam, triazolam), and pimozide are generally contraindicated with strong CYP3A4 inhibitors.
Restrictions Lapatinib is available **only** at specialty pharmacies through a restricted-access program, Tykerb® CARES. Information is available at www.tykerbcares.com or 1-866-489-5372.
Dosage Summary
Oral:
Children: Dosage not established
Adults: 1250 mg once daily

Dosage Forms Excipient information presented when available (limited, particularly for generics); consult specific product labeling.
Tablet:
Tykerb®: 250 mg

◆ **Lapatinib Ditosylate** *see* Lapatinib *on page 898*
◆ **Lariam®** *see* Mefloquine *on page 976*
◆ **Lasix®** *see* Furosemide *on page 699*
◆ **L-asparaginase** *see* Asparaginase *on page 142*
◆ ***l*-Bunolol Hydrochloride** *see* Levobunolol *on page 907*
◆ **LCM** *see* Lacosamide *on page 885*
◆ **L-Deoxythymidine** *see* Telbivudine *on page 1541*
◆ **L-Deprenyl** *see* Selegiline *on page 1466*
◆ **LDP-341** *see* Bortezomib *on page 192*
◆ **Leena™** *see* Ethinyl Estradiol and Norethindrone *on page 597*

Leflunomide (le FLOO noh mide)

U.S. Brand Names Arava®
Canadian Brand Names Apo-Leflunomide®; Arava®; Novo-Leflunomide
Mexican Brand Names Arava
Pharmacologic Category Antirheumatic, Disease Modifying
Use Treatment of active rheumatoid arthritis; indicated to reduce signs and symptoms, and to retard structural damage and improve physical function
Orphan drug: Prevention of acute and chronic rejection in recipients of solid organ transplants
Unlabeled/Investigational Use Treatment of cytomegalovirus (CMV) disease
Effect on Mental Status May cause dizziness, malaise, anxiety, depression, or insomnia
Effect on Psychiatric Treatment May rarely cause leukopenia, caution with clozapine and carbamazepine
Dosage Summary
Oral:
Children: Dosage not established
Adults: Initial: 100 mg/day for 3 days followed by 20 mg/day (may decrease to 10 mg/day if necessary). Maintenance range: 10-20 mg/day
Note: Dosing has been described for off-label uses which differs from approved dosing.
Dosage Forms Excipient information presented when available (limited, particularly for generics); consult specific product labeling.
Tablet (Arava®): 10 mg, 20 mg

◆ **Legatrin PM® [OTC]** *see* Acetaminophen and Diphenhydramine *on page 35*

Lenalidomide (le na LID oh mide)

Medication Safety Issues
High alert medication: The Institute for Safe Medication Practices (ISMP) includes this medication among its list of drug classes which have a heightened risk of causing significant patient harm when used in error.
U.S. Brand Names Revlimid®
Canadian Brand Names Revlimid®
Index Terms CC-5013; IMid-3; NSC-703813
Pharmacologic Category Angiogenesis Inhibitor; Antineoplastic Agent; Immunomodulator, Systemic
Use Treatment of myelodysplastic syndrome (MDS) in patients with deletion 5q (del 5q) cytogenetic abnormality; treatment of multiple myeloma
Unlabeled/Investigational Use Treatment of metastatic malignant melanoma; treatment of myelofibrosis
Effect on Mental Status Dizziness and fatigue are common; may cause insomnia or depression (check thyroid function tests)
Effect on Psychiatric Treatment Hematologic side effects are common; concomitant use with clozapine and carbamazepine are best avoided. GI side effects are common; concomitant use with SSRIs, lithium, valproic acid, and carbamazepine may produce additive effects. May cause hypothyroidism; concomitant use with lithium may produce additive effects.
Restrictions Lenalidomide is approved for marketing in the U.S. only under a Food and Drug Administration (FDA) approved, restricted distribution program

called RevAssist[SM] (www.REVLIMID.com or 1-888-423-5436). In Canada, distribution is restricted through RevAid[SM] (www.RevAid.ca or 1-888-738-2431). Physicians, pharmacies, and patients must be registered; a maximum 28-day supply may be dispensed; a new prescription is required each time it is filled; pregnancy testing is required for females of childbearing potential.

An FDA-approved medication guide must be distributed when dispensing an outpatient prescription (new or refill) where this medication is to be used without direct supervision of a healthcare provider. Medication guides are available at http://www.fda.gov/cder/Offices/ODS/medication_guides.htm.

Dosage Summary

Oral:

Children: Dosage not established

Adults: 10 once daily **or** 25 mg once daily for 21 of 28 days

Dosage Forms Excipient information presented when available (limited, particularly for generics); consult specific product labeling.

Capsule:

Revlimid®: 5 mg, 10 mg, 15 mg, 25 mg

Lepirudin (leh puh ROO din)

Medication Safety Issues

High alert medication: The Institute for Safe Medication Practices (ISMP) includes this medication among its list of drugs which have a heightened risk of causing significant patient harm when used in error.

U.S. Brand Names Refludan®

Canadian Brand Names Refludan®

Index Terms Lepirudin (rDNA); Recombinant Hirudin

Pharmacologic Category Anticoagulant, Thrombin Inhibitor

Use Indicated for anticoagulation in patients with heparin-induced thrombocytopenia (HIT) and associated thromboembolic disease in order to prevent further thromboembolic complications

Unlabeled/Investigational Use Investigational: Prevention or reduction of ischemic complications associated with unstable angina

Effect on Mental Status None reported

Effect on Psychiatric Treatment Contraindicated in patients with a recent stroke

Dosage Summary Note: Dosing is weight-based, however, patients weighing >110 kg should not receive doses greater than the recommended dose for a patient weighing 110 kg (44 mg bolus and initial maximal infusion rate of 16.5 mg/hour).

I.V.:

Children: Dosage not established

Adults: Bolus: 0.2-0.4 mg/kg; Infusion: 0.1-0.15 mg/kg/hour (maximum: 0.21 mg/kg/hour); **Note:** Initial bolus dose may be omitted unless acute HITTS

Dosage Forms Excipient information presented when available (limited, particularly for generics); consult specific product labeling.

Injection, powder for reconstitution: 50 mg

◆ **Lepirudin (rDNA)** *see* Lepirudin *on page 900*

◆ **Lescol®** *see* Fluvastatin *on page 676*

◆ **Lescol® XL** *see* Fluvastatin *on page 676*

◆ **Lessina™** *see* Ethinyl Estradiol and Levonorgestrel *on page 595*

Letrozole (LET roe zole)

Medication Safety Issues

Sound-alike/look-alike issues:

Femara® may be confused with Famvir®, femhrt®, Provera®

Letrozole may be confused with anastrozole

U.S. Brand Names Femara®

Canadian Brand Names Femara®

Mexican Brand Names Femara

Index Terms CGS-20267; NSC-719345

Pharmacologic Category Antineoplastic Agent, Aromatase Inhibitor

Use For use in postmenopausal women in the adjuvant treatment of hormone receptor positive early breast cancer, extended adjuvant treatment of early breast cancer after 5 years of tamoxifen, advanced breast cancer with disease progression following antiestrogen therapy, hormone receptor positive or hormone receptor unknown, locally-advanced, or metastatic breast cancer

Unlabeled/Investigational Use Treatment of ovarian (epithelial) cancer, endometrial cancer

Effect on Mental Status May cause drowsiness or dizziness

Effect on Psychiatric Treatment None reported

Dosage Summary

Oral:

Children: Dosage not established

Adults (females): 2.5 mg once daily

Dosage Forms Excipient information presented when available (limited, particularly for generics); consult specific product labeling.

Tablet:

Femara®: 2.5 mg

◆ **Leukeran®** *see* Chlorambucil *on page 315*

◆ **Leukine®** *see* Sargramostim *on page 1462*

Leuprolide (loo PROE lide)

Medication Safety Issues

Sound-alike/look-alike issues:

Lupron® may be confused with Nuprin®

Lupron Depot®-3 Month may be confused with Lupron Depot-Ped®

U.S. Brand Names Eligard®; Lupron Depot-Ped®; Lupron Depot®; Lupron®; Viadur® [DSC]

Canadian Brand Names Eligard®; Lupron®; Lupron® Depot®; Viadur®

Mexican Brand Names Lorelin; Lucrin Depot; Prelar Depot

Index Terms Abbott-43818; Leuprolide Acetate; Leuprorelin Acetate; TAP-144

Pharmacologic Category Antineoplastic Agent, Gonadotropin-Releasing Hormone Agonist; Gonadotropin Releasing Hormone Agonist

Use Palliative treatment of advanced prostate cancer; management of endometriosis; treatment of anemia caused by uterine leiomyomata (fibroids); central precocious puberty

Unlabeled/Investigational Use Treatment of breast, ovarian, and endometrial cancer; infertility; prostatic hyperplasia

Effect on Mental Status Depression is common; may cause drowsiness, dizziness, or insomnia

Effect on Psychiatric Treatment None reported

Dosage Summary

I.M.:

Children ≤25 kg: Lupron® Depot-Ped®: 0.3 mg/kg/dose **or** 7.5 mg every 28 days (minimum dose: 7.5 mg)

Children >25-37.5 kg: Lupron® Depot-Ped®: 0.3 mg/kg/dose **or** 11.25 mg every 28 days (minimum dose: 7.5 mg)

Children >37.5 kg: Lupron® Depot-Ped®: 0.3 mg/kg/dose **or** 15 mg every 28 days (minimum dose: 7.5 mg)

Adults:

Lupron Depot®: 3.75 **or** 7.5 mg/dose once monthly

Lupron Depot®-3: 11.25 mg **or** 22.5 mg once every 3 months **or** 11.25 as a single dose

Lupron Depot®-4: 30 mg every 4 months

SubQ:

Children: Lupron®: Initial: 50 mcg/kg/day; titrate dose upward by 10 mcg/kg/day if down-regulation is not achieved

Adults:

Eligard®: 7.5 mg monthly **or** 22.5 mg every 3 months **or** 30 mg every 4 months **or** 45 mg every 6 months

Lupron®: 1 mg/day

Viadur®: 65 mg implanted every 12 months

Dosage Forms Excipient information presented when available (limited, particularly for generics); consult specific product labeling. [DSC] = Discontinued product

Implant, subcutaneous:

Viadur®: 65 mg [released over 12 months; packaged with administration kit] [DSC]

Injection, solution, as acetate: 5 mg/mL (2.8 mL)

Lupron®: 5 mg/mL (2.8 mL) [contains benzyl alcohol; packaged with syringes and alcohol swabs]

Injection, powder for reconstitution, as acetate [depot formulation]:
Eligard®:
7.5 mg [released over 1 month; contains polylactide-co-glycolide]
22.5 mg [released over 3 months; contains polylactide-co-glycolide]
30 mg [released over 4 months; contains polylactide-co-glycolide]
45 mg [released over 6 months; contains polylactide-co-glycolide]
Lupron Depot®: 3.75 mg, 7.5 mg [released over 1 month; contains polysorbate 80, polylactide-co-glycolide]
Lupron Depot®-3 Month: 11.25 mg, 22.5 mg [released over 3 months; contains polysorbate 80, polylactide-co-glycolide]
Lupron Depot®-4 Month: 30 mg [released over 4 months; contains polysorbate 80, polylactide-co-glycolide]
Lupron Depot-Ped®: 7.5 mg, 11.25 mg, 15 mg [released over 1 month; contains polysorbate 80, polylactide-co-glycolide]

◆ **Leuprolide Acetate** *see* Leuprolide *on page 901*
◆ **Leuprorelin Acetate** *see* Leuprolide *on page 901*
◆ **Leurocristine Sulfate** *see* VinCRIStine *on page 1673*
◆ **Leustatin®** *see* Cladribine *on page 360*

Levalbuterol (leve al BYOO ter ole)

Medication Safety Issues
Sound-alike/look-alike issues:
Xopenex® may be confused with Xanax®

U.S. Brand Names Xopenex HFA™; Xopenex®

Canadian Brand Names Xopenex®

Index Terms Levalbuterol Hydrochloride; Levalbuterol Tartrate; R-albuterol

Pharmacologic Category Beta$_2$-Adrenergic Agonist

Generic Available No

Use Treatment or prevention of bronchospasm in children and adults with reversible obstructive airway disease

Effect on Mental Status May cause nervousness, anxiety, and dizziness; may rarely cause insomnia

Effect on Psychiatric Treatment Effects of anxiolytics may be ameliorated; cardiac effects may be potentiated with MAO inhibitors and TCAs

Pregnancy Risk Factor C

Pregnancy Considerations Teratogenic effects were not observed in animal studies; however, racemic albuterol was teratogenic in some species. There are no adequate and well-controlled studies in pregnant women. This drug should be used during pregnancy only if benefit exceeds risk. Use caution if needed for bronchospasm during labor and delivery; has potential to interfere with uterine contractions.

Lactation Excretion in breast milk unknown/use caution

Contraindications Hypersensitivity to levalbuterol, albuterol, or any component of the formulation

Warnings/Precautions Optimize anti-inflammatory treatment before initiating maintenance treatment with levalbuterol. Do not use as a component of chronic therapy without an anti-inflammatory agent. Only the mildest form of asthma (Step 1 and/or exercise-induced) would not require concurrent use based upon asthma guidelines. Patient must be instructed to seek medical attention in cases where acute symptoms are not relieved or a previous level of response is diminished. The need to increase frequency of use may indicate deterioration of asthma, and treatment must not be delayed. A spacer device or valved holding chamber is recommended when using a metered-dose inhaler.

Use caution in patients with cardiovascular disease (arrhythmia or hypertension or HF), convulsive disorders, diabetes, glaucoma, hyperthyroidism, or hypokalemia. Beta-agonists may cause elevation in blood pressure, heart rate, and result in CNS stimulation/excitation. Beta$_2$-agonists may increase risk of arrhythmia, increase serum glucose, or decrease serum potassium.

Immediate hypersensitivity reactions (urticaria, angioedema, rash, bronchospasm) have been reported. Do not exceed recommended dose; serious adverse events including fatalities, have been associated with excessive use of inhaled sympathomimetics. Rarely, paradoxical bronchospasm may occur with use of inhaled bronchodilating agents; this should be distinguished from inadequate response. Use with caution during labor and delivery. Safety and efficacy have not been established in patients <4 years of age.

Adverse Reactions

>10%:

Endocrine & metabolic: Serum glucose increased, serum potassium decreased

Neuromuscular & skeletal: Tremor (≤7%)

Respiratory: Rhinitis (3% to 11%)

Miscellaneous: Viral infection (7% to 12%)

>2% to 10%:

Central nervous system: Headache (8% to 12%), nervousness (3% to 10%), dizziness (1% to 3%), anxiety (≤3%), migraine (≤3%), weakness (3%)

Cardiovascular: Tachycardia (~3%)

Dermatologic: Rash (≤8%)

Gastrointestinal: Diarrhea (2% to 6%), dyspepsia (1% to 3%)

Neuromuscular & skeletal: Leg cramps (≤3%)

Respiratory: Asthma (9%), pharyngitis (3% to 10%), cough (1% to 4%), sinusitis (1% to 4%), nasal edema (1% to 3%)

Miscellaneous: Flu-like syndrome (1% to 4%), accidental injury (≤3%)

<2% (Limited to important or life-threatening): Abnormal ECG, acne, anaphylaxis, angina, angioedema, arrhythmia, atrial fibrillation, chest pain, chills, constipation, conjunctivitis, cough, diaphoresis, dysmenorrhea, dyspnea, epistaxis, extrasystole, gastroenteritis, hematuria, hyper-/hypotension, hypoesthesia (hand), hypokalemia, insomnia, itching eyes, lymphadenopathy, myalgia, nausea, oropharyngeal dryness, paresthesia, supraventricular arrhythmia, syncope, vaginal moniliasis, vertigo, vomiting, wheezing, xerostomia

Note: Immediate hypersensitivity reactions have occurred (including angioedema, oropharyngeal edema, urticaria, and anaphylaxis).

Drug Interactions

Alpha-/Beta-Blockers: May diminish the therapeutic effect of Beta2-Agonists. *Risk D: Consider therapy modification*

Atomoxetine: May enhance the tachycardic effect of Beta2-Agonists. *Risk C: Monitor therapy*

Beta-Blockers (Beta1 Selective): May diminish the bronchodilatory effect of Beta2-Agonists. Of particular concern with nonselective beta-blockers or higher doses of the beta1 selective beta-blockers. *Risk C: Monitor therapy*

Beta-Blockers (Nonselective): May diminish the bronchodilatory effect of Beta2-Agonists. *Risk D: Consider therapy modification*

Betahistine: May diminish the therapeutic effect of Beta2-Agonists. *Risk C: Monitor therapy*

Cannabinoids: May enhance the tachycardic effect of Sympathomimetics. *Risk C: Monitor therapy*

MAO Inhibitors: May enhance the adverse/toxic effect of Beta2-Agonists. *Risk C: Monitor therapy*

Sympathomimetics: May enhance the adverse/toxic effect of other Sympathomimetics. *Risk C: Monitor therapy*

Tricyclic Antidepressants: May enhance the adverse/toxic effect of Beta2-Agonists. *Risk C: Monitor therapy*

Stability

Aerosol: Store at room temperature of 20°C to 25°C (68°F to 77°F); protect from freezing and direct sunlight. Store with mouthpiece down. Discard after 200 actuations.

Solution for nebulization: Store in protective foil pouch at room temperature of 20°C to 25°C (68°F to 77°F). Protect from light and excessive heat. Vials should be used within 2 weeks after opening protective pouch. Use within 1 week and protect from light if removed from pouch. Vials of concentrated solution should be used immediately after removing from protective pouch. Concentrated solution should be diluted with 2.5 mL NS prior to use.

Mechanism of Action Relaxes bronchial smooth muscle by action on beta$_2$-receptors with little effect on heart rate

Pharmacodynamics/Kinetics

Onset of action (as measured by a 15% increase in FEV$_1$):

Aerosol: 5.5-10.2 minutes

Peak effect: ~77 minutes

Nebulization: 10-17 minutes

Peak effect: 1.5 hours

Duration (as measured by a 15% increase in FEV$_1$):

Aerosol: 3-4 hours (up to 6 hours in some patients)

Nebulization: 5-6 hours (up to 8 hours in some patients)

Absorption: A portion of inhaled dose is absorbed to systemic circulation

Half-life elimination: 3.3-4 hours

Time to peak, serum:

Aerosol: Children: 0.8 hours, Adults: 0.5 hours

Nebulization: Children: 0.3-0.6 hours, Adults: 0.2 hours

Dosage

Metered-dose inhaler (45 mcg/puff):
  Children 5-11 years:
    Bronchospasm, quick relief: 1-2 puffs every 4-6 hours as needed
    Exacerbation of asthma (acute, severe) *(NIH Guidelines, 2007)*: 4-8 puffs every 20 minutes for 3 doses, then every 1-4 hours as needed
  Children ≥12 years and Adults:
    Bronchospasm, quick relief: 1-2 puffs every 4-6 hours
    Exacerbation of asthma (acute, severe) *(NIH Guidelines, 2007)*: 4-8 puffs every 20 minutes for up to 4 hours, then every 1-4 hours as needed
Solution for nebulization:
  Children: ≤4 years:
    Bronchospasm, quick relief *(NIH Guidelines, 2007)*: 0.31-1.25 mg every 4-6 hours as needed
    Exacerbation of asthma (acute, severe) *(NIH Guidelines, 2007)*: 0.075 mg/kg (minimum: 1.25 mg) every 20 minutes for 3 doses, then 0.075-0.15 mg/kg (maximum: 5 mg) every 1-4 hours as needed
  Children 5-11 years:
    Bronchospasm, quick relief: 0.31-0.63 mg every 8 hours as needed
    Exacerbation of asthma (acute severe) *(NIH Guidelines, 2007)*: 0.075 mg/kg (minimum: 1.25 mg) every 20 minutes for 3 doses, then 0.075-0.15 mg/kg (maximum: 5 mg) every 1-4 hours as needed
  Children ≥12 years and Adults:
    Bronchospasm, quick relief: 0.63-1.25 mg every 8 hours as needed
    Exacerbation of asthma (acute, severe) *(NIH Guidelines, 2007)*: 1.25-2.5 mg every 20 minutes for 3 doses, then 1.25-5 mg every 1-4 hours as needed
Elderly: Only a small number of patients have been studied. Although greater sensitivity of some elderly patients cannot be ruled out, no overall differences in safety or effectiveness were observed. An initial dose of 0.63 mg should be used in all patients >65 years of age.

Administration Inhalation:

Metered-dose inhaler: Shake well before use; prime with 4 test sprays prior to first use or if inhaler has not been use of more than 3 days. Clean actuator (mouthpiece) weekly. A spacer device or valved holding chamber is recommended when using a metered-dose inhaler.

Solution for nebulization: Safety and efficacy were established when administered with the following nebulizers: PARI LC Jet™, PARI LC Plus™, as well as the following compressors: PARI Master®, Dura-Neb® 2000, and Dura-Neb® 3000. Concentrated solution should be diluted prior to use. Blow-by administration is not recommended, use a mask device if patient unable to hold mouthpiece in mouth for administration.

Monitoring Parameters Asthma symptoms; FEV_1, peak flow, and/or other pulmonary function tests; heart rate, blood pressure, CNS stimulation; arterial blood gases (if condition warrants); serum potassium, serum glucose (in selected patients)

Dosage Forms Excipient information presented when available (limited, particularly for generics); consult specific product labeling.

Note: Strength expressed as base.

Aerosol, for oral inhalation, as tartrate:
  Xopenex HFA™: 45 mcg/actuation (15 g) [200 actuations; chlorofluorocarbon free]
Solution for nebulization, as hydrochloride [preservative free]:
  Xopenex®: 0.31 mg/3 mL (24s); 0.63 mg/3 mL (24s); 1.25 mg/3 mL (24s)
Solution for nebulization, as hydrochloride [concentrate; preservative free]:
  Xopenex®: 1.25 mg/0.5 mL (30s)

◆ **Levalbuterol Hydrochloride** *see* Levalbuterol *on page 902*

◆ **Levalbuterol Tartrate** *see* Levalbuterol *on page 902*

◆ **Levall™** *see* Carbetapentane, Guaifenesin, and Phenylephrine *on page 274*

◆ **Levall 5.0 [DSC]** *see* Hydrocodone, Phenylephrine, and Guaifenesin *on page 783*

◆ **Levall G** *see* Guaifenesin and Pseudoephedrine *on page 744*

◆ **Levaquin®** *see* Levofloxacin *on page 913*

◆ **Levarterenol Bitartrate** *see* Norepinephrine *on page 1150*

◆ **Levatol®** *see* Penbutolol *on page 1238*

◆ **Levbid®** *see* Hyoscyamine *on page 799*

◆ **Levemir®** *see* Insulin Detemir *on page 825*

Levetiracetam (lee va tye RA se tam)

Medication Safety Issues

Sound-alike/look-alike issues:

Keppra® may be confused with Keppra XR™

Levetiracetam may be confused with levofloxacin

Potential for dispensing errors between Keppra® and Kaletra® (lopinavir/ritonavir)

Related Information

Anticonvulsants By Seizure Type *on page 1759*

U.S. Brand Names Keppra XR™; Keppra®

Canadian Brand Names Apo-Levetiracetam; CO Levetiracetam; DOM-Levetiracetam; Keppra®; PHL-Levetiracetam; PMS-Levetiracetam

Mexican Brand Names Keppra

Pharmacologic Category Anticonvulsant, Miscellaneous

Generic Available Yes: Tablet

Use Adjunctive therapy in the treatment of partial onset, myoclonic, and/or primary generalized tonic-clonic seizures

Unlabeled/Investigational Use Bipolar disorder

Effect on Mental Status Associated with somnolence and fatigue, psychosis, hallucinations, psychotic depression, and other behavioral symptoms (agitation, anger, aggression, irritability, hostility, anxiety, apathy, emotional lability, depersonalization, and depression)

Effect on Psychiatric Treatment May cause leukopenia, neutropenia, pancytopenia, and thrombocytopenia; use caution with clozapine, carbamazepine, and valproic acid

Pregnancy Risk Factor C

Pregnancy Considerations Developmental toxicities were observed in animal studies. There are no adequate and well-controlled studies in pregnant women. Two registries are available for women exposed to levetiracetam during pregnancy:

Antiepileptic Drug Pregnancy Registry (888-233-2334 or http://www.mgh.harvard.edu/aed/)

Keppra® pregnancy registry (888-537-7734 or http://www.keppra.com)

Lactation Enters breast milk/not recommended

Contraindications Hypersensitivity to levetiracetam or any component of the formulation

Warnings/Precautions Psychotic symptoms (psychosis, hallucinations) and behavioral symptoms (including aggression, anger, anxiety, depersonalization, depression, personality disorder) may occur; incidence may be increased in children. Dose reduction may be required. Levetiracetam should be withdrawn gradually to minimize the potential of increased seizure frequency. Use caution with renal impairment; dosage adjustment may be necessary. Weakness, dizziness, and somnolence occur mostly during the first month of therapy. Although rare, decreases in red blood cell counts, hemoglobin, hematocrit, white blood cell counts and neutrophils have been observed. Safety and efficacy in children <4 years of age (oral formulation) or <16 years (I.V. formulation and extended release tablets) have not been established.

Adverse Reactions

>10%:

Central nervous system: Behavioral symptoms (agitation, aggression, anger, anxiety, apathy, depersonalization, depression, emotional lability, hostility, hyperkinesias, irritability, nervousness, neurosis and personality disorder: adults 5% to 13%; children 5% to 38%), somnolence (8% to 23%), headache (14%), hostility (2% to 12%)

Gastrointestinal: Vomiting (15%), anorexia (3% to 13%)

Neuromuscular & skeletal: Weakness (9% to 15%)

Respiratory: Pharyngitis (6% to 14%), rhinitis (4% to 13%), cough (2% to 11%)

Miscellaneous: Accidental injury (17%), infection (2% to 13%)

1% to 10%:

Cardiovascular: Facial edema (2%)

Central nervous system: Fatigue (10%), nervousness (4% to 10%), dizziness (5% to 9%), personality disorder (8%), pain (6% to 7%), agitation (6%), irritability (6% to 7%), emotional lability (2% to 6%), mood swings (5%), depression (3% to 5%), vertigo (3% to 5%), ataxia (3%), amnesia (2%), anxiety (2%), confusion (2%)

Dermatologic: Bruising (4%), pruritus (2%), rash (2%), skin discoloration (2%)

Endocrine & metabolic: Dehydration (2%)

Gastrointestinal: Diarrhea (8%), nausea (5%), gastroenteritis (4%), constipation (3%)

Genitourinary: Urine abnormality (2%)

Hematologic: Leukocytes decreased (2% to 3%)

Neuromuscular & skeletal: Neck pain (2% to 8%), paresthesia (2%), reflexes increased (2%)

Ocular: Conjunctivitis (3%), diplopia (2%), amblyopia (2%)

Otic: Ear pain (2%)

Renal: Albuminuria (4%)

Respiratory: Influenza (5%), asthma (2%), sinusitis (2%)

Miscellaneous: Flu-like syndrome (3% to 8%), viral infection (2%)

<1% (Limited to important or life-threatening): Alopecia, anemia, catatonia, hematocrit decreased, hemoglobin decreased, hepatic failure, hepatitis, leukopenia, LFTs abnormal, neutropenia, pancreatitis, pancytopenia (with bone marrow suppression), psychotic symptoms, red blood cells decreased, suicide attempt, suicide behavior, suicide ideation, thrombocytopenia, weight loss

Drug Interactions

Alcohol (Ethyl): CNS Depressants may enhance the CNS depressant effect of Alcohol (Ethyl). *Risk C: Monitor therapy*

CNS Depressants: May enhance the adverse/toxic effect of other CNS Depressants. *Risk C: Monitor therapy*

Ketorolac: May diminish the therapeutic effect of Anticonvulsants. *Risk C: Monitor therapy*

Mefloquine: May diminish the therapeutic effect of Anticonvulsants. Mefloquine may decrease the serum concentration of Anticonvulsants. Management: Mefloquine is contraindicated in persons with a history of convulsions. If anticonvulsant is being used for another indication monitor response to treatment closely, as concurrent mefloquine may decrease response to treatment. *Risk D: Consider therapy modification*

Ethanol/Nutrition/Herb Interactions

Ethanol: Avoid ethanol (may increase CNS depression).

Food: Food may delay, but does not affect the extent of absorption.

Stability

Oral solution, tablets: Store at 25°C (77°F); excursions permitted to 15°C to 30°C (59°F to 86°F).

Injection solution: Store at 25°C (77°F); excursions permitted to 15°C to 30°C (59°F to 86°F). Must dilute dose in 100 mL of NS, LR, or D_5W. Admixed solution is stable for 24 hours in PVC bags kept at room temperature.

Mechanism of Action The precise mechanism by which levetiracetam exerts its antiepileptic effect is unknown. However, several studies have suggested the mechanism may involve one or more of the following central pharmacologic effects: inhibition of voltage-dependent N-type calcium channels; facilitation of GABA-ergic inhibitory transmission through displacement of negative modulators; reduction of delayed rectifier potassium current; and/or binding to synaptic proteins which modulate neurotransmitter release.

Pharmacodynamics/Kinetics

Absorption: Oral: Rapid and almost complete

Distribution: V_d: Similar to total body water

Protein binding: <10%

Metabolism: Not extensive; primarily by enzymatic hydrolysis; forms metabolites (inactive)

Bioavailability: 100%

Half-life elimination: ~6-8 hours; extended release tablet: ~7 hours; half-life increased in renal dysfunction

Time to peak, plasma: Oral: Immediate release: ~1 hour; Extended release: ~4 hours

Excretion: Urine (66% as unchanged drug)

Dosage

Oral:

Children 4-15 years: Partial onset seizures: Immediate release: 10 mg/kg/dose given twice daily; may increase every 2 weeks by 10 mg/kg/dose to a maximum of 30 mg/kg/dose twice daily

Children 6-15 years: Tonic-clonic seizures: Immediate release: Initial: 10 mg/kg dose given twice daily; may increase every 2 weeks by 10 mg/kg/dose to the recommended dose of 30 mg/kg twice daily. Efficacy of doses >60 mg/kg/day has not been established.

Children ≥12 years and Adults: Myoclonic seizures: Immediate release: Initial: 500 mg twice daily; may increase every 2 weeks by 500 mg/dose to the recommended dose of 1500 mg twice daily. Efficacy of doses >3000 mg/day has not been established.

Children ≥16 years and Adults:
Partial onset seizure:
Immediate release: Initial: 500 mg twice daily; may increase every 2 weeks by 500 mg/dose to a maximum of 1500 mg twice daily. Doses >3000 mg/day have been used in trials; however, there is no evidence of increased benefit.
Extended release: Initial: 1000 mg once daily; may increase every 2 weeks by 1000 mg/day to a maximum of 3000 mg once daily.
Tonic-clonic seizures: Immediate release: Initial: 500 mg twice daily; may increase every 2 weeks by 500 mg/dose to the recommended dose of 1500 mg twice daily. Efficacy of doses >3000 mg/day has not been established.
Bipolar disorder (unlabeled use): Immediate release: Initial: 500 mg twice daily; if tolerated, increase by 500 mg twice daily; dose may be increased every 3 days until target dose of 3000 mg/day is reached; maximum: 4000 mg/day
Adults: Loading dose (unlabeled): Immediate release: Initial doses of 1500-2000 mg have been well-tolerated (Koubeissi, 2008; Betts, 2000), although the necessity of a loading dose has not been established
I.V.: Children ≥16 years and Adults: Partial onset seizure: Initial: 500 mg twice daily; may increase every 2 weeks by 500 mg/dose to a maximum of 1500 mg twice daily. Doses >3000 mg/day have been used in trials; however, there is no evidence of increased benefit.
Note: When switching from oral to I.V. formulations, the total daily dose should be the same.

Dosing adjustment in renal impairment: Adults:
Immediate release and I.V. formulations:
Cl_{cr} >80 mL/minute: 500-1500 mg every 12 hours
Cl_{cr} 50-80 mL/minute: 500-1000 mg every 12 hours
Cl_{cr} 30-50 mL/minute: 250-750 mg every 12 hours
Cl_{cr} <30 mL/minute: 250-500 mg every 12 hours
End-stage renal disease patients using dialysis: 500-1000 mg every 24 hours; a supplemental dose of 250-500 mg following dialysis is recommended

Extended release tablets:
Cl_{cr} >80 mL/minute: 1000-3000 mg every 24 hours
Cl_{cr} 50-80 mL/minute: 1000-2000 mg every 24 hours
Cl_{cr} 30-50 mL/minute: 500-1500 mg every 24 hours
Cl_{cr} <30 mL/minute: 500-1000 mg every 24 hours

Dosing adjustment in hepatic impairment: No adjustment required
Dietary Considerations May be taken with or without food.
Administration
I.V.: Infuse over 15 minutes
Oral: May be taken with or without food.
Oral solution: Should be administered with a calibrated measuring device (not a household teaspoon or tablespoon)
Tablet (immediate release and extended release): Only administer as whole tablet; do not crush, break or chew.
Dosage Forms Excipient information presented when available (limited, particularly for generics); consult specific product labeling.
Injection, solution:
Keppra®: 100 mg/mL (5 mL)
Solution, oral:
Keppra®: 100 mg/mL (480 mL) [dye free; grape flavor]
Tablet: 250 mg, 500 mg, 750 mg
Keppra®: 250 mg, 500 mg, 750 mg, 1000 mg
Tablet, extended release:
Keppra XR™: 500 mg

◆ **Levitra®** *see* Vardenafil *on page 1654*
◆ **Levlen®** *see* Ethinyl Estradiol and Levonorgestrel *on page 595*
◆ **Levlite™** *see* Ethinyl Estradiol and Levonorgestrel *on page 595*

Levobunolol (lee voe BYOO noe lole)

Medication Safety Issues
Sound-alike/look-alike issues:
Levobunolol may be confused with levocabastine
Betagan® may be confused with Betadine®, Betoptic® S

International issues:

Betagan® may be confused with Betagon® which is a brand name for mepindolol in Italy

U.S. Brand Names Betagan®

Canadian Brand Names Apo-Levobunolol®; Betagan®; Novo-Levobunolol; Optho-Bunolol®; PMS-Levobunolol; Sandoz-Levobunolol

Mexican Brand Names Betagan

Index Terms *l*-Bunolol Hydrochloride; Levobunolol Hydrochloride

Pharmacologic Category Beta-Adrenergic Blocker, Nonselective; Ophthalmic Agent, Antiglaucoma

Use To lower intraocular pressure in chronic open-angle glaucoma or ocular hypertension

Effect on Mental Status May cause dizziness

Effect on Psychiatric Treatment May increase the effects of oral beta-blockers

Dosage Summary

Ophthalmic:

Children: Dosage not established

Adults: Instill 1 drop in the affected eye(s) 1-2 times/day

Dosage Forms Excipient information presented when available (limited, particularly for generics); consult specific product labeling.

Solution, ophthalmic, as hydrochloride: 0.25% (5 mL, 10 mL); 0.5% (5 mL, 10 mL, 15 mL) [contains benzalkonium chloride and sodium metabisulfite]

Betagan®: 0.25% (5 mL, 10 mL); 0.5% (2 mL, 5 mL, 10 mL, 15 mL) [contains benzalkonium chloride and sodium metabisulfite]

◆ **Levobunolol Hydrochloride** *see* Levobunolol *on page 907*

Levobupivacaine (LEE voe byoo PIV a kane)

Medication Safety Issues

High alert medication: The Institute for Safe Medication Practices (ISMP) includes this medication (epidural administration) among its list of drug classes which have a heightened risk of causing significant patient harm when used in error.

U.S. Brand Names Chirocaine® [DSC]

Canadian Brand Names Chirocaine®

Mexican Brand Names Quirocaine

Pharmacologic Category Local Anesthetic

Use Production of local or regional anesthesia for surgery and obstetrics, and for postoperative pain management

Effect on Mental Status May cause anxiety, dizziness or somnolence; may rarely cause confusion

Effect on Psychiatric Treatment Fluvoxamine and nefazodone may increase the levels of levobupivacaine; carbamazepine and barbiturates may lower levels

Dosage Summary

Epidural:

Children: Dosage not established

Adults:

C-section: 100-150 mg of 0.5% solution

Labor analgesia: 25-50 mg of 0.25% solution

Postoperative pain: Infusion: 5-25 mg/hour of 0.125%-0.25% concentration

Surgery: 50-150 mg of 0.5%-0.75% solution

Infiltration (local):

Children: Dosage not established

Adults: 150 mg of 0.25% solution

Ophthalmic:

Children: Dosage not established

Adults: 37.5-112.5 mg of 0.75% solution

Peripheral nerve:

Children: Dosage not established

Adults: 1-2 mg/kg (75-150 mg) of 0.25%-0.5% solution

Dosage Forms Excipient information presented when available (limited, particularly for generics); consult specific product labeling. [DSC] = Discontinued product

Injection, solution [preservative free]: 2.5 mg/mL (10 mL, 30 mL); 5 mg/mL (10 mL, 30 mL); 7.5 mg/mL (10 mL, 30 mL) [DSC]

Levocabastine (LEE voe kab as teen)

Medication Safety Issues

Sound-alike/look-alike issues:

Levocabastine may be confused with levobunolol, levocarnitine
Livostin® may be confused with lovastatin

International issues:

Livostin® may be confused with Limoxin® which is a brand name for amoxicillin in Mexico

Livostin® may be confused with Lovastin® which is a brand name for lovastatin in Malaysia and Poland

U.S. Brand Names Livostin® [DSC]

Canadian Brand Names Livostin®

Mexican Brand Names Livostin

Index Terms Levocabastine Hydrochloride

Pharmacologic Category Histamine H_1 Antagonist; Histamine H_1 Antagonist, Second Generation

Use Treatment of allergic conjunctivitis

Effect on Mental Status May cause drowsiness

Effect on Psychiatric Treatment None reported

Dosage Summary

Ophthalmic:

Children <12 years: Dosage not established
Children ≥12 years: Instill 1 drop in affected eye(s) 4 times/day
Adults: Instill 1 drop in affected eye(s) 4 times/day

Dosage Forms Excipient information presented when available (limited, particularly for generics); consult specific product labeling. [DSC] = Discontinued product

Suspension, ophthalmic: 0.05% (5 mL, 10 mL) [contains benzalkonium chloride] [DSC]

◆ **Levocabastine Hydrochloride** *see* Levocabastine *on page 909*

Levocetirizine (LEE vo se TI ra zeen)

Medication Safety Issues

Sound-alike/look-alike issues:

Levocetirizine may be confused with cetirizine

U.S. Brand Names Xyzal®

Mexican Brand Names Xusal; Zyxem

Index Terms Levocetirizine Dihydrochloride

Pharmacologic Category Histamine H_1 Antagonist; Histamine H_1 Antagonist, Second Generation

Generic Available No

Use Relief of symptoms of perennial and seasonal allergic rhinitis; treatment of skin manifestations (uncomplicated) of chronic idiopathic urticaria

Effect on Mental Status May cause CNS depression; use with caution. Rare reports of aggression and agitation.

Effect on Psychiatric Treatment Acetylcholinesterase inhibitors may diminish the therapeutic effect of levocetirizine. Conversely, levocetirizine may diminish the therapeutic effect of centrally-acting acetylcholinesterase inhibitors. May cause anticholinergic and sedative adverse effects; concomitant use with psychotropics with anticholinergic or sedative activity may produce additive effects. Antihistamines may enhance the arrhythmogenic effect of phenothiazine antipsychotic agents.

Pregnancy Risk Factor B

Pregnancy Considerations Levocetirizine was not shown to be teratogenic in animal studies. There are no adequate and well-controlled studies in pregnant women. Use during pregnancy only if clearly needed.

Lactation Excretion in breast milk unknown/not recommended

Contraindications Hypersensitivity to levocetirizine, cetirizine, or any component of the formulation; end-stage renal disease; hemodialysis; children 6-11 years of age with renal impairment

Warnings/Precautions Use with caution in adults with mild-to-moderate renal impairment; dosage adjustments may be needed. Use is contraindicated in end-stage renal disease (Cl_{cr} <10 mL/minute), patients undergoing hemodialysis, and in children 6-11 years of age with renal impairment (levocetirizine is excreted primarily by the kidneys). Use with caution in the elderly. May cause drowsiness; use caution performing tasks which require alertness (eg, operating machinery or driving). Not FDA approved for use in children <6 years of age.

Adverse Reactions

1% to 10%:

Central nervous system: Somnolence (3% to 6%), fever (children 4%), fatigue (1% to 4%)

Gastrointestinal: Xerostomia (2% to 3%)

Neuromuscular & skeletal: Weakness (2%)

Respiratory: Nasopharyngitis (4% to 6%), cough (children 3%), epistaxis (children 2%), pharyngitis (1% to 2%)

<1% (Limited to important or life-threatening): Aggression, agitation, anaphylaxis, angioneurotic edema, bilirubin increased, dyspnea, fixed-drug eruption, hepatitis, hypersensitivity, myalgia, nausea, palpitation, pruritus, rash, seizure, syncope, transaminases increased, urticaria, visual disturbances, weight gain

The following potentially-severe adverse reactions have been reported with cetirizine and, therefore, may also occur with levocetirizine: Cholestasis, glomuleronephritis, hallucination, hypotension (severe), orofacial dyskinesia, suicidal ideation

Drug Interactions

Acetylcholinesterase Inhibitors (Central): Anticholinergics may diminish the therapeutic effect of Acetylcholinesterase Inhibitors (Central). Acetylcholinesterase Inhibitors (Central) may diminish the therapeutic effect of Anticholinergics. If the anticholinergic action is a side effect of the agent, the result may be beneficial. *Risk C: Monitor therapy*

Alcohol (Ethyl): CNS Depressants may enhance the CNS depressant effect of Alcohol (Ethyl). *Risk C: Monitor therapy*

Amphetamines: May diminish the sedative effect of Antihistamines. *Risk C: Monitor therapy*

Anticholinergics: May enhance the adverse/toxic effect of other Anticholinergics. **Exceptions:** Paliperidone. *Risk C: Monitor therapy*

Betahistine: Antihistamines may diminish the therapeutic effect of Betahistine. *Risk C: Monitor therapy*

CNS Depressants: May enhance the adverse/toxic effect of other CNS Depressants. *Risk C: Monitor therapy*

Pramlintide: May enhance the anticholinergic effect of Anticholinergics. These effects are specific to the GI tract. *Risk D: Consider therapy modification*

Ethanol/Nutrition/Herb Interactions Ethanol: Avoid ethanol (may increase CNS depression).

Stability Store at room temperature of 20°C to 25°C (68°F to 77°F); excursions permitted to 15°C to 30°C (59°F to 86°F).

Mechanism of Action Levocetirizine is an antihistamine which selectively competes with histamine for H_1-receptor sites on effector cells in the gastrointestinal tract, blood vessels, and respiratory tract. Levocetirizine, the active enantiomer of cetirizine, has twice the binding affinity at the H1-receptor compared to cetirizine.

Pharmacodynamics/Kinetics

Onset: 1 hour

Duration: 24 hours

Absorption: Rapid and extensive

Distribution: 0.4 L/kg

Protein binding: 91% to 92%

Metabolism: Minimal (<14%); via aromatic oxidation, N and O-dealkylation (via CYPA4), and taurine conjugation

Half-life elimination: Children: ~6 hours; Adults: ~8-9 hours; Renal impairment: 11-34 hours; End-stage renal disease: 46 hours

Time to peak, plasma: Children: 1.2 hours; Adults: Oral solution: 0.5 hours, Tablet: 0.9 hours

Excretion: Urine (85%); feces (13%)

Dosage Oral: Allergic rhinitis, chronic urticaria:

Children 6-11 years: 2.5 mg once daily (in the evening); maximum: 2.5 mg/day

Children ≥12 years and Adults: 5 mg once daily (in the evening); some patients may experience relief of symptoms with 2.5 mg once daily

Elderly: Refer to adult dosing; dosing should begin at the lower end of the dosing range

Dosage adjustments in renal impairment:

Children 6-11 years with renal impairment: Contraindicated

Children ≥12 and Adults:

Cl_{cr} 50-80 mL/minute: 2.5 mg once daily

Cl_{cr} 30-50 mL/minute: 2.5 mg once every other day

Cl_{cr} 10-30 mL/minute: 2.5 mg twice weekly (every 3 or 4 days)
Cl_{cr} <10 mL/minute, hemodialysis patients: Contraindicated

Dosage adjustments in hepatic impairment: No adjustment required.

Dietary Considerations May be taken with or without food.

Administration Administer in the evening. May be administered with or without food.

Monitoring Parameters Creatinine clearance (prior to treatment for dosing adjustment)

Dosage Forms Excipient information presented when available (limited, particularly for generics); consult specific product labeling.

Solution, oral, as dihydrochloride:
Xyzal®: 0.5 mg/mL (150 mL)

Tablet, as dihydrochloride [scored]:
Xyzal®: 5 mg

◆ **Levocetirizine Dihydrochloride** *see* Levocetirizine *on page 909*

◆ **Levodopa and Carbidopa** *see* Carbidopa and Levodopa *on page 277*

Levodopa, Carbidopa, and Entacapone

(lee voe DOE pa, kar bi DOE pa, & en TA ka pone)

Related Information

Antiparkinsonian Agents *on page 1767*

U.S. Brand Names Stalevo®

Index Terms Carbidopa, Levodopa, and Entacapone; Entacapone, Carbidopa, and Levodopa

Pharmacologic Category Anti-Parkinson's Agent, COMT Inhibitor; Anti-Parkinson's Agent, Dopamine Agonist

Generic Available No

Use Treatment of idiopathic Parkinson's disease

Pregnancy Risk Factor C

Pregnancy Considerations Teratogenic effects were observed with levodopa, carbidopa, and entacapone in animal studies. There are case reports of levodopa crossing the placenta in humans. There are no adequate and well-controlled studies in pregnant women. Use during pregnancy only if potential benefit exceeds risks.

Lactation Excretion in breast milk unknown/use caution

Contraindications Hypersensitivity to levodopa, carbidopa, entacapone, or any component of the formulation; use of nonselective MAO inhibitor therapy with or within prior 14 days; narrow-angle glaucoma; undiagnosed skin lesions or history of melanoma

Warnings/Precautions Use caution with severe cardiovascular disease, chronic wide-angle glaucoma, biliary obstruction, and severe renal or hepatic dysfunction. Use with caution when interpreting plasma/urine catecholamine levels; falsely diagnosed pheochromocytoma has been rarely reported. Severe cases or rhabdomyolysis have been reported. Use caution with history of peptic ulcer; risk of gastrointestinal hemorrhage may be increased. Use caution with history of psychoses; observe all patients closely for development of depression with concomitant suicidal tendencies. May cause hallucinations.

Dopamine agonists have been associated with compulsive behaviors and/or loss of impulse control, which has manifested as pathological gambling, libido increases (hypersexuality), and/or binge eating. Causality has not been established, and controversy exists as to whether this phenomenon is related to the underlying disease, prior behaviors/addictions and/or drug therapy. Dose reduction or discontinuation of therapy has been reported to reverse these behaviors in some, but not all cases.

Ergot-derived dopamine agonists have also been associated with fibrotic complications (eg, retroperitoneal fibrosis, pleural thickening, and pulmonary infiltrates); monitor closely for signs and symptoms of fibrosis. Use caution with agents metabolized by COMT (eg, epinephrine, dopamine, methyldopa) regardless of route of administration; effects may be enhanced when used with entacapone. Withdrawal or significant dosage reduction after long-term use may be associated with a neuroleptic malignant-like syndrome; avoid abrupt dose reductions or discontinuation. May cause or exacerbate dyskinesias. May cause syncope; incidence may be increased in patients with documented hypotension. Safety and efficacy have not been established in pediatric patients.

Adverse Reactions See individual agents.

Drug Interactions

Alcohol (Ethyl): CNS Depressants may enhance the CNS depressant effect of Alcohol (Ethyl). *Risk C: Monitor therapy*

Antipsychotics (Atypical): May diminish the therapeutic effect of Anti-Parkinson's Agents (Dopamine Agonist). *Risk D: Consider therapy modification*

Antipsychotics (Typical): May diminish the therapeutic effect of Anti-Parkinson's Agents (Dopamine Agonist). *Risk D: Consider therapy modification*

CNS Depressants: May enhance the adverse/toxic effect of other CNS Depressants. *Risk C: Monitor therapy*

COMT Substrates: COMT Inhibitors may decrease the metabolism of COMT Substrates. *Risk C: Monitor therapy*

Iron Salts: May decrease the absorption of Levodopa. Only applies to oral iron preparations. **Exceptions:** Ferric Gluconate; Iron Dextran Complex; Iron Sucrose. *Risk D: Consider therapy modification*

MAO Inhibitors: Levodopa may enhance the adverse/toxic effect of MAO Inhibitors. Of particular concern is the development of hypertensive reactions when levodopa is used with nonselective MAOI. *Risk D: Consider therapy modification*

MAO Inhibitors: COMT Inhibitors may enhance the adverse/toxic effect of MAO Inhibitors. *Risk D: Consider therapy modification*

Methionine: May diminish the therapeutic effect of Levodopa. Probably only with large doses of methionine. Data was generated using 4.5gm daily. *Risk D: Consider therapy modification*

Metoclopramide: May diminish the therapeutic effect of Anti-Parkinson's Agents (Dopamine Agonist). *Risk C: Monitor therapy*

Phenytoin: May diminish the therapeutic effect of Levodopa. *Risk C: Monitor therapy*

Pyridoxine: May diminish the therapeutic effect of Levodopa. *Risk D: Consider therapy modification*

Sapropterin: May enhance the adverse/toxic effect of Levodopa. *Risk C: Monitor therapy*

Ethanol/Nutrition/Herb Interactions Food: High-protein diets and increased stomach acid may delay absorption of levodopa. Iron may decrease bioavailability of levodopa. Entacapone has been reported to chelate iron and decreasing serum iron levels were noted in clinical trials; however, clinically significant anemia has not been observed.

Stability Store at controlled room temperature of 25°C (77°F).

Mechanism of Action

Levodopa: The metabolic precursor of dopamine, a chemical depleted in Parkinson's disease. Levodopa is able to circulate in the plasma and cross the blood-brain-barrier (BBB), where it is converted by striatal enzymes to dopamine.

Carbidopa: Inhibits the peripheral plasma breakdown of levodopa by inhibiting its decarboxylation; increases available levodopa at the BBB

Entacapone: A reversible and selective inhibitor of catechol-O-methyltransferase (COMT). Alters the pharmacokinetics of levodopa, resulting in more sustained levodopa serum levels and increased concentrations available for absorption across the BBB.

Pharmacodynamics/Kinetics See individual agents.

Dosage Oral: Adults: Parkinson's disease:

Note: All strengths of Stalevo® contain a carbidopa/levodopa ratio of 1:4 plus entacapone 200 mg.

Dose should be individualized based on therapeutic response; doses may be adjusted by changing strength or adjusting interval. Fractionated doses are not recommended and only 1 tablet should be given at each dosing interval; maximum daily dose: 8 tablets of Stalevo® 50, 75, 100, 125, or 150, **or** 6 tablets of Stalevo® 200.

Patients previously treated with carbidopa/levodopa immediate release tablets (ratio of 1:4):

With current entacapone therapy: May switch directly to corresponding strength of combination tablet. No data available on transferring patients from controlled release preparations or products with a 1:10 ratio of carbidopa/levodopa.

Without entacapone therapy:

If current levodopa dose is >600 mg/day: Levodopa dose reduction may be required when adding entacapone to therapy; therefore, titrate dose using individual products first (carbidopa/levodopa immediate release with a ratio of 1:4 plus entacapone 200 mg); then transfer to combination product once stabilized.

If current levodopa dose is <600 mg without dyskinesias: May transfer to corresponding dose of combination product; monitor, dose reduction of levodopa may be required.

Dosage adjustment in renal impairment: Use caution with severe renal impairment; specific dosing recommendations not available

Dosage adjustment in hepatic impairment: Use with caution; specific dosing recommendations not available

Dietary Considerations May take with or without food. Distribute protein intake throughout the day to avoid fluctuations in levodopa absorption. Separate dosing of iron supplements and multivitamins with minerals.

Administration Swallow tablet whole; do not crush, break, or chew. Only 1 tablet should be administered at each dosing interval.

Monitoring Parameters Signs and symptoms of Parkinson's disease; liver function tests, renal function; blood pressure, mental status; signs and symptoms of neuroleptic malignant syndrome if abrupt discontinuation required (as with surgery); serum iron (if signs of anemia); IOP (in patients with wide-angle glaucoma)

Test Interactions False-negative reaction using glucose-oxidase tests for glucosuria; false-positive urine ketones; false diagnosis for pheochromocytoma (rare) based on plasma and urine levels of catecholamines

Dosage Forms Excipient information presented when available (limited, particularly for generics); consult specific product labeling.

Tablet:

Stalevo® 50: Levodopa 50 mg, carbidopa 12.5 mg, and entacapone 200 mg

Stalevo® 75: Levodopa 75 mg, carbidopa 18.75 mg, and entacapone 200 mg

Stalevo® 100: Levodopa 100 mg, carbidopa 25 mg, and entacapone 200 mg

Stelevo® 125: Levodopa 125 mg, carbidopa 31.25 mg, and entacapone 200 mg

Stalevo® 150: Levodopa 150 mg, carbidopa 37.5 mg, and entacapone 200 mg

Stalevo® 200: Levodopa 200 mg, carbidopa 50 mg, and entacapone 200 mg

◆ **Levo-Dromoran®** *see* Levorphanol *on page 919*

Levofloxacin (lee voe FLOKS a sin)

Medication Safety Issues

Sound-alike/look-alike issues:

Levaquin® may be confused with Levoxyl®, Levsin/SL®, Lovenox®

Levofloxacin may be confused with levetiracetam, levodopa, levothyroxine

U.S. Brand Names Iquix®; Levaquin®; Quixin®

Canadian Brand Names Levaquin®; Novo-Levofloxacin

Mexican Brand Names Cina; Elequine; Flevox; Ovelquin; Ran-Levo; Tavanic; Voflaxin

Pharmacologic Category Antibiotic, Quinolone; Respiratory Fluoroquinolone

Generic Available No

Use

Systemic: Treatment of community-acquired pneumonia, including multidrug resistant strains of *S. pneumoniae* (MDRSP); nosocomial pneumonia; chronic bronchitis (acute bacterial exacerbation); acute bacterial sinusitis; prostatitis, urinary tract infection (uncomplicated or complicated); acute pyelonephritis; skin or skin structure infections (uncomplicated or complicated); reduce incidence or disease progression of inhalational anthrax (postexposure)

Ophthalmic: Treatment of bacterial conjunctivitis caused by susceptible organisms (Quixin™ 0.5% ophthalmic solution); treatment of corneal ulcer caused by susceptible organisms (Iquix® 1.5% ophthalmic solution)

Unlabeled/Investigational Use Diverticulitis, enterocolitis (*Shigella* spp.), epididymitis (nongonococcal), gonococcal infections, Legionnaires' disease, peritonitis, PID

Note: As of April 2007, the CDC no longer recommends the use of fluoroquinolones for the treatment of gonococcal disease.

Effect on Mental Status May cause agitation, anxiety, confusion, depression, dizziness, hallucinations, insomnia, nervousness, paranoia, and sedation

Effect on Psychiatric Treatment May cause leukopenia; use caution with clozapine and carbamazepine; inhibits CYP1A2 isoenzyme; caution with clozapine and other psychotropics; monitor for adverse effects

Restrictions

An FDA-approved patient medication guide is available and must be distributed when dispensing an outpatient prescription (new or refill) where this medication is to be used without direct supervision of a healthcare provider. Medication guides are available at http://www.fda.gov/cder/Offices/ODS/medication_guides.htm.

Pregnancy Risk Factor C

Pregnancy Considerations Adverse events have been observed in some animal studies; therefore, the manufacturer classifies levofloxacin as pregnancy category C. Levofloxacin crosses the placenta. Quinolone exposure during human pregnancy has been reported with other agents (see Ciprofloxacin, Ofloxacin, and Norfloxacin monographs). To date, no specific teratogenic effect or increased pregnancy risk has been identified; however, because of concerns of cartilage damage in immature animals exposed to quinolones and the limited levofloxacin specific data, levofloxacin should only be used during pregnancy if a safer option is not available.

Lactation Enters breast milk/not recommended

Contraindications Hypersensitivity to levofloxacin, any component of the formulation, or other quinolones

Warnings/Precautions

Systemic: [U.S. Boxed Warning]: There have been reports of tendon inflammation and/or rupture with quinolone antibiotics; risk may be increased with concurrent corticosteroids, organ transplant recipients, and in patients >60 years of age. Rupture of the Achilles tendon sometimes requiring surgical repair has been reported most frequently; but other tendon sites (eg, rotator cuff, biceps) have also been reported. Strenuous physical activity, rheumatoid arthritis, and renal impairment may be an independent risk factor for tendonitis. Discontinue at first sign of tendon inflammation or pain. May occur even after discontinuation of therapy. Use with caution in patients with rheumatoid arthritis; may increase risk of tendon rupture. Systemic use is only recommended in children <18 years of age for the prevention of inhalational anthrax (postexposure); increased incidence of musculoskeletal disorders (eg, arthralgia, tendon rupture) has been observed in children; CNS stimulation may occur (tremor, restlessness, confusion, and very rarely hallucinations or seizures). Potential for seizures, although very rare, may be increased with concomitant NSAID therapy. Use with caution in individuals at risk of seizures, with known or suspected CNS disorders or renal dysfunction. Avoid excessive sunlight and take precautions to limit exposure (eg, loose fitting clothing, sunscreen); may cause moderate-to-severe phototoxicity reactions. Discontinue use if photosensitivity occurs.

Rare cases of torsade de pointes have been reported in patients receiving levofloxacin. Use caution in patients with known prolongation of QT interval, bradycardia, hypokalemia, hypomagnesemia, or in those receiving concurrent therapy with Class Ia or Class III antiarrhythmics.

Severe hypersensitivity reactions, including anaphylaxis, have occurred with quinolone therapy. Reactions may present as typical allergic symptoms after a single dose, or may manifest as severe idiosyncratic dermatologic, vascular, pulmonary, renal, hepatic, and/or hematologic events, usually after multiple doses. Prompt discontinuation of drug should occur if skin rash or other symptoms arise. Prolonged use may result in fungal or bacterial superinfection, including *C. difficile*-associated diarrhea (CDAD) and pseudomembranous colitis; CDAD has been observed >2 months postantibiotic treatment. Peripheral neuropathies have been linked to levofloxacin use; discontinue if numbness, tingling, or weakness develops. Quinolones may exacerbate myasthenia gravis. Unrelated to hypersensitivity, severe hepatotoxicity (including acute hepatitis and fatalities) has been reported. Elderly patients may be at greater risk. Discontinue therapy immediately if signs and symptoms of hepatitis occur. Hemolytic reactions may (rarely) occur with quinolone use in patients with latent or actual G6PD deficiency.

Fluoroquinolones have been associated with the development of serious, and sometimes fatal, hypoglycemia, most often in elderly diabetics, but also in patients without diabetes. This occurred most frequently with gatifloxacin (no longer available systemically) but may occur at a lower frequency with other quinolones.

Ophthalmic solution: For topical use only. Do not inject subconjunctivally or introduce into anterior chamber of the eye. Contact lenses should not be worn during treatment for bacterial conjunctivitis. Safety and efficacy in children <1 year of age (Quixin™) or <6 years of age (Iquix®) have not been established. **Note:** Indications for ophthalmic solutions are product concentration-specific and should not be used interchangeably.

Adverse Reactions

1% to 10%:

Cardiovascular: Chest pain (1%), edema (1%)

Central nervous system: Headache (6%), insomnia (4%), dizziness (3%), fatigue (1%), pain (1%)

Dermatologic: Rash (2%), pruritus (1%)

Gastrointestinal: Taste disturbance (8% to 10% [ophthalmic]), nausea (7%), diarrhea (5%), constipation (3%), abdominal pain (2%), dyspepsia (2%), vomiting (2%)

Genitourinary: Vaginitis (1%)

Local: Injection site reaction (1%)

Ocular (with ophthalmic solution use): Decreased vision (transient), foreign body sensation, transient ocular burning, ocular pain or discomfort, photophobia

Respiratory: Pharyngitis (4%), dyspnea (1%)

Miscellaneous: Moniliasis (1%)

<1% (Limited to important or life-threatening):

Systemic: Acute renal failure, agitation, agranulocytosis; allergic reaction (including anaphylaxis, angioedema, pneumonitis rash, pneumonitis, and serum sickness); anaphylactoid reaction, arrhythmia (including atrial/ventricular tachycardia/fibrillation and torsade de pointes), aplastic anemia, arthralgia, ascites, bradycardia, bronchospasm, carcinoma, cardiac failure, cholecystitis, cholelithiasis, confusion, depression, EEG abnormalities, encephalopathy, eosinophilia, erythema multiforme, GI hemorrhage, granulocytopenia, hallucination, heart block, hemolytic anemia, hemoptysis, hepatic failure (some fatal), hepatitis, hyper-/hypoglycemia, hyperkalemia, hyperkinesias, hyper-/hypotension, infection, INR increased, intestinal obstruction, intracranial hypertension, involuntary muscle contractions, jaundice, leukocytosis, leukopenia, leukorrhea, lymphadenopathy, MI, migraine, multiple organ failure, myalgia, nephritis (interstitial), palpitation, pancreatitis, pancytopenia, paralysis, paresthesia, peripheral neuropathy, photosensitivity (<0.1%), pleural effusion, pneumonitis, postural hypotension, prothrombin time increased/decreased, pseudomembraneous colitis, psychosis, pulmonary edema, pulmonary embolism, purpura, QT_c prolongation, respiratory depression, rhabdomyolysis, seizure, skin disorder, somnolence, speech disorder, Stevens-Johnson syndrome, stupor, suicide attempt/ideation, syncope, tendonitis, tendon rupture, tongue edema, toxic epidermal necrolysis, transaminases increased, thrombocythemia, thrombocytopenia, tremor, urticaria, WBC abnormality

Ophthalmic solution: Allergic reaction, lid edema, ocular dryness, ocular itching

Drug Interactions

Alfuzosin: May enhance the QTc-prolonging effect of QTc-Prolonging Agents. *Risk C: Monitor therapy*

Antacids: May decrease the absorption of Quinolone Antibiotics. Of concern only with oral administration of quinolones. **Exceptions:** Sodium Bicarbonate. *Risk D: Consider therapy modification*

Calcium Salts: May decrease the absorption of Quinolone Antibiotics. Of concern only with oral administration of both agents. **Exceptions:** Calcium Chloride. *Risk D: Consider therapy modification*

Ciprofloxacin: May enhance the QTc-prolonging effect of QTc-Prolonging Agents. *Risk C: Monitor therapy*

Corticosteroids (Systemic): Quinolone Antibiotics may enhance the adverse/toxic effect of Corticosteroids (Systemic). Risk of tendon-related side effects, including tendonitis and rupture, may be enhanced. *Risk C: Monitor therapy*

Didanosine: May decrease the absorption of Quinolone Antibiotics. Of concern only with oral administration of both agents (excludes enteric coated formulation of didanosine). *Risk D: Consider therapy modification*

Gadobutrol: May enhance the QTc-prolonging effect of QTc-Prolonging Agents. *Risk D: Consider therapy modification*

Insulin: May enhance the hyperglycemic effect of Quinolone Antibiotics. Insulin may enhance the hypoglycemic effect of Quinolone Antibiotics. *Risk C: Monitor therapy*

Iron Salts: May decrease the absorption of Quinolone Antibiotics. Of concern only with oral administration of both agents. **Exceptions:** Ferric Gluconate; Iron Dextran Complex; Iron Sucrose. *Risk D: Consider therapy modification*

Magnesium Salts: May decrease the absorption of Quinolone Antibiotics. Of concern only with oral administration of both agents. *Risk D: Consider therapy modification*

Mycophenolate: Quinolone Antibiotics may decrease the serum concentration of Mycophenolate. Specifically, quinolones may decrease concentrations of the active metabolite of mycophenolate. *Risk C: Monitor therapy*

Nilotinib: May enhance the QTc-prolonging effect of QTc-Prolonging Agents. *Risk X: Avoid combination*

Nonsteroidal Anti-Inflammatory Agents: May enhance the neuroexcitatory and/or seizure-potentiating effect of Quinolone Antibiotics. *Risk C: Monitor therapy*

Probenecid: May increase the serum concentration of Quinolone Antibiotics. *Risk C: Monitor therapy*

QTc-Prolonging Agents: May enhance the adverse/toxic effect of other QTc-Prolonging Agents. Their effects can be additive, causing life-threatening ventricular arrhythmias. *Risk D: Consider therapy modification*

Quinapril: May decrease the absorption of Quinolone Antibiotics. Of concern only with oral administration of quinolones. *Risk D: Consider therapy modification*

Sevelamer: May decrease the absorption of Quinolone Antibiotics. *Risk D: Consider therapy modification*

Sucralfate: May decrease the absorption of Quinolone Antibiotics. Of concern only with oral administration of quinolones. *Risk D: Consider therapy modification*

Sulfonylureas: Quinolone Antibiotics may enhance the hyperglycemic effect of Sulfonylureas. Quinolone Antibiotics may enhance the hypoglycemic effect of Sulfonylureas. *Risk C: Monitor therapy*

Tetrabenazine: QTc-Prolonging Agents may enhance the QTc-prolonging effect of Tetrabenazine. *Risk X: Avoid combination*

Thioridazine: QTc-Prolonging Agents may enhance the QTc-prolonging effect of Thioridazine. *Risk X: Avoid combination*

Typhoid Vaccine: Antibiotics may diminish the therapeutic effect of Typhoid Vaccine. Only the live attenuated Ty21a strain is affected. *Risk D: Consider therapy modification*

Vitamin K Antagonists (eg, warfarin): Quinolone Antibiotics may enhance the anticoagulant effect of Vitamin K Antagonists. *Risk C: Monitor therapy*

Zinc Salts: May decrease the absorption of Quinolone Antibiotics. Of concern only with oral administration of both agents. *Risk D: Consider therapy modification*

Ziprasidone: QTc-Prolonging Agents may enhance the QTc-prolonging effect of Ziprasidone. The risk of a severe arrhythmia may be increased. *Risk X: Avoid combination*

Stability

Solution for injection:

Vial: Store at room temperature. Protect from light. When diluted to 5 mg/mL in a compatible I.V. fluid, solution is stable for 72 hours when stored at room temperature; stable for 14 days when stored under refrigeration. When frozen, stable for 6 months; do not refreeze. Do not thaw in microwave or by bath immersion.

Premixed: Store at ≤25°C (77°F); do not freeze. Brief exposure to 40°C (104°F) does not affect product. Protect from light.

Tablet, oral solution: Store at 25°C (77°F); excursions permitted to 15°C to 30°C (59°F to 86°F).

Ophthalmic solution: Store at 15°C to 25°C (59°F to 77°F).

Mechanism of Action As the S (-) enantiomer of the fluoroquinolone, ofloxacin, levofloxacin, inhibits DNA-gyrase in susceptible organisms thereby inhibits relaxation of supercoiled DNA and promotes breakage of DNA strands. DNA gyrase (topoisomerase II), is an essential bacterial enzyme that maintains the superhelical structure of DNA and is required for DNA replication and transcription, DNA repair, recombination, and transposition.

Pharmacodynamics/Kinetics

Absorption: Rapid and complete

Distribution: V_d: 74-112 L; CSF concentrations ~15% of serum levels; high concentrations are achieved in prostate, lung, and gynecological tissues, sinus, saliva

Protein binding: ~24% to 38%; primarily to albumin

Metabolism: Minimally hepatic

Bioavailability: ~99%

Half-life elimination: ~6-8 hours

Time to peak, serum: Oral: 1-2 hours

Excretion: Urine (~87% as unchanged drug, <5% as metabolites); feces (<4%)

Dosage Note: Sequential therapy (intravenous to oral) may be instituted based on prescriber's discretion.

Usual dosage range:

Children ≥1 year: Ophthalmic: 1-2 drops every 2-6 hours

Adults:

Ophthalmic: 1-2 drops every 2-6 hours

Oral, I.V.: 250-500 mg every 24 hours; severe or complicated infections: 750 mg every 24 hours

Indication-specific dosing:

Children ≥1 year and Adults: Ophthalmic:

Conjunctivitis (0.5% ophthalmic solution):

Treatment day 1 and day 2: Instill 1-2 drops into affected eye(s) every 2 hours while awake, up to 8 times/day

Treatment day 3 through day 7: Instill 1-2 drops into affected eye(s) every 4 hours while awake, up to 4 times/day

Children ≥6 years and Adults: Ophthalmic:

Corneal ulceration (1.5% ophthalmic solution):

Treatment day 1 through day 3: Instill 1-2 drops into affected eye(s) every 30 minutes to 2 hours while awake and 4-6 hours after retiring

Treatment day 4 through completion: Instill 1-2 drops into affected eye(s) every 1-4 hours while awake

Children ≥6 months and Adults: Oral, I.V.

Anthrax (inhalational, postexposure):

≤50 kg: 8 mg/kg every 12 hours for 60 days (do not exceed 250 mg/dose), beginning as soon as possible after exposure

>50 kg and Adults: 500 mg every 24 hours for 60 days, beginning as soon as possible after exposure

Adults: Oral, I.V.:

Chronic bronchitis (acute bacterial exacerbation): 500 mg every 24 hours for at least 7 days

Diverticulitis, peritonitis (unlabeled use): 750 mg every 24 hours for 7-10 days; use adjunctive metronidazole therapy

Dysenteric enterocolitis, *Shigella* spp. (unlabeled use): 500 mg every 24 hours for 3-5 days

Epididymitis, nongonococcal (unlabeled use): 500 mg once daily for 10 days

Gonococcal infection (unlabeled use):

Cervicitis, urethritis: 250 mg for one dose with azithromycin or doxycycline; **Note:** As of April 2007, the CDC no longer recommends the use of fluoroquinolones for the treatment of uncomplicated gonococcal disease.

Disseminated infection: 250 mg I.V. once daily; 24 hours after symptoms improve may change to 500 mg orally every 24 hours to complete total therapy of 7 days; **Note:** As of April 2007, the CDC no longer recommends the use of fluoroquinolones for the treatment of more serious gonococcal disease, unless no other options exist and susceptibility can be confirmed via culture.

Pelvic inflammatory disease (unlabeled use): 500 mg once daily for 14 days with or without adjunctive metronidazole; **Note:** The CDC recommends use only if standard cephalosporin therapy is not feasible and community prevalence of quinolone-resistant gonococcal organisms is low. Culture sensitivity must be confirmed.

Pneumonia:

Community-acquired: 500 mg every 24 hours for 7-14 days or 750 mg every 24 hours for 5 days (efficacy of 5-day regimen for MDRSP not established)

Nosocomial: 750 mg every 24 hours for 7-14 days

Prostatitis (chronic bacterial): 500 mg every 24 hours for 28 days

Sinusitis (acute bacterial): 500 mg every 24 hours for 10-14 days or 750 mg every 24 hours for 5 days

Skin and skin structure infections:

Uncomplicated: 500 mg every 24 hours for 7-10 days

Complicated: 750 mg every 24 hours for 7-14 days

Traveler's diarrhea (unlabeled use): 500 mg for one dose

Urinary tract infections:

Uncomplicated: 250 mg once daily for 3 days

Complicated, including pyelonephritis: 250 mg once daily for 10 days **or** 750 mg once daily for 5 days

Dosing adjustment in renal impairment:

Normal renal function dosing of 750 mg/day:

Cl_{cr} 20-49 mL/minute: Administer 750 mg every 48 hours

Cl_{cr} 10-19 mL/minute: Administer 750 mg initial dose, followed by 500 mg every 48 hours

Hemodialysis/CAPD: Administer 750 mg initial dose, followed by 500 mg every 48 hours

Normal renal function dosing of 500 mg/day:

Cl_{cr} 20-49 mL/minute: Administer 500 mg initial dose, followed by 250 mg every 24 hours

Cl_{cr} 10-19 mL/minute: Administer 500 mg initial dose, followed by 250 mg every 48 hours

Hemodialysis/CAPD: Administer 500 mg initial dose, followed by 250 mg every 48 hours

Normal renal function dosing of 250 mg/day:

Cl_{cr} 20-49 mL/minute: No dosage adjustment required

Cl_{cr} 10-19 mL/minute: Administer 250 mg every 48 hours (except in uncomplicated UTI, where no dosage adjustment is required)

Hemodialysis/CAPD: No information available

CRRT: **Note:** Clearance dependent on filter type, flow rates, and other variables.

CVVH/CVVHD/CVVHDF: Alternative recommendations exist:

500 mg every 48 hours **or**

250 mg every 24 hours (**Note:** This regimen has been shown to be equivalent to 500 mg/day in normal renal function. Appropriateness of this regimen for target dosing equal to 750 mg/day is not known.)

Dietary Considerations Tablets may be taken without regard to meals. Oral solution should be administered on an empty stomach (1 hour before or 2 hours after a meal). Take 2 hours before or 2 hours after multiple vitamins, antacids, or other products containing magnesium, aluminum, iron, or zinc.

Administration

Oral: Tablets may be administered without regard to meals. Oral solution should be administered 1 hour before or 2 hours after meals. Maintain adequate hydration of patient to prevent crystalluria.

I.V.: Infuse 250-500 mg I.V. solution over 60 minutes; infuse 750 mg I.V. solution over 90 minutes. Too rapid of infusion can lead to hypotension. Avoid administration through an intravenous line with a solution containing multivalent cations (eg, magnesium, calcium). Maintain adequate hydration of patient to prevent crystalluria.

Monitoring Parameters Evaluation of organ system functions (renal, hepatic, ophthalmologic, and hematopoietic) is recommended periodically during therapy; the possibility of crystalluria should be assessed; WBC and signs of infection

Test Interactions Some quinolones may produce a false-positive urine screening result for opiates using commercially-available immunoassay kits. This has been demonstrated most consistently for levofloxacin and ofloxacin, but other quinolones have shown cross-reactivity in certain assay kits. Confirmation of positive opiate screens by more specific methods should be considered.

Dosage Forms Excipient information presented when available (limited, particularly for generics); consult specific product labeling.

Infusion [premixed in D_5W]:

Levaquin®: 250 mg (50 mL); 500 mg (100 mL); 750 mg (150 mL)

Injection, solution [preservative free]

Levaquin®: 25 mg/mL (20 mL, 30 mL)

Solution, ophthalmic [drops]:

Iquix®: 1.5% (5 mL)

Quixin®: 0.5% (5 mL) [contains benzalkonium chloride]

Solution, oral:

Levaquin®: 25 mg/mL (480 mL) [contains benzyl alcohol]

Tablet, oral:

Levaquin®: 250 mg, 500 mg, 750 mg

Levaquin® Leva-Pak: 750 mg (5s)

◆ **Levomepromazine** *see* Methotrimeprazine *on page 1015*

Levonorgestrel (LEE voe nor jes trel)

U.S. Brand Names Mirena®; Plan B® [RX/OTC]

Canadian Brand Names Mirena®; Norplant® Implant; Plan B™

Mexican Brand Names Postinor-2

Index Terms LNg 20

Pharmacologic Category Contraceptive; Progestin

Use

Intrauterine device (IUD): Prevention of pregnancy

Oral: Emergency contraception following unprotected intercourse or possible contraceptive failure

Unlabeled/Investigational Use IUD: Idiopathic menorrhagia; protection against endometrial hyperplasia in menopausal women using estrogen

Effect on Mental Status May cause nervousness or dizziness

Effect on Psychiatric Treatment Carbamazepine may decrease the effects of levonorgestrel

Restrictions Plan B® is approved for OTC use by women ≥18 years of age and available by prescription only for women ≤17 years of age. Sales of Plan B® will be limited to pharmacies or healthcare clinics with a valid license to distribute prescription products. Because there will be one package for both OTC and prescription use, pharmacies are required to keep the product behind the counter.

Dosage Summary

Intrauterine:

Children: Not for use prior to menarche

Adults: Insert into uterine cavity, releases 20 mcg/day over 5 years

Oral:

Children: Not for use prior to menarche

Adults: One 0.75 mg tablet as soon as possible within 72 hours of unprotected sexual intercourse, repeat once 12 hours after the first dose

Dosage Forms Excipient information presented when available (limited, particularly for generics); consult specific product labeling.

Intrauterine device:

Mirena®: 52 mg/unit [releases levonorgestrel 20 mcg/day]

Tablet:

Plan B®: 0.75 mg

◆ **Levonorgestrel and Ethinyl Estradiol** *see* Ethinyl Estradiol and Levonorgestrel *on page 595*

◆ **Levophed®** *see* Norepinephrine *on page 1150*

◆ **Levora®** *see* Ethinyl Estradiol and Levonorgestrel *on page 595*

Levorphanol (lee VOR fa nole)

Medication Safety Issues

High alert medication: The Institute for Safe Medication Practices (ISMP) includes this medication among its list of drug classes which have a heightened risk of causing significant patient harm when used in error.

Related Information

Narcotic / Opioid Analgesics *on page 1789*

U.S. Brand Names Levo-Dromoran®

Index Terms Levorphan Tartrate; Levorphanol Tartrate

Pharmacologic Category Analgesic, Opioid

Use Relief of moderate to severe pain; also used parenterally for preoperative sedation and an adjunct to nitrous oxide/oxygen anesthesia

Effect on Mental Status Drowsiness and dizziness are common; may cause nervousness, restlessness, or confusion; may rarely cause depression, hallucinations, or paradoxical CNS stimulation

Effect on Psychiatric Treatment Concurrent use with psychotropics may produce additive sedation

Restrictions C-II

Dosage Summary

I.M.:

Children: Dosage not established

Adults: 1-2 mg every 6-8 hours as needed **or** 1-2 mg/dose 60-90 minutes prior to surgery

I.V.:

Children: Dosage not established

Adults: Up to 1 mg/dose every 3-6 hours as needed

Oral:

Children: Dosage not established

Adults: 2-4 mg every 6-8 hours as needed

SubQ:

Children: Dosage not established

Adults: 1-2 mg every 6-8 hours as needed **or** 1-2 mg/dose 60-90 minutes prior to surgery

Dosage Forms Excipient information presented when available (limited, particularly for generics); consult specific product labeling.

Injection, solution, as tartrate: 2 mg/mL (1 mL, 10 mL)

Tablet, as tartrate: 2 mg

◆ **Levorphanol Tartrate** *see* Levorphanol *on page 919*

◆ **Levorphan Tartrate** *see* Levorphanol *on page 919*

◆ **Levothroid®** *see* Levothyroxine *on page 920*

Levothyroxine (lee voe thye ROKS een)

Medication Safety Issues

Sound-alike/look-alike issues:

Levothyroxine may be confused with levofloxacin, liothyronine

Levoxyl® may be confused with Lanoxin®, Levaquin®, Luvox®

Synthroid® may be confused with Symmetrel®

To avoid errors due to misinterpretation of a decimal point, always express dosage in mcg (**not** mg).

Significant differences exist between oral and I.V. dosing. Use caution when converting from one route of administration to another.

U.S. Brand Names Levothroid®; Levoxyl®; Synthroid®; Tirosint™; Unithroid®

Canadian Brand Names Eltroxin®; Gen-Levothyroxine; Levothyroxine Sodium; Synthroid®

Mexican Brand Names Cynocuatro; Eutirox; Levhexal; Tiroidine

Index Terms *L*-Thyroxine Sodium; Levothyroxine Sodium; T_4

Pharmacologic Category Thyroid Product

Generic Available Yes: Excludes capsule

Use Replacement or supplemental therapy in hypothyroidism; pituitary TSH suppression

Effect on Mental Status May rarely cause nervousness or insomnia

Effect on Psychiatric Treatment Used to augment antidepressants; TCAs may increase toxic potential of both drugs

Pregnancy Risk Factor A

Pregnancy Considerations Untreated maternal hypothyroidism may have adverse effects on fetal growth and development and is associated with higher rate of complications (spontaneous abortion, pre-eclampsia, stillbirth, premature delivery). Treatment should not be discontinued during pregnancy. TSH levels should be monitored during each trimester and 6-8 weeks postpartum. Increased doses may be needed during pregnancy.

Lactation Enters breast milk/compatible

Contraindications Hypersensitivity to levothyroxine sodium or any component of the formulation; recent MI or thyrotoxicosis; uncorrected adrenal insufficiency

Warnings/Precautions [U.S. Boxed Warning]: Ineffective and potentially toxic for weight reduction. High doses may produce serious or even life-threatening toxic effects particularly when used with some anorectic drugs. Use with caution and reduce dosage in patients with angina pectoris or other cardiovascular disease; decrease initial dose. Use cautiously in the elderly since they may be more likely to have compromised cardiovascular functions. Patients with adrenal insufficiency, myxedema, diabetes mellitus and insipidus may have symptoms exaggerated or aggravated. Chronic hypothyroidism predisposes patients to coronary artery disease. Long-term therapy can decrease bone mineral density. Levoxyl® may rapidly swell and disintegrate causing choking or gagging (should be administered with a full glass of water); use caution in patients with dysphagia or other swallowing disorders.

Adverse Reactions Frequency not defined.

Cardiovascular: Angina, arrhythmia, blood pressure increased, cardiac arrest, flushing, heart failure, MI, palpitation, pulse increased, tachycardia

Central nervous system: Anxiety, emotional lability, fatigue, fever, headache, hyperactivity, insomnia, irritability, nervousness, pseudotumor cerebri (children), seizure (rare)

Dermatologic: Alopecia

Endocrine & metabolic: Fertility impaired, menstrual irregularities

Gastrointestinal: Abdominal cramps, appetite increased, diarrhea, vomiting, weight loss

Hepatic: Liver function tests increased

Neuromuscular & skeletal: Bone mineral density decreased, muscle weakness, tremor, slipped capital femoral epiphysis (children)

Respiratory: Dyspnea

Miscellaneous: Diaphoresis, heat intolerance, hypersensitivity (to inactive ingredients, symptoms include urticaria, pruritus, rash, flushing, angioedema, GI symptoms, fever, arthralgia, serum sickness, wheezing)

Levoxyl®: Choking, dysphagia, gagging

Drug Interactions

Bile Acid Sequestrants: May decrease the absorption of Thyroid Products. *Risk C: Monitor therapy*

CarBAMazepine: May decrease the serum concentration of Thyroid Products. *Risk C: Monitor therapy*

Estrogen Derivatives: May diminish the therapeutic effect of Thyroid Products. *Risk C: Monitor therapy*

Ferrous Sulfate: May decrease the serum concentration of Levothyroxine. *Risk D: Consider therapy modification*

Orlistat: May decrease the serum concentration of Levothyroxine. *Risk C: Monitor therapy*

Phenytoin: May increase the metabolism of Thyroid Products. Phenytoin may also displace thyroid hormones from protein binding sites. *Risk C: Monitor therapy*

Raloxifene: May decrease the absorption of Levothyroxine. *Risk D: Consider therapy modification*

Rifampin: May decrease the serum concentration of Thyroid Products. *Risk C: Monitor therapy*

Sodium Iodide I131: Thyroid Products may diminish the therapeutic effect of Sodium Iodide I131. *Risk X: Avoid combination*

Sucralfate: May decrease the serum concentration of Levothyroxine. *Risk C: Monitor therapy*

Theophylline Derivatives: Thyroid Products may increase the metabolism of Theophylline Derivatives. **Exceptions:** Dyphylline. *Risk C: Monitor therapy*

Vitamin K Antagonists (eg, warfarin): Thyroid Products may enhance the anticoagulant effect of Vitamin K Antagonists. *Risk D: Consider therapy modification*

Ethanol/Nutrition/Herb Interactions Food: Taking levothyroxine with enteral nutrition may cause reduced bioavailability and may lower serum thyroxine levels leading to signs or symptoms of hypothyroidism. Soybean flour (infant formula), cottonseed meal, walnuts, and dietary fiber may decrease absorption of levothyroxine from the GI tract.

Stability

Tablet: Store at room temperature of 15°C to 30°C (59°F to 86°F). Protect from light and moisture.

Injection: Store at room temperature of 15°C to 30°C (59°F to 86°F). Dilute vials for injection with 5 mL normal saline. Reconstituted concentrations for the 200 mcg and 500 mcg vials are 40 mcg/mL and 100 mcg/mL, respectively. Shake well. Reconstituted solutions should be used immediately and any unused portions discarded.

Mechanism of Action Exact mechanism of action is unknown; however, it is believed the thyroid hormone exerts its many metabolic effects through control of DNA transcription and protein synthesis; involved in normal metabolism, growth, and development; promotes gluconeogenesis, increases utilization and mobilization of glycogen stores, and stimulates protein synthesis, increases basal metabolic rate

Pharmacodynamics/Kinetics

Onset of action: Therapeutic: Oral: 3-5 days; I.V. 6-8 hours

Peak effect: I.V.: 24 hours

Absorption: Oral: Erratic (40% to 80%); may be decreased by age and specific foods and drugs

Protein binding: >99%

Metabolism: Hepatic to triiodothyronine (active)

Time to peak, serum: 2-4 hours

Half-life elimination: Euthyroid: 6-7 days; Hypothyroid: 9-10 days; Hyperthyroid: 3-4 days

Excretion: Urine and feces; decreases with age

Dosage Doses should be adjusted based on clinical response and laboratory parameters.

Oral:

Children: Hypothyroidism:

Newborns: Initial: 10-15 mcg/kg/day. Lower doses of 25 mcg/day should be considered in newborns at risk for cardiac failure. Newborns with T_4 levels <5 mcg/dL should be started at 50 mcg/day. Adjust dose at 4- to 6-week intervals.

Infants and Children: Dose based on body weight and age as listed below. Children with severe or chronic hypothyroidism should be started at 25 mcg/day; adjust dose by 25 mcg every 2-4 weeks. In older children, hyperactivity may be decreased by starting with 1/4 of the recommended dose and increasing by 1/4 dose each week until the full replacement dose is reached. Refer to adult dosing once growth and puberty are complete.

0-3 months: 10-15 mcg/kg/day

3-6 months: 8-10 mcg/kg/day

6-12 months: 6-8 mcg/kg/day

1-5 years: 5-6 mcg/kg/day

6-12 years: 4-5 mcg/kg/day
>12 years: 2-3 mcg/kg/day

Adults:

Hypothyroidism: 1.7 mcg/kg/day in otherwise healthy adults <50 years old, children in whom growth and puberty are complete, and older adults who have been recently treated for hyperthyroidism or who have been hypothyroid for only a few months. Titrate dose every 6 weeks. Average full replacement dose is 100-125 mcg/day for a 70 kg adult; usual doses are ≤200 mcg/day; doses ≥300 mcg/day are rare (consider poor compliance, malabsorption, and/or drug interactions). **Note:** For patients >50 years or patients with cardiac disease, refer to Elderly dosing.

Severe hypothyroidism: Initial: 12.5-25 mcg/day; adjust dose by 25 mcg/day every 2-4 weeks as appropriate; **Note:** Oral agents are not recommended for myxedema (see I.V. dosing).

Subclinical hypothyroidism (if treated): 1 mcg/kg/day

TSH suppression:

Well-differentiated thyroid cancer: Highly individualized; Doses >2 mcg/kg/day may be needed to suppress TSH to <0.1 mU/L. High-risk tumors may need a target level of <0.01 mU/L for TSH suppression.

Benign nodules and nontoxic multinodular goiter: Goal TSH suppression: 0.1-0.5 mU/L (benign nodules) and 0.5-1 mU/L (multinodular goiter)

Elderly: Hypothyroidism:

>50 years without cardiac disease **or** <50 years with cardiac disease: Initial: 25-50 mcg/day; adjust dose at 6- to 8-week intervals as needed

>50 years with cardiac disease: Initial: 12.5-25 mcg/day; adjust dose by 12.5-25 mcg increments at 4- to 6-week intervals. (**Note:** Many clinicians prefer to adjust at 6- to 8-week intervals.)

Note: Elderly patients may require <1 mcg/kg/day

I.M., I.V.: Children, Adults, Elderly: Hypothyroidism: 50% of the oral dose

I.V.:

Adults: Myxedema coma or stupor: 200-500 mcg, then 100-300 mcg the next day if necessary; smaller doses should be considered in patients with cardiovascular disease

Elderly: Myxedema coma: Refer to adult dosing; lower doses may be needed

Dietary Considerations Should be taken on an empty stomach, at least 30 minutes before food.

Administration

Oral: Administer in the morning on an empty stomach, at least 30 minutes before food. Tablets may be crushed and suspended in 1-2 teaspoonfuls of water; suspension should be used immediately. Levoxyl® should be administered with a full glass of water to prevent gagging (due to tablet swelling).

Parenteral: Dilute vial with 5 mL normal saline; use immediately after reconstitution; should not be admixed with other solutions

Monitoring Parameters Thyroid function test (serum thyroxine, thyrotropin concentrations), resin triiodothyronine uptake (rT_3U), free thyroxine index (FTI), T_4, TSH, heart rate, blood pressure, clinical signs of hypo- and hyperthyroidism; TSH is the most reliable guide for evaluating adequacy of thyroid replacement dosage. TSH may be elevated during the first few months of thyroid replacement despite patients being clinically euthyroid. In cases where T_4 remains low and TSH is within normal limits, an evaluation of "free" (unbound) T_4 is needed to evaluate further increase in dosage

Infants: Monitor closely for cardiac overload, arrhythmias, and aspiration from avid suckling

Infants/children: Monitor closely for under/overtreatment. Undertreatment may decrease intellectual development and linear growth, and lead to poor school performance due to impaired concentration and slowed mentation. Overtreatment may adversely affect brain maturation, accelerate bone age (leading to premature closure of the epiphyses and reduced adult height); craniosynostosis has been reported in infants. Treated children may experience a period of catch-up growth. Monitor TSH and total or free T_4 at 2 and 4 weeks after starting treatment; every 1-2 months for first year of life; every 2-3 months during years 1-3; every 3-12 months until growth completed.

Adults: Monitor TSH every 6-8 weeks until normalized; 8-12 weeks after dosage changes; every 6-12 months throughout therapy

Reference Range Pediatrics: Cord T_4 and values in the first few weeks are much higher, falling over the first months and years. ≥10 years: ~5.8-11 mcg/dL (SI: 75-142 nmol/L). Borderline low: ≤4.5-5.7 mcg/dL (SI: 58-73 nmol/L); low: ≤4.4 mcg/dL (SI: 57 nmol/L); results <2.5 mcg/dL (SI: <32 nmol/L) are strong evidence for hypothyroidism.

Approximate adult normal range: 4-12 mcg/dL (SI: 51-154 nmol/L). Borderline high: 11.1-13 mcg/dL (SI: 143-167 nmol/L); high: ≥13.1 mcg/dL (SI: 169 nmol/L). Normal range is increased in women on birth control pills (5.5-12 mcg/dL); normal range in pregnancy: ~5.5-16 mcg/dL (SI: ~71-206 nmol/L). TSH: 0.4-10 (for those ≥80 years) mIU/L; T_4: 4-12 mcg/dL (SI: 51-154 nmol/L); T_3 (RIA) (total T_3): 80-230 ng/dL (SI: 1.2-3.5 nmol/L); T_4 free (free T_4): 0.7-1.8 ng/dL (SI: 9-23 pmol/L).

Test Interactions Many drugs may have effects on thyroid function tests (see Additional Information). Pregnancy, infectious hepatitis, and acute intermittent porphyria may increase TBG concentrations; nephrosis, severe hypoproteinemia, severe liver disease, and acromegaly may decrease TBG concentrations.

Additional Information Equivalent doses: The following statement on relative potency of thyroid products is included in a joint statement by American Thyroid Association (ATA), American Association of Clinical Endocrinologists (AACE) and The Endocrine Society (TES): For purposes of conversion, levothyroxine sodium (T_4) 100 mcg is usually considered equivalent to desiccated thyroid 60 mg, thyroglobulin 60 mg, or liothyronine sodium (T_3) 25 mcg. However, these are rough guidelines only and do not obviate the careful re-evaluation of a patient when switching thyroid hormone preparations, including a change from one brand of levothyroxine to another. Joint position statement is available at http://www.thyroid.org/professionals/advocacy/04_12_08_thyroxine.html.

Note: Several medications have effects on thyroid production or conversion. The impact in thyroid replacement has not been specifically evaluated, but patient response should be monitored:

Methimazole: Decreases thyroid hormone secretion, while propylthiouracil decrease thyroid hormone secretion and decreases conversion of T_4 to T_3.

Beta-adrenergic antagonists: Decrease conversion of T_4 to T_3 (dose related, propranolol ≥160 mg/day); patients may be clinically euthyroid.

Iodide, iodine-containing radiographic contrast agents may decrease thyroid hormone secretion; may also increase thyroid hormone secretion, especially in patients with Graves' disease.

Other agents reported to impact on thyroid production/conversion include aminoglutethimide, amiodarone, chloral hydrate, diazepam, ethionamide, interferon-alpha, interleukin-2, lithium, lovastatin (case report), glucocorticoids (dose-related), mercaptopurine, sulfonamides, thiazide diuretics, and tolbutamide.

In addition, a number of medications have been noted to cause transient depression in TSH secretion, which may complicate interpretation of monitoring tests for levothyroxine, including corticosteroids, octreotide, and dopamine. Metoclopramide may increase TSH secretion

Dosage Forms Excipient information presented when available (limited, particularly for generics); consult specific product labeling.

Capsule, soft gelatin, as sodium:

Tirosint™: 13 mcg, 25 mcg, 50 mcg, 75 mcg, 100 mcg, 125 mcg, 150 mcg

Injection, powder for reconstitution, as sodium: 0.2 mg, 0.5 mg

Tablet, as sodium: 25 mcg, 50 mcg, 75 mcg, 88 mcg, 100 mcg, 112 mcg, 125 mcg, 137 mcg, 150 mcg, 175 mcg, 200 mcg, 300 mcg

Levothroid®: 25 mcg, 50 mcg, 75 mcg, 88 mcg, 100 mcg, 112 mcg, 125 mcg, 137 mcg, 150 mcg, 175 mcg, 200 mcg, 300 mcg

Levoxyl®: 25 mcg, 50 mcg, 75 mcg, 88 mcg, 100 mcg, 112 mcg, 125 mcg, 137 mcg, 150 mcg, 175 mcg, 200 mcg

Synthroid®: 25 mcg, 50 mcg, 75 mcg, 88 mcg, 100 mcg, 112 mcg, 125 mcg, 137 mcg, 150 mcg, 175 mcg, 200 mcg, 300 mcg

Unithroid®: 25 mcg, 50 mcg, 75 mcg, 88 mcg, 100 mcg, 112 mcg, 125 mcg, 150 mcg, 175 mcg, 200 mcg, 300 mcg

- **Levothyroxine Sodium** *see* Levothyroxine *on page 920*
- **Levoxyl®** *see* Levothyroxine *on page 920*
- **Levsin®** *see* Hyoscyamine *on page 799*
- **Levsin®/SL** *see* Hyoscyamine *on page 799*
- **Lexapro®** *see* Escitalopram *on page 564*
- **Lexiva®** *see* Fosamprenavir *on page 689*
- **Lexxel® [DSC]** *see* Enalapril and Felodipine *on page 536*
- **LFA-3/IgG(1) Fusion Protein, Human** *see* Alefacept *on page 58*
- **LHRH** *see* Gonadorelin *on page 734*
- **LH-RH Agonist** *see* Histrelin *on page 769*
- ***l*-Hyoscyamine Sulfate** *see* Hyoscyamine *on page 799*

- ◆ **Lialda™** *see* Mesalamine *on page 994*
- ◆ **Librax®** ***[reformulation]*** **[DSC]** *see* Chlordiazepoxide and Methscopolamine *on page 319*
- ◆ **Librax®** ***[original formulation]*** *see* Clidinium and Chlordiazepoxide *on page 362*
- ◆ **Librium®** *see* ChlordiazePOXIDE *on page 316*
- ◆ **LidaMantle®** *see* Lidocaine *on page 924*

Lidocaine (LYE doe kane)

Medication Safety Issues

High alert medication: The Institute for Safe Medication Practices (ISMP) includes this medication (epidural administration; I.V. formulation) among its list of drugs which have a heightened risk of causing significant patient harm when used in error.

Transdermal patch may contain conducting metal (eg, aluminum); remove patch prior to MRI.

International issues:

Lidpen® may be confused with Linoten® which is a brand name for pamidronate in Spain

U.S. Brand Names Akten™; Anestacon®; Anestafoam™ [OTC]; Band-Aid® Hurt-Free™ Antiseptic Wash [OTC]; Burn Jel® [OTC]; Burn-O-Jel [OTC]; Burnamycin [OTC]; L-M-X™ 4 [OTC]; L-M-X™ 5 [OTC]; LidaMantle®; Lidoderm®; LTA® 360; Premjact® [OTC]; Solarcaine® Aloe Extra Burn Relief [OTC]; Topicaine® [OTC]; Unburn®; Xylocaine®; Xylocaine® MPF; Xylocaine® Viscous; Zilactin-L® [OTC]; Zingo™

Canadian Brand Names Betacaine®; Lidodan™; Lidoderm®; Xylocaine®; Xylocard®; Zilactin®

Mexican Brand Names Betacaine; Hipoden; Sensipharma; Sunicaine; Uvega; Xylocaina

Index Terms Lidocaine Hydrochloride; Lignocaine Hydrochloride

Pharmacologic Category Analgesic, Topical; Antiarrhythmic Agent, Class Ib; Local Anesthetic; Local Anesthetic, Ophthalmic

Use Local anesthetic and acute treatment of ventricular arrhythmias (such as from myocardial infarction or cardiac manipulation)

Intradermal: To provide local anesthesia prior to venipuncture or peripheral I.V. cannulation

Ophthalmic: To provide local anesthesia to ocular surface during ophthalmologic procedures

Rectal: Temporary relief of pain and itching due to anorectal disorders

Topical: Local anesthetic for use in laser, cosmetic, and outpatient surgeries; minor burns, cuts, and abrasions of the skin

Lidoderm® Patch: Relief of allodynia (painful hypersensitivity) and chronic pain in postherpetic neuralgia

Unlabeled/Investigational Use ACLS guidelines (not considered drug of choice): Stable monomorphic VT (preserved ventricular function), polymorphic VT (preserved ventricular function), drug-induced monomorphic VT

Effect on Mental Status May rarely cause agitation, anxiety, euphoria, or hallucinations

Effect on Psychiatric Treatment None reported

Dosage Summary

E.T.:

Children: 2-3 mg/kg; flush with 5 mL of NS and follow with 5 assisted manual ventilations

Adults (loading dose only): 2-2.5 times the I.V. bolus dose

I.O.:

Children: Loading dose: 1 mg/kg, may repeat 0.5-1 mg/kg (maximum 100 mg); Infusion: 20-50 mcg/kg/minute

Adults: Dosage not established

I.V.:

Children: Loading dose: 1 mg/kg (maximum 100 mg), may repeat 0.5-1 mg/kg; Infusion: 20-50 mcg/kg/minute

Adults: Bolus: 1-1.5 mg/kg, may repeat 0.5-0.75 mg/kg up to a total of 3 mg/kg; Infusion: 1-4 mg/minute

Local injection:

Children: Varies with procedure, degree of anesthesia needed, vascularity of tissue, duration of anesthesia required, and physical condition of patient (maximum: 4.5 mg/kg/dose); do not repeat within 2 hours

Adults: Varies with procedure, degree of anesthesia needed, vascularity of tissue, duration of anesthesia required, and physical condition of patient (maximum: 4.5 mg/kg/dose); do not repeat within 2 hours

Ophthalmic:

Children: 2 drops to ocular surface; may repeat to maintain effect

Adults: 2 drops to ocular surface; may repeat to maintain effect

Topical:

Cream:

Children <2 years: LidaMantle®: Apply to affected area 2-3 times/day as needed

Children 2-12 years:

LidaMantle®: Apply to affected area 2-3 times/day as needed

L-M-X™ 4: Apply 1/4 inch thick layer to intact skin, remove once adequate anesthetic effect obtained

Children ≥12 years:

LidaMantle®: Apply to affected area 2-3 times/day as needed

L-M-X™ 4: Apply 1/4 inch thick layer to intact skin, remove once adequate anesthetic effect obtained

L-M-X™ 5: Apply to clean, dry area or using applicator, insert rectally, ≤6 times/day

Adults:

LidaMantle®: Apply to affected area 2-3 times/day as needed

L-M-X™ 4: Apply 1/4 inch thick layer to intact skin, remove once adequate anesthetic effect obtained

L-M-X™ 5: Apply to clean, dry area or using applicator, insert rectally, ≤6 times/day

Gel, ointment, solution:

Children: Dosage not established

Adults: Apply to affected area ≤3 times/day as needed (maximum: 4.5 mg/kg/dose; 300 mg/dose)

Jelly:

Children <10 years: Dosage not established

Children ≥10 years: Dose varies with age and weight (maximum: 4.5 mg/kg/dose)

Adults: 5-30 mL (maximum: 30 mL (600mg)/12 hour period)

Liquid:

Children <5 years: Dosage not established

Children ≥5 years: Apply to affected area every 6 hours as needed

Adults: Apply to affected area every 6 hours as needed

Patch:

Children: Dosage not established

Adults: Apply up to 3 patches in a single application for up to 12 hours in any 24-hour period.

Intradermal:

Children <3 years: Dosage not established

Children 3-18 years: Zingo™: 0.5 mg to site of venipuncture or peripheral I.V. cannulation, 1-3 minutes prior to procedure

Adults: Dosage not established

Dosage Forms Excipient information presented when available (limited, particularly for generics); consult specific product labeling. [DSC] = Discontinued product

Aerosol, topical [foam]:

Anestafoam™: 4% (30 g) [contains benzalkonium chloride and benzyl alcohol]

Cream, rectal (L-M-X™ 5): 5% (15 g) [contains benzyl alcohol; packaged with applicator]; (30 g) [contains benzyl alcohol]

Cream, topical (L-M-X™ 4): 4% (5 g) [contains benzyl alcohol; packaged with Tegaderm™ dressing]; (15 g, 30 g) [contains benzyl alcohol]

Cream, topical, as hydrochloride: 3% (30 g)

LidaMantle®: 3% (30 g, 85 g)

Gel, ophthalmic:

Akten™: 3.5% (5 mL) [preservative free]

Gel, topical:

Burn-O-Jel: 0.5% (90 g)

Topicaine®: 4% (10 g, 30 g, 113 g) [contains alcohol 35%, benzyl alcohol, aloe vera, and jojoba]

Gel, topical, as hydrochloride:

Burn Jel®: 2% (3.5 g, 120 g)

Solarcaine® Aloe Extra Burn Relief: 0.5% (113 g, 226 g) [contains aloe vera gel and tartrazine]

Unburn®: 2.5% (3.5 g, 59 mL, 118 mL) [contains vitamin E]

Infusion, as hydrochloride [premixed in D_5W]: 0.4% [4 mg/mL] (250 mL, 500 mL); 0.8% [8 mg/mL] (250 mL, 500 mL)
Injection, solution, as hydrochloride: 0.5% [5 mg/mL] (50 mL); 1% [10 mg/mL] (2 mL, 10 mL, 20 mL, 30 mL, 50 mL); 2% [20 mg/mL] (2 mL, 5 mL, 20 mL, 50 mL)
Xylocaine®: 0.5% [5 mg/mL] (50 mL); 1% [10 mg/mL] (10 mL, 20 mL, 50 mL); 2% [20 mg/mL] (1.8 mL, 10 mL, 20 mL, 50 mL)
Injection, solution, as hydrochloride [preservative free]: 0.5% [5 mg/mL] (50 mL); 1% [10 mg/mL] (2 mL, 5 mL, 30 mL); 1.5% [15 mg/mL] (20 mL); 2% [20 mg/mL] (2 mL, 5 mL, 10 mL); 4% [40 mg/mL] (5 mL)
Xylocaine®: 10% [100 mg/mL] (5 mL) [for ventricular arrhythmias]
Xylocaine® MPF: 0.5% [5 mg/mL] (50 mL); 1% [10 mg/mL] (2 mL, 5 mL, 10 mL, 30 mL); 1.5% [15 mg/mL] (10 mL, 20 mL); 2% [20 mg/mL] (2 mL, 5 mL, 10 mL); 4% [40 mg/mL] (5 mL)
Injection, solution, as hydrochloride [premixed in $D_{7.5}W$, preservative free]: 5% (2 mL)
Xylocaine® MPF: 1.5% (2 mL) [DSC]
Jelly, topical, as hydrochloride: 2% (5 mL, 30 mL)
Anestacon®: 2% (15 mL) [contains benzalkonium chloride]
Xylocaine®: 2% (5 mL, 30 mL)
Liquid, topical (Zilactin®-L): 2.5% (7.5 mL)
Lotion, topical, as hydrochloride (LidaMantle®): 3% (177 mL)
Ointment, topical: 5% (37 g, 50 g)
Powder, intradermal, as hydrochloride:
Zingo™: 0.5 mg
Solution, topical, as hydrochloride: 4% [40 mg/mL] (50 mL)
Band-Aid® Hurt-Free™ Antiseptic Wash: 2% (180 mL)
LTA® 360: 4% [40 mg/mL] (4 mL) [packaged with cannula for laryngotracheal administration]
Xylocaine®: 4% [40 mg/mL] (50 mL)
Solution, viscous, as hydrochloride: 2% [20 mg/mL] (20 mL, 100 mL)
Xylocaine® Viscous: 2% [20 mg/mL] (100 mL, 450 mL)
Spray, topical:
Burnamycin: 0.5% (60 mL) [contains aloe vera gel and menthol]
Premjact®: 9.6% (13 mL)
Solarcaine® Aloe Extra Burn Relief: 0.5% (127 g) [contains aloe vera]
Transdermal system, topical (Lidoderm®): 5% (30s)

- ◆ **Lidocaine Hydrochloride** *see* Lidocaine *on page 924*
- ◆ **Lidoderm®** *see* Lidocaine *on page 924*
- ◆ **Lignocaine Hydrochloride** *see* Lidocaine *on page 924*
- ◆ **Limbitrol®** *see* Amitriptyline and Chlordiazepoxide *on page 94*
- ◆ **Limbitrol® DS** *see* Amitriptyline and Chlordiazepoxide *on page 94*
- ◆ **Limbrel™** *see* Flavocoxid *on page 633*
- ◆ **Lincocin®** *see* Lincomycin *on page 926*

Lincomycin (lin koe MYE sin)

Medication Safety Issues
Sound-alike/look-alike issues:
Lincocin® may be confused with Cleocin®, Indocin®, Minocin®
International issues:
Lincocin® may be confused with Lidosen® which is a brand name for lidocaine in Italy
Lincocin® may be confused with Limoxin® which is a brand name for amoxicillin in Mexico

U.S. Brand Names Lincocin®
Canadian Brand Names Lincocin®
Mexican Brand Names Libiocid; Lincocin; Princol
Index Terms Lincomycin Hydrochloride
Pharmacologic Category Antibiotic, Lincosamide
Use Treatment of serious susceptible bacterial infections, mainly those caused by streptococci, pneumococci, and staphylococci resistant to other agents
Effect on Mental Status May cause dizziness
Effect on Psychiatric Treatment May cause granulocytopenia; use caution with clozapine and carbamazepine
Dosage Summary
I.M.:
Children ≤1 month: Dosage not established

Children >1 month: 10 mg/kg every 12-24 hours
Adults: 600 mg every 12-24 hours

I.V.:

Children ≤1 month: Dosage not established
Children >1 month: 10-20 mg/kg/day divided every 8-12 hours
Adults: 600 mg to 1 g every 8-12 hours (maximum: 8 g/day)

Subconjunctival injection:

Children: Dosage not established
Adults: 75 mg

Dosage Forms Excipient information presented when available (limited, particularly for generics); consult specific product labeling.

Injection, solution, as hydrochloride: 300 mg/mL (2 mL, 10 mL) [contains benzyl alcohol]

◆ **Lincomycin Hydrochloride** *see* Lincomycin *on page 926*

Lindane (LIN dane)

Canadian Brand Names Hexit™; PMS-Lindane

Mexican Brand Names Herklin

Index Terms Benzene Hexachloride; Gamma Benzene Hexachloride; Hexachlorocyclohexane

Pharmacologic Category Antiparasitic Agent, Topical; Pediculocide; Scabicidal Agent

Use Treatment of *Sarcoptes scabiei* (scabies), *Pediculus capitis* (head lice), and *Phthirus pubis* (crab lice); FDA recommends reserving lindane as a second-line agent or with inadequate response to other therapies

Effect on Mental Status May cause dizziness or restlessness

Effect on Psychiatric Treatment May cause aplastic anemia; use caution with clozapine and carbamazepine

Restrictions An FDA-approved medication guide must be distributed when dispensing an outpatient prescription (new or refill) where this medication is to be used without direct supervision of a healthcare provider. Medication guides are available at http://www.fda.gov/cder/Offices/ODS/medication_guides.htm.

Dosage Summary

Topical:

Lotion:

Children: Apply a thin layer and massage onto skin from the neck to the toes; bathe and remove drug after 8-12 hours

Adults: Apply a thin layer and massage onto skin from the neck to the toes; bathe and remove drug after 8-12 hours

Shampoo:

Children: Apply to dry hair and massage for 4 minutes; add small quantities of water until lather forms, then rinse thoroughly and comb with a fine tooth comb to remove nits (maximum: 60 mL)

Adults: Apply to dry hair and massage for 4 minutes; add small quantities of water until lather forms, then rinse thoroughly and comb with a fine tooth comb to remove nits (maximum: 60 mL)

Dosage Forms Excipient information presented when available (limited, particularly for generics); consult specific product labeling.

Lotion, topical: 1% (60 mL)
Shampoo, topical: 1% (60 mL) [contains alcohol 0.5%]

Linezolid (li NE zoh lid)

Medication Safety Issues

Sound-alike/look-alike issues:

Zyvox® may be confused with Ziox™, Zosyn®, Zovirax®

U.S. Brand Names Zyvox®

Canadian Brand Names Zyvoxam®

Mexican Brand Names Zyvoxam

Pharmacologic Category Antibiotic, Oxazolidinone

Use Treatment of vancomycin-resistant *Enterococcus faecium* (VRE) infections, nosocomial pneumonia caused by *Staphylococcus aureus* including MRSA or *Streptococcus pneumoniae* (including multidrug-resistant strains [MDRSP]), complicated and uncomplicated skin and skin structure infections (including diabetic foot infections without concomitant osteomyelitis), and community-acquired pneumonia caused by susceptible gram-positive organisms

Effect on Mental Status May cause insomnia and dizziness

Effect on Psychiatric Treatment Has mild MAO inhibitor properties and has the potential to have the same interactions as other MAO inhibitors; thrombocytopenia has been reported and may be dependent on duration of therapy (generally >2 weeks of treatment), caution with valproic acid; avoid use with serotonergic agents such as TCAs, venlafaxine, trazodone, sibutramine, meperidine, dextromethorphan, and SSRIs; may cause leukopenia, use caution with clozapine and carbamazepine

Dosage Summary

I.V.:

Preterm neonates (<34 weeks gestational age): 10 mg/kg every 8-12 hours
Children ≤11 years: 10 mg/kg every 8 hours
Children ≥12 years: 600 mg every 12 hours
Adults: 600 mg every 12 hours

Oral:

Preterm neonates (<34 weeks gestational age): 10 mg/kg every 8-12 hours
Children <5 years: 10 mg/kg every 8 hours
Children 5-11 years: 10 mg/kg every 8-12 hours
Children ≥12 years: 400-600 mg every 12 hours
Adults: 400-600 mg every 12 hours

Dosage Forms Excipient information presented when available (limited, particularly for generics); consult specific product labeling.

Infusion [premixed]:

Zyvox®: 200 mg (100 mL) [contains sodium 1.7 mEq]; 600 mg (300 mL) [contains sodium 5 mEq]

Powder for oral suspension:

Zyvox®: 20 mg/mL (150 mL) [contains phenylalanine 20 mg/5 mL, sodium benzoate, and sodium 0.4 mEq/5 mL; orange flavor]

Tablet:

Zyvox®: 600 mg [contains sodium 0.1 mEq/tablet]

◆ **Lioresal®** *see* Baclofen *on page 168*

Liothyronine (lye oh THYE roe neen)

Medication Safety Issues

Sound-alike/look-alike issues:

Liothyronine may be confused with levothyroxine

T3 is an error-prone abbreviation (mistaken as acetaminophen and codeine [ie, Tylenol® #3])

U.S. Brand Names Cytomel®; Triostat®

Canadian Brand Names Cytomel®

Mexican Brand Names Cynomel; Triyotex

Index Terms Liothyronine Sodium; Sodium *L*-Triiodothyronine; T_3 Sodium (error-prone abbreviation)

Pharmacologic Category Thyroid Product

Generic Available Yes: Injection

Use

Oral: Replacement or supplemental therapy in hypothyroidism; management of nontoxic goiter; a diagnostic aid

I.V.: Treatment of myxedema coma/precoma

Effect on Mental Status May cause nervousness or insomnia

Effect on Psychiatric Treatment Used to augment antidepressants

Pregnancy Risk Factor A

Pregnancy Considerations Untreated hypothyroidism may have adverse effects on fetal growth and development, and is associated with higher rate of complications; treatment should not be discontinued during pregnancy.

Lactation Enters breast milk (small amounts)/compatible

Contraindications Hypersensitivity to liothyronine sodium or any component of the formulation; undocumented or uncorrected adrenal insufficiency; recent myocardial infarction or thyrotoxicosis; artificial rewarming (injection)

Warnings/Precautions [U.S. Boxed Warning]: Ineffective and potentially toxic for weight reduction. High doses may produce serious or even life-threatening toxic effects particularly when used with some anorectic drugs. Use with extreme caution in patients with angina pectoris or other cardiovascular disease (including hypertension) or coronary artery disease. Use with caution in elderly patients since they may be more likely to have compromised cardiovascular function. Patients with adrenal insufficiency, myxedema, diabetes mellitus and insipidus may have symptoms exaggerated or aggravated. Thyroid replacement requires periodic assessment of thyroid status. Chronic hypothyroidism predisposes patients to coronary artery disease.

Adverse Reactions

1% to 10%: Cardiovascular: Arrhythmia (6%), tachycardia (3%), cardiopulmonary arrest (2%), hypotension (2%), MI (2%)

<1% (Limited to important or life-threatening): Allergic skin reactions, angina, CHF, fever, hypertension, phlebitis, twitching

Drug Interactions

Bile Acid Sequestrants: May decrease the absorption of Thyroid Products. *Risk C: Monitor therapy*

CarBAMazepine: May decrease the serum concentration of Thyroid Products. *Risk C: Monitor therapy*

Estrogen Derivatives: May diminish the therapeutic effect of Thyroid Products. *Risk C: Monitor therapy*

Phenytoin: May increase the metabolism of Thyroid Products. Phenytoin may also displace thyroid hormones from protein binding sites. *Risk C: Monitor therapy*

Rifampin: May decrease the serum concentration of Thyroid Products. *Risk C: Monitor therapy*

Sodium Iodide I131: Thyroid Products may diminish the therapeutic effect of Sodium Iodide I131. *Risk X: Avoid combination*

Theophylline Derivatives: Thyroid Products may increase the metabolism of Theophylline Derivatives. **Exceptions:** Dyphylline. *Risk C: Monitor therapy*

Vitamin K Antagonists (eg, warfarin): Thyroid Products may enhance the anticoagulant effect of Vitamin K Antagonists. *Risk D: Consider therapy modification*

Stability Vials must be stored under refrigeration at 2°C to 8°C (36°F to 46°F). Store tablets at 15°C to 30°C (59°F to 86°F).

Mechanism of Action Exact mechanism of action is unknown; however, it is believed the thyroid hormone exerts its many metabolic effects through control of DNA transcription and protein synthesis; involved in normal metabolism, growth, and development; promotes gluconeogenesis, increases utilization and mobilization of glycogen stores, and stimulates protein synthesis, increases basal metabolic rate

Pharmacodynamics/Kinetics

Onset of action: 2-4 hours

Peak response: 2-3 days

Absorption: Oral: Well absorbed (95% in 4 hours)

Half-life elimination: 2.5 days

Excretion: Urine

Dosage Doses should be adjusted based on clinical response and laboratory parameters.

Children: Congenital hypothyroidism: Oral: 5 mcg/day increase by 5 mcg every 3-4 days until the desired response is achieved. Usual maintenance dose: 20 mcg/day for infants, 50 mcg/day for children 1-3 years of age, and adult dose for children >3 years.

Adults:

Hypothyroidism: Oral: 25 mcg/day increase by increments of 12.5-25 mcg/day every 1-2 weeks to a maximum of 100 mcg/day; usual maintenance dose: 25-75 mcg/day.

Patients with cardiovascular disease: Refer to Elderly dosing.

T_3 suppression test: Oral: 75-100 mcg/day for 7 days; use lowest dose for elderly

Myxedema: Oral: Initial: 5 mcg/day; increase in increments of 5-10 mcg/day every 1-2 weeks. When 25 mcg/day is reached, dosage may be increased at intervals of 5-25 mcg/day every 1-2 weeks. Usual maintenance dose: 50-100 mcg/day.

Myxedema coma: I.V.: 25-50 mcg

Patients with known or suspected cardiovascular disease: 10-20 mcg

Note: Normally, at least 4 hours should be allowed between doses to adequately assess therapeutic response and no more than 12 hours should elapse between doses to avoid fluctuations in hormone levels. Oral therapy should be resumed as soon as the clinical situation has been stabilized and the patient is able to take oral medication. If levothyroxine rather than liothyronine sodium is used in initiating oral therapy, the physician should bear in mind that there is a delay of several days in the onset of levothyroxine activity and that I.V. therapy should be discontinued gradually.

Simple (nontoxic) goiter: Oral: Initial: 5 mcg/day; increase by 5-10 mcg every 1-2 weeks; after 25 mcg/day is reached, may increase dose by 12.5-25 mcg. Usual maintenance dose: 75 mcg/day

Elderly: Oral: 5 mcg/day; increase by 5 mcg/day every 2 weeks

Administration I.V.: For I.V. use only; **do not administer I.M. or SubQ**
Administer doses at least 4 hours, and no more than 12 hours, apart
Resume oral therapy as soon as the clinical situation has been stabilized and the patient is able to take oral medication
When switching to tablets, discontinue the injectable, initiate oral therapy at a low dosage and increase gradually according to response
If **levothyroxine** is used for oral therapy, there is a delay of several days in the onset of activity; therefore, discontinue I.V. therapy gradually.

Monitoring Parameters T_3, TSH, heart rate, blood pressure, renal function, clinical signs of hypo- and hyperthyroidism; TSH is the most reliable guide for evaluating adequacy of thyroid replacement dosage. TSH may be elevated during the first few months of thyroid replacement despite patients being clinically euthyroid. In cases where T_4 remains low and TSH is within normal limits, an evaluation of "free" (unbound) T_4 is needed to evaluate further increase in dosage.

Reference Range Free T_3, serum: 250-390 pg/dL; TSH: 0.4 and up to 10 (≥80 years) mIU/L; remains normal in pregnancy

Additional Information Equivalent doses: The following statement on relative potency of thyroid products is included in a joint statement by American Thyroid Association (ATA), American Association of Clinical Endocrinologists (AACE) and The Endocrine Society (TES): For purposes of conversion, levothyroxine sodium (T_4) 100 mcg is usually considered equivalent to desiccated thyroid 60 mg, thyroglobulin 60 mg, or liothyronine sodium (T_3) 25 mcg. However, these are rough guidelines only and do not obviate the careful re-evaluation of a patient when switching thyroid hormone preparations, including a change from one brand of levothyroxine to another. Joint position statement is available at http://www.thyroid.org/professionals/advocacy/04_12_08_thyroxine.html.

A synthetic form of *L*-Triiodothyronine (T_3) can be used in patients allergic to products derived from pork or beef.

Note: Several medications have effects on thyroid production or conversion. The impact in thyroid replacement has not been specifically evaluated, but patient response should be monitored:

Methimazole: Decreases thyroid hormone secretion, while propylthiouracil decrease thyroid hormone secretion and decreases conversion of T_4 to T_3.
Beta-adrenergic antagonists: Decrease conversion of T_4 to T_3 (dose related, propranolol ≥160 mg/day); patients may be clinically euthyroid.
Iodide, iodine-containing radiographic contrast agents may decrease thyroid hormone secretion; may also increase thyroid hormone secretion, especially in patients with Graves' disease.
Other agents reported to impact on thyroid production/conversion include aminoglutethimide, amiodarone, chloral hydrate, diazepam, ethionamide, interferon-alpha, interleukin-2, lithium, lovastatin (case report), glucocorticoids (dose-related), mercaptopurine, sulfonamides, thiazide diuretics, and tolbutamide.

In addition, a number of medications have been noted to cause transient depression in TSH secretion, which may complicate interpretation of monitoring tests for thyroid hormones, including corticosteroids, octreotide, and dopamine. Metoclopramide may increase TSH secretion.

Dosage Forms Excipient information presented when available (limited, particularly for generics); consult specific product labeling.
Injection, solution: 10 mcg/mL (1 mL)
Triostat®: 10 mcg/mL (1 mL) [contains ethanol 6.8%]
Tablet, oral:
Cytomel®: 5 mcg, 25 mcg, 50 mcg

◆ **Liothyronine Sodium** *see* Liothyronine *on page 928*

Liotrix (LYE oh triks)

Medication Safety Issues
Sound-alike/look-alike issues:
Liotrix may be confused with Klotrix®
Thyrolar® may be confused with Theolair™, Thyrogen®, Thytropar®

U.S. Brand Names Thyrolar®

Canadian Brand Names Thyrolar®

Index Terms T_3/T_4 Liotrix

Pharmacologic Category Thyroid Product

Use Replacement or supplemental therapy in hypothyroidism (uniform mixture of T_4:T_3 in 4:1 ratio by weight); little advantage to this product exists and cost is not justified

Effect on Mental Status May cause nervousness or insomnia

Effect on Psychiatric Treatment None reported

Dosage Summary

Oral:

Children 0-6 months: 8-10 mcg/kg **or** 25-50 mcg/day

Children 6-12 months: 6-8 mcg/kg **or** 50-75 mcg/day

Children 1-5 years: 5-6 mcg/kg **or** 75-100 mcg/day

Children 6-12 years: 4-5 mcg/kg **or** 100-150 mcg/day

Children >12 years: 2-3 mcg/kg **or** >150 mcg/day

Adults: Initial: 15-30 mg/day (lower dose in cardiovascualr impairment and elderly); Usual maintenance: 60-120 mg/day; **Note:** Titration is recommended

Elderly: Initial: 15 mg, adjust dose at 2- to 4-week intervals by increments of 15 mg

Dosage Forms Excipient information presented when available (limited, particularly for generics); consult specific product labeling.

Tablet:

1/4 [levothyroxine sodium 12.5 mcg and liothyronine sodium 3.1 mcg]
1/2 [levothyroxine sodium 25 mcg and liothyronine sodium 6.25 mcg]
1 [levothyroxine sodium 50 mcg and liothyronine sodium 12.5 mcg]
2 [levothyroxine sodium 100 mcg and liothyronine sodium 25 mcg]
3 [levothyroxine sodium 150 mcg and liothyronine sodium 37.5 mcg]

- ◆ **Lipitor®** *see* Atorvastatin *on page 153*
- ◆ **Lipofen™** *see* Fenofibrate *on page 620*
- ◆ **Liposomal DAUNOrubicin** *see* DAUNOrubicin Citrate (Liposomal) *on page 421*
- ◆ **Liposomal DOXOrubicin** *see* DOXOrubicin (Liposomal) *on page 508*
- ◆ **Liquadd™** *see* Dextroamphetamine *on page 441*
- ◆ **Liquibid-D®** *see* Guaifenesin and Phenylephrine *on page 742*
- ◆ **Liquid Antidote** *see* Charcoal *on page 312*
- ◆ **Liqui-Doss® [OTC] [DSC]** *see* Mineral Oil *on page 1055*
- ◆ **Liquid Paraffin** *see* Mineral Oil *on page 1055*

Lisdexamfetamine (lis dex am FET a meen)

Medication Safety Issues

Sound-alike/look-alike issues:

Vyvanse™ may be confused with Vytorin®, Glucovance®, Vivactil®

Related Information

Stimulant Agents Used for ADHD *on page 1797*

U.S. Brand Names Vyvanse™

Index Terms Lisdexamfetamine Dimesylate; Lisdexamphetamine; NRP104

Pharmacologic Category Stimulant

Generic Available No

Use Treatment of attention-deficit/hyperactivity disorder (ADHD)

Restrictions C-II

An FDA-approved medication guide must be distributed when dispensing an outpatient prescription (new or refill) where this medication is to be used without direct supervision of a healthcare provider. Medication guides are available at http://www.fda.gov/cder/Offices/ODS/medication_guides.htm.

Pregnancy Risk Factor C

Pregnancy Considerations Animal studies have shown that amphetamines may cause embryotoxic and teratogenic effects and that pre- or early postnatal exposure to amphetamines may lead to lasting changes in behavior, including impaired learning, memory, and motor skills, as well as changes to libido. There are no adequate and well-controlled studies in pregnant women. No reproductive studies have been performed with lisdexamfetamine. Infants born to mothers dependent on amphetamines are more likely to arrive prematurely with low birth weight and may experience withdrawal symptoms including irritation, restlessness, anxiousness, weakness, listlessness, or lethargy.

Lactation Enters breast milk/not recommended

Contraindications Known hypersensitivity or idiosyncratic reaction sympathomimetic amines; advanced arteriosclerosis, symptomatic cardiovascular disease, moderate-to-severe hypertension; hyperthyroidism; glaucoma; agitated states; history of drug abuse; concurrent use or within 2 weeks of use of MAO inhibitors

Warnings/Precautions [U.S. Boxed Warning]: Use has been associated with serious cardiovascular events including sudden death in patients

with pre-existing structural cardiac abnormalities or other serious heart problems (sudden death in children and adolescents; sudden death, stroke and MI in adults. Use of this product should be avoided in the patients with known serious structural cardiac abnormalities, cardiomyopathy, serious heart rhythm abnormalities, coronary artery disease (adults), or other serious cardiac problems that could increase the risk of sudden death that these conditions alone carry. Patients should be carefully evaluated for these cardiac disorders prior to initiation of therapy.

Use with caution in patients with psychiatric or seizure disorders. May exacerbate symptoms of behavior and thought disorder in psychotic patients. Stimulants may unmask tics in individuals with coexisting Tourette's syndrome. **[U.S. Boxed Warning]: Potential for drug dependency exists; prolonged use may lead to drug dependency.** Use is contraindicated is patients with history of ethanol or drug abuse. Prescriptions should be written for the smallest quantity consistent with good patient care to minimize the possibility of overdose. Abrupt discontinuation following high doses or for prolonged periods may result in symptoms for withdrawal. Recommended to be used as part of a comprehensive treatment program for attention deficit disorders. Safety and efficacy of long-term use have not yet been established. Safety and efficacy in children <6 years of age or children >12 years of age have not been established. Amphetamines are not recommended in children <3 years of age. Appetite suppression may occur; monitor weight during therapy, particularly in children. Use of stimulants has been associated with slowing of growth rate; monitor growth rate during treatment. Treatment interruption may be necessary in patients who are not growing or gaining weight as expected.

Adverse Reactions

>10%:

Central nervous system: Headache (children 12%), insomnia (19% to 27%; 4% [initially])

Gastrointestinal: Appetite decreased (27% to 39%), xerostomia (children 5%; adults 26%), abdominal pain (children 12%)

1% to 10%:

Cardiovascular: Blood pressure increased (adults 3%), heart rate increased (adults 2%)

Central nervous system: Irritability (children 10%), anxiety (adults 6%), dizziness (children 5%), jitteriness (adults 4%), affect lability (children 3%), agitation (adults 3%), restlessness (adults 3%), fever (children: 2%), somnolence (children 2%), tic (children 2%)

Dermatologic: Hyperhidrosis (adults 3%), rash (children 3%)

Gastrointestinal: Vomiting (children 9%), weight loss (children 9%), diarrhea (adults 7%), nausea (6% to 7%), anorexia (adult: 5%)

Neuromuscular & skeletal: Tremor (adults 2%)

Respiratory: Dyspnea (adults 2%)

Additional adverse reaction associated with amphetamines; frequency not defined.

Cardiovascular: Cardiomyopathy, hypertension, MI, palpitation, sudden death, tachycardia

Central nervous system: Depression, dyskinesia, dysphoria, euphoria, exacerbation of motor and phonic tics, Tourette's syndrome, overstimulation, psychotic episodes, seizure, stroke

Dermatologic: Angioedema, Stevens-Johnson syndrome, toxic epidermal necrolysis, urticaria

Endocrine & metabolic: Libido changes

Gastrointestinal: Abnormal taste, constipation

Genitourinary: Impotence

Miscellaneous: Anaphylaxis

Drug Interactions

Alkalinizing Agents: May decrease the excretion of Amphetamines. *Risk D: Consider therapy modification*

Ammonium Chloride: May decrease the serum concentration of Amphetamines. This effect is likely due to an enhanced excretion of amphetamines in the urine. *Risk C: Monitor therapy*

Analgesics (Opioid): Amphetamines may enhance the analgesic effect of Analgesics (Opioid). *Risk C: Monitor therapy*

Antacids: May decrease the excretion of Amphetamines. *Risk C: Monitor therapy*

Antihistamines: Amphetamines may diminish the sedative effect of Antihistamines. *Risk C: Monitor therapy*

Antipsychotics: May diminish the stimulatory effect of Amphetamines. *Risk C: Monitor therapy*

Cannabinoids: May enhance the tachycardic effect of Sympathomimetics. *Risk C: Monitor therapy*

Carbonic Anhydrase Inhibitors: May decrease the excretion of Amphetamines. **Exceptions:** Brinzolamide; Dorzolamide. *Risk C: Monitor therapy*

Ethosuximide: Amphetamines may diminish the therapeutic effect of Ethosuximide. Amphetamines may decrease the serum concentration of Ethosuximide. *Risk C: Monitor therapy*

Gastrointestinal Acidifying Agents: May decrease the serum concentration of Amphetamines. *Risk C: Monitor therapy*

Lithium: May diminish the stimulatory effect of Amphetamines. *Risk C: Monitor therapy*

MAO Inhibitors: May enhance the hypertensive effect of Amphetamines. *Risk X: Avoid combination*

Methenamine: May decrease the serum concentration of Amphetamines. This effect is likely due to an enhanced excretion of amphetamines in the urine. *Risk C: Monitor therapy*

PHENobarbital: Amphetamines may decrease the serum concentration of PHENobarbital. *Risk C: Monitor therapy*

Phenytoin: Amphetamines may decrease the serum concentration of Phenytoin. *Risk C: Monitor therapy*

Sympathomimetics: May enhance the adverse/toxic effect of other Sympathomimetics. *Risk C: Monitor therapy*

Tricyclic Antidepressants: May enhance the stimulatory effect of Amphetamines. Tricyclic Antidepressants may also potentiate the cardiovascular effects of Amphetamines. *Risk C: Monitor therapy*

Ethanol/Nutrition/Herb Interactions

Ethanol: Avoid ethanol (may increase CNS depression).

Food: High-fat meal prolongs T_{max} by ~1 hour.

Stability Store at controlled room temperature of 25°C (77°F) excursions permitted to 15°C to 30°C (59°F to 86°F). Protect from light.

Mechanism of Action Lisdexamfetamine dimesylate is a prodrug that is converted to the active component dextroamphetamine (a noncatecholamine, sympathomimetic amine); CNS stimulant effects are thought to result from the interference of norepinephrine and dopamine reuptake into presynaptic neurons as well as increasing their release from nerve terminals; inhibits the actions of monoamine oxidase; peripheral actions include increase in systolic and diastolic blood pressure as well as weak bronchodilator and respiratory stimulant action.

Pharmacodynamics/Kinetics

Absorption: Rapid

Distribution: Dextroamphetamine: V_d: Adults: 3.5-4.6 L/kg; distributes into CNS; mean CSF concentrations are 80% of plasma; enters breast milk

Metabolism: Non-CYP-mediated hepatic or intestinal metabolism to dextroamphetamine and l-lysine

Half-life elimination: Lisdexamfetamine: <1 hour; Dextroamphetamine: 10-13 hours

Time to peak, serum: T_{max}: Lisdexamfetamine: ~1 hour; Dextroamphetamine: ~3.5 hours

Excretion: Urine (96%, 42% as amphetamine-related compounds, 2% as lisdexamfetamine, 25% hippuric acid); feces (minimal)

Dosage Oral: Individualize dosage based on patient need and response to therapy. Administer at the lowest effective dose.

Children: 6-12 years and Adults: Initial: 30 mg once daily in the morning; may increase in increments of 10 mg or 20 mg/day at weekly intervals until optimal response is obtained; maximum: 70 mg/day

Dietary Considerations May be taken with or without food.

Administration Administer in the morning with or without food; swallow capsule whole, do not chew; capsule may be opened and the contents dissolved in glass of water; consume the resulting solution immediately; do not store solution.

Monitoring Parameters Cardiac evaluation should be completed on any patient who develops chest pain, unexplained syncope, and any symptom of cardiac disease during treatment with stimulants; growth and CNS activity in all patients

When used for the treatment of ADHD, thoroughly evaluate for cardiovascular risk. Monitor heart rate, blood pressure, and consider obtaining ECG prior to initiation (Vetter, 2008).

Test Interactions Amphetamines may interfere with urinary steroid determinations.

Dosage Forms
Capsule, as dimesylate:
Vyvanse™: 20 mg, 30 mg, 40 mg, 50 mg, 60 mg, 70 mg

- **Lisdexamfetamine Dimesylate** *see* Lisdexamfetamine *on page 931*
- **Lisdexamphetamine** *see* Lisdexamfetamine *on page 931*

Lisinopril (lyse IN oh pril)

Medication Safety Issues
Sound-alike/look-alike issues:
Lisinopril may be confused with fosinopril, Lioresal®, Risperdal®
Prinivil® may be confused with Plendil®, Pravachol®, Prevacid®, Prilosec®, Proventil®
Zestril® may be confused with Desyrel®, Restoril®, Vistaril®, Zetia®, Zostrix®

International issues:
Acepril® [Denmark] may be confused with Accupril® which is a brand name for quinapril in the U.S.
Acepril®: Brand name for enalapril in Hungary and Switzerland; brand name for captopril in Great Britain
Carace® [Ireland; Great Britain] may be confused with Carac™ which is a brand name for fluorouracil in the U.S.
Zetril® may be confused with Nostril® which is a brand name for chlorhexidine/cetrimonium in France

Related Information
Angiotensin Agents *on page 1754*

U.S. Brand Names Prinivil®; Zestril®

Canadian Brand Names Apo-Lisinopril®; CO Lisinopril; Gen-Lisinopril; Novo-Lisinopril; PMS-Lisinopril; Prinivil®; Ran-Lisinopril; ratio-Lisinopril; Riva-Lisinopril; Zestril®

Mexican Brand Names Alfaken; Dosteril; Fersivag; Pesatril; Prinivil; Zestril

Pharmacologic Category Angiotensin-Converting Enzyme (ACE) Inhibitor

Generic Available Yes

Use Treatment of hypertension, either alone or in combination with other antihypertensive agents; adjunctive therapy in treatment of heart failure (HF); treatment of acute myocardial infarction (MI) within 24 hours in hemodynamically-stable patients to improve survival

Effect on Mental Status May cause dizziness or fatigue; may rarely cause sedation, insomnia, or depression

Effect on Psychiatric Treatment May cause neutropenia; use caution with clozapine and carbamazepine; may decrease lithium clearance resulting in an increase in serum lithium levels and potential lithium toxicity; monitor serum lithium levels

Pregnancy Risk Factor C (1st trimester); D (2nd and 3rd trimesters)

Pregnancy Considerations Due to adverse events observed in some animal studies, lisinopril is considered pregnancy category C during the first trimester. Based on human data, lisinopril is considered pregnancy category D if used during the second and third trimesters (per the manufacturer; however, one study suggests that fetal injury may occur at anytime during pregnancy). Lisinopril crosses the placenta. First trimester exposure to ACE inhibitors may cause major congenital malformations. An increased risk of cardiovascular and/or central nervous system malformations was observed in one study; however, an increased risk of teratogenic events was not observed in other studies. Second and third trimester use of an ACE inhibitor is associated with oligohydramnios. Oligohydramnios due to decreased fetal renal function may lead to fetal limb contractures, craniofacial deformation, and hypoplastic lung development. The use of ACE inhibitors during the second and third trimesters is also associated with anuria, hypotension, renal failure (reversible or irreversible), skull hypoplasia, and death in the fetus/neonate. Chronic maternal hypertension itself is also associated with adverse events in the fetus/infant. ACE inhibitors are not recommended during pregnancy to treat maternal hypertension or heart failure. Those who are planning a pregnancy should be considered for other medication options if an ACE inhibitor is currently prescribed or the ACE inhibitor should be discontinued as soon as possible once pregnancy is detected. The exposed fetus should be monitored for fetal growth, amniotic fluid volume, and organ formation. Infants exposed to an ACE inhibitor *in utero*, especially during the second and third trimester, should be monitored for hyperkalemia, hypotension, and oliguria.

[U.S. Boxed Warning]: Based on human data, ACE inhibitors can cause injury and death to the developing fetus when used in the second and third trimesters. ACE inhibitors should be discontinued as soon as possible once pregnancy is detected.

Lactation Excretion in breast milk unknown/not recommended

Contraindications Hypersensitivity to lisinopril or any component of the formulation; angioedema related to previous treatment with an ACE inhibitor; patients with idiopathic or hereditary angioedema

Warnings/Precautions Anaphylactic reactions may occur rarely with ACE inhibitors. At any time during treatment (especially following first dose), angioedema may occur rarely with ACE inhibitors; it may involve the head and neck (potentially compromising airway) or the intestine (presenting with abdominal pain). African-Americans may be at an increased risk. Prolonged frequent monitoring may be required especially if tongue, glottis, or larynx are involved as they are associated with airway obstruction. Patients with a history of airway surgery may have a higher risk of airway obstruction. Aggressive early and appropriate management is critical. Use in patients with idiopathic or hereditary angioedema or previous angioedema associated with ACE inhibitor therapy is contraindicated. Severe anaphylactoid reactions may be seen during hemodialysis (eg, CVVHD) with high-flux dialysis membranes (eg, AN69), and rarely, during low density lipoprotein apheresis with dextran sulfate cellulose. Rare cases of anaphylactoid reactions have been reported in patients undergoing sensitization treatment with hymenoptera (bee, wasp) venom while receiving ACE inhibitors.

Symptomatic hypotension with or without syncope can occur with ACE inhibitors (usually with the first several doses); effects are most often observed in volume depleted patients; correct volume depletion prior to initiation; close monitoring of patient is required especially with initial dosing and dosing increases; blood pressure must be lowered at a rate appropriate for the patient's clinical condition. Initiation of therapy in patients with ischemic heart disease or cerebrovascular disease warrants close observation due to the potential consequences posed by falling blood pressure (eg, MI, stroke). Use with caution in hypertrophic cardiomyopathy with outflow tract obstruction, severe aortic stenosis, or before, during, or immediately after major surgery. **[U.S. Boxed Warning]: Based on human data, ACEIs can cause injury and death to the developing fetus when used in the second and third trimesters. ACEIs should be discontinued as soon as possible once pregnancy is detected.**

Hyperkalemia may occur with ACE inhibitors; risk factors include renal dysfunction, diabetes mellitus, concomitant use of potassium-sparing diuretics, potassium supplements, and/or potassium-containing salts. Use cautiously, if at all, with these agents and monitor potassium closely. Cough may occur with ACE inhibitors. Other causes of cough should be considered (eg, pulmonary congestion in patients with heart failure) and excluded prior to discontinuation.

May be associated with deterioration of renal function and/or increases in serum creatinine, particularly in patients with low renal blood flow (eg, renal artery stenosis, heart failure) whose glomerular filtration rate (GFR) is dependent on efferent arteriolar vasoconstriction by angiotensin II; deterioration may result in oliguria, acute renal failure, and progressive azotemia. Small increases in serum creatinine may occur following initiation; consider discontinuation only in patients with progressive and/or significant deterioration in renal function. Use with caution in patients with unstented unilateral/bilateral renal artery stenosis. When unstented bilateral renal artery stenosis is present, use is generally avoided due to the elevated risk of deterioration in renal function unless possible benefits outweigh risks.

Rare toxicities associated with ACE inhibitors include cholestatic jaundice (which may progress to fulminant hepatic necrosis), agranulocytosis, neutropenia, or leukopenia with myeloid hypoplasia. Patients with collagen vascular diseases (especially with concomitant renal impairment) or renal impairment alone may be at increased risk for hematologic toxicity; periodically monitor CBC with differential in these patients. Safety and efficacy have not been established in children <6 years of age or children with a Cl_{cr} ≤30 mL/minute.

Adverse Reactions Note: Frequency ranges include data from hypertension and heart failure trials. Higher rates of adverse reactions have generally been noted in patients with CHF. However, the frequency of adverse effects associated with placebo is also increased in this population.

1% to 10%:

Cardiovascular: Orthostatic effects (1%), hypotension (1% to 4%)

Central nervous system: Headache (4% to 6%), dizziness (5% to 12%), fatigue (3%)
Dermatologic: Rash (1% to 2%)
Endocrine & metabolic: Hyperkalemia (2% to 5%)
Gastrointestinal: Diarrhea (3% to 4%), nausea (2%), vomiting (1%), abdominal pain (2%)
Genitourinary: Impotence (1%)
Hematologic: Decreased hemoglobin (small)
Neuromuscular & skeletal: Chest pain (3%), weakness (1%)
Renal: BUN increased (2%); deterioration in renal function (in patients with bilateral renal artery stenosis or hypovolemia); serum creatinine increased (often transient)
Respiratory: Cough (4% to 9%), upper respiratory infection (1% to 2%)

<1% (Limited to important or life-threatening): Acute renal failure, alopecia, anaphylactoid reactions, angioedema, anuria, arrhythmia, arthralgia, arthritis, asthma, ataxia, azotemia, bilirubin increased, bone marrow suppression, bronchospasm, cardiac arrest, cutaneous pseudolymphoma, decreased libido, gout, hemolytic anemia, hepatic necrosis, hepatitis, hyponatremia, leukopenia, jaundice (cholestatic), MI, neutropenia, oliguria, orthostatic hypotension, pancreatitis, paresthesia, pemphigus, peripheral neuropathy, photosensitivity, pleural effusion, pulmonary embolism, pulmonary infiltrates, SIADH, Stevens-Johnson syndrome, stroke, syncope, systemic lupus erythematosus, thrombocytopenia, TIA, toxic epidermal necrolysis, transaminases increased, tremor, urticaria, vasculitis, vertigo, vision loss, volume overload, vomiting, weight gain/loss, wheezing, xerostomia

Drug Interactions

Allopurinol: ACE Inhibitors may enhance the potential for allergic or hypersensitivity reactions to Allopurinol. *Risk D: Consider therapy modification*

Angiotensin II Receptor Blockers: May enhance the adverse/toxic effect of ACE Inhibitors. *Risk C: Monitor therapy*

Antacids: May decrease the serum concentration of ACE Inhibitors. *Risk C: Monitor therapy*

Aprotinin: May diminish the antihypertensive effect of ACE Inhibitors. *Risk C: Monitor therapy*

AzaTHIOprine: ACE Inhibitors may enhance the neutropenic effect of AzaTHIOprine. *Risk C: Monitor therapy*

CycloSPORINE: ACE Inhibitors may enhance the nephrotoxic effect of CycloSPORINE. *Risk D: Consider therapy modification*

Diazoxide: May enhance the hypotensive effect of Antihypertensives. *Risk C: Monitor therapy*

Eplerenone: May enhance the hyperkalemic effect of ACE Inhibitors. *Risk C: Monitor therapy*

Ferric Gluconate: ACE Inhibitors may enhance the adverse/toxic effect of Ferric Gluconate. *Risk C: Monitor therapy*

Gold Sodium Thiomalate: ACE Inhibitors may enhance the adverse/toxic effect of Gold Sodium Thiomalate. An increased risk of nitritoid reactions has been appreciated. *Risk C: Monitor therapy*

Herbs (Hypertensive Properties): May diminish the antihypertensive effect of Antihypertensives. *Risk C: Monitor therapy*

Herbs (Hypotensive Properties): May enhance the hypotensive effect of Antihypertensives. *Risk C: Monitor therapy*

Lithium: ACE Inhibitors may increase the serum concentration of Lithium. *Risk D: Consider therapy modification*

Loop Diuretics: May enhance the hypotensive effect of ACE Inhibitors. Specifically, postural hypotension which can accompany ACE Inhibitor initiation. Loop Diuretics may enhance the nephrotoxic effect of ACE Inhibitors. *Risk C: Monitor therapy*

Methylphenidate: May diminish the antihypertensive effect of Antihypertensives. *Risk C: Monitor therapy*

Nonsteroidal Anti-Inflammatory Agents: May diminish the antihypertensive effect of ACE Inhibitors. *Risk C: Monitor therapy*

Potassium Salts: May enhance the hyperkalemic effect of ACE Inhibitors. *Risk C: Monitor therapy*

Potassium-Sparing Diuretics: May enhance the hyperkalemic effect of ACE Inhibitors. *Risk C: Monitor therapy*

Prostacyclin Analogues: May enhance the hypotensive effect of Antihypertensives. *Risk C: Monitor therapy*

RiTUXimab: Antihypertensives may enhance the hypotensive effect of RiTUXimab. *Risk D: Consider therapy modification*

Salicylates: May diminish the antihypertensive effect of ACE Inhibitors. They may also diminish other beneficial pharmacodynamic effects desired for the treatment of CHF. The effects are likely dose-related. 100 mg doses aspirin appear to cause no problems, whereas 300 mg doses appear to significantly affect ACE Inhibitor efficacy. *Risk C: Monitor therapy*

Sirolimus: May enhance the adverse/toxic effect of ACE Inhibitors. *Risk C: Monitor therapy*

Temsirolimus: May enhance the adverse/toxic effect of ACE Inhibitors. *Risk C: Monitor therapy*

Thiazide Diuretics: May enhance the hypotensive effect of ACE Inhibitors. Specifically, postural hypotension which can accompany ACE Inhibitor initiation. Thiazide Diuretics may enhance the nephrotoxic effect of ACE Inhibitors. *Risk C: Monitor therapy*

Trimethoprim: May enhance the hyperkalemic effect of ACE Inhibitors. *Risk C: Monitor therapy*

Ethanol/Nutrition/Herb Interactions

Food: Potassium-containing salt substitutes may increase risk of hyperkalemia.

Herb/Nutraceutical: Avoid bayberry, blue cohosh, cayenne, ephedra, ginger, ginseng (American), kola, licorice (may worsen hypertension). Avoid black cohosh, California poppy, coleus, golden seal, hawthorn, mistletoe, periwinkle, quinine, shepherd's purse (may have increased antihypertensive effect).

Mechanism of Action Competitive inhibitor of angiotensin-converting enzyme (ACE); prevents conversion of angiotensin I to angiotensin II, a potent vasoconstrictor; results in lower levels of angiotensin II which causes an increase in plasma renin activity and a reduction in aldosterone secretion; a CNS mechanism may also be involved in hypotensive effect as angiotensin II increases adrenergic outflow from CNS; vasoactive kallikreins may be decreased in conversion to active hormones by ACE inhibitors, thus reducing blood pressure

Pharmacodynamics/Kinetics

Onset of action: 1 hour

Peak effect: Hypotensive: Oral: ~6 hours

Duration: 24 hours

Absorption: Well absorbed; unaffected by food

Protein binding: 25%

Metabolism: Not metabolized

Bioavailability: Decreased with NYHA Class II-IV heart failure

Half-life elimination: 11-12 hours

Time to peak: ~7 hours

Excretion: Primarily urine (as unchanged drug)

Dosage Oral:

Hypertension:

Children ≥6 years: Initial: 0.07 mg/kg once daily (up to 5 mg); increase dose at 1- to 2-week intervals; doses >0.61 mg/kg or >40 mg have not been evaluated.

Adults: Usual dosage range (JNC 7): 10-40 mg/day

Not maintained on diuretic: Initial: 10 mg/day

Maintained on diuretic: Initial: 5 mg/day

Note: Antihypertensive effect may diminish toward the end of the dosing interval especially with doses of 10 mg/day. An increased dose may aid in extending the duration of antihypertensive effect. Doses up to 80 mg/day have been used, but do not appear to give greater effect.

Elderly: Initial: 2.5-5 mg/day; increase doses 2.5-5 mg/day at 1- to 2-week intervals; maximum daily dose: 40 mg

Patients taking diuretics should have them discontinued 2-3 days prior to initiating lisinopril if possible. Restart diuretic after blood pressure is stable if needed. If diuretic cannot be discontinued prior to therapy, begin with 5 mg with close supervision until stable blood pressure. In patients with hyponatremia (<130 mEq/L), start dose at 2.5 mg/day

Heart failure: Adults: Initial: 2.5-5 mg once daily; then increase by no more than 10 mg increments at intervals no less than 2 weeks to a maximum daily dose of 40 mg. Usual maintenance: 5-40 mg/day as a single dose. Target dose: 20-40 mg once daily (ACC/AHA 2005 Heart Failure Guidelines)

Note: If patient has hyponatremia (serum sodium <130 meq/L) or renal impairment (Cl_{cr} <30 mL/minute or creatinine >3 mg/dL), then initial dose should be 2.5 mg/day

Acute myocardial infarction (within 24 hours in hemodynamically stable patients): Oral: 5 mg immediately, then 5 mg at 24 hours, 10 mg at 48 hours, and 10 mg every day thereafter for 6 weeks. Patients should continue to receive standard treatments such as thrombolytics, aspirin, and beta-blockers.

Dosing adjustment in renal impairment:
Hypertension:
Adults: Initial doses should be modified and upward titration should be cautious, based on response (maximum: 40 mg/day)
Cl_{cr} >30 mL/minute: Initial: 10 mg/day
Cl_{cr} 10-30 mL/minute: Initial: 5 mg/day
Hemodialysis: Initial: 2.5 mg/day; dialyzable (50%)
Children: Use in not recommended in pediatric patients with GFR <30 mL/minute/1.73 m^2
Heart failure: Adults: Cl_{cr} <30 mL/minute or creatinine >3 mg/dL): Initial: 2.5 mg/day

Dietary Considerations Use potassium-containing salt substitutes cautiously in patients with diabetes, patients with renal dysfunction, or those maintained on potassium supplements or potassium-sparing diuretics.

Administration Watch for hypotensive effects within 1-3 hours of first dose or new higher dose.

Monitoring Parameters BUN, serum creatinine, renal function, WBC, and potassium; if patient has collagen vascular disease and/or renal impairment, periodically monitor CBC with differential

Test Interactions May cause false-positive results in urine acetone determinations using sodium nitroprusside reagent

Dosage Forms Excipient information presented when available (limited, particularly for generics); consult specific product labeling.
Tablet: 2.5 mg, 5 mg, 10 mg, 20 mg, 30 mg, 40 mg
Prinivil®: 5 mg, 10 mg, 20 mg
Zestril®: 2.5 mg, 5 mg, 10 mg, 20 mg, 30 mg, 40 mg

Lisinopril and Hydrochlorothiazide

(lyse IN oh pril & hye droe klor oh THYE a zide)

U.S. Brand Names Prinzide®; Zestoretic®

Canadian Brand Names Apo-Lisinopril/Hctz; Gen-Lisinopril/Hctz; Novo-Lisinopril/Hctz; Prinzide®; Sandoz Lisinopril/Hctz; Zestoretic®

Mexican Brand Names Prinzide; Zestoretic

Index Terms Hydrochlorothiazide and Lisinopril

Pharmacologic Category Angiotensin-Converting Enzyme (ACE) Inhibitor; Diuretic, Thiazide

Use Treatment of hypertension

Effect on Mental Status May cause dizziness or fatigue; may rarely cause sedation, insomnia, or depression

Effect on Psychiatric Treatment May cause neutropenia; use caution with clozapine and carbamazepine; may decrease lithium clearance resulting in an increase in serum lithium levels and potential lithium toxicity; monitor serum lithium levels

Dosage Summary
Oral:
Children: Dosage not established
Adults: Lisinopril 10-80 mg and hydrochlorothiazide 12.5-50 mg once daily (lisinopril doses >40 mg may not provide additional efficacy)

Dosage Forms Excipient information presented when available (limited, particularly for generics); consult specific product labeling. [DSC] = Discontinued product
Tablet: 10/12.5: Lisinopril 10 mg and hydrochlorothiazide 12.5 mg; 20/12.5: Lisinopril 20 mg and hydrochlorothiazide 12.5 mg; 20/25: Lisinopril 20 mg and hydrochlorothiazide 25 mg
Prinizide®:
10/12.5: Lisinopril 10 mg and hydrochlorothiazide 12.5 mg
20/12.5: Lisinopril 20 mg and hydrochlorothiazide 12.5 mg [DSC]
20/25: Lisinopril 20 mg and hydrochlorothiazide 25 mg
Zestoretic®:
10/12.5: Lisinopril 10 mg and hydrochlorothiazide 12.5 mg
20/12.5: Lisinopril 20 mg and hydrochlorothiazide 12.5 mg
20/25: Lisinopril 20 mg and hydrochlorothiazide 25 mg

◆ **Lispro Insulin** *see* Insulin Lispro *on page 832*

Lithium (LITH ee um)

Medication Safety Issues
Sound-alike/look-alike issues:
Eskalith® may be confused with Estratest®

Lithobid® may be confused with Levbid®, Lithostat®

Do not confuse **mEq** (milliequivalent) with **mg** (milligram). **Note:** 8 mEq lithium carbonate equals 300 mg lithium carbonate. Dosage should be written in **mg** (milligrams) to avoid confusion. Check prescriptions for unusually high volumes of the syrup for dosing errors.

Related Information

Adverse Effects of Approved Mood Stabilizers / Anticonvulsants *on page 1751*

Agents Approved for Bipolar Disorder *on page 1752*

Liquid Compatibility of Antidepressants, Antipsychotics, and Mood Stabilizers *on page 1788*

U.S. Brand Names Eskalith CR® [DSC]; Eskalith® [DSC]; Lithobid®

Canadian Brand Names Apo-Lithium® Carbonate; Apo-Lithium® Carbonate SR; Carbolith™; Duralith®; Lithane™; PMS-Lithium Carbonate; PMS-Lithium Citrate

Mexican Brand Names Carbolit; Litheum 300

Index Terms Lithium Carbonate; Lithium Citrate

Pharmacologic Category Antimanic Agent

Generic Available Yes

Use Management of bipolar disorders; treatment of mania in individuals with bipolar disorder (maintenance treatment prevents or diminishes intensity of subsequent episodes)

Unlabeled/Investigational Use Potential augmenting agent for antidepressants; aggression, post-traumatic stress disorder, conduct disorder in children

Mental Health Comment Lithium remains the gold standard for bipolar disorder. It is most useful for the management of euphoric mania and least effective for the mixed and rapid-cycling types of bipolar disorder. Among patients treated for bipolar disorder, risk of suicide attempt and suicide death is lower during treatment with lithium than during treatment with divalproex (Goodwin, 2003). Fine hand tremor associated with lithium therapy may be treated with propranolol. Incidence of hypothyroidism secondary to lithium therapy is 7% to 8% with a 9:1 female to male ratio. Diabetes insipidus may be treated with a thiazide diuretic (hydrochlorothiazide 25-50 mg/day) or amiloride (5-10 mg twice daily). The thiazide diuretics are thought to work by decreasing intracellular volume via sodium depletion, thereby enhancing reabsorption of sodium and water proximally leading to a decrease in fluid volume to the distal convoluted tubule and collecting duct which increases sodium reabsorption and decreases water excretion. Leukocytosis (without a left shift) begins in the first week of lithium therapy, peaks at 2 weeks.

Goodwin GM and Young AH, "The British Association for Psychopharmacology Guidelines for Treatment of Bipolar Disorder: A Summary," *J Psychopharmacol*, 2003, 17(4 Suppl):3-6.

Pregnancy Risk Factor D

Pregnancy Considerations Cardiac malformations in the infant, including Ebstein's anomaly, are associated with use of lithium during the first trimester of pregnancy. Nontoxic effects to the newborn include shallow respiration, hypotonia, lethargy, cyanosis, diabetes insipidus, thyroid depression, and nontoxic goiter when lithium is used near term. Efforts should be made to avoid lithium use during the first trimester; if an alternative therapy is not appropriate, the lowest possible dose of lithium should be used throughout the pregnancy. Fetal echocardiography and ultrasound to screen for anomalies should be conducted between 16-20 weeks of gestation. Lithium levels should be monitored in the mother and may need to be adjusted following delivery.

Lactation Enters breast milk/contraindicated

Contraindications Hypersensitivity to lithium or any component of the formulation; avoid use in patients with severe cardiovascular or renal disease, or with severe debilitation, dehydration, or sodium depletion; pregnancy

Warnings/Precautions [U.S. Boxed Warning]: Lithium toxicity is closely related to serum levels and can occur at therapeutic doses; serum lithium determinations are required to monitor therapy. Use with caution in patients with thyroid disease, mild-moderate renal impairment, or mild-moderate cardiovascular disease. Use caution in patients receiving medications which alter sodium excretion (eg, diuretics, ACE inhibitors, NSAIDs), or in patients with significant fluid loss (protracted sweating, diarrhea, or prolonged fever); temporary reduction or cessation of therapy may be warranted. Some elderly patients may be extremely sensitive to the effects of lithium, see Dosage and Reference Range. Chronic therapy results in diminished renal concentrating ability (nephrogenic DI); this is usually reversible when lithium is discontinued. Changes in renal function should be monitored, and re-evaluation of treatment may be necessary. Use caution in patients at risk of suicide (suicidal thoughts or behavior).

Use with caution in patients receiving neuroleptic medications - a syndrome resembling NMS has been associated with concurrent therapy. Lithium may impair the patient's alertness, affecting the ability to operate machinery or driving a vehicle. Neuromuscular-blocking agents should be administered with caution; the response may be prolonged.

Higher serum concentrations may be required and tolerated during an acute manic phase; however, the tolerance decreases when symptoms subside. Normal fluid and salt intake must be maintained during therapy.

Safety and efficacy have not been established in children <12 years of age.

Adverse Reactions Frequency not defined.

Cardiovascular: Cardiac arrhythmia, hypotension, sinus node dysfunction, flattened or inverted T waves (reversible), edema, bradycardia, syncope

Central nervous system: Dizziness, vertigo, slurred speech, blackout spells, seizure, sedation, restlessness, confusion, psychomotor retardation, stupor, coma, dystonia, fatigue, lethargy, headache, pseudotumor cerebri, slowed intellectual functioning, tics

Dermatologic: Dry or thinning of hair, folliculitis, alopecia, exacerbation of psoriasis, rash

Endocrine & metabolic: Euthyroid goiter and/or hypothyroidism, hyperthyroidism, hyperglycemia, diabetes insipidus

Gastrointestinal: Polydipsia, anorexia, nausea, vomiting, diarrhea, xerostomia, metallic taste, weight gain, salivary gland swelling, excessive salivation

Genitourinary: Incontinence, polyuria, glycosuria, oliguria, albuminuria

Hematologic: Leukocytosis

Neuromuscular & skeletal: Tremor, muscle hyperirritability, ataxia, choreoathetoid movements, hyperactive deep tendon reflexes, myasthenia gravis (rare)

Ocular: Nystagmus, blurred vision, transient scotoma

Miscellaneous: Coldness and painful discoloration of fingers and toes

Drug Interactions

ACE Inhibitors: May increase the serum concentration of Lithium. *Risk D: Consider therapy modification*

Amphetamines: Lithium may diminish the stimulatory effect of Amphetamines. *Risk C: Monitor therapy*

Angiotensin II Receptor Blockers: May increase the serum concentration of Lithium. Management: Lithium dosage reductions will likely be needed following the addition of an angiotensin II receptor antagonist. *Risk D: Consider therapy modification*

Antipsychotics: Lithium formulations may enhance the neurotoxic effect of Antipsychotics. Lithium formulations may decrease the serum concentration of Antipsychotics. Specifically noted with chlorpromazine. *Risk C: Monitor therapy*

Calcium Channel Blockers (Nondihydropyridine): May enhance the neurotoxic effect of Lithium. Calcium Channel Blockers (Nondihydropyridine) may increase the serum concentration of Lithium. Decreased or unaltered lithium concentrations have also been reported with this combination. *Risk C: Monitor therapy*

CarBAMazepine: May enhance the adverse/toxic effect of Lithium. *Risk C: Monitor therapy*

Desmopressin: Lithium may diminish the therapeutic effect of Desmopressin. Desmopressin may increase the serum concentration of Lithium. *Risk C: Monitor therapy*

MAO Inhibitors: May enhance the adverse/toxic effect of Lithium. **Exceptions:** Moclobemide. *Risk C: Monitor therapy*

Methyldopa: May enhance the adverse/toxic effect of Lithium. This may occur without notable changes in serum lithium concentrations. *Risk C: Monitor therapy*

Neuromuscular-Blocking Agents: Lithium may enhance the neuromuscular-blocking effect of Neuromuscular-Blocking Agents. *Risk C: Monitor therapy*

Nonsteroidal Anti-Inflammatory Agents: May increase the serum concentration of Lithium. **Exceptions:** Sulindac. *Risk D: Consider therapy modification*

Phenytoin: May enhance the adverse/toxic effect of Lithium. *Risk C: Monitor therapy*

Potassium Iodide: May enhance the adverse/toxic effect of Lithium. Specifically the hypothyroid/goiter-potentiating effects. *Risk C: Monitor therapy*

Selective Serotonin Reuptake Inhibitors: May enhance the adverse/toxic effect of Lithium. *Risk C: Monitor therapy*

Serotonin Modulators: May enhance the adverse/toxic effect of other Serotonin Modulators. The development of serotonin syndrome may occur. *Risk D: Consider therapy modification*

Sibutramine: May enhance the serotonergic effect of Serotonin Modulators. This may cause serotonin syndrome. *Risk X: Avoid combination*

Sodium Bicarbonate: May increase the excretion of Lithium. *Risk C: Monitor therapy*

Sodium Chloride: May increase the excretion of Lithium. *Risk C: Monitor therapy*

Theophylline Derivatives: May increase the excretion of Lithium. **Exceptions:** Dyphylline. *Risk C: Monitor therapy*

Thiazide Diuretics: May decrease the excretion of Lithium. *Risk D: Consider therapy modification*

Tricyclic Antidepressants: Lithium may enhance the neurotoxic effect of Tricyclic Antidepressants. *Risk C: Monitor therapy*

Ethanol/Nutrition/Herb Interactions Food: Lithium serum concentrations may be increased if taken with food. Limit caffeine.

Mechanism of Action Alters cation transport across cell membrane in nerve and muscle cells and influences reuptake of serotonin and/or norepinephrine; second messenger systems involving the phosphatidylinositol cycle are inhibited; postsynaptic D2 receptor supersensitivity is inhibited

Pharmacodynamics/Kinetics

Absorption: Rapid and complete

Distribution: V_d: Initial: 0.3-0.4 L/kg; V_{dss}: 0.7-1 L/kg; crosses placenta; enters breast milk at 35% to 50% the concentrations in serum; distribution is complete in 6-10 hours

CSF, liver concentrations: 1/3 to 1/2 of serum concentration

Erythrocyte concentration: ~1/2 of serum concentration

Heart, lung, kidney, muscle concentrations: Equivalent to serum concentration

Saliva concentration: 2-3 times serum concentration

Thyroid, bone, brain tissue concentrations: Increase 50% over serum concentrations

Protein binding: Not protein bound

Metabolism: Not metabolized

Bioavailability: Not affected by food; Capsule, immediate release tablet: 95% to 100%; Extended release tablet: 60% to 90%; Syrup: 100%

Half-life elimination: 18-24 hours; can increase to more than 36 hours in elderly or with renal impairment

Time to peak, serum: Nonsustained release: ~0.5-2 hours; slow release: 4-12 hours; syrup: 15-60 minutes

Excretion: Urine (90% to 98% as unchanged drug); sweat (4% to 5%); feces (1%)

Clearance: 80% of filtered lithium is reabsorbed in the proximal convoluted tubules; therefore, clearance approximates 20% of GFR or 20-40 mL/minute

Dosage Oral: Monitor serum concentrations and clinical response (efficacy and toxicity) to determine proper dose

Children 6-12 years:

Bipolar disorder (unlabeled use): 15-60 mg/kg/day in 3-4 divided doses; dose not to exceed usual adult dosage

Conduct disorder (unlabeled use): 15-30 mg/kg/day in 3-4 divided doses; dose not to exceed usual adult dosage

Adults: Bipolar disorder: 900-2400 mg/day in 3-4 divided doses or 900-1800 mg/day (sustained release) in 2 divided doses

Elderly: Bipolar disorder: Initial dose: 300 mg once or twice daily; increase weekly in increments of 300 mg/day, monitoring levels; rarely need >900-1200 mg/day

Dosing adjustment in renal impairment:

Cl_{cr} 10-50 mL/minute: Administer 50% to 75% of normal dose

Cl_{cr} <10 mL/minute: Administer 25% to 50% of normal dose

Hemodialysis: Dialyzable (50% to 100%); 4-7 times more efficient than peritoneal dialysis

Child/Adolescent Considerations Information regarding the safety and effectiveness of lithium carbonate in children <12 years of age is not available; its use in this population group is not recommended.

Dietary Considerations May be taken with meals to avoid GI upset; have patient drink 2-3 L of water daily.

Administration Administer with meals to decrease GI upset. Slow release tablets must be swallowed whole; do not crush or chew.

Monitoring Parameters Serum lithium every 4-5 days during initial therapy; draw lithium serum concentrations 8-12 hours postdose; renal, thyroid, and cardiovascular function; fluid status; serum electrolytes; CBC with differential, urinalysis; monitor for signs of toxicity; beta-hCG pregnancy test for all females not known to be sterile

Reference Range Levels should be obtained twice weekly until both patient's clinical status and levels are stable then levels may be obtained every 1-3 months

Timing of serum samples: Draw trough just before next dose (8-12 hours after previous dose)

Therapeutic levels:

Acute mania: 0.6-1.2 mEq/L (SI: 0.6-1.2 mmol/L)

Protection against future episodes in most patients with bipolar disorder: 0.8-1 mEq/L (SI: 0.8-1.0 mmol/L); a higher rate of relapse is described in subjects who are maintained at <0.4 mEq/L (SI: 0.4 mmol/L)

Elderly patients can usually be maintained at lower end of therapeutic range (0.6-0.8 mEq/L)

Toxic concentration: >1.5 mEq/L (SI: >2 mmol/L)

Adverse effect levels:

GI complaints/tremor: 1.5-2 mEq/L

Confusion/somnolence: 2-2.5 mEq/L

Seizures/death: >2.5 mEq/L

Dosage Forms Excipient information presented when available (limited, particularly for generics); consult specific product labeling. [DSC] = Discontinued product

Capsule, as carbonate: 150 mg, 300 mg, 600 mg

Eskalith®: 300 mg [contains benzyl alcohol] [DSC]

Solution, as citrate: 300 mg/5 mL (5 mL, 500 mL) [equivalent to amount of lithium in lithium carbonate]

Syrup, as citrate: 300 mg/5 mL (480 mL) [equivalent to amount of lithium in lithium carbonate]

Tablet, as carbonate: 300 mg

Tablet, controlled release, as carbonate: 450 mg

Eskalith CR®: 450 mg [DSC]

Tablet, slow release, as carbonate: 300 mg

Lithobid®: 300 mg

- ◆ **Lithium Carbonate** *see* Lithium *on page 938*
- ◆ **Lithium Citrate** *see* Lithium *on page 938*
- ◆ **Lithobid®** *see* Lithium *on page 938*
- ◆ **Little Colds® Multi-Symptom Cold Formula [OTC] [DSC]** *see* Acetaminophen, Dextromethorphan, and Phenylephrine *on page 42*
- ◆ **Little Fevers™ [OTC]** *see* Acetaminophen *on page 30*
- ◆ **Little Noses® Decongestant [OTC]** *see* Phenylephrine *on page 1273*
- ◆ **Live Attenuated Influenza Vaccine (LAIV)** *see* Influenza Virus Vaccine *on page 820*
- ◆ **Live Smallpox Vaccine** *see* Smallpox Vaccine *on page 1493*
- ◆ **Livostin® [DSC]** *see* Levocabastine *on page 909*
- ◆ **L-methylfolate** *see* Methylfolate *on page 1022*
- ◆ **LNg 20** *see* Levonorgestrel *on page 918*
- ◆ **Locoid®** *see* Hydrocortisone *on page 785*
- ◆ **Locoid Lipocream®** *see* Hydrocortisone *on page 785*
- ◆ **Lodosyn®** *see* Carbidopa *on page 276*

Lodoxamide (loe DOKS a mide)

Medication Safety Issues

International issues:

Thilomide® [Turkey] may be confused with Thalomid® which is a brand name for thalidomide in the U.S.

U.S. Brand Names Alomide®

Canadian Brand Names Alomide®

Mexican Brand Names Alomide

Index Terms Lodoxamide Tromethamine

Pharmacologic Category Mast Cell Stabilizer

Use Treatment of vernal keratoconjunctivitis, vernal conjunctivitis, and vernal keratitis

Effect on Mental Status May cause drowsiness or dizziness

Effect on Psychiatric Treatment None reported

Dosage Summary

Ophthalmic:

Children <2 years: Dosage not established

Children ≥2 years: Instill 1-2 drops in eye(s) 4 times/day

Adults: Instill 1-2 drops in eye(s) 4 times/day

Dosage Forms Excipient information presented when available (limited, particularly for generics); consult specific product labeling.

Solution, ophthalmic: 0.1% (10 mL) [contains benzalkonium chloride]

◆ **Lodoxamide Tromethamine** *see* Lodoxamide *on page 942*

◆ **Lodrane® [DSC]** *see* Brompheniramine and Pseudoephedrine *on page 206*

◆ **Lodrane® 12D** *see* Brompheniramine and Pseudoephedrine *on page 206*

◆ **Lodrane® 12 Hour** *see* Brompheniramine *on page 205*

◆ **Lodrane® 24** *see* Brompheniramine *on page 205*

◆ **Lodrane® 24D** *see* Brompheniramine and Pseudoephedrine *on page 206*

◆ **Lodrane® D** *see* Brompheniramine and Pseudoephedrine *on page 206*

◆ **Lodrane® XR** *see* Brompheniramine *on page 205*

◆ **Loestrin®** *see* Ethinyl Estradiol and Norethindrone *on page 597*

◆ **Loestrin® 24 Fe** *see* Ethinyl Estradiol and Norethindrone *on page 597*

◆ **Loestrin® Fe** *see* Ethinyl Estradiol and Norethindrone *on page 597*

◆ **Lofibra®** *see* Fenofibrate *on page 620*

◆ **LoHist-12** *see* Brompheniramine *on page 205*

◆ **LoHist 12D** *see* Brompheniramine and Pseudoephedrine *on page 206*

◆ **LoHist-D** *see* Chlorpheniramine and Pseudoephedrine *on page 325*

◆ **LoHist LQ** *see* Brompheniramine and Pseudoephedrine *on page 206*

◆ **LoHist PD** *see* Brompheniramine and Pseudoephedrine *on page 206*

◆ **L-OHP** *see* Oxaliplatin *on page 1191*

◆ **Lomotil®** *see* Diphenoxylate and Atropine *on page 486*

Lomustine (loe MUS teen)

Medication Safety Issues

Sound-alike/look-alike issues:

Lomustine may be confused with carmustine

High alert medication: The Institute for Safe Medication Practices (ISMP) includes this medication among its list of drugs which have a heightened risk of causing significant patient harm when used in error.

Lomustine should only be administered as a single dose once every 6 weeks; serious errors have occurred when lomustine was inadvertently administered daily.

U.S. Brand Names CeeNU®

Canadian Brand Names CeeNU®

Mexican Brand Names CEENU

Index Terms CCNU; NSC-79037

Pharmacologic Category Antineoplastic Agent, Alkylating Agent

Use Treatment of brain tumors and Hodgkin's disease

Unlabeled/Investigational Use Non-Hodgkin's lymphoma, melanoma, renal carcinoma, lung cancer, colon cancer

Effect on Mental Status May rarely cause sedation or disorientation

Effect on Psychiatric Treatment Myelosuppression is common; avoid usage with clozapine and carbamazepine; concurrent use with phenobarbital may result in diminished efficacy of both drugs

Dosage Summary

Oral:

Children: 75-150 mg/m^2 as a single dose once every 6 weeks

Adults: 100-130 mg/m^2 as a single dose once every 6 weeks

Dosage Forms Excipient information presented when available (limited, particularly for generics); consult specific product labeling. [DSC] = Discontinued product

Capsule:

CeeNU®: 10 mg, 40 mg, 100 mg

Capsule [dose pack]:

CeeNU®: 10 mg (2s); 40 mg (2s); 100 mg (2s) [DSC]

◆ **Lonox®** *see* Diphenoxylate and Atropine *on page 486*

◆ **Lo/Ovral®** *see* Ethinyl Estradiol and Norgestrel *on page 601*

Loperamide (loe PER a mide)

Medication Safety Issues
Sound-alike/look-alike issues:
Imodium® A-D may be confused with Indocin®, Ionamin®

U.S. Brand Names Diamode [OTC]; Imodium® A-D [OTC]; K-Pek II [OTC]; Kao-Paverin® [OTC]

Canadian Brand Names Apo-Loperamide®; Diarr-Eze; Dom-Loperamide; Imodium®; Loperacap; Novo-Loperamide; PMS-Loperamine; Rhoxal-Loperamide; Rho®-Loperamine; Riva-Loperamide; Sandoz-Loperamide

Mexican Brand Names Diaperol; Imodium; Lomotil

Index Terms Loperamide Hydrochloride

Pharmacologic Category Antidiarrheal

Use Treatment of chronic diarrhea associated with inflammatory bowel disease; acute nonspecific diarrhea; increased volume of ileostomy discharge
OTC labeling: Control of symptoms of diarrhea, including Traveler's diarrhea

Unlabeled/Investigational Use Cancer treatment-induced diarrhea (eg, irinotecan induced); chronic diarrhea caused by bowel resection

Effect on Mental Status May cause drowsiness or dizziness

Effect on Psychiatric Treatment Concurrent use with psychotropics may produce additive sedation and dry mouth

Dosage Summary
Oral:
Children <2 years: Dosage not established
Children 2-5 years (13-20 kg): Acute diarrhea: Initial: 1 mg 3 times/day for first 24 hours; Maintenance: 0.1 mg/kg after each loose stool
Children 6-8 years (20-30 kg):
Acute diarrhea: Initial: 2 mg twice daily for first 24 hours; Maintenance: 0.1 mg/kg after each loose stool
Traveler's diarrhea: 2 mg after first loose stool, followed by 1 mg after each subsequent stool (maximum: 4 mg/day)
Children 8-12 years (>30 kg): Acute diarrhea: Initial: 2 mg 3 times/day for first 24 hours; Maintenance: 0.1 mg/kg after each loose stool
Children 9-11 years: Traveler's diarrhea: 2 mg after first loose stool, followed by 1 mg after each subsequent stool (maximum: 6 mg/day)
Children ≥12 years: Traveler's diarrhea: Initial: 4 mg after first loose stool, followed by 2 mg after each subsequent stool (maximum: 8 mg/day)
Adults:
Acute diarrhea: Initial: 4 mg followed by 2 mg after each loose stool (maximum: 16 mg/day)
Chronic diarrhea: 4-8 mg/day in divided doses
Traveler's diarrhea: Initial: 4 mg after first loose stool, followed by 2 mg after each subsequent stool (maximum: 8 mg/day)

Dosage Forms Excipient information presented when available (limited, particularly for generics); consult specific product labeling.
Caplet, as hydrochloride: 2 mg
Diamode, Imodium® A-D, Kao-Paverin®: 2 mg
Capsule, as hydrochloride: 2 mg
Liquid, oral, as hydrochloride: 1 mg/5 mL (5 mL, 10 mL, 120 mL)
Imodium® A-D: 1 mg/5 mL (60 mL, 120 mL) [contains alcohol, sodium benzoate, benzoic acid; cherry mint flavor]
Imodium® A-D [new formulation]: 1 mg/7.5 mL (60 mL, 120 mL, 360 mL) [contains sodium 10 mg/30 mL, sodium benzoate; creamy mint flavor]
Tablet, as hydrochloride: 2 mg
K-Pek II: 2 mg

Loperamide and Simethicone (loe PER a mide & sye METH i kone)

U.S. Brand Names Imodium® Advanced

Index Terms Simethicone and Loperamide Hydrochloride

Pharmacologic Category Antidiarrheal; Antiflatulent

Use Control of symptoms of diarrhea and gas (bloating, pressure, and cramps)

Effect on Mental Status May cause drowsiness or dizziness

Effect on Psychiatric Treatment Concurrent use with psychotropics may produce additive sedation and dry mouth

Dosage Summary
Oral:
Children <6 years or <48 lbs: Dosage not established

Children 6-8 years (48-59 lbs): 1 caplet/tablet after first loose stool, followed by 1/2 caplet/tablet with each subsequent loose stool (maximum: 2 caplets or tablets/24 hours)

Children 9-11 years (60-95 lbs): 1 caplet/tablet after first loose stool, followed by 1/2 caplet/tablet with each subsequent loose stool (maximum: 3 caplets or tablets/24 hours)

Children ≥12 years: 1 caplet/tablet after each loose stool (maximum: 4 caplets or tablets/24 hours)

Adults: 1 caplet/tablet after each loose stool (maximum: 4 caplets or tablets/24 hours)

Dosage Forms Excipient information presented when available (limited, particularly for generics); consult specific product labeling.

Caplet: Loperamide hydrochloride 2 mg and simethicone 125 mg

Tablet, chewable: Loperamide hydrochloride 2 mg and simethicone 125 mg [mint flavor]

◆ **Loperamide Hydrochloride** *see* Loperamide *on page 944*

◆ **Lopid®** *see* Gemfibrozil *on page 711*

Lopinavir and Ritonavir (loe PIN a veer & rit ON uh veer)

Medication Safety Issues

Sound-alike/look-alike issues:

Potential for dispensing errors between Kaletra™ and Keppra® (levetiracetam)

Administration issues:

Children's doses are based on weight and calculated by milligrams of lopinavir. Care should be taken to accurately calculate the dose. The oral solution contains lopinavir 80 mg and ritonavir 20 mg per one mL. Children <12 years of age (and ≤40 kg) who are not taking certain concomitant antiretroviral medications will receive <5 mL of solution per dose.

U.S. Brand Names Kaletra®

Canadian Brand Names Kaletra®

Mexican Brand Names Kaletra

Index Terms Ritonavir and Lopinavir

Pharmacologic Category Antiretroviral Agent, Protease Inhibitor

Use Treatment of HIV infection in combination with other antiretroviral agents

Effect on Mental Status May cause abnormal dreams, agitation, amnesia, anxiety, ataxia, confusion, dizziness, emotional lability, insomnia, nervousness, somnolence, and abnormal thinking

Effect on Psychiatric Treatment Contraindicated with ergot derivatives, midazolam, pimozide, and triazolam. Avoid concurrent use with St John's wort; may lead to loss of virologic response and/or resistance. Dyslipidemia is common; use caution with clozapine, olanzapine, and quetiapine. Diarrhea is common; use caution with lithium, valproic acid, and SSRIs. Increased LFTs is common; use caution with olanzapine and valproic acid. May cause hyperglycemia; use caution with clozapine and olanzapine. May cause thrombocytopenia; use caution with valproic acid. Carbamazepine, phenytoin, and phenobarbital may decrease levels of lopinavir. Ritonavir may increase levels of zolpidem. The solution contains ethanol; use caution with disulfiram.

Dosage Summary

Oral:

Children <14 days: Dosage not established

Children 14 days to 6 months: Lopinavir 16 mg/kg or 300 mg/m2 twice daily

Children 6 months to 18 years and <15 kg: 12 mg lopinavir/kg twice daily (maximum dose: Lopinavir 400 mg/ritonavir 100 mg)

Children 6 months to 18 years and 15-40 kg: 10 mg lopinavir/kg twice daily (maximum dose: Lopinavir 400 mg/ritonavir 100 mg)

Children 6 months to 18 years and >40 kg: Lopinavir 400 mg/ritonavir 100 mg twice daily

Adults: Lopinavir 400 mg/ritonavir 100 mg twice daily **or** lopinavir 800 mg/ritonavir 200 mg once daily

Note: Dose adjustments may be needed for therapy-experienced patients or those taking amprenavir, efavirenz, fosamprenavir, maraviroc, nelfinavir, nevirapine, or saquinavir.

Dosage Forms Excipient information presented when available (limited, particularly for generics); consult specific product labeling.

Solution, oral:

Kaletra®: Lopinavir 80 mg and ritonavir 20 mg per mL (160 mL) [contains alcohol 42.4%]

Tablet:
Kaletra®:
Lopinavir 100 mg and ritonavir 25 mg
Lopinavir 200 mg and ritonavir 50 mg

◆ **Lopremone** *see* Protirelin *on page 1363*
◆ **Lopressor®** *see* Metoprolol *on page 1036*
◆ **Lopressor HCT®** *see* Metoprolol and Hydrochlorothiazide *on page 1040*
◆ **Lorabid® [DSC]** *see* Loracarbef *on page 946*

Loracarbef (lor a KAR bef)

Medication Safety Issues
Sound-alike/look-alike issues:
Lorabid® may be confused with Levbid®, Lopid®, Lortab®, Slo-bid™

U.S. Brand Names Lorabid® [DSC]

Canadian Brand Names Lorabid®

Mexican Brand Names Carbac; Lorabid

Pharmacologic Category Antibiotic, Carbacephem

Use Treatment of infections caused by susceptible organisms involving the upper and lower respiratory tract, uncomplicated skin and skin structure, and urinary tract (including uncomplicated pyelonephritis)

Effect on Mental Status May cause nervousness; cephalosporins reported to cause illusions, delusion, depersonalization, and euphoria

Effect on Psychiatric Treatment May cause neutropenia; use caution with clozapine and carbamazepine

Dosage Summary
Oral:
Children <6 months: Dosage not established
Children 6 months to 12 years: 7.5-15 mg/kg twice daily
Children ≥13 years: 200-400 mg every 12-24 hours
Adults: 200-400 mg every 12-24 hours

Dosage Forms Excipient information presented when available (limited, particularly for generics); consult specific product labeling. [DSC] = Discontinued product
Capsule:
Lorabid®: 200 mg, 400 mg [DSC]
Powder for oral suspension:
Lorabid®: 100 mg/5 mL (100 mL); 200 mg/5 mL (100 mL) [strawberry bubble gum flavor] [DSC]

◆ **Loradamed [OTC]** *see* Loratadine *on page 946*

Loratadine (lor AT a deen)

Medication Safety Issues
Sound-alike/look-alike issues:
Claritin® may be confused with clarithromycin

U.S. Brand Names Alavert™ Allergy Relief 24-Hour [OTC]; Alavert™ [OTC]; Allergy Relief [OTC]; Claritin® 24 Hour Allergy [OTC]; Claritin® Children's Allergy [OTC]; Claritin® Children's [OTC]; Claritin® Hives Relief [OTC]; Dimetapp® ND Children's [OTC]; Loradamed [OTC]; Tavist® ND ALLERGY [OTC]

Canadian Brand Names Apo-Loratadine®; Claritin®; Claritin® Kids

Mexican Brand Names Albatrina; Clarityne; Curyken; Dimegan; Dymaten; Efectine; Inigrin; Laritol; Lertamine; Lorimox; Lotan; Neoalexil; Sensibit; Vincidal

Pharmacologic Category Histamine H_1 Antagonist; Histamine H_1 Antagonist, Second Generation

Generic Available Yes

Use Relief of nasal and non-nasal symptoms of seasonal allergic rhinitis; treatment of chronic idiopathic urticaria

Effect on Mental Status Drowsiness is common; may cause anxiety or depression

Effect on Psychiatric Treatment None reported

Pregnancy Risk Factor B

Pregnancy Considerations Loratadine was not found to be teratogenic in animal studies. There are no adequate and well-controlled studies in pregnant woman; use during pregnancy only if clearly needed.

Lactation Enters breast milk/not recommended (AAP rates "compatible")

Contraindications Hypersensitivity to loratadine or any component of the formulation

Warnings/Precautions Use with caution in patients with liver or renal impairment; dosage adjustment recommended. Safety and efficacy in children <2 years of age have not been established. Some products may contain phenylalanine.

Adverse Reactions

Adults:

Central nervous system: Headache (12%), somnolence (8%), fatigue (4%)

Gastrointestinal: Xerostomia (3%)

Children:

Central nervous system: Nervousness (4% ages 6-12 years), fatigue (3% ages 6-12 years, 2% to 3% ages 2-5 years), malaise (2% ages 6-12 years)

Dermatologic: Rash (2% to 3% ages 2-5 years)

Gastrointestinal: Abdominal pain (2% ages 6-12 years), stomatitis (2% to 3% ages 2-5 years)

Neuromuscular & skeletal: Hyperkinesia (3% ages 6-12 years)

Ocular: Conjunctivitis (2% ages 6-12 years)

Respiratory: Wheezing (4% ages 6-12 years), dysphonia (2% ages 6-12 years), upper respiratory infection (2% ages 6-12 years), epistaxis (2% to 3% ages 2-5 years), pharyngitis (2% to 3% ages 2-5 years)

Miscellaneous: Flu-like syndrome (2% to 3% ages 2-5 years), viral infection (2% to 3% ages 2-5 years)

Adults and Children: <2% (Limited to important or life-threatening): Abnormal hepatic function, agitation, alopecia, altered lacrimation, altered micturition, altered salivation, altered taste, amnesia, anaphylaxis, angioneurotic edema, anorexia, arthralgia, back pain, blepharospasm, blurred vision, breast enlargement, breast pain, bronchospasm, chest pain, confusion, depression, dizziness, dysmenorrhea, dyspnea, erythema multiforme, hemoptysis, hepatic necrosis, hepatitis, hypotension, impaired concentration, impotence, insomnia, irritability, jaundice, menorrhagia, migraine, nausea, palpitation, paresthesia, paroniria, peripheral edema, photosensitivity, pruritus, purpura, rigors, seizure, supraventricular tachyarrhythmia, syncope, tachycardia, tremor, urinary discoloration, urticaria, thrombocytopenia, vaginitis, vertigo, vomiting, weight gain

Metabolism/Transport Effects Substrate (minor) of CYP2D6, 3A4; **Inhibits** CYP2C8 (weak), 2C19 (moderate), 2D6 (weak)

Drug Interactions

Acetylcholinesterase Inhibitors (Central): Anticholinergics may diminish the therapeutic effect of Acetylcholinesterase Inhibitors (Central). Acetylcholinesterase Inhibitors (Central) may diminish the therapeutic effect of Anticholinergics. If the anticholinergic action is a side effect of the agent, the result may be beneficial. *Risk C: Monitor therapy*

Alcohol (Ethyl): CNS Depressants may enhance the CNS depressant effect of Alcohol (Ethyl). *Risk C: Monitor therapy*

Amphetamines: May diminish the sedative effect of Antihistamines. *Risk C: Monitor therapy*

Anticholinergics: May enhance the adverse/toxic effect of other Anticholinergics. **Exceptions:** Paliperidone. *Risk C: Monitor therapy*

Betahistine: Antihistamines may diminish the therapeutic effect of Betahistine. *Risk C: Monitor therapy*

CNS Depressants: May enhance the adverse/toxic effect of other CNS Depressants. *Risk C: Monitor therapy*

P-Glycoprotein Inducers: May decrease the serum concentration of P-Glycoprotein Substrates. P-glycoprotein inducers may also further limit the distribution of p-glycoprotein substrates to specific cells/tissues/organs where p-glycoprotein is present in large amounts (e.g., brain, T-lymphocytes, testes, etc.). *Risk C: Monitor therapy*

P-Glycoprotein Inhibitors: May increase the serum concentration of P-Glycoprotein Substrates. P-glycoprotein inhibitors may also enhance the distribution of p-glycoprotein substrates to specific cells/tissues/organs where p-glycoprotein is present in large amounts (e.g., brain, T-lymphocytes, testes, etc.). *Risk C: Monitor therapy*

Pramlintide: May enhance the anticholinergic effect of Anticholinergics. These effects are specific to the GI tract. *Risk D: Consider therapy modification*

Ethanol/Nutrition/Herb Interactions

Ethanol: Avoid ethanol (although sedation is limited with loratadine, may increase risk of CNS depression).

Food: Increases bioavailability and delays peak.

Herb/Nutraceutical: St John's wort may decrease loratadine levels.

Stability Store at 2°C to 25°C (36°F to 77°F).

Rapidly-disintegrating tablets: Use within 6 months of opening foil pouch, and immediately after opening individual tablet blister. Store in a dry place.

Mechanism of Action Long-acting tricyclic antihistamine with selective peripheral histamine H_1-receptor antagonistic properties

Pharmacodynamics/Kinetics

Onset of action: 1-3 hours

Peak effect: 8-12 hours

Duration: >24 hours

Absorption: Rapid

Distribution: Significant amounts enter breast milk

Metabolism: Extensively hepatic via CYP2D6 and 3A4 to active metabolite

Half-life elimination: 12-15 hours

Excretion: Urine (40%) and feces (40%) as metabolites

Dosage Oral: Seasonal allergic rhinitis, chronic idiopathic urticaria:

Children 2-5 years: 5 mg once daily

Children ≥6 years and Adults: 10 mg once daily

Elderly: Peak plasma levels are increased; elimination half-life is slightly increased; specific dosing adjustments are not available

Dosage adjustment in renal impairment: Cl_{cr} ≤30 mL/minute:

Children 2-5 years: 5 mg every other day

Children ≥6 years and Adults: 10 mg every other day

Dosage adjustment in hepatic impairment: Elimination half-life increases with severity of disease

Children 2-5 years: 5 mg every other day

Children ≥6 years and Adults: 10 mg every other day

Dietary Considerations Take on an empty stomach. Alavert® and Dimetapp® Children's ND contain phenylalanine 8.4 mg per 10 mg tablet. Claritin® Children's Allergy 5 mg contains phenylalanine 1.4 mg per tablet.

Administration Take on an empty stomach.

Dosage Forms Excipient information presented when available (limited, particularly for generics); consult specific product labeling.

Solution, oral: 5 mg/5 mL (120 mL)

Syrup, oral: 1 mg/mL (120 mL)

Allergy Relief: 1 mg/mL (120 mL)

Claritin® Children's: 5 mg/5 mL (60 mL, 120 mL) [alcohol free, dye free, sugar free; contains propylene glycol, sodium benzoate, and sodium 6 mg/5 mL; grape flavor]

Claritin® Children's Allergy: 1 mg/mL (120 mL) [alcohol free, dye free; contains propylene glycol and sodium benzoate; fruit flavor]

Tablet, oral: 10 mg

Alavert™: 10 mg

Claritin® 24 Hour Allergy: 10 mg

Claritin® Hives Relief: 10 mg

Loradamed: 10 mg

Tavist® ND ALLERGY: 10 mg

Tablet, chewable, oral:

Claritin® Children's Allergy: 5 mg [contains phenylalanine 1.4 mg/tablet; grape flavor]

Tablet, orally disintegrating, oral:

Alavert™ Allergy Relief 24-Hour: 10 mg [contains phenylalanine 8.4 mg/tablet]

Dimetapp® ND Children's: 10 mg [contains phenylalanine 8.4 mg/tablet]

Loratadine and Pseudoephedrine

(lor AT a deen & soo doe e FED rin)

U.S. Brand Names Alavert™ Allergy and Sinus [OTC]; Claritin-D® 12 Hour Allergy & Congestion [OTC]; Claritin-D® 24 Hour Allergy & Congestion [OTC]

Canadian Brand Names Chlor-Tripolon ND®; Claritin® Extra; Claritin® Liberator

Mexican Brand Names Clariflu; Clarifriol; Clarityne; Dimegan D; Gralddep; Lertamine D; Lorimox; Sensibit; Theraflu

Index Terms Pseudoephedrine and Loratadine

Pharmacologic Category Alpha/Beta Agonist; Histamine H_1 Antagonist; Histamine H_1 Antagonist, Second Generation

Use Temporary relief of symptoms of seasonal allergic rhinitis, other upper respiratory allergies, or the common cold

Effect on Mental Status Dizziness, drowsiness, nervousness, and insomnia are common; may cause anxiety or depression; may rarely cause hallucinations

Effect on Psychiatric Treatment Contraindicated with MAO inhibitors

Dosage Summary

Oral:

Children <12 years: Dosage not established

Children ≥12 years:

Alavert™ Allergy and Sinus, Claritin-D® 24-Hour: 1 tablet every 24 hours

Claritin-D® 12-Hour: 1 tablet every 12 hours

Adults:

Alavert™ Allergy and Sinus, Claritin-D® 24-Hour: 1 tablet every 24 hours

Claritin-D® 12-Hour: 1 tablet every 12 hours

Dosage Forms Excipient information presented when available (limited, particularly for generics); consult specific product labeling.

Tablet, extended release: Loratadine 10 mg and pseudoephedrine sulfate 240 mg

Alavert™ Allergy and Sinus: Loratadine 5 mg and pseudoephedrine sulfate 120 mg

Claritin-D® 12 Hour Allergy & Congestion: Loratadine 5 mg and pseudoephedrine sulfate 120 mg [contains calcium 30 mg/tablet]

Claritin-D® 24 Hour Allergy & Congestion: Loratadine 10 mg and pseudoephedrine sulfate 240 mg [contains calcium 25 mg/tablet]

LORazepam (lor A ze pam)

Medication Safety Issues

Sound-alike/look-alike issues:

LORazepam may be confused with ALPRAZolam, clonazePAM, diazepam, temazepam

Ativan® may be confused with Atarax®, Atgam®, Avitene®

Injection dosage form contains propylene glycol. Monitor for toxicity when administering continuous lorazepam infusions.

Related Information

Benzodiazepines *on page 1774*

CMS: Long-Term Care Facility Thresholds *on page 1815*

Discontinuation of Psychotropic Drugs *on page 1839*

U.S. Brand Names Ativan®; Lorazepam Intensol®

Canadian Brand Names Apo-Lorazepam®; Ativan®; Lorazepam Injection, USP; Novo-Lorazepam; Nu-Loraz; PHL-Lorazepam; PMS-Lorazepam; Riva-Lorazepam

Mexican Brand Names Ativan

Pharmacologic Category Benzodiazepine

Generic Available Yes

Use

Oral: Management of anxiety disorders or short-term (≤4 months) relief of the symptoms of anxiety or anxiety associated with depressive symptoms

I.V.: Status epilepticus, preanesthesia for desired amnesia

Unlabeled/Investigational Use Ethanol detoxification; insomnia; psychogenic catatonia; partial complex seizures; agitation (I.V.); antiemetic adjunct

Mental Health Comment In 2007, the FDA requested that all manufacturers of sedative-hypnotic drug products revise labeling to include a greater emphasis on the risks of adverse effects. These risks include severe allergic reactions (anaphylaxis, angioedema) and complex sleep-related behaviors, which may include sleep-driving (driving while not fully awake and with no memory of the event), making phone calls, and preparing and eating food while asleep.

There are two subtypes of GABA receptors (GABA-A and GABA-B) and three different benzodiazepine receptors (Bz_1, Bz_2, and Bz_3). Benzodiazepine receptors and effects appear to be linked to the GABA-A receptors. Benzodiazepines do not bind to GABA-B receptors. The role of GABA-B receptors is unclear. Benzodiazepines have no specificity for benzodiazepine receptor subtypes.

Lorazepam is a short half-life benzodiazepine. Duration of action after a single dose is determined by redistribution rather than metabolism. Tolerance develops to the sedative, hypnotic, and anticonvulsant effects. It does not develop to the anxiolytic or skeletal muscle relaxing effects. Psychological and physical dependence may occur with prolonged use of benzodiazepines. The onset of withdrawal symptoms is usually seen on the first day without drug and lasts 5-7 days in patients receiving short half-life benzodiazepines, whereas, the onset occurs after 5 days with a duration of 10-14 days after abrupt discontinuance of long half-life benzodiazepines. Risk factors for abuse include personal or family history of substance abuse and personality disorder.

Lorazepam is rapidly and completely absorbed after I.M. injection; undergoes phase II metabolism and, therefore, is less likely to be affected in patients with hepatic dysfunction.

Restrictions C-IV

Pregnancy Risk Factor D

Pregnancy Considerations Teratogenic effects have been observed in some animal studies. Lorazepam crosses the human placenta. Respiratory depression, withdrawal symptoms, or hypotonia may occur if administered late in pregnancy or near the time of delivery.

Lactation Enters breast milk/not recommended (AAP rates "of concern")

Contraindications Hypersensitivity to lorazepam or any component of the formulation (cross-sensitivity with other benzodiazepines may exist); acute narrow-angle glaucoma; sleep apnea (parenteral); intra-arterial injection of parenteral formulation; severe respiratory insufficiency (except during mechanical ventilation)

Warnings/Precautions Use with caution in elderly or debilitated patients, patients with hepatic disease (including alcoholics) or renal impairment. Use with caution in patients with respiratory disease (COPD or sleep apnea) or limited pulmonary reserve, or impaired gag reflex. Initial doses in elderly or debilitated patients should be at the lower end of the dosing range. May worsen hepatic encephalopathy.

Causes CNS depression (dose-related) resulting in sedation, dizziness, confusion, or ataxia which may impair physical and mental capabilities. Patients must be cautioned about performing tasks which require mental alertness (eg, operating machinery or driving). Use with caution in patients receiving other CNS depressants or psychoactive agents. Effects with other sedative drugs or ethanol may be potentiated. Benzodiazepines have been associated with falls and traumatic injury and should be used with extreme caution in patients who are at risk of these events (especially the elderly).

Lorazepam may cause anterograde amnesia. Paradoxical reactions, including hyperactive or aggressive behavior have been reported with benzodiazepines, particularly in adolescent/pediatric or psychiatric patients. Does not have analgesic, antidepressant, or antipsychotic properties.

Use caution in patients with depression, particularly if suicidal risk may be present. Pre-existing depression may worsen or emerge during therapy. Not recommended for use in primary depressive or psychotic disorders. Use with caution in patients with a history of drug dependence, alcoholism, or significant personality disorders. Benzodiazepines have been associated with dependence and acute withdrawal symptoms on discontinuation or reduction in dose. Acute withdrawal, including seizures, may be precipitated after administration of flumazenil to patients receiving long-term benzodiazepine therapy.

As a hypnotic agent, should be used only after evaluation of potential causes of sleep disturbance. Failure of sleep disturbance to resolve after 7-10 days may indicate psychiatric or medical illness. A worsening of insomnia or the emergence of new abnormalities of thought or behavior may represent unrecognized psychiatric or medical illness and requires immediate and careful evaluation.

The parenteral formulation of lorazepam contains polyethylene glycol and propylene glycol which have resulted in toxicity during high dose and/or longer term infusions. Also contains benzyl alcohol; avoid in neonates.

Safety and efficacy have not been established in children <12 years of age.

Adverse Reactions

>10%:
- Central nervous system: Sedation
- Respiratory: Respiratory depression

1% to 10%:
- Cardiovascular: Hypotension
- Central nervous system: Confusion, dizziness, akathisia, ataxia, headache, depression, disorientation, amnesia
- Dermatologic: Dermatitis, rash
- Gastrointestinal: Weight gain/loss, nausea, changes in appetite
- Neuromuscular & skeletal: Weakness
- Ocular: Visual disturbances
- Respiratory: Nasal congestion, hyperventilation, apnea

<1% or frequency not defined (Limited to important or life-threatening): Asthenia, blood dyscrasias, disinhibition, euphoria, fatigue, increased salivation, menstrual irregularities, physical and psychological dependence

(with prolonged use), reflex slowing, polyethylene glycol or propylene glycol poisoning (prolonged I.V. infusion), suicidal ideation, seizure, vertigo

Drug Interactions

Alcohol (Ethyl): CNS Depressants may enhance the CNS depressant effect of Alcohol (Ethyl). *Risk C: Monitor therapy*

Clozapine: Benzodiazepines may enhance the adverse/toxic effect of Clozapine. *Risk D: Consider therapy modification*

CNS Depressants: May enhance the adverse/toxic effect of other CNS Depressants. *Risk C: Monitor therapy*

Loxapine: May enhance the adverse/toxic effect of LORazepam. Specifically, prolonged stupor, respiratory depression, and/or hypotension. *Risk C: Monitor therapy*

Phenytoin: Benzodiazepines may increase the serum concentration of Phenytoin. Short-term exposure to benzodiazepines may not present as much risk as chronic therapy. *Risk C: Monitor therapy*

Probenecid: May decrease the metabolism of LORazepam. *Risk D: Consider therapy modification*

Theophylline Derivatives: May diminish the therapeutic effect of Benzodiazepines. *Risk D: Consider therapy modification*

Valproic Acid: May decrease the metabolism of LORazepam. *Risk D: Consider therapy modification*

Ethanol/Nutrition/Herb Interactions

Ethanol: Avoid or limit ethanol (may increase CNS depression).

Herb/Nutraceutical: Avoid valerian, St John's wort, kava kava, gotu kola (may increase CNS depression).

Stability

I.V.: Intact vials should be refrigerated. Protect from light. Do not use discolored or precipitate-containing solutions. May be stored at room temperature for up to 60 days. Parenteral admixture is stable at room temperature (25°C) for 24 hours. Dilute I.V. dose with equal volume of compatible diluent (D_5W, NS, SWI).

Infusion: Use 2 mg/mL injectable vial to prepare; there may be deceased stability when using 4 mg/mL vial. Dilute ≤1 mg/mL and mix in glass bottle. Precipitation may develop. Can also be administered undiluted via infusion.

Tablet: Store at room temperature.

Mechanism of Action Binds to stereospecific benzodiazepine receptors on the postsynaptic GABA neuron at several sites within the central nervous system, including the limbic system, reticular formation. Enhancement of the inhibitory effect of GABA on neuronal excitability results by increased neuronal membrane permeability to chloride ions. This shift in chloride ions results in hyperpolarization (a less excitable state) and stabilization.

Pharmacodynamics/Kinetics

Onset of action:

Hypnosis: I.M.: 20-30 minutes

Sedation: I.V.: 5-20 minutes

Anticonvulsant: I.V.: 5 minutes, oral: 30-60 minutes

Duration: 6-8 hours

Absorption: Oral, I.M.: Prompt

Distribution:

V_d: Neonates: 0.76 L/kg, Adults: 1.3 L/kg; crosses placenta; enters breast milk

Protein binding: 85%; free fraction may be significantly higher in elderly

Metabolism: Hepatic to inactive compounds

Bioavailability: Oral: 90%

Half-life elimination: Neonates: 40.2 hours; Older children: 10.5 hours; Adults: 12.9 hours; Elderly: 15.9 hours; End-stage renal disease: 32-70 hours

Time to peak: Oral: 2 hours

Excretion: Urine; feces (minimal)

Dosage

Antiemetic (unlabeled use):

Children 2-15 years: I.V.: 0.05 mg/kg (up to 2 mg/dose) prior to chemotherapy

Adults: Oral, I.V. (**Note:** May be administered sublingually; not a labeled route): 0.5-2 mg every 4-6 hours as needed

Anxiety and sedation (unlabeled in children except for oral use in children >12 years):

Infants and Children: Oral, I.M., I.V.: Usual: 0.05 mg/kg/dose (range: 0.02-0.09 mg/kg) every 4-8 hours

I.V.: May use smaller doses (eg, 0.01-0.03 mg/kg) and repeat every 20 minutes, as needed to titrate to effect

Adults: Oral: 1-10 mg/day in 2-3 divided doses; usual dose: 2-6 mg/day in divided doses

Elderly: 0.5-4 mg/day; initial dose not to exceed 2 mg

Insomnia: Adults: Oral: 2-4 mg at bedtime
Preoperative: Adults:
I.M.: 0.05 mg/kg administered 2 hours before surgery (maximum: 4 mg/dose)
I.V.: 0.044 mg/kg 15-20 minutes before surgery (usual maximum: 2 mg/dose)
Preprocedural anxiety (dental use): Adults: Oral: 1-2 mg 1 hour before procedure
Operative amnesia: Adults: I.V.: Up to 0.05 mg/kg (maximum: 4 mg/dose)
Sedation (preprocedure): Infants and Children (unlabeled):
Oral, I.M., I.V.: Usual: 0.05 mg/kg (range: 0.02-0.09 mg/kg)
I.V.: May use smaller doses (eg, 0.01-0.03 mg/kg) and repeat every 20 minutes, as needed to titrate to effect
Status epilepticus: I.V.:
Infants and Children (unlabeled): 0.05-0.1 mg/kg slow I.V. over 2-5 minutes; do not exceed 4 mg/single dose; may repeat second dose of 0.05 mg/kg slow I.V. in 5-10 minutes if needed
Adolescents: 0.07 mg/kg slow I.V. over 2-5 minutes; maximum: 4 mg/dose; may repeat in 5-10 minutes
Adults: 4 mg/dose slow I.V. over 2-5 minutes; may repeat in 5-10 minutes; usual maximum dose: 8 mg
Rapid tranquilization of agitated patient (administer every 30-60 minutes): Adults:
Oral: 1-2 mg
I.M.: 0.5-1 mg
Average total dose for tranquilization: Oral, I.M.: 4-8 mg
Agitation in the ICU patient (unlabeled): Adults:
I.V.: 0.02-0.06 mg/kg every 2-6 hours
I.V. infusion: 0.01-0.1 mg/kg/hour
Concurrent use of probenecid or valproic acid: Reduce lorazepam dose by 50%

Dosage adjustment in renal impairment: I.V.: Risk of propylene glycol toxicity. Monitor closely if using for prolonged periods of time or at high doses.
Dosage adjustment in hepatic impairment: Use cautiously.

Administration May be administered by I.M., I.V., or orally
I.M.: Should be administered deep into the muscle mass
I.V.: Do not exceed 2 mg/minute or 0.05 mg/kg over 2-5 minutes; dilute I.V. dose with equal volume of compatible diluent (D_5W, NS, SWI). Avoid intra-arterial administration. Monitor I.V. site for extravasation.

Monitoring Parameters Respiratory and cardiovascular status, blood pressure, heart rate, symptoms of anxiety

Reference Range Therapeutic: 50-240 ng/mL (SI: 156-746 nmol/L)

Additional Information Oral doses >0.09 mg/kg produced increased ataxia without increased sedative benefit vs lower doses; preferred anxiolytic when I.M. route needed. Abrupt discontinuation after sustained use (generally >10 days) may cause withdrawal symptoms.

Dosage Forms Excipient information presented when available (limited, particularly for generics); consult specific product labeling.
Injection, solution: 2 mg/mL (1 mL, 10 mL); 4 mg/mL (1 mL, 10 mL)
Ativan®: 2 mg/mL (1 mL, 10 mL); 4 mg/mL (1 mL, 10 mL) [contains benzyl alcohol, polyethylene glycol, and propylene glycol]
Solution, oral concentrate:
Lorazepam Intensol®: 2 mg/mL (30 mL) [alcohol free, dye free]
Tablet: 0.5 mg, 1 mg, 2 mg
Ativan®: 0.5 mg, 1 mg, 2 mg

◆ **Lorazepam Intensol®** *see* LORazepam *on page 949*
◆ **Lorcet® 10/650** *see* Hydrocodone and Acetaminophen *on page 777*
◆ **Lorcet® Plus** *see* Hydrocodone and Acetaminophen *on page 777*
◆ **Lortab®** *see* Hydrocodone and Acetaminophen *on page 777*

Losartan (loe SAR tan)

Medication Safety Issues
Sound-alike/look-alike issues:
Cozaar® may be confused with Colace®, Coreg®, Hyzaar®, Zocor®
Losartan may be confused with valsartan

Related Information
Angiotensin Agents *on page 1754*

U.S. Brand Names Cozaar®
Canadian Brand Names Cozaar®
Mexican Brand Names Cozaar

Index Terms DuP 753; Losartan Potassium; MK594

Pharmacologic Category Angiotensin II Receptor Blocker

Generic Available No

Use Treatment of hypertension (HTN); treatment of diabetic nephropathy in patients with type 2 diabetes mellitus (noninsulin dependent, NIDDM) and a history of hypertension; stroke risk reduction in patients with HTN and left ventricular hypertrophy (LVH)

Unlabeled/Investigational Use To slow the rate of progression of aortic-root dilation in pediatric patients with Marfan's syndrome

Effect on Mental Status May cause dizziness or insomnia; may rarely cause anxiety, confusion, depression, and sleep disorders

Effect on Psychiatric Treatment Barbiturates may decrease the effects of losartan

Pregnancy Risk Factor C (1st trimester); D (2nd and 3rd trimesters)

Pregnancy Considerations Medications which act on the renin-angiotensin system are reported to have the following fetal/neonatal effects: Hypotension, neonatal skull hypoplasia, anuria, renal failure, and death; oligohydramnios is also reported. These effects are reported to occur with exposure during the second and third trimesters. There are no adequate and well-controlled studies in pregnant women. **[U.S. Boxed Warning]: Based on human data, drugs that act on the angiotensin system can cause injury and death to the developing fetus when used in the second and third trimesters. Angiotensin receptor blockers should be discontinued as soon as possible once pregnancy is detected.**

Lactation Excretion in breast milk unknown/not recommended

Contraindications Hypersensitivity to losartan or any component of the formulation

Warnings/Precautions [U.S. Boxed Warning]: Based on human data, drugs that act on the angiotensin system can cause injury and death to the developing fetus when used in the second and third trimesters. Angiotensin receptor blockers should be discontinued as soon as possible once pregnancy is detected. Avoid use or use a much smaller dose in patients who are volume-depleted; correct depletion first. Use with caution in patients with significant aortic/mitral stenosis. May cause hyperkalemia; avoid potassium supplementation unless specifically required by healthcare provider. May be associated with deterioration of renal function and/or increases in serum creatinine, particularly in patients with low renal blood flow (eg, renal artery stenosis, heart failure) whose glomerular filtration rate (GFR) is dependent on efferent arteriolar vasoconstriction by angiotensin II. Use caution in patients with unstented unilateral/bilateral renal artery stenosis. When unstented bilateral renal artery stenosis is present, use is generally avoided due to the elevated risk of deterioration in renal function unless possible benefits outweigh risks. Use with caution with pre-existing renal insufficiency. AUCs of losartan (not the active metabolite) are about 50% greater in patients with Cl_{cr} <30 mL/minute and are doubled in hemodialysis patients.

At any time during treatment (especially following first dose), angioedema may occur rarely; may involve the head and neck (potentially compromising airway) or the intestine (presenting with abdominal pain). Patients with idiopathic or hereditary angioedema or previous angioedema associated with ACE-inhibitor therapy may be at an increased risk. Prolonged frequent monitoring may be required, especially if tongue, glottis, or larynx are involved, as they are associated with airway obstruction. Patients with a history of airway surgery may have a higher risk of airway obstruction. Aggressive early management is critical; intramuscular (I.M.) administration of epinephrine may be necessary.

When used to reduce the risk of stroke in patients with HTN and LVH, may not be effective in African-American population. Use caution with hepatic dysfunction, dose adjustment may be needed. Safety and efficacy have not been established in children <6 years of age.

Adverse Reactions

Note: The incidence of some adverse reactions varied based on the underlying disease state. Notations are made, where applicable, for data derived from trials conducted in diabetic nephropathy and hypertensive patients, respectively.

>10%:

Cardiovascular: Chest pain (12% diabetic nephropathy)
Central nervous system: Fatigue (14% diabetic nephropathy)
Endocrine: Hypoglycemia (14% diabetic nephropathy)
Gastrointestinal: Diarrhea (2% hypertension to 15% diabetic nephropathy)
Genitourinary: Urinary tract infection (13% diabetic nephropathy)

Hematologic: Anemia (14% diabetic nephropathy)
Neuromuscular & skeletal: Weakness (14% diabetic nephropathy), back pain (2% hypertension to 12% diabetic nephropathy)
Respiratory: Cough (≤3% to 11%; similar to placebo; incidence higher in patients with previous cough related to ACE inhibitor therapy)

1% to 10%:
Cardiovascular: Hypotension (7% diabetic nephropathy), orthostatic hypotension (4% hypertension to 4% diabetic nephropathy), first-dose hypotension (dose related: <1% with 50 mg, 2% with 100 mg)
Central nervous system: Dizziness (4%), hypoesthesia (5% diabetic nephropathy), fever (4% diabetic nephropathy), insomnia (1%)
Dermatology: Cellulitis (7% diabetic nephropathy)
Endocrine: Hyperkalemia (<1% hypertension to 7% diabetic nephropathy)
Gastrointestinal: Gastritis (5% diabetic nephropathy), weight gain (4% diabetic nephropathy), dyspepsia (1% to 4%), abdominal pain (2%), nausea (2%)
Neuromuscular & skeletal: Muscular weakness (7% diabetic nephropathy), knee pain (5% diabetic nephropathy), leg pain (1% to 5%), muscle cramps (1%), myalgia (1%)
Respiratory: Bronchitis (10% diabetic nephropathy), upper respiratory infection (8%), nasal congestion (2%), sinusitis (1% hypertension to 6% diabetic nephropathy)
Miscellaneous: Infection (5% diabetic nephropathy), flu-like syndrome (10% diabetic nephropathy)

<1% (Limited to important or life-threatening): Acute psychosis with paranoid delusions, ageusia, allergic reaction, alopecia, anaphylactic reactions, anemia, angina, angioedema, anorexia, anxiety, arrhythmia, arthralgia, arthritis, ataxia, AV block (second degree), bilirubin increased, blurred vision, bradycardia, bronchitis, BUN increased, confusion, conjunctivitis, constipation, CVA, depression, dermatitis, dysgeusia, dyspnea, ecchymosis, epistaxis, erythroderma, erythema, facial edema, fever, flatulence, flushing, gastritis, gout, hematocrit decreased, hemoglobin decreased, Henoch-Schönlein purpura, hepatitis, hyperkalemia, hyponatremia, hypotension, impotence, joint swelling, maculopapular rash, myositis, memory impairment, MI, migraine, muscle weakness, nervousness, orthostatic effects, pancreatitis, paresthesia, peripheral neuropathy, pharyngitis, photosensitivity, pruritus, rash, rhabdomyolysis, rhinitis, serum creatinine increased, sleep disorder, somnolence, syncope, tachycardia, taste perversion, thrombocytopenia, tinnitus, transaminases increased, tremor, urinary frequency, urticaria, vasculitis, ventricular arrhythmia, vertigo, visual acuity decreased, vomiting, xerostomia

Metabolism/Transport Effects Substrate (major) of CYP2C9, 3A4; **Inhibits** CYP1A2 (weak), 2C8 (moderate), 2C9 (moderate), 2C19 (weak), 3A4 (weak)

Drug Interactions

ACE Inhibitors: Angiotensin II Receptor Blockers may enhance the adverse/toxic effect of ACE Inhibitors. *Risk C: Monitor therapy*

Antifungal Agents (Azole Derivatives, Systemic): May decrease the metabolism of Losartan. *Risk C: Monitor therapy*

CYP2C8 Substrates (High risk): CYP2C8 Inhibitors (Moderate) may decrease the metabolism of CYP2C8 Substrates (High risk). *Risk C: Monitor therapy*

CYP2C9 Inducers (Highly Effective): May increase the metabolism of CYP2C9 Substrates (High risk). *Risk C: Monitor therapy*

CYP2C9 Inhibitors (Moderate): May decrease the metabolism of CYP2C9 Substrates (High risk). *Risk C: Monitor therapy*

CYP2C9 Inhibitors (Strong): May decrease the metabolism of CYP2C9 Substrates (High risk). *Risk D: Consider therapy modification*

CYP2C9 Substrates (High risk): CYP2C9 Inhibitors (Moderate) may decrease the metabolism of CYP2C9 Substrates (High risk). *Risk C: Monitor therapy*

CYP3A4 Inducers (Strong): May increase the metabolism of CYP3A4 Substrates. *Risk C: Monitor therapy*

Deferasirox: May decrease the serum concentration of CYP3A4 Substrates. *Risk C: Monitor therapy*

Diazoxide: May enhance the hypotensive effect of Antihypertensives. *Risk C: Monitor therapy*

Eplerenone: May enhance the hyperkalemic effect of Angiotensin II Receptor Blockers. *Risk C: Monitor therapy*

Fluconazole: May decrease the metabolism of Losartan. *Risk C: Monitor therapy*

Herbs (CYP3A4 Inducers): May increase the metabolism of CYP3A4 Substrates. *Risk C: Monitor therapy*

Herbs (Hypertensive Properties): May diminish the antihypertensive effect of Antihypertensives. *Risk C: Monitor therapy*

Herbs (Hypoglycemic Properties): May enhance the hypoglycemic effect of Hypoglycemic Agents. *Risk C: Monitor therapy*

Herbs (Hypotensive Properties): May enhance the hypotensive effect of Antihypertensives. *Risk C: Monitor therapy*

Lithium: Angiotensin II Receptor Blockers may increase the serum concentration of Lithium. Management: Lithium dosage reductions will likely be needed following the addition of an angiotensin II receptor antagonist. *Risk D: Consider therapy modification*

Methylphenidate: May diminish the antihypertensive effect of Antihypertensives. *Risk C: Monitor therapy*

Nonsteroidal Anti-Inflammatory Agents: May diminish the therapeutic effect of Angiotensin II Receptor Blockers. The combination of these two agents may also significantly decrease glomerular filtration and renal function. *Risk C: Monitor therapy*

Potassium Salts: May enhance the hyperkalemic effect of Angiotensin II Receptor Blockers. *Risk C: Monitor therapy*

Potassium-Sparing Diuretics: Angiotensin II Receptor Blockers may enhance the hyperkalemic effect of Potassium-Sparing Diuretics. *Risk C: Monitor therapy*

Prostacyclin Analogues: May enhance the hypotensive effect of Antihypertensives. *Risk C: Monitor therapy*

Rifamycin Derivatives: May increase the metabolism of Angiotensin II Receptor Blockers. *Risk C: Monitor therapy*

RiTUXimab: Antihypertensives may enhance the hypotensive effect of RiTUXimab. *Risk D: Consider therapy modification*

Trimethoprim: May enhance the hyperkalemic effect of Angiotensin II Receptor Blockers. *Risk C: Monitor therapy*

Ethanol/Nutrition/Herb Interactions Herb/Nutraceutical: St John's wort may decrease levels of losartan. Avoid bayberry, blue cohosh, ginseng (American), kola, licorice (may worsen hypertension). Avoid black cohosh; california poppy; coleus; golden seal; hawthorn; mistletoe; periwinkle; quinine; shepherd's purse (may increase risk for hypotension). Hypoglycemic effects of losartan may be enhanced by alfalfa; aloe; bilberry; bitter melon; burdock; celery; damiana; fenugreek; garcinia; garlic; ginger; ginseng (American); gymnema; marshmallow; stinging nettle.

Stability Store at 15°C to 30°C (59°F to 86°F). Protect from light.

Mechanism of Action As a selective and competitive, nonpeptide angiotensin II receptor antagonist, losartan blocks the vasoconstrictor and aldosterone-secreting effects of angiotensin II; losartan interacts reversibly at the AT1 and AT2 receptors of many tissues and has slow dissociation kinetics; its affinity for the AT1 receptor is 1000 times greater than the AT2 receptor. Angiotensin II receptor antagonists may induce a more complete inhibition of the renin-angiotensin system than ACE inhibitors, they do not affect the response to bradykinin, and are less likely to be associated with nonrenin-angiotensin effects (eg, cough and angioedema). Losartan increases urinary flow rate and in addition to being natriuretic and kaliuretic, increases excretion of chloride, magnesium, uric acid, calcium, and phosphate.

Pharmacodynamics/Kinetics

Onset of action: 6 hours

Distribution: V_d: Losartan: 34 L; E-3174: 12 L; does not cross blood brain barrier

Protein binding, plasma: High

Metabolism: Hepatic (14%) via CYP2C9 and 3A4 to active metabolite, E-3174 (40 times more potent than losartan); extensive first-pass effect

Bioavailability: 25% to 33%; AUC of E-3174 is four times greater than that of losartan

Half-life elimination: Losartan: 1.5-2 hours; E-3174: 6-9 hours

Time to peak, serum: Losartan: 1 hour; E-3174: 3-4 hours

Excretion: Urine (4% as unchanged drug, 6% as active metabolite)

Clearance: Plasma: Losartan: 600 mL/minute; Active metabolite: 50 mL/minute

Dosage Oral:

Hypertension:

Children 6-16 years:

U.S. labeling: 0.7 mg/kg once daily (maximum: 50 mg/day); doses >1.4 mg/kg (maximum: 100 mg) have not been studied

Canadian labeling:

≥20 kg to <50 kg: 25 mg once daily (maximum: 50 mg once daily)

≥50 kg: 50 mg once daily (maximum: 100 mg once daily)

Adults: Usual starting dose: 50 mg once daily; can be administered once or twice daily with total daily doses ranging from 25-100 mg

Patients receiving diuretics or with intravascular volume depletion: Usual initial dose: 25 mg once daily

Aortic-root dilation with Marfan's syndrome (unlabeled use): Children 14 months to 16 years: Initial: 0.6 mg/kg/day; can be increased to a maximum of 1.4 mg/kg/day (not to exceed adult maximum of 100 mg/day)

Nephropathy in patients with type 2 diabetes and hypertension: Adults: Initial: 50 mg once daily; can be increased to 100 mg once daily based on blood pressure response

Stroke reduction (HTN with LVH): Adults: 50 mg once daily (maximum daily dose: 100 mg); may be used in combination with a thiazide diuretic

Dosing adjustment in renal impairment:

Children: Use is not recommended if GFR <30 mL/minute/1.73m^2

Adults: No adjustment necessary.

Dosing adjustment in hepatic impairment:

Children 6-16 years:

U.S. labeling: No specific dosing recommendations are provided in the approved labeling, however it may be advisable to initiate therapy at a reduced dosage.

Canadian labeling: Use is not recommended.

Adults: Reduce the initial dose to 25 mg/day

Dietary Considerations May be taken with or without food.

Administration May be administered with or without food.

Monitoring Parameters Supine blood pressure, electrolytes, serum creatinine, BUN, urinalysis, symptomatic hypotension and tachycardia, CBC

Dosage Forms Excipient information presented when available (limited, particularly for generics); consult specific product labeling.

Tablet, oral, as potassium:

Cozaar®: 25 mg [contains potassium 2.12 mg (0.054 mEq)]

Cozaar®: 50 mg [contains potassium 4.24 mg (0.108 mEq)]

Cozaar®: 100 mg [contains potassium 8.48 mg (0.216 mEq)]

Losartan and Hydrochlorothiazide

(loe SAR tan & hye droe klor oh THYE a zide)

Medication Safety Issues

Sound-alike/look-alike issues:

Hyzaar® may be confused with Cozaar®

U.S. Brand Names Hyzaar®

Canadian Brand Names Hyzaar®; Hyzaar® DS

Mexican Brand Names Hyzaar

Index Terms Hydrochlorothiazide and Losartan

Pharmacologic Category Angiotensin II Receptor Blocker; Diuretic, Thiazide

Use Treatment of hypertension; stroke risk reduction in patients with HTN and left ventricular hypertrophy (LVH)

Effect on Mental Status May cause dizziness or insomnia; may rarely cause anxiety, confusion, depression, and sleep disorders

Effect on Psychiatric Treatment Barbiturates may decrease the effects of losartan; may decrease lithium clearance resulting in an increase in serum lithium levels and potential lithium toxicity; monitor serum lithium levels

Dosage Summary

Oral:

Children: Dosage not established

Adults: Losartan 50-100 mg and hydrochlorothiazide 12.5-50 mg once daily

Dosage Forms Excipient information presented when available (limited, particularly for generics); consult specific product labeling.

Tablet:

Hyzaar® 50-12.5: Losartan potassium 50 mg and hydrochlorothiazide 12.5 mg

Hyzaar® 100-12.5: Losartan potassium 100 mg and hydrochlorothiazide 12.5 mg

Hyzaar® 100-25: Losartan potassium 100 mg and hydrochlorothiazide 25 mg

◆ **Losartan Potassium** *see* Losartan *on page 952*

◆ **Lotensin®** *see* Benazepril *on page 178*

◆ **Lotensin® HCT** *see* Benazepril and Hydrochlorothiazide *on page 179*

◆ **Lotrel®** *see* Amlodipine and Benazepril *on page 104*

Lovastatin (LOE va sta tin)

Medication Safety Issues

Sound-alike/look-alike issues:

Lovastatin may be confused with Leustatin®, Livostin®, Lotensin®

Mevacor® may be confused with Mivacron®

International issues:

Lovacol® [Chile and Finland] may be confused with Levatol® which is a brand name for penbutolol in the U.S.

Lovastin® [Poland] may be confused with Livostin® which is a brand name for levocabastine in the U.S.

Related Information

Lipid-Lowering Agents *on page 1786*

U.S. Brand Names Altoprev®; Mevacor®

Canadian Brand Names Apo-Lovastatin®; CO Lovastatin; Gen-Lovastatin; Mevacor®; Novo-Lovastatin; Nu-Lovastatin; PMS-Lovastatin; RAN™-Lovastatin; ratio-Lovastatin; Riva-Lovastatin; Sandoz-Lovastatin

Mexican Brand Names Dilucid; Liperol; Mevacor; Sidevar

Index Terms Mevinolin; Monacolin K

Pharmacologic Category Antilipemic Agent, HMG-CoA Reductase Inhibitor

Generic Available Yes: Immediate release tablet

Use

Adjunct to dietary therapy to decrease elevated serum total and LDL-cholesterol concentrations in primary hypercholesterolemia

Primary prevention of coronary artery disease (patients without symptomatic disease with average to moderately elevated total and LDL-cholesterol and below average HDL-cholesterol); slow progression of coronary atherosclerosis in patients with coronary heart disease

Adjunct to dietary therapy in adolescent patients (10-17 years of age, females >1 year postmenarche) with heterozygous familial hypercholesterolemia having LDL >189 mg/dL, **or** LDL >160 mg/dL with positive family history of premature cardiovascular disease (CVD), **or** LDL >160 mg/dL with the presence of at least two other CVD risk factors

Effect on Mental Status May cause dizziness

Effect on Psychiatric Treatment None reported

Pregnancy Risk Factor X

Pregnancy Considerations Cholesterol biosynthesis may be important in fetal development. Contraindicated in pregnancy. Administer to women of childbearing potential only when conception is highly unlikely and patients have been informed of potential hazards.

Lactation Excretion unknown/contraindicated

Contraindications Hypersensitivity to lovastatin or any component of the formulation; active liver disease; unexplained persistent elevations of serum transaminases; pregnancy; breast-feeding

Warnings/Precautions Secondary causes of hyperlipidemia should be ruled out prior to therapy. Liver function must be monitored by periodic laboratory assessment. Rhabdomyolysis with or without acute renal failure has occurred. Risk is dose-related and is increased with concurrent use of lipid-lowering agents which may cause rhabdomyolysis (gemfibrozil, fibric acid derivatives, or niacin at doses ≥1 g/day) or during concurrent use with potent CYP3A4 inhibitors. Avoid concurrent use of azole antifungals, macrolide antibiotics, and protease inhibitors. Use caution/limit dose with amiodarone, cyclosporine, danazol, gemfibrozil (or other fibrates), lipid-lowering doses of niacin, or verapamil. Monitor closely if used with other drugs associated with myopathy (eg, colchicine). Patients should be instructed to report unexplained muscle pain or weakness; lovastatin should be discontinued if myopathy is suspected/confirmed. Temporarily discontinue in any patient experiencing an acute or serious condition predisposing to renal failure secondary to rhabdomyolysis. Based upon current evidence, HMG-CoA reductase inhibitor therapy should be continued in the perioperative period unless risk outweighs cardioprotective benefit. Use with caution in patients with advanced age, these patients are predisposed to myopathy. Use with caution in patients who consume large amounts of ethanol or have a history of liver disease. Safety and efficacy of the immediate release tablet have not been evaluated in prepubertal patients, patients <10 years of age, or doses >40 mg/day in appropriately-selected adolescents; extended release tablets have not been studied in patients <20 years of age.

Adverse Reactions Percentages as reported with immediate release tablets; similar adverse reactions seen with extended release tablets.

>10%: Neuromuscular & skeletal: Increased CPK (>2x normal) (11%)

1% to 10%:

Central nervous system: Headache (2% to 3%), dizziness (0.5% to 1%)

Dermatologic: Rash (0.8% to 1%)

Gastrointestinal: Abdominal pain (2% to 3%), constipation (2% to 4%), diarrhea (2% to 3%), dyspepsia (1% to 2%), flatulence (4% to 5%), nausea (2% to 3%)

Neuromuscular & skeletal: Myalgia (2% to 3%), weakness (1% to 2%), muscle cramps (0.6% to 1%)

Ocular: Blurred vision (0.8% to 1%)

<1% (Limited to important or life-threatening): Acid regurgitation, alopecia, arthralgia, chest pain, dermatomyositis, eye irritation, insomnia, leg pain, paresthesia, pruritus, vomiting, xerostomia

Additional class-related events or case reports (not necessarily reported with lovastatin therapy): Alkaline phosphatase increased, alopecia, alteration in taste, anaphylaxis, angioedema, anorexia, anxiety, arthritis, cataracts, chills, cholestatic jaundice, cirrhosis, CPK increased (>10x normal), depression, dryness of skin/mucous membranes, dyspnea, eosinophilia, erectile dysfunction, erythema multiforme, ESR increased, facial paresis, fatty liver, fever, flushing, fulminant hepatic necrosis, GGT increased, gynecomastia, hemolytic anemia, hepatitis, hepatoma, hyperbilirubinemia, hypersensitivity reaction, impaired extraocular muscle movement, impotence, leukopenia, libido decreased, malaise, memory loss, myopathy, nail changes, nodules, ophthalmoplegia, pancreatitis, paresthesia, peripheral nerve palsy, peripheral neuropathy, photosensitivity, polymyalgia rheumatica, positive ANA, pruritus, psychic disturbance, purpura, rash, renal failure (secondary to rhabdomyolysis), rhabdomyolysis, skin discoloration, Stevens-Johnson syndrome, systemic lupus erythematosus-like syndrome, thrombocytopenia, thyroid dysfunction, toxic epidermal necrolysis, transaminases increased, tremor, urticaria, vasculitis, vertigo, vomiting

Metabolism/Transport Effects **Substrate** of CYP3A4 (major); **Inhibits** CYP2C9 (weak), 2D6 (weak), 3A4 (weak)

Drug Interactions

Amiodarone: May decrease the metabolism of HMG-CoA Reductase Inhibitors. Management: Dose of simvastatin should not exceed 20 mg/day during concurrent therapy. *Risk D: Consider therapy modification*

Antifungal Agents (Azole Derivatives, Systemic): May decrease the metabolism of HMG-CoA Reductase Inhibitors. *Risk D: Consider therapy modification*

Bosentan: May increase the metabolism of HMG-CoA Reductase Inhibitors. *Risk C: Monitor therapy*

Calcium Channel Blockers (Nondihydropyridine): May decrease the metabolism of HMG-CoA Reductase Inhibitors. *Risk D: Consider therapy modification*

Colchicine: May enhance the myopathic (rhabdomyolysis) effect of HMG-CoA Reductase Inhibitors. Colchicine may increase the serum concentration of HMG-CoA Reductase Inhibitors. *Risk D: Consider therapy modification*

CycloSPORINE: May increase the serum concentration of HMG-CoA Reductase Inhibitors. *Risk D: Consider therapy modification*

CYP3A4 Inducers (Strong): May increase the metabolism of CYP3A4 Substrates. *Risk C: Monitor therapy*

CYP3A4 Inhibitors (Moderate): May decrease the metabolism of CYP3A4 Substrates. *Risk C: Monitor therapy*

CYP3A4 Inhibitors (Strong): May decrease the metabolism of CYP3A4 Substrates. *Risk D: Consider therapy modification*

Danazol: May decrease the metabolism of HMG-CoA Reductase Inhibitors. *Risk C: Monitor therapy*

DAPTOmycin: HMG-CoA Reductase Inhibitors may enhance the adverse/toxic effect of DAPTOmycin. Specifically, the risk of skeletal muscle toxicity may be increased. Management: Consider temporarily stopping HMG-CoA reductase inhibitor therapy prior to daptomycin. If used together, regular (i.e., at least weekly) monitoring of CPK concentrations is recommended. *Risk D: Consider therapy modification*

Dasatinib: May increase the serum concentration of CYP3A4 Substrates. *Risk C: Monitor therapy*

Deferasirox: May decrease the serum concentration of CYP3A4 Substrates. *Risk C: Monitor therapy*

Etravirine: May decrease the serum concentration of HMG-CoA Reductase Inhibitors. This applies to atorvastatin, lovastatin and simvastatin. Conversely, levels of fluvastatin may be increased. Management: Dose adjustment of the HMG-CoA reductase inhibitor may be warranted. No interaction is expected with rosuvastatin or pravastatin. *Risk C: Monitor therapy*

Fenofibrate: May enhance the adverse/toxic effect of HMG-CoA Reductase Inhibitors. *Risk C: Monitor therapy*

Fluconazole: May decrease the metabolism of HMG-CoA Reductase Inhibitors. *Risk D: Consider therapy modification*

Gemfibrozil: May enhance the myopathic (rhabdomyolysis) effect of HMG-CoA Reductase Inhibitors. Gemfibrozil may increase the serum concentration of HMG-CoA Reductase Inhibitors. *Risk D: Consider therapy modification*

Grapefruit Juice: May decrease the metabolism of HMG-CoA Reductase Inhibitors. *Risk D: Consider therapy modification*

Macrolide Antibiotics: May decrease the metabolism of HMG-CoA Reductase Inhibitors. **Exceptions:** Azithromycin; Dirithromycin [Off Market]; Spiramycin. *Risk D: Consider therapy modification*

Nefazodone: May decrease the metabolism of HMG-CoA Reductase Inhibitors. *Risk D: Consider therapy modification*

Niacin: May enhance the adverse/toxic effect of HMG-CoA Reductase Inhibitors. *Risk C: Monitor therapy*

Niacinamide: May enhance the adverse/toxic effect of HMG-CoA Reductase Inhibitors. *Risk C: Monitor therapy*

P-Glycoprotein Inducers: May decrease the serum concentration of P-Glycoprotein Substrates. P-glycoprotein inducers may also further limit the distribution of p-glycoprotein substrates to specific cells/tissues/organs where p-glycoprotein is present in large amounts (e.g., brain, T-lymphocytes, testes, etc.). *Risk C: Monitor therapy*

P-Glycoprotein Inhibitors: May increase the serum concentration of P-Glycoprotein Substrates. P-glycoprotein inhibitors may also enhance the distribution of p-glycoprotein substrates to specific cells/tissues/organs where p-glycoprotein is present in large amounts (e.g., brain, T-lymphocytes, testes, etc.). *Risk C: Monitor therapy*

Phenytoin: May increase the metabolism of HMG-CoA Reductase Inhibitors. *Risk D: Consider therapy modification*

Protease Inhibitors: May increase the serum concentration of HMG-CoA Reductase Inhibitors. Limited data suggest pravastatin may slightly decrease protease inhibitor concentrations. Management: Lovastatin and simvastatin are contraindicated with many protease inhibitors; use lowest possible HMG-CoA reductase inhibitor dose and monitor for signs and symptoms of rhabdomyolysis if these agents are used concomitantly. *Risk D: Consider therapy modification*

Rifamycin Derivatives: May increase the metabolism of HMG-CoA Reductase Inhibitors. *Risk D: Consider therapy modification*

Sildenafil: May decrease the metabolism of HMG-CoA Reductase Inhibitors. *Risk D: Consider therapy modification*

St Johns Wort: May increase the metabolism of HMG-CoA Reductase Inhibitors. *Risk C: Monitor therapy*

Vitamin K Antagonists (eg, warfarin): HMG-CoA Reductase Inhibitors may enhance the anticoagulant effect of Vitamin K Antagonists. *Risk C: Monitor therapy*

Ethanol/Nutrition/Herb Interactions

Ethanol: Avoid excessive ethanol consumption (due to potential hepatic effects).

Food: Food **decreases** the bioavailability of lovastatin extended release tablets and **increases** the bioavailability of lovastatin immediate release tablets. Lovastatin serum concentrations may be increased if taken with grapefruit juice; avoid concurrent intake of large quantities (>1 quart/day). Red yeast rice contains an estimated 2.4 mg lovastatin per 600 mg rice.

Herb/Nutraceutical: St John's wort may decrease lovastatin levels.

Stability

Tablet, immediate release: Store between 5°C to 30°C (41°F to 86°F). Protect from light

Tablet, extended release: Store between 20°C to 25°C (68°F to 77°F). Avoid excessive heat and humidity.

Mechanism of Action Lovastatin acts by competitively inhibiting 3-hydroxyl-3-methylglutaryl-coenzyme A (HMG-CoA) reductase, the enzyme that catalyzes the rate-limiting step in cholesterol biosynthesis

Pharmacodynamics/Kinetics

Onset of action: LDL-cholesterol reductions: 3 days

Absorption: 30%; increased with extended release tablets when taken in the fasting state

Protein binding: 95%

Metabolism: Hepatic; extensive first-pass effect; hydrolyzed to B-hydroxy acid (active)

Bioavailability: Increased with extended release tablets

Half-life elimination: 1.1-1.7 hours

Time to peak, serum: 2-4 hours

Excretion: Feces (~80% to 85%); urine (10%)

Dosage Oral:

Adolescents 10-17 years: Immediate release tablet:

LDL reduction <20%: Initial: 10 mg/day with evening meal

LDL reduction ≥20%: Initial: 20 mg/day with evening meal

Usual range: 10-40 mg with evening meal, then adjust dose at 4-week intervals

Adults: Initial: 20 mg with evening meal, then adjust at 4-week intervals; maximum dose: 80 mg/day immediate release tablet **or** 60 mg/day extended release tablet

Dosage modification/limits based on concurrent therapy:

Cyclosporine and other immunosuppressant drugs: Initial dose: 10 mg/day with a maximum recommended dose of 20 mg/day

Concurrent therapy with fibrates, danazol, and/or lipid-lowering doses of niacin (>1 g/day): Maximum recommended dose: 20 mg/day. Concurrent use with fibrates should be avoided unless risk to benefit favors use.

Concurrent therapy with amiodarone or verapamil: Maximum recommended dose: 40 mg/day of regular release or 20 mg/day with extended release.

Dosage adjustment in renal impairment: Cl_{cr} <30 mL/minute: Use doses >20 mg/day with caution.

Dietary Considerations Before initiation of therapy, patients should be placed on a standard cholesterol-lowering diet for 6 weeks and the diet should be continued during drug therapy. Avoid intake of large quantities of grapefruit juice (≥1 quart/day); may increase toxicity. Red yeast rice contains an estimated 2.4 mg lovastatin per 600 mg rice.

Administration Administer immediate release tablet with meals. Administer extended release tablet at bedtime; do not crush or chew.

Monitoring Parameters

Obtain baseline LFTs and total cholesterol profile. LFTs should also be assessed prior to upwards dosage adjustment to ≥40 mg daily or when otherwise indicated clinically. Enzyme levels should be followed periodically thereafter as clinically warranted.

Reference Range NCEP classification of pediatric patients with familial history of hypercholesterolemia or premature CVD: Acceptable total cholesterol: <170 mg/dL, LDL: <110 mg/dL

Test Interactions Altered thyroid function tests

Dosage Forms Excipient information presented when available (limited, particularly for generics); consult specific product labeling.

Tablet: 10 mg, 20 mg, 40 mg

Mevacor®: 20 mg, 40 mg

Tablet, extended release:

Altoprev®: 20 mg, 40 mg, 60 mg

◆ **Lovastatin and Niacin** *see* Niacin and Lovastatin *on page 1127*

◆ **Lovaza®** *see* Omega-3-Acid Ethyl Esters *on page 1175*

◆ **Lovenox®** *see* Enoxaparin *on page 537*

◆ **Low-Molecular-Weight Iron Dextran (INFeD®)** *see* Iron Dextran Complex *on page 857*

◆ **Low-Ogestrel®** *see* Ethinyl Estradiol and Norgestrel *on page 601*

Loxapine (LOKS a peen)

Medication Safety Issues

Sound-alike/look-alike issues:

Loxitane® may be confused with Lexapro®, Soriatane®

International issues:

Loxitane® may be confused with Lexotan® which is a brand name for bromazepam in multiple international markets

Related Information

Anticholinergic Effects of Common Psychotropics *on page 1758*

Antipsychotic Agents *on page 1769*

CMS: Long-Term Care Facility Thresholds *on page 1815*

Discontinuation of Psychotropic Drugs *on page 1839*

Liquid Compatibility of Antidepressants, Antipsychotics, and Mood Stabilizers *on page 1788*

U.S. Brand Names Loxitane®

Canadian Brand Names Apo-Loxapine®; Loxapac® IM; Nu-Loxapine; PMS-Loxapine

Index Terms Loxapine Succinate; Oxilapine Succinate

Pharmacologic Category Antipsychotic Agent, Typical

Generic Available Yes

Use Management of psychotic disorders

Unlabeled/Investigational Use Psychosis/agitation related to Alzheimer's dementia

Mental Health Comment Loxapine is not commonly used. Older antipsychotic medications (chlorpromazine, haloperidol), which do not meet specific criteria for "atypical" antipsychotics, are often referred to as typical antipsychotics. They are associated with the troubling side effect, EPS. However, it is commonly believed that in order for a drug to treat psychosis, it must block dopamine is some manner.

Common side effects include sedation and neuroleptic effect (reduced initiative, interest in the environment, and display of emotion or affect). All **typical** antipsychotics are considered to be equally effective if given in equipotent doses. An inverse relationship exists between intrinsic antimuscarinic activity and propensity to cause extrapyramidal side effects. If dystonia or pseudoparkinsonism occurs, antiparkinsonian agents should be considered. If akathisia occurs, beta-blockers (eg, propranolol), benzodiazepines, or antiparkinsonian agents should be considered. Tardive dyskinesia (TD) secondary to typical antipsychotics has an estimated incidence of 3% to 5% per year for the first 5 years of treatment. After this time period, the incidence is estimated to be 2% to 3% per year. Prevalence rates are ~15% to 20%. Female gender and age constitute risk factors for TD. Indeed, prevalence rates have been reported to be as high as 70% in elderly females. No specific treatment exists for TD, however, patients are often initiated on/switched to an atypical antipsychotic because of their lower incidence to cause TD and hopes of suppression.

Typical antipsychotics are usually only indicated for schizophrenia, but are generally effective for mania and psychosis and/or behavioral syndromes secondary to other mental conditions. Nonpsychiatric uses include Tourette's syndrome, Huntington's disease, and occasionally, intractable hiccups, pruritus, nausea, and vomiting.

These drugs are thought to exert their antipsychotic activity by blocking dopamine D_2 receptors in the mesolimbic dopaminergic pathway. Side effects are often related to their ability to antagonize dopamine receptors in the nigrostriatal and tuberoinfundibular pathways.

Coadministration of two or more antipsychotics does not generally improve clinical response and may increase the potential for adverse effects.

In 2008, the FDA issued a warning regarding increased mortality risk with typical **and** atypical antipsychotic drugs when used in elderly patients with dementia-related psychosis.

Pregnancy Risk Factor C

Lactation Excretion in breast milk unknown/not recommended

Contraindications Hypersensitivity to loxapine or any component of the formulation; severe CNS depression; coma

Warnings/Precautions Elderly patients with dementia-related psychosis treated with antipsychotics are at an increased risk of death compared to placebo. An increased incidence of cerebrovascular adverse events (including fatalities) has been reported in elderly patients with dementia-related psychosis. Loxapine is not approved for this indication.May alter cardiac conduction; life-threatening arrhythmias have occurred with therapeutic doses of antipsychotics. Avoid use in patients with underlying QT prolongation, in those taking medicines that prolong the QT interval, or cause polymorphic ventricular tachycardia; monitor ECG closely for dose-related QT effects. Myelosuppression (eg, leukopenia, agranulocytosis) has been observed with antipsychotic use; check blood counts periodically and discontinue at first signs of blood dyscrasias. Antipsychotic use has been associated with esophageal dysmotility and aspiration; use with caution in patients at risk of pneumonia (ie, Alzheimer's disease). May cause extrapyramidal symptoms (EPS), including pseudoparkinsonism, acute dystonic reactions, akathisia, and tardive dyskinesia (risk of these reactions is high relative to other neuroleptics). Risk of dystonia (and possibly other EPS) may be greater with increased doses, use of conventional antipsychotics, males, and younger patients. Use may be associated with NMS; monitor for mental status changes, fever, muscle rigidity, and/or autonomic instability (risk may be increased in patients with Parkinson's disease or Lewy body dementia). May cause orthostatic hypotension; use with caution in patients at risk of this effect or in those who would not tolerate transient hypotensive episodes (cerebrovascular disease, cardiovascular disease, hypovolemia, or concurrent medication use which may predispose to hypotension/bradycardia). May be associated with pigmentary retinopathy. May be sedating, use with caution in disorders where CNS depression is a feature; patients must be cautioned about performing tasks which require mental alertness (eg, operating machinery or driving). Impaired core body temperature regulation may occur; caution with strenuous exercise, heat exposure, dehydration, and concomitant medication possessing anticholinergic effects.

May be sedating, use with caution in disorders where CNS depression is a feature; patients must be cautioned about performing tasks which require mental alertness (eg, operating machinery or driving). May cause anticholinergic effects (constipation, xerostomia, blurred vision, urinary retention); use with caution in patients with decreased gastrointestinal motility, paralytic ileus, urinary retention, BPH, xerostomia, or visual problems. Relative to other antipsychotics, loxapine has a low potency of cholinergic blockade. May mask toxicity of other drugs or conditions (eg, intestinal obstruction, Reye's syndrome, brain tumor) due to antiemetic effects.

Use with caution in patients with severe cardiovascular disease, narrow-angle glaucoma, hepatic impairment, myasthenia gravis, Parkinson's disease, breast cancer or other prolactin-dependent tumors, renal impairment, respiratory disease, or seizure disorder. Safety and efficacy have not been established in children.

Adverse Reactions Frequency not defined.

Cardiovascular: Abnormal T waves with prolonged ventricular repolarization, arrhythmia, hyper-/hypotension, orthostatic hypotension, tachycardia, syncope

Central nervous system: Agitation, altered central temperature regulation, ataxia, confusion, dizziness, drowsiness, extrapyramidal reactions (akathisia, akinesia, dystonia, pseudoparkinsonism, tardive dyskinesia), faintness, headache, insomnia, lightheadedness, neuroleptic malignant syndrome (NMS), seizure, slurred speech, tension

Dermatologic: Alopecia, dermatitis, photosensitivity, pruritus, rash, seborrhea

Endocrine & metabolic: Amenorrhea, enlargement of breasts, galactorrhea, gynecomastia, menstrual irregularity

Gastrointestinal: Adynamic ileus, constipation, nausea, polydipsia, vomiting, weight gain/loss, xerostomia

Genitourinary: Sexual dysfunction, urinary retention

Hematologic: Agranulocytosis, leukopenia, thrombocytopenia

Neuromuscular & skeletal: Weakness

Ocular: Blurred vision

Respiratory: Nasal congestion

Drug Interactions

Acetylcholinesterase Inhibitors (Central): May enhance the neurotoxic (central) effect of Antipsychotics. Severe extrapyramidal symptoms have occurred in some patients. *Risk C: Monitor therapy*

Alcohol (Ethyl): CNS Depressants may enhance the CNS depressant effect of Alcohol (Ethyl). *Risk C: Monitor therapy*

Alfuzosin: May enhance the QTc-prolonging effect of QTc-Prolonging Agents. *Risk C: Monitor therapy*

Amphetamines: Antipsychotics may diminish the stimulatory effect of Amphetamines. *Risk C: Monitor therapy*

Anticholinergics: May enhance the adverse/toxic effect of other Anticholinergics. **Exceptions:** Paliperidone. *Risk C: Monitor therapy*

Anti-Parkinson's Agents (Dopamine Agonist): Antipsychotics (Typical) may diminish the therapeutic effect of Anti-Parkinson's Agents (Dopamine Agonist). *Risk D: Consider therapy modification*

Ciprofloxacin: May enhance the QTc-prolonging effect of QTc-Prolonging Agents. *Risk C: Monitor therapy*

CNS Depressants: May enhance the adverse/toxic effect of other CNS Depressants. *Risk C: Monitor therapy*

Gadobutrol: May enhance the QTc-prolonging effect of QTc-Prolonging Agents. *Risk D: Consider therapy modification*

Lithium formulations: May enhance the neurotoxic effect of Antipsychotics. Lithium formulations may decrease the serum concentration of Antipsychotics. Specifically noted with chlorpromazine. *Risk C: Monitor therapy*

LORazepam: Loxapine may enhance the adverse/toxic effect of LORazepam. Specifically, prolonged stupor, respiratory depression, and/or hypotension. *Risk C: Monitor therapy*

Nilotinib: May enhance the QTc-prolonging effect of QTc-Prolonging Agents. *Risk X: Avoid combination*

Pramlintide: May enhance the anticholinergic effect of Anticholinergics. These effects are specific to the GI tract. *Risk D: Consider therapy modification*

QTc-Prolonging Agents: May enhance the adverse/toxic effect of other QTc-Prolonging Agents. Their effects can be additive, causing life-threatening ventricular arrhythmias. *Risk D: Consider therapy modification*

Tetrabenazine: May enhance the adverse/toxic effect of Antipsychotics. *Risk C: Monitor therapy*

Thioridazine: QTc-Prolonging Agents may enhance the QTc-prolonging effect of Thioridazine. *Risk X: Avoid combination*

Ziprasidone: QTc-Prolonging Agents may enhance the QTc-prolonging effect of Ziprasidone. The risk of a severe arrhythmia may be increased. *Risk X: Avoid combination*

Ethanol/Nutrition/Herb Interactions

Ethanol: Avoid ethanol (may increase CNS depression).

Herb/Nutraceutical: Avoid kava kava, gotu kola, valerian, St John's wort (may increase CNS depression).

Stability Protect from light. Dispense in amber or opaque vials.

Mechanism of Action Loxapine is a dibenzoxazepine antipsychotic which blocks postsynaptic mesolimbic D_1 and D_2 receptors in the brain, and also possesses serotonin 5-HT_2 blocking activity

Pharmacodynamics/Kinetics

Onset of action: Neuroleptic: Oral: 20-30 minutes

Peak effect: 1.5-3 hours

Duration: ~12 hours

Metabolism: Hepatic to glucuronide conjugates

Half-life elimination: Biphasic: Initial: 5 hours; Terminal: 12-19 hours

Excretion: Urine; feces (small amounts)

Dosage Oral:

Adults: 10 mg twice daily, increase dose until psychotic symptoms are controlled; usual dose range: 20-100 mg/day in divided doses 2-4 times/day; dosages >250 mg/day are not recommended

Elderly: 20-60 mg/day

Monitoring Parameters Vital signs, orthostatic blood pressures 3-5 days after initiation of therapy or a dose increase; lipid profile, fasting blood glucose/Hgb A_{1c}; BMI; mental status, abnormal involuntary movement scale (AIMS), extrapyramidal symptoms (EPS)

Test Interactions False-positives for phenylketonuria, amylase, uroporphyrins, urobilinogen

Dosage Forms Excipient information presented when available (limited, particularly for generics); consult specific product labeling.

Capsule, as succinate: 5 mg, 10 mg, 25 mg, 50 mg

- **Loxapine Succinate** *see* Loxapine *on page 960*
- **Loxitane®** *see* Loxapine *on page 960*
- **L-PAM** *see* Melphalan *on page 983*
- **LRH** *see* Gonadorelin *on page 734*
- **L-Sarcolysin** *see* Melphalan *on page 983*
- **LTA® 360** *see* Lidocaine *on page 924*
- **LTG** *see* LamoTRIgine *on page 889*
- **Lu-26-054** *see* Escitalopram *on page 564*

Lubiprostone (loo bi PROS tone)

U.S. Brand Names Amitiza®

Index Terms RU 0211; SPI 0211

Pharmacologic Category Chloride Channel Activator; Gastrointestinal Agent, Miscellaneous

Use Treatment of chronic idiopathic constipation; treatment of irritable bowel syndrome with constipation in adult women

Effect on Mental Status May cause insomnia, dizziness, depression, or anxiety

Effect on Psychiatric Treatment Nausea and diarrhea are common; concomitant use with SSRIs, lithium, valproic acid, and carbamazepine may produce additive effects

Dosage Summary

Oral:

Children: Dosage not established

Adults (females): 8 mcg twice daily **or** 24 mcg twice daily

Adults (males): 24 mcg twice daily

Dosage Forms Excipient information presented when available (limited, particularly for generics); consult specific product labeling.

Capsule, softgel:

Amitiza®: 8 mcg, 24 mcg

◆ **Ludiomil** *see* Maprotiline *on page 968*
◆ **Lufyllin®** *see* Dyphylline *on page 521*
◆ **Lufyllin®-GG** *see* Dyphylline and Guaifenesin *on page 522*
◆ **Lugol's Solution** *see* Potassium Iodide and Iodine *on page 1317*
◆ **Luminal® Sodium** *see* PHENobarbital *on page 1265*
◆ **Lunesta®** *see* Eszopiclone *on page 589*
◆ **LupiCare® Dandruff [OTC]** *see* Salicylic Acid *on page 1454*
◆ **LupiCare® Psoriasis [OTC]** *see* Salicylic Acid *on page 1454*
◆ **LupiCare® Psoriasis Scalp [OTC] [DSC]** *see* Salicylic Acid *on page 1454*
◆ **Lupron®** *see* Leuprolide *on page 901*
◆ **Lupron Depot®** *see* Leuprolide *on page 901*
◆ **Lupron Depot-Ped®** *see* Leuprolide *on page 901*
◆ **Lupulus** *see* Hops *(Humulus lupulus) on page 770*
◆ **LuSonal™** *see* Phenylephrine *on page 1273*
◆ **Luteinizing Hormone Releasing Hormone** *see* Gonadorelin *on page 734*
◆ **Lutera™** *see* Ethinyl Estradiol and Levonorgestrel *on page 595*

Lutropin Alfa (LOO troe pin AL fa)

U.S. Brand Names Luveris®
Mexican Brand Names Luver-I.S.
Index Terms r-hLH; Recombinant Human Luteinizing Hormone
Pharmacologic Category Gonadotropin; Ovulation Stimulator
Use Stimulation of follicular development in infertile hypogonadotropic hypogonadal (HH) women with profound luteinizing hormone (LH) deficiency; to be used in combination with follitropin alfa
Effect on Mental Status May cause fatigue
Effect on Psychiatric Treatment May cause GI side effects; concurrent use with SSRIs, lithium, or valproic acid may produce additive GI effects
Dosage Summary
SubQ:
Children: Dosage not established
Adults (females): 75 int. units daily (maximum duration: 14 days)
Dosage Forms Excipient information presented when available (limited, particularly for generics); consult specific product labeling.
Injection, powder for reconstitution:
Luveris®: 75 int. units [contains sucrose; packaged with SWFI]

◆ **Luveris®** *see* Lutropin Alfa *on page 964*
◆ **Luvox** *see* Fluvoxamine *on page 678*
◆ **Luvox® CR** *see* Fluvoxamine *on page 678*
◆ **Luxiq®** *see* Betamethasone *on page 184*
◆ **LY139603** *see* Atomoxetine *on page 151*
◆ **LY146032** *see* DAPTOmycin *on page 418*
◆ **LY170053** *see* OLANZapine *on page 1160*
◆ **LY231514** *see* Pemetrexed *on page 1238*
◆ **LY248686** *see* DULoxetine *on page 516*
◆ **LY2148568** *see* Exenatide *on page 609*
◆ **Lybrel™** *see* Ethinyl Estradiol and Levonorgestrel *on page 595*
◆ **Lymphocyte Immune Globulin** *see* Antithymocyte Globulin (Equine) *on page 126*
◆ **Lymphocyte Mitogenic Factor** *see* Aldesleukin *on page 58*
◆ **Lyrica®** *see* Pregabalin *on page 1332*
◆ **Lysodren®** *see* Mitotane *on page 1061*
◆ **Maalox® [OTC]** *see* Aluminum Hydroxide, Magnesium Hydroxide, and Simethicone *on page 78*
◆ **Maalox® Max [OTC]** *see* Aluminum Hydroxide, Magnesium Hydroxide, and Simethicone *on page 78*
◆ **Maalox® Regular Chewable [OTC]** *see* Calcium Carbonate *on page 254*
◆ **Maalox® Total Stomach Relief® [OTC]** *see* Bismuth *on page 189*

◆ **Macrobid®** *see* Nitrofurantoin *on page 1147*
◆ **Macrodantin®** *see* Nitrofurantoin *on page 1147*
◆ **Macugen®** *see* Pegaptanib *on page 1235*
◆ **Mag 64™ [OTC]** *see* Magnesium Chloride *on page 965*

Magaldrate and Simethicone (MAG al drate & sye METH i kone)

Medication Safety Issues
Sound-alike/look-alike issues:
Riopan Plus® may be confused with Repan®

U.S. Brand Names Riopan Plus® Double Strength [OTC] [DSC]; Riopan Plus® [OTC] [DSC]

Index Terms Simethicone and Magaldrate

Pharmacologic Category Antacid; Antiflatulent

Use Relief of hyperacidity associated with peptic ulcer, gastritis, peptic esophagitis, and hiatal hernia which are accompanied by symptoms of gas

Effect on Mental Status None reported

Effect on Psychiatric Treatment Constipation is common; concurrent use with psychotropics may produce additive effects

Dosage Summary
Oral:
Children: Dosage not established
Adults: 5-10 mL (540-1080 mg magaldrate) between meals and at bedtime

Dosage Forms Excipient information presented when available (limited, particularly for generics); consult specific product labeling. [DSC] = Discontinued product
Suspension, oral: Magaldrate 540 mg and simethicone 20 mg per 5 mL (360 mL)
Riopan Plus®: Magaldrate 540 mg and simethicone 20 mg per 5 mL (360 mL) [DSC]
Riopan Plus® Double Strength: Magaldrate 1080 mg and simethicone 40 mg per 5 mL (360 mL) [DSC]

◆ **Mag-Caps [OTC]** *see* Magnesium Oxide *on page 966*
◆ **Mag Delay® [OTC]** *see* Magnesium Chloride *on page 965*
◆ **MagGel™ [OTC]** *see* Magnesium Oxide *on page 966*
◆ **Magnacet™** *see* Oxycodone and Acetaminophen *on page 1205*

Magnesium Chloride (mag NEE zhum KLOR ide)

U.S. Brand Names Chloromag®; Mag 64™ [OTC]; Mag Delay® [OTC]; Slow-Mag® [OTC]

Mexican Brand Names Solural

Pharmacologic Category Electrolyte Supplement, Oral; Electrolyte Supplement, Parenteral; Magnesium Salt

Use Correction or prevention of hypomagnesemia; dietary supplement

Effect on Mental Status May cause somnolence

Effect on Psychiatric Treatment Concurrent use with psychotropics may produce additive sedation

Dosage Summary
I.V.:
Children <50 kg: 0.3-0.5 mEq/kg/day
Children >50 kg: 10-30 mEq/day
Adults: 8-24 mEq/day added to TPN
Oral: RDA (elemental magnesium):
Children:
1-3 years: 80 mg/day
4-8 years: 130 mg/day
9-13 years: 240 mg/day
14-18 years:
Female: 360 mg/day
Pregnant female: 400 mg/day
Male: 410 mg/day
Adults:
19-30 years:
Female: 310 mg/day
Pregnant female: 350 mg/day
Male: 400 mg/day

≥31 years:
Female: 320 mg/day
Pregnant female: 360 mg/day
Male: 420 mg/day

Dosage Forms Excipient information presented when available (limited, particularly for generics); consult specific product labeling.

Injection, solution: 200 mg/mL [1.97 mEq/mL] (50 mL)
Chloromag®: 200 mg/mL [1.97 mEq/mL] (50 mL)

Tablet [enteric coated]:
Slow-Mag®: Elemental magnesium 64 mg [contains elemental calcium 106 mg]

Tablet, delayed release:
Mag 64™, Mag Delay®: Magnesium chloride hexahydrate 535 mg [equivalent to elemental magnesium 64 mg; contains elemental calcium 110 mg]

- **Magnesium Hydroxide, Aluminum Hydroxide, and Simethicone** *see* Aluminum Hydroxide, Magnesium Hydroxide, and Simethicone *on page 78*
- **Magnesium Hydroxide and Calcium Carbonate** *see* Calcium Carbonate and Magnesium Hydroxide *on page 256*
- **Magnesium Hydroxide, Famotidine, and Calcium Carbonate** *see* Famotidine, Calcium Carbonate, and Magnesium Hydroxide *on page 614*

Magnesium Oxide (mag NEE zhum OKS ide)

U.S. Brand Names Mag-Caps [OTC]; Mag-Ox® 400 [OTC]; MagGel™ [OTC]; Uro-Mag® [OTC]

Pharmacologic Category Electrolyte Supplement, Oral; Magnesium Salt

Use Electrolyte replacement

Effect on Mental Status May rarely cause depression

Effect on Psychiatric Treatment None reported

Dosage Summary

Oral: RDA (elemental magnesium):

Children:
1-3 years: 80 mg/day
4-8 years: 130 mg/day
9-13 years: 240 mg/day
14-18 years:
Female: 360 mg/day
Pregnant female: 400 mg/day
Male: 410 mg/day

Adults:
19-30 years:
Female: 310 mg/day
Pregnant female: 350 mg/day
Male: 400 mg/day
≥31 years:
Female: 320 mg/day
Pregnant female: 360 mg/day
Male: 420 mg/day

Dosage Forms Excipient information presented when available (limited, particularly for generics); consult specific product labeling.

Caplet: 250 mg

Capsule:
Mag-Caps: Elemental magnesium 85 mg
Uro-Mag®: 140 mg [magnesium 7 mEq; equivalent to elemental magnesium 84.5 mg]

Capsule, softgel:
MagGel™: 600 mg [magnesium 28.64 mEq; equivalent to elemental magnesium 348 mg]

Tablet: 400 mg [magnesium 20 mEq; equivalent to elemental magnesium 242 mg], 500 mg
Mag-Ox® 400: 400 mg [magnesium 20 mEq; equivalent to elemental magnesium 242 mg]

Magnesium Sulfate (mag NEE zhum SUL fate)

Medication Safety Issues

Sound-alike/look-alike issues:
Magnesium sulfate may be confused with manganese sulfate, morphine sulfate

$MgSO_4$ is an error-prone abbreviation (mistaken as morphine sulfate)

High alert medication: The Institute for Safe Medication Practices (ISMP) includes this medication (I.V. formulation) among its list of drugs which have a heightened risk of causing significant patient harm when used in error.

Mexican Brand Names Cholal modificado; Kiddi Pharmaton; Vivioptal Junior

Index Terms Epsom Salts; $MgSO_4$ (error-prone abbreviation)

Pharmacologic Category Anticonvulsant, Miscellaneous; Electrolyte Supplement, Parenteral; Magnesium Salt

Use Treatment and prevention of hypomagnesemia; prevention and treatment of seizures in severe pre-eclampsia or eclampsia, pediatric acute nephritis; torsade de pointes; treatment of cardiac arrhythmias (VT/VF) caused by hypomagnesemia; soaking aid

Unlabeled/Investigational Use
Asthma exacerbation (life-threatening)

Effect on Mental Status May cause sedation or CNS depression

Effect on Psychiatric Treatment Concurrent use with psychotropics may produce additive CNS depression

Dosage Summary

I.V.:

Children:

Hypomagnesemia: 25-50 mg/kg/dose; maximum single dose: 2000 mg; may also administer I.O.

TPN:

<50 kg: 0.3-0.5 mEq elemental magnesium/kg/day

>50 kg: 10-30 mEq elemental magnesium/day

Adults:

Hypomagnesemia, torsade de pointes: 1-2 g, followed by 0.5-1 g/hour continuous infusion

Eclampsia, pre-eclampsia (severe): 4-5 g infusion; followed by a 1-2 g/hour continous infusion; or may follow with I.M. doses of 4-5 g in each buttock every 4 hours. **Note:** Initial infusion may be given over 3-4 minutes if eclampsia is severe; ACOG guidelines recommend infusion over 15-20 minutes. Maximum: 40 g/24 hours.

TPN: 8-24 mEq elemental magnesium/day

Oral:

Children:

RDA:

1-3 years: 80 mg elemental magnesium/day

4-8 years: 130 mg elemental magnesium/day

9-13 years: 240 mg elemental magnesium/day

14-18 years

Female: 360 mg elemental magnesium/day

Pregnant female: 400 mg elemental magnesium/day

Male: 410 mg elemental magnesium/day

Adults:

RDA:

19-30 years:

Female: 310 mg elemental magnesium/day

Pregnant female: 350 mg elemental magnesium/day

Male: 400 mg elemental magnesium/day

≥31 years:

Female: 320 mg elemental magnesium/day

Pregnant female: 360 mg elemental magnesium/day

Male: 420 mg elemental magnesium/day

I.M.:

Children: Dosage not established

Adults: Hypomagnesemia: 1-4 g/day in divided doses

Topical:

Children: Dosage not established

Adults: Soaking aid: Dissolve 2 cupfuls of powder per gallon of warm water

Dosage Forms Excipient information presented when available (limited, particularly for generics); consult specific product labeling.

Infusion [premixed in D_5W]: 10 mg/mL (100 mL); 20 mg/mL (500 mL)

Infusion [premixed in water for injection]: 40 mg/mL (100 mL, 500 mL, 1000 mL); 80 mg/mL (50 mL)

Injection, solution: 500 mg/mL (2 mL, 10 mL, 20 mL, 50 mL)

Powder, oral/topical: Magnesium sulfate USP (227 g, 454 g, 480 g, 1810 g, 1920 g, 2720 g)

◆ **Magnevist®** *see* Gadopentetate Dimeglumine *on page 705*

◆ **Mag-Ox® 400 [OTC]** *see* Magnesium Oxide *on page 966*

- **Ma Huang** *see* Ephedra *(Ephedra sinica) on page 541*
- **Malarone®** *see* Atovaquone and Proguanil *on page 157*
- **Mandrake** *see* Podophyllum Resin *on page 1309*

Mannitol (MAN i tole)

Medication Safety Issues

Sound-alike/look-alike issues:

Osmitrol® may be confused with esmolol

U.S. Brand Names Osmitrol®; Resectisol®

Canadian Brand Names Osmitrol®

Mexican Brand Names Photoderm Max Bio

Index Terms *D*-Mannitol

Pharmacologic Category Diuretic, Osmotic; Genitourinary Irrigant

Use Reduction of increased intracranial pressure associated with cerebral edema; promotion of diuresis in the prevention and/or treatment of oliguria or anuria due to acute renal failure; reduction of increased intraocular pressure; promoting urinary excretion of toxic substances; genitourinary irrigant in transurethral prostatic resection or other transurethral surgical procedures

Effect on Mental Status May cause dizziness

Effect on Psychiatric Treatment Has been used to treat lithium toxicity/overdose but its overall effect in lowering serum lithium level is minimum; if toxicity is severe, hemodialysis is the treatment of choice

Dosage Summary

I.V.:

Children: Initial: 0.25-1 g/kg; Maintenance: 0.25-0.5 g/kg every 4-6 hours

Adults:

Diuresis: Initial: 0.5-1 g/kg; Maintenance: 0.25-0.5 g/kg every 4-6 hours (usually 20-200 g/day)

Intracranial pressure/cerebral edema: 0.25-1.5 g/kg as 15-20% solution; maintain serum osmolality 310 to <320 mOsm/kg

Preoperative: 1.5-2 g/kg prior to surgery

Prevention/treatment oliguria: 50-100 g dose

Transurethral:

Children: Dosage not established

Adults: Use urogenital solution as required for irrigation

Dosage Forms Excipient information presented when available (limited, particularly for generics); consult specific product labeling.

Injection, solution: 5% [50 mg/mL] (1000 mL); 10% [100 mg/mL] (500 mL, 1000 mL); 15% [150 mg/mL] (500 mL); 20% [200 mg/mL] (150 mL, 250 mL, 500 mL); 25% [250 mg/mL] (50 mL)

Osmitrol®: 5% [50 mg/mL] (1000 mL); 10% [100 mg/mL] (500 mL, 1000 mL); 15% [150 mg/mL] (500 mL); 20% [200 mg/mL] (250 mL, 500 mL)

Solution, urogenital (Resectisol®): 5% [50 mg/mL] (2000 mL, 4000 mL)

- **Mapap [OTC]** *see* Acetaminophen *on page 30*
- **Mapap Children's [OTC]** *see* Acetaminophen *on page 30*
- **Mapap Extra Strength [OTC]** *see* Acetaminophen *on page 30*
- **Mapap Infants [OTC]** *see* Acetaminophen *on page 30*
- **Mapap® Multi-Symptom Cold [OTC]** *see* Acetaminophen, Dextromethorphan, and Phenylephrine *on page 42*
- **Mapap® Sinus Congestion and Pain Daytime [OTC]** *see* Acetaminophen and Phenylephrine *on page 36*
- **Mapap Sinus Maximum Strength [OTC]** *see* Acetaminophen and Pseudoephedrine *on page 37*

Maprotiline (ma PROE ti leen)

Medication Safety Issues

Sound-alike/look-alike issues:

Ludiomil may be confused with Lamictal®, lamotrigine, Lomotil®

Related Information

Anticholinergic Effects of Common Psychotropics *on page 1758*

Antidepressant Agents *on page 1760*

Antidepressant Receptor Profile *on page 1764*

Discontinuation of Psychotropic Drugs *on page 1839*

Canadian Brand Names Novo-Maprotiline

Mexican Brand Names Ludiomil

Index Terms Ludiomil; Maprotiline Hydrochloride

Pharmacologic Category Antidepressant, Tetracyclic

Generic Available Yes

Use Treatment of depression and anxiety associated with depression

Unlabeled/Investigational Use Bulimia; duodenal ulcers; enuresis; urinary symptoms of multiple sclerosis; pain; panic attacks; tension headache; cocaine withdrawal

Restrictions An FDA-approved medication guide concerning the use of antidepressants in children, adolescents, and young adults must be distributed when dispensing an outpatient prescription (new or refill) where this medication is to be used without direct supervision of a healthcare provider. Medication guides are available at http://www.fda.gov/cder/Offices/ODS/medication_guides.htm. Dispense to parents or guardians of children and adolescents receiving this medication.

Pregnancy Risk Factor B

Contraindications Hypersensitivity to maprotiline or any component of the formulation; use of MAO inhibitors within 14 days; use in a patient during the acute recovery phase of MI

Warnings/Precautions **[U.S. Boxed Warning]: Antidepressants increase the risk of suicidal thinking and behavior in children, adolescents, and young adults (18-24 years of age) with major depressive disorder (MDD) and other psychiatric disorders;** consider risk prior to prescribing. Short-term studies did not show an increased risk in patients >24 years of age and showed a decreased risk in patients ≥65 years. Closely monitor for clinical worsening, suicidality, or unusual changes in behavior; the patient's family or caregiver should be instructed to closely observe the patient and communicate condition with healthcare provider. A medication guide should be dispensed with each prescription. **Maprotiline is not FDA approved for use in children.**

The possibility of a suicide attempt is inherent in major depression and may persist until remission occurs. Monitor for worsening of depression or suicidality, especially during initiation of therapy (generally first 1-2 months) or with dose increases or decreases. Use caution in high-risk patients. Worsening depression and severe abrupt suicidality that are not part of the presenting symptoms may require discontinuation or modification of drug therapy. The patient's family or caregiver should be alerted to monitor patients for the emergence of suicidality and associated behaviors (such as agitation, irritability, hostility, impulsivity, and hypomania) and call healthcare provider.

May worsen psychosis in some patients or precipitate a shift to mania or hypomania in patients with bipolar disorder. Patients presenting with depressive symptoms should be screened for bipolar disorder. Monotherapy in patients with bipolar disorder should be avoided. **Maprotiline is not FDA approved for the treatment of bipolar depression.**

Maprotiline has a high risk of sedation relative to other antidepressants. Sedation is common, and may result in impaired performance of tasks requiring alertness (eg, operating machinery or driving). Sedative effects may be additive with other CNS depressants and/or ethanol.

The risk of orthostatic hypotension and/or cardiac conduction abnormalities is moderate relative to other antidepressants. Use with caution in patients with a history of cardiovascular disease (including previous MI, stroke, tachycardia, or conduction abnormalities). The degree of anticholinergic blockade produced by this agent is moderate relative to other cyclic antidepressants, however, caution should still be used in patients with urinary retention, benign prostatic hyperplasia, narrow-angle glaucoma, xerostomia, visual problems, constipation, or history of bowel obstruction.

Consider discontinuing, when possible, prior to elective surgery. Therapy should not be abruptly discontinued in patients receiving high doses for prolonged periods. Use caution in patients with a previous seizure disorder or condition predisposing to seizures such as brain damage, alcoholism, or concurrent therapy with other drugs which lower the seizure threshold. May increase the risks associated with electroconvulsive therapy. Use with caution in hyperthyroid patients or those receiving thyroid supplementation. Use with caution in patients with hepatic or renal dysfunction and in elderly patients.

Adverse Reactions

>10%:

Central nervous system: Drowsiness

Gastrointestinal: Xerostomia

1% to 10%:

Central nervous system: Insomnia, nervousness, anxiety, agitation, dizziness, fatigue, headache

Gastrointestinal: Constipation, nausea
Neuromuscular & skeletal: Tremor, weakness
Ocular: Blurred vision

<1% (Limited to important or life-threatening): Accommodation disturbances, akathisia, arrhythmia, ataxia, confusion, delusions, disorientation, dysarthria, dysphagia, extrapyramidal symptoms (EPS), hallucinations, heart block, hyper-/hypotension, impotence, mania, photosensitivity, rash, seizure, syncope, tinnitus, urinary retention, vomiting

Metabolism/Transport Effects **Substrate** of CYP2D6 (major)

Drug Interactions

Acetylcholinesterase Inhibitors (Central): Anticholinergics may diminish the therapeutic effect of Acetylcholinesterase Inhibitors (Central). Acetylcholinesterase Inhibitors (Central) may diminish the therapeutic effect of Anticholinergics. If the anticholinergic action is a side effect of the agent, the result may be beneficial. *Risk C: Monitor therapy*

Alcohol (Ethyl): CNS Depressants may enhance the CNS depressant effect of Alcohol (Ethyl). *Risk C: Monitor therapy*

Alfuzosin: May enhance the QTc-prolonging effect of QTc-Prolonging Agents. *Risk C: Monitor therapy*

Anticholinergics: May enhance the adverse/toxic effect of other Anticholinergics. **Exceptions:** Paliperidone. *Risk C: Monitor therapy*

Ciprofloxacin: May enhance the QTc-prolonging effect of QTc-Prolonging Agents. *Risk C: Monitor therapy*

CNS Depressants: May enhance the adverse/toxic effect of other CNS Depressants. *Risk C: Monitor therapy*

CYP2D6 Inhibitors (Moderate): May decrease the metabolism of CYP2D6 Substrates. *Risk C: Monitor therapy*

CYP2D6 Inhibitors (Strong): May decrease the metabolism of CYP2D6 Substrates. *Risk D: Consider therapy modification*

Darunavir: May increase the serum concentration of CYP2D6 Substrates. *Risk C: Monitor therapy*

Gadobutrol: May enhance the QTc-prolonging effect of QTc-Prolonging Agents. *Risk D: Consider therapy modification*

MAO Inhibitors: Maprotiline may enhance the adverse/toxic effect of MAO Inhibitors. *Risk X: Avoid combination*

Nilotinib: May enhance the QTc-prolonging effect of QTc-Prolonging Agents. *Risk X: Avoid combination*

Pramlintide: May enhance the anticholinergic effect of Anticholinergics. These effects are specific to the GI tract. *Risk D: Consider therapy modification*

QTc-Prolonging Agents: May enhance the adverse/toxic effect of other QTc-Prolonging Agents. Their effects can be additive, causing life-threatening ventricular arrhythmias. *Risk D: Consider therapy modification*

Serotonin Modulators: May enhance the adverse/toxic effect of other Serotonin Modulators. The development of serotonin syndrome may occur. *Risk D: Consider therapy modification*

Sibutramine: May enhance the serotonergic effect of Serotonin Modulators. This may cause serotonin syndrome. *Risk X: Avoid combination*

Sulfonylureas: Cyclic Antidepressants may enhance the hypoglycemic effect of Sulfonylureas. *Risk C: Monitor therapy*

Tetrabenazine: QTc-Prolonging Agents may enhance the QTc-prolonging effect of Tetrabenazine. *Risk X: Avoid combination*

Thioridazine: QTc-Prolonging Agents may enhance the QTc-prolonging effect of Thioridazine. *Risk X: Avoid combination*

Ziprasidone: QTc-Prolonging Agents may enhance the QTc-prolonging effect of Ziprasidone. The risk of a severe arrhythmia may be increased. *Risk X: Avoid combination*

Ethanol/Nutrition/Herb Interactions Ethanol: Avoid ethanol (may increase CNS depression).

Mechanism of Action Traditionally believed to increase the synaptic concentration of norepinephrine in the central nervous system by inhibition of their reuptake by the presynaptic neuronal membrane. However, additional receptor effects have been found including desensitization of adenyl cyclase, down regulation of beta-adrenergic receptors, and down regulation of serotonin receptors.

Pharmacodynamics/Kinetics

Absorption: Slow
Protein binding: 88%
Metabolism: Hepatic to active and inactive compounds
Half-life elimination, serum: 27-58 hours (mean: 43 hours)
Time to peak, serum: Within 12 hours
Excretion: Urine (70%); feces (30%)

Dosage Oral:

Adults: Depression/anxiety: 75 mg/day to start, increase by 25 mg every 2 weeks up to 150-225 mg/day; given in 3 divided doses or in a single daily dose

Elderly: Depression/anxiety: Initial: 25 mg at bedtime, increase by 25 mg every 3 days for inpatients and weekly for outpatients if tolerated; usual maintenance dose: 50-75 mg/day, higher doses may be necessary in nonresponders

Monitoring Parameters Monitor blood pressure and pulse rate prior to and during initial therapy; evaluate mood and somatic complaints, suicidal ideation (especially at the beginning of therapy or when doses are increased or decreased); monitor appetite and weight; ECG in older adults

Additional Information Odorless, bitter tasting; seizures are rarely seen 5-30 hours postdrug ingestion.

Dosage Forms Excipient information presented when available (limited, particularly for generics); consult specific product labeling.

Tablet, as hydrochloride: 25 mg, 50 mg, 75 mg

◆ **Maprotiline Hydrochloride** *see* Maprotiline *on page 968*

Maraviroc (mah RAV er rock)

U.S. Brand Names Selzentry™

Canadian Brand Names Celsentri™

Index Terms UK-427,857

Pharmacologic Category Antiretroviral Agent, CCR5 Antagonist

Use Treatment of CCR5-tropic HIV-1 infection, in combination with other antiretroviral agents in treatment-experienced patients with evidence of viral replication and HIV-1 strains resistant to multiple antiretroviral therapy

Effect on Mental Status May cause dizziness, insomnia, or depression

Effect on Psychiatric Treatment May produce postural hypotension; concomitant use with psychotropic agents may produce additive effects. May cause neutropenia; use caution with clozapine and carbamazepine. High potential for drug-drug interactions. Carbamazepine, phenobarbital, and phenytoin may decrease the levels/effects of maraviroc; dosage adjustment of maraviroc may be recommended. Nefazodone may increase the levels/effects of maraviroc; dosage adjustment of maraviroc may be recommended. St John's wort may decrease levels of maraviroc and lead to possible resistance; concurrent use is not recommended.

Restrictions An FDA-approved medication guide is available at http://www.-selzentry.com/content/SELZENTRY_MedicationGuide.pdf; distribute to each patient to whom this medication is dispensed.

Dosage Summary

Oral:

Children <16 years: Dosage not established

Children ≥16 years: 300 mg twice daily; adjusted dosage: 150 mg twice daily **or** 600 mg twice daily

Adults: 300 mg twice daily; adjusted dosage: 150 mg twice daily **or** 600 mg twice daily

Dosage Forms Excipient information presented when available (limited, particularly for generics); consult specific product labeling.

Tablet:

Selzentry™: 150 mg, 300 mg

◆ **Marcaine®** *see* Bupivacaine *on page 211*

◆ **Marcaine® Spinal** *see* Bupivacaine *on page 211*

◆ **Marezine® [OTC]** *see* Cyclizine *on page 405*

◆ **Margesic® H** *see* Hydrocodone and Acetaminophen *on page 777*

◆ **Marinol®** *see* Dronabinol *on page 512*

◆ **Mark 1™** *see* Atropine and Pralidoxime *on page 159*

◆ **Marplan®** *see* Isocarboxazid *on page 858*

◆ ***Matricaria chamomilla*** *see* Chamomile, German *(Matricaria chamomilla, Matricaria recutita) on page 310*

◆ ***Matricaria recutita*** *see* Chamomile, German *(Matricaria chamomilla, Matricaria recutita) on page 310*

◆ **Matulane®** *see* Procarbazine *on page 1340*

◆ **Mavik®** *see* Trandolapril *on page 1608*

◆ **Maxair™ Autohaler™** *see* Pirbuterol *on page 1305*

◆ **Maxalt®** *see* Rizatriptan *on page 1437*

◆ **Maxalt-MLT®** *see* Rizatriptan *on page 1437*

◆ **Maxidex®** *see* Dexamethasone *on page 436*

◆ **Maxidone®** *see* Hydrocodone and Acetaminophen *on page 777*

◆ **Maxifed®** *see* Guaifenesin and Pseudoephedrine *on page 744*

◆ **Maxifed DM** *see* Guaifenesin, Pseudoephedrine, and Dextromethorphan *on page 748*

◆ **Maxifed DMX** *see* Guaifenesin, Pseudoephedrine, and Dextromethorphan *on page 748*

◆ **Maxifed-G®** *see* Guaifenesin and Pseudoephedrine *on page 744*

◆ **Maximum D3®** *see* Cholecalciferol *on page 341*

◆ **Maxiphen DM** *see* Guaifenesin, Dextromethorphan, and Phenylephrine *on page 746*

◆ **Maxipime®** *see* Cefepime *on page 294*

◆ **Maxi-Tuss HC®** *see* Phenylephrine, Hydrocodone, and Chlorpheniramine *on page 1277*

◆ **Maxi-Tuss HCG [DSC]** *see* Hydrocodone and Guaifenesin *on page 779*

◆ **Maxi-Tuss HCX** *see* Phenylephrine, Hydrocodone, and Chlorpheniramine *on page 1277*

◆ **Maxzide®** *see* Hydrochlorothiazide and Triamterene *on page 776*

◆ **Maxzide®-25** *see* Hydrochlorothiazide and Triamterene *on page 776*

◆ **May Apple** *see* Podophyllum Resin *on page 1309*

◆ **Maybush** *see* Hawthorn *(Crataegus oxyacantha) on page 758*

◆ **MCV4** *see* Meningococcal Polysaccharide (Groups A / C / Y and W-135) Diphtheria Toxoid Conjugate Vaccine *on page 985*

◆ **MDL 73,147EF** *see* Dolasetron *on page 493*

Measles, Mumps, Rubella, and Varicella Virus Vaccine

(MEE zels, mumpz, roo BEL a, & var i SEL a VYE rus vak SEEN)

U.S. Brand Names ProQuad®

Index Terms MMR-V; MMRV; Mumps, Rubella, Varicella, and Measles Vaccine; Rubella, Varicella, Measles, and Mumps Vaccine; Varicella, Measles, Mumps, and Rubella Vaccine

Pharmacologic Category Vaccine, Live (Viral)

Use To provide simultaneous active immunization against measles, mumps, rubella, and varicella

Effect on Mental Status May cause irritability; may rarely cause insomnia or malaise

Effect on Psychiatric Treatment None reported

Dosage Summary

SubQ:

Children <12 months: Dosage not established

Children 12 months to 12 years: 0.5 mL as a single dose

Children >12 years: Dosage not established

Adults: Dosage not established

Dosage Forms Excipient information presented when available (limited, particularly for generics); consult specific product labeling.

Injection, powder for reconstitution [preservative free]:

ProQuad®: Measles virus ≥3.00 log_{10} $TCID_{50}$, mumps virus ≥4.3 log_{10} $TCID_{50}$, rubella virus ≥3.00 log_{10} $TCID_{50}$, and varicella virus ≥3.99 log_{10} PFU [contains albumin (human), bovine serum, chicken egg protein, gelatin, neomycin, sorbitol, and sucrose (≤21 mg/vial)]

◆ **Mebaral®** *see* Mephobarbital *on page 988*

Mebendazole (me BEN da zole)

U.S. Brand Names Vermox® [DSC]

Canadian Brand Names Vermox®

Mexican Brand Names L-Ombrix; Mebedal; Mebendazol; Mebensole; Revapol; Vermin-Dazol; Vermox; Vertizole

Pharmacologic Category Anthelmintic

Use Treatment of pinworms (*Enterobius vermicularis*), whipworms (*Trichuris trichiura*), roundworms (*Ascaris lumbricoides*), and hookworms (*Ancylostoma duodenale*)

Effect on Mental Status May cause dizziness

Effect on Psychiatric Treatment Carbamazepine may decrease the effects of mebendazole; may rarely cause neutropenia; use caution with clozapine and carbamazepine

Dosage Summary

Oral:

Children <2 years: Dosage not established

Children ≥2 years: 100 mg as a single dose or twice daily **or** 200 mg twice daily

Adults: 100 mg as a single dose or twice daily **or** 200 mg twice daily

Dosage Forms Excipient information presented when available (limited, particularly for generics); consult specific product labeling.

Tablet, chewable: 100 mg

Mecamylamine (mek a MIL a meen)

Medication Safety Issues

Sound-alike/look-alike issues:

Mecamylamine may be confused with mesalamine

U.S. Brand Names Inversine®

Canadian Brand Names Inversine®

Index Terms Mecamylamine Hydrochloride

Pharmacologic Category Ganglionic Blocking Agent

Use Treatment of moderately severe to severe hypertension and in uncomplicated malignant hypertension

Unlabeled/Investigational Use Tourette's syndrome

Effect on Mental Status May cause drowsiness, confusion, or depression

Effect on Psychiatric Treatment None reported

Dosage Summary

Oral:

Children: Dosage not established

Adults: Initial: 2.5 mg twice daily; Average dose: 25 mg/day in 3 divided doses; **Note:** Titration is recommended

Dosage Forms Excipient information presented when available (limited, particularly for generics); consult specific product labeling.

Tablet, as hydrochloride: 2.5 mg

◆ **Mecamylamine Hydrochloride** *see* Mecamylamine *on page 973*

Mecasermin (mek a SER min)

U.S. Brand Names Increlex™; Iplex™ [DSC]

Index Terms Mecasermin (rDNA Origin) ; Mecasermin Rinfabate; Recombinant Human Insulin-Like Growth Factor-1; rhIGF-1; rhIGF-1/rhIGFBP-3

Pharmacologic Category Growth Hormone

Use Treatment of growth failure in children with severe primary insulin-like growth factor-1 deficiency (IGF-1 deficiency; primary IGFD), or with growth hormone (GH) gene deletions who have developed neutralizing antibodies to GH

Effect on Mental Status May cause dizziness

Effect on Psychiatric Treatment None reported

Dosage Summary

SubQ:

Children <2 years: Dosage not established

Children 2-<3 years: Increlex™: Initial: 0.04-0.08 mg/kg twice daily; Maintenance: 0.04-0.12 mg/kg twice daily

Children ≥3 years:

Increlex™: Initial: 0.04-0.08 mg/kg twice daily; Maintenance: 0.04-0.12 mg/kg twice daily

Iplex™: Initial: 0.5 mg/kg once daily; Maintenance: 0.5-2 mg/kg once daily

Adults: Dosage not established

Dosage Forms Excipient information presented when available (limited, particularly for generics); consult specific product labeling.

Injection, solution:

Increlex™: 10 mg/mL (4 mL) [contains benzyl alcohol]

Injection, solution, as rinfabate [preservative free]:

Iplex™: 36 mg/0.6 mL (0.6 mL) [DSC]

◆ **Mecasermin (rDNA Origin)** *see* Mecasermin *on page 973*

◆ **Mecasermin Rinfabate** *see* Mecasermin *on page 973*

Mechlorethamine (me klor ETH a meen)

Medication Safety Issues

High alert medication: The Institute for Safe Medication Practices (ISMP) includes this medication among its list of drugs which have a heightened risk of causing significant patient harm when used in error.

U.S. Brand Names Mustargen®

Canadian Brand Names Mustargen®

Mexican Brand Names Mustargen

Index Terms Chlorethazine; Chlorethazine Mustard; HN_2; Mechlorethamine Hydrochloride; Mustine; Nitrogen Mustard; NSC-762

Pharmacologic Category Antineoplastic Agent, Alkylating Agent (Nitrogen Mustard)

Use Hodgkin's disease; non-Hodgkin's lymphoma; intracavitary injection for treatment of metastatic tumors; pleural and other malignant effusions; topical treatment of mycosis fungoides

Effect on Mental Status May cause dizziness

Effect on Psychiatric Treatment Leukopenia is common; avoid use with clozapine and carbamazepine

Dosage Forms Excipient information presented when available (limited, particularly for generics); consult specific product labeling.

Injection, powder for reconstitution, as hydrochloride: 10 mg

◆ **Mechlorethamine Hydrochloride** *see* Mechlorethamine *on page 974*

Meclizine (MEK li zeen)

Medication Safety Issues

Sound-alike/look-alike issues:

Antivert® may be confused with Axert™

U.S. Brand Names Antivert®; Bonine® [OTC]; Dramamine® Less Drowsy Formula [OTC]; Medi-Meclizine [OTC]

Canadian Brand Names Bonamine™; Bonine®

Mexican Brand Names Bonadoxina

Index Terms Meclizine Hydrochloride; Meclozine Hydrochloride

Pharmacologic Category Antiemetic; Histamine H_1 Antagonist; Histamine H_1 Antagonist, First Generation

Use Prevention and treatment of symptoms of motion sickness; management of vertigo with diseases affecting the vestibular system

Effect on Mental Status Drowsiness is common; may cause dizziness or nervousness; may rarely cause sedation or depression

Effect on Psychiatric Treatment Concurrent use with psychotropic may produce additive sedation and dry mouth

Dosage Summary

Oral:

Children ≤12 years: Dosage not established

Children >12 years: 12.5-50 mg 1 hour before travel, may repeat every 12-24 hours if needed **or** 25-100 mg/day in divided doses

Adults: 12.5-50 mg 1 hour before travel, may repeat every 12-24 hours if needed **or** 25-100 mg/day in divided doses

Dosage Forms Excipient information presented when available (limited, particularly for generics); consult specific product labeling.

Tablet, as hydrochloride: 12.5 mg, 25 mg

Antivert®: 12.5 mg, 25 mg, 50 mg

Dramamine® Less Drowsy Formula: 25 mg

Medi-Meclizine: 25 mg

Tablet, chewable, as hydrochloride (Bonine®): 25 mg

◆ **Meclizine Hydrochloride** *see* Meclizine *on page 974*

Meclofenamate (me kloe fen AM ate)

Related Information

Nonsteroidal Anti-Inflammatory Agents *on page 1792*

Canadian Brand Names Meclomen®

Index Terms Meclofenamate Sodium

Pharmacologic Category Nonsteroidal Anti-inflammatory Drug (NSAID), Oral

Use Treatment of inflammatory disorders, arthritis, mild to moderate pain, dysmenorrhea

Effect on Mental Status Dizziness is common; may cause drowsiness, confusion, hallucinations, or depression

Effect on Psychiatric Treatment May rarely cause agranulocytosis; use caution with clozapine or carbamazepine; may decrease lithium clearance resulting in an increase in serum lithium levels and potential lithium toxicity; monitor serum lithium levels

Restrictions An FDA-approved medication guide must be distributed when dispensing an oral outpatient prescription (new or refill) where this medication is to be used without direct supervision of a healthcare provider. Medication guides are available at http://www.fda.gov/cder/Offices/ODS/medication_guides.htm.

Dosage Summary

Oral:

Children ≤14 years: Dosage not established

Children >14 years: 50-100 mg every 4-6 hours (maximum: 400 mg/day)

Adults: 50-100 mg every 4-6 hours (maximum: 400 mg/day)

Dosage Forms Excipient information presented when available (limited, particularly for generics); consult specific product labeling.

Capsule, as sodium: 50 mg, 100 mg

- ◆ **Meclofenamate Sodium** *see* Meclofenamate *on page 974*
- ◆ **Meclozine Hydrochloride** *see* Meclizine *on page 974*
- ◆ **Medent-DM** *see* Guaifenesin, Pseudoephedrine, and Dextromethorphan *on page 748*
- ◆ **Medent LD** *see* Guaifenesin and Pseudoephedrine *on page 744*
- ◆ **Medicinal Carbon** *see* Charcoal *on page 312*
- ◆ **Medicinal Charcoal** *see* Charcoal *on page 312*
- ◆ **Medicone® Suppositories [OTC]** *see* Phenylephrine *on page 1273*
- ◆ **Medigesic®** *see* Butalbital, Acetaminophen, and Caffeine *on page 229*
- ◆ **Medi-Meclizine [OTC]** *see* Meclizine *on page 974*
- ◆ **Medi-Phenyl [OTC]** *see* Phenylephrine *on page 1273*
- ◆ **Mediproxen [OTC]** *see* Naproxen *on page 1102*
- ◆ **Medi-Synal [OTC]** *see* Acetaminophen and Pseudoephedrine *on page 37*
- ◆ **Medrol®** *see* MethylPREDNISolone *on page 1029*

MedroxyPROGESTERone (me DROKS ee proe JES te rone)

Medication Safety Issues

Sound-alike/look-alike issues:

MedroxyPROGESTERone may be confused with hydroxyprogesterone, methylPREDNISolone, methylTESTOSTERone

Provera® may be confused with Covera®, Femara®, Parlodel®, Premarin®

The injection dosage form is available in different formulations. Carefully review prescriptions to assure the correct formulation and route of administration.

U.S. Brand Names Depo-Provera®; Depo-Provera® Contraceptive; depo-subQ provera 104™; Provera®

Canadian Brand Names Alti-MPA; Apo-Medroxy®; Depo-Prevera®; Depo-Provera®; Gen-Medroxy; Novo-Medrone; Provera-Pak; Provera®

Mexican Brand Names Megestron; Provera

Index Terms Acetoxymethylprogesterone; Medroxyprogesterone Acetate; Methylacetoxyprogesterone; MPA

Pharmacologic Category Contraceptive; Progestin

Use Endometrial carcinoma or renal carcinoma; secondary amenorrhea or abnormal uterine bleeding due to hormonal imbalance; reduction of endometrial hyperplasia in nonhysterectomized postmenopausal women receiving conjugated estrogens; prevention of pregnancy; management of endometriosis-associated pain

Effect on Mental Status May cause dizziness, headache, depression, insomnia, nervousness, irritability, and mood disturbances

Effect on Psychiatric Treatment The Women's Health Initiative (WHI) Memory Study reported an increased risk of developing dementia in postmenopausal women ≥65 years of age during 4 years of treatment with oral conjugated equine estrogens and medroxyprogesterone acetate relative to placebo (1.8% vs 0.9%). Relative risk was 2.05 (95% CI 1.21-3.48). Therefore, estrogens and progestins should not be used for the prevention of dementia. The WHI also reported an increased risk of stroke (29 vs 21 per 10,000 women-years) compared to women receiving placebo. The increase in risk was observed after the first year and persisted. May cause hypertriglyceridemia; monitor in patients receiving antipsychotics especially clozapine, olanzapine, and quetiapine.

Dosage Summary

I.M.:

Children: Dosage not established

Adolescents: Contraceptive: 150 mg every 3 months

Adults:

Carcinoma: 400-1000 mg/week

Contraceptive: 150 mg every 3 months

Oral:

Children: Dosage not established

Adolescents: 5-10 mg once daily

Adults: 5-10 mg once daily

SubQ:

Children: Dosage not established

Adolescents: 104 mg every 3 months (every 12-14 weeks)

Adults: 104 mg every 3 months (every 12-14 weeks)

Dosage Forms Excipient information presented when available (limited, particularly for generics); consult specific product labeling.

Injection, suspension, as acetate: 150 mg/mL (1 mL)

Depo-Provera®: 400 mg/mL (2.5 mL)

Depo-Provera® Contraceptive: 150 mg/mL (1 mL) [prefilled syringe or vial]

depo-subQ provera 104™: 104 mg/0.65 mL (0.65 mL) [prefilled syringe]

Tablet, as acetate: 2.5 mg, 5 mg, 10 mg

Provera®: 2.5 mg, 5 mg, 10 mg

◆ **Medroxyprogesterone Acetate** *see* MedroxyPROGESTERone *on page 975*

◆ **Medroxyprogesterone and Estrogens (Conjugated)** *see* Estrogens (Conjugated/Equine) and Medroxyprogesterone *on page 583*

Mefenamic Acid (me fe NAM ik AS id)

Medication Safety Issues

Sound-alike/look-alike issues:

Ponstel® may be confused with Pronestyl®

Related Information

Nonsteroidal Anti-Inflammatory Agents *on page 1792*

U.S. Brand Names Ponstel®

Canadian Brand Names Apo-Mefenamic®; Dom-Mefenamic Acid; Mefenamic-250; Nu-Mefenamic; PMS-Mefenamic Acid; Ponstan®

Mexican Brand Names Ponstan-500

Pharmacologic Category Nonsteroidal Anti-inflammatory Drug (NSAID), Oral

Use Short-term relief of mild to moderate pain including primary dysmenorrhea

Effect on Mental Status Dizziness is common; may cause nervousness, may rarely cause confusion, hallucination, or depression

Effect on Psychiatric Treatment May rarely cause agranulocytosis; use caution with clozapine or carbamazepine; may decrease lithium clearance resulting in an increase in serum lithium levels and potential lithium toxicity; monitor serum lithium levels

Restrictions An FDA-approved medication guide must be distributed when dispensing an oral outpatient prescription (new or refill) where this medication is to be used without direct supervision of a healthcare provider. Medication guides are available at http://www.fda.gov/cder/Offices/ODS/medication_guides.htm.

Dosage Summary

Oral:

Children ≤14 years: Dosage not established

Children >14 years: 500 mg to start then 250 mg every 4 hours as needed (maximum therapy: 1 week)

Adults: 500 mg to start then 250 mg every 4 hours as needed (maximum therapy: 1 week)

Dosage Forms Excipient information presented when available (limited, particularly for generics); consult specific product labeling.

Capsule: 250 mg

Ponstel®: 250 mg

Mefloquine (ME floe kwin)

U.S. Brand Names Lariam®

Canadian Brand Names Apo-Mefloquine®; Lariam®

Index Terms Mefloquine Hydrochloride

Pharmacologic Category Antimalarial Agent

Use Treatment of acute malarial infections and prevention of malaria

Effect on Mental Status May cause anxiety, agitation, confusion, paranoia, depression, hallucinations, and psychotic behavior. Case reports of suicide and suicidal ideation have been reported.

Effect on Psychiatric Treatment Contraindicated with ziprasidone. Concurrent use with valproic acid may alter valproate blood levels; monitor levels. Contraindicated in patients with active depression, recent history of depression, generalized anxiety disorder, psychosis, schizophrenia, or with a history of convulsions. In patients taking anticonvulsants (valproic acid, carbamazepine) the concomitant use of mefloquine may reduce seizure control by lowering plasma concentrations.

Restrictions An FDA-approved medication guide and wallet card must be distributed when dispensing an outpatient prescription (new or refill) to prevent malaria where this medication is to be used without direct supervision of a healthcare provider. Medication guides are available at http://www.fda.gov/cder/Offices/ODS/medication_guides.htm.

Dosage Summary

Oral:

Children <6 months and ≤5 kg: Dosage not established

Children ≥6 months and >5 kg: Prophylaxis: 5 mg/kg/once weekly (maximum: 250 mg/dose); Treatment: 20-25 mg/kg in 2 divided doses, taken 6-8 hours apart (maximum: 1250 mg)

Adults: Prophylaxis: 1 tablet (250 mg) once weekly; Treatment: 5 tablets (1250 mg) as a single dose

Dosage Forms Excipient information presented when available (limited, particularly for generics); consult specific product labeling.

Tablet, as hydrochloride: 250 mg [equivalent to 228 mg base]

Lariam®: 250 mg [equivalent to 228 mg base]

◆ **Mefloquine Hydrochloride** *see* Mefloquine *on page 976*

◆ **Megace®** *see* Megestrol *on page 977*

◆ **Megace® ES** *see* Megestrol *on page 977*

Megestrol (me JES trole)

Medication Safety Issues

Sound-alike/look-alike issues:

Megace® may be confused with Reglan®

U.S. Brand Names Megace®; Megace® ES

Canadian Brand Names Apo-Megestrol®; Megace®; Megace® OS; Nu-Megestrol

Mexican Brand Names Mestrel

Index Terms 5071-1DL(6); Megestrol Acetate; NSC-71423

Pharmacologic Category Antineoplastic Agent, Hormone; Appetite Stimulant; Progestin

Use Palliative treatment of breast and endometrial carcinoma; treatment of anorexia, cachexia, or unexplained significant weight loss in patients with AIDS

Effect on Mental Status May cause insomnia or depression

Effect on Psychiatric Treatment May rarely cause myelosuppression; use caution with clozapine and carbamazepine

Dosage Summary

Oral:

Children: Dosage not established

Adults (females): Tablet: 40-320 mg/day in divided doses

Adults (males/females): Suspension: 400-800 mg/day [Megace®] **or** 625 mg/day [Megace® ES]

Dosage Forms Excipient information presented when available (limited, particularly for generics); consult specific product labeling.

Suspension, oral, as acetate: 40 mg/mL (10 mL, 20 mL, 240 mL, 480 mL)

Megace®: 40 mg/mL (240 mL) [contains ethanol 0.06% and sodium benzoate; lemon-lime flavor]

Megace® ES: 125 mg/mL (150 mL) [contains ethanol 0.06% and sodium benzoate; lemon-lime flavor]

Tablet, as acetate: 20 mg, 40 mg

◆ **Megestrol Acetate** *see* Megestrol *on page 977*

Melatonin (mel ah TOE nin)

Natural Product Category Nutraceutical

Synonyms N-acetyl-5-methoxytryptamine

Dosage Oral: 0.5-10 mg/day taken at night

Reported Uses

ADHD (sleep disorders) (Van der Heijden, 2007; Weiss, 2006)

Alzheimer's disease (sleep disorders) (Brusco, 1998; Cardinali, 2002; Singer, 1997)

Autism (sleep disorders) (Garstang, 2006)

Benzodiazepine tapering (Cardinali, 2002; Dagan, 1997; Garfinkel, 1999; Rasmussen, 1997)

Bipolar disorder (Leibenluft, 1997; Robertson, 1997)

Cancer (Barni, 1995; Lissoni, 1995; Lissoni, 2001; Neri, 1998; Todisco, 2001)

Cardioprotection (Dominguez-Rodriguez, 2007)

Chemotheraphy adverse effects (Barni, 1996; Lissoni, 1996; Lissoni, 1997; Lissoni, 1997; Viviani, 1990)

Depression (sleep disturbances) (Dalton, 2000; deVries, 1997; Dolberg, 1998; Kripke, 2003)

Dyspepsia (Klupińska, 2007)

Glaucoma (Samples, 1988; Viggiano, 1994)

Glycemic control (Hussain, 2006)

Headache prevention (Claustrat, 1997; Gagnier, 2001; Leone, 1996; Nagtegaal, 1998)

HIV/AIDS (Lissoni, 1995)

Hypertension (Birau, 1981; Cagnacci, 1997; Zaslavskaia, 1999; Zaslavskaia, 2000; Zaslavaskaia, 2000); nocturnal hypertension (Cagnacci, 2005; Grossman, 2006)

Insomnia (Zhdanova, 2001; Zisapel, 1999)

Irritable bowel syndrome (Saha, 2007)

Jet lag (Suhner, 1998)

Nocturia (Sugaya, 2007)

Oxidative stress in dialysis patients (preventive) (Herrera, 2001)

Parkinson's disease (Antolin, 2002; Bordet, 2003; Shaw, 1973)

Periodic limb movement disorder (Kunz, 2001)

Preoperative sedation/anxiolysis (Naguib, 1999; Naguib, 2000; Naguib, 2003; Naguib, 2003)

Rett syndrome (McArthur, 1998; Miyamoto, 1999)

Sarcoidosis, chronic (Pignone, 2006)

Schizophrenia (sleep disorders) (Shamir, 2000; Shamir, 2000; Suresh Kumar, 2007)

Seasonal affective disorder (SAD) (Avery, 1998; Leppanmaki, 2003; Lewy, 1998; Sherer, 1985; Wirz-Justice, 1990)

Sedation (children) (Schmidt, 2007)

Seizure disorders (Brueske, 1981; Fauteck, 1999; Jan, 1999; Molina-Carballo, 1997; Rufo-Campos, 2002; Siddiqui, 2001)

Skin damage (Bangha, 1996, Bangha, 1997; Dreher, 1998; Fischer, 1999)

Sleep disturbances (Sack, 2000)

Stroke (Adams, 2002; Chaudhary, 2003; Gupta, 2002; Pei, 2002; Pei, 2002; Pei, 2003; Pei, 2003; Reiter, 2003)

Tardive dyskinesia (Bhattacharya, 2002; Naidu, 2003; Naidu, 2003; Nelson, 2003; Shamir, 2000; Shamir, 2001)

Thrombocytopenia (Barni, 1996; Lissoni, 1995; Lissoni, 1995; Lissoni, 1997; Lissoni, 1999; Lissoni, 2001)

Tinnitus (sleep disorders) (Megwalu, 2006)

Summary Melatonin appears to be the primary sleep-regulating hormone of the body. It is secreted in concert with normal day/night cycles. Adults experience about a 37% decline in daily melatonin output between 20 and 70 years of age. It has been used by individuals suffering from insomnia, particularly when adjusting to shift-work cycles or jet lag.

Effect on Mental Status May cause drowsiness, giddiness, or dysphoria

Effect on Psychiatric Treatment Combined use with psychotropics may produce additive CNS depression. Fluvoxamine may increase the bioavailability of melatonin.

Pharmacology Melatonin is a hormone secreted from the pineal gland in a 24-hour circadian rhythm, regulating the normal sleep/wake cycle. As a supplement, melatonin has both phase-shifting and sleep-promoting properties. In addition to promoting sleep, physiologic roles of melatonin include regulation of the secretion of growth hormone and gonadotropic hormones. It also possesses antioxidant activity.

Warnings and Interactions No known toxicity or serious side effects reported; however, long-term human studies have not been conducted. Excessive dosages may cause morning sedation or drowsiness.

Use with caution in individuals with a history of bleeding, hemostatic disorders, or drug-related hemostatic problems; in individuals taking anticoagulant medications, including warfarin, aspirin, aspirin-containing products, NSAIDs, or antiplatelet agents (eg, ticlopidine, clopidogrel, dipyridamole); and in individuals taking antidiabetic agents. Melatonin may reduce glucose tolerance and insulin sensitivity.

Symptoms of Deficiency Insomnia and other sleep disturbances

Reported Interactions

Drug/Nutrient Interactions: Drugs that deplete vitamin B_6 may inhibit the body's ability to synthesize melatonin from the tryptophan-serotonin-melatonin pathway. These include oral contraceptives, estrogen, hydralazine, loop diuretics, penicillamine, and theophylline. In addition, beta-blockers and benzodiazepines may deplete melatonin by enzyme inhibition. Isoniazid alters B_6 metabolism, limiting formation of melatonin. Theoretically, effects may be additive with medications which cause CNS sedation, including alcohol. Melatonin may reduce glucose tolerance and insulin sensitivity and may interact with antidiabetic agents or insulin.

In vitro data suggests this product may inhibit the CYP1A2 isoenzyme. Theoretically, it may affect the disposition of the following medications: Theophylline, caffeine, clozapine, haloperidol, tacrine, and other medications influenced by this enzyme system. Other *in vitro* data suggests melatonin may also affect the disposition of the CYP2C9 isoenzyme. Therefore, it may affect the disposition of the following medications: NSAIDs, phenytoin, warfarin, zafirlukast, and others affected by this isoenzyme. Melatonin may interact with calcium channel blockers.

Nutrient/Nutrient Interactions: A deficiency of pyridoxine inhibits the synthesis of melatonin.

References

Adams JD Jr, Yang J, Mishra LC, et al, "Effects of Ashwagandha in a Rat Model of Stroke," *Altern Ther Health Med*, 2002, 8(5):18-9.

Antolin I, Mayo JC, Sainz RM, et al, "Protective Effect of Melatonin in a Chronic Experimental Model of Parkinson's Disease," *Brain Res*, 2002, 943(2):163-73.

Avery D, Lenz M, and Landis C, "Guidelines for Prescribing Melatonin," *Ann Med*, 1998, 30 (1):122-30.

Bangha E, Elsner P, and Kistler GS, "Suppression of UV-Induced Erythema by Topical Treatment With Melatonin (N-Acetyl-5-Methoxytryptamine). A Dose Response Study," *Arch Dermatol Res*, 1996, 288(9):522-6.

Bangha E, Elsner P, and Kistler GS, "Suppression of UV-Induced Erythema by Topical Treatment With Melatonin (N-Acetyl-5-Methoxytryptamine). Influence of the Application Time Point," *Dermatology*, 1997, 195(3):248-52.

Barni S, Lissoni P, Cazzaniga M, et al, "A Randomized Study of Low-Dose Subcutaneous Interleukin-2 Plus Melatonin Versus Supportive Care Alone in Metastatic Colorectal Cancer Patients Progressing Under 5-Fluorouracil and Folates," *Oncology*, 1995, 52 (3):243-5.

Barni S, Lissoni P, Paolorossi F, et al, "Prevention of Chemotherapy-Induced Thrombocytopenia by the Pineal Hormore Melatonin (MLT)," *Proc Annu Meet Am Soc Clin Oncol*, 1996, 15:528.

Bhattacharya SK, Bhattacharya D, Sairam K, et al, "Effect of *Withania somnifera* Glycowithanolides on a Rat Model of Tardive Dyskinesia," *Phytomedicine*, 2002, 9 (2):167-70.

Birau N, Petersen U, Meyer C, et al, "Hypotensive Effect of Melatonin in Essential Hypertension," *IRCS Med Sci*, 1981, 9:905-6.

Bordet R, Devos D, Brique S, et al, "Study of Circadian Melatonin Secretion Pattern at Different Stages of Parkinson's Disease," *Clin Neuropharmacol*, 2003, 26(2):65-72.

Brueske V, Allen J, Kepic T, et al, "Melatonin Inhibition of Seizure Activity in Man," *Electroencephalog Clin Neurophysiol*, 1981, 51:20.

Brusco LI, Marquez M, and Cardinali DP, "Monozygotic Twins With Alzheimer's Disease Treated With Melatonin: Case Report," *J Pineal Res*, 1998, 25(4):260-3.

Cagnacci A, Arangino S, Angiolucci M, et al, "Potentially Beneficial Cardiovascular Effects of Melatonin Administration in Women," *J Pineal Res*, 1997, 22(1):16-9.

Cagnacci A, Cannoletta M, Renzi A, et al, "Prolonged Melatonin Administration Decreases Nocturnal Blood Pressure in Women," *Am J Hypertens*, 2005, 18(12 Pt 1):1614-8.

Cardinali DP, Brusco LI, Liberczuk C, et al, "The Use of Melatonin in Alzheimer's Disease," *Neuro Endocrinol Lett*, 2002, 23 Suppl 1:20-3.

Cardinali DP, Gvozdenovich E, Kaplan MR, et al, "A Double Blind-Placebo Controlled Study on Melatonin Efficacy to Reduce Anxiolytic Benzodiazepine Use in the Elderly," *Neuro Endocrinol Lett*, 2002, 23(1):55-60.

Chaudhary G, Sharma U, Jagannathan NR, et al, "Evaluation of *Withania somnifera* in a Middle Cerebral Artery Occlusion Model of Stroke in Rats," *Clin Exp Pharmacol Physiol*, 2003, 30(5-6):399-404.

Claustrat B, Brun J, Geoffriau M, et al, "Nocturnal Plasma Melatonin Profile and Melatonin Kinetics During Infusion in Status Migrainosus," *Cephalalgia*, 1997, 17(4):511-7.

Dagan Y, Zisapel N, Nof D, et al, "Rapid Reversal of Tolerance to Benzodiazepine Hypnotics by Treatment With Oral Melatonin: A Case Report," *Eur Neuropsychopharmacol*, 1997, 7 (2):157-60.

Dalton EJ, Rotondi D, Levitan RD, et al, "Use of Slow-Release Melatonin in Treatment-Resistant Depression," *J Psychiatry Neurosci*, 2000, 25(1):48-52.

deVries MW and Peeters FP, "Melatonin as a Therapeutic Agent in the Treatment of Sleep Disturbance in Depression," *J Nerv Ment Dis*, 1997, 185(3):201-2.

Dolberg OT, Hirschmann S, and Grunhaus L, "Melatonin for the Treatment of Sleep Disturbances in Major Depressive Disorder," *Am J Psychiatry*, 1998, 155(8):1119-21.

Dominguez-Rodriguez A, Abreu-Gonzalez P, Garcia-Gonzalez MJ, et al, "A Unicenter, Randomized, Double-Blind, Parallel-Group, Placebo-Controlled Study of Melatonin as an Adjunct in Patients With Acute Myocardial Infarction Undergoing Primary Angioplasty the Melatonin Adjunct in the Acute Myocardial Infarction Treated With Angioplasty (MARIA) Trial: Study Design and Rationale," *Contemp Clin Trials*, 2007, 28(4):532-9.

Dreher F, Gabard B, Schwindt DA, et al, "Topical Melatonin in Combination With Vitamins E and C Protects Skin From Ultraviolet-Induced Erythema: A Human Study *in vivo*," *Br J Dermatol*, 1998, 139(2):332-9.

Fauteck J, Schmidt H, Lerchl A, et al, "Melatonin in Epilepsy: First Results of Replacement Therapy and First Clinical Results," *Biol Signals Recept*, 1999, 8(1-2):105-10.

Fischer T, Bangha E, Elsner P, et al, "Suppression of UV-Induced Erythema by Topical Treatment With Melatonin. Influence of the Application Time Point," *Biol Signals Recept*, 1999, 8(1-2):132-5.

Gagnier JJ, "The Therapeutic Potential of Melatonin in Migraines and Other Headache Types," *Altern Med Rev*, 2001, 6(4):383-9.

Garfinkel D, Zisapel N, Wainstein J, et al, "Facilitation of Benzodiazepine Discontinuation by Melatonin: A New Clinical Approach," *Arch Intern Med*, 1999, 159(20):2456-60.

Garstang J and Wallis M, "Randomized Controlled Trial of Melatonin for Children With Autistic Spectrum Disorders and Sleep Problems," *Child Care Health Dev*, 2006, 32 (5):585-9.

Grossman E, Laudon M, Yalcin R, et al, "Melatonin Reduces Night Blood Pressure in Patients With Nocturnal Hypertension," *Am J Med*, 2006, 119(10):898-902.

Gupta YK, Chaudhary G, and Sinha K, "Enhanced Protection by Melatonin and Meloxicam Combination in a Middle Cerebral Artery Occlusion Model of Acute Ischemic Stroke in Rat," *Can J Physiol Pharmacol*, 2002, 80(3):210-7.

Herrera J, Nava M, Romero F, et al, "Melatonin Prevents Oxidative Stress Resulting From Iron and Erythropoietin Administration," *Am J Kidney Dis*, 2001, 37(4):750-7.

Hussain SA, Khadim HM, Khalaf BH, et al, "Effects of Melatonin and Zinc on Glycemic Control in Type 2 Diabetic Patients Poorly Controlled With Metformin," *Saudi Med J*, 2006, 27(10):1483-8.

Jan JE, Connolly MB, Hamilton D, et al, "Melatonin Treatment of Non-Epileptic Myoclonus in Children," *Dev Med Child Neurol*, 1999, 41(4):255-9.

Klupińska G, Poplawski T, Drzewoski J, et al, "Therapeutic Effect of Melatonin in Patients With Functional Dyspepsia," *J Clin Gastroenterol*, 2007, 41(3):270-4.

Kripke DF, Youngstedt SD, Rex KM, et al, "Melatonin Excretion With Affect Disorders Over Age 60," *Psychiatry Res*, 2003, 118(1):47-54.

Kunz D and Bes F, "Exogenous Melatonin in Periodic Limb Movement Disorder: An Open Clinical Trial and a Hypothesis," *Sleep*, 2001, 24(2):183-7.

Leibenluft E, Feldman-Naim S, Turner EH, et al, "Effects of Exogenous Melatonin Administration and Withdrawal in Five Patients With Rapid-Cycling Bipolar Disorder," *J Clin Psychiatry*, 1997, 58(9):383-8.

Leone M, D'Amico D, Moschiano F, et al, "Melatonin Versus Placebo in the Prophylaxis of Cluster Headache: A Double-Blind Pilot Study With Parallel Groups," *Cephalalgia*, 1996, 16(7):494-6.

Leppamaki S, Partonen T, Vakkuri O, et al, "Effect of Controlled-Release Melatonin on Sleep Quality, Mood, and Quality of Life in Subjects With Seasonal or Weather-Associated Changes in Mood and Behaviour," *Eur Neuropsychopharmacol*, 2003, 13(3):137-45.

Lewy AJ, Bauer VK, Cutler NL, et al, "Melatonin Treatment of Winter Depression: A Pilot Study," *Psychiatry Res*, 1998, 77(1):57-61.

Lissoni P, Ardizzoia A, Barni S, et al, "Randomized Study of Tamoxifen Alone Versus Tamoxifen Plus Melatonin in Estrogen Receptor-Negative Heavily Pretreated Metastatic Breast Cancer Patients," *Oncology Reports*, 1995, 2:871-3.

Lissoni P, Barni S, Brivio F, et al, "A Biological Study on the Efficacy of Low-Dose Subcutaneous Interleukin-2 Plus Melatonin in the Treatment of Cancer-Related Thrombocytopenia," *Oncology*, 1995, 52(5):360-2.

Lissoni P, Barni S, Brivio F, et al, "Treatment of Cancer-Related Thrombocytopenia by Low-Dose Subcutaneous Interleukin-2 Plus the Pineal Hormone Melatonin: A Biological Phase II Study," *J Biol Regul Homeost Agents*, 1995, 9(2):52-4.

Lissoni P, Bucovec R, Bonfanti A, et al, "Thrombopoietic Properties of 5-Methoxytryptamine Plus Melatonin Versus Melatonin Alone in the Treatment of Cancer-Related Thrombocytopenia," *J Pineal Res*, 2001, 30(2):123-6.

Lissoni P, Cazzaniga M, Tancini G, et al, "Reversal of Clinical Resistance to LHRH Analogue in Metastatic Prostate Cancer by the Pineal Hormone Melatonin: Efficacy of LHRH Analogue Plus Melatonin in Patients Progressing on LHRH Analogue Alone," *Eur Urol*, 1997, 31(2):178-81.

Lissoni P, Paolorossi F, Tancini G, et al, "Is There a Role for Melatonin in the Treatment of Neoplastic Cachexia?," *Eur J Cancer*, 1996, 32A(8):1340-3.

Lissoni P, Rovelli F, Malugani F, et al, "Anti-Angiogenic Activity of Melatonin in Advanced Cancer Patients," *Neuro Endocrinol Lett*, 2001, 22(1):45-7.

Lissoni P, Tancini G, Barni S, et al, "Treatment of Cancer Chemotherapy-Induced Toxicity With the Pineal Hormone Melatonin," *Support Care Cancer*, 1997, 5(2):126-9.

Lissoni P, Tancini G, Paolorossi F, et al, "Chemoneuroendocrine Therapy of Metastatic Breast Cancer With Persistent Thrombocytopenia With Weekly Low-Dose Epirubicin Plus Melatonin: A Phase II Study," *J Pineal Res*, 1999, 26(3):169-73.

Lissoni P, Vigore L, Rescaldani R, et al, "Neuroimmunotherapy With Low-Dose Subcutaneous Interleukin-2 Plus Melatonin in AIDS Patients With CD4 Cell Number Below 200/ mm^3: A Biological Phase-II Study," *J Biol Regul Homeost Agents*, 1995, 9(4):155-8.

Lusardi P, Piazza E, and Fogari R, "Cardiovascular Effects of Melatonin in Hypertensive Patients Well Controlled by Nifedipine: A 24-Hour Study," *Br J Clin Pharmacol*, 2000, 49 (5):423-7.

McArthur AJ and Budden SS, "Sleep Dysfunction in Rett Syndrome: A Trial of Exogenous Melatonin Treatment," *Dev Med Child Neurol*, 1998, 40(3):186-92.

Megwalu UC, Finnell JE, and Piccirillo JF, "The Effects of Melatonin on Tinnitus and Sleep," *Otolaryngol Head Neck Surg*, 2006, 134(2):210-3.

Miyamoto A, Oki J, Takahashi S, et al, "Serum Melatonin Kinetics and Long-Term Melatonin Treatment for Sleep Disorders in Rett Syndrome," *Brain Dev*, 1999, 21(1):59-62.

Molina-Carballo A, Munoz-Hoyos A, Reiter RJ, et al, "Utility of High Doses of Melatonin as Adjunctive Anticonvulsant Therapy in a Child With Severe Myoclonic Epilepsy: Two Years' Experience," *J Pineal Res*, 1997, 23(2):97-105.

Nagtegaal JE, Smits MG, Swart AC, et al, "Melatonin-Responsive Headache in Delayed Sleep Phase Syndrome: Preliminary Observations," *Headache*, 1998, 38(4):303-7.

Naguib M and Samarkandi AH, "Premedication With Melatonin: A Double-Blind, Placebo-Controlled Comparison With Midazolam," *Br J Anaesth*, 1999, 82(6):875-80.

Naguib M and Samarkandi AH, "The Comparative Dose-Response Effects of Melatonin and Midazolam for Premedication of Adult Patients: A Double-Blinded, Placebo-Controlled Study," *Anesth Analg*, 2000, 91(2):473-9.

Naguib M, Hammond DL, Schmid PG 3rd, et al, "Pharmacological Effects of Intravenous Melatonin: Comparative Studies With Thiopental and Propofol," *Br J Anaesth*, 2003, 90 (4):504-7.

Naguib M, Schmid PG 3rd, and Baker MT, "The Electroencephalographic Effects of I.V. Anesthetic Doses of Melatonin: Comparative Studies With Thiopental and Propofol," *Anesth Analg*, 2003, 97(1):238-43.

Naidu PS, Singh A, and Kulkarni SK, "Effect of *Withania somnifera* Root Extract on Haloperidol-Induced Orofacial Dyskinesia: Possible Mechanisms of Action," *J Med Food*, 2003, 6(2):107-14.

Naidu PS, Singh A, Kaur P, et al, "Possible Mechanism of Action in Melatonin Attenuation of Haloperidol-Induced Orofacial Dyskinesia," *Pharmacol Biochem Behav*, 2003, 74 (3):641-8.

Natural Standard Research Collaboration, Chief Editors: Ulbricht C, Basch E, *Natural Standard Herb and Supplement Reference - Evidence-Based Clinical Reviews*, USA: Elsevier/Mosby, 2005.

Nelson LA, McGuire JM, and Hausafus SN, "Melatonin for the Treatment of Tardive Dyskinesia," *Ann Pharmacother*, 2003, 37(7-8):1128-31.

Neri B, de Leonardis V, Gemelli MT, et al, "Melatonin as Biological Response Modifier in Cancer Patients," *Anticancer Res*, 1998, 18(2B):1329-32.

Pei Z, Fung PC, and Cheung RT, "Melatonin Reduces Nitric Oxide Level During Ischemia But Not Blood-Brain Barrier Breakdown During Reperfusion in a Rat Middle Cerebral Artery Occlusion Stroke Model," *J Pineal Res*, 2003, 34(2):110-8.

Pei Z, Ho HT, and Cheung RT, "Pretreatment With Melatonin Reduces Volume of Cerebral Infarction in a Permanent Middle Cerebral Artery Occlusion Stroke Model in the Rat," *Neurosci Lett*, 2002, 318(3):141-4.

Pei Z, Pang SF, and Cheung RT, "Administration of Melatonin After Onset of Ischemia Reduces the Volume of Cerebral Infarction in a Rat Middle Cerebral Artery Occlusion Stroke Model," *Stroke*, 2003, 34(3):770-5.

Pei Z, Pang SF, and Cheung RT, "Pretreatment With Melatonin Reduces Volume of Cerebral Infarction in a Rat Middle Cerebral Artery Occlusion Stroke Model," *J Pineal Res*, 2002, 32 (3):168-72.

Pignone AM, Rosso AD, Fiori G, et al, "Melatonin Is a Safe and Effective Treatment for Chronic Pulmonary and Extrapulmonary Sarcoidosis," *J Pineal Res*, 2006, 41(2):95-100.

Rasmussen P, "A Role of Phytotherapy Treatment of Benzodiazepine and Opiate Drug Withdrawal," *The European Journal of Herbal Medicine*, 1997, 3(1):11-21.

Reiter RJ, Sainz RM, Lopez-Burillo S, et al, "Melatonin Ameliorates Neurologic Damage and Neurophysiologic Deficits in Experimental Models of Stroke," *Ann N Y Acad Sci*, 2003, 993:35-47.

Robertson JM and Tanguay PE, "Case Study: The Use of Melatonin in a Boy With Refractory Bipolar Disorder," *J Am Acad Child Adolesc Psychiatry*, 1997, 36(6):822-5.

Rufo-Campos M, "Melatonin and Epilepsy," *Rev Neurol*, 2002, 35(1 Suppl):S51-8.

Sack RL, Brandes RW, Kendall AR, et al, "Entrainment of Free-Running Circadian Rhythms by Melatonin in Blind People," *N Engl J Med*, 2000, 343(15):1070-7.

Saha L, Malhotra S, Rana S, et al, "A Preliminary Study of Melatonin in Irritable Bowel Syndrome," *J Clin Gastroenterol*, 2007, 41(1):29-32.

Samples JR, Krause G, and Lewy AJ, "Effect of Melatonin on Intraocular Pressure," *Curr Eye Res*, 1988, 7(7):649-53.

Schmidt CM, Knief A, Deuster D, et al, "Melatonin Is a Useful Alternative to Sedation in Children Undergoing Brainstem Audiometry With an Age Dependent Success Rate - A Field Report of 250 Investigations," *Neuropediatrics*, 2007, 38(1):2-4.

Shamir E, Barak Y, Plopsky I, et al, "Is Melatonin Treatment Effective for Tardive Dyskinesia?," *J Clin Psychiatry*, 2000, 61(8):556-8.

Shamir E, Barak Y, Shalman I, et al, "Melatonin Treatment for Tardive Dyskinesia: A Double-Blind, Placebo-Controlled, Crossover Study," *Arch Gen Psychiatry*, 2001, 58(11):1049-52.

Shamir E, Laudon M, Barak Y, et al, "Melatonin Improves Sleep Quality of Patients With Chronic Schizophrenia," *J Clin Psychiatry*, 2000, 61(5):373-7.

Shamir E, Rotenberg VS, Laudon M, et al, "First-Night Effect of Melatonin Treatment in Patients With Chronic Schizophrenia," *J Clin Psychopharmacol*, 2000, 20(6):691-4.

Shaw KM, Stern GM, and Sandler M, "Melatonin and Parkinsonism," *Lancet*, 1973, 1 (7797):271.

Sherer MA, Weingartner H, James SP, et al, "Effects of Melatonin on Performance Testing in Patients With Seasonal Affective Disorder," *Neurosci Lett*, 1985, 58(3):277-82.

Siddiqui MA, Nazmi AS, Karim S, et al, "Effect of Melatonin and Valproate in Epilepsy and Depression," *Indian J Pharmacol*, 2001, 33:378-81.

Singer CM, Moffit MT, Colling ED, et al, "Low Dose Melatonin Administration and Nocturnal Activity Levels in Patients With Alzheimer's Disease," *Sleep Res*, 1997, 26:752.

Sugaya K, Nishijima S, Miyazato M, et al, "Effects of Melatonin and Rilmazafone on Nocturia in the Elderly," *J Int Med Res*, 2007, 35(5):685-91.

Suhner A, Schlagenhauf P, Johnson R, et al, "Comparative Study to Determine the Optimal Melatonin Dosage Form for the Alleviation of Jet Lag," *Chronobiol Int*, 1998, 15(6):655-66.

Suresh Kumar PN, Andrade C, Bhakta SG, et al, "Melatonin in Schizophrenic Outpatients With Insomnia: A Double-Blind, Placebo-Controlled Study," *J Clin Psychiatry*, 2007, 68 (2):237-41.

Todisco M, Casaccia P, and Rossi N, "Cyclophosphamide Plus Somatostatin, Bromocriptin, Retinoids, Melatonin and ACTH in the Treatment of Low-Grade Non-Hodgkin's Lymphomas at Advanced Stage: Results of a Phase II Trial," *Cancer Biother Radiopharm*, 2001, 16(2):171-7.

Van der Heijden KB, Smits MG, Van Someren EJ, et al, "Effect of Melatonin on Sleep, Behavior, and Cognition in ADHD and Chronic Sleep-Onset Insomnia," *J Am Acad Child Adolesc Psychiatry*, 2007, 46(2):233-41.

Viggiano SR, Koskela TK, Klee GG, et al, "The Effect of Melatonin on Aqueous Humor Flow in Humans During the Day," *Ophthalmology*, 1994, 101(2):326-31.

Viviani S, Negretti E, Orazi A, et al, "Preliminary Studies on Melatonin in the Treatment of Myelodysplastic Syndromes Following Cancer Chemotherapy," *J Pineal Res*, 1990, 8 (4):347-54.

Von Bahr C, Ursing C, Yasui N, et al, "Fluvoxamine But Not Citalopram Increases Serum Melatonin in Healthy Subjects - An Indication That Cytochrome P450 CYP1A2 and CYP2C19 Hydroxylate Melatonin," *Eur J Clin Pharmacol*, 2000, 56(2):123-7.

Weiss MD, Wasdell MB, Bomben MM, et al, "Sleep Hygiene and Melatonin Treatment for Children and Adolescents With ADHD and Initial Insomnia," *J Am Acad Child Adolesc Psychiatry*, 2006, 45(5):512-9.

Wirz-Justice A, Graw P, Krauchi K, et al, "Morning or Night-Time Melatonin Is Ineffective in Seasonal Affective Disorder," *J Psychiatr Res*, 1990, 24(2):129-37.

Zaslavskaia RM, Biiasilov NS, Akhmetov KZh, et al, "Capozide-50 Alone and in Combination With Melatonin in Therapy of Hypertension," *Klin Med (Mosk)*, 2000, 78(11):39-41.

Zaslavskaia RM, Komarov FI, Shakirova AN, et al, "Effect of Moxonidine Monotherapy and in Combination With Melatonin on Hemodynamic Parameters in Patients With Arterial Hypertension," *Klin Med (Mosk)*, 2000, 78(4):41-4.

Zaslavskaia RM, Shakirova AN, Komarov FI, et al, "Effects of Melatonin Alone and in Combination With Aceten on Chronostructure of Diurnal Hemodynamic Rhythms in Patients With Hypertension Stage II," *Ter Arkh*, 1999, 71(12):21-4.

Zhdanova IV, Wurtman RJ, Regan MM, et al "Melatonin Treatment for Age-Related Insomnia," *J Clin Endocrinol Metab*, 2001, 86(10):4727-30.

Zisapel N, "The Use of Melatonin for the Treatment of Insomnia," *Biol Signals Recept*, 1999, 8(1-2):84-9.

Meloxicam (mel OKS i kam)

Related Information

Nonsteroidal Anti-Inflammatory Agents *on page 1792*

U.S. Brand Names Mobic®

Canadian Brand Names Apo-Meloxicam®; CO Meloxicam; Gen-Meloxicam; Mobicox®; Mobic®; Novo-Meloxicam; PMS-Meloxicam

Mexican Brand Names Aflamid; Exel; Loxibest; Melosteral; Mobicox

Pharmacologic Category Nonsteroidal Anti-inflammatory Drug (NSAID), Oral

Use Relief of signs and symptoms of osteoarthritis, rheumatoid arthritis, and juvenile rheumatoid arthritis (JRA)

Effect on Mental Status May cause dizziness; may rarely cause abnormal dreams, anxiety, confusion, depression, nervousness, and somnolence

Effect on Psychiatric Treatment Rare reports of agranulocytosis, use caution with clozapine and carbamazepine; lithium levels can be increased; avoid concurrent use if possible or monitor lithium levels and adjust dose. When NSAID is stopped, lithium will need adjustment again.

Restrictions An FDA-approved medication guide must be distributed when dispensing an oral outpatient prescription (new or refill) where this medication is to be used without direct supervision of a healthcare provider. Medication guides are available at http://www.fda.gov/cder/Offices/ODS/medication_guides.htm.

Dosage Summary

Oral:

Children <2 years: Dosage not established

Children ≥2 years: 0.125 mg/kg/day (maximum: 7.5 mg/day)

Adults: Initial: 7.5 mg once daily; maintenance: 7.5-15 mg once daily (maximum: 15 mg/day)

Dosage Forms Excipient information presented when available (limited, particularly for generics); consult specific product labeling.

Suspension: 7.5 mg/5 mL (100 mL)

Mobic®: 7.5 mg/5 mL (100 mL) [contains sodium benzoate; raspberry flavor]

Tablet: 7.5 mg, 15 mg

Mobic®: 7.5 mg, 15 mg

Melphalan (MEL fa lan)

Medication Safety Issues

Sound-alike/look-alike issues:

Melphalan may be confused with Mephyton®, Myleran®

Alkeran® may be confused with Alferon®, Leukeran®, Myleran®

High alert medication: The Institute for Safe Medication Practices (ISMP) includes this medication among its list of drugs which have a heightened risk of causing significant patient harm when used in error.

U.S. Brand Names Alkeran®

Canadian Brand Names Alkeran®

Mexican Brand Names Alkeran

Index Terms L-PAM; L-Sarcolysin; NSC-8806; Phenylalanine Mustard

Pharmacologic Category Antineoplastic Agent, Alkylating Agent

Use Palliative treatment of multiple myeloma and nonresectable epithelial ovarian carcinoma

Unlabeled/Investigational Use Treatment of neuroblastoma, rhabdomyosarcoma, breast cancer; part of an induction regimen for marrow and stem cell transplantation

Effect on Mental Status None reported

Effect on Psychiatric Treatment Myelosuppression is common; avoid concurrent use with clozapine and carbamazepine

Dosage Forms Excipient information presented when available (limited, particularly for generics); consult specific product labeling.

Injection, powder for reconstitution: 50 mg [diluent contains ethanol and propylene glycol]

Tablet: 2 mg

Memantine (me MAN teen)

U.S. Brand Names Namenda™

Canadian Brand Names Ebixa®

Mexican Brand Names Ebixa

Index Terms Memantine Hydrochloride

Pharmacologic Category N-Methyl-D-Aspartate Receptor Antagonist

Generic Available No

Use Treatment of moderate-to-severe dementia of the Alzheimer's type

Unlabeled/Investigational Use Treatment of mild-to-moderate vascular dementia; mild cognitive impairment

Pregnancy Risk Factor B

Pregnancy Considerations Teratogenic effects were not observed in animal studies. There are no studies in pregnant women.

Lactation Excretion in breast milk unknown/use caution

Contraindications Hypersensitivity to memantine or any component of the formulation

Warnings/Precautions Use caution with seizure disorders or severe hepatic impairment. Caution with use in severe renal impairment; dose adjustment recommended. Clearance is significantly reduced by alkaline urine; use caution with medications, dietary changes, or patient conditions which may alter urine pH.

Adverse Reactions

1% to 10%:

Cardiovascular: Hypertension (4%), cardiac failure, syncope, cerebrovascular accident, transient ischemic attack

Central nervous system: Dizziness (7%), confusion (6%), headache (6%), hallucinations (3%), pain (3%), somnolence (3%), fatigue (2%), aggressive reaction, ataxia, vertigo

Dermatologic: Rash

Gastrointestinal: Constipation (5%), vomiting (3%), weight loss

Genitourinary: Micturition

Hematologic: Anemia
Hepatic: Alkaline phosphatase increased
Neuromuscular & skeletal: Back pain (3%), hypokinesia
Ocular: Cataract, conjunctivitis
Respiratory: Cough (4%), dyspnea (2%), pneumonia

<1% (Limited to important or life-threatening): Allergic reaction, AV block, cerebral infarction, dyskinesia, dysphagia, hepatic failure, hyperlipidemia, hypoglycemia, ileus, NMS, pancreatitis, renal failure, QT prolongation, seizure, Stevens-Johnson syndrome, sudden death, tardive dyskinesia, thrombocytopenia

Drug Interactions

Carbonic Anhydrase Inhibitors: May decrease the excretion of Memantine. *Risk C: Monitor therapy*

Sodium Bicarbonate: May decrease the excretion of Memantine. *Risk C: Monitor therapy*

Stability Store at controlled room temperature of 15°C to 30°C (59°F to 86°F).

Mechanism of Action Glutamate, the primary excitatory amino acid in the CNS, may contribute to the pathogenesis of Alzheimer's disease (AD) by overstimulating various glutamate receptors leading to excitotoxicity and neuronal cell death. Memantine is an uncompetitive antagonist of the N-methyl-D-aspartate (NMDA) type of glutamate receptors, located ubiquitously throughout the brain. Under normal physiologic conditions, the (unstimulated) NMDA receptor ion channel is blocked by magnesium ions, which are displaced after agonist-induced depolarization. Pathologic or excessive receptor activation, as postulated to occur during AD, prevents magnesium from reentering and blocking the channel pore resulting in a chronically open state and excessive calcium influx. Memantine binds to the intra-pore magnesium site, but with longer dwell time, and thus functions as an effective receptor blocker only under conditions of excessive stimulation; memantine does not affect normal neurotransmission.

Pharmacodynamics/Kinetics

Distribution: 9-11 L/kg
Protein binding: 45%
Metabolism: Forms 3 metabolites (minimal activity)
Half-life elimination: Terminal: 60-80 hours; severe renal impairment (Cl_{cr} 5-29 mL/minute): 117-156 hours
Time to peak, serum: 3-7 hours
Excretion: Urine (57% to 82% unchanged); excretion reduced by alkaline urine pH

Dosage Oral: Adults:

Alzheimer's disease: Initial: 5 mg/day; increase dose by 5 mg/day to a target dose of 20 mg/day; wait at least 1 week between dosage changes. Doses >5 mg/day should be given in 2 divided doses.

Suggested titration: 5 mg/day for ≥1 week; 5 mg twice daily for ≥1 week; 15 mg/day given in 5 mg and 10 mg separated doses for ≥1 week; then 10 mg twice daily

Mild-to-moderate vascular dementia (unlabeled use): 10 mg twice daily

Dosage adjustment in renal impairment:

Mild-to-moderate impairment: No adjustment required
Severe impairment: Cl_{cr} 5-29 mL/minute): 5 mg twice daily

Dietary Considerations May be taken with or without food.

Dosage Forms Excipient information presented when available (limited, particularly for generics); consult specific product labeling.

Solution, oral: 2 mg/mL (360 mL) [alcohol free, dye free, sugar free; peppermint flavor]

Tablet, as hydrochloride: 5 mg, 10 mg

Combination package [titration pack contains two separate tablet formulations]: Memantine hydrochloride 5 mg (28s) and memantine hydrochloride 10 mg (21s)

◆ **Memantine Hydrochloride** *see* Memantine *on page 983*

◆ **Menactra®** *see* Meningococcal Polysaccharide (Groups A / C / Y and W-135) Diphtheria Toxoid Conjugate Vaccine *on page 985*

◆ **Menest®** *see* Estrogens, Esterified *on page 587*

Meningococcal Polysaccharide (Groups A / C / Y and W-135) Diphtheria Toxoid Conjugate Vaccine

(me NIN joe kok al pol i SAK a ride groops aye, see, why & dubl yoo won thur tee fyve dif THEER ee a TOKS oyds KON joo gate vak SEEN)

Medication Safety Issues

Administration issue:

Menactra® (MCV4) should be administered by intramuscular (I.M.) injection only. Inadvertent subcutaneous (SubQ) administration has been reported; possibly due to confusion of this product with Menomume® (MPSV4), also a meningococcal polysaccharide vaccine, which is administered by the SubQ route.

U.S. Brand Names Menactra®

Index Terms MCV4; Quadrivalent Meningococcal Conjugate Vaccine

Pharmacologic Category Vaccine

Use Provide active immunization of children and adults (2-55 years of age) against invasive meningococcal disease caused by *N. meningitidis* serogroups A, C, Y, and W-135

The ACIP recommends routine vaccination of all persons 11-18 years of age at the earliest opportunity. Adolescents should be vaccinated at the 11-12 year visit. For adolescents not previously vaccinated, vaccine should be administered prior to high school entry (~15 years of age).

The ACIP also recommends vaccination for persons at increased risk for meningococcal disease. (MCV4 is preferred for persons aged 2-55 years; MPSV4 may be used if MCV4 is not available). Persons at increased risk include:

College freshmen living in dormitories

Microbiologists routinely exposed to isolates of *N. meningitides*

Military recruits

Persons traveling to or who reside in countries where *N. meningitides* is hyperendemic or epidemic, particularly if contact with local population will be prolonged

Persons with terminal complement component deficiencies

Persons with anatomic or functional asplenia

Use is also recommended during meningococcal outbreaks caused by vaccine preventable serogroups.

Effect on Mental Status Malaise and fatigue are common

Effect on Psychiatric Treatment Diarrhea is common; concomitant use with SSRIs may produce additive effects

Dosage Summary

I.M.

Children <2 years: Dosage not established

Children ≥2 years: 0.5 mL as a single dose

Adolescents 11-18 years: 0.5 mL as a single dose

Adults ≤55 years: 0.5 mL as a single dose

Adults >55 years: Dosage not established

Dosage Forms Excipient information presented when available (limited, particularly for generics); consult specific product labeling.

Injection, solution [MCV4; preservative free]:

Menactra®: 4 mcg each of polysaccharide antigen groups A, C, Y, and W-135 [bound to diphtheria toxoid 48 mcg] per 0.5 mL [contains natural rubber/natural latex in packaging of vials]

Meningococcal Polysaccharide Vaccine (Groups A / C / Y and W-135)

(me NIN joe kok al pol i SAK a ride vak SEEN groops aye, see, why & dubl yoo won thur tee fyve)

Medication Safety Issues

Administration issue:

Menomume® (MPSV4) should be administered by subcutaneous (SubQ) injection. Menactra® (MCV4), also a meningococcal polysaccharide vaccine, is to be administered by intramuscular (I.M.) injection only.

U.S. Brand Names Menomune®-A/C/Y/W-135

Index Terms MPSV4; Quadrivalent Meningococcal Conjugate Vaccine

Pharmacologic Category Vaccine

Use Provide active immunity to meningococcal serogroups contained in the vaccine

The ACIP recommends routine vaccination for persons at increased risk for meningococcal disease. (Use of MPSV4 is recommended in children 2-10 years and adults >55 years. MCV4 is preferred for persons aged 11-55 years; MPSV4 may be used if MCV4 is not available). Persons at increased risk include:

College freshmen living in dormitories

Microbiologists routinely exposed to isolates of *N. meningitides*

Military recruits

Persons traveling to or who reside in countries where *N. meningitides* is hyperendemic or epidemic, particularly if contact with local population will be prolonged

Persons with terminal complement component deficiencies

Persons with anatomic or functional asplenia

Use is also recommended during meningococcal outbreaks caused by vaccine preventable serogroups.

Effect on Mental Status May cause drowsiness

Effect on Psychiatric Treatment None reported

Dosage Summary

SubQ:

Children <2 years: Not usually recommended

Children ≥2 years: 0.5 mL as a single dose

Adults: 0.5 mL as a single dose

Dosage Forms Excipient information presented when available (limited, particularly for generics); consult specific product labeling.

Injection, powder for reconstitution [MPSV4]:

Menomune®-A/C/Y/W-135: 50 mcg each of polysaccharide antigen groups A, C, Y, and W-135 per 0.5 mL dose [contains lactose 2.5-5 mg/0.5 mL, natural rubber/natural latex in packaging, thimerosal in diluent for multidose vial]

◆ **Menomune®-A/C/Y/W-135** *see* Meningococcal Polysaccharide Vaccine (Groups A / C / Y and W-135) *on page 985*

◆ **Menostar®** *see* Estradiol *on page 576*

Mepenzolate (me PEN zoe late)

Medication Safety Issues

Sound-alike/look-alike issues:

Cantil® may be confused with Bentyl®

U.S. Brand Names Cantil® [DSC]

Canadian Brand Names Cantil®

Index Terms Mepenzolate Bromide

Pharmacologic Category Anticholinergic Agent; Antispasmodic Agent, Gastrointestinal

Use Adjunctive treatment of peptic ulcer disease

Effect on Mental Status May rarely cause confusion, amnesia, drowsiness, nervousness, or insomnia

Effect on Psychiatric Treatment Concurrent use with psychotropics may produce additive drowsiness or anticholinergic side effects (dry mouth)

Dosage Summary

Oral:

Children: Dosage not established

Adults: 25-50 mg 4 times/day with meals and at bedtime

Dosage Forms Excipient information presented when available (limited, particularly for generics); consult specific product labeling. [DSC] = Discontinued product

Tablet, as bromide: 25 mg [contains tartrazine] [DSC]

◆ **Mepenzolate Bromide** *see* Mepenzolate *on page 986*

◆ **Mepergan** *see* Meperidine and Promethazine *on page 987*

Meperidine (me PER i deen)

Medication Safety Issues

Avoid the use of meperidine for pain control, especially in elderly and renally-compromised patients (Institute for Safe Medication Practices [ISMP], 2007)

Sound-alike/look-alike issues:

Meperidine may be confused with meprobamate

Demerol® may be confused with Demulen®, Desyrel®, dicumarol, Dilaudid®, Dymelor®, Pamelor®

High alert medication: The Institute for Safe Medication Practices (ISMP) includes this medication among its list of drug classes which have a heightened risk of causing significant patient harm when used in error.

Related Information

Narcotic / Opioid Analgesics *on page 1789*

U.S. Brand Names Demerol®; Meperitab®

Canadian Brand Names Demerol®

Mexican Brand Names Demerol HCl

Index Terms Isonipecaine Hydrochloride; Meperidine Hydrochloride; Pethidine Hydrochloride

Pharmacologic Category Analgesic, Opioid

Use Management of moderate-to-severe pain; adjunct to anesthesia and preoperative sedation

Unlabeled/Investigational Use

Reduce postoperative shivering; reduce rigors from amphotericin

Effect on Mental Status Sedation is common; may cause nervousness or confusion; may rarely produce depression, hallucinations, or paradoxical CNS stimulation

Effect on Psychiatric Treatment Sedation is common; may cause nervousness or confusion; may rarely produce depression, hallucinations, or paradoxical CNS stimulation

Restrictions C-II

Dosage Summary

I.M.:

Children: 1-1.5 mg/kg/dose every 3-4 hours as needed **or** 1-2 mg/kg as a single dose preoperatively (maximum: 100 mg/dose)

Adults: Initial: 50-75 mg every 3-4 hours as needed **or** 50-100 mg as a single dose preoperatively

Elderly: 25 mg every 4 hours

I.V.:

Children: 1-1.5 mg/kg/dose every 3-4 hours as needed **or** 1-2 mg as a single dose preoperatively (maximum: 100 mg/dose)

Adults: Initial: 5-10 mg every 5 minutes as needed

Oral:

Children: 1-1.5 mg/kg/dose every 3-4 hours as needed (maximum: 100 mg/dose)

Adults: Initial: 50 mg every 3-4 hours as needed; Maintenance: 50-150 mg every 2-4 hours as needed

Elderly: 50 mg every 4 hours

SubQ:

Children: 1-1.5 mg/kg/dose every 3-4 hours as needed **or** 1-2 mg as a single dose preoperatively (maximum: 100 mg/dose)

Adults: Initial: 50-75 mg every 3-4 hours as needed **or** 50-100 mg as a single dose preoperatively

Dosage Forms Excipient information presented when available (limited, particularly for generics); consult specific product labeling. [DSC] = Discontinued product

Injection, solution, as hydrochloride [ampul]: 25 mg/0.5 mL (0.5 mL); 25 mg/mL (1 mL); 50 mg/mL (1 mL, 1.5 mL, 2 mL); 75 mg/mL (1 mL); 100 mg/mL (1 mL)

Injection, solution, as hydrochloride [prefilled syringe]: 25 mg/mL (1 mL); 50 mg/mL (1 mL); 75 mg/mL (1 mL); 100 mg/mL (1 mL)

Injection, solution, as hydrochloride [for PCA pump]: 10 mg/mL (30 mL, 50 mL, 60 mL)

Injection, solution, as hydrochloride [vial]: 25 mg/mL (1 mL); 50 mg/mL (1 mL, 30 mL); 75 mg/mL (1 mL); 100 mg/mL (1 mL, 20 mL) [may contain sodium metabisulfite]

Solution, oral, as hydrochloride: 50 mg/5 mL (500 mL)

Syrup, as hydrochloride:

Demerol®: 50 mg/5 mL (480 mL) [contains benzoic acid; banana flavor] [DSC]

Tablet, as hydrochloride: 50 mg, 100 mg

Demerol®, Meperitab®: 50 mg, 100 mg

Meperidine and Promethazine (me PER i deen & proe METH a zeen)

Medication Safety Issues

Sound-alike/look-alike issues:

Mepergan may be confused with meprobamate

High alert medication: The Institute for Safe Medication Practices (ISMP) includes this medication among its list of drug classes which have a heightened risk of causing significant patient harm when used in error.

Index Terms Mepergan; Promethazine and Meperidine

Pharmacologic Category Analgesic Combination (Opioid)

Use Management of moderate pain

Effect on Mental Status Sedation is common; may cause nervousness or confusion; may rarely produce depression, hallucinations, or paradoxical CNS stimulation

Effect on Psychiatric Treatment CYP2D6 enzyme substrate; may aggravate the adverse effects of MAO inhibitors, fluoxetine, and other serotonin uptake inhibitors. CNS depressants, tricyclic antidepressants, and phenothiazines may potentiate the effects of meperidine. Phenothiazines inhibit the ability of bromocriptine to lower serum prolactin concentrations; benztropine (and other anticholinergics) may inhibit the therapeutic response to promethazine and excess anticholinergic effects may occur.

Restrictions C-II

Dosage Summary

Oral:

Children: Dosage not established

Adults: One capsule every 4-6 hours as needed

Dosage Forms Excipient information presented when available (limited, particularly for generics); consult specific product labeling.

Capsule: Meperidine hydrochloride 50 mg and promethazine hydrochloride 25 mg

◆ **Meperidine Hydrochloride** *see* Meperidine *on page 986*

◆ **Meperitab®** *see* Meperidine *on page 986*

Mephobarbital (me foe BAR bi tal)

Medication Safety Issues

Sound-alike/look-alike issues:

Mephobarbital may be confused with methocarbamol

Mebaral® may be confused with Medrol®, Mellaril®, Tegretol®

U.S. Brand Names Mebaral®

Canadian Brand Names Mebaral®

Index Terms Methylphenobarbital

Pharmacologic Category Barbiturate

Generic Available No

Use Sedative; treatment of grand mal and petit mal epilepsy

Effect on Mental Status Dizziness and drowsiness are common; may cause confusion, nervousness, depression, nightmares, or insomnia; may rarely cause hallucinations

Effect on Psychiatric Treatment May rarely cause agranulocytosis; use caution with clozapine and carbamazepine; may induce hepatic enzymes resulting in an increase or decrease effect of concurrent psychotropic; monitor to altered response

Restrictions C-IV

Pregnancy Risk Factor D

Contraindications Hypersensitivity to mephobarbital, other barbiturates, or any component of the formulation; pre-existing CNS depression; respiratory depression; severe uncontrolled pain; history of porphyria; pregnancy

Adverse Reactions

>10%: Central nervous system: Dizziness, "hangover" effect, lightheadedness, somnolence

1% to 10%:

Central nervous system: Confusion, faint feeling, headache, insomnia, mental depression, nervousness, nightmares, unusual excitement

Gastrointestinal: Constipation, nausea, vomiting

<1% (Limited to important or life-threatening): Agranulocytosis, angioedema, dependence, exfoliative dermatitis, hallucinations, hypotension, megaloblastic anemia, respiratory depression, skin rash, Stevens-Johnson syndrome, thrombocytopenia, thrombophlebitis

Metabolism/Transport Effects Substrate of CYP2B6 (minor), 2C9 (minor), 2C19 (major); **Inhibits** CYP2C19 (weak); **Induces** CYP2A6 (weak)

Drug Interactions

Acetaminophen: Barbiturates may increase the metabolism of Acetaminophen. This may 1) diminish the effect of acetaminophen; and 2) increase the risk of liver damage. *Risk C: Monitor therapy*

Alcohol (Ethyl): CNS Depressants may enhance the CNS depressant effect of Alcohol (Ethyl). *Risk C: Monitor therapy*

Beta-Blockers: Barbiturates may decrease the serum concentration of Beta-Blockers. **Exceptions:** Atenolol; Levobunolol; Metipranolol; Nadolol. *Risk C: Monitor therapy*

Calcium Channel Blockers: Barbiturates may increase the metabolism of Calcium Channel Blockers. **Exceptions:** Clevidipine. *Risk D: Consider therapy modification*

Chloramphenicol: May decrease the metabolism of Barbiturates. Barbiturates may increase the metabolism of Chloramphenicol. *Risk D: Consider therapy modification*

CNS Depressants: May enhance the adverse/toxic effect of other CNS Depressants. *Risk C: Monitor therapy*

Contraceptive (Progestins): Barbiturates may diminish the therapeutic effect of Contraceptive (Progestins). Contraceptive failure is possible. *Risk D: Consider therapy modification*

Corticosteroids (Systemic): Barbiturates may increase the metabolism of Corticosteroids (Systemic). *Risk C: Monitor therapy*

CycloSPORINE: Barbiturates may increase the metabolism of CycloSPORINE. *Risk D: Consider therapy modification*

CYP2C19 Inducers (Strong): May increase the metabolism of CYP2C19 Substrates. *Risk C: Monitor therapy*

CYP2C19 Inhibitors (Moderate): May decrease the metabolism of CYP2C19 Substrates. *Risk C: Monitor therapy*

CYP2C19 Inhibitors (Strong): May decrease the metabolism of CYP2C19 Substrates. *Risk D: Consider therapy modification*

Disopyramide: Barbiturates may increase the metabolism of Disopyramide. *Risk D: Consider therapy modification*

Doxycycline: Barbiturates may decrease the serum concentration of Doxycycline. *Risk D: Consider therapy modification*

Etoposide: Barbiturates may increase the metabolism of Etoposide. *Risk C: Monitor therapy*

Etoposide Phosphate: Barbiturates may decrease the serum concentration of Etoposide Phosphate. Barbiturates may increase the metabolism, via CYP isoenzymes, of etoposide phosphate. *Risk C: Monitor therapy*

Felbamate: May increase the serum concentration of Barbiturates. *Risk C: Monitor therapy*

Griseofulvin: Barbiturates may decrease the absorption of Griseofulvin. *Risk D: Consider therapy modification*

LamoTRIgine: Barbiturates may increase the metabolism of LamoTRIgine. *Risk D: Consider therapy modification*

Meperidine: Barbiturates may enhance the CNS depressant effect of Meperidine. *Risk C: Monitor therapy*

Methadone: Barbiturates may increase the metabolism of Methadone. *Risk D: Consider therapy modification*

Oral Contraceptive (Estrogens): Barbiturates may diminish the therapeutic effect of Oral Contraceptive (Estrogens). Contraceptive failure is possible. *Risk D: Consider therapy modification*

Primidone: May enhance the adverse/toxic effect of Barbiturates. Primidone is converted to phenobarbital, and thus becomes additive with existing barbiturate therapy. *Risk C: Monitor therapy*

Propafenone: Barbiturates may increase the metabolism of Propafenone. *Risk D: Consider therapy modification*

Pyridoxine: May increase the metabolism of Barbiturates. Apparent in high pyridoxine doses (eg, 200 mg/day) *Risk C: Monitor therapy*

QuiNIDine: Barbiturates may increase the metabolism of QuiNIDine. *Risk D: Consider therapy modification*

Rifamycin Derivatives: May increase the metabolism of Barbiturates. *Risk C: Monitor therapy*

Teniposide: Barbiturates may increase the metabolism of Teniposide. *Risk C: Monitor therapy*

Theophylline Derivatives: Barbiturates may increase the metabolism of Theophylline Derivatives. **Exceptions:** Dyphylline. *Risk C: Monitor therapy*

Tricyclic Antidepressants: Barbiturates may increase the metabolism of Tricyclic Antidepressants. *Risk D: Consider therapy modification*

Valproic Acid: May decrease the metabolism of Barbiturates. Barbiturates may decrease the serum concentration of Valproic Acid. *Risk C: Monitor therapy*

Vitamin K Antagonists (eg, warfarin): Barbiturates may increase the metabolism of Vitamin K Antagonists. *Risk D: Consider therapy modification*

Voriconazole: Barbiturates may decrease the serum concentration of Voriconazole. *Risk X: Avoid combination*

Mechanism of Action Increases seizure threshold in the motor cortex; depresses monosynaptic and polysynaptic transmission in the CNS

Pharmacodynamics/Kinetics

Onset of action: 20-60 minutes

Duration: 6-8 hours

Absorption: ~50%

Half-life elimination, serum: 34 hours

Dosage Oral:

Epilepsy:

Children: 6-12 mg/kg/day in 2-4 divided doses

Adults: 200-600 mg/day in 2-4 divided doses

Sedation:

Children:

<5 years: 16-32 mg 3-4 times/day

>5 years: 32-64 mg 3-4 times/day

Adults: 32-100 mg 3-4 times/day

Dosing adjustment in renal or hepatic impairment: Use with caution and reduce dosages

Dietary Considerations High doses of pyridoxine may decrease drug effect; barbiturates may increase the metabolism of vitamin D & K; dietary requirements of vitamin D, K, C, B_{12}, folate and calcium may be increased with long-term use.

Dosage Forms Excipient information presented when available (limited, particularly for generics); consult specific product labeling.

Tablet: 32 mg, 50 mg, 100 mg

◆ **Mephyton®** *see* Phytonadione *on page 1289*

Mepivacaine (me PIV a kane)

Medication Safety Issues

Sound-alike/look-alike issues:

Mepivacaine may be confused with bupivacaine

Polocaine® may be confused with prilocaine

High alert medication: The Institute for Safe Medication Practices (ISMP) includes this medication (epidural administration) among its list of drug classes which have a heightened risk of causing significant patient harm when used in error.

U.S. Brand Names Carbocaine®; Polocaine®; Polocaine® Dental; Polocaine® MPF; Scandonest® 3% Plain

Canadian Brand Names Carbocaine®; Polocaine®

Mexican Brand Names Lentocaine

Index Terms Mepivacaine Hydrochloride

Pharmacologic Category Local Anesthetic

Use Local or regional analgesia; anesthesia by local infiltration, peripheral and central neural techniques including epidural and caudal blocks; **not** for use in spinal anesthesia

Effect on Mental Status May rarely cause anxiety, restlessness, confusion, drowsiness

Effect on Psychiatric Treatment None reported

Dosage Summary

Brachial, cervical, intercostal, pudenal nerve block:

Children: Dosage not established

Adults: 5-40 mL of 1% solution **or** 5-20 mL of 2% solution (maximum: 400 mg)

Caudal and epidural block (preservative free solutions only):

Children: Dosage not established

Adults: 15-30 mL of 1% solution (maximum: 300 mg) **or** 10-25 mL of 1.5% solution (maximum: 375 mg) **or** 10-20 mL of a 2% solution (maximum: 400 mg)

Dental anesthesia:

Children: Dosage not established

Adults: 54 mg (1.8 mL) as a 3% solution (single site) **or** 270 mg (9 mL) as a 3% solution (entire oral cavity) (maximum: 400 mg)

Infiltration:

Children: Dosage not established

Adults: Up to 40 mL of 1% solution (maximum: 400 mg)

Local injection:

Children <3 years or <14 kg: Dose varies; only concentrations less than 2% should be used (maximum: 5-6 mg/kg)

Children ≥3 years or ≥14 kg: Dose varies (maximum: 5-6 mg/kg)

Adults: Dose varies (maximum: 400 mg/dose; 1000 mg/day)

Paracervical block:

Children: Dosage not established

Adults: Up to 20 mL (both sides) of 1% solution (maximum: 200 mg)

Therapeutic block:

Children: Dosage not established

Adults: 1-5 mL of 1% solution (maximum: 50 mg) or 1-5 mL of 2% solution (maximum: 100 mg)

Transvaginal block:

Children: Dosage not established

Adults: Up to 30 mL (both sides) of a 1% solution (maximum: 300 mg)

Dosage Forms Excipient information presented when available (limited, particularly for generics); consult specific product labeling.

Injection, solution, as hydrochloride [contains methylparabens]:

Carbocaine®: 1% (50 mL); 2% (50 mL)

Polocaine®: 1% (50 mL); 2% (50 mL)

Scandonest® 3% Plain: 3% (1.7 mL) [dental cartridge]

Injection, solution, as hydrochloride [preservative free]:

Carbocaine®: 1% (30 mL); 1.5% (30 mL); 2% (20 mL); 3% (1.8 mL) [dental cartridge]

Polocaine® Dental: 3% (1.8 mL) [dental cartridge]

Polocaine® MPF: 1% (30 mL); 1.5% (30 mL); 2% (20 mL)

◆ **Mepivacaine Hydrochloride** *see* Mepivacaine *on page 990*

Meprobamate (me proe BA mate)

Medication Safety Issues

Sound-alike/look-alike issues:

Meprobamate may be confused with Mepergan, meperidine

Equanil may be confused with Elavil®

U.S. Brand Names Miltown® [DSC]

Canadian Brand Names Novo-Mepro

Index Terms Equanil

Pharmacologic Category Antianxiety Agent, Miscellaneous

Generic Available Yes

Use Management of anxiety disorders

Unlabeled/Investigational Use Demonstrated value for muscle contraction, headache, premenstrual tension, external sphincter spasticity, muscle rigidity, opisthotonos-associated with tetanus

Restrictions C-IV

Pregnancy Risk Factor D

Lactation Enters breast milk/not recommended

Contraindications Hypersensitivity to meprobamate, related compounds (including carisoprodol), or any component of the formulation; acute intermittent porphyria; pre-existing CNS depression; narrow-angle glaucoma; severe uncontrolled pain; pregnancy

Warnings/Precautions Physical and psychological dependence and abuse may occur; abrupt cessation may precipitate withdrawal. Use with caution in patients with depression or suicidal tendencies, or in patients with a history of drug abuse. May cause CNS depression, which may impair physical or mental abilities. Patients must be cautioned about performing tasks which require mental alertness (eg, operating machinery or driving). Effects with other sedative drugs or ethanol may be potentiated. Safety and efficacy have not been established in children <6 years of age; allergic reaction may occur in patients with history of dermatological condition (usually by fourth dose). Use with caution in patients with renal or hepatic impairment, or with a history of seizures. Use caution in the elderly as it may cause confusion, cognitive impairment, or excessive sedation.

Adverse Reactions Frequency not defined.

Cardiovascular: Syncope, peripheral edema, palpitation, tachycardia, arrhythmia

Central nervous system: Drowsiness, ataxia, dizziness, paradoxical excitement, confusion, slurred speech, headache, euphoria, chills, vertigo, paresthesia, overstimulation

Dermatologic: Rashes, purpura, dermatitis, Stevens-Johnson syndrome, petechiae, ecchymosis

Gastrointestinal: Diarrhea, vomiting, nausea

Hematologic: Leukopenia, eosinophilia, agranulocytosis, aplastic anemia

Neuromuscular & skeletal: Weakness

Ocular: Blurred vision, impairment of accommodation

Renal: Renal failure
Respiratory: Wheezing, dyspnea, bronchospasm, angioneurotic edema

Drug Interactions
There are no known significant interactions.

Ethanol/Nutrition/Herb Interactions
Ethanol: Avoid ethanol (may increase CNS depression).
Herb/Nutraceutical: Avoid valerian, St John's wort, kava kava, gotu kola (may increase CNS depression).

Mechanism of Action Affects the thalamus and limbic system; also appears to inhibit multineuronal spinal reflexes

Pharmacodynamics/Kinetics
Onset of action: Sedation: ~1 hour
Distribution: Crosses placenta; enters breast milk
Metabolism: Hepatic
Half-life elimination: 10 hours
Excretion: Urine (8% to 20% as unchanged drug); feces (10% as metabolites)

Dosage Oral:
Children 6-12 years: Anxiety: 100-200 mg 2-3 times/day
Adults: Anxiety: 400 mg 3-4 times/day, up to 2400 mg/day
Dosing interval in renal impairment:
Cl_{cr} 10-50 mL/minute: Administer every 9-12 hours
Cl_{cr} <10 mL/minute: Administer every 12-18 hours
Hemodialysis: Moderately dialyzable (20% to 50%)
Dosing adjustment in hepatic impairment: Probably necessary in patients with liver disease

Monitoring Parameters Mental status

Reference Range Therapeutic: 6-12 mcg/mL (SI: 28-55 µmol/L); Toxic: >60 mcg/mL (SI: >275 µmol/L)

Additional Information Withdrawal should be gradual over 1-2 weeks. Benzodiazepine and buspirone are better choices for treatment of anxiety disorders.

Dosage Forms Excipient information presented when available (limited, particularly for generics); consult specific product labeling. [DSC] = Discontinued product
Tablet: 200 mg, 400 mg [DSC]
Miltown®: 200 mg, 400 mg [DSC]

Meprobamate and Aspirin (me proe BA mate & AS pir in)

U.S. Brand Names Equagesic®
Canadian Brand Names 292 MEP®
Index Terms Aspirin and Meprobamate
Pharmacologic Category Antianxiety Agent, Miscellaneous; Salicylate
Use Adjunct to the short-term treatment of pain in patients with skeletal-muscular disease exhibiting tension and/or anxiety
Effect on Mental Status Sedation is common
Effect on Psychiatric Treatment May cause leukopenia; use caution with clozapine and carbamazepine; may displace valproic acid from binding sites resulting in an increase of unbound drug; monitor for toxicity; meprobamate is a CNS depressant; monitor for additive effects with concurrent psychotropic use
Restrictions C-IV
Dosage Summary
Oral:
Children <12 years: Dosage not established
Children ≥12 years: 1-2 tablets 3-4 times/day for up to 10 days
Adults: 1-2 tablet 3-4 times/day for up to 10 days

Dosage Forms Excipient information presented when available (limited, particularly for generics); consult specific product labeling.
Tablet:
Equagesic®: Meprobamate 200 mg and aspirin 325 mg

◆ **Mepron®** *see* Atovaquone *on page 157*

Mequinol and Tretinoin (ME kwi nole & TRET i noyn)

U.S. Brand Names Solagé®
Canadian Brand Names Solagé®
Index Terms Solage; Tretinoin and Mequinol
Pharmacologic Category Retinoic Acid Derivative; Vitamin A Derivative; Vitamin, Topical

Use Treatment of solar lentigines; the efficacy of using Solagé® daily for >24 weeks has not been established

Effect on Mental Status None reported

Effect on Psychiatric Treatment Photosensitizing drugs such as psychotropics can further increase sun sensitivity; avoid concurrent use

Dosage Summary

Topical:

Children: Dosage not established

Adults: Apply twice daily, separate application by at least 8 hours

Dosage Forms Excipient information presented when available (limited, particularly for generics); consult specific product labeling.

Liquid, topical:

Solagé®: Mequinol 2% and tretinoin 0.01% (30 mL) [contains alcohol 78%; dispensed in applicator bottle]

Mercaptopurine (mer kap toe PYOOR een)

Medication Safety Issues

Sound-alike/look-alike issues:

Purinethol® may be confused with propylthiouracil

High alert medication: The Institute for Safe Medication Practices (ISMP) includes this medication among its list of drugs which have a heightened risk of causing significant patient harm when used in error.

To avoid potentially serious dosage errors, the terms "6-mercaptopurine" or "6-MP" should be avoided; use of these terms has been associated with sixfold overdosages.

Azathioprine is metabolized to mercaptopurine; concurrent use of these commercially-available products has resulted in profound myelosuppression.

U.S. Brand Names Purinethol®

Canadian Brand Names Purinethol®

Mexican Brand Names Purinethol

Index Terms 6-Mercaptopurine (error-prone abbreviation); 6-MP (error-prone abbreviation); NSC-755

Pharmacologic Category Antineoplastic Agent, Antimetabolite; Immunosuppressant Agent

Use Treatment (maintenance and induction) of acute lymphoblastic leukemia (ALL)

Unlabeled/Investigational Use Steroid-sparing agent for corticosteroid-dependent Crohn's disease (CD) and ulcerative colitis (UC); maintenance of remission in CD; fistulizing Crohn's disease

Effect on Mental Status None reported

Effect on Psychiatric Treatment May cause leukopenia; use caution with clozapine or carbamazepine

Dosage Summary

Oral:

Children: Induction: 2.5-5 mg/kg/day **or** 70-100 mg/m^2/day given once daily; Maintenance: 1.5-2.5 mg/kg/day **or** 50-75 mg/m^2/day given once daily

Adults: Induction: 2.5-5 mg/kg/day (100-200 mg); Maintenance: 1.5-2.5 mg/kg/day **or** 80-100 mg/m^2/day given once daily

Dosage Forms Excipient information presented when available (limited, particularly for generics); consult specific product labeling.

Tablet [scored]: 50 mg

◆ **6-Mercaptopurine (error-prone abbreviation)** *see* Mercaptopurine *on page 993*

◆ **Mercapturic Acid** *see* Acetylcysteine *on page 47*

◆ **Meridia®** *see* Sibutramine *on page 1479*

Meropenem (mer oh PEN em)

Medication Safety Issues

Sound-alike/look-alike issues:

Meropenem may be confused with ertapenem, imipenem, metronidazole.

U.S. Brand Names Merrem® I.V.

Canadian Brand Names Merrem®

Mexican Brand Names Merrem

Pharmacologic Category Antibiotic, Carbapenem

Use Treatment of intra-abdominal infections (complicated appendicitis and peritonitis); treatment of bacterial meningitis in pediatric patients ≥3 months of age caused by *S. pneumoniae*, *H. influenzae*, and *N. meningitidis*; treatment of complicated skin and skin structure infections caused by susceptible organisms

Unlabeled/Investigational Use *Burkholderia pseudomallei* (melioidosis), febrile neutropenia, liver abscess, meningitis (adults), otitis externa, pneumonia, urinary tract infections

Effect on Mental Status May rarely cause agitation, confusion, insomnia, hallucinations, or depression

Effect on Psychiatric Treatment None reported

Dosage Summary

I.V.:

Neonates (postnatal age 0-7 days): 20 mg/kg/dose every 12 hours

Neonates (postnatal age >7 days and 1200-2000 g): 20 mg/kg/dose every 12 hours

Neonates (postnatal age >7 days and >2000 g): 20 mg/kg/dose every 8 hours

Children ≥3 months and <50 kg: 10-40 mg/kg every 8 hours (maximum: 2 g every 8 hours)

Children ≥50 kg: 500 mg to 2 g every 8 hours

Adults: 500 mg to 2 g every 8 hours

Dosage Forms Excipient information presented when available (limited, particularly for generics); consult specific product labeling.

Injection, powder for reconstitution:

Merrem® I.V: 500 mg [contains sodium 45.1 mg as sodium carbonate (1.96 mEq)]; 1 g [contains sodium 90.2 mg as sodium carbonate (3.92 mEq)]

◆ **Merrem® I.V.** *see* Meropenem *on page 993*

Mesalamine (me SAL a meen)

Medication Safety Issues

Sound-alike/look-alike issues:

Mesalamine may be confused with mecamylamine

Asacol® may be confused with Ansaid®, Os-Cal®

Lialda™ may be confused with Aldara®

U.S. Brand Names Asacol®; Canasa®; Lialda™; Pentasa®; Rowasa®

Canadian Brand Names Asacol®; Asacol® 800; Mesasal®; Mezavant®; Novo-5 ASA; Pendo-5 ASA; Pentasa®; Quintasa®; Rowasa®; Salofalk®

Mexican Brand Names Asacol

Index Terms 5-Aminosalicylic Acid; 5-ASA; Fisalamine; Mesalazine

Pharmacologic Category 5-Aminosalicylic Acid Derivative

Use

Oral: Treatment and maintenance of remission of mildly- to moderately-active ulcerative colitis

Rectal: Treatment of active mild-to-moderate distal ulcerative colitis, proctosigmoiditis, or proctitis

Effect on Mental Status Malaise is common

Effect on Psychiatric Treatment None reported

Dosage Summary

Oral:

Children: Dosage not established

Adults:

Capsule: 1 g 4 times/day

Tablet:

Asacol®: 800 mg 3 times/day

Lialda™, Mezavant®: 2.4-4.8 g once daily

Rectal:

Children: Dosage not established

Adults:

Retention enema: 60 mL (4 g) at bedtime, retained overnight (~8 hours)

Suppository: Insert 1000 mg at bedtime; **Note:** Suppositories should be retained for at least 1-3 hours to achieve maximum benefit

Dosage Forms Excipient information presented when available (limited, particularly for generics); consult specific product labeling. [CAN] = Canadian brand name

Capsule, controlled release:

Pentasa®: 250 mg, 500 mg

Suppository, rectal:

Canasa®: 1000 mg [contains saturated vegetable fatty acid esters]

Suspension, rectal: 4 g/60 mL (7s, 28s) [contains potassium metabisulfite and sodium benzoate]

Rowasa®: 4 g/60 mL (7s, 28s) [contains potassium metabisulfite and sodium benzoate]

Tablet, delayed release [enteric coated]:
Asacol®: 400 mg
Lialda™: 1.2 g
Tablet, delayed and extended release:
Mezavant® [CAN]: 1.2 g [not available in U.S.]

◆ **Mesalazine** *see* Mesalamine *on page 994*

Mesna (MES na)

U.S. Brand Names Mesnex®
Canadian Brand Names Mesnex®; Uromitexan
Mexican Brand Names Mescryo; Mesnil; Mesodal; Uroprot
Index Terms Sodium 2-Mercaptoethane Sulfonate
Pharmacologic Category Antidote
Use Orphan drug: Prevention of hemorrhagic cystitis induced by ifosfamide
Unlabeled/Investigational Use Prevention of hemorrhagic cystitis induced by cyclophosphamide
Effect on Mental Status May cause malaise
Effect on Psychiatric Treatment None reported
Dosage Forms Excipient information presented when available (limited, particularly for generics); consult specific product labeling.
Injection, solution: 100 mg/mL (10 mL) [contains benzyl alcohol]
Tablet: 400 mg

◆ **Mesnex®** *see* Mesna *on page 995*
◆ **Mestinon®** *see* Pyridostigmine *on page 1374*
◆ **Mestinon® Timespan®** *see* Pyridostigmine *on page 1374*

Mestranol and Norethindrone (MES tra nole & nor eth IN drone)

Medication Safety Issues
Sound-alike/look-alike issues:
Norinyl® may be confused with Nardil®
U.S. Brand Names Necon® 1/50; Norinyl® 1+50; Ortho-Novum® 1/50 [DSC]
Canadian Brand Names Ortho-Novum® 1/50
Mexican Brand Names Norace
Index Terms Norethindrone and Mestranol; Ortho Novum 1/50
Pharmacologic Category Contraceptive; Estrogen and Progestin Combination
Use Prevention of pregnancy
Unlabeled/Investigational Use Treatment of hypermenorrhea (menorrhagia); pain associated with endometriosis; dysmenorrhea; dysfunctional uterine bleeding
Effect on Mental Status May cause anxiety or depression
Effect on Psychiatric Treatment Hepatic metabolism of TCAs, benzodiazepines (oxidatively metabolized) and beta-blockers may be decreased by oral contraceptives; monitor increased/toxic effects; may increase the clearance of benzodiazepines (glucuronidation); barbiturates may increase the metabolism of oral contraceptives resulting in decreased effectiveness
Dosage Summary
Oral:
21 tablet package:
Children prior to menarche: Dosage not established
Children (menarche): 1 tablet daily for 21 days, followed by 7 days off
Adults: 1 tablet daily for 21 days, followed by 7 days off
28 tablet package:
Children prior to menarche: Dosage not established
Children (menarche): 1 tablet daily without interruption
Adults: 1 tablet daily without interruption
Dosage Forms Excipient information presented when available (limited, particularly for generics); consult specific product labeling.
Tablet, monophasic formulations:
Necon® 1/50: Norethindrone 1 mg and mestranol 0.05 mg [21 light blue tablets and 7 white inactive tablets] (28s)
Norinyl® 1+50: Norethindrone 1 mg and mestranol 0.05 mg [21 white tablets and 7 orange inactive tablets] (28s)
Ortho-Novum® 1/50: Norethindrone 1 mg and mestranol 0.05 mg [21 yellow tablets and 7 green inactive tablets] (28s) [DSC]

- **Metacortandralone** *see* PrednisoLONE *on page 1326*
- **Metadate® CD** *see* Methylphenidate *on page 1024*
- **Metadate® ER** *see* Methylphenidate *on page 1024*
- **Metaglip™** *see* Glipizide and Metformin *on page 729*
- **123 Meta-Iodobenzylguanidine Sulfate** *see* Iobenguane I 123 *on page 849*

Metaproterenol (met a proe TER e nol)

Medication Safety Issues

Sound-alike/look-alike issues:

Metaproterenol may be confused with metipranolol, metoprolol

Alupent® may be confused with Atrovent®

U.S. Brand Names Alupent®

Canadian Brand Names Apo-Orciprenaline®; ratio-Orciprenaline®; Tanta-Orciprenaline®

Index Terms Metaproterenol Sulfate; Orciprenaline Sulfate

Pharmacologic Category $Beta_2$-Adrenergic Agonist

Use Bronchodilator in reversible airway obstruction due to asthma or COPD; because of its delayed onset of action (1 hour) and prolonged effect (4 or more hours), this may not be the drug of choice for assessing response to a bronchodilator

Effect on Mental Status Nervousness is common; may cause dizziness, restlessness, or insomnia

Effect on Psychiatric Treatment Concurrent use with TCAs and MAO inhibitors may result in additive toxicity

Dosage Summary

Inhalation:

Children ≤12 years: Dosage not established

Children >12 years: 2-3 inhalations every 3-4 hours (maximum: 12 inhalations/day)

Adults: 2-3 inhalations every 3-4 hours (maximum: 12 inhalations/day)

Nebulizer:

Infants: 0.01-0.02 mL/kg of 5% solution diluted in 2-3 mL normal saline every 4-6 hours (minimum: 0.1 mL/dose; maximum: 0.3 mL/dose)

Children: 0.01-0.02 mL/kg of 5% solution diluted in 2-3 mL normal saline every 4-6 hours (minimum: 0.1 mL/dose; maximum: 0.3 mL/dose)

Adolescents: 5-20 breaths of full strength 5% metaproterenol **or** 0.2 to 0.3 mL 5% metaproterenol in 2.5-3 mL normal saline every 4-6 hours

Adults: 5-20 breaths of full strength 5% metaproterenol **or** 0.2 to 0.3 mL 5% metaproterenol in 2.5-3 mL normal saline every 4-6 hours

Oral:

Children <2 years: 0.4 mg/kg/dose 3-4 times/day (every 8-12 hours for infants)

Children 2-6 years: 1-2.6 mg/kg/day divided every 6 hours

Children 6-9 years: 10 mg/dose 3-4 times/day

Children >9 years: 20 mg 3-4 times/day

Adults: 20 mg 3-4 times/day

Elderly: Initial: 10 mg 3-4 times/day, may increase to 20 mg 3-4 times/day

Dosage Forms Excipient information presented when available (limited, particularly for generics); consult specific product labeling.

Aerosol for oral inhalation, as sulfate:

Alupent®: 0.65 mg/inhalation (14 g) [contains chlorofluorocarbon; 200 doses]

Solution for nebulization, as sulfate [preservative free]: 0.4% [4 mg/mL] (2.5 mL); 0.6% [6 mg/mL] (2.5 mL)

Syrup, as sulfate: 10 mg/5 mL (480 mL)

Tablet, as sulfate: 10 mg, 20 mg

- **Metaproterenol Sulfate** *see* Metaproterenol *on page 996*

Metaxalone (me TAKS a lone)

Medication Safety Issues

Sound-alike/look-alike issues:

Metaxalone may be confused with metolazone

U.S. Brand Names Skelaxin®

Canadian Brand Names Skelaxin®

Pharmacologic Category Skeletal Muscle Relaxant

Use Relief of discomfort associated with acute, painful musculoskeletal conditions

Effect on Mental Status Drowsiness and dizziness are common; may cause paradoxical stimulation

Effect on Psychiatric Treatment May cause leukopenia; use caution with clozapine and carbamazepine; concurrent use with psychotropics may produce additive sedation

Dosage Summary

Oral:

Children ≤12 years: Dosage not established

Children >12 years: 800 mg 3-4 times/day

Adults: 800 mg 3-4 times/day

Dosage Forms Excipient information presented when available (limited, particularly for generics); consult specific product labeling. [DSC] = Discontinued product

Tablet: 400 mg [DSC], 800 mg

MetFORMIN (met FOR min)

Medication Safety Issues

Sound-alike/look-alike issues:

MetFORMIN may be confused with metroNIDAZOLE

Glucophage® may be confused with Glucotrol®, Glutofac®

U.S. Brand Names Fortamet®; Glucophage®; Glucophage® XR; Glumetza™; Riomet®

Canadian Brand Names Alti-Metformin; Apo-Metformin®; BCI-Metformin; Gen-Metformin; Glucophage®; Glumetza™; Glycon; Novo-Metformin; Nu-Metformin; PMS-Metformin; RAN™-Metformin; ratio-Metformin; Rho®-Metformin; Sandoz-Metformin FC

Mexican Brand Names Dabex; Dimefor; Glucophage

Index Terms Metformin Hydrochloride

Pharmacologic Category Antidiabetic Agent, Biguanide

Generic Available Yes: Excludes solution

Use Management of type 2 diabetes mellitus (noninsulin dependent, NIDDM) as monotherapy when hyperglycemia cannot be managed with diet and exercise alone. In adults, may be used concomitantly with a sulfonylurea or insulin to improve glycemic control.

Unlabeled/Investigational Use Gestational diabetes mellitus (GDM); polycystic ovary syndrome (PCOS)

Effect on Mental Status None reported

Effect on Psychiatric Treatment May cause leukopenia; use caution with clozapine and carbamazepine; concurrent use with psychotropics may produce additive sedation

Pregnancy Risk Factor B

Pregnancy Considerations Adverse events have not been observed in animal studies; therefore, metformin is classified as pregnancy category B. Metformin has been found to cross the placenta in levels which may be comparable to those found in the maternal plasma. Pharmacokinetic studies suggest that clearance of metformin may be increased during pregnancy and dosing may need adjusted in some women when used during the third trimester.

Fetal, neonatal, and maternal outcomes have been evaluated following maternal use of metformin for the treatment of GDM and type 2 diabetes. Available information suggests that metformin use during pregnancy may be safe as long as good glycemic control is maintained; however, many studies used metformin during the second or third trimester only. Maternal hyperglycemia can be associated with adverse effects in the fetus, including macrosomia, neonatal hyperglycemia, and hyperbilirubinemia; the risk of congenital malformations is increased when the Hb A_{1c} is above the normal range. Diabetes can also be associated with adverse effects in the mother. Poorly-treated diabetes may cause end-organ damage that may negatively affect obstetric outcomes. Physiologic glucose levels should be maintained prior to and during pregnancy to decrease the risk of adverse events in the mother and the fetus. Until additional safety and efficacy data are obtained, the use of oral agents is generally not recommended as routine management of GDM or type 2 diabetes mellitus during pregnancy. Insulin is the drug of choice for the control of diabetes mellitus during pregnancy.

Metformin has also been evaluated for the treatment of PCOS, a syndrome which may exhibit oligomenorrhea and in some women, hyperinsulinemia. When used to treat infertility related to PCOS, current guidelines restrict the use of metformin to women with glucose intolerance.

Lactation Enters breast milk/not recommended

Contraindications Hypersensitivity to metformin or any component of the formulation; renal disease or renal dysfunction (serum creatinine ≥1.5 mg/dL in males or ≥1.4 mg/dL in females) or abnormal creatinine clearance from any cause, including shock, acute myocardial infarction, or septicemia; acute or chronic metabolic acidosis with or without coma (including diabetic ketoacidosis)

Note: Temporarily discontinue in patients undergoing radiologic studies in which intravascular iodinated contrast media are utilized.

Warnings/Precautions [U.S. Boxed Warning]: Lactic acidosis is a rare, but potentially severe consequence of therapy with metformin. Lactic acidosis should be suspected in any patient with diabetes receiving metformin with evidence of acidosis but without evidence of ketoacidosis. Discontinue metformin in clinical situations predisposing to hypoxemia, including conditions such as cardiovascular collapse, respiratory failure, acute myocardial infarction, acute congestive heart failure, and septicemia. Use caution in patients with congestive heart failure requiring pharmacologic management, particularly in patients with unstable or acute CHF; risk of lactic acidosis may be increased secondary to hypoperfusion.

Metformin is substantially excreted by the kidney. The risk of accumulation and lactic acidosis increases with the degree of impairment of renal function. Patients with renal function below the limit of normal for their age should not receive metformin. In elderly patients, renal function should be monitored regularly; should not be initiated in patients ≥80 years of age unless normal renal function is confirmed. Use of concomitant medications that may affect renal function (ie, affect tubular secretion) may also affect metformin disposition. Metformin should be withheld in patients with dehydration and/or prerenal azotemia. Therapy should be suspended for any surgical procedures (resume only after normal intake resumed and normal renal function is verified). Therapy should be temporarily discontinued prior to or at the time of intravascular administration of iodinated contrast media (potential for acute alteration in renal function). Metformin should be withheld for 48 hours after the radiologic study and restarted only after renal function has been confirmed as normal. It may be necessary to discontinue metformin and administer insulin if the patient is exposed to stress (fever, trauma, infection, surgery).

Avoid use in patients with impaired liver function. Patient must be instructed to avoid excessive acute or chronic ethanol use; ethanol may potentiate metformin's effect on lactate metabolism. Administration of oral antidiabetic drugs has been reported to be associated with increased cardiovascular mortality; metformin does not appear to share this risk. Safety and efficacy of metformin have been established for use in children ≥10 years of age; the extended release preparation is for use in patients ≥17 years of age.

Insoluble tablet shell of Glumetza™ 1000 mg extended release tablet may remain intact and be visible in the stool. Other extended released tablets (Fortamet®, Glucophage® XR, Glumetza™ 500 mg) may appear in the stool as a soft mass resembling the tablet.

Adverse Reactions

>10%:

- Gastrointestinal: Diarrhea (10% to 53%), nausea/vomiting (7% to 26%), flatulence (12%)
- Neuromuscular & skeletal: Weakness (9%)

1% to 10%:

- Cardiovascular: Chest discomfort, flushing, palpitation
- Central nervous system: Headache (6%), chills, dizziness, lightheadedness
- Dermatologic: Rash
- Endocrine & metabolic: Hypoglycemia
- Gastrointestinal: Indigestion (7%), abdominal discomfort (6%), abdominal distention, abnormal stools, constipation, dyspepsia/ heartburn, taste disorder
- Neuromuscular & skeletal: Myalgia
- Respiratory: Dyspnea, upper respiratory tract infection
- Miscellaneous: Decreased vitamin B_{12} levels (7%), increased diaphoresis, flu-like syndrome, nail disorder

<1% (Limited to important or life-threatening): Lactic acidosis, leukocytoclastic vasculitis, megaloblastic anemia, pneumonitis

Drug Interactions

Cephalexin: May increase the serum concentration of MetFORMIN. *Risk C: Monitor therapy*

Cimetidine: May decrease the excretion of MetFORMIN. *Risk C: Monitor therapy*

Corticosteroids (Orally Inhaled): May diminish the hypoglycemic effect of Antidiabetic Agents. In some instances, corticosteroid-mediated HPA axis suppression has led to episodes of acute adrenal crisis, which may manifest as enhanced hypoglycemia, particularly in the setting of insulin or other antidiabetic agent use. *Risk C: Monitor therapy*

Corticosteroids (Systemic): May diminish the hypoglycemic effect of Antidiabetic Agents. In some instances, corticosteroid-mediated HPA axis suppression has led to episodes of acute adrenal crisis, which may manifest as enhanced hypoglycemia, particularly in the setting of insulin or other antidiabetic agent use. *Risk C: Monitor therapy*

Iodinated Contrast Agents: May enhance the adverse/toxic effect of MetFORMIN. Renal dysfunction that may be caused by iodinated contrast agents may lead to metformin-associated lactic acidosis. *Risk D: Consider therapy modification*

Luteinizing Hormone-Releasing Hormone Analogs: May diminish the therapeutic effect of Antidiabetic Agents. *Risk C: Monitor therapy*

Pegvisomant: May enhance the hypoglycemic effect of Antidiabetic Agents. *Risk C: Monitor therapy*

Somatropin: May diminish the hypoglycemic effect of Antidiabetic Agents. *Risk D: Consider therapy modification*

Ethanol/Nutrition/Herb Interactions

Ethanol: Avoid or limit ethanol (incidence of lactic acidosis may be increased; may cause hypoglycemia).

Food: Food decreases the extent and slightly delays the absorption. May decrease absorption of vitamin B_{12} and/or folic acid.

Herb/Nutraceutical: Caution with chromium, garlic, gymnema (may cause hypoglycemia).

Stability

Oral solution: Store at 15°C to 30°C (59°F to 86°F).

Tablets: Store at 20°C to 25°C (68°F to 77°F); excursion permitted to 15°C to 30°C (59°F to 86°F). Protect from light and moisture.

Mechanism of Action Decreases hepatic glucose production, decreasing intestinal absorption of glucose and improves insulin sensitivity (increases peripheral glucose uptake and utilization)

Pharmacodynamics/Kinetics

Onset of action: Within days; maximum effects up to 2 weeks

Distribution: V_d: 654 ± 358 L; partitions into erythrocytes

Protein binding: Negligible

Metabolism: Not metabolized by the liver

Bioavailability: Absolute: Fasting: 50% to 60%

Half-life elimination: Plasma: 4-9 hours

Time to peak, serum: Immediate release: 2-3 hours; Extended release: 7 hours (range: 4-8 hours)

Excretion: Urine (90% as unchanged drug; active secretion)

Dosage Type 2 diabetes management: **Note:** Allow 1-2 weeks between dose titrations: Generally, clinically significant responses are not seen at doses <1500 mg daily; however, a lower recommended starting dose and gradual increased dosage is recommended to minimize gastrointestinal symptoms.

Immediate release tablet or solution: Oral:

Children 10-16 years: Initial: 500 mg twice daily; increases in daily dosage should be made in increments of 500 mg at weekly intervals, given in divided doses, up to a maximum of 2000 mg/day

Chidlren ≥17 years and Adults: Initial: 500 mg twice daily **or** 850 mg once daily; increase dosage incrementally.

Incremental dosing recommendations based on dosage form:

500 mg tablet: One tablet/day at weekly intervals

850 mg tablet: One tablet/day every other week

Oral solution: 500 mg twice daily every other week

Doses of up to 2000 mg/day may be given twice daily. If a dose >2000 mg/day is required, it may be better tolerated in three divided doses. Maximum recommended dose 2550 mg/day.

Extended release tablet: Oral: **Note:** If glycemic control is not achieved at maximum dose, may divide dose and administer twice daily.

Children ≥17 years and Adults:

Fortamet®: Initial: 1000 mg once daily; dosage may be increased by 500 mg weekly; maximum dose: 2500 mg once daily

Glucophage® XR: Initial: 500 mg once daily; dosage may be increased by 500 mg weekly; maximum dose: 2000 mg once daily

Adults: Glumetza™: Initial: 1000 mg once daily; dosage may be increased by 500 mg weekly; maximum dose: 2000 mg once daily

Elderly: The initial and maintenance dosing should be conservative, due to the potential for decreased renal function. Generally, elderly patients should not be titrated to the maximum dose of metformin. Do not use in patients ≥80 years of age unless normal renal function has been established.

Transfer from other antidiabetic agents: No transition period is generally necessary except when transferring from chlorpropamide. When transferring from chlorpropamide, care should be exercised during the first 2 weeks because of the prolonged retention of chlorpropamide in the body, leading to overlapping drug effects and possible hypoglycemia.

Concomitant metformin and oral sulfonylurea therapy: If patients have not responded to 4 weeks of the maximum dose of metformin monotherapy, consider a gradual addition of an oral sulfonylurea, even if prior primary or secondary failure to a sulfonylurea has occurred. Continue metformin at the maximum dose. If adequate response has not occurred following 3 months of metformin and sulfonylurea combination therapy, consider switching to insulin with or without metformin.

Failed sulfonylurea therapy: Patients with prior failure on glyburide may be treated by gradual addition of metformin. Initiate with glyburide 20 mg and metformin 500 mg daily. Metformin dosage may be increased by 500 mg/day at weekly intervals, up to a maximum metformin dose (dosage of glyburide maintained at 20 mg/day).

Concomitant metformin and insulin therapy: Initial: 500 mg metformin once daily, continue current insulin dose; increase by 500 mg metformin weekly until adequate glycemic control is achieved

Maximum daily dose: Immediate release and solution: 2550 mg metformin; Extended release: 2000-2500 mg (varies by product)

Decrease insulin dose 10% to 25% when FPG <120 mg/dL; monitor and make further adjustments as needed

Dosing adjustment/comments in renal impairment: The plasma and blood half-life of metformin is prolonged and the renal clearance is decreased in proportion to the decrease in creatinine clearance. Per the manufacturer, metformin is contraindicated in the presence of renal dysfunction defined as a serum creatinine >1.5 mg/dL in males, or >1.4 mg/dL in females and in patients with abnormal clearance. Clinically, it has been recommended that metformin be avoided in patients with Cl_{cr} <60-70 mL/minute (DeFronzo, 1999).

Dosing adjustment in hepatic impairment: Avoid metformin; liver disease is a risk factor for the development of lactic acidosis during metformin therapy.

Dietary Considerations Drug may cause GI upset; take with food (to decrease GI upset). Take at the same time each day. Dietary modification based on ADA recommendations is a part of therapy. Monitor for signs and symptoms of vitamin B_{12} and/or folic acid deficiency; supplementation may be required.

Administration Extended release dosage form should be swallowed whole; do not crush, break, or chew; administer with food (to decrease GI upset). Administer Fortamet® with a glass of water.

Monitoring Parameters Urine for glucose and ketones, fasting blood glucose, and hemoglobin A_{1c}. Initial and periodic monitoring of hematologic parameters (eg, hemoglobin/hematocrit and red blood cell indices) and renal function should be performed, at least annually. Check vitamin B_{12} and folate if anemia is present.

Reference Range Recommendations for glycemic control in adults with diabetes:

Hb A_{1c}: <7%

Preprandial capillary plasma glucose: 70-130 mg/dL

Peak postprandial capillary blood glucose: <180 mg/dL

Blood pressure: <130/80 mm Hg

Dosage Forms Excipient information presented when available (limited, particularly for generics); consult specific product labeling.

Solution, oral, as hydrochloride:

Riomet®: 100 mg/mL (118 mL, 473 mL) [contains saccharin; cherry flavor]

Tablet, as hydrochloride: 500 mg, 850 mg, 1000 mg

Glucophage®: 500 mg, 850 mg, 1000 mg

Tablet, extended release, as hydrochloride: 500 mg, 750 mg

Fortamet®: 500 mg, 1000 mg

Glucophage® XR: 500 mg

Glumetza™: 500 mg, 1000 mg

◆ **Metformin and Glipizide** *see* Glipizide and Metformin *on page 729*

◆ **Metformin and Glyburide** *see* Glyburide and Metformin *on page 733*

◆ **Metformin and Repaglinide** *see* Repaglinide and Metformin *on page 1412*

- **Metformin and Rosiglitazone** *see* Rosiglitazone and Metformin *on page 1449*
- **Metformin and Sitagliptin** *see* Sitagliptin and Metformin *on page 1492*
- **Metformin Hydrochloride** *see* MetFORMIN *on page 997*
- **Metformin Hydrochloride and Pioglitazone Hydrochloride** *see* Pioglitazone and Metformin *on page 1301*
- **Metformin Hydrochloride and Rosiglitazone Maleate** *see* Rosiglitazone and Metformin *on page 1449*

Methadone (METH a done)

Medication Safety Issues

Sound-alike/look-alike issues:

Methadone may be confused with dexmethylphenidate, Mephyton®, methylphenidate, Metadate® CD, and Metadate® ER

High alert medication: The Institute for Safe Medication Practices (ISMP) includes this medication among its list of drug classes which have a heightened risk of causing significant patient harm when used in error.

Related Information

Addiction Treatments *on page 1817*

Narcotic / Opioid Analgesics *on page 1789*

U.S. Brand Names Dolophine®; Methadone Diskets®; Methadone Intensol™; Methadose®

Canadian Brand Names Metadol™

Mexican Brand Names Rubidexol

Index Terms Methadone Hydrochloride

Pharmacologic Category Analgesic, Opioid

Generic Available Yes

Use Management of moderate-to-severe pain; detoxification and maintenance treatment of opioid addiction (if used for detoxification and maintenance treatment of narcotic addiction, it must be part of an FDA-approved program)

Restrictions C-II

When used for treatment of opioid addiction: May only be dispensed in accordance to guidelines established by the Substance Abuse and Mental Health Services Administration's (SAMHSA) Center for Substance Abuse Treatment (CSAT). Regulations regarding methadone use may vary by state and/or country. Obtain advice from appropriate regulatory agencies and/or consult with pain management/palliative care specialists.

Note: Regulatory Exceptions to the General Requirement to Provide Opioid Agonist Treatment (per manufacturer's labeling):

1. During inpatient care, when the patient was admitted for any condition other than concurrent opioid addiction, to facilitate the treatment of the primary admitting diagnosis.
2. During an emergency period of no longer than 3 days while definitive care for the addiction is being sought in an appropriately licensed facility.

Pregnancy Risk Factor C/D (prolonged use or high doses at term)

Pregnancy Considerations Teratogenic effects have been observed in some, but not all, animal studies. Data collected by the Teratogen Information System are complicated by maternal use of illicit drugs, nutrition, infection, and psychosocial circumstances. However, pregnant women in methadone treatment programs are reported to have improved fetal outcomes compared to pregnant women using illicit drugs. Methadone can be detected in the amniotic fluid, cord plasma, and newborn urine. Fetal growth, birth weight, length, and/or head circumference may be decreased in infants born to narcotic-addicted mothers treated with methadone during pregnancy. Growth deficits do not appear to persist; however, decreased performance on psychometric and behavioral tests has been found to continue into childhood. Abnormal fetal nonstress tests have also been reported. Withdrawal symptoms in the neonate may be observed up to 2-4 weeks after delivery. The manufacturer states that methadone should be used during pregnancy only if clearly needed. Because methadone clearance in pregnant women is increased and half-life is decreased during the 2nd and 3rd trimesters of pregnancy, withdrawal symptoms may be observed in the mother; dosage of methadone may need increased or dosing interval decreased during pregnancy.

Lactation Enters breast milk/not recommended (AAP rates "compatible")

Contraindications Hypersensitivity to methadone or any component of the formulation; respiratory depression (in the absence of resuscitative equipment or in an unmonitored setting); acute bronchial asthma or hypercarbia; paralytic ileus; concurrent use of selegiline

Warnings/Precautions An opioid-containing analgesic regimen should be tailored to each patient's needs and based upon the type of pain being treated (acute versus chronic), the route of administration, degree of tolerance for opioids (naive versus chronic user), age, weight, and medical condition. The optimal analgesic dose varies widely among patients. Doses should be titrated to pain relief/prevention. Patients maintained on stable doses of methadone may need higher and/or more frequent doses in case of acute pain (eg, postoperative pain, physical trauma). Methadone is ineffective for the relief of anxiety.

[U.S. Boxed Warning]: May prolong the QT_c interval and increase risk for torsade de pointes. Patients should be informed of the potential arrhythmia risk, evaluated for any history of structural heart disease, arrhythmia, syncope, and for existence of potential drug interactions including drugs that possess QT_c interval-prolonging properties, promote hypokalemia, hypomagnesemia, or hypocalcemia, or reduce elimination of methadone (eg, CYP3A4 inhibitors). Obtain baseline ECG for all patients and risk stratify according to QT_c interval (see Monitoring Parameters). Use with caution in patients at risk for QT_c prolongation, with medications known to prolong the QT_c interval, promote electrolyte depletion, or inhibit CYP3A4, or history of conduction abnormalities. QT_c interval prolongation and torsade de pointes may be associated with doses >100 mg/day, but have also been observed with lower doses. May cause severe hypotension; use caution with severe volume depletion or other conditions which may compromise maintenance of normal blood pressure. Use caution with cardiovascular disease or patients predisposed to dysrhythmias.

[U.S. Boxed Warning]: May cause respiratory depression. Use caution in patients with respiratory disease or pre-existing respiratory conditions (eg, severe obesity, asthma, COPD, sleep apnea, CNS depression). Because the respiratory effects last longer than the analgesic effects, slow titration is required. Use extreme caution during treatment initiation, dose titration and conversion from other opioid agonists. Incomplete cross tolerance may occur; patients tolerant to other mu opioid agonists may not be tolerant to methadone. Abrupt cessation may precipitate withdrawal symptoms.

May cause CNS depression, which may impair physical or mental abilities. Patients must be cautioned about performing tasks which require mental alertness (eg, operating machinery or driving). Effects with other sedative drugs or ethanol may be potentiated. Use with caution in patients with depression or suicidal tendencies, or in patients with a history of drug abuse. Tolerance or psychological and physical dependence may occur with prolonged use.

Use with caution in patients with head injury or increased intracranial pressure. May obscure diagnosis or clinical course of patients with acute abdominal conditions. Elderly may be more susceptible to adverse effects (eg, CNS, respiratory, gastrointestinal). Decrease initial dose and use caution in the elderly or debilitated; with hyper/hypothyroidism, morbid obesity, adrenal insufficiency, prostatic hyperplasia, or urethral stricture; or with severe renal or hepatic failure. Use with caution in patients with biliary tract dysfunction; acute pancreatitis may cause constriction of sphincter of Oddi. Safety and efficacy have not been established in children. **[U.S. Boxed Warning]: For oral administration only;** excipients to deter use by injection are contained in tablets.

[U.S. Boxed Warning]: When used for treatment of narcotic addiction: May only be dispensed by opioid treatment programs certified by the Substance Abuse and Mental Health Services Administration (SAMHSA) and certified by the designated state authority. Exceptions include inpatient treatment of other conditions and emergency period (not >3 days) while definitive substance abuse treatment is being sought.

Adverse Reactions Frequency not defined. During prolonged administration, adverse effects may decrease over several weeks; however, constipation and sweating may persist.

Cardiovascular: Arrhythmia, bigeminal rhythms, bradycardia, cardiac arrest, cardiomyopathy, ECG changes, edema, extrasystoles, faintness, flushing, heart failure, hypotension, palpitation,peripheral vasodilation, phlebitis, orthostatic hypotension, QT interval prolonged, shock, syncope, tachycardia, torsade de pointes, T-wave inversion, ventricular fibrillation, ventricular tachycardia,

Central nervous system: Agitation, confusion, disorientation, dizziness, drowsiness, dysphoria, euphoria, hallucination, headache, insomnia, lightheadedness, sedation, seizure

Dermatologic: Hemorrhagic urticaria, pruritus, rash, urticaria

Endocrine & metabolic: Antidiuretic effect, amenorrhea, hypokalemia, hypomagnesemia, libido decreased

Gastrointestinal: Abdominal pain, anorexia, biliary tract spasm, constipation, glossitis, nausea, stomach cramps, vomiting, weight gain, xerostomia

Genitourinary: Impotence, urinary retention or hesitancy

Hematologic: Thrombocytopenia (reversible, reported in patients with chronic hepatitis)

Neuromuscular & skeletal: Weakness

Local: I.M./SubQ injection: Erythema, pain, swelling; I.V. injection: Hemorrhagic urticaria (rare), pruritus, urticaria, rash

Ocular: Miosis, visual disturbances

Respiratory: Pulmonary edema, respiratory depression, respiratory arrest

Miscellaneous: Death, diaphoresis, physical and psychological dependence

Metabolism/Transport Effects Substrate of CYP2C9 (minor), 2C19 (minor), 2D6 (minor), 3A4 (major); **Inhibits** CYP2D6 (moderate), 3A4 (weak)

Drug Interactions

Alcohol (Ethyl): CNS Depressants may enhance the CNS depressant effect of Alcohol (Ethyl). *Risk C: Monitor therapy*

Alfuzosin: May enhance the QTc-prolonging effect of QTc-Prolonging Agents. *Risk C: Monitor therapy*

Alvimopan: Analgesics (Opioid) may enhance the adverse/toxic effect of Alvimopan. This is most notable for patients receiving long-term (i.e., more than 7 days) opiates prior to alvimopan initiation. Management: Alvimopan is contraindicated in patients receiving therapeutic doses of opioids for more than 7 consecutive days immediately prior to alvimopan initiation. *Risk D: Consider therapy modification*

Ammonium Chloride: May increase the excretion of Analgesics (Opioid). *Risk C: Monitor therapy*

Amphetamines: May enhance the analgesic effect of Analgesics (Opioid). *Risk C: Monitor therapy*

Antifungal Agents (Azole Derivatives, Systemic): May increase the serum concentration of Methadone. *Risk C: Monitor therapy*

Antipsychotic Agents (Phenothiazines): May enhance the hypotensive effect of Analgesics (Opioid). *Risk C: Monitor therapy*

Barbiturates: May increase the metabolism of Methadone. *Risk D: Consider therapy modification*

CarBAMazepine: May increase the metabolism of Methadone. *Risk D: Consider therapy modification*

Ciprofloxacin: May enhance the QTc-prolonging effect of QTc-Prolonging Agents. *Risk C: Monitor therapy*

CNS Depressants: May enhance the adverse/toxic effect of other CNS Depressants. *Risk C: Monitor therapy*

Codeine: CYP2D6 Inhibitors (Moderate) may diminish the therapeutic effect of Codeine. These CYP2D6 inhibitors may prevent the metabolic conversion of codeine to its active metabolite morphine. *Risk C: Monitor therapy*

CYP2D6 Substrates: CYP2D6 Inhibitors (Moderate) may decrease the metabolism of CYP2D6 Substrates. **Exceptions:** Tamoxifen. *Risk C: Monitor therapy*

CYP3A4 Inducers (Strong): May increase the metabolism of CYP3A4 Substrates. *Risk C: Monitor therapy*

CYP3A4 Inhibitors (Moderate): May decrease the metabolism of CYP3A4 Substrates. *Risk C: Monitor therapy*

CYP3A4 Inhibitors (Strong): May decrease the metabolism of CYP3A4 Substrates. *Risk D: Consider therapy modification*

Dasatinib: May increase the serum concentration of CYP3A4 Substrates. *Risk C: Monitor therapy*

Deferasirox: May decrease the serum concentration of CYP3A4 Substrates. *Risk C: Monitor therapy*

Desmopressin: Analgesics (Opioid) may enhance the adverse/toxic effect of Desmopressin. *Risk C: Monitor therapy*

Didanosine: Methadone may decrease the serum concentration of Didanosine. *Risk C: Monitor therapy*

Etravirine: May decrease the serum concentration of Methadone. *Risk C: Monitor therapy*

Gadobutrol: May enhance the QTc-prolonging effect of QTc-Prolonging Agents. *Risk D: Consider therapy modification*

Herbs (CYP3A4 Inducers): May increase the metabolism of CYP3A4 Substrates. *Risk C: Monitor therapy*

Nebivolol: CYP2D6 Inhibitors (Moderate) may increase the serum concentration of Nebivolol. *Risk C: Monitor therapy*

Nilotinib: May enhance the QTc-prolonging effect of QTc-Prolonging Agents. *Risk X: Avoid combination*

Pegvisomant: Analgesics (Opioid) may diminish the therapeutic effect of Pegvisomant. *Risk C: Monitor therapy*

Phenytoin: May increase the metabolism of Methadone. *Risk C: Monitor therapy*

Protease Inhibitors: May decrease the metabolism of Methadone. **Exceptions:** Atazanavir; Indinavir. *Risk C: Monitor therapy*

QTc-Prolonging Agents: May enhance the adverse/toxic effect of other QTc-Prolonging Agents. Their effects can be additive, causing life-threatening ventricular arrhythmias. *Risk D: Consider therapy modification*

Reverse Transcriptase Inhibitors (Non-Nucleoside): May increase the metabolism of Methadone. **Exceptions:** Delavirdine; Etravirine. *Risk D: Consider therapy modification*

Rifamycin Derivatives: May increase the metabolism of Methadone. **Exceptions:** Rifabutin. *Risk C: Monitor therapy*

Selective Serotonin Reuptake Inhibitors: May decrease the metabolism of Methadone. Fluvoxamine appears to be the only interacting SSRI. *Risk D: Consider therapy modification*

Selective Serotonin Reuptake Inhibitors: Analgesics (Opioid) may enhance the serotonergic effect of Selective Serotonin Reuptake Inhibitors. This may cause serotonin syndrome. *Risk C: Monitor therapy*

Succinylcholine: May enhance the bradycardic effect of Analgesics (Opioid). *Risk C: Monitor therapy*

Tamoxifen: CYP2D6 Inhibitors (Moderate) may decrease the metabolism of Tamoxifen. Specifically, CYP2D6 inhibitors may decrease the formation of highly potent active metabolites. *Risk D: Consider therapy modification*

Tetrabenazine: QTc-Prolonging Agents may enhance the QTc-prolonging effect of Tetrabenazine. *Risk X: Avoid combination*

TraMADol: CYP2D6 Inhibitors (Moderate) may diminish the therapeutic effect of TraMADol. These CYP2D6 inhibitors may prevent the metabolic conversion of tramadol to its active metabolite that accounts for much of its opioid-like effects. *Risk C: Monitor therapy*

Zidovudine: Methadone may increase the serum concentration of Zidovudine. *Risk C: Monitor therapy*

Ziprasidone: QTc-Prolonging Agents may enhance the QTc-prolonging effect of Ziprasidone. The risk of a severe arrhythmia may be increased. *Risk X: Avoid combination*

Ethanol/Nutrition/Herb Interactions

Ethanol: Avoid ethanol (may increase CNS effects). Watch for sedation.

Herb/Nutraceutical: Avoid St John's wort (may decrease methadone levels; may increase CNS depression). Avoid valerian, kava kava, gotu kola (may increase CNS depression). Methadone is metabolized by CYP3A4 in the intestines; avoid concurrent use of grapefruit juice.

Stability

Injection: Store at controlled room temperature of 15°C to 30°C (59°F to 86°F). Protect from light.

Oral concentrate, oral solution, tablet: Store at controlled room temperature of 15°C to 30°C (59°F to 86°F).

Mechanism of Action Binds to opiate receptors in the CNS, causing inhibition of ascending pain pathways, altering the perception of and response to pain; produces generalized CNS depression

Pharmacodynamics/Kinetics

Onset of action: Oral: Analgesic: 0.5-1 hour; Parenteral: 10-20 minutes

Peak effect: Parenteral: 1-2 hours; Oral: continuous dosing: 3-5 days

Duration of analgesia: Oral: 4-8 hours, increases to 22-48 hours with repeated doses

Distribution: V_{dss}: 1-8 L/kg

Protein binding: 85% to 90%

Metabolism: Hepatic; N-demethylation primarily via CYP3A4, CYP2B6, and CYP2C19 to inactive metabolites

Bioavailability: Oral: 36% to 100%

Half-life elimination: 8-59 hours; may be prolonged with alkaline pH, decreased during pregnancy

Time to peak, plasma: 1-7.5 hours

Excretion: Urine (<10% as unchanged drug); increased with urine pH <6

Dosage Regulations regarding methadone use may vary by state and/or country. Obtain advice from appropriate regulatory agencies and/or consult with pain management/palliative care specialists. **Note:** These are guidelines and do not represent the maximum doses that may be required in all patients. Methadone accumulates with repeated doses and dosage may need reduction after 3-5 days to prevent CNS depressant effects. Some patients may benefit from every 8-12 hour dosing interval for chronic pain management. Doses should be titrated to appropriate effects.

Children (unlabeled use):

Pain (analgesia):

Oral: Initial: 0.1-0.2 mg/kg 4-8 hours initially for 2-3 doses, then every 6-12 hours as needed. Dosing interval may range from 4-12 hours during initial therapy; decrease in dose or frequency may be required (~ days 2-5) due to accumulation with repeated doses (maximum dose: 5-10 mg)

I.V.: 0.1 mg/kg every 4-8 hours initially for 2-3 doses, then every 6-12 hours as needed. Dosing interval may range from 4-12 hours during initial therapy; decrease in dose or frequency may be required (~ days 2-5) due to accumulation with repeated doses (maximum dose: 5-8 mg)

Iatrogenic narcotic dependency: Oral: General guidelines: Initial: 0.05-0.1 mg/kg/dose every 6 hours; increase by 0.05 mg/kg/dose until withdrawal symptoms are controlled; after 24-48 hours, the dosing interval can be lengthened to every 12-24 hours; to taper dose, wean by 0.05 mg/kg/day; if withdrawal symptoms recur, taper at a slower rate

Adults:

Acute pain (moderate-to-severe):

Oral: Opioid-naive: Initial: 2.5-10 mg every 8-12 hours; more frequent administration may be required during initiation to maintain adequate analgesia. Dosage interval may range from 4-12 hours, since duration of analgesia is relatively short during the first days of therapy, but increases substantially with continued administration.

Chronic pain (opioid-tolerant): **Conversion from oral morphine to oral methadone:**

Daily oral morphine dose <100 mg: Estimated daily oral methadone dose: 20% to 30% of total daily morphine dose

Daily oral morphine dose 100-300 mg: Estimated daily oral methadone dose: 10% to 20% of total daily morphine dose

Daily oral morphine dose 300-600 mg: Estimated daily oral methadone dose: 8% to 12% of total daily morphine dose

Daily oral morphine dose 600-1000 mg: Estimated daily oral methadone dose: 5% to 10% of total daily morphine dose.

Daily oral morphine dose >1000 mg: Estimated daily oral methadone dose: <5% of total daily morphine dose.

Note: The total daily methadone dose should then be divided to reflect the intended dosing schedule.

I.V.: Manufacturers labeling: Initial: 2.5-10 mg every 8-12 hours in opioid-naive patients; titrate slowly to effect; may also be administered by SubQ or I.M. injection

Conversion from oral methadone to parenteral methadone dose: Initial dose: Parenteral:Oral ratio: 1:2 (eg, 5 mg parenteral methadone equals 10 mg oral methadone)

Detoxification: Oral:

Initial: A single dose of 20-30 mg is generally sufficient to suppress symptoms. Should not exceed 30 mg; lower doses should be considered in patients with low tolerance at initiation (eg, absence of opioids ≥5 days); an additional 5-10 mg of methadone may be provided if withdrawal symptoms have not been suppressed or if symptoms reappear after 2-4 hours; total daily dose on the first day should not exceed 40 mg, unless the program physician documents in the patient's record that 40 mg did not control opiate abstinence symptoms.

Maintenance: Titrate to a dosage which attenuates craving, blocks euphoric effects of other opiates, and tolerance to sedative effect of methadone. Usual range: 80-120 mg/day (titration should occur cautiously)

Withdrawal: Dose reductions should be <10% of the maintenance dose, every 10-14 days

Detoxification (short-term): Oral:

Initial: Titrate to ~40 mg/day in divided doses to achieve stabilization, may continue 40 mg dose for 2-3 days

Maintenance: Titrate to a dosage which prevents/attenuates euphoric effects of self-administered opioids, reduces drug craving, and withdrawal symptoms are prevented for 24 hours.

Withdrawal: Requires individualization. Decrease daily or every other day, keeping withdrawal symptoms tolerable; hospitalized patients may tolerate a 20% reduction/day; ambulatory patients may require a slower reduction

Dosage adjustment during pregnancy: Methadone dose may need to be increased, or the dosing interval decreased; see Pregnancy Considerations - use should be reserved for cases where the benefits clearly outweigh the risks

Dosage adjustment for toxicity:

QT_c >450-499 msecs: Monitor QT_c more frequently

QT_c ≥500 msecs: Consider discontinuation or reducing methadone dose

Dosage adjustment in renal impairment: Cl_{cr} <10 mL/minute: Administer 50% to 75% of normal dose

Dosage adjustment in hepatic impairment: Avoid in severe liver disease

Administration Oral dose for detoxification and maintenance may be administered in fruit juice or water. Dispersible tablet should not be chewed or swallowed; add to liquid and allow to dissolve before administering. May rinse if residual remains.

Monitoring Parameters Obtain baseline ECG (evaluate QT_c interval), within 30 days of initiation, and then annually for all patients receiving methadone. Increase ECG monitoring if patient receiving >100 mg/day or if unexplained syncope or seizure occurs while on methadone (Krantz, 2008).

If before or at anytime during therapy:

QT_c >450-499 msecs: Discuss potential risks and benefits; monitor QT_c more frequently

QT_c ≥500 msecs: Consider discontinuation or reducing methadone dose **or** eliminate factors promoting QT_c prolongation (eg, potassium-wasting drugs) **or** use alternative therapy (eg, buprenorphine)

Pain relief, respiratory and mental status, blood pressure

Reference Range Prevention of opiate withdrawal: Therapeutic: 100-400 ng/mL (SI: 0.32-1.29 µmol/L); Toxic: >2 mcg/mL (SI: >6.46 µmol/L)

Test Interactions Some quinolones may produce a false-positive urine screening result for opiates using commercially-available immunoassay kits. This has been demonstrated most consistently for levofloxacin and ofloxacin, but other quinolones have shown cross-reactivity in certain assay kits. Confirmation of positive opiate screens by more specific methods should be considered.

Dosage Forms Excipient information presented when available (limited, particularly for generics); consult specific product labeling.

Injection, solution, as hydrochloride: 10 mg/mL (20 mL)

Solution, oral, as hydrochloride: 5 mg/5 mL (500 mL); 10 mg/5 mL (500 mL) [contains alcohol 8%; citrus flavor]

Solution, oral, as hydrochloride [concentrate]: 10 mg/mL (946 mL)
- Methadone Intensol™: 10 mg/mL (30 mL)
- Methadose®: 10 mg/mL (1000 mL) [cherry flavor]
- Methadose®: 10 mg/mL (1000 mL) [dye free, sugar free, unflavored]

Tablet, as hydrochloride: 5 mg, 10 mg
- Dolophine®: 5 mg, 10 mg
- Methadose®: 5 mg, 10 mg [DSC]

Tablet, dispersible, as hydrochloride: 40 mg
- Methadose®: 40 mg
- Methadone Diskets®: 40 mg [orange-pineapple flavor]

◆ **Methadone Diskets®** *see* Methadone *on page 1001*

◆ **Methadone Hydrochloride** *see* Methadone *on page 1001*

◆ **Methadone Intensol™** *see* Methadone *on page 1001*

◆ **Methadose®** *see* Methadone *on page 1001*

◆ **Methaminodiazepoxide Hydrochloride** *see* ChlordiazePOXIDE *on page 316*

Methamphetamine (meth am FET a meen)

Medication Safety Issues

Sound-alike/look-alike issues:

Desoxyn® may be confused with digoxin

Related Information

Stimulant Agents Used for ADHD *on page 1797*

U.S. Brand Names Desoxyn®

Canadian Brand Names Desoxyn®

Index Terms Desoxyephedrine Hydrochloride; Methamphetamine Hydrochloride

Pharmacologic Category Anorexiant; Stimulant; Sympathomimetic

Generic Available Yes

Use Treatment of attention-deficit/hyperactivity disorder (ADHD); exogenous obesity (short-term adjunct)

Unlabeled/Investigational Use Narcolepsy

Restrictions C-II

An FDA-approved medication guide must be distributed when dispensing an outpatient prescription (new or refill) where this medication is to be used without direct supervision of a healthcare provider. Medication guides are available at http://www.fda.gov/cder/drug/infopage/ADHD/default.htm.

Pharmacotherapy for weight loss is recommended only for obese patients with a body mass index ≥30 kg/m^2, or ≥27 kg/m^2 in the presence of other risk factors such as hypertension, diabetes, and/or dyslipidemia or a high waist circumference; therapy should be used in conjunction with a comprehensive weight management program. Rule out organic causes of obesity (eg, untreated hypothyroidism) prior to use.

Note: Methamphetamine is not approved for long-term use. The limited usefulness of medications in this class should be weighed against possible risks associated with their use. Consult weight loss guidelines for current pharmacotherapy recommendations.

Pregnancy Risk Factor C

Pregnancy Considerations Teratogenic and embryocidal effects have been observed in animal studies. Infants may deliver prematurely and suffer withdrawal symptoms. There are no adequate and well-controlled studies in pregnant women.

Lactation Enters breast milk/contraindicated

Contraindications Hypersensitivity to methamphetamine, any component of the formulation, or idiosyncrasy to amphetamines or other sympathomimetic amines; patients with advanced arteriosclerosis, symptomatic cardiovascular disease, moderate-to-severe hypertension, hyperthyroidism, glaucoma, agitated states; patients with a history of drug abuse; use during or within 14 days following MAO inhibitor therapy; stimulant medications are contraindicated for use in children with attention-deficit/hyperactivity disorders and concomitant Tourette's syndrome or tics

Warnings/Precautions Use has been associated with serious cardiovascular events including sudden death in patients with pre-existing structural cardiac abnormalities or other serious heart problems (sudden death in children and adolescents; sudden death, stroke and MI in adults). These products should be avoided in the patients with known serious structural cardiac abnormalities, cardiomyopathy, serious heart rhythm abnormalities, or other serious cardiac problems that could increase the risk of sudden death that these conditions alone carry. Patients should be carefully evaluated for cardiac disease prior to initiation of therapy. Use with caution in patients with hypertension and other cardiovascular conditions that might be exacerbated by increases in blood pressure or heart rate. Use is contraindicated in patients with moderate to severe hypertension. Amphetamines may impair the ability to engage in potentially hazardous activities. Difficulty in accommodation and blurred vision has been reported with the use of stimulants.

Use with caution in patients with psychiatric disorders, diabetes, or seizure disorders,. May exacerbate symptoms of behavior and thought disorder in psychotic patients. Stimulants may unmask tics in individuals with coexisting Tourette's syndrome **[U.S. Boxed Warning]: Potential for drug dependency exists; prolonged use may lead to drug dependency.** Use is contraindicated in patients with history of ethanol or drug abuse. Prescriptions should be written for the smallest quantity consistent with good patient care to minimize possibility of overdose. **[U.S. Boxed Warning]: Use in weight reduction programs only when alternative therapy has been ineffective.** Abrupt discontinuation following high doses or for prolonged periods may result in symptoms for withdrawal. Discontinue if satisfactory weight loss has not occurred within the first 4 weeks of treatment, or if tolerance develops. Safety and efficacy have not been established in children <12 years of age for obesity. Use of stimulants has been associated with suppression of growth; monitor growth rate during treatment.

Adverse Reactions Frequency not defined.

Cardiovascular: Hypertension, tachycardia, palpitation

Central nervous system: Restlessness, headache, exacerbation of motor and phonic tics and Tourette's syndrome, dizziness, psychosis, dysphoria, overstimulation, euphoria, insomnia

Dermatologic: Rash, urticaria

Endocrine & metabolic: Change in libido

Gastrointestinal: Diarrhea, nausea, vomiting, stomach cramps, constipation, anorexia, weight loss, xerostomia, unpleasant taste

Genitourinary: Impotence

Neuromuscular & skeletal: Tremor

Miscellaneous: Suppression of growth in children, tolerance and withdrawal with prolonged use

Metabolism/Transport Effects Substrate of CYP2D6 (major)

Drug Interactions

Alkalinizing Agents: May decrease the excretion of Amphetamines. *Risk D: Consider therapy modification*

Ammonium Chloride: May decrease the serum concentration of Amphetamines. This effect is likely due to an enhanced excretion of amphetamines in the urine. *Risk C: Monitor therapy*

Analgesics (Opioid): Amphetamines may enhance the analgesic effect of Analgesics (Opioid). *Risk C: Monitor therapy*

Antacids: May decrease the excretion of Amphetamines. *Risk C: Monitor therapy*

Antihistamines: Amphetamines may diminish the sedative effect of Antihistamines. *Risk C: Monitor therapy*

Antipsychotics: May diminish the stimulatory effect of Amphetamines. *Risk C: Monitor therapy*

Cannabinoids: May enhance the tachycardic effect of Sympathomimetics. *Risk C: Monitor therapy*

Carbonic Anhydrase Inhibitors: May decrease the excretion of Amphetamines. **Exceptions:** Brinzolamide; Dorzolamide. *Risk C: Monitor therapy*

CYP2D6 Inhibitors (Moderate): May decrease the metabolism of CYP2D6 Substrates. *Risk C: Monitor therapy*

CYP2D6 Inhibitors (Strong): May decrease the metabolism of CYP2D6 Substrates. *Risk D: Consider therapy modification*

Darunavir: May increase the serum concentration of CYP2D6 Substrates. *Risk C: Monitor therapy*

Ethosuximide: Amphetamines may diminish the therapeutic effect of Ethosuximide. Amphetamines may decrease the serum concentration of Ethosuximide. *Risk C: Monitor therapy*

Gastrointestinal Acidifying Agents: May decrease the serum concentration of Amphetamines. *Risk C: Monitor therapy*

Lithium: May diminish the stimulatory effect of Amphetamines. *Risk C: Monitor therapy*

MAO Inhibitors: May enhance the hypertensive effect of Amphetamines. *Risk X: Avoid combination*

Methenamine: May decrease the serum concentration of Amphetamines. This effect is likely due to an enhanced excretion of amphetamines in the urine. *Risk C: Monitor therapy*

PHENobarbital: Amphetamines may decrease the serum concentration of PHENobarbital. *Risk C: Monitor therapy*

Phenytoin: Amphetamines may decrease the serum concentration of Phenytoin. *Risk C: Monitor therapy*

Sympathomimetics: May enhance the adverse/toxic effect of other Sympathomimetics. *Risk C: Monitor therapy*

Tricyclic Antidepressants: May enhance the stimulatory effect of Amphetamines. Tricyclic Antidepressants may also potentiate the cardiovascular effects of Amphetamines. *Risk C: Monitor therapy*

Ethanol/Nutrition/Herb Interactions

Ethanol: Avoid ethanol (may cause CNS depression).

Food: Amphetamine serum levels may be altered if taken with acidic food, juices, or vitamin C. Avoid caffeine.

Herb/Nutraceutical: Avoid ephedra (may cause hypertension or arrhythmias).

Stability Store below 30°C (86°F). Protect from light.

Mechanism of Action A sympathomimetic amine related to ephedrine and amphetamine with CNS stimulant activity; peripheral actions include elevation of systolic and diastolic blood pressure and weak bronchodilator and respiratory stimulant action

Pharmacodynamics/Kinetics

Absorption: Rapid from GI tract

Metabolism: Hepatic; forms metabolite

Half-life elimination: 4-5 hours

Excretion: Urine primarily (dependent on urine pH)

Dosage Oral:

Children ≥6 years and Adults: ADHD: 5 mg 1-2 times/day; may increase by 5 mg increments at weekly intervals until optimum response is achieved, usually 20-25 mg/day

Children ≥12 years and Adults: Exogenous obesity: 5 mg 30 minutes before each meal; treatment duration should not exceed a few weeks

Dietary Considerations Most effective when combined with a low calorie diet and behavior modification counseling.

Monitoring Parameters Heart rate, respiratory rate, blood pressure, CNS activity, body weight (BMI); growth rate in children

When used for the treatment of ADHD, thoroughly evaluate for cardiovascular risk. Monitor heart rate, blood pressure, and consider obtaining ECG prior to initiation (Vetter, 2008).

Reference Range

Adult classification of weight by BMI (kg/m^2):

Underweight: <18.5
Normal: 18.5-24.9
Overweight: 25-29.9
Obese, class I: 30-34.9
Obese, class II: 35-39.9
Extreme obesity (class III): ≥40

Waist circumference: In adults with a BMI of 25-34.9 kg/m^2, high-risk waist circumference is defined as:

Men >102 cm (>40 in)
Women >88 cm (>35 in)

Additional Information Illicit methamphetamine may contain lead; alkalinizing urine can result in longer methamphetamine half-life and elevated blood level; ephedrine is a precursor in the illicit manufacture of methamphetamine; ephedrine is extracted by dissolving ephedrine tablets in water or alcohol (50,000 tablets can result in 1 kg of ephedrine); conversion to methamphetamine occurs at a rate of 50% to 70% of the weight of ephedrine. 3,4-methylene dioxymethamphetamine (slang: XTC, Ecstasy, Adam) affects the serotonergic, dopaminergic, and noradrenergic pathways. As such, it can cause the serotonin syndrome associated with malignant hyperthermia and rhabdomyolysis.

Dosage Forms Excipient information presented when available (limited, particularly for generics); consult specific product labeling.

Tablet, as hydrochloride: 5 mg

◆ **Methamphetamine Hydrochloride** *see* Methamphetamine *on page 1006*

Methazolamide (meth a ZOE la mide)

Medication Safety Issues

Sound-alike/look-alike issues:

Methazolamide may be confused with methenamine, metolazone
Neptazane® may be confused with Nesacaine®

Canadian Brand Names Apo-Methazolamide®

Pharmacologic Category Carbonic Anhydrase Inhibitor; Diuretic, Carbonic Anhydrase Inhibitor; Ophthalmic Agent, Antiglaucoma

Use Adjunctive treatment of open-angle or secondary glaucoma; short-term therapy of narrow-angle glaucoma when delay of surgery is desired

Effect on Mental Status Sedation is common; may cause dizziness or depression

Effect on Psychiatric Treatment May rarely cause bone marrow suppression; use caution with clozapine and carbamazepine; may increase lithium excretion but overall effect is minimal; if lithium toxicity is severe, hemodialysis is the treatment of choice

Dosage Summary

Oral:

Children: Dosage not established
Adults: 50-100 mg 2-3 times/day

Dosage Forms Excipient information presented when available (limited, particularly for generics); consult specific product labeling.

Tablet: 25 mg, 50 mg

Methenamine, Phenyl Salicylate, Methylene Blue, Benzoic Acid, and Hyoscyamine

(meth EN a meen, fen nil sa LIS i late, METH i leen bloo, ben ZOE ik AS id & hye oh SYE a meen)

U.S. Brand Names Prosed®/DS

Index Terms Benzoic Acid, Methenamine, Methylene Blue, Phenyl Salicylate, and Hyoscyamine; Hyoscyamine, Methenamine, Benzoic Acid, Phenyl Salicylate, and Methylene Blue; Methylene Blue, Methenamine, Benzoic Acid, Phenyl Salicylate, and Hyoscyamine; Phenyl Salicylate, Methenamine, Methylene Blue, Benzoic Acid, and Hyoscyamine

Pharmacologic Category Antibiotic, Miscellaneous

Use Urinary tract discomfort secondary to hypermotility resulting from infection or diagnostic procedures

Effect on Mental Status May cause dizziness

Effect on Psychiatric Treatment May cause anticholinergic side effects; concomitant use with psychotropic agents may produce additive effects

Dosage Summary

Oral:

Children ≤12 years: Dosage not established

Children >12 years: Must be individualized

Adults: One tablet 4 times/day

Dosage Forms Excipient information presented when available (limited, particularly for generics); consult specific product labeling.

Tablet, oral:

Prosed®/DS: Methenamine 81.6 mg, phenyl salicylate 36.2 mg, methylene blue 10.8 mg, benzoic acid 9 mg, hyoscyamine sulfate 0.12 mg

Methenamine, Sodium Biphosphate, Phenyl Salicylate, Methylene Blue, and Hyoscyamine

(meth EN a meen, SOW dee um bye FOS fate, fen nil sa LIS i late, METH i leen bloo, & hye oh SYE a meen)

U.S. Brand Names Urelle®; Urimar-T; Uta®; Utira™-C

Index Terms Hyoscyamine, Methenamine, Sodium Biphosphate, Phenyl Salicylate, and Methylene Blue; Methylene Blue, Methenamine, Sodium Biphosphate, Phenyl Salicylate, and Hyoscyamine; Phenyl Salicylate, Methenamine, Methylene Blue, Sodium Biphosphate, and Hyoscyamine; Sodium Biphosphate, Methenamine, Methylene Blue, Phenyl Salicylate, and Hyoscyamine

Pharmacologic Category Antibiotic, Miscellaneous

Use Treatment of symptoms of irritative voiding; relief of local symptoms associated with urinary tract infections; relief of urinary tract symptoms caused by diagnostic procedures

Effect on Mental Status May cause dizziness

Effect on Psychiatric Treatment May cause anticholinergic side effects which may be additive with psychotropics

Dosage Summary

Oral:

Children ≤6 years: Dosage not established

Children >6 years: Must be individualized

Adults: One tablet 4 times/day

Dosage Forms Excipient information presented when available (limited, particularly for generics); consult specific product labeling.

Capsule, oral:

Uta®: Methenamine 120 mg, sodium biphosphate 40.8 mg, phenyl salicylate 36 mg, methylene blue 10 mg, hyoscyamine sulfate 0.12 mg

Tablet, oral:

Urelle®: Methenamine 81 mg, sodium biphosphate 40.8 mg, phenyl salicylate 32.4 mg, methylene blue 10.8 mg, hyoscyamine sulfate 0.12 mg

Urimar-T: Methenamine 81.6 mg, sodium biphosphate 40.8 mg, phenyl salicylate 36.2 mg, methylene blue 10.8 mg, hyoscyamine sulfate 0.12 mg

Utira™-C: Methenamine 81.6 mg, sodium biphosphate 40.8 mg, phenyl salicylate 36.2 mg, methylene blue 10.8 mg, hyoscyamine sulfate 0.12 mg

◆ **Methergine®** *see* Methylergonovine *on page 1022*

Methimazole (meth IM a zole)

Medication Safety Issues

Sound-alike/look-alike issues:

Methimazole may be confused with metolazone

U.S. Brand Names Northyx™; Tapazole®

Canadian Brand Names Dom-Methimazole; PHL-Methimazole; Tapazole®

Index Terms Thiamazole

Pharmacologic Category Antithyroid Agent; Thioamide

Use Palliative treatment of hyperthyroidism, return the hyperthyroid patient to a normal metabolic state prior to thyroidectomy, and to control thyrotoxic crisis that may accompany thyroidectomy

Effect on Mental Status May cause dizziness or drowsiness

Effect on Psychiatric Treatment Leukopenia is common; use caution with clozapine and carbamazepine; concurrent use with lithium may increase the effects on the thyroid

Dosage Summary

Oral:

Children: Initial: 0.4-0.7 mg/kg/day **or** 15-20 mg/m²/day in 3 divided doses (approximately every 8 hours); Maintenance: 0.2 mg/kg/day **or** 1/3 to 2/3 of the initial dose in 3 divided doses, approximately every 8 hours (maximum: 30 mg/day)

Adults: Initial: 15-60 mg/day in 3 divided doses (approximately every 8 hours); Maintenance: 5-15 mg/day in 1-3 divided doses (approximately every 8 hours)

Dosage Forms Excipient information presented when available (limited, particularly for generics); consult specific product labeling.

Tablet: 5 mg, 10 mg, 20 mg

Northyx™: 5 mg, 10 mg, 15 mg, 20 mg

Tapazole®: 5 mg, 10 mg

◆ **Methitest™** *see* MethylTESTOSTERone *on page 1030*

Methocarbamol (meth oh KAR ba mole)

Medication Safety Issues

Sound-alike/look-alike issues:

Methocarbamol may be confused with mephobarbital

Robaxin® may be confused with ribavirin, Rubex®

U.S. Brand Names Robaxin®

Canadian Brand Names Robaxin®

Mexican Brand Names Rexivin

Pharmacologic Category Skeletal Muscle Relaxant

Use Treatment of muscle spasm associated with acute painful musculoskeletal conditions; supportive therapy in tetanus

Effect on Mental Status Drowsiness and dizziness are common

Effect on Psychiatric Treatment May rarely cause leukopenia; use caution with clozapine and carbamazepine; concurrent use with psychotropics may produce additive sedation

Dosage Summary

I.M.:

Children <16 years: Dosage not established

Children ≥16 years: 1 g every 8 hours (maximum therapy: 3 consecutive days)

Adults: 1 g every 8 hours (maximum therapy: 3 consecutive days)

I.V.:

Children <16 years (recommended only for tetanus): 15 mg/kg/dose **or** 500 mg/m²/dose every 6 hours if needed (maximum: 1.8 g/m²/day for 3 days)

Children ≥16 years: 15 mg/kg/dose **or** 500 mg/m²/dose every 6 hours if needed (maximum: 1.8 g/m²/day for 3 days) **or** 1 g every 8 hours (maximum therapy: 3 consecutive days)

Adults: 1-3 g every 6 hours **or** 1 g every 8 hours (maximum therapy: 3 consecutive days)

Oral:

Children <16 years: Dosage not established

Children ≥16 years: Initial: 1.5 g 4 times/day for 2-3 days (maximum: 8 g/day); Maintenance: 4-4.5 g/day in 3-6 divided doses

Adults: Initial: 1.5 g 4 times/day for 2-3 days (maximum: 8 g/day); Maintenance: 4-4.5 g/day in 3-6 divided doses

Elderly: Initial: 500 mg 4 times/day; Maintenance: Titrate to response

Dosage Forms Excipient information presented when available (limited, particularly for generics); consult specific product labeling.

Injection, solution: 100 mg/mL (10 mL) [in polyethylene glycol; vial stopper contains latex]

Tablet: 500 mg, 750 mg

Methohexital (meth oh HEKS i tal)

Medication Safety Issues

Sound-alike/look-alike issues:

Brevital® may be confused with Brevibloc®

High alert medication: The Institute for Safe Medication Practices (ISMP) includes this medication among its list of drugs which have a heightened risk of causing significant patient harm when used in error.

U.S. Brand Names Brevital® Sodium

Canadian Brand Names Brevital®

Index Terms Methohexital Sodium

Pharmacologic Category Barbiturate; General Anesthetic

Generic Available No

Use For induction of anesthesia prior to the use of other general anesthetic agents; as an adjunct to subpotent inhalational anesthetic agents for short surgical procedures; for short surgical, diagnostic, or therapeutic procedures associated with minimal painful stimuli

Additional indications for adults: For use with other parenteral agents, usually narcotic analgesics, to supplement subpotent inhalational anesthetic agents for longer surgical procedures; as an agent to induce a hypnotic state

Unlabeled/Investigational Use Wada test

Effect on Mental Status Drowsiness is common

Effect on Psychiatric Treatment Used as induction anesthesia for electroconvulsive therapy (ECT); concurrent use with psychotropics may produce additive CNS depression

Restrictions C-IV

Pregnancy Risk Factor B

Pregnancy Considerations Animal studies have not shown fetal or maternal harm. There are no adequate and well-controlled studies in pregnant women. Methohexital crosses the placenta. Use only if potential benefit outweighs risk to fetus.

Lactation Enters breast milk/use caution

Contraindications Hypersensitivity to barbiturates, methohexital, or any component of the formulation; porphyria (latent or manifest); patients in whom general anesthesia is contraindicated

Warnings/Precautions Use with caution in patients with liver impairment, renal impairment, cardiovascular disease (including heart failure), severe anemia, extreme obesity, or seizure disorder, the elderly and children. May cause hypotension; use with caution in hemodynamically unstable patients (hypotension or shock) or severe hypertension. May cause respiratory depression; use with caution in patients with pulmonary disease. Use with caution in patients with asthma and chronic obstructive pulmonary disease. Use with extreme caution in patients with ongoing status asthmaticus; hiccups, coughing, laryngospasm, and muscle twitching have occurred impairing ventilation.

Postmarketing studies have indicated that the use of hypnotic/sedative agents for sleep has been associated with hypersensitivity reactions including anaphylaxis as well as angioedema. Effects with other sedative drugs or ethanol may be potentiated. Repeated dosing or continuous infusions may cause cumulative effects. Ensure patient has intravenous access; extravasation or intra-arterial injection causes necrosis. **[U.S. Boxed Warning]: Should only be administered in hospitals or ambulatory care settings with continuous monitoring of respiratory function; resuscitative drugs, age- and size-appropriate and intubation equipment and trained personnel experienced in handling their use should be readily available. For deeply sedated patients, a healthcare provider other than the individual performing the procedure should be present to continuously monitor the patient.**

Adverse Reactions Frequency not defined.

Cardiovascular: Cardiorespiratory arrest, circulatory depression, hypotension, peripheral vascular collapse, tachycardia

Central nervous system: Anxiety, emergence delirium, headache, restlessness, seizure

Dermatologic: Erythema, pruritus, urticaria

Gastrointestinal: Abdominal pain, nausea, salivation, vomiting

Hepatic: Transaminases increased

Local: Injection site pain, nerve injury adjacent to injection site, thrombophlebitis

Neuromuscular & skeletal: Involuntary muscle movement, radial nerve palsy, rigidity, tremor, twitching

Respiratory: Apnea, bronchospasm, cough, dyspnea, hiccups, laryngospasm, respiratory depression, rhinitis

Miscellaneous: Anaphylaxis (rare)

Drug Interactions

Acetaminophen: Barbiturates may increase the metabolism of Acetaminophen. This may 1) diminish the effect of acetaminophen; and 2) increase the risk of liver damage. *Risk C: Monitor therapy*

Alcohol (Ethyl): CNS Depressants may enhance the CNS depressant effect of Alcohol (Ethyl). *Risk C: Monitor therapy*

Beta-Blockers: Barbiturates may decrease the serum concentration of Beta-Blockers. **Exceptions:** Atenolol; Levobunolol; Metipranolol; Nadolol. *Risk C: Monitor therapy*

Calcium Channel Blockers: Barbiturates may increase the metabolism of Calcium Channel Blockers. **Exceptions:** Clevidipine. *Risk D: Consider therapy modification*

Chloramphenicol: May decrease the metabolism of Barbiturates. Barbiturates may increase the metabolism of Chloramphenicol. *Risk D: Consider therapy modification*

CNS Depressants: May enhance the adverse/toxic effect of other CNS Depressants. *Risk C: Monitor therapy*

Contraceptive (Progestins): Barbiturates may diminish the therapeutic effect of Contraceptive (Progestins). Contraceptive failure is possible. *Risk D: Consider therapy modification*

Corticosteroids (Systemic): Barbiturates may increase the metabolism of Corticosteroids (Systemic). *Risk C: Monitor therapy*

CycloSPORINE: Barbiturates may increase the metabolism of CycloSPORINE. *Risk D: Consider therapy modification*

Disopyramide: Barbiturates may increase the metabolism of Disopyramide. *Risk D: Consider therapy modification*

Doxycycline: Barbiturates may decrease the serum concentration of Doxycycline. *Risk D: Consider therapy modification*

Etoposide: Barbiturates may increase the metabolism of Etoposide. *Risk C: Monitor therapy*

Etoposide Phosphate: Barbiturates may decrease the serum concentration of Etoposide Phosphate. Barbiturates may increase the metabolism, via CYP isoenzymes, of etoposide phosphate. *Risk C: Monitor therapy*

Felbamate: May increase the serum concentration of Barbiturates. *Risk C: Monitor therapy*

LamoTRIgine: Barbiturates may increase the metabolism of LamoTRIgine. *Risk D: Consider therapy modification*

Meperidine: Barbiturates may enhance the CNS depressant effect of Meperidine. *Risk C: Monitor therapy*

Methadone: Barbiturates may increase the metabolism of Methadone. *Risk D: Consider therapy modification*

Oral Contraceptive (Estrogens): Barbiturates may diminish the therapeutic effect of Oral Contraceptive (Estrogens). Contraceptive failure is possible. *Risk D: Consider therapy modification*

Primidone: May enhance the adverse/toxic effect of Barbiturates. Primidone is converted to phenobarbital, and thus becomes additive with existing barbiturate therapy. *Risk C: Monitor therapy*

Propafenone: Barbiturates may increase the metabolism of Propafenone. *Risk D: Consider therapy modification*

Pyridoxine: May increase the metabolism of Barbiturates. Apparent in high pyridoxine doses (eg, 200 mg/day) *Risk C: Monitor therapy*

QuiNIDine: Barbiturates may increase the metabolism of QuiNIDine. *Risk D: Consider therapy modification*

Rifamycin Derivatives: May increase the metabolism of Barbiturates. *Risk C: Monitor therapy*

Teniposide: Barbiturates may increase the metabolism of Teniposide. *Risk C: Monitor therapy*

Theophylline Derivatives: Barbiturates may increase the metabolism of Theophylline Derivatives. **Exceptions:** Dyphylline. *Risk C: Monitor therapy*

Tricyclic Antidepressants: Barbiturates may increase the metabolism of Tricyclic Antidepressants. *Risk D: Consider therapy modification*

Valproic Acid: May decrease the metabolism of Barbiturates. Barbiturates may decrease the serum concentration of Valproic Acid. *Risk C: Monitor therapy*

Vitamin K Antagonists (eg, warfarin): Barbiturates may increase the metabolism of Vitamin K Antagonists. *Risk D: Consider therapy modification*

Stability Do not dilute with solutions containing bacteriostatic agents. Solutions should be freshly prepared and used promptly. Store at 20°C to 25°C (68°F to 77°F). Reconstituted solutions are chemically stable at room temperature for 24 hours; 0.2% (2 mg/mL) solutions in D_5W or NS are stable at room temperature for 24 hours.

Reconstitution:

For a 1% (10 mg/mL) solution:

500 mg vial: Dilute with 50 mL with SWFI (preferred), D_5W, or NS

2.5 g vial: Dilute with 15 mL of SWFI (preferred), D_5W, or NS, then add to 235 mL for a total volume of 250 mL

For a 5% (50 mg/mL) solution:

500 mg vial: Dilute with 10 mL of SWFI (preferred), D_5W, or NS

2.5 g vial: Dilute with 50 mL of SWFI (preferred), D_5W, or NS

For a 10% (100 mg/mL) solution:
500 mg vial: Dilute with 5 mL of SWFI (Pomeranz, 2000)
2.5 g vial: Dilute with 25 mL of SWFI (Pomeranz, 2000)
For continuous I.V. anesthesia: Prepare a 0.2% (2 mg/mL) solution by adding 500 mg to 250 mL of D_5W or NS. Do not dilute with SWFI (use of SWFI to make the 0.2% solution will result in extreme hypotonicity).

Mechanism of Action Ultra short-acting I.V. barbiturate anesthetic

Pharmacodynamics/Kinetics
Onset of action: I.V.: Immediate; I.M. (pediatrics): 2-10 minutes; Rectal (pediatrics): 5-15 minutes
Duration: Single dose: I.V.: 10-20 minutes; Rectal: 45 minutes
Metabolism: Hepatic via demethylation and oxidation
Excretion: Urine

Dosage Doses must be titrated to effect.
Infants <1 month: Safety and efficacy not established
Infants ≥1 month and Children:
Anesthesia induction:
I.M.: 6.6-10 mg/kg of a 5% solution
Rectal: Usual: 25 mg/kg of a 1% solution
I.V. (unlabeled dose): 1-2 mg/kg/dose of a 1% solution
Procedural sedation (unlabeled dose):
I.V.: Initial: 0.5 mg/kg given immediately prior to procedure; if sedation not adequate, repeat 0.5 mg/kg to a maximum total dose of 2 mg/kg
Rectal: 25 mg/kg of a 10% (100 mg/mL) solution given 5-15 minutes prior to procedure; maximum dose 500 mg
Adults: I.V.:
Induction: 1-1.5 mg/kg; maintenance: 50-120 mcg/kg/minute (or 20-40 mg every 4-7 minutes)
Wada test (unlabeled): 2-4 mg
Dosing adjustment/comments in hepatic impairment: Lower dosage and monitor closely

Administration
I.V.: Dilute to a maximum concentration of 1% for I.V. use
Induction and maintenance of anesthesia: 1% (10 mg/mL) solution is administered I.V. at a rate of ~1 mL/5 seconds or ~2 mg/second
Wada testing: Dilution of 0.1% (1 mg/mL) has been used; administer I.V. at a rate of 1 mg/second
Continuous I.V. infusion: Use 0.2% (2 mg/mL) solution
I.M. administration: Use 5% (50 mg/mL) solution
Rectal administration: Use 1% (10 mg/mL) solution; 10% (100 mg/mL) solution has also been used (Pomeranz, 2000)

Monitoring Parameters Respiratory status (for conscious sedation, includes pulse oximetry), cardiovascular status, CNS status (when used for procedures monitor sedation score); cardiac monitor and blood pressure monitor required

Dosage Forms Excipient information presented when available (limited, particularly for generics); consult specific product labeling.
Injection, powder for reconstitution, as sodium:
Brevital® Sodium: 500 mg, 2.5 g

◆ **Methohexital Sodium** *see* Methohexital *on page 1011*

Methotrexate (meth oh TREKS ate)

Medication Safety Issues
Sound-alike/look-alike issues:
Methotrexate may be confused with metolazone, mitoxantrone
MTX is an error-prone abbreviation (mistaken as mitoxantrone)

High alert medication: The Institute for Safe Medication Practices (ISMP) includes this medication among its list of drugs which have a heightened risk of causing significant patient harm when used in error.
Errors have occurred (resulting in death) when methotrexate was administered as "daily" dose instead of the recommended "weekly" dose.

International issues:
Trexall™ may be confused with Truxal® which is a brand name for chlorprothixene in Belgium
Trexall™ may be confused with Trexol® which is a brand name for tramadol in Mexico

U.S. Brand Names Rheumatrex® Dose Pack®; Trexall™

Canadian Brand Names Apo-Methotrexate®; ratio-Methotrexate

Mexican Brand Names Atrexel; Ledertrexate; Medsatrexate; Otaxem; Texate; Trixilem

Index Terms Amethopterin; Methotrexate Sodium; MTX (error-prone abbreviation) ; NSC-740

Pharmacologic Category Antineoplastic Agent, Antimetabolite (Antifolate); Antirheumatic, Disease Modifying

Use Treatment of trophoblastic neoplasms; leukemias; psoriasis; rheumatoid arthritis (RA), including polyarticular-course juvenile rheumatoid arthritis (JRA); breast, head and neck, and lung carcinomas; osteosarcoma; soft-tissue sarcomas; carcinoma of gastrointestinal tract, esophagus, testes; lymphomas

Unlabeled/Investigational Use Treatment and maintenance of remission in Crohn's disease; ectopic pregnancy

Effect on Mental Status May cause drowsiness or dizziness

Effect on Psychiatric Treatment Leukopenia is common; avoid clozapine and carbamazepine

Dosage Summary **Note:** Doses between 100-500 mg/m^2 may require leucovorin rescue in some patients

I.M.:

Children: 5-30 mg/m^2 once weekly or every 2 weeks

Adults: 15-30 mg/day for 5 days **or** 25-50 mg/m^2 once weekly **or** 5-50 mg once weekly **or** 15-37.5 mg twice weekly **or** 50 mg/m^2 as a single dose

I.V.:

Children: 10-18,000 mg/m^2 bolus dosing or continuous infusion over 6-42 hours

Adults: 11-1500 mg/m^2 on a specified number of days every 3-4 weeks **or** 25-50 mg/m^2 once weekly **or** 8-12 g/m^2 weekly for 2-4 weeks **or** 50 mg/m^2 as a single dose

Intrathecal:

Children ≤3 months: 3 mg/dose **or** 10-15 mg/m^2 (maximum: 15 mg/dose)

Children 4-11 months: 6 mg/dose **or** 10-15 mg/m^2 (maximum: 15 mg/dose)

Children 1 year: 8 mg/dose **or** 10-15 mg/m^2 (maximum: 15 mg/dose)

Children 2 years: 10 mg/dose **or** 10-15 mg/m^2 (maximum: 15 mg/dose)

Children ≥3 years: 12 mg/dose **or** 10-15 mg/m^2 (maximum: 15 mg/dose)

Adults: Dosage not established

Oral:

Children: 5-30 mg/m^2 once weekly or every 2 weeks **or** 0.3-1 mg/kg once weekly

Adults: 15-30 mg/day for 5 days **or** 25-50 mg/m^2 once weekly **or** 5-50 mg once weekly **or** 15-37.5 mg twice weekly

Dosage Forms Excipient information presented when available (limited, particularly for generics); consult specific product labeling.

Injection, powder for reconstitution [preservative free]: 20 mg, 1 g

Injection, solution: 25 mg/mL (2 mL, 10 mL) [contains benzyl alcohol]

Injection, solution [preservative free]: 25 mg/mL (2 mL, 4 mL, 8 mL, 10 mL, 40 mL)

Tablet: 2.5 mg

Trexall™: 5 mg, 7.5 mg, 10 mg, 15 mg

Tablet, as sodium [dose pack] (Rheumatrex® Dose Pack): 2.5 mg (4 cards with 2, 3, 4, 5, or 6 tablets each)

◆ **Methotrexate Sodium** *see* Methotrexate *on page 1014*

Methotrimeprazine (meth oh trye MEP ra zeen)

Canadian Brand Names Apo-Methoprazine®; Novo-Meprazine; Nozinan®; PMS-Methotrimeprazine

Mexican Brand Names Sinogan

Index Terms Levomepromazine; Methotrimeprazine Hydrochloride

Pharmacologic Category Analgesic, Nonopioid

Generic Available No

Use Treatment of schizophrenia or psychosis; management of pain, including pain caused by neuralgia or cancer; adjunct to general anesthesia; management of nausea and vomiting; sedation

Unlabeled/Investigational Use Bipolar disorder, agitation

Effect on Mental Status Is a phenothiazine; dizziness and extrapyramidal symptoms are common; may rarely cause neuroleptic malignant syndrome

Effect on Psychiatric Treatment Contraindicated with MAO inhibitors and patient with hypersensitivity to phenothiazines; may rarely cause agranulocytosis; use caution with clozapine and carbamazepine

Restrictions Not available in U.S.

Pregnancy Risk Factor C

Contraindications Hypersensitivity to methotrimeprazine, phenothiazines, or any component of the formulation; severe cardiac or hepatic disease; hematologic disorders (blood dyscrasia); history of convulsive disorders; severe CNS depression or coma; concurrent use of MAO inhibitors

Warnings/Precautions May be sedating; use with caution in disorders where CNS depression is a feature. May impair physical or mental abilities; patients must cautioned about performing tasks which require mental alertness (eg, operating machinery or driving). Effects with other sedative drugs or ethanol may be potentiated. Use with caution in Parkinson's disease; hemodynamic instability; bone marrow suppression; predisposition to seizures; and in severe cardiac, hepatic, renal, or respiratory disease. Caution in breast cancer or other prolactin-dependent tumors (may elevate prolactin levels). May alter temperature regulation or mask toxicity of other drugs due to antiemetic effects. May alter cardiac conduction; life-threatening arrhythmias have occurred with therapeutic doses of phenothiazines. May cause orthostatic hypotension; use with caution in patients at risk of hypotension or where transient hypotensive episodes would be poorly tolerated (cardiovascular disease or cerebrovascular disease). Hypotension may occur following administration, particularly when parenteral form is used or in high dosages.

Phenothiazines may cause anticholinergic effects (constipation, xerostomia, blurred vision, urinary retention); therefore, they should be used with caution in patients with decreased gastrointestinal motility, urinary retention, BPH, xerostomia, or visual problems. Conditions which also may be exacerbated by cholinergic blockade include narrow-angle glaucoma (screening is recommended) and worsening of myasthenia gravis. May cause extrapyramidal symptoms and/or tardive dyskinesia. May be associated with neuroleptic malignant syndrome (NMS).

Adverse Reactions Note: Frequencies not defined; some reactions listed are based on reports for other agents in this same pharmacologic class, and may not be specifically reported for methotrimeprazine.

Cardiovascular: Hypotension, orthostatic hypotension, tachycardia, QT_c prolongation (rare)

Central nervous system: Extrapyramidal symptoms (pseudoparkinsonism, akathisia, dystonias, tardive dyskinesia), dizziness, seizure, headache, drowsiness, neuroleptic malignant syndrome (NMS), impairment of temperature regulation

Dermatologic: Photosensitivity (rare), rash

Endocrine & metabolic: Gynecomastia, weight gain, menstrual irregularity, libido (changes in)

Gastrointestinal: Constipation, vomiting, nausea, xerostomia, ileus

Genitourinary: Difficulty in urination, ejaculatory disturbances, incontinence, polyuria, ejaculating dysfunction, priapism

Hematologic: Agranulocytosis (rare), leukopenia, eosinophilia, hemolytic anemia, thrombocytopenic purpura, pancytopenia

Hepatic: Cholestatic jaundice, hepatotoxicity

Miscellaneous: Diaphoresis

Metabolism/Transport Effects Inhibits CYP2D6

Drug Interactions Inhibits CYP2D6 (moderate)

Acetylcholinesterase inhibitors (central): May increase the risk of antipsychotic-related extrapyramidal symptoms; monitor.

Aluminum salts: May decrease the absorption of phenothiazines; monitor.

Amphetamines: Efficacy may be diminished by antipsychotics; in addition, amphetamines may increase psychotic symptoms; avoid concurrent use.

Anticholinergics: May inhibit the therapeutic response to phenothiazines and excess anticholinergic effects may occur; includes benztropine, trihexyphenidyl, biperiden, and drugs with significant anticholinergic activity (TCAs, antihistamines, disopyramide).

Antihypertensives: Concurrent use of phenothiazines with an antihypertensive may produce additive hypotensive effects (particularly orthostasis).

Bromocriptine: Phenothiazines inhibit the ability of bromocriptine to lower serum prolactin concentrations.

CNS depressants: Sedative effects may be additive with phenothiazines. If a patient is receiving methotrimeprazine, the dose of a barbiturate or narcotic should be reduced by 50%. Monitor for increased effects of benzodiazepines, ethanol and other sedative agents.

CYP2D6 substrates: Methotrimeprazine may increase the levels/effects of CYP2D6 substrates. Example substrates include amphetamines, selected beta-blockers, dextromethorphan, fluoxetine, lidocaine, mirtazapine, nefazodone, paroxetine, risperidone, ritonavir, thioridazine, tricyclic antidepressants, and venlafaxine.

CYP2D6 prodrug substrates: Methotrimeprazine may decrease the levels/effects of CYP2D6 prodrug substrates. Example prodrug substrates include codeine, hydrocodone, oxycodone, and tramadol.

Epinephrine: Low potency antipsychotics may diminish the pressor effects of epinephrine.

Guanethidine and guanadrel: Antihypertensive effects may be inhibited by phenothiazines.

Levodopa: Phenothiazines may inhibit the antiparkinsonian effect of levodopa; avoid this combination.

Lithium: Phenothiazines may produce neurotoxicity with lithium; this is a rare effect.

MAO inhibitors: Concurrent use of MAO inhibitors may result in toxicity; these combinations are best avoided.

Metoclopramide: May increase extrapyramidal symptoms (EPS) or risk.

Phenytoin: May reduce serum levels of phenothiazines; phenothiazines may increase phenytoin serum levels.

Polypeptide antibiotics: Rare cases of respiratory paralysis have been reported with concurrent use of phenothiazines.

Propranolol: Serum concentrations of phenothiazines may be increased; propranolol also increases phenothiazine concentrations.

Sulfadoxine-pyrimethamine: May increase phenothiazine concentrations.

Trazodone: Phenothiazines and trazodone may produce additive hypotensive effects.

Tricyclic antidepressants: Concurrent use may produce increased toxicity or altered therapeutic response.

Valproic acid: Serum levels may be increased by phenothiazines.

Ethanol/Nutrition/Herb Interactions

Ethanol: Avoid ethanol (may increase CNS depression).

Food: Limit caffeine.

Herb/Nutraceutical: Avoid dong quai, St John's wort (may also cause photosensitization). Avoid kava kava, gotu kola, valerian, St John's wort (may increase CNS depression).

Stability Injection: Protect from light.

Mechanism of Action Dopamine antagonist; also binds alpha-1, alpha-2, and serotonin receptors

Pharmacodynamics/Kinetics

Onset of action: Injection: 1 hour

Duration of action: 2-4 hours

Bioavailability: 50%

Time to peak, serum: I.M.: 0.5-1.5 hours; Oral: 1-3 hours

Half-life elimination: 30 hours

Dosage

Children >2 years:

- Oral: 0.25 mg/kg/day in 2-3 divided doses; may increase gradually based on response.
  - Maximum dose: 40 mg/day in children <12 years
- I.M.: 0.06-0.125 mg/kg/day in 1-3 divided doses

Adults:

- Oral:
  - Anxiety, mild-moderate pain: 6-25 mg/day in 3 divided doses
  - Psychoses, severe pain: 50-75 mg/day in 2-3 divided doses; titrate to effect (doses up to 1000 mg/day or greater have been used in treatment of some patients with psychoses). If higher dosages are used to initiate therapy (100-200 mg/day), patients should be restricted to bed for the first few days of therapy.
  - Sedative: 10-25 mg at bedtime
- I.M.:
  - Psychoses, severe pain: 75-100 mg (administered in 3-4 deep I.M. injections)
  - Analgesia (postoperative): 10-25 mg every 8 hours (2.5-7.5 mg every 4-6 hours is suggested postoperatively if residual effects of anesthetic may be present)
  - Premedication: 10-25 mg every 8 hours (final preoperative dose may be 25-50 mg administered ~1 hour prior to surgery)
- I.V.: During surgical procedures/labor: 20-50 mcg/minute (some patients may require up to 100 mcg/minute)
- SubQ (continuous infusion): Palliative care: 25-200 mcg/day (via syringe driver)

Dosing adjustment/comments in renal/hepatic disease: Administer cautiously although no specific guidelines are available.

Monitoring Parameters Liver function should be obtained at baseline and every 2-3 months during therapy.

Additional Information Not available in U.S.

Dosage Forms Excipient information presented when available (limited, particularly for generics); consult specific product labeling.

Injection, solution, as hydrochloride: 25 mg/mL (1 mL)
Solution, oral: 5 mg/mL (500 mL) [contains ethanol 2%]
Solution, oral drops: 40 mg/mL (100 mL) [contains ethanol 16.5%]
Tablet, as maleate: 2 mg, 5 mg, 25 mg, 50 mg

◆ **Methotrimeprazine Hydrochloride** *see* Methotrimeprazine *on page 1015*

Methoxsalen (meth OKS a len)

Medication Safety Issues

Sound-alike/look-alike issues:

Methoxsalen soft gelatin capsules (Oxsoralen-Ultra®) may be confused with methoxsalen hard gelatin capsules (8-MOP®, Oxsoralen®); bioavailability and photosensitization onset differ between the two products.

U.S. Brand Names 8-MOP®; Oxsoralen-Ultra®; Oxsoralen®; Uvadex®

Canadian Brand Names Oxsoralen-Ultra®; Oxsoralen®; Ultramop™; Uvadex®

Mexican Brand Names Meladinina

Index Terms 8-Methoxypsoralen; 8-MOP; Methoxypsoralen

Pharmacologic Category Psoralen

Use

Oral: Symptomatic control of severe, recalcitrant disabling psoriasis; repigmentation of idiopathic vitiligo; palliative treatment of skin manifestations of cutaneous T-cell lymphoma (CTCL)
Topical: Repigmentation of idiopathic vitiligo
Extracorporeal: Palliative treatment of skin manifestations of CTCL

Effect on Mental Status May cause nervousness, dizziness, or depression

Effect on Psychiatric Treatment Concurrent use with psychotropics may produce additive photosensitivity

Dosage Summary

Extracorporeal:

Children: Dosage not established

Adults: 200 mcg injected into photoactivation bag for two consecutive days every 4 weeks for a minimum of 7 treatment cycles; may accelerate to two consecutive days every 2 weeks if skin score worsens (eg, increases from baseline) after assessment during the fourth treatment cycle. If skin score improves by 25% after 4 consecutive weeks of accelerated therapy, may resume regular treatment schedule. Maximum: 20 accelerated therapy cycles.

Oral:

Children: Dosage not established

Adults:

Psoriasis: Initial: 10-70 mg 1.5-2 hours prior to UVA light exposure, may repeat 2-3 times/week (48 hours between doses); dose based on patient's weight. **Note:** Dosage may be increased (one time) by 10 mg after 15th treatment if minimal or no response. Maintenance: When 95% psoriasis clearing achieved, may begin 1 treatment every week for at least 2 treatments; followed by 1 treatment every 2 weeks for at least 2 treatments; then every 3 weeks for at least 2 treatments then as needed to maintain response while minimizing UVA exposure.

Vitiligo: 20 mg 2-4 hours prior to UVA light exposure, may repeat based on erythema and tenderness of skin; do not give on 2 consecutive days

Topical:

Children ≤12 years: Dosage not established

Children >12 years: Lotion is applied prior to UVA light exposure, usually no more than once weekly

Adults: Lotion is applied prior to UVA light exposure, usually no more than once weekly

Dosage Forms Excipient information presented when available (limited, particularly for generics); consult specific product labeling.

Capsule:
8-MOP®: 10 mg [hard-gelatin capsule]
Oxsoralen-Ultra®: 10 mg [soft-gelatin capsule]

Lotion (Oxsoralen®): 1% (30 mL) [contains alcohol 71%]

Solution, for extracorporeal administration (Uvadex®): 20 mcg/mL (10 mL) **[not for injection]**

◆ **Methoxypsoralen** *see* Methoxsalen *on page 1018*

◆ **8-Methoxypsoralen** *see* Methoxsalen *on page 1018*

Methscopolamine (meth skoe POL a meen)

Medication Safety Issues

International issues:

Pamine® may be confused with Pemine® which is a brand name for penicillamine in Italy

U.S. Brand Names Pamine®; Pamine® Forte

Canadian Brand Names Pamine®

Index Terms Methscopolamine Bromide

Pharmacologic Category Anticholinergic Agent

Use Adjunctive therapy in the treatment of peptic ulcer

Effect on Mental Status May rarely cause drowsiness, confusion, amnesia, or nervousness

Effect on Psychiatric Treatment Concurrent use with psychotropics may produce additive sedation and dry mouth

Dosage Summary

Oral:

Children: Dosage not established

Adults: 2.5-5 mg twice daily

Dosage Forms Excipient information presented when available (limited, particularly for generics); consult specific product labeling.

Tablet, as bromide: 2.5 mg, 5 mg

Pamine®: 2.5 mg [lactose free]

Pamine® Forte: 5 mg [lactose free; dosepak]

◆ **Methscopolamine and Pseudoephedrine** *see* Pseudoephedrine and Methscopolamine *on page 1370*

◆ **Methscopolamine Bromide** *see* Methscopolamine *on page 1019*

◆ **Methscopolamine, Chlorpheniramine, and Pseudoephedrine** *see* Chlorpheniramine, Pseudoephedrine, and Methscopolamine *on page 334*

◆ **Methscopolamine Nitrate and Chlordiazepoxide Hydrochloride** *see* Chlordiazepoxide and Methscopolamine *on page 319*

◆ **Methscopolamine Nitrate, Chlorpheniramine Maleate, and Phenylephrine Hydrochloride** *see* Chlorpheniramine, Phenylephrine, and Methscopolamine *on page 329*

◆ **Methscopolamine, Pseudoephedrine, and Chlorpheniramine** *see* Chlorpheniramine, Pseudoephedrine, and Methscopolamine *on page 334*

Methsuximide (meth SUKS i mide)

Medication Safety Issues

Sound-alike/look-alike issues:

Methsuximide may be confused with ethosuximide

U.S. Brand Names Celontin®

Canadian Brand Names Celontin®

Pharmacologic Category Anticonvulsant, Succinimide

Generic Available No

Use Control of absence (petit mal) seizures that are refractory to other drugs

Unlabeled/Investigational Use Partial complex (psychomotor) seizures

Pregnancy Risk Factor C

Contraindications Hypersensitivity to succinimides or any component of the formulation

Warnings/Precautions Use with caution in patients with hepatic or renal disease. Abrupt withdrawal of the drug may precipitate absence status. Methsuximide may increase tonic-clonic seizures in patients with mixed seizure disorders. Methsuximide must be used in combination with other anticonvulsants in patients with both absence and tonic-clonic seizures. Effects with other sedative drugs or ethanol may be potentiated. Consider evaluation of blood counts in patients with signs/symptoms of infection. Succinimides have been associated with severe blood dyscrasias and cases of systemic lupus erythematosus.

Adverse Reactions Frequency not defined.

Cardiovascular: Hyperemia

Central nervous system: Ataxia, dizziness, drowsiness, headache, aggressiveness, mental depression, irritability, nervousness, insomnia, confusion, psychosis, suicidal behavior, auditory hallucinations

Dermatologic: Stevens-Johnson syndrome, rash, urticaria, pruritus

Gastrointestinal: Anorexia, nausea, vomiting, weight loss, diarrhea, epigastric and abdominal pain, constipation

Genitourinary: Proteinuria, hematuria (microscopic); cases of blood dyscrasias have been reported with succinimides

Hematologic: Leukopenia, pancytopenia, eosinophilia, monocytosis

Neuromuscular & skeletal: Cases of systemic lupus erythematosus have been reported

Ocular: Blurred vision, photophobia, peripheral edema

Metabolism/Transport Effects **Substrate** of CYP2C19 (major); **Inhibits** CYP2C19 (weak)

Drug Interactions

Alcohol (Ethyl): CNS Depressants may enhance the CNS depressant effect of Alcohol (Ethyl). *Risk C: Monitor therapy*

CNS Depressants: May enhance the adverse/toxic effect of other CNS Depressants. *Risk C: Monitor therapy*

CYP2C19 Inducers (Strong): May increase the metabolism of CYP2C19 Substrates. *Risk C: Monitor therapy*

CYP2C19 Inhibitors (Moderate): May decrease the metabolism of CYP2C19 Substrates. *Risk C: Monitor therapy*

CYP2C19 Inhibitors (Strong): May decrease the metabolism of CYP2C19 Substrates. *Risk D: Consider therapy modification*

Ketorolac: May diminish the therapeutic effect of Anticonvulsants. *Risk C: Monitor therapy*

Mefloquine: May diminish the therapeutic effect of Anticonvulsants. Mefloquine may decrease the serum concentration of Anticonvulsants. Management: Mefloquine is contraindicated in persons with a history of convulsions. If anticonvulsant is being used for another indication monitor response to treatment closely, as concurrent mefloquine may decrease response to treatment. *Risk D: Consider therapy modification*

Stability Protect from high temperature.

Mechanism of Action Increases the seizure threshold and suppresses paroxysmal spike-and-wave pattern in absence seizures; depresses nerve transmission in the motor cortex

Pharmacodynamics/Kinetics

Metabolism: Hepatic; rapidly demethylated to N-desmethylmethsuximide (active metabolite)

Half-life elimination: 2-4 hours

Time to peak, serum: Within 1-3 hours

Excretion: Urine (<1% as unchanged drug)

Dosage Oral:

Children: Anticonvulsant: Initial: 10-15 mg/kg/day in 3-4 divided doses; increase weekly up to maximum of 30 mg/kg/day

Adults: Anticonvulsant: 300 mg/day for the first week; may increase by 300 mg/day at weekly intervals up to 1.2 g/day in 2-4 divided doses/day

Monitoring Parameters CBC, hepatic function tests, urinalysis

Dosage Forms Excipient information presented when available (limited, particularly for generics); consult specific product labeling.

Capsule: 150 mg, 300 mg

Methyclothiazide (meth i kloe THYE a zide)

Medication Safety Issues

Sound-alike/look-alike issues:

Enduron® may be confused with Empirin®, Imuran®, Inderal®

U.S. Brand Names Enduron® [DSC]

Canadian Brand Names Aquatensen®; Enduron®

Pharmacologic Category Diuretic, Thiazide

Use Management of mild to moderate hypertension; treatment of edema in congestive heart failure and nephrotic syndrome

Effect on Mental Status May cause drowsiness

Effect on Psychiatric Treatment May rarely cause agranulocytosis; use caution with clozapine and carbamazepine; may cause photosensitivity; use psychotropics with caution; may decrease lithium clearance resulting in an increase in serum lithium levels and potential lithium toxicity; monitor serum lithium levels

Dosage Summary

Oral:

Children: Dosage not established

Adults: 2.5-10 mg once daily

Dosage Forms Excipient information presented when available (limited, particularly for generics); consult specific product labeling.

Tablet: 5 mg

◆ **Methylacetoxyprogesterone** *see* MedroxyPROGESTERone *on page 975*

Methyldopa (meth il DOE pa)

Medication Safety Issues

Sound-alike/look-alike issues:

Methyldopa may be confused with L-dopa, levodopa

Canadian Brand Names Apo-Methyldopa®; Nu-Medopa

Mexican Brand Names Aldomet

Index Terms Aldomet; Methyldopate Hydrochloride

Pharmacologic Category Alpha-Adrenergic Inhibitor; Alpha$_2$-Adrenergic Agonist

Use Management of moderate to severe hypertension

Effect on Mental Status May cause drowsiness, dizziness, anxiety, nightmares, or depression

Effect on Psychiatric Treatment Contraindicated with MAO inhibitors; may rarely cause leukopenia; use caution with clozapine and carbamazepine; associated with lithium toxicity; use alternative antihypertensive agent; methyldopa may interact with psychotropics; monitor blood pressure and clinical status

Dosage Summary

I.V.:

Children: 5-10 mg/kg/dose every 6-8 hours (maximum: 65 mg/kg/day; 3 g/day)

Adults: 250-500 mg every 6-8 hours (maximum: 1 g every 6 hours)

Oral:

Children: Initial: 10 mg/kg/day in 2-4 divided doses; Maintenance: Up to 65 mg/kg/day (maximum: 3 g/day)

Adults: Initial: 250 mg 2-3 times/day; Maintenance: 250-1000 mg/day in 2 divided doses (maximum: 3 g/day)

Elderly: Initial: 125 mg 1-2 times/day; increase by 125 mg every 2-3 days as needed

Dosage Forms Excipient information presented when available (limited, particularly for generics); consult specific product labeling.

Injection, solution, as methyldopate hydrochloride: 50 mg/mL (5 mL) [contains sodium bisulfite]

Tablet: 250 mg, 500 mg

Methyldopa and Hydrochlorothiazide
(meth il DOE pa & hye droe klor oh THYE a zide)

Medication Safety Issues

Sound-alike/look-alike issues:

Aldoril® may be confused with Aldoclor®, Aldomet®, Elavil®

U.S. Brand Names Aldoril®

Canadian Brand Names Apo-Methazide®

Index Terms Hydrochlorothiazide and Methyldopa

Pharmacologic Category Alpha$_2$-Adrenergic Agonist; Diuretic, Thiazide

Use Management of moderate-to-severe hypertension

Effect on Mental Status May cause drowsiness, dizziness, anxiety, nightmares, or depression

Effect on Psychiatric Treatment Contraindicated with MAO inhibitors; may rarely cause leukopenia; use caution with clozapine and carbamazepine; associated with lithium toxicity; use alternative antihypertensive agent; methyldopa may interact with psychotropics; monitor blood pressure and clinical status; thiazides may decrease lithium clearance resulting in an increase in serum lithium levels and potential lithium toxicity; monitor serum lithium levels

Dosage Summary

Oral:

Children: Dosage not established

Adults: 1 tablet 2-3 times/day (maximum: 50 mg/day [hydrochlorothiazide]; 3 g/day [methyldopa])

Dosage Forms Excipient information presented when available (limited, particularly for generics); consult specific product labeling.

Tablet:
Methyldopa 250 mg and hydrochlorothiazide 15 mg
Methyldopa 250 mg and hydrochlorothiazide 25 mg
Aldoril® 25: Methyldopa 250 mg and hydrochlorothiazide 25 mg

◆ **Methyldopate Hydrochloride** *see* Methyldopa *on page 1021*

◆ **Methylene Blue, Methenamine, Benzoic Acid, Phenyl Salicylate, and Hyoscyamine** *see* Methenamine, Phenyl Salicylate, Methylene Blue, Benzoic Acid, and Hyoscyamine *on page 1009*

◆ **Methylene Blue, Methenamine, Sodium Biphosphate, Phenyl Salicylate, and Hyoscyamine** *see* Methenamine, Sodium Biphosphate, Phenyl Salicylate, Methylene Blue, and Hyoscyamine *on page 1010*

◆ **Methylergometrine Maleate** *see* Methylergonovine *on page 1022*

Methylergonovine (meth il er goe NOE veen)

Medication Safety Issues

Sound-alike/look-alike issues:
Methylergonovine and terbutaline parenteral dosage forms look similar. Due to their contrasting indications, use care when administering these agents.

U.S. Brand Names Methergine®

Canadian Brand Names Methergine®

Mexican Brand Names Methergin

Index Terms Methylergometrine Maleate; Methylergonovine Maleate

Pharmacologic Category Ergot Derivative

Use Prevention and treatment of postpartum and postabortion hemorrhage caused by uterine atony or subinvolution

Effect on Mental Status May rarely cause dizziness or hallucinations

Effect on Psychiatric Treatment None reported

Dosage Summary

I.M.:
Children: Dosage not established
Adults: 0.2 mg after delivery of anterior shoulder, after delivery of placenta, or during puerperium; may repeat every 2-4 hours

I.V.:
Children: Dosage not established
Adults: 0.2 mg after delivery of anterior shoulder, after delivery of placenta, or during puerperium; may repeat every 2-4 hours

Oral:
Children: Dosage not established
Adults: 0.2 mg 3-4 times/day in the puerperium for 2-7 days

Dosage Forms Excipient information presented when available (limited, particularly for generics); consult specific product labeling.

Injection, solution, as maleate: 0.2 mg/mL (1 mL)
Methergine®: 0.2 mg/mL (1 mL)
Tablet, as maleate:
Methergine®: 0.2 mg

◆ **Methylergonovine Maleate** *see* Methylergonovine *on page 1022*

Methylfolate (meth il FO late)

U.S. Brand Names Deplin™

Index Terms 6(S)-5-methyltetrahydrofolate; 6(S)-5-MTHF; L-methylfolate

Pharmacologic Category Dietary Supplement

Use Medicinal food for management of patients with low plasma and/or low red blood cell folate

Mental Health Comment Pilot studies have explored the potential to improve response to antidepressant treatment with the addition of folate, a water-soluble B vitamin. Alpert et al, evaluated the efficacy of methylfolate as an adjunctive treatment in 22 adults with major depression who had an inadequate response to SSRI therapy in an 8 week prospective trial. Leucovorin (folinic acid), which is metabolized to methylfolate, was added to SSRI therapy at 15-30 mg/day. Hamilton Depression Rating Scale scores decrease significantly (p <0.01) in the 16 completers. Thirty-one percent of the completers and 27% of the intent-to-treat sample achieved response and 19% of the completers and 18% of the intent-to-treat sample achieved remission.

In support of the finding by Alpert et al, assessed the relationship between serum folate, vitamin B_{12}, homocysteine levels, and clinical response in patients with major depression who had previously failed to respond to open treatment with fluoxetine 20 mg/day. Low serum folate levels but not elevated homocysteine or low vitamin B_{12} levels were associated with poorer response to treatment. The response rate for patients with and without low folate levels was 7.1% and 44.7% respectively.

In part two of the above study, Papakostas et al, evaluated the relationship between serum folate, vitamin B_{12}, and homocysteine levels on the rate of relapse in outpatients with remitted major depression during a 28-week continuation phase of treatment with fluoxetine. Low serum folate levels but not elevated homocysteine or low vitamin B_{12} levels were associated with relapse during continuation treatment with fluoxetine. The relapse rate for patients with and without low folate levels was 42.9% and 3.2% respectively.

Further study is necessary to determine to role of methylfolate in the management of major depressive disorder.

Alpert JE, Mischoulon D, Rubenstein GE, et al, "Folinic Acid (Leucovorin) as an Adjunctive Treatment for SSRI-Refractory Depression," *Ann Clin Psychiatry*, 2002, 14(1):33-8.

Papakostas GI, Petersen T, Mischoulon D, et al, "Serum Folate, Vitamin B_{12}, and Homocysteine in Major Depressive Disorder, Part 2: Predictors of Relapse During the Continuation Phase of Pharmacotherapy," *J Clin Psychiatry*, 2004, 65(8):1096-8.

Dosage Summary

Oral:

Children: Dosage not established

Adults: 7.5 mg daily

Dosage Forms Excipient information presented when available (limited, particularly for generics); consult specific product labeling.

Tablet:

Deplin™: L-methylfolate 7.5 mg [gluten free, lactose free, sugar free, yeast free]

◆ **Methylin®** *see* Methylphenidate *on page 1024*

◆ **Methylin® ER** *see* Methylphenidate *on page 1024*

◆ **Methylmorphine** *see* Codeine *on page 394*

Methylnaltrexone (meth il nal TREKS one)

Medication Safety Issues

Sound-alike/look-alike issues:

Methylnaltrexone may be confused with naltrexone

U.S. Brand Names Relistor™

Index Terms Methylnaltrexone Bromide; N-methylnaltrexone Bromide

Pharmacologic Category Gastrointestinal Agent, Miscellaneous; Opioid Antagonist, Peripherally-Acting

Use Treatment of opioid-induced constipation in patients with advanced illness receiving palliative care with inadequate response to conventional laxative regimens

Effect on Mental Status May cause dizziness

Effect on Psychiatric Treatment GI side effects are common; concomitant use with SSRIs, lithium, carbamazepine, or valproic acid may produce additive effects.

Dosage Summary

SubQ:

Children: Dosage not established

Adults <38 kg: 0.15 mg/kg (round dose up to nearest 0.1 mL of volume) every other day as needed (maximum: 1 dose/24 hours)

Adults 38 to <62 kg: 8 mg every other day as needed (maximum: 1 dose/24 hours)

Adults 62-114 kg: 12 mg every other day as needed (maximum: 1 dose/24 hours)

Adults >114 kg: 0.15 mg/kg (round dose up to nearest 0.1 mL of volume) every other day as needed (maximum: 1 dose/24 hours)

Dosage Forms Excipient information presented when available (limited, particularly for generics); consult specific product labeling.

Injection, solution:

Relistor™: 12 mg/0.6 mL (0.6 mL) [contains edetate calcium disodium]

◆ **Methylnaltrexone Bromide** *see* Methylnaltrexone *on page 1023*

Methylphenidate (meth il FEN i date)

Medication Safety Issues

Sound-alike/look-alike issues:

Metadate® CD may be confused with Metadate® ER

Metadate® ER may be confused with Metadate® CD, methadone

Methylphenidate may be confused with methadone

Ritalin® may be confused with Ismelin®, Rifadin®, ritodrine

Related Information

Clozapine-Induced Side Effects *on page 1818*

Stimulant Agents Used for ADHD *on page 1797*

U.S. Brand Names Concerta®; Daytrana™; Metadate® CD; Metadate® ER; Methylin®; Methylin® ER; Ritalin-SR®; Ritalin®; Ritalin® LA

Canadian Brand Names Apo-Methylphenidate®; Apo-Methylphenidate® SR; Biphentin®; Concerta®; PMS-Methylphenidate; Riphenidate; Ritalin®; Ritalin® SR

Mexican Brand Names Concerta; Ritalin; Tradea

Index Terms Methylphenidate Hydrochloride

Pharmacologic Category Central Nervous System Stimulant

Generic Available Yes: Immediate release tablet, extended release tablet, sustained release tablet

Use Treatment of attention-deficit/hyperactivity disorder (ADHD); symptomatic management of narcolepsy

Unlabeled/Investigational Use Depression (especially elderly or medically ill)

Restrictions C-II

An FDA-approved medication guide must be distributed when dispensing an outpatient prescription (new or refill) where this medication is to be used without direct supervision of a healthcare provider. Medication guides are available at http://www.fda.gov/cder/Offices/ODS/medication_guides.htm.

Pregnancy Risk Factor C

Pregnancy Considerations Animal studies have shown teratogenic effects to the fetus. There are no adequate and well-controlled studies in pregnant women. Do not use in women of childbearing age unless the potential benefit outweighs the possible risk.

Lactation Enters breast milk/use caution

Contraindications Hypersensitivity to methylphenidate, any component of the formulation, or idiosyncratic reactions to sympathomimetic amines; marked anxiety, tension, and agitation; glaucoma; use during or within 14 days following MAO inhibitor therapy; family history or diagnosis of Tourette's syndrome or tics

Metadate® CD and Metadate® ER: Additional contraindications: Severe hypertension, heart failure, arrhythmia, hyperthyroidism, recent MI or angina; concomitant use of halogenated anesthetics

Warnings/Precautions CNS stimulant use has been associated with serious cardiovascular events including sudden death in patients with pre-existing structural cardiac abnormalities or other serious heart problems (sudden death in children and adolescents; sudden death, stroke, and MI in adults). These products should be avoided in patients with known serious structural cardiac abnormalities, cardiomyopathy, serious heart rhythm abnormalities, or other serious cardiac problems that could further increase their risk of sudden death. Patients should be carefully evaluated for cardiac disease prior to initiation of therapy. Use of stimulants can cause an increase in blood pressure (average 2-4 mm Hg) and increases in heart rate (average 3-6 bpm), although some patients may have larger than average increases. Use caution with hypertension, hyperthyroidism, or other cardiovascular conditions that might be exacerbated by increases in blood pressure or heart rate. Some products are contraindicated in patients with heart failure, arrhythmias, severe hypertension, hyperthyroidism, angina, or recent MI.

Has demonstrated value as part of a comprehensive treatment program for ADHD. Use with caution in patients with bipolar disorder (may induce mixed/manic episode). May exacerbate symptoms of behavior and thought disorder in psychotic patients; new onset psychosis or mania may occur with stimulant use; observe for symptoms of aggression and/or hostility. Use caution with seizure disorders (may reduce seizure threshold). Use caution in patients with history of ethanol or drug abuse. May exacerbate symptoms of behavior and thought disorder in psychotic patients. **[U.S. Boxed Warning]: Potential for drug dependency exists - avoid abrupt discontinuation in patients who have received for prolonged periods.** Visual disturbances have been reported (rare). Not labeled for use in children <6 years of age. Use of stimulants has been associated with suppression of growth in children; monitor growth rate during treatment.

Concerta® should not be used in patients with esophageal motility disorders or pre-existing severe gastrointestinal narrowing (small bowel disease, short gut syndrome, history of peritonitis, cystic fibrosis, chronic intestinal pseudo-obstruction, Meckel's diverticulum). Metadate® CD and Metadate® ER contain sucrose and lactose, respectively; avoid administration in hereditary galactose intolerance, Lapp lactase deficiency, or glucose-galactose malabsorption. Concomitant use with halogenated anesthetics is contraindicated; may cause sudden elevations in blood pressure; if surgery is planned, do not administer Metadate® CD or Metadate® ER on the day of surgery. Transdermal system may cause allergic contact sensitization, characterized by intense local reactions (edema, papules); sensitization may subsequently manifest systemically with other routes of methylphenidate administration; monitor closely. Avoid exposure of application site to any direct external heat sources (eg, hair dryers, heating pads, electric blankets); may increase risk of overdose. Efficacy of transdermal methylphenidate therapy for >7 weeks has not been established.

Adverse Reactions

Transdermal system: Frequency of adverse events as reported in trials of 7-week duration. Incidence of some events higher with extended use.

>10%:

Central nervous system: Headache (long-term use in children: 28%), insomnia (13%; long-term use in children: 30%)

Gastrointestinal: Appetite decreased (26%), nausea (12%)

Miscellaneous: Viral infection (long-term use in children: 28%)

1% to 10%:

Central nervous system: Tic (7%), emotional instability (6%)

Gastrointestinal: Vomiting (10%), weight loss (9%), anorexia (5%; long-term use in children: 46%)

Local: Application site reaction

Respiratory: Nasal congestion (6%) nasopharyngitis (5%)

Postmarketing and/or case reports (limited to important or life-threatening): Allergic contact sensitization, anaphylaxis, angioedema, hallucinations, seizures

All dosage forms: Frequency not defined:

Cardiovascular: Angina, cardiac arrhythmia, cerebral arteritis, cerebral occlusion, hyper-/hypotension, MI, murmur, palpitation, pulse increased/decreased, Raynaud's phenomenon, tachycardia

Central nervous system: Aggression, agitation, anger, anxiety, confusional state, depression, dizziness, drowsiness, fatigue, fever, headache, hypervigilance, insomnia, irritability, lethargy, mood alterations, nervousness, neuroleptic malignant syndrome (NMS) (rare), restlessness, stroke, tension, Tourette's syndrome (rare), toxic psychosis, tremor, vertigo

Dermatologic: Alopecia, erythema multiforme, exfoliative dermatitis, hyperhidrosis, rash, urticaria

Endocrine & metabolic: Dysmenorrhea, growth retardation, libido decreased

Gastrointestinal: Abdominal pain, anorexia, appetite decreased, bruxism, constipation, diarrhea, dyspepsia, nausea, vomiting, weight loss, xerostomia

Genitourinary: Erectile dysfunction

Hematologic: Anemia, leukopenia, pancytopenia, thrombocytopenic purpura, thrombocytopenia

Hepatic: Bilirubin increased, liver function tests abnormal, hepatic coma, transaminases increased

Neuromuscular & skeletal: Arthralgia, dyskinesia, muscle tightness, paresthesia

Ocular: Blurred vision, dry eyes, mydriasis, visual accommodation disturbance

Renal: Necrotizing vasculitis

Respiratory: Cough increased, dyspnea, pharyngitis, pharyngolaryngeal pain, rhinitis, sinusitis, upper respiratory tract infection

Miscellaneous: Accidental injury, hypersensitivity reactions

Postmarketing and/or case reports: Alkaline phosphatase increased, angina pectoris, bradycardia, chest pain, diplopia, disorientation, extrasystole, mydriasis; hypersensitivity reactions (eg, angioedema, anaphylactic reactions, auricular swelling, bullous conditions, exfoliative conditions, urticaria, pruritus, rash, eruptions, exanthemas); muscle twitching, hallucinations, mania, erythema, seizure, supraventricular tachycardia, ventricular extrasystole

Metabolism/Transport Effects Inhibits CYP2D6 (weak)

Drug Interactions

Antihypertensives: Methylphenidate may diminish the antihypertensive effect of Antihypertensives. *Risk C: Monitor therapy*

Cannabinoids: May enhance the tachycardic effect of Sympathomimetics. *Risk C: Monitor therapy*

CloNIDine: Methylphenidate may enhance the adverse/toxic effect of CloNIDine. *Risk C: Monitor therapy*

Inhalational Anesthetics: Methylphenidate may enhance the hypertensive effect of Inhalational Anesthetics. *Risk X: Avoid combination*

MAO Inhibitors: May enhance the hypertensive effect of Methylphenidate. *Risk X: Avoid combination*

Phenytoin: Methylphenidate may decrease the metabolism of Phenytoin. *Risk C: Monitor therapy*

Sympathomimetics: May enhance the adverse/toxic effect of other Sympathomimetics. *Risk C: Monitor therapy*

Tricyclic Antidepressants: Methylphenidate may decrease the metabolism of Tricyclic Antidepressants. *Risk C: Monitor therapy*

Ethanol/Nutrition/Herb Interactions

Ethanol: Avoid ethanol (may cause CNS depression).

Food: Food may increase oral absorption; Concerta® formulation is not affected. Food delays early peak and high-fat meals increase C_{max} and AUC of Metadate® CD formulation.

Herb/Nutraceutical: Avoid ephedra (may cause hypertension or arrhythmias) and yohimbe (also has CNS stimulatory activity).

Stability

Capsule, *extended release:* Store at controlled room temperature of 20°C to 25°C (68°F to 77°F). Protect from light.

Solution: Store at controlled room temperature of 20°C to 25°C (68°F to 77°F).

Tablet:

Chewable: Store at controlled room temperature of 20°C to 25°C (68°F to 77°F). Protect from light and moisture.

Extended and sustained release: Store at controlled room temperature of 20°C to 25°C (68°F to 77°F). Protect from light and moisture.

Immediate release: Store at controlled room temperature of 20°C to 25°C (68°F to 77°F). Protect from light and moisture.

Osmotic controlled release (Concerta®): Store at controlled room temperature of 25°C; excursions permitted to 15°C to 30°C (59°F to 86°F). Protect from humidity.

Transdermal system: Store at controlled room temperature of 20°C to 25°C (68°F to 77°F). Keep patches stored in protective pouch. Once tray is opened, use patches within 2 months. Do not refrigerate or freeze.

Mechanism of Action Mild CNS stimulant; blocks the reuptake of norepinephrine and dopamine into presynaptic neurons; appears to stimulate the cerebral cortex and subcortical structures similar to amphetamines

Pharmacodynamics/Kinetics

Onset of action: Peak effect:

Immediate release tablet: Cerebral stimulation: ~2 hours

Extended release capsule (Metadate® CD): Biphasic; initial peak similar to immediate release product, followed by second rising portion (corresponding to extended release portion)

Sustained release tablet: 4-7 hours

Osmotic release tablet (Concerta®): Initial: 1-2 hours

Transdermal: ~2 hours; may be expedited by the application of external heat

Duration: Immediate release tablet: 3-6 hours; Sustained release tablet: 8 hours; Extended release tablet: Methylin® ER, Metadate® ER: 8 hours, Concerta®: 12 hours

Absorption:

Oral: Readily absorbed

Transdermal: Absorption increased when applied to inflamed skin or exposed to heat. Absorption is continuous for 9 hours after application.

Metabolism: Hepatic via de-esterification to minimally active metabolite

Half-life elimination: *d*-methylphenidate: 3-4 hours; *l*-methylphenidate: 1-3 hours

Time to peak: Concerta®: C_{max}: 6-8 hours; Daytrana™: 7.5-10.5 hours

Excretion: Urine (90% as metabolites and unchanged drug)

Dosage

ADHD:

Oral:

Immediate release products Children ≥6 years and Adults: Initial: 5 mg/dose (~0.3 mg/kg/dose) given twice daily before breakfast and lunch;

increase by 5-10 mg/day (0.2 mg/kg/day) at weekly intervals; maximum dose: 60 mg/day (2 mg/kg/day). **Note:** Discontinue periodically to re-evaluate or if no improvement occurs within 1 month.

Extended release products:

Children ≥6 years and Adults:

Metadate® ER, Methylin® ER, Ritalin® SR: May be given in place of immediate release products, once the daily dose is titrated and the titrated 8-hour dosage corresponds to sustained or extended release tablet size; maximum: 60 mg/day

Metadate® CD, Ritalin® LA: Initial: 20 mg once daily; may be adjusted in 10-20 mg increments at weekly intervals; maximum: 60 mg/day

Children 6-12 years and Adolescents 13-17 years: *Concerta®:*

Patients not currently taking methylphenidate: Initial dose: 18 mg once daily in the morning

Patients currently taking methylphenidate: **Note:** Initial dose: Dosing based on current regimen and clinical judgment; suggested dosing listed below:

- Patients taking methylphenidate 5 mg 2-3 times/day: 18 mg once every morning
- Patients taking methylphenidate 10 mg 2-3 times/day: 36 mg once every morning
- Patients taking methylphenidate 15 mg 2-3 times/day: 54 mg once every morning

Dose adjustment: May increase dose in increments of 18 mg; dose may be adjusted at weekly intervals. A dosage strength of 27 mg is available for situations in which a dosage between 18-36 mg is desired. Maximum dose should not exceed 2 mg/kg/day **or** 54 mg/day in children 6-12 years or 72 mg/day in children 13-17 years.

Adults: *Concerta®:*

Patients not currently taking methylphenidate: Initial dose: 18-36 mg once daily in the morning

Patients currently taking methylphenidate: **Note:** Initial dose: Dosing based on current regimen and clinical judgment; suggested dosing listed below:

- Patients taking methylphenidate 5 mg 2-3 times/day: 18 mg once every morning
- Patients taking methylphenidate 10 mg 2-3 times/day: 36 mg once every morning
- Patients taking methylphenidate 15 mg 2-3 times/day: 54 mg once every morning
- Patients taking methylphenidate 20 mg 2-3 times/day: 72 mg once every morning

Dose adjustment: May increase dose in increments of 18 mg; dose may be adjusted at weekly intervals. A dosage strength of 27 mg is available for situations in which a dosage between 18-36 mg is desired. Maximum dose should not exceed 72 mg/day.

Transdermal (Daytrana™): Children ≥6 years: Initial: 10 mg patch once daily; remove up to 9 hours after application. Titrate based on response and tolerability; may increase to next transdermal dose no more frequently than every week. **Note:** Application should occur 2 hours prior to desired effect. Drug absorption may continue for a period of time after patch removal; patients converting from another formulation of methylphenidate should be initiated at 10 mg regardless of their previous dose and titrated as needed due to the differences in bioavailability of the transdermal formulation.

Narcolepsy: Oral: Adults: 10 mg 2-3 times/day, up to 60 mg/day

Depression (unlabeled use): Oral: Adults: Initial: 2.5 mg every morning before 9 AM; dosage may be increased by 2.5-5 mg every 2-3 days as tolerated to a maximum of 20 mg/day; may be divided (ie, 7 AM and 12 noon), but should not be given after noon; do not use sustained release product

Dietary Considerations Should be taken 30-45 minutes before meals. Concerta® is not affected by food and should be taken with water, milk, or juice. Metadate® CD should be taken before breakfast. Metadate® ER should be taken before breakfast and lunch. Methylin® chewable tablets contain phenylalanine 0.42 mg/methylphenidate 2.5 mg.

Administration

Oral: Do not crush or allow patient to chew sustained or extended release dosage form. To effectively avoid insomnia, dosing should be completed by noon.

Concerta®: Administer dose once daily in the morning. May be taken with or without food, but must be taken with water, milk, or juice.

Metadate® CD, Ritalin® LA: Capsules may be opened and the contents sprinkled onto a small amount (equal to 1 tablespoon) of applesauce. Swallow applesauce without chewing. Do not crush or chew capsule contents.

Methylin® chewable tablet: Administer with at least 8 ounces of water or other fluid.

Topical: Transdermal (Daytrana™): Apply to clean, dry, non-oily, intact skin to the hip area, avoiding the waistline. Apply at the same time each day to alternating hips. Press firmly for 30 seconds to ensure proper adherence. Avoid exposure of application site to external heat source, which may increase the amount of drug absorbed. Do not use a patch that has been damaged or torn; do not cut patch. If patch should dislodge, may replace with new patch (to different site) but total wear time should not exceed 9 hours; do not reapply with dressings, tape, or common adhesives. Patch may be removed early if a shorter duration of effect is desired or if late day side effects occur. Wash hands with soap and water after handling. Avoid touching the sticky side of the patch. If patch removal is difficult, an oil-based product (eg, petroleum jelly, olive oil) may be applied to the patch edges to aid removal; never apply acetone-based products (eg, nail polish remover) to patch. Dispose of used patch by folding adhesive side onto itself, and discard in toilet or appropriate lidded container.

Monitoring Parameters Blood pressure, heart rate, signs and symptoms of depression, aggression, or hostility; CBC, differential and platelet counts, liver function tests; growth rate in children, signs of central nervous system stimulation

Transdermal: Signs of worsening erythema, blistering or edema which does not improve within 24 hours of patch removal, or spreads beyond patch site.

When used for the treatment of ADHD, thoroughly evaluate for cardiovascular risk. Monitor heart rate, blood pressure, and consider obtaining ECG prior to initiation (Vetter, 2008).

Additional Information Treatment with methylphenidate may include "drug holidays" or periodic discontinuation in order to assess the patient's requirements and to decrease tolerance and limit suppression of linear growth and weight. Specific patients may require 3 doses/day for treatment of ADHD (ie, additional dose at 4 PM).

Concerta® is an osmotic controlled release formulation (OROS®) of methylphenidate. The tablet has an immediate-release overcoat that provides an initial dose of methylphenidate within 1 hour. The overcoat covers a trilayer core. The trilayer core is composed of two layers containing the drug and excipients, and one layer of osmotic components. As water from the gastrointestinal tract enters the core, the osmotic components expand and methylphenidate is released.

Metadate® CD capsules contain a mixture of immediate release and extended release beads, designed to release 30% of the dose immediately and 70% over an extended period.

Ritalin® LA uses a combination of immediate release and enteric coated, delayed release beads.

Dosage Forms Excipient information presented when available (limited, particularly for generics); consult specific product labeling. [DSC] = Discontinued product

Capsule, extended release, oral, as hydrochloride [bi-modal release]:

Metadate CD®: 10 mg [contains sucrose; 3 mg immediate release, 7 mg extended release]

Metadate CD®: 20 mg [contains sucrose; 6 mg immediate release, 14 mg extended release]

Metadate CD®: 30 mg [contains sucrose; 9 mg immediate release, 21 mg extended release]

Metadate CD®: 40 mg [contains sucrose; 12 mg immediate release, 28 mg extended release]

Metadate CD®: 50 mg [contains sucrose; 15 mg immediate release, 35 mg extended release]

Metadate CD®: 60 mg [contains sucrose; 18 mg immediate release, 42 mg extended release]

Ritalin LA®: 10 mg [5 mg immediate release, 5 mg extended release]

Ritalin LA®: 20 mg [10 mg immediate release, 10 mg extended release]

Ritalin LA®: 30 mg [15 mg immediate release, 15 mg extended release]

Ritalin LA®: 40 mg [20 mg immediate release, 20 mg extended release]

Solution, oral, as hydrochloride:
Methylin®: 5 mg/5 mL (500 mL) [grape flavor]; 10 mg/5 mL (500 mL) [grape flavor]
Tablet, as hydrochloride: 5 mg, 10 mg, 20 mg
Methylin®, Ritalin®: 5 mg, 10 mg, 20 mg
Tablet, chewable, as hydrochloride:
Methylin®: 2.5 mg [contains phenylalanine 0.42 mg; grape flavor]; 5 mg [contains phenylalanine 0.84 mg; grape flavor]; 10 mg [contains phenylalanine 1.68 mg; grape flavor]
Tablet, extended release, as hydrochloride: 20 mg
Metadate® ER: 10 mg [contains lactose]; 20 mg [contains lactose]
Methylin® ER: 10 mg, 20 mg
Tablet, extended release, as hydrochloride [bi-modal release]:
Concerta®: 18 mg [4 mg immediate release, 14 mg extended release]
Concerta®: 27 mg [6 mg immediate release, 21 mg extended release]
Concerta®: 36 mg [8 mg immediate release, 28 mg extended release]
Concerta®: 54 mg [12 mg immediate release, 42 mg extended release]
Tablet, sustained release, as hydrochloride: 20 mg
Ritalin-SR®: 20 mg [dye free]
Transdermal system [once-daily patch]:
Daytrana™: 10 mg/9 hours (10s [DSC], 30s) [12.5 cm^2, total methylphenidate 27.5 mg]
Daytrana™: 15 mg/9 hours (10s [DSC], 30s) [18.75 cm^2, total methylphenidate 41.3 mg]
Daytrana™: 20 mg/9 hours (10s [DSC], 30s) [25 cm^2, total methylphenidate 55 mg]
Daytrana™: 30 mg/9 hours (10s [DSC], 30s) [37.5 cm^2, total methylphenidate 82.5 mg]

- ◆ **Methylphenidate Hydrochloride** *see* Methylphenidate *on page 1024*
- ◆ **Methylphenobarbital** *see* Mephobarbital *on page 988*
- ◆ **Methylphenoxy-Benzene Propanamine** *see* Atomoxetine *on page 151*
- ◆ **Methylphenyl Isoxazolyl Penicillin** *see* Oxacillin *on page 1190*
- ◆ **Methylphytyl Napthoquinone** *see* Phytonadione *on page 1289*

MethylPREDNISolone (meth il pred NIS oh lone)

Medication Safety Issues
Sound-alike/look-alike issues:
MethylPREDNISolone may be confused with medroxyPROGESTERone, predniSONE
Depo-Medrol® may be confused with Solu-Medrol®
Medrol® may be confused with Mebaral®
Solu-Medrol® may be confused with Depo-Medrol®, Solu-Cortef®

International issues:
Medor® may be confused with Medral® which is a brand name for omeprazole in Mexico

Related Information
Corticosteroids *on page 1780*

U.S. Brand Names Depo-Medrol®; Medrol®; Solu-Medrol®

Canadian Brand Names Depo-Medrol®; Medrol®; Methylprednisolone Acetate; Solu-Medrol®

Mexican Brand Names Advantan; Cryosolona; Depo-Medrol; Predlitem; Solu-Medrol

Index Terms 6-α-Methylprednisolone; A-Methapred; Methylprednisolone Acetate; Methylprednisolone Sodium Succinate

Pharmacologic Category Corticosteroid, Systemic

Use Primarily as an anti-inflammatory or immunosuppressant agent in the treatment of a variety of diseases including those of hematologic, allergic, inflammatory, neoplastic, and autoimmune origin. Prevention and treatment of graft-versus-host disease following allogeneic bone marrow transplantation.

Effect on Mental Status Nervousness and insomnia are common; may rarely cause delirium, mood swings, euphoria, or hallucinations

Effect on Psychiatric Treatment Barbiturates may increase the clearance of methylprednisolone

Dosage Summary Note: Dosing should be based on the lesser of ideal body weight or actual body weight. Only sodium succinate may be given I.V.

I.M.:
Acetate:
Children: Dosage not established

Adults: 10-80 mg every 1-2 weeks
Sodium succinate:
Children: 0.5-1.7 mg/kg/day **or** 5-25 mg/m²/day divided every 6-12 hours; "Pulse" therapy: 15-30 mg/kg/dose over ≥30 minutes given once daily for 3 days
Adults: 10-80 mg once daily

I.V. (sodium succinate):
Note: Dosage varies considerably by indication; ranges listed are representative.
Children: 0.5-4 mg/kg/day **or** 5-25 mg/m²/day divided every 6-12 hours; "Pulse" therapy: 15-30 mg/kg/dose over ≥30 minutes given once daily for 3 days or every other day for 6 doses.
Spinal cord injury: 30 mg/kg over 15 minutes, followed in 45 minutes by a continuous infusion of 5.4 mg/kg/hour for 23 hours.
Adults: 10-60 mg/dose at intervals depending on clinical response **or** 2 mg/kg/dose, then 0.5-1 mg/kg/dose every 6 hours **or** 1 g/day for 3 days **or** 1 mg/kg/day or 40 mg/day (whichever dose is higher), for 4 days **or** 30 mg/kg every 4-6 hours for 48 hours
Spinal cord injury: 30 mg/kg over 15 minutes, followed in 45 minutes by a continuous infusion of 5.4 mg/kg/hour for 23 hours [spinal cord injury]

Intra-articular (acetate):
Children: Dosage not established
Adults: Large joints: 20-80 mg; Small joints: 4-10 mg

Intralesional (acetate):
Children: Dosage not established
Adults: 20-60 mg every 1-5 weeks

Oral:
Children: 0.5-1.7 mg/kg/day **or** 5-25 mg/m²/day divided every 6-12 hours; "Pulse" therapy: 15-30 mg/kg/dose once daily for 3 days
Adults: 2-60 mg/day in 1-4 divided doses

Dosage Forms Excipient information presented when available (limited, particularly for generics); consult specific product labeling.
Injection, powder for reconstitution, as sodium succinate: 40 mg, 125 mg, 500 mg, 1 g [strength expressed as base]
Solu-Medrol®: 40 mg, 125 mg, 500 mg, 1 g, 2 g [contains benzyl alcohol (in diluent); strength expressed as base]
Solu-Medrol®: 500 mg, 1 g
Injection, suspension, as acetate: 40 mg/mL (5 mL, 10 mL); 80 mg/mL (5 mL)
Depo-Medrol®: 20 mg/mL (5 mL); 40 mg/mL (5 mL); 80 mg/mL (5 mL) [contains benzyl alcohol; strength expressed as base]
Depo-Medrol®: 40 mg/mL (1 mL); 80 mg/mL (1 mL)
Tablet: 4 mg
Medrol®: 2 mg, 4 mg, 8 mg, 16 mg, 32 mg
Tablet, dose-pack: 4 mg (21s)
Medrol® Dosepak™: 4 mg (21s)

- **6-α-Methylprednisolone** *see* MethylPREDNISolone *on page 1029*
- **Methylprednisolone Acetate** *see* MethylPREDNISolone *on page 1029*
- **Methylprednisolone Sodium Succinate** *see* MethylPREDNISolone *on page 1029*
- **4-Methylpyrazole** *see* Fomepizole *on page 685*

MethylTESTOSTERone (meth il tes TOS te rone)

Medication Safety Issues
Sound-alike/look-alike issues:
MethylTESTOSTERone may be confused with medroxyPROGESTERone
Virilon® may be confused with Verelan®

U.S. Brand Names Android®; Methitest™; Testred®; Virilon®

Pharmacologic Category Androgen

Use
Male: Hypogonadism; delayed puberty; impotence and climacteric symptoms
Female: Palliative treatment of metastatic breast cancer

Effect on Mental Status None reported

Effect on Psychiatric Treatment May cause leukopenia; use caution with clozapine and carbamazepine

Restrictions C-III

Dosage Summary
Buccal:
Children: Dosage not established

Adults: 5-100 mg/day

Oral:

Children: Dosage not established

Adults: 10-200 mg/day

Dosage Forms Excipient information presented when available (limited, particularly for generics); consult specific product labeling.

Capsule (Android®, Testred®, Virilon®): 10 mg

Tablet (Methitest™): 10 mg

Metipranolol (met i PRAN oh lol)

Medication Safety Issues

Sound-alike/look-alike issues:

Metipranolol may be confused with metaproterenol

International issues:

Betanol® [Monaco] may be confused with Beta-Val® which is a brand name for betamethasone in the U.S.

Betanol® [Monaco] may be confused with Patanol® which is a brand name for olopatadine in the U.S.

Betanol® [Monaco] may be confused with Betimol® which is a brand name for timolol in the U.S.

U.S. Brand Names OptiPranolol®

Canadian Brand Names OptiPranolol®

Index Terms Metipranolol Hydrochloride

Pharmacologic Category Beta-Adrenergic Blocker, Nonselective; Ophthalmic Agent, Antiglaucoma

Use Agent for lowering intraocular pressure in patients with chronic open-angle glaucoma

Effect on Mental Status None reported

Effect on Psychiatric Treatment May produce CNS depression; concurrent use with psychotropic agents may produce additive effects

Dosage Summary

Ophthalmic:

Children: Dosage not established

Adults: Instill 1 drop into affected eye(s) twice daily

Dosage Forms Excipient information presented when available (limited, particularly for generics); consult specific product labeling.

Solution, ophthalmic: 0.3% (5 mL, 10 mL) [contains benzalkonium chloride]

◆ **Metipranolol Hydrochloride** *see* Metipranolol *on page 1031*

Metoclopramide (met oh KLOE pra mide)

Medication Safety Issues

Sound-alike/look-alike issues:

Metoclopramide may be confused with metolazone

Reglan® may be confused with Megace®, Regonol®, Renagel®

U.S. Brand Names Reglan®

Canadian Brand Names Apo-Metoclop®; Metoclopramide Hydrochloride Injection; Nu-Metoclopramide

Mexican Brand Names Carnotprim; Dirpasid; Meclomid; Plasil; Polcotec

Pharmacologic Category Antiemetic; Gastrointestinal Agent, Prokinetic

Generic Available Yes

Use

Oral: Symptomatic treatment of diabetic gastric stasis; gastroesophageal reflux

I.V., I.M.: Symptomatic treatment of diabetic gastric stasis; postpyloric placement of enteral feeding tubes; prevention and/or treatment of nausea and vomiting associated with chemotherapy, or postsurgery; to stimulate gastric emptying and intestinal transit of barium during radiological examination

Effect on Mental Status Drowsiness and restlessness are common; may cause insomnia or depression. Depression has occurred in patients with and without a prior history of depression. Symptoms have ranged from mild to severe, and have included suicidal ideation and suicide. Metoclopramide is a D_2 blocker; may cause extrapyramidal symptoms especially when used in high dosages (dystonia) or in the elderly (tardive dyskinesia). Dystonic reactions occur in approximately 1 in 500 patients with the usual adult dosage of 30-40 mg/day. These reactions are usually seen during the first 1-2 days of therapy with metoclopramide, occurring more frequently in pediatric patients and adults <30 years of age, and are more frequent when higher doses are used in prophylaxis of vomiting due to cancer chemotherapy. NMS has rarely been reported.

Effect on Psychiatric Treatment Anticholinergics may antagonize metoclopramide's effects; concurrent use with psychotropic may produce additive sedation

Pregnancy Risk Factor B

Pregnancy Considerations Crosses the placenta; available evidence suggests safe use during pregnancy.

Lactation Enters breast milk/use caution

Contraindications Hypersensitivity to metoclopramide or any component of the formulation; GI obstruction, perforation or hemorrhage; pheochromocytoma; history of seizures

Warnings/Precautions Use caution with a history of mental illness; has been associated with extrapyramidal symptoms (EPS) and depression. The frequency of EPS is higher in pediatric patients and adults <30 years of age; risk is increased at higher dosages. Extrapyramidal reactions typically occur within the initial 24-48 hours of treatment. Use caution with concurrent use of other drugs associated with EPS. Use caution in the elderly and with Parkinson's disease; may have increased risk of tardive dyskinesia. Neuroleptic malignant syndrome (NMS) has been reported (rarely) with metoclopramide. Use lowest recommended doses initially; may cause transient increase in serum aldosterone; use caution in patients who are at risk of fluid overload (HF, cirrhosis). Use caution in patients with hypertension or following surgical anastomosis/closure. Patients with NADH-cytochrome b5 reductase deficiency are at increased risk of methemoglobinemia and/or sulfhemoglobinemia. Abrupt discontinuation may (rarely) result in withdrawal symptoms (dizziness, headache, nervousness). Use caution and adjust dose in renal impairment.

Adverse Reactions Frequency not always defined.

Cardiovascular: AV block, bradycardia, CHF, fluid retention, flushing (following high I.V. doses), hyper-/hypotension, supraventricular tachycardia

Central nervous system: Drowsiness (~10% to 70%; dose related), fatigue (~10%), restlessness (~10%), acute dystonic reactions (<1% to 25%; dose and age related), akathisia, confusion, depression, dizziness, hallucinations (rare), headache, insomnia, neuroleptic malignant syndrome (rare), Parkinsonian-like symptoms, suicidal ideation, seizure, tardive dyskinesia

Dermatologic: Angioneurotic edema (rare), rash, urticaria

Endocrine & metabolic: Amenorrhea, galactorrhea, gynecomastia, impotence

Gastrointestinal: Diarrhea, nausea

Genitourinary: Incontinence, urinary frequency

Hematologic: Agranulocytosis, leukopenia, neutropenia, porphyria

Hepatic: Hepatotoxicity (rare)

Ocular: Visual disturbance

Respiratory: Bronchospasm, laryngeal edema (rare)

Miscellaneous: Allergic reactions, methemoglobinemia, sulfhemoglobinemia

Metabolism/Transport Effects Substrate (minor) of CYP1A2, 2D6; **Inhibits** CYP2D6 (weak)

Drug Interactions

Anti-Parkinson's Agents (Dopamine Agonist): Metoclopramide may diminish the therapeutic effect of Anti-Parkinson's Agents (Dopamine Agonist). *Risk C: Monitor therapy*

CycloSPORINE: Metoclopramide may increase the absorption of CycloSPORINE. *Risk C: Monitor therapy*

Sertraline: Metoclopramide may enhance the adverse/toxic effect of Sertraline. Specifically, the risk of serotonin syndrome may be increased. *Risk C: Monitor therapy*

Venlafaxine: Metoclopramide may enhance the adverse/toxic effect of Venlafaxine. Specifically, the risk of serotonin syndrome may be increased. *Risk C: Monitor therapy*

Ethanol/Nutrition/Herb Interactions Ethanol: Avoid ethanol (may increase CNS depression).

Stability

Injection: Store intact vial at controlled room temperature. Injection is photosensitive and should be protected from light during storage. Parenteral admixtures in D_5W or NS are stable for at least 24 hours and do not require light protection if used within 24 hours.

Tablet: Store at controlled room temperature.

Mechanism of Action Blocks dopamine receptors and (when given in higher doses) also blocks serotonin receptors in chemoreceptor trigger zone of the CNS; enhances the response to acetylcholine of tissue in upper GI tract causing enhanced motility and accelerated gastric emptying without stimulating gastric, biliary, or pancreatic secretions; increases lower esophageal sphincter tone

Pharmacodynamics/Kinetics

Onset of action: Oral: 0.5-1 hour; I.V.: 1-3 minutes; I.M.: 10-15 minutes
Duration: Therapeutic: 1-2 hours, regardless of route
Distribution: V_d: 2-4 L/kg
Protein binding: 30%
Bioavailability: Oral: 65% to 95%
Half-life elimination: Normal renal function: 4-6 hours (may be dose dependent)
Time to peak, serum: Oral: 1-2 hours
Excretion: Urine (~85%)

Dosage

Children:
- Gastroesophageal reflux (unlabeled use): Oral: 0.1-0.2 mg/kg/dose 4 times/day
- Antiemetic (chemotherapy-induced emesis) (unlabeled): I.V.: 1-2 mg/kg 30 minutes before chemotherapy and every 2-4 hours
- Postpyloric feeding tube placement: I.V.:
  - <6 years: 0.1 mg/kg
  - 6-14 years: 2.5-5 mg
  - >14 years: Refer to adult dosing.

Adults:
- Gastroesophageal reflux: Oral: 10-15 mg/dose up to 4 times/day 30 minutes before meals or food and at bedtime; single doses of 20 mg are occasionally needed for provoking situations. Treatment >12 weeks has not been evaluated.
- Diabetic gastric stasis:
  - Oral: 10 mg 30 minutes before each meal and at bedtime
  - I.M., I.V. (for severe symptoms): 10 mg over 1-2 minutes; 10 days of I.V. therapy may be necessary for best response
- Chemotherapy-induced emesis:
  - I.V.: 1-2 mg/kg 30 minutes before chemotherapy and repeated every 2 hours for 2 doses, then every 3 hours for 3 doses (manufacturer labeling)
    - Alternate dosing (with or without diphenhydramine):
      - Moderate emetic risk chemotherapy: 0.5 mg/kg every 6 hours on days 2-4
      - Low and minimal risk chemotherapy: 1-2 mg/kg every 3-4 hours
      - Breakthrough treatment: 1-2 mg/kg every 3-4 hours
  - Oral (unlabeled use; with or without diphenhydramine):
    - Moderate emetic risk chemotherapy: 0.5 mg/kg every 6 hours or 20 mg 4 times/day on days 2-4
    - Low and minimal risk chemotherapy: 20-40 mg every 4-6 hours
    - Breakthrough treatment: 20-40 mg every 4-6 hours
- Postoperative nausea and vomiting: I.M., I.V.: 10-20 mg near end of surgery
- Postpyloric feeding tube placement, radiological exam: I.V.: 10 mg

Elderly:
- Gastroesophageal reflux: Oral: 5 mg 4 times/day (30 minutes before meals or food and at bedtime); increase dose to 10 mg 4 times/day if no response at lower dose
- Gastrointestinal hypomotility:
  - Oral: Initial: 5 mg 30 minutes before meals and at bedtime; increase if necessary to 10 mg doses
  - I.V.: Initiate at 5 mg over 1-2 minutes; increase to 10 mg if necessary
- Postoperative nausea and vomiting: I.M., I.V.: 5 mg near end of surgery; may repeat dose if necessary

Dosing adjustment in renal impairment: Cl_{cr} <40 mL/minute: Administer at 50% of normal dose

Hemodialysis: Not dialyzable (0% to 5%); supplemental dose is not necessary

Administration Injection solution may be given I.M., direct I.V. push, short infusion (15-30 minutes), or continuous infusion; lower doses (≤10 mg) of metoclopramide can be given I.V. push undiluted over 1-2 minutes; higher doses to be given IVPB over at least 15 minutes; continuous SubQ infusion and rectal administration have been reported. **Note:** Rapid I.V. administration may be associated with a transient (but intense) feeling of anxiety and restlessness, followed by drowsiness.

Monitoring Parameters Dystonic reactions; signs of hypoglycemia in patients using insulin and those being treated for gastroparesis; agitation, and onfusion

Test Interactions Increased aminotransferase [ALT/AST] (S), increased amylase (S)

Dosage Forms Excipient information presented when available (limited, particularly for generics); consult specific product labeling.

Injection, solution [preservative free]: 5 mg/mL (2 mL)
- Reglan®: 5 mg/mL (2 mL, 10 mL, 30 mL)

Solution, oral: 5 mg/5 mL (10 mL, 480 mL)
Tablet: 5 mg, 10 mg
Reglan®: 5 mg, 10 mg

Metolazone (me TOLE a zone)

Medication Safety Issues
Sound-alike/look-alike issues:
Metolazone may be confused with metaxalone, methazolamide, methimazole, methotrexate, metoclopramide, metoprolol, minoxidil
Zaroxolyn® may be confused with Zarontin®

U.S. Brand Names Zaroxolyn®

Canadian Brand Names Zaroxolyn®

Pharmacologic Category Diuretic, Thiazide-Related

Generic Available Yes

Use Management of mild to moderate hypertension; treatment of edema in congestive heart failure and nephrotic syndrome, impaired renal function

Effect on Mental Status Dizziness is common; may cause drowsiness

Effect on Psychiatric Treatment May rarely cause agranulocytosis; use caution with clozapine and carbamazepine; may decrease lithium clearance resulting in an increase in serum lithium levels and potential lithium toxicity; monitor serum lithium levels

Pregnancy Risk Factor B (manufacturer); D (expert analysis)

Pregnancy Considerations Teratogenic effects were not observed in animal studies. Metolazone crosses the placenta and appears in cord blood. Hypoglycemia, hypokalemia, hyponatremia, jaundice, and thrombocytopenia are reported as complications to the fetus or newborn following maternal use of thiazide diuretics.

Lactation Enters breast milk/not recommended

Contraindications Hypersensitivity to metolazone, any component of the formulation, other thiazides, and sulfonamide derivatives; anuria; hepatic coma; pregnancy (expert analysis)

Warnings/Precautions Electrolyte disturbances (hypokalemia, hypochloremic alkalosis, hyponatremia) can occur. Large or prolonged fluid and electrolyte losses may occur with concomitant furosemide administration. Use with caution in severe hepatic dysfunction; hepatic encephalopathy can be caused by electrolyte disturbances. Gout can be precipitate in certain patients with a history of gout, a familial predisposition to gout, or chronic renal failure. Cautious use in patients with prediabetes or diabetes; may see a change in glucose control. Can cause SLE exacerbation or activation. Use caution in severe renal impairment. Use with caution in patients with moderate or high cholesterol concentrations. Photosensitization may occur.

Chemical similarities are present among sulfonamides, sulfonylureas, carbonic anhydrase inhibitors, thiazides, and loop diuretics (except ethacrynic acid). Use in patients with thiazide or sulfonamide allergy is specifically contraindicated in product labeling, however, a risk of cross-reaction exists in patients with allergy to any of these compounds; avoid use when previous reaction has been severe. Discontinue if signs of hypersensitivity are noted.

Adverse Reactions Frequency not defined.
Cardiovascular: Chest pain/discomfort, necrotizing angiitis, orthostatic hypotension, palpitation, syncope, venous thrombosis, vertigo, volume depletion
Central nervous system: chills, depression, dizziness, drowsiness, fatigue, headache, lightheadedness, restlessness
Dermatologic: Petechiae, photosensitivity, pruritus, purpura, rash, skin necrosis, Stevens-Johnson syndrome, toxic epidermal necrolysis, urticaria
Endocrine & metabolic: Gout attacks, hypercalcemia, hyperglycemia, hyperuricemia, hypochloremia, hypochloremic alkalosis, hypokalemia, hypomagnesemia, hyponatremia, hypophosphatemia
Gastrointestinal: Abdominal bloating, abdominal pain, anorexia, constipation, diarrhea, epigastric distress, nausea, pancreatitis, vomiting, xerostomia
Genitourinary: Impotence
Hematologic: Agranulocytosis, aplastic/hypoplastic anemia, hemoconcentration, leukopenia, thrombocytopenia
Hepatic: Cholestatic jaundice, hepatitis
Neuromuscular & skeletal: Joint pain, muscle cramps/spasm, neuropathy, paresthesia, weakness
Ocular: Blurred vision (transient)
Renal: BUN increased, glucosuria

Drug Interactions

ACE Inhibitors: Thiazide Diuretics may enhance the hypotensive effect of ACE Inhibitors. Specifically, postural hypotension which can accompany ACE Inhibitor initiation. Thiazide Diuretics may enhance the nephrotoxic effect of ACE Inhibitors. *Risk C: Monitor therapy*

Allopurinol: Thiazide Diuretics may enhance the potential for allergic or hypersensitivity reactions to Allopurinol. Thiazide Diuretics may increase the serum concentration of Allopurinol. Specifically, Thiazide Diuretics may increase the concentration of Oxypurinolol, an active metabolite of Allopurinol. *Risk C: Monitor therapy*

Bile Acid Sequestrants: May decrease the absorption of Thiazide Diuretics. The diuretic response is likewise decreased. *Risk D: Consider therapy modification*

Calcitriol: Thiazide Diuretics may enhance the hypercalcemic effect of Calcitriol. *Risk C: Monitor therapy*

Calcium Salts: Thiazide Diuretics may decrease the excretion of Calcium Salts. Continued concomitant use can also result in metabolic alkalosis. *Risk C: Monitor therapy*

Corticosteroids (Orally Inhaled): May enhance the hypokalemic effect of Thiazide Diuretics. *Risk C: Monitor therapy*

Corticosteroids (Systemic): May enhance the hypokalemic effect of Thiazide Diuretics. *Risk C: Monitor therapy*

Dofetilide: Thiazide Diuretics may enhance the QTc-prolonging effect of Dofetilide. Thiazide Diuretics may increase the serum concentration of Dofetilide. *Risk D: Consider therapy modification*

Herbs (Hypertensive Properties): May diminish the antihypertensive effect of Antihypertensives. *Risk C: Monitor therapy*

Herbs (Hypotensive Properties): May enhance the hypotensive effect of Antihypertensives. *Risk C: Monitor therapy*

Lithium: Thiazide Diuretics may decrease the excretion of Lithium. *Risk D: Consider therapy modification*

Methylphenidate: May diminish the antihypertensive effect of Antihypertensives. *Risk C: Monitor therapy*

Nonsteroidal Anti-Inflammatory Agents: May diminish the therapeutic effect of Thiazide Diuretics. *Risk C: Monitor therapy*

Prostacyclin Analogues: May enhance the hypotensive effect of Antihypertensives. *Risk C: Monitor therapy*

RiTUXimab: Antihypertensives may enhance the hypotensive effect of RiTUXimab. *Risk D: Consider therapy modification*

Ethanol/Nutrition/Herb Interactions

Ethanol: May potentiate hypotensive effect of metazolone.

Herb/Nutraceutical: Avoid dong quai if using for hypertension (has estrogenic activity). Avoid dong quai, St John's wort (may also cause photosensitization). Avoid ephedra, yohimbe, ginseng (may worsen hypertension). Avoid natural licorice. Avoid garlic (may have increased antihypertensive effect).

Mechanism of Action Inhibits sodium reabsorption in the distal tubules causing increased excretion of sodium and water, as well as, potassium and hydrogen ions

Pharmacodynamics/Kinetics

Onset of action: Diuresis: ~60 minutes

Duration: ≥24 hours

Absorption: Incomplete

Distribution: Crosses placenta; enters breast milk

Protein binding: 95%

Half-life elimination: 20 hours

Excretion: Urine (80%); bile (10%)

Dosage Oral:

Adults:

Edema: 2.5-20 mg/dose every 24 hours (ACC/AHA 2005 Heart Failure Guidelines)

Hypertension: 2.5-5 mg/dose every 24 hours

Elderly: Initial: 2.5 mg/day or every other day

Dosage adjustment in renal impairment: Dialysis: Not dialyzable (0% to 5%) via hemo- or peritoneal dialysis; supplemental dose is not necessary

Dietary Considerations Should be taken after breakfast; may require potassium supplementation

Administration May be taken with food or milk. Take early in day to avoid nocturia. Take the last dose of multiple doses no later than 6 PM unless instructed otherwise.

Monitoring Parameters Serum electrolytes (potassium, sodium, chloride, bicarbonate), renal function, blood pressure (standing, sitting/supine)

Additional Information Metolazone 5 mg is approximately equivalent to hydrochlorothiazide 50 mg.

Dosage Forms Excipient information presented when available (limited, particularly for generics); consult specific product labeling.

Tablet: 2.5 mg, 5 mg, 10 mg

Zaroxolyn®: 2.5 mg, 5 mg, 10 mg

Metoprolol (me toe PROE lole)

Medication Safety Issues

Sound-alike/look-alike issues:

Metoprolol may be confused with metaproterenol, metolazone, misoprostol

Toprol-XL® may be confused with Tegretol®, Tegretol®-XR, Topamax®

High alert medication: The Institute for Safe Medication Practices (ISMP) includes this medication among its list of drugs which have a heightened risk of causing significant patient harm when used in error.

Significant differences exist between oral and I.V. dosing. Use caution when converting from one route of administration to another.

Related Information

Beta-Blockers *on page 1776*

U.S. Brand Names Lopressor®; Toprol-XL®

Canadian Brand Names Apo-Metoprolol®; Betaloc®; Betaloc® Durules®; Dom-Metoprolol; Gen-Metoprolol; Lopressor®; Metoprolol Tartrate Injection, USP; Metoprolol-25; Novo-Metoprolol; Nu-Metop; PHL-Metoprolol; PMS-Metoprolol; Sandoz-Metoprolol; Toprol-XL®

Mexican Brand Names Lopresor; Mezelol; Nipresol; Promiced; Seloken-Zok

Index Terms Metoprolol Succinate; Metoprolol Tartrate

Pharmacologic Category Beta Blocker, $Beta_1$ Selective

Generic Available Yes

Use Treatment of angina pectoris, hypertension, or hemodynamically-stable acute myocardial infarction

Extended release: Treatment of angina pectoris or hypertension; to reduce mortality/hospitalization in patients with heart failure (stable NYHA Class II or III) already receiving ACE inhibitors, diuretics, and/or digoxin

Unlabeled/Investigational Use Treatment of ventricular arrhythmias, atrial ectopy; migraine prophylaxis, essential tremor, aggressive behavior (not recommended for dementia-associated aggression); prevention of myocardial infarction, atrial fibrillation, and atrial flutter; symptomatic treatment of hypertrophic obstructive cardiomyopathy

Effect on Mental Status Sedation and dizziness are common; may cause depression; may rarely cause insomnia, confusion, amnesia, or nightmares

Effect on Psychiatric Treatment Barbiturates may decrease the effects of metoprolol; beta-blockers may increase the effects of psychotropics; monitor clinical status for potential changes

Pregnancy Risk Factor C (manufacturer); D (2nd and 3rd trimesters - expert analysis)

Pregnancy Considerations Teratogenic effects were not observed in animal studies. Metoprolol crosses the placenta. Maternal use of beta-blockers has been associated with fetal bradycardia, hypotension, and IUGR; IUGR is probably related to maternal hypertension. Available evidence suggests beta-blockers are generally safe during pregnancy (JNC 7). Cases of neonatal hypoglycemia have been reported following maternal use of beta-blockers at parturition. Information specific to metoprolol is limited.

Lactation Enters breast milk/use caution (AAP rates "compatible")

Contraindications Note: Contraindications are indication-specific.

Hypersensitivity to metoprolol, any component of the formulation, or other beta-blockers; additionally:

Hypertension and angina: Sick sinus syndrome (except in patients with a functioning artificial pacemaker); severe peripheral arterial disease; pheochromocytoma (without alpha blockade)

Myocardial infarction: Severe sinus bradycardia (heart rate <45 beats/minute); significant first-degree heart block (P-R interval ≥0.24 seconds); second- and third-degree heart block; systolic blood pressure <100 mm Hg; moderate-to-severe cardiac failure; cardiogenic shock

Warnings/Precautions [U.S. Boxed Warning]: Beta-blocker therapy should not be withdrawn abruptly (particularly in patients with CAD), but gradually tapered over 1-2 weeks to avoid acute tachycardia, hypertension, and/or ischemia. Consider pre-existing conditions such as sick sinus syndrome before initiating. Metoprolol commonly produces mild first-degree heart block (P-R interval >0.2-0.24 sec). May also produce severe first- (P-R interval ≥0.26 sec), second-, or third-degree heart block. Patients with acute MI (especially right ventricular MI) have a high risk of developing heart block of varying degrees. If severe heart block occurs, metoprolol should be discontinued and measures to increase heart rate should be employed. Symptomatic hypotension may occur with use. Use caution in patients with PVD (can aggravate arterial insufficiency). Use caution with concurrent use of beta-blockers and either verapamil or diltiazem; bradycardia or heart block can occur; avoid concurrent I.V. use of both agents.

In general, beta-blockers should be avoided in patients with bronchospastic disease. Metoprolol, with B_1 selectivity, should be used cautiously in bronchospastic disease with close monitoring. Use cautiously in patients with diabetes because it can mask prominent hypoglycemic symptoms. Use caution in hyperthyroidism since beta-blockade may mask signs of thyrotoxicosis. Use caution with hepatic dysfunction. Use with caution in patients with myasthenia gravis or psychiatric disease (may cause CNS depression). Use caution with inhalation anesthetic agents which may decrease myocardial function. Use of beta-blockers may unmask cardiac failure in patients without a history of dysfunction. Adequate alpha-blockade is required prior to use of any beta-blocker for patients with untreated pheochromocytoma. Use caution with history of severe anaphylaxis to allergens; patients taking beta-blockers may become more sensitive to repeated allergen challenges. Treatment of anaphylaxis (eg, epinephrine) in patients taking beta-blockers may be ineffective or promote undesirable effects. Safety and efficacy have not been established in children <1 year of age.

Extended release: Use with caution in patients with compensated heart failure; monitor for a worsening of heart failure.

Adverse Reactions Frequency may not be defined.

Cardiovascular: Hypotension (1% to 27%), bradycardia (2% to 16%), first-degree heart block (P-R interval ≥0.26 sec; 5%), arterial insufficiency (usually Raynaud type; 1%), chest pain (1%), CHF (1%), edema (peripheral; 1%), palpitation (1%), syncope (1%)

Central nervous system: Dizziness (2% to 10%), fatigue (1% to 10%), depression (5%), confusion, hallucinations, headache, insomnia, memory loss (short-term), nightmares, sleep disturbances, somnolence, vertigo

Dermatology: Pruritus (5%), rash (5%), photosensitivity, psoriasis exacerbated

Endocrine & metabolic: Libido decreased, Peyronie's disease (<1%), diabetes exacerbated

Gastrointestinal: Diarrhea (5%), constipation (1%), flatulence (1%), gastrointestinal pain (1%), heartburn (1%), nausea (1%), xerostomia (1%), vomiting

Hematologic: Claudication

Neuromuscular & skeletal: Musculoskeletal pain

Ocular: Blurred vision, visual disturbances

Otic: Tinnitus

Respiratory: Dyspnea (1% to 3%), bronchospasm (1%), wheezing (1%), rhinitis

Miscellaneous: Cold extremities (1%)

Postmarketing and/or case reports: Agranulocytosis, alkaline phosphatase increased, alopecia (reversible), arthralgia, arthritis, anxiety, cardiogenic shock, diaphoresis increased, dry eyes, gangrene, hepatitis, HDL decreased, impotence, jaundice, lactate dehydrogenase increased, nervousness, paresthesia, retroperitoneal fibrosis, second-degree heart block, taste disturbance, third-degree heart block, thrombocytopenia, transaminases increased, triglycerides increased, urticaria, vomiting, weight gain

Other events reported with beta-blockers: Catatonia, emotional lability, fever, hypersensitivity reactions, laryngospasm, nonthrombocytopenic purpura, respiratory distress, thrombocytopenic purpura

Metabolism/Transport Effects **Substrate** of CYP2C19 (minor), 2D6 (major); **Inhibits** CYP2D6 (weak)

Drug Interactions

Acetylcholinesterase Inhibitors: May enhance the bradycardic effect of Beta-Blockers. *Risk C: Monitor therapy*

Alpha-/Beta-Agonists (Direct-Acting): Beta-Blockers may enhance the vasopressor effect of Alpha-/Beta-Agonists (Direct-Acting). Epinephrine used as a local anesthetic for dental procedures will not likely cause clinically relevant problems. **Exceptions:** Dipivefrin. *Risk D: Consider therapy modification*

Alpha1-Blockers: Beta-Blockers may enhance the orthostatic effect of Alpha1-Blockers. The risk associated with ophthalmic products is probably less than systemic products. *Risk D: Consider therapy modification*

Alpha2-Agonists: Beta-Blockers may enhance the rebound hypertensive effect of Alpha2-Agonists. This effect can occur when the $alpha_2$-agonist is abruptly withdrawn. **Exceptions:** Apraclonidine; Brimonidine. *Risk D: Consider therapy modification*

Aminoquinolines (Antimalarial): May decrease the metabolism of Beta-Blockers. *Risk C: Monitor therapy*

Amiodarone: May enhance the bradycardic effect of Beta-Blockers. Possibly to the point of cardiac arrest. Amiodarone may increase the serum concentration of Beta-Blockers. *Risk C: Monitor therapy*

Anilidopiperidine Opioids: May enhance the bradycardic effect of Beta-Blockers. Anilidopiperidine Opioids may enhance the hypotensive effect of Beta-Blockers. *Risk C: Monitor therapy*

Antipsychotic Agents (Phenothiazines): May enhance the hypotensive effect of Beta-Blockers. Beta-Blockers may decrease the metabolism of Antipsychotic Agents (Phenothiazines). Antipsychotic Agents (Phenothiazines) may decrease the metabolism of Beta-Blockers. *Risk C: Monitor therapy*

Barbiturates: May decrease the serum concentration of Beta-Blockers. *Risk C: Monitor therapy*

Beta2-Agonists: Beta-Blockers (Beta1 Selective) may diminish the bronchodilatory effect of Beta2-Agonists. Of particular concern with nonselective beta-blockers or higher doses of the beta1 selective beta-blockers. *Risk C: Monitor therapy*

Calcium Channel Blockers (Nondihydropyridine): May enhance the hypotensive effect of Beta-Blockers. Bradycardia and signs of heart failure have also been reported. Calcium Channel Blockers (Nondihydropyridine) may increase the serum concentration of Beta-Blockers. *Risk C: Monitor therapy*

Cardiac Glycosides: Beta-Blockers may enhance the bradycardic effect of Cardiac Glycosides. *Risk C: Monitor therapy*

CYP2D6 Inhibitors (Moderate): May decrease the metabolism of CYP2D6 Substrates. *Risk C: Monitor therapy*

CYP2D6 Inhibitors (Strong): May decrease the metabolism of CYP2D6 Substrates. *Risk D: Consider therapy modification*

Darunavir: May increase the serum concentration of CYP2D6 Substrates. *Risk C: Monitor therapy*

Diazoxide: May enhance the hypotensive effect of Antihypertensives. *Risk C: Monitor therapy*

Dipyridamole: May enhance the bradycardic effect of Beta-Blockers. *Risk C: Monitor therapy*

Disopyramide: May enhance the bradycardic effect of Beta-Blockers. *Risk C: Monitor therapy*

Herbs (Hypertensive Properties): May diminish the antihypertensive effect of Antihypertensives. *Risk C: Monitor therapy*

Herbs (Hypotensive Properties): May enhance the hypotensive effect of Antihypertensives. *Risk C: Monitor therapy*

Insulin: Beta-Blockers may enhance the hypoglycemic effect of Insulin. *Risk C: Monitor therapy*

Lidocaine: Beta-Blockers may decrease the metabolism of Lidocaine. *Risk C: Monitor therapy*

Methacholine: Beta-Blockers may enhance the adverse/toxic effect of Methacholine. *Risk X: Avoid combination*

Methylphenidate: May diminish the antihypertensive effect of Antihypertensives. *Risk C: Monitor therapy*

Midodrine: Beta-Blockers may enhance the bradycardic effect of Midodrine. *Risk C: Monitor therapy*

Nonsteroidal Anti-Inflammatory Agents: May diminish the antihypertensive effect of Beta-Blockers. *Risk C: Monitor therapy*

Propafenone: May decrease the metabolism of Beta-Blockers. Propafenone possesses some independent beta blocking activity. *Risk C: Monitor therapy*

Propoxyphene: May decrease the metabolism of Beta-Blockers. *Risk C: Monitor therapy*

Prostacyclin Analogues: May enhance the hypotensive effect of Antihypertensives. *Risk C: Monitor therapy*

QuiNIDine: May decrease the metabolism of Beta-Blockers. *Risk C: Monitor therapy*

Reserpine: May enhance the hypotensive effect of Beta-Blockers. *Risk C: Monitor therapy*

Rifamycin Derivatives: May decrease the serum concentration of Beta-Blockers. **Exceptions:** Rifabutin. *Risk C: Monitor therapy*

RiTUXimab: Antihypertensives may enhance the hypotensive effect of RiTUXimab. *Risk D: Consider therapy modification*

Selective Serotonin Reuptake Inhibitors: May enhance the bradycardic effect of Beta-Blockers. **Exceptions:** Fluvoxamine. *Risk C: Monitor therapy*

Theophylline Derivatives: Beta-Blockers (Beta1 Selective) may diminish the bronchodilatory effect of Theophylline Derivatives. This is true at higher beta-blockers doses where cardioselectivity is lost. *Risk C: Monitor therapy*

Ethanol/Nutrition/Herb Interactions

Food: Food increases absorption. Metoprolol serum levels may be increased if taken with food.

Herb/Nutraceutical: Avoid bayberry, blue cohosh, cayenne, ephedra, ginger, ginseng (American), gotu kola, licorice, (may worsen hypertension). Avoid black cohosh, California poppy, coleus, golden seal, hawthorn, mistletoe, periwinkle, quinine, shepherd's purse (may have increased antihypertensive effect).

Stability

Injection: Store at controlled room temperature of 25°C (77°F). Protect from light.

Tablet: Store at controlled room temperature of 25°C (77°F). Protect from moisture.

Mechanism of Action Selective inhibitor of $beta_1$-adrenergic receptors; competitively blocks $beta_1$-receptors, with little or no effect on $beta_2$-receptors at doses <100 mg; does not exhibit any membrane stabilizing or intrinsic sympathomimetic activity

Pharmacodynamics/Kinetics

Onset of action: Peak effect: Oral: 1.5-4 hours; I.V.: 20 minutes (when infused over 10 minutes)

Duration: Oral: Immediate release: 10-20 hours, Extended release: ~24 hours; I.V.: 5-8 hours

Absorption: 95%, rapid and complete

Protein binding: 12% to albumin

Metabolism: Extensively hepatic via CYP2D6; significant first-pass effect (~50%)

Bioavailability: Oral: ~50%

Half-life elimination: 3-8 hours (dependent on rate of CYP2D6 metabolism)

Excretion: Urine (<5% to 10% as unchanged drug)

Dosage

Children: Hypertension: Oral:

1-17 years: Immediate release tablet: (National High Blood Pressure Education Program Working Group on High Blood Pressure in Children and Adolescents, 2004): Initial: 1-2 mg/kg/day; maximum 6 mg/kg/day (≤200 mg/day); administer in 2 divided doses

≥6 years: Extended release tablet: Initial: 1 mg/kg once daily (maximum initial dose: 50 mg/day). Adjust dose based on patient response (maximum: 2 mg/kg/day or 200 mg/day)

Adults:

Hypertension: Oral: 100-450 mg/day in 2-3 divided doses, begin with 50 mg twice daily and increase doses at weekly intervals to desired effect; usual dosage range (JNC 7): 50-100 mg/day

Extended release: Initial: 25-100 mg/day (maximum: 400 mg/day)

Angina, SVT, MI prophylaxis: Oral: 100-450 mg/day in 2-3 divided doses, begin with 50 mg twice daily and increase doses at weekly intervals to desired effect

Extended release: Initial: 100 mg/day (maximum: 400 mg/day)

Hypertension/ventricular rate control: I.V. (in patients having nonfunctioning GI tract): Initial: 1.25-5 mg every 6-12 hours; titrate initial dose to response. Initially, low doses may be appropriate to establish response; however, up to 15 mg every 3-6 hours has been employed.

Congestive heart failure: Oral (extended release): Initial: 25 mg once daily (reduce to 12.5 mg once daily in NYHA class higher than class II); may double dosage every 2 weeks as tolerated (maximum: 200 mg/day)

Myocardial infarction (acute): I.V.: 5 mg every 2 minutes for 3 doses in early treatment of myocardial infarction; thereafter give 50 mg orally every 6 hours 15 minutes after last I.V. dose and continue for 48 hours; then administer a maintenance dose of 100 mg twice daily.

Elderly: Initiate at the lower end of the dosage range

Note: Switching dosage forms:

When switching from immediate release metoprolol to extended release, the same total daily dose of metoprolol should be used.

When switching between oral and intravenous dosage forms, equivalent beta-blocking effect is achieved when doses in a 2.5:1 (Oral:I.V.) ratio is used.

Dosing adjustment in renal impairment: No adjustment required.

Dosing adjustment in hepatic impairment: Reduced dose may be necessary ▶

Dietary Considerations Regular tablets should be taken with food. Extended release tablets may be taken without regard to meals.

Administration

Oral: Extended release tablets may be divided in half; do not crush or chew.

I.V.: When administered acutely for cardiac treatment, monitor ECG and blood pressure. May administer by rapid infusion (I.V. push) over 1 minute or by slow infusion (ie, 5-10 mg of metoprolol in 50 mL of fluid) over ~30 minutes. Necessary monitoring for surgical patients who are unable to take oral beta-blockers (prolonged ileus) has not been defined. Some institutions require monitoring of baseline and postinfusion heart rate and blood pressure when a patient's response to beta-blockade has not been characterized (ie, the patient's initial dose or following a change in dose). Consult individual institutional policies and procedures.

Monitoring Parameters Acute cardiac treatment: Monitor ECG and blood pressure with I.V. administration; heart rate and blood pressure with oral administration

Dosage Forms Excipient information presented when available (limited, particularly for generics); consult specific product labeling.

Injection, solution, as tartrate: 1 mg/mL (5 mL)

Lopressor®: 1 mg/mL (5 mL)

Tablet, as tartrate: 25 mg, 50 mg, 100 mg

Lopressor®: 50 mg, 100 mg

Tablet, extended release, as succinate: 25 mg, 50 mg, 100 mg, 200 mg [expressed as mg equivalent to tartrate]

Toprol-XL®: 25 mg, 50 mg, 100 mg, 200 mg [expressed as mg equivalent to tartrate]

Metoprolol and Hydrochlorothiazide

(me toe PROE lole & hye droe klor oh THYE a zide)

U.S. Brand Names Lopressor HCT®

Mexican Brand Names Selopres Zok

Index Terms Hydrochlorothiazide and Metoprolol; Hydrochlorothiazide and Metoprolol Tartrate; Metoprolol Tartrate and Hydrochlorothiazide

Pharmacologic Category Beta Blocker, $Beta_1$ Selective; Diuretic, Thiazide

Use Treatment of hypertension (not recommended for initial treatment)

Effect on Mental Status May cause dizziness, drowsiness, or abnormal dreams

Effect on Psychiatric Treatment Hydrochlorothiazide decreases lithium clearance resulting in an increase in serum lithium levels and potential for lithium toxicity; monitor lithium levels. Beta-blockers may increase the effects of psychotropics; monitor clinical status for potential changes.

Dosage Summary

Oral:

Children: Dosage not established

Adults: Metoprolol 50-100 mg and hydrochlorothiazide 25-50 mg administered daily as single or 2 divided doses (maximum: 50 mg/day [hydrochlorothiazide])

Dosage Forms Excipient information presented when available (limited, particularly for generics); consult specific product labeling.

Tablet:

50/25: Metoprolol tartrate 50 mg and hydrochlorothiazide 25 mg

100/25: Metoprolol tartrate 100 mg and hydrochlorothiazide 25 mg

100/50: Metoprolol tartrate 100 mg and hydrochlorothiazide 50 mg

◆ **Metoprolol Succinate** *see* Metoprolol *on page 1036*

◆ **Metoprolol Tartrate** *see* Metoprolol *on page 1036*

◆ **Metoprolol Tartrate and Hydrochlorothiazide** *see* Metoprolol and Hydrochlorothiazide *on page 1040*

◆ **MetroCream®** *see* MetroNIDAZOLE *on page 1040*

◆ **MetroGel®** *see* MetroNIDAZOLE *on page 1040*

◆ **MetroGel-Vaginal®** *see* MetroNIDAZOLE *on page 1040*

◆ **MetroLotion®** *see* MetroNIDAZOLE *on page 1040*

MetroNIDAZOLE (met roe NYE da zole)

Medication Safety Issues

Sound-alike/look-alike issues:

MetroNIDAZOLE may be confused with meropenem, metFORMIN

U.S. Brand Names Flagyl ER®; Flagyl®; MetroCream®; MetroGel-Vaginal®; MetroGel®; MetroLotion®; Noritate®; Vandazole™

Canadian Brand Names Apo-Metronidazole®; Flagyl®; Florazole® ER; MetroCream®; Metrogel®; Nidagel™; Noritate®; Trikacide

Mexican Brand Names Amebidal; Elyzol-S; Epaq; Flagenase; Flagyl; MetroCream; MetroGel; Otrozol; Vertisal

Index Terms Metronidazole Hydrochloride

Pharmacologic Category Amebicide; Antibiotic, Miscellaneous; Antibiotic, Topical; Antiprotozoal, Nitroimidazole

Generic Available Yes: Capsule, cream, gel, infusion, lotion, tablet

Use Treatment of susceptible anaerobic bacterial and protozoal infections in the following conditions: Amebiasis, symptomatic and asymptomatic trichomoniasis; skin and skin structure infections; CNS infections; intra-abdominal infections (as part of combination regimen); systemic anaerobic infections; treatment of antibiotic-associated pseudomembranous colitis (AAPC), bacterial vaginosis; as part of a multidrug regimen for *H. pylori* eradication to reduce the risk of duodenal ulcer recurrence

Topical: Treatment of inflammatory lesions and erythema of rosacea

Unlabeled/Investigational Use Crohn's disease

Effect on Mental Status Dizziness is common; case reports of depression, insomnia, confusion, panic, delusions, hallucinations, exacerbation of schizophrenia

Effect on Psychiatric Treatment May rarely cause leukopenia; use caution with clozapine and carbamazepine; may decrease lithium clearance resulting in an increase in serum lithium levels and potential lithium toxicity; monitor serum lithium levels

Pregnancy Risk Factor B (may be contraindicated in 1st trimester)

Pregnancy Considerations Crosses the placenta (carcinogenic in rats); contraindicated for the treatment of trichomoniasis during the first trimester of pregnancy, unless alternative treatment is inadequate. Until safety and efficacy for other indications have been established, use only during pregnancy when the benefit to the mother outweighs the potential risk to the fetus.

Lactation Enters breast milk/not recommended (AAP rates "of concern")

Contraindications Hypersensitivity to metronidazole, nitroimidazole derivatives, or any component of the formulation; pregnancy (1st trimester - found to be carcinogenic in rats)

Warnings/Precautions Use with caution in patients with liver impairment due to potential accumulation, blood dyscrasias; history of seizures, CHF, or other sodium retaining states; reduce dosage in patients with severe liver impairment, CNS disease, and consider dosage reduction in longer-term therapy with severe renal failure (Cl_{cr} <10 mL/minute); if *H. pylori* is not eradicated in patients being treated with metronidazole in a regimen, it should be assumed that metronidazole-resistance has occurred and it should not again be used; seizures and neuropathies have been reported especially with increased doses and chronic treatment; if this occurs, discontinue therapy. **[U.S. Boxed Warning]: Possibly carcinogenic based on animal data.** Prolonged use may result in fungal or bacterial superinfection, including *C. difficile*-associated diarrhea (CDAD) and pseudomembranous colitis; CDAD has been observed >2 months postantibiotic treatment.

Adverse Reactions

Systemic: Frequency not defined:

Cardiovascular: Flattening of the T-wave, flushing

Central nervous system: Ataxia, confusion, coordination impaired, dizziness, fever, headache, insomnia, irritability, seizure, vertigo

Dermatologic: Erythematous rash, urticaria

Endocrine & metabolic: Disulfiram-like reaction, dysmenorrhea, libido decreased

Gastrointestinal: Nausea (~12%), anorexia, abdominal cramping, constipation, diarrhea, furry tongue, glossitis, proctitis, stomatitis, unusual/metallic taste, vomiting, xerostomia

Genitourinary: Cystitis, darkened urine (rare), dysuria, incontinence, polyuria, vaginitis

Hematologic: Neutropenia (reversible), thrombocytopenia (reversible, rare)

Neuromuscular & skeletal: Peripheral neuropathy, weakness

Respiratory: Nasal congestion, rhinitis, sinusitis, pharyngitis

Miscellaneous: Flu-like syndrome, moniliasis

Topical: Frequency not defined:

Central nervous system: Headache

Dermatologic: Burning, contact dermatitis, dryness, erythema, irritation, pruritus, rash

Gastrointestinal: Unusual/metallic taste, nausea, constipation

Local: Local allergic reaction
Neuromuscular & skeletal: Tingling/numbness of extremities
Ocular: Eye irritation

Vaginal:

>10%: Genitourinary: Vaginal discharge (12%)

1% to 10%:

Central nervous system: Headache (5%), dizziness (2%)
Gastrointestinal: Gastrointestinal discomfort (7%), nausea and/or vomiting (4%), unusual/metallic taste (2%), diarrhea (1%)
Genitourinary: Vaginitis (10%), vulva/vaginal irritation (9%), pelvic discomfort (3%)
Hematologic: WBC increased (2%)

<1%: Abdominal bloating, abdominal gas, darkened urine, depression, fatigue, itching, rash, thirst, xerostomia

Metabolism/Transport Effects Inhibits CYP2C9 (weak), 3A4 (moderate)

Drug Interactions

Alcohol (Ethyl): MetroNIDAZOLE may enhance the adverse/toxic effect of Alcohol (Ethyl). A disulfiram-like reaction may occur. *Risk C: Monitor therapy*

Amprenavir: MetroNIDAZOLE may enhance the adverse/toxic effect of Amprenavir. This is specifically related to the propylene glycol contained in amprenavir oral solution, not capsules. *Risk X: Avoid combination*

Busulfan: MetroNIDAZOLE may increase the serum concentration of Busulfan. *Risk D: Consider therapy modification*

Calcineurin Inhibitors: MetroNIDAZOLE may decrease the metabolism of Calcineurin Inhibitors. *Risk C: Monitor therapy*

CYP3A4 Substrates: CYP3A4 Inhibitors (Moderate) may decrease the metabolism of CYP3A4 Substrates. *Risk C: Monitor therapy*

Disulfiram: May enhance the adverse/toxic effect of MetroNIDAZOLE. *Risk D: Consider therapy modification*

Eplerenone: CYP3A4 Inhibitors (Moderate) may increase the serum concentration of Eplerenone. Management: A lower starting dose of eplerenone (25 mg once daily) is recommended in patients with hypertension who are also taking drugs that are moderate inhibitors of CYP3A4. *Risk D: Consider therapy modification*

Maraviroc: CYP3A4 Inhibitors may increase the serum concentration of Maraviroc. *Risk D: Consider therapy modification*

Mebendazole: May enhance the adverse/toxic effect of MetroNIDAZOLE. Particularly the risk for Stevens-Johnson Syndrome or Toxic Epidermal Necrolysis may be increased. *Risk D: Consider therapy modification*

Mycophenolate: MetroNIDAZOLE may decrease the serum concentration of Mycophenolate. Specifically, metronidazole may decrease concentrations of the active metabolite of mycophenolate. *Risk C: Monitor therapy*

Pimecrolimus: CYP3A4 Inhibitors (Moderate) may decrease the metabolism of Pimecrolimus. *Risk C: Monitor therapy*

Ranolazine: CYP3A4 Inhibitors (Moderate) may increase the serum concentration of Ranolazine. Management: Limit the ranolazine dose to a maximum of 500mg twice daily in patients concurrently receiving moderate CYP3A4 inhibitors (e.g., diltiazem, verapamil, erythromycin, etc.). *Risk D: Consider therapy modification*

Salmeterol: CYP3A4 Inhibitors (Moderate) may increase the serum concentration of Salmeterol. *Risk C: Monitor therapy*

Tipranavir: MetroNIDAZOLE may enhance the adverse/toxic effect of Tipranavir. *Risk C: Monitor therapy*

Typhoid Vaccine: Antibiotics may diminish the therapeutic effect of Typhoid Vaccine. Only the live attenuated Ty21a strain is affected. *Risk D: Consider therapy modification*

Vitamin K Antagonists (eg, warfarin): MetroNIDAZOLE may decrease the metabolism of Vitamin K Antagonists. *Risk D: Consider therapy modification*

Ethanol/Nutrition/Herb Interactions

Ethanol: The manufacturer recommends to avoid all ethanol or any ethanol-containing drugs (may cause disulfiram-like reaction characterized by flushing, headache, nausea, vomiting, sweating, or tachycardia).

Food: Peak antibiotic serum concentration lowered and delayed, but total drug absorbed not affected.

Stability Metronidazole injection should be stored at 15°C to 30°C and protected from light. Product may be refrigerated but crystals may form. Crystals redissolve on warming to room temperature. Prolonged exposure to light will cause a darkening of the product. However, short-term exposure to normal room light does not adversely affect metronidazole stability. Direct sunlight should be avoided. Stability of parenteral admixture at room temperature (25°C): Out of overwrap stability: 30 days.

Standard diluent: 500 mg/100 mL NS.

Mechanism of Action After diffusing into the organism, interacts with DNA to cause a loss of helical DNA structure and strand breakage resulting in inhibition of protein synthesis and cell death in susceptible organisms

Pharmacodynamics/Kinetics

Absorption: Oral: Well absorbed; Topical: Concentrations achieved systemically after application of 1 g topically are 10 times less than those obtained after a 250 mg oral dose

Distribution: To saliva, bile, seminal fluid, breast milk, bone, liver, and liver abscesses, lung and vaginal secretions; crosses placenta and blood-brain barrier

CSF:blood level ratio: Normal meninges: 16% to 43%; Inflamed meninges: 100%

Protein binding: <20%

Metabolism: Hepatic (30% to 60%)

Half-life elimination: Neonates: 25-75 hours; Others: 6-8 hours, prolonged with hepatic impairment; End-stage renal disease: 21 hours

Time to peak, serum: Oral: Immediate release: 1-2 hours

Excretion: Urine (20% to 40% as unchanged drug); feces (6% to 15%)

Dosage

Infants and Children:

Amebiasis: Oral: 35-50 mg/kg/day in divided doses every 8 hours for 10 days

Trichomoniasis: Oral: 15-30 mg/kg/day in divided doses every 8 hours for 7 days

Anaerobic infections:

Oral: 15-35 mg/kg/day in divided doses every 8 hours

I.V.: 30 mg/kg/day in divided doses every 6 hours

Clostridium difficile (antibiotic-associated colitis): Oral: 20 mg/kg/day divided every 6 hours

Maximum dose: 2 g/day

Adults:

Anaerobic infections (diverticulitis, intra-abdominal, peritonitis, cholangitis, or abscess): Oral, I.V.: 500 mg every 6-8 hours, not to exceed 4 g/day

Acne rosacea: Topical:

0.75%: Apply and rub a thin film twice daily, morning and evening, to entire affected areas after washing. Significant therapeutic results should be noticed within 3 weeks. Clinical studies have demonstrated continuing improvement through 9 weeks of therapy.

1%: Apply thin film to affected area once daily

Amebiasis: Oral: 500-750 mg every 8 hours for 5-10 days

Antibiotic-associated pseudomembranous colitis: Oral: 250-500 mg 3-4 times/day for 10-14 days

Note: Due to the emergence of a new strain of *C. difficile*, some clinicians recommend converting to oral vancomycin therapy if the patient does not show a clear clinical response after 2 days of metronidazole therapy.

Giardiasis: 500 mg twice daily for 5-7 days

Helicobacter pylori eradication: Oral: 250-500 mg with meals and at bedtime for 14 days; requires combination therapy with at least one other antibiotic and an acid-suppressing agent (proton pump inhibitor or H_2 blocker)

Bacterial vaginosis or vaginitis due to *Gardnerella*, *Mobiluncus*:

Oral: 500 mg twice daily (regular release) or 750 mg once daily (extended release tablet) for 7 days

Vaginal: 1 applicatorful (~37.5 mg metronidazole) intravaginally once or twice daily for 5 days; apply once in morning and evening if using twice daily, if daily, use at bedtime

Trichomoniasis: Oral: 250 mg every 8 hours for 7 days **or** 375 mg twice daily for 7 days **or** 2 g as a single dose

Elderly: Use lower end of dosing recommendations for adults, do not administer as a single dose

Dosing adjustment in renal impairment: Cl_{cr} <10 mL/minute, but not on dialysis: Recommendations vary: To reduce possible accumulation in patients receiving multiple doses, consider reduction to 50% of dose or every 12 hours; **Note:** Dosage reduction is unnecessary in short courses of therapy. Clinical recommendations and practice vary. Some references do not recommend reduction at any level of renal impairment (Lamp, 1999).

Hemodialysis: Extensively removed by hemodialysis and peritoneal dialysis (50% to 100%); dosage reduction not recommended; administer full dose posthemodialysis

Peritoneal dialysis: Dose as for Cl_{cr} <10 mL/minute

Continuous arteriovenous or venovenous hemofiltration: Administer usual dose

Dosing adjustment/comments in hepatic disease: Unchanged in mild liver disease; reduce dosage in severe liver disease

Dietary Considerations Take on an empty stomach. Drug may cause GI upset; if GI upset occurs, take with food. Extended release tablets should be taken on an empty stomach (1 hour before or 2 hours after meals). Sodium content of 500 mg (I.V.): 322 mg (14 mEq). The manufacturer recommends that ethanol be avoided during treatment and for 3 days after therapy is complete.

Administration

Oral: May be taken with food to minimize stomach upset. Extended release tablets should be taken on an empty stomach (1 hour before or 2 hours after meals).

Topical: No disulfiram-like reactions have been reported after **topical** application, although metronidazole can be detected in the blood. Apply to clean, dry skin. Cosmetics may be used after application (wait at least 5 minutes after using lotion).

Test Interactions May interfere with AST, ALT, triglycerides, glucose, and LDH testing

Dosage Forms Excipient information presented when available (limited, particularly for generics); consult specific product labeling.

Capsule: 375 mg
  Flagyl®: 375 mg
Cream, topical: 0.75% (45 g)
  MetroCream®: 0.75% (45 g) [contains benzyl alcohol]
  Noritate®: 1% (60 g)
Gel, topical: 0.75% (45 g)
  MetroGel®: 1% (46 g, 60 g) [60 g tube also packaged in a kit with Cetaphil® skin cleanser]
Gel, vaginal: 0.75% (70 g)
  MetroGel-Vaginal®, Vandazole™: 0.75% (70 g)
Infusion [premixed iso-osmotic sodium chloride solution]: 500 mg (100 mL)
Lotion, topical: 0.75% (60 mL)
  MetroLotion®: 0.75% (60 mL) [contains benzyl alcohol]
Tablet: 250 mg, 500 mg
  Flagyl®: 250 mg, 500 mg
Tablet, extended release:
  Flagyl® ER: 750 mg

- **Metronidazole, Bismuth Subcitrate Potassium, and Tetracycline** *see* Bismuth, Metronidazole, and Tetracycline *on page 190*
- **Metronidazole, Bismuth Subsalicylate, and Tetracycline** *see* Bismuth, Metronidazole, and Tetracycline *on page 190*
- **Metronidazole Hydrochloride** *see* MetroNIDAZOLE *on page 1040*

Metyrosine (me TYE roe seen)

Medication Safety Issues

Sound-alike/look-alike issues:
  Metyrosine may be confused with metyrapone

U.S. Brand Names Demser®

Canadian Brand Names Demser®

Index Terms AMPT; OGMT

Pharmacologic Category Tyrosine Hydroxylase Inhibitor

Use Short-term management of pheochromocytoma before surgery, long-term management when surgery is contraindicated or when chronic malignant pheochromocytoma exists

Effect on Mental Status Drowsiness and extrapyramidal symptoms are common; may cause depression, hallucinations, or confusion

Effect on Psychiatric Treatment Concurrent use with antipsychotics may increase the risk of extrapyramidal symptoms

Dosage Summary

Oral:

Children ≤12 years: Dosage not established

Children >12 years: Initial: 250 mg 4 times/day; Maintenance: 2-3 g/day in 4 divided doses (maximum: 4 g/day)

Adults: Initial: 250 mg 4 times/day; Maintenance: 2-3 g/day in 4 divided doses (maximum: 4 g/day)

Dosage Forms Excipient information presented when available (limited, particularly for generics); consult specific product labeling.

Capsule: 250 mg

- **Mevacor®** *see* Lovastatin *on page 956*

- **Mevinolin** *see* Lovastatin *on page 956*

Mexiletine (meks IL e teen)

U.S. Brand Names Mexitil® [DSC]
Canadian Brand Names Novo-Mexiletine
Pharmacologic Category Antiarrhythmic Agent, Class Ib
Use Management of serious ventricular arrhythmias; suppression of PVCs
Unlabeled/Investigational Use Diabetic neuropathy
Effect on Mental Status Dizziness and nervousness are common; may cause confusion and insomnia
Effect on Psychiatric Treatment May rarely cause agranulocytosis; use caution with clozapine and carbamazepine; barbiturates may decrease the effects of mexiletine; monitor
Dosage Summary
Oral:
Children: Dosage not established
Adults: Initial: 200 mg every 8 hours; Maintenance: 200-300 mg every 8 hours (maximum: 1.2 g/day)
Dosage Forms Excipient information presented when available (limited, particularly for generics); consult specific product labeling. [DSC] = Discontinued product
Capsule, as hydrochloride: 150 mg, 200 mg, 250 mg
Mexitil®: 150 mg, 200 mg, 250 mg [DSC]

- **Mexitil® [DSC]** *see* Mexiletine *on page 1045*
- **M-FA-142** *see* Amonafide *on page 108*
- **$MgSO_4$ (error-prone abbreviation)** *see* Magnesium Sulfate *on page 966*
- **Miacalcin®** *see* Calcitonin *on page 253*
- **Mi-Acid [OTC]** *see* Aluminum Hydroxide, Magnesium Hydroxide, and Simethicone *on page 78*
- **Mi-Acid™ Double Strength [OTC]** *see* Calcium Carbonate and Magnesium Hydroxide *on page 256*
- **Mi-Acid Maximum Strength [OTC]** *see* Aluminum Hydroxide, Magnesium Hydroxide, and Simethicone *on page 78*

Micafungin (mi ka FUN gin)

U.S. Brand Names Mycamine®
Canadian Brand Names Mycamine®
Index Terms Micafungin Sodium
Pharmacologic Category Antifungal Agent, Parenteral; Echinocandin
Use Treatment of esophageal candidiasis; *Candida* prophylaxis in patients undergoing hematopoietic stem cell transplant (HSCT); treatment of candidemia, acute disseminated candidiasis, and other *Candida* infections (peritonitis and abscesses)
Unlabeled/Investigational Use Treatment of infections due to *Aspergillus* spp; prophylaxis of HIV-related esophageal candidiasis
Effect on Mental Status May cause delirium, dizziness, or sedation
Effect on Psychiatric Treatment None reported
Dosage Summary
I.V.:
Children: Dosage not established
Adults: Prophylaxis: 50 mg daily; Treatment: 100-150 mg daily
Dosage Forms Excipient information presented when available (limited, particularly for generics); consult specific product labeling.
Injection, powder for reconstitution, as sodium [preservative-free]:
Mycamine®: 50 mg, 100 mg [contains lactose]

- **Micafungin Sodium** *see* Micafungin *on page 1045*
- **Micardis®** *see* Telmisartan *on page 1542*
- **Micardis® HCT** *see* Telmisartan and Hydrochlorothiazide *on page 1544*
- **MICRhoGAM®** *see* Rh_o(D) Immune Globulin *on page 1415*
- **Microgestin™** *see* Ethinyl Estradiol and Norethindrone *on page 597*
- **Microgestin™ Fe** *see* Ethinyl Estradiol and Norethindrone *on page 597*
- **microK®** *see* Potassium Chloride *on page 1315*
- **microK® 10** *see* Potassium Chloride *on page 1315*

- **Micronase®** *see* GlyBURIDE *on page 730*
- **Microzide®** *see* Hydrochlorothiazide *on page 773*

Midazolam (MID aye zoe lam)

Medication Safety Issues

Sound-alike/look-alike issues:

Versed may be confused with VePesid®, Vistaril®

High alert medication: The Institute for Safe Medication Practices (ISMP) includes this medication among its list of drugs which have a heightened risk of causing significant patient harm when used in error.

Related Information

Benzodiazepines *on page 1774*

Discontinuation of Psychotropic Drugs *on page 1839*

Canadian Brand Names Apo-Midazolam®; Midazolam Injection

Mexican Brand Names Dormicum; Midozor; Relacum

Index Terms Midazolam Hydrochloride; Versed

Pharmacologic Category Benzodiazepine

Generic Available Yes

Use Preoperative sedation and provides conscious sedation prior to diagnostic or radiographic procedures; ICU sedation (continuous infusion); intravenous anesthesia (induction); intravenous anesthesia (maintenance)

Unlabeled/Investigational Use Anxiety, status epilepticus

Mental Health Comment In 2007, the FDA requested that all manufacturers of sedative-hypnotic drug products revise labeling to include a greater emphasis on the risks of adverse effects. These risks include severe allergic reactions (anaphylaxis, angioedema) and complex sleep-related behaviors, which may include sleep-driving (driving while not fully awake and with no memory of the event), making phone calls, and preparing and eating food while asleep.

There are two subtypes of GABA receptors (GABA-A and GABA-B) and three different benzodiazepine receptors (Bz_1, Bz_2, and Bz_3). Benzodiazepine receptors and effects appear to be linked to the GABA-A receptors. Benzodiazepines do not bind to GABA-B receptors. The role of GABA-B receptors is unclear. Benzodiazepines have no specificity for benzodiazepine receptor subtypes.

Midazolam is a short half-life benzodiazepine and may be of benefit in patients where a rapidly and short-acting agent is desired (acute agitation). Duration of action after a single dose is determined by redistribution rather than metabolism. Tolerance develops to the sedative, hypnotic, and anticonvulsant effects. It does not develop to the anxiolytic or skeletal muscle relaxing effects. Psychological and physical dependence may occur with prolonged use of benzodiazepines. The onset of withdrawal symptoms is usually seen on the first day without drug and lasts 5-7 days in patients receiving short half-life benzodiazepines, whereas, the onset occurs after 5 days with a duration of 10-14 days after abrupt discontinuance of long half-life benzodiazepines. Risk factors for abuse include personal or family history of substance abuse and personality disorder.

Midazolam is rapidly and completely absorbed after I.M. injection.

Restrictions C-IV

Pregnancy Risk Factor D

Pregnancy Considerations Midazolam has been found to cross the placenta; not recommended for use during pregnancy.

Lactation Enters breast milk/not recommended (AAP rates "of concern")

Contraindications Hypersensitivity to midazolam or any component of the formulation, including benzyl alcohol (cross-sensitivity with other benzodiazepines may exist); parenteral form is not for intrathecal or epidural injection; narrow-angle glaucoma; concurrent use of potent inhibitors of CYP3A4 (amprenavir, atazanavir, or ritonavir); pregnancy

Warnings/Precautions **[U.S. Boxed Warning]: May cause severe respiratory depression, respiratory arrest, or apnea. Use with extreme caution, particularly in noncritical care settings.** Appropriate resuscitative equipment and qualified personnel must be available for administration and monitoring. Initial dosing must be cautiously titrated and individualized, particularly in elderly or debilitated patients, patients with hepatic impairment (including alcoholics), or in renal impairment, particularly if other CNS depressants (including opiates) are used concurrently. **[U.S. Boxed Warning]: Initial doses in elderly or debilitated patients should be conservative; as little as 1 mg, but not to exceed 2.5 mg.** Use with caution in patients with respiratory disease or impaired gag reflex. Use during upper airway procedures may increase risk of hypoventilation. Prolonged responses have been noted following extended administration by continuous infusion (possibly due to metabolite accumulation) or in the presence of drugs which inhibit midazolam metabolism.

Causes CNS depression (dose-related) resulting in sedation, dizziness, confusion, or ataxia which may impair physical and mental capabilities. Patients must be cautioned about performing tasks which require mental alertness (eg, operating machinery or driving). A minimum of 1 day should elapse after midazolam administration before attempting these tasks. Use with caution in patients receiving other CNS depressants or psychoactive agents. Effects with other sedative drugs or ethanol may be potentiated. Benzodiazepines have been associated with falls and traumatic injury and should be used with extreme caution in patients who are at risk of these events (especially the elderly).

May cause hypotension - hemodynamic events are more common in pediatric patients or patients with hemodynamic instability. Hypotension and/or respiratory depression may occur more frequently in patients who have received opioid analgesics. Use with caution in obese patients, chronic renal failure, and HF. Does not protect against increases in heart rate or blood pressure during intubation. Should not be used in shock, coma, or acute alcohol intoxication. **[U.S. Boxed Warning]: Parenteral form contains benzyl alcohol; avoid rapid injection in neonates or prolonged infusions.** Avoid intra-arterial administration or extravasation of parenteral formulation.

Midazolam causes anterograde amnesia. Paradoxical reactions, including hyperactive or aggressive behavior have been reported with benzodiazepines, particularly in adolescent/pediatric or psychiatric patients. Does not have analgesic, antidepressant, or antipsychotic properties.

Benzodiazepines have been associated with dependence and acute withdrawal symptoms on discontinuation or reduction in dose. Acute withdrawal, including seizures, may be precipitated after administration of flumazenil to patients receiving long-term benzodiazepine therapy.

Adverse Reactions As reported in adults unless otherwise noted:

>10%: Respiratory: Decreased tidal volume and/or respiratory rate decrease, apnea (3% children)

1% to 10%:

- Cardiovascular: Hypotension (3% children)
- Central nervous system: Drowsiness (1%), oversedation, headache (1%), seizure-like activity (1% children)
- Gastrointestinal: Nausea (3%), vomiting (3%)
- Local: Pain and local reactions at injection site (4% I.M., 5% I.V.; severity less than diazepam)
- Ocular: Nystagmus (1% children)
- Respiratory: Cough (1%)
- Miscellaneous: Physical and psychological dependence with prolonged use, hiccups (4%, 1% children), paradoxical reaction (2% children)

<1% (Limited to important or life-threatening): Agitation, amnesia, bigeminy, bronchospasm, emergence delirium, euphoria, hallucinations, laryngospasm, rash

Metabolism/Transport Effects Substrate of CYP2B6 (minor), 3A4 (major); **Inhibits** CYP2C8 (weak), 2C9 (weak), 3A4 (weak)

Drug Interactions

Alcohol (Ethyl): CNS Depressants may enhance the CNS depressant effect of Alcohol (Ethyl). *Risk C: Monitor therapy*

Antifungal Agents (Azole Derivatives, Systemic): May decrease the metabolism of Benzodiazepines (metabolized by oxidation). *Risk D: Consider therapy modification*

Aprepitant: May increase the serum concentration of Benzodiazepines (metabolized by oxidation). *Risk C: Monitor therapy*

Atorvastatin: May increase the serum concentration of Midazolam. *Risk C: Monitor therapy*

Calcium Channel Blockers (Nondihydropyridine): May decrease the metabolism of Benzodiazepines (metabolized by oxidation). *Risk D: Consider therapy modification*

CarBAMazepine: May increase the metabolism of Benzodiazepines (metabolized by oxidation). *Risk C: Monitor therapy*

Cimetidine: May decrease the metabolism of Benzodiazepines (metabolized by oxidation). *Risk C: Monitor therapy*

Clozapine: Benzodiazepines may enhance the adverse/toxic effect of Clozapine. *Risk D: Consider therapy modification*

CNS Depressants: May enhance the adverse/toxic effect of other CNS Depressants. *Risk C: Monitor therapy*

CYP3A4 Inducers (Strong): May increase the metabolism of CYP3A4 Substrates. *Risk C: Monitor therapy*

CYP3A4 Inhibitors (Moderate): May decrease the metabolism of CYP3A4 Substrates. *Risk C: Monitor therapy*

CYP3A4 Inhibitors (Strong): May decrease the metabolism of CYP3A4 Substrates. *Risk D: Consider therapy modification*

Dasatinib: May increase the serum concentration of CYP3A4 Substrates. *Risk C: Monitor therapy*

Deferasirox: May decrease the serum concentration of CYP3A4 Substrates. *Risk C: Monitor therapy*

Disulfiram: May decrease the metabolism of Benzodiazepines (metabolized by oxidation). *Risk C: Monitor therapy*

Efavirenz: May increase the serum concentration of Midazolam. *Risk X: Avoid combination*

Fluconazole: May decrease the metabolism of Benzodiazepines (metabolized by oxidation). *Risk D: Consider therapy modification*

Fosaprepitant: May increase the serum concentration of Benzodiazepines (metabolized by oxidation). Specifically, the active metabolite aprepitant is likely responsible for this effect. *Risk C: Monitor therapy*

Grapefruit Juice: May decrease the metabolism of Benzodiazepines (metabolized by oxidation). *Risk D: Consider therapy modification*

Isoniazid: May decrease the metabolism of Benzodiazepines (metabolized by oxidation). *Risk C: Monitor therapy*

Macrolide Antibiotics: May decrease the metabolism of Benzodiazepines (metabolized by oxidation). **Exceptions:** Azithromycin; Dirithromycin [Off Market]; Spiramycin. *Risk D: Consider therapy modification*

Nefazodone: May decrease the metabolism of Benzodiazepines (metabolized by oxidation). *Risk D: Consider therapy modification*

Oral Contraceptive (Estrogens): May decrease the metabolism of Benzodiazepines (metabolized by oxidation). *Risk C: Monitor therapy*

Oral Contraceptive (Progestins): May decrease the metabolism of Benzodiazepines (metabolized by oxidation). *Risk C: Monitor therapy*

Phenytoin: Benzodiazepines may increase the serum concentration of Phenytoin. Short-term exposure to benzodiazepines may not present as much risk as chronic therapy. *Risk C: Monitor therapy*

Protease Inhibitors: May decrease the metabolism of Benzodiazepines (metabolized by oxidation). Management: Amprenavir, atazanavir, darunavir, indinavir, nelfinavir, ritonavir, and tipranavir are contraindicated with midazolam and triazolam according to each protease inhibitor 's prescribing information. *Risk D: Consider therapy modification*

Proton Pump Inhibitors: May increase the serum concentration of Benzodiazepines (metabolized by oxidation). **Exceptions:** Lansoprazole; Pantoprazole; Rabeprazole. *Risk C: Monitor therapy*

Rifamycin Derivatives: May increase the metabolism of Benzodiazepines (metabolized by oxidation). *Risk D: Consider therapy modification*

Selective Serotonin Reuptake Inhibitors: May decrease the metabolism of Benzodiazepines (metabolized by oxidation). **Exceptions:** Citalopram; Escitalopram; PARoxetine; Sertraline. *Risk C: Monitor therapy*

St Johns Wort: May increase the metabolism of Benzodiazepines (metabolized by oxidation). *Risk C: Monitor therapy*

Theophylline Derivatives: May diminish the therapeutic effect of Benzodiazepines. *Risk D: Consider therapy modification*

Ethanol/Nutrition/Herb Interactions

Ethanol: Avoid ethanol (may increase CNS depression).

Food: Grapefruit juice may increase serum concentrations of midazolam; avoid concurrent use with oral form.

Herb/Nutraceutical: Avoid concurrent use with St John's wort (may decrease midazolam levels, may increase CNS depression). Avoid concurrent use with valerian, kava kava, gotu kola (may increase CNS depression).

Stability The manufacturer states that midazolam, at a final concentration of 0.5 mg/mL, is stable for up to 24 hours when diluted with D_5W or NS. A final concentration of 1 mg/mL in NS has been documented to be stable for up to 10 days (McMullen, 1995). Admixtures do not require protection from light for short-term storage.

Mechanism of Action Binds to stereospecific benzodiazepine receptors on the postsynaptic GABA neuron at several sites within the central nervous system, including the limbic system, reticular formation. Enhancement of the inhibitory effect of GABA on neuronal excitability results by increased neuronal membrane permeability to chloride ions. This shift in chloride ions results in hyperpolarization (a less excitable state) and stabilization.

Pharmacodynamics/Kinetics

Onset of action: I.M.: Sedation: ~15 minutes; I.V.: 1-5 minutes
  Peak effect: I.M.: 0.5-1 hour
Duration: I.M.: Up to 6 hours; Mean: 2 hours
Absorption: Oral: Rapid
Distribution: V_d: 0.8-2.5 L/kg; increased with congestive heart failure (CHF) and chronic renal failure
Protein binding: 95%
Metabolism: Extensively hepatic via CYP3A4
Bioavailability: Mean: 45%
Half-life elimination: 1-4 hours; prolonged with cirrhosis, congestive heart failure, obesity, and elderly
Excretion: Urine (as glucuronide conjugated metabolites); feces (~2% to 10%)

Dosage The dose of midazolam needs to be individualized based on the patient's age, underlying diseases, and concurrent medications. Decrease dose (by ~30%) if narcotics or other CNS depressants are administered concomitantly. **Personnel and equipment needed for standard respiratory resuscitation should be immediately available during midazolam administration.**

Children <6 years may require higher doses and closer monitoring than older children; calculate dose on ideal body weight
Conscious sedation for procedures or preoperative sedation:
  Oral: 0.25-0.5 mg/kg as a single dose preprocedure, up to a maximum of 20 mg; administer 30-45 minutes prior to procedure. Children <6 years or less cooperative patients may require as much as 1 mg/kg as a single dose; 0.25 mg/kg may suffice for children 6-16 years of age.
  Intranasal (not an approved route): 0.2 mg/kg (up to 0.4 mg/kg in some studies), to a maximum of 15 mg; may be administered 30-45 minutes prior to procedure
  I.M.: 0.1-0.15 mg/kg 30-60 minutes before surgery or procedure; range 0.05-0.15 mg/kg; doses up to 0.5 mg/kg have been used in more anxious patients; maximum total dose: 10 mg
  I.V.:
    Infants <6 months: Limited information is available in nonintubated infants; dosing recommendations not clear; infants <6 months are at higher risk for airway obstruction and hypoventilation; titrate dose in small increments to desired effect; monitor carefully
    Infants 6 months to Children 5 years: Initial: 0.05-0.1 mg/kg; titrate dose carefully; total dose of 0.6 mg/kg may be required; usual maximum total dose: 6 mg
    Children 6-12 years: Initial: 0.025-0.05 mg/kg; titrate dose carefully; total doses of 0.4 mg/kg may be required; usual maximum total dose: 10 mg
    Children 12-16 years: Dose as adults; usual maximum total dose: 10 mg
  Conscious sedation during mechanical ventilation: Children: Loading dose: 0.05-0.2 mg/kg, followed by initial continuous infusion: 0.06-0.12 mg/kg/hour (1-2 mcg/kg/minute); titrate to the desired effect; usual range: 0.4-6 mcg/kg/minute
  Status epilepticus refractory to standard therapy (unlabeled use): Infants >2 months and Children: Loading dose: 0.15 mg/kg followed by a continuous infusion of 0.06 mg/kg/hour; titrate dose upward every 5 minutes until clinical seizure activity is controlled; mean infusion rate required in 24 children was 0.14 mg/kg/hour (2.3 mcg/kg/minute) with a range of 0.06-1.1 mg/kg/hour

Adults:
  Preoperative sedation:
    I.M.: 0.07-0.08 mg/kg 30-60 minutes prior to surgery/procedure; usual dose: 5 mg; **Note:** Reduce dose in patients with COPD, high-risk patients, patients ≥60 years of age, and patients receiving other narcotics or CNS depressants
    I.V.: 0.02-0.04 mg/kg; repeat every 5 minutes as needed to desired effect or up to 0.1-0.2 mg/kg
    Intranasal (not an approved route): 0.2 mg/kg (up to 0.4 mg/kg in some studies); administer 30-45 minutes prior to surgery/procedure
  Conscious sedation: I.V.: Initial: 0.5-2 mg slow I.V. over at least 2 minutes; slowly titrate to effect by repeating doses every 2-3 minutes if needed; usual total dose: 2.5-5 mg; use decreased doses in elderly
    Healthy Adults <60 years: Some patients respond to doses as low as 1 mg; no more than 2.5 mg should be administered over a period of 2 minutes. Additional doses of midazolam may be administered after a 2-minute waiting period and evaluation of sedation after each dose increment. A total dose >5 mg is generally not needed. If narcotics or other CNS

depressants are administered concomitantly, the midazolam dose should be reduced by 30%.

Anesthesia: I.V.:

Induction:

Unpremedicated patients: 0.3-0.35 mg/kg (up to 0.6 mg/kg in resistant cases)

Premedicated patients: 0.15-0.35 mg/kg

Maintenance: 0.05-0.3 mg/kg as needed, or continuous infusion 0.25-1.5 mcg/kg/minute

Sedation in mechanically-ventilated patients: I.V. continuous infusion: 100 mg in 250 mL D_5W or NS (if patient is fluid-restricted, may concentrate up to a maximum of 0.5 mg/mL); initial dose: 0.02-0.08 mg/kg (~1 mg to 5 mg in 70 kg adult) initially and either repeated at 5-15 minute intervals until adequate sedation is achieved or continuous infusion rates of 0.04-0.2 mg/kg/hour and titrate to reach desired level of sedation

Refractory status epilepticus (unlabeled use): I.V.: Initial: 0.2 mg/kg bolus, then 0.05-0.6 mg/kg/hour

Elderly: I.V.: Conscious sedation: Initial: 0.5 mg slow I.V.; give no more than 1.5 mg in a 2-minute period; if additional titration is needed, give no more than 1 mg over 2 minutes, waiting another 2 or more minutes to evaluate sedative effect; a total dose of >3.5 mg is rarely necessary

Dosage adjustment in renal impairment:

Hemodialysis: Supplemental dose is not necessary

Peritoneal dialysis: Significant drug removal is unlikely based on physiochemical characteristics

Dietary Considerations Injection: Sodium content of 1 mL: 0.14 mEq

Administration

Intranasal: Administer using a 1 mL needleless syringe into the nostrils over 15 seconds; use the 5 mg/mL injection; 1/2 of the dose may be administered to each nostril

Oral: Do not mix with any liquid (such as grapefruit juice) prior to administration

Parenteral:

I.M.: Administer deep I.M. into large muscle.

I.V.: Administer by slow I.V. injection over at least 2-5 minutes at a concentration of 1-5 mg/mL or by I.V. infusion. Continuous infusions should be administered via an infusion pump.

Monitoring Parameters Respiratory and cardiovascular status, blood pressure, blood pressure monitor required during I.V. administration

Additional Information Abrupt discontinuation after sustained use (generally >10 days) may cause withdrawal symptoms. For neonates, since both concentrations of the injection contain 1% benzyl alcohol, use the 5 mg/mL injection and dilute to 0.5 mg/mL with SWI without preservatives to decrease the amount of benzyl alcohol delivered to the neonate; with continuous infusion, midazolam may accumulate in peripheral tissues; use lowest effective infusion rate to reduce accumulation effects; midazolam is 3-4 times as potent as diazepam; paradoxical reactions associated with midazolam use in children (eg, agitation, restlessness, combativeness) have been successfully treated with flumazenil (Massanari, 1997).

Dosage Forms Excipient information presented when available (limited, particularly for generics); consult specific product labeling.

Injection, solution: 1 mg/mL (2 mL, 5 mL, 10 mL); 5 mg/mL (1 mL, 2 mL, 5 mL, 10 mL) [contains benzyl alcohol 1%]

Injection, solution [preservative free]: 1 mg/mL (2 mL, 5 mL); 5 mg/mL (1 mL, 2 mL)

Syrup: 2 mg/mL (118 mL) [contains sodium benzoate; cherry flavor]

◆ **Midazolam Hydrochloride** *see* Midazolam *on page 1046*

Midodrine (MI doe dreen)

Medication Safety Issues

Sound-alike/look-alike issues:

ProAmatine® may be confused with protamine

U.S. Brand Names ProAmatine®

Canadian Brand Names Amatine®; Apo-Midodrine®

Index Terms Midodrine Hydrochloride

Pharmacologic Category $Alpha_1$ Agonist

Use Orphan drug: Treatment of symptomatic orthostatic hypotension

Unlabeled/Investigational Use Investigational: Management of urinary incontinence

Effect on Mental Status May cause anxiety, dizziness, confusion, or insomnia

Effect on Psychiatric Treatment None reported

Dosage Summary

Oral:

Children: Dosage not established

Adults: 10 mg 3 times/day (maximum: 40 mg/day)

Dosage Forms Excipient information presented when available (limited, particularly for generics); consult specific product labeling.

Tablet, as hydrochloride: 2.5 mg, 5 mg, 10 mg

ProAmatine®: 2.5 mg, 5 mg, 10 mg [scored]

◆ **Midodrine Hydrochloride** *see* Midodrine *on page 1050*

◆ **Midol® Cramp and Body Aches [OTC]** *see* Ibuprofen *on page 803*

◆ **Midol® Extended Relief** *see* Naproxen *on page 1102*

◆ **Midrin®** *see* Acetaminophen, Isometheptene, and Dichloralphenazone *on page 45*

◆ **Midsummer Daisy** *see* Feverfew *(Tanacetum parthenium) on page 628*

◆ **Mifeprex®** *see* Mifepristone *on page 1051*

Mifepristone (mi FE pris tone)

Medication Safety Issues

Sound-alike/look-alike issues:

Mifeprex® may be confused with Mirapex®

Mifepristone may be confused with misoprostol

High alert medication: The Institute for Safe Medication Practices (ISMP) includes this medication among its list of drug classes which have a heightened risk of causing significant patient harm when used in error.

U.S. Brand Names Mifeprex®

Index Terms RU-38486; RU-486

Pharmacologic Category Abortifacient; Antineoplastic Agent, Hormone Antagonist; Antiprogestin

Use Medical termination of intrauterine pregnancy, through day 49 of pregnancy. Patients may need treatment with misoprostol and possibly surgery to complete therapy

Unlabeled/Investigational Use Treatment of unresectable meningioma; has been studied in the treatment of breast cancer, ovarian cancer, and adrenal cortical carcinoma

Effect on Mental Status May cause dizziness, fatigue, insomnia, or anxiety

Effect on Psychiatric Treatment Gastrointestinal side effects are common; use caution with lithium, valproic acid, and SSRIs. Fluoxetine, fluvoxamine, and nefazodone may increase mifepristone serum levels and/or toxicity; monitor. Carbamazepine, phenobarbital, and St John's wort may increase the metabolism of mifepristone, resulting in decreased mifepristone levels and/or effect; monitor.

Restrictions Investigators wishing to obtain the agent for use in oncology patients must apply for a patient-specific IND from the FDA. Mifepristone will be supplied only to licensed physicians who sign and return a "Prescriber's Agreement." Distribution of mifepristone will be subject to specific requirements imposed by the distributor. Mifepristone will **not** be available to the public through licensed pharmacies. An FDA-approved medication guide must be distributed when dispensing an outpatient prescription (new or refill) where this medication is to be used without direct supervision of a healthcare provider. Medication guides are available at http://www.fda.gov/cder/Offices/ODS/medication_guides.htm.

Not available in Canada

Dosage Summary

Oral:

Children: Not for use prior to menarche

Adults:

Day 1: 600 mg (three 200 mg tablets) taken as a single dose under physician supervision

Day 3: 400 mcg (two 200 mcg tablets) of misoprostol if abortion had not occurred

Elderly: Dosage not established

Dosage Forms Excipient information presented when available (limited, particularly for generics); consult specific product labeling.

Tablet: 200 mg

- **Migergot** *see* Ergotamine and Caffeine *on page 554*

Miglitol (MIG li tol)

U.S. Brand Names Glyset®

Canadian Brand Names Glyset®

Mexican Brand Names Diastabol

Pharmacologic Category Antidiabetic Agent, Alpha-Glucosidase Inhibitor

Generic Available No

Use Type 2 diabetes mellitus (noninsulin-dependent, NIDDM):

Monotherapy adjunct to diet to improve glycemic control in patients with type 2 diabetes mellitus (noninsulin-dependent, NIDDM) whose hyperglycemia cannot be managed with diet alone

Combination therapy with a sulfonylurea when diet plus either miglitol or a sulfonylurea alone do not result in adequate glycemic control. The effect of miglitol to enhance glycemic control is additive to that of sulfonylureas when used in combination.

Effect on Mental Status None reported

Effect on Psychiatric Treatment GI side effects are common; concomitant use with SSRIs, carbamazepine, valproic acid, and lithium may produce additive effects

Pregnancy Risk Factor B

Pregnancy Considerations Adverse events have not been reported in animal reproduction studies; therefore, miglitol is classified as pregnancy category B. Information specific to the use of miglitol during pregnancy has not been located. Maternal hyperglycemia can be associated with adverse effects in the fetus, including macrosomia, neonatal hyperglycemia, and hyperbilirubinemia; the risk of congenital malformations is increased when the Hb A_{1c} is above the normal range. Diabetes can also be associated with adverse effects in the mother. Poorly-treated diabetes may cause end-organ damage that may in turn negatively affect obstetric outcomes. Physiologic glucose levels should be maintained prior to and during pregnancy to decrease the risk of adverse events in the mother and the fetus. Until additional safety and efficacy data are obtained, the use of oral agents is generally not recommended as routine management of GDM or type 2 diabetes mellitus during pregnancy. Insulin is the drug of choice for the control of diabetes mellitus during pregnancy.

Lactation Enters breast milk (small amounts)/not recommended

Contraindications Hypersensitivity to miglitol or any of component of the formulation; diabetic ketoacidosis; inflammatory bowel disease; colonic ulceration; partial intestinal obstruction or predisposition to intestinal obstruction; chronic intestinal diseases associated with marked disorders of digestion or absorption or with conditions that may deteriorate as a result of increased gas formation in the intestine

Warnings/Precautions GI symptoms are the most common reactions. The incidence of abdominal pain and diarrhea tend to diminish considerably with continued treatment. Long-term clinical trials in patients with diabetes with significant renal dysfunction (serum creatinine >2 mg/dL) have not been conducted. Treatment of these patients is not recommended. In combination with a sulfonylurea will cause a further lowering of blood glucose and may increase the hypoglycemic potential of the sulfonylurea. It may be necessary to discontinue miglitol and administer insulin if the patient is exposed to stress (ie, fever, trauma, infection, surgery). Safety and efficacy have not been established in children.

Adverse Reactions

>10%: Gastrointestinal: Flatulence (41.5%), diarrhea (28.7%), abdominal pain (11.7%)

1% to 10%: Dermatologic: Rash (4.3%)

Drug Interactions

Corticosteroids (Orally Inhaled): May diminish the hypoglycemic effect of Antidiabetic Agents. In some instances, corticosteroid-mediated HPA axis suppression has led to episodes of acute adrenal crisis, which may manifest as enhanced hypoglycemia, particularly in the setting of insulin or other antidiabetic agent use. *Risk C: Monitor therapy*

Corticosteroids (Systemic): May diminish the hypoglycemic effect of Antidiabetic Agents. In some instances, corticosteroid-mediated HPA axis suppression has led to episodes of acute adrenal crisis, which may manifest as enhanced hypoglycemia, particularly in the setting of insulin or other antidiabetic agent use. *Risk C: Monitor therapy*

Herbs (Hypoglycemic Properties): May enhance the hypoglycemic effect of Hypoglycemic Agents. *Risk C: Monitor therapy*

Luteinizing Hormone-Releasing Hormone Analogs: May diminish the therapeutic effect of Antidiabetic Agents. *Risk C: Monitor therapy*

Pegvisomant: May enhance the hypoglycemic effect of Antidiabetic Agents. *Risk C: Monitor therapy*

Somatropin: May diminish the hypoglycemic effect of Antidiabetic Agents. *Risk D: Consider therapy modification*

Mechanism of Action In contrast to sulfonylureas, miglitol does not enhance insulin secretion; the antihyperglycemic action of miglitol results from a reversible inhibition of membrane-bound intestinal alpha-glucosidases which hydrolyze oligosaccharides and disaccharides to glucose and other monosaccharides in the brush border of the small intestine. In patients with diabetes, this enzyme inhibition results in delayed glucose absorption and lowering of postprandial hyperglycemia.

Pharmacodynamics/Kinetics

Absorption: Saturable at high doses: 25 mg dose: Completely absorbed; 100 mg dose: 50% to 70% absorbed

Distribution: V_d: 0.18 L/kg

Protein binding: <4%

Metabolism: None

Half-life elimination: ~2 hours

Time to peak: 2-3 hours

Excretion: Urine (as unchanged drug)

Dosage Adults: Oral: 25 mg 3 times/day with the first bite of food at each meal; the dose may be increased to 50 mg 3 times/day after 4-8 weeks; maximum recommended dose: 100 mg 3 times/day

Dosing adjustment in renal impairment: Miglitol is primarily excreted by the kidneys; there is little information of miglitol in patients with a Cl_{cr} <25 mL/minute

Dosing adjustment in hepatic impairment: No adjustment necessary

Administration Should be taken orally at the start (with the first bite) of each main meal

Monitoring Parameters Monitor therapeutic response by periodic blood glucose tests; measurement of glycosylated hemoglobin is recommended for the monitoring of long-term glycemic control

Reference Range Recommendations for glycemic control in adults with diabetes:

Hb A_{1c}: <7%

Preprandial capillary plasma glucose: 70-130 mg/dL

Peak postprandial capillary blood glucose: <180 mg/dL

Blood pressure: <130/80 mm Hg

Dosage Forms Excipient information presented when available (limited, particularly for generics); consult specific product labeling.

Tablet: 25 mg, 50 mg, 100 mg

Miglustat (MIG loo stat)

U.S. Brand Names Zavesca®

Canadian Brand Names Zavesca®

Index Terms OGT-918

Pharmacologic Category Enzyme Inhibitor

Generic Available No

Use Treatment of mild-to-moderate type 1 Gaucher disease when enzyme replacement therapy is not a therapeutic option

Effect on Mental Status Dizziness is common

Effect on Psychiatric Treatment GI side effects are common; use caution with SSRIs

Pregnancy Risk Factor X

Pregnancy Considerations Decreased fetus weight, fetal loss, and difficult or delayed births were observed in animal studies. Women with reproduction potential should use effective contraception during therapy. In addition, adverse effects on spermatogenesis and reduced fertility were observed in male animal studies. The manufacturer recommends that male patients use reliable contraception during therapy and for 3 months following treatment.

Lactation Excretion in breast milk unknown/not recommended

Contraindications Hypersensitivity to miglustat or any component of the formulation; pregnancy

Warnings/Precautions Diarrhea observed in the majority of patients, many also reported weight loss. Incidence decreases over time; foods with high carbohydrate content should be avoided. If symptoms persist, patients should be evaluated for underlying GI disease. Peripheral neuropathy has been reported with use and neurologic monitoring is required. Weigh risk versus benefit of therapy if patient develops numbness and tingling. Tremor or exacerbations of existing tremor may occur; may resolve over time or respond to dosage reduction. Use caution in renal impairment; dosage adjustments recommended. Not recommended in patients with severe impairment. Miglustat increases the clearance of imiglucerase; combination therapy is not indicated. Safety and efficacy in severe type 1 Gaucher disease have not been established.

Adverse Reactions Percentages reported from open-label, uncontrolled monotherapy trials.

>10%:

Central nervous system: Headache (21% to 22%), dizziness (up to 11%)

Gastrointestinal: Diarrhea (89% to 100%), weight loss (39% to 67%), abdominal pain (18% to 67%), flatulence (29% to 50%), nausea (8% to 22%), vomiting (4% to 11%)

Neuromuscular & skeletal: Tremor (11% to 30%), weakness (17%), leg cramps (4% to 11%)

Ocular: Visual disturbances (up to 17%)

1% to 10%:

Central nervous system: Memory impairment (8%), migraine (up to 6%)

Endocrine & metabolic: Menstrual disorder (up to 6%)

Gastrointestinal: Constipation (8%), xerostomia (8%), bloating (up to 8%), anorexia (up to 7%), dyspepsia (up to 7%), epigastric pain (up to 6%)

Hematologic: Thrombocytopenia (6% to 7%)

Neuromuscular & skeletal: Paresthesia (up to 7%)

Drug Interactions

There are no known significant interactions.

Ethanol/Nutrition/Herb Interactions

Food: Food decreases the rate, but not the extent, of absorption.

Stability Store at controlled room temperature of 20°C to 25°C (68°F to 77°F).

Mechanism of Action Miglustat competitively and reversibly inhibits the enzyme needed to produce glycosphingolipids and decreases the rate of glycosphingolipid glucosylceramide formation. Glucosylceramide accumulates in type 1 Gaucher disease, causing complications specific to this disease.

Pharmacodynamics/Kinetics

Distribution: V_d: 83-105 L

Protein binding: No binding to plasma proteins

Metabolism: No evidence of metabolism in humans

Bioavailability: 97%

Half-life elimination: 6-7 hours

Time to peak, plasma: 2-2.5 hours

Excretion: Urine (as unchanged drug)

Dosage Oral: Adults: Type 1 Gaucher disease: 100 mg 3 times/day; dose may be reduced to 100 mg 1-2 times/day in patients with adverse effects (ie, tremor, GI distress)

Dosage adjustment in renal impairment:

Cl_{cr} 50-75 mL/minute: 100 mg twice daily

Cl_{cr} 30-50 mL/minute: 100 mg once daily

Cl_{cr} <30 mL/minute: Not recommended

Dietary Considerations May be taken with or without food. Patients with diarrhea should avoid foods with high carbohydrate content.

Administration Capsules should be swallowed whole and taken at the same time each day. May be taken with or without food.

Monitoring Parameters Neurologic evaluations baseline and repeated every 6 months; adverse effects; weight

Dosage Forms Excipient information presented when available (limited, particularly for generics); consult specific product labeling.

Capsule:

Zavesca®: 100 mg

◆ **Migquin [DSC]** *see* Acetaminophen, Isometheptene, and Dichloralphenazone *on page 45*

◆ **Migranal®** *see* Dihydroergotamine *on page 470*

◆ **Migratine** *see* Acetaminophen, Isometheptene, and Dichloralphenazone *on page 45*

◆ **Migrazone® [DSC]** *see* Acetaminophen, Isometheptene, and Dichloralphenazone *on page 45*

◆ **Migrin-A [DSC]** *see* Acetaminophen, Isometheptene, and Dichloralphenazone *on page 45*

◆ **Mild-C® [OTC]** *see* Ascorbic Acid *on page 141*

◆ **Millipred™** *see* PrednisoLONE *on page 1326*

Milrinone (MIL ri none)

Medication Safety Issues

Sound-alike/look-alike issues:

Primacor® may be confused with Primaxin®

High alert medication: The Institute for Safe Medication Practices (ISMP) includes this medication among its list of drugs which have a heightened risk of causing significant patient harm when used in error.

U.S. Brand Names Primacor®

Canadian Brand Names Milrinone Lactate Injection; Primacor®

Mexican Brand Names Primacor

Index Terms Milrinone Lactate

Pharmacologic Category Phosphodiesterase Enzyme Inhibitor

Use Short-term I.V. therapy of acutely-decompensated heart failure

Unlabeled/Investigational Use Inotropic therapy for patients unresponsive to other acute heart failure therapies (eg, dobutamine); outpatient inotropic therapy for heart transplant candidates; palliation of symptoms in end-stage heart failure patients who cannot otherwise be discharged from the hospital and are not transplant candidates

Effect on Mental Status None reported

Effect on Psychiatric Treatment May cause hypotension; concurrent use with a psychotropic may further this risk; monitor. May rarely cause thrombocytopenia; use caution with valproic acid; monitor.

Dosage Summary

I.V.:

Children: Dosage not established

Adults: Loading dose (optional): 50 mcg/kg; Maintenance: 0.375-0.75 mcg/kg/minute

Dosage Forms Excipient information presented when available (limited, particularly for generics); consult specific product labeling. [DSC] = Discontinued product

Infusion [premixed in D_5W]: 200 mcg/mL (100 mL, 200 mL)

Primacor®: 200 mcg/mL (200 mL)

Injection, solution: 1 mg/mL (10 mL, 20 mL, 50 mL)

◆ **Milrinone Lactate** *see* Milrinone *on page 1055*

◆ **Miltown® [DSC]** *see* Meprobamate *on page 991*

Mineral Oil (MIN er al oyl)

U.S. Brand Names Fleet® Mineral Oil Enema [OTC]; Kondremul® [OTC]; Liqui-Doss® [OTC] [DSC]

Mexican Brand Names Fleet enema para Adulto

Index Terms Heavy Mineral Oil; Liquid Paraffin; White Mineral Oil

Pharmacologic Category Laxative, Lubricant

Use Temporary relief of occasional constipation, relief of fecal impaction; removal of barium sulfate residues following barium administration

Effect on Mental Status None reported

Effect on Psychiatric Treatment Patients with Parkinson's and Alzheimer's disease who have difficulty swallowing and are at an increased risk for aspiration may develop lipid pneumonitis.

Dosage Summary

Oral:

Children <1 year: Dosage not established

Children ≥1 year: Disimpaction: 15-30 mL per year of age (maximum: 240 mL/day); Maintenance: 1-3 mL/kg/day

Children 6-11 years:

Kondremul®: 10-25 mL/day

Liqui-Doss®: 5-15 mL at bedtime

Children ≥12 years:

Kondremul®: 30-75 mL/day

Liqui-Doss®: 15-45 mL at bedtime

Adults:

Kondremul®: 30-75 mL/day

Liqui-Doss®: 15-45 mL at bedtime

Rectal:

Children <2 years: Dosage not established

Children 2-12 years: 59 mL as a single dose

Children ≥12 years: 118 mL as a single dose
Adults: 118 mL as a single dose

Dosage Forms Excipient information presented when available (limited, particularly for generics); consult specific product labeling.
Liquid, oral:
Liqui-Doss®: 13.5 mL/15 mL (480 mL) [self-emulsifying oily liquid; alcohol free, sugar free] [DSC]
Microemulsion, oral:
Kondremul®: 2.5 mL/5 mL (480 mL) [sugar free; mint flavor]
Oil, rectal [enema]:
Fleet® Mineral Oil: 100% (118 mL)
Oil, oral: 100% (30 mL, 480 mL, 3840 mL)
Oil, topical: 100% (480 mL) [light]

- **Minipress®** *see* Prazosin *on page 1325*
- **Minitran™** *see* Nitroglycerin *on page 1147*
- **Minizide® [DSC]** *see* Prazosin and Polythiazide *on page 1325*
- **Minocin® PAC** *see* Minocycline *on page 1056*

Minocycline (mi noe SYE kleen)

Medication Safety Issues
Sound-alike/look-alike issues:
Dynacin® may be confused with Dyazide®, Dynabac®, DynaCirc®, Dynapen®
Minocin® may be confused with Indocin®, Lincocin®, Minizide®, Mithracin®, niacin

U.S. Brand Names Dynacin®; Minocin® PAC; myrac™; Solodyn™

Canadian Brand Names Alti-Minocycline; Apo-Minocycline®; Gen-Minocycline; Minocin®; Novo-Minocycline; PMS-Minocycline; Rhoxal-minocycline; Sandoz-Minocycline

Mexican Brand Names Micromycin; Minocin

Index Terms Minocycline Hydrochloride

Pharmacologic Category Antibiotic, Tetracycline Derivative

Use Treatment of susceptible bacterial infections of both gram-negative and gram-positive organisms; treatment of anthrax (inhalational, cutaneous, and gastrointestinal); moderate-to-severe acne; meningococcal (asymptomatic) carrier state; Rickettsial diseases (including Rocky Mountain spotted fever, Q fever); nongonococcal urethritis, gonorrhea; acute intestinal amebiasis
Extended release (Solodyn™): Only indicated for treatment of inflammatory lesions of non-nodular moderate-to-severe acne

Unlabeled/Investigational Use Rheumatoid arthritis (patients with low disease activity of short duration)

Effect on Psychiatric Treatment Barbiturates and carbamazepine may decrease the effects of tetracyclines; tetracyclines may decrease lithium clearance resulting in an increase in serum lithium levels and potential lithium toxicity; monitor serum lithium levels. No data documenting these effects with minocycline; use caution.

Dosage Summary
Oral:
Children ≤8 years: Dosage not established
Children >8 years: 4 mg/kg initially, followed by 2 mg/kg/dose every 12 hours
Children ≥12 years: Solodyn™: 45-135 mg once daily (weight based)
Adults: 200 mg initially, followed by 100 mg every 12 hours **or** 50-100 mg twice daily (acne)
Solodyn™: 45-135 mg once daily (weight based)

Dosage Forms Excipient information presented when available (limited, particularly for generics); consult specific product labeling. [DSC] = Discontinued product
Capsule: 50 mg, 75 mg, 100 mg
Dynacin®: 75 mg [DSC], 100 mg [DSC]
Capsule, pellet filled: 50 mg, 100 mg
Minocin® PAC: 50 mg, 100 mg [packaged with wipes, serum, and masque]
Tablet: 50 mg, 75 mg, 100 mg
Dynacin®, myrac™: 50 mg, 75 mg, 100 mg
Tablet, extended release:
Solodyn™: 45 mg, 90 mg, 135 mg

- **Minocycline Hydrochloride** *see* Minocycline *on page 1056*

Minoxidil (mi NOKS i dil)

Medication Safety Issues

Sound-alike/look-alike issues:

Minoxidil may be confused with metolazone, midodrine, Minipress®, Minocin®, Monopril®, Noxafil®

International issues:

Noxidil® [Thailand] may be confused with Noxafil® which is a brand name for posaconazole in the U.S.

U.S. Brand Names Rogaine® Extra Strength for Men [OTC]; Rogaine® for Men [OTC]; Rogaine® for Women [OTC]

Canadian Brand Names Apo-Gain®; Loniten®; Minox; Rogaine®

Mexican Brand Names Regaine

Pharmacologic Category Topical Skin Product; Vasodilator, Direct-Acting

Use Management of severe hypertension (usually in combination with a diuretic and beta-blocker); treatment (topical formulation) of alopecia androgenetica in males and females

Effect on Mental Status May cause dizziness

Effect on Psychiatric Treatment May rarely cause leukopenia; use caution with clozapine and carbamazepine

Dosage Summary

Oral:

Children <12 years: Initial: 0.1-0.2 mg/kg once daily (maximum: 5 mg/day); Usual dosage range: 0.25-1 mg/kg/day in 1-2 divided doses (maximum: 50 mg/day); **Note:** Titration is recommended

Children ≥12 years: Initial: 5 mg once daily; Usual dosage range: 2.5-80 mg/day in 1-2 divided doses (maximum: 100 mg/day); **Note:** Titration is recommended

Adults: Initial: 5 mg once daily; Usual dosage range: 2.5-80 mg/day in 1-2 divided doses (maximum: 100 mg/day); **Note:** Titration is recommended

Elderly: Initial: 2.5 mg once daily; increase gradually

Topical:

Children: Dosage not established

Adults: Apply twice daily

Dosage Forms Excipient information presented when available (limited, particularly for generics); consult specific product labeling. [DSC] = Discontinued product

Aerosol, topical [foam]:

Rogaine for Men®: 5% (60 g)

Solution, topical: 2% (60 mL); 5% (60 mL)

Rogaine® for Men: (60 mL) [DSC] [supplied with dropper applicator]

Rogaine® for Women: 2% (60 mL) [supplied with dropper applicator]

Rogaine® Extra Strength for Men: 5% (60 mL) [supplied with dropper applicator]

Tablet: 2.5 mg, 10 mg

- ◆ **Mintab DM** *see* Guaifenesin and Dextromethorphan *on page 739*
- ◆ **Mintezol®** *see* Thiabendazole *on page 1567*
- ◆ **Mintox Extra Strength [OTC]** *see* Aluminum Hydroxide, Magnesium Hydroxide, and Simethicone *on page 78*
- ◆ **Mintox Plus [OTC]** *see* Aluminum Hydroxide, Magnesium Hydroxide, and Simethicone *on page 78*
- ◆ **Mintuss DR** *see* Chlorpheniramine, Phenylephrine, and Dextromethorphan *on page 327*
- ◆ **Mintuss G [DSC]** *see* Hydrocodone, Phenylephrine, and Guaifenesin *on page 783*
- ◆ **Mintuss HC** *see* Phenylephrine, Hydrocodone, and Chlorpheniramine *on page 1277*
- ◆ **Mintuss MS** *see* Phenylephrine, Hydrocodone, and Chlorpheniramine *on page 1277*
- ◆ **Miochol®-E** *see* Acetylcholine *on page 47*
- ◆ **Mirapex®** *see* Pramipexole *on page 1318*
- ◆ **Mircette®** *see* Ethinyl Estradiol and Desogestrel *on page 592*
- ◆ **Mirena®** *see* Levonorgestrel *on page 918*

Mirtazapine (mir TAZ a peen)

Medication Safety Issues

Sound-alike/look-alike issues:

Remeron® may be confused with Premarin®, Zemuron®

International issues:

Avanza® [Australia] may be confused with Albenza® which is a brand name for albendazole in the U.S.

Avanza® [Australia] may be confused with Avandia® which is a brand name for rosiglitazone in the U.S.

Remeron® my be confused with Reneuron® which is a brand name for fluoxetine in Spain

Related Information

Antidepressant Agents *on page 1760*
Antidepressant Receptor Profile *on page 1764*

U.S. Brand Names Remeron SolTab®; Remeron®

Canadian Brand Names CO Mirtazapine; Gen-Mirtazapine; Novo-Mirtazapine; PMS-Mirtazapine; ratio-Mirtazapine; Remeron®; Remeron® RD; Rhoxal-mirtazapine; Rhoxal-mirtazapine FC; Riva-Mirtazapine; Sandoz-Mirtazapine; Sandoz-Mirtazapine FC

Mexican Brand Names Remeron

Pharmacologic Category Antidepressant, Alpha-2 Antagonist

Generic Available Yes

Use Treatment of depression

Restrictions An FDA-approved medication guide concerning the use of antidepressants in children, adolescents, and young adults must be distributed when dispensing an outpatient prescription (new or refill) where this medication is to be used without direct supervision of a healthcare provider. Medication guides are available at http://www.fda.gov/cder/Offices/ODS/medication_guides.htm. Dispense to parents or guardians of children and adolescents receiving this medication.

Pregnancy Risk Factor C

Pregnancy Considerations Animal studies did not show teratogenic effects, however, there was an increase in fetal loss and decrease in birth weight; use during pregnancy only if clearly needed.

Lactation Excretion in breast milk unknown/not recommended

Contraindications Hypersensitivity to mirtazapine or any component of the formulation; use of MAO inhibitors within 14 days

Warnings/Precautions [U.S. Boxed Warning]: Antidepressants increase the risk of suicidal thinking and behavior in children, adolescents, and young adults (18-24 years of age) with major depressive disorder (MDD) and other psychiatric disorders; consider risk prior to prescribing. Short-term studies did not show an increased risk in patients >24 years of age and showed a decreased risk in patients ≥65 years. Closely monitor for clinical worsening, suicidality, or unusual changes in behavior; the patient's family or caregiver should be instructed to closely observe the patient and communicate condition with healthcare provider. A medication guide should be dispensed with each prescription. **Mirtazapine is not FDA approved for use in children.**

The possibility of a suicide attempt is inherent in major depression and may persist until remission occurs. Monitor for worsening of depression or suicidality, especially during initiation of therapy (generally first 1-2 months) or with dose increases or decreases. Use caution in high-risk patients. Worsening depression and severe abrupt suicidality that are not part of the presenting symptoms may require discontinuation or modification of drug therapy. The patient's family or caregiver should be alerted to monitor patients for the emergence of suicidality and associated behaviors (such as agitation, irritability, hostility, impulsivity, and hypomania) and call healthcare provider.

May worsen psychosis in some patients or precipitate a shift to mania or hypomania in patients with bipolar disorder. Patients presenting with depressive symptoms should be screened for bipolar disorder. Monotherapy in patients with bipolar disorder should be avoided. **Mirtazapine is not FDA approved for the treatment of bipolar depression.**

Discontinue immediately if signs and symptoms of neutropenia/agranulocytosis occur. May cause sedation, resulting in impaired performance of tasks requiring alertness (eg, operating machinery or driving). Sedative effects may be additive with other CNS depressants and/or ethanol. The degree of sedation is moderate-high relative to other antidepressants. The risks of orthostatic hypotension or anticholinergic effects are low relative to other antidepressants.

The incidence of sexual dysfunction with mirtazapine is generally lower than with SSRIs. Potential for severe reaction when used with MAO inhibitors; autonomic instability, coma, death, delirium, diaphoresis, hyperthermia, mental status changes/agitation, muscular rigidity, myoclonus, neuroleptic malignant syndrome features, and seizures may occur.

May increase appetite and stimulate weight gain. Weight gain of >7% of body weight reported in 7.5% of patients treated with mirtazapine compared to 0% for placebo; 8% of patients receiving mirtazapine discontinued treatment due to the weight gain. In an 8-week pediatric clinical trial, 49% of mirtazapine-treated patients had a weight gain of at least 7% (mean increase 4 kg) as compared to 5.7% of placebo-treated patients (mean increase 1 kg). May increase serum cholesterol and triglyceride levels.

Use caution in patients with a previous seizure disorder or condition predisposing to seizures such as brain damage, alcoholism, or concurrent therapy with other drugs which lower the seizure threshold. Use with caution in patients with hepatic or renal dysfunction and in elderly patients. SolTab® formulation contains phenylalanine.

Adverse Reactions

>10%:

Central nervous system: Somnolence (54%)

Endocrine & metabolic: Cholesterol increased

Gastrointestinal: Constipation (13%), xerostomia (25%), appetite increased (17%), weight gain (12%; weight gain of >7% reported in 8% of adults, ≤49% of pediatric patients)

1% to 10%:

Cardiovascular: Hypertension, vasodilatation, peripheral edema (2%), edema (1%)

Central nervous system: Dizziness (7%), abnormal dreams (4%), abnormal thoughts (3%), confusion (2%), malaise

Endocrine & metabolic: Triglycerides increased

Gastrointestinal: Vomiting, anorexia, abdominal pain

Genitourinary: Urinary frequency (2%)

Neuromuscular & skeletal: Myalgia (2%), back pain (2%), arthralgia, tremor (2%), weakness (8%)

Respiratory: Dyspnea (1%)

Miscellaneous: Flu-like syndrome (5%), thirst (<1%)

<1% (Limited to important or life-threatening): Agranulocytosis, dehydration, liver function test increases, lymphadenopathy, neutropenia, orthostatic hypotension, seizure (1 case reported), torsade de pointes (1 case reported), weight loss

Metabolism/Transport Effects **Substrate** of CYP1A2 (major), 2C9 (minor), 2D6 (major), 3A4 (major); **Inhibits** CYP1A2 (weak), 3A4 (weak)

Drug Interactions

Alcohol (Ethyl): CNS Depressants may enhance the CNS depressant effect of Alcohol (Ethyl). *Risk C: Monitor therapy*

Alpha2-Agonists: Antidepressants (Alpha2-Antagonist) may diminish the hypotensive effect of Alpha2-Agonists. **Exceptions:** Apraclonidine; Brimonidine. *Risk D: Consider therapy modification*

CNS Depressants: May enhance the adverse/toxic effect of other CNS Depressants. *Risk C: Monitor therapy*

CYP1A2 Inducers (Strong): May increase the metabolism of CYP1A2 Substrates. *Risk C: Monitor therapy*

CYP1A2 Inhibitors (Moderate): May decrease the metabolism of CYP1A2 Substrates. *Risk C: Monitor therapy*

CYP1A2 Inhibitors (Strong): May decrease the metabolism of CYP1A2 Substrates. *Risk D: Consider therapy modification*

CYP2D6 Inhibitors (Moderate): May decrease the metabolism of CYP2D6 Substrates. *Risk C: Monitor therapy*

CYP2D6 Inhibitors (Strong): May decrease the metabolism of CYP2D6 Substrates. *Risk D: Consider therapy modification*

CYP3A4 Inducers (Strong): May increase the metabolism of CYP3A4 Substrates. *Risk C: Monitor therapy*

CYP3A4 Inhibitors (Moderate): May decrease the metabolism of CYP3A4 Substrates. *Risk C: Monitor therapy*

CYP3A4 Inhibitors (Strong): May decrease the metabolism of CYP3A4 Substrates. *Risk D: Consider therapy modification*

Darunavir: May increase the serum concentration of CYP2D6 Substrates. *Risk C: Monitor therapy*

Dasatinib: May increase the serum concentration of CYP3A4 Substrates. *Risk C: Monitor therapy*

Deferasirox: May decrease the serum concentration of CYP3A4 Substrates. *Risk C: Monitor therapy*

Herbs (CYP3A4 Inducers): May increase the metabolism of CYP3A4 Substrates. *Risk C: Monitor therapy*

MAO Inhibitors: May enhance the neurotoxic (central) effect of Mirtazapine. *Risk X: Avoid combination*

Serotonin Modulators: May enhance the adverse/toxic effect of other Serotonin Modulators. The development of serotonin syndrome may occur. *Risk D: Consider therapy modification*

Sibutramine: May enhance the serotonergic effect of Serotonin Modulators. This may cause serotonin syndrome. *Risk X: Avoid combination*

Ethanol/Nutrition/Herb Interactions

Ethanol: Avoid ethanol (may increase CNS depression).

Herb/Nutraceutical: Avoid St John's wort (may decrease mirtazapine levels). Avoid valerian, St John's wort, SAMe, kava kava (may increase CNS depression).

Stability Store at controlled room temperature.

SolTab®: Protect from light and moisture. Use immediately upon opening tablet blister.

Mechanism of Action Mirtazapine is a tetracyclic antidepressant that works by its central presynaptic alpha$_2$-adrenergic antagonist effects, which results in increased release of norepinephrine and serotonin. It is also a potent antagonist of 5-HT$_2$ and 5-HT$_3$ serotonin receptors and H1 histamine receptors and a moderate peripheral alpha$_1$-adrenergic and muscarinic antagonist; it does not inhibit the reuptake of norepinephrine or serotonin.

Pharmacodynamics/Kinetics

Protein binding: 85%

Metabolism: Extensively hepatic via CYP1A2, 2C9, 2D6, 3A4 and via demethylation and hydroxylation

Bioavailability: 50%

Half-life elimination: 20-40 hours; hampered with renal or hepatic impairment

Time to peak, serum: 2 hours

Excretion: Urine (75%) and feces (15%) as metabolites

Dosage

Treatment of depression: Adults: Oral: Initial: 15 mg nightly, titrate up to 15-45 mg/day with dose increases made no more frequently than every 1-2 weeks; there is an inverse relationship between dose and sedation

Elderly: Decreased clearance seen (40% males, 10% females); no specific dosage adjustment recommended by manufacturer

Alzheimer's dementia-related depression: Initial: 7.5 mg at bedtime; may increase at 7.5-15 mg increments to 45-60 mg/day

Dosage adjustment in renal impairment:

Cl_{cr} 11-39 mL/minute: 30% decreased clearance

Cl_{cr} <10 mL/minute: 50% decreased clearance

Dosage adjustment in hepatic impairment: Clearance decreased by 30%

Dietary Considerations Remeron SolTab® contains phenylalanine: 2.6 mg per 15 mg tablet; 5.2 mg per 30 mg tablet; 7.8 mg per 45 mg tablet

Administration SolTab®: Open blister pack and place tablet on the tongue. Do not split tablet. Tablet is formulated to dissolve on the tongue without water.

Monitoring Parameters Patients should be monitored for signs of agranulocytosis or severe neutropenia such as sore throat, stomatitis or other signs of infection or a low WBC; mental status for depression, suicidal ideation (especially at the beginning of therapy or when doses are increased or decreased), anxiety, social functioning, mania, panic attacks; lipid profile

Additional Information Note: At least 14 days should elapse between discontinuation of an MAO inhibitor and initiation of therapy with mirtazapine; at least 14 days should be allowed after discontinuing mirtazapine before starting an MAO inhibitor.

Dosage Forms Excipient information presented when available (limited, particularly for generics); consult specific product labeling.

Tablet: 7.5 mg, 15 mg, 30 mg, 45 mg

Remeron®: 15 mg, 30 mg, 45 mg

Tablet, orally disintegrating: 15 mg, 30 mg

Remeron SolTab®:

15 mg [contains phenylalanine 2.6 mg/tablet; orange flavor]

30 mg [contains phenylalanine 5.2 mg/tablet; orange flavor]

45 mg [contains phenylalanine 7.8 mg/tablet; orange flavor]

◆ **Misoprostol and Diclofenac** *see* Diclofenac and Misoprostol *on page 458*

Mitomycin (mye toe MYE sin)

Medication Safety Issues

Sound-alike/look-alike issues:

Mitomycin may be confused with mithramycin, mitotane, mitoxantrone

High alert medication: The Institute for Safe Medication Practices (ISMP) includes this medication among its list of drugs which have a heightened risk of causing significant patient harm when used in error.

Canadian Brand Names Mutamycin®

Mexican Brand Names Mitotie

Index Terms Mitomycin-C; Mitomycin-X; MTC; NSC-26980

Pharmacologic Category Antineoplastic Agent, Antibiotic

Use Treatment of adenocarcinoma of stomach or pancreas, bladder cancer, breast cancer, or colorectal cancer

Unlabeled/Investigational Use Prevention of excess scarring in glaucoma filtration procedures in patients at high risk of bleb failure

Effect on Mental Status May cause drowsiness

Effect on Psychiatric Treatment Myelosuppression is common; avoid with clozapine and carbamazepine

Dosage Summary

I.V.:

Children (unlabeled use): 20 mg/m^2 every 6-8 weeks as a single agent **or** 10 mg/m^2 every 6-8 weeks as combination therapy

Adults: 20 mg/m^2 every 6-8 weeks as a single agent **or** 10 mg/m^2 every 6-8 weeks as combination therapy

Dosage Forms Excipient information presented when available (limited, particularly for generics); consult specific product labeling.

Injection, powder for reconstitution: 5 mg, 20 mg, 40 mg

◆ **Mitomycin-X** *see* Mitomycin *on page 1061*

◆ **Mitomycin-C** *see* Mitomycin *on page 1061*

Mitotane (MYE toe tane)

Medication Safety Issues

Sound-alike/look-alike issues:

Mitotane may be confused with mitomycin

High alert medication: The Institute for Safe Medication Practices (ISMP) includes this medication among its list of drugs which have a heightened risk of causing significant patient harm when used in error.

U.S. Brand Names Lysodren®

Canadian Brand Names Lysodren®

Index Terms NSC-38721; o,p'-DDD

Pharmacologic Category Antineoplastic Agent, Miscellaneous

Use Treatment of adrenocortical carcinoma

Unlabeled/Investigational Use Treatment of Cushing's syndrome

Effect on Mental Status Dizziness and depression are common; may cause sedation, irritability, or confusion

Effect on Psychiatric Treatment May cause myelosuppression; use caution with clozapine and carbamazepine; concurrent use with psychotropics may produce additive sedation

Dosage Summary

Oral:

Children (unlabeled use): 1-2 g/day in divided doses increasing gradually (maximum: 7 g/day)

Adults: Initial: 2-6 g/day in divided doses, then increase incrementally to 9-10 g/day in 3-4 divided doses (maximum: 18 g/day)

Dosage Forms Excipient information presented when available (limited, particularly for generics); consult specific product labeling.

Tablet [scored]:

Lysodren®: 500 mg

Mitoxantrone (mye toe ZAN trone)

Medication Safety Issues

Sound-alike/look-alike issues:

Mitoxantrone may be confused with methotrexate, mitomycin, Mutamycin®

High alert medication: The Institute for Safe Medication Practices (ISMP) includes this medication among its list of drug classes which have a heightened risk of causing significant patient harm when used in error.

U.S. Brand Names Novantrone®

Canadian Brand Names Mitoxantrone Injection®; Novantrone®

Mexican Brand Names Mitoxgen; Mitroxone

Index Terms CL-232315; DHAD; DHAQ; Dihydroxyanthracenedione Dihydrochloride; Mitoxantrone Hydrochloride; Mitozantrone; NSC-301739

Pharmacologic Category Antineoplastic Agent, Anthracenedione

Use Treatment of acute nonlymphocytic leukemias, prostate cancer, lymphoma, secondary progressive or relapsing-remitting multiple sclerosis (MS)

Unlabeled/Investigational Use Treatment of pediatric acute leukemias, pediatric sarcoma

Effect on Mental Status May cause drowsiness

Effect on Psychiatric Treatment May cause myelosuppression; use caution with clozapine and carbamazepine

Dosage Summary

I.V.:

Children: Dosage not established

Adults: 12 mg/m^2/day once daily for 2-3 days **or** 12-14 mg/m^2 every 3-4 weeks **or** 2-4 mg/m^2/day for 5 days **or** 12 mg/m^2 every 3 months [multiple sclerosis] (maximum lifetime cumulative dose: 140 mg/m^2)

Dosage Forms Excipient information presented when available (limited, particularly for generics); consult specific product labeling. [DSC] = Discontinued product

Injection, solution [concentrate; preservative free]: 2 mg/mL (10 mL, 12.5 mL, 15 mL, 20 mL)

Novantrone®: 2 mg/mL (10 mL, 15 mL [DSC])

- **Mitoxantrone Hydrochloride** *see* Mitoxantrone *on page 1061*
- **Mitozantrone** *see* Mitoxantrone *on page 1061*
- **MK383** *see* Tirofiban *on page 1586*
- **MK-0431** *see* SitaGLIPtin *on page 1491*
- **MK462** *see* Rizatriptan *on page 1437*
- **MK 0517** *see* Fosaprepitant *on page 690*
- **MK-0518** *see* Raltegravir *on page 1393*
- **MK594** *see* Losartan *on page 952*
- **MK0826** *see* Ertapenem *on page 557*
- **MK 869** *see* Aprepitant *on page 130*
- **MLN341** *see* Bortezomib *on page 192*
- **MMF** *see* Mycophenolate *on page 1087*
- **MMR-V** *see* Measles, Mumps, Rubella, and Varicella Virus Vaccine *on page 972*
- **MMRV** *see* Measles, Mumps, Rubella, and Varicella Virus Vaccine *on page 972*
- **Moban®** *see* Molindone *on page 1069*
- **Mobic®** *see* Meloxicam *on page 982*

Moclobemide (moe KLOE be mide)

Canadian Brand Names Apo-Moclobemide®; Dom-Moclobemide; Manerix®; Novo-Moclobemide; Nu-Moclobemide; PMS-Moclobemide

Mexican Brand Names Aurorex; Feraken

Pharmacologic Category Antidepressant, Monoamine Oxidase Inhibitor, Reversible

Generic Available Yes

Use Symptomatic relief of depressive illness

Restrictions Not available in U.S.

Pregnancy Risk Factor Not available

Pregnancy Considerations Safety has not been established, use only if benefits outweigh the risks.

Lactation Enters breast milk/use caution

Contraindications Hypersensitivity to moclobemide or any component of the formulation; uncontrolled hypertension; hepatic disease; confusional states; concurrent use of sympathomimetics (and related compounds), MAO inhibitors, meperidine, tricyclic antidepressants, serotonergic drugs (including SSRIs) - do not use within 5 weeks of fluoxetine discontinuation or 2 weeks of other antidepressant discontinuation; general anesthesia, local vasoconstrictors;

spinal anesthesia (hypotension may be exaggerated). Not approved for use in patients <18 years of age.

Warnings/Precautions The possibility of a suicide attempt is inherent in major depression and may persist until remission occurs. Use caution in high-risk patients during initiation of therapy. Prescriptions should be written for the smallest quantity consistent with good patient care. Use caution in patients with thyrotoxicosis, pheochromocytoma, and renal dysfunction. Use caution in patients receiving concurrent CNS depressants, ethanol, or buspirone. Severe reactions may occur if MAO inhibitors and serotonergic agents, including SSRIs are used concurrently. Discontinue 2 days prior to local or general anesthesia. Use caution in hepatic impairment (dose adjustment required). Dietary restriction of tyramine does not appear to be necessary for patients receiving moclobemide (patients must be informed of signs/symptoms of reaction).

Adverse Reactions

1% to 10%:

Cardiovascular: Tachycardia (4%), hypotension (3%)

Central nervous system: Headache (8%), sleep disturbance (7%), dizziness (7%), agitation (5%), nervousness (5%), somnolence (4%), sedation (4%), anxiety (3%)

Endocrine & metabolic: Appetite increased (1%)

Gastrointestinal: Xerostomia (9%), nausea (5%), constipation (4%), diarrhea (2%), abdominal pain (2%), vomiting (2%)

Neuromuscular & skeletal: Weakness (1%)

Ocular: Blurred vision (2%)

Miscellaneous: Diaphoresis increased (2%)

<1% (Limited to important or life-threatening): Aggression, allergic reaction, angina, bradycardia, confusion, disorientation, delusions, dysarthria, dyspnea, extrapyramidal reactions, hallucinations, hypertension, mania, migraine, paresthesia, pruritus, rash, urticaria, visual disturbances

Metabolism/Transport Effects Substrate (major) of CYP2C19, 2D6; **Inhibits** CYP1A2 (weak), 2C19 (weak), 2D6 (weak)

Drug Interactions

Acetylcholinesterase Inhibitors (Central): Anticholinergics may diminish the therapeutic effect of Acetylcholinesterase Inhibitors (Central). Acetylcholinesterase Inhibitors (Central) may diminish the therapeutic effect of Anticholinergics. If the anticholinergic action is a side effect of the agent, the result may be beneficial. *Risk C: Monitor therapy*

Alcohol (Ethyl): CNS Depressants may enhance the CNS depressant effect of Alcohol (Ethyl). *Risk C: Monitor therapy*

Alpha-/Beta-Agonists (Direct-Acting): MAO Inhibitors may enhance the vasopressor effect of Alpha-/Beta-Agonists (Direct-Acting). Primarily with oral administration of phenylephrine. **Exceptions:** Dipivefrin. *Risk D: Consider therapy modification*

Alpha-/Beta-Agonists (Indirect-Acting): MAO Inhibitors may enhance the hypertensive effect of Alpha-/Beta-Agonists (Indirect-Acting). *Risk X: Avoid combination*

Alpha1-Agonists: MAO Inhibitors may enhance the hypertensive effect of Alpha1-Agonists. *Risk X: Avoid combination*

Alpha2-Agonists (Ophthalmic): MAO Inhibitors may enhance the hypertensive effect of Alpha2-Agonists (Ophthalmic). *Risk X: Avoid combination*

Altretamine: May enhance the orthostatic effect of MAO Inhibitors. *Risk C: Monitor therapy*

Amphetamines: MAO Inhibitors may enhance the hypertensive effect of Amphetamines. *Risk X: Avoid combination*

Anilidopiperidine Opioids: May enhance the serotonergic effect of MAO Inhibitors. This could result in serotonin syndrome. Management: Avoid use of fentanyl (and other anilidopiperidine opioids when possible) in patients who have used a monoamine oxidase inhibitor within the past 14 days due to reports of unpredictable but severe adverse effects. *Risk D: Consider therapy modification*

Anticholinergics: May enhance the adverse/toxic effect of other Anticholinergics. **Exceptions:** Paliperidone. *Risk C: Monitor therapy*

Antidepressants (Serotonin/Norepinephrine Reuptake Inhibitor): MAO Inhibitors may enhance the serotonergic effect of Antidepressants (Serotonin/Norepinephrine Reuptake Inhibitor). This may cause serotonin syndrome. *Risk X: Avoid combination*

Atomoxetine: MAO Inhibitors may enhance the neurotoxic (central) effect of Atomoxetine. *Risk X: Avoid combination*

Beta2-Agonists: MAO Inhibitors may enhance the adverse/toxic effect of Beta2-Agonists. *Risk C: Monitor therapy*

BuPROPion: MAO Inhibitors may enhance the neurotoxic (central) effect of BuPROPion. *Risk X: Avoid combination*

BusPIRone: May enhance the adverse/toxic effect of MAO Inhibitors. Elevated blood pressure has been reported. *Risk X: Avoid combination*

Cimetidine: May decrease the metabolism of Moclobemide. *Risk D: Consider therapy modification*

CNS Depressants: May enhance the adverse/toxic effect of other CNS Depressants. *Risk C: Monitor therapy*

COMT Inhibitors: May enhance the adverse/toxic effect of MAO Inhibitors. *Risk D: Consider therapy modification*

Cyclobenzaprine: May enhance the serotonergic effect of MAO Inhibitors. This could result in serotonin syndrome. *Risk X: Avoid combination*

CYP2C19 Inducers (Strong): May increase the metabolism of CYP2C19 Substrates. *Risk C: Monitor therapy*

CYP2C19 Inhibitors (Moderate): May decrease the metabolism of CYP2C19 Substrates. *Risk C: Monitor therapy*

CYP2C19 Inhibitors (Strong): May decrease the metabolism of CYP2C19 Substrates. *Risk D: Consider therapy modification*

CYP2D6 Inhibitors (Moderate): May decrease the metabolism of CYP2D6 Substrates. *Risk C: Monitor therapy*

CYP2D6 Inhibitors (Strong): May decrease the metabolism of CYP2D6 Substrates. *Risk D: Consider therapy modification*

Darunavir: May increase the serum concentration of CYP2D6 Substrates. *Risk C: Monitor therapy*

Dexmethylphenidate: MAO Inhibitors may enhance the hypertensive effect of Dexmethylphenidate. *Risk X: Avoid combination*

Dextromethorphan: MAO Inhibitors may enhance the serotonergic effect of Dextromethorphan. This may cause serotonin syndrome. *Risk X: Avoid combination*

Levodopa: May enhance the adverse/toxic effect of MAO Inhibitors. Of particular concern is the development of hypertensive reactions when levodopa is used with nonselective MAOI. *Risk D: Consider therapy modification*

Linezolid: MAO Inhibitors may enhance the adverse/toxic effect of Linezolid. *Risk X: Avoid combination*

Maprotiline: May enhance the adverse/toxic effect of MAO Inhibitors. *Risk X: Avoid combination*

Meperidine: MAO Inhibitors may enhance the serotonergic effect of Meperidine. This may cause serotonin syndrome. *Risk X: Avoid combination*

Methyldopa: MAO Inhibitors may enhance the adverse/toxic effect of Methyldopa. *Risk X: Avoid combination*

Methylphenidate: MAO Inhibitors may enhance the hypertensive effect of Methylphenidate. *Risk X: Avoid combination*

Mirtazapine: MAO Inhibitors may enhance the neurotoxic (central) effect of Mirtazapine. *Risk X: Avoid combination*

Pramlintide: May enhance the anticholinergic effect of Anticholinergics. These effects are specific to the GI tract. *Risk D: Consider therapy modification*

Propoxyphene: May enhance the adverse/toxic effect of MAO Inhibitors. Specifically, the risk of serotonin syndrome or other serotonergic adverse events may be increased. *Risk X: Avoid combination*

Rauwolfia Alkaloids: MAO Inhibitors may enhance the adverse/toxic effect of Rauwolfia Alkaloids. Existing MAOI therapy can result in paradoxical effects of added rauwolfia alkaloids (eg, excitation, hypertension). *Risk D: Consider therapy modification*

Selective Serotonin Reuptake Inhibitors: MAO Inhibitors may enhance the serotonergic effect of Selective Serotonin Reuptake Inhibitors. This may cause serotonin syndrome. *Risk X: Avoid combination*

Serotonin 5-HT1D Receptor Agonists: MAO Inhibitors may decrease the metabolism of Serotonin 5-HT1D Receptor Agonists. Management: If MAO inhibitor therapy is required, naratriptan, eletriptan or frovatriptan may be a suitable 5-HT1D agonist to employ. **Exceptions:** Eletriptan; Frovatriptan; Naratriptan. *Risk X: Avoid combination*

Serotonin Modulators: May enhance the adverse/toxic effect of other Serotonin Modulators. The development of serotonin syndrome may occur. *Risk D: Consider therapy modification*

Sibutramine: May enhance the serotonergic effect of Serotonin Modulators. This may cause serotonin syndrome. *Risk X: Avoid combination*

Tetrabenazine: May enhance the adverse/toxic effect of MAO Inhibitors. *Risk X: Avoid combination*

TraMADol: May enhance the neuroexcitatory and/or seizure-potentiating effect of MAO Inhibitors. *Risk D: Consider therapy modification*

Tricyclic Antidepressants: MAO Inhibitors may enhance the serotonergic effect of Tricyclic Antidepressants. This may cause serotonin syndrome. *Risk X: Avoid combination*

Ethanol/Nutrition/Herb Interactions
Ethanol: Avoid ethanol (may increase CNS depression).
Food: Dietary restriction of tyramine does not appear to be necessary.
Herb/Nutraceutical: Avoid valerian, St John's wort, SAMe, ginseng. Avoid ginkgo (may lead to MAO inhibitor toxicity). Avoid ephedra, yohimbe (can cause hypertension). Avoid kava (may increase CNS depression).

Stability Store at 15°C to 30°C (59°F to 86°F).

Mechanism of Action Moclobemide is a benzamide derivative which acts as a short-acting reversible inhibitor of monoamine oxidase (MAO), which inhibits the metabolism (deamination) of serotonin, norepinephrine, and dopamine. It has a relative specificity for the A subtype of monoamine oxidase (MAO type A). Its action leads to increased concentrations of these neurotransmitters, which may account for the antidepressant activity of moclobemide.

Pharmacodynamics/Kinetics
Absorption: 98% from GI tract
Distribution: 1.2 L/kg
Protein binding: ~50% to albumin
Metabolism: Oxidative reactions
Half-life elimination: Terminal: 1-2 hours
Excretion: Urine (95%, as metabolites)

Dosage Oral: Adults: Initial: 300 mg/day in 2 divided doses; increase gradually to maximum of 600 mg/day; **Note:** Individual patient response may allow a reduction in daily dose in long-term therapy.
Dosage adjustment in hepatic impairment: Decrease daily dose by 1/3 to 1/2

Dietary Considerations Should be taken immediately after meals. Manufacturer states no special dietary restrictions are required; may be taken with tyramine-containing foods. However, patients should be instructed to recognize occipital headache, palpitations, neck stiffness, or other signs of a severe reaction.

Administration Administer immediately after meals.

Monitoring Parameters Blood pressure, warning signs of suicide

Additional Information Not available in U.S.

Dosage Forms Excipient information presented when available (limited, particularly for generics); consult specific product labeling. [CAN] = Canadian brand name
Tablet: 150 mg, 300 mg
Alti-Moclobemide [CAN], Apo-Moclobemide® [CAN], Dom-Moclobemide® [CAN], Manerix®e [CAN], Novo-Moclobemidee [CAN], Nu-Moclobemidee [CAN], PMS-Moclobemide [CAN]: 150 mg, 300 mg [not available in the U.S.]

Modafinil (moe DAF i nil)

U.S. Brand Names Provigil®

Canadian Brand Names Alertec®; Provigil®

Mexican Brand Names Modiodal

Pharmacologic Category Stimulant

Generic Available No

Use Improve wakefulness in patients with excessive daytime sleepiness associated with narcolepsy and shift work sleep disorder (SWSD); adjunctive therapy for obstructive sleep apnea/hypopnea syndrome (OSAHS)

Unlabeled/Investigational Use Attention-deficit/hyperactivity disorder (ADHD); treatment of fatigue in MS and other disorders

Restrictions C-IV

Pregnancy Risk Factor C

Pregnancy Considerations Embryotoxic effects have been observed in some, but not all animal studies. There are no adequate and well-controlled studies in pregnant women; use only when the potential risk of drug therapy is outweighed by the drug's benefits. Efficacy of steroidal contraceptives may be decreased; alternate means of contraception should be considered during therapy and for 1 month after modafinil is discontinued.

Lactation Excretion in breast milk unknown/use caution

Contraindications Hypersensitivity to modafinil, armodafinil, or any component of the formulation

Warnings/Precautions For use following complete evaluation of sleepiness and in conjunction with other standard treatments (eg, CPAP). The degree of sleepiness should be reassessed frequently; some patients may not return to a normal level of wakefulness. Use is not recommended with a history of angina, cardiac ischemia, recent history of myocardial infarction, left ventricular hypertrophy, or patients with mitral valve prolapse who have developed mitral valve prolapse syndrome with previous CNS stimulant use.

Serious and life-threatening rashes (including Stevens-Johnson syndrome and toxic epidermal necrolysis) have been reported with modafinil. Most cases have occurred within the first 5 weeks of therapy, however rare cases have occurred after long-term use. No risk factors have been identified to predict occurrence or severity. Patients should be advised to discontinue at first sign of rash. In addition, rare cases of multiorgan hypersensitivity reactions in association with modafinil use, and lone cases of angioedema and anaphylactoid reactions with armodafinil, have been reported. Signs and symptoms are diverse, reflecting the involvement of specific organs. Patients typically present with fever and rash associated with organ-system dysfunction. Patients should be advised to report any signs and symptoms related to these effects; discontinuation of therapy is recommended.

Caution should be exercised when modafinil is given to patients with a history of psychosis; may impair the ability to engage in potentially hazardous activities. Stimulants may unmask tics in individuals with coexisting Tourette's syndrome. Use caution with renal or hepatic impairment (dosage adjustment in hepatic dysfunction is recommended). Safety and efficacy have not been established in children <16 years of age (U.S. labeling) or <18 years of age (Canadian labeling).

Adverse Reactions

>10%:

Central nervous system: Headache (34%, dose related)

Gastrointestinal: Nausea (11%)

1% to 10%:

Cardiovascular: Chest pain (3%), hypertension (3%), palpitation (2%), tachycardia (2%), vasodilation (2%), edema (1%)

Central nervous system: Nervousness (7%), dizziness (5%), depression (2%), anxiety (5%; dose related), insomnia (5%), somnolence (2%), chills (1%), agitation (1%), confusion (1%), emotional lability (1%), vertigo (1%)

Dermatologic: Rash (1%; includes some severe cases requiring hospitalization)

Gastrointestinal: Diarrhea (6%), dyspepsia (5%), xerostomia (4%), anorexia (4%), constipation (2%), flatulence (1%), mouth ulceration (1%), taste perversion (1%)

Genitourinary: Abnormal urine (1%), hematuria (1%), pyuria (1%)

Hematologic: Eosinophilia (1%)

Hepatic: LFTs abnormal (2%)

Neuromuscular & skeletal: Back pain (6%), paresthesia (2%), dyskinesia (1%), hyperkinesia (1%), hypertonia (1%), neck rigidity (1%), tremor (1%)

Ocular: Amblyopia (1%), eye pain (1%), vision abnormal (1%)

Respiratory: Pharyngitis (4%), rhinitis (7%), lung disorder (2%), asthma (1%), epistaxis (1%)

Miscellaneous: Diaphoresis

Postmarketing and/or case reports: Agranulocytosis, anaphylactic reaction, angioedema, DRESS syndrome, erythema multiforme, hypersensitivity syndrome (multiorgan), mania, psychosis, Stevens-Johnson syndrome, toxic epidermal necrolysis

Metabolism/Transport Effects **Substrate** of CYP3A4 (major); **Inhibits** CYP1A2 (weak), 2A6 (weak), 2C9 (weak), 2C19 (strong), 2E1 (weak), 3A4 (weak); **Induces** CYP1A2 (weak), 2B6 (weak), 3A4 (weak)

Drug Interactions

Cannabinoids: May enhance the tachycardic effect of Sympathomimetics. *Risk C: Monitor therapy*

CYP2C19 Substrates: CYP2C19 Inhibitors (Strong) may decrease the metabolism of CYP2C19 Substrates. *Risk D: Consider therapy modification*

CYP3A4 Inducers (Strong): May increase the metabolism of CYP3A4 Substrates. *Risk C: Monitor therapy*

CYP3A4 Inhibitors (Moderate): May decrease the metabolism of CYP3A4 Substrates. *Risk C: Monitor therapy*

CYP3A4 Inhibitors (Strong): May decrease the metabolism of CYP3A4 Substrates. *Risk D: Consider therapy modification*

Dasatinib: May increase the serum concentration of CYP3A4 Substrates. *Risk C: Monitor therapy*

Deferasirox: May decrease the serum concentration of CYP3A4 Substrates. *Risk C: Monitor therapy*

Herbs (CYP3A4 Inducers): May increase the metabolism of CYP3A4 Substrates. *Risk C: Monitor therapy*

Maraviroc: CYP3A4 Inducers may decrease the serum concentration of Maraviroc. *Risk D: Consider therapy modification*

Oral Contraceptive (Estrogens): Modafinil may decrease the serum concentration of Oral Contraceptive (Estrogens). *Risk D: Consider therapy modification*

Sympathomimetics: May enhance the adverse/toxic effect of other Sympathomimetics. *Risk C: Monitor therapy*

Ethanol/Nutrition/Herb Interactions

Ethanol: Avoid or limit ethanol.

Food: Delays absorption, but does not affect bioavailability.

Mechanism of Action The exact mechanism of action is unclear, it does not appear to alter the release of dopamine or norepinephrine, it may exert its stimulant effects by decreasing GABA-mediated neurotransmission, although this theory has not yet been fully evaluated; several studies also suggest that an intact central alpha-adrenergic system is required for modafinil's activity; the drug increases high-frequency alpha waves while decreasing both delta and theta wave activity, and these effects are consistent with generalized increases in mental alertness

Pharmacodynamics/Kinetics Modafinil is a racemic compound (10% *d*-isomer and 90% *l*-isomer at steady state) whose enantiomers have different pharmacokinetics

Distribution: V_d: 0.9 L/kg

Protein binding: 60%, primarily to albumin

Metabolism: Hepatic; multiple pathways including CYP3A4

Half-life elimination: Effective half-life: 15 hours; Steady-state: 2-4 days

Time to peak, serum: 2-4 hours

Excretion: Urine (as metabolites, <10% as unchanged drug)

Dosage Oral:

Children: ADHD (unlabeled use): 50-100 mg once daily

Adults:

ADHD (unlabeled use): 100-300 mg once daily

Narcolepsy, obstructive sleep apnea/hypopnea syndrome (OSAHS): Initial: 200 mg as a single daily dose in the morning

Shift work sleep disorder (SWSD): Initial: 200 mg as a single dose taken ~1 hour prior to start of work shift

Note: Doses of 400 mg/day, given as a single dose, have been well tolerated, but there is no consistent evidence that this dose confers additional benefit.

Elderly: Elimination of modafinil and its metabolites may be reduced as a consequence of aging and as a result, consider initiating dose at 100 mg once daily.

Dosing adjustment in renal impairment: Safety and efficacy have not been established in severe renal impairment.

Dosing adjustment in hepatic impairment: Dose should be reduced to one-half of that recommended for patients with normal liver function.

Child/Adolescent Considerations Across three large randomized, double-blind, placebo-controlled trials, a total of 638 children and adolescents (range: 6-17 years of age) with ADHD were treated with modafanil (170-425 mg once daily) or placebo for 7-9 weeks (Biederman, 2005; Greenhill, 2006; Swanson, 2006). Modafanil treatment was associated with significant decreases in the ADHD-RS-IV scores compared relative to baseline and significantly compared to placebo (p<0.0001) for all three studies. Despite the demonstrated efficacy, these studies revealed a high rate of serious dermatological reactions (including Stevens-Johnson syndrome) in these patients.

Biederman J, Swanson JM, Wigal SB, et al, "Efficacy and Safety of Modafinil Film-Coated Tablets in Children and Adolescents With Attention-Deficit/Hyperactivity Disorder: Results of a Randomized, Double-Blind, Placebo-Controlled, Flexible-Dose Study," *Pediatrics*, 2005, 116(6):e777-84.

Greenhill LL, Biederman J, Boellner SW, et al, "A Randomized, Double-Blind, Placebo-Controlled Study of Modafinil Film-Coated Tablets in Children and Adolescents With Attention-Deficit/Hyperactivity Disorder," *J Am Acad Child Adolesc Psychiatry*, 2006, 45(5):503-11.

Swanson JM, Greenhill LL, Lopez FA, et al, "Modafinil Film-Coated Tablets in Children and Adolescents With Attention-Deficit/Hyperactivity Disorder: Results of a Randomized, Double-Blind, Placebo-Controlled, Fixed-Dose Study Followed by Abrupt Discontinuation," *J Clin Psychiatry*, 2006, 67 (1):137-47.

Monitoring Parameters Levels of sleepiness; blood pressure in patients with hypertension

When used for the treatment of ADHD, thoroughly evaluate for cardiovascular risk. Monitor heart rate, blood pressure, and consider obtaining ECG prior to initiation (Vetter, 2008).

Dosage Forms Excipient information presented when available (limited, particularly for generics); consult specific product labeling.
Tablet:
Provigil®: 100 mg, 200 mg

◆ **Modicon®** *see* Ethinyl Estradiol and Norethindrone *on page 597*

Moexipril (mo EKS i pril)

Medication Safety Issues
Sound-alike/look-alike issues:
Moexipril may be confused with Monopril®

Related Information
Angiotensin Agents *on page 1754*

U.S. Brand Names Univasc®

Index Terms Moexipril Hydrochloride

Pharmacologic Category Angiotensin-Converting Enzyme (ACE) Inhibitor

Use Treatment of hypertension, alone or in combination with thiazide diuretics

Effect on Mental Status May cause drowsiness or dizziness; may rarely cause anxiety or mood changes

Effect on Psychiatric Treatment May cause neutropenia; use caution with clozapine and carbamazepine; may decrease lithium clearance resulting in an increase in serum lithium levels and potential lithium toxicity; monitor serum lithium levels

Dosage Summary

Oral:
Children: Dosage not established
Adults: Initial: 3.75-7.5 mg once daily; Maintenance: 7.5-30 mg/day in 1 or 2 divided doses

Dosage Forms Excipient information presented when available (limited, particularly for generics); consult specific product labeling.
Tablet, as hydrochloride [scored]: 7.5 mg, 15 mg
Univasc®: 7.5 mg, 15 mg

Moexipril and Hydrochlorothiazide
(mo EKS i pril & hye droe klor oh THYE a zide)

U.S. Brand Names Uniretic®

Canadian Brand Names Uniretic®

Index Terms Hydrochlorothiazide and Moexipril

Pharmacologic Category Angiotensin-Converting Enzyme (ACE) Inhibitor; Diuretic, Thiazide

Use Treatment of hypertension; not indicated for initial treatment of hypertension

Effect on Mental Status May cause drowsiness or dizziness; may rarely cause anxiety or mood changes

Effect on Psychiatric Treatment Thiazides and ACE inhibitors may decrease lithium clearance resulting in an increase in serum lithium levels and potential lithium toxicity; monitor serum lithium levels; may cause neutropenia; use caution with clozapine and carbamazepine

Dosage Summary

Oral:
Children: Dosage not established
Adults: 7.5-30 mg of moexipril/day and ≤50 mg hydrochlorothiazide/day in a single or divided dose

Dosage Forms Excipient information presented when available (limited, particularly for generics); consult specific product labeling.
Tablet [scored]:
7.5/12.5: Moexipril hydrochloride 7.5 mg and hydrochlorothiazide 12.5 mg
15/12.5: Moexipril hydrochloride 15 mg and hydrochlorothiazide 12.5 mg
15/25: Moexipril hydrochloride 15 mg and hydrochlorothiazide 25 mg
Uniretic®:
7.5/12.5: Moexipril hydrochloride 7.5 mg and hydrochlorothiazide 12.5 mg
15/12.5: Moexipril hydrochloride 15 mg and hydrochlorothiazide 12.5 mg
15/25: Moexipril hydrochloride 15 mg and hydrochlorothiazide 25 mg

◆ **Moexipril Hydrochloride** *see* Moexipril *on page 1068*

Molindone (moe LIN done)

Medication Safety Issues

Sound-alike/look-alike issues:

Molindone may be confused with Mobidin®

Moban® may be confused with Mobidin®, Modane®

Related Information

Anticholinergic Effects of Common Psychotropics *on page 1758*
Antipsychotic Agents *on page 1769*
CMS: Long-Term Care Facility Thresholds *on page 1815*
Discontinuation of Psychotropic Drugs *on page 1839*

U.S. Brand Names Moban®

Canadian Brand Names Moban®

Index Terms Molindone Hydrochloride

Pharmacologic Category Antipsychotic Agent, Typical

Generic Available No

Use Management of schizophrenia

Unlabeled/Investigational Use Management of psychotic disorders; behavioral symptoms associated with dementia (elderly); psychosis/agitation related to Alzheimer's dementia

Mental Health Comment Molindone is not commonly used, and is an intermediate-potency antipsychotic. Older antipsychotic medications (chlorpromazine, haloperidol), which do not meet specific criteria for "atypical" antipsychotics, are often referred to as typical antipsychotics. They are associated with the troubling side effect, EPS. However, it is commonly believed that in order for a drug to treat psychosis, it must block dopamine is some manner.

Common side effects include sedation and neuroleptic effect (reduced initiative, interest in the environment, and display of emotion or affect). All **typical** antipsychotics are considered to be equally effective if given in equipotent doses. An inverse relationship exists between intrinsic antimuscarinic activity and propensity to cause extrapyramidal side effects. If dystonia or pseudoparkinsonism occurs, antiparkinsonian agents should be considered. If akathisia occurs, beta-blockers (eg, propranolol), benzodiazepines, or antiparkinsonian agents should be considered. Tardive dyskinesia (TD) secondary to typical antipsychotics has an estimated incidence of 3% to 5% per year for the first 5 years of treatment. After this time period, the incidence is estimated to be 2% to 3% per year. Prevalence rates are ~15% to 20%. Female gender and age constitute risk factors for TD. Indeed, prevalence rates have been reported to be as high as 70% in elderly females. No specific treatment exists for TD, however, patients are often initiated on/switched to an atypical antipsychotic because of their lower incidence to cause TD and hopes of suppression.

Typical antipsychotics are usually only indicated for schizophrenia, but are generally effective for mania and psychosis and/or behavioral syndromes secondary to other mental conditions. Nonpsychiatric uses include Tourette's syndrome, Huntington's disease, and occasionally, intractable hiccups, pruritus, nausea, and vomiting.

These drugs are thought to exert their antipsychotic activity by blocking dopamine D_2 receptors in the mesolimbic dopaminergic pathway. Side effects are often related to their ability to antagonize dopamine receptors in the nigrostriatal and tuberoinfundibular pathways.

Coadministration of two or more antipsychotics does not generally improve clinical response and may increase the potential for adverse effects.

In 2008, the FDA issued a warning regarding increased mortality risk with typical **and** atypical antipsychotic drugs when used in elderly patients with dementia-related psychosis.

Pregnancy Risk Factor C

Lactation Excretion in breast milk unknown

Contraindications Hypersensitivity to molindone or any component of the formulation (cross-reactivity between phenothiazines may occur); severe CNS depression; coma

Warnings/Precautions [U.S. Boxed Warning]: Elderly patients with dementia-related psychosis treated with antipsychotics are at an increased risk of death compared to placebo. An increased incidence of cerebrovascular adverse events (including fatalities) has been reported in elderly patients with dementia-related psychosis. Molindone is not approved for this indication.May alter cardiac conduction; life-threatening arrhythmias have occurred with therapeutic doses of antipsychotics. Avoid use in patients with underlying QT prolongation, in those taking medicines that prolong the QT interval, or cause polymorphic ventricular tachycardia; monitor ECG closely for dose-related QT effects. Myelosuppression (eg, leukopenia, agranulocytosis) has been observed with antipsychotic use; check blood counts periodically and discontinue at first signs of blood dyscrasias. Antipsychotic use has been associated with esophageal dysmotility and aspiration; use with caution in patients at risk of pneumonia (ie, Alzheimer's disease). May cause extrapyramidal symptoms (EPS), including pseudoparkinsonism, acute dystonic reactions, akathisia, and tardive dyskinesia (risk of these reactions is high relative to other neuroleptics). Risk of dystonia (and possibly other EPS) may be greater with increased doses, use of conventional antipsychotics, males, and younger patients. Use may be associated with NMS; monitor for mental status changes, fever, muscle rigidity, and/or autonomic instability (risk may be increased in patients with Parkinson's disease or Lewy body dementia). May rarely cause orthostatic hypotension; use with caution in patients at risk of this effect or in those who would not tolerate transient hypotensive episodes (cerebrovascular disease, cardiovascular disease, hypovolemia, or concurrent medication use which may predispose to hypotension/bradycardia). May be associated with pigmentary retinopathy. Impaired core body temperature regulation may occur; caution with strenuous exercise, heat exposure, dehydration, and concomitant medication possessing anticholinergic effects.

May be sedating, use with caution in disorders where CNS depression is a feature; patients must be cautioned about performing tasks which require mental alertness (eg, operating machinery or driving). May cause anticholinergic effects (constipation, xerostomia, blurred vision, urinary retention); use with caution in patients with decreased gastrointestinal motility, paralytic ileus, urinary retention, BPH, xerostomia, or visual problems. Relative to other neuroleptics, molindone has a low potency of cholinergic blockade. May mask toxicity of other drugs or conditions (eg, intestinal obstruction, Reye's syndrome, brain tumor) due to antiemetic effects.

Use with caution in patients with severe cardiovascular disease, hepatic impairment, Parkinson's disease, breast cancer or other prolactin-dependent tumors, renal impairment, respiratory disease, or seizure disorder. Initiate therapy at a reduced dose in the elderly and debilitated patients; may be more susceptible to adverse effects. Due to calcium sulfate content in the tablet, concomitant use may decrease the absorption of phenytoin and tetracyclines.

Adverse Reactions Frequency not defined.

Cardiovascular: Arrhythmia, orthostatic hypotension, tachycardia, T wave changes (transient; rare)

Central nervous system: Central temperature regulation altered, drowsiness, euphoria, extrapyramidal reactions (akathisia, pseudoparkinsonism, dystonia, tardive dyskinesia), hyperactivity, mental depression, neuroleptic malignant syndrome (NMS), restlessness, sedation, seizure

Dermatologic: Rash

Endocrine & metabolic: Amenorrhea, change in menstrual periods, galactorrhea, gynecomastia, libido increased

Gastrointestinal: Constipation, nausea, salivation, weight gain (minimal compared to other antipsychotics), weight loss, xerostomia

Genitourinary: Priapism, urinary retention

Hematologic: Leukopenia (rare), leukocytosis (rare)

Hepatic: Liver function tests altered (rare)

Ocular: Blurred vision, lens opacities, retinal pigmentation

Drug Interactions

Acetylcholinesterase Inhibitors (Central): May enhance the neurotoxic (central) effect of Antipsychotics. Severe extrapyramidal symptoms have occurred in some patients. *Risk C: Monitor therapy*

Alcohol (Ethyl): CNS Depressants may enhance the CNS depressant effect of Alcohol (Ethyl). *Risk C: Monitor therapy*

Amphetamines: Antipsychotics may diminish the stimulatory effect of Amphetamines. *Risk C: Monitor therapy*

Anticholinergics: May enhance the adverse/toxic effect of other Anticholinergics. **Exceptions:** Paliperidone. *Risk C: Monitor therapy*

Anti-Parkinson's Agents (Dopamine Agonist): Antipsychotics (Typical) may diminish the therapeutic effect of Anti-Parkinson's Agents (Dopamine Agonist). *Risk D: Consider therapy modification*

CNS Depressants: May enhance the adverse/toxic effect of other CNS Depressants. *Risk C: Monitor therapy*

Lithium formulations: May enhance the neurotoxic effect of Antipsychotics. Lithium formulations may decrease the serum concentration of Antipsychotics. Specifically noted with chlorpromazine. *Risk C: Monitor therapy*

Pramlintide: May enhance the anticholinergic effect of Anticholinergics. These effects are specific to the GI tract. *Risk D: Consider therapy modification*

Tetrabenazine: May enhance the adverse/toxic effect of Antipsychotics. *Risk C: Monitor therapy*

Ethanol/Nutrition/Herb Interactions

Ethanol: Avoid ethanol (may increase CNS depression).

Herb/Nutraceutical: Avoid kava kava, gotu kola, valerian, St John's wort (may increase CNS depression).

Stability Store at controlled room temperature of 25°C (77°F). Protect from light.

Mechanism of Action Molindone is a dihydroindoline antipsychotic whose mechanism of action mimics that of chlorpromazine; however, it produces more extrapyramidal symptoms and less sedation than chlorpromazine

Pharmacodynamics/Kinetics

Metabolism: Hepatic

Half-life elimination: 1.5 hours

Time to peak, serum: ~1.5 hours

Excretion: Urine and feces (90%) within 24 hours

Dosage Oral:

Children: Schizophrenia/psychoses (unlabeled use):

- 3-5 years: 1-2.5 mg/day in 4 divided doses
- 5-12 years: 0.5-1 mg/kg/day in 4 divided doses

Adults: Schizophrenia/psychoses:

- Initial: 50-75 mg/day, may increase to 100 mg/day in 3-4 days; may further increase dose gradually to maximum of 225 mg/day
- Maintenance: 5-15 mg (mild symptoms) or 10-25 mg (moderate symptoms) 3-4 times/day (up to 225 mg/day may be required in severe cases)

Elderly: Behavioral symptoms associated with dementia (unlabeled use): Initial: 5-10 mg 1-2 times/day; increase at 4- to 7-day intervals by 5-10 mg/day; increase dosing intervals (bid, tid, etc) as necessary to control response or side effects.

Monitoring Parameters Vital signs; lipid profile, fasting blood glucose/Hgb A_{1c}; BMI; mental status, abnormal involuntary movement scale (AIMS), extrapyramidal symptoms (EPS)

Dosage Forms Excipient information presented when available (limited, particularly for generics); consult specific product labeling.

Tablet, as hydrochloride: 5 mg, 10 mg, 25 mg, 50 mg

◆ **Molindone Hydrochloride** *see* Molindone *on page 1069*

Mometasone (moe MET a sone)

Medication Safety Issues

Sound-alike/look-alike issues:

Elocon® lotion may be confused with ophthalmic solutions. Manufacturer's labeling emphasizes the product is **NOT** for use in the eyes.

Related Information

Corticosteroids *on page 1780*

U.S. Brand Names Asmanex® Twisthaler®; Elocon®; Nasonex®

Canadian Brand Names Elocom®; Nasonex®; PMS-Mometasone; ratio-Mometasone; Taro-Mometasone

Mexican Brand Names Elica; Elomet; Elovent Twisthaler; Rinelon; Uniclar

Index Terms Mometasone Furoate

Pharmacologic Category Corticosteroid, Inhalant (Oral); Corticosteroid, Nasal; Corticosteroid, Topical

Generic Available Yes: Cream, lotion, ointment

Use Relief of the inflammatory and pruritic manifestations of corticosteroid-responsive dermatoses (medium potency topical corticosteroid); treatment of nasal symptoms of seasonal and perennial allergic rhinitis; prevention of nasal symptoms associated with seasonal allergic rhinitis; treatment of nasal polyps in adults; maintenance treatment of asthma as prophylactic therapy or as a supplement in asthma patients requiring oral corticosteroids for the purpose of decreasing or eliminating the oral corticosteroid requirement

Effect on Mental Status May cause depression, dizziness, euphoria, fatigue, insomnia, mood swings, and personality changes; may cause exacerbation of pre-existing psychiatric conditions

Effect on Psychiatric Treatment None reported

Pregnancy Risk Factor C

Pregnancy Considerations There are no adequate and well-controlled studies using topical or inhaled mometasone during pregnancy. However, teratogenicity and intrauterine growth retardation has been reported in animal studies with some topical steroids. Avoid use of large amounts for long periods of time during pregnancy. Hypoadrenalism may occur in infants born to women receiving corticosteroids during pregnancy. Monitor these infants closely after birth. Following oral inhalation, <1% of a single 400 mcg dose is available systemically in the mother; inhaled corticosteroids are considered first-line agents for the treatment of persistent of asthma during pregnancy.

Lactation Excretion in breast milk unknown/use caution

Contraindications Hypersensitivity to mometasone or any component of the formulation; treatment of acute bronchospasm (oral inhaler)

Warnings/Precautions May cause hypercorticism or suppression of hypothalamic-pituitary-adrenal (HPA) axis, particularly in younger children or in patients receiving high doses for prolonged periods. HPA axis suppression may lead to adrenal crisis. Withdrawal and discontinuation of a corticosteroid should be done slowly and carefully. Particular care is required when patients are transferred from systemic corticosteroids to inhaled products due to possible adrenal insufficiency or withdrawal from steroids, including an increase in allergic symptoms. Patients receiving >20 mg per day of prednisone (or equivalent) may be most susceptible. Fatalities have occurred due to adrenal insufficiency in asthmatic patients during and after transfer from systemic corticosteroids to aerosol steroids; aerosol steroids do not provide the systemic steroid needed to treat patients having trauma, surgery, or infections. When transferring to oral inhaler, previously-suppressed allergic conditions (rhinitis, conjunctivitis, eczema) may be unmasked.

Bronchospasm may occur with wheezing after inhalation; if this occurs stop steroid and treat with a fast-acting bronchodilator. Supplemental steroids (oral or parenteral) may be needed during stress or severe asthma attacks. Not to be used in status asthmaticus or for the relief of acute bronchospasm. Corticosteroid use may cause psychiatric disturbances, including depression, euphoria, insomnia, mood swings, and personality changes. Pre-existing psychiatric conditions may be exacerbated by corticosteroid use. Prolonged use of corticosteroids may also increase the incidence of secondary infection, mask acute infection (including fungal infections), prolong or exacerbate viral infections, or limit response to vaccines. Exposure to chickenpox should be avoided; corticosteroids should not be used to treat ocular herpes simplex. Corticosteroids should not be used for cerebral malaria or viral hepatitis. Close observation is required in patients with latent tuberculosis and/or TB reactivity; restrict use in active TB (only in conjunction with antituberculosis treatment). Prolonged treatment with corticosteroids has been associated with the development of Kaposi's sarcoma (case reports); if noted, discontinuation of therapy should be considered.

Use with caution in patients with thyroid disease, hepatic impairment, renal impairment, cardiovascular disease, diabetes, glaucoma, cataracts, myasthenia gravis, patients with or who are at risk for osteoporosis, patients at risk for seizures, or GI diseases (diverticulitis, peptic ulcer, ulcerative colitis) due to perforation risk. Use caution following acute MI (corticosteroids have been associated with myocardial rupture). Because of the risk of adverse effects, systemic corticosteroids should be used cautiously in the elderly in the smallest possible effective dose for the shortest duration. Avoid nasal corticosteroid use in patients with recent nasal septal ulcers, nasal surgery or nasal trauma until healing has occurred.

Orally-inhaled and intranasal corticosteroids may cause a reduction in growth velocity in pediatric patients (~1 centimeter per year [range: 0.3-1.8 cm per year] and related to dose and duration of exposure). To minimize the systemic effects of orally-inhaled and intranasal corticosteroids, each patient should be titrated to the lowest effective dose. Growth should be routinely monitored in pediatric patients. Prior to use, the dose and duration of treatment should be based on the risk versus benefit for each individual patient. In general, use the smallest effective dose for the shortest duration of time to minimize adverse events. A gradual tapering of dose may be required prior to discontinuing therapy. There have been reports of systemic corticosteroid withdrawal symptoms (eg, joint/muscle pain, lassitude, depression) when withdrawing inhalation therapy.

Adverse Reactions

Nasal/oral inhalation:

>10%:

Central nervous system: Headache (17% to 26%), fatigue (oral inhalation 1% to 13%), depression (oral inhalation 11%)

Neuromuscular & skeletal: Musculoskeletal pain (1% to 22%), arthralgia (oral inhalation 13%)

Respiratory: Rhinitis (2% to 20%), upper respiratory infection (5% to 15%), pharyngitis (8% to 13%), cough (nasal inhalation 7% to 13%), epistaxis (1% to 11%)

Miscellaneous: Viral infection (nasal inhalation 8% to 14%), oral candidiasis (oral inhalation 4% to 22%)

1% to 10%:

Cardiovascular: Chest pain

Central nervous system: Pain

Gastrointestinal: Abdominal pain, anorexia, dry throat (oral inhalation), diarrhea, dyspepsia, flatulence, gastroenteritis, nausea, vomiting

Genitourinary: Dysmenorrhea

Neuromuscular & skeletal: Back pain, myalgia

Ocular: Conjunctivitis

Otic: Earache, otitis media

Respiratory: Asthma, bronchitis, dysphonia, nasal irritation, sinusitis, wheezing

Miscellaneous: Accidental injury, flu-like syndrome

<1% (Limited to important or life-threatening): Anaphylaxis, angioedema, growth suppression, nasal candidiasis, nasal burning and irritation, nasal septal perforation, nasal ulcers, oral candidiasis (nasal inhalation), smell disturbance (rare), taste disturbance (rare)

Topical:

1% to 10%: Dermatologic: Bacterial skin infection, burning, furunculosis, pruritus, skin atrophy, tingling/stinging

<1% (Limited to important or life-threatening): Folliculitis, glucocorticoid levels decreased (pediatric patients), moniliasis, paresthesia, rosacea, skin depigmentation, skin atrophy

Cataract formation, reduction in growth velocity, and HPA axis suppression have been reported with other corticosteroids

Metabolism/Transport Effects **Substrate** of CYP3A4 (minor)

Drug Interactions

Corticorelin: Corticosteroids may diminish the therapeutic effect of Corticorelin. Specifically, the plasma ACTH response to corticorelin may be blunted by recent or current corticosteroid therapy. *Risk C: Monitor therapy*

Stability

Cream: Store between 2°C to 25°C (36°F to 77°F).

Lotion: Store between 2°C to 30°C (36°F to 86°F).

Nasal spray: Store at room temperature of 15°C to 30°C (59°F to 86°F). Protect from light.

Ointment: Store at room temperature of 15°C to 30°C (59°F to 86°F).

Oral Inhaler: Store at room temperature of 25°C (77°F). Discard when oral dose counter reads "00" (or 45 days after opening the foil pouch).

Mechanism of Action May depress the formation, release, and activity of endogenous chemical mediators of inflammation (kinins, histamine, liposomal enzymes, prostaglandins). Leukocytes and macrophages may have to be present for the initiation of responses mediated by the above substances. Inhibits the margination and subsequent cell migration to the area of injury, and also reverses the dilatation and increased vessel permeability in the area resulting in decreased access of cells to the sites of injury.

Pharmacodynamics/Kinetics

Absorption:

Nasal inhalation: Mometasone furoate monohydrate: Undetectable in plasma

Ointment: 0.7%; increased by occlusive dressings

Oral inhalation: Systemic absorption <1%

Protein binding: Mometasone furoate: 98% to 99%

Metabolism: Mometasone furoate: Hepatic via CYP3A4; forms metabolite

Half-life elimination: Oral inhalation: 5 hours

Excretion: Feces, bile, urine

Dosage

Oral inhalation:

Children 4-11 years: 110 mcg once daily in the evening (maximum 110 mcg/day)

Children ≥12 years and Adults: Previous therapy:

Bronchodilators or inhaled corticosteroids: Initial: 1 inhalation (220 mcg) daily (maximum 2 inhalations or 440 mcg/day); may be given in the evening or in divided doses twice daily

Oral corticosteroids: Initial: 440 mcg twice daily (maximum 880 mcg/day); prednisone should be reduced no faster than 2.5 mg/day on a weekly basis, beginning after at least 1 week of mometasone furoate use

NIH Asthma Guidelines (NIH, 2007): Children ≥12 years and Adults:

"Low" dose: 220 mcg/day

"Medium" dose: 440 mcg/day

"High" dose: >440 mcg/day

Note: Maximum effects may not be evident for 1-2 weeks or longer; dose should be titrated to effect, using the lowest possible dose

Nasal spray:

Allergic rhinitis:

Children 2-11 years: 1 spray (50 mcg) in each nostril daily

Children ≥12 years and Adults: 2 sprays (100 mcg) in each nostril daily; when used for the prevention of allergic rhinitis, treatment should begin 2-4 weeks prior to pollen season

Nasal polyps: Adults: 2 sprays (100 mcg) in each nostril twice daily; 2 sprays (100 mcg) once daily may be effective in some patients

Topical: Apply sparingly, do not use occlusive dressings. Therapy should be discontinued when control is achieved; if no improvement is seen in 2 weeks, reassessment of diagnosis may be necessary.

Cream, ointment: Children ≥2 years and Adults: Apply a thin film to affected area once daily; do not use in pediatric patients for longer than 3 weeks

Lotion: Children ≥12 years and Adults: Apply a few drops to affected area once daily

Dietary Considerations Asmanex® Twisthaler® contains lactose.

Administration

Nasal spray: Prior to first use, prime pump by actuating 10 times or until fine spray appears; may store for a maximum of 1 week without repriming. Spray should be administered once or twice daily, at a regular interval. Shake well prior to use.

Oral inhalation: Exhale fully prior to bringing the Twisthaler® up to the mouth. Place between lips and inhale quickly and deeply. Do not breathe out through the inhaler. Remove inhaler and hold breath for 10 seconds if possible.

Topical: Apply sparingly; avoid eyes, face, underarms, and groin. Do not wrap or bandage affected area.

Monitoring Parameters HPA axis suppression

Asthma: FEV_1, peak flow, and/or other pulmonary function tests

Dosage Forms Excipient information presented when available (limited, particularly for generics); consult specific product labeling.

Cream, topical, as furoate: 0.1% (15 g, 45 g)

Elocon®: 0.1% (15 g, 45 g)

Lotion, topical, as furoate: 0.1% (30 mL, 60 mL)

Elocon®: 0.1% (30 mL, 60 mL) [contains isopropyl alcohol 40%]

Ointment, topical, as furoate: 0.1% (15 g, 45 g)

Elocon®: 0.1% (15 g, 45 g)

Powder for oral inhalation, as furoate:

Asmanex® Twisthaler®: 110 mcg (30 units) [contains lactose; delivers 100 mcg/actuation]; 220 mcg (14 units, 30 units, 60 units, 120 units) [contains lactose; delivers 200 mcg/actuation]

Suspension, intranasal, as furoate [spray]:

Nasonex®: 50 mcg/spray (17 g) [delivers 120 sprays; contains benzalkonium chloride]

◆ **Mometasone Furoate** *see* Mometasone *on page 1071*

◆ **Monacolin K** *see* Lovastatin *on page 956*

◆ **Monoclonal Antibody** *see* Muromonab-CD3 *on page 1086*

◆ **Monodox®** *see* Doxycycline *on page 509*

◆ **Monoket®** *see* Isosorbide Mononitrate *on page 869*

◆ **MonoNessa™** *see* Ethinyl Estradiol and Norgestimate *on page 600*

◆ **Mononine®** *see* Factor IX *on page 612*

◆ **Monopril®** *see* Fosinopril *on page 691*

◆ **Monopril-HCT®** *see* Fosinopril and Hydrochlorothiazide *on page 692*

Montelukast (mon te LOO kast)

Medication Safety Issues

Sound-alike/look-alike issues:

Singulair® may be confused with Sinequan®

U.S. Brand Names Singulair®

Canadian Brand Names Singulair®

Mexican Brand Names Singulair

Index Terms Montelukast Sodium

Pharmacologic Category Leukotriene-Receptor Antagonist

Generic Available No

Use Prophylaxis and chronic treatment of asthma; relief of symptoms of seasonal allergic rhinitis and perennial allergic rhinitis; prevention of exercise-induced bronchospasm

Unlabeled/Investigational Use Acute asthma

Effect on Mental Status May cause dizziness or drowsiness

Effect on Psychiatric Treatment Barbiturates may decrease the effects of montelukast; CYP3A4 substrate; nefazodone may increase effects

Pregnancy Risk Factor B

Pregnancy Considerations Montelukast was not teratogenic in animal studies, however, there are no adequate and well-controlled studies in pregnant women. Use during pregnancy only if clearly needed. Based on limited data, structural defects have been reported in neonates exposed to montelukast *in utero*, however, a specific pattern and relationship to montelukast has not been established. Healthcare providers should report any prenatal exposures to the montelukast pregnancy registry at (800) 986-8999.

Lactation Excretion in breast milk unknown/use caution

Contraindications Hypersensitivity to montelukast or any component of the formulation

Warnings/Precautions Montelukast is not FDA approved for use in the reversal of bronchospasm in acute asthma attacks, including status asthmaticus; some clinicians, however, support its use (Cylly, 2003; Camargo, 2003; Ferreira, 2001). Advise patients to have appropriate rescue medication available. Appropriate clinical monitoring and caution are recommended when systemic corticosteroid reduction is considered in patients receiving montelukast. Inform phenylketonuric patients that the chewable tablet contains phenylalanine. Safety and efficacy in children <6 months of age have not been established.

In rare cases, patients on therapy with montelukast may present with systemic eosinophilia, sometimes presenting with clinical features of vasculitis consistent with Churg-Strauss syndrome, a condition which is often treated with systemic corticosteroid therapy. Healthcare providers should be alert to eosinophilia, vasculitic rash, worsening pulmonary symptoms, cardiac complications, and/or neuropathy presenting in their patients. A causal association between montelukast and these underlying conditions has not been established. Montelukast will not interrupt bronchoconstrictor response to aspirin or other NSAIDs; aspirin sensitive asthmatics should continue to avoid these agents.

Adverse Reactions (As reported in adults)

1% to 10%:

- Central nervous system: Dizziness (2%), fatigue (2%), fever (2%)
- Dermatologic: Rash (2%)
- Gastrointestinal: Abdominal pain (3%), dyspepsia (2%), dental pain (2%), gastroenteritis (2%)
- Hepatic: AST increased (2%)
- Neuromuscular & skeletal: Weakness (2%)
- Respiratory: Cough (3%), nasal congestion (2%)

<1% (Limited to important or life-threatening): Aggression, agitation, anaphylaxis, angioedema, arthralgia, behavior/mood changes, bleeding tendency, bruising, cholestasis (rare), Churg-Strauss syndrome (rare), depression, diarrhea, dream abnormalities, drowsiness, dyspepsia, edema, eosinophilia (systemic; rare), erythema nodosum, hallucinations, hepatic eosinophilic infiltration (rare); hepatitis (mixed pattern, hepatocellular, and cholestatic); hypersensitivity, hypoesthesia, insomnia, irritability, muscle cramps, myalgia, nausea, palpitation, pancreatitis (rare), paresthesia, pruritus, psychomotor hyperactivity, restlessness, seizure (rare), suicidal thinking/behavior (suicidality), suicide, tremor, urticaria, vasculitis (rare), vomiting

Metabolism/Transport Effects Substrate (major) of CYP2C9, 3A4; **Inhibits** CYP2C8 (weak), 2C9 (weak)

Drug Interactions

CYP2C9 Inducers (Highly Effective): May increase the metabolism of CYP2C9 Substrates (High risk). *Risk C: Monitor therapy*

CYP2C9 Inhibitors (Moderate): May decrease the metabolism of CYP2C9 Substrates (High risk). *Risk C: Monitor therapy*

CYP2C9 Inhibitors (Strong): May decrease the metabolism of CYP2C9 Substrates (High risk). *Risk D: Consider therapy modification*

CYP3A4 Inducers (Strong): May increase the metabolism of CYP3A4 Substrates. *Risk C: Monitor therapy*

Deferasirox: May decrease the serum concentration of CYP3A4 Substrates. *Risk C: Monitor therapy*

Herbs (CYP3A4 Inducers): May increase the metabolism of CYP3A4 Substrates. *Risk C: Monitor therapy*

Ethanol/Nutrition/Herb Interactions Herb/Nutraceutical: St John's wort may decrease montelukast levels.

Stability Store at room temperature of 15°C to 30°C (59°F to 86°F). Protect from moisture and light.

Granules: Use within 15 minutes of opening packet.

Mechanism of Action Selective leukotriene receptor antagonist that inhibits the cysteinyl leukotriene receptor. Cysteinyl leukotrienes and leukotriene receptor occupation have been correlated with the pathophysiology of asthma, including airway edema, smooth muscle contraction, and altered cellular activity associated with the inflammatory process, which contribute to the signs and symptoms of asthma. Cysteinyl leukotrienes are also released from the nasal mucosa following allergen exposure leading to symptoms associated with allergic rhinitis.

Pharmacodynamics/Kinetics

Duration: >24 hours

Absorption: Rapid

Distribution: V_d: 8-11 L

Protein binding, plasma: >99%

Metabolism: Extensively hepatic via CYP3A4 and 2C9

Bioavailability: Tablet: 10 mg: Mean: 64%; 5 mg: 63% to 73%

Half-life elimination, plasma: Mean: 2.7-5.5 hours

Time to peak, serum: Tablet: 10 mg: 3-4 hours; 5 mg: 2-2.5 hours; 4 mg: 2 hours

Excretion: Feces (86%); urine (<0.2%)

Dosage Oral:

Children:

6-11 months: Asthma (unlabeled use): 4 mg (oral granules) once daily, taken in the evening

6-23 months: Perennial allergic rhinitis: 4 mg (oral granules) once daily

12-23 months: Asthma: 4 mg (oral granules) once daily, taken in the evening

2-5 years: Asthma, seasonal or perennial allergic rhinitis: 4 mg (chewable tablet or oral granules) once daily, taken in the evening

6-14 years: Asthma, seasonal or perennial allergic rhinitis: 5 mg (chewable tablet) once daily, taken in the evening

Children ≥15 years and Adults:

Asthma, seasonal or perennial allergic rhinitis: 10 mg/day, taken in the evening

Asthma, acute (unlabeled use): 10 mg as a single dose administered with first-line therapy

Bronchoconstriction, exercise-induced (prevention): 10 mg at least 2 hours prior to exercise; additional doses should not be administered within 24 hours. Daily administration to prevent exercise-induced bronchoconstriction has not been evaluated.

Dosing adjustment in renal impairment: No adjustment necessary

Dosing adjustment in hepatic impairment: Mild-to-moderate: No adjustment necessary. Patients with severe hepatic disease were **not** studied.

Dietary Considerations Tablet, chewable: 4 mg strength contains phenylalanine 0.674 mg; 5 mg strength contains phenylalanine 0.842 mg

Administration When treating asthma, administer dose in the evening. Patients with allergic rhinitis may individualize administration time. Granules may be administered directly in the mouth or mixed with applesauce, carrots, rice, ice cream, baby formula, or breast milk; do not add to any other liquids. Administer within 15 minutes of opening packet.

Monitoring Parameters Mood or behavior changes, including suicidal thinking/behavior

Dosage Forms Excipient information presented when available (limited, particularly for generics); consult specific product labeling.

Granules:

Singulair®: 4 mg/packet (30s)

Tablet:

Singulair®: 10 mg

Tablet, chewable:

Singulair®: 4 mg [contains phenylalanine 0.674 mg; cherry flavor]; 5 mg [contains phenylalanine 0.842 mg; cherry flavor]

◆ **Montelukast Sodium** *see* Montelukast *on page 1074*

◆ **Monurol®** *see* Fosfomycin *on page 691*

◆ **8-MOP** *see* Methoxsalen *on page 1018*

◆ **8-MOP®** *see* Methoxsalen *on page 1018*

Moricizine (mor I siz een)

Medication Safety Issues

Sound-alike/look-alike issues:

Ethmozine® may be confused with Erythrocin®, erythromycin

U.S. Brand Names Ethmozine® [DSC]

Canadian Brand Names Ethmozine®

Index Terms Moricizine Hydrochloride

Pharmacologic Category Antiarrhythmic Agent, Class I

Use Treatment of ventricular tachycardia and life-threatening ventricular arrhythmias

Unlabeled/Investigational Use PVCs, complete and nonsustained ventricular tachycardia, atrial arrhythmias

Effect on Mental Status Dizziness is common; may cause sedation or insomnia; may rarely cause anxiety, confusion, amnesia

Effect on Psychiatric Treatment Use caution with TCAs may produce QT prolongation

Dosage Summary

Oral:

Children: Dosage not established

Adults: 200-300 mg every 8 hours

Dosage Forms Excipient information presented when available (limited, particularly for generics); consult specific product labeling. [DSC] = Discontinued product

Tablet, as hydrochloride:

Ethmozine®: 200 mg, 250 mg, 300 mg [DSC]

◆ **Moricizine Hydrochloride** *see* Moricizine *on page 1077*

◆ **Morning After Pill** *see* Ethinyl Estradiol and Norgestrel *on page 601*

Morphine Sulfate (MOR feen SUL fate)

Medication Safety Issues

Sound-alike/look-alike issues:

Morphine may be confused with HYDROmorphone

Morphine sulfate may be confused with magnesium sulfate

MS Contin® may be confused with Oxycontin®

MSO_4 and MS are error-prone abbreviations (mistaken as magnesium sulfate)

Avinza® may be confused with Evista®, Invanz®

Roxanol™ may be confused with OxyFast®, Roxicet™, Roxicodone®

High alert medication: The Institute for Safe Medication Practices (ISMP) includes this medication (I.V. formulation) among its list of drug classes which have a heightened risk of causing significant patient harm when used in error.

Use care when prescribing and/or administering morphine solutions. These products are available in different concentrations. Always prescribe dosage in mg; **not** by volume (mL).

Use caution when selecting a morphine formulation for use in neurologic infusion pumps (eg, Medtronic delivery systems). The product should be appropriately labeled as "preservative-free" and suitable for intraspinal use via continuous infusion. In addition, the product should be formulated in a pH range that is compatible with the device operation specifications.

Significant differences exist between oral and I.V. dosing. Use caution when converting from one route of administration to another.

Related Information

Hallucinogenic Drugs *on page 1783*

Narcotic / Opioid Analgesics *on page 1789*

U.S. Brand Names Astramorph/PF™; Avinza®; DepoDur®; Duramorph®; Infumorph®; Kadian®; MS Contin®; Oramorph SR®; Roxanol™

Canadian Brand Names Doloral; Kadian®; M-Eslon®; M.O.S.-SR®; M.O.S.-Sulfate®; M.O.S.® 10; M.O.S.® 20; M.O.S.® 30; Morphine HP®; Morphine LP® Epidural; MS Contin®; MS-IR®; Novo-Morphine SR; PMS-Morphine Sulfate SR; Ratio-Morphine; Ratio-Morphine SR; Statex®; Zomorph®

Mexican Brand Names Anafil; Graten

Index Terms MS (error-prone abbreviation and should not be used) ; MSO_4 (error-prone abbreviation and should not be used)

Pharmacologic Category Analgesic, Opioid

Generic Available Yes: Excludes capsule, controlled release tablet, sustained release tablet, extended release liposomal suspension for injection

Use Relief of moderate to severe acute and chronic pain; relief of pain of myocardial infarction; relief of dyspnea of acute left ventricular failure and pulmonary edema; preanesthetic medication

DepoDur®: Epidural (lumbar) single-dose management of surgical pain

Infumorph®: Used in continuous microinfusion devices for intrathecal or epidural administration in treatment of intractable chronic pain

Controlled, extended, or sustained release products: Only intended/indicated for use when repeated doses for an extended period of time are required. The 100 mg and 200 mg tablets or capsules of Kadian®, MS Contin®, and morphine sulfate controlled-release tablets and the 60 mg, 90 mg, and 120 mg capsules of Avinza® should only be used in opioid-tolerant patients.

Effect on Mental Status Sedation is common; may cause dysphoric reactions, toxic psychosis, dizziness, euphoria, anxiety, restlessness, confusion, and depression; may rarely cause insomnia

Effect on Psychiatric Treatment May cause severe hypotension in patients receiving phenothiazines; monitor blood pressure. The depressant effects of morphine are potentiated by alcohol and psychotropic medications. Use of typical antipsychotics with neuraxial morphine may increase the risk of respiratory depression.

Restrictions C-II

Pregnancy Risk Factor C/D (prolonged use or high doses at term)

Pregnancy Considerations Morphine crosses the placenta. The frequency of congenital malformations has not been reported to be greater than expected in children from mothers treated with morphine during pregnancy. Reduced growth and behavioral abnormalities in offspring have been observed in animal studies. Neonates born to mothers receiving chronic opioids during pregnancy should be monitored for neonatal withdrawal syndrome.

DepoDur® may be used in women undergoing cesarean section following clamping of the umbilical cord; not for use in vaginal labor and delivery.

Lactation Enters breast milk/use caution (AAP rates "compatible")

Contraindications Note: Some contraindications are product specific. For details, please see detailed product prescribing information.

Hypersensitivity to morphine sulfate or any component of the formulation; severe respiratory depression (without resuscitative equipment); acute or severe asthma; known or suspected paralytic ileus; sustained release products are not recommended with gastrointestinal obstruction or in acute/postoperative pain; pregnancy (prolonged use or high doses at term). Oral solutions contraindicated in patients with heart failure due to chronic lung disease, cardiac arrhythmias, head injuries, brain tumors, acute alcoholism, deliriums tremens, seizure disorders, Injectable solution contraindicated during labor when a premature birth is anticipated. Some products contraindicated in patients with head injuries or increased intracranial pressure. DepoDur® contraindicated in circulatory shock and upper airway obstruction. MS Contin® and Kadian® contraindicated in patients with hypercarbia. Some immediate release formulations (tablets and solution) contraindicated in post biliary tract surgery, suspected surgical abdomen, surgical anastomosis, MAO inhibitor use (concurrent or within 14 days), general CNS depression.

Warnings/Precautions An opioid-containing analgesic regimen should be tailored to each patient's needs and based upon the type of pain being treated (acute versus chronic), the route of administration, degree of tolerance for opioids (naive versus chronic user), age, weight, and medical condition. The optimal analgesic dose varies widely among patients. Doses should be titrated to pain relief/prevention. When used as an epidural injection, monitor for delayed sedation. **[U.S. Boxed Warning]: Healthcare provider should be alert to problems of abuse, misuse, and diversion.**

May cause respiratory depression; use with caution in patients (particularly elderly or debilitated) with impaired respiratory function, morbid obesity, adrenal insufficiency, prostatic hyperplasia, urinary stricture, renal impairment, or severe hepatic dysfunction and in patients with hypersensitivity reactions to other phenanthrene derivative opioid agonists (codeine, hydrocodone, hydromorphone, levorphanol, oxycodone, oxymorphone). Use with caution in patients with biliary tract dysfunction; acute pancreatitis may cause constriction of sphincter of Oddi. Some preparations contain sulfites which may cause allergic reactions; infants <3 months of age are more susceptible to respiratory depression, use with caution and generally in reduced doses in this age group.

May cause CNS depression, which may impair physical or mental abilities; patients must be cautioned about performing tasks which require mental alertness (eg, operating machinery or driving). Effects may be potentiated when used with other sedative drugs or ethanol. May cause hypotension in patients with acute myocardial infarction, volume depletion, or concurrent drug therapy which may exaggerate vasodilation. Use with extreme caution in patients with head injury, intracranial lesions, or elevated intracranial pressure; exaggerated elevation of ICP may occur. May cause seizures if high doses are used; use with caution in patients with seizure disorders. Tolerance or drug dependence may result from extended use. Concurrent use of agonist/antagonist analgesics may precipitate withdrawal symptoms and/or reduced analgesic efficacy in patients following prolonged therapy with mu opioid agonists. Abrupt discontinuation following prolonged use may also lead to withdrawal symptoms. Elderly may be particularly susceptible to adverse effects of narcotics. May obscure diagnosis or clinical course of patients with acute abdominal conditions.

Extended or sustained-release formulations:

[U.S. Boxed Warning]: Extended or sustained release dosage forms should not be crushed or chewed. Controlled-, extended-, or sustained-release products are not intended for "as needed (PRN)" use. **MS Contin® 100 or 200 mg tablets and Kadian® 100 mg or 200 mg capsules are for use only in opioid-tolerant patients.** Avinza®, Kadian®, MS Contin®: **[U.S. Boxed Warning]: Indicated for the management of moderate-to-severe pain when around the clock pain control is needed for an extended time period.**

[U.S. Boxed Warning]: Avinza®: Do not administer with alcoholic beverages or ethanol-containing products, which may disrupt extended-release characteristic of product.

Injections: Note: Products are designed for administration by specific routes (I.V., intrathecal, epidural). Use caution when prescribing, dispensing, or administering to use formulations only by intended route(s).

[U.S. Boxed Warning]: Duramorph®: Due to the risk of severe and/or sustained cardiopulmonary depressant effects of Duramorph® must be administered in a fully equipped and staffed environment. Naloxone injection should be immediately available. Patient should remain in this environment for at least 24 hours following the initial dose.

[U.S. Boxed Warning]: Intrathecal dosage is usually 1/10 that of epidural dosage.

Infumorph® solutions are **for use in microinfusion devices only**; not for I.V., I.M., or SubQ administration, or for single-dose administration.

When used as an epidural injection, monitor for delayed sedation.

DepoDur®: **For lumbar administration only.** Intrathecal administration has resulted in prolonged respiratory depression. Freezing may adversely affect modified-release mechanism of drug; check freeze indicator within carton prior to administration.

Adverse Reactions Note: Individual patient differences are unpredictable, and percentage may differ in acute pain (surgical) treatment. Reactions may be dose, formulation, and/or route dependent.

Frequency not defined:

- Cardiovascular: Circulatory depression, flushing, shock
- Central nervous system: Physical and psychological dependence, sedation
- Endocrine & metabolic: Antidiuretic hormone release

>10%:

- Cardiovascular: Bradycardia, hypotension
- Central nervous system: Drowsiness (9% to 48%; tolerance usually develops to drowsiness with regular dosing for 1-2 weeks), dizziness (6% to 20%), fever (<3% to >10%), confusion, headache (following epidural or intrathecal use)
- Dermatologic: Pruritus (may be dose related)
- Gastrointestinal: Xerostomia (78%), constipation (9% to 40%; tolerance develops very slowly if at all), nausea (7% to 28%; tolerance usually develops to nausea and vomiting with chronic use), vomiting
- Genitourinary: Urinary retention (16%; may be prolonged, up to 20 hours, following epidural or intrathecal use)
- Hematologic: Anemia (following intrathecal use)
- Local: Pain at injection site
- Neuromuscular & skeletal: Weakness
- Respiratory: Oxygen saturation decreased
- Miscellaneous: Histamine release

1% to 10%:

Cardiovascular: Atrial fibrillation (<3%), chest pain (<3%), edema, hypertension, palpitation, peripheral edema, syncope, tachycardia, vasodilation

Central nervous system: Amnesia, agitation, anxiety, apathy, ataxia, chills, coma, delirium, depression, dream abnormalities, euphoria, false sense of well being, hallucination, hypoesthesia, insomnia, lethargy, malaise, nervousness, restlessness, seizure, slurred speech, somnolence, vertigo

Dermatologic: Dry skin, rash, urticaria

Endocrine & metabolic: Gynecomastia (<3%), hypokalemia, hyponatremia, libido decreased

Gastrointestinal: Abdominal distension, abdominal pain, anorexia, biliary colic, diarrhea, dyspepsia, dysphagia, flatulence, gastroenteritis, GERD, GI irritation, paralytic ileus, rectal disorder, taste perversion, weight loss

Genitourinary: Bladder spasm, dysuria, ejaculation abnormal, impotence, urination decreased

Hematologic: Leukopenia (<3%), thrombocytopenia (<3%), hematocrit decreased

Hepatic: Liver function tests increased

Neuromuscular & skeletal: Arthralgia, back pain, bone pain, foot drop, gait abnormalities, paresthesia, rigors, skeletal muscle rigidity, tremor

Ocular: Amblyopia, conjunctivitis, eye pain, vision problems/disturbance

Renal: Oliguria

Respiratory: Asthma, atelectasis, dyspnea, hiccups, hypercapnia, hypoxia, pulmonary edema (noncardiogenic), respiratory depression, rhinitis

Miscellaneous: Diaphoresis, flu-like syndrome, infection, thirst, voice alteration, withdrawal syndrome

<1% (Limited to important or life-threatening): Amenorrhea, anaphylaxis, apnea, biliary tract spasm, blurred vision, bronchospasm, cardiac arrest, cough reflex decreased, dehydration, diplopia, disorientation, hemorrhagic urticaria, intestinal obstruction, intracranial pressure increased, laryngospasm, menstrual irregularities, miosis, myoclonus, nystagmus, paradoxical CNS stimulation, respiratory arrest, sepsis, urinary tract spasm, thermal dysregulation, toxic psychoses

Metabolism/Transport Effects Substrate of CYP2D6 (minor)

Drug Interactions

Alcohol (Ethyl): CNS Depressants may enhance the CNS depressant effect of Alcohol (Ethyl). *Risk C: Monitor therapy*

Alvimopan: Analgesics (Opioid) may enhance the adverse/toxic effect of Alvimopan. This is most notable for patients receiving long-term (i.e., more than 7 days) opiates prior to alvimopan initiation. Management: Alvimopan is contraindicated in patients receiving therapeutic doses of opioids for more than 7 consecutive days immediately prior to alvimopan initiation. *Risk D: Consider therapy modification*

Ammonium Chloride: May increase the excretion of Analgesics (Opioid). *Risk C: Monitor therapy*

Amphetamines: May enhance the analgesic effect of Analgesics (Opioid). *Risk C: Monitor therapy*

Antipsychotic Agents (Phenothiazines): May enhance the hypotensive effect of Analgesics (Opioid). *Risk C: Monitor therapy*

CNS Depressants: May enhance the adverse/toxic effect of other CNS Depressants. *Risk C: Monitor therapy*

Desmopressin: Analgesics (Opioid) may enhance the adverse/toxic effect of Desmopressin. *Risk C: Monitor therapy*

Pegvisomant: Analgesics (Opioid) may diminish the therapeutic effect of Pegvisomant. *Risk C: Monitor therapy*

Rifamycin Derivatives: May decrease the serum concentration of Morphine Sulfate. *Risk C: Monitor therapy*

Selective Serotonin Reuptake Inhibitors: Analgesics (Opioid) may enhance the serotonergic effect of Selective Serotonin Reuptake Inhibitors. This may cause serotonin syndrome. *Risk C: Monitor therapy*

Succinylcholine: May enhance the bradycardic effect of Analgesics (Opioid). *Risk C: Monitor therapy*

Trovafloxacin: Morphine Sulfate may decrease the serum concentration of Trovafloxacin. *Risk D: Consider therapy modification*

Ethanol/Nutrition/Herb Interactions

Ethanol: Avoid ethanol, including alcoholic beverages or ethanol-containing products (may increase CNS depression).

Avinza®: Alcoholic beverages or ethanol-containing products may disrupt extended-release formulation resulting in rapid release of entire morphine dose.

Food: Administration of oral morphine solution with food may increase bioavailability (ie, a report of 34% increase in morphine AUC when morphine oral solution followed a high-fat meal). The bioavailability of Avinza®, Oramorph SR®, or Kadian® does not appear to be affected by food.

Herb/Nutraceutical: Avoid valerian, St John's wort, kava kava, gotu kola (may increase CNS depression).

Stability

Capsule, sustained release (Avinza®, Kadian®): Store at 25°C (77°F); excursions permitted to 15°C to 30°C (59°F to 86°F). Protect from light and moisture.

Injection: Store at controlled room temperature of 20°C to 25°C (68°F to 77°F); do not freeze. Protect from light. Degradation depends on pH and presence of oxygen; relatively stable in pH ≤4; darkening of solutions indicate degradation. Usual concentration for continuous I.V. infusion: 0.1-1 mg/mL in D_5W.

DepoDur®: Store under refrigeration at 2°C to 8°C (36°F to 46°F); keep vials in carton during refrigeration; do not freeze. Check freeze indicator before administration; do not administer if bulb is pink or purple. May store at room temperature for up to 30 days in sealed, unopened vials. DepoDur® may be diluted in preservative-free NS to a volume of 5 mL. Gently invert to suspend particles prior to removal from vial. Once vial is opened, use within 4 hours.

Oral solution: Store at controlled room temperature of 25°C (68°F to 77°F). Do not freeze.

Suppositories: Store at controlled room temperature 25°C (77°F). Protect from light.

Tablet, extended release: Store at controlled room temperature of 25°C (77°F).

Tablet, immediate release: Store at controlled room temperature of 25°C (77°F). Protect from moisture.

Mechanism of Action Binds to opiate receptors in the CNS, causing inhibition of ascending pain pathways, altering the perception of and response to pain; produces generalized CNS depression

Pharmacodynamics/Kinetics

Onset of action (patient dependent; dosing must be individualized): Oral (immediate release): ~30 minutes; I.V.: 5-10 minutes

Duration (patient dependent; dosing must be individualized): Pain relief:

Immediate release formulations: 4 hours

Extended release capsule and tablet: 8-24 hours (formulation dependent)

Extended release epidural injection (DepoDur®): >48 hours

Absorption: Variable

Distribution: V_d: 3-4 L/kg; binds to opioid receptors in the CNS and periphery (eg, GI tract)

Protein binding: 30% to 35%

Metabolism: Hepatic via conjugation with glucuronic acid primarily to morphine-6-glucoronide (active analgesic) morphine-3-glucuronide (inactive as analgesic); minor metabolites include morphine-3-6-diglucuronide; other minor metabolites include normorphine (active) and morphine 3-ethereal sulfate

Bioavailability: Oral: 17% to 33% (first-pass effect limits oral bioavailability; oral: parenteral effectiveness reportedly varies from 1:6 in opioid naive patients to 1:3 with chronic use)

Half-life elimination: Adults: 2-4 hours (immediate release forms)

Time to peak, plasma: Avinza®: 30 minutes (maintained for 24 hours); Kadian®: ~10 hours; Oramorph® SR: ~4 hours

Excretion: Urine (primarily as morphine-3-glucuronide, ~2% to 12% excreted unchanged); feces (~7% to 10%). It has been suggested that accumulation of morphine-6-glucuronide might cause toxicity with renal insufficiency. All of the metabolites (ie, morphine-3-glucuronide, morphine-6-glucuronide, and normorphine) have been suggested as possible causes of neurotoxicity (eg, myoclonus).

Dosage Note: These are guidelines and do not represent the doses that may be required in all patients. Doses and dosage intervals should be titrated to pain relief/prevention.

Children >6 months and <50 kg: Acute pain (moderate-to-severe):

Oral (immediate release formulations): 0.15-0.3 mg/kg every 3-4 hours as needed

I.M., I.V.: 0.1-0.2 mg/kg every 3-4 hours as needed

I.V. infusion: Range: 10-60 mcg/kg/hour

Adults:

Acute pain (moderate-to-severe):

Oral (immediate release formulations): Opiate-naive: Initial: 10 mg every 4 hours as needed; patients with prior opiate exposure may require higher initial doses: usual dosage range: 10-30 mg every 4 hours as needed

I.M., SubQ: **Note:** Repeated SubQ administration causes local tissue irritation, pain, and induration.
Initial: Opiate-naive: 5-10 mg every 4 hours as needed; patients with prior opiate exposure may require higher initial doses; usual dosage range: 5-20 mg every 4 hours as needed
Rectal: 10-20 mg every 3-4 hours
I.V.: Initial: Opiate-naive: 2.5-5 mg every 3-4 hours; patients with prior opiate exposure may require higher initial doses. **Note:** Repeated doses (up to every 5 minutes if needed) in small increments (eg, 1-4 mg) may be preferred to larger and less frequent doses.
Acute myocardial infarction, analgesia (ACC/AHA 2004 guidelines): Initial management: 2-4 mg, give 2-8 mg every 5-15 minutes as needed.
Critically-ill patients (unlabeled dose): 0.7-10 mg (based on 70 kg patient) **or** 0.01-0.15 mg/kg every 1-2 hours as needed. **Note:** More frequent dosing may be needed (eg, mechanically-ventilated patients).
I.V., SubQ continuous infusion: 0.8-10 mg/hour; usual range: Up to 80 mg/hour
Continuous infusion: Usual dosage range: 5-35 mg/hour (based on 70 kg patient) **or** 0.07-0.5 mg/kg/hour
Patient-controlled analgesia (PCA): (Opiate-naive: Consider lower end of dosing range):
Usual concentration: 1 mg/mL
Demand dose: Usual: 1 mg; range: 0.5-2.5 mg
Lockout interval: 5-10 minutes
Intrathecal (I.T.): **Note:** Administer with extreme caution and in reduced dosage to geriatric or debilitated patients. I.T. dose is usually 1/10 that of epidural dosage.
Opioid-naive: 0.2-1 mg/dose (may provide adequate relief for 24 hours); repeat doses are **not** recommended
Continuous microinfusion (Infumorph®): Initial: 0.2-1 mg/day
Opioid-tolerant: 1-10 mg/day
Continuous microinfusion (Infumorph®): Initial: 1-10 mg/day, titrate to effect; usual maximum is ~20 mg/day
Epidural: Pain management: **Note:** Administer with extreme caution and in reduced dosage to geriatric or debilitated patients. Vigilant monitoring is particularly important in these patients.
Single-dose (Astromorph/PF™, Duramorph®): Initial: 5 mg, if pain relief not achieved in 1 hour, careful administration of 1-2 mg at intervals sufficient to assess effectiveness may be given; maximum: 10 mg/24 hours
Infusion: Bolus dose: 1-6 mg; infusion rate: 0.1-0.2 mg/hour; maximum dose: 10 mg/24 hours
Continuous microinfusion (Infumorph®):
Opioid-naive: Initial: 0.2-1 mg/day
Opioid-tolerant: Initial: 1-10 mg/day, titrate to effect; usual maximum is ~20 mg/day

Surgical anesthesia: Epidural: Single-dose (extended release, DepoDur®): Lumbar epidural only; not recommended in patients <18 years of age:
Cesarean section: 10 mg (after clamping umbilical cord)
Lower abdominal/pelvic surgery: 10-15 mg
Major orthopedic surgery of lower extremity: 15 mg
For DepoDur®: To minimize the pharmacokinetic interaction resulting in higher peak serum concentrations of morphine, administer the test dose of the local anesthetic at least 15 minutes prior to DepoDur® administration. Use of DepoDur® with epidural local anesthetics has not been studied. Other medications should not be administered into the epidural space for at least 48 hours after administration of DepoDur®.
Note: Some patients may benefit from a 20 mg dose, however, the incidence of adverse effects may be increased.

Chronic pain: Note: Patients taking opioids chronically may become tolerant and require doses higher than the usual dosage range to maintain the desired effect. Tolerance can be managed by appropriate dose titration. There is no optimal or maximal dose for morphine in chronic pain. The appropriate dose is one that relieves pain throughout its dosing interval without causing unmanageable side effects.
Oral: Controlled-, extended-, or sustained-release formulations: A patient's morphine requirement should be established using prompt-release formulations. Conversion to long-acting products may be considered when chronic, continuous treatment is required. Higher dosages should be reserved for use only in opioid-tolerant patients.
Capsules, extended release (Avinza®): Daily dose administered once daily (for best results, administer at same time each day)

Capsules, sustained release (Kadian®): Daily dose administered once daily or in 2 divided doses daily (every 12 hours)

Tablets, controlled release (MS Contin®), sustained release (Oramorph SR®), or extended release: Daily dose divided and administered every 8 or every 12 hours

Elderly or debilitated patients: Use with caution; may require dose reduction

Dosing adjustment in renal impairment:

Cl_{cr} 10-50 mL/minute: Children and Adults: Administer at 75% of normal dose

Cl_{cr} <10 mL/minute: Children and Adults: Administer at 50% of normal dose

Intermittent HD:

Children: Administer 50% of normal dose

Adults: No dosage adjustment necessary

Peritoneal dialysis: Children: Administer 50% of normal dose

CRRT: Children and Adults: Administer 75% of normal dose, titrate

Dosing adjustment/comments in hepatic disease: Unchanged in mild liver disease; substantial extrahepatic metabolism may occur; excessive sedation may occur in cirrhosis

Dietary Considerations Morphine may cause GI upset; take with food if GI upset occurs. Be consistent when taking morphine with or without meals.

Administration

Oral: Do not crush controlled release drug product, swallow whole. Kadian® and Avinza® can be opened and sprinkled on applesauce; do not crush or chew the beads. Contents of Kadian® capsules may be opened and sprinkled over 10 mL water and flushed through prewetted 16F gastrostomy tube; do not administer Kadian® through nasogastric tube.

I.V.: When giving morphine I.V. push, it is best to first dilute in 4-5 mL of sterile water, and then to administer slowly (eg, 15 mg over 3-5 minutes)

Epidural: Use preservative-free solutions

Epidural, extended release liposomal suspension (DepoDur®): Intended for lumbar administration only. Thoracic administration has not been studied. May be administered undiluted or diluted up to 5 mL total volume in preservative-free NS. Do not use an in-line filter during administration. Not for I.V., I.M., or intrathecal administration.

Resedation may occur following epidural administration; this may be delayed ≥48 hours in patients receiving extended-release (DepoDur®) injections.

Administration of an epidural test dose (lidocaine 1.5% and epinephrine 1:200,000) may affect the release of morphine from the liposomal preparation. Delaying the dose for an interval of at least 15 minutes following the test dose minimizes this pharmacokinetic interaction. Except for a test dose, other epidural local anesthetics or medications should not be administered epidurally before or after this product for a minimum of 48 hours.

Intrathecal: Use preservative-free solutions

Monitoring Parameters Pain relief, respiratory and mental status, blood pressure

Astromorph/PF™, Duramorph®, Infumorph®: Patients should be observed in a fully-equipped and staffed environment for at least 24 hours following initiation, and as appropriate for the first several days after catheter implantation.

DepoDur®: Patient should be monitored for at least 48 hours following administration.

Reference Range Therapeutic: Surgical anesthesia: 65-80 ng/mL (SI: 227-280 nmol/L); Toxic: 200-5000 ng/mL (SI: 700-17,500 nmol/L)

Test Interactions Some quinolones may produce a false-positive urine screening result for opiates using commercially-available immunoassay kits. This has been demonstrated most consistently for levofloxacin and ofloxacin, but other quinolones have shown cross-reactivity in certain assay kits. Confirmation of positive opiate screens by more specific methods should be considered.

Dosage Forms Excipient information presented when available (limited, particularly for generics); consult specific product labeling. [DSC] = Discontinued product; [CAN] Canadian brand name

Capsule, extended release:

Avinza®: 30 mg, 60 mg, 90 mg, 120 mg

Kadian®: 10 mg, 20 mg, 30 mg, 50 mg, 60 mg, 80 mg, 100 mg, 200 mg

Infusion [premixed in D_5W]: 1 mg/mL (100 mL, 250 mL)

Injection, extended release liposomal suspension [lumbar epidural injection, preservative free]:

DepoDur®: 10 mg/mL (1 mL, 1.5 mL, 2 mL)

Injection, solution: 2 mg/mL (1 mL); 4 mg/mL (1 mL); 5 mg/mL (1 mL); 8 mg/mL (1 mL); 10 mg/0.7 mL (0.7 mL); 10 mg/mL (1 mL, 10 mL); 15 mg/mL (1 mL,

20 mL); 25 mg/mL (4 mL, 10 mL, 20 mL, 40 mL, 50 mL, 100 mL, 250 mL); 50 mg/mL (20 mL, 40 mL) [some preparations contain sodium metabisulfite]
Injection, solution [epidural, intrathecal, or I.V. infusion; preservative free]:
Astramorph/PF™: 0.5 mg/mL (2 mL, 10 mL); 1 mg/mL (2 mL, 10 mL)
Duramorph®: 0.5 mg/mL (10 mL); 1 mg/mL (10 mL)
Injection, solution [epidural or intrathecal infusion via microinfusion device; preservative free]:
Infumorph®: 10 mg/mL (20 mL); 25 mg/mL (20 mL)
Injection, solution [I.V. infusion via PCA pump]: 0.5 mg/mL (30 mL); 1 mg/mL (30 mL, 50 mL); 2 mg/mL (30 mL); 5 mg/mL (30 mL, 50 mL)
Injection, solution [preservative free]: 0.5 mg/mL (10 mL); 1 mg/mL (10 mL); 25 mg/mL (4 mL, 10 mL, 20 mL)
Solution, oral: 10 mg/5 mL (5 mL, 100 mL, 500 mL); 20 mg/5 mL (100 mL, 500 mL); 20 mg/mL (30 mL, 120 mL, 240 mL)
Doloral [CAN]: 1 mg/mL (10 mL, 250 mL, 500 mL); 5 mg/mL (10 mL, 250 mL, 500 mL) [not available in U.S.]
Solution, oral [concentrate]: 5 mg/0.25 mL (0.25 mL) [DSC]; 10 mg/0.5 mL (0.5 mL) [DSC]; 20 mg/mL (1 mL, 15 ml, 30 mL, 120 mL, 240 mL)
Roxanol™: 20 mg/mL (30 mL, 120 mL); 100 mg/5 mL (240 mL)
Suppository, rectal: 5 mg (12s), 10 mg (12s), 20 mg (12s), 30 mg (12s)
Tablet: 10 mg [DSC], 15 mg, 30 mg
Tablet, controlled release:
MS Contin®: 15 mg, 30 mg, 60 mg, 100 mg, 200 mg
Tablet, extended release: 15 mg, 30 mg, 60 mg, 100 mg, 200 mg
Tablet, sustained release:
Oramorph SR®: 15 mg, 30 mg, 60 mg, 100 mg

◆ **Mosco® Callus & Corn Remover [OTC]** *see* Salicylic Acid *on page 1454*
◆ **Motofen® [DSC]** *see* Difenoxin and Atropine *on page 462*
◆ **Motrin® [DSC]** *see* Ibuprofen *on page 803*
◆ **Motrin® Children's [OTC]** *see* Ibuprofen *on page 803*
◆ **Motrin® IB [OTC]** *see* Ibuprofen *on page 803*
◆ **Motrin® Infants' [OTC]** *see* Ibuprofen *on page 803*
◆ **Motrin® Junior [OTC]** *see* Ibuprofen *on page 803*
◆ **MoviPrep®** *see* Polyethylene Glycol-Electrolyte Solution *on page 1310*

Moxifloxacin (moxs i FLOKS a sin)

Medication Safety Issues
Sound-alike/look-alike issues:
Avelox® may be confused with Avonex®

International issues:
Vigamox™ may be confused with Fisamox® which is a brand name for amoxicillin in Australia

U.S. Brand Names Avelox®; Avelox® I.V.; Vigamox™
Canadian Brand Names Avelox®; Avelox® I.V.; Vigamox™
Mexican Brand Names Avelox; Vigamoxi
Index Terms Moxifloxacin Hydrochloride
Pharmacologic Category Antibiotic, Ophthalmic; Antibiotic, Quinolone; Respiratory Fluoroquinolone
Use Treatment of mild-to-moderate community-acquired pneumonia, including multidrug-resistant *Streptococcus pneumoniae* (MDRSP); acute bacterial exacerbation of chronic bronchitis; acute bacterial sinusitis; complicated and uncomplicated skin and skin structure infections; complicated intra-abdominal infections; bacterial conjunctivitis (ophthalmic formulation)
Unlabeled/Investigational Use *Legionella*
Effect on Mental Status May cause dizziness, insomnia; may rarely produce abnormal thinking, agitation, anorexia, anxiety, asthenia, ataxia, confusion, depersonalization, depression, euphoria, hallucination, hostility, nervousness, panic attacks, paranoia, psychosis, sedation, somnolence, or stress
Effect on Psychiatric Treatment Contraindicated with ziprasidone; may have potential to prolong QT interval; should avoid in patients with uncorrected hypokalemia, or concurrent administration of other medications known to prolong the QT interval (antipsychotics and tricyclic antidepressants)
Restrictions
An FDA-approved patient medication guide is available and must be distributed when dispensing an outpatient prescription (new or refill) where this medication is to be used without direct supervision of a healthcare provider. Medication

guides are available at http://www.fda.gov/cder/Offices/ODS/medication_guides.htm.

Dosage Summary

I.V.:

Children: Dosage not established

Adults: 400 mg every 24 hours

Ophthalmic:

Children <1 year: Dosage not established

Children ≥1 year: Instill 1 drop into affected eye(s) 3 times/day

Adults: Instill 1 drop into affected eye(s) 3 times/day

Oral:

Children: Dosage not established

Adults: 400 mg every 24 hours

Dosage Forms Excipient information presented when available (limited, particularly for generics); consult specific product labeling.

Infusion [premixed in sodium chloride 0.8%] (Avelox® I.V.): 400 mg (250 mL)

Solution, ophthalmic (Vigamox™): 0.5% (3 mL)

Tablet:

Avelox®: 400 mg

Avelox® ABC Pack [unit-dose pack]: 400 mg (5s)

- **Moxifloxacin Hydrochloride** *see* Moxifloxacin *on page 1084*
- **4-MP** *see* Fomepizole *on page 685*
- **MPA** *see* MedroxyPROGESTERone *on page 975*
- **MPA** *see* Mycophenolate *on page 1087*
- **MPA and Estrogens (Conjugated)** *see* Estrogens (Conjugated/Equine) and Medroxyprogesterone *on page 583*
- **6-MP (error-prone abbreviation)** *see* Mercaptopurine *on page 993*
- **MPSV4** *see* Meningococcal Polysaccharide Vaccine (Groups A / C / Y and W-135) *on page 985*
- **MS Contin®** *see* Morphine Sulfate *on page 1077*
- **MS (error-prone abbreviation and should not be used)** *see* Morphine Sulfate *on page 1077*
- **MSO_4 (error-prone abbreviation and should not be used)** *see* Morphine Sulfate *on page 1077*
- **MTC** *see* Mitomycin *on page 1061*
- **MTX (error-prone abbreviation)** *see* Methotrexate *on page 1014*
- **Mucinex® [OTC]** *see* GuaiFENesin *on page 737*
- **Mucinex®-D [OTC]** *see* Guaifenesin and Pseudoephedrine *on page 744*
- **Mucinex® D Maximum Strength [OTC]** *see* Guaifenesin and Pseudoephedrine *on page 744*
- **Mucinex®, Children's [OTC]** *see* GuaiFENesin *on page 737*
- **Mucinex® Children's Cough [OTC]** *see* Guaifenesin and Dextromethorphan *on page 739*
- **Mucinex®, Children's Mini-Melts™ [OTC]** *see* GuaiFENesin *on page 737*
- **Mucinex® DM [OTC]** *see* Guaifenesin and Dextromethorphan *on page 739*
- **Mucinex® DM Maximum Strength [OTC]** *see* Guaifenesin and Dextromethorphan *on page 739*
- **Mucinex® Full force™ [OTC]** *see* Oxymetazoline *on page 1208*
- **Mucinex®, Junior Mini-Melts™ [OTC]** *see* GuaiFENesin *on page 737*
- **Mucinex® Maximum Strength [OTC]** *see* GuaiFENesin *on page 737*
- **Mucinex® moisture smart™ [OTC]** *see* Oxymetazoline *on page 1208*
- **Mucomyst** *see* Acetylcysteine *on page 47*
- **Multitargeted Antifolate** *see* Pemetrexed *on page 1238*
- **Mumps, Rubella, Varicella, and Measles Vaccine** *see* Measles, Mumps, Rubella, and Varicella Virus Vaccine *on page 972*

Mupirocin (myoo PEER oh sin)

Medication Safety Issues

Sound-alike/look-alike issues:

Bactroban® may be confused with bacitracin, baclofen, Bactrim™

U.S. Brand Names Bactroban®; Bactroban® Nasal; Centany™ [DSC]

Canadian Brand Names Bactroban®

Mexican Brand Names Bactroban; Sinpebac

Index Terms Mupirocin Calcium; Pseudomonic Acid A
Pharmacologic Category Antibiotic, Topical
Use
Intranasal: Eradication of nasal colonization with MRSA in adult patients and healthcare workers
Topical: Treatment of impetigo or secondary infected traumatic skin lesions due to *S. aureus* and *S. pyogenes*
Unlabeled/Investigational Use Intranasal: Surgical prophylaxis to prevent wound infections
Effect on Mental Status May cause dizziness
Effect on Psychiatric Treatment None reported
Dosage Summary
Intranasal:
Children <12 years: Dosage not established
Children ≥12 years: Approximately one-half of the ointment from the single-use tube should be applied into one nostril and the other half into the other nostril twice daily
Adults: Approximately one-half of the ointment from the single-use tube should be applied into one nostril and the other half into the other nostril twice daily
Topical:
Children ≥2 months: Ointment: Apply to affected area 3 times/day [impetigo]
Children ≥ 3 months: Cream: Apply to affected area 3 times/day for 10 days [secondary skin infections]
Adults: Apply to affected area 3 times/day
Dosage Forms Excipient information presented when available (limited, particularly for generics); consult specific product labeling. [DSC] = Discontinued product
Note: Strength expressed as base
Cream, topical, as calcium:
Bactroban®: 2% (15 g, 30 g) [contains benzyl alcohol]
Ointment, intranasal, as calcium:
Bactroban® Nasal: 2% (1 g) [single-use tube]
Ointment, topical: 2% (0.9 g, 22 g)
Bactroban®: 2% (22 g) [contains polyethylene glycol]
Centany™: 2% (15 g) [DSC]

◆ **Mupirocin Calcium** *see* Mupirocin *on page 1085*
◆ **Murine® Tears Plus [OTC]** *see* Tetrahydrozoline *on page 1560*

Muromonab-CD3 (myoo roe MOE nab see dee three)

U.S. Brand Names Orthoclone OKT® 3
Canadian Brand Names Orthoclone OKT® 3
Mexican Brand Names Orthoclone OKT3
Index Terms Monoclonal Antibody; OKT3
Pharmacologic Category Immunosuppressant Agent
Use Treatment of acute allograft rejection in renal transplant patients; treatment of acute hepatic, and kidney rejection episodes resistant to conventional treatment
Unlabeled/Investigational Use Treatment of acute pancreas rejection episodes resistant to conventional treatment
Effect on Mental Status Dizziness is common; may rarely cause sedation, confusion, or hallucinations
Effect on Psychiatric Treatment None reported
Dosage Summary
I.V.:
Children <30 kg: 2.5 mg once daily
Children >30 kg: 5 mg once daily
Adults: 5 mg once daily
Dosage Forms Excipient information presented when available (limited, particularly for generics); consult specific product labeling.
Injection, solution: 1 mg/mL (5 mL) [contains sodium 43 mg/5 mL]

◆ **Muse®** *see* Alprostadil *on page 77*
◆ **Mustargen®** *see* Mechlorethamine *on page 974*
◆ **Mustine** *see* Mechlorethamine *on page 974*
◆ **Mutterkraut** *see* Feverfew *(Tanacetum parthenium) on page 628*
◆ **M.V.I.®-12** *see* Vitamins (Multiple/Injectable) *on page 1677*

- ◆ **M.V.I. Adult™** *see* Vitamins (Multiple/Injectable) *on page 1677*
- ◆ **M.V.I® Pediatric** *see* Vitamins (Multiple/Injectable) *on page 1677*
- ◆ **Myambutol®** *see* Ethambutol *on page 592*
- ◆ **Mycamine®** *see* Micafungin *on page 1045*
- ◆ **Mycobutin®** *see* Rifabutin *on page 1418*

Mycophenolate (mye koe FEN oh late)

U.S. Brand Names CellCept®; Myfortic®

Canadian Brand Names CellCept®; Myfortic®

Mexican Brand Names Myfortic

Index Terms MMF; MPA; Mycophenolate Mofetil; Mycophenolate Sodium; Mycophenolic Acid

Pharmacologic Category Immunosuppressant Agent

Use Prophylaxis of organ rejection concomitantly with cyclosporine and corticosteroids in patients receiving allogeneic renal (CellCept®, Myfortic®), cardiac (CellCept®), or hepatic (CellCept®) transplants

Unlabeled/Investigational Use Treatment of rejection in liver transplant patients unable to tolerate tacrolimus or cyclosporine due to neurotoxicity; mild rejection in heart transplant patients; treatment of moderate-severe psoriasis; treatment of proliferative lupus nephritis; treatment of myasthenia gravis; prevention and treatment of graft-versus-host disease (GVHD)

Effect on Mental Status Dizziness and insomnia are common

Effect on Psychiatric Treatment Leukopenia is common; avoid clozapine and carbamazepine

Dosage Summary

I.V.:

Children: Dosage not established

Adults: 1-1.5 g twice daily

Oral:

Cellcept®:

Children (suspension): 600 mg/m^2/dose twice daily (maximum: 1 g twice daily)

Children with BSA 1.25-1.5 m^2: 750 mg capsule twice daily

Children with BSA >1.5 m^2: 1 g capsule or tablet twice daily

Adults: 1-1.5 g twice daily

Myfortic®:

Children with BSA <1.19 m^2: Use of this formulation is not recommended

Children with BSA 1.19-1.58 m^2: 540 mg twice daily (maximum: 1080 mg/day)

Children with BSA >1.58 m^2: 720 mg twice daily (maximum: 1440 mg/day)

Adults: 720 mg twice daily

Dosage Forms Excipient information presented when available (limited, particularly for generics); consult specific product labeling.

Capsule, as mofetil:

CellCept®: 250 mg

Injection, powder for reconstitution, as mofetil hydrochloride:

CellCept®: 500 mg [contains polysorbate 80]

Powder for oral suspension, as mofetil:

CellCept®: 200 mg/mL (225 mL) [provides 175 mL suspension following reconstitution; contains phenylalanine 0.56 mg/mL; mixed fruit flavor]

Tablet, as mofetil:

CellCept®: 500 mg [may contain ethyl alcohol]

Tablet, delayed release, as mycophenolic acid:

Myfortic®: 180 mg, 360 mg [formulated as a sodium salt]

- ◆ **Mycophenolate Mofetil** *see* Mycophenolate *on page 1087*
- ◆ **Mycophenolate Sodium** *see* Mycophenolate *on page 1087*
- ◆ **Mycophenolic Acid** *see* Mycophenolate *on page 1087*
- ◆ **MyDex** *see* Guaifenesin and Phenylephrine *on page 742*
- ◆ **Mydfrin®** *see* Phenylephrine *on page 1273*
- ◆ **Mydral™** *see* Tropicamide *on page 1636*
- ◆ **Mydriacyl®** *see* Tropicamide *on page 1636*
- ◆ **Myfortic®** *see* Mycophenolate *on page 1087*
- ◆ **MyHist-DM** *see* Phenylephrine, Pyrilamine, and Dextromethorphan *on page 1278*
- ◆ **MyHist-PD** *see* Chlorpheniramine, Pyrilamine, and Phenylephrine *on page 335*

- **MyKidz Iron 10™** *see* Ferrous Sulfate *on page 627*
- **Mylanta® Children's [OTC]** *see* Calcium Carbonate *on page 254*
- **Mylanta® Gelcaps® [OTC]** *see* Calcium Carbonate and Magnesium Hydroxide *on page 256*
- **Mylanta® Liquid [OTC]** *see* Aluminum Hydroxide, Magnesium Hydroxide, and Simethicone *on page 78*
- **Mylanta® Maximum Strength Liquid [OTC]** *see* Aluminum Hydroxide, Magnesium Hydroxide, and Simethicone *on page 78*
- **Mylanta® Supreme [OTC]** *see* Calcium Carbonate and Magnesium Hydroxide *on page 256*
- **Mylanta® Ultra [OTC]** *see* Calcium Carbonate and Magnesium Hydroxide *on page 256*
- **Myleran®** *see* Busulfan *on page 226*
- **Mylocel™** *see* Hydroxyurea *on page 796*
- **Mylotarg®** *see* Gemtuzumab Ozogamicin *on page 713*
- **Myobloc®** *see* Botulinum Toxin Type B *on page 197*
- **Myochrysine®** *see* Gold Sodium Thiomalate *on page 734*
- **Myphetane DX** *see* Brompheniramine, Pseudoephedrine, and Dextromethorphan *on page 208*
- **myrac™** *see* Minocycline *on page 1056*
- **Mysoline®** *see* Primidone *on page 1336*
- **Mytelase®** *see* Ambenonium *on page 82*
- **Mytussin® AC** *see* Guaifenesin and Codeine *on page 738*
- **Mytussin® DAC** *see* Guaifenesin, Pseudoephedrine, and Codeine *on page 747*
- **N-0923** *see* Rotigotine *on page 1449*
- **NAAK** *see* Atropine and Pralidoxime *on page 159*
- **Nabi-HB®** *see* Hepatitis B Immune Globulin *on page 762*

Nabilone (NA bi lone)

U.S. Brand Names Cesamet®

Canadian Brand Names Cesamet™

Pharmacologic Category Antiemetic

Generic Available No

Use Treatment of nausea and vomiting associated with cancer chemotherapy

Effect on Mental Status Dizziness, drowsiness, and euphoria are common; may cause depression; may rarely cause confusion and hallucinations

Effect on Psychiatric Treatment Concurrent use with psychotropic may produce additive sedation

Restrictions C-II

Pregnancy Risk Factor C

Pregnancy Considerations Animal studies did not demonstrate teratogenic effects; however, dose-related decreased fetal weights and increased fetal resorptions were observed. There are no adequate and well-controlled studies in pregnant women. Use during pregnancy only if clearly needed.

Lactation Excretion in breast milk unknown/not recommended

Contraindications Nausea and vomiting not secondary to cancer chemotherapy

Warnings/Precautions May affect CNS function; use with caution in the elderly and those with pre-existing CNS depression. May cause additive CNS effects with sedatives, hypnotics, or other psychoactive agents; patients must be cautioned about performing tasks which require mental alertness (eg, operating machinery or driving). Use caution with current or previous history of mental illness; cannabinoid use may reveal symptoms of psychiatric disorders. Psychiatric adverse reactions may persist for up to 3 days after discontinuing treatment. Has potential for abuse and or dependence, use caution in patients with substance abuse history or potential. May cause tachycardia and orthostatic hypotension; use caution with cardiovascular disease. Safety and efficacy in children have not been established.

Adverse Reactions

>10%:

Central nervous system: Dizziness, drowsiness, vertigo, euphoria, clumsiness

Gastrointestinal: Xerostomia

1% to 10%:

Cardiovascular: Orthostatic hypotension

Central nervous system: Ataxia, depression
Ocular: Blurred vision

Drug Interactions CNS depression is potentiated with ethanol

Ethanol/Nutrition/Herb Interactions Ethanol: Avoid ethanol (may increase CNS depression).

Stability Store at room temperature between 15°C and 30°C (59°F and 86°F).

Mechanism of Action Not fully characterized; antiemetic activity may be due to effect on cannabinoid receptors (CB1) within the central nervous system.

Pharmacodynamics/Kinetics

Absorption: Rapid and complete
Distribution: ~12.5 L/kg
Metabolism: To several active metabolites by oxidation and stereospecific enzyme reduction; CYP450 enzymes may also be involved
Half-life elimination: Parent compound: 2 hours; Metabolites: 35 hours
Time to peak, serum: Within 2 hours
Excretion: Feces (~60%); renal (~24%)

Dosage Oral:

Children >4 years:
<18 kg: 0.5 mg twice daily
18-30 kg: 1 mg twice daily
>30 kg: 1 mg 3 times/day

Adults: 1-2 mg twice daily beginning 1-3 hours before chemotherapy is administered and continuing around-the-clock until 1 dose after chemotherapy is completed; maximum daily dose: 6 mg divided in 3 doses

Administration Initial dose should be given 1-3 hours before chemotherapy; may be given 2-3 times a day during the entire chemotherapy course and for up to 48 hours after the last dose of chemotherapy; a dose of 1-2 mg the night before chemotherapy may be useful.

Monitoring Parameters Blood pressure, heart rate; signs and symptoms of excessive use, abuse, or misuse

Dosage Forms Capsule: 1 mg

◆ **nab-Paclitaxel** *see* Paclitaxel (Protein Bound) *on page 1214*

Nabumetone (na BYOO me tone)

Related Information

Nonsteroidal Anti-Inflammatory Agents *on page 1792*

Canadian Brand Names Apo-Nabumetone®; Gen-Nabumetone; Novo-Nabumetone; Relafen®; Rhoxal-nabumetone; Sandoz-Nabumetone

Mexican Brand Names Relifex

Index Terms Relafen

Pharmacologic Category Nonsteroidal Anti-inflammatory Drug (NSAID), Oral

Use Management of osteoarthritis and rheumatoid arthritis

Unlabeled/Investigational Use Moderate pain

Effect on Mental Status Dizziness is common; may cause nervousness; may rarely cause insomnia, confusion, depression, or hallucinations

Effect on Psychiatric Treatment May rarely cause agranulocytosis; use caution with clozapine and carbamazepine; may decrease lithium clearance resulting in an increase in serum lithium levels and potential lithium toxicity; monitor serum lithium levels

Restrictions An FDA-approved medication guide must be distributed when dispensing an oral outpatient prescription (new or refill) where this medication is to be used without direct supervision of a healthcare provider. Medication guides are available at http://www.fda.gov/cder/Offices/ODS/medication_guides.htm.

Dosage Summary Note: Patients <50 kg are less likely to require doses >1000 mg/day.

Oral:

Children: Dosage not established

Adults: 1000 mg/day in 1-2 divided doses (maximum: 2000 mg/day)

Dosage Forms Excipient information presented when available (limited, particularly for generics); consult specific product labeling. [DSC] = Discontinued product

Tablet: 500 mg, 750 mg
Relafen®: 500 mg, 750 mg [DSC]

◆ **NAC** *see* Acetylcysteine *on page 47*
◆ **N-acetyl-5-methoxytryptamine** *see* Melatonin *on page 978*
◆ ***N*-Acetyl-L-cysteine** *see* Acetylcysteine *on page 47*

◆ ***N*-Acetylcysteine** *see* Acetylcysteine *on page 47*

◆ **N-Acetyl-P-Aminophenol** *see* Acetaminophen *on page 30*

Nadolol (NAY doe lol)

Medication Safety Issues

Sound-alike/look-alike issues:

Nadolol may be confused with Mandol®

Corgard® may be confused with Cognex®, Coreg®

Related Information

Beta-Blockers *on page 1776*

U.S. Brand Names Corgard®

Canadian Brand Names Alti-Nadolol; Apo-Nadol®; Corgard®; Novo-Nadolol

Mexican Brand Names Corgard

Pharmacologic Category Beta-Adrenergic Blocker, Nonselective

Generic Available Yes

Use Treatment of hypertension and angina pectoris; prophylaxis of migraine headaches

Unlabeled/Investigational Use Primary and secondary prophylaxis of variceal hemorrhage

Effect on Mental Status May cause drowsiness, dizziness, depression, insomnia, or confusion

Effect on Psychiatric Treatment Barbiturates may decrease the effects of beta-blockers; has been used to treat akathisia; propranolol preferred; concurrent use with antipsychotics may potentiate antihypertensive effect or antipsychotic blood levels; use with MAO inhibitors may cause bradycardia; effects of benzodiazepines may be increased by beta-blockers; monitor for clinical changes

Pregnancy Risk Factor C

Pregnancy Considerations No data available on crossing the placenta. Beta-blockers have been associated with bradycardia, hypotension, and IUGR; IUGR is probably related to maternal hypertension. Alternative beta-blockers are preferred for use during pregnancy due to limited data and prolonged half-life. Cases of neonatal hypoglycemia have been reported following maternal use of beta-blockers at parturition or during breast-feeding. Monitor breast-fed infant for symptoms of beta-blockade.

Lactation Enters breast milk/use caution (AAP rates "compatible")

Contraindications Hypersensitivity to nadolol or any component of the formulation; bronchial asthma; sinus bradycardia; sinus node dysfunction; heart block greater than first degree (except in patients with a functioning artificial pacemaker); cardiogenic shock; uncompensated cardiac failure

Warnings/Precautions Consider pre-existing conditions such as sick sinus syndrome before initiating. Administer only with extreme caution in patients with compensated heart failure, monitor for a worsening of the condition. Efficacy in heart failure has not been established for nadolol. **[U.S. Boxed Warning]: Beta-blocker therapy should not be withdrawn abruptly (particularly in patients with CAD), but gradually tapered to avoid acute tachycardia, hypertension, and/or ischemia.** Use caution with concurrent use of beta-blockers and either verapamil or diltiazem; bradycardia or heart block can occur. In general, patients with bronchospastic disease should not receive beta-blockers. Nadolol, if used at all, should be used cautiously in bronchospastic disease with close monitoring. Use cautiously in diabetics because it can mask prominent hypoglycemic symptoms. Use cautiously in the renally impaired (dosage adjustments are required). Use with caution in patients with myasthenia gravis, peripheral vascular disease, or psychiatric disease (may cause CNS depression). Use care with anesthetic agents which decrease myocardial function. Adequate alpha-blockade is required prior to use of any beta-blocker for patients with untreated pheochromocytoma. Use caution with history of severe anaphylaxis to allergens; patients taking beta-blockers may become more sensitive to repeated challenges. Treatment of anaphylaxis (eg, epinephrine) in patients taking beta-blockers may be ineffective or promote undesirable effects. Safety and efficacy have not been established in children.

Adverse Reactions

>10%:

Central nervous system: Drowsiness, insomnia

Endocrine & metabolic: Decreased sexual ability

1% to 10%:

Cardiovascular: Bradycardia, palpitation, edema, CHF, reduced peripheral circulation

Central nervous system: Mental depression

Gastrointestinal: Diarrhea or constipation, nausea, vomiting, stomach discomfort

Respiratory: Bronchospasm

Miscellaneous: Cold extremities

<1% (Limited to important or life-threatening): Arrhythmias, chest pain, confusion (especially in the elderly), depression, dyspnea, hallucinations, leukopenia, orthostatic hypotension, thrombocytopenia

Drug Interactions

Acetylcholinesterase Inhibitors: May enhance the bradycardic effect of Beta-Blockers. *Risk C: Monitor therapy*

Alpha-/Beta-Agonists (Direct-Acting): Beta-Blockers may enhance the vasopressor effect of Alpha-/Beta-Agonists (Direct-Acting). Epinephrine used as a local anesthetic for dental procedures will not likely cause clinically relevant problems. **Exceptions:** Dipivefrin. *Risk D: Consider therapy modification*

Alpha1-Blockers: Beta-Blockers may enhance the orthostatic effect of Alpha1-Blockers. The risk associated with ophthalmic products is probably less than systemic products. *Risk D: Consider therapy modification*

Alpha2-Agonists: Beta-Blockers may enhance the rebound hypertensive effect of Alpha2-Agonists. This effect can occur when the alpha2-agonist is abruptly withdrawn. **Exceptions:** Apraclonidine; Brimonidine. *Risk D: Consider therapy modification*

Amiodarone: May enhance the bradycardic effect of Beta-Blockers. Possibly to the point of cardiac arrest. Amiodarone may increase the serum concentration of Beta-Blockers. *Risk C: Monitor therapy*

Anilidopiperidine Opioids: May enhance the bradycardic effect of Beta-Blockers. Anilidopiperidine Opioids may enhance the hypotensive effect of Beta-Blockers. *Risk C: Monitor therapy*

Beta2-Agonists: Beta-Blockers (Nonselective) may diminish the bronchodilatory effect of Beta2-Agonists. *Risk D: Consider therapy modification*

Calcium Channel Blockers (Nondihydropyridine): May enhance the hypotensive effect of Beta-Blockers. Bradycardia and signs of heart failure have also been reported. Calcium Channel Blockers (Nondihydropyridine) may increase the serum concentration of Beta-Blockers. *Risk C: Monitor therapy*

Cardiac Glycosides: Beta-Blockers may enhance the bradycardic effect of Cardiac Glycosides. *Risk C: Monitor therapy*

Diazoxide: May enhance the hypotensive effect of Antihypertensives. *Risk C: Monitor therapy*

Dipyridamole: May enhance the bradycardic effect of Beta-Blockers. *Risk C: Monitor therapy*

Disopyramide: May enhance the bradycardic effect of Beta-Blockers. *Risk C: Monitor therapy*

Herbs (Hypertensive Properties): May diminish the antihypertensive effect of Antihypertensives. *Risk C: Monitor therapy*

Herbs (Hypotensive Properties): May enhance the hypotensive effect of Antihypertensives. *Risk C: Monitor therapy*

Insulin: Beta-Blockers may enhance the hypoglycemic effect of Insulin. *Risk C: Monitor therapy*

Lidocaine: Beta-Blockers may decrease the metabolism of Lidocaine. *Risk C: Monitor therapy*

Methacholine: Beta-Blockers may enhance the adverse/toxic effect of Methacholine. *Risk X: Avoid combination*

Methylphenidate: May diminish the antihypertensive effect of Antihypertensives. *Risk C: Monitor therapy*

Midodrine: Beta-Blockers may enhance the bradycardic effect of Midodrine. *Risk C: Monitor therapy*

Nonsteroidal Anti-Inflammatory Agents: May diminish the antihypertensive effect of Beta-Blockers. *Risk C: Monitor therapy*

P-Glycoprotein Inducers: May decrease the serum concentration of P-Glycoprotein Substrates. P-glycoprotein inducers may also further limit the distribution of p-glycoprotein substrates to specific cells/tissues/organs where p-glycoprotein is present in large amounts (e.g., brain, T-lymphocytes, testes, etc.). *Risk C: Monitor therapy*

P-Glycoprotein Inhibitors: May increase the serum concentration of P-Glycoprotein Substrates. P-glycoprotein inhibitors may also enhance the distribution of p-glycoprotein substrates to specific cells/tissues/organs where p-glycoprotein is present in large amounts (e.g., brain, T-lymphocytes, testes, etc.). *Risk C: Monitor therapy*

Prostacyclin Analogues: May enhance the hypotensive effect of Antihypertensives. *Risk C: Monitor therapy*

Reserpine: May enhance the hypotensive effect of Beta-Blockers. *Risk C: Monitor therapy*

RiTUXimab: Antihypertensives may enhance the hypotensive effect of RiTUXimab. *Risk D: Consider therapy modification*

Theophylline Derivatives: Beta-Blockers (Nonselective) may diminish the bronchodilatory effect of Theophylline Derivatives. *Risk D: Consider therapy modification*

Ethanol/Nutrition/Herb Interactions Herb/Nutraceutical: Avoid dong quai if using for hypertension (has estrogenic activity). Avoid ephedra, garlic, yohimbe, ginseng (may worsen hypertension). Avoid natural licorice (causes sodium and water retention and increases potassium loss).

Mechanism of Action Competitively blocks response to $beta_1$- and $beta_2$-adrenergic stimulation; does not exhibit any membrane stabilizing or intrinsic sympathomimetic activity. Nonselective beta-adrenergic blockers (propranolol, nadolol) reduce portal pressure by producing splanchnic vasoconstriction ($beta_2$ effect) thereby reducing portal blood flow.

Pharmacodynamics/Kinetics

Duration: 17-24 hours

Absorption: 30% to 40%

Distribution: Concentration in human breast milk is 4.6 times higher than serum

Protein binding: 28%

Half-life elimination: Adults: 10-24 hours; prolonged with renal impairment; End-stage renal disease: 45 hours

Time to peak, serum: 2-4 hours

Excretion: Urine (as unchanged drug)

Dosage Oral:

Adults: Initial: 40 mg/day, increase dosage gradually by 40-80 mg increments at 3- to 7-day intervals until optimum clinical response is obtained with profound slowing of heart rate; doses up to 160-240 mg/day in angina and 240-320 mg/day in hypertension may be necessary.

Hypertension: Usual dosage range (JNC 7): 40-120 mg once daily

Variceal hemorrhage prophylaxis (unlabeled use; Garcia-Tsao, 2007):

Primary prophylaxis: Initial: 40 mg once daily; adjust to maximal tolerated dose. **Note:** Risk factors for hemorrhage include Child-Pugh class B/C or variceal red wale markings on endoscopy.

Secondary prophylaxis: Initial: 40 mg once daily; adjust to maximal tolerated dose

Elderly: Initial: 20 mg/day; increase doses by 20 mg increments at 3- to 7-day intervals; usual dosage range: 20-240 mg/day.

Dosing adjustment in renal impairment:

Cl_{cr} 31-40 mL/minute: Administer every 24-36 hours or administer 50% of normal dose.

Cl_{cr} 10-30 mL/minute: Administer every 24-48 hours or administer 50% of normal dose.

Cl_{cr} <10 mL/minute: Administer every 40-60 hours or administer 25% of normal dose.

Hemodialysis: Moderately dialyzable (20% to 50%); administer dose post-dialysis or administer 40 mg supplemental dose.

Peritoneal dialysis: Supplemental dose is not necessary.

Dosing adjustment/comments in hepatic disease: Reduced dose probably necessary.

Dietary Considerations May be taken without regard to meals.

Dosage Forms Excipient information presented when available (limited, particularly for generics); consult specific product labeling. [DSC] = Discontinued product

Tablet: 20 mg, 40 mg, 80 mg

Corgard®: 20 mg, 40 mg, 80 mg, 120 mg [DSC], 160 mg [DSC]

Nadolol and Bendroflumethiazide

(NAY doe lol & ben droe floo meth EYE a zide)

U.S. Brand Names Corzide®

Index Terms Bendroflumethiazide and Nadolol

Pharmacologic Category Beta Blocker, Nonselective; Diuretic, Thiazide

Use Treatment of hypertension; combination product should not be used for initial therapy

Effect on Mental Status May cause drowsiness, dizziness, depression, insomnia, or confusion

Effect on Psychiatric Treatment Barbiturates may decrease the effects of beta-blockers. Nadolol has been used to treat akathisia; propranolol preferred. Concurrent use with antipsychotics may potentiate antihypertensive effect or antipsychotic blood levels. Use with MAO inhibitors may cause bradycardia. Effects of benzodiazepines may be increased by beta-blockers; monitor for clinical changes. There are rare reports of agranulocytosis with bendroflumethiazide; use caution with clozapine, carbamazepine, and mirtazapine. May decrease lithium clearance resulting in an increase in serum lithium levels and potential lithium toxicity; monitor.

Dosage Summary

Oral:

Children: Dosage not established

Adults: Initial: Nadolol 40 mg and bendroflumethiazide 5 mg once daily; Maintenance: Nadolol 40-80 mg and bendroflumethiazide 5 mg once daily

Dosage Forms Excipient information presented when available (limited, particularly for generics); consult specific product labeling.

Tablet: Nadolol 40 mg and bendroflumethiazide 5 mg; nadolol 80 mg and bendroflumethiazide 5 mg

Corzide® 40/5: Nadolol 40 mg and bendroflumethiazide 5 mg [scored]

Corzide® 80/5: Nadolol 80 mg and bendroflumethiazide 5 mg [scored]

Nafarelin (naf a REL in)

Medication Safety Issues

Sound-alike/look-alike issues:

Nafarelin may be confused with Anafranil®, enalapril

U.S. Brand Names Synarel®

Canadian Brand Names Synarel®

Mexican Brand Names Synarel

Index Terms Nafarelin Acetate

Pharmacologic Category Gonadotropin Releasing Hormone Agonist

Use Treatment of endometriosis, including pain and reduction of lesions; treatment of central precocious puberty (CPP; gonadotropin-dependent precocious puberty) in children of both sexes

Effect on Mental Status Emotional lability is common; may cause insomnia

Effect on Psychiatric Treatment None reported

Dosage Summary

Nasal:

Children: 2 sprays (400 mcg) into each nostril in the morning and evening, may increase to 3 sprays (600 mcg) into alternating nostrils 3 times/day

Adults: 1 spray (200 mcg) in 1 nostril each morning and the other nostril each evening starting on days 2-4 of menstrual cycle for 6 month

Dosage Forms Excipient information presented when available (limited, particularly for generics); consult specific product labeling.

Solution, intranasal [spray]:

Synarel®: 2 mg/mL (8 mL) [200 mcg/spray: 60 metered sprays; contains benzalkonium chloride]

◆ **Nafarelin Acetate** *see* Nafarelin *on page 1093*

Nafcillin (naf SIL in)

Canadian Brand Names Nallpen®; Unipen®

Index Terms Ethoxynaphthamido Penicillin Sodium; Nafcillin Sodium; Nallpen; Sodium Nafcillin

Pharmacologic Category Antibiotic, Penicillin

Use Treatment of infections such as osteomyelitis, septicemia, endocarditis, and CNS infections caused by susceptible strains of staphylococci species

Effect on Mental Status Penicillins reported to cause apprehension, illusions, hallucinations, depersonalization, agitation, insomnia, and encephalopathy

Effect on Psychiatric Treatment May cause neutropenia; use caution with clozapine and carbamazepine

Dosage Summary

I.M.:

Neonates 1200-2000 g, <7 days: 50 mg/kg/day divided every 12 hours

Neonates >2000 g, <7 days: 75 mg/kg/day divided every 8 hours

Neonates 1200-2000 g, ≥7 days: 75 mg/kg/day divided every 8 hours

Neonates >2000 g, ≥7 days: 100-140 mg/kg/day divided every 6 hours

Children: 25 mg/kg twice daily

Adults: 500 mg every 4-6 hours

I.V.:

Neonates 1200-2000 g, <7 days: 50 mg/kg/day divided every 12 hours

Neonates >2000 g, <7 days: 75 mg/kg/day divided every 8 hours

Neonates 1200-2000 g, ≥7 days: 75 mg/kg/day divided every 8 hours

Neonates >2000 g, ≥7 days: 100-140 mg/kg/day divided every 6 hours

Children: 50-200 mg/kg/day in divided every 4-6 hours (maximum: 12 g/day)
Adults: 500-2000 mg every 4-6 hours

Dosage Forms Excipient information presented when available (limited, particularly for generics); consult specific product labeling.
Infusion [premixed iso-osmotic dextrose solution]: 1 g (50 mL); 2 g (100 mL)
Injection, powder for reconstitution, as sodium: 1 g, 2 g, 10 g

- **Nafcillin Sodium** *see* Nafcillin *on page 1093*
- **Nafidimide** *see* Amonafide *on page 108*
- **Naglazyme™** *see* Galsulfase *on page 708*
- **NaHCO$_3$** *see* Sodium Bicarbonate *on page 1494*

Nalbuphine (NAL byoo feen)

Medication Safety Issues
Sound-alike/look-alike issues:
Nubain® may be confused with Navane®, Nebcin®

High alert medication: The Institute for Safe Medication Practices (ISMP) includes this medication among its list of drug classes which have a heightened risk of causing significant patient harm when used in error.

Related Information
Narcotic / Opioid Analgesics *on page 1789*

U.S. Brand Names Nubain®

Mexican Brand Names Bufigen; Nalcryn SP

Index Terms Nalbuphine Hydrochloride

Pharmacologic Category Analgesic, Opioid

Use Relief of moderate to severe pain; preoperative analgesia, postoperative and surgical anesthesia, and obstetrical analgesia during labor and delivery

Unlabeled/Investigational Use Opioid-induced pruritus

Effect on Mental Status Drowsiness is common; may cause dizziness; may rarely cause restlessness, nervousness, confusion, depression, or hallucinations

Effect on Psychiatric Treatment Concurrent use with psychotropic may produce additive sedation

Dosage Summary

I.M.:
Children <1 year: Dosage not established
Children ≥1 year (unlabeled use): 0.1-0.2 mg/kg every 3-4 hours as needed (maximum: 20 mg/dose; 160 mg/day)
Adults: 10 mg/70 kg every 3-6 hours (maximum 20 mg/dose; 160 mg/day)

I.V.:
Children <1 year: Dosage not established
Children ≥1 year (unlabeled use): 0.1-0.2 mg/kg every 3-4 hours as needed (maximum: 20 mg/dose; 160 mg/day)
Adults: 10 mg/70 kg every 3-6 hours (maximum 20 mg/dose; 160 mg/day) **or** 0.3-3 mg/kg over 10-15 minutes, then 0.25-0.5 mg/kg as required for anesthesia **or** 2.5-5 mg (1-2 doses)

SubQ:
Children <1 year: Dosage not established
Children ≥1 year (unlabeled use): 0.1-0.2 mg/kg every 3-4 hours as needed (maximum: 20 mg/dose; 160 mg/day)
Adults: 10 mg/70 kg every 3-6 hours (maximum 20 mg/dose; 160 mg/day)

Dosage Forms Excipient information presented when available (limited, particularly for generics); consult specific product labeling. [DSC] = Discontinued product
Injection, solution, as hydrochloride: 10 mg/mL (10 mL); 20 mg/mL (10 mL)
Nubain®: 10 mg/mL (10 mL) [DSC]; 20 mg/mL (10 mL)
Injection, solution, as hydrochloride [preservative free]: 10 mg/mL (1 mL); 20 mg/mL (1 mL)
Nubain®: 10 mg/mL (1 mL); 20 mg/mL (1 mL)

- **Nalbuphine Hydrochloride** *see* Nalbuphine *on page 1094*
- **Nalex®-A** *see* Chlorpheniramine, Phenylephrine, and Phenyltoloxamine *on page 331*
- **Nalex A 12** *see* Chlorpheniramine, Pyrilamine, and Phenylephrine *on page 335*
- **Nalfon®** *see* Fenoprofen *on page 623*
- **Nallpen** *see* Nafcillin *on page 1093*
- ***N*-allylnoroxymorphine Hydrochloride** *see* Naloxone *on page 1097*

Nalmefene (NAL me feen)

Medication Safety Issues

Sound-alike/look-alike issues:

Revex® may be confused with Nimbex®, ReVia®, Rubex®

Color-coded ampuls denote indication-specific concentrations:

Blue-labeled ampul (for postoperative use) contains 1 mL (100 mcg/mL)

Green-labeled ampul (for overdose management) contains 2 mL (1 mg/mL)

International issues:

Revex® may be confused with Brivex® which is a brand name for brivudine in Switzerland

Revex® may be confused with Rubex® which is a brand name for ascorbic acid in Ireland

U.S. Brand Names Revex® [DSC]

Index Terms Nalmefene Hydrochloride

Pharmacologic Category Antidote; Opioid Antagonist

Generic Available No

Use Complete or partial reversal of opioid drug effects, including respiratory depression induced by natural or synthetic opioids; reversal of postoperative opioid depression; management of known or suspected opioid overdose

Effect on Mental Status May cause dizziness; may rarely cause agitation, confusion, depression, nervousness, and sedation

Effect on Psychiatric Treatment May precipitate opioid withdrawal in dependent patients

Pregnancy Risk Factor B

Pregnancy Considerations Animal studies have not demonstrated fetal harm or fertility impairment. There are no adequate and well-controlled studies in pregnant women. Use only if clearly needed.

Lactation Excretion in breast milk unknown/use caution

Contraindications Hypersensitivity to nalmefene or any component of the formulation

Warnings/Precautions May induce symptoms of acute withdrawal in opioid-dependent patients; recurrence of respiratory depression is possible if the opioid involved is long-acting; observe patients until there is no reasonable risk of recurrent respiratory depression. Nalmefene is structurally similar to both naltrexone and naloxone; patients with hypersensitivity to these agents may also react to nalmefene. Concurrent use of flumazenil and nalmefene may increase the risk of seizures. Safety and efficacy have not been established in children. Avoid abrupt reversal of opioid effects in patients of high cardiovascular risk or who have received potentially cardiotoxic drugs. Pulmonary edema and cardiovascular instability have been reported in association with abrupt reversal with other narcotic antagonists. Animal studies indicate nalmefene may not completely reverse buprenorphine-induced respiratory depression. Use caution with renal impairment. Excessive dosages should be avoided after use of opiates in surgery. Abrupt postoperative reversal may result in nausea, vomiting, sweating, tachycardia, hypertension, seizures, and other cardiovascular events (including pulmonary edema and arrhythmias). Discharged patients who are opioid-dependent may attempt to override the narcotic-blocking effect of nalmefene. Patients are at a greater risk of overdose when nalmefene wears off if megadosing of opiates has occurred. Adequate duration of monitoring should be provided.

Two products are available at different concentrations. A blue-labeled ampul contains a 100 mcg/mL solution of nalmefene and is intended for postoperative use. A green-labeled ampul contains a 1 mg/mL (**10** times as concentrated; **20** times as much drug) and is intended to be used for the management of an overdose.

Adverse Reactions

>10%: Gastrointestinal: Nausea (18%)

1% to 10%:

Cardiovascular: Tachycardia (5%), hypertension (5%), hypotension (1%), vasodilation (1%)

Central nervous system: Fever (3%), dizziness (3%), headache (1%), chills (1%)

Gastrointestinal: Vomiting (9%)

Miscellaneous: Postoperative pain (4%)

<1% (Limited to important or life-threatening): Agitation, arrhythmia, AST increased, bradycardia, confusion, depression, diarrhea, myoclonus, nervousness, pharyngitis, pruritus, pulmonary edema, somnolence, tremor, urinary retention, withdrawal syndrome, xerostomia

Drug Interactions
There are no known significant interactions.

Stability Store at controlled room temperature.

Mechanism of Action As a 6-methylene analog of naltrexone, nalmefene acts as a competitive antagonist at opioid receptor sites, preventing or reversing the respiratory depression, sedation, and hypotension induced by opiates; no pharmacologic activity of its own (eg, opioid agonist activity) has been demonstrated

Pharmacodynamics/Kinetics
Onset of action: I.M., SubQ: 5-15 minutes
Distribution: V_d: 8.6 L/kg; rapid
Protein binding: 45%
Metabolism: Hepatic via glucuronide conjugation to metabolites with little or no activity
Bioavailability: I.M., SubQ: 100%
Half-life elimination: 10.8 hours
Time to peak, serum: Serum: I.M.: 2.3 hours; I.V.: <2 minutes; SubQ: 1.5 hours
Excretion: Feces (17%); urine (<5% as unchanged drug)
Clearance: 0.8 L/hour/kg

Dosage I.M., I.V., SubQ:
Reversal of postoperative opioid depression: Blue-labeled product (100 mcg/mL): Titrate to reverse the undesired effects of opioids; initial dose for nonopioid dependent patients: 0.25 mcg/kg followed by 0.25 mcg/kg incremental doses at 2- to 5-minute intervals; after a total dose >1 mcg/kg, further therapeutic response is unlikely
Note: In patients with increased cardiovascular risks, dilute 1:1 in NS or SWFI, and initiate/titrate with 0.1 mcg/kg doses.
Management of known/suspected opioid overdose: **Note:** I.V. route is preferred. Green-labeled product (1 mg/mL): Adults:
Nonopioid-dependent patients: 0.5 mg/70 kg; may repeat with 1 mg/70 kg in 2-5 minutes; further increase beyond a total dose of 1.5 mg/70 kg will not likely result in improved response and may result in cardiovascular stress and precipitated withdrawal syndrome
Opioid-dependent patients: Administer a challenge dose of 0.1 mg/70 kg; if no withdrawal symptoms are observed in 2 minutes, give 0.5 mg/70 kg; may repeat with 1 mg/70 kg in 2-5 minutes; further increase beyond a total dose of 1.5 mg/70 kg will not likely result in improved response and may result in cardiovascular stress and precipitated withdrawal syndrome
Note: If recurrence of respiratory depression is noted, dose may again be titrated to clinical effect using incremental doses.
Note: If I.V. access is lost or not readily obtainable, a single SubQ or I.M. dose of 1 mg may be effective in 5-15 minutes.
Dosing adjustment in renal impairment: Not necessary with single use, however, slow administration (over 60 seconds) of incremental doses is recommended to minimize hypertension and dizziness
Dosing adjustment in hepatic impairment: No adjustment necessary with single use.

Administration Check dosage strength carefully before use to avoid error. Slow administration (over 60 seconds) of incremental doses is recommended to minimize hypertension and dizziness in renal patients. Dilute drug (1:1) with diluent and use smaller doses in patients known to be at increased cardiovascular risk. May be administered via I.M. or SubQ routes if I.V. access is not feasible. A single SubQ or I.M. dose of 1 mg may be effective in 5-15 minutes.

Monitoring Parameters Symptoms of withdrawal; neurological status, oxygenation, pain, vital signs

Additional Information Proper steps should be used to prevent use of the incorrect dosage strength. The goal of treatment in the postoperative setting is to achieve reversal of excessive opioid effects without inducing a complete reversal and acute pain.

If opioid dependence is suspected, nalmefene should only be used in opioid overdose if the likelihood of overdose is high based on history or the clinical presentation of respiratory depression with concurrent pupillary constriction is present.

Dosage Forms Excipient information presented when available (limited, particularly for generics); consult specific product labeling.
Injection, solution:
Revex®: 100 mcg/mL (1 mL) [blue label]; 1 mg/mL (2 mL) [green label] [DSC]

◆ **Nalmefene Hydrochloride** *see* Nalmefene *on page 1095*

Naloxone (nal OKS one)

Medication Safety Issues

Sound-alike/look-alike issues:

Naloxone may be confused with naltrexone

Narcan® may be confused with Marcaine®, Norcuron®

International issues:

Narcan® may be confused with Marcen® which is a brand name for ketazolam in Spain

Canadian Brand Names Naloxone Hydrochloride Injection®

Mexican Brand Names Narcanti

Index Terms *N*-allylnoroxymorphine Hydrochloride; Naloxone Hydrochloride; Narcan

Pharmacologic Category Antidote; Opioid Antagonist

Generic Available Yes

Use

Complete or partial reversal of opioid depression, including respiratory depression, induced by natural and synthetic opioids, including heroin, morphine, propoxyphene, methadone, and certain mixed agonist-antagonist analgesics: nalbuphine, pentazocine, and butorphanol

Diagnosis of suspected opioid dependence or acute opioid overdose

Adjunctive agent to increase blood pressure in the management of septic shock

Unlabeled/Investigational Use Opioid-induced pruritus

Pregnancy Risk Factor C

Pregnancy Considerations Consider benefit to the mother and the risk to the fetus before administering to a pregnant woman who is known or suspected to be opioid dependent. May precipitate withdrawal in both the mother and fetus.

Lactation Excretion in breast milk unknown/not recommended

Contraindications Hypersensitivity to naloxone or any component of the formulation

Warnings/Precautions Due to an association between naloxone and acute pulmonary edema, use with caution in patients with cardiovascular disease or in patients receiving medications with potential adverse cardiovascular effects (eg, hypotension, pulmonary edema, or arrhythmias). Administration of naloxone causes the release of catecholamines; may precipitate acute withdrawal or unmask pain in those who regularly take opioids. Excessive dosages should be avoided after use of opiates in surgery. Abrupt post-operative reversal may result in nausea, vomiting, sweating, tachycardia, hypertension, seizures, and other cardiovascular events (including pulmonary edema and arrhythmias). May precipitate withdrawal symptoms in patients addicted to opiates, including pain, hypertension, sweating, agitation, irritability; in neonates: shrill cry, failure to feed; carefully titrate dose to reverse hypoventilation; do not fully awaken patient or reverse analgesic effect (postoperative patient). Use caution in patients with history of seizures; avoid use in treatment of meperidine-induced seizures. Recurrence of respiratory depression is possible if the opioid involved is long-acting; observe patients until there is no reasonable risk of recurrent respiratory depression.

Adverse Reactions Adverse reactions are related to reversing dependency and precipitating withdrawal. Withdrawal symptoms are the result of sympathetic excess. Adverse events occur secondarily to reversal (withdrawal) of narcotic analgesia and sedation.

Central nervous system: Narcotic withdrawal

Drug Interactions

There are no known significant interactions.

Stability Store at 25°C (77°F). Protect from light. Stable in 0.9% sodium chloride and D_5W at 4 mcg/mL for 24 hours.

Mechanism of Action Pure opioid antagonist that competes and displaces narcotics at opioid receptor sites

Pharmacodynamics/Kinetics

Onset of action: Endotracheal, I.M., SubQ: 2-5 minutes; I.V.: ~2 minutes

Duration: ~30-120 minutes depending on route of administration; I.V. has a shorter duration of action than I.M. administration; since naloxone's action is shorter than that of most opioids, repeated doses are usually needed

Distribution: Crosses placenta

Metabolism: Primarily hepatic via glucuronidation

Half-life elimination: Neonates: 3-4 hours; Adults: 0.5-1.5 hours

Excretion: Urine (as metabolites)

Dosage Note: I.M., I.V. (preferred), and SubQ routes are available. Endotracheal administration is the least desirable and is supported by only anecdotal evidence (case report) (ACLS guidelines, 2005):

Infants and Children: Postoperative reversal: 0.01 mg/kg; may repeat every 2-3 minutes as needed based on response (adequate ventilation without significant pain)

Children:

Opioid intoxication: Respiratory depression:

I.V.:

Birth (including premature infants) to 5 years or <20 kg: Initial: 0.1 mg/kg (maximum dose: 2 mg); repeat every 2-3 minutes if needed (*Drugs for Pediatric Emergencies*, 1998)

>5 years or ≥20 kg: 2 mg/dose; if no response, repeat every 2-3 minutes (*Drugs for Pediatric Emergencies*, 1998)

Continuous infusion: I.V.: If continuous infusion is required, calculate dosage/hour based on effective intermittent dose used and duration of adequate response seen **or** use 2/3 of the initial effective naloxone bolus on an hourly basis; titrate dose (typically 0.04-0.16 mg/kg/hour for 2-5 days in children); 1/2 of the initial bolus dose should be readministered 15 minutes after initiation of the continuous infusion to prevent a drop in naloxone levels; increase infusion rate as needed to assure adequate ventilation and prevent withdrawal symptoms

Adults:

Opioid intoxication: Respiratory depression: I.V.: 0.4-2 mg; may need to repeat doses every 2-3 minutes; after reversal, may need to readminister dose(s) at a later interval (ie, 20-60 minutes) depending on type/duration of opioid. If no response is observed after 10 mg, consider other causes of respiratory depression. **Note:** Opioid-dependent patients may require lower doses (0.1 mg) titrated incrementally to avoid precipitating acute withdrawal.

Continuous infusion: I.V.: Calculate dosage/hour based on effective intermittent dose used and duration of adequate response seen **or** use 2/3 of the initial effective naloxone bolus on an hourly basis (typically 0.25-6.25 mg/hour); 1/2 of the initial bolus dose should be readministered 15 minutes after initiation of the continuous infusion to prevent a drop in naloxone levels; adjust infusion rate as needed to assure adequate ventilation and prevent withdrawal symptoms

Opioid-dependent patients being treated for cancer pain (unlabeled; NCCN guidelines, 2008): I.V.: 0.04-0.08 mg (40-80 mcg) slow I.V. push; administer every 30-60 seconds until improvement in symptoms, if no response is observed after total naloxone dose 1 mg, consider other causes of respiratory depression. **Note:** May dilute 0.4 mg/mL (1 mL) ampule into 9 mL of normal saline for a total volume of 10 mL to achieve a 0.04 mg/mL (40 mcg/mL) concentration.

Postoperative reversal: I.V.: 0.1-0.2 mg every 2-3 minutes until desired response (adequate ventilation and alertness without significant pain). **Note:** Repeat doses may be needed within 1-2 hour intervals depending on type, dose, and timing of the last dose of opioid administered.

Opioid-induced pruritus (unlabeled use): I.V. infusion: 0.25 mcg/kg/hour; **Note:** Monitor pain control; verify that the naloxone is not reversing analgesia.

Administration

Endotracheal: There is only anecdotal support for this route of administration. May require a slightly higher dose than used in other routes. Dilute to 1-2 mL with normal saline; flush with 5 cc of saline and then administer 5 ventilations

Intratracheal: Dilute to 1-2 mL with normal saline

I.V. push: Administer over 30 seconds as undiluted preparation **or** (unlabeled) administer as diluted preparation slow I.V. push by diluting 0.4 mg (1 mL) ampul with 9 mL of normal saline for a total volume of 10 mL to achieve a concentration of 0.04 mg/mL

I.V. continuous infusion: Dilute to 4 mcg/mL in D_5W or normal saline

Monitoring Parameters Respiratory rate, heart rate, blood pressure, temperature, level of consciousness, ABGs or pulse oximetry

Additional Information May contain methyl and propylparabens

Dosage Forms Excipient information presented when available (limited, particularly for generics); consult specific product labeling.

Injection, solution, as hydrochloride: 0.4 mg/mL (1 mL, 10 mL)

Injection, solution, as hydrochloride [preservative free]: 0.4 mg/mL (1 mL); 1 mg/mL (2 mL)

◆ **Naloxone and Buprenorphine** *see* Buprenorphine and Naloxone *on page 215*

- **Naloxone Hydrochloride** *see* Naloxone *on page 1097*
- **Naloxone Hydrochloride and Pentazocine Hydrochloride** *see* Pentazocine *on page 1243*
- **Naloxone Hydrochloride Dihydrate and Buprenorphine Hydrochloride** *see* Buprenorphine and Naloxone *on page 215*

Naltrexone (nal TREKS one)

Medication Safety Issues

Sound-alike/look-alike issues:

Naltrexone may be confused with methylnaltrexone, naloxone

ReVia® may be confused with Revatio®, Revex®

Administration issues: Vivitrol™: For intramuscular (I.M.) gluteal injection only

Related Information

Addiction Treatments *on page 1817*

U.S. Brand Names Depade®; ReVia®; Vivitrol™

Canadian Brand Names ReVia®

Mexican Brand Names Re-Via

Index Terms Naltrexone Hydrochloride

Pharmacologic Category Antidote; Opioid Antagonist

Generic Available Yes: Tablet

Use Treatment of ethanol dependence; blockade of the effects of exogenously administered opioids

Pregnancy Risk Factor C

Pregnancy Considerations Evidence of early fetal loss has been observed in animal studies with oral naltrexone. There are no adequate and well-controlled studies in pregnant women.

Lactation Enters breast milk/not recommended

Contraindications Hypersensitivity to naltrexone or any component of the formulation; narcotic dependence or current use of opioid analgesics; acute opioid withdrawal; failure to pass Narcan® challenge or positive urine screen for opioids; acute hepatitis; liver failure

Warnings/Precautions

[U.S. Boxed Warning]: Dose-related hepatocellular injury is possible; the margin of separation between the apparent safe and hepatotoxic doses appears to be ≤ fivefold.

May precipitate withdrawal symptoms in patients addicted to opiates; patients should be opioid-free for a minimum of 7-10 days; use naloxone challenge test to confirm. Use with caution in patients with hepatic or renal impairment. Patients may respond to lower opioid doses than previously used. This could result in potentially life-threatening opioid intoxication. Use of naltrexone does not eliminate or diminish withdrawal symptoms. Warn patients that attempts to overcome opioid blockade could lead to fatal overdose. Suicidal thoughts and depression have been reported; monitor closely. Cases of eosinophilic pneumonia have been reported; monitor for hypoxia and dyspnea. Use with caution in patients with a history of bleeding disorders (including thrombocytopenia) and/or patients on anticoagulant therapy; bleeding/hematoma may occur from I.M. administration. Serious injection site reactions (eg, cellulitis, induration, hematoma, abscess, necrosis) have been reported with use. Patients should report injection site pain, swelling, bruising, pruritus, or redness that does not improve (or worsens) within 2 weeks; consider surgical consult for worsening reactions. For I.M. use only; do not administer I.V., SubQ, or into fatty tissue; may increase the risk of injection site reactions. Vehicle used in injectable (polylactide-co-glycolide microspheres) has rarely been associated with retinal artery occlusion in patients with abnormal arteriovenous anastomosis. Safety and efficacy in children have not been established.

Adverse Reactions Combined reporting of adverse events from oral and injectable formulations:

>10%:

Cardiovascular: Syncope (13%)

Central nervous system: Headache (25%), insomnia (14%), dizziness (13%), anxiety (12%), somnolence (4%), nervousness, fatigue

Gastrointestinal: Nausea (33%), vomiting (14%), appetite decreased (14%), diarrhea (13%), abdominal pain (11%), abdominal cramping

Local: Injection site reaction (69%; includes bruising, induration, nodules, pain, pruritus, swelling, tenderness)

Neuromuscular & skeletal: Arthralgia (12%), CPK increased (11%)

Respiratory: Upper respiratory tract infection (13%), pharyngitis (11%)

1% to 10%:

Central nervous system: Depression (8%), suicidal thoughts (1%), energy increased, feeling down

Dermatologic: Rash (6%)

Endocrine & metabolic: Polydipsia

Gastrointestinal: Dry mouth (5%)

Genitourinary: Delayed ejaculation, impotency

Hepatic: AST increased (2%)

Neuromuscular & skeletal: Muscle cramps (8%), back pain (6%)

<1% (Limited to important or life-threatening): ALT increased, angina, atrial fibrillation, blood pressure increased, cerebral aneurysm, chest pain, chest tightness, CHF, cholecystitis, cholelithiasis, colitis, COPD, dehydration, delirium, disorientation, DVT, dyspnea, eosinophilic pneumonia, euphoria, GI hemorrhage, hallucinations, hypercholesterolemia, hypersensitivity reaction (includes angioedema and urticaria), hypertension, influenza, ischemic stroke, leukocytosis, lymphadenopathy, MI, narcotic withdrawal, palpitation, paralytic ileus, paranoia, PE, perirectal abscess, pneumonia, pyrexia, rigors, seizure, suicide attempts, tachycardia, thrombocytopenia, tooth abscess, UTI

Drug Interactions

There are no known significant interactions.

Stability

Injection: Store unopened kit at 2°C to 8°C (36°F to 46°F). Kit may be kept at room temperature of ≤25°C (77°F) for ≤7 days prior to use; do not freeze.

Tablet: Store at 20°C to 25°C (68°F to 77°F).

Mechanism of Action Naltrexone (a pure opioid antagonist) is a cyclopropyl derivative of oxymorphone similar in structure to naloxone and nalorphine (a morphine derivative); it acts as a competitive antagonist at opioid receptor sites, showing the highest affinity for mu receptors.

Pharmacodynamics/Kinetics

Duration: Oral: 50 mg: 24 hours; 100 mg: 48 hours; 150 mg: 72 hours; I.M.: 4 weeks

Absorption: Oral: Almost complete

Distribution: V_d: 19 L/kg; widely throughout the body but considerable interindividual variation exists

Protein binding: 21%

Metabolism: Noncytochrome-mediated dehydrogenase conversion to 6-beta-naltrexol and related minor metabolites; Oral: Extensive first-pass effect

Half-life elimination: Oral: 4 hours; 6-beta-naltrexol: 13 hours; I.M.: naltrexone and 6-beta-naltrexol: 5-10 days

Time to peak, serum: Oral: ~60 minutes; I.M.: Biphasic: 2 hours (first peak), 2-3 days (second peak)

Excretion: Primarily urine (as metabolites and unchanged drug)

Dosage Adults: Do not give until patient is opioid-free for 7-10 days as determined by urinalysis

Oral: Alcohol dependence, opioid antidote: 25 mg; if no withdrawal signs within 1 hour give another 25 mg; maintenance regimen is flexible, variable and individualized (50 mg/day to 100-150 mg 3 times/week for 12 weeks); up to 800 mg/day has been tolerated in a small number of healthy adults without an adverse effect

I.M.: Alcohol dependence: 380 mg once every 4 weeks

Dosage adjustment in renal impairment: Use caution. No adjustment needed in mild impairment. Not adequately studied in moderate-to-severe renal impairment.

Dosage adjustment in hepatic impairment: Use caution. An increase in naltrexone AUC of approximately five- and 10-fold in patients with compensated or decompensated liver cirrhosis respectively, compared with normal liver function has been reported No adjustment required with mild-to-moderate hepatic impairment. Not adequately studied in severe hepatic impairment.

Administration If there is any question of occult opioid dependence, perform a naloxone challenge test; do not attempt treatment until naloxone challenge is negative.

Oral: To minimize adverse gastrointestinal effects, administer with food or antacids or after meals; advise patient not to self-administer opiates while receiving naltrexone therapy.

I.M.: Vivitrol™: Administer I.M. into the upper outer quadrant of the gluteal area; use provided 1.5 inch 20-gauge needle for administration. Avoid inadvertent injection into a blood vessel; do not administer I.V., SubQ, or into fatty tissue (the risk of serious injection site reaction is increased if given SubQ or into fatty tissue. Injection should alternate between the two buttocks. Do not substitute any components of the dose-pack.

Monitoring Parameters For narcotic withdrawal; liver function tests; injection site reactions

Test Interactions May cause cross-reactivity with some opioid immunoassay methods.

Dosage Forms Excipient information presented when available (limited, particularly for generics); consult specific product labeling.

Injection, microspheres for suspension, extended release:

Vivitrol™: 380 mg [contains polylactide-co-glycolide; packaged with diluent, syringe, needles, and safety device]

Tablet, as hydrochloride: 50 mg

Depade®: 25 mg, 50 mg, 100 mg

ReVia®: 50 mg

◆ **Naltrexone Hydrochloride** *see* Naltrexone *on page 1099*

◆ **Namenda™** *see* Memantine *on page 983*

Nandrolone (NAN droe lone)

Canadian Brand Names Deca-Durabolin®; Durabolin®

Mexican Brand Names Deca-Durabolin

Index Terms Nandrolone Decanoate; Nandrolone Phenpropionate

Pharmacologic Category Androgen

Use Control of metastatic breast cancer; management of anemia of renal insufficiency

Effect on Mental Status May cause insomnia

Effect on Psychiatric Treatment None reported

Restrictions C-III

Dosage Summary

I.M.:

Decanoate:

Children <2 years: Dosage not established

Children 2-13 years: 25-50 mg every 3-4 weeks

Adults: Female: 50-100 mg/week; Male: 100-200 mg/week

Phenpropionate:

Children: Dosage not established

Adults: 50-100 mg/week

Dosage Forms Excipient information presented when available (limited, particularly for generics); consult specific product labeling.

Injection, solution, as decanoate [in sesame oil]: 100 mg/mL (2 mL); 200 mg/mL (1 mL) [contains benzyl alcohol] [DSC]

◆ **Nandrolone Decanoate** *see* Nandrolone *on page 1101*

◆ **Nandrolone Phenpropionate** *see* Nandrolone *on page 1101*

Naphazoline (naf AZ oh leen)

U.S. Brand Names AK-Con™; Albalon® [DSC]; Clear eyes® for Dry Eyes and ACR Relief [OTC]; Clear eyes® for Dry Eyes and Redness Relief [OTC]; Clear eyes® Redness Relief [OTC]; Clear eyes® Seasonal Relief [OTC]; Naphcon® [OTC]; Privine® [OTC]

Canadian Brand Names Naphcon Forte®; Vasocon®

Mexican Brand Names Afazol Grin; Alphadinal; Celunaf; Gotinal

Index Terms Naphazoline Hydrochloride

Pharmacologic Category Alpha$_1$ Agonist; Imidazoline Derivative; Ophthalmic Agent, Vasoconstrictor

Use Topical ocular vasoconstrictor; temporary relief of nasal congestion associated with the common cold, upper respiratory allergies or sinusitis; relief of redness of the eye due to minor irritation

Effect on Mental Status May cause nervousness or dizziness

Effect on Psychiatric Treatment TCAs and MAO inhibitors may potentiate the pressor response of decongestants; monitor for changes in response

Dosage Summary

Nasal:

Children <12 years: Dosage not established

Children ≥12 years: Instill 1-2 drops or sprays of 0.05% every 6 hours if needed (maximum duration: 3 days)

Adults: Instill 1-2 drops or sprays of 0.05% every 6 hours if needed (maximum duration: 3 days)

Ophthalmic:

Children: Dosage not established

Adults:
0.1% (prescription): 1-2 drops into conjuctival sac every 3-4 hours as needed
0.012% or 0.025% (OTC): 1-2 drops into affected eye(s) up to 4 times a day (maximum duration: 3 days)

Dosage Forms Excipient information presented when available (limited, particularly for generics); consult specific product labeling.
Solution, intranasal, as hydrochloride [drops]:
Privine®: 0.05% (25 mL)
Solution, intranasal, as hydrochloride [spray]:
Privine®: 0.05% (20 mL)
Solution, ophthalmic, as hydrochloride:
AK-Con™, Albalon® [DSC]: 0.1% (15 mL) [contains benzalkonium chloride]
Clear eyes® for Dry Eyes and ACR Relief: 0.025% (15 mL) [contains hypromellose, and zinc sulfate]
Clear eyes® for Dry Eyes and Redness Relief: 0.012% (15 mL) [contains hypromellose, glycerin and benzalkonium chloride]
Clear eyes® Redness Relief: 0.012% (6 mL, 15 mL, 30 mL) [contains glycerin and benzalkonium chloride]
Clear eyes® Seasonal Relief: 0.012% (15 mL, 30 mL) [contains glycerin, zinc sulfate and benzalkonium chloride]
Naphcon®: 0.012% (15 mL) [contains benzalkonium chloride]

Naphazoline and Pheniramine (naf AZ oh leen & fen NIR a meen)

Medication Safety Issues
Sound-alike/look-alike issues:
Visine® may be confused with Visken®

U.S. Brand Names Naphcon-A® [OTC]; Opcon-A® [OTC]; Visine-A® [OTC]

Canadian Brand Names Naphcon-A®; Visine® Advanced Allergy

Index Terms Pheniramine and Naphazoline

Pharmacologic Category Histamine H_1 Antagonist; Histamine H_1 Antagonist, First Generation; Ophthalmic Agent, Vasoconstrictor

Use Treatment of ocular congestion, irritation, and itching

Effect on Mental Status May cause nervousness or dizziness

Effect on Psychiatric Treatment TCAs and MAO inhibitors may potentiate the pressor response of decongestants; monitor for changes in response

Dosage Summary
Ophthalmic:
Children <6 years: Dosage not established
Children ≥6 years: 1-2 drops up to 4 times/day
Adults: 1-2 drops up to 4 times/day

Dosage Forms Excipient information presented when available (limited, particularly for generics); consult specific product labeling.
Solution, ophthalmic:
Naphcon-A®: Naphazoline hydrochloride 0.025% and pheniramine maleate 0.3% (5 mL) [contains benzalkonium chloride; 2 bottles/box], (15 mL) [contains benzalkonium chloride]
Opcon-A®: Naphazoline hydrochloride 0.027% and pheniramine maleate 0.3% (15 mL) [contains benzalkonium chloride]
Visine-A®: Naphazoline hydrochloride 0.025% and pheniramine maleate 0.3% (15 mL) [contains benzalkonium chloride]

- ◆ **Naphazoline Hydrochloride** *see* Naphazoline *on page 1101*
- ◆ **Naphcon® [OTC]** *see* Naphazoline *on page 1101*
- ◆ **Naphcon-A® [OTC]** *see* Naphazoline and Pheniramine *on page 1102*
- ◆ **NapraPAC™** *see* Lansoprazole and Naproxen *on page 897*
- ◆ **Naprelan®** *see* Naproxen *on page 1102*
- ◆ **Naprosyn®** *see* Naproxen *on page 1102*

Naproxen (na PROKS en)

Medication Safety Issues
Sound-alike/look-alike issues:
Naproxen may be confused with Natacyn®, Nebcin®
Aleve® may be confused with Alesse®
Anaprox® may be confused with Anaspaz®, Avapro®
Naprelan® may be confused with Naprosyn®
Naprosyn® may be confused with Naprelan®, Natacyn®, Nebcin®

International issues:

Flogen® [Mexico] may be confused with Flovent® which is a brand name for fluticasone in the U.S.

Flogen® [Mexico] may be confused with Floxin® which is a brand name for ofloxacin in the U.S.

Related Information

Nonsteroidal Anti-Inflammatory Agents *on page 1792*

U.S. Brand Names Aleve® [OTC]; Anaprox®; Anaprox® DS; EC-Naprosyn®; Mediproxen [OTC]; Midol® Extended Relief; Naprelan®; Naprosyn®; Pamprin® Maximum Strength All Day Relief [OTC]

Canadian Brand Names Anaprox®; Anaprox® DS; Apo-Napro-Na DS®; Apo-Napro-Na®; Apo-Naproxen EC®; Apo-Naproxen SR®; Apo-Naproxen®; Gen-Naproxen EC; Naprosyn®; Naxen®; Naxen® EC; Novo-Naproc EC; Novo-Naprox; Novo-Naprox Sodium; Novo-Naprox Sodium DS; Novo-Naprox SR; Nu-Naprox; PMS-Naproxen EC; Riva-Naproxen; Sab-Naproxen

Mexican Brand Names Naprodil; Naxen; Novaxen

Index Terms Naproxen Sodium

Pharmacologic Category Nonsteroidal Anti-inflammatory Drug (NSAID), Oral

Generic Available Yes

Use Management of ankylosing spondylitis, osteoarthritis, and rheumatoid disorders (including juvenile rheumatoid arthritis); acute gout; mild-to-moderate pain; tendonitis, bursitis; dysmenorrhea; fever

Effect on Mental Status Dizziness is common; may cause nervousness; may rarely cause drowsiness, confusion, insomnia, depression, or hallucinations

Effect on Psychiatric Treatment May rarely cause agranulocytosis; use caution with clozapine and carbamazepine; may decrease lithium clearance resulting in an increase in serum lithium levels and potential lithium toxicity; monitor serum lithium levels

Restrictions An FDA-approved medication guide must be distributed when dispensing an oral outpatient prescription (new or refill) where this medication is to be used without direct supervision of a healthcare provider. Medication guides are available at http://www.fda.gov/cder/Offices/ODS/medication_guides.htm.

Pregnancy Risk Factor C/D (3rd trimester)

Lactation Enters breast milk/not recommended (AAP rates "compatible")

Contraindications Hypersensitivity to naproxen, aspirin, other NSAIDs, or any component of the formulation; perioperative pain in the setting of coronary artery bypass graft (CABG) surgery

Warnings/Precautions **[U.S. Boxed Warning]: NSAIDs are associated with an increased risk of adverse cardiovascular thrombotic events, including MI, stroke, and new onset or worsening of pre-existing hypertension.** Risk may be increased with duration of use or pre-existing cardiovascular risk factors or disease. Carefully evaluate individual cardiovascular risk profiles prior to prescribing. Use caution with fluid retention, heart failure, or hypertension. Use the lowest effective dose for the shortest duration of time, consistent with individual patient goals, to reduce risk of cardiovascular or GI adverse events. Alternate therapies should be considered for patients at high risk. Concurrent administration of ibuprofen, and potentially other nonselective NSAIDs, may interfere with aspirin's cardioprotective effect. **[U.S. Boxed Warning]: Use is contraindicated for treatment of perioperative pain in the setting of coronary artery bypass graft (CABG) surgery.** Risk of MI and stroke may be increased with use following CABG surgery.

[U.S. Boxed Warning]: NSAIDs may increase risk of gastrointestinal irritation, inflammation, ulceration, bleeding, and perforation. These events may occur at any time during therapy and without warning. Use caution with a history of GI disease (bleeding or ulcers), concurrent therapy with aspirin, anticoagulants and/or corticosteroids, smoking, use of alcohol, the elderly or debilitated patients.

May increase the risk of aseptic meningitis, especially in patients with systemic lupus erythematosus (SLE) and mixed connective tissue disorders. Platelet adhesion and aggregation may be decreased; may prolong bleeding time; patients with coagulation disorders or who are receiving anticoagulants should be monitored closely. Anemia may occur; patients on long-term NSAID therapy should be monitored for anemia. NSAID use may compromise existing renal function; dose-dependent decreases in prostaglandin synthesis may result from NSAID use, reducing renal blood flow which may cause renal decompensation. Patients with impaired renal function, dehydration, heart failure, liver dysfunction, those taking diuretics, and ACE inhibitors, and the elderly are at greater risk of renal toxicity. Rehydrate patient before starting therapy; monitor renal function closely. Not recommended for use in patients with advanced renal disease. Long-term NSAID use may result in renal papillary necrosis.

NSAIDs may cause serious skin adverse events including exfoliative dermatitis, Stevens-Johnson Syndrome (SJS) and toxic epidermal necrolysis (TEN); discontinue use at first sign of skin rash or hypersensitivity. Anaphylactoid reactions may occur, even without prior exposure; patients with "aspirin triad" (bronchial asthma, aspirin intolerance, rhinitis) may be at increased risk. Do not use in patients who experience bronchospasm, asthma, rhinitis, or urticaria with NSAID or aspirin therapy. Use caution in other forms of asthma.

Use with caution in patients with decreased hepatic function. Closely monitor patients with any abnormal LFT. Severe hepatic reactions (eg, fulminant hepatitis, liver failure) have occurred with NSAID use, rarely; discontinue if signs or symptoms of liver disease develop, or if systemic manifestations occur.

The elderly are at increased risk for adverse effects (especially peptic ulceration, CNS effects, renal toxicity) from NSAIDs even at low doses.

Withhold for at least 4-6 half-lives prior to surgical or dental procedures. Safety and efficacy have not been established in children <2 years of age.

OTC labeling: Prior to self-medication, patients should contact healthcare provider if they have had recurring stomach pain or upset, ulcers, bleeding problems, high blood pressure, heart or kidney disease, other serious medical problems, are currently taking a diuretic, or are ≥60 years of age. Recommended dosages should not be exceeded, due to an increased risk of GI bleeding. Consuming ≥3 alcoholic beverages/day or taking longer than recommended may increase the risk of GI bleeding. Not for self-medication (OTC use) in children <12 years of age.

Adverse Reactions

1% to 10%:

Cardiovascular: Edema (3% to 9%), palpitations (<3%)

Central nervous system: Dizziness (3% to 9%), drowsiness (3% to 9%), headache (3% to 9%), lightheadedness (<3%), vertigo (<3%)

Dermatologic: Pruritus (3% to 9%), skin eruption (3% to 9%), ecchymosis (3% to 9%), purpura (<3%), rash

Endocrine & metabolic: Fluid retention (3% to 9%)

Gastrointestinal: Abdominal pain (3% to 9%), constipation (3% to 9%), nausea (3% to 9%), heartburn (3% to 9%), diarrhea (<3%), dyspepsia (<3%), stomatitis (<3%), flatulence, gross bleeding/perforation, indigestion, ulcers, vomiting

Genitourinary: Abnormal renal function

Hematologic: Hemolysis (3% to 9%), ecchymosis (3% to 9%), anemia, bleeding time increased

Hepatic: LFTs increased

Ocular: Visual disturbances (<3%)

Otic: Tinnitus (3% to 9%), hearing disturbances (<3%)

Respiratory: Dyspnea (3% to 9%)

Miscellaneous: Diaphoresis (<3%), thirst (<3%)

<1% (Limited to important or life-threatening): Agranulocytosis, alopecia, anaphylactic/anaphylactoid reaction, angioneurotic edema, arrhythmia, aseptic meningitis, asthma, blurred vision, cognitive dysfunction, colitis, coma, confusion, CHF, conjunctivitis, cystitis, depression, dream abnormalities, dysuria, eosinophilia, eosinophilic pneumonitis, erythema multiforme, exfoliative dermatitis, glossitis, granulocytopenia, hallucinations, hematemesis, hepatitis, hyper-/hypoglycemia, hyper-/hypotension, infection, interstitial nephritis, melena, jaundice, leukopenia, liver failure, lymphadenopathy, menstrual disorders, malaise, MI, muscle weakness, myalgia, oliguria, pancreatitis, pancytopenia, paresthesia, photosensitivity, pneumonia, polyuria, proteinuria, pyrexia, rectal bleeding, renal failure, renal papillary necrosis, respiratory depression, sepsis, Stevens-Johnson syndrome, tachycardia, seizure, syncope, thrombocytopenia, toxic epidermal necrolysis ulcerative stomatitis, vasculitis

Metabolism/Transport Effects Substrate (minor) of CYP1A2, 2C9

Drug Interactions

ACE Inhibitors: Nonsteroidal Anti-Inflammatory Agents may diminish the antihypertensive effect of ACE Inhibitors. *Risk C: Monitor therapy*

Aminoglycosides: Nonsteroidal Anti-Inflammatory Agents may decrease the excretion of Aminoglycosides. Data only in premature infants. *Risk C: Monitor therapy*

Angiotensin II Receptor Blockers: Nonsteroidal Anti-Inflammatory Agents may diminish the therapeutic effect of Angiotensin II Receptor Blockers. The combination of these two agents may also significantly decrease glomerular filtration and renal function. *Risk C: Monitor therapy*

Anticoagulants: Nonsteroidal Anti-Inflammatory Agents may enhance the anticoagulant effect of Anticoagulants. *Risk C: Monitor therapy*

Antidepressants (Serotonin/Norepinephrine Reuptake Inhibitor): May enhance the antiplatelet effect of NSAID (Nonselective). *Risk C: Monitor therapy*

Antidepressants (Tricyclic, Tertiary Amine): May enhance the antiplatelet effect of NSAID (Nonselective). *Risk C: Monitor therapy*

Antiplatelet Agents: Nonsteroidal Anti-Inflammatory Agents may enhance the adverse/toxic effect of Antiplatelet Agents. An increased risk of bleeding may occur. *Risk C: Monitor therapy*

Beta-Blockers: Nonsteroidal Anti-Inflammatory Agents may diminish the antihypertensive effect of Beta-Blockers. **Exceptions:** Levobunolol; Metipranolol. *Risk C: Monitor therapy*

Bile Acid Sequestrants: May decrease the absorption of Nonsteroidal Anti-Inflammatory Agents. *Risk D: Consider therapy modification*

Bisphosphonate Derivatives: Nonsteroidal Anti-Inflammatory Agents may enhance the adverse/toxic effect of Bisphosphonate Derivatives. Both an increased risk of gastrointestinal ulceration and an increased risk of nephrotoxicity are of concern. *Risk C: Monitor therapy*

Corticosteroids (Systemic): May enhance the adverse/toxic effect of NSAID (Nonselective). *Risk C: Monitor therapy*

CycloSPORINE: Nonsteroidal Anti-Inflammatory Agents may enhance the nephrotoxic effect of CycloSPORINE. Nonsteroidal Anti-Inflammatory Agents may increase the serum concentration of CycloSPORINE. *Risk D: Consider therapy modification*

Desmopressin: Nonsteroidal Anti-Inflammatory Agents may enhance the adverse/toxic effect of Desmopressin. *Risk C: Monitor therapy*

Eplerenone: Nonsteroidal Anti-Inflammatory Agents may diminish the antihypertensive effect of Eplerenone. *Risk C: Monitor therapy*

Herbs (Anticoagulant/Antiplatelet Properties) (eg, Alfalfa, Anise, Bilberry): May enhance the adverse/toxic effect of Nonsteroidal Anti-Inflammatory Agents. Bleeding may occur. *Risk D: Consider therapy modification*

HydrALAZINE: Nonsteroidal Anti-Inflammatory Agents may diminish the antihypertensive effect of HydrALAZINE. *Risk C: Monitor therapy*

Ketorolac: May enhance the adverse/toxic effect of Nonsteroidal Anti-Inflammatory Agents. *Risk X: Avoid combination*

Lithium: Nonsteroidal Anti-Inflammatory Agents may increase the serum concentration of Lithium. *Risk D: Consider therapy modification*

Loop Diuretics: Nonsteroidal Anti-Inflammatory Agents may diminish the diuretic effect of Loop Diuretics. *Risk C: Monitor therapy*

Methotrexate: Nonsteroidal Anti-Inflammatory Agents may decrease the excretion of Methotrexate. *Risk D: Consider therapy modification*

Nonsteroidal Anti-Inflammatory Agents: May enhance the adverse/toxic effect of other Nonsteroidal Anti-Inflammatory Agents. *Risk C: Monitor therapy*

Pemetrexed: NSAID (Nonselective) may decrease the excretion of Pemetrexed. *Risk D: Consider therapy modification*

Probenecid: May increase the serum concentration of Nonsteroidal Anti-Inflammatory Agents. *Risk C: Monitor therapy*

Quinolone Antibiotics: Nonsteroidal Anti-Inflammatory Agents may enhance the neuroexcitatory and/or seizure-potentiating effect of Quinolone Antibiotics. *Risk C: Monitor therapy*

Salicylates: NSAID (Nonselective) may enhance the antiplatelet effect of Salicylates. NSAID (Nonselective) may diminish the cardioprotective effect of Salicylates. Salicylates may decrease the serum concentration of NSAID (Nonselective). **Exceptions:** Choline Magnesium Trisalicylate. *Risk D: Consider therapy modification*

Selective Serotonin Reuptake Inhibitors: May enhance the antiplatelet effect of NSAID (Nonselective). *Risk D: Consider therapy modification*

Thiazide Diuretics: Nonsteroidal Anti-Inflammatory Agents may diminish the therapeutic effect of Thiazide Diuretics. *Risk C: Monitor therapy*

Thrombolytic Agents: Nonsteroidal Anti-Inflammatory Agents may enhance the adverse/toxic effect of Thrombolytic Agents. An increased risk of bleeding may occur. *Risk C: Monitor therapy*

Treprostinil: May enhance the adverse/toxic effect of Nonsteroidal Anti-Inflammatory Agents. Bleeding may occur. *Risk C: Monitor therapy*

Vancomycin: Nonsteroidal Anti-Inflammatory Agents may decrease the excretion of Vancomycin. *Risk C: Monitor therapy*

Vitamin K Antagonists (eg, warfarin): NSAID (Nonselective) may enhance the anticoagulant effect of Vitamin K Antagonists. *Risk D: Consider therapy modification*

Ethanol/Nutrition/Herb Interactions

Ethanol: Avoid ethanol (may enhance gastric mucosal irritation).

Food: Naproxen absorption rate/levels may be decreased if taken with food.

Herb/Nutraceutical: Avoid alfalfa, anise, bilberry, bladderwrack, bromelain, cat's claw, celery, chamomile, coleus, cordyceps, dong quai, evening primrose, fenugreek, feverfew, garlic, ginger, ginkgo biloba, ginseng (American, Panax, Siberian), grapeseed, green tea, guggul, horse chestnut seed, horseradish, licorice, prickly ash, red clover, reishi, SAMe (S-adenosylmethionine), sweet clover, turmeric, white willow (all have additional antiplatelet activity).

Stability Store oral suspension and tablet at 15°C to 30°C (59°F to 86°F).

Mechanism of Action Reversibly inhibits cyclooxygenase-1 and 2 (COX-1 and 2) enzymes, which result in decreased formation of prostaglandin precursors; has antipyretic, analgesic, and anti-inflammatory properties

Pharmacodynamics/Kinetics

Onset of action: Analgesic: 1 hour; Anti-inflammatory:~2 weeks

Peak effect: Anti-inflammatory: 2-4 weeks

Duration: Analgesic: ≤7 hours; Anti-inflammatory: ≤12 hours

Absorption: Almost 100%

Protein binding: >99%; increased free fraction in elderly

Half-life elimination: Normal renal function: 12-17 hours; End-stage renal disease: No change

Time to peak, serum: 1-4 hours

Excretion: Urine (95%)

Dosage Note: Dosage expressed as naproxen base; 200 mg naproxen base is equivalent to 220 mg naproxen sodium.

Oral:

Children >2 years: Juvenile arthritis: 10 mg/kg/day in 2 divided doses

Adults:

Gout, acute: Initial: 750 mg, followed by 250 mg every 8 hours until attack subsides. **Note:** EC-Naprosyn® is not recommended.

Migraine, acute (unlabeled use): Initial: 500-750 mg.; an additional 250-500 mg may be given if needed (maximum: 1250 mg in 24 hours). **Note:** EC-Naprosyn® is not recommended.

Pain (mild-to-moderate), dysmenorrhea, acute tendonitis, bursitis: Initial: 500 mg, then 250 mg every 6-8 hours; maximum: 1250 mg/day naproxen base

Rheumatoid arthritis, osteoarthritis, and ankylosing spondylitis: 500-1000 mg/day in 2 divided doses; may increase to 1.5 g/day of naproxen base for limited time period

OTC labeling: Pain/fever:

Children ≥12 years and Adults ≤65 years: 200 mg naproxen base every 8-12 hours; if needed, may take 400 mg naproxen base for the initial dose; maximum: 600 mg naproxen base/24 hours

Adults >65 years: 200 mg naproxen base every 12 hours

Dosing adjustment in renal impairment: Cl_{cr} <30 mL/minute: use is not recommended

Dietary Considerations Drug may cause GI upset, bleeding, ulceration, perforation; take with food or milk to minimize GI upset.

Administration Administer with food, milk, or antacids to decrease GI adverse effects

Suspension: Shake suspension well before administration.

Tablet, extended release: Swallow tablet whole; do not break, crush, or chew.

Monitoring Parameters Occult blood loss, periodic liver function test, CBC, BUN, serum creatinine; urine output

Test Interactions Naproxen may interfere with 5-HIAA urinary assays; due to an interaction with m-dinitrobenzene, naproxen should be discontinued 72 hours before adrenal function testing if the Porter-Silber test is used.

Dosage Forms Excipient information presented when available (limited, particularly for generics); consult specific product labeling.

Caplet, as sodium: 220 mg [equivalent to naproxen 200 mg and sodium 20 mg]

Aleve®, Midol® Extended Relief, Pamprin® Maximum Strength All Day Relief: 220 mg [equivalent to naproxen 200 mg and sodium 20 mg]

Capsule, liquid gel, as sodium:

Aleve®: 220 mg [equivalent to naproxen 200 mg and sodium 20 mg]

Gelcap, as sodium:

Aleve®: 220 mg [equivalent to naproxen 200 mg and sodium 20 mg]

Suspension, oral: 125 mg/5 mL (500 mL)

Naprosyn®: 125 mg/5 mL (480 mL) [contains sodium 39 mg (1.5 mEq/5 mL); orange-pineapple flavor]

Tablet: 250 mg, 375 mg, 500 mg

Naprosyn®: 250 mg, 375 mg, 500 mg

Tablet, as sodium: 220 mg [equivalent to naproxen 200 mg and sodium 20 mg]; 275 mg [equivalent to naproxen 250 mg and sodium 25 mg]; 550 mg [equivalent to naproxen 500 mg and sodium 50 mg]
Aleve®: 220 mg [equivalent to naproxen 200 mg and sodium 20 mg]
Anaprox®: 275 mg [equivalent to naproxen 250 mg and sodium 25 mg]
Anaprox® DS: 550 mg [equivalent to naproxen 500 mg and sodium 50 mg]
Mediproxen: 220 mg [equivalent to naproxen 200 mg and sodium 20 mg]
Tablet, controlled release, as sodium: 550 mg [equivalent to naproxen 500 mg and sodium 50 mg]
Naprelan®: 412.5 mg [equivalent to naproxen 375 mg and sodium 37.5 mg]; 550 mg [equivalent to naproxen 500 mg and sodium 50 mg]
Tablet, delayed release, enteric coated: 375 mg, 500 mg
EC-Naprosyn®: 375 mg, 500 mg
Tablet, extended release, as sodium: 550 mg [equivalent to naproxen 500 mg and sodium 50 mg]

◆ **Naproxen and Lansoprazole** *see* Lansoprazole and Naproxen *on page 897*

Naproxen and Pseudoephedrine

(na PROKS en & soo doe e FED rin)

U.S. Brand Names Aleve® Cold & Sinus [OTC] [DSC]; Aleve® Sinus & Headache [OTC] [DSC]; Aleve®-D Sinus & Cold [OTC]; Aleve®-D Sinus & Headache [OTC]

Index Terms Naproxen Sodium and Pseudoephedrine; Pseudoephedrine and Naproxen

Pharmacologic Category Decongestant/Analgesic

Use Temporary relief of cold, sinus, and flu symptoms (including nasal congestion, sinus congestion/pressure, headache, minor body aches and pains, and fever)

Effect on Mental Status May cause dizziness, drowsiness, confusion, insomnia, depression, or hallucinations

Effect on Psychiatric Treatment Contraindicated with or within 2 weeks of discontinuing an MAO inhibitor. May decrease lithium clearance resulting in an increase in serum lithium levels and potential lithium toxicity; monitor serum lithium levels.

Dosage Summary

Oral:

Children <12 years: Dosage not established
Children ≥12 years: One caplet every 12 hours (maximum: 2 caplets/day)
Adults: One caplet every 12 hours (maximum: 2 caplets/day)

Dosage Forms Excipient information presented when available (limited, particularly for generics); consult specific product labeling. [DSC] = Discontinued product

Caplet, extended release:
Aleve® Cold & Sinus [DSC], Aleve® Sinus & Headache [DSC], Aleve®-D Sinus & Cold, Aleve®-D Sinus & Headache: Naproxen sodium 220 mg [equivalent to naproxen 200 mg and sodium 20 mg] and pseudoephedrine hydrochloride 120 mg

◆ **Naproxen and Sumatriptan** *see* Sumatriptan and Naproxen *on page 1530*

◆ **Naproxen Sodium** *see* Naproxen *on page 1102*

◆ **Naproxen Sodium and Pseudoephedrine** *see* Naproxen and Pseudoephedrine *on page 1107*

◆ **Naproxen Sodium and Sumatriptan** *see* Sumatriptan and Naproxen *on page 1530*

◆ **Naproxen Sodium and Sumatriptan Succinate** *see* Sumatriptan and Naproxen *on page 1530*

Naratriptan (NAR a trip tan)

Medication Safety Issues

Sound-alike/look-alike issues:
Amerge® may be confused with Altace®, Amaryl®

Related Information

Antimigraine Drugs: 5-HT_1 Receptor Agonists *on page 1766*

U.S. Brand Names Amerge®

Canadian Brand Names Amerge®

Mexican Brand Names Naramig

Index Terms Naratriptan Hydrochloride

Pharmacologic Category Antimigraine Agent; Serotonin 5-$HT_{1B, 1D}$ Receptor Agonist

Generic Available No

Use Treatment of acute migraine headache with or without aura

Effect on Mental Status May cause drowsiness, dizziness, or fatigue; may rarely cause panic reactions or hallucinations

Effect on Psychiatric Treatment SSRIs may cause hyper-reflexia, weakness, or lack of coordination when used with naratriptan; these combinations should be avoided

Pregnancy Risk Factor C

Pregnancy Considerations There are no adequate and well-controlled studies using naratriptan in pregnant women. Use only if potential benefit to the mother outweighs the potential risk to the fetus. A pregnancy registry has been established to monitor outcomes of women exposed to naratriptan during pregnancy (800-336-2176). In animal studies, administration was associated with embryolethality, fetal abnormalities, and pup mortality and growth retardation. Tremors were observed in the offspring of female rats when exposed to naratriptan late in gestation.

Lactation Excretion in breast milk unknown/use caution

Contraindications Hypersensitivity to naratriptan or any component of the formulation; cerebrovascular, peripheral vascular disease (ischemic bowel disease), ischemic heart disease (angina pectoris, history of myocardial infarction, or proven silent ischemia); or in patients with symptoms consistent with ischemic heart disease, coronary artery vasospasm, or Prinzmetal's angina; uncontrolled hypertension or patients who have received within 24 hours another 5-HT agonist (sumatriptan, zolmitriptan) or ergotamine-containing product; patients with known risk factors associated with coronary artery disease; patients with severe hepatic or renal disease (Cl_{cr} <15 mL/minute); do not administer naratriptan to patients with hemiplegic or basilar migraine

Warnings/Precautions Use only if there is a clear diagnosis of migraine. Do not give to patients with risk factors for CAD until a cardiovascular evaluation has been performed; if evaluation is satisfactory, the healthcare provider should administer the first dose and cardiovascular status should be periodically re-evaluated. Cardiac events (coronary artery vasospasm, transient ischemia, myocardial infarction, ventricular tachycardia/fibrillation, cardiac arrest, and death), cerebral/subarachnoid hemorrhage, stroke, peripheral vascular ischemia, and colonic ischemia have been reported with 5-HT_1 agonist administration. Significant elevation in blood pressure, including hypertensive crisis, has also been reported on rare occasions in patients with and without a history of hypertension. If the patient does not respond to the first dose, re-evaluate the diagnosis of migraine before trying a second dose. Safety and efficacy have not been established in children <18 years of age.

Adverse Reactions

1% to 10%:

Central nervous system: Dizziness, drowsiness, malaise/fatigue

Gastrointestinal: Nausea, vomiting

Neuromuscular & skeletal: Paresthesia

Miscellaneous: Pain or pressure in throat or neck

<1% (Limited to important or life-threatening): Allergic reaction, atrial fibrillation, atrial flutter, coronary artery vasospasm, hallucinations, MI, PR prolongation, premature ventricular contractions, QT_c prolongation, seizure, ventricular fibrillation, ventricular tachycardia

Drug Interactions

Ergot Derivatives: May enhance the vasoconstricting effect of Serotonin 5-HT1D Receptor Agonists. Serotonin 5-HT1D Receptor Agonists may enhance the vasoconstricting effect of Ergot Derivatives. *Risk X: Avoid combination*

Serotonin Modulators: May enhance the adverse/toxic effect of other Serotonin Modulators. The development of serotonin syndrome may occur. *Risk D: Consider therapy modification*

Sibutramine: May enhance the serotonergic effect of Serotonin Modulators. This may cause serotonin syndrome. *Risk X: Avoid combination*

Mechanism of Action The therapeutic effect for migraine is due to serotonin agonist activity

Pharmacodynamics/Kinetics

Onset of action: 30 minutes

Absorption: Well absorbed

Protein binding, plasma: 28% to 31%

Metabolism: Hepatic via CYP

Bioavailability: 70%

Time to peak: 2-3 hours

Excretion: Urine

Dosage

Adults: Oral: 1-2.5 mg at the onset of headache; it is recommended to use the lowest possible dose to minimize adverse effects. If headache returns or does not fully resolve, the dose may be repeated after 4 hours; do not exceed 5 mg in 24 hours.

Elderly: Not recommended for use in the elderly

Dosing in renal impairment:

Cl_{cr} 18-39 mL/minute: Initial: 1 mg; do not exceed 2.5 mg in 24 hours

Cl_{cr} <15 mL/minute: Do not use

Dosing in hepatic impairment: Contraindicated in patients with severe liver failure; maximum dose: 2.5 mg in 24 hours for patients with mild or moderate liver failure; recommended starting dose: 1 mg

Administration Do **not** crush or chew tablet; swallow whole with water.

Dosage Forms Excipient information presented when available (limited, particularly for generics); consult specific product labeling.

Tablet: 1 mg, 2.5 mg

- **Naratriptan Hydrochloride** *see* Naratriptan *on page 1107*
- **Narcan** *see* Naloxone *on page 1097*
- **Nardil®** *see* Phenelzine *on page 1261*
- **Nasacort® AQ** *see* Triamcinolone *on page 1617*
- **NasalCrom® [OTC]** *see* Cromolyn *on page 402*
- **Nasarel®** *see* Flunisolide *on page 646*
- **Nasatab® LA** *see* Guaifenesin and Pseudoephedrine *on page 744*
- **Nascobal®** *see* Cyanocobalamin *on page 404*
- **Nasex-G** *see* Guaifenesin and Phenylephrine *on page 742*
- **Nasofed™** *see* Pseudoephedrine *on page 1367*
- **Nasonex®** *see* Mometasone *on page 1071*
- **Nasop12™** *see* Phenylephrine *on page 1273*

Natalizumab (na ta LIZ u mab)

U.S. Brand Names Tysabri®

Canadian Brand Names Tysabri®

Index Terms AN100226; Anti-4 Alpha Integrin; IgG4-Kappa Monoclonal Antibody

Pharmacologic Category Gastrointestinal Agent, Miscellaneous; Monoclonal Antibody, Selective Adhesion-Molecule Inhibitor

Generic Available No

Use

U.S. labeling: Monotherapy for the treatment of relapsing forms of multiple sclerosis; treatment of moderately- to severely-active Crohn's disease

Canada labeling: Treatment of relapsing forms of multiple sclerosis

Effect on Mental Status Sedation is common; may cause depression, suicidal ideation has been reported; use caution in patients with a history of depression; monitor for depressive symptoms

Effect on Psychiatric Treatment Concomitant use with psychotropic agents may produce additive effects; monitor

Restrictions Patients must be enrolled in the Tysabri® Outreach Unified Commitment to Health (TOUCH™) Prescribing Program (800-456-2255) to receive natalizumab (MS-TOUCH™ for multiple sclerosis or CD-TOUCH™ for Crohn's disease). Healthcare providers must also register with the program in order to prescribe, dispense or administer natalizumab. Treatment must be reauthorized every 6 months. Natalizumab is available only through infusion centers registered with the TOUCH™ program; infusion center information is available at 1-800-456-2255.

Medication guides are available at http://www.fda.gov/cder/Offices/ODS/MG/natalizumabMG.pdf and should be provided to every patient prior to initiation of therapy.

Pregnancy Risk Factor C

Pregnancy Considerations Adverse events have been observed in animal studies. There are no adequate and well-controlled studies in pregnant women. Use only if clearly needed. Pregnant women exposed to natalizumab should be enrolled in the Tysabri® Pregnancy Exposure Registry (800-456-2255).

Lactation Excretion in breast milk unknown/not recommended

Contraindications Hypersensitivity to natalizumab, murine proteins, or any component of the formulation; current or history of progressive multifocal leukoencephalopathy (PML)

Canada labeling: Additional contraindications (not in U.S. labeling): Immunocompromised patients as a result of immunosuppressant or antineoplastic therapy, or immunodeficiencies (eg, HIV, leukemia, lymphoma)

Warnings/Precautions [U.S. Boxed Warning]: Increased risk of developing fatal or disabling progressive multifocal leukoencephalopathy (PML), an opportunistic infection caused by the JC virus; patients must be routinely monitored for signs of PML with baseline and periodic MRI evaluations; access to and provision of therapy requires registration of patients and healthcare providers; with the TOUCH™ prescribing program; concurrent immunomodulator therapy or immunosuppression may be risk factors for the development of PML, however, PML has also been reported with natalizumab monotherapy. Use may be associated with an increased risk of infections, including opportunistic infections and serious herpes infections (rare, postmarketing reports; concurrent use of antineoplastic, immunosuppressant [including short-course corticosteroids], or immunomodulating agents may increase this risk). In the presence of a serious herpes infection, discontinue therapy until successful resolution of the infection. A brain MRI scan (baseline) should be obtained prior to initiating therapy in MS patients and should be considered in Crohn's patients. Use should be restricted to patients with inadequate response to or intolerant to other therapies for Crohn's disease or multiple sclerosis.

During clinical studies, up to 24% of patients experienced an infusion-related reaction; serious systemic hypersensitivity reactions occurred in ≤1% of patients. Severe reactions, including anaphylaxis, occur rarely. Patients treated with brief initial courses of therapy (≤3 infusions) followed by an extended interruption in therapy (≥3 months) may be at an increased risk for hypersensitivity reactions following reinitiation of therapy. Retreatment is not recommended in patients developing hypersensitivity reactions. Infusion-related reactions may occur more frequently in patients with antibody to natalizumab. Antibody formation (which occurs in about 10% of patients) is associated with a decrease in natalizumab levels and a decrease in the efficacy of natalizumab. The Canadian labeling recommends antibody testing in patients who have received brief initial courses of natalizumab therapy followed by an extended interruption in therapy.

Natalizumab should not be used in combination with immunosuppressants or tumor necrosis factor (TNF) inhibitors in patients with Crohn's disease; aminosalicylates may be used concurrently with natalizumab. For patients who begin treatment while on chronic oral corticosteroids, begin tapering oral steroids when the onset of natalizumab therapeutic benefit is observed; discontinue use if patient cannot be tapered off of oral corticosteroids within 6 months of therapy initiation. If additional concomitant corticosteroids are required and exceed 3 months/year (in addition to initial corticosteroid taper), consider discontinuing therapy.

Hepatotoxicity, including transaminase and bilirubin elevation, has been reported with use; may occur as early as 6 days after the first dose; may recur with treatment rechallenge; discontinue with jaundice or signs/symptoms of hepatic injury. Use caution in patients with a history of depression; closely monitor. Safety and efficacy have not been established in chronic progressive multiple sclerosis, for therapy >2 years, or in children (<18 years of age).

Adverse Reactions

>10%:

Central nervous system: Headache (32% to 38%), fatigue (10% to 27%), depression (≤19%)

Dermatologic: Rash (6% to 12%)

Gastrointestinal: Nausea (≤17%), gastroenteritis (≤11%), abdominal discomfort (≤11%)

Genitourinary: Urinary tract infection (3% to 21%)

Neuromuscular & skeletal: Arthralgia (8% to 19%), extremity pain (16%), back pain (≤12%)

Respiratory: Upper respiratory infection (≤22%), lower respiratory infection (≤17%)

Miscellaneous: Infusion-related reaction (11% to 24%), influenza (≤12%), flu-like syndrome (≤11%)

1% to 10%:

Cardiovascular: Peripheral edema (5% to 6%), chest discomfort (≤5%)

Central nervous system: Vertigo (≤6%), dysesthesia (3%), syncope (≤2%), somnolence (≤2%)
Dermatologic: Dermatitis (≤7%), pruritus (≤4%), urticaria (≤2%), dry skin (≤1%)
Endocrine & metabolic: Menstrual irregularities (≤5%), dysmenorrhea (2% to 6%), amenorrhea (≤2%), ovarian cyst (≤2%)
Gastrointestinal: Diarrhea (10%), dyspepsia (≤5%), abdominal pain (≤4%), constipation (≤4%), flatulence (≤3%), aphthous stomatitis (≤2%), weight changes (≤2%), cholelithiasis (≤1%), gingival infection (1%)
Genitourinary: Vaginitis/vaginal infections (4% to 10%), urinary frequency (≤9%), urinary incontinence (≤4%)
Hematologic: Hematoma (1%)
Hepatic: Transaminase increased (≤5%)
Local: Bleeding at injection site (≤3%)
Neuromuscular & skeletal: Muscle cramp (≤5%), tremor (1% to 3%), rigors (≤3%), joint swelling (≤2%)
Respiratory: Sinusitis (≤8%), cough (≤7%), tonsillitis (≤7%), pharyngolaryngeal pain (≤6%), epistaxis (2%)
Miscellaneous: Antibody formation (9% to 10%), tooth infection (≤9%), herpes infection (≤8%), viral infection (≤7%), hypersensitivity reactions (acute: 2% to 4%; serious acute: ≤1%; delayed: ≤5%), toothache (≤4%), serious infection (2% to 3%), night sweats (≤1%)

<1% (Limited to important or life-threatening): Acne, agitation, anaphylaxis/anaphylactoid reactions, anemia, angina, appendicitis, bilirubin increased, bronchopulmonary aspergillosis, *Burkholderia cepacia*, Crohn's disease exacerbation, cryptosporidial gastroenteritis, cytomegalovirus hepatitis, dizziness, dyspnea, erythema. fever, flushing, hemoglobin decreased (mild, transient), hepatotoxicity, herpes encephalitis, herpes meningitis, hypotension, joint stiffness, lethargy, leukocytosis, nasopharyngitis, opportunistic infections (including progressive multifocal leukoencephalopathy [PML], meningitis, and bronchopulmonary infections), muscle spasms, muscle weakness, onychorrhexis, paresis, petechiae, pharyngitis, *Pneumocystis jiroveci* pneumonia, pneumonia, psychomotor hyperactivity, pulmonary *Mycobacterium avium intracellulare*, suicidal ideation, tachycardia, thrombocytopenia, thrombophlebitis, varicella pneumonia, vasodilatation

Drug Interactions

Echinacea: May diminish the therapeutic effect of Immunosuppressants. *Risk D: Consider therapy modification*

Immunosuppressants: May enhance the adverse/toxic effect of Natalizumab. Specifically, the risk of concurrent infection may be increased. *Risk X: Avoid combination*

Trastuzumab: May enhance the neutropenic effect of Immunosuppressants. *Risk C: Monitor therapy*

Vaccines (Inactivated): Immunosuppressants may diminish the therapeutic effect of Vaccines (Inactivated). *Risk C: Monitor therapy*

Vaccines (Live): Immunosuppressants may enhance the adverse/toxic effect of Vaccines (Live). Vaccinal infections may develop. Immunosuppressants may also decrease therapeutic response to vaccines. *Risk X: Avoid combination*

Stability Store concentrated solution under refrigeration between 2°C to 8°C (36°F to 46°F); do not freeze. Protect from light. Do not shake. Dilute natalizumab 300 mg in NS 100 mL to a final concentration of 2.6 mg/mL. Gently invert to mix; do not shake. Following dilution, may store refrigerated for use within up to 8 hours.

Mechanism of Action Natalizumab is a monoclonal antibody against the alpha-4 subunit of integrin molecules. These molecules are important to adhesion and migration of cells from the vasculature into inflamed tissue. Natalizumab blocks integrin association with vascular receptors, limiting adhesion and transmigration of leukocytes. Efficacy in specific disorders may be related to reduction in specific inflammatory cell populations in target tissues. In multiple sclerosis, efficacy may be related to blockade of T-lymphocyte migration into the central nervous system; treatment results in a decreased frequency of relapse. In Crohn's disease, natalizumab decreases inflammation by binding to alpha-4 integrin, blocking adhesion and migration of leukocytes in the gut.

Pharmacodynamics/Kinetics

Distribution: Crohn's disease: 2.4-8 L; Multiple sclerosis: 3.8-7.6 L

Half-life elimination: Crohn's disease: 3-17 days; Multiple sclerosis: 7-15 days

Dosage I.V.: Adults:

Multiple sclerosis: 300 mg infused over 1 hour every 4 weeks

Crohn's disease: 300 mg infused over 1 hour every 4 weeks; discontinue if therapeutic benefit is not observed within initial 12 weeks of therapy

Concomitant use with corticosteroids: For patients who begin treatment while on chronic oral corticosteroids, begin tapering oral steroids when the onset of natalizumab therapeutic benefit is observed; discontinue use if patient cannot be tapered off of oral corticosteroids within 6 months of therapy initiation. If additional concomitant corticosteroids are required and exceed 3 months/year (in addition to initial corticosteroid taper), consider discontinuing therapy.

Dosage adjustment in renal impairment: Not studied

Dosage adjustment in hepatic impairment: Not studied. Discontinue use with jaundice or signs/symptoms of hepatic injury.

Administration Solution may be warmed to room temperature prior to administration. Diluted solution should be infused over 1 hour; do not administer by I.V. bolus or push. Patients should be closely monitored for signs and symptoms of hypersensitivity during the infusion and for at least 1 hour after the infusion is complete. The infusion should be discontinued if a reaction occurs, and treatment of the reaction should be instituted. Following infusion, flush line with NS.

Monitoring Parameters Monitor for hypersensitivity reactions during, and for 1 hour after, infusion; signs and symptoms of hepatotoxicity (eg, serum transaminases, bilirubin)

Baseline brain MRI scan; if PML is suspected, obtain gadolinium-enhanced brain MRI scan and CSF analysis for JC viral DNA. Evaluate for signs or symptoms of progressive multifocal leukoencephalopathy (focal neurologic deficits, which may present as hemiparesis, visual field deficits, cognitive impairment, aphasia, ataxia, and/or cranial nerve deficits) at 3 and 6 months after first infusion; every 6 months thereafter. **Note:** Transient and reversible leukocytosis (excluding neutrophils) and mildly reduced hemoglobin may occur with treatment and may require ~4 months for return to baseline values after the last dose.

Canadian labeling recommends antibody testing in patients who have received brief initial courses of natalizumab therapy followed by an extended interruption in therapy.

Additional Information

U.S. patients and healthcare providers (eg, pharmacies, physicians) must register with the TOUCH Program (800-456-2255) to ensure the safe and appropriate use of natalizumab. Enrollment in the program insures that participants acknowledge and adhere to the following requirements:

Healthcare providers/prescribers: Ability to diagnose, including management or referral of potential PML complications; educate patients on program enrollment procedures, including risk/benefit of treatment; file appropriate program paperwork with manufacturer; report serious infections to manufacturer and FDA; evaluate patient response to therapy and assess appropriateness of continued treatment.

Patients: Understand medication guide; promptly report worsening symptoms (including hypersensitivity); inform other healthcare providers of their therapy with natalizumab.

Canadian patients are encouraged to enroll in the Canadian Tysabri® Care Program™ (888)-827-2827, a patient registry for those prescribed natalizumab.

Dosage Forms Excipient information presented when available (limited, particularly for generics); consult specific product labeling.

Injection, solution [preservative free]:

Tysabri®: 300 mg/15 mL (15 mL) [contains polysorbate-80]

Nateglinide (na te GLYE nide)

Medication Safety Issues

High alert medication: The Institute for Safe Medication Practices (ISMP) includes this medication among its list of drug classes which have a heightened risk of causing significant patient harm when used in error.

U.S. Brand Names Starlix®

Canadian Brand Names Starlix®

Mexican Brand Names Starlix

Pharmacologic Category Antidiabetic Agent, Meglitinide Derivative

Generic Available No

Use Management of type 2 diabetes mellitus (noninsulin dependent, NIDDM) as monotherapy when hyperglycemia cannot be managed by diet and exercise alone; in combination with metformin or a thiazolidinedione to lower blood glucose in patients whose hyperglycemia cannot be controlled by exercise, diet, or a single agent alone

Effect on Mental Status May cause dizziness

Effect on Psychiatric Treatment May cause weight gain; psychotropics may produce additive effects. Beta-blockers and MAO inhibitors may potentiate the hypoglycemic effects of nateglinide. May cause flu-like symptoms; take this into consideration if also concerned about SSRI discontinuation syndrome.

Pregnancy Risk Factor C

Pregnancy Considerations Adverse events have been observed in animal reproduction studies; therefore, nateglinide is classified as pregnancy category C. Information describing the effects of nateglinide on pregnancy outcomes is limited. Maternal hyperglycemia can be associated with adverse effects in the fetus, including macrosomia, neonatal hyperglycemia, and hyperbilirubinemia; the risk of congenital malformations is increased when the Hb A_{1c} is above the normal range. Diabetes can also be associated with adverse effects in the mother. Poorly-treated diabetes may cause end-organ damage that may in turn negatively affect obstetric outcomes. Physiologic glucose levels should be maintained prior to and during pregnancy to decrease the risk of adverse events in the mother and the fetus. Until additional safety and efficacy data are obtained, the use of oral agents is generally not recommended as routine management of GDM or type 2 diabetes mellitus during pregnancy. Insulin is the drug of choice for the control of diabetes mellitus during pregnancy.

Lactation Excretion in breast milk unknown/not recommended

Contraindications Hypersensitivity to nateglinide or any component of the formulation; diabetic ketoacidosis, with or without coma (treat with insulin); type 1 diabetes mellitus (insulin dependent, IDDM)

Warnings/Precautions Use with caution in patients with moderate-to-severe hepatic impairment. Use caution in severe renal dysfunction, elderly, malnourished, or patients with adrenal/pituitary dysfunction; may be more susceptible to glucose-lowering effects. All oral hypoglycemic agents are capable of producing hypoglycemia. Proper patient selection, dosage, and instructions to the patients are important to avoid hypoglycemic episodes. It may be necessary to discontinue nateglinide and administer insulin if the patient is exposed to stress (ie, fever, trauma, infection, surgery). Indicated for adjunctive therapy with metformin; not to be used as a substitute for metformin monotherapy. Combination treatment with sulfonylureas is not recommended (no additional benefit). Patients not adequately controlled on oral agents which stimulate insulin release (eg, glyburide) should not be switched to nateglinide or have nateglinide added to therapy. Safety and efficacy in pediatric patients have not been established.

Adverse Reactions As reported with nateglinide monotherapy:

1% to 10%:

Central nervous system: Dizziness (4%)

Endocrine & metabolic: Hypoglycemia (2%), increased uric acid

Gastrointestinal: Weight gain

Neuromuscular & skeletal: Arthropathy (3%)

Respiratory: Upper respiratory infection (10%)

Miscellaneous: Flu-like syndrome (4%)

Postmarketing and/or case reports: Cholestatic hepatitis, jaundice, liver enzymes increased, rash, pruritus, urticaria

Metabolism/Transport Effects **Substrate** (major) of CYP2C9, 3A4; **Inhibits** CYP2C9 (weak)

Drug Interactions

Corticosteroids (Orally Inhaled): May diminish the hypoglycemic effect of Antidiabetic Agents. In some instances, corticosteroid-mediated HPA axis suppression has led to episodes of acute adrenal crisis, which may manifest as enhanced hypoglycemia, particularly in the setting of insulin or other antidiabetic agent use. *Risk C: Monitor therapy*

Corticosteroids (Systemic): May diminish the hypoglycemic effect of Antidiabetic Agents. In some instances, corticosteroid-mediated HPA axis suppression has led to episodes of acute adrenal crisis, which may manifest as enhanced hypoglycemia, particularly in the setting of insulin or other antidiabetic agent use. *Risk C: Monitor therapy*

CYP2C9 Inducers (Highly Effective): May increase the metabolism of CYP2C9 Substrates (High risk). *Risk C: Monitor therapy*

CYP2C9 Inhibitors (Moderate): May decrease the metabolism of CYP2C9 Substrates (High risk). *Risk C: Monitor therapy*

CYP2C9 Inhibitors (Strong): May decrease the metabolism of CYP2C9 Substrates (High risk). *Risk D: Consider therapy modification*

CYP3A4 Inducers (Strong): May increase the metabolism of CYP3A4 Substrates. *Risk C: Monitor therapy*

CYP3A4 Inhibitors (Moderate): May decrease the metabolism of CYP3A4 Substrates. *Risk C: Monitor therapy*

CYP3A4 Inhibitors (Strong): May decrease the metabolism of CYP3A4 Substrates. *Risk D: Consider therapy modification*

Dasatinib: May increase the serum concentration of CYP3A4 Substrates. *Risk C: Monitor therapy*

Deferasirox: May decrease the serum concentration of CYP3A4 Substrates. *Risk C: Monitor therapy*

Herbs (CYP3A4 Inducers): May increase the metabolism of CYP3A4 Substrates. *Risk C: Monitor therapy*

Herbs (Hypoglycemic Properties): May enhance the hypoglycemic effect of Hypoglycemic Agents. *Risk C: Monitor therapy*

Luteinizing Hormone-Releasing Hormone Analogs: May diminish the therapeutic effect of Antidiabetic Agents. *Risk C: Monitor therapy*

Pegvisomant: May enhance the hypoglycemic effect of Antidiabetic Agents. *Risk C: Monitor therapy*

Somatropin: May diminish the hypoglycemic effect of Antidiabetic Agents. *Risk D: Consider therapy modification*

Ethanol/Nutrition/Herb Interactions

Ethanol: Avoid ethanol (increased risk of hypoglycemia).

Food: Rate of absorption is decreased and time to T_{max} is delayed when taken with food. Food does not affect AUC. Multiple peak plasma concentrations may be observed if fasting. Not affected by composition of meal.

Herb/Nutraceutical: Avoid alfalfa, aloe, bilberry, bitter melon, burdock, celery, damiana, fenugreek, garcinia, garlic, ginger, ginseng (American), gymnema, marshmallow, and stinging nettle (may enhance the hypoglycemic effects of antidiabetic agents). St. John's wort may decrease the levels/effect of nateglinide.

Stability Store at 25°C (77°F).

Mechanism of Action A phenylalanine derivative, nonsulfonylurea hypoglycemic agent used in the management of type 2 diabetes mellitus (noninsulin dependent, NIDDM); stimulates insulin release from the pancreatic beta cells to reduce postprandial hyperglycemia; amount of insulin release is dependent upon existing glucose levels

Pharmacodynamics/Kinetics

Onset of action: Insulin secretion: ~20 minutes

Peak effect: 1 hour

Duration: 4 hours

Absorption: Rapid

Distribution: 10 L

Protein binding: 98%, primarily to albumin

Metabolism: Hepatic via hydroxylation followed by glucuronide conjugation via CYP2C9 (70%) and CYP3A4 (30%) to metabolites

Bioavailability: 73%

Half-life elimination: 1.5 hours

Time to peak: ≤1 hour

Excretion: Urine (83%, 16% as unchanged drug); feces (10%)

Dosage

Adults: Management of type 2 diabetes mellitus: Oral: Initial and maintenance dose: 120 mg 3 times/day, 1-30 minutes before meals; may be given alone or in combination with metformin or a thiazolidinedione; patients close to Hb A_{1c} goal may be started at 60 mg 3 times/day

Elderly: No changes in safety and efficacy were seen in patients ≥65 years; however, some elderly patients may show increased sensitivity to dosing

Dosage adjustment in renal impairment: No specific dosage adjustment is recommended for patients with mild-to-severe renal disease; patients on dialysis showed reduced medication exposure and plasma protein binding. Patients with severe renal dysfunction are more susceptible to glucose-lowering effect; use with caution.

Dosage adjustment in hepatic impairment: Increased serum levels seen with mild hepatic insufficiency; no dosage adjustment is needed. Has not been studied in patients with moderate to severe liver disease; use with caution.

Dietary Considerations Nateglinide should be taken 1-30 minutes prior to meals. Scheduled dose should not be taken if meal is missed. Dietary modification based on ADA recommendations is a part of therapy. Decreases blood glucose concentration. Hypoglycemia may occur. Must be able to recognize symptoms of hypoglycemia (palpitations, sweaty palms, lightheadedness).

Administration Patients who are anorexic or NPO will need to have their dose held to avoid hypoglycemia.

Monitoring Parameters Glucose and Hb A_{1c} levels, weight, lipid profile

Reference Range Recommendations for glycemic control in adults with diabetes:

Hb A_{1c}: <7%

Preprandial capillary plasma glucose: 70-130 mg/dL

Peak postprandial capillary blood glucose: <180 mg/dL

Blood pressure: <130/80 mm Hg

Additional Information An increase in weight was seen in nateglinide monotherapy, which was not seen when used in combination with metformin.

Dosage Forms Excipient information presented when available (limited, particularly for generics); consult specific product labeling.

Tablet:

Starlix®: 60 mg, 120 mg

- ◆ **Natrecor®** *see* Nesiritide *on page 1123*
- ◆ **Natriuretic Peptide** *see* Nesiritide *on page 1123*
- ◆ **Nature-Throid™** *see* Thyroid, Desiccated *on page 1579*
- ◆ **Navane®** *see* Thiothixene *on page 1576*
- ◆ **Navelbine®** *see* Vinorelbine *on page 1674*
- ◆ **NC-722665** *see* Bicalutamide *on page 188*

Nebivolol (ne BIV oh lole)

U.S. Brand Names Bystolic™

Index Terms Nebivolol Hydrochloride

Pharmacologic Category Beta Blocker, $Beta_1$ Selective

Use Treatment of hypertension, alone or in combination with other agents

Unlabeled/Investigational Use Heart failure

Effect on Mental Status May cause CNS depression, fatigue, dizziness, or insomnia

Effect on Psychiatric Treatment Acetylcholinesterase inhibitors and SSRIs may enhance the bradycardic effect of beta-blockers; monitor. Amphetamines may diminish the antihypertensive effect of beta-blockers. Chlorpromazine, fluoxetine, paroxetine, pergolide, and ropinirole may increase the levels/effects of nebivolol.

Dosage Summary

Oral:

Children ≤18 years: Dosage not established

Adults: Initial: 5 mg once daily; Maintenance: 5-40 mg once daily

Dosage Forms Excipient information presented when available (limited, particularly for generics); consult specific product labeling.

Tablet:

Bystolic™: 2.5 mg, 5 mg, 10 mg

- ◆ **Nebivolol Hydrochloride** *see* Nebivolol *on page 1115*
- ◆ **NebuPent®** *see* Pentamidine *on page 1242*
- ◆ **Necon® 0.5/35** *see* Ethinyl Estradiol and Norethindrone *on page 597*
- ◆ **Necon® 1/35** *see* Ethinyl Estradiol and Norethindrone *on page 597*
- ◆ **Necon® 1/50** *see* Mestranol and Norethindrone *on page 995*
- ◆ **Necon® 7/7/7** *see* Ethinyl Estradiol and Norethindrone *on page 597*
- ◆ **Necon® 10/11** *see* Ethinyl Estradiol and Norethindrone *on page 597*

Nedocromil (ne doe KROE mil)

U.S. Brand Names Alocril®; Tilade® [DSC]

Canadian Brand Names Alocril®; Tilade®

Mexican Brand Names Irtan

Index Terms Nedocromil Sodium

Pharmacologic Category Mast Cell Stabilizer

Use

Aerosol: Maintenance therapy in patients with mild to moderate bronchial asthma

Ophthalmic: Treatment of itching associated with allergic conjunctivitis

Effect on Mental Status May cause dizziness or drowsiness

Effect on Psychiatric Treatment None reported

Dosage Summary

Inhalation:

Children <6 years: Dosage not established

Children ≥6 years: 2 inhalations 2-4 times/day

Adults: 2 inhalations 2-4 times/day

Ophthalmic:

Children <3 years: Dosage not established

Children ≥3 years: 1-2 drops in each eye twice daily

Adults: 1-2 drops in each eye twice daily

Dosage Forms Excipient information presented when available (limited, particularly for generics); consult specific product labeling. [DSC] = Discontinued product

Aerosol for oral inhalation, as sodium:

Tilade®: 1.75 mg/activation (16.2 g; at least 104 inhalations) [DSC]

Solution, ophthalmic, as sodium:

Alocril®: 2% (5 mL) [contains benzalkonium chloride]

◆ **Nedocromil Sodium** *see* Nedocromil *on page 1115*

Nefazodone (nef AY zoe done)

Medication Safety Issues

Sound-alike/look-alike issues:

Serzone® may be confused with selegiline, Serentil®, Seroquel®, sertraline

Related Information

Antidepressant Agents *on page 1760*

Antidepressant Receptor Profile *on page 1764*

Index Terms Nefazodone Hydrochloride; Serzone

Pharmacologic Category Antidepressant, Serotonin Reuptake Inhibitor/Antagonist

Generic Available Yes

Use Treatment of depression

Unlabeled/Investigational Use Post-traumatic stress disorder

Mental Health Comment Due to its $5\text{-}HT_2$ antagonistic activity, nefazodone is associated with a low incidence of sexual dysfunction. Nefazodone may be useful for individuals with post-traumatic stress disorder. Nefazodone has a lower incidence of sedation and orthostasis than trazodone, primarily related to its noradrenergic activity.

Restrictions An FDA-approved medication guide concerning the use of antidepressants in children, adolescents, and young adults must be distributed when dispensing an outpatient prescription (new or refill) where this medication is to be used without direct supervision of a healthcare provider. Medication guides are available at http://www.fda.gov/cder/Offices/ODS/medication_guides.htm. Dispense to parents or guardians of children and adolescents receiving this medication.

Pregnancy Risk Factor C

Pregnancy Considerations Nefazodone is classified as pregnancy category C due to adverse effects observed in animal studies. When nefazodone is taken during pregnancy, an increased risk of major malformations has not been observed in the small number of pregnancies studied. The long-term effects on neurobehavior have not been evaluated.

Women treated for major depression and who are euthymic prior to pregnancy are more likely to experience a relapse when medication is discontinued as compared to pregnant women who continue taking antidepressant medications. Therapy during pregnancy should be individualized; treatment of depression during pregnancy should incorporate the clinical expertise of the mental health clinician, obstetrician, primary healthcare provider, and pediatrician. If treatment during pregnancy is required, consider tapering therapy during the third trimester to prevent potential withdrawal symptoms in the infant. If this is done and the woman is considered to be at risk of relapse from her major depressive disorder, the medication can be restarted following delivery.

Lactation Enters breast milk/use caution

Contraindications Hypersensitivity to nefazodone, related compounds (phenylpiperazines), or any component of the formulation; liver injury due to previous nefazodone treatment, active liver disease, or elevated serum transaminases; concurrent use or use of MAO inhibitors within previous 14 days; use in a patient during the acute recovery phase of MI; concurrent use with carbamazepine, cisapride, or pimozide; concurrent therapy with triazolam or alprazolam is generally contraindicated (dosage must be reduced by 75% for triazolam and 50% for alprazolam; such reductions may not be possible with available dosage forms).

Warnings/Precautions [U.S. Boxed Warning]: Antidepressants increase the risk of suicidal thinking and behavior in children, adolescents, and young adults (18-24 years of age) with major depressive disorder (MDD) and other psychiatric disorders; consider risk prior to prescribing. Short-term studies did not show an increased risk in patients >24 years of age and showed a decreased risk in patients ≥65 years. Closely monitor for clinical worsening, suicidality, or unusual changes in behavior; the patient's family or caregiver should be instructed to closely observe the patient and communicate condition with healthcare provider. A medication guide should be dispensed with each prescription. **Nefazodone is not FDA approved for use in children.**

The possibility of a suicide attempt is inherent in major depression and may persist until remission occurs. Monitor for worsening of depression or suicidality, especially during initiation of therapy (generally first 1-2 months) or with dose increases or decreases. Use caution in high-risk patients. Worsening depression and severe abrupt suicidality that are not part of the presenting symptoms may require discontinuation or modification of drug therapy. The patient's family or caregiver should be alerted to monitor patients for the emergence of suicidality and associated behaviors (such as agitation, irritability, hostility, impulsivity, and hypomania) and call healthcare provider.

May worsen psychosis in some patients or precipitate a shift to mania or hypomania in patients with bipolar disorder. Patients presenting with depressive symptoms should be screened for bipolar disorder. Monotherapy in patients with bipolar disorder should be avoided. **Nefazodone is not FDA approved for the treatment of bipolar depression.**

Cases of life-threatening hepatic failure have been reported (risk should be considered when choosing an agent for the treatment of depression); discontinue if clinical signs or symptoms suggest liver failure. May cause sedation, resulting in impaired performance of tasks requiring alertness (eg, operating machinery or driving). May increase the risks associated with electroconvulsive therapy. Consider discontinuing, when possible, prior to elective surgery. Therapy should not be abruptly discontinued in patients receiving high doses for prolonged periods. Rare reports of priapism have occurred. The incidence of sexual dysfunction with nefazodone is generally lower than with SSRIs.

The risk of sedation, conduction disturbances, orthostatic hypotension, or anticholinergic effects are very low relative to other antidepressants. Use with caution in patients with a history of cardiovascular disease (including previous MI, stroke, tachycardia, or conduction abnormalities). Use with caution in patients with urinary retention, benign prostatic hyperplasia, narrow-angle glaucoma, xerostomia, visual problems, constipation, or history of bowel obstruction (due to anticholinergic effects).

Use caution in patients with a previous seizure disorder or condition predisposing to seizures such as brain damage, alcoholism, or concurrent therapy with other drugs which lower the seizure threshold. Use with caution in patients with renal dysfunction and in elderly patients.

Adverse Reactions

>10%:

- Central nervous system: Headache, drowsiness, insomnia, agitation, dizziness
- Gastrointestinal: Xerostomia, nausea, constipation
- Neuromuscular & skeletal: Weakness

1% to 10%:

- Cardiovascular: Bradycardia, hypotension, peripheral edema, postural hypotension, vasodilation
- Central nervous system: Chills, fever, incoordination, lightheadedness, confusion, memory impairment, abnormal dreams, decreased concentration, ataxia, psychomotor retardation, tremor
- Dermatologic: Pruritus, rash
- Endocrine & metabolic: Breast pain, impotence, libido decreased
- Gastrointestinal: Gastroenteritis, vomiting, dyspepsia, diarrhea, increased appetite, thirst, taste perversion
- Genitourinary: Urinary frequency, urinary retention
- Hematologic: Hematocrit decreased
- Neuromuscular & skeletal: Arthralgia, hypertonia, paresthesia, neck rigidity, tremor
- Ocular: Blurred vision (9%), abnormal vision (7%), eye pain, visual field defect

Otic: Tinnitus
Respiratory: Bronchitis, cough, dyspnea, pharyngitis
Miscellaneous: Flu syndrome, infection

<1% (Limited to important or life-threatening): Allergic reaction, angioedema, AV block, galactorrhea, gynecomastia, hallucinations, hepatic failure, hepatic necrosis, hepatitis, hyponatremia, impotence, increased prolactin, leukopenia, liver function tests (abnormal), photosensitivity, priapism, rhabdomyolysis (with lovastatin/simvastatin), seizure, serotonin syndrome, Stevens-Johnson syndrome, thrombocytopenia

Metabolism/Transport Effects Substrate (major) of CYP2D6, 3A4; **Inhibits** CYP1A2 (weak), 2B6 (weak), 2C8 (weak), 2D6 (weak), 3A4 (strong)

Drug Interactions

Alcohol (Ethyl): CNS Depressants may enhance the CNS depressant effect of Alcohol (Ethyl). *Risk C: Monitor therapy*

Alfuzosin: CYP3A4 Inhibitors (Strong) may increase the serum concentration of Alfuzosin. *Risk X: Avoid combination*

Alosetron: CYP3A4 Inhibitors (Strong) may increase the serum concentration of Alosetron. *Risk C: Monitor therapy*

Benzodiazepines (metabolized by oxidation): Nefazodone may decrease the metabolism of Benzodiazepines (metabolized by oxidation). *Risk D: Consider therapy modification*

BusPIRone: May enhance the serotonergic effect of Antidepressants (Serotonin Reuptake Inhibitor/Antagonist). This may cause serotonin syndrome. *Risk C: Monitor therapy*

Cardiac Glycosides: Nefazodone may increase the serum concentration of Cardiac Glycosides. *Risk C: Monitor therapy*

Ciclesonide: CYP3A4 Inhibitors (Strong) may increase the serum concentration of Ciclesonide. Specifically, concentrations of the active des-ciclesonide metabolite may be increased. *Risk C: Monitor therapy*

Cisapride: Nefazodone may decrease the metabolism of Cisapride. *Risk X: Avoid combination*

Clozapine: Nefazodone may decrease the metabolism of Clozapine. *Risk C: Monitor therapy*

CNS Depressants: May enhance the adverse/toxic effect of other CNS Depressants. *Risk C: Monitor therapy*

CYP2D6 Inhibitors (Moderate): May decrease the metabolism of CYP2D6 Substrates. *Risk C: Monitor therapy*

CYP2D6 Inhibitors (Strong): May decrease the metabolism of CYP2D6 Substrates. *Risk D: Consider therapy modification*

CYP3A4 Inducers (Strong): May increase the metabolism of CYP3A4 Substrates. *Risk C: Monitor therapy*

CYP3A4 Inhibitors (Moderate): May decrease the metabolism of CYP3A4 Substrates. *Risk C: Monitor therapy*

CYP3A4 Inhibitors (Strong): May decrease the metabolism of CYP3A4 Substrates. *Risk D: Consider therapy modification*

CYP3A4 Substrates: CYP3A4 Inhibitors (Strong) may decrease the metabolism of CYP3A4 Substrates. *Risk D: Consider therapy modification*

Dabigatran Etexilate: P-Glycoprotein Inducers may decrease the serum concentration of Dabigatran Etexilate. *Risk C: Monitor therapy*

Darunavir: May increase the serum concentration of CYP2D6 Substrates. *Risk C: Monitor therapy*

Dasatinib: May increase the serum concentration of CYP3A4 Substrates. *Risk C: Monitor therapy*

Deferasirox: May decrease the serum concentration of CYP3A4 Substrates. *Risk C: Monitor therapy*

Eplerenone: CYP3A4 Inhibitors (Strong) may increase the serum concentration of Eplerenone. *Risk X: Avoid combination*

Herbs (CYP3A4 Inducers): May increase the metabolism of CYP3A4 Substrates. *Risk C: Monitor therapy*

HMG-CoA Reductase Inhibitors: Nefazodone may decrease the metabolism of HMG-CoA Reductase Inhibitors. **Exceptions:** Fluvastatin; Pravastatin; Rosuvastatin. *Risk D: Consider therapy modification*

Ixabepilone: CYP3A4 Inhibitors (Strong) may increase the serum concentration of Ixabepilone. *Risk D: Consider therapy modification*

Maraviroc: CYP3A4 Inhibitors may increase the serum concentration of Maraviroc. *Risk D: Consider therapy modification*

Nilotinib: CYP3A4 Inhibitors (Strong) may increase the serum concentration of Nilotinib. *Risk X: Avoid combination*

Nisoldipine: CYP3A4 Inhibitors (Strong) may increase the serum concentration of Nisoldipine. *Risk X: Avoid combination*

P-Glycoprotein Substrates: P-Glycoprotein Inducers may decrease the serum concentration of P-Glycoprotein Substrates. P-glycoprotein inducers may also further limit the distribution of p-glycoprotein substrates to specific cells/tissues/organs where p-glycoprotein is present in large amounts (e.g., brain, T-lymphocytes, testes, etc.). *Risk C: Monitor therapy*

Pimecrolimus: CYP3A4 Inhibitors (Strong) may decrease the metabolism of Pimecrolimus. *Risk C: Monitor therapy*

Pimozide: Nefazodone may decrease the metabolism of Pimozide. *Risk X: Avoid combination*

Protease Inhibitors: May decrease the metabolism of Nefazodone. *Risk C: Monitor therapy*

Ranolazine: CYP3A4 Inhibitors (Strong) may increase the serum concentration of Ranolazine. *Risk X: Avoid combination*

Rivaroxaban: CYP3A4 Inhibitors (Strong) may increase the serum concentration of Rivaroxaban. *Risk X: Avoid combination*

Salmeterol: CYP3A4 Inhibitors (Strong) may increase the serum concentration of Salmeterol. *Risk X: Avoid combination*

Selective Serotonin Reuptake Inhibitors: May enhance the serotonergic effect of Antidepressants (Serotonin Reuptake Inhibitor/Antagonist). This may cause serotonin syndrome. *Risk C: Monitor therapy*

Serotonin Modulators: May enhance the adverse/toxic effect of other Serotonin Modulators. The development of serotonin syndrome may occur. *Risk D: Consider therapy modification*

Sibutramine: May enhance the serotonergic effect of Serotonin Modulators. This may cause serotonin syndrome. *Risk X: Avoid combination*

Sorafenib: CYP3A4 Inhibitors (Strong) may increase the serum concentration of Sorafenib. *Risk C: Monitor therapy*

Tacrolimus: Antidepressants (Serotonin Reuptake Inhibitor/Antagonist) may decrease the metabolism of Tacrolimus. *Risk D: Consider therapy modification*

Ethanol/Nutrition/Herb Interactions

Ethanol: Avoid ethanol (may increase CNS depression).

Food: Nefazodone absorption may be delayed and bioavailability may be decreased if taken with food.

Herb/Nutraceutical: Avoid valerian, St John's wort, SAMe, kava kava (may increase risk of serotonin syndrome and/or excessive sedation).

Stability Store at room temperature, below 40°C (104°F) in a tight container.

Mechanism of Action Inhibits neuronal reuptake of serotonin and norepinephrine; also blocks 5-HT_2 and alpha_1 receptors; has no significant affinity for alpha_2, beta-adrenergic, 5-HT_{1A}, cholinergic, dopaminergic, or benzodiazepine receptors

Pharmacodynamics/Kinetics

Onset of action: Therapeutic: Up to 6 weeks

Distribution: V_d: 0.22-0.87 L/kg

Protein binding: >99%

Metabolism: Hepatic to three active metabolites: Triazoledione, hydroxynefazodone, and m-chlorophenylpiperazine (mCPP)

Bioavailability: 20% (variable)

Half-life elimination: Parent drug: 2-4 hours; active metabolites persist longer

Time to peak, serum: 1 hour, prolonged in presence of food

Excretion: Primarily urine (as metabolites); feces

Dosage Oral:

Children and Adolescents (unlabeled use): Depression: Target dose: 300-400 mg/day (mean: 3.4 mg/kg)

Adults: Depression: 200 mg/day, administered in 2 divided doses initially, with a range of 300-600 mg/day in 2 divided doses thereafter

Child/Adolescent Considerations Seven treatment-refractory and very comorbid children and adolescents (mean age: 12.4 years) with a juvenile mood disorder were treated with a mean daily dose of 357 mg (3.4 mg/kg) for 13 weeks (Wilens, 1997).

Wilens TE, Spencer TJ, Biederman J, et al, "Case Study: Nefazodone for Juvenile Mood Disorders," *J Am Acad Child Adolesc Psychiatry*, 1997, 36 (4):481-5.

Administration Dosing after meals may decrease lightheadedness and postural hypotension, but may also decrease absorption and therefore effectiveness.

Monitoring Parameters If AST/ALT increase >3 times ULN, the drug should be discontinued and not reintroduced; mental status for depression, suicidal ideation (especially at the beginning of therapy or when doses are increased or decreased), anxiety, social functioning, mania, panic attacks

Reference Range Therapeutic plasma levels have not yet been defined

Additional Information May cause less sexual dysfunction than other antidepressants. Women and elderly receiving single doses attain significant higher peak concentrations than male volunteers.

Dosage Forms Excipient information presented when available (limited, particularly for generics); consult specific product labeling.

Tablet, as hydrochloride: 50 mg, 100 mg, 150 mg, 200 mg, 250 mg

◆ **Nefazodone Hydrochloride** *see* Nefazodone *on page 1116*

Nelarabine (nel AY re been)

Medication Safety Issues

High alert medication: The Institute for Safe Medication Practices (ISMP) includes this medication among its list of drugs which have a heightened risk of causing significant patient harm when used in error.

U.S. Brand Names Arranon®

Canadian Brand Names Atriance™

Index Terms 2-Amino-6-Methoxypurine Arabinoside; 506U78; GW506U78

Pharmacologic Category Antineoplastic Agent, Antimetabolite

Use Treatment of relapsed or refractory T-cell acute lymphoblastic leukemia (ALL) and T-cell lymphoblastic lymphoma

Unlabeled/Investigational Use CML (Philadelphia chromosome positive) T-Cell blast phase

Effect on Mental Status May cause amnesia, confusion, depression, dizziness, fatigue, insomnia, somnolence, and coma

Effect on Psychiatric Treatment GI side effects are common; concomitant use with SSRIs, lithium, valproic acid, and carbamazepine may produce additive effects. Hematologic side effects are common; use caution with clozapine.

Dosage Summary

I.V.:

Children: 650 mg/m^2/day on days 1 through 5; repeat every 21 days

Adults: 1500 mg/m^2/day on days 1, 3, and 5; repeat every 21 days

Dosage Forms Excipient information presented when available (limited, particularly for generics); consult specific product labeling. [CAN] = Canadian brand name

Injection, solution:

Arranon®: 5 mg/mL (50 mL)

Atriance™ [CAN]: 5 mg/ml (50 mL)

Nelfinavir (nel FIN a veer)

Medication Safety Issues

Sound-alike/look-alike issues:

Nelfinavir may be confused with nevirapine

Viracept® may be confused with Viramune®

U.S. Brand Names Viracept®

Canadian Brand Names Viracept®

Mexican Brand Names Viracept

Index Terms NFV

Pharmacologic Category Antiretroviral Agent, Protease Inhibitor

Use In combination with other antiretroviral therapy in the treatment of HIV infection

Effect on Mental Status May cause dizziness, anxiety, insomnia, difficulty concentrating, depression, and suicidal ideation

Effect on Psychiatric Treatment May rarely cause leukopenia; use caution with clozapine and carbamazepine; concurrent use with midazolam and triazolam may produce oversedation; barbiturates and carbamazepine may decrease the effectiveness of nelfinavir. Concomitant use of nelfinavir and St John's wort is not recommended. Coadministration of protease inhibitors (nelfinavir) with St John's wort is expected to substantially decrease protease inhibitor serum concentrations leading to a loss of virologic response and possible resistance to nelfinavir or to the class of protease inhibitors. Concomitant use with trazodone may increase plasma levels of trazodone; monitor for nausea, dizziness, hypotension, and syncope; consider using a lower dose of trazodone.

Dosage Summary

Oral:

Children <2 years: Dosage not established

Children 2-13 years: 45-55 mg/kg twice daily **or** 25-35 mg/kg 3 times/day (maximum: 2500 mg/day)

Adults: 750 mg 3 times/day **or** 1250 mg twice daily with meals

Dosage Forms Excipient information presented when available (limited, particularly for generics); consult specific product labeling.

Powder, oral:

Viracept®: 50 mg/g (144 g) [contains phenylalanine 11.2 mg/g]

Tablet:

Viracept®: 250 mg, 625 mg

- **Nembutal®** *see* PENTobarbital *on page 1247*
- **Neo DM** *see* Chlorpheniramine, Phenylephrine, and Dextromethorphan *on page 327*
- **Neofrin™** *see* Phenylephrine *on page 1273*
- **NeoProfen®** *see* Ibuprofen *on page 803*
- **Neoral®** *see* CycloSPORINE *on page 409*
- **Neosar** *see* Cyclophosphamide *on page 408*

Neostigmine (nee oh STIG meen)

Medication Safety Issues

Sound-alike/look-alike issues:

Prostigmin® may be confused with physostigmine

U.S. Brand Names Prostigmin®

Canadian Brand Names Prostigmin®

Mexican Brand Names Prostigmine

Index Terms Neostigmine Bromide; Neostigmine Methylsulfate

Pharmacologic Category Acetylcholinesterase Inhibitor

Generic Available Yes: Injection

Use Diagnosis and treatment of myasthenia gravis; prevention and treatment of postoperative bladder distention and urinary retention; reversal of the effects of nondepolarizing neuromuscular-blocking agents after surgery

Effect on Mental Status May rarely cause drowsiness, restlessness, or agitation

Effect on Psychiatric Treatment None reported

Pregnancy Risk Factor C

Lactation Excretion in breast milk unknown/not recommended

Contraindications Hypersensitivity to neostigmine, bromides, or any component of the formulation; GI or GU obstruction

Warnings/Precautions Does **not** antagonize and may prolong the Phase I block of depolarizing muscle relaxants (eg, succinylcholine). Use with caution in patients with epilepsy, asthma, bradycardia, hyperthyroidism, cardiac arrhythmias, or peptic ulcer; not generally recommended for use in patients with vagotonia. Adequate facilities should be available for cardiopulmonary resuscitation when testing and adjusting dose for myasthenia gravis. Have atropine and epinephrine ready to treat hypersensitivity reactions. Overdosage may result in cholinergic crisis, this must be distinguished from myasthenic crisis. Anticholinesterase insensitivity can develop for brief or prolonged periods.

Adverse Reactions Frequency not defined.

Cardiovascular: Arrhythmias (especially bradycardia), hypotension, tachycardia, AV block, nodal rhythm, nonspecific ECG changes, cardiac arrest, syncope, flushing

Central nervous system: Convulsions, dysarthria, dysphonia, dizziness, loss of consciousness, drowsiness, headache

Dermatologic: Skin rash, thrombophlebitis (I.V.), urticaria

Gastrointestinal: Hyperperistalsis, nausea, vomiting, salivation, diarrhea, stomach cramps, dysphagia, flatulence

Genitourinary: Urinary urgency

Neuromuscular & skeletal: Weakness, fasciculations, muscle cramps, spasms, arthralgia

Ocular: Small pupils, lacrimation

Respiratory: Increased bronchial secretions, laryngospasm, bronchiolar constriction, respiratory muscle paralysis, dyspnea, respiratory depression, respiratory arrest, bronchospasm

Miscellaneous: Diaphoresis (increased), anaphylaxis, allergic reactions

Drug Interactions

Beta-Blockers: Acetylcholinesterase Inhibitors may enhance the bradycardic effect of Beta-Blockers. **Exceptions:** Levobunolol; Metipranolol. *Risk C: Monitor therapy*

Cholinergic Agonists: Acetylcholinesterase Inhibitors may enhance the adverse/toxic effect of Cholinergic Agonists. *Risk C: Monitor therapy*

Corticosteroids (Systemic): May enhance the adverse/toxic effect of Acetylcholinesterase Inhibitors. Increased muscular weakness may occur. *Risk C: Monitor therapy*

Ginkgo Biloba: May enhance the adverse/toxic effect of Acetylcholinesterase Inhibitors. *Risk C: Monitor therapy*

Neuromuscular-Blocking Agents (Nondepolarizing): Acetylcholinesterase Inhibitors may diminish the neuromuscular-blocking effect of Neuromuscular-Blocking Agents (Nondepolarizing). Acetylcholinesterase Inhibitors may decrease the metabolism of Neuromuscular-Blocking Agents (Nondepolarizing). This is only true for mivacurium in which case the neuromuscular blocking effects might be prolonged. *Risk C: Monitor therapy*

Succinylcholine: Acetylcholinesterase Inhibitors may enhance the neuromuscular-blocking effect of Succinylcholine. *Risk C: Monitor therapy*

Mechanism of Action Inhibits destruction of acetylcholine by acetylcholinesterase which facilitates transmission of impulses across myoneural junction

Pharmacodynamics/Kinetics

Onset of action: I.M.: 20-30 minutes; I.V.: 1-20 minutes

Duration: I.M.: 2.5-4 hours; I.V.: 1-2 hours

Absorption: Oral: Poor, <2%

Metabolism: Hepatic

Half-life elimination: Normal renal function: 0.5-2.1 hours; End-stage renal disease: Prolonged

Excretion: Urine (50% as unchanged drug)

Dosage

Myasthenia gravis: Diagnosis: I.M.:
- Children: 0.04 mg/kg as a single dose
- Adults: 0.02 mg/kg as a single dose

Myasthenia gravis: Treatment:
- Children:
  - Oral: 2 mg/kg/day divided every 3-4 hours
  - I.M., I.V., SubQ: 0.01-0.04 mg/kg every 2-4 hours
- Adults:
  - Oral: 15 mg/dose every 3-4 hours up to 375 mg/day maximum; interval between doses must be individualized to maximal response
  - I.M., I.V., SubQ: 0.5-2.5 mg every 1-3 hours up to 10 mg/24 hours maximum

Reversal of nondepolarizing neuromuscular blockade after surgery in conjunction with atropine (must administer atropine several minutes prior to neostigmine): I.V.:
- Infants: 0.025-0.1 mg/kg/dose
- Children: 0.025-0.08 mg/kg/dose
- Adults: 0.5-2.5 mg; total dose not to exceed 5 mg

Bladder atony: Adults: I.M., SubQ:
- Prevention: 0.25 mg every 4-6 hours for 2-3 days
- Treatment: 0.5-1 mg every 3 hours for 5 doses after bladder has emptied

Dosing adjustment in renal impairment:
- Cl_{cr} 10-50 mL/minute: Administer 50% of normal dose
- Cl_{cr} <10 mL/minute: Administer 25% of normal dose

Administration May be administered undiluted by slow I.V. injection over several minutes

Additional Information In the diagnosis of myasthenia gravis, all anticholinesterase medications should be discontinued for at least 8 hours before administering neostigmine.

Dosage Forms Excipient information presented when available (limited, particularly for generics); consult specific product labeling.

Injection, solution, as methylsulfate: 0.5 mg/mL (1 mL, 10 mL); 1 mg/mL (10 mL)

Tablet, as bromide: 15 mg

◆ **Neostigmine Bromide** *see* Neostigmine *on page 1121*

◆ **Neostigmine Methylsulfate** *see* Neostigmine *on page 1121*

◆ **Neo-Synephrine® 12 Hour [OTC]** *see* Oxymetazoline *on page 1208*

◆ **Neo-Synephrine® 12 Hour Extra Moisturizing [OTC]** *see* Oxymetazoline *on page 1208*

◆ **Neo-Synephrine® Extra Strength [OTC]** *see* Phenylephrine *on page 1273*

- **Neo-Synephrine® Injection** *see* Phenylephrine *on page 1273*
- **Neo-Synephrine® Mild [OTC]** *see* Phenylephrine *on page 1273*
- **Neo-Synephrine® Regular Strength [OTC]** *see* Phenylephrine *on page 1273*
- **Nephro-Calci® [OTC]** *see* Calcium Carbonate *on page 254*
- **Nephro-Fer® [OTC]** *see* Ferrous Fumarate *on page 626*
- **Nerve Agent Antidote Kit** *see* Atropine and Pralidoxime *on page 159*

Nesiritide (ni SIR i tide)

Medication Safety Issues

High alert medication: The Institute for Safe Medication Practices (ISMP) includes this medication among its list of drugs which have a heightened risk of causing significant patient harm when used in error.

International issues:

Natrecor® may be confused with Nitrocor® which is a brand name for nitroglycerin in Chile and Italy

U.S. Brand Names Natrecor®

Canadian Brand Names Natrecor®

Index Terms B-type Natriuretic Peptide (Human); hBNP; Natriuretic Peptide

Pharmacologic Category Natriuretic Peptide, B-Type, Human; Vasodilator

Use Treatment of acutely decompensated congestive heart failure (CHF) in patients with dyspnea at rest or with minimal activity

Effect on Mental Status May cause sedation, insomnia, anxiety, or confusion

Effect on Psychiatric Treatment May cause hypotension; use caution with antipsychotics and TCAs. May cause cardiac conduction abnormalities; use caution with TCAs and ziprasidone.

Dosage Summary

I.V.:

Children: Dosage not established

Adults: Bolus: 2 mcg/kg; Infusion: Initial: 0.01 mcg/kg/minute (maximum: 0.03 mcg/kg/minute); **Note:** Titration is recommended

Dosage Forms Excipient information presented when available (limited, particularly for generics); consult specific product labeling.

Injection, powder for reconstitution:

Natrecor®: 1.5 mg

- **Neulasta®** *see* Pegfilgrastim *on page 1236*
- **Neumega®** *see* Oprelvekin *on page 1184*
- **Neupogen®** *see* Filgrastim *on page 632*
- **Neupro® [DSC]** *see* Rotigotine *on page 1449*
- **Neurontin®** *see* Gabapentin *on page 702*
- **Neut®** *see* Sodium Bicarbonate *on page 1494*
- **NeuTrexin® [DSC]** *see* Trimetrexate *on page 1629*
- **Neutrogena® Advanced Solutions™ [OTC]** *see* Salicylic Acid *on page 1454*
- **Neutrogena® Blackhead Eliminating™ 2-in-1 Foaming Pads [OTC]** *see* Salicylic Acid *on page 1454*
- **Neutrogena® Blackhead Eliminating™ Astringent [OTC] [DSC]** *see* Salicylic Acid *on page 1454*
- **Neutrogena® Blackhead Eliminating™ Daily Scrub [OTC]** *see* Salicylic Acid *on page 1454*
- **Neutrogena® Blackhead Eliminating™ Treatment Mask [OTC] [DSC]** *see* Salicylic Acid *on page 1454*
- **Neutrogena® Body Clear® [OTC]** *see* Salicylic Acid *on page 1454*
- **Neutrogena® Clear Pore™ Oil-Controlling Astringent [OTC]** *see* Salicylic Acid *on page 1454*
- **Neutrogena® Oil-Free Acne Wash [OTC]** *see* Salicylic Acid *on page 1454*
- **Neutrogena® Oil-Free Acne Wash 60 Second Mask Scrub [OTC]** *see* Salicylic Acid *on page 1454*
- **Neutrogena® Oil-Free Acne Wash Cream Cleanser [OTC]** *see* Salicylic Acid *on page 1454*
- **Neutrogena® Oil-Free Acne Wash Foam Cleanser [OTC]** *see* Salicylic Acid *on page 1454*
- **Neutrogena® Rapid Clear® Acne Defense [OTC]** *see* Salicylic Acid *on page 1454*

- **Neutrogena® Rapid Clear® Acne Eliminating [OTC]** *see* Salicylic Acid *on page 1454*

Nevirapine (ne VYE ra peen)

Medication Safety Issues

Sound-alike/look-alike issues:

Nevirapine may be confused with nelfinavir

Viramune® may be confused with Viracept®

U.S. Brand Names Viramune®

Canadian Brand Names Viramune®

Mexican Brand Names Viramune

Index Terms NVP

Pharmacologic Category Antiretroviral Agent, Reverse Transcriptase Inhibitor (Non-nucleoside)

Use In combination therapy with other antiretroviral agents for the treatment of HIV-1

Effect on Mental Status None reported

Effect on Psychiatric Treatment Neutropenia is common; avoid clozapine and carbamazepine

Restrictions An FDA-approved medication guide must be distributed when dispensing an outpatient prescription (new or refill) where this medication is to be used without direct supervision of a healthcare provider. Medication guides are available at http://www.fda.gov/cder/Offices/ODS/medication_guides.htm.

Dosage Summary

Oral:

Infants (AIDSinfo guidelines): 2 mg/kg as a single dose between birth and 72 hours if mother received intrapartum dose of nevirapine. If maternal dose was given ≤2 hours prior to delivery, administer infant dose as soon as possible following birth

Infants ≥15 days and Children: 150 mg/m^2 once daily for first 14 days (maximum dose: 200 mg/day); increase dose to 150 mg/m^2 twice daily if no rash or untoward effects (maximum dose: ≤400 mg/day). Children ≤8 years of age: May require 200 mg/m^2 twice daily.

Adolescents: Initial: 200 mg once daily for first 14 days; Maintenance: 200 mg twice daily with other antiretrovirals

Adults: Initial: 200 mg once daily for first 14 days; Maintenance: 200 mg twice daily with other antiretrovirals

Pregnant women: 200 mg as a single dose at onset of labor

Dosage Forms Excipient information presented when available (limited, particularly for generics); consult specific product labeling.

Suspension, oral:

Viramune®: 50 mg/5 mL (240 mL)

Tablet:

Viramune®: 200 mg

- **Nexavar®** *see* Sorafenib *on page 1501*
- **Nexium®** *see* Esomeprazole *on page 570*
- **Nexphen PD** *see* Guaifenesin and Phenylephrine *on page 742*
- **NFV** *see* Nelfinavir *on page 1120*

Niacin (NYE a sin)

Medication Safety Issues

Sound-alike/look-alike issues:

Niacin may be confused with Minocin®, Niaspan®, Nispan®

Niaspan® may be confused with niacin

Nicobid® may be confused with Nitro-Bid®

International issues:

Niacor® may be confused with Nacor® which is a brand name for enalapril in Spain

Related Information

Lipid-Lowering Agents *on page 1786*

U.S. Brand Names Niacin-Time®; Niacor®; Niaspan®; Slo-Niacin® [OTC]

Canadian Brand Names Niaspan®

Mexican Brand Names Pepevit

Index Terms Nicotinic Acid; Vitamin B_3

Pharmacologic Category Antilipemic Agent, Miscellaneous; Vitamin, Water Soluble

Generic Available Yes

Use Adjunctive treatment of dyslipidemias (types IIa and IIb or primary hypercholesterolemia) to lower the risk of recurrent MI and/or slow progression of coronary artery disease, including combination therapy with other anti-dyslipidemic agents when additional triglyceride-lowering or HDL-increasing effects are desired; treatment of hypertriglyceridemia in patients at risk of pancreatitis; treatment of peripheral vascular disease and circulatory disorders; treatment of pellagra; dietary supplement

Effect on Mental Status May cause dizziness, insomnia, or nervousness

Effect on Psychiatric Treatment None reported

Pregnancy Risk Factor A/C (dose exceeding RDA recommendation)

Pregnancy Considerations Animal reproduction studies have not been conducted. It is unknown whether or not niacin at lipid-lowering doses is harmful to the developing fetus. If a woman becomes pregnant while receiving niacin for primary hypercholesterolemia, niacin should be discontinued. If a woman becomes pregnant while receiving niacin for hypertriglyceridemia, the benefits and risks of continuing niacin should be assessed on an individual basis.

Lactation Enters breast milk/consult prescriber

Contraindications Hypersensitivity to niacin, niacinamide, or any component of the formulation; active hepatic disease or significant or unexplained hepatic dysfunction; active peptic ulcer; arterial hemorrhage

Warnings/Precautions Use caution in heavy ethanol users, unstable angina or MI, diabetes (may interfere with glucose control), renal disease, active gallbladder disease (can exacerbate), gout, past history of hepatic disease, or with anticoagulants (may slightly increase prothrombin time). Rare cases of rhabdomyolysis have occurred during concomitant use with HMG-CoA reductase inhibitors. With concurrent use or if symptoms suggestive of myopathy occur, monitor creatinine phosphokinase (CPK) and potassium. Immediate and extended or sustained release products are not interchangeable. Cases of severe hepatotoxicity have occurred when immediate release (crystalline) niacin products have been substituted with sustained-release (modified release, timed-release) niacin products at equivalent doses. Patients should be initiated with low doses (eg, 500 mg at bedtime) with titration to achieve desired response. Flushing is common and can be attenuated with a gradual increase in dose, and/or by taking aspirin or an NSAID 30-60 minutes before dosing. Compliance is enhanced with twice-daily dosing. Prior to initiation, secondary causes for hypercholesterolemia (eg, poorly controlled diabetes mellitus, hypothyroidism) should be excluded; management with diet and other nonpharmacologic measures (eg, exercise or weight reduction) should be attempted prior to initiation.

Adverse Reactions Frequency not defined.

Cardiovascular: Arrhythmias, atrial fibrillation, edema, flushing, hypotension, orthostasis, palpitation, syncope (rare), tachycardia

Central nervous system: Chills, dizziness, headache, insomnia, migraine, nervousness, pain

Dermatologic: Acanthosis nigricans, dry skin, hyperpigmentation, maculopapular rash, pruritus, rash, urticaria

Endocrine & metabolic: Glucose tolerance decreased, gout, phosphorous levels decreased, hyperuricemia

Gastrointestinal: Abdominal pain, diarrhea, dyspepsia, eructation, flatulence, nausea, peptic ulcers, vomiting

Hematologic: Platelet counts decreased

Hepatic: Hepatic necrosis (rare), jaundice, transaminases increased (dose-related), prothrombin time increased

Neuromuscular & skeletal: Leg cramps, myalgia, myasthenia, myopathy (with concurrent HMG-CoA reductase inhibitor), paresthesia, rhabdomyolysis (with concurrent HMG-CoA reductase inhibitor; rare), weakness

Ocular: Cystoid macular edema, toxic amblyopia

Respiratory: Dyspnea

Miscellaneous: Diaphoresis, hypersensitivity reactions (rare)

Drug Interactions

Bile Acid Sequestrants: May decrease the absorption of Niacin. *Risk D: Consider therapy modification*

HMG-CoA Reductase Inhibitors: Niacin may enhance the adverse/toxic effect of HMG-CoA Reductase Inhibitors. *Risk C: Monitor therapy*

Ethanol/Nutrition/Herb Interactions Ethanol: Avoid heavy use; avoid use around niacin dose.

Stability

Niaspan®: Store at room temperature of 20°C to 25°C (68°F to 77°F).

Niacor®: Store at controlled room temperature of 15°C to 30°C (59°F to 86°F).

Mechanism of Action Component of two coenzymes which is necessary for tissue respiration, lipid metabolism, and glycogenolysis; inhibits the synthesis of very low density lipoproteins (VLDL) and low density lipoproteins (LDL); may also increase the rate of chylomicron triglyceride removal from plasma.

Pharmacodynamics/Kinetics

Absorption: Rapid and extensive (60% to 76%)

Distribution: Mainly to hepatic, renal, and adipose tissue

Metabolism: Extensive first-pass effects; converted to nicotinamide adenine dinucleotide, nicotinuric acid, and other metabolites

Half-life elimination: 20-45 minutes

Time to peak, serum: Immediate release formulation: 30-60 minutes; extended release formulation: 4-5 hours

Excretion: Urine 60% to 88% (unchanged drug and metabolites)

Dosage Note: Formulations of niacin (regular release versus extended release) are not interchangeable.

Children: Oral:
- Pellagra: 50-100 mg/dose 3 times/day
- Recommended daily allowances:
  - 0-0.5 years: 5 mg/day
  - 0.5-1 year: 6 mg/day
  - 1-3 years: 9 mg/day
  - 4-6 years: 12 mg/day
  - 7-10 years: 13 mg/day

Children and Adolescents: Recommended daily allowances:
- Male:
  - 11-14 years: 17 mg/day
  - 15-18 years: 20 mg/day
  - 19-24 years: 19 mg/day
- Female: 11-24 years: 15 mg/day

Adults: Oral:
- Recommended daily allowances:
  - Male: 25-50 years: 19 mg/day; >51 years: 15 mg/day
  - Female: 25-50 years: 15 mg/day; >51 years: 13 mg/day
- Hyperlipidemia: Usual target dose: Regular release: 1.5-6 g/day in 3 divided doses with or after meals using a dosage titration schedule. Extended release: 500 mg to 2 g once daily at bedtime.
  - Regular release formulation (Niacor®): Initial: 250 mg once daily (with evening meal); increase frequency and/or dose every 4-7 days to desired response or first-level therapeutic dose (1.5-2 g/day in 2-3 divided doses); after 2 months, may increase at 2- to 4-week intervals to 3 g/day in 3 divided doses (maximum dose: 6 g/day in 3 divided doses)
  - Extended release formulation (Niaspan®): Initial: 500 mg at bedtime for 4 weeks, then 1 g at bedtime for 4 weeks; adjust dose to response and tolerance; can increase to a maximum of 2 g/day, but only at 500 mg/day at 4-week intervals
  - With lovastatin: Recommended initial dose: 20 mg/day; Maximum lovastatin dose: 40 mg/day
- Pellagra: 50-100 mg 3-4 times/day, maximum: 500 mg/day
- Niacin deficiency: 10-20 mg/day, maximum: 100 mg/day

Dosage adjustment in renal impairment: Use with caution

Dosage adjustment in hepatic impairment: Contraindicated in patients with significant or unexplained hepatic dysfunction, active liver disease or unexplained transaminase elevations.

Dosage adjustment for hepatic toxicity: Transaminases rise ≥3 times ULN, either persistent or if symptoms of nausea, fever, and/or malaise occur: Discontinue therapy.

Dietary Considerations Should be taken with meal; low-fat meal if treating hyperlipidemia. Avoid hot drinks around the time of niacin dose.

Administration Administer with food. Administer Niaspan® at bedtime. Niaspan® tablet strengths are not interchangeable. When switching from immediate release tablet, initiate Niaspan® at lower dose and titrate. Long-acting forms should not be crushed, broken, or chewed. Do not substitute long-acting forms for immediate release ones.

Monitoring Parameters Blood glucose (in diabetic patients); CPK and serum potassium (if on concurrent HMG-CoA reductase inhibitor); liver function tests pretreatment, every 6-12 weeks for first year, then periodically (approximately every 6 months), monitor liver function more frequently if history of transaminase elevation with prior use; lipid profile; platelets; PT (if on anticoagulants); uric acid (if predisposed to gout); phosphorus (if predisposed to hypophosphatemia)

Test Interactions False elevations in some fluorometric determinations of plasma or urinary catecholamines; false-positive urine glucose (Benedict's reagent)

Dosage Forms Excipient information presented when available (limited, particularly for generics); consult specific product labeling.
Capsule, extended release: 125 mg, 250 mg, 400 mg, 500 mg
Capsule, timed release: 250 mg, 500 mg
Tablet: 50 mg, 100 mg, 250 mg, 500 mg
Niacor®: 500 mg
Tablet, controlled release (Slo-Niacin®): 250 mg, 500 mg, 750 mg
Tablet, extended release (Niaspan®): 500 mg, 750 mg, 1000 mg
Tablet, timed release: 250 mg, 500 mg, 750 mg, 1000 mg
Niacin-Time®: 500 mg

Niacin and Lovastatin (NYE a sin & LOE va sta tin)

Medication Safety Issues
Sound-alike/look-alike issues:
Advicor® may be confused with Advair, Altocor™

U.S. Brand Names Advicor®

Canadian Brand Names Advicor®

Index Terms Lovastatin and Niacin

Pharmacologic Category Antilipemic Agent, HMG-CoA Reductase Inhibitor; Antilipemic Agent, Miscellaneous

Use For use when treatment with both extended-release niacin and lovastatin is appropriate in combination with a standard cholesterol-lowering diet:
Extended-release niacin: Adjunctive treatment of dyslipidemias (types IIa and IIb or primary hypercholesterolemia) to lower the risk of recurrent MI and/or slow progression of coronary artery disease, including combination therapy with other antidyslipidemic agents when additional triglyceride-lowering or HDL-increasing effects are desired; treatment of hypertriglyceridemia in patients at risk of pancreatitis
Lovastatin: Treatment of primary hypercholesterolemia (Frederickson types IIa and IIb); primary and secondary prevention of cardiovascular disease

Effect on Mental Status May cause dizziness; may rarely cause anxiety and depression

Effect on Psychiatric Treatment Concurrent use with fluvoxamine or nefazodone may increase the risk of myopathy and/or rhabdomyolysis. May rarely cause leukopenia and thrombocytopenia; use caution with clozapine, carbamazepine, and valproic acid.

Dosage Summary
Oral:
Children: Dosage not established
Adults: Initial: Niacin 500 mg/lovastatin 20 mg at bedtime; Maintenance: Up to niacin 2000 mg/lovastatin 40 mg at bedtime; **Note:** Titration is recommended

Dosage Forms Excipient information presented when available (limited, particularly for generics); consult specific product labeling.
Tablet, variable release (Advicor®):
500/20: Niacin 500 mg [extended release] and lovastatin 20 mg [immediate release] [contains polysorbate 80]
750/20: Niacin 750 mg [extended release] and lovastatin 20 mg [immediate release] [contains polysorbate 80]
1000/20: Niacin 1000 mg [extended release] and lovastatin 20 mg [immediate release] [contains polysorbate 80]
1000/40: Niacin 1000 mg [extended release] and lovastatin 40 mg [immediate release] [contains polysorbate 80]

Niacin and Simvastatin (NYE a sin & sim va STAT in)

Medication Safety Issues
International issue:
Simcor® is also a brand name for simvastatin in Indonesia.

Related Information
Hyperlipidemia Management *on page 1821*
Lipid-Lowering Agents *on page 1786*

U.S. Brand Names Simcor®

Index Terms Simvastatin and Niacin

Pharmacologic Category Antilipemic Agent, HMG-CoA Reductase Inhibitor; Antilipemic Agent, Miscellaneous

Use Treatment of primary hypercholesterolemia, mixed dyslipidemia (types IIa and IIb), or hypertriglyceridemia (type IV hyperlipidemia) in combination with standard cholesterol-lowering diet when simvastatin or niacin monotherapy is inadequate

Effect on Mental Status May cause depression, dizziness, nervousness, or insomnia

Effect on Psychiatric Treatment Moderate-to-strong inhibitors of CYP3A4 (eg, nefazodone, caffeine, desipramine, haloperidol, sertraline, and verapamil) may elevate simvastatin levels and the risk of myopathy and renal failure. St John's wort may decrease simvastatin levels; monitor.

Dosage Summary

Oral:

Children: Dosage not established

Adults: Initial: Niacin 500 mg/simvastatin 20 mg once daily; may increase by not more than 500 mg (niacin) at 4-week intervals; Maintenance: Niacin 1000 mg/simvastatin 20 mg to niacin 2000 mg/simvastatin 40 mg once daily (maximum: niacin 2000 mg/simvastatin 40 mg once daily)

Dosage Forms Excipient information presented when available (limited, particularly for generics); consult specific product labeling.

Tablet, variable release:

Simcor®:

500/20: Niacin 500 mg [extended release] and simvastatin 20 mg [immediate release]

750/20: Niacin 750 mg [extended release] and simvastatin 20 mg [immediate release]

1000/20: Niacin 1000 mg [extended release] and simvastatin 20 mg [immediate release]

◆ **Niacin-Time®** *see* Niacin *on page 1124*

◆ **Niacor®** *see* Niacin *on page 1124*

◆ **Niaspan®** *see* Niacin *on page 1124*

NiCARdipine (nye KAR de peen)

Medication Safety Issues

Sound-alike/look-alike issues:

NiCARdipine may be confused with niacinamide, NIFEdipine, niMODipine

Cardene® may be confused with Cardizem®, Cardura®, codeine

International issues:

Cardene® may be confused with Cardem® which is a brand name for celiprolol in Spain

Cardene® may be confused with Cardin® which is a brand name for methyldopa in Brazil and a brand name for simvastatin in Poland

Significant differences exist between oral and I.V. dosing. Use caution when converting from one route of administration to another.

Related Information

Calcium Channel Blockers *on page 1778*

U.S. Brand Names Cardene®; Cardene® I.V.; Cardene® SR

Mexican Brand Names Ridene

Index Terms Nicardipine Hydrochloride

Pharmacologic Category Calcium Channel Blocker

Generic Available Yes: Capsule, injection

Use Chronic stable angina (immediate-release product only); management of hypertension (immediate and sustained release); parenteral only for short-term use when oral treatment is not feasible

Unlabeled/Investigational Use Congestive heart failure, control of blood pressure in acute ischemic stroke and spontaneous intracranial hemorrhage, postoperative hypertension associated with carotid endarterectomy, perioperative hypertension, prevention of migraine headaches, subarachnoid hemorrhage associated cerebral vasospasm

Effect on Mental Status Drowsiness and dizziness are common; may rarely cause insomnia

Effect on Psychiatric Treatment Concurrent use with propranolol may increase AV nodal effects

Pregnancy Risk Factor C

Pregnancy Considerations Crosses the placenta; may exhibit tocolytic effect

Lactation Enters breast milk/not recommended

Contraindications Hypersensitivity to nicardipine or any component of the formulation; advanced aortic stenosis

Warnings/Precautions Symptomatic hypotension with or without syncope can rarely occur; blood pressure must be lowered at a rate appropriate for the patient's clinical condition. Reflex tachycardia may occur resulting in angina and/or MI in patients with obstructive coronary disease especially in the absence of concurrent beta blockade. The most common side effect is peripheral edema (dose-dependent); occurs within 2-3 weeks of starting therapy. Use with caution in CAD (can cause increase in angina), HF (can worsen heart failure symptoms), aortic stenosis (may reduce coronary perfusion resulting in ischemia), and hypertrophic cardiomyopathy with outflow tract obstruction. Peripheral infusion sites (for I.V. therapy) should be changed every 12 hours. Titrate I.V. dose cautiously in patients with HF, renal or hepatic dysfunction. Use the I.V. form cautiously in patients with portal hypertension (can cause increase in hepatic pressure gradient). Initiate at the low end of the dosage range in the elderly. Concurrent use of fentanyl anesthesia may result in hypotension. Abrupt withdrawal may cause rebound angina in patients with CAD. Safety and efficacy have not been established in pediatric patients.

Adverse Reactions

1% to 10%:

Cardiovascular: Cardiovascular: Flushing (6% to 10%), peripheral edema (dose related; 6% to 8%), hypotension (I.V. 6%), increased angina (dose related; 6%), palpitation (3% to 4%), tachycardia (1% to 4%), vasodilation (1% to 5%), chest pain (I.V. 1%), ECG abnormal (I.V. 1%), extrasystoles (I.V. 1%), hemopericardium (I.V. 1%), hypertension (I.V. 1%), orthostasis (1%), supraventricular tachycardia (I.V. 1%), syncope (1%), ventricular extrasystoles (I.V. 1%), ventricular tachycardia (I.V. 1%)

Central nervous system: Headache (6% to 15%), dizziness (1% to 7%), hypoesthesia (1%), intracranial hemorrhage (1%) pain (1%), somnolence (1%)

Dermatologic: Rash (1%)

Endocrine & metabolic: Hypokalemia (I.V. 1%)

Gastrointestinal: Nausea (2% to 5%), vomiting (I.V. 5%), dyspepsia (oral 2%), abdominal pain (I.V. 1%), dry mouth (1%)

Genitourinary: Polyuria (1%)

Local: Injection site pain (I.V. 1%), injection site reaction (I.V. 1%)

Neuromuscular & skeletal: Weakness (1% to 6%), myalgia (1%), paresthesia (1%)

Renal: Hematuria (1%)

Respiratory: Dyspnea (1%)

Miscellaneous: Diaphoresis (1%)

<1% (Limited to important or life-threatening): Allergic reaction, confusion, constipation, deep vein thrombophlebitis; ECG effects (AV block, inverted T wave, ST segment depression); gingival hyperplasia, hypertonia, hypophosphatemia, insomnia, malaise, nervousness, nocturia, parotitis, thrombocytopenia, tinnitus, tremor

Metabolism/Transport Effects **Substrate** of CYP1A2 (minor), 2C9 (minor), 2D6 (minor), 2E1 (minor), 3A4 (major); **Inhibits** CYP2C9 (strong), 2C19 (moderate), 2D6 (moderate), 3A4 (strong)

Drug Interactions

Alosetron: CYP3A4 Inhibitors (Strong) may increase the serum concentration of Alosetron. *Risk C: Monitor therapy*

Alpha1-Blockers: May enhance the hypotensive effect of Calcium Channel Blockers. *Risk C: Monitor therapy*

Antifungal Agents (Azole Derivatives, Systemic): May decrease the metabolism of Calcium Channel Blockers. *Risk D: Consider therapy modification*

Barbiturates: May increase the metabolism of Calcium Channel Blockers. *Risk D: Consider therapy modification*

Calcium Channel Blockers (Nondihydropyridine): May enhance the hypotensive effect of Calcium Channel Blockers (Dihydropyridine). Calcium Channel Blockers (Nondihydropyridine) may decrease the metabolism of Calcium Channel Blockers (Dihydropyridine). *Risk C: Monitor therapy*

Calcium Salts: May diminish the therapeutic effect of Calcium Channel Blockers. *Risk C: Monitor therapy*

CarBAMazepine: May increase the metabolism of Calcium Channel Blockers (Dihydropyridine). *Risk C: Monitor therapy*

Ciclesonide: CYP3A4 Inhibitors (Strong) may increase the serum concentration of Ciclesonide. Specifically, concentrations of the active des-ciclesonide metabolite may be increased. *Risk C: Monitor therapy*

Codeine: CYP2D6 Inhibitors (Moderate) may diminish the therapeutic effect of Codeine. These CYP2D6 inhibitors may prevent the metabolic conversion of codeine to its active metabolite morphine. *Risk C: Monitor therapy*

CycloSPORINE: May decrease the metabolism of Calcium Channel Blockers (Dihydropyridine). Nicardipine may likewise inhibit the metabolism of cyclosporine. Cyclosporine dosage adjustments might be needed. *Risk C: Monitor therapy*

CYP2C19 Substrates: CYP2C19 Inhibitors (Moderate) may decrease the metabolism of CYP2C19 Substrates. *Risk C: Monitor therapy*

CYP2C9 Substrates (High risk): CYP2C9 Inhibitors (Strong) may decrease the metabolism of CYP2C9 Substrates (High risk). *Risk D: Consider therapy modification*

CYP2D6 Substrates: CYP2D6 Inhibitors (Moderate) may decrease the metabolism of CYP2D6 Substrates. **Exceptions:** Tamoxifen. *Risk C: Monitor therapy*

CYP3A4 Inducers (Strong): May increase the metabolism of CYP3A4 Substrates. *Risk C: Monitor therapy*

CYP3A4 Inhibitors (Moderate): May decrease the metabolism of CYP3A4 Substrates. *Risk C: Monitor therapy*

CYP3A4 Inhibitors (Strong): May decrease the metabolism of CYP3A4 Substrates. *Risk D: Consider therapy modification*

CYP3A4 Substrates: CYP3A4 Inhibitors (Strong) may decrease the metabolism of CYP3A4 Substrates. *Risk D: Consider therapy modification*

Dabigatran Etexilate: P-Glycoprotein Inhibitors may increase the serum concentration of Dabigatran Etexilate. *Risk X: Avoid combination*

Dasatinib: May increase the serum concentration of CYP3A4 Substrates. *Risk C: Monitor therapy*

Deferasirox: May decrease the serum concentration of CYP3A4 Substrates. *Risk C: Monitor therapy*

Diazoxide: May enhance the hypotensive effect of Antihypertensives. *Risk C: Monitor therapy*

Eplerenone: CYP3A4 Inhibitors (Strong) may increase the serum concentration of Eplerenone. *Risk X: Avoid combination*

Fluconazole: May decrease the metabolism of Calcium Channel Blockers. *Risk C: Monitor therapy*

Grapefruit Juice: May decrease the metabolism of Calcium Channel Blockers. *Risk C: Monitor therapy*

Herbs (CYP3A4 Inducers): May increase the metabolism of CYP3A4 Substrates. *Risk C: Monitor therapy*

Herbs (Hypertensive Properties): May diminish the antihypertensive effect of Antihypertensives. *Risk C: Monitor therapy*

Herbs (Hypotensive Properties): May enhance the hypotensive effect of Antihypertensives. *Risk C: Monitor therapy*

Ixabepilone: CYP3A4 Inhibitors (Strong) may increase the serum concentration of Ixabepilone. *Risk D: Consider therapy modification*

Macrolide Antibiotics: May decrease the metabolism of Calcium Channel Blockers. **Exceptions:** Azithromycin; Dirithromycin [Off Market]; Spiramycin. *Risk D: Consider therapy modification*

Magnesium Salts: Calcium Channel Blockers may enhance the adverse/toxic effect of Magnesium Salts. Magnesium Salts may enhance the hypotensive effect of Calcium Channel Blockers. *Risk C: Monitor therapy*

Maraviroc: CYP3A4 Inhibitors may increase the serum concentration of Maraviroc. *Risk D: Consider therapy modification*

Methylphenidate: May diminish the antihypertensive effect of Antihypertensives. *Risk C: Monitor therapy*

Nafcillin: May increase the metabolism of Calcium Channel Blockers. *Risk D: Consider therapy modification*

Neuromuscular-Blocking Agents (Nondepolarizing): Calcium Channel Blockers may enhance the neuromuscular-blocking effect of Neuromuscular-Blocking Agents (Nondepolarizing). *Risk C: Monitor therapy*

Nilotinib: CYP3A4 Inhibitors (Strong) may increase the serum concentration of Nilotinib. *Risk X: Avoid combination*

Nisoldipine: CYP3A4 Inhibitors (Strong) may increase the serum concentration of Nisoldipine. *Risk X: Avoid combination*

Nitroprusside: Calcium Channel Blockers may enhance the hypotensive effect of Nitroprusside. *Risk C: Monitor therapy*

P-Glycoprotein Inducers: May decrease the serum concentration of P-Glycoprotein Substrates. P-glycoprotein inducers may also further limit the distribution of p-glycoprotein substrates to specific cells/tissues/organs where p-glycoprotein is present in large amounts (e.g., brain, T-lymphocytes, testes, etc.). *Risk C: Monitor therapy*

P-Glycoprotein Inhibitors: May increase the serum concentration of P-Glycoprotein Substrates. P-glycoprotein inhibitors may also enhance the distribution of p-glycoprotein substrates to specific cells/tissues/organs where p-glycoprotein is present in large amounts (e.g., brain, T-lymphocytes, testes, etc.). *Risk C: Monitor therapy*

P-Glycoprotein Substrates: P-Glycoprotein Inhibitors may increase the serum concentration of P-Glycoprotein Substrates. P-glycoprotein inhibitors may also enhance the distribution of p-glycoprotein substrates to specific cells/tissues/organs where p-glycoprotein is present in large amounts (e.g., brain, T-lymphocytes, testes, etc.). *Risk C: Monitor therapy*

Phenytoin: Calcium Channel Blockers may decrease the metabolism of Phenytoin. *Risk D: Consider therapy modification*

Pimecrolimus: CYP3A4 Inhibitors (Strong) may decrease the metabolism of Pimecrolimus. *Risk C: Monitor therapy*

Prostacyclin Analogues: May enhance the hypotensive effect of Antihypertensives. *Risk C: Monitor therapy*

Protease Inhibitors: May decrease the metabolism of Calcium Channel Blockers (Dihydropyridine). *Risk D: Consider therapy modification*

QuiNIDine: Calcium Channel Blockers (Dihydropyridine) may decrease the serum concentration of QuiNIDine. *Risk C: Monitor therapy*

Quinupristin: May decrease the metabolism of Calcium Channel Blockers. *Risk C: Monitor therapy*

Ranolazine: CYP3A4 Inhibitors (Strong) may increase the serum concentration of Ranolazine. *Risk X: Avoid combination*

Rifamycin Derivatives: May increase the metabolism of Calcium Channel Blockers. This primarily affects oral forms of calcium channel blockers. *Risk D: Consider therapy modification*

RiTUXimab: Antihypertensives may enhance the hypotensive effect of RiTUXimab. *Risk D: Consider therapy modification*

Rivaroxaban: P-Glycoprotein Inhibitors may increase the serum concentration of Rivaroxaban. *Risk X: Avoid combination*

Rivaroxaban: CYP3A4 Inhibitors (Strong) may increase the serum concentration of Rivaroxaban. *Risk X: Avoid combination*

Salmeterol: CYP3A4 Inhibitors (Strong) may increase the serum concentration of Salmeterol. *Risk X: Avoid combination*

Sorafenib: CYP3A4 Inhibitors (Strong) may increase the serum concentration of Sorafenib. *Risk C: Monitor therapy*

Tacrolimus: Calcium Channel Blockers (Dihydropyridine) may increase the serum concentration of Tacrolimus. *Risk C: Monitor therapy*

Tamoxifen: CYP2D6 Inhibitors (Moderate) may decrease the metabolism of Tamoxifen. Specifically, CYP2D6 inhibitors may decrease the formation of highly potent active metabolites. *Risk D: Consider therapy modification*

Thioridazine: CYP2D6 Inhibitors may decrease the metabolism of Thioridazine. *Risk X: Avoid combination*

Topotecan: P-Glycoprotein Inhibitors may increase the serum concentration of Topotecan. *Risk X: Avoid combination*

TraMADol: CYP2D6 Inhibitors (Moderate) may diminish the therapeutic effect of TraMADol. These CYP2D6 inhibitors may prevent the metabolic conversion of tramadol to its active metabolite that accounts for much of its opioid-like effects. *Risk C: Monitor therapy*

Ethanol/Nutrition/Herb Interactions

Ethanol: Avoid ethanol (may increase CNS depression).

Food: Nicardipine average peak concentrations may be decreased if taken with food. Serum concentrations/toxicity of nicardipine may be increased by grapefruit juice; avoid concurrent use.

Herb/Nutraceutical: St John's wort may decrease levels. Avoid bayberry, blue cohosh, cayenne, ephedra, ginger, ginseng (American), kola, licorice (may worsen hypertension). Avoid black cohosh, California poppy, coleus, golden seal, hawthorn, mistletoe, periwinkle, quinine, shepherd's purse (may have increased antihypertensive effect).

Stability

I.V.:

Premixed bags: Store at controlled room temperature of 20°C to 25°C (68°F to 77°F) . Protect from light and excessive heat. Do not freeze.

Vials: Store at controlled room temperature of 20°C to 25°C (68°F to 77°F). Diluted solutions are stable for 24 hours at room temperature. Protect from light. Dilute 25 mg ampul with 240 mL of compatible solution to provide a 250 mL total volume solution and a final concentration of 0.1 mg/mL.

Oral (Cardene®, Cardene SR®): Store at 15°C to 30°C (59°F to 86°F). Protect from light. Freezing does not affect stability.

Mechanism of Action Inhibits calcium ion from entering the "slow channels" or select voltage-sensitive areas of vascular smooth muscle and myocardium during depolarization, producing a relaxation of coronary vascular smooth muscle and coronary vasodilation; increases myocardial oxygen delivery in patients with vasospastic angina

Pharmacodynamics/Kinetics

Onset of action: Oral: 0.5-2 hours; I.V.: 10 minutes; Hypotension: ~20 minutes

Duration:
I.V.: ≤8 hours
Oral: Immediate release capsules: ≤8 hours; Sustained release capsules: 8-12 hours
Absorption: Oral: ~100%
Protein binding: >95%
Metabolism: Hepatic; CYP3A4 substrate (major); extensive first-pass effect (saturable)
Bioavailability: 35%
Half-life elimination: 2-4 hours
Time to peak, serum: Oral: Immediate release: 30-120 minutes; Sustained release: 60-240 minutes
Excretion: Urine (49% to 60% as metabolites); feces (43% as metabolites)

Dosage

Adults:
Oral:
Immediate release: Initial: 20 mg 3 times/day; usual: 20-40 mg 3 times/day (allow 3 days between dose increases)
Sustained release: Initial: 30 mg twice daily, titrate up to 60 mg twice daily
Note: The total daily dose of immediate-release product may not automatically be equivalent to the daily sustained-release dose; use caution in converting.
I.V.:
Acute hypertension: Initial: 5 mg/hour increased by 2.5 mg/hour every 15 minutes to a maximum of 15 mg/hour; consider reduction to 3 mg/hour after response is achieved. Monitor and titrate to lowest dose necessary to maintain stable blood pressure.
Substitution for oral therapy (approximate equivalents):
20 mg every 8 hours oral, equivalent to 0.5 mg/hour I.V. infusion
30 mg every 8 hours oral, equivalent to 1.2 mg/hour I.V. infusion
40 mg every 8 hours oral, equivalent to 2.2 mg/hour I.V. infusion
Elderly: Initiate at the low end of the dosage range. Specific guidelines for adjustment of nicardipine are not available, but careful monitoring is warranted and adjustment may be necessary.

Dosing adjustment in renal impairment: Titrate dose beginning with 20 mg 3 times/day (immediate release capsule) or 30 mg twice daily (sustained release capsule). Specific guidelines for adjustment of nicardipine are not available, but careful monitoring is warranted and adjustment may be necessary.

Dosing adjustment in hepatic impairment: Starting dose: 20 mg twice daily (immediate release) with titration. Specific guidelines for adjustment of nicardipine are not available, but careful monitoring is warranted and adjustment may be necessary.

Administration

Oral: The total daily dose of immediate-release product may not automatically be equivalent to the daily sustained-release dose; use caution in converting. Do not chew or crush the sustained release formulation, swallow whole. Do not open or cut capsules.
I.V.:
Ampuls must be diluted before use. Administer as a slow continuous infusion.
Premixed bags: No further dilution needed. For single use only, discard any unused portion. Use only if solution is clear; the manufacturer recommends not to admix or run in the same line as other medications.

Dosage Forms Excipient information presented when available (limited, particularly for generics); consult specific product labeling.
Capsule, oral, as hydrochloride: 20 mg, 30 mg
Cardene®: 20 mg, 30 mg
Capsule, sustained release, oral, as hydrochloride:
Cardene® SR: 30 mg, 45 mg, 60 mg
Infusion, premixed in iso-osmotic dextrose, as hydrochloride:
Cardene® IV: 20 mg (200 mL)
Infusion, premixed in iso-osmotic sodium chloride, as hydrochloride:
Cardene® IV: 20 mg (200 mL)
Injection, solution, as hydrochloride: 2.5 mg/mL (10 mL)
Cardene® IV: 2.5 mg/mL (10 mL)

◆ **Nicardipine Hydrochloride** *see* NiCARdipine *on page 1128*
◆ **NicoDerm® CQ® [OTC]** *see* Nicotine *on page 1133*
◆ **Nicorette® [OTC]** *see* Nicotine *on page 1133*

Nicotine (nik oh TEEN)

Medication Safety Issues

Sound-alike/look-alike issues:

NicoDerm® may be confused with Nitroderm

Nicorette® may be confused with Nordette®

Transdermal patch may contain conducting metal (eg, aluminum); remove patch prior to MRI.

Related Information

Addiction Treatments *on page 1817*

U.S. Brand Names Commit® [OTC]; NicoDerm® CQ® [OTC]; Nicorette® [OTC]; Nicotrol® Inhaler; Nicotrol® NS; Thrive™ [OTC]

Canadian Brand Names Habitrol®; Nicoderm®; Nicorette®; Nicorette® Plus; Nicotrol®

Mexican Brand Names Nicotinell TTS; Niquitin

Index Terms Habitrol

Pharmacologic Category Smoking Cessation Aid

Generic Available Yes: Transdermal patch and gum

Use Treatment to aid smoking cessation for the relief of nicotine withdrawal symptoms (including nicotine craving)

Unlabeled/Investigational Use Management of ulcerative colitis (transdermal)

Pregnancy Risk Factor D (nasal)

Pregnancy Considerations Nicotine is teratogenic in animal studies. Nicotine exposure via cigarette smoke may cause increased ectopic pregnancy, low birth weight, increased risk of spontaneous abortion, increased perinatal mortality; increased aortic blood flow, increased heart rate, decreased uterine blood flow, and decreased breathing have been reported in the fetus. Smoking during pregnancy is associated with sudden infant death syndrome (SIDS), an increased risk of asthma, infantile colic, and childhood obesity. Women who are pregnant should be encouraged not to smoke. The use of nicotine replacement products to aid in smoking cessation has not been adequately studied in pregnant women (amount of nicotine exposure is varied). Nonpharmacologic treatments are recommended. If the benefits of nicotine replacement therapy outweigh the unknown risks, products with intermittent dosing are suggested to be tried first. If a patch is used, it is suggested to remove it overnight while sleeping to decrease fetal exposure.

Lactation Excretion in breast milk unknown/use caution

Contraindications Hypersensitivity to nicotine or any component of the formulation; patients who are smoking during the postmyocardial infarction period; patients with life-threatening arrhythmias, or severe or worsening angina pectoris; active temporomandibular joint disease (gum); pregnancy; not for use in nonsmokers

Warnings/Precautions Use caution in patients with hyperthyroidism, pheochromocytoma, or insulin-dependent diabetes. Use with caution in oropharyngeal inflammation and in patients with history of esophagitis, peptic ulcer, coronary artery disease, serious cardiac arrhythmias, vasospastic disease, angina, hypertension, hyperthyroidism, pheochromocytoma, diabetes, severe renal dysfunction, and hepatic dysfunction. The inhaler should be used with caution in patients with bronchospastic disease (other forms of nicotine replacement may be preferred). Use of nasal product is not recommended with chronic nasal disorders (eg, allergy, rhinitis, nasal polyps, and sinusitis). Transdermal patch may contain conducting metal (eg, aluminum); remove patch prior to MRI. Cautious use of topical nicotine in patiens with certain skin diseases. Hypersensitivity to the topical products can occur. Dental problems may be worsened by chewing the gum. Urge patients to stop smoking completely when initiating therapy. Safety and efficacy have not been established in pediatric patients.

Adverse Reactions

Nasal spray/inhaler:

>10%:

Central nervous system: Headache (18% to 26%)

Gastrointestinal: Inhaler: Mouth/throat irritation (66%), dyspepsia (18%)

Respiratory: Inhaler: Cough (32%), rhinitis (23%)

1% to 10%:

Dermatologic: Acne (3%)

Endocrine & metabolic: Dysmenorrhea (3%)

Gastrointestinal: Flatulence (4%), gum problems (4%), diarrhea, hiccup, nausea, taste disturbance, tooth disorder

Neuromuscular & skeletal: Back pain (6%), arthralgia (5%), jaw/neck pain

Respiratory: Sinusitis
Miscellaneous: Withdrawal symptoms
<1% (Limited to important or life-threatening): Allergy, amnesia, aphasia, bronchitis, bronchospasm, edema, migraine, numbness, pain, purpura, rash, sputum increased, vision abnormalities, xerostomia

Adverse events previously reported in prescription labeling for chewing gum, lozenge and/or transdermal systems. Frequency not defined; may be product or dose specific:
Central nervous system: Concentration impaired, depression, dizziness, headache, insomnia, nervousness, pain
Gastrointestinal: Aphthous stomatitis, constipation, cough, diarrhea, dyspepsia, flatulence, gingival bleeding, glossitis, hiccups, jaw pain, nausea, salivation increased, stomatitis, taste perversion, tooth disorder, ulcerative stomatitis, xerostomia
Dermatologic: Rash
Local: Application site reaction, local edema, local erythema
Neuromuscular & skeletal: Arthralgia, myalgia, paresthesia
Respiratory: Cough, sinusitis
Miscellaneous: Allergic reaction, diaphoresis

Metabolism/Transport Effects Substrate (minor) of CYP1A2, 2A6, 2B6, 2C9, 2C19, 2D6, 2E1, 3A4; **Inhibits** CYP2A6 (weak), 2E1 (weak)

Drug Interactions

Adenosine: Nicotine may enhance the AV-blocking effect of Adenosine. Nicotine may enhance the tachycardic effect of Adenosine. *Risk C: Monitor therapy*

Cimetidine: May decrease the metabolism of Nicotine. *Risk C: Monitor therapy*

Ethanol/Nutrition/Herb Interactions Food: Lozenge: Acidic foods/beverages decrease absorption of nicotine.

Stability Nicotrol®: Store inhaler cartridge at room temperature not to exceed 30°C (86°F). Protect cartridges from light.

Mechanism of Action Nicotine is one of two naturally-occurring alkaloids which exhibit their primary effects via autonomic ganglia stimulation. The other alkaloid is lobeline which has many actions similar to those of nicotine but is less potent. Nicotine is a potent ganglionic and central nervous system stimulant, the actions of which are mediated via nicotine-specific receptors. Biphasic actions are observed depending upon the dose administered. The main effect of nicotine in small doses is stimulation of all autonomic ganglia; with larger doses, initial stimulation is followed by blockade of transmission. Biphasic effects are also evident in the adrenal medulla; discharge of catecholamines occurs with small doses, whereas prevention of catecholamines release is seen with higher doses as a response to splanchnic nerve stimulation. Stimulation of the central nervous system (CNS) is characterized by tremors and respiratory excitation. However, convulsions may occur with higher doses, along with respiratory failure secondary to both central paralysis and peripheral blockade to respiratory muscles.

Pharmacodynamics/Kinetics

Onset of action: Intranasal: More closely approximate the time course of plasma nicotine levels observed after cigarette smoking than other dosage forms
Duration: Transdermal: 24 hours
Absorption: Transdermal: Slow
Metabolism: Hepatic, primarily to cotinine ($^1/_5$ as active)
Half-life elimination: 4 hours
Time to peak, serum: Transdermal: 8-9 hours
Excretion: Urine
Clearance: Renal: pH dependent

Dosage

Smoking deterrent: Patients should be advised to completely stop smoking upon initiation of therapy.

Oral:

Gum: Chew 1 piece of gum when urge to smoke, up to 24 pieces/day. Patients who smoke <25 cigarettes/day should start with 2-mg strength; patients smoking ≥25 cigarettes/day should start with the 4-mg strength. Use according to the following 12-week dosing schedule:
Weeks 1-6: Chew 1 piece of gum every 1-2 hours; to increase chances of quitting, chew at least 9 pieces/day during the first 6 weeks
Weeks 7-9: Chew 1 piece of gum every 2-4 hours
Weeks 10-12: Chew 1 piece of gum every 4-8 hours

Inhaler: Usually 6 to 16 cartridges per day; best effect was achieved by frequent continuous puffing (20 minutes); recommended duration of treatment is 3 months, after which patients may be weaned from the inhaler by gradual reduction of the daily dose over 6-12 weeks

Lozenge: Patients who smoke their first cigarette within 30 minutes of waking should use the 4 mg strength; otherwise the 2 mg strength is recommended. Use according to the following 12-week dosing schedule:

Weeks 1-6: One lozenge every 1-2 hours

Weeks 7-9: One lozenge every 2-4 hours

Weeks 10-12: One lozenge every 4-8 hours

Note: Use at least 9 lozenges/day during first 6 weeks to improve chances of quitting; do not use more than one lozenge at a time (maximum: 5 lozenges every 6 hours, 20 lozenges/day)

Topical:

Transdermal patch: Apply new patch every 24 hours to nonhairy, clean, dry skin on the upper body or upper outer arm; each patch should be applied to a different site. **Note:** Adjustment may be required during initial treatment (move to higher dose if experiencing withdrawal symptoms; lower dose if side effects are experienced).

NicoDerm CQ®:

Patients smoking ≥10 cigarettes/day: Begin with **step 1** (21 mg/day) for 6 weeks, followed by **step 2** (14 mg/day) for 2 weeks; finish with **step 3** (7 mg/day) for 2 weeks

Patients smoking <10 cigarettes/day: Begin with **step 2** (14 mg/day) for 6 weeks, followed by **step 3** (7 mg/day) for 2 weeks

Note: Patients receiving >600 mg/day of cimetidine: Decrease to the next lower patch size

Note: Benefits of use of nicotine transdermal patches beyond 3 months have not been demonstrated.

Ulcerative colitis (unlabeled use): Transdermal: Titrated to 22-25 mg/day

Nasal: Spray: 1-2 sprays/hour; do not exceed more than 5 doses (10 sprays) per hour [maximum: 40 doses/day (80 sprays); each dose (2 sprays) contains 1 mg of nicotine]

Dietary Considerations

Commit®: Each lozenge contains phenylalanine 3.4 mg and sodium 18 mg.

Nicorette®: Fresh mint and fruit chill flavors: The 2-mg strength contains calcium 94 mg/gum and sodium 11 mg/gum. The 4-mg strength contains calcium 94 mg/gum and sodium 13 mg/gum.

Administration

Gum: Should be chewed slowly to avoid jaw ache and to maximize benefit. Chew slowly until it tingles, then park gum between cheek and gum until tingle is gone; repeat process until most of tingle is gone (~30 minutes).

Lozenge: Should not be chewed or swallowed; allow to dissolve slowly (~20-30 minutes)

Transdermal patch: Do not cut patch; causes rapid evaporation, rendering the patch useless

Monitoring Parameters Heart rate and blood pressure periodically during therapy; discontinue therapy if signs of nicotine toxicity occur (eg, severe headache, dizziness, mental confusion, disturbed hearing and vision, abdominal pain; rapid, weak and irregular pulse; salivation, nausea, vomiting, diarrhea, cold sweat, weakness); therapy should be discontinued if rash develops; discontinuation may be considered if other adverse effects of patch occur such as myalgia, arthralgia, abnormal dreams, insomnia, nervousness, dry mouth, sweating

Additional Information A cigarette has 10-25 mg nicotine.

Dosage Forms Excipient information presented when available (limited, particularly for generics); consult specific product labeling.

Gum, chewing, as polacrilex: 2 mg (20s, 50s, 110s); 4 mg (20s, 50s, 110s)

Nicorette®:

2 mg (48s, 50s, 108s, 110s, 168s, 170s, 192s, 200s, 216s) [original and mint flavors]; (48s, 108s, 110s) [orange flavor]; (40s, 100s) [contains calcium 94 mg/gum and sodium 11 mg/gum; fresh mint and fruit chill flavors]

4 mg (48s, 50s, 108s, 110s, 168s, 170s, 192s, 200s, 216s) [original and mint flavors]; (48s, 108s, 110s) [orange flavor]; (40s, 100s) [contains calcium 94 mg/gum and sodium 13 mg/gum; fresh mint and fruit chill flavors]

Thrive™:

2 mg (40s) [gluten free, sucrose free; mint flavor]

4 mg (40s) [gluten free, sucrose free; mint flavor]

Lozenge, as polacrilex:
Commit®:
2 mg (48s, 72s, 84s, 168s) [contains phenylalanine 3.4 mg/lozenge, sodium 18 mg/lozenge; mint flavor]; (108s) [contains phenylalanine 3.4 mg/lozenge, sodium 18 mg/lozenge; original flavor]
4 mg (48s, 72s, 84s, 168s, 192s) [contains phenylalanine 3.4 mg/lozenge, sodium 18 mg/lozenge; mint flavor]; (108s) [contains phenylalanine 3.4 mg/lozenge, sodium 18 mg/lozenge; original flavor]
Oral inhalation system:
Nicotrol® Inhaler: 10 mg cartridge (168s) [cartridge delivers nicotine 4 mg; each unit consists of 5 mouthpieces, 28 storage trays each containing 6 cartridges, and 1 storage case]
Solution, intranasal [spray]:
Nicotrol® NS: 10 mg/mL (10 mL) [delivers 0.5 mg/spray; 200 sprays]
Transdermal system, topical: 7 mg/24 (30s); 14 mg/24 hours (30s); 21 mg/24 hours (30s)
NicoDerm® CQ®: 7 mg/24 hours (14s) [step 3; available in tan or clear patch]; 14 mg/24 hours (14s) [step 2; available in tan or clear patch]; 21 mg/24 hours (7s, 14s) [step 1; available in tan or clear patch]

- **Nicotinic Acid** *see* Niacin *on page 1124*
- **Nicotrol® Inhaler** *see* Nicotine *on page 1133*
- **Nicotrol® NS** *see* Nicotine *on page 1133*
- **Nicoumalone** *see* Acenocoumarol *on page 30*
- **Nifediac™ CC** *see* NIFEdipine *on page 1136*
- **Nifedical™ XL** *see* NIFEdipine *on page 1136*

NIFEdipine (nye FED i peen)

Medication Safety Issues
Sound-alike/look-alike issues:
NIFEdipine may be confused with niCARdipine, niMODipine, nisoldipine
Procardia XL® may be confused with Cartia® XT

International issues:
Nipin® [Italy and Singapore] may be confused with Nipent® which is a brand name for pentostatin in the U.S.

Related Information
Anticholinergic Effects of Common Psychotropics *on page 1758*
Calcium Channel Blockers *on page 1778*

U.S. Brand Names Adalat® CC; Afeditab™ CR; Nifediac™ CC; Nifedical™ XL; Procardia XL®; Procardia®

Canadian Brand Names Adalat® XL®; Apo-Nifed PA®; Apo-Nifed®; Novo-Nifedin; Nu-Nifed; Procardia®

Mexican Brand Names Adalat; Cordilat; Nifar-GB; Nifedigel; Nifezzard; Noviken LP

Pharmacologic Category Calcium Channel Blocker

Generic Available Yes

Use Angina and hypertension (sustained release only), pulmonary hypertension

Effect on Mental Status Dizziness is common; may cause nervousness, sedation, or mood changes

Effect on Psychiatric Treatment May cause leukopenia; use caution with clozapine and carbamazepine; concurrent use with propranolol may increase AV nodal effects; barbiturates may decrease effects of nifedipine

Pregnancy Risk Factor C

Pregnancy Considerations Use in pregnancy only when clearly needed and when the benefits outweigh the potential hazard to the fetus. No data on crossing the placenta. Hypotension, IUGR reported. IUGR probably related to maternal hypertension. May exhibit tocolytic effects. Available evidence suggests safe use during pregnancy.

Lactation Enters breast milk/compatible

Contraindications Hypersensitivity to nifedipine or any component of the formulation; immediate release preparation for treatment of urgent or emergent hypertension; acute MI

Warnings/Precautions Symptomatic hypotension with or without syncope can rarely occur; blood pressure must be lowered at a rate appropriate for the patient's clinical condition. **The use of sublingual short-acting nifedipine in hypertensive emergencies and urgencies is neither safe nor effective and SHOULD BE ABANDONED!** Serious adverse events (eg, cerebrovascular ischemia, syncope, stroke, acute myocardial infarction, and fetal distress) have been reported in relation to such use.

Blood pressure lowering should be done at a rate appropriate for the patient's condition. Rapid drops in blood pressure can lead to arterial insufficiency. Increased angina and/or MI has occurred with initiation or dosage titration of calcium channel blockers. Severe hypotension may occur in patients taking immediate release concurrently with beta-blockers when undergoing CABG with high dose fentanyl anesthesia. When considering surgery with high dose fentanyl, may consider withdrawing nifedipine (>36 hours) before surgery if possible.

The most common side effect is peripheral edema; occurs within 2-3 weeks of starting therapy. Reflex tachycardia may occur with use. Use with caution in HF or severe aortic stenosis (especially with concomitant beta-adrenergic blocker), severe left ventricular dysfunction, renal impairment, hypertrophic cardiomyopathy (especially obstructive), concomitant therapy with beta-blockers or digoxin, and edema. Use caution in patients with severe hepatic impairment (may need dosage adjustment). Mild and transient elevations in liver function enzymes may be apparent within 8 weeks of therapy initiation. Abrupt withdrawal may cause rebound angina in patients with CAD. The elderly may be more susceptible to adverse effects. Avoid use of extended release tablets (Procardia XL®) in patients with known stricture/narrowing of the GI tract.

Adverse Reactions

>10%:

Cardiovascular: Flushing (10% to 25%), peripheral edema (dose related 7% to 10%; up to 50%)

Central nervous system: Dizziness/lightheadedness/giddiness (10% to 27%), headache (10% to 23%)

Gastrointestinal: Nausea/heartburn (10% to 11%)

Neuromuscular & skeletal: Weakness (10% to 12%)

≥1% to 10%:

Cardiovascular: Palpitation (≤2% to 7%), transient hypotension (dose related 5%), CHF (2%)

Central nervous system: Nervousness/mood changes (≤2% to 7%), shakiness (≤2%), jitteriness (≤2%), sleep disturbances (≤2%), difficulties in balance (≤2%), fever (≤2%), chills (≤2%)

Dermatologic: Dermatitis (≤2%), pruritus (≤2%), urticaria (≤2%)

Endocrine & metabolic: Sexual difficulties (≤2%)

Gastrointestinal: Diarrhea (≤2%), constipation (≤2%), cramps (≤2%), flatulence (≤2%), gingival hyperplasia (≤10%)

Neuromuscular & skeletal: Muscle cramps/tremor (≤2% to 8%), inflammation (≤2%), joint stiffness (≤2%)

Ocular: Blurred vision (≤2%)

Respiratory: Cough/wheezing (6%), nasal congestion/sore throat (≤2% to 6%), chest congestion (≤2%), dyspnea (≤2%)

Miscellaneous: Diaphoresis (≤2%)

<1% (Limited to important or life-threatening): Agranulocytosis, allergic hepatitis, angina, angioedema, aplastic anemia, arthritis with positive ANA, bezoars (sustained-release preparations), cerebral ischemia, depression, erythema multiforme, erythromelalgia, exfoliative dermatitis, extrapyramidal symptoms, fever, gingival hyperplasia, gynecomastia, leukopenia, memory dysfunction, paranoid syndrome, photosensitivity, purpura, Stevens-Johnson syndrome, syncope, thrombocytopenia, tinnitus, transient blindness

Reported with use of sublingual short-acting nifedipine: Acute MI, cerebrovascular ischemia, ECG changes, fetal distress, heart block, severe hypotension, sinus arrest, stroke, syncope

Metabolism/Transport Effects **Substrate** of CYP2D6 (minor), 3A4 (major); **Inhibits** CYP1A2 (moderate), 2C9 (weak), 2D6 (weak), 3A4 (weak)

Drug Interactions

Alcohol (Ethyl): May increase the serum concentration of NIFEdipine. *Risk C: Monitor therapy*

Alpha1-Blockers: May enhance the hypotensive effect of Calcium Channel Blockers. *Risk C: Monitor therapy*

Antifungal Agents (Azole Derivatives, Systemic): May decrease the metabolism of Calcium Channel Blockers. *Risk D: Consider therapy modification*

Barbiturates: May increase the metabolism of Calcium Channel Blockers. *Risk D: Consider therapy modification*

Calcium Channel Blockers (Nondihydropyridine): May enhance the hypotensive effect of Calcium Channel Blockers (Dihydropyridine). Calcium Channel Blockers (Nondihydropyridine) may decrease the metabolism of Calcium Channel Blockers (Dihydropyridine). *Risk C: Monitor therapy*

Calcium Salts: May diminish the therapeutic effect of Calcium Channel Blockers. *Risk C: Monitor therapy*

CarBAMazepine: May increase the metabolism of Calcium Channel Blockers (Dihydropyridine). *Risk C: Monitor therapy*

Cimetidine: May decrease the metabolism of Calcium Channel Blockers. *Risk D: Consider therapy modification*

Cisapride: May increase the serum concentration of NIFEdipine. Reported with sustained release nifedipine product. *Risk C: Monitor therapy*

CycloSPORINE: May decrease the metabolism of Calcium Channel Blockers (Dihydropyridine). Nicardipine may likewise inhibit the metabolism of cyclosporine. Cyclosporine dosage adjustments might be needed. *Risk C: Monitor therapy*

CYP1A2 Substrates: CYP1A2 Inhibitors (Moderate) may decrease the metabolism of CYP1A2 Substrates. *Risk C: Monitor therapy*

CYP3A4 Inducers (Strong): May increase the metabolism of CYP3A4 Substrates. *Risk C: Monitor therapy*

CYP3A4 Inhibitors (Moderate): May decrease the metabolism of CYP3A4 Substrates. *Risk C: Monitor therapy*

CYP3A4 Inhibitors (Strong): May decrease the metabolism of CYP3A4 Substrates. *Risk D: Consider therapy modification*

Dasatinib: May increase the serum concentration of CYP3A4 Substrates. *Risk C: Monitor therapy*

Deferasirox: May decrease the serum concentration of CYP3A4 Substrates. *Risk C: Monitor therapy*

Diazoxide: May enhance the hypotensive effect of Antihypertensives. *Risk C: Monitor therapy*

Fluconazole: May decrease the metabolism of Calcium Channel Blockers. *Risk C: Monitor therapy*

Grapefruit Juice: May decrease the metabolism of Calcium Channel Blockers. *Risk C: Monitor therapy*

Herbs (CYP3A4 Inducers): May increase the metabolism of CYP3A4 Substrates. *Risk C: Monitor therapy*

Herbs (Hypertensive Properties): May diminish the antihypertensive effect of Antihypertensives. *Risk C: Monitor therapy*

Herbs (Hypotensive Properties): May enhance the hypotensive effect of Antihypertensives. *Risk C: Monitor therapy*

Macrolide Antibiotics: May decrease the metabolism of Calcium Channel Blockers. **Exceptions:** Azithromycin; Dirithromycin [Off Market]; Spiramycin. *Risk D: Consider therapy modification*

Magnesium Salts: Calcium Channel Blockers may enhance the adverse/toxic effect of Magnesium Salts. Magnesium Salts may enhance the hypotensive effect of Calcium Channel Blockers. *Risk C: Monitor therapy*

Methylphenidate: May diminish the antihypertensive effect of Antihypertensives. *Risk C: Monitor therapy*

Nafcillin: May increase the metabolism of Calcium Channel Blockers. *Risk D: Consider therapy modification*

Neuromuscular-Blocking Agents (Nondepolarizing): Calcium Channel Blockers may enhance the neuromuscular-blocking effect of Neuromuscular-Blocking Agents (Nondepolarizing). *Risk C: Monitor therapy*

Nitroprusside: Calcium Channel Blockers may enhance the hypotensive effect of Nitroprusside. *Risk C: Monitor therapy*

Phenytoin: Calcium Channel Blockers may decrease the metabolism of Phenytoin. *Risk D: Consider therapy modification*

Prostacyclin Analogues: May enhance the hypotensive effect of Antihypertensives. *Risk C: Monitor therapy*

Protease Inhibitors: May decrease the metabolism of Calcium Channel Blockers (Dihydropyridine). *Risk D: Consider therapy modification*

QuiNIDine: Calcium Channel Blockers (Dihydropyridine) may decrease the serum concentration of QuiNIDine. *Risk C: Monitor therapy*

Quinupristin: May decrease the metabolism of Calcium Channel Blockers. *Risk C: Monitor therapy*

Rifamycin Derivatives: May increase the metabolism of Calcium Channel Blockers. This primarily affects oral forms of calcium channel blockers. *Risk D: Consider therapy modification*

RiTUXimab: Antihypertensives may enhance the hypotensive effect of RiTUXimab. *Risk D: Consider therapy modification*

Tacrolimus: Calcium Channel Blockers (Dihydropyridine) may increase the serum concentration of Tacrolimus. *Risk C: Monitor therapy*

VinCRIStine: NIFEdipine may decrease the excretion of VinCRIStine. *Risk C: Monitor therapy*

Ethanol/Nutrition/Herb Interactions

Ethanol: Avoid ethanol (may increase CNS depression and may increase the effects of nifedipine). Monitor.

Food: Nifedipine serum levels may be decreased if taken with food. Food may decrease the rate but not the extent of absorption of Procardia XL®. Increased therapeutic and vasodilator side effects, including severe hypotension and myocardial ischemia, may occur if nifedipine is taken by patients ingesting grapefruit.

Herb/Nutraceutical: St John's wort may decrease nifedipine levels. Avoid dong quai if using for hypertension (has estrogenic activity). Avoid ephedra, yohimbe, ginseng (may worsen hypertension). Avoid garlic (may have increased antihypertensive effect).

Mechanism of Action Inhibits calcium ion from entering the "slow channels" or select voltage-sensitive areas of vascular smooth muscle and myocardium during depolarization, producing a relaxation of coronary vascular smooth muscle and coronary vasodilation; increases myocardial oxygen delivery in patients with vasospastic angina

Pharmacodynamics/Kinetics

Onset of action: Immediate release: ~20 minutes

Protein binding (concentration dependent): 92% to 98%

Metabolism: Hepatic to inactive metabolites

Bioavailability: Capsule: 40% to 77%; Sustained release: 65% to 89% relative to immediate release capsules

Half-life elimination: Adults: Healthy: 2-5 hours, Cirrhosis: 7 hours; Elderly: 6.7 hours

Excretion: Urine (as metabolites)

Dosage Oral:

Children:

Hypertrophic cardiomyopathy: 0.6-0.9 mg/kg/24 hours in 3-4 divided doses

Hypertension: Children 1-17 years: Extended release tablet: Initial: 0.25-0.5 mg/kg/day once daily or in 2 divided doses; maximum: 3 mg/kg/day up to 120 mg/day

Adults: (**Note:** When switching from immediate release to sustained release formulations, total daily dose will start the same)

Initial: 30 mg once daily as sustained release formulation, or if indicated, 10 mg 3 times/day as capsules

Usual dose: 10-30 mg 3 times/day as capsules or 30-60 mg once daily as sustained release

Maximum dose: 120-180 mg/day

Increase sustained release at 7- to 14-day intervals

Hemodialysis: Supplemental dose is not necessary.

Peritoneal dialysis effects: Supplemental dose is not necessary.

Dosing adjustment in hepatic impairment: Reduce oral dose by 50% to 60% in patients with cirrhosis.

Dietary Considerations Avoid grapefruit juice with all products.

Immediate release: Capsule is rapidly absorbed orally if it is administered without food, but may result in vasodilator side effects; if flushing is problematic, administration with low-fat meals may decrease. In general, can take with or without food.

Extended release: Adalat®CC, Afeditab™ CR, Nifediac™ CC: Take on an empty stomach (manufacturer recommendation). Other extended release products may not have this recommendation; consult product labeling.

Administration

Immediate release: In general, may be administered with or without food.

Extended release: Tablets should be swallowed whole; do not crush or chew.

Adalat®CC, Afeditab™ CR, Nifediac™ CC: Administer on an empty stomach (per manufacturer). Other extended release products may not have this recommendation; consult product labeling.

Monitoring Parameters Heart rate, blood pressure, signs and symptoms of CHF, peripheral edema

Additional Information When measuring smaller doses from the liquid-filled capsules, consider the following concentrations (for Procardia®) 10 mg capsule = 10 mg/0.34 mL; 20 mg capsule = 20 mg/0.45 mL; may be used preoperative to treat hypertensive urgency.

Considerable attention has been directed to potential increases in mortality and morbidity when short-acting nifedipine is used in treating hypertension. The rapid reduction in blood pressure may precipitate adverse cardiovascular events. At this time, there is no indication for the use of short-acting calcium channel blocker therapy. Nifedipine also has potent negative inotropic effects and can worsen heart failure.

Dosage Forms Excipient information presented when available (limited, particularly for generics); consult specific product labeling.

Capsule, softgel: 10 mg, 20 mg
Procardia®: 10 mg
Tablet, extended release: 30 mg, 60 mg, 90 mg
Adalat® CC, Procardia XL®: 30 mg, 60 mg, 90 mg
Afeditab™ CR, Nifedical™ XL: 30 mg, 60 mg
Nifediac™ CC: 30 mg, 60 mg, 90 mg [90 mg tablet contains tartrazine]

◆ **Niferex® [OTC]** *see* Polysaccharide-Iron Complex *on page 1313*

◆ **Niftolid** *see* Flutamide *on page 667*

◆ **Nilandron®** *see* Nilutamide *on page 1140*

Nilotinib (nye LOE ti nib)

Medication Safety Issues

Sound-alike/look-alike issues:
Nilotinib may be confused with nilutamide

High alert medication: The Institute for Safe Medication Practices (ISMP) includes this medication among its list of drug classes which have a heightened risk of causing significant patient harm when used in error.

U.S. Brand Names Tasigna®

Index Terms AMN107; Nilotinib Hydrochloride Monohydrate

Pharmacologic Category Antineoplastic Agent, Tyrosine Kinase Inhibitor

Use Treatment of Philadelphia chromosome-positive chronic myelogenous leukemia (Ph+ CML) in chronic and accelerated phase (refractory or intolerant to prior therapy, including imatinib)

Unlabeled/Investigational Use Treatment of Ph+ acute lymphoblastic leukemia (ALL), systemic mastocytosis (with c-kit activation), hypereosinophilic syndrome

Effect on Mental Status Fatigue is common; may cause dizziness and insomnia

Effect on Psychiatric Treatment Nilotinib may decrease the levels/effects of CYP2B6 substrates (eg, bupropion, promethazine, selegiline, and sertraline). Nilotinib may alter (increase or decrease) the levels/effects of CYP2C9 substrates (eg, fluoxetine, phenytoin). May decrease the levels/effects of active metabolites generated by CYP2D6 (eg, codeine and tramadol). May increase the levels/effects of CYP2D6 substrates (eg, amphetamines, select beta-blockers, dextromethorphan, fluoxetine, mirtazapine, nefazodone, paroxetine, risperidone, thioridazine, tricyclic antidepressants, and venlafaxine). Carbamazepine, phenobarbital, and phenytoin may decrease the levels/effects of nilotinib; avoid concurrent use. Avoid concurrent use with nefazodone. Nilotinib may increase the levels/effects of CYP3A4 substrates (eg, benzodiazepines, mirtazapine, nefazodone, and venlafaxine). Avoid concurrent use of nilotinib with other drugs which may prolong QT interval (includes thioridazine and ziprasidone); may increase the risk of potentially-fatal arrhythmias. GI side effects are common; use caution with SSRIs, lithium, and carbamazepine. Hematologic side effects are common; use caution with clozapine, carbamazepine, and valproic acid.

Dosage Summary

Oral:

Children: Dosage not established
Adults: 400 mg twice daily

Dosage Forms Excipient information presented when available (limited, particularly for generics); consult specific product labeling.

Capsule:
Tasigna®: 200 mg

◆ **Nilotinib Hydrochloride Monohydrate** *see* Nilotinib *on page 1140*

Nilutamide (ni LOO ta mide)

Medication Safety Issues

Sound-alike/look-alike issues:
Nilutamide may be confused with nilotinib

U.S. Brand Names Nilandron®

Canadian Brand Names Anandron®

Mexican Brand Names Anandron

Index Terms NSC-684588; RU-23908

Pharmacologic Category Antiandrogen; Antineoplastic Agent, Antiandrogen

Use Treatment of metastatic prostate cancer
Effect on Mental Status Insomnia is common; may cause dizziness or depression
Effect on Psychiatric Treatment None reported
Dosage Summary
Oral:
Children: Dosage not established
Adults: Initial: 300 mg once daily for 30 days; Maintenance: 150 mg once daily
Dosage Forms Excipient information presented when available (limited, particularly for generics); consult specific product labeling.
Tablet: 150 mg

◆ **Nimbex®** *see* Cisatracurium *on page 353*

NiMODipine (nye MOE di peen)

Medication Safety Issues
Sound-alike/look-alike issues:
NiMODipine may be confused with niCARdipine, NIFEdipine, nisoldipine

Administration issues: **For oral administration only.** For patients unable to swallow a capsule, the drug should be dispensed in an oral syringe labeled **"for oral use only."** Nimodipine has inadvertently been administered I.V. when withdrawn from capsules into a syringe for subsequent nasogastric administration. Severe cardiovascular adverse events, including fatalities, have resulted. Employ precautions against such an event.
Related Information
Calcium Channel Blockers *on page 1778*
U.S. Brand Names Nimotop®
Canadian Brand Names Nimotop®
Mexican Brand Names Kenzolol; Nimotop
Pharmacologic Category Calcium Channel Blocker
Generic Available Yes
Use Spasm following subarachnoid hemorrhage from ruptured intracranial aneurysms regardless of the patients neurological condition postictus (Hunt and Hess grades I-V)
Effect on Mental Status May cause dizziness; may rarely cause depression
Effect on Psychiatric Treatment None reported
Pregnancy Risk Factor C
Pregnancy Considerations Use in pregnancy only when clearly needed and when the benefits outweigh the potential hazard to the fetus. Teratogenic and embryotoxic effects have been demonstrated in small animals. No well-controlled studies have been conducted in pregnant women.
Lactation Enters breast milk/not recommended
Contraindications Hypersensitivity to nimodipine or any component of the formulation
Warnings/Precautions Increased angina and/or MI has occurred with initiation or dosage titration of calcium channel blockers. The most common side effect is peripheral edema; occurs within 2-3 weeks of starting therapy. Reflex tachycardia may occur with use. Symptomatic hypotension with or without syncope can rarely occur; blood pressure must be lowered at a rate appropriate for the patient's clinical condition. Use caution in hepatic impairment. Intestinal pseudo-obstruction and ileus have been reported during the use of nimodipine. Use caution in patients with decreased GI motility of a history of bowel obstruction. Use caution when treating patients with hypertrophic cardiomyopathy. Safety and efficacy have not been established in children.

[U.S. Boxed Warning]: Nimodipine has inadvertently been administered I.V. when withdrawn from capsules into a syringe for subsequent nasogastric administration. Severe cardiovascular adverse events, including fatalities, have resulted; precautions should be employed against such an event.
Adverse Reactions
1% to 10%:
Cardiovascular: Reductions in systemic blood pressure (1% to 8%)
Central nervous system: Headache (1% to 4%)
Dermatologic: Rash (1% to 2%)
Gastrointestinal: Diarrhea (2% to 4%), abdominal discomfort (2%)
<1% (Limited to important or life-threatening): Anemia, CHF, deep vein thrombosis, depression, disseminated intravascular coagulation, dyspnea,

ECG abnormalities, GI hemorrhage, hemorrhage, hepatitis, jaundice, neurological deterioration, rebound vasospasm, thrombocytopenia, vomiting

Metabolism/Transport Effects Substrate of CYP3A4 (major)

Drug Interactions

Alpha1-Blockers: May enhance the hypotensive effect of Calcium Channel Blockers. *Risk C: Monitor therapy*

Antifungal Agents (Azole Derivatives, Systemic): May decrease the metabolism of Calcium Channel Blockers. *Risk D: Consider therapy modification*

Barbiturates: May increase the metabolism of Calcium Channel Blockers. *Risk D: Consider therapy modification*

Calcium Channel Blockers (Nondihydropyridine): May enhance the hypotensive effect of Calcium Channel Blockers (Dihydropyridine). Calcium Channel Blockers (Nondihydropyridine) may decrease the metabolism of Calcium Channel Blockers (Dihydropyridine). *Risk C: Monitor therapy*

Calcium Salts: May diminish the therapeutic effect of Calcium Channel Blockers. *Risk C: Monitor therapy*

CarBAMazepine: May increase the metabolism of Calcium Channel Blockers (Dihydropyridine). *Risk C: Monitor therapy*

Cimetidine: May decrease the metabolism of Calcium Channel Blockers. *Risk D: Consider therapy modification*

CycloSPORINE: May decrease the metabolism of Calcium Channel Blockers (Dihydropyridine). Nicardipine may likewise inhibit the metabolism of cyclosporine. Cyclosporine dosage adjustments might be needed. *Risk C: Monitor therapy*

CYP3A4 Inducers (Strong): May increase the metabolism of CYP3A4 Substrates. *Risk C: Monitor therapy*

CYP3A4 Inhibitors (Moderate): May decrease the metabolism of CYP3A4 Substrates. *Risk C: Monitor therapy*

CYP3A4 Inhibitors (Strong): May decrease the metabolism of CYP3A4 Substrates. *Risk D: Consider therapy modification*

Dasatinib: May increase the serum concentration of CYP3A4 Substrates. *Risk C: Monitor therapy*

Deferasirox: May decrease the serum concentration of CYP3A4 Substrates. *Risk C: Monitor therapy*

Diazoxide: May enhance the hypotensive effect of Antihypertensives. *Risk C: Monitor therapy*

Fluconazole: May decrease the metabolism of Calcium Channel Blockers. *Risk C: Monitor therapy*

Grapefruit Juice: May decrease the metabolism of Calcium Channel Blockers. *Risk C: Monitor therapy*

Herbs (CYP3A4 Inducers): May increase the metabolism of CYP3A4 Substrates. *Risk C: Monitor therapy*

Herbs (Hypertensive Properties): May diminish the antihypertensive effect of Antihypertensives. *Risk C: Monitor therapy*

Herbs (Hypotensive Properties): May enhance the hypotensive effect of Antihypertensives. *Risk C: Monitor therapy*

Macrolide Antibiotics: May decrease the metabolism of Calcium Channel Blockers. **Exceptions:** Azithromycin; Dirithromycin [Off Market]; Spiramycin. *Risk D: Consider therapy modification*

Magnesium Salts: Calcium Channel Blockers may enhance the adverse/toxic effect of Magnesium Salts. Magnesium Salts may enhance the hypotensive effect of Calcium Channel Blockers. *Risk C: Monitor therapy*

Methylphenidate: May diminish the antihypertensive effect of Antihypertensives. *Risk C: Monitor therapy*

Nafcillin: May increase the metabolism of Calcium Channel Blockers. *Risk D: Consider therapy modification*

Neuromuscular-Blocking Agents (Nondepolarizing): Calcium Channel Blockers may enhance the neuromuscular-blocking effect of Neuromuscular-Blocking Agents (Nondepolarizing). *Risk C: Monitor therapy*

Nitroprusside: Calcium Channel Blockers may enhance the hypotensive effect of Nitroprusside. *Risk C: Monitor therapy*

Phenytoin: Calcium Channel Blockers may decrease the metabolism of Phenytoin. *Risk D: Consider therapy modification*

Prostacyclin Analogues: May enhance the hypotensive effect of Antihypertensives. *Risk C: Monitor therapy*

Protease Inhibitors: May decrease the metabolism of Calcium Channel Blockers (Dihydropyridine). *Risk D: Consider therapy modification*

QuiNIDine: Calcium Channel Blockers (Dihydropyridine) may decrease the serum concentration of QuiNIDine. *Risk C: Monitor therapy*

Quinupristin: May decrease the metabolism of Calcium Channel Blockers. *Risk C: Monitor therapy*

Rifamycin Derivatives: May increase the metabolism of Calcium Channel Blockers. This primarily affects oral forms of calcium channel blockers. *Risk D: Consider therapy modification*

RiTUXimab: Antihypertensives may enhance the hypotensive effect of RiTUXimab. *Risk D: Consider therapy modification*

Tacrolimus: Calcium Channel Blockers (Dihydropyridine) may increase the serum concentration of Tacrolimus. *Risk C: Monitor therapy*

Ethanol/Nutrition/Herb Interactions

Food: Nimodipine has shown a 1.5-fold increase in bioavailability when taken with grapefruit juice; avoid concurrent use.

Herb/Nutraceutical: St John's wort may decrease levels. Avoid dong quai if using for hypertension (has estrogenic activity). Avoid ephedra, yohimbe, ginseng (may worsen hypertension). Avoid garlic (may have increased antihypertensive effect).

Mechanism of Action Nimodipine shares the pharmacology of other calcium channel blockers; animal studies indicate that nimodipine has a greater effect on cerebral arterials than other arterials; this increased specificity may be due to the drug's increased lipophilicity and cerebral distribution as compared to nifedipine; inhibits calcium ion from entering the "slow channels" or select voltage sensitive areas of vascular smooth muscle and myocardium during depolarization

Pharmacodynamics/Kinetics

Protein binding: >95%

Metabolism: Extensively hepatic

Bioavailability: 13%

Half-life elimination: 1-2 hours; prolonged with renal impairment

Time to peak, serum: ~1 hour

Excretion: Urine (50%) and feces (32%) within 4 days

Dosage Note: Capsules and contents are for oral administration **ONLY.**

Adults: Oral: 60 mg every 4 hours for 21 days, start therapy within 96 hours after subarachnoid hemorrhage.

Dialysis: Not removed by hemo- or peritoneal dialysis; supplemental dose is not necessary.

Dosing adjustment in hepatic impairment: Reduce dosage to 30 mg every 4 hours in patients with liver failure.

Administration For oral administration **ONLY.** If the capsules cannot be swallowed, the liquid may be removed by making a hole in each end of the capsule with an 18-gauge needle and extracting the contents into a syringe. If administered via NG tube, follow with a flush of 30 mL NS.

Dosage Forms Excipient information presented when available (limited, particularly for generics); consult specific product labeling.

Capsule, liquid filled: 30 mg

Nimotop®: 30 mg

- **Nimotop®** *see* NiMODipine *on page 1141*
- **Ninjin** *see* Ginseng, Panax *(Panax ginseng) on page 718*
- **Nipent®** *see* Pentostatin *on page 1250*
- **Niravam™** *see* ALPRAZolam *on page 72*

Nisoldipine (nye SOL di peen)

Medication Safety Issues

Sound-alike/look-alike issues:

Nisoldipine may be confused with NIFEdipine, niMODipine

Related Information

Calcium Channel Blockers *on page 1778*

U.S. Brand Names Sular®

Pharmacologic Category Calcium Channel Blocker

Generic Available Yes: Extended release tablet

Use Management of hypertension, alone or in combination with other antihypertensive agents

Effect on Mental Status May cause dizziness

Effect on Psychiatric Treatment None reported

Pregnancy Risk Factor C

Pregnancy Considerations Animal studies have demonstrated fetotoxic but not teratogenic effects. There are no adequate and well-controlled studies in pregnant women. Use during pregnancy only if potential benefit to the mother outweighs potential risk to the fetus.

Lactation Excretion in breast milk unknown/not recommended

Contraindications Hypersensitivity to nisoldipine, any component of the formulation, or other dihydropyridine calcium channel blockers

Warnings/Precautions With initiation or dosage titration of dihydropyridine calcium channel blockers, reflex tachycardia may occur resulting in angina and/or MI in patients with obstructive coronary disease especially in the absence of concurrent beta-blockade. Use with caution in patients with severe aortic stenosis, HF, and hypertrophic cardiomyopathy with outflow tract obstruction. Use with caution in hepatic impairment; lower starting dose required. The most common side effect is peripheral edema; occurs within 2-3 weeks of starting therapy. Symptomatic hypotension with or without syncope can rarely occur; blood pressure must be lowered at a rate appropriate for the patient's clinical condition. Contains tartrazine, which may cause allergic reactions in certain individuals (eg, aspirin hypersensitivity). Use with caution in patients >65 years of age; lower starting dose recommended. Safety and efficacy have not been established in children.

Adverse Reactions

>10%:

Cardiovascular: Peripheral edema (dose related; 7% to 27%)

Central nervous system: Headache (22%)

1% to 10%:

Cardiovascular: Vasodilation (4%), palpitation (3%), angina exacerbation (2%), chest pain (2%)

Central nervous system: Dizziness (3% to 7%)

Dermatologic: Rash (2%)

Gastrointestinal: Nausea (2%)

Respiratory: Pharyngitis (5%), sinusitis (3%)

<1% (Limited to important or life-threatening): Alopecia, amblyopia, amnesia, anemia, angina, anxiety, arthralgia, arthritis, asthma, ataxia, atrial fibrillation, blepharitis, BUN increased, bruising, cellulitis, cerebral ischemia, chills, colitis, confusion, conjunctivitis, cough, creatinine increased, creatine kinase increased, CVA, depression, diabetes mellitus, diaphoresis, diarrhea, dyspepsia, dysphagia, dyspnea, dysuria, end inspiratory wheeze, epistaxis, exfoliative dermatitis, facial edema, fever, first-degree AV block, flu-like syndrome, fungal dermatitis, gastritis, gastrointestinal hemorrhage, gingival hyperplasia, glaucoma, glossitis, gout, gynecomastia, heart failure, hematuria, hepatomegaly, herpes simplex, herpes zoster; hypersensitivity reaction (eg, angioedema, shortness of breath, tachycardia, chest tightness, hypotension, and rash); hyper-/hypotension, hypertonia, hypoesthesia, hypokalemia, jugular venous distention, keratoconjunctivitis, laryngitis, leg cramps, leukopenia, libido decreased, liver function tests abnormal, maculopapular rash, malaise, melena, migraine, mouth ulceration, myalgia, myasthenia, MI, myositis, nervousness, nocturia, nonprotein nitrogen increased, otitis media, paresthesia, petechiae, photosensitivity, pleural effusion, postural hypotension, pruritus, pustular rash, rales, retinal detachment, skin discoloration, skin ulcer, somnolence, supraventricular tachycardia, syncope, systolic ejection murmur, temporary unilateral loss of vision, tenosynovitis, thyroiditis, tinnitus, tremor; T-wave abnormalities on ECG (flattening, inversion, nonspecific changes); urinary frequency, urticaria, vaginal hemorrhage, vaginitis, venous insufficiency, ventricular extrasystoles, vertigo, vision abnormal, vitreous floater, weight gain/loss, xerostomia

Metabolism/Transport Effects **Substrate** of CYP3A4 (major); **Inhibits** CYP1A2 (weak), 3A4 (weak)

Drug Interactions

Alpha1-Blockers: May enhance the hypotensive effect of Calcium Channel Blockers. *Risk C: Monitor therapy*

Antifungal Agents (Azole Derivatives, Systemic): May decrease the metabolism of Calcium Channel Blockers. *Risk D: Consider therapy modification*

Barbiturates: May increase the metabolism of Calcium Channel Blockers. *Risk D: Consider therapy modification*

Calcium Channel Blockers (Nondihydropyridine): May enhance the hypotensive effect of Calcium Channel Blockers (Dihydropyridine). Calcium Channel Blockers (Nondihydropyridine) may decrease the metabolism of Calcium Channel Blockers (Dihydropyridine). *Risk C: Monitor therapy*

Calcium Salts: May diminish the therapeutic effect of Calcium Channel Blockers. *Risk C: Monitor therapy*

CarBAMazepine: May increase the metabolism of Calcium Channel Blockers (Dihydropyridine). *Risk C: Monitor therapy*

Cimetidine: May decrease the metabolism of Calcium Channel Blockers. *Risk D: Consider therapy modification*

CycloSPORINE: May decrease the metabolism of Calcium Channel Blockers (Dihydropyridine). Nicardipine may likewise inhibit the metabolism of cyclosporine. Cyclosporine dosage adjustments might be needed. *Risk C: Monitor therapy*

CYP3A4 Inducers (Strong): May decrease the serum concentration of Nisoldipine. *Risk X: Avoid combination*

CYP3A4 Inhibitors (Moderate): May decrease the metabolism of CYP3A4 Substrates. *Risk C: Monitor therapy*

CYP3A4 Inhibitors (Strong): May increase the serum concentration of Nisoldipine. *Risk X: Avoid combination*

Dasatinib: May increase the serum concentration of CYP3A4 Substrates. *Risk C: Monitor therapy*

Deferasirox: May decrease the serum concentration of CYP3A4 Substrates. *Risk C: Monitor therapy*

Diazoxide: May enhance the hypotensive effect of Antihypertensives. *Risk C: Monitor therapy*

Fluconazole: May decrease the metabolism of Calcium Channel Blockers. *Risk C: Monitor therapy*

Grapefruit Juice: May decrease the metabolism of Calcium Channel Blockers. *Risk C: Monitor therapy*

Herbs (CYP3A4 Inducers): May increase the metabolism of CYP3A4 Substrates. *Risk C: Monitor therapy*

Herbs (Hypertensive Properties): May diminish the antihypertensive effect of Antihypertensives. *Risk C: Monitor therapy*

Herbs (Hypotensive Properties): May enhance the hypotensive effect of Antihypertensives. *Risk C: Monitor therapy*

Macrolide Antibiotics: May decrease the metabolism of Calcium Channel Blockers. **Exceptions:** Azithromycin; Dirithromycin [Off Market]; Spiramycin. *Risk D: Consider therapy modification*

Magnesium Salts: Calcium Channel Blockers may enhance the adverse/toxic effect of Magnesium Salts. Magnesium Salts may enhance the hypotensive effect of Calcium Channel Blockers. *Risk C: Monitor therapy*

Methylphenidate: May diminish the antihypertensive effect of Antihypertensives. *Risk C: Monitor therapy*

Nafcillin: May increase the metabolism of Calcium Channel Blockers. *Risk D: Consider therapy modification*

Neuromuscular-Blocking Agents (Nondepolarizing): Calcium Channel Blockers may enhance the neuromuscular-blocking effect of Neuromuscular-Blocking Agents (Nondepolarizing). *Risk C: Monitor therapy*

Nitroprusside: Calcium Channel Blockers may enhance the hypotensive effect of Nitroprusside. *Risk C: Monitor therapy*

Phenytoin: Calcium Channel Blockers may decrease the metabolism of Phenytoin. *Risk D: Consider therapy modification*

Prostacyclin Analogues: May enhance the hypotensive effect of Antihypertensives. *Risk C: Monitor therapy*

Protease Inhibitors: May decrease the metabolism of Calcium Channel Blockers (Dihydropyridine). *Risk D: Consider therapy modification*

Quinupristin: May decrease the metabolism of Calcium Channel Blockers. *Risk C: Monitor therapy*

Rifamycin Derivatives: May increase the metabolism of Calcium Channel Blockers. This primarily affects oral forms of calcium channel blockers. *Risk D: Consider therapy modification*

RiTUXimab: Antihypertensives may enhance the hypotensive effect of RiTUXimab. *Risk D: Consider therapy modification*

Tacrolimus: Calcium Channel Blockers (Dihydropyridine) may increase the serum concentration of Tacrolimus. *Risk C: Monitor therapy*

Ethanol/Nutrition/Herb Interactions

Food: Nisoldipine bioavailability may be increased if taken with high-lipid foods or with grapefruit juice. Avoid grapefruit products before and after dosing.

Herb/Nutraceutical: Avoid St John's wort (may decrease nisoldipine levels). Avoid bayberry, blue cohosh, cayenne, ephedra, ginger, ginseng (American), kola, licorice (may worsen hypertension). Avoid black cohosh, California poppy, coleus, golden seal, hawthorn, mistletoe, periwinkle, quinine, shepherd's purse (may have increased antihypertensive effect).

Stability Store at controlled room temperature of 20°C to 25°C (68°F to 77°F). Protect from light; protect from moisture.

Mechanism of Action As a dihydropyridine calcium channel blocker, structurally similar to nifedipine, nisoldipine impedes the movement of calcium ions into vascular smooth muscle and cardiac muscle. Dihydropyridines are potent vasodilators and are not as likely to suppress cardiac contractility and slow cardiac conduction as other calcium antagonists such as verapamil and diltiazem; nisoldipine is 5-10 times as potent a vasodilator as nifedipine.

Pharmacodynamics/Kinetics

Duration: >24 hours

Absorption: Well absorbed
Protein binding: >99%
Metabolism: Extensively hepatic; 1 active metabolite (10% of parent); first-pass effect
Bioavailability: ~5%
Half-life elimination: 9-18 hours
Time to peak: 4-14 hours
Excretion: Urine (as metabolites)

Dosage Oral:

Adults: Initial: 17 mg once daily, then increase by 8.5 mg/week (or longer intervals) to attain adequate control of blood pressure; usual dose range: 17-34 mg once daily; doses >34 mg once daily are not recommended.

Elderly: Initial dose: 8.5 mg/day, increase by 8.5 mg/week (or longer intervals) to attain adequate blood pressure control

Dosage adjustment in hepatic impairment: A starting dose not exceeding 8.5 mg/day is recommended.

Dietary Considerations Take on an empty stomach (1 hour before or 2 hours after a meal).

Administration Administer at the same time each day to ensure minimal fluctuation of serum levels. Avoid high-fat diet. Administer on an empty stomach (1 hour before or 2 hours after a meal). Swallow whole; do not crush, break, split, or chew.

Monitoring Parameters Blood pressure, heart rate

Dosage Forms Excipient information presented when available (limited, particularly for generics); consult specific product labeling.

Tablet, extended release [original formulation]: 20 mg, 30 mg, 40 mg
Sular®: 10 mg, 20 mg, 30 mg 40 mg [DSC]

Tablet, extended release [Geomatrix® delivery system]:
Sular®: 8.5 mg; 17 mg [contains tartrazine]; 25.5 mg, 34 mg

◆ **Nitalapram** *see* Citalopram *on page 354*

Nitazoxanide (nye ta ZOX a nide)

U.S. Brand Names Alinia®

Mexican Brand Names Daxon; Dexidex; Kidonax; Pacovanton; Paramix

Index Terms NTZ

Pharmacologic Category Antiprotozoal

Use Treatment of diarrhea caused by *Cryptosporidium parvum* or *Giardia lamblia*

Effect on Mental Status May rarely cause dizziness

Effect on Psychiatric Treatment None reported

Dosage Summary

Oral:

Children <1 year: Dosage not established
Children 1-3 years: 100 mg every 12 hours
Children 4-11 years: 200 mg every 12 hours
Children ≥12 years: 500 mg every 12 hours
Adults: 500 mg every 12 hours

Dosage Forms Excipient information presented when available (limited, particularly for generics); consult specific product labeling.

Powder for suspension, oral: 100 mg/5 mL (60 mL) [contains sucrose 1.48 g/5 mL, sodium benzoate; strawberry flavor]

Tablet: 500 mg
Alinia® 3-Day Therapy Packs™ [unit-dose pack]: 500 mg (6s)

Nitisinone (ni TIS i known)

U.S. Brand Names Orfadin®

Pharmacologic Category 4-Hydroxyphenylpyruvate Dioxygenase Inhibitor

Use Treatment of hereditary tyrosinemia type 1 (HT-1); to be used with dietary restriction of tyrosine and phenylalanine

Effect on Mental Status May rarely cause nervousness

Effect on Psychiatric Treatment May cause leukopenia and thrombocytopenia; use caution with clozapine, carbamazepine, and valproic acid

Restrictions Distributed by Rare Disease Therapeutics, Inc (contact 615-399-0700)

Dosage Summary Note: Must be used in conjunction with a low protein diet restricted in tyrosine and phenylalanine

Oral:

Children: 1 mg/kg/day in divided doses 1 hour before meals

Adults: 1 mg/kg/day in divided doses 1 hour before meals

Dosage Forms Excipient information presented when available (limited, particularly for generics); consult specific product labeling.

Capsule: 2 mg, 5 mg, 10 mg

- **Nitrek® [DSC]** *see* Nitroglycerin *on page 1147*
- **4′-Nitro-3′-Trifluoromethylisobutyrantide** *see* Flutamide *on page 667*
- **Nitro-Bid®** *see* Nitroglycerin *on page 1147*
- **Nitro-Dur®** *see* Nitroglycerin *on page 1147*

Nitrofurantoin (nye troe fyoor AN toyn)

Medication Safety Issues

International issues:

Macrobid® may be confused with Mikrozid® which is a brand name for ethanol/propanol combination in Great Britain

U.S. Brand Names Furadantin®; Macrobid®; Macrodantin®

Canadian Brand Names Apo-Nitrofurantoin®; Macrobid®; Macrodantin®; Novo-Furantoin

Mexican Brand Names Furadantina; Macrodantina

Pharmacologic Category Antibiotic, Miscellaneous

Use Prevention and treatment of urinary tract infections caused by susceptible strains of *E. coli, S. aureus, Enterococcus, Klebsiella,* and *Enterobacter*

Effect on Mental Status May cause drowsiness or dizziness

Effect on Psychiatric Treatment Concurrent use with anticholinergic/antiparkinsonian medications may increase the absorption of nitrofurantoin

Dosage Summary

Oral:

Children ≤1 month: Dosage not established

Children >1 month: Furadantin®, Macrodantin®: 5-7 mg/kg/day divided every 6 hours (maximum: 400 mg/day) (treatment) **or** 1-2 mg/kg/day divided every 12-24 hours (maximum: 100 mg/day) (prophylaxis)

Children >12 years: Macrobid®: 100 mg twice daily for 7 days

Adults: Furadantin®, Macrodantin®: 50-100 mg/dose every 6 hours (treatment) **or** 50-100 mg/dose at bedtime (prophylaxis); Macrobid®: 100 mg twice daily (treatment)

Dosage Forms Excipient information presented when available (limited, particularly for generics); consult specific product labeling.

Capsule [macrocrystal]: 50 mg, 100 mg

Macrodantin®: 25 mg, 50 mg, 100 mg

Capsule [macrocrystal/monohydrate]: 100 mg [nitrofurantoin macrocrystal 25% and nitrofurantoin monohydrate 75%]

Macrobid®: 100 mg [nitrofurantoin macrocrystal 25% and nitrofurantoin monohydrate 75%]

Suspension, oral:

Furadantin®: 25 mg/5 mL (470 mL)

- **Nitrogen Mustard** *see* Mechlorethamine *on page 974*

Nitroglycerin (nye troe GLI ser in)

Medication Safety Issues

Sound-alike/look-alike issues:

Nitroglycerin may be confused with nitroprusside
Nitro-Bid® may be confused with Nicobid®
Nitroderm may be confused with NicoDerm®
Nitrol® may be confused with Nizoral®
Nitrostat® may be confused with Nilstat®, nystatin

Nitroglycerin transdermal patches should be removed prior to defibrillation or MRI study.

International issues:

Nitrocor® [Chile and Italy] may be confused with Natrecor® which is a brand name for nesiritide in the U.S.

Nitrocor® [Chile and Italy] may be confused with Nutracort® which is a brand name for hydrocortisone in the U.S.

Nitro-Dur® may be confused with Nitrocor® [Chile and Italy]

U.S. Brand Names Minitran™; Nitrek® [DSC]; Nitro-Bid®; Nitro-Dur®; Nitrolingual®; NitroQuick®; Nitrostat®; NitroTime®

Canadian Brand Names Gen-Nitro; Minitran™; Nitro-Dur®; Nitroglycerin Injection, USP; Nitrol®; Nitrostat™; Rho®-Nitro; Transderm-Nitro®; Trinipatch® 0.2; Trinipatch® 0.4; Trinipatch® 0.6

Mexican Brand Names Nitradisc

Index Terms Glyceryl Trinitrate; Nitroglycerol; NTG

Pharmacologic Category Vasodilator

Use Treatment of angina pectoris; I.V. for congestive heart failure (especially when associated with acute myocardial infarction); pulmonary hypertension; hypertensive emergencies occurring perioperatively (especially during cardiovascular surgery)

Unlabeled/Investigational Use Esophageal spastic disorders (sublingual)

Effect on Mental Status May cause dizziness

Effect on Psychiatric Treatment None reported, but monitor for hypotension if receiving a psychotropic

Dosage Summary

I.V.:

Children: Initial: 0.25-0.5 mcg/kg/minute Maintenance: 1-3 mcg/kg/minute maximum: 5 mcg/kg/minute); **Note:** Titration is recommended

Adults: Initial: 5 mcg/minute; Maintenance: 20-200 mcg/minute; **Note:** Titration is recommended

Oral:

Children: Dosage not established

Adults: 2.5-9 mg 2-4 times/day (maximum: 104 mg/day)

Sublingual:

Children: Dosage not established

Adults: 0.2-0.6 mg every 5 minutes for maximum of 3 doses in 15 minutes **or** 5-10 minutes prior to activities which may provoke an attack

Topical:

Children: Dosage not established

Adults:

Ointment: Apply 0.5" to 2" every 6 hours with a nitrate free interval of ~10-12 hours

Patch: Initial: 0.2-0.4 mg/hour for 12-14 hours; Maintenance: 0.2-0.8 mg/hour for 12-14 hours; **Note:** Titration is recommended

Translingual:

Children: Dosage not established

Adults: 1-2 sprays under tongue every 3-5 minutes for maximum of 3 doses in 15 minutes **or** 5-10 minutes prior to activities which may provoke an attack

Dosage Forms Excipient information presented when available (limited, particularly for generics); consult specific product labeling.

Capsule, extended release: 2.5 mg, 6.5 mg, 9 mg

Nitro-Time®: 2.5 mg, 6.5 mg, 9 mg

Infusion [premixed in D_5W]: 25 mg (250 mL) [0.1 mg/mL]; 50 mg (250 mL) [0.2 mg/mL]; 50 mg (500 mL) [0.1 mg/mL]; 100 mg (250 mL) [0.4 mg/mL]; 200 mg (500 mL) [0.4 mg/mL]

Injection, solution: 5 mg/mL (5 mL, 10 mL) [contains ethanol and propylene glycol]

Ointment, topical:

Nitro-Bid®: 2% [20 mg/g] (1 g, 30 g, 60 g)

Solution, translingual [spray]:

Nitrolingual®: 0.4 mg/metered spray (4.9 g) [contains ethanol 20%; 60 metered sprays]; (12 g) [contains ethanol 20%; 200 metered sprays]; (16.9 g) [contains ethanol 20%; 260 metered sprays]

Tablet, sublingual: 0.3 mg, 0.4 mg, 0.6 mg

NitroQuick®, Nitrostat®: 0.3 mg, 0.4 mg, 0.6 mg

Transdermal system [once-daily patch]: 0.1 mg/hour (30s); 0.2 mg/hour (30s); 0.4 mg/hour (30s); 0.6 mg/hour (30s)

Minitran™: 0.1 mg/hour (30s); 0.2 mg/hour (30s); 0.4 mg/hour (30s); 0.6 mg/hour (30s)

Nitrek®: 0.2 mg/hour (30s); 0.4 mg/hour (30s); 0.6 mg/hour (30s) [DSC]

Nitro-Dur®: 0.1 mg/hour (30s); 0.2 mg/hour (30s); 0.3 mg/hour (30s); 0.4 mg/hour (30s); 0.6 mg/hour (30s); 0.8 mg/hour (30s)

◆ **Nitroglycerol** *see* Nitroglycerin *on page 1147*

◆ **Nitrolingual®** *see* Nitroglycerin *on page 1147*

◆ **Nitropress®** *see* Nitroprusside *on page 1149*

Nitroprusside (nye troe PRUS ide)

Medication Safety Issues

Sound-alike/look-alike issues:

Nitroprusside may be confused with nitroglycerin

High alert medication: The Institute for Safe Medication Practices (ISMP) includes this medication among its list of drugs which have a heightened risk of causing significant patient harm when used in error.

U.S. Brand Names Nitropress®

Mexican Brand Names Nitan

Index Terms Nitroprusside Sodium; Sodium Nitroferricyanide; Sodium Nitroprusside

Pharmacologic Category Vasodilator

Use Management of hypertensive crises; congestive heart failure; used for controlled hypotension to reduce bleeding during surgery

Effect on Mental Status May cause restlessness, disorientation, or psychosis

Effect on Psychiatric Treatment None reported, but monitor for hypotension if receiving a psychotropic

Dosage Summary

I.V.:

Children: Infusion: Initial: 1 mcg/kg/minute; Usual dose: 3 mcg/kg/minute (maximum: 5 mcg/kg/minute); **Note:** Titration is recommended

Adults: Infusion: Initial: 0.3-0.5 mcg/kg/minute; Usual dose: 3 mcg/kg/minute (maximum: 10 mcg/kg/minute); **Note:** Titration is recommended

Dosage Forms Excipient information presented when available (limited, particularly for generics); consult specific product labeling.

Injection, solution, as sodium: 25 mg/mL (2 mL)

◆ **Nitroprusside Sodium** *see* Nitroprusside *on page 1149*

◆ **NitroQuick®** *see* Nitroglycerin *on page 1147*

◆ **Nitrostat®** *see* Nitroglycerin *on page 1147*

◆ **NitroTime®** *see* Nitroglycerin *on page 1147*

Nizatidine (ni ZA ti deen)

Medication Safety Issues

Sound-alike/look-alike issues:

Axid® may be confused with Ansaid®

International issues:

Tazac® [Australia] may be confused with Tiazac® which is a brand name for diltiazem in the U.S.

U.S. Brand Names Axid®; Axid® AR [OTC]

Canadian Brand Names Apo-Nizatidine®; Axid®; Gen-Nizatidine; Novo-Nizatidine; Nu-Nizatidine; PMS-Nizatidine

Mexican Brand Names Axid

Pharmacologic Category Histamine H_2 Antagonist

Use Treatment and maintenance of duodenal ulcer; treatment of benign gastric ulcer; treatment of gastroesophageal reflux disease (GERD); OTC tablet used for the prevention of meal-induced heartburn, acid indigestion, and sour stomach

Unlabeled/Investigational Use Part of a multidrug regimen for *H. pylori* eradication to reduce the risk of duodenal ulcer recurrence

Effect on Mental Status May cause dizziness or drowsiness; may rarely cause insomnia

Effect on Psychiatric Treatment May rarely cause agranulocytosis; use caution with clozapine and carbamazepine

Dosage Summary

Oral:

Children <12 years (unlabeled use): 10 mg/kg/day in 2 divided doses

Children ≥12 years: 150 mg twice daily

Adults: 150 mg twice daily **or** 300 mg at bedtime **or** 75 mg twice daily (OTC dosing)

Dosage Forms Excipient information presented when available (limited, particularly for generics); consult specific product labeling.

Capsule:

Axid®: 150 mg, 300 mg [DSC]

Solution, oral:

Axid®: 15 mg/mL (120 mL, 480 mL) [bubble gum flavor]

Tablet:

Axid® AR: 75 mg

- ◆ **Nizoral®** *see* Ketoconazole *on page 876*
- ◆ **Nizoral® A-D [OTC]** *see* Ketoconazole *on page 876*
- ◆ **N-Methylhydrazine** *see* Procarbazine *on page 1340*
- ◆ **N-methylnaltrexone Bromide** *see* Methylnaltrexone *on page 1023*
- ◆ **No Doz® Maximum Strength [OTC]** *see* Caffeine *on page 250*
- ◆ **NoHist** *see* Chlorpheniramine and Phenylephrine *on page 323*
- ◆ **NoHist-A** *see* Chlorpheniramine, Phenylephrine, and Phenyltoloxamine *on page 331*
- ◆ **Nora-BE™** *see* Norethindrone *on page 1150*
- ◆ **Noradrenaline** *see* Norepinephrine *on page 1150*
- ◆ **Noradrenaline Acid Tartrate** *see* Norepinephrine *on page 1150*
- ◆ **Norco®** *see* Hydrocodone and Acetaminophen *on page 777*
- ◆ **Nordeoxyguanosine** *see* Ganciclovir *on page 708*
- ◆ **Nordette®** *see* Ethinyl Estradiol and Levonorgestrel *on page 595*
- ◆ **Norditropin®** *see* Somatropin *on page 1499*
- ◆ **Norditropin® NordiFlex®** *see* Somatropin *on page 1499*
- ◆ **Norel DM™** *see* Chlorpheniramine, Phenylephrine, and Dextromethorphan *on page 327*
- ◆ **norel® EX** *see* Guaifenesin and Phenylephrine *on page 742*
- ◆ **Norelgestromin and Ethinyl Estradiol** *see* Ethinyl Estradiol and Norelgestromin *on page 597*

Norepinephrine (nor ep i NEF rin)

Medication Safety Issues

High alert medication: The Institute for Safe Medication Practices (ISMP) includes this medication among its list of drugs which have a heightened risk of causing significant patient harm when used in error.

U.S. Brand Names Levophed®

Canadian Brand Names Levophed®

Index Terms Levarterenol Bitartrate; Noradrenaline; Noradrenaline Acid Tartrate; Norepinephrine Bitartrate

Pharmacologic Category Alpha/Beta Agonist

Use Treatment of shock which persists after adequate fluid volume replacement

Effect on Mental Status May cause anxiety, dizziness, or insomnia

Effect on Psychiatric Treatment Monitor for increased pressor effect when used with TCAs, MAO inhibitors, and antihistamines

Dosage Summary Note: Norepinephrine dosage is stated in terms of norepinephrine base and intravenous formulation is norepinephrine bitartrate (Norepinephrine bitartrate 2 mg = norepinephrine base 1 mg)

I.V.:

Children: Initial: 0.05-0.1 mcg/kg/minute; Maintenance: Titrate to desired effect (maximum: 2 mcg/kg/minute)

Adults: Initial: 0.5-1 mcg/minute; Maintenance: 0.5-30 mcg/minute; **Note:** Titration is recommended

Dosage Forms Excipient information presented when available (limited, particularly for generics); consult specific product labeling.

Injection, solution, as bitartrate: 1 mg/mL (4 mL) [contains sodium metabisulfite]

- ◆ **Norepinephrine Bitartrate** *see* Norepinephrine *on page 1150*

Norethindrone (nor ETH in drone)

Medication Safety Issues

Sound-alike/look-alike issues:

Micronor® may be confused with miconazole, Micronase®

U.S. Brand Names Aygestin®; Camila™; Errin™; Jolivette™; Nor-QD®; Nora-BE™; Ortho Micronor®

Canadian Brand Names Micronor®; Norlutate®

Mexican Brand Names Ortho-Novum

Index Terms Norethindrone Acetate; Norethisterone

Pharmacologic Category Contraceptive; Progestin

Use Treatment of amenorrhea; abnormal uterine bleeding; endometriosis; prevention of pregnancy

Effect on Mental Status May cause insomnia or depression

Effect on Psychiatric Treatment None reported

Dosage Summary

Oral:

Norethindrone:

Children (premenarche): Dosage not established

Children (postmenarche): Contraception: 0.35 mg every day

Adults: Contraception: 0.35 mg every day

Norethindrone acetate:

Children: Dosage not established

Adolescents:

Amenorrhea and abnormal uterine bleeding: 2.5-10 mg once daily for 5-10 days during the second half of the menstrual cycle

Endometriosis: Initial: 5 mg/day for 14 days; Maintenance: 15 mg/day; **Note:** Titration is recommended

Adults:

Amenorrhea and abnormal uterine bleeding: 2.5-10 mg once daily for 5-10 days during the second half of the menstrual cycle

Endometriosis: Initial: 5 mg/day for 14 days; Maintenance: 15 mg/day; **Note:** Titration is recommended

Dosage Forms Excipient information presented when available (limited, particularly for generics); consult specific product labeling.

Tablet:

Camila™, Errin™, Jolivette™, Ortho Micronor®, Nora-BE™, Nor-QD®: 0.35 mg

Tablet, as acetate:

Aygestin®: 5 mg

◆ **Norethindrone Acetate** *see* Norethindrone *on page 1150*

◆ **Norethindrone Acetate and Ethinyl Estradiol** *see* Ethinyl Estradiol and Norethindrone *on page 597*

◆ **Norethindrone and Estradiol** *see* Estradiol and Norethindrone *on page 579*

◆ **Norethindrone and Mestranol** *see* Mestranol and Norethindrone *on page 995*

◆ **Norethisterone** *see* Norethindrone *on page 1150*

◆ **Norflex™** *see* Orphenadrine *on page 1186*

Norfloxacin (nor FLOKS a sin)

Medication Safety Issues

Sound-alike/look-alike issues:

Norfloxacin may be confused with Norflex™, Noroxin®

Noroxin® may be confused with Neurontin®, Norflex™, norfloxacin

U.S. Brand Names Noroxin®

Canadian Brand Names Apo-Norflox®; CO Norfloxacin; Norfloxacine®; Noroxin® ; Novo-Norfloxacin; PMS-Norfloxacin; Riva-Norfloxacin

Mexican Brand Names Floxacin; Noroxin; Noroxin Oftalmico; Oranor

Pharmacologic Category Antibiotic, Quinolone

Use Uncomplicated and complicated urinary tract infections caused by susceptible gram-negative and gram-positive bacteria; sexually-transmitted disease (eg, uncomplicated urethral and cervical gonorrhea) caused by *N. gonorrhoeae*; prostatitis due to *E. coli*

Note: As of April 2007, the CDC no longer recommends the use of fluoroquinolones for the treatment of gonococcal disease.

Effect on Mental Status May cause dizziness, drowsiness, or insomnia; quinolones reported to cause restlessness, hallucinations, euphoria, depression, panic, and paranoia

Effect on Psychiatric Treatment Inhibits CYP1A2 isoenzyme; use caution with clozapine and other psychotropics; monitor for adverse effects

Restrictions An FDA-approved patient medication guide is available and must be distributed when dispensing an outpatient prescription (new or refill) where this medication is to be used without direct supervision of a healthcare provider. Medication guides are available at http://www.fda.gov/cder/Offices/ODS/medication_guides.htm.

Dosage Summary

Oral:

Children: Dosage not established

Adults: 400 mg every 12 hours **or** 800 mg as a single dose

Dosage Forms Excipient information presented when available (limited, particularly for generics); consult specific product labeling.

Tablet:

Noroxin®: 400 mg

- **Norgesic™ [DSC]** *see* Orphenadrine, Aspirin, and Caffeine *on page 1187*
- **Norgesic™ Forte [DSC]** *see* Orphenadrine, Aspirin, and Caffeine *on page 1187*
- **Norgestimate and Estradiol** *see* Estradiol and Norgestimate *on page 580*
- **Norgestimate and Ethinyl Estradiol** *see* Ethinyl Estradiol and Norgestimate *on page 600*
- **Norgestrel and Ethinyl Estradiol** *see* Ethinyl Estradiol and Norgestrel *on page 601*
- **Norinyl® 1+35** *see* Ethinyl Estradiol and Norethindrone *on page 597*
- **Norinyl® 1+50** *see* Mestranol and Norethindrone *on page 995*
- **Noritate®** *see* MetroNIDAZOLE *on page 1040*
- **Noroxin®** *see* Norfloxacin *on page 1151*
- **Norpace®** *see* Disopyramide *on page 488*
- **Norpace® CR** *see* Disopyramide *on page 488*
- **Norpramin®** *see* Desipramine *on page 426*
- **Nor-QD®** *see* Norethindrone *on page 1150*
- **Nortemp Children's [OTC]** *see* Acetaminophen *on page 30*
- **Northyx™** *see* Methimazole *on page 1010*
- **Nortrel™** *see* Ethinyl Estradiol and Norethindrone *on page 597*
- **Nortrel™ 7/7/7** *see* Ethinyl Estradiol and Norethindrone *on page 597*

Nortriptyline (nor TRIP ti leen)

Medication Safety Issues

Sound-alike/look-alike issues:

Aventyl® HCl may be confused with Bentyl®

Nortriptyline may be confused with amitriptyline, desipramine, Norpramin®

Pamelor® may be confused with Demerol®, Dymelor®, Panlor® DC

Related Information

Anticholinergic Effects of Common Psychotropics *on page 1758*

Antidepressant Agents *on page 1760*

Antidepressant Receptor Profile *on page 1764*

Discontinuation of Psychotropic Drugs *on page 1839*

U.S. Brand Names Pamelor®

Canadian Brand Names Alti-Nortriptyline; Apo-Nortriptyline®; Aventyl®; Gen-Nortriptyline; Norventyl; Novo-Nortriptyline; Nu-Nortriptyline; PMS-Nortriptyline

Index Terms Nortriptyline Hydrochloride

Pharmacologic Category Antidepressant, Tricyclic (Secondary Amine)

Generic Available Yes: Excludes solution

Use Treatment of symptoms of depression

Unlabeled/Investigational Use Chronic pain, anxiety disorders, enuresis, attention-deficit/hyperactivity disorder (ADHD); adjunctive therapy for smoking cessation

Mental Health Comment Tricyclic antidepressants may be classified as tertiary (amitriptyline, doxepin, clomipramine, imipramine, trimipramine) or secondary amines (nortriptyline, desipramine, protriptyline). The tertiary amines are not recommended to treat depression in the elderly. If a TCA is used in the elderly, it should be a secondary amine. The tertiary amines are commonly used in low dosages for various conditions associated with pain. Toxicity is generally dose dependent. Relatively small overdoses (1-week supply) can be potentially fatal.

Plasma concentrations correlate with clinical response. A curvilinear relationship exists.

Restrictions An FDA-approved medication guide concerning the use of antidepressants in children, adolescents, and young adults must be distributed when dispensing an outpatient prescription (new or refill) where this medication is to be used without direct supervision of a healthcare provider. Medication guides are available at http://www.fda.gov/cder/Offices/ODS/medication_guides.htm. Dispense to parents or guardians of children and adolescents receiving this medication.

Lactation Enters breast milk/contraindicated (AAP rates "of concern")

Contraindications Hypersensitivity to nortriptyline and similar chemical class, or any component of the formulation; use of MAO inhibitors within 14 days; use in a patient during the acute recovery phase of MI

Warnings/Precautions **[U.S. Boxed Warning]: Antidepressants increase the risk of suicidal thinking and behavior in children, adolescents, and young adults (18-24 years of age) with major depressive disorder (MDD) and other psychiatric disorders;** consider risk prior to prescribing. Short-term studies did not show an increased risk in patients >24 years of age and showed a decreased risk in patients ≥65 years. Closely monitor for clinical worsening, suicidality, or unusual changes in behavior; the patient's family or caregiver should be instructed to closely observe the patient and communicate condition with healthcare provider. A medication guide should be dispensed with each prescription. **Nortriptyline is not FDA approved for use in children.**

The possibility of a suicide attempt is inherent in major depression and may persist until remission occurs. Monitor for worsening of depression or suicidality, especially during initiation of therapy (generally first 1-2 months) or with dose increases or decreases. Use caution in high-risk patients. Worsening depression and severe abrupt suicidality that are not part of the presenting symptoms may require discontinuation or modification of drug therapy. The patient's family or caregiver should be alerted to monitor patients for the emergence of suicidality and associated behaviors (such as agitation, irritability, hostility, impulsivity, and hypomania) and call healthcare provider.

May worsen psychosis in some patients or precipitate a shift to mania or hypomania in patients with bipolar disorder. Patients presenting with depressive symptoms should be screened for bipolar disorder. Monotherapy in patients with bipolar disorder should be avoided. **Nortriptyline is not FDA approved for the treatment of bipolar depression.**

TCAs may rarely cause bone marrow suppression; monitor for any signs of infection and obtain CBC if symptoms (eg, fever, sore throat) evident. The risk of sedation and orthostatic effects are low relative to other antidepressants. However, nortriptyline may result in impaired performance of tasks requiring alertness (eg, operating machinery or driving). Sedative effects may be additive with other CNS depressants and/or ethanol. The degree of anticholinergic blockade produced by this agent is moderate relative to other cyclic antidepressants, however, caution should still be used in patients with urinary retention, benign prostatic hyperplasia, narrow-angle glaucoma, xerostomia, visual problems, constipation, or history of bowel obstruction. May cause orthostatic hypotension (risk is low relative to other antidepressants) or conduction disturbances. Use with caution in patients with a history of cardiovascular disease (including previous MI, stroke, tachycardia, or conduction abnormalities). The risk conduction abnormalities with this agent is moderate relative to other antidepressants.

Consider discontinuing, when possible, prior to elective surgery. Therapy should not be abruptly discontinued in patients receiving high doses for prolonged periods. May alter glucose regulation - use caution in patients with diabetes. Use caution in patients with a previous seizure disorder or condition predisposing to seizures such as brain damage, alcoholism, or concurrent therapy with other drugs which lower the seizure threshold. May increase the risks associated with electroconvulsive therapy. Use with caution in hyperthyroid patients or those receiving thyroid supplementation. Use with caution in patients with hepatic or renal dysfunction and in elderly patients.

Adverse Reactions Frequency not defined.

Cardiovascular: Arrhythmia, flushing, heart block, hypertension, MI, palpitation, postural hypotension, tachycardia

Central nervous system: Agitation, anxiety, ataxia, confusion, delirium, delusions, disorientation, dizziness, drowsiness, EEG changes, exacerbation of psychosis, extrapyramidal symptoms, fatigue, hallucinations, headache, hypomania, incoordination, insomnia, nightmares, panic, restlessness, seizure

Dermatologic: Alopecia, itching, petechiae, photosensitivity, rash, urticaria

Endocrine & metabolic: Blood sugar increases/decreases, breast enlargement, galactorrhea, gynecomastia, increase or decrease in libido, sexual dysfunction, SIADH

Gastrointestinal: Abdominal cramps, anorexia, black tongue, constipation, diarrhea, epigastric distress, nausea, paralytic ileus, stomatitis, taste disturbance, vomiting, weight gain/loss, xerostomia

Genitourinary: Delayed micturition, impotence, nocturia, polyuria, testicular edema, urinary retention

Hematologic: Agranulocytosis (rare), eosinophilia, purpura, thrombocytopenia

Hepatic: Cholestatic jaundice, transaminases increased
Neuromuscular & skeletal: Numbness, paresthesia, peripheral neuropathy, tingling, tremor, weakness
Ocular: Blurred vision, disturbances in accommodation, eye pain, mydriasis
Otic: Tinnitus
Miscellaneous: Allergic reactions (eg, general edema or of the face/tongue), diaphoresis (excessive), withdrawal symptoms

Metabolism/Transport Effects Substrate of CYP1A2 (minor), 2C19 (minor), 2D6 (major), 3A4 (minor); **Inhibits** CYP2D6 (weak), 2E1 (weak)

Drug Interactions

Acetylcholinesterase Inhibitors (Central): Anticholinergics may diminish the therapeutic effect of Acetylcholinesterase Inhibitors (Central). Acetylcholinesterase Inhibitors (Central) may diminish the therapeutic effect of Anticholinergics. If the anticholinergic action is a side effect of the agent, the result may be beneficial. *Risk C: Monitor therapy*

Alcohol (Ethyl): CNS Depressants may enhance the CNS depressant effect of Alcohol (Ethyl). *Risk C: Monitor therapy*

Alfuzosin: May enhance the QTc-prolonging effect of QTc-Prolonging Agents. *Risk C: Monitor therapy*

Alpha-/Beta-Agonists (Direct-Acting): Tricyclic Antidepressants may enhance the vasopressor effect of Alpha-/Beta-Agonists (Direct-Acting). **Exceptions:** Dipivefrin. *Risk D: Consider therapy modification*

Alpha1-Agonists: Tricyclic Antidepressants may enhance the vasopressor effect of Alpha1-Agonists. *Risk D: Consider therapy modification*

Alpha2-Agonists: Tricyclic Antidepressants may diminish the antihypertensive effect of Alpha2-Agonists. **Exceptions:** Apraclonidine; Brimonidine. *Risk D: Consider therapy modification*

Altretamine: May enhance the orthostatic effect of Tricyclic Antidepressants. *Risk C: Monitor therapy*

Amphetamines: Tricyclic Antidepressants may enhance the stimulatory effect of Amphetamines. Tricyclic Antidepressants may also potentiate the cardiovascular effects of Amphetamines. *Risk C: Monitor therapy*

Anticholinergics: May enhance the adverse/toxic effect of other Anticholinergics. **Exceptions:** Paliperidone. *Risk C: Monitor therapy*

Barbiturates: May increase the metabolism of Tricyclic Antidepressants. *Risk D: Consider therapy modification*

Beta2-Agonists: Tricyclic Antidepressants may enhance the adverse/toxic effect of Beta2-Agonists. *Risk C: Monitor therapy*

BuPROPion: May decrease the metabolism of Tricyclic Antidepressants. *Risk C: Monitor therapy*

CarBAMazepine: May increase the metabolism of Tricyclic Antidepressants. *Risk C: Monitor therapy*

Cimetidine: May decrease the metabolism of Tricyclic Antidepressants. *Risk C: Monitor therapy*

Cinacalcet: May increase the serum concentration of Tricyclic Antidepressants. *Risk C: Monitor therapy*

Ciprofloxacin: May enhance the QTc-prolonging effect of QTc-Prolonging Agents. *Risk C: Monitor therapy*

CNS Depressants: May enhance the adverse/toxic effect of other CNS Depressants. *Risk C: Monitor therapy*

CYP2D6 Inhibitors (Moderate): May decrease the metabolism of CYP2D6 Substrates. *Risk C: Monitor therapy*

CYP2D6 Inhibitors (Strong): May decrease the metabolism of CYP2D6 Substrates. *Risk D: Consider therapy modification*

Darunavir: May increase the serum concentration of CYP2D6 Substrates. *Risk C: Monitor therapy*

Desmopressin: Tricyclic Antidepressants may enhance the adverse/toxic effect of Desmopressin. *Risk C: Monitor therapy*

Dexmethylphenidate: May decrease the metabolism of Tricyclic Antidepressants. *Risk C: Monitor therapy*

DULoxetine: May decrease the metabolism of Tricyclic Antidepressants. *Risk C: Monitor therapy*

Gadobutrol: May enhance the QTc-prolonging effect of QTc-Prolonging Agents. *Risk D: Consider therapy modification*

Lithium: May enhance the neurotoxic effect of Tricyclic Antidepressants. *Risk C: Monitor therapy*

MAO Inhibitors: May enhance the serotonergic effect of Tricyclic Antidepressants. This may cause serotonin syndrome. *Risk X: Avoid combination*

Methylphenidate: May decrease the metabolism of Tricyclic Antidepressants. *Risk C: Monitor therapy*

Nilotinib: May enhance the QTc-prolonging effect of QTc-Prolonging Agents. *Risk X: Avoid combination*

Pramlintide: May enhance the anticholinergic effect of Anticholinergics. These effects are specific to the GI tract. *Risk D: Consider therapy modification*

Propoxyphene: May enhance the CNS depressant effect of Tricyclic Antidepressants. *Risk C: Monitor therapy*

Protease Inhibitors: May increase the serum concentration of Tricyclic Antidepressants. *Risk C: Monitor therapy*

QTc-Prolonging Agents: May enhance the adverse/toxic effect of other QTc-Prolonging Agents. Their effects can be additive, causing life-threatening ventricular arrhythmias. *Risk D: Consider therapy modification*

QuiNIDine: Tricyclic Antidepressants may enhance the QTc-prolonging effect of QuiNIDine. QuiNIDine may decrease the metabolism of Tricyclic Antidepressants. *Risk D: Consider therapy modification*

Selective Serotonin Reuptake Inhibitors: May decrease the metabolism of Tricyclic Antidepressants. *Risk D: Consider therapy modification*

Serotonin Modulators: May enhance the adverse/toxic effect of other Serotonin Modulators. The development of serotonin syndrome may occur. *Risk D: Consider therapy modification*

Sibutramine: May enhance the serotonergic effect of Serotonin Modulators. This may cause serotonin syndrome. *Risk X: Avoid combination*

St Johns Wort: May increase the metabolism of Tricyclic Antidepressants. The risk of serotonin syndrome may theoretically be increased. *Risk D: Consider therapy modification*

Sulfonylureas: Cyclic Antidepressants may enhance the hypoglycemic effect of Sulfonylureas. *Risk C: Monitor therapy*

Terbinafine: May decrease the metabolism of Tricyclic Antidepressants. *Risk D: Consider therapy modification*

Tetrabenazine: QTc-Prolonging Agents may enhance the QTc-prolonging effect of Tetrabenazine. *Risk X: Avoid combination*

Thioridazine: QTc-Prolonging Agents may enhance the QTc-prolonging effect of Thioridazine. *Risk X: Avoid combination*

TraMADol: Tricyclic Antidepressants may enhance the neuroexcitatory and/or seizure-potentiating effect of TraMADol. *Risk C: Monitor therapy*

Valproic Acid: May increase the serum concentration of Tricyclic Antidepressants. *Risk C: Monitor therapy*

Vitamin K Antagonists (eg, warfarin): Tricyclic Antidepressants may enhance the anticoagulant effect of Vitamin K Antagonists. *Risk C: Monitor therapy*

Ziprasidone: QTc-Prolonging Agents may enhance the QTc-prolonging effect of Ziprasidone. The risk of a severe arrhythmia may be increased. *Risk X: Avoid combination*

Ethanol/Nutrition/Herb Interactions

Ethanol: Avoid ethanol (may increase CNS depression).

Herb/Nutraceutical: Avoid valerian, St John's wort, SAMe, kava kava (may increase risk of serotonin syndrome and/or excessive sedation).

Stability Store at 20°C to 25°C (68°F to 77°F). Protect from light.

Mechanism of Action Traditionally believed to increase the synaptic concentration of serotonin and/or norepinephrine in the central nervous system by inhibition of their reuptake by the presynaptic neuronal membrane. However, additional receptor effects have been found including desensitization of adenyl cyclase, down regulation of beta-adrenergic receptors, and down regulation of serotonin receptors.

Pharmacodynamics/Kinetics

Onset of action: Therapeutic: 1-3 weeks

Distribution: V_d: 21 L/kg

Protein binding: 93% to 95%

Metabolism: Primarily hepatic; extensive first-pass effect

Half-life elimination: 28-31 hours

Time to peak, serum: 7-8.5 hours

Excretion: Urine (as metabolites and small amounts of unchanged drug); feces (small amounts)

Dosage Oral:

Nocturnal enuresis: Children (unlabeled use): 10-20 mg/day; titrate to a maximum of 40 mg/day

Depression: Children (unlabeled use): 1-3 mg/kg/day

Depression:

Adults: 25 mg 3-4 times/day up to 150 mg/day; doses may be given once daily

Elderly: Initial: 30-50 mg/day, given as a single daily dose or in divided doses. **Note:** Nortriptyline is one of the best tolerated TCAs in the elderly)

Myofascial pain, neuralgia, burning mouth syndrome (dental use): Adults: Initial: 10-25 mg at bedtime; dosage may be increased by 25 mg/day weekly, if tolerated; usual maintenance dose: 75 mg as a single bedtime dose or 2 divided doses

Chronic urticaria, angioedema, nocturnal pruritus (unlabeled use): Adults: Oral: 75 mg/day

Smoking cessation (unlabeled use): Adults: 25-75 mg/day beginning 10-14 days before "quit" day; continue therapy for ≥12 weeks after "quit" day

Dosing adjustment in hepatic impairment: Lower doses and slower titration dependent on individualization of dosage is recommended

Monitoring Parameters Blood pressure and pulse rate (ECG, cardiac monitoring) prior to and during initial therapy in older adults; weight; blood levels are useful for therapeutic monitoring; suicidal ideation (especially at the beginning of therapy or when doses are increased or decreased)

Reference Range

Plasma levels do not always correlate with clinical effectiveness

Therapeutic: 50-150 ng/mL (SI: 190-570 nmol/L)

Toxic: >500 ng/mL (SI: >1900 nmol/L)

Dosage Forms Excipient information presented when available (limited, particularly for generics); consult specific product labeling.

Capsule: 10 mg, 25 mg, 50 mg, 75 mg

Pamelor®: 10 mg, 25 mg, 50 mg, 75 mg [may contain benzyl alcohol; 50 mg may also contain sodium bisulfite]

Solution:

Pamelor®: 10 mg/5 mL (473 mL) [contains ethanol 4% and benzoic acid]

- **Nortriptyline Hydrochloride** *see* Nortriptyline *on page 1152*
- **Norvasc®** *see* AmLODIPine *on page 100*
- **Norvir®** *see* Ritonavir *on page 1433*
- **Novahistine DH** *see* Dihydrocodeine, Chlorpheniramine, and Phenylephrine *on page 469*
- **Novantrone®** *see* Mitoxantrone *on page 1061*
- **Novarel®** *see* Chorionic Gonadotropin (Human) *on page 342*
- **Novocain®** *see* Procaine *on page 1340*
- **Novolin® 70/30** *see* Insulin NPH and Insulin Regular *on page 836*
- **Novolin® N** *see* Insulin NPH *on page 835*
- **Novolin® R** *see* Insulin Regular *on page 838*
- **NovoLog®** *see* Insulin Aspart *on page 822*
- **NovoLog® Mix 70/30** *see* Insulin Aspart Protamine and Insulin Aspart *on page 824*
- **Noxafil®** *see* Posaconazole *on page 1314*
- **NPH Insulin** *see* Insulin NPH *on page 835*
- **NPH Insulin and Regular Insulin** *see* Insulin NPH and Insulin Regular *on page 836*
- **NRP104** *see* Lisdexamfetamine *on page 931*
- **NRS® [OTC]** *see* Oxymetazoline *on page 1208*
- **NSC-740** *see* Methotrexate *on page 1014*
- **NSC-750** *see* Busulfan *on page 226*
- **NSC-752** *see* Thioguanine *on page 1569*
- **NSC-755** *see* Mercaptopurine *on page 993*
- **NSC-762** *see* Mechlorethamine *on page 974*
- **NSC-3053** *see* DACTINomycin *on page 415*
- **NSC-3088** *see* Chlorambucil *on page 315*
- **NSC-8806** *see* Melphalan *on page 983*
- **NSC-13875** *see* Altretamine *on page 78*
- **NSC-15200** *see* Gallium Nitrate *on page 707*
- **NSC-26271** *see* Cyclophosphamide *on page 408*
- **NSC-26980** *see* Mitomycin *on page 1061*
- **NSC-27640** *see* Floxuridine *on page 634*
- **NSC-38721** *see* Mitotane *on page 1061*
- **NSC-49842** *see* VinBLAStine *on page 1672*
- **NSC-63878** *see* Cytarabine *on page 412*
- **NSC-66847** *see* Thalidomide *on page 1561*
- **NSC-67574** *see* VinCRIStine *on page 1673*
- **NSC-71423** *see* Megestrol *on page 977*
- **NSC-77213** *see* Procarbazine *on page 1340*

◆ **NSC-79037** *see* Lomustine *on page 943*
◆ **NSC-82151** *see* DAUNOrubicin Hydrochloride *on page 421*
◆ **NSC-85998** *see* Streptozocin *on page 1510*
◆ **NSC-89199** *see* Estramustine *on page 580*
◆ **NSC-102816** *see* AzaCITIDine *on page 161*
◆ **NSC-105014** *see* Cladribine *on page 360*
◆ **NSC-106977 (*Erwinia*)** *see* Asparaginase *on page 142*
◆ **NSC-109229 (*E. coli*)** *see* Asparaginase *on page 142*
◆ **NSC-109724** *see* Ifosfamide *on page 809*
◆ **NSC-122758** *see* Tretinoin, Oral *on page 1617*
◆ **NSC-123127** *see* DOXOrubicin *on page 507*
◆ **NSC-125066** *see* Bleomycin *on page 192*
◆ **NSC-125973** *see* Paclitaxel *on page 1213*
◆ **NSC-127716** *see* Decitabine *on page 422*
◆ **NSC-147834** *see* Flutamide *on page 667*
◆ **NSC-169780** *see* Dexrazoxane *on page 441*
◆ **NSC-218321** *see* Pentostatin *on page 1250*
◆ **NSC-241240** *see* CARBOplatin *on page 281*
◆ **NSC-256439** *see* IDArubicin *on page 809*
◆ **NSC-256942** *see* Epirubicin *on page 545*
◆ **NSC-266046** *see* Oxaliplatin *on page 1191*
◆ **NSC-301739** *see* Mitoxantrone *on page 1061*
◆ **NSC-308847** *see* Amonafide *on page 108*
◆ **NSC-312887** *see* Fludarabine *on page 641*
◆ **NSC-352122** *see* Trimetrexate *on page 1629*
◆ **NSC-362856** *see* Temozolomide *on page 1547*
◆ **NSC-367982** *see* Interferon Alfa-2a *on page 844*
◆ **NSC-373364** *see* Aldesleukin *on page 58*
◆ **NSC-377523** *see* Interferon Alfa-2b *on page 844*
◆ **NSC-409962** *see* Carmustine *on page 284*
◆ **NSC-603071** *see* Aminocamptothecin *on page 86*
◆ **NSC-606864** *see* Goserelin *on page 735*
◆ **NSC606869** *see* Clofarabine *on page 367*
◆ **NSC-609699** *see* Topotecan *on page 1602*
◆ **NSC-613327** *see* Gemcitabine *on page 710*
◆ **NSC-613795** *see* Sargramostim *on page 1462*
◆ **NSC-614629** *see* Filgrastim *on page 632*
◆ **NSC-616348** *see* Irinotecan *on page 856*
◆ **NSC-628503** *see* Docetaxel *on page 491*
◆ **NSC-644468** *see* Deferoxamine *on page 423*
◆ **NSC-644954** *see* Pegaspargase *on page 1235*
◆ **NSC-671663** *see* Octreotide *on page 1158*
◆ **NSC-673089** *see* Paclitaxel *on page 1213*
◆ **NSC-681239** *see* Bortezomib *on page 192*
◆ **NSC-683864** *see* Temsirolimus *on page 1547*
◆ **NSC-684588** *see* Nilutamide *on page 1140*
◆ **NSC-687451** *see* RiTUXimab *on page 1434*
◆ **NSC-688097** *see* Trastuzumab *on page 1613*
◆ **NSC-697732** *see* DAUNOrubicin Citrate (Liposomal) *on page 421*
◆ **NSC-698037** *see* Pemetrexed *on page 1238*
◆ **NSC-701852** *see* Vorinostat *on page 1678*
◆ **NSC-703813** *see* Lenalidomide *on page 899*
◆ **NSC-704865** *see* Bevacizumab *on page 187*
◆ **NSC-706363** *see* Arsenic Trioxide *on page 140*
◆ **NSC-706725** *see* Raloxifene *on page 1391*
◆ **NSC-712227** *see* DOXOrubicin (Liposomal) *on page 508*
◆ **NSC-712807** *see* Capecitabine *on page 263*

- **NSC-714692** *see* Cetuximab *on page 310*
- **NSC-714744** *see* Denileukin Diftitox *on page 425*
- **NSC-715055** *see* Gefitinib *on page 709*
- **NSC-715969** *see* Alemtuzumab *on page 59*
- **NSC-716051** *see* Imatinib *on page 810*
- **NSC-718781** *see* Erlotinib *on page 556*
- **NSC-719344** *see* Anastrozole *on page 125*
- **NSC-719345** *see* Letrozole *on page 900*
- **NSC-720568** *see* Gemtuzumab Ozogamicin *on page 713*
- **NSC-721517** *see* Zoledronic Acid *on page 1702*
- **NSC-721631** *see* Rasburicase *on page 1407*
- **NSC-722623** *see* Ibandronate *on page 801*
- **NSC-722848** *see* Oprelvekin *on page 1184*
- **NSC-724223** *see* Epoetin Alfa *on page 546*
- **NSC-724577** *see* Anagrelide *on page 124*
- **NSC-724772** *see* Sorafenib *on page 1501*
- **NSC-725961** *see* Pegfilgrastim *on page 1236*
- **NSC-727989** *see* Lapatinib *on page 898*
- **NSC-728729** *see* InFLIXimab *on page 819*
- **NSC-729969** *see* Darbepoetin Alfa *on page 419*
- **NSC-732517** *see* Dasatinib *on page 420*
- **NSC-736511** *see* Sunitinib *on page 1530*
- **NSC-736631** *see* Paclitaxel (Protein Bound) *on page 1214*
- **NSC-742319** *see* Panitumumab *on page 1221*
- **NTG** *see* Nitroglycerin *on page 1147*
- ***N*-trifluoroacetyladriamycin-14-valerate** *see* Valrubicin *on page 1649*
- **NTZ** *see* Nitazoxanide *on page 1146*
- **Nubain®** *see* Nalbuphine *on page 1094*
- **Nucofed®** *see* Pseudoephedrine and Codeine *on page 1368*
- **Nucofed® Expectorant [DSC]** *see* Guaifenesin, Pseudoephedrine, and Codeine *on page 747*
- **Nucofed® Pediatric Expectorant [DSC]** *see* Guaifenesin, Pseudoephedrine, and Codeine *on page 747*
- **Nu-Iron® 150 [OTC]** *see* Polysaccharide-Iron Complex *on page 1313*
- **NuLev™ [DSC]** *see* Hyoscyamine *on page 799*
- **NuLYTELY®** *see* Polyethylene Glycol-Electrolyte Solution *on page 1310*
- **Nupercainal® Hydrocortisone Cream [OTC]** *see* Hydrocortisone *on page 785*
- **Nutracort®** *see* Hydrocortisone *on page 785*
- **Nutralox® [OTC]** *see* Calcium Carbonate *on page 254*
- **Nutropin®** *see* Somatropin *on page 1499*
- **Nutropin AQ®** *see* Somatropin *on page 1499*
- **NuvaRing®** *see* Ethinyl Estradiol and Etonogestrel *on page 594*
- **Nuvigil™** *see* Armodafinil *on page 138*
- **NVP** *see* Nevirapine *on page 1124*
- **Nytol® Quick Caps [OTC]** *see* DiphenhydrAMINE *on page 481*
- **Nytol® Quick Gels [OTC]** *see* DiphenhydrAMINE *on page 481*
- **NāSop™ [DSC]** *see* Phenylephrine *on page 1273*
- **Nōstrilla® [OTC]** *see* Oxymetazoline *on page 1208*
- **OCBZ** *see* OXcarbazepine *on page 1195*
- **Occlusal®-HP [OTC]** *see* Salicylic Acid *on page 1454*
- **Ocella™** *see* Ethinyl Estradiol and Drospirenone *on page 593*

Octreotide (ok TREE oh tide)

Medication Safety Issues

Sound-alike/look-alike issues:

Sandostatin® may be confused with Sandimmune®, Sandostatin LAR®, sargramostim, simvastatin

U.S. Brand Names Sandostatin LAR®; Sandostatin®

Canadian Brand Names Octreotide Acetate Injection; Octreotide Acetate Omega; Sandostatin LAR®; Sandostatin®
Mexican Brand Names Cryostatin; Nomactril; Proclose; Sandostatina
Index Terms NSC-671663; Octreotide Acetate
Pharmacologic Category Antidiarrheal; Antidote; Somatostatin Analog
Use Control of symptoms in patients with metastatic carcinoid and vasoactive intestinal peptide-secreting tumors (VIPomas); treatment of acromegaly
Unlabeled/Investigational Use AIDS-associated secretory diarrhea (including *Cryptosporidiosis*); control of bleeding of esophageal varices; second-line treatment for thymic malignancies; Cushing's syndrome (ectopic); insulinomas; glucagonoma; small bowel fistulas; pancreatic tumors; gastrinoma; postgastrectomy dumping syndrome; chemotherapy-induced diarrhea; graft-versus-host disease (GVHD) induced diarrhea; Zollinger-Ellison syndrome; congenital hyperinsulinism; hypothalamic obesity; treatment of hypoglycemia secondary to sulfonylurea poisoning (as an adjunct to dextrose)
Effect on Mental Status May cause drowsiness, dizziness, or depression; may rarely cause anxiety
Effect on Psychiatric Treatment None reported
Dosage Summary

I.M.:
Children: Dosage not established
Adults: Depot: 20 mg every 4 weeks (maximum: 40 mg every 2 weeks)

I.V.:
Children (unlabeled use): 1-10 mcg/kg every 12 hours
Adults: 50-1500 mcg/day in 2-4 divided doses

SubQ:
Children (unlabeled use): 1-10 mcg/kg every 12 hours **or** 3-40 mcg/kg/day
Adults: 50-1500 mcg/day in 2-4 divided doses

Dosage Forms Excipient information presented when available (limited, particularly for generics); consult specific product labeling.
Injection, microspheres for suspension, as acetate [depot formulation]:
Sandostatin LAR®: 10 mg, 20 mg, 30 mg [contains polylactide-co-glycolide; packaged with diluent and syringe]
Injection, solution, as acetate: 0.2 mg/mL (5 mL); 1 mg/mL (5 mL)
Sandostatin®: 0.2 mg/mL (5 mL); 1 mg/mL (5 mL)
Injection, solution, as acetate [preservative free]: 0.05 mg/mL (1 mL); 0.1 mg/mL (1 mL); 0.5 mg/mL (1 mL)
Sandostatin®: 0.05 mg/mL (1 mL); 0.1 mg/mL (1 mL); 0.5 mg/mL (1 mL)

- ◆ **Octreotide Acetate** *see* Octreotide *on page 1158*
- ◆ **Ocufen®** *see* Flurbiprofen *on page 667*
- ◆ **Ocuflox®** *see* Ofloxacin *on page 1159*
- ◆ **OcuNefrin™ [OTC]** *see* Phenylephrine *on page 1273*
- ◆ **O-desmethylvenlafaxine** *see* Desvenlafaxine *on page 433*
- ◆ **ODV** *see* Desvenlafaxine *on page 433*
- ◆ **Off-Ezy® Wart Remover [OTC] [DSC]** *see* Salicylic Acid *on page 1454*

Ofloxacin (oh FLOKS a sin)

Medication Safety Issues
Sound-alike/look-alike issues:
Floxin® may be confused with Flexeril®
Ocuflox® may be confused with Occlusal®-HP, Ocufen®

International issues:
Floxin® may be confused with Flogen® which is a brand name for naproxen in Mexico
Floxin® may be confused with Fluoxin® which is a brand name for fluoxetine in the Czech Republic and Romania
Floxin® may be confused with Flexin® which is a brand name for orphenadrine in Israel and indomethacin in Great Britain

U.S. Brand Names Floxin®; Ocuflox®
Canadian Brand Names Apo-Ofloxacin® ; Apo-Oflox®; Floxin®; Novo-Ofloxacin; Ocuflox®; PMS-Ofloxacin
Mexican Brand Names Bactocin; Floxil; Floxstat; Ocuflox
Index Terms Floxin Otic Singles
Pharmacologic Category Antibiotic, Quinolone
Use Quinolone antibiotic for the treatment of acute exacerbations of chronic bronchitis, community-acquired pneumonia, skin and skin structure infections (uncomplicated), urethral and cervical gonorrhea (acute, uncomplicated),

urethritis and cervicitis (nongonococcal), mixed infections of the urethra and cervix, pelvic inflammatory disease (acute), cystitis (uncomplicated), urinary tract infections (complicated), prostatitis

Note: As of April 2007, the CDC no longer recommends the use of fluoroquinolones for the treatment of gonococcal disease.

Ophthalmic: Treatment of superficial ocular infections involving the conjunctiva or cornea due to strains of susceptible organisms

Otic: Otitis externa, chronic suppurative otitis media, acute otitis media

Unlabeled/Investigational Use Epididymitis (nongonococcal), leprosy, Traveler's diarrhea

Effect on Mental Status May cause drowsiness, dizziness, nervousness, or insomnia; quinolones reported to cause restlessness, hallucinations, euphoria, depression, panic, and paranoia

Effect on Psychiatric Treatment Inhibits CYP1A2 isoenzyme; use caution with clozapine and other psychotropics; monitor for adverse effects

Restrictions An FDA-approved patient medication guide is available and must be distributed when dispensing an outpatient prescription (new or refill) where this medication is to be used without direct supervision of a healthcare provider. Medication guides are available at http://www.fda.gov/cder/Offices/ODS/medication_guides.htm.

Dosage Summary

Ophthalmic:

Children ≤1 year: Dosage not established

Children >1 year: Initial: 1-2 drops every 30 minutes to 4 hours; Maintenance: 1-2 drops every 4-6 hours

Adults: Initial: 1-2 drops every 30 minutes to 4 hours; Maintenance: 1-2 drops every 4-6 hours

Oral:

Children: Dosage not established

Adults: 200-400 mg every 12 hours

Otic:

Children <6 months: Dosage not established

Children ≥6 months to 12 years: 5 drops daily

Children >12 years: 10 drops once or twice daily

Adults: 10 drops once or twice daily

Dosage Forms Excipient information presented when available (limited, particularly for generics); consult specific product labeling.

Solution, ophthalmic [drops]: 0.3% (5 mL, 10 mL)

Ocuflox®: 0.3% (5 mL) [contains benzalkonium chloride]

Solution, otic [drops]: 0.3% (5 mL, 10 mL)

Floxin®: 0.3% (5 mL, 10 mL) [contains benzalkonium chloride]

Floxin® Otic Singles™: 0.3% (0.25 mL) [contains benzalkonium chloride; packaged as 2 single-dose containers per pouch, 10 pouches per carton, total net volume 5 mL]

Tablet: 200 mg, 300 mg, 400 mg

- **Ogen®** *see* Estropipate *on page 588*
- **Ogestrel®** *see* Ethinyl Estradiol and Norgestrel *on page 601*
- **OGMT** *see* Metyrosine *on page 1044*
- **OGT-918** *see* Miglustat *on page 1053*
- **9-OH-risperidone** *see* Paliperidone *on page 1215*
- **OKT3** *see* Muromonab-CD3 *on page 1086*

OLANZapine (oh LAN za peen)

Medication Safety Issues

Sound-alike/look-alike issues:

OLANZapine may be confused with olsalazine, QUEtiapine

Zyprexa® may be confused with Celexa™, Zyrtec®

Related Information

Agents Approved for Bipolar Disorder *on page 1752*

Antipsychotic Agents *on page 1769*

Antipsychotic Receptor Profile *on page 1772*

Atypical Antipsychotics *on page 1773*

CMS: Long-Term Care Facility Thresholds *on page 1815*

Discontinuation of Psychotropic Drugs *on page 1839*

U.S. Brand Names Zyprexa®; Zyprexa® Zydis®

Canadian Brand Names Novo-Olanzapine; Zyprexa®; Zyprexa® Zydis®

Mexican Brand Names Zyprexa

Index Terms LY170053; Zyprexa Zydis

Pharmacologic Category Antimanic Agent; Antipsychotic Agent, Atypical

Generic Available No

Use Treatment of the manifestations of schizophrenia; treatment of acute or mixed mania episodes associated with Bipolar I Disorder (as monotherapy or in combination with lithium or valproate); maintenance treatment of bipolar disorder; acute agitation (patients with schizophrenia or bipolar mania)

Unlabeled/Investigational Use Treatment of psychosis/schizophrenia in children or adolescents; chronic pain; prevention of chemotherapy-associated delayed nausea or vomiting; psychosis/agitation related to Alzheimer's dementia

Mental Health Comment Olanzapine is an antipsychotic agent of a class often referred to as atypical. It should be noted that the definition of the term "atypical" is not universally agreed upon. Some prefer to describe antipsychotics based on their pharmacological properties. A common feature of all definitions used to describe "atypical" antipsychotics is the lack of significant acute or subacute EPS, at dosages generally associated with antipsychotic actions. Other experts have included definitions of atypicality that include a) failure to increase serum prolactin levels; b) superior efficacy for positive, negative, and cognitive symptoms; and c) lack of evidence of tardive dyskinesia or dystonia following chronic administration. Olanzapine meets most of these criteria, but is associated with dose-dependent EPS. Fortunately, if doses are kept within the approved dosage range (5-20 mg/day), EPS is low.

Tardive dyskinesia (TD) secondary to **typical** antipsychotics has an estimated incidence of 3% to 5% per year for the first 5 years of treatment. The incidence of TD associated with the atypical antipsychotics is estimated to be 0.5% to 1%. It is not clear if this estimate represents a risk associated with mental illness or to what extent drug therapy can be implicated. Atypical antipsychotics appear less likely to cause tardive dyskinesia than typical antipsychotics (fluphenazine, haloperidol).

Coadministration of two or more antipsychotics does not generally improve clinical response and may increase the potential for adverse effects.

In 2008, the FDA issued a warning regarding increased mortality risk with typical **and** atypical antipsychotic drugs when used in elderly patients with dementia-related psychosis.

Pregnancy Risk Factor C

Pregnancy Considerations No evidence of teratogenicity reported in animal studies. However, fetal toxicity and prolonged gestation have been observed. There are no adequate and well-controlled studies in pregnant women.

Lactation Enters breast milk/not recommended

Contraindications Hypersensitivity to olanzapine or any component of the formulation

Warnings/Precautions **[U.S. Boxed Warning]: Elderly patients with dementia-related psychosis treated with atypical antipsychotics are at an increased risk of death compared to placebo.** An increased incidence of cerebrovascular adverse events (including fatalities) has been reported in elderly patients with dementia-related psychosis. Olanzapine is not approved for this indication.

Moderate to highly sedating, use with caution in disorders where CNS depression is a feature; patients must be cautioned about performing tasks which require mental alertness (eg, operating machinery or driving). Use caution in patients with cardiac disease. Use with caution in Parkinson's disease, predisposition to seizures, or severe hepatic or renal disease. Life-threatening arrhythmias have occurred with therapeutic doses of some neuroleptics. May induce orthostatic hypotension; use caution with history of cardiovascular disease. Esophageal dysmotility and aspiration have been associated with antipsychotic use; use with caution in patients at risk of aspiration pneumonia. Caution in breast cancer or other prolactin-dependent tumors (elevates prolactin levels). Significant weight gain (>7% of baseline weight) may occur; monitor waist circumference and BMI. Impaired core body temperature regulation may occur; caution with strenuous exercise, heat exposure, dehydration, and concomitant medication possessing anticholinergic effects.

May cause anticholinergic effects; use with caution in patients with decreased gastrointestinal motility, urinary retention, BPH, xerostomia, glaucoma, or myasthenia gravis. Relative to other neuroleptics, olanzapine has a moderate potency of cholinergic blockade. May cause extrapyramidal symptoms (EPS), although risk of these reactions is lower relative to other neuroleptics. Risk of dystonia (and probably other EPS) may be greater with increased doses, use of conventional antipsychotics, males, and younger patients. May be associated with neuroleptic malignant syndrome (NMS). May cause extreme and life-threatening hyperglycemia; use with caution in patients with diabetes or other disorders of glucose regulation; monitor. Olanzapine levels may be lower in patients who smoke, requiring dosage adjustment.

The possibility of a suicide attempt is inherent in psychotic illness or bipolar disorder; use caution in high-risk patients during initiation of therapy. Prescriptions should be written for the smallest quantity consistent with good patient care. Safety and efficacy in pediatric patients have not been established.

Intramuscular administration: Patients should remain recumbent if drowsy/dizzy until hypotension, bradycardia, and/or hypoventilation has been ruled out. Concurrent use of I.M./I.V. benzodiazepines is not recommended (fatalities have been reported, though causality not determined).

Adverse Reactions

>10%:

Central nervous system: Somnolence (6% to 39% dose dependent), extrapyramidal symptoms (15% to 32% dose dependent), insomnia (up to 12%), dizziness (4% to 18%)

Gastrointestinal: Dyspepsia (7% to 11%), constipation (9% to 11%), weight gain (5% to 6%, has been reported as high as 40%), xerostomia (9% to 22% dose dependent)

Neuromuscular & skeletal: Weakness (2% to 20% dose dependent)

Miscellaneous: Accidental injury (12%)

1% to 10%:

Cardiovascular: Postural hypotension (1% to 5%), tachycardia (up to 3%), peripheral edema (up to 3%), chest pain (up to 3%), hyper-/hypotension (up to 2%)

Central nervous system: Personality changes (8%), speech disorder (7%), fever (up to 6%), abnormal dreams, euphoria, amnesia, delusions, emotional lability, mania, schizophrenia

Dermatologic: Bruising (up to 5%)

Endocrine & metabolic: Cholesterol increased, prolactin increased

Gastrointestinal: Nausea (up to 9% dose dependent), appetite increased (3% to 6%), vomiting (up to 4%), flatulence, salivation increased, thirst

Genitourinary: Incontinence (up to 2%), UTI (up to 2%), vaginitis

Hepatic: ALT increased (2%)

Local: Injection site pain (I.M. administration)

Neuromuscular & skeletal: Tremor (1% to 7% dose dependent), abnormal gait (6%), back pain (up to 5%), joint/extremity pain (up to 5%), akathisia (3% to 5% dose dependent), hypertonia (up to 3%), articulation impairment (up to 2%), falling (particularly in older patients), joint stiffness, paresthesia, twitching

Ocular: Amblyopia (up to 3%), conjunctivitis

Respiratory: Rhinitis (up to 7%), cough (up to 6%), pharyngitis (up to 4%), dyspnea

Miscellaneous: Dental pain, diaphoresis, flu-like syndrome

<1% (Limited to important or life-threatening): Acidosis, akinesia, albuminuria, anaphylactoid reaction, anemia, angioedema, apnea, arteritis, asthma, ataxia, atelectasis, atrial fibrillation, AV block, cerebrovascular accident, coma, confusion, congestive heart failure, deafness, diabetes mellitus, diabetic acidosis, diabetic coma, dyskinesia, dysphagia, dystonia, dysuria, encephalopathy, facial paralysis, glaucoma, gynecomastia, heart arrest, heart block, heart failure, hematuria, hemoptysis, hemorrhage (eye, rectal, subarachnoid, vaginal), hepatitis, hyper-/hypoglycemia, hyper-/hypokalemia, hyperlipemia, hyper-/hyponatremia, hyperuricemia, hyper-/hypoventilation, hypoesthesia, hypokinesia, hypoproteinemia, hypoxia, jaundice, ileus, ketosis, leukocytosis (eosinophilia), leukopenia, liver damage (cholestatic or mixed), liver fatty deposit, lung edema, lymphadenopathy, menstrual irregularities, migraine, myasthenia, myopathy, neuralgia, neuroleptic malignant syndrome, neuropathy, neutropenia, osteoporosis, pancreatitis, paralysis, priapism, pulmonary embolus, rhabdomyolysis, seizure, stridor, sudden death, suicide attempt, syncope, tardive dyskinesia, thrombocythemia, thrombocytopenia, tongue edema, venous thrombotic events, vomiting, withdrawal syndrome

Metabolism/Transport Effects Substrate of CYP1A2 (major), 2D6 (minor); **Inhibits** CYP1A2 (weak), 2C9 (weak), 2C19 (weak), 2D6 (weak), 3A4 (weak)

Drug Interactions

Acetylcholinesterase Inhibitors (Central): May enhance the neurotoxic (central) effect of Antipsychotics. Severe extrapyramidal symptoms have occurred in some patients. *Risk C: Monitor therapy*

Alcohol (Ethyl): CNS Depressants may enhance the CNS depressant effect of Alcohol (Ethyl). *Risk C: Monitor therapy*

Amphetamines: Antipsychotics may diminish the stimulatory effect of Amphetamines. *Risk C: Monitor therapy*

Anticholinergics: May enhance the adverse/toxic effect of other Anticholinergics. **Exceptions:** Paliperidone. *Risk C: Monitor therapy*

Anti-Parkinson's Agents (Dopamine Agonist): Antipsychotics (Atypical) may diminish the therapeutic effect of Anti-Parkinson's Agents (Dopamine Agonist). *Risk D: Consider therapy modification*

CNS Depressants: May enhance the adverse/toxic effect of other CNS Depressants. *Risk C: Monitor therapy*

CYP1A2 Inducers (Strong): May increase the metabolism of CYP1A2 Substrates. *Risk C: Monitor therapy*

CYP1A2 Inhibitors (Moderate): May decrease the metabolism of CYP1A2 Substrates. *Risk C: Monitor therapy*

CYP1A2 Inhibitors (Strong): May decrease the metabolism of CYP1A2 Substrates. *Risk D: Consider therapy modification*

Fluvoxamine: May decrease the metabolism of OLANZapine. *Risk D: Consider therapy modification*

LamoTRIgine: May enhance the sedative effect of OLANZapine. *Risk C: Monitor therapy*

Lithium formulations: May enhance the neurotoxic effect of Antipsychotics. Lithium formulations may decrease the serum concentration of Antipsychotics. Specifically noted with chlorpromazine. *Risk C: Monitor therapy*

Pramlintide: May enhance the anticholinergic effect of Anticholinergics. These effects are specific to the GI tract. *Risk D: Consider therapy modification*

Tetrabenazine: May enhance the adverse/toxic effect of Antipsychotics. *Risk C: Monitor therapy*

Ethanol/Nutrition/Herb Interactions

Ethanol: Avoid ethanol (may increase CNS depression).

Herb/Nutraceutical: Avoid dong quai, St John's wort (may also cause photosensitization). Avoid kava kava, gotu kola, valerian, St John's wort (may increase CNS depression).

Stability

Injection, powder for reconstitution: Store at room temperature 15°C to 30°C (59°F to 86°F); do not freeze. Protect from light. Reconstitute 10 mg vial with 2.1 mL SWFI. Resulting solution is ~5 mg/mL. Use immediately (within 1 hour) following reconstitution. Discard any unused portion.

Tablet and orally-disintegrating tablet: Store at room temperature of 15°C to 30°C (59°F to 86°F). Protect from light and moisture.

Mechanism of Action Olanzapine is a second generation thienobenzodiazepine antipsychotic which displays potent antagonism of serotonin 5-HT_{2A} and 5-HT_{2C}, dopamine D_{1-4}, histamine H_1 and alpha$_1$-adrenergic receptors. Olanzapine shows moderate antagonism of 5-HT_3 and muscarinic M_{1-5} receptors, and weak binding to GABA-A, BZD, and beta-adrenergic receptors. Although the precise mechanism of action in schizophrenia and bipolar disorder is not known, the efficacy of olanzapine is thought to be mediated through combined antagonism of dopamine and serotonin type 2 receptor sites.

Pharmacodynamics/Kinetics

Absorption:

I.M.: Rapidly absorbed

Oral: Well absorbed; not affected by food; tablets and orally-disintegrating tablets are bioequivalent

Distribution: V_d: Extensive, 1000 L

Protein binding, plasma: 93% bound to albumin and alpha$_1$-glycoprotein

Metabolism: Highly metabolized via direct glucuronidation and cytochrome P450 mediated oxidation (CYP1A2, CYP2D6); 40% removed via first pass metabolism

Bioavailability: >57%

Half-life elimination: 21-54 hours; ~1.5 times greater in elderly

Time to peak, plasma: Maximum plasma concentrations after I.M. administration are 5 times higher than maximum plasma concentrations produced by an oral dose.

I.M.: 15-45 minutes

Oral: ~6 hours

Excretion: Urine (57%, 7% as unchanged drug); feces (30%)

Clearance: 40% increase in olanzapine clearance in smokers; 30% decrease in females

Dosage

Children: Schizophrenia/bipolar disorder (unlabeled use): Oral: Initial: 2.5 mg/day; titrate as necessary to 20 mg/day (0.12-0.29 mg/kg/day)

Adults:

Schizophrenia: Oral: Initial: 5-10 mg once daily (increase to 10 mg once daily within 5-7 days); thereafter, adjust by 5 mg/day at 1-week intervals, up to a recommended maximum of 20 mg/day. Maintenance: 10-20 mg once daily. **Note:** Doses of 30-50 mg/day have been used; however, doses >10 mg/day have not demonstrated better efficacy, and safety and efficacy of doses >20 mg/day have not been evaluated.

Bipolar I acute mixed or manic episodes: Oral:

Monotherapy: Initial: 10-15 mg once daily; increase by 5 mg/day at intervals of not less than 24 hours. Maintenance: 5-20 mg/day; recommended maximum dose: 20 mg/day.

Combination therapy (with lithium or valproate): Initial: 10 mg once daily; dosing range: 5-20 mg/day

Agitation (acute, associated with bipolar I mania or schizophrenia): I.M.: Initial dose: 5-10 mg (a lower dose of 2.5 mg may be considered when clinical factors warrant); additional doses (2.5-10 mg) may be considered; however, 2-4 hours should be allowed between doses to evaluate response (maximum total daily dose: 30 mg, per manufacturer's recommendation)

Prevention of chemotherapy-associated delayed nausea or vomiting (unlabeled use; in combination with a corticosteroid and serotonin [$5HT_3$] antagonist): Oral: 10 mg once daily for 3-5 days, beginning on day 1 of chemotherapy **or** 5 mg once daily for 2 days before chemotherapy, followed by 10 mg once daily (beginning on the day of chemotherapy) for 3-8 days

Elderly: Oral, I.M.: Consider lower starting dose of 2.5-5 mg/day for elderly or debilitated patients; may increase as clinically indicated and tolerated with close monitoring of orthostatic blood pressure

Psychosis/agitation related to Alzheimer's dementia (unlabeled use): Initial: 1.25-5 mg/day; if necessary, gradually increase as tolerated not to exceed 10 mg/day

Dosage adjustment in renal impairment: No adjustment required. Not removed by dialysis.

Dosage adjustment in hepatic impairment: Dosage adjustment may be necessary, however, there are no specific recommendations. Monitor closely.

Child/Adolescent Considerations Five hospitalized children 6-11 years of age with varying diagnoses were treated with a mean daily dose of 7.5 mg/day (2.5-10 mg/day) or 0.22 mg/kg/day (0.12-0.29 mg/kg/day) for a mean of 32 days (Krishnamoorthy, 1998). Seven adolescents 12-17 years of age with DSM-IV bipolar disorder, manic episode were treated with a mean dose of 11 mg/day or 0.146 ± 0.086 mg/kg/day (Soutullo, 1999).

Krishnamoorthy J and King BH, "Open-Label Olanzapine Treatment in Five Preadolescent Children," *J Child Adolesc Psychopharmacol*, 1998, 8 (2):107-13.

Soutullo CA, Sorter MT, Foster KD, et al, "Olanzapine in the Treatment of Adolescent Acute Mania: A Report of Seven Cases," *J Affect Disord*, 1999, 53(3):279-83.

Schizophrenia: Olanzapine has shown modest efficacy in pediatric schizophrenia, although treatment effects appear inferior to clozapine. However, the more favorable safety profile (compared to clozapine) may justify its continued use in this patient population.

In an open-label, single-arm pilot study, 8 children/adolescents (mean age: 15.3 years) diagnosed with childhood-onset schizophrenia (DSM-III-R) that was refractory to two prior typical neuroleptic regimens were evaluated for efficacy on olanzapine therapy for 8 weeks (Kumra, 1998). Rating instruments included the CGI, SANS, SAPS, and BPRS scales. In a separate study, a cohort of 15 children who received clozapine for 6 weeks was used as a comparative control group. Overall, olanzapine was well tolerated and did not cause any hematologic, EEG, or epileptogenic adverse effects, whereas 4 patients on clozapine required prophylactic anticonvulsant treatment. Body weight increases did not differ significantly between groups. Olanzapine dosing was initiated at 2.5 mg every other day (<40 kg) or every day (>40 kg), and titrated every 5-9 days by 2.5-5 mg up to a maximum of 20 mg/day. By the 6th week of treatment, the mean daily olanzapine dose was 17.5 mg (range: 12.5-20 mg) or 0.27 mg/kg. After 8 weeks of treatment, improvements relative to baseline were noted in each of the rating scales, ranging from 6% to 33%. However, the magnitude of response as measured by these scales was approximately threefold lower than the improvements seen with clozapine (using the same instruments) at the 6-week mark. Further, none of the olanzapine treated patients were rated as responders (based on standard criteria) at 6 weeks of therapy, and only 3 (38%) were responsive or partially responsive at 8 weeks.

In comparison, 8 (53%) of clozapine-receiving patients were considered responders at the 6-week time point.

A double-blind, randomized, 8 week trial of olanzapine compared to clozapine was conducted in children/adolescents aged 7-16 years who met DSM-IV criteria for treatment-refractory schizophrenia (Shaw, 2006). The primary outcome measures were the CGI-S and SANS/SAPS scales. Patients randomized to olanzapine (n=13) were 12.8 years of age on average and received an average daily dose of 18.1 mg (20 mg/day maximum). Clozapine patients (n=12) were 11.7 years of age and received a mean daily dose of 387 mg (900 mg/day maximum). Side effects were reported more frequently in the clozapine arm (55 events) compared to the olanzapine arm (28 events, $p<0.001$), including significantly more cardiovascular events noted. Body weight increases and incidence of neutropenia did not differ significantly between groups. Relative to baseline antipsychotic-free scores, patients receiving clozapine showed improvements in the assessment scales of 23% to 48%, compared to 15% to 29% for olanzapine treated patients. Based on differential treatment effects, this equated to a 2.5-fold greater treatment effect in the clozapine arm.

Kumra S, Jacobsen LK, Lenane M, et al, "Childhood-Onset Schizophrenia: An Open-Label Study of Olanzapine in Adolescents," *J Am Acad Child Adolesc Psychiatry*, 1998, 37(4):377-85.

Shaw P, Sporn A, Gogtay N, et al, "Childhood-Onset Schizophrenia: A Double-Blind, Randomized Clozapine-Olanzapine Comparison," *Arch Gen Psychiatry*, 2006, 63(7):721-30.

Dietary Considerations Tablets may be taken with or without food. Zyprexa® Zydis®: 5 mg tablet contains phenylalanine 0.34 mg; 10 mg tablet contains phenylalanine 0.45 mg; 15 mg tablet contains phenylalanine 0.67 mg; 20 mg tablet contains phenylalanine 0.9 mg.

Administration

Injection: For I.M. administration only; do not administer injection intravenously; inject slowly, deep into muscle. If dizziness and/or drowsiness are noted, patient should remain recumbent until examination indicates postural hypotension and/or bradycardia are not a problem. Concurrent use of I.M/I.V. benzodiazepines is not recommended (fatalities have been reported, though causality not determined).

Tablet: May be administered with or without food.

Orally-disintegrating: Remove from foil blister by peeling back (do not push tablet through the foil); place tablet in mouth immediately upon removal; tablet dissolves rapidly in saliva and may be swallowed with or without liquid. May be administered with or without food/meals.

Monitoring Parameters Vital signs; fasting lipid profile and fasting blood glucose/Hgb A_{1c} (prior to treatment, at 3 months, then annually); periodic assessment of hepatic transaminases (in patients with hepatic disease); BMI, personal/family history of obesity, waist circumference; orthostatic blood pressure; mental status, abnormal involuntary movement scale (AIMS), extrapyramidal symptoms (EPS). Weight should be assessed prior to treatment, at 4 weeks, 8 weeks, 12 weeks, and then at quarterly intervals. Consider titrating to a different antipsychotic agent for a weight gain ≥5% of the initial weight.

Dosage Forms Excipient information presented when available (limited, particularly for generics); consult specific product labeling.

Injection, powder for reconstitution (Zyprexa® IntraMuscular): 10 mg [contains lactose 50 mg]

Tablet (Zyprexa®): 2.5 mg, 5 mg, 7.5 mg, 10 mg, 15 mg, 20 mg

Tablet, orally disintegrating (Zyprexa® Zydis®): 5 mg [contains phenylalanine 0.34 mg/tablet], 10 mg [contains phenylalanine 0.45 mg/tablet], 15 mg [contains phenylalanine 0.67 mg/tablet], 20 mg [contains phenylalanine 0.9 mg/tablet]

Olanzapine and Fluoxetine (oh LAN za peen & floo OKS e teen)

Related Information

Agents Approved for Bipolar Disorder *on page 1752*

U.S. Brand Names Symbyax®

Index Terms Fluoxetine and Olanzapine; Olanzapine and Fluoxetine Hydrochloride

Pharmacologic Category Antidepressant, Selective Serotonin Reuptake Inhibitor; Antipsychotic Agent, Atypical

Generic Available No

Use Treatment of depressive episodes associated with bipolar disorder

Mental Health Comment A small trial has demonstrated the olanzapine and fluoxetine combination formulation to be efficacious for the treatment of bipolar depression. However, in the clinical setting, this fixed-drug combination is uncommonly used due to inability to titrate individual components.

In 2008, the FDA issued a warning regarding increased mortality risk with typical **and** atypical antipsychotic drugs when used in elderly patients with dementia-related psychosis.

Restrictions An FDA-approved medication guide concerning the use of antidepressants in children, adolescents, and young adults must be distributed when dispensing an outpatient prescription (new or refill) where this medication is to be used without direct supervision of a healthcare provider. Medication guides are available at http://www.fda.gov/cder/Offices/ODS/medication_guides.htm. Dispense to parents or guardians of children and adolescents receiving this medication.

Pregnancy Risk Factor C

Pregnancy Considerations A decrease in fetal weight, testicular degeneration and atrophy, depletion of epididymal sperm, and infertility in males was reported in some animal reproduction studies using this combination. Use during pregnancy is not recommended. Refer to individual agents for additional information.

Lactation Enters breast milk/not recommended

Contraindications Hypersensitivity to olanzapine, fluoxetine, or any component of the formulation; patients currently receiving MAO inhibitors, thioridazine, pimozide, or mesoridazine; treatment within 14 days of MAO therapy

Warnings/Precautions See individual agents.

Adverse Reactions As reported with combination product (also see individual agents):

>10%:

Central nervous system: Somnolence (21% to 22%)

Gastrointestinal: Weight gain (17% to 21%), diarrhea (8% to 19%), appetite increased (13% to 16%), xerostomia (11% to 16%)

Neuromuscular & skeletal: Weakness (13% to 15%)

1% to 10%:

Cardiovascular: Peripheral edema (4% to 8%), edema (up to 5%), hypertension (2%), tachycardia (2%), vasodilation

Central nervous system: Thinking abnormal (6%), fever (3% to 4%), amnesia (1% to 3%), personality disorder (1% to 2%), sleep disorder (1% to 2%), speech disorder (up to 2%), chills, migraine

Dermatologic: Photosensitivity

Endocrine & metabolic: Ejaculation abnormal (2% to 7%), impotence (2% to 4%), libido decreased (2% to 4%), anorgasmia (1% to 3%), breast pain, menorrhagia

Gastrointestinal: Tooth disorder (1% to 2%), salivation increased, taste perversion, thirst, weight loss

Genitourinary: Urinary frequency, urinary incontinence, urinary tract infection

Neuromuscular & skeletal: Tremor (8% to 9%), twitching (2% to 6%), arthralgia (3% to 5%), hyperkinesias (1% to 2%), joint disorder (1% to 2%), bruising, neck pain/rigidity

Ocular: Amblyopia (4% to 5%), vision abnormal

Otic: Ear pain (1% to 2%), otitis media (up to 2%), tinnitus

Respiratory: Pharyngitis (4% to 6%), dyspnea (1% to 2%), bronchitis, lung disorder

Frequency not defined: Alkaline phosphate increased, cholesterol increased, GGT increased, hemoglobin decreased, prolactin increased, uric acid increased

Postmarketing (limited to significant or life-threatening): Acidosis, acute brain syndrome, anemia, angina pectoris, apnea, arrhythmia (various), asthma, ataxia, behavioral/personality changes (eg, hostility, emotional lability), bilirubinemia, bradycardia, breast carcinoma, bundle branch block, cellulitis, cerebral ischemia, cholelithiasis, coagulation disorder, colitis, coma, confusion, congestive heart failure, conjunctivitis, creatinine increased, deafness, dehydration, dystonia, emphysema, exfoliative dermatitis, extrapyramidal syndrome, eye hemorrhage, fatty liver, gastrointestinal hemorrhage, hematuria, hemoptysis, hepatomegaly, hyperkalemia, hyperlipemia, hyperprolactinemia, hyperventilation, hypoesthesia, hypoglycemia, hypokalemia, hyponatremia, hypokinesia, hypotension, hypothyroidism, incontinence, intestinal obstruction, jaundice, kidney calculus, leukocytosis, leukopenia, liver damage (cholestatic or mixed), lymphadenopathy, maculopapular rash, menopause, menstrual disorders, myasthenia, myocardial infarct, myoclonus, myopathy, neoplasm, neuralgia, osteoporosis, ovarian disorder, pancreatitis, pelvic pain, peptic ulcer, periodontal abscess, peripheral vascular disorder, pneumonia, purpura, QT interval increased, rheumatoid arthritis, seizure, subarachnoid hemorrhage, suicide attempt, tendinous contracture, tenosynovitis, thrombocythemia, transaminases increased, T-wave inverted, urination impaired, uterine fibroids enlarged, vesiculobullous rash, withdrawal syndrome

Drug Interactions

Acetylcholinesterase Inhibitors (Central): May enhance the neurotoxic (central) effect of Antipsychotics. Severe extrapyramidal symptoms have occurred in some patients. *Risk C: Monitor therapy*

Alcohol (Ethyl): CNS Depressants may enhance the CNS depressant effect of Alcohol (Ethyl). *Risk C: Monitor therapy*

Alfuzosin: May enhance the QTc-prolonging effect of QTc-Prolonging Agents. *Risk C: Monitor therapy*

Alpha-/Beta-Blockers: Selective Serotonin Reuptake Inhibitors may decrease the metabolism of Alpha-/Beta-Blockers. *Risk C: Monitor therapy*

Amphetamines: Antipsychotics may diminish the stimulatory effect of Amphetamines. *Risk C: Monitor therapy*

Analgesics (Opioid): May enhance the serotonergic effect of Selective Serotonin Reuptake Inhibitors. This may cause serotonin syndrome. *Risk C: Monitor therapy*

Anticholinergics: May enhance the adverse/toxic effect of other Anticholinergics. **Exceptions:** Paliperidone. *Risk C: Monitor therapy*

Anticoagulants: Antiplatelet Agents may enhance the anticoagulant effect of Anticoagulants. *Risk C: Monitor therapy*

Antidepressants (Serotonin Reuptake Inhibitor/Antagonist): Selective Serotonin Reuptake Inhibitors may enhance the serotonergic effect of Antidepressants (Serotonin Reuptake Inhibitor/Antagonist). This may cause serotonin syndrome. *Risk C: Monitor therapy*

Anti-Parkinson's Agents (Dopamine Agonist): Antipsychotics (Atypical) may diminish the therapeutic effect of Anti-Parkinson's Agents (Dopamine Agonist). *Risk D: Consider therapy modification*

Antiplatelet Agents: May enhance the anticoagulant effect of other Antiplatelet Agents. *Risk C: Monitor therapy*

Aspirin: Selective Serotonin Reuptake Inhibitors may enhance the antiplatelet effect of Aspirin. *Risk C: Monitor therapy*

Benzodiazepines (metabolized by oxidation): Selective Serotonin Reuptake Inhibitors may decrease the metabolism of Benzodiazepines (metabolized by oxidation). *Risk C: Monitor therapy*

Beta-Blockers: Selective Serotonin Reuptake Inhibitors may enhance the bradycardic effect of Beta-Blockers. **Exceptions:** Acebutolol; Atenolol; Carteolol; Esmolol; Levobunolol; Metipranolol; Nadolol; Penbutolol. *Risk C: Monitor therapy*

BusPIRone: May enhance the serotonergic effect of Selective Serotonin Reuptake Inhibitors. This may cause serotonin syndrome. Selective Serotonin Reuptake Inhibitors may decrease the metabolism of BusPIRone. *Risk C: Monitor therapy*

CarBAMazepine: Selective Serotonin Reuptake Inhibitors may decrease the metabolism of CarBAMazepine. Specifically those SSRIs that inhibit CYP3A4 isoenzymes. CarBAMazepine may increase the metabolism of Selective Serotonin Reuptake Inhibitors. Specifically those agents metabolized via CYP1A2, 2C, and/or 3A4 isoenzymes. *Risk D: Consider therapy modification*

Cimetidine: May decrease the metabolism of Selective Serotonin Reuptake Inhibitors. *Risk D: Consider therapy modification*

Ciprofloxacin: May enhance the QTc-prolonging effect of QTc-Prolonging Agents. *Risk C: Monitor therapy*

Clozapine: Selective Serotonin Reuptake Inhibitors may decrease the metabolism of Clozapine. *Risk D: Consider therapy modification*

CNS Depressants: May enhance the adverse/toxic effect of other CNS Depressants. *Risk C: Monitor therapy*

CYP1A2 Inducers (Strong): May increase the metabolism of CYP1A2 Substrates. *Risk C: Monitor therapy*

CYP1A2 Inhibitors (Moderate): May decrease the metabolism of CYP1A2 Substrates. *Risk C: Monitor therapy*

CYP1A2 Inhibitors (Strong): May decrease the metabolism of CYP1A2 Substrates. *Risk D: Consider therapy modification*

CYP1A2 Substrates: CYP1A2 Inhibitors (Moderate) may decrease the metabolism of CYP1A2 Substrates. *Risk C: Monitor therapy*

CYP2C19 Substrates: CYP2C19 Inhibitors (Moderate) may decrease the metabolism of CYP2C19 Substrates. *Risk C: Monitor therapy*

CYP2C9 Inducers (Highly Effective): May increase the metabolism of CYP2C9 Substrates (High risk). *Risk C: Monitor therapy*

CYP2C9 Inhibitors (Moderate): May decrease the metabolism of CYP2C9 Substrates (High risk). *Risk C: Monitor therapy*

CYP2C9 Inhibitors (Strong): May decrease the metabolism of CYP2C9 Substrates (High risk). *Risk D: Consider therapy modification*

CYP2D6 Inhibitors (Moderate): May decrease the metabolism of CYP2D6 Substrates. *Risk C: Monitor therapy*

CYP2D6 Inhibitors (Strong): May decrease the metabolism of CYP2D6 Substrates. *Risk D: Consider therapy modification*

CYP2D6 Substrates: CYP2D6 Inhibitors (Strong) may decrease the metabolism of CYP2D6 Substrates. **Exceptions:** Tamoxifen. *Risk D: Consider therapy modification*

Cyproheptadine: May diminish the therapeutic effect of Selective Serotonin Reuptake Inhibitors. *Risk C: Monitor therapy*

Darunavir: May increase the serum concentration of CYP2D6 Substrates. *Risk C: Monitor therapy*

Dasatinib: May enhance the anticoagulant effect of Antiplatelet Agents. *Risk C: Monitor therapy*

Desmopressin: Selective Serotonin Reuptake Inhibitors may enhance the adverse/toxic effect of Desmopressin. *Risk C: Monitor therapy*

Dextromethorphan: Selective Serotonin Reuptake Inhibitors may enhance the adverse/toxic effect of Dextromethorphan. *Risk D: Consider therapy modification*

Drotrecogin Alfa: Antiplatelet Agents may enhance the adverse/toxic effect of Drotrecogin Alfa. Bleeding may occur. *Risk D: Consider therapy modification*

Fluvoxamine: May decrease the metabolism of OLANZapine. *Risk D: Consider therapy modification*

Gadobutrol: May enhance the QTc-prolonging effect of QTc-Prolonging Agents. *Risk D: Consider therapy modification*

Galantamine: Selective Serotonin Reuptake Inhibitors may decrease the metabolism of Galantamine. *Risk C: Monitor therapy*

Haloperidol: Selective Serotonin Reuptake Inhibitors may decrease the metabolism of Haloperidol. *Risk C: Monitor therapy*

Herbs (Anticoagulant/Antiplatelet Properties) (eg, Alfalfa, Anise, Bilberry): May enhance the adverse/toxic effect of Antiplatelet Agents. Bleeding may occur. *Risk D: Consider therapy modification*

Ibritumomab: Antiplatelet Agents may enhance the adverse/toxic effect of Ibritumomab. Both agents may contribute to impaired platelet function and an increased risk of bleeding. *Risk C: Monitor therapy*

LamoTRIgine: May enhance the sedative effect of OLANZapine. *Risk C: Monitor therapy*

Lithium: Selective Serotonin Reuptake Inhibitors may enhance the adverse/toxic effect of Lithium. *Risk C: Monitor therapy*

Lithium formulations: May enhance the neurotoxic effect of Antipsychotics. Lithium formulations may decrease the serum concentration of Antipsychotics. Specifically noted with chlorpromazine. *Risk C: Monitor therapy*

Macrolide Antibiotics: May decrease the metabolism of Selective Serotonin Reuptake Inhibitors. **Exceptions:** Azithromycin; Dirithromycin [Off Market]; Spiramycin. *Risk C: Monitor therapy*

MAO Inhibitors: May enhance the serotonergic effect of Selective Serotonin Reuptake Inhibitors. This may cause serotonin syndrome. *Risk X: Avoid combination*

Methadone: Selective Serotonin Reuptake Inhibitors may decrease the metabolism of Methadone. Fluvoxamine appears to be the only interacting SSRI. *Risk D: Consider therapy modification*

Mexiletine: Selective Serotonin Reuptake Inhibitors may decrease the metabolism of Mexiletine. *Risk D: Consider therapy modification*

Nilotinib: May enhance the QTc-prolonging effect of QTc-Prolonging Agents. *Risk X: Avoid combination*

NSAID (COX-2 Inhibitor): Selective Serotonin Reuptake Inhibitors may enhance the antiplatelet effect of NSAID (COX-2 Inhibitor). *Risk D: Consider therapy modification*

NSAID (Nonselective): Selective Serotonin Reuptake Inhibitors may enhance the antiplatelet effect of NSAID (Nonselective). *Risk D: Consider therapy modification*

Omega-3-Acid Ethyl Esters: May enhance the antiplatelet effect of Antiplatelet Agents. *Risk C: Monitor therapy*

Pentosan Polysulfate Sodium: May enhance the adverse/toxic effect of Antiplatelet Agents. Specifically, the risk of bleeding may be increased by concurrent use of these agents. *Risk C: Monitor therapy*

Phenytoin: Selective Serotonin Reuptake Inhibitors may decrease the metabolism of Phenytoin. *Risk D: Consider therapy modification*

Pimozide: Selective Serotonin Reuptake Inhibitors may enhance the adverse/toxic effect of Pimozide. *Risk X: Avoid combination*

Pramlintide: May enhance the anticholinergic effect of Anticholinergics. These effects are specific to the GI tract. *Risk D: Consider therapy modification*

Propafenone: Selective Serotonin Reuptake Inhibitors may decrease the metabolism of Propafenone. *Risk D: Consider therapy modification*

Prostacyclin Analogues: May enhance the antiplatelet effect of Antiplatelet Agents. *Risk C: Monitor therapy*

QTc-Prolonging Agents: May enhance the adverse/toxic effect of other QTc-Prolonging Agents. Their effects can be additive, causing life-threatening ventricular arrhythmias. *Risk D: Consider therapy modification*

QuiNIDine: Selective Serotonin Reuptake Inhibitors may decrease the metabolism of QuiNIDine. Fluvoxamine appears to be the only SSRI of concern. *Risk D: Consider therapy modification*

Risperidone: Selective Serotonin Reuptake Inhibitors may decrease the metabolism of Risperidone. *Risk C: Monitor therapy*

Salicylates: Antiplatelet Agents may enhance the adverse/toxic effect of Salicylates. Increased risk of bleeding may result. *Risk C: Monitor therapy*

Serotonin Modulators: May enhance the adverse/toxic effect of other Serotonin Modulators. The development of serotonin syndrome may occur. *Risk D: Consider therapy modification*

Sibutramine: May enhance the serotonergic effect of Serotonin Modulators. This may cause serotonin syndrome. *Risk X: Avoid combination*

Tamoxifen: CYP2D6 Inhibitors (Strong) may decrease the metabolism of Tamoxifen. Specifically, strong CYP2D6 inhibitors may decrease the formation of highly potent active metabolites. *Risk X: Avoid combination*

Tetrabenazine: May enhance the adverse/toxic effect of Antipsychotics. *Risk C: Monitor therapy*

Thioridazine: QTc-Prolonging Agents may enhance the QTc-prolonging effect of Thioridazine. *Risk X: Avoid combination*

Thioridazine: CYP2D6 Inhibitors may decrease the metabolism of Thioridazine. *Risk X: Avoid combination*

Thrombolytic Agents: Antiplatelet Agents may enhance the anticoagulant effect of Thrombolytic Agents. *Risk C: Monitor therapy*

Tositumomab and Iodine I 131 Tositumomab: Antiplatelet Agents may enhance the adverse/toxic effect of Tositumomab and Iodine I 131 Tositumomab. Specifically, the risk of bleeding-related adverse events may be increased. *Risk C: Monitor therapy*

TraMADol: Selective Serotonin Reuptake Inhibitors may enhance the neuroexcitatory and/or seizure-potentiating effect of TraMADol. TraMADol may enhance the serotonergic effect of Selective Serotonin Reuptake Inhibitors. This may cause serotonin syndrome. *Risk D: Consider therapy modification*

Tricyclic Antidepressants: Selective Serotonin Reuptake Inhibitors may decrease the metabolism of Tricyclic Antidepressants. *Risk D: Consider therapy modification*

Tryptophan: May enhance the serotonergic effect of Selective Serotonin Reuptake Inhibitors. This may cause serotonin syndrome. *Risk D: Consider therapy modification*

Vitamin K Antagonists (eg, warfarin): Selective Serotonin Reuptake Inhibitors may enhance the anticoagulant effect of Vitamin K Antagonists. *Risk C: Monitor therapy*

Ziprasidone: QTc-Prolonging Agents may enhance the QTc-prolonging effect of Ziprasidone. The risk of a severe arrhythmia may be increased. *Risk X: Avoid combination*

Ethanol/Nutrition/Herb Interactions See individual agents.

Stability Store at controlled room temperature of 15°C to 30°C (59°F to 86°F). Protect from moisture.

Mechanism of Action Olanzapine is a second generation thienobenzodiazepine antipsychotic which displays potent antagonism of serotonin 5-HT_{2A} and 5-HT_{2C}, dopamine D_{1-4}, histamine H_1 and alpha$_1$-adrenergic receptors. Olanzapine shows moderate antagonism of 5-HT_3 and muscarinic M_{1-5} receptors, and weak binding to GABA-A, BZD, and beta-adrenergic receptors. Fluoxetine inhibits CNS neuron serotonin reuptake; minimal or no effect on reuptake of norepinephrine or dopamine; does not significantly bind to alpha-adrenergic, histamine, or cholinergic receptors. The enhanced antidepressant effect of the combination may be due to synergistic increases in serotonin, norepinephrine, and dopamine.

Pharmacodynamics/Kinetics See individual agents.

Dosage Oral:

Adults: Depression associated with bipolar disorder: Initial: Olanzapine 3-6 mg/fluoxetine 25 mg once daily in the evening. Dosing range: Olanzapine 6-12 mg/fluoxetine 25-50 mg. Lower doses (olanzapine 3 mg/fluoxetine 25 mg) should be used in patients predisposed to hypotension, in hepatic impairment, with combined factors for reduced metabolism (females, the elderly, nonsmokers), or enhanced sensitivity to olanzapine; use caution in dose adjustments in these patients. Safety of daily doses of olanzapine >18 mg/fluoxetine >75 mg have not been evaluated.

Elderly: Initial: Olanzapine 3-6 mg/fluoxetine 25 mg once daily in the evening; use caution adjusting dose (metabolism may be decreased). Safety and efficacy have not been established in patients >65 years of age.

Dosage adjustment in hepatic impairment: Initial: Olanzapine 6 mg/fluoxetine 25 mg once daily in the evening; use caution adjusting dose (metabolism may be decreased).

Dietary Considerations May be taken with or without food.

Administration Capsules should be taken once daily in the evening; may be taken with or without food

Monitoring Parameters Vital signs; lipid profile, fasting blood glucose/Hgb A_{1c}; BMI; mental status; abnormal involuntary movement scale (AIMS), extrapyramidal symptoms (EPS); signs and symptoms of depression, anxiety, suicidal ideation (especially at the beginning of therapy or when doses are increased or decreased), sleep; liver function tests in patients with hepatic disease

Dosage Forms Excipient information presented when available (limited, particularly for generics); consult specific product labeling.

Capsule:

Symbyax® 3/25: Olanzapine 3 mg and fluoxetine 25 mg
Symbyax® 6/25: Olanzapine 6 mg and fluoxetine 25 mg
Symbyax® 6/50: Olanzapine 6 mg and fluoxetine 50 mg
Symbyax® 12/25: Olanzapine 12 mg and fluoxetine 25 mg
Symbyax® 12/50: Olanzapine 12 mg and fluoxetine 50 mg

◆ **Olanzapine and Fluoxetine Hydrochloride** *see* Olanzapine and Fluoxetine *on page 1165*

Olmesartan (ole me SAR tan)

Related Information

Angiotensin Agents *on page 1754*

U.S. Brand Names Benicar®

Mexican Brand Names Almetec

Index Terms Olmesartan Medoxomil

Pharmacologic Category Angiotensin II Receptor Blocker

Generic Available No

Use Treatment of hypertension with or without concurrent use of other antihypertensive agents

Effect on Mental Status May cause dizziness

Effect on Psychiatric Treatment May cause hyperglycemia and hypertriglyceridemia; combined use with psychotropics (atypical antipsychotics and mirtazapine) may produce additive effects; may cause diarrhea, these effects may be additive with concurrent use of SSRIs, lithium, or valproate. May cause flu-like symptoms, take this into consideration if also concerned about SSRI discontinuation syndrome. Combined use with lithium may produce lithium toxicity; monitor lithium levels.

Pregnancy Risk Factor C (1st trimester); D (2nd and 3rd trimesters)

Pregnancy Considerations Medications which act on the renin-angiotensin system are reported to have the following fetal/neonatal effects: Hypotension, neonatal skull hypoplasia, anuria, renal failure, and death; oligohydramnios is also reported. These effects are reported to occur with exposure during the second and third trimesters. There are no adequate and well-controlled studies in pregnant women. **[U.S. Boxed Warning]: Based on human data, drugs that act on the angiotensin system can cause injury and death to the developing fetus when used in the second and third trimesters. Angiotensin receptor blockers should be discontinued as soon as possible once pregnancy is detected.**

Lactation Excretion in breast milk unknown/contraindicated

Contraindications Hypersensitivity to olmesartan or any component of the formulation

Warnings/Precautions **[U.S. Boxed Warning]: Based on human data, drugs that act on the angiotensin system can cause injury and death to**

the developing fetus when used in the second and third trimesters. Angiotensin receptor blockers should be discontinued as soon as possible once pregnancy is detected. May cause hyperkalemia; avoid potassium supplementation unless specifically required by healthcare provider. Avoid use or use a smaller dose in patients who are volume depleted; correct depletion first. May be associated with deterioration of renal function and/or increases in serum creatinine, particularly in patients with low renal blood flow (eg, renal artery stenosis, heart failure) whose glomerular filtration rate (GFR) is dependent on efferent arteriolar vasoconstriction by angiotensin II. Use with caution in unstented unilateral/bilateral renal artery stenosis. When unstented bilateral renal artery stenosis is present, use is generally avoided due to the elevated risk of deterioration in renal function unless possible benefits outweigh risks. Use with caution with pre-existing renal insufficiency; significant aortic/mitral stenosis. Safety and efficacy in pediatric patients have not been established.

Adverse Reactions

1% to 10%:

Central nervous system: Dizziness (3%), headache
Endocrine & metabolic: Hyperglycemia, hypertriglyceridemia
Gastrointestinal: Diarrhea
Neuromuscular & skeletal: Back pain, CPK increased
Renal: Hematuria
Respiratory: Bronchitis, pharyngitis, rhinitis, sinusitis
Miscellaneous: Flu-like syndrome

<1% (Limited to important or life-threatening): Abdominal pain, acute renal failure, alopecia, angioedema, arthralgia, arthritis, bilirubin increased, chest pain, dyspepsia, facial edema, fatigue, gastroenteritis, hypercholesterolemia, hyperkalemia, hyperlipidemia, hyperuricemia, insomnia, liver enzymes increased, myalgia, nausea, pain, peripheral edema, pruritus, rash, rhabdomyolysis, serum creatinine increased, skeletal pain, tachycardia, urinary tract infection, urticaria, vertigo, vomiting

Drug Interactions

ACE Inhibitors: Angiotensin II Receptor Blockers may enhance the adverse/toxic effect of ACE Inhibitors. *Risk C: Monitor therapy*

Diazoxide: May enhance the hypotensive effect of Antihypertensives. *Risk C: Monitor therapy*

Eplerenone: May enhance the hyperkalemic effect of Angiotensin II Receptor Blockers. *Risk C: Monitor therapy*

Herbs (Hypertensive Properties): May diminish the antihypertensive effect of Antihypertensives. *Risk C: Monitor therapy*

Herbs (Hypotensive Properties): May enhance the hypotensive effect of Antihypertensives. *Risk C: Monitor therapy*

Lithium: Angiotensin II Receptor Blockers may increase the serum concentration of Lithium. Management: Lithium dosage reductions will likely be needed following the addition of an angiotensin II receptor antagonist. *Risk D: Consider therapy modification*

Methylphenidate: May diminish the antihypertensive effect of Antihypertensives. *Risk C: Monitor therapy*

Nonsteroidal Anti-Inflammatory Agents: May diminish the therapeutic effect of Angiotensin II Receptor Blockers. The combination of these two agents may also significantly decrease glomerular filtration and renal function. *Risk C: Monitor therapy*

Potassium Salts: May enhance the hyperkalemic effect of Angiotensin II Receptor Blockers. *Risk C: Monitor therapy*

Potassium-Sparing Diuretics: Angiotensin II Receptor Blockers may enhance the hyperkalemic effect of Potassium-Sparing Diuretics. *Risk C: Monitor therapy*

Prostacyclin Analogues: May enhance the hypotensive effect of Antihypertensives. *Risk C: Monitor therapy*

RiTUXimab: Antihypertensives may enhance the hypotensive effect of RiTUXimab. *Risk D: Consider therapy modification*

Trimethoprim: May enhance the hyperkalemic effect of Angiotensin II Receptor Blockers. *Risk C: Monitor therapy*

Ethanol/Nutrition/Herb Interactions

Food: Does not affect olmesartan bioavailability.

Herb/Nutraceutical: Avoid bayberry, blue cohosh, cayenne, ephedra, ginger, ginseng (American), kola, licorice (may worsen hypertension). Avoid black cohosh, California poppy, coleus, golden seal, hawthorn, mistletoe, periwinkle, quinine, shepherd's purse (may have increased antihypertensive effect).

Stability Store at 20°C to 25°C (68°F to 77°F).

Mechanism of Action As a selective and competitive, nonpeptide angiotensin II receptor antagonist, olmesartan blocks the vasoconstrictor and aldosterone-secreting effects of angiotensin II; olmesartan interacts reversibly at the AT1 and AT2 receptors of many tissues and has slow dissociation kinetics; its affinity for the AT1 receptor is 12,500 times greater than the AT2 receptor. Angiotensin II receptor antagonists may induce a more complete inhibition of the renin-angiotensin system than ACE inhibitors, they do not affect the response to bradykinin, and are less likely to be associated with nonrenin-angiotensin effects (eg, cough and angioedema). Olmesartan increases urinary flow rate and, in addition to being natriuretic and kaliuretic, increases excretion of chloride, magnesium, uric acid, calcium, and phosphate.

Pharmacodynamics/Kinetics

Distribution: 17 L; does not cross the blood-brain barrier (animal studies)

Protein binding: 99%

Metabolism: Olmesartan medoxomil is hydrolyzed in the GI tract to active olmesartan. No further metabolism occurs.

Bioavailability: 26%

Half-life elimination: Terminal: 13 hours

Time to peak: 1-2 hours

Excretion: All as unchanged drug: Feces (50% to 65%); urine (35% to 50%)

Dosage Oral:

Adults: Initial: Usual starting dose is 20 mg once daily; if initial response is inadequate, may be increased to 40 mg once daily after 2 weeks. May administer with other antihypertensive agents if blood pressure inadequately controlled with olmesartan. Consider lower starting dose in patients with possible depletion of intravascular volume (eg, patients receiving diuretics).

Elderly: No dosage adjustment necessary

Dosage adjustment in renal impairment: No specific guidelines for dosage adjustment; patients undergoing hemodialysis have not been studied.

Dosage adjustment in hepatic impairment: No adjustment necessary.

Dietary Considerations May be taken with or without food.

Administration May be administered with or without food.

Monitoring Parameters Blood pressure, serum potassium

Dosage Forms Excipient information presented when available (limited, particularly for generics); consult specific product labeling.

Tablet, as medoxomil:

Benicar®: 5 mg, 20 mg, 40 mg

◆ **Olmesartan and Amlodipine** *see* Amlodipine and Olmesartan *on page 104*

Olmesartan and Hydrochlorothiazide

(ole me SAR tan & hye droe klor oh THYE a zide)

U.S. Brand Names Benicar HCT®

Index Terms Hydrochlorothiazide and Olmesartan Medoxomil; Olmesartan Medoxomil and Hydrochlorothiazide

Pharmacologic Category Angiotensin II Receptor Blocker; Diuretic, Thiazide

Use Treatment of hypertension (not recommended for initial treatment)

Effect on Mental Status May cause dizziness

Effect on Psychiatric Treatment May cause hyperglycemia and hypertriglyceridemia; combined use with psychotropics (atypical antipsychotics and mirtazapine) may produce additive effects. May cause diarrhea, these effects may be additive with concurrent use of SSRIs, lithium, or valproate. May cause flu-like symptoms, take this into consideration if also concerned about SSRI discontinuation syndrome. Combined use with lithium may produce lithium toxicity; monitor lithium levels.

Dosage Summary

Oral:

Children: Dosage not established

Adults: Olmesartan 20-40 mg and hydrochlorothiazide 12.5-25 mg once daily (maximum: 25 mg/day [hydrochlorothiazide]; 40 mg/day [olmesartan])

Dosage Forms Excipient information presented when available (limited, particularly for generics); consult specific product labeling.

Tablet:

20/12.5: Olmesartan medoxomil 20 mg and hydrochlorothiazide 12.5 mg

40/12.5: Olmesartan medoxomil 40 mg and hydrochlorothiazide 12.5 mg

40/25: Olmesartan medoxomil 40 mg and hydrochlorothiazide 25 mg

◆ **Olmesartan Medoxomil** *see* Olmesartan *on page 1170*

◆ **Olmesartan Medoxomil and Hydrochlorothiazide** *see* Olmesartan and Hydrochlorothiazide *on page 1172*

Olsalazine (ole SAL a zeen)

Medication Safety Issues

Sound-alike/look-alike issues:

Olsalazine may be confused with OLANZapine

Dipentum® may be confused with Dilantin®

U.S. Brand Names Dipentum®

Canadian Brand Names Dipentum®

Index Terms Olsalazine Sodium

Pharmacologic Category 5-Aminosalicylic Acid Derivative

Generic Available No

Use Maintenance of remission of ulcerative colitis in patients intolerant to sulfasalazine

Effect on Mental Status May cause drowsiness or depression

Effect on Psychiatric Treatment None reported

Pregnancy Risk Factor C

Pregnancy Considerations Animal studies have demonstrated fetal developmental toxicities. There are no well-controlled studies in pregnant women. Use during pregnancy only if clearly necessary.

Lactation Enters breast milk/not recommended

Contraindications Hypersensitivity to olsalazine, salicylates, or any component of the formulation

Warnings/Precautions Diarrhea is a common adverse effect of olsalazine. May exacerbate symptoms of colitis. Use with caution in patients with renal or hepatic impairment. Use with caution in elderly patients. Use with caution in patients with severe allergies or asthma. Safety and efficacy have not been established in children.

Adverse Reactions

>10%: Gastrointestinal: Diarrhea (11% to 17%; dose related)

1% to 10%:

Central nervous system: Headache (5%), depression (2%). fatigue (2%), vertigo (1%)

Dermatologic: Rash (2%), pruritus (1%)

Gastrointestinal: Abdominal pain/cramps (10%), heartburn (2%), nausea (5%), stomatitis (1%), vomiting (1%)

Neuromuscular & skeletal: Arthralgia (4%)

Respiratory: Upper respiratory infection (2%)

Postmarketing and/or case reports: Alopecia, angioedema, aplastic anemia, bilirubin increase, blood dyscrasias, blood in stool, blurred vision, bronchospasm, cholestatic jaundice, chills, cirrhosis, dyspnea, dysuria, eosinophilia, erythema, erythema nodosum, fever, heart block (second degree), hematuria, hemolytic anemia, hepatitis, hepatic failure, hepatic necrosis, hypertension, impotence, interstitial nephritis, interstitial pneumonia, jaundice, Kawasaki-like syndrome, leukopenia, lymphopenia, menorrhagia, muscle cramps, myalgia, myocarditis, nephritic syndrome, neutropenia, orthostatic hypotension, pancreatitis, pancytopenia, paresthesia, pericarditis, peripheral edema, photosensitivity, proteinuria, rectal bleeding, rigors, tachycardia, thrombocytopenia, tinnitus, transaminase increase, tremor, urinary frequency, xerostomia

Drug Interactions

Cardiac Glycosides: 5-ASA Derivatives may decrease the absorption of Cardiac Glycosides. *Risk C: Monitor therapy*

Thiopurine Analogs: 5-ASA Derivatives may decrease the metabolism of Thiopurine Analogs. *Risk C: Monitor therapy*

Varicella Virus-Containing Vaccines: 5-ASA Derivatives may enhance the adverse/toxic effect of Varicella Virus-Containing Vaccines. The primary concern is the potential development of Reye 's Syndrome, a condition that has been associated with the use of salicylates in children with varicella infections. *Risk D: Consider therapy modification*

Mechanism of Action Mesalamine (5-aminosalicylic acid) is the active component of olsalazine; the specific mechanism of action of mesalamine is unknown; however, it is thought that it modulates local chemical mediators of the inflammatory response, especially leukotrienes, and is also postulated to be a free radical scavenger or an inhibitor of tumor necrosis factor (TNF); action appears topical rather than systemic.

Pharmacodynamics/Kinetics

Absorption: <3%; very little intact olsalazine is systemically absorbed

Protein binding, plasma: >99%

Metabolism: Primarily via colonic bacteria to active drug, 5-aminosalicylic acid

Half-life elimination: 56 minutes

Time to peak: ~1 hour
Excretion: Primarily feces

Dosage Adults: Oral: 1 g/day in 2 divided doses

Dietary Considerations Take with food, increases residence of drug in body.

Administration Administer with food in evenly divided doses.

Monitoring Parameters CBC, hepatic function, renal function; stool frequency

Test Interactions Increased ALT, AST (S), GGT, LDH, alkaline phosphatase, bilirubin

Dosage Forms Excipient information presented when available (limited, particularly for generics); consult specific product labeling.
Capsule, as sodium: 250 mg

◆ **Olsalazine Sodium** *see* Olsalazine *on page 1173*

◆ **Omacor® [DSC]** *see* Omega-3-Acid Ethyl Esters *on page 1175*

Omalizumab (oh mah lye ZOO mab)

U.S. Brand Names Xolair®

Canadian Brand Names Xolair®

Index Terms rhuMAb-E25

Pharmacologic Category Monoclonal Antibody, Anti-Asthmatic

Use Treatment of moderate-to-severe, persistent allergic asthma not adequately controlled with inhaled corticosteroids

Effect on Mental Status May cause dizziness and fatigue

Effect on Psychiatric Treatment None reported

Restrictions An FDA-approved medication guide is available at http://www.fda.gov/cder/Offices/ODS/medication_guides.htm; distribute to each patient to whom this medication is dispensed.

Dosage Summary

SubQ: Dose is based on pretreatment IgE serum levels and body weight.

IgE ≥30-100 int. units/mL:
- *Children <12 years:* Dosage not established
- *Children ≥12 years and 30-90 kg:* 150 mg every 4 weeks
- *Children ≥12 years and >90-150 kg:* 300 mg every 4 weeks
- *Adults 30-90 kg:* 150 mg every 4 weeks
- *Adults >90-150 kg:* 300 mg every 4 weeks

IgE >100-200 int. units/mL:
- *Children <12 years:* Dosage not established
- *Children ≥12 years and 30-90 kg:* 300 mg every 4 weeks
- *Children ≥12 years and >90-150 kg:* 225 mg every 2 weeks
- *Adults 30-90 kg:* 300 mg every 4 weeks
- *Adults >90-150 kg:* 225 mg every 2 weeks

IgE >200-300 int. units/mL:
- *Children <12 years:* Dosage not established
- *Children ≥12 years and 30-60 kg:* 300 mg every 4 weeks
- *Children ≥12 years and >60-90 kg:* 225 mg every 2 weeks
- *Children ≥12 years and >90-150 kg:* 300 mg every 2 weeks
- *Adults 30-60 kg:* 300 mg every 4 weeks
- *Adults >60-90 kg:* 225 mg every 2 weeks
- *Adults >90-150 kg:* 300 mg every 2 weeks

IgE >300-400 int. units/mL:
- *Children <12 years:* Dosage not established
- *Children ≥12 years and 30-70 kg:* 225 mg every 2 weeks
- *Children ≥12 years and >70-90 kg:* 300 mg every 2 weeks
- *Children ≥12 years and >90 kg:* Do not administer dose
- *Adults 30-70 kg:* 225 mg every 2 weeks
- *Adults >70-90 kg:* 300 mg every 2 weeks
- *Adults >90 kg:* Do not administer dose

IgE >400-500 int. units/mL:
- *Children <12 years:* Dosage not established
- *Children ≥12 years and 30-70 kg:* 300 mg every 2 weeks
- *Children ≥12 years and >70-90 kg:* 375 mg every 2 weeks
- *Children ≥12 years and >90 kg:* Do not administer dose
- *Adults 30-70 kg:* 300 mg every 2 weeks
- *Adults >70-90 kg:* 375 mg every 2 weeks
- *Adults >90 kg:* Do not administer

IgE >500-600 int. units/mL:
- *Children <12 years:* Dosage not established
- Children ≥12 years and 30-60 kg: 300 mg every 2 weeks
- *Children ≥12 years and >60-70 kg:* 375 mg every 2 weeks
- *Children ≥12 years and >70 kg:* Do not administer dose

Adults 30-60 kg: 300 mg every 2 weeks
Adults >60-70 kg: 375 mg every 2 weeks
Adults >70 kg: Do not administer dose
IgE >600-700 int. units/mL:
Children <12 years: Dosage not established
Children ≥12 years and 30-60 kg: 375 mg every 2 weeks
Children ≥12 years and >60 kg: Do not administer dose
Adults 30-60 kg: 375 mg every 2 weeks
Adults >60 kg: Do not administer dose

Dosage Forms Excipient information presented when available (limited, particularly for generics); consult specific product labeling.
Injection, powder for reconstitution [preservative free]:
Xolair®: 150 mg [contains sucrose 145.5 g]

Omega-3-Acid Ethyl Esters (oh MEG a three AS id ETH il ES ters)

Medication Safety Issues
Sound-alike/look-alike issues:
Omacor® may be confused with Amicar®

U.S. Brand Names Lovaza®; Omacor® [DSC]

Index Terms Ethyl Esters of Omega-3 Fatty Acids; Fish Oil

Pharmacologic Category Antilipemic Agent, Miscellaneous

Use Lovaza®: Adjunct to diet therapy in the treatment of hypertriglyceridemia (≥500 mg/dL)

Note: A number of OTC formulations containing omega-3 fatty acids are marketed as nutritional supplements; these do not have FDA-approved indications and may not contain the same amounts of the active ingredient.

Unlabeled/Investigational Use Lovaza®: Treatment of IgA nephropathy

Effect on Mental Status May cause flu-like syndrome; rule out antidepressant withdrawal syndrome

Effect on Psychiatric Treatment May prolong bleeding time; concomitant use with SSRIs may produce additive effects; monitor. Beta-blockers may decrease the effects of omega-3-acid ethyl esters; monitor.

Pregnancy Risk Factor C

Pregnancy Considerations In some animal studies, embryocidal and maternal effects have been observed at high doses. There are no adequate or well-controlled studies in pregnant women. Use during pregnancy only if potential benefit outweighs possible risk.

Lactation Excretion in breast milk unknown/use caution

Contraindications Hypersensitivity to omega-3-acid ethyl esters or any component of the formulation

Warnings/Precautions Use with caution in patients with known allergy or sensitivity to fish. Should be used as an adjunct to diet therapy and exercise and only in those with very high triglyceride levels (≥500 mg/dL). Treatment of primary metabolic disorders (eg, diabetes, thyroid disease) and/or evaluation of the patient's medication regimen for possible etiologic agents should be completed prior to a decision to initiate therapy. Secondary causes of hyperlipidemia should be ruled out prior to therapy. If triglyceride levels do not adequately respond after 2 months of treatment with omega-3-acid ethyl esters, discontinue treatment. ALT may be increased without ALT increasing. May increase LDL levels; periodically monitor LDL levels. Prolongation of bleeding time has been observed in some clinical studies; use with caution in patients with coagulopathy or in those receiving therapeutic anticoagulation; monitor INR. Safety and efficacy have not been established in children (<18 years of age).

Adverse Reactions
Cardiovascular: Angina (1%)
Central nervous system: Pain (2%)
Dermatologic: Rash (2%)
Gastrointestinal: Eructation (5%), dyspepsia (3%), taste perversion (3%)
Neuromuscular & skeletal: Back pain (2%)
Miscellaneous: Flu-like syndrome (4%), infection (4%)
<1% (Limited to important or life-threatening): Abdominal distention, alopecia, anorexia, appetite increased, arrhythmia, arthralgia, arthritis, asthma, body odor, bronchitis, cardiac arrest, cataract, chest pain, chills, colitis, constipation, cough, depression, diaphoresis, dizziness, dysphagia, dyspnea, eczema, edema, emotional lability, epididymitis, epistaxis, facial paralysis, fecal incontinence, fever, fracture, fungal infection, gastritis, gastroenteritis, GI disorder, hyperglycemia, hyperlipemia, hypertension, impotence, insomnia, intestinal obstruction, laryngitis, LDL increased, liver transaminases increased, lymphadenopathy, malaise, melena, MI, migraine, myalgia,

myocardial ischemia, neck pain, neoplasm, pancreatitis, peripheral vascular disorder, pharyngitis, pneumonia, pruritus, rheumatoid arthritis, rhinitis, sinusitis, sudden death, suicide, syncope, tachycardia, tendon disorder, tenesmus, vasodilatation, vertigo, viral infection, vomiting, weakness, xerostomia

Drug Interactions

Antiplatelet Agents: Omega-3-Acid Ethyl Esters may enhance the antiplatelet effect of Antiplatelet Agents. *Risk C: Monitor therapy*

Warfarin: Omega-3-Acid Ethyl Esters may enhance the anticoagulant effect of Warfarin. *Risk C: Monitor therapy*

Ethanol/Nutrition/Herb Interactions

Ethanol: Monitor ethanol use (alcohol use may increase triglycerides).

Stability Store at controlled room temperature of 25°C (77°F); do not freeze.

Mechanism of Action Mechanism has not been completely defined. Possible mechanisms include inhibition of acyl CoA:1,2 diacylglycerol acyltransferase, increased hepatic beta-oxidation, a reduction in the hepatic synthesis of triglycerides, or an increase in plasma lipoprotein lipase activity.

Dosage Oral: Adults:

Hypertriglyceridemia: 4 g/day as a single daily dose or in 2 divided doses

Treatment of IgA nephropathy (unlabeled use): 4 g/day

Dosage adjustment in renal impairment: No dosage adjustment required.

Dietary Considerations May be taken with or without food. Dietary modification is important in the control of severe hypertriglyceridemia. Maintain standard cholesterol-lowering diet during therapy..

Administration May be administered with or without food.

Monitoring Parameters Triglycerides and other lipids (LDL-C) should be monitored at baseline and periodically. Hepatic transaminase levels, particularly ALT, should be monitored periodically.

Additional Information

Due to reports of prescribing errors associated with the similarity between Omacor® and Amicar,® (aminocaproic acid) the name Omacor® has been changed to Lovaza®. The size, strength, ingredients, and dose all remain the same

Dosage Forms Excipient information presented when available (limited, particularly for generics); consult specific product labeling. [DSC] = Discontinued product

Capsule:

Lovaza®, Omacor® [DSC]: 1 g [contains EPA ~465 mg and DHA ~375 mg]

Omeprazole (oh MEP ra zole)

Medication Safety Issues

Sound-alike/look-alike issues:

Prilosec® may be confused with Plendil®, Prevacid®, predniSONE, prilocaine, Prinivil®, Proventil®, Prozac®

International issues:

Norpramin®: Brand name for desipramine in the U.S.

U.S. Brand Names Prilosec OTC™ [OTC]; Prilosec®

Canadian Brand Names Apo-Omeprazole®; Losec MUPS®; Losec®; ratio-Omeprazole; Sandoz Omeprazole

Mexican Brand Names Aleprozil; Azoran; Domer; Inhibitron; Losec; Mopral; Olexin; Prazidec; Suifac; Ulsen; Vulcasid

Pharmacologic Category Proton Pump Inhibitor; Substituted Benzimidazole

Generic Available Yes

Use Short-term (4-8 weeks) treatment of active duodenal ulcer disease or active benign gastric ulcer; treatment of heartburn and other symptoms associated with gastroesophageal reflux disease (GERD); short-term (4-8 weeks) treatment of endoscopically-diagnosed erosive esophagitis; maintenance healing of erosive esophagitis; long-term treatment of pathological hypersecretory conditions; as part of a multidrug regimen for *H. pylori* eradication to reduce the risk of duodenal ulcer recurrence

OTC labeling: Short-term treatment of frequent, uncomplicated heartburn occurring ≥2 days/week

Unlabeled/Investigational Use Healing NSAID-induced ulcers; prevention of NSAID-induced ulcers

Effect on Mental Status May cause dizziness, agitation, aggression, depression, confusion, insomnia, nervousness, anxiety, or hallucinations; may rarely cause sedation

Effect on Psychiatric Treatment May inhibit the metabolism of diazepam; monitor for increased sedation

Pregnancy Risk Factor C

Pregnancy Considerations Crosses the placenta; congenital abnormalities have been reported sporadically following omeprazole use during pregnancy. Based on data collected by the Teratogen Information System (TERIS), it was concluded that therapeutic doses used during pregnancy would be unlikely to pose a substantial teratogenic risk (quantity/quality of data: fair). Because the possibility of harm still exists, the manufacturer recommends use during pregnancy only if the potential benefit to the mother outweighs the possible risk to the fetus.

Lactation Enters breast milk/not recommended

Contraindications Hypersensitivity to omeprazole, substituted benzimidazoles (ie, esomeprazole, lansoprazole, pantoprazole, rabeprazole), or any component of the formulation

Warnings/Precautions Relief of symptoms does not preclude the presence of a gastric malignancy. Atrophic gastritis (by biopsy) has been noted with long-term omeprazole therapy. In long-term (2-year) studies in rats, omeprazole produced a dose-related increase in gastric carcinoid tumors. While available endoscopic evaluations and histologic examinations of biopsy specimens from human stomachs have not detected a risk from short-term exposure to omeprazole, further human data on the effect of sustained hypochlorhydria and hypergastrinemia is needed to rule out the possibility of an increased risk for the development of tumors in humans receiving long-term therapy. Bioavailability may be increased in the elderly, Asian population, and with hepatic dysfunction. Safety and efficacy have not been established in children <2 years of age. When used for self-medication (OTC), do not use for >14 days. Treatment should not be repeated more often than every 4 months. OTC and oral suspension are not approved for use in children <18 years of age.

Adverse Reactions

1% to 10%:

Central nervous system: Headache (3% to 7%), dizziness (2%)

Dermatologic: Rash (2%)

Gastrointestinal: Diarrhea (3% to 4%), abdominal pain (2% to 5%), nausea (2% to 4%), vomiting (2% to 3%), flatulence (≤3%), acid regurgitation (2%), constipation (1% to 2%), taste perversion

Neuromuscular & skeletal: Weakness (1%), back pain (1%)

Respiratory: Upper respiratory infection (2%), cough (1%)

<1% (Limited to important or life-threatening; adverse event occurrence may vary based on formulation): Abdominal swelling, abnormal dreams, aggression, agitation, agranulocytosis, alkaline phosphatase increased, allergic reactions, alopecia, ALT increased, AST increased, anaphylaxis, anemia, angina, angioedema, anorexia, anxiety, apathy, atrophic gastritis, benign gastric polyps, bilirubin increased, blurred vision, bradycardia, chest pain, cholestatic hepatitis, confusion, creatinine increased, depression, diaphoresis, double vision, dry skin, epistaxis, erythema multiforme, esophageal candidiasis, fatigue, fecal discoloration, fever, gastroduodenal carcinoids, GGT increased, glycosuria, gynecomastia, hallucinations, hematuria, hemifacial dysesthesia, hemolytic anemia, hepatic encephalopathy, hepatic failure, hepatic necrosis, hepatitis, hepatocellular hepatitis, hyperhidrosis, hypertension, hypoglycemia, hyponatremia, insomnia, interstitial nephritis, irritable colon, jaundice, joint pain, leg pain, leukocytosis, leukopenia, liver disease (hepatocellular, cholestatic, mixed), malaise, microscopic pyuria, mucosal atrophy (tongue), muscle cramps, muscle weakness, myalgia, nervousness, neutropenia, ocular irritation, optic atrophy, optic neuritis, optic neuropathy (anterior ischemic), pain, palpitation, pancreatitis, pancytopenia, paresthesia, peripheral edema, petechiae, pharyngeal pain, photosensitivity, pneumothorax, proteinuria, pruritus, psychic disturbance, purpura, rash, skin inflammation, somnolence, Stevens-Johnson syndrome, stomatitis, tachycardia, taste perversion, testicular pain, thrombocytopenia, tinnitus, toxic epidermal necrolysis, tremor, urinary frequency, urinary tract infection, urticaria, vertigo, weight gain, xerophthalmia, xerostomia

Metabolism/Transport Effects Substrate of CYP2A6 (minor), 2C9 (minor), 2C19 (major), 2D6 (minor), 3A4 (major); **Inhibits** CYP1A2 (weak), 2C9 (moderate), 2C19 (strong), 2D6 (weak), 3A4 (weak); **Induces** CYP1A2 (weak)

Drug Interactions

Antifungal Agents (Azole Derivatives, Systemic): Proton Pump Inhibitors may decrease the absorption of Antifungal Agents (Azole Derivatives, Systemic). **Exceptions:** Miconazole. *Risk D: Consider therapy modification*

Atazanavir: Proton Pump Inhibitors may decrease the absorption of Atazanavir. *Risk D: Consider therapy modification*

Benzodiazepines (metabolized by oxidation): Proton Pump Inhibitors may increase the serum concentration of Benzodiazepines (metabolized by oxidation). *Risk C: Monitor therapy*

Cilostazol: Omeprazole may enhance the adverse/toxic effect of Cilostazol. *Risk D: Consider therapy modification*

Clopidogrel: Proton Pump Inhibitors may diminish the therapeutic effect of Clopidogrel. This appears to be due to reduced formation of the active clopidogrel metabolite. *Risk C: Monitor therapy*

Clozapine: Omeprazole may decrease the serum concentration of Clozapine. Omeprazole may increase the serum concentration of Clozapine. *Risk C: Monitor therapy*

CYP2C19 Inducers (Strong): May increase the metabolism of CYP2C19 Substrates. *Risk C: Monitor therapy*

CYP2C19 Substrates: CYP2C19 Inhibitors (Strong) may decrease the metabolism of CYP2C19 Substrates. *Risk D: Consider therapy modification*

CYP2C9 Substrates (High risk): CYP2C9 Inhibitors (Moderate) may decrease the metabolism of CYP2C9 Substrates (High risk). *Risk C: Monitor therapy*

Dabigatran Etexilate: Proton Pump Inhibitors may decrease the serum concentration of Dabigatran Etexilate. *Risk C: Monitor therapy*

Dasatinib: Proton Pump Inhibitors may decrease the absorption of Dasatinib. *Risk D: Consider therapy modification*

Erlotinib: Proton Pump Inhibitors may decrease the serum concentration of Erlotinib. *Risk X: Avoid combination*

Indinavir: Proton Pump Inhibitors may decrease the absorption of Indinavir. *Risk C: Monitor therapy*

Iron Salts: Proton Pump Inhibitors may decrease the absorption of Iron Salts. **Exceptions:** Ferric Gluconate; Iron Dextran Complex; Iron Sucrose. *Risk C: Monitor therapy*

Methotrexate: Proton Pump Inhibitors may decrease the excretion of Methotrexate. Antirheumatic doses of methotrexate probably hold minimal risk. *Risk C: Monitor therapy*

Mycophenolate: Proton Pump Inhibitors may decrease the serum concentration of Mycophenolate. Specifically, concentrations of the active mycophenolic acid may be reduced. *Risk C: Monitor therapy*

Nelfinavir: Omeprazole may decrease the serum concentration of Nelfinavir. *Risk C: Monitor therapy*

Phenytoin: Proton Pump Inhibitors may increase the serum concentration of Phenytoin. *Risk C: Monitor therapy*

Saquinavir: Proton Pump Inhibitors may increase the serum concentration of Saquinavir. *Risk C: Monitor therapy*

Tipranavir: May decrease the serum concentration of Proton Pump Inhibitors. These data are derived from studies with Ritonavir-boosted Tipranavir. *Risk C: Monitor therapy*

Warfarin: Proton Pump Inhibitors may increase the serum concentration of Warfarin. *Risk C: Monitor therapy*

Ethanol/Nutrition/Herb Interactions

Ethanol: Avoid ethanol (may cause gastric mucosal irritation).

Food: Food delays absorption.

Stability Store at 15°C to 30°C (59°F to 86°F). Protect from light.

Mechanism of Action Proton pump inhibitor; suppresses gastric basal and stimulated acid secretion by inhibiting the parietal cell H+/K+ ATP pump

Pharmacodynamics/Kinetics

Onset of action: Antisecretory: ~1 hour

Peak effect: 0.5-3.5 hours

Duration: Up to 72 hours

Protein binding: ~95%

Metabolism: Extensively hepatic to inactive metabolites

Bioavailability: Oral: ~30% to 40%; increased in Asian patients and patients with hepatic dysfunction

Half-life elimination: Delayed release capsule: 0.5-1 hour

Excretion: Urine (77% as metabolites, very small amount as unchanged drug); feces

Dosage Oral:

Children ≥2 years: GERD or other acid-related disorders:

<20 kg: 10 mg once daily

≥20 kg: 20 mg once daily

Adults:

Active duodenal ulcer: 20 mg/day for 4-8 weeks

Gastric ulcers: 40 mg/day for 4-8 weeks

Symptomatic GERD: 20 mg/day for up to 4 weeks

Erosive esophagitis: 20 mg/day for 4-8 weeks; maintenance of healing: 20 mg/day for up to 12 months total therapy (including treatment period of 4-8 weeks)

Helicobacter pylori eradication: Dose varies with regimen: 20 mg once daily **or** 40 mg/day as single dose or in 2 divided doses; requires combination therapy with antibiotics

Pathological hypersecretory conditions: Initial: 60 mg once daily; doses up to 120 mg 3 times/day have been administered; administer daily doses >80 mg in divided doses

Frequent heartburn (OTC labeling): 20 mg/day for 14 days; treatment may be repeated after 4 months if needed

Dosage adjustment in hepatic impairment: Specific guidelines are not available; bioavailability is increased with chronic liver disease

Dietary Considerations Should be taken on an empty stomach; best if taken before breakfast.

Administration

Capsule: Should be swallowed whole; do not chew or crush. Best if taken before breakfast. Delayed release capsule may be opened and contents added to applesauce. Administration via NG tube should be in an acidic juice.

Tablet: Should be swallowed whole; do not crush or chew.

Dosage Forms Excipient information presented when available (limited, particularly for generics); consult specific product labeling.

Capsule, delayed release: 10 mg, 20 mg, 40 mg

Prilosec®: 10 mg, 20 mg, 40 mg

Tablet, delayed release: 20 mg

Prilosec OTC™: 20 mg

Omeprazole and Sodium Bicarbonate

(oh ME pray zol & SOW dee um bye KAR bun ate)

U.S. Brand Names Zegerid®

Pharmacologic Category Proton Pump Inhibitor; Substituted Benzimidazole

Use Short-term (4-8 weeks) treatment of active duodenal ulcer disease or active benign gastric ulcer; treatment of heartburn and other symptoms associated with gastroesophageal reflux disease (GERD); short-term (4-8 weeks) treatment of endoscopically-diagnosed erosive esophagitis; maintenance healing of erosive esophagitis; reduction of risk of upper gastrointestinal bleeding in critically-ill patients

Effect on Mental Status May cause dizziness, agitation, aggression, depression, confusion, insomnia, nervousness, anxiety, or hallucinations; may rarely cause sedation

Effect on Psychiatric Treatment May inhibit the metabolism of diazepam; monitor for increased sedation

Dosage Summary Oral: Both strengths of Zegerid® capsule and powder for oral suspension have identical sodium bicarbonate content, respectively. Do not substitute two 20 mg capsules/packets for one 40 mg dose.

Children: Dosage not established

Adults: 20-40 mg/day (may be given in 2 divided doses)

Dosage Forms Excipient information presented when available (limited, particularly for generics); consult specific product labeling.

Capsule, immediate release:

Zegerid®: 20 mg, 40 mg [both strengths contain sodium bicarbonate 1100 mg, equivalent to sodium 300 mg (13 mEq) per capsule]

Powder for oral suspension:

Zegerid®: 20 mg/packet (30s), 40 mg/packet (30s) [both strengths contain sodium bicarbonate 1680 mg, equivalent to sodium 460 mg per packet]

- **Omnaris™** *see* Ciclesonide *on page 343*
- **Omnicef®** *see* Cefdinir *on page 293*
- **OMNIhist® II L.A.** *see* Chlorpheniramine, Phenylephrine, and Methscopolamine *on page 329*
- **Omnipred™** *see* PrednisoLONE *on page 1326*
- **Omnitrope™** *see* Somatropin *on page 1499*
- **Oncaspar®** *see* Pegaspargase *on page 1235*
- **Oncovin** *see* VinCRIStine *on page 1673*

Ondansetron (on DAN se tron)

Medication Safety Issues

Sound-alike/look-alike issues:

Ondansetron may be confused with dolasetron, granisetron, palonosetron

Zofran® may be confused with Zantac®, Zosyn®

U.S. Brand Names Zofran®; Zofran® ODT

Canadian Brand Names Apo-Ondansetron®; Gen-Ondansetron; Novo-Ondansetron; Ondansetron Injection; Ondansetron-Omega; PHL-Ondansetron; PMS-Ondansetron; ratio-Ondansetron; Sandoz-Ondansetron; Zofran®; Zofran® ODT

Mexican Brand Names Danac; Lartron; Zofran

Index Terms GR38032R; Ondansetron Hydrochloride

Pharmacologic Category Antiemetic; Selective 5-HT_3 Receptor Antagonist

Generic Available Yes

Use Prevention of nausea and vomiting associated with moderately- to highly-emetogenic cancer chemotherapy; radiotherapy in patients receiving total body irradiation or fractions to the abdomen; prevention of postoperative nausea and vomiting (PONV); treatment of PONV if no prophylactic dose received

Unlabeled/Investigational Use Treatment of early-onset alcoholism; hyperemesis gravidarum

Effect on Mental Status May cause dizziness

Effect on Psychiatric Treatment Barbiturates and carbamazepine may increase the metabolism of ondansetron; monitor for diminished effects

Pregnancy Risk Factor B

Pregnancy Considerations Teratogenic effects were not observed in animal studies; however, there are no adequate and well-controlled studies in pregnant women. Use of ondansetron for the treatment of nausea and vomiting of pregnancy (NVP) has been evaluated. Additional studies are needed to determine safety to the fetus, particularly during the first trimester. Based on preliminary data, use is generally reserved for severe NVP (hyperemesis gravidarum) or when conventional treatments are not effective.

Lactation Excretion in breast milk unknown/use caution

Contraindications Hypersensitivity to ondansetron, other selective 5-HT_3 antagonists, or any component of the formulation

Warnings/Precautions Ondansetron should be used on a scheduled basis, not on an "as needed" (PRN) basis, since data support the use of this drug only in the prevention of nausea and vomiting (due to antineoplastic therapy) and not in the rescue of nausea and vomiting. Ondansetron should only be used in the first 24-48 hours of chemotherapy. Data do not support any increased efficacy of ondansetron in delayed nausea and vomiting. Does not stimulate gastric or intestinal peristalsis; may mask progressive ileus and/or gastric distension. Use with caution in patients allergic to other 5-HT_3 receptor antagonists; cross-reactivity has been reported.

Use with caution in patients with congenital long QT syndrome or other risk factors for QT prolongation (eg, medications known to prolong QT interval, electrolyte abnormalities, and cumulative high-dose anthracycline therapy). 5-HT_3 antagonists have been associated with a number of dose-dependent increases in ECG intervals (eg, PR, QRS duration, QT/QT_c, JT), usually occurring 1-2 hours after I.V. administration. In general, these changes are not clinically relevant, however, when used in conjunction with other agents that prolong these intervals, arrhythmia may occur. When used with agents that prolong the QT interval (eg, Class I and III antiarrhythmics), clinically relevant QT interval prolongation may occur resulting in torsade de pointes. I.V. formulations of 5-HT_3 antagonists have more association with ECG interval changes, compared to oral formulations.

Orally-disintegrating tablets contain phenylalanine. Safety and efficacy for children <1 month of age have not been established.

Adverse Reactions Note: Percentages reported in adult patients.

>10%:

Central nervous system: Headache (9% to 27%), malaise/fatigue (9% to 13%)

Gastrointestinal: Constipation (6% to 11%)

1% to 10%:

Central nervous system: Drowsiness (8%), fever (2% to 8%), dizziness (4% to 7%), anxiety (6%), cold sensation (2%)

Dermatologic: Pruritus (2% to 5%), rash (1%)

Gastrointestinal: Diarrhea (2% to 7%)

Genitourinary: Gynecological disorder (7%), urinary retention (5%)

Hepatic: ALT increased (1% to 5%), AST increased (1% to 5%)
Local: Injection site reaction (4%; pain, redness, burning)
Neuromuscular & skeletal: Paresthesia (2%)
Respiratory: Hypoxia (9%)

<1% (Limited to important or life-threatening): Anaphylactoid reactions, anaphylaxis, angina, angioedema, arrhythmia, blindness (transient/following infusion; lasting ≤48 hours), blurred vision (transient/following infusion), bradycardia, bronchospasm, cardiopulmonary arrest, dyspnea, dystonic reaction, ECG changes, electrocardiographic alterations (second-degree heart block and ST-segment depression), extrapyramidal symptoms, flushing, grand mal seizure, hiccups, hypersensitivity reaction, hypokalemia, hypotension, laryngeal edema, laryngospasm, oculogyric crisis, palpitation, premature ventricular contractions (PVC), QT interval increased, shock, stridor, supraventricular tachycardia, syncope, tachycardia, urticaria, vascular occlusive events, ventricular arrhythmia

Metabolism/Transport Effects Substrate of CYP1A2 (minor), 2C9 (minor), 2D6 (minor), 2E1 (minor), 3A4 (major); **Inhibits** CYP1A2 (weak), 2C9 (weak), 2D6 (weak)

Drug Interactions

Apomorphine: Antiemetics (5HT3 Antagonists) may enhance the hypotensive effect of Apomorphine. *Risk X: Avoid combination*

CYP3A4 Inducers (Strong): May increase the metabolism of CYP3A4 Substrates. *Risk C: Monitor therapy*

Deferasirox: May decrease the serum concentration of CYP3A4 Substrates. *Risk C: Monitor therapy*

Herbs (CYP3A4 Inducers): May increase the metabolism of CYP3A4 Substrates. *Risk C: Monitor therapy*

P-Glycoprotein Inducers: May decrease the serum concentration of P-Glycoprotein Substrates. P-glycoprotein inducers may also further limit the distribution of p-glycoprotein substrates to specific cells/tissues/organs where p-glycoprotein is present in large amounts (e.g., brain, T-lymphocytes, testes, etc.). *Risk C: Monitor therapy*

P-Glycoprotein Inhibitors: May increase the serum concentration of P-Glycoprotein Substrates. P-glycoprotein inhibitors may also enhance the distribution of p-glycoprotein substrates to specific cells/tissues/organs where p-glycoprotein is present in large amounts (e.g., brain, T-lymphocytes, testes, etc.). *Risk C: Monitor therapy*

Rifamycin Derivatives: May increase the metabolism of Antiemetics (5HT3 Antagonists). *Risk C: Monitor therapy*

Ethanol/Nutrition/Herb Interactions

Food: Food increases the extent of absorption. The C_{max} and T_{max} do not change much.

Herb/Nutraceutical: St John's wort may decrease ondansetron levels.

Stability

Oral solution: Store between 15°C and 30°C (59°F and 86°F). Protect from light.

Premixed bag: Store between 2°C and 30°C (36°F and 86°F). Protect from light.

Tablet: Store between 2°C and 30°C (36°F and 86°F).

Vial: Store between 2°C and 30°C (36°F and 86°F). Protect from light. Prior to I.V. infusion, dilute in 50 mL D_5W or NS. Solution is stable for 48 hours at room temperature.

Mechanism of Action Selective 5-HT_3-receptor antagonist, blocking serotonin, both peripherally on vagal nerve terminals and centrally in the chemoreceptor trigger zone

Pharmacodynamics/Kinetics

Onset of action: ~30 minutes

Distribution: V_d: Children: 1.7-3.7 L/kg; Adults: 2.2-2.5 L/kg

Protein binding, plasma: 70% to 76%

Metabolism: Extensively hepatic via hydroxylation, followed by glucuronide or sulfate conjugation; CYP1A2, CYP2D6, and CYP3A4 substrate; some demethylation occurs

Bioavailability: Oral: 56% to 71%; Rectal: 58% to 74%

Half-life elimination: Children <15 years: 2-7 hours; Adults: 3-6 hours
Mild-to-moderate hepatic impairment: Adults: 12 hours
Severe hepatic impairment (Child-Pugh C): Adults: 20 hours

Time to peak: Oral: ~2 hours

Excretion: Urine (44% to 60% as metabolites, 5% to 10% as unchanged drug); feces (~25%)

Dosage Note: Studies in adults have shown a single daily dose of 8-12 mg I.V. or 8-24 mg orally to be as effective as mg/kg dosing, and should be considered for **all** patients whose mg/kg dose exceeds 8-12 mg I.V.; oral solution and ODT formulations are bioequivalent to corresponding doses of tablet formulation

Children:

I.V.:

Prevention of chemotherapy-induced emesis: 6 months to 18 years: 0.15 mg/kg/dose administered 30 minutes prior to chemotherapy, 4 and 8 hours after the first dose **or** 0.45 mg/kg/day as a single dose

Prevention of postoperative nausea and vomiting: 1 month to 12 years:

≤40 kg: 0.1 mg/kg as a single dose

>40 kg: 4 mg as a single dose

Oral: Prevention of chemotherapy-induced emesis:

4-11 years: 4 mg 30 minutes before chemotherapy; repeat 4 and 8 hours after initial dose, then 4 mg every 8 hours for 1-2 days after chemotherapy completed

≥12 years: Refer to adult dosing.

Adults:

I.V.:

Prevention of chemotherapy-induced emesis:

0.15 mg/kg 3 times/day beginning 30 minutes prior to chemotherapy **or**

0.45 mg/kg once daily **or**

8-10 mg 1-2 times/day **or**

24 mg or 32 mg once daily

Treatment of hyperemesis gravidum (unlabeled use): 8 mg administered over 15 minutes every 12 hours **or** 1 mg/hour infused continuously for up to 24 hours

I.M., I.V.: Postoperative nausea and vomiting: 4 mg as a single dose approximately 30 minutes before the end of anesthesia, or as treatment if vomiting occurs after surgery

Note: Repeat doses given in response to inadequate control of nausea/ vomiting from preoperative doses are generally ineffective.

Oral:

Chemotherapy-induced emesis:

Highly-emetogenic agents/single-day therapy: 24 mg given 30 minutes prior to the start of therapy

Moderately-emetogenic agents: 8 mg every 12 hours beginning 30 minutes before chemotherapy, continuously for 1-2 days after chemotherapy completed

Total body irradiation: 8 mg 1-2 hours before daily each fraction of radiotherapy

Single high-dose fraction radiotherapy to abdomen: 8 mg 1-2 hours before irradiation, then 8 mg every 8 hours after first dose for 1-2 days after completion of radiotherapy

Daily fractionated radiotherapy to abdomen: 8 mg 1-2 hours before irradiation, then 8 mg 8 hours after first dose for each day of radiotherapy

Postoperative nausea and vomiting: 16 mg given 1 hour prior to induction of anesthesia

Treatment of hyperemesis gravidum (unlabeled use): 8 mg every 12 hours

Elderly: No dosing adjustment required

Dosage adjustment in renal impairment: No dosing adjustment required

Dosage adjustment in hepatic impairment: Severe liver disease (Child-Pugh C): Maximum daily dose: 8 mg

Dietary Considerations Take without regard to meals.

Orally-disintegrating tablet contains <0.03 mg phenylalanine

Administration

Oral: Oral dosage forms should be administered 30 minutes prior to chemotherapy; 1-2 hours before radiotherapy; 1 hour prior to the induction of anesthesia.

Orally-disintegrating tablets: Do not remove from blister until needed. Peel backing off the blister, do not push tablet through. Using dry hands, place tablet on tongue and allow to dissolve. Swallow with saliva.

I.M.: Should be administered undiluted.

I.V.:

IVPB: Dilute in 50 mL D_5W or NS. Infuse over 15-30 minutes; 24-hour continuous infusions have been reported, but are rarely used.

Chemotherapy-induced nausea and vomiting: Give first dose 30 minutes prior to beginning chemotherapy.

I.V. push: Prevention of postoperative nausea and vomiting: Single doses may be administered I.V. injection over 2-5 minutes as undiluted solution.

Monitoring Parameters Closely monitor patients <4 months of age

Dosage Forms Excipient information presented when available (limited, particularly for generics); consult specific product labeling. [DSC] = Discontinued product

Infusion, premixed in D_5 [preservative free]: 32 mg (50 mL)
Zofran®: 32 mg (50 mL) [DSC]
Injection, solution: 2 mg/mL (2 mL, 20 mL)
Zofran®: 2 mg/mL (2 mL, 20 mL)
Injection, solution [preservative free]: 2 mg/mL (2 mL)
Solution, oral: 4 mg/5 mL (50 mL)
Zofran®: 4 mg/5 mL (50 mL) [contains sodium benzoate; strawberry flavor]
Tablet: 4 mg; 8 mg
Zofran®: 4 mg; 8 mg
Tablet, orally disintegrating: 4 mg; 8 mg
Zofran® ODT: 4 mg, 8 mg [each strength contains phenylalanine <0.03 mg/tablet; strawberry flavor]

- ◆ **Ondansetron Hydrochloride** *see* Ondansetron *on page 1180*
- ◆ **One Gram C [OTC]** *see* Ascorbic Acid *on page 141*
- ◆ **ONTAK®** *see* Denileukin Diftitox *on page 425*
- ◆ **Onxol®** *see* Paclitaxel *on page 1213*
- ◆ **Opana®** *see* Oxymorphone *on page 1210*
- ◆ **Opana® ER** *see* Oxymorphone *on page 1210*
- ◆ **OPC-13013** *see* Cilostazol *on page 344*
- ◆ **OPC-14597** *see* Aripiprazole *on page 133*
- ◆ **OP-CCK** *see* Sincalide *on page 1489*
- ◆ **Opcon-A® [OTC]** *see* Naphazoline and Pheniramine *on page 1102*
- ◆ **Ophthetic®** *see* Proparacaine *on page 1352*
- ◆ **Opium and Belladonna** *see* Belladonna and Opium *on page 174*

Opium Tincture (OH pee um TING chur)

Medication Safety Issues

Sound-alike/look-alike issues:
Opium tincture may be confused with camphorated tincture of opium (paregoric)

High alert medication: The Institute for Safe Medication Practices (ISMP) includes this medication among its list of drugs which have a heightened risk of causing significant patient harm when used in error.

Use care when prescribing opium tincture; each mL contains the equivalent of morphine 10 mg; paregoric contains the equivalent of morphine 0.4 mg/mL

DTO is an error-prone abbreviation (mistaken as Diluted Tincture of Opium; dose equivalency of paregoric)

Index Terms DTO (error-prone abbreviation); Opium Tincture, Deodorized

Pharmacologic Category Analgesic, Opioid; Antidiarrheal

Use Treatment of diarrhea or relief of pain

Effect on Mental Status Dizziness and drowsiness are common; may cause restlessness; may rarely cause insomnia or depression

Effect on Psychiatric Treatment Concurrent use with psychotropics may alter the analgesic effects of opioids; monitor for altered response

Restrictions C-II

Dosage Summary

Oral: Note: Opium tincture 10% contains morphine 10 mg/mL. Use caution in ordering, dispensing, and/or administering.
Children: 0.005-0.02 mL/kg/dose every 3-4 hours (maximum: 0.06 mL/kg/day [diarrhea])
Adults: 0.3-1.5 mL/dose every 2-6 hours (maximum: 6 mL/day [diarrhea])

Dosage Forms Excipient information presented when available (limited, particularly for generics); consult specific product labeling.
Liquid: 10% (120 mL, 480 mL) [0.6 mL equivalent to morphine 6 mg; contains alcohol 19%]

- ◆ **Opium Tincture, Deodorized** *see* Opium Tincture *on page 1183*

Oprelvekin (oh PREL ve kin)

Medication Safety Issues

Sound-alike/look-alike issues:

Oprelvekin may be confused with aldesleukin, Proleukin®

Neumega® may be confused with Neulasta®, Neupogen®

U.S. Brand Names Neumega®

Mexican Brand Names Neumega

Index Terms IL-11; Interleukin-11; NSC-722848; Recombinant Human Interleukin-11; Recombinant Interleukin-11; rhIL-11; rIL-11

Pharmacologic Category Biological Response Modulator; Human Growth Factor

Use Prevention of severe thrombocytopenia; reduce the need for platelet transfusions following myelosuppressive chemotherapy

Effect on Mental Status Dizziness, insomnia, and fatigue are common

Effect on Psychiatric Treatment Anemia is common; use caution with clozapine and carbamazepine

Dosage Summary

SubQ:

Children (unlabeled use): 75-100 mcg/kg once daily; **Note:** A safe and effective dose for use in children has not been established by the manufacturer.

Adults: 50 mcg/kg once daily

Dosage Forms Excipient information presented when available (limited, particularly for generics); consult specific product labeling.

Injection, powder for reconstitution:

Neumega®: 5 mg [packaged with diluent]

- ◆ **Opti-Clear [OTC]** *see* Tetrahydrozoline *on page 1560*
- ◆ **Optigene® 3 [OTC] [DSC]** *see* Tetrahydrozoline *on page 1560*
- ◆ **OptiPranolol®** *see* Metipranolol *on page 1031*
- ◆ **Optivar®** *see* Azelastine *on page 162*
- ◆ **o,p'-DDD** *see* Mitotane *on page 1061*
- ◆ **Oracea™** *see* Doxycycline *on page 509*
- ◆ **Oramorph SR®** *see* Morphine Sulfate *on page 1077*
- ◆ **Oranyl [OTC]** *see* Pseudoephedrine *on page 1367*
- ◆ **Oranyl Plus [OTC]** *see* Acetaminophen and Pseudoephedrine *on page 37*
- ◆ **Orap®** *see* Pimozide *on page 1290*
- ◆ **Orapred®** *see* PrednisoLONE *on page 1326*
- ◆ **Orapred ODT™** *see* PrednisoLONE *on page 1326*
- ◆ **OraVerse™** *see* Phentolamine *on page 1272*
- ◆ **Orciprenaline Sulfate** *see* Metaproterenol *on page 996*
- ◆ **Orencia®** *see* Abatacept *on page 22*
- ◆ **Orfadin®** *see* Nitisinone *on page 1146*
- ◆ **Organidin® NR** *see* GuaiFENesin *on page 737*

Orlistat (OR li stat)

Medication Safety Issues

Sound-alike/look-alike issues:

Xenical® may be confused with Xeloda®

U.S. Brand Names Alli™ [OTC]; Xenical®

Canadian Brand Names Xenical®

Mexican Brand Names Xenical

Pharmacologic Category Lipase Inhibitor

Generic Available No

Use Management of obesity, including weight loss and weight management when used in conjunction with a reduced-calorie diet; reduce the risk of weight regain after prior weight loss; indicated for obese patients with an initial body mass index (BMI) ≥30 kg/m^2 or ≥27 kg/m^2 in the presence of other risk factors; see Body Mass Index on page 1746 in the Appendix

Effect on Mental Status May cause anxiety, fatigue, and sleep disorders

Effect on Psychiatric Treatment None reported; be vigilant for abuse in patients with anorexia nervosa or bulimia

Pregnancy Risk Factor B

Pregnancy Considerations There are no adequate and well-controlled studies of orlistat in pregnant women. Because animal reproductive studies are not always predictive of human response, orlistat is not recommended for use during pregnancy. Teratogenicity studies were conducted in rats and rabbits at doses up to 800 mg/kg/day. Neither study showed embryotoxicity or teratogenicity. This dose is 23 and 47 times the daily human dose calculated on a body surface area basis for rats and rabbits, respectively.

Lactation Excretion in breast milk unknown/not recommended

Contraindications Hypersensitivity to orlistat or any component of the formulation; chronic malabsorption syndrome or cholestasis

Warnings/Precautions Patients should be advised to adhere to dietary guidelines; gastrointestinal adverse events may increase if taken with a diet high in fat (>30% total daily calories from fat). The daily intake of fat should be distributed over three main meals. If taken with any one meal very high in fat, the possibility of gastrointestinal effects increases. Patients should be counseled to take a multivitamin supplement that contains fat-soluble vitamins to ensure adequate nutrition because orlistat has been shown to reduce the absorption of some fat-soluble vitamins and beta-carotene. Some patients may develop increased levels of urinary oxalate following treatment; caution should be exercised when prescribing it to patients with a history of hyperoxaluria or calcium oxalate nephrolithiasis. As with any weight-loss agent, the potential exists for misuse in appropriate patient populations (eg, patients with anorexia nervosa or bulimia). Safety and efficacy have not been established in children <12 years of age. Safety and efficacy with >4 years of use have not been established.

OTC labeling: Prior to use, patients should contact their healthcare provider if they have ever had kidney stones, gall bladder disease, or pancreatitis. Patients taking medications for diabetes or thyroid disease, anticoagulants, or other weight-loss products should consult their healthcare provider or pharmacist. Patients who have had an organ transplant should not use orlistat. If severe and/or continuous abdominal pain occurs, use should be discontinued and healthcare provider consulted.

Adverse Reactions

>10%:

- Central nervous system: Headache (31%)
- Gastrointestinal: Oily spotting (27%), abdominal pain/discomfort (26%), flatus with discharge (24%), fecal urgency (22%), fatty/oily stool (20%), oily evacuation (12%), defecation increased (11%)
- Neuromuscular & skeletal: Back pain (14%)
- Respiratory: Upper respiratory infection (38%)

1% to 10%:

- Central nervous system: Fatigue (7%), anxiety (5%), sleep disorder (4%)
- Dermatologic: Dry skin (2%)
- Endocrine & metabolic: Menstrual irregularities (10%)
- Gastrointestinal: Fecal incontinence (8%), nausea (8%), infectious diarrhea (5%), rectal pain/discomfort (5%), vomiting (4%)
- Neuromuscular & skeletal: Arthritis (5%), myalgia (4%)
- Otic: Otitis (4%)

<1% (Limited to important or life-threatening): Abdominal distension, allergic reactions, anaphylaxis, angioedema, bronchitis, bronchospasm, bullous eruption, cholelithiasis (may be caused by weight loss), hepatitis (causal relationship not established), hypoglycemia (in patients with diabetes), pancreatitis, pruritus, rash, transaminases increased, urticaria

Drug Interactions

Amiodarone: Orlistat may decrease the absorption of Amiodarone. *Risk C: Monitor therapy*

Levothyroxine: Orlistat may decrease the serum concentration of Levothyroxine. *Risk C: Monitor therapy*

Warfarin: Orlistat may enhance the anticoagulant effect of Warfarin. *Risk C: Monitor therapy*

Ethanol/Nutrition/Herb Interactions

Fat-soluble vitamins: Absorption of vitamins A, D, E, and K may be decreased by orlistat. A multivitamin containing the fat-soluble vitamins (A, D, E, and K) should be administered once daily at least 2 hours before or after orlistat.

Stability Store at 15°C to 30°C (59°F to 86°F).

Mechanism of Action A reversible inhibitor of gastric and pancreatic lipases, thus inhibiting absorption of dietary fats by 30% (at doses of 120 mg 3 times/day).

Pharmacodynamics/Kinetics

Onset: 24-48 hours

Duration of action: 48-72 hours
Absorption: Minimal
Metabolism: Metabolized within the gastrointestinal wall; forms inactive metabolites
Excretion: Feces (97%, 83% as unchanged drug); urine (<2%)

Dosage Oral:
Children ≥12 years and Adults (Xenical®): 120 mg 3 times/day with each main meal containing fat (during or up to 1 hour after the meal); omit dose if meal is occasionally missed or contains no fat.
Adults (Alli™): OTC labeling: 60 mg 3 times/day with each main meal containing fat

Dietary Considerations Multivitamin supplements that contain fat-soluble vitamins should be taken once daily at least 2 hours before or after the administration of orlistat (ie, bedtime). Distribute the daily intake of fat over 3 main meals. Gastrointestinal effects of orlistat may increase if taken with any 1 meal very high in fat.

Dosage Forms Excipient information presented when available (limited, particularly for generics); consult specific product labeling.
Capsule:
Alli™: 60 mg
Xenical®: 120 mg

- **Ornex® *[OTC]*** *see* Acetaminophen and Pseudoephedrine *on page 37*
- **Ornex® Maximum Strength *[OTC]*** *see* Acetaminophen and Pseudoephedrine *on page 37*

Orphenadrine (or FEN a dreen)

Medication Safety Issues
Sound-alike/look-alike issues:
Norflex™ may be confused with norfloxacin, Noroxin®
International issues:
Flexin® [Israel] may be confused with Floxin® which is a brand name for ofloxacin in the U.S.
Flexin® [Israel]: Brand name for indomethacin in Great Britain

U.S. Brand Names Norflex™

Canadian Brand Names Norflex™; Orphenace®; Rhoxal-orphendrine

Mexican Brand Names Norflex

Index Terms Orphenadrine Citrate

Pharmacologic Category Anti-Parkinson's Agent, Anticholinergic; Skeletal Muscle Relaxant

Generic Available Yes

Use Treatment of muscle spasm associated with acute painful musculoskeletal conditions

Effect on Mental Status Drowsiness and dizziness are common; may rarely cause hallucinations

Effect on Psychiatric Treatment May rarely cause aplastic anemia; use caution with clozapine and carbamazepine; has been used to treat tardive dyskinesia and augment typical antipsychotics; clozapine is a better option; concurrent use with psychotropics may produce additive sedation

Pregnancy Risk Factor C

Pregnancy Considerations Animal reproduction studies have not been conducted. There are no adequate and well-controlled studies in pregnant women. Use during pregnancy only if clearly needed.

Lactation Excretion in breast milk unknown/use caution

Contraindications Hypersensitivity to orphenadrine or any component of the formulation; glaucoma; GI obstruction, stenosing peptic ulcer; prostatic hypertrophy, bladder neck obstruction; cardiospasm; myasthenia gravis

Warnings/Precautions Use with caution in patients with HF, cardiac decompensation, coronary insufficiency, tachycardia or cardiac arrhythmias. May cause CNS depression, which may impair physical or mental abilities. Potential for abuse; use with caution in patients with history of drug abuse. Solution for injection contains sodium bisulfite which may cause allergic reaction in some individuals. Has not been evaluated for continuous long-term use; monitor closely. Safety and efficacy in children have not been established.

Adverse Reactions Frequency not defined.
Cardiovascular: Palpitation, tachycardia
Central nervous system: Agitation, drowsiness, dizziness, euphoria, hallucination, headache, mental confusion
Dermatologic: Pruritus, urticaria

Gastrointestinal: Constipation, gastric irritation, nausea, vomiting, xerostomia
Genitourinary: Urination hesitancy, urinary retention
Hematologic: Aplastic anemia (rare)
Neuromuscular & skeletal: Tremor, weakness
Ocular: Blurred vision, intraocular pressure increased, nystagmus, pupil dilation
Respiratory: Nasal congestion
Miscellaneous: Anaphylactic reaction (injection, rare), hypersensitivity

Metabolism/Transport Effects **Substrate** (minor) of CYP1A2, 2B6, 2D6, 3A4; **Inhibits** CYP1A2 (weak), 2A6 (weak), 2B6 (weak), 2C9 (weak), 2C19 (weak), 2D6 (weak), 2E1 (weak), 3A4 (weak)

Drug Interactions

Acetylcholinesterase Inhibitors (Central): Anticholinergics may diminish the therapeutic effect of Acetylcholinesterase Inhibitors (Central). Acetylcholinesterase Inhibitors (Central) may diminish the therapeutic effect of Anticholinergics. If the anticholinergic action is a side effect of the agent, the result may be beneficial. *Risk C: Monitor therapy*

Alcohol (Ethyl): CNS Depressants may enhance the CNS depressant effect of Alcohol (Ethyl). *Risk C: Monitor therapy*

Anticholinergics: May enhance the adverse/toxic effect of other Anticholinergics. **Exceptions:** Paliperidone. *Risk C: Monitor therapy*

Cannabinoids: Anticholinergic Agents may enhance the tachycardic effect of Cannabinoids. *Risk C: Monitor therapy*

CNS Depressants: May enhance the adverse/toxic effect of other CNS Depressants. *Risk C: Monitor therapy*

Potassium Chloride: Anticholinergic Agents may enhance the ulcerogenic effect of Potassium Chloride. *Risk D: Consider therapy modification*

Pramlintide: May enhance the anticholinergic effect of Anticholinergics. These effects are specific to the GI tract. *Risk D: Consider therapy modification*

Secretin: Anticholinergic Agents may diminish the stimulatory effect of Secretin. *Risk D: Consider therapy modification*

Ethanol/Nutrition/Herb Interactions

Ethanol: Avoid ethanol (may increase CNS depression).

Herb/Nutraceutical: Avoid valerian, St John's wort, kava kava, gotu kola (may increase CNS depression).

Stability Store at 15°C to 30°C (59°F to 86°F). Protect injection solution from light.

Mechanism of Action Indirect skeletal muscle relaxant thought to work by central atropine-like effects; has some euphorigenic and analgesic properties

Pharmacodynamics/Kinetics

Onset of effect: Peak effect: Oral: 2-4 hours
Duration: 4-6 hours
Protein binding: 20%
Metabolism: Extensively hepatic
Half-life elimination: 14-16 hours
Excretion: Primarily urine (8% as unchanged drug)

Dosage

Adults:
  Oral: 100 mg twice daily
  I.M., I.V.: 60 mg every 12 hours
Elderly: Use caution; generally not recommended for use in the elderly

Administration Do not crush sustained release drug product.

Dosage Forms Excipient information presented when available (limited, particularly for generics); consult specific product labeling.

Injection, solution, as citrate: 30 mg/mL (2 mL)
  Norflex™: 30 mg/mL (2 mL) [contains sodium bisulfite]
Tablet, extended release, as citrate: 100 mg

Orphenadrine, Aspirin, and Caffeine

(or FEN a dreen, AS pir in, & KAF een)

Medication Safety Issues

Sound-alike/look-alike issues:
  Norgesic™ Forte may be confused with Norgesic 40®

U.S. Brand Names Norgesic™ Forte [DSC]; Norgesic™ [DSC]; Orphengesic Forte [DSC]; Orphengesic [DSC]

Canadian Brand Names Norgesic™; Norgesic™ Forte

Index Terms Aspirin, Orphenadrine, and Caffeine; Caffeine, Orphenadrine, and Aspirin

Pharmacologic Category Skeletal Muscle Relaxant

Use Relief of discomfort associated with skeletal muscular conditions

Effect on Mental Status Drowsiness and dizziness are common; may rarely cause hallucinations

Effect on Psychiatric Treatment May rarely cause aplastic anemia; use caution with clozapine and carbamazepine; concurrent use with psychotropics may produce additive sedation

Dosage Summary

Oral:

Children: Dosage not established

Adults: 1-2 tablets 3-4 times/day

Elderly: Use not recommended

Dosage Forms Excipient information presented when available (limited, particularly for generics); consult specific product labeling. [DSC] = Discontinued product

Tablet: Orphenadrine citrate 25 mg, aspirin 385 mg, and caffeine 30 mg; orphenadrine citrate 50 mg, aspirin 770 mg, and caffeine 60 mg

Norgesic™, Orphengesic: Orphenadrine citrate 25 mg, aspirin 385 mg, and caffeine 30 mg [DSC]

Norgesic™ Forte, Orphengesic Forte: Orphenadrine citrate 50 mg, aspirin 770 mg, and caffeine 60 mg [DSC]

◆ **Orphenadrine Citrate** *see* Orphenadrine *on page 1186*

◆ **Orphengesic [DSC]** *see* Orphenadrine, Aspirin, and Caffeine *on page 1187*

◆ **Orphengesic Forte [DSC]** *see* Orphenadrine, Aspirin, and Caffeine *on page 1187*

◆ **Ortho Cept** *see* Ethinyl Estradiol and Desogestrel *on page 592*

◆ **Ortho-Cept®** *see* Ethinyl Estradiol and Desogestrel *on page 592*

◆ **Orthoclone OKT® 3** *see* Muromonab-CD3 *on page 1086*

◆ **Ortho Cyclen** *see* Ethinyl Estradiol and Norgestimate *on page 600*

◆ **Ortho-Cyclen®** *see* Ethinyl Estradiol and Norgestimate *on page 600*

◆ **Ortho Est** *see* Estropipate *on page 588*

◆ **Ortho-Est®** *see* Estropipate *on page 588*

◆ **Ortho-Evra** *see* Ethinyl Estradiol and Norelgestromin *on page 597*

◆ **Ortho Evra®** *see* Ethinyl Estradiol and Norelgestromin *on page 597*

◆ **Ortho Micronor®** *see* Norethindrone *on page 1150*

◆ **Ortho Novum** *see* Ethinyl Estradiol and Norethindrone *on page 597*

◆ **Ortho-Novum®** *see* Ethinyl Estradiol and Norethindrone *on page 597*

◆ **Ortho Novum 1/50** *see* Mestranol and Norethindrone *on page 995*

◆ **Ortho-Novum® 1/50 [DSC]** *see* Mestranol and Norethindrone *on page 995*

◆ **Ortho Prefest** *see* Estradiol and Norgestimate *on page 580*

◆ **Ortho Tri Cyclen** *see* Ethinyl Estradiol and Norgestimate *on page 600*

◆ **Ortho Tri-Cyclen®** *see* Ethinyl Estradiol and Norgestimate *on page 600*

◆ **Ortho Tri-Cyclen® Lo** *see* Ethinyl Estradiol and Norgestimate *on page 600*

◆ **Os-Cal® 500 [OTC] [DSC]** *see* Calcium Carbonate *on page 254*

Oseltamivir (oh sel TAM i vir)

Medication Safety Issues

Sound-alike/look-alike issues:

Tamiflu® may be confused with Thera-Flu®

U.S. Brand Names Tamiflu®

Canadian Brand Names Tamiflu®

Mexican Brand Names Tamiflu

Pharmacologic Category Antiviral Agent; Neuraminidase Inhibitor

Generic Available No

Use Treatment of uncomplicated acute illness due to influenza (A or B) infection in children ≥1 year of age and adults who have been symptomatic for no more than 2 days; prophylaxis against influenza (A or B) infection in children ≥1 year of age and adults

The Advisory Committee on Immunization Practices (ACIP) recommends that **treatment** be considered for the following:

- Persons hospitalized with laboratory confirmed influenza (may also have benefit if started >48 hours after onset of illness).
- Persons with laboratory confirmed influenza pneumonia.
- Persons with laboratory confirmed influenza and bacterial infections.

- Persons with laboratory confirmed influenza and who are at higher risk for influenza complications.
- Persons presenting for care within 48 hours of laboratory confirmed influenza onset and who want to decrease duration and/or severity of their symptoms or decrease the risk of transmission to those at high risk for complications.

The ACIP recommends that **prophylaxis** be considered for the following:

- Persons at high risk for influenza infection during the first 2 weeks following vaccination (eg, children <9 years and not previously vaccinated) if the virus is circulating in the community.
- Persons at high risk for influenza infection, but the vaccination is contraindicated.
- Unvaccinated family members or healthcare providers with prolonged exposure to or close contact with high-risk persons, unvaccinated persons, or infants <6 months of age.
- Persons at high risk for influenza infection, their family members and close contacts, and healthcare workers when the circulating strain of influenza is not matched with the vaccine.
- Persons with immune deficiency or those who may not respond to vaccination.
- Unvaccinated staff and persons during response to an outbreak in a closed institutional setting that has patients at high risk for infection (eg, extended care facilities).

Effect on Mental Status May cause insomnia

Effect on Psychiatric Treatment None reported

Pregnancy Risk Factor C

Pregnancy Considerations There are insufficient human data to determine the risk to a pregnant woman or developing fetus. Studies evaluating the effects on embryo-fetal development in rats and rabbits showed a dose-dependent increase in the rates of minor skeleton abnormalities in exposed offspring. The rate of each abnormality remained within the background rate of occurrence in the species studied.

Lactation Enters breast milk/not recommended

Contraindications Hypersensitivity to oseltamivir or any component of the formulation

Warnings/Precautions Oseltamivir is not a substitute for the influenza virus vaccine. Use caution with renal impairment; dosage adjustment is required for creatinine clearance <30 mL/minute. Also consider primary or concomitant bacterial infections. Safety and efficacy for use in severe hepatic impairment or for treatment or prophylaxis in immunocompromised patients have not been established. Efficacy has not been established if treatment begins >40 hours after the onset of symptoms or in the treatment of patients with chronic cardiac and/or respiratory disease. Rare but severe hypersensitivity reactions (anaphylaxis, severe dermatologic reactions) have been associated with use. Rare occurrences of neuropsychiatric events (including confusion, delirium, hallucinations, and/or self-injury) have been reported from postmarketing surveillance (primarily in pediatric patients); direct causation is difficult to establish (influenza infection may also be associated with behavioral and neurologic changes). Monitor closely for signs of any unusual behavior. Safety and efficacy in children (<1 year of age) have not been established.

Adverse Reactions

>10%: Gastrointestinal: Vomiting (2% to 15%)

1% to 10%: Gastrointestinal: Nausea (3% to 10%), abdominal pain (2% to 5%)

<1% (Limited to important or life-threatening): Allergy, anaphylactic/anaphylactoid reaction, arrhythmia, confusion, dermatitis, diabetes aggravation, eczema, erythema multiforme, hepatitis, liver function tests abnormal, neuropsychiatric events (self-injury, confusion, delirium), rash, seizure, Stevens-Johnson syndrome, swelling of face or tongue, toxic epidermal necrolysis, urticaria

Drug Interactions

Influenza Virus Vaccine: Antiviral Agents (Influenza A and B) may diminish the therapeutic effect of Influenza Virus Vaccine. This only pertains to live, attentuated influenza virus vaccine. *Risk D: Consider therapy modification*

Stability

Capsules: Store at 25°C (77°F).

Oral suspension: Store powder for suspension at 25°C (77°F). Reconstitute with 23 mL of water (to make 25 mL total suspension). Once reconstituted, store suspension under refrigeration at 2°C to 8°C (36°F to 46°F); do not freeze. Use within 10 days of preparation.

Mechanism of Action Oseltamivir, a prodrug, is hydrolyzed to the active form, oseltamivir carboxylate (OC). OC inhibits influenza virus neuraminidase, an enzyme known to cleave the budding viral progeny from its cellular envelope attachment point (neuraminic acid) just prior to release.

Pharmacodynamics/Kinetics

Absorption: Well absorbed

Distribution: V_d: 23-26 L (oseltamivir carboxylate)

Protein binding, plasma: Oseltamivir carboxylate: 3%; Oseltamivir: 42%

Metabolism: Hepatic (90%) to oseltamivir carboxylate; neither the parent drug nor active metabolite has any effect on the cytochrome P450 system

Bioavailability: 75% as oseltamivir carboxylate

Half-life elimination: Oseltamivir: 1-3 hours; Oseltamivir carboxylate: 6-10 hours

Excretion: Urine (>90% as oseltamivir carboxylate); feces

Dosage Oral:

Treatment: Initiate treatment within 2 days of onset of symptoms; duration of treatment: 5 days:

Children: 1-12 years:

≤15 kg: 30 mg twice daily

>15 kg to ≤23 kg: 45 mg twice daily

>23 kg to ≤40 kg: 60 mg twice daily

>40 kg: 75 mg twice daily

Adolescents ≥13 years and Adults: 75 mg twice daily

Prophylaxis: Initiate treatment within 2 days of contact with an infected individual; duration of treatment: 10 days

Children: 1-12 years:

≤15 kg: 30 mg once daily

>15 kg to ≤23 kg: 45 mg once daily

>23 kg to ≤40 kg: 60 mg once daily

>40 kg: 75 mg once daily

Adolescents ≥13 years and Adults: 75 mg once daily. During community outbreaks, dosing is 75 mg once daily. May be used for up to 6 weeks; duration of protection lasts for length of dosing period

Dosage adjustment in renal impairment: Adults:

Cl_{cr} 10-30 mL/minute:

Treatment: Reduce dose to 75 mg once daily for 5 days

Prophylaxis: 75 mg every other day or 30 mg once daily

CAPD (unlabeled dose): 30 mg once weekly (Robson, 2006)

Hemodialysis (unlabeled dose): 30 mg after every other session (Robson, 2006)

Dosage adjustment in hepatic impairment: No adjustment required in mild-to-moderate hepatic impairment. Safety and kinetics in patients with severe hepatic impairment have not been evaluated.

Dietary Considerations Take with or without food; take with food to improve tolerance.

Administration Capsules may be opened and mixed with sweetened liquid (eg, chocolate syrup).

Monitoring Parameters Signs or symptoms of unusual behavior, including attempts at self-injury, confusion, and/or delirium

Additional Information In clinical studies of the influenza virus, 1.3% of post-treatment isolates in adults and adolescents and 8.6% of isolates in children had decreased neuraminidase susceptibility *in vitro* to oseltamivir carboxylate.

Dosage Forms Excipient information presented when available (limited, particularly for generics); consult specific product labeling.

Capsule, as phosphate:

Tamiflu®: 30 mg, 45 mg, 75 mg

Powder for oral suspension:

Tamiflu®: 12 mg/mL (25 mL) [contains sodium benzoate; tutti-frutti flavor]

- **OSI-774** *see* Erlotinib *on page 556*
- **Osmitrol®** *see* Mannitol *on page 968*
- **OTFC (Oral Transmucosal Fentanyl Citrate)** *see* FentaNYL *on page 624*
- **Otrivin® [OTC] [DSC]** *see* Xylometazoline *on page 1687*
- **Otrivin® Pediatric [OTC] [DSC]** *see* Xylometazoline *on page 1687*
- **Ovcon®** *see* Ethinyl Estradiol and Norethindrone *on page 597*
- **Ovidrel®** *see* Chorionic Gonadotropin (Recombinant) *on page 343*

Oxacillin (oks a SIL in)

Index Terms Methylphenyl Isoxazolyl Penicillin; Oxacillin Sodium

Pharmacologic Category Antibiotic, Penicillin

Use Treatment of infections such as osteomyelitis, septicemia, endocarditis, and CNS infections caused by susceptible strains of *Staphylococcus*

Effect on Mental Status Penicillins reported to cause apprehension, illusions, hallucinations, depersonalization, agitation, insomnia, and encephalopathy

Effect on Psychiatric Treatment May cause neutropenia; use caution with clozapine and carbamazepine

Dosage Summary

I.M.:

Children: 100-200 mg/kg/day in divided doses every 6 hours (maximum: 12 g/day)

Adults: 250-2000 mg every 4-6 hours

I.V.:

Children: 100-200 mg/kg/day in divided doses every 6 hours (maximum: 12 g/day)

Adults: 250-2000 mg every 4-6 hours

Dosage Forms Excipient information presented when available (limited, particularly for generics); consult specific product labeling.

Infusion [premixed iso-osmotic dextrose solution]: 1 g (50 mL); 2 g (50 mL)

Injection, powder for reconstitution: 1 g, 2 g, 10 g

◆ **Oxacillin Sodium** *see* Oxacillin *on page 1190*

Oxaliplatin (ox AL i pla tin)

Medication Safety Issues

Sound-alike/look-alike issues:

Oxaliplatin may be confused with Aloxi®, carboplatin

High alert medication: The Institute for Safe Medication Practices (ISMP) includes this medication among its list of drug classes which have a heightened risk of causing significant patient harm when used in error.

U.S. Brand Names Eloxatin®

Canadian Brand Names Eloxatin®

Mexican Brand Names Eloxatin; Olipcis; Riptam

Index Terms Diaminocyclohexane Oxalatoplatinum; L-OHP; NSC-266046

Pharmacologic Category Antineoplastic Agent, Alkylating Agent; Antineoplastic Agent, Platinum Analog

Use Treatment of stage III colon cancer and advanced colorectal cancer

Unlabeled/Investigational Use Treatment of esophageal cancer, gastric cancer, head and neck cancer, non-Hodgkin's lymphoma, ovarian cancer, pancreatic cancer

Effect on Mental Status Fatigue is common; may cause insomnia and dizziness

Effect on Psychiatric Treatment GI side effects are common; use caution with SSRIs. Hematologic side effects are common; use caution with clozapine, carbamazepine, and valproic acid

Dosage Summary

I.V.:

Children: Dosage not established

Adults: 85 mg/m^2 every 2 weeks **or** 20-25 mg/m^2 days 1-5 every 3 weeks **or** 100-130 mg/m^2 every 2-3 weeks

Dosage Forms Excipient information presented when available (limited, particularly for generics); consult specific product labeling. [CAN] = Canadian availability; not available in U.S.

Injection, solution [preservative free]:

Eloxatin®: 5 mg/mL (10 mL, 20 mL, 40 mL)

Injection, powder for reconstitution [preservative free]:

Eloxatin® [CAN]: 50 mg [contains lactose], 100 mg [contains lactose] [not available in U.S.]

◆ **Oxandrin®** *see* Oxandrolone *on page 1191*

Oxandrolone (oks AN droe lone)

U.S. Brand Names Oxandrin®

Pharmacologic Category Androgen

Generic Available Yes

Use Adjunctive therapy to promote weight gain after weight loss following extensive surgery, chronic infections, or severe trauma, and in some patients who, without definite pathophysiologic reasons, fail to gain or to maintain normal weight; to offset protein catabolism with prolonged corticosteroid administration; relief of bone pain associated with osteoporosis

Effect on Mental Status May cause insomnia

Effect on Psychiatric Treatment None reported

Restrictions C-III

Pregnancy Risk Factor X

Pregnancy Considerations Masculinization of the fetus has been reported.

Lactation Excretion in breast milk unknown/not recommended

Contraindications Hypersensitivity to oxandrolone or any component of the formulation; nephrosis; carcinoma of breast or prostate; hypercalcemia; pregnancy

Warnings/Precautions **[U.S. Boxed Warning]: Anabolic steroids may cause peliosis hepatis or liver cell tumors which may not be apparent until liver failure or intra-abdominal hemorrhage develops.** Discontinue in case of cholestatic hepatitis with jaundice or abnormal liver function tests. Use caution with concomitant warfarin therapy; warfarin dose may need significantly decreased. **[U.S. Boxed Warning]: May cause blood lipid changes with increased risk of arteriosclerosis.** Use with caution in elderly patients, they may be at greater risk for prostatic hyperplasia, fluid retention, and transaminase elevations. Use with caution in patients with cardiac, renal, or hepatic disease; COPD; diabetes; or epilepsy. Use with caution in patients with breast cancer; may cause hypercalcemia by stimulating osteolysis. Discontinue with evidence of mild virilization in women. May accelerate bone maturation without producing compensatory gain in linear growth in children; in prepubertal children perform radiographic examination of the hand and wrist every 6 months to determine the rate of bone maturation and to assess the effect of treatment on the epiphyseal centers.

Adverse Reactions Frequency not defined.

Cardiovascular: Edema

Central nervous system: Depression, excitation, insomnia

Dermatologic: Acne (females and prepubertal males)

Also reported in females: Hirsutism, male-pattern baldness

Endocrine & metabolic: Electrolyte imbalances, glucose intolerance, gonadotropin secretion inhibited, gynecomastia, HDL decreased, LDL increased

Also reported in females: Clitoral enlargement, menstrual irregularities

Genitourinary:

Prepubertal males: Increased or persistent erections, penile enlargement

Postpubertal males: Bladder irritation, epididymitis, impotence, oligospermia, priapism (chronic), testicular atrophy, testicular function

Hepatic: Alkaline phosphatase increased, ALT increased, AST increased, bilirubin increased, cholestatic jaundice, hepatic necrosis (rare), hepatocellular neoplasms, peliosis hepatis (with long-term therapy)

Neuromuscular & skeletal: CPK increased, premature closure of epiphyses (in children)

Renal: Creatinine excretion increased

Miscellaneous: Bromsulfophthalein retention, habituation, voice alteration (deepening, in females)

Drug Interactions

CycloSPORINE: Androgens may enhance the hepatotoxic effect of CycloSPORINE. Androgens may increase the serum concentration of CycloSPORINE. *Risk D: Consider therapy modification*

Vitamin K Antagonists (eg, warfarin): Androgens may enhance the anticoagulant effect of Vitamin K Antagonists. *Risk D: Consider therapy modification*

Mechanism of Action Synthetic testosterone derivative with similar androgenic and anabolic actions

Pharmacodynamics/Kinetics Half-life elimination: 10-13 hours

Dosage

Children: Total daily dose: ≤0.1 mg/kg **or** ≤0.045 mg/lb

Adults: 2.5-20 mg in divided doses 2-4 times/day based on individual response; a course of therapy of 2-4 weeks is usually adequate. This may be repeated intermittently as needed.

Elderly: 5 mg twice daily

Dosing adjustment in renal impairment: Caution is recommended because of the propensity of oxandrolone to cause edema and water retention

Dosing adjustment in hepatic impairment: Caution is advised but there are not specific guidelines for dosage reduction

Monitoring Parameters Liver function tests, cholesterol profile, hemoglobin/hematocrit; INR/PT in patients on anticoagulant therapy

Children: Radiographs of left wrist every 6 months (to assess bone maturation)

Adult females: Signs of virilization (deepening voice, hirsutism, acne, clitoromegaly); urine and serum calcium in women with breast cancer

Test Interactions May suppress factors II, V, VII, and X; may increase PT; may decrease thyroxine-binding globulin and radioactive iodine uptake

Dosage Forms Excipient information presented when available (limited, particularly for generics); consult specific product labeling.

Tablet: 2.5 mg, 10 mg

Oxandrin®: 2.5 mg, 10 mg

Oxaprozin (oks a PROE zin)

Medication Safety Issues

Sound-alike/look-alike issues:

Daypro® may be confused with Diupres®

Oxaprozin may be confused with oxazepam

Related Information

Nonsteroidal Anti-Inflammatory Agents *on page 1792*

U.S. Brand Names Daypro®

Canadian Brand Names Apo-Oxaprozin®; Daypro®

Pharmacologic Category Nonsteroidal Anti-inflammatory Drug (NSAID), Oral

Use Acute and long-term use in the management of signs and symptoms of osteoarthritis and rheumatoid arthritis; juvenile rheumatoid arthritis

Effect on Mental Status Dizziness is common; may cause nervousness; may rarely cause drowsiness, confusion, insomnia, or depression

Effect on Psychiatric Treatment May rarely cause agranulocytosis; use caution with clozapine and carbamazepine; may decrease lithium clearance resulting in an increase in serum lithium levels and potential lithium toxicity; monitor serum lithium levels

Restrictions An FDA-approved medication guide must be distributed when dispensing an oral outpatient prescription (new or refill) where this medication is to be used without direct supervision of a healthcare provider. Medication guides are available at http://www.fda.gov/cder/Offices/ODS/medication_guides.htm.

Dosage Summary

Oral:

Children <6 years: Dosage not established

Children 6-16 years and 22-31 kg: 600 mg once daily

Children 6-16 years and 32-54 kg: 900 mg once daily

Children 6-16 years and ≥55 kg: 1200 mg once daily

Adults: 600-1200 mg once daily (maximum: 1200 mg/day [<50 kg]; 1800 mg/day or 26 mg/kg/day (whichever lower) [>50 kg])

Dosage Forms Excipient information presented when available (limited, particularly for generics); consult specific product labeling.

Tablet: 600 mg

Oxazepam (oks A ze pam)

Medication Safety Issues

Sound-alike/look-alike issues:

Oxazepam may be confused with oxaprozin, quazepam

Serax® may be confused with Eurax®, Urex®, Zyrtec®

International issues:

Murelax® [Australia] may be confused with Miralax™ which is a brand name for polyethylene glycol 3350 in the U.S.

Related Information

Benzodiazepines *on page 1774*

CMS: Long-Term Care Facility Thresholds *on page 1815*

Discontinuation of Psychotropic Drugs *on page 1839*

U.S. Brand Names Serax®

Canadian Brand Names Apo-Oxazepam®; Bio-Oxazepam; Novoxapram®; Oxpam®; Oxpram®; PMS-Oxazepam; Riva-Oxazepam

Pharmacologic Category Benzodiazepine

Generic Available Yes: Capsule

Use Treatment of anxiety; management of ethanol withdrawal

Unlabeled/Investigational Use Anticonvulsant in management of simple partial seizures; hypnotic

Mental Health Comment In 2007, the FDA requested that all manufacturers of sedative-hypnotic drug products revise labeling to include a greater emphasis on the risks of adverse effects. These risks include severe allergic reactions (anaphylaxis, angioedema) and complex sleep-related behaviors, which may include sleep-driving (driving while not fully awake and with no memory of the event), making phone calls, and preparing and eating food while asleep.

There are two subtypes of GABA receptors (GABA-A and GABA-B) and three different benzodiazepine receptors (Bz_1, Bz_2, and Bz_3). Benzodiazepine receptors and effects appear to be linked to the GABA-A receptors. Benzodiazepines do not bind to GABA-B receptors. The role of GABA-B receptors is unclear. Benzodiazepines have no specificity for benzodiazepine receptor subtypes.

Oxazepam is a short half-life benzodiazepine. Duration of action after a single dose is determined by redistribution rather than metabolism. Tolerance develops to the sedative, hypnotic, and anticonvulsant effects. It does not develop to the anxiolytic or skeletal muscle relaxing effects. Psychological and physical dependence may occur with prolonged use of benzodiazepines. The onset of withdrawal symptoms is usually seen on the first day without drug and lasts 5-7 days in patients receiving short half-life benzodiazepines, whereas, the onset occurs after 5 days with a duration of 10-14 days after abrupt discontinuance of long half-life benzodiazepines. Risk factors for abuse include personal or family history of substance abuse and personality disorder. Oxazepam undergoes phase II metabolism and, therefore, is less likely to be affected in patients with hepatic dysfunction.

Restrictions C-IV

Pregnancy Risk Factor D

Lactation Enters breast milk/not recommended

Contraindications Hypersensitivity to oxazepam or any component of the formulation (cross-sensitivity with other benzodiazepines may exist); narrow-angle glaucoma (not in product labeling, however, benzodiazepines are contraindicated); not indicated for use in the treatment of psychosis; pregnancy

Warnings/Precautions May cause hypotension (rare) - use with caution in patients with cardiovascular or cerebrovascular disease, or in patients who would not tolerate transient decreases in blood pressure. Serax® 15 contains tartrazine; Safety and efficacy in established in pediatric patients <6 years of age; dose has not been established between 6-12 years of age.

Use with caution in elderly or debilitated patients, patients with hepatic disease (including alcoholics), or renal impairment. Use with caution in patients with respiratory disease or impaired gag reflex. Avoid use in patients with sleep apnea.

Causes CNS depression (dose-related) resulting in sedation, dizziness, confusion, or ataxia which may impair physical and mental capabilities. Patients must be cautioned about performing tasks which require mental alertness (eg, operating machinery or driving). Use with caution in patients receiving other CNS depressants or psychoactive agents. Benzodiazepines have been associated with falls and traumatic injury and should be used with extreme caution in patients who are at risk of these events (especially the elderly).

Use caution in patients with depression, particularly if suicidal risk may be present. Use with caution in patients with a history of drug dependence. Benzodiazepines have been associated with dependence and acute withdrawal symptoms on discontinuation or reduction in dose. Acute withdrawal, including seizures, may be precipitated after administration of flumazenil to patients receiving long-term benzodiazepine therapy.

Benzodiazepines have been associated with anterograde amnesia. Paradoxical reactions, including hyperactive or aggressive behavior have been reported with benzodiazepines, particularly in adolescent/pediatric or psychiatric patients. Does not have analgesic, antidepressant, or antipsychotic properties.

Adverse Reactions Frequency not defined.

Cardiovascular: Syncope (rare), edema

Central nervous system: Drowsiness, ataxia, dizziness, vertigo, memory impairment, headache, paradoxical reactions (excitement, stimulation of effect), lethargy, amnesia, euphoria

Dermatologic: Rash

Endocrine & metabolic: Decreased libido, menstrual irregularities

Genitourinary: Incontinence

Hematologic: Leukopenia, blood dyscrasias

Hepatic: Jaundice

Neuromuscular & skeletal: Dysarthria, tremor, reflex slowing

Ocular: Blurred vision, diplopia

Miscellaneous: Drug dependence

Drug Interactions

Alcohol (Ethyl): CNS Depressants may enhance the CNS depressant effect of Alcohol (Ethyl). *Risk C: Monitor therapy*

Clozapine: Benzodiazepines may enhance the adverse/toxic effect of Clozapine. *Risk D: Consider therapy modification*

CNS Depressants: May enhance the adverse/toxic effect of other CNS Depressants. *Risk C: Monitor therapy*

Phenytoin: Benzodiazepines may increase the serum concentration of Phenytoin. Short-term exposure to benzodiazepines may not present as much risk as chronic therapy. *Risk C: Monitor therapy*

Theophylline Derivatives: May diminish the therapeutic effect of Benzodiazepines. *Risk D: Consider therapy modification*

Ethanol/Nutrition/Herb Interactions

Ethanol: Avoid ethanol (may increase CNS depression).

Herb/Nutraceutical: Avoid valerian, St John's wort, kava kava, gotu kola (may increase CNS depression).

Mechanism of Action Binds to stereospecific benzodiazepine receptors on the postsynaptic GABA neuron at several sites within the central nervous system, including the limbic system, reticular formation. Enhancement of the inhibitory effect of GABA on neuronal excitability results by increased neuronal membrane permeability to chloride ions. This shift in chloride ions results in hyperpolarization (a less excitable state) and stabilization.

Pharmacodynamics/Kinetics

Absorption: Almost complete

Protein binding: 86% to 99%

Metabolism: Hepatic to inactive compounds (primarily as glucuronides)

Half-life elimination: 2.8-5.7 hours

Time to peak, serum: 2-4 hours

Excretion: Urine (as unchanged drug (50%) and metabolites)

Dosage Oral:

Adults:

Anxiety: 10-30 mg 3-4 times/day

Ethanol withdrawal: 15-30 mg 3-4 times/day

Hypnotic: 15-30 mg

Elderly: Oral: Anxiety: 10 mg 2-3 times/day; increase gradually as needed to a total of 30-45 mg/day. Dose titration should be slow to evaluate sensitivity.

Hemodialysis: Not dialyzable (0% to 5%)

Administration Administer orally in divided doses

Monitoring Parameters Respiratory and cardiovascular status

Reference Range Therapeutic: 0.2-1.4 mcg/mL (SI: 0.7-4.9 μmol/L)

Additional Information Not intended for management of anxieties and minor distresses associated with everyday life. Treatment longer than 4 months should be re-evaluated to determine the patient's need for the drug. Abrupt discontinuation after sustained use (generally >10 days) may cause withdrawal symptoms.

Dosage Forms Excipient information presented when available (limited, particularly for generics); consult specific product labeling.

Capsule: 10 mg, 15 mg, 30 mg

Tablet: 15 mg [contains tartrazine]

OXcarbazepine (ox car BAZ e peen)

Medication Safety Issues

Sound-alike/look-alike issues:

OXcarbazepine may be confused with carBAMazepine

Related Information

Anticonvulsants By Seizure Type *on page 1759*

U.S. Brand Names Trileptal®

Canadian Brand Names Trileptal®

Mexican Brand Names Actinium; Deprectal; Oxetol; Trileptal

Index Terms GP 47680; OCBZ

Pharmacologic Category Anticonvulsant, Miscellaneous

Generic Available Yes: Tablet

Use Monotherapy or adjunctive therapy in the treatment of partial seizures in adults and children ≥4 years of age with epilepsy; adjunctive therapy in the treatment of partial seizures in children ≥2 years of age with epilepsy

Unlabeled/Investigational Use Bipolar disorder; treatment of neuropathic pain

Mental Health Comment Oxcarbazepine has been associated with psychomotor slowing, difficulty with concentration, speech or language problems, sedation, ataxia, and gait disturbances. Because this agent is the 10-keto analog of carbamazepine, it is often considered useful for the management of bipolar disorder. However, there is a paucity of research data supporting this usage.

Pregnancy Risk Factor C

Pregnancy Considerations Oxcarbazepine crosses the human placenta. Teratogenic effects have been observed in animal studies. There are no adequate and well-controlled studies in pregnant women; however, oxcarbazepine is structurally related to carbamazepine (teratogenic in humans); use during pregnancy only if the benefit to the mother outweighs the potential risk to the fetus. Nonhormonal forms of contraception should be used during therapy.

Lactation Enters breast milk/not recommended

Contraindications Hypersensitivity to oxcarbazepine or any component of the formulation

Warnings/Precautions Clinically-significant hyponatremia (sodium <125 mmol/L) can develop during oxcarbazepine use. Rare cases of anaphylaxis and angioedema have been reported, even after initial dosing; permanently discontinue should symptoms occur. Use caution in patients with previous hypersensitivity to carbamazepine (cross-sensitivity occurs in 25% to 30%). Potentially serious, sometimes fatal, dermatologic reactions (eg, Stevens-Johnson, toxic epidermal necrolysis) and multiorgan hypersensitivity reactions have been reported in adults and children; monitor for signs and symptoms of skin reactions and possible disparate manifestations associated with lymphatic, hepatic, renal, and/or hematologic organ systems; discontinuation and conversion to alternate therapy may be required. As with all antiepileptic drugs, oxcarbazepine should be withdrawn gradually to minimize the potential of increased seizure frequency. Use of oxcarbazepine has been associated with CNS-related adverse events, most significant of these were cognitive symptoms including psychomotor slowing, difficulty with concentration, speech or language problems, somnolence or fatigue, and coordination abnormalities, including ataxia and gait disturbances. Effects with other sedative drugs or ethanol may be potentiated. Single-dose studies show that half-life of the primary active metabolite is prolonged 3-4 fold and AUC is doubled in patients with Cl_{cr} <30 mL/minute; dose adjustment required in these patients. May reduce the efficacy of oral contraceptives (nonhormonal contraceptive measures are recommended). Safety and efficacy in children <2 years of age have not been established.

Adverse Reactions As reported in adults with doses of up to 2400 mg/day (includes patients on monotherapy, adjunctive therapy, and those not previously on AEDs); incidence in children was similar.

>10%:

- Central nervous system: Dizziness (22% to 49%), somnolence (20% to 36%), headache (13% to 32%), ataxia (5% to 31%), fatigue (12% to 15%), vertigo (6% to 15%)
- Gastrointestinal: Vomiting (7% to 36%), nausea (15% to 29%), abdominal pain (10% to 13%)
- Neuromuscular & skeletal: Abnormal gait (5% to 17%), tremor (3% to 16%)
- Ocular: Diplopia (14% to 40%), nystagmus (7% to 26%), abnormal vision (4% to 14%)

1% to 10%:

- Cardiovascular: Hypotension (1% to 2%), leg edema (1% to 2%)
- Central nervous system: Nervousness (2% to 5%), amnesia (4%), abnormal thinking (2% to 4%), insomnia (2% to 4%), speech disorder (1% to 3%), EEG abnormalities (2%), abnormal feelings (1% to 2%), agitation (1% to 2%), confusion (1% to 2%)
- Dermatologic: Rash (4%), acne (1% to 2%)
- Endocrine & metabolic: Hyponatremia (1% to 3%)
- Gastrointestinal: Diarrhea (5% to 7%), dyspepsia (5% to 6%), constipation (2% to 6%), gastritis (1% to 2%), weight gain (1% to 2%)
- Neuromuscular & skeletal: Weakness (3% to 6%), back pain (4%), falling down (4%), abnormal coordination (1% to 4%), dysmetria (1% to 3%), sprains/strains (2%), muscle weakness (1% to 2%)
- Ocular: Abnormal accommodation (2%)
- Respiratory: Upper respiratory tract infection (7%), rhinitis (2% to 5%), chest infection (4%), epistaxis (4%), sinusitis (4%)

Postmarketing and/or case reports (limited to important or life-threatening): Aggressive reaction, amylase increased, anaphylaxis, angioedema, aphasia, asthma, aura, biliary pain, blood in stool, bradycardia, bruising, cardiac failure, cataract, cerebral hemorrhage, chest pain, cholelithiasis, colitis, conjunctival hemorrhage, consciousness decreased, convulsions aggravated, delirium, delusion, duodenal ulcer, dysphagia, dysphonia, dyspnea, dystonia, dysuria, emotional lability, enteritis, erythema multiforme, erythematosus rash, esophagitis, eye edema, extrapyramidal disorder, facial rash, gastric ulcer, GGT increased, gingival bleeding, hematuria, hemianopia, hemiplegia, hematemesis, hot flushes, hyper-/hypoglycemia, hyper-/hypokinesia, hyper-/hyporeflexia, hypersensitivity reaction, hyper-/hypotonia, hypertension, hypocalcemia, hypochondrium pain, hypoesthesia, hypokalemia, hysteria, intermenstrual bleeding, laryngismus, leukopenia, leukorrhea, lipase increased, liver enzymes elevated, maculopapular rash, manic reaction, migraine, menorrhagia, multiorgan hypersensitivity (eosinophilia, arthralgia, rash, fever, lymphadenopathy), muscle contractions (involuntary), mydriasis, neuralgia, oculogyric crisis, otitis externa, palpitation, pancreatitis, panic disorder, paralysis, paroniria, photophobia, photosensitivity reaction, pleurisy, postural hypotension, priapism, purpura, psychosis, ptosis, rectal hemorrhage, renal calculus, renal pain, rigors, scotoma, sialoadenitis, Stevens-Johnson syndrome, stupor, suicidal behavior/ideation, syncope, systemic lupus erythematosus, tachycardia, tetany, thrombocytopenia, toxic epidermal necrolysis, ulcerative stomatitis, urinary tract pain, urticaria, vitiligo, weight loss, xerophthalmia

Metabolism/Transport Effects **Inhibits** CYP2C19 (weak); **Induces** CYP3A4 (strong)

Drug Interactions

CYP3A4 Substrates: CYP3A4 Inducers (Strong) may increase the metabolism of CYP3A4 Substrates. *Risk C: Monitor therapy*

Maraviroc: CYP3A4 Inducers may decrease the serum concentration of Maraviroc. *Risk D: Consider therapy modification*

Nilotinib: CYP3A4 Inducers (Strong) may decrease the serum concentration of Nilotinib. *Risk X: Avoid combination*

Nisoldipine: CYP3A4 Inducers (Strong) may decrease the serum concentration of Nisoldipine. *Risk X: Avoid combination*

Oral Contraceptive (Estrogens): OXcarbazepine may decrease the serum concentration of Oral Contraceptive (Estrogens). Contraceptive failure is possible. *Risk D: Consider therapy modification*

Oral Contraceptive (Progestins): OXcarbazepine may decrease the serum concentration of Oral Contraceptive (Progestins). Contraceptive failure is possible. *Risk D: Consider therapy modification*

PHENobarbital: May decrease the serum concentration of OXcarbazepine. *Risk C: Monitor therapy*

Phenytoin: May decrease the serum concentration of OXcarbazepine. OXcarbazepine may increase the serum concentration of Phenytoin. *Risk C: Monitor therapy*

Ranolazine: CYP3A4 Inducers (Strong) may decrease the serum concentration of Ranolazine. *Risk X: Avoid combination*

Sorafenib: CYP3A4 Inducers (Strong) may decrease the serum concentration of Sorafenib. *Risk D: Consider therapy modification*

Valproic Acid: May decrease the serum concentration of OXcarbazepine. *Risk C: Monitor therapy*

Ethanol/Nutrition/Herb Interactions

Ethanol: Avoid ethanol (may increase CNS depression).

Herb/Nutraceutical: St John's wort may decrease oxcarbazepine levels. Avoid evening primrose (seizure threshold decreased). Avoid valerian, St John's wort, kava kava, gotu kola.

Stability Store tablets and suspension at 25°C (77°F). Use suspension within 7 weeks of first opening container.

Mechanism of Action Pharmacological activity results from both oxcarbazepine and its monohydroxy metabolite (MHD). Precise mechanism of anticonvulsant effect has not been defined. Oxcarbazepine and MHD block voltage-sensitive sodium channels, stabilizing hyperexcited neuronal membranes, inhibiting repetitive firing, and decreasing the propagation of synaptic impulses. These actions are believed to prevent the spread of seizures. Oxcarbazepine and MHD also increase potassium conductance and modulate the activity of high-voltage activated calcium channels.

Pharmacodynamics/Kinetics

Absorption: Complete; food has no affect on rate or extent

Distribution: MHD: V_d: 49 L

Protein binding, serum: MHD: 40%

Metabolism: Hepatic to 10-monohydroxy metabolite (MHD; active); MHD is further glucuronidated or oxidized to a 10,11-dihydroxy metabolite (DHD; inactive)

Bioavailability: Decreased in children <8 years; increased in elderly >60 years

Half-life elimination: Parent drug: 2 hours; MHD: 9 hours; renal impairment (Cl_{cr} 30 mL/minute): MHD: 19 hours

Clearance of MHD is increased in younger children (~80% in children 2-4 years of age) and approaches that of adults by ~13 years of age

Time to peak, serum (median): Tablets: 4.5 hours; oral suspension: 6 hours

Excretion: Urine (95%, <1% as unchanged oxcarbazepine, 27% as unchanged MHD, 49% as MHD glucuronides); feces (<4%)

Dosage Oral:

Children 2-3 years:

Adjunctive therapy: 8-10 mg/kg/day, not to exceed 600 mg/day, given in 2 divided daily doses. Maintenance dose should be achieved over 2 weeks, and is dependent upon patient weight.

<20 kg: Consider initiating dose at 16-20 mg/kg/day; maximum maintenance dose should be achieved over 2-4 weeks and should not exceed 60 mg/kg/day

Children 4-16 years:

Adjunctive therapy: 8-10 mg/kg/day, not to exceed 600 mg/day, given in 2 divided daily doses. Maintenance dose should be achieved over 2 weeks, and is dependent upon patient weight, according to the following:

20-29 kg: 900 mg/day in 2 divided doses
29.1-39 kg: 1200 mg/day in 2 divided doses
>39 kg: 1800 mg/day in 2 divided doses

Children 4-16 years:

Conversion to monotherapy: Oxcarbazepine 8-10 mg/kg/day in twice daily divided doses, while simultaneously initiating the reduction of the dose of the concomitant antiepileptic drug; the concomitant drug should be withdrawn over 3-6 weeks. Oxcarbazepine dose may be increased by a maximum of 10 mg/kg/day at weekly intervals. See below for recommended total daily dose by weight.

Initiation of monotherapy: Oxcarbazepine should be initiated at 8-10 mg/kg/day in twice daily divided doses; doses may be titrated by 5 mg/kg/day every third day. See below for recommended total daily dose by weight.

Range of maintenance doses by weight during monotherapy:

20 kg: 600-900 mg/day
25-30 kg: 900-1200 mg/day
35-40 kg: 900-1500 mg/day
45 kg: 1200-1500 mg/day
50-55 kg: 1200-1800 mg/day
60-65 kg: 1200-2100 mg/day
70 kg: 1500-2100 mg/day

Adults:

Adjunctive therapy: Initial: 300 mg twice daily; dose may be increased by as much as 600 mg/day at weekly intervals; recommended daily dose: 1200 mg/day in 2 divided doses. Although daily doses >1200 mg/day were somewhat more efficacious, most patients were unable to tolerate 2400 mg/day (due to CNS effects).

Conversion to monotherapy: Oxcarbazepine 600 mg/day in twice daily divided doses while simultaneously initiating the reduction of the dose of the concomitant antiepileptic drug. The concomitant dosage should be withdrawn over 3-6 weeks, while the maximum dose of oxcarbazepine should be reached in about 2-4 weeks. Recommended daily dose: 2400 mg/day.

Initiation of monotherapy: Oxcarbazepine should be initiated at a dose of 600 mg/day in twice daily divided doses; doses may be titrated upward by 300 mg/day every third day to a final dose of 1200 mg/day given in 2 daily divided doses

Dosing adjustment in renal impairment: Cl_{cr} <30 mL/minute: Therapy should be initiated at one-half the usual starting dose (300 mg/day in adults) and increased slowly to achieve the desired clinical response

Dosing adjustment in hepatic impairment: Adjustment not needed for mild-to-moderate impairment. No data in patients with severe impairment.

Dietary Considerations May be taken with or without food.

Administration Suspension: Prior to using for the first time, firmly insert the plastic adapter provided with the bottle. Cover adapter with child-resistant cap when not in use. Shake bottle for at least 10 seconds, remove child-resistant cap, and insert the oral dosing syringe provided to withdraw appropriate dose. Dose may be taken directly from oral syringe or may be mixed in a small glass of water immediately prior to swallowing. Rinse syringe with warm water after use and allow to dry thoroughly. Discard any unused portion after 7 weeks of first opening bottle.

Monitoring Parameters Seizure frequency, serum sodium (particularly during first 3 months of therapy), symptoms of CNS depression (dizziness, headache, somnolence). Additional serum sodium monitoring recommended during maintenance treatment in patients receiving other medications known to decrease sodium levels, in patients with signs/symptoms of hyponatremia, and in patients with an increase in seizure frequency or severity.

Test Interactions Thyroid function tests may depress serum T_4 without affecting T_3 levels or TSH.

Dosage Forms Excipient information presented when available (limited, particularly for generics); consult specific product labeling.

Suspension, oral:

Trileptal®: 300 mg/5 mL (250 mL) [contains ethanol; packaged with oral syringe]

Tablet: 150 mg, 300 mg, 600 mg

Trileptal®: 150 mg, 300 mg, 600 mg

- ◆ **Oxilapine Succinate** *see* Loxapine *on page 960*
- ◆ **Oxpentifylline** *see* Pentoxifylline *on page 1251*
- ◆ **Oxsoralen®** *see* Methoxsalen *on page 1018*
- ◆ **Oxsoralen-Ultra®** *see* Methoxsalen *on page 1018*

Oxybutynin (oks i BYOO ti nin)

Medication Safety Issues

Sound-alike/look-alike issues:

Oxybutynin may be confused with OxyContin®

Ditropan® may be confused with Detrol®, diazepam, Diprivan®, dithranol

Transdermal patch may contain conducting metal (eg, aluminum); remove patch prior to MRI.

Related Information

Clozapine-Induced Side Effects *on page 1818*

U.S. Brand Names Ditropan®; Ditropan® XL; Oxytrol®

Canadian Brand Names Apo-Oxybutynin®; Ditropan®; Ditropan® XL; Gen-Oxybutynin; Novo-Oxybutynin; Nu-Oxybutyn; Oxytrol®; PMS-Oxybutynin; Riva-Oxybutynin; Uromax®

Mexican Brand Names Inprax; Lyrinel; Nefryl; Tavor

Index Terms Oxybutynin Chloride

Pharmacologic Category Antispasmodic Agent, Urinary

Generic Available Yes: Excludes transdermal patch

Use Antispasmodic for neurogenic bladder (urgency, frequency, urge incontinence)

Effect on Mental Status Drowsiness is common; may cause insomnia or dizziness

Effect on Psychiatric Treatment Concurrent use with psychotropics may produce additive sedation and anticholinergic side effects (dry mouth)

Pregnancy Risk Factor B

Pregnancy Considerations Teratogenic effects were not observed in animal studies. There are no adequate and well-controlled studies in pregnant women; use during pregnancy only if clearly needed.

Lactation Excretion in breast milk unknown/use caution

Contraindications Hypersensitivity to oxybutynin or any component of the formulation; untreated glaucoma; urinary retention; gastric retention or conditions with severely decreased GI motility

Warnings/Precautions Use with caution in patients with bladder outflow obstruction, angle-closure glaucoma (treated), hyperthyroidism, reflux esophagitis (including concurrent therapy with oral bisphosphonates or drugs which may increase the risk of esophagitis), heart disease, hepatic or renal disease, prostatic hyperplasia, autonomic neuropathy, ulcerative colitis (may cause ileus and toxic megacolon), hypertension, hiatal hernia, myasthenia gravis, dementia, ulcerative colitis, or intestinal atony. Caution should be used in elderly due to anticholinergic activity (eg, confusion, constipation, blurred vision, and tachycardia). May increase the risk of heat prostration. May cause anticholinergic effects (agitation, confusion, hallucinations, somnolence) which may require dose reduction or discontinuation of therapy. May cause CNS depression, which may impair physical or mental abilities; patients must be cautioned about performing tasks which require mental alertness (eg, operating machinery or driving).

The extended release formulation consists of drug within a nondeformable matrix; following drug release/absorption, the matrix/shell is expelled in the stool. The use of nondeformable products in patients with known stricture/narrowing of the GI tract has been associated with symptoms of obstruction.

Transdermal patch may contain conducting metal (eg, aluminum); remove patch prior to MRI.

Adverse Reactions

Oral:

>10%:

Central nervous system: Dizziness (4% to 17%), somnolence (2% to 14%)

Gastrointestinal: Xerostomia (29% to 71%; dose related), constipation (7% to 15%), nausea (2% to 12%)

5% to 10%:

Central nervous system: Headache (6% to 10%), pain (4% to 7%), nervousness (1% to 7%), insomnia (1% to 6%)

Gastrointestinal: Diarrhea (7% to 9%), dyspepsia (6% to 7%)

Genitourinary: Urinary hesitation (9%), urinary tract infection (5% to 7%), urinary retention (6%)

Neuromuscular & skeletal: Weakness (3% to 7%)

Ocular: Blurred vision (1% to 10%), dry eyes (3% to 6%)

Respiratory: Rhinitis (2% to 6%)

1% to <5% (Limited to important or life-threatening): Abdominal pain, agitation, aptyalism, arrhythmia, arthralgia, asthma, back pain, bronchitis, confusion, convulsion, cough, cycloplegia, cystitis, depression, dry skin, dry throat, dysgeusia, dysphagia, dysuria, edema, eructation, extremity pain, eye irritation, fatigue, flank pain, flatulence, fluid retention, flushing, fungal infection, gastrointestinal reflux disease, GI motility decreased, hallucination, hoarseness, hyperglycemia, hyper-/hypotension, impotence, keratoconjunctivitis sicca, loose stools, mydriasis, nasal congestion, nasal dryness, nasopharyngitis, pain, palpitation, pharyngolaryngeal pain, pollakiuria, pruritus, psychotic disorder, rash, sinus congestion, sinus headache, sweating decreased, tachycardia, thirst, tongue coated, upper respiratory tract infection, vomiting

Transdermal:

>10%: Local: Application site reaction (17%), pruritus (14%)

1% to 10%:

Gastrointestinal: Xerostomia (4% to 10%), diarrhea (3%), constipation (3%)

Genitourinary: Dysuria (2%)

Local: Erythema (6% to 8%), vesicles (3%), rash (3%)

Ocular: Vision changes (3%)

Postmarketing and/or case reports: Cardiac arrhythmia, cycloplegia, hallucinations, lactation suppressed, myocarditis, impotence, seizure, sweating decreased, tachycardia

Metabolism/Transport Effects **Substrate** of CYP3A4 (minor); **Inhibits** CYP2C8 (weak), 2D6 (weak), 3A4 (weak)

Drug Interactions

Acetylcholinesterase Inhibitors (Central): Anticholinergics may diminish the therapeutic effect of Acetylcholinesterase Inhibitors (Central). Acetylcholinesterase Inhibitors (Central) may diminish the therapeutic effect of Anticholinergics. If the anticholinergic action is a side effect of the agent, the result may be beneficial. *Risk C: Monitor therapy*

Anticholinergics: May enhance the adverse/toxic effect of other Anticholinergics. **Exceptions:** Paliperidone. *Risk C: Monitor therapy*

Cannabinoids: Anticholinergic Agents may enhance the tachycardic effect of Cannabinoids. *Risk C: Monitor therapy*

Potassium Chloride: Anticholinergic Agents may enhance the ulcerogenic effect of Potassium Chloride. *Risk D: Consider therapy modification*

Pramlintide: May enhance the anticholinergic effect of Anticholinergics. These effects are specific to the GI tract. *Risk D: Consider therapy modification*

Secretin: Anticholinergic Agents may diminish the stimulatory effect of Secretin. *Risk D: Consider therapy modification*

Ethanol/Nutrition/Herb Interactions Ethanol: Use ethanol with caution (may increase CNS depression and toxicity). Watch for sedation.

Stability Store at controlled room temperature. Protect syrup from light. Keep transdermal patch in sealed pouch.

Mechanism of Action Direct antispasmodic effect on smooth muscle, also inhibits the action of acetylcholine on smooth muscle (exhibits 1/5 the anticholinergic activity of atropine, but is 4-10 times the antispasmodic activity); does not block effects at skeletal muscle or at autonomic ganglia; increases bladder capacity, decreases uninhibited contractions, and delays desire to void, therefore, decreases urgency and frequency

Pharmacodynamics/Kinetics

Onset of action: Oral: 30-60 minutes

Peak effect: 3-6 hours

Duration: 6-10 hours (up to 24 hours for extended release oral formulation)
Absorption: Oral: Rapid and well absorbed; Transdermal: High
Distribution: I.V.: V_d: 193 L
Metabolism: Hepatic via CYP3A4; Oral: High first-pass metabolism (not with I.V. or transdermal use); forms active and inactive metabolites
Bioavailability: Oral: ~6%
Half-life elimination: I.V.: ~2 hours (parent drug), 7-8 hours (metabolites)
Time to peak, serum: Oral: ~60 minutes; Transdermal: 24-48 hours
Excretion: Urine, as metabolites and unchanged drug (<0.1%)

Dosage

Oral:

Children:

1-5 years (unlabeled use): 0.2 mg/kg/dose 2-4 times/day
>5 years: 5 mg twice daily, up to 5 mg 3 times/day maximum
>6 years: Extended release: 5 mg once daily; adjust dose in 5 mg increments; maximum dose: 20 mg/day

Adults: 5 mg 2-3 times/day up to 5 mg 4 times/day maximum

Extended release: Initial: 5-10 mg once daily, adjust dose in 5 mg increments at weekly intervals; maximum: 30 mg daily

Elderly: Regular release: Initial dose: 2.5 mg 2-3 times/day; increase as needed to 5 mg 2-3 times/day

Transdermal: Adults: Apply one 3.9 mg/day patch twice weekly (every 3-4 days)

Note: Should be discontinued periodically to determine whether the patient can manage without the drug and to minimize resistance to the drug

Dietary Considerations Food causes a slight delay in the absorption of the oral solution and bioavailability is increased by ~25%. Absorption of the extended release tablet is not affected by food.

Administration

Oral: Immediate release tablets and solution should be administered on an empty stomach with water. Extended release tablets may be taken with or without food and must be swallowed whole; do not crush, divide, or chew.

Transdermal: Apply to clean, dry skin on abdomen, hip, or buttock. Select a new site for each new system (avoid reapplication to same site within 7 days).

Monitoring Parameters Incontinence episodes, postvoid residual (PVR)

Test Interactions May suppress the wheal and flare reactions to skin test antigens.

Dosage Forms Excipient information presented when available (limited, particularly for generics); consult specific product labeling.

Syrup, as chloride: 5 mg/5 mL (473 mL)
Ditropan®: 5 mg/5 mL (473 mL)

Tablet, as chloride: 5 mg
Ditropan®: 5 mg

Tablet, extended release, as chloride: 5 mg, 10 mg, 15 mg
Ditropan® XL: 5 mg, 10 mg, 15 mg

Transdermal system:
Oxytrol®: 3.9 mg/day (8s) [39 cm^2; total oxybutynin 36 mg]

◆ **Oxybutynin Chloride** *see* Oxybutynin *on page 1199*

OxyCODONE (oks i KOE done)

Medication Safety Issues

Sound-alike/look-alike issues:

OxyCODONE may be confused with HYDROcodone, OxyContin®, oxymorphone
OxyContin® may be confused with MS Contin®, oxybutynin
OxyFast® may be confused with Roxanol™
Roxicodone® may be confused with Roxanol™

High alert medication: The Institute for Safe Medication Practices (ISMP) includes this medication among its list of drug classes which have a heightened risk of causing significant patient harm when used in error.

Related Information

Narcotic / Opioid Analgesics *on page 1789*

U.S. Brand Names ETH-Oxydose™; OxyContin®; OxyFast®; OxyIR®; Roxicodone®

Canadian Brand Names Oxy.IR®; OxyContin®; Supeudol®

Mexican Brand Names Plexicodim

Index Terms Dihydrohydroxycodeinone; Oxycodone Hydrochloride

Pharmacologic Category Analgesic, Opioid

Generic Available Yes

Use Management of moderate-to-severe pain, normally used in combination with nonopioid analgesics

OxyContin® is indicated for around-the-clock management of moderate-to-severe pain when an analgesic is needed for an extended period of time.

Effect on Mental Status Drowsiness and dizziness are common; may cause agitation, confusion, amnesia, depression, emotional lability, hallucinations, and malaise

Effect on Psychiatric Treatment Concurrent use with psychotropics may cause additive sedation; use lower doses of both agents. Oxycodone may cause severe hypotension after concurrent administration with drugs which compromise vasomotor tone (eg, phenothiazines); monitor blood pressure.

Restrictions C-II

Pregnancy Risk Factor B/D (prolonged use or high doses at term)

Pregnancy Considerations Should be used in pregnancy only if clearly needed. Use of narcotics during pregnancy may produce physical dependence in the neonate; respiratory depression may occur in the newborn if narcotics are used prior to delivery (especially high doses).

Lactation Enters breast milk/use caution

Contraindications Hypersensitivity to oxycodone or any component of the formulation; significant respiratory depression; hypercarbia; acute or severe bronchial asthma; OxyContin® is also contraindicated in paralytic ileus (known or suspected); pregnancy (prolonged use or high doses at term)

Warnings/Precautions May cause CNS depression, which may impair physical or mental abilities; patients must be cautioned about performing tasks which require mental alertness (eg, operating machinery or driving). Effects may be potentiated when used with other sedative drugs or ethanol. Use with caution in patients with hypersensitivity reactions to other phenanthrene derivative opioid agonists (morphine, hydrocodone, hydromorphone, levorphanol, oxymorphone), respiratory diseases including asthma, emphysema, or COPD. Use with caution in pancreatitis or biliary tract disease, acute alcoholism (including delirium tremens), morbid obesity, adrenocortical insufficiency, history of seizure disorders, CNS depression/coma, kyphoscoliosis (or other skeletal disorder which may alter respiratory function), hypothyroidism (including myxedema), prostatic hyperplasia, urethral stricture, and toxic psychosis. May obscure diagnosis or clinical course of patients with acute abdominal conditions.

Use with caution in the elderly, debilitated, severe hepatic or renal function. Hemodynamic effects (hypotension, orthostasis) may be exaggerated in patients with hypovolemia, concurrent vasodilating drugs, or in patients with head injury. Respiratory depressant effects and capacity to elevate CSF pressure may be exaggerated in presence of head injury, other intracranial lesion, or pre-existing intracranial pressure.

Use the oral concentrate formulation with caution in patients with latex sensitivity; dropper dispenser contains dry, natural rubber. Concurrent use of agonist/antagonist analgesics may precipitate withdrawal symptoms and/or reduced analgesic efficacy in patients following prolonged therapy with mu opioid agonists. Abrupt discontinuation following prolonged use may also lead to withdrawal symptoms.

[U.S. Boxed Warning]: Healthcare provider should be alert to problems of abuse, misuse, and diversion. Tolerance or drug dependence may result from extended use.

Controlled-release formulations:

[U.S. Boxed Warning]: OxyContin® is not intended for use as an "as needed" analgesic or for immediately-postoperative pain management (should be used postoperatively only if the patient has received it prior to surgery or if severe, persistent pain is anticipated). **[U.S. Boxed Warning]: Do NOT crush, break, or chew controlled-release tablets;** 60 mg, 80 mg, and 160 mg strengths are for use only in opioid-tolerant patients.

Adverse Reactions

>10%:

Central nervous system: Somnolence (23% to 24%), dizziness (13% to 16%)

Dermatologic: Pruritus (12% to 13%)

Gastrointestinal: Nausea (23% to 27%), constipation (23% to 26%), vomiting (12% to 14%)

1% to 10%:

Cardiovascular: Postural hypotension (1% to 5%)

Central nervous system: Headache (7% to 8%), abnormal dreams (1% to 5%), anxiety (1% to 5%), chills (1% to 5%), confusion (1% to 5%), euphoria (1% to 5%), fever (1% to 5%), insomnia (1% to 5%), nervousness (1% to 5%), thought abnormalities (1% to 5%)

Dermatologic: Rash (1% to 5%)

Gastrointestinal: Xerostomia (6% to 7%), abdominal pain (1% to 5%), anorexia (1% to 5%), diarrhea (1% to 5%), dyspepsia (1% to 5%), gastritis (1% to 5%)

Neuromuscular & skeletal: Weakness (6% to 7%), twitching (1% to 5%)

Respiratory: Dyspnea (1% to 5%), hiccups (1% to 5%)

Miscellaneous: Diaphoresis (5% to 6%)

<1% (Limited to important or life-threatening): Agitation, amenorrhea, amnesia, anaphylaxis, anaphylactoid reaction, appetite increased, chest pain, cough, dehydration, depression, dysphagia, dysuria, edema, emotional lability, eructation, exfoliative dermatitis, facial edema, hallucinations, hematuria, histamine release, hyperkinesia, hypoesthesia, hyponatremia, hypotonia, ileus, impotence, intracranial pressure increased, libido decreased, malaise, migraine, paradoxical CNS stimulation, paralytic ileus, paresthesia, pharyngitis, physical dependence, polyuria, psychological dependence, seizure, SIADH, speech disorder, ST segment depression, stomatitis, stupor, syncope, tablet in stool (OxyCodone®), taste perversion, thirst, tinnitus, tremor, urinary retention, urticaria, vasodilation, vertigo, vision change, voice alteration, withdrawal syndrome

Metabolism/Transport Effects Substrate (minor) of CYP2D6, 3A

Drug Interactions

Alcohol (Ethyl): CNS Depressants may enhance the CNS depressant effect of Alcohol (Ethyl). *Risk C: Monitor therapy*

Alvimopan: Analgesics (Opioid) may enhance the adverse/toxic effect of Alvimopan. This is most notable for patients receiving long-term (i.e., more than 7 days) opiates prior to alvimopan initiation. Management: Alvimopan is contraindicated in patients receiving therapeutic doses of opioids for more than 7 consecutive days immediately prior to alvimopan initiation. *Risk D: Consider therapy modification*

Ammonium Chloride: May increase the excretion of Analgesics (Opioid). *Risk C: Monitor therapy*

Amphetamines: May enhance the analgesic effect of Analgesics (Opioid). *Risk C: Monitor therapy*

Antipsychotic Agents (Phenothiazines): May enhance the hypotensive effect of Analgesics (Opioid). *Risk C: Monitor therapy*

CNS Depressants: May enhance the adverse/toxic effect of other CNS Depressants. *Risk C: Monitor therapy*

Desmopressin: Analgesics (Opioid) may enhance the adverse/toxic effect of Desmopressin. *Risk C: Monitor therapy*

Pegvisomant: Analgesics (Opioid) may diminish the therapeutic effect of Pegvisomant. *Risk C: Monitor therapy*

Selective Serotonin Reuptake Inhibitors: Analgesics (Opioid) may enhance the serotonergic effect of Selective Serotonin Reuptake Inhibitors. This may cause serotonin syndrome. *Risk C: Monitor therapy*

Succinylcholine: May enhance the bradycardic effect of Analgesics (Opioid). *Risk C: Monitor therapy*

Ethanol/Nutrition/Herb Interactions

Ethanol: Avoid ethanol (may increase CNS depression).

Food: When taken with a high-fat meal, peak concentration is 25% greater following a single OxyContin® 160 mg tablet as compared to two 80 mg tablets.

Herb/Nutraceutical: Avoid valerian, St John's wort, kava kava, gotu kola (may increase CNS depression).

Stability Store at 15°C to 30°C (59°F to 86°F). Protect from light.

Mechanism of Action Binds to opiate receptors in the CNS, causing inhibition of ascending pain pathways, altering the perception of and response to pain; produces generalized CNS depression

Pharmacodynamics/Kinetics

Onset of action: Pain relief: 10-15 minutes

Peak effect: 0.5-1 hour

Duration: Immediate release: 3-6 hours; Controlled release: ≤12 hours

Distribution: V_d: 2.6 L/kg; distributed to skeletal muscle, liver, intestinal tract, lungs, spleen, brain, and breast milk

Protein binding: ~45%

Metabolism: Hepatically via CYP3A4 to noroxycodone (has weak analgesic), noroxymorphone, and alpha- and beta-noroxycodol. CYP2D6 mediated metabolism produces oxymorphone (has analgesic activity; low plasma concentrations), alpha- and beta-oxymorphol.

Bioavailability: Controlled release, immediate release: 60% to 87%
Half-life elimination: Immediate release: 2-3 hours; controlled release: ~5 hours
Excretion: Urine (~19% as parent; > 64% as metabolites)

Dosage Oral:

Children: Immediate release:
- 6-12 years: 1.25 mg every 6 hours as needed
- >12 years: 2.5 mg every 6 hours as needed

Adults:
- Immediate release: 5 mg every 6 hours as needed
- Controlled release:
  - Opioid naive: 10 mg every 12 hours
  - Concurrent CNS depressants: Reduce usual dose by 1/3 to 1/2
  - Conversion from transdermal fentanyl: For each 25 mcg/hour transdermal dose, substitute 10 mg controlled release oxycodone every 12 hours; should be initiated 18 hours after the removal of the transdermal fentanyl patch
  - Currently on opioids: Use standard conversion chart to convert daily dose to oxycodone equivalent. Divide daily dose in 2 (for twice-daily dosing, usually every 12 hours) and round down to nearest dosage form.
  - **Note:** 60 mg, 80 mg, or 160 mg tablets are for use **only** in opioid-tolerant patients. Special safety considerations must be addressed when converting to OxyContin® doses ≥160 mg every 12 hours. Dietary caution must be taken when patients are initially titrated to 160 mg tablets. Using different strengths to obtain the same daily dose is equivalent (eg, four 40 mg tablets, two 80 mg tablets, one 160 mg tablet); all produce similar blood levels.

Multiplication factors for converting the daily dose of current oral opioid to the daily dose of oral oxycodone:

Current opioid mg/day dose x factor = Oxycodone mg/day dose

Codeine mg/day oral dose **x** 0.15 = Oxycodone mg/day dose
Hydrocodone mg/day oral dose **x** 0.9 = Oxycodone mg/day dose
Hydromorphone mg/day oral dose **x** 4 = Oxycodone mg/day dose
Levorphanol mg/day oral dose **x** 7.5 = Oxycodone mg/day dose
Meperidine mg/day oral dose **x** 0.1 = Oxycodone mg/day dose
Methadone mg/day oral dose **x** 1.5 = Oxycodone mg/day dose
Morphine mg/day oral dose **x** 0.5 = Oxycodone mg/day dose

Note: Divide the oxycodone mg/day dose into the appropriate dosing interval for the specific form being used.

Dosing adjustment in hepatic impairment: Reduce dosage in patients with severe liver disease

Dietary Considerations Instruct patient to avoid high-fat meals when taking OxyContin® 160 mg tablets.

Administration Do not crush, break, or chew controlled-release tablets; 60 mg, 80 mg, and 160 mg tablets are for use **only** in opioid-tolerant patients. Do not administer OxyContin® 160 mg tablet with a high-fat meal. Controlled release tablets are not indicated for rectal administration; increased risk of adverse events due to better rectal absorption.

Monitoring Parameters Pain relief, respiratory and mental status, blood pressure

Reference Range Blood level of 5 mg/L associated with fatality

Test Interactions Some quinolones may produce a false-positive urine screening result for opiates using commercially-available immunoassay kits. This has been demonstrated most consistently for levofloxacin and ofloxacin, but other quinolones have shown cross-reactivity in certain assay kits. Confirmation of positive opiate screens by more specific methods should be considered.

Additional Information Prophylactic use of a laxative should be considered. OxyContin® 60 mg, 80 mg, and 160 mg tablets are for use in opioid-tolerant patients only.

Dosage Forms Excipient information presented when available (limited, particularly for generics); consult specific product labeling.

Capsule, immediate release, as hydrochloride: 5 mg
- OxyIR®: 5 mg

Liquid, oral, as hydrochloride [concentrate]:
- Roxicodone®: 20 mg/mL (30 mL) [contains sodium benzoate]

Solution, oral, as hydrochloride: 5 mg/5 mL (500 mL)
- Roxicodone®: 5 mg/5 mL (5 mL, 500 mL) [contains ethanol]

Solution, oral, as hydrochloride [concentrate]: 20 mg/mL (30 mL)
- ETH-Oxydose™: 20 mg/mL (1 mL, 30 mL) [contains sodium benzoate; berry flavor]

OxyFast®: 20 mg/mL (30 mL) [contains natural rubber/natural latex in packaging and sodium benzoate]

Tablet, as hydrochloride: 5 mg, 10 mg, 15 mg, 20 mg, 30 mg

Roxicodone®: 5 mg, 15 mg, 30 mg

Tablet, controlled release, as hydrochloride:

OxyContin®: 10 mg, 15 mg, 20 mg, 30 mg, 40 mg, 60 mg, 80 mg, 160 mg

Tablet, extended release, as hydrochloride: 10 mg, 20 mg, 40 mg, 80 mg [DSC]

Oxycodone and Acetaminophen

(oks i KOE done & a seet a MIN oh fen)

Medication Safety Issues

Sound-alike/look-alike issues:

Endocet® may be confused with Indocid®

Percocet® may be confused with Fioricet®, Percodan®

Roxicet™ may be confused with Roxanol™

Tylox® may be confused with Trimox®, Tylenol®, Wymox®, Xanax®

High alert medication: The Institute for Safe Medication Practices (ISMP) includes this medication among its list of drug classes which have a heightened risk of causing significant patient harm when used in error.

Duplicate therapy issues: This product contains acetaminophen, which may be a component of other combination products. Do not exceed the maximum recommended daily dose of acetaminophen.

U.S. Brand Names Endocet®; Magnacet™; Percocet®; Primalev™; Roxicet™; Roxicet™ 5/500; Tylox®

Canadian Brand Names Endocet®; Oxycocet®; Percocet®; Percocet®-Demi; PMS-Oxycodone-Acetaminophen

Index Terms Acetaminophen and Oxycodone

Pharmacologic Category Analgesic, Opioid

Generic Available Yes: Excludes caplet and solution

Use Management of moderate-to-severe pain

Effect on Mental Status Drowsiness and fatigue are common. May cause restlessness, nervousness, or confusion; may rarely cause hallucinations, depression, or paradoxical CNS stimulation.

Effect on Psychiatric Treatment Concurrent use with psychotropics may cause additive sedation; use lower doses of both agents. Oxycodone may cause severe hypotension after concurrent administration with drugs which compromise vasomotor tone (eg, phenothiazines); monitor blood pressure.

Restrictions C-II

Pregnancy Risk Factor C/D (prolonged periods or high doses at term)

Pregnancy Considerations Use of narcotics during pregnancy may produce physical dependence in the neonate; respiratory depression may occur in the newborn if narcotics are used prior to delivery (especially high doses).

Lactation Enters breast milk/use caution

Contraindications Hypersensitivity to oxycodone, acetaminophen, or any component of the formulation; severe respiratory depression (in absence of resuscitative equipment or ventilatory support); pregnancy (prolonged periods or high doses at term)

Warnings/Precautions Use with caution in patients with hypersensitivity reactions to other phenanthrene-derivative opioid agonists (morphine, codeine, hydrocodone, hydromorphone, levorphanol, oxymorphone); respiratory diseases including asthma, emphysema, COPD; severe liver or renal insufficiency; hypothyroidism; Addison's disease; seizure disorder; toxic psychosis; morbid obesity; CNS depression/coma; biliary tract impairment; prostatic hyperplasia; or urethral stricture. May obscure diagnosis or clinical course of patients with acute abdominal conditions. Some preparations contain sulfites which may cause allergic reactions. May be habit-forming. Causes sedation; caution must be used in performing tasks which require alertness (eg, operating machinery or driving). Effects may be potentiated when used with other sedative drugs or ethanol. May cause hypotension. Concurrent use of agonist/antagonist analgesics may precipitate withdrawal symptoms and/or reduced analgesic efficacy in patients following prolonged therapy with mu opioid agonists. Abrupt discontinuation following prolonged use may also lead to withdrawal symptoms.

Use with caution in patients with head injury and increased intracranial pressure (respiratory depressant effects increased and may also elevate CSF pressure).

Enhanced analgesia has been seen in elderly and debilitated patients on therapeutic doses of narcotics. Duration of action may be increased in the elderly. The elderly may be particularly susceptible to the CNS depressant and constipating effects of narcotics.

May cause severe hepatic toxicity on acute overdose; in addition, chronic daily dosing in adults has resulted in liver damage in some patients. Use with caution in patients with alcoholic liver disease; consuming ≥3 alcoholic drinks/day may increase the risk of liver damage. Use with caution in patients with known G6PD deficiency. Limit acetaminophen dose to <4 g/day.

Adverse Reactions Frequency not defined (also see individual agents): Allergic reaction, constipation, dizziness, dysphoria, euphoria, lightheadedness, nausea, pruritus, respiratory depression, sedation, skin rash, vomiting

Metabolism/Transport Effects

Oxycodone: **Substrate** (minor) of CYP2D6, 3A

Acetaminophen: **Substrate** (minor) of CYP1A2, 2A6, 2C9, 2D6, 2E1, 3A4

Drug Interactions

Alcohol (Ethyl): CNS Depressants may enhance the CNS depressant effect of Alcohol (Ethyl). *Risk C: Monitor therapy*

Alvimopan: Analgesics (Opioid) may enhance the adverse/toxic effect of Alvimopan. This is most notable for patients receiving long-term (i.e., more than 7 days) opiates prior to alvimopan initiation. Management: Alvimopan is contraindicated in patients receiving therapeutic doses of opioids for more than 7 consecutive days immediately prior to alvimopan initiation. *Risk D: Consider therapy modification*

Ammonium Chloride: May increase the excretion of Analgesics (Opioid). *Risk C: Monitor therapy*

Amphetamines: May enhance the analgesic effect of Analgesics (Opioid). *Risk C: Monitor therapy*

Anticonvulsants (Hydantoin): May increase the metabolism of Acetaminophen. This may 1) diminish the effect of acetaminophen; and 2) increase the risk of liver damage. *Risk C: Monitor therapy*

Antipsychotic Agents (Phenothiazines): May enhance the hypotensive effect of Analgesics (Opioid). *Risk C: Monitor therapy*

Barbiturates: May increase the metabolism of Acetaminophen. This may 1) diminish the effect of acetaminophen; and 2) increase the risk of liver damage. *Risk C: Monitor therapy*

CarBAMazepine: May increase the metabolism of Acetaminophen. This may 1) diminish the effect of acetaminophen; and 2) increase the risk of liver damage. *Risk C: Monitor therapy*

Cholestyramine Resin: May decrease the absorption of Acetaminophen. Effect is minimal if cholestyramine is administered 1 hour after acetaminophen. *Risk D: Consider therapy modification*

CNS Depressants: May enhance the adverse/toxic effect of other CNS Depressants. *Risk C: Monitor therapy*

Desmopressin: Analgesics (Opioid) may enhance the adverse/toxic effect of Desmopressin. *Risk C: Monitor therapy*

Imatinib: May increase the serum concentration of Acetaminophen. *Risk D: Consider therapy modification*

Isoniazid: May enhance the adverse/toxic effect of Acetaminophen. *Risk C: Monitor therapy*

Pegvisomant: Analgesics (Opioid) may diminish the therapeutic effect of Pegvisomant. *Risk C: Monitor therapy*

Selective Serotonin Reuptake Inhibitors: Analgesics (Opioid) may enhance the serotonergic effect of Selective Serotonin Reuptake Inhibitors. This may cause serotonin syndrome. *Risk C: Monitor therapy*

Succinylcholine: May enhance the bradycardic effect of Analgesics (Opioid). *Risk C: Monitor therapy*

Vitamin K Antagonists (eg, warfarin): Acetaminophen may enhance the anticoagulant effect of Vitamin K Antagonists. Most likely with daily acetaminophen doses >1.3 g for >1 week. *Risk C: Monitor therapy*

Ethanol/Nutrition/Herb Interactions Ethanol: May have additive CNS depression. In addition, excessive intake of ethanol may increase the risk of acetaminophen-induced hepatotoxicity. Avoid ethanol or limit to <3 drinks/day.

Stability Store at controlled room temperature of 20°C to 25°C (68°F to 77°F). Protect from moisture.

Mechanism of Action

Oxycodone, as with other narcotic (opiate) analgesics, blocks pain perception in the cerebral cortex by binding to specific receptor molecules (opiate receptors) within the neuronal membranes of synapses. This binding results in a decreased synaptic chemical transmission throughout the CNS thus inhibiting the flow of pain sensations into the higher centers. Mu and kappa are the two subtypes of the opiate receptor to which oxycodone binds to cause analgesia.

Acetaminophen inhibits the synthesis of prostaglandins in the CNS and peripherally blocks pain impulse generation; produces antipyresis from inhibition of hypothalamic heat-regulating center.

Pharmacodynamics/Kinetics See individual agents.

Dosage Oral: Doses should be given every 4-6 hours as needed and titrated to appropriate analgesic effects. **Note:** Initial dose is based on the **oxycodone** content; however, the maximum daily dose is based on the **acetaminophen** content.

Children: Maximum acetaminophen dose: Children <45 kg: 90 mg/kg/day; children >45 kg: 4 g/day

Mild-to-moderate pain: Initial dose, **based on oxycodone content:** 0.05-0.1 mg/kg/dose

Severe pain: Initial dose, **based on oxycodone content:** 0.3 mg/kg/dose

Adults:

Mild-to-moderate pain: Initial dose, **based on oxycodone content:** 2.5-5 mg

Severe pain: Initial dose, **based on oxycodone content:** 10-30 mg. Do not exceed acetaminophen 4 g/day.

Elderly: Doses should be titrated to appropriate analgesic effects: Initial dose, **based on oxycodone content:** 2.5-5 mg every 6 hours. Do not exceed acetaminophen 4 g/day.

Dosage adjustment in hepatic impairment: Dose should be reduced in patients with severe liver disease.

Monitoring Parameters Monitor for pain relief, respiratory and mental status, blood pressure, constipation

Dosage Forms Excipient information presented when available (limited, particularly for generics); consult specific product labeling.

Caplet:

Roxicet™ 5/500: Oxycodone hydrochloride 5 mg and acetaminophen 500 mg

Capsule: 5/500: Oxycodone hydrochloride 5 mg and acetaminophen 500 mg

Tylox®: 5/500: Oxycodone hydrochloride 5 mg and acetaminophen 500 mg [contains sodium benzoate and sodium metabisulfite]

Solution, oral:

Roxicet™: Oxycodone hydrochloride 5 mg and acetaminophen 325 mg per 5 mL (5 mL, 500 mL) [contains alcohol <0.5%]

Tablet: 5/325: Oxycodone hydrochloride 5 mg and acetaminophen 325 mg; 7.5/325: Oxycodone hydrochloride 7.5 mg and acetaminophen 325 mg; 7.5/500: Oxycodone hydrochloride 7.5 mg and acetaminophen 500 mg; 10/325: Oxycodone hydrochloride 10 mg and acetaminophen 325 mg; 10/650: Oxycodone hydrochloride 10 mg and acetaminophen 650 mg

Endocet® 5/325 [scored]: Oxycodone hydrochloride 5 mg and acetaminophen 325 mg

Endocet® 7.5/325: Oxycodone hydrochloride 7.5 mg and acetaminophen 325 mg

Endocet® 7.5/500: Oxycodone hydrochloride 7.5 mg and acetaminophen 500 mg

Endocet® 10/325: Oxycodone hydrochloride 10 mg and acetaminophen 325 mg

Endocet® 10/650: Oxycodone hydrochloride 10 mg and acetaminophen 650 mg

Magnacet™ 2.5/400: Oxycodone hydrochloride 2.5 mg and acetaminophen 400 mg

Magnacet™ 5/400: Oxycodone hydrochloride 5 mg and acetaminophen 400 mg

Magnacet™ 7.5/400: Oxycodone hydrochloride 7.5 mg and acetaminophen 400 mg

Magnacet™ 10/400: Oxycodone hydrochloride 10 mg and acetaminophen 400 mg

Percocet® 2.5/325: Oxycodone hydrochloride 2.5 mg and acetaminophen 325 mg

Percocet® 5/325 [scored]: Oxycodone hydrochloride 5 mg and acetaminophen 325 mg

Percocet® 7.5/325: Oxycodone hydrochloride 7.5 mg and acetaminophen 325 mg

Percocet® 7.5/500: Oxycodone hydrochloride 7.5 mg and acetaminophen 500 mg

Percocet® 10/325: Oxycodone hydrochloride 10 mg and acetaminophen 325 mg

Percocet® 10/650: Oxycodone hydrochloride 10 mg and acetaminophen 650 mg
Primalev™ 2.5/300: Oxycodone hydrochloride 2.5 mg and acetaminophen 300 mg
Primalev™ 5/300: Oxycodone hydrochloride 5 mg and acetaminophen 300 mg
Primalev™ 7.5/300: Oxycodone hydrochloride 7.5 mg and acetaminophen 300 mg
Primalev™ 10/300: Oxycodone hydrochloride 10 mg and acetaminophen 300 mg
Roxicet™ [scored]: Oxycodone hydrochloride 5 mg and acetaminophen 325 mg

Oxycodone and Aspirin (oks i KOE done & AS pir in)

Medication Safety Issues
Sound-alike/look-alike issues:
Percodan® may be confused with Decadron®, Percocet®, Percogesic®, Periactin®

High alert medication: The Institute for Safe Medication Practices (ISMP) includes this medication among its list of drug classes which have a heightened risk of causing significant patient harm when used in error.

U.S. Brand Names Endodan®; Percodan®
Canadian Brand Names Endodan®; Oxycodan®; Percodan®
Index Terms Aspirin and Oxycodone
Pharmacologic Category Analgesic, Opioid
Use Management of moderate-to-severe pain
Effect on Mental Status Drowsiness and fatigue are common. May cause agitation, anxiety, lethargy, mental impairment, restlessness, nervousness, or confusion; may rarely cause hallucinations, depression, or paradoxical CNS stimulation.
Effect on Psychiatric Treatment Concurrent use with psychotropics may cause additive sedation; use lower doses of both agents. Oxycodone may cause severe hypotension after concurrent administration with drugs which compromise vasomotor tone (eg, phenothiazines); monitor blood pressure. May cause GI side effects which may be further exacerbated with concurrent SSRI, lithium, or valproic acid use; monitor. May cause platelet abnormalities which may be further exacerbated with concurrent SSRI use; monitor. Salicylate can displace phenytoin and valproic acid leading to a decrease in phenytoin and an increase in valproic acid levels; monitor.
Restrictions C-II
Dosage Summary
Oral:
Children: 0.05-0.3 mg/kg/dose (based on oxycodone content) every 6 hours as needed (maximum: 5 mg/dose [oxycodone]; 4 g/day [aspirin])
Adults: 1 tablet every 6 hours as needed (maximum: 12 tablets/day)
Dosage Forms Excipient information presented when available (limited, particularly for generics); consult specific product labeling.
Tablet: Oxycodone hydrochloride 4.5 mg, oxycodone terephthalate 0.38 mg, and aspirin 325 mg
Endodan®, Percodan®: Oxycodone hydrochloride 4.8355 mg and aspirin 325 mg

◆ **Oxycodone Hydrochloride** *see* OxyCODONE *on page 1201*
◆ **OxyContin®** *see* OxyCODONE *on page 1201*
◆ **OxyFast®** *see* OxyCODONE *on page 1201*
◆ **OxyIR®** *see* OxyCODONE *on page 1201*

Oxymetazoline (oks i met AZ oh leen)

Medication Safety Issues
Sound-alike/look-alike issues:
Oxymetazoline may be confused with oxymetholone
Afrin® may be confused with aspirin
Visine® may be confused with Visken®
U.S. Brand Names 4-Way® 12 Hour [OTC]; Afrin® Extra Moisturizing [OTC]; Afrin® Original [OTC]; Afrin® Severe Congestion [OTC]; Afrin® Sinus [OTC]; Dristan™ 12-Hour [OTC]; Duramist® Plus [OTC]; Duration® [OTC] [DSC]; Genasal [OTC]; Mucinex® Full force™ [OTC]; Mucinex® moisture smart™

[OTC]; Neo-Synephrine® 12 Hour Extra Moisturizing [OTC]; Neo-Synephrine® 12 Hour [OTC]; NRS® [OTC]; Nōstrilla® [OTC]; Vicks Sinex® 12 Hour Ultrafine Mist [OTC]; Vicks Sinex® 12 Hour [OTC]; Vicks® Early Defense™ [OTC]; Visine® L.R. [OTC]

Canadian Brand Names Claritin® Allergic Decongestant; Dristan® Long Lasting Nasal; Drixoral® Nasal

Mexican Brand Names Afrin; Collifrin; Iliadin; Oximetazolina; Oxylin Liquifilm; Visine A. D.

Index Terms Oxymetazoline Hydrochloride

Pharmacologic Category Adrenergic Agonist Agent; Imidazoline Derivative; Vasoconstrictor

Use Adjunctive therapy of middle ear infections, associated with acute or chronic rhinitis, the common cold, sinusitis, hay fever, or other allergies

Ophthalmic: Relief of redness of eye due to minor eye irritations

Effect on Mental Status None reported

Effect on Psychiatric Treatment May increase toxicity if used with MAO inhibitors (hypertension)

Dosage Summary

Intranasal:

Children <6 years: Dosage not established

Children ≥6 years: Instill 2-3 sprays into each nostril twice daily

Adults: Instill 2-3 sprays into each nostril twice daily

Ophthalmic:

Children <6 years: Dosage not established

Children ≥6 years: Instill 1-2 drops in affected eye(s) every 6 hours as needed

Adults: Instill 1-2 drops in affected eye(s) every 6 hours as needed

Dosage Forms Excipient information presented when available (limited, particularly for generics); consult specific product labeling. [DSC] = Discontinued product

Gel, intranasal, as hydrochloride [spray]:

Vicks® Early Defense™: 0.05% (14.7 mL) [microgel; contains benzyl alcohol and menthol]

Solution, intranasal, as hydrochloride [spray]: 0.05% (15 mL, 30 mL)

Afrin® Extra Moisturizing: 0.05% (15 mL) [contains benzyl alcohol and glycerin; regular or no drip formula]

Afrin® Original: 0.05% (15 mL, 30 mL) [contains benzalkonium chloride]

Afrin® Original: 0.05% (15 mL) [contains benzyl alcohol and benzalkonium chloride; no drip formula]

Afrin® Severe Congestion: 0.05% (15 mL) [contains benzyl alcohol and menthol; regular or no drip formula]

Afrin® Sinus: 0.05% (15 mL) [contains benzyl alcohol, benzalkonium chloride, camphor, phenol; regular or no drip formula]

Dristan™ 12-Hour: 0.05% (15 mL) [contains benzyl alcohol and benzalkonium chloride]

Duramist® Plus, Neo-Synephrine® 12 Hour, Nōstrilla®, Vicks Sinex® 12 Hour Ultrafine Mist, Vicks Sinex® 12 Hour, 4-Way® 12 Hour: 0.05% (15 mL) [contains benzalkonium chloride]

Duration®: 0.05% (30 mL) [contains benzalkonium chloride] [DSC]

Genasal, NRS®: 0.05% (15 mL, 30 mL) [contains benzalkonium chloride]

Mucinex® Full force™: 0.05% (22 mL) [contains benzalkonium chloride, camphor, and menthol]

Mucinex® moisture smart™: 0.05% (22 mL) [contains benzalkonium chloride and glycerin]

Neo-Synephrine® 12 Hour Extra Moisturizing: 0.05% (15 mL) [contains glycerin]

Solution, ophthalmic, as hydrochloride:

Visine® L.R.: 0.025% (15 mL, 30 mL) [contains benzalkonium chloride]

◆ **Oxymetazoline Hydrochloride** *see* Oxymetazoline *on page 1208*

Oxymetholone (oks i METH oh lone)

Medication Safety Issues

Sound-alike/look-alike issues:

Oxymetholone may be confused with oxymetazoline, oxymorphone

U.S. Brand Names Anadrol®-50

Pharmacologic Category Anabolic Steroid

Use Treatment of anemias caused by deficient red cell production
Effect on Mental Status May cause insomnia
Effect on Psychiatric Treatment None reported
Restrictions C-III
Dosage Summary
Oral:
Children: 1-5 mg/kg once daily
Adults: 1-5 mg/kg once daily

Dosage Forms Excipient information presented when available (limited, particularly for generics); consult specific product labeling.
Tablet:
Anadrol®-50: 50 mg

Oxymorphone (oks i MOR fone)

Medication Safety Issues
Sound-alike/look-alike issues:
Oxymorphone may be confused with oxycodone, oxymetholone

High alert medication: The Institute for Safe Medication Practices (ISMP) includes this medication among its list of drug classes which have a heightened risk of causing significant patient harm when used in error.

Related Information
Narcotic / Opioid Analgesics *on page 1789*

U.S. Brand Names Opana®; Opana® ER
Index Terms Oxymorphone Hydrochloride
Pharmacologic Category Analgesic, Opioid
Generic Available No
Use
Parenteral: Management of moderate-to-severe pain and preoperatively as a sedative and/or supplement to anesthesia
Oral, regular release: Management of moderate-to-severe pain
Oral, extended release: Management of moderate-to-severe pain in patients requiring around-the-clock opioid treatment for an extended period of time

Effect on Mental Status Drowsiness and dizziness are common; may cause nervousness, restlessness or confusion; may rarely cause depression or hallucinations

Effect on Psychiatric Treatment Psychotropics may alter the analgesic effects of opioids; monitor for change in pain relief

Restrictions C-II

Pregnancy Risk Factor C/D (prolonged use or high doses at term)

Pregnancy Considerations Teratogenic effects were not observed in animal studies, however, decreased fetal weight, decreased litter size, increased stillbirths, and increased neonatal death were noted. Chronic opioid use during pregnancy may lead to a withdrawal syndrome in the neonate. Symptoms include irritability, hyperactivity, loss of sleep pattern, abnormal crying, tremor, vomiting, diarrhea, weight loss, or failure to gain weight. Opioid analgesics are considered pregnancy risk factor D if used for prolonged periods or in larger doses near term.

Lactation Excretion in breast milk unknown/use caution

Contraindications Hypersensitivity to oxymorphone, other morphine analogs (phenanthrene derivatives), or any component of the formulation; paralytic ileus (known or suspected); increased intracranial pressure; moderate-to-severe hepatic impairment; severe respiratory depression (unless in monitored setting with resuscitative equipment); acute/severe bronchial asthma; hypercarbia; pregnancy (prolonged use or high doses at term).

Note: Injection formulation is also contraindicated in the treatment of upper airway obstruction and pulmonary edema due to a chemical respiratory irritant.

Warnings/Precautions An opioid-containing analgesic regimen should be tailored to each patient's needs and based upon the type of pain being treated (acute versus chronic), the route of administration, degree of tolerance for opioids (naive versus chronic user), age, weight, and medical condition. The optimal analgesic dose varies widely among patients. Doses should be titrated to pain relief/prevention.

May cause CNS depression, which may impair physical or mental abilities; patients must be cautioned about performing tasks which require mental alertness (eg, operating machinery or driving). Effects may be potentiated when used with other sedative drugs or ethanol. Use with caution in patients with hypersensitivity reactions to other phenanthrene-derivative opioid agonists (codeine, hydrocodone, hydromorphone, levorphanol, oxycodone). May cause respiratory depression. Use extreme caution in patients with COPD or other chronic respiratory conditions characterized by hypoxia, hypercapnia, or diminished respiratory reserve (myxedema, cor pulmonale, kyphoscoliosis, obstructive sleep apnea, severe obesity). Use with caution in patients (particularly elderly or debilitated) with impaired respiratory function, adrenal disease, morbid obesity, thyroid dysfunction, prostatic hyperplasia, or renal impairment. Use caution in mild hepatic dysfunction; use is contraindicated in moderate-to-severe hepatic impairment. Use only with extreme caution (if at all) in patients with head injury or increased intracranial pressure (ICP); potential to elevate ICP and/or blunt papillary response may be greatly exaggerated in these patients. Use with caution in biliary tract disease or acute pancreatitis (may cause constriction of sphincter of Oddi). May obscure diagnosis or clinical course of patients with acute abdominal conditions.

Oxymorphone shares the toxic potential of opiate agonists and usual precautions of opiate agonist therapy should be observed; may cause hypotension in patients with acute myocardial infarction, volume depletion, or concurrent drug therapy which may exaggerate vasodilation. The elderly may be particularly susceptible to adverse effects of narcotics. Safety and efficacy have not been established in children <18 years of age.

[U.S. Boxed Warning]: Healthcare provider should be alert to problems of abuse, misuse, and diversion. Tolerance or drug dependence may result from extended use. Use caution in patients with a history of drug dependence or abuse. Abrupt discontinuation may precipitate withdrawal syndrome.

Extended release formulation:

[U.S. Boxed Warnings]: Opana® ER is an extended release oral formulation of oxymorphone and is not suitable for use as an "as needed" analgesic. Tablets should not be broken, chewed, dissolved, or crushed; tablets should be swallowed whole. Opana® ER is intended for use in long-term, continuous management of moderate to severe chronic pain. It is not indicated for use in the immediate postoperative period (12-24 hours). **[U.S. Boxed Warning]: The coingestion of ethanol or ethanol-containing medications with Opana® ER may result in accelerated release of drug from the dosage form, abruptly increasing plasma levels, which may have fatal consequences.**

Adverse Reactions

Frequency not defined.

Cardiovascular: Bradycardia, cardiac shock, flushing, hypotension, orthostatic hypotension, palpitation, peripheral vasodilation, shock, tachycardia

Central nervous system: Agitation, amnesia, anorexia, anxiety, CNS depression, coma, confusion, convulsion, dizziness, drowsiness, dysphoria, euphoria, fatigue, fever, hallucinations, headache, insomnia, intracranial pressure increased, malaise, mental depression, mental impairment, nervousness, restlessness, paradoxical CNS stimulation

Dermatologic: Pruritus, urticaria, rash

Endocrine & metabolic: Antidiuretic hormone release, weight loss

Gastrointestinal: Abdominal pain, appetite depression, biliary tract spasm, constipation, dehydration, dry mouth, dyspepsia, flatulence, nausea, paralytic ileus, stomach cramps, vomiting, xerostomia

Genitourinary: Urination decreased, urinary retention, urinary tract spasm

Local: Pain/reaction at injection site

Neuromuscular & skeletal: Weakness

Ocular: Blurred vision, diplopia, miosis

Renal: Oliguria

Respiratory: Apnea, bronchospasm, cyanosis, dyspnea, hypoventilation, laryngeal edema, laryngeal spasm, respiratory depression

Miscellaneous: Diaphoresis, histamine release, physical and psychological dependence

Drug Interactions

Alcohol (Ethyl): CNS Depressants may enhance the CNS depressant effect of Alcohol (Ethyl). *Risk C: Monitor therapy*

Alvimopan: Analgesics (Opioid) may enhance the adverse/toxic effect of Alvimopan. This is most notable for patients receiving long-term (i.e., more than 7 days) opiates prior to alvimopan initiation. Management: Alvimopan is contraindicated in patients receiving therapeutic doses of opioids for more than 7 consecutive days immediately prior to alvimopan initiation. *Risk D: Consider therapy modification*

Ammonium Chloride: May increase the excretion of Analgesics (Opioid). *Risk C: Monitor therapy*

Amphetamines: May enhance the analgesic effect of Analgesics (Opioid). *Risk C: Monitor therapy*

Antipsychotic Agents (Phenothiazines): May enhance the hypotensive effect of Analgesics (Opioid). *Risk C: Monitor therapy*

CNS Depressants: May enhance the adverse/toxic effect of other CNS Depressants. *Risk C: Monitor therapy*

Desmopressin: Analgesics (Opioid) may enhance the adverse/toxic effect of Desmopressin. *Risk C: Monitor therapy*

Pegvisomant: Analgesics (Opioid) may diminish the therapeutic effect of Pegvisomant. *Risk C: Monitor therapy*

Selective Serotonin Reuptake Inhibitors: Analgesics (Opioid) may enhance the serotonergic effect of Selective Serotonin Reuptake Inhibitors. This may cause serotonin syndrome. *Risk C: Monitor therapy*

Succinylcholine: May enhance the bradycardic effect of Analgesics (Opioid). *Risk C: Monitor therapy*

Ethanol/Nutrition/Herb Interactions

Ethanol: Avoid ethanol (may increase CNS depression). Ethanol ingestion with extended-release tablets is specifically contraindicated due to possible accelerated release and potentially fatal overdose.

Food: When taken orally with a high-fat meal, peak concentration is 38% to 50% greater. Both immediate-release and extended-release tablets should be taken 1 hour before or 2 hours after eating.

Herb/Nutraceutical: Avoid valerian, St John's wort, kava kava, gotu kola (may increase CNS depression).

Stability Injection solution, tablet: Store at 15°C to 30°C (59°F to 86°F).

Mechanism of Action Oxymorphone hydrochloride (Numorphan®) is a potent narcotic analgesic with uses similar to those of morphine. The drug is a semisynthetic derivative of morphine (phenanthrene derivative) and is closely related to hydromorphone chemically (Dilaudid®).

Pharmacodynamics/Kinetics

Onset of action: Parenteral: 5-10 minutes

Duration: Analgesic: Parenteral: 3-6 hours

Distribution: V_d: I.V.: 1.94-4.22 L/kg

Protein binding: 10% to 12%

Metabolism: Hepatic via glucuronidation to active and inactive metabolites

Bioavailability: Oral: 10%

Half-life elimination: Oral: Immediate release: 7-9 hours; Extended release: 9-11 hours

Excretion: Urine (<1% as unchanged drug); feces

Dosage Adults: **Note:** Dosage must be individualized.

I.M., SubQ: Initial: 1-1.5 mg; may repeat every 4-6 hours as needed

Labor analgesia: I.M.: 0.5-1 mg

I.V.: Initial: 0.5 mg

Oral:

Immediate release:

Opioid-naive: 10-20 mg every 4-6 hours as needed. Initial dosages as low as 5 mg may be considered in selected patients and/or patients with renal impairment. Dosage adjustment should be based on level of analgesia, side effects, and pain intensity. Initiation of therapy with initial dose >20 mg is **not** recommended.

Currently on stable dose of parenteral oxymorphone: ~10 times the daily parenteral requirement. The calculated amount should be divided and given in 4-6 equal doses.

Currently on other opioids: Use standard conversion chart to convert daily dose to oxymorphone equivalent. Generally start with 1/2 the calculated daily oxymorphone dosage and administered in divided doses every 4-6 hours.

Extended release (Opana® ER):

Opioid-naive: Initial: 5 mg every 12 hours. Supplemental doses of immediate-release oxymorphone may be used as "rescue" medication as dosage is titrated.

Note: Continued requirement for supplemental dosing may be used to titrate the dose of extended-release continuous therapy. Adjust therapy incrementally, by 5-10 mg every 12 hours at intervals of every 3-7 days. Ideally, basal dosage may be titrated to generally mild pain or no pain with the regular use of fewer than 2 supplemental doses per 24 hours.

Currently on stable dose of parenteral oxymorphone: Approximately 10 times the daily parenteral requirement. The calculated amount should be given in 2 divided doses (every 12 hours).

Currently on opioids: Use conversion chart (see Note below) to convert daily dose to oxymorphone equivalent. Generally start with 1/2 the calculated daily oxymorphone dosage. Divide daily dose in 2 (for every 12-hour dosing) and round down to nearest dosage form. **Note:** Per manufacturer, the following approximate oral dosages are equivalent to oxymorphone 10 mg:

Hydrocodone 20 mg
Oxycodone 20 mg
Methadone 20 mg
Morphine 30 mg

Conversion of stable dose of immediate-release oxymorphone to extended-release oxymorphone: Administer 1/2 of the daily dose of immediate-release oxymorphone (Opana®) as the extended-release formulation (Opana® ER) every 12 hours

Elderly: Initiate dosing at the lower end of the dosage range

Dosing adjustment in renal impairment: Cl_{cr} <50 mL/minute: Reduce initial dosage of oral formulations (bioavailability increased 57% to 65%). Begin therapy at lowest dose and titrate carefully.

Dosing adjustment in hepatic impairment: Generally, contraindicated for use in patients with moderate-to-severe liver disease. Initiate with lowest possible dose and titrate slowly in mild impairment.

Dietary Considerations Immediate release and extended release tablets should be taken 1 hour before or 2 hours after eating.

Administration Administer immediate release and extended release tablets 1 hour before or 2 hours after eating. Opana® ER tablet should be swallowed; do not break, crush, or chew.

Monitoring Parameters Respiratory rate, heart rate, blood pressure, CNS activity

Test Interactions Some quinolones may produce a false-positive urine screening result for opiates using commercially-available immunoassay kits. This has been demonstrated most consistently for levofloxacin and ofloxacin, but other quinolones have shown cross-reactivity in certain assay kits. Confirmation of positive opiate screens by more specific methods should be considered. May cause elevation in amylase (due to constriction of the sphincter of Oddi).

Dosage Forms Excipient information presented when available (limited, particularly for generics); consult specific product labeling.

Injection, solution, as hydrochloride:
Opana®: 1 mg/mL (1 mL)
Tablet, as hydrochloride:
Opana®: 5 mg, 10 mg
Tablet, extended release, as hydrochloride:
Opana®: ER: 5 mg, 7.5 mg, 10 mg, 15 mg, 20 mg, 30 mg, 40 mg

◆ **Oxymorphone Hydrochloride** *see* Oxymorphone *on page 1210*
◆ **Oxytrol®** *see* Oxybutynin *on page 1199*
◆ **Oysco 500 [OTC]** *see* Calcium Carbonate *on page 254*
◆ **Oyst-Cal 500 [OTC]** *see* Calcium Carbonate *on page 254*
◆ **P-V Tussin Tablet [DSC]** *see* Hydrocodone and Pseudoephedrine *on page 781*
◆ **P-071** *see* Cetirizine *on page 307*
◆ **Pacerone®** *see* Amiodarone *on page 89*

Paclitaxel (pac li TAKS el)

Medication Safety Issues

Sound-alike/look-alike issues:
Paclitaxel may be confused with paroxetine, Paxil®
Paclitaxel (conventional) may be confused with paclitaxel (protein-bound)
Taxol® may be confused with Abraxane®, Paxil®, Taxotere®

High alert medication: The Institute for Safe Medication Practices (ISMP) includes this medication among its list of drugs which have a heightened risk of causing significant patient harm when used in error.

U.S. Brand Names Onxol® ; Taxol®

Canadian Brand Names Apo-Paclitaxel®; Taxol®

Mexican Brand Names Aclixel; Asotax; Bristaxol; Cryoxet; Praxel

Index Terms NSC-125973; NSC-673089

Pharmacologic Category Antineoplastic Agent, Antimicrotubular; Antineoplastic Agent, Natural Source (Plant) Derivative; Antineoplastic Agent, Taxane Derivative

Use Treatment of breast, nonsmall cell lung, and ovarian cancers; treatment of AIDS-related Kaposi's sarcoma (KS)

Unlabeled/Investigational Use Treatment of bladder, cervical, prostate, small cell lung, and head and neck cancers; treatment of (unknown primary) adenocarcinoma

Effect on Mental Status None reported

Effect on Psychiatric Treatment May cause neutropenia; use caution with clozapine and carbamazepine

Dosage Summary

I.V.:

Children: Dosage not established

Adults: 135-250 mg/m^2 over 3 hours every 3 weeks **or** 135 mg/m^2 over 24 hours every 3 weeks **or** 50-80 mg/m^2 over 1-3 hours weekly **or** 1.4-4 mg/m^2/day continuous infusion for 14 days every 4 weeks **or** 100 mg/m^2 over 3 hours every 2 weeks

Dosage Forms Excipient information presented when available (limited, particularly for generics); consult specific product labeling.

Injection, solution: 6 mg/mL (5 mL, 16.7 mL, 25 mL, 50 mL) [contains ethanol and purified Cremophor® EL (polyoxyethylated castor oil)]

Onxol® : 6 mg/mL (5 mL, 25 mL, 50 mL) [contains ethanol and purified Cremophor® EL (polyoxyethylated castor oil)]

Taxol®: 6 mg/mL (5 mL [DSC], 16.7 mL, 50 mL) [contains ethanol and purified Cremophor® EL (polyoxyethylated castor oil)]

Paclitaxel (Protein Bound) (pac li TAKS el PROE teen bownd)

Medication Safety Issues

Sound-alike/look-alike issues:

Paclitaxel (protein bound) may be confused with paclitaxel (conventional)

Abraxane® may be confused with Paxil®, Taxol®, Taxotere®

High alert medication: The Institute for Safe Medication Practices (ISMP) includes this medication among its list of drug classes which have a heightened risk of causing significant patient harm when used in error.

U.S. Brand Names Abraxane®

Index Terms ABI-007; Albumin-Bound Paclitaxel; nab-Paclitaxel; NSC-736631; Protein-Bound Paclitaxel

Pharmacologic Category Antineoplastic Agent, Antimicrotubular; Antineoplastic Agent, Natural Source (Plant) Derivative; Antineoplastic Agent, Taxane Derivative

Use Treatment of relapsed or refractory breast cancer

Effect on Mental Status None reported

Effect on Psychiatric Treatment ECG abnormalities are common; avoid use with ziprasidone, pimozide, thioridazine, and mesoridazine. GI side effects are common; concomitant use with SSRIs, lithium, or valproic acid may produce additive effects. Neutropenia is common; use caution with clozapine, carbamazepine, and valproic acid. Carbamazepine, phenobarbital, and phenytoin may reduce the effects of paclitaxel.

Dosage Summary

I.V.:

Children: Dosage not established

Adults: 260 mg/m^2 every 3 weeks

Dosage Forms Excipient information presented when available (limited, particularly for generics); consult specific product labeling.

Injection, powder for reconstitution:

Abraxane®: 100 mg [contains albumin (human)]

- **Pain Eze [OTC]** *see* Acetaminophen *on page 30*
- **Pain-Off [OTC]** *see* Acetaminophen, Aspirin, and Caffeine *on page 39*
- **Palgic®** *see* Carbinoxamine *on page 280*
- **Palgic®-D [DSC]** *see* Carbinoxamine and Pseudoephedrine *on page 280*
- **Palgic®-DS [DSC]** *see* Carbinoxamine and Pseudoephedrine *on page 280*

Palifermin (pal ee FER min)

U.S. Brand Names Kepivance™

Index Terms AMJ 9701; rHu-KGF

Pharmacologic Category Keratinocyte Growth Factor

Use Decrease the incidence and severity of severe oral mucositis associated with hematologic malignancies in patients receiving myelotoxic therapy requiring hematopoietic stem cell support

Effect on Mental Status None reported

Effect on Psychiatric Treatment Edema is common; rule out lithium as a cause. Rash is common; monitor, especially if receiving lamotrigine.

Dosage Summary

I.V.:

Children: Dosage not established

Adults: 60 mcg/kg/day for 3 consecutive days before and after myelotoxic therapy; total of 6 doses

Dosage Forms Excipient information presented when available (limited, particularly for generics); consult specific product labeling.

Injection, powder for reconstitution [preservative free]: 6.25 mg [contains mannitol 50 mg, sucrose 25 mg]

Paliperidone (pal ee PER i done)

Related Information

Antipsychotic Agents *on page 1769*

Antipsychotic Receptor Profile *on page 1772*

Atypical Antipsychotics *on page 1773*

U.S. Brand Names Invega®

Canadian Brand Names Invega®

Index Terms 9-hydroxy-risperidone; 9-OH-risperidone

Pharmacologic Category Antipsychotic Agent, Atypical

Generic Available No

Use Treatment of schizophrenia

Unlabeled/Investigational Use Psychosis/agitation related to Alzheimer's dementia

Mental Health Comment Paliperidone is an antipsychotic agent of a class often referred to as atypical. It should be noted that the definition of the term "atypical" is not universally agreed upon. Some prefer to describe antipsychotics based on their pharmacological properties. A common feature of all definitions used to describe "atypical" antipsychotics is the lack of significant acute or subacute EPS, at dosages generally associated with antipsychotic actions. Other experts have included definitions of atypicality that include a) failure to increase serum prolactin levels; b) superior efficacy for positive, negative, and cognitive symptoms; and c) lack of evidence of tardive dyskinesia or dystonia following chronic administration. Paliperidone is associated with a dose dependent increase in EPS; however, there was no difference compared with placebo in the incidence of any EPS symptoms at doses ≤6 mg/day.

Tardive dyskinesia (TD) secondary to **typical** antipsychotics has an estimated incidence of 3% to 5% per year for the first 5 years of treatment. The incidence of TD associated with the atypical antipsychotics is estimated to be 0.5% to 1%. It is not clear if this estimate represents a risk associated with mental illness or to what extent drug therapy can be implicated. Atypical antipsychotics appear less likely to cause tardive dyskinesia than typical antipsychotics (fluphenazine, haloperidol).

Coadministration of two or more antipsychotics does not generally improve clinical response and may increase the potential for adverse effects.

In 2008, the FDA issued a warning regarding increased mortality risk with typical **and** atypical antipsychotic drugs when used in elderly patients with dementia-related psychosis.

Pregnancy Risk Factor C

Pregnancy Considerations Animal studies with risperidone indicate an increase in fetal mortality. There are no adequate and well-controlled studies in pregnant women. Reversible EPS symptoms were noted in neonates following maternal use of risperidone during the last trimester.

Lactation Enters breast milk/use caution

Contraindications Hypersensitivity to paliperidone, risperidone, or any component of the formulation

Warnings/Precautions **[U.S. Boxed Warning]: Elderly patients with dementia-related psychosis treated with atypical antipsychotics are at an increased risk of death compared to placebo.** An increased incidence of cerebrovascular adverse events (including fatalities) has been reported in elderly patients with dementia-related psychosis. Paliperidone has not been studied in this clinical population and is not approved for the treatment of dementia-related psychosis.

Compared with risperidone, paliperidone is low to moderately sedating; use with caution in disorders where CNS depression is a feature. Use caution in patients with predisposition to seizures. Use with caution in renal dysfunction; dose reduction recommended. Esophageal dysmotility and aspiration have been associated with antipsychotic use; use with caution in patients at risk of aspiration pneumonia (eg, Alzheimer's disease). Elevates prolactin levels; use with caution in breast cancer or other prolactin-dependent tumors. May alter temperature regulation. May mask toxicity of other drugs or conditions (eg intestinal obstruction, Reyes syndrome, brain tumor) due to antiemetic effects.

May cause orthostasis. Use with caution in patients with cardiovascular diseases (eg, heart failure, history of myocardial infarction or ischemia, cerebrovascular disease, conduction abnormalities). Use caution in patients receiving medications for hypertension (orthostatic effects may be exacerbated) or in patients with hypovolemia or dehydration. May alter cardiac conduction; life-threatening arrhythmias have occurred with therapeutic doses of neuroleptics. Avoid use in combination with QT_c-prolonging drugs. Avoid use in patients with congenital long-QT syndrome and in patients with history of cardiac arrhythmia.

May cause extrapyramidal symptoms (EPS), including pseudoparkinsonism, acute dystonic reactions, akathisia, and tardive dyskinesia (risk of these reactions is low relative to other neuroleptics, and is dose dependent). Risk of dystonia (and probably other EPS) may be greater with increased doses, use of conventional antipsychotics, males, and younger patients. Risk of neuroleptic malignant syndrome (NMS) may be increased in patients with Parkinson's disease or Lewy body dementia; monitor for symptoms of confusion, obtundation, postural instability and extrapyramidal symptoms. May cause hyperglycemia; in some cases may be extreme and associated with ketoacidosis, hyperosmolar coma, or death. Use with caution in patients with diabetes (or risk factors) or other disorders of glucose regulation; monitor for worsening of glucose control. Significant weight gain has been observed with antipsychotic therapy; incidence varies with product. Monitor waist circumference and BMI.

The possibility of a suicide attempt is inherent in psychotic illness or bipolar disorder; use caution in high-risk patients during initiation of therapy. Prescriptions should be written for the smallest quantity consistent with good patient care.

Formulation consists of drug within a nonabsorbable shell that is expelled and may be visible in the stool. Use is not recommended in patients with preexisting severe gastrointestinal narrowing disorders. Patients with upper GI tract alterations in transit time may have increased or decreased bioavailability of paliperidone. Do not use in patients unable to swallow the tablet whole.

Safety and efficacy have not been established in patients <18 years of age.

Adverse Reactions

>10%:

Cardiovascular: Tachycardia (12% to 14%)

Central nervous system: Headache (11% to 14%), somnolence (6% to 11% dose dependent)

1% to 10%:

Cardiovascular: Orthostatic hypotension (1% to 4% dose dependent), bundle branch block (<1% to 3%), AV block (first degree ≤2%), arrhythmia (≤2%)

Central nervous system: Akathisia (3% to 10% dose dependent), EPS (2% to 7% dose dependent), parkinsonism (≤7% dose dependent), dizziness (4% to 6%), dystonia (1% to 5% dose dependent), hypertonia (1% to 4% dose dependent), fatigue (1% to 2%)

Endocrine & metabolic: Weight gain (6% to 9% dose dependent)

Gastrointestinal: Salivation increased (≤4% dose dependent), xerostomia (1% to 3%), abdominal pain (1% to 3%)

Neuromuscular & skeletal: Hyperkinesia (3% to 10% dose dependent), dyskinesia (3% to 9% dose dependent), tremor (3% to 4%), weakness (≤2%)

<1% (Limited to important or life-threatening): Anaphylactic reaction, bradycardia, edema, hyperglycemia, ischemia, neuroleptic malignant syndrome, palpitation, prolactin increased, QT_c interval prolongation, sedation, seizure, syncope, tardive dyskinesia, tongue swelling

Drug Interactions

Acetylcholinesterase Inhibitors (Central): May enhance the neurotoxic (central) effect of Antipsychotics. Severe extrapyramidal symptoms have occurred in some patients. *Risk C: Monitor therapy*

Alcohol (Ethyl): CNS Depressants may enhance the CNS depressant effect of Alcohol (Ethyl). *Risk C: Monitor therapy*

Amphetamines: Antipsychotics may diminish the stimulatory effect of Amphetamines. *Risk C: Monitor therapy*

Anti-Parkinson's Agents (Dopamine Agonist): Antipsychotics (Atypical) may diminish the therapeutic effect of Anti-Parkinson's Agents (Dopamine Agonist). *Risk D: Consider therapy modification*

CarBAMazepine: May decrease the serum concentration of Paliperidone. *Risk C: Monitor therapy*

CNS Depressants: May enhance the adverse/toxic effect of other CNS Depressants. *Risk C: Monitor therapy*

Itraconazole: May decrease the metabolism of Paliperidone. *Risk C: Monitor therapy*

Lithium formulations: May enhance the neurotoxic effect of Antipsychotics. Lithium formulations may decrease the serum concentration of Antipsychotics. Specifically noted with chlorpromazine. *Risk C: Monitor therapy*

P-Glycoprotein Inducers: May decrease the serum concentration of P-Glycoprotein Substrates. P-glycoprotein inducers may also further limit the distribution of p-glycoprotein substrates to specific cells/tissues/organs where p-glycoprotein is present in large amounts (e.g., brain, T-lymphocytes, testes, etc.). *Risk C: Monitor therapy*

P-Glycoprotein Inhibitors: May increase the serum concentration of P-Glycoprotein Substrates. P-glycoprotein inhibitors may also enhance the distribution of p-glycoprotein substrates to specific cells/tissues/organs where p-glycoprotein is present in large amounts (e.g., brain, T-lymphocytes, testes, etc.). *Risk C: Monitor therapy*

Tetrabenazine: May enhance the adverse/toxic effect of Antipsychotics. *Risk C: Monitor therapy*

Ethanol/Nutrition/Herb Interactions

Ethanol: Avoid ethanol (may increase CNS depression).

Herb/Nutraceutical: Avoid kava kava, gotu kola, valerian, St John's wort (may increase CNS depression).

Stability Store at controlled room temperature of ≤25°C (77°F); excursions permitted to 15°C to 30°C (59°F to 86°F). Protect from moisture.

Mechanism of Action Paliperidone is considered a benzisoxazole atypical antipsychotic as it is the primary active metabolite of risperidone. As with other atypical antipsychotics, it's therapeutic efficacy is believed to result from mixed central serotonergic and dopaminergic antagonism. The addition of serotonin antagonism to dopamine antagonism (classic neuroleptic mechanism) is thought to improve negative symptoms of psychoses and reduce the incidence of extrapyramidal side effects. Similar to risperidone, paliperidone demonstrates high affinity to α_1, D_2, H_1, and 5-HT_{2C} receptors, and low affinity for muscarinic and 5-HT_{1A} receptors. In contrast to risperidone, paliperidone displays nearly 10-fold lower affinity for α_2 and 5-HT_{2A} receptors, and nearly three- to fivefold less affinity for 5-HT_{1A} and 5-HT_{1D}, respectively.

Pharmacodynamics/Kinetics

Distribution: V_d: 487 L

Protein binding: 74%

Metabolism: Hepatic via CYP2D6 and 3A4 (limited role in elimination); minor metabolism (<10% each) via dealkylation, hydroxylation, dehydrogenation, and benzisoxazole scission

Bioavailability: 28%

Half-life elimination: 23 hours; 24-51 hours with renal impairment (Cl_{cr} <80 mL/minute)

Time to peak, plasma: ~24 hours

Excretion: Urine (80%); feces (11%)

Dosage Oral:

Adults: Schizophrenia: Usual: 6 mg once daily in the morning; titration not required, though some may benefit from higher or lower doses. If exceeding 6 mg/day, increases of 3 mg/day are recommended no more frequently than every 5 days, up to a maximum of 12 mg/day. Some patients may require only 3 mg/day.

Dosage adjustment in renal impairment:

Mild impairment (Cl_{cr} 50 to <80 mL/minute): Initial: 3 mg once daily; may increase to maximal dose of 6 mg/day if needed

Moderate-to-severe impairment (Cl_{cr} 10-49 mL/minute): Initial: 1.5 mg once daily; may increase to maximal dose of 3 mg/day if needed

Severe impairment (Cl_{cr} <10 mL/minute): Has not been studied; not recommended

Dosage adjustment in hepatic impairment: No adjustment necessary for mild-to-moderate (Child-Pugh class A and B) impairment. Not studied in severe impairment.

Dietary Considerations May be taken with or without food.

Administration May be administered with or without food. Extended release tablets should be swallowed whole with liquids; do not crush, chew, or divide.

Monitoring Parameters Vital signs; fasting lipid profile and fasting blood glucose/Hgb A_{1c} (prior to treatment, at 3 months, then annually), prolactin levels; BMI, personal/family history of obesity, diabetes, waist circumference; blood pressure; mental status, abnormal involuntary movement scale (AIMS), extrapyramidal symptoms; orthostatic blood pressure changes for 3-5 days after starting or increasing dose. Weight should be assessed prior to treatment, at 4 weeks, 8 weeks, 12 weeks, and then at quarterly intervals. Consider titrating to a different antipsychotic agent for a weight gain ≥5% of the initial weight.

Additional Information Invega® is an extended release tablet based on the OROS® osmotic delivery system. Water from the GI tract enters through a semipermeable membrane coating the tablet, solubilizing the drug into a gelatinous form which, through hydrophilic expansion, is then expelled through laser-drilled holes in the coating.

Dosage Forms Excipient information presented when available (limited, particularly for generics); consult specific product labeling. [CAN] = Canadian availability; not available in U.S.

Tablet, extended-release:

Invega®: 1.5 mg, 3 mg, 6 mg, 9 mg [osmotic controlled release]

Invega® [CAN]: 12 mg [osmotic controlled release, not available in the U.S.]

Palivizumab (pah li VIZ u mab)

Medication Safety Issues

Sound-alike/look-alike issues:

Synagis® may be confused with Synalgos®-DC, Synvisc®

U.S. Brand Names Synagis®

Canadian Brand Names Synagis®

Mexican Brand Names Synagis

Pharmacologic Category Monoclonal Antibody

Use Prevention of serious lower respiratory tract disease caused by respiratory syncytial virus (RSV) in infants and children at high risk of RSV disease

Effect on Mental Status May rarely cause nervousness

Effect on Psychiatric Treatment May cause anemia; use caution with clozapine and carbamazepine

Dosage Summary

I.M.:

Children <2 years: 15 mg/kg monthly throughout RSV season

Children >2 years: Dosage not established

Adults: Dosage not established

Dosage Forms Excipient information presented when available (limited, particularly for generics); consult specific product labeling.

Injection, solution [preservative free]:

Synagis®: 100 mg/mL (0.5 mL, 1 mL)

◆ **Palmer's® Skin Success Acne Cleanser [OTC]** *see* Salicylic Acid *on page 1454*

Palonosetron (pal oh NOE se tron)

Medication Safety Issues

Sound-alike/look-alike issues:

Aloxi® may be confused with Eloxatin®, oxaliplatin

Palonosetron may be confused with dolasetron, granisetron, ondansetron

U.S. Brand Names Aloxi®

Mexican Brand Names Onicit

Index Terms Palonosetron Hydrochloride; RS-25259; RS-25259-197

Pharmacologic Category Antiemetic; Selective 5-HT_3 Receptor Antagonist

Generic Available No

Use Prevention of chemotherapy-associated nausea and vomiting; indicated for prevention of acute (highly-emetogenic therapy) as well as acute and delayed (moderately-emetogenic therapy) nausea and vomiting; prevention of postoperative nausea and vomiting (PONV)

Effect on Mental Status May cause anxiety and dizziness; may rarely cause euphoria, insomnia, or sedation

Effect on Psychiatric Treatment Use caution with thioridazine and ziprasidone; combined use may cause QT prolongation

Pregnancy Risk Factor B

Pregnancy Considerations Teratogenic effects were not observed in animal studies. There are no adequate and well-controlled studies in pregnant women; use during pregnancy only if clearly needed.

Lactation Excretion in breast milk unknown/not recommended

Contraindications Hypersensitivity to palonosetron or any component of the formulation

Warnings/Precautions Use caution in patients allergic to other 5-HT_3 receptor antagonists; cross-reactivity is possible. Some selective 5-HT_3 receptor antagonists have been associated with dose-dependent increases in ECG intervals (eg, PR, QRS duration, QT/QT_c, JT), usually occurring 1-2 hours after I.V. administration. In general, these changes are not clinically relevant, however, when these agents are used in conjunction with other agents that prolong these intervals, arrhythmia may occur. When used with agents that prolong the QT interval (eg, Class I and III antiarrhythmics), clinically relevant QT interval prolongation could result in torsade de pointes. A number of trials have shown that 5-HT_3 antagonists produce QT interval prolongation to variable degrees. Use with caution in patients at risk of QT prolongation and/or ventricular arrhythmia. Reduction in heart rate may also occur with the 5-HT_3 antagonists. Use with caution in patients with congenital long QT syndrome or other risk factors for QT prolongation (eg, medications known to prolong QT interval, electrolyte abnormalities, and cumulative high dose anthracycline therapy).

Not intended for treatment of nausea and vomiting or for chronic continuous therapy. **For chemotherapy, should be used on a scheduled basis, not on an "as needed" (PRN) basis,** since data support the use of this drug only in the prevention of nausea and vomiting (due to antineoplastic therapy) and not in the rescue of nausea and vomiting. For PONV, may use for low expectation of PONV if it is essential to avoid nausea and vomiting in the postoperative period; use is not recommended if there is little expectation of nausea and vomiting. Safety and efficacy in children have not been established.

Adverse Reactions Adverse events may vary according to indication.

1% to 10%:

- Cardiovascular: QT prolongation (chemotherapy-associated <1%; PONV 1% to 5%), bradycardia (chemotherapy-associated 1%), hypotension (≤1%), sinus bradycardia (≤1%), tachycardia (nonsustained) (≤1%)
- Central nervous system: Headache (chemotherapy-associated 5% to 9%), anxiety (1%), dizziness (≤1%)
- Dermatologic: Pruritus (≤1%)
- Endocrine & metabolic: Hyperkalemia (1%)
- Gastrointestinal: Constipation (2% to 5%), diarrhea (1%), flatulence (≤1%)
- Genitourinary: Urinary retention (≤1%)
- Hepatic: ALT or AST increased (≤1%; transient)
- Neuromuscular & skeletal: Weakness (1%)

<1% (Limited to important or life-threatening): Abdominal pain, allergic dermatitis, amblyopia, anorexia, appetite decreased, arrhythmia, arthralgia, bilirubin increased (transient), dyspepsia, edema (generalized), electrolyte fluctuations, euphoric mood, extrasystoles, eye irritation, fatigue, fever, flu-like syndrome, glycosuria, hiccups, hot flash, hyperglycemia, hypersensitivity (rare), hypersomnia, hyper-/hypotension, hypokalemia, hypoventilation, injection site reactions (burning/discomfort/induration/pain; rare), insomnia, intestinal hypomotility, laryngospasm, metabolic acidosis, motion sickness, myocardial ischemia, paresthesia, platelets decreased, rash, salivation increased, sinus arrhythmia, sinus tachycardia, somnolence, supraventricular extrasystoles, tinnitus, T-wave amplitude decreased, vein discoloration, vein distention, ventricular extrasystoles, xerostomia

Metabolism/Transport Effects Substrate (minor) of CYP1A2, 2D6, 3A4

Drug Interactions

Apomorphine: Antiemetics (5HT3 Antagonists) may enhance the hypotensive effect of Apomorphine. *Risk X: Avoid combination*

Stability Store intact vials at room temperature of 20°C to 25°C (68°F to 77°F); excursions permitted to 15°C to 30°C (59°F to 86°F); do not freeze. Protect from light. Solutions of 5 mcg/mL and 30 mcg/mL in NS, D_5W, $D_5$1/2NS, and D_5LR injection are stable for 48 hours at room temperature and 14 days under refrigeration.

Mechanism of Action Selective 5-HT_3 receptor antagonist, blocking serotonin, both on vagal nerve terminals in the periphery and centrally in the chemoreceptor trigger zone

Pharmacodynamics/Kinetics

Distribution: V_d: 8.3 ± 2.5 L/kg

Protein binding: ~62%

Metabolism: ~50% metabolized via CYP enzymes (and likely other pathways) to relatively inactive metabolites (N-oxide-palonosetron and 6-S-hydroxy-palonosetron); CYP1A2, 2D6, and 3A4 contribute to its metabolism
Half-life elimination: Terminal: ~40 hours
Excretion: Urine (80%, 40% as unchanged drug)

Dosage I.V.: Adults:
Chemotherapy-associated nausea and vomiting: 0.25 mg 30 minutes prior to the start of chemotherapy administration, day 1 of each cycle
Breakthrough: Palonosetron has not been shown to be effective in terminating nausea or vomiting once it occurs and should not be used for this purpose.
PONV: 0.075 mg immediately prior to anesthesia induction
Elderly: No dosage adjustment necessary
Dosage adjustment in renal/hepatic impairment: No dosage adjustment necessary

Administration I.V.: Flush I.V. line with NS prior to and following administration.
Chemotherapy-associated nausea and vomiting: Infuse over 30 seconds, 30 minutes prior to the start of chemotherapy
PONV: Infuse over 10 seconds immediately prior to anesthesia induction

Dosage Forms Excipient information presented when available (limited, particularly for generics); consult specific product labeling.
Injection, solution:
Aloxi®: 0.05 mg/mL (1.5 mL, 5 mL) [contains edetate disodium]

- **Palonosetron Hydrochloride** *see* Palonosetron *on page 1218*
- **2-PAM** *see* Pralidoxime *on page 1318*
- **Pamelor®** *see* Nortriptyline *on page 1152*

Pamidronate (pa mi DROE nate)

Medication Safety Issues
Sound-alike/look-alike issues:
Aredia® may be confused with Adriamycin, Meridia®

International issues:
Linoten® [Spain] may be confused with Lidopen® which is a brand name for lidocaine in the U.S.

U.S. Brand Names Aredia®

Canadian Brand Names Aredia®; Pamidronate Disodium®; Rhoxal-pamidronate

Mexican Brand Names Pamisol

Index Terms Pamidronate Disodium

Pharmacologic Category Antidote; Bisphosphonate Derivative

Use Treatment of hypercalcemia associated with malignancy; treatment of osteolytic bone lesions associated with multiple myeloma or metastatic breast cancer; moderate to severe Paget's disease of bone

Unlabeled/Investigational Use Treatment of pediatric osteoporosis, treatment of osteogenesis imperfecta

Effect on Mental Status May cause drowsiness

Effect on Psychiatric Treatment May rarely cause leukopenia; use caution with clozapine and carbamazepine. Bisphosphonates, including pamidronate, have been associated with renal toxicity manifested as deterioration of renal function and potential renal failure. Use caution in patients receiving lithium.

Dosage Summary
I.V.:
Children: Dosage not established
Adults: 60-90 mg as a single dose, may repeat every 3-4 weeks **or** 30 mg daily for 3 consecutive days

Dosage Forms Excipient information presented when available (limited, particularly for generics); consult specific product labeling.
Injection, powder for reconstitution, as disodium: 30 mg, 90 mg
Aredia®: 30 mg, 90 mg
Injection, solution: 3 mg/mL (10 mL); 6 mg/mL (10 mL); 9 mg/mL (10 mL)

- **Pamidronate Disodium** *see* Pamidronate *on page 1220*
- **Pamine®** *see* Methscopolamine *on page 1019*
- **Pamine® Forte** *see* Methscopolamine *on page 1019*
- **p-Aminoclonidine** *see* Apraclonidine *on page 129*
- **Pamprin® Maximum Strength All Day Relief [OTC]** *see* Naproxen *on page 1102*

- ◆ ***Panax ginseng*** *see* Ginseng, Panax *(Panax ginseng) on page 718*
- ◆ **Pancof® [DSC]** *see* Pseudoephedrine, Dihydrocodeine, and Chlorpheniramine *on page 1371*
- ◆ **Pancof®-EXP** *see* Dihydrocodeine, Pseudoephedrine, and Guaifenesin *on page 469*
- ◆ **Pancof-XP [DSC]** *see* Hydrocodone and Guaifenesin *on page 779*
- ◆ **Pandel®** *see* Hydrocortisone *on page 785*
- ◆ **Panhematin®** *see* Hemin *on page 760*

Panitumumab (pan i TOOM yoo mab)

U.S. Brand Names Vectibix®

Canadian Brand Names Vectibix®

Index Terms ABX-EGF; NSC-742319; rHuMAb-EGFr

Pharmacologic Category Antineoplastic Agent, Monoclonal Antibody; Epidermal Growth Factor Receptor (EGFR) Inhibitor

Use Monotherapy in treatment of refractory (EGFR-expressing) metastatic colorectal cancer

Effect on Mental Status Fatigue is common

Effect on Psychiatric Treatment GI side effects are common; concomitant use with lithium, valproic acid, carbamazepine, and SSRIs may produce additive effects

Dosage Summary

I.V.:

Children: Dosage not established

Adults: 6 mg/kg every 2 weeks

Dosage Forms Excipient information presented when available (limited, particularly for generics); consult specific product labeling.

Injection, solution [preservative free]:

Vectibix®: 20 mg/mL (5 mL, 10 mL, 20 mL)

- ◆ **Panlor® DC** *see* Acetaminophen, Caffeine, and Dihydrocodeine *on page 39*
- ◆ **Panlor® SS** *see* Acetaminophen, Caffeine, and Dihydrocodeine *on page 39*
- ◆ **Panretin®** *see* Alitretinoin *on page 66*

Pantoprazole (pan TOE pra zole)

Medication Safety Issues

Sound-alike/look-alike issues:

Protonix® may be confused with Lotronex®, Lovenox®, protamine

Vials containing Protonix® I.V. for injection are not recommended for use with spiked I.V. system adaptors. Nurses and pharmacists have reported breakage of the glass vials during attempts to connect spiked I.V. system adaptors, which may potentially result in injury to healthcare professionals.

International issues:

Protonix® may be confused with Pretanix® which is a brand name for indapamide in Hungary

U.S. Brand Names Protonix®

Canadian Brand Names Apo-Pantoprazole; Pantoloc®; Pantoloc® M; Panto™ I.V.; PMS-Pantoprazole; Protonix®; Ran-Pantoprazole

Mexican Brand Names Ciproton; Kuppam; Leminter; Pantozol; Pauly; Peucetol; Prozolan; Regad; Tecta; Unigastrozol; Zolpra; Zurcal

Pharmacologic Category Proton Pump Inhibitor; Substituted Benzimidazole

Generic Available Yes: Delayed release tablet

Use

Oral: Treatment and maintenance of healing of erosive esophagitis associated with GERD; reduction in relapse rates of daytime and nighttime heartburn symptoms in GERD; hypersecretory disorders associated with Zollinger-Ellison syndrome or other GI hypersecretory disorders

I.V.: Short-term treatment (7-10 days) of patients with gastroesophageal reflux disease (GERD) and a history of erosive esophagitis; hypersecretory disorders associated with Zollinger-Ellison syndrome or other neoplastic disorders

Unlabeled/Investigational Use Peptic ulcer disease, active ulcer bleeding (parenteral formulation); adjunct treatment with antibiotics for *Helicobacter pylori* eradication; stress-ulcer prophylaxis in the critically-ill

Effect on Mental Status May cause anxiety or dizziness; may rarely produce confusion, depression, dysarthria, hallucinations, nervousness, or somnolence ▶

Effect on Psychiatric Treatment None reported

Pregnancy Risk Factor B

Pregnancy Considerations Teratogenic effects were not observed in animal studies. There are no adequate and well-controlled studies in pregnant women. Use in pregnancy only if clearly needed.

Lactation Enters breast milk/not recommended

Contraindications Hypersensitivity to pantoprazole, substituted benzamidazoles (eg, esomeprazole, lansoprazole, omeprazole, rabeprazole), or any component of the formulation

Warnings/Precautions Relief of symptoms does not preclude the presence of a gastric malignancy. Long-term pantoprazole therapy (especially in patients who were *H. pylori* positive) has caused biopsy-proven atrophic gastritis. No reports of enterochromaffin-like (ECL) cell carcinoids, dysplasia, or neoplasia such as those seen in rodent studies have occurred in humans. Not indicated for maintenance therapy; safety and efficacy for use beyond 16 weeks have not been established. Prolonged treatment (typically >3 years) may lead to vitamin B_{12} malabsorption and subsequent deficiency. Intravenous preparation contains edetate sodium (EDTA); use caution in patients who are at risk for zinc deficiency if other EDTA-containing solutions are coadministered.

Adverse Reactions

≥1%:

Cardiovascular: Chest pain

Central nervous system: Headache (2% to 9%), insomnia (≤1%), anxiety, dizziness, migraine, pain

Dermatologic: Rash (≤2%)

Endocrine & metabolic: Hyperglycemia (≤1%), hyperlipidemia

Gastrointestinal: Diarrhea (2% to 6%), flatulence (2% to 4%), abdominal pain (1% to 4%), nausea (≤2%), vomiting (≤2%), eructation (≤1%), constipation, dyspepsia, gastroenteritis, rectal disorder

Genitourinary: Urinary frequency, UTI

Hepatic: Liver function tests abnormal (≤2%)

Local: Injection site reaction (includes thrombophlebitis and abscess)

Neuromuscular & skeletal: Arthralgia, back pain, hypertonia, neck pain, weakness

Respiratory: Bronchitis, cough, dyspnea, pharyngitis, rhinitis, sinusitis, upper respiratory tract infection

Miscellaneous: Flu syndrome, infection

<1% (Limited to important or life-threatening): Abnormal dreams, acne, albuminuria, alkaline phosphatase increased, allergic reaction, alopecia, anaphylaxis, anemia, angioedema, angina pectoris, anorexia, aphthous stomatitis, appetite increased, arrhythmia, asthma exacerbation, atrial fibrillation/flutter, atrophic gastritis, balanitis, biliary pain, blurred vision, bone pain, breast pain, bursitis, cataract, CHF, chills, cholecystitis, cholelithiasis, CPK increased, colitis, confusion, contact dermatitis, creatinine increased, cystitis, deafness, decreased reflexes, dehydration, depression, diabetes mellitus, diaphoresis, diplopia, duodenitis, dysarthria, dysmenorrhea, dysphagia, dysuria, ecchymosis, ECG abnormality, eczema, eosinophilia, epididymitis, epistaxis, erythema multiforme, esophagitis, extraocular palsy, facial edema, fever, fungal dermatitis, gastrointestinal carcinoma, gastrointestinal hemorrhage, gastrointestinal moniliasis, generalized edema, GGT increased, gingivitis, glaucoma, glossitis, glycosuria, goiter, gout, halitosis, hallucinations, heat stroke, hematemesis, hematuria, hemorrhage, hepatic failure, hepatitis, hernia, herpes simplex, herpes zoster, hiccup, hyperbilirubinemia, hyperesthesia, hyper-/hypotension, hyperkinesia, hyperuricemia, hypokinesia, impaired urination, impotence, interstitial nephritis, jaundice, kidney calculus, kidney pain, laryngitis, leg cramps, leukocytosis, leukopenia, libido decreased, lichenoid dermatitis, maculopapular rash, malaise, melena, mouth ulceration, myalgia, myocardial infarction, myocardial ischemia, neoplasm, nervousness, neuralgia, neuritis, nocturia, optic neuropathy (including anterior ischemic), otitis externa, palpitation, pancreatitis, pancytopenia, paresthesia, periodontal abscess, periodontitis, photosensitivity, pneumonia, pruritus, pyelonephritis, rectal hemorrhage, retinal vascular disorder, rhabdomyolysis, salivation increased, scrotal edema, seizure, skin ulcer, somnolence, Stevens-Johnson syndrome, stomach ulcer, stomatitis, syncope, tachycardia, taste perversion, tenosynovitis, thrombocytopenia, thrombosis, tinnitus, tongue discoloration, toxic epidermal necrolysis, tremor, urethral pain, urethritis, urticaria, vaginitis, vasodilation, vertigo, vision abnormal, weight changes, xerostomia

Metabolism/Transport Effects Substrate of CYP2C19 (major), 2C9 (minor), 2D6 (minor), 3A4 (minor); **Inhibits** 2C9 (weak); **Induces** CYP1A2 (weak), 3A4 (weak)

Drug Interactions

Antifungal Agents (Azole Derivatives, Systemic): Proton Pump Inhibitors may decrease the absorption of Antifungal Agents (Azole Derivatives, Systemic). **Exceptions:** Miconazole. *Risk D: Consider therapy modification*

Atazanavir: Proton Pump Inhibitors may decrease the absorption of Atazanavir. *Risk D: Consider therapy modification*

Clopidogrel: Proton Pump Inhibitors may diminish the therapeutic effect of Clopidogrel. This appears to be due to reduced formation of the active clopidogrel metabolite. *Risk C: Monitor therapy*

CYP2C19 Inducers (Strong): May increase the metabolism of CYP2C19 Substrates. *Risk C: Monitor therapy*

Dabigatran Etexilate: Proton Pump Inhibitors may decrease the serum concentration of Dabigatran Etexilate. *Risk C: Monitor therapy*

Dasatinib: Proton Pump Inhibitors may decrease the absorption of Dasatinib. *Risk D: Consider therapy modification*

Erlotinib: Proton Pump Inhibitors may decrease the serum concentration of Erlotinib. *Risk X: Avoid combination*

Indinavir: Proton Pump Inhibitors may decrease the absorption of Indinavir. *Risk C: Monitor therapy*

Iron Salts: Proton Pump Inhibitors may decrease the absorption of Iron Salts. **Exceptions:** Ferric Gluconate; Iron Dextran Complex; Iron Sucrose. *Risk C: Monitor therapy*

Methotrexate: Proton Pump Inhibitors may decrease the excretion of Methotrexate. Antirheumatic doses of methotrexate probably hold minimal risk. *Risk C: Monitor therapy*

Mycophenolate: Proton Pump Inhibitors may decrease the serum concentration of Mycophenolate. Specifically, concentrations of the active mycophenolic acid may be reduced. *Risk C: Monitor therapy*

Saquinavir: Proton Pump Inhibitors may increase the serum concentration of Saquinavir. *Risk C: Monitor therapy*

Tipranavir: May decrease the serum concentration of Proton Pump Inhibitors. These data are derived from studies with Ritonavir-boosted Tipranavir. *Risk C: Monitor therapy*

Topotecan: BCRP/ABCG2 Inhibitors may increase the serum concentration of Topotecan. *Risk D: Consider therapy modification*

Ethanol/Nutrition/Herb Interactions

Ethanol: Avoid ethanol (may cause gastric mucosal irritation).

Herb/Nutraceutical: Prolonged treatment (typically >3 years) may lead to vitamin B_{12} malabsorption and subsequent deficiency.

Stability

Oral: Store tablet and oral suspension at controlled room temperature of 20°C to 25°C (68°F to 77°F).

I.V.: Prior to reconstitution, store at controlled room temperature of 20°C to 25°C (68°F to 77°F). Protect from light. Reconstitute with 10 mL NS (final concentration 4 mg/mL). Reconstituted solution may be given intravenously (over 2 minutes) or may be added to 100 mL D_5W, NS, or LR (for 15-minute infusion). When reconstituted, solution is stable up to 96 hours at room temperature (Johnson, 2005). The preparation should be stored at 3°C to 5°C (37°F to 41°F) if it is stored beyond 48 hours to minimize discoloration. If further diluting in 100 mL of D_5W, LR, or NS, dilute within 6 hours of reconstitution. Diluted solution is stable at room temperature for up to 24 hours from the time of initial reconstitution; protection from light is not required.

Mechanism of Action Suppresses gastric acid secretion by inhibiting the parietal cell H^+/K^+ ATP pump

Pharmacodynamics/Kinetics

Absorption: Rapid, well absorbed

Distribution: V_d: 11-24 L

Protein binding: 98%, primarily to albumin

Metabolism: Extensively hepatic; CYP2C19 (demethylation), CYP3A4; no evidence that metabolites have pharmacologic activity

Bioavailability: 77%

Half-life elimination: 1 hour; increased to 3.5-10 hours with CYP2C19 deficiency

Time to peak: Oral: 2.5 hours

Excretion: Urine (71%); feces (18%)

Dosage

Oral:

Children ≥5 years (unlabeled use): GERD, erosive esophagitis associated with GERD: 20-40 mg once daily

Adults:

Erosive esophagitis associated with GERD:

Treatment: 40 mg once daily for up to 8 weeks; an additional 8 weeks may be used in patients who have not healed after an 8-week course

Maintenance of healing: 40 mg once daily

Note: Lower doses (20 mg once daily) have been used successfully in mild GERD treatment and maintenance of healing

Hypersecretory disorders (including Zollinger-Ellison): Initial: 40 mg twice daily; adjust dose based on patient needs; doses up to 240 mg/day have been administered

Helicobacter pylori eradication (unlabeled use): Doses up to 40 mg twice daily have been used as part of combination therapy

I.V.:

Erosive esophagitis associated with GERD: 40 mg once daily for 7-10 days

Hypersecretory disorders: 80 mg twice daily; adjust dose based on acid output measurements; 160-240 mg/day in divided doses has been used for a limited period (up to 7 days)

Prevention of rebleeding in peptic ulcer bleed (unlabeled use): 80 mg, followed by 8 mg/hour infusion for 72 hours. **Note:** A daily infusion of 40 mg does not raise gastric pH sufficiently to enhance coagulation in active GI bleeds.

Elderly: Dosage adjustment not required

Dosage adjustment in renal impairment: Not required; pantoprazole is not removed by hemodialysis

Dosage adjustment in hepatic impairment: Not required

Dietary Considerations

Oral: May be taken with or without food; best if taken before breakfast.

I.V.: Due to EDTA in preparation, zinc supplementation may be needed in patients prone to zinc deficiency.

Administration

I.V.: Flush I.V. line before and after administration. In-line filter not required.

2-minute infusion: The volume of reconstituted solution (4 mg/mL) to be injected may be administered intravenously over at least 2 minutes.

15-minute infusion: Infuse over 15 minutes at a rate not to exceed 7 mL/minute (3 mg/minute).

Oral:

Tablet: Should be swallowed whole, do not crush or chew. Best if taken before breakfast.

Delayed-release oral suspension: Should only be administered in apple juice or applesauce and taken ~30 minutes before a meal. Do not administer with any other liquid (eg, water) or foods.

Oral administration in **applesauce**: Sprinkle intact granules on 1 tablespoon of applesauce and swallow within 10 minutes of preparation.

Oral administration in **apple juice**: Empty intact granules into 5 mL of apple juice (~1 teaspoonful), stir for 5 seconds, and swallow immediately after preparation. Rinse container once or twice with apple juice and swallow immediately.

Nasogastric tube administration: Separate the plunger from the barrel of a 60 mL catheter tip syringe and connect to a ≥16 French nasogastric tube. Holding the syringe attached to the tubing as high as possible, empty the contents of the packet into barrel of the syringe, add 10 mL of apple juice and gently tap/shake the barrel of the syringe to help empty the syringe. Add an additional 10 mL of apple juice and gently tap/shake the barrel to help rinse. Repeat rinse with at least 2 -10 mL aliquots of apple juice. No granules should remain in the syringe.

Monitoring Parameters Hypersecretory disorders: Acid output measurements, target level <10 mEq/hour (<5 mEq/hour if prior gastric acid-reducing surgery)

Test Interactions False-positive urine screening tests for tetrahydrocannabinol (THC) have been noted in patients receiving proton pump inhibitors, including pantoprazole.

Dosage Forms Excipient information presented when available (limited, particularly for generics); consult specific product labeling. [CAN] = Canadian brand name

Note: Strength expressed as base

Granules for suspension, delayed release, enteric coated, as sodium, oral:

Protonix®: 40 mg/packet (30s)

Injection, powder for reconstitution, as sodium:

Protonix®: 40 mg [contains edetate sodium 1 mg]

Tablet, delayed release, as sodium: 20 mg, 40 mg

Protonix®: 20 mg, 40 mg

Tablet, enteric coated, as magnesium:
Pantoloc® M [CAN]: 40 mg [not available in the U.S.]

Papaverine (pa PAV er een)

U.S. Brand Names Para-Time SR®
Index Terms Papaverine Hydrochloride; Pavabid [DSC]
Pharmacologic Category Vasodilator
Use Oral: Relief of peripheral and cerebral ischemia associated with arterial spasm and myocardial ischemia complicated by arrhythmias
Unlabeled/Investigational Use Investigational: Parenteral: Various vascular spasms associated with muscle spasms as in myocardial infarction, angina, peripheral and pulmonary embolism, peripheral vascular disease, angiospastic states, and visceral spasm (ureteral, biliary, and GI colic); testing for impotence
Effect on Mental Status May cause drowsiness or dizziness
Effect on Psychiatric Treatment May decrease the effects of levodopa
Dosage Summary
I.M.:
Children: 6 mg/kg/day in 4 divided doses
Adults: 30-65 mg, may repeat every 3 hours
I.V.:
Children: 6 mg/kg/day in 4 divided doses
Adults: 30-65 mg, may repeat every 3 hours
Oral:
Children: Dosage not established
Adults: 150-300 mg every 12 hours **or** 150 mg every 8 hours
Dosage Forms Excipient information presented when available (limited, particularly for generics); consult specific product labeling.
Capsule, sustained release, as hydrochloride: 150 mg
Para-Time SR®: 150 mg
Injection, solution, as hydrochloride: 30 mg/mL (2 mL, 10 mL)

- **Papaverine Hydrochloride** *see* Papaverine *on page 1225*
- **Para-Aminosalicylate Sodium** *see* Aminosalicylic Acid *on page 88*
- **Paracetamol** *see* Acetaminophen *on page 30*
- **Parafon Forte® DSC** *see* Chlorzoxazone *on page 341*
- **Parathyroid Hormone (1-34)** *see* Teriparatide *on page 1553*
- **Para-Time SR®** *see* Papaverine *on page 1225*
- **Parcaine™** *see* Proparacaine *on page 1352*
- **Parcopa™** *see* Carbidopa and Levodopa *on page 277*

Paregoric (par e GOR ik)

Medication Safety Issues
Sound-alike/look-alike issues:
Camphorated tincture of opium is an error-prone synonym (mistaken as opium tincture)
Paregoric may be confused with Percogesic®

High alert medication: The Institute for Safe Medication Practices (ISMP) includes this medication among its list of drug classes which have a heightened risk of causing significant patient harm when used in error.

Use care when prescribing opium tincture; each mL contains the equivalent of morphine 10 mg; paregoric contains the equivalent of morphine 0.4 mg/mL
Index Terms Camphorated Tincture of Opium (error-prone synonym)
Pharmacologic Category Analgesic, Opioid
Use Treatment of diarrhea or relief of pain; neonatal opiate withdrawal
Effect on Mental Status Drowsiness and dizziness are common; may cause restlessness; may rarely cause insomnia or depression
Effect on Psychiatric Treatment Concurrent use with psychotropics may produce additive sedation
Restrictions C-III
Dosage Summary
Oral:
Neonates: 3-6 drops every 3-6 hours as needed **or** 0.2-0.7 mL every 3 hours; **Note:** Titration is recommended
Children: 0.25-0.5 mL/kg 1-4 times/day
Adults: 5-10 mL 1-4 times/day

Dosage Forms Excipient information presented when available (limited, particularly for generics); consult specific product labeling.
Liquid, oral: Morphine equivalent 2 mg/5 mL (473 mL) [equivalent to opium 20 mg powder; contains alcohol 45% and benzoic acid]

Paricalcitol (pah ri KAL si tole)

U.S. Brand Names Zemplar®
Canadian Brand Names Zemplar®
Mexican Brand Names Zemplar
Pharmacologic Category Vitamin D Analog
Use
I.V.: Prevention and treatment of secondary hyperparathyroidism associated with stage 5 chronic kidney disease (CKD)
Oral: Prevention and treatment of secondary hyperparathyroidism associated with stage 3 and 4 CKD
Effect on Mental Status May cause dizziness
Effect on Psychiatric Treatment None reported
Dosage Summary
I.V.:
Children <5 years: Dosage not established
Children ≥5 years: 0.04-0.24 mcg/kg (2.8-16.8 mcg) every other day during dialysis
Adults: 0.04-0.24 mcg/kg (2.8-16.8 mcg) every other day during dialysis
Oral:
Children: Dosage not established
Adults: 1-2 mcg/day **or** 2 mcg or 4 mcg 3 times/week
Dosage Forms Excipient information presented when available (limited, particularly for generics); consult specific product labeling.
Capsule, gelatin: 1 mcg, 2 mcg, 4 mcg [contains alcohol and coconut or palm kernel oil]
Injection, solution: 2 mcg/mL (1 mL); 5 mcg/mL (1 mL, 2 mL) [contains alcohol 20% v/v and propylene glycol 30% v/v]

◆ **Pariprazole** *see* Rabeprazole *on page 1389*
◆ **Parlodel®** *see* Bromocriptine *on page 202*
◆ **Parlodel® SnapTabs®** *see* Bromocriptine *on page 202*
◆ **Parnate®** *see* Tranylcypromine *on page 1609*

Paromomycin (par oh moe MYE sin)

U.S. Brand Names Humatin® [DSC]
Canadian Brand Names Humatin®
Index Terms Paromomycin Sulfate
Pharmacologic Category Amebicide
Use Treatment of acute and chronic intestinal amebiasis; hepatic coma
Unlabeled/Investigational Use Treatment of cryptosporidiosis
Effect on Mental Status May cause dizziness
Effect on Psychiatric Treatment None reported
Dosage Summary
Oral:
Children: 11 mg/kg every 15 minutes for 4 doses **or** 25-35 mg/kg/day in 3 divided doses **or** 45 mg/kg once daily
Adults: 25-35 mg/kg/day in 3 divided doses **or** 4 g/day in 2-4 divided doses **or** 45 mg/kg once daily
Dosage Forms Excipient information presented when available (limited, particularly for generics); consult specific product labeling. [DSC] = Discontinued product
Capsule: 250 mg
Humatin®: 250 mg [DSC]

◆ **Paromomycin Sulfate** *see* Paromomycin *on page 1226*

PARoxetine (pa ROKS e teen)

Medication Safety Issues
Sound-alike/look-alike issues:
PARoxetine may be confused with FLUoxetine, paclitaxel, pyridoxine
Paxil® may be confused with Doxil®, paclitaxel, Plavix®, Taxol®

Related Information

Antidepressant Agents *on page 1760*
Antidepressant Receptor Profile *on page 1764*
Discontinuation of Psychotropic Drugs *on page 1839*
Liquid Compatibility of Antidepressants, Antipsychotics, and Mood Stabilizers *on page 1788*
Selective Serotonin Reuptake Inhibitors (SSRIs) CYP Profile *on page 1793*
Selective Serotonin Reuptake Inhibitors (SSRIs) FDA-Approved Indication(s) *on page 1794*
Selective Serotonin Reuptake Inhibitors (SSRIs) Pharmacokinetics *on page 1795*
Selective Serotonin Reuptake Inhibitors (SSRIs) Receptor Profile *on page 1796*

U.S. Brand Names Paxil CR®; Paxil®; Pexeva®

Canadian Brand Names Apo-Paroxetine®; CO Paroxetine; Gen-Paroxetine; Novo-Paroxetine; Paxil CR®; Paxil®; PMS-Paroxetine; ratio-Paroxetine; Rhoxal-paroxetine; Sandoz-Paroxetine

Mexican Brand Names Aropax; Paxil

Index Terms Paroxetine Hydrochloride; Paroxetine Mesylate

Pharmacologic Category Antidepressant, Selective Serotonin Reuptake Inhibitor

Generic Available Yes

Use Treatment of major depressive disorder (MDD); treatment of panic disorder with or without agoraphobia; obsessive-compulsive disorder (OCD); social anxiety disorder (social phobia); generalized anxiety disorder (GAD); post-traumatic stress disorder (PTSD); premenstrual dysphoric disorder (PMDD)

Unlabeled/Investigational Use May be useful in eating disorders, impulse control disorders, self-injurious behavior; vasomotor symptoms of menopause; treatment of depression and obsessive-compulsive disorder (OCD) in children; treatment of mild dementia-associated agitation in nonpsychotic patients

Mental Health Comment The SSRIs as a class are generally considered to be safe and equally effective. For the management of depression, these drugs display a flat dose-response curve. Allow sufficient dose-response time (6-12 weeks). Differences lie in approved indications, receptor profiles, pharmacokinetics, and cytochrome P450 activity profile. Subtle differences exist in adverse effect profiles. All SSRIs have the potential to cause sexual dysfunction. Among the SSRIs, paroxetine is felt to be the most sedating and anticholinergic. Discontinuation syndromes may be more severe with paroxetine compared to other SSRIs. It also has been associated with more long-term weight gain (Marks, 2008).

Marks DM, Park MH, Ham BJ, et al, "Paroxetine: Safety and Tolerability Issues," *Expert Opin Drug Saf*, 2008, 7(6):783-94.

Restrictions An FDA-approved medication guide concerning the use of antidepressants in children, adolescents, and young adults must be distributed when dispensing an outpatient prescription (new or refill) where this medication is to be used without direct supervision of a healthcare provider. Medication guides are available at http://www.fda.gov/cder/Offices/ODS/medication_guides.htm. Dispense to parents or guardians of children and adolescents receiving this medication.

Pregnancy Risk Factor D

Pregnancy Considerations Due to adverse events observed in human studies, paroxetine is classified as pregnancy category D. Paroxetine crosses the placenta. The risk of cardiovascular and other congenital malformations may be higher with paroxetine than with other antidepressants. Nonteratogenic effects in the newborn following SSRI exposure late in the third trimester include respiratory distress, cyanosis, apnea, seizures, temperature instability, feeding difficulty, vomiting, hypoglycemia, hypo- or hypertonia, hyper-reflexia, jitteriness, irritability, constant crying, and tremor. An increased risk of low birth weight, lower APGAR scores, and blunted behavioral response to pain for a prolonged period after delivery has also been reported. Exposure to SSRIs after the twentieth week of gestation has been associated with persistent pulmonary hypertension of the newborn (PPHN). Adverse effects may be due to toxic effects of the SSRI or drug withdrawal due to discontinuation. The long-term effects of *in utero* SSRI exposure on infant development and behavior are not known.

Due to pregnancy-induced physiologic changes, women who are pregnant may require increased doses of paroxetine to achieve euthymia. Women treated for major depression and who are euthymic prior to pregnancy are more likely to experience a relapse when medication is discontinued as compared to pregnant women who continue taking antidepressant medications. The ACOG recommends that therapy with SSRIs or SNRIs during pregnancy be individualized; treatment of depression during pregnancy should incorporate the clinical expertise of the mental health clinician, obstetrician, primary healthcare provider, and pediatrician (ACOG, 2007). The ACOG also recommend that therapy with paroxetine be avoided during pregnancy if possible and that fetuses exposed in early pregnancy be assessed with a fetal echocardiography. If treatment during pregnancy is required, consider tapering therapy during the third trimester in order to prevent withdrawal symptoms in the infant. If this is done and the woman is considered to be at risk from her major depressive disorder, the medication can be restarted following delivery, although the dose should be readjusted to that required before pregnancy.

Lactation Enters breast milk/use caution (AAP rates "of concern")

Contraindications Hypersensitivity to paroxetine or any component of the formulation; use with or within 14 days of MAO inhibitors; concurrent use with thioridazine or pimozide

Warnings/Precautions **[U.S. Boxed Warning]: Antidepressants increase the risk of suicidal thinking and behavior in children, adolescents, and young adults (18-24 years of age) with major depressive disorder (MDD) and other psychiatric disorders;** consider risk prior to prescribing. Short-term studies did not show an increased risk in patients >24 years of age and showed a decreased risk in patients ≥65 years. Closely monitor patients for clinical worsening, suicidality, or unusual changes in behavior, particularly during the initial 1-2 months of therapy or during periods of dosage adjustments (increases or decreases); the patient's family or caregiver should be instructed to closely observe the patient and communicate condition with healthcare provider. A medication guide concerning the use of antidepressants should be dispensed with each prescription. **Paroxetine is not FDA approved for use in children.**

The possibility of a suicide attempt is inherent in major depression and may persist until remission occurs. Patients treated with antidepressants (for any indication) should be observed for clinical worsening and suicidality, especially during the initial few months of a course of drug therapy, or at times of dose changes, either increases or decreases. Use caution in high-risk patients. Worsening depression and severe abrupt suicidality that are not part of the presenting symptoms may require discontinuation or modification of drug therapy. The patient's family or caregiver should be alerted to monitor patients for the emergence of suicidality and associated behaviors (such as agitation, irritability, hostility, impulsivity, and hypomania) and call healthcare provider.

May worsen psychosis in some patients or precipitate a shift to mania or hypomania in patients with bipolar disorder. Patients presenting with depressive symptoms should be screened for bipolar disorder. Monotherapy in patients with bipolar disorder should be avoided. **Paroxetine is not FDA approved for the treatment of bipolar depression.**

Potential for severe reaction when used with MAO inhibitors, SSRIs/SNRIs or triptans; serotonin syndrome (hyperthermia, muscular rigidity, mental status changes/agitation, autonomic instability) may occur; concurrent use with MAO inhibitors contraindicated. May increase the risks associated with electroconvulsive therapy. Has a low potential to impair cognitive or motor performance - caution operating hazardous machinery or driving. Symptoms of agitation and/or restlessness may occur during initial few weeks of therapy. Low potential for sedation or anticholinergic effects relative to cyclic antidepressants.

Use caution in patients with a previous seizure disorder or condition predisposing to seizures such as brain damage, alcoholism, or concurrent therapy with other drugs which lower the seizure threshold. Use with caution in patients with hepatic dysfunction and in elderly patients. May cause hyponatremia/SIADH (elderly at increased risk); volume depletion (diuretics may increase risk). Use caution with concomitant use of NSAIDs, ASA, or other drugs that affect coagulation; the risk of bleeding may be potentiated. Use with caution in patients with renal insufficiency or other concurrent illness (due to limited experience); dose reduction recommended with severe renal impairment. May cause or exacerbate sexual dysfunction. Use caution in patients with narrow-angle glaucoma. Avoid use in the first trimester of pregnancy.

Upon discontinuation of paroxetine therapy, gradually taper dose and monitor for discontinuation symptoms (eg, dizziness, dysphoric mood, irritability, agitation, confusion, paresthesias). If intolerable symptoms occur following a decrease in dosage or upon discontinuation of therapy, then resuming the previous dose with a more gradual taper should be considered. Safety and efficacy in children have not been established.

Adverse Reactions Frequency varies by dose and indication. Adverse reactions reported as a composite of all indications.

>10%:

Central nervous system: Somnolence (15% to 24%), insomnia (11% to 24%), headache (17% to 18%), dizziness (6% to 14%)

Endocrine & metabolic: Libido decreased (3% to 15%)

Gastrointestinal: Nausea (19% to 26%), xerostomia (9% to 18%), constipation (5% to 16%), diarrhea (9% to 12%)

Genitourinary: Ejaculatory disturbances (10% to 28%)

Neuromuscular & skeletal: Weakness (12% to 22%), tremor (4% to 11%)

Miscellaneous: Diaphoresis (5% to 14%)

1% to 10%:

Cardiovascular: Vasodilation (2% to 4%), chest pain (3%), palpitation (2% to 3%), hypertension (≥1%), tachycardia (≥1%)

Central nervous system: Nervousness (4% to 9%), anxiety (5%), agitation (3% to 5%), abnormal dreams (3% to 4%), concentration impaired (3% to 4%), yawning (2% to 4%), depersonalization (up to 3%), amnesia (2%), emotional lability (≥1%), vertigo (≥1%), confusion (1%), chills (2%)

Dermatologic: Rash (2% to 3%), pruritus (≥1%)

Endocrine & metabolic: Orgasmic disturbance (2% to 9%), dysmenorrhea (5%)

Gastrointestinal: Anorexia, appetite decreased (5% to 9%), dyspepsia (2% to 5%), flatulence (4%), abdominal pain (4%), appetite increased (2% to 4%), vomiting (2% to 3%), taste perversion (2%), weight gain (≥1%)

Genitourinary: Impotence (2% to 9%), genital disorder (female 2% to 9%), urinary frequency (2% to 3%), urinary tract infection (2%)

Neuromuscular & skeletal: Paresthesia (4%), myalgia (2% to 4%), back pain (3%), myoclonus (2% to 3%), myopathy (2%), myasthenia (1%), arthralgia (≥1%)

Ocular: Blurred vision (4%), abnormal vision (2% to 4%)

Otic: Tinnitus (≥1%)

Respiratory: Respiratory disorder (up to 7%), pharyngitis (4%), sinusitis (up to 4%), rhinitis (3%)

Miscellaneous: Infection (5% to 6%)

<1%, postmarketing, and/or case reports (limited to important or life-threatening): Acute renal failure, adrenergic syndrome, akinesia, alkaline phosphatase increased, allergic reaction, anaphylaxis, anemias (various), angina pectoris, angioedema, aphasia, aphthous stomatitis, arrhythmias (atrial and ventricular), arthrosis, asthma, behavioral disturbances (various), bilirubinemia, bleeding time increased, blood dyscrasias, bloody diarrhea, bradycardia, bronchitis, bulimia, BUN increased, bundle branch block, cardiospasm, cataract, cellulitis, cerebral ischemia, cerebrovascular accident, cholelithiasis, colitis, congestive heart failure, creatinine phosphokinase increased, deafness, dehydration, delirium, diabetes mellitus, drug dependence, dyskinesia, dysphagia, dyspnea, dystonia, ecchymosis, eclampsia, electrolyte abnormalities, emphysema, erythema, exfoliative dermatitis, extrapyramidal syndrome, fecal impactions, fungal dermatitis, gamma globulins increased, gastroenteritis, glaucoma, goiter, Guillain-Barré syndrome, hallucinations, hematemesis, hematoma, hemorrhage, hemoptysis, hepatic necrosis, hepatitis, hypercholesteremia, hyper-/hypoglycemia, hyper-/hypothyroidism, hypotension, ileus, intestinal obstruction, jaundice, ketosis, lactic dehydrogenase increased, liver function tests abnormal, low cardiac output, lung fibrosis, lymphadenopathy, meningitis, MI, migraine, myelitis, myocardial ischemia, neuroleptic malignant syndrome, neuropathy, osteoporosis, pancreatitis, pancytopenia, peptic ulcer, peritonitis, phlebitis, pneumonia, platelet count abnormalities, pulmonary edema, pulmonary embolus, pulmonary hypertension, seizure, sepsis, serotonin syndrome, status epilepticus, suicidal tendencies, syncope, tetany, thrombophlebitis, thrombosis, tongue edema, torsade de pointes, toxic epidermal necrolysis, vasculitic syndrome

Metabolism/Transport Effects **Substrate** of CYP2D6 (major); **Inhibits** CYP1A2 (weak), 2B6 (moderate), 2C9 (weak), 2C19 (weak), 2D6 (strong), 3A4 (weak)

Drug Interactions

Alcohol (Ethyl): CNS Depressants may enhance the CNS depressant effect of Alcohol (Ethyl). *Risk C: Monitor therapy*

Alpha-/Beta-Blockers: Selective Serotonin Reuptake Inhibitors may decrease the metabolism of Alpha-/Beta-Blockers. *Risk C: Monitor therapy*

Amprenavir: May decrease the serum concentration of PARoxetine. *Risk C: Monitor therapy*

Analgesics (Opioid): May enhance the serotonergic effect of Selective Serotonin Reuptake Inhibitors. This may cause serotonin syndrome. *Risk C: Monitor therapy*

Anticoagulants: Antiplatelet Agents may enhance the anticoagulant effect of Anticoagulants. *Risk C: Monitor therapy*

Antidepressants (Serotonin Reuptake Inhibitor/Antagonist): Selective Serotonin Reuptake Inhibitors may enhance the serotonergic effect of Antidepressants (Serotonin Reuptake Inhibitor/Antagonist). This may cause serotonin syndrome. *Risk C: Monitor therapy*

Antiplatelet Agents: May enhance the anticoagulant effect of other Antiplatelet Agents. *Risk C: Monitor therapy*

Aspirin: Selective Serotonin Reuptake Inhibitors may enhance the antiplatelet effect of Aspirin. *Risk C: Monitor therapy*

Atomoxetine: PARoxetine may decrease the metabolism of Atomoxetine. *Risk D: Consider therapy modification*

Beta-Blockers: Selective Serotonin Reuptake Inhibitors may enhance the bradycardic effect of Beta-Blockers. **Exceptions:** Acebutolol; Atenolol; Carteolol; Esmolol; Levobunolol; Metipranolol; Nadolol; Penbutolol. *Risk C: Monitor therapy*

BusPIRone: May enhance the serotonergic effect of Selective Serotonin Reuptake Inhibitors. This may cause serotonin syndrome. Selective Serotonin Reuptake Inhibitors may decrease the metabolism of BusPIRone. *Risk C: Monitor therapy*

CarBAMazepine: Selective Serotonin Reuptake Inhibitors may decrease the metabolism of CarBAMazepine. Specifically those SSRIs that inhibit CYP3A4 isoenzymes. CarBAMazepine may increase the metabolism of Selective Serotonin Reuptake Inhibitors. Specifically those agents metabolized via CYP1A2, 2C, and/or 3A4 isoenzymes. *Risk D: Consider therapy modification*

Cimetidine: May decrease the metabolism of Selective Serotonin Reuptake Inhibitors. *Risk D: Consider therapy modification*

Clozapine: Selective Serotonin Reuptake Inhibitors may decrease the metabolism of Clozapine. *Risk D: Consider therapy modification*

CNS Depressants: May enhance the adverse/toxic effect of other CNS Depressants. *Risk C: Monitor therapy*

CYP2B6 Substrates: CYP2B6 Inhibitors (Moderate) may decrease the metabolism of CYP2B6 Substrates. *Risk C: Monitor therapy*

CYP2D6 Inhibitors (Moderate): May decrease the metabolism of CYP2D6 Substrates. *Risk C: Monitor therapy*

CYP2D6 Inhibitors (Strong): May decrease the metabolism of CYP2D6 Substrates. *Risk D: Consider therapy modification*

CYP2D6 Substrates: CYP2D6 Inhibitors (Strong) may decrease the metabolism of CYP2D6 Substrates. **Exceptions:** Tamoxifen. *Risk D: Consider therapy modification*

Cyproheptadine: May diminish the therapeutic effect of Selective Serotonin Reuptake Inhibitors. *Risk C: Monitor therapy*

Darunavir: May decrease the serum concentration of PARoxetine. *Risk C: Monitor therapy*

Dasatinib: May enhance the anticoagulant effect of Antiplatelet Agents. *Risk C: Monitor therapy*

Desmopressin: Selective Serotonin Reuptake Inhibitors may enhance the adverse/toxic effect of Desmopressin. *Risk C: Monitor therapy*

Dextromethorphan: Selective Serotonin Reuptake Inhibitors may enhance the adverse/toxic effect of Dextromethorphan. *Risk D: Consider therapy modification*

Drotrecogin Alfa: Antiplatelet Agents may enhance the adverse/toxic effect of Drotrecogin Alfa. Bleeding may occur. *Risk D: Consider therapy modification*

DULoxetine: PARoxetine may decrease the metabolism of DULoxetine. *Risk C: Monitor therapy*

Fosamprenavir: May decrease the serum concentration of PARoxetine. The active metabolite amprenavir is likely responsible for this effect. *Risk C: Monitor therapy*

Galantamine: Selective Serotonin Reuptake Inhibitors may decrease the metabolism of Galantamine. *Risk C: Monitor therapy*

Haloperidol: Selective Serotonin Reuptake Inhibitors may decrease the metabolism of Haloperidol. *Risk C: Monitor therapy*

Herbs (Anticoagulant/Antiplatelet Properties) (eg, Alfalfa, Anise, Bilberry): May enhance the adverse/toxic effect of Antiplatelet Agents. Bleeding may occur. *Risk D: Consider therapy modification*

Ibritumomab: Antiplatelet Agents may enhance the adverse/toxic effect of Ibritumomab. Both agents may contribute to impaired platelet function and an increased risk of bleeding. *Risk C: Monitor therapy*

Lithium: Selective Serotonin Reuptake Inhibitors may enhance the adverse/toxic effect of Lithium. *Risk C: Monitor therapy*

MAO Inhibitors: May enhance the serotonergic effect of Selective Serotonin Reuptake Inhibitors. This may cause serotonin syndrome. *Risk X: Avoid combination*

Methadone: Selective Serotonin Reuptake Inhibitors may decrease the metabolism of Methadone. Fluvoxamine appears to be the only interacting SSRI. *Risk D: Consider therapy modification*

Mexiletine: Selective Serotonin Reuptake Inhibitors may decrease the metabolism of Mexiletine. *Risk D: Consider therapy modification*

NSAID (COX-2 Inhibitor): Selective Serotonin Reuptake Inhibitors may enhance the antiplatelet effect of NSAID (COX-2 Inhibitor). *Risk D: Consider therapy modification*

NSAID (Nonselective): Selective Serotonin Reuptake Inhibitors may enhance the antiplatelet effect of NSAID (Nonselective). *Risk D: Consider therapy modification*

Omega-3-Acid Ethyl Esters: May enhance the antiplatelet effect of Antiplatelet Agents. *Risk C: Monitor therapy*

Pentosan Polysulfate Sodium: May enhance the adverse/toxic effect of Antiplatelet Agents. Specifically, the risk of bleeding may be increased by concurrent use of these agents. *Risk C: Monitor therapy*

Pimozide: Selective Serotonin Reuptake Inhibitors may enhance the adverse/toxic effect of Pimozide. *Risk X: Avoid combination*

Propafenone: Selective Serotonin Reuptake Inhibitors may decrease the metabolism of Propafenone. *Risk D: Consider therapy modification*

Prostacyclin Analogues: May enhance the antiplatelet effect of Antiplatelet Agents. *Risk C: Monitor therapy*

Risperidone: Selective Serotonin Reuptake Inhibitors may decrease the metabolism of Risperidone. *Risk C: Monitor therapy*

Salicylates: Antiplatelet Agents may enhance the adverse/toxic effect of Salicylates. Increased risk of bleeding may result. *Risk C: Monitor therapy*

Serotonin Modulators: May enhance the adverse/toxic effect of other Serotonin Modulators. The development of serotonin syndrome may occur. *Risk D: Consider therapy modification*

Sibutramine: May enhance the serotonergic effect of Serotonin Modulators. This may cause serotonin syndrome. *Risk X: Avoid combination*

Tamoxifen: CYP2D6 Inhibitors (Strong) may decrease the metabolism of Tamoxifen. Specifically, strong CYP2D6 inhibitors may decrease the formation of highly potent active metabolites. *Risk X: Avoid combination*

Tetrabenazine: CYP2D6 Inhibitors (Strong) may increase the serum concentration of Tetrabenazine. Specifically, concentrations of the active alpha- and beta-dihydrotetrabenazine metabolites may be increased. Management: Tetrabenazine dose should be reduced by 50% when starting a strong CYP2D6 inhibitor. Maximum tetrabenazine dose is 50mg/day when used with a strong CYP2D6 inhibitor. *Risk D: Consider therapy modification*

Thioridazine: CYP2D6 Inhibitors may decrease the metabolism of Thioridazine. *Risk X: Avoid combination*

Thrombolytic Agents: Antiplatelet Agents may enhance the anticoagulant effect of Thrombolytic Agents. *Risk C: Monitor therapy*

Tositumomab and Iodine I 131 Tositumomab: Antiplatelet Agents may enhance the adverse/toxic effect of Tositumomab and Iodine I 131 Tositumomab. Specifically, the risk of bleeding-related adverse events may be increased. *Risk C: Monitor therapy*

TraMADol: Selective Serotonin Reuptake Inhibitors may enhance the neuroexcitatory and/or seizure-potentiating effect of TraMADol. TraMADol may enhance the serotonergic effect of Selective Serotonin Reuptake Inhibitors. This may cause serotonin syndrome. *Risk D: Consider therapy modification*

Tricyclic Antidepressants: Selective Serotonin Reuptake Inhibitors may decrease the metabolism of Tricyclic Antidepressants. *Risk D: Consider therapy modification*

Tryptophan: May enhance the serotonergic effect of Selective Serotonin Reuptake Inhibitors. This may cause serotonin syndrome. *Risk D: Consider therapy modification*

Vitamin K Antagonists (eg, warfarin): Selective Serotonin Reuptake Inhibitors may enhance the anticoagulant effect of Vitamin K Antagonists. *Risk C: Monitor therapy*

Ethanol/Nutrition/Herb Interactions

Ethanol: Avoid ethanol (may increase CNS depression).

Food: Peak concentration is increased, but bioavailability is not significantly altered by food.

Herb/Nutraceutical: Avoid valerian, St John's wort, SAMe, kava kava.

Stability

Suspension: Store at ≤25°C (≤77°F).

Tablet: Store at 15°C to 30°C (59°F to 86°F).

Mechanism of Action Paroxetine is a selective serotonin reuptake inhibitor, chemically unrelated to tricyclic, tetracyclic, or other antidepressants;

presumably, the inhibition of serotonin reuptake from brain synapse stimulated serotonin activity in the brain

Pharmacodynamics/Kinetics

Onset of action: Depression: The onset of action is within a week; however, individual response varies greatly and full response may not be seen until 8-12 weeks after initiation of treatment.

Absorption: Completely absorbed following oral administration

Distribution: V_d: 8.7 L/kg (3-28 L/kg)

Protein binding: 93% to 95%

Metabolism: Extensively hepatic via CYP2D6 enzymes; primary metabolites are formed via oxidation and methylation of parent drug, with subsequent glucuronide/sulfate conjugation; nonlinear pharmacokinetics (via 2D6 saturation) may be seen with higher doses and longer duration of therapy. Metabolites exhibit ~2% potency of parent compound. C_{min} concentrations are 70% to 80% greater in the elderly compared to nonelderly patients; clearance is also decreased.

Half-life elimination: 21 hours (3-65 hours)

Time to peak: Immediate release: 5.2 hours; controlled release: 6-10 hours

Excretion: Urine (64%, 2% as unchanged drug); feces (36% primarily via bile, <1% as unchanged drug)

Dosage Oral:

Children:

Depression (unlabeled use; not recommended by FDA): Initial: 10 mg/day and adjusted upward on an individual basis to 20 mg/day

Obsessive-compulsive disorder (unlabeled use): Initial: 10 mg/day and titrate up as necessary to 60 mg/day

Self-injurious behavior (unlabeled use): 20 mg/day

Social anxiety disorder (unlabeled use): 2.5-15 mg/day

Adults:

Major depressive disorder:

Paxil®, Pexeva®: Initial: 20 mg once daily, preferably in the morning; increase if needed by 10 mg/day increments at intervals of at least 1 week; maximum dose: 50 mg/day

Paxil CR®: Initial: 25 mg once daily; increase if needed by 12.5 mg/day increments at intervals of at least 1 week; maximum dose: 62.5 mg/day

Generalized anxiety disorder (Paxil®, Pexeva®): Initial: 20 mg once daily, preferably in the morning (if dose is increased, adjust in increments of 10 mg/day at 1-week intervals); doses of 20-50 mg/day were used in clinical trials, however, no greater benefit was seen with doses >20 mg.

Obsessive-compulsive disorder (Paxil®, Pexeva™): Initial: 20 mg once daily, preferably in the morning; increase if needed by 10 mg/day increments at intervals of at least 1 week; recommended dose: 40 mg/day; range: 20-60 mg/day; maximum dose: 60 mg/day

Panic disorder:

Paxil®, Pexeva®: Initial: 10 mg once daily, preferably in the morning; increase if needed by 10 mg/day increments at intervals of at least 1 week; recommended dose: 40 mg/day; range: 10-60 mg/day; maximum dose: 60 mg/day

Paxil CR®: Initial: 12.5 mg once daily; increase if needed by 12.5 mg/day at intervals of at least 1 week; maximum dose: 75 mg/day

Premenstrual dysphoric disorder (Paxil CR®): Initial: 12.5 mg once daily in the morning; may be increased to 25 mg/day; dosing changes should occur at intervals of at least 1 week. May be given daily throughout the menstrual cycle or limited to the luteal phase.

Post-traumatic stress disorder (Paxil®): Initial: 20 mg once daily, preferably in the morning; increase if needed by 10 mg/day increments at intervals of at least 1 week; range: 20-50 mg. Limited data suggest doses of 40 mg/day were not more efficacious than 20 mg/day.

Social anxiety disorder:

Paxil®: Initial: 20 mg once daily, preferably in the morning; recommended dose: 20 mg/day; range: 20-60 mg/day; doses >20 mg may not have additional benefit

Paxil CR®: Initial: 12.5 mg once daily, preferably in the morning; may be increased by 12.5 mg/day at intervals of at least 1 week; maximum dose: 37.5 mg/day

Vasomotor symptoms of menopause (unlabeled use, Paxil CR®): 12.5-25 mg/day

Elderly:

Paxil®, Pexeva®: Initial: 10 mg/day; increase if needed by 10 mg/day increments at intervals of at least 1 week; maximum dose: 40 mg/day

Paxil CR®; Initial: 12.5 mg/day; increase if needed by 12.5 mg/day increments at intervals of at least 1 week; maximum dose: 50 mg/day

Note: Upon discontinuation of paroxetine therapy, gradually taper dose:

Paxil®, Pexeva®: 10 mg/day at weekly intervals; when 20 mg/day dose is reached, continue for 1 week before treatment is discontinued. Some patients may need to be titrated to 10 mg/day for 1 week before discontinuation.

Paxil CR®: Patients receiving 37.5 mg/day in clinical trials had their dose decreased by 12.5 mg/day to a dose of 25 mg/day and remained at a dose of 25 mg/day for 1 week before treatment was discontinued.

Dosage adjustment in renal impairment: Adults:

Cl_{cr} <30 mL/minute: Mean plasma concentration is ~4 times that seen in normal function.

Cl_{cr} 30-60 mL/minute: Plasma concentration is 2 times that seen in normal function.

Paxil®, Pexeva®: Initial: 10 mg/day; increase if needed by 10 mg/day increments at intervals of at least 1 week; maximum dose: 40 mg/day

Paxil CR®: Initial: 12.5 mg/day; increase if needed by 12.5 mg/day increments at intervals of at least 1 week; maximum dose: 50 mg/day

Dosage adjustment in severe hepatic impairment: Adults: In hepatic dysfunction, plasma concentration is 2 times that seen in normal function.

Paxil®, Pexeva®: Initial: 10 mg/day; increase if needed by 10 mg/day increments at intervals of at least 1 week; maximum dose: 40 mg/day

Paxil CR®: Initial: 12.5 mg/day; increase if needed by 12.5 mg/day increments at intervals of at least 1 week; maximum dose: 50 mg/day

Child/Adolescent Considerations

Depression: Paroxetine was shown to be effective and generally well tolerated in a recent randomized, double-blind, placebo-controlled parallel-design study; 275 adolescents (12-18 years of age) with major depression were randomized to receive paroxetine, imipramine, or placebo; 93 patients (mean age: 14.8 ± 1.6 years) received paroxetine at initial doses of 20 mg/day given in the morning; doses were increased if needed at week 5 to 30 mg/day (given in divided doses) and at weeks 6-8 to 40 mg/day (given in divided doses); 48% of patients remained at the initial starting dose of 20 mg/day; mean optimal daily dose: 28 ± 8.54 mg (Keller, 2001). Paroxetine was shown to be effective and well tolerated in an open label clinical trial in 45 children <14 years of age (mean: 10.7 ± 2 years) with major depression (Rey-Sanchoz, 1997). Doses were initiated at 10 mg/day and adjusted upward on an individual basis with a mean dose of 16.2 mg/day used for an average of 8.4 months. Further studies are needed.

Obsessive-compulsive disorder (OCD): Twenty OCD outpatients 8-17 years of age were treated with daily doses ranging from 10-60 mg/day for 12 weeks (Rosenberg, 1999). A randomized, double-blind, placebo-controlled trial with paroxetine was conducted in 207 pediatric patients (aged 7-17 years) meeting DSM-IV criteria for OCD (Geller et al, 2004). Patients received 10-50 mg/day paroxetine or placebo for 10 weeks and change from baseline of the Children's Yale-Brown Obsessive-Compulsive Scale was assessed as the primary endpoint. In the intent-to-treat population, paroxetine was associated with a significant adjusted mean difference improvement (-3.45; 95% CI: -5.6 to -1.29, p =0.002) compared to placebo. Side effects were generally mild to moderate, with 10% and 3% of paroxetine- and placebo-receiving patients, respectively, discontinuing due to adverse events.

Self-injurious behavior: A 15-year old autistic male with self-injurious behavior was successfully treated with 20 mg/day (Snead, 1994). Further studies are needed.

Social anxiety disorder: A small case series reported the effective use of paroxetine in 5 pediatric patients with social phobia [2 children (7 and 11 years of age) and 3 adolescents (16, 17, and 18 years of age)]; comorbid diagnoses (obsessive compulsive disorder and/or dysthymia) existed in 3 patients; doses were adjusted on an individual basis; the 7-year old was started on 2.5 mg/day and increased to 5 mg/day after 4 weeks; the 11-year old was started on 5 mg/day and the dose was titrated upwards by 5 mg/day increments every 3-4 weeks to 15 mg/day; adolescents were started on 20 mg/day (Mancini, 1999); further studies are needed. In a 16-week trial of pediatric patients (aged 8-17 years) presenting with social anxiety disorder, 163 were randomized to receive paroxetine (10-50 mg/day) and 156 to receive placebo (Wagner et al, 2004). From the intent-to-treat analysis, 77.6% of paroxetine patients responded (achievement of Clinical Global Impression-Improvement score of 1 or 2) compared to 38.3% of placebo patients (odds ratio: 7.02, p <0.001). Adverse events occurred in 5% of paroxetine-receiving patients (twice the placebo rate) and consisted mainly of insomnia, decreased appetite and vomiting.

A recent report described the SSRI discontinuation syndrome in 6 children; the syndrome was similar to that reported in adults (Diler, 2002).

Diler RS and Avci A, "Selective Serotonin Reuptake Inhibitor Discontinuation Syndrome in Children: Six Case Reports," *Current Therapeutic Research*, 2002, 63(3):188-97.

Geller DA, Wagner KD, Emslie G, et al, "Paroxetine Treatment in Children and Adolescents with Obsessive-Compulsive Disorder: A Randomized, multi-center, Double-Blind, Placebo-Controlled Trial," *J Am Acad Child Adolesc Psychiatry*, 2004, 43(11):1387-96.

Keller MB, Ryan ND, Strober M, et al, "Efficacy of Paroxetine in the Treatment of Adolescent Major Depression: A Randomized, Controlled Trial," *J Am Acad Child Adolesc Psychiatry*, 2001, 40(7):762-72.

Mancini C, Van Ameringen M, Oakman JM, et al, "Serotonergic Agents in the Treatment of Social Phobia in Children and Adolescents: A Case Series," *Depress Anxiety*, 1999, 10(1):33-9.

Rey-Sanchez F and Guitierrez-Cassares JR, "Paroxetine in Children With Major Depressive Disorder: An Open Trial," *J Am Acad Child Adolesc Psychiatry*, 1997, 36(10):1443-7.

Rosenberg DR, Stewart CM, Fitzgerald KD, et al, "Paroxetine Open-Label Treatment of Pediatric Outpatients With Obsessive-Compulsive Disorder," *J Am Acad Child Adolesc Psychiatry*, 1999, 38(9):1180-5.

Snead RW, Boon F, and Presberg J, "Paroxetine for Self-Injurious Behavior," *J Am Acad Child Adolesc Psychiatry*, 1994, 33(6):909-10.

Wagner KD, Berard R, Stein MB, et al, "A Multicenter, Randomized, Double-Blind, Placebo-Controlled Trial of Paroxetine in Children and Adolescents With Social Anxiety Disorder," *Arch Gen Psychiatry*, 2004, 61(11):1153-62.

Dietary Considerations May be taken with or without food.

Administration May be administered with or without food. Do not crush, break, or chew controlled release tablets.

Monitoring Parameters Mental status for depression, suicidal ideation (especially at the beginning of therapy or when doses are increased or decreased), anxiety, social functioning, mania, panic attacks; akathisia

Additional Information Paxil CR® incorporates a degradable polymeric matrix (Geomatrix™) to control dissolution rate over a period of 4-5 hours. An enteric coating delays the start of drug release until tablets have left the stomach.

Dosage Forms Excipient information presented when available (limited, particularly for generics); consult specific product labeling.

Note: Strength expressed as base:

Suspension, oral, as hydrochloride: 10 mg/5 mL (250 mL)
 Paxil®: 10 mg/5 mL (250 mL) [orange flavor]

Tablet, as hydrochloride: 10 mg, 20 mg, 30 mg, 40 mg
 Paxil®: 10 mg, 20 mg, 30 mg, 40 mg

Tablet, as mesylate:
 Pexeva®: 10 mg, 20 mg, 30 mg, 40 mg

Tablet, controlled release, as hydrochloride: 37.5 mg
 Paxil CR®: 12.5 mg, 25 mg, 37.5 mg

Tablet, extended release, as hydrochloride: 12.5 mg, 25 mg

◆ **Paroxetine Hydrochloride** *see* PARoxetine *on page 1226*

◆ **Paroxetine Mesylate** *see* PARoxetine *on page 1226*

◆ **PAS** *see* Aminosalicylic Acid *on page 88*

◆ **Paser®** *see* Aminosalicylic Acid *on page 88*

◆ **Pavabid [DSC]** *see* Papaverine *on page 1225*

◆ **Paxil®** *see* PARoxetine *on page 1226*

◆ **Paxil CR®** *see* PARoxetine *on page 1226*

◆ **PCA (error-prone abbreviation)** *see* Procainamide *on page 1339*

◆ **PCE®** *see* Erythromycin *on page 557*

◆ **P Chlor GG** *see* Chlorpheniramine, Phenylephrine, and Guaifenesin *on page 329*

◆ **PCM** *see* Chlorpheniramine, Phenylephrine, and Methscopolamine *on page 329*

◆ **PCM Allergy [DSC]** *see* Chlorpheniramine, Phenylephrine, and Methscopolamine *on page 329*

◆ **PCV7** *see* Pneumococcal Conjugate Vaccine, 7-Valent *on page 1308*

◆ **PD-Cof** *see* Chlorpheniramine, Phenylephrine, and Dextromethorphan *on page 327*

◆ **PD-Hist-D** *see* Chlorpheniramine and Phenylephrine *on page 323*

- **PediaCare® Infants' Decongestant & Cough [OTC] [DSC]** *see* Pseudoephedrine and Dextromethorphan *on page 1369*
- **PediaCare® Infants' Long-Acting Cough [OTC] [DSC]** *see* Dextromethorphan *on page 448*
- **Pediacof® [DSC]** *see* Chlorpheniramine, Phenylephrine, Codeine, and Potassium Iodide *on page 332*
- **PediaHist DM** *see* Brompheniramine, Pseudoephedrine, and Dextromethorphan *on page 208*
- **Pediapred®** *see* PrednisoLONE *on page 1326*
- **Pedia Relief™ [OTC]** *see* Chlorpheniramine, Pseudoephedrine, and Dextromethorphan *on page 333*
- **Pedia Relief Cough and Cold [OTC]** *see* Pseudoephedrine and Dextromethorphan *on page 1369*
- **Pedia Relief Infants [OTC]** *see* Pseudoephedrine and Dextromethorphan *on page 1369*
- **Pediarix®** *see* Diphtheria, Tetanus Toxoids, Acellular Pertussis, Hepatitis B (Recombinant), and Poliovirus (Inactivated) Vaccine *on page 487*
- **PediaTan™** *see* Chlorpheniramine *on page 321*
- **PediaTan™ D** *see* Chlorpheniramine and Phenylephrine *on page 323*
- **Pediatex™-D [DSC]** *see* Carbinoxamine and Pseudoephedrine *on page 280*
- **PedvaxHIB®** *see* *Haemophilus* b Conjugate Vaccine *on page 753*
- **PEG-L-asparaginase** *see* Pegaspargase *on page 1235*
- **Peganone®** *see* Ethotoin *on page 604*

Pegaptanib (peg AP ta nib)

U.S. Brand Names Macugen®
Canadian Brand Names Macugen®
Index Terms EYE001; Pegaptanib Sodium
Pharmacologic Category Ophthalmic Agent; Vascular Endothelial Growth Factor (VEGF) Inhibitor
Use Treatment of neovascular (wet) age-related macular degeneration (AMD)
Effect on Mental Status May cause dizziness
Effect on Psychiatric Treatment Blurred vision and GI side effects are common. Concomitant use with psychotropics with high anticholinergic load may produce additive effects; monitor. Concomitant use with SSRIs, lithium, or valproic acid may produce additive effects; monitor.
Dosage Summary
Intravitreous:
Children: Dosage not established
Adults: 0.3 mg into affected eye every 6 weeks
Dosage Forms Excipient information presented when available (limited, particularly for generics); consult specific product labeling.
Injection, solution [preservative free]: 0.3 mg/90 µL (90 µL) [prefilled syringe]

- **Pegaptanib Sodium** *see* Pegaptanib *on page 1235*

Pegaspargase (peg AS par jase)

Medication Safety Issues
Sound-alike/look-alike issues:
Pegaspargase may be confused with asparaginase

High alert medication: The Institute for Safe Medication Practices (ISMP) includes this medication among its list of drugs which have a heightened risk of causing significant patient harm when used in error.
U.S. Brand Names Oncaspar®
Index Terms NSC-644954; PEG-L-asparaginase
Pharmacologic Category Antineoplastic Agent, Miscellaneous
Use Treatment of acute lymphocytic leukemia (ALL); treatment of ALL with previous hypersensitivity to native L-asparaginase
Effect on Mental Status Drowsiness is common
Effect on Psychiatric Treatment May cause pancytopenia; use caution with clozapine and carbamazepine
Dosage Summary
I.M.:
Children with BSA <0.6 m^2: 82.5 int. units/kg every 14 days

Children with BSA ≥0.6 m^2: 2500 int. units/m^2 every 14 days
Adults: 2500 int. units/m^2 every 14 days

I.V.:
Children with BSA <0.6 m^2: 82.5 int. units/kg every 14 days
Children with BSA ≥0.6 m^2: 2500 int. units/m^2 every 14 days
Adults: 2500 int. units/m^2 every 14 days

Dosage Forms Excipient information presented when available (limited, particularly for generics); consult specific product labeling.
Injection, solution [preservative free]:
Oncaspar®: 750 units/mL (5 mL)

◆ **Pegasys®** *see* Peginterferon Alfa-2a *on page 1236*

Pegfilgrastim (peg fil GRA stim)

Medication Safety Issues
Sound-alike/look-alike issues:
Neulasta® may be confused with Neumega® and Lunesta™

U.S. Brand Names Neulasta®

Canadian Brand Names Neulasta®

Index Terms G-CSF (PEG Conjugate); Granulocyte Colony Stimulating Factor (PEG Conjugate); NSC-725961; SD/01

Pharmacologic Category Colony Stimulating Factor

Use To decrease the incidence of infection, by stimulation of granulocyte production, in patients with nonmyeloid malignancies receiving myelosuppressive therapy associated with a significant risk of febrile neutropenia

Effect on Mental Status None reported

Effect on Psychiatric Treatment Lithium may potentiate release of neutrophils from bone marrow

Dosage Summary

SubQ:
Children: Dosage not established
Adolescents >45 kg: 6 mg once per chemotherapy cycle
Adults: 6 mg once per chemotherapy cycle

Dosage Forms Excipient information presented when available (limited, particularly for generics); consult specific product labeling.
Injection, solution [preservative free]:
Neulasta®: 10 mg/mL (0.6 mL) [prefilled syringe; needle cover contains latex]

Peginterferon Alfa-2a (peg in ter FEER on AL fa too aye)

U.S. Brand Names Pegasys®

Canadian Brand Names Pegasys®

Mexican Brand Names Pegasys

Index Terms Interferon Alfa-2a (PEG Conjugate); Pegylated Interferon Alfa-2a

Pharmacologic Category Interferon

Use Treatment of chronic hepatitis C (CHC), alone or in combination with ribavirin, in patients with compensated liver disease and histological evidence of cirrhosis (Child-Pugh class A) and patients with clinically-stable HIV disease; treatment of patients with HBeAg positive and HBeAg negative chronic hepatitis B with compensated liver disease and evidence of viral replication and liver inflammation

Effect on Mental Status Severe psychiatric adverse effects (including depression, suicidal ideation, and suicide attempt) may occur. May also cause sedation, anxiety, emotional lability, irritability, insomnia, dizziness, and impaired concentration.

Effect on Psychiatric Treatment Contraindicated in those with severe psychiatric disorder. Gastrointestinal side effects are common; use caution with SSRIs, valproic acid, and lithium. Flu-like symptoms are common; take this into consideration if also concerned about SSRI discontinuation syndrome. A case of agranulocytosis has been reported with concurrent use of clozapine; monitor.

Restrictions An FDA-approved medication guide must be distributed when dispensing an outpatient prescription (new or refill) where this medication is to be used without direct supervision of a healthcare provider. Medication guides are available at http://www.fda.gov/cder/Offices/ODS/medication_guides.htm.

Dosage Summary

SubQ:
Children: Dosage not established
Adults: 180 mcg once weekly

Dosage Forms Excipient information presented when available (limited, particularly for generics); consult specific product labeling.
Injection solution:
Pegasys®
180 mcg/0.5 mL (0.5 mL) [prefilled syringe; contains benzyl alcohol and polysorbate 80; packaged with needles and alcohol swabs]
180 mcg/mL (1 mL) [vial; contains benzyl alcohol and polysorbate 80]

Peginterferon Alfa-2b (peg in ter FEER on AL fa too bee)

Medication Safety Issues
Sound-alike/look-alike issues:
Peginterferon alfa-2b may be confused with interferon alfa-2a, interferon alfa-2b, interferon alfa-n3, peginterferon alfa-2a
PegIntron™ may be confused with Intron® A

International issues:
Peginterferon alfa-2b may be confused with interferon alpha multi-subtype which is available in international markets

U.S. Brand Names PegIntron™
Canadian Brand Names PegIntron™
Mexican Brand Names Pegtron
Index Terms Interferon Alfa-2b (PEG Conjugate); Pegylated Interferon Alfa-2b
Pharmacologic Category Interferon
Use Treatment of chronic hepatitis C (as monotherapy or in combination with ribavirin) in adult patients who have never received alfa interferons and have compensated liver disease
Unlabeled/Investigational Use Treatment of advanced melanoma
Effect on Mental Status Severe psychiatric adverse effects (including depression, suicidal ideation, and suicide attempt) may occur. May also cause sedation, anxiety, emotional lability, irritability, insomnia, dizziness, and impaired concentration.
Effect on Psychiatric Treatment Contraindicated in those with severe psychiatric disorder. Gastrointestinal side effects are common; use caution with SSRIs, valproic acid, and lithium. Flu-like symptoms are common; take this into consideration if also concerned about SSRI discontinuation syndrome. A case of agranulocytosis has been reported with concurrent use of clozapine; monitor.
Restrictions An FDA-approved medication guide must be distributed when dispensing an outpatient prescription (new or refill) where this medication is to be used without direct supervision of a healthcare provider. Medication guides are available at http://www.fda.gov/cder/Offices/ODS/medication_guides.htm.
Dosage Summary
SubQ:
Children: Dosage not established
Adults: 1 mcg/kg/week
Adults ≤45 kg: 40 mcg once weekly
Adults 46-56 kg: 50 mcg once weekly
Adults 57-72 kg: 64 mcg once weekly
Adults 73-88 kg: 80 mcg once weekly
Adults 89-106 kg: 96 mcg once weekly
Adults 107-136 kg: 120 mcg once weekly
Adults 137-160 kg: 150 mcg once weekly
Dosage Forms Excipient information presented when available (limited, particularly for generics); consult specific product labeling.
Injection, powder for reconstitution [preservative free]:
PegIntron™: 50 mcg, 80 mcg, 120 mcg, 150 mcg [contains polysorbate 80 and sucrose]
PegIntron™ Redipen®: 50 mcg, 80 mcg, 120 mcg, 150 mcg [contains polysorbate 80 and sucrose]

◆ **PegIntron™** *see* Peginterferon Alfa-2b *on page 1237*

Pegvisomant (peg VI soe mant)

U.S. Brand Names Somavert®
Canadian Brand Names Somavert®
Index Terms B2036-PEG
Pharmacologic Category Growth Hormone Receptor Antagonist
Use Treatment of acromegaly in patients resistant to or unable to tolerate other therapies

Effect on Mental Status May cause dizziness

Effect on Psychiatric Treatment GI side effects are common; use caution with SSRIs. Increased dose of pegvisomant may be needed in patients receiving opioids.

Dosage Summary

SubQ:

Children: Dosage not established

Adults: Initial loading dose: 40 mg; Maintenance: 10-30 mg/day (maximum: 30 mg/day). **Note:** Titration is recommended

Dosage Forms Excipient information presented when available (limited, particularly for generics); consult specific product labeling.

Injection, powder for reconstitution [preservative free]:

Somavert®: 10 mg, 15 mg, 20 mg [vial stopper contains latex; packaged with SWFI]

- **Pegylated Interferon Alfa-2a** *see* Peginterferon Alfa-2a *on page 1236*
- **Pegylated Interferon Alfa-2b** *see* Peginterferon Alfa-2b *on page 1237*
- **Pegylated Liposomal DOXOrubicin** *see* DOXOrubicin (Liposomal) *on page 508*
- **PE-Hist DM** *see* Chlorpheniramine, Phenylephrine, and Dextromethorphan *on page 327*

Pemetrexed (pem e TREKS ed)

Medication Safety Issues

High alert medication: The Institute for Safe Medication Practices (ISMP) includes this medication among its list of drug classes which have a heightened risk of causing significant patient harm when used in error.

U.S. Brand Names Alimta®

Canadian Brand Names Alimta®

Mexican Brand Names Alimta

Index Terms LY231514; Multitargeted Antifolate; NSC-698037; Pemetrexed Disodium

Pharmacologic Category Antineoplastic Agent, Antimetabolite; Antineoplastic Agent, Antimetabolite (Antifolate)

Use Treatment of malignant pleural mesothelioma; treatment of locally advanced or metastatic nonsquamous nonsmall cell lung cancer (NSCLC)

Unlabeled/Investigational Use Treatment of bladder cancer

Effect on Mental Status Fatigue and depression are common

Effect on Psychiatric Treatment Gastrointestinal side effects are common; these effects may be additive with concurrent use of SSRIs, acetylcholinesterase inhibitors, aripiprazole, or ziprasidone. Hematologic adverse effects are common; use caution with clozapine, carbamazepine, valproate, mirtazapine. Sedation is common; concurrent use with psychotropics may produce additive effects.

Dosage Summary

I.V.:

Children: Dosage not established

Adults: 500 mg/m^2 on day 1 of each 21-day cycle

Dosage Forms Excipient information presented when available (limited, particularly for generics); consult specific product labeling.

Injection, powder for reconstitution:

Alimta®: 100 mg, 500 mg

- **Pemetrexed Disodium** *see* Pemetrexed *on page 1238*

Penbutolol (pen BYOO toe lole)

Medication Safety Issues

Sound-alike/look-alike issues:

Levatol® may be confused with Lipitor®

International issues:

Levatol® may be confused with Lovacol® which is a brand name for lovastatin in Chile, Finland, and France

Related Information

Beta-Blockers *on page 1776*

U.S. Brand Names Levatol®

Canadian Brand Names Levatol®

Index Terms Penbutolol Sulfate

Pharmacologic Category Beta Blocker With Intrinsic Sympathomimetic Activity

Use Treatment of mild to moderate arterial hypertension

Effect on Mental Status May cause dizziness or depression; may rarely cause insomnia, confusion, or nightmares

Effect on Psychiatric Treatment Concurrent use with phenothiazines may potentiate hypotensive effects of penbutolol

Dosage Summary

Oral:

Children: Dosage not established

Adults: Initial: 20 mg once daily; Maintenance: 10-40 mg once daily (maximum: 80 mg/day)

Dosage Forms Excipient information presented when available (limited, particularly for generics); consult specific product labeling.

Tablet, as sulfate: 20 mg

- ◆ **Penbutolol Sulfate** *see* Penbutolol *on page 1238*
- ◆ **Pendex** *see* Guaifenesin and Phenylephrine *on page 742*

Penicillamine (pen i SIL a meen)

Medication Safety Issues

Sound-alike/look-alike issues:

Penicillamine may be confused with penicillin

Depen® may be confused with Endal®

International issues:

Depen® may be confused with Depon® which is a brand name for acetaminophen in Greece

Depen® may be confused with Dipen® which is a brand name for diltiazem in Greece

Pemine® [Italy] may be confused with Pamine® which is a brand name for methscopolamine in the U.S.

U.S. Brand Names Cuprimine®; Depen®

Canadian Brand Names Cuprimine®; Depen®

Mexican Brand Names Adalken

Index Terms D-3-Mercaptovaline; D-Penicillamine; β,β-Dimethylcysteine

Pharmacologic Category Chelating Agent

Use Treatment of Wilson's disease, cystinuria; adjunctive treatment of rheumatoid arthritis

Unlabeled/Investigational Use Chelation therapy for the treatment of lead poisoning (third-line agent); treatment of arsenic poisoning

Effect on Mental Status May cause anxiety, agitation, visual and psychic disturbances

Effect on Psychiatric Treatment May cause aplastic anemia; use caution with clozapine and carbamazepine. May cause dystonia. May cause thrombocytopenia; monitor in patients receiving valproate.

Dosage Summary

Oral:

Children <12 years: 20 mg/kg/day in 2-3 divided doses **or** 30 mg/kg/day in 4 divided doses (maximum: 1 g/day)

Children ≥12 years: 30 mg/kg/day in 4 divided doses

Adults: 250-4000 mg/day divided every 6 hours

Dosage Forms Excipient information presented when available (limited, particularly for generics); consult specific product labeling.

Capsule:

Cuprimine®: 250 mg

Tablet:

Depen®: 250 mg

Penicillin G Benzathine (pen i SIL in jee BENZ a theen)

Medication Safety Issues

Sound-alike/look-alike issues:

Penicillin may be confused with penicillamine

Bicillin® may be confused with Wycillin®

Bicillin® C-R (penicillin G benzathine and penicillin G procaine) may be confused with Bicillin® L-A (penicillin G benzathine). Penicillin G benzathine is the only product currently approved for the treatment of syphilis. Administration of penicillin G benzathine and penicillin G procaine combination instead of Bicillin® L-A may result in inadequate treatment response.

Penicillin G benzathine may only be administered by deep intramuscular injection; intravenous administration of penicillin G benzathine has been associated with cardiopulmonary arrest and death.

U.S. Brand Names Bicillin® L-A

Canadian Brand Names Bicillin® L-A

Mexican Brand Names Benzetacil

Index Terms Benzathine Benzylpenicillin; Benzathine Penicillin G; Benzylpenicillin Benzathine

Pharmacologic Category Antibiotic, Penicillin

Use Active against some gram-positive organisms, few gram-negative organisms such as *Neisseria gonorrhoeae*, and some anaerobes and spirochetes; used in the treatment of syphilis; used only for the treatment of mild to moderately severe infections caused by organisms susceptible to low concentrations of penicillin G or for prophylaxis of infections caused by these organisms

Effect on Mental Status May rarely cause drowsiness or confusion; penicillins reported to cause apprehension, illusions, hallucinations, depersonalization, agitation, insomnia, and encephalopathy

Effect on Psychiatric Treatment None reported

Dosage Summary

I.M.:

Neonates >1200 g: 50,000 units/kg as a single dose

Children: 25,000-50,000 units/kg as a single dose (maximum: 2.4 million units/dose)

Adults: 1.2-2.4 million units as a single dose

Dosage Forms Excipient information presented when available (limited, particularly for generics); consult specific product labeling.

Injection, suspension [prefilled syringe]: 600,000 units/mL (1 mL, 2 mL, 4 mL)

Penicillin G Benzathine and Penicillin G Procaine

(pen i SIL in jee BENZ a theen & pen i SIL in jee PROE kane)

Medication Safety Issues

Bicillin® C-R (penicillin G benzathine and penicillin G procaine) may be confused with Bicillin® L-A (penicillin G benzathine). Penicillin G benzathine is the only product currently approved for the treatment of syphilis. Administration of penicillin G benzathine and penicillin G procaine combination instead of Bicillin® L-A may result in inadequate treatment response.

Penicillin G benzathine may only be administered by deep intramuscular injection; intravenous administration of penicillin G benzathine has been associated with cardiopulmonary arrest and death.

Sound-alike/look-alike issues:

Penicillin may be confused with penicillamine

Bicillin® may be confused with Wycillin®

U.S. Brand Names Bicillin® C-R; Bicillin® C-R 900/300

Index Terms Penicillin G Procaine and Benzathine Combined

Pharmacologic Category Antibiotic, Penicillin

Use May be used in specific situations in the treatment of streptococcal infections

Effect on Mental Status May rarely cause drowsiness or confusion

Effect on Psychiatric Treatment None reported

Dosage Summary

I.M.:

Children <14 kg: 600,000 units as a single dose

Children 14-27 kg: 900,000 units to 1.2 million units as a single dose

Children >27 kg: 2.4 million units as a single dose

Adults: 2.4 million units as a single dose

Dosage Forms Excipient information presented when available (limited, particularly for generics); consult specific product labeling. [DSC] = Discontinued product

Injection, suspension [prefilled syringe]:

Bicillin® C-R:

600,000 units: Penicillin G benzathine 300,000 units and penicillin G procaine 300,000 units per 1 mL (1 mL) [DSC]

1,200,000 units: Penicillin G benzathine 600,000 units and penicillin G procaine 600,000 units per 2 mL (2 mL)

2,400,000 units: Penicillin G benzathine 1,200,000 units and penicillin G procaine 1,200,000 units per 4 mL (4 mL) [DSC]

Bicillin® C-R 900/300: 1,200,000 units: Penicillin G benzathine 900,000 units and penicillin G procaine 300,000 units per 2 mL (2 mL)

Penicillin G, Parenteral, Aqueous

(pen i SIL in jee, pa REN ter al, AYE kwee us)

Medication Safety Issues

Sound-alike/look-alike issues:

Penicillin may be confused with penicillamine

U.S. Brand Names Pfizerpen®

Canadian Brand Names Crystapen®

Mexican Brand Names Pengesod; Sodipen

Index Terms Benzylpenicillin Potassium; Benzylpenicillin Sodium; Crystalline Penicillin; Penicillin G Potassium; Penicillin G Sodium

Pharmacologic Category Antibiotic, Penicillin

Use Treatment of infections (including sepsis, pneumonia, pericarditis, endocarditis, meningitis, anthrax) caused by susceptible organisms; active against some gram-positive organisms, generally not *Staphylococcus aureus*; some gram-negative organisms such as *Neisseria gonorrhoeae*, and some anaerobes and spirochetes

Effect on Mental Status May rarely cause drowsiness or confusion

Effect on Psychiatric Treatment None reported

Dosage Summary

I.M.:

Infants >1 month: 100,000-400,000 units/kg/day in divided doses every 4-6 hours (maximum: 24 million units/day)

Children: 100,000-400,000 units/kg/day in divided doses every 4-6 hours (maximum: 24 million units/day)

Adults: 2-30 million units/day in divided doses every 4-6 hours

I.V.:

Infants >1 month: 100,000-400,000 units/kg/day in divided doses every 4-6 hours (maximum: 24 million units/day)

Children: 100,000-400,000 units/kg/day in divided doses every 4-6 hours (maximum: 24 million units/day)

Adults: 2-30 million units/day in divided doses every 4-6 hours

Dosage Forms Excipient information presented when available (limited, particularly for generics); consult specific product labeling.

Infusion, as potassium [premixed iso-osmotic dextrose solution, frozen]: 1 million units (50 mL), 2 million units (50 mL), 3 million units (50 mL) [contains sodium 1.02 mEq and potassium 1.7 mEq per 1 million units]

Injection, powder for reconstitution, as potassium (Pfizerpen®): 5 million units, 20 million units [contains sodium 6.8 mg (0.3 mEq) and potassium 65.6 mg (1.68 mEq) per 1 million units]

Injection, powder for reconstitution, as sodium: 5 million units [contains sodium 1.68 mEq per 1 million units]

◆ **Penicillin G Potassium** *see* Penicillin G, Parenteral, Aqueous *on page 1241*

Penicillin G Procaine (pen i SIL in jee PROE kane)

Medication Safety Issues

Sound-alike/look-alike issues:

Penicillin G procaine may be confused with penicillin V potassium

Wycillin® may be confused with Bicillin®

Canadian Brand Names Pfizerpen-AS®; Wycillin®

Mexican Brand Names Benzetacil; Hidrociclina

Index Terms APPG; Aqueous Procaine Penicillin G; Procaine Benzylpenicillin; Procaine Penicillin G; Wycillin [DSC]

Pharmacologic Category Antibiotic, Penicillin

Use Treatment of moderately-severe infections due to *Treponema pallidum* and other penicillin G-sensitive microorganisms that are susceptible to low, but prolonged serum penicillin concentrations; anthrax due to *Bacillus anthracis* (postexposure) to reduce the incidence or progression of disease following exposure to aerolized *Bacillus anthracis*

Effect on Mental Status May rarely cause drowsiness, confusion, or CNS stimulation

Effect on Psychiatric Treatment None reported

Dosage Summary

I.M.:

Children: 25,000-50,000 units/kg/day in divided doses 1-2 times/day; (maximum: 4.8 million units/day)

Adults: 0.6-4.8 million units/day in divided doses every 12-24 hours

Dosage Forms Excipient information presented when available (limited, particularly for generics); consult specific product labeling.

Injection, suspension: 600,000 units/mL (1 mL, 2 mL)

◆ **Penicillin G Procaine and Benzathine Combined** *see* Penicillin G Benzathine and Penicillin G Procaine *on page 1240*

◆ **Penicillin G Sodium** *see* Penicillin G, Parenteral, Aqueous *on page 1241*

Penicillin V Potassium (pen i SIL in vee poe TASS ee um)

Medication Safety Issues

Sound-alike/look-alike issues:

Penicillin V procaine may be confused with penicillin G potassium

Canadian Brand Names Apo-Pen VK®; Novo-Pen-VK; Nu-Pen-VK

Mexican Brand Names Anapenil; Pen-Vi-K; Pota-Vi-Kin

Index Terms Pen VK; Phenoxymethyl Penicillin

Pharmacologic Category Antibiotic, Penicillin

Use Treatment of infections caused by susceptible organisms involving the respiratory tract, otitis media, sinusitis, skin, and urinary tract; prophylaxis in rheumatic fever

Effect on Mental Status Penicillins reported to cause apprehension, illusions, hallucinations, depersonalization, agitation, insomnia, and encephalopathy

Effect on Psychiatric Treatment None reported

Dosage Summary

Oral:

Children <12 years: 25-50 mg/kg/day divided every 6-8 hours (maximum: 3 g/day)

Children ≥12 years: 125-500 mg every 6-8 hours

Adults: 125-500 mg every 6-8 hours

Dosage Forms Excipient information presented when available (limited, particularly for generics); consult specific product labeling.

Note: 250 mg = 400,000 units

Powder for oral solution: 125 mg/5 mL (100 mL, 200 mL); 250 mg/5 mL (100 mL, 200 mL)

Tablet: 250 mg, 500 mg

◆ **Pentahydrate** *see* Sodium Thiosulfate *on page 1497*

◆ **Pentam-300®** *see* Pentamidine *on page 1242*

Pentamidine (pen TAM i deen)

U.S. Brand Names NebuPent®; Pentam-300®

Canadian Brand Names Pentamidine Isetionate for Injection

Mexican Brand Names Pentam 300

Index Terms Pentamidine Isethionate

Pharmacologic Category Antibiotic, Miscellaneous

Use Treatment and prevention of pneumonia caused by *Pneumocystis carinii* (PCP)

Unlabeled/Investigational Use Treatment of trypanosomiasis and visceral leishmaniasis

Effect on Mental Status Sedation and dizziness are common; may cause confusion or hallucinations

Effect on Psychiatric Treatment Contraindicated with ziprasidone. May cause leukopenia; use caution with clozapine and carbamazepine.

Dosage Summary

I.M.:

Children: 4 mg/kg once daily, every 2 weeks or monthly

Adults: 4 mg/kg once daily

I.V.:

Children: 4 mg/kg once daily, every 2 weeks or monthly

Adults: 4 mg/kg once daily

Inhalation:

Children <5 years: 8 mg/kg/dose has been used

Children ≥5 years: 300 mg/dose given every 3-4 weeks

Adults: 300 mg every 4 weeks

Dosage Forms Excipient information presented when available (limited, particularly for generics); consult specific product labeling.

Injection, powder for reconstitution, as isethionate [preservative free]:
Pentam-300®: 300 mg

Powder for solution, for nebulization, as isethionate [preservative free]:
NebuPent®: 300 mg

◆ **Pentamidine Isethionate** *see* Pentamidine *on page 1242*

◆ **Pentasa®** *see* Mesalamine *on page 994*

Pentazocine (pen TAZ oh seen)

Medication Safety Issues

High alert medication: The Institute for Safe Medication Practices (ISMP) includes this medication among its list of drug classes which have a heightened risk of causing significant patient harm when used in error.

Related Information

Narcotic / Opioid Analgesics *on page 1789*

U.S. Brand Names Talwin®; Talwin® Nx

Canadian Brand Names Talwin®

Index Terms Naloxone Hydrochloride and Pentazocine Hydrochloride; Pentazocine Hydrochloride; Pentazocine Hydrochloride and Naloxone Hydrochloride; Pentazocine Lactate

Pharmacologic Category Analgesic, Opioid

Generic Available Yes: Tablet

Use

Talwin®: Relief of moderate-to-severe pain; has also been used as a sedative prior to surgery and as a supplement to surgical anesthesia

Talwin® Nx: Relief of moderate-to-severe pain; indicated for oral use only

Effect on Mental Status Drowsiness and euphoria are common; may cause restlessness or nightmares; may rarely cause confusion, depression, or hallucinations

Effect on Psychiatric Treatment Concurrent use with psychotropics may produce additive effects or toxicity; may cause withdrawal in patients currently dependent on narcotics

Restrictions C-IV

Pregnancy Risk Factor C/D (prolonged use or high doses at term)

Pregnancy Considerations Pentazocine was not found to be teratogenic in animal studies. Pentazocine and naloxone have been shown to cross the human placenta. Use should be avoided during labor and delivery of premature infants. Abstinence syndromes in the newborn have been reported after long-term use of pentazocine during pregnancy. Other adverse effects in the newborn have been reported following abuse of pentazocine during pregnancy; these effects may be due to pentazocine, other drugs abused, the mother's lifestyle, or a combination of all factors.

Lactation Excretion in breast milk unknown/use caution

Contraindications Hypersensitivity to pentazocine, naloxone, or any component of the formulation

Warnings/Precautions May cause CNS depression, which may impair physical or mental abilities; patients must be cautioned about performing tasks which require mental alertness (eg, operating machinery or driving). Effects may be potentiated when used with other sedative drugs or ethanol. Use with caution in seizure-prone patients, acute myocardial infarction, patients undergoing biliary tract impairment, thyroid dysfunction, prostatic hyperplasia/urinary stricture, patients with respiratory, adrenal insufficiency, morbid obesity, renal and hepatic dysfunction, head trauma, increased intracranial pressure, and patients with a history of prior opioid dependence or abuse; pentazocine may precipitate opiate withdrawal symptoms in patients who have been receiving opiates regularly; injection contains sulfites which may cause allergic reaction; tolerance or drug dependence may result from extended use. May cause hypotension; use with caution in patients with hypovolemia, cardiovascular disease (including acute MI), or drugs which may exaggerate hypotensive effects (including phenothiazines or general anesthetics). May obscure diagnosis or clinical course of patients with acute abdominal conditions. Abrupt discontinuation may result in withdrawal symptoms; taper dose to decrease risk of withdrawal symptoms. **[U.S. Boxed Warning]: Talwin® Nx is intended for oral administration only; severe vascular reactions have resulted from misuse by injection**. Severe sclerosis has occurred at the injection-site following multiple injections; rotate sites of injection. Use with caution in the elderly and debilitated patients; may be more sensitive to adverse effects.

Safety and efficacy have not been established in children <1 year of age (Talwin®) and <12 years of age (Talwin® Nx).

Adverse Reactions Frequency not defined.

Cardiovascular: Circulatory depression, facial edema, flushing, hypotension, shock, syncope, tachycardia

Central nervous system: Chills, CNS depression, confusion, disorientation, dizziness, drowsiness, euphoria, excitement, hallucinations, headache, insomnia, irritability, lightheadedness, malaise, nightmares, sedation

Dermatologic: Dermatitis, erythema multiforme, pruritus, rash, Stevens-Johnson syndrome, toxic epidermal necrolysis, urticaria

Gastrointestinal: Abdominal distress, anorexia, constipation, diarrhea, nausea, vomiting, xerostomia

Genitourinary: Urinary retention

Hematologic: Decreased WBCs, eosinophilia

Local: Tissue damage and irritation with I.M./SubQ use

Neuromuscular & skeletal: Paresthesia, tremor, weakness

Ocular: Blurred vision, miosis

Otic: Tinnitus

Respiratory: Dyspnea, respiratory depression (rare)

Miscellaneous: Anaphylaxis, diaphoresis, physical and psychological dependence

Drug Interactions

Alcohol (Ethyl): CNS Depressants may enhance the CNS depressant effect of Alcohol (Ethyl). *Risk C: Monitor therapy*

Alvimopan: Analgesics (Opioid) may enhance the adverse/toxic effect of Alvimopan. This is most notable for patients receiving long-term (i.e., more than 7 days) opiates prior to alvimopan initiation. Management: Alvimopan is contraindicated in patients receiving therapeutic doses of opioids for more than 7 consecutive days immediately prior to alvimopan initiation. *Risk D: Consider therapy modification*

Ammonium Chloride: May increase the excretion of Analgesics (Opioid). *Risk C: Monitor therapy*

Amphetamines: May enhance the analgesic effect of Analgesics (Opioid). *Risk C: Monitor therapy*

Antipsychotic Agents (Phenothiazines): May enhance the hypotensive effect of Analgesics (Opioid). *Risk C: Monitor therapy*

CNS Depressants: May enhance the adverse/toxic effect of other CNS Depressants. *Risk C: Monitor therapy*

Desmopressin: Analgesics (Opioid) may enhance the adverse/toxic effect of Desmopressin. *Risk C: Monitor therapy*

Pegvisomant: Analgesics (Opioid) may diminish the therapeutic effect of Pegvisomant. *Risk C: Monitor therapy*

Selective Serotonin Reuptake Inhibitors: Analgesics (Opioid) may enhance the serotonergic effect of Selective Serotonin Reuptake Inhibitors. This may cause serotonin syndrome. *Risk C: Monitor therapy*

Succinylcholine: May enhance the bradycardic effect of Analgesics (Opioid). *Risk C: Monitor therapy*

Ethanol/Nutrition/Herb Interactions Ethanol: Avoid ethanol (may increase CNS depression).

Stability

Injection: Store at 20°C to 25°C (68°F to 77°F); do not freeze. Protect from heat.

Tablet: Store at 25°C (77°F); excursions permitted between 15°C to 30°C (59°F to 86°F).

Mechanism of Action

Pentazocine: Binds to opiate receptors in the CNS, causing inhibition of ascending pain pathways, altering the perception of and response to pain; produces generalized CNS depression; partial agonist-antagonist

Naloxone: Pure opioid antagonist that competes for and displaces narcotics at opioid receptor sites in CNS

Pharmacodynamics/Kinetics

Onset of action: Oral, I.M., SubQ: 15-20 minutes; I.V.: 2-3 minutes

Duration: Oral: 4-5 hours; Parenteral: 2-3 hours

Protein binding: 60%

Metabolism: Hepatic via oxidative and glucuronide conjugation pathways; extensive first-pass effect

Bioavailability: Oral: ~20%; increased to 60% to 70% with cirrhosis

Half-life elimination: 2-3 hours; prolonged with hepatic impairment

Excretion: Urine (small amounts as unchanged drug)

Dosage

Preoperative/preanesthetic: Children 1-16 years: I.M.: 0.5 mg/kg

Analgesia:
Children: I.M.:
5-8 years: 15 mg
8-14 years: 30 mg
Children >12 years and Adults: Oral: 50 mg every 3-4 hours; may increase to 100 mg/dose if needed, but should not exceed 600 mg/day (maximum: 12 tablets/day)
Adults:
I.M., SubQ: 30-60 mg every 3-4 hours; do not exceed 60 mg/dose (maximum: 360 mg/day)
I.V.: 30 mg every 3-4 hours; do not exceed 30 mg/dose (maximum: 360 mg/day)
Elderly: Elderly patients may be more sensitive to the analgesic and sedating effects. The elderly may also have impaired renal function. If needed, dosing should be started at the lower end of dosing range and adjust dose for renal function.

Dosing adjustment in renal impairment:
Cl_{cr} 10-50 mL/minute: Administer 75% of normal dose
Cl_{cr} <10 mL/minute: Administer 50% of normal dose

Dosing adjustment in hepatic impairment: Reduce dose or avoid use in patients with liver disease

Administration Rotate injection site for I.M.; avoid intra-arterial injection; avoid SubQ use unless absolutely necessary (may cause tissue damage)

Monitoring Parameters Relief of pain, respiratory and mental status, blood pressure

Additional Information Talwin® Nx: If tablet misused as an injection, the naloxone component will prevent the effect of pentazocine.

Dosage Forms Excipient information presented when available (limited, particularly for generics); consult specific product labeling.
Injection, solution:
Talwin®: 30 mg/mL (1 mL, 10 mL) [10 mL size contains sodium bisulfite]
Tablet: Pentazocine 50 mg and naloxone 0.5 mg
Talwin® Nx: Pentazocine 50 mg and naloxone 0.5 mg

Pentazocine and Acetaminophen

(pen TAZ oh seen & a seet a MIN oh fen)

Medication Safety Issues
Sound-alike/look-alike issues:
Talacen® may be confused with Tegison®, Timoptic®, Tinactin®
International issues:
Talacen® may be confused with Talliton® which is a brand name for carvedilol in Hungary

High alert medication: The Institute for Safe Medication Practices (ISMP) includes this medication among its list of drug classes which have a heightened risk of causing significant patient harm when used in error.

Duplicate therapy issues: This product contains acetaminophen, which may be a component of other combination products. Do not exceed the maximum recommended daily dose of acetaminophen.

U.S. Brand Names Talacen®

Index Terms Acetaminophen and Pentazocine; Pentazocine Hydrochloride and Acetaminophen

Pharmacologic Category Analgesic Combination (Opioid)

Generic Available Yes

Use Relief of mild to moderate pain

Restrictions C-IV

Pregnancy Risk Factor C/D (prolonged use or high doses at term)

Pregnancy Considerations Pentazocine was not found to be teratogenic in animal studies. Pentazocine and acetaminophen cross the placenta in humans. Use should be avoided during labor and delivery of premature infants. Abstinence syndromes in the newborn have been reported after long-term use of pentazocine during pregnancy. Other adverse effects in the newborn have been reported following abuse of pentazocine during pregnancy; these effects may be due to pentazocine, other drugs abused, the mother's lifestyle, or a combination of all factors.

Lactation Excretion in breast milk unknown/use caution

Contraindications Hypersensitivity to pentazocine, acetaminophen, or any component of the formulation

Warnings/Precautions Contains sodium metabisulfite; may cause allergic-type reactions; potential for elevating CSF pressure due to respiratory effects which may be exaggerated in presence of head injury, intracranial lesions, or pre-existing increase in intracranial lesions. May cause CNS depression, which may impair physical or mental abilities; patients must be cautioned about performing tasks which require mental alertness (eg, operating machinery or driving). Effects may be potentiated when used with other sedative drugs or ethanol. May cause severe hepatic toxicity on acute overdose; in addition, chronic daily dosing in adults has resulted in liver damage in some patients. May cause psychological and physical dependence. May obscure diagnosis or clinical course of patients with acute abdominal conditions. Use with caution in patients with respiratory depression, G6PD deficiency, biliary tract impairment, prostatic hyperplasia, urinary stricture, ethanol abuse, CNS depression, coma, severely limited respiratory reserve, severe bronchial asthma, other obstructive respiratory conditions or cyanosis, impaired renal or hepatic function, patients prone to seizures. Use with caution in elderly or debilitated patients. Abrupt discontinuation may result in withdrawal symptoms; taper dose to decrease risk of withdrawal symptoms. Pentazocine may precipitate opiate withdrawal symptoms in patients who have been receiving opiates regularly. Limit acetaminophen dose to <4 g/day.

Adverse Reactions Adverse reactions attributed to pentazocine 50 mg. Frequency not defined.

Cardiovascular: Flushing, hypotension, syncope, tachycardia

Central nervous system: Chills, confusion, depression, disorientation, dizziness, drowsiness, euphoria, excitement, hallucinations, headache, insomnia, irritability, lightheadedness, sedation

Dermatologic: Erythema multiforme, rash, Stevens-Johnson syndrome, toxic epidermal necrolysis, urticaria

Gastrointestinal: Abdominal distress, anorexia, biliary spasm, constipation, diarrhea, nausea, vomiting

Genitourinary: Urinary retention

Hematologic: Agranulocytosis, eosinophilia, hemolytic anemia, thrombocytopenic purpura, WBCs decreased

Neuromuscular & skeletal: Paresthesia, tremor, weakness

Ocular: Blurred vision

Otic: Tinnitus

Respiratory: Respiratory depression

Miscellaneous: Anaphylaxis, diaphoresis, facial edema

Drug Interactions

Alcohol (Ethyl): CNS Depressants may enhance the CNS depressant effect of Alcohol (Ethyl). *Risk C: Monitor therapy*

Alvimopan: Analgesics (Opioid) may enhance the adverse/toxic effect of Alvimopan. This is most notable for patients receiving long-term (i.e., more than 7 days) opiates prior to alvimopan initiation. Management: Alvimopan is contraindicated in patients receiving therapeutic doses of opioids for more than 7 consecutive days immediately prior to alvimopan initiation. *Risk D: Consider therapy modification*

Ammonium Chloride: May increase the excretion of Analgesics (Opioid). *Risk C: Monitor therapy*

Amphetamines: May enhance the analgesic effect of Analgesics (Opioid). *Risk C: Monitor therapy*

Anticonvulsants (Hydantoin): May increase the metabolism of Acetaminophen. This may 1) diminish the effect of acetaminophen; and 2) increase the risk of liver damage. *Risk C: Monitor therapy*

Antipsychotic Agents (Phenothiazines): May enhance the hypotensive effect of Analgesics (Opioid). *Risk C: Monitor therapy*

Barbiturates: May increase the metabolism of Acetaminophen. This may 1) diminish the effect of acetaminophen; and 2) increase the risk of liver damage. *Risk C: Monitor therapy*

CarBAMazepine: May increase the metabolism of Acetaminophen. This may 1) diminish the effect of acetaminophen; and 2) increase the risk of liver damage. *Risk C: Monitor therapy*

Cholestyramine Resin: May decrease the absorption of Acetaminophen. Effect is minimal if cholestyramine is administered 1 hour after acetaminophen. *Risk D: Consider therapy modification*

CNS Depressants: May enhance the adverse/toxic effect of other CNS Depressants. *Risk C: Monitor therapy*

Desmopressin: Analgesics (Opioid) may enhance the adverse/toxic effect of Desmopressin. *Risk C: Monitor therapy*

Imatinib: May increase the serum concentration of Acetaminophen. *Risk D: Consider therapy modification*

Isoniazid: May enhance the adverse/toxic effect of Acetaminophen. *Risk C: Monitor therapy*

Pegvisomant: Analgesics (Opioid) may diminish the therapeutic effect of Pegvisomant. *Risk C: Monitor therapy*

Selective Serotonin Reuptake Inhibitors: Analgesics (Opioid) may enhance the serotonergic effect of Selective Serotonin Reuptake Inhibitors. This may cause serotonin syndrome. *Risk C: Monitor therapy*

Succinylcholine: May enhance the bradycardic effect of Analgesics (Opioid). *Risk C: Monitor therapy*

Vitamin K Antagonists (eg, warfarin): Acetaminophen may enhance the anticoagulant effect of Vitamin K Antagonists. Most likely with daily acetaminophen doses >1.3 g for >1 week. *Risk C: Monitor therapy*

Ethanol/Nutrition/Herb Interactions

Ethanol: Avoid ethanol (may increase CNS depression).

Herb/Nutraceutical: Avoid valerian, St John's wort, kava kava, gotu kola (may increase CNS depression).

Stability Store at 25°C (77°F); excursions permitted to 15°C to 30°C (59°F to 86°F).

Mechanism of Action

Pentazocine: Binds to opiate receptors in the CNS, causing inhibition of ascending pain pathways, altering the perception of and response to pain; produces generalized CNS depression; partial agonist-antagonist

Acetaminophen: Inhibits the synthesis of prostaglandins in the central nervous system and peripherally blocks pain impulse generation

Pharmacodynamics/Kinetics See individual agents.

Dosage Oral: Adults: Analgesic: 1 caplet every 4 hours (maximum: 6 caplets/day)

Dosage Forms Excipient information presented when available (limited, particularly for generics); consult specific product labeling.

Caplet:

Talacen®: Pentazocine 25 mg and acetaminophen 650 mg [contains sodium metabisulfite]

Tablet: Pentazocine 25 mg and acetaminophen 650 mg

◆ **Pentazocine Hydrochloride** *see* Pentazocine *on page 1243*

◆ **Pentazocine Hydrochloride and Acetaminophen** *see* Pentazocine and Acetaminophen *on page 1245*

◆ **Pentazocine Hydrochloride and Naloxone Hydrochloride** *see* Pentazocine *on page 1243*

◆ **Pentazocine Lactate** *see* Pentazocine *on page 1243*

PENTobarbital (pen toe BAR bi tal)

Medication Safety Issues

Sound-alike/look-alike issues:

PENTobarbital may be confused with PHENobarbital

Nembutal® may be confused with Myambutol®

U.S. Brand Names Nembutal®

Canadian Brand Names Nembutal® Sodium

Index Terms Pentobarbital Sodium

Pharmacologic Category Anticonvulsant, Barbiturate; Barbiturate

Generic Available No

Use Sedative/hypnotic; preanesthetic; high-dose barbiturate coma for treatment of increased intracranial pressure or status epilepticus unresponsive to other therapy

Restrictions C-II

Pregnancy Risk Factor D

Lactation Enters breast milk/contraindicated

Contraindications Hypersensitivity to barbiturates or any component of the formulation; marked hepatic impairment; dyspnea or airway obstruction; porphyria; pregnancy

Warnings/Precautions Tolerance to hypnotic effect can occur; do not use for >2 weeks to treat insomnia. Potential for drug dependency exists, abrupt cessation may precipitate withdrawal, including status epilepticus in epileptic patients. Do not administer to patients in acute pain. Use caution in elderly, debilitated, renally impaired, hepatic dysfunction, or pediatric patients. May cause paradoxical responses, including agitation and hyperactivity, particularly in acute pain and pediatric patients. Use with caution in patients with depression or suicidal tendencies, or in patients with a history of drug abuse. Tolerance, psychological and physical dependence may occur with prolonged use.

May cause CNS depression, which may impair physical or mental abilities. Patients must be cautioned about performing tasks which require mental alertness (eg, operating machinery or driving). Effects with other sedative drugs or ethanol may be potentiated. Use of this agent as a hypnotic in the elderly is not recommended due to its long half-life and potential for physical and psychological dependence.

May cause respiratory depression or hypotension, particularly when administered intravenously. Use with caution in hemodynamically unstable patients or patients with respiratory disease. High doses (loading doses of 15-35 mg/kg given over 1-2 hours) have been utilized to induce pentobarbital coma, but these higher doses often cause hypotension requiring vasopressor therapy.

Adverse Reactions Frequency not defined.

Cardiovascular: Bradycardia, hypotension, syncope

Central nervous system: Drowsiness, lethargy, CNS excitation or depression, impaired judgment, "hangover" effect, confusion, somnolence, agitation, hyperkinesia, ataxia, nervousness, headache, insomnia, nightmares, hallucinations, anxiety, dizziness

Dermatologic: Rash, exfoliative dermatitis, Stevens-Johnson syndrome

Gastrointestinal: Nausea, vomiting, constipation

Hematologic: Agranulocytosis, thrombocytopenia, megaloblastic anemia

Local: Pain at injection site, thrombophlebitis with I.V. use

Renal: Oliguria

Respiratory: Laryngospasm, respiratory depression, apnea (especially with rapid I.V. use), hypoventilation

Miscellaneous: Gangrene with inadvertent intra-arterial injection

Metabolism/Transport Effects **Induces** CYP2A6 (strong), 3A4 (strong)

Drug Interactions

Acetaminophen: Barbiturates may increase the metabolism of Acetaminophen. This may 1) diminish the effect of acetaminophen; and 2) increase the risk of liver damage. *Risk C: Monitor therapy*

Alcohol (Ethyl): CNS Depressants may enhance the CNS depressant effect of Alcohol (Ethyl). *Risk C: Monitor therapy*

Beta-Blockers: Barbiturates may decrease the serum concentration of Beta-Blockers. **Exceptions:** Atenolol; Levobunolol; Metipranolol; Nadolol. *Risk C: Monitor therapy*

Calcium Channel Blockers: Barbiturates may increase the metabolism of Calcium Channel Blockers. **Exceptions:** Clevidipine. *Risk D: Consider therapy modification*

Carbonic Anhydrase Inhibitors: May enhance the adverse/toxic effect of Anticonvulsants (Barbiturate). Specifically, osteomalacia and rickets. **Exceptions:** Brinzolamide; Dorzolamide. *Risk C: Monitor therapy*

Chloramphenicol: May decrease the metabolism of Barbiturates. Barbiturates may increase the metabolism of Chloramphenicol. *Risk D: Consider therapy modification*

CNS Depressants: May enhance the adverse/toxic effect of other CNS Depressants. *Risk C: Monitor therapy*

Contraceptive (Progestins): Barbiturates may diminish the therapeutic effect of Contraceptive (Progestins). Contraceptive failure is possible. *Risk D: Consider therapy modification*

Corticosteroids (Systemic): Barbiturates may increase the metabolism of Corticosteroids (Systemic). *Risk C: Monitor therapy*

CycloSPORINE: Barbiturates may increase the metabolism of CycloSPORINE. *Risk D: Consider therapy modification*

CYP2A6 Substrates: CYP2A6 Inducers (Strong) may increase the metabolism of CYP2A6 Substrates. *Risk C: Monitor therapy*

CYP3A4 Substrates: CYP3A4 Inducers (Strong) may increase the metabolism of CYP3A4 Substrates. *Risk C: Monitor therapy*

Disopyramide: Barbiturates may increase the metabolism of Disopyramide. *Risk D: Consider therapy modification*

Doxycycline: Barbiturates may decrease the serum concentration of Doxycycline. *Risk D: Consider therapy modification*

Etoposide: Barbiturates may increase the metabolism of Etoposide. *Risk C: Monitor therapy*

Etoposide Phosphate: Barbiturates may decrease the serum concentration of Etoposide Phosphate. Barbiturates may increase the metabolism, via CYP isoenzymes, of etoposide phosphate. *Risk C: Monitor therapy*

Felbamate: May increase the serum concentration of Barbiturates. *Risk C: Monitor therapy*

Griseofulvin: Barbiturates may decrease the absorption of Griseofulvin. *Risk D: Consider therapy modification*

Ketorolac: May diminish the therapeutic effect of Anticonvulsants. *Risk C: Monitor therapy*

LamoTRIgine: Barbiturates may increase the metabolism of LamoTRIgine. *Risk D: Consider therapy modification*

Maraviroc: CYP3A4 Inducers may decrease the serum concentration of Maraviroc. *Risk D: Consider therapy modification*

Mefloquine: May diminish the therapeutic effect of Anticonvulsants. Mefloquine may decrease the serum concentration of Anticonvulsants. Management: Mefloquine is contraindicated in persons with a history of convulsions. If anticonvulsant is being used for another indication monitor response to treatment closely, as concurrent mefloquine may decrease response to treatment. *Risk D: Consider therapy modification*

Meperidine: Barbiturates may enhance the CNS depressant effect of Meperidine. *Risk C: Monitor therapy*

Methadone: Barbiturates may increase the metabolism of Methadone. *Risk D: Consider therapy modification*

Nilotinib: CYP3A4 Inducers (Strong) may decrease the serum concentration of Nilotinib. *Risk X: Avoid combination*

Oral Contraceptive (Estrogens): Barbiturates may diminish the therapeutic effect of Oral Contraceptive (Estrogens). Contraceptive failure is possible. *Risk D: Consider therapy modification*

Primidone: May enhance the adverse/toxic effect of Barbiturates. Primidone is converted to phenobarbital, and thus becomes additive with existing barbiturate therapy. *Risk C: Monitor therapy*

Propafenone: Barbiturates may increase the metabolism of Propafenone. *Risk D: Consider therapy modification*

Pyridoxine: May increase the metabolism of Barbiturates. Apparent in high pyridoxine doses (eg, 200 mg/day) *Risk C: Monitor therapy*

QuiNIDine: Barbiturates may increase the metabolism of QuiNIDine. *Risk D: Consider therapy modification*

Ranolazine: CYP3A4 Inducers (Strong) may decrease the serum concentration of Ranolazine. *Risk X: Avoid combination*

Rifamycin Derivatives: May increase the metabolism of Barbiturates. *Risk C: Monitor therapy*

Sorafenib: CYP3A4 Inducers (Strong) may decrease the serum concentration of Sorafenib. *Risk D: Consider therapy modification*

Teniposide: Barbiturates may increase the metabolism of Teniposide. *Risk C: Monitor therapy*

Theophylline Derivatives: Barbiturates may increase the metabolism of Theophylline Derivatives. **Exceptions:** Dyphylline. *Risk C: Monitor therapy*

Tricyclic Antidepressants: Barbiturates may increase the metabolism of Tricyclic Antidepressants. *Risk D: Consider therapy modification*

Valproic Acid: May decrease the metabolism of Barbiturates. Barbiturates may decrease the serum concentration of Valproic Acid. *Risk C: Monitor therapy*

Vitamin K Antagonists (eg, warfarin): Barbiturates may increase the metabolism of Vitamin K Antagonists. *Risk D: Consider therapy modification*

Ethanol/Nutrition/Herb Interactions Ethanol: Avoid ethanol (may increase CNS depression).

Stability Protect from freezing. Aqueous solutions are not stable; a commercially available vehicle (containing propylene glycol) is more stable. When mixed with an acidic solution, precipitate may form. Use only clear solution.

Mechanism of Action Short-acting barbiturate with sedative, hypnotic, and anticonvulsant properties. Barbiturates depress the sensory cortex, decrease motor activity, alter cerebellar function, and produce drowsiness, sedation, and hypnosis. In high doses, barbiturates exhibit anticonvulsant activity; barbiturates produce dose-dependent respiratory depression.

Pharmacodynamics/Kinetics

Onset of action: I.M.: 10-15 minutes; I.V.: ~1 minute

Duration: I.V.: 15 minutes

Distribution: V_d: Children: 0.8 L/kg; Adults: 1 L/kg

Protein binding: 35% to 55%

Metabolism: Extensively hepatic via hydroxylation and oxidation pathways

Half-life elimination: Terminal: Children: 25 hours; Adults: Healthy: 22 hours (range: 15-50 hours)

Excretion: Urine (<1% as unchanged drug)

Dosage

Children:

Hypnotic: I.M.: 2-6 mg/kg; maximum: 100 mg/dose

Preoperative/preprocedure sedation: ≥6 months:

Note: Limited information is available for infants <6 months of age.

I.M.: 2-6 mg/kg; maximum: 100 mg/dose

I.V.: 1-3 mg/kg to a maximum of 100 mg until asleep

Conscious sedation prior to a procedure: Children 5-12 years: I.V.: 2 mg/kg 5-10 minutes before procedures, may repeat one time

Adolescents: Conscious sedation: I.V.: 100 mg prior to a procedure

Children and Adults: Barbiturate coma in head injury patients: I.V.: Loading dose: 5-10 mg/kg given slowly over 1-2 hours; monitor blood pressure and respiratory rate; Maintenance infusion: Initial: 1 mg/kg/hour; may increase to 2-3 mg/kg/hour; maintain burst suppression on EEG

Status epilepticus: I.V.: **Note**: Intubation required; monitor hemodynamics

Children: Loading dose: 5-15 mg/kg given slowly over 1-2 hours; maintenance infusion: 0.5-5 mg/kg/hour

Adults: Loading dose: 10-20 mg/kg given slowly over 1-2 hours; maintenance infusion: 0.5-3 mg/kg/hour

Adults:

Hypnotic:

I.M.: 150-200 mg

I.V.: Initial: 100 mg, may repeat every 1-3 minutes up to 200-500 mg total dose

Preoperative sedation: I.M.: 150-200 mg

Dosing adjustment in hepatic impairment: Reduce dosage in patients with severe liver dysfunction

Administration Pentobarbital may be administered by deep I.M. or slow I.V. injection.

I.M.: No more than 5 mL (250 mg) should be injected at any one site because of possible tissue irritation.

I.V.: I.V. push doses can be given undiluted, but should be administered no faster than 50 mg/minute; parenteral solutions are highly alkaline; avoid extravasation; avoid rapid I.V. administration >50 mg/minute; avoid intra-arterial injection

Monitoring Parameters Respiratory status (for conscious sedation, includes pulse oximetry), cardiovascular status, CNS status; cardiac monitor and blood pressure monitor required

Reference Range

Therapeutic:

Hypnotic: 1-5 mcg/mL (SI: 4-22 μmol/L)

Coma: 10-50 mcg/mL (SI: 88-221 μmol/L)

Toxic: >10 mcg/mL (SI: >44 μmol/L)

Dosage Forms Excipient information presented when available (limited, particularly for generics); consult specific product labeling.

Injection, solution, as sodium: 50 mg/mL (20 mL, 50 mL) [contains alcohol 10% and propylene glycol 40%]

◆ **Pentobarbital Sodium** *see* PENTobarbital *on page 1247*

Pentosan Polysulfate Sodium

(PEN toe san pol i SUL fate SOW dee um)

Medication Safety Issues

Sound-alike/look-alike issues:

Pentosan may be confused with pentostatin

Elmiron® may be confused with Imuran®

U.S. Brand Names Elmiron®

Canadian Brand Names Elmiron®

Index Terms PPS

Pharmacologic Category Analgesic, Urinary

Use Orphan drug: Relief of bladder pain or discomfort due to interstitial cystitis

Effect on Mental Status May cause dizziness

Effect on Psychiatric Treatment May cause anemia and leukopenia; use caution with clozapine and carbamazepine

Dosage Summary

Oral:

Children: Dosage not established

Adults: 100 mg 3 times/day, 1 hour before or 2 hours after meals

Dosage Forms Excipient information presented when available (limited, particularly for generics); consult specific product labeling.

Capsule: 100 mg

Pentostatin (pen toe STAT in)

Medication Safety Issues

Sound-alike/look-alike issues:

Pentostatin may be confused with pentamidine, pentosan

High alert medication: The Institute for Safe Medication Practices (ISMP) includes this medication among its list of drug classes which have a heightened risk of causing significant patient harm when used in error.

International issues:

Nipent® may be confused with Nipin® which is a brand name for nifedipine in Italy and Singapore

U.S. Brand Names Nipent®

Canadian Brand Names Nipent®

Index Terms 2′-Deoxycoformycin; Co-Vidarabine; dCF; Deoxycoformycin; NSC-218321

Pharmacologic Category Antineoplastic Agent, Antibiotic; Antineoplastic Agent, Antimetabolite (Purine Antagonist)

Use Treatment of hairy cell leukemia

Unlabeled/Investigational Use Treatment of cutaneous T-cell lymphoma, chronic lymphocytic leukemia (CLL), and acute and chronic graft-versus-host-disease (GVHD)

Effect on Mental Status Sedation is common; may cause anxiety, confusion, insomnia, depression

Effect on Psychiatric Treatment Leukopenia is common; avoid clozapine and carbamazepine

Dosage Summary

I.V.:

Children: Dosage not established

Adults: 4 mg/m^2 every 2 weeks

Dosage Forms Excipient information presented when available (limited, particularly for generics); consult specific product labeling.

Injection, powder for reconstitution [preservative free]: 10 mg [contains mannitol 50 mg]

Nipent®: 10 mg [contains mannitol 50 mg]

◆ **Pentothal®** *see* Thiopental *on page 1570*

Pentoxifylline (pen toks IF i lin)

Medication Safety Issues

Sound-alike/look-alike issues:

Pentoxifylline may be confused with tamoxifen

Trental® may be confused with Bentyl®, Tegretol®, Trandate®

U.S. Brand Names Pentoxil®; Trental®

Canadian Brand Names Albert® Pentoxifylline; Apo-Pentoxifylline SR®; Nu-Pentoxifylline SR; ratio-Pentoxifylline; Trental®

Mexican Brand Names Artelife; Duplat; Fixoten; Kentadin; Peridane; Profiben; Sufisal; Trental; Vantoxyl; Xipen

Index Terms Oxpentifylline

Pharmacologic Category Blood Viscosity Reducer Agent

Use Treatment of intermittent claudication on the basis of chronic occlusive arterial disease of the limbs; may improve function and symptoms, but not intended to replace more definitive therapy

Unlabeled/Investigational Use AIDS patients with increased TNF, CVA, cerebrovascular diseases, diabetic atherosclerosis, diabetic neuropathy, gangrene, hemodialysis shunt thrombosis, vascular impotence, cerebral malaria, septic shock, sickle cell syndromes, vasculitis, and venous leg ulcers

Effect on Mental Status May cause anxiety, confusion, depression, dizziness, or rarely agitation

Effect on Psychiatric Treatment May cause seizures; use with caution with concomitant use of clozapine, which is associated with dose-dependent risk of seizures

Dosage Summary

Oral:

Children: Dosage not established

Adults: 400 mg 2-3 times/day with meals

Dosage Forms Excipient information presented when available (limited, particularly for generics); consult specific product labeling.

Tablet, controlled release:

Trental®: 400 mg

Tablet, extended release: 400 mg

Pentoxil®: 400 mg

◆ **Pentoxil®** *see* Pentoxifylline *on page 1251*

◆ **Pen VK** *see* Penicillin V Potassium *on page 1242*

- **Pepcid®** *see* Famotidine *on page 613*
- **Pepcid® AC [OTC]** *see* Famotidine *on page 613*
- **Pepcid® AC Maximum Strength [OTC]** *see* Famotidine *on page 613*
- **Pepcid® Complete [OTC]** *see* Famotidine, Calcium Carbonate, and Magnesium Hydroxide *on page 614*
- **Peptic Relief [OTC]** *see* Bismuth *on page 189*
- **Pepto-Bismol® [OTC]** *see* Bismuth *on page 189*
- **Pepto-Bismol® Maximum Strength [OTC]** *see* Bismuth *on page 189*
- **Pepto Relief [OTC]** *see* Bismuth *on page 189*
- **Percocet®** *see* Oxycodone and Acetaminophen *on page 1205*
- **Percodan®** *see* Oxycodone and Aspirin *on page 1208*
- **Percogesic® [OTC]** *see* Acetaminophen and Phenyltoloxamine *on page 36*
- **Percogesic® Extra Strength [OTC]** *see* Acetaminophen and Diphenhydramine *on page 35*
- **Perforomist™** *see* Formoterol *on page 686*
- **Periactin** *see* Cyproheptadine *on page 410*

Periciazine (per ee CYE ah zeen)

Canadian Brand Names Neuleptil®

Index Terms Pericyazine

Pharmacologic Category Antipsychotic Agent, Typical, Phenothiazine, Piperidine

Use Adjunctive therapy in selected psychotic patients to control prevailing hostility, impulsivity, or aggression

Mental Health Comment In 2008, the FDA issued a warning regarding increased mortality risk with typical **and** atypical antipsychotic drugs when used in elderly patients with dementia-related psychosis.

Restrictions Not available in U.S.

Pregnancy Considerations Teratogenic effects were observed in some animal studies. Safety and efficacy have not been established in pregnant women.

Contraindications Hypersensitivity to periciazine, phenothiazine derivatives, or any component of the formulation; severe CNS depression including acute intoxication with CNS depressant medications; subcortical brain damage; hepatic dysfunction; circulatory collapse; severely-depressed patients; bone marrow suppression; blood dyscrasias; coma; patients receiving spinal or regional anesthesia

Warnings/Precautions Check blood counts periodically and discontinue at first signs of blood dyscrasias; use is contraindicated in patients with bone marrow suppression. May be sedating; use with caution in disorders where CNS depression is a feature (risk may be lower than with other phenothiazines); caution patients about performing tasks which require mental alertness. Use with caution in Parkinson's disease (may be more sensitive to adverse effects), hemodynamic instability, and predisposition to seizures. Esophageal dysmotility and aspiration have been associated with antipsychotic use; use with caution in patients at risk of pneumonia (eg, Alzheimer's disease). Use with caution in breast cancer or other prolactin-dependent tumors (may elevate prolactin levels). May alter temperature regulation; use caution with strenuous exercise, heat exposure, dehydration, and concomitant medication possessing anticholinergic effects. May mask toxicity of other drugs or conditions (eg, intestinal obstruction, Reye's syndrome, brain tumor) due to antiemetic effects.

Use caution in cardiovascular disease. May alter cardiac conduction (life-threatening arrhythmias have occurred with therapeutic doses of phenothiazines); relative risk with periciazine has not been established, although rare cases of QT_c prolongation have been reported. May cause orthostatic hypotension; use with caution in patients at risk of this effect or those who would not tolerate transient hypotensive episodes (cerebrovascular disease, cardiovascular disease, or other medications which may predispose). Phenothiazines have been associated with worsening of pheochromocytoma and mitral valve prolapse; use caution.

Phenothiazines may cause anticholinergic effects (confusion, agitation, constipation, xerostomia, blurred vision, urinary retention); therefore, use with caution in patients with decreased gastrointestinal motility, urinary retention, BPH, xerostomia, or visual problems. Conditions which also may be exacerbated by cholinergic blockade include narrow-angle glaucoma (screening is recommended) and worsening of myasthenia gravis.

May cause extrapyramidal symptoms, including pseudoparkinsonism, acute dystonic reactions, akathisia, and tardive dyskinesia. May be associated with neuroleptic malignant syndrome (NMS); monitor for mental status changes, fever, muscle rigidity, and/or autonomic instability (risk may be increased in patients with Parkinson's disease or Lewy body dementia). Prolonged therapy may cause pigmentary retinopathy, corneal deposits, and/or changes in skin pigmentation. Use with caution in the elderly; risk for developing tardive dyskinesia is increased.

Adverse Reactions Frequency not defined; listing includes adverse reactions reported with other agents from the phenothiazine class.

Cardiovascular: AV block, cardiac arrest, ECG changes, edema, hypotension, paroxysmal atrial tachycardia, QT_c prolongation, syncope, tachycardia

Central nervous system; Aggressive behavior, agitation, anxiety, bizarre dreams, cerebral edema, depression, dizziness, drowsiness, EEG changes, excitement; extrapyramidal symptoms (tremor, akathisia, dystonia, dyskinesia, oculogyric, opisthotonos, hyper-reflexia, pseudo-Parkinsonism, rigidity, sialorrhea); fatigue, fever, headache, insomnia, paradoxical psychosis, restlessness, seizures, sleep disturbance, tardive dyskinesia

Dermatologic: Angioedema, dermatitis, eczema, epithelial keratopathy, erythema, exfoliative dermatitis, photosensitivity, pruritus, rash, seborrhea, skin pigmentation (prolonged therapy), urticaria

Endocrine & metabolic: Anorexia, appetite increased, delayed ovulation, galactorrhea, gynecomastia, libido changes, menstrual irregularities, thirst, weight changes

Gastrointestinal: Adynamic ileus, constipation, fecal impaction, nausea, salivation, vomiting, xerostomia

Genitourinary: Bladder paralysis, impotence, incontinence, polyuria, urinary retention

Hematologic: Agranulocytosis, anemia, eosinophilia, leukopenia, pancytopenia, thrombocytopenia

Hepatic: Cholestasis, cholestatic jaundice, jaundice

Ocular: Blurred vision, corneal deposits (prolonged therapy), glaucoma, lenticular deposits, pigmentary retinopathy (prolonged therapy)

Respiratory: Nasal congestion, pneumonia, pneumonitis

Miscellaneous: Diaphoresis increased, lupus-like syndrome

Metabolism/Transport Effects No published data on CYP metabolism. Based on structural analysis, may be a substrate of CYP2D6 and 3A4.

Drug Interactions No published data on CYP metabolism. Based on structural analysis, may be a substrate of CYP2D6 and 3A4.

Aluminum salts: May decrease the absorption of phenothiazines; monitor.

Amphetamines: Efficacy may be diminished by antipsychotics; in addition, amphetamines may increase psychotic symptoms; avoid concurrent use.

Anticholinergics: May inhibit the therapeutic response to phenothiazines and excess anticholinergic effects may occur; includes benztropine, trihexyphenidyl, biperiden, and drugs with significant anticholinergic activity (TCAs, antihistamines, disopyramide).

Antihypertensives: Concurrent use of phenothiazines with an antihypertensive may produce additive hypotensive effects (particularly orthostasis).

Beta-blockers: May increase the risk of arrhythmia; serum concentrations of phenothiazines may be increased; propranolol also increases phenothiazine concentrations; may also occur with pindolol. Propranolol and pindolol are contraindicated.

Bromocriptine: Phenothiazines inhibit the ability of bromocriptine to lower serum prolactin concentrations.

Carvedilol: Serum concentrations may be increased, leading to hypotension and bradycardia; avoid concurrent use.

CNS depressants: Sedative effects may be additive with phenothiazines; monitor for increased effect; includes barbiturates, benzodiazepines, opioid analgesics, ethanol, and other sedative agents.

CYP2D6 inhibitors: May increase the levels/effects of Periciazine. Example inhibitors include chlorpromazine, delavirdine, fluoxetine, miconazole, paroxetine, pergolide, quinidine, quinine, ritonavir, and ropinirole. Other piperidine phenothiazines (thioridazine) are contraindicated with inhibitors of this enzyme.

CYP3A4 inhibitors: May increase the levels/effects of Periciazine. Example inhibitors include azole antifungals, clarithromycin, diclofenac, doxycycline, erythromycin, imatinib, isoniazid, nefazodone, nicardipine, propofol, protease inhibitors, quinidine,telithromycin, and verapamil.

Epinephrine: Low potency antipsychotics may diminish the pressor effects of epinephrine.

Guanethidine and guanadrel: Antihypertensive effects may be inhibited by phenothiazines.

Levodopa: Phenothiazines may inhibit the antiparkinsonian effect of levodopa; avoid this combination.

Lithium: Phenothiazines may produce neurotoxicity with lithium; this is a rare effect.

Metoclopramide: May increase extrapyramidal symptoms (EPS) or risk.

Phenytoin: May reduce serum levels of phenothiazines; phenothiazines may increase phenytoin serum levels.

Polypeptide antibiotics (eg, bacitracin): Rare cases of respiratory paralysis have been reported with concurrent use of phenothiazines.

Potassium-depleting agents: May increase the risk of serious arrhythmias with phenothiazines; includes many diuretics, aminoglycosides, and amphotericin; monitor serum potassium closely.

QT_c-prolonging agents: Effects on QT_c interval may be additive with phenothiazines, increasing the risk of malignant arrhythmias; includes type Ia antiarrhythmics, TCAs, and some quinolone antibiotics (moxifloxacin). These agents are contraindicated with other piperidine phenothiazines (thioridazine).

Sulfadoxine-pyrimethamine: May increase phenothiazine concentrations.

Trazodone: Phenothiazines and trazodone may produce additive hypotensive effects.

Tricyclic antidepressants: Concurrent use may produce increased toxicity or altered therapeutic response.

Valproic acid: Serum levels may be increased by phenothiazines.

Ethanol/Nutrition/Herb Interactions

Ethanol: Avoid ethanol (may increase CNS depression).

Herb/Nutraceutical: Avoid kava kava, valerian, St John's wort, gotu kola (may increase CNS depression). Avoid dong quai, St John's wort (may also cause photosensitization). Cigarette smoking may decrease the serum concentrations of periciazine.

Stability Store at room temperature of 20°C to 25°C (68°F to 77°F). Protect from light.

Mechanism of Action Blocks postsynaptic mesolimbic dopaminergic receptors in the brain; depresses the release of hypothalamic and hypophyseal hormones.

Dosage Oral:

Children >5 years: 2.5-10 mg in the morning, followed by 5-30 mg in the evening. In general, lower dosage should be used on initiation and gradually increased based on effect and tolerance.

Adults: 5-20 mg in the morning, followed by 10-40 mg in the evening. In dividing doses, it is suggested that the larger dose should be administered in the evening. In general, lower dosage should be used on initiation and gradually increased based on effect and tolerance.

Elderly: Initial daily dose should be ~5 mg/day. May be increased gradually based on effect and tolerance. Also see adult dosing.

Dosage adjustment in renal impairment: No dosage adjustment required.

Monitoring Parameters Vital signs; serum potassium and magnesium, lipid profile, waist circumference, fasting blood glucose/Hgb A_{1c}; BMI; mental status, abnormal involuntary movement scale (AIMS); periodic eye exam and evaluation of renal and liver function tests (long-term therapy).

Based on experience with other piperidine phenothiazines: Consider baseline and periodic ECG; do not initiate if QT_c >450 msec.

Test Interactions Phenothiazines have been reported to cause false-positive pregnancy tests.

Dosage Forms Excipient information presented when available (limited, particularly for generics); consult specific product labeling. [CAN] = Canadian brand name

Capsule:

Neuleptil® [CAN]: 5 mg, 10 mg, 20 mg [not available in the U.S.]

Solution, oral drops:

Neuleptil® [CAN]: 10 mg/mL (100 mL) [contains ethanol 12% and sucrose 250 mg/mL [not available in the U.S.]

◆ **Peri-Colace® [OTC]** *see* Docusate and Senna *on page 491*

◆ **Pericyazine** *see* Periciazine *on page 1252*

Perindopril Erbumine (per IN doe pril er BYOO meen)

Related Information

Angiotensin Agents *on page 1754*

U.S. Brand Names Aceon®

Canadian Brand Names Apo-Perindopril®; Coversyl®

Mexican Brand Names Coversyl

Pharmacologic Category Angiotensin-Converting Enzyme (ACE) Inhibitor

Use Treatment of hypertension; reduction of cardiovascular mortality or nonfatal myocardial infarction in patients with stable coronary artery disease

Unlabeled/Investigational Use To delay the progression of nephropathy and reduce risks of cardiovascular events in hypertensive patients with type 1 or 2 diabetes mellitus

Effect on Mental Status May cause dizziness or fatigue; may rarely cause sedation, insomnia, or depression

Effect on Psychiatric Treatment May cause neutropenia; use caution with clozapine and carbamazepine; may decrease lithium clearance resulting in an increase in serum lithium levels and potential lithium toxicity; monitor serum lithium levels

Dosage Summary

Oral:

Children: Dosage not established

Adults: Initial: 2-4 mg once daily; Maintenance: 4-8 mg/day in 1-2 divided doses (maximum: 16 mg/day)

Elderly >65 to 70 years: Initial: 4 mg/day; Maintenance: 8 mg/day

Elderly >70 years: Initial: 2-4 mg/day; Maintenance: 8 mg/day

Dosage Forms Excipient information presented when available (limited, particularly for generics); consult specific product labeling.

Tablet: 2 mg, 4 mg, 8 mg

◆ **Periostat®** *see* Doxycycline *on page 509*

Perphenazine (per FEN a zeen)

Medication Safety Issues

Sound-alike/look-alike issues:

Trilafon® may be confused with Tri-Levlen®

Related Information

Anticholinergic Effects of Common Psychotropics *on page 1758*

Antipsychotic Agents *on page 1769*

CMS: Long-Term Care Facility Thresholds *on page 1815*

Discontinuation of Psychotropic Drugs *on page 1839*

Canadian Brand Names Apo-Perphenazine®

Mexican Brand Names Leptopsique

Pharmacologic Category Antiemetic; Antipsychotic Agent, Typical, Phenothiazine

Generic Available Yes

Use Treatment of schizophrenia; severe nausea and vomiting

Unlabeled/Investigational Use Ethanol withdrawal; behavioral symptoms associated with dementia (elderly); Tourette's syndrome; Huntington's chorea; spasmodic torticollis; Reye's syndrome; psychosis; psychosis/agitation related to Alzheimer's dementia

Mental Health Comment Perphenazine is an intermediate-potency antipsychotic. Older antipsychotic medications (chlorpromazine, haloperidol), which do not meet specific criteria for "atypical" antipsychotics, are often referred to as typical antipsychotics. They are associated with the troubling side effect, EPS. However, it is commonly believed that in order for a drug to treat psychosis, it must block dopamine is some manner.

Common side effects include sedation and neuroleptic effect (reduced initiative, interest in the environment, and display of emotion or affect). All **typical** antipsychotics are considered to be equally effective if given in equipotent doses. An inverse relationship exists between intrinsic antimuscarinic activity and propensity to cause extrapyramidal side effects. If dystonia or pseudoparkinsonism occurs, antiparkinsonian agents should be considered. If akathisia occurs, beta-blockers (eg, propranolol), benzodiazepines, or antiparkinsonian agents should be considered. Tardive dyskinesia (TD) secondary to typical antipsychotics has an estimated incidence of 3% to 5% per year for the first 5 years of treatment. After this time period, the incidence is estimated to be 2% to 3% per year. Prevalence rates are approximately 15% to 20%. Female gender and age constitute risk factors for TD. Indeed, prevalence rates have been reported to be as high as 70% in elderly females. No specific treatment exists for TD, however, patients are often initiated on/switched to an atypical antipsychotic because of their lower incidence to cause TD and hopes of suppression.

Typical antipsychotics are usually only indicated for schizophrenia, but are generally effective for mania and psychosis and/or behavioral syndromes ▶

secondary to other mental conditions. Nonpsychiatric uses include Tourette's syndrome, Huntington's disease, and occasionally, intractable hiccups, pruritus, nausea, and vomiting.

These drugs are thought to exert their antipsychotic activity by blocking dopamine D_2 receptors in the mesolimbic dopaminergic pathway. Side effects are often related to their ability to antagonize dopamine receptors in the nigrostriatal and tuberoinfundibular pathways.

Coadministration of two or more antipsychotics does not generally improve clinical response and may increase the potential for adverse effects.

In 2008, the FDA issued a warning regarding increased mortality risk with typical **and** atypical antipsychotic drugs when used in elderly patients with dementia-related psychosis.

Pregnancy Risk Factor C

Lactation Enters breast milk/not recommended (AAP rates "of concern")

Contraindications Hypersensitivity to perphenazine or any component of the formulation (cross-reactivity between phenothiazines may occur); severe CNS depression (comatose or patients receiving large doses of CNS depressants); subcortical brain damage; bone marrow suppression; blood dyscrasias; liver damage

Warnings/Precautions Elderly patients with dementia-related psychosis treated with antipsychotics are at an increased risk of death compared to placebo. An increased incidence of cerebrovascular adverse events (including fatalities) has been reported in elderly patients with dementia-related psychosis. Perphenazine is not approved for this indication.

May cause hypotension. May be sedating, use with caution in disorders where CNS depression is a feature. Use with caution in depressed patients. Use with caution in Parkinson's disease. Caution in patients with hemodynamic instability; predisposition to seizures; severe cardiac, hepatic, renal, or respiratory disease. Esophageal dysmotility and aspiration have been associated with antipsychotic use; use with caution in patients at risk of pneumonia (eg, Alzheimer's disease). Caution in breast cancer or other prolactin-dependent tumors (may elevate prolactin levels). May alter temperature regulation or mask toxicity of other drugs due to antiemetic effects. May alter cardiac conduction - life-threatening arrhythmias have occurred with therapeutic doses of phenothiazines. May cause orthostatic hypotension; use with caution in patients at risk of this effect or those who would tolerate transient hypotensive episodes (cerebrovascular disease, cardiovascular disease, or other medications which may predispose). Check blood counts periodically and discontinue at first signs of blood dyscrasias; use is contraindicated in patients with bone marrow suppression.

Phenothiazines may cause anticholinergic effects (confusion, agitation, constipation, xerostomia, blurred vision, urinary retention); therefore, they should be used with caution in patients with decreased gastrointestinal motility, urinary retention, BPH, xerostomia, or visual problems. Conditions which also may be exacerbated by cholinergic blockade include narrow-angle glaucoma (screening is recommended) and worsening of myasthenia gravis. Relative to other neuroleptics, perphenazine has a low potency of cholinergic blockade. Use with caution in patients with reduced functional alleles of CYP2D6. Poor metabolizers may have higher plasma concentrations at usual doses, increasing risk for adverse reactions.

May cause extrapyramidal reactions (EPS), including pseudoparkinsonism, acute dystonic reactions, akathisia, and tardive dyskinesia (risk of these reactions is moderate-high relative to other neuroleptics). Risk of dystonia (and possibly other EPS) may be greater with increased doses, use of conventional antipsychotics, males, and younger patients.May be associated with neuroleptic malignant syndrome (NMS) or pigmentary retinopathy. May cause photosensitization.

Adverse Reactions Frequency not defined.

Cardiovascular: Bradycardia, cardiac arrest, ECG changes, hyper-/hypotension, orthostatic hypotension, pallor, peripheral edema, sudden death, tachycardia

Central nervous system: Bizarre dreams, catatonic-like states, cerebral edema, dizziness, drowsiness, extrapyramidal symptoms (pseudoparkinsonism, akathisia, dystonias, tardive dyskinesia), faintness, headache, hyperactivity, hyperpyrexia, impairment of temperature regulation, insomnia, lethargy, neuroleptic malignant syndrome (NMS), nocturnal confusion, paradoxical excitement, paranoid reactions, restlessness, seizure

Dermatologic: Discoloration of skin (blue-gray), photosensitivity, rash

Endocrine & metabolic: Amenorrhea, breast enlargement, hyper-/hypoglycemia, galactorrhea, lactation, libido changes, gynecomastia, menstrual irregularity, parotid swelling (rare), SIADH

Gastrointestinal: Adynamic ileus, anorexia, appetite increased, constipation, diarrhea, fecal impaction, obstipation, nausea, salivation, stomach pain, vomiting, weight gain, xerostomia

Genitourinary: Bladder paralysis, ejaculatory disturbances, incontinence, polyuria, priapism, urinary retention

Hematologic: Agranulocytosis, eosinophilia, hemolytic anemia, leukopenia, pancytopenia, thrombocytopenic purpura

Hepatic: Hepatotoxicity, jaundice

Neuromuscular & skeletal: Muscle weakness, tremor

Ocular: Blurred vision, cornea and lens changes, epithelial keratopathies, glaucoma, mydriasis, myosis, pigmentary photophobia, retinopathy

Renal: Glycosuria

Respiratory: Nasal congestion

Miscellaneous: Allergic reactions, diaphoresis, systemic lupus erythematosus-like syndrome

Metabolism/Transport Effects Substrate of CYP1A2 (minor), 2C9 (minor), 2C19 (minor), 2D6 (major), 3A4 (minor); **Inhibits** CYP1A2 (weak), 2D6 (weak)

Drug Interactions

Acetylcholinesterase Inhibitors (Central): May enhance the neurotoxic (central) effect of Antipsychotics. Severe extrapyramidal symptoms have occurred in some patients. *Risk C: Monitor therapy*

Alcohol (Ethyl): CNS Depressants may enhance the CNS depressant effect of Alcohol (Ethyl). *Risk C: Monitor therapy*

Amphetamines: Antipsychotics may diminish the stimulatory effect of Amphetamines. *Risk C: Monitor therapy*

Analgesics (Opioid): Antipsychotic Agents (Phenothiazines) may enhance the hypotensive effect of Analgesics (Opioid). *Risk C: Monitor therapy*

Antacids: May decrease the absorption of Antipsychotic Agents (Phenothiazines). *Risk C: Monitor therapy*

Anticholinergics: May enhance the adverse/toxic effect of other Anticholinergics. **Exceptions:** Paliperidone. *Risk C: Monitor therapy*

Antimalarial Agents: May increase the serum concentration of Antipsychotic Agents (Phenothiazines). *Risk C: Monitor therapy*

Anti-Parkinson's Agents (Dopamine Agonist): Antipsychotics (Typical) may diminish the therapeutic effect of Anti-Parkinson's Agents (Dopamine Agonist). *Risk D: Consider therapy modification*

Beta-Blockers: Antipsychotic Agents (Phenothiazines) may enhance the hypotensive effect of Beta-Blockers. Beta-Blockers may decrease the metabolism of Antipsychotic Agents (Phenothiazines). Antipsychotic Agents (Phenothiazines) may decrease the metabolism of Beta-Blockers. **Exceptions:** Atenolol; Levobunolol; Metipranolol; Nadolol. *Risk C: Monitor therapy*

CNS Depressants: May enhance the adverse/toxic effect of other CNS Depressants. *Risk C: Monitor therapy*

CYP2D6 Inhibitors (Moderate): May decrease the metabolism of CYP2D6 Substrates. *Risk C: Monitor therapy*

CYP2D6 Inhibitors (Strong): May decrease the metabolism of CYP2D6 Substrates. *Risk D: Consider therapy modification*

Darunavir: May increase the serum concentration of CYP2D6 Substrates. *Risk C: Monitor therapy*

Lithium formulations: May enhance the neurotoxic effect of Antipsychotics. Lithium formulations may decrease the serum concentration of Antipsychotics. Specifically noted with chlorpromazine. *Risk C: Monitor therapy*

Pramlintide: May enhance the anticholinergic effect of Anticholinergics. These effects are specific to the GI tract. *Risk D: Consider therapy modification*

Tetrabenazine: May enhance the adverse/toxic effect of Antipsychotics. *Risk C: Monitor therapy*

Ethanol/Nutrition/Herb Interactions

Ethanol: Avoid ethanol (may increase CNS depression).

Herb/Nutraceutical: Avoid kava kava, gotu kola, valerian, St John's wort (may increase CNS depression).

Stability Store at controlled room temperature of 20°C to 25°C (68°F to 77°F). Protect from light.

Mechanism of Action Perphenazine is a piperazine phenothiazine antipsychotic which blocks postsynaptic mesolimbic dopaminergic receptors in the brain; exhibits alpha-adrenergic blocking effect and depresses the release of hypothalamic and hypophyseal hormones

Pharmacodynamics/Kinetics

Absorption: Oral: Well absorbed

Distribution: Crosses placenta

Metabolism: Extensively hepatic to metabolites via sulfoxidation, hydroxylation, dealkylation, and glucuronidation

Half-life elimination: Perphenazine: 9-12 hours; 7-hydroxyperphenazine: 10-19 hours

Time to peak, serum: Perphenazine: 1-3 hours; 7-hydroxyperphenazine: 2-4 hours

Excretion: Urine and feces

Dosage Oral: Adults:

Schizophrenia/psychoses:

Nonhospitalized: Initial: 4-8 mg 3 times/day; reduce dose as soon as possible to minimum effective dosage (maximum: 64 mg/day)

Hospitalized: 8-16 mg 2-4 times/day (maximum: 64 mg/day)

Nausea/vomiting: 8-16 mg/day in divided doses (maximum: 24 mg/day)

Elderly: Behavioral symptoms associated with dementia (unlabeled use): Initial: 2-4 mg 1-2 times/day; increase at 4- to 7-day intervals by 2-4 mg/day. Increase dose intervals (bid, tid, etc) as necessary to control behavior response or side effects. Maximum daily dose: 32 mg; gradual increase (titration) and bedtime administration may prevent some side effects or decrease their severity.

Hemodialysis: Not dialyzable (0% to 5%)

Dosing adjustment in hepatic impairment: Dosage reductions should be considered in patients with liver disease although no specific guidelines are available

Monitoring Parameters Vital signs; lipid profile, fasting blood glucose/Hgb A_{1c}, baseline liver and kidney function, CBC prior to and periodically during therapy; BMI; mental status, abnormal involuntary movement scale (AIMS), extrapyramidal symptoms (EPS)

Reference Range 2-6 nmol/L

Dosage Forms Excipient information presented when available (limited, particularly for generics); consult specific product labeling.

Tablet: 2 mg, 4 mg, 8 mg, 16 mg

- **Perphenazine and Amitriptyline Hydrochloride** *see* Amitriptyline and Perphenazine *on page 98*
- **Persantine®** *see* Dipyridamole *on page 488*
- **Pethidine Hydrochloride** *see* Meperidine *on page 986*
- **Pexeva®** *see* PARoxetine *on page 1226*
- **PFA** *see* Foscarnet *on page 690*
- **Pfizerpen®** *see* Penicillin G, Parenteral, Aqueous *on page 1241*
- **PGE_1** *see* Alprostadil *on page 77*
- **PGE_2** *see* Dinoprostone *on page 480*
- **PGI_2** *see* Epoprostenol *on page 547*
- **PGX** *see* Epoprostenol *on page 547*
- **Phanasin® [OTC]** *see* GuaiFENesin *on page 737*
- **Phanasin® Diabetic Choice [OTC]** *see* GuaiFENesin *on page 737*
- **Phanatuss® DM [OTC]** *see* Guaifenesin and Dextromethorphan *on page 739*
- **Phanatuss® HC [DSC]** *see* Hydrocodone and Guaifenesin *on page 779*
- **Phenabid®** *see* Chlorpheniramine and Phenylephrine *on page 323*
- **Phenabid DM®** *see* Chlorpheniramine, Phenylephrine, and Dextromethorphan *on page 327*
- **Phenadoz™** *see* Promethazine *on page 1347*
- **Phenagesic [OTC]** *see* Acetaminophen and Phenyltoloxamine *on page 36*
- **PhenaVent™ [DSC]** *see* Guaifenesin and Phenylephrine *on page 742*
- **PhenaVent™ D [DSC]** *see* Guaifenesin and Phenylephrine *on page 742*
- **PhenaVent™ LA [DSC]** *see* Guaifenesin and Phenylephrine *on page 742*
- **PhenaVent™ Ped [DSC]** *see* Guaifenesin and Phenylephrine *on page 742*

Phenazopyridine (fen az oh PEER i deen)

Medication Safety Issues

Sound-alike/look-alike issues:

Phenazopyridine may be confused with phenoxybenzamine

Pyridium® may be confused with Dyrenium®, Perdiem®, pyridoxine, pyrithione

U.S. Brand Names AZO-Gesic® [OTC]; AZO-Standard® Maximum Strength [OTC]; AZO-Standard® [OTC]; Baridium® [OTC]; Prodium® [OTC]; Pyridium®; ReAzo [OTC]; Uristat® [OTC] [DSC]; UTI Relief® [OTC]

Canadian Brand Names Phenazo™

Mexican Brand Names Pirimir

Index Terms Phenazopyridine Hydrochloride; Phenylazo Diamino Pyridine Hydrochloride

Pharmacologic Category Analgesic, Urinary

Use Symptomatic relief of urinary burning, itching, frequency and urgency in association with urinary tract infection or following urologic procedures

Effect on Mental Status May cause dizziness

Effect on Psychiatric Treatment None reported

Dosage Summary

Oral:

Children: 12 mg/kg/day in 3 divided doses after meals

Adults: 100-200 mg 3 times/day after meals

Dosage Forms Excipient information presented when available (limited, particularly for generics); consult specific product labeling. [DSC] = Discontinued product

Tablet, as hydrochloride: 100 mg, 200 mg

AZO-Gesic®, Prodium®, ReAzo; Uristat® [DSC]: 95 mg

AZO-Standard®: 95 mg [gluten free]

AZO Standard® Maximum Strength: 97.5 mg [gluten free]

Baridium®, UTI Relief®: 97.2 mg

Pyridium®: 100 mg, 200 mg

◆ **Phenazopyridine Hydrochloride** *see* Phenazopyridine *on page 1258*

◆ **Phencarb GG** *see* Carbetapentane, Guaifenesin, and Phenylephrine *on page 274*

Phendimetrazine (fen dye ME tra zeen)

Medication Safety Issues

Sound-alike/look-alike issues:

Bontril PDM® may be confused with Bentyl®

U.S. Brand Names Bontril PDM®; Bontril® Slow-Release

Canadian Brand Names Bontril®; Plegine®; Statobex®

Index Terms Phendimetrazine Tartrate

Pharmacologic Category Anorexiant; Sympathomimetic

Generic Available Yes

Use Short-term (few weeks) adjunct in exogenous obesity

Restrictions C-III

Pharmacotherapy for weight loss is recommended only for obese patients with a body mass index ≥30 kg/m^2, or ≥27 kg/m^2 in the presence of other risk factors such as hypertension, diabetes, and/or dyslipidemia or a high waist circumference; therapy should be used in conjunction with a comprehensive weight management program. Rule out organic causes of obesity (eg, untreated hypothyroidism) prior to use.

Note: Phendimetrazine is not approved for long-term use. The limited usefulness of medications in this class should be weighed against possible risks associated with their use. Consult weight loss guidelines for current pharmacotherapy recommendations.

Pregnancy Risk Factor C

Pregnancy Considerations Reproduction studies have not been conducted.

Lactation Excretion in breast milk unknown/not recommended

Contraindications Hypersensitivity or idiosyncrasy to phendimetrazine or other sympathomimetic amines or any component of the formulation; advanced arteriosclerosis, symptomatic cardiovascular disease; pulmonary hypertension; moderate and severe hypertension; hyperthyroidism; glaucoma; highly nervous or agitated states, history of drug abuse; use with other CNS stimulants; during or within 14 days following MAO inhibitor therapy

Warnings/Precautions The use of some anorexigens has been associated with the development of valvular heart disease. Avoid stimulants in patients with known serious structural cardiac abnormalities, cardiomyopathy, serious heart rhythm abnormalities, or other serious cardiac problems that could increase the risk of sudden death that these conditions alone carry. Caution should be used in patients with mild hypertension and other cardiovascular conditions that might be exacerbated by increases in blood pressure or heart rate.

Primary pulmonary hypertension (PPH), a rare and frequently fatal disease of the lungs, has been found to occur with increased frequency in patients receiving some anorexigens.

Use caution with diabetes; antidiabetic agent requirements may be altered with anorexigens and concomitant dietary restrictions. Stimulants may unmask tics in individuals with coexisting Tourette's syndrome. Use caution with seizure disorders. Phendimetrazine is pharmacologically related to the amphetamines, which have a high abuse potential; prolonged use may lead to dependency. Prescriptions should be written for the smallest quantity consistent with good patient care to minimize possibility of overdose. Amphetamines may impair the ability to engage in potentially hazardous activities.

Not recommended for use in patients who used other anorectic agents within the past year. Discontinue if satisfactory weight loss has not occurred within the first 4 weeks of treatment, or if tolerance develops. Safety and efficacy have not been established for use with other weight loss medications including over-the-counter or herbal products. Safety and efficacy have not been established in children.

Adverse Reactions Frequency not defined.

Cardiovascular: Flushing, hypertension, palpitation, tachycardia

Central nervous system: Agitation, dizziness, headache, insomnia, overstimulation, psychosis, restlessness

Endocrine & metabolic: Changes in libido

Gastrointestinal: Constipation, diarrhea, nausea, stomach pain, xerostomia

Genitourinary: Dysuria, urinary frequency

Neuromuscular & skeletal: Tremor

Ocular: Blurred vision, mydriasis

Miscellaneous: Diaphoresis, tachyphylaxis

Postmarketing and/or case reports: Dilated cardiomyopathy

Drug Interactions

Alkalinizing Agents: May decrease the excretion of Amphetamines. *Risk D: Consider therapy modification*

Ammonium Chloride: May decrease the serum concentration of Amphetamines. This effect is likely due to an enhanced excretion of amphetamines in the urine. *Risk C: Monitor therapy*

Analgesics (Opioid): Amphetamines may enhance the analgesic effect of Analgesics (Opioid). *Risk C: Monitor therapy*

Antacids: May decrease the excretion of Amphetamines. *Risk C: Monitor therapy*

Antihistamines: Amphetamines may diminish the sedative effect of Antihistamines. *Risk C: Monitor therapy*

Antipsychotics: May diminish the stimulatory effect of Amphetamines. *Risk C: Monitor therapy*

Cannabinoids: May enhance the tachycardic effect of Sympathomimetics. *Risk C: Monitor therapy*

Carbonic Anhydrase Inhibitors: May decrease the excretion of Amphetamines. **Exceptions:** Brinzolamide; Dorzolamide. *Risk C: Monitor therapy*

Ethosuximide: Amphetamines may diminish the therapeutic effect of Ethosuximide. Amphetamines may decrease the serum concentration of Ethosuximide. *Risk C: Monitor therapy*

Gastrointestinal Acidifying Agents: May decrease the serum concentration of Amphetamines. *Risk C: Monitor therapy*

Lithium: May diminish the stimulatory effect of Amphetamines. *Risk C: Monitor therapy*

MAO Inhibitors: May enhance the hypertensive effect of Amphetamines. *Risk X: Avoid combination*

Methenamine: May decrease the serum concentration of Amphetamines. This effect is likely due to an enhanced excretion of amphetamines in the urine. *Risk C: Monitor therapy*

PHENobarbital: Amphetamines may decrease the serum concentration of PHENobarbital. *Risk C: Monitor therapy*

Phenytoin: Amphetamines may decrease the serum concentration of Phenytoin. *Risk C: Monitor therapy*

Sympathomimetics: May enhance the adverse/toxic effect of other Sympathomimetics. *Risk C: Monitor therapy*

Tricyclic Antidepressants: May enhance the stimulatory effect of Amphetamines. Tricyclic Antidepressants may also potentiate the cardiovascular effects of Amphetamines. *Risk C: Monitor therapy*

Mechanism of Action Phendimetrazine is a sympathomimetic amine with pharmacologic properties similar to the amphetamines. The mechanism of action in reducing appetite appears to be secondary to CNS effects, including stimulation of the hypothalamus to release norepinephrine.

Pharmacodynamics/Kinetics
Metabolism: Forms 2 metabolites
Half-life elimination: Bontril® PDM: ~2 hours; Bontril® Slow Release: ~10 hours
Excretion: Urine

Dosage Adults: Oral:
Capsule: 105 mg once daily in the morning before breakfast
Tablet: 17.5-35 mg 2 or 3 times daily, 1 hour before meals (maximum: 70 mg 3 times/day)

Dietary Considerations Most effective when combined with a low calorie diet and behavior modification counseling.

Administration
Capsule: Administer 30-60 minutes before morning meal
Tablet: Administer 1 hour before meals

Monitoring Parameters Baseline cardiac evaluation (for preexisting valvular heart disease, pulmonary hypertension); echocardiogram during therapy; weight, waist circumference; blood pressure

Reference Range
Adult classification of weight by BMI (kg/m^2):
Underweight: <18.5
Normal: 18.5-24.9
Overweight: 25-29.9
Obese, class I: 30-34.9
Obese, class II: 35-39.9
Extreme obesity (class III): ≥40
Waist circumference: In adults with a BMI of 25-34.9 kg/m^2, high-risk waist circumference is defined as:
Men >102 cm (>40 in)
Women >88 cm (>35 in)

Dosage Forms Excipient information presented when available (limited, particularly for generics); consult specific product labeling.
Capsule, slow release, as tartrate: 105 mg
Bontril® Slow Release: 105 mg
Tablet, as tartrate: 35 mg
Bontril PDM®: 35 mg

◆ **Phendimetrazine Tartrate** *see* Phendimetrazine *on page 1259*

Phenelzine (FEN el zeen)

Medication Safety Issues
Sound-alike/look-alike issues:
Phenelzine may be confused with phenytoin
Nardil® may be confused with Norinyl®

Related Information
Antidepressant Agents *on page 1760*
Tyramine Content of Foods *on page 1848*

U.S. Brand Names Nardil®

Canadian Brand Names Nardil®

Index Terms Phenelzine Sulfate

Pharmacologic Category Antidepressant, Monoamine Oxidase Inhibitor

Generic Available No

Use Symptomatic treatment of atypical, nonendogenous, or neurotic depression

Unlabeled/Investigational Use Selective mutism

Mental Health Comment Not commonly used due to a required low tyramine diet and drug-drug interactions. It is estimated that 20 mg of tranylcypromine = 40 mg of isocarboxazid = 45 mg phenelzine. Phenelzine and isocarboxazid are hydrazine MAO inhibitors and tranylcypromine is a nonhydrazine. These drugs produce irreversible inhibition of MAO inhibitors. The half-life for regeneration is 2-3 days. Therefore, a 2-week period is required when switching from an MAO inhibitor to another antidepressant.

While hypertension and hypertensive crisis are risks associated with MAO inhibitor therapy, orthostatic hypotension may also occur. Orthostasis associated with MAO inhibitor therapy is not related to $alpha_1$-adrenergic receptor blockade. The "false transmitter" concept is used to explain this side effect. This concept states that MAO inhibitors promote gradual accumulation in sympathetic nerve ending of amines lacking direct sympathomimetic activity (octopamine) at the expense of the normal synaptic transmitter, norepinephrine. Since octopamine has little ability to activate either alpha- or beta-adrenergic receptors, a functional impairment of sympathetic neurotransmission occurs.

The MAO inhibitors are usually reserved for patients who do not tolerate or respond to other antidepressants. The brain activity of monoamine oxidase increases with age and even more so in patients with Alzheimer's disease. Therefore, the MAO inhibitors may have an increased role in patients with Alzheimer's disease who are depressed. Phenelzine is less stimulating than tranylcypromine.

Restrictions An FDA-approved medication guide concerning the use of antidepressants in children, adolescents, and young adults must be distributed when dispensing an outpatient prescription (new or refill) where this medication is to be used without direct supervision of a healthcare provider. Medication guides are available at http://www.fda.gov/cder/Offices/ODS/medication_guides.htm. Dispense to parents or guardians of children and adolescents receiving this medication.

Pregnancy Risk Factor C

Lactation Excretion in breast milk unknown/not recommended

Contraindications Hypersensitivity to phenelzine or any component of the formulation; congestive heart failure; pheochromocytoma; abnormal liver function tests or history of hepatic disease; renal disease or severe renal impairment

Concurrent use of sympathomimetics (including amphetamines, cocaine, dopamine, epinephrine, methylphenidate, norepinephrine, or phenylephrine) and related compounds (methyldopa, levodopa, phenylalanine, tryptophan, or tyrosine), as well as ophthalmic $alpha_2$-agonists (apraclonidine, brimonidine); may result in hypertensive reactions

CNS depressants, cyclobenzaprine, dextromethorphan, ethanol, meperidine, bupropion, or buspirone; may result in delirium, excitation, hyperpyrexia, seizures, and coma.

At least 2 weeks should elapse between the discontinuation of serotoninergic agents (including SNRIs, SSRIs, and tricyclics) and other MAO inhibitors and the initiation of phenelzine. At least 5 weeks should elapse between the discontinuation of fluoxetine and the initiation of phenelzine. In all cases, a sufficient amount of time must be allowed for the clearance of the serotoninergic agent and any active metabolites prior to the initiation of phenelzine.

At least 2 weeks should elapse between the discontinuation of phenelzine and the initiation of the following agents: Serotoninergic agents (including SNRIs, SSRIs, fluoxetine, and tricyclics), bupropion, buspirone, and other antidepressants.

General anesthesia, spinal anesthesia (hypotension may be exaggerated). Use caution with local anesthetics containing sympathomimetic agents. Phenelzine should be discontinued ≥10 days prior to elective surgery.

Foods high in tyramine or dopamine content; foods and/or supplements containing tyrosine, phenylalanine, tryptophan, or caffeine; may result in hypertensive reactions

Warnings/Precautions **[U.S. Boxed Warning]: Antidepressants increase the risk of suicidal thinking and behavior in children, adolescents, and young adults (18-24 years of age) with major depressive disorder (MDD) and other psychiatric disorders;** consider risk prior to prescribing. Short-term studies did not show an increased risk in patients >24 years of age and showed a decreased risk in patients ≥65 years. Closely monitor for clinical worsening, suicidality, or unusual changes in behavior; the patient's family or caregiver should be instructed to closely observe the patient and communicate condition with healthcare provider. Such observation would generally include at least weekly face-to-face contact with patients or their family members or caregivers during the first 4 weeks of treatment, then every other week visits for the next 4 weeks, then at 12 weeks, and as clinically indicated beyond 12 weeks. Additional contact by telephone may be appropriate between face-to-face visits. Adults treated with antidepressants should be observed similarly for clinical worsening and suicidality, especially during the initial few months of a course of drug therapy, or at times of dose changes, either increases or decreases. A medication guide should be dispensed with each prescription. Phenelzine is not generally considered a first-line agent for the treatment of depression; phenelzine is typically used in patients who have failed to respond to other treatments. **Phenelzine is not FDA approved for the treatment of depression in children ≤16 years of age.**

The possibility of a suicide attempt is inherent in major depression and may persist until remission occurs. Monitor for worsening of depression or suicidality, especially during initiation of therapy (generally first 1-2 months) or with dose increases or decreases. Worsening depression and severe abrupt suicidality that are not part of the presenting symptoms may require discontinuation or modification of drug therapy. Use caution in high-risk patients during initiation of therapy. Prescriptions should be written for the smallest quantity consistent with good patient care. The patient's family or caregiver should be alerted to monitor patients for the emergence of suicidality and associated behaviors such as anxiety, agitation, panic attacks, insomnia, irritability, hostility, impulsivity, akathisia, hypomania, and mania; patients should be instructed to notify their healthcare provider if any of these symptoms or worsening depression occur.

May worsen psychosis in some patients or precipitate a shift to mania or hypomania in patients with bipolar disorder. Monotherapy in patients with bipolar disorder should be avoided. Patients presenting with depressive symptoms should be screened for bipolar disorder. Phenelzine is not FDA approved for the treatment of bipolar depression.

Sensitization to the effects of insulin may occur; monitor blood glucose closely in patients with diabetes. Use with caution in patients who have glaucoma, or hyperthyroidism. Hypertensive crisis may occur with tyramine-, tryptophan-, or dopamine-containing foods. Phentolamine is recommended for the treatment of hypertensive crisis. Do not use with other MAO inhibitors or antidepressants. Avoid products containing sympathomimetic stimulants or dextromethorphan. Concurrent use with antihypertensive agents may lead to exaggeration of hypotensive effects. May cause orthostatic hypotension; use with caution in patients with hypotension or patients who would not tolerate transient hypotensive episodes (cardiovascular or cerebrovascular disease); effects may be additive with other agents which cause orthostasis. Use with caution in patients at risk of seizures, or in patients receiving other drugs which may lower seizure threshold. Discontinue at least 48 hours prior to myelography. May increase the risks associated with electroconvulsive therapy. Consider discontinuing, when possible, prior to elective surgery.

Adverse Reactions Frequency not defined.

Cardiovascular: Edema, orthostatic hypotension

Central nervous system: Anxiety (acute), ataxia, coma, delirium, dizziness, drowsiness, fatigue, fever, headache, hyper-reflexia, mania, seizure, sleep disturbances, twitching

Dermatologic: Pruritus, rash

Endocrine & metabolic: Decreased sexual ability (anorgasmia, ejaculatory disturbances, impotence), hypermetabolic syndrome, hypernatremia

Gastrointestinal: Constipation, weight gain, xerostomia

Genitourinary: Urinary retention

Hematologic: Leukopenia

Hepatic: Hepatitis, jaundice, necrotizing hepatocellular necrosis (rare)

Neuromuscular & skeletal: Lupus-like syndrome, myoclonia, tremor, weakness

Ocular: Blurred vision, glaucoma

Miscellaneous: Diaphoresis, transient cardiac or respiratory depression (following ECT), withdrawal syndrome (nausea, vomiting, malaise)

Respiratory: Edema (glottis)

Drug Interactions

Acetylcholinesterase Inhibitors (Central): Anticholinergics may diminish the therapeutic effect of Acetylcholinesterase Inhibitors (Central). Acetylcholinesterase Inhibitors (Central) may diminish the therapeutic effect of Anticholinergics. If the anticholinergic action is a side effect of the agent, the result may be beneficial. *Risk C: Monitor therapy*

Alcohol (Ethyl): CNS Depressants may enhance the CNS depressant effect of Alcohol (Ethyl). *Risk C: Monitor therapy*

Alpha-/Beta-Agonists (Direct-Acting): MAO Inhibitors may enhance the vasopressor effect of Alpha-/Beta-Agonists (Direct-Acting). Primarily with oral administration of phenylephrine. **Exceptions:** Dipivefrin. *Risk D: Consider therapy modification*

Alpha-/Beta-Agonists (Indirect-Acting): MAO Inhibitors may enhance the hypertensive effect of Alpha-/Beta-Agonists (Indirect-Acting). *Risk X: Avoid combination*

Alpha1-Agonists: MAO Inhibitors may enhance the hypertensive effect of Alpha1-Agonists. *Risk X: Avoid combination*

Alpha2-Agonists (Ophthalmic): MAO Inhibitors may enhance the hypertensive effect of Alpha2-Agonists (Ophthalmic). *Risk X: Avoid combination*

Altretamine: May enhance the orthostatic effect of MAO Inhibitors. *Risk C: Monitor therapy*

Amphetamines: MAO Inhibitors may enhance the hypertensive effect of Amphetamines. *Risk X: Avoid combination*

Anilidopiperidine Opioids: May enhance the serotonergic effect of MAO Inhibitors. This could result in serotonin syndrome. Management: Avoid use of fentanyl (and other anilidopiperidine opioids when possible) in patients who have used a monoamine oxidase inhibitor within the past 14 days due to reports of unpredictable but severe adverse effects. *Risk D: Consider therapy modification*

Anticholinergics: May enhance the adverse/toxic effect of other Anticholinergics. **Exceptions:** Paliperidone. *Risk C: Monitor therapy*

Antidepressants (Serotonin/Norepinephrine Reuptake Inhibitor): MAO Inhibitors may enhance the serotonergic effect of Antidepressants (Serotonin/Norepinephrine Reuptake Inhibitor). This may cause serotonin syndrome. *Risk X: Avoid combination*

Atomoxetine: MAO Inhibitors may enhance the neurotoxic (central) effect of Atomoxetine. *Risk X: Avoid combination*

Beta2-Agonists: MAO Inhibitors may enhance the adverse/toxic effect of Beta2-Agonists. *Risk C: Monitor therapy*

BuPROPion: MAO Inhibitors may enhance the neurotoxic (central) effect of BuPROPion. *Risk X: Avoid combination*

BusPIRone: May enhance the adverse/toxic effect of MAO Inhibitors. Elevated blood pressure has been reported. *Risk X: Avoid combination*

CNS Depressants: May enhance the adverse/toxic effect of other CNS Depressants. *Risk C: Monitor therapy*

COMT Inhibitors: May enhance the adverse/toxic effect of MAO Inhibitors. *Risk D: Consider therapy modification*

Cyclobenzaprine: May enhance the serotonergic effect of MAO Inhibitors. This could result in serotonin syndrome. *Risk X: Avoid combination*

Dexmethylphenidate: MAO Inhibitors may enhance the hypertensive effect of Dexmethylphenidate. *Risk X: Avoid combination*

Dextromethorphan: MAO Inhibitors may enhance the serotonergic effect of Dextromethorphan. This may cause serotonin syndrome. *Risk X: Avoid combination*

Levodopa: May enhance the adverse/toxic effect of MAO Inhibitors. Of particular concern is the development of hypertensive reactions when levodopa is used with nonselective MAOI. *Risk D: Consider therapy modification*

Linezolid: MAO Inhibitors may enhance the adverse/toxic effect of Linezolid. *Risk X: Avoid combination*

Lithium: MAO Inhibitors may enhance the adverse/toxic effect of Lithium. *Risk C: Monitor therapy*

Maprotiline: May enhance the adverse/toxic effect of MAO Inhibitors. *Risk X: Avoid combination*

Meperidine: MAO Inhibitors may enhance the serotonergic effect of Meperidine. This may cause serotonin syndrome. *Risk X: Avoid combination*

Methyldopa: MAO Inhibitors may enhance the adverse/toxic effect of Methyldopa. *Risk X: Avoid combination*

Methylphenidate: MAO Inhibitors may enhance the hypertensive effect of Methylphenidate. *Risk X: Avoid combination*

Mirtazapine: MAO Inhibitors may enhance the neurotoxic (central) effect of Mirtazapine. *Risk X: Avoid combination*

Pramlintide: May enhance the anticholinergic effect of Anticholinergics. These effects are specific to the GI tract. *Risk D: Consider therapy modification*

Propoxyphene: May enhance the adverse/toxic effect of MAO Inhibitors. Specifically, the risk of serotonin syndrome or other serotonergic adverse events may be increased. *Risk X: Avoid combination*

Rauwolfia Alkaloids: MAO Inhibitors may enhance the adverse/toxic effect of Rauwolfia Alkaloids. Existing MAOI therapy can result in paradoxical effects of added rauwolfia alkaloids (eg, excitation, hypertension). *Risk D: Consider therapy modification*

Selective Serotonin Reuptake Inhibitors: MAO Inhibitors may enhance the serotonergic effect of Selective Serotonin Reuptake Inhibitors. This may cause serotonin syndrome. *Risk X: Avoid combination*

Serotonin 5-HT1D Receptor Agonists: MAO Inhibitors may decrease the metabolism of Serotonin 5-HT1D Receptor Agonists. Management: If MAO inhibitor therapy is required, naratriptan, eletriptan or frovatriptan may be a suitable 5-HT1D agonist to employ. **Exceptions:** Eletriptan; Frovatriptan; Naratriptan. *Risk X: Avoid combination*

Serotonin Modulators: May enhance the adverse/toxic effect of other Serotonin Modulators. The development of serotonin syndrome may occur. *Risk D: Consider therapy modification*

Sibutramine: May enhance the serotonergic effect of Serotonin Modulators. This may cause serotonin syndrome. *Risk X: Avoid combination*

Succinylcholine: Phenelzine may enhance the neuromuscular-blocking effect of Succinylcholine. *Risk D: Consider therapy modification*

Tetrabenazine: May enhance the adverse/toxic effect of MAO Inhibitors. *Risk X: Avoid combination*

TraMADol: May enhance the neuroexcitatory and/or seizure-potentiating effect of MAO Inhibitors. *Risk D: Consider therapy modification*

Tricyclic Antidepressants: MAO Inhibitors may enhance the serotonergic effect of Tricyclic Antidepressants. This may cause serotonin syndrome. *Risk X: Avoid combination*

Ethanol/Nutrition/Herb Interactions

Ethanol: Avoid ethanol (based on CNS depressant effects and potential tyramine content)

Food: Concurrent ingestion of foods rich in tyramine may cause sudden and severe high blood pressure (hypertensive crisis). Avoid tyramine-containing foods with MAO-Is. Food's freshness is also an important concern; improperly stored or spoiled food can create an environment where tyramine concentrations may increase.

Herb/Nutraceuticals: Avoid supplements containing caffeine, tyrosine, tryptophan or phenylalanine. Ingestion of large quantities may increase the risk of severe side effects (eg, hypertensive reactions, serotonin syndrome).

Stability Protect from light.

Mechanism of Action Thought to act by increasing endogenous concentrations of norepinephrine, dopamine, and serotonin through inhibition of the enzyme (monoamine oxidase) responsible for the breakdown of these neurotransmitters

Pharmacodynamics/Kinetics

Onset of action: Therapeutic: 2-4 weeks; geriatric patients receiving an average of 55 mg/day developed a mean platelet MAO activity inhibition of about 85%.

Duration: May continue to have a therapeutic effect and interactions 2 weeks after discontinuing therapy

Absorption: Well absorbed

Metabolism: Oxidized via monoamine oxidase (primary pathway) and acetylation (minor pathway)

Half-life elimination: 11 hours

Excretion: Urine (primarily as metabolites and unchanged drug)

Dosage Oral:

Children: Selective mutism (unlabeled use): 30-60 mg/day

Adults: Depression: 15 mg 3 times/day; may increase to 60-90 mg/day during early phase of treatment, then reduce dose for maintenance therapy slowly after maximum benefit is obtained; takes 2-4 weeks for a significant response to occur

Elderly: Depression: Initial: 7.5 mg/day; increase by 7.5-15 mg/day every 3-4 days as tolerated; usual therapeutic dose: 15-60 mg/day in 3-4 divided doses

Child/Adolescent Considerations Four children 5.5-7 years of age, diagnosed with selective mutism were treated with 30-60 mg/day for 24-60 weeks (Golwyn, 1999).

Golwyn DH and Sevlie CP, "Phenelzine Treatment of Selective Mutism in Four Prepubertal Children," *J Child Adolesc Psychopharmacol*, 1999, 9(2):109-13.

Monitoring Parameters Blood pressure, heart rate; diet, weight; mood (if depressive symptoms), suicidal ideation (especially during the initial months of therapy or when doses are increased or decreased)

Additional Information Pyridoxine deficiency has occurred; symptoms include numbness and edema of hands; may respond to supplementation.

Dosage Forms Excipient information presented when available (limited, particularly for generics); consult specific product labeling.

Tablet: 15 mg

◆ **Phenelzine Sulfate** *see* Phenelzine *on page 1261*

◆ **Phenergan®** *see* Promethazine *on page 1347*

◆ **Pheniramine and Naphazoline** *see* Naphazoline and Pheniramine *on page 1102*

PHENobarbital (fee noe BAR bi tal)

Medication Safety Issues

Sound-alike/look-alike issues:

PHENobarbital may be confused with PENTobarbital

Luminal® may be confused with Tuinal®

Related Information

Anticonvulsants By Seizure Type *on page 1759*

U.S. Brand Names Luminal® Sodium

Canadian Brand Names PMS-Phenobarbital

Mexican Brand Names Alepsal

Index Terms Phenobarbital Sodium; Phenobarbitone; Phenylethylmalonylurea

Pharmacologic Category Anticonvulsant, Barbiturate; Barbiturate

Generic Available Yes

Use Management of generalized tonic-clonic (grand mal) and partial seizures; sedative

Unlabeled/Investigational Use Febrile seizures in children; may also be used for prevention and treatment of neonatal hyperbilirubinemia and lowering of bilirubin in chronic cholestasis; neonatal seizures; management of sedative/hypnotic withdrawal

Restrictions C-IV

Pregnancy Risk Factor D

Pregnancy Considerations Crosses the placenta. Cardiac defect reported; hemorrhagic disease of newborn due to fetal vitamin K depletion may occur; may induce maternal folic acid deficiency; withdrawal symptoms observed in infant following delivery. Epilepsy itself, number of medications, genetic factors, or a combination of these probably influence the teratogenicity of anticonvulsant therapy. Benefit:risk ratio usually favors continued use during pregnancy and breast-feeding.

Lactation Enters breast milk/not recommended (AAP recommends use "with caution")

Contraindications Hypersensitivity to barbiturates or any component of the formulation; marked hepatic impairment; dyspnea or airway obstruction; porphyria; pregnancy

Warnings/Precautions Potential for drug dependency exists, abrupt cessation may precipitate withdrawal, including status epilepticus in epileptic patients. Do not administer to patients in acute pain. Use caution in elderly, debilitated, renally or hepatic dysfunction, and pediatric patients. May cause paradoxical responses, including agitation and hyperactivity, particularly in acute pain and pediatric patients. Use with caution in patients with depression or suicidal tendencies, or in patients with a history of drug abuse. Tolerance, psychological and physical dependence may occur with prolonged use. May cause CNS depression, which may impair physical or mental abilities. Effects with other sedative drugs or ethanol may be potentiated. May cause respiratory depression or hypotension, particularly when administered intravenously. Use with caution in hemodynamically unstable patients (hypovolemic shock, CHF) or patients with respiratory disease. Due to its long half-life and risk of dependence, phenobarbital is not recommended as a sedative in the elderly. Use has been associated with cognitive deficits in children. Use with caution in patients with hypoadrenalism.

Adverse Reactions Frequency not defined.

Cardiovascular: Bradycardia, hypotension, syncope

Central nervous system: Drowsiness, lethargy, CNS excitation or depression, impaired judgment, "hangover" effect, confusion, somnolence, agitation, hyperkinesia, ataxia, nervousness, headache, insomnia, nightmares, hallucinations, anxiety, dizziness

Dermatologic: Rash, exfoliative dermatitis, Stevens-Johnson syndrome

Gastrointestinal: Nausea, vomiting, constipation

Hematologic: Agranulocytosis, thrombocytopenia, megaloblastic anemia

Local: Pain at injection site, thrombophlebitis with I.V. use

Renal: Oliguria

Respiratory: Laryngospasm, respiratory depression, apnea (especially with rapid I.V. use), hypoventilation

Miscellaneous: Gangrene with inadvertent intra-arterial injection

Metabolism/Transport Effects Substrate of CYP2C9 (minor), 2C19 (major), 2E1 (minor); **Induces** CYP1A2 (strong), 2A6 (strong), 2B6 (strong), 2C8 (strong), 2C9 (strong), 3A4 (strong)

Drug Interactions

Acetaminophen: Barbiturates may increase the metabolism of Acetaminophen. This may 1) diminish the effect of acetaminophen; and 2) increase the risk of liver damage. *Risk C: Monitor therapy*

Alcohol (Ethyl): CNS Depressants may enhance the CNS depressant effect of Alcohol (Ethyl). *Risk C: Monitor therapy*

Aminocamptothecin: PHENobarbital may decrease the serum concentration of Aminocamptothecin. *Risk C: Monitor therapy*

Amphetamines: May decrease the serum concentration of PHENobarbital. *Risk C: Monitor therapy*

Bendamustine: CYP1A2 Inducers (Strong) may decrease the serum concentration of Bendamustine. Concentrations of active metabolites may be increased. *Risk C: Monitor therapy*

Beta-Blockers: Barbiturates may decrease the serum concentration of Beta-Blockers. **Exceptions:** Atenolol; Levobunolol; Metipranolol; Nadolol. *Risk C: Monitor therapy*

Calcium Channel Blockers: Barbiturates may increase the metabolism of Calcium Channel Blockers. **Exceptions:** Clevidipine. *Risk D: Consider therapy modification*

Carbonic Anhydrase Inhibitors: May enhance the adverse/toxic effect of Anticonvulsants (Barbiturate). Specifically, osteomalacia and rickets. **Exceptions:** Brinzolamide; Dorzolamide. *Risk C: Monitor therapy*

Chloramphenicol: May decrease the metabolism of Barbiturates. Barbiturates may increase the metabolism of Chloramphenicol. *Risk D: Consider therapy modification*

CNS Depressants: May enhance the adverse/toxic effect of other CNS Depressants. *Risk C: Monitor therapy*

Contraceptive (Progestins): Barbiturates may diminish the therapeutic effect of Contraceptive (Progestins). Contraceptive failure is possible. *Risk D: Consider therapy modification*

Corticosteroids (Systemic): Barbiturates may increase the metabolism of Corticosteroids (Systemic). *Risk C: Monitor therapy*

CycloSPORINE: Barbiturates may increase the metabolism of CycloSPORINE. *Risk D: Consider therapy modification*

CYP1A2 Substrates: CYP1A2 Inducers (Strong) may increase the metabolism of CYP1A2 Substrates. *Risk C: Monitor therapy*

CYP2A6 Substrates: CYP2A6 Inducers (Strong) may increase the metabolism of CYP2A6 Substrates. *Risk C: Monitor therapy*

CYP2B6 Substrates: CYP2B6 Inducers (Strong) may increase the metabolism of CYP2B6 Substrates. *Risk C: Monitor therapy*

CYP2C19 Inducers (Strong): May increase the metabolism of CYP2C19 Substrates. *Risk C: Monitor therapy*

CYP2C19 Inhibitors (Moderate): May decrease the metabolism of CYP2C19 Substrates. *Risk C: Monitor therapy*

CYP2C19 Inhibitors (Strong): May decrease the metabolism of CYP2C19 Substrates. *Risk D: Consider therapy modification*

CYP2C8 Substrates (High risk): CYP2C8 Inducers (Highly Effective) may increase the metabolism of CYP2C8 Substrates (High risk). *Risk C: Monitor therapy*

CYP2C9 Substrates (High risk): CYP2C9 Inducers (Highly Effective) may increase the metabolism of CYP2C9 Substrates (High risk). *Risk C: Monitor therapy*

CYP3A4 Substrates: CYP3A4 Inducers (Strong) may increase the metabolism of CYP3A4 Substrates. *Risk C: Monitor therapy*

Darunavir: PHENobarbital may decrease the serum concentration of Darunavir. *Risk X: Avoid combination*

Disopyramide: Barbiturates may increase the metabolism of Disopyramide. *Risk D: Consider therapy modification*

Doxycycline: Barbiturates may decrease the serum concentration of Doxycycline. *Risk D: Consider therapy modification*

Etoposide: Barbiturates may increase the metabolism of Etoposide. *Risk C: Monitor therapy*

Etoposide Phosphate: Barbiturates may decrease the serum concentration of Etoposide Phosphate. Barbiturates may increase the metabolism, via CYP isoenzymes, of etoposide phosphate. *Risk C: Monitor therapy*

Etravirine: PHENobarbital may decrease the serum concentration of Etravirine. Management: The manufacturer of etravirine states these drugs should not be used in combination *Risk X: Avoid combination*

Felbamate: May increase the serum concentration of Barbiturates. *Risk C: Monitor therapy*

Folic Acid: May decrease the serum concentration of PHENobarbital. *Risk C: Monitor therapy*

Griseofulvin: Barbiturates may decrease the absorption of Griseofulvin. *Risk D: Consider therapy modification*

Ketorolac: May diminish the therapeutic effect of Anticonvulsants. *Risk C: Monitor therapy*

Lacosamide: PHENobarbital may decrease the serum concentration of Lacosamide. *Risk C: Monitor therapy*

LamoTRIgine: Barbiturates may increase the metabolism of LamoTRIgine. *Risk D: Consider therapy modification*

Leucovorin-Levoleucovorin: May decrease the serum concentration of PHENobarbital. *Risk C: Monitor therapy*

Maraviroc: CYP3A4 Inducers may decrease the serum concentration of Maraviroc. *Risk D: Consider therapy modification*

Mefloquine: May diminish the therapeutic effect of Anticonvulsants. Mefloquine may decrease the serum concentration of Anticonvulsants. Management: Mefloquine is contraindicated in persons with a history of convulsions. If anticonvulsant is being used for another indication monitor response to treatment closely, as concurrent mefloquine may decrease response to treatment. *Risk D: Consider therapy modification*

Meperidine: Barbiturates may enhance the CNS depressant effect of Meperidine. *Risk C: Monitor therapy*

Methadone: Barbiturates may increase the metabolism of Methadone. *Risk D: Consider therapy modification*

Methylfolate: May decrease the serum concentration of PHENobarbital. *Risk C: Monitor therapy*

Nilotinib: CYP3A4 Inducers (Strong) may decrease the serum concentration of Nilotinib. *Risk X: Avoid combination*

Oral Contraceptive (Estrogens): Barbiturates may diminish the therapeutic effect of Oral Contraceptive (Estrogens). Contraceptive failure is possible. *Risk D: Consider therapy modification*

OXcarbazepine: PHENobarbital may decrease the serum concentration of OXcarbazepine. *Risk C: Monitor therapy*

Primidone: May enhance the adverse/toxic effect of Barbiturates. Primidone is converted to phenobarbital, and thus becomes additive with existing barbiturate therapy. *Risk C: Monitor therapy*

Propafenone: Barbiturates may increase the metabolism of Propafenone. *Risk D: Consider therapy modification*

Pyridoxine: May increase the metabolism of Barbiturates. Apparent in high pyridoxine doses (eg, 200 mg/day) *Risk C: Monitor therapy*

QuiNIDine: Barbiturates may increase the metabolism of QuiNIDine. *Risk D: Consider therapy modification*

Ranolazine: CYP3A4 Inducers (Strong) may decrease the serum concentration of Ranolazine. *Risk X: Avoid combination*

Rifamycin Derivatives: May increase the metabolism of Barbiturates. *Risk C: Monitor therapy*

Sorafenib: CYP3A4 Inducers (Strong) may decrease the serum concentration of Sorafenib. *Risk D: Consider therapy modification*

Teniposide: Barbiturates may increase the metabolism of Teniposide. *Risk C: Monitor therapy*

Theophylline Derivatives: Barbiturates may increase the metabolism of Theophylline Derivatives. **Exceptions:** Dyphylline. *Risk C: Monitor therapy*

Tipranavir: PHENobarbital may decrease the serum concentration of Tipranavir. Tipranavir may decrease the serum concentration of PHENobarbital. *Risk D: Consider therapy modification*

Tricyclic Antidepressants: Barbiturates may increase the metabolism of Tricyclic Antidepressants. *Risk D: Consider therapy modification*

Valproic Acid: May decrease the metabolism of Barbiturates. Barbiturates may decrease the serum concentration of Valproic Acid. *Risk C: Monitor therapy*

Vitamin K Antagonists (eg, warfarin): Barbiturates may increase the metabolism of Vitamin K Antagonists. *Risk D: Consider therapy modification*

Voriconazole: Barbiturates may decrease the serum concentration of Voriconazole. *Risk X: Avoid combination*

Ethanol/Nutrition/Herb Interactions

Ethanol: Avoid ethanol (may increase CNS depression).

Food: May cause decrease in vitamin D and calcium.

Herb/Nutraceutical: Avoid evening primrose (seizure threshold decreased). Avoid valerian, St John's wort, kava kava, gotu kola (may increase CNS depression).

Stability Protect elixir from light. Not stable in aqueous solutions; use only clear solutions. Do not add to acidic solutions; precipitation may occur.

Mechanism of Action Long-acting barbiturate with sedative, hypnotic, and anticonvulsant properties. Barbiturates depress the sensory cortex, decrease motor activity, alter cerebellar function, and produce drowsiness, sedation, and hypnosis. In high doses, barbiturates exhibit anticonvulsant activity; barbiturates produce dose-dependent respiratory depression.

Pharmacodynamics/Kinetics

Onset of action: Oral: Hypnosis: 20-60 minutes; I.V.: ~5 minutes

Peak effect: I.V.: ~30 minutes

Duration: Oral: 6-10 hours; I.V.: 4-10 hours

Absorption: Oral: 70% to 90%

Protein binding: 20% to 45%; decreased in neonates

Metabolism: Hepatic via hydroxylation and glucuronide conjugation

Half-life elimination: Neonates: 45-500 hours; Infants: 20-133 hours; Children: 37-73 hours; Adults: 53-140 hours

Time to peak, serum: Oral: 1-6 hours

Excretion: Urine (20% to 50% as unchanged drug)

Dosage

Children:

Sedation: Oral: 2 mg/kg 3 times/day

Hypnotic: I.M., I.V., SubQ: 3-5 mg/kg at bedtime
Preoperative sedation: Oral, I.M., I.V.: 1-3 mg/kg 1-1.5 hours before procedure
Adults:
Sedation: Oral, I.M.: 30-120 mg/day in 2-3 divided doses
Hypnotic: Oral, I.M., I.V., SubQ: 100-320 mg at bedtime
Preoperative sedation: I.M.: 100-200 mg 1-1.5 hours before procedure

Anticonvulsant: Status epilepticus: **Loading dose:** I.V.:
Infants and Children: 10-20 mg/kg in a single or divided dose; in select patients may administer additional 5 mg/kg/dose every 15-30 minutes until seizure is controlled or a total dose of 40 mg/kg is reached
Adults: 300-800 mg initially followed by 120-240 mg/dose at 20-minute intervals until seizures are controlled or a total dose of 1-2 g
Anticonvulsant maintenance dose: Oral, I.V.:
Infants: 5-8 mg/kg/day in 1-2 divided doses
Children:
1-5 years: 6-8 mg/kg/day in 1-2 divided doses
5-12 years: 4-6 mg/kg/day in 1-2 divided doses
Children >12 years and Adults: 1-3 mg/kg/day in divided doses or 50-100 mg 2-3 times/day
Sedative/hypnotic withdrawal (unlabeled use): Initial daily requirement is determined by substituting phenobarbital 30 mg for every 100 mg pentobarbital used during tolerance testing; then daily requirement is decreased by 10% of initial dose

Dosing interval in renal impairment: Cl_{cr} <10 mL/minute: Administer every 12-16 hours
Hemodialysis: Moderately dialyzable (20% to 50%)
Dosing adjustment/comments in hepatic disease: Increased side effects may occur in severe liver disease; monitor plasma levels and adjust dose accordingly

Dietary Considerations Vitamin D: Loss in vitamin D due to malabsorption; increase intake of foods rich in vitamin D. Supplementation of vitamin D and/or calcium may be necessary. Sodium content of injection (65 mg, 1 mL): 6 mg (0.3 mEq).

Administration Avoid rapid I.V. administration >50 mg/minute; avoid intra-arterial injection; parenteral solutions are highly alkaline; avoid extravasation

Monitoring Parameters Phenobarbital serum concentrations, mental status, CBC, LFTs, seizure activity

Reference Range
Therapeutic:
Infants and children: 15-30 mcg/mL (SI: 65-129 μmol/L)
Adults: 20-40 mcg/mL (SI: 86-172 μmol/L)
Toxic: >40 mcg/mL (SI: >172 μmol/L)
Toxic concentration: Slowness, ataxia, nystagmus: 35-80 mcg/mL (SI: 150-344 μmol/L)
Coma with reflexes: 65-117 mcg/mL (SI: 279-502 μmol/L)
Coma without reflexes: >100 mcg/mL (SI: >430 μmol/L)

Test Interactions Assay interference of LDH

Additional Information Injectable solutions contain propylene glycol.

Dosage Forms Excipient information presented when available (limited, particularly for generics); consult specific product labeling.
Elixir: 20 mg/5 mL (5 mL, 7.5 mL, 15 mL, 480 mL) [contains alcohol]
Injection, solution, as sodium: 65 mg/mL (1 mL); 130 mg/mL (1 mL) [contains alcohol and propylene glycol]
Luminal® Sodium: 60 mg/mL (1 mL); 130 mg/mL (1 mL) [contains alcohol 10% and propylene glycol]
Tablet: 15 mg, 30 mg, 60 mg, 100 mg

- ◆ **Phenobarbital, Belladonna, and Ergotamine Tartrate** *see* Belladonna, Phenobarbital, and Ergotamine *on page 175*
- ◆ **Phenobarbital, Hyoscyamine, Atropine, and Scopolamine** *see* Hyoscyamine, Atropine, Scopolamine, and Phenobarbital *on page 800*
- ◆ **Phenobarbital Sodium** *see* PHENobarbital *on page 1265*
- ◆ **Phenobarbitone** *see* PHENobarbital *on page 1265*

Phenoxybenzamine (fen oks ee BEN za meen)

Medication Safety Issues

Sound-alike/look-alike issues:

Phenoxybenzamine may be confused with phenazopyridine

U.S. Brand Names Dibenzyline®

Canadian Brand Names Dibenzyline®

Index Terms Phenoxybenzamine Hydrochloride

Pharmacologic Category $Alpha_1$ Blocker; Antidote

Use Symptomatic management of pheochromocytoma

Unlabeled/Investigational Use Micturition problems associated with neurogenic bladder, functional outlet obstruction, and partial prostate obstruction; treatment of hypertensive crisis caused by sympathomimetic amines

Effect on Mental Status May cause sedation, confusion, or dizziness

Effect on Psychiatric Treatment Concurrent use with low potency antipsychotics, TCAs and MAO inhibitors may produce additive hypotension

Dosage Summary

Oral:

Children (unlabeled use): Initial: 0.25-1 mg/kg/day, increase slowly to blood pressure control (maximum: 10 mg/day)

Adults: Initial: 10 mg twice daily; Maintenance: 10-40 mg 1-3 times/day (maximum: 240 mg/day)

Dosage Forms Excipient information presented when available (limited, particularly for generics); consult specific product labeling.

Capsule, as hydrochloride:

Dibenzyline®: 10 mg [contains benzyl alcohol]

◆ **Phenoxybenzamine Hydrochloride** *see* Phenoxybenzamine *on page 1270*

◆ **Phenoxymethyl Penicillin** *see* Penicillin V Potassium *on page 1242*

Phentermine (FEN ter meen)

Medication Safety Issues

Sound-alike/look-alike issues:

Phentermine may be confused with phentolamine, phenytoin

Ionamin® may be confused with Imodium®

U.S. Brand Names Adipex-P®; Ionamin®

Canadian Brand Names Ionamin®

Mexican Brand Names Sinpet

Index Terms Phentermine Hydrochloride

Pharmacologic Category Anorexiant; Sympathomimetic

Generic Available Yes: Capsule (excludes resin complex capsule), tablet

Use Short-term adjunct in a regimen of weight reduction based on exercise, behavioral modification, and caloric reduction in the management of exogenous obesity for patients with an initial body mass index ≥30 kg/m^2 or ≥27 kg/m^2 in the presence of other risk factors (diabetes, hypertension); see Body Mass Index on page 1746 in the Appendix

Restrictions C-IV

Pharmacotherapy for weight loss is recommended only for obese patients with a body mass index ≥30 kg/m^2, or ≥27 kg/m^2 in the presence of other risk factors such as hypertension, diabetes, and/or dyslipidemia or a high waist circumference; therapy should be used in conjunction with a comprehensive weight management program. Rule out organic causes of obesity (eg, untreated hypothyroidism) prior to use.

Note: Phentermine is not approved for long-term use. The limited usefulness of medications in this class should be weighed against possible risks associated with their use. Consult weight loss guidelines for current pharmacotherapy recommendations.

Pregnancy Risk Factor C

Pregnancy Considerations Reproduction studies have not been conducted.

Contraindications Hypersensitivity or idiosyncrasy to phentermine or other sympathomimetic amines or any component of the formulation; advanced arteriosclerosis, cardiovascular disease, moderate-to-severe hypertension; pulmonary hypertension; hyperthyroidism, glaucoma, agitated states, patients with a history of drug abuse; use during or within 14 days following MAO inhibitor therapy

Warnings/Precautions Primary pulmonary hypertension (PPH), a rare and frequently fatal pulmonary disease, has been reported to occur in patients receiving a combination of phentermine and fenfluramine or dexfenfluramine. The possibility of an association between PPH and the use of phentermine alone cannot be ruled out. The use of phenteramine has been associated with the development of valvular heart disease. Avoid stimulants in patients with known serious structural cardiac abnormalities, cardiomyopathy, serious heart rhythm abnormalities, or other serious cardiac problems that could increase the risk of sudden death that these conditions alone carry. Caution should be used in patients with hypertension and other cardiovascular conditions that might be exacerbated by increases in blood pressure or heart rate.

Use caution with diabetes; antidiabetic agent requirements may be altered with anorexigens and concomitant dietary restrictions. Stimulants may unmask tics in individuals with coexisting Tourette's syndrome. Use caution with seizure disorders. Phentermine is pharmacologically related to the amphetamines, which have a high abuse potential; prolonged use may lead to dependency. Prescriptions should be written for the smallest quantity consistent with good patient care to minimize possibility of overdose. Amphetamines may impair the ability to engage in potentially hazardous activities.

Not recommended for use in patients who used other anorectic agents within the past year. Discontinue if satisfactory weight loss has not occurred within the first 4 weeks of treatment, or if tolerance develops. Safety and efficacy have not been established for use with other weight loss medications including over-the-counter or herbal products. Safety and efficacy have not been established in children ≤16 years of age.

Adverse Reactions Frequency not defined.

Cardiovascular: Hypertension, palpitation, primary pulmonary hypertension and/or regurgitant cardiac valvular disease, tachycardia

Central nervous system: Dizziness, dysphoria, euphoria, headache, insomnia, overstimulation, psychosis, restlessness

Dermatologic: Urticaria

Endocrine & metabolic: Changes in libido

Gastrointestinal: Constipation, diarrhea, unpleasant taste, xerostomia

Genitourinary: Impotence

Neuromuscular & skeletal: Tremor

Drug Interactions

Alkalinizing Agents: May decrease the excretion of Amphetamines. *Risk D: Consider therapy modification*

Ammonium Chloride: May decrease the serum concentration of Amphetamines. This effect is likely due to an enhanced excretion of amphetamines in the urine. *Risk C: Monitor therapy*

Analgesics (Opioid): Amphetamines may enhance the analgesic effect of Analgesics (Opioid). *Risk C: Monitor therapy*

Antacids: May decrease the excretion of Amphetamines. *Risk C: Monitor therapy*

Antihistamines: Amphetamines may diminish the sedative effect of Antihistamines. *Risk C: Monitor therapy*

Antipsychotics: May diminish the stimulatory effect of Amphetamines. *Risk C: Monitor therapy*

Cannabinoids: May enhance the tachycardic effect of Sympathomimetics. *Risk C: Monitor therapy*

Carbonic Anhydrase Inhibitors: May decrease the excretion of Amphetamines. **Exceptions:** Brinzolamide; Dorzolamide. *Risk C: Monitor therapy*

Ethosuximide: Amphetamines may diminish the therapeutic effect of Ethosuximide. Amphetamines may decrease the serum concentration of Ethosuximide. *Risk C: Monitor therapy*

Gastrointestinal Acidifying Agents: May decrease the serum concentration of Amphetamines. *Risk C: Monitor therapy*

Lithium: May diminish the stimulatory effect of Amphetamines. *Risk C: Monitor therapy*

MAO Inhibitors: May enhance the hypertensive effect of Amphetamines. *Risk X: Avoid combination*

Methenamine: May decrease the serum concentration of Amphetamines. This effect is likely due to an enhanced excretion of amphetamines in the urine. *Risk C: Monitor therapy*

PHENobarbital: Amphetamines may decrease the serum concentration of PHENobarbital. *Risk C: Monitor therapy*

Phenytoin: Amphetamines may decrease the serum concentration of Phenytoin. *Risk C: Monitor therapy*

Sympathomimetics: May enhance the adverse/toxic effect of other Sympathomimetics. *Risk C: Monitor therapy*

Tricyclic Antidepressants: May enhance the stimulatory effect of Amphetamines. Tricyclic Antidepressants may also potentiate the cardiovascular effects of Amphetamines. *Risk C: Monitor therapy*

Mechanism of Action Phentermine is a sympathomimetic amine with pharmacologic properties similar to the amphetamines. The mechanism of action in reducing appetite appears to be secondary to CNS effects, including stimulation of the hypothalamus to release norepinephrine.

Pharmacodynamics/Kinetics

Duration: Resin produces more prolonged clinical effects

Absorption: Well absorbed; resin absorbed slower

Excretion: Primarily urine

Dosage Oral: Children >16 years and Adults: Obesity:

Phentermine hydrochloride: 18.75-37.5 mg/ day

Phentermine resin: 15-30 mg/day

Dietary Considerations Most effective when combined with a low calorie diet and behavior modification counseling.

Administration

Phentermine hydrochloride: Administer before breakfast or 1-2 hours after breakfast. Tablets may be divided in half and dose may be given in 2 divided doses. Avoid late evening administration.

Phentermine resin: Administer before breakfast or 10-14 hours before retiring. Swallow capsules whole.

Monitoring Parameters Weight, waist circumference; blood pressure

Reference Range

Adult classification of weight by BMI (kg/m^2):

- Underweight: <18.5
- Normal: 18.5-24.9
- Overweight: 25-29.9
- Obese, class I: 30-34.9
- Obese, class II: 35-39.9
- Extreme obesity (class III): ≥40

Waist circumference: In adults with a BMI of 25-34.9 kg/m^2, high-risk waist circumference is defined as:

- Men >102 cm (>40 in)
- Women >88 cm (>35 in)

Dosage Forms Excipient information presented when available (limited, particularly for generics); consult specific product labeling.

Capsule, as hydrochloride: 15 mg, 30 mg, 37.5 mg

- Adipex-P®: 37.5 mg

Capsule, resin complex:

- Ionamin®: 15 mg

Tablet, as hydrochloride: 37.5 mg

- Adipex-P®: 37.5 mg

◆ **Phentermine Hydrochloride** *see* Phentermine *on page 1270*

Phentolamine (fen TOLE a meen)

Medication Safety Issues

Sound-alike/look-alike issues:

Phentolamine may be confused with phentermine, Ventolin®

U.S. Brand Names OraVerse™

Canadian Brand Names Regitine®; Rogitine®

Index Terms Phentolamine Mesylate; Regitine [DSC]

Pharmacologic Category Alpha$_1$ Blocker

Use Diagnosis of pheochromocytoma and treatment of hypertension associated with pheochromocytoma or other forms of hypertension caused by excess sympathomimetic amines; as treatment of dermal necrosis after extravasation of drugs with alpha-adrenergic effects (norepinephrine, dopamine, epinephrine)

OraVerse™: Reversal of soft tissue anesthesia and the associated functional deficits resulting from a local dental anesthetic containing a vasoconstrictor

Unlabeled/Investigational Use Treatment of pralidoxime-induced hypertension

Effect on Mental Status May cause dizziness

Effect on Psychiatric Treatment Concurrent use with psychotropics may produce additive hypotension; treatment of choice for hypertensive crisis secondary to MAO inhibitors

Dosage Summary

I.M.:

Children: 0.05-0.1 mg/kg/dose as a single dose 1-2 hours before procedure, repeat as needed every 2-4 hours (maximum: 5 mg/dose)

Adults: 5 mg as a single dose 1-2 hours before procedure, may repeat as needed every 2-4 hours

I.V.:

Children: 0.05-0.1 mg/kg/dose as a single dose 1-2 hours before procedure, repeat as needed every 2-4 hours (maximum: 5 mg/dose)

Adults: 5 mg as a single dose 1-2 hours before procedure, may repeat as needed every 2-4 hours **or** 5-20 mg (hypertensive crisis)

Submucosal injection:

Children <15 kg and <12 years: Dosage not established

Children 15-30 kg and <12 years: 0.2 mg (maximum)

Children >30 kg and <12 years: 0.4 mg (maximum)

Children >30 kg and ≥12 years: 0.2 mg to 0.8 mg (depending on number of cartridges of anesthesia)

Adults: 0.2 mg to 0.8 mg (depending on number of cartridges of anesthesia)

SubQ:

Children: Infiltrate area with a small amount (eg, 1 mL) of solution (made by diluting 5-10 mg in 10 mL of NS) within 12 hours of extravasation (maximum: 0.1-0.2 mg/kg **or** 5 mg total)

Adults: Infiltrate area with a small amount (eg, 1 mL) of solution (made by diluting 5-10 mg in 10 mL of NS) within 12 hours of extravasation (maximum: 0.1-0.2 mg/kg **or** 5 mg total)

Dosage Forms Excipient information presented when available (limited, particularly for generics); consult specific product labeling.

Injection, powder for reconstitution, as mesylate: 5 mg

Injection, solution, as mesylate [preservative free]:

OraVerse™: 0.4 mg/1.7 mL (1.7 mL) [contains edetate disodium; dental cartridge]

◆ **Phentolamine Mesylate** *see* Phentolamine *on page 1272*

◆ **Phenylalanine Mustard** *see* Melphalan *on page 983*

◆ **Phenylazo Diamino Pyridine Hydrochloride** *see* Phenazopyridine *on page 1258*

Phenylephrine (fen il EF rin)

Medication Safety Issues

Sound-alike/look-alike issues:

Mydfrin® may be confused with Midrin®

High alert medication: The Institute for Safe Medication Practices (ISMP) includes this medication among its list of drugs which have a heightened risk of causing significant patient harm when used in error.

U.S. Brand Names 4 Way® Fast Acting [OTC]; 4 Way® Menthol [OTC]; 4 Way® No Drip [OTC]; AK-Dilate®; Altafrin; Anu-Med [OTC]; Dimetapp® Toddler's [OTC]; Formulation R™ [OTC]; Little Noses® Decongestant [OTC]; LuSonal™; Medi-Phenyl [OTC]; Medicone® Suppositories [OTC]; Mydfrin®; Nasop12™; Neo-Synephrine® Extra Strength [OTC]; Neo-Synephrine® Injection; Neo-Synephrine® Mild [OTC]; Neo-Synephrine® Regular Strength [OTC]; Neofrin™; NāSop™ [DSC]; OcuNefrin™ [OTC]; Preparation H® [OTC]; Rectacaine [OTC]; Relief® [OTC] [DSC]; Rhinall [OTC]; Sudafed PE™ [OTC]; Triaminic® Infant Thin Strips® Decongestant [OTC] [DSC]; Triaminic® Thin Strips® Cold [OTC]; Tronolane® Suppository [OTC]; Tur-bi-kal® [OTC]; Vicks® Sinex® Nasal Spray [OTC]; Vicks® Sinex® UltraFine Mist [OTC]

Canadian Brand Names Dionephrine®; Mydfrin®; Neo-Synephrine®

Mexican Brand Names Afrinex infantil; Bregamin; Bremagan Flu; Coldaid; Flavit AV; Fluviatol NF

Index Terms Phenylephrine Hydrochloride; Phenylephrine Tannate

Pharmacologic Category Alpha/Beta Agonist; Ophthalmic Agent, Antiglaucoma; Ophthalmic Agent, Mydriatic

Use Treatment of hypotension, vascular failure in shock; as a vasoconstrictor in regional analgesia; as a mydriatic in ophthalmic procedures and treatment of wide-angle glaucoma; supraventricular tachycardia

For OTC use as symptomatic relief of nasal and nasopharyngeal mucosal congestion, treatment of hemorrhoids, relief of redness of the eye due to irritation

Effect on Mental Status May cause anxiety or restlessness

Effect on Psychiatric Treatment Concurrent use with MAO inhibitors may result in hypertensive crisis; avoid combination

Dosage Summary

I.V.:

Children: Bolus: 5-20 mcg/kg/dose every 10-15 minutes as needed; Infusion: 0.1-0.5 mcg/kg/minute

Adults: Bolus: 0.1-0.5 mg/dose every 10-15 minutes as needed (maximum: 0.5 mg); Infusion: 0.4-9.1 mcg/kg/minute **or** 40-360 mcg/minute

Intranasal:

Children <2 years: Dosage not established

Children 2-6 years: Instill 1 drop every 2-4 hours of 0.125% solution as needed (maximum: 3 continuous days of therapy)

Children 6-12 years: Instill 1-2 sprays or drops every 4 hours of 0.25% solution as needed (maximum: 3 continuous days)

Children >12 years: Instill 1-2 sprays or drops every 4 hours of 0.25% to 0.5% solution as needed (maximum: 3 continuous days)

Adults: Instill 1-2 sprays or drops every 4 hours of 0.25% to 1% solution as needed (maximum: 3 continuous days)

Ophthalmic:

Infants <1 year: Instill 1 drop of 2.5% 15-30 minutes before procedures

Children ≥1 year: Instill 1 drop of 2.5% or 10% solution, may repeat in 10-60 minutes as needed

Adults: Instill 1 drop of 2.5% or 10% solution, may repeat in 10-60 minutes as needed **or** 1-2 drops of 0.12% solution up to 4 times/day [OTC dosing] (maximum: 72 hours)

Oral:

Children <6 years: Dosage not established

Children 6-12 years: Hydrochloride salt: 10 mg every 4 hours; Tannate salt: 1/2 to 1 tablet (5-10 mg) every 12 hours

Children >12 years: Hydrochloride salt: 10-20 mg every 4 hours; Tannate salt: 1-2 tablets (10-20 mg) every 12 hours

Adults: Hydrochloride salt: 10-20 mg every 4 hours; Tannate salt: 1-2 tablets (10-20 mg) every 12 hours

Rectal:

Children ≤12 years: Dosage not established

Children >12 years: Cream/ointment: Apply up to 4 times/day; Suppository: Insert 1 up to 4 times/day

Adults: Cream/ointment: Apply up to 4 times/day; Suppository: Insert 1 up to 4 times/day

Dosage Forms Excipient information presented when available (limited, particularly for generics); consult specific product labeling. [DSC] = Discontinued product

Cream, rectal, as hydrochloride:

Formulation R™: 0.25% (54 g) [contains sodium benzoate]

Filmstrip, orally disintegrating, as hydrochloride:

Sudafed PE™: 10 mg (5s, 10s) [contains phenylalanine 1 mg/strip; cherry menthol flavor]

Triaminic® Infant Thin Strips® Decongestant: 1.25 mg [mixed berry flavor] [DSC]

Triaminic® Thin Strips® Cold: 2.5 mg [raspberry flavor]

Injection, solution, as hydrochloride: 1% [10 mg/mL] (1 mL, 5 mL, 10 mL) [may contain sodium metabisulfite]

Neo-Synephrine®: 1% (1 mL) [contains sodium metabisulfite]

Liquid, oral, as hydrochloride:

LuSonal™: 7.5 mg/5 mL (480 mL) [contains phenylalanine; strawberry flavor]

Liquid, oral, as hydrochloride [drops]:

Dimetapp® Toddler's: 1.25 mg/0.8 mL (15 mL) [alcohol free; contains sodium benzoate; grape flavor]

Ointment, rectal, as hydrochloride:

Formulation R™, Preparation H®: 0.25% (30 g, 60 g) [contains benzoic acid]

Rectacaine: 0.25% (30 g)

Solution, intranasal, as hydrochloride [drops]:

Little Noses® Decongestant: 0.125% (15 mL) [contains benzalkonium chloride]

Neo-Synephrine® Extra Strength: 1% (15 mL) [contains benzalkonium chloride]

Neo-Synephrine® Regular Strength: 0.5% (15 mL) [contains benzalkonium chloride]

Rhinall: 0.25% (30 mL) [contains benzalkonium chloride and sodium bisulfite]

Tur-bi-kal®: 0.17% (30 mL) [contains benzalkonium chloride]

Solution, intranasal, as hydrochloride [spray]:

4 Way® Fast Acting: 1% (15 mL, 30 mL) [contains benzalkonium chloride]

4 Way® Menthol: 1% (15 mL) [contains benzalkonium chloride and menthol]

4 Way® No Drip: 1% (15 mL) [contains benzalkonium chloride]

Neo-Synephrine® Extra Strength: 1% (15 mL) [contains benzalkonium chloride]
Neo-Synephrine® Mild: 0.25% (15 mL) [contains benzalkonium chloride]
Neo-Synephrine® Regular Strength: 0.5% (15 mL) [contains benzalkonium chloride]
Rhinall: 0.25% (40 mL) [contains benzalkonium chloride and sodium bisulfite]
Vicks® Sinex®, Vicks® Sinex® UltraFine Mist: 0.5% (15 mL) [contains benzalkonium chloride]

Solution, ophthalmic, as hydrochloride: 2.5% (2 mL, 3 mL, 5 mL, 15 mL) [may contain sodium bisulfite]
AK-Dilate®: 2.5% (2 mL, 15 mL); 10% (5 mL) [contains benzyl alcohol]
Altrafrin: 0.12% (15 mL) [OTC]; 2.5% (15 mL) [RX; contains benzalkonium chloride]; 10% (5 mL) [RX; contains benzalkonium chloride]
Mydfrin®: 2.5% (3 mL, 5 mL) [contains sodium bisulfite]
Neofrin™: 2.5% (15 mL); 10% (15 mL)
OcuNefrin™: 0.12% (15 mL)
Relief®: 0.12% (15 mL) [contains benzalkonium chloride] [DSC]

Suppository, rectal, as hydrochloride: 0.25% (12s)
Anu-Med: 0.25% (12s)
Formulation R™, Preparation H®: 0.25% (12s, 24s, 48s)
Medicone®, Tronolane®: 0.25% (12s, 24s)
Rectacaine: 0.25% (12s)

Suspension, oral, as tannate:
NāSop™: 7.5 mg/5 mL (120 mL) [orange flavor] [DSC]

Tablet, chewable, as tannate:
Nasop12™: 10 mg [grape flavor]

Tablet, as hydrochloride: 10 mg
Medi-Phenyl: 5 mg
Sudafed PE™: 10 mg

Tablet, orally dissolving, as hydrochloride:
NāSop™: 10 mg [contains phenylalanine 4 mg/tablet; bubble gum flavor] [DSC]

- **Phenylephrine CM** *see* Chlorpheniramine, Phenylephrine, and Methscopolamine *on page 329*
- **Phenylephrine, Acetaminophen, and Dextromethorphan** *see* Acetaminophen, Dextromethorphan, and Phenylephrine *on page 42*
- **Phenylephrine and Chlorpheniramine** *see* Chlorpheniramine and Phenylephrine *on page 323*
- **Phenylephrine and Cyclopentolate** *see* Cyclopentolate and Phenylephrine *on page 407*
- **Phenylephrine and Diphenhydramine** *see* Diphenhydramine and Phenylephrine *on page 485*
- **Phenylephrine and Promethazine** *see* Promethazine and Phenylephrine *on page 1350*

Phenylephrine and Pyrilamine (fen il EF rin & peer IL a meen)

U.S. Brand Names Aldex®D; AllanVan-S [DSC]; Deconsal® CT; K-Tan 4 [DSC]; K-Tan [DSC]; Pyrilafen Tannate-12™; Ry-T-12; Ryna-12 S®; Ryna®-12; Rynesa 12S; V-Tann™ [DSC]; Viravan® [DSC]

Index Terms Pyrilamine Tannate and Phenylephrine Tannate

Pharmacologic Category Alpha/Beta Agonist; Histamine H_1 Antagonist; Histamine H_1 Antagonist, First Generation

Use Symptomatic relief of nasal congestion and discharge associated with the common cold, sinusitis, allergic rhinitis, and other respiratory tract conditions

Effect on Mental Status May cause sedation, dysphoria, euphoria, insomnia, anxiety, excitability, nervousness, fatigue, or depression

Effect on Psychiatric Treatment Contraindicated with MAO inhibitors. Concurrent use with psychotropic agents may result in additive sedative and/or anticholinergic effects; monitor. May cause seizures; monitor in patients receiving clozapine. May rarely be associated with agranulocytosis; use caution with clozapine, carbamazepine, and mirtazapine. May cause thrombocytopenia; monitor in patients receiving valproic acid.

Dosage Summary

Oral:

Children <2 years: Dosage not established
Children 2-6 years: 2.5 mL of the suspension or 1/2 tablet every 12 hours
Children 6-12 years: 5 mL of the suspension or 1/2 to 1 tablet every 12 hours
Children >12 years: 5-10 mL of the suspension or 1-2 tablets every 12 hours
Adults: 5-10 mL of the suspension or 1-2 tablets every 12 hours

Dosage Forms Excipient information presented when available (limited, particularly for generics); consult specific product labeling. [DSC] = Discontinued product

Suspension:

Aldex®D: Phenylephrine hydrochloride 5 mg and pyrilamine maleate 16 mg (480 mL) [contains tannic acid to provide a tannate suspension; contains sodium benzoate; grape flavor]

AllanVan-S: Phenylephrine tannate 12.5 mg and pyrilamine tannate 30 mg per 5 mL (120 mL, 480 mL) [contains sodium benzoate; grape flavor] [DSC]

K-Tan 4: Phenylephrine tannate 5 mg and pyrilamine tannate 30 mg per 5 mL (120 mL) [contains benzoic acid; strawberry-currant flavor] [DSC]

Pyrilafen Tannate-12™: Phenylephrine tannate 5 mg and pyrilamine tannate 30 mg per 5 mL (120 mL, 480 mL [DSC]) [strawberry-black currant flavor]

Ryna-12 S®: Phenylephrine tannate 5 mg and pyrilamine tannate 30 mg per 5 mL (120 mL) [contains benzoic acid; strawberry-currant flavor]

Rynesa 12S: Phenylephrine tannate 5 mg and pyrilamine tannate 30 mg per 5 mL (120 mL, 480 mL) [contains sodium benzoate; cherry berry flavor]

Ry-T-12: Phenylephrine tannate 5 mg and pyrilamine tannate 30 mg per 5 mL (120 mL, 480 mL) [contains benzoic acid]

V-Tann™: Phenylephrine tannate 12.5 mg and pyrilamine tannate 30 mg per 5 mL (120 mL, 480 mL) [alcohol free, dye free, gluten free; contains sodium benzoate; grape flavor] [DSC]

Viravan®: Phenylephrine tannate 12.5 mg and pyrilamine tannate 30 mg per 5 mL (120 mL, 480 mL) [contains sodium benzoate; grape flavor] [DSC]

Tablet:

K-Tan [DSC], Ryna®-12: Phenylephrine tannate 25 mg and pyrilamine tannate 60 mg

Tablet, chewable:

Deconsal® CT: Phenylephrine hydrochloride 10 mg and pyrilamine maleate 16 mg [dye free; grape flavor]

Viravan®: Phenylephrine tannate 25 mg and pyrilamine tannate 30 mg [dye free; grape flavor] [DSC]

- **Phenylephrine, Chlorpheniramine, and Carbetapentane** *see* Carbetapentane, Phenylephrine, and Chlorpheniramine *on page 274*
- **Phenylephrine, Chlorpheniramine, and Dextromethorphan** *see* Chlorpheniramine, Phenylephrine, and Dextromethorphan *on page 327*
- **Phenylephrine, Chlorpheniramine, and Dihydrocodeine** *see* Dihydrocodeine, Chlorpheniramine, and Phenylephrine *on page 469*
- **Phenylephrine, Chlorpheniramine, and Guaifenesin** *see* Chlorpheniramine, Phenylephrine, and Guaifenesin *on page 329*
- **Phenylephrine, Chlorpheniramine, and Phenyltoloxamine** *see* Chlorpheniramine, Phenylephrine, and Phenyltoloxamine *on page 331*
- **Phenylephrine, Chlorpheniramine, Codeine, and Potassium Iodide** *see* Chlorpheniramine, Phenylephrine, Codeine, and Potassium Iodide *on page 332*
- **Phenylephrine, Dextromethorphan, and Acetaminophen** *see* Acetaminophen, Dextromethorphan, and Phenylephrine *on page 42*
- **Phenylephrine, Diphenhydramine, and Hydrocodone** *see* Hydrocodone, Phenylephrine, and Diphenhydramine *on page 782*
- **Phenylephrine, Ephedrine, Chlorpheniramine, and Carbetapentane** *see* Chlorpheniramine, Ephedrine, Phenylephrine, and Carbetapentane *on page 326*
- **Phenylephrine, Guaifenesin, and Hydrocodone** *see* Hydrocodone, Phenylephrine, and Guaifenesin *on page 783*
- **Phenylephrine Hydrochloride** *see* Phenylephrine *on page 1273*
- **Phenylephrine Hydrochloride, Acetaminophen, and Diphenhydramine** *see* Acetaminophen, Diphenhydramine, and Phenylephrine *on page 44*
- **Phenylephrine Hydrochloride and Acetaminophen** *see* Acetaminophen and Phenylephrine *on page 36*
- **Phenylephrine Hydrochloride and Diphenhydramine Hydrochloride** *see* Diphenhydramine and Phenylephrine *on page 485*
- **Phenylephrine Hydrochloride and Guaifenesin** *see* Guaifenesin and Phenylephrine *on page 742*
- **Phenylephrine Hydrochloride, Carbetapentane Citrate, and Guaifenesin** *see* Carbetapentane, Guaifenesin, and Phenylephrine *on page 274*

- **Phenylephrine Hydrochloride, Chlorpheniramine maleate, Dextromethorphan Hydrobromide, and Guaifenesin** *see* Dextromethorphan, Chlorpheniramine, Phenylephrine, and Guaifenesin *on page 450*
- **Phenylephrine Hydrochloride, Guaifenesin, and Dextromethorphan Hydrobromide** *see* Guaifenesin, Dextromethorphan, and Phenylephrine *on page 746*
- **Phenylephrine Hydrochloride, Hydrocodone Bitartrate, and Chlorpheniramine Maleate** *see* Phenylephrine, Hydrocodone, and Chlorpheniramine *on page 1277*

Phenylephrine, Hydrocodone, and Chlorpheniramine

(fen il EF rin, hye droe KOE done, & klor fen IR a meen)

U.S. Brand Names B-Tuss™; Coughtuss; Cytuss HC; De-Chlor HC; DroTuss-CP; ED-TLC; ED-Tuss HC; Histinex® HC; Hydro PC II Plus; Hydro-PC II; Hydron CP; Maxi-Tuss HCX; Maxi-Tuss HC®; Mintuss HC; Mintuss MS; PolyTussin HD; Relacon-HC; Rindal HD Plus; Triant-HC™

Index Terms Chlorpheniramine, Phenylephrine, and Hydrocodone; Dihydrocodeine Bitartrate, Phenylephrine Hydrochloride, and Chlorpheniramine Maleate; Hydrocodone, Phenylephrine, and Chlorpheniramine; Phenylephrine Hydrochloride, Hydrocodone Bitartrate, and Chlorpheniramine Maleate

Pharmacologic Category Alpha/Beta Agonist; Analgesic, Opioid; Antitussive; Histamine H_1 Antagonist; Histamine H_1 Antagonist, First Generation

Use Symptomatic relief of cough and congestion associated with the common cold, sinusitis, or acute upper respiratory tract infections

Effect on Mental Status May cause anxiety, restlessness, and sedation; may rarely cause hallucinations

Effect on Psychiatric Treatment Contraindicated with MAO inhibitors; concurrent use with psychotropics may result in additive sedation; may result in loss of pain control if used with fluoxetine or paroxetine

Restrictions C-III

Dosage Summary Note: Dosing is product specific, see individual products

Oral:

Children <2 years: Dosage not established

Children 2-6 years: 1.25-2.5 mL every 6 hours (maximum: 10 mL/day)

Children 6-12 years:

2.5 mL every 4 hours (maximum: 15 mL/24 hours) **or** 5 mL every 4 hours (maximum: 20 mL/24 hours) or 2.5-5 mL every 6 hours

Children >12 years: 5-10 mL every 4-6 hours (maximum: 40 mL/day)

Adults: 5-10 mL every 4-6 hours (maximum: 40 mL/day)

Dosage Forms Excipient information presented when available (limited, particularly for generics); consult specific product labeling.

Liquid:

B-Tuss™: Phenylephrine hydrochloride 5 mg, hydrocodone bitartrate 5 mg, and chlorpheniramine maleate 2 mg per 5 mL (480 mL) [alcohol free, sugar free; candy apple flavor]

Coughtuss: Phenylephrine hydrochloride 5 mg, hydrocodone bitartrate 5 mg, and chlorpheniramine maleate 2 mg per 5 mL (480 mL) [alcohol free, sugar free; candy apple flavor]

De-Chlor HC: Phenylephrine hydrochloride 10 mg, hydrocodone bitartrate 2.5 mg, and chlorpheniramine maleate 2 mg per 5 mL (480 mL) [cherry flavor]

DroTuss-CP: Phenylephrine hydrochloride 5 mg, hydrocodone bitartrate 5 mg, and chlorpheniramine maleate 2 mg per 5 mL (480 mL) [alcohol free, sugar free; candy apple flavor]

ED-Tuss HC: Phenylephrine hydrochloride 10 mg, hydrocodone bitartrate 3.5 mg, and chlorpheniramine maleate 4 mg per 5 mL (480 mL)

ED-TLC: Phenylephrine hydrochloride 5 mg, hydrocodone bitartrate 1.67 mg, and chlorpheniramine maleate 2 mg per 5 mL (480 mL)

Hydron CP: Phenylephrine hydrochloride 10 mg, hydrocodone bitartrate 5 mg, and chlorpheniramine maleate 2 mg per 5 mL (480 mL) [pineapple-orange flavor]

Hydro PC II Plus: Phenylephrine hydrochloride 7.5 mg, hydrocodone bitartrate 3.5 mg, and chlorpheniramine maleate 2 mg per 5 mL (480 mL) [strawberry flavor]

Maxi-Tuss HCX: Phenylephrine hydrochloride 12 mg, hydrocodone bitartrate 6 mg and chlorpheniramine maleate 2 mg per 5 mL (480 mL) [alcohol free, sugar free; contains aspartame; vanilla bean flavor]

Relacon-HC: Phenylephrine hydrochloride 10 mg, hydrocodone bitartrate 3.5 mg, and chlorpheniramine maleate 2.5 mg per 5 mL (480 mL) [raspberry flavor]

Triant-HC™: Phenylephrine hydrocloride 5 mg, hydrocodone bitartrate 1.67 mg, and chlorpheniramine maleate 2 mg per 5 mL (480 mL) [alcohol free, sugar free; strawberry flavor]

Syrup:

Cytuss HC: Phenylephrine hydrochloride 5 mg, hydrocodone bitartrate 2.5 mg, and chlorpheniramine maleate 2 mg per 5 mL (480 mL) [peach flavor]

Histinex® HC: Phenylephrine hydrochloride 5 mg, hydrocodone bitartrate 2.5 mg, and chlorpheniramine maleate 2 mg per 5 mL (480 mL, 960 mL) [alcohol free, sugar free; contains sodium benzoate]

Hydro-PC II: Phenylephrine hydrochloride 7.5 mg, hydrocodone bitartrate 2 mg, and chlorpheniramine maleate 2 mg per 5 mL (480 mL) [strawberry flavor]

Maxi-Tuss HC®: Phenylephrine hydrochloride 10 mg, hydrocodone bitartrate 2.5 mg, and chlorpheniramine maleate 4 mg per 5 mL (480 mL) [orange flavor]

Mintuss HC: Phenylephrine hydrochloride 10 mg, hydrocodone bitartrate 2.5 mg, and chlorpheniramine maleate 2 mg per 5 mL (480 mL) [alcohol free; contains sodium benzoate; black cherry flavor]

Mintuss MS: Phenylephrine hydrochloride 10 mg, hydrocodone bitartrate 5 mg, and chlorpheniramine maleate 2 mg per 5 mL (480 mL) [alcohol free; contains sodium benzoate; orange flavor]

PolyTussin HD: Phenylephrine hydrochloride 5 mg, hydrocodone bitartrate 6 mg, and chlorpheniramine maleate 2 mg per 5 mL (480 mL) [alcohol free, sugar free]

Rindal HD Plus: Phenylephrine hydrochloride 7.5 mg, hydrocodone bitartrate 3.5 mg, and chlorpheniramine maleate 2 mg per 5 mL (480 mL) [alcohol free, sugar free; contains sodium benzoate; black raspberry flavor]

◆ **Phenylephrine, Promethazine, and Codeine** *see* Promethazine, Phenylephrine, and Codeine *on page 1350*

Phenylephrine, Pyrilamine, and Dextromethorphan

(fen il EF rin, peer IL a meen, & deks troe meth OR fan)

U.S. Brand Names Aldex® DM; AllanVan-DM; Codal-DM [OTC]; codimal® DM [OTC]; Codituss DM [OTC]; MyHist-DM; Poly-Hist DM; Tannate-V-DM; Viravan®-DM

Index Terms Dextromethorphan Tannate, Pyrilamine Tannate, and Phenylephrine Tannate; Pyrilamine Maleate, Dextromethorphan Hydrobromide, and Phenylephrine Hydrochloride

Pharmacologic Category Alpha/Beta Agonist; Antitussive; Histamine H_1 Antagonist; Histamine H_1 Antagonist, First Generation

Use Symptomatic relief of cough, nasal congestion, and discharge associated with the common cold, sinusitis, allergic rhinitis, and other respiratory tract conditions

Effect on Mental Status Sedation is common; may cause anxiety, excitability, dysphoria, euphoria, insomnia, nervousness, fatigue, or depression

Effect on Psychiatric Treatment Contraindicated with MAO inhibitors. Concurrent use with psychotropic agents may result in additive sedative and/or anticholinergic effects; monitor. May cause seizures; monitor in patients receiving clozapine. May rarely be associated with agranulocytosis; use caution with clozapine, carbamazepine, and mirtazapine. May cause thrombocytopenia; monitor in patients receiving valproic acid.

Dosage Summary

Oral:

Children <2 years: Dosage not established

Children 2-6 years: Viravan®-DM: 2.5 mL of the suspension **or** 1/2 tablet every 12 hours

Children 6-12 years:

Codimal® DM: 5 mL every 4 hours (maximum: 30 mL/day)

Viravan®-DM: 5 mL of the suspension **or** 1/2 to 1 tablet every 12 hours

Children >12 years:

Codimal® DM: 10 mL every 4 hours (maximum: 60 mL/day)

Viravan®-DM: 5-10 mL of the suspension **or** 1-2 tablets every 12 hours

Adults:

Codimal® DM: 10 mL every 4 hours (maximum: 60 mL/day)

Viravan®-DM: 5-10 mL of the suspension **or** 1-2 tablets every 12 hours

Dosage Forms Excipient information presented when available (limited, particularly for generics); consult specific product labeling.

Liquid:

MyHist-DM: Phenylephrine hydrochloride 7.5 mg, pyrilamine maleate 12.5 mg, and dextromethorphan hydrochloride 15 mg per 5 mL (480 mL) [alcohol free, dye free, sugar free; grape flavor]

Suspension:

AllanVan-DM, Tannate-V-DM, Viravan®-DM: Phenylephrine tannate 12.5 mg, pyrilamine tannate 30 mg, and dextromethorphan tannate 25 mg per 5 mL (480 mL) [contains sodium benzoate; grape flavor]

Aldex® DM: Phenylephrine hydrochloride 5 mg, pyrilamine maleate 16 mg, and dextromethorphan hydrochloride 15 mg per 5 mL (480 mL) [contains tannic acid to provide a tannate suspension; contains sodium benzoate; grape flavor]

Syrup:

Codal-DM: Phenylephrine hydrochloride 5 mg, pyrilamine maleate 8.33 mg, and dextromethorphan hydrobromide 10 mg (480 mL) [cherry flavor]

codimal® DM: Phenylephrine hydrochloride 5 mg, pyrilamine maleate 8.33 mg, and dextromethorphan hydrobromide 10 mg (120 mL, 480 mL) [alcohol free, dye free, sugar free; contains benzoic acid]

Codituss DM: Phenylephrine hydrochloride 5 mg, pyrilamine maleate 8.33 mg, and dextromethorphan hydrobromide 10 mg (120 mL, 480 mL) [alcohol free, dye free, sugar free; cherry punch flavor]

Poly Hist DM: Phenylephrine hydrochloride 7.5 mg, pyrilamine maleate 8.33 mg, and dextromethorphan hydrobromide 10 mg (480 mL) [alcohol free, dye free, sugar free; grape flavor]

Tablet, chewable [scored]:

Deconsal® DM: Phenylephrine hydrochloride 10 mg, pyrilamine maleate 16 mg, and dextromethorphan hydrobromide 15 mg [dye free; grape flavor]

Viravan®-DM: Phenylephrine tannate 25 mg, pyrilamine tannate 30 mg, and dextromethorphan tannate 25 mg [dye free; grape flavor]

Phenylephrine, Pyrilamine, and Guaifenesin

(fen il EF rin, peer IL a meen, & gwye FEN e sin)

U.S. Brand Names Ryna-12X®

Index Terms Guaifenesin, Pyrilamine Tannate, and Phenylephrine Tannate; Pyrilamine Tannate, Guaifenesin, and Phenylephrine Tannate

Pharmacologic Category Alpha/Beta Agonist; Decongestant; Expectorant; Histamine H_1 Antagonist; Histamine H_1 Antagonist, First Generation

Use

Symptomatic relief of cough, nasal congestion, and discharge associated with the common cold, sinusitis, allergic rhinitis, and other respiratory tract conditions

Effect on Mental Status May cause sedation, nervousness, restlessness, or dizziness

Effect on Psychiatric Treatment Contraindicated with or within 14 days of MAO inhibitor treatment. May cause CNS depression, concurrent use with psychotropics may produce additive effects.

Dosage Summary

Oral:

Children <2 years: Dosage not established

Children 2-6 years: 2.5-5 mL of the suspension every 12 hours

Children 6-11 years: 5-10 mL of the suspension **or** 1/2 to 1 tablet every 12 hours

Children ≥12 years: 1-2 tablets every 12 hours

Adults: 1-2 tablets every 12 hours

Dosage Forms Excipient information presented when available (limited, particularly for generics); consult specific product labeling.

Suspension:

Ryna-12X®: Phenylephrine tannate 5 mg, pyrilamine tannate 30 mg, and guaifenesin 100 mg per 5 mL (120 mL) [contains benzoic acid; grape flavor]

Tablet [scored]:

Ryna-12X®: Phenylephrine tannate 25 mg, pyrilamine tannate 60 mg, and guaifenesin 200 mg

◆ **Phenylephrine Tannate** *see* Phenylephrine *on page 1273*

◆ **Phenylephrine Tannate and Carbetapentane Tannate** *see* Carbetapentane and Phenylephrine *on page 273*

◆ **Phenylephrine Tannate and Diphenhydramine Tannate** *see* Diphenhydramine and Phenylephrine *on page 485*

◆ **Phenylephrine Tannate, Carbetapentane Tannate, and Pyrilamine Tannate** *see* Carbetapentane, Phenylephrine, and Pyrilamine *on page 275*

- **Phenylephrine Tannate, Chlorpheniramine Tannate, and Methscopolamine Nitrate** *see* Chlorpheniramine, Phenylephrine, and Methscopolamine *on page 329*
- **Phenylethylmalonylurea** *see* PHENobarbital *on page 1265*
- **Phenylgesic [OTC]** *see* Acetaminophen and Phenyltoloxamine *on page 36*
- **Phenyl Salicylate, Methenamine, Methylene Blue, Benzoic Acid, and Hyoscyamine** *see* Methenamine, Phenyl Salicylate, Methylene Blue, Benzoic Acid, and Hyoscyamine *on page 1009*
- **Phenyl Salicylate, Methenamine, Methylene Blue, Sodium Biphosphate, and Hyoscyamine** *see* Methenamine, Sodium Biphosphate, Phenyl Salicylate, Methylene Blue, and Hyoscyamine *on page 1010*
- **Phenyltoloxamine, Chlorpheniramine, and Phenylephrine** *see* Chlorpheniramine, Phenylephrine, and Phenyltoloxamine *on page 331*
- **Phenyltoloxamine Citrate and Acetaminophen** *see* Acetaminophen and Phenyltoloxamine *on page 36*
- **Phenytek®** *see* Phenytoin *on page 1280*

Phenytoin (FEN i toyn)

Medication Safety Issues

Sound-alike/look-alike issues:

Phenytoin may be confused with phenelzine, phentermine

Dilantin® may be confused with Dilaudid®, diltiazem, Dipentum®

High alert medication: The Institute for Safe Medication Practices (ISMP) includes this medication (I.V. formulation) among its list of drug classes which have a heightened risk of causing significant patient harm when used in error.

International issues:

Dilantin® may be confused with Dolantine® which is a brand name for pethidine in Belgium and Switzerland

Related Information

Anticonvulsants By Seizure Type *on page 1759*

U.S. Brand Names Dilantin®; Phenytek®

Canadian Brand Names Dilantin®

Mexican Brand Names Epamin; Fenidantoin S; Fenitron; Fomiken; Hidantoína

Index Terms Diphenylhydantoin; DPH; Phenytoin Sodium; Phenytoin Sodium, Extended; Phenytoin Sodium, Prompt

Pharmacologic Category Antiarrhythmic Agent, Class Ib; Anticonvulsant, Hydantoin

Generic Available Yes: Excludes chewable tablet

Use Management of generalized tonic-clonic (grand mal), complex partial seizures; prevention of seizures following head trauma/neurosurgery

Pregnancy Risk Factor D

Pregnancy Considerations Phenytoin crosses the placenta. Congenital malformations (including a pattern of malformations termed the "fetal hydantoin syndrome" or "fetal anticonvulsant syndrome") have been reported in infants. Isolated cases of malignancies (including neuroblastoma) and coagulation defects in the neonate following delivery have also been reported. Epilepsy itself, the number of medications, genetic factors, or a combination of these probably influence the teratogenicity of anticonvulsant therapy.

Total plasma concentrations of phenytoin are decreased by 56% in the mother during pregnancy; unbound plasma (free) concentrations are decreased by 31%. Because protein binding is decreased, monitoring of unbound plasma concentrations is recommended. Concentrations should be monitored through the 8th week postpartum. The use of folic acid throughout pregnancy and vitamin K during the last month of pregnancy is recommended.

A pregnancy registry is available for women exposed to antiepileptic drug (including phenytoin) at the Genetics and Teratology Unit Massachusetts General Hospital, 1-888-233-2334.

Lactation Enters breast milk/not recommended (AAP rates "compatible")

Contraindications Hypersensitivity to phenytoin, other hydantoins, or any component of the formulation; pregnancy

Warnings/Precautions May increase frequency of petit mal seizures; I.V. form may cause hypotension, skin necrosis at I.V. site; avoid I.V. administration in small veins; use with caution in patients with porphyria; discontinue if rash or lymphadenopathy occurs; a spectrum of hematologic effects have been reported with use (eg, neutropenia, leukopenia, thrombocytopenia, pancytopenia, and anemias); use with caution in patients with hepatic dysfunction, sinus bradycardia, S-A block, or AV block; use with caution in elderly or debilitated patients, or in any condition associated with low serum albumin levels, which will increase the free fraction of phenytoin in the serum and, therefore, the pharmacologic response. Sedation, confusional states, or cerebellar dysfunction (loss of motor coordination) may occur at higher total serum concentrations, or at lower total serum concentrations when the free fraction of phenytoin is increased. Effects with other sedative drugs or ethanol may be potentiated. Abrupt withdrawal may precipitate status epilepticus. Severe reactions, including toxic epidermal necrolysis and Stevens-Johnson syndromes, although rarely reported, have resulted in fatalities; drug should be discontinued if there are any signs of rash. Patients of Asian descent with the variant *HLA-B*1502* may be at an increased risk of developing Stevens-Johnson syndrome and/or toxic epidermal necrolysis.

Adverse Reactions I.V. effects: Hypotension, bradycardia, cardiac arrhythmia, cardiovascular collapse (especially with rapid I.V. use), venous irritation and pain, thrombophlebitis

Effects not related to plasma phenytoin concentrations: Hypertrichosis, gingival hypertrophy, thickening of facial features, carbohydrate intolerance, folic acid deficiency, peripheral neuropathy, vitamin D deficiency, osteomalacia, systemic lupus erythematosus

Concentration-related effects: Nystagmus, blurred vision, diplopia, ataxia, slurred speech, dizziness, drowsiness, lethargy, coma, rash, fever, nausea, vomiting, gum tenderness, confusion, mood changes, folic acid depletion, osteomalacia, hyperglycemia

Related to elevated concentrations:

>20 mcg/mL: Far lateral nystagmus

>30 mcg/mL: 45° lateral gaze nystagmus and ataxia

>40 mcg/mL: Decreased mentation

>100 mcg/mL: Death

Cardiovascular: Hypotension, bradycardia, cardiac arrhythmia, cardiovascular collapse

Central nervous system: Psychiatric changes, slurred speech, dizziness, drowsiness, headache, insomnia

Dermatologic: Rash

Gastrointestinal: Constipation, nausea, vomiting, gingival hyperplasia, enlargement of lips

Hematologic: Leukopenia, thrombocytopenia, agranulocytosis

Hepatic: Hepatitis

Local: Thrombophlebitis

Neuromuscular & skeletal: Tremor, peripheral neuropathy, paresthesia

Ocular: Diplopia, nystagmus, blurred vision

Rarely seen effects: Blood dyscrasias, coarsening of facial features, dyskinesias, hepatitis, hypertrichosis, lymphadenopathy, lymphoma, pseudolymphoma, SLE-like syndrome, Stevens-Johnson syndrome, toxic epidermal necrolysis, venous irritation and pain

Metabolism/Transport Effects Substrate of CYP2C9 (major), 2C19 (major), 3A4 (minor); **Induces** CYP2B6 (strong), 2C8 (strong), 2C9 (strong), 2C19 (strong), 3A4 (strong)

Drug Interactions

Acetaminophen: Anticonvulsants (Hydantoin) may increase the metabolism of Acetaminophen. This may 1) diminish the effect of acetaminophen; and 2) increase the risk of liver damage. *Risk C: Monitor therapy*

Alcohol (Ethyl): CNS Depressants may enhance the CNS depressant effect of Alcohol (Ethyl). *Risk C: Monitor therapy*

Aminocamptothecin: Phenytoin may decrease the serum concentration of Aminocamptothecin. *Risk C: Monitor therapy*

Amiodarone: Phenytoin may increase the metabolism of Amiodarone. Amiodarone may decrease the metabolism of Phenytoin. *Risk C: Monitor therapy*

Amphetamines: May decrease the serum concentration of Phenytoin. *Risk C: Monitor therapy*

Amprenavir: Phenytoin may increase the serum concentration of Amprenavir. Amprenavir may decrease the serum concentration of Phenytoin. *Risk C: Monitor therapy*

Antacids: May decrease the serum concentration of Anticonvulsants (Hydantoin). *Risk C: Monitor therapy*

Antifungal Agents (Azole Derivatives, Systemic): May increase the serum concentration of Phenytoin. Phenytoin may decrease the serum concentration of Antifungal Agents (Azole Derivatives, Systemic). **Exceptions:** Miconazole. *Risk D: Consider therapy modification*

Benzodiazepines: May increase the serum concentration of Phenytoin. Short-term exposure to benzodiazepines may not present as much risk as chronic therapy. **Exceptions:** ALPRAZolam. *Risk C: Monitor therapy*

Calcium Channel Blockers: May decrease the metabolism of Phenytoin. **Exceptions:** Clevidipine. *Risk D: Consider therapy modification*

Capecitabine: May increase the serum concentration of Phenytoin. *Risk D: Consider therapy modification*

CarBAMazepine: May increase the metabolism of Phenytoin. Phenytoin may increase the metabolism of CarBAMazepine. CarBAMazepine may decrease the metabolism of Phenytoin. Possibly by competitive inhibition at sites of metabolism. *Risk D: Consider therapy modification*

Carbonic Anhydrase Inhibitors: May enhance the adverse/toxic effect of Anticonvulsants (Hydantoin). Specifically, osteomalacia and rickets. **Exceptions:** Brinzolamide; Dorzolamide. *Risk C: Monitor therapy*

Caspofungin: Inducers of Drug Clearance may decrease the serum concentration of Caspofungin. Management: Consider using an increased caspofungin dose of 70 mg daily in adults (or 70 mg/m^2, up to a maximum of 70 mg, daily in pediatric patients) when coadministered with known inducers of drug clearance. *Risk D: Consider therapy modification*

Chloramphenicol: May decrease the metabolism of Anticonvulsants (Hydantoin). Anticonvulsants (Hydantoin) may decrease the serum concentration of Chloramphenicol. Increased chloramphenicol concentrations have also been seen. *Risk D: Consider therapy modification*

Cimetidine: May decrease the metabolism of Anticonvulsants (Hydantoin). *Risk D: Consider therapy modification*

Ciprofloxacin: May decrease the serum concentration of Phenytoin. *Risk C: Monitor therapy*

Clozapine: Phenytoin may increase the metabolism of Clozapine. *Risk C: Monitor therapy*

CNS Depressants: May enhance the adverse/toxic effect of other CNS Depressants. *Risk C: Monitor therapy*

Colesevelam: May decrease the serum concentration of Phenytoin. *Risk D: Consider therapy modification*

Contraceptive (Progestins): Phenytoin may diminish the therapeutic effect of Contraceptive (Progestins). Contraceptive failure is possible. *Risk D: Consider therapy modification*

CycloSPORINE: Phenytoin may increase the metabolism of CycloSPORINE. *Risk D: Consider therapy modification*

CYP2B6 Substrates: CYP2B6 Inducers (Strong) may increase the metabolism of CYP2B6 Substrates. *Risk C: Monitor therapy*

CYP2C19 Inducers (Strong): May increase the metabolism of CYP2C19 Substrates. *Risk C: Monitor therapy*

CYP2C19 Inhibitors (Moderate): May decrease the metabolism of CYP2C19 Substrates. *Risk C: Monitor therapy*

CYP2C19 Inhibitors (Strong): May decrease the metabolism of CYP2C19 Substrates. *Risk D: Consider therapy modification*

CYP2C19 Substrates: CYP2C19 Inducers (Strong) may increase the metabolism of CYP2C19 Substrates. *Risk C: Monitor therapy*

CYP2C8 Substrates (High risk): CYP2C8 Inducers (Highly Effective) may increase the metabolism of CYP2C8 Substrates (High risk). *Risk C: Monitor therapy*

CYP2C9 Inducers (Highly Effective): May increase the metabolism of CYP2C9 Substrates (High risk). *Risk C: Monitor therapy*

CYP2C9 Inhibitors (Moderate): May decrease the metabolism of CYP2C9 Substrates (High risk). *Risk C: Monitor therapy*

CYP2C9 Inhibitors (Strong): May decrease the metabolism of CYP2C9 Substrates (High risk). *Risk D: Consider therapy modification*

CYP2C9 Substrates (High risk): CYP2C9 Inducers (Highly Effective) may increase the metabolism of CYP2C9 Substrates (High risk). *Risk C: Monitor therapy*

CYP3A4 Substrates: CYP3A4 Inducers (Strong) may increase the metabolism of CYP3A4 Substrates. *Risk C: Monitor therapy*

Darunavir: Phenytoin may decrease the serum concentration of Darunavir. *Risk X: Avoid combination*

Dexmethylphenidate: May decrease the metabolism of Phenytoin. *Risk C: Monitor therapy*

Diazoxide: May decrease the serum concentration of Phenytoin. Total phenytoin concentrations may be affected more than free phenytoin concentrations. *Risk C: Monitor therapy*

Disopyramide: Phenytoin may increase the metabolism of Disopyramide. *Risk D: Consider therapy modification*

Disulfiram: May decrease the metabolism of Phenytoin. *Risk D: Consider therapy modification*

Doxycycline: Phenytoin may decrease the serum concentration of Doxycycline. *Risk D: Consider therapy modification*

Efavirenz: Phenytoin may decrease the serum concentration of Efavirenz. Efavirenz may increase the serum concentration of Phenytoin. *Risk D: Consider therapy modification*

Etoposide: Phenytoin may increase the metabolism of Etoposide. *Risk C: Monitor therapy*

Etoposide Phosphate: Phenytoin may decrease the serum concentration of Etoposide Phosphate. Phenytoin may increase the metabolism, via CYP isoenzymes, of etoposide phosphate. *Risk C: Monitor therapy*

Etravirine: Phenytoin may decrease the serum concentration of Etravirine. Management: The manufacturer of etravirine states these drugs should not be used in combination *Risk X: Avoid combination*

Felbamate: Phenytoin may increase the metabolism of Felbamate. Felbamate may increase the serum concentration of Phenytoin. *Risk D: Consider therapy modification*

Floxuridine: May increase the serum concentration of Phenytoin. *Risk D: Consider therapy modification*

Fluconazole: May decrease the metabolism of Phenytoin. *Risk D: Consider therapy modification*

Flunarizine: Phenytoin may decrease the serum concentration of Flunarizine. *Risk C: Monitor therapy*

Fluorouracil: May increase the serum concentration of Phenytoin. *Risk D: Consider therapy modification*

Folic Acid: May decrease the serum concentration of Phenytoin. *Risk C: Monitor therapy*

Fosamprenavir: May decrease the serum concentration of Phenytoin. The active amprenavir metabolite is likely responsible for this effect. Phenytoin may increase the serum concentration of Fosamprenavir. Specifically, phenytoin may increase the concentration of the active metabolite amprenavir. *Risk C: Monitor therapy*

HMG-CoA Reductase Inhibitors: Phenytoin may increase the metabolism of HMG-CoA Reductase Inhibitors. **Exceptions:** Rosuvastatin. *Risk D: Consider therapy modification*

Irinotecan: Phenytoin may increase the metabolism of Irinotecan. *Risk D: Consider therapy modification*

Isoniazid: May decrease the metabolism of Phenytoin. *Risk D: Consider therapy modification*

Ketorolac: May diminish the therapeutic effect of Anticonvulsants. *Risk C: Monitor therapy*

Lacosamide: Phenytoin may decrease the serum concentration of Lacosamide. *Risk C: Monitor therapy*

LamoTRIgine: Phenytoin may increase the metabolism of LamoTRIgine. *Risk D: Consider therapy modification*

Leucovorin-Levoleucovorin: May decrease the serum concentration of Phenytoin. *Risk C: Monitor therapy*

Levodopa: Phenytoin may diminish the therapeutic effect of Levodopa. *Risk C: Monitor therapy*

Lithium: Phenytoin may enhance the adverse/toxic effect of Lithium. *Risk C: Monitor therapy*

Loop Diuretics: Phenytoin may diminish the diuretic effect of Loop Diuretics. *Risk C: Monitor therapy*

Lopinavir: Phenytoin may decrease the serum concentration of Lopinavir. Lopinavir may decrease the serum concentration of Phenytoin. Management: The manufacturer of lopinavir/ritonavir recommends avoiding once-daily administration if used together with phenytoin. *Risk D: Consider therapy modification*

Maraviroc: CYP3A4 Inducers may decrease the serum concentration of Maraviroc. *Risk D: Consider therapy modification*

Mebendazole: Phenytoin may decrease the serum concentration of Mebendazole. *Risk C: Monitor therapy*

Mefloquine: May diminish the therapeutic effect of Anticonvulsants. Mefloquine may decrease the serum concentration of Anticonvulsants. Management: Mefloquine is contraindicated in persons with a history of convulsions. If anticonvulsant is being used for another indication monitor response to treatment closely, as concurrent mefloquine may decrease response to treatment. *Risk D: Consider therapy modification*

Meperidine: Phenytoin may increase the metabolism of Meperidine. *Risk C: Monitor therapy*

Methadone: Phenytoin may increase the metabolism of Methadone. *Risk C: Monitor therapy*

Methylfolate: May decrease the serum concentration of Phenytoin. *Risk C: Monitor therapy*

Methylphenidate: May decrease the metabolism of Phenytoin. *Risk C: Monitor therapy*

Metyrapone: Phenytoin may increase the metabolism of Metyrapone. The oral metyrapone test would thus be unreliable unless the metapyrone dosage was substantially increased (eg, 750 mg every 2 hours). *Risk D: Consider therapy modification*

Mexiletine: Phenytoin may increase the metabolism of Mexiletine. *Risk C: Monitor therapy*

Nilotinib: CYP3A4 Inducers (Strong) may decrease the serum concentration of Nilotinib. *Risk X: Avoid combination*

Oral Contraceptive (Estrogens): Phenytoin may diminish the therapeutic effect of Oral Contraceptive (Estrogens). Contraceptive failure is possible. *Risk D: Consider therapy modification*

OXcarbazepine: Phenytoin may decrease the serum concentration of OXcarbazepine. OXcarbazepine may increase the serum concentration of Phenytoin. *Risk C: Monitor therapy*

Primidone: Phenytoin may increase the metabolism of Primidone. The ratio of primidone:phenobarbital is thus changed. *Risk C: Monitor therapy*

Proton Pump Inhibitors: May increase the serum concentration of Phenytoin. **Exceptions:** Esomeprazole; Lansoprazole; Pantoprazole; Rabeprazole. *Risk C: Monitor therapy*

Pyridoxine: May increase the metabolism of Phenytoin. This is most apparent in high pyridoxine doses (eg, 80 mg to 200 mg daily) *Risk C: Monitor therapy*

QUEtiapine: Phenytoin may increase the metabolism of QUEtiapine. *Risk D: Consider therapy modification*

QuiNIDine: Phenytoin may increase the metabolism of QuiNIDine. *Risk D: Consider therapy modification*

Ranolazine: CYP3A4 Inducers (Strong) may decrease the serum concentration of Ranolazine. *Risk X: Avoid combination*

Rifamycin Derivatives: May increase the metabolism of Phenytoin. *Risk D: Consider therapy modification*

Ritonavir: Phenytoin may decrease the serum concentration of Ritonavir. Ritonavir may decrease the serum concentration of Phenytoin. *Risk D: Consider therapy modification*

Selective Serotonin Reuptake Inhibitors: May decrease the metabolism of Phenytoin. **Exceptions:** PARoxetine. *Risk D: Consider therapy modification*

Sirolimus: Phenytoin may increase the metabolism of Sirolimus. *Risk D: Consider therapy modification*

Sorafenib: CYP3A4 Inducers (Strong) may decrease the serum concentration of Sorafenib. *Risk D: Consider therapy modification*

Sulfonamide Derivatives: May decrease the metabolism of Phenytoin. *Risk C: Monitor therapy*

Tacrolimus: Phenytoin may increase the metabolism of Tacrolimus. Tacrolimus may increase the serum concentration of Phenytoin. *Risk C: Monitor therapy*

Temsirolimus: Phenytoin may decrease the serum concentration of Temsirolimus. Concentrations of the active metabolite, sirolimus, are also likely to be decreased (and maybe to an even greater degree). Management: Temsirolimus prescribing information recommends against coadministration with strong CYP3A4 inducers such as phenytoin; however, if concurrent therapy is necessary, an increase in temsirolimus dose to 50 mg/week should be considered. *Risk D: Consider therapy modification*

Teniposide: Phenytoin may increase the metabolism of Teniposide. *Risk C: Monitor therapy*

Theophylline Derivatives: Phenytoin may increase the metabolism of Theophylline Derivatives. Theophylline Derivatives may decrease the serum concentration of Phenytoin. **Exceptions:** Dyphylline. *Risk C: Monitor therapy*

Thyroid Products: Phenytoin may increase the metabolism of Thyroid Products. Phenytoin may also displace thyroid hormones from protein binding sites. *Risk C: Monitor therapy*

Ticlopidine: May decrease the metabolism of Phenytoin. *Risk D: Consider therapy modification*

Tipranavir: Phenytoin may decrease the serum concentration of Tipranavir. Tipranavir may decrease the serum concentration of Phenytoin. *Risk D: Consider therapy modification*

Topiramate: May decrease the metabolism of Phenytoin. Phenytoin may increase the metabolism of Topiramate. *Risk C: Monitor therapy*

Trimethoprim: May decrease the metabolism of Phenytoin. *Risk C: Monitor therapy*

Valproic Acid: Phenytoin may increase the metabolism of Valproic Acid. A hepatotoxic metabolite of valproic acid may result. Valproic Acid may decrease the serum concentration of Phenytoin. Continued therapy usually yields a normalization (or slight increase) of serum phenytoin concentrations. Free phenytoin concentrations, however, tend to remain relatively stable (possibly increased with continued therapy). *Risk C: Monitor therapy*

Vecuronium: Phenytoin may decrease the serum concentration of Vecuronium. *Risk C: Monitor therapy*

Vigabatrin: May decrease the serum concentration of Phenytoin. *Risk C: Monitor therapy*

Vitamin K Antagonists (eg, warfarin): Phenytoin may enhance the anticoagulant effect of Vitamin K Antagonists. Vitamin K Antagonists may increase the serum concentration of Phenytoin. *Risk D: Consider therapy modification*

Zonisamide: Phenytoin may increase the metabolism of Zonisamide. *Risk C: Monitor therapy*

Ethanol/Nutrition/Herb Interactions

Ethanol:

Acute use: Avoid or limit ethanol (inhibits metabolism of phenytoin). Watch for sedation.

Chronic use: Avoid or limit ethanol (stimulates metabolism of phenytoin).

Food: Phenytoin serum concentrations may be altered if taken with food. If taken with enteral nutrition, phenytoin serum concentrations may be decreased. Tube feedings decrease bioavailability; hold tube feedings 1-2 hours before and 1-2 hours after phenytoin administration. May decrease calcium, folic acid, and vitamin D levels.

Herb/Nutraceutical: Avoid evening primrose (seizure threshold decreased). Avoid valerian, St John's wort, kava kava, gotu kola (may increase CNS depression).

Stability

Capsule, tablet: Store below 30°C (86°F). Protect from light and moisture.

Oral suspension: Store at room temperature of 20°C to 25°C (68°F to 77°F); do not freeze. Protect from light.

Solution for injection: Store at room temperature of 15°C to 30°C (59°F to 86°F). Use only clear solutions free of precipitate and haziness; slightly yellow solutions may be used. Precipitation may occur if solution is refrigerated and may dissolve at room temperature.

Further dilution of the solution for I.V. infusion is controversial and no consensus exists as to the optimal concentration and length of stability. Stability is concentration and pH dependent. Based on limited clinical consensus, NS or LR are recommended diluents. Dilutions of 1-10 mg/mL have been used and should be administered as soon as possible after preparation (some recommend to discard if not used within 4 hours). Do not refrigerate.

Mechanism of Action Stabilizes neuronal membranes and decreases seizure activity by increasing efflux or decreasing influx of sodium ions across cell membranes in the motor cortex during generation of nerve impulses; prolongs effective refractory period and suppresses ventricular pacemaker automaticity, shortens action potential in the heart

Pharmacodynamics/Kinetics

Onset of action: I.V.: ~0.5-1 hour

Absorption: Oral: Slow

Distribution: V_d:

Neonates: Premature: 1-1.2 L/kg; Full-term: 0.8-0.9 L/kg

Infants: 0.7-0.8 L/kg

Children: 0.7 L/kg

Adults: 0.6-0.7 L/kg

Protein binding:

Neonates: ≥80% (≤20% free)

Infants: ≥85% (≤15% free)

Adults: 90% to 95%

Others: Decreased protein binding

Disease states resulting in a decrease in serum albumin concentration: Burns, hepatic cirrhosis, nephrotic syndrome, pregnancy, cystic fibrosis

Disease states resulting in an apparent decrease in affinity of phenytoin for serum albumin: Renal failure, jaundice (severe), other drugs (displacers), hyperbilirubinemia (total bilirubin >15 mg/dL), Cl_{cr} <25 mL/minute (unbound fraction is increased two- to threefold in uremia)

Metabolism: Follows dose-dependent capacity-limited (Michaelis-Menten) pharmacokinetics with increased V_{max} in infants >6 months of age and children versus adults; major metabolite (via oxidation), HPPA, undergoes enterohepatic recirculation

Bioavailability: Form dependent
Half-life elimination: Oral: 22 hours (range: 7-42 hours)
Time to peak, serum (form dependent): Oral: Extended-release capsule: 4-12 hours; Immediate release preparation: 2-3 hours
Excretion: Urine (<5% as unchanged drug); as glucuronides
Clearance: Highly variable, dependent upon intrinsic hepatic function and dose administered; increased clearance and decreased serum concentrations with febrile illness

Dosage

Status epilepticus: I.V.:

Infants and Children: Loading dose: 15-20 mg/kg in a single or divided dose; maintenance dose: Initial: 5 mg/kg/day in 2 divided doses; usual doses:
- 6 months to 3 years: 8-10 mg/kg/day
- 4-6 years: 7.5-9 mg/kg/day
- 7-9 years: 7-8 mg/kg/day
- 10-16 years: 6-7 mg/kg/day, some patients may require every 8 hours dosing

Adults: Loading dose: Manufacturer recommends 10-15 mg/kg, however, 15-20 mg/kg is generally recommended; maximum rate: 50 mg/minute

Anticonvulsant: Children and Adults: Oral:

Loading dose: 15-20 mg/kg; based on phenytoin serum concentrations and recent dosing history; administer oral loading dose in 3 divided doses given every 2-4 hours to decrease GI adverse effects and to ensure complete oral absorption; maintenance dose: same as I.V.

Neurosurgery (prophylactic): 100-200 mg at approximately 4-hour intervals during surgery and during the immediate postoperative period

Dosage adjustment in obesity: Adults: Loading dose: Use adjusted body weight (ABW) (Abernethy, 1985)

ABW = [(Actual body weight – IBW) x 1.33] + IBW

Maximum loading dose: 2000 mg (Erstad, 2004)

Maintenance doses should be based on ideal body weight, conventional daily doses with adjustments based upon therapeutic drug monitoring and clinical effectiveness. (Abernethy, 1985; Erstad, 2002; Erstad, 2004)

Dosing adjustment/comments in renal impairment or hepatic disease: Safe in usual doses in mild liver disease; clearance may be substantially reduced in cirrhosis and plasma level monitoring with dose adjustment advisable. Free phenytoin levels should be monitored closely.

Dietary Considerations

Folic acid: Phenytoin may decrease mucosal uptake of folic acid; to avoid folic acid deficiency and megaloblastic anemia, some clinicians recommend giving patients on anticonvulsants prophylactic doses of folic acid and cyanocobalamin. However, folate supplementation may increase seizures in some patients (dose dependent). Discuss with healthcare provider prior to using any supplements.

Calcium: Hypocalcemia has been reported in patients taking prolonged high-dose therapy with an anticonvulsant. Some clinicians have given an additional 4000 units/week of vitamin D (especially in those receiving poor nutrition and getting no sun exposure) to prevent hypocalcemia.

Vitamin D: Phenytoin interferes with vitamin D metabolism and osteomalacia may result; may need to supplement with vitamin D

Tube feedings: Tube feedings decrease phenytoin absorption. To avoid decreased serum levels with continuous NG feeds, hold feedings for 1-2 hours prior to and 1-2 hours after phenytoin administration, if possible. There is a variety of opinions on how to administer phenytoin with enteral feedings. Be **consistent** throughout therapy.

Sodium content of 1 g injection: 88 mg (3.8 mEq)

Administration

Oral: Suspension: Shake well prior to use. Absorption is impaired when phenytoin suspension is given concurrently to patients who are receiving continuous nasogastric feedings. A method to resolve this interaction is to divide the daily dose of phenytoin and withhold the administration of nutritional supplements for 1-2 hours before and after each phenytoin dose.

I.M.: Although approved for I.M. use, I.M. administration is not recommended due to erratic absorption and pain on injection. Fosphenytoin may be considered.

I.V.: Vesicant. Fosphenytoin may be considered for loading in patients who are in status epilepticus, hemodynamically unstable, or develop hypotension/bradycardia with I.V. administration of phenytoin. Phenytoin may be administered by IVP or IVPB administration. The maximum rate of I.V. administration is 50 mg/minute. Highly sensitive patients (eg, elderly, patients with pre-existing cardiovascular conditions) should receive phenytoin more slowly (eg, 20 mg/minute). An in-line 0.22-5 micron filter is recommended for IVPB solutions due to the high potential for precipitation of the solution. Avoid extravasation. Following I.V. administration, NS should be injected through the same needle or I.V. catheter to prevent irritation.

pH: 10.0-12.3

SubQ: SubQ administration is not recommended because of the possibility of local tissue damage (due to high pH).

Monitoring Parameters Blood pressure, vital signs (with I.V. use); plasma phenytoin level, CBC, liver function. **Note:** If available, free phenytoin concentrations should be obtained in patients with renal impairment and/or hypoalbuminemia. If free phenytoin levels are unavailable, the adjusted total level is based upon equations in adult patients.

Reference Range Timing of serum samples: Because it is slowly absorbed, peak blood levels may occur 4-8 hours after ingestion of an oral dose. The serum half-life varies with the dosage and the drug follows Michaelis-Menten kinetics. The average adult half-life is about 24 hours. Steady-state concentrations are reached in 5-10 days.

Children and Adults: Toxicity is measured clinically, and some patients require levels outside the suggested therapeutic range

Therapeutic range:

Total phenytoin: 10-20 mcg/mL (children and adults), 8-15 mcg/mL (neonates)

Concentrations of 5-10 mcg/mL may be therapeutic for some patients but concentrations <5 mcg/mL are not likely to be effective

50% of patients show decreased frequency of seizures at concentrations >10 mcg/mL

86% of patients show decreased frequency of seizures at concentrations >15 mcg/mL

Add another anticonvulsant if satisfactory therapeutic response is not achieved with a phenytoin concentration of 20 mcg/mL

Free phenytoin: 1-2.5 mcg/mL

Total phenytoin:

Toxic: >30 mcg/mL (SI: <120-200 µmol/L)

Lethal: >100 mcg/mL (SI: >400 µmol/L)

When to draw levels: This is dependent on the disease state being treated and the clinical condition of the patient

Key points:

Slow absorption of extended capsules and prolonged half-life minimize fluctuations between peak and trough concentrations, timing of sampling not crucial

Trough concentrations are generally recommended for routine monitoring. Daily levels are not necessary and may result in incorrect dosage adjustments. If it is determined essential to monitor free phenytoin concentrations, concomitant monitoring of total phenytoin concentrations is not necessary and expensive.

After a loading dose: If rapid therapeutic levels are needed, initial levels may be drawn after 1 hour (I.V. loading dose) or within 24 hours (oral loading dose) to aid in determining maintenance dose or need to reload.

Rapid achievement: Draw within 2-3 days of therapy initiation to ensure that the patient's metabolism is not remarkably different from that which would be predicted by average literature-derived pharmacokinetic parameters; early levels should be used cautiously in design of new dosing regimens

Second concentration: Draw within 6-7 days with subsequent doses of phenytoin adjusted accordingly

If plasma concentrations have not changed over a 3- to 5-day period, monitoring interval may be increased to once weekly in the acute clinical setting

In stable patients requiring long-term therapy, generally monitor levels at 3- to 12-month intervals

Adjustment of serum concentration: See tables on next page.

Note: Although it is ideal to obtain free phenytoin concentrations to assess serum concentrations in patients with hypoalbuminemia or renal failure (Cl_{cr} ≤10 mL/minute), it may not always be possible. If free phenytoin concentrations are unavailable, the following equations may be utilized in adult patients.

Adjustment of Serum Concentration in Adults With Low Serum Albumin

Measured Total Phenytoin Concentration (mcg/mL)	Patient's Serum Albumin (g/dL)			
	3.5	3	2.5	2
	Adjusted Total Phenytoin Concentration (mcg/mL)[1]			
5	6	7	8	10
10	13	14	17	20
15	19	21	25	30

[1]Adjusted concentration = measured total concentration divided by [(0.2 x albumin) + 0.1].

Adjustment of Serum Concentration in Adults With Renal Failure (Cl_{cr} ≤10 mL/min)

Measured Total Phenytoin Concentration (mcg/mL)	Patient's Serum Albumin (g/dL)				
	4	3.5	3	2.5	2
	Adjusted Total Phenytoin Concentration (mcg/mL)[1]				
5	10	11	13	14	17
10	20	22	25	29	33
15	30	33	38	43	50

[1]Adjusted concentration = measured total concentration divided by [(0.1 x albumin) + 0.1].

Dosage Forms Excipient information presented when available (limited, particularly for generics); consult specific product labeling.

Capsule, extended release, as sodium: 100 mg
- Dilantin®: 30 mg [contains sodium benzoate], 100 mg
- Phenytek®: 200 mg, 300 mg

Capsule, prompt release, as sodium: 100 mg

Injection, solution, as sodium: 50 mg/mL (2 mL, 5 mL) [contains alcohol and propylene glycol]

Suspension, oral: 100 mg/4 mL (4 mL); 125 mg/5 mL (240 mL)
- Dilantin®: 125 mg/5 mL (240 mL) [contains alcohol <0.6%, sodium benzoate; orange vanilla flavor]

Tablet, chewable:
- Dilantin®: 50 mg

- ◆ **Phenytoin Sodium** *see* Phenytoin *on page 1280*
- ◆ **Phenytoin Sodium, Extended** *see* Phenytoin *on page 1280*
- ◆ **Phenytoin Sodium, Prompt** *see* Phenytoin *on page 1280*
- ◆ **Phlemex** *see* Guaifenesin and Dextromethorphan *on page 739*
- ◆ **PhosLo®** *see* Calcium Acetate *on page 254*
- ◆ **Phosphonoformate** *see* Foscarnet *on page 690*
- ◆ **Phosphonoformic Acid** *see* Foscarnet *on page 690*
- ◆ **Photofrin®** *see* Porfimer *on page 1314*
- ◆ **Phrenilin®** *see* Butalbital and Acetaminophen *on page 236*
- ◆ **Phrenilin® Forte** *see* Butalbital and Acetaminophen *on page 236*
- ◆ **Phrenilin® with Caffeine and Codeine** *see* Butalbital, Acetaminophen, Caffeine, and Codeine *on page 232*
- ◆ ***p*-Hydroxyampicillin** *see* Amoxicillin *on page 112*
- ◆ **Phylloquinone** *see* Phytonadione *on page 1289*

Physostigmine (fye zoe STIG meen)

Medication Safety Issues

Sound-alike/look-alike issues:
- Physostigmine may be confused with Prostigmin®, pyridostigmine

Canadian Brand Names Eserine®; Isopto® Eserine

Index Terms Eserine Salicylate; Physostigmine Salicylate; Physostigmine Sulfate

Pharmacologic Category Acetylcholinesterase Inhibitor

Use Reverse toxic, life-threatening delirium caused by atropine, diphenhydramine, dimenhydrinate, *Atropa belladonna* (deadly nightshade), or jimson weed (*Datura* spp)

Effect on Mental Status May cause restlessness, nervousness, or hallucinations

Effect on Psychiatric Treatment None reported

Dosage Summary

I.M.:

Children: Dosage not established

Adults: Initial: 0.5-2 mg, repeat every 20 minutes until response or adverse effects occur; repeat 1-4 mg every 30-60 minutes as life-threatening symptoms recur

I.V.: Note: Administer slowly over 5 minutes to prevent respiratory distress and seizures. Continuous infusions of physostigmine should never be used.

Children: 0.01-0.03 mg/kg/dose, may repeat after 5-10 minutes (maximum total dose: 2 mg)

Adults: Initial: 0.5-2 mg, repeat every 20 minutes until response or adverse effects occur; repeat 1-4 mg every 30-60 minutes as life-threatening symptoms recur

Dosage Forms Excipient information presented when available (limited, particularly for generics); consult specific product labeling.

Injection, solution, as salicylate: 1 mg/mL (2 mL) [contains benzyl alcohol and sodium metabisulfite]

◆ **Physostigmine Salicylate** *see* Physostigmine *on page 1288*

◆ **Physostigmine Sulfate** *see* Physostigmine *on page 1288*

◆ **Phytomenadione** *see* Phytonadione *on page 1289*

Phytonadione (fye toe na DYE one)

Medication Safety Issues

Sound-alike/look-alike issues:

Mephyton® may be confused with melphalan, methadone

U.S. Brand Names Mephyton®

Canadian Brand Names AquaMEPHYTON®; Konakion; Mephyton®

Mexican Brand Names Konakion MM

Index Terms Methylphytyl Napthoquinone; Phylloquinone; Phytomenadione; Vitamin K_1

Pharmacologic Category Vitamin, Fat Soluble

Use Prevention and treatment of hypoprothrombinemia caused by coumarin derivative-induced or other drug-induced vitamin K deficiency, hypoprothrombinemia caused by malabsorption or inability to synthesize vitamin K; hemorrhagic disease of the newborn

Unlabeled/Investigational Use Treatment of hypoprothrombinemia caused by anticoagulant rodenticides

Effect on Mental Status May rarely cause dizziness

Effect on Psychiatric Treatment None reported

Dosage Summary

I.M.:

Newborns: Prophylaxis: 0.5-1 mg within 1 hour of birth; Treatment: 1 mg/dose/day

Children: Dosage not established

Adults: Initial: 2.5-25 mg per dose (usual: 5-10 mg; maximum 50 mg)

I.V.:

Children: Dosage not established

Adults: Initial: 2.5-25 mg per dose (usual: 5-10 mg; maximum 50 mg

Oral:

Children <1 years: Dosage not established

Children 1-3 years: RDA: 30 mcg/day

Children 4-8 years: RDA: 55 mcg/day

Children 9-13 years: RDA: 60 mcg/day

Children 14-18 years: RDA: 75 mcg/day

Adults: Initial: 2.5-25 mg per dose (usual: 5-10 mg; maximum 50 mg)

SubQ:

Newborns: 1 mg/dose/day

Children: Dosage not established

Adults: Initial: 2.5-25 mg per dose (usual: 5-10 mg; maximum 50 mg

Dosage Forms Excipient information presented when available (limited, particularly for generics); consult specific product labeling.

Injection, aqueous colloidal: 2 mg/mL (0.5 mL); 10 mg/mL (1 mL)

Tablet: 100 mcg [OTC]
Mephyton®: 5 mg

- ◆ **Pidorubicin** *see* Epirubicin *on page 545*
- ◆ **Pidorubicin Hydrochloride** *see* Epirubicin *on page 545*

Pilocarpine (pye loe KAR peen)

Medication Safety Issues

Sound-alike/look-alike issues:

Isopto® Carpine may be confused with Isopto® Carbachol
Salagen® may be confused with Salacid®, selegiline

International issues:

Salagen® may be confused with Poagen® which is a brand name for grass pollen extract in Portugal

U.S. Brand Names Isopto® Carpine; Pilopine HS®; Salagen®

Canadian Brand Names Diocarpine; Isopto® Carpine; Pilopine HS®; Salagen®

Mexican Brand Names Caliprene; Dretinof

Index Terms Pilocarpine Hydrochloride

Pharmacologic Category Cholinergic Agonist; Ophthalmic Agent, Antiglaucoma; Ophthalmic Agent, Miotic

Use

Ophthalmic: Management of chronic simple glaucoma, chronic and acute angle-closure glaucoma

Oral: Symptomatic treatment of xerostomia caused by salivary gland hypofunction resulting from radiotherapy for cancer of the head and neck or Sjögren's syndrome

Unlabeled/Investigational Use Counter effects of cycloplegics

Effect on Mental Status None reported

Effect on Psychiatric Treatment Pilocarpine may antagonize the effects of anticholinergics and produce cardiac conduction abnormalities in patients receiving beta-blockers

Dosage Summary

Ophthalmic:

Children: Dosage not established

Adults:

Gel: Instill 0.5" ribbon once daily at bedtime
Solution: Instill 1-2 drops up to 6 times/day

Oral:

Children: Dosage not established

Adults: 5 mg 3-4 times/day (maximum: 30 mg/day)

Dosage Forms Excipient information presented when available (limited, particularly for generics); consult specific product labeling.

Gel, ophthalmic, as hydrochloride (Pilopine HS®): 4% (4 g) [contains benzalkonium chloride]

Solution, ophthalmic, as hydrochloride: 0.5% (15 mL); 1% (2 mL, 15 mL); 2% (2 mL, 15 mL); 3% (15 mL); 4% (2 mL, 15 mL); 6% (15 mL) [may contain benzalkonium chloride]

Isopto® Carpine: 1% (15 mL); 2% (15 mL); 4% (15 mL) [contains benzalkonium chloride]

Tablet, as hydrochloride: 5 mg, 7.5 mg

Salagen®: 5 mg, 7.5 mg

- ◆ **Pilocarpine Hydrochloride** *see* Pilocarpine *on page 1290*
- ◆ **Pilopine HS®** *see* Pilocarpine *on page 1290*

Pimozide (PI moe zide)

Related Information

Antipsychotic Agents *on page 1769*
CMS: Long-Term Care Facility Thresholds *on page 1815*
Discontinuation of Psychotropic Drugs *on page 1839*

U.S. Brand Names Orap®

Canadian Brand Names Apo-Pimozide®; Orap®

Pharmacologic Category Antipsychotic Agent, Typical

Generic Available No

Use Suppression of severe motor and phonic tics in patients with Tourette's disorder who have failed to respond satisfactorily to standard treatment

Unlabeled/Investigational Use Psychosis; reported use in individuals with delusions focused on physical symptoms (ie, preoccupation with parasitic infestation); Huntington's chorea; psychosis/agitation related to Alzheimer's dementia

Mental Health Comment Older antipsychotic medications (chlorpromazine, haloperidol), which do not meet specific criteria for "atypical antipsychotics", are often referred to as typical antipsychotics. They are associated with the troubling side effect, EPS. However, it is commonly believed that in order for a drug to treat psychosis, it must block dopamine is some manner.

Common side effects include sedation and neuroleptic effect (reduced initiative, interest in the environment, and display of emotion or affect). All **typical** antipsychotics are considered to be equally effective if given in equipotent doses. An inverse relationship exists between intrinsic antimuscarinic activity and propensity to cause extrapyramidal side effects. If dystonia or pseudoparkinsonism occurs, antiparkinsonian agents should be considered. If akathisia occurs, beta-blockers (eg, propranolol), benzodiazepines, or antiparkinsonian agents should be considered. Tardive dyskinesia (TD) secondary to typical antipsychotics has an estimated incidence of 3% to 5% per year for the first 5 years of treatment. After this time period, the incidence is estimated to be 2% to 3% per year. Prevalence rates are ~15% to 20%. Female gender and age constitute risk factors for TD. No specific treatment exists for TD, however, patients are often initiated on/switched to an atypical antipsychotic because of their lower incidence to cause TD and hopes of suppression.

Typical antipsychotics are usually only indicated for schizophrenia, but are generally effective for mania and psychosis and/or behavioral syndromes secondary to other mental conditions. Nonpsychiatric uses include Tourette's syndrome, Huntington's disease, and occasionally, intractable hiccups, pruritus, nausea, and vomiting.

These drugs are thought to exert their antipsychotic activity by blocking dopamine D_2 receptors in the mesolimbic dopaminergic pathway. Side effects are often related to their ability to antagonize dopamine receptors in the nigrostriatal and tuberoinfundibular pathways.

Coadministration of two or more antipsychotics does not generally improve clinical response and may increase the potential for adverse effects.

In 2008, the FDA issued a warning regarding increased mortality risk with typical **and** atypical antipsychotic drugs when used in elderly patients with dementia-related psychosis.

Pregnancy Risk Factor C

Lactation Excretion in breast milk unknown

Contraindications Hypersensitivity to pimozide or any component of the formulation; severe CNS depression; coma; history of dysrhythmia; prolonged QT syndrome; concurrent use with QT_c-prolonging agents; hypokalemia or hypomagnesemia; concurrent use of drugs that are inhibitors of CYP3A4, including concurrent use of azole antifungals, fluvoxamine, macrolide antibiotics (such as clarithromycin or erythromycin [**Note:** The manufacturer lists azithromycin and dirithromycin in its list of contraindicated macrolides; however, these drugs do not inhibit CYP3A4 and are not expected to interact with pimozide]), mesoridazine, nefazodone, protease inhibitors (ie, atazanavir, indinavir, nelfinavir, ritonavir, saquinavir), sertraline, thioridazine, zileuton, and ziprasidone; simple tics other than Tourette's

Warnings/Precautions Elderly patients with dementia-related psychosis treated with antipsychotics are at an increased risk of death compared to placebo. An increased incidence of cerebrovascular adverse events (including fatalities) has been reported in elderly patients with dementia-related psychosis. Pimozide is not approved for this indication.May alter cardiac conduction; life-threatening arrhythmias have occurred with therapeutic doses of antipsychotics. Avoid use in patients with underlying QT prolongation, in those taking medicines that prolong the QT interval, or cause polymorphic ventricular tachycardia; monitor ECG closely for dose-related QT effects. Sudden unexplained deaths have occurred in patients taking high doses (>10 mg). Myelosuppression (eg, leukopenia, agranulocytosis) has been observed with antipsychotic use; check blood counts periodically and discontinue at first signs of blood dyscrasias. Antipsychotic use has been associated with esophageal dysmotility and aspiration; use with caution in patients at risk of pneumonia (ie, Alzheimer's disease). May cause extrapyramidal symptoms (EPS), including pseudoparkinsonism, acute dystonic reactions, akathisia, and tardive dyskinesia (risk of these reactions is high relative to other neuroleptics). Risk of dystonia (and possibly other EPS) may be greater with increased doses, use of conventional antipsychotics, males, and younger patients. Use may be associated with NMS; monitor for mental status changes, fever, muscle rigidity, and/or autonomic instability (risk may be increased in patients with Parkinson's disease or Lewy body dementia). May cause orthostatic hypotension; use with caution in patients at risk of this effect or in those who would not tolerate transient hypotensive episodes (cerebrovascular disease, cardiovascular disease, hypovolemia, or concurrent medication use which may predispose to hypotension/bradycardia). May be associated with pigmentary retinopathy. May be sedating, use with caution in disorders where CNS depression is a feature; patients must be cautioned about performing tasks which require mental alertness (eg, operating machinery or driving). Impaired core body temperature regulation may occur; caution with strenuous exercise, heat exposure, dehydration, and concomitant medication possessing anticholinergic effects.

May be sedating, use with caution in disorders where CNS depression is a feature; patients must be cautioned about performing tasks which require mental alertness (eg, operating machinery or driving). May cause anticholinergic effects (constipation, xerostomia, blurred vision, urinary retention); use with caution in patients with decreased gastrointestinal motility, paralytic ileus, urinary retention, BPH, xerostomia, or visual problems. Relative to neuroleptics, pimozide has a moderate potency of cholinergic blockade. May mask toxicity of other drugs or conditions (eg, intestinal obstruction, Reye's syndrome, brain tumor) due to antiemetic effects.

Use with caution in patients with severe cardiovascular disease, narrow-angle glaucoma, hepatic impairment, myasthenia gravis, Parkinson's disease, breast cancer or other prolactin-dependent tumors, renal impairment, respiratory disease, or seizure disorder.

Adverse Reactions

Frequencies >1% reported in adults (limited data) and/or children with Tourette's disorder:

Cardiovascular: Abnormal ECG (3%)

Central nervous system: Somnolence (up to 28% in children), sedation (14%), akathisia (8%), nervousness (1% to 8%), drowsiness (7%), hyperkinesias (6%), insomnia (2%), depression (2%), headache (1%)

Dermatologic: Rash (8%)

Gastrointestinal: Xerostomia (25%), constipation (20%), increased salivation (14%), diarrhea (5%), thirst (5%), appetite increased (5%), taste disturbance (5%), dysphagia (3%)

Genitourinary: Impotence (15%)

Neuromuscular & skeletal: Weakness (22%), muscle tightness (15%), rigidity (10%), myalgia (3%), torticollis (3%), tremor (3%)

Ocular: Visual disturbance (6% to 20%), accommodation decreased (20%)

Miscellaneous: Speech disorder (10%)

Frequency not established (reported in disorders other than Tourette's disorder): Blood dyscrasias, breast edema, chest pain, dizziness, extrapyramidal symptoms (akathisia, akinesia, dystonia, pseudoparkinsonism, tardive dyskinesia); facial edema, gingival hyperplasia (case report), hyper-/hypotension, hyponatremia, jaundice, libido decreased, neuroleptic malignant syndrome, orthostatic hypotension, palpitation, periorbital edema, postural hypotension, QT_c prolongation, seizure, tachycardia, ventricular arrhythmia, vomiting, weight gain/loss

Metabolism/Transport Effects Substrate (major) of CYP1A2, 3A4; **Inhibits** CYP2C19 (weak), 2D6 (weak), 2E1 (weak), 3A4 (weak)

Drug Interactions

Acetylcholinesterase Inhibitors (Central): May enhance the neurotoxic (central) effect of Antipsychotics. Severe extrapyramidal symptoms have occurred in some patients. *Risk C: Monitor therapy*

Alcohol (Ethyl): CNS Depressants may enhance the CNS depressant effect of Alcohol (Ethyl). *Risk C: Monitor therapy*

Alfuzosin: May enhance the QTc-prolonging effect of QTc-Prolonging Agents. *Risk C: Monitor therapy*

Amphetamines: Antipsychotics may diminish the stimulatory effect of Amphetamines. *Risk C: Monitor therapy*

Anticholinergics: May enhance the adverse/toxic effect of other Anticholinergics. **Exceptions:** Paliperidone. *Risk C: Monitor therapy*

Antifungal Agents (Azole Derivatives, Systemic): May decrease the metabolism of Pimozide. *Risk X: Avoid combination*

Anti-Parkinson's Agents (Dopamine Agonist): Antipsychotics (Typical) may diminish the therapeutic effect of Anti-Parkinson's Agents (Dopamine Agonist). *Risk D: Consider therapy modification*

Aprepitant: May increase the serum concentration of Pimozide. *Risk X: Avoid combination*

Ciprofloxacin: May enhance the QTc-prolonging effect of QTc-Prolonging Agents. *Risk C: Monitor therapy*

CNS Depressants: May enhance the adverse/toxic effect of other CNS Depressants. *Risk C: Monitor therapy*

CYP1A2 Inducers (Strong): May increase the metabolism of CYP1A2 Substrates. *Risk C: Monitor therapy*

CYP1A2 Inhibitors (Moderate): May decrease the metabolism of CYP1A2 Substrates. *Risk C: Monitor therapy*

CYP1A2 Inhibitors (Strong): May decrease the metabolism of CYP1A2 Substrates. *Risk D: Consider therapy modification*

CYP3A4 Inducers (Strong): May increase the metabolism of CYP3A4 Substrates. *Risk C: Monitor therapy*

CYP3A4 Inhibitors (Moderate): May decrease the metabolism of CYP3A4 Substrates. *Risk C: Monitor therapy*

CYP3A4 Inhibitors (Strong): May decrease the metabolism of CYP3A4 Substrates. *Risk D: Consider therapy modification*

Dasatinib: May increase the serum concentration of CYP3A4 Substrates. *Risk C: Monitor therapy*

Deferasirox: May decrease the serum concentration of CYP3A4 Substrates. *Risk C: Monitor therapy*

Efavirenz: May enhance the arrhythmogenic effect of Pimozide. *Risk X: Avoid combination*

Fosaprepitant: May increase the serum concentration of Pimozide. The active metabolite aprepitant is likely responsible for this effect. *Risk X: Avoid combination*

Gadobutrol: May enhance the QTc-prolonging effect of QTc-Prolonging Agents. *Risk D: Consider therapy modification*

Herbs (CYP3A4 Inducers): May increase the metabolism of CYP3A4 Substrates. *Risk C: Monitor therapy*

Lithium formulations: May enhance the neurotoxic effect of Antipsychotics. Lithium formulations may decrease the serum concentration of Antipsychotics. Specifically noted with chlorpromazine. *Risk C: Monitor therapy*

Macrolide Antibiotics: May decrease the metabolism of Pimozide. QTc prolongation is a risk. **Exceptions:** Azithromycin; Dirithromycin [Off Market]; Spiramycin. *Risk X: Avoid combination*

Nefazodone: May decrease the metabolism of Pimozide. *Risk X: Avoid combination*

Nilotinib: May enhance the QTc-prolonging effect of QTc-Prolonging Agents. *Risk X: Avoid combination*

Pramlintide: May enhance the anticholinergic effect of Anticholinergics. These effects are specific to the GI tract. *Risk D: Consider therapy modification*

Protease Inhibitors: May decrease the metabolism of Pimozide. *Risk X: Avoid combination*

QTc-Prolonging Agents: May enhance the adverse/toxic effect of other QTc-Prolonging Agents. Their effects can be additive, causing life-threatening ventricular arrhythmias. *Risk D: Consider therapy modification*

Selective Serotonin Reuptake Inhibitors: May enhance the adverse/toxic effect of Pimozide. *Risk X: Avoid combination*

Tetrabenazine: May enhance the adverse/toxic effect of Antipsychotics. *Risk C: Monitor therapy*

Thioridazine: QTc-Prolonging Agents may enhance the QTc-prolonging effect of Thioridazine. *Risk X: Avoid combination*

Ziprasidone: QTc-Prolonging Agents may enhance the QTc-prolonging effect of Ziprasidone. The risk of a severe arrhythmia may be increased. *Risk X: Avoid combination*

Ethanol/Nutrition/Herb Interactions

Ethanol: Avoid ethanol (may increase CNS depression).

Food: Pimozide serum concentration may be increased when taken with grapefruit juice; avoid concurrent use.

Herb/Nutraceutical: St John's wort may decrease pimozide levels. Avoid kava kava, gotu kola, valerian, St John's wort (may increase CNS depression).

Mechanism of Action Pimozide, a diphenylbutylperidine antipsychotic, is a potent centrally-acting dopamine-receptor antagonist resulting in its characteristic neuroleptic effects

Pharmacodynamics/Kinetics

Absorption: 50%

Protein binding: 99%

Metabolism: Hepatic; significant first-pass effect

Half-life elimination: 50 hours

Time to peak, serum: 6-8 hours

Excretion: Urine

Dosage Oral: **Note:** An ECG should be performed baseline and periodically thereafter, especially during dosage adjustment:

Children ≤12 years: Tourette's disorder: Initial: 0.05 mg/kg preferably once at bedtime; may be increased every third day; usual range: 2-4 mg/day; do not exceed 10 mg/day (0.2 mg/kg/day)

Children >12 years and Adults: Tourette's disorder: Initial: 1-2 mg/day in divided doses, then increase dosage as needed every other day; range is usually 7-16 mg/day, maximum dose: 10 mg/day or 0.2 mg/kg/day are not generally recommended

Note: Sudden unexpected deaths have occurred in patients taking doses >10 mg. Therefore, dosages exceeding 10 mg/day are generally not recommended.

Dosing adjustment in hepatic impairment: Reduction of dose is necessary in patients with liver disease

Child/Adolescent Considerations Twenty-two children 7-16 years of age with Tourette's disorder were treated with a mean dose of 3.4 mg/day (Sallee, 1997). Twenty-four patients with Tourette's disorder were treated with 2.9 mg/day (Bruggeman, 2001).

Bruggeman R, van der Linden C, Buitelaar JK, et al, "Risperidone Versus Pimozide in Tourette's Disorder: A Comparative Double-Blind Parallel-Group Study," *J Clin Psychiatry*, 2001, 62(1):50-6.

Sallee FR, Nesbitt L, Jackson C, et al, "Relative Efficacy of Haloperidol and Pimozide in Children and Adolescents With Tourette's Disorder," *Am J Psychiatry*, 1997, 154(8):1057-62.

Monitoring Parameters ECG should be performed baseline and periodically thereafter, especially during dosage adjustment; vital signs; lipid profile, fasting blood glucose/Hgb A_{1c}; BMI; mental status, abnormal involuntary movement scale (AIMS), extrapyramidal symptoms (EPS)

Additional Information Less sedation, but pimozide is more likely to cause acute extrapyramidal symptoms than chlorpromazine.

Dosage Forms Excipient information presented when available (limited, particularly for generics); consult specific product labeling.

Tablet: 1 mg, 2 mg

◆ **Pin-X® [OTC]** *see* Pyrantel Pamoate *on page 1373*

Pindolol (PIN doe lole)

Medication Safety Issues

Sound-alike/look-alike issues:

Pindolol may be confused with Parlodel®, Plendil®

Visken® may be confused with Visine®

Related Information

Beta-Blockers *on page 1776*

Canadian Brand Names Apo-Pindol®; Gen-Pindolol; Novo-Pindol; Nu-Pindol; PMS-Pindolol; Visken®

Mexican Brand Names Visken

Pharmacologic Category Beta Blocker With Intrinsic Sympathomimetic Activity

Generic Available Yes

Use Treatment of hypertension, alone or in combination with other agents

Unlabeled/Investigational Use Potential augmenting agent for antidepressants; ventricular arrhythmias/tachycardia, antipsychotic-induced akathisia, situational anxiety; aggressive behavior associated with dementia

Effect on Mental Status Insomnia is common; may cause dizziness, fatigue, nervousness, or nightmares; may rarely cause depression or hallucinations

Effect on Psychiatric Treatment Has been used as an augmentive agent to the SSRIs for the treatment of depression; barbiturates may decrease the effects of beta-blockers

Pregnancy Risk Factor B

Pregnancy Considerations Adverse events were not observed in animal studies. Pindolol crosses the human placenta. Beta-blockers have been associated with bradycardia, hypotension, and IUGR; IUGR is probably related to maternal hypertension. Available evidence suggests beta-blockers are generally safe during pregnancy (JNC 7).

Lactation Enters breast milk/not recommended

Contraindications Bronchial asthma; cardiogenic shock; heart block (2nd or 3rd degree) except in patients with a functioning artificial pacemaker; overt cardiac failure; severe bradycardia

Warnings/Precautions Consider pre-existing conditions such as sick sinus syndrome before initiating. Use with caution in patients with inadequate myocardial function, undergoing anesthesia, bronchospastic disease, myasthenia gravis, peripheral vascular disease, renal impairment, psychiatric disease (may cause CNS depression) or impaired hepatic function. Use with caution in patients with diabetes mellitus; may potentiate hypoglycemia and/or mask signs and symptoms. Beta-blockers with intrinsic sympathomimetic activity (including pindolol) do not appear to be of benefit in HF. If use is warranted with compensated HF, use with caution and monitor for a worsening of the condition. If condition worsens, consider temporary discontinuation or dosage reduction of pindolol. Beta-blocker therapy should not be withdrawn abruptly (particularly in patients with CAD), but gradually tapered to avoid acute tachycardia, hypertension, and/or ischemia. Adequate alpha-blockade is required prior to use of any beta-blocker for patients with untreated pheochromocytoma. Use caution with history of severe anaphylaxis to allergens; patients taking beta-blockers may become more sensitive to repeated challenges. Treatment of anaphylaxis (eg, epinephrine) in patients taking beta-blockers may be ineffective or promote undesirable effects. Use with caution in patients receiving anesthetic agents which decrease myocardial function (eg, ether, cyclopropane and trichloroethylene). Use with caution in patients on concurrent verapamil or diltiazem; bradycardia or heart block may occur. Safety and efficacy have not been established in children.

Adverse Reactions

1% to 10%:

Cardiovascular: Edema (6%), chest pain (3%), bradycardia (≤2%), heart block (≤2%), hypotension (≤2%), syncope (≤2%), tachycardia (≤2%), palpitation (≤1%)

Central nervous system: Insomnia (10%), dizziness (9%), fatigue (8%), nervousness (7%), nightmares/vivid dreams (5%), anxiety (≤2%), lethargy (≤2%)

Dermatologic: Hyperhidrosis (≤2%), pruritus (1%)

Gastrointestinal: Nausea (5%), diarrhea (≤2%), vomiting (≤2%), weight gain (≤2%)

Genitourinary: Impotence (≤2%)

Hematologic: Claudication (≤2%)

Hepatic: AST/ALT increased (7%)

Neuromuscular & skeletal: Muscle pain (10%), arthralgia (7%), weakness (4%), paresthesia (3%), muscle cramps (3%)

Ocular: Burning eyes (≤2%), visual disturbances (≤2%), eye discomfort (≤2%)

Renal: Polyuria (≤2%)

Respiratory: Dyspnea (5%), wheezing (≤2%)

Miscellaneous: Cold extremities (≤2%)

<1% (Limited to important or life-threatening): Alkaline phosphatase increased, hallucination, heart failure, lactic acid dehydrogenase increased, uric acid increased

Other adverse reactions (noted with other beta-adrenergic-blocking agents that should be considered potential adverse events with pindolol): Agranulocytosis, alopecia, catatonia, clouded sensorium, disorientation, emotional lability, fever, intensification of pre-existing AV block, ischemic colitis, laryngospasm, mental depression, mesenteric artery thrombosis, nonthrombocytopenic purpura, Peyronie's disease, rash (erythematous), respiratory distress, short-term memory loss, thrombocytopenic purpura

Metabolism/Transport Effects **Substrate** of CYP2D6 (major); **Inhibits** CYP2D6 (weak)

Drug Interactions

Acetylcholinesterase Inhibitors: May enhance the bradycardic effect of Beta-Blockers. *Risk C: Monitor therapy*

Alpha-/Beta-Agonists (Direct-Acting): Beta-Blockers may enhance the vasopressor effect of Alpha-/Beta-Agonists (Direct-Acting). Epinephrine used as a local anesthetic for dental procedures will not likely cause clinically relevant problems. **Exceptions:** Dipivefrin. *Risk D: Consider therapy modification*

Alpha1-Blockers: Beta-Blockers may enhance the orthostatic effect of Alpha1-Blockers. The risk associated with ophthalmic products is probably less than systemic products. *Risk D: Consider therapy modification*

Alpha2-Agonists: Beta-Blockers may enhance the rebound hypertensive effect of Alpha2-Agonists. This effect can occur when the alpha$_2$-agonist is abruptly withdrawn. **Exceptions:** Apraclonidine; Brimonidine. *Risk D: Consider therapy modification*

Aminoquinolines (Antimalarial): May decrease the metabolism of Beta-Blockers. *Risk C: Monitor therapy*

Amiodarone: May enhance the bradycardic effect of Beta-Blockers. Possibly to the point of cardiac arrest. Amiodarone may increase the serum concentration of Beta-Blockers. *Risk C: Monitor therapy*

Anilidopiperidine Opioids: May enhance the bradycardic effect of Beta-Blockers. Anilidopiperidine Opioids may enhance the hypotensive effect of Beta-Blockers. *Risk C: Monitor therapy*

Antipsychotic Agents (Phenothiazines): May enhance the hypotensive effect of Beta-Blockers. Beta-Blockers may decrease the metabolism of Antipsychotic Agents (Phenothiazines). Antipsychotic Agents (Phenothiazines) may decrease the metabolism of Beta-Blockers. *Risk C: Monitor therapy*

Barbiturates: May decrease the serum concentration of Beta-Blockers. *Risk C: Monitor therapy*

Beta2-Agonists: Beta-Blockers (Nonselective) may diminish the bronchodilatory effect of Beta2-Agonists. *Risk D: Consider therapy modification*

Calcium Channel Blockers (Nondihydropyridine): May enhance the hypotensive effect of Beta-Blockers. Bradycardia and signs of heart failure have also been reported. Calcium Channel Blockers (Nondihydropyridine) may increase the serum concentration of Beta-Blockers. *Risk C: Monitor therapy*

Cardiac Glycosides: Beta-Blockers may enhance the bradycardic effect of Cardiac Glycosides. *Risk C: Monitor therapy*

Diazoxide: May enhance the hypotensive effect of Antihypertensives. *Risk C: Monitor therapy*

Dipyridamole: May enhance the bradycardic effect of Beta-Blockers. *Risk C: Monitor therapy*

Disopyramide: May enhance the bradycardic effect of Beta-Blockers. *Risk C: Monitor therapy*

Herbs (Hypertensive Properties): May diminish the antihypertensive effect of Antihypertensives. *Risk C: Monitor therapy*

Herbs (Hypotensive Properties): May enhance the hypotensive effect of Antihypertensives. *Risk C: Monitor therapy*

Insulin: Beta-Blockers may enhance the hypoglycemic effect of Insulin. *Risk C: Monitor therapy*

Lidocaine: Beta-Blockers may decrease the metabolism of Lidocaine. *Risk C: Monitor therapy*

Methacholine: Beta-Blockers may enhance the adverse/toxic effect of Methacholine. *Risk X: Avoid combination*

Methylphenidate: May diminish the antihypertensive effect of Antihypertensives. *Risk C: Monitor therapy*

Midodrine: Beta-Blockers may enhance the bradycardic effect of Midodrine. *Risk C: Monitor therapy*

Nonsteroidal Anti-Inflammatory Agents: May diminish the antihypertensive effect of Beta-Blockers. *Risk C: Monitor therapy*

Propafenone: May decrease the metabolism of Beta-Blockers. Propafenone possesses some independent beta blocking activity. *Risk C: Monitor therapy*

Propoxyphene: May decrease the metabolism of Beta-Blockers. *Risk C: Monitor therapy*

Prostacyclin Analogues: May enhance the hypotensive effect of Antihypertensives. *Risk C: Monitor therapy*

QuiNIDine: May decrease the metabolism of Beta-Blockers. *Risk C: Monitor therapy*

Reserpine: May enhance the hypotensive effect of Beta-Blockers. *Risk C: Monitor therapy*

Rifamycin Derivatives: May decrease the serum concentration of Beta-Blockers. **Exceptions:** Rifabutin. *Risk C: Monitor therapy*

RiTUXimab: Antihypertensives may enhance the hypotensive effect of RiTUXimab. *Risk D: Consider therapy modification*

Selective Serotonin Reuptake Inhibitors: May enhance the bradycardic effect of Beta-Blockers. **Exceptions:** Fluvoxamine. *Risk C: Monitor therapy*

Theophylline Derivatives: Beta-Blockers (Nonselective) may diminish the bronchodilatory effect of Theophylline Derivatives. *Risk D: Consider therapy modification*

Ethanol/Nutrition/Herb Interactions Herb/Nutraceutical: Avoid bayberry, blue cohosh, cayenne, ephedra, ginger, ginseng (American), kola, and licorice (may worsen hypertension). Avoid black cohosh, california poppy, coleus, golden seal, hawthorn, mistletoe, periwinkle, quinine, and shepherd's purse (may increase antihypertensive effect).

Stability Store below 30°C (86°F). Protect from light.

Mechanism of Action Blocks both beta$_1$- and beta$_2$-receptors and has mild intrinsic sympathomimetic activity; pindolol has negative inotropic and chronotropic effects and can significantly slow AV nodal conduction. Augmentive action of antidepressants thought to be mediated via a serotonin 1A autoreceptor antagonism.

Pharmacodynamics/Kinetics
Absorption: Rapid, 50% to 95%
Distribution: V_d: ~2 L/kg
Protein binding: 40%
Metabolism: Hepatic (60% to 65%) to conjugates
Half-life elimination: 3-4 hours; prolonged with advanced age, and cirrhosis (range: 2.5-30 hours)
Time to peak, serum: ~1 hour
Excretion: Urine (35% to 40% as unchanged drug); feces (6% to 9%)

Dosage Oral:
Adults:
Hypertension: Initial: 5 mg twice daily, increase as necessary by 10 mg/day every 3-4 weeks (maximum daily dose: 60 mg); usual dose range (JNC 7): 10-40 mg twice daily
Antidepressant augmentation (unlabeled use): 2.5 mg 3 times/day
Elderly: Initial: 5 mg once daily, increase as necessary by 5 mg/day every 3-4 weeks

Dosing adjustment in renal impairment: Use with caution. Clearance significantly decreased in uremic patients. Dosage reduction may be necessary.

Dosage adjustment in hepatic impairment: Use with caution. Elimination half-life in cirrhotic patients may be 10 times as long compared to normal patients. Dosage reduction is necessary in severely impaired.

Dietary Considerations May be taken without regard to meals.

Monitoring Parameters Blood pressure, heart rate, respiratory function

Dosage Forms Excipient information presented when available (limited, particularly for generics); consult specific product labeling.
Tablet: 5 mg, 10 mg

◆ **Pink Bismuth** *see* Bismuth *on page 189*

Pioglitazone (pye oh GLI ta zone)

Medication Safety Issues
Sound-alike/look-alike issues:
Actos® may be confused with Actidose®, Actonel®

U.S. Brand Names Actos®

Canadian Brand Names Actos®; Apo-Pioglitazone; CO Pioglitazone; Gen-Pioglitazone; Novo-Pioglitazone; PMS-Pioglitazone; ratio-Pioglitazone; Sandoz-Pioglitazone; SPEF-Pioglitazone

Mexican Brand Names Actos; Zactos

Pharmacologic Category Antidiabetic Agent, Thiazolidinedione

Generic Available No

Use
Type 2 diabetes mellitus (noninsulin dependent, NIDDM), monotherapy: Adjunct to diet and exercise, to improve glycemic control
Type 2 diabetes mellitus (noninsulin dependent, NIDDM), combination therapy with sulfonylurea, metformin, or insulin: When diet, exercise, and a single agent alone does not result in adequate glycemic control

Unlabeled/Investigational Use
Polycystic ovary syndrome (PCOS)

Effect on Mental Status May cause fatigue

Effect on Psychiatric Treatment Weight gain is common; caution with atypical antipsychotics; nefazodone and other CYP3A4 inhibitors may decrease the metabolism of pioglitazone; glucose may need to be checked more frequently

Pregnancy Risk Factor C

Pregnancy Considerations Pioglitazone is classified as pregnancy category C due to adverse effects observed in animal studies. The use of pioglitazone in pregnant women is limited to very few case reports where pregnancy occurred during treatment for polycystic ovarian syndrome (PCOS); details concerning fetal outcomes are limited. Thiazolidinediones may cause ovulation in anovulatory premenopausal women, increasing the risk of pregnancy; adequate contraception in premenopausal women is recommended. Maternal hyperglycemia can be associated with adverse effects in the fetus, including macrosomia, neonatal hyperglycemia, and hyperbilirubinemia; the risk of congenital malformations is increased when the Hb A_{1c} is above the normal range. Diabetes can also be associated with adverse effects in the mother. Poorly-treated diabetes may cause end-organ damage that may in turn negatively affect obstetric outcomes. Physiologic glucose levels should be maintained prior to and during pregnancy to decrease the risk of adverse events in the mother and the fetus. Until additional safety and efficacy data are obtained, the use of oral agents is generally not recommended as routine management of GDM or type 2 diabetes mellitus during pregnancy. Insulin is the drug of choice for the control of diabetes mellitus during pregnancy.

Lactation Excretion in breast milk unknown/not recommended

Contraindications Hypersensitivity to pioglitazone or any component of the formulation; NYHA Class III/IV heart failure (initiation of therapy)

Warnings/Precautions [U.S. Boxed Warning]: Thiazolidinediones, including pioglitazone, may cause or exacerbate heart failure; closely monitor for signs and symptoms of heart failure (eg, rapid weight gain, dyspnea, edema), particularly after initiation or dose increases. Not recommended for use in any patient with symptomatic heart failure; initiation of therapy is contraindicated in patients with NYHA class III or IV heart failure. If used in patients with NYHA class II (systolic heart failure), initiate at lowest dosage and monitor closely. Use with caution in patients with edema; may increase plasma volume and/or cause fluid retention. Dose reduction or discontinuation is recommended if heart failure suspected. Dose-related weight gain observed with use; mechanism unknown but likely associated with fluid retention and fat accumulation.

Should not be used in diabetic ketoacidosis. Mechanism requires the presence of insulin; therefore use in type 1 diabetes is not recommended. Use with caution in premenopausal, anovulatory women - may result in a resumption of ovulation, increasing the risk of pregnancy. Use with caution in patients with anemia (may reduce hemoglobin and hematocrit). Increased incidence of bone fractures in females treated with pioglitazone; majority of fractures occurred in the lower limb and distal upper limb.

Use with caution in patients with elevated transaminases (AST or ALT); do not initiate in patients with active liver disease of ALT >2.5 times the upper limit of normal at baseline. During therapy, if ALT >3 times the upper limit of normal, reevaluate levels promptly and discontinue if elevation persists or if jaundice occurs at any time during use. Idiosyncratic hepatotoxicity has been reported with another thiazolidinedione agent (troglitazone); avoid use in patients who previously experienced jaundice during troglitazone therapy. Monitoring should include periodic determinations of liver function. Use caution with pre-existing macular edema or diabetic retinopathy. Postmarketing reports of new-onset or worsening diabetic macular edema with decreased visual acuity has been reported. Safety and efficacy have not been established in children.

Adverse Reactions

>10%:

Cardiovascular: Edema (5%; in combination trials with sulfonlyureas or insulin, the incidence of edema was as high as 15%)

Respiratory: Upper respiratory tract infection (13%)

1% to 10%:

Cardiovascular: Heart failure (requiring hospitalization; up to 6% in patients with prior macrovascular disease)

Central nervous system: Headache (9%), fatigue (4%)

Gastrointestinal: Tooth disorder (5%)

Hematologic: Anemia (≤2%)

Neuromuscular & skeletal: Myalgia (5%)

Respiratory: Sinusitis (6%), pharyngitis (5%)

<1% (Limited to important or life-threatening): Bladder cancer, blurred vision, CPK increased, dyspnea (associated with weight gain and/or edema), fractures (females; usually in distal upper limbs or distal lower limbs), hepatic failure (very rare), hepatitis, macular edema (new onset or worsening), transaminases increased, visual acuity decreased

Frequency not defined: HDL-cholesterol increased, hematocrit/hemoglobin decreased, hypoglycemia (in combination trials with sulfonylureas or insulin), serum triglycerides decreased, weight gain/loss

Metabolism/Transport Effects Substrate of CYP2C8 (major), 3A4 (minor); **Inhibits** CYP2C8 (moderate), 2C9 (weak), 2C19 (weak), 2D6 (moderate); **Induces** CYP3A4 (weak)

Drug Interactions

Bile Acid Sequestrants: May decrease the absorption of Antidiabetic Agents (Thiazolidinedione). *Risk D: Consider therapy modification*

Codeine: CYP2D6 Inhibitors (Moderate) may diminish the therapeutic effect of Codeine. These CYP2D6 inhibitors may prevent the metabolic conversion of codeine to its active metabolite morphine. *Risk C: Monitor therapy*

Corticosteroids (Orally Inhaled): May diminish the hypoglycemic effect of Antidiabetic Agents. In some instances, corticosteroid-mediated HPA axis suppression has led to episodes of acute adrenal crisis, which may manifest as enhanced hypoglycemia, particularly in the setting of insulin or other antidiabetic agent use. *Risk C: Monitor therapy*

Corticosteroids (Systemic): May diminish the hypoglycemic effect of Antidiabetic Agents. In some instances, corticosteroid-mediated HPA axis suppression has led to episodes of acute adrenal crisis, which may manifest as enhanced hypoglycemia, particularly in the setting of insulin or other antidiabetic agent use. *Risk C: Monitor therapy*

CYP2C8 Inducers (Highly Effective): May increase the metabolism of CYP2C8 Substrates (High risk). *Risk C: Monitor therapy*

CYP2C8 Inhibitors (Moderate): May decrease the metabolism of CYP2C8 Substrates (High risk). *Risk C: Monitor therapy*

CYP2C8 Inhibitors (Strong): May decrease the metabolism of CYP2C8 Substrates (High risk). *Risk D: Consider therapy modification*

CYP2C8 Substrates (High risk): CYP2C8 Inhibitors (Moderate) may decrease the metabolism of CYP2C8 Substrates (High risk). *Risk C: Monitor therapy*

CYP2D6 Substrates: CYP2D6 Inhibitors (Moderate) may decrease the metabolism of CYP2D6 Substrates. **Exceptions:** Tamoxifen. *Risk C: Monitor therapy*

Gemfibrozil: May decrease the metabolism of Antidiabetic Agents (Thiazolidinedione). *Risk C: Monitor therapy*

Herbs (Hypoglycemic Properties): May enhance the hypoglycemic effect of Hypoglycemic Agents. *Risk C: Monitor therapy*

Insulin: May enhance the fluid-retaining effect of Antidiabetic Agents (Thiazolidinedione). *Risk C: Monitor therapy*

Luteinizing Hormone-Releasing Hormone Analogs: May diminish the therapeutic effect of Antidiabetic Agents. *Risk C: Monitor therapy*

Maraviroc: CYP3A4 Inducers may decrease the serum concentration of Maraviroc. *Risk D: Consider therapy modification*

Nebivolol: CYP2D6 Inhibitors (Moderate) may increase the serum concentration of Nebivolol. *Risk C: Monitor therapy*

Pegvisomant: May enhance the hypoglycemic effect of Antidiabetic Agents. *Risk C: Monitor therapy*

Pregabalin: May enhance the fluid-retaining effect of Antidiabetic Agents (Thiazolidinedione). *Risk C: Monitor therapy*

Rifampin: May increase the metabolism of Antidiabetic Agents (Thiazolidinedione). *Risk C: Monitor therapy*

Somatropin: May diminish the hypoglycemic effect of Antidiabetic Agents. *Risk D: Consider therapy modification*

Tamoxifen: CYP2D6 Inhibitors (Moderate) may decrease the metabolism of Tamoxifen. Specifically, CYP2D6 inhibitors may decrease the formation of highly potent active metabolites. *Risk D: Consider therapy modification*

Thioridazine: CYP2D6 Inhibitors may decrease the metabolism of Thioridazine. *Risk X: Avoid combination*

TraMADol: CYP2D6 Inhibitors (Moderate) may diminish the therapeutic effect of TraMADol. These CYP2D6 inhibitors may prevent the metabolic conversion of tramadol to its active metabolite that accounts for much of its opioid-like effects. *Risk C: Monitor therapy*

Trimethoprim: May decrease the metabolism of Antidiabetic Agents (Thiazolidinedione). *Risk C: Monitor therapy*

Ethanol/Nutrition/Herb Interactions

Ethanol: Caution with ethanol (may cause hypoglycemia).

Food: Peak concentrations are delayed when administered with food, but the extent of absorption is not affected. Pioglitazone may be taken without regard to meals.

Herb/Nutraceutical: Caution with alfalfa, aloe, bilberry, bitter melon, burdock, celery, damiana, fenugreek, garcinia, garlic, ginger, ginseng (American), gymnema, marshmallow, and stinging nettle (may cause hypoglycemia).

Mechanism of Action Thiazolidinedione antidiabetic agent that lowers blood glucose by improving target cell response to insulin, without increasing pancreatic insulin secretion. It has a mechanism of action that is dependent on the presence of insulin for activity. Pioglitazone is a potent and selective agonist for peroxisome proliferator-activated receptor-gamma (PPARgamma). Activation of nuclear PPARgamma receptors influences the production of a number of gene products involved in glucose and lipid metabolism. PPARgamma is abundant in the cells within the renal collecting tubules; fluid retention results from stimulation by thiazolidinediones which increases sodium reabsorption.

Pharmacodynamics/Kinetics

Onset of action: Delayed

Peak effect: Glucose control: Several weeks

Distribution: V_{ss} (apparent): 0.63 L/kg

Protein binding: 99.8%; primarily to albumin

Metabolism: Hepatic (99%) via CYP2C8 and 3A4 to both active and inactive metabolites
Half-life elimination: Parent drug: 3-7 hours; Total: 16-24 hours
Time to peak: ~2 hours; delayed with food
Excretion: Urine (15% to 30%) and feces as metabolites

Dosage Oral:
Adults:
Monotherapy: Initial: 15-30 mg once daily; if response is inadequate, the dosage may be increased in increments up to 45 mg once daily; maximum recommended dose: 45 mg once daily
Combination therapy: Maximum recommended dose: 45 mg/day
With sulfonylureas: Initial: 15-30 mg once daily; dose of sulfonylurea should be reduced if the patient reports hypoglycemia
With metformin: Initial: 15-30 mg once daily; it is unlikely that the dose of metformin will need to be reduced due to hypoglycemia
With insulin: Initial: 15-30 mg once daily; dose of insulin should be reduced by 10% to 25% if the patient reports hypoglycemia or if the plasma glucose falls to <100 mg/dL.
Dosage adjustment in patients with CHF (NYHA Class II) in mono- or combination therapy: Initial: 15 mg once daily; may be increased after several months of treatment, with close attention to heart failure symptoms
Elderly: No dosage adjustment is recommended in elderly patients.
Dosage adjustment in renal impairment: No dosage adjustment is required.
Dosage adjustment in hepatic impairment: Clearance is significantly lower in hepatic impairment (Child-Pugh Grade B/C). Therapy should not be initiated if the patient exhibits active liver disease or increased transaminases (>2.5 times ULN) at baseline. During treatment if ALT levels elevate >3 times ULN, the test should be repeated as soon as possible. If ALT levels remain >3 times ULN or if the patient is jaundiced, therapy should be discontinued.

Dietary Considerations Management of type 2 diabetes mellitus (noninsulin dependent, NIDDM) should include diet control. May be taken without regard to meals.

Administration May be administered without regard to meals

Monitoring Parameters Hemoglobin A_{1c}, serum glucose; signs and symptoms of heart failure; liver enzymes prior to initiation and periodically during treatment (per clinician judgment). If the ALT is increased to >2.5 times the upper limit of normal, liver function testing should be performed more frequently until the levels return to normal or pretreatment values. Patients with an elevation in ALT >3 times the upper limit of normal should be rechecked as soon as possible. If the ALT levels remain >3 times the upper limit of normal, therapy with pioglitazone should be discontinued. Routine ophthalmic exams are recommended; patients reporting visual deterioration should have a prompt referral to an ophthalmologist and consideration should be given to discontinuing pioglitazone.

Reference Range Recommendations for glycemic control in adults with diabetes:
Hb A_{1c}: <7%
Preprandial capillary plasma glucose: 70-130 mg/dL
Peak postprandial capillary blood glucose: <180 mg/dL
Blood pressure: <130/80 mm Hg

Dosage Forms Excipient information presented when available (limited, particularly for generics); consult specific product labeling.
Tablet:
Actos®: 15 mg, 30 mg, 45 mg

Pioglitazone and Glimepiride

(pye oh GLI ta zone & GLYE me pye ride)

Medication Safety Issues
High alert medication: The Institute for Safe Medication Practices (ISMP) includes this medication among its list of drugs which have a heightened risk of causing significant patient harm when used in error.

U.S. Brand Names Duetact™

Index Terms Glimepiride and Pioglitazone; Glimepiride and Pioglitazone Hydrochloride

Pharmacologic Category Antidiabetic Agent, Sulfonylurea; Antidiabetic Agent, Thiazolidinedione; Hypoglycemic Agent, Oral

Use Management of type 2 diabetes mellitus (noninsulin dependent, NIDDM) as an adjunct to diet and exercise

Effect on Mental Status May cause fatigue

Effect on Psychiatric Treatment Weight gain is common; use caution with atypical antipsychotics. Nefazodone and other CYP3A4 inhibitors may decrease the metabolism of pioglitazone; glucose may need to be checked more frequently. Phenothiazines and TCAs may antagonize hypoglycemic effects of glimepiride; MAO inhibitors and TCAs may enhance hypoglycemic effects.

Dosage Summary

Oral:

Children: Dosage not established

Adults:

Patients inadequately controlled on **glimepiride** alone: Initial dose: Pioglitazone 30 mg and glimepiride 2-4 mg once daily (maximum: 45 mg/day [pioglitazone]; 8 mg/day [glimepiride])

Patients inadequately controlled on **pioglitazone** alone: Initial dose: Pioglitazone 30 mg and glimepiride 2 mg once daily (maximum: 45 mg/day [pioglitazone]; 8 mg/day [glimepiride])

Elderly: Initial: Glimepiride 1 mg/day prior to initiating Duetact™

Dosage Forms Excipient information presented when available (limited, particularly for generics); consult specific product labeling.

Tablet:

Duetact™:

30 mg/2 mg: Pioglitazone 30 mg and glimepiride 2 mg

30 mg/4 mg: Pioglitazone 30 mg and glimepiride 4 mg

Pioglitazone and Metformin (pye oh GLI ta zone & met FOR min)

U.S. Brand Names Actoplus Met™

Index Terms Metformin Hydrochloride and Pioglitazone Hydrochloride

Pharmacologic Category Antidiabetic Agent, Biguanide; Antidiabetic Agent, Thiazolidinedione

Use Management of type 2 diabetes mellitus (noninsulin dependent, NIDDM)

Effect on Mental Status May cause dizziness

Effect on Psychiatric Treatment May cause weight gain; concomitant use with psychotropic agents may produce additive effects; monitor. May cause GI side effects, which when combined with lithium, SSRIs, valproic acid, or carbamazepine may produce additive effects.

Dosage Summary

Oral:

Children: Dosage not established

Adults: Pioglitazone 15-45 mg/day and metformin 500-2550 mg/day in divided doses with meals (maximum: 45 mg/day [pioglitazone]; 2550 mg/day [metformin])

Elderly ≥80 years: Do not use unless normal renal function has been established

Dosage Forms Excipient information presented when available (limited, particularly for generics); consult specific product labeling.

Tablet:

Actoplus Met™:

15/500: Pioglitazone 15 mg and metformin hydrochloride 500 mg

15/850: Pioglitazone 15 mg and metformin hydrochloride 850 mg

Piperacillin (pi PER a sil in)

Canadian Brand Names Piperacillin for Injection, USP

Index Terms Piperacillin Sodium

Pharmacologic Category Antibiotic, Penicillin

Use Treatment of susceptible infections such as septicemia, acute and chronic respiratory tract infections, skin and soft tissue infections, and urinary tract infections due to susceptible strains of *Pseudomonas*, *Proteus*, and *Escherichia coli* and *Enterobacter*; active against some streptococci and some anaerobic bacteria; febrile neutropenia (as part of combination regimen)

Effect on Mental Status May cause drowsiness or confusion; penicillins reported to cause apprehension, illusions, hallucinations, depersonalization, agitation, encephalopathy, and insomnia

Effect on Psychiatric Treatment May cause leukopenia, neutropenia, pancytopenia, and agranulocytosis; monitor patients receiving clozapine, carbamazepine, or valproic acid therapy.

Dosage Summary

I.M.:

Neonates: 100 mg/kg every 12 hours

Children: 200-300 mg/kg/day in divided doses every 4-6 hours

Adults: 2-4 g/dose every 4-6 hours (maximum: 24 g/day)

I.V.:

Neonates: 100 mg/kg every 12 hours

Children: 200-300 mg/kg/day in divided doses every 4-6 hours

Adults: 2-4 g/dose every 4-6 hours (maximum: 24 g/day)

Dosage Forms Excipient information presented when available (limited, particularly for generics); consult specific product labeling.

Injection, powder for reconstitution: 2 g, 3 g, 4 g, 40 g

Piperacillin and Tazobactam Sodium

(pi PER a sil in & ta zoe BAK tam SOW dee um)

Medication Safety Issues

Sound-alike/look-alike issues:

Zosyn® may be confused with Zofran®, Zyvox®

U.S. Brand Names Zosyn®

Canadian Brand Names Tazocin®

Mexican Brand Names Tasovak; Tazocin

Index Terms Piperacillin Sodium and Tazobactam Sodium; Tazobactam and Piperacillin

Pharmacologic Category Antibiotic, Penicillin

Use Treatment of moderate-to-severe infections caused by susceptible organisms, including infections of the lower respiratory tract (community-acquired pneumonia, nosocomial pneumonia); urinary tract; uncomplicated and complicated skin and skin structures; gynecologic (endometritis, pelvic inflammatory disease); bone and joint infections; intra-abdominal infections (appendicitis with rupture/abscess, peritonitis); and septicemia. Tazobactam expands activity of piperacillin to include beta-lactamase producing strains of *S. aureus*, *H. influenzae*, *Bacteroides*, and other gram-negative bacteria.

Effect on Mental Status May cause insomnia, dizziness or agitation; may rarely cause confusion; penicillins reported to cause apprehension, illusions, hallucinations, depersonalization, agitation, encephalopathy, and insomnia

Effect on Psychiatric Treatment None reported

Dosage Summary

I.V.:

Children 2-8 months: 80 mg/kg every 8 hours (appendicitis, peritonitis; dosing based on piperacillin component)

Children ≥9 months and ≤40 kg: 100 mg/kg every 8 hours (appendicitis, peritonitis; dosing based on piperacillin component)

Children >40 kg: 4.5 g every 8 hour **or** 3.375 every 6 hours (appendicitis, peritonitis)

Adults: 3.375 g every 6 hours **or** 4.5 g every 6-8 hours; maximum: 18 g/day

Dosage Forms Excipient information presented when available (limited, particularly for generics); consult specific product labeling.

Note: 8:1 ratio of piperacillin sodium/tazobactam sodium

Infusion [premixed iso-osmotic solution, frozen]:

2.25 g: Piperacillin 2 g and tazobactam 0.25 g (50 mL) [contains sodium 5.58 mEq (128 mg) and EDTA]

3.375 g: Piperacillin 3 g and tazobactam 0.375 g (50 mL) [contains sodium 8.38 mEq (192 mg) and EDTA]

4.5 g: Piperacillin 4 g and tazobactam 0.5 g (50 mL) [contains sodium 11.17 mEq (256 mg) and EDTA]

Injection, powder for reconstitution:

2.25 g: Piperacillin 2 g and tazobactam 0.25 g [contains sodium 5.58 mEq (128 mg) and EDTA]

3.375 g: Piperacillin 3 g and tazobactam 0.375 g [contains sodium 8.38 mEq (192 mg) and EDTA]

4.5 g: Piperacillin 4 g and tazobactam 0.5 g [contains sodium 11.17 mEq (256 mg) and EDTA]

40.5 g: Piperacillin 36 g and tazobactam 4.5 g [contains sodium 100.4 mEq (2304 mg) and EDTA; bulk pharmacy vial]

◆ **Piperacillin Sodium** *see* Piperacillin *on page 1301*

◆ **Piperacillin Sodium and Tazobactam Sodium** *see* Piperacillin and Tazobactam Sodium *on page 1302*

Piperazine (PI per a zeen)

Canadian Brand Names Entacyl®

Index Terms Piperazine Citrate

Pharmacologic Category Anthelmintic

Use Treatment of pinworm and roundworm infections (used as an alternative to first-line agents, mebendazole, or pyrantel pamoate)

Effect on Mental Status May cause dizziness

Effect on Psychiatric Treatment May cause seizures; use caution with high-dose clozapine

Dosage Summary

Oral:

Children: 65-75 mg/kg once daily (maximum: 3.5 g/day; exceptions occur [indication specific])

Adults: 65 mg/kg once daily **or** 3.5 g once daily (maximum: 3.5 g/day; exceptions occur [indication specific])

Dosage Forms Excipient information presented when available (limited, particularly for generics); consult specific product labeling.

Piperazine citrate is available from Panorama Pharmacy (1-800-247-9767).

◆ **Piperazine Citrate** *see* Piperazine *on page 1303*

◆ **Piperazine Estrone Sulfate** *see* Estropipate *on page 588*

◆ ***Piper methysticum*** *see* Kava Kava *(Piper methysticum) on page 874*

Pipotiazine (pip oh TYE a zeen)

Canadian Brand Names Piportil® L_4

Mexican Brand Names Piportil L4

Index Terms Pipotiazine Palmitate

Pharmacologic Category Antipsychotic Agent, Typical, Phenothiazine, Piperidine

Generic Available No

Use Management of schizophrenia

Mental Health Comment Coadministration of two or more antipsychotics does not generally improve clinical response and may increase the potential for adverse effects.

In 2008, the FDA issued a warning regarding increased mortality risk with typical **and** atypical antipsychotic drugs when used in elderly patients with dementia-related psychosis.

Restrictions Not available in U.S.

Pregnancy Considerations Safety and efficacy in pregnant women have not been established.

Lactation Excretion in breast milk unknown/not recommended

Contraindications Hypersensitivity to pipotiazine, phenothiazine derivatives, or any component of the formulation (cross-reactivity between phenothiazines may occur); severe CNS depression; subcortical brain damage; hepatic or renal dysfunction; circulatory collapse; severe hypotension; severely depressed patients; high doses of hypnotics; bone marrow suppression; blood dyscrasias; coma; pheochromocytoma

Other piperidine phenothiazines (ie, thioridazine) are contraindicated for use in combination with other drugs that are known to prolong the QT_c interval; in patients with congenital long QT syndrome or a history of cardiac arrhythmias. In addition, these drugs are contraindicated with concurrent use with medications that inhibit the metabolism of phenothiazines (fluoxetine, paroxetine, fluvoxamine, propranolol, pindolol), and in patients known to have genetic defect leading to reduced levels of activity of CYP2D6. The metabolism and adverse effect profile of pipotiazine have not been adequately characterized to evaluate whether these contraindications also apply to this drug. They are not labeled contraindications (per Canadian product monograph).

Warnings/Precautions Avoid use in patients with known allergy to sesame oil or similar compounds. Check blood counts periodically and discontinue at first signs of blood dyscrasias; use is contraindicated in patients with bone marrow suppression. May be sedating, use with caution in disorders where CNS depression is a feature (risk may be lower than with other phenothiazines). Use with caution in Parkinson's disease; hemodynamic instability; bone marrow suppression; predisposition to seizures; severe cardiac or respiratory disease. Esophageal dysmotility and aspiration have been associated with antipsychotic use; use with caution in patients at risk of pneumonia (eg, Alzheimer's disease).

Caution in breast cancer or other prolactin-dependent tumors (may elevate prolactin levels). May alter temperature regulation or mask toxicity of other drugs due to antiemetic effects.

Use with caution in patients with cardiovascular disease. May cause orthostatic hypotension (risk may be low relative to other phenothiazines); use with caution in patients at risk of this effect or those who would not tolerate transient hypotensive episodes (cerebrovascular disease, cardiovascular disease, or other medications which may predispose).

Phenothiazines may cause anticholinergic effects (confusion, agitation, constipation, xerostomia, blurred vision, urinary retention); therefore, they should be used with caution in patients with decreased gastrointestinal motility, urinary retention, BPH, xerostomia, or visual problems. Conditions which also may be exacerbated by cholinergic blockade include narrow-angle glaucoma (screening is recommended) and worsening of myasthenia gravis.

May cause extrapyramidal symptoms, including pseudoparkinsonism, acute dystonic reactions, akathisia, and tardive dyskinesia. May be associated with neuroleptic malignant syndrome (NMS). Prolonged therapy may cause pigmentary retinopathy, corneal deposits, and/or changes in skin pigmentation. Adverse effects of depot injections may be prolonged. Use with caution in the elderly. Safety and efficacy in pediatric patients have not been established.

Adverse Reactions Frequency not defined.

Cardiovascular: Cardiac arrest, ECG changes, edema, hypotension, QT_c prolongation, syncope, tachycardia

Central nervous system: Agitation, anxiety, bizarre dreams, cerebral edema, depression, dizziness, drowsiness, EEG changes, excitement, extrapyramidal symptoms (akathisia, dyskinesia, dystonia, hyper-reflexia, oculogyric crisis, opisthotonos, pseudoparkinsonism, rigidity, sialorrhea, tremor), fatigue, fever, headache, insomnia, paradoxical psychosis, restlessness, seizure, sleep disturbance, tardive dyskinesia

Dermatologic: Angioedema, eczema, epithelial keratopathy erythema, exfoliative dermatitis, dermatitis, photosensitivity, pruritus, rash, seborrhea, skin pigmentation (prolonged therapy), urticaria

Endocrine & metabolic: Anorexia, appetite increased, galactorrhea, gynecomastia, libido (changes in), menstrual irregularities, thirst, weight changes

Gastrointestinal: Adynamic ileus, cholestasis, constipation, fecal impaction, jaundice nausea, salivation, vomiting, xerostomia

Genitourinary: Bladder paralysis, impotence, incontinence, polyuria, urinary retention

Hematologic: Agranulocytosis, anemia, eosinophilia, leukopenia, pancytopenia, thrombocytopenia

Ocular: Blurred vision, corneal deposits (prolonged therapy), glaucoma, lenticular deposits, pigmentary retinopathy (prolonged therapy)

Respiratory: Nasal congestion, pneumonia, pneumonitis

Miscellaneous: Diaphoresis iincreased, lupus-like syndrome

Metabolism/Transport Effects No published data on CYP metabolism. Based on structural analysis, pipotiazine may be a substrate of CYP2D6 and 3A4.

Drug Interactions

Analgesics (Opioid): Antipsychotic Agents (Phenothiazines) may enhance the hypotensive effect of Analgesics (Opioid). *Risk C: Monitor therapy*

Antacids: May decrease the absorption of Antipsychotic Agents (Phenothiazines). *Risk C: Monitor therapy*

Antimalarial Agents: May increase the serum concentration of Antipsychotic Agents (Phenothiazines). *Risk C: Monitor therapy*

Beta-Blockers: Antipsychotic Agents (Phenothiazines) may enhance the hypotensive effect of Beta-Blockers. Beta-Blockers may decrease the metabolism of Antipsychotic Agents (Phenothiazines). Antipsychotic Agents (Phenothiazines) may decrease the metabolism of Beta-Blockers. **Exceptions:** Atenolol; Levobunolol; Metipranolol; Nadolol. *Risk C: Monitor therapy*

CYP2D6 Inhibitors (Moderate): May decrease the metabolism of CYP2D6 Substrates. *Risk C: Monitor therapy*

CYP2D6 Inhibitors (Strong): May decrease the metabolism of CYP2D6 Substrates. *Risk D: Consider therapy modification*

CYP3A4 Inducers (Strong): May increase the metabolism of CYP3A4 Substrates. *Risk C: Monitor therapy*

CYP3A4 Inhibitors (Moderate): May decrease the metabolism of CYP3A4 Substrates. *Risk C: Monitor therapy*

CYP3A4 Inhibitors (Strong): May decrease the metabolism of CYP3A4 Substrates. *Risk D: Consider therapy modification*

Darunavir: May increase the serum concentration of CYP2D6 Substrates. *Risk C: Monitor therapy*

Dasatinib: May increase the serum concentration of CYP3A4 Substrates. *Risk C: Monitor therapy*

Deferasirox: May decrease the serum concentration of CYP3A4 Substrates. *Risk C: Monitor therapy*

Herbs (CYP3A4 Inducers): May increase the metabolism of CYP3A4 Substrates. *Risk C: Monitor therapy*

Ethanol/Nutrition/Herb Interactions

Ethanol: Avoid ethanol (may increase CNS depression).

Herb/Nutraceutical: Avoid kava kava, valerian, St John's wort, gotu kola (may increase CNS depression). Avoid dong quai, St John's wort (may also cause photosensitization).

Stability Store at room temperature of 20°C to 25°C (68°F to 77°F). Protect from light.

Mechanism of Action Blocks postsynaptic mesolimbic dopaminergic receptors in the brain; depresses the release of hypothalamic and hypophyseal hormones. Relative to other piperidine phenothiazines, pipotiazine appears to be less sedating, with less potential to potentiate other CNS depressants, and may possess a lower propensity to cause hypotension. However, it has a relatively high propensity for cause extrapyramidal reactions.

Pharmacodynamics/Kinetics

Onset: I.M.: 2-3 days

Duration: 3-6 weeks

Dosage Adults: I.M.: Initial (dosage must be individualized): 50-100 mg; may be increased in 25 mg increments every 2-3 weeks. Optimal dosage and interval must be determined by individual response. Usual maintenance dose: 75-150 mg every 4 weeks; range: 25-250 mg every 3-4 weeks. A lower dose at a shorter interval (eg, every 3 weeks) may be preferred to higher doses every 4 weeks.

Elderly ≥50 years: Initial dosage <50 mg is recommended

Administration Administer using at least a 21-gauge needle for injection.

Monitoring Parameters Vital signs; serum potassium and magnesium, lipid profile evaluation of renal and liver function tests (long-term therapy), fasting blood glucose/Hgb A_{1c}; waist circumference, BMI; mental status, abnormal involuntary movement scale (AIMS); periodic eye exam

Based on experience with other piperidine phenothiazines: consider baseline and periodic ECG, do not initiate if QT_c >450 msec

Test Interactions Phenothiazines have been reported to cause false positive pregnancy tests.

Dosage Forms Excipient information presented when available (limited, particularly for generics); consult specific product labeling. [CAN] = Canadian brand name

Injection, oil:

Piportil® L_4: 25 mg/mL (1 mL) [contains sesame oil]; 50 mg/mL (1 mL, 2 mL) [contains sesame oil]

◆ **Pipotiazine Palmitate** *see* Pipotiazine *on page 1303*

Pirbuterol (peer BYOO ter ole)

U.S. Brand Names Maxair™ Autohaler™

Index Terms Pirbuterol Acetate

Pharmacologic Category $Beta_2$-Adrenergic Agonist

Generic Available No

Use Prevention and treatment of reversible bronchospasm including asthma

Effect on Mental Status Nervousness and restlessness are common; may cause dizziness; may rarely cause insomnia

Effect on Psychiatric Treatment Concurrent use with TCAs and MAO inhibitors may results in increased toxicity; monitor

Pregnancy Risk Factor C

Lactation Excretion in breast milk unknown

Contraindications Hypersensitivity to pirbuterol, albuterol, or any component of the formulation

Warnings/Precautions Optimize anti-inflammatory treatment before initiating maintenance treatment with pirbuterol. Do not use as a component of chronic therapy without an anti-inflammatory agent. Only the mildest form of asthma (Step 1 and/or exercise-induced) would not require concurrent use based upon asthma guidelines. Patient must be instructed to seek medical attention in cases where acute symptoms are not relieved or a previous level of response is diminished. The need to increase frequency of use may indicate deterioration of asthma, and treatment must not be delayed.

Use caution in patients with cardiovascular disease (arrhythmia or hypertension or CHF), convulsive disorders, diabetes, glaucoma, hyperthyroidism, or hypokalemia. Beta-agonists may cause elevation in blood pressure, heart rate, and result in CNS stimulation/excitation. Beta$_2$-agonists may increase risk of arrhythmia, increase serum glucose, or decrease serum potassium.

Do not exceed recommended dose; serious adverse events including fatalities, have been associated with excessive use of inhaled sympathomimetics. Rarely, paradoxical bronchospasm may occur with use of inhaled bronchodilating agents; this should be distinguished from inadequate response. All patients should utilize a spacer device when using a metered-dose inhaler. Safety and efficacy have not been established in children <12 years of age.

Adverse Reactions

>10%:

Central nervous system: Nervousness, restlessness

Endocrine & metabolic: Serum glucose increased, serum potassium decreased

Neuromuscular & skeletal: Trembling

1% to 10%:

Cardiovascular: Tachycardia, palpitation

Central nervous system: Headache, dizziness, lightheadedness

Gastrointestinal: Taste changes, vomiting, nausea

<1% (Limited to important or life-threatening): Arrhythmias, chest pain, hypertension, hypokalemia, insomnia, paradoxical bronchospasm

Drug Interactions

Alpha-/Beta-Blockers: May diminish the therapeutic effect of Beta2-Agonists. *Risk D: Consider therapy modification*

Atomoxetine: May enhance the tachycardic effect of Beta2-Agonists. *Risk C: Monitor therapy*

Beta-Blockers (Beta1 Selective): May diminish the bronchodilatory effect of Beta2-Agonists. Of particular concern with nonselective beta-blockers or higher doses of the beta1 selective beta-blockers. *Risk C: Monitor therapy*

Beta-Blockers (Nonselective): May diminish the bronchodilatory effect of Beta2-Agonists. *Risk D: Consider therapy modification*

Betahistine: May diminish the therapeutic effect of Beta2-Agonists. *Risk C: Monitor therapy*

Cannabinoids: May enhance the tachycardic effect of Sympathomimetics. *Risk C: Monitor therapy*

MAO Inhibitors: May enhance the adverse/toxic effect of Beta2-Agonists. *Risk C: Monitor therapy*

Sympathomimetics: May enhance the adverse/toxic effect of other Sympathomimetics. *Risk C: Monitor therapy*

Tricyclic Antidepressants: May enhance the adverse/toxic effect of Beta2-Agonists. *Risk C: Monitor therapy*

Stability Store between 15°C and 30°C (59°F and 86°F).

Mechanism of Action Pirbuterol is a beta$_2$-adrenergic agonist with a similar structure to albuterol, specifically a pyridine ring has been substituted for the benzene ring in albuterol. The increased beta$_2$ selectivity of pirbuterol results from the substitution of a tertiary butyl group on the nitrogen of the side chain, which additionally imparts resistance of pirbuterol to degradation by monoamine oxidase and provides a lengthened duration of action in comparison to the less selective previous beta-agonist agents.

Pharmacodynamics/Kinetics

Onset of action: Peak effect: Therapeutic: Oral: 2-3 hours with peak serum concentration of 6.2-9.8 mcg/L; Inhalation: 0.5-1 hour

Half-life elimination: 2-3 hours

Metabolism: Hepatic

Excretion: Urine (10% as unchanged drug)

Dosage Children ≥12 years and Adults: 2 inhalations every 4-6 hours for prevention; two inhalations at an interval of at least 1-3 minutes, followed by a third inhalation in treatment of bronchospasm, not to exceed 12 inhalations/day

Administration Inhalation: Shake inhaler well before use.

Monitoring Parameters Respiratory rate; FEV$_1$, peak flow, and/or other pulmonary function tests; blood pressure, heart rate; CNS stimulation; serum glucose, serum potassium

Dosage Forms Excipient information presented when available (limited, particularly for generics); consult specific product labeling.

Aerosol for oral inhalation, as acetate:

Maxair™ Autohaler™: 200 mcg/actuation (14 g) [400 actuations; contains chlorofluorocarbons]

◆ **Pirbuterol Acetate** *see* Pirbuterol *on page 1305*

Piroxicam (peer OKS i kam)

Medication Safety Issues

International issues:

Flogene® [Brazil] may be confused with Florone® which is a brand name for diflorasone in the U.S.

Related Information

Nonsteroidal Anti-Inflammatory Agents *on page 1792*

U.S. Brand Names Feldene®

Canadian Brand Names Apo-Piroxicam®; Gen-Piroxicam; Novo-Pirocam; Nu-Pirox; Pexicam®

Mexican Brand Names Brucam; Edecam; Facicam; Feldene; Genoldene; Pirox; Zuparex

Pharmacologic Category Nonsteroidal Anti-inflammatory Drug (NSAID), Oral

Use Symptomatic treatment of acute and chronic rheumatoid arthritis and osteoarthritis

Unlabeled/Investigational Use Ankylosing spondylitis

Effect on Mental Status Dizziness is common; may cause nervousness; may rarely cause drowsiness, confusion, depression, or hallucinations

Effect on Psychiatric Treatment May rarely cause agranulocytosis; use caution with clozapine and carbamazepine; may decrease lithium clearance resulting in an increase in serum lithium levels and potential lithium toxicity; monitor serum lithium levels

Restrictions An FDA-approved medication guide must be distributed when dispensing an oral outpatient prescription (new or refill) where this medication is to be used without direct supervision of a healthcare provider. Medication guides are available at http://www.fda.gov/cder/Offices/ODS/medication_guides.htm.

Dosage Summary

Oral:

Children (unlabeled use): 0.2-0.3 mg/kg once daily (maximum: 15 mg/day)

Adults: 10-20 mg once daily (maximum: 20 mg/day: higher doses used with increased frequency of adverse effects)

Elderly: Initial: 10 mg every other day has been used (maximum: 20 mg/day)

Dosage Forms Excipient information presented when available (limited, particularly for generics); consult specific product labeling.

Capsule: 10 mg, 20 mg

◆ ***p*-Isobutylhydratropic Acid** *see* Ibuprofen *on page 803*

Pizotifen (pi ZOE ti fen)

Canadian Brand Names Sandomigran DS®; Sandomigran®

Index Terms Pizotifen Malate

Pharmacologic Category Serotonin and Histamine Antagonist

Generic Available No

Use Migraine prophylaxis

Restrictions Not available in U.S.

Pregnancy Risk Factor Not available

Pregnancy Considerations Use only if potential benefit to the mother outweighs possible risk to the fetus.

Contraindications Hypersensitivity to pizotifen or any component of the formulation; concurrent use of MAO inhibitors; gastric outlet obstruction (pyloroduodenal obstruction, stenosing pyloric ulcer)

Warnings/Precautions Not for use in acute treatment of migraine attacks. May cause sedation; effects may be additive with other CNS depressants or ethanol. Patients must be cautioned to avoid operating machinery or driving until effects are known. Although anticholinergic effects are limited, use with caution in patients intolerant to anticholinergic agents, including tricyclic antidepressants, phenothiazines, or cyproheptadine. Use with caution in patients with narrow angle glaucoma, myasthenia gravis, bladder outlet obstruction (BPH), or other disorders in which anticholinergic effects may be poorly tolerated. Use caution in renal or hepatic disease/insufficiency, diabetes, cardiovascular disease, or in obese patients. Therapeutic response may require several weeks of therapy. Avoid abrupt discontinuation; taper dosage over 2 weeks prior to discontinuation. Tolerance may develop in some patients. Consider drug-free period after several months of treatment. Safety and efficacy have not been established in children <12 years of age.

Adverse Reactions Frequency not defined.

Cardiovascular: Edema, hypotension

Central nervous system: Drowsiness, dizziness, headache, fatigue, confusion, depression, nervousness
Endocrine & metabolic: Increased appetite, weight gain
Gastrointestinal: Nausea, xerostomia, epigastric distress
Genitourinary: Impotence
Neuromuscular & skeletal: Weakness, muscle pain

Drug Interactions

Acetylcholinesterase Inhibitors (Central): Anticholinergics may diminish the therapeutic effect of Acetylcholinesterase Inhibitors (Central). Acetylcholinesterase Inhibitors (Central) may diminish the therapeutic effect of Anticholinergics. If the anticholinergic action is a side effect of the agent, the result may be beneficial. *Risk C: Monitor therapy*

Alcohol (Ethyl): CNS Depressants may enhance the CNS depressant effect of Alcohol (Ethyl). *Risk C: Monitor therapy*

Amphetamines: May diminish the sedative effect of Antihistamines. *Risk C: Monitor therapy*

Anticholinergics: May enhance the adverse/toxic effect of other Anticholinergics. **Exceptions:** Paliperidone. *Risk C: Monitor therapy*

Betahistine: Antihistamines may diminish the therapeutic effect of Betahistine. *Risk C: Monitor therapy*

CNS Depressants: May enhance the adverse/toxic effect of other CNS Depressants. *Risk C: Monitor therapy*

Pramlintide: May enhance the anticholinergic effect of Anticholinergics. These effects are specific to the GI tract. *Risk D: Consider therapy modification*

Ethanol/Nutrition/Herb Interactions

Ethanol: Avoid ethanol (may increase CNS depression).
Herb/Nutraceutical: Avoid valerian, St John's wort, kava kava, gotu kola (may increase CNS depression).

Mechanism of Action Serotonin and histamine antagonist; mechanism of action in migraine prophylaxis has not been fully elucidated

Pharmacodynamics/Kinetics

Onset: May require several weeks of therapy
Half-life elimination: 26 hours
Time to peak: 5-7 hours

Dosage Oral: Children ≥12 years and Adults: Migraine prophylaxis: Initial: 0.5 mg at bedtime; increase gradually to 0.5 mg 3 times/day; usual dosage range: 1-6 mg/day

Note: Therapeutic response may require several weeks of therapy. Do not discontinue abruptly (reduce gradually over 2-week period).

Monitoring Parameters Hepatic function tests (prolonged use)

Additional Information Not available in U.S.

Dosage Forms Excipient information presented when available (limited, particularly for generics); consult specific product labeling. [CAN] = Canadian brand name

Tablet:
Sandomigran® [CAN]: 0.5 mg [pizotifen malate 0.73 mg]

Tablet, double strength:
Sandomigran® DS [CAN]: 1 mg [pizotifen malate 1.46 mg]

- **Pizotifen Malate** *see* Pizotifen *on page 1307*
- **Plan B® [RX/OTC]** *see* Levonorgestrel *on page 918*
- **Plaquenil®** *see* Hydroxychloroquine *on page 796*
- **Plavix®** *see* Clopidogrel *on page 380*
- **Plendil®** *see* Felodipine *on page 617*
- **Pletal®** *see* Cilostazol *on page 344*
- **PMPA** *see* Tenofovir *on page 1549*
- **Pneumococcal 7-Valent Conjugate Vaccine** *see* Pneumococcal Conjugate Vaccine, 7-Valent *on page 1308*

Pneumococcal Conjugate Vaccine, 7-Valent

(noo moe KOK al KON ju gate vak SEEN, seven vay lent)

Medication Safety Issues

Sound-alike/look-alike issues:
Prevnar® may be confused with PREVEN®

U.S. Brand Names Prevnar®

Canadian Brand Names Prevnar®

Index Terms Diphtheria CRM_{197} Protein; PCV7; Pneumococcal 7-Valent Conjugate Vaccine

Pharmacologic Category Vaccine

Use Immunization of infants and toddlers against *Streptococcus pneumoniae* infection caused by serotypes included in the vaccine

Advisory Committee on Immunization Practices (ACIP) guidelines also recommend PCV7 for use in:

All children 2-23 months

Children ≥2-59 months with cochlear implants

Children ages 24-59 months with: Sickle cell disease (including other sickle cell hemoglobinopathies, asplenia, splenic dysfunction), HIV infection, immunocompromising conditions (congenital immunodeficiencies, renal failure, nephrotic syndrome, diseases associated with immunosuppressive or radiation therapy, solid organ transplant), chronic illnesses (cardiac disease, cerebrospinal fluid leaks, diabetes mellitus, pulmonary disease excluding asthma unless on high dose corticosteroids)

Consider use in all children 24-59 months with priority given to:

Children 24-35 months

Children 24-59 months who are of Alaska native, American Indian, or African-American descent

Children 24-59 months who attend group day care centers

Effect on Mental Status Irritability, drowsiness, and restlessness are common

Effect on Psychiatric Treatment May lessen the effects of anxiolytics

Dosage Forms Excipient information presented when available (limited, particularly for generics); consult specific product labeling.

Injection, suspension:

Prevnar®: 2 mcg of each capsular saccharide for serotypes 4, 9V, 14, 18C, 19F, and 23F, and 4 mcg of serotype 6B [bound to diphtheria CRM_{197} protein ~20 mcg] per 0.5 mL (0.5 mL) [contains aluminum, natural rubber/natural latex in packaging, soy, and yeast]

Pneumococcal Polysaccharide Vaccine (Polyvalent)

(noo moe KOK al pol i SAK a ride vak SEEN, pol i VAY lent)

U.S. Brand Names Pneumovax® 23

Canadian Brand Names Pneumo 23™; Pneumovax® 23

Index Terms 23-Valent Pneumococcal Polysaccharide Vaccine; 23PS; PPV23

Pharmacologic Category Vaccine

Use Children ≥2 years of age and adults who are at increased risk of pneumococcal disease and its complications because of underlying health conditions (including patients with cochlear implants); routine use in older adults >50 years of age, including all those ≥65 years

Current Advisory Committee on Immunization Practices (ACIP) guidelines recommend **pneumococcal 7-valent conjugate vaccine (PCV7)** be used for children 2-23 months of age and, in certain situations, children up to 59 months of age

Effect on Mental Status May cause malaise

Effect on Psychiatric Treatment None reported

Dosage Forms Excipient information presented when available (limited, particularly for generics); consult specific product labeling.

Injection, solution:

Pneumovax® 23: 25 mcg each of 23 capsular polysaccharide isolates/0.5 mL (0.5 mL, 2.5 mL)

- ◆ **Pneumotussin® [DSC]** *see* Hydrocodone and Guaifenesin *on page 779*
- ◆ **Pneumovax® 23** *see* Pneumococcal Polysaccharide Vaccine (Polyvalent) *on page 1309*
- ◆ **PNU-140690E** *see* Tipranavir *on page 1586*
- ◆ **Podocon-25®** *see* Podophyllum Resin *on page 1309*
- ◆ **Podophyllin** *see* Podophyllum Resin *on page 1309*

Podophyllum Resin (po DOF fil um REZ in)

U.S. Brand Names Podocon-25®

Canadian Brand Names Podofilm®

Mexican Brand Names Podofilia No. 2

Index Terms Mandrake; May Apple; Podophyllin

Pharmacologic Category Keratolytic Agent

Use Topical treatment of benign growths including external genital and perianal warts, papillomas, fibroids; compound benzoin tincture generally is used as the medium for topical application

Effect on Mental Status None reported

Effect on Psychiatric Treatment May rarely cause leukopenia, use caution with clozapine and carbamazepine

Dosage Summary

Topical:

Children: 10-25% solution applied 1-5 times/day

Adults: 10-25% solution applied 1-5 times/day

Dosage Forms Excipient information presented when available (limited, particularly for generics); consult specific product labeling.

Liquid, topical: 25% (15 mL) [in benzoin tincture]

◆ **Polocaine®** *see* Mepivacaine *on page 990*

◆ **Polocaine® Dental** *see* Mepivacaine *on page 990*

◆ **Polocaine® MPF** *see* Mepivacaine *on page 990*

Polyethylene Glycol-Electrolyte Solution

(pol i ETH i leen GLY kol ee LEK troe lite soe LOO shun)

Medication Safety Issues

Sound-alike/look-alike issues:

GoLYTELY® may be confused with NuLYTELY®

NuLYTELY® may be confused with GoLYTELY®

U.S. Brand Names Colyte®; GoLYTELY®; MoviPrep®; NuLYTELY®; TriLyte®

Canadian Brand Names Colyte™; Klean-Prep®; PegLyte®

Index Terms Electrolyte Lavage Solution

Pharmacologic Category Laxative, Osmotic

Generic Available Yes

Use Bowel cleansing prior to GI examination

Unlabeled/Investigational Use Whole bowel irrigation (WBI) in the following toxic ingestions: Packets of illicit drugs (body packers, body stuffers), potentially toxic sustained-release or enteric-coated agents, substantial amounts of iron (AACT, 2004)

Effect on Mental Status None reported

Effect on Psychiatric Treatment Oral medications should not be administered within 1 hour of start of therapy

Pregnancy Risk Factor C

Pregnancy Considerations Reproduction studies have not been conducted in animals or in humans.

Lactation Excretion in breast milk unknown/use caution

Contraindications Hypersensitivity to polyethylene glycol or any component of the formulation; ileus, gastrointestinal obstruction, gastric retention, bowel perforation, toxic colitis, toxic megacolon

Warnings/Precautions Seizures associated with electrolyte abnormalities (eg, hyponatremia, hypokalemia) have occurred. Use caution with concomitant administration of medications that alter electrolyte balance or in patients with underlying hyponatremia. Do not add flavorings, unless provided by the manufacturer, as additional ingredients before use; observe unconscious or semiconscious patients with impaired gag reflex or those who are otherwise prone to regurgitation or aspiration during administration; use with caution in patients with severe ulcerative colitis. Evaluate patients with symptoms of bowel obstruction (nausea, vomiting, abdominal pain or distension) prior to use.

MoviPrep®: May be safer to use in patients who cannot tolerate fluid load (eg, heart failure, renal insufficiency, ascites). Use cautiously in patients with G6PD deficiency. Contains phenylalanine.

Adverse Reactions

>10%:

Central nervous system: Malaise (18% to 27%)

Gastrointestinal: Abdominal distension (<60%), anal irritation (<52%), nausea (14% to 47%), abdominal pain (13% to 39%), vomiting (7% to 12%)

Neuromuscular & skeletal: Rigors (34%)

Miscellaneous: Thirst (<47%)

1% to 10%:

Central nervous system: Dizziness (7%), headache (2%)

Gastrointestinal: Dyspepsia (1% to 3%)

Frequency not defined, postmarketing, and/or case reports: Abdominal cramps, abdominal fullness, allergic reactions, anaphylaxis, aspiration, asystole, bloating, chest tightness, dehydration (children), dermatitis, dyspnea (acute), esophageal perforation, facial edema, flatulence, hypersensitivity reactions, hypokalemia (children), Mallory-Weiss tear, pulmonary edema, rash, rhinorrhea, seizure, throat tightness, upper GI bleeding, urticaria

Drug Interactions

There are no known significant interactions.

Stability

CoLyte®, GoLYTELY®, NuLYTELY®, TriLyte®: Store at controlled room temperature of 25°C (77°F) before reconstitution. Use within 48 hours of preparation; refrigerate reconstituted solution; tap water may be used for preparation of the solution; shake container vigorously several times to ensure dissolution of powder.

MoviPrep®: Store at controlled room temperature of 25°C (77°F) before reconstitution. Mix the contents of pouch A and pouch B (one each) in container provided. Add 1 L of lukewarm water; mix the solution until dissolved. Repeat mixing procedure if second liter is needed. Refrigerate reconstituted solution. Use within 24 hours of preparation.

Mechanism of Action Induces catharsis by strong electrolyte and osmotic effects

Pharmacodynamics/Kinetics Onset of effect: Oral: ~1-2 hours

Dosage

Oral:

Children ≥6 months: Bowel cleansing prior to GI exam (CoLyte®, GoLYTELY®, NuLYTELY®, TriLyte®): 25 mL/kg/hour (some studies have used up to 40 mL/kg/hour) for 4-10 hours (until rectal effluent is clear). Maximum total dose: 4 L. **Note:** The solution may be given via nasogastric tube to patients who are unwilling or unable to drink the solution. Patients <2 years should be monitored closely.

Adults: Bowel cleansing prior to GI exam:

CoLyte®, GoLYTELY®, NuLYTELY®, TriLyte®: 240 mL (8 oz) every 10 minutes, until 4 L are consumed or the rectal effluent is clear; rapid drinking of each portion is preferred to drinking small amounts continuously. Ideally, patients should fast for ~3-4 hours prior to administration; absolutely no solid food for at least 2 hours before the solution is given. **Note:** The solution may be given via nasogastric tube to patients who are unwilling or unable to drink the solution.

MoviPrep®: Administer 2 L total with an additional 1 L of clear fluid prior to colonoscopy as follows:

Split dose: Evening before colonoscopy: 240 mL (8 oz) every 15 minutes until 1 L is consumed. Then drink 16 oz of clear liquid. On the morning of the colonoscopy, repeat process with second liter over 1 hour and then drink 16 oz of clear liquid at least 1 hour before the procedure.

Full dose: Evening before colonoscopy (~6 PM): 240 mL (8 oz every 15 minutes) until 1 L is consumed; 90 minutes later (~7:30 PM), repeat dose. Then drink 32 oz of clear liquid.

Nasogastric tube (CoLyte®, GoLYTELY®, NuLYTELY®, TriLyte®):

Bowel cleansing prior to GI exam:

Children ≥6 months: 25 mL/kg/hour until rectal effluent is clear.

Adults: Bowel cleansing prior to GI exam: 20-30 mL/minute (1.2-1.8 L/hour); the first bowel movement should occur ~1 hour after the start of administration.

Toxic ingestion (unlabeled use; AACT, 2004):

Children ≥9 months to 6 years: 500 mL/hour until rectal effluent is clear

Children 6-12 years: 1000 mL/hour until rectal effluent is clear

Adolescents and Adults: 1500-2000 mL/hour until rectal effluent is clear

Note: May take several hours for the rectal effluent to become clear. Duration may be extended if evidence of continued presence of toxins in GI tract (eg, radiographic evidence or ongoing elimination of toxins)

Dietary Considerations

CoLyte®, GoLYTELY®, NuLYTELY®, TriLyte®: Ideally, the patient should fast for ~3-4 hours prior to administration, but in no case should solid food be given for at least 2 hours before the solution is given. Some products contain aspartame which is metabolized to phenylalanine.

MoviPrep®: Patient should not eat solid food from start of solution administration until after colonoscopy. Patient may have clear liquid soup/plain yogurt for dinner; finish at least 1 hour before start of colon prep.

Administration Oral: Rapid drinking of each portion is preferred to drinking small amounts continuously. Do not add flavorings, unless provided by the manufacturer, as additional ingredients before use. Chilled solution often more palatable. Oral medications should not be administered within 1 hour of start of therapy.

Monitoring Parameters Electrolytes, serum glucose, BUN, urine osmolality; children <2 years of age should be monitored for hypoglycemia, dehydration, hypokalemia

Dosage Forms Excipient information presented when available (limited, particularly for generics); consult specific product labeling.

Powder, for oral solution: PEG 3350 240 g, sodium sulfate 22.72 g, sodium bicarbonate 6.72 g, sodium chloride 5.84 g, and potassium chloride 2.98 g (4000 mL)

Colyte®: PEG 3350 240 g, sodium sulfate 22.72 g, sodium bicarbonate 6.72 g, sodium chloride 5.84 g, and potassium chloride 2.98 g (4000 mL) [available with citrus berry, lemon lime, cherry, orange, and pineapple flavor packets]

GoLYTELY®:

PEG 3350 236 g, sodium sulfate 22.74 g, sodium bicarbonate 6.74 g, sodium chloride 5.86 g, and potassium chloride 2.97 g (4000 mL) [regular and pineapple flavor]

PEG 3350 227.1 g, sodium sulfate 21.5 g, sodium bicarbonate 6.36 g, sodium chloride 5.53 g, and potassium chloride 2.82 g per packet (1s) [regular flavor; makes 1 gallon of solution after mixing]

MoviPrep®: Pouch A: PEG 3350 100g, sodium sulfate 7.5 g, sodium chloride 2.69 g, potassium chloride 1.015 g; Pouch B: Ascorbic acid 4.7 g, sodium ascorbate 5.9 g (1000 mL) [contains phenylalanine 2.33 mg/treatment; lemon flavor; packaged with 2 of Pouch A and 2 of Pouch B in carton and a disposable reconstitution container]

NuLYTELY®: PEG 3350 420 g, sodium bicarbonate 5.72 g, sodium chloride 11.2 g, and potassium chloride 1.48 (4000 mL) [cherry, lemon-lime, orange, and pineapple flavors]

TriLyte®: PEG 3350 420 g, sodium bicarbonate 5.72 g, sodium chloride 11.2 g, and potassium chloride 1.48 g (4000 mL) [supplied with flavor packets]

◆ **Poly-Hist DM** *see* Phenylephrine, Pyrilamine, and Dextromethorphan *on page 1278*

◆ **Poly Hist Forte®** *see* Chlorpheniramine, Pyrilamine, and Phenylephrine *on page 335*

◆ **Poly Hist PD** *see* Chlorpheniramine, Pyrilamine, and Phenylephrine *on page 335*

◆ **Poly-Iron 150 [OTC]** *see* Polysaccharide-Iron Complex *on page 1313*

Polymyxin B (pol i MIKS in bee)

Medication Safety Issues

High alert medication: The Institute for Safe Medication Practices (ISMP) includes this medication (intrathecal administration) among its list of drug classes which have a heightened risk of causing significant patient harm when used in error.

U.S. Brand Names Poly-Rx

Mexican Brand Names Alosol; Biodexan Ofteno; Cortisporin Otico; Dexsul; Glubacida; Maxitrol; Neobacigrin; Neosporin; Polixin; Septilisin; Synalar; Syntex; Tribiot; Trioftín

Index Terms Polymyxin B Sulfate

Pharmacologic Category Antibiotic, Irrigation; Antibiotic, Miscellaneous

Use Treatment of acute infections caused by susceptible strains of *Pseudomonas aeruginosa*; used occasionally for gut decontamination; parenteral use of polymyxin B has mainly been replaced by less toxic antibiotics, reserved for life-threatening infections caused by organisms resistant to the preferred drugs (eg, pseudomonal meningitis - intrathecal administration)

Effect on Mental Status May rarely cause irritability, drowsiness, or ataxia

Effect on Psychiatric Treatment None reported

Dosage Summary

I.M.:

Children <2 years: Up to 40,000 units/kg/day divided every 6 hours

Children ≥2 years: 25,000-30,000 units/kg/day divided every 4-6 hours (maximum: 2,000,000 units/day)

Adults: 25,000-30,000 units/kg/day divided every 4-6 hours (maximum: 2,000,000 units/day)

I.V.:

Children <2 years: Up to 40,000 units/kg/day divided every 12 hours

Children ≥2 years: 15,000-25,000 units/kg/day divided every 12 hours (maximum: 2,000,000 units/day)

Adults: 15,000-25,000 units/kg/day divided every 12 hours (maximum: 2,000,000 units/day)

Intrathecal:
Children <2 years: 20,000 units/day for 3-4 days, then 25,000 units every other day
Children ≥2 years: 50,000 units/day for 3-4 days, then every other day
Adults: 50,000 units/day for 3-4 days, then every other day

Irrigation:
Children: Dosage not established
Adults:
Bladder: 20 mg (equal to 200,000 units) added to 1 L of normal saline as continuous irrigant or rinse
Topical: 500,000 units/L of normal saline (maximum: 2 million units/day)

Ophthalmic:
Children ≥2 years: Initial: 1-3 drops/hour; Reduce to 1-2 drops 4-6 times/day based on response
*Adults:*Initial: 1-3 drops/hour; Reduce to 1-2 drops 4-6 times/day based on response

Otic:
Children: 1-2 drops 3-4 times/day
Adults: 1-2 drops 3-4 times/day

Dosage Forms Excipient information presented when available (limited, particularly for generics); consult specific product labeling.
Injection, powder for reconstitution: 500,000 units
Powder [for prescription compounding]:
Poly-Rx: 100 million units (13 g)

- **Polymyxin B Sulfate** *see* Polymyxin B *on page 1312*
- **Poly-Rx** *see* Polymyxin B *on page 1312*

Polysaccharide-Iron Complex (pol i SAK a ride-EYE ern KOM pleks)

Medication Safety Issues
Sound-alike/look-alike issues:
Niferex® may be confused with Nephrox®

U.S. Brand Names Ferrex 150 [OTC]; Niferex® [OTC]; Nu-Iron® 150 [OTC]; Poly-Iron 150 [OTC]; ProFe [OTC]

Index Terms Iron-Polysaccharide Complex

Pharmacologic Category Iron Salt

Use Prevention and treatment of iron-deficiency anemias

Effect on Mental Status None reported

Effect on Psychiatric Treatment Constipation is common, concurrent use with psychotropic may produce additive effects

Dosage Summary

Oral:
Children <6 years: Dosage not established
Children ≥6 years: 50-100 mg once daily or in divided doses
Adults: 100-300 mg/day in 1-2 divided doses

Dosage Forms Excipient information presented when available (limited, particularly for generics); consult specific product labeling.
Capsule: Elemental iron 150 mg
Ferrex 150, Nu-Iron® 150: Elemental iron 150 mg
Niferex®: Elemental iron 60 mg
Poly-Iron 150: Elemental iron 150 mg [contains tartrazine]
ProFe: Elemental iron 180 mg
Elixir:
Niferex®: Elemental iron 100 mg/5 mL (240 mL) [contains alcohol 10%; dye free, sugar free]

Polythiazide (pol i THYE a zide)

U.S. Brand Names Renese®

Pharmacologic Category Diuretic, Thiazide

Use Adjunctive therapy in treatment of edema and hypertension

Effect on Mental Status May cause drowsiness

Effect on Psychiatric Treatment May decrease lithium clearance resulting in an increase in serum lithium levels and potential lithium toxicity; monitor serum lithium levels

Dosage Summary

Oral:
Children: Dosage not established
Adults: 1-4 mg/day

Dosage Forms Tablet: 2 mg

◆ **Polythiazide and Prazosin** *see* Prazosin and Polythiazide *on page 1325*
◆ **Poly Tussin DM** *see* Chlorpheniramine, Phenylephrine, and Dextromethorphan *on page 327*
◆ **PolyTussin HD** *see* Phenylephrine, Hydrocodone, and Chlorpheniramine *on page 1277*
◆ **Ponstel®** *see* Mefenamic Acid *on page 976*
◆ **Pontocaine®** *see* Tetracaine *on page 1557*
◆ **Pontocaine® Niphanoid®** *see* Tetracaine *on page 1557*

Porfimer (POR fi mer)

Medication Safety Issues

High alert medication: The Institute for Safe Medication Practices (ISMP) includes this medication among its list of drug classes which have a heightened risk of causing significant patient harm when used in error.

U.S. Brand Names Photofrin®

Canadian Brand Names Photofrin®

Index Terms CL-184116; Dihematoporphyrin Ether; Porfimer Sodium

Pharmacologic Category Antineoplastic Agent, Miscellaneous

Use Palliation in patients with obstructing (partial or complete) esophageal cancer; treatment of microinvasive endobronchial nonsmall cell lung cancer (NSCLC); reduction of obstruction and palliation in patients with obstructing (partial or complete) NSCLC; ablation of high-grade dysplasia in Barrett's esophagus

Unlabeled/Investigational Use Treatment of gastric cancer (obstruction); treatment of actinic keratoses and low-risk basal and squamous cell skin cancers

Effect on Mental Status Insomnia is common; may cause anxiety or confusion

Effect on Psychiatric Treatment May cause anemia; use caution with clozapine and carbamazepine; concurrent use with psychotropics may increase the risk of photosensitivity reactions

Dosage Summary

I.V.:

Children: Dosage not established

Adults: 2 mg/kg, followed by exposure to the appropriate laser light

Dosage Forms Excipient information presented when available (limited, particularly for generics); consult specific product labeling.

Injection, powder for reconstitution, as sodium:

Photofrin®: 75 mg

◆ **Porfimer Sodium** *see* Porfimer *on page 1314*
◆ **Portia™** *see* Ethinyl Estradiol and Levonorgestrel *on page 595*

Posaconazole (poe sa KON a zole)

Medication Safety Issues

Sound-alike/look-alike issues:

Noxafil® may be confused with minoxidil

International issues:

Noxafil® may be confused with Noxidil® which is a brand name for minoxidil in Thailand

U.S. Brand Names Noxafil®

Canadian Brand Names Spriafil®

Index Terms SCH 56592

Pharmacologic Category Antifungal Agent, Oral

Use Prophylaxis of invasive *Aspergillus* and *Candida* infections in severely-immunocompromised patients [eg, hematopoietic stem cell transplant (HSCT) recipients with graft-versus-host disease (GVHD) or those with prolonged neutropenia secondary to chemotherapy for hematologic malignancies]; treatment of oropharyngeal candidiasis (including patients refractory to itraconazole and/or fluconazole)

Unlabeled/Investigational Use Salvage therapy of refractory invasive fungal infections; mucormycosis

Effect on Mental Status May cause dizziness, fatigue, or insomnia

Effect on Psychiatric Treatment Contraindicated with pimozide and ergot alkaloids. Diarrhea and other GI side effects are common and may be worse with combined use of lithium, valproic acid, carbamazepine, or SSRIs. May cause neutropenia; use caution with clozapine. May cause thrombocytopenia; use caution with valproic acid. May increase level of some benzodiazepines, mirtazapine, nefazodone, or venlafaxine; monitor for increased effects and/or toxicity.

Dosage Summary

Oral:

Children <13 years: Dosage not established

Children ≥13 years: 100-800 mg/day; doses >100 mg/day are given in 2-3 divided doses

Adults: 100-800 mg/day; doses >100 mg/day are given in 2-3 divided doses

Dosage Forms Excipient information presented when available (limited, particularly for generics); consult specific product labeling.

Suspension, oral:

Noxafil®: 40 mg/mL (123 mL) [contains sodium benzoate; delivers 105 mL of suspension; cherry flavor; packaged with calibrated dosing spoon]

◆ **Post Peel Healing Balm [OTC]** *see* Hydrocortisone *on page 785*

Potassium Bicarbonate and Potassium Citrate

(poe TASS ee um bye KAR bun ate & poe TASS ee um SIT rate)

Medication Safety Issues

Sound-alike/look-alike issues:

Klor-Con® may be confused with Klaron®, K-Lor®

U.S. Brand Names Effer-K™; K-Lyte®; K-Lyte® DS; Klor-Con®/EF

Index Terms Potassium Bicarbonate and Potassium Citrate (Effervescent)

Pharmacologic Category Electrolyte Supplement, Oral

Use Treatment or prevention of hypokalemia

Effect on Mental Status May rarely cause confusion

Effect on Psychiatric Treatment None reported

Dosage Summary

Oral:

Children: 1-4 mEq/kg/day in divided doses

Adults: Prevention: 16-24 mEq/day in 2-4 divided doses; Treatment: 40-100 mEq/day in 2-4 divided doses

Dosage Forms Excipient information presented when available (limited, particularly for generics); consult specific product labeling.

Tablet, effervescent:

Effer-K™: Potassium 25 mEq [cherry berry, lemon citrus, orange, or unflavored]

Klor-Con®/EF: Potassium 25 mEq [sugar free; orange flavor]

K-Lyte®: Potassium 25 mEq [orange flavor]

K-Lyte® DS: Potassium 50 mEq [orange flavor]

◆ **Potassium Bicarbonate and Potassium Citrate (Effervescent)** *see* Potassium Bicarbonate and Potassium Citrate *on page 1315*

Potassium Chloride (poe TASS ee um KLOR ide)

Medication Safety Issues

Sound-alike/look-alike issues:

Kaon-Cl-10® may be confused with kaolin

KCl may be confused with HCl

K-Lor® may be confused with Klor-Con®

Klor-Con® may be confused with Klaron®, K-Lor®

microK® may be confused with Micronase®

High alert medication: The Institute for Safe Medication Practices (ISMP) includes this medication (I.V. formulation) among its list of drugs which have a heightened risk of causing significant patient harm when used in error.

Per JCAHO recommendations, concentrated electrolyte solutions should not be available in patient care areas.

Consider special storage requirements for intravenous potassium salts; I.V. potassium salts have been administered IVP in error, leading to fatal outcomes.

U.S. Brand Names K-Lor®; K-Tab®; Kaon-Cl-10®; Kay Ciel® [DSC]; Klor-Con®; Klor-Con® 10; Klor-Con® 8; Klor-Con® M; Klor-Con®/25; microK®; microK® 10

Canadian Brand Names Apo-K®; K-10®; K-Dur®; K-Lor®; K-Lyte®/Cl; Micro-K Extencaps®; Roychlor®; Slo-Pot; Slow-K®

Mexican Brand Names Corpotasin; K-Dur; Kelefusin

Index Terms KCl

Pharmacologic Category Electrolyte Supplement, Oral; Electrolyte Supplement, Parenteral

Use Treatment or prevention of hypokalemia

Effect on Mental Status None reported

Effect on Psychiatric Treatment May cause GI side effects; concomitant use with SSRIs, carbamazepine, valproic acid, and lithium may produce additive effects. Anticholinergic agents (many psychotropics possess anticholinergic activity) may enhance the ulcerogenic effects of potassium chloride.

Dosage Summary

I.V.:

Children: Initial: 0.5-1 mEq/kg/dose (maximum dose 40 mEq); repeat as needed based on lab values

Adults: Intermittent infusion: ≤10 mEq/hour; repeat as needed based on lab values (maximum: 200 mEq/day)

Oral:

Children: 1-2 mEq/kg/day in 1-2 divided doses or as needed based on lab values

Adults: 40-100 mEq/day in divided doses or as needed based on lab values

Dosage Forms Excipient information presented when available (limited, particularly for generics); consult specific product labeling. [DSC] = Discontinued product

Capsule, extended release, microencapsulated: 8 mEq [600 mg]; 10 mEq [750 mg]
- microK®: 8 mEq [600 mg]
- microK® 10: 10 mEq [750 mg]

Infusion [premixed in D_5W]: 20 mEq (1000 mL); 30 mEq (1000 mL); 40 mEq (1000 mL)

Infusion [premixed in D_5W and LR]: 20 mEq (1000 mL); 30 mEq (1000 mL); 40 mEq (1000 mL)

Infusion [premixed in D_5W and sodium chloride 0.2%]: 5 mEq (250 mL); 10 mEq (500 mL, 1000 mL); 20 mEq (1000 mL); 30 mEq (1000 mL); 40 mEq (1000 mL)

Infusion [premixed in D_5W and sodium chloride 0.225%: 10 mEq (500 mL, 1000 mL); 20 mEq (1000 mL); 30 mEq (1000 mL); 40 mEq (1000 mL)

Infusion [premixed in D_5W and sodium chloride 0.3%]: 10 mEq (500 mL); 20 mEq (1000 mL)

Infusion [premixed in D_5W and sodium chloride 0.33%]: 10 mEq (500 mL); 20 mEq (1000 mL)

Infusion [premixed in D_5W and sodium chloride 0.45%]: 10 mEq (500 mL, 1000 mL); 20 mEq (1000 mL); 30 mEq (1000 mL); 40 mEq (1000 mL)

Infusion [premixed in D_5W and NS]: 20 mEq (1000 mL); 40 mEq (1000 mL)

Infusion [premixed in $D_{10}W$ and sodium chloride 0.2%]: 5 mEq (250 mL)

Infusion [premixed in sodium chloride 0.45%]: 20 mEq (1000 mL); 40 mEq (1000 mL)

Infusion [premixed in NS]: 20 mEq (1000 mL); 40 mEq (1000 mL)

Infusion [premixed in SWFI; highly concentrated]: 10 mEq (50 mL, 100 mL); 20 mEq (50 mL, 100 mL); 30 mEq (100 mL); 40 mEq (100 mL)

Injection, solution [concentrate]: 2 mEq/mL (5 mL, 10 mL, 15 mL, 20 mL, 30 mL, 250 mL, 500 mL)

Powder, for oral solution: 20 mEq/packet (30s, 100s, 1000s)
- K-Lor™: 20 mEq/packet (30s, 100s) [fruit flavor]
- Kay Ciel® 10%: 20 mEq/packet (30s, 100s) [sugar free] [DSC]
- Klor-Con®: 20 mEq/packet (30s, 100s) [sugar free; fruit flavor]
- Klor-Con®/25: 25 mEq/packet (30s, 100s) [sugar free; fruit flavor]

Solution, oral: 20 mEq/15 mL (15 mL, 30 mL, 480 mL, 3840 mL); 40 mEq/15 mL (15 mL, 480 mL)

Tablet, extended release: 8 mEq [600 mg]; 10 mEq [750 mg]; 20 mEq [1500 mg]
- K-Tab®: 10 mEq [750 mg]
- Kaon-Cl® 10: 10 mEq [750 mg]

Tablet, extended release, microencapsulated: 10 mEq, 20 mEq
- Klor-Con® M10: 10 mEq [750 mg]
- Klor-Con® M15: 15 mEq [1125 mg; scored]
- Klor-Con® M20: 20 mEq [1500 mg; scored]

Tablet, extended release, wax matrix: 8 mEq, 10 mEq
- Klor-Con® 8: 8 mEq [600 mg]
- Clor-Con® 10: 10 mEq [750 mg]

Potassium Iodide (poe TASS ee um EYE oh dide)

Medication Safety Issues

Sound-alike/look-alike issues:

Potassium iodide products, including saturated solution of potassium iodide (SSKI®) may be confused with potassium iodide and iodine (Strong Iodide Solution or Lugol's solution)

U.S. Brand Names Iosat™ [OTC]; SSKI®; ThyroSafe™ [OTC]; ThyroShield™ [OTC]

Index Terms KI

Pharmacologic Category Antithyroid Agent; Expectorant

Use Expectorant for the symptomatic treatment of chronic pulmonary diseases complicated by mucous; reduce thyroid vascularity prior to thyroidectomy and management of thyrotoxic crisis; block thyroidal uptake of radioactive isotopes of iodine in a radiation emergency or other exposure to radioactive iodine

Unlabeled/Investigational Use Lymphocutaneous and cutaneous sporotrichosis

Effect on Mental Status None reported

Effect on Psychiatric Treatment Concurrent use with lithium may produce additive hypothyroid effects

Dosage Summary

Oral:

Infants <1 month:

Iosat™, ThyroSafe™, ThyroShield™: 16.25 mg once daily

SSKI®: 150-250 mg (3-5 drops) 3 times/day

Infants 1-12 month:

Iosat™, ThyroSafe™, ThyroShield™: 32.5 mg once daily

SSKI®: 150-250 mg (3-5 drops) 3 times/day

Children 1-3 years:

Iosat™, ThyroSafe™, ThyroShield™: 32.5 mg once daily

SSKI®: 50-500 mg (1-10 drops) 3 times/day

Children 3-18 years:

Iosat™, ThyroSafe™, ThyroShield™: 65 mg once daily **or** 130 mg once daily if >68 kg

SSKI®: 50-500 mg (1-10 drops) 3 times/day

Adults:

Iosat™, ThyroSafe™, ThyroShield™: 130 mg once daily

SSKI®: 50-600 mg 3-4 times/day

Dosage Forms Excipient information presented when available (limited, particularly for generics); consult specific product labeling.

Solution, oral:

SSKI®: 1 g/mL (30 mL, 240 mL) [contains sodium thiosulfate]

ThyroShield™: 65 mg/mL (30 mL) [black raspberry flavor]

Tablet:

Iosat™: 130 mg

ThyroSafe™: 65 mg [equivalent to iodine 50 mg]

Potassium Iodide and Iodine

(poe TASS ee um EYE oh dide & EYE oh dine)

Medication Safety Issues

Sound-alike/look-alike issues:

Potassium iodide and iodine (Strong Iodide Solution or Lugol's solution) may be confused with potassium iodide products, including saturated solution of potassium iodide (SSKI®)

Index Terms Lugol's Solution; Strong Iodine Solution

Pharmacologic Category Antithyroid Agent

Use Reduce thyroid vascularity prior to thyroidectomy and management of thyrotoxic crisis; block thyroidal uptake of radioactive isotopes of iodine in a radiation emergency or other exposure to radioactive iodine

Effect on Mental Status May cause drowsiness or confusion

Effect on Psychiatric Treatment Concurrent use with lithium may produce additive hypothyroid effects

Dosage Summary

Oral:

Children:

Preoperative thyroidectomy: 0.1-0.3 mL (3-5 drops) 3 times/day, administer for 10 days before surgery

Thyrotoxic crisis: 1 mL 3 times/day

Adults:
Preoperative thyroidectomy: 0.1-0.3 mL (3-5 drops) 3 times/day, administer for 10 days before surgery
Thyrotoxic crisis: 1 mL 3 times/day

Dosage Forms Excipient information presented when available (limited, particularly for generics); consult specific product labeling.
Solution, oral: Potassium iodide 100 mg/mL and iodine 50 mg/mL (480 mL)
Solution, topical: Potassium iodide 100 mg/mL and iodine 50 mg/mL (8 mL)

◆ **Potassium Iodide, Chlorpheniramine, Phenylephrine, and Codeine** *see* Chlorpheniramine, Phenylephrine, Codeine, and Potassium Iodide *on page 332*

◆ **PPS** *see* Pentosan Polysulfate Sodium *on page 1250*

◆ **PPV23** *see* Pneumococcal Polysaccharide Vaccine (Polyvalent) *on page 1309*

Pralidoxime (pra li DOKS eem)

Medication Safety Issues
Sound-alike/look-alike issues:
Pralidoxime may be confused with pramoxine, pyridoxine
Protopam® may be confused with Proloprim®, protamine, Protropin®

U.S. Brand Names Protopam®

Canadian Brand Names Protopam®

Index Terms 2-PAM; 2-Pyridine Aldoxime Methochloride; Pralidoxime Chloride

Pharmacologic Category Antidote

Use Reverse muscle paralysis caused by toxic exposure to organophosphate anticholinesterase pesticides and chemicals; control of overdose of anticholinesterase medications used to treat myasthenia gravis (ambenonium, neostigmine, pyridostigmine)

Unlabeled/Investigational Use Treatment of nerve agent toxicity (chemical warfare) in combination with atropine

Effect on Mental Status May cause dizziness or drowsiness

Effect on Psychiatric Treatment Avoid with phenothiazines; effects of barbiturates may be increased

Dosage Summary
I.M.:
Children: 20-50 mg/kg/dose, repeat in 1-2 hours if muscle weakness has not been relieved, then at 8- to 12-hour intervals if cholinergic signs recur
Adults: 1-2 g; repeat in 1 hour if muscle weakness has not been relieved, then at 8- to 12-hour intervals if cholinergic signs recur **or** 1-2 g followed by increments of 250 mg every 5 minutes until response is observed
I.V.:
Children: 20-50 mg/kg/dose; repeat in 1-2 hours if muscle weakness has not been relieved, then at 8- to 12-hour intervals if cholinergic signs recur
Adults: 1-2 g; repeat in 1 hour if muscle weakness has not been relieved, then at 8- to 12-hour intervals if cholinergic signs recur **or** 1-2 g followed by increments of 250 mg every 5 minutes until response is observed

Dosage Forms Excipient information presented when available (limited, particularly for generics); consult specific product labeling.
Injection, powder for reconstitution, as chloride:
Protopam®: 1 g
Injection, solution: 300 mg/mL (2 mL) [contains benzyl alcohol; prefilled auto injector]

◆ **Pralidoxime and Atropine** *see* Atropine and Pralidoxime *on page 159*

◆ **Pralidoxime Chloride** *see* Pralidoxime *on page 1318*

Pramipexole (pra mi PEKS ole)

Medication Safety Issues
Sound-alike/look-alike issues:
Mirapex® may be confused with Mifeprex®, MiraLax™

Related Information
Antiparkinsonian Agents *on page 1767*

U.S. Brand Names Mirapex®

Canadian Brand Names Apo-Pramipexole; Mirapex®; Novo-Pramipexole; PMS-Pramipexole

Mexican Brand Names Sifrol

Pharmacologic Category Anti-Parkinson's Agent, Dopamine Agonist

Generic Available No

Use Treatment of the signs and symptoms of idiopathic Parkinson's disease; treatment of moderate-to-severe primary Restless Legs Syndrome (RLS)

Unlabeled/Investigational Use Treatment of depression

Pregnancy Risk Factor C

Pregnancy Considerations Early embryonic loss and postnatal growth inhibition were observed in animal studies. There are no adequate and well-controlled studies in pregnant women.

Lactation Excretion in breast milk unknown/not recommended

Contraindications Hypersensitivity to pramipexole or any component of the formulation

Warnings/Precautions Caution should be taken in patients with renal insufficiency; dose adjustment necessary. Caution in patients with pre-existing dyskinesias; may be exacerbated. May cause orthostatic hypotension; Parkinson's disease patients appear to have an impaired capacity to respond to a postural challenge. Use with caution in patients at risk of hypotension or where transient hypotensive episodes would be poorly tolerated. Parkinson's patients being treated with dopaminergic agonists ordinarily require careful monitoring for signs and symptoms of postural hypotension, especially during dose escalation. May cause hallucinations.

Dopamine agonists have been associated with compulsive behaviors and/or loss of impulse control, which has manifested as pathological gambling, libido increases (hypersexuality), and/or binge eating. Causality has not been established, and controversy exists as to whether this phenomenon is related to the underlying disease, prior behaviors/addictions and/or drug therapy. Dose reduction or discontinuation of therapy has been reported to reverse these behaviors in some, but not all cases.

Dopaminergic agents have been associated with a syndrome resembling neuroleptic malignant syndrome on abrupt withdrawal or significant dosage reduction after long-term use. Ergot-derived dopamine agonists have also been associated with fibrotic complications (eg, retroperitoneal fibrosis, pleural thickening, and pulmonary infiltrates). Although pramipexole is not an ergot, there have been postmarketing reports of possible fibrotic complications with pramipexole; monitor closely for signs and symptoms of fibrosis.

Pramipexole has been associated with somnolence, particularly at higher dosages (>1.5 mg/day). In addition, patients have been reported to fall asleep during activities of daily living, including driving, while taking this medication. Whether these patients exhibited somnolence prior to these events is not clear. Patients should be advised of this issue and factors which may increase risk (sleep disorders, other sedating medications, or concomitant medications which increase pramipexole concentrations) and instructed to report daytime somnolence or sleepiness to the prescriber. Patients should use caution in performing activities which require alertness (driving or operating machinery), and to avoid other medications which may cause CNS depression, including ethanol.

Pathologic degenerative changes were observed in the retinas of albino rats during studies with this agent, but were not observed in the retinas of albino mice or in other species. The significance of these data for humans remains uncertain. Augmentation (earlier onset of symptoms in the evening/afternoon, increase and/or spread of symptoms to other extremities) or rebound (shifting of symptoms to early morning hours) may occur in some RLS patients. Safety and efficacy have not been established in children.

Adverse Reactions Parkinson's disease (PD) unless identified as RLS:

>10%:

- Cardiovascular: Postural hypotension (dose related; PD 53%)
- Central nervous system: Dizziness (PD 25%), headache (RLS 16%), somnolence (dose related; RLS 6%; PD 9% to 22%), insomnia (RLS 13%; PD 17% to 27%), hallucinations (PD 9% to 17%), abnormal dreams (RLS up to 8%)
- Gastrointestinal: Nausea (dose related; RLS: 5% to 27%; PD 28%), constipation (dose related; RLS: 4%; PD 10% to 14%)
- Neuromuscular & skeletal: Weakness (PD 10% to 14%), dyskinesia (PD 47%), EPS

1% to 10%:

- Cardiovascular: Edema, syncope, tachycardia, chest pain
- Central nervous system: Malaise, confusion (PD 4% to 10%), amnesia (dose related), dystonias, akathisia, thinking abnormalities, myoclonus, hyperesthesia, paranoia, fever
- Endocrine & metabolic: Decreased libido

Gastrointestinal: Anorexia, diarrhea (RLS 3% to7%), dysphagia, weight loss, xerostomia (up to 7%)
Genitourinary: Urinary frequency (PD 6%), impotence, urinary incontinence
Neuromuscular & skeletal: Muscle twitching, leg cramps, arthritis, bursitis, myasthenia, gait abnormalities, hypertonia
Ocular: Vision abnormalities
Respiratory: Dyspnea, nasal congestion (RLS up to 6%), rhinitis
Miscellaneous: Influenza (RLS 3%)

<1% (Limited to important or life-threatening): Augmentation (RLS ~20% but similar to placebo), compulsive gambling, liver transaminases increased, rebound (RLS), rhabdomyolysis, tolerance (RLS)
Reported with dopamine agonists: Impulsive/compulsive behaviors (eg, pathological gambling, hypersexuality, binge eating)

Frequency not defined, dose related: Falling asleep during activities of daily living

Drug Interactions

Alcohol (Ethyl): CNS Depressants may enhance the CNS depressant effect of Alcohol (Ethyl). *Risk C: Monitor therapy*

Antipsychotics (Atypical): May diminish the therapeutic effect of Anti-Parkinson's Agents (Dopamine Agonist). *Risk D: Consider therapy modification*

Antipsychotics (Typical): May diminish the therapeutic effect of Anti-Parkinson's Agents (Dopamine Agonist) *Risk D: Consider therapy modification*

CNS Depressants: May enhance the adverse/toxic effect of other CNS Depressants. *Risk C: Monitor therapy*

Metoclopramide: May diminish the therapeutic effect of Anti-Parkinson's Agents (Dopamine Agonist). *Risk C: Monitor therapy*

Ethanol/Nutrition/Herb Interactions

Ethanol: Avoid ethanol (may increase CNS depression).

Food: Food intake does not affect the extent of drug absorption, although the time to maximal plasma concentration is delayed by 60 minutes when taken with a meal.

Herb/Nutraceutical: Avoid valerian, St John's wort, SAMe, kava kava (may increase risk of serotonin syndrome and/or excessive sedation).

Stability Store at 15°C to 30°C (59°F to 86°F). Protect from light.

Mechanism of Action Pramipexole is a nonergot dopamine agonist with specificity for the D_2 subfamily dopamine receptor, and has also been shown to bind to D_3 and D_4 receptors. By binding to these receptors, it is thought that pramipexole can stimulate dopamine activity on the nerves of the striatum and substantia nigra.

Pharmacodynamics/Kinetics

Absorption: Rapid
Distribution: V_d: 500 L
Protein binding: 15%
Bioavailability: >90%
Half-life elimination: ~8 hours; Elderly: 12-14 hours
Time to peak, serum: ~2 hours
Excretion: Urine (90% as unchanged drug)

Dosage Oral: Adults:

Parkinson's disease: Initial: 0.375 mg/day given in 3 divided doses, increase gradually by 0.125 mg/dose every 5-7 days; range: 1.5-4.5 mg/day

Restless legs syndrome: Initial: 0.125 mg once daily 2-3 hours before bedtime. Dose may be doubled every 4-7 days up to 0.5 mg/day. Maximum dose: 0.5 mg/day (manufacturer's recommendation).

Note: Most patients require <0.5 mg/day, but higher doses have been used (2 mg/day). If augmentation occurs, dose earlier in the day.

Dosage adjustment in renal impairment: Use caution; renally-eliminated

Parkinson's disease:

Cl_{cr} 35-59 mL/minute: Initial: 0.125 mg twice daily (maximum dose: 1.5 mg twice daily)

Cl_{cr} 15-34 mL/minute: Initial: 0.125 mg once daily (maximum dose: 1.5 mg once daily)

Cl_{cr} <15 mL/minute (or hemodialysis patients): Not adequately studied

Restless legs syndrome:

Cl_{cr} 20-60 mL/minute: Duration between titration should be increased to 14 days

Cl_{cr} <20 mL/minute: Not adequately studied

Dietary Considerations May be taken with food to decrease nausea.

Administration Doses should be titrated gradually in all patients to avoid the onset of intolerable side effects. The dosage should be increased to achieve a maximum therapeutic effect, balanced against the side effects of dyskinesia, hallucinations, somnolence, and dry mouth.

Monitoring Parameters Monitor for improvement in symptoms of Parkinson's disease (eg, mentation, behavior, daily living activities, motor examinations), blood pressure, body weight changes, and heart rate

Dosage Forms Excipient information presented when available (limited, particularly for generics); consult specific product labeling. [CAN] = Canadian product

Tablet, as dihydrochloride monohydrate: 0.25 mg [CAN; generic not available in U.S.], 0.5 mg [CAN; generic not available in U.S.], 1 mg [CAN; generic not available in U.S.], 1.5 mg [CAN; generic not available in U.S.]

Mirapex®: 0.125 mg, 0.25 mg, 0.5 mg, 0.75 mg, 1 mg, 1.5 mg

Pramlintide (PRAM lin tide)

Medication Safety Issues

High alert medication: The Institute for Safe Medication Practices (ISMP) includes this medication among its list of drug classes which have a heightened risk of causing significant patient harm when used in error.

Dosing: The concentration of this product is 600 micrograms (mcg)/mL. Manufacturer recommended dosing ranges from 15 mcg to 120 mcg, which corresponds to injectable volumes of 0.025 mL to 0.2 mL. Patients and healthcare providers should exercise caution when administering this product to avoid inadvertent calculation of the dose based on "units," which could result in a sixfold overdose.

U.S. Brand Names Symlin®

Index Terms Pramlintide Acetate

Pharmacologic Category Amylinomimetic; Antidiabetic Agent

Use

Adjunctive treatment with mealtime insulin in type 1 diabetes mellitus (insulin dependent, IDDM) patients who have failed to achieve desired glucose control despite optimal insulin therapy

Adjunctive treatment with mealtime insulin in type 2 diabetes mellitus (noninsulin dependent, NIDDM) patients who have failed to achieve desired glucose control despite optimal insulin therapy, with or without concurrent sulfonylurea and/or metformin

Effect on Mental Status May cause dizziness or fatigue

Effect on Psychiatric Treatment GI side effects are common; concomitant use with SSRIs, lithium, and valproic acid may produce additive effects. Psychotropics with anticholinergic properties may produce synergistic impairment of gastric motility if used with pramlintide.

Restrictions An FDA-approved medication guide must be distributed when dispensing an outpatient prescription (new or refill) where this medication is to be used without direct supervision of a healthcare provider. Medication guides are available at http://www.fda.gov/cder/Offices/ODS/medication_guides.htm.

Dosage Summary

SubQ:

Children: Dosage not established

Adults:

Type 1 diabetes mellitus (insulin dependent, IDDM): Initial: 15 mcg immediately prior to meals; Target dose: 30-60 mcg prior to meals; **Note:** Titration is recommended

Type 2 diabetes mellitus (noninsulin dependent, NIDDM): Initial: 60 mcg immediately prior to meals, after 3-7 days increase to 120 mcg prior to meals

Dosage Forms Excipient information presented when available (limited, particularly for generics); consult specific product labeling.

Injection, solution, as acetate:

Symlin®: 600 mcg/mL (5 mL); 1000 mcg/mL (1.5 mL) [60 pen-injector]; 1000 mcg/mL (2.7 mL) [120 pen-injector]

- **Pramlintide Acetate** *see* Pramlintide *on page 1321*
- **PrandiMet™** *see* Repaglinide and Metformin *on page 1412*
- **Prandin®** *see* Repaglinide *on page 1409*
- **Pravachol®** *see* Pravastatin *on page 1321*

Pravastatin (prav a STAT in)

Medication Safety Issues

Sound-alike/look-alike issues:

Pravachol® may be confused with Prevacid®, Prinivil®, propranolol

Related Information
Lipid-Lowering Agents *on page 1786*

U.S. Brand Names Pravachol®

Canadian Brand Names Apo-Pravastatin®; CO Pravastatin; Novo-Pravastatin; PMS-Pravastatin; Pravachol®; ratio-Pravastatin; Riva-Pravastatin; Sandoz-Pravastatin

Mexican Brand Names Astin; Brakhor; Brufincol; Col-Alphar; Colpradin; Emipastin; Genoestatina; Kenstatin; Loretsin; Novina; Pravacol; Tissulest

Index Terms Pravastatin Sodium

Pharmacologic Category Antilipemic Agent, HMG-CoA Reductase Inhibitor

Generic Available Yes

Use Use with dietary therapy for the following:

Primary prevention of coronary events: In hypercholesterolemic patients without established coronary heart disease to reduce cardiovascular morbidity (myocardial infarction, coronary revascularization procedures) and mortality.

Secondary prevention of cardiovascular events in patients with established coronary heart disease: To slow the progression of coronary atherosclerosis; to reduce cardiovascular morbidity (myocardial infarction, coronary vascular procedures) and to reduce mortality; to reduce the risk of stroke and transient ischemic attacks

Hyperlipidemias: Reduce elevations in total cholesterol, LDL-C, apolipoprotein B, and triglycerides (elevations of 1 or more components are present in Fredrickson type IIa, IIb, III, and IV hyperlipidemias)

Heterozygous familial hypercholesterolemia (HeFH): In pediatric patients, 8-18 years of age, with HeFH having LDL-C ≥190 mg/dL **or** LDL ≥160 mg/dL with positive family history of premature cardiovascular disease (CVD) or 2 or more CVD risk factors in the pediatric patient

Effect on Mental Status May cause dizziness

Effect on Psychiatric Treatment None reported

Pregnancy Risk Factor X

Pregnancy Considerations Cholesterol biosynthesis may be important in fetal development. Contraindicated in pregnancy. Administer to women of child-bearing potential only when conception is highly unlikely and patients have been informed of potential hazards.

Lactation Enters breast milk/contraindicated

Contraindications Hypersensitivity to pravastatin or any component of the formulation; active liver disease; unexplained persistent elevations of serum transaminases; pregnancy; breast-feeding

Warnings/Precautions Secondary causes of hyperlipidemia should be ruled out prior to therapy. Liver function must be monitored by periodic laboratory assessment. Rhabdomyolysis with acute renal failure has occurred. Risk may be increased with concurrent use of other drugs which may cause rhabdomyolysis (including colchicine, gemfibrozil, fibric acid derivatives, or niacin at doses ≥1 g/day). Temporarily discontinue in any patient experiencing an acute or serious condition predisposing to renal failure secondary to rhabdomyolysis. Based upon current evidence, HMG-CoA reductase inhibitor therapy should be continued in the perioperative period unless risk outweighs cardioprotective benefit. Use with caution in patients with advanced age, these patients are predisposed to myopathy. Use caution in patients with previous liver disease or heavy ethanol use. Treatment in patients <8 years of age is not recommended.

Adverse Reactions As reported in short-term trials; safety and tolerability with long-term use were similar to placebo

1% to 10%:

Cardiovascular: Chest pain (4%)

Central nervous system: Headache (2% to 6%), fatigue (4%), dizziness (1% to 3%)

Dermatologic: Rash (4%)

Gastrointestinal: Nausea/vomiting (7%), diarrhea (6%), heartburn (3%)

Hepatic: Transaminases increased (>3x normal on two occasions - 1%)

Neuromuscular & skeletal: Myalgia (2%)

Respiratory: Cough (3%)

Miscellaneous: Influenza (2%)

<1% (Limited to important or life-threatening): Allergy, lens opacity, libido change, memory impairment, muscle weakness, neuropathy, paresthesia, taste disturbance, tremor, vertigo

Postmarketing and/or case reports: Anaphylaxis, angioedema, cholestatic jaundice, cirrhosis, cranial nerve dysfunction, dermatomyositis, erythema multiforme, ESR increase, fulminant hepatic necrosis, gynecomastia, hemolytic anemia, hepatitis, hepatoma, lupus erythematosus-like syndrome, myopathy, pancreatitis, peripheral nerve palsy, polymyalgia rheumatica, positive ANA, purpura, rhabdomyolysis, Stevens-Johnson syndrome, vasculitis

Additional class-related events or case reports (not necessarily reported with pravastatin therapy): Angioedema, cataracts, depression, dyspnea, eosinophilia, erectile dysfunction, facial paresis, hypersensitivity reaction, impaired extraocular muscle movement, impotence, leukopenia, malaise, memory loss, ophthalmoplegia, paresthesia, peripheral neuropathy, photosensitivity, psychic disturbance, skin discoloration, thrombocytopenia, thyroid dysfunction, toxic epidermal necrolysis, transaminases increased, vomiting

Metabolism/Transport Effects **Substrate** of CYP3A4 (minor); **Inhibits** CYP2C9 (weak), 2D6 (weak), 3A4 (weak)

Drug Interactions

Antifungal Agents (Azole Derivatives, Systemic): May decrease the metabolism of HMG-CoA Reductase Inhibitors. *Risk D: Consider therapy modification*

Colchicine: May enhance the myopathic (rhabdomyolysis) effect of HMG-CoA Reductase Inhibitors. Colchicine may increase the serum concentration of HMG-CoA Reductase Inhibitors. *Risk D: Consider therapy modification*

CycloSPORINE: May increase the serum concentration of HMG-CoA Reductase Inhibitors. *Risk D: Consider therapy modification*

DAPTOmycin: HMG-CoA Reductase Inhibitors may enhance the adverse/toxic effect of DAPTOmycin. Specifically, the risk of skeletal muscle toxicity may be increased. Management: Consider temporarily stopping HMG-CoA reductase inhibitor therapy prior to daptomycin. If used together, regular (i.e., at least weekly) monitoring of CPK concentrations is recommended. *Risk D: Consider therapy modification*

Fenofibrate: May enhance the adverse/toxic effect of HMG-CoA Reductase Inhibitors. *Risk C: Monitor therapy*

Gemfibrozil: May enhance the myopathic (rhabdomyolysis) effect of HMG-CoA Reductase Inhibitors. Gemfibrozil may increase the serum concentration of HMG-CoA Reductase Inhibitors. *Risk D: Consider therapy modification*

Niacin: May enhance the adverse/toxic effect of HMG-CoA Reductase Inhibitors. *Risk C: Monitor therapy*

Niacinamide: May enhance the adverse/toxic effect of HMG-CoA Reductase Inhibitors. *Risk C: Monitor therapy*

P-Glycoprotein Inducers: May decrease the serum concentration of P-Glycoprotein Substrates. P-glycoprotein inducers may also further limit the distribution of p-glycoprotein substrates to specific cells/tissues/organs where p-glycoprotein is present in large amounts (e.g., brain, T-lymphocytes, testes, etc.). *Risk C: Monitor therapy*

P-Glycoprotein Inhibitors: May increase the serum concentration of P-Glycoprotein Substrates. P-glycoprotein inhibitors may also enhance the distribution of p-glycoprotein substrates to specific cells/tissues/organs where p-glycoprotein is present in large amounts (e.g., brain, T-lymphocytes, testes, etc.). *Risk C: Monitor therapy*

Phenytoin: May increase the metabolism of HMG-CoA Reductase Inhibitors. *Risk D: Consider therapy modification*

Protease Inhibitors: May increase the serum concentration of HMG-CoA Reductase Inhibitors. Limited data suggest pravastatin may slightly decrease protease inhibitor concentrations. Management: Lovastatin and simvastatin are contraindicated with many protease inhibitors; use lowest possible HMG-CoA reductase inhibitor dose and monitor for signs and symptoms of rhabdomyolysis if these agents are used concomitantly. *Risk D: Consider therapy modification*

Rifamycin Derivatives: May increase the metabolism of HMG-CoA Reductase Inhibitors. *Risk D: Consider therapy modification*

Vitamin K Antagonists (eg, warfarin): HMG-CoA Reductase Inhibitors may enhance the anticoagulant effect of Vitamin K Antagonists. *Risk C: Monitor therapy*

Ethanol/Nutrition/Herb Interactions

Ethanol: Consumption of large amounts of ethanol may increase the risk of liver damage with HMG-CoA reductase inhibitors.

Food: Red yeast rice contains an estimated 2.4 mg lovastatin per 600 mg rice.

Herb/Nutraceutical: St John's wort may decrease pravastatin levels.

Stability Store at 25°C (77°F); excursions permitted to 15°C to 30°C (59°F to 86°F). Protect from moisture and light.

Mechanism of Action Pravastatin is a competitive inhibitor of 3-hydroxy-3-methylglutaryl coenzyme A (HMG-CoA) reductase, which is the rate-limiting enzyme involved in *de novo* cholesterol synthesis.

Pharmacodynamics/Kinetics

Onset of action: Several days

Peak effect: 4 weeks

Absorption: Rapidly absorbed; average absorption 34%
Protein binding: 50%
Metabolism: Hepatic to at least two metabolites
Bioavailability: 17%
Half-life elimination: ~2-3 hours
Time to peak, serum: 1-1.5 hours
Excretion: Feces (70%); urine (≤20%, 8% as unchanged drug)

Dosage Oral: **Note:** Doses should be individualized according to the baseline LDL-cholesterol levels, the recommended goal of therapy, and patient response; adjustments should be made at intervals of 4 weeks or more; doses may need adjusted based on concomitant medications

Children: HeFH:

8-13 years: 20 mg/day

14-18 years: 40 mg/day

Dosage adjustment for pravastatin based on concomitant cyclosporine: Refer to adult dosing section

Adults: Hyperlipidemias, primary prevention of coronary events, secondary prevention of cardiovascular events: Initial: 40 mg once daily; titrate dosage to response; usual range: 10-80 mg; (maximum dose: 80 mg once daily)

Dosage adjustment for pravastatin based on concomitant cyclosporine: Initial: 10 mg/day, titrate with caution (maximum dose: 20 mg/day)

Elderly: No specific dosage recommendations. Clearance is reduced in the elderly, resulting in an increase in AUC between 25% to 50%. However, substantial accumulation is not expected.

Dosing adjustment in renal impairment: Initial: 10 mg/day

Dosing adjustment in hepatic impairment: Initial: 10 mg/day

Dietary Considerations May be taken without regard to meals. Before initiation of therapy, patients should be placed on a standard cholesterol-lowering diet for 6 weeks and the diet should be continued during drug therapy. Red yeast rice contains an estimated 2.4 mg lovastatin per 600 mg rice.

Administration May be taken without regard to meals.

Monitoring Parameters Obtain baseline LFTs and total cholesterol profile; creatine phosphokinase due to possibility of myopathy. Repeat LFTs prior to elevation of dose. May be measured when clinically indicated and/or periodically thereafter.

Dosage Forms Excipient information presented when available (limited, particularly for generics); consult specific product labeling.

Tablet, as sodium: 10 mg, 20 mg, 40 mg, 80 mg

Pravachol®: 10 mg; 20 mg [DSC]; 40 mg, 80 mg

- **Pravastatin and Aspirin** *see* Aspirin and Pravastatin *on page 146*
- **Pravastatin Sodium** *see* Pravastatin *on page 1321*
- **Pravigard™ PAC [DSC]** *see* Aspirin and Pravastatin *on page 146*

Praziquantel (pray zi KWON tel)

U.S. Brand Names Biltricide®

Canadian Brand Names Biltricide®

Mexican Brand Names Cesol; Cisticid

Pharmacologic Category Anthelmintic

Use All stages of schistosomiasis caused by all *Schistosoma* species pathogenic to humans; clonorchiasis and opisthorchiasis

Unlabeled/Investigational Use Cysticercosis and many intestinal tapeworms

Effect on Mental Status May cause dizziness or drowsiness

Effect on Psychiatric Treatment None reported

Dosage Summary

Oral:

Children ≤4 years: Dosage not established

Children >4 years: 20 mg/kg/dose 2-3 times/day for 1 day at 4- to 6-hour intervals **or** 25 mg/kg 3 times/day for 1 day

Adults: 20 mg/kg/dose 2-3 times/day for 1 day at 4- to 6-hour intervals **or** 25 mg/kg 3 times/day for 1 day

Dosage Forms Excipient information presented when available (limited, particularly for generics); consult specific product labeling.

Tablet [tri-scored]: 600 mg

Prazosin (PRAZ oh sin)

Medication Safety Issues

Sound-alike/look-alike issues:

Prazosin may be confused with predniSONE

International issues:

Prazac® [Denmark] may be confused with Prozac® which is a brand name for fluoxetine in the U.S.

Prazepam [multiple international markets] may be confused with prazosin.

U.S. Brand Names Minipress®

Canadian Brand Names Apo-Prazo®; Minipress®; Novo-Prazin; Nu-Prazo

Mexican Brand Names Minipres

Index Terms Furazosin; Prazosin Hydrochloride

Pharmacologic Category Alpha$_1$ Blocker

Use Treatment of hypertension

Unlabeled/Investigational Use Post-traumatic stress disorder (PTSD); benign prostatic hyperplasia; Raynaud's syndrome

Effect on Mental Status Dizziness is common; may cause drowsiness or nervousness; may rarely cause nightmares

Effect on Psychiatric Treatment Concurrent use with low potency antipsychotics and TCAs may increase risk of postural hypotension

Dosage Summary

Oral:

Children (unlabeled use): Initial: 0.05-0.1 mg/kg/day in 3 divided doses; maximum: 0.5 mg/kg/day

Adults: Initial: 1 mg/dose 2-3 times/day; Maintenance: 3-15 mg/day in divided doses 2-4 times/day (maximum: 20 mg/day) **or** 10-20 mg once, may repeat in 30 minutes

Elderly: Initial: 1 mg 1-2 times/day

Dosage Forms Excipient information presented when available (limited, particularly for generics); consult specific product labeling.

Capsule, as hydrochloride: 1 mg, 2 mg, 5 mg

Prazosin and Polythiazide (PRAZ oh sin & pol i THYE a zide)

Medication Safety Issues

Sound-alike/look-alike issues:

Minizide® may be confused with Minocin®

U.S. Brand Names Minizide® [DSC]

Index Terms Polythiazide and Prazosin

Pharmacologic Category Alpha$_1$ Blocker; Diuretic, Thiazide

Use Management of mild-to-moderate hypertension

Effect on Mental Status Dizziness is common; may cause drowsiness or nervousness; may rarely cause nightmares

Effect on Psychiatric Treatment Concurrent use with low potency antipsychotics and TCAs may increase risk of postural hypotension; may decrease lithium clearance resulting in an increase in serum lithium levels and potential lithium toxicity; monitor serum lithium levels

Dosage Summary

Oral:

Children: Dosage not established

Adults: Initial: 1 capsule 2-3 times/day; Maintenance: Increase slowly to prazosin 20 mg/day and polythiazide 1-4 mg/day

Dosage Forms Excipient information presented when available (limited, particularly for generics); consult specific product labeling. [DSC] = Discontinued product

Capsule:

Minizide® 1: Prazosin 1 mg and polythiazide 0.5 mg [DSC]

Minizide® 2: Prazosin 2 mg and polythiazide 0.5 mg [DSC]

Minizide® 5: Prazosin 5 mg and polythiazide 0.5 mg [DSC]

- **Prazosin Hydrochloride** *see* Prazosin *on page 1325*
- **Precedex™** *see* Dexmedetomidine *on page 438*
- **Precose®** *see* Acarbose *on page 25*
- **Pred Forte®** *see* PrednisoLONE *on page 1326*
- **Pred Mild®** *see* PrednisoLONE *on page 1326*

PrednisoLONE (pred NISS oh lone)

Medication Safety Issues

Sound-alike/look-alike issues:

PrednisoLONE may be confused with predniSONE

Pediapred® may be confused with Pediazole®

Related Information

Anticholinergic Effects of Common Psychotropics *on page 1758*

Corticosteroids *on page 1780*

U.S. Brand Names Econopred® Plus [DSC]; Millipred™; Omnipred™; Orapred ODT™; Orapred®; Pediapred®; Pred Forte®; Pred Mild®; Prelone®

Canadian Brand Names Diopred®; Hydeltra T.B.A.®; Inflamase® Mild; Novo-Prednisolone; Ophtho-Tate®; Pediapred®; Pred Forte®; Pred Mild®; Sab-Prenase

Mexican Brand Names Fisopred; Meticortelone; Pred Un; Pred-NF; Prednefrin SF; Sophipren Ofteno

Index Terms Deltahydrocortisone; Metacortandralone; Prednisolone Acetate; Prednisolone Acetate, Ophthalmic; Prednisolone Sodium Phosphate; Prednisolone Sodium Phosphate, Ophthalmic

Pharmacologic Category Corticosteroid, Ophthalmic; Corticosteroid, Systemic

Use Treatment of palpebral and bulbar conjunctivitis; corneal injury from chemical, radiation, thermal burns, or foreign body penetration; endocrine disorders, rheumatic disorders, collagen diseases, dermatologic diseases, allergic states, ophthalmic diseases, respiratory diseases, hematologic disorders, neoplastic diseases, edematous states, and gastrointestinal diseases; resolution of acute exacerbations of multiple sclerosis; management of fulminating or disseminated tuberculosis and trichinosis; acute or chronic solid organ rejection

Effect on Mental Status Nervousness and insomnia are common; may rarely cause delirium, mood swings, euphoria, and hallucinations

Effect on Psychiatric Treatment Barbiturates and carbamazepine may decrease corticosteroid effectiveness

Dosage Summary

Ophthalmic:

Children: Initial: Instill 1-2 drops into conjunctival sac every hour during day, every 2 hours at night; Maintenance: 1 drop every 4 hours

Adults: Initial: Instill 1-2 drops into conjunctival sac every hour during day, every 2 hours at night; Maintenance: 1 drop every 4 hours

Oral:

Note: Oral dosage expressed in terms of prednisolone base.

Children: 1-2 mg/kg/day divided 1-2 times/day **or** 0.1-2 mg/kg/day divided 1-4 times/day **or** Nephrotic syndrome: Initial: 2 mg/kg/day **or** 60 mg/m^2/day (maximum: 80 mg/day) in divided doses 3-4 times/day until urine is protein free for 3 consecutive days (maximum: 28 days); followed by 1-1.5 mg/kg/dose **or** 40 mg/m^2/dose given every other day for 4 weeks; Maintenance (frequent relapses: 0.5-1 mg/kg/dose given every other day for 3-6 months

Adults: 5-60 mg/day **or** 200 mg/day for 1 week followed by 80 mg every other day for 1 month

Dosage Forms Excipient information presented when available (limited, particularly for generics); consult specific product labeling. [DSC] = Discontinued product

Solution, ophthalmic, as sodium phosphate: 1% (5 mL, 10 mL, 15 mL) [contains benzalkonium chloride]

Solution, oral, as base: Prednisolone 15 mg/5 mL (240 mL, 480 mL)

Solution, oral, as sodium phosphate: Prednisolone base 5 mg/5 mL (120 mL, 240 mL); prednisolone base 15 mg/5 mL (240 mL)

Millipred™: 13.4 mg/5 mL (237 mL) [equivalent to prednisolone base 10 mg/5 mL; dye free; grape flavor]

Orapred®: 20 mg/5 mL (20 mL, 240 mL) [equivalent to prednisolone base 15 mg/5 mL; dye free; contains alcohol 2%, sodium benzoate; grape flavor]

Pediapred®: 6.7 mg/5 mL (120 mL) [equivalent to prednisolone base 5 mg/5 mL; dye free; raspberry flavor]

Suspension, ophthalmic, as acetate: 1% (5 mL, 10 mL, 15 mL)

Econopred® Plus [DSC], Omnipred™: 1% (5 mL, 10 mL) [contains benzalkonium chloride]

Pred Forte®: 1% (1 mL, 5 mL, 10 mL, 15 mL) [contains benzalkonium chloride and sodium bisulfite]

Pred Mild®: 0.12% (5 mL, 10 mL) [contains benzalkonium chloride and sodium bisulfite]

Syrup, as base: 5 mg/5 mL (120 mL); 15 mg/5 mL (5 mL [DSC], 240 mL, 480 mL)
Prelone®: 15 mg/5 mL (240 mL, 480 mL) [contains alcohol 5%, benzoic acid; cherry flavor]
Tablet, as base: 5 mg
Tablet, orally disintegrating, as sodium phosphate [strength expressed as base]:
Orapred ODT™: 10 mg, 15 mg, 30 mg [grape flavor]

◆ **Prednisolone Acetate** *see* PrednisoLONE *on page 1326*
◆ **Prednisolone Acetate, Ophthalmic** *see* PrednisoLONE *on page 1326*
◆ **Prednisolone and Sulfacetamide** *see* Sulfacetamide and Prednisolone *on page 1516*
◆ **Prednisolone Sodium Phosphate** *see* PrednisoLONE *on page 1326*
◆ **Prednisolone Sodium Phosphate, Ophthalmic** *see* PrednisoLONE *on page 1326*

PredniSONE (PRED ni sone)

Medication Safety Issues
Sound-alike/look-alike issues:
PredniSONE may be confused with methylPREDNISolone, Pramosone®, prazosin, prednisoLONE, Prilosec®, primidone, promethazine

Related Information
Corticosteroids *on page 1780*

U.S. Brand Names PredniSONE Intensol™; Sterapred®; Sterapred® DS
Canadian Brand Names Apo-Prednisone®; Novo-Prednisone; Winpred™
Mexican Brand Names Ednapron; Meticorten; Norapred; Prednidib
Index Terms Deltacortisone; Deltadehydrocortisone
Pharmacologic Category Corticosteroid, Systemic
Generic Available Yes
Use Treatment of a variety of diseases, including:
Allergic states (including adjunctive treatment of anaphylaxis)
Autoimmune disorders (including systemic lupus erythematosus [SLE])
Collagen diseases
Dermatologic conditions/diseases
Edematous states (including nephrotic syndrome)
Endocrine disorders
Gastrointestinal diseases
Hematologic disorders (including idiopathic thrombocytopenia purpura [ITP])
Multiple sclerosis exacerbations
Neoplastic diseases
Ophthalmic diseases
Respiratory diseases (including acute asthma exacerbation)
Rheumatic disorders (including rheumatoid arthritis)
Trichinosis with neurologic or myocardial involvement
Tuberculous meningitis

Unlabeled/Investigational Use Adjunctive therapy for *Pneumocystis jiroveci* (formerly *carinni*) pneumonia (PCP); autoimmune hepatitis; adjunctive therapy for pain management in immunocompetent patients with herpes zoster; tuberculosis (severe, paradoxical reactions)

Effect on Mental Status Nervousness and insomnia are common; may rarely cause delirium, mood swings, euphoria, and hallucinations

Effect on Psychiatric Treatment Barbiturates and carbamazepine may decrease corticosteroid effectiveness

Pregnancy Considerations Adverse events have been observed with corticosteroids in animal reproduction studies. Prednisone and prednisolone cross the human placenta. In the mother, prednisone is converted to the active metabolite prednisolone by the liver. Prior to reaching the fetus, prednisolone is converted by placental enzymes back to prednisone. As a result, the level of prednisone remaining in the maternal serum and reaching the fetus are similar, however, the amount of prednisolone reaching the fetus is ~8-10 times lower than the maternal serum concentration (healthy women at term). Some studies have shown an association between first trimester prednisone use and oral clefts; adverse events in the fetus/neonate have been noted in case reports following large doses of systemic corticosteroids during pregnancy. Pregnant women exposed to prednisone for antirejection therapy following a transplant may contact the National Transplantation Pregnancy Registry (NTPR) at 215-955-4820. Women exposed to prednisone during pregnancy for the

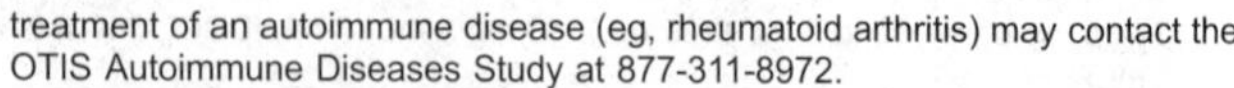

treatment of an autoimmune disease (eg, rheumatoid arthritis) may contact the OTIS Autoimmune Diseases Study at 877-311-8972.

Lactation Enters breast milk/AAP rates "compatible"

Contraindications Hypersensitivity to any component of the formulation; systemic fungal infections; administration of live or live attenuated vaccines with immunosuppressive doses of prednisone

Warnings/Precautions May cause hypercorticism or suppression of hypothalamic-pituitary-adrenal (HPA) axis, particularly in younger children or in patients receiving high doses for prolonged periods. HPA axis suppression may lead to adrenal crisis. Withdrawal and discontinuation of a corticosteroid should be done slowly and carefully. Particular care is required when patients are transferred from systemic corticosteroids to inhaled products due to possible adrenal insufficiency or withdrawal from steroids, including an increase in allergic symptoms. Patients receiving >20 mg per day of prednisone (or equivalent) may be most susceptible. Fatalities have occurred due to adrenal insufficiency in asthmatic patients during and after transfer from systemic corticosteroids to aerosol steroids; aerosol steroids do **not** provide the systemic steroid needed to treat patients having trauma, surgery, or infections.

Acute myopathy has been reported with high dose corticosteroids, usually in patients with neuromuscular transmission disorders; may involve ocular and/or respiratory muscles; monitor creatine kinase; recovery may be delayed. Prolonged use of corticosteroids may increase the incidence of secondary infection, mask acute infection (including fungal infections), prolong or exacerbate viral infections, or limit response to vaccines. Exposure to chickenpox should be avoided. Corticosteroids should not be used to treat ocular herpes simplex or cerebral malaria. Close observation is required in patients with latent tuberculosis and/or TB reactivity; restrict use in active TB (only in conjunction with antituberculosis treatment). Prolonged treatment with corticosteroids has been associated with the development of Kaposi's sarcoma (case reports); if noted, discontinuation of therapy should be considered. Prolonged use may cause posterior subcapsular cataracts, glaucoma (with possible nerve damage) and may increase the risk for ocular infections. Corticosteroid use may cause psychiatric disturbances, including depression, euphoria, insomnia, mood swings, and personality changes. Pre-existing psychiatric conditions may be exacerbated by corticosteroid use.

Use with caution in patients with HF, diabetes, GI diseases (diverticulitis, peptic ulcer, ulcerative colitis; due to risk of perforation), hepatic impairment, myasthenia gravis, MI, patients with or who are at risk for osteoporosis, seizure disorders or thyroid disease. May affect growth velocity; growth should be routinely monitored in pediatric patients.

Prior to use, the dose and duration of treatment should be based on the risk versus benefit for each individual patient. In general, use the smallest effective dose for the shortest duration of time to minimize adverse events. A gradual tapering of dose may be required prior to discontinuing therapy.

Adverse Reactions

Frequency not defined.

Cardiovascular: Congestive heart failure (in susceptible patients), hypertension

Central nervous system: Emotional instability, headache, intracranial pressure increased (with papilledema), psychic derangements (including euphoria, insomnia, mood swings, personality changes, severe depression), seizure, vertigo

Dermatologic: Bruising, facial erythema, petechiae, thin fragile skin, urticaria, wound healing impaired

Endocrine & metabolic: Adrenocortical and pituitary unresponsiveness (in times of stress), carbohydrate intolerance, Cushing's syndrome, diabetes mellitus, fluid retention, growth suppression (in children), hypokalemic alkalosis, hypothyroidism enhanced, menstrual irregularities, negative nitrogen balance due to protein catabolism, potassium loss, sodium retention

Gastrointestinal: Abdominal distension, pancreatitis, peptic ulcer (with possible perforation and hemorrhage), ulcerative esophagitis

Hepatic: ALT increased, AST increased, alkaline phosphatase increased

Neuromuscular & skeletal: Aseptic necrosis of femoral and humeral heads, muscle mass loss, muscle weakness, osteoporosis, pathologic fracture of long bones, steroid myopathy, tendon rupture (particularly Achilles tendon), vertebral compression fractures

Ocular: Exophthalmos, glaucoma, intraocular pressure increased, posterior subcapsular cataracts

Miscellaneous: Allergic reactions, anaphylactic reactions, diaphoresis, hypersensitivity reactions, infections, Kaposi's sarcoma

Metabolism/Transport Effects **Substrate** of CYP3A4 (minor); **Induces** CYP2C19 (weak), 3A4 (weak)

Drug Interactions

Acetylcholinesterase Inhibitors: Corticosteroids (Systemic) may enhance the adverse/toxic effect of Acetylcholinesterase Inhibitors. Increased muscular weakness may occur. *Risk C: Monitor therapy*

Aminoglutethimide: May increase the metabolism of Corticosteroids (Systemic). *Risk C: Monitor therapy*

Amphotericin B: Corticosteroids (Systemic) may enhance the hypokalemic effect of Amphotericin B. *Risk C: Monitor therapy*

Antacids: May decrease the bioavailability of Corticosteroids (Oral). *Risk D: Consider therapy modification*

Antidiabetic Agents: Corticosteroids (Systemic) may diminish the hypoglycemic effect of Antidiabetic Agents. In some instances, corticosteroid-mediated HPA axis suppression has led to episodes of acute adrenal crisis, which may manifest as enhanced hypoglycemia, particularly in the setting of insulin or other antidiabetic agent use. *Risk C: Monitor therapy*

Antifungal Agents (Azole Derivatives, Systemic): May decrease the metabolism of Corticosteroids (Systemic). *Risk C: Monitor therapy*

Aprepitant: May increase the serum concentration of Corticosteroids (Systemic). *Risk D: Consider therapy modification*

Barbiturates: May increase the metabolism of Corticosteroids (Systemic). *Risk C: Monitor therapy*

Bile Acid Sequestrants: May decrease the absorption of Corticosteroids (Oral). *Risk C: Monitor therapy*

Calcitriol: Corticosteroids (Systemic) may diminish the therapeutic effect of Calcitriol. *Risk C: Monitor therapy*

Calcium Channel Blockers (Nondihydropyridine): May decrease the metabolism of Corticosteroids (Systemic). *Risk C: Monitor therapy*

Corticorelin: Corticosteroids may diminish the therapeutic effect of Corticorelin. Specifically, the plasma ACTH response to corticorelin may be blunted by recent or current corticosteroid therapy. *Risk C: Monitor therapy*

CycloSPORINE: Corticosteroids (Systemic) may increase the serum concentration of CycloSPORINE. CycloSPORINE may increase the serum concentration of Corticosteroids (Systemic). *Risk C: Monitor therapy*

Echinacea: May diminish the therapeutic effect of Immunosuppressants. *Risk D: Consider therapy modification*

Estrogen Derivatives: May increase the serum concentration of Corticosteroids (Systemic). *Risk C: Monitor therapy*

Fluconazole: May decrease the metabolism of Corticosteroids (Systemic). *Risk C: Monitor therapy*

Fosaprepitant: May increase the serum concentration of Corticosteroids (Systemic). The active metabolite aprepitant is likely responsible for this effect. *Risk D: Consider therapy modification*

Isoniazid: Corticosteroids (Systemic) may decrease the serum concentration of Isoniazid. *Risk C: Monitor therapy*

Loop Diuretics: Corticosteroids (Systemic) may enhance the hypokalemic effect of Loop Diuretics. *Risk C: Monitor therapy*

Macrolide Antibiotics: May decrease the metabolism of Corticosteroids (Systemic). **Exceptions:** Azithromycin; Dirithromycin [Off Market]; Spiramycin. *Risk D: Consider therapy modification*

Maraviroc: CYP3A4 Inducers may decrease the serum concentration of Maraviroc. *Risk D: Consider therapy modification*

Natalizumab: Immunosuppressants may enhance the adverse/toxic effect of Natalizumab. Specifically, the risk of concurrent infection may be increased. *Risk X: Avoid combination*

Neuromuscular-Blocking Agents (Nondepolarizing): May enhance the adverse neuromuscular effect of Corticosteroids (Systemic). Increased muscle weakness, possibly progressing to polyneuropathies and myopathies, may occur. *Risk D: Consider therapy modification*

NSAID (COX-2 Inhibitor): Corticosteroids (Systemic) may enhance the adverse/toxic effect of NSAID (COX-2 Inhibitor). *Risk C: Monitor therapy*

NSAID (Nonselective): Corticosteroids (Systemic) may enhance the adverse/toxic effect of NSAID (Nonselective). *Risk C: Monitor therapy*

Primidone: May increase the metabolism of Corticosteroids (Systemic). *Risk C: Monitor therapy*

Quinolone Antibiotics: May enhance the adverse/toxic effect of Corticosteroids (Systemic). Risk of tendon-related side effects, including tendonitis and rupture, may be enhanced. *Risk C: Monitor therapy*

Rifamycin Derivatives: May increase the metabolism of Corticosteroids (Systemic). *Risk C: Monitor therapy*

Salicylates: May enhance the adverse/toxic effect of Corticosteroids (Systemic). These specifically include gastrointestinal ulceration and bleeding. Corticosteroids (Systemic) may decrease the serum concentration of Salicylates. Withdrawal of corticosteroids may result in salicylate toxicity. *Risk C: Monitor therapy*

Somatropin: May diminish the therapeutic effect of PredniSONE. Growth hormone may reduce the conversion of prednisone to the active prednisolone metabolite. *Risk D: Consider therapy modification*

Thiazide Diuretics: Corticosteroids (Systemic) may enhance the hypokalemic effect of Thiazide Diuretics. *Risk C: Monitor therapy*

Trastuzumab: May enhance the neutropenic effect of Immunosuppressants. *Risk C: Monitor therapy*

Vaccines (Inactivated): Immunosuppressants may diminish the therapeutic effect of Vaccines (Inactivated). *Risk C: Monitor therapy*

Vaccines (Live): Immunosuppressants may enhance the adverse/toxic effect of Vaccines (Live). Vaccinal infections may develop. Immunosuppressants may also decrease therapeutic response to vaccines. *Risk X: Avoid combination*

Warfarin: Corticosteroids (Systemic) may enhance the anticoagulant effect of Warfarin. *Risk C: Monitor therapy*

Ethanol/Nutrition/Herb Interactions

Ethanol: Avoid ethanol (may increase gastric mucosal irritation)

Food: Prednisone interferes with calcium absorption. Limit caffeine.

Herb/Nutraceutical: St John's wort may decrease prednisone levels. Avoid cat's claw, echinacea (have immunostimulant properties).

Mechanism of Action Decreases inflammation by suppression of migration of polymorphonuclear leukocytes and reversal of increased capillary permeability; suppresses the immune system by reducing activity and volume of the lymphatic system; suppresses adrenal function at high doses. Antitumor effects may be related to inhibition of glucose transport, phosphorylation, or induction of cell death in immature lymphocytes. Antiemetic effects are thought to occur due to blockade of cerebral innervation of the emetic center via inhibition of prostaglandin synthesis.

Pharmacodynamics/Kinetics

Absorption: 50% to 90% (may be altered in IBS or hyperthyroidism)

Protein binding (concentration dependent): 65% to 91%

Metabolism: Hepatically converted from prednisone (inactive) to prednisolone (active); may be impaired with hepatic dysfunction

Half-life elimination: Normal renal function: ~3.5 hours

Excretion: Urine (small portion)

Dosage Oral:

General dosing range: Children and Adults: Initial: 5-60 mg/day: **Note:** Dose depends upon condition being treated and response of patient; dosage for infants and children should be based on severity of the disease and response of the patient rather than on strict adherence to dosage indicated by age, weight, or body surface area. Consider alternate day therapy for long-term therapy. Discontinuation of long-term therapy requires gradual withdrawal by tapering the dose.

Prednisone taper (other regimens also available):

Day 1: 30 mg divided as 10 mg before breakfast, 5 mg at lunch, 5 mg at dinner, 10 mg at bedtime

Day 2: 5 mg at breakfast, 5 mg at lunch, 5 mg at dinner, 10 mg at bedtime

Day 3: 5 mg 4 times/day (with meals and at bedtime)

Day 4: 5 mg 3 times/day (breakfast, lunch, bedtime)

Day 5: 5 mg 2 times/day (breakfast, bedtime)

Day 6: 5 mg before breakfast

Indication-specific dosing:

Children:

Acute asthma (NIH guidelines, 2007):

0-11 years 1-2 mg/kg/day for 3-10 days (maximum: 60 mg/day)

≥12 years: Refer to Adults dosing

Autoimmune hepatitis (unlabeled use; Czaja 2002): Initial treatment: 2 mg/kg/day for 2 weeks (maximum: 60 mg/day), followed by a taper over 6-8 weeks to a dose of 0.1-0.2 mg/kg/day or 5 mg/day

Nephrotic syndrome (Pediatric Nephrology Panel recommendations [Hogg, 2000]): Initial: 2 mg/kg/day or 60 mg/m^2/day given every day in 1-3 divided doses (maximum: 80 mg/day) until urine is protein free or for 4-6 weeks; followed by maintenance dose: 2 mg/kg/dose or 40 mg/m^2/dose given every other day in the morning; gradually taper and discontinue after 4-6 weeks. **Note:** No definitive treatment guidelines exist. Dosing is dependant on institution protocols and individual response.

PCP pneumonia (AIDSinfo guidelines, 2008): 1 mg/kg twice daily for 5 days, *followed by* 0.5-1 mg/kg twice daily for 5 days, *followed by* 0.5 mg/kg once daily for 11-21 days

Adolescents and Adults:

PCP pneumonia (AIDSinfo guidelines, 2008): Note: Begin within 72 hours of PCP therapy: 40 mg twice daily for 5 days, *followed by* 40 mg once daily for 5 days, *followed by* 20 mg once daily for 11 days or until antimicrobial regimen is completed

Adults:

Acute asthma (NIH guidelines, 2007): 40-60 mg per day for 3-10 days; administer as single or 2divided doses

Anaphylaxis, adjunctive treatment (Lieberman 2005): 0.5 mg/kg

Antineoplastic: Usual range: 10 mg/day to 100 mg/m^2/day (depending on indication). **Note:** Details concerning dosing in combination regimens should also be consulted.

Autoimmune hepatitis (unlabeled use; Czaja 2002): Initial treatment: 60 mg/day for 1 week, *followed by* 40 mg/day for 1 week, *then* 30 mg/day for 2 weeks, *then* 20 mg/day. Half this dose should be given when used in combination with azathioprine

Herpes zoster (unlabeled use; Dworkin 2007): 60 mg/day for 7 days, *followed by* 30 mg/day for 7 days, *then* 15 mg/day for 7 days

Idiopathic thrombocytopenia purpura (American Society of Hematology 1997): 1-2 mg/kg/day

Rheumatoid arthritis (American College of Rheumatology 2002): ≤10 mg/day

Systemic lupus erythematosus (American College of Rheumatology 1999):

Mild SLE: ≤10 mg/day

Refractory or severe organ-threatening disease: 20-60 mg/day

Thyrotoxicosis (type II amiodarone induced; unlabeled use): 30-40 mg/day for 7-14 days, gradually taper over 3 months

Tuberculosis, severe, paradoxical reactions (unlabeled use, AIDS info guidelines 2008): 1 mg/kg/day, gradually reduce after 1-2 weeks

Elderly: Use the lowest effective dose

Dosing adjustment in hepatic impairment: Prednisone is inactive and must be metabolized by the liver to prednisolone. This conversion may be impaired in patients with liver disease, however, prednisolone levels are observed to be higher in patients with severe liver failure than in normal patients. Therefore, compensation for the inadequate conversion of prednisone to prednisolone occurs.

Dosing adjustment in hyperthyroidism: Prednisone dose may need to be increased to achieve adequate therapeutic effects

Hemodialysis: Supplemental dose is not necessary

Peritoneal dialysis: Supplemental dose is not necessary

Dietary Considerations Should be taken after meals or with food or milk; may require increased dietary intake of pyridoxine, vitamin C, vitamin D, folate, calcium, and phosphorus; may require decreased dietary intake of sodium

Administration Administer with food to decrease gastrointestinal upset

Monitoring Parameters Blood pressure, blood glucose, electrolytes

Following prolonged use: Bone mass density, growth in children, signs and symptoms of infection, cataract formation

Test Interactions Decreased response to skin tests

Additional Information Tapering of corticosteroids after a short course of therapy (<7-10 days) is generally not required unless the disease/inflammatory process is slow to respond. Tapering after prolonged exposure is dependent upon the individual patient, duration of corticosteroid treatments, and size of steroid dose. Recovery of the HPA axis may require several months. Subtle but important HPA axis suppression may be present for as long as several months after a course of as few as 10-14 days duration. Testing of HPA axis (cosyntropin) may be required, and signs/symptoms of adrenal insufficiency should be monitored in patients with a history of use.

Dosage Forms Excipient information presented when available (limited, particularly for generics); consult specific product labeling.

Solution, oral: 1 mg/mL (5 mL, 120 mL, 500 mL) [contains alcohol 5%, sodium benzoate; peppermint vanilla flavor]

Solution, oral [concentrate]:

PredniSONE Intensol™: 5 mg/mL (30 mL) [contains alcohol 30%]

Tablet: 1 mg, 2.5 mg, 5 mg, 10 mg, 20 mg, 50 mg

Sterapred®: 5 mg [supplied as 21 tablet 6-day unit-dose package or 48 tablet 12-day unit-dose package]

Sterapred® DS: 10 mg [supplied as 21 tablet 6-day unit-dose package or 48 tablet 12-day unit-dose package]

◆ **PredniSONE Intensol™** *see* PredniSONE *on page 1327*

◆ **Prefest™** *see* Estradiol and Norgestimate *on page 580*

Pregabalin (pre GAB a lin)

U.S. Brand Names Lyrica®
Canadian Brand Names Lyrica®
Mexican Brand Names Lyrica
Index Terms CI-1008; S-(+)-3-isobutylgaba
Pharmacologic Category Analgesic, Miscellaneous; Anticonvulsant, Miscellaneous
Generic Available No
Use Management of pain associated with diabetic peripheral neuropathy; management of postherpetic neuralgia; adjunctive therapy for partial-onset seizure disorder in adults; management of fibromyalgia
Restrictions C-V
Pregnancy Risk Factor C
Pregnancy Considerations Increased incidence of fetal abnormalities, particularly skeletal malformations, were observed in animal studies. Male-mediated teratogenicity has been observed in animal studies; implications in humans are not defined. Impaired male and female fertility has been noted in animal studies. There are no adequate and well-controlled studies in pregnant women. Use only when potential benefit to the mother outweighs possible risk to the fetus.
Lactation Excretion in breast milk unknown/not recommended
Contraindications Hypersensitivity to pregabalin or any component of the formulation
Warnings/Precautions Angioedema has been reported; may be life threatening; use with caution in patients with a history of angioedema episodes. Concurrent use with other drugs known to cause angioedema (eg, ACE inhibitors) may increase risk. Hypersensitivity reactions, including skin redness, blistering, hives, rash, dyspnea and wheezing have been reported; discontinue treatment of hypersensitivity occurs. May cause CNS depression and/or dizziness, which may impair physical or mental abilities. Patients must be cautioned about performing tasks which require mental alertness (eg, operating machinery or driving). Effects with other sedative drugs or ethanol may be potentiated. Visual disturbances (blurred vision, decreased acuity and visual field changes) have been associated with pregabalin therapy; patients should be instructed to notify their physician if these effects are noted.

Pregabalin has been associated with increases in CPK and rare cases of rhabdomyolysis. Patients should be instructed to notify their prescriber if unexplained muscle pain, tenderness, or weakness, particularly if fever and/or malaise are associated with these symptoms. Use may be associated with weight gain and peripheral edema; use caution in patients with congestive heart failure, hypertension, or diabetes. Effect on weight gain/edema may be additive to thiazolidinedione antidiabetic agent; particularly in patients with prior cardiovascular disease. May decrease platelet count or prolong PR interval.

Has been noted to be tumorigenic (increased incidence of hemangiosarcoma) in animal studies; significance of these findings in humans is unknown. Pregabalin has been associated with discontinuation symptoms following abrupt cessation, and increases in seizure frequency (when used as an antiepileptic) may occur. Should not be discontinued abruptly; dosage tapering over at least 1 week is recommended. Use caution in renal impairment; dosage adjustment required. Safety and efficacy have not been established in pediatric patients.
Adverse Reactions Note: Frequency of adverse effects may be influenced by dose or concurrent therapy. In add-on trials in epilepsy, frequency of CNS and adverse effects were higher than those reported in pain management trials. Range noted below is inclusive of all trials.
>10%:
Cardiovascular: Peripheral edema (up to 16%)
Central nervous system: Dizziness (8% to 45%), somnolence (4% to 28%), ataxia (up to 20%), headache (up to 14%)
Gastrointestinal: Weight gain (up to 16%), xerostomia (1% to 15%)
Neuromuscular & skeletal: Tremor (up to 11%)
Ocular: Blurred vision (1% to 12%), diplopia (up to 12%)
Miscellaneous: Infection (up to 14%), accidental injury (2% to 11%)

1% to 10%:

Cardiovascular: Chest pain (up to 4%), edema (up to 6%)

Central nervous system: Neuropathy (up to 9%), thinking abnormal (up to 9%), fatigue (up to 8%), confusion (up to 7%), euphoria (up to 7%), speech disorder (up to 7%), attention disturbance (up to 6%), incoordination (up to 6%), amnesia (up to 6%), pain (up to 5%), memory impaired (up to 4%), vertigo (up to 4%), feeling abnormal (up to 3%), hypoesthesia (up to 3%), anxiety (up to 2%), depression (up to 2%), disorientation (up to 2%), lethargy (up to 2%), fever (≥1%), depersonalization (≥1%), hypertonia (≥1%), stupor (≥1%), nervousness (up to 1%)

Dermatologic: Facial edema (up to 3%), bruising (≥1%), pruritus (≥1%)

Endocrine & metabolic: Fluid retention (up to 3%), hypoglycemia (up to 3%), libido decreased (≥1%)

Gastrointestinal: Constipation (up to 10%), appetite increased (up to 7%), flatulence (up to 3%), vomiting (up to 3%), abdominal distension (up to 2%), abdominal pain (≥1%), gastroenteritis (≥1%)

Genitourinary: Incontinence (up to 2%), anorgasmia (≥1%), impotence (≥1%), urinary frequency (≥1%)

Hematologic: Thrombocytopenia (3%)

Neuromuscular & skeletal: Balance disorder (up to 9%), abnormal gait (up to 8%), weakness (up to 7%), arthralgia (up to 6%), twitching (up to 5%), back pain (up to 4%), muscle spasm (up to 4%), myoclonus (up to 4%), paresthesia (>2%), CPK increased (2%), leg cramps (≥1%), myalgia (≥1%), myasthenia (up to 1%)

Ocular: Visual abnormalities (up to 5%), visual field defect (≥2%), eye disorder (up to 2%), nystagmus (>2%), conjunctivitis (≥1%)

Otic: Otitis media (≥1%), tinnitus (≥1%)

Respiratory: Sinusitis (up to 7%), dyspnea (up to 3%), bronchitis (up to 3%), pharyngolaryngeal pain (up to 3%)

Miscellaneous: Flu-like syndrome (up to 2%), allergic reaction (≥1%)

<1% (Limited to important or life-threatening): Abscess, acute renal failure, addiction (rare), agitation, albuminuria, anaphylactoid reaction, anemia, angioedema, aphasia, aphthous stomatitis, apnea, ascites, atelectasis, blepharitis, blindness, bronchiolitis, cellulitis, cerebellar syndrome, cervicitis, chills, cholecystitis, cholelithiasis, chondrodystrophy, circumoral paresthesia, cogwheel rigidity, colitis, coma, corneal ulcer, crystalluria (urate), delirium, delusions, diarrhea, dysarthria, dysautonomia, dyskinesia, dysphagia, dystonia, dysuria, encephalopathy, eosinophilia, esophageal ulcer, esophagitis, exfoliative dermatitis, extraocular palsy, extrapyramidal syndrome, gastritis, GI hemorrhage, glomerulitis, glucose tolerance decreased, granuloma, Guillain-Barré syndrome, hallucinations, heart failure, hematuria, hostility, hyper-/hypokinesia; hypersensitivity (including skin redness, blistering, hives, rash, dyspnea, and wheezing); hypotension, hypotonia, intracranial hypertension, laryngismus, leukopenia, leukorrhea, leukocytosis, lymphadenopathy, manic reaction, melena, myelofibrosis, nausea, nephritis, neuralgia, ocular hemorrhage, oliguria, optic atrophy, pancreatitis, papilledema, paranoid reaction, pelvic pain, periodontal abscess, peripheral neuritis, polycythemia, postural hypotension, prothrombin decreased, psychotic depression, ptosis, pulmonary edema, pulmonary fibrosis, purpura, pyelonephritis, rectal hemorrhage, renal calculus, retinal edema, retinal vascular disorder, retroperitoneal fibrosis, rhabdomyolysis, schizophrenic reaction, shock, skin necrosis, skin ulcer, spasm (generalized), ST depression, Stevens-Johnson syndrome, subcutaneous nodule, suicide, suicide attempt, syncope, thrombocythemia, thrombophlebitis, tongue edema, torticollis, trismus, uveitis, ventricular fibrillation

Drug Interactions

Alcohol (Ethyl): CNS Depressants may enhance the CNS depressant effect of Alcohol (Ethyl). *Risk C: Monitor therapy*

Antidiabetic Agents (Thiazolidinedione): Pregabalin may enhance the fluid-retaining effect of Antidiabetic Agents (Thiazolidinedione). *Risk C: Monitor therapy*

CNS Depressants: May enhance the adverse/toxic effect of other CNS Depressants. *Risk C: Monitor therapy*

Ketorolac: May diminish the therapeutic effect of Anticonvulsants. *Risk C: Monitor therapy*

Mefloquine: May diminish the therapeutic effect of Anticonvulsants. Mefloquine may decrease the serum concentration of Anticonvulsants. Management: Mefloquine is contraindicated in persons with a history of convulsions. If anticonvulsant is being used for another indication monitor response to treatment closely, as concurrent mefloquine may decrease response to treatment. *Risk D: Consider therapy modification*

Ethanol/Nutrition/Herb Interactions

Ethanol: Avoid ethanol (may increase CNS depression).

Herb/Nutraceutical: Avoid valerian, St John's wort, kava kava, gotu kola (may increase CNS depression).

Stability Store at 15°C to 30°C (59°F to 86°F).

Mechanism of Action Binds to alpha$_2$-delta subunit of voltage-gated calcium channels within the CNS, inhibiting excitatory neurotransmitter release. Although structurally related to GABA, it does not bind to GABA or benzodiazepine receptors. Exerts antinociceptive and anticonvulsant activity. Decreases symptoms of painful peripheral neuropathies and, as adjunctive therapy in partial seizures, decreases the frequency of seizures.

Pharmacodynamics/Kinetics

Onset: Pain management: Effects may be noted as early as the first week of therapy.

Distribution: V_d: 0.5 L/kg

Protein binding: 0%

Metabolism: Negligible

Bioavailability: >90%

Half-life elimination: 6.3 hours

Time to peak, plasma: 1.5 hours (3 hours with food)

Excretion: Urine (90% as unchanged drug; minor metabolites)

Dosage Oral: Adults:

Fibromyalgia: Initial: 150 mg/day in divided doses (75 mg 2 times/day); may be increased to 300 mg/day (150 mg 2 times/day) within 1 week based on tolerability and effect; may be further increased to 450 mg/day (225 mg 2 times/day). Maximum dose: 450 mg/day (dosages up to 600 mg/day were evaluated with no significant additional benefit and an increase in adverse effects)

Neuropathic pain (diabetes-associated): Initial: 150 mg/day in divided doses (50 mg 3 times/day); may be increased within 1 week based on tolerability and effect; maximum dose: 300 mg/day (dosages up to 600 mg/day were evaluated with no significant additional benefit and an increase in adverse effects)

Postherpetic neuralgia: Initial: 150 mg/day in divided doses (75 mg 2 times/day or 50 mg 3 times/day); may be increased to 300 mg/day within 1 week based on tolerability and effect; further titration (to 600 mg/day) after 2-4 weeks may be considered in patients who do not experience sufficient relief of pain provided they are able to tolerate pregabalin. Maximum dose: 600 mg/day

Partial-onset seizures (adjunctive therapy): Initial: 150 mg per day in divided doses (75 mg 2 times/day or 50 mg 3 times/day); may be increased based on tolerability and effect (optimal titration schedule has not been defined). Maximum dose: 600 mg/day

Discontinuing therapy: Pregabalin should not be abruptly discontinued; taper dosage over at least 1 week

Dosage adjustment in renal impairment: In renally-impaired patients, dosage adjustment depends on renal function and daily dosage.

Pregabalin Renal Impairment Dosing

Cl_{cr} (mL/minute)	Total Pregabalin Daily Dose (mg/day)				Dosing Frequency
≥60	150	300	450	600	2-3 divided doses
30-60	75	150	225	300	2-3 divided doses
15-30	25-50	75	100-150	150	1-2 divided doses
<15	25	25-50	50-75	75	Single daily dose

Posthemodialysis supplementary dosage (as a single additional dose):

25 mg/day schedule: Single supplementary dose of 25 mg **or** 50 mg
25-50 mg/day schedule: Single supplementary dose of 50 mg **or** 75 mg
50-75 mg/day schedule: Single supplementary dose of 75 mg **or** 100 mg
75 mg/day schedule: Single supplementary dose of 100 mg **or** 150 mg

Dietary Considerations May be taken with or without food.

Administration May be administered with or without food.

Monitoring Parameters Measures of efficacy (pain intensity/seizure frequency); degree of sedation; symptoms of myopathy or ocular disturbance; weight gain/edema; CPK; skin integrity (in patients with diabetes).

Dosage Forms Excipient information presented when available (limited, particularly for generics); consult specific product labeling.
Capsule:
Lyrica®: 25 mg, 50 mg, 75 mg, 100 mg, 150 mg, 200 mg, 225 mg, 300 mg

- **Pregnenedione** *see* Progesterone *on page 1345*
- **Pregnyl®** *see* Chorionic Gonadotropin (Human) *on page 342*
- **Prelone®** *see* PrednisoLONE *on page 1326*
- **Premarin®** *see* Estrogens (Conjugated/Equine) *on page 582*
- **Premjact® [OTC]** *see* Lidocaine *on page 924*
- **Premphase®** *see* Estrogens (Conjugated/Equine) and Medroxyprogesterone *on page 583*
- **Prempro™** *see* Estrogens (Conjugated/Equine) and Medroxyprogesterone *on page 583*
- **Preparation H® [OTC]** *see* Phenylephrine *on page 1273*
- **Preparation H® Hydrocortisone [OTC]** *see* Hydrocortisone *on page 785*
- **Prepidil®** *see* Dinoprostone *on page 480*
- **Pretz-D® [OTC]** *see* EPHEDrine *on page 542*
- **Prevacid®** *see* Lansoprazole *on page 894*
- **Prevacid® NapraPAC™** *see* Lansoprazole and Naproxen *on page 897*
- **Prevacid® SoluTab™** *see* Lansoprazole *on page 894*
- **Prevalite®** *see* Cholestyramine Resin *on page 341*
- **Previfem™** *see* Ethinyl Estradiol and Norgestimate *on page 600*
- **Prevnar®** *see* Pneumococcal Conjugate Vaccine, 7-Valent *on page 1308*
- **Prevpac®** *see* Lansoprazole, Amoxicillin, and Clarithromycin *on page 897*
- **Prezista®** *see* Darunavir *on page 420*
- **Prialt®** *see* Ziconotide *on page 1695*
- **Priftin®** *see* Rifapentine *on page 1420*
- **Prilosec®** *see* Omeprazole *on page 1176*
- **Prilosec OTC™ [OTC]** *see* Omeprazole *on page 1176*
- **Primaclone** *see* Primidone *on page 1336*
- **Primacor®** *see* Milrinone *on page 1055*
- **Primalev™** *see* Oxycodone and Acetaminophen *on page 1205*

Primaquine (PRIM a kween)

Medication Safety Issues
Sound-alike/look-alike issues:
Primaquine may be confused with primidone

Index Terms Primaquine Phosphate; Prymaccone

Pharmacologic Category Aminoquinoline (Antimalarial)

Use Prevention of relapse of *P. vivax* malaria

Unlabeled/Investigational Use Prevention of relapse of *P. ovale* malaria; treatment of *Pneumocystis jiroveci* pneumonia (PCP); prevention of chloroquine-resistant malaria

Effect on Mental Status None reported

Effect on Psychiatric Treatment Contraindicated in patients receiving clozapine or carbamazepine

Dosage Summary Note: Dosage expressed as mg of base (15 mg base = 26.3 mg primaquine phosphate)

Oral:

Children: 0.5 mg/kg once daily for 14 days (maximum dose: 30 mg/day); alternative regimen (recommended for mild G6PD deficiency): 45 mg once weekly for 8 weeks

Adults: 30 mg once daily for 14 days; alternative regimen (recommended for mild G6PD deficiency): 45 mg once weekly for 8 weeks

Dosage Forms Excipient information presented when available (limited, particularly for generics); consult specific product labeling.
Tablet, as phosphate: 26.3 mg [15 mg base]

- **Primaquine Phosphate** *see* Primaquine *on page 1335*
- **Primatene® Mist [OTC]** *see* EPINEPHrine *on page 543*
- **Primaxin®** *see* Imipenem and Cilastatin *on page 812*

Primidone (PRI mi done)

Medication Safety Issues

Sound-alike/look-alike issues:

Primidone may be confused with predniSONE, primaquine

Related Information

Anticonvulsants By Seizure Type *on page 1759*

U.S. Brand Names Mysoline®

Canadian Brand Names Apo-Primidone®

Index Terms Desoxyphenobarbital; Primaclone

Pharmacologic Category Anticonvulsant, Miscellaneous; Barbiturate

Generic Available Yes

Use Management of grand mal, psychomotor, and focal seizures

Unlabeled/Investigational Use Benign familial tremor (essential tremor)

Pregnancy Risk Factor D

Pregnancy Considerations Crosses the placenta. Dysmorphic facial features; hemorrhagic disease of newborn due to fetal vitamin K depletion, maternal folic acid deficiency may occur. Epilepsy itself, number of medications, genetic factors, or a combination of these probably influence the teratogenicity of anticonvulsant therapy. Benefit:risk ratio usually favors continued use during pregnancy.

Lactation Enters breast milk/not recommended (AAP recommends use "with caution")

Contraindications Hypersensitivity to primidone, phenobarbital, or any component of the formulation; porphyria; pregnancy

Warnings/Precautions Use with caution in patients with renal or hepatic impairment, pulmonary insufficiency; abrupt withdrawal may precipitate status epilepticus. Potential for drug dependency exists. Do not administer to patients in acute pain. Use caution in elderly, debilitated, or pediatric patients - may cause paradoxical responses. May cause CNS depression, which may impair physical or mental abilities. Patients must cautioned about performing tasks which require mental alertness (eg, operating machinery or driving). Effects with other sedative drugs or ethanol may be potentiated. Use with caution in patients with depression or suicidal tendencies, or in patients with a history of drug abuse. Tolerance or psychological and physical dependence may occur with prolonged use. Primidone's metabolite, phenobarbital, has been associated with cognitive deficits in children. Use with caution in patients with hypoadrenalism.

Adverse Reactions Frequency not defined.

Central nervous system: Drowsiness, vertigo, ataxia, lethargy, behavior change, fatigue, hyperirritability

Dermatologic: Rash

Gastrointestinal: Nausea, vomiting, anorexia

Genitourinary: Impotence

Hematologic: Agranulocytopenia, agranulocytosis, anemia

Ocular: Diplopia, nystagmus

Metabolism/Transport Effects Metabolized to phenobarbital; **Induces** CYP1A2 (strong), 2B6 (strong), 2C8 (strong), 2C9 (strong), 3A4 (strong)

Drug Interactions

Alcohol (Ethyl): CNS Depressants may enhance the CNS depressant effect of Alcohol (Ethyl). *Risk C: Monitor therapy*

Barbiturates: Primidone may enhance the adverse/toxic effect of Barbiturates. Primidone is converted to phenobarbital, and thus becomes additive with existing barbiturate therapy. *Risk C: Monitor therapy*

Bendamustine: CYP1A2 Inducers (Strong) may decrease the serum concentration of Bendamustine. Concentrations of active metabolites may be increased. *Risk C: Monitor therapy*

Carbonic Anhydrase Inhibitors: May enhance the adverse/toxic effect of Primidone. Specifically, osteomalacia and rickets. Carbonic Anhydrase Inhibitors may decrease the serum concentration of Primidone. **Exceptions:** Brinzolamide; Dorzolamide. *Risk C: Monitor therapy*

CNS Depressants: May enhance the adverse/toxic effect of other CNS Depressants. *Risk C: Monitor therapy*

Corticosteroids (Systemic): Primidone may increase the metabolism of Corticosteroids (Systemic). *Risk C: Monitor therapy*

CYP1A2 Substrates: CYP1A2 Inducers (Strong) may increase the metabolism of CYP1A2 Substrates. *Risk C: Monitor therapy*

CYP2B6 Substrates: CYP2B6 Inducers (Strong) may increase the metabolism of CYP2B6 Substrates. *Risk C: Monitor therapy*

CYP2C8 Substrates (High risk): CYP2C8 Inducers (Highly Effective) may increase the metabolism of CYP2C8 Substrates (High risk). *Risk C: Monitor therapy*

CYP2C9 Substrates (High risk): CYP2C9 Inducers (Highly Effective) may increase the metabolism of CYP2C9 Substrates (High risk). *Risk C: Monitor therapy*

CYP3A4 Substrates: CYP3A4 Inducers (Strong) may increase the metabolism of CYP3A4 Substrates. *Risk C: Monitor therapy*

Felbamate: May increase the serum concentration of Primidone. Specifically, the concentration of its metabolite, phenobarbital. *Risk C: Monitor therapy*

Folic Acid: May decrease the serum concentration of Primidone. Additionally, folic acid may decrease concentrations of active metabolites of primidone (e.g., phenobarbital). *Risk C: Monitor therapy*

Ketorolac: May diminish the therapeutic effect of Anticonvulsants. *Risk C: Monitor therapy*

LamoTRIgine: Primidone may increase the metabolism of LamoTRIgine. *Risk D: Consider therapy modification*

Leucovorin-Levoleucovorin: May decrease the serum concentration of Primidone. Additionally, leucovorin/levoleucovorin may decrease concentrations of active metabolites of primidone (e.g., phenobarbital). *Risk C: Monitor therapy*

Maraviroc: CYP3A4 Inducers may decrease the serum concentration of Maraviroc. *Risk D: Consider therapy modification*

Mefloquine: May diminish the therapeutic effect of Anticonvulsants. Mefloquine may decrease the serum concentration of Anticonvulsants. Management: Mefloquine is contraindicated in persons with a history of convulsions. If anticonvulsant is being used for another indication monitor response to treatment closely, as concurrent mefloquine may decrease response to treatment. *Risk D: Consider therapy modification*

Methylfolate: May decrease the serum concentration of Primidone. *Risk C: Monitor therapy*

Nilotinib: CYP3A4 Inducers (Strong) may decrease the serum concentration of Nilotinib. *Risk X: Avoid combination*

Nisoldipine: CYP3A4 Inducers (Strong) may decrease the serum concentration of Nisoldipine. *Risk X: Avoid combination*

Phenytoin: May increase the metabolism of Primidone. The ratio of primidone: phenobarbital is thus changed. *Risk C: Monitor therapy*

QuiNIDine: Primidone may increase the metabolism of QuiNIDine. *Risk D: Consider therapy modification*

Ranolazine: CYP3A4 Inducers (Strong) may decrease the serum concentration of Ranolazine. *Risk X: Avoid combination*

Sorafenib: CYP3A4 Inducers (Strong) may decrease the serum concentration of Sorafenib. *Risk D: Consider therapy modification*

Valproic Acid: May decrease the metabolism of Primidone. More specifically, the metabolism of phenobarbital, primidone's primary active metabolite, would be decreased. Primidone may decrease the serum concentration of Valproic Acid. *Risk C: Monitor therapy*

Ethanol/Nutrition/Herb Interactions

Ethanol: Avoid ethanol (may increase CNS depression).

Food: Protein-deficient diets increase duration of action of primidone.

Herb/Nutraceutical: Avoid valerian, St John's wort, kava kava, gotu kola (may increase CNS depression).

Stability Protect from light.

Mechanism of Action Decreases neuron excitability, raises seizure threshold similar to phenobarbital; primidone has two active metabolites, phenobarbital and phenylethylmalonamide (PEMA); PEMA may enhance the activity of phenobarbital

Pharmacodynamics/Kinetics

Absorption: 60% to 80%

Distribution: Adults: V_d: 0.6 L/kg

Protein binding: 30%

Metabolism: Hepatic to phenobarbital (active) by oxidation and to phenylethylmalonamide (PEMA; active) by scission of the heterocyclic ring

Half-life elimination (age dependent): Primidone: Mean: 5-15 hours (variable); PEMA: 16 hours (variable)

Time to peak, serum: ~3 hours (variable)

Excretion: Urine (40% as unchanged drug; the remainder is unconjugated PEMA, phenobarbital and its metabolites)

Dosage Oral:

Children <8 years: Initial: 50-125 mg/day given at bedtime; increase by 50-125 mg/day increments every 3-7 days; usual dose: 10-25 mg/kg/day in divided doses 3-4 times/day

Children ≥8 years and Adults: Initial: 125-250 mg/day at bedtime; increase by 125-250 mg/day every 3-7 days; usual dose: 750-1500 mg/day in divided doses 3-4 times/day with maximum dosage of 2 g/day

Adults: Essential tremor (unlabeled use): 750 mg early in divided doses

Dosing interval in renal impairment:

Cl_{cr} 50-80 mL/minute: Administer every 8 hours

Cl_{cr} 10-50 mL/minute: Administer every 8-12 hours

Cl_{cr} <10 mL/minute: Administer every 12-24 hours

Hemodialysis: Moderately dialyzable (20% to 50%); administer dose post-dialysis or administer supplemental 30% dose

Dietary Considerations Folic acid: Low erythrocyte and CSF folate concentrations. Megaloblastic anemia has been reported. To avoid folic acid deficiency and megaloblastic anemia, some clinicians recommend giving patients on anticonvulsants prophylactic doses of folic acid and cyanocobalamin.

Monitoring Parameters Serum primidone and phenobarbital concentration, CBC, neurological status. Due to CNS effects, monitor closely when initiating drug in elderly. Monitor CBC at 6-month intervals to compare with baseline obtained at start of therapy. Since elderly metabolize phenobarbital at a slower rate than younger adults, it is suggested to measure both primidone and phenobarbital levels together.

Reference Range Therapeutic: Children <5 years: 7-10 mcg/mL (SI: 32-46 µmol/L); Adults: 5-12 mcg/mL (SI: 23-55 µmol/L); toxic effects rarely present with levels <10 mcg/mL (SI: 46 µmol/L) if phenobarbital concentrations are low. Dosage of primidone is adjusted with reference mostly to the phenobarbital level; Toxic: >15 mcg/mL (SI: >69 µmol/L)

Dosage Forms Excipient information presented when available (limited, particularly for generics); consult specific product labeling.

Tablet: 50 mg, 250 mg [generic tablet may contain sodium benzoate]

Dosage forms available in Canada: Tablet: 125 mg, 250 mg. **Note:** 50 mg tablet is **not** available in Canada.

- **Primsol®** *see* Trimethoprim *on page 1629*
- **Prinivil®** *see* Lisinopril *on page 934*
- **Prinzide®** *see* Lisinopril and Hydrochlorothiazide *on page 938*
- **Priscoline® [DSC]** *see* Tolazoline *on page 1592*
- **Pristinamycin** *see* Quinupristin and Dalfopristin *on page 1388*
- **Pristiq™** *see* Desvenlafaxine *on page 433*
- **Privine® [OTC]** *see* Naphazoline *on page 1101*
- **ProAir™ HFA** *see* Albuterol *on page 54*
- **ProAmatine®** *see* Midodrine *on page 1050*

Probenecid (proe BEN e sid)

Medication Safety Issues

Sound-alike/look-alike issues:

Probenecid may be confused with Procanbid®

Canadian Brand Names Benuryl™

Mexican Brand Names Benecid Valdecasas

Index Terms Benemid [DSC]

Pharmacologic Category Uricosuric Agent

Use Prevention of hyperuricemia associated with gout or gouty arthritis; prolongation and elevation of beta-lactam plasma levels

Effect on Mental Status May cause dizziness

Effect on Psychiatric Treatment May rarely cause leukopenia; use caution with clozapine and carbamazepine

Dosage Summary

Oral:

Children <2 years: Contraindicated

Children 2-14 years: Prolong penicillin serum levels: Initial: 25 mg/kg then 40 mg/kg/day given 4 times/day (maximum: 500 mg/dose)

Children >45 kg: Gonorrhea: 1 g as a single dose

Adults:

Gonorrhea, PID: 1 g as a single dose

Gout: Initial: 250 mg twice daily (maximum: 2-3 g/day)

Neurosyphilis: 500 mg 4 times/day for 10-14 days

Prolong PCN levels: 500 mg 4 times/day

Dosage Forms Excipient information presented when available (limited, particularly for generics); consult specific product labeling.

Tablet: 500 mg

◆ **Probenecid and Colchicine** *see* Colchicine and Probenecid *on page 398*

Procainamide (pro KANE a mide)

Medication Safety Issues

Sound-alike/look-alike issues:

Procanbid® may be confused with probenecid

Pronestyl® may be confused with Ponstel®

High alert medication: The Institute for Safe Medication Practices (ISMP) includes this medication among its list of drugs which have a heightened risk of causing significant patient harm when used in error.

PCA is an error-prone abbreviation (mistaken as patient controlled analgesia)

U.S. Brand Names Procanbid® [DSC]

Canadian Brand Names Apo-Procainamide®; Procainamide Hydrochloride Injection, USP; Procan® SR; Pronestyl®-SR

Index Terms PCA (error-prone abbreviation); Procainamide Hydrochloride; Procaine Amide Hydrochloride

Pharmacologic Category Antiarrhythmic Agent, Class Ia

Use Treatment of ventricular tachycardia (VT), premature ventricular contractions, paroxysmal atrial tachycardia (PSVT), and atrial fibrillation (AF); prevent recurrence of ventricular tachycardia, paroxysmal supraventricular tachycardia, atrial fibrillation or flutter

Unlabeled/Investigational Use

ACLS guidelines:

Stable monomorphic VT (EF >40%, no CHF)

Stable wide complex tachycardia, likely VT (EF >40%, no CHF, patient stable)

Atrial fibrillation or flutter, including pre-excitation syndrome (EF >40%, no CHF)

AV reentrant, narrow complex tachycardia (eg, reentrant SVT) [preserved ventricular function]

PALS guidelines: Tachycardia with pulses and poor perfusion (possible VT)

Effect on Mental Status May cause dizziness, confusion, depression, or hallucinations

Effect on Psychiatric Treatment Contraindicated with ziprasidone. May rarely cause agranulocytosis; use caution with clozapine and carbamazepine. Concurrent use with phenothiazines, TCAs, or beta-blockers may produce AV block.

Dosage Summary

I.M.:

Children: 50 mg/kg/day divided into doses of 1/8 to 1/4 every 3-6 hours

Adults: 0.5-1 g every 4-8 hours

I.V.:

Children: Loading dose: 3-6 mg/kg/dose over 5 minutes (maximum: 100 mg/dose), may repeat every 5-10 minutes to maximum of 15 mg/kg/load; Infusion: 20-80 mcg/kg/minute (maximum: 2 g/day)

Adults: Loading dose: 15-18 mg/kg administered as slow infusion over 25-30 minutes **or** 100-200 mg/dose repeated every 5 minutes as needed (maximum total dose: 1 g); Infusion: 1-4 mg/minute

Oral:

Extended release:

Children: Dosage not established

Adults: 500 mg to 1 g every 6 hours **or** 1000-2500 mg every 12 hours (Procanbid®)

Immediate release:

Children: 15-50 mg/kg/day divided every 3-6 hours

Adults: 250-500 mg/dose every 3-6 hours

Dosage Forms Excipient information presented when available (limited, particularly for generics); consult specific product labeling. [DSC] = Discontinued product

Capsule, as hydrochloride: 250 mg, 500 mg [DSC]

Injection, solution, as hydrochloride: 100 mg/mL (10 mL); 500 mg/mL (2 mL) [contains sodium metabisulfite]

Tablet, extended release, as hydrochloride: 750 mg [DSC]

Procanbid®: 500 mg, 1000 mg [DSC]

◆ **Procainamide Hydrochloride** *see* Procainamide *on page 1339*

Procaine (PROE kane)

Medication Safety Issues

High alert medication: The Institute for Safe Medication Practices (ISMP) includes this medication (epidural administration) among its list of drug classes which have a heightened risk of causing significant patient harm when used in error.

U.S. Brand Names Novocain®

Index Terms Procaine Hydrochloride

Pharmacologic Category Local Anesthetic

Use Produces spinal anesthesia

Effect on Mental Status None reported

Effect on Psychiatric Treatment If used with a vasoconstrictor, the effects of MAO inhibitors may be enhanced

Dosage Summary

Injection:

Children: Dosage not established

Adults: Dose varies with procedure, desired depth, and duration of anesthesia, desired muscle relaxation, vascularity of tissues, physical condition, and age of patient. Total dose (range): 50-200 mg

Dosage Forms Excipient information presented when available (limited, particularly for generics); consult specific product labeling.

Injection, solution, as hydrochloride:

Novocain®: 10% (2 mL) [contains sodium bisulfite]

◆ **Procaine Amide Hydrochloride** *see* Procainamide *on page 1339*

◆ **Procaine Benzylpenicillin** *see* Penicillin G Procaine *on page 1241*

◆ **Procaine Hydrochloride** *see* Procaine *on page 1340*

◆ **Procaine Penicillin G** *see* Penicillin G Procaine *on page 1241*

◆ **Procanbid® [DSC]** *see* Procainamide *on page 1339*

Procarbazine (proe KAR ba zeen)

Medication Safety Issues

Sound-alike/look-alike issues:

Procarbazine may be confused with dacarbazine

Matulane® may be confused with Modane®

High alert medication: The Institute for Safe Medication Practices (ISMP) includes this medication among its list of drugs which have a heightened risk of causing significant patient harm when used in error.

U.S. Brand Names Matulane®

Canadian Brand Names Matulane®; Natulan®

Index Terms Benzmethyzin; N-Methylhydrazine; NSC-77213; Procarbazine Hydrochloride

Pharmacologic Category Antineoplastic Agent, Alkylating Agent

Use Treatment of Hodgkin's disease

Unlabeled/Investigational Use Treatment of non-Hodgkin's lymphoma, brain tumors, melanoma, lung cancer, multiple myeloma

Effect on Mental Status Dizziness, nervousness, insomnia, confusion, mania, depression, and hallucinations are common

Effect on Psychiatric Treatment May cause myelosuppression; use caution with clozapine and carbamazepine; procarbazine possesses MAO inhibitor activity; avoid with antidepressants, narcotics, phenothiazines, and foods containing tyramine

Dosage Summary Note: Manufacturer states that the dose is based on patient's ideal weight if the patient is obese or has abnormal fluid retention. Other studies suggest that ideal body weight may not be necessary

Children: 12.5 mg/kg/day every other day for 4 doses **or** 100 mg/m^2/day for 14 days and repeated every 4 weeks **or** doses as high as 100-200 mg/m2/day once daily (neuroblastoma/medulloblastoma)

Adults: Initial: 2-4 mg/kg/day in single or divided doses for 7 days then increase dose to 4-6 mg/kg/day; Maintenance: 1-2 mg/kg/day

Dosage Forms Excipient information presented when available (limited, particularly for generics); consult specific product labeling.

Capsule, as hydrochloride:

Matulane®: 50 mg

◆ **Procarbazine Hydrochloride** *see* Procarbazine *on page 1340*

- **Procardia®** *see* NIFEdipine *on page 1136*
- **Procardia XL®** *see* NIFEdipine *on page 1136*
- **Procetofene** *see* Fenofibrate *on page 620*
- **Prochieve®** *see* Progesterone *on page 1345*

Prochlorperazine (proe klor PER a zeen)

Medication Safety Issues

Sound-alike/look-alike issues:

Prochlorperazine may be confused with chlorproMAZINE

Compazine® may be confused with Copaxone®, Coumadin®

CPZ (occasional abbreviation for Compazine®) is an error-prone abbreviation (mistaken as chlorpromazine)

Related Information

CMS: Long-Term Care Facility Thresholds *on page 1815*

U.S. Brand Names Compro™

Canadian Brand Names Apo-Prochlorperazine®; Compazine®; Nu-Prochlor; Stemetil®

Index Terms Chlormeprazine; Compazine; Prochlorperazine Edisylate; Prochlorperazine Maleate

Pharmacologic Category Antiemetic; Antipsychotic Agent, Typical, Phenothiazine

Generic Available Yes: Injection, tablet, suppository

Use Management of nausea and vomiting; psychotic disorders including schizophrenia; anxiety

Unlabeled/Investigational Use Behavioral syndromes in dementia; psychosis/agitation related to Alzheimer's dementia

Mental Health Comment While structurally a phenothiazine, this agent has limited antipsychotic activity and should not be used as such.

In 2008, the FDA issued a warning regarding increased mortality risk with typical **and** atypical antipsychotic drugs when used in elderly patients with dementia-related psychosis.

Pregnancy Considerations Crosses the placenta. Isolated reports of congenital anomalies, however, some included exposures to other drugs. Jaundice, extrapyramidal signs, hyper-/hyporeflexes have been noted in newborns. Available evidence with use of occasional low doses suggests safe use during pregnancy.

Lactation Excretion in breast milk unknown/use caution

Contraindications Hypersensitivity to prochlorperazine or any component of the formulation (cross-reactivity between phenothiazines may occur); severe CNS depression; coma; pediatric surgery; Reye's syndrome; should not be used in children <2 years of age or <9 kg

Warnings/Precautions Elderly patients with dementia-related psychosis treated with antipsychotics are at an increased risk of death compared to placebo. An increased incidence of cerebrovascular adverse events (including fatalities) has been reported in elderly patients with dementia-related psychosis. Prochlorperazine is not approved for this indication.

May be sedating; use with caution in disorders where CNS depression is a feature. May obscure intestinal obstruction or brain tumor. May impair physical or mental abilities. Effects with other sedative drugs or ethanol may be potentiated. Use with caution in Parkinson's disease; hemodynamic instability; bone marrow suppression; predisposition to seizures; subcortical brain damage; and in severe cardiac, hepatic, renal or respiratory disease. Caution in breast cancer or other prolactin-dependent tumors. May alter temperature regulation or mask toxicity of other drugs. Use caution with exposure to heat. May alter cardiac conduction. May cause orthostatic hypotension. Hypotension may occur following administration, particularly when parenteral form is used or in high dosages. Antipsychotic use has been associated with esophageal dysmotility and aspiration; use with caution in patients at risk of pneumonia (ie, Alzheimer's disease). May be associated with pigmentary retinopathy.

Phenothiazines may cause anticholinergic effects; therefore, they should be used with caution in patients with decreased gastrointestinal motility, urinary retention, BPH, xerostomia, or visual problems. Conditions which also may be exacerbated by cholinergic blockade include narrow-angle glaucoma (screening is recommended) and worsening of myasthenia gravis. May cause extrapyramidal symptoms (EPS), including pseudoparkinsonism, acute dystonic reactions, akathisia, and tardive dyskinesia (risk of these reactions is high relative to other neuroleptics). Risk of dystonia (and possibly other EPS) may be greater with increased doses, use of conventional antipsychotics, males, and younger patients. Use caution in the elderly. Children with acute illness or dehydration are more susceptible to neuromuscular reactions; use cautiously. May be associated with neuroleptic malignant syndrome (NMS).

Adverse Reactions Reported with prochlorperazine or other phenothiazines. Frequency not defined

Cardiovascular: Cardiac arrest, hypotension, peripheral edema, Q-wave distortions, T-wave distortions

Central nervous system: Agitation, catatonia, cerebral edema, cough reflex suppressed, dizziness, drowsiness, fever (mild - I.M.), headache, hyperactivity, hyperpyrexia, impairment of temperature regulation, insomnia, neuroleptic malignant syndrome (NMS), paradoxical excitement, restlessness, seizure

Dermatologic: Angioedema, contact dermatitis, discoloration of skin (blue-gray), epithelial keratopathy, erythema, eczema, exfoliative dermatitis (injectable), itching, photosensitivity, rash, skin pigmentation, urticaria

Endocrine & metabolic: Amenorrhea, breast enlargement, galactorrhea, gynecomastia, glucosuria, hyperglycemia, hypoglycemia, lactation, libido (changes in), menstrual irregularity, SIADH

Gastrointestinal: Appetite increased, atonic colon, constipation, ileus, nausea, weight gain, xerostomia

Genitourinary: Ejaculating dysfunction, ejaculatory disturbances, impotence, incontinence, polyuria, priapism, urinary retention, urination difficulty

Hematologic: Agranulocytosis, aplastic anemia, eosinophilia, hemolytic anemia, leukopenia, pancytopenia, thrombocytopenic purpura

Hepatic: Biliary stasis, cholestatic jaundice, hepatotoxicity

Neuromuscular & skeletal: Dystonias (torticollis, opisthotonos, carpopedal spasm, trismus, oculogyric crisis, protusion of tongue); extrapyramidal symptoms (pseudoparkinsonism, akathisia, dystonias, tardive dyskinesia); SLE-like syndrome, tremor

Ocular: blurred vision, cornea and lens changes, lenticular/corneal deposits, miosis, mydriasis, pigmentary retinopathy

Respiratory: Asthma, laryngeal edema, nasal congestion

Miscellaneous: Allergic reactions, diaphoresis

Drug Interactions

Acetylcholinesterase Inhibitors (Central): May enhance the neurotoxic (central) effect of Antipsychotics. Severe extrapyramidal symptoms have occurred in some patients. *Risk C: Monitor therapy*

Alcohol (Ethyl): CNS Depressants may enhance the CNS depressant effect of Alcohol (Ethyl). *Risk C: Monitor therapy*

Amphetamines: Antipsychotics may diminish the stimulatory effect of Amphetamines. *Risk C: Monitor therapy*

Analgesics (Opioid): Antipsychotic Agents (Phenothiazines) may enhance the hypotensive effect of Analgesics (Opioid). *Risk C: Monitor therapy*

Antacids: May decrease the absorption of Antipsychotic Agents (Phenothiazines). *Risk C: Monitor therapy*

Anticholinergics: May enhance the adverse/toxic effect of other Anticholinergics. **Exceptions:** Paliperidone. *Risk C: Monitor therapy*

Antimalarial Agents: May increase the serum concentration of Antipsychotic Agents (Phenothiazines). *Risk C: Monitor therapy*

Anti-Parkinson's Agents (Dopamine Agonist): Antipsychotics (Typical) may diminish the therapeutic effect of Anti-Parkinson's Agents (Dopamine Agonist). *Risk D: Consider therapy modification*

Beta-Blockers: Antipsychotic Agents (Phenothiazines) may enhance the hypotensive effect of Beta-Blockers. Beta-Blockers may decrease the metabolism of Antipsychotic Agents (Phenothiazines). Antipsychotic Agents (Phenothiazines) may decrease the metabolism of Beta-Blockers. **Exceptions:** Atenolol; Levobunolol; Metipranolol; Nadolol. *Risk C: Monitor therapy*

CNS Depressants: May enhance the adverse/toxic effect of other CNS Depressants. *Risk C: Monitor therapy*

Lithium formulations: May enhance the neurotoxic effect of Antipsychotics. Lithium formulations may decrease the serum concentration of Antipsychotics. Specifically noted with chlorpromazine. *Risk C: Monitor therapy*

Pramlintide: May enhance the anticholinergic effect of Anticholinergics. These effects are specific to the GI tract. *Risk D: Consider therapy modification*

Tetrabenazine: May enhance the adverse/toxic effect of Antipsychotics. *Risk C: Monitor therapy*

Ethanol/Nutrition/Herb Interactions

Ethanol: Avoid ethanol (may increase CNS depression).

Food: Limit caffeine.

Herb/Nutraceutical: Avoid dong quai, St John's wort (may also cause photosensitization). Avoid kava kava, gotu kola, valerian, St John's wort (may increase CNS depression).

Stability

Injection: Store at <30°C (<86°F); do not freeze. Protect from light. Clear or slightly yellow solutions may be used.

I.V. infusion: Injection may be diluted in 50-100 mL NS or D_5W.

Suppository, tablet: Store at 15°C to 30°C (59°F to 86°F). Protect from light.

Mechanism of Action Prochlorperazine is a piperazine phenothiazine antipsychotic which blocks postsynaptic mesolimbic dopaminergic D_1 and D_2 receptors in the brain, including the chemoreceptor trigger zone; exhibits a strong alpha-adrenergic and anticholinergic blocking effect and depresses the release of hypothalamic and hypophyseal hormones; believed to depress the reticular activating system, thus affecting basal metabolism, body temperature, wakefulness, vasomotor tone and emesis

Pharmacodynamics/Kinetics

Onset of action: Oral: 30-40 minutes; I.M.: 10-20 minutes; Rectal: ~60 minutes

Peak antiemetic effect: I.V.: 30-60 minutes

Duration: Rectal: 12 hours; Oral: 3-4 hours; I.M., I.V.: Adults: 4-6 hours; I.M.: Children: 12 hours

Distribution: V_d: 1400-1548 L; crosses placenta; enters breast milk

Metabolism: Primarily hepatic; N-desmethyl prochlorperazine (major active metabolite)

Bioavailability: Oral: 12.5%

Half-life elimination: Oral: 3-5 hours; I.V.: ~7 hours

Dosage

Antiemetic: Children (therapy >1 day usually not required): **Note:** Not recommended for use in children <9 kg or <2 years:

Oral, rectal: >9 kg: 0.4 mg/kg/24 hours in 3-4 divided doses; **or**

9-13 kg: 2.5 mg every 12-24 hours as needed; maximum: 7.5 mg/day

13.1-17 kg: 2.5 mg every 8-12 hours as needed; maximum: 10 mg/day

17.1-37 kg: 2.5 mg every 8 hours or 5 mg every 12 hours as needed; maximum: 15 mg/day

I.M.: 0.13 mg/kg/dose; change to oral as soon as possible

Antiemetic: Adults:

Oral (tablet): 5-10 mg 3-4 times/day; usual maximum: 40 mg/day; larger doses may rarely be required

I.M. (deep): 5-10 mg every 3-4 hours; usual maximum: 40 mg/day

I.V.: 2.5-10 mg; maximum 10 mg/dose or 40 mg/day; may repeat dose every 3-4 hours as needed

Rectal: 25 mg twice daily

Surgical nausea/vomiting: Adults: **Note:** Should not exceed 40 mg/day

I.M.: 5-10 mg 1-2 hours before induction or to control symptoms during or after surgery; may repeat once if necessary

I.V. (administer slow IVP <5 mg/minute): 5-10 mg 15-30 minutes before induction or to control symptoms during or after surgery; may repeat once if necessary

Rectal (unlabeled use): 25 mg

Antipsychotic:

Children 2-12 years (not recommended in children <9 kg or <2 years):

Oral, rectal: 2.5 mg 2-3 times/day; do not give more than 10 mg the first day; increase dosage as needed to maximum daily dose of 20 mg for 2-5 years and 25 mg for 6-12 years

I.M.: 0.13 mg/kg/dose; change to oral as soon as possible

Adults:

Oral: 5-10 mg 3-4 times/day; titrate dose slowly every 2-3 days; doses up to 150 mg/day may be required in some patients for treatment of severe disturbances

I.M.: Initial: 10-20 mg; if necessary repeat initial dose every 1-4 hours to gain control; more than 3-4 doses are rarely needed. If parenteral administration is still required; give 10-20 mg every 4-6 hours; change to oral as soon as possible.

Nonpsychotic anxiety: Oral (tablet): Adults: Usual dose: 15-20 mg/day in divided doses; do not give doses >20 mg/day or for longer than 12 weeks

Elderly: Behavioral symptoms associated with dementia (unlabeled use): Initial: 2.5-5 mg 1-2 times/day; increase dose at 4- to 7-day intervals by 2.5-5 mg/day; increase dosing intervals (twice daily, 3 times/day, etc) as necessary to control response or side effects; maximum daily dose should probably not exceed 75 mg in elderly; gradual increases (titration) may prevent some side effects or decrease their severity

Dietary Considerations Increase dietary intake of riboflavin; should be administered with food or water. Rectal suppositories may contain coconut and palm oil.

Administration May be administered orally, I.M., or I.V.

I.M.: Inject by deep IM into outer quadrant of buttocks.

I.V.: Doses should be given as a short (~30 minute) infusion to avoid orthostatic hypotension; administer at ≤5 mg/minute

Monitoring Parameters Vital signs; lipid profile, fasting blood glucose/Hgb A_{1c}; BMI; mental status, abnormal involuntary movement scale (AIMS); periodic ophthalmic exams (if chronically used); extrapyramidal symptoms (EPS)

Test Interactions False-positives for phenylketonuria, pregnancy, urinary amylase, uroporphyrins, urobilinogen

Additional Information Not recommended as an antipsychotic due to inferior efficacy compared to other phenothiazines.

Dosage Forms Excipient information presented when available (limited, particularly for generics); consult specific product labeling.

Injection, solution, as edisylate: 5 mg/mL (2 mL, 10 mL) [contains benzyl alcohol]

Suppository, rectal: 25 mg (12s) [may contain coconut and palm oil]

Compro™: 25 mg (12s) [contains coconut and palm oils]

Tablet, as maleate: 5 mg, 10 mg [strength expressed as base]

- ◆ **Prochlorperazine Edisylate** *see* Prochlorperazine *on page 1341*
- ◆ **Prochlorperazine Maleate** *see* Prochlorperazine *on page 1341*
- ◆ **Procrit®** *see* Epoetin Alfa *on page 546*
- ◆ **Proctocort®** *see* Hydrocortisone *on page 785*
- ◆ **ProctoCream® HC** *see* Hydrocortisone *on page 785*
- ◆ **Proctofene** *see* Fenofibrate *on page 620*
- ◆ **Procto-Kit™** *see* Hydrocortisone *on page 785*
- ◆ **Procto-Pak™** *see* Hydrocortisone *on page 785*
- ◆ **Proctosert** *see* Hydrocortisone *on page 785*
- ◆ **Proctosol-HC®** *see* Hydrocortisone *on page 785*
- ◆ **Proctozone-HC™** *see* Hydrocortisone *on page 785*

Procyclidine (proe SYE kli deen)

Medication Safety Issues

Sound-alike/look-alike issues:

Kemadrin® may be confused with Coumadin®

Related Information

Antiparkinsonian Agents *on page 1767*

U.S. Brand Names Kemadrin® [DSC]

Canadian Brand Names PMS-Procyclidine

Index Terms Procyclidine Hydrochloride

Pharmacologic Category Anti-Parkinson's Agent, Anticholinergic; Anticholinergic Agent

Generic Available No

Use Relieves symptoms of parkinsonian syndrome and drug-induced extrapyramidal symptoms

Pregnancy Risk Factor C

Lactation Excretion in breast milk unknown/not recommended

Contraindications Hypersensitivity to procyclidine or any component of the formulation; angle-closure glaucoma; myasthenia gravis; safe use in children not established

Warnings/Precautions Use with caution in hot weather or during exercise. Elderly patients frequently develop increased sensitivity and require strict dosage regulation - side effects may be more severe in elderly patients with atherosclerotic changes. Use with caution in patients with tachycardia, cardiac arrhythmias, hypertension, hypotension, prostatic hyperplasia (especially in the elderly) or any tendency toward urinary retention, liver or kidney disorders and obstructive disease of the GI or GU tract. When given in large doses or to susceptible patients, may cause weakness and inability to move particular muscle groups. May be associated with confusion or hallucinations (generally at higher dosages); intensification of symptoms or toxic psychosis may occur in patients with mental disorders. May cause CNS depression, which may impair physical or mental abilities; patients must be cautioned about performing tasks which require mental alertness (eg, operating machinery or driving). Safety and efficacy have not been established in children.

Adverse Reactions Frequency not defined.

Cardiovascular: Palpitation, tachycardia

Central nervous system: Ataxia, confusion, drowsiness, fatigue, giddiness, headache, lightheadedness, loss of memory

Dermatologic: Dry skin, photosensitivity, rash

Gastrointestinal: Constipation, dry throat, epigastric distress, nausea, vomiting, xerostomia

Genitourinary: Difficult urination

Neuromuscular & skeletal: Weakness

Ocular: Blurred vision, increased intraocular pain, mydriasis

Respiratory: Dry nose

Miscellaneous: Diaphoresis decreased

Drug Interactions

Acetylcholinesterase Inhibitors (Central): Anticholinergics may diminish the therapeutic effect of Acetylcholinesterase Inhibitors (Central). Acetylcholinesterase Inhibitors (Central) may diminish the therapeutic effect of Anticholinergics. If the anticholinergic action is a side effect of the agent, the result may be beneficial. *Risk C: Monitor therapy*

Anticholinergics: May enhance the adverse/toxic effect of other Anticholinergics. **Exceptions:** Paliperidone. *Risk C: Monitor therapy*

Cannabinoids: Anticholinergic Agents may enhance the tachycardic effect of Cannabinoids. *Risk C: Monitor therapy*

Potassium Chloride: Anticholinergic Agents may enhance the ulcerogenic effect of Potassium Chloride. *Risk D: Consider therapy modification*

Pramlintide: May enhance the anticholinergic effect of Anticholinergics. These effects are specific to the GI tract. *Risk D: Consider therapy modification*

Secretin: Anticholinergic Agents may diminish the stimulatory effect of Secretin. *Risk D: Consider therapy modification*

Ethanol/Nutrition/Herb Interactions Ethanol: Avoid ethanol.

Mechanism of Action Thought to act by blocking excess acetylcholine at cerebral synapses; many of its effects are due to its pharmacologic similarities with atropine; it exerts an antispasmodic effect on smooth muscle, is a potent mydriatic; inhibits salivation

Pharmacodynamics/Kinetics

Onset of action: 30-40 minutes

Duration: 4-6 hours

Dosage Adults: Oral: 2.5 mg 3 times/day after meals; if tolerated, gradually increase dose, maximum of 20 mg/day if necessary

Dosing adjustment in hepatic impairment: Decrease dose to a twice daily dosing regimen

Dietary Considerations Should be taken after meals to minimize stomach upset.

Administration Should be administered after meals to minimize stomach upset.

Monitoring Parameters Symptoms of EPS or Parkinson's disease, pulse, anticholinergic effects (ie, CNS, bowel and bladder function)

Dosage Forms Excipient information presented when available (limited, particularly for generics); consult specific product labeling. [DSC] = Discontinued product

Tablet, as hydrochloride:

Kemadrin®: 5 mg [scored] [DSC]

- ◆ **Procyclidine Hydrochloride** *see* Procyclidine *on page 1344*
- ◆ **Prodium® [OTC]** *see* Phenazopyridine *on page 1258*
- ◆ **ProFe [OTC]** *see* Polysaccharide-Iron Complex *on page 1313*
- ◆ **Profen II® [DSC]** *see* Guaifenesin and Pseudoephedrine *on page 744*
- ◆ **Profen II DM®** *see* Guaifenesin, Pseudoephedrine, and Dextromethorphan *on page 748*
- ◆ **Profen Forte™ DM** *see* Guaifenesin, Pseudoephedrine, and Dextromethorphan *on page 748*
- ◆ **Profilnine® SD** *see* Factor IX Complex (Human) *on page 612*

Progesterone (proe JES ter one)

U.S. Brand Names Crinone®; Endometrin®; First™-Progesterone VGS; Prochieve®; Prometrium®

Canadian Brand Names Crinone®; Prometrium®

Mexican Brand Names Gepromi; Geslutin; Utrogestan

Index Terms Pregnenedione; Progestin

Pharmacologic Category Progestin

Use

Oral: Prevention of endometrial hyperplasia in nonhysterectomized, postmenopausal women who are receiving conjugated estrogen tablets; secondary amenorrhea

I.M.: Amenorrhea; abnormal uterine bleeding due to hormonal imbalance

Intravaginal gel: Part of assisted reproductive technology (ART) for infertile women with progesterone deficiency; secondary amenorrhea

Vaginal tablet: Part of ART for infertile women with progesterone deficiency

Effect on Mental Status May cause insomnia or depression

Effect on Psychiatric Treatment None reported

Dosage Summary

I.M.:

Children: Dosage not established

Adults (females): 5-10 mg/day for 6 doses

Intravaginal:

Children: Dosage not established

Adults (females):

ART: 90 mg (8% gel) once or twice daily or 100 mg (vaginal tablet) 2-3 times/day

Secondary amenorrhea: 45 mg (4% gel) every other day, may increase to 90 mg (8% gel) every other day if needed (maximum: 6 doses)

Oral:

Children: Dosage not established

Adults (females):

Amenorrhea: 400 mg once daily in the evening for 10 days

Endometrial hyperplasia prevention: 200 mg once daily in the evening for 12 days sequentially per 28-day cycle

Dosage Forms Excipient information presented when available (limited, particularly for generics); consult specific product labeling.

Capsule:

Prometrium®: 100 mg, 200 mg [contains peanut oil]

Gel, vaginal:

Crinone®: 8% (1.45 g) [90 mg/dose; contains palm oil; 6 or 18 prefilled applicators]

Prochieve®: 4% (1.45 g) [45 mg/dose; contains palm oil; 6 prefilled applicators]; 8% (1.45 g) [90 mg/dose; contains palm oil; 6 or 18 prefilled applicators]

Injection, oil: 50 mg/mL (10 mL) [contains benzyl alcohol 10%, sesame oil]

Powder, for prescription compounding [micronized]: Progesterone USP (10 g, 25 g, 100 g, 1000 g)

Powder, for prescription compounding [wettable]: Progesterone USP (10 g, 25 g, 100 g, 1000 g)

First™-Progesterone VGS 25: Progesterone USP (0.75 g) [makes 30 progesterone 25 mg vaginal suppositories; kit contains fatty acid base, suppository mold, stirrer, filling tool, guide plate, mold cover with dispensing tool]

First™-Progesterone VGS 50: Progesterone USP (1.5 g) [makes 30 progesterone 50 mg vaginal suppositories; kit contains fatty acid base, suppository mold, stirrer, filling tool, guide plate, mold cover with dispensing tool]

First™-Progesterone VGS 100: Progesterone USP (3 g) [makes 30 progesterone 100 mg vaginal suppositories; kit contains fatty acid base, suppository mold, stirrer, filling tool, guide plate, mold cover with dispensing tool]

First™-Progesterone VGS 200: Progesterone USP (6 g) [makes 30 progesterone 200 mg vaginal suppositories; kit contains fatty acid base, suppository mold, stirrer, filling tool, guide plate, mold cover with dispensing tool]

First™-Progesterone VGS 400: Progesterone USP (12 g) [makes 30 progesterone 400 mg vaginal suppositories; kit contains fatty acid base, suppository mold, stirrer, filling tool, guide plate, mold cover with dispensing tool]

Tablet, vaginal:

Endometrin®: 100 mg (21s) [packaged with applicators]

◆ **Progestin** *see* Progesterone *on page 1345*

◆ **Proglycem®** *see* Diazoxide *on page 456*

◆ **Prograf®** *see* Tacrolimus *on page 1533*

◆ **Proguanil and Atovaquone** *see* Atovaquone and Proguanil *on page 157*

◆ **Proguanil Hydrochloride and Atovaquone** *see* Atovaquone and Proguanil *on page 157*

- **Proleukin®** *see* Aldesleukin *on page 58*
- **Prolex®-D [DSC]** *see* Guaifenesin and Phenylephrine *on page 742*
- **Prolex®-PD [DSC]** *see* Guaifenesin and Phenylephrine *on page 742*
- **Promacet** *see* Butalbital and Acetaminophen *on page 236*

Promethazine (proe METH a zeen)

Medication Safety Issues

Sound-alike/look-alike issues:

Promethazine may be confused with chlorproMAZINE, predniSONE, promazine

Phenergan® may be confused with Phenaphen®, Phrenilin®, Theragran®

High alert medication: The Institute for Safe Medication Practices (ISMP) includes this medication (I.V. formulation) among its list of drugs which have a heightened risk of causing significant patient harm when used in error.

Administration issues:

To prevent or minimize tissue damage during I.V. administration, the Institute for Safe Medication Practices (ISMP) has the following recommendations:

Limit concentration available to the 25 mg/mL product
Consider limiting initial doses to 6.25-12.5 mg
Further dilute the 25 mg/mL strength into 10-20 mL NS
Administer through a large bore vein (not hand or wrist)
Administer via running I.V. line at port furthest from patient's vein
Consider administering over 10-15 minutes
Instruct patients to report immediately signs of pain or burning

U.S. Brand Names Phenadoz™; Phenergan®; Promethegan™

Canadian Brand Names Bioniche Promethazine; Histantil; Phenergan®; PMS-Promethazine

Index Terms Promethazine Hydrochloride

Pharmacologic Category Antiemetic; Histamine H_1 Antagonist; Histamine H_1 Antagonist, First Generation

Generic Available Yes

Use Symptomatic treatment of various allergic conditions; antiemetic; motion sickness; sedative; postoperative pain (adjunctive therapy); anesthetic (adjunctive therapy); anaphylactic reactions (adjunctive therapy)

Pregnancy Risk Factor C

Pregnancy Considerations Teratogenic effects were not observed in animal studies. Crosses the placenta. Possible respiratory depression if drug is administered near time of delivery; behavioral changes, EEG alterations, impaired platelet aggregation reported with use during labor.

Lactation Excretion in breast milk unknown/use caution

Contraindications Hypersensitivity to promethazine or any component of the formulation (cross-reactivity between phenothiazines may occur); coma; treatment of lower respiratory tract symptoms, including asthma; children <2 years of age

Warnings/Precautions [U.S. Boxed Warning]: Respiratory fatalities have been reported in children <2 years of age. In children ≥2 years, use the lowest possible dose; other drugs with respiratory depressant effects should be avoided. Not for SubQ or intra-arterial administration. Injection may contain sodium metabisulfite. I.M. is the preferred route of parenteral administration. I.V. use has been associated with severe tissue damage; discontinue immediately if burning or pain occurs with administration. May be sedating; use with caution in disorders where CNS depression is a feature. May impair physical or mental abilities; patients must be cautioned about performing tasks which require mental alertness. Use with caution in Parkinson's disease; hemodynamic instability; bone marrow suppression; subcortical brain damage; and in severe cardiac, hepatic, renal, or respiratory disease. Avoid use in Reye's syndrome. May lower seizure threshold; use caution in persons with seizure disorders or in persons using narcotics or local anesthetics which may also affect seizure threshold. May alter temperature regulation or mask toxicity of other drugs due to antiemetic effects. May alter cardiac conduction (life-threatening arrhythmias have occurred with therapeutic doses of phenothiazines). May cause orthostatic hypotension; use with caution in patients at risk of hypotension or where transient hypotensive episodes would be poorly tolerated (cardiovascular disease or cerebrovascular disease).

Phenothiazines may cause anticholinergic effects; therefore, they should be used with caution in patients with decreased gastrointestinal motility, urinary retention, BPH, xerostomia, or visual problems. Conditions which also may be exacerbated by cholinergic blockade include narrow-angle glaucoma (screening is recommended) and worsening of myasthenia gravis. May cause extrapyramidal symptoms, including pseudoparkinsonism, acute dystonic reactions, akathisia, and tardive dyskinesia. May be associated with neuroleptic malignant syndrome (NMS).

Adverse Reactions

Cardiovascular: Bradycardia, hypertension, nonspecific QT changes, postural hypotension, tachycardia

Central nervous system: Akathisia, catatonic states, confusion, delirium, disorientation, dizziness, drowsiness, dystonias, euphoria, excitation, extrapyramidal symptoms, fatigue, hallucinations, hysteria, insomnia, lassitude, nervousness, neuroleptic malignant syndrome, nightmares, pseudoparkinsonism, sedation, seizure, somnolence, tardive dyskinesia

Dermatologic: Angioneurotic edema, dermatitis, photosensitivity, skin pigmentation (slate gray), urticaria

Endocrine & metabolic: Amenorrhea, breast engorgement, gynecomastia, hyper-/hypoglycemia, lactation

Gastrointestinal: Constipation, nausea, vomiting, xerostomia

Genitourinary: Ejaculatory disorder, impotence, urinary retention

Hematologic: Agranulocytosis, aplastic anemia, eosinophilia, hemolytic anemia, leukopenia, thrombocytopenia, thrombocytopenic purpura

Hepatic: Jaundice

Local: Venous thrombosis; injection site reactions (burning, erythema, pain, edema)

Neuromuscular & skeletal: Incoordination, tremor

Ocular: Blurred vision, corneal and lenticular changes, diplopia, epithelial keratopathy, pigmentary retinopathy

Otic: Tinnitus

Respiratory: Apnea, asthma, nasal congestion, respiratory depression

Metabolism/Transport Effects **Substrate** (major) of CYP2B6, 2D6; **Inhibits** CYP2D6 (weak)

Drug Interactions

Acetylcholinesterase Inhibitors (Central): Anticholinergics may diminish the therapeutic effect of Acetylcholinesterase Inhibitors (Central). Acetylcholinesterase Inhibitors (Central) may diminish the therapeutic effect of Anticholinergics. If the anticholinergic action is a side effect of the agent, the result may be beneficial. *Risk C: Monitor therapy*

Anticholinergics: May enhance the adverse/toxic effect of other Anticholinergics. **Exceptions:** Paliperidone. *Risk C: Monitor therapy*

CYP2B6 Inducers (Strong): May increase the metabolism of CYP2B6 Substrates. *Risk C: Monitor therapy*

CYP2B6 Inhibitors (Moderate): May decrease the metabolism of CYP2B6 Substrates. *Risk C: Monitor therapy*

CYP2B6 Inhibitors (Strong): May decrease the metabolism of CYP2B6 Substrates. *Risk D: Consider therapy modification*

CYP2D6 Inhibitors (Moderate): May decrease the metabolism of CYP2D6 Substrates. *Risk C: Monitor therapy*

CYP2D6 Inhibitors (Strong): May decrease the metabolism of CYP2D6 Substrates. *Risk D: Consider therapy modification*

Darunavir: May increase the serum concentration of CYP2D6 Substrates. *Risk C: Monitor therapy*

Pramlintide: May enhance the anticholinergic effect of Anticholinergics. These effects are specific to the GI tract. *Risk D: Consider therapy modification*

Serotonin Modulators: May enhance the adverse/toxic effect of other Serotonin Modulators. The development of serotonin syndrome may occur. *Risk D: Consider therapy modification*

Sibutramine: May enhance the serotonergic effect of Serotonin Modulators. This may cause serotonin syndrome. *Risk X: Avoid combination*

Ethanol/Nutrition/Herb Interactions

Ethanol: Avoid ethanol (may increase CNS depression).

Herb/Nutraceutical: Avoid valerian, St John's wort, kava kava, gotu kola (may increase CNS depression).

Stability

Injection: Prior to dilution, store at room temperature. Protect from light. Solutions in NS or D_5W are stable for 24 hours at room temperature.

Suppositories: Store refrigerated at 2°C to 8°C (36°F to 46°F).

Tablets: Store at room temperature. Protect from light.

Mechanism of Action Blocks postsynaptic mesolimbic dopaminergic receptors in the brain; exhibits a strong alpha-adrenergic blocking effect and depresses the release of hypothalamic and hypophyseal hormones; competes with histamine for the H_1-receptor; reduces stimuli to the brainstem reticular system

Pharmacodynamics/Kinetics

Onset of action: I.M.: ~20 minutes; I.V.: 3-5 minutes

Peak effect: C_{max}: 9.04 ng/mL (suppository); 19.3 ng/mL (syrup)
Duration: 2-6 hours
Absorption:
I.M.: Bioavailability may be greater than with oral or rectal administration
Oral: Rapid and complete; large first pass effect limits systemic bioavailability
Distribution: V_d: 171 L
Protein binding: 93%
Metabolism: Hepatic; primarily oxidation; forms metabolites
Half-life elimination: 9-16 hours
Time to maximum serum concentration: 4.4 hours (syrup); 6.7-8.6 hours (suppositories)
Excretion: Primarily urine and feces (as inactive metabolites)

Dosage
Children ≥2 years:
Allergic conditions: Oral, rectal: 0.1 mg/kg/dose (maximum: 12.5 mg) every 6 hours during the day and 0.5 mg/kg/dose (maximum: 25 mg) at bedtime as needed
Antiemetic: Oral, I.M., I.V., rectal: 0.25-1 mg/kg 4-6 times/day as needed (maximum: 25 mg/dose)
Motion sickness: Oral, rectal: 0.5 mg/kg/dose 30 minutes to 1 hour before departure, then every 12 hours as needed (maximum dose: 25 mg twice daily)
Sedation: Oral, I.M., I.V., rectal: 0.5-1 mg/kg/dose every 6 hours as needed (maximum: 50 mg/dose)
Adults:
Allergic conditions (including allergic reactions to blood or plasma):
Oral, rectal: 25 mg at bedtime **or** 12.5 mg before meals and at bedtime (range: 6.25-12.5 mg 3 times/day)
I.M., I.V.: 25 mg, may repeat in 2 hours when necessary; switch to oral route as soon as feasible
Antiemetic: Oral, I.M., I.V., rectal: 12.5-25 mg every 4-6 hours as needed
Motion sickness: Oral, rectal: 25 mg 30-60 minutes before departure, then every 12 hours as needed
Sedation: Oral, I.M., I.V., rectal: 12.5-50 mg/dose

Dietary Considerations Increase dietary intake of riboflavin.

Administration Formulations available for oral, rectal, I.M./I.V.; not for SubQ or intra-arterial administration. Administer I.M. into deep muscle (preferred route of administration). I.V. administration is **not** the preferred route; severe tissue damage may occur. Solution for injection should be administered in a maximum concentration of 25 mg/mL (more dilute solutions are recommended). Administer via running I.V. line at port furthest from patient's vein, or through a large bore vein (not hand or wrist). Consider administering over 10-15 minutes (maximum: 25 mg/minute). Discontinue immediately if burning or pain occurs with administration.

Monitoring Parameters Relief of symptoms, mental status

Test Interactions Alters the flare response in intradermal allergen tests; hCG-based pregnancy tests may result in false-negatives or false-positives; increased serum glucose may be seen with glucose tolerance tests

Dosage Forms Excipient information presented when available (limited, particularly for generics); consult specific product labeling. [DSC] = Discontinued product
Injection, solution, as hydrochloride: 25 mg/mL (1 mL); 50 mg/mL (1 mL)
Phenergan®: 25 mg/mL (1 mL); 50 mg/mL (1 mL) [contains sodium metabisulfite]
Suppository, rectal, as hydrochloride: 12.5 mg, 25 mg, 50 mg
Phenadoz™: 12.5 mg, 25 mg
Phenergan®: 25 mg, 50 mg [DSC]
Promethegan™: 12.5 mg, 25 mg, 50 mg
Syrup, as hydrochloride: 6.25 mg/5 mL (120 mL, 480 mL) [contains alcohol]
Tablet, as hydrochloride: 12.5 mg, 25 mg, 50 mg
Phenergan®: 25 mg [DSC]

Promethazine and Codeine (proe METH a zeen & KOE deen)

Index Terms Codeine and Promethazine

Pharmacologic Category Alpha/Beta Agonist; Analgesic, Opioid; Histamine H_1 Antagonist; Histamine H_1 Antagonist, First Generation

Use Temporary relief of coughs and upper respiratory symptoms associated with allergy or the common cold

Effect on Mental Status May cause drowsiness

Effect on Psychiatric Treatment Concurrent use with psychotropics may produce additive sedation

Restrictions C-V

Dosage Summary

Oral:

Children <16 years: Dosage not established

Children ≥16 years: 5 mL every 4-6 hours (maximum: 30 mL/24 hours)

Adults: 5 mL every 4-6 hours (maximum: 30 mL/24 hours)

Dosage Forms Excipient information presented when available (limited, particularly for generics); consult specific product labeling.

Syrup: Promethazine hydrochloride 6.25 mg and codeine phosphate 10 mg per 5 mL (120 mL, 473 mL) [contains alcohol]

Promethazine and Dextromethorphan

(proe METH a zeen & deks troe meth OR fan)

Index Terms Dextromethorphan and Promethazine

Pharmacologic Category Antitussive; Histamine H_1 Antagonist; Histamine H_1 Antagonist, First Generation

Use Temporary relief of coughs and upper respiratory symptoms associated with allergy or the common cold

Effect on Mental Status May cause drowsiness

Effect on Psychiatric Treatment Concurrent use with psychotropics may produce additive sedation

Dosage Summary

Oral:

Children <2 years: Dosage not established

Children 2-6 years: 1.25-2.5 mL every 4-6 hours (maximum: 10 mL/day)

Children 6-12 years: 2.5-5 mL every 4-6 hours (maximum: 20 mL/day)

Adults: 5 mL every 4-6 hours (maximum: 30 mL/day)

Dosage Forms Excipient information presented when available (limited, particularly for generics); consult specific product labeling.

Syrup: Promethazine hydrochloride 6.25 mg and dextromethorphan hydrobromide 15 mg per 5 mL (120 mL, 480 mL) [contains alcohol 7%]

◆ **Promethazine and Meperidine** *see* Meperidine and Promethazine *on page 987*

Promethazine and Phenylephrine

(proe METH a zeen & fen il EF rin)

Index Terms Phenylephrine and Promethazine

Pharmacologic Category Alpha/Beta Agonist; Histamine H_1 Antagonist; Histamine H_1 Antagonist, First Generation

Use Temporary relief of upper respiratory symptoms associated with allergy or the common cold

Effect on Mental Status May cause drowsiness

Effect on Psychiatric Treatment Concurrent use with psychotropics may produce additive sedation

Dosage Summary

Oral:

Children <2 years: Dosage not established

Children 2-6 years: 1.25-2.5 mL every 4-6 hours (maximum: 7.5 mL/day)

Children 6-12 years: 2.5-5 mL every 4-6 hours (maximum: 30 mL/day)

Children >12 years: 5 mL every 4-6 hours (maximum: 30 mL/day)

Adults: 5 mL every 4-6 hours (maximum: 30 mL/day)

Dosage Forms Excipient information presented when available (limited, particularly for generics); consult specific product labeling.

Syrup: Promethazine hydrochloride 6.25 mg and phenylephrine hydrochloride 5 mg per 5 mL (473 mL) [contains alcohol]

◆ **Promethazine Hydrochloride** *see* Promethazine *on page 1347*

Promethazine, Phenylephrine, and Codeine

(proe METH a zeen, fen il EF rin, & KOE deen)

Index Terms Codeine, Promethazine, and Phenylephrine; Phenylephrine, Promethazine, and Codeine

Pharmacologic Category Alpha/Beta Agonist; Analgesic, Opioid; Antitussive; Histamine H_1 Agonist; Histamine H_1 Antagonist, First Generation

Use Temporary relief of coughs and upper respiratory symptoms including nasal congestion associated with allergy or the common cold

Effect on Mental Status May cause drowsiness

Effect on Psychiatric Treatment Concurrent use with psychotropics may produce additive sedation

Restrictions C-V

Dosage Summary

Oral:

Children <16 years: Dosage not established

Children ≥16 years: 5 mL every 4-6 hours (maximum: 30 mL/day)

Adults: 5 mL every 4-6 hours (maximum: 30 mL/day)

Dosage Forms Excipient information presented when available (limited, particularly for generics); consult specific product labeling.

Syrup: Promethazine hydrochloride 6.25 mg, phenylephrine hydrochloride 5 mg, and codeine phosphate 10 mg per 5 mL (480 mL) [contains alcohol and sodium benzoate]

◆ **Promethegan™** *see* Promethazine *on page 1347*

◆ **Prometrium®** *see* Progesterone *on page 1345*

Propafenone (pro PAF en one)

U.S. Brand Names Rythmol®; Rythmol® SR

Canadian Brand Names Apo-Propafenone®; PMS-Propafenone; Rythmol® Gen-Propafenone

Mexican Brand Names Nistaken; Norfenon

Index Terms Propafenone Hydrochloride

Pharmacologic Category Antiarrhythmic Agent, Class Ic

Use Treatment of life-threatening ventricular arrhythmias

Rythmol® SR: Maintenance of normal sinus rhythm in patients with symptomatic atrial fibrillation

Unlabeled/Investigational Use Supraventricular tachycardias, including those patients with Wolff-Parkinson-White syndrome

Effect on Mental Status Dizziness and drowsiness are common; may cause anxiety

Effect on Psychiatric Treatment May rarely cause agranulocytosis; use caution with clozapine and carbamazepine; use TCAs with caution; may cause QT prolongation

Dosage Summary

Oral:

Extended release:

Children: Dosage not established

Adults: Initial: 225 mg every 12 hours; Maintenance: 225-425 mg every 12 hours

Immediate release:

Children: Dosage not established

Adults: Initial: 150 mg every 8 hours; Maintenance: 150-300 mg every 8 hours

Dosage Forms Excipient information presented when available (limited, particularly for generics); consult specific product labeling.

Capsule, extended release, as hydrochloride (Rythmol® SR): 225 mg, 325 mg, 425 mg [contains soy lecithin]

Tablet, as hydrochloride (Rythmol®): 150 mg, 225 mg, 300 mg

◆ **Propafenone Hydrochloride** *see* Propafenone *on page 1351*

Propantheline (proe PAN the leen)

Index Terms Propantheline Bromide

Pharmacologic Category Anticholinergic Agent

Use Adjunctive treatment of peptic ulcer, irritable bowel syndrome, pancreatitis, ureteral and urinary bladder spasm; reduce duodenal motility during diagnostic radiologic procedures

Effect on Mental Status May cause drowsiness, confusion, amnesia, nervousness, or insomnia

Effect on Psychiatric Treatment Concurrent use with psychotropics may produce additive sedation or anticholinergic side effects (dry mouth)

Dosage Summary

Oral:

Children: 1-3 mg/kg/day in 3-6 divided doses

Adults: 15 mg 3 times/day before meals or food and 30 mg at bedtime

Dosage Forms Excipient information presented when available (limited, particularly for generics); consult specific product labeling.
Tablet, as bromide: 15 mg [contains lactose 23.2 mg]

◆ **Propantheline Bromide** *see* Propantheline *on page 1351*

Proparacaine (proe PAR a kane)

Medication Safety Issues
Sound-alike/look-alike issues:
Proparacaine may be confused with propoxyphene
U.S. Brand Names Alcaine®; Ophthetic®; Parcaine™
Canadian Brand Names Alcaine®; Diocaine®
Index Terms Proparacaine Hydrochloride; Proxymetacaine
Pharmacologic Category Local Anesthetic, Ophthalmic
Use Anesthesia for tonometry, gonioscopy; suture removal from cornea; removal of corneal foreign body; cataract extraction, glaucoma surgery; short operative procedure involving the cornea and conjunctiva
Effect on Mental Status May rarely produce CNS depression
Effect on Psychiatric Treatment None reported
Dosage Summary
Ophthalmic:
Children: Instill 1-2 drops of 0.5% solution in eye just prior to procedure **or** instill 1 drop of 0.5% solution in eye every 5-10 minutes for 5-7 doses
Adults: Instill 1-2 drops of 0.5% solution in eye just prior to procedure **or** instill 1 drop of 0.5% solution in eye every 5-10 minutes for 5-7 doses
Dosage Forms Excipient information presented when available (limited, particularly for generics); consult specific product labeling.
Solution, ophthalmic, as hydrochloride: 0.5% (15 mL) [contains benzalkonium chloride]
Alcaine®: 0.5% (15 mL) [contains benzalkonium chloride]
Ophthetic®: 0.5% (15 mL) [contains benzalkonium chloride]
Parcaine™: 0.5% (15 mL) [contains benzalkonium chloride]

◆ **Proparacaine Hydrochloride** *see* Proparacaine *on page 1352*
◆ **Proplex® T [DSC]** *see* Factor IX Complex (Human) *on page 612*

Propofol (PROE po fole)

Medication Safety Issues
Sound-alike/look-alike issues:
Diprivan® may be confused with Diflucan®, Ditropan®

High alert medication: The Institute for Safe Medication Practices (ISMP) includes this medication among its list of drugs which have a heightened risk of causing significant patient harm when used in error.
U.S. Brand Names Diprivan®
Canadian Brand Names Diprivan®
Mexican Brand Names Diprivan; Indofol; Recofol
Pharmacologic Category General Anesthetic
Use Induction of anesthesia for inpatient or outpatient surgery in patients ≥3 years of age; maintenance of anesthesia for inpatient or outpatient surgery in patients >2 months of age; in adults, for induction and maintenance of monitored anesthesia care sedation during procedures; sedation in intubated, mechanically-ventilated ICU patients
Unlabeled/Investigational Use Postoperative antiemetic; refractory delirium tremens (case reports); moderate sedation (conscious sedation)
Effect on Mental Status May cause dizziness
Effect on Psychiatric Treatment Concurrent use with psychotropics may produce additive CNS depression and respiratory depression; monitor and adjust dosages as needed
Dosage Summary
I.V.:
Children <2 months: Dosage not established
Children:
Induction (3-16 years):
ASA-PS 1 or 2: 2.5-3.5 mg/kg over 20-30 seconds
ASA-PS 3 or 4: Use lower dose

Maintenance (2 months to 16 years):
ASA-PS 1 or 2: Initial: 200-300 mcg/kg/minute, decrease after 30 minutes; Infusion: 125-300 mcg/kg/minute; **Note:** Children ≤5 years may require higher infusion rates compared to older children

Adults:
Induction:
ASA-PS 1 or 2, <55 years:
General anesthesia: 2-2.5 mg/kg (~40 mg every 10 seconds)
Monitored anesthesia care sedation: 100-150 mcg/kg/minute for 3-5 minutes **or** 0.5 mg/kg over 3-5 minutes
Elderly, debilitated, ASA-PS 3 or 4:
General anesthesia: 1-1.5 mg/kg (~20 mg every 10 seconds until onset of induction); do not use rapid bolus dose (single or repeated)
Elderly, debilitated, ASA-PS 3 or 4, neurosurgical:
Monitored anesthesia care sedation: Use 80% of healthy adult dose; do not use rapid bolus doses (single or repeated)
Cardiac anesthesia: 0.5-1.5 mg/kg (~20 mg every 10 seconds until onset of induction)
Neurosurgical anesthesia: 1-2 mg/kg (~20 mg every 10 seconds until onset of induction)
Maintenance:
ASA-PS 1 or 2, <55 years:
General anesthesia: 100-200 mcg/kg/minute for 10-15 minutes, then decrease by 30% to 50%; Usual rate: 50-100 mcg/kg/minute **or** 25-50 mg increments as needed
Monitored anesthesia care sedation: 25-75 mcg/kg/minute **or** 10-20 mg incremental boluses
Elderly, debilitated, ASA-PS 3 or 4:
General anesthesia: 50-100 mcg/kg/minute
Elderly, debilitated, ASA-PS 3 or 4, neurosurgical:
Monitored anesthesia care sedation: Use 80% of healthy adult dose; do not use rapid bolus doses (single or repeated)
Cardiac anesthesia: 50-150 mcg/kg/minute
Neurosurgical anesthesia: 100-200 mcg/kg/minute

Adults (mechanically-ventilated): ICU sedation: Initial: 5 mcg/kg/minute; Maintenance: 5-80 mcg/kg/minute; **Note:** Titration is recommended

Elderly, debilitated, ASA-PS 3 or 4 (mechanically-ventilated): ICU sedation: Use 80% of healthy adult dose; do not use rapid bolus doses (single or repeated)

Dosage Forms Excipient information presented when available (limited, particularly for generics); consult specific product labeling.
Injection, emulsion: 10 mg/mL (20 mL, 50 mL, 100 mL) [products may contain egg lecithin, and soybean oil; may contain benzyl alcohol, sodium benzoate, or sodium metabisulfite]
Diprivan®: 10 mg/mL (20 mL, 50 mL, 100 mL) [contains egg lecithin, soybean oil, and disodium edetate]

Propoxyphene (proe POKS i feen)

Medication Safety Issues
Sound-alike/look-alike issues:
Propoxyphene may be confused with proparacaine
Darvon® may be confused with Devrom®, Diovan®
Darvon-N® may be confused with Darvocet-N®

High alert medication: The Institute for Safe Medication Practices (ISMP) includes this medication among its list of drug classes which have a heightened risk of causing significant patient harm when used in error.

Related Information
Narcotic / Opioid Analgesics *on page 1789*

U.S. Brand Names Darvon-N®; Darvon®

Canadian Brand Names 642® Tablet; Darvon-N®

Index Terms Dextropropoxyphene; Propoxyphene Hydrochloride; Propoxyphene Napsylate

Pharmacologic Category Analgesic, Opioid

Use Management of mild to moderate pain

Effect on Mental Status Dizziness, drowsiness, insomnia, and paradoxical excitement are common; may cause nervousness, restlessness, confusion; may rarely cause depression or hallucinations

Effect on Psychiatric Treatment Concurrent use with psychotropics may produce additive sedation as well as increase their serum levels; monitor for altered clinical response or preferably, use a different analgesic

Restrictions C-IV

Dosage Summary

Oral:

Hydrochloride:

Children: Doses not well established; 2-3 mg/kg/day divided every 6 hours has been used

Adults: 65 mg every 3-4 hours as needed (maximum: 390 mg/day)

Elderly: 65 mg every 4-6 hours as needed

Napsylate:

Children: Dosage not established

Adults: 100 mg every 4 hours as needed (maximum: 600 mg/day)

Elderly: 100 mg every 4-6 hours as needed

Dosage Forms Excipient information presented when available (limited, particularly for generics); consult specific product labeling.

Capsule, as hydrochloride: 65 mg

Darvon®: 65 mg

Tablet, as napsylate:

Darvon-N®: 100 mg

Propoxyphene and Acetaminophen

(proe POKS i feen & a seet a MIN oh fen)

Medication Safety Issues

Sound-alike/look-alike issues:

Darvocet-N® may be confused with Darvon-N®

High alert medication: The Institute for Safe Medication Practices (ISMP) includes this medication among its list of drug classes which have a heightened risk of causing significant patient harm when used in error.

Duplicate therapy issues: This product contains acetaminophen, which may be a component of other combination products. Do not exceed the maximum recommended daily dose of acetaminophen.

U.S. Brand Names Balacet 325™; Darvocet A500®; Darvocet-N® 100; Darvocet-N® 50

Canadian Brand Names Darvocet-N® 100; Darvocet-N® 50

Index Terms Acetaminophen and Propoxyphene; Propoxyphene Hydrochloride and Acetaminophen; Propoxyphene Napsylate and Acetaminophen

Pharmacologic Category Analgesic Combination (Opioid)

Use Management of mild to moderate pain

Effect on Mental Status Dizziness, drowsiness, insomnia, and paradoxical excitement are common; may cause nervousness, restlessness, confusion; may rarely cause depression or hallucinations

Effect on Psychiatric Treatment Concurrent use with psychotropics may produce additive sedation as well as increase their serum levels; monitor for altered clinical response or preferably, use a different analgesic

Restrictions C-IV

Dosage Summary

Oral:

Propoxyphene hydrochloride and acetaminophen 65/650 mg:

Children: Dosage not established

Adults: 1 tablet every 4 hours as needed (maximum: 4 g/day [acetaminophen]; 390 mg/day propoxyphene hydrochloride])

Propoxyphene napsylate and acetaminophen:

Children: Dosage not established

Adults:

Darvocet A500™, Darvocet-N® 100: 1 tablet every 4 hours as needed (maximum: 4 g/day [acetaminophen]; 600 mg/day [propoxyphene napsylate])

Darvocet-N® 50: 1-2 tablets every 4 hours as needed (maximum: 4 g/day [acetaminophen]; 600 mg/day [propoxyphene napsylate])

Dosage Forms Excipient information presented when available (limited, particularly for generics); consult specific product labeling.

Tablet, 50/325:

Darvocet-N® 50: Propoxyphene napsylate 50 mg and acetaminophen 325 mg

Tablet, 65/650: Propoxyphene hydrochloride 65 mg and acetaminophen 650 mg

Tablet, 100/325:

Balacet 325™: Propoxyphene napsylate 100 mg and acetaminophen 325 mg

Tablet, 100/500: Propoxyphene hydrochloride 100 mg and acetaminophen 500 mg

Darvocet A500®: Propoxyphene napsylate 100 mg and acetaminophen 500 mg

Tablet, 100/650: Propoxyphene napsylate 100 mg and acetaminophen 650 mg

Darvocet-N® 100: Propoxyphene napsylate 100 mg and acetaminophen 650 mg

Propoxyphene, Aspirin, and Caffeine

(proe POKS i feen, AS pir in, & KAF een)

Medication Safety Issues

Sound-alike/look-alike issues:

Darvon® may be confused with Devrom®, Diovan®

High alert medication: The Institute for Safe Medication Practices (ISMP) includes this medication among its list of drug classes which have a heightened risk of causing significant patient harm when used in error.

U.S. Brand Names Darvon® Compound [DSC]

Index Terms Aspirin, Caffeine, and Propoxyphene; Caffeine, Propoxyphene, and Aspirin; Propoxyphene Hydrochloride, Aspirin, and Caffeine

Pharmacologic Category Analgesic Combination (Opioid)

Use Treatment of mild-to-moderate pain

Effect on Mental Status Dizziness, drowsiness, insomnia, and paradoxical excitement are common; may cause nervousness, restlessness, confusion; may rarely cause depression or hallucinations

Effect on Psychiatric Treatment Concurrent use with psychotropics may produce additive sedation as well as increase their serum levels; monitor for altered clinical response or preferably, use a different analgesic

Restrictions C-IV

Dosage Summary

Oral:

Children: Dosing not established

Adults: One capsule (propoxyphene 65 mg/aspirin 389 mg/caffeine 32.4 mg) every 4 hours as needed (maximum: 390 mg/day [propoxyphene])

Dosage Forms Excipient information presented when available (limited, particularly for generics); consult specific product labeling. [DSC] = Discontinued product

Capsule (Darvon® Compound 65): Propoxyphene hydrochloride 65 mg, aspirin 389 mg, and caffeine 32.4 mg [DSC]

◆ **Propoxyphene Hydrochloride** *see* Propoxyphene *on page 1353*

◆ **Propoxyphene Hydrochloride and Acetaminophen** *see* Propoxyphene and Acetaminophen *on page 1354*

◆ **Propoxyphene Hydrochloride, Aspirin, and Caffeine** *see* Propoxyphene, Aspirin, and Caffeine *on page 1355*

◆ **Propoxyphene Napsylate** *see* Propoxyphene *on page 1353*

◆ **Propoxyphene Napsylate and Acetaminophen** *see* Propoxyphene and Acetaminophen *on page 1354*

Propranolol (proe PRAN oh lole)

Medication Safety Issues

Sound-alike/look-alike issues:

Propranolol may be confused with Pravachol®, Propulsid®

Inderal® may be confused with Adderall®, Enduron®, Enduronyl®, Imdur®, Imuran®, Inderide®, Isordil®, Toradol®

Inderal® 40 may be confused with Enduronyl® Forte

High alert medication: The Institute for Safe Medication Practices (ISMP) includes this medication among its list of drugs which have a heightened risk of causing significant patient harm when used in error.

Significant differences exist between oral and I.V. dosing. Use caution when converting from one route of administration to another.

International issues:

Inderal® may be confused with Indiaral® which is a brand name for loperamide in France

Related Information

Beta-Blockers *on page 1776*

Clozapine-Induced Side Effects *on page 1818*

Nonbenzodiazepine Anxiolytics and Hypnotics *on page 1791*

U.S. Brand Names Inderal®; Inderal® LA; InnoPran XL™

Canadian Brand Names Apo-Propranolol®; Dom-Propranolol; Inderal®; Inderal®-LA; Novo-Pranol; Nu-Propranolol; PMS-Propranolol; Propranolol Hydrochloride Injection, USP

Mexican Brand Names Colliprol; Inderalici; Pranidol

Index Terms Propranolol Hydrochloride

Pharmacologic Category Antiarrhythmic Agent, Class II; Beta-Adrenergic Blocker, Nonselective

Generic Available Yes

Use Management of hypertension; angina pectoris; pheochromocytoma; essential tremor; supraventricular arrhythmias (such as atrial fibrillation and flutter, AV nodal re-entrant tachycardias), ventricular tachycardias (catecholamine-induced arrhythmias, digoxin toxicity); prevention of myocardial infarction; migraine headache prophylaxis; symptomatic treatment of hypertrophic subaortic stenosis (hypertrophic obstructive cardiomyopathy)

Unlabeled/Investigational Use Tremor due to Parkinson's disease; ethanol withdrawal; aggressive behavior (not recommended for dementia-associated aggression), anxiety, schizophrenia; antipsychotic-induced akathisia; primary and secondary prophylaxis of variceal hemorrhage; acute panic; thyrotoxicosis; tetralogy of Fallot (TOF) hypercyanotic spells

Effect on Mental Status Fatigue and malaise are common and often mistaken for depression; may also cause dizziness, confusion, insomnia, or hallucinations

Effect on Psychiatric Treatment Low-dose propranolol is considered by many to be the drug of choice for akathisia. Concurrent use with psychotropic drugs may produce additive hypotensive effects; monitor blood pressure. Cutaneous reactions, including Stevens-Johnson syndrome, have been reported with use of propranolol; use caution with lamotrigine or valproic combination as combined usage with propranolol has been associated with these reactions.

Pregnancy Risk Factor C (manufacturer); D (2nd and 3rd trimesters - expert analysis)

Pregnancy Considerations Embryotoxicity has been observed in some animal studies. Propranolol crosses the placenta. Beta-blockers have been associated with bradycardia, hypotension, and IUGR. IUGR is probably related to maternal hypertension. Available evidence suggests beta-blockers are generally safe during pregnancy (JNC 7). Neonatal hypoglycemia, respiratory depression and congenital abnormalities have been reported following maternal use of beta-blockers.

Lactation Enters breast milk/use caution (AAP rates "compatible")

Contraindications Hypersensitivity to propranolol, beta-blockers, or any component of the formulation; uncompensated congestive heart failure (unless the failure is due to tachyarrhythmias being treated with propranolol), cardiogenic shock, severe sinus bradycardia or heart block (2nd or 3rd degree), severe hyperactive airway disease (asthma or COPD)

Warnings/Precautions Consider pre-existing conditions such as sick sinus syndrome before initiating. Administer cautiously in compensated heart failure and monitor for a worsening of the condition (efficacy of propranolol in HF has not been demonstrated). Beta-blocker therapy should not be withdrawn abruptly (particularly in patients with CAD), but gradually tapered to avoid acute tachycardia, hypertension, and/or ischemia. Use caution in patient with peripheral vascular disease (PVD). Use caution with concurrent use of beta-blockers and either verapamil or diltiazem; bradycardia or heart block can occur. Avoid concurrent I.V. use of both agents.

Use cautiously in patients with diabetes because it can mask prominent hypoglycemic symptoms. Use caution in hyperthyroidism since beta-blockade may mask signs of thyrotoxicosis. May alter thyroid-function tests. Use with caution in myasthenia gravis or psychiatric disease (may cause CNS depression). Use cautiously in renal and hepatic dysfunction; dosage adjustment required in hepatic impairment. Use care with anesthetic agents which decrease myocardial function. In general, patients with bronchospastic disease should not receive beta-blockers; if used at all, should be used cautiously with close monitoring. Adequate alpha-blockade is required prior to use of any beta-blocker for patients with untreated pheochromocytoma. Use caution with history of severe anaphylaxis to allergens; patients taking beta-blockers may become more sensitive to repeated challenges. Treatment of anaphylaxis (eg, epinephrine) in patients taking beta-blockers may be ineffective or promote undesirable effects. Safety and efficacy in children have not been established.

Adverse Reactions Frequency not defined.

Cardiovascular: Angina, arterial insufficiency, AV conduction disturbance increased, bradycardia, cardiogenic shock, CHF, hypotension, impaired myocardial contractility, mesenteric arterial thrombosis (rare), Raynaud's syndrome, syncope

Central nervous system: Amnesia, catatonia, cognitive dysfunction, confusion, depression, dizziness, emotional lability, fatigue, hallucinations, hypersomnolence, insomnia, lethargy, lightheadedness, psychosis, vertigo, vivid dreams

Dermatologic: Alopecia, contact dermatitis, cutaneous ulcers, eczematous eruptions, erythema multiforme, exfoliative dermatitis, hyperkeratosis, nail changes, oculomucocutaneous reactions, pruritus, psoriasiform eruptions, rash, Stevens-Johnson syndrome, toxic epidermal necrolysis, ulcers, ulcerative lichenoid, urticaria

Endocrine & metabolic: Hyper-/hypoglycemia, hyperkalemia, hyperlipidemia

Gastrointestinal: Anorexia, cramping, constipation, diarrhea, ischemic colitis, nausea, stomach discomfort, vomiting

Genitourinary: Impotence, interstitial nephritis (rare), oliguria (rare), Peyronie's disease, proteinuria (rare)

Hematologic: Agranulocytosis, nonthrombocytopenic purpura, thrombocytopenia, thrombocytopenic purpura

Hepatic: Alkaline phosphatase increased, transaminases increased

Neuromuscular & skeletal: Arthropathy, carpal tunnel syndrome (rare), myotonus, paresthesia, polyarthritis, weakness

Ocular: Hyperemia of the conjunctiva, mydriasis, visual acuity decreased, visual disturbances, xerophthalmia

Renal: BUN increased

Respiratory: Bronchospasm, dyspnea, laryngospasm, pharyngitis, pulmonary edema, respiratory distress, wheezing

Miscellaneous: Anaphylactic/anaphylactoid allergic reaction, cold extremities, lupus-like syndrome (rare)

Metabolism/Transport Effects **Substrate** of CYP1A2 (major), 2C19 (minor), 2D6 (major), 3A4 (minor); **Inhibits** CYP1A2 (weak), 2D6 (weak)

Drug Interactions

Acetylcholinesterase Inhibitors: May enhance the bradycardic effect of Beta-Blockers. *Risk C: Monitor therapy*

Alcohol (Ethyl): May decrease the serum concentration of Propranolol. Alcohol (Ethyl) may increase the serum concentration of Propranolol. *Risk C: Monitor therapy*

Alpha-/Beta-Agonists (Direct-Acting): Beta-Blockers may enhance the vasopressor effect of Alpha-/Beta-Agonists (Direct-Acting). Epinephrine used as a local anesthetic for dental procedures will not likely cause clinically relevant problems. **Exceptions:** Dipivefrin. *Risk D: Consider therapy modification*

Alpha1-Blockers: Beta-Blockers may enhance the orthostatic effect of Alpha1-Blockers. The risk associated with ophthalmic products is probably less than systemic products. *Risk D: Consider therapy modification*

Alpha2-Agonists: Beta-Blockers may enhance the rebound hypertensive effect of Alpha2-Agonists. This effect can occur when the alpha$_2$-agonist is abruptly withdrawn. **Exceptions:** Apraclonidine; Brimonidine. *Risk D: Consider therapy modification*

Aminoquinolines (Antimalarial): May decrease the metabolism of Beta-Blockers. *Risk C: Monitor therapy*

Amiodarone: May enhance the bradycardic effect of Beta-Blockers. Possibly to the point of cardiac arrest. Amiodarone may increase the serum concentration of Beta-Blockers. *Risk C: Monitor therapy*

Anilidopiperidine Opioids: May enhance the bradycardic effect of Beta-Blockers. Anilidopiperidine Opioids may enhance the hypotensive effect of Beta-Blockers. *Risk C: Monitor therapy*

Antipsychotic Agents (Phenothiazines): May enhance the hypotensive effect of Beta-Blockers. Beta-Blockers may decrease the metabolism of Antipsychotic Agents (Phenothiazines). Antipsychotic Agents (Phenothiazines) may decrease the metabolism of Beta-Blockers. *Risk C: Monitor therapy*

Barbiturates: May decrease the serum concentration of Beta-Blockers. *Risk C: Monitor therapy*

Beta2-Agonists: Beta-Blockers (Nonselective) may diminish the bronchodilatory effect of Beta2-Agonists. *Risk D: Consider therapy modification*

Calcium Channel Blockers (Nondihydropyridine): May enhance the hypotensive effect of Beta-Blockers. Bradycardia and signs of heart failure have also been reported. Calcium Channel Blockers (Nondihydropyridine) may increase the serum concentration of Beta-Blockers. *Risk C: Monitor therapy*

Cardiac Glycosides: Beta-Blockers may enhance the bradycardic effect of Cardiac Glycosides. *Risk C: Monitor therapy*

CYP1A2 Inducers (Strong): May increase the metabolism of CYP1A2 Substrates. *Risk C: Monitor therapy*

CYP1A2 Inhibitors (Moderate): May decrease the metabolism of CYP1A2 Substrates. *Risk C: Monitor therapy*

CYP1A2 Inhibitors (Strong): May decrease the metabolism of CYP1A2 Substrates. *Risk D: Consider therapy modification*

CYP2D6 Inhibitors (Moderate): May decrease the metabolism of CYP2D6 Substrates. *Risk C: Monitor therapy*

CYP2D6 Inhibitors (Strong): May decrease the metabolism of CYP2D6 Substrates. *Risk D: Consider therapy modification*

Dabigatran Etexilate: P-Glycoprotein Inhibitors may increase the serum concentration of Dabigatran Etexilate. *Risk X: Avoid combination*

Darunavir: May increase the serum concentration of CYP2D6 Substrates. *Risk C: Monitor therapy*

Diazoxide: May enhance the hypotensive effect of Antihypertensives. *Risk C: Monitor therapy*

Dipyridamole: May enhance the bradycardic effect of Beta-Blockers. *Risk C: Monitor therapy*

Disopyramide: May enhance the bradycardic effect of Beta-Blockers. *Risk C: Monitor therapy*

Fluvoxamine: May increase the serum concentration of Propranolol. Management: Use a lower initial propranolol dose and be cautious with propranolol dose titration. *Risk D: Consider therapy modification*

Herbs (Hypertensive Properties): May diminish the antihypertensive effect of Antihypertensives. *Risk C: Monitor therapy*

Herbs (Hypotensive Properties): May enhance the hypotensive effect of Antihypertensives. *Risk C: Monitor therapy*

Insulin: Beta-Blockers may enhance the hypoglycemic effect of Insulin. *Risk C: Monitor therapy*

Lidocaine: Beta-Blockers may decrease the metabolism of Lidocaine. *Risk C: Monitor therapy*

Methacholine: Beta-Blockers may enhance the adverse/toxic effect of Methacholine. *Risk X: Avoid combination*

Methylphenidate: May diminish the antihypertensive effect of Antihypertensives. *Risk C: Monitor therapy*

Midodrine: Beta-Blockers may enhance the bradycardic effect of Midodrine. *Risk C: Monitor therapy*

Nonsteroidal Anti-Inflammatory Agents: May diminish the antihypertensive effect of Beta-Blockers. *Risk C: Monitor therapy*

P-Glycoprotein Substrates: P-Glycoprotein Inhibitors may increase the serum concentration of P-Glycoprotein Substrates. P-glycoprotein inhibitors may also enhance the distribution of p-glycoprotein substrates to specific cells/tissues/organs where p-glycoprotein is present in large amounts (e.g., brain, T-lymphocytes, testes, etc.). *Risk C: Monitor therapy*

Propafenone: May decrease the metabolism of Beta-Blockers. Propafenone possesses some independent beta blocking activity. *Risk C: Monitor therapy*

Propoxyphene: May decrease the metabolism of Beta-Blockers. *Risk C: Monitor therapy*

Prostacyclin Analogues: May enhance the hypotensive effect of Antihypertensives. *Risk C: Monitor therapy*

QuiNIDine: May decrease the metabolism of Beta-Blockers. *Risk C: Monitor therapy*

Reserpine: May enhance the hypotensive effect of Beta-Blockers. *Risk C: Monitor therapy*

Rifamycin Derivatives: May decrease the serum concentration of Beta-Blockers. **Exceptions:** Rifabutin. *Risk C: Monitor therapy*

RiTUXimab: Antihypertensives may enhance the hypotensive effect of RiTUXimab. *Risk D: Consider therapy modification*

Rivaroxaban: P-Glycoprotein Inhibitors may increase the serum concentration of Rivaroxaban. *Risk X: Avoid combination*

Selective Serotonin Reuptake Inhibitors: May enhance the bradycardic effect of Beta-Blockers. **Exceptions:** Fluvoxamine. *Risk C: Monitor therapy*

Serotonin 5-HT1D Receptor Agonists: Propranolol may increase the serum concentration of Serotonin 5-HT1D Receptor Agonists. **Exceptions:** Almotriptan; Eletriptan; Frovatriptan; Naratriptan; SUMAtriptan; Zolmitriptan. *Risk D: Consider therapy modification*

Theophylline Derivatives: Beta-Blockers (Nonselective) may diminish the bronchodilatory effect of Theophylline Derivatives. *Risk D: Consider therapy modification*

Topotecan: P-Glycoprotein Inhibitors may increase the serum concentration of Topotecan. *Risk X: Avoid combination*

Zileuton: May increase the serum concentration of Propranolol. *Risk C: Monitor therapy*

Ethanol/Nutrition/Herb Interactions

Ethanol: Ethanol may increase or decrease plasma levels of propranolol. Reports are variable and have shown both enhanced as well as inhibited hepatic metabolism (of propranolol). Caution advised with consumption of alcohol and monitor for heart rate and/or blood pressure changes.

Food: Propranolol serum levels may be increased if taken with food. Protein-rich foods may increase bioavailability; a change in diet from high carbohydrate/low protein to low carbohydrate/high protein may result in increased oral clearance.

Cigarette: Smoking may decrease plasma levels of propranolol by increasing metabolism.

Herb/Nutraceutical: Avoid dong quai if using for hypertension (has estrogenic activity). Avoid bayberry, blue cohosh, cayenne, ephedra, ginger, ginseng (american), gotu kola, licorice, yohimbe (may worsen hypertension). Avoid black cohosh, california poppy, coleus, garlic, golden seal, hawthorn, mistletoe, periwinkle, quinine, shepherd's purse (have antihypertensive activity, may cause hypotension).

Stability

Injection: Store at 20°C to 25°C (68°F to 77°F); protect from freezing or excessive heat. Once diluted, propranolol is stable for 24 hours at room temperature in D_5W or NS. Protect from light. Solution has a maximum stability at pH of 3 and decomposes rapidly in alkaline pH.

Capsule, tablet: Store at 20°C to 25°C (68°F to 77°F); protect from freezing or excessive heat. Protect from light and moisture.

Mechanism of Action Nonselective beta-adrenergic blocker (class II antiarrhythmic); competitively blocks response to $beta_1$- and $beta_2$-adrenergic stimulation which results in decreases in heart rate, myocardial contractility, blood pressure, and myocardial oxygen demand. Nonselective beta-adrenergic blockers (propranolol, nadolol) reduce portal pressure by producing splanchnic vasoconstriction ($beta_2$ effect) thereby reducing portal blood flow.

Pharmacodynamics/Kinetics

Onset of action: Beta-blockade: Oral: 1-2 hours

Duration: Immediate release: 6-12 hours; Extended-release formulations: ~24-27 hours

Distribution: V_d: 4 L/kg in adults; crosses placenta; small amounts enter breast milk

Protein binding: Newborns: 68%; Adults: 90%

Metabolism: Hepatic to active and inactive compounds; extensive first-pass effect

Bioavailability: 30% to 40%

Half-life elimination: Neonates and Infants: Possible increased half-life; Children: 3.9-6.4 hours; Adults: Immediate release formulation: 3-6 hours; Extended-release formulations: 8-10 hours

Time to peak: Immediate release: 1-4 hours; Extended-release formulations: ~6-14 hours

Excretion: Urine (96% to 99%)

Dosage

Akathisia (unlabeled use): Oral: Adults: 30-120 mg/day in 2-3 divided doses

Essential tremor: Oral: Adults: 40 mg twice daily initially; maintenance doses: Usually 120-320 mg/day

Hypertension:

Oral:

Children (unlabeled use): Initial: 0.5-1 mg/kg/day in divided doses every 6-12 hours; increase gradually every 5-7 days; maximum: 16 mg/kg/24 hours

Adults: Initial: 40 mg twice daily; increase dosage every 3-7 days; usual dose: 120-240 mg divided in 2-3 doses/day; maximum daily dose: 640 mg; usual dosage range (JNC 7): 40-160 mg/day in 2 divided doses

Extended release formulations:

Inderal® LA: Initial: 80 mg once daily; usual maintenance: 120-160 mg once daily; maximum daily dose: 640 mg; usual dosage range (JNC 7): 60-180 mg/day once daily

InnoPran XL™: Initial: 80 mg once daily at bedtime; if initial response is inadequate, may be increased at 2-3 week intervals to a maximum dose of 120 mg

Hypertrophic subaortic stenosis: Oral: Adults: 20-40 mg 3-4 times/day

Inderal® LA: 80-160 mg once daily

Migraine headache prophylaxis: Oral:

Children (unlabeled use): Initial: 2-4 mg/kg/day **or**

≤35 kg: 10-20 mg 3 times/day

>35 kg: 20-40 mg 3 times/day

Adults: Initial: 80 mg/day divided every 6-8 hours; increase by 20-40 mg/dose every 3-4 weeks to a maximum of 160-240 mg/day given in divided doses every 6-8 hours; if satisfactory response not achieved within 6 weeks of starting therapy, drug should be withdrawn gradually over several weeks

Inderal® LA: Initial: 80 mg once daily; effective dose range: 160-240 mg once daily

Post-MI mortality reduction: Oral: Adults: Initial: 40 mg 3 times/day; usual dosage range: 180-240 mg/day in 3-4 divided doses

Pheochromocytoma: Oral: Adults: 30-60 mg/day in divided doses

Stable angina: Oral: Adults: 80-320 mg/day in doses divided 2-4 times/day

Inderal® LA: Initial: 80 mg once daily; maximum dose: 320 mg once daily

Tachyarrhythmias:

Oral:

Children (unlabeled use): Initial: 0.5-1 mg/kg/day in divided doses every 6-8 hours; titrate dosage upward every 3-7 days; usual dose: 2-6 mg/kg/day; higher doses may be needed; do not exceed 16 mg/kg/day or 60 mg/day

Adults: 10-30 mg/dose every 6-8 hours

Elderly: Initial: 10 mg twice daily; increase dosage every 3-7 days; usual dosage range: 10-320 mg given in 2 divided doses

I.V.:

Children (unlabeled use): 0.01-0.1 mg/kg/dose slow IVP over 10 minutes; maximum dose: 1 mg for infants; 3 mg for children

Adults: 1-3 mg/dose slow IVP; repeat every 2-5 minutes up to a total of 5 mg; titrate initial dose to desired response

or

0.1 mg/kg divided into 3 equal doses given at 2-3 minute intervals. May repeat total dose in 2 minutes if necessary (ACLS guidelines, 2005)

Note: Once response achieved or maximum dose administered, additional doses should not be given for at least 4 hours.

Elderly: Use caution; initiate at lower end of the dosing range.

Hypercyanotic spells (TOF) (unlabeled use): Children:

Oral: Palliation: Initial: 1 mg/kg/day every 6 hours; if ineffective, may increase dose after 1 week by 1 mg/kg/day to a maximum of 5 mg/kg/day; if patient becomes refractory, may increase slowly to a maximum of 10-15 mg/kg/day. Allow 24 hours between dosing changes.

I.V.: 0.01-0.2 mg/kg/dose infused over 10 minutes; maximum dose: 5 mg

Thyrotoxicosis (unlabeled use):

Oral:

Children: 2 mg/kg/day, divided every 6-8 hours, titrate to effective dose

Adolescents and Adults: Oral: 10-40 mg/dose every 6 hours

I.V.: Adults: 1-3 mg/dose slow IVP as a single dose

Variceal hemorrhage prophylaxis (unlabeled use; Garcia-Tsao, 2007): Oral: Adults:

Primary prophylaxis: Initial: 20 mg twice daily; adjust to maximal tolerated dose. **Note:** Risk factors for hemorrhage include Child-Pugh class B/C or variceal red wale markings on endoscopy.

Secondary prophylaxis: Initial: 20 mg twice daily; adjust to maximal tolerated dose

Dosing adjustment in renal impairment:

Not dialyzable (0% to 5%); supplemental dose is not necessary.

Peritoneal dialysis effects: Supplemental dose is not necessary.

Dosing adjustment in hepatic disease: Marked slowing of heart rate may occur in chronic liver disease with conventional doses; low initial dose and regular heart rate monitoring

Dietary Considerations Tablets (immediate release) should be taken on an empty stomach; capsules (extended release) may be taken with or without food, but should always be taken consistently (with food or on an empty stomach)

Administration I.V. dose is much smaller than oral dose. When administered acutely for cardiac treatment, monitor ECG and blood pressure. May administer by rapid infusion (I.V. push) at a rate of 1 mg/minute or by slow infusion over ~30 minutes. Necessary monitoring for surgical patients who are unable to take oral beta-blockers (prolonged ileus) has not been defined. Some institutions require monitoring of baseline and postinfusion heart rate and blood pressure when a patient's response to beta-blockade has not been characterized (ie, the patient's initial dose or following a change in dose). Consult individual institutional policies and procedures. Do not crush long-acting oral forms.

Monitoring Parameters Acute cardiac treatment: Monitor ECG, heart rate, and blood pressure with I.V. administration; heart rate and blood pressure with oral administration

Reference Range Therapeutic: 50-100 ng/mL (SI: 190-390 nmol/L) at end of dose interval

Dosage Forms Excipient information presented when available (limited, particularly for generics); consult specific product labeling. [DSC] = Discontinued product

Capsule, extended release, as hydrochloride: 60 mg, 80 mg, 120 mg, 160 mg
 InnoPran XL™: 80 mg, 120 mg

Capsule, sustained release, as hydrochloride:
 Inderal® LA: 60 mg, 80 mg, 120 mg, 160 mg

Injection, solution, as hydrochloride: 1 mg/mL (1 mL)
 Inderal®: 1 mg/mL (1 mL)

Solution, oral, as hydrochloride: 4 mg/mL (500 mL); 8 mg/mL (500 mL) [strawberry-mint flavor; contains alcohol 0.6%]

Tablet, as hydrochloride: 10 mg, 20 mg, 40 mg, 60 mg, 80 mg
 Inderal®: 10 mg, 20 mg, 40 mg; 60 mg [DSC]

Propranolol and Hydrochlorothiazide

(proe PRAN oh lole & hye droe klor oh THYE a zide)

Medication Safety Issues

Sound-alike/look-alike issues:
 Inderide® may be confused with Inderal®

U.S. Brand Names Inderide®

Index Terms Hydrochlorothiazide and Propranolol

Pharmacologic Category Beta Blocker, Nonselective; Diuretic, Thiazide

Use Management of hypertension

Effect on Mental Status Propranolol may cause fatigue and malaise which are commonly mistaken for depression; may also cause dizziness, confusion, insomnia, or hallucinations

Effect on Psychiatric Treatment Concurrent use with psychotropic drugs may produce additive hypotensive effects; monitor blood pressure. May decrease lithium clearance resulting in an increase in serum lithium levels and potential lithium toxicity; monitor serum lithium levels. Cutaneous reactions, including Stevens-Johnson syndrome, have been reported with use of propranolol; use caution with lamotrigine or valproic combination as combined usage with propranolol has been associated with these reactions.

Dosage Summary

Oral:

Children: Dosage not established

Adults: Propranolol 80-160 mg/day and hydrochlorothiazide 12.5-50 mg/day in 2 divided doses

Dosage Forms Excipient information presented when available (limited, particularly for generics); consult specific product labeling.

Tablet: Propranolol hydrochloride 40 mg and hydrochlorothiazide 25 mg; propranolol hydrochloride 80 mg and hydrochlorothiazide 25 mg
 Inderide®: 40/25: Propranolol hydrochloride 40 mg and hydrochlorothiazide 25 mg

- ◆ **Propranolol Hydrochloride** *see* Propranolol *on page 1355*
- ◆ **Proprinal [OTC]** *see* Ibuprofen *on page 803*
- ◆ **Proprinal® Cold and Sinus [OTC]** *see* Pseudoephedrine and Ibuprofen *on page 1369*
- ◆ **Propulsid®** *see* Cisapride *U.S. - Available Via Limited-Access Protocol Only on page 353*
- ◆ **2-Propylpentanoic Acid** *see* Valproic Acid and Derivatives *on page 1642*

Propylthiouracil (proe pil thye oh YOOR a sil)

Medication Safety Issues

Sound-alike/look-alike issues:
 Propylthiouracil may be confused with Purinethol®
 PTU is an error-prone abbreviation (mistaken as mercaptopurine [Purinethol®; 6-MP])

Canadian Brand Names Propyl-Thyracil®

Index Terms PTU (error-prone abbreviation)

Pharmacologic Category Antithyroid Agent; Thioamide

Use Palliative treatment of hyperthyroidism as an adjunct to ameliorate hyperthyroidism in preparation for surgical treatment or radioactive iodine therapy; management of thyrotoxic crisis

Effect on Mental Status May cause dizziness or drowsiness

Effect on Psychiatric Treatment Leukopenia is common; avoid clozapine and carbamazepine

Dosage Summary

Oral:

Children <6 years: Initial: 5-7 mg/kg/day **or** 150-200 mg/m^2/day in divided doses every 8 hours; Maintenance: 1/3 to 2/3 of the initial dose in divided doses every 8-12 hours

Children 6-10 years: Initial: 5-7 mg/kg/day **or** 150-200 mg/m^2/day **or** 50-150 mg/day in divided doses every 8 hours; Maintenance: 1/3 to 2/3 of the initial dose in divided doses every 8-12 hours

Children >10 years: Initial: 5-7 mg/kg/day **or** 150-200 mg/m^2/day **or** 150-300 mg/day in divided doses every 8 hours; Maintenance: 1/3 to 2/3 of the initial dose in divided doses every 8-12 hours

Adults: Initial: 300-450 mg/day divided every 8 hours; Maintenance: 100-150 mg/day divided every 8-12 hours (maximum: 1200 mg/day)

Elderly: Initial: 150-300 mg/day divided every 8 hours; Maintenance: 100-150 mg/day divided every 8-12 hours

Dosage Forms Excipient information presented when available (limited, particularly for generics); consult specific product labeling.

Tablet: 50 mg

- **2-Propylvaleric Acid** *see* Valproic Acid and Derivatives *on page 1642*
- **ProQuad®** *see* Measles, Mumps, Rubella, and Varicella Virus Vaccine *on page 972*
- **Proquin® XR** *see* Ciprofloxacin *on page 346*
- **Prosed®/DS** *see* Methenamine, Phenyl Salicylate, Methylene Blue, Benzoic Acid, and Hyoscyamine *on page 1009*
- **ProSom® [DSC]** *see* Estazolam *on page 574*
- **Prostacyclin** *see* Epoprostenol *on page 547*
- **Prostacyclin PGI$_2$** *see* Iloprost *on page 810*
- **Prostaglandin E$_1$** *see* Alprostadil *on page 77*
- **Prostaglandin E$_2$** *see* Dinoprostone *on page 480*
- **Prostaglandin F$_2$** *see* Carboprost Tromethamine *on page 282*
- **Prostigmin®** *see* Neostigmine *on page 1121*
- **Prostin E$_2$®** *see* Dinoprostone *on page 480*
- **Prostin VR Pediatric®** *see* Alprostadil *on page 77*

Protamine Sulfate (PROE ta meen SUL fate)

Medication Safety Issues

Sound-alike/look-alike issues:

Protamine may be confused with ProAmatine®, Protonix®, Protopam®, Protropin®

Pharmacologic Category Antidote

Use Treatment of heparin overdosage; neutralize heparin during surgery or dialysis procedures

Unlabeled/Investigational Use Treatment of low molecular weight heparin (LMWH) overdose

Effect on Mental Status May cause drowsiness

Effect on Psychiatric Treatment None reported

Dosage Summary

I.V.:

Children: 1 mg of protamine neutralizes 90 USP units of heparin (lung) and 115 USP units of heparin (intestinal) (maximum dose: 50 mg); **Note:** Dosage should be adjusted depending on the duration since heparin administration

Adults: 1 mg of protamine neutralizes 90 USP units of heparin (lung) and 115 USP units of heparin (intestinal) (maximum dose: 50 mg); **Note:** Dosage should be adjusted depending on the duration since heparin administration

Dosage Forms Excipient information presented when available (limited, particularly for generics); consult specific product labeling.

Injection, solution, as sulfate [preservative free]: 10 mg/mL (5 mL, 25 mL)

- **Protein-Bound Paclitaxel** *see* Paclitaxel (Protein Bound) *on page 1214*
- **Prothrombin Complex Concentrate** *see* Factor IX Complex (Human) *on page 612*

Protirelin (proe TYE re lin)

U.S. Brand Names Thyrel® TRH [DSC]

Canadian Brand Names Relefact® TRH

Index Terms Lopremone; Thyrotropin Releasing Hormone; TRH

Pharmacologic Category Diagnostic Agent

Use Adjunct in the diagnostic assessment of thyroid function, and an adjunct to other diagnostic procedures in patients with pituitary or hypothalamic dysfunction; also causes release of prolactin from the pituitary and is used to detect defective control of prolactin secretion

Effect on Mental Status Dizziness is common; may cause anxiety

Effect on Psychiatric Treatment None reported

Dosage Summary

I.V.:

Infants and Children <6 years: Experience limited, but doses of 7 mcg/kg have been administered

Children 6-16 years: 7 mcg/kg (maximum: 500 mcg)

Adults: 200-500 mcg

Dosage Forms Excipient information presented when available (limited, particularly for generics); consult specific product labeling.

Injection, solution: 500 mcg/mL (1 mL)

◆ **Protonix®** *see* Pantoprazole *on page 1221*

◆ **Protopam®** *see* Pralidoxime *on page 1318*

◆ **Protopic®** *see* Tacrolimus *on page 1533*

Protriptyline (proe TRIP ti leen)

Medication Safety Issues

Sound-alike/look-alike issues:

Vivactil® may be confused with Vyvanse™

Related Information

Antidepressant Agents *on page 1760*

Antidepressant Receptor Profile *on page 1764*

Discontinuation of Psychotropic Drugs *on page 1839*

U.S. Brand Names Vivactil®

Index Terms Protriptyline Hydrochloride

Pharmacologic Category Antidepressant, Tricyclic (Secondary Amine)

Generic Available Yes

Use Treatment of depression

Mental Health Comment Tricyclic antidepressants may be classified as tertiary (amitriptyline, doxepin, clomipramine, imipramine, trimipramine) or secondary amines (nortriptyline, desipramine, protriptyline). The tertiary amines are not recommended to treat depression in the elderly. If a TCA is used in the elderly, it should be a secondary amine. The tertiary amines are commonly used in low dosages for various conditions associated with pain. Toxicity is generally dose dependent. Relatively small overdoses (1-week supply) can be potentially fatal. Protriptyline is thought to have stimulating properties.

Restrictions An FDA-approved medication guide concerning the use of antidepressants in children, adolescents, and young adults must be distributed when dispensing an outpatient prescription (new or refill) where this medication is to be used without direct supervision of a healthcare provider. Medication guides are available at http://www.fda.gov/cder/Offices/ODS/medication_guides.htm. Dispense to parents or guardians of children and adolescents receiving this medication.

Pregnancy Risk Factor C

Lactation Excretion in breast milk unknown/not recommended

Contraindications Hypersensitivity to protriptyline (cross-reactivity to other cyclic antidepressants may occur) or any component of the formulation; use of MAO inhibitors within 14 days; use of cisapride; use in a patient during the acute recovery phase of MI

Warnings/Precautions **[U.S. Boxed Warning]: Antidepressants increase the risk of suicidal thinking and behavior in children, adolescents, and young adults (18-24 years of age) with major depressive disorder (MDD) and other psychiatric disorders;** consider risk prior to prescribing. Short-term studies did not show an increased risk in patients >24 years of age and showed a decreased risk in patients ≥65 years. Closely monitor for clinical worsening, suicidality, or unusual changes in behavior; the patient's family or caregiver should be instructed to closely observe the patient and communicate condition with healthcare provider. A medication guide should be dispensed with each prescription. **Protriptyline is FDA approved for the treatment of depression in adolescents.**

The possibility of a suicide attempt is inherent in major depression and may persist until remission occurs. Monitor for worsening of depression or suicidality, especially during initiation of therapy (generally first 1-2 months) or with dose increases or decreases. Use caution in high-risk patients. Worsening depression and severe abrupt suicidality that are not part of the presenting symptoms may require discontinuation or modification of drug therapy. The patient's family or caregiver should be alerted to monitor patients for the emergence of suicidality and associated behaviors (such as agitation, irritability, hostility, impulsivity, and hypomania) and call healthcare provider.

May worsen psychosis in some patients or precipitate a shift to mania or hypomania in patients with bipolar disorder. Patients presenting with depressive symptoms should be screened for bipolar disorder. Monotherapy in patients with bipolar disorder should be avoided. **Protriptyline is not FDA approved for the treatment of bipolar depression.**

TCAs may rarely cause bone marrow suppression; monitor for any signs of infection and obtain CBC if symptoms (eg, fever, sore throat) evident. Although the degree of sedation is low relative to other antidepressant agents, protriptyline may cause sedation, resulting in impaired performance of tasks requiring alertness (eg, operating machinery or driving). Sedative effects may be additive with other CNS depressants and/or ethanol. Protriptyline may aggravate aggressive behavior. Consider discontinuing, when possible, prior to elective surgery. Therapy should not be abruptly discontinued in patients receiving high doses for prolonged periods. May alter glucose regulation - use with caution in patients with diabetes.

May cause orthostatic hypotension or conduction abnormalities (risks are moderate relative to other antidepressants). Use with caution in patients with a history of cardiovascular disease (including previous MI, stroke, tachycardia, or conduction abnormalities). The degree of anticholinergic blockade produced by this agent is moderate relative to other cyclic antidepressants; however, caution should still be used in patients with urinary retention, benign prostatic hyperplasia, narrow-angle glaucoma, xerostomia, visual problems, constipation, or history of bowel obstruction.

Hyperpyrexia has been observed with TCAs in combination with anticholinergics and/or neuroleptics, particularly during hot weather. Use caution in patients with a previous seizure disorder or condition predisposing to seizures such as brain damage, alcoholism, or concurrent therapy with other drugs which lower the seizure threshold. May increase the risks associated with electroconvulsive therapy. Use with caution in hyperthyroid patients or those receiving thyroid supplementation. Use with caution in patients with hepatic or renal dysfunction and in elderly patients.

Adverse Reactions Frequency not defined.

Cardiovascular: Arrhythmias, heart block, hyper-/hypotension, MI, palpitation, stroke, tachycardia

Central nervous system: agitation, anxiety, ataxia, confusion, delirium, delusions, dizziness, drowsiness, EPS, exacerbation of psychosis, fatigue, hallucinations, headache, hypomania, incoordination, insomnia, nightmares, panic, restlessness, seizure

Dermatologic: Alopecia, itching, petechiae, photosensitivity, rash, urticaria

Endocrine & metabolic: Breast enlargement, galactorrhea, gynecomastia, increased or decreased libido, syndrome of inappropriate ADH secretion (SIADH)

Gastrointestinal: Anorexia, constipation, decreased lower esophageal sphincter tone may cause GE reflux, diarrhea, heartburn, increased appetite, nausea, trouble with gums, unpleasant taste, vomiting, weight gain/loss, xerostomia

Genitourinary: Difficult urination, impotence, testicular edema

Hematologic: Agranulocytosis, eosinophilia, leukopenia, purpura, thrombocytopenia

Hepatic: Cholestatic jaundice, increased liver enzymes

Neuromuscular & skeletal: Fine muscle tremor, numbness, tingling, tremor, weakness

Ocular: Blurred vision, eye pain, increased intraocular pressure

Otic: Tinnitus

Miscellaneous: Allergic reactions, excessive diaphoresis

Metabolism/Transport Effects Substrate of CYP2D6 (major)

Drug Interactions

Acetylcholinesterase Inhibitors (Central): Anticholinergics may diminish the therapeutic effect of Acetylcholinesterase Inhibitors (Central). Acetylcholinesterase Inhibitors (Central) may diminish the therapeutic effect of Anticholinergics. If the anticholinergic action is a side effect of the agent, the result may be beneficial. *Risk C: Monitor therapy*

Alcohol (Ethyl): CNS Depressants may enhance the CNS depressant effect of Alcohol (Ethyl). *Risk C: Monitor therapy*

Alfuzosin: May enhance the QTc-prolonging effect of QTc-Prolonging Agents. *Risk C: Monitor therapy*

Alpha-/Beta-Agonists (Direct-Acting): Tricyclic Antidepressants may enhance the vasopressor effect of Alpha-/Beta-Agonists (Direct-Acting). **Exceptions:** Dipivefrin. *Risk D: Consider therapy modification*

Alpha1-Agonists: Tricyclic Antidepressants may enhance the vasopressor effect of Alpha1-Agonists. *Risk D: Consider therapy modification*

Alpha2-Agonists: Tricyclic Antidepressants may diminish the antihypertensive effect of Alpha2-Agonists. **Exceptions:** Apraclonidine; Brimonidine. *Risk D: Consider therapy modification*

Altretamine: May enhance the orthostatic effect of Tricyclic Antidepressants. *Risk C: Monitor therapy*

Amphetamines: Tricyclic Antidepressants may enhance the stimulatory effect of Amphetamines. Tricyclic Antidepressants may also potentiate the cardiovascular effects of Amphetamines. *Risk C: Monitor therapy*

Anticholinergics: May enhance the adverse/toxic effect of other Anticholinergics. **Exceptions:** Paliperidone. *Risk C: Monitor therapy*

Barbiturates: May increase the metabolism of Tricyclic Antidepressants. *Risk D: Consider therapy modification*

Beta2-Agonists: Tricyclic Antidepressants may enhance the adverse/toxic effect of Beta2-Agonists. *Risk C: Monitor therapy*

CarBAMazepine: May increase the metabolism of Tricyclic Antidepressants. *Risk C: Monitor therapy*

Cimetidine: May decrease the metabolism of Tricyclic Antidepressants. *Risk C: Monitor therapy*

Cinacalcet: May increase the serum concentration of Tricyclic Antidepressants. *Risk C: Monitor therapy*

Ciprofloxacin: May enhance the QTc-prolonging effect of QTc-Prolonging Agents. *Risk C: Monitor therapy*

Cisapride: Protriptyline may enhance the arrhythmogenic effect of Cisapride. *Risk X: Avoid combination*

CNS Depressants: May enhance the adverse/toxic effect of other CNS Depressants. *Risk C: Monitor therapy*

CYP2D6 Inhibitors (Moderate): May decrease the metabolism of CYP2D6 Substrates. *Risk C: Monitor therapy*

CYP2D6 Inhibitors (Strong): May decrease the metabolism of CYP2D6 Substrates. *Risk D: Consider therapy modification*

Darunavir: May increase the serum concentration of CYP2D6 Substrates. *Risk C: Monitor therapy*

Desmopressin: Tricyclic Antidepressants may enhance the adverse/toxic effect of Desmopressin. *Risk C: Monitor therapy*

Dexmethylphenidate: May decrease the metabolism of Tricyclic Antidepressants. *Risk C: Monitor therapy*

DULoxetine: May decrease the metabolism of Tricyclic Antidepressants. *Risk C: Monitor therapy*

Gadobutrol: May enhance the QTc-prolonging effect of QTc-Prolonging Agents. *Risk D: Consider therapy modification*

Lithium: May enhance the neurotoxic effect of Tricyclic Antidepressants. *Risk C: Monitor therapy*

MAO Inhibitors: May enhance the serotonergic effect of Tricyclic Antidepressants. This may cause serotonin syndrome. *Risk X: Avoid combination*

Methylphenidate: May decrease the metabolism of Tricyclic Antidepressants. *Risk C: Monitor therapy*

Nilotinib: May enhance the QTc-prolonging effect of QTc-Prolonging Agents. *Risk X: Avoid combination*

Pramlintide: May enhance the anticholinergic effect of Anticholinergics. These effects are specific to the GI tract. *Risk D: Consider therapy modification*

Propoxyphene: May enhance the CNS depressant effect of Tricyclic Antidepressants. *Risk C: Monitor therapy*

Protease Inhibitors: May increase the serum concentration of Tricyclic Antidepressants. *Risk C: Monitor therapy*

QTc-Prolonging Agents: May enhance the adverse/toxic effect of other QTc-Prolonging Agents. Their effects can be additive, causing life-threatening ventricular arrhythmias. *Risk D: Consider therapy modification*

QuiNIDine: Tricyclic Antidepressants may enhance the QTc-prolonging effect of QuiNIDine. QuiNIDine may decrease the metabolism of Tricyclic Antidepressants. *Risk D: Consider therapy modification*

Selective Serotonin Reuptake Inhibitors: May decrease the metabolism of Tricyclic Antidepressants. *Risk D: Consider therapy modification*

Serotonin Modulators: May enhance the adverse/toxic effect of other Serotonin Modulators. The development of serotonin syndrome may occur. *Risk D: Consider therapy modification*

Sibutramine: May enhance the serotonergic effect of Serotonin Modulators. This may cause serotonin syndrome. *Risk X: Avoid combination*

St Johns Wort: May increase the metabolism of Tricyclic Antidepressants. The risk of serotonin syndrome may theoretically be increased. *Risk D: Consider therapy modification*

Sulfonylureas: Cyclic Antidepressants may enhance the hypoglycemic effect of Sulfonylureas. *Risk C: Monitor therapy*

Terbinafine: May decrease the metabolism of Tricyclic Antidepressants. *Risk D: Consider therapy modification*

Tetrabenazine: QTc-Prolonging Agents may enhance the QTc-prolonging effect of Tetrabenazine. *Risk X: Avoid combination*

Thioridazine: QTc-Prolonging Agents may enhance the QTc-prolonging effect of Thioridazine. *Risk X: Avoid combination*

TraMADol: Tricyclic Antidepressants may enhance the neuroexcitatory and/or seizure-potentiating effect of TraMADol. *Risk C: Monitor therapy*

Valproic Acid: May increase the serum concentration of Tricyclic Antidepressants. *Risk C: Monitor therapy*

Vitamin K Antagonists (eg, warfarin): Tricyclic Antidepressants may enhance the anticoagulant effect of Vitamin K Antagonists. *Risk C: Monitor therapy*

Ziprasidone: QTc-Prolonging Agents may enhance the QTc-prolonging effect of Ziprasidone. The risk of a severe arrhythmia may be increased. *Risk X: Avoid combination*

Ethanol/Nutrition/Herb Interactions

Ethanol: Avoid ethanol (may increase CNS depression).

Food: Grapefruit juice may inhibit the metabolism of some TCAs and clinical toxicity may result.

Herb/Nutraceutical: Avoid valerian, St John's wort, SAMe, kava kava (may increase risk of serotonin syndrome and/or excessive sedation).

Mechanism of Action Increases the synaptic concentration of serotonin and/or norepinephrine in the central nervous system by inhibition of their reuptake by the presynaptic neuronal membrane

Pharmacodynamics/Kinetics

Distribution: Crosses placenta

Protein binding: 92%

Metabolism: Extensively hepatic via N-oxidation, hydroxylation, and glucuronidation; first-pass effect (10% to 25%)

Half-life elimination: 54-92 hours (average: 74 hours)

Time to peak, serum: 24-30 hours

Excretion: Urine

Dosage Oral:

Adolescents: 15-20 mg/day

Adults: 15-60 mg/day in 3-4 divided doses

Elderly: Initial: 5-10 mg/day; increase every 3-7 days by 5-10 mg; usual dose: 15-20 mg/day

Dietary Considerations May be taken with food to decrease GI distress.

Administration Make any dosage increase in the morning dose

Monitoring Parameters Monitor for cardiac abnormalities in elderly patients receiving doses >20 mg; suicidal ideation (especially at the beginning of therapy or when doses are increased or decreased)

Reference Range Therapeutic: 70-250 ng/mL (SI: 266-950 nmol/L); Toxic: >500 ng/mL (SI: >1900 nmol/L)

Dosage Forms Excipient information presented when available (limited, particularly for generics); consult specific product labeling.

Tablet, as hydrochloride: 5 mg, 10 mg

Vivactil®: 5 mg, 10 mg

◆ **Protriptyline Hydrochloride** *see* Protriptyline *on page 1363*

◆ **Proventil® [DSC]** *see* Albuterol *on page 54*

◆ **Proventil® HFA** *see* Albuterol *on page 54*

◆ **Provera®** *see* MedroxyPROGESTERone *on page 975*

- **Provigil®** *see* Modafinil *on page 1065*
- **Proxymetacaine** *see* Proparacaine *on page 1352*
- **Prozac®** *see* FLUoxetine *on page 650*
- **Prozac® Weekly™** *see* FLUoxetine *on page 650*
- **PRP-OMP** *see Haemophilus* b Conjugate Vaccine *on page 753*
- **PRP-T** *see Haemophilus* b Conjugate Vaccine *on page 753*
- **Prudoxin™** *see* Doxepin *on page 502*
- **Prymaccone** *see* Primaquine *on page 1335*
- **P&S® [OTC]** *see* Salicylic Acid *on page 1454*
- **23PS** *see* Pneumococcal Polysaccharide Vaccine (Polyvalent) *on page 1309*
- **PS-341** *see* Bortezomib *on page 192*
- **Pseudacarb™** *see* Carbetapentane and Pseudoephedrine *on page 273*

Pseudoephedrine (soo doe e FED rin)

Medication Safety Issues

Sound-alike/look-alike issues:

Dimetapp® may be confused with Dermatop®, Dimetabs®, Dimetane®

Sudafed® may be confused with Sufenta®

U.S. Brand Names Genaphed® [OTC]; Kidkare Decongestant [OTC]; Nasofed™; Oranyl [OTC]; Silfedrine Children's [OTC]; Sudafed® 12 Hour [OTC]; Sudafed® 24 Hour [OTC]; Sudafed® Children's [OTC]; Sudafed® Maximum Strength Nasal Decongestant [OTC]; Sudo-Tab® [OTC]; SudoGest [OTC]; Unifed [OTC]

Canadian Brand Names Balminil Decongestant; Benylin® D for Infants; Contac® Cold 12 Hour Relief Non Drowsy; Drixoral® ND; Eltor®; PMS-Pseudoephedrine; Pseudofrin; Robidrine®; Sudafed® Decongestant

Mexican Brand Names Sudafed

Index Terms *d*-Isoephedrine Hydrochloride; Pseudoephedrine Hydrochloride; Pseudoephedrine Sulfate

Pharmacologic Category Alpha/Beta Agonist

Use Temporary symptomatic relief of nasal congestion due to common cold, upper respiratory allergies, and sinusitis; also promotes nasal or sinus drainage

Effect on Mental Status Dizziness, drowsiness, nervousness, and insomnia are common; may rarely cause hallucinations

Effect on Psychiatric Treatment Contraindicated with MAO inhibitors

Dosage Summary

Oral:

Hydrochloride salt:

Immediate release:

Children <2 years: 4 mg/kg/day divided every 6 hours

Children 2-5 years: 15 mg every 4-6 hours (maximum: 60 mg/day)

Children 6-12 years: 30 mg every 4-6 hours (maximum: 120 mg/day)

Adults: 30-60 mg every 4-6 hours (maximum: 240 mg/day)

Sustained release:

Children: Dosage not established

Adults: 120 mg every 12 hours (maximum: 240 mg/day)

Tannate salt:

Children <2 years: Dosage not established

Children 2-5 years: 1.25-2.5 mL (12.5-25 mg) every 12 hours

Children 6-11 years: 2.5-5 mL (25-50 mg) every 12 hours

Children ≥12 years: 5-10 mL (50-100 mg) every 12 hours

Adults: 5-10 mL (50-100 mg) every 12 hours

Dosage Forms Excipient information presented when available (limited, particularly for generics); consult specific product labeling.

Caplet, extended release, as hydrochloride:

Sudafed® 12 Hour: 120 mg

Liquid, as hydrochloride: 30 mg/5 mL (120 mL)

Silfedrine Children's: 15 mg/5 mL (120 mL, 480 mL) [alcohol and sugar free; grape flavor]

Sudafed® Children's: 15 mg/5 mL (120 mL) [alcohol and sugar free; contains sodium benzoate; grape flavor]

Unifed: 30 mg/5 mL (120 mL, 480 mL, 3840 mL)

Liquid, oral, as hydrochloride [drops]:

Kidkare Decongestant: 7.5 mg/0.8 mL (30 mL) [alcohol free; contains benzoic acid and sodium benzoate; cherry flavor]

Suspension, oral, as tannate:
Nasofed™: 50 mg/5 mL (118 mL) [contains phenylalanine 7 mg/5 mL, propylene glycol; strawberry flavor]
Syrup, as hydrochloride: 30 mg/5 mL (118 mL, 473 mL)
Tablet, as hydrochloride: 30 mg, 60 mg
Genaphed®, Oranyl, Sudafed®, Sudo-Tab®: 30 mg
SudoGest: 30 mg, 60 mg
Tablet, chewable, as hydrochloride:
Sudafed® Children's: 15 mg [sugar free; contains phenylalanine 0.78 mg/tablet; orange flavor]
Tablet, extended release, as hydrochloride:
Sudafed® 24 Hour: 240 mg

- **Pseudoephedrine, Acetaminophen, and Chlorpheniramine** *see* Acetaminophen, Chlorpheniramine, and Pseudoephedrine *on page 40*
- **Pseudoephedrine, Acetaminophen, and Dextromethorphan** *see* Acetaminophen, Dextromethorphan, and Pseudoephedrine *on page 43*
- **Pseudoephedrine and Acetaminophen** *see* Acetaminophen and Pseudoephedrine *on page 37*
- **Pseudoephedrine and Brompheniramine** *see* Brompheniramine and Pseudoephedrine *on page 206*
- **Pseudoephedrine and Carbetapentane** *see* Carbetapentane and Pseudoephedrine *on page 273*
- **Pseudoephedrine and Carbinoxamine** *see* Carbinoxamine and Pseudoephedrine *on page 280*
- **Pseudoephedrine and Chlorpheniramine** *see* Chlorpheniramine and Pseudoephedrine *on page 325*

Pseudoephedrine and Codeine (soo doe e FED rin & KOE deen)

U.S. Brand Names Nucofed®

Index Terms Codeine and Pseudoephedrine; Codeine Phosphate and Pseudoephedrine Hydrochloride; Pseudoephedrine Hydrochloride and Codeine Phosphate

Pharmacologic Category Antitussive/Decongestant

Use Temporary symptomatic relief of congestion and cough due to upper respiratory infections including common cold, bronchitis, sinusitis, and influenza

Effect on Mental Status May cause sedation, dizziness, insomnia, nervousness, and restlessness

Effect on Psychiatric Treatment May cause CNS depression; concurrent use with psychotropics, valerian, kava kava, and gotu kola may produce additive effects. Codeine may cause psychological and physical dependence; use caution in patients with a history of substance abuse. St John's wort may decrease codeine levels.

Restrictions C-III

Dosage Summary

Oral:

Children <12 years: Dosage not established
Children ≥12 years: One capsule every 6 hours as needed (maximum: 4 capsules/24 hours)
Adults: One capsule every 6 hours as needed (maximum: 4 capsules/24 hours)

Dosage Forms Excipient information presented when available (limited, particularly for generics); consult specific product labeling.

Capsule:
Nucofed®: Pseudoephedrine hydrochloride 60 mg and codeine phosphate 20 mg

- **Pseudoephedrine and Desloratadine** *see* Desloratadine and Pseudoephedrine *on page 431*
- **Pseudoephedrine and Dexbrompheniramine** *see* Dexbrompheniramine and Pseudoephedrine *on page 437*

Pseudoephedrine and Dextromethorphan

(soo doe e FED rin & deks troe meth OR fan)

U.S. Brand Names Pedia Relief Cough and Cold [OTC]; Pedia Relief Infants [OTC]; PediaCare® Infants' Decongestant & Cough [OTC] [DSC]; Sudafed® Children's Cold & Cough [OTC]; SudoGest Children's [OTC]

Canadian Brand Names Balminil DM D; Benylin® DM-D; Koffex DM-D; Novahistex® DM Decongestant; Novahistine® DM Decongestant; Robitussin® Childrens Cough & Cold

Index Terms Dextromethorphan and Pseudoephedrine

Pharmacologic Category Antitussive/Decongestant

Use Temporary symptomatic relief of nasal congestion and cough due to common cold, hay fever, upper respiratory allergies

Effect on Mental Status Dizziness, drowsiness, nervousness, and insomnia are common; may rarely cause hallucinations

Effect on Psychiatric Treatment Contraindicated with MAO inhibitors

Dosage Summary

Oral:

Children <2 years: Dosage not established

Children 2-6 years: 15 mg (based on pseudoephedrine) every 4-6 hours (maximum: 60 mg/day)

Children 6-12 years: 30 mg (based on pseudoephedrine) every 4-6 hours (maximum: 120 mg/day)

Children ≥12 years: 60 mg (based on pseudoephedrine) every 4-6 hours (maximum: 240 mg/day)

Adults: 60 mg (based on pseudoephedrine) every 4-6 hours (maximum: 240 mg/day)

Dosage Forms Excipient information presented when available (limited, particularly for generics); consult specific product labeling. [DSC] = Discontinued product

Liquid:

Sudafed® Children's Cold & Cough: Pseudoephedrine hydrochloride 15 mg and dextromethorphan hydrobromide 5 mg per 5 mL (120 mL) [alcohol free, sugar free; contains sodium benzoate; cherry berry flavor]

Liquid, oral [drops]:

PediaCare® Infants' Decongestant & Cough: Pseudoephedrine hydrochloride 7.5 mg and dextromethorphan hydrobromide 2.5 mg per 0.8 mL (15 mL) [alcohol free; contains sodium benzoate; cherry flavor] [DSC]

Pedia Relief Infants: Pseudoephedrine hydrochloride 7.5 mg and dextromethorphan hydrobromide 2.5 mg per 0.8 mL (15 mL) [cherry flavor]

Syrup:

Pedia Relief Cough and Cold: Pseudoephedrine hydrochloride 15 mg and dextromethorphan hydrobromide 7.5 mg per 5 mL (120 mL) [cherry flavor]

SudoGest Children's: Pseudoephedrine hydrochloride 15 mg and dextromethorphan hydrobromide 5 mg per 5 mL (120 mL)

◆ **Pseudoephedrine and Diphenhydramine** *see* Diphenhydramine and Pseudoephedrine *on page 486*

◆ **Pseudoephedrine and Fexofenadine** *see* Fexofenadine and Pseudoephedrine *on page 631*

◆ **Pseudoephedrine and Guaifenesin** *see* Guaifenesin and Pseudoephedrine *on page 744*

Pseudoephedrine and Ibuprofen

(soo doe e FED rin & eye byoo PROE fen)

U.S. Brand Names Advil® Cold & Sinus [OTC]; Advil® Cold, Children's [OTC] [DSC]; Proprinal® Cold and Sinus [OTC]

Canadian Brand Names Advil® Cold & Sinus; Children's Advil® Cold; Sudafed® Sinus Advance

Index Terms Ibuprofen and Pseudoephedrine

Pharmacologic Category Decongestant/Analgesic

Use For temporary relief of cold, sinus and flu symptoms (including nasal congestion, sinus pressure, headache, minor body aches and pains, and fever)

Effect on Mental Status Dizziness, drowsiness, nervousness, and insomnia are common; may rarely cause hallucinations, insomnia, confusion, or depression

Effect on Psychiatric Treatment Contraindicated with MAO inhibitors; may rarely cause agranulocytosis; use caution with clozapine and carbamazepine;

may decrease lithium clearance resulting in an increase in serum lithium levels and potential lithium toxicity; monitor serum lithium levels

Dosage Summary

Oral:

Children <12 years: Dosage not established

Children ≥12 years: 1-2 doses (ibuprofen 200 mg and pseudoephedrine 30 mg per dose) every 4-6 hours as needed (maximum: 6 doses/day)

Adults: 1-2 doses (ibuprofen 200 mg and pseudoephedrine 30 mg per dose) every 4-6 hours as needed (maximum: 6 doses/day)

Dosage Forms Excipient information presented when available (limited, particularly for generics); consult specific product labeling. [DSC] = Discontinued product

Caplet:

Advil® Cold and Sinus, Proprinal® Cold and Sinus: Pseudoephedrine hydrochloride 30 mg and ibuprofen 200 mg

Capsule, liquid filled:

Advil® Cold and Sinus: Pseudoephedrine hydrochloride 30 mg and ibuprofen 200 mg [solubilized ibuprofen as free acid and potassium salt; contains potassium 20 mg/capsule and coconut oil]

Suspension:

Advil® Cold, Children's: Pseudoephedrine hydrochloride 15 mg and ibuprofen 100 mg per 5 mL (120 mL) [alcohol free; contains sodium 3 mg/5 mL and sodium benzoate; grape flavor] [DSC]

◆ **Pseudoephedrine and Loratadine** *see* Loratadine and Pseudoephedrine *on page 948*

Pseudoephedrine and Methscopolamine

(soo doe e FED rin & meth skoe POL a meen)

U.S. Brand Names AlleRx™-D; Amdry-D; Extendryl PSE

Index Terms Methscopolamine and Pseudoephedrine; Pseudoephedrine hydrochloride and Methscopolamine Nitrate

Pharmacologic Category Decongestant/Anticholingeric Combination

Use Relief of symptoms of allergic rhinitis, vasomotor rhinitis, sinusitis, and the common cold

Effect on Mental Status May cause sedation, anxiety, dizziness, drowsiness, excitability, hallucinations, insomnia, irritability, nervousness, and restlessness

Effect on Psychiatric Treatment Contraindicated with or within 14 days of MAO inhibitor therapy. Concomitant use with psychotropics may produce additive anticholinergic and sedative effects especially in the elderly.

Dosage Summary

Oral:

Children <12 years: Dosage not established

Children ≥12 years: One tablet every 12 hours (maximum: 2 tablets/24 hours)

Adults: One tablet every 12 hours (maximum: 2 tablets/24 hours)

Dosage Forms Excipient information presented when available (limited, particularly for generics); consult specific product labeling.

Tablet: Pseudoephedrine hydrochloride 120 mg and methscopolamine nitrate 2.5 mg

Allerx™-D, Amdry-D: Pseudoephedrine hydrochloride 120 mg and methscopolamine nitrate 2.5 mg

Tablet, extended release:

Extendryl PSE: Pseudoephedrine hydrochloride 120 mg and methscopolamine nitrate 2.5 mg

◆ **Pseudoephedrine and Naproxen** *see* Naproxen and Pseudoephedrine *on page 1107*

◆ **Pseudoephedrine and Triprolidine** *see* Triprolidine and Pseudoephedrine *on page 1634*

◆ **Pseudoephedrine, Chlorpheniramine, and Acetaminophen** *see* Acetaminophen, Chlorpheniramine, and Pseudoephedrine *on page 40*

◆ **Pseudoephedrine, Chlorpheniramine, and Codeine** *see* Chlorpheniramine, Pseudoephedrine, and Codeine *on page 332*

◆ **Pseudoephedrine, Chlorpheniramine, and Dextromethorphan** *see* Chlorpheniramine, Pseudoephedrine, and Dextromethorphan *on page 333*

◆ **Pseudoephedrine, Chlorpheniramine, and Dihydrocodeine** *see* Pseudoephedrine, Dihydrocodeine, and Chlorpheniramine *on page 1371*

◆ **Pseudoephedrine, Codeine, and Triprolidine** *see* Triprolidine, Pseudoephedrine, and Codeine *on page 1635*

- **Pseudoephedrine, Dextromethorphan, and Acetaminophen** *see* Acetaminophen, Dextromethorphan, and Pseudoephedrine *on page 43*
- **Pseudoephedrine, Dextromethorphan, and Guaifenesin** *see* Guaifenesin, Pseudoephedrine, and Dextromethorphan *on page 748*

Pseudoephedrine, Dihydrocodeine, and Chlorpheniramine

(soo doe e FED rin, dye hye droe KOE deen, & klor fen IR a meen)

U.S. Brand Names Coldcough; DiHydro-CP; Hydro-Tussin™ DHC [DSC]; Pancof® [DSC]; Uni-Cof [DSC]

Index Terms Chlorpheniramine, Pseudoephedrine, and Dihydrocodeine; Dihydrocodeine Bitartrate, Pseudoephedrine Hydrochloride, and Chlorpheniramine Maleate; Pseudoephedrine, Chlorpheniramine, and Dihydrocodeine

Pharmacologic Category Alpha/Beta Agonist; Analgesic, Opioid; Antitussive; Histamine H_1 Antagonist; Histamine H_1 Antagonist, First Generation

Use Temporary relief of cough, congestion, and sneezing due to colds, respiratory infections, or hay fever

Effect on Mental Status Sedation is common

Effect on Psychiatric Treatment Contraindicated with or within 14 days of MAO inhibitor therapy. Fluoxetine, paroxetine, and ropinirole may decrease the effects of dihydrocodeine. Nefazodone may increase the effects of chlorpheniramine. Concomitant use with psychotropics may produce additive sedative and anticholinergic effects.

Mental Health Comment May cause paradoxical excitation in some patients. Chlorpheniramine is highly sedative and anticholinergic. Alternative therapy should be considered in the elderly.

Restrictions C-III

Dosage Summary

Oral:

Children <2 years: Dosage not established
Children 2-6 years: 1.25-2.5 mL every 4-6 hours (maximum: 4 doses/day)
Children 6-12 years: 2.5-5 mL every 4-6 hours (maximum: 4 doses/day)
Children >12 years: 5-10 mL every 4-6 hours (maximum: 4 doses/day)
Adults: 5-10 mL every 4-6 hours (maximum: 4 doses/day)

Dosage Forms Excipient information presented when available (limited, particularly for generics); consult specific product labeling. [DSC] = Discontinued product

Syrup:

Coldcough, Hydro-Tussin™ DHC [DSC], Pancof® [DSC], Uni-Cof [DSC]: Pseudoephedrine hydrochloride 15 mg, dihydrocodeine bitartrate 7.5 mg, and chlorpheniramine maleate 2 mg per 5 mL (480 mL) [alcohol free, dye free, sugar free; grape flavor]

DiHydro-CP: Pseudoephedrine hydrochloride 15 mg, dihydrocodeine bitartrate 7.5 mg, and chlorpheniramine maleate 2 mg per 5 mL (480 mL) [grape flavor]

- **Pseudoephedrine, Guaifenesin, and Codeine** *see* Guaifenesin, Pseudoephedrine, and Codeine *on page 747*
- **Pseudoephedrine Hydrochloride** *see* Pseudoephedrine *on page 1367*
- **Pseudoephedrine Hydrochloride and Acrivastine** *see* Acrivastine and Pseudoephedrine *on page 48*
- **Pseudoephedrine Hydrochloride and Cetirizine Hydrochloride** *see* Cetirizine and Pseudoephedrine *on page 309*
- **Pseudoephedrine Hydrochloride and Codeine Phosphate** *see* Pseudoephedrine and Codeine *on page 1368*
- **Pseudoephedrine Hydrochloride and Hydrocodone Bitartrate** *see* Hydrocodone and Pseudoephedrine *on page 781*
- **Pseudoephedrine hydrochloride and Methscopolamine Nitrate** *see* Pseudoephedrine and Methscopolamine *on page 1370*
- **Pseudoephedrine Hydrochloride, Guaifenesin, and Dihydrocodeine Bitartrate** *see* Dihydrocodeine, Pseudoephedrine, and Guaifenesin *on page 469*
- **Pseudoephedrine Hydrochloride, Hydrocodone Bitartrate, and Chlorpheniramine Maleate** *see* Pseudoephedrine, Hydrocodone, and Chlorpheniramine *on page 1372*
- **Pseudoephedrine Hydrochloride, Methscopolamine Nitrate, and Chlorpheniramine Maleate** *see* Chlorpheniramine, Pseudoephedrine, and Methscopolamine *on page 334*

◆ **Pseudoephedrine, Hydrocodone, and Carbinoxamine** *see* Hydrocodone, Carbinoxamine, and Pseudoephedrine *on page 782*

Pseudoephedrine, Hydrocodone, and Chlorpheniramine

(soo doe e FED rin, hye droe KOE done, & klor fen IR a meen)

U.S. Brand Names Atuss® HD [DSC]; Coldcough HC [DSC]; Detuss [DSC]; Hydron PSC [DSC]; Hyphed [DSC]

Canadian Brand Names Vasophrinic DH

Index Terms Chlorpheniramine, Pseudoephedrine, and Hydrocodone; Hydrocodone, Chlorpheniramine, and Pseudoephedrine; Pseudoephedrine Hydrochloride, Hydrocodone Bitartrate, and Chlorpheniramine Maleate

Pharmacologic Category Alpha/Beta Agonist; Analgesic, Opioid; Antitussive; Histamine H_1 Antagonist; Histamine H_1 Antagonist, First Generation

Use Temporary relief of cough, congestion, and sneezing due to colds, respiratory infections, or hay fever

Effect on Mental Status May cause dizziness, drowsiness, nervousness, insomnia, and sedation; may rarely cause hallucinations

Effect on Psychiatric Treatment Contraindicated with MAO inhibitors; concurrent use with psychotropics may produce additive sedation and dry mouth; may result in loss of pain control if used with fluoxetine and paroxetine

Restrictions C-III

Dosage Summary

Oral:

Children <2 years: Dosage not established

Children 2-6 years:

Hydro-Tussin™ HC: 1.25-2.5 mL every 4-6 hours (maximum: 4 doses/day)

Histinex® PV, P-V-Tussin®: 2.5 mL every 4-6 hours (maximum: 4 doses/day)

Children 6-12 years:

Histinex® PV, P-V-Tussin®: 5 mL **or** 1/2 tablet every 4-6 hours (maximum: 4 doses/day)

Hydro-Tussin™ HC: 2.5-5 mL **or** 1/2 tablet every 4-6 hours (maximum: 4 doses/day

Children >12 years:

Histinex® PV, P-V-Tussin®: 10 mL **or** 1 tablet every 4-6 hours (maximum: 4 doses/day)

Hydro-Tussin™ HC: 5-10 mL **or** 1 tablet every 4-6 hours; do not exceed 4 doses in 24 hours

Adults:

Histinex® PV, P-V-Tussin®: 10 mL **or** 1 tablet every 4-6 hours (maximum: 4 doses/day)

Hydro-Tussin™ HC: 5-10 mL **or** 1 tablet every 4-6 hours; do not exceed 4 doses in 24 hours

Dosage Forms Excipient information presented when available (limited, particularly for generics); consult specific product labeling. [DSC] = Discontinued product

Capsule, variable release:

Atuss® HD: Pseudoephedrine hydrochloride 30 mg [sustained release], hydrocodone bitartrate 5 mg [immediate release], and chlorpheniramine maleate 2 mg [sustained release] [DSC]

Liquid:

Detuss: Pseudoephedrine hydrochloride 30 mg, hydrocodone bitartrate 5 mg, and chlorpheniramine maleate 2 mg per 5 mL (480 mL) [alcohol free; vanilla flavor] [DSC]

Hydron PSC: Pseudoephedrine hydrochloride 30 mg, hydrocodone bitartrate 5 mg, and chlorpheniramine maleate 2 mg per 5 mL (480 mL) [vanilla flavor] [DSC]

Syrup:

Coldcough HC: Pseudoephedrine hydrochloride 15 mg, hydrocodone bitartrate 3 mg, and chlorpheniramine maleate 2 mg per 5 mL (480 mL) [alcohol free, dye free, sugar free; grape flavor] [DSC]

Hyphed: Pseudoephedrine hydrochloride 30 mg, hydrocodone bitartrate 2.5 mg, and chlorpheniramine maleate 2 mg per 5 mL (480 mL) [contains alcohol 5%; raspberry flavor] [DSC]

◆ **Pseudoephedrine, Hydrocodone, and Guaifenesin** *see* Hydrocodone, Pseudoephedrine, and Guaifenesin *on page 784*

◆ **Pseudoephedrine, Methscopolamine, and Chlorpheniramine** *see* Chlorpheniramine, Pseudoephedrine, and Methscopolamine *on page 334*

◆ **Pseudoephedrine Sulfate** *see* Pseudoephedrine *on page 1367*

- **Pseudoephedrine Tannate, Dextromethorphan Tannate, and Brompheniramine Tannate** *see* Brompheniramine, Pseudoephedrine, and Dextromethorphan *on page 208*
- **Pseudoephedrine, Triprolidine, and Codeine** *see* Triprolidine, Pseudoephedrine, and Codeine *on page 1635*
- **Pseudo GG TR** *see* Guaifenesin and Pseudoephedrine *on page 744*
- **Pseudo Max** *see* Guaifenesin and Pseudoephedrine *on page 744*
- **Pseudo Max DMX** *see* Guaifenesin, Pseudoephedrine, and Dextromethorphan *on page 748*
- **Pseudomonic Acid A** *see* Mupirocin *on page 1085*
- **Pseudovent™ [DSC]** *see* Guaifenesin and Pseudoephedrine *on page 744*
- **Pseudovent™ 400 [DSC]** *see* Guaifenesin and Pseudoephedrine *on page 744*
- **Pseudovent™ DM [DSC]** *see* Guaifenesin, Pseudoephedrine, and Dextromethorphan *on page 748*
- **Pseudovent™-Ped [DSC]** *see* Guaifenesin and Pseudoephedrine *on page 744*
- **P-Tann D** *see* Chlorpheniramine and Phenylephrine *on page 323*
- **Pteroylglutamic Acid** *see* Folic Acid *on page 684*
- **PTU (error-prone abbreviation)** *see* Propylthiouracil *on page 1361*
- **Pulmicort Flexhaler™** *see* Budesonide *on page 210*
- **Pulmicort Respules®** *see* Budesonide *on page 210*
- **Purinethol®** *see* Mercaptopurine *on page 993*
- **Purple Coneflower** *see* Echinacea *(Echinacea purpurea, Echinacea angustifolia) on page 523*
- **Pylera™** *see* Bismuth, Metronidazole, and Tetracycline *on page 190*

Pyrantel Pamoate (pi RAN tel PAM oh ate)

U.S. Brand Names Pin-X® [OTC]; Reese's® Pinworm Medicine [OTC]

Canadian Brand Names Combantrin™

Pharmacologic Category Anthelmintic

Use Treatment of pinworms (*Enterobius vermicularis*) and roundworms (*Ascaris lumbricoides*)

Unlabeled/Investigational Use Treatment of whipworms (*Trichuris trichiura*) and hookworms (*Ancylostoma duodenale*)

Effect on Mental Status May cause dizziness, drowsiness, or insomnia

Effect on Psychiatric Treatment None reported

Dosage Summary

Oral:

Children: 11 mg/kg as a single dose (maximum: 1 g/dose); repeat in 2 weeks for pinworm (dose is expressed as pyrantel base)

Adults: 11 mg/kg as a single dose (maximum: 1 g/dose); repeat in 2 weeks for pinworm (dose is expressed as pyrantel base)

Dosage Forms Excipient information presented when available (limited, particularly for generics); consult specific product labeling.

Caplet, as pamoate:

Reese's® Pinworm Medicine: 180 mg [equivalent to pyrantel base 62.5 mg/tablet]

Suspension, oral as pamoate:

Pin-X®: 144 mg/mL (30 mL, 60 mL) [equivalent to pyrantel base 50 mg/mL; sugar free; contains sodium benzoate; caramel flavor]

Reese's® Pinworm Medicine: 144 mg/mL (30 mL) [equivalent to pyrantel base 50 mg/mL]

Tablet, chewable, as pamoate:

Pin-X®: 720.5 mg [equivalent to pyrantel base 250 mg/tablet; contains aspartame; orange flavor]

Pyrazinamide (peer a ZIN a mide)

Canadian Brand Names Tebrazid™

Mexican Brand Names Rifater

Index Terms Pyrazinoic Acid Amide

Pharmacologic Category Antitubercular Agent

Use Adjunctive treatment of tuberculosis in combination with other antituberculosis agents

Effect on Mental Status May cause drowsiness

Effect on Psychiatric Treatment None reported

Dosage Summary

Note: Dosing in adults is based on lean body weight.

Oral:

Children: 15-30 mg/kg once daily (maximum: 2 g/day) **or** 50 mg/kg/dose twice weekly (maximum: 4 g/dose)

Adults 40-55 kg: 1000 mg (15-30 mg/kg) once daily **or** 2000 mg (50 mg/kg) twice weekly **or** 1500 mg (25-30 mg/kg) three times/week

Adults: 56-75 kg: 1500 mg (15-30 mg/kg) once daily **or** 3000 mg (50 mg/kg) twice weekly **or** 2500 mg (25-30 mg/kg) three times/week

Adults 76-90 kg: 2000 mg (15-30 mg/kg) once daily (maximum: 2 g/day) **or** 4000 mg (50 mg/kg) twice weekly (maximum: 4000 mg/dose) **or** 3000 mg (25-30 mg/kg) three times/week (maximum: 3000 mg/dose)

Elderly: Start with a lower daily dose (15 mg/kg) and increase as tolerated

Dosage Forms Excipient information presented when available (limited, particularly for generics); consult specific product labeling.

Tablet: 500 mg

◆ **Pyrazinamide, Rifampin, and Isoniazid** *see* Rifampin, Isoniazid, and Pyrazinamide *on page 1419*

◆ **Pyrazinoic Acid Amide** *see* Pyrazinamide *on page 1373*

◆ **Pyri-500 [OTC]** *see* Pyridoxine *on page 1376*

◆ **2-Pyridine Aldoxime Methochloride** *see* Pralidoxime *on page 1318*

◆ **Pyridium®** *see* Phenazopyridine *on page 1258*

Pyridostigmine (peer id oh STIG meen)

Medication Safety Issues

Sound-alike/look-alike issues:

Pyridostigmine may be confused with physostigmine

Mestinon® may be confused with Metatensin®

Regonol® may be confused with Reglan®, Renagel®

U.S. Brand Names Mestinon®; Mestinon® Timespan®; Regonol®

Canadian Brand Names Mestinon®; Mestinon®-SR

Mexican Brand Names Mestinon

Index Terms Pyridostigmine Bromide

Pharmacologic Category Acetylcholinesterase Inhibitor

Generic Available Yes: Tablet

Use Symptomatic treatment of myasthenia gravis; antidote for nondepolarizing neuromuscular blockers

Military use: Pretreatment for Soman nerve gas exposure

Effect on Mental Status May rarely cause dysphoria or drowsiness

Effect on Psychiatric Treatment None reported; but mouth watering is common and may be additive to the sialorrhea associated with clozapine therapy

Pregnancy Risk Factor B

Pregnancy Considerations Safety has not been established for use during pregnancy. The potential benefit to the mother should outweigh the potential risk to the fetus. When pyridostigmine is needed in myasthenic mothers, giving dose parenterally 1 hour before completion of the second stage of labor may facilitate delivery and protect the neonate during the immediate postnatal state.

Lactation Enters breast milk/compatible

Contraindications Hypersensitivity to pyridostigmine, bromides, or any component of the formulation; GI or GU obstruction

Warnings/Precautions Use with caution in patients with epilepsy, asthma, bradycardia, hyperthyroidism, cardiac arrhythmias, or peptic ulcer; adequate facilities should be available for cardiopulmonary resuscitation when testing and adjusting dose for myasthenia gravis; have atropine and epinephrine ready to treat hypersensitivity reactions; overdosage may result in cholinergic crisis, this must be distinguished from myasthenic crisis; anticholinesterase insensitivity can develop for brief or prolonged periods. Regonol® injection contains 1% benzyl alcohol as the preservative (not intended for use in newborns). **[U.S. Boxed Warning]: Regonol® injection must be administered by trained personnel.**

Adverse Reactions Frequency not defined.

Cardiovascular: Arrhythmias (especially bradycardia), AV block, cardiac arrest, decreased carbon monoxide, flushing, hypotension, nodal rhythm, nonspecific ECG changes, syncope, tachycardia

Central nervous system: Convulsions, dizziness, drowsiness, dysphonia, headache, loss of consciousness
Dermatologic: Skin rash, thrombophlebitis (I.V.), urticaria
Gastrointestinal: Abdominal pain, diarrhea, dysphagia, flatulence, hyperperistalsis, nausea, salivation, stomach cramps, vomiting
Genitourinary: Urinary urgency
Neuromuscular & skeletal: Arthralgia, dysarthria, fasciculations, muscle cramps, myalgia, spasms, weakness
Ocular: Amblyopia, lacrimation, small pupils
Respiratory: Bronchial secretions increased, bronchiolar constriction, bronchospasm, dyspnea, laryngospasm, respiratory arrest, respiratory depression, respiratory muscle paralysis
Miscellaneous: Allergic reactions, anaphylaxis, diaphoresis increased

Drug Interactions

Beta-Blockers: Acetylcholinesterase Inhibitors may enhance the bradycardic effect of Beta-Blockers. **Exceptions:** Levobunolol; Metipranolol. *Risk C: Monitor therapy*
Cholinergic Agonists: Acetylcholinesterase Inhibitors may enhance the adverse/toxic effect of Cholinergic Agonists. *Risk C: Monitor therapy*
Corticosteroids (Systemic): May enhance the adverse/toxic effect of Acetylcholinesterase Inhibitors. Increased muscular weakness may occur. *Risk C: Monitor therapy*
Ginkgo Biloba: May enhance the adverse/toxic effect of Acetylcholinesterase Inhibitors. *Risk C: Monitor therapy*
Methocarbamol: May diminish the therapeutic effect of Pyridostigmine. *Risk C: Monitor therapy*
Neuromuscular-Blocking Agents (Nondepolarizing): Acetylcholinesterase Inhibitors may diminish the neuromuscular-blocking effect of Neuromuscular-Blocking Agents (Nondepolarizing). Acetylcholinesterase Inhibitors may decrease the metabolism of Neuromuscular-Blocking Agents (Nondepolarizing). This is only true for mivacurium in which case the neuromuscular blocking effects might be prolonged. *Risk C: Monitor therapy*
Succinylcholine: Acetylcholinesterase Inhibitors may enhance the neuromuscular-blocking effect of Succinylcholine. *Risk C: Monitor therapy*

Stability

Injection: Protect from light.
Tablet:
30 mg: Store under refrigeration at 2°C to 8°C (36°F to 46°F). Protect from light. Stable at room temperature for up to 3 months.
Mestinon®: Store at 25°C (77°F). Protect from moisture.

Mechanism of Action Inhibits destruction of acetylcholine by acetylcholinesterase which facilitates transmission of impulses across myoneural junction

Pharmacodynamics/Kinetics

Onset of action: Oral, I.M.: 15-30 minutes; I.V. injection: 2-5 minutes
Duration: Oral: Up to 6-8 hours (due to slow absorption); I.V.: 2-3 hours
Absorption: Oral: Very poor
Distribution: 19 ± 12 L
Metabolism: Hepatic
Bioavailability: 10% to 20%
Half-life elimination: 1-2 hours; Renal failure: ≤6 hours
Excretion: Urine (80% to 90% as unchanged drug)

Dosage

Myasthenia gravis:
Oral:
Children: 7 mg/kg/24 hours divided into 5-6 doses
Adults: Highly individualized dosing ranges: 60-1500 mg/day, usually 600 mg/day divided into 5-6 doses, spaced to provide maximum relief
Sustained release formulation: Highly individualized dosing ranges: 180-540 mg once or twice daily (doses separated by at least 6 hours); **Note:** Most clinicians reserve sustained release dosage form for bedtime dose only.
I.M., slow I.V. push:
Children: 0.05-0.15 mg/kg/dose
Adults: To supplement oral dosage pre- and postoperatively during labor and postpartum, during myasthenic crisis, or when oral therapy is impractical: ~1/30th of oral dose; observe patient closely for cholinergic reactions
or
I.V. infusion: Initial: 2 mg/hour with gradual titration in increments of 0.5-1 mg/hour, up to a maximum rate of 4 mg/hour

Pretreatment for Soman nerve gas exposure (military use): Oral: Adults: 30 mg every 8 hours beginning several hours prior to exposure; discontinue at first sign of nerve agent exposure, then begin atropine and pralidoxime

Reversal of nondepolarizing muscle relaxants: **Note:** Atropine sulfate (0.6-1.2 mg) I.V. immediately prior to pyridostigmine to minimize side effects: I.V.:

Children: Dosing range: 0.1-0.25 mg/kg/dose*

Adults: 0.1-0.25 mg/kg/dose; 10-20 mg is usually sufficient*

*Full recovery usually occurs ≤15 minutes, but ≥30 minutes may be required

Dosage adjustment in renal dysfunction: Lower dosages may be required due to prolonged elimination; no specific recommendations have been published

Administration Do **not** crush sustained release tablet.

Monitoring Parameters Observe for cholinergic reactions, particularly when administered I.V.

Test Interactions Increased aminotransferase [ALT/AST] (S), increased amylase (S)

Dosage Forms Excipient information presented when available (limited, particularly for generics); consult specific product labeling.

Injection, solution, as bromide:

Regonol®: 5 mg/mL (2 mL) [contains benzyl alcohol]

Syrup, as bromide:

Mestinon®: 60 mg/5 mL (480 mL) [raspberry flavor; contains alcohol 5%, sodium benzoate]

Tablet, as bromide: 60 mg

Mestinon®: 60 mg

Tablet, sustained release, as bromide:

Mestinon® Timespan®: 180 mg

◆ **Pyridostigmine Bromide** *see* Pyridostigmine *on page 1374*

Pyridoxine (peer i DOKS een)

Medication Safety Issues

Sound-alike/look-alike issues:

Pyridoxine may be confused with paroxetine, pralidoxime, Pyridium®

Related Information

Anticonvulsants By Seizure Type *on page 1759*

U.S. Brand Names Aminoxin [OTC]; Pyri-500 [OTC]

Mexican Brand Names Bedoyecta; Dodemina; Dolo Bedoyecta; Dolvifen; Incremin con hierro; M. V. I. 12; Natele; Nuro-B; Pharmaton; Poly-B con Vitamina C; Trineurovita

Index Terms Pyridoxine Hydrochloride; Vitamin B_6

Pharmacologic Category Vitamin, Water Soluble

Use Prevention and treatment of vitamin B_6 deficiency, pyridoxine-dependent seizures in infants

Unlabeled/Investigational Use Treatment and prophylaxis of neurological toxicities (ie, seizures, coma) associated with isoniazid, hydrazine, and Gyromitrin-containing mushroom (false morel) overdose/toxicity

Effect on Mental Status None reported

Effect on Psychiatric Treatment May decrease the effects of levodopa and phenobarbital

Dosage Summary

I.M.:

Infants: Deficiency: 10-100 mg

Children:

Hydrazine toxicity: 25 mg/kg in divided doses

INH toxicity: Dose equal to the amount of INH ingested (5 g if ingested dose unknown)

Adults:

Hydrazine toxicity: 25 mg/kg in divided doses

INH toxicity: Dose equal to the amount of INH ingested (5 g if ingested dose unknown)

I.V.:

Infants: Deficiency: 10-100 mg

Children:

Hydrazine toxicity: 25 mg/kg in divided doses

INH toxicity: Dose equal to the amount of INH ingested (5 g if ingested dose unknown)

Adults:

Hydrazine toxicity: 25 mg/kg in divided doses

INH toxicity: Dose equal to the amount of INH ingested (5 g if ingested dose unknown)

Oral:

Infants: Deficiency: 2-100 mg/day

Children:

Deficiency: 1.5-25 mg/day

Neuritis: Prophylaxis: 1-2 mg/kg/day; Treatment: 10-50 mg/day

Adults:

Deficiency: 10-20 mg/day

Neuritis: Prophylaxis: 25-100 mg/day; Treatment: 100-200 mg/day

SubQ:

Infants: Deficiency: 10-100 mg

Children: Dosage not established

Adults: Dosage not established

Dosage Forms Excipient information presented when available (limited, particularly for generics); consult specific product labeling.

Capsule, as hydrochloride: 50 mg, 250 mg

Aminoxin: 20 mg

Injection, solution, as hydrochloride: 100 mg/mL (1 mL)

Liquid, oral, as hydrochloride: 200 mg/5 mL (120 mL)

Tablet, as hydrochloride: 25 mg, 50 mg, 100 mg, 250 mg, 500 mg

Tablet, sustained release, as hydrochloride:

Pyri-500: 500 mg

- ◆ **Pyridoxine and Doxylamine** *see* Doxylamine and Pyridoxine *on page 511*
- ◆ **Pyridoxine Hydrochloride** *see* Pyridoxine *on page 1376*
- ◆ **Pyrilafen Tannate-12™** *see* Phenylephrine and Pyrilamine *on page 1275*
- ◆ **Pyrilamine Maleate, Dextromethorphan Hydrobromide, and Phenylephrine Hydrochloride** *see* Phenylephrine, Pyrilamine, and Dextromethorphan *on page 1278*
- ◆ **Pyrilamine, Phenylephrine, and Carbetapentane** *see* Carbetapentane, Phenylephrine, and Pyrilamine *on page 275*
- ◆ **Pyrilamine Tannate and Phenylephrine Tannate** *see* Phenylephrine and Pyrilamine *on page 1275*
- ◆ **Pyrilamine Tannate, Guaifenesin, and Phenylephrine Tannate** *see* Phenylephrine, Pyrilamine, and Guaifenesin *on page 1279*

Pyrimethamine (peer i METH a meen)

Medication Safety Issues

Sound-alike/look-alike issues:

Daraprim® may be confused with Dantrium®, Daranide®

U.S. Brand Names Daraprim®

Canadian Brand Names Daraprim®

Mexican Brand Names Daraprim

Pharmacologic Category Antimalarial Agent

Use Prophylaxis of malaria due to susceptible strains of plasmodia; used in conjunction with quinine and sulfadiazine for the treatment of uncomplicated attacks of chloroquine-resistant *P. falciparum* malaria; used in conjunction with fast-acting schizonticide to initiate transmission control and suppression cure; synergistic combination with sulfonamide in treatment of toxoplasmosis

Effect on Mental Status May rarely cause drowsiness, insomnia, or depression

Effect on Psychiatric Treatment May cause leukopenia; use caution with clozapine and carbamazepine; mild hepatotoxicity associated with concurrent usage of lorazepam

Dosage Forms Excipient information presented when available (limited, particularly for generics); consult specific product labeling.

Tablet: 25 mg

- ◆ **Pyrimethamine and Sulfadoxine** *see* Sulfadoxine and Pyrimethamine *on page 1517*
- ◆ **QDALL® [DSC]** *see* Chlorpheniramine and Pseudoephedrine *on page 325*
- ◆ **QDALL® AR** *see* Chlorpheniramine *on page 321*
- ◆ **Quadrivalent Meningococcal Conjugate Vaccine** *see* Meningococcal Polysaccharide (Groups A / C / Y and W-135) Diphtheria Toxoid Conjugate Vaccine *on page 985*

◆ **Quadrivalent Meningococcal Conjugate Vaccine** *see* Meningococcal Polysaccharide Vaccine (Groups A / C / Y and W-135) *on page 985*

◆ **Quad Tann®** *see* Chlorpheniramine, Ephedrine, Phenylephrine, and Carbetapentane *on page 326*

◆ **Quad Tann® Pediatric** *see* Chlorpheniramine, Ephedrine, Phenylephrine, and Carbetapentane *on page 326*

◆ **Qualaquin™** *see* QuiNINE *on page 1388*

◆ **Quartuss™** *see* Dextromethorphan, Chlorpheniramine, Phenylephrine, and Guaifenesin *on page 450*

◆ **Quasense™** *see* Ethinyl Estradiol and Levonorgestrel *on page 595*

Quazepam (KWAZ e pam)

Medication Safety Issues

Sound-alike/look-alike issues:

Quazepam may be confused with oxazepam

Related Information

Benzodiazepines *on page 1774*

CMS: Long-Term Care Facility Thresholds *on page 1815*

Discontinuation of Psychotropic Drugs *on page 1839*

U.S. Brand Names Doral®

Canadian Brand Names Doral®

Pharmacologic Category Benzodiazepine

Generic Available No

Use Treatment of insomnia

Mental Health Comment In 2007, the FDA requested that all manufacturers of sedative-hypnotic drug products revise labeling to include a greater emphasis on the risks of adverse effects. These risks include severe allergic reactions (anaphylaxis, angioedema) and complex sleep-related behaviors, which may include sleep-driving (driving while not fully awake and with no memory of the event), making phone calls, and preparing and eating food while asleep.

There are two subtypes of GABA receptors (GABA-A and GABA-B) and three different benzodiazepine receptors (Bz_1, Bz_2, and Bz_3). Benzodiazepine receptors and effects appear to be linked to the GABA-A receptors. Benzodiazepines do not bind to GABA-B receptors. The role of GABA-B receptors is unclear. Benzodiazepines have no specificity for benzodiazepine receptor subtypes.

Quazepam is a long half-life benzodiazepine. Duration of action after a single dose is determined by redistribution rather than metabolism. Tolerance develops to the sedative, hypnotic, and anticonvulsant effects. It does not develop to the anxiolytic or skeletal muscle relaxing effects. Psychological and physical dependence may occur with prolonged use of benzodiazepines. The onset of withdrawal symptoms is usually seen on the first day without drug and lasts 5-7 days in patients receiving short half-life benzodiazepines, whereas, the onset occurs after 5 days with a duration of 10-14 days after abrupt discontinuance of long half-life benzodiazepines. Risk factors for abuse include personal or family history of substance abuse and personality disorder.

Restrictions C-IV

Pregnancy Risk Factor X

Pregnancy Considerations Adverse events were observed in animal studies. An increased risk of congenital malformations has been observed with other benzodiazepines following exposure during the 1st trimester. Withdrawal symptoms in the neonate and neonatal flaccidity have been reported following maternal use of benzodiazepines during pregnancy. Use during pregnancy is contraindicated.

Lactation Enters breast milk/not recommended (AAP rates "of concern")

Contraindications Hypersensitivity to quazepam, other benzodiazepines, or any component of the formulation; sleep apnea; pregnancy

Note: Product labeling does not include narrow-angle glaucoma; however, use in narrow-angle glaucoma is contraindicated with other benzodiazepines.

Warnings/Precautions Should be used only after evaluation of potential causes of sleep disturbance. Failure of sleep disturbance to resolve after 7-10 days may indicate psychiatric or medical illness. A worsening of insomnia or the emergence of new abnormalities of thought or behavior may represent unrecognized psychiatric or medical illness and requires immediate and careful evaluation. Use with caution in elderly or debilitated patients, patients with hepatic disease (including alcoholics), or renal impairment. Use with caution in patients with respiratory disease or impaired gag reflex. Avoid use in patients with sleep apnea.

Causes CNS depression (dose related) resulting in sedation, dizziness, confusion, or ataxia which may impair physical and mental capabilities. Patients must be cautioned about performing tasks which require mental alertness (operating machinery or driving). Use with caution in patients receiving other CNS depressants or psychoactive agents. Postmarketing studies have indicated that the use of hypnotic/sedative agents for sleep has been associated with hypersensitivity reactions including anaphylaxis as well as angioedema. An increased risk for hazardous sleep-related activities such as sleep-driving; cooking and eating food, and making phone calls while asleep have also been noted. Effects with other sedative drugs or ethanol may be potentiated. Benzodiazepines have been associated with falls and traumatic injury and should be used with extreme caution in patients who are at risk of these events (especially the elderly).

Use caution in patients with depression, particularly if suicidal risk may be present. Use with caution in patients with a history of drug dependence. Benzodiazepines have been associated with dependence and acute withdrawal symptoms on discontinuation or reduction in dose. Acute withdrawal, including seizures, may be precipitated after administration of flumazenil to patients receiving long-term benzodiazepine therapy.

Benzodiazepines have been associated with anterograde amnesia. Paradoxical reactions, including hyperactive or aggressive behavior have been reported with benzodiazepines, particularly in adolescent/pediatric or psychiatric patients. Does not have analgesic, antidepressant, or antipsychotic properties. Use lowest effective dose. Safety and efficacy have not been established in pediatric patients.

Adverse Reactions

>10%: Central nervous system: Daytime drowsiness (12%)

<10%:

Central nervous system: Headache (5%), dizziness (2%), fatigue (2%)

Gastrointestinal: Xerostomia (2%), dyspepsia (1%)

Frequency not defined. **Note:** Asterisked (*) reactions are those reported with benzodiazepines.

Cardiovascular: Palpitation

Central nervous system: Abnormal thinking, agitation, amnesia, anxiety, apathy, ataxia, confusion, depression, dystonia*, euphoria, hallucinations*, hyper-/hypokinesia, incoordination, irritability*, malaise, memory impairment*, nervousness, nightmare, paranoid reaction, sleep disturbances*, slurred speech*, speech disorder, stimulation*

Dermatologic: Dermatitis*, pruritus, rash

Endocrine & metabolic: Libido decreased, menstrual irregularities*

Gastrointestinal: Abdominal pain, abnormal taste perception, anorexia, appetite increased/decreased*, constipation, diarrhea, nausea

Genitourinary: Impotence, incontinence, urinary retention*

Hematologic: Blood dyscrasias

Hepatic: Jaundice*, SGOT increased

Neuromuscular & skeletal: Dysarthria*, muscle cramps*, muscle spasticity*, reflex slowing*, rigidity*, tremor, weakness

Ocular: Abnormal vision, blurred vision*, cataract

Miscellaneous: Drug dependence, withdrawal*

Postmarketing and/or case reports: Anaphylaxis, angioedema, complex sleep-related behavior (sleep-driving, cooking or eating food, making phone calls)

Metabolism/Transport Effects **Substrate** of CYP2C19 (major), and CYP3A4 (major)

Drug Interactions

Alcohol (Ethyl): CNS Depressants may enhance the CNS depressant effect of Alcohol (Ethyl). *Risk C: Monitor therapy*

Aprepitant: May increase the serum concentration of Benzodiazepines (metabolized by oxidation). *Risk C: Monitor therapy*

Calcium Channel Blockers (Nondihydropyridine): May decrease the metabolism of Benzodiazepines (metabolized by oxidation). *Risk D: Consider therapy modification*

CarBAMazepine: May increase the metabolism of Benzodiazepines (metabolized by oxidation). *Risk C: Monitor therapy*

Cimetidine: May decrease the metabolism of Benzodiazepines (metabolized by oxidation). *Risk C: Monitor therapy*

Clozapine: Benzodiazepines may enhance the adverse/toxic effect of Clozapine. *Risk D: Consider therapy modification*

CNS Depressants: May enhance the adverse/toxic effect of other CNS Depressants. *Risk C: Monitor therapy*

Disulfiram: May decrease the metabolism of Benzodiazepines (metabolized by oxidation). *Risk C: Monitor therapy*

Fluconazole: May decrease the metabolism of Benzodiazepines (metabolized by oxidation). *Risk D: Consider therapy modification*

Fosaprepitant: May increase the serum concentration of Benzodiazepines (metabolized by oxidation). Specifically, the active metabolite aprepitant is likely responsible for this effect. *Risk C: Monitor therapy*

Grapefruit Juice: May decrease the metabolism of Benzodiazepines (metabolized by oxidation). *Risk D: Consider therapy modification*

Isoniazid: May decrease the metabolism of Benzodiazepines (metabolized by oxidation). *Risk C: Monitor therapy*

Macrolide Antibiotics: May decrease the metabolism of Benzodiazepines (metabolized by oxidation). **Exceptions:** Azithromycin; Dirithromycin [Off Market]; Spiramycin. *Risk D: Consider therapy modification*

Nefazodone: May decrease the metabolism of Benzodiazepines (metabolized by oxidation). *Risk D: Consider therapy modification*

Oral Contraceptive (Estrogens): May decrease the metabolism of Benzodiazepines (metabolized by oxidation). *Risk C: Monitor therapy*

Oral Contraceptive (Progestins): May decrease the metabolism of Benzodiazepines (metabolized by oxidation). *Risk C: Monitor therapy*

Phenytoin: Benzodiazepines may increase the serum concentration of Phenytoin. Short-term exposure to benzodiazepines may not present as much risk as chronic therapy. *Risk C: Monitor therapy*

Protease Inhibitors: May decrease the metabolism of Benzodiazepines (metabolized by oxidation). Management: Amprenavir, atazanavir, darunavir, indinavir, nelfinavir, ritonavir, and tipranavir are contraindicated with midazolam and triazolam according to each protease inhibitor 's prescribing information. *Risk D: Consider therapy modification*

Proton Pump Inhibitors: May increase the serum concentration of Benzodiazepines (metabolized by oxidation). **Exceptions:** Lansoprazole; Pantoprazole; Rabeprazole. *Risk C: Monitor therapy*

Rifamycin Derivatives: May increase the metabolism of Benzodiazepines (metabolized by oxidation). *Risk D: Consider therapy modification*

Selective Serotonin Reuptake Inhibitors: May decrease the metabolism of Benzodiazepines (metabolized by oxidation). **Exceptions:** Citalopram; Escitalopram; PARoxetine; Sertraline. *Risk C: Monitor therapy*

St Johns Wort: May increase the metabolism of Benzodiazepines (metabolized by oxidation). *Risk C: Monitor therapy*

Theophylline Derivatives: May diminish the therapeutic effect of Benzodiazepines. *Risk D: Consider therapy modification*

Ethanol/Nutrition/Herb Interactions

Ethanol: Avoid ethanol (may increase CNS depression).

Food: Grapefruit juice may decrease the metabolism of quazepam.

Herb/Nutraceutical: Avoid St John's wort (may increase the metabolism of quazepam).

Stability Store at controlled room temperature of 20°C to 25°C (68°F to 77°F).

Mechanism of Action Binds to stereospecific benzodiazepine receptors on the postsynaptic GABA neuron at several sites within the central nervous system, including the limbic system, reticular formation. Enhancement of the inhibitory effect of GABA on neuronal excitability results by increased neuronal membrane permeability to chloride ions. This shift in chloride ions results in hyperpolarization (a less excitable state) and stabilization.

Pharmacodynamics/Kinetics

Absorption: Rapid

Protein binding: >95%

Metabolism: Hepatic; forms metabolites (active)- 2-oxoquasepam and N-desalkyl-2-oxoquazepam

Half-life elimination, serum: Quazepam, 2-oxoquasepam: 39 hours; N-desalkyl-2-oxoquazepam: 73 hours

Time to peak, plasma: ~2 hours

Excretion: Urine (31%, only trace amounts as unchanged drug); feces (23%)

Dosage Adults: Oral: Initial: 15 mg at bedtime; in some patients, the dose may be reduced to 7.5 mg after a few nights

Elderly: Dosing should be cautious; begin at lower end of dosing range (ie, 7.5 mg)

Dosing adjustment in hepatic impairment: Dose reduction may be necessary

Monitoring Parameters Respiratory and cardiovascular status; mental status

Additional Information More likely than short-acting benzodiazepine to cause daytime sedation and fatigue. Classified as a long-acting benzodiazepine hypnotic (eg, flurazepam), this long duration of action may prevent withdrawal symptoms when therapy is discontinued. Abrupt discontinuation after sustained use (generally >10 days) may cause withdrawal symptoms.

Dosage Forms Excipient information presented when available (limited, particularly for generics); consult specific product labeling.

Tablet:

Doral®: 15 mg

◆ **Quelicin®** *see* Succinylcholine *on page 1511*

◆ **Questran®** *see* Cholestyramine Resin *on page 341*

◆ **Questran® Light** *see* Cholestyramine Resin *on page 341*

QUEtiapine (kwe TYE a peen)

Medication Safety Issues

Sound-alike/look-alike issues:

QUEtiapine may be confused with OLANZapine

Seroquel® may be confused with Serentil®, Serzone®, Sinequan®

Related Information

Agents Approved for Bipolar Disorder *on page 1752*

Antipsychotic Agents *on page 1769*

Antipsychotic Receptor Profile *on page 1772*

Atypical Antipsychotics *on page 1773*

Clozapine-Induced Side Effects *on page 1818*

CMS: Long-Term Care Facility Thresholds *on page 1815*

Discontinuation of Psychotropic Drugs *on page 1839*

U.S. Brand Names Seroquel®; Seroquel® XR

Canadian Brand Names Seroquel®; Seroquel® XR

Mexican Brand Names Seroquel

Index Terms Quetiapine Fumarate

Pharmacologic Category Antipsychotic Agent, Atypical

Generic Available No

Use Treatment of schizophrenia; treatment of acute manic episodes associated with bipolar disorder (as monotherapy or in combination with lithium or divalproex); maintenance treatment of bipolar disorder (in combination with lithium or divalproex); treatment of depressive episodes associated with bipolar disorder

Unlabeled/Investigational Use Autism, psychosis (children); psychosis/agitation related to Alzheimer's dementia

Mental Health Comment Quetiapine is an antipsychotic agent of a class often referred to as atypical. It should be noted that the definition of the term "atypical" is not universally agreed upon. Some prefer to describe antipsychotics based on their pharmacological properties. A common feature of all definitions used to describe "atypical" antipsychotics is the lack of significant acute or subacute EPS, at dosages generally associated with antipsychotic actions. Other experts have included definitions of atypicality that include a) failure to increase serum prolactin levels; b) superior efficacy for positive, negative, and cognitive symptoms; and c) lack of evidence of tardive dyskinesia or dystonia following chronic administration.

Clinically, the dosage range for quetiapine is large and depends on what is being targeted. The general dose range for GAD and depression is low (50-300 mg/day), bipolar mania and depression is 300-600 mg/day, while dosages for schizophrenia can range from 300-1200 mg/day.

Tardive dyskinesia (TD) secondary to **typical** antipsychotics has an estimated incidence of 3% to 5% per year for the first 5 years of treatment. The incidence of TD associated with the atypical antipsychotics is estimated to be 0.5% to 1%. It is not clear if this estimate represents a risk associated with mental illness or to what extent drug therapy can be implicated. Atypical antipsychotics appear less likely to cause tardive dyskinesia than typical antipsychotics (fluphenazine, haloperidol).

Coadministration of two or more antipsychotics does not generally improve clinical response and may increase the potential for adverse effects.

In 2008, the FDA issued a warning regarding increased mortality risk with typical **and** atypical antipsychotic drugs when used in elderly patients with dementia-related psychosis.

Restrictions An FDA-approved medication guide concerning the use of antidepressants in children, adolescents, and young adults must be distributed when dispensing an outpatient prescription (new or refill) where this medication is to be used without direct supervision of a healthcare provider. Medication guides are available at http://www.fda.gov/cder/drug/antidepressants/MG_template.pdf. Dispense to parents or guardians of children and adolescents receiving this medication.

Pregnancy Risk Factor C

Lactation Excretion in breast milk unknown/not recommended

Contraindications Hypersensitivity to quetiapine or any component of the formulation

Warnings/Precautions [U.S. Boxed Warning]: Antidepressants increase the risk of suicidal thinking and behavior in children, adolescents, and young adults (18-24 years of age) with major depressive disorder (MDD) and other psychiatric disorders; consider risk prior to prescribing. Short-term studies did not show an increased risk in patients >24 years of age and showed a decreased risk in patients ≥65 years. Closely monitor all patients for clinical worsening, suicidality, or unusual changes in behavior; particularly during the initial 1-2 months of therapy or during periods of dosage adjustments (increased or decreases); the patient's family or caregiver should be instructed to closely observe the patient and communicate condition with healthcare provider. A medication guide concerning the use of antidepressants should be dispensed with each prescription. **Quetiapine is not FDA approved for use in children.**

[U.S. Boxed Warning]: Elderly patients with dementia-related psychosis treated with atypical antipsychotics are at an increased risk of death compared to placebo. An increased incidence of cerebrovascular adverse events (including fatalities) has been reported in elderly patients with dementia-related psychosis. Quetiapine is not approved for this indication.

May be sedating, use with caution in disorders where CNS depression is a feature. Use with caution in Parkinson's disease. May induce orthostatic hypotension associated with dizziness, tachycardia, and, in some cases, syncope, especially during the initial dose titration period. Should be used with particular caution in patients with known cardiovascular disease (history of MI or ischemic heart disease, heart failure, or conduction abnormalities), cerebrovascular disease, or conditions that predispose to hypotension. Esophageal dysmotility and aspiration have been associated with antipsychotic use; use with caution in patients at risk of aspiration pneumonia (eg, Alzheimer's disease). Development of cataracts has been observed in animal studies, therefore, lens examinations should be made upon initiation of therapy and every 6 months thereafter. Leukopenia, neutropenia, and agranulocytosis (sometimes fatal) have been reported in clinical trials and postmarketing reports; presence of risk factors (eg, pre-existing low WBC or history of drug-induced leuko-/neutropenia) should prompt periodic blood count assessment and discontinuation at first signs of blood dyscrasias.

Due to anticholinergic effects, use with caution in patients with decreased gastrointestinal motility, urinary retention, BPH, xerostomia, visual problems, narrow-angle glaucoma (screening is recommended), and myasthenia gravis. Relative to other antipsychotics, quetiapine has a moderate potency of cholinergic blockade. May cause extrapyramidal symptoms (EPS), pseudoparkinsonism, and/or tardive dyskinesia. Risk of dystonia (and probably other EPS) may be greater with increased doses, use of conventional antipsychotics, males, and younger patients. Impaired core body temperature regulation may occur; caution with strenuous exercise, heat exposure, dehydration, and concomitant medication possessing anticholinergic effects. Neuroleptic malignant syndrome (NMS) is a potentially fatal symptom complex that has been reported in association with administration of antipsychotic drugs. Clinical manifestations of NMS are hyperpyrexia, muscle rigidity, altered mental status, and evidence of autonomic instability (irregular pulse or blood pressure, tachycardia, diaphoresis, and cardiac dysrhythmia). Management of NMS should include immediate discontinuation of antipsychotic drugs and other drugs not essential to concurrent therapy, intensive symptomatic treatment and medication monitoring, and treatment of any concomitant medical problems for which specific treatment are available.

Use caution in patients with a history of seizures. May cause decreases in total free thyroxine, elevations of liver enzymes, cholesterol levels, and/or triglyceride increases.

May cause hyperglycemia; in some cases may be extreme and associated with ketoacidosis, hyperosmolar coma, or death. Use with caution in patients with diabetes or other disorders of glucose regulation; monitor for worsening of glucose control. Significant weight gain has been observed with antipsychotic therapy; incidence varies with product. Monitor waist circumference and BMI.

Adverse Reactions

>10%:

Central nervous system: Somnolence (12% to 34%), sedation (13% to 30%), headache (17% to 21%), agitation (6% to 20%), dizziness (9% to 18%), extrapyramidal symptoms (8% to 12%)

Endocrine & metabolic: Triglycerides increased (14% to 23%), cholesterol increased (9% to 16%)

Gastrointestinal: Xerostomia (9% to 44%), weight gain (dose-related; <5% to 23%)

1% to 10%:

Cardiovascular: Orthostatic hypotension (4% to 7%), tachycardia (≤6%), palpitation (≥1%), peripheral edema (≥1%), syncope (≤1%)

Central nervous system: Fatigue (10%), pain (7%), lethargy (5%), akathisia (<5%), fever (2% to <5%), dystonia (<5%), tardive dyskinesia (<5%), anxiety (4%)

Dermatologic: Rash (4% to <5%)

Endocrine & metabolic: Hyperglycemia (≥200 mg/dL post glucose challenge or fasting glucose ≥126 mg/dL, 4%)

Gastrointestinal: Constipation (6% to 10%), dyspepsia (dose-related; 5% to 7%), abdominal pain (dose-related; 4% to 7%), vomiting (5% to 6%), appetite increased (≤5%), drooling (<5%), dysphagia (<5%), gastroenteritis (2%), anorexia (≥1%)

Hematologic: Leukopenia (<5%)

Hepatic: Transaminases increased (1% to 6%), GGT increased (1%)

Neuromuscular & skeletal: Weakness (5% to 10%), tremor (≤8%), back pain (3% to 5%), dysarthria (<5%), hypertonia (≥1%)

Ocular: Blurred vision (<5%), amblyopia (2%)

Respiratory: Pharyngitis (4% to 6%), nasal congestion (≤5%), rhinitis (3%), cough (≥1%), dyspnea (≥1%)

Miscellaneous: Diaphoresis (≥1%), flu-like syndrome (≥1%)

<1% (Limited to important or life-threatening): Abnormal dreams, acute renal failure, agranulocytosis, alkaline phosphatase increased, amnesia, anaphylactic reaction, anaphylaxis, anemia, angina, asthma, bradycardia, bundle branch block, cardiomyopathy, cataract formation, cerebral ischemia, cerebrovascular accident, CHF, confusion, creatinine increased, dehydration, diabetes mellitus, eosinophilia, epistaxis, exfoliative dermatitis, dysuria, hallucinations, hypoglycemia, hyper-/hypothyroidism, hypersensitivity, hypertonia, hypokalemia, hyponatremia, involuntary movements, leukocytosis, lymphadenopathy, myocarditis, neuroleptic malignant syndrome, neutropenia, pancreatitis, pneumonia, priapism, QRS duration increased, QT prolongation, rectal bleeding, restless leg syndrome, rhabdomyolysis, seizure, SIADH, Stevens-Johnson syndrome, ST segment elevation, suicide attempt, thrombocytopenia, tinnitus, T-wave abnormal, T-wave inversion, urinary retention, vertigo

Metabolism/Transport Effects Substrate of CYP2D6 (minor), 3A4 (major)

Drug Interactions

Acetylcholinesterase Inhibitors (Central): May enhance the neurotoxic (central) effect of Antipsychotics. Severe extrapyramidal symptoms have occurred in some patients. *Risk C: Monitor therapy*

Alcohol (Ethyl): CNS Depressants may enhance the CNS depressant effect of Alcohol (Ethyl). *Risk C: Monitor therapy*

Alfuzosin: May enhance the QTc-prolonging effect of QTc-Prolonging Agents. *Risk C: Monitor therapy*

Amphetamines: Antipsychotics may diminish the stimulatory effect of Amphetamines. *Risk C: Monitor therapy*

Anticholinergics: May enhance the adverse/toxic effect of other Anticholinergics. **Exceptions:** Paliperidone. *Risk C: Monitor therapy*

Anti-Parkinson's Agents (Dopamine Agonist): Antipsychotics (Atypical) may diminish the therapeutic effect of Anti-Parkinson's Agents (Dopamine Agonist). *Risk D: Consider therapy modification*

Ciprofloxacin: May enhance the QTc-prolonging effect of QTc-Prolonging Agents. *Risk C: Monitor therapy*

CNS Depressants: May enhance the adverse/toxic effect of other CNS Depressants. *Risk C: Monitor therapy*

CYP3A4 Inducers (Strong): May increase the metabolism of CYP3A4 Substrates. *Risk C: Monitor therapy*

CYP3A4 Inhibitors (Moderate): May decrease the metabolism of CYP3A4 Substrates. *Risk C: Monitor therapy*

CYP3A4 Inhibitors (Strong): May decrease the metabolism of CYP3A4 Substrates. *Risk D: Consider therapy modification*

Dasatinib: May increase the serum concentration of CYP3A4 Substrates. *Risk C: Monitor therapy*

Deferasirox: May decrease the serum concentration of CYP3A4 Substrates. *Risk C: Monitor therapy*

Gadobutrol: May enhance the QTc-prolonging effect of QTc-Prolonging Agents. *Risk D: Consider therapy modification*

Herbs (CYP3A4 Inducers): May increase the metabolism of CYP3A4 Substrates. *Risk C: Monitor therapy*

Lithium formulations: May enhance the neurotoxic effect of Antipsychotics. Lithium formulations may decrease the serum concentration of Antipsychotics. Specifically noted with chlorpromazine. *Risk C: Monitor therapy*

Nilotinib: May enhance the QTc-prolonging effect of QTc-Prolonging Agents. *Risk X: Avoid combination*

Phenytoin: May increase the metabolism of QUEtiapine. *Risk D: Consider therapy modification*

Pramlintide: May enhance the anticholinergic effect of Anticholinergics. These effects are specific to the GI tract. *Risk D: Consider therapy modification*

QTc-Prolonging Agents: May enhance the adverse/toxic effect of other QTc-Prolonging Agents. Their effects can be additive, causing life-threatening ventricular arrhythmias. *Risk D: Consider therapy modification*

Tetrabenazine: May enhance the adverse/toxic effect of Antipsychotics. *Risk C: Monitor therapy*

Thioridazine: QTc-Prolonging Agents may enhance the QTc-prolonging effect of Thioridazine. *Risk X: Avoid combination*

Ziprasidone: QTc-Prolonging Agents may enhance the QTc-prolonging effect of Ziprasidone. The risk of a severe arrhythmia may be increased. *Risk X: Avoid combination*

Ethanol/Nutrition/Herb Interactions

Ethanol: Avoid ethanol (may cause excessive impairment in cognition/motor function).

Food: In healthy volunteers, administration of quetiapine (immediate release) with food resulted in an increase in the peak serum concentration and AUC (each by ~15%) compared to the fasting state. Administration of the extended release with a high-fat meal (~800-1000 calories) resulted in an increase in peak serum concentration by 44% to 52% and AUC by 20% to 22% for the 50 mg and 300 mg tablets; administration with a light meal had no significant effect on the C_{max} or AUC.

Herb/Nutraceutical: St John's wort may decrease quetiapine levels. Avoid valerian, St John's wort, kava kava, gotu kola (may increase CNS depression).

Stability Store at controlled room temperature of 25°C (77°F).

Mechanism of Action Quetiapine is a dibenzothiazepine atypical antipsychotic. It has been proposed that this drug's antipsychotic activity is mediated through a combination of dopamine type 2 (D_2) and serotonin type 2 ($5\text{-}HT_2$) antagonism. It is an antagonist at multiple neurotransmitter receptors in the brain: serotonin $5\text{-}HT_{1A}$ and $5\text{-}HT_2$, dopamine D_1 and D_2, histamine H_1, and adrenergic alpha$_1$- and alpha$_2$- receptors; but appears to have no appreciable affinity at cholinergic muscarinic and benzodiazepine receptors.

Antagonism at receptors other than dopamine and $5\text{-}HT_2$ with similar receptor affinities may explain some of the other effects of quetiapine. The drug's antagonism of histamine H_1-receptors may explain the somnolence observed with it. The drug's antagonism of adrenergic alpha$_1$-receptors may explain the orthostatic hypotension observed with it.

Pharmacodynamics/Kinetics

Absorption: Rapidly absorbed following oral administration

Distribution: V_d: 6-14 L/kg; V_{dss}: ~2 days

Protein binding, plasma: 83%

Metabolism: Primarily hepatic; via CYP3A4; forms the metabolite N-desalkyl quetiapine (active) and two inactive metabolites

Bioavailability: 9% ± 4%; tablet is 100% bioavailable relative to solution

Half-life elimination: Mean: Terminal: Quetiapine: ~6 hours; N-desalkyl quetiapine: 9-12 hours

Time to peak, plasma: 1.5 hours

Excretion: Urine (73% as metabolites, <1% as unchanged drug); feces (20%)

Dosage Oral:

Children and Adolescents:

Autism (unlabeled use): 100-350 mg/day (1.6-5.2 mg/kg/day)

Psychosis and mania (unlabeled use): Initial: 25 mg twice daily; titrate as necessary to 450 mg/day

Adults:

Bipolar disorder:

Depression: Immediate release tablet: Initial: 50 mg/day the first day; increase to 100 mg/day on day 2, further increasing by 100 mg/day each day to a target of 300 mg/day by day 4. Further increases up to 600 mg/day by day 8 have been evaluated in clinical trials, but no additional antidepressant efficacy was noted.

Mania: Immediate release tablet: Initial: 50 mg twice daily on day 1, increase dose in increments of 100 mg/day to 200 mg twice daily on day 4; may increase to a target dose of 800 mg/day by day 6 at increments ≤200 mg/day. Usual dosage range: 400-800 mg/day.

Maintenance therapy: 200-400 mg twice daily with lithium or divalproex; **Note:** Average time of stabilization was 15 weeks in clinical trials.

Schizophrenia/psychoses:

Immediate release tablet: Initial: 25 mg twice daily; increase in increments of 25-50 mg 2-3 times/day on the second and third day, if tolerated, to a target dose of 300-400 mg/day in 2-3 divided doses by day 4. Make further adjustments as needed at intervals of at least 2 days in adjustments of 25-50 mg twice daily. Usual maintenance range: 300-800 mg/day.

Extended release tablet: Initial: 300 mg once daily; increase in increments of up to 300 mg/day (in intervals of ≥1 day). For dosage requirements <200 mg during initial titration, the immediate release formulation should be used. Usual maintenance range: 400-800 mg/day.

Note: Dose reductions should be attempted periodically to establish lowest effective dose in patients with psychosis. Patients being restarted after 1 week of no drug need to be titrated as above.

Elderly: 40% lower mean oral clearance of quetiapine in adults >65 years of age; higher plasma levels expected and, therefore, dosage adjustment may be needed; elderly patients usually require 50-200 mg/day with a slower titration schedule. Begin titration with immediate release formulation, increase dose by 25-50 mg/day to effective dose, based on clinical response and tolerability. May transition to extended release formulation (at equivalent total daily dose) when effective dose has been reached. See "Note" in adult dosing.

Psychosis/agitation related to Alzheimer's dementia (unlabeled use): Initial: 12.5-50 mg/day; if necessary, gradually increase as tolerated not to exceed 200-300 mg/day

Dosing comments in renal insufficiency: 25% lower mean oral clearance of quetiapine than normal subjects; however, plasma concentrations similar to normal subjects receiving the same dose; no dosage adjustment required

Dosing comments in hepatic insufficiency: 30% lower mean oral clearance of quetiapine than normal subjects; higher plasma levels expected in hepatically impaired subjects; dosage adjustment may be needed

Initial: 25 mg/day, increase dose by 25-50 mg/day to effective dose, based on clinical response and tolerability to patient. Begin titration with immediate-release formulation; may transition to extended-release formulation (at equivalent total daily dose) when effective dose has been reached.

Child/Adolescent Considerations Six children with autistic disorder (mean age: 10.9 years) received 100-350 mg/day (1.6-5.2 mg/kg/day; Martin, 1999). Ten patients with DSM-IV chronic or intermittent psychotic disorders (12.3-15.9 years of age) received quetiapine twice daily starting at 25 mg and reaching 400 mg by day 20. The trial ended on day 23 (McConville, 2000). Thirty manic or mixed bipolar I adolescents (12-18 years of age) received quetiapine 25 mg twice daily with titration to 450 mg/day by day 7 (DelBello, 2001).

DelBello MP, Schwiers ML, Rosenberg HL, et al, "Quetiapine as Adjunctive Treatment for Adolescent Mania," Poster presented at Fourth International Conference on Bipolar Disorder, Pittsburgh, PA: Jun 14.

Martin A, Koenig K, Scahill L, et al, "Open-Label Quetiapine in the Treatment of Children and Adolescents With Autistic Disorder," *J Child Adolesc Psychopharmacol*, 1999, 9(2):99-107.

McConville BJ, Arvanitis LA, Thyrum PT, et al, "Pharmacokinetics, Tolerability, and Clinical Effectiveness of Quetiapine Fumarate: An Open-Label Trial in Adolescents With Psychotic Disorders," *J Clin Psychiatry*, 2000, 61 (4):252-60.

Dietary Considerations

Immediate-release tablet: May be taken with or without food.

Extended release tablet: Take without food or with a light meal (≤300 calories).

Administration

Immediate release tablet: May be administered with or without food.

Extended release tablet: Administer without food or with a light meal (≤300 calories), preferably in the evening. Swallow tablet whole; do not break, crush, or chew.

Monitoring Parameters Vital signs; fasting lipid profile and fasting blood glucose/Hgb A_{1c} (prior to treatment, at 3 months, then annually); CBC frequently during first few months of therapy in patients with pre-existing low WBC or a history of drug-induced leukopenia/neutropenia; BMI, personal/family history of obesity, waist circumference; blood pressure; mental status, abnormal involuntary movement scale (AIMS). Weight should be assessed prior to treatment, at 4 weeks, 8 weeks, 12 weeks, and then at quarterly intervals. Consider titrating to a different antipsychotic agent for a weight gain ≥5% of the initial weight. Patients should have eyes checked for cataracts every 6 months while on this medication. Observe for new or worsening depression, anxiety, irritability, aggression, or other symptoms of unusual behavior, mood, or suicidal ideation (especially at the beginning of therapy or when doses are increased or decreased).

Dosage Forms Excipient information presented when available (limited, particularly for generics); consult specific product labeling. [CAN] = Canadian availability; not available in U.S.

Tablet:

Seroquel®: 25 mg, 50 mg, 100 mg, 200 mg, 300 mg, 400 mg

Tablet, extended release:

Seroquel® XR: 50 mg [CAN] (not available in U.S.), 200 mg, 300 mg, 400 mg

◆ **Quetiapine Fumarate** *see* QUEtiapine *on page 1381*

◆ **Quibron® [DSC]** *see* Theophylline and Guaifenesin *on page 1567*

◆ **Quinalbarbitone Sodium** *see* Secobarbital *on page 1464*

Quinapril (KWIN a pril)

Medication Safety Issues

Sound-alike/look-alike issues:

Accupril® may be confused with Accolate®, Accutane®, AcipHex®, Monopril®

International issues:

Accupril® may be confused with Acepril® which is a brand name for lisinopril in Denmark, a brand name for enalapril in Hungary and Switzerland, and a brand name for captopril in Great Britain

Related Information

Angiotensin Agents *on page 1754*

U.S. Brand Names Accupril®

Canadian Brand Names Accupril®; GD-Quinapril

Mexican Brand Names Accupril; Acupril

Index Terms Quinapril Hydrochloride

Pharmacologic Category Angiotensin-Converting Enzyme (ACE) Inhibitor

Use Treatment of hypertension; treatment of heart failure

Unlabeled/Investigational Use Treatment of left ventricular dysfunction after myocardial infarction; pediatric hypertension; to delay the progression of nephropathy and reduce risks of cardiovascular events in hypertensive patients with type 1 or 2 diabetes mellitus

Effect on Mental Status May cause dizziness or drowsiness; may rarely cause insomnia or depression

Effect on Psychiatric Treatment May cause neutropenia; use caution with clozapine and carbamazepine; may decrease lithium clearance resulting in an increase in serum lithium levels and potential lithium toxicity; monitor serum lithium levels

Dosage Summary

Oral:

Children (unlabeled use): Initial 5-10 mg once daily; maximum: 80 mg/day

Adults: Initial: 5-20 mg/day in 1-2 divided doses; Maintenance: 10-40 mg/day in 1-2 divided doses

Elderly: Initial: 2.5-5 mg/day; Maintenance: 10-40 mg/day

Dosage Forms Excipient information presented when available (limited, particularly for generics); consult specific product labeling.

Tablet: 5 mg, 10 mg, 20 mg, 40 mg

Accupril®: 5 mg, 10 mg, 20 mg, 40 mg

Quinapril and Hydrochlorothiazide

(KWIN a pril & hye droe klor oh THYE a zide)

U.S. Brand Names Accuretic®; Quinaretic

Canadian Brand Names Accuretic®

Index Terms Hydrochlorothiazide and Quinapril

Pharmacologic Category Angiotensin-Converting Enzyme (ACE) Inhibitor; Diuretic, Thiazide

Use Treatment of hypertension (not for initial therapy)

Effect on Mental Status May cause dizziness or drowsiness; may rarely cause insomnia or depression

Effect on Psychiatric Treatment May cause neutropenia; use caution with clozapine and carbamazepine. May decrease lithium clearance, resulting in an increase in serum lithium levels and potential lithium toxicity; monitor serum lithium levels.

Dosage Summary

Oral:

Children: Dosage not established

Adults: Initial: 10-20 mg quinapril and 12.5 mg hydrochlorothiazide once daily; Maintenance: 5-40 mg quinapril and 6.25-25 mg hydrochlorothiazide once daily

Dosage Forms Excipient information presented when available (limited, particularly for generics); consult specific product labeling.

Tablet:

10/12.5: Quinapril 10 mg and hydrochlorothiazide 12.5 mg

20/12.5: Quinapril 20 mg and hydrochlorothiazide 12.5 mg

20/25: Quinapril 20 mg and hydrochlorothiazide 25 mg

Accuretic® 10/12.5, Quinaretic 10/12.5: Quinapril 10 mg and hydrochlorothiazide 12.5 mg

Accuretic® 20/12.5, Quinaretic 20/12.5: Quinapril 20 mg and hydrochlorothiazide 12.5 mg

Accuretic® 20/25, Quinaretic 20/25: Quinapril 20 mg and hydrochlorothiazide 25 mg

◆ **Quinapril Hydrochloride** *see* Quinapril *on page 1386*

◆ **Quinaretic** *see* Quinapril and Hydrochlorothiazide *on page 1386*

QuiNIDine (KWIN i deen)

Medication Safety Issues

Sound-alike/look-alike issues:

QuiNIDine may be confused with cloNIDine, quiNINE, Quinora®

High alert medication: The Institute for Safe Medication Practices (ISMP) includes this medication (I.V. formulation) among its list of drug classes which have a heightened risk of causing significant patient harm when used in error.

Canadian Brand Names Apo-Quinidine®; BioQuin® Durules™; Novo-Quinidin; Quinate®

Index Terms Quinidine Gluconate; Quinidine Polygalacturonate; Quinidine Sulfate

Pharmacologic Category Antiarrhythmic Agent, Class Ia

Use Prophylaxis after cardioversion of atrial fibrillation and/or flutter to maintain normal sinus rhythm; prevent recurrence of paroxysmal supraventricular tachycardia, paroxysmal AV junctional rhythm, paroxysmal ventricular tachycardia, paroxysmal atrial fibrillation, and atrial or ventricular premature contractions; has activity against *Plasmodium falciparum* malaria

Effect on Mental Status May cause dizziness; may rarely cause confusion or delirium

Effect on Psychiatric Treatment Contraindicated with ziprasidone. May cause anemia; use caution with clozapine and carbamazepine. Concurrent use with TCAs may raise serum levels or produce AV block; avoid combination. Concurrent use with beta-blockers may increase bradycardia.

Dosage Summary Note: Dosage expressed in terms of the salt: 267 mg of quinidine gluconate = 200 mg of quinidine sulfate.

I.M.:

Children: Test dose: 2 mg/kg **or** 60 mg/m^2

Adults: Test dose: 200 mg, then 400 mg every 4-6 hours

I.V.:

Children: 2-10 mg/kg/dose every 3-6 hours as needed; **Note:** This route not recommended

Adults: 200-400 mg/dose

Oral:

Gluconate:

Children: Dosage not established

Adults: 324-972 mg every 8-12 hours

Sulfate:

Children: Initial: 6 mg/kg every 4-6 hours **or** 15-60 mg/kg/day in 4-5 divided doses; Usual: 30 mg/kg/day in 5 divided doses **or** 900 mg/m^2/day in 5 divided doses

Adults: 100-600 mg/dose every 4-6 hours (maximum: 4 g/day)

Dosage Forms Excipient information presented when available (limited, particularly for generics); consult specific product labeling.

Injection, solution, as gluconate: 80 mg/mL (10 mL) [equivalent to quinidine base 50 mg/mL]

Tablet, as sulfate: 200 mg, 300 mg

Tablet, extended release, as gluconate: 324 mg [equivalent to quinidine base 202 mg]

Tablet, extended release, as sulfate: 300 mg [equivalent to quinidine base 249 mg]

- **Quinidine Gluconate** *see* QuiNIDine *on page 1387*
- **Quinidine Polygalacturonate** *see* QuiNIDine *on page 1387*
- **Quinidine Sulfate** *see* QuiNIDine *on page 1387*

QuiNINE (KWYE nine)

Medication Safety Issues

Sound-alike/look-alike issues:

QuiNINE may be confused with quiNIDine

U.S. Brand Names Qualaquin™

Canadian Brand Names Apo-Quinine®; Novo-Quinine; Quinine-Odan™

Index Terms Quinine Sulfate

Pharmacologic Category Antimalarial Agent

Use In conjunction with other antimalarial agents, treatment of uncomplicated chloroquine-resistant *P. falciparum* malaria

Unlabeled/Investigational Use Treatment of *Babesia microti* infection in conjunction with clindamycin

Note: Prevention/treatment of nocturnal leg cramps (unapproved) removed following FDA-issued warning regarding severe adverse events (eg, cardiac arrhythmias, thrombocytopenia, and severe hypersensitivity reactions) and potentially serious drug interactions associated with quinine; use not justified in this condition.

Effect on Mental Status None reported

Effect on Psychiatric Treatment Barbiturates and carbamazepine may decrease serum concentrations of quinine; CYP2D6 inhibitor; may interact with TCAs or beta-blockers; monitor

Dosage Summary

Oral:

Children: 30 mg/kg/day divided every 8 hours

Adults: 648 mg every 8 hours

Dosage Forms Excipient information presented when available (limited, particularly for generics); consult specific product labeling. [DSC] = Discontinued product

Capsule, as sulfate: 325 mg [DSC]

Qualaquin™: 324 mg

Tablet, as sulfate: 260 mg [DSC]

- **Quinine Sulfate** *see* QuiNINE *on page 1388*

Quinupristin and Dalfopristin (kwi NYOO pris tin & dal FOE pris tin)

U.S. Brand Names Synercid®

Canadian Brand Names Synercid®

Index Terms Pristinamycin; RP-59500

Pharmacologic Category Antibiotic, Streptogramin

Use Treatment of serious or life-threatening infections associated with vancomycin-resistant *Enterococcus faecium* bacteremia; treatment of complicated skin and skin structure infections caused by methcillin-susceptible *Staphylococcus aureus* or *Streptococcus pyogenes*

Has been studied in the treatment of a variety of infections caused by *Enterococcus faecium* (not *E. fecalis*) including vancomycin-resistant strains. May also be effective in the treatment of serious infections caused by *Staphylococcus* species including those resistant to methicillin.

Effect on Mental Status May rarely cause anxiety, confusion, or insomnia

Effect on Psychiatric Treatment May rarely produce pancytopenia; caution with clozapine and carbamazepine

Dosage Summary
I.V.:
Children (limited information): 7.5 mg/kg/dose every 8 hours
Adults: 7.5 mg/kg every 8-12 hours

Dosage Forms Excipient information presented when available (limited, particularly for generics); consult specific product labeling.
Injection, powder for reconstitution:
Synercid®: 500 mg: Quinupristin 150 mg and dalfopristin 350 mg

◆ **Quixin®** *see* Levofloxacin *on page 913*
◆ **QVAR®** *see* Beclomethasone *on page 171*
◆ **R 14-15** *see* Erlotinib *on page 556*

Rabeprazole (ra BEP ra zole)

Medication Safety Issues
Sound-alike/look-alike issues:
AcipHex® may be confused with Acephen®, Accupril®, Aricept®, pHisoHex®
Rabeprazole may be confused with aripiprazole,donepezil, lansoprazole, omeprazole, raloxifene

U.S. Brand Names AcipHex®

Canadian Brand Names AcipHex®; Novo-Rabeprazole EC; Pariet®; Ran-Rabeprazole

Mexican Brand Names Pariet

Index Terms Pariprazole

Pharmacologic Category Proton Pump Inhibitor; Substituted Benzimidazole

Generic Available No

Use Short-term (4-8 weeks) treatment and maintenance of erosive or ulcerative gastroesophageal reflux disease (GERD); symptomatic GERD; short-term (up to 4 weeks) treatment of duodenal ulcers; long-term treatment of pathological hypersecretory conditions, including Zollinger-Ellison syndrome; *H. pylori* eradication (in combination with amoxicillin and clarithromycin)
Canadian labeling: Additional uses (not in U.S. labeling): Treatment of nonerosive reflux disease (NERD); treatment of gastric ulcers

Unlabeled/Investigational Use Maintenance of duodenal ulcer

Effect on Mental Status May cause insomnia, anxiety, dizziness, depression, nervousness, somnolence, vertigo, convulsions, abnormal dreams; may rarely cause agitation, amnesia, confusion, extrapyramidal syndrome

Effect on Psychiatric Treatment None reported

Pregnancy Risk Factor B

Pregnancy Considerations Not shown to be teratogenic in animal studies, however, adequate and well-controlled studies have not been done in humans; use during pregnancy only if clearly needed

Lactation Excretion in breast milk unknown/not recommended

Contraindications Hypersensitivity to rabeprazole, substituted benzimidazoles (ie, esomeprazole, lansoprazole, omeprazole, pantoprazole), or any component of the formulation

Warnings/Precautions Use caution in severe hepatic impairment. Relief of symptoms with rabeprazole does not preclude the presence of a gastric malignancy. Safety and efficacy have not been established in patients <12 years of age.

Adverse Reactions
1% to 10%:
Central nervous system: Pain (3%), headache (2% to 5%)
Gastrointestinal: Diarrhea (3%), flatulence (3%), constipation (2%), nausea (2%)
Respiratory: Pharyngitis (3%)
Miscellaneous: Infection (2%)

<1% (Limited to important or life-threatening): Abdomen enlarged, abdominal pain, abnormal stools, abnormal vision, agitation, agranulocytosis, albuminuria, allergic reaction, alopecia, amblyopia, anaphylaxis, anemia, angina pectoris, angioedema, anorexia, apnea, arrhythmia, arthralgia, arthritis, ascites, asthma, bloody diarrhea, bone pain, bradycardia, breast enlargement, bullous and other drug eruptions of skin, bundle branch block, bursitis, cataract, cellulitis, cerebral hemorrhage, chest pain substernal, cholangitis, cholecystitis, cholelithiasis, colitis, coma, constipation, contact dermatitis, convulsions, corneal opacity, CPK increased, cystitis, deafness, delirium, depression, diaphoresis, diabetes mellitus, diplopia, disorientation, dizziness, duodenitis, dysmenorrhea, dyspepsia, dysphagia, dyspnea, dysuria, edema, electrocardiogram abnormal, embolus, epistaxis, erythema multiforme,

esophageal stenosis, esophagitis, extrapyramidal syndrome, eye hemorrhage, facial edema, fever, flatulence, fungal dermatitis, gastritis, gastroenteritis, gastrointestinal hemorrhage, gingivitis, glaucoma, glossitis, gout, gynecomastia, hematuria, hemolytic anemia, hepatic encephalopathy, hepatic cirrhosis, hepatic enzymes increased, hepatitis, hepatoma, hernia, hyperammonemia, hypercholesteremia, hyperglycemia, hyperkinesia, hyperlipemia, hypertension, hyper-/hypothyroidism, hypertonia, hypokalemia, hyponatremia, hypoxia, impotence, injection site hemorrhage/pain/reaction, insomnia, interstitial nephritis, interstitial pneumonia, jaundice, kidney calculus, leukocytosis, leukopenia, leukorrhea, liver fatty deposit, lymphadenopathy, malaise, melena, menorrhagia, metrorrhagia, MI, migraine, myalgia, nausea, neck rigidity, nervousness, neuralgia, neuropathy, neutropenia, orchitis, palpitation, pancreatitis, pancytopenia, paresthesia, peripheral edema, photosensitivity, polycystic kidney, polyuria, proctitis, pruritus, PSA increased, psoriasis, pulmonary embolus, QT_c prolongation, rash, rectal hemorrhage, retinal degeneration, rhabdomyolysis, salivary gland enlargement, sinus bradycardia, skin discoloration, somnolence, Stevens-Johnson syndrome, stomatitis, strabismus, sudden death, supraventricular tachycardia, syncope, tachycardia, taste abnormal, thrombocytopenia, thrombophlebitis, thrombosis, thirst (rare) tinnitus, toxic epidermal necrolysis, tremor, TSH increased, ulcerative colitis, urinary incontinence, urticaria, vasodilation, ventricular arrhythmias, vertigo, vomiting, weakness, weight gain/loss, xerostomia

Metabolism/Transport Effects Substrate (major) of CYP2C19, 3A4; **Inhibits** CYP2C8 (moderate), 2C19 (moderate), 2DC (weak), 3A4 (weak)

Drug Interactions

Antifungal Agents (Azole Derivatives, Systemic): Proton Pump Inhibitors may decrease the absorption of Antifungal Agents (Azole Derivatives, Systemic). **Exceptions:** Miconazole. *Risk D: Consider therapy modification*

Atazanavir: Proton Pump Inhibitors may decrease the absorption of Atazanavir. *Risk D: Consider therapy modification*

Clopidogrel: Proton Pump Inhibitors may diminish the therapeutic effect of Clopidogrel. This appears to be due to reduced formation of the active clopidogrel metabolite. *Risk C: Monitor therapy*

CYP2C19 Inducers (Strong): May increase the metabolism of CYP2C19 Substrates. *Risk C: Monitor therapy*

CYP2C19 Substrates: CYP2C19 Inhibitors (Moderate) may decrease the metabolism of CYP2C19 Substrates. *Risk C: Monitor therapy*

CYP2C8 Substrates (High risk): CYP2C8 Inhibitors (Moderate) may decrease the metabolism of CYP2C8 Substrates (High risk). *Risk C: Monitor therapy*

CYP3A4 Inducers (Strong): May increase the metabolism of CYP3A4 Substrates. *Risk C: Monitor therapy*

Dabigatran Etexilate: Proton Pump Inhibitors may decrease the serum concentration of Dabigatran Etexilate. *Risk C: Monitor therapy*

Dasatinib: Proton Pump Inhibitors may decrease the absorption of Dasatinib. *Risk D: Consider therapy modification*

Deferasirox: May decrease the serum concentration of CYP3A4 Substrates. *Risk C: Monitor therapy*

Erlotinib: Proton Pump Inhibitors may decrease the serum concentration of Erlotinib. *Risk X: Avoid combination*

Herbs (CYP3A4 Inducers): May increase the metabolism of CYP3A4 Substrates. *Risk C: Monitor therapy*

Indinavir: Proton Pump Inhibitors may decrease the absorption of Indinavir. *Risk C: Monitor therapy*

Iron Salts: Proton Pump Inhibitors may decrease the absorption of Iron Salts. **Exceptions:** Ferric Gluconate; Iron Dextran Complex; Iron Sucrose. *Risk C: Monitor therapy*

Methotrexate: Proton Pump Inhibitors may decrease the excretion of Methotrexate. Antirheumatic doses of methotrexate probably hold minimal risk. *Risk C: Monitor therapy*

Mycophenolate: Proton Pump Inhibitors may decrease the serum concentration of Mycophenolate. Specifically, concentrations of the active mycophenolic acid may be reduced. *Risk C: Monitor therapy*

Saquinavir: Proton Pump Inhibitors may increase the serum concentration of Saquinavir. *Risk C: Monitor therapy*

Tipranavir: May decrease the serum concentration of Proton Pump Inhibitors. These data are derived from studies with Ritonavir-boosted Tipranavir. *Risk C: Monitor therapy*

Ethanol/Nutrition/Herb Interactions

Ethanol: Avoid ethanol (may cause gastric mucosal irritation).

Food: High-fat meals may delay absorption, but C_{max} and AUC are not altered.

Herb/Nutraceutical: St John's wort may increase the metabolism and thus decrease the levels/effects of rabeprazole.

Stability Store at 25°C (77°F). Protect from moisture.

Mechanism of Action Potent proton pump inhibitor; suppresses gastric acid secretion by inhibiting the parietal cell H+/K+ ATP pump

Pharmacodynamics/Kinetics

Onset of action: Within 1 hour

Duration: 24 hours

Absorption: Oral: Well absorbed within 1 hour

Protein binding, serum: ~96%

Metabolism: Hepatic via CYP3A and 2C19 to inactive metabolites

Bioavailability: Oral: ~52%

Half-life elimination (dose dependent): 1-2 hours

Time to peak, plasma: 2-5 hours

Excretion: Urine (90% primarily as thioether carboxylic acid metabolites); remainder in feces

Dosage Oral:

Children ≥12 years: *U.S. labeling:* Short-term treatment of GERD: 20 mg once daily for ≤8 weeks

Adults >18 years and Elderly:

Erosive/ulcerative GERD: Treatment: 20 mg once daily for 4-8 weeks; if inadequate response, may repeat up to an additional 8 weeks; maintenance: 20 mg once daily

Canadian labeling: 20 mg once daily for 4 weeks; if inadequate response, may repeat for an additional 4 weeks (lack of symptom control after 4 weeks warrants further evaluation); maintenance: 10 mg once daily (maximum: 20 mg once daily)

Symptomatic GERD: Treatment: 20 mg once daily for 4 weeks; if inadequate response, may repeat for an additional 4 weeks

Canadian labeling: 10 mg once daily (maximum: 20 mg once daily) for 4 weeks; lack of symptom control after 4 weeks warrants further evaluation

Duodenal ulcer: 20 mg/day before breakfast for 4 weeks; additional therapy may be required for some patients

Gastric ulcers (*Canadian labeling*): 20 mg once daily up to 6 weeks; additional therapy may be required for some patients

H. pylori eradication: 20 mg twice daily for 7 days; to be administered with amoxicillin 1000 mg and clarithromycin 500 mg, also given twice daily for 7 days.

Hypersecretory conditions: 60 mg once daily; dose may need to be adjusted as necessary. Doses as high as 100 mg once daily and 60 mg twice daily have been used, and continued as long as necessary (up to 1 year in some patients).

NERD (*Canadian labeling*): Treatment: 10 mg (maximum: 20 mg once daily) for 4 weeks; lack of symptom control after 4 weeks warrants further evaluation

Dosage adjustment in renal impairment: No dosage adjustment required

Dosage adjustment in hepatic impairment:

Mild to moderate: Elimination decreased; no dosage adjustment required

Severe: Use caution

Dietary Considerations May be taken with or without food; best if taken before breakfast.

Administration May be administered with or without food; best if taken before breakfast. Do not crush, split, or chew tablet. May be administered with an antacid.

Dosage Forms Excipient information presented when available (limited, particularly for generics); consult specific product labeling. [CAN] = Canadian brand name

Tablet, delayed release, enteric coated, as sodium:

AcipHex®: 20 mg

Pariet® [CAN]: 10 mg, 20 mg

- ◆ **Racepinephrine** *see* EPINEPHrine *on page 543*
- ◆ **R-albuterol** *see* Levalbuterol *on page 902*
- ◆ **Ralix** *see* Chlorpheniramine, Phenylephrine, and Methscopolamine *on page 329*

Raloxifene (ral OKS i feen)

Medication Safety Issues

Sound-alike/look-alike issues:

Evista® may be confused with Avinza™

U.S. Brand Names Evista®

Canadian Brand Names Evista®

Mexican Brand Names Evista

Index Terms Keoxifene Hydrochloride; NSC-706725; Raloxifene Hydrochloride

Pharmacologic Category Selective Estrogen Receptor Modulator (SERM)

Generic Available No

Use Prevention and treatment of osteoporosis in postmenopausal women; risk reduction for invasive breast cancer in postmenopausal women with osteoporosis and in postmenopausal women with high risk for invasive breast cancer

Effect on Mental Status May cause insomnia or depression

Effect on Psychiatric Treatment None reported

Pregnancy Risk Factor X

Pregnancy Considerations Animal studies have demonstrated teratogenicity and fetal loss. There are no adequate and well-controlled studies in pregnant women. Raloxifene should not be used by pregnant women or by women planning to become pregnant in the immediate future.

Lactation Excretion in breast milk unknown/contraindicated

Contraindications History of or current venous thromboembolic disorders (including DVT, PE, and retinal vein thrombosis); pregnancy; breast-feeding

Warnings/Precautions Hazardous agent - use appropriate precautions for handling and disposal. **[U.S. Boxed Warning]: May increase the risk for DVT or PE;** use with caution in patients at high risk for venous thromboembolism; the risk for DVT and PE are higher in the first 4 months of treatment. Discontinue at least 72 hours prior to and during prolonged immobilization (postoperative recovery or prolonged bedrest). Use is contraindicated with a history of or current venous thromboembolic disorders. **[U.S. Boxed Warning]: The risk of death due to stroke may be increased in women with coronary heart disease or in women at risk for coronary events;** use with caution in patients with cardiovascular disease. Not be used for the prevention of cardiovascular disease. Use caution with moderate-to-severe renal dysfunction, hepatic impairment, unexplained uterine bleeding, and in women with a history of elevated triglycerides in response to treatment with oral estrogens (or estrogen/progestin). Safety with concomitant estrogen therapy has not been established. Safety and efficacy in premenopausal women or men have not been established. Not indicated for treatment of invasive breast cancer, to reduce the risk of recurrence of invasive breast cancer or to reduce the risk of noninvasive breast cancer. The efficacy (for breast cancer risk reduction) in women with inherited BRCA1 and BRCA1 mutations has not been established.

Adverse Reactions Note: Raloxifene has been associated with increased risk of thromboembolism (DVT, PE) and superficial thrombophlebitis; risk is similar to reported risk of HRT

>10%:

- Cardiovascular: Peripheral edema (3% to 14%)
- Endocrine & metabolic: Hot flashes (8% to 29%)
- Neuromuscular & skeletal: Arthralgia (11% to 16%), leg cramps/muscle spasm (6% to 12%)
- Miscellaneous: Flu syndrome (14% to 15%), infection (11% to 15%)

1% to 10%:

- Cardiovascular: Chest pain (3% to 4%), syncope (2%), varicose vein (2%), venous thromboembolism (1% to 2%)
- Central nervous system: Headache (9%), depression (6%), insomnia (6%), vertigo (4%), fever (3% to 4%), migraine (2%), hypoesthesia (≤2%)
- Dermatologic: Rash (6%)
- Endocrine & metabolic: Breast pain (4%)
- Gastrointestinal: Nausea (8% to 9%), weight gain (9%), abdominal pain (7%), diarrhea (7%), dyspepsia (6%), vomiting (3% to 5%), flatulence (2% to 3%), cholelithiasis (≤3%), gastroenteritis (≤3%)
- Genitourinary: Vaginal bleeding (6%), cystitis (3% to 5%), urinary tract infection (4%), vaginitis (4%), leukorrhea (3%), urinary tract disorder (3%), uterine disorder (3%), vaginal hemorrhage (3%), endometrial disorder (≤3%)
- Neuromuscular & skeletal: Myalgia (8%), arthritis (4%), tendon disorder (4%), neuralgia (≤2%)
- Ocular: Conjunctivitis (2%)
- Respiratory: Bronchitis (10%), rhinitis (10%), sinusitis (8% to 10%), cough (6% to 9%), pharyngitis (5% to 8%), pneumonia (3%), laryngitis (≤2%)
- Miscellaneous: Diaphoresis (3%)

<1% (Limited to important or life-threatening): Apolipoprotein A1 increased, apolipoprotein B decreased, death related to VTE, fibrinogen decreased, hypertriglyceridemia (in women with a history of increased triglycerides in

response to oral estrogens), intermittent claudication, LDL cholesterol decreased, lipoprotein decreased, muscle spasm, retinal vein occlusion, stroke related to VTE, superficial thrombophlebitis, total serum cholesterol decreased

Drug Interactions

Bile Acid Sequestrants: May decrease the absorption of Raloxifene. *Risk D: Consider therapy modification*

Levothyroxine: Raloxifene may decrease the absorption of Levothyroxine. *Risk D: Consider therapy modification*

Ethanol/Nutrition/Herb Interactions Ethanol: Avoid ethanol (may increase risk of osteoporosis).

Stability Store between 15°C to 30°C (59°F to 86°F).

Mechanism of Action A selective estrogen receptor modulator (SERM), meaning that it affects some of the same receptors that estrogen does, but not all, and in some instances, it antagonizes or blocks estrogen; it acts like estrogen to prevent bone loss and has the potential to block some estrogen effects in the breast and uterine tissues. Raloxifene decreases bone resorption, increasing bone mineral density and decreasing fracture incidence.

Pharmacodynamics/Kinetics

Onset of action: 8 weeks

Absorption: Rapid; ~60%

Distribution: 2348 L/kg

Protein binding: >95% to albumin and α-glycoprotein; does not bind to sex-hormone-binding globulin

Metabolism: Hepatic, extensive first-pass effect; metabolized to glucuronide conjugates

Bioavailability: ~2%

Half-life elimination: 28-33 hours

Excretion: Primarily feces; urine (<0.2% as unchanged drug; <6% as glucuronide conjugates)

Dosage Adults: Females: Oral:

Osteoporosis: 60 mg/day

Invasive breast cancer risk reduction: 60 mg/day

Dosage adjustment in hepatic impairment: Child-Pugh class A: Plasma concentrations were higher and correlated with total bilirubin. Safety and efficacy in hepatic insufficiency have not been established.

Dietary Considerations Supplemental calcium or vitamin D may be required if dietary intake is not adequate.

Administration May be administered any time of the day without regard to meals.

Monitoring Parameters Bone mineral density (BMD), CBC, lipid profile; adequate diagnostic measures, including endometrial sampling, if indicated, should be performed to rule out malignancy in all cases of undiagnosed abnormal vaginal bleeding

Additional Information The decrease in estrogen-related adverse effects with the selective estrogen-receptor modulators in general and raloxifene in particular should improve compliance and decrease the incidence of cardiovascular events and fractures while not increasing breast cancer.

Dosage Forms Excipient information presented when available (limited, particularly for generics); consult specific product labeling.

Tablet, as hydrochloride:

Evista®: 60 mg

◆ **Raloxifene Hydrochloride** *see* Raloxifene *on page 1391*

Raltegravir (ral TEG ra vir)

U.S. Brand Names Isentress™

Canadian Brand Names Isentress™

Index Terms MK-0518

Pharmacologic Category Antiretroviral Agent, Integrase Inhibitor

Use Treatment of HIV-1 infection in combination with other antiretroviral agents in treatment-experienced patients with virus that shows multidrug resistance and active replication

Effect on Mental Status May cause fatigue, dizziness, or insomnia. Rarely associated with anxiety, depression, abnormal dreams, irritability, and somnolence.

Effect on Psychiatric Treatment May cause elevation in lipid panel; concomitant use with atypical antipsychotics may produce additive effects. St John's wort may decrease the serum levels/effects of raltegravir.

Dosage Summary

Oral:

Children <16 years: Dosage not established

Adolescents ≥16 years: 400 mg twice daily

Adults: 400 mg twice daily

Dosage Forms Excipient information presented when available (limited, particularly for generics); consult specific product labeling.

Tablet:

Isentress™: 400 mg

Ramelteon (ra MEL tee on)

Medication Safety Issues

Sound-alike/look-alike issues:

Rozerem™ may be confused with Razadyne™

Related Information

CMS: Long-Term Care Facility Thresholds *on page 1815*

Nonbenzodiazepine Anxiolytics and Hypnotics *on page 1791*

U.S. Brand Names Rozerem™

Index Terms TAK-375

Pharmacologic Category Hypnotic, Nonbenzodiazepine

Generic Available No

Use Treatment of insomnia characterized by difficulty with sleep onset

Mental Health Comment In 2007, the FDA requested that all manufacturers of sedative-hypnotic drug products revise labeling to include a greater emphasis on the risks of adverse effects. These risks include severe allergic reactions (anaphylaxis, angioedema) and complex sleep-related behaviors, which may include sleep-driving (driving while not fully awake and with no memory of the event), making phone calls, and preparing and eating food while asleep.

Pregnancy Risk Factor C

Pregnancy Considerations Animal studies have demonstrated teratogenic effects. May cause disturbances of reproductive hormonal regulation (eg, disruption of menses or decreased libido). There are no adequate and well-controlled studies in pregnant women.

Lactation Excretion in breast mik unknown/not recommended

Contraindications Hypersensitivity to ramelteon or any component of the formulation; severe hepatic impairment; concurrent use with fluvoxamine

Warnings/Precautions Symptomatic treatment of insomnia should be initiated only after careful evaluation of potential causes of sleep disturbance. Failure of sleep disturbance to resolve after a reasonable period of treatment may indicate psychiatric and/or medical illness. Because of the rapid onset of action, administer immediately prior to bedtime or after the patient has gone to bed and is having difficulty falling asleep. Hypnotics/sedatives have been associated with abnormal thinking and behavior changes including decreased inhibition, aggression, bizarre behavior, agitation, hallucinations, and depersonalization. These changes may occur unpredictably and may indicate previously unrecognized psychiatric disorders; evaluate appropriately. Postmarketing studies have indicated that the use of hypnotic/sedative agents for sleep has been associated with hypersensitivity reactions including anaphylaxis as well as angioedema. An increased risk for hazardous sleep-related activities such as sleep-driving; cooking and eating food, and making phone calls while asleep have also been noted. Use caution with pre-existing depression or other psychiatric conditions. Caution when using with other CNS depressants; avoid engaging in hazardous activities or activities requiring mental alertness. Not recommended for use in patients with severe sleep apnea or COPD. Use caution with moderate hepatic impairment. May cause disturbances of hormonal regulation. Use caution when administered concomitantly with strong CYP1A2 inhibitors. Safety and efficacy in pediatric patients have not been established.

Adverse Reactions 1% to 10%:

Central nervous system: Headache (7%, same as placebo), somnolence (5%), dizziness (5%), fatigue (4%), insomnia worsened (3%), depression (2%)

Endocrine & metabolic: Serum cortisol decreased (1%)

Gastrointestinal: Nausea (3%), diarrhea (2%, same as placebo), taste perversion (2%)

Neuromuscular & skeletal: Myalgia (2%), arthralgia (2%)

Respiratory: Upper respiratory infection (3%; 2% with placebo)

Miscellaneous: Influenza (1%)

Postmarketing and/or case reports: Anaphylaxis, angioedema, complex sleep-related behavior (sleep-driving, cooking or eating food, making phone calls), prolactin levels increased, testosterone levels decreased

Metabolism/Transport Effects Substrate of CYP1A2 (major), CYP3A4 (minor), CYP2C family (minor)

Drug Interactions

Alcohol (Ethyl): CNS Depressants may enhance the CNS depressant effect of Alcohol (Ethyl). *Risk C: Monitor therapy*

Antifungal Agents (Azole Derivatives, Systemic): May decrease the metabolism of Ramelteon. *Risk C: Monitor therapy*

CNS Depressants: May enhance the adverse/toxic effect of other CNS Depressants. *Risk C: Monitor therapy*

CYP1A2 Inhibitors (Moderate): May decrease the metabolism of CYP1A2 Substrates. *Risk C: Monitor therapy*

CYP1A2 Inhibitors (Strong): May decrease the metabolism of CYP1A2 Substrates. *Risk D: Consider therapy modification*

Fluconazole: May decrease the metabolism of Ramelteon. *Risk C: Monitor therapy*

Fluvoxamine: May decrease the metabolism of Ramelteon. *Risk X: Avoid combination*

Rifamycin Derivatives: May increase the metabolism of Ramelteon. *Risk C: Monitor therapy*

Ethanol/Nutrition/Herb Interactions

Ethanol: Avoid ethanol (may increase CNS depression).

Food: Taking with high-fat meal delays T_{max} and increases AUC (~31%); do not take with high-fat meal.

Stability Store at 15°C to 30°C (59°F to 86°F).

Mechanism of Action Potent, selective agonist of melatonin receptors MT_1 and MT_2 (with little affinity for MT_3) within the suprachiasmic nucleus of the hypothalamus, an area responsible for determination of circadian rhythms and synchronization of the sleep-wake cycle. Agonism of MT_1 is thought to preferentially induce sleepiness, while MT_2 receptor activation preferentially influences regulation of circadian rhythms. Ramelteon is eightfold more selective for MT_1 than MT_2 and exhibits nearly sixfold higher affinity for MT_1 than melatonin, presumably allowing for enhanced effects on sleep induction.

Pharmacodynamics/Kinetics

Onset of action: 30 minutes

Absorption: Rapid; high-fat meal delays T_{max} and increases AUC (~31%)

Distribution: 74 L

Protein binding: 82%

Metabolism: Extensive first-pass effect; oxidative metabolism primarily through CYP1A2 and to a lesser extent through CYP2C and CYP3A4; forms active metabolite (M-II)

Bioavailability: Absolute: 1.8%

Half-life elimination: Ramelteon: 1-2.6 hours; M-II: 2-5 hours

Time to peak, plasma: Median: 0.5-1.5 hours

Excretion: Primarily as metabolites: Urine (84%); feces (4%)

Dosage

Oral: Adults: One 8 mg tablet within 30 minutes of bedtime

Dosage adjustment in renal impairment: No dosage adjustment required

Dosage adjustment in hepatic impairment: No adjustment required for mild-to-moderate impairment. Avoid use with severe impairment.

Dietary Considerations Taking with high-fat meal delays T_{max} and increases AUC (~31%); do not take with high-fat meal.

Administration Do not administer with a high-fat meal.

Dosage Forms Excipient information presented when available (limited, particularly for generics); consult specific product labeling.

Tablet: 8 mg

Ramipril (RA mi pril)

Medication Safety Issues

Sound-alike/look-alike issues:

Ramipril may be confused with enalapril, Monopril®

Altace® may be confused with alteplase, Amaryl®, Amerge®, Artane®

International issues:

Altace® may be confused with Altace® HCT which is a brand name for ramipril/hydrochlorothiazide combination product in Canada

Related Information

Angiotensin Agents *on page 1754*

U.S. Brand Names Altace®

Canadian Brand Names Altace®; Apo-Ramipril®; CO Ramipril; Novo-Ramipril; ratio-Ramipril; Sandoz-Ramipril

Mexican Brand Names Tritace

Pharmacologic Category Angiotensin-Converting Enzyme (ACE) Inhibitor

Generic Available Yes: Capsule

Use Treatment of hypertension, alone or in combination with thiazide diuretics; treatment of left ventricular dysfunction after MI; to reduce risk of MI, stroke, and death in patients at increased risk for these events

Unlabeled/Investigational Use Treatment of heart failure; to delay the progression of nephropathy and reduce risks of cardiovascular events in hypertensive patients with type 1 or 2 diabetes mellitus

Effect on Mental Status May cause dizziness or drowsiness; may rarely cause nervousness, amnesia, insomnia, or depression

Effect on Psychiatric Treatment May cause neutropenia; use caution with clozapine and carbamazepine; may decrease lithium clearance resulting in an increase in serum lithium levels and potential lithium toxicity; monitor serum lithium levels

Pregnancy Risk Factor C (1st trimester); D (2nd and 3rd trimesters)

Pregnancy Considerations Due to adverse events observed in some animal studies, ramipril is considered pregnancy category C during the first trimester. Based on human data, ramipril is considered pregnancy category D if used during the second and third trimesters (per the manufacturer; however, one study suggests that fetal injury may occur at anytime during pregnancy). Ramipril crosses the placenta. First trimester exposure to ACE inhibitors may cause major congenital malformations. An increased risk of cardiovascular and/or central nervous system malformations was observed in one study; however, an increased risk of teratogenic events was not observed in other studies. Second and third trimester use of an ACE inhibitor is associated with oligohydramnios. Oligohydramnios due to decreased fetal renal function may lead to fetal limb contractures, craniofacial deformation, and hypoplastic lung development. The use of ACE inhibitors during the second and third trimesters is also associated with anuria, hypotension, renal failure (reversible or irreversible), skull hypoplasia, and death in the fetus/neonate. Chronic maternal hypertension itself is also associated with adverse events in the fetus/infant. ACE inhibitors are not recommended during pregnancy to treat maternal hypertension or heart failure. Those who are planning a pregnancy should be considered for other medication options if an ACE inhibitor is currently prescribed or the ACE inhibitor should be discontinued as soon as possible once pregnancy is detected. The exposed fetus should be monitored for fetal growth, amniotic fluid volume, and organ formation. Infants exposed to an ACE inhibitor *in utero*, especially during the second and third trimester, should be monitored for hyperkalemia, hypotension, and oliguria.

[U.S. Boxed Warning]: Based on human data, ACE inhibitors can cause injury and death to the developing fetus when used in the second and third trimesters. ACE inhibitors should be discontinued as soon as possible once pregnancy is detected.

Lactation Excretion in breast milk unknown/not recommended

Contraindications Hypersensitivity to ramipril or any component of the formulation; prior hypersensitivity (including angioedema) to ACE inhibitors

Warnings/Precautions Anaphylactic reactions may occur rarely with ACE inhibitors. At any time during treatment (especially following first dose) angioedema may occur rarely with ACE inhibitors; it may involve the head and neck (potentially compromising airway) or the intestine (presenting with abdominal pain). African-Americans and patients with idiopathic or hereditary angioedema may be at an increased risk. Prolonged frequent monitoring may be required especially if tongue, glottis, or larynx are involved as they are associated with airway obstruction. Patients with a history of airway surgery may have a higher risk of airway obstruction. Aggressive early and appropriate management is critical. Use in patients with previous angioedema associated with ACE inhibitor therapy is contraindicated. Severe anaphylactoid reactions may be seen during hemodialysis (eg, CVVHD) with high-flux dialysis membranes (eg, AN69), and rarely, during low density lipoprotein apheresis with dextran sulfate cellulose. Rare cases of anaphylactoid reactions have been reported in patients undergoing sensitization treatment with hymenoptera (bee, wasp) venom while receiving ACE inhibitors.

Symptomatic hypotension with or without syncope can occur with ACE inhibitors (usually with the first several doses); effects are most often observed in volume-depleted patients; close monitoring of patient is required especially with initial dosing and dosing increases; blood pressure must be lowered at a rate appropriate for the patient's clinical condition. Initiation of therapy in patients with ischemic heart disease or cerebrovascular disease warrants close observation due to the potential consequences posed by falling blood pressure (eg, MI, stroke). Use with caution in hypertrophic cardiomyopathy with outflow tract obstruction, severe aortic stenosis, or before, during, or immediately after major surgery. **[U.S. Boxed Warning]: Based on human data, ACEIs can cause injury and death to the developing fetus when used in the second and third trimesters. ACEIs should be discontinued as soon as possible once pregnancy is detected.**

Hyperkalemia may occur with ACE inhibitors; risk factors include renal dysfunction, diabetes mellitus, concomitant use of potassium-sparing diuretics, potassium supplements, and/or potassium containing salts. Use cautiously, if at all, with these agents and monitor potassium closely. Cough may occur with ACE inhibitors. Other causes of cough should be considered (eg, pulmonary congestion in patients with heart failure) and excluded prior to discontinuation.

May be associated with deterioration of renal function and/or increases in serum creatinine, particularly in patients with low renal blood flow (eg, renal artery stenosis, heart failure) whose glomerular filtration rate (GFR) is dependent on efferent arteriolar vasoconstriction by angiotensin II; deterioration may result in oliguria, acute renal failure, and progressive azotemia. Small increases in serum creatinine may occur following initiation; consider discontinuation only in patients with progressive and/or significant deterioration in renal function. Use with caution in patients with unstented unilateral/bilateral renal artery stenosis. When unstented bilateral renal artery stenosis is present, use is generally avoided due to the elevated risk of deterioration in renal function unless possible benefits outweigh risks.

Rare toxicities associated with ACE inhibitors include cholestatic jaundice (which may progress to fulminant hepatic necrosis), agranulocytosis, neutropenia, or leukopenia with myeloid hypoplasia. Patients with collagen vascular diseases (especially with concomitant renal impairment) or renal impairment alone may be at increased risk for hematologic toxicity; periodically monitor CBC with differential in these patients. Safety and efficacy have not been established in children.

Adverse Reactions Note: Frequency ranges include data from hypertension and heart failure trials. Higher rates of adverse reactions have generally been noted in patients with CHF. However, the frequency of adverse effects associated with placebo is also increased in this population.

>10%: Respiratory: Cough (increased) (7% to 12%)

1% to 10%:

- Cardiovascular: Hypotension (11%), angina (up to 3%), postural hypotension (2%), syncope (up to 2%)
- Central nervous system: Headache (1% to 5%), dizziness (2% to 4%), fatigue (2%), vertigo (up to 2%)
- Endocrine & metabolic: Hyperkalemia (1% to 10%)
- Gastrointestinal: Nausea/vomiting (1% to 2%)
- Neuromuscular & skeletal: Chest pain (noncardiac) (1%)
- Renal: Renal dysfunction (1%), serum creatinine increased (1% to 2%), BUN increased (<1% to 3%); transient increases of creatinine and/or BUN may occur more frequently
- Respiratory: Cough (estimated 1% to 10%)

<1% (Limited to important or life-threatening): Agitation, agranulocytosis, amnesia, anaphylactoid reaction, angioedema, arrhythmia, bone marrow depression, convulsions, depression, dysphagia, dyspnea, edema, eosinophilia, erythema multiforme, hearing loss, hemolytic anemia, hepatitis, hypersensitivity reactions (urticaria, rash, fever), impotence, insomnia, myalgia, MI, neuropathy, onycholysis, pancreatitis, pancytopenia, paresthesia, pemphigoid, pemphigus, photosensitivity, proteinuria, somnolence, Stevens-Johnson syndrome, symptomatic hypotension, thrombocytopenia, toxic epidermal necrolysis

Worsening of renal function may occur in patients with bilateral renal artery stenosis or in hypovolemia. In addition, a syndrome which may include fever, myalgia, arthralgia, interstitial nephritis, vasculitis, rash, eosinophilia and positive ANA, and elevated ESR has been reported with ACE inhibitors. Risk of pancreatitis and/or agranulocytosis may be increased in patients with collagen vascular disease or renal impairment.

Drug Interactions

Allopurinol: ACE Inhibitors may enhance the potential for allergic or hypersensitivity reactions to Allopurinol. *Risk D: Consider therapy modification*

Angiotensin II Receptor Blockers: May enhance the adverse/toxic effect of ACE Inhibitors. *Risk C: Monitor therapy*

Antacids: May decrease the serum concentration of ACE Inhibitors. *Risk C: Monitor therapy*

Aprotinin: May diminish the antihypertensive effect of ACE Inhibitors. *Risk C: Monitor therapy*

AzaTHIOprine: ACE Inhibitors may enhance the neutropenic effect of AzaTHIOprine. *Risk C: Monitor therapy*

CycloSPORINE: ACE Inhibitors may enhance the nephrotoxic effect of CycloSPORINE. *Risk D: Consider therapy modification*

Diazoxide: May enhance the hypotensive effect of Antihypertensives. *Risk C: Monitor therapy*

Eplerenone: May enhance the hyperkalemic effect of ACE Inhibitors. *Risk C: Monitor therapy*

Ferric Gluconate: ACE Inhibitors may enhance the adverse/toxic effect of Ferric Gluconate. *Risk C: Monitor therapy*

Gold Sodium Thiomalate: ACE Inhibitors may enhance the adverse/toxic effect of Gold Sodium Thiomalate. An increased risk of nitritoid reactions has been appreciated. *Risk C: Monitor therapy*

Herbs (Hypertensive Properties): May diminish the antihypertensive effect of Antihypertensives. *Risk C: Monitor therapy*

Herbs (Hypotensive Properties): May enhance the hypotensive effect of Antihypertensives. *Risk C: Monitor therapy*

Lithium: ACE Inhibitors may increase the serum concentration of Lithium. *Risk D: Consider therapy modification*

Loop Diuretics: May enhance the hypotensive effect of ACE Inhibitors. Specifically, postural hypotension which can accompany ACE Inhibitor initiation. Loop Diuretics may enhance the nephrotoxic effect of ACE Inhibitors. *Risk C: Monitor therapy*

Methylphenidate: May diminish the antihypertensive effect of Antihypertensives. *Risk C: Monitor therapy*

Nonsteroidal Anti-Inflammatory Agents: May diminish the antihypertensive effect of ACE Inhibitors. *Risk C: Monitor therapy*

Potassium Salts: May enhance the hyperkalemic effect of ACE Inhibitors. *Risk C: Monitor therapy*

Potassium-Sparing Diuretics: May enhance the hyperkalemic effect of ACE Inhibitors. *Risk C: Monitor therapy*

Prostacyclin Analogues: May enhance the hypotensive effect of Antihypertensives. *Risk C: Monitor therapy*

RiTUXimab: Antihypertensives may enhance the hypotensive effect of RiTUXimab. *Risk D: Consider therapy modification*

Salicylates: May diminish the antihypertensive effect of ACE Inhibitors. They may also diminish other beneficial pharmacodynamic effects desired for the treatment of CHF. The effects are likely dose-related. 100 mg doses aspirin appear to cause no problems, whereas 300 mg doses appear to significantly affect ACE Inhibitor efficacy. *Risk C: Monitor therapy*

Sirolimus: May enhance the adverse/toxic effect of ACE Inhibitors. *Risk C: Monitor therapy*

Temsirolimus: May enhance the adverse/toxic effect of ACE Inhibitors. *Risk C: Monitor therapy*

Thiazide Diuretics: May enhance the hypotensive effect of ACE Inhibitors. Specifically, postural hypotension which can accompany ACE Inhibitor initiation. Thiazide Diuretics may enhance the nephrotoxic effect of ACE Inhibitors. *Risk C: Monitor therapy*

Trimethoprim: May enhance the hyperkalemic effect of ACE Inhibitors. *Risk C: Monitor therapy*

Ethanol/Nutrition/Herb Interactions Herb/Nutraceutical: Avoid bayberry, blue cohosh, cayenne, ephedra, ginger, ginseng (American), kola, licorice (may worsen hypertension). Avoid black cohosh, California poppy, coleus, golden seal, hawthorn, mistletoe, periwinkle, quinine, shepherd's purse (may have increased antihypertensive effect).

Stability Store at controlled room temperature.

Mechanism of Action Ramipril is an ACE inhibitor which prevents the formation of angiotensin II from angiotensin I and exhibits pharmacologic effects that are similar to captopril. Ramipril must undergo enzymatic saponification by esterases in the liver to its biologically active metabolite, ramiprilat. The pharmacodynamic effects of ramipril result from the high-affinity, competitive, reversible binding of ramiprilat to angiotensin-converting enzyme, thus preventing the formation of the potent vasoconstrictor angiotensin II. This isomerized enzyme-inhibitor complex has a slow rate of dissociation, which results in high potency and a long duration of action; a CNS mechanism may also be involved in the hypotensive effect as angiotensin II increases adrenergic outflow from CNS; vasoactive kallikreins may be decreased in conversion to active hormones by ACE inhibitors, thus reducing blood pressure

Pharmacodynamics/Kinetics
Onset of action: 1-2 hours
Duration: 24 hours
Absorption: Well absorbed (50% to 60%)
Distribution: Plasma levels decline in a triphasic fashion; rapid decline is a distribution phase to peripheral compartment, plasma protein and tissue ACE (half-life: 2-4 hours); 2nd phase is an apparent elimination phase representing the clearance of free ramiprilat (half-life: 9-18 hours); and final phase is the terminal elimination phase representing the equilibrium phase between tissue binding and dissociation
Protein binding:
Ramipril: 73%
Ramiprilat: 56%
Metabolism: Hepatic to the active form, ramiprilat
Bioavailability:
Ramipril: 28%
Ramiprilat: 44%
Half-life elimination: Ramiprilat: Effective: 13-17 hours; Terminal: >50 hours
Time to peak, serum:
Ramipril: ~1 hour
Ramiprilat: 2-4 hours
Excretion: Urine (60%) and feces (40%) as parent drug and metabolites

Dosage Adults: Oral:
Hypertension: 2.5-5 mg once daily, maximum: 20 mg/day
Reduction in risk of MI, stroke, and death from cardiovascular causes: Initial: 2.5 mg once daily for 1 week, then 5 mg once daily for the next 3 weeks, then increase as tolerated to 10 mg once daily (may be given as divided dose)
Heart failure postmyocardial infarction: Initial: 2.5 mg twice daily titrated upward, if possible, to 5 mg twice daily.
Heart failure (unlabeled use): Initial: 1.25-2.5 mg once daily; target dose: 10 mg once daily (ACC/AHA 2005 Heart Failure Guidelines)
Note: The dose of any concomitant diuretic should be reduced. If the diuretic cannot be discontinued, initiate therapy with 1.25 mg. After the initial dose, the patient should be monitored carefully until blood pressure has stabilized.
Dosing adjustment in renal impairment:
Cl_{cr} <40 mL/minute: Administer 25% of normal dose.
Renal failure and hypertension: Administer 1.25 mg once daily, titrated upward as possible.
Renal failure and heart failure: Administer 1.25 mg once daily, increasing to 1.25 mg twice daily up to 2.5 mg twice daily as tolerated.

Administration Capsule is usually swallowed whole, but may be may be mixed in water, apple juice, or applesauce.

Monitoring Parameters Blood pressure; serum creatinine and potassium; if patient has collagen vascular disease and/or renal impairment, periodically monitor CBC with differential

Test Interactions Increases BUN, creatinine, potassium, positive Coombs' [direct]; decreases cholesterol (S); may cause false-positive results in urine acetone determinations using sodium nitroprusside reagent

Dosage Forms Excipient information presented when available (limited, particularly for generics); consult specific product labeling.
Capsule: 1.25 mg, 2.5 mg, 5 mg, 10 mg
Altace®: 1.25 mg, 2.5 mg, 5 mg, 10 mg
Tablet:
Altace®: 1.25 mg, 2.5 mg, 5 mg, 10 mg

◆ **Ranexa®** *see* Ranolazine *on page 1403*
◆ **Raniclor™** *see* Cefaclor *on page 291*

Ranitidine (ra NI ti deen)

Medication Safety Issues
Sound-alike/look-alike issues:
Ranitidine may be confused with amantadine, rimantadine
Zantac® may be confused with Xanax®, Zarontin®, Zofran®, Zyrtec®

International issues:
Antagon®: Brand name for astemizole in Mexico; brand name for ganirelix in the U.S.

Related Information
Anticholinergic Effects of Common Psychotropics *on page 1758*

U.S. Brand Names Zantac 150™ [OTC]; Zantac 75® [OTC]; Zantac®; Zantac® EFFERdose®

Canadian Brand Names Acid Reducer; Acid Reducer Maximum Strength Non Prescription; Alti-Ranitidine; Apo-Ranitidine®; BCI-Ranitidine; CO Ranitidine; Dom-Ranitidine; Gen-Ranidine; Novo-Ranidine; Nu-Ranit; PMS-Ranitidine; Ranitidine Injection, USP; Ratio-Ranitidine; Rhoxal-Ranitidine; Riva-Ranitidine; Sandoz-Ranitidine; ScheinPharm Ranitidine; Zantac 75®; Zantac Maximum Strength Non-Prescription; Zantac®

Mexican Brand Names Acloral; Azantac; Galidrin; Iqfadina; Ranisen

Index Terms Ranitidine Hydrochloride

Pharmacologic Category Histamine H_2 Antagonist

Generic Available Yes: Excludes effervescent tablet

Use

Zantac®: Short-term and maintenance therapy of duodenal ulcer, gastric ulcer, gastroesophageal reflux, active benign ulcer, erosive esophagitis, and pathological hypersecretory conditions; as part of a multidrug regimen for *H. pylori* eradication to reduce the risk of duodenal ulcer recurrence

Zantac 75® [OTC]: Relief of heartburn, acid indigestion, and sour stomach

Unlabeled/Investigational Use Recurrent postoperative ulcer, upper GI bleeding, prevention of acid-aspiration pneumonitis during surgery, and prevention of stress-induced ulcers

Effect on Mental Status May cause drowsiness or dizziness

Effect on Psychiatric Treatment May rarely cause agranulocytosis; use caution with clozapine and carbamazepine; concurrent use with diazepam may reduce diazepam's effectiveness

Pregnancy Risk Factor B

Pregnancy Considerations Ranitidine crosses the placenta, teratogenic effects to the fetus have not been reported in animal studies. Use with caution during pregnancy.

Lactation Enters breast milk/use caution

Contraindications Hypersensitivity to ranitidine or any component of the formulation

Warnings/Precautions Ranitidine has been associated with confusional states (rare). Use with caution in patients with hepatic impairment; use with caution in renal impairment, dosage modification required. Avoid use in patients with history of acute porphyria (may precipitate attacks); long-term therapy may be associated with vitamin B_{12} deficiency. Symptoms of GI distress may be associated with a variety of conditions; symptomatic response to H_2 antagonists does not rule out the potential for significant pathology (eg, malignancy). EFFERdose® formulation contains phenylalanine. Safety and efficacy of ranitidine have not been established for pediatric patients <1 month of age

Adverse Reactions Frequency not defined (limited to important or life-threatening):

Cardiovascular: Arrhythmias, vasculitis

Central nervous system: Dizziness, hallucinations, headache, mental confusion, somnolence, vertigo

Dermatologic: Erythema multiforme, rash

Gastrointestinal: Pancreatitis

Hematologic: Acquired hemolytic anemia, agranulocytosis, aplastic anemia, granulocytopenia, leukopenia, pancytopenia, thrombocytopenia

Hepatic: Hepatic failure

Respiratory: Pneumonia (causal relationship not established)

Miscellaneous: Anaphylaxis, hypersensitivity reactions

Metabolism/Transport Effects Substrate (minor) of CYP1A2, 2C19, 2D6; **Inhibits** CYP1A2 (weak), 2D6 (weak)

Drug Interactions

Antifungal Agents (Azole Derivatives, Systemic): H2-Antagonists may decrease the absorption of Antifungal Agents (Azole Derivatives, Systemic). **Exceptions:** Miconazole; Voriconazole. *Risk D: Consider therapy modification*

Atazanavir: H2-Antagonists may decrease the absorption of Atazanavir. *Risk D: Consider therapy modification*

Cefpodoxime: H2-Antagonists may decrease the absorption of Cefpodoxime. Separate oral doses by at least 2 hours. *Risk C: Monitor therapy*

Cefuroxime: H2-Antagonists may decrease the absorption of Cefuroxime. Separate oral doses by at least 2 hours. *Risk C: Monitor therapy*

Dasatinib: H2-Antagonists may decrease the absorption of Dasatinib. *Risk D: Consider therapy modification*

Erlotinib: H2-Antagonists may decrease the serum concentration of Erlotinib. *Risk X: Avoid combination*

Fosamprenavir: H2-Antagonists may decrease the serum concentration of Fosamprenavir. Cimetidine may also inhibit the metabolism of the active metabolite amprenavir, making its effects on fosamprenavir/amprenavir concentrations difficult to predict. *Risk C: Monitor therapy*

Iron Salts: H2-Antagonists may decrease the absorption of Iron Salts. **Exceptions:** Ferric Gluconate; Iron Dextran Complex; Iron Sucrose. *Risk C: Monitor therapy*

P-Glycoprotein Inducers: May decrease the serum concentration of P-Glycoprotein Substrates. P-glycoprotein inducers may also further limit the distribution of p-glycoprotein substrates to specific cells/tissues/organs where p-glycoprotein is present in large amounts (e.g., brain, T-lymphocytes, testes, etc.). *Risk C: Monitor therapy*

P-Glycoprotein Inhibitors: May increase the serum concentration of P-Glycoprotein Substrates. P-glycoprotein inhibitors may also enhance the distribution of p-glycoprotein substrates to specific cells/tissues/organs where p-glycoprotein is present in large amounts (e.g., brain, T-lymphocytes, testes, etc.). *Risk C: Monitor therapy*

Saquinavir: H2-Antagonists may increase the serum concentration of Saquinavir. *Risk C: Monitor therapy*

Ethanol/Nutrition/Herb Interactions

Ethanol: Avoid ethanol (may cause gastric mucosal irritation).

Food: Does not interfere with absorption of ranitidine.

Stability

Injection: Vials: Store between 4°C to 30°C (39°F to 86°F). Protect from light. Solution is a clear, colorless to yellow solution; slight darkening does not affect potency.

Premixed bag: Store between 2°C to 25°C (36°F to 77°F). Protect from light.

EFFERdose® formulations: Store between 2°C to 30°C (36°F to 86°F).

Syrup: Store between 4°C to 25°C (39°F to 77°F). Protect from light.

Tablet: Store in dry place, between 15°C to 30°C (59°F to 86°F). Protect from light.

Vials can be mixed with NS or D_5W; solutions are stable for 48 hours at room temperature.

Intermittent bolus injection: Dilute to maximum of 2.5 mg/mL.

Intermittent infusion: Dilute to maximum of 0.5 mg/mL.

Mechanism of Action Competitive inhibition of histamine at H_2-receptors of the gastric parietal cells, which inhibits gastric acid secretion, gastric volume, and hydrogen ion concentration are reduced. Does not affect pepsin secretion, pentagastrin-stimulated intrinsic factor secretion, or serum gastrin.

Pharmacodynamics/Kinetics

Absorption: Oral: 50%

Distribution: Normal renal function: V_d: 1.7 L/kg; Cl_{cr} 25-35 mL/minute: 1.76 L/kg minimally penetrates the blood-brain barrier; enters breast milk

Protein binding: 15%

Metabolism: Hepatic to N-oxide, S-oxide, and N-desmethyl metabolites

Bioavailability: Oral: 48%

Half-life elimination:

Oral: Normal renal function: 2.5-3 hours; Cl_{cr} 25-35 mL/minute: 4.8 hours

I.V.: Normal renal function: 2-2.5 hours

Time to peak, serum: Oral: 2-3 hours; I.M.: ≤15 minutes

Excretion: Urine: Oral: 30%, I.V.: 70% (as unchanged drug); feces (as metabolites)

Dosage

Children 1 month to 16 years:

Duodenal and gastric ulcer:

Oral:

Treatment: 2-4 mg/kg/day divided twice daily; maximum treatment dose: 300 mg/day

Maintenance: 2-4 mg/kg once daily; maximum maintenance dose: 150 mg/day

I.V.: 2-4 mg/kg/day divided every 6-8 hours; maximum: 200 mg/day

GERD and erosive esophagitis:

Oral: 5-10 mg/kg/day divided twice daily; maximum: GERD: 300 mg/day, erosive esophagitis: 600 mg/day

I.V. (unlabeled): 2-4 mg/kg/day divided every 6-8 hours; maximum: 200 mg/day **or as an alternative**

Continuous infusion: Initial: 1 mg/kg/dose for one dose followed by infusion of 0.08-0.17 mg/kg/hour or 2-4 mg/kg/day

Children ≥12 years: Prevention of heartburn: Oral: Zantac 75® [OTC]: 75 mg 30-60 minutes before eating food or drinking beverages which cause heartburn; maximum: 150 mg/24 hours; do not use for more than 14 days

Adults:

Duodenal ulcer: Oral: Treatment: 150 mg twice daily, or 300 mg once daily after the evening meal or at bedtime; maintenance: 150 mg once daily at bedtime

Helicobacter pylori eradication: 150 mg twice daily; requires combination therapy

Pathological hypersecretory conditions:

Oral: 150 mg twice daily; adjust dose or frequency as clinically indicated; doses of up to 6 g/day have been used

I.V.: Continuous infusion for Zollinger-Ellison: 1 mg/kg/hour; measure gastric acid output at 4 hours, if >10 mEq or if patient is symptomatic, increase dose in increments of 0.5 mg/kg/hour; doses of up to 2.5 mg/kg/hour have been used

Gastric ulcer, benign: Oral: 150 mg twice daily; maintenance: 150 mg once daily at bedtime

Erosive esophagitis: Oral: Treatment: 150 mg 4 times/day; maintenance: 150 mg twice daily

Prevention of heartburn: Oral: Zantac 75® [OTC]: 75 mg 30-60 minutes before eating food or drinking beverages which cause heartburn; maximum: 150 mg in 24 hours; do not use for more than 14 days

Patients not able to take oral medication:

I.M.: 50 mg every 6-8 hours

I.V.: Intermittent bolus or infusion: 50 mg every 6-8 hours

Continuous I.V. infusion: 6.25 mg/hour

Elderly: Ulcer healing rates and incidence of adverse effects are similar in the elderly, when compared to younger patients; dosing adjustments not necessary based on age alone

Dosing adjustment in renal impairment: Adults: Cl_{cr} <50 mL/minute:

Oral: 150 mg every 24 hours; adjust dose cautiously if needed

I.V.: 50 mg every 18-24 hours; adjust dose cautiously if needed

Hemodialysis: Adjust dosing schedule so that dose coincides with the end of hemodialysis

Dosing adjustment/comments in hepatic disease: Patients with hepatic impairment may have minor changes in ranitidine half-life, distribution, clearance, and bioavailability; dosing adjustments not necessary, monitor

Dietary Considerations Oral dosage forms may be taken with or without food.

Zantac® EFFERdose®: Effervescent tablet 25 mg contains sodium 1.33 mEq/tablet and phenylalanine 2.81 mg/tablet

Administration

Ranitidine injection may be administered I.M. or I.V.:

I.M.: Injection is administered undiluted

I.V.: Must be diluted; may be administered IVP or IVPB or continuous I.V. infusion

IVP: Ranitidine (usually 50 mg) should be diluted to a total of 20 mL with NS or D_5W and administered over at least 5 minutes

IVPB: Administer over 15-20 minutes

Continuous I.V. infusion: Administer at 6.25 mg/hour and titrate dosage based on gastric pH by continuous infusion over 24 hours

EFFERdose®: Should not be chewed, swallowed whole, or dissolved on tongue: 25 mg tablet: Dissolve in at least 5 mL (1 teaspoonful) of water; wait until completely dissolved before administering

Monitoring Parameters AST, ALT, serum creatinine; when used to prevent stress-related GI bleeding, measure the intragastric pH and try to maintain pH >4; signs and symptoms of peptic ulcer disease, occult blood with GI bleeding, monitor renal function to correct dose; monitor for side effects

Test Interactions False-positive urine protein using Multistix®, gastric acid secretion test, skin test allergen extracts, serum creatinine, urine protein test

Dosage Forms Excipient information presented when available (limited, particularly for generics); consult specific product labeling.

Capsule 150 mg, 300 mg

Infusion [premixed in NaCl 0.45%; preservative free]:

Zantac®: 50 mg (50 mL)

Injection, solution: 25 mg/mL (2 mL, 6 mL)

Zantac®: 25 mg/mL (2 mL, 6 mL, 40 mL) [contains phenol 0.5% as preservative]

Syrup: 15 mg/mL (5 mL, 10 mL, 473 mL)

Zantac®: 15 mg/mL (473 mL) [contains alcohol 7.5%; peppermint flavor]

Tablet: 75 mg [OTC], 150 mg, 300 mg

Zantac®: 150 mg, 300 mg

Zantac 75®: 75 mg

Zantac 150™: 150 mg

Tablet, for solution, oral [effervescent]:
Zantac® EFFERdose®: 25 mg [contains phenylalanine 2.81 mg/tablet, sodium 1.33 mEq/tablet, sodium benzoate]

◆ **Ranitidine Hydrochloride** *see* Ranitidine *on page 1399*

Ranolazine (ra NOE la zeen)

Medication Safety Issues
Sound-alike/look-alike issues:
Ranexa™ may be confused with Celexa®
U.S. Brand Names Ranexa®
Pharmacologic Category Cardiovascular Agent, Miscellaneous
Use Treatment of chronic angina
Effect on Mental Status May cause dizziness
Effect on Psychiatric Treatment Contraindicated with QT_c-prolonging agents including amitriptyline, chlorpromazine, domperidone, droperidol, fluoxetine, flupenthixol, haloperidol, imipramine, loxapine, mesoridazine, pimozide, quetiapine, thioridazine, thiothixene, ziprasidone, and zuclopenthixol. Also contraindicated with strong or moderate CYP3A4 inhibitors such as nefazodone. Carbamazepine may reduce the levels and/or effects of ranolazine.
Dosage Summary
Oral:
Children: Dosage not established
Adults: Initial: 500 mg twice daily; Maintenance: 500-1000 mg twice daily (maximum: 2000 mg/day)
Dosage Forms Excipient information presented when available (limited, particularly for generics); consult specific product labeling.
Tablet, extended release:
Ranexa®: 500 mg, 1000 mg

◆ **Rapamune®** *see* Sirolimus *on page 1490*
◆ **Raphon [OTC]** *see* EPINEPHrine *on page 543*
◆ **Raptiva®** *see* Efalizumab *on page 526*

Rasagiline (ra SA ji leen)

Medication Safety Issues
Sound-alike/look-alike issues:
Azilect® may be confused with Aricept®
Related Information
Antiparkinsonian Agents *on page 1767*
U.S. Brand Names Azilect®
Index Terms AGN 1135; Rasagiline Mesylate; TVP-1012
Pharmacologic Category Anti-Parkinson's Agent, MAO Type B Inhibitor
Generic Available No
Use Initial monotherapy or as adjunct to levodopa in the treatment of idiopathic Parkinson's disease
Mental Health Comment

Adverse effects: Rasagiline is a second generation MAO type B selective inhibitor derived from the propargylamine class of compounds from which selegiline originates. However, unlike selegiline, the parent structure of rasagiline is not an amphetamine derivative, nor is it metabolized to an amphetamine-like structure. This structural difference may differentiate rasagiline from selegiline in terms of an overall lower incidence of psychiatric and vasoactive side effects (eg, hallucinations, orthostasis).

Selective MAO inhibition: Comparable to selegiline, rasagiline has been shown in both *in vitro* and *in vivo* animal model investigations to inhibit MAO-B (by 50%) approximately 17- to 65-fold more selectively than MAO-A. However, >80% inhibition of MAO-B is regarded as necessary for therapeutic benefit. As selectivity is lost in a dose-dependent manner, higher dosages needed to achieve this target may compromise selectivity. *In vivo* animal data show that ≥80% inhibition of MAO-B was achieved by rasagiline doses in rats which were 10-fold higher than the therapeutic human dose (on a mg/kg basis). At this dose level, rasagiline retained nearly fourfold selectivity for MAO-B. The extent of selectivity for MAO-B given higher doses and/or extended durations of exposure in humans is not known. Given the lack of clinical data fully characterizing the effects of rasagiline on gut MAO-A activity at therapeutically effective doses, there remains a warning on the dietary consumption of tyramine-containing foods.

Pregnancy Risk Factor C

Pregnancy Considerations Animal studies have documented decreased offspring survival and birth weight. An increased incidence of teratogenic effects, embryo-fetal deaths, and cardiovascular abnormalities were also noted with rasagiline in combination with levodopa/carbidopa. There are no adequate and well-controlled studies in pregnant women.

Lactation Excretion in breast milk unknown/use caution

Contraindications Hypersensitivity to rasagiline or any component of the formulation; concomitant use of amphetamine, tramadol, propoxyphene, methadone, dextromethorphan, St John's wort, mirtazapine, cyclobenzaprine, or sympathomimetic amines (eg, pseudoephedrine, ephedrine); use of meperidine or other MAO inhibitor within 14 days of rasagiline; elective surgery requiring general anesthesia, local anesthesia containing sympathomimetic vasoconstrictors; patients with pheochromocytoma

Warnings/Precautions

Cardiovascular system: Hypertensive crisis may occur with tyramine, tryptophan, or dopamine-containing foods; avoid for at least 2 weeks following discontinuation of rasagiline. May cause orthostatic hypotension, particularly in combination with levodopa; use with caution in patients with hypotension or patients who would not tolerate transient hypotensive episodes (cardiovascular or cerebrovascular disease); orthostasis is usually most problematic during first 2 months of therapy and tends to abate thereafter. Due to the potential for hemodynamic instability, patients should not undergo elective surgery requiring general anesthesia and should avoid local anesthesia containing sympathomimetic vasoconstrictors within 14 days of discontinuing rasagiline. If surgery is required, benzodiazepines, mivacurium, fentanyl, morphine or codeine may be used cautiously.

Central nervous system: May cause hallucinations; signs of severe CNS toxicity (some fatal), including hyperpyrexia, hyperthermia, rigidity, altered mental status, seizure and coma have been reported with selective and nonselective MAO inhibitor use in combination with antidepressants. Do not use within 5 weeks of fluoxetine discontinuation; do not initiate tricyclic, SSRI or SNRI therapy within 2 weeks of discontinuing rasagiline. Addition to levodopa therapy may result in exacerbation of dyskinesias, requiring a reduction in levodopa dosage.

Dermatologic: Risk of melanoma may be increased with rasagiline, although increased risk has been associated with Parkinson's disease itself; patients should have regular and frequent skin examinations.

Organ dysfunction: Use caution in mild hepatic impairment; dose reduction recommended. Do not use with moderate to severe hepatic impairment.

Safety and efficacy in pediatric patients have not been established.

Adverse Reactions Unless otherwise noted, the following adverse reactions are as reported for monotherapy. Spectrum of adverse events was generally similar with adjunctive (levodopa) therapy, though the incidence tended to be higher.

>10%:

Central nervous system: Dyskinesia (18% adjunct therapy), headache (14%)

Gastrointestinal: Nausea (10% to 12% adjunct therapy)

1% to 10%:

Cardiovascular: Postural hypotension (6% to 9% adjunct therapy; dose dependent), bundle branch block angina, chest pain, syncope

Central nervous system: Depression (5%), hallucinations (4% to 5% adjunct therapy), fever (3%), malaise (2%), vertigo (2%), anxiety, dizziness

Dermatologic: Bruising (2%), alopecia, skin carcinoma, vesiculobullous rash

Endocrine & metabolic: Impotence, libido decreased

Gastrointestinal: Constipation (4% to 9% adjunct therapy), weight loss (2% to 9% adjunct therapy; dose dependent), dyspepsia (7%), xerostomia (2% to 6% adjunct therapy; dose dependent), gastroenteritis (3%), anorexia, diarrhea, gastrointestinal hemorrhage, vomiting

Genitourinary: Hematuria, urinary incontinence

Hematologic: Leukopenia

Hepatic: Liver function tests increased

Neuromuscular & skeletal: Arthralgia (7%), neck pain (2%), arthritis (2%), paresthesia (2%), abnormal gait, hyperkinesias, hypertonia, neuropathy, tremor, weakness

Ocular: Conjunctivitis (3%)

Renal: Albuminuria

Respiratory: Rhinitis (3%), asthma, cough increased

Miscellaneous: Fall (5%), flu-like syndrome (5%), allergic reaction

<1% (Limited to important or life-threatening): Acute kidney failure, aphasia, apnea, atrial arrhythmia, bigeminy, blepharitis, blindness, bone necrosis, cerebral hemorrhage, cerebral ischemia, circumoral paresthesia, deafness, deep thrombophlebitis, delirium, diplopia, dysautonomia, dysesthesia, emphysema, esophageal ulcer, exfoliative dermatitis, facial paralysis, glaucoma, gynecomastia, heart failure, hematemesis, hemiplegia, hemorrhage (various locations), hostility, hypocalcemia, incoordination, interstitial pneumonia, intestinal obstruction, intestinal perforation, intestinal stenosis, jaundice, keratitis, kidney calculus, large intestine perforation, laryngismus, larynx edema, leukoderma, leukorrhea, lung fibrosis, macrocytic anemia, manic depressive reaction, mania, megacolon, menstrual abnormalities, MI, muscle atrophy, myelitis, neuralgia, neuritis, neurosis, nocturia, paranoid reaction, parosmia, personality disorder, pleural effusion, pneumothorax, polyuria, psychosis, psychotic depression, ptosis, purpura, retinal degeneration, retinal detachment, seizure, stomach ulcer, strabismus, stupor, thrombocythemia, thrombosis, tongue edema, urinary disorders, vaginal moniliasis, ventricular fibrillation, ventricular tachycardia, vestibular disorder, visual field defect

Metabolism/Transport Effects Substrate of CYP1A2 (major)

Drug Interactions

Alpha-/Beta-Agonists (Direct-Acting): MAO Inhibitors may enhance the vasopressor effect of Alpha-/Beta-Agonists (Direct-Acting). Primarily with oral administration of phenylephrine. **Exceptions:** Dipivefrin. *Risk D: Consider therapy modification*

Alpha-/Beta-Agonists (Indirect-Acting): MAO Inhibitors may enhance the hypertensive effect of Alpha-/Beta-Agonists (Indirect-Acting). *Risk X: Avoid combination*

Alpha1-Agonists: MAO Inhibitors may enhance the hypertensive effect of Alpha1-Agonists. *Risk X: Avoid combination*

Alpha2-Agonists (Ophthalmic): MAO Inhibitors may enhance the hypertensive effect of Alpha2-Agonists (Ophthalmic). *Risk X: Avoid combination*

Altretamine: May enhance the orthostatic effect of MAO Inhibitors. *Risk C: Monitor therapy*

Amphetamines: MAO Inhibitors may enhance the hypertensive effect of Amphetamines. *Risk X: Avoid combination*

Anilidopiperidine Opioids: May enhance the serotonergic effect of MAO Inhibitors. This could result in serotonin syndrome. Management: Avoid use of fentanyl (and other anilidopiperidine opioids when possible) in patients who have used a monoamine oxidase inhibitor within the past 14 days due to reports of unpredictable but severe adverse effects. *Risk D: Consider therapy modification*

Antidepressants (Serotonin/Norepinephrine Reuptake Inhibitor): MAO Inhibitors may enhance the serotonergic effect of Antidepressants (Serotonin/Norepinephrine Reuptake Inhibitor). This may cause serotonin syndrome. *Risk X: Avoid combination*

Atomoxetine: MAO Inhibitors may enhance the neurotoxic (central) effect of Atomoxetine. *Risk X: Avoid combination*

Beta2-Agonists: MAO Inhibitors may enhance the adverse/toxic effect of Beta2-Agonists. *Risk C: Monitor therapy*

BuPROPion: MAO Inhibitors may enhance the neurotoxic (central) effect of BuPROPion. *Risk X: Avoid combination*

BusPIRone: May enhance the adverse/toxic effect of MAO Inhibitors. Elevated blood pressure has been reported. *Risk X: Avoid combination*

COMT Inhibitors: May enhance the adverse/toxic effect of MAO Inhibitors. *Risk D: Consider therapy modification*

Cyclobenzaprine: May enhance the serotonergic effect of MAO Inhibitors. This could result in serotonin syndrome. *Risk X: Avoid combination*

CYP1A2 Inducers (Strong): May increase the metabolism of CYP1A2 Substrates. *Risk C: Monitor therapy*

CYP1A2 Inhibitors (Moderate): May decrease the metabolism of CYP1A2 Substrates. *Risk C: Monitor therapy*

CYP1A2 Inhibitors (Strong): May decrease the metabolism of CYP1A2 Substrates. *Risk D: Consider therapy modification*

Dexmethylphenidate: MAO Inhibitors may enhance the hypertensive effect of Dexmethylphenidate. *Risk X: Avoid combination*

Dextromethorphan: MAO Inhibitors may enhance the serotonergic effect of Dextromethorphan. This may cause serotonin syndrome. *Risk X: Avoid combination*

Levodopa: May enhance the adverse/toxic effect of MAO Inhibitors. Of particular concern is the development of hypertensive reactions when levodopa is used with nonselective MAOI. *Risk D: Consider therapy modification*

Linezolid: MAO Inhibitors may enhance the adverse/toxic effect of Linezolid. *Risk X: Avoid combination*

Lithium: MAO Inhibitors may enhance the adverse/toxic effect of Lithium. *Risk C: Monitor therapy*

Maprotiline: May enhance the adverse/toxic effect of MAO Inhibitors. *Risk X: Avoid combination*

Meperidine: MAO Inhibitors may enhance the serotonergic effect of Meperidine. This may cause serotonin syndrome. *Risk X: Avoid combination*

Methyldopa: MAO Inhibitors may enhance the adverse/toxic effect of Methyldopa. *Risk X: Avoid combination*

Methylphenidate: MAO Inhibitors may enhance the hypertensive effect of Methylphenidate. *Risk X: Avoid combination*

Mirtazapine: MAO Inhibitors may enhance the neurotoxic (central) effect of Mirtazapine. *Risk X: Avoid combination*

Propoxyphene: May enhance the adverse/toxic effect of MAO Inhibitors. Specifically, the risk of serotonin syndrome or other serotonergic adverse events may be increased. *Risk X: Avoid combination*

Rauwolfia Alkaloids: MAO Inhibitors may enhance the adverse/toxic effect of Rauwolfia Alkaloids. Existing MAOI therapy can result in paradoxical effects of added rauwolfia alkaloids (eg, excitation, hypertension). *Risk D: Consider therapy modification*

Selective Serotonin Reuptake Inhibitors: MAO Inhibitors may enhance the serotonergic effect of Selective Serotonin Reuptake Inhibitors. This may cause serotonin syndrome. *Risk X: Avoid combination*

Serotonin 5-HT1D Receptor Agonists: MAO Inhibitors may decrease the metabolism of Serotonin 5-HT1D Receptor Agonists. Management: If MAO inhibitor therapy is required, naratriptan, eletriptan or frovatriptan may be a suitable 5-HT1D agonist to employ. **Exceptions:** Eletriptan; Frovatriptan; Naratriptan. *Risk X: Avoid combination*

Serotonin Modulators: May enhance the adverse/toxic effect of other Serotonin Modulators. The development of serotonin syndrome may occur. *Risk D: Consider therapy modification*

Sibutramine: May enhance the serotonergic effect of Serotonin Modulators. This may cause serotonin syndrome. *Risk X: Avoid combination*

Tetrabenazine: May enhance the adverse/toxic effect of MAO Inhibitors. *Risk X: Avoid combination*

TraMADol: May enhance the neuroexcitatory and/or seizure-potentiating effect of MAO Inhibitors. *Risk D: Consider therapy modification*

Tricyclic Antidepressants: MAO Inhibitors may enhance the serotonergic effect of Tricyclic Antidepressants. This may cause serotonin syndrome. *Risk X: Avoid combination*

Ethanol/Nutrition/Herb Interactions

Ethanol: Avoid ethanol. Avoid beverages containing tyramine (hearty red wine and beer).

Food: Concurrent ingestion of foods rich in tyramine may cause sudden and severe high blood pressure (hypertensive crisis). Avoid tyramine-containing foods with MAO-Is. Food's freshness is also an important concern; improperly stored or spoiled food can create an environment where tyramine concentrations may increase.

Herb/Nutraceutical: Avoid valerian, St John's wort, SAMe, kava kava (may increase risk of serotonin syndrome and/or excessive sedation); Avoid supplements containing caffeine, tyrosine, tryptophan, or phenylalanine. Ingestion of large quantities may increase the risk of severe side effects (eg, hypertensive reactions, serotonin syndrome).

Stability Store at 15°C to 30°C (59°F to 86°F).

Mechanism of Action Potent, irreversible and selective inhibitor of brain monoamine oxidase (MAO) type B, which plays a major role in the catabolism of dopamine. Inhibition of dopamine depletion in the striatal region of the brain reduces the symptomatic motor deficits of Parkinson's disease. There is also experimental evidence of rasagiline conferring neuroprotective effects (antioxidant, antiapoptotic), which may delay onset of symptoms and progression of neuronal deterioration.

Pharmacodynamics/Kinetics

Onset of action: Therapeutic: Within 1 hour

Duration: ~1 week (irreversible inhibition); may require ~14-40 days for complete restoration of (brain) MAO-B activity

Absorption: Rapid

Protein binding: 88% to 94%

Metabolism: Hepatic N-dealkylation and/or hydroxylation via CYP1A2 to multiple inactive metabolites (nonamphetamine derivatives)

Distribution: V_{dss}: 87 L

Bioavailability: 36%

Half-life elimination: ~1.3-3 hours (no correlation with biologic effect due to irreversible inhibition)
Time to peak, plasma: 30 minutes to 1 hour
Excretion: Urine (62%, >99% as metabolites); feces (7%)

Dosage Oral: Adults: Parkinson's disease:
Monotherapy: 1 mg once daily
Adjunctive therapy with levodopa: Initial: 0.5 mg once daily; may increase to 1 mg once daily based on response and tolerability
Note: When added to existing levodopa therapy, a dose reduction of levodopa may be required to avoid exacerbation of dyskinesias; typical dose reductions of ~9% to 13% were employed in clinical trials

Dose reduction with concomitant ciprofloxacin or other CYP1A2 inhibitors: 0.5 mg once daily

Dosage adjustment in renal impairment:
Mild impairment: No adjustment necessary
Moderate-to-severe impairment: No data available
Dosage adjustment in hepatic impairment:
Mild impairment (Child-Pugh ≤6): 0.5 mg once daily
Moderate-to-severe impairment: Not recommended

Dietary Considerations Avoid tyramine-containing foods/beverages. Some examples include aged or matured cheese, air-dried or cured meats (including sausages and salamis), fava or broad bean pods, tap/draft beers, Marmite concentrate, sauerkraut, soy sauce and other soybean condiments.

Monitoring Parameters Blood pressure; symptoms of parkinsonism; general mood and behavior (increased anxiety, or presence of mania or agitation); skin examination for presence of melanoma (higher incidence in Parkinson's patients- drug causation not established)

Additional Information When adding rasagiline to levodopa/carbidopa, the dose of the latter can usually be decreased. Studies are investigating the use of rasagiline in early Parkinson's disease to slow the progression of the disease.

Dosage Forms Excipient information presented when available (limited, particularly for generics); consult specific product labeling.
Tablet:
Azilect®: 0.5 mg, 1 mg

◆ **Rasagiline Mesylate** *see* Rasagiline *on page 1403*

Rasburicase (ras BYOOR i kayse)

U.S. Brand Names Elitek™
Canadian Brand Names Fasturtec®
Index Terms NSC-721631; Recombinant Urate Oxidase
Pharmacologic Category Enzyme; Enzyme, Urate-Oxidase (Recombinant)
Use Initial management of uric acid levels in pediatric patients with leukemia, lymphoma, and solid tumor malignancies receiving anticancer therapy expected to result in tumor lysis and elevation of plasma uric acid
Unlabeled/Investigational Use Prevention and treatment of malignancy-associated hyperuricemia in adults
Effect on Mental Status None reported
Effect on Psychiatric Treatment GI side effects are common; use caution with SSRIs. May cause neutropenia; use caution with clozapine.
Dosage Summary
I.V.:
Children: 0.15 mg/kg **or** 0.2 mg/kg once daily
Adults: Dosage not established
Dosage Forms Excipient information presented when available (limited, particularly for generics); consult specific product labeling.
Injection, powder for reconstitution:
Elitek™: 1.5 mg [packaged with three 1 mL ampuls of diluent]; 7.5 mg [packaged with 5 mL of diluent]

◆ **rATG** *see* Antithymocyte Globulin (Rabbit) *on page 126*
◆ **Razadyne™** *see* Galantamine *on page 705*
◆ **Razadyne™ ER** *see* Galantamine *on page 705*
◆ **ReAzo [OTC]** *see* Phenazopyridine *on page 1258*
◆ **Rebetol®** *see* Ribavirin *on page 1417*
◆ **Rebetron®** *see* Interferon Alfa-2b and Ribavirin *on page 846*
◆ **Rebif®** *see* Interferon Beta-1a *on page 848*

- **Reclast®** *see* Zoledronic Acid *on page 1702*
- **Reclipsen™** *see* Ethinyl Estradiol and Desogestrel *on page 592*
- **Recombinant Hirudin** *see* Lepirudin *on page 900*
- **Recombinant Human Insulin-Like Growth Factor-1** *see* Mecasermin *on page 973*
- **Recombinant Human Interleukin-11** *see* Oprelvekin *on page 1184*
- **Recombinant Human Luteinizing Hormone** *see* Lutropin Alfa *on page 964*
- **Recombinant Human Parathyroid Hormone (1-34)** *see* Teriparatide *on page 1553*
- **Recombinant Interleukin-11** *see* Oprelvekin *on page 1184*
- **Recombinant N-Acetylgalactosamine 4-Sulfatase** *see* Galsulfase *on page 708*
- **Recombinant Urate Oxidase** *see* Rasburicase *on page 1407*
- **Recombivax HB®** *see* Hepatitis B Vaccine *on page 764*
- **Rectacaine [OTC]** *see* Phenylephrine *on page 1273*
- **Reese's® Pinworm Medicine [OTC]** *see* Pyrantel Pamoate *on page 1373*
- **Refenesen™ [OTC]** *see* GuaiFENesin *on page 737*
- **Refenesen™ 400 [OTC]** *see* GuaiFENesin *on page 737*
- **Refenesen™ DM [OTC]** *see* Guaifenesin and Dextromethorphan *on page 739*
- **Refenesen™ PE [OTC]** *see* Guaifenesin and Phenylephrine *on page 742*
- **Refenesen Plus [OTC]** *see* Guaifenesin and Pseudoephedrine *on page 744*
- **Refludan®** *see* Lepirudin *on page 900*
- **Regitine [DSC]** *see* Phentolamine *on page 1272*
- **Reglan®** *see* Metoclopramide *on page 1031*
- **Regonol®** *see* Pyridostigmine *on page 1374*
- **Regular Insulin** *see* Insulin Regular *on page 838*
- **Relacon-DM NR** *see* Guaifenesin, Pseudoephedrine, and Dextromethorphan *on page 748*
- **Relacon-HC** *see* Phenylephrine, Hydrocodone, and Chlorpheniramine *on page 1277*
- **Relafen** *see* Nabumetone *on page 1089*
- **Relenza®** *see* Zanamivir *on page 1693*
- **Relief® [OTC] [DSC]** *see* Phenylephrine *on page 1273*
- **Relistor™** *see* Methylnaltrexone *on page 1023*
- **Relpax®** *see* Eletriptan *on page 528*
- **Remeron®** *see* Mirtazapine *on page 1058*
- **Remeron SolTab®** *see* Mirtazapine *on page 1058*
- **Remicade®** *see* InFLIXimab *on page 819*

Remifentanil (rem i FEN ta nil)

Medication Safety Issues

Sound-alike/look-alike issues:

Remifentanil may be confused with alfentanil

High alert medication: The Institute for Safe Medication Practices (ISMP) includes this medication among its list of drug classes which have a heightened risk of causing significant patient harm when used in error.

Related Information

Narcotic / Opioid Analgesics *on page 1789*

U.S. Brand Names Ultiva®

Canadian Brand Names Ultiva®

Mexican Brand Names Ultiva

Index Terms GI87084B

Pharmacologic Category Analgesic, Opioid; Anilidopiperidine Opioid

Use Analgesic for use during the induction and maintenance of general anesthesia; for continued analgesia into the immediate postoperative period; analgesic component of monitored anesthesia

Unlabeled/Investigational Use Management of pain in mechanically-ventilated patients

Effect on Mental Status May cause dizziness or agitation

Effect on Psychiatric Treatment None reported

Restrictions C-II

Dosage Summary **Note:** Dose should be based on ideal body weight (IBW) in obese patients (>30% over IBW)

I.V.:

Infants Birth to 2 months: With nitrous oxide 70%: Infusion: 0.4-1 mcg/kg/minute; Supplemental bolus dose: ≤1 mcg/kg

Children 1-12 years: Anesthesia (with halothane, sevoflurane, or isoflurane): Infusion: 0.05-1.3 mcg/kg/minute; Bolus: 1 mcg/kg every 2-5 minutes; **Note:** Titration is recommended

Adults:

Induction of anesthesia: 0.5-1 mcg/kg/minute (1 mcg/kg/minute for coronary bypass)

Maintenance of anesthesia: **Note:** Supplemental boluses of 0.5-1 mcg/kg every 2-5 minutes may be given

Coronary bypass: 0.125-4 mcg/kg/minute

With isoflurane or propofol: 0.05-2 mcg/kg/minute

With nitrous oxide (60%): 0.1-2 mcg/kg/minute

Postoperative: 0.025-0.2 mcg/kg/minute; Coronary bypass or ICU: 0.05-1 mcg/kg/minute

Analgesic component of monitored anesthesia care: Alone: Bolus: 1 mcg/kg; Infusion: 0.025-0.2 mcg/kg/minute; With midazolam: Bolus: 0.5 mcg/kg; Infusion: 0.025-0.2 mcg/kg/minute; **Note:** Supplemental oxygen is recommended

Elderly: Doses should be decreased by 1/2 and titrated

Dosage Forms Excipient information presented when available (limited, particularly for generics); consult specific product labeling.

Injection, powder for reconstitution: 1 mg, 2 mg, 5 mg [contains glycine 15 mg]

◆ **Reminyl® [DSC]** *see* Galantamine *on page 705*

◆ **Renese®** *see* Polythiazide *on page 1313*

Repaglinide (re PAG li nide)

Medication Safety Issues

Sound-alike/look-alike issues:

Prandin® may be confused with Avandia®

High alert medication: The Institute for Safe Medication Practices (ISMP) includes this medication among its list of drug classes which have a heightened risk of causing significant patient harm when used in error.

U.S. Brand Names Prandin®

Canadian Brand Names GlucoNorm®; Prandin®

Mexican Brand Names NovoNorm

Pharmacologic Category Antidiabetic Agent, Meglitinide Derivative

Generic Available No

Use Management of type 2 diabetes mellitus (noninsulin dependent, NIDDM) as an adjunct to diet and exercise; may be used in combination with metformin or thiazolidinediones

Effect on Mental Status None reported

Effect on Psychiatric Treatment Repaglinide is a CYP3A4 substrate; monitor glucose when used with an enzyme inducer (carbamazepine, barbiturates) or an inhibitor (nefazodone, fluvoxamine)

Pregnancy Risk Factor C

Pregnancy Considerations Adverse events have been observed in some animal studies; therefore, repaglinide is classified as pregnancy category C. Information describing the effects of repaglinide on pregnancy outcomes is limited. Maternal hyperglycemia can be associated with adverse effects in the fetus, including macrosomia, neonatal hyperglycemia, and hyperbilirubinemia; the risk of congenital malformations is increased when the Hb A_{1c} is above the normal range. Diabetes can also be associated with adverse effects in the mother. Poorly-treated diabetes may cause end-organ damage that may in turn negatively affect obstetric outcomes. Physiologic glucose levels should be maintained prior to and during pregnancy to decrease the risk of adverse events in the mother and the fetus. Until additional safety and efficacy data are obtained, the use of oral agents is generally not recommended as routine management of GDM or type 2 diabetes mellitus during pregnancy. Insulin is the drug of choice for the control of diabetes mellitus during pregnancy.

Lactation Excretion in breast milk unknown/not recommended

Contraindications Hypersensitivity to repaglinide or any component of the formulation; diabetic ketoacidosis, with or without coma (treat with insulin); type 1 diabetes (insulin dependent, IDDM)

Warnings/Precautions Use with caution in patients with moderate-to-severe hepatic impairment. Use caution in severe renal dysfunction, elderly, malnourished, or patients with adrenal/pituitary dysfunction; may be more susceptible to glucose-lowering effects. May cause hypoglycemia; appropriate patient selection, dosage, and patient education are important to avoid hypoglycemic episodes. It may be necessary to discontinue repaglinide and administer insulin if the patient is exposed to stress (fever, trauma, infection, surgery). Theoretically, repaglinide may increase cardiovascular events as observed in some studies using sulfonylureas, but there are no long-term studies assessing this concern. Not indicated for use in combination with NPH insulin as there have been case reports of myocardial ischemia; further evaluation required to assess the safety of this combination. Safety and efficacy have not been established in pediatric patients.

Adverse Reactions

>10%:

Central nervous system: Headache (9% to 11%)

Endocrine & metabolic: Hypoglycemia (16% to 31%)

Respiratory: Upper respiratory tract infection (10% to 16%)

1% to 10%:

Cardiovascular: Ischemia (4%), chest pain (2% to 3%)

Gastrointestinal: Diarrhea (4% to 5%), constipation (2% to 3%), tooth disorder (≤2%)

Genitourinary: Urinary tract infection (2% to 3%)

Neuromuscular & skeletal: Arthralgia (3% to 6%), back pain (5% to 6%)

Respiratory: Sinusitis (3% to 6%), bronchitis (2% to 6%)

Miscellaneous: Allergy (1% to 2%)

<1% (Limited to important or life-threatening): Alopecia, anaphylactoid reaction, arrhythmias, ECG abnormal, hemolytic anemia, hepatic dysfunction (severe), hepatitis, hypertension, jaundice, leukopenia, liver function tests increased, MI, palpitation, pancreatitis, Stevens-Johnson syndrome, thrombocytopenia

Metabolism/Transport Effects Substrate of CYP2C8 (major), 3A4 (major)

Drug Interactions

Antifungal Agents (Azole Derivatives, Systemic): May increase the serum concentration of Repaglinide. Management: Concurrent use of an azole antifungal with both repaglinide and gemfibrozil should be avoided. *Risk C: Monitor therapy*

Corticosteroids (Orally Inhaled): May diminish the hypoglycemic effect of Antidiabetic Agents. In some instances, corticosteroid-mediated HPA axis suppression has led to episodes of acute adrenal crisis, which may manifest as enhanced hypoglycemia, particularly in the setting of insulin or other antidiabetic agent use. *Risk C: Monitor therapy*

Corticosteroids (Systemic): May diminish the hypoglycemic effect of Antidiabetic Agents. In some instances, corticosteroid-mediated HPA axis suppression has led to episodes of acute adrenal crisis, which may manifest as enhanced hypoglycemia, particularly in the setting of insulin or other antidiabetic agent use. *Risk C: Monitor therapy*

CycloSPORINE: May increase the serum concentration of Repaglinide. *Risk C: Monitor therapy*

CYP2C8 Inducers (Highly Effective): May increase the metabolism of CYP2C8 Substrates (High risk). *Risk C: Monitor therapy*

CYP2C8 Inhibitors (Moderate): May decrease the metabolism of CYP2C8 Substrates (High risk). *Risk C: Monitor therapy*

CYP2C8 Inhibitors (Strong): May decrease the metabolism of CYP2C8 Substrates (High risk). *Risk D: Consider therapy modification*

CYP3A4 Inducers (Strong): May increase the metabolism of CYP3A4 Substrates. *Risk C: Monitor therapy*

CYP3A4 Inhibitors (Moderate): May decrease the metabolism of CYP3A4 Substrates. *Risk C: Monitor therapy*

CYP3A4 Inhibitors (Strong): May decrease the metabolism of CYP3A4 Substrates. *Risk D: Consider therapy modification*

Dasatinib: May increase the serum concentration of CYP3A4 Substrates. *Risk C: Monitor therapy*

Deferasirox: May decrease the serum concentration of CYP3A4 Substrates. *Risk C: Monitor therapy*

Gemfibrozil: May increase the serum concentration of Repaglinide. The addition of itraconazole may augment the effect of gemfibrozil on repaglinide. Management: Consider alternative therapy combinations to avoid this potentially significant interaction. Avoid concurrent use when also used with a CYP3A4 inhibitor. *Risk D: Consider therapy modification*

Herbs (CYP3A4 Inducers): May increase the metabolism of CYP3A4 Substrates. *Risk C: Monitor therapy*

Herbs (Hypoglycemic Properties): May enhance the hypoglycemic effect of Hypoglycemic Agents. *Risk C: Monitor therapy*

Luteinizing Hormone-Releasing Hormone Analogs: May diminish the therapeutic effect of Antidiabetic Agents. *Risk C: Monitor therapy*

Macrolide Antibiotics: May increase the serum concentration of Repaglinide. **Exceptions:** Azithromycin; Dirithromycin [Off Market]; Spiramycin. *Risk C: Monitor therapy*

Pegvisomant: May enhance the hypoglycemic effect of Antidiabetic Agents. *Risk C: Monitor therapy*

Rifamycin Derivatives: May increase the metabolism of Repaglinide. *Risk C: Monitor therapy*

Somatropin: May diminish the hypoglycemic effect of Antidiabetic Agents. *Risk D: Consider therapy modification*

Trimethoprim: May decrease the metabolism of Repaglinide. *Risk C: Monitor therapy*

Ethanol/Nutrition/Herb Interactions

Ethanol: Avoid ethanol (may cause hypoglycemia).

Food: When given with food, the AUC of repaglinide is decreased.

Herb/Nutraceutical: St John's wort may decrease repaglinide levels. Avoid gymnema, garlic (may cause hypoglycemia).

Stability Do not store above 25°C (77°F). Protect from moisture.

Mechanism of Action Nonsulfonylurea hypoglycemic agent of the meglitinide class (the nonsulfonylurea moiety of glyburide) used in the management of type 2 diabetes mellitus; stimulates insulin release from the pancreatic beta cells

Pharmacodynamics/Kinetics

Onset of action: Single dose: Increased insulin levels: ~15-60 minutes

Duration: 4-6 hours

Absorption: Rapid and complete

Distribution: V_d: 31 L

Protein binding, plasma: >98% to albumin

Metabolism: Hepatic via CYP3A4 and CYP2C8 isoenzymes and glucuronidation to inactive metabolites

Bioavailability: Mean absolute: ~56%

Half-life elimination: ~1 hour

Time to peak, plasma: ~1 hour

Excretion: Within 96 hours: Feces (~90%, <2% as parent drug); Urine (~8%)

Dosage Adults: Oral: Should be taken within 15 minutes of the meal, but time may vary from immediately preceding the meal to as long as 30 minutes before the meal

Initial: For patients not previously treated or whose Hb A_{1c} is <8%, the starting dose is 0.5 mg before each meal. For patients previously treated with blood glucose-lowering agents whose Hb A_{1c} is ≥8%, the initial dose is 1 or 2 mg before each meal.

Dose adjustment: Determine dosing adjustments by blood glucose response, usually fasting blood glucose. Double the preprandial dose up to 4 mg until satisfactory blood glucose response is achieved. At least 1 week should elapse to assess response after each dose adjustment.

Dose range: 0.5-4 mg taken with meals. Repaglinide may be dosed preprandial 2, 3, or 4 times/day in response to changes in the patient's meal pattern. Maximum recommended daily dose: 16 mg.

Patients receiving other oral hypoglycemic agents: When repaglinide is used to replace therapy with other oral hypoglycemic agents, it may be started the day after the final dose is given. Observe patients carefully for hypoglycemia because of potential overlapping of drug effects. When transferred from longer half-life sulfonylureas (eg, chlorpropamide), close monitoring may be indicated for up to ≥1 week.

Combination therapy: If repaglinide monotherapy does not result in adequate glycemic control, metformin or a thiazolidinedione may be added. Or, if metformin or thiazolidinedione therapy does not provide adequate control, repaglinide may be added. The starting dose and dose adjustments for combination therapy are the same as repaglinide monotherapy. Carefully adjust the dose of each drug to determine the minimal dose required to achieve the desired pharmacologic effect. Failure to do so could result in an increase in the incidence of hypoglycemic episodes. Use appropriate monitoring of FPG and Hb A_{1c} measurements to ensure that the patient is not subjected to excessive drug exposure or increased probability of secondary drug failure. If glucose is not achieved after a suitable trial of combination therapy, consider discontinuing these drugs and using insulin.

Dosing adjustment in renal impairment:

Cl_{cr} 40-80 mL/minute (mild to moderate renal dysfunction): Initial dosage adjustment does not appear to be necessary.

Cl_{cr} 20-40 mL/minute: Initiate 0.5 mg with meals; titrate carefully.

Cl_{cr} <20 mL/minute: Not studied.

Dosing adjustment in hepatic impairment: Use conservative initial and maintenance doses. Use longer intervals between dosage adjustments.

Dietary Considerations Administer repaglinide 15-30 minutes before meals. Dietary modification based on ADA recommendations is a part of therapy. May cause hypoglycemia. Must be able to recognize symptoms of hypoglycemia (palpitations, tachycardia, sweaty palms, diaphoresis, lightheadedness).

Administration Administer repaglinide 15-30 minutes before meals. Patients who are anorexic or NPO, may need to have their dose held to avoid hypoglycemia. Patients consuming extra meals should be instructed to add a dose for the extra meal.

Monitoring Parameters Monitor fasting blood glucose (periodically) and glycosylated hemoglobin (Hb A_{1c}) levels (every 3 months) with a goal of decreasing these levels towards the normal range. During dose adjustment, fasting glucose can be used to determine response.

Reference Range Recommendations for glycemic control in adults with diabetes:

Hb A_{1c}: <7%

Preprandial capillary plasma glucose: 70-130 mg/dL

Peak postprandial capillary blood glucose: <180 mg/dL

Blood pressure: <130/80 mm Hg

Dosage Forms Excipient information presented when available (limited, particularly for generics); consult specific product labeling.

Tablet:

Prandin®: 0.5 mg, 1 mg, 2 mg

Repaglinide and Metformin (re PAG li nide & met FOR min)

Medication Safety Issues

Sound-alike/look-alike issues:

PrandiMet™ may be confused with Avandamet®, Prandin®

High alert medication: The Institute for Safe Medication Practices (ISMP) includes this medication among its list of drug classes which have a heightened risk of causing significant patient harm when used in error.

U.S. Brand Names PrandiMet™

Index Terms Metformin and Repaglinide; Repaglinide and Metformin Hydrochloride

Pharmacologic Category Antidiabetic Agent, Biguanide; Antidiabetic Agent, Meglitinide Derivative; Hypoglycemic Agent, Oral

Use Management of type 2 diabetes mellitus (noninsulin dependent, NIDDM), as an adjunct to diet and exercise, in patients currently receiving or not adequately controlled on metformin and/or a meglitinide

Effect on Mental Status None reported

Effect on Psychiatric Treatment Repaglinide is a CYP3A4 substrate; monitor glucose when used with an enzyme inducer (carbamazepine, barbiturates) or an inhibitor (nefazodone, fluvoxamine). St John's wort may decrease repaglinide levels.

Dosage Summary

Oral:

Children: Dosage not established

Adults: Repaglinide 1-2 mg and metformin 500 mg 2-3 times daily with meals (maximum single dose: 4 mg/dose [repaglinide], 1000 mg/dose [metformin]; maximum daily dose: 10 mg/day [repaglinide], 2500 mg/day [metformin])

Dosage Forms Excipient information presented when available (limited, particularly for generics); consult specific product labeling.

Tablet:

PrandiMet™:

1/500: Repaglinide 1 mg and metformin hydrochloride 500 mg

2/500: Repaglinide 2 mg and metformin hydrochloride 500 mg

◆ **Repaglinide and Metformin Hydrochloride** *see* Repaglinide and Metformin *on page 1412*

◆ **Repan®** *see* Butalbital, Acetaminophen, and Caffeine *on page 229*

- **Reprexain®** *see* Hydrocodone and Ibuprofen *on page 780*
- **Requa® Activated Charcoal [OTC]** *see* Charcoal *on page 312*
- **Requip®** *see* Ropinirole *on page 1440*
- **Requip® XL™** *see* Ropinirole *on page 1440*
- **Rescon®** *see* Chlorpheniramine, Phenylephrine, and Methscopolamine *on page 329*
- **Rescon® MX** *see* Chlorpheniramine, Phenylephrine, and Methscopolamine *on page 329*
- **Rescon DM [OTC]** *see* Chlorpheniramine, Pseudoephedrine, and Dextromethorphan *on page 333*
- **Rescon GG [OTC]** *see* Guaifenesin and Phenylephrine *on page 742*
- **Rescon-Jr®** *see* Chlorpheniramine and Phenylephrine *on page 323*
- **Rescriptor®** *see* Delavirdine *on page 424*
- **Resectisol®** *see* Mannitol *on page 968*

Reserpine (re SER peen)

Medication Safety Issues

Sound-alike/look-alike issues:

Reserpine may be confused with Risperdal®, risperidone

Pharmacologic Category Central Monoamine-Depleting Agent; Rauwolfia Alkaloid

Generic Available Yes

Use Management of mild-to-moderate hypertension; treatment of agitated psychotic states (schizophrenia)

Unlabeled/Investigational Use Management of tardive dyskinesia

Effect on Mental Status May cause dizziness, nightmares, and drowsiness; high dose may cause depression, anxiety, or psychosis

Effect on Psychiatric Treatment Contraindicated in depression and with MAO inhibitors. Discontinue reserpine 7 days before ECT. Combined use with CNS depressants may produce additive effects. TCAs may diminish reserpine's antihypertensive effects.

Pregnancy Risk Factor C

Lactation Enters breast milk/use caution

Contraindications Hypersensitivity to reserpine or any component of the formulation; active peptic ulcer disease, ulcerative colitis; history of mental depression (especially with suicidal tendencies); patients receiving electroconvulsive therapy (ECT)

Warnings/Precautions Use with caution in patients with impaired renal function, inflammatory bowel disease, asthma, Parkinson's disease, gallstones, or history of peptic ulcer disease, and the elderly. At high doses, significant mental depression, anxiety, or psychosis may occur (uncommon at dosages <0.25 mg/day). May cause orthostatic hypotension; use with caution in patients at risk of hypotension or in patients where transient hypotensive episodes would be poorly tolerated (cardiovascular disease or cerebrovascular disease). Avoid concurrent use of MAO inhibitors and/or drugs with MAO-inhibiting properties. Discontinue reserpine 7 days before electroshock therapy. Some products may contain tartrazine.

Adverse Reactions Frequency not defined.

Cardiovascular: Arrhythmia, bradycardia, chest pain, hypotension, peripheral edema, PVC, syncope

Central nervous system: Dizziness, drowsiness, dull sensorium, fatigue, headache, mental depression, nightmares, nervousness, parkinsonism, paradoxical anxiety

Dermatologic: Flushing of skin, pruritus, purpura, rash

Endocrine & metabolic: Gynecomastia, weight gain

Gastrointestinal: Anorexia, diarrhea, dry mouth, gastric acid secretion increased, nausea, salivation increased, vomiting

Genitourinary: Impotence, libido decreased

Hematologic: Thrombocytopenia purpura

Neuromuscular & skeletal: Muscle ache

Ocular: Blurred vision, optic atrophy

Respiratory: Dyspnea, epistaxis, nasal congstion

Drug Interactions

Alcohol (Ethyl): CNS Depressants may enhance the CNS depressant effect of Alcohol (Ethyl). *Risk C: Monitor therapy*

Amphetamines: Gastrointestinal Acidifying Agents may decrease the serum concentration of Amphetamines. *Risk C: Monitor therapy*

Beta-Blockers: Reserpine may enhance the hypotensive effect of Beta-Blockers. *Risk C: Monitor therapy*

CNS Depressants: May enhance the adverse/toxic effect of other CNS Depressants. *Risk C: Monitor therapy*

Dabigatran Etexilate: P-Glycoprotein Inhibitors may increase the serum concentration of Dabigatran Etexilate. *Risk X: Avoid combination*

Diazoxide: May enhance the hypotensive effect of Antihypertensives. *Risk C: Monitor therapy*

Herbs (Hypertensive Properties): May diminish the antihypertensive effect of Antihypertensives. *Risk C: Monitor therapy*

Herbs (Hypotensive Properties): May enhance the hypotensive effect of Antihypertensives. *Risk C: Monitor therapy*

MAO Inhibitors: May enhance the adverse/toxic effect of Rauwolfia Alkaloids. Existing MAOI therapy can result in paradoxical effects of added rauwolfia alkaloids (eg, excitation, hypertension). *Risk D: Consider therapy modification*

Methylphenidate: May diminish the antihypertensive effect of Antihypertensives. *Risk C: Monitor therapy*

P-Glycoprotein Substrates: P-Glycoprotein Inhibitors may increase the serum concentration of P-Glycoprotein Substrates. P-glycoprotein inhibitors may also enhance the distribution of p-glycoprotein substrates to specific cells/tissues/organs where p-glycoprotein is present in large amounts (e.g., brain, T-lymphocytes, testes, etc.). *Risk C: Monitor therapy*

Prostacyclin Analogues: May enhance the hypotensive effect of Antihypertensives. *Risk C: Monitor therapy*

RiTUXimab: Antihypertensives may enhance the hypotensive effect of RiTUXimab. *Risk D: Consider therapy modification*

Rivaroxaban: P-Glycoprotein Inhibitors may increase the serum concentration of Rivaroxaban. *Risk X: Avoid combination*

Tetrabenazine: Reserpine may enhance the adverse/toxic effect of Tetrabenazine. *Risk X: Avoid combination*

Topotecan: P-Glycoprotein Inhibitors may increase the serum concentration of Topotecan. *Risk X: Avoid combination*

Ethanol/Nutrition/Herb Interactions

Ethanol: Avoid ethanol (may increase CNS depression).

Herb/Nutraceutical: Avoid dong quai if using for hypertension (has estrogenic activity). Avoid ephedra, yohimbe (may worsen hypertension). Avoid valerian, St John's wort, kava kava, gotu kola (may increase CNS depression). Avoid garlic (may have increased antihypertensive effect).

Stability Protect oral dosage forms from light.

Mechanism of Action Reduces blood pressure via depletion of sympathetic biogenic amines (norepinephrine and dopamine); this also commonly results in sedative effects

Pharmacodynamics/Kinetics

Onset of action: Antihypertensive: 3-6 days

Duration: 2-6 weeks

Absorption: ~40%

Distribution: Crosses placenta; enters breast milk

Protein binding: 96%

Metabolism: Extensively hepatic (>90%)

Half-life elimination: 50-100 hours

Excretion: Feces (30% to 60%); urine (10%)

Dosage Note: When used for management of hypertension, full antihypertensive effects may take as long as 3 weeks.

Oral:

Children: Hypertension: 0.01-0.02 mg/kg/24 hours divided every 12 hours; maximum dose: 0.25 mg/day (not recommended in children)

Adults:

Hypertension:

Manufacturer's labeling: Initial: 0.5 mg/day for 1-2 weeks; maintenance: 0.1-0.25 mg/day

Note: Clinically, the need for a "loading" period (as recommended by the manufacturer) is not well supported, and alternative dosing is preferred.

Alternative dosing (unlabeled): Initial: 0.1 mg once daily; adjust as necessary based on response.

Usual dose range (JNC 7): 0.05-0.25 mg once daily; 0.1 mg every other day may be given to achieve 0.05 mg once daily

Schizophrenia (labeled use) or tardive dyskinesia (unlabeled use): Dosing recommendations vary; initial dose recommendations generally range from 0.05-0.25 mg (although manufacturer recommends 0.5 mg once daily initially in schizophrenia). May be increased in increments of 0.1-0.25 mg; maximum dose in tardive dyskinesia: 5 mg/day.

Elderly: Initial: 0.05 mg once daily, increasing by 0.05 mg every week as necessary

Dosing adjustment in renal impairment: Cl_{cr} <10 mL/minute: Avoid use

Dialysis: Not removed by hemo or peritoneal dialysis; supplemental dose is not necessary

Monitoring Parameters Blood pressure, standing and sitting/supine

Additional Information Adverse effects are usually dose related, mild, and infrequent when administered for the management of hypertension.

Dosage Forms Excipient information presented when available (limited, particularly for generics); consult specific product labeling.

Tablet: 0.1 mg, 0.25 mg

- **Respa®-1st** *see* Guaifenesin and Pseudoephedrine *on page 744*
- **Respa-DM®** *see* Guaifenesin and Dextromethorphan *on page 739*
- **Respahist®** *see* Brompheniramine and Pseudoephedrine *on page 206*
- **Respaire®-60 SR [DSC]** *see* Guaifenesin and Pseudoephedrine *on page 744*
- **Respaire®-120 SR [DSC]** *see* Guaifenesin and Pseudoephedrine *on page 744*
- **Respa® PE [DSC]** *see* Guaifenesin and Phenylephrine *on page 742*
- **Respi-Tann™** *see* Carbetapentane and Pseudoephedrine *on page 273*
- **Restasis®** *see* CycloSPORINE *on page 409*
- **Restoril®** *see* Temazepam *on page 1545*
- **Retrovir®** *see* Zidovudine *on page 1695*
- **Revatio®** *see* Sildenafil *on page 1482*
- **Revex® [DSC]** *see* Nalmefene *on page 1095*
- **ReVia®** *see* Naltrexone *on page 1099*
- **Revlimid®** *see* Lenalidomide *on page 899*
- **Reyataz®** *see* Atazanavir *on page 147*
- **rhASB** *see* Galsulfase *on page 708*
- **r-hCG** *see* Chorionic Gonadotropin (Recombinant) *on page 343*
- **Rheumatrex® Dose Pack®** *see* Methotrexate *on page 1014*
- **r-h α-GAL** *see* Agalsidase Beta *on page 52*
- **RhIG** *see* $Rh_o(D)$ Immune Globulin *on page 1415*
- **rhIGF-1** *see* Mecasermin *on page 973*
- **rhIGF-1/rhIGFBP-3** *see* Mecasermin *on page 973*
- **rhIL-11** *see* Oprelvekin *on page 1184*
- **Rhinacon A** *see* Chlorpheniramine, Phenylephrine, and Phenyltoloxamine *on page 331*
- **Rhinall [OTC]** *see* Phenylephrine *on page 1273*
- **Rhinocort® Aqua®** *see* Budesonide *on page 210*
- **RhinoFlex™** *see* Acetaminophen and Phenyltoloxamine *on page 36*
- **RhinoFlex 650** *see* Acetaminophen and Phenyltoloxamine *on page 36*
- **r-hLH** *see* Lutropin Alfa *on page 964*
- **Rho(D) Immune Globulin (Human)** *see* $Rh_o(D)$ Immune Globulin *on page 1415*

$Rh_o(D)$ Immune Globulin (ar aych oh (dee) i MYUN GLOB yoo lin)

U.S. Brand Names HyperRHO™ S/D Full Dose; HyperRHO™ S/D Mini Dose; MICRhoGAM®; RhoGAM®; Rhophylac®; WinRho® SDF

Canadian Brand Names WinRho® SDF

Mexican Brand Names Probi RHO (D)

Index Terms RhIG; Rho(D) Immune Globulin (Human); RhoIGIV; RhoIVIM

Pharmacologic Category Immune Globulin

Use

Suppression of Rh isoimmunization: Use in the following situations when an $Rh_o(D)$-negative individual is exposed to $Rh_o(D)$-positive blood: During delivery of an $Rh_o(D)$-positive infant; abortion; amniocentesis; chorionic villus sampling; ruptured tubal pregnancy; abdominal trauma; hydatidiform mole; transplacental hemorrhage. Used when the mother is $Rh_o(D)$ negative, the father of the child is either $Rh_o(D)$ positive or $Rh_o(D)$ unknown, the baby is either $Rh_o(D)$ positive or $Rh_o(D)$ unknown.

Transfusion: Suppression of Rh isoimmunization in $Rh_o(D)$-negative individuals transfused with $Rh_o(D)$ antigen-positive RBCs or blood components containing $Rh_o(D)$ antigen-positive RBCs

Treatment of idiopathic thrombocytopenic purpura (ITP): Used in the following nonsplenectomized Rh_o(D) positive individuals: Children with acute or chronic ITP, adults with chronic ITP, children and adults with ITP secondary to HIV infection

Effect on Mental Status May cause dizziness and sedation

Effect on Psychiatric Treatment None reported

Dosage Summary

I.M.:

Children:

Transfusion: 12 mcg/mL Rho(D) positive whole blood **or** 24 mcg/mL Rho(D) positive red blood cell exposure; administer 1200 mcg every 12 hours until the total dose is received.

Adults:

Rho(D) suppression: 50 mcg, 120 mcg, or 300 mcg as a single dose

Transfusion: 12 mcg/mL Rho(D) positive whole blood **or** 24 mcg/mL Rho(D) positive red blood cell exposure; administer 1200 mcg every 12 hours until the total dose is received.

I.V.:

Children:

ITP: Initial: 25-50 mcg/kg as a single injection, or can be given as a divided dose on separate days; Maintenance: 25-60 mcg/kg based on platelet and hemoglobin levels

Transfusion: 9 mcg/mL Rho(D) positive whole blood **or** 18 mcg/mL Rho(D) positive red blood cell exposure; administer 600 mcg every 8 hours until the total dose is received.

Adults:

ITP: Initial: 25-50 mcg/kg as a single injection, or can be given as a divided dose on separate days; Maintenance: 25-60 mcg/kg based on platelet and hemoglobin levels

Rho(D) suppression: 50 mcg, 120 mcg, or 300 mcg as a single dose

Transfusion: 9 mcg/mL Rho(D) positive whole blood **or** 18 mcg/mL Rho(D) positive red blood cell exposure; administer 600 mcg every 8 hours until the total dose is received.

Dosage Forms Excipient information presented when available (limited, particularly for generics); consult specific product labeling. [DSC] = Discontinued product

Injection, solution [preservative free]:

HyperRHO™ S/D Full Dose: 300 mcg [for I.M. use only]

HyperRHO™ S/D Mini Dose: 50 mcg [for I.M. use only]

MICRhoGAM®: 50 mcg [for I.M. use only; contains polysorbate 80]

RhoGAM®: 300 mcg [for I.M. use only; contains polysorbate 80]

Rhophylac®: 300 mcg/2 mL (2 mL) [1500 int. units; for I.M. or I.V. use; contains human albumin]

WinRho® SDF:

120 mcg/~0.5 mL (~0.5 mL) [600 int. units; contains maltose and polysorbate 80; for I.M. or I.V. use] [DSC]

300 mcg/~1.3 mL (~1.3 mL) [1500 int. units; contains maltose and polysorbate 80; for I.M. or I.V. use]

500 mcg/~2.2 mL (~2.2 mL) [2500 int. units; contains maltose and polysorbate 80; for I.M. or I.V. use]

1000 mcg/~4.4 mL (~4.4 mL) [5000 int. units; contains maltose and polysorbate 80; for I.M. or I.V. use]

3000 mcg/~13 mL (~13 mL) [15,000 int. units; contains maltose and polysorbate 80; for I.M. or I.V. use]

- **RhoGAM®** *see* Rh_o(D) Immune Globulin *on page 1415*
- **RhoIGIV** *see* Rh_o(D) Immune Globulin *on page 1415*
- **RhoIVIM** *see* Rh_o(D) Immune Globulin *on page 1415*
- **Rhophylac®** *see* Rh_o(D) Immune Globulin *on page 1415*
- **rhPTH(1-34)** *see* Teriparatide *on page 1553*
- ***r*HuEPO-α** *see* Epoetin Alfa *on page 546*
- **rhuGM-CSF** *see* Sargramostim *on page 1462*
- **rHu-KGF** *see* Palifermin *on page 1214*
- **rhuMAb-E25** *see* Omalizumab *on page 1174*
- **rHuMAb-EGFr** *see* Panitumumab *on page 1221*
- **rhuMAb-VEGF** *see* Bevacizumab *on page 187*
- **RibaPak™** *see* Ribavirin *on page 1417*
- **Ribasphere®** *see* Ribavirin *on page 1417*

Ribavirin (rye ba VYE rin)

Medication Safety Issues

Sound-alike/look-alike issues:

Ribavirin may be confused with riboflavin, rifampin, Robaxin®

U.S. Brand Names Copegus®; Rebetol®; RibaPak™; Ribasphere®; Virazole®

Canadian Brand Names Virazole®

Mexican Brand Names Copegus; Desiken; Probirina; Trivorin; Vilona; Virazide

Index Terms RTCA; Tribavirin

Pharmacologic Category Antiviral Agent

Use

Inhalation: Treatment of patients with respiratory syncytial virus (RSV) infections; specially indicated for treatment of severe lower respiratory tract RSV infections in patients with an underlying compromising condition (prematurity, bronchopulmonary dysplasia and other chronic lung conditions, congenital heart disease, immunodeficiency, immunosuppression), and recent transplant recipients

Oral capsule:

In combination with interferon alfa-2b (Intron® A) injection for the treatment of chronic hepatitis C in patients with compensated liver disease who have relapsed after alpha interferon therapy or were previously untreated with alpha interferons

In combination with peginterferon alfa-2b (PEG-Intron®) injection for the treatment of chronic hepatitis C in patients with compensated liver disease who were previously untreated with alpha interferons

Oral solution: In combination with interferon alfa 2b (Intron® A) injection for the treatment of chronic hepatitis C in patients with compensated liver disease who were previously untreated with alpha interferons or patients who have relapsed after alpha interferon therapy

Oral tablet: In combination with peginterferon alfa-2a (Pegasys®) injection for the treatment of chronic hepatitis C in patients with compensated liver disease who were previously untreated with alpha interferons (includes patients with histological evidence of cirrhosis [Child-Pugh class A] and patients with clinically-stable HIV disease)

Unlabeled/Investigational Use Used in other viral infections including influenza A and B and adenovirus

Effect on Mental Status When used in combination with interferon alfa-2A or alfa-2b: Dizziness and drowsiness are common; may rarely cause delirium. Severe psychiatric disorders, including depression and suicidal behavior, have been associated with the use of some interferons. Careful neuropsychiatric monitoring is recommended.

Effect on Psychiatric Treatment When used in combination with interferon alfa-2A or alfa-2b: May cause leukopenia; use caution with clozapine and carbamazepine; concurrent use with psychotropics may produce additive sedation and dry mouth

Restrictions An FDA-approved medication guide must be distributed when dispensing an outpatient prescription (new or refill) for treatment of hepatitis C where this medication is to be used without direct supervision of a healthcare provider. Medication guides are available at http://www.fda.gov/cder/Offices/ODS/medication_guides.htm.

Dosage Summary

Inhalation:

Children: RSV: 20 mg/mL (6 g in 300 mL) solution administered with Viratek® small particle aerosol generator; continuous: 12-18 hours/day

Adults: Dosage not established

Oral:

Children <3 years: Dosage not established

Children ≥3 years and ≤25 kg: 15 mg/kg/day in 2 divided doses in combination with interferon alfa-2b

Children ≥3 years and 26-36 kg: 400 mg/day in 2 divided doses in combination with interferon alfa-2b

Children ≥3 years and 37-49 kg: 600 mg/day (200 mg in the morning and 400 mg in the evening) in combination with interferon alfa-2b

Children ≥3 years and 50-61 kg: 800 mg/day (400 mg in the morning and evening) in combination with interferon alfa-2b

Children ≥3 years and >61 kg but <75 kg: 1000 mg/day (400 mg in the morning and 600 mg in the evening) in combination with interferon alfa-2b

Adults ≤75 kg: 400 mg in the morning, then 600 mg in the evening in combination with interferon alfa-2b **or** 800 mg/day **or** 1000 mg/day in 2 divided doses in combination with peginterferon alfa-2a

Adults >75 kg: 600 mg in the morning, then 600 mg in the evening in combination with interferon alfa-2b **or** 800 mg/day **or** 1200 mg/day in 2 divided doses in combination with peginterferon alfa-2a

Dosage Forms Excipient information presented when available (limited, particularly for generics); consult specific product labeling.

Capsule: 200 mg
  Rebetol®, Ribasphere®: 200 mg
Combination package [dose pack]:
  RibaPak™ 400/600 [each package contains]:
    Tablet: 400 mg (7s)
    Tablet: 600 mg (2s)
Powder for solution, for nebulization:
  Virazole®: 6 g (1s) [reconstituted product contains ribavirin 20 mg/mL]
Solution, oral:
  Rebetol®: 40 mg/mL (100 mL) [contains propylene glycol and sodium benzoate; bubble-gum flavor]
Tablet: 200 mg
  Copegus®: 200 mg
  Ribasphere®: 200 mg, 400 mg, 600 mg
Tablet [dose pack]:
  RibaPak™: 400 mg (14s); 600 mg (14s)

◆ **Ribavirin and Interferon Alfa-2b Combination Pack** *see* Interferon Alfa-2b and Ribavirin *on page 846*

◆ **Ridaura®** *see* Auranofin *on page 160*

Rifabutin (rif a BYOO tin)

Medication Safety Issues

Sound-alike/look-alike issues:
  Rifabutin may be confused with rifampin

U.S. Brand Names Mycobutin®

Canadian Brand Names Mycobutin®

Index Terms Ansamycin

Pharmacologic Category Antibiotic, Miscellaneous; Antitubercular Agent

Use Prevention of disseminated *Mycobacterium avium* complex (MAC) in patients with advanced HIV infection

Unlabeled/Investigational Use Utilized in multidrug regimens for treatment of MAC

Effect on Mental Status May rarely cause insomnia

Effect on Psychiatric Treatment Neutropenia is common; avoid clozapine and carbamazepine; rifabutin is a hepatic enzyme inducer; monitor for altered clinical effects when used concurrently with psychotropics

Dosage Summary

Oral:
  Children ≤1 year: Dosage not established
  Children >1 year: 5 mg/kg once daily
  Adults: 300 mg once daily

Dosage Forms Excipient information presented when available (limited, particularly for generics); consult specific product labeling.

Capsule: 150 mg

◆ **Rifadin®** *see* Rifampin *on page 1418*

◆ **Rifamate®** *see* Rifampin and Isoniazid *on page 1419*

◆ **Rifampicin** *see* Rifampin *on page 1418*

Rifampin (rif AM pin)

Medication Safety Issues

Sound-alike/look-alike issues:
  Rifadin® may be confused with Rifater®, Ritalin®
  Rifampin may be confused with ribavirin, rifabutin, Rifamate®, rifapentine, rifaximin

U.S. Brand Names Rifadin®

Canadian Brand Names Rifadin®; Rofact™

Mexican Brand Names Rifadin; Rimactan

Index Terms Rifampicin

Pharmacologic Category Antibiotic, Miscellaneous; Antitubercular Agent

Use Management of active tuberculosis in combination with other agents; elimination of meningococci from the nasopharynx in asymptomatic carriers

Unlabeled/Investigational Use Prophylaxis of *Haemophilus influenzae* type b infection; *Legionella* pneumonia; used in combination with other anti-infectives in the treatment of staphylococcal infections; treatment of *M. leprae* infections

Effect on Mental Status May cause drowsiness, dizziness, confusion, behavioral changes, or ataxia; report of cognitive disturbances, delusions, and hallucinations

Effect on Psychiatric Treatment May cause leukopenia; use caution with clozapine and carbamazepine; rifampin is a potent hepatic enzyme inducer; monitor for altered clinical effects when used concurrently with psychotropics

Dosage Summary

I.V.:

Children <12 years: 10-20 mg/kg/day in 1-2 divided doses **or** 10-20 mg/kg twice weekly (maximum: 600 mg/day)

Children ≥12 years: 10-20 mg/kg/day in 1-2 divided doses

Adults: 10 mg/kg/day **or** 10 mg/kg 2-3 times/week **or** 600 mg every 12-24 hours

Oral:

Children <12 years: 10-20 mg/kg/day in 1-2 divided doses **or** 10-20 mg/kg twice weekly (maximum: 600 mg/day)

Children ≥12 years: 10 mg/kg/day **or** 10 mg/kg 2-3 times/week **or** 600 mg every 12-24 hours

Adults: 10 mg/kg/day **or** 10 mg/kg 2-3 times/week **or** 600 mg every 12-24 hours

Dosage Forms Excipient information presented when available (limited, particularly for generics); consult specific product labeling.

Capsule: 150 mg, 300 mg

Injection, powder for reconstitution: 600 mg

Rifampin and Isoniazid (rif AM pin & eye soe NYE a zid)

Medication Safety Issues

Sound-alike/look-alike issues:

Rifamate® may be confused with rifampin

U.S. Brand Names IsonaRif™; Rifamate®

Canadian Brand Names Rifamate®

Mexican Brand Names Rifinah

Index Terms Isoniazid and Rifampin

Pharmacologic Category Antibiotic, Miscellaneous

Use Management of active tuberculosis; see individual agents for additional information

Effect on Mental Status Rifampin may cause drowsiness, dizziness, confusion, behavioral changes, or ataxia; report of cognitive disturbances, delusions, and hallucinations; isoniazid may cause drowsiness or dizziness; may rarely cause depression or psychosis; reports of insomnia, restlessness, disorientation, hallucinations, delusions, obsessive-compulsive symptoms, and exacerbation of schizophrenia

Effect on Psychiatric Treatment May cause leukopenia; use caution with clozapine and carbamazepine; rifampin is a potent hepatic enzyme inducer; monitor for altered clinical effects when used concurrently with psychotropics; isoniazid may impair the metabolism of carbamazepine and oxidatively metabolized benzodiazepines; monitor for adverse effects

Dosage Summary

Oral:

Children: Dosage not established

Adults: 2 capsules/day

Dosage Forms Excipient information presented when available (limited, particularly for generics); consult specific product labeling.

Capsule:

IsonaRif™, Rifamate®: 300/150: Rifampin 300 mg and isoniazid 150 mg

Rifampin, Isoniazid, and Pyrazinamide

(rif AM pin, eye soe NYE a zid, & peer a ZIN a mide)

Medication Safety Issues

Sound-alike/look-alike issues:

Rifater® may be confused with Rifadin®

U.S. Brand Names Rifater®

Canadian Brand Names Rifater®

Index Terms Isoniazid, Rifampin, and Pyrazinamide; Pyrazinamide, Rifampin, and Isoniazid

Pharmacologic Category Antibiotic, Miscellaneous

Use Initial phase, short-course treatment of pulmonary tuberculosis; see individual agents for additional information

Effect on Mental Status Rifampin may cause drowsiness, dizziness, confusion, behavioral changes, or ataxia; report of cognitive disturbances, delusions, and hallucinations; isoniazid may cause drowsiness or dizziness; may rarely cause depression or psychosis; reports of insomnia, restlessness, disorientation, hallucinations, delusions, obsessive-compulsive symptoms, and exacerbation of schizophrenia

Effect on Psychiatric Treatment May cause leukopenia; use caution with clozapine and carbamazepine; rifampin is a potent hepatic enzyme inducer; monitor for altered clinical effects when used concurrently with psychotropics; isoniazid may impair the metabolism of carbamazepine and oxidatively metabolized benzodiazepines; monitor for adverse effects

Dosage Summary

Oral:

Children: Dosage not established
Adults ≤44 kg: 4 tablets once daily
Adults 45-54 kg: 5 tablets once daily
Adults ≥55 kg: 6 tablets once daily

Dosage Forms Excipient information presented when available (limited, particularly for generics); consult specific product labeling.
Tablet: Rifampin 120 mg, isoniazid 50 mg, and pyrazinamide 300 mg

Rifapentine (rif a PEN teen)

Medication Safety Issues
Sound-alike/look-alike issues:
Rifapentine may be confused with rifampin

U.S. Brand Names Priftin®

Canadian Brand Names Priftin®

Pharmacologic Category Antitubercular Agent

Use Treatment of pulmonary tuberculosis; rifapentine must always be used in conjunction with at least one other antituberculosis drug to which the isolate is susceptible; it may also be necessary to add a third agent (either streptomycin or ethambutol) until susceptibility is known.

Effect on Mental Status May cause dizziness or drowsiness; has rarely been associated with aggression

Effect on Psychiatric Treatment May cause neutropenia; use caution with clozapine and carbamazepine; rifapentine is an inducer of CYP3A4; monitor of altered clinical effects with barbiturates, benzodiazepines, phenytoin, beta-blockers, haloperidol and TCAs.

Dosage Summary Note: Rifapentine should not be used alone; initial phase should include a 3- to 4-drug regimen.

Oral:

Children: Dosage not established
Adults: 600 mg once or twice weekly

Dosage Forms Excipient information presented when available (limited, particularly for generics); consult specific product labeling.
Tablet: 150 mg

◆ **Rifater®** *see* Rifampin, Isoniazid, and Pyrazinamide *on page 1419*

Rifaximin (rif AX i min)

Medication Safety Issues
Sound-alike/look-alike issues:
Rifaximin may be confused with rifampin

U.S. Brand Names Xifaxan™

Mexican Brand Names Flonorm

Pharmacologic Category Antibiotic, Miscellaneous

Use Treatment of travelers' diarrhea caused by noninvasive strains of *E. coli*

Effect on Mental Status May cause abnormal dreams, insomnia, or fatigue

Effect on Psychiatric Treatment None reported

Dosage Summary

Oral:

Children <12 years: Dosage not established
Children ≥12 years: 200 mg 3 times/day
Adults: 200 mg 3 times/day

Dosage Forms Excipient information presented when available (limited, particularly for generics); consult specific product labeling.
Tablet: 200 mg

- **rIFN-A** *see* Interferon Alfa-2a *on page 844*
- **rIFN beta-1a** *see* Interferon Beta-1a *on page 848*
- **rIFN beta-1b** *see* Interferon Beta-1b *on page 848*
- **rIL-11** *see* Oprelvekin *on page 1184*
- **Rilutek®** *see* Riluzole *on page 1421*

Riluzole (RIL yoo zole)

U.S. Brand Names Rilutek®

Canadian Brand Names Rilutek®

Mexican Brand Names Rilutek

Index Terms 2-Amino-6-Trifluoromethoxy-benzothiazole; RP-54274

Pharmacologic Category Glutamate Inhibitor

Generic Available No

Use Treatment of amyotrophic lateral sclerosis (ALS); riluzole can extend survival or time to tracheostomy

Effect on Mental Status May cause agitation, depression, dizziness, insomnia, malaise, or somnolence

Effect on Psychiatric Treatment May cause neutropenia; use caution with clozapine and carbamazepine. GI side effects are common; concomitant use with SSRIs, carbamazepine, valproic acid, and lithium may produce additive effects. Riluzole is a CYP1A2 substrate; cigarette smoking may increase metabolism of riluzole.

Pregnancy Risk Factor C

Pregnancy Considerations Impaired fertility, decreased implantation, increased intrauterine death, and adverse effects on offspring growth and viability were observed in animal studies. There are no adequate or well-controlled studies in pregnant women.

Lactation Excretion in breast milk unknown/not recommended

Contraindications Severe hypersensitivity reactions to riluzole or any component of the formulation

Warnings/Precautions Among 4000 patients given riluzole for ALS, there were 3 cases of marked neutropenia (ANC <500/mm^3), all seen within the first 2 months of treatment. Use with caution in patients with concomitant renal insufficiency. Use with caution in patients with current evidence or history of abnormal liver function; do not administer if baseline liver function tests are elevated. May cause elevations in transaminases (usually transient); discontinue if jaundice develops. The elderly, female, or Japanese patients may have decreased clearance of riluzole; use with caution. May cause dizziness or somnolence; caution should be used performing tasks which require alertness (operating machinery or driving). Safety and efficacy have not been established in children.

Adverse Reactions

>10%:

Gastrointestinal: Nausea (12% to 21%)

Neuromuscular & skeletal: Weakness (15% to 20%)

Respiratory: Lung function decreased (10% to 16%)

1% to 10%:

Cardiovascular: Edema, hypertension, tachycardia

Central nervous system: Agitation, circumoral paresthesia, depression, dizziness, headache, insomnia, malaise, somnolence, tremor, vertigo

Dermatologic: Alopecia, eczema, pruritus

Gastrointestinal: Abdominal pain, anorexia, diarrhea, dyspepsia, flatulence, oral moniliasis, stomatitis, vomiting

Hepatic: Liver function tests increased

Neuromuscular & skeletal: Arthralgia, back pain

Respiratory: Cough increased, rhinitis, sinusitis

Miscellaneous: Aggravation reaction

<1% (Limited to important or life-threatening): Exfoliative dermatitis, neutropenia, postural hypertension, seizure

Metabolism/Transport Effects Substrate of CYP1A2 (major)

Drug Interactions

CYP1A2 Inducers (Strong): May increase the metabolism of CYP1A2 Substrates. *Risk C: Monitor therapy*

Ethanol/Nutrition/Herb Interactions

Ethanol: Avoid ethanol (due to CNS depression and possible risk of liver toxicity).

Food: A high-fat meal decreases absorption of riluzole (decreasing AUC by 20% and peak blood levels by 45%). Charbroiled food may increase riluzole elimination.

Stability Store at 20°C to 25°C (68°F to 77°F). Protect from bright light.

Mechanism of Action Mechanism of action is not known. Pharmacologic properties include inhibitory effect on glutamate release, inactivation of voltage-dependent sodium channels; and ability to interfere with intracellular events that follow transmitter binding at excitatory amino acid receptors

Pharmacodynamics/Kinetics

Absorption: 90%; high-fat meal decreases AUC by 20% and peak blood levels by 45%

Protein binding, plasma: 96%, primarily to albumin and lipoproteins

Metabolism: Extensively hepatic to six major and a number of minor metabolites via CYP1A2 dependent hydroxylation and glucuronidation

Bioavailability: Oral: Absolute: 60%

Half-life elimination: 12 hours

Excretion: Urine (90%; 85% as metabolites, 2% as unchanged drug) and feces (5%) within 7 days

Dosage Adults: Oral: 50 mg every 12 hours; no increased benefit can be expected from higher daily doses, but adverse events are increased

Dosage adjustment in smoking: Cigarette smoking is known to induce CYP1A2; patients who smoke cigarettes would be expected to eliminate riluzole faster. There is no information, however, on the effect of, or need for, dosage adjustment in these patients.

Dosage adjustment in special populations: Females and Japanese patients may possess a lower metabolic capacity to eliminate riluzole compared with male and Caucasian subjects, respectively

Dosage adjustment in renal impairment: Use with caution in patients with concomitant renal insufficiency

Dosage adjustment in hepatic impairment: Use with caution in patients with current evidence or history of abnormal liver function indicated by significant abnormalities in serum transaminase, bilirubin or GGT levels. Baseline elevations of several LFTs (especially elevated bilirubin) should preclude use of riluzole.

Dietary Considerations Take at least 1 hour before, or 2 hours after, a meal.

Administration Administer at the same time each day, 1 hour before or 2 hours after a meal.

Monitoring Parameters Monitor serum aminotransferases including ALT levels before and during therapy. Evaluate serum ALT levels every month during the first 3 months of therapy, every 3 months during the remainder of the first year and periodically thereafter. Evaluate ALT levels more frequently in patients who develop elevations. Maximum increases in serum ALT usually occurred within 3 months after the start of therapy and were usually transient when <5 times ULN (upper limits of normal).

In trials, if ALT levels were <5 times ULN, treatment continued and ALT levels usually returned to below 2 times ULN within 2-6 months. There is no experience with continued treatment of ALS patients once ALT values exceed 5 times ULN.

If a decision is made to continue treatment in patients when the ALT exceeds 5 times ULN, frequent monitoring (at least weekly) of complete liver function is recommended. Discontinue treatment if ALT exceeds 10 times ULN or if clinical jaundice develops. Monitor temperature, especially during first 2 months of therapy.

Dosage Forms Excipient information presented when available (limited, particularly for generics); consult specific product labeling.

Tablet: 50 mg

Rimantadine (ri MAN ta deen)

Medication Safety Issues

Sound-alike/look-alike issues:

Rimantadine may be confused with amantadine, ranitidine, Rimactane®

Flumadine® may be confused with fludarabine, flunisolide, flutamide

U.S. Brand Names Flumadine®

Canadian Brand Names Flumadine®

Mexican Brand Names Gabirol

Index Terms Rimantadine Hydrochloride

Pharmacologic Category Antiviral Agent, Adamantane

Generic Available Yes: Tablet

Use Prophylaxis (adults and children >1 year of age) and treatment (adults) of influenza A viral infection (per manufacturer labeling; also refer to current ACIP guidelines for recommendations during current flu season)

Note: In certain circumstances, the ACIP recommends use of rimantadine in combination with oseltamivir for the treatment or prophylaxis of influenza A infection when resistance to oseltamivir is suspected.

Effect on Mental Status May cause dizziness, anxiety, confusion, insomnia, restlessness, irritability, or hallucinations

Effect on Psychiatric Treatment None reported

Pregnancy Risk Factor C

Pregnancy Considerations Animal data suggest embryotoxicity, maternal toxicity, and offspring mortality at doses 7-11 times the recommended human dose. There are no adequate and well-controlled studies in pregnant women.

Lactation Excretion in breast milk unknown/ not recommended

Contraindications Hypersensitivity to drugs of the adamantine class, including rimantadine and amantadine, or any component of the formulation

Warnings/Precautions Use with caution in patients with renal and hepatic dysfunction; avoid use, if possible, in patients with recurrent and eczematoid dermatitis, uncontrolled psychosis, or severe psychoneurosis. An increase in seizure incidence may occur in patients with seizure disorders; discontinue drug if seizures occur; resistance may develop during treatment; viruses exhibit cross-resistance between amantadine and rimantadine. Due to increased resistance, the ACIP has recommended that rimantadine and amantadine no longer be used for the treatment or prophylaxis of influenza A in the United States until susceptibility has been re-established; consult current guidelines.

Adverse Reactions

1% to 10%:

Central nervous system: Dizziness (1% to 2%), insomnia (2% to 3%), concentration impaired (2%), anxiety (1%), fatigue (1%), headache (1%), nervousness (1% to 2%)

Gastrointestinal: Nausea (3%), anorexia (2%), vomiting (2%), xerostomia (2%), abdominal pain (1%)

Neuromuscular & skeletal: Weakness (1%)

<1% (Limited to important or life-threatening): Agitation, ataxia, bronchospasm, cardiac failure, confusion, convulsions, cough, depression, diarrhea, dyspepsia, dyspnea, euphoria, gait abnormality, hallucinations, heart block, hyperkinesias, hypertension, lactation, palpitation, pallor, parosmia, pedal edema, rash, somnolence, syncope, tachycardia, taste alteration, tinnitus, tremor

Drug Interactions

Influenza Virus Vaccine: Antiviral Agents (Influenza A and B) may diminish the therapeutic effect of Influenza Virus Vaccine. This only pertains to live, attentuated influenza virus vaccine. *Risk D: Consider therapy modification*

Ethanol/Nutrition/Herb Interactions Food: Food does not affect rate or extent of absorption

Stability Store at 15°C to 30°C (59°F to 86°F).

Mechanism of Action Exerts its inhibitory effect on three antigenic subtypes of influenza A virus (H1N1, H2N2, H3N2) early in the viral replicative cycle, possibly inhibiting the uncoating process; it has no activity against influenza B virus and is two- to eightfold more active than amantadine

Pharmacodynamics/Kinetics

Onset of action: Antiviral activity: No data exist establishing a correlation between plasma concentration and antiviral effect

Absorption: Tablet and syrup formulations are equally absorbed

Metabolism: Extensively hepatic

Half-life elimination: 25.4 hours; prolonged in elderly

Time to peak: 6 hours

Excretion: Urine (<25% as unchanged drug)

Clearance: Hemodialysis does not contribute to clearance

Dosage Oral:

Prophylaxis:

Children 1-10 years: 5 mg/kg/day; maximum: 150 mg/day

Children >10 years and Adults: 100 mg twice daily

Elderly: 100 mg/day in nursing home patients or all elderly patients who may experience adverse effects using the adult dose

Treatment:

Adults: 100 mg twice daily

Elderly: 100 mg once daily in patients ≥65 years

Dosage adjustment in renal impairment:
Cl_{cr} >10 mL/minute: Dose adjustment not required
Cl_{cr} ≤10 mL/minute: 100 mg/day

Dosage adjustment in hepatic impairment: Severe dysfunction: 100 mg/day

Administration Initiation of rimantadine within 48 hours of the onset of influenza A illness halves the duration of illness and significantly reduces the duration of viral shedding and increased peripheral airways resistance; continue therapy for 5-7 days after symptoms begin

Monitoring Parameters Monitor for CNS or GI effects in elderly or patients with renal or hepatic impairment

Dosage Forms Excipient information presented when available (limited, particularly for generics); consult specific product labeling. [DSC] = Discontinued product
Syrup, as hydrochloride:
Flumadine®: 50 mg/5 mL (240 mL) [raspberry flavor] [DSC]
Tablet, as hydrochloride: 100 mg
Flumadine®: 100 mg

◆ **Rimantadine Hydrochloride** *see* Rimantadine *on page 1422*
◆ **Rimso-50®** *see* Dimethyl Sulfoxide *on page 480*
◆ **Rinate™ Pediatric** *see* Chlorpheniramine and Phenylephrine *on page 323*
◆ **Rindal HD Plus** *see* Phenylephrine, Hydrocodone, and Chlorpheniramine *on page 1277*
◆ **Rindal HPD [DSC]** *see* Hydrocodone, Phenylephrine, and Diphenhydramine *on page 782*
◆ **Riomet®** *see* MetFORMIN *on page 997*
◆ **Riopan Plus® [OTC] [DSC]** *see* Magaldrate and Simethicone *on page 965*
◆ **Riopan Plus® Double Strength [OTC] [DSC]** *see* Magaldrate and Simethicone *on page 965*

Risedronate (ris ED roe nate)

Medication Safety Issues
Sound-alike/look-alike issues:
Actonel® may be confused with Actos®

U.S. Brand Names Actonel®

Canadian Brand Names Actonel®

Mexican Brand Names Actonel

Index Terms Risedronate Sodium

Pharmacologic Category Bisphosphonate Derivative

Use Treatment of Paget's disease of the bone; treatment and prevention of glucocorticoid-induced osteoporosis; treatment and prevention of osteoporosis in postmenopausal women; treatment of osteoporosis in men

Effect on Mental Status May cause depression, insomnia, anxiety, and dizziness

Effect on Psychiatric Treatment Nausea and diarrhea are common; concomitant use with SSRIs, lithium, valproic acid, or carbamazepine may produce additive effects

Dosage Summary
Oral:
Children: Dosage not established
Adults: 5 mg once daily **or** 35 mg once weekly **or** one 75 mg tablet taken on 2 consecutive days once a month (total of 2 tablets/month) **or** 150 mg once a month **or** 30 mg once daily (Paget's disease)

Dosage Forms Excipient information presented when available (limited, particularly for generics); consult specific product labeling.
Tablet, as sodium:
Actonel®: 5 mg, 30 mg, 35 mg, 75 mg, 150 mg

Risedronate and Calcium (ris ED roe nate & KAL see um)

Medication Safety Issues
Sound-alike/look-alike issues:
Actonel® may be confused with Actos®

U.S. Brand Names Actonel® and Calcium

Index Terms Calcium and Risedronate; Risedronate Sodium and Calcium Carbonate

Pharmacologic Category Bisphosphonate Derivative; Calcium Salt

Use Treatment and prevention of osteoporosis in postmenopausal women

Effect on Mental Status May cause depression, insomnia, anxiety, and dizziness

Effect on Psychiatric Treatment Nausea and diarrhea are common; concomitant use with SSRIs, lithium, valproic acid, or carbamazepine may produce additive effects

Dosage Summary

Oral:

Children: Dosage not established

Adults: Calcium carbonate: 1250 mg (500 mg elemental calcium) once daily on days 2-7 of 7-day treatment cycle; Risedronate: 35 mg once weekly on day 1 or 7 day treatment cycle

Dosage Forms Excipient information presented when available (limited, particularly for generics); consult specific product labeling.

Combination package [each package contains]:

Tablet (Actonel®): Risedronate 35 mg (4s)

Tablet: Calcium carbonate 1250 mg (24s) [equivalent to elemental calcium 500 mg]

◆ **Risedronate Sodium** *see* Risedronate *on page 1424*

◆ **Risedronate Sodium and Calcium Carbonate** *see* Risedronate and Calcium *on page 1424*

◆ **Risperdal®** *see* Risperidone *on page 1425*

◆ **Risperdal M-Tab** *see* Risperidone *on page 1425*

◆ **Risperdal® M-Tab®** *see* Risperidone *on page 1425*

◆ **Risperdal® Consta®** *see* Risperidone *on page 1425*

Risperidone (ris PER i done)

Medication Safety Issues

Sound-alike/look-alike issues:

Risperidone may be confused with reserpine

Risperdal® may be confused with lisinopril, reserpine

Related Information

Agents Approved for Bipolar Disorder *on page 1752*

Antipsychotic Agents *on page 1769*

Antipsychotic Receptor Profile *on page 1772*

Atypical Antipsychotics *on page 1773*

CMS: Long-Term Care Facility Thresholds *on page 1815*

Discontinuation of Psychotropic Drugs *on page 1839*

Liquid Compatibility of Antidepressants, Antipsychotics, and Mood Stabilizers *on page 1788*

U.S. Brand Names Risperdal®; Risperdal® Consta®; Risperdal® M-Tab®

Canadian Brand Names Apo-Risperidone®; CO Risperidone; Dom-Risperidone; Gen-Risperidone; Novo-Risperidone; PHL-Risperidone; PMS-Risperidone ODT; Ran-Risperidone; Ratio-Risperidone; Risperdal®; Risperdal® Consta®; Risperdal® M-Tab®; Riva-Risperidone; Sandoz Risperidone

Mexican Brand Names Risperdal; Ñorispez

Index Terms Risperdal M-Tab

Pharmacologic Category Antimanic Agent; Antipsychotic Agent, Atypical

Generic Available Yes: Tablet

Use Treatment of schizophrenia; treatment of acute mania or mixed episodes associated with bipolar I disorder (as monotherapy in children or adults, or in combination with lithium or valproate in adults); treatment of irritability/aggression associated with autistic disorder

Unlabeled/Investigational Use Treatment of Tourette's disorder; treatment of pervasive developmental disorder; psychosis/agitation related to Alzheimer's dementia

Mental Health Comment Risperidone is an antipsychotic agent of a class often referred to as atypical. It should be noted that the definition of the term "atypical" is not universally agreed upon. Some prefer to describe antipsychotics based on their pharmacological properties. A common feature of all definitions used to describe "atypical" antipsychotics is the lack of significant acute or subacute EPS, at dosages generally associated with antipsychotic actions. Other experts have included definitions of atypicality that include a) failure to increase serum prolactin levels; b) superior efficacy for positive, negative, and cognitive symptoms; and c) lack of evidence of tardive dyskinesia or dystonia following chronic administration.

Risperidone is associated with a dose dependent increase in EPS. Optimal dosage for most patients is ~4 mg/day. EPS is low when dosed ≤6 mg/day. Dosages >6 mg/day give a clinical picture similar to haloperidol.

Tardive dyskinesia (TD) secondary to **typical** antipsychotics has an estimated incidence of 3% to 5% per year for the first 5 years of treatment. The incidence of TD associated with the atypical antipsychotics is estimated to be 0.5% to 1%. It is not clear if this estimate represents a risk associated with mental illness or to what extent drug therapy can be implicated. Atypical antipsychotics appear less likely to cause tardive dyskinesia than typical antipsychotics (fluphenazine, haloperidol).

Coadministration of two or more antipsychotics does not generally improve clinical response and may increase the potential for adverse effects.

The long acting dosage form of risperidone is formed by cross-linking polylactide and glycolide molecules into a polymer, then exposing that polymer to risperidone to create microspheres that are 25-150 microns in diameter. The microspheres must be suspended in the water-based diluent (provided in the kit) prior to injection. Since the microspheres may not be uniformly distributed in the diluent, the entire contents of the vial must be injected to ensure accurate dosing (dividing a dose is not accurately possible). Further, the bore of the needle (included in the kit) is Teflon® coated to prevent destruction of the microspheres and loss of drug due to sticking to the interior surface during injection.

Approximately 1% of the drug is released for the first 3 weeks after an injection. Therefore, one must overlap with oral therapy for at least 3 weeks and often 4-6 weeks or longer. This dosage form is not amenable to loading dose strategies. However, it is water-based (as opposed to oil) and is associated with less pain after injection than haloperidol decanoate or fluphenazine decanoate. The vials can be stored at room temperature for ≤7 days total prior to reconstitution and should be stored in a refrigerator until the day of injection.

In 2008, the FDA issued a warning regarding increased mortality risk with typical **and** atypical antipsychotic drugs when used in elderly patients with dementia-related psychosis.

Pregnancy Risk Factor C

Pregnancy Considerations Animal studies indicate an increase in fetal mortality. Reversible EPS symptoms were noted in neonates following use of risperidone during the last trimester. Agenesis of the corpus callosum has also been noted in one case report. There are no adequate and well-controlled studies in pregnant women. When using Risperdal® Consta®, patients should notify healthcare provider if they become or intend to become pregnant during therapy or within 12 weeks of last injection. Risperidone may cause hyperprolactinemia, which may decrease reproductive function in both males and females.

Lactation Enters breast milk/not recommended

Contraindications Hypersensitivity to risperidone or any component of the formulation

Warnings/Precautions [U.S. Boxed Warning]: Elderly patients with dementia-related psychosis treated with atypical antipsychotics are at an increased risk of death compared to placebo. An increased incidence of cerebrovascular adverse events (including fatalities) has been reported in elderly patients with dementia-related psychosis. Risperidone is not approved for the treatment of dementia-related psychosis.

Low to moderately sedating, use with caution in disorders where CNS depression is a feature. Use with caution in Parkinson's disease. Caution in patients with predisposition to seizures; or severe cardiac disease. Use with caution in renal or hepatic dysfunction; dose reduction recommended. Esophageal dysmotility and aspiration have been associated with antipsychotic use; use with caution in patients at risk of aspiration pneumonia (ie, Alzheimer's disease). Elevates prolactin levels; effects seen in adults and children. Use with caution in breast cancer or other prolactin-dependent tumors. May alter temperature regulation. May mask toxicity of other drugs or conditions (eg intestinal obstruction, Reyes syndrome, brain tumor) due to antiemetic effects.

Use with caution in patients with cardiovascular diseases (eg, heart failure, history of myocardial infarction or ischemia, cerebrovascular disease, conduction abnormalities). May cause orthostatic hypotension; use with caution in patients at risk of this effect (eg, concurrent medication use which may predispose to hypotension/bradycardia or presence of hypovolemia) or in those who would not tolerate transient hypotensive episodes. May alter cardiac conduction (low risk relative to other neuroleptics); life-threatening arrhythmias have occurred with therapeutic doses of neuroleptics.

May cause anticholinergic effects (confusion, agitation, constipation, xerostomia, blurred vision, urinary retention); therefore, they should be used with caution in patients with decreased gastrointestinal motility, urinary retention, BPH, xerostomia, or visual problems. Conditions which also may be exacerbated by cholinergic blockade include narrow-angle glaucoma (screening is recommended) and worsening of myasthenia gravis. Relative to other neuroleptics, risperidone has a low potency of cholinergic blockade.

May cause extrapyramidal symptoms (EPS), including pseudoparkinsonism, acute dystonic reactions, akathisia, and tardive dyskinesia (risk of these reactions is low relative to other neuroleptics, and is dose dependent). Risk of dystonia (and probably other EPS) may be greater with increased doses, use of conventional antipsychotics, males, and younger patients. Risk of neuroleptic malignant syndrome (NMS) may be increased in patients with Parkinson's disease or Lewy body dementia; monitor for symptoms of confusion, obtundation, postural instability and extrapyramidal symptoms. May cause hyperglycemia; in some cases may be extreme and associated with ketoacidosis, hyperosmolar coma, or death. Use with caution in patients with diabetes or other disorders of glucose regulation; monitor for worsening of glucose control. Significant weight gain has been observed with antipsychotic therapy; incidence varies with product. Monitor waist circumference and BMI. Rare cases of priapism have been reported.

The possibility of a suicide attempt is inherent in psychotic illness or bipolar disorder; use caution in high-risk patients during initiation of therapy. Prescriptions should be written for the smallest quantity consistent with good patient care. Safety and efficacy have not been established in children <5 years of age. Long-term effects on growth or sexual maturation have not been evaluated. Vehicle used in injectable (polylactide-co-glycolide microspheres) has rarely been associated with retinal artery occlusion in patients with abnormal arteriovenous anastomosis.

Adverse Reactions

The frequency of adverse effects is reported as absolute percentages and is not based upon net frequencies as compared to placebo. Actual frequency may be dependant upon dose and/or indication. Events are reported from placebo controlled studies and not with combination therapy. Unless otherwise noted, frequency of adverse effects is reported for the oral formulation in adults.

>10%:

Central nervous system: Somnolence (adults 5% to 14%; children 12% to 67%), fatigue (adults 1% to 3%; children 18% to 42%), Parkinsonism (adults 12% to 20%; children 2% to 16%), fever (adults 1% to 2%; children 20%), dystonia (adults 5% to 11%; children 9% to 18%), anxiety (adults 2% to 16%; children ≤16%), dizziness (adults 4% to 10%; children 7% to 16%)

Dermatologic: Rash (adults 2% to 4%; children ≤11%)

Gastrointestinal: Appetite increased (children 4% to 49%), vomiting (children 10% to 25%), salivation increased (adults 1% to 3%; children ≤22%), constipation (adults 8% to 9%; children 21%), abdominal pain (adults 3% to 4%; children 15% to 18%), nausea (adults 4% to 9%; children 8% to 16%), dyspepsia (adults 4% to 10%; children 5% to 16%), xerostomia (adults ≤4%; children 13%)

Genitourinary: Urinary incontinence (children ≤22%)

Neuromuscular & skeletal: Tremor (adults 6%; children 10% to 12%)

Respiratory: Rhinitis (adults 7% to 11%; children 13% to 36%), upper respiratory infection (adults 2% to 3%; children 34%), cough (adults 3%; children 34%)

1% to 10%:

Cardiovascular: Tachycardia (adults 1% to 5%; children ≤7%), chest pain (1% to 3%), creatine phosphokinase increased (≤2%), postural hypotension (≤2%), arrhythmia (≤1%), edema (≤1%), hypotension (≤1%), syncope (≤1%)

Central nervous system: Akathisia (adults 5% to 9%; children ≤10%), automatism (children 7%), confusion (children 5%)

Dermatologic: Seborrhea (up to 2%), acne (1%)

Endocrine & metabolic: Lactation nonpuerperal (adults 1%; children 2% to 5%), ejaculation failure (≤1%)

Gastrointestinal: Diarrhea (adults ≤3%; children 7% to 8%), anorexia (adults ≤2%; children 8%), weight gain (adults ≤1% children 5%)

Genitourinary: Urinary tract infection (≤3%)

Hematologic: Anemia (≥1% I.M. injection; ≤1% oral)

Hepatic: Transaminases increased (≥1% I.M. injection; 1% oral)

Neuromuscular & skeletal: Dyskinesia (adults 1%, children 7%), myalgia (≤2%), arthralgia (2% to 3%), back pain (2% to 3%), weakness (1%)
Ocular: Abnormal vision (adults 1% to 3%; children 4% to 7%)
Otic: Earache (1%)
Respiratory: Epistaxis (≤2%), dyspnea (adults 2%; children 2% to 5%)

≤1% (Limited to important or life-threatening): Agranulocytosis, allergic reaction, amenorrhea, amnesia, anaphylactic reaction, anemias (oral formulations), angina pectoris, angioedema, antidiuretic hormone disorder, aphasia, apnea, ascites, aspiration, asthma, atrial fibrillation, AV block, bronchospasm, cachexia, catatonic reaction, cerebrovascular accident, cerebrovascular disorder, cholecystitis, cholelithiasis, cholestatic hepatitis, cholinergic syndrome, coma, dehydration, delirium, depression, diabetes mellitus, diabetic ketoacidosis, diverticulitis, dysphagia, esophagitis, esophageal dysmotility, fecal incontinence, flu-like syndrome, gastroenteritis, hematemesis, hematuria, hemorrhage, hepatic failure, hepatocellular damage, hyper-/hypoglycemia, hyperphosphatemia, hypertriglyceridemia, hyperuricemia, hypokalemia, hyponatremia, hypoproteinemia, intestinal obstruction, jaundice, leukocytosis, leukopenia, leukorrhea, lymphadenopathy, mastitis, menstrual irregularities, migraine, myocardial infarction, myocarditis, palpitation, pancreatitis, Pelger-Huët anomaly, pituitary adenomas, pneumonia, precocious puberty, premature atrial contractions, priapism, pulmonary embolism, purpura, QT_c prolongation, RBC disorders, renal insufficiency, retinal artery occlusion (I.M. formulation), rigors, sarcoidosis, skin exfoliation, skin ulceration, ST depression, stomatitis, stridor, stroke, superficial phlebitis, synostosis, T wave inversions, thrombocytopenia, thrombophlebitis, thrombotic thrombocytopenic purpura, tinnitus, tongue discoloration, tongue edema, tongue paralysis, torticollis, transient ischemic attack, urinary retention, urticaria, ventricular extrasystoles, ventricular tachycardia, water intoxication, withdrawal syndrome, xerophthalmia

Metabolism/Transport Effects **Substrate** of CYP2D6 (major), 3A4 (minor); **Inhibits** CYP2D6 (weak), 3A4 (weak)

Drug Interactions

Acetylcholinesterase Inhibitors (Central): May enhance the neurotoxic (central) effect of Antipsychotics. Severe extrapyramidal symptoms have occurred in some patients. *Risk C: Monitor therapy*

Alcohol (Ethyl): CNS Depressants may enhance the CNS depressant effect of Alcohol (Ethyl). *Risk C: Monitor therapy*

Alfuzosin: May enhance the QTc-prolonging effect of QTc-Prolonging Agents. *Risk C: Monitor therapy*

Amphetamines: Antipsychotics may diminish the stimulatory effect of Amphetamines. *Risk C: Monitor therapy*

Anticholinergics: May enhance the adverse/toxic effect of other Anticholinergics. **Exceptions:** Paliperidone. *Risk C: Monitor therapy*

Anti-Parkinson's Agents (Dopamine Agonist): Antipsychotics (Atypical) may diminish the therapeutic effect of Anti-Parkinson's Agents (Dopamine Agonist). *Risk D: Consider therapy modification*

CarBAMazepine: May decrease the serum concentration of Risperidone. *Risk C: Monitor therapy*

Ciprofloxacin: May enhance the QTc-prolonging effect of QTc-Prolonging Agents. *Risk C: Monitor therapy*

CNS Depressants: May enhance the adverse/toxic effect of other CNS Depressants. *Risk C: Monitor therapy*

CYP2D6 Inhibitors (Moderate): May decrease the metabolism of CYP2D6 Substrates. *Risk C: Monitor therapy*

CYP2D6 Inhibitors (Strong): May decrease the metabolism of CYP2D6 Substrates. *Risk D: Consider therapy modification*

Darunavir: May increase the serum concentration of CYP2D6 Substrates. *Risk C: Monitor therapy*

Gadobutrol: May enhance the QTc-prolonging effect of QTc-Prolonging Agents. *Risk D: Consider therapy modification*

Lithium formulations: May enhance the neurotoxic effect of Antipsychotics. Lithium formulations may decrease the serum concentration of Antipsychotics. Specifically noted with chlorpromazine. *Risk C: Monitor therapy*

Nilotinib: May enhance the QTc-prolonging effect of QTc-Prolonging Agents. *Risk X: Avoid combination*

Pramlintide: May enhance the anticholinergic effect of Anticholinergics. These effects are specific to the GI tract. *Risk D: Consider therapy modification*

QTc-Prolonging Agents: May enhance the adverse/toxic effect of other QTc-Prolonging Agents. Their effects can be additive, causing life-threatening ventricular arrhythmias. *Risk D: Consider therapy modification*

Selective Serotonin Reuptake Inhibitors: May decrease the metabolism of Risperidone. **Exceptions:** Fluvoxamine. *Risk C: Monitor therapy*

Tetrabenazine: May enhance the adverse/toxic effect of Antipsychotics. *Risk C: Monitor therapy*

Thioridazine: QTc-Prolonging Agents may enhance the QTc-prolonging effect of Thioridazine. *Risk X: Avoid combination*

Valproic Acid: May enhance the adverse/toxic effect of Risperidone. Generalized edema has developed. *Risk C: Monitor therapy*

Verapamil: May increase the serum concentration of Risperidone. *Risk C: Monitor therapy*

Ziprasidone: QTc-Prolonging Agents may enhance the QTc-prolonging effect of Ziprasidone. The risk of a severe arrhythmia may be increased. *Risk X: Avoid combination*

Ethanol/Nutrition/Herb Interactions

Ethanol: Avoid ethanol (may increase CNS depression).

Herb/Nutraceutical: Avoid kava kava, gotu kola, valerian, St John's wort (may increase CNS depression).

Stability

Injection: Risperdal® Consta®: Store in refrigerator at 2°C to 8°C (36°F to 46°F) and protect from light. May be stored at room temperature of 25°C (77°F) for up to 7 days prior to administration. Bring to room temperature prior to reconstitution. Reconstitute with provided diluent only. Shake vigorously to mix; will form thick, milky suspension. Following reconstitution, store at room temperature and use within 6 hours. If suspension settles prior to use, shake vigorously to resuspend.

Oral solution, tablet: Store at 15°C to 25°C (59°F to 77°F). Protect from light and moisture. Keep orally-disintegrating tablets sealed in foil pouch until ready to use. Do not freeze solution.

Mechanism of Action Risperidone is a benzisoxazole atypical antipsychotic with mixed serotonin-dopamine antagonist activity that binds to 5-HT_2-receptors in the CNS and in the periphery with a very high affinity; binds to dopamine-D_2 receptors with less affinity. The binding affinity to the dopamine-D_2 receptor is 20 times lower than the 5-HT_2 affinity. The addition of serotonin antagonism to dopamine antagonism (classic neuroleptic mechanism) is thought to improve negative symptoms of psychoses and reduce the incidence of extrapyramidal side effects. $Alpha_1$, $alpha_2$ adrenergic, and histaminergic receptors are also antagonized with high affinity. Risperidone has low to moderate affinity for 5-HT_{1C}, 5-HT_{1D}, and 5-HT_{1A} receptors, weak affinity for D_1 and no affinity for muscarinics or $beta_1$ and $beta_2$ receptors

Pharmacodynamics/Kinetics

Absorption:

- Oral: Rapid and well absorbed; food does not affect rate or extent
- Injection: <1% absorbed initially; main release occurs at ~3 weeks and is maintained from 4-6 weeks

Distribution: V_d: 1-2 L/kg

Protein binding, plasma: Risperidone 90%; 9-hydroxyrisperidone: 77%

Metabolism: Extensively hepatic via CYP2D6 to 9-hydroxyrisperidone (similar pharmacological activity as risperidone); *N*-dealkylation is a second minor pathway

Bioavailability: Solution: 70%; Tablet: 66%; orally-disintegrating tablets and oral solution are bioequivalent to tablets

Half-life elimination: Active moiety (risperidone and its active metabolite 9-hydroxyrisperidone)

- Oral: 20 hours (mean)
  - Extensive metabolizers: Risperidone: 3 hours; 9-hydroxyrisperidone: 21 hours
  - Poor metabolizers: Risperidone: 20 hours; 9-hydroxyrisperidone: 30 hours
- Injection: 3-6 days; related to microsphere erosion and subsequent absorption of risperidone

Time to peak, plasma: Oral: Risperidone: Within 1 hour; 9-hydroxyrisperidone: Extensive metabolizers: 3 hours; Poor metabolizers: 17 hours

Excretion: Urine (70%); feces (15%)

Dosage

Oral:

- Children ≥5 years and Adolescents: Autism:
  - <15 kg: Use with caution; specific dosing recommendations not available
  - <20 kg: Initial: 0.25 mg/day; may increase dose to 0.5 mg/day after ≥4 days, maintain dose for ≥14 days. In patients not achieving sufficient clinical response, may increase dose by 0.25 mg/day in ≥2-week intervals. Therapeutic effect reached plateau at 1 mg/day in clinical trials. Following clinical response, consider gradually lowering dose. May be administered once daily or in divided doses twice daily.
  - ≥20 kg: Initial: 0.5 mg/day; may increase dose to 1 mg/day after ≥4 days, maintain dose for ≥14 days. In patients not achieving sufficient clinical

response, may increase dose by 0.5 mg/day in ≥2-week intervals. Therapeutic effect reached plateau at 2.5 mg/day (3 mg/day in children >45 kg) in clinical trials. Following clinical response, consider gradually lowering dose. May be administered once daily or in divided doses twice daily.

Children and Adolescents:

Pervasive developmental disorder (unlabeled use): Initial: 0.25 mg twice daily; titrate up 0.25 mg/day every 5-7 days; optimal dose range: 0.75-3 mg/day

Schizophrenia: Adolescents 13-17 years: Initial: 0.5 mg once daily; dose may be adjusted in increments of 0.5-1 mg/day at intervals ≥24 hours to a dose of 3 mg/day. Doses ranging from 1-6 mg/day have been evaluated, however, doses >3 mg/day do not confer additional benefit and are associated with increased adverse events.

Bipolar disorder: Children and Adolescents 10-17 years: Initial: 0.5 mg once daily; dose may be adjusted in increments of 0.5-1 mg/day at intervals ≥24 hours to a dose of 2.5 mg/day. Doses ranging from 0.5-6 mg/day have been evaluated, however doses >2.5 mg/day do not confer additional benefit and are associated with increased adverse events.

Tourette's disorder (unlabeled use): Initial: 0.5 mg; titrate to 2-4 mg/day

Adults:

Schizophrenia:

Initial: 1 mg twice daily; may be increased by 1-2 mg/day at intervals ≥24 hours to a target dose of 6 mg/day; usual range: 4-8 mg/day; may be given as a single daily dose once maintenance dose is achieved; daily dosages >6 mg do not appear to confer any additional benefit, and the incidence of extrapyramidal symptoms is higher than with lower doses. Further dose adjustments should be made in increments/decrements of 1-2 mg/day on a weekly basis. Dose range studied in clinical trials: 4-16 mg/day.

Maintenance: Target dose: 4 mg once daily (range 2-8 mg/day)

Bipolar mania:

Initial: 2-3 mg once daily; if needed, adjust dose by 1 mg/day in intervals ≥24 hours; dosing range: 1-6 mg/day

Maintenance: No dosing recommendation available for treatment >3 weeks duration.

Elderly:

Oral: A starting dose of 0.5 mg twice daily, and titration should progress slowly in increments of no more than 0.5 mg twice daily; increases to dosages >1.5 mg twice daily should occur at intervals of ≥1 week.

Psychosis/agitation related to Alzheimer's dementia (unlabeled use): Initial: 0.25-1 mg/day; if necessary, gradually increase as tolerated not to exceed 1.5-2 mg/day

I.M. (Risperdal® Consta®): A lower initial dose of 12.5 mg may be appropriate.

Note: Additional monitoring of renal function and orthostatic blood pressure may be warranted. If once-a-day dosing in the elderly or debilitated patient is considered, a twice daily regimen should be used to titrate to the target dose, and this dose should be maintained for 2-3 days prior to attempts to switch to a once-daily regimen.

I.M.: Adults: Schizophrenia (Risperdal® Consta®): 25 mg every 2 weeks; some patients may benefit from larger doses; maximum dose not to exceed 50 mg every 2 weeks. Dosage adjustments should not be made more frequently than every 4 weeks. A lower initial dose of 12.5 mg may be appropriate in some patients.

Note: Oral risperidone (or other antipsychotic) should be administered with the initial injection of Risperdal® Consta® and continued for 3 weeks (then discontinued) to maintain adequate therapeutic plasma concentrations prior to main release phase of risperidone from injection site. When switching from depot administration to a short-acting formulation, administer short-acting agent in place of the next regularly-scheduled depot injection.

Dosing adjustment in renal impairment:

Oral: Starting dose of 0.5 mg twice daily; titration should progress slowly in increments of no more than 0.5 mg twice daily; increases to dosages >1.5 mg twice daily should occur at intervals of ≥1 week. Clearance of the active moiety is decreased by 60% in patients with moderate-to-severe renal disease compared to healthy subjects.

I.M.: An initial dose of 12.5 mg may be considered

Dosing adjustment in hepatic impairment:

Oral: Starting dose of 0.5 mg twice daily; titration should progress slowly in increments of no more than 0.5 mg twice daily; increases to dosages

>1.5 mg twice daily should occur at intervals of ≥1 week. The mean free fraction of risperidone in plasma was increased by 35% in patients with hepatic impairment compared to healthy subjects.

I.M.: An initial dose of 12.5 mg may be considered

Child/Adolescent Considerations

Aggression: In a randomized, double-blind, placebo-controlled study, 10 children and adolescents 6-14 years of age (mean: 9.2 ± 2.9 years) with conduct disorder and prominent aggressive behavior received risperidone in the following doses: Patients <50 kg: Initial: 0.25 mg once daily; doses were increased as needed by 0.25 mg/day increments each week to a maximum of 1.5 mg/day; patients ≥50 kg: Initial: 0.5 mg once daily; doses were increased as needed by 0.5 mg/day increments each week to a maximum of 3 mg/day; final dose: 0.75-1.5 mg/day; mean: 0.028 ± 0.004 mg/kg/day (Findling, 2000). In another randomized, double-blind, placebo-controlled study, 19 adolescents (mean age: 14 ± 1.5 years; 7 with borderline IQ and 6 with mild mental retardation) received initial risperidone doses of 0.5 mg twice daily; doses were increased as needed by 1 mg/day increments up to a planned maximum of 5 mg twice daily; final doses: Range: 1.5-4 mg/day (0.019-0.08 mg/kg/day); mean: 2.9 mg/day (0.044 mg/kg/day); the authors recommend the following initial doses for clinical practice: Patients <25 kg: 0.25 mg/day; patients ≥25 kg: 0.5 mg/day (Buitelaar, 2001).

In an open trial, 26 children and adolescents 10-18 years of age (mean: 15 ± 1.9 years) with a borderline IQ (n=19) or mild mental retardation (n=5) received initial risperidone doses of 0.5 mg/day; doses were increased by 0.5-1 mg/day increments every 3 days up to a planned maximum of 6 mg/day and given in twice daily doses; final dose: 0.5-4 mg/day; mean: 2.1 ± 1 mg/day (Buitelaar, 2000). Eleven children and adolescents 5.5-16 years of age (mean: 9.8 years) with mood disorders and aggressive behavior received risperidone in titrated doses in an open trial; final dose: 0.75-2.5 mg/day given in 2-3 divided doses (Schreier, 1998).

Autism: A multicenter double-blind, placebo-controlled trial of risperidone in children and adolescents 5-17 years of age (mean: 8.8 ± 2.7 years) with autism and serious behavioral problems demonstrated the short-term efficacy of risperidone for the treatment of aggression, tantrums, or self-injurious behavior. The following doses were used: Children 15-20 kg: Initial: 0.25 mg/day. Children 20-45 kg: Initial: 0.5 mg at bedtime on days 1-3 and 0.5 mg twice daily on day 4; dose was gradually increased in 0.5 mg increments to a maximum dose of 2.5 mg/day. Children >45 kg: Maximum dose: 3.5 mg/day; mean effective dose: 1.8 ± 0.7 mg/day (range: 0.5-3.5 mg/day) (McCracken, 2002).

In an open-labeled prospective study, 10 boys 4.5-10.8 years of age (mean: 7.2 ± 2.2 years) with autistic disorder were started on risperidone 0.5 mg/day; final dose: range: 1-2.5 mg/day (0.03-0.08 mg/kg/day); mean: 1.3 ± 0.5 mg/day (0.05 ± 0.2 mg/kg/day) (Nicolson, 1998). In an open clinical trial, 6 children 5-9 years of age (mean: 7.33 years) with autistic disorder were started on risperidone monotherapy 0.25 mg at bedtime; final dose: range: 0.75-1.5 mg/day (0.03-0.06 mg/kg/day); mean: 1.1 mg (0.04 mg/kg/day) (Findling, 1997).

Bipolar disorder: In a retrospective chart review, 28 children and adolescents 4-17 years of age (mean: 10.4 ± 3.8 years) were treated for bipolar disorder; optimal mean dose: 1.7 ± 1.3 mg/day (Frazier 1999).

Pervasive developmental disorders (PDDs): In a prospective open-labeled study, children and adolescents 5-18 years of age (mean 10.2 ± 3.7 years) were treated for PDDs (11 with autistic disorder) with initial doses of 0.5 mg at night; optimal dose: 1-4 mg/day (mean: 1.8 ± 1 mg/day) (McDougle, 1997). Fourteen children and adolescents 9-17 years of age (mean: 12.7 ± 4 years) were treated in an open case series, for PDDs (4 with autistic disorder) with initial doses of 0.25 mg twice daily; optimal dose: 0.75-1.5 mg/day given in divided doses (Fisman, 1996). In an open trial, 6 children and adolescents 7-14 years of age (mean: 10.7 ± 3.3 years) were treated for PDDs (5 with autistic disorder; all 6 with severe behavioral problems) with initial doses of 0.5 mg once or twice daily; optimal dose: 1-6 mg/day (mean 2.7 ± 2.2 mg/day) (Perry, 1997). Twenty children and adolescents (age: 8-17 years) with developmental disorders refractory to previous psychotropic agents were treated in an open clinical trial with risperidone; final doses: 1.5-10 mg/day; responders: 1-4 mg/day; non-responders: 4.5-10 mg/day (Hardan, 1996).

Schizophrenia: In a prospective, open-labeled pilot study, 10 children and adolescents 11-18 years of age (mean: 15.1 years) were treated for schizophrenia with initial doses of 1 mg twice daily; final dose: Range: 4-10 mg/day (0.05-0.17 mg/kg/day); mean: 6.6 mg/day (0.095 mg/kg/day)

(Armenteros, 1997). In a retrospective study, 16 children and adolescents 9-20 years of age (mean: 14.9 ± 2.73 years) were treated for psychotic disorders with initial doses of 1 mg twice daily; optimal dose: 2-10 mg/day (mean: 5.9 ± 2.8 mg/day) divided and given in 2-3 doses/day (Grcevich, 1996).

Tourette's syndrome: In a multicenter, double-blind, parallel-group comparative study, 50 patients 11-50 years of age were treated for Tourette's syndrome with risperidone versus pimozide; final dose: 0.5-6 mg/day (mean: 3.8 mg/day) (Bruggeman, 2001).

Seven children and adolescents 11-16 years of age (mean: 12.9 ± 1.9 years) were treated in a prospective open-labeled trial for chronic tic disorders (5 with Tourette's syndrome) with initial doses of 0.5 mg at bedtime; final dose: 1-2.5 mg/day (Lombroso, 1995). In a retrospective review, 28 children and adolescents 5-18 years of age (mean 11.1 ± 3.6 years) with Tourette's syndrome and aggressive behavior were treated with risperidone; final dose: 0.5-9 mg/day (mean: 2 mg/day) (Sandor, 2000).

Armenteros JL, Whitaker AH, Welikson M, et al, "Risperidone in Adolescents With Schizophrenia: An Open Pilot Study," *J Am Acad Child Adolesc Psychiatry*, 1997, 36(5):694-700.

Bruggeman R, van der Linden C, Buitelaar JK, et al, "Risperidone Versus Pimozide in Tourette's Disorder: A Comparative Double-Blind Parallel-Group Study," *J Clin Psychiatry*, 2001, 62(1):50-6.

Buitelaar JK, "Open-Label Treatment With Risperidone of 26 Psychiatrically-Hospitalized Children and Adolescents With Mixed Diagnoses and Aggressive Behavior," *J Child Adolesc Psychopharmacol*, 2000, 10(1):19-26.

Buitelaar JK, van der Gaag RJ, Cohen-Kettenis P, et al, "A Randomized Controlled Trial of Risperidone in the Treatment of Aggression in Hospitalized Adolescents With Subaverage Cognitive Abilities," *J Clin Psychiatry*, 2001, 62 (4):239-48.

Findling RL, Maxwell K, and Wiznitzer M, "An Open Clinical Trial of Risperidone Monotherapy in Young Children With Autistic Disorder," *Psychopharmacol Bull*, 1997, 33(1):155-9.

Findling RL, McNamara NK, Branicky LA, et al, "A Double-Blind Pilot Study of Risperidone in the Treatment of Conduct Disorder," *J Am Acad Child Adolesc Psychiatry*, 2000, 39(4):509-16.

Fisman S and Steele M, "Use of Risperidone in Pervasive Developmental Disorders: A Case Series," *J Child Adolesc Psychopharmacol*, 1996, 6 (3):177-90.

Frazier JA, Meyer MC, Biederman J, et al, "Risperidone Treatment for Juvenile Bipolar Disorder: A Retrospective Chart Review," *J Am Acad Child Adolesc Psychiatry*, 1999, 38(8):960-5.

Grcevich SJ, Findling RL, Rowane WA, et al, "Risperidone in the Treatment of Children and Adolescents With Schizophrenia: A Retrospective Study," *J Child Adolesc Psychopharmacol*, 1996, 6(4):251-7.

Hardan A, Johnson K, Johnson C, et al, "Case Study: Risperidone Treatment of Children and Adolescents With Developmental Disorders," *J Am Acad Child Adolesc Psychiatry*, 1996, 35(11):1551-6.

Lombroso PJ, Scahill L, King RA, et al, "Risperidone Treatment of Children and Adolescents With Chronic Tic Disorders: A Preliminary Report," *J Am Acad Child Adolesc Psychiatry*, 1995, 34(9):1147-52.

McCracken JT, McGough J, Shah B, et al, "Risperidone in Children With Autism and Serious Behavioral Problems," *N Engl J Med*, 2002, 347(5):314-21.

McDougle CJ, Holmes JP, Bronson MR, et al, "Risperidone Treatment of Children and Adolescents With Pervasive Developmental Disorders: A Prospective Open-Label Study," *J Am Acad Child Adolesc Psychiatry*, 1997, 36(5):685-93.

Nicolson R, Awad G, and Sloman L, "An Open Trial of Risperidone in Young Autistic Children," *J Am Acad Child Adolesc Psychiatry*, 1998, 37(4):372-6.

Perry R, Pataki C, Munoz-Silva DM, et al, "Risperidone in Children and Adolescents With Pervasive Developmental Disorder: Pilot Trial and Follow-Up," *J Child Adolesc Psychopharmacol*, 1997, 7(3):167-79.

Sandor P and Stephens RJ, "Risperidone Treatment of Aggressive Behavior in Children With Tourette Syndrome," *J Clin Psychopharmacol*, 2000, 20 (6):710-2.

Schreier HA, "Risperidone for Young Children With Mood Disorders and Aggressive Behavior," *J Child Adolesc Psychopharmacol*, 1998, 8(1):49-59.

Dietary Considerations May be taken with or without food. Risperdal® M-Tabs® contain phenylalanine.

Administration

Oral:

Oral solution can be mixed with water, coffee, orange juice, or low-fat milk, but is **not compatible** with cola or tea. May be administered with or without food.

In children or adolescents experiencing somnolence, half the daily dose may be administered twice daily **or** the once-daily dose may be administered at bedtime.

When reinitiating treatment after discontinuation, the initial titration schedule should be followed.

Risperdal® M-Tabs® should not be removed from blister pack until administered. Using dry hands, place immediately on tongue. Tablet will dissolve within seconds, and may be swallowed with or without liquid. Do not split or chew.

I.M.: Risperdal® Consta® should be administered into the upper outer quadrant of the gluteal area. Avoid inadvertent injection into vasculature. Injection should alternate between the two buttocks. Do not combine two different dosage strengths into one single administration. Do not substitute any components of the dose-pack; administer with needle provided.

Monitoring Parameters Vital signs; fasting lipid profile and fasting blood glucose/Hgb A_{1c} (prior to treatment, at 3 months, then annually); BMI, personal/family history of obesity, waist circumference; blood pressure; mental status, abnormal involuntary movement scale (AIMS), extrapyramidal symptoms; orthostatic blood pressure changes for 3-5 days after starting or increasing dose. Weight should be assessed prior to treatment, at 4 weeks, 8 weeks, 12 weeks, and then at quarterly intervals. Consider titrating to a different antipsychotic agent for a weight gain ≥5% of the initial weight.

Additional Information Risperdal® Consta® is an injectable formulation of risperidone using the extended release Medisorb® drug-delivery system; small polymeric microspheres degrade slowly, releasing the medication at a controlled rate.

Dosage Forms Excipient information presented when available (limited, particularly for generics); consult specific product labeling.

Injection, microspheres for reconstitution, extended release:

Risperdal® Consta®: 12.5 mg, 25 mg, 37.5 mg, 50 mg [contains polylactide-co-glycolide; supplied in a dose-pack containing vial with active ingredient in microsphere formulation, prefilled syringe with diluent, needle-free vial access device, and safety needle]

Solution, oral:

Risperdal®: 1 mg/mL (30 mL) [contains benzoic acid]

Tablet: 0.25 mg, 0.5 mg, 1 mg, 2 mg, 3 mg, 4 mg

Risperdal®: 0.25 mg, 0.5 mg, 1 mg, 2 mg, 3 mg, 4 mg

Tablet, orally disintegrating:

Risperdal® M-Tabs®: 0.5 mg [contains phenylalanine 0.14 mg]; 1 mg [contains phenylalanine 0.28 mg]; 2 mg [contains phenylalanine 0.42 mg]; 3 mg [contains phenylalanine 0.63 mg]; 4 mg [contains phenylalanine 0.84 mg]

◆ **Ritalin®** *see* Methylphenidate *on page 1024*

◆ **Ritalin® LA** *see* Methylphenidate *on page 1024*

◆ **Ritalin-SR®** *see* Methylphenidate *on page 1024*

Ritonavir (ri TOE na veer)

Medication Safety Issues

Sound-alike/look-alike issues:

Ritonavir may be confused with Retrovir®

Norvir® may be confused with Norvasc®

U.S. Brand Names Norvir®

Canadian Brand Names Norvir®; Norvir® SEC

Mexican Brand Names Kaletra

Pharmacologic Category Antiretroviral Agent, Protease Inhibitor

Use Treatment of HIV infection; should always be used as part of a multidrug regimen (at least three antiretroviral agents); may be used as a pharmacokinetic "booster" for other protease inhibitors

Effect on Mental Status May cause abnormal dreams, agitation, amnesia, aphasia, confusion, depersonalization, emotional lability, euphoria, hallucinations, mania, nervousness, and sleep disturbances

Effect on Psychiatric Treatment Contraindicated with pimozide, midazolam, and triazolam (may use temazepam or lorazepam). Concomitant use of ritonavir and St John's wort is not recommended. Coadministration of protease inhibitors (ritonavir) with St John's wort is expected to substantially decrease protease inhibitor serum concentrations leading to a loss of virologic response and possible resistance to ritonavir or to the class of protease inhibitors. Ritonavir may increase the levels of many antidepressants, including TCAs, SSRIs, bupropion, and trazodone. Use cautiously and monitor closely for adverse effects.

Ritonavir oral solution contains alcohol and can produce a disulfiram-like reaction when coadministered with disulfiram. Ritonavir affects anticonvulsants in opposite directions depending on the anticonvulsants. Ritonavir may increase levels of carbamazepine, clonazepam, and ethosuximide with concomitant use while combined use with divalproex, lamotrigine and phenytoin may result in lower serum concentrations. Be mindful of the anticonvulsant used. A dose increase or decrease may be needed. Check serum levels, and monitor for adverse reactions.

A dose decrease may be needed when coadministered with antipsychotics (includes perphenazine, risperidone, thioridazine); sedative/hypnotics (includes buspirone, clorazepate, diazepam, estazolam, flurazepam, and zolpidem); and stimulants (includes methamphetamine). Monitor for dose-dependent adverse reactions.

Dosage Summary

Oral:

Children <1 month: Dosage not established

Children >1 month: Initial: 250 mg/m^2 twice daily; Maintenance: 350-400 mg/m^2 twice daily (maximum dose: 1200 mg/day); **Note:** Titration is recommended

Adults: 600 mg twice daily; Booster with other protease inhibitors: 100-400 mg/day; **Note:** Titration is recommended

Dosage Forms Excipient information presented when available (limited, particularly for generics); consult specific product labeling.

Capsule, soft gelatin:

Norvir®: 100 mg [contains ethanol and polyoxyl 35 castor oil]

Solution:

Norvir®: 80 mg/mL (240 mL) [contains ethanol, polyoxyl 35 castor oil, and propylene glycol; peppermint and caramel flavor]

◆ **Ritonavir and Lopinavir** *see* Lopinavir and Ritonavir *on page 945*

◆ **Rituxan®** *see* RiTUXimab *on page 1434*

RiTUXimab (ri TUK si mab)

Medication Safety Issues

Sound-alike/look-alike issues:

Rituxan® may be confused with Remicade®

RiTUXimab may be confused with inFLIXimab

High alert medication: The Institute for Safe Medication Practices (ISMP) includes this medication among its list of drug classes which have a heightened risk of causing significant patient harm when used in error.

The rituximab dose for rheumatoid arthritis is a flat dose (1000 mg) and is not based on body surface area (BSA).

U.S. Brand Names Rituxan®

Canadian Brand Names Rituxan®

Mexican Brand Names Mabthera

Index Terms Anti-CD20 Monoclonal Antibody; C2B8 Monoclonal Antibody; IDEC-C2B8; NSC-687451

Pharmacologic Category Antineoplastic Agent, Monoclonal Antibody; Monoclonal Antibody

Use Treatment of low-grade or follicular CD20-positive, B-cell non-Hodgkin's lymphoma (NHL); treatment of diffuse large B-cell CD20-positive NHL; treatment of moderately- to severely-active rheumatoid arthritis (RA) in combination with methotrexate

Unlabeled/Investigational Use Treatment of autoimmune hemolytic anemia (AIHA) in children; chronic immune thrombocytopenic purpura (ITP); chronic lymphocytic leukemia (CLL); small lymphocytic lymphoma (SLL); pemphigus vulgaris, Waldenström's macroglobulinemia (WM); treatment of systemic autoimmune diseases (other than rheumatoid arthritis); treatment of refractory chronic graft-versus-host disease (GVHD)

Effect on Mental Status May cause dizziness or depression

Effect on Psychiatric Treatment Leukopenia is common; avoid concurrent use with clozapine or carbamazepine

Restrictions An FDA-approved medication guide is available; distribute to each patient to whom this medication is dispensed.

Dosage Summary Note: Pretreatment with acetaminophen and an antihistamine is recommended.

I.V.:

Children (unlabeled use): 375 mg/m^2 once weekly for 2-4 doses

Adults: Infusion: 375 mg/m^2 once weekly for 4 or 8 doses **or** 100 mg/m^2 I.V. day 1, then 375 mg/m^2 3 times/week for 11 doses **or** 1000 mg on days 1 and 15 in combination with methotrexate **or** 375 mg/m^2 on day 1 of each chemotherapy cycle for up to 8 doses **or** 250 mg/m^2 I.V. day 1, repeat in 7-9 days with ibritumomab

Dosage Forms Excipient information presented when available (limited, particularly for generics); consult specific product labeling.

Injection, solution [preservative free]:

Rituxan®: 10 mg/mL (10 mL, 50 mL) [contains polysorbate 80]

Rivastigmine (ri va STIG meen)

U.S. Brand Names Exelon®

Canadian Brand Names Exelon®

Mexican Brand Names Exelon

Index Terms ENA 713; Rivastigmine Tartrate; SDZ ENA 713

Pharmacologic Category Acetylcholinesterase Inhibitor (Central)

Generic Available No

Use Treatment of mild-to-moderate dementia associated with Alzheimer's disease or Parkinson's disease

Unlabeled/Investigational Use Severe dementia associated with Alzheimer's disease; Lewy body dementia

Pregnancy Risk Factor B

Pregnancy Considerations Teratogenic effects were not observed in animal studies. There are no adequate and well-controlled studies in pregnant women. Should be used only if the benefit outweighs the potential risk to the fetus.

Lactation Excretion in breast milk unknown/use caution

Contraindications Hypersensitivity to rivastigmine, other carbamate derivatives (eg, neostigmine, pyridostigmine, physostigmine), or any component of the formulation

Warnings/Precautions Significant nausea, vomiting, anorexia, and weight loss are associated with use; occurs more frequently in women and during the titration phase. Nausea and/or vomiting may be severe, particularly at doses higher than recommended. Monitor weight during therapy. Therapy should be initiated at lowest dose and titrated; if treatment is interrupted for more than several days, reinstate at the lowest daily dose. Cholinesterase inhibitors may have vagotonic effects which may cause bradycardia and/or heart block with or without a history of cardiac disease. Alzheimer's treatment guidelines consider bradycardia to be a relative contraindication for use of centrally-active cholinesterase inhibitors. Use caution in patients with a history of peptic ulcer disease or concurrent NSAID use. Use caution in patients undergoing anesthesia who will receive succinylcholine-type muscle relaxation, patients with sick-sinus syndrome, bradycardia or supraventricular conduction conditions, urinary obstruction, seizure disorders, or pulmonary conditions such as asthma or COPD. Use caution in patients with low body weight (<50 kg) due to increased risk of adverse reactions. Safety and efficacy in children have not been established.

Adverse Reactions Note: Many concentration-related effects are reported at a lower frequency by transdermal route.

>10%:

Central nervous system: Dizziness (2% to 21%), headache (3% to 17%)

Gastrointestinal: Nausea (7% to 47%), vomiting (6% to 31%), diarrhea (5% to 19%), anorexia (3% to 17%), abdominal pain (1% to 13%)

1% to 10%:

Cardiovascular: Syncope (3%), hypertension (3%)

Central nervous system: Fatigue (2% to 9%), insomnia (1% to 9%), confusion (8%), depression (4% to 6%), anxiety (2% to 5%), malaise (5%), somnolence (4% to 5%), hallucinations (4%), aggressiveness (3%), parkinsonism symptoms worsening (2% to 3%), vertigo (≤2%)

Gastrointestinal: Dyspepsia (9%), constipation (5%), flatulence (4%), weight loss (3% to 8%), eructation (2%), dehydration (2%)

Genitourinary: Urinary tract infection (1% to 7%)

Neuromuscular & skeletal: Weakness (2% to 6%), tremor (1%; up to 10% in Parkinson's patients)

Respiratory: Rhinitis (4%)

Miscellaneous: Diaphoresis (4%), flu-like syndrome (3%)

<1% (Limited to important or life-threatening symptoms; reactions may be at a similar frequency to placebo): Abnormal hepatic function, acute renal failure, albuminuria, allergy, anemia, angina, aphasia, apnea, apraxia, ataxia, atrial fibrillation, AV block, bradycardia, bronchospasm, bundle branch block, cachexia, cardiac arrest, cardiac failure, chest pain, cholecystitis, diplopia, diverticulitis, dysphagia, dyspnea, dysphonia, edema, esophagitis, extrasystoles, fecal incontinence, gastritis, gastroesophageal reflux, GGT increased, glaucoma, hematuria, hot flashes, hyper-/hypoglycemia, hypercholesterolemia, hyper-/hypokinesia, hypertonia, hypokalemia, hyponatremia, hypotension (including postural), hypothermia, hypothyroidism, intestinal obstruction, intracranial hemorrhage, mastitis, MI, migraine, neuralgia, palpitation, pancreatitis, paresthesia, periorbital or facial edema, peripheral ischemia, peripheral neuropathy, pneumonia, pruritus, psychiatric disorders (eg, delirium, depersonalization, psychosis, emotional lability, suicidal ideation or tendencies), rash, retinopathy, rigors, seizure, sick-sinus syndrome, sudden cardiac death, supraventricular tachycardia, thrombocytopenia, thrombophlebitis, thrombosis, transient ischemic attack, ulcerative stomatitis, urinary incontinence, urticaria, vasovagal syncope

Drug Interactions

Anticholinergics: May diminish the therapeutic effect of Acetylcholinesterase Inhibitors (Central). Acetylcholinesterase Inhibitors (Central) may diminish the therapeutic effect of Anticholinergics. If the anticholinergic action is a side effect of the agent, the result may be beneficial. **Exceptions:** Paliperidone. *Risk C: Monitor therapy*

Antipsychotics: Acetylcholinesterase Inhibitors (Central) may enhance the neurotoxic (central) effect of Antipsychotics. Severe extrapyramidal symptoms have occurred in some patients. *Risk C: Monitor therapy*

Beta-Blockers: Acetylcholinesterase Inhibitors may enhance the bradycardic effect of Beta-Blockers. **Exceptions:** Levobunolol; Metipranolol. *Risk C: Monitor therapy*

Cholinergic Agonists: Acetylcholinesterase Inhibitors may enhance the adverse/toxic effect of Cholinergic Agonists. *Risk C: Monitor therapy*

Corticosteroids (Systemic): May enhance the adverse/toxic effect of Acetylcholinesterase Inhibitors. Increased muscular weakness may occur. *Risk C: Monitor therapy*

Ginkgo Biloba: May enhance the adverse/toxic effect of Acetylcholinesterase Inhibitors. *Risk C: Monitor therapy*

Neuromuscular-Blocking Agents (Nondepolarizing): Acetylcholinesterase Inhibitors may diminish the neuromuscular-blocking effect of Neuromuscular-Blocking Agents (Nondepolarizing). Acetylcholinesterase Inhibitors may decrease the metabolism of Neuromuscular-Blocking Agents (Nondepolarizing). This is only true for mivacurium in which case the neuromuscular blocking effects might be prolonged. *Risk C: Monitor therapy*

Succinylcholine: Acetylcholinesterase Inhibitors may enhance the neuromuscular-blocking effect of Succinylcholine. *Risk C: Monitor therapy*

Ethanol/Nutrition/Herb Interactions

Smoking: Nicotine increases the clearance of rivastigmine by 23%.

Ethanol: Avoid ethanol (due to risk of sedation; may increase GI irritation).

Food: Food delays absorption by 90 minutes, lowers C_{max} by 30% and increases AUC by 30%.

Herb/Nutraceutical: Avoid ginkgo biloba (may increase cholinergic effects).

Stability

Oral: Store at 15°C to 30°C (59°F to 86°F); do not freeze. Store solution in an upright position.

Transdermal patch: Store at 15°C to 30°C (59°F to 86°F). Patches should be kept in sealed pouch until use.

Mechanism of Action A deficiency of cortical acetylcholine is thought to account for some of the symptoms of Alzheimer's disease and the dementia of Parkinson's disease; rivastigmine increases acetylcholine in the central nervous system through reversible inhibition of its hydrolysis by cholinesterase

Pharmacodynamics/Kinetics

Duration: Anticholinesterase activity (CSF): ~10 hours (6 mg oral dose)

Absorption: Oral: Fasting: Rapid and complete within 1 hour

Distribution: V_d: 1.8-2.7 L/kg; penetrates blood-brain barrier (CSF levels are ~40% of plasma levels following oral administration)

Protein binding: 40%

Metabolism: Extensively via cholinesterase-mediated hydrolysis in the brain; metabolite undergoes N-demethylation and/or sulfate conjugation hepatically; CYP minimally involved; linear kinetics at 3 mg twice daily, but nonlinear at higher doses

Bioavailability: Oral: 36% to 40%

Half-life elimination: Oral: 1.5 hours; Transdermal patch: 3 hours (after removal)
Time to peak: Oral: 1 hour; Transdermal patch: 10-16 hours following first dose
Excretion: Urine (97% as metabolites); feces (0.4%)

Dosage Adults:

Oral: **Note:** Exelon® oral solution and capsules are bioequivalent.

Mild-to-moderate Alzheimer's dementia: Initial: 1.5 mg twice daily; may increase by 3 mg/day (1.5 mg/dose) every 2 weeks based on tolerability (maximum recommended dose: 6 mg twice daily)

Note: If GI adverse events occur, discontinue treatment for several doses then restart at the same or next lower dosage level; antiemetics have been used to control GI symptoms. If treatment is interrupted for longer than several days, restart the treatment at the lowest dose and titrate as previously described.

Mild-to-moderate Parkinson's-related dementia: Initial: 1.5 mg twice daily; may increase by 3 mg/day (1.5 mg/dose) every 4 weeks based on tolerability (maximum recommended dose: 6 mg twice daily)

Transdermal patch: Mild-to-moderate Alzheimer's- or Parkinson's-related dementia:

Initial: 4.6 mg/24 hours; if well tolerated, may be increased (after at least 4 weeks) to 9.5 mg/24 hours (recommended effective dose)

Maintenance: 9.5 mg/24 hours (maximum dose: 9.5 mg/24 hours)

Note: If intolerance is noted (nausea, vomiting), patch should be removed and treatment interrupted for several days and restarted at the same or lower dosage. If interrupted for more than several days, reinitiate at lowest dosage and increase to maintenance dose after 4 weeks.

Conversion from oral therapy: If oral daily dose <6 mg, switch to 4.6 mg/24 hours patch; if oral daily dose 6-12 mg, switch to 9.5 mg/24 hours patch. Apply patch on the next day following last oral dose.

Elderly: Following oral administration, clearance is significantly lower in patients >60 years of age, but dosage adjustments are not recommended. Age was not associated with exposure in patients treated transdermally. Titrate dose to individual's tolerance.

Dosage adjustment in renal impairment: Dosage adjustments are not recommended, however, titrate the dose to the individual's tolerance.

Dosage adjustment in hepatic impairment: Clearance is significantly reduced in mild to moderately impaired patients. Although dosage adjustments are not recommended, use lowest possible dose and titrate according to individual's tolerance. Consider intervals of >2 weeks between dosage adjustments.

Dietary Considerations Capsules should be taken with meals.

Administration

Oral: Should be administered with meals (breakfast or dinner). Capsule should be swallowed whole. Liquid form is available for patients who cannot swallow capsules (can be swallowed directly from syringe or mixed with water, soda, or cold fruit juice). Stir well and drink within 4 hours of mixing.

Topical: Apply transdermal patch to upper or lower back (alternatively, nay apply to upper arm or chest). Avoid reapplication to same spot of skin for 14 days (may rotate sections of back, for example). Do not apply to red, irritated, or broken skin. Avoid areas of recent application of lotion or powder. After removal, fold patch to press adhesive surfaces together, and discard. Avoid eye contact; wash hands after handling patch. Replace patch every 24 hours. Avoid exposing the patch to external sources of heat (eg, sauna, excessive light) for prolonged periods of time.

Monitoring Parameters Cognitive function at periodic intervals (MMSE), symptoms of GI intolerance, weight

Dosage Forms Excipient information presented when available (limited, particularly for generics); consult specific product labeling.

Capsule:

Exelon®: 1.5 mg, 3 mg, 4.5 mg, 6 mg

Solution, oral:

Exelon®: 2 mg/mL (120 mL) [contains sodium benzoate]

Transdermal system [once-daily patch]:

Exelon®: 4.6 mg/24 hours (30s) [5 cm^2; contains rivastigmine 9 mg]; 9.5 mg/24 hours (30s) [10 cm^2; contains rivastigmine 18 mg]

◆ **Rivastigmine Tartrate** *see* Rivastigmine *on page 1435*

Rizatriptan (rye za TRIP tan)

Related Information

Antimigraine Drugs: 5-HT_1 Receptor Agonists *on page 1766*

U.S. Brand Names Maxalt-MLT®; Maxalt®

Canadian Brand Names Maxalt RPD™; Maxalt™

Mexican Brand Names Maxalt

Index Terms MK462

Pharmacologic Category Antimigraine Agent; Serotonin 5-$HT_{1B,\ 1D}$ Receptor Agonist

Generic Available No

Use Acute treatment of migraine with or without aura

Effect on Mental Status Drowsiness and dizziness are common

Effect on Psychiatric Treatment Contraindicated with other serotonin agonists (SSRIs) and MAO inhibitors

Pregnancy Risk Factor C

Pregnancy Considerations There are no adequate and well-controlled studies using rizatriptan in pregnant women. Use only if potential benefit to the mother outweighs the potential risk to the fetus. A pregnancy registry has been established to monitor outcomes of women exposed to rizatriptan during pregnancy (800-986-8999). In some animal studies, administration was associated with decreased weight gain, developmental toxicity and increased mortality in the offspring. Teratogenic effects were not observed.

Lactation Excretion in breast milk unknown/use caution

Contraindications Hypersensitivity to rizatriptan or any component of the formulation; documented ischemic heart disease or Prinzmetal's angina; uncontrolled hypertension; basilar or hemiplegic migraine; during or within 2 weeks of MAO inhibitors; during or within 24 hours of treatment with another 5-HT_1 agonist, or an ergot-containing or ergot-type medication (eg, methysergide, dihydroergotamine)

Warnings/Precautions Only indicated for treatment of acute migraine; if a patient does not respond to the first dose, the diagnosis of migraine should be reconsidered. Coronary artery vasospasm, transient ischemia, myocardial infarction, ventricular tachycardia/fibrillation, cardiac arrest, and death have been reported with 5-HT_1 agonist administration. Patients who experience sensations of chest pain/pressure/tightness or symptoms suggestive of angina following dosing should be evaluated for coronary artery disease or Prinzmetal's angina before receiving additional doses. Should not be given to patients who have risk factors for CAD (eg, hypertension, hypercholesterolemia, smoker, obesity, diabetes, strong family history of CAD, menopause, male >40 years of age) without adequate cardiac evaluation. Patients with suspected CAD should have cardiovascular evaluation to rule out CAD before considering use; if cardiovascular evaluation "is satisfactory", first dose should be given in the healthcare provider's office. Periodic evaluation of cardiovascular status should be done in all patients. Significant elevation in blood pressure, including hypertensive crisis, has also been reported on rare occasions in patients with and without a history of hypertension. Cerebral/subarachnoid hemorrhage, stroke, peripheral vascular ischemia, and colonic ischemia have been reported with 5-HT_1 agonist administration.

Use with caution in elderly or patients with hepatic or renal impairment (including dialysis patients). Symptoms of agitation, confusion, hallucinations, hyper-reflexia, myoclonus, shivering, and tachycardia may occur with concomitant proserotonergic drugs (eg, SSRIs/SNRIs or triptans) or agents which reduce rizatriptan's metabolism. Concurrent use of serotonin precursors (eg, tryptophan) is not recommended. Safety and efficacy have not been established in children <18 years of age. Maxalt-MLT® tablets contain phenylalanine.

Adverse Reactions

1% to 10%:

Cardiovascular: Systolic/diastolic blood pressure increases (5-10 mm Hg), chest pain (5%), palpitation

Central nervous system: Dizziness, drowsiness, fatigue (13% to 30%, dose related)

Dermatologic: Skin flushing

Endocrine & metabolic: Mild increase in growth hormone, hot flashes

Gastrointestinal: Abdominal pain, dry mouth (<5%), nausea

Respiratory: Dyspnea

<1% (Limited to important or life-threatening): Akinesia, angina, angioedema, arrhythmia, bradycardia, bradykinesia, decreased mental activity, myalgia, myocardial ischemia, MI, neck pain/stiffness, neurological/psychiatric abnormalities, pruritus, stroke, syncope, tachycardia, tinnitus, toxic epidermal necrolysis, wheezing

Drug Interactions

Ergot Derivatives: May enhance the vasoconstricting effect of Serotonin 5-HT1D Receptor Agonists. Serotonin 5-HT1D Receptor Agonists may enhance the vasoconstricting effect of Ergot Derivatives. *Risk X: Avoid combination*

MAO Inhibitors: May decrease the metabolism of Serotonin 5-HT1D Receptor Agonists. Management: If MAO inhibitor therapy is required, naratriptan, eletriptan or frovatriptan may be a suitable 5-HT1D agonist to employ. *Risk X: Avoid combination*

Propranolol: May increase the serum concentration of Serotonin 5-HT1D Receptor Agonists. *Risk D: Consider therapy modification*

Serotonin Modulators: May enhance the adverse/toxic effect of other Serotonin Modulators. The development of serotonin syndrome may occur. *Risk D: Consider therapy modification*

Sibutramine: May enhance the serotonergic effect of Serotonin Modulators. This may cause serotonin syndrome. *Risk X: Avoid combination*

Ethanol/Nutrition/Herb Interactions Food: Food delays absorption.

Stability Store in blister pack until administration.

Mechanism of Action Selective agonist for serotonin (5-HT_{1D} receptor) in cranial arteries to cause vasoconstriction and reduce sterile inflammation associated with antidromic neuronal transmission correlating with relief of migraine

Pharmacodynamics/Kinetics

Onset of action: ~30 minutes

Duration: 14-16 hours

Protein binding: 14%

Metabolism: Via monoamine oxidase-A; first-pass effect

Bioavailability: 40% to 50%

Half-life elimination: 2-3 hours

Time to peak: 1-1.5 hours

Excretion: Urine (82%, 8% to 16% as unchanged drug); feces (12%)

Dosage Note: In patients with risk factors for coronary artery disease, following adequate evaluation to establish the absence of coronary artery disease, the initial dose should be administered in a setting where response may be evaluated (physician's office or similarly staffed setting). ECG monitoring may be considered.

Oral: 5-10 mg, repeat after 2 hours if significant relief is not attained; maximum: 30 mg in a 24-hour period (use 5 mg dose in patients receiving propranolol with a maximum of 15 mg in 24 hours)

Note: For orally-disintegrating tablets (Maxalt-MLT®): Patient should be instructed to place tablet on tongue and allow to dissolve. Dissolved tablet will be swallowed with saliva.

Dietary Considerations Orally-disintegrating tablet contains phenylalanine (1.05 mg per 5 mg tablet, 2.10 mg per 10 mg tablet).

Monitoring Parameters Headache severity, signs/symptoms suggestive of angina; consider monitoring blood pressure, heart rate, and/or ECG with first dose in patients with likelihood of unrecognized coronary disease, such as patients with significant hypertension, hypercholesterolemia, obese patients, patients with diabetes, smokers with other risk factors or strong family history of coronary artery disease

Dosage Forms Excipient information presented when available (limited, particularly for generics); consult specific product labeling.

Tablet:

Maxalt®: 5 mg, 10 mg

Tablet, orally disintegrating:

Maxalt-MLT®: 5 mg [contains phenylalanine 1.05 mg/tablet; peppermint flavor]; 10 mg [contains phenylalanine 2.1 mg/tablet; peppermint flavor]

◆ **rLFN-α2** *see* Interferon Alfa-2b *on page 844*

◆ **R-modafinil** *see* Armodafinil *on page 138*

◆ **Ro 5488** *see* Tretinoin, Oral *on page 1617*

◆ **Robafen® AC** *see* Guaifenesin and Codeine *on page 738*

◆ **Robafen DM [OTC]** *see* Guaifenesin and Dextromethorphan *on page 739*

◆ **Robafen DM Clear [OTC]** *see* Guaifenesin and Dextromethorphan *on page 739*

◆ **Robaxin®** *see* Methocarbamol *on page 1011*

◆ **Robinul®** *see* Glycopyrrolate *on page 734*

◆ **Robinul® Forte** *see* Glycopyrrolate *on page 734*

◆ **Robitussin® [OTC]** *see* GuaiFENesin *on page 737*

- **Robitussin® Children's Cough & Cold Long-Acting [OTC]** *see* Dextromethorphan and Chlorpheniramine *on page 449*
- **Robitussin® Cold and Cough CF [OTC]** *see* Guaifenesin, Dextromethorphan, and Phenylephrine *on page 746*
- **Robitussin® Cough and Allergy [OTC]** *see* Chlorpheniramine, Phenylephrine, and Dextromethorphan *on page 327*
- **Robitussin® Cough and Cold [OTC]** *see* Guaifenesin, Pseudoephedrine, and Dextromethorphan *on page 748*
- **Robitussin® Cough and Cold CF [OTC]** *see* Guaifenesin, Pseudoephedrine, and Dextromethorphan *on page 748*
- **Robitussin® Cough and Cold Infant CF [OTC]** *see* Guaifenesin, Pseudoephedrine, and Dextromethorphan *on page 748*
- **Robitussin® Cough and Cold Nighttime [OTC]** *see* Chlorpheniramine, Phenylephrine, and Dextromethorphan *on page 327*
- **Robitussin® Cough and Congestion [OTC]** *see* Guaifenesin and Dextromethorphan *on page 739*
- **Robitussin® Cough & Cold Long-Acting [OTC]** *see* Dextromethorphan and Chlorpheniramine *on page 449*
- **Robitussin® CoughGels™ [OTC]** *see* Dextromethorphan *on page 448*
- **Robitussin® DM [OTC]** *see* Guaifenesin and Dextromethorphan *on page 739*
- **Robitussin® DM Infant [OTC] [DSC]** *see* Guaifenesin and Dextromethorphan *on page 739*
- **Robitussin® Maximum Strength Cough [OTC]** *see* Dextromethorphan *on page 448*
- **Robitussin® Night Time Cough & Cold [OTC]** *see* Diphenhydramine and Phenylephrine *on page 485*
- **Robitussin® Pediatric Cold and Cough CF [OTC]** *see* Guaifenesin, Dextromethorphan, and Phenylephrine *on page 746*
- **Robitussin® Pediatric Cough [OTC]** *see* Dextromethorphan *on page 448*
- **Robitussin® Pediatric Cough and Cold Nighttime [OTC]** *see* Chlorpheniramine, Phenylephrine, and Dextromethorphan *on page 327*
- **Robitussin® Sugar Free Cough [OTC]** *see* Guaifenesin and Dextromethorphan *on page 739*
- **Rocephin®** *see* CefTRIAXone *on page 300*
- **Roferon®-A [DSC]** *see* Interferon Alfa-2a *on page 844*
- **Rogaine® Extra Strength for Men [OTC]** *see* Minoxidil *on page 1057*
- **Rogaine® for Men [OTC]** *see* Minoxidil *on page 1057*
- **Rogaine® for Women [OTC]** *see* Minoxidil *on page 1057*
- **Rolaids® [OTC]** *see* Calcium Carbonate and Magnesium Hydroxide *on page 256*
- **Rolaids® Extra Strength [OTC]** *see* Calcium Carbonate and Magnesium Hydroxide *on page 256*
- **Rolaids® Softchews [OTC]** *see* Calcium Carbonate *on page 254*
- **Romazicon®** *see* Flumazenil *on page 644*
- **Romilar® AC** *see* Guaifenesin and Codeine *on page 738*
- **Romycin®** *see* Erythromycin *on page 557*
- **Rondec®** *see* Chlorpheniramine and Phenylephrine *on page 323*
- **Rondec®-DM** *see* Chlorpheniramine, Phenylephrine, and Dextromethorphan *on page 327*

Ropinirole (roe PIN i role)

Medication Safety Issues

Sound-alike/look-alike issues:

Requip® may be confused with Reglan®

Ropinirole may be confused with ropivacaine

Related Information

Antiparkinsonian Agents *on page 1767*

U.S. Brand Names Requip®; Requip® XL™

Canadian Brand Names Requip®

Index Terms Ropinirole Hydrochloride

Pharmacologic Category Anti-Parkinson's Agent, Dopamine Agonist

Generic Available Yes: Excludes combination package, extended-release tablets

Use Treatment of idiopathic Parkinson's disease; in patients with early Parkinson's disease who were not receiving concomitant levodopa therapy as well as in patients with advanced disease on concomitant levodopa; treatment of moderate-to-severe primary Restless Legs Syndrome (RLS)

Pregnancy Risk Factor C

Pregnancy Considerations Teratogenic effects have been observed in animal studies. There are no adequate and well-controlled studies in pregnant women; use only if potential benefit outweighs the risk to the fetus.

Lactation Excretion in breast milk unknown/not recommended

Contraindications Hypersensitivity to ropinirole or any component of the formulation

Warnings/Precautions Syncope, sometimes associated with bradycardia, was observed in association with ropinirole in both early Parkinson's disease (without levodopa) patients and advanced Parkinson's disease (with levodopa) patients. Dopamine agonists appear to impair the systemic regulation of blood pressure resulting in postural hypotension, especially during dose escalation. Parkinson's disease patients appear to have an impaired capacity to respond to a postural challenge; use with caution in patients at risk of hypotension (ie, those receiving antihypertensive drugs) or where transient hypotensive episodes would be poorly tolerated (cardiovascular disease or cerebrovascular disease). Parkinson's patients being treated with dopaminergic agonists ordinarily require careful monitoring for signs and symptoms of postural hypotension, especially during dose escalation, and should be informed of this risk. May cause hallucinations; risk may be increased in the elderly. Use with caution in patients with pre-existing dyskinesia, severe hepatic or renal dysfunction. Avoid use in patients with a major psychotic disorder; may exacerbate psychosis.

Patients treated with ropinirole have reported falling asleep while engaging in activities of daily living; this has been reported to occur without significant warning signs. Monitor for daytime somnolence or pre-existing sleep disorder; caution with concomitant sedating medication; discontinue if significant daytime sleepiness or episodes of falling asleep occur. Patients must be cautioned about performing tasks which require mental alertness (eg, operating machinery or driving). Use with caution in patients receiving other CNS depressants or psychoactive agents. Effects with other sedative drugs or ethanol may be potentiated.

Dopamine agonists have been associated with compulsive behaviors and/or loss of impulse control, which has manifested as pathological gambling, libido increases (hypersexuality), and/or binge eating. Causality has not been established, and controversy exists as to whether this phenomenon is related to the underlying disease, prior behaviors/addictions and/or drug therapy. Dose reduction or discontinuation of therapy has been reported to reverse these behaviors in some, but not all cases.

Some patients treated for RLS may experience worsening of symptoms in the early morning hours (rebound) or an increase and/or spread of daytime symptoms (augmentation); clinical management of these phenomena has not been evaluated in controlled clinical trials. Pathologic degenerative changes were observed in the retinas of albino rats during studies with this agent, but were not observed in the retinas of albino mice or in other species. The significance of these data for humans remains uncertain.

Other dopaminergic agents have been associated with a syndrome resembling neuroleptic malignant syndrome on withdrawal or significant dosage reduction after long-term use. Risk of fibrotic complications (eg, pleural effusion/fibrosis, interstitial lung disease) and melanoma has been reported in patients receiving ropinirole; drug causation has not been established. Safety and efficacy have not been established in children.

Adverse Reactions

Data inclusive of trials in early Parkinson's disease (without levodopa) and Restless Legs Syndrome:

>10%:

Cardiovascular: Syncope (1% to 12%)

Central nervous system: Somnolence (11% to 40%), dizziness (6% to 40%), fatigue (8% to 11%)

Gastrointestinal: Nausea (immediate release: 40% to 60%; extended release: 19%), vomiting (11% to 12%)

Miscellaneous: Viral infection (11%)

1% to 10%:

Cardiovascular: Dependent/leg edema (2% to 7%), orthostasis (1% to 6%), hypertension (5%), chest pain (4%), flushing (3%), palpitation (3%), peripheral ischemia (2% to 3%), atrial fibrillation (2%), extrasystoles (2%), hypotension (2%), tachycardia (2%)

Central nervous system: Pain (3% to 8%), headache (extended release: 6%), confusion (5%), hallucinations (up to 5%; dose related), hypoesthesia (4%), amnesia (3%), malaise (3%), yawning (3%), concentration impaired (2%), vertigo (2%)

Dermatologic: Hyperhidrosis (3%)

Gastrointestinal: Constipation (≥5%), dyspepsia (4% to 10%), abdominal pain (3% to 7%), xerostomia (3% to 5%), diarrhea (5%), anorexia (4%), flatulence (3%)

Genitourinary: Urinary tract infection (5%), impotence (3%)

Hepatic: Alkaline phosphatase increased (3%)

Neuromuscular & skeletal: Weakness (6%), arthralgia (4%), muscle cramps (3%), paresthesia (3%), hyperkinesia (2%)

Ocular: Abnormal vision (6%), xerophthalmia (2%)

Respiratory: Pharyngitis (6% to 9%), rhinitis (4%), sinusitis (4%), bronchitis (3%), dyspnea (3%), influenza (3%), cough (3%), nasal congestion (2%)

Miscellaneous: Diaphoresis increased (3% to 6%)

Advanced Parkinson's disease (with levodopa):

>10%:

Central nervous system: Dizziness (immediate release: 26%; extended-release: 8%), somnolence (immediate release: 20%, extended release: 7%), headache (17%)

Gastrointestinal: Nausea (immediate release: 30%; extended-release: 11%)

Neuromuscular & skeletal: Dyskinesias (immediate release: 34%; extended-release: 13%; dose related)

1% to 10%:

Cardiovascular: Hypotension (2% to 5%; including orthostatic), peripheral edema (4%), syncope (3%), hypertension (3%; dose related)

Central nervous system: Hallucinations (7% to 10%; dose related), confusion (9%), anxiety (2% to 6%), amnesia (5%), nervousness (5%), pain (5%), vertigo (4%), abnormal dreaming (3%), paresis (3%), aggravated parkinsonism, insomnia

Gastrointestinal: Abdominal pain (6% to 9%), vomiting (7%), constipation (4% to 6%), diarrhea (3% to 5%), xerostomia (2% to 5%), dysphagia (2%), flatulence (2%), salivation increased (2%), weight loss (2%)

Genitourinary: Urinary tract infection (6%), pyuria (2%), urinary incontinence (2%)

Hematologic: Anemia (2%)

Neuromuscular & skeletal: Falls (2% to 10%; dose related), arthralgia (7%), tremor (6%), hypokinesia (5%), paresthesia (5%), arthritis (3%), back pain (3%)

Ocular: Diplopia (2%)

Respiratory: Upper respiratory tract infection (9%), dyspnea (3%)

Miscellaneous: Injury, diaphoresis increased (7%), viral infection, increased drug level (7%)

Other adverse effects (all phase 2/3 trials for Parkinson's disease and Restless Leg Syndrome):

≥1%: Asthma, BUN increased, depression, gastroenteritis, gastrointestinal reflux, irritability, migraine, muscle spasm, myalgia, neck pain, neuralgia, osteoarthritis, pharyngolaryngeal pain, rash, rigors, sleep disorder, tendonitis

<1% (Limited to important or life-threatening): Abnormal coordination, acidosis, agitation, aneurysm, angina, aphasia, behavioral disorders, bradycardia, bundle branch block, cardiac arrest, cardiac failure, cardiac valvulopathy, cardiomegaly, cellulitis, cholecystitis, cholelithiasis, choreoathetosis, colitis, coma, conjunctival hemorrhage, dehydration, diabetes mellitus, diverticulitis, Dupuytren's contracture, dysphonia, electrolyte disturbances, eosinophilia, extrapyramidal symptoms, gangrene, gastrointestinal hemorrhage, gastrointestinal ulceration, glaucoma, goiter, gynecomastia, hematuria, hemiparesis, hemiplegia, hepatitis (ischemic), hyperbilirubinemia, hypercholesterolemia, hyper-/hypothyroidism, hyper-/hypotonia, hypoglycemia, hyponatremia, hyperphosphatemia, hyperuricemia; impulsive/compulsive behaviors (eg, pathological gambling, hypersexuality, binge eating); infections (bacterial, viral or fungal); interstitial lung disease, intestinal obstruction, leukocytosis, leukopenia, limb embolism, liver enzymes increased, lymphadenopathy, lymphedema, lymphocytosis, lymphopenia, menstrual abnormalities, mitral insufficiency, MI, neoplasms (various), pancreatitis, paralysis, peripheral neuropathy, photosensitivity, pleural

effusion, pleural fibrosis, proteinuria, psychiatric disorders, pulmonary edema, pulmonary embolism, renal calculus, renal failure (acute), seizure, sepsis, SIADH, skin disorders, stomatitis, stupor, subarachnoid hemorrhage, suicide attempt, SVT, thrombocytopenia, thrombosis, tinnitus, tongue edema, torticollis, urticaria, vagina/uterine hemorrhage, ventricular tachycardia, visual disturbances

Metabolism/Transport Effects **Substrate** of CYP1A2 (major), 3A4 (minor); **Inhibits** CYP1A2 (weak)

Drug Interactions

Antipsychotics (Atypical): May diminish the therapeutic effect of Anti-Parkinson's Agents (Dopamine Agonist). *Risk D: Consider therapy modification*

Antipsychotics (Typical): May diminish the therapeutic effect of Anti-Parkinson's Agents (Dopamine Agonist). *Risk D: Consider therapy modification*

Ciprofloxacin: May decrease the metabolism of Ropinirole. *Risk C: Monitor therapy*

CYP1A2 Inducers (Strong): May increase the metabolism of CYP1A2 Substrates. *Risk C: Monitor therapy*

CYP1A2 Inhibitors (Moderate): May decrease the metabolism of CYP1A2 Substrates. *Risk C: Monitor therapy*

CYP1A2 Inhibitors (Strong): May decrease the metabolism of CYP1A2 Substrates. *Risk D: Consider therapy modification*

Estrogen Derivatives: May increase the serum concentration of Ropinirole. *Risk C: Monitor therapy*

Metoclopramide: May diminish the therapeutic effect of Anti-Parkinson's Agents (Dopamine Agonist). *Risk C: Monitor therapy*

Ethanol/Nutrition/Herb Interactions

Ethanol: Avoid ethanol (may increase CNS depression).

Herb/Nutraceutical: Avoid kava kava, gotu kola, valerian, St John's wort (may increase CNS depression).

Stability Store at controlled room temperature of 20°C to 25°C (68°F to 77°F). Protect from light.

Mechanism of Action Ropinirole has a high relative *in vitro* specificity and full intrinsic activity at the D_2 and D_3 dopamine receptor subtypes, binding with higher affinity to D_3 than to D_2 or D_4 receptor subtypes; relevance of D_3 receptor binding in Parkinson's disease is unknown. Ropinirole has moderate *in vitro* affinity for opioid receptors. Ropinirole and its metabolites have negligible *in vitro* affinity for dopamine D_1, 5-HT_1, 5-HT_2, benzodiazepine, GABA, muscarinic, $alpha_1$-, $alpha_2$-, and beta-adrenoreceptors. Although precise mechanism of action of ropinirole is unknown, it is believed to be due to stimulation of postsynaptic dopamine D_2-type receptors within the caudate putamen in the brain. Ropinirole caused decreases in systolic and diastolic blood pressure at doses >0.25 mg. The mechanism of ropinirole-induced postural hypotension is believed to be due to D_2-mediated blunting of the noradrenergic response to standing and subsequent decrease in peripheral vascular resistance.

Pharmacodynamics/Kinetics

Absorption: Not affected by food

Distribution: V_d: 525 L

Protein binding: 40%

Metabolism: Extensively hepatic via CYP1A2 to inactive metabolites; first-pass effect

Bioavailability: Absolute: 45% to 55%

Half-life elimination: ~6 hours

Time to peak: Immediate release: ~1-2 hours; Extended release: 6-10 hours; T_{max} increased by 2.5-3 hours when drug taken with food

Excretion: Urine (<10% as unchanged drug, 60% as metabolites)

Clearance: Reduced by 15% to 30% in patients >65 years of age

Dosage Oral: Adults:

Parkinson's disease:

Immediate release tablet: The dosage should be increased to achieve a maximum therapeutic effect, balanced against the principal side effects of nausea, dizziness, somnolence and dyskinesia. Recommended starting dose is 0.25 mg 3 times/day; based on individual patient response, the dosage should be titrated with weekly increments as described below:

- Week 1: 0.25 mg 3 times/day; total daily dose: 0.75 mg
- Week 2: 0.5 mg 3 times/day; total daily dose: 1.5 mg
- Week 3: 0.75 mg 3 times/day; total daily dose: 2.25 mg
- Week 4: 1 mg 3 times/day; total daily dose: 3 mg

Note: After week 4, if necessary, daily dosage may be increased by 1.5 mg/day on a weekly basis up to a dose of 9 mg/day, and then by up to 3 mg/day weekly to a total of 24 mg/day

Parkinson's disease discontinuation taper: Ropinirole should be gradually tapered over 7 days as follows: reduce frequency of administration from 3 times daily to twice daily for 4 days, then reduce to once daily for remaining 3 days.

Extended release tablet: Initial: 2 mg once daily for 1-2 weeks, followed by increases of 2 mg/day at weekly or longer intervals based on therapeutic response and tolerability (maximum: 24 mg/day); **Note:** When discontinuing gradually taper over 7 days.

Restless legs syndrome: Immediate release tablets: Initial: 0.25 mg once daily 1-3 hours before bedtime. Dose may be increased after 2 days to 0.5 mg daily, and after 7 days to 1 mg daily. Dose may be further titrated upward in 0.5 mg increments every week until reaching a daily dose of 3 mg during week 6. If symptoms persist or reappear, the daily dose may be increased to a maximum of 4 mg beginning week 7.

Note: Doses up to 4 mg per day may be discontinued without tapering.

Converting from ropinirole immediate release tablets to ropinirole extended-release tablets: Choose a once daily extended-release dose that most closely matches current immediate-release daily dose.

Dosage adjustment in renal impairment: No adjustment needed in patients with moderate renal impairment (Cl_{cr} 30-50 mL/minute); has not been studied in patients with severe impairment.

Removal by hemodialysis is unlikely.

Dosage adjustment in hepatic impairment: Titrate with caution; has not been studied.

Dietary Considerations May be taken with or without food; taking with food may reduce nausea.

Administration May be administered with or without food; taking with food may reduce nausea. Swallow extended-release tablet whole; do not crush, split, or chew.

Monitoring Parameters

Blood pressure (orthostatic); daytime alertness

Additional Information If therapy with a drug known to be a potent inhibitor of CYP1A2 is stopped or started during treatment with ropinirole, adjustment of ropinirole dose may be required. Ropinirole binds to melanin-containing tissues (ie, eyes, skin) in pigmented rats. After a single dose, long-term retention of drug was demonstrated, with a half-life in the eye of 20 days; not known if ropinirole accumulates in these tissues over time.

Dosage Forms Excipient information presented when available (limited, particularly for generics); consult specific product labeling. [DSC] = Discontinued product

Combination package:

Requip® [starter kit; contents per each administration card]: Tablet: 0.25 mg (2s), 0.5 mg (5s), 1 mg (7s) [DSC]

Tablet: 0.25 mg, 0.5 mg, 1 mg, 2 mg, 3 mg, 4 mg, 5 mg

Requip®: 0.25 mg, 0.5 mg, 1 mg, 2 mg, 3 mg, 4 mg, 5 mg

Tablet, extended-release:

Requip® XL™: 2 mg, 4 mg, 8 mg

◆ **Ropinirole Hydrochloride** *see* Ropinirole *on page 1440*

Rosiglitazone (roh si GLI ta zone)

Medication Safety Issues

Sound-alike/look-alike issues:

Avandia® may be confused with Avalide®, Coumadin®, Prandin®

International issues:

Avandia® may be confused with Avanza® which is a brand name for mirtazapine in Australia

U.S. Brand Names Avandia®

Canadian Brand Names Avandia®

Mexican Brand Names Avandia

Pharmacologic Category Antidiabetic Agent, Thiazolidinedione

Generic Available No

Use Type 2 diabetes mellitus (noninsulin dependent, NIDDM):

Monotherapy: Improve glycemic control as an adjunct to diet and exercise

Note: Canadian labeling approves use as monotherapy only when metformin is contraindicated or not tolerated.

Combination therapy: **Note:** Use when diet, exercise, and a single agent do not result in adequate glycemic control.

U.S. labeling: In combination with a sulfonylurea, metformin, or sulfonylurea plus metformin

Canadian labeling: In combination with metformin; in combination with a sulfonylurea only when metformin use is contraindicated or not tolerated

Unlabeled/Investigational Use Polycystic ovary syndrome (PCOS)

Effect on Mental Status May cause headache and fatigue

Effect on Psychiatric Treatment Weight gain is common; caution with atypical antipsychotics

Restrictions An FDA-approved medication guide must be distributed when dispensing an outpatient prescription (new or refill) where this medication is to be used without direct supervision of a healthcare provider. Medication guides are available at http://www.fda.gov/cder/Offices/ODS/medication_guides.htm.

Pregnancy Risk Factor C

Pregnancy Considerations Rosiglitazone is classified as pregnancy category C due to adverse effects observed in initial animal studies. Rosiglitazone has been found to cross the placenta during the first trimester of pregnancy. Inadvertent use early in pregnancy has not shown adverse fetal effects although in the majority of cases, the medication was stopped as soon as pregnancy was detected. Thiazolidinediones may cause ovulation in anovulatory premenopausal women, increasing the risk of pregnancy; adequate contraception in premenopausal women is recommended. Maternal hyperglycemia can be associated with adverse effects in the fetus, including macrosomia, neonatal hyperglycemia, and hyperbilirubinemia; the risk of congenital malformations is increased when the Hb A_{1c} is above the normal range. Diabetes can also be associated with adverse effects in the mother. Poorly-treated diabetes may cause end-organ damage that may in turn negatively affect obstetric outcomes. Physiologic glucose levels should be maintained prior to and during pregnancy to decrease the risk of adverse events in the mother and the fetus. Until additional safety and efficacy data are obtained, the use of oral agents is generally not recommended as routine management of GDM or type 2 diabetes mellitus during pregnancy. Insulin is the drug of choice for the control of diabetes mellitus during pregnancy.

Lactation Excretion in breast milk unknown/not recommended

Contraindications

U.S. labeling: NYHA Class III/IV heart failure (initiation of therapy)

Canadian labeling: Hypersensitivity to rosiglitazone or any component of the formulation; any stage of heart failure (eg, NYHA Class I, II, III, IV); serious hepatic impairment; pregnancy

Warnings/Precautions [U.S. Boxed Warning]: Thiazolidinediones, including rosiglitazone, may cause or exacerbate congestive heart failure; closely monitor for signs/symptoms of congestive heart failure (eg, rapid weight gain, dyspnea, edema), particularly after initiation or dose increases. Not recommended for use in any patient with symptomatic heart failure. In the U.S., initiation of therapy is contraindicated in patients with NYHA class III or IV heart failure; in Canada use is contraindicated in patients with any stage of heart failure (NYHA Class I, II, III, IV). Use with caution in patients with edema; may increase plasma volume and/or cause fluid retention, leading to heart failure. Dose-related weight gain observed with use; mechanism unknown but likely associated with fluid retention and fat accumulation. Use may also be associated with an increased risk of angina and MI. Use caution in patients at risk for cardiovascular events and monitor closely. Discontinue if any deterioration in cardiac status occurs.

Should not be used in diabetic ketoacidosis. Mechanism requires the presence of insulin; therefore, use in type 1 diabetes (insulin dependent, IDDM) is not recommended. Combination therapy with other hypoglycemic agents may increase risk for hypoglycemic events; dose reduction with the concomitant agent may be warranted. Concomitant use with nitrates is not recommended due to increased risk of myocardial ischemia. Avoid use with insulin due to an increased risk of edema, congestive heart failure, and myocardial ischemic events.

Use with caution in patients with elevated transaminases (AST or ALT); do not initiate in patients with active liver disease or ALT >2.5 times ULN at baseline; evaluate patients with ALT ≤2.5 times ULN at baseline or during therapy for cause of enzyme elevation; during therapy, if ALT >3 times ULN, reevaluate levels promptly and discontinue if elevation persists or if jaundice occurs at any time during use. Idiosyncratic hepatotoxicity has been reported with another thiazolidinedione agent (troglitazone); avoid use in patients who previously experienced jaundice during troglitazone therapy. Monitoring should include periodic determinations of liver function. Increased incidence of bone fractures in females treated with rosiglitazone observed during analysis of long-term trial;

majority of fractures occurred in the upper arm, hand, and foot (differing from the hip or spine fractures usually associated with postmenopausal osteoporosis). May decrease hemoglobin/hematocrit and/or WBC count (slight); effects may be related to increased plasma volume and/or dose related; use with caution in patients with anemia.

Rosiglitazone has been associated with new onset and/or worsening of macular edema in patients with diabetes. Rosiglitazone should be used with caution in patients with a pre-existing macular edema or diabetic retinopathy. Discontinuation of rosiglitazone should be considered in any patient who reports visual deterioration. In addition, ophthalmological consultation should be initiated in these patients. Use with caution in premenopausal, anovulatory women; may result in resumption of ovulation, increasing the risk of pregnancy. Safety and efficacy in pediatric patients have not been established.

Additional Canadian warnings (not included in U.S. labeling): If glycemic control is inadequate, rosiglitazone may be added to metformin or a sulfonylurea (if metformin use is contraindicated or not tolerated); use of triple therapy (rosiglitazone in combination with both metformin and a sulfonylurea) is not indicated due to increased risks of heart failure and fluid retention.

Adverse Reactions Note: The rate of certain adverse reactions (eg, anemia, edema, hypoglycemia) may be higher with some combination therapies.

>10%: Endocrine & metabolic: HDL-cholesterol increased, LDL-cholesterol increased, total cholesterol increased, weight gain

1% to 10%:

Cardiovascular: Edema (5%), hypertension (4%); heart failure/CHF (up to 2% to 3% in patients receiving insulin; incidence likely higher in patients with pre-existing HF; myocardial ischemia (3%; incidence likely higher in patients with preexisting CAD)

Central nervous system: Headache (6%)

Endocrine & metabolic: Hypoglycemia (1% to 3%; combination therapy with insulin: 12% to 14%)

Gastrointestinal: Diarrhea (3%)

Hematologic: Anemia (2%)

Neuromuscular & skeletal: Fractures (up to 9%; incidence greater in females; usually upper arm, hand, or foot), arthralgia (5%), back pain (4% to 5%)

Respiratory: Upper respiratory tract infection (4% to 10%), nasopharyngitis (6%)

Miscellaneous: Injury (8%)

<1% (Limited to important or life-threatening): Anaphylaxis, angina, angioedema, bilirubin increased, blurred vision, cardiac arrest, dyspnea, coronary artery disease, coronary thrombosis, hematocrit decreased, hemoglobin decreased, hepatic failure, hepatitis, HDL-cholesterol decreased, jaundice (reversible), macular edema, MI, pleural effusion, pruritus, pulmonary edema, rash, Stevens-Johnson syndrome, thrombocytopenia, transaminases increased, urticaria, visual acuity decreased, weight gain (rapid, excessive; usually due to fluid accumulation), WBC count decreased

Note: Rare cases of hepatocellular injury have been reported in men in their 60s within 2-3 weeks after initiation of rosiglitazone therapy. LFTs in these patients revealed severe hepatocellular injury which responded with rapid improvement of liver function and resolution of symptoms upon discontinuation of rosiglitazone. Patients were also receiving other potentially hepatotoxic medications (Al-Salman, 2000; Freid, 2000).

Metabolism/Transport Effects Substrate of CYP2C8 (major), 2C9 (minor); **Inhibits** CYP2C8 (moderate), 2C9 (weak), 2C19 (weak), 2D6 (weak)

Drug Interactions

Bile Acid Sequestrants: May decrease the absorption of Antidiabetic Agents (Thiazolidinedione). *Risk D: Consider therapy modification*

Corticosteroids (Orally Inhaled): May diminish the hypoglycemic effect of Antidiabetic Agents. In some instances, corticosteroid-mediated HPA axis suppression has led to episodes of acute adrenal crisis, which may manifest as enhanced hypoglycemia, particularly in the setting of insulin or other antidiabetic agent use. *Risk C: Monitor therapy*

Corticosteroids (Systemic): May diminish the hypoglycemic effect of Antidiabetic Agents. In some instances, corticosteroid-mediated HPA axis suppression has led to episodes of acute adrenal crisis, which may manifest as enhanced hypoglycemia, particularly in the setting of insulin or other antidiabetic agent use. *Risk C: Monitor therapy*

CYP2C8 Inducers (Highly Effective): May increase the metabolism of CYP2C8 Substrates (High risk). *Risk C: Monitor therapy*

CYP2C8 Inhibitors (Moderate): May decrease the metabolism of CYP2C8 Substrates (High risk). *Risk C: Monitor therapy*

CYP2C8 Inhibitors (Strong): May decrease the metabolism of CYP2C8 Substrates (High risk). *Risk D: Consider therapy modification*

CYP2C8 Substrates (High risk): CYP2C8 Inhibitors (Moderate) may decrease the metabolism of CYP2C8 Substrates (High risk). *Risk C: Monitor therapy*

Gemfibrozil: May decrease the metabolism of Antidiabetic Agents (Thiazolidinedione). *Risk C: Monitor therapy*

Herbs (Hypoglycemic Properties): May enhance the hypoglycemic effect of Hypoglycemic Agents. *Risk C: Monitor therapy*

Insulin: May enhance the fluid-retaining effect of Antidiabetic Agents (Thiazolidinedione). *Risk C: Monitor therapy*

Luteinizing Hormone-Releasing Hormone Analogs: May diminish the therapeutic effect of Antidiabetic Agents. *Risk C: Monitor therapy*

Pegvisomant: May enhance the hypoglycemic effect of Antidiabetic Agents. *Risk C: Monitor therapy*

Pregabalin: May enhance the fluid-retaining effect of Antidiabetic Agents (Thiazolidinedione). *Risk C: Monitor therapy*

Rifampin: May increase the metabolism of Antidiabetic Agents (Thiazolidinedione). *Risk C: Monitor therapy*

Somatropin: May diminish the hypoglycemic effect of Antidiabetic Agents. *Risk D: Consider therapy modification*

Trimethoprim: May decrease the metabolism of Antidiabetic Agents (Thiazolidinedione). *Risk C: Monitor therapy*

Vasodilators (Organic Nitrates): May enhance the adverse/toxic effect of Rosiglitazone. Specifically, a greater risk of myocardial ischemia was reported for users of this combination in a meta-analysis. Management: Consider alternatives to this combination when possible. Rosiglitazone prescribing information states that the combination of rosiglitazone and a nitrate is not recommended. *Risk D: Consider therapy modification*

Ethanol/Nutrition/Herb Interactions

Ethanol: Avoid ethanol (may cause hypoglycemia).

Food: Peak concentrations are lower by 28% and delayed when administered with food, but these effects are not believed to be clinically significant.

Herb/Nutraceutical: Avoid alfalfa, aloe, bilberry, bitter melon, burdock, celery, damiana, fenugreek, garcinia, garlic, ginger, ginseng (American), gymnema, marshmallow, stinging nettle (may cause hypoglycemia).

Stability Store at 15°C to 30°C (59°F to 86°F). Protect from light.

Mechanism of Action Thiazolidinedione antidiabetic agent that lowers blood glucose by improving target cell response to insulin, without increasing pancreatic insulin secretion. It has a mechanism of action that is dependent on the presence of insulin for activity. Rosiglitazone is an agonist for peroxisome proliferator-activated receptor-gamma (PPARgamma). Activation of nuclear PPARgamma receptors influences the production of a number of gene products involved in glucose and lipid metabolism. Thiazolidinedione antidiabetic agent that lowers blood glucose by improving target cell response to insulin, without increasing pancreatic insulin secretion. It has a mechanism of action that is dependent on the presence of insulin for activity. PPARgamma is abundant in the cells within the renal collecting tubules; fluid retention results from stimulation by thiazolidinediones which increases sodium reabsorption.

Pharmacodynamics/Kinetics

Onset of action: Delayed; Maximum effect: Up to 12 weeks

Distribution: V_{dss} (apparent): 17.6 L

Protein binding: 99.8%; primarily albumin

Metabolism: Hepatic (99%) via CYP2C8; minor metabolism via CYP2C9

Bioavailability: 99%

Half-life elimination: 3-4 hours

Time to peak, plasma: 1 hour; delayed with food

Excretion: Urine (64%) and feces (23%) as metabolites

Dosage Oral:

Adults: **Note:** All patients should be initiated at the lowest recommended dose.

Monotherapy: Initial: 4 mg daily as a single daily dose or in divided doses twice daily. If response is inadequate after 8-12 weeks of treatment, the dosage may be increased to 8 mg daily as a single daily dose or in divided doses twice daily. In clinical trials, the 4 mg twice-daily regimen resulted in the greatest reduction in fasting plasma glucose and Hb A_{1c}.

Combination therapy: When adding rosiglitazone to existing therapy, continue current dose(s) of previous agents:

U.S. labeling: With sulfonylureas or metformin (or sulfonylurea plus metformin): Initial: 4 mg daily as a single daily dose or in divided doses twice daily. If response is inadequate after 8-12 weeks of treatment, the dosage may be increased to 8 mg daily as a single daily dose or in divided doses twice daily. Reduce dose of sulfonylurea if hypoglycemia occurs. It is unlikely that the dose of metformin will need to be reduced due to hypoglycemia.

Canadian labeling:

With metformin: Initial: 4 mg daily as a single daily dose or in divided doses twice daily. If response is inadequate after 8-12 weeks of treatment, the dosage may be increased to 8 mg daily as a single daily dose or in divided doses twice daily.

With a sulfonylurea: 4 mg daily as a single daily dose or in divided doses twice daily. Dose should not exceed 4 mg daily when using in combination with a sulfonylurea. Reduce dose of sulfonylurea if hypoglycemia occurs.

Elderly: No dosage adjustment is recommended

Dosage adjustment in renal impairment: No dosage adjustment is required

Dosage comment in hepatic impairment: Clearance is significantly lower in hepatic impairment. Therapy should not be initiated if the patient exhibits active liver disease or increased transaminases (ALT >2.5 times the upper limit of normal) at baseline.

Dietary Considerations Management of type 2 diabetes mellitus (noninsulin dependent, NIDDM) should include diet control. May be taken without regard to meals.

Monitoring Parameters Hemoglobin A_{1c}, fasting serum glucose; signs and symptoms of fluid retention or heart failure; liver enzymes (prior to initiation of therapy, then periodically thereafter); ophthalmic exams. Evaluate patients with ALT ≤2.5 times ULN at baseline or during therapy for cause of enzyme elevation. Patients with an elevation in ALT >3 times ULN should be rechecked as soon as possible. If the ALT levels remain >3 times ULN, therapy with rosiglitazone should be discontinued.

Reference Range Recommendations for glycemic control in adults with diabetes:

Hb A_{1c}: <7%

Preprandial capillary plasma glucose: 70-130 mg/dL

Peak postprandial capillary blood glucose: <180 mg/dL

Dosage Forms Excipient information presented when available (limited, particularly for generics); consult specific product labeling.

Tablet:

Avandia®: 2 mg, 4 mg, 8 mg

Rosiglitazone and Glimepiride

(roh si GLI ta zone & GLYE me pye ride)

Medication Safety Issues

High alert medication: The Institute for Safe Medication Practices (ISMP) includes this medication among its list of drugs which have a heightened risk of causing significant patient harm when used in error.

U.S. Brand Names Avandaryl™

Index Terms Glimepiride and Rosiglitazone Maleate

Pharmacologic Category Antidiabetic Agent, Sulfonylurea; Antidiabetic Agent, Thiazolidinedione

Use Management of type 2 diabetes mellitus (noninsulin dependent, NIDDM) as an adjunct to diet and exercise

Effect on Mental Status May cause headache and fatigue

Effect on Psychiatric Treatment May rarely cause agranulocytosis; use caution with clozapine and carbamazepine. Phenothiazines, atypical antipsychotics, and TCAs may antagonize glimepiride hypoglycemic effects; MAO inhibitors and TCAs may enhance hypoglycemic effects. Weight gain is common; caution with atypical antipsychotics, valproic acid, and lithium.

Dosage Summary

Oral:

Children: Dosage not established

Adults: Initial: Rosiglitazone 4 mg and glimepiride 1-2 mg once daily; Maintenance: Rosiglitazone 4-8 mg and glimepiride 1-4 mg once daily; **Note:** Titration is recommended

Elderly: Initial: Rosiglitazone 4 mg and glimepiride 1 mg once daily; **Note:** Titration is recommended

Dosage Forms Excipient information presented when available (limited, particularly for generics); consult specific product labeling.

Tablet:

Avandaryl™ 4 mg/1 mg: Rosiglitazone maleate 4 mg and glimepiride 1 mg
Avandaryl™ 4 mg/2 mg: Rosiglitazone maleate 4 mg and glimepiride 2 mg
Avandaryl™ 4 mg/4 mg: Rosiglitazone maleate 4 mg and glimepiride 4 mg
Avandaryl™ 8 mg/2 mg: Rosiglitazone maleate 8 mg and glimepiride 2 mg
Avandaryl™ 8 mg/4 mg: Rosiglitazone maleate 8 mg and glimepiride 4 mg

Rosiglitazone and Metformin (roh si GLI ta zone & met FOR min)

Medication Safety Issues
Sound-alike/look-alike issues:
Avandamet® may be confused with Anzemet®

U.S. Brand Names Avandamet®

Canadian Brand Names Avandamet®

Index Terms Metformin and Rosiglitazone; Metformin Hydrochloride and Rosiglitazone Maleate; Rosiglitazone Maleate and Metformin Hydrochloride

Pharmacologic Category Antidiabetic Agent, Biguanide; Antidiabetic Agent, Thiazolidinedione

Use Management of type 2 diabetes mellitus (noninsulin dependent, NIDDM) as an adjunct to diet and exercise in patients where dual rosiglitazone and metformin therapy is appropriate

Effect on Mental Status May cause fatigue

Effect on Psychiatric Treatment May cause weight gain; concurrent use with psychotropics may produce additive weight gain

Dosage Summary

Oral:

Children: Dosage not established

Adults: Initial: Rosiglitazone 2 mg and metformin 500 mg once or twice daily; may increase by 2 mg/500 mg per day after 4 weeks (maximum: rosiglitazone 8 mg/day; metformin 2000 mg/day)

Elderly ≥80 years: Do not use unless normal renal function has been established

Dosage Forms Excipient information presented when available (limited, particularly for generics); consult specific product labeling. [DSC] = Discontinued product

Tablet:

Avandamet®: 1/500: Rosiglitazone 1 mg and metformin hydrochloride 500 mg [DSC]

Avandamet®: 2/500: Rosiglitazone 2 mg and metformin hydrochloride 500 mg

Avandamet®: 4/500: Rosiglitazone 4 mg and metformin hydrochloride 500 mg

Avandamet®: 2/1000: Rosiglitazone 2 mg and metformin hydrochloride 1000 mg

Avandamet®: 4/1000: Rosiglitazone 4 mg and metformin hydrochloride 1000 mg

◆ **Rosiglitazone Maleate and Metformin Hydrochloride** *see* Rosiglitazone and Metformin *on page 1449*

Rotigotine (roe TIG oh teen)

Medication Safety Issues
Sound-alike/look-alike issues:
Neupro® may be confused with Neupogen®

Transdermal patch contains metal (eg, aluminum); remove patch prior to MRI.

Related Information
Antiparkinsonian Agents *on page 1767*

U.S. Brand Names Neupro® [DSC]

Index Terms N-0923

Pharmacologic Category Anti-Parkinson's Agent, Dopamine Agonist

Generic Available No

Use Treatment of the signs and symptoms of early-stage idiopathic Parkinson's disease

Pregnancy Risk Factor C

Pregnancy Considerations Fetal death and adverse effects on embryo-fetal development were observed in some, but not all animal studies. There are no adequate and well-controlled studies in pregnant women.

Lactation Excretion in breast milk unknown/not recommended

Contraindications Hypersensitivity to rotigotine or any component of the formulation

Warnings/Precautions Use commonly associated with somnolence. In addition, patients falling asleep during activities of daily living, including driving, have also been reported and may occur without significant warning signs. Monitor for daytime somnolence or pre-existing sleep disorder. Patients must be cautioned about performing tasks which require mental alertness (eg, operating machinery or driving). Use with caution in patients receiving other CNS depressants or psychoactive agents; discontinue if significant daytime sleepiness or episodes of falling asleep occur. Effects with other sedative drugs or ethanol may be potentiated.

Dopamine agonists may cause orthostatic hypotension and syncope; Parkinson's disease patients appear to have an impaired capacity to respond to a postural challenge. Use with caution in patients at risk of hypotension (such as those receiving antihypertensive drugs) or where transient hypotensive episodes would be poorly tolerated (cardiovascular disease or cerebrovascular disease). Parkinson's patients being treated with dopaminergic agonists ordinarily require careful monitoring for signs and symptoms of postural hypotension, especially during dose escalation, and should be informed of this risk. Therapy has also been associated with inconsistent increases in blood pressure, increased heart rate (average increase of 2-4 bpm), and fluid retention.

Dopamine agonists have been associated with compulsive behaviors and/or loss of impulse control, which has manifested as pathological gambling, libido increases (hypersexuality), and/or binge eating. Causality has not been established, and controversy exists as to whether this phenomenon is related to the underlying disease, prior behaviors/addictions and/or drug therapy. Dose reduction or discontinuation of therapy has been reported to reverse these behaviors in some, but not all cases.

Use with caution in patients with pre-existing dyskinesia; therapy may exacerbate. Therapy may also cause hallucinations. Risk for melanoma development is increased in Parkinson's disease patients; drug causation or factors contributing to risk have not been established. Other dopaminergic agents have been associated with a syndrome resembling neuroleptic malignant syndrome on withdrawal and/or significant dosage reduction. Taper treatment when discontinuing therapy; do not stop abruptly. Rare cases of pleural, retroperitoneal fibrosis and/or cardiac valvulopathy have been reported in patients treated with ergot-derived dopamine agonists, generally with prolonged use. The potential of rotigotine, a nonergot-derived dopamine agonist, to cause similar fibrotic complications is unknown.

Patch contains aluminum; remove patch prior to magnetic resonance imaging or cardioversion to avoid skin burns. Patch also contains sodium metabisulfite which may cause allergic reaction in susceptible individuals. Patients should be instructed to rotate application sites to reduce incidence of application site reactions. Reactions increasing in severity, spreading outside of application site or persistent reactions (lasting longer than several days) prompt assessment and any generalized skin reaction require discontinuation of therapy. Patients should be instructed to avoid patch exposure to heat sources; heat application may result in several fold increases in drug absorption. Safety and effectiveness have not been established in children <18 years of age.

Adverse Reactions

>10%:

- Central nervous system: Somnolence (13% to 25%), dizziness (18%), headache (14%), insomnia (6% to 14%)
- Gastrointestinal: Nausea (34% to 48%), vomiting (10% to 20%)
- Local: Application site reactions (21% to 37%)

1% to 10%:

- Cardiovascular: Sinus tachycardia (9%), peripheral edema (7%), orthostatic hypotension (5% to 7%), hypertension (3%), syncope
- Central nervous system: Fatigue (8%), abnormal dreams (2% to 5%), hallucination (≤3%), vertigo (3%), ataxia, confusion, fever, hypoesthesia, malaise
- Dermatologic: Erythematous rash (2% to 6%), contact dermatitis, pruritus, purpura
- Endocrine & metabolic: Hypoglycemia (7%)
- Gastrointestinal: Constipation (dose related; 5%), dyspepsia (4%), anorexia (dose related; 3%), xerostomia (3%), weight gain (3%), weight loss (≤2%)
- Genitourinary: Urinary tract infection (3%), urinary incontinence
- Hematologic: Hemoglobin decreased
- Hepatic: Albumin decreased, GGT increased
- Neuromuscular & skeletal: Back pain (6%), arthralgia (4%), myalgia (≤2%), abnormal gait, hypertonia, leg pain, neuralgia, paresthesia
- Ocular: Vision changes (dose related; 3%)
- Respiratory: Sinusitis (3%)
- Miscellaneous: Accident (5%), diaphoresis increased (4%)

<1% (Limited to important or life-threatening): Allergic reaction, appetite increased, atrial fibrillation, AV block, BUN increased, bundle branch block, flushing, heart failure, hot flashes, hyperesthesia, impotence, paranoia, psychosis, photopsia, rigors, saliva increased, seizure, sexual urgency, thrombocytopenia, tinnitus, ventricular arrhythmia, ventricular tachycardia

Reported with dopamine agonists: Impulsive/compulsive behaviors (eg, pathological gambling, hypersexuality, binge eating)

Drug Interactions

Alcohol (Ethyl): CNS Depressants may enhance the CNS depressant effect of Alcohol (Ethyl). *Risk C: Monitor therapy*

Antipsychotics (Atypical): May diminish the therapeutic effect of Anti-Parkinson's Agents (Dopamine Agonist). *Risk D: Consider therapy modification*

Antipsychotics (Typical): May diminish the therapeutic effect of Anti-Parkinson's Agents (Dopamine Agonist). *Risk D: Consider therapy modification*

CNS Depressants: May enhance the adverse/toxic effect of other CNS Depressants. *Risk C: Monitor therapy*

Metoclopramide: May diminish the therapeutic effect of Anti-Parkinson's Agents (Dopamine Agonist). *Risk C: Monitor therapy*

Ethanol/Nutrition/Herb Interactions Ethanol: Avoid ethanol (may increase CNS depression).

Stability Store at 15°C to 30°C (59°F to 86°F). Store in original pouch until application.

Mechanism of Action Rotigotine is a nonergot dopamine agonist with specificity for D_3-, D_2-, and D_1-dopamine receptors. Although the precise mechanism of action of rotigotine is unknown, it is believed to be due to stimulation of postsynaptic dopamine D_2-type auto receptors within the substantia nigra in the brain, leading to improved dopaminergic transmission in the motor areas of the basal ganglia, notably the caudate nucleus/putamen regions.

Pharmacodynamics/Kinetics

Distribution: V_d: 84 L/kg

Protein binding: ~90%

Metabolism: Extensive conjugation and N-dealkylation

Half-life elimination: After removal of patch: ~5-7 hours

Time to peak, plasma: 15-18 hours; can occur 4-27 hours post application

Excretion: Urine (~71% as metabolites, <1% as unchanged drug); feces (~11%)

Dosage Topical: Transdermal: Adults: Initial: Apply 2 mg/24 hours patch once daily; may increase by 2 mg/24 hours weekly, based on clinical response and tolerability (maximum: 6 mg/24 hours)

Dosage reductions or discontinuation: Decrease by 2 mg/24 hours every other day

Note: In clinical trials, the lowest effective dose was 4 mg/24 hours and doses >6 mg/24 hours did not provide any additional therapeutic benefit and increased incidence of adverse effects

Dosage adjustment in renal impairment: Severe impairment (Cl_{cr} 15-29 mL/minute): No dosage adjustment required

Dosage adjustment in hepatic impairment:

Moderate hepatic impairment (Child-Pugh class B): No dosage adjustment required

Severe hepatic impairment: Not studied

Administration Inspect patches for formation of crystals. Do not use if crystallization is present. Apply to clean, dry, hairless area of skin on the front of the abdomen, thigh, hip, flank, shoulder, or upper arm at approximately the same time daily. Remove from pouch immediately before use and press patch firmly in place on skin for 20-30 seconds. Application sites should be rotated on a daily basis. Do not apply to same application site for more than once every 14 days or apply patch to oily, irritated or damaged skin. Avoid exposing patch to external heat sources (eg, heating pad, electric blanket, heat lamp, hot tub). If applied to hairy area, shave ≥3 days prior to applying patch. If patch detaches, immediately apply a new one to a new site.

Monitoring Parameters Blood pressure (orthostatic); daytime alertness; periodic skin evaluations (melanoma development)

Dosage Forms Excipient information presented when available (limited, particularly for generics); consult specific product labeling. [DSC] = Discontinued product

Transdermal system [once-daily patch]:

Neupro®:

2 mg/24 hours (7s, 30s) [10 cm^2, total rotigotine 4.5 mg; contains sodium metabisulfite] [DSC]

4 mg/24 hours (7s, 30s) [20 cm^2, total rotigotine 9 mg; contains sodium metabisulfite] [DSC]

6 mg/24 hours (7s, 30s) [30 cm^2, total rotigotine 13.5 mg; contains sodium metabisulfite] [DSC]

- ◆ **Rowasa®** *see* Mesalamine *on page 994*
- ◆ **Roxanol™** *see* Morphine Sulfate *on page 1077*
- ◆ **Roxicet™** *see* Oxycodone and Acetaminophen *on page 1205*
- ◆ **Roxicet™ 5/500** *see* Oxycodone and Acetaminophen *on page 1205*
- ◆ **Roxicodone®** *see* OxyCODONE *on page 1201*
- ◆ **Rozerem™** *see* Ramelteon *on page 1394*
- ◆ **RP-6976** *see* Docetaxel *on page 491*
- ◆ **RP-54274** *see* Riluzole *on page 1421*
- ◆ **RP-59500** *see* Quinupristin and Dalfopristin *on page 1388*
- ◆ **(R,R)-Formoterol L-Tartrate** *see* Arformoterol *on page 131*
- ◆ **RS-25259** *see* Palonosetron *on page 1218*
- ◆ **RS-25259-197** *see* Palonosetron *on page 1218*
- ◆ **R-Tanna** *see* Chlorpheniramine and Phenylephrine *on page 323*
- ◆ **R-Tanna Pediatric** *see* Chlorpheniramine and Phenylephrine *on page 323*
- ◆ **RTCA** *see* Ribavirin *on page 1417*
- ◆ **RU 0211** *see* Lubiprostone *on page 963*
- ◆ **RU-486** *see* Mifepristone *on page 1051*
- ◆ **RU-23908** *see* Nilutamide *on page 1140*
- ◆ **RU-38486** *see* Mifepristone *on page 1051*
- ◆ **Rubella, Varicella, Measles, and Mumps Vaccine** *see* Measles, Mumps, Rubella, and Varicella Virus Vaccine *on page 972*
- ◆ **Rubex® [DSC]** *see* DOXOrubicin *on page 507*
- ◆ **Rubidomycin Hydrochloride** *see* DAUNOrubicin Hydrochloride *on page 421*
- ◆ **RUF 331** *see* Rufinamide *on page 1452*

Rufinamide (roo FIN a mide)

Related Information

Anticonvulsants by Seizure Type *on page 1759*

U.S. Brand Names Banzel™

Index Terms CGP 33101; E 2080; RUF 331; Xilep

Pharmacologic Category Anticonvulsant, Triazole Derivative

Generic Available No

Use Adjunctive therapy in the treatment of generalized seizures of Lennox-Gastaut syndrome

Restrictions An FDA-approved patient medication guide is available and must be distributed when dispensing an outpatient prescription (new or refill) where this medication is to be used without direct supervision of a healthcare provider. Medication guides are available at http://www.fda.gov/cder/Offices/ODS/medication_guides.htm.

Pregnancy Risk Factor C

Pregnancy Considerations Adverse effects were seen in animal studies. There are no adequate and well-controlled studies in pregnant women; use during pregnancy only if clearly needed. Hormonal contraceptives may be less effective with concurrent rufinamide use; additional forms of nonhormonal contraceptives should be used.

Lactation Excretion in breast milk unknown/not recommended

Contraindications Patients with familial short QT syndrome

Warnings/Precautions Has been associated with shortening of the QT interval. Use caution in patients receiving concurrent medications that shorten the QT interval. Contraindicated in patients with familial short-QT syndrome. Use has been associated with CNS-related adverse events, most significant of these were cognitive symptoms (including somnolence or fatigue) and coordination abnormalities (including ataxia, dizziness, and gait disturbances). Caution patients about performing tasks which require mental alertness (eg, operating machinery or driving). Effects with other sedative drugs or ethanol may be potentiated. Potentially serious, sometimes fatal, multiorgan hypersensitivity reactions have been reported with some antiepileptic drugs, including rufinamide; monitor for signs and symptoms of possible disparate manifestations associated with lymphatic, hepatic, renal, and/or hematologic organ systems; gradual discontinuation and conversion to alternate therapy may be required. Closely monitor any patient who develops a rash; instruct patients to report any rash associated with fever.

Antiepileptics may increase the risk of suicidal ideation. Monitor patients closely for unusual changes in mood or behavior, worsening depression, or suicidal behavior or thoughts. Caregivers and families should also be educated to watch for these signs and symptoms and notify healthcare provider if signs/symptoms develop. Use with caution in patients with mild to moderate hepatic impairment; use in not recommended in patients with severe hepatic impairment. Concurrent use with hormonal contraceptives may lead to contraceptive failure. Anticonvulsants should not be discontinued abruptly because of the possibility of increasing seizure frequency; therapy should be withdrawn gradually to minimize the potential of increased seizure frequency, unless safety concerns require a more rapid withdrawal. Reducing dose by ~25% every two days was effective in trials.

Adverse Reactions

>10%:

Cardiovascular: QT shortening (46% to 65%; dose related)

Central nervous system: Headache (16% to 27%), somnolence (11% to 24%), dizziness (3% to 19%), fatigue (9% to 16%)

Gastrointestinal: Vomiting (5% to 17%), nausea (7% to 12%)

1% to 10%:

Central nervous system: Ataxia (4 % to 5%), seizure (children 5%), status epilepticus (up to 4%), aggression (children 3%), anxiety (adults 3%), attention disturbance (children 3%), hyperactivity (children 3%), vertigo (adults 3%)

Dermatologic: Rash (children 4%), pruritus (children 3%)

Gastrointestinal: Appetite decreased (≥1% to 5%), abdominal pain (3%), constipation (adults 3%), dyspepsia (adults 3%), appetite increased (≥1%)

Hematologic: Leukopenia (≤4%), anemia (≥1%)

Neuromuscular & skeletal: Tremor (adults 6%), back pain (adults 3%), gait disturbance (1% to 3%)

Ocular: Diplopia (4% to 9%), blurred vision (adults 6%), nystagmus (adults 6%)

Otic: Otitis media (children 3%)

Renal: Pollakiuria (≥1%)

Respiratory: Nasopharyngitis (≥5%), bronchitis (children 3%), sinusitis (children 3%)

Miscellaneous: Influenza (children 5%)

<1% (Limited to important or life-threatening): Atrioventricular block (first degree), bundle branch block (right), dysuria, enuresis, hematuria, incontinence, iron-deficiency anemia, lymphadenopathy, nephrolithiasis, neutropenia, nocturia, polyuria, thrombocytopenia, urinary incontinence

In addition, multiorgan hypersensitivity (including rash, urticaria, facial edema, fever, eosinophilia, stuporous state, severe hepatitis, LFTs increased) has been reported.

Ethanol/Nutrition/Herb Interactions

Ethanol: Avoid ethanol (may increase CNS depression).

Food: Food increases the absorption of rufinamide.

Herb/Nutraceutical: Avoid evening primrose (seizure threshold decreased).

Stability Store at 25°C (77°F); excursions permitted to 15°C to 30°C (59°F to 86°F). Protect from moisture.

Mechanism of Action A triazole-derivative antiepileptic whose exact mechanism is unknown. *In vitro*, it prolongs the inactive state of the sodium channels, thereby limiting repetitive firing of sodium-dependent action potentials mediating anticonvulsant effects.

Pharmacodynamics/Kinetics

Absorption: Slow; extensive ≥85%; increased with food

Distribution: V_d: ~50 L

Protein binding: 34%, primarily to albumin

Metabolism: Extensively via carboxylesterase-mediated hydrolysis of the carboxylamide group to CGP 47292 (inactive metabolite); weak inhibitor of CYP2E1 and weak inducer of CYP3A4

Bioavailability: Extent decreased with increased dose

Half-life elimination: ~6-10 hours

Time to peak, plasma: 4-6 hours

Excretion: Urine (85%, ~66% as CGP 47292, <2% as unchanged drug)

Dosage Oral: Lennox-Gastaut (adjunctive):

Children ≥4 years: Initial: 10 mg/kg/day in 2 equally divided doses; increase dose by ~10 mg/kg/day every other day to a target dose of 45 mg/kg/day or 3200 mg/day (whichever is lower) in 2 equally divided doses

Adults: Initial: 400-800 mg/day in 2 equally divided doses; increase dose by 400-800 mg/day every 2 days until maximum daily dose: 3200 mg/day in 2 equally divided doses

Dosage adjustment in renal impairment: Cl_{cr} <30 mL/minute: No dosage adjustment needed

Hemodialysis: No specific guidelines available; consider dosage adjustment for loss of drug

Dosage adjustment in hepatic impairment:

Mild-to-moderate impairment: Use caution

Severe impairment: Use in severe impairment has not been studied and is not recommended

Dietary Considerations Take with food.

Administration Administer with food. Tablets may be split in half or crushed.

Monitoring Parameters Seizure (frequency and duration); serum levels of concurrent anticonvulsants

Dosage Forms Excipient information presented when available (limited, particularly for generics); consult specific product labeling.

Tablet:

Banzel™: 200 mg, 400 mg

- **Ru-Hist Forte** *see* Chlorpheniramine, Pyrilamine, and Phenylephrine *on page 335*
- **Ru-Tuss DM** *see* Guaifenesin, Pseudoephedrine, and Dextromethorphan *on page 748*
- **Rutuss Jr** *see* Guaifenesin and Pseudoephedrine *on page 744*
- **Ryna®-12** *see* Phenylephrine and Pyrilamine *on page 1275*
- **Ryna-12 S®** *see* Phenylephrine and Pyrilamine *on page 1275*
- **Ryna-12X®** *see* Phenylephrine, Pyrilamine, and Guaifenesin *on page 1279*
- **Rynatan®** *see* Chlorpheniramine and Phenylephrine *on page 323*
- **Rynatan® Pediatric** *see* Chlorpheniramine and Phenylephrine *on page 323*
- **Rynatuss®** *see* Chlorpheniramine, Ephedrine, Phenylephrine, and Carbetapentane *on page 326*
- **Rynesa 12S** *see* Phenylephrine and Pyrilamine *on page 1275*
- **Ry-T-12** *see* Phenylephrine and Pyrilamine *on page 1275*
- **Rythmol®** *see* Propafenone *on page 1351*
- **Rythmol® SR** *see* Propafenone *on page 1351*
- **S2® [OTC]** *see* EPINEPHrine *on page 543*
- **S-(+)-3-isobutylgaba** *see* Pregabalin *on page 1332*
- **6(S)-5-methyltetrahydrofolate** *see* Methylfolate *on page 1022*
- **6(S)-5-MTHF** *see* Methylfolate *on page 1022*
- **S-4661** *see* Doripenem *on page 498*
- **S-adenosylmethionine** *see* SAMe (S-adenosyl methionine) *on page 1460*
- **Safe Tussin® DM [OTC]** *see* Guaifenesin and Dextromethorphan *on page 739*
- **SAHA** *see* Vorinostat *on page 1678*
- **Saizen®** *see* Somatropin *on page 1499*
- **SalAc® [OTC]** *see* Salicylic Acid *on page 1454*
- **Sal-Acid® [OTC]** *see* Salicylic Acid *on page 1454*
- **Salactic® [OTC]** *see* Salicylic Acid *on page 1454*
- **Salagen®** *see* Pilocarpine *on page 1290*
- **Salbutamol** *see* Albuterol *on page 54*
- **Salbutamol and Ipratropium** *see* Ipratropium and Albuterol *on page 854*
- **Salbutamol Sulphate** *see* Albuterol *on page 54*
- **Salex®** *see* Salicylic Acid *on page 1454*
- **Salicylazosulfapyridine** *see* Sulfasalazine *on page 1522*

Salicylic Acid (sal i SIL ik AS id)

Medication Safety Issues

Sound-alike/look-alike issues:

Occlusal®-HP may be confused with Ocuflox®

Transdermal patch may contain conducting metal (eg, aluminum); remove patch prior to MRI.

U.S. Brand Names Akurza; Aliclen™; Beta Sal® [OTC]; Compound W® One-Step Wart Remover for Feet [OTC]; Compound W® One-Step Wart Remover for Kids [OTC]; Compound W® One-Step Wart Remover [OTC]; Compound W® [OTC]; Dermarest® Psoriasis Medicated Moisturizer [OTC]; Dermarest® Psoriasis Medicated Scalp Treatment [OTC]; Dermarest® Psoriasis Medicated Shampoo/Conditioner [OTC]; Dermarest® Psoriasis Medicated Skin Treatment [OTC]; Dermarest® Psoriasis Overnight Treatment [OTC]; Dermarest® Psoriasis Scalp Treatment Mousse [OTC] [DSC]; DHS™ Sal [OTC]; Freezone® [OTC]; Fung-O® [OTC]; Gordofilm® [OTC]; Hydrisalic™ [OTC]; Ionil Plus® [OTC]; Ionil® [OTC]; Keralyt® [OTC]; LupiCare® Dandruff [OTC]; LupiCare® Psoriasis Scalp [OTC] [DSC]; LupiCare® Psoriasis [OTC]; Mosco® Callus & Corn Remover [OTC]; Neutrogena® Advanced Solutions™ [OTC]; Neutrogena® Blackhead Eliminating™ 2-in-1 Foaming Pads [OTC]; Neutrogena® Blackhead Eliminating™ Astringent [OTC] [DSC]; Neutrogena® Blackhead Eliminating™ Daily Scrub [OTC]; Neutrogena® Blackhead Eliminating™ Treatment Mask [OTC] [DSC]; Neutrogena® Body Clear® [OTC]; Neutrogena® Clear Pore™ Oil-Controlling Astringent [OTC]; Neutrogena® Oil-Free Acne Wash 60 Second Mask Scrub [OTC]; Neutrogena® Oil-Free Acne Wash Cream Cleanser [OTC]; Neutrogena® Oil-Free Acne Wash Foam Cleanser [OTC]; Neutrogena® Oil-Free Acne Wash [OTC]; Neutrogena® Rapid Clear® Acne Defense [OTC]; Neutrogena® Rapid Clear® Acne Eliminating [OTC]; Occlusal®-HP [OTC]; Off-Ezy® Wart Remover [OTC] [DSC]; P&S® [OTC]; Palmer's® Skin Success Acne Cleanser [OTC]; Sal-Acid® [OTC]; Sal-Plant® [OTC]; Salactic® [OTC]; SalAc® [OTC]; Salex®; Salex™ [DSC]; Salitop™; Stridex® Essential Care® [OTC]; Stridex® Facewipes To Go® [OTC]; Stridex® Maximum Strength [OTC]; Stridex® Sensitive Skin [OTC]; Tinamed® Corn and Callus Remover [OTC]; Tinamed® Wart Remover [OTC]; Trans-Ver-Sal® [OTC]; Wart-Off® Maximum Strength [OTC]

Canadian Brand Names Duofilm®; Duoforte® 27; Occlusal™-HP; Sebcur®; Soluver®; Soluver® Plus; Trans-Plantar®; Trans-Ver-Sal®

Pharmacologic Category Acne Products; Keratolytic Agent; Topical Skin Product, Acne

Use Topically for its keratolytic effect in controlling seborrheic dermatitis or psoriasis of body and scalp, dandruff, and other scaling dermatoses; also used to remove warts, corns, and calluses; acne

Effect on Mental Status May cause confusion

Effect on Psychiatric Treatment None reported

Dosage Summary

Topical:

Children <12 years: Consult specific product labeling

Children ≥12 years: Apply 1-4 times/day as directed; Consult specific product labeling

Adults: Apply 1-4 times/day as directed; Consult specific product labeling

Dosage Forms Excipient information presented when available (limited, particularly for generics); consult specific product labeling. [DSC] = Discontinued product

Aerosol, topical [foam]:

Dermarest® Psoriasis Scalp Treatment Mousse: 3% (90 mL) [DSC]

Bar, topical [soap]: 2%

Cloth, topical:

Neutrogena® Oil-Free Acne Wash: 2% (30s)

Cream, topical: 6% (400 g)

Akurza: 6% (340 g)

LupiCare® Psoriasis Scalp: 2% (113 g, 227 g) [DSC]

LupiCare™ Psoriasis: 2% (56 g [DSC]; 227 g)

Neutrogena® Oil-Free Acne Wash Cream Cleanser: 2% (200 mL) [contains ethanol]

Salex®: 6% (400 g [DSC]; 454 g)

Salex™: 6% (400 g) [DSC]

Salitop™: 6% (400 g) [contains ethanol]

Gel, topical:

Compound W®: 17.6% (7 g) [contains ethanol 67.5%]

Dermarest® Psoriasis Medicated Scalp Treatment: 3% (118 mL)

Dermarest® Psoriasis Medicated Skin Treatment: 3% (118 mL)

Dermarest® Psoriasis Overnight Treatment: 3% (56.7 g)

Hydrisalic®: 6% (28 g) [contains ethanol]

Keralyt®: 3% (30 g); 6% (40 g) [contains ethanol 21%]

Neutrogena® Oil-Free Acne Wash: 2% (177 mL) [contains tartrazine]

Neutrogena® Rapid Clear® Acne Eliminating: 2% (15 mL) [contains ethanol 38%]

Sal-Plant®: 17% (14 g) [contains isopropyl alcohol]

Gel, topical [mask]:
Neutrogena® Blackhead Eliminating™ Treatment Mask: 0.5% (56 g) [DSC]
Gel, topical [peel]:
Neutrogena® Advanced Solutions™: 2% (40 g)
Liquid, topical: 17% (14.8 mL)
Compound W®: 17.6% (9 mL) [contains ethanol 21.2%]
Freezone®: 17.6% (9.3 mL) [contains ethanol]
Fung-O®: 17% (15 mL) [contains ethanol 2%]
Gordofilm: 16.7% (15 mL)
Mosco® Callus & Corn Remover: 17.6% (9 mL) [contains ethanol 27%]
Neutrogena® Blackhead Eliminating™ Astringent: 0.5% (250 mL) [contains ethanol 35%] [DSC]
Neutrogena® Blackhead Eliminating™ Daily Scrub: 2% (125 mL)
Neutrogena® Clear Pore™ Oil-Controlling Astringent: 2% (236 mL) [contains ethanol 45%]
Occlusal®-HP: 17% (10 mL)
Off-Ezy® Wart Remover: 17% (13.3 mL) [DSC]
Palmer's® Skin Success Acne Cleanser: 0.5% (240 mL) [contains aloe, vitamin E]
Salactic®: 17% (15 mL) [contains isopropyl alcohol]
Tinamed® Corn and Callus Remover: 17% (15 mL)
Tinamed® Wart Remover: 17% (15 mL)
Wart-Off® Maximum Strength: 17% (13 mL) [contains ethanol]
Liquid, topical [body scrub with microbeads]:
Neutrogena® Body Clear®: 2% (250 mL) [contains tartrazine]
Liquid, topical [body wash]:
Neutrogena® Body Clear®: 2% (250 mL) [contains tartrazine]
Liquid, topical [cleanser]:
SalAc®: 2% (177 mL) [contains benzyl alcohol]
Liquid, topical [foam]:
Neutrogena® Oil-Free Acne Wash Foam Cleanser: 2% (150 mL)
Liquid, topical [mask/wash]:
Neutrogena® Oil-Free Acne Wash 60 Second Mask Scrub: 1% (170 g) [ethanol free]
Lotion, topical: 6% (414 mL, 420 mL)
Akurza: 6% (355 mL)
Dermarest® Psoriasis Medicated Moisturizer: 2% (118 mL)
Neutrogena® Rapid Clear® Acne Defense: 2% (50 mL) [contains ethanol]
Salex®: 6% (237 mL; 414 mL [DSC])
Salex™: 6% (414 mL) [DSC]
Salitop™: 6% (414 mL) [contains ethanol]
Pad, topical:
Neutrogena® Blackhead Eliminating™ 2-in-1 Foaming Pads: 0.5% (28s)
Stridex® Essential Care®: 1% (55s) [ethanol free; contains vitamin A, vitamin E]
Stridex® Facewipes To Go™: 0.5% (32s) [contains aloe, ethanol 28%]
Stridex® Maximum Strength: 2% (55s, 90s) [ethanol free]
Stridex® Sensitive Skin: 0.5% (55s, 90s) [ethanol free]
Patch, topical:
Compound W® One-Step Wart Remover for Feet: 40% (20s)
Compound W® One-Step Wart Remover: 40% (14s)
Compound W® One-Step Wart Remover for Kids: 40% (12s)
Trans-Ver-Sal®: 15% (10s, 25s) [20 mm PlantarPatch]
Trans-Ver-Sal®: 15% (15s, 40s) [contains propylene glycol]
Trans-Ver-Sal®: 15% (12s, 40s) [contains propylene glycol; 12 mm AdultPatch]
Plaster, topical:
Sal-Acid®: 40% (14s) [applied as plaster-impregnated bandages]
Shampoo, topical: 6% (177 mL)
Aliclen™, Salex®: 6% (177 mL)
Beta Sal®: 3% (480 mL)
DHS™ Sal: 3% (120 mL)
Ionil Plus®: 2% (240 mL) [conditioning shampoo]
Ionil®: 2% (120 mL; 240 mL, 480 mL, 960 mL [DSC])
LupiCare® Dandruff: 2% (237 mL)
LupiCare® Psoriasis: 2% (118 mL [DSC]; 237 mL)
P&S®: 2% (118 mL, 236 mL)
Shampoo/conditioner, topical:
Dermarest® Psoriasis Medicated Shampoo/Conditioner: 3% (236 mL)

◆ **Salicylsalicylic Acid** *see* Salsalate *on page 1459*

◆ **Salitop™** *see* Salicylic Acid *on page 1454*

Salmeterol (sal ME te role)

Medication Safety Issues

Sound-alike/look-alike issues:

Salmeterol may be confused with Salbutamol

Serevent® may be confused with Serentil®

U.S. Brand Names Serevent® Diskus®

Canadian Brand Names Serevent® Diskhaler® Disk; Serevent® Diskus®

Mexican Brand Names Serevent

Index Terms Salmeterol Xinafoate

Pharmacologic Category Beta2-Adrenergic Agonist, Long-Acting; Beta$_2$-Adrenergic Agonist

Generic Available No

Use Maintenance treatment of asthma; prevention of bronchospasm with reversible obstructive airway disease, including patients with symptoms of nocturnal asthma; prevention of exercise-induced bronchospasm; maintenance treatment of bronchospasm associated with COPD

Effect on Mental Status May cause nervousness, dizziness, hyperactivity, or insomnia

Effect on Psychiatric Treatment Salmeterol is a sympathomimetic; use MAO inhibitors and TCAs with caution

Restrictions An FDA-approved medication guide must be distributed when dispensing an outpatient prescription (new or refill) where this medication is to be used without direct supervision of a healthcare provider. Medication guides are available at http://www.fda.gov/cder/Offices/ODS/medication_guides.htm.

Pregnancy Risk Factor C

Pregnancy Considerations Animal studies have demonstrated (dose-dependent) teratogenicity. There are no adequate and well-controlled studies in pregnant women. Beta-agonists may interfere with uterine contractility if administered during labor. Use only if clearly needed.

Lactation Enters breast milk/use caution

Contraindications Hypersensitivity to salmeterol or any component of the formulation

Warnings/Precautions

Asthma treatment: [U.S. Boxed Warning]: Long-acting beta$_2$-agonists may increase the risk of asthma-related deaths. In a large, randomized clinical trial (SMART, 2006), salmeterol was associated with an increase in asthma-related deaths (when added to usual asthma therapy); risk may be greater in African-American patients versus Caucasians. Should only be used as adjuvant therapy in patients not adequately controlled on inhaled corticosteroids or whose disease requires two maintenance therapies. Do **not** use for acute asthmatic symptoms. Short-acting beta$_2$-agonist (eg, albuterol) should be used for acute symptoms and symptoms occurring between treatments. Do **not** initiate in patients with significantly worsening or acutely deteriorating asthma; reports of severe (sometimes fatal) respiratory events have been reported when salmeterol has been initiated in this situation. Salmeterol is not a substitute for inhaled or oral corticosteroids. Corticosteroids should not be stopped or reduced when salmeterol is initiated. During the initiation of salmeterol watch for signs of worsening asthma. Patients must be instructed to use short-acting beta$_2$-agonists (eg, albuterol) for acute asthmatic or COPD symptoms and to seek medical attention in cases where acute symptoms are not relieved or a previous level of response is diminished. The need to increase frequency of use of short-acting beta$_2$-agonist may indicate deterioration of asthma, and treatment must not be delayed. Salmeterol should not be used more than twice daily; do not use with other long-acting beta$_2$-agonists.

Concurrent diseases: Use caution in patients with cardiovascular disease (eg, arrhythmia, hypertension, or HF), seizure disorders, diabetes, glaucoma, hyperthyroidism, hepatic impairment, or hypokalemia. Beta-agonists may cause elevation in blood pressure, heart rate, CNS stimulation/excitation, increased risk of arrhythmia, increase serum glucose, or decrease serum potassium.

Adverse events: Immediate hypersensitivity reactions (urticaria, angioedema, rash, bronchospasm) have been reported. There have been reports of laryngeal spasm, irritation, swelling (stridor, choking) with use. Salmeterol should not be used more than twice daily; do not exceed recommended dose; do not use with other long-acting beta$_2$-agonists; serious adverse events have been associated with excessive use of inhaled sympathomimetics. Rarely, paradoxical bronchospasm may occur with use of inhaled bronchodilating agents; this should be distinguished from inadequate response. Powder for oral inhalation contains lactose; very rare anaphylactic reactions have been reported in patients with severe milk protein allergy.

Safety and efficacy have not been established in children <4 years of age.

Adverse Reactions

>10%:

Central nervous system: Headache (13% to 17%)

Neuromuscular & skeletal: Pain (1% to 12%)

1% to 10%:

Cardiovascular: Hypertension (4%), edema (1% to 3%), pallor

Central nervous system: Dizziness (4%), sleep disturbance (1% to 3%), fever (1% to 3%), anxiety (1% to 3%), migraine (1% to 3%)

Dermatologic: Rash (1% to 4%), contact dermatitis (1% to 3%), eczema (1% to 3%), urticaria (3%), photodermatitis (1% to 2%)

Endocrine & metabolic: Hyperglycemia (1% to 3%)

Gastrointestinal: Throat irritation (7%), nausea (1% to 3%), dyspepsia (1% to 3%), dental pain (1% to 3%), gastrointestinal infection (1% to 3%), oropharyngeal candidiasis (1% to 3%), xerostomia (1% to 3%)

Neuromuscular & skeletal: Muscular cramps/spasm (3%), articular rheumatism (1% to 3%), arthralgia (1% to 3%), joint pain (1% to 3%), muscular stiffness (1% to 3%), paresthesia (1% to 3%), rigidity (1% to 3%)

Ocular: Keratitis/conjunctivitis (1% to 3%)

Respiratory: Nasal congestion (4% to 9%), tracheitis/bronchitis (7%), pharyngitis (≤6%), cough (5%), influenza (5%), viral respiratory tract infection (5%), sinusitis (4% to 5%), rhinitis (4% to 5%), asthma (3% to 4%)

<1% (Limited to important or life-threatening): Abdominal pain, agitation, aggression, anaphylactic reaction (Diskus®: severe milk allergy), angioedema, aphonia, arrhythmia, atrial fibrillation, bronchospasm and immediate bronchospasm, cataracts, chest congestion, chest tightness, choking, contusions, Cushing syndrome, Cushingoid features, depression, dysmenorrhea, dyspnea, earache, ecchymoses, edema (facial, oropharyngeal), eosinophilic conditions, glaucoma, growth velocity reduction in children/adolescents, hypercorticism, hypersensitivity reaction (immediate and delayed), hypokalemia, hypothyroidism, intraocular pressure increased, laryngeal spasm/irritation, irregular menstruation, myositis, osteoporosis, pallor, paradoxical tracheitis, paranasal sinus pain, PID, restlessness, stridor, supraventricular tachycardia, syncope, tremor, vaginal candidiasis, vaginitis, vulvovaginitis, rare cases of vasculitis (Churg-Strauss syndrome), ventricular tachycardia, weight gain

Metabolism/Transport Effects Substrate of CYP3A4 (major)

Drug Interactions

Alpha-/Beta-Blockers: May diminish the therapeutic effect of Beta2-Agonists. *Risk D: Consider therapy modification*

Atomoxetine: May enhance the tachycardic effect of Beta2-Agonists. *Risk C: Monitor therapy*

Beta-Blockers (Beta1 Selective): May diminish the bronchodilatory effect of Beta2-Agonists. Of particular concern with nonselective beta-blockers or higher doses of the beta1 selective beta-blockers. *Risk C: Monitor therapy*

Beta-Blockers (Nonselective): May diminish the bronchodilatory effect of Beta2-Agonists. *Risk D: Consider therapy modification*

Betahistine: May diminish the therapeutic effect of Beta2-Agonists. *Risk C: Monitor therapy*

Cannabinoids: May enhance the tachycardic effect of Sympathomimetics. *Risk C: Monitor therapy*

CYP3A4 Inhibitors (Moderate): May increase the serum concentration of Salmeterol. *Risk C: Monitor therapy*

CYP3A4 Inhibitors (Strong): May increase the serum concentration of Salmeterol. *Risk X: Avoid combination*

MAO Inhibitors: May enhance the adverse/toxic effect of Beta2-Agonists. *Risk C: Monitor therapy*

Sympathomimetics: May enhance the adverse/toxic effect of other Sympathomimetics. *Risk C: Monitor therapy*

Tricyclic Antidepressants: May enhance the adverse/toxic effect of Beta2-Agonists. *Risk C: Monitor therapy*

Stability Inhalation powder: Store at controlled room temperature 20°C to 25°C (68°F to 77°F) in a dry place away from direct heat or sunlight. Stable for 6 weeks after removal from foil pouch.

Mechanism of Action Relaxes bronchial smooth muscle by selective action on $beta_2$-receptors with little effect on heart rate; salmeterol acts locally in the lung.

Pharmacodynamics/Kinetics

Onset of action: Asthma: 30-48 minutes, COPD: 2 hours

Peak effect: Asthma: 3 hours, COPD: 2-5 hours

Duration: 12 hours
Absorption: Systemic: Inhalation: Undetectable to poor
Protein binding: 96%
Metabolism: Hepatic; hydroxylated via CYP3A4
Half-life elimination: 5.5 hours
Time to peak, serum: ~20 minutes
Excretion: Feces (60%), urine (25%)

Dosage Inhalation, powder (50 mcg/inhalation):
Asthma, maintenance and prevention: Children ≥4 years and Adults: One inhalation twice daily (~12 hours apart); maximum: 1 inhalation twice daily
Exercise-induced asthma, prevention: Children ≥4 years and Adults: One inhalation at least 30 minutes prior to exercise; additional doses should not be used for 12 hours; should not be used in individuals already receiving salmeterol twice daily
COPD maintenance: Adults: One inhalation twice daily (~12 hours apart); maximum: 1 inhalation twice daily
Dosage adjustment in hepatic impairment: No dosage adjustment required; manufacturer suggests close monitoring of patients with hepatic impairment.

Dietary Considerations Powder for oral inhalation contains lactose; very rare anaphylactic reactions have been reported in patients with severe milk protein allergy.

Administration Inhalation: **Not** to be used for the relief of acute attacks. Not for use with a spacer device. Administer with Diskus® in a level, horizontal position. Do not wash mouthpiece; Diskus® should be kept dry.

Monitoring Parameters FEV_1, peak flow, and/or other pulmonary function tests; blood pressure, heart rate; CNS stimulation. Monitor for increased use of short-acting $beta_2$-agonist inhalers; may be marker of a deteriorating asthma condition.

Dosage Forms Excipient information presented when available (limited, particularly for generics); consult specific product labeling. [CAN] = Canadian brand name
Powder for oral inhalation:
Serevent® Diskus®: Salmeterol xinafoate 50 mcg (28s, 60s) [delivers 50 mcg/inhalation; contains lactose]
Serevent® Diskhaler® Disk [CAN]: Salmeterol xinafoate 50 mcg (60s) [delivers 50 mcg/inhalation; contains lactose] [not available in U.S]

◆ **Salmeterol and Fluticasone** *see* Fluticasone and Salmeterol *on page 674*
◆ **Salmeterol Xinafoate** *see* Salmeterol *on page 1457*
◆ **Sal-Plant® [OTC]** *see* Salicylic Acid *on page 1454*

Salsalate (SAL sa late)

Medication Safety Issues
Sound-alike/look-alike issues:
Salsalate may be confused with sucralfate, sulfasalazine

Related Information
Nonsteroidal Anti-Inflammatory Agents *on page 1792*

U.S. Brand Names Amigesic® [DSC]

Canadian Brand Names Amigesic®; Salflex®

Index Terms Disalicylic Acid; Salicylsalicylic Acid

Pharmacologic Category Salicylate

Use Treatment of minor pain or fever; arthritis

Effect on Mental Status May cause drowsiness; may rarely cause nervousness or insomnia

Effect on Psychiatric Treatment May rarely cause leukopenia; use caution with clozapine and carbamazepine

Dosage Summary
Oral:
Children: Dosage not established
Adults: 3 g/day in 2-3 divided doses

Dosage Forms Excipient information presented when available (limited, particularly for generics); consult specific product labeling. [DSC] = Discontinued product
Tablet: 500 mg, 750 mg
Amigesic®: 500 mg [DSC], 750 mg [DSC]

◆ **Sal-Tropine™** *see* Atropine *on page 158*

SAMe (S-adenosyl methionine)

Natural Product Category Nutraceutical

Synonyms AdoMet; S-adenosylmethionine

Dosage

Oral: 400-1600 mg/day

I.V.: 150-1600 mg/day

Active Forms S-adenosyl methionine

Reported Uses

Attention-deficit hyperactivity disorder (ADHD) (Shekim, 1990)

Cardiovascular disease (Loehrer, 1996)

Cholestasis (Frezza, 1984; Frezza, 1987; Frezza, 1990; Lafuenti, 1988; Qin, 2000)

Depression (Bressa, 1994; Fava, 1995; Kagan, 1990; Rosenbaum, 1990)

Fibromyalgia (Jacobsen, 1991)

Headache (pharmacologic activity)

Insomnia (Sitaram, 1995)

Liver disease (Miglio, 1975)

Osteoarthritis (di Padova, 1987)

Rheumatoid arthritis (Polli, 1975)

Summary S-adenosyl methionine (SAMe) is formed from the essential amino acid methionine. It is a cofactor in three important biochemical pathways, and is synthesized throughout the body. Due to the nature and scope of biochemical reactions that it regulates, SAMe has been investigated for its effects in depression, fibromyalgia, arthritis, and cardiovascular disease.

Effect on Mental Status May cause mania, hypomania, anxiety, and restlessness

Effect on Psychiatric Treatment Not recommended for patients with bipolar disorder; may potentiate antidepressants (combined use is discouraged)

Pharmacology SAMe is involved in several primary biochemical pathways. It functions as a methyl donor in synthetic pathways which form nucleic acids (DNA and RNA), proteins, phospholipids, and neurotransmitters. The role of SAMe in phospholipid synthesis may influence membrane fluidity. It has also been noted to protect neuronal anoxia and promote myelination of nerve fibers. It is involved in trans-sulfuration reactions, regulating formation of sulfur-containing amino acids such as cysteine, glutathione, and taurine. Of note, glutathione is an important antioxidant, involved in the detoxification of a number of physiologic and environmental toxins. SAMe is also a cofactor in the synthesis of polyamines, which include spermidine, puescine, and spermine. Polyamines are essential for cellular growth and differentiation by virtue of their effects on gene expression, protein phosphorylation, neuron regeneration, and the DNA repair.

Warnings and Interactions Minor side effects, including dry mouth, nausea, and restlessness, are occasionally reported. Use caution when combining SAMe with other antidepressants, tryptophan, or 5-HTP. SAMe is not effective for the depressive symptoms associated with bipolar disorder.

SAMe has been reported to block platelet aggregation *in vitro* (De la Cruz, 1997; De la Cruz, 1997); contraindicated in individuals with active bleeding (eg, peptic ulcer, intracranial bleeding). Use with caution in individuals with a history of bleeding, hemostatic disorders, or drug-related hemostatic problems and in individuals taking anticoagulant medications, including warfarin, aspirin, aspirin-containing products, NSAIDs, or antiplatelet agents (eg, ticlopidine, clopidogrel, dipyridamole). Discontinue use prior to dental or surgical procedures (generally at least 14 days before).

Symptoms of Deficiency A specific deficiency syndrome has not been adequately defined. As an essential cofactor in multiple biochemical pathways, a wide variety of symptoms are potentially related to a deficiency in SAMe.

Reported Interactions

Drug/Nutrient Interactions: May potentiate activity and/or toxicities of MAO inhibitors, tricyclic antidepressants, or SSRIs (not documented); intravenous SAMe may cause additive effects with oral hypoglycemics; may have a synergistic effect with ursodeoxycholic acid

Nutrient/Nutrient Interactions: May potentiate the antidepressant effects of 5-HTP, tryptophan, and St John's wort

References

Binder T, Salaj P, Zima T, et al, "Randomized Prospective Comparative Study of Ursodeoxycholic Acid and S-Adenosyl-L-Methionine in the Treatment of Intrahepatic Cholestasis of Pregnancy," *J Perinat Med*, 2006, 34(5):383-91.

Bressa GM, "S-Adenosyl-L-Methionine (SAMe) as Antidepressant: Meta-Analysis of Clinical Studies," *Acta Neurol Scand*, Suppl 1994, 154:7-14.

De la Cruz JP, Gonzalez-Correa JA, Martin-Aurioles E, et al, "Effects of S-Adenosyl-L-Methionine on Platelet Thromboxane and Vascular Prostacyclin," *Biochem Pharmacol*, 1997, 53(11):1761-3.

De la Cruz JP, Merida M, Gonzalez-Correa JA, et al, "Effects of S-Adenosyl-L-Methionine on Blood Platelet Activation," *Gen Pharmacol*, 1997, 29(4):651-5.

di Padova C, "S-Adenosylmethionine in the Treatment of Osteoarthritis. Review of the Clinical Studies," *Am J Med*, 1987, 83(5A):60-5.

Fava M, Giannelli A, Rapisarda V, et al, "Rapidity of Onset of the Antidepressant Effect of Parenteral S-Adenosyl-L-Methionine," *Psychiatry Res*, 1995, 56(3):295-7.

Frezza M, Centini G, Cammareri G, et al, "S-Adenosylmethionine for the Treatment of Intrahepatic Cholestasis of Pregnancy. Results of a Controlled Clinical Trial," *Hepatogastroenterology*, 1990, 37(2 Suppl):122-5.

Frezza M, Di Padova C, and Italian Study Group for SAMe, "Multicenter Placebo Controlled Clinical Trial of Intravenous and Oral S-Adenosyl-L-Methionine (SAMe) in Cholestatic Patients With Liver Disease," *Hepatology*, 1987, 7(5):1105.

Frezza M, Pozzato G, Chiesa L, el al, "Reversal of Intrahepatic Cholestasis of Pregnancy in Women After High Dose S-Adenosyl-L-Methionine Administration," *Hepatology*, 1984, 4 (2):274-8.

Jacobsen S, Danneskiold-Samsoe B, and Anderson BB, "Oral S-Adenosylmethionine in Primary Fibromyalgia. Double-Blind Clinical Evaluation," *Scand J Rheumatol*, 1991, 20 (4):294-302.

Kagan BL, Sultzer DL, Rosenlicht, et al, "Oral S-Adenosylmethionine in Depression: A Randomized, Double-Blind, Placebo-Controlled Trial," *Am J Psychiatry*, 1990, 147 (5):591-5.

Lafuenti G, Plotti G, Nicolanti G, et al, "Evaluation of the Obstetrical Risk in Pregnant Women With Intrahepatic Cholestasis Treated With S-Adenosyl-L-Methionine," *Recenti Prog Med*, 1988, 79(10):420-3.

Loehrer FM, Angst CP, Haefeli WE, et al, "Low Whole-Blood S-Adenosylmethionine and Correlation Between 5-Methyltetrahydrofolate and Homocysteine in Coronary Artery Disease," *Arterioscler Thromb Vasc Biol*, 1996, 16(6):727-33.

Miglio F, Stefanini GF, Corazza GR, et al, "Double-Blind Studies of the Therapeutic Action of S-Adenosylmethionine (SAMe) in Oral Administration, in Liver Cirrhosis and Other Chronic Hepatitides," *Minerva Med*, 1975, 66(33):1595-9.

Natural Standard Research Collaboration, Chief Editors: Ulbricht C, Basch E, *Natural Standard Herb and Supplement Reference - Evidence-Based Clinical Reviews*, USA: Elsevier/Mosby, 2005.

Polli E, Cortellareo M, Parrini L, et al, "Pharmacological and Clinical Aspects of S-Adenosylmethionine (SAMe) in Primary Degenerative Arthropathy," *Minerva Med*, 1975, 66(83):4443-59.

Qin B, Guo S, Zhao Y, et al, "A Trial of Ademetionine in the Treatment of Intrahepatic Biliary Stasis Viral Hepatitis," *Zhonghua Gan Zang Bing Za Zhi*, 2000, 8(3):158-60.

Rosenbaum JF, Fava M, Falk WE, et al, "The Antidepressant Potential of Oral S-Adenosyl-L-Methionine," *Acta Psychiatr Scand*, 1990, 81(5):432-6.

Shekim WO, Antun F, Hanna GL, et al, "S-Adenosyl-L-Methionine (SAM) in Adults With ADHD, RS: Preliminary Results From an Open Trial," *Psychopharmacol Bull*, 1990, 26 (2):249-53.

Sitaram BR, Sitaram M, Traut M, et al, "Nyctohemeral Rhythm in the Levels of S-Adenosylmethionine in the Rat Pineal Gland and Its Relationship to Melatonin Biosynthesis," *J Neurochem*, 1995, 65(4):1887-94.

◆ **Sanctura®** *see* Trospium *on page 1636*

◆ **Sanctura® XR** *see* Trospium *on page 1636*

◆ **Sancuso®** *see* Granisetron *on page 736*

◆ **Sandimmune®** *see* CycloSPORINE *on page 409*

◆ **Sandostatin®** *see* Octreotide *on page 1158*

◆ **Sandostatin LAR®** *see* Octreotide *on page 1158*

Saquinavir (sa KWIN a veer)

Medication Safety Issues

Sound-alike/look-alike issues:

Saquinavir may be confused with Sinequan®

U.S. Brand Names Invirase®

Canadian Brand Names Invirase®

Mexican Brand Names Fortovase

Index Terms Saquinavir Mesylate

Pharmacologic Category Antiretroviral Agent, Protease Inhibitor

Use Treatment of HIV infection; used in combination with at least two other antiretroviral agents

Effect on Mental Status May rarely cause confusion or ataxia; report of acute paranoia reaction to saquinavir

Effect on Psychiatric Treatment Contraindicated with triazolam and midazolam; barbiturates and carbamazepine may increase the metabolism of saquinavir. Concomitant use of saquinavir and St John's wort is not recommended. Coadministration of protease inhibitors (saquinavir) with St John's wort is expected to substantially decrease protease inhibitor serum concentrations leading to a loss of virologic response and possible resistance to saquinavir or to the class of protease inhibitors.

Dosage Summary

Oral:

Children ≤16 years: Dosage not established

Children >16 years: 1000 mg (with ritonavir 100 mg) twice daily; **Note:** Saquinavir (Invirase®) should not be used in "unboosted regimens."

Adults: 1000 mg (with ritonavir 100 mg) twice daily; **Note:** Saquinavir (Invirase®) should not be used in "unboosted regimens."

Dosage Forms Excipient information presented when available (limited, particularly for generics); consult specific product labeling.

Capsule:

Invirase®: 200 mg [contains lactose 63.3 mg/capsule]

Tablet:

Invirase®: 500 mg

◆ **Saquinavir Mesylate** *see* Saquinavir *on page 1461*

◆ **Sarafem®** *see* FLUoxetine *on page 650*

Sargramostim (sar GRAM oh stim)

Medication Safety Issues

Sound-alike/look-alike issues:

Leukine® may be confused with Leukeran®, leucovorin

Related Information

Clozapine-Induced Side Effects *on page 1818*

U.S. Brand Names Leukine®

Canadian Brand Names Leukine®

Index Terms GM-CSF; Granulocyte-Macrophage Colony Stimulating Factor; NSC-613795; rhuGM-CSF

Pharmacologic Category Colony Stimulating Factor

Use

Acute myelogenous leukemia (AML) following induction chemotherapy in older adults (≥55 years of age) to shorten time to neutrophil recovery and to reduce the incidence of severe and life-threatening infections and infections resulting in death

Bone marrow transplant (allogeneic or autologous) failure or engraftment delay

Myeloid reconstitution after allogeneic bone marrow transplantation

Myeloid reconstitution after autologous bone marrow transplantation: Non-Hodgkin's lymphoma (NHL), acute lymphoblastic leukemia (ALL), Hodgkin's lymphoma

Peripheral stem cell transplantation: Mobilization and myeloid reconstitution following autologous peripheral stem cell transplantation

Effect on Mental Status May cause drowsiness

Effect on Psychiatric Treatment May be used to treat clozapine-induced agranulocytosis; lithium may potentiate the release of neutrophils; use with caution

Dosage Summary

I.V.:

Children: Infusion: 250 mcg/m^2/day (maximum: 500 mcg/m^2 /day)

Adults: Infusion: 250 mcg/m^2/day (maximum: 500 mcg/m^2/day)

SubQ:

Children: 250 mcg/m^2 once daily

Adults: 250 mcg/m^2 once daily

Dosage Forms Excipient information presented when available (limited, particularly for generics); consult specific product labeling.

Injection, powder for reconstitution:

Leukine®: 250 mcg [contains sucrose 10 mg/mL]

Injection, solution:

Leukine®: 500 mcg/mL (1 mL) [contains benzyl alcohol and sucrose 10 mg/mL]

◆ **Sarnol®-HC [OTC]** *see* Hydrocortisone *on page 785*

◆ **SB-265805** *see* Gemifloxacin *on page 712*

◆ **SC 33428** *see* IDArubicin *on page 809*

◆ **Scandonest® 3% Plain** *see* Mepivacaine *on page 990*

◆ **SCH 13521** *see* Flutamide *on page 667*

◆ **SCH 56592** *see* Posaconazole *on page 1314*

- **S-Citalopram** *see* Escitalopram *on page 564*
- **Scopace™** *see* Scopolamine Derivatives *on page 1463*
- **Scopolamine Base** *see* Scopolamine Derivatives *on page 1463*
- **Scopolamine Butylbromide** *see* Scopolamine Derivatives *on page 1463*

Scopolamine Derivatives (skoe POL a meen dah RIV ah tives)

Medication Safety Issues
Transdermal patch may contain conducting metal (eg, aluminum); remove patch prior to MRI.

U.S. Brand Names Isopto® Hyoscine; Scopace™; Transderm Scōp®

Canadian Brand Names Buscopan®; Transderm-V®

Index Terms Hyoscine Butylbromide; Hyoscine Hydrobromide; Scopolamine Base; Scopolamine Butylbromide; Scopolamine Hydrobromide

Pharmacologic Category Anticholinergic Agent

Use

Scopolamine base:

Transdermal: Prevention of nausea/vomiting associated with motion sickness and recovery from anesthesia and surgery

Scopolamine hydrobromide:

Injection: Preoperative medication to produce amnesia, sedation, tranquilization, antiemetic effects, and decrease salivary and respiratory secretions

Ophthalmic: Produce cycloplegia and mydriasis; treatment of iridocyclitis

Oral: Symptomatic treatment of postencephalitic parkinsonism and paralysis agitans; in spastic states; inhibits excessive motility and hypertonus of the gastrointestinal tract in such conditions as the irritable colon syndrome, mild dysentery, diverticulitis, pylorospasm, and cardiospasm

Scopolamine butylbromide [not available in the U.S.]:

Oral/injection: Treatment of smooth muscle spasm of the genitourinary or gastrointestinal tract; injection may also be used to prior to radiological/diagnostic procedures to prevent spasm

Effect on Mental Status May cause drowsiness; may rarely cause confusion or amnesia

Effect on Psychiatric Treatment May decrease the effects of levodopa; concurrent use with psychotropics may produce additive sedation of anticholinergic side effects (dry mouth)

Dosage Summary

I.M.:

Children <6 months: Dosage not established
Children 6 months to 3 years: 0.1-0.15 mg
Children 3-6 years: 0.2-0.3 mg
Adults: 0.3-0.65 mg (single dose) **or** 0.6 mg 3-4 times/day

I.V.:

Children <6 months: Dosage not established
Children 6 months to 3 years: 0.1-0.15 mg
Children 3-6 years: 0.2-0.3 mg
Adults: 0.3-0.65 mg (single dose) **or** 0.6 mg 3-4 times/day

Ophthalmic:

Children: Instill 1 drop (0.25%) to eye(s) up to 3 times/day
Adults: Instill 1-2 drops (0.25%) up to 4 times/day

Oral:

Children: Dosage not established
Adults: 0.4-0.8 mg as a single dose or every 8-12 hours as needed.

SubQ:

Children <6 months: Dosage not established
Children 6 months to 3 years: 0.1-0.15 mg
Children 3-6 years: 0.2-0.3 mg
Adults: 0.3-0.65 mg (single dose) **or** 0.6 mg 3-4 times/day

Transdermal:

Children: Dosage not established
Adults: Apply 1 patch behind ear at least 4 hours prior to exposure and every 3 days as needed

Dosage Forms Excipient information presented when available (limited, particularly for generics); consult specific product labeling. [CAN] = Canadian brand name

Injection, solution, as hydrobromide: 0.4 mg/mL (1 mL)

Injection, solution, as hyoscine-N-butylbromide:
Buscopan® [CAN]: 20 mg/mL [not available in U.S.]

Solution, ophthalmic, as hydrobromide:
Isopto® Hyoscine: 0.25% (5 mL) [contains benzalkonium chloride]
Tablet, as hyoscine-N-butylbromide:
Buscopan® [CAN]: 10 mg [not available in U.S.]
Tablet, soluble, as hydrobromide:
Scopace™: 0.4 mg
Transdermal system:
Transderm Scōp®: 1.5 mg (4s, 10s, 24s) [releases ~1 mg over 72 hours]

◆ **Scopolamine Hydrobromide** *see* Scopolamine Derivatives *on page 1463*
◆ **Scopolamine, Hyoscyamine, Atropine, and Phenobarbital** *see* Hyoscyamine, Atropine, Scopolamine, and Phenobarbital *on page 800*
◆ **Scot-Tussin DM® Cough Chasers [OTC] [DSC]** *see* Dextromethorphan *on page 448*
◆ **Scot-Tussin® DM Maximum Strength [OTC]** *see* Dextromethorphan and Chlorpheniramine *on page 449*
◆ **Scot-Tussin® Expectorant [OTC]** *see* GuaiFENesin *on page 737*
◆ **Scot-Tussin® Senior [OTC]** *see* Guaifenesin and Dextromethorphan *on page 739*
◆ **SD/01** *see* Pegfilgrastim *on page 1236*
◆ **SDX-105** *see* Bendamustine *on page 179*
◆ **SDZ ENA 713** *see* Rivastigmine *on page 1435*
◆ **Seasonale®** *see* Ethinyl Estradiol and Levonorgestrel *on page 595*
◆ **Seasonique™** *see* Ethinyl Estradiol and Levonorgestrel *on page 595*

Secobarbital (see koe BAR bi tal)

Medication Safety Issues
Sound-alike/look-alike issues:
Seconal® may be confused with Sectral®

U.S. Brand Names Seconal®

Index Terms Quinalbarbitone Sodium; Secobarbital Sodium

Pharmacologic Category Barbiturate

Generic Available No

Use Preanesthetic agent; short-term treatment of insomnia

Mental Health Comment In 2007, the FDA requested that all manufacturers of sedative-hypnotic drug products revise labeling to include a greater emphasis on the risks of adverse effects. These risks include severe allergic reactions (anaphylaxis, angioedema) and complex sleep-related behaviors, which may include sleep-driving (driving while not fully awake and with no memory of the event), making phone calls, and preparing and eating food while asleep.

Restrictions C-II

Pregnancy Risk Factor D

Lactation Enters breast milk/use caution (AAP rates "compatible")

Contraindications Hypersensitivity to barbiturates or any component of the formulation; marked hepatic impairment; dyspnea or airway obstruction; porphyria; pregnancy

Warnings/Precautions Should be used only after evaluation of potential causes of sleep disturbance. Failure of sleep disturbance to resolve after 7-10 days may indicate psychiatric or medical illness. Potential for drug dependency exists, abrupt cessation may precipitate withdrawal, including status epilepticus in epileptic patients. Do not administer to patients in acute pain. Use caution in elderly, debilitated, renally impaired, or pediatric patients. May cause paradoxical responses, including agitation and hyperactivity, particularly in acute pain and pediatric patients. Use with caution in patients with depression or suicidal tendencies, or in patients with a history of drug abuse. Tolerance, psychological and physical dependence may occur with prolonged use. Use with caution in patients with hepatic function impairment. May cause CNS depression, which may impair physical or mental abilities. Patients must cautioned about performing tasks which require mental alertness (eg, operating machinery or driving). Postmarketing studies have indicated that the use of hypnotic/sedative agents for sleep has been associated with hypersensitivity reactions including anaphylaxis as well as angioedema. An increased risk for hazardous sleep-related activities such as sleep-driving; cooking and eating food, and making phone calls while asleep have also been noted. Effects with other sedative drugs or ethanol may be potentiated. May cause respiratory depression or hypotension, Use with caution in patients with cardiovascular or respiratory disease.

Adverse Reactions Frequency not defined.

Cardiovascular: Hypotension

Central nervous system: Dizziness, lightheadedness, "hangover" effect, drowsiness, CNS depression, fever, confusion, mental depression, unusual excitement, nervousness, faint feeling, headache, insomnia, nightmares, hallucinations

Dermatologic: Exfoliative dermatitis, rash, Stevens-Johnson syndrome

Gastrointestinal: Nausea, vomiting, constipation

Hematologic: Agranulocytosis, megaloblastic anemia, thrombocytopenia, thrombophlebitis, urticaria

Local: Pain at injection site

Respiratory: Apnea, laryngospasm, respiratory depression

Postmarketing and/or case reports: Anaphylaxis, angioedema, complex sleep-related behavior (sleep-driving, cooking or eating food, making phone calls)

Metabolism/Transport Effects Induces CYP2A6 (strong), 2C8 (strong), 2C9 (strong)

Drug Interactions

Acetaminophen: Barbiturates may increase the metabolism of Acetaminophen. This may 1) diminish the effect of acetaminophen; and 2) increase the risk of liver damage. *Risk C: Monitor therapy*

Alcohol (Ethyl): CNS Depressants may enhance the CNS depressant effect of Alcohol (Ethyl). *Risk C: Monitor therapy*

Beta-Blockers: Barbiturates may decrease the serum concentration of Beta-Blockers. **Exceptions:** Atenolol; Levobunolol; Metipranolol; Nadolol. *Risk C: Monitor therapy*

Calcium Channel Blockers: Barbiturates may increase the metabolism of Calcium Channel Blockers. **Exceptions:** Clevidipine. *Risk D: Consider therapy modification*

Chloramphenicol: May decrease the metabolism of Barbiturates. Barbiturates may increase the metabolism of Chloramphenicol. *Risk D: Consider therapy modification*

CNS Depressants: May enhance the adverse/toxic effect of other CNS Depressants. *Risk C: Monitor therapy*

Contraceptive (Progestins): Barbiturates may diminish the therapeutic effect of Contraceptive (Progestins). Contraceptive failure is possible. *Risk D: Consider therapy modification*

Corticosteroids (Systemic): Barbiturates may increase the metabolism of Corticosteroids (Systemic). *Risk C: Monitor therapy*

CycloSPORINE: Barbiturates may increase the metabolism of CycloSPORINE. *Risk D: Consider therapy modification*

CYP2A6 Substrates: CYP2A6 Inducers (Strong) may increase the metabolism of CYP2A6 Substrates. *Risk C: Monitor therapy*

CYP2C8 Substrates (High risk): CYP2C8 Inducers (Highly Effective) may increase the metabolism of CYP2C8 Substrates (High risk). *Risk C: Monitor therapy*

CYP2C9 Substrates (High risk): CYP2C9 Inducers (Highly Effective) may increase the metabolism of CYP2C9 Substrates (High risk). *Risk C: Monitor therapy*

Disopyramide: Barbiturates may increase the metabolism of Disopyramide. *Risk D: Consider therapy modification*

Doxycycline: Barbiturates may decrease the serum concentration of Doxycycline. *Risk D: Consider therapy modification*

Etoposide: Barbiturates may increase the metabolism of Etoposide. *Risk C: Monitor therapy*

Etoposide Phosphate: Barbiturates may decrease the serum concentration of Etoposide Phosphate. Barbiturates may increase the metabolism, via CYP isoenzymes, of etoposide phosphate. *Risk C: Monitor therapy*

Felbamate: May increase the serum concentration of Barbiturates. *Risk C: Monitor therapy*

Griseofulvin: Barbiturates may decrease the absorption of Griseofulvin. *Risk D: Consider therapy modification*

LamoTRIgine: Barbiturates may increase the metabolism of LamoTRIgine. *Risk D: Consider therapy modification*

Meperidine: Barbiturates may enhance the CNS depressant effect of Meperidine. *Risk C: Monitor therapy*

Methadone: Barbiturates may increase the metabolism of Methadone. *Risk D: Consider therapy modification*

Oral Contraceptive (Estrogens): Barbiturates may diminish the therapeutic effect of Oral Contraceptive (Estrogens). Contraceptive failure is possible. *Risk D: Consider therapy modification*

Primidone: May enhance the adverse/toxic effect of Barbiturates. Primidone is converted to phenobarbital, and thus becomes additive with existing barbiturate therapy. *Risk C: Monitor therapy*

Propafenone: Barbiturates may increase the metabolism of Propafenone. *Risk D: Consider therapy modification*

Pyridoxine: May increase the metabolism of Barbiturates. Apparent in high pyridoxine doses (eg, 200 mg/day) *Risk C: Monitor therapy*

QuiNIDine: Barbiturates may increase the metabolism of QuiNIDine. *Risk D: Consider therapy modification*

Rifamycin Derivatives: May increase the metabolism of Barbiturates. *Risk C: Monitor therapy*

Teniposide: Barbiturates may increase the metabolism of Teniposide. *Risk C: Monitor therapy*

Theophylline Derivatives: Barbiturates may increase the metabolism of Theophylline Derivatives. **Exceptions:** Dyphylline. *Risk C: Monitor therapy*

Tricyclic Antidepressants: Barbiturates may increase the metabolism of Tricyclic Antidepressants. *Risk D: Consider therapy modification*

Valproic Acid: May decrease the metabolism of Barbiturates. Barbiturates may decrease the serum concentration of Valproic Acid. *Risk C: Monitor therapy*

Vitamin K Antagonists (eg, warfarin): Barbiturates may increase the metabolism of Vitamin K Antagonists. *Risk D: Consider therapy modification*

Ethanol/Nutrition/Herb Interactions

Ethanol: Avoid ethanol (may increase CNS depression).

Herb/Nutraceutical: Avoid valerian, St John's wort, kava kava, gotu kola (may increase CNS depression).

Mechanism of Action Depresses CNS activity by binding to barbiturate site at GABA-receptor complex enhancing GABA activity, depressing reticular activity system; higher doses may be gabamimetic

Pharmacodynamics/Kinetics

Onset of hypnosis: 15-30 minutes

Duration: 3-4 hours with 100 mg dose

Distribution: 1.5 L/kg; crosses the placenta; appears in breast milk

Protein binding: 45% to 60%

Metabolism: Hepatic, by microsomal enzyme system

Half-life elimination: 15-40 hours, mean: 28 hours

Time to peak, serum: Within 2-4 hours

Excretion: Urine (as inactive metabolites, small amounts as unchanged drug)

Dosage Oral:

Children:

Preoperative sedation: 2-6 mg/kg (maximum dose: 100 mg/dose) 1-2 hours before procedure

Sedation: 6 mg/kg/day divided every 8 hours

Adults:

Hypnotic: Usual: 100 mg/dose at bedtime; range: 100-200 mg/dose

Preoperative sedation: 100-300 mg 1-2 hours before procedure

Monitoring Parameters Blood pressure, heart rate, respiratory rate, CNS status

Dosage Forms Excipient information presented when available (limited, particularly for generics); consult specific product labeling.

Capsule, as sodium: 100 mg

◆ **Secobarbital Sodium** *see* Secobarbital *on page 1464*

◆ **Seconal®** *see* Secobarbital *on page 1464*

◆ **Sectral®** *see* Acebutolol *on page 27*

◆ **Sedapap®** *see* Butalbital and Acetaminophen *on page 236*

Selegiline (se LE ji leen)

Medication Safety Issues

Sound-alike/look-alike issues:

Selegiline may be confused with Salagen®, Serentil®, sertraline, Serzone®, Stelazine®

Eldepryl® may be confused with Elavil®, enalapril

Zelapar™ may be confused with zaleplon, Zemplar®

Related Information

Antidepressant Agents *on page 1760*

Antiparkinsonian Agents *on page 1767*

U.S. Brand Names Eldepryl®; Emsam®; Zelapar™

Canadian Brand Names Apo-Selegiline®; Gen-Selegiline; Novo-Selegiline; Nu-Selegiline

Mexican Brand Names Niar

Index Terms Deprenyl; L-Deprenyl; Selegiline Hydrochloride

Pharmacologic Category Anti-Parkinson's Agent, MAO Type B Inhibitor; Antidepressant, Monoamine Oxidase Inhibitor

Generic Available Yes: Capsule, tablet

Use Adjunct in the management of parkinsonian patients in which levodopa/carbidopa therapy is deteriorating (oral products); treatment of major depressive disorder (transdermal product)

Unlabeled/Investigational Use Early Parkinson's disease; attention-deficit/hyperactivity disorder (ADHD); negative symptoms of schizophrenia; extrapyramidal symptoms

Mental Health Comment Selegiline is a selective MAO-B inhibitor when used in low oral doses (≤10 mg/day). The patch formulation inhibits both MAO-A and MAO-B inhibitors. When using the 6 mg/day patch, no special diet is required; however, when using the 9 mg/day or 12 mg/day patch a tyramine-restricted diet should be utilized.

Restrictions An FDA-approved medication guide concerning the use of antidepressants in children, adolescents, and young adults must be distributed when dispensing a transdermal selegiline outpatient prescription (new or refill) where this medication is to be used without direct supervision of a healthcare provider. Medication guides are available at http://www.fda.gov/cder/Offices/ODS/medication_guides.htm. Dispense to parents or guardians of children and adolescents receiving this medication.

Pregnancy Risk Factor C

Pregnancy Considerations Teratogenic and adverse behavioral events were noted in animal studies. There are no adequate and well-controlled studies in pregnant women.

Lactation Excretion in breast milk unknown/use caution

Contraindications Hypersensitivity to selegiline or any component of the formulation; concomitant use of meperidine

Orally disintegrating tablet: Additional contraindications: Concomitant use of dextromethorphan, methadone, propoxyphene, tramadol, oral selegiline, other MAO inhibitors

Transdermal: Additional contraindications: Pheochromocytoma; concomitant use of bupropion, selective or dual serotonin reuptake inhibitors (including SSRIs and SNRIs), tricyclic antidepressants, buspirone, tramadol, propoxyphene, methadone, dextromethorphan, St. John's wort, mirtazapine, cyclobenzaprine, oral selegiline and other MAO inhibitors; carbamazepine, and oxcarbazepine; elective surgery requiring general anesthesia, local anesthesia containing sympathomimetic vasoconstrictors; sympathomimetics (and related compounds); foods high in tyramine content; supplements containing tyrosine, phenylalanine, tryptophan, or caffeine

Warnings/Precautions

Oral: MAO-B selective inhibition should not pose a problem with tyramine-containing products as long as the typical oral doses are employed, however, rare reactions have been reported. Increased risk of nonselective MAO inhibition occurs with oral capsule/tablet doses >10 mg/day or orally disintegrating tablet doses >2.5 mg/day. Use of oral selegiline with tricyclic antidepressants and SSRIs has also been associated with rare reactions and should generally be avoided. Addition to levodopa therapy may result in exacerbation of levodopa adverse effects, requiring a reduction in levodopa dosage.

Transdermal: Nonselective MAO inhibition occurs with transdermal delivery and is necessary for antidepressant efficacy. Hypertensive crisis as a result of ingesting tyramine-rich foods is always a concern with nonselective MAO inhibition. Although transdermal delivery minimizes inhibition of MAO-A in the gut, there is limited data with higher transdermal doses; dietary restrictions are recommended with doses >6 mg/24 hours.

Transdermal: **[U.S. Boxed Warning]: Antidepressants increase the risk of suicidal thinking and behavior in children, adolescents, and young adults (18-24 years of age) with major depressive disorder (MDD) and other psychiatric disorders;** consider risk prior to prescribing. Short-term studies did not show an increased risk in patients >24 years of age and showed a decreased risk in patients ≥65 years. Closely monitor patients for worsening of depression, suicidality and/or associated behaviors, particularly during the initial 1-2 months of therapy or during periods of dosage adjustments (increases or decreases); the patient's family or caregiver should be instructed to closely observe the patient and communicate condition with healthcare provider. A medication guide concerning the use of antidepressants should be dispensed with each prescription. **Transdermal selegiline is not FDA approved for use in children <12 years of age.**

Transdermal: The possibility of a suicide attempt is inherit in major depression and may persist until remission occurs. Patients treated with antidepressants (for any indication) should be observed for clinical worsening and suicidality, especially during the initial few months of a course of drug therapy, or at times of dose changes, either increases or decreases. Use caution in high-risk patients. Worsening depression and severe abrupt suicidality that are not part of the presenting symptoms may require discontinuation or modification of drug therapy. Use caution in high-risk patients during initiation of therapy. The patient's family or caregiver should be alerted to monitor patients for the emergence of suicidality and associated behaviors (such as agitation, irritability, hostility, and hypomania) and call healthcare provider.

Transdermal selegiline may worsen psychosis in some patients or precipitate a shift to mania or hypomania in patients with bipolar disorder. Monotherapy in patients with bipolar disorder should be avoided. Patients presenting with depressive symptoms should be screened for bipolar disorder. **Selegiline is not FDA approved for the treatment of bipolar depression.**

Adverse Reactions Unless otherwise noted, the percentage of adverse events is reported for the transdermal patch (**Note:** ODT = orally disintegrating tablet, Oral = capsule/tablet)

>10%:

Central nervous system: Headache (18%; ODT 7%; oral 2%), insomnia (12%; ODT 7%), dizziness (ODT 11%; oral 7%)

Gastrointestinal: Nausea (ODT 11%; oral 10%)

Local: Application site reaction (24%)

1% to 10%:

Cardiovascular: Hypotension (including postural 3% to 10%), chest pain (≥1%; ODT 2%), hypertension (≥1%), peripheral edema (≥1%)

Central nervous system: Pain (ODT 8%), hallucinations (ODT 4%; oral 3%), confusion (ODT 4%; oral 3%), headache (ODT 7%; oral 2%), ataxia (ODT 3%), somnolence (ODT 3%), agitation (≥1%), amnesia (≥1%), paresthesia (≥1%), thinking abnormal (≥1%), depression (<1%; ODT 2%)

Dermatologic: Rash (4%), ecchymosis (ODT 2%), bruising (≥1%), pruritus (≥1%), acne (≥1%)

Endocrine & metabolic: Weight loss (5%), hypokalemia (ODT 2%), sexual side effects (≤1%)

Gastrointestinal: Diarrhea (9%; ODT 2%), xerostomia (8%; ODT 4%), stomatitis (ODT 5%), abdominal pain (oral 4%), dyspepsia (4%; ODT 5%), constipation (≥1%; ODT 4%), flatulence (≥1%; ODT 2%), anorexia (≥1%), gastroenteritis (≥1%), taste perversion (≥1%; ODT 2%), vomiting (≥1%; ODT 3%), tooth disorder (ODT 2%), dysphagia (ODT 2%)

Genitourinary: Dysmenorrhea (≥1%), metrorrhagia (≥1%), UTI (≥1%), urinary frequency (≥1%)

Neuromuscular & skeletal: Dyskinesia (ODT 6%), back pain (ODT 5%), ataxia (<1%; ODT 3%), leg cramps (ODT 3%), myalgia (≥1%; ODT 3%), neck pain (≥1%), tremor (<1%; ODT 3%)

Otic: Tinnitus (≥1%)

Respiratory: Rhinitis (ODT 7%), pharyngitis (3%; ODT 4%), sinusitis (3%), cough (≥1%), bronchitis (≥1%), dyspnea (<1%; ODT 3%)

Miscellaneous: Diaphoresis (≥1%)

Oral and/or transdermal patch: <1% or frequency not defined (limited to important or life-threatening): Abnormal liver function tests, alkaline phosphatase increased, appetite increased, arrhythmia, asthma, ataxia, atrial fibrillation, bacterial infection, behavior/mood changes, bilirubinemia, bradycardia, bradykinesia, breast neoplasm (female), breast pain, chorea, circumoral paresthesia, colitis, dehydration, delusions, dental caries, depersonalization, depression, emotional lability, epistaxis, eructation, euphoria, face edema, fever, fungal infection, gastritis, generalized spasm, glossitis, heat stroke, hematuria (female), hernia, hostility, hypercholesterolemia, hyperesthesia, hyperglycemia, hyperkinesias, hypertonia, hypoglycemic reaction, hyponatremia, kidney calculus (female), lactate dehydrogenase increased, laryngismus, leukocytosis, leukopenia, libido increased, loss of balance, lymphadenopathy, maculopapular rash, manic reaction, melena, migraine, moniliasis, myasthenia, myocardial infarct, myoclonus, neoplasia, neurosis, osteoporosis, otitis external, palpitation, paranoid reaction, parasitic infection, parosmia, pelvic pain, periodontal abscess, peripheral vascular disorder, pneumonia, polyuria (female), prostatic hyperplasia, rectal hemorrhage, salivation increased, skin hypertrophy, skin benign neoplasm, suicide attempt, syncope, tachycardia, tenosynovitis, tongue edema, twitching, urinary retention, urinary urgency (male and female), urination impaired (male), urticaria, vaginal hemorrhage, vaginal moniliasis, vaginitis, vasodilatation, vertigo, vesiculobullous rash, viral infection, visual field defect

Metabolism/Transport Effects Substrate of CYP1A2 (minor), 2A6 (minor), 2B6 (major), 2C8 (minor), 2C19 (minor), 2D6 (minor), 3A4 (minor); **Inhibits** CYP1A2 (weak), 2A6 (weak), 2C9 (weak), 2C19 (weak), 2D6 (weak), 2E1 (weak), 3A4 (weak)

Drug Interactions

Alpha-/Beta-Agonists (Direct-Acting): MAO Inhibitors may enhance the vasopressor effect of Alpha-/Beta-Agonists (Direct-Acting). Primarily with oral administration of phenylephrine. **Exceptions:** Dipivefrin. *Risk D: Consider therapy modification*

Alpha-/Beta-Agonists (Indirect-Acting): MAO Inhibitors may enhance the hypertensive effect of Alpha-/Beta-Agonists (Indirect-Acting). *Risk X: Avoid combination*

Alpha1-Agonists: MAO Inhibitors may enhance the hypertensive effect of Alpha1-Agonists. *Risk X: Avoid combination*

Alpha2-Agonists (Ophthalmic): MAO Inhibitors may enhance the hypertensive effect of Alpha2-Agonists (Ophthalmic). *Risk X: Avoid combination*

Altretamine: May enhance the orthostatic effect of MAO Inhibitors. *Risk C: Monitor therapy*

Amphetamines: MAO Inhibitors may enhance the hypertensive effect of Amphetamines. *Risk X: Avoid combination*

Anilidopiperidine Opioids: May enhance the serotonergic effect of MAO Inhibitors. This could result in serotonin syndrome. Management: Avoid use of fentanyl (and other anilidopiperidine opioids when possible) in patients who have used a monoamine oxidase inhibitor within the past 14 days due to reports of unpredictable but severe adverse effects. *Risk D: Consider therapy modification*

Antidepressants (Serotonin/Norepinephrine Reuptake Inhibitor): MAO Inhibitors may enhance the serotonergic effect of Antidepressants (Serotonin/Norepinephrine Reuptake Inhibitor). This may cause serotonin syndrome. *Risk X: Avoid combination*

Atomoxetine: MAO Inhibitors may enhance the neurotoxic (central) effect of Atomoxetine. *Risk X: Avoid combination*

Beta2-Agonists: MAO Inhibitors may enhance the adverse/toxic effect of Beta2-Agonists. *Risk C: Monitor therapy*

BuPROPion: MAO Inhibitors may enhance the neurotoxic (central) effect of BuPROPion. *Risk X: Avoid combination*

BusPIRone: May enhance the adverse/toxic effect of MAO Inhibitors. Elevated blood pressure has been reported. *Risk X: Avoid combination*

COMT Inhibitors: May enhance the adverse/toxic effect of MAO Inhibitors. *Risk D: Consider therapy modification*

Cyclobenzaprine: May enhance the serotonergic effect of MAO Inhibitors. This could result in serotonin syndrome. *Risk X: Avoid combination*

CYP2B6 Inducers (Strong): May increase the metabolism of CYP2B6 Substrates. *Risk C: Monitor therapy*

CYP2B6 Inhibitors (Moderate): May decrease the metabolism of CYP2B6 Substrates. *Risk C: Monitor therapy*

CYP2B6 Inhibitors (Strong): May decrease the metabolism of CYP2B6 Substrates. *Risk D: Consider therapy modification*

Dexmethylphenidate: MAO Inhibitors may enhance the hypertensive effect of Dexmethylphenidate. *Risk X: Avoid combination*

Dextromethorphan: MAO Inhibitors may enhance the serotonergic effect of Dextromethorphan. This may cause serotonin syndrome. *Risk X: Avoid combination*

Levodopa: May enhance the adverse/toxic effect of MAO Inhibitors. Of particular concern is the development of hypertensive reactions when levodopa is used with nonselective MAOI. *Risk D: Consider therapy modification*

Linezolid: MAO Inhibitors may enhance the adverse/toxic effect of Linezolid. *Risk X: Avoid combination*

Lithium: MAO Inhibitors may enhance the adverse/toxic effect of Lithium. *Risk C: Monitor therapy*

Maprotiline: May enhance the adverse/toxic effect of MAO Inhibitors. *Risk X: Avoid combination*

Meperidine: MAO Inhibitors may enhance the serotonergic effect of Meperidine. This may cause serotonin syndrome. *Risk X: Avoid combination*

Methyldopa: MAO Inhibitors may enhance the adverse/toxic effect of Methyldopa. *Risk X: Avoid combination*

Methylphenidate: MAO Inhibitors may enhance the hypertensive effect of Methylphenidate. *Risk X: Avoid combination*

Mirtazapine: MAO Inhibitors may enhance the neurotoxic (central) effect of Mirtazapine. *Risk X: Avoid combination*

Oral Contraceptive (Estrogens): May increase the serum concentration of Selegiline. *Risk D: Consider therapy modification*

Oral Contraceptive (Progestins): May increase the serum concentration of Selegiline. *Risk D: Consider therapy modification*

Propoxyphene: May enhance the adverse/toxic effect of MAO Inhibitors. Specifically, the risk of serotonin syndrome or other serotonergic adverse events may be increased. *Risk X: Avoid combination*

Rauwolfia Alkaloids: MAO Inhibitors may enhance the adverse/toxic effect of Rauwolfia Alkaloids. Existing MAOI therapy can result in paradoxical effects of added rauwolfia alkaloids (eg, excitation, hypertension). *Risk D: Consider therapy modification*

Selective Serotonin Reuptake Inhibitors: MAO Inhibitors may enhance the serotonergic effect of Selective Serotonin Reuptake Inhibitors. This may cause serotonin syndrome. *Risk X: Avoid combination*

Serotonin 5-HT1D Receptor Agonists: MAO Inhibitors may decrease the metabolism of Serotonin 5-HT1D Receptor Agonists. Management: If MAO inhibitor therapy is required, naratriptan, eletriptan or frovatriptan may be a suitable 5-HT1D agonist to employ. **Exceptions:** Eletriptan; Frovatriptan; Naratriptan. *Risk X: Avoid combination*

Serotonin Modulators: May enhance the adverse/toxic effect of other Serotonin Modulators. The development of serotonin syndrome may occur. *Risk D: Consider therapy modification*

Sibutramine: May enhance the serotonergic effect of Serotonin Modulators. This may cause serotonin syndrome. *Risk X: Avoid combination*

Tetrabenazine: May enhance the adverse/toxic effect of MAO Inhibitors. *Risk X: Avoid combination*

TraMADol: May enhance the neuroexcitatory and/or seizure-potentiating effect of MAO Inhibitors. *Risk D: Consider therapy modification*

Tricyclic Antidepressants: MAO Inhibitors may enhance the serotonergic effect of Tricyclic Antidepressants. This may cause serotonin syndrome. *Risk X: Avoid combination*

Ethanol/Nutrition/Herb Interactions

Ethanol: Avoid ethanol (based on CNS depressant effects and potential tyramine content)

Food: Concurrent ingestion of foods rich in tyramine may cause sudden and severe high blood pressure (hypertensive crisis). Avoid tyramine-containing foods with MAO-Is. Food's freshness is also an important concern; improperly stored or spoiled food can create an environment where tyramine concentrations may increase.

Herb/Nutraceuticals: Avoid valerian, St John's wort, SAMe, kava kava. Avoid supplements containing caffeine, tryptophan, or phenylalanine. Ingestion of large quantities may increase the risk of severe side effects (eg, hypertensive reactions, serotonin syndrome).

Stability

Capsule, tablet: Store at controlled room temperature 15°C to 30°C (59°F to 86°F).

Orally-disintegrating tablet: Store at controlled room temperature 15°C to 30°C (59°F to 86°F). Use within 3 months of opening pouch and immediately after opening individual blister.

Transdermal: Store at 20°C to 25°C (68°F to 77°F).

Mechanism of Action Potent, irreversible inhibitor of monoamine oxidase (MAO). Plasma concentrations achieved via administration of oral dosage forms in recommended doses confer selective inhibition of MAO type B, which plays a major role in the metabolism of dopamine; selegiline may also increase dopaminergic activity by interfering with dopamine reuptake at the synapse. When administered transdermally in recommended doses, selegiline achieves higher blood levels and effectively inhibits both MAO-A and MAO-B, which blocks catabolism of other centrally-active biogenic amine neurotransmitters.

Pharmacodynamics/Kinetics

Onset of action: Therapeutic: Oral: Within 1 hour

Duration: Oral: 24-72 hours

Absorption:

- Orally disintegrating tablet: Rapid; greater bioavailability than capsule/tablet
- Transdermal: 25% to 30% (of total selegiline content) over 24 hours

Protein binding: ~90%

Metabolism: Hepatic, primarily via CYP2B6 to active (N-desmethylselegiline, amphetamine, methamphetamine) and inactive metabolites

Half-life elimination: Oral: 10 hours; Transdermal: 18-25 hours

Excretion: Urine (primarily metabolites); feces

Dosage

Capsule/tablet:

Children and Adolescents: ADHD (unlabeled use): 5-15 mg/day

Adults: Parkinson's disease: 5 mg twice daily with breakfast and lunch or 10 mg in the morning

Elderly: Parkinson's disease: Initial: 5 mg in the morning, may increase to a total of 10 mg/day

Orally disintegrating tablet (Zelapar™): Adults: Parkinson's disease: Initial 1.25 mg daily for at least 6 weeks; may increase to 2.5 mg daily based on clinical response (maximum: 2.5 mg daily)

Transdermal (Emsam®): Depression:

Adults: Initial: 6 mg/24 hours once daily; may titrate based on clinical response in increments of 3 mg/day every 2 weeks up to a maximum of 12 mg/24 hours

Elderly: 6 mg/24 hours

Dosage adjustment in renal impairment: No adjustment necessary.

Dosage adjustment in hepatic impairment: No adjustment necessary in mild-moderate hepatic impairment.

Child/Adolescent Considerations Twenty-nine children 6-18 years of age (mean: 11.2 years) with ADHD refractory to conventional treatments received an average daily dose of 8.1 mg (5-15 mg/day) for an average of 6.7 months (Jankovic, 1993).

Two randomized, double-blind, placebo-controlled trials have shown selegiline to be as effective, and possibly better tolerated, than methylphenidate in the treatment of children (n=68, range: 4-15 years of age) with ADHD (Akhondzadeh, 2003; Mohammadi, 2004).

Akhondzadeh S, Tavakolian R, Davari-Ashtiani R, et al, "Selegiline in the Treatment of Attention Deficit Hyperactivity Disorder in Children: A Double Blind and Randomized Trial," *Prog Neuropsychopharmacol Biol Psychiatry*, 2003, 27(5):841-5.

Jankovic J, "Deprenyl in Attention Deficit Associated With Tourette's Syndrome," *Arch Neurol*, 1993, 50(3):286-8.

Mohammadi MR, Ghanizadeh A, Alaghband-Rad J, et al, "Selegiline in Comparison With Methylphenidate in Attention Deficit Hyperactivity Disorder Children and Adolescents in a Double-Blind, Randomized Clinical Trial," *J Child Adolesc Psychopharmacol*, 2004, 14(3):418-25.

Dietary Considerations Avoid tyramine-containing foods/beverages. Some examples include aged or matured cheese, air-dried or cured meats (including sausages and salamis), fava or broad bean pods, tap/draft beers, Marmite concentrate, sauerkraut, soy sauce and other soybean condiments.

Emsam® 9 mg/24 hours or 12 mg/24 hours: Avoid tyramine-rich foods or beverages beginning the first day of treatment or for 2 weeks after discontinuation or dose reduction to 6 mg/24 hours.

Zelapar™: Phenylalanine 1.25 mg per 1.25 mg tablet; do not take with food or liquid

Administration

Oral: Orally disintegrating tablet (Zelapar™): Take in morning before breakfast; place on top of tongue and allow to dissolve. Avoid food or liquid 5 minutes before and after administration.

Topical: Transdermal (Emsam®): Apply to clean, dry, intact skin to the upper torso (below the neck and above the waist), upper thigh, or outer surface of the upper arm. Avoid exposure of application site to external heat source, which may increase the amount of drug absorbed. Apply at the same time each day and rotate application sites. Wash hands with soap and water after handling. Avoid touching the sticky side of the patch.

Monitoring Parameters Blood pressure; symptoms of parkinsonism; general mood and behavior (increased anxiety, presence of mania or agitation); suicidal ideation (especially at the beginning of therapy or when doses are increased or decreased)

Additional Information When adding selegiline to levodopa/carbidopa, the dose of the latter can usually be decreased.

Dosage Forms Excipient information presented when available (limited, particularly for generics); consult specific product labeling.

Capsule, oral, as hydrochloride: 5 mg

Eldepryl®: 5 mg

Tablet, oral, as hydrochloride: 5 mg

Tablet, orally-disintegrating:

Zelapar™: 1.25 mg [contains phenylalanine 1.25 mg/tablet]

Transdermal system, topical [once-daily patch]:
Emsam®: 6 mg/24 hours (30s) [20 cm^2, total selegiline 20 mg]; 9 mg/24 hours (30s) [30 cm^2, total selegiline 30 mg]; 12 mg/24 hours (30s) [40 cm^2, total selegiline 40 mg]

- ◆ **Selegiline Hydrochloride** *see* Selegiline *on page 1466*
- ◆ **Selfemra™** *see* FLUoxetine *on page 650*
- ◆ **Selzentry™** *see* Maraviroc *on page 971*
- ◆ **Semprex®-D** *see* Acrivastine and Pseudoephedrine *on page 48*
- ◆ **Senna and Docusate** *see* Docusate and Senna *on page 491*
- ◆ **Senna-S** *see* Docusate and Senna *on page 491*
- ◆ **Senokot-S® [OTC]** *see* Docusate and Senna *on page 491*
- ◆ **SenoSol™-SS [OTC]** *see* Docusate and Senna *on page 491*
- ◆ **Sensipar®** *see* Cinacalcet *on page 345*
- ◆ **Sensorcaine®** *see* Bupivacaine *on page 211*
- ◆ **Sensorcaine®-MPF** *see* Bupivacaine *on page 211*
- ◆ **Sensorcaine®-MPF Spinal** *see* Bupivacaine *on page 211*
- ◆ **Septra®** *see* Sulfamethoxazole and Trimethoprim *on page 1517*
- ◆ **Septra® DS** *see* Sulfamethoxazole and Trimethoprim *on page 1517*
- ◆ **Serax®** *see* Oxazepam *on page 1193*
- ◆ **Serevent® Diskus®** *see* Salmeterol *on page 1457*
- ◆ **Seromycin®** *see* CycloSERINE *on page 408*
- ◆ **Serophene®** *see* ClomiPHENE *on page 368*
- ◆ **Seroquel®** *see* QUEtiapine *on page 1381*
- ◆ **Seroquel® XR** *see* QUEtiapine *on page 1381*
- ◆ **Serostim®** *see* Somatropin *on page 1499*

Sertraline (SER tra leen)

Medication Safety Issues

Sound-alike/look-alike issues:

Sertraline may be confused with selegiline, Serentil®

Zoloft® may be confused with Zocor®

Related Information

Antidepressant Agents *on page 1760*
Antidepressant Receptor Profile *on page 1764*
Discontinuation of Psychotropic Drugs *on page 1839*
Liquid Compatibility of Antidepressants, Antipsychotics, and Mood Stabilizers *on page 1788*
Selective Serotonin Reuptake Inhibitors (SSRIs) CYP Profile *on page 1793*
Selective Serotonin Reuptake Inhibitors (SSRIs) FDA-Approved Indication(s) *on page 1794*
Selective Serotonin Reuptake Inhibitors (SSRIs) Pharmacokinetics *on page 1795*
Selective Serotonin Reuptake Inhibitors (SSRIs) Receptor Profile *on page 1796*

U.S. Brand Names Zoloft®

Canadian Brand Names Apo-Sertraline®; CO Sertraline; Dom-Sertraline; Gen-Sertraline; GMD-Sertraline; Novo-Sertraline; Nu-Sertraline; PHL-Sertraline; PMS-Sertraline; ratio-Sertraline; Rhoxal-sertraline; Riva-Sertraline; Sandoz-Sertraline; Zoloft®

Mexican Brand Names Aleval; Altruline; Aluprex; Prosertin; Serolux; Sertex

Index Terms Sertraline Hydrochloride

Pharmacologic Category Antidepressant, Selective Serotonin Reuptake Inhibitor

Generic Available Yes

Use Treatment of major depression; obsessive-compulsive disorder (OCD); panic disorder; post-traumatic stress disorder (PTSD); premenstrual dysphoric disorder (PMDD); social anxiety disorder

Unlabeled/Investigational Use Eating disorders; generalized anxiety disorder (GAD); impulse control disorders; treatment of mild dementia-associated agitation in nonpsychotic patients

Mental Health Comment The SSRIs as a class are generally considered to be safe and equally effective. Allow sufficient dose-response time (6-12 weeks). Differences lie in approved indications, receptor profiles, pharmacokinetics, and cytochrome P450 activity profile. Subtle differences exist in adverse effect profiles. All SSRIs have the potential to cause sexual dysfunction. Among the SSRIs, sertraline is felt to be associated with the most GI side effects.

Restrictions An FDA-approved medication guide concerning the use of antidepressants in children, adolescents, and young adults must be distributed when dispensing an outpatient prescription (new or refill) where this medication is to be used without direct supervision of a healthcare provider. Medication guides are available at http://www.fda.gov/cder/Offices/ODS/medication_guides.htm. Dispense to parents or guardians of children and adolescents receiving this medication.

Pregnancy Risk Factor C

Pregnancy Considerations Due to adverse effects observed in animal studies, sertraline is classified as pregnancy category C. Sertraline crosses the human placenta. Nonteratogenic effects in the newborn following SSRI exposure late in the third trimester include respiratory distress, cyanosis, apnea, seizures, temperature instability, feeding difficulty, vomiting, hypoglycemia, hypo- or hypertonia, hyper-reflexia, jitteriness, irritability, constant crying, and tremor. An increased risk of low birth weight, lower APGAR scores, and blunted behavioral response to pain for a prolonged period after delivery has also been reported. Exposure to SSRIs after the twentieth week of gestation has been associated with persistent pulmonary hypertension of the newborn (PPHN). Adverse effects may be due to toxic effects of the SSRI or drug discontinuation. The long-term effects of *in utero* SSRI exposure on infant development and behavior are not known.

Due to pregnancy-induced physiologic changes, women who are pregnant may require increased doses of sertraline to achieve euthymia. Women treated for major depression and who are euthymic prior to pregnancy are more likely to experience a relapse when medication is discontinued as compared to pregnant women who continue taking antidepressant medications. The ACOG recommends that therapy with SSRIs or SNRIs during pregnancy be individualized; treatment of depression during pregnancy should incorporate the clinical expertise of the mental health clinician, obstetrician, primary healthcare provider, and pediatrician (ACOG, 2007). If treatment during pregnancy is required, consider tapering therapy during the third trimester in order to prevent withdrawal symptoms in the infant. If this is done and the woman is considered to be at risk from her major depressive disorder, the medication can be restarted following delivery, although the dose should be readjusted to that required before pregnancy.

Lactation Enters breast milk/use caution (AAP rates "of concern")

Contraindications Hypersensitivity to sertraline or any component of the formulation; use of MAO inhibitors within 14 days; concurrent use of pimozide; concurrent use of sertraline oral concentrate with disulfiram

Warnings/Precautions [U.S. Boxed Warning]: Antidepressants increase the risk of suicidal thinking and behavior in children, adolescents, and young adults (18-24 years of age) with major depressive disorder (MDD) and other psychiatric disorders; consider risk prior to prescribing. Short-term studies did not show an increased risk in patients >24 years of age and showed a decreased risk in patients ≥65 years. Closely monitor patients for clinical worsening, suicidality, or unusual changes in behavior, particularly during the initial 1-2 months of therapy or during periods of dosage adjustments (increases or decreases); the patient's family or caregiver should be instructed to closely observe the patient and communicate condition with healthcare provider. A medication guide concerning the use of antidepressants should be dispensed with each prescription. **Sertraline is not FDA approved for use in children with major depressive disorder (MDD). However, it is approved for the treatment of obsessive-compulsive disorder (OCD) in children ≥6 years of age.**

The possibility of a suicide attempt is inherent in major depression and may persist until remission occurs. Use caution in high-risk patients. Worsening depression and severe abrupt suicidality that are not part of the presenting symptoms may require discontinuation or modification of drug therapy. The patient's family or caregiver should be alerted to monitor patients for the emergence of suicidality and associated behaviors (such as agitation, irritability, hostility, impulsivity, and hypomania) and call healthcare provider.

May worsen psychosis in some patients or precipitate a shift to mania or hypomania in patients with bipolar disorder. Patients presenting with depressive symptoms should be screened for bipolar disorder. Monotherapy in patients with bipolar disorder should be avoided. **Sertraline is not FDA approved for the treatment of bipolar depression.**

The potential for severe reaction exists when used with MAO inhibitors, SSRIs/SNRIs or triptans; serotonin syndrome (hyperthermia, muscular rigidity, mental status changes/agitation, autonomic instability) may occur; concomitant use with MAO inhibitors is contraindicated. Has a very low potential to impair cognitive or motor performance. However, caution patients regarding activities requiring alertness until response to sertraline is known. Does not appear to potentiate the effects of alcohol, however, ethanol use is not advised.

Use caution in patients with a previous seizure disorder or condition predisposing to seizures such as brain damage, alcoholism, or concurrent therapy with other drugs which lower the seizure threshold. May increase the risks associated with electroconvulsive therapy. Use with caution in patients with hepatic or renal dysfunction and in elderly patients. May cause hyponatremia/SIADH (elderly at increased risk); volume depletion (diuretics may increase risk). Use with caution in patients with renal insufficiency or other concurrent illness (due to limited experience). Sertraline acts as a mild uricosuric; use with caution in patients at risk of uric acid nephropathy. Use caution with concomitant use of NSAIDs, ASA, or other drugs that affect coagulation; the risk of bleeding may be potentiated. Use with caution in patients where weight loss is undesirable. May cause or exacerbate sexual dysfunction.

Use oral concentrate formulation with caution in patients with latex sensitivity; dropper dispenser contains dry natural rubber. Monitor growth in pediatric patients. Discontinuation symptoms (eg, dysphoric mood, irritability, agitation, confusion, anxiety, insomnia, hypomania) may occur upon abrupt discontinuation. Taper dose when discontinuing therapy.

Adverse Reactions

>10%:

Central nervous system: Dizziness, fatigue, headache, insomnia, somnolence

Endocrine & metabolic: Libido decreased

Gastrointestinal: Anorexia, diarrhea, nausea, xerostomia

Genitourinary: Ejaculatory disturbances

Neuromuscular & skeletal: Tremors

Miscellaneous: Diaphoresis

1% to 10%:

Cardiovascular: Chest pain, palpitation

Central nervous system: Agitation, anxiety, hypoesthesia, malaise, nervousness, pain

Dermatologic: Rash

Endocrine & metabolic: Impotence

Gastrointestinal: Appetite increased, constipation, dyspepsia, flatulence, vomiting, weight gain

Neuromuscular & skeletal: Back pain, hypertonia, myalgia, paresthesia, weakness

Ocular: Visual difficulty, abnormal vision

Otic: Tinnitus

Respiratory: Rhinitis

Miscellaneous: Yawning

<1% (Limited to important or life-threatening): Abdominal pain, acute renal failure, agranulocytosis, allergic reaction, anaphylactoid reaction, angioedema, aplastic anemia, atrial arrhythmia, AV block, bilirubin increased, blindness, bradycardia, cataract, dystonia, extrapyramidal symptoms, galactorrhea, gum hyperplasia, gynecomastia, hallucinations, hepatic failure, hepatitis, hepatomegaly, hyperglycemia, hyperprolactinemia, hypothyroidism, jaundice, leukopenia, lupus-like syndrome, micturition disorders, neuroleptic malignant syndrome, oculogyric crisis, serotonin syndrome, SIADH, Stevens-Johnson syndrome (and other severe dermatologic reactions), optic neuritis, pancreatitis (rare), photosensitivity, priapism, psychosis, PT/INR increased, pulmonary hypertension, QT_c prolongation, serum sickness, thrombocytopenia, torsade de pointes, transaminases increased, vasculitis, ventricular tachycardia

Additional adverse reactions reported in pediatric patients (frequency >2%): Aggressiveness, epistaxis, hyperkinesia, purpura, sinusitis, urinary incontinence

Metabolism/Transport Effects Substrate of CYP2B6 (minor), 2C9 (minor), 2C19 (major), 2D6 (major), 3A4 (minor); **Inhibits** CYP1A2 (weak), 2B6 (moderate), 2C8 (weak), 2C9 (weak), 2C19 (moderate), 2D6 (moderate), 3A4 (moderate)

Drug Interactions

Alcohol (Ethyl): CNS Depressants may enhance the CNS depressant effect of Alcohol (Ethyl). *Risk C: Monitor therapy*

Alpha-/Beta-Blockers: Selective Serotonin Reuptake Inhibitors may decrease the metabolism of Alpha-/Beta-Blockers. *Risk C: Monitor therapy*

Analgesics (Opioid): May enhance the serotonergic effect of Selective Serotonin Reuptake Inhibitors. This may cause serotonin syndrome. *Risk C: Monitor therapy*

Anticoagulants: Antiplatelet Agents may enhance the anticoagulant effect of Anticoagulants. *Risk C: Monitor therapy*

Antidepressants (Serotonin Reuptake Inhibitor/Antagonist): Selective Serotonin Reuptake Inhibitors may enhance the serotonergic effect of Antidepressants (Serotonin Reuptake Inhibitor/Antagonist). This may cause serotonin syndrome. *Risk C: Monitor therapy*

Antiplatelet Agents: May enhance the anticoagulant effect of other Antiplatelet Agents. *Risk C: Monitor therapy*

Aspirin: Selective Serotonin Reuptake Inhibitors may enhance the antiplatelet effect of Aspirin. *Risk C: Monitor therapy*

Beta-Blockers: Selective Serotonin Reuptake Inhibitors may enhance the bradycardic effect of Beta-Blockers. **Exceptions:** Acebutolol; Atenolol; Carteolol; Esmolol; Levobunolol; Metipranolol; Nadolol; Penbutolol. *Risk C: Monitor therapy*

BusPIRone: May enhance the serotonergic effect of Selective Serotonin Reuptake Inhibitors. This may cause serotonin syndrome. Selective Serotonin Reuptake Inhibitors may decrease the metabolism of BusPIRone. *Risk C: Monitor therapy*

CarBAMazepine: Selective Serotonin Reuptake Inhibitors may decrease the metabolism of CarBAMazepine. Specifically those SSRIs that inhibit CYP3A4 isoenzymes. CarBAMazepine may increase the metabolism of Selective Serotonin Reuptake Inhibitors. Specifically those agents metabolized via CYP1A2, 2C, and/or 3A4 isoenzymes. *Risk D: Consider therapy modification*

Cimetidine: May decrease the metabolism of Selective Serotonin Reuptake Inhibitors. *Risk D: Consider therapy modification*

Clozapine: Selective Serotonin Reuptake Inhibitors may decrease the metabolism of Clozapine. *Risk D: Consider therapy modification*

CNS Depressants: May enhance the adverse/toxic effect of other CNS Depressants. *Risk C: Monitor therapy*

CYP2B6 Substrates: CYP2B6 Inhibitors (Moderate) may decrease the metabolism of CYP2B6 Substrates. *Risk C: Monitor therapy*

CYP2C19 Substrates: CYP2C19 Inhibitors (Moderate) may decrease the metabolism of CYP2C19 Substrates. *Risk C: Monitor therapy*

CYP2D6 Inhibitors (Moderate): May decrease the metabolism of CYP2D6 Substrates. *Risk C: Monitor therapy*

CYP2D6 Inhibitors (Strong): May decrease the metabolism of CYP2D6 Substrates. *Risk D: Consider therapy modification*

CYP2D6 Substrates: CYP2D6 Inhibitors (Moderate) may decrease the metabolism of CYP2D6 Substrates. **Exceptions:** Tamoxifen. *Risk C: Monitor therapy*

CYP3A4 Substrates: CYP3A4 Inhibitors (Moderate) may decrease the metabolism of CYP3A4 Substrates. *Risk C: Monitor therapy*

Cyproheptadine: May diminish the therapeutic effect of Selective Serotonin Reuptake Inhibitors. *Risk C: Monitor therapy*

Darunavir: May decrease the serum concentration of Sertraline. *Risk C: Monitor therapy*

Dasatinib: May enhance the anticoagulant effect of Antiplatelet Agents. *Risk C: Monitor therapy*

Desmopressin: Selective Serotonin Reuptake Inhibitors may enhance the adverse/toxic effect of Desmopressin. *Risk C: Monitor therapy*

Dextromethorphan: Selective Serotonin Reuptake Inhibitors may enhance the adverse/toxic effect of Dextromethorphan. *Risk D: Consider therapy modification*

Disulfiram: May enhance the adverse/toxic effect of Sertraline. This is specifically related to sertraline oral concentrate due to its alcohol content (12%). Management: Sertraline Oral Concentrate contains 12% alcohol, and its use should be avoided with disulfiram. *Risk X: Avoid combination*

Drotrecogin Alfa: Antiplatelet Agents may enhance the adverse/toxic effect of Drotrecogin Alfa. Bleeding may occur. *Risk D: Consider therapy modification*

Efavirenz: May decrease the serum concentration of Sertraline. *Risk C: Monitor therapy*

Eplerenone: CYP3A4 Inhibitors (Moderate) may increase the serum concentration of Eplerenone. Management: A lower starting dose of eplerenone (25 mg once daily) is recommended in patients with hypertension who are also taking drugs that are moderate inhibitors of CYP3A4. *Risk D: Consider therapy modification*

Galantamine: Selective Serotonin Reuptake Inhibitors may decrease the metabolism of Galantamine. *Risk C: Monitor therapy*

Haloperidol: Selective Serotonin Reuptake Inhibitors may decrease the metabolism of Haloperidol. *Risk C: Monitor therapy*

Herbs (Anticoagulant/Antiplatelet Properties) (eg, Alfalfa, Anise, Bilberry): May enhance the adverse/toxic effect of Antiplatelet Agents. Bleeding may occur. *Risk D: Consider therapy modification*

Ibritumomab: Antiplatelet Agents may enhance the adverse/toxic effect of Ibritumomab. Both agents may contribute to impaired platelet function and an increased risk of bleeding. *Risk C: Monitor therapy*

Lithium: Selective Serotonin Reuptake Inhibitors may enhance the adverse/toxic effect of Lithium. *Risk C: Monitor therapy*

Macrolide Antibiotics: May decrease the metabolism of Selective Serotonin Reuptake Inhibitors. **Exceptions:** Azithromycin; Dirithromycin [Off Market]; Spiramycin. *Risk C: Monitor therapy*

MAO Inhibitors: May enhance the serotonergic effect of Selective Serotonin Reuptake Inhibitors. This may cause serotonin syndrome. *Risk X: Avoid combination*

Maraviroc: CYP3A4 Inhibitors may increase the serum concentration of Maraviroc. *Risk D: Consider therapy modification*

Methadone: Selective Serotonin Reuptake Inhibitors may decrease the metabolism of Methadone. Fluvoxamine appears to be the only interacting SSRI. *Risk D: Consider therapy modification*

Metoclopramide: May enhance the adverse/toxic effect of Sertraline. Specifically, the risk of serotonin syndrome may be increased. *Risk C: Monitor therapy*

NSAID (COX-2 Inhibitor): Selective Serotonin Reuptake Inhibitors may enhance the antiplatelet effect of NSAID (COX-2 Inhibitor). *Risk D: Consider therapy modification*

NSAID (Nonselective): Selective Serotonin Reuptake Inhibitors may enhance the antiplatelet effect of NSAID (Nonselective). *Risk D: Consider therapy modification*

Omega-3-Acid Ethyl Esters: May enhance the antiplatelet effect of Antiplatelet Agents. *Risk C: Monitor therapy*

Pentosan Polysulfate Sodium: May enhance the adverse/toxic effect of Antiplatelet Agents. Specifically, the risk of bleeding may be increased by concurrent use of these agents. *Risk C: Monitor therapy*

Phenytoin: Selective Serotonin Reuptake Inhibitors may decrease the metabolism of Phenytoin. *Risk D: Consider therapy modification*

Pimecrolimus: CYP3A4 Inhibitors (Moderate) may decrease the metabolism of Pimecrolimus. *Risk C: Monitor therapy*

Pimozide: Selective Serotonin Reuptake Inhibitors may enhance the adverse/toxic effect of Pimozide. *Risk X: Avoid combination*

Propafenone: Selective Serotonin Reuptake Inhibitors may decrease the metabolism of Propafenone. *Risk D: Consider therapy modification*

Prostacyclin Analogues: May enhance the antiplatelet effect of Antiplatelet Agents. *Risk C: Monitor therapy*

Ranolazine: CYP3A4 Inhibitors (Moderate) may increase the serum concentration of Ranolazine. Management: Limit the ranolazine dose to a maximum of 500mg twice daily in patients concurrently receiving moderate CYP3A4 inhibitors (e.g., diltiazem, verapamil, erythromycin, etc.). *Risk D: Consider therapy modification*

Risperidone: Selective Serotonin Reuptake Inhibitors may decrease the metabolism of Risperidone. *Risk C: Monitor therapy*

Salicylates: Antiplatelet Agents may enhance the adverse/toxic effect of Salicylates. Increased risk of bleeding may result. *Risk C: Monitor therapy*

Salmeterol: CYP3A4 Inhibitors (Moderate) may increase the serum concentration of Salmeterol. *Risk C: Monitor therapy*

Serotonin Modulators: May enhance the adverse/toxic effect of other Serotonin Modulators. The development of serotonin syndrome may occur. *Risk D: Consider therapy modification*

Sibutramine: May enhance the serotonergic effect of Serotonin Modulators. This may cause serotonin syndrome. *Risk X: Avoid combination*

Tamoxifen: CYP2D6 Inhibitors (Moderate) may decrease the metabolism of Tamoxifen. Specifically, CYP2D6 inhibitors may decrease the formation of highly potent active metabolites. *Risk D: Consider therapy modification*

Thioridazine: CYP2D6 Inhibitors may decrease the metabolism of Thioridazine. *Risk X: Avoid combination*

Thrombolytic Agents: Antiplatelet Agents may enhance the anticoagulant effect of Thrombolytic Agents. *Risk C: Monitor therapy*

Tositumomab and Iodine I 131 Tositumomab: Antiplatelet Agents may enhance the adverse/toxic effect of Tositumomab and Iodine I 131 Tositumomab. Specifically, the risk of bleeding-related adverse events may be increased. *Risk C: Monitor therapy*

TraMADol: Selective Serotonin Reuptake Inhibitors may enhance the neuroexcitatory and/or seizure-potentiating effect of TraMADol. TraMADol may enhance the serotonergic effect of Selective Serotonin Reuptake Inhibitors. This may cause serotonin syndrome. *Risk D: Consider therapy modification*

Tricyclic Antidepressants: Selective Serotonin Reuptake Inhibitors may decrease the metabolism of Tricyclic Antidepressants. *Risk D: Consider therapy modification*

Tryptophan: May enhance the serotonergic effect of Selective Serotonin Reuptake Inhibitors. This may cause serotonin syndrome. *Risk D: Consider therapy modification*

Vitamin K Antagonists (eg, warfarin): Selective Serotonin Reuptake Inhibitors may enhance the anticoagulant effect of Vitamin K Antagonists. *Risk C: Monitor therapy*

Ethanol/Nutrition/Herb Interactions

Ethanol: Avoid ethanol (may increase CNS depression).

Food: Sertraline average peak serum levels may be increased if taken with food.

Herb/Nutraceutical: Avoid valerian, St John's wort, kava kava, gotu kola (may increase CNS depression).

Stability Tablets and oral solution should be stored at controlled room temperature of 15°C to 30°C (59°F to 86°F).

Mechanism of Action Antidepressant with selective inhibitory effects on presynaptic serotonin (5-HT) reuptake and only very weak effects on norepinephrine and dopamine neuronal uptake. *In vitro* studies demonstrate no significant affinity for adrenergic, cholinergic, GABA, dopaminergic, histaminergic, serotonergic, or benzodiazepine receptors.

Pharmacodynamics/Kinetics

Onset of action: Depression: The onset of action is within a week, however, individual response varies greatly and full response may not be seen until 8-12 weeks after initiation of treatment.

Absorption: Slow

Protein binding: 98%

Metabolism: Hepatic; may involve CYP2C19 and CYP2D6; extensive first pass metabolism; forms metabolite N-desmethylsertraline

Bioavailability: Bioavailability of tablets and solution are equivalent

Half-life elimination: Sertraline: 26 hours; N-desmethylsertraline: 66 hours (range: 62-104 hours)

Time to peak, plasma: Sertraline: 4.5-8.4 hours

Excretion: Urine and feces

Dosage Oral:

Children and Adolescents: Obsessive-compulsive disorder:

6-12 years: Initial: 25 mg once daily

13-17 years: Initial: 50 mg once daily

Note: May increase daily dose, at intervals of not less than 1 week, to a maximum of 200 mg/day. If somnolence is noted, give at bedtime.

Adults:

Depression/obsessive-compulsive disorder: Oral: Initial: 50 mg/day (see "Note" above)

Panic disorder, post-traumatic stress disorder, social anxiety disorder: Initial: 25 mg once daily; increase to 50 mg once daily after 1 week (see "Note" above)

Premenstrual dysphoric disorder: 50 mg/day either daily throughout menstrual cycle **or** limited to the luteal phase of menstrual cycle, depending on physician assessment. Patients not responding to 50 mg/day may benefit from dose increases (50 mg increments per menstrual cycle) up to 150 mg/day when dosing throughout menstrual cycle **or** up to 100 mg day when dosing during luteal phase only. If a 100 mg/day dose has been established with luteal phase dosing, a 50 mg/day titration step for 3 days should be utilized at the beginning of each luteal phase dosing period.

Elderly: Depression/obsessive-compulsive disorder: Start treatment with 25 mg/day in the morning and increase by 25 mg/day increments every 2-3 days if tolerated to 50-100 mg/day; additional increases may be necessary; maximum dose: 200 mg/day. **Note:** Patients with Alzheimer's dementia-related depression may require a lower starting dosage of 12.5 mg/day, with titration intervals of 1-2 weeks, up to 150-200 mg/day maximum.

Dosage adjustment/comment in renal impairment: Multiple-dose pharmacokinetics are unaffected by renal impairment.

Hemodialysis: Not removed by hemodialysis

Dosage adjustment/comment in hepatic impairment: Sertraline is extensively metabolized by the liver; caution should be used in patients with hepatic impairment; a lower dose or less frequent dosing should be used.

Child/Adolescent Considerations Twenty-nine children (6-12 years of age) and 32 adolescents (13-17 years of age) with major depression, obsessive-compulsive disorder, or both, received 25-200 mg/day (Alderman, 1998). Fifty-three children (6-12 years of age) and 39 adolescents (13-17 years of age) with obsessive-compulsive disorder (OCD) received up to 200 mg/day (March, 1998).

The efficacy of sertraline in the treatment of OCD was demonstrated in a 12-week, multicenter, placebo-controlled study with 187 outpatients 6-17 years of age. The safety of sertraline use in children and adolescents (6-18 years of age) was evaluated in a 12-week, multicenter, placebo-controlled study with 187 outpatients (6-17 years of age), and in a flexible dose, 52-week open extension study of 137 patients (6-18 years of age), who had completed the initial 12-week, double-blind, placebo-controlled study. Sertraline was administered at doses of either 25 mg/day (children 6-12 years of age) or 50 mg/day (adolescents 13-18 years of age). The dose was then titrated in weekly 25 mg/day or 50 mg/day increments, respectively, to a maximum dose of 200 mg/day based upon clinical response. The mean dose for completers was 157 mg/day. In the acute 12-week pediatric study and in the 52 week study, sertraline had an adverse event profile generally similar to that observed in adults (Zoloft® package insert, Pfizer, November, 2001).

A recent report describes 5 children (8-15 years of age) who developed epistaxis (n=4) or bruising (n=1) while receiving sertraline (Lake, 2000). Another recent report describes the SSRI discontinuation syndrome in 6 children; the syndrome was similar to that reported in adults (Diler, 2002).

Alderman J, Wolkow R, Chung M, et al, "Sertraline Treatment of Children and Adolescents With Obsessive-Compulsive Disorder or Depression: Pharmacokinetics, Tolerability, and Efficacy," *J Am Acad Child Adolesc Psychiatry*, 1998, 37(4):386-94.

Diler RS and Avci A, "Selective Serotonin Reuptake Inhibitor Discontinuation Syndrome in Children: Six Case Reports," *Current Therapeutic Reseach*, 2002, 63(3):188-97.

Lake MB, Birmaher B, Wassick S, et al, "Bleeding and Selective Serotonin Reuptake Inhibitors in Childhood and Adolescence," *J Child Adolesc Psychopharmacol*, 2000, 10(1):35-8.

March JS, Biederman J, Wolkow R, et al, "Sertraline in Children and Adolescents With Obsessive-Compulsive Disorder: A Multicenter Randomized Controlled Trial," *JAMA*, 1998, 280(20):1752-6.

Administration Oral concentrate: Must be diluted before use. Immediately before administration, use the dropper provided to measure the required amount of concentrate; mix with 4 ounces (1/2 cup) of water, ginger ale, lemon/lime soda, lemonade, or orange juice **only**. Do not mix with any other liquids than these. The dose should be taken immediately after mixing; do not mix in advance. A slight haze may appear after mixing; this is normal. **Note:** Use with caution in patients with latex sensitivity; dropper dispenser contains dry natural rubber.

Monitoring Parameters Monitor nutritional intake and weight; mental status for depression, suicidal ideation (especially at the beginning of therapy or when doses are increased or decreased), anxiety, social functioning, mania, panic attacks; akathisia; growth in pediatric patients

Dosage Forms Excipient information presented when available (limited, particularly for generics); consult specific product labeling.

Solution, oral [concentrate]: 20 mg/mL (60 mL)

Zoloft®: 20 mg/mL (60 mL) [contains alcohol 12%; dropper contains dry natural rubber]

Tablet: 25 mg, 50 mg, 100 mg

Zoloft®: 25 mg, 50 mg, 100 mg

◆ **Sertraline Hydrochloride** *see* Sertraline *on page 1472*

◆ **Serzone** *see* Nefazodone *on page 1116*

◆ **Setwall** *see* Valerian *(Valeriana officinalis) on page 1641*

Sevoflurane (see voe FLOO rane)

Medication Safety Issues

Sound-alike/look-alike issues:

Ultane® may be confused with Ultram®

High alert medication: The Institute for Safe Medication Practices (ISMP) includes this medication among its list of drug classes which have a heightened risk of causing significant patient harm when used in error.

U.S. Brand Names Sojourn™; Ultane®

Canadian Brand Names Sevorane® AF

Mexican Brand Names Sevorane

Pharmacologic Category General Anesthetic, Inhalation

Use Induction and maintenance of general anesthesia

Effect on Mental Status May cause agitation, somnolence, or dizziness

Effect on Psychiatric Treatment None reported

Dosage Summary

Inhalation:

Neonates 0-1 month (full-term): 3.3% in O_2

Infants 1-<6 months: 3% in O_2

Children 6 months to <3 years: 2.8% in O_2; 2% in 60% N_20/40% O_2

Children 3-12 years: 2.5% in O_2

Adults 25 years: 2.6% in O_2; 1.4% in 65% N_20/35% O_2

Adults 40 years: 2.1% in O_2; 1.1% in 65% N_20/35% O_2

Adults 60 years: 1.7% in O_2; 0.9% in 65% N_20/35% O_2

Adults 80 years: 1.4% in O_2; 0.7% in 65% N_20/35% O_2

Dosage Forms Excipient information presented when available (limited, particularly for generics); consult specific product labeling.

Liquid for inhalation: 100% (250 mL)

Sojourn™, Ultane®: 100% (250 mL)

- ◆ **Shanzha Rou** *see* Hawthorn *(Crataegus oxyacantha) on page 758*
- ◆ **Siberian Ginseng** *see* Ginseng, Siberian *(Eleutherococcus senticosus) on page 720*

Sibutramine (si BYOO tra meen)

Medication Safety Issues

Sound-alike/look-alike issues:

Meridia® may be confused with Aredia®

U.S. Brand Names Meridia®

Canadian Brand Names Meridia®

Mexican Brand Names Ectiva; Raductil; Reductil

Index Terms Sibutramine Hydrochloride Monohydrate

Pharmacologic Category Anorexiant; Sympathomimetic

Generic Available No

Use Management of obesity

Restrictions C-IV

Pharmacotherapy for weight loss is recommended only for obese patients with a body mass index ≥30 kg/m^2, or ≥27 kg/m^2 in the presence of other risk factors such as hypertension, diabetes, and/or dyslipidemia or a high waist circumference; therapy should be used in conjunction with a comprehensive weight management program. Rule out organic causes of obesity (eg, untreated hypothyroidism) prior to use.

Pregnancy Risk Factor C

Pregnancy Considerations Teratogenic effects were not observed in animal studies except at doses also causing maternal toxicity. There are no adequate and well-controlled studies in pregnant women. Use in pregnancy is not recommended.

Lactation Excretion in breast milk unknown/not recommended

Contraindications Hypersensitivity to sibutramine or any component of the formulation; during or within 2 weeks of MAO inhibitors or concomitant centrally-acting appetite suppressants; anorexia nervosa, bulimia nervosa; poorly-controlled or uncontrolled hypertension, coronary artery disease, CHF arrhythmia; stroke

Warnings/Precautions The use of some anorexigens has been associated with the development of valvular heart disease. Avoid use in patients with known serious structural cardiac abnormalities, cardiomyopathy, serious heart rhythm abnormalities, or other serious cardiac problems that could increase the risk of sudden death that these conditions alone carry.

May cause increase in blood pressure or pulse rate. For patients experiencing a sustained increase in blood pressure or pulse, dose reduction or discontinuation should be considered. Caution should be used in patients with hypertension and other cardiovascular conditions that might be exacerbated by increases in blood pressure or heart rate. Should not be used in patients with coronary artery disease, HF, arrhythmia, or stroke.

Primary pulmonary hypertension (PPH), a rare and frequently fatal disease of the lungs, has been found to occur with increased frequency in patients receiving some anorexigens. Although not reported in clinical trials, it is possible that sibutramine may share this potential, and patients should be monitored closely.

Use with caution in mild-moderate renal impairment or hepatic dysfunction, seizure disorder, gallstones, narrow-angle glaucoma, and elderly patients; not for use in patients with severe renal or hepatic impairment. Use caution with diabetes; antidiabetic agent requirements may be altered with anorexigens and concomitant dietary restrictions. Avoid concurrent use with other serotonergic agents, due to the risk of developing serotonin syndrome. Rare cases of bleeding have been reported; use caution in patients with bleeding disorders. Stimulants may unmask tics in individuals with coexisting Tourette's syndrome. Rare reports of depression, suicide and suicidal ideation have been documented; use caution and monitor closely in patients with history of psychiatric symptoms. May impair the ability to engage in potentially hazardous activities. Safety and efficacy have not been established in children <16 years of age.

Adverse Reactions

>10%:

Central nervous system: Headache (30%), insomnia (11%)

Gastrointestinal: Xerostomia (17%), anorexia (13%), constipation (12%)

1% to 10%:

Cardiovascular: Tachycardia (3%), vasodilation (2%), hypertension (2%), palpitation (2%), chest pain (2%)

Central nervous system: Dizziness (7%), nervousness (5%), anxiety (5%), depression (4%), somnolence (2%), CNS stimulation (2%), emotional lability (1%)

Dermatologic: Rash (4%)

Endocrine & metabolic: Dysmenorrhea (4%)

Gastrointestinal: Appetite increased (9%), nausea (6%), abdominal pain (5%), dyspepsia (5%), gastritis (2%), taste perversion (2%)

Genitourinary: Vaginal *Monilia* (1%)

Hepatic: Abnormal LFTs (2%)

Neuromuscular & skeletal: Back pain (8%), weakness (6%), arthralgia (6%), neck pain (2%), myalgia (2%), paresthesia (2%), tenosynovitis (1%), joint disorder (1%)

Otic: Ear disorder (2%)

Respiratory: Pharyngitis (10%), rhinitis (10%), sinusitis (5%), cough (4%)

Miscellaneous: Flu-like syndrome (8%), diaphoresis (3%), allergic reactions (2), thirst (2%)

<1%: Bruising

Frequency not defined:

Cardiovascular: Peripheral edema

Central nervous system: Thinking abnormal, agitation, fever

Dermatologic: Pruritus

Endocrine & metabolic: Menstrual disorders/irregularities

Gastrointestinal: Diarrhea, flatulence, gastroenteritis, tooth disorder

Neuromuscular & skeletal: Arthritis, hypertonia, leg cramps

Ocular: Amblyopia

Respiratory: Bronchitis, dyspnea

Postmarketing and/or case reports (frequency not defined; limited to important or life-threatening): Amnesia, anaphylactic shock, anaphylactoid reaction, anemia, angina, angioedema, arrhythmia, arthrosis, atrial fibrillation, blurred vision, cardiac arrest, cerebrovascular accident, CHF, cholecystitis, cholelithiasis, GI hemorrhage, goiter, hematuria, hyper-/hypoglycemia, hyper-/hypothyroidism, hypersensitivity reaction, impotence, interstitial nephritis, intestinal obstruction, intraocular pressure increased, leukopenia, lymphadenopathy, mania, mouth/stomach ulcer, mydriasis, photosensitivity, seizure, serotonin syndrome, stroke, suicidal ideation, syncope, thrombocytopenia, tongue edema, torsade de pointes, Tourette's syndrome, urinary retention, urticaria, transient ischemic attack, vascular headache, ventricular arrhythmia, vertigo

Metabolism/Transport Effects **Substrate** of CYP3A4 (major)

Drug Interactions

Cannabinoids: May enhance the tachycardic effect of Sympathomimetics. *Risk C: Monitor therapy*

CYP3A4 Inhibitors (Moderate): May decrease the metabolism of CYP3A4 Substrates. *Risk C: Monitor therapy*

CYP3A4 Inhibitors (Strong): May decrease the metabolism of CYP3A4 Substrates. *Risk D: Consider therapy modification*

Dasatinib: May increase the serum concentration of CYP3A4 Substrates. *Risk C: Monitor therapy*

Ergot Derivatives: Sibutramine may enhance the serotonergic effect of Ergot Derivatives. This may cause serotonin syndrome. *Risk X: Avoid combination*

Serotonin Modulators: Sibutramine may enhance the serotonergic effect of Serotonin Modulators. This may cause serotonin syndrome. *Risk X: Avoid combination*

Sympathomimetics: May enhance the adverse/toxic effect of other Sympathomimetics. *Risk C: Monitor therapy*

Ethanol/Nutrition/Herb Interactions

Ethanol: Avoid excess ethanol ingestion.

Herb/Nutraceutical: St John's wort and SAMe may decrease sibutramine levels.

Stability Store at room temperature of 15°C to 30°C (59°F to 86°F).

Mechanism of Action Sibutramine and its two primary metabolites block the neuronal uptake of norepinephrine, serotonin, and (to a lesser extent) dopamine. There is no monoamine-releasing (or depleting) activity.

Pharmacodynamics/Kinetics

Absorption: 77%; rapid

Protein binding, plasma: Parent drug and metabolites: >94%

Metabolism: Hepatic; undergoes first-pass metabolism via CYP3A4; forms two primary metabolites (M_1 and M_2; active)

Half-life elimination: Sibutramine: 1 hour; Metabolites: M_1: 14 hours; M_2: 16 hours

Time to peak: Sibutramine: 1.2 hours; Metabolites (M_1 and M_2): 3-4 hours

Excretion: Primarily urine (77% as inactive metabolites); feces

Dosage Children ≥16 years and Adults:

Initial: 10 mg once daily; after 4 weeks may titrate up to 15 mg once daily as needed and tolerated (may be used for up to 2 years, per manufacturer labeling)

Maintenance: 5-15 mg once daily

Dosage adjustment in renal/hepatic impairment: Should not be used in patients with severe renal or hepatic impairment

Dietary Considerations Sibutramine, as an appetite suppressant, is the most effective when combined with a low calorie diet and behavior modification counseling.

Administration May take with or without food.

Monitoring Parameters Weight, waist circumference, blood pressure, heart rate. Do initial blood pressure and heart rate evaluation and then monitor regularly during therapy. If patient has sustained increases in either blood pressure or pulse rate, consider discontinuing or reducing the dose of the drug.

Reference Range

Adult classification of weight by BMI (kg/m^2):

Underweight: <18.5

Normal: 18.5-24.9

Overweight: 25-29.9

Obese, class I: 30-34.9

Obese, class II: 35-39.9

Extreme obesity (class III): ≥40

Waist circumference: In adults with a BMI of 25-34.9 kg/m^2, high-risk waist circumference is defined as:

Men >102 cm (>40 in)

Women >88 cm (>35 in)

Additional Information Physicians should carefully evaluate patients for history of drug abuse and follow such patients closely, observing them for signs of misuse or abuse (eg, development of tolerance, excessive increases of doses, drug seeking behavior).

Dosage Forms Excipient information presented when available (limited, particularly for generics); consult specific product labeling.

Capsule, as hydrochloride:

Meridia®: 5 mg, 10 mg, 15 mg

- **Sibutramine Hydrochloride Monohydrate** *see* Sibutramine *on page 1479*
- **Siladryl® Allergy [OTC]** *see* DiphenhydrAMINE *on page 481*
- **Silafed® [OTC]** *see* Triprolidine and Pseudoephedrine *on page 1634*
- **Silapap® Children's [OTC]** *see* Acetaminophen *on page 30*
- **Silapap® Infants [OTC]** *see* Acetaminophen *on page 30*
- **Sildec [DSC]** *see* Carbinoxamine and Pseudoephedrine *on page 280*
- **Sildec PE [DSC]** *see* Chlorpheniramine and Phenylephrine *on page 323*
- **Sildec PE-DM** *see* Chlorpheniramine, Phenylephrine, and Dextromethorphan *on page 327*
- **Sildec Syrup** *see* Brompheniramine and Pseudoephedrine *on page 206*

Sildenafil (sil DEN a fil)

Medication Safety Issues

Sound-alike/look-alike issues:

Revatio® may be confused with ReVia®

Sildenafil may be confused with silodosin, tadalafil, vardenafil

Viagra® may be confused with Allegra®, Vaniqa™

U.S. Brand Names Revatio®; Viagra®

Canadian Brand Names Viagra®

Mexican Brand Names Viagra

Index Terms UK92480

Pharmacologic Category Phosphodiesterase-5 Enzyme Inhibitor

Generic Available No

Use

Revatio®: Treatment of pulmonary arterial hypertension (WHO Group I)

Viagra®: Treatment of erectile dysfunction (ED)

Unlabeled/Investigational Use Pulmonary arterial hypertension in children

Effect on Mental Status May cause dizziness

Effect on Psychiatric Treatment Useful for psychotropic-induced sexual dysfunction

Pregnancy Risk Factor B

Pregnancy Considerations Teratogenic effects were not observed in animal studies. There are no adequate and well-controlled studies in pregnant women. Less than 0.001% appears in the semen.

Lactation Excretion in breast milk unknown/use caution

Contraindications Hypersensitivity to sildenafil or any component of the formulation; concurrent use (regularly/intermittently) of organic nitrates in any form (eg, nitroglycerin, isosorbide dinitrate)

Warnings/Precautions Decreases in blood pressure may occur due to vasodilator effects; use with caution in patients with left ventricular outflow obstruction (aortic stenosis or hypertrophic obstructive cardiomyopathy); may be more sensitive to hypotensive actions. Concurrent use with alpha-adrenergic antagonist therapy or substantial ethanol consumption may cause symptomatic hypotension; patients should be hemodynamically stable prior to initiating therapy at the lowest possible dose. Use with caution in patients with hypotension (<90/50 mm Hg); uncontrolled hypertension (>170/110 mm Hg); life-threatening arrhythmias, stroke or MI within the last 6 months; cardiac failure or coronary artery disease causing unstable angina; safety and efficacy have not been studied in these patients. There is a degree of cardiac risk associated with sexual activity; therefore, physicians should consider the cardiovascular status of their patients prior to initiating any treatment for erectile dysfunction.

Sildenafil should be used with caution in patients with anatomical deformation of the penis (angulation, cavernosal fibrosis, or Peyronie's disease) and in patients who have conditions which may predispose them to priapism (sickle cell anemia, multiple myeloma, leukemia). All patients should be instructed to seek medical attention if erection persists >4 hours.

Vision loss may occur rarely and be a sign of nonarteritic anterior ischemic optic neuropathy (NAION). Risk may be increased with history of vision loss. Other risk factors for NAION include low cup-to-disc ratio ("crowded disc"), coronary artery disease, diabetes, hypertension, hyperlipidemia, smoking, and age >50 years. May cause dose-related impairment of color discrimination. Use caution in patients with retinitis pigmentosa; a minority have genetic disorders of retinal phosphodiesterases (no safety information available). Sudden decrease or loss of hearing has been reported rarely; hearing changes may be accompanied by tinnitus and dizziness. A direct relationship between therapy and vision or hearing loss has not been determined.

The potential underlying causes of erectile dysfunction should be evaluated prior to treatment. The safety and efficacy of sildenafil with other treatments for erectile dysfunction have not been established; use is not recommended. Efficacy with concurrent bosentan therapy has not been evaluated; use with caution. Use with caution in patients taking strong CYP3A4 inhibitors or alpha-blockers. Concomitant use with all forms of nitrates is contraindicated. If nitrate administration is medically necessary, it is not known when nitrates can be safely administered following the use of sildenafil (per manufacturer); the ACC/AHA 2007 guidelines supports administration of nitrates only if 24 hours have elapsed.

Use caution in patients with bleeding disorders or with active peptic ulcer disease; safety and efficacy have not been established. Use with caution in the elderly, or patients with renal or hepatic dysfunction; dose adjustment may be needed.

Adverse Reactions Based upon normal doses for either indication. (Adverse effects such as flushing, diarrhea, myalgia, and visual disturbances may be increased with doses >100 mg/24 hours.)

>10%:

Central nervous system: Headache (16% to 46%)

Gastrointestinal: Dyspepsia (7% to 17%; dose related)

2% to 10%:

Cardiovascular: Flushing (10%)

Central nervous system: Insomnia (≤7%), pyrexia (6%), dizziness (2%)

Dermatologic: Erythema (6%), rash (2%)

Gastrointestinal: Diarrhea (3% to 9%), gastritis (≤3%)

Genitourinary: Urinary tract infection (3%)

Hepatic: LFTs increased

Neuromuscular & skeletal: Myalgia (≤7%), paresthesia (≤3%)

Ocular: Abnormal vision (color changes, blurred vision, or increased sensitivity to light 3% to 11%; dose related)

Respiratory: Epistaxis (9% to 13%), dyspnea exacerbated (≤7%), nasal congestion (4%), rhinitis (4%), sinusitis (3%)

<2% (Limited to important or life-threatening): Allergic reaction, amnesia (transient global), anemia, angina pectoris, anorgasmia, asthma, AV block, cardiac arrest, cardiomyopathy, cataract, cerebral thrombosis, cerebrovascular hemorrhage, colitis, cystitis, depression, dysphagia, edema, exfoliative dermatitis, eye hemorrhage, gout, hearing decreased, hearing loss, heart failure, hematuria, hemorrhage, hyper-/hypoglycemia, hypernatremia, hyper-/hypotension, hyperuricemia, intracerebral hemorrhage, intraocular pressure increased, leukopenia, migraine, myocardial ischemia, MI, myasthenia, mydriasis, neuralgia, nonarteritic ischemic optic neuropathy (NAION), palpitation, postural hypotension, priapism, pulmonary hemorrhage, rectal hemorrhage, retinal vascular disease or bleeding, seizure, shock, stomatitis, subarachnoid hemorrhage, syncope, tachycardia, tendon rupture, TIA, urinary incontinence, ventricular arrhythmia, vertigo, visual field loss, vitreous detachment/traction, vomiting

Metabolism/Transport Effects **Substrate** of CYP2C9 (minor), 3A4 (major); **Inhibits** CYP1A2 (weak), 2C9 (weak), 2C19 (weak), 2D6 (weak), 2E1 (weak), 3A4 (weak)

Drug Interactions

Alpha1-Blockers: Phosphodiesterase 5 Inhibitors may enhance the hypotensive effect of Alpha1-Blockers. **Exceptions:** Dapiprazole [Off Market]. *Risk D: Consider therapy modification*

Antifungal Agents (Azole Derivatives, Systemic): May decrease the metabolism of Phosphodiesterase 5 Inhibitors. *Risk D: Consider therapy modification*

Bosentan: May increase the metabolism of Sildenafil. Sildenafil may increase the serum concentration of Bosentan. *Risk C: Monitor therapy*

CYP3A4 Inhibitors (Moderate): May decrease the metabolism of CYP3A4 Substrates. *Risk C: Monitor therapy*

CYP3A4 Inhibitors (Strong): May decrease the metabolism of CYP3A4 Substrates. *Risk D: Consider therapy modification*

Dasatinib: May increase the serum concentration of CYP3A4 Substrates. *Risk C: Monitor therapy*

Etravirine: May decrease the serum concentration of Phosphodiesterase 5 Inhibitors. Management: No empiric dosage adjustments are recommended with concomitant therapy; however, dose of the phosphodiesterase inhibitor may need to be altered based on clinical response. *Risk C: Monitor therapy*

HMG-CoA Reductase Inhibitors: Sildenafil may decrease the metabolism of HMG-CoA Reductase Inhibitors. **Exceptions:** Fluvastatin; Pravastatin; Rosuvastatin. *Risk D: Consider therapy modification*

Macrolide Antibiotics: May decrease the metabolism of Phosphodiesterase 5 Inhibitors. **Exceptions:** Azithromycin; Dirithromycin [Off Market]; Spiramycin. *Risk D: Consider therapy modification*

Protease Inhibitors: May decrease the metabolism of Phosphodiesterase 5 Inhibitors. Management: Dose restrictions for tadalafil, and/or sildenafil and vardenafil are recommended in combination with ritonavir, atazanavir, indinavir, darunavir and saquinavir. Consult specific prescribing information for detailed recommendations. *Risk D: Consider therapy modification*

Sapropterin: May enhance the hypotensive effect of Phosphodiesterase 5 Inhibitors. *Risk C: Monitor therapy*

Vasodilators (Organic Nitrates): Phosphodiesterase 5 Inhibitors may enhance the vasodilatory effect of Vasodilators (Organic Nitrates). *Risk X: Avoid combination*

Ethanol/Nutrition/Herb Interactions

Food: Amount and rate of absorption of sildenafil is reduced when taken with a high-fat meal. Serum concentrations/toxicity may be increased with grapefruit juice; avoid concurrent use.

Herb/Nutraceutical: St John's wort may decrease sildenafil levels.

Stability Store tablets at controlled room temperature of 25°C (77°F); excursions permitted to 15°C to 30°C (59°F to 86°F).

Mechanism of Action

Erectile dysfunction: Does not directly cause penile erections, but affects the response to sexual stimulation. The physiologic mechanism of erection of the penis involves release of nitric oxide (NO) in the corpus cavernosum during sexual stimulation. NO then activates the enzyme guanylate cyclase, which results in increased levels of cyclic guanosine monophosphate (cGMP), producing smooth muscle relaxation and inflow of blood to the corpus cavernosum. Sildenafil enhances the effect of NO by inhibiting phosphodiesterase type 5 (PDE-5), which is responsible for degradation of cGMP in the corpus cavernosum; when sexual stimulation causes local release of NO, inhibition of PDE-5 by sildenafil causes increased levels of cGMP in the corpus cavernosum, resulting in smooth muscle relaxation and inflow of blood to the corpus cavernosum; at recommended doses, it has no effect in the absence of sexual stimulation.

Pulmonary arterial hypertension (PAH): Inhibits phosphodiesterase type 5 (PDE-5) in smooth muscle of pulmonary vasculature where PDE-5 is responsible for the degradation of cyclic guanosine monophosphate (cGMP). Increased cGMP concentration results in pulmonary vasculature relaxation; vasodilation in the pulmonary bed and the systemic circulation (to a lesser degree) may occur.

Pharmacodynamics/Kinetics

Onset of action: ~60 minutes

Duration: 2-4 hours

Absorption: Rapid; slower with a high-fat meal

Distribution: V_{dss}: 105 L

Protein binding, plasma: ~96%

Metabolism: Hepatic via CYP3A4 (major) and CYP2C9 (minor route); forms metabolite (active)

Bioavailability: 40%

Half-life elimination: 4 hours

Time to peak: 30-120 minutes; delayed by 60 minutes with a high-fat meal

Excretion: Feces (80%); urine (13%)

Dosage Oral:

Children ≥1 month: Pulmonary arterial hypertension (unlabeled use): 0.25-2 mg/kg/dose every 4-6 hours. Most reports used 0.5 mg/kg/dose and titrated up to 2 mg/kg/dose

Adults:

Erectile dysfunction (Viagra®): Usual dose: 50 mg once daily 1 hour (range: 30 minutes to 4 hours) before sexual activity; dosing range: 25-100 mg once daily

Pulmonary arterial hypertension (Revatio®): Pulmonary arterial hypertension (Revatio®): 20 mg 3 times/day, taken 4-6 hours apart

Elderly >65 years: Use with caution

Revatio®: Refer to adult dosing.

Viagra®: Starting dose of 25 mg should be considered.

Dosage considerations for patients stable on alpha-blockers: Viagra®: Initial 25 mg

Dosage adjustment for concomitant use of potent CYP34A inhibitors:

Revatio®:

Erythromycin, saquinavir: No dosage adjustment

Itraconazole, ketoconazole, ritonavir: Not recommended

Viagra®:
Erythromycin, itraconazole, ketoconazole, saquinavir: Starting dose of 25 mg should be considered
Ritonavir: Maximum: 25 mg every 48 hours

Dosage adjustment in renal impairment:
Revatio®: Dose adjustment not necessary
Viagra®: Cl_{cr} <30 mL/minute: Starting dose of 25 mg should be considered

Dosage adjustment in hepatic impairment:
Revatio®: Child-Pugh class A and B: Dose adjustment not necessary
Viagra®: Child-Pugh class A and B: Starting dose of 25 mg should be considered; not studied in severe impairment (Child-Pugh class C)

Administration
Revatio®: Administer tablets at least 4-6 hours apart
Viagra®: Administer orally 30 minutes to 4 hours before sexual activity

Additional Information Sildenafil is ~10 times more selective for PDE-5 as compared to PDE6. This enzyme is found in the retina and is involved in phototransduction. At higher plasma levels, interference with PDE6 is believed to be the basis for changes in color vision noted in some patients.

Dosage Forms Excipient information presented when available (limited, particularly for generics); consult specific product labeling.
Tablet:
Revatio®: 20 mg
Viagra®: 25 mg, 50 mg, 100 mg

- **Silexin [OTC]** *see* Guaifenesin and Dextromethorphan *on page 739*
- **Silfedrine Children's [OTC]** *see* Pseudoephedrine *on page 1367*
- **Silphen® [OTC]** *see* DiphenhydrAMINE *on page 481*
- **Silphen DM® [OTC]** *see* Dextromethorphan *on page 448*
- **Sil-Tex** *see* Guaifenesin and Phenylephrine *on page 742*
- **Siltussin DAS [OTC]** *see* GuaiFENesin *on page 737*
- **Siltussin DM [OTC]** *see* Guaifenesin and Dextromethorphan *on page 739*
- **Siltussin DM DAS [OTC]** *see* Guaifenesin and Dextromethorphan *on page 739*
- **Siltussin SA [OTC]** *see* GuaiFENesin *on page 737*
- **Silvadene®** *see* Silver Sulfadiazine *on page 1485*
- **Silver Apricot** *see* Ginkgo *(Ginkgo biloba) on page 715*

Silver Sulfadiazine (SIL ver sul fa DYE a zeen)

U.S. Brand Names Silvadene®; SSD®; SSD® AF; Thermazene®
Canadian Brand Names Flamazine®
Mexican Brand Names Silvadene
Pharmacologic Category Antibiotic, Topical
Use Prevention and treatment of infection in second and third degree burns
Effect on Mental Status None reported
Effect on Psychiatric Treatment May cause leukopenia; use caution with clozapine and carbamazepine

Dosage Summary
Topical:
Children: Apply to a thickness of 1/16" once or twice daily
Adults: Apply to a thickness of 1/16" once or twice daily

Dosage Forms Excipient information presented when available (limited, particularly for generics); consult specific product labeling.
Cream, topical: 1% (25 g, 50 g, 85 g, 400 g)
Silvadene®, Thermazene®: 1% (20 g, 50 g, 85 g, 400 g, 1000 g)
SSD®: 1% (25 g, 50 g, 85 g, 400 g)
SSD® AF: 1% (50 g, 400 g)

- **Simcor®** *see* Niacin and Simvastatin *on page 1127*
- **Simethicone, Aluminum Hydroxide, and Magnesium Hydroxide** *see* Aluminum Hydroxide, Magnesium Hydroxide, and Simethicone *on page 78*
- **Simethicone and Loperamide Hydrochloride** *see* Loperamide and Simethicone *on page 944*
- **Simethicone and Magaldrate** *see* Magaldrate and Simethicone *on page 965*
- **Simply Sleep® [OTC]** *see* DiphenhydrAMINE *on page 481*
- **Simuc [DSC]** *see* Guaifenesin and Phenylephrine *on page 742*
- **Simuc-DM** *see* Guaifenesin and Dextromethorphan *on page 739*

◆ **Simulect®** *see* Basiliximab *on page 171*

Simvastatin (sim va STAT in)

Medication Safety Issues
Sound-alike/look-alike issues:
Zocor® may be confused with Cozaar®, Yocon®, Zoloft®

International issues:
Cardin® [Poland] may be confused with Cardene® which is a brand name for nicardipine in the U.S.
Cardin® [Poland] may be confused with Cardem® which is a brand name for celiprolol in Spain

Related Information
Lipid-Lowering Agents *on page 1786*

U.S. Brand Names Zocor®

Canadian Brand Names Apo-Simvastatin®; CO Simvastatin; Dom-Simvastatin; Gen-Simvastatin; Novo-Simvastatin; Nu-Simvastatin; PHL-Simvastatin; PMS-Simvastatin; ratio-Simvastatin; Riva-Simvastatin; Sandoz-Simvastatin; Taro-Simvastatin; Zocor®

Mexican Brand Names Colesken; Pusarat; Simlo; Simplaqor; Tulip; Zeid; Zocor; Zorced

Pharmacologic Category Antilipemic Agent, HMG-CoA Reductase Inhibitor

Generic Available Yes

Use Used with dietary therapy for the following:
Secondary prevention of cardiovascular events in hypercholesterolemic patients with established coronary heart disease (CHD) or at high risk for CHD: To reduce cardiovascular morbidity (myocardial infarction, coronary revascularization procedures) and mortality; to reduce the risk of stroke and transient ischemic attacks
Hyperlipidemias: To reduce elevations in total cholesterol, LDL-C, apolipoprotein B, and triglycerides, and increase HDL-C in patients with primary hypercholesterolemia (elevations of 1 or more components are present in Fredrickson type IIa, IIb, III, and IV hyperlipidemias); treatment of homozygous familial hypercholesterolemia
Heterozygous familial hypercholesterolemia (HeFH): In adolescent patients (10-17 years of age, females >1 year postmenarche) with HeFH having LDL-C ≥190 mg/dL **or** LDL ≥160 mg/dL with positive family history of premature cardiovascular disease (CVD), or 2 or more CVD risk factors in the adolescent patient

Effect on Mental Status May cause drowsiness

Effect on Psychiatric Treatment Rhabdomyolysis with acute renal failure has occurred; risk is increased with concurrent use of fluvoxamine nefazodone and verapamil

Pregnancy Risk Factor X

Pregnancy Considerations Cholesterol biosynthesis may be important in fetal development. Contraindicated in pregnancy. Administer to women of child-bearing potential only when conception is highly unlikely and patients have been informed of potential hazards. If pregnancy occurs during treatment, discontinue simvastatin immediately.

Lactation Excretion in breast milk unknown/contraindicated

Contraindications Hypersensitivity to simvastatin or any component of the formulation; active liver disease; unexplained persistent elevations of serum transaminases; pregnancy; breast-feeding

Warnings/Precautions Secondary causes of hyperlipidemia should be ruled out prior to therapy. Liver function must be monitored by laboratory assessment. Rhabdomyolysis with acute renal failure has occurred. Risk is dose-related and is increased with concurrent use of lipid-lowering agents which may cause rhabdomyolysis (gemfibrozil, fibric acid derivatives, or niacin at doses ≥1 g/day), during concurrent use with danazol or strong CYP3A4 inhibitors (including amiodarone, clarithromycin, cyclosporine, erythromycin, telithromycin, itraconazole, ketoconazole, nefazodone, grapefruit juice in large quantities, verapamil, or protease inhibitors such as indinavir, nelfinavir, or ritonavir). Monitor closely if used with other drugs associated with myopathy (eg, colchicine). Weigh the risk versus benefit when combining any of these drugs with simvastatin. Do not initiate simvastatin-containing treatment in a patient with pre-existing therapy of cyclosporine or danazol, unless the patient has previously demonstrated tolerance to ≥5 mg/day simvastatin. Temporarily discontinue in any patient experiencing an acute or serious major medical or surgical condition which may increase the risk of rhabdomyolysis. Discontinue temporarily for elective surgical procedures. Based upon current evidence,

HMG-CoA reductase inhibitor therapy should be continued in the perioperative period unless risk outweighs cardioprotective benefit. Use caution in patients with renal insufficiency. Use with caution in patients with advanced age, these patients are predisposed to myopathy. Use with caution in patients who consume large amounts of ethanol or have a history of liver disease. Use is contraindicated with active liver disease and with unexplained transaminase elevations. Safety and efficacy have not been established in patients <10 years of age or in premenarcheal girls.

Adverse Reactions

1% to 10%:

Gastrointestinal: Constipation (2%), flatulence (1% to 2%), dyspepsia (1%)

Hepatic: Transaminases increased (>3x ULN; 1%)

Neuromuscular & skeletal: CPK elevation (>3x normal on one or more occasions; 5%)

Respiratory: Upper respiratory infection (2%)

<1% (Limited to important or life-threatening): Abdominal pain, depression, dermatomyositis, diarrhea, dizziness, fatigue, headache, hypotension, insomnia, lichen planus, muscle pain, muscle tenderness, muscle weakness, myopathy, nausea, photosensitivity, pruritus, thrombocytopenia, vertigo, weakness

Additional class-related events or case reports (not necessarily reported with simvastatin therapy): Alopecia, alkaline phosphatase increased, alteration in taste, alopecia, anaphylaxis, angioedema, anorexia, anxiety, arthralgia, arthritis, bilirubin increased, cataracts, chills, cholestatic jaundice, cirrhosis, decreased libido, depression, dermatomyositis, dryness of skin/mucous membranes, dyspnea, eosinophilia, erectile dysfunction/impotence, erythema multiforme, facial paresis, fatty liver, fever, flushing, fulminant hepatic necrosis, gynecomastia, hemolytic anemia, hepatic failure, hepatitis, hepatoma, hyperbilirubinemia, hypersensitivity reaction, impaired extraocular muscle movement, increased alkaline phosphatase, increased CPK (>10x normal), increased ESR, increased GGT, leukopenia, malaise, memory loss, myopathy, nail changes, nodules, ophthalmoplegia, pancreatitis, paresthesia, peripheral nerve palsy, peripheral neuropathy, photosensitivity, polymyalgia rheumatica, positive ANA, pruritus, psychic disturbance, purpura, rash, renal failure (secondary to rhabdomyolysis), rhabdomyolysis, skin discoloration, Stevens-Johnson syndrome, systemic lupus erythematosus-like syndrome, thrombocytopenia, thyroid dysfunction, toxic epidermal necrolysis, transaminases increased, tremor, urticaria, vasculitis, vertigo, vomiting

Metabolism/Transport Effects **Substrate** of CYP3A4 (major); **Inhibits** CYP2C8 (weak), 2C9 (weak), 2D6 (weak)

Drug Interactions

Amiodarone: May decrease the metabolism of HMG-CoA Reductase Inhibitors. Management: Dose of simvastatin should not exceed 20 mg/day during concurrent therapy. *Risk D: Consider therapy modification*

Antifungal Agents (Azole Derivatives, Systemic): May decrease the metabolism of HMG-CoA Reductase Inhibitors. *Risk D: Consider therapy modification*

Bosentan: May increase the metabolism of HMG-CoA Reductase Inhibitors. *Risk C: Monitor therapy*

Calcium Channel Blockers (Nondihydropyridine): May decrease the metabolism of HMG-CoA Reductase Inhibitors. *Risk D: Consider therapy modification*

Colchicine: May enhance the myopathic (rhabdomyolysis) effect of HMG-CoA Reductase Inhibitors. Colchicine may increase the serum concentration of HMG-CoA Reductase Inhibitors. *Risk D: Consider therapy modification*

CycloSPORINE: May increase the serum concentration of HMG-CoA Reductase Inhibitors. *Risk D: Consider therapy modification*

CYP3A4 Inducers (Strong): May increase the metabolism of CYP3A4 Substrates. *Risk C: Monitor therapy*

CYP3A4 Inhibitors (Moderate): May decrease the metabolism of CYP3A4 Substrates. *Risk C: Monitor therapy*

CYP3A4 Inhibitors (Strong): May decrease the metabolism of CYP3A4 Substrates. *Risk D: Consider therapy modification*

Danazol: May decrease the metabolism of HMG-CoA Reductase Inhibitors. *Risk C: Monitor therapy*

DAPTOmycin: HMG-CoA Reductase Inhibitors may enhance the adverse/toxic effect of DAPTOmycin. Specifically, the risk of skeletal muscle toxicity may be increased. Management: Consider temporarily stopping HMG-CoA reductase inhibitor therapy prior to daptomycin. If used together, regular (i.e., at least weekly) monitoring of CPK concentrations is recommended. *Risk D: Consider therapy modification*

Dasatinib: May increase the serum concentration of CYP3A4 Substrates. *Risk C: Monitor therapy*

Deferasirox: May decrease the serum concentration of CYP3A4 Substrates. *Risk C: Monitor therapy*

Etravirine: May decrease the serum concentration of HMG-CoA Reductase Inhibitors. This applies to atorvastatin, lovastatin and simvastatin. Conversely, levels of fluvastatin may be increased. Management: Dose adjustment of the HMG-CoA reductase inhibitor may be warranted. No interaction is expected with rosuvastatin or pravastatin. *Risk C: Monitor therapy*

Fenofibrate: May enhance the adverse/toxic effect of HMG-CoA Reductase Inhibitors. *Risk C: Monitor therapy*

Fluconazole: May decrease the metabolism of HMG-CoA Reductase Inhibitors. *Risk D: Consider therapy modification*

Gemfibrozil: May enhance the myopathic (rhabdomyolysis) effect of HMG-CoA Reductase Inhibitors. Gemfibrozil may increase the serum concentration of HMG-CoA Reductase Inhibitors. *Risk D: Consider therapy modification*

Grapefruit Juice: May decrease the metabolism of HMG-CoA Reductase Inhibitors. *Risk D: Consider therapy modification*

Imatinib: May decrease the metabolism of Simvastatin. *Risk C: Monitor therapy*

Macrolide Antibiotics: May decrease the metabolism of HMG-CoA Reductase Inhibitors. **Exceptions:** Azithromycin; Dirithromycin [Off Market]; Spiramycin. *Risk D: Consider therapy modification*

Nefazodone: May decrease the metabolism of HMG-CoA Reductase Inhibitors. *Risk D: Consider therapy modification*

Niacin: May enhance the adverse/toxic effect of HMG-CoA Reductase Inhibitors. *Risk C: Monitor therapy*

Niacinamide: May enhance the adverse/toxic effect of HMG-CoA Reductase Inhibitors. *Risk C: Monitor therapy*

Phenytoin: May increase the metabolism of HMG-CoA Reductase Inhibitors. *Risk D: Consider therapy modification*

Protease Inhibitors: May increase the serum concentration of HMG-CoA Reductase Inhibitors. Limited data suggest pravastatin may slightly decrease protease inhibitor concentrations. Management: Lovastatin and simvastatin are contraindicated with many protease inhibitors; use lowest possible HMG-CoA reductase inhibitor dose and monitor for signs and symptoms of rhabdomyolysis if these agents are used concomitantly. *Risk D: Consider therapy modification*

Ranolazine: May increase the serum concentration of Simvastatin. *Risk C: Monitor therapy*

Rifamycin Derivatives: May increase the metabolism of HMG-CoA Reductase Inhibitors. *Risk D: Consider therapy modification*

Sildenafil: May decrease the metabolism of HMG-CoA Reductase Inhibitors. *Risk D: Consider therapy modification*

St Johns Wort: May increase the metabolism of HMG-CoA Reductase Inhibitors. *Risk C: Monitor therapy*

Vitamin K Antagonists (eg, warfarin): HMG-CoA Reductase Inhibitors may enhance the anticoagulant effect of Vitamin K Antagonists. *Risk C: Monitor therapy*

Ethanol/Nutrition/Herb Interactions

Ethanol: Avoid excessive ethanol consumption (due to potential hepatic effects).

Food: Simvastatin serum concentration may be increased when taken with grapefruit juice; avoid concurrent intake of large quantities (>1 quart/day). Red yeast rice contains an estimated 2.4 mg lovastatin per 600 mg rice.

Herb/Nutraceutical: St John's wort may decrease simvastatin levels.

Stability Tablets should be stored in tightly-closed containers at temperatures between 5°C to 30°C (41°F to 86°F).

Mechanism of Action Simvastatin is a methylated derivative of lovastatin that acts by competitively inhibiting 3-hydroxy-3-methylglutaryl-coenzyme A (HMG-CoA) reductase, the enzyme that catalyzes the rate-limiting step in cholesterol biosynthesis

Pharmacodynamics/Kinetics

Onset of action: >3 days

Peak effect: 2 weeks

Absorption: 85%

Protein binding:~95%

Metabolism: Hepatic via CYP3A4; extensive first-pass effect

Bioavailability: <5%

Half-life elimination: Unknown

Time to peak: 1.3-2.4 hours

Excretion: Feces (60%); urine (13%)

Dosage Oral: **Note:** Doses should be individualized according to the baseline LDL-cholesterol levels, the recommended goal of therapy, and the patient's response; adjustments should be made at intervals of 4 weeks or more; doses may need adjusted based on concomitant medications

Children 10-17 years (females >1 year postmenarche): HeFH: 10 mg once daily in the evening; range: 10-40 mg/day (maximum: 40 mg/day)

Dosage adjustment for simvastatin with concomitant amiodarone, cyclosporine, danazol, gemfibrozil, or verapamil: Refer to drug-specific dosing in adult dosing section

Adults:

Homozygous familial hypercholesterolemia: 40 mg once daily in the evening **or** 80 mg/day (given as 20 mg, 20 mg, and 40 mg evening dose)

Prevention of cardiovascular events, hyperlipidemias: 20-40 mg once daily in the evening; range: 5-80 mg/day

Patients requiring only moderate reduction of LDL-cholesterol may be started at 10 mg once daily

Patients requiring reduction of >45% in low-density lipoprotein (LDL) cholesterol may be started at 40 mg once daily in the evening

Patients with CHD or at high risk for CHD: Dosing should be started at 40 mg once daily in the evening; simvastatin should be started simultaneously with diet therapy.

Dosage adjustment with concomitant medications:

Cyclosporine or danazol: Initial: 5 mg simvastatin, should **not** exceed 10 mg/day

Gemfibrozil: Simvastatin dose should **not** exceed 10 mg/day

Amiodarone or verapamil: Simvastatin dose should **not** exceed 20 mg/day

Dosing adjustment/comments in renal impairment: Because simvastatin does not undergo significant renal excretion, modification of dose should not be necessary in patients with mild to moderate renal insufficiency.

Severe renal impairment: Cl_{cr} <10 mL/minute: Initial: 5 mg/day with close monitoring.

Dietary Considerations Red yeast rice contains an estimated 2.4 mg lovastatin per 600 mg rice.

Administration May be taken without regard to meals. Administer in the evening for maximal efficacy.

Monitoring Parameters Creatine phosphokinase levels due to possibility of myopathy; serum cholesterol (total and fractionated)

Obtain liver function tests prior to initiation, dose, and thereafter when clinically indicated. Patients titrated to the 80 mg dose should be tested prior to initiation and 3 months after initiating the 80 mg dose. Thereafter, periodic monitoring (ie, semiannually) is recommended for the first year of treatment. Patients with elevated transaminase levels should have a second (confirmatory) test and frequent monitoring until values normalize. Discontinue if increase in ALT/AST is persistently >3 times ULN.

Dosage Forms Excipient information presented when available (limited, particularly for generics); consult specific product labeling. [DSC] = Discontinued product

Tablet: 5 mg, 10 mg, 20 mg, 40 mg, 80 mg

Zocor®: 5 mg [DSC]; 10 mg, 20 mg, 40 mg, 80 mg

- ◆ **Simvastatin and Ezetimibe** *see* Ezetimibe and Simvastatin *on page 611*
- ◆ **Simvastatin and Niacin** *see* Niacin and Simvastatin *on page 1127*
- ◆ **Sina-12X** *see* Guaifenesin and Phenylephrine *on page 742*

Sincalide (SIN ka lide)

U.S. Brand Names Kinevac®

Index Terms C8-CCK; OP-CCK

Pharmacologic Category Diagnostic Agent

Use Postevacuation cholecystography; gallbladder bile sampling; stimulate pancreatic secretion for analysis; accelerate the transit of barium through the small bowel

Effect on Mental Status May cause dizziness

Effect on Psychiatric Treatment None reported

Dosage Summary

I.M.:

Children: Dosage not established

Adults: 0.1 mcg/kg

I.V.:

Children: Dosage not established

Adults: 0.02-0.04 mcg/kg over 30-60 seconds, may repeat **or** 0.02 mcg/kg over 30 minutes **or** 0.12 mcg/kg in 30 or 100 mL of NS over 30-50 minutes

Dosage Forms Excipient information presented when available (limited, particularly for generics); consult specific product labeling.

Injection, powder for reconstitution: 5 mcg [contains sodium metabisulfite]

- **Sinemet®** *see* Carbidopa and Levodopa *on page 277*
- **Sinemet® CR** *see* Carbidopa and Levodopa *on page 277*
- **Sinequan® [DSC]** *see* Doxepin *on page 502*
- **Singulair®** *see* Montelukast *on page 1074*
- **Sinutab® Non-Drying [OTC]** *see* Guaifenesin and Pseudoephedrine *on page 744*
- **Sinutab® Sinus [OTC]** *see* Acetaminophen and Phenylephrine *on page 36*
- **Sinutab® Sinus Allergy Maximum Strength [OTC]** *see* Acetaminophen, Chlorpheniramine, and Pseudoephedrine *on page 40*
- **SINUtuss® DM** *see* Guaifenesin, Dextromethorphan, and Phenylephrine *on page 746*
- **SINUvent® PE** *see* Guaifenesin and Phenylephrine *on page 742*
- **Sirdalud®** *see* TiZANidine *on page 1587*

Sirolimus (sir OH li mus)

Medication Safety Issues

Sound-alike/look-alike issues:

Rapamune® may be confused with Rapaflo®

Sirolimus may be confused with tacrolimus, temsirolimus

U.S. Brand Names Rapamune®

Canadian Brand Names Rapamune®

Mexican Brand Names Rapamune

Pharmacologic Category Immunosuppressant Agent; mTOR Kinase Inhibitor

Use Prophylaxis of organ rejection in patients receiving renal transplants, in combination with corticosteroids and cyclosporine (cyclosporine may be withdrawn in low-to-moderate immunological risk patients after 2-4 months, in conjunction with an increase in sirolimus dosage; in high-risk patients, use in combination with cyclosporine and corticosteroids is recommended for the first year)

Unlabeled/Investigational Use Prophylaxis of organ rejection in heart transplant recipients; immunosuppression in peripheral stem cell/bone marrow transplantation

Effect on Mental Status Insomnia is common; may cause anxiety, confusion, depression, emotional lability, and somnolence

Effect on Psychiatric Treatment Leukopenia is common; use caution with clozapine and carbamazepine; nefazodone may increase serum levels of sirolimus

Dosage Summary

Oral:

Children <13 years: Dosage not established

Children ≥13 years and <40 kg: Low-to-moderate risk: Loading dose: 3 mg/m^2 on day 1; Maintenance: 1 mg/m^2/day; titrate to therapeutic dose based on levels

Children ≥13 years and ≥40 kg: Low-to-moderate risk: Loading dose: 6 mg on day 1; Maintenance: 2 mg/day; titrate to therapeutic dose based on levels; maximum daily dose: 40 mg; may divide larger doses (including loading dose) over 2 days

Adults <40 kg: Low-to-moderate risk: Loading dose: 3 mg/m^2 on day 1; Maintenance: 1 mg/m^2/day; titrate to therapeutic dose based on levels; maximum dose in 1 day: 40 mg; if required dose is >40 mg (due to loading dose), divide over 2 days

Adults ≥40 kg: Low-to-moderate risk: Loading dose: 6 mg on day 1; Maintenance: 2 mg/day; titrate to therapeutic dose based on levels; maximum daily dose: 40 mg; may divide larger doses (including loading dose) over 2 days; High risk: Loading dose: Up to 15 mg on day 1; maintenance: 5 mg/day; titrate to therapeutic dose based on levels; maximum dose in 1 day: 40 mg; if required dose is >40 mg (due to loading dose) divide over 2 days

Dosage Forms Excipient information presented when available (limited, particularly for generics); consult specific product labeling.

Solution, oral:
Rapamune®: 1 mg/mL (60 mL) [contains ethanol 1.5% to 2.5%; packaged with oral syringes and a carrying case]
Tablet:
Rapamune®: 1 mg, 2 mg

SitaGLIPtin (sit a GLIP tin)

Medication Safety Issues
Sound-alike/look-alike issues:
Januvia™ may be confused with Jantoven™
SitaGLIPtin may be confused with SUMAtriptan

U.S. Brand Names Januvia™

Mexican Brand Names Januvia

Index Terms MK-0431; Sitagliptin Phosphate

Pharmacologic Category Antidiabetic Agent, Dipeptidyl Peptidase IV (DPP-IV) Inhibitor

Generic Available No

Use
U.S. labeling: Management of type 2 diabetes mellitus (noninsulin dependent, NIDDM) as an adjunct to diet and exercise as monotherapy or in combination therapy with other antidiabetic agents
Canadian labeling: Management of NIDDM in combination with metformin therapy, diet, and exercise. **Note:** Use as monotherapy is not approved in Canadian labeling.

Effect on Mental Status None reported

Effect on Psychiatric Treatment May produce GI side effects; concomitant use with SSRIs, carbamazepine, valproic acid, and lithium may produce additive effects

Pregnancy Risk Factor B

Pregnancy Considerations Adverse events have not been observed in animal reproduction studies; therefore, sitagliptan is classified as pregnancy category B. There are no adequate and well controlled studies in pregnant women. Maternal hyperglycemia can be associated with adverse effects in the fetus, including macrosomia, neonatal hyperglycemia, and hyperbilirubinemia; the risk of congenital malformations is increased when the Hb A_{1c} is above the normal range. Diabetes can also be associated with adverse effects in the mother. Poorly-treated diabetes may cause end-organ damage that may in turn negatively affect obstetric outcomes. Physiologic glucose levels should be maintained prior to and during pregnancy to decrease the risk of adverse events in the mother and the fetus. Until additional safety and efficacy data are obtained, the use of oral agents is generally not recommended as routine management of GDM or type 2 diabetes mellitus during pregnancy. Insulin is the drug of choice for the control of diabetes mellitus during pregnancy. Health professionals are encouraged to report any prenatal exposure to sitagliptin by contacting Merck's pregnancy registry (1-800-986-8999).

Lactation Excretion in breast milk unknown/use caution

Contraindications Serious hypersensitivity (eg, anaphylaxis, angioedema) or any component of the formulation; type 1 diabetes mellitus (insulin dependent, IDDM), diabetic ketoacidosis

Warnings/Precautions Use caution when used in conjunction with sulfonylureas; risk of hypoglycemia is increased. Monitor blood glucose closely; dosage adjustments of the sulfonylurea may be necessary. Use with caution in patients with moderate-to-severe renal dysfunction and end-stage renal disease (ESRD) requiring hemodialysis or peritoneal dialysis; dosing adjustment required. Rare hypersensitivity reactions, including anaphylaxis, angioedema, and/or severe dermatologic reactions such as Stevens-Johnson syndrome, have been reported in postmarketing surveillance; discontinue if signs/symptoms of hypersensitivity reactions occur. Safety and efficacy have not been established in children <18 years of age.

Adverse Reactions
1% to 10%:
Gastrointestinal: Diarrhea (3%), abdominal pain (2%), nausea (1%)
Respiratory: Nasopharyngitis (5%)
Postmarketing and/or case reports: Anaphylaxis, angioedema, exfoliative dermatitis, hypoglycemia (risk increased in conjunction with sulfonylureas), hypersensitivity, rash, serum creatinine increased, Stevens-Johnson syndrome, urticaria, white blood cells increased

Metabolism/Transport Effects Substrate (minor) of CYP2C8, 3A4

Drug Interactions
There are no known significant interactions.

Stability Store at 20°C to 25°C (68°F to 77°F).

Mechanism of Action Sitagliptin inhibits dipeptidyl peptidase IV (DPP-IV) enzyme resulting in prolonged active incretin levels. Incretin hormones (eg, glucagon-like peptide-1 [GLP-1] and glucose-dependent insulinotropic polypeptide [GIP]) regulate glucose homeostasis by increasing insulin synthesis and release from pancreatic beta cells and decreasing glucagon secretion from pancreatic alpha cells. Decreased glucagon secretion results in decreased hepatic glucose production. Under normal physiologic circumstances, incretin hormones are released by the intestine throughout the day and levels are increased in response to a meal; incretin hormones are rapidly inactivated by the DPP-IV enzyme.

Pharmacodynamics/Kinetics

Absorption: Rapid

Distribution: ~198 L

Protein binding: 38%

Metabolism: Not extensively metabolized; minor metabolism via CYP3A4 and 2C8 to metabolites (inactive) suggested by *in vitro* studies

Bioavailability: ~87%

Half-life elimination: 12 hours

Time to peak, plasma: 1-4 hours

Excretion: Urine 87% (79% as unchanged drug, 16% as metabolites); feces 13%

Dosage Oral: Adults: Type 2 diabetes: 100 mg once daily

Concomitant use with sulfonylureas: Reduced dose of sulfonylurea may be needed

Dosage adjustment in renal impairment:

Cl_{cr} ≥50 mL/minute: No adjustment required

Cl_{cr} ≥30 to <50 mL/minute: 50 mg once daily

S_{cr}: Males: >1.7 to ≤3.0 mg/dL; Females: >1.5 to ≤2.5 mg/dL: 50 mg once daily

Cl_{cr}<30 mL/minute: 25 mg once daily

S_{cr}: Males: >3.0 mg/dL; Females: >2.5 mg/dL: 25 mg once daily

ESRD requiring hemodialysis or peritoneal dialysis: 25 mg once daily; administered without regard to timing of hemodialysis

Dosage adjustment in hepatic impairment:

Mild-to-moderate impairment (Child-Pugh score 7-9): No dosage adjustment required

Severe impairment (Child-Pugh score >9): Not studied

Dietary Considerations May be taken with or without food.

Administration May be administered with or without food.

Monitoring Parameters Hgb A_{1C} and serum glucose; renal function prior to initiation and periodically during treatment.

Reference Range Recommendations for glycemic control in adults with diabetes:

Hb A_{1c}: <7%

Preprandial capillary plasma glucose: 70-130 mg/dL

Peak postprandial capillary blood glucose: <180 mg/dL

Blood pressure: <130/80 mm Hg

Dosage Forms Excipient information presented when available (limited, particularly for generics); consult specific product labeling.

Tablet:

Januvia™: 25 mg, 50 mg, 100 mg

Sitagliptin and Metformin (sit a GLIP tin & met FOR min)

Medication Safety Issues

Sound-alike/look-alike issues:

Janumet™ may be confused with Jantoven™

U.S. Brand Names Janumet™

Index Terms Metformin and Sitagliptin; Sitagliptin Phosphate and Metformin Hydrochloride

Pharmacologic Category Antidiabetic Agent, Biguanide; Antidiabetic Agent, Dipeptidyl Peptidase IV (DPP-IV) Inhibitor; Hypoglycemic Agent, Oral

Use Management of type 2 diabetes mellitus (noninsulin dependent, NIDDM) in patients not adequately controlled on metformin or sitagliptin monotherapy and as an adjunct to diet and exercise

Effect on Mental Status May cause dizziness

Effect on Psychiatric Treatment GI side effects are common; concurrent use with lithium, carbamazepine, valproic acid, and SSRIs may produce additive effects.

Dosage Summary

Oral:

Children: Dosage not established

Adults: Sitagliptin 50 mg and metformin 500-1000 mg twice daily (maximum: 100 mg/day [sitagliptin], 2000 mg/day [metformin])

Elderly <80 years: Initial and maintenance dosing should be conservative, due to the potential for decreased renal function

Elderly ≥80 years: Do not use unless normal renal function has been established

Dosage Forms Excipient information presented when available (limited, particularly for generics); consult specific product labeling.

Tablet:

Janumet™:

50/500: Sitagliptin 50 mg and metformin hydrochloride 500 mg

50/1000: Sitagliptin 50 mg and metformin hydrochloride 1000 mg

- **Sitagliptin Phosphate** *see* SitaGLIPtin *on page 1491*
- **Sitagliptin Phosphate and Metformin Hydrochloride** *see* Sitagliptin and Metformin *on page 1492*
- **SJW** *see* St John's Wort *(Hypericum perforatum) on page 1506*
- **Skelaxin®** *see* Metaxalone *on page 996*
- **Skelid®** *see* Tiludronate *on page 1583*
- **SKF 104864** *see* Topotecan *on page 1602*
- **SKF 104864-A** *see* Topotecan *on page 1602*
- **Sleep-ettes D [OTC]** *see* DiphenhydrAMINE *on page 481*
- **Sleepinal® [OTC]** *see* DiphenhydrAMINE *on page 481*
- **Slo-Niacin® [OTC]** *see* Niacin *on page 1124*
- **Slow FE® [OTC]** *see* Ferrous Sulfate *on page 627*
- **Slow-Mag® [OTC]** *see* Magnesium Chloride *on page 965*

Smallpox Vaccine (SMAL poks vak SEEN)

U.S. Brand Names ACAM2000™

Index Terms Dried Smallpox Vaccine; Live Smallpox Vaccine; Vaccinia Vaccine

Pharmacologic Category Vaccine

Use Active immunization against vaccinia virus, the causative agent of smallpox in persons determined to be at risk for smallpox infection. The ACIP recommends vaccination of laboratory workers at risk of exposure from cultures or contaminated animals which may be a source of vaccinia or related Orthopoxviruses capable of causing infections in humans (monkeypox, cowpox, or variola). The ACIP also recommends that consideration be given for vaccination in healthcare workers having contact with clinical specimens, contaminated material, or patients receiving vaccinia or recombinant vaccinia viruses. ACIP recommends revaccination every 10 years. The Armed Forces recommend vaccination of certain personnel categories. Recommendations for use in response to bioterrorism are regularly updated by the CDC, and may be found at www.cdc.gov.

Effect on Mental Status Fatigue is common; may rarely cause encephalitis and encephalopathy

Effect on Psychiatric Treatment None reported

Restrictions The smallpox vaccine is not available for general public use. All supplies are currently owned by the federal government for inclusion in the Strategic National Stockpile. In October 2002, the FDA approved the licensing of the stockpile of smallpox vaccine. This approval allows the vaccine to be distributed and administered in the event of a smallpox attack. The bulk of current supplies have been designated for use by the U.S. military. Additionally, laboratory workers who may be at risk of exposure may require vaccination. Bioterrorism experts have proposed immunization of first responders (including police, fire, and emergency workers), but these plans may not be implemented until additional stocks of vaccine are licensed.

ACAM2000™ is subject to a Risk Minimization Action Plan (RiskMAP) which includes mandatory adverse event reporting, risk management evaluation, and education for both healthcare providers administering the vaccine and patients. Patients who receive the vaccine must be given an FDA-approved medication guide which is available at http://www.fda.gov/cber/label/acam2000pi.pdf.

Dosage Summary

Scarification:

Children <12 months: Dosage not established

Children ≥12 months: ACAM2000™: Emergency conditions only: A single drop of vaccine suspension and 15 needle punctures into superficial skin for both primary vaccination and revaccination.

Adults: ACAM2000™: A single drop of vaccine suspension and 15 needle punctures into superficial skin for both primary vaccination and revaccination

Dosage Forms Excipient information presented when available (limited, particularly for generics); consult specific product labeling. [DSC] = Discontinued product

Injection, powder for reconstitution [purified monkey cell source]:

ACAM2000™: 1-5 x 10^8 plaque-forming units per mL [contains polymyxin B, neomycin (trace amounts) and human albumin; packed with diluent, tuberculin syringes for reconstitution, and 100 bifurcated needles for administration]

- ◆ **Small Wolf** *see* Hops *(Humulus lupulus) on page 770*
- ◆ **SMZ-TMP** *see* Sulfamethoxazole and Trimethoprim *on page 1517*
- ◆ **(+)-(*S*)-*N*-Methyl-γ-(1-naphthyloxy)-2-thiophenepropylamine Hydrochloride** *see* DULoxetine *on page 516*
- ◆ **Sodium 2-Mercaptoethane Sulfonate** *see* Mesna *on page 995*
- ◆ **Sodium 4-Hydroxybutyrate** *see* Sodium Oxybate *on page 1495*
- ◆ **Sodium *L*-Triiodothyronine** *see* Liothyronine *on page 928*
- ◆ **Sodium Acid Carbonate** *see* Sodium Bicarbonate *on page 1494*
- ◆ **Sodium Aurothiomalate** *see* Gold Sodium Thiomalate *on page 734*
- ◆ **Sodium Benzoate and Caffeine** *see* Caffeine *on page 250*

Sodium Bicarbonate (SOW dee um bye KAR bun ate)

U.S. Brand Names Brioschi® [OTC]; Neut®

Mexican Brand Names Betsol "Z"

Index Terms Baking Soda; $NaHCO_3$; Sodium Acid Carbonate; Sodium Hydrogen Carbonate

Pharmacologic Category Alkalinizing Agent; Antacid; Electrolyte Supplement, Oral; Electrolyte Supplement, Parenteral

Use Management of metabolic acidosis; gastric hyperacidity; as an alkalinization agent for the urine; treatment of hyperkalemia; management of overdose of certain drugs, including tricyclic antidepressants and aspirin

Unlabeled/Investigational Use Prevention of contrast-induced nephropathy (CIN)

Effect on Mental Status None reported

Effect on Psychiatric Treatment May decrease serum lithium levels due to increased clearance but overall effect is minimal; does not offer much benefit in lithium overdose; if lithium toxicity is severe, dialysis is the treatment of choice

Dosage Summary

I.V.:

Children: 0.5-1 mEq/kg/dose repeated every 10 minutes or as indicated by arterial blood gases **or** HCO_3^- (mEq) = 0.3 x weight (kg) x base deficit (mEq/L), administer 1/2 dose initially, then remaining 1/2 dose over the next 24 hours **or** 2-5 mEq/kg I.V. infusion over 4-8 hours

Adults: Initial: 1 mEq/kg/dose or 50 mEq one time; Maintenance: 0.5 mEq/kg/dose every 10 minutes or as indicated by arterial blood gases **or** HCO_3^- (mEq) = 0.3 x weight (kg) x base deficit (mEq/L), administer 1/2 dose initially, then remaining 1/2 dose over the next 24 hours **or** 2-5 mEq/kg I.V. infusion over 4-8 hours

Oral:

Children: 1-10 mEq/kg/day as a single dose **or** divided every 4-6 hours

Adults <60 years: 0.5-200 mEq/kg/day in 4-5 divided doses **or** 325 mg to 2 g 1-4 times/day (maximum: 16 g [200 mEq] day)

Adults ≥60 years: 0.5-100 mEq/kg/day in 4-6 divided doses **or** 325 mg to 2 g 1-4 times/day (maximum: 8 g [100 mEq] day)

Dosage Forms Excipient information presented when available (limited, particularly for generics); consult specific product labeling.

Granules, for solution, oral [effervescent]:

Brioschi®: 2.69 g/packet (12s) [contains sodium 770 mg/packet; lemon flavor]; 2.69 g/capful (120 g, 240 g) [contains sodium 770 mg/capful; lemon flavor]

Infusion [premixed in water for injection]: 5% (500 mL) [5.95 mEq/10 mL]

Injection, solution:

4.2% (10 mL) [5 mEq/10 mL]

7.5% (50 mL) [8.92 mEq/10 mL]
8.4% (10 mL, 50 mL, 250 mL, 500 mL) [10 mEq/10 mL]
Neut®: 4% (5 mL) [2.4 mEq/5 mL; contains edetate disodium]
Powder: Sodium bicarbonate USP (120 g, 480 g) [contains sodium 30 mEq per 1/2 teaspoon]
Tablet: 325 mg [3.8 mEq]; 650 mg [7.6 mEq]

- **Sodium Biphosphate, Methenamine, Methylene Blue, Phenyl Salicylate, and Hyoscyamine** *see* Methenamine, Sodium Biphosphate, Phenyl Salicylate, Methylene Blue, and Hyoscyamine *on page 1010*
- **Sodium Diuril®** *see* Chlorothiazide *on page 321*
- **Sodium Etidronate** *see* Etidronate Disodium *on page 605*
- **Sodium Ferric Gluconate** *see* Ferric Gluconate *on page 626*
- **Sodium Hydrogen Carbonate** *see* Sodium Bicarbonate *on page 1494*
- **Sodium Hyposulfate** *see* Sodium Thiosulfate *on page 1497*
- **Sodium Nafcillin** *see* Nafcillin *on page 1093*
- **Sodium Nitroferricyanide** *see* Nitroprusside *on page 1149*
- **Sodium Nitroprusside** *see* Nitroprusside *on page 1149*

Sodium Oxybate (SOW dee um ox i BATE)

U.S. Brand Names Xyrem®

Canadian Brand Names Xyrem®

Index Terms 4-Hydroxybutyrate; Gamma Hydroxybutyric Acid; GHB; Sodium 4-Hydroxybutyrate

Pharmacologic Category Central Nervous System Depressant

Generic Available No

Use Treatment of cataplexy and daytime sleepiness in patients with narcolepsy

Restrictions C-I (illicit use); C-III (medical use)

Sodium oxybate oral solution will be available only to prescribers enrolled in the Xyrem® Patient Success Program® and dispensed to the patient through the designated centralized pharmacy (1-866-997-3688). Prior to dispensing the first prescription, prescribers will be sent educational materials to be reviewed with the patient and enrollment forms for the postmarketing surveillance program. Patients must be seen at least every 3 months; prescriptions can be written for a maximum of 3 months (the first prescription may only be written for a 1-month supply).

An FDA-approved medication guide must be distributed when dispensing an outpatient prescription (new or refill) where this medication is to be used without direct supervision of a healthcare provider. Medication guides are available at http://www.fda.gov/cder/Offices/ODS/medication_guides.htm.

Pregnancy Risk Factor B

Pregnancy Considerations Reproduction studies in animals have not shown teratogenic effects. However, there are no well-controlled studies in pregnant women. Use during pregnancy only if clearly needed. Past use during labor and delivery as an anesthetic has shown a slight decrease in Apgar scores due to sleepiness in the neonate.

Lactation Excretion in breast milk unknown/use caution

Contraindications Hypersensitivity to sodium oxybate or any component of the formulation; ethanol and other CNS depressants; semialdehyde dehydrogenase deficiency

Warnings/Precautions [U.S. Boxed Warning]: Sodium oxybate is a CNS depressant with abuse potential; it should not be used with ethanol or other CNS depressants. Seizures, respiratory depression, decreases in level of consciousness, coma, and death have been reported when used for nonprescription purposes. Due to the rapid onset of CNS depressant effects, doses should be administered only at bedtime and while the patient is sitting up in bed. May impair respiratory drive; use caution with compromised respiratory function. Most patients (~80%) in clinical trials were also treated with stimulants; therefore, an independent assessment of the effects of sodium oxybate is lacking. May cause confusion, psychosis, paranoia, hallucinations, agitation, and depression; use caution with history of depression or suicide attempt. May cause sleepwalking, urinary, and/or fecal incontinence. Use caution with hepatic dysfunction. Contains significant amounts of sodium; use caution with heart failure, hypertension, or compromised renal function.

Patients should be instructed not to engage in hazardous activities requiring mental alertness for at least 6 hours after taking this medication and that CNS effects may carryover to the next day. Tolerance to sodium oxybate, or withdrawal following its discontinuation, have not been clearly defined in controlled clinical trials, but have been reported at larger doses used for illicit purposes. Safety and efficacy have not been established in patients <16 years of age.

[U.S. Boxed Warning]: Sodium oxybate oral solution will be available only to prescribers enrolled in the Xyrem® Patient Success Program® and dispensed to the patient through the designated centralized pharmacy (1-866-997-3688).

Adverse Reactions

>10%:

Central nervous system: Dizziness (8% to 37%), headache (9% to 37%), pain (9% to 20%), somnolence (1% to 14%), confusion (3% to 17%), sleep disorder (6% to 14%)

Gastrointestinal: Nausea (8% to 40%), vomiting (2% to 23%), abdominal pain (3% to 11%)

Genitourinary: Urinary incontinence (<1% to 14%, usually nocturnal), enuresis (3% to 17%), cystitis, metrorrhagia, urinary frequency

Miscellaneous: Diaphoresis (3% to 11%)

1% to 10%:

Cardiovascular: Hypertension (6%), chest pain, edema

Central nervous system: Disorientation (up to 9%), inebriation (up to 9%), concentration decreased (3% to 9%), dream abnormality (3% to 9%), sleepwalking (4% to 7%), depression (3% to 6%), amnesia (3% to 6%), anxiety (3% to 6%), thinking abnormality (3% to 6%), lethargy (up to 6%), insomnia (5%), agitation, ataxia, chills, fatigue, malaise, memory impairment, nervousness, pyrexia, seizure, stupor, tremor, vertigo

Dermatologic: Hyperhidrosis (3% to 6%), pruritus, rash

Endocrine & metabolic: Dysmenorrhea (3% to 6%)

Gastrointestinal: Dyspepsia (6% to 9%), diarrhea (6% to 8%), abdominal pain (6%), nausea and vomiting (6%), anorexia, constipation, tooth ache, weight gain

Hepatic: Alkaline phosphatase increased, hypercholesteremia, hypocalcemia

Neuromuscular & skeletal: Hypoesthesia (6%), weakness (6% to 8%), myasthenia (3% to 6%), pain (3% to 6%), arthritis, leg cramps, myalgia

Ocular: Amblyopia (6%), blurred vision (6%)

Otic: Tinnitus (6%), ear pain

Renal: Albuminuria, hematuria

Respiratory: Pharyngitis (6% to 8%), rhinitis (8%), nasopharyngitis (3% to 8%), infection (3% to 6%), bronchitis, cough, dyspnea

Miscellaneous: Infection (3% to 6%), viral infection (3% to 9%), allergic reaction, flu-like syndrome

<1% (Limited to important or life-threatening): Abdominal distension, accident, acne, affect lability, akathisia, ALT/AST increased, allergic reaction, alopecia, anemia, apathy, apnea, arthritis, asthma, bilirubinemia, bronchitis, bruising, coma, conjunctivitis, contusion, contact dermatitis, creatinine increased, dehydration, depersonalization, dysgeusia, dysphagia, edema, epistaxis, eructation, euphoria, eye irritation, eye pain, eye redness, eye swelling, fall, fecal incontinence, flatulence, fracture, gastroinesophageal reflux disease, gait abnormal, hangover, hematuria, hiccups, hypersensitivity, hyperuricemia, hyperglycemia, hypernatremia, hypertonia, hypotension, infection, injury, keratoconjunctivitis sicca, laceration, leukocytosis, leukopenia, libido decreased, lymphadenopathy, mental impairment, migraine, miosis, mouth ulceration, myoclonus, neck rigidity, neuralgia, night sweats, paralysis, paranoia, polyarthritis, polycythemia, positive ANA test, proteinuria, psychomotor activity, restless leg syndrome, rosacea, salivary hypersecretion, sinusitis, snoring, stomatitis, suicidal behavior/thoughts, suicidal attempts, syncope, tachycardia, taste loss, tendonitis, thirst, urinary urgency, urticaria

Drug Interactions

There are no known significant interactions.

Ethanol/Nutrition/Herb Interactions

Ethanol: Avoid ethanol (increases CNS depression).

Food: High-fat meal decreases bioavailability, delays absorption, and decreases peak serum level.

Herb/Nutraceutical: Avoid any products that may cause CNS depression (eg, kava kava or valerian).

Stability Store at controlled room temperature of 15°C to 30°C (59°F to 86°F) in the original bottle and in a safe and secure place (may need to be locked up). Prepare both doses prior to bedtime and place safely near bed, out of reach of pets and children. Each dose should be diluted with 2 ounces of water in the child-resistant dosing cups. Once diluted, solutions should be used within 24 hours.

Mechanism of Action Sodium oxybate is derived from gamma aminobutyric acid (GABA) and acts as an inhibitory chemical transmitter in the brain. May function through specific receptors for gamma hydroxybutyrate (GHB) and GABA (B).

Pharmacodynamics/Kinetics

Absorption: Rapid

Distribution: 190-384 mL/kg

Protein binding: <1%

Metabolism: Primarily via the Krebs cycle to form water and carbon dioxide; secondarily via beta oxidation; significant first-pass effect; no active metabolites; metabolic pathways are saturable

Bioavailability: 25%

Half-life elimination: 30-60 minutes

Time to peak: 30-75 minutes

Excretion: Primarily pulmonary (as carbon dioxide); urine (<5% unchanged drug)

Dosage Oral:

Children ≥16 years and Adults: Narcolepsy: Initial: 4.5 g/day, in 2 equal doses; first dose to be given at bedtime after the patient is in bed, and second dose to be given 2.5-4 hours later. Dose may be increased or adjusted in 2-week intervals; average dose: 6-9 g/day (maximum: 9 g/day)

Elderly: Safety and efficacy have not been studied in patients >65 years.

Dosage adjustment in renal impairment: Adjustment not necessary; consider sodium content

Dosage adjustment in hepatic impairment: Decrease starting dose to half and titrate doses carefully in patients with liver dysfunction. Elimination half-life significantly longer in patients with Child's class C liver dysfunction.

Dietary Considerations Take on an empty stomach; separate last meal (or food) and first dose by several hours; try to take at similar time each day. Xyrem® 500 mg/mL contains sodium 91 mg/mL.

Administration Take on an empty stomach; separate last meal (or food) and first dose by several hours; try to take at similar time each day. Doses should be administered while patient is sitting up in bed. Both doses should be prepared prior to bedtime. The first dose is taken at bedtime and the second dose is taken 2.5-4 hours later; an alarm clock may need to be set for the second dose. After taking the dose, patient is to lie down and remain in bed.

Monitoring Parameters Signs and symptoms of depression, drug abuse

Additional Information Sodium oxybate is a known substance of abuse. When used illegally, it has been referred to as a "date-rape drug". Street names include Liquid Ecstasy, Liquid X, Liquid E, Georgia Home Boy, Grievous Bodily Harm, G-Riffick, Soap, Scoop, Salty Water, Somatomax, and Organic Quaalude. As part of the FDA approval for prescription use, all patients and prescribers must be enrolled in a program designed to restrict its distribution and to provide postmarketing evaluations. Detailed instructions for the use of sodium oxybate will be provided to the patient and healthcare provider prior dispensing the first dose.

Dosage Forms Excipient information presented when available (limited, particularly for generics); consult specific product labeling.

Solution, oral:

Xyrem®: 500 mg/mL (180 mL) [contains sodium 91 mg/mL; supplied in a kit containing bottle adapter, two dosing cups, and oral syringe (as measuring device)]

◆ **Sodium PAS** *see* Aminosalicylic Acid *on page 88*

Sodium Thiosulfate (SOW dee um thye oh SUL fate)

U.S. Brand Names Versiclear™

Index Terms Disodium Thiosulfate Pentahydrate; Pentahydrate; Sodium Hyposulfate; Sodium Thiosulphate; Thiosulfuric Acid Disodium Salt

Pharmacologic Category Antidote

Use

Parenteral: Used alone or with sodium nitrite or amyl nitrite in cyanide poisoning; reduce the risk of nephrotoxicity associated with cisplatin therapy; treatment of cyanide poisoning due to nitroprusside

Topical: Treatment of tinea versicolor

Unlabeled/Investigational Use Management of I.V. extravasation

Effect on Mental Status May cause coma, CNS depression secondary to thiocyanate intoxication, psychosis, or confusion

Effect on Psychiatric Treatment CNS depressant effect of psychotropics may be potentiated; monitor

Dosage Summary

I.V.:

Children: 7 g/m^2 (maximum dose: 12.5 g) given over 10 minutes; may repeat at 1/2 the original dose if symptoms return **or** 12 g/m^2 over 6 hours or 9 g/m^2 I.V. push followed by 1.2 g/m^2 continuous infusion for 6 hours

Adults: 12.5 g, may repeat at half dose if needed **or** 0.95-1.95 mL/kg (maximum: 50 mL) **or** 12 g/m^2 over 6 hours or 9 g/m^2 I.V. push followed by 1.2 g/m^2 continuous infusion for 6 hours

Topical:

Children: Apply a thin layer (20% to 25%) to affected areas twice daily

Adults: Apply a thin layer (20% to 25%) to affected areas twice daily

Dosage Forms Excipient information presented when available (limited, particularly for generics); consult specific product labeling.

Injection, solution [preservative free]: 100 mg/mL (10 mL); 250 mg/mL (50 mL)

Lotion: Sodium thiosulfate 25% and salicylic acid 1% (120 mL) [contains isopropyl alcohol 10%]

- **Sodium Thiosulphate** *see* Sodium Thiosulfate *on page 1497*
- **Sojourn™** *see* Sevoflurane *on page 1479*
- **Solage** *see* Mequinol and Tretinoin *on page 992*
- **Solagé®** *see* Mequinol and Tretinoin *on page 992*
- **Solaraze®** *see* Diclofenac *on page 457*
- **Solarcaine® Aloe Extra Burn Relief [OTC]** *see* Lidocaine *on page 924*
- **Solia™** *see* Ethinyl Estradiol and Desogestrel *on page 592*

Solifenacin (sol i FEN a sin)

Medication Safety Issues

Sound-alike/look-alike issues:

VESIcare® may be confused with Visicol®

U.S. Brand Names VESIcare®

Index Terms Solifenacin Succinate; YM905

Pharmacologic Category Anticholinergic Agent

Use Treatment of overactive bladder with symptoms of urinary frequency, urgency, or urge incontinence

Effect on Mental Status May cause depression, sedation, or dizziness

Effect on Psychiatric Treatment Dry mouth and constipation are common; concomitant use with psychotropic agents may produce additive effects; monitor. Carbamazepine, phenobarbital, phenytoin, and St John's wort may decrease levels of solifenacin while nefazodone may increase the levels of solifenacin; monitor.

Dosage Summary

Oral:

Children: Dosage not established

Adults: 5-10 mg/day

Dosage Forms Excipient information presented when available (limited, particularly for generics); consult specific product labeling.

Tablet, as succinate:

VESIcare®: 5 mg, 10 mg

- **Solifenacin Succinate** *see* Solifenacin *on page 1498*
- **Solodyn™** *see* Minocycline *on page 1056*
- **Soltamox™ [DSC]** *see* Tamoxifen *on page 1537*
- **Solu-Cortef®** *see* Hydrocortisone *on page 785*
- **Solu-Medrol®** *see* MethylPREDNISolone *on page 1029*
- **Soma®** *see* Carisoprodol *on page 283*
- **Soma** *see* Ephedra *(Ephedra sinica) on page 541*
- **Soma® Compound** *see* Carisoprodol and Aspirin *on page 284*
- **Soma® Compound w/Codeine [DSC]** *see* Carisoprodol, Aspirin, and Codeine *on page 284*
- **Somatrem** *see* Somatropin *on page 1499*

Somatropin (soe ma TROE pin)

Medication Safety Issues

Sound-alike/look-alike issues:

Somatrem may be confused with somatropin

Somatropin may be confused with somatrem, sumatriptan

International issues:

Genotropin® may be confused with Genatropine® which is a brand name for atropine in France

U.S. Brand Names Genotropin Miniquick®; Genotropin®; Humatrope®; Norditropin®; Norditropin® NordiFlex®; Nutropin AQ®; Nutropin®; Omnitrope™; Saizen®; Serostim®; Tev-Tropin®; Zorbtive®

Canadian Brand Names Humatrope®; Nutropine®; Nutropin® AQ; Saizen®; Serostim®

Mexican Brand Names Humatrope; Saizen; Serostim

Index Terms hGH; Human Growth Hormone; Somatrem

Pharmacologic Category Growth Hormone

Use

Children:

Treatment of growth failure due to inadequate endogenous growth hormone secretion (Genotropin®, Humatrope®, Norditropin®, Nutropin®, Nutropin AQ®, Omnitrope™, Saizen®, Tev-Tropin®)

Treatment of short stature associated with Turner syndrome (Genotropin®, Humatrope®, Norditropin®, Nutropin®, Nutropin AQ®)

Treatment of Prader-Willi syndrome (Genotropin®)

Treatment of growth failure associated with chronic renal insufficiency (CRI) up until the time of renal transplantation (Nutropin®, Nutropin AQ®)

Treatment of growth failure in children born small for gestational age who fail to manifest catch-up growth by 2 years of age (Genotropin®) or by 2-4 years of age (Norditropin®)

Treatment of idiopathic short stature (nongrowth hormone-deficient short stature) defined by height standard deviation score (SDS) less than or equal to -2.25 and growth rate not likely to attain normal adult height (Genotropin®, Humatrope®, Nutropin®, Nutropin AQ®)

Treatment of short stature or growth failure associated with short stature homeobox gene (SHOX) deficiency (Humatrope®)

Treatment of short stature associated with Noonan syndrome (Norditropin®)

Adults:

HIV patients with wasting or cachexia with concomitant antiviral therapy (Serostim®)

Replacement of endogenous growth hormone in patients with adult growth hormone deficiency who meet both of the following criteria (Genotropin®, Humatrope®, Norditropin®, Nutropin®, Nutropin AQ®, Omnitrope™, Saizen®):

Biochemical diagnosis of adult growth hormone deficiency by means of a subnormal response to a standard growth hormone stimulation test (peak growth hormone ≤5 mcg/L). Confirmatory testing may not be required in patients with congenital/genetic growth hormone deficiency or multiple pituitary hormone deficiencies due to organic diseases.

and

Adult-onset: Patients who have adult growth hormone deficiency whether alone or with multiple hormone deficiencies (hypopituitarism) as a result of pituitary disease, hypothalamic disease, surgery, radiation therapy, or trauma

or

Childhood-onset: Patients who were growth hormone deficient during childhood, confirmed as an adult before replacement therapy is initiated

Treatment of short-bowel syndrome (Zorbtive®)

Unlabeled/Investigational Use Investigational: Congestive heart failure; pediatric HIV patients with wasting/cachexia (Serostim®); HIV-associated adipose redistribution syndrome (HARS) (Serostim®)

Effect on Mental Status May cause aggression (in pediatric patients with Prader-Willi syndrome)

Effect on Psychiatric Treatment Contraindicated in pediatric patients with Prader-Willi syndrome who are severely obese or have severe respiratory impairment; fatalities have been reported.

Dosage Summary Note: Use caution: Dosage is indication and formulation specific; individualize dose

I.M.:

Children:

Growth hormone deficiency:

Humatrope®: Weekly dosage: 0.18 mg/kg; maximum replacement dose: 0.3 mg/kg/week; dosing should be divided into equal doses given 3 times/week on alternating days, 6 times/week, or daily

Saizen®: 0.18 mg/kg/week in divided doses administered daily **or** as 0.06 mg/kg/dose administered 3 times/week **or** as 0.03 mg/kg/dose administered 6 times/week

Adults: Dosage not established

SubQ:

Children:

Chronic renal insufficiency: Nutropin®, Nutropin® AQ: Weekly dosage: 0.35 mg/kg divided into daily injections; continue until the time of renal transplantation

Growth hormone deficiency:

Genotropin®, Omnitrope™: Weekly dosage: 0.16-0.24 mg/kg divided into 6-7 daily doses

Humatrope®: Weekly dosage: 0.18 mg/kg; maximum replacement dose: 0.3 mg/kg/week; dosing should be divided into equal doses given 3 times/week on alternating days, 6 times/week, or daily

Norditropin®: 0.024-0.034 mg/kg/day, 6-7 times/week

Nutropin®, Nutropin® AQ: Weekly dosage: 0.3 mg/kg divided into daily doses; pubertal patients: ≤0.7 mg/kg/week divided daily

Tev-Tropin®: Up to 0.1 mg/kg administered 3 times/week

Saizen®: 0.18 mg/kg/week in divided doses administered daily **or** as 0.06 mg/kg/dose administered 3 times/week **or** as 0.03 mg/kg/dose administered 6 times/week

Idiopathic short stature:

Gentropin®: SubQ: Weekly dosage: 0.47 mg/kg divided into equal doses 6-7 times per week

Humatrope®: Weekly dosage: 0.37 mg/kg divided into equal doses 6-7 times per week

Nutropin®, Nutropin AQ®: Weekly dosage: Up to 0.3 mg/kg divided into daily doses

Prader-Willi syndrome: Genotropin®: Weekly dosage: 0.24 mg/kg divided into 6-7 doses

Small for gestational age:

Genotropin®: Weekly dosage: 0.48 mg/kg divided into 6-7 doses

Norditropin®: SubQ: Up to 0.067 mg/kg/day

Turner syndrome:

Genotropin®: Weekly dosage: 0.33 mg/kg divided into 6-7 doses

Humatrope®, Nutropin®, Nutropin® AQ: Weekly dosage: ≤0.375 mg/kg divided into equal doses 3-7 times per week

Norditropin®: Up to 0.067 mg/kg/day

SHOX deficiency: Humatrope®: 0.35 mg/kg/week divided into equal daily doses

Noonan syndrome: Norditropin®: SubQ: Up to 0.066 mg/kg/day

Adults:

Growth hormone deficiency: **Note:** To minimize adverse events in older or overweight patients, reduced dosages may be necessary. During therapy, dosage should be decreased if required by the occurrence of side effects or excessive IGF-I levels.

Genotropin®, Omnitrope™: Weekly dosage: ≤0.04 mg/kg divided into 6-7 daily doses; dose may be increased at 4- to 8-week intervals according to individual requirements, to a maximum of 0.08 mg/kg/week

Humatrope®: ≤0.006 mg/kg/day; dose may be increased according to individual requirements, up to a maximum of 0.0125 mg/kg/day

Norditropin®: Initial dose ≤0.004 mg/kg/day; after 6 weeks of therapy, may increase dose to 0.016 mg/kg/day

Nutropin®, Nutropin® AQ: ≤0.006 mg/kg/day; dose may be increased according to individual requirements, up to a maximum of 0.025 mg/kg/day in patients <35 years of age, or up to a maximum of 0.0125 mg/kg/day in patients ≥35 years of age

Saizen®: ≤0.005 mg/kg/day; dose may be increased to not more than 0.01 mg/kg/day after 4 weeks, based on individual requirements.

HIV patients with wasting or cachexia (Serostim®): SubQ: 0.1 mg/kg once daily at bedtime (maximum: 6 mg/day)

Short-bowel syndrome (Zorbtive®): 0.1 mg/kg once daily for 4 weeks (maximum: 8 mg/day)

Dosage Forms Excipient information presented when available (limited, particularly for generics); consult specific product labeling.

Injection, powder for reconstitution [rDNA origin]:

Genotropin®: 5.8 mg [~15 int. units/mL; delivers 5 mg/mL; contains m-cresol]; 13.8 mg [~36 int. units/mL; delivers 12 mg/mL; contains m-cresol]

Genotropin Miniquick® [preservative free]: 0.2 mg, 0.4 mg, 0.6 mg, 0.8 mg, 1 mg, 1.2 mg, 1.4 mg, 1.6 mg, 1.8 mg, 2 mg [each strength delivers 0.25 mL]

Humatrope®: 5 mg [15 int. units], 6 mg [18 int. units], 12 mg [36 int. units], 24 mg [72 int. units]

Nutropin®: 5 mg [~15 int. units; packaged with diluent containing benzyl alcohol]; 10 mg [~30 int. units; packaged with diluent containing benzyl alcohol]

Omnitrope™: 5.8 mg [~17.4 int. units; packaged with diluent containing benzyl alcohol]

Saizen®: 5 mg [~15 int. units; contains sucrose 34.2 mg; packaged with diluent containing benzyl alcohol]; 8.8 mg [~26.4 int. units; contains sucrose 60.2 mg; packaged with diluent containing benzyl alcohol]

Serostim®: 4 mg [~12 int. units; contains sucrose 27.3 mg; packaged with diluent containing benzyl alcohol; 5 mg [~15 int. units; contains sucrose 34.2 mg]; 6 mg [~18 int. units; contains sucrose 41 mg]; 8.8 mg [~26.4 int. units; contains sucrose 60.19 mg; packaged with diluent containing benzyl alcohol]

Tev-Tropin®: 5 mg [15 int. units/mL; packaged with diluent containing benzyl alcohol]

Zorbtive®: 8.8 mg [~26.4 int. units; contains sucrose 60.19 mg; packaged with diluent containing benzyl alcohol]

Injection, solution [rDNA origin]:

Norditropin®: 5 mg/1.5 mL (1.5 mL); 15 mg/1.5 mL (1.5 mL)

Norditropin® NordiFlex®: 5 mg/1.5 mL (1.5 mL); 10 mg/1.5 mL (1.5 mL); 15 mg/1.5 mL (1.5 mL)

Nutropin AQ®: 5 mg/mL (2 mL) [~15 int. units/mL]

Omnitrope™: 5 mg/1.5 mL (1.5 mL); 10 mg/1.5 mL (1.5 mL)

◆ **Somavert®** *see* Pegvisomant *on page 1237*

◆ **Sominex® [OTC]** *see* DiphenhydrAMINE *on page 481*

◆ **Sominex® Maximum Strength [OTC]** *see* DiphenhydrAMINE *on page 481*

◆ **Somnote®** *see* Chloral Hydrate *on page 313*

◆ **Sonata®** *see* Zaleplon *on page 1691*

Sorafenib (sor AF e nib)

Medication Safety Issues

Sound-alike/look-alike issues:

Nexavar® may be confused with Nexium®

Sorafenib may be confused with sunitinib

High alert medication: The Institute for Safe Medication Practices (ISMP) includes this medication among its list of drug classes which have a heightened risk of causing significant patient harm when used in error.

U.S. Brand Names Nexavar®

Canadian Brand Names Nexavar®

Mexican Brand Names Nexavar

Index Terms BAY 43-9006; NSC-724772; Sorafenib Tosylate

Pharmacologic Category Antineoplastic Agent, Tyrosine Kinase Inhibitor; Vascular Endothelial Growth Factor (VEGF) Inhibitor

Use Treatment of advanced renal cell cancer (RCC), unresectable hepatocellular cancer (HCC)

Unlabeled/Investigational Use Treatment of advanced thyroid cancer

Effect on Mental Status Sedation is common; may cause depression

Effect on Psychiatric Treatment GI side effects are common; concomitant use with SSRIs, lithium, valproic acid may produce additive effects. Sedative effects may be additive if used in combination with psychotropics. May cause neutropenia, thrombocytopenia, or leukopenia; use caution with clozapine, carbamazepine, and valproic acid. Avoid concurrent use with St John's wort.

Dosage Summary

Oral:

Children: Dosage not established

Adults: 400 mg twice daily

Dosage Forms Excipient information presented when available (limited, particularly for generics); consult specific product labeling.

Tablet, as tosylate:
Nexavar®: 200 mg

- **Sorafenib Tosylate** *see* Sorafenib *on page 1501*
- **Sorine®** *see* Sotalol *on page 1502*

Sotalol (SOE ta lole)

Medication Safety Issues
Sound-alike/look-alike issues:
Sotalol may be confused with Stadol®
Betapace® may be confused with Betapace AF®
Betapace AF® may be confused with Betapace®

Related Information
Beta-Blockers *on page 1776*

U.S. Brand Names Betapace AF®; Betapace®; Sorine®

Canadian Brand Names Alti-Sotalol; Apo-Sotalol®; Betapace AF®; CO Sotalol; Gen-Sotalol; Lin-Sotalol; Novo-Sotalol; Nu-Sotalol; PMS-Sotalol; Rho®-Sotalol; Riva-Sotalol; Rylosol; Sotacor®

Index Terms Sotalol Hydrochloride

Pharmacologic Category Antiarrhythmic Agent, Class II; Antiarrhythmic Agent, Class III; Beta-Adrenergic Blocker, Nonselective

Use Treatment of documented ventricular arrhythmias (ie, sustained ventricular tachycardia), that in the judgment of the physician are life-threatening; maintenance of normal sinus rhythm in patients with symptomatic atrial fibrillation and atrial flutter who are currently in sinus rhythm. Manufacturer states substitutions should not be made for Betapace AF® since Betapace AF® is distributed with a patient package insert specific for atrial fibrillation/flutter.

Effect on Mental Status Dizziness and drowsiness are common; may cause confusion, anxiety, or depression

Effect on Psychiatric Treatment Contraindicated with ziprasidone. May rarely cause leukopenia; use caution with clozapine and carbamazepine. Barbiturates may decrease the effects of beta-blockers; beta-blockers may alter the effects antipsychotics; monitor for altered response.

Dosage Summary

Oral:

Children ≤2 years: Dosage should be adjusted (decreased) by plotting of the child's age on a logarithmic scale; **Note:** Refer to manufacturer's package labeling

Children >2 years: Initial: 90 mg/m^2/day in 3 divided doses; Maintenance: 90-180 mg/m^2/day in 3 divided doses (maximum: 180 mg/m^2/day)

Adults: Initial: 80 mg twice daily; Maintenance: 240-320 mg/day in 2-3 divided doses (maximum: 320 mg/day [exceptions occur-indication specific])

Dosage Forms Excipient information presented when available (limited, particularly for generics); consult specific product labeling.

Tablet, as hydrochloride: 80 mg, 80 mg [artrial fibrillation], 120 mg, 120 mg [artrial fibrillation], 160 mg, 160 mg [artrial fibrillation], 240 mg
Betapace®: 80 mg, 120 mg, 160 mg, 240 mg
Betapace AF®: 80 mg, 120 mg, 160 mg [artrial fibrillation]
Sorine®: 80 mg, 120 mg, 160 mg, 240 mg

- **Sotalol Hydrochloride** *see* Sotalol *on page 1502*
- **Sotret®** *see* Isotretinoin *on page 871*
- **Spacol [DSC]** *see* Hyoscyamine *on page 799*
- **Spacol T/S [DSC]** *see* Hyoscyamine *on page 799*
- **Spastrin® [DSC]** *see* Belladonna, Phenobarbital, and Ergotamine *on page 175*
- **SPD417** *see* CarBAMazepine *on page 265*

Spectinomycin (spek ti noe MYE sin)

Medication Safety Issues
Sound-alike/look-alike issues:
Trobicin® may be confused with tobramycin

U.S. Brand Names Trobicin® [DSC]

Index Terms Spectinomycin Hydrochloride

Pharmacologic Category Antibiotic, Miscellaneous

Use Treatment of uncomplicated gonorrhea
Effect on Mental Status May cause dizziness
Effect on Psychiatric Treatment None reported
Dosage Summary
I.M.:
Children <45 kg: 40 mg/kg/dose as a single dose
Children ≥45 kg: 2-4 g as a single dose **or** 2 g every 12 hours
Adults: 2-4 g as a single dose **or** 2 g every 12 hours
Dosage Forms Excipient information presented when available (limited, particularly for generics); consult specific product labeling.
Injection, powder for reconstitution, as hydrochloride:
Trobicin®: 2 g [diluent contains benzyl alcohol] [DSC]

- **Spectinomycin Hydrochloride** *see* Spectinomycin *on page 1502*
- **Spectracef®** *see* Cefditoren *on page 293*
- **SPI 0211** *see* Lubiprostone *on page 963*

Spironolactone (speer on oh LAK tone)

Medication Safety Issues
Sound-alike/look-alike issues:
Aldactone® may be confused with Aldactazide®

International issues:
Aldactone®: Brand name for potassium canrenoate in Austria, Czech Republic, Germany, and Hungary
U.S. Brand Names Aldactone®
Canadian Brand Names Aldactone®; Novo-Spiroton
Mexican Brand Names Aldactone; Vivitar
Pharmacologic Category Diuretic, Potassium-Sparing; Selective Aldosterone Blocker
Generic Available Yes
Use Management of edema associated with excessive aldosterone excretion; hypertension; congestive heart failure; primary hyperaldosteronism; hypokalemia; cirrhosis of liver accompanied by edema or ascites
Unlabeled/Investigational Use Female acne (adjunctive therapy); hirsutism; hypertension (pediatric); diuretic (pediatric)
Effect on Mental Status May cause drowsiness, dizziness, nervousness, or confusion
Effect on Psychiatric Treatment Has been used to treat lithium-related edema
Pregnancy Risk Factor C/D in pregnancy-induced hypertension (per expert analysis)
Pregnancy Considerations Teratogenic effects were not observed in animal studies; however, doses used were less than or equal to equivalent doses in humans. The antiandrogen effects of spironolactone have been shown to cause feminization of the male fetus in animal studies. Two case reports did not demonstrate this effect in humans however, the authors caution that adequate data is lacking. Diuretics are generally avoided in pregnancy due to the theoretical risk that decreased plasma volume may cause placental insufficiency. Diuretics should not be used during pregnancy in the presence of reduced placental perfusion (eg, pre-eclampsia, intrauterine growth restriction).
Lactation Enters breast milk/not recommended (AAP rates "compatible")
Contraindications Hypersensitivity to spironolactone or any component of the formulation; anuria; acute renal insufficiency; significant impairment of renal excretory function; hyperkalemia; pregnancy (pregnancy-induced hypertension - per expert analysis)
Warnings/Precautions Avoid potassium supplements, potassium-containing salt substitutes, a diet rich in potassium, or other drugs that can cause hyperkalemia. Excess amounts can lead to profound diuresis with fluid and electrolyte loss; close medical supervision and dose evaluation are required. Watch for and correct electrolyte disturbances; adjust dose to avoid dehydration. In cirrhosis, avoid electrolyte and acid/base imbalances that might lead to hepatic encephalopathy. Gynecomastia is related to dose and duration of therapy. Discontinue use prior to adrenal vein catheterization. When evaluating a heart failure patient for spironolactone treatment, creatinine should be ≤2.5 mg/dL in men or ≤2 mg/dL in women and potassium <5 mEq/L. **[U.S. Boxed Warning]: Shown to be a tumorigen in chronic toxicity animal studies. Avoid unnecessary use.**
Adverse Reactions Incidence of adverse events is not always reported (mean daily dose 26 mg).

Cardiovascular: Edema (2%, placebo 2%)

Central nervous system: Disorders (23%, placebo 21%) which may include drowsiness, lethargy, headache, mental confusion, drug fever, ataxia, fatigue

Dermatologic: Maculopapular, erythematous cutaneous eruptions, urticaria, hirsutism, eosinophilia

Endocrine & metabolic: Gynecomastia (men 9%; placebo 1%), breast pain (men 2%; placebo 0.1%), serious hyperkalemia (2%, placebo 1%), hyponatremia, dehydration, hyperchloremic metabolic acidosis (in decompensated hepatic cirrhosis), impotence, menstrual irregularities, amenorrhea, postmenopausal bleeding

Gastrointestinal: Disorders (29%, placebo 29%) which may include anorexia, nausea, cramping, diarrhea, gastric bleeding, ulceration, gastritis, vomiting

Hematologic: Agranulocytosis

Hepatic: Cholestatic/hepatocellular toxicity

Renal: Increased BUN concentration

Miscellaneous: Deepening of the voice, anaphylactic reaction, breast cancer

Drug Interactions

ACE Inhibitors: Potassium-Sparing Diuretics may enhance the hyperkalemic effect of ACE Inhibitors. *Risk C: Monitor therapy*

Ammonium Chloride: Potassium-Sparing Diuretics may enhance the adverse/toxic effect of Ammonium Chloride. Specifically the risk of systemic acidosis. *Risk D: Consider therapy modification*

Angiotensin II Receptor Blockers: May enhance the hyperkalemic effect of Potassium-Sparing Diuretics. *Risk C: Monitor therapy*

Cardiac Glycosides: Potassium-Sparing Diuretics may diminish the therapeutic effect of Cardiac Glycosides. Specifically, the inotropic effects. *Risk C: Monitor therapy*

Diazoxide: May enhance the hypotensive effect of Antihypertensives. *Risk C: Monitor therapy*

Drospirenone: May enhance the hyperkalemic effect of Potassium-Sparing Diuretics. *Risk C: Monitor therapy*

Eplerenone: May enhance the hyperkalemic effect of Potassium-Sparing Diuretics. Management: This combination is contraindicated in patients receiving eplerenone for treatment of hypertension. *Risk D: Consider therapy modification*

Herbs (Hypertensive Properties): May diminish the antihypertensive effect of Antihypertensives. *Risk C: Monitor therapy*

Herbs (Hypotensive Properties): May enhance the hypotensive effect of Antihypertensives. *Risk C: Monitor therapy*

Methylphenidate: May diminish the antihypertensive effect of Antihypertensives. *Risk C: Monitor therapy*

Mitotane: Potassium-Sparing Diuretics may diminish the therapeutic effect of Mitotane. High dose diuretics (eg, Cushings syndrome) may present significantly higher risk than low doses (eg, CHF). *Risk D: Consider therapy modification*

Potassium Salts: May enhance the hyperkalemic effect of Potassium-Sparing Diuretics. *Risk D: Consider therapy modification*

Prostacyclin Analogues: May enhance the hypotensive effect of Antihypertensives. *Risk C: Monitor therapy*

QuiNIDine: Potassium-Sparing Diuretics may diminish the therapeutic effect of QuiNIDine. *Risk C: Monitor therapy*

RiTUXimab: Antihypertensives may enhance the hypotensive effect of RiTUXimab. *Risk D: Consider therapy modification*

Ethanol/Nutrition/Herb Interactions

Food: Food increases absorption.

Herb/Nutraceutical: Avoid natural licorice (due to mineralocorticoid activity)

Stability Protect from light.

Mechanism of Action Competes with aldosterone for receptor sites in the distal renal tubules, increasing sodium chloride and water excretion while conserving potassium and hydrogen ions; may block the effect of aldosterone on arteriolar smooth muscle as well

Pharmacodynamics/Kinetics

Duration of action: 2-3 days

Protein binding: 91% to 98%

Metabolism: Hepatic to multiple metabolites, including canrenone (active)

Half-life elimination: 78-84 minutes

Time to peak, serum: 1-3 hours (primarily as the active metabolite)

Excretion: Urine and feces

Dosage To reduce delay in onset of effect, a loading dose of 2 or 3 times the daily dose may be administered on the first day of therapy. Oral:

Children:

Diuretic, hypertension (unlabeled use): Children 1-17 years: Initial: 1 mg/kg/day divided every 12-24 hours (maximum dose: 3.3 mg/kg/day, up to 100 mg/day)

Diagnosis of primary aldosteronism (unlabeled use): 125-375 mg/m^2/day in divided doses

Adults:

Edema, hypokalemia: 25-200 mg/day in 1-2 divided doses

Hypertension (JNC 7): 25-50 mg/day in 1-2 divided doses

Diagnosis of primary aldosteronism: 100-400 mg/day in 1-2 divided doses

Acne in women (unlabeled use): 25-200 mg once daily

Hirsutism in women (unlabeled use): 50-200 mg/day in 1-2 divided doses

CHF, severe (with ACE inhibitor and a loop diuretic ± digoxin): 12.5-25 mg/day; maximum daily dose: 50 mg (higher doses may occasionallly be used). In the RALES trial, 25 mg every other day was the lowest maintenance dose possible.

Note: If potassium >5.4 mEq/L, consider dosage reduction.

Elderly: Initial: 25-50 mg/day in 1-2 divided doses, increasing by 25-50 mg every 5 days as needed.

Dosing interval in renal impairment:

Cl_{cr} 10-50 mL/minute: Administer every 12-24 hours.

Cl_{cr} <10 mL/minute: Avoid use.

Dietary Considerations Should be taken with food to decrease gastrointestinal irritation and to increase absorption. Excessive potassium intake (eg, salt substitutes, low-salt foods, bananas, nuts) should be avoided.

Monitoring Parameters Blood pressure, serum electrolytes (potassium, sodium), renal function, I & O ratios and daily weight throughout therapy

CHF: Potassium levels and renal function should be checked in 3 days and 1 week after initiation, then every 2-4 weeks for 3-12 months, then every 3-6 months.

Test Interactions May cause false elevation in serum digoxin concentrations measured by RIA

Additional Information Maximum diuretic effect may be delayed 2-3 days and maximum hypertensive effects may be delayed 2-3 weeks.

Dosage Forms Excipient information presented when available (limited, particularly for generics); consult specific product labeling.

Tablet: 25 mg, 50 mg, 100 mg

- ◆ **Spironolactone and Hydrochlorothiazide** *see* Hydrochlorothiazide and Spironolactone *on page 776*
- ◆ **SPM 927** *see* Lacosamide *on page 885*
- ◆ **Sporanox®** *see* Itraconazole *on page 872*
- ◆ **SPP100** *see* Aliskiren *on page 65*
- ◆ **Sprintec™** *see* Ethinyl Estradiol and Norgestimate *on page 600*
- ◆ **Sprycel®** *see* Dasatinib *on page 420*
- ◆ **Sronyx™** *see* Ethinyl Estradiol and Levonorgestrel *on page 595*
- ◆ **SSD®** *see* Silver Sulfadiazine *on page 1485*
- ◆ **SSD® AF** *see* Silver Sulfadiazine *on page 1485*
- ◆ **SSKI®** *see* Potassium Iodide *on page 1317*
- ◆ **Stadol® [DSC]** *see* Butorphanol *on page 247*
- ◆ **Staflex** *see* Acetaminophen and Phenyltoloxamine *on page 36*
- ◆ **Stagesic™** *see* Hydrocodone and Acetaminophen *on page 777*
- ◆ **Stalevo®** *see* Levodopa, Carbidopa, and Entacapone *on page 911*
- ◆ **Starlix®** *see* Nateglinide *on page 1112*
- ◆ **Statuss™ DM** *see* Chlorpheniramine, Phenylephrine, and Dextromethorphan *on page 327*

Stavudine (STAV yoo deen)

Medication Safety Issues

Sound-alike/look-alike issues:

Zerit® may be confused with Ziac®

U.S. Brand Names Zerit®

Canadian Brand Names Zerit®

Mexican Brand Names Landstav; Ranstar; Zerit

Index Terms d4T

Pharmacologic Category Antiretroviral Agent, Reverse Transcriptase Inhibitor (Nucleoside)

Use Treatment of HIV infection in combination with other antiretroviral agents

Effect on Mental Status May cause drowsiness, insomnia, anxiety, or depression

Effect on Psychiatric Treatment May cause neutropenia; use caution with clozapine and carbamazepine; concurrent use with lithium may increase the risk of peripheral neuropathy

Dosage Summary

Oral:

Newborns (Birth to 13 days): 0.5 mg/kg every 12 hours

Children >14 days and <30 kg: 1 mg/kg every 12 hours

Children ≥30 kg: 30 mg every 12 hours

Adults <60 kg: 30 mg every 12 hours

Adults ≥60 kg: 40 mg every 12 hours

Dosage Forms Excipient information presented when available (limited, particularly for generics); consult specific product labeling.

Capsule:

Zerit®: 15 mg, 20 mg, 30 mg, 40 mg

Powder for solution, oral:

Zerit®: 1 mg/mL (200 mL) [dye free; contains sucrose 50 mg/mL; fruit flavor]

◆ **Stavzor™** *see* Valproic Acid and Derivatives *on page 1642*

◆ **Sterapred®** *see* PredniSONE *on page 1327*

◆ **Sterapred® DS** *see* PredniSONE *on page 1327*

◆ **STI-571** *see* Imatinib *on page 810*

◆ **Stimate®** *see* Desmopressin *on page 431*

St John's Wort *(Hypericum perforatum)*

Natural Product Category Herb

Synonyms *Hypericum perforatum*; Hyperforin; Hypericum; SJW

Plant Part Flowering buds

Dosage and Standardization Note: Use varies with route of administration; see Reported Uses

Oral: 300 mg 3 times/day, standardized to contain 0.3% to 0.5% hypericin and/or 3% to 5% hyperforin per dose; minimum of 4-6 weeks of therapy is recommended before results may be seen.

Topical: Apply oil extract as needed to affected area

Reported Uses

Antibacterial, anti-inflammatory (topical: minor wounds, infections, bruises, muscle soreness, and sprains) (Newall, 1996)

Antiviral (Miller, 1998)

Atopic dermatitis (Schempp, 2003; Schempp, 2003)

Climacteric symptoms (combination therapy) (Chung, 2007; Uebelhack, 2006)

Depression (mild to moderate only) (Randløv, 2006), depression (children) (Findling, 2003; Hubner, 2001; Kobak, 2003), seasonal affective disorder (SAD) (Kasper, 1997; Stevinson, 2000) melancholia, stress, and anxiety (Cott, 1998; Gaster, 2000; Harrer, 1999; Hippius, 1998; Lenoir, 1999; Linde, 1996; Volz, 1997; Vorbach, 1997; Woelk, 2000), major depression (Kasper, 2006)

No reported benefit (Hypericum Depression Trial Study Group, 2002; Shelton, 2001)

Obsessive-compulsive disorder (OCD) (Kobak, 2005; Simeon, 2005)

Perimenopausal symptoms (Steger, 1985; Taylor, 2000)

Premenstrual syndrome (PMS) (Grube, 1999; Hicks, 2004)

Smoking cessation (Lawvere, 2006)

Contradictory study (Barnes, 2006)

Social phobia (Wheatley, 1999)

Somatoform disorders (Maisenbacher, 1992; Muller, 2004)

Summary St John's wort has been used in Europe for centuries for mild to moderate depression. It has attracted attention as a natural alternative to current prescription therapies in the United States. Comparative trials with tricyclic antidepressants have been favorable, and comparative trials with SSRIs are ongoing. St John's wort has also been used as a topical preparation to accelerate wound and burn healing, and to improve muscle soreness/stiffness and neuralgia.

A study in JAMA found St John's wort no more effective than placebo or a prescription antidepressant (sertraline) for moderate to severe depression (Shelton, 2001). There are many questions surrounding methodology and study groups; St John's wort has previously been shown to be effective in mild forms of depression.

Effect on Mental Status May cause mania and drowsiness

Effect on Psychiatric Treatment Usefulness of St John's wort in severe depression has not been demonstrated. May alter actions of MAO inhibitors, SSRIs, TCAs; combined use is not recommended. Use with caution in bipolar disorder; may potentiate mania.

Pharmacology St John's wort is a perennial flowering plant, which grows in many areas of the world, including Europe and the United States. The activity has been correlated to the hypericin component of the plant. It is believed to act through a variety of mechanisms, including inhibition of cortisol secretion, blockade of catabolic hormones (such as IL-6), and increased concentrations of central nervous system neurotransmitters, including serotonin. It may have mild MAO-inhibiting activity, but this does not appear to be its major mechanism of action. St John's wort may amplify the response to serotonin following receptor binding.

Additionally, hypericin and xanthones have been claimed to have antiviral activity, including activity in HIV, by stimulating an increase in T killer cell activity.

Recent research suggests that hyperforin and hypericin content varies in many commercially available St John's wort products. Therefore, users are encouraged to use the same brand on a regular basis, and **not** switch between brands, to help ensure consistency in response (Wurglics, 2001).

Warnings and Interactions May be associated with hypertensive crisis (Patel, 2002) or mania (Moses, 2000).

Theoretical Cautions and Contraindications St John's wort is contraindicated in pregnancy (based on animal studies) (Grush 1998). Use with caution in individuals taking digoxin (may alter levels of this medication) (Johne 1999). It is not for use in severe depression. Use with caution in individuals taking other antidepressants (Gordon, 1998). Based on its pharmacologic activity, St John's wort may alter the actions of monoamine oxidase (MAO) inhibitors, tricyclic antidepressants, and selective serotonin reuptake inhibitors (SSRIs) (Bennett, 1998; Chatterjee, 1998). May elevate hepatic transaminases (noted animal studies at high doses) (Brockmoller, 1990). May cause photosensitivity (based on animal studies and a human clinical trial) (Brockmoller, 1997). Use with caution in individuals on reserpine (effects may be antagonized by St John's wort) (Okpanyi, 1987). Use with caution in individuals on narcotic medications (based on animal studies, may enhance sedation from these drugs) (Okpanyi, 1987).

May cause drowsiness (mild). Based on pharmacologic activity, use with caution while driving or operating machinery. Use caution in individuals taking sedative medications (eg, anxiolytics, benzodiazepines). Effects may be additive with other CNS depressants or natural products with sedative properties.

Antidepressant therapy may precipitate a shift to mania or hypomania in individuals with bipolar affective disorder (Schneck, 1998).

Three patients experienced mania after short-term St John's wort use. All returned to normal after discontinuing the product.

St John's wort may induce the cytochrome P450 enzyme system, although there is conflicting information about this claim. Specifically, data indicates probable interactions between St John's wort and the HIV-1 protease inhibitor indinavir (Piscitelli, 2000) and between St John's wort and the antirejection medication cyclosporine (Ruschitzka, 2000). Additionally, enzyme induction may result in decreased estrogen levels in individuals taking oral contraceptives (Yue, 2000). While the FDA has issued a public health advisory regarding this issue, the authors recommend considerable caution be exercised before adding St John's wort to any medication regimen containing a cytochrome P-450 3A substrate.

St John's wort may cause an increase in thyroid-stimulating hormone (Ferko, 2001; Hauben, 2002).

General Warnings Use all herbal supplements with extreme caution in children <2 years of age and in pregnancy or lactation. Some herbs are contraindicated in pregnancy or lactation; make sure to observe warnings. Use with caution in individuals on medication and with pre-existing medical conditions. Always review for potential herb-drug interactions (HDIs) and other warnings (see ▶

Reported Interactions). Large and prolonged doses may increase the potential for adverse effects. Herbs may cause transient adverse effects such as nausea, vomiting, and GI distress due to a variety of chemical constituents. Use caution in individuals having known allergies to plants.

Theoretical Interactions Do not use St John's wort in combination with any prescription medication unless reviewed in advance with your healthcare provider. Specific medication examples reported to interact with St John's wort include: Antirejection medications, HIV-1 protease inhibitors, oral contraceptives, cardiac glycosides, other antidepressants, sedatives (including narcotics), sibutramine, migraine medications, lithium, anesthetic agents, photosensitizers, thyroid medications, other medications altered by a specific liver enzyme system, and anything that affects the neurotransmitter serotonin.

Reported Interactions Imatinib (Gleevec®) (Frye, 2004), indinavir (Piscitelli, 2000), and possibly other HIV-1 protease inhibitors; antirejection medications, specifically cyclosporine and tacrolimus (Ruschitzka, 2000); antifungal agents, specifically voriconazole (Rengelshausen, 2005); benzodiazepines, specifically quazepam (Kawaguchi, 2004); calcium channel blockers, specifically verapamil (Tannergren, 2004); histamine antagonists, specifically fexofenadine (Dresser, 2003; Wang, 2002); opioids, specifically methadone (Eich-Hochli, 2003); mycophenolic acid (Mai, 2003); and simvastatin (Eggertsen, 2007). Any medication metabolized by the cytochrome P450 isoenzyme 3A system should not be used in combination with St John's wort unless under the supervision of a physician.

References

Barnes J, Barber N, Wheatley D, et al, "A Pilot Randomised, Open, Uncontrolled, Clinical Study of Two Dosages of St John's Wort (*Hypericum perforatum*) Herb Extract (LI-160) as an Aid to Motivational/Behavioural Support in Smoking Cessation," *Planta Med*, 2006, 72 (4):378-82.

Bennett DA Jr, Phun L, Polk JF, et al, "Neuropharmacology of St John's Wort (*Hypericum*)," *Ann Pharmacother*, 1998, 32(11):1201-8.

Brockmoller J, Reum T, Bauer S, et al, "Hypericin and Pseudohypericin: Pharmacokinetics and Effects of Photosensitivity in Humans," *Pharmacopsychiatry*, 1997, 30(Supp 2):94-101.

Chatterjee SS, Bhattacharya SK, Wonnemann M, et al, "Hyperforin as a Possible Antidepressant Component of *Hypericum* Extracts," *Life Sci*, 1998, 63(6):499-510.

Chung DJ, Kim HY, Park KH, et al, "Black Cohosh and St John's Wort (GYNO-Plus) for Climacteric Symptoms," *Yonsei Med J*, 2007, 48(2):289-94.

Cott JM and Fugh-Berman A, "Is St John's Wort (*Hypericum perforatum*) an Effective Antidepressant?" *J Nerv Ment Dis*, 1998, 186(8):500-1.

Dresser GK, Schwarz UI, Wilkinson GR, et al, "Coordinate Induction of Both Cytochrome P4503A and MDR1 by St John's Wort in Healthy Subjects," *Clin Pharmacol Ther*, 2003, 73 (1):41-50.

Eggertsen R, Andreasson A, and Andrén L, "Effects of Treatment With a Commercially Available St John's Wort Product (Movina) on Cholesterol Levels in Patients With Hypercholesterolemia Treated With Simvastatin," *Scand J Prim Health Care*, 2007, 25 (3):154-9.

Eich-Hochli D, Oppliger R, Golay KP, et al, "Methadone Maintenance Treatment and St. John's Wort - A Case Report," *Pharmacopsychiatry*, 2003, 36(1):35-7.

Ferko N and Levine MA, "Evaluation of the Association Between St John's Wort and Elevated Thyroid-Stimulating Hormone," *Pharmacotherapy*, 2001, 21(12):1574-8.

Findling RL, McNamara NK, O'Riordan MA, et al, "An Open-Label Pilot Study of St. John's Wort in Juvenile Depression," *J Am Acad Child Adolesc Psychiatry*, 2003, 42(8):908-14.

Frye RF, Fitzgerald SM, Lagattuta TF, et al, "Effect of St John's Wort on Imatinib Mesylate Pharmacokinetics," P96 American Society for Clinical Pharmacology and Therapeutics, PDII-B-4, February 2004.

Gaster B and Holroyd J, "St John's Wort for Depression: A Systematic Review," *Arch Intern Med*, 2000, 160(2):152-6.

Goldman P, "Herbal Medicines Today and the Roots of Modern Pharmacology," *Ann Intern Med*, 2001, 135(8 Pt 1):594-600.

Gordon JB, "SSRIs and St John's Wort: Possible Toxicity?" *Am Fam Physician*, 1998, 57 (5):950,953.

Grube B, Walper A, and Wheatley D, "St. John's Wort Extract: Efficacy for Menopausal Symptoms of Psychological Origin," *Adv Ther*, 1999, 16(4):177-86.

Grush LR, Nierenberg A, Keefe B, et al, "St John's Wort During Pregnancy," *JAMA*, 1998, 280(18):1566.

Harrer G, Schmidt U, Kuhn U, et al, "Comparison of Equivalence Between the St John's Wort Extract LoHyp-57 and Fluoxetine," *Arzneimittelforschung*, 1999, 49(4):289-96.

Hauben M, "The Association of St John's Wort With Elevated Thyroid-Stimulating Hormone," *Pharmacotherapy*, 2002, 22(5):673-5.

Hicks SM, Walker AF, Gallagher J, et al, "The Significance of 'Nonsignificance' in Randomized Controlled Studies: A Discussion Inspired by a Double-Blinded Study on St. John's Wort (*Hypericum perforatum* L.) for Premenstrual Symptoms," *J Altern Complement Med*, 2004, 10(6):925-32.

Hippius H, "St John's Wort (*Hypericum perforatum*) - A Herbal Antidepressant," *Curr Med Res Opin*, 1998, 14(3):171-84.

Hubner WD and Kirste T, "Experience With St John's Wort (*Hypericum perforatum*) in Children Under 12 Years With Symptoms of Depression and Psychovegetative Disturbances," *Phytother Res*, 2001, 15(4):367-70.

Hypericum Depression Trial Study Group, "Effect of *Hypericum perforatum* (St John's Wort) in Major Depressive Disorder: A Randomized Controlled Trial," *JAMA*, 2002, 287 (14):1807-14.

Johne A, Brockmoller J, Bauer S, et al, "Pharmacokinetic Interaction of Digoxin With an Herbal Extract from St John's Wort," *Clin Pharmacol Ther*, 1999, 66(4):338-45.

Kasper S, Anghelescu IG, Szegedi A, et al, "Superior Efficacy of St John's Wort Extract WS 5570 Compared to Placebo in Patients With Major Depression: A Randomized, Double-Blind, Placebo-Controlled, Multi-Center Trial [ISRCTN77277298]," *BMC Med*, 2006, 4:14.

Kasper S, "Treatment of Seasonal Affective Disorder (SAD) With *Hypericum* Extract," *Pharmacopsychiatry*, 1997, 2(30 Suppl):89-93.

Kawaguchi A, Ohmori M, Tsuruoka S, et al, "Drug Interaction Between St John's Wort and Quazepam," *Br J Clin Pharmacol*, 2004, 58(4):403-10.

Kobak KA, Taylor L, Futterer R, et al, "St. John's Wort in Generalized Anxiety Disorder: Three More Case Reports," *J Clin Psychopharmacol*, 2003, 23(5):531-2.

Kobak KA, Taylor LV, Bystritsky A, et al, "St John's Wort Versus Placebo in Obsessive-Compulsive Disorder: Results From a Double-Blind Study," *Int Clin Psychopharmacol*, 2005, 20(6):299-304.

Lawvere S, Mahoney MC, Cummings KM, et al, "A Phase II Study of St John's Wort for Smoking Cessation," *Complement Ther Med*, 2006, 14(3):175-84.

Lenoir S, Degenring FH, and Saller R, "A Double-Blind Randomised Trial to Investigate Three Different Concentrations of a Standardised Fresh Plant Extract Obtained From the Shoot Tips of *Hypericum perforatum* L," *Phytomedicine*, 1999, 6(3):141-6.

Linde K, Ramirez G, Mulrow CD, et al, "St John's Wort for Depression - An Overview and Meta-Analysis of Randomised Clinical Trials," *BMJ*, 1996 313(7052):253-8.

Mai I, Stormer E, Bauer S, et al, "Impact of St John's Wort Treatment on the Pharmacokinetics of Tacrolimus and Mycophenolic Acid in Renal Transplant Patients," *Nephrol Dial Transplant*, 2003, 18(4):819-22.

Maisenbacher HJ and Kuhn U, "The Therapy of Depressions in Practice: Results of a Post-Marketing Surveillance Study With Herba Hyperici," *Natura Medica*, 1992, 7(5):394-9.

Miller AL, "St John's Wort (*Hypericum perforatum*): Clinical Effects on Depression and Other Conditions," *Altern Med Rev*, 1998, 3(1):18-26.

Moses EL and Mallinger AG, "St John's Wort: Three Cases of Possible Mania Induction," *J Clin Psychopharmacol*, 2000, 20(1):115-7.

Muller T, Mannel M, Murck H, et al, "Treatment of Somatoform Disorders With St. John's Wort: A Randomized, Double-Blind and Placebo-Controlled Trial," *Psychosom Med*, 2004, 66(4):538-47.

Natural Standard Research Collaboration, Chief Editors: Ulbricht C, Basch E, *Natural Standard Herb and Supplement Reference - Evidence-Based Clinical Reviews*, USA: Elsevier/Mosby, 2005.

Newall CA, Anderson LA, and Phillipson JD, *Herbal Medicines: A Guide for Health Care Professionals*, London, England: The Pharmaceutical Press, 1996, 250-2.

Okpanyi SN and Weischer ML, "Animal Experiments on the Psychotropic Action of a *Hypericum* Extract," *Arzneimittelforschung*, 1987, 37(1):10-3.

Patel S, Robinson R and Burk M, "Hypertensive Crisis Associated With St John's Wort," *Am J Med*, 2002, 112(6):507-8.

Piscitelli SC, Burstein AH, Chaitt D, et al, "Indinavir Concentration and St John's Wort," *Lancet*, 2000, 355:547-8.

Randløv C, Mehlsen J, Thomsen CF, et al, "The Efficacy of St John's Wort in Patients With Minor Depressive Symptoms or Dysthymia - a Double-Blind Placebo-Controlled Study," *Phytomedicine*, 2006, 13(4):215-21.

Rengelshausen J, Banfield M, Riedel KD, et al, "Opposite Effects of Short-Term and Long-Term St John's Wort Intake on Voriconazole Pharmacokinetics," *Clin Pharmacol Ther*, 2005, 78(1):25-33.

Ruschitzka F, Meier PJ, Turina M, et al, "Acute Heart Transplant Rejection Due to St John's Wort," *Lancet*, 2000, 355:548-9.

Schempp CM, Hezel S, and Simon JC, "Topical Treatment of Atopic Dermatitis With *Hypericum* Cream. A Randomised, Placebo-Controlled, Double-Blind Half-Side Comparison Study," *Hautarzt*, 2003, 54(3):248-53.

Schempp CM, Winghofer B, Muller K, et al, "Effect of Oral Administration of *Hypericum perforatum* Extract (St. John's Wort) on Skin Erythema and Pigmentation Induced by UVB, UVA, Visible Light and Solar Simulated Radiation," *Phytother Res*, 2003, 17(2):141-6.

Schneck C, "St John's Wort and Hypomania," *J Clin Psychiatry*, 1998 59(12):689.

Shelton RC, Keller MB, Gelenberg A, et al, "Effectiveness of St John's Wort in Major Depression: A Randomized Controlled Trial," *JAMA*, 2001, 285(15):1978-86.

Simeon J, Nixon MK, Milin R, et al, "Open-Label Pilot Study of St. John's Wort in Adolescent Depression," *J Child Adolesc Psychopharmacol*, 2005, 15(2):293-301.

Steger W, "Depressive Verstimmungen," *Z Allg Med*, 1985, 61:914-8.

Stevinson C and Ernst E, "A Pilot Study of *Hypericum perforatum* for the Treatment of Premenstrual Syndrome," *BJOG*, 2000, 107(7):870-6.

Tannergren C, Engman H, Knutson L, et al, "St John's Wort Decreases the Bioavailability of R- and S-Verapamil Through Induction of the First-Pass Metabolism," *Clin Pharmacol Ther*, 2004, 75(4):298-309.

Taylor LH and Kobak KA, "An Open-Label Trial of St. John's Wort (*Hypericum perforatum*) in Obsessive-Compulsive Disorder," *J Clin Psychiatry*, 2000, 61(8):575-8.

Uebelhack R, Blohmer JU, Graubaum HJ, et al, "Black Cohosh and St John's Wort for Climacteric Complaints: A Randomized Trial," *Obstet Gynecol*, 2006, 107:247-55.

Volz HP, "Controlled Clinical Trials of *Hypericum* Extracts in Depressed Patients - An Overview," *Pharmacopsychiatry*, 1997, 30(Suppl 2):72-6.

Vorbach EU, Arnoldt KH, and Hubner WD, "Efficacy and Tolerability of St John's Wort Extract LI 160 Versus Imipramine in Patients With Severe Depressive Episodes According to ICD-10," *Pharmacopsychiatry*, 1997, Suppl 2:81-5.

Wang Z, Hamman MA, Huang SM, et al, "Effect of St John's Wort on the Pharmacokinetics of Fexofenadine," *Clin Pharmacol Ther*, 2002, 71(6):414-20.

Wheatley D, "Hypericum in Seasonal Affective Disorder (SAD)," *Curr Med Res Opin*, 1999, 15(1):33-7.

Woelk H, "Comparison of St John's Wort and Imipramine for Treating Depression: Randomised Controlled Trial," *BMJ*, 2000, 321(7260):536-9.

Wurglics M, Westerhoff K, Kaunzinger A, et al, "Comparison of German St John's Wort Products According to Hyperforin and Total Hypericin Content," *J Am Pharm Assoc (Wash)*, 2001, 41(4):560-6.

Yue QY, Bergquist C, and Gerden B, "Safety of St John's Wort," *Lancet*, 2000, 355 (9203):576-7.

◆ **St. Joseph® Adult Aspirin [OTC]** *see* Aspirin *on page 143*

◆ **Strattera®** *see* Atomoxetine *on page 151*

Streptomycin (strep toe MYE sin)

Medication Safety Issues
Sound-alike/look-alike issues:
Streptomycin may be confused with streptozocin

Mexican Brand Names Estrepto-Monaxin

Index Terms Streptomycin Sulfate

Pharmacologic Category Antibiotic, Aminoglycoside; Antitubercular Agent

Use Part of combination therapy of active tuberculosis; used in combination with other agents for treatment of streptococcal or enterococcal endocarditis, mycobacterial infections, plague, tularemia, and brucellosis

Effect on Mental Status May cause drowsiness

Effect on Psychiatric Treatment None reported

Dosage Summary

I.M.:

Children: 20-40 mg/kg given daily or 2-3 times/week (maximum: 1 g/day)

Adults: Tuberculosis: 15 mg/kg/day **or** 25-30 mg/kg 2-3 times/week; Other indications: 1-4 g/day in 2 divided doses

Elderly: 10 mg/kg/day (maximum: 750 mg/day)

I.V.:

Children: 20-40 mg/kg/day **or** 20-40 mg/kg twice weekly **or** 25-30 mg/kg 3 times/week (maximum: 1 g/day)

Adults: 1-4 g/day in 2 divided doses

Dosage Forms Excipient information presented when available (limited, particularly for generics); consult specific product labeling.
Injection, powder for reconstitution: 1 g

◆ **Streptomycin Sulfate** *see* Streptomycin *on page 1510*

Streptozocin (strep toe ZOE sin)

Medication Safety Issues
Sound-alike/look-alike issues:
Streptozocin may be confused with streptomycin

High alert medication: The Institute for Safe Medication Practices (ISMP) includes this medication among its list of drugs which have a heightened risk of causing significant patient harm when used in error.

U.S. Brand Names Zanosar®

Canadian Brand Names Zanosar®

Index Terms NSC-85998

Pharmacologic Category Antineoplastic Agent, Alkylating Agent

Use Treatment of metastatic islet cell carcinoma of the pancreas, carcinoid tumor and syndrome, Hodgkin's disease, palliative treatment of colorectal cancer

Effect on Mental Status May cause lethargy, confusion, or depression

Effect on Psychiatric Treatment May cause leukopenia; use caution with clozapine and carbamazepine; renal dysfunction occurs commonly with streptozocin; will need to monitor and adjust lithium and gabapentin doses

Dosage Summary

I.V.:

Children: 1-1.5 g/m^2 weekly for 6 weeks followed by a 4-week rest period **or** 0.5-1 g/m^2 for 5 consecutive days as combination therapy followed by a 4- to 6-week rest period

Adults: 1-1.5 g/m^2 weekly for 6 weeks followed by a 4-week rest period **or** 0.5-1 g/m^2 for 5 consecutive days as combination therapy followed by a 4- to 6-week rest period

Dosage Forms Excipient information presented when available (limited, particularly for generics); consult specific product labeling.
Injection, powder for reconstitution: 1 g

- ◆ **Striant®** *see* Testosterone *on page 1553*
- ◆ **Stridex® Essential Care® [OTC]** *see* Salicylic Acid *on page 1454*
- ◆ **Stridex® Facewipes To Go® [OTC]** *see* Salicylic Acid *on page 1454*
- ◆ **Stridex® Maximum Strength [OTC]** *see* Salicylic Acid *on page 1454*
- ◆ **Stridex® Sensitive Skin [OTC]** *see* Salicylic Acid *on page 1454*
- ◆ **Stromectol®** *see* Ivermectin *on page 873*
- ◆ **Strong Iodine Solution** *see* Potassium Iodide and Iodine *on page 1317*
- ◆ **SU11248** *see* Sunitinib *on page 1530*
- ◆ **Suberoylanilide Hydroxamic Acid** *see* Vorinostat *on page 1678*
- ◆ **Sublimaze®** *see* FentaNYL *on page 624*
- ◆ **Suboxone®** *see* Buprenorphine and Naloxone *on page 215*
- ◆ **Subutex®** *see* Buprenorphine *on page 212*

Succimer (SUKS si mer)

U.S. Brand Names Chemet®
Canadian Brand Names Chemet®
Index Terms DMSA
Pharmacologic Category Antidote
Use Treatment of lead poisoning in children with serum lead levels >45 mcg/dL
Unlabeled/Investigational Use
Treatment of lead poisoning in symptomatic adults
Effect on Mental Status May cause drowsiness or dizziness
Effect on Psychiatric Treatment None reported
Dosage Summary
Oral:
Children: 10 mg/kg(or 350 mg/m^2/dose) every 8-12 hours (maximum: 500 mg/dose)
Adults (unlabeled): 10 mg/kg (or 350 mg/m^2/dose) every 8-12 hours (maximum: 500 mg/dose)
Dosage Forms Excipient information presented when available (limited, particularly for generics); consult specific product labeling.
Capsule:
Chemet®:100 mg

Succinylcholine (suks in il KOE leen)

Medication Safety Issues
High alert medication: The Institute for Safe Medication Practices (ISMP) includes this medication among its list of drugs which have a heightened risk of causing significant patient harm when used in error.
U.S. Brand Names Anectine®; Quelicin®
Canadian Brand Names Quelicin®
Mexican Brand Names Anectine
Index Terms Succinylcholine Chloride; Suxamethonium Chloride
Pharmacologic Category Neuromuscular Blocker Agent, Depolarizing
Generic Available No
Use Adjunct to general anesthesia to facilitate both rapid sequence and routine endotracheal intubation and to relax skeletal muscles during surgery; to reduce the intensity of muscle contractions of pharmacologically- or electrically-induced convulsions; does not relieve pain or produce sedation
Effect on Mental Status None reported
Effect on Psychiatric Treatment MAO inhibitors may prolong the effects of succinylcholine
Pregnancy Risk Factor C
Pregnancy Considerations Reproduction studies have not been conducted. Small amounts cross the placenta. Sensitivity to succinylcholine may be increased due to a ~24% decrease in plasma cholinesterase activity during pregnancy and several days postpartum.
Lactation Excretion in breast milk unknown/use caution
Contraindications Hypersensitivity to succinylcholine or any component of the formulation; personal or familial history of malignant hyperthermia; myopathies associated with elevated serum creatine phosphokinase (CPK) values; acute ▶

phase of injury following major burns, multiple trauma, extensive denervation of skeletal muscle or upper motor neuron injury

Warnings/Precautions [U.S. Boxed Warning]: Use caution in children and adolescents. Acute rhabdomyolysis with hyperkalemia, ventricular arrhythmias and cardiac arrest have been reported (rarely) in children with undiagnosed skeletal muscle myopathy. Use in children should be reserved for emergency intubation or where immediate airway control is necessary. Use with caution in patients with pre-existing hyperkalemia, extensive or severe burns; severe hyperkalemia may develop in patients with chronic abdominal infections, burn injuries, children with skeletal muscle myopathy, subarachnoid hemorrhage, or conditions which cause degeneration of the nervous system. Alkalosis, hypercalcemia, demyelinating lesions, peripheral neuropathies, denervation, infection, muscle trauma, and diabetes mellitus may result in antagonism of neuromuscular blockade. Electrolyte abnormalities, severe hyponatremia, severe hypocalcemia, severe hypokalemia, hypermagnesemia, neuromuscular diseases, acidosis, acute intermittent porphyria, Eaton-Lambert syndrome, myasthenia gravis, renal failure, and hepatic failure may result in potentiation of neuromuscular blockade. May increase vagal tone.

Succinylcholine is metabolized by plasma cholinesterase; use with caution (if at all) in patients suspected of being homozygous for the atypical plasma cholinesterase gene.

Use with caution in patients with extensive or severe burns; risk of hyperkalemia is increased following injury. May increase intraocular pressure; use caution with narrow angle glaucoma or penetrating eye injuries. Risk of bradycardia may be increased with second dose and may occur more in children. Use may be associated with acute onset of malignant hyperthermia; risk may be increased with concomitant administration of volatile anesthetics. Use with caution in the elderly; effects and duration are more variable.

Maintenance of an adequate airway and respiratory support is critical. Should be administered by adequately trained individuals familiar with its use.

Adverse Reactions

Frequency not defined.

Cardiovascular: Arrhythmias, bradycardia (higher with second dose, more frequent in children), cardiac arrest, hyper-/hypotension, tachycardia

Dermatologic: Rash

Endocrine & metabolic: Hyperkalemia

Gastrointestinal: Salivation (excessive)

Neuromuscular & skeletal: Jaw rigidity, muscle fasciculation, postoperative muscle pain, rhabdomyolysis (with possible myoglobinuric acute renal failure)

Ocular: Intraocular pressure increased

Renal: Acute renal failure (secondary to rhabdomyolysis)

Respiratory: Apnea, respiratory depression (prolonged)

Miscellaneous: Anaphylaxis, malignant hyperthermia

Postmarketing and/or case reports: Acute quadriplegic myopathy syndrome (prolonged use), myositis ossificans (prolonged use)

Drug Interactions

Acetylcholinesterase Inhibitors: May enhance the neuromuscular-blocking effect of Succinylcholine. *Risk C: Monitor therapy*

Aminoglycosides: May enhance the respiratory depressant effect of Neuromuscular-Blocking Agents. *Risk C: Monitor therapy*

Analgesics (Opioid): Succinylcholine may enhance the bradycardic effect of Analgesics (Opioid). *Risk C: Monitor therapy*

Botulinum Toxin Type A: Neuromuscular-Blocking Agents may enhance the neuromuscular-blocking effect of Botulinum Toxin Type A. *Risk C: Monitor therapy*

Botulinum Toxin Type B: Neuromuscular-Blocking Agents may enhance the neuromuscular-blocking effect of Botulinum Toxin Type B. *Risk C: Monitor therapy*

Capreomycin: May enhance the neuromuscular-blocking effect of Neuromuscular-Blocking Agents. *Risk C: Monitor therapy*

Cardiac Glycosides: Neuromuscular-Blocking Agents may enhance the arrhythmogenic effect of Cardiac Glycosides. *Risk C: Monitor therapy*

Colistimethate: May enhance the neuromuscular-blocking effect of Neuromuscular-Blocking Agents. *Risk D: Consider therapy modification*

Cyclophosphamide: May decrease the metabolism of Succinylcholine. *Risk D: Consider therapy modification*

Echothiophate Iodide: May decrease the metabolism of Succinylcholine. *Risk D: Consider therapy modification*

Lincosamide Antibiotics: May enhance the neuromuscular-blocking effect of Neuromuscular-Blocking Agents. *Risk C: Monitor therapy*

Lithium: May enhance the neuromuscular-blocking effect of Neuromuscular-Blocking Agents. *Risk C: Monitor therapy*

Loop Diuretics: May diminish the neuromuscular-blocking effect of Neuromuscular-Blocking Agents. Loop Diuretics may enhance the neuromuscular-blocking effect of Neuromuscular-Blocking Agents. *Risk C: Monitor therapy*

Magnesium Salts: May enhance the neuromuscular-blocking effect of Neuromuscular-Blocking Agents. Only of concern in patients with increased serum magnesium concentrations. *Risk C: Monitor therapy*

Phenelzine: May enhance the neuromuscular-blocking effect of Succinylcholine. *Risk D: Consider therapy modification*

Polymyxin B: May enhance the neuromuscular-blocking effect of Neuromuscular-Blocking Agents. *Risk D: Consider therapy modification*

Procainamide: May enhance the neuromuscular-blocking effect of Neuromuscular-Blocking Agents. *Risk C: Monitor therapy*

QuiNIDine: May enhance the neuromuscular-blocking effect of Neuromuscular-Blocking Agents. *Risk C: Monitor therapy*

Tetracycline Derivatives: May enhance the neuromuscular-blocking effect of Neuromuscular-Blocking Agents. *Risk C: Monitor therapy*

Vancomycin: May enhance the neuromuscular-blocking effect of Neuromuscular-Blocking Agents. *Risk C: Monitor therapy*

Stability Refrigerate at 2°C to 8°C (36°F to 46°F); however, stable for ≤3 months unrefrigerated (25°C). May dilute to a final concentration of 1-2 mg/mL. Do not mix with alkaline solutions (pH > 8.5). Stability of parenteral admixture (1-2 mg/mL) at refrigeration temperature (4°C) is 24 hours in D_5W or NS.

Mechanism of Action Acts similar to acetylcholine, produces depolarization of the motor endplate at the myoneural junction which causes sustained flaccid skeletal muscle paralysis produced by state of accommodation that developes in adjacent excitable muscle membranes

Pharmacodynamics/Kinetics

Onset of action: I.M.: 2-3 minutes; I.V.: Complete muscular relaxation: 30-60 seconds

Duration: I.M.: 10-30 minutes; I.V.: 4-6 minutes with single administration

Metabolism: Rapidly hydrolyzed by plasma pseudocholinesterase

Excretion: Urine

Dosage I.M., I.V.: Dose to effect; doses will vary due to interpatient variability; use ideal body weight for obese patients

I.M.: Children and Adults: Up to 3-4 mg/kg, total dose should not exceed 150 mg

I.V.:

Children: **Note:** Because of the risk of malignant hyperthermia, use of continuous infusions is not recommended in infants and children

Smaller Children: Intermittent: Initial: 2 mg/kg/dose one time; maintenance: 0.3-0.6 mg/kg/ dose every 5-10 minutes as needed

Older Children and Adolescents: Intermittent: Initial: 1 mg/kg/dose one time; maintenance: 0.3-0.6 mg/kg every 5-10 minutes as needed

Adults: Initial:

Short surgical procedures: 0.6 mg/kg (range 0.3-1.1 mg/kg)

Long surgical procedures:

Continuous infusion: 2.5-4.3 mg/minute; adjust dose based on response

Intermittent: Initial: 0.3-1.1 mg/kg; maintenance: 0.04-0.07 mg/kg/dose as required

Note: Initial dose of succinylcholine must be increased when nondepolarizing agent pretreatment used because of the antagonism between succinylcholine and nondepolarizing neuromuscular-blocking agents.

Dose adjustment with reduced plasma cholinesterase activity: Administer a test dose of 5-10 mg to evaluate sensitivity, or cautiously administer 1 mg/mL by slow I.V. infusion to produce neuromuscular blockade

Dosing adjustment in hepatic impairment: Dose should be decreased in patients with severe liver disease

Administration May be administered by rapid I.V. injection without further dilution. I.M. injections should be made deeply, preferably high into deltoid muscle; use only when I.V. access is not available.

Monitoring Parameters Monitor cardiac, blood pressure, and oxygenation during administration; temperature, serum potassium and calcium, assisted ventilator status; neuromuscular function with a peripheral nerve stimulator

Dosage Forms Excipient information presented when available (limited, particularly for generics); consult specific product labeling.

Injection, solution, as chloride:

Anectine®: 20 mg/mL (10 mL)

Quelicin®: 20 mg/mL (10 mL)
Injection, solution, as chloride [preservative free]:
Quelicin®: 100 mg/mL (10 mL)

◆ **Succinylcholine Chloride** *see* Succinylcholine *on page 1511*

◆ **Suclor™** *see* Chlorpheniramine and Pseudoephedrine *on page 325*

Sucralfate (soo KRAL fate)

Medication Safety Issues
Sound-alike/look-alike issues:
Sucralfate may be confused with salsalate
Carafate® may be confused with Cafergot®

U.S. Brand Names Carafate®

Canadian Brand Names Novo-Sucralate; Nu-Sucralate; PMS-Sucralate; Sulcrate®; Sulcrate® Suspension Plus

Mexican Brand Names Unival

Index Terms Aluminum Sucrose Sulfate, Basic

Pharmacologic Category Gastrointestinal Agent, Miscellaneous

Generic Available Yes

Use Short-term (≤8 weeks) management of duodenal ulcers; maintenance therapy for duodenal ulcers

Unlabeled/Investigational Use Gastric ulcers; suspension may be used topically for treatment of stomatitis due to cancer chemotherapy and other causes of esophageal and gastric erosions; GERD, esophagitis; treatment of NSAID mucosal damage; prevention of stress ulcers; postsclerotherapy for esophageal variceal bleeding

Effect on Mental Status May cause drowsiness, dizziness, or insomnia

Effect on Psychiatric Treatment None reported

Pregnancy Risk Factor B

Pregnancy Considerations Teratogenic effects were not observed in animal studies. Sucralfate is only minimally absorbed following oral administration.

Lactation Excretion in breast milk unknown/use caution

Contraindications Hypersensitivity to sucralfate or any component of the formulation

Warnings/Precautions Because sucralfate acts locally at the ulcer site, successful therapy with sucralfate should not be expected to alter the posthealing frequency of recurrence or the severity of duodenal ulceration. Use with caution in patients with chronic renal failure; sucralfate is an aluminum complex, small amounts of aluminum are absorbed following oral administration. Excretion of aluminum may be decreased in patients with chronic renal failure. Because of the potential for sucralfate to alter the absorption of some drugs, separate administration (take other medication 2 hours before sucralfate) should be considered when alterations in bioavailability are believed to be critical. Safety and efficacy have not been established in children.

Adverse Reactions
1% to 10%: Gastrointestinal: Constipation (2%)
<1% (Limited to important or life-threatening): Back pain, bezoar formation, diarrhea, dizziness, flatulence, headache, gastric discomfort; hypersensitivity (urticaria, angioedema, facial swelling, laryngospasm, respiratory difficulty, rhinitis); indigestion, insomnia, nausea, pruritus, rash, sleepiness, vertigo, vomiting, xerostomia

Drug Interactions
Antifungal Agents (Azole Derivatives, Systemic): Sucralfate may decrease the absorption of Antifungal Agents (Azole Derivatives, Systemic). **Exceptions:** Miconazole. *Risk C: Monitor therapy*
Levothyroxine: Sucralfate may decrease the serum concentration of Levothyroxine. *Risk C: Monitor therapy*
Phosphate Supplements: Sucralfate may decrease the absorption of Phosphate Supplements. *Risk D: Consider therapy modification*
Quinolone Antibiotics: Sucralfate may decrease the absorption of Quinolone Antibiotics. Of concern only with oral administration of quinolones. *Risk D: Consider therapy modification*

Ethanol/Nutrition/Herb Interactions Food: Sucralfate may interfere with absorption of vitamin A, vitamin D, vitamin E, and vitamin K.

Stability Suspension: Shake well. Store at 20°C to 25°C (68°F to 77°F); do **not** freeze.

Mechanism of Action Forms a complex by binding with positively charged proteins in exudates, forming a viscous paste-like, adhesive substance. This selectively forms a protective coating that acts locally to protect the gastric lining against peptic acid, pepsin, and bile salts.

Pharmacodynamics/Kinetics

Onset of action: Paste formation and ulcer adhesion: 1-2 hours

Duration: Up to 6 hours

Absorption: Oral: <5%

Distribution: Acts locally at ulcer sites; unbound in GI tract to aluminum and sucrose octasulfate

Metabolism: None

Excretion: Urine (small amounts as unchanged compounds)

Dosage Oral:

Children (unlabeled use): Doses of 40-80 mg/kg/day divided every 6 hours have been used

Stomatitis (unlabeled use): 5-10 mL (1 g/10 mL suspension), swish and spit or swish and swallow 4 times/day

Adults:

Stress ulcer (unlabeled use):

Prophylaxis: 1 g 4 times/day

Treatment: 1 g every 4 hours

Duodenal ulcer:

Treatment: 1 g 4 times/day on an empty stomach and at bedtime for 4-8 weeks, or alternatively 2 g twice daily; treatment is recommended for 4-8 weeks in adults

Maintenance: Prophylaxis: 1 g twice daily

Stomatitis (unlabeled use): 10 mL (1 g/10 mL suspension), swish and spit or swish and swallow 4 times/day

Dosage comment in renal impairment: Aluminum salt is minimally absorbed (<5%), however, may accumulate in renal failure

Dietary Considerations Administer with water on an empty stomach.

Administration Tablet may be broken or dissolved in water before ingestion. Administer with water on an empty stomach.

Dosage Forms Excipient information presented when available (limited, particularly for generics); consult specific product labeling.

Suspension, oral: 1 g/10 mL (10 mL)

Carafate®: 1 g/10 mL (420 mL)

Tablet: 1 g

Carafate®: 1 g

- ◆ **Sudafed® 12 Hour [OTC]** *see* Pseudoephedrine *on page 1367*
- ◆ **Sudafed® 24 Hour [OTC]** *see* Pseudoephedrine *on page 1367*
- ◆ **Sudafed® Children's [OTC]** *see* Pseudoephedrine *on page 1367*
- ◆ **Sudafed® Children's Cold & Cough [OTC]** *see* Pseudoephedrine and Dextromethorphan *on page 1369*
- ◆ **Sudafed® Maximum Strength Nasal Decongestant [OTC]** *see* Pseudoephedrine *on page 1367*
- ◆ **Sudafed® Maximum Strength Sinus Nighttime [OTC] [DSC]** *see* Triprolidine and Pseudoephedrine *on page 1634*
- ◆ **Sudafed® Multi-Symptom Sinus and Cold [OTC]** *see* Acetaminophen and Pseudoephedrine *on page 37*
- ◆ **Sudafed PE™ [OTC]** *see* Phenylephrine *on page 1273*
- ◆ **Sudafed PE® Nighttime Cold [OTC]** *see* Acetaminophen, Diphenhydramine, and Phenylephrine *on page 44*
- ◆ **Sudafed PE® Severe Cold [OTC]** *see* Acetaminophen, Diphenhydramine, and Phenylephrine *on page 44*
- ◆ **Sudafed PE® Sinus & Allergy [OTC]** *see* Chlorpheniramine and Phenylephrine *on page 323*
- ◆ **Sudafed PE® Sinus Headache [OTC]** *see* Acetaminophen and Phenylephrine *on page 36*
- ◆ **Sudafed® Sinus & Allergy [OTC]** *see* Chlorpheniramine and Pseudoephedrine *on page 325*
- ◆ **SudaHist®** *see* Chlorpheniramine and Pseudoephedrine *on page 325*
- ◆ **Sudal® 12** *see* Chlorpheniramine and Pseudoephedrine *on page 325*
- ◆ **SudaTex-DM** *see* Guaifenesin, Pseudoephedrine, and Dextromethorphan *on page 748*
- ◆ **SudaTex-G** *see* Guaifenesin and Pseudoephedrine *on page 744*
- ◆ **SudoGest [OTC]** *see* Pseudoephedrine *on page 1367*

- **SudoGest Children's [OTC]** *see* Pseudoephedrine and Dextromethorphan *on page 1369*
- **Sudo-Tab® [OTC]** *see* Pseudoephedrine *on page 1367*
- **Sufenta®** *see* SUFentanil *on page 1516*

SUFentanil (soo FEN ta nil)

Medication Safety Issues
Sound-alike/look-alike issues:
SUFentanil may be confused with alfentanil, fentaNYL
Sufenta® may be confused with Alfenta®, Sudafed®, Survanta®

High alert medication: The Institute for Safe Medication Practices (ISMP) includes this medication among its list of drugs which have a heightened risk of causing significant patient harm when used in error.

Related Information
Narcotic / Opioid Analgesics *on page 1789*

U.S. Brand Names Sufenta®

Canadian Brand Names Sufentanil Citrate Injection, USP; Sufenta®

Index Terms Sufentanil Citrate

Pharmacologic Category Analgesic, Opioid; Anilidopiperidine Opioid; General Anesthetic

Use Analgesic supplement in maintenance of balanced general anesthesia; primary anesthetic for induction and maintenance of anesthesia in patients undergoing major surgical procedures; epidural anesthetic in conjunction with bupivacaine in labor and delivery

Effect on Mental Status Drowsiness is common; may cause confusion; may rarely cause delirium or depression

Effect on Psychiatric Treatment Concurrent use with psychotropics may produce additive sedation

Restrictions C-II

Dosage Summary Note: In obese patients (ie, >20% above ideal body weight), use lean body weight to determine dosage

I.V.:
Children <2 years: Dosage not established
Children 2-12 years: 10-25 mcg/kg with 100% O_2; Maintenance: Up to 1-2 mcg/kg total dose
Adults: 1-2 mcg/kg with N_2O/O_2; Maintenance: 5-20 mcg/kg as needed

Epidural:
Children: Dosage not established
Adults: 10-15 mcg (maximum: 3 doses)

Dosage Forms Excipient information presented when available (limited, particularly for generics); consult specific product labeling.
Injection, solution [preservative free]: 50 mcg/mL (1 mL, 2 mL, 5 mL)
Sufenta®: 50 mcg/mL (1 mL, 2 mL, 5 mL)

- **Sufentanil Citrate** *see* SUFentanil *on page 1516*
- **Sular®** *see* Nisoldipine *on page 1143*
- **Sulbactam and Ampicillin** *see* Ampicillin and Sulbactam *on page 122*

Sulfacetamide and Prednisolone
(sul fa SEE ta mide & pred NIS oh lone)

Medication Safety Issues
Sound-alike/look-alike issues:
Blephamide® may be confused with Bleph®-10

U.S. Brand Names Blephamide®

Canadian Brand Names Blephamide®; Dioptimyd®

Mexican Brand Names Blefamide SF; Blefamide SOP; Metimyd

Index Terms Prednisolone and Sulfacetamide

Pharmacologic Category Antibiotic/Corticosteroid, Ophthalmic

Use Steroid-responsive inflammatory ocular conditions in which a corticosteroid is indicated and where infection is present or there is a risk of infection

Effect on Mental Status May rarely cause dizziness or psychosis

Effect on Psychiatric Treatment None reported

Dosage Summary

Ophthalmic:
Children <6 years: Dosage not established
Children ≥6 years:
Ointment: Apply ~1/2 inch ribbon 3-4 times/day and 1-2 times at night

Solution, suspension: Instill 2 drops every 4 hours

Adults:

Ointment: Apply ~1/2 inch ribbon 3-4 times/day and 1-2 times at night

Solution, suspension: Instill 2 drops every 4 hours

Dosage Forms Excipient information presented when available (limited, particularly for generics); consult specific product labeling.

Ointment, ophthalmic:

Blephamide®: Sulfacetamide sodium 10% and prednisolone acetate 0.2% (3.5 g)

Solution, ophthalmic [drops]: Sulfacetamide sodium 10% and prednisolone sodium phosphate 0.25% (5 mL, 10 mL)

Suspension, ophthalmic [drops]:

Blephamide®: Sulfacetamide sodium 10% and prednisolone acetate 0.2% (5 mL, 10 mL) [contains benzalkonium chloride]

SulfADIAZINE (sul fa DYE a zeen)

Medication Safety Issues

Sound-alike/look-alike issues:

SulfaDIAZINE may be confused with sulfasalazine, sulfiSOXAZOLE

Pharmacologic Category Antibiotic, Sulfonamide Derivative

Use Treatment of urinary tract infections and nocardiosis; adjunctive treatment in toxoplasmosis; uncomplicated attack of malaria

Unlabeled/Investigational Use Rheumatic fever prophylaxis

Effect on Mental Status Dizziness is common; sulfonamides reported to cause restlessness, irritability, depression, euphoria, disorientation, panic, hallucinations, and delusions

Effect on Psychiatric Treatment Photosensitivity is common; use caution with concurrent psychotropics; may cause granulocytopenia; caution with clozapine and carbamazepine

Dosage Forms Excipient information presented when available (limited, particularly for generics); consult specific product labeling.

Tablet: 500 mg

Sulfadoxine and Pyrimethamine

(sul fa DOKS een & peer i METH a meen)

U.S. Brand Names Fansidar®

Index Terms Pyrimethamine and Sulfadoxine

Pharmacologic Category Antimalarial Agent

Use Treatment of *Plasmodium falciparum* malaria in patients in whom chloroquine resistance is suspected; malaria prophylaxis for travelers to areas where chloroquine-resistant malaria is endemic

Effect on Mental Status Sulfonamides reported to cause restlessness, irritability, depression, euphoria, disorientation, panic, hallucinations, and delusions

Effect on Psychiatric Treatment Photosensitivity is common; use caution with concurrent psychotropics; may cause leukopenia; caution with clozapine and carbamazepine

Dosage Summary

Oral:

Children <2 months: Dosage not established

Children 2-11 months: 1/4 tablet as a single dose

Children 1-3 years: 1/2 tablet as a single dose

Children 4-8 years: 1 tablet as a single dose

Children 9-14 years: 2 tablets as a single dose

Children >14 years: 3 tablets as a single dose

Adults: 3 tablets as a single dose

Dosage Forms Excipient information presented when available (limited, particularly for generics); consult specific product labeling.

Tablet: Sulfadoxine 500 mg and pyrimethamine 25 mg

Sulfamethoxazole and Trimethoprim

(sul fa meth OKS a zole & trye METH oh prim)

Medication Safety Issues

Sound-alike/look-alike issues:

Bactrim™ may be confused with bacitracin, Bactine®, Bactroban®

Co-trimoxazole may be confused with clotrimazole

Septra® may be confused with Ceptaz®, Sectral®

Septra® DS may be confused with Semprex®-D

U.S. Brand Names Bactrim™; Bactrim™ DS; Septra®; Septra® DS; Sulfatrim®

Canadian Brand Names Apo-Sulfatrim®; Apo-Sulfatrim® DS; Apo-Sulfatrim® Pediatric; Novo-Trimel; Novo-Trimel D.S.; Nu-Cotrimox; Septra® Injection

Mexican Brand Names Anitrim; Bactelan; Bacteric; Bactiver; Bactrim; Bactropin; Brogamax; Dibaprim; Ectaprim; Metoxiprim; Octex; Septrin; Servitrim; Soltrim; Sulfoid Trimetho; Timexole; Trimetoger; Trimexazol

Index Terms Co-Trimoxazole; SMZ-TMP; Sulfatrim; TMP-SMZ; Trimethoprim and Sulfamethoxazole

Pharmacologic Category Antibiotic, Miscellaneous; Antibiotic, Sulfonamide Derivative

Generic Available Yes

Use

Oral treatment of urinary tract infections due to *E. coli*, *Klebsiella* and *Enterobacter* sp, *M. morganii*, *P. mirabilis* and *P. vulgaris*; acute otitis media in children; acute exacerbations of chronic bronchitis in adults due to susceptible strains of *H. influenzae* or *S. pneumoniae*; treatment and prophylaxis of *Pneumocystis jiroveci* pneumonitis (PCP); traveler's diarrhea due to enterotoxigenic *E. coli*; treatment of enteritis caused by *Shigella flexneri* or *Shigella sonnei*

I.V. treatment or severe or complicated infections when oral therapy is not feasible, for documented PCP, empiric treatment of PCP in immune compromised patients; treatment of documented or suspected shigellosis, typhoid fever, *Nocardia asteroides* infection, or other infections caused by susceptible bacteria

Unlabeled/Investigational Use Cholera and *Salmonella*-type infections and nocardiosis; chronic prostatitis; as prophylaxis in neutropenic patients with *P. jiroveci* infections, in leukemia patients, and in patients following renal transplantation, to decrease incidence of PCP; treatment of *Cyclospora* infection, typhoid fever, *Nocardia asteroides* infection; prophylaxis against urinary tract infection

Effect on Mental Status Rarely may cause depression, hallucination, or confusion; sulfonamides may cause euphoria, restlessness, irritability, disorientation, panic, and delusions

Effect on Psychiatric Treatment May rarely cause granulocytopenia; use caution with clozapine and carbamazepine

Pregnancy Risk Factor C/D (at term - expert analysis)

Pregnancy Considerations Do not use at term to avoid kernicterus in the newborn; use during pregnancy only if risks outweigh the benefits since folic acid metabolism may be affected.

Lactation Enters breast milk/contraindicated (AAP rates "compatible with restrictions")

Contraindications Hypersensitivity to any sulfa drug, trimethoprim, or any component of the formulation; megaloblastic anemia due to folate deficiency; infants <2 months of age; marked hepatic damage or severe renal disease (if patient not monitored); pregnancy (at term); breast-feeding

Warnings/Precautions Use with caution in patients with G6PD deficiency, impaired renal or hepatic function or potential folate deficiency (malnourished, chronic anticonvulsant therapy, or elderly); maintain adequate hydration to prevent crystalluria; adjust dosage in patients with renal impairment. Injection vehicle contains benzyl alcohol and sodium metabisulfite.

Chemical similarities are present among sulfonamides, sulfonylureas, carbonic anhydrase inhibitors, thiazides, and loop diuretics (except ethacrynic acid). Use in patients with sulfonamide allergy is specifically contraindicated in product labeling, however, a risk of cross-reaction exists in patients with allergy to any of these compounds; avoid use when previous reaction has been severe.

Fatalities associated with severe reactions including Stevens-Johnson syndrome, toxic epidermal necrolysis, hepatic necrosis, agranulocytosis, aplastic anemia and other blood dyscrasias; discontinue use at first sign of rash or serious adverse reactions. Elderly patients appear at greater risk for more severe adverse reactions. May cause hypoglycemia, particularly in malnourished, or patients with renal or hepatic impairment. Use with caution in patients with porphyria or thyroid dysfunction. Slow acetylators may be more prone to adverse reactions. Caution in patients with allergies or asthma. May cause hyperkalemia (associated with high doses of trimethoprim). Incidence of adverse effects appears to be increased in patients with AIDS. Prolonged use may result in fungal or bacterial superinfection, including *C. difficile*-associated diarrhea (CDAD) and pseudomembranous colitis; CDAD has been observed >2 months postantibiotic treatment.

Adverse Reactions The most common adverse reactions include gastrointestinal upset (nausea, vomiting, anorexia) and dermatologic reactions (rash or urticaria). Rare, life-threatening reactions have been associated with co-trimoxazole, including severe dermatologic reactions, blood dyscrasias, and hepatotoxic reactions. Most other reactions listed are rare, however, frequency cannot be accurately estimated.

Cardiovascular: Allergic myocarditis

Central nervous system: Apathy, aseptic meningitis, ataxia, chills, depression, fatigue, fever, hallucinations, headache, insomnia, kernicterus (in neonates), nervousness, peripheral neuritis, seizure, vertigo

Dermatologic: Photosensitivity, pruritus, rash, skin eruptions, urticaria; rare reactions include erythema multiforme, exfoliative dermatitis, Henoch-Schönlein purpura, Stevens-Johnson syndrome, and toxic epidermal necrolysis

Endocrine & metabolic: Hyperkalemia (generally at high dosages), hypoglycemia (rare), hyponatremia

Gastrointestinal: Abdominal pain, anorexia, diarrhea, glottis, nausea, pancreatitis, pseudomembranous colitis, stomatitis, vomiting

Hematologic: Agranulocytosis, aplastic anemia, eosinophilia, hemolysis (with G6PD deficiency), hemolytic anemia, hypoprothrombinemia, leukopenia, megaloblastic anemia, methemoglobinemia, neutropenia, thrombocytopenia

Hepatic: Hepatotoxicity (including hepatitis, cholestasis, and hepatic necrosis), hyperbilirubinemia, transaminases increased

Neuromuscular & skeletal: Arthralgia, myalgia, rhabdomyolysis, weakness

Otic: Tinnitus

Renal: BUN increased, crystalluria, diuresis (rare), interstitial nephritis, nephrotoxicity (in association with cyclosporine), renal failure, serum creatinine increased, toxic nephrosis (with anuria and oliguria)

Respiratory: Cough, dyspnea, pulmonary infiltrates

Miscellaneous: Allergic reaction, anaphylaxis, angioedema, periarteritis nodosa (rare), serum sickness, systemic lupus erythematosus (rare)

Metabolism/Transport Effects

Sulfamethoxazole: **Substrate** of CYP2C9 (major), 3A4 (minor); **Inhibits** CYP2C9 (moderate)

Trimethoprim: **Substrate** (major) of CYP2C9, 3A4; **Inhibits** CYP2C8 (moderate), 2C9 (moderate)

Drug Interactions

ACE Inhibitors: Trimethoprim may enhance the hyperkalemic effect of ACE Inhibitors. *Risk C: Monitor therapy*

Angiotensin II Receptor Blockers: Trimethoprim may enhance the hyperkalemic effect of Angiotensin II Receptor Blockers. *Risk C: Monitor therapy*

Antidiabetic Agents (Thiazolidinedione): Trimethoprim may decrease the metabolism of Antidiabetic Agents (Thiazolidinedione). *Risk C: Monitor therapy*

AzaTHIOprine: Sulfamethoxazole may enhance the myelosuppressive effect of AzaTHIOprine. *Risk C: Monitor therapy*

AzaTHIOprine: Trimethoprim may enhance the myelosuppressive effect of AzaTHIOprine. *Risk C: Monitor therapy*

CycloSPORINE: Sulfonamide Derivatives may enhance the nephrotoxic effect of CycloSPORINE. Sulfonamide Derivatives may decrease the serum concentration of CycloSPORINE. *Risk C: Monitor therapy*

CYP2C8 Substrates (High risk): CYP2C8 Inhibitors (Moderate) may decrease the metabolism of CYP2C8 Substrates (High risk). *Risk C: Monitor therapy*

CYP2C9 Inducers (Highly Effective): May increase the metabolism of CYP2C9 Substrates (High risk). *Risk C: Monitor therapy*

CYP2C9 Inhibitors (Moderate): May decrease the metabolism of CYP2C9 Substrates (High risk). *Risk C: Monitor therapy*

CYP2C9 Inhibitors (Strong): May decrease the metabolism of CYP2C9 Substrates (High risk). *Risk D: Consider therapy modification*

CYP2C9 Substrates (High risk): CYP2C9 Inhibitors (Moderate) may decrease the metabolism of CYP2C9 Substrates (High risk). *Risk C: Monitor therapy*

CYP3A4 Inducers (Strong): May increase the metabolism of CYP3A4 Substrates. *Risk C: Monitor therapy*

Dapsone: Trimethoprim may increase the serum concentration of Dapsone. Dapsone may increase the serum concentration of Trimethoprim. *Risk C: Monitor therapy*

Deferasirox: May decrease the serum concentration of CYP3A4 Substrates. *Risk C: Monitor therapy*

Dofetilide: Trimethoprim may decrease the excretion of Dofetilide. *Risk X: Avoid combination*

Herbs (CYP3A4 Inducers): May increase the metabolism of CYP3A4 Substrates. *Risk C: Monitor therapy*

LamiVUDine: Trimethoprim may decrease the excretion of LamiVUDine. *Risk C: Monitor therapy*

Leucovorin-Levoleucovorin: May diminish the therapeutic effect of Trimethoprim. *Risk D: Consider therapy modification*

Methotrexate: Sulfonamide Derivatives may enhance the adverse/toxic effect of Methotrexate. *Risk D: Consider therapy modification*

Methotrexate: Trimethoprim may enhance the adverse/toxic effect of Methotrexate. *Risk D: Consider therapy modification*

Phenytoin: Sulfonamide Derivatives may decrease the metabolism of Phenytoin. *Risk C: Monitor therapy*

Phenytoin: Trimethoprim may decrease the metabolism of Phenytoin. *Risk C: Monitor therapy*

Procainamide: Trimethoprim may decrease the excretion of Procainamide. *Risk D: Consider therapy modification*

Procaine: May diminish the therapeutic effect of Sulfonamide Derivatives. *Risk X: Avoid combination*

Repaglinide: Trimethoprim may decrease the metabolism of Repaglinide. *Risk C: Monitor therapy*

Sulfonylureas: Sulfonamide Derivatives may enhance the hypoglycemic effect of Sulfonylureas. *Risk C: Monitor therapy*

Typhoid Vaccine: Antibiotics may diminish the therapeutic effect of Typhoid Vaccine. Only the live attenuated Ty21a strain is affected. *Risk D: Consider therapy modification*

Vitamin K Antagonists (eg, warfarin): Sulfonamide Derivatives may enhance the anticoagulant effect of Vitamin K Antagonists. *Risk D: Consider therapy modification*

Ethanol/Nutrition/Herb Interactions Herb/Nutraceutical: Avoid dong quai; St John's wort (may diminish effects and also cause photosensitization).

Stability

Injection: Store at room temperature; do not refrigerate. Less soluble in more alkaline pH. Protect from light. Solution must be diluted prior to administration. Following dilution, store at room temperature; do not refrigerate. Manufacturer recommended dilutions and stability of parenteral admixture at room temperature (25°C):

5 mL/125 mL D_5W; stable for 6 hours.

5 mL/100 mL D_5W; stable for 4 hours.

5 mL/75 mL D_5W; stable for 2 hours.

Studies have also confirmed limited stability in NS; detailed references should be consulted.

Suspension, tablet: Store at controlled room temperature of 15°C to 25°C (59°F to 77°F). Protect from light.

Mechanism of Action Sulfamethoxazole interferes with bacterial folic acid synthesis and growth via inhibition of dihydrofolic acid formation from para-aminobenzoic acid; trimethoprim inhibits dihydrofolic acid reduction to tetrahydrofolate resulting in sequential inhibition of enzymes of the folic acid pathway

Pharmacodynamics/Kinetics

Absorption: Oral: Almost completely, 90% to 100%

Protein binding: SMX: 68%, TMP: 45%

Metabolism: SMX: N-acetylated and glucuronidated; TMP: Metabolized to oxide and hydroxylated metabolites

Half-life elimination: SMX: 9 hours, TMP: 6-17 hours; both are prolonged in renal failure

Time to peak, serum: Within 1-4 hours

Excretion: Both are excreted in urine as metabolites and unchanged drug

Effects of aging on the pharmacokinetics of both agents has been variable; increase in half-life and decreases in clearance have been associated with reduced creatinine clearance

Dosage Dosage recommendations are based on the trimethoprim component. Double-strength tablets are equivalent to sulfamethoxazole 800 mg and trimethoprim 160 mg.

Usual dosage ranges:

Children >2 months:

Mild-to-moderate infections: Oral: 8-12 mg TMP/kg/day in divided doses every 12 hours

Serious infection:

Oral: 20 mg TMP/kg/day in divided doses every 6 hours

I.V.: 8-12 mg TMP/kg/day in divided doses every 6 hours

Adults:
- Oral: One double strength tablet (sulfamethoxazole 800 mg; trimethoprim 160 mg) every 12-24 hours
- I.V.: 8-20 mg TMP/kg/day divided every 6-12 hours

Indication-specifc dosing:

Children >2 months:

Acute otitis media: Oral: 8 mg TMP/kg/day in divided doses every 12 hours for 10 days. **Note:** Recommended by the American Academy of Pediatrics as an alternative agent in penicillin-allergic patients at a dose of 6-10 mg TMP/kg/day (AOM guidelines, 2004).

Urinary tract infection:

Treatment:
- Oral: 6-12 mg TMP/kg/day in divided doses every 12 hours
- I.V.: 8-10 mg TMP/kg/day in divided doses every 6, 8, or 12 hours for up to 14 days with serious infections

Prophylaxis: Oral: 2 mg TMP/kg/dose daily or 5 mg TMP/kg/dose twice weekly

Pneumocystis jiroveci:

Treatment: Oral, I.V.: 15-20 mg TMP/kg/day in divided doses every 6-8 hours

Prophylaxis: Oral, 150 mg TMP/m^2/day in divided doses every 12 hours for 3 days/week; dose should not exceed trimethoprim 320 mg and sulfamethoxazole 1600 mg daily

Alternative prophylaxis dosing schedules include:

150 mg TMP/m^2/day as a single daily dose 3 times/week on consecutive days

or

150 mg TMP/m^2/day in divided doses every 12 hours administered 7 days/week

or

150 mg TMP/m^2/day in divided doses every 12 hours administered 3 times/week on alternate days

Shigellosis:
- Oral: 8 mg TMP/kg/day in divided doses every 12 hours for 5 days
- I.V.: 8-10 mg TMP/kg/day in divided doses every 6, 8, or 12 hours for up to 5 days

***Cyclospora* (unlabeled use):** Oral, I.V.: 5 mg TMP/kg twice daily for 7-10 days

Adults:

Urinary tract infection:

Oral: One double-strength tablet every 12 hours

Duration of therapy: Uncomplicated: 3-5 days; Complicated: 7-10 days

Pyelonephritis: 14 days

Prostatitis: Acute: 2 weeks; Chronic: 2-3 months

I.V.: 8-10 mg TMP/kg/day in divided doses every 6, 8, or 12 hours for up to 14 days with severe infections

Chronic bronchitis (acute): Oral: One double-strength tablet every 12 hours for 10-14 days

Meningitis (bacterial): I.V.: 10-20 mg TMP/kg/day in divided doses every 6-12 hours

Shigellosis:
- Oral: One double strength tablet every 12 hours for 5 days
- I.V.: 8-10 mg TMP/kg/day in divided doses every 6, 8, or 12 hours for up to 5 days

Travelers' diarrhea: Oral: One double strength tablet every 12 hours for 5 days

Sepsis: I.V.: 20 TMP/kg/day divided every 6 hours

***Pneumocystis jiroveci*:**
- Prophylaxis: Oral: 1 double strength tablet daily or 3 times/week
- Treatment: Oral, I.V.: 15-20 mg TMP/kg/day in 3-4 divided doses

Cyclospora (unlabeled use): Oral, I.V.: 160 mg TMP twice daily for 7-10 days. **Note:** AIDS patients: Oral: 1 double strength tablet 2-4 times/day for 10 days, then 1 double strength tablet 3 times/week for 10 weeks (Verdier, 2000 and Pape, 1994).

Nocardia (unlabeled use): Oral, I.V.:
- Cutaneous infections: 5-10 mg TMP/kg/day in 2-4 divided doses
- Severe infections (pulmonary/cerebral): 15 mg TMP/kg/day in 2-4 divided doses for 3-4 weeks, then 10 mg TMP/kg/day in 2-4 divided doses. Treatment duration is controversial; an average of 7 months has been reported.

Note: Therapy for severe infection may be initiated I.V. and converted to oral therapy (frequently converted to approximate dosages of oral solid dosage forms: 2 DS tablets every 8-12 hours). Although not widely available, sulfonamide levels should be considered in patients with questionable absorption, at risk for dose-related toxicity, or those with poor therapeutic response.

Dosing adjustment in renal impairment: Oral, I.V.:
Cl_{cr} 15-30 mL/minute: Administer 50% of recommended dose
Cl_{cr} <15 mL/minute: Use is not recommended

Dietary Considerations Should be taken with 8 oz of water.

Administration
I.V.: Infuse over 60-90 minutes, must dilute well before giving; may be given less diluted in a central line; not for I.M. injection
Oral: May be taken with or without food. Administer with at least 8 ounces of water.

Monitoring Parameters Perform culture and sensitivity testing prior to initiating therapy; CBC, serum potassium, creatinine, BUN

Test Interactions Increased creatinine (Jaffé alkaline picrate reaction); increased serum methotrexate by dihydrofolate reductase method

Dosage Forms Excipient information presented when available (limited, particularly for generics); consult specific product labeling. **Note:** The 5:1 ratio (SMX:TMP) remains constant in all dosage forms.
Injection, solution: Sulfamethoxazole 80 mg and trimethoprim 16 mg per mL (5 mL, 10 mL, 30 mL)
Suspension, oral: Sulfamethoxazole 200 mg and trimethoprim 40 mg per 5 mL (480 mL)
Sulfatrim®: Sulfamethoxazole 200 mg and trimethoprim 40 mg per 5 mL (100 mL, 480 mL) [contains alcohol ≤0.5% propylene glycol; cherry flavor]
Tablet: Sulfamethoxazole 400 mg and trimethoprim 80 mg
Bactrim™: Sulfamethoxazole 400 mg and trimethoprim 80 mg
Septra®: Sulfamethoxazole 400 mg and trimethoprim 80 mg
Tablet, double strength: Sulfamethoxazole 800 mg and trimethoprim 160 mg
Bactrim™ DS: Sulfamethoxazole 800 mg and trimethoprim 160 mg
Septra® DS: Sulfamethoxazole 800 mg and trimethoprim 160 mg

Sulfasalazine (sul fa SAL a zeen)

Medication Safety Issues
Sound-alike/look-alike issues:
Sulfasalazine may be confused with salsalate, sulfaDIAZINE, sulfiSOXAZOLE
Azulfidine® may be confused with Augmentin®, azaTHIOprine

U.S. Brand Names Azulfidine®; Azulfidine® EN-tabs®; Sulfazine; Sulfazine EC

Canadian Brand Names Alti-Sulfasalazine; Salazopyrin En-Tabs®; Salazopyrin®

Mexican Brand Names Azulfidina

Index Terms Salicylazosulfapyridine

Pharmacologic Category 5-Aminosalicylic Acid Derivative

Use Management of ulcerative colitis; enteric coated tablets are also used for rheumatoid arthritis (including juvenile rheumatoid arthritis) in patients who inadequately respond to analgesics and NSAIDs

Unlabeled/Investigational Use Ankylosing spondylitis, collagenous colitis, Crohn's disease, psoriasis, psoriatic arthritis, juvenile chronic arthritis

Effect on Mental Status Dizziness is common; sulfonamides reported to cause restlessness, irritability, depression, euphoria, disorientation, panic, hallucinations, and delusions

Effect on Psychiatric Treatment Photosensitivity is common; use caution with concurrent psychotropics; may cause leukopenia; caution with clozapine and carbamazepine

Dosage Summary
Oral:
Delayed release:
Children <6 years: Dosage not established
Children ≥6 years: Initial: 1/4 to 1/3 of expected maintenance dose; Maintenance: 30-50 mg/kg/day in 2 divided doses (maximum: 2 g/day); **Note:** Titration is recommended
Adults: Initial: 0.5-1 g/day; Maintenance: 2 g/day in 2 divided doses (maximum: 3 g/day); **Note:** Titration is recommended
Immediate release:
Children <2 years: Dosage not established

Children ≥2 years: Initial: 40-60 mg/kg/day in 3-6 divided doses; Maintenance: 20-30 mg/kg/day in 4 divided doses

Adults: Initial: 1 g 3-4 times/day; Maintenance: 2 g/day in divided doses

Dosage Forms Excipient information presented when available (limited, particularly for generics); consult specific product labeling.

Tablet: 500 mg

Azulfidine®, Sulfazine: 500 mg

Tablet, delayed release, enteric coated: 500 mg

Azulfidine® EN-tabs®, Sulfazine EC: 500 mg

◆ **Sulfatrim** *see* Sulfamethoxazole and Trimethoprim *on page 1517*

◆ **Sulfatrim®** *see* Sulfamethoxazole and Trimethoprim *on page 1517*

◆ **Sulfazine** *see* Sulfasalazine *on page 1522*

◆ **Sulfazine EC** *see* Sulfasalazine *on page 1522*

SulfiSOXAZOLE (sul fi SOKS a zole)

Medication Safety Issues

Sound-alike/look-alike issues:

SulfiSOXAZOLE may be confused with sulfaDIAZINE, sulfamethoxazole, sulfasalazine

Gantrisin® may be confused with Gastrosed™

U.S. Brand Names Gantrisin®

Canadian Brand Names Novo-Soxazole; Sulfizole®

Index Terms Sulfisoxazole Acetyl; Sulphafurazole

Pharmacologic Category Antibiotic, Sulfonamide Derivative

Use Treatment of urinary tract infections, otitis media, *Chlamydia*; nocardiosis

Effect on Mental Status Dizziness is common; sulfonamides reported to cause restlessness, irritability, depression, euphoria, disorientation, panic, hallucinations, and delusions

Effect on Psychiatric Treatment Photosensitivity is common; use caution with concurrent psychotropics; may cause leukopenia; caution with clozapine and carbamazepine

Dosage Summary

Oral:

Children ≤2 months: Dosage not established

Children >2 months: Initial: 75 mg/kg as a single dose; Maintenance: 120-150 mg/kg/day divided every 4-6 hours (maximum: 6 g/day)

Adults: Initial: 2-4 g as a single dose; Maintenance: 4-8 g/day divided every 4-6 hours

Dosage Forms Excipient information presented when available (limited, particularly for generics); consult specific product labeling.

Suspension, oral [pediatric]

Gantrisin®: 500 mg/5 mL (480 mL) [contains alcohol 0.3%; raspberry flavor]

◆ **Sulfisoxazole Acetyl** *see* SulfiSOXAZOLE *on page 1523*

◆ **Sulfisoxazole and Erythromycin** *see* Erythromycin and Sulfisoxazole *on page 563*

Sulindac (SUL in dak)

Medication Safety Issues

Sound-alike/look-alike issues:

Clinoril® may be confused with Cleocin®, Clozaril®, Oruvail®

Related Information

Nonsteroidal Anti-Inflammatory Agents *on page 1792*

U.S. Brand Names Clinoril®

Canadian Brand Names Apo-Sulin®; Novo-Sundac; Nu-Sundac

Mexican Brand Names Brurem; Clinoril; Clison; Renidac; Vindacin

Pharmacologic Category Nonsteroidal Anti-inflammatory Drug (NSAID), Oral

Generic Available Yes

Use Management of inflammatory diseases including osteoarthritis, rheumatoid arthritis, acute gouty arthritis, ankylosing spondylitis, acute painful shoulder (bursitis/tendonitis)

Effect on Mental Status Dizziness is common; may cause nervousness; may rarely cause drowsiness, confusion, insomnia, hallucinations, or depression

Effect on Psychiatric Treatment May rarely cause agranulocytosis; use caution with clozapine and carbamazepine; may decrease lithium clearance (evidence suggest that this effect may be less than with other NSAIDs) resulting in an increase in serum lithium levels and potential lithium toxicity; monitor serum lithium levels

Restrictions An FDA-approved medication guide must be distributed when dispensing an oral outpatient prescription (new or refill) where this medication is to be used without direct supervision of a healthcare provider. Medication guides are available at http://www.fda.gov/cder/Offices/ODS/medication_guides.htm.

Pregnancy Risk Factor C/D (3rd trimester)

Pregnancy Considerations Animal studies have not documented teratogenic effects. However, known effects of NSAIDs suggest the potential for premature ductus arteriosus closure, particularly in late pregnancy.

Lactation Excretion in breast milk unknown/not recommended

Contraindications Hypersensitivity or allergic-type reactions to sulindac, aspirin, other NSAIDs, or any component of the formulation; perioperative pain in the setting of coronary artery bypass graft (CABG) surgery

Warnings/Precautions [U.S. Boxed Warning]: NSAIDs are associated with an increased risk of adverse cardiovascular thrombotic events, including MI, stroke, and new onset or worsening of pre-existing hypertension. Use caution with fluid retention, heart failure, or hypertension. Concurrent administration of ibuprofen, and potentially other nonselective NSAIDs, may interfere with aspirin's cardioprotective effect. NSAID use may compromise existing renal function; dose-dependent decreases in prostaglandin synthesis may result from NSAID use, reducing renal blood flow which may cause renal decompensation. Patients with impaired renal function, dehydration, heart failure, liver dysfunction, those taking diuretics, and ACE inhibitors, and the elderly are at greater risk of renal toxicity. Rehydrate patient before starting therapy; monitor renal function closely. Not recommended for use in patients with advanced renal disease. Long-term NSAID use may result in renal papillary necrosis. Use caution in patients with renal lithiasis; sulindac metabolites have been reported as components of renal stones. Use hydration in patients with a history of renal stones. Use with caution in patients with decreased hepatic function. May require dosage adjustment in hepatic dysfunction; sulfide and sulfone metabolites may accumulate. **[U.S. Boxed Warning]: Use is contraindicated for treatment of perioperative pain in the setting of coronary artery bypass graft (CABG) surgery.** Risk of MI and stroke may be increased with use following CABG surgery.

[U.S. Boxed Warning]: NSAIDs may increase risk of gastrointestinal irritation, inflammation, ulceration, bleeding, and perforation. Use the lowest effective dose for the shortest duration of time, consistent with individual patient goals, to reduce risk of cardiovascular or GI adverse events. Pancreatitis has been reported; discontinue with suspected pancreatitis.

Platelet adhesion and aggregation may be decreased, may prolong bleeding time; patients with coagulation disorders or who are receiving anticoagulants should be monitored closely. Anemia may occur; patients on long-term NSAID therapy should be monitored for anemia. NSAIDs may cause serious skin adverse events including exfoliative dermatitis, Stevens-Johnson syndrome (SJS) and toxic epidermal necrolysis (TEN); discontinue use at first sign of skin rash or hypersensitivity. Anaphylactoid reactions may occur. Do not use in patients who experience bronchospasm, asthma, rhinitis, or urticaria with NSAID or aspirin therapy. Use caution in other forms of asthma. May increase the risk of aseptic meningitis, especially in patients with systemic lupus erythematosus (SLE) and mixed connective tissue disorders. Safety and efficacy have not been established in children.

Withhold for at least 4-6 half-lives prior to surgical or dental procedures.

Adverse Reactions

1% to 10%:

Cardiovascular: Edema (1% to 3%)

Central nervous system: Dizziness (3% to 9%), headache (3% to 9%), nervousness (1% to 3%)

Dermatologic: Rash (3% to 9%), pruritus (1% to 3%)

Gastrointestinal: GI pain (10%), constipation (3% to 9%), diarrhea (3% to 9%), dyspepsia (3% to 9%), nausea (3% to 9%), abdominal cramps (1% to 3%), anorexia (1% to 3%), flatulence (1% to 3%), vomiting (1% to 3%)

Otic: Tinnitus (1% to 3%)

<1% (Limited to important or life-threatening): Agranulocytosis, ageusia, alopecia, anaphylaxis, angioneurotic edema, aplastic anemia, arrhythmia, aseptic meningitis, bitter taste, blurred vision, bone marrow depression, bronchial spasm, bruising, CHF, cholestasis, colitis, conjunctivitis, crystalluria, depression, dry mucous membranes, dyspnea, dysuria, epistaxis, erythema multiforme, exfoliative dermatitis, fever, gastritis, GI bleeding, GI perforation,

glossitis, gynecomastia, hearing decreased, hematuria, hemolytic anemia, hepatitis, hepatic failure, hyperglycemia, hyperkalemia, hypersensitivity reaction, hypersensitivity syndrome (includes chills, diaphoresis, fever, flushing), hypersensitivity vasculitis, hypertension, insomnia, intestinal stricture, interstitial nephritis, jaundice, leukopenia, liver function abnormal, metallic taste, necrotizing fascitis, nephrotic syndrome, neuritis, neutropenia, palpitation, pancreatitis, paresthesia, peptic ulcer, photosensitivity, proteinuria, psychosis, purpura, renal calculi, renal failure, renal impairment, retinal disturbances, seizure, somnolence, Stevens-Johnson syndrome, stomatitis, syncope, thrombocytopenia, toxic epidermal necrolysis, urine discoloration, vaginal bleeding, vertigo, visual disturbance, weakness

Drug Interactions

ACE Inhibitors: Nonsteroidal Anti-Inflammatory Agents may diminish the antihypertensive effect of ACE Inhibitors. *Risk C: Monitor therapy*

Aminoglycosides: Nonsteroidal Anti-Inflammatory Agents may decrease the excretion of Aminoglycosides. Data only in premature infants. *Risk C: Monitor therapy*

Angiotensin II Receptor Blockers: Nonsteroidal Anti-Inflammatory Agents may diminish the therapeutic effect of Angiotensin II Receptor Blockers. The combination of these two agents may also significantly decrease glomerular filtration and renal function. *Risk C: Monitor therapy*

Anticoagulants: Nonsteroidal Anti-Inflammatory Agents may enhance the anticoagulant effect of Anticoagulants. *Risk C: Monitor therapy*

Antidepressants (Serotonin/Norepinephrine Reuptake Inhibitor): May enhance the antiplatelet effect of NSAID (Nonselective). *Risk C: Monitor therapy*

Antidepressants (Tricyclic, Tertiary Amine): May enhance the antiplatelet effect of NSAID (Nonselective). *Risk C: Monitor therapy*

Antiplatelet Agents: Nonsteroidal Anti-Inflammatory Agents may enhance the adverse/toxic effect of Antiplatelet Agents. An increased risk of bleeding may occur. *Risk C: Monitor therapy*

Beta-Blockers: Nonsteroidal Anti-Inflammatory Agents may diminish the antihypertensive effect of Beta-Blockers. **Exceptions:** Levobunolol; Metipranolol. *Risk C: Monitor therapy*

Bile Acid Sequestrants: May decrease the absorption of Nonsteroidal Anti-Inflammatory Agents. *Risk D: Consider therapy modification*

Bisphosphonate Derivatives: Nonsteroidal Anti-Inflammatory Agents may enhance the adverse/toxic effect of Bisphosphonate Derivatives. Both an increased risk of gastrointestinal ulceration and an increased risk of nephrotoxicity are of concern. *Risk C: Monitor therapy*

Corticosteroids (Systemic): May enhance the adverse/toxic effect of NSAID (Nonselective). *Risk C: Monitor therapy*

CycloSPORINE: Nonsteroidal Anti-Inflammatory Agents may enhance the nephrotoxic effect of CycloSPORINE. Nonsteroidal Anti-Inflammatory Agents may increase the serum concentration of CycloSPORINE. *Risk D: Consider therapy modification*

Desmopressin: Nonsteroidal Anti-Inflammatory Agents may enhance the adverse/toxic effect of Desmopressin. *Risk C: Monitor therapy*

Dimethyl Sulfoxide: May decrease the metabolism of Sulindac. Specifically, the concentrations of the active sulfide metabolite are decreased. *Risk C: Monitor therapy*

Eplerenone: Nonsteroidal Anti-Inflammatory Agents may diminish the antihypertensive effect of Eplerenone. *Risk C: Monitor therapy*

Herbs (Anticoagulant/Antiplatelet Properties) (eg, Alfalfa, Anise, Bilberry): May enhance the adverse/toxic effect of Nonsteroidal Anti-Inflammatory Agents. Bleeding may occur. *Risk D: Consider therapy modification*

HydrALAZINE: Nonsteroidal Anti-Inflammatory Agents may diminish the antihypertensive effect of HydrALAZINE. *Risk C: Monitor therapy*

Ketorolac: May enhance the adverse/toxic effect of Nonsteroidal Anti-Inflammatory Agents. *Risk X: Avoid combination*

Loop Diuretics: Nonsteroidal Anti-Inflammatory Agents may diminish the diuretic effect of Loop Diuretics. *Risk C: Monitor therapy*

Methotrexate: Nonsteroidal Anti-Inflammatory Agents may decrease the excretion of Methotrexate. *Risk D: Consider therapy modification*

Nonsteroidal Anti-Inflammatory Agents: May enhance the adverse/toxic effect of other Nonsteroidal Anti-Inflammatory Agents. *Risk C: Monitor therapy*

Pemetrexed: NSAID (Nonselective) may decrease the excretion of Pemetrexed. *Risk D: Consider therapy modification*

Probenecid: May increase the serum concentration of Nonsteroidal Anti-Inflammatory Agents. *Risk C: Monitor therapy*

Quinolone Antibiotics: Nonsteroidal Anti-Inflammatory Agents may enhance the neuroexcitatory and/or seizure-potentiating effect of Quinolone Antibiotics. *Risk C: Monitor therapy*

Salicylates: NSAID (Nonselective) may enhance the antiplatelet effect of Salicylates. NSAID (Nonselective) may diminish the cardioprotective effect of Salicylates. Salicylates may decrease the serum concentration of NSAID (Nonselective). **Exceptions:** Choline Magnesium Trisalicylate. *Risk D: Consider therapy modification*

Selective Serotonin Reuptake Inhibitors: May enhance the antiplatelet effect of NSAID (Nonselective). *Risk D: Consider therapy modification*

Thiazide Diuretics: Nonsteroidal Anti-Inflammatory Agents may diminish the therapeutic effect of Thiazide Diuretics. *Risk C: Monitor therapy*

Thrombolytic Agents: Nonsteroidal Anti-Inflammatory Agents may enhance the adverse/toxic effect of Thrombolytic Agents. An increased risk of bleeding may occur. *Risk C: Monitor therapy*

Treprostinil: May enhance the adverse/toxic effect of Nonsteroidal Anti-Inflammatory Agents. Bleeding may occur. *Risk C: Monitor therapy*

Vancomycin: Nonsteroidal Anti-Inflammatory Agents may decrease the excretion of Vancomycin. *Risk C: Monitor therapy*

Vitamin K Antagonists (eg, warfarin): NSAID (Nonselective) may enhance the anticoagulant effect of Vitamin K Antagonists. *Risk D: Consider therapy modification*

Ethanol/Nutrition/Herb Interactions

Ethanol: Avoid ethanol (may enhance gastric mucosal irritation).

Herb/Nutraceutical: Avoid alfalfa, anise, bilberry, bladderwrack, bromelain, cat's claw, celery, chamomile, coleus, cordyceps, dong quai, evening primrose, fenugreek, feverfew, garlic, ginger, ginkgo biloba, ginseng (American, Panax, Siberian), grapeseed, green tea, guggul, horse chestnut seed, horseradish, licorice, prickly ash, red clover, reishi, SAMe (S-adenosylmethionine), sweet clover, turmeric, white willow (all have additional antiplatelet activity).

Stability Store at room temperature of 15°C to 30°C (59°F to 86°F).

Mechanism of Action Reversibly inhibits cyclooxygenase-1 and 2 (COX-1 and 2) enzymes, which result in decreased formation of prostaglandin precursors; has antipyretic, analgesic, and anti-inflammatory properties

Pharmacodynamics/Kinetics

Absorption: 90%

Protein binding: Sulindac, sulfone, and sulfide metabolites: 93% to 98% primarily to albumin

Distribution: Crosses blood-brain barrier (brain concentrations <4% of plasma concentrations) and placental barriers

Metabolism: Hepatic; prodrug metabolized to sulfide metabolite (active) for therapeutic effects and to sulfone metabolites (inactive); parent and inactive sulfone metabolite undergo extensive enterohepatic recirculation

Half-life elimination: Parent drug: ~8 hours; Active metabolite: ~16 hours

Excretion: Urine (~50%, primarily as inactive metabolites, <1% as active metabolite); feces (~25%, primarily as metabolites)

Dosage Oral:

Children: Dose not established

Adults: **Note:** Maximum daily dose: 400 mg

Osteoarthritis, rheumatoid arthritis, ankylosing spondylitis: 150 mg twice daily

Acute painful shoulder (bursitis/tendonitis): 200 mg twice daily; usual treatment: 7-14 days

Acute gouty arthritis: 200 mg twice daily; usual treatment: 7 days

Dosing adjustment in renal impairment: Not recommended with advanced renal impairment; if required, decrease dose and monitor closely

Dosing adjustment in hepatic impairment: Dose reduction is necessary; discontinue if abnormal liver function tests occur

Dietary Considerations Drug may cause GI upset, bleeding, ulceration, perforation; take with food or milk to minimize GI upset.

Administration Should be administered with food or milk.

Monitoring Parameters Liver enzymes, BUN, serum creatinine, CBC, blood pressure; signs and symptoms of GI bleeding; ophthalmic exam (if ocular complaints develop during treatment)

Test Interactions Increased chloride (S), increased sodium (S), increased bleeding time

Dosage Forms Excipient information presented when available (limited, particularly for generics); consult specific product labeling.

Tablet: 150 mg, 200 mg

Clinoril®: 200 mg

◆ **Sulphafurazole** *see* SulfiSOXAZOLE *on page 1523*

SUMAtriptan (soo ma TRIP tan SUKS i nate)

Medication Safety Issues

Sound-alike/look-alike issues:

SUMAtriptan may be confused with sitaGLIPtin, somatropin, zolmitriptan

International issues:

Imitrex® may be confused with Nitrex® which is a brand name for isosorbide mononitrate in Italy

Related Information

Antimigraine Drugs: 5-HT_1 Receptor Agonists *on page 1766*

U.S. Brand Names Imitrex®

Canadian Brand Names Apo-Sumatriptan®; CO Sumatriptan; Dom-Sumatriptan; Gen-Sumatriptan; Imitrex®; Imitrex® DF; Imitrex® Nasal Spray; Novo-Sumatriptan; PHL-Sumatriptan; PMS-Sumatriptan; ratio-Sumatriptan; Rhoxal-sumatriptan; Riva-Sumatriptan; Sandoz-Sumatriptan; Sumatryx

Mexican Brand Names Fermig; Imigran; Nograine; Tebegran

Index Terms Sumatriptan Succinate

Pharmacologic Category Antimigraine Agent; Serotonin $5\text{-HT}_{1B,\ 1D}$ Receptor Agonist

Generic Available Yes: Injection

Use

Oral, SubQ: Acute treatment of migraine with or without aura

SubQ: Acute treatment of cluster headache episodes

Effect on Mental Status Dizziness is common; may cause drowsiness

Effect on Psychiatric Treatment Contraindicated with other serotonin agonists (SSRIs) and MAO inhibitors

Pregnancy Risk Factor C

Pregnancy Considerations There are no adequate and well-controlled studies using sumatriptan in pregnant women. Use only if potential benefit to the mother outweighs the potential risk to the fetus. A pregnancy registry has been established to monitor outcomes of women exposed to sumatriptan during pregnancy (800-336-2176). Preliminary data from the registry do not suggest a greater risk of birth defects than the general population and so far a specific pattern of malformations has not been identified. However, sample sizes are small and studies are ongoing. In some (but not all) animal studies, administration was associated with embryolethality, fetal malformations and pup mortality.

Lactation Enters breast milk/use caution (AAP rates "compatible")

Contraindications Hypersensitivity to sumatriptan or any component of the formulation; patients with ischemic heart disease or signs or symptoms of ischemic heart disease (including Prinzmetal's angina, angina pectoris, myocardial infarction, silent myocardial ischemia); cerebrovascular syndromes (including strokes, transient ischemic attacks); peripheral vascular syndromes (including ischemic bowel disease); uncontrolled hypertension; use within 24 hours of ergotamine derivatives; use within 24 hours of another 5-HT_1 agonist; concurrent administration or within 2 weeks of discontinuing an MAO inhibitor, specifically MAO type A inhibitors; management of hemiplegic or basilar migraine; prophylactic treatment of migraine; severe hepatic impairment; not for I.V. administration

Warnings/Precautions Sumatriptan is indicated only in patients ≥18 years of age with a clear diagnosis of migraine or cluster headache. Cardiac events (coronary artery vasospasm, transient ischemia, myocardial infarction, ventricular tachycardia/fibrillation, cardiac arrest and death), cerebral/subarachnoid hemorrhage, and stroke have been reported with 5-HT_1 agonist administration. Do not give to patients with risk factors for CAD until a cardiovascular evaluation has been performed; if evaluation is satisfactory, the healthcare provider should administer the first dose and cardiovascular status should be periodically evaluated.

Significant elevation in blood pressure, including hypertensive crisis, has also been reported on rare occasions in patients with and without a history of hypertension. Vasospasm-related reactions have been reported other than coronary artery vasospasm. Peripheral vascular ischemia and colonic ischemia with abdominal pain and bloody diarrhea have occurred. Use with caution in patients with a history of seizure disorder or in patients with a lowered seizure threshold. Use with caution in patients with hepatic impairment. Symptoms of agitation, confusion, hallucinations, hyper-reflexia, myoclonus, shivering, and tachycardia (serotonin syndrome) may occur with concomitant proserotonergic drugs (ie, SSRIs/SNRIs or triptans) or agents which reduce sumatriptan's metabolism. Concurrent use of serotonin precursors (eg, tryptophan) is not recommended. Safety and efficacy in pediatric patients have not been established.

Adverse Reactions

Injection:

>10%:

Central nervous system: Dizziness (12%), warm/hot sensation (11%)

Local: Pain at injection site (59%)

Neuromuscular & skeletal: Paresthesia (14%)

1% to 10%:

Cardiovascular: Chest pain/tightness/heaviness/pressure (2% to 3%), hyper-/hypotension (1%)

Central nervous system: Burning (7%), feeling of heaviness (7%), flushing (7%), pressure sensation (7%), feeling of tightness (5%), drowsiness (3%), malaise/fatigue (1%), feeling strange (2%), headache (2%), tight feeling in head (2%), cold sensation (1%), anxiety (1%)

Gastrointestinal: Abdominal discomfort (1%), dysphagia (1%)

Neuromuscular & skeletal: Neck, throat, and jaw pain/tightness/pressure (2% to 5%), mouth/tongue discomfort (5%), weakness (5%), myalgia (2%); muscle cramps (1%), numbness (5%)

Ocular: Vision alterations (1%)

Respiratory: Throat discomfort (3%), nasal disorder/discomfort (2%)

Miscellaneous: Diaphoresis (2%)

Nasal spray:

>10%: Gastrointestinal: Bad taste (13% to 24%), nausea (11% to 13%), vomiting (11% to 13%)

1% to 10%:

Central nervous system: Dizziness (1% to 2%)

Respiratory: Nasal disorder/discomfort (2% to 4%), throat discomfort (1% to 2%)

Tablet:

1% to 10%:

Cardiovascular: Chest pain/tightness/heaviness/pressure (1% to 2%), hyper-/hypotension (1%), palpitation (1%), syncope (1%)

Central nervous system: Burning (1%), dizziness (>1%), drowsiness (>1%), malaise/fatigue (2% to 3%), headache (>1%), nonspecified pain (1% to 2%, placebo 1%), vertigo (<1% to 2%), migraine (>1%), sleepiness (>1%)

Gastrointestinal: Diarrhea (1%), nausea (>1%), vomiting (>1%), hyposalivation (>1%)

Genitourinary: Hematuria (1%)

Hematologic: Hemolytic anemia (1%)

Neuromuscular & skeletal: Neck, throat, and jaw pain/tightness/pressure (2% to 3%), paresthesia (3% to 5%), myalgia (1%), numbness (1%)

Otic: Ear hemorrhage (1%), hearing loss (1%), sensitivity to noise (1%), tinnitus (1%)

Respiratory: Allergic rhinitis (1%), dyspnea (1%), nasal inflammation (1%), nose/throat hemorrhage (1%), sinusitis (1%), upper respiratory inflammation (1%)

Miscellaneous: Hypersensitivity reactions (1%), nonspecified pressure/tightness/heaviness (1% to 3%, placebo 2%); warm/cold sensation (2% to 3%, placebo 2%)

Route unspecified: <1%: Postmarketing and uncontrolled studies (limited to important or life-threatening): Abdominal aortic aneurysm, abdominal discomfort, abnormal menstrual cycle, abnormal/elevated liver function tests, accommodation disorders, acute renal failure, agitation, anaphylactoid reaction, anaphylaxis, anemia, angioneurotic edema, arrhythmia, atrial fibrillation, bronchospasm, cerebral ischemia, cerebrovascular accident, convulsions, deafness, death, decreased appetite, dental pain, diarrhea, dyspeptic symptoms, dysphagia, dystonic reaction, ECG changes, fluid disturbances (including retention), flushing, gastrointestinal pain, hallucinations, heart block, hematuria, hemolytic anemia, hiccups, hypersensitivity reactions, intestinal obstruction, intracranial pressure increased, ischemic colitis, joint ache, muscle stiffness, nose/throat hemorrhage, numbness of tongue, optic neuropathy (ischemic), pancytopenia, paresthesia, phlebitis, photosensitivity, Prinzmetal's angina, pruritus, psychomotor disorders, pulmonary embolism, rash, Raynaud syndrome, sensation changes, shock, subarachnoid hemorrhage, swallowing disorders, syncope, thrombocytopenia, thrombophlebitis, thrombosis, transient myocardial ischemia, TSH increased, vasculitis, vision loss, xerostomia

Drug Interactions

Ergot Derivatives: May enhance the vasoconstricting effect of Serotonin 5-HT1D Receptor Agonists. Serotonin 5-HT1D Receptor Agonists may enhance the vasoconstricting effect of Ergot Derivatives. *Risk X: Avoid combination*

MAO Inhibitors: May decrease the metabolism of Serotonin 5-HT1D Receptor Agonists. Management: If MAO inhibitor therapy is required, naratriptan, eletriptan or frovatriptan may be a suitable 5-HT1D agonist to employ. *Risk X: Avoid combination*

Serotonin Modulators: May enhance the adverse/toxic effect of other Serotonin Modulators. The development of serotonin syndrome may occur. *Risk D: Consider therapy modification*

Sibutramine: May enhance the serotonergic effect of Serotonin Modulators. This may cause serotonin syndrome. *Risk X: Avoid combination*

Stability Store at 2°C to 20°C (36°F to 86°F). Protect from light.

Mechanism of Action Selective agonist for serotonin (5-HT_{1D} receptor) in cranial arteries to cause vasoconstriction and reduces sterile inflammation associated with antidromic neuronal transmission correlating with relief of migraine

Pharmacodynamics/Kinetics

Onset of action: ~30 minutes

Distribution: V_d: 2.4 L/kg

Protein binding: 14% to 21%

Metabolism: Hepatic, primarily via MAO-A isoenzyme

Bioavailability: SubQ: 97% ± 16% of that following I.V. injection; Oral: 15%

Half-life elimination: Injection, tablet: 2.5 hours; Nasal spray: 2 hours

Time to peak, serum: 5-20 minutes

Excretion:

Injection: Urine (38% as indole acetic acid metabolite, 22% as unchanged drug)

Nasal spray: Urine (42% as indole acetic acid metabolite, 3% as unchanged drug)

Tablet: Urine (60% as indole acetic acid metabolite, 3% as unchanged drug); feces (40%)

Dosage Adults:

Oral: A single dose of 25 mg, 50 mg, or 100 mg (taken with fluids). If a satisfactory response has not been obtained at 2 hours, a second dose may be administered. Results from clinical trials show that initial doses of 50 mg and 100 mg are more effective than doses of 25 mg, and that 100 mg doses do not provide a greater effect than 50 mg and may have increased incidence of side effects. Although doses of up to 300 mg/day have been studied, the total daily dose should not exceed 200 mg. The safety of treating an average of >4 headaches in a 30-day period have not been established.

Intranasal: A single dose of 5 mg, 10 mg, or 20 mg administered in one nostril. A 10 mg dose may be achieved by administering a single 5 mg dose in each nostril. If headache returns, the dose may be repeated once after 2 hours, not to exceed a total daily dose of 40 mg. The safety of treating an average of >4 headaches in a 30-day period has not been established.

SubQ: Up to 6 mg; if side effects are dose-limiting, lower doses may be used. A second injection may be administered at least 1 hour after the initial dose, but not more than 2 injections in a 24-hour period.

Dosage adjustment in renal impairment: Dosage adjustment not necessary

Dosage adjustment in hepatic impairment: Bioavailability of oral sumatriptan is increased with liver disease. If treatment is needed, do not exceed single doses of 50 mg. The nasal spray has not been studied in patients with hepatic impairment, however, because the spray does not undergo first-pass metabolism, levels would not be expected to alter. Use of all dosage forms is contraindicated with severe hepatic impairment.

Administration

Oral: Should be taken with fluids as soon as symptoms appear

Injection solution: For SubQ administration; do not administer I.V.; may cause coronary vasospasm. An autoinjection device (STATdose System®) is available for use with the 4 mg and 6 mg cartridges.

Dosage Forms Excipient information presented when available (limited, particularly for generics); consult specific product labeling. **Note:** Strength expressed as sumatriptan base

Injection, solution, as succinate: 8 mg/mL (0.5 mL); 12 mg/mL (0.5 mL)

Imitrex®: 8 mg/mL (0.5 mL); 12 mg/mL (0.5 mL)

Solution, intranasal [spray]:
Imitrex®: 5 mg/0.1 mL device (6s); 20 mg/0.1 mL device (6s)
Tablet, as succinate:
Imitrex®: 25 mg, 50 mg, 100 mg

Sumatriptan and Naproxen (soo ma TRIP tan & na PROKS en)

Medication Safety Issues
Sound-alike/look-alike issues:
Naproxen may be confused with Natacyn®, Nebcin®, neomycin, niacin
SUMAtriptan may be confused with somatropin, zolmitriptan
Treximet™ may be confused with Trexall™

U.S. Brand Names Treximet™

Index Terms Naproxen and Sumatriptan; Naproxen Sodium and Sumatriptan; Naproxen Sodium and Sumatriptan Succinate; Sumatriptan Succinate and Naproxen; Sumatriptan Succinate and Naproxen Sodium

Pharmacologic Category Antimigraine Agent; Nonsteroidal Anti-inflammatory Drug (NSAID), Oral; Serotonin 5-$HT_{1B, 1D}$ Receptor Agonist

Use Acute treatment of migraine with or without aura

Effect on Mental Status May cause drowsiness or dizziness. May rarely cause drowsiness, confusion, insomnia, depression, or hallucinations

Effect on Psychiatric Treatment Contraindicated with other serotonin agonists (SSRIs/SNRIs) and MAO inhibitors. Naproxen may decrease lithium clearance resulting in an increase in serum lithium levels and potential lithium toxicity; monitor serum lithium levels. SSRIs may enhance the antiplatelet effects of naproxen.

Restrictions
An FDA-approved medication guide must be distributed when dispensing an oral outpatient prescription (new or refill) where this medication is to be used without direct supervision of a healthcare provider. Medication guides are available at http://www.fda.gov/cder/Offices/ODS/medication_guides.htm.

Dosage Summary
Oral:
Children: Dosage not established
Adults: 1 tablet (sumatriptan 85 mg and naproxen 500 mg). If a satisfactory response has not been obtained at 2 hours, a second dose may be administered (maximum: 2 tablets/24 hours)

Dosage Forms Excipient information presented when available (limited, particularly for generics); consult specific product labeling.
Tablet:
Treximet™ 85/500: Sumatriptan 85 mg and naproxen sodium 500 mg [contains sodium 61.2 mg/tablet (~2.7 mEq/tablet)]

◆ **Sumatriptan Succinate** *see* SUMAtriptan *on page 1527*
◆ **Sumatriptan Succinate and Naproxen** *see* Sumatriptan and Naproxen *on page 1530*
◆ **Sumatriptan Succinate and Naproxen Sodium** *see* Sumatriptan and Naproxen *on page 1530*
◆ **Summer's Eve® SpecialCare™ Medicated Anti-Itch Cream [OTC] [DSC]** *see* Hydrocortisone *on page 785*

Sunitinib (su NIT e nib)

Medication Safety Issues
Sound-alike/look-alike issues:
Sunitinib may be confused with sorafenib
High alert medication: The Institute for Safe Medication Practices (ISMP) includes this medication among its list of drug classes which have a heightened risk of causing significant patient harm when used in error.

U.S. Brand Names Sutent®

Canadian Brand Names Sutent®

Index Terms NSC-736511; SU11248; Sunitinib Malate

Pharmacologic Category Antineoplastic Agent, Tyrosine Kinase Inhibitor; Vascular Endothelial Growth Factor (VEGF) Inhibitor

Use Treatment of gastrointestinal stromal tumor (GIST) intolerance to or disease progression on imatinib; treatment of advanced renal cell cancer (RCC)

Effect on Mental Status Fatigue and dizziness are common

Effect on Psychiatric Treatment GI side effects are common; combined use with lithium, valproic acid, carbamazepine, and SSRIs may produce an additive risk. Neutropenia and thrombocytopenia are common; concomitant use with clozapine, carbamazepine, and valproic acid may produce additive risks. Carbamazepine and St John's wort may reduce the effectiveness of sunitinib.

Dosage Summary Note: Dosage modifications should be done in increments of 12.5 mg; individualize based on safety and tolerability

Oral:

Children: Dosage not established

Adults: 50 mg once daily for 4 weeks of a 6-week treatment cycle

Dosage Forms Excipient information presented when available (limited, particularly for generics); consult specific product labeling.

Capsule:

Sutent®: 12.5 mg, 25 mg, 50 mg

◆ **Sunitinib Malate** *see* Sunitinib *on page 1530*

◆ **Supprelin® LA** *see* Histrelin *on page 769*

◆ **Suprax®** *see* Cefixime *on page 294*

◆ **Surmontil®** *see* Trimipramine *on page 1630*

◆ **Sustiva®** *see* Efavirenz *on page 526*

◆ **Sutent®** *see* Sunitinib *on page 1530*

◆ **Su-Tuss DM** *see* Guaifenesin and Dextromethorphan *on page 739*

◆ **Su-Tuss®-HD [DSC]** *see* Hydrocodone, Pseudoephedrine, and Guaifenesin *on page 784*

◆ **Suxamethonium Chloride** *see* Succinylcholine *on page 1511*

◆ **Symax SL** *see* Hyoscyamine *on page 799*

◆ **Symax SR** *see* Hyoscyamine *on page 799*

◆ **Symbyax®** *see* Olanzapine and Fluoxetine *on page 1165*

◆ **Symlin®** *see* Pramlintide *on page 1321*

◆ **Symmetrel®** *see* Amantadine *on page 79*

◆ **SymTan™ [DSC]** *see* Hydrocodone and Pseudoephedrine *on page 781*

◆ **Synacthen** *see* Cosyntropin *on page 402*

◆ **Synagis®** *see* Palivizumab *on page 1218*

◆ **Synalgos®-DC** *see* Dihydrocodeine, Aspirin, and Caffeine *on page 468*

◆ **Synarel®** *see* Nafarelin *on page 1093*

◆ **Synercid®** *see* Quinupristin and Dalfopristin *on page 1388*

◆ **Syntest D.S. [DSC]** *see* Estrogens (Esterified) and Methyltestosterone *on page 587*

◆ **Syntest H.S. [DSC]** *see* Estrogens (Esterified) and Methyltestosterone *on page 587*

◆ **Synthroid®** *see* Levothyroxine *on page 920*

◆ **Syprine®** *see* Trientine *on page 1623*

◆ **Syrup of Ipecac** *see* Ipecac Syrup *on page 851*

◆ **T_3 Sodium (error-prone abbreviation)** *see* Liothyronine *on page 928*

◆ **T_3/T_4 Liotrix** *see* Liotrix *on page 930*

◆ **T_4** *see* Levothyroxine *on page 920*

◆ **T-20** *see* Enfuvirtide *on page 537*

◆ **Tabloid®** *see* Thioguanine *on page 1569*

Tacrine (TAK reen)

Medication Safety Issues

Sound-alike/look-alike issues:

Cognex® may be confused with Corgard®

International issues:

Cognex® may be confused with Codex® which is a brand name for *Saccharomyces boulardii* in Italy

U.S. Brand Names Cognex®

Index Terms Tacrine Hydrochloride; Tetrahydroaminoacrine; THA

Pharmacologic Category Acetylcholinesterase Inhibitor (Central)

Generic Available No

Use Treatment of mild-to-moderate dementia of the Alzheimer's type

Unlabeled/Investigational Use Lewy body dementia

Pregnancy Risk Factor C

Lactation Excretion in breast milk unknown/not recommended

Contraindications Hypersensitivity to tacrine, acridine derivatives, or any component of the formulation; patients previously treated with tacrine who developed jaundice

Warnings/Precautions The use of tacrine has been associated with elevations in serum transaminases; serum transaminases (specifically ALT) must be monitored throughout therapy; use extreme caution in patients with current evidence of a history of abnormal liver function tests. Cholinesterase inhibitors may have vagotonic effects which may cause bradycardia and/or heart block with or without a history of cardiac disease. Alzheimer's treatment guidelines consider bradycardia to be a relative contraindication for use of centrally-active cholinesterase inhibitors. Use caution in patients with urinary tract obstruction (bladder outlet obstruction or prostatic hyperplasia), asthma, and sick-sinus syndrome, bradycardia, or conduction abnormalities (tacrine may cause bradycardia and/or heart block). Also, patients with cardiovascular disease, asthma, or peptic ulcer should use cautiously. Use with caution in patients with a history of seizures. May cause nausea, vomiting, or loose stools. Abrupt discontinuation or dosage decrease may worsen cognitive function. May be associated with neutropenia. May exaggerate neuromuscular blockade effects of depolarizing neuromuscular-blocking agents like succinylcholine. Safety and efficacy have not been established in children.

Adverse Reactions

>10%:

Central nervous system: Dizziness, headache

Gastrointestinal: Diarrhea, nausea, vomiting

Miscellaneous: Transaminases increased

1% to 10%:

Cardiovascular: Flushing

Central nervous system: Ataxia, confusion, depression, fatigue, insomnia, somnolence

Dermatologic: Rash

Gastrointestinal: Abdominal pain, anorexia, constipation, dyspepsia, flatulence, weight loss

Neuromuscular & skeletal: Myalgia, tremor

Respiratory: Rhinitis

Metabolism/Transport Effects **Substrate** of CYP1A2 (major); **Inhibits** CYP1A2 (weak)

Drug Interactions

Anticholinergics: May diminish the therapeutic effect of Acetylcholinesterase Inhibitors (Central). Acetylcholinesterase Inhibitors (Central) may diminish the therapeutic effect of Anticholinergics. If the anticholinergic action is a side effect of the agent, the result may be beneficial. **Exceptions:** Paliperidone. *Risk C: Monitor therapy*

Antipsychotics: Acetylcholinesterase Inhibitors (Central) may enhance the neurotoxic (central) effect of Antipsychotics. Severe extrapyramidal symptoms have occurred in some patients. *Risk C: Monitor therapy*

Beta-Blockers: Acetylcholinesterase Inhibitors may enhance the bradycardic effect of Beta-Blockers. **Exceptions:** Levobunolol; Metipranolol. *Risk C: Monitor therapy*

Cholinergic Agonists: Acetylcholinesterase Inhibitors may enhance the adverse/toxic effect of Cholinergic Agonists. *Risk C: Monitor therapy*

Corticosteroids (Systemic): May enhance the adverse/toxic effect of Acetylcholinesterase Inhibitors. Increased muscular weakness may occur. *Risk C: Monitor therapy*

CYP1A2 Inhibitors (Moderate): May decrease the metabolism of CYP1A2 Substrates. *Risk C: Monitor therapy*

CYP1A2 Inhibitors (Strong): May decrease the metabolism of CYP1A2 Substrates. *Risk D: Consider therapy modification*

Fluvoxamine: May decrease the metabolism of Tacrine. *Risk D: Consider therapy modification*

Ginkgo Biloba: May enhance the adverse/toxic effect of Acetylcholinesterase Inhibitors. *Risk C: Monitor therapy*

Neuromuscular-Blocking Agents (Nondepolarizing): Acetylcholinesterase Inhibitors may diminish the neuromuscular-blocking effect of Neuromuscular-Blocking Agents (Nondepolarizing). Acetylcholinesterase Inhibitors may decrease the metabolism of Neuromuscular-Blocking Agents

(Nondepolarizing). This is only true for mivacurium in which case the neuromuscular blocking effects might be prolonged. *Risk C: Monitor therapy*

Succinylcholine: Acetylcholinesterase Inhibitors may enhance the neuromuscular-blocking effect of Succinylcholine. *Risk C: Monitor therapy*

Theophylline Derivatives: Tacrine may decrease the metabolism of Theophylline Derivatives. **Exceptions:** Dyphylline. *Risk C: Monitor therapy*

Ethanol/Nutrition/Herb Interactions Food: Food decreases bioavailability.

Mechanism of Action Centrally-acting cholinesterase inhibitor. It elevates acetylcholine in cerebral cortex by slowing the degradation of acetylcholine.

Pharmacodynamics/Kinetics

Absorption: Oral: Rapid

Distribution: V_d: Mean: 349 L; reduced by food

Protein binding, plasma: 55%

Metabolism: Extensively by CYP450 to multiple metabolites; first pass effect

Bioavailability: Absolute: 17%

Half-life elimination, serum: 2-4 hours; Steady-state: 24-36 hours

Time to peak, plasma: 1-2 hours

Dosage Adults: Initial: 10 mg 4 times/day; may increase by 40 mg/day adjusted every 6 weeks; maximum: 160 mg/day; best administered separate from meal times.

Dose adjustment based upon transaminase elevations:

ALT ≤3 times ULN*: Continue titration

ALT >3 to ≤5 times ULN*: Decrease dose by 40 mg/day, resume when ALT returns to normal

ALT >5 times ULN*: Stop treatment, may rechallenge upon return of ALT to normal

*ULN = upper limit of normal

Patients with clinical jaundice confirmed by elevated total bilirubin (>3 mg/dL) should not be rechallenged with tacrine

Dietary Considerations Give with food if GI side effects are intolerable.

Monitoring Parameters ALT levels and other liver enzymes weekly for at least the first 18 weeks, then monitor once every 3 months

Reference Range In clinical trials, serum concentrations >20 ng/mL were associated with a much higher risk of development of symptomatic adverse effects

Dosage Forms Excipient information presented when available (limited, particularly for generics); consult specific product labeling.

Capsule, as hydrochloride: 10 mg, 20 mg, 30 mg, 40 mg

◆ **Tacrine Hydrochloride** *see* Tacrine *on page 1531*

Tacrolimus (ta KROE li mus)

Medication Safety Issues

Sound-alike/look-alike issues:

Prograf® may be confused with Gengraf®, Prozac®

Tacrolimus may be confused with sirolimus, temsirolimus

U.S. Brand Names Prograf®; Protopic®

Canadian Brand Names Advagraf™; Prograf®; Protopic®

Mexican Brand Names Limustin; Proalid; Prograf; Protopic

Index Terms FK506

Pharmacologic Category Immunosuppressant Agent; Topical Skin Product

Use

Oral/injection: Potent immunosuppressive drug used in heart, kidney, or liver transplant recipients

Topical: Moderate-to-severe atopic dermatitis in patients not responsive to conventional therapy or when conventional therapy is not appropriate

Unlabeled/Investigational Use Potent immunosuppressive drug used in lung, small bowel transplant recipients; immunosuppressive drug for peripheral stem cell/bone marrow transplantation

Effect on Mental Status Insomnia is common

Effect on Psychiatric Treatment Contraindicated with ziprasidone; barbiturates and carbamazepine may decrease the effects of tacrolimus

Restrictions An FDA-approved medication guide must be distributed when dispensing the outpatient prescription (new or refill) for tacrolimus ointment where this medication is to be used without direct supervision of a healthcare provider. Medication guides are available at http://www.fda.gov/cder/Offices/ODS/medication_guides.htm.

Dosage Summary

I.V.:

Children: 0.03-0.05 mg/kg/day as a continuous infusion

Adults: 0.03-0.05 mg/kg/day as a continuous infusion

Oral:

Children: 0.15-0.2 mg/kg/day in divided doses every 12 hours

Adults: 0.1-0.2 mg/kg/day in divided doses every 12 hours

Topical:

Children <2 years: Dosage not established

Children ≥2 years: Apply 0.03% to affected area twice daily

Adults: Apply minimum amount of 0.03% or 0.1% to affected area twice daily

Dosage Forms Excipient information presented when available (limited, particularly for generics); consult specific product labeling.

Capsule (Prograf®): 0.5 mg, 1 mg, 5 mg

Injection, solution (Prograf®): 5 mg/mL (1 mL) [contains dehydrated alcohol 80% and polyoxyl 60 hydrogenated castor oil]

Ointment, topical (Protopic®): 0.03% (30 g, 60 g, 100 g); 0.1% (30 g, 60 g, 100 g)

Tadalafil (tah DA la fil)

Medication Safety Issues

Sound-alike/look-alike issues:

Tadalafil may be confused with sildenafil, vardenafil

U.S. Brand Names Cialis®

Canadian Brand Names Cialis®

Mexican Brand Names Cialis

Index Terms GF196960

Pharmacologic Category Phosphodiesterase-5 Enzyme Inhibitor

Generic Available No

Use Treatment of erectile dysfunction (ED)

Effect on Mental Status May cause dizziness, insomnia, or fatigue

Effect on Psychiatric Treatment Concurrent use with antidepressants (eg, TCAs) and antipsychotics may produce significant hypotension secondary to alpha-receptor blockade; alpha-blockers contraindicated with tadalafil (except tamsulosin). Nefazodone may increase levels of tadalafil; dosage adjustment needed.

Pregnancy Risk Factor B

Pregnancy Considerations Teratogenic events were not reported in animal reproduction studies. Postnatal development and pup survival was decreased at some doses. Tadalafil is not indicated for use in women. Less than 0.0005% is found in the semen of healthy males.

Lactation Excretion in breast milk unknown

Contraindications Concurrent use (regularly/intermittently) of organic nitrates in any form (eg, nitroglycerin, isosorbide dinitrate)

Warnings/Precautions There is a degree of cardiac risk associated with sexual activity; therefore, physicians should consider the cardiovascular status of their patients prior to initiating any treatment for erectile dysfunction. Use with caution in patients with hypotension (<90/50 mm Hg), uncontrolled hypertension (>170/100 mm Hg), NYHA class II-IV heart failure within the last 6 months, uncontrolled arrhythmias, stroke within the last 6 months, MI within the last 3 months; safety and efficacy have not been studied in these patients. Use caution in patients with left ventricular outflow obstruction (eg, aortic stenosis). Concurrent use with alpha-adrenergic antagonist therapy or substantial alcohol consumption may cause symptomatic hypotension; patients should be hemodynamically stable prior to initiating tadalafil therapy at the lowest possible dose. Use caution in patients receiving strong CYP3A4 inhibitors, the elderly, or those with hepatic impairment or renal impairment; dosage adjustment/limitation is needed. Use caution in patients with bleeding disorders or peptic ulcer disease.

Agents for the treatment of erectile dysfunction should be used with caution in patients with anatomical deformation of the penis (angulation, cavernosal fibrosis, or Peyronie's disease), or in patients who have conditions which may predispose them to priapism (sickle cell anemia, multiple myeloma, leukemia). All patients should be instructed to seek immediate medical attention if erection persists >4 hours. The safety and efficacy of tadalafil with other treatments for erectile dysfunction have not been studied and are, therefore, not recommended as combination therapy.

Rare cases of nonarteritic anterior ischemic optic neuropathy (NAION) have been reported; risk may be increased with history of vision loss. Other risk factors for NAION include heart disease, diabetes, hypertension, smoking, age >50 years, or history of certain eye problems. Sudden decrease or loss of hearing has been reported rarely; hearing changes may be accompanied by tinnitus and dizziness. A direct relationship between therapy and vision or hearing loss has not been determined.

Patients with genetic retinal disorders (eg, retinitis pigmentosa) were not evaluated in clinical trials; use is not recommended. Safety and efficacy in children ≤18 years of age have not been established.

Adverse Reactions Similar adverse events are reported with once-daily dosing, but are generally lower than with doses used as needed.

>10%: Central nervous system: Headache (3% to 15%)

2% to 10%:

Cardiovascular: Flushing (1% to 3%), hypertension (1% to 3%)

Gastrointestinal: Dyspepsia (3% to 10%)

Neuromuscular & skeletal: Back pain (3% to 6%), CPK increased (2%), myalgia (1% to 4%), limb pain (1% to 3%)

Respiratory: Upper respiratory tract infection (3% to 4%), cough (2% to 4%), nasal congestion (2% to 4%)

<2% (Limited to important or life-threatening): Abdominal pain (upper), amnesia (transient global), angina pectoris, arthralgia, blurred vision, chest pain, color perception change, color vision decreased, conjunctival hyperemia, conjunctivitis, diaphoresis, diarrhea, dizziness, dysphagia, dyspnea, epistaxis, esophagitis, exfoliative dermatitis, eye pain, eyelid swelling, facial edema, fatigue, gastritis, gastroesophageal reflux, hearing decreased, hearing loss, hepatic enzymes increased, hyper-/hypotension, hypoesthesia, GGTP increased, insomnia, lacrimation, migraine, MI, nausea, neck pain, nonarteritic ischemic optic neuropathy, pain, palpitation, paresthesia, pharyngitis, photophobia, postural hypotension, priapism (reported with drugs in this class), pruritus, rash, retinal artery occlusion, retinal vein occlusion, seizure, somnolence, Stevens-Johnson syndrome, stroke, sudden cardiac death, syncope, tachycardia, tinnitus, urinary tract infection, urticaria, vertigo, visual changes (color vision), visual field loss, vomiting, weakness, xerostomia

Metabolism/Transport Effects **Substrate of** CYP3A4 (major)

Drug Interactions

Alpha1-Blockers: Phosphodiesterase 5 Inhibitors may enhance the hypotensive effect of Alpha1-Blockers. **Exceptions:** Dapiprazole [Off Market]. *Risk D: Consider therapy modification*

Antifungal Agents (Azole Derivatives, Systemic): May decrease the metabolism of Phosphodiesterase 5 Inhibitors. *Risk D: Consider therapy modification*

CYP3A4 Inhibitors (Moderate): May decrease the metabolism of CYP3A4 Substrates. *Risk C: Monitor therapy*

CYP3A4 Inhibitors (Strong): May decrease the metabolism of CYP3A4 Substrates. *Risk D: Consider therapy modification*

Dasatinib: May increase the serum concentration of CYP3A4 Substrates. *Risk C: Monitor therapy*

Etravirine: May decrease the serum concentration of Phosphodiesterase 5 Inhibitors. Management: No empiric dosage adjustments are recommended with concomitant therapy; however, dose of the phosphodiesterase inhibitor may need to be altered based on clinical response. *Risk C: Monitor therapy*

Macrolide Antibiotics: May decrease the metabolism of Phosphodiesterase 5 Inhibitors. **Exceptions:** Azithromycin; Dirithromycin [Off Market]; Spiramycin. *Risk D: Consider therapy modification*

Protease Inhibitors: May decrease the metabolism of Phosphodiesterase 5 Inhibitors. Management: Dose restrictions for tadalafil, and/or sildenafil and vardenafil are recommended in combination with ritonavir, atazanavir, indinavir, darunavir and saquinavir. Consult specific prescribing information for detailed recommendations. *Risk D: Consider therapy modification*

Sapropterin: May enhance the hypotensive effect of Phosphodiesterase 5 Inhibitors. *Risk C: Monitor therapy*

Vasodilators (Organic Nitrates): Phosphodiesterase 5 Inhibitors may enhance the vasodilatory effect of Vasodilators (Organic Nitrates). *Risk X: Avoid combination*

Ethanol/Nutrition/Herb Interactions

Ethanol: Substantial consumption of ethanol may increase the risk of hypotension and orthostasis. Lower ethanol consumption has not been associated with significant changes in blood pressure or increase in orthostatic symptoms.

Food: Rate and extent of absorption are not affected by food. Grapefruit juice may increase serum levels/toxicity of tadalafil. When used on an as-needed basis, do not give more than a single 10 mg dose of tadalafil more frequently than every 72 hours in patients who regularly consume grapefruit juice. When used on a once-daily basis, the dose of tadalafil should not exceed 2.5 mg/day in patients who regularly consume grapefruit juice.

Herb/Nutraceutical: St John's wort: Use caution with concomitant use.

Stability Store at controlled room temperature of 25°C (77°F); excursions permitted to 15°C to 30°C (59°F to 86°F).

Mechanism of Action Does not directly cause penile erections, but affects the response to sexual stimulation. The physiologic mechanism of erection of the penis involves release of nitric oxide (NO) in the corpus cavernosum during sexual stimulation. NO then activates the enzyme guanylate cyclase, which results in increased levels of cyclic guanosine monophosphate (cGMP), producing smooth muscle relaxation and inflow of blood to the corpus cavernosum. Tadalafil enhances the effect of NO by inhibiting phosphodiesterase type 5 (PDE-5), which is responsible for degradation of cGMP in the corpus cavernosum; when sexual stimulation causes local release of NO, inhibition of PDE-5 by tadalafil causes increased levels of cGMP in the corpus cavernosum, resulting in smooth muscle relaxation and inflow of blood to the corpus cavernosum. At recommended doses, it has no effect in the absence of sexual stimulation.

Pharmacodynamics/Kinetics

Onset: Within 1 hour

Duration: Up to 36 hours

Distribution: V_d: 63 L

Protein binding: 94%

Metabolism: Hepatic, via CYP3A4 to metabolites (inactive)

Half-life elimination: 17.5 hours

Time to peak, plasma: ~2 hours (range: 30 minutes to 6 hours)

Excretion: Feces (61%, as metabolites); urine (36%, as metabolites)

Dosage Oral: Erectile dysfunction:

Adults:

As-needed dosing: 10 mg at least 30 minutes prior to anticipated sexual activity (dosing range: 5-20 mg); to be given as one single dose and not given more than once daily. **Note:** Erectile function may be improved for up to 36 hours following a single dose; adjust dose.

Once-daily dosing: 2.5 mg once daily (dosing range: 2.5-5 mg/day) to be given at approximately the same time daily without regard to timing of sexual activity

Elderly: No dose adjustment for patients >65 years of age; use with caution in patients with concomitant medications or renal/hepatic impairment

Dosing adjustment with concomitant medications:

Alpha$_1$-blockers: If stabilized on either alpha-blockers or tadalafil therapy, initiate new therapy with the other agent at the lowest possible dose.

CYP3A4 inhibitors: Dose reduction of tadalafil is recommended with strong CYP3A4 inhibitors. When used on an as-needed basis, the dose of tadalafil should not exceed 10 mg, and tadalafil should not be taken more frequently than once every 72 hours. When used on a once-daily basis, the dose of tadalafil should not exceed 2.5 mg. Examples of such inhibitors include amprenavir, atazanavir, clarithromycin, conivaptan, delavirdine, diclofenac, fosamprenavir, imatinib, indinavir, isoniazid, itraconazole, ketoconazole, miconazole, nefazodone, nelfinavir, nicardipine, propofol, quinidine, ritonavir, and telithromycin.

Dosage adjustment in renal impairment:

As-needed use:

Cl_{cr} 51-80 mL/minute: Dosage adjustment not required

Cl_{cr} 31-50 mL/minute: Initial dose 5 mg once daily; maximum dose 10 mg not to be given more frequently than every 48 hours

Cl_{cr} <30 mL/minute and on hemodialysis: Maximum dose 5 mg not to be given more frequently than every 72 hours

Once-daily use:

Cl_{cr} 51-80 mL/minute: Dosage adjustment not required

Cl_{cr} 31-50 mL/minute: Dose adjustment not needed

Cl_{cr} <30 mL/minute and on hemodialysis: Use not recommended

Dosage adjustment in hepatic impairment:

As-needed use:

Mild-to-moderate hepatic impairment (Child-Pugh class A or B): Use with caution; dose should not exceed 10 mg once daily

Severe hepatic impairment (Child-Pugh class C): Use is not recommended

Once-daily use:

Mild-to-moderate hepatic impairment (Child-Pugh class A or B): Use with caution

Severe hepatic impairment: Use is not recommended

Dietary Considerations May be taken with or without food.

Administration May be administered with or without food, prior to anticipated sexual activity. When used on an as-needed basis, should be taken at least

30 minutes prior to sexual activity. When used on a once-daily basis, should be taken at the same time each day, without regard to timing of sexual activity.

Monitoring Parameters Monitor for response and adverse effects.

Dosage Forms Excipient information presented when available (limited, particularly for generics); consult specific product labeling.

Tablet:

Cialis®: 2.5 mg, 5 mg, 10 mg, 20 mg

- **Tagamet® HB 200 [OTC]** *see* Cimetidine *on page 345*
- **TAK-375** *see* Ramelteon *on page 1394*
- **Talacen®** *see* Pentazocine and Acetaminophen *on page 1245*
- **Talwin®** *see* Pentazocine *on page 1243*
- **Talwin® Nx** *see* Pentazocine *on page 1243*
- **Tambocor™** *see* Flecainide *on page 633*
- **Tamiflu®** *see* Oseltamivir *on page 1188*

Tamoxifen (ta MOKS i fen)

Medication Safety Issues

Sound-alike/look-alike issues:

Tamoxifen may be confused with pentoxifylline, Tambocor™

U.S. Brand Names Soltamox™ [DSC]

Canadian Brand Names Apo-Tamox®; Gen-Tamoxifen; Nolvadex®; Nolvadex®-D; Novo-Tamoxifen; Tamofen®

Mexican Brand Names Nolvadex; Tecnofen

Index Terms ICI-46474; Tamoxifen Citrate

Pharmacologic Category Antineoplastic Agent, Estrogen Receptor Antagonist; Selective Estrogen Receptor Modulator (SERM)

Use Treatment of metastatic (female and male) breast cancer; adjuvant treatment of breast cancer; reduce risk of invasive breast cancer in women with ductal carcinoma *in situ* (DCIS); reduce the incidence of breast cancer in women at high risk

Unlabeled/Investigational Use Treatment of mastalgia, gynecomastia, melanoma and desmoid tumors; induction of ovulation; treatment of precocious puberty in females, secondary to McCune-Albright syndrome

Effect on Mental Status May cause dizziness, drowsiness, or confusion

Effect on Psychiatric Treatment May cause leukopenia; use caution with clozapine and carbamazepine

Restrictions An FDA-approved medication guide must be distributed when dispensing the outpatient prescription (new or refill) to females for breast cancer prevention or treatment of ductal carcinoma *in situ* where this medication is to be used without direct supervision of a healthcare provider. Medication guides are available at http://www.fda.gov/cder/Offices/ODS/medication_guides.htm.

Dosage Summary

Oral:

Children: Dosage not established

Adults: 20-40 mg/day in 1-2 divided doses

Dosage Forms Excipient information presented when available (limited, particularly for generics); consult specific product labeling. [DSC] = Discontinued product

Solution, oral:

Soltamox™: 10 mg/5 mL (150 mL) [sugar free; licorice flavor] [DSC]

Tablet: 10 mg, 20 mg

- **Tamoxifen Citrate** *see* Tamoxifen *on page 1537*

Tamsulosin (tam SOO loe sin)

Medication Safety Issues

Sound-alike/look-alike issues:

Flomax® may be confused with Flonase®, Flovent®, Foltx®, Fosamax®, Volmax®

Tamsulosin may be confused with tacrolimus, tamoxifen, terazosin

International issues:

Flomax®: Brand name for morniflumate in Italy

Flomax® may be confused with Flomox® which is a brand name for cefcapene in Japan

U.S. Brand Names Flomax®

Canadian Brand Names Flomax®; Flomax® CR; Gen-Tamsulosin; Novo-Tamsulosin; Ran-Tamsulosin; ratio-Tamsulosin; Sandoz-Tamsulosin

Mexican Brand Names Secotex

Index Terms Tamsulosin Hydrochloride

Pharmacologic Category $Alpha_1$ Blocker

Generic Available No

Use Treatment of signs and symptoms of benign prostatic hyperplasia (BPH)

Unlabeled/Investigational Use Symptomatic treatment of bladder outlet obstruction or dysfunction

Effect on Mental Status Dizziness is common; may cause drowsiness or insomnia

Effect on Psychiatric Treatment None reported

Pregnancy Risk Factor B

Pregnancy Considerations Teratogenic effects were not observed in animal studies, however, tamsulosin is not approved for use in women.

Contraindications Hypersensitivity to tamsulosin or any component of the formulation

Warnings/Precautions Not intended for use as an antihypertensive drug. May cause significant orthostatic hypotension and syncope, especially with first dose; anticipate a similar effect if therapy is interrupted for a few days, if dosage is rapidly increased, or if another antihypertensive drug (particularly vasodilators) or a PDE-5 inhibitor (eg, sildenafil, tadalafil, vardenafil) is introduced. "First-dose" orthostatic hypotension may occur 4-8 hours after dosing; may be dose related. Patients should be cautioned about performing hazardous tasks when starting new therapy or adjusting dosage upward. Discontinue if symptoms of angina occur or worsen. Rule out prostatic carcinoma before beginning therapy with tamsulosin. Intraoperative floppy iris syndrome has been observed in cataract surgery patients who were on or were previously treated with $alpha_1$-blockers; causality has not been established and there appears to be no benefit in discontinuing alpha-blocker therapy prior to surgery. Priapism has been associated with use (rarely). Rarely, patients with a sulfa allergy have also developed an allergic reaction to tamsulosin; avoid use when previous reaction has been severe. Not indicated for use in women or children.

Adverse Reactions

>10%:

- Cardiovascular: Orthostatic hypotension (6 % to 19%)
- Central nervous system: Headache (19% to 21%), dizziness (15% to 17%)
- Genitourinary: Abnormal ejaculation (8% to 18%)
- Respiratory: Rhinitis (13% to 18%)
- Miscellaneous: Infection (9% to 11%)

1% to 10%:

- Cardiovascular: Chest pain (4%)
- Central nervous system: Somnolence (3% to 4%), insomnia (1% to 2%), vertigo (≤1%)
- Endocrine & metabolic: Libido decreased (1% to 2%)
- Gastrointestinal: Diarrhea (4% to 6%), nausea (3% to 4%), tooth disorder (1% to 2%)
- Neuromuscular & skeletal: Weakness (8% to 9%), back pain (7% to 8%)
- Ocular: Blurred vision (≤2%)
- Respiratory: Pharyngitis (5% to 6%), cough (3% to 5%), sinusitis (2% to 4%)

<1% (Limited to important or life-threatening): Allergic reactions (angioedema, pruritus, rash, urticaria, respiratory symptoms); constipation, hypotension, intraoperative floppy iris syndrome, orthostasis (symptomatic), palpitation, priapism, skin desquamation, syncope, transaminases increased, vomiting

Metabolism/Transport Effects Substrate (major) of CYP2D6, 3A4

Drug Interactions

Alfuzosin: Alpha1-Blockers may enhance the antihypertensive effect of Alfuzosin. Risk of orthostatic hypotension or syncope may be increased. Alfuzosin may enhance the antihypertensive effect of Alpha1-Blockers. *Risk X: Avoid combination*

Alpha1-Blockers: May enhance the antihypertensive effect of Tamsulosin. Risk of orthostatic hypotension or syncope may be increased. Tamsulosin may enhance the antihypertensive effect of Alpha1-Blockers. *Risk X: Avoid combination*

Beta-Blockers: May enhance the orthostatic effect of Alpha1-Blockers. The risk associated with ophthalmic products is probably less than systemic products. **Exceptions:** Levobunolol; Metipranolol. *Risk D: Consider therapy modification*

Calcium Channel Blockers: Alpha1-Blockers may enhance the hypotensive effect of Calcium Channel Blockers. *Risk C: Monitor therapy*

CYP2D6 Inhibitors (Moderate): May decrease the metabolism of CYP2D6 Substrates. *Risk C: Monitor therapy*

CYP2D6 Inhibitors (Strong): May decrease the metabolism of CYP2D6 Substrates. *Risk D: Consider therapy modification*

CYP3A4 Inducers (Strong): May increase the metabolism of CYP3A4 Substrates. *Risk C: Monitor therapy*

CYP3A4 Inhibitors (Moderate): May decrease the metabolism of CYP3A4 Substrates. *Risk C: Monitor therapy*

CYP3A4 Inhibitors (Strong): May decrease the metabolism of CYP3A4 Substrates. *Risk D: Consider therapy modification*

Darunavir: May increase the serum concentration of CYP2D6 Substrates. *Risk C: Monitor therapy*

Dasatinib: May increase the serum concentration of CYP3A4 Substrates. *Risk C: Monitor therapy*

Deferasirox: May decrease the serum concentration of CYP3A4 Substrates. *Risk C: Monitor therapy*

Diazoxide: May enhance the hypotensive effect of Antihypertensives. *Risk C: Monitor therapy*

Herbs (CYP3A4 Inducers): May increase the metabolism of CYP3A4 Substrates. *Risk C: Monitor therapy*

Herbs (Hypertensive Properties): May diminish the antihypertensive effect of Antihypertensives. *Risk C: Monitor therapy*

Herbs (Hypotensive Properties): May enhance the hypotensive effect of Antihypertensives. *Risk C: Monitor therapy*

Methylphenidate: May diminish the antihypertensive effect of Antihypertensives. *Risk C: Monitor therapy*

Phosphodiesterase 5 Inhibitors: May enhance the hypotensive effect of Alpha1-Blockers. *Risk D: Consider therapy modification*

Prostacyclin Analogues: May enhance the hypotensive effect of Antihypertensives. *Risk C: Monitor therapy*

RiTUXimab: Antihypertensives may enhance the hypotensive effect of RiTUXimab. *Risk D: Consider therapy modification*

Ethanol/Nutrition/Herb Interactions

Food: Fasting increases bioavailability by 30% and peak concentration 40% to 70%.

Herb/Nutraceutical: St John's wort: May decrease the levels/effects of tamsulosin. Avoid herbs with hypotensive properties (black cohosh, California poppy, coleus, golden seal, hawthorn, mistletoe, periwinkle, quinine, Shepherd's purse); may enhance the hypotensive effect of tamsulosin. Avoid saw palmetto (due to limited experience with this combination).

Stability Store at room temperature of 25°C (77°F); excursions permitted to 15°C to 30°C (59°F to 86°F).

Mechanism of Action Tamsulosin is an antagonist of $alpha_{1A}$-adrenoreceptors in the prostate. Smooth muscle tone in the prostate is mediated by $alpha_{1A}$-adrenoreceptors; blocking them leads to relaxation of smooth muscle in the bladder neck and prostate causing an improvement of urine flow and decreased symptoms of BPH. Approximately 75% of the $alpha_1$-receptors in the prostate are of the $alpha_{1A}$ subtype.

Pharmacodynamics/Kinetics

Absorption: >90%

Protein binding: 94% to 99%, primarily to $alpha_1$ acid glycoprotein (AAG)

Metabolism: Hepatic via CYP3A4 and 2D6; metabolites undergo extensive conjugation to glucuronide or sulfate

Bioavailability: Fasting: 30% increase

Distribution: V_d: 16 L

Steady-state: By the fifth day of once-daily dosing

Half-life elimination: Healthy volunteers: 9-13 hours; Target population: 14-15 hours

Time to peak: Fasting: 4-5 hours; With food: 6-7 hours

Excretion: Urine (76%, <10% as unchanged drug); feces (21%)

Dosage Oral: Adults:

BPH: 0.4 mg once daily ~30 minutes after the same meal each day; dose may be increased after 2-4 weeks to 0.8 mg once daily in patients who fail to respond. If therapy is interrupted for several days, restart with 0.4 mg once daily.

Bladder outlet obstruction (unlabeled use): 0.4 mg once daily ~30 minutes after the same meal each day

Dosage adjustment in renal impairment:

Cl_{cr} ≥10 mL/minute: No adjustment needed

Cl_{cr} <10 mL/minute: Not studied

Dosage adjustment in hepatic impairment:

Mild-to-moderate impairment: No adjustment needed

Severe impairment: Not studied

Dietary Considerations Take once daily, 30 minutes after the same meal each day.

Administration Administer 30 minutes after the same meal each day. Capsules should be swallowed whole; do not crush, chew, or open.

Dosage Forms Excipient information presented when available (limited, particularly for generics); consult specific product labeling.

Capsule, as hydrochloride:

Flomax®: 0.4 mg

- ◆ **Tamsulosin Hydrochloride** *see* Tamsulosin *on page 1537*
- ◆ ***Tanacetum parthenium*** *see* Feverfew *(Tanacetum parthenium) on page 628*
- ◆ **TanaCof-XR** *see* Brompheniramine *on page 205*
- ◆ **Tanafed DMX™** *see* Chlorpheniramine, Pseudoephedrine, and Dextromethorphan *on page 333*
- ◆ **Tannate-V-DM** *see* Phenylephrine, Pyrilamine, and Dextromethorphan *on page 1278*
- ◆ **Tannate 12 S** *see* Carbetapentane and Chlorpheniramine *on page 272*
- ◆ **Tannate PD-DM** *see* Chlorpheniramine, Pseudoephedrine, and Dextromethorphan *on page 333*
- ◆ **Tannate Pediatric** *see* Chlorpheniramine and Phenylephrine *on page 323*
- ◆ **Tannic-12 [DSC]** *see* Carbetapentane and Chlorpheniramine *on page 272*
- ◆ **Tannic-12 S** *see* Carbetapentane and Chlorpheniramine *on page 272*
- ◆ **Tannihist-12 D [DSC]** *see* Carbetapentane, Phenylephrine, and Pyrilamine *on page 275*
- ◆ **Tannihist-12 RF [DSC]** *see* Carbetapentane and Chlorpheniramine *on page 272*
- ◆ **TAP-144** *see* Leuprolide *on page 901*
- ◆ **Tapazole®** *see* Methimazole *on page 1010*
- ◆ **Tarceva®** *see* Erlotinib *on page 556*
- ◆ **Targretin®** *see* Bexarotene *on page 187*
- ◆ **Tarka®** *see* Trandolapril and Verapamil *on page 1608*
- ◆ **Tasigna®** *see* Nilotinib *on page 1140*
- ◆ **Tasmar®** *see* Tolcapone *on page 1593*
- ◆ **Tavist® Allergy [OTC]** *see* Clemastine *on page 361*
- ◆ **Tavist® ND ALLERGY [OTC]** *see* Loratadine *on page 946*
- ◆ **Taxol®** *see* Paclitaxel *on page 1213*
- ◆ **Taxotere®** *see* Docetaxel *on page 491*

Tazarotene (taz AR oh teen)

U.S. Brand Names Avage™; Tazorac®

Canadian Brand Names Tazorac®

Mexican Brand Names Suretin

Pharmacologic Category Acne Products; Keratolytic Agent; Topical Skin Product, Acne

Use Topical treatment of facial acne vulgaris; topical treatment of stable plaque psoriasis of up to 20% body surface area involvement; mitigation (palliation) of facial skin wrinkling, facial mottled hyper-/hypopigmentation, and benign facial lentigines

Effect on Mental Status None reported

Effect on Psychiatric Treatment Use caution with drugs known to cause photosensitivity (psychotropics), effects may be augmented

Dosage Summary

Topical:

Children <12 years: Dosage not established

Children ≥12 years: Apply a thin film **or** 2 mg/cm^2 once daily, in the evening

Adults: Apply a thin film **or** 2 mg/cm^2 once daily, in the evening

Dosage Forms Excipient information presented when available (limited, particularly for generics); consult specific product labeling.

Cream:

Avage™: 0.1% (30 g) [contains benzyl alcohol]

Tazorac®: 0.05% (30 g, 60 g); 0.1% (30 g, 60 g) [contains benzyl alcohol]

Gel (Tazorac®): 0.05% (30 g, 100 g); 0.1% (30 g, 100 g) [contains benzyl alcohol]

- **Tazicef®** *see* Ceftazidime *on page 298*
- **Tazobactam and Piperacillin** *see* Piperacillin and Tazobactam Sodium *on page 1302*
- **Tazorac®** *see* Tazarotene *on page 1540*
- **Taztia XT™** *see* Diltiazem *on page 473*
- **3TC** *see* LamiVUDine *on page 888*
- **T-Cell Growth Factor** *see* Aldesleukin *on page 58*
- **TCGF** *see* Aldesleukin *on page 58*
- **TCN** *see* Tetracycline *on page 1558*
- **TDF** *see* Tenofovir *on page 1549*

Tegaserod (teg a SER od)

U.S. Brand Names Zelnorm®

Canadian Brand Names Zelnorm® [DSC]

Mexican Brand Names Zelmac

Index Terms HTF919; Tegaserod Maleate

Pharmacologic Category Serotonin 5-HT_4 Receptor Agonist

Use Emergency treatment of irritable bowel syndrome with constipation (IBS-C) and chronic idiopathic constipation (CIC) in women (<55 years of age) in which no alternative therapy exists

Effect on Mental Status May cause dizziness and headache; may rarely cause depression, mood lability, and insomnia

Effect on Psychiatric Treatment GI side effects are common; use caution with SSRIs

Restrictions Available in U.S. under an emergency investigational new drug (IND) process. Emergency situations are defined as immediately life-threatening or requiring hospitalization. Physicians with patients who may qualify can contact the FDA's Division of Drug Information via email (druginfo@fda.hhs.gov), by calling (301-796-3400), or at http://www.fda.gov/cder. The FDA may either deny the request or authorize shipment of Zelnorm® by Novartis. Additional information can be found at http://www.zelnorm.com or http://www.fda.gov/cder/drug/infopage/zelnorm/default.htm

Dosage Summary

Oral:

Children: Dosage not established

Adults:

Females <55 years of age: 6 mg twice daily, before meals

Females ≥55 years of age: Use is contraindicated.

Dosage Forms Excipient information presented when available (limited, particularly for generics); consult specific product labeling.

Tablet:

Zelnorm®: 2 mg, 6 mg

- **Tegaserod Maleate** *see* Tegaserod *on page 1541*
- **Tegretol®** *see* CarBAMazepine *on page 265*
- **Tegretol®-XR** *see* CarBAMazepine *on page 265*
- **Tekturna®** *see* Aliskiren *on page 65*
- **Tekturna HCT®** *see* Aliskiren and Hydrochlorothiazide *on page 66*

Telbivudine (tel BI vyoo deen)

U.S. Brand Names Tyzeka™

Canadian Brand Names Sebivo®

Index Terms L-Deoxythymidine

Pharmacologic Category Antiretroviral Agent, Reverse Transcriptase Inhibitor (Nucleoside)

Use Treatment of chronic hepatitis B with evidence of viral replication and either persistent transaminase elevations or histologically-active disease

Effect on Mental Status Fatigue and malaise are common; may cause dizziness or insomnia

Effect on Psychiatric Treatment May cause myopathy with serum creatine kinase elevations, weeks to months after initiation; consider this when evaluating patients for neuroleptic malignant syndrome and malignant hyperthermia. May cause neutropenia; use caution with clozapine and carbamazepine.

Dosage Summary

Oral:

Children <16 years: Dosage not established.

Children ≥16 years: 600 mg once daily

Adults: 600 mg once daily

Dosage Forms Excipient information presented when available (limited, particularly for generics); consult specific product labeling.

Tablet:

Tyzeka™: 600 mg

◆ **Teldrin® HBP [OTC]** *see* Chlorpheniramine *on page 321*

Telithromycin (tel ith roe MYE sin)

U.S. Brand Names Ketek®

Canadian Brand Names Ketek®

Mexican Brand Names Ketek

Index Terms HMR 3647

Pharmacologic Category Antibiotic, Ketolide

Use Treatment of community-acquired pneumonia (mild-to-moderate) caused by susceptible strains of *Streptococcus pneumoniae* (including multidrug-resistant isolates), *Haemophilus influenzae*, *Chlamydophila pneumoniae*, *Moraxella catarrhalis*, and *Mycoplasma pneumoniae*

Effect on Mental Status May cause dizziness, fatigue, somnolence, or insomnia; may rarely cause nervousness, tremor, and abnormal dreams

Effect on Psychiatric Treatment May prolong QT_c interval; use caution with thioridazine and ziprasidone. Gastrointestinal side effects are common; these effects may be additive with concomitant use of SSRIs, lithium, and valproic acid. Telithromycin may increase the effects of alprazolam, carbamazepine, ergot alkaloids, midazolam, mirtazapine, nefazodone, pimozide, triazolam, and venlafaxine. Concomitant use with ergots, midazolam, pimozide, or triazolam is generally contraindicated. Nefazodone may increase the effects of telithromycin. Carbamazepine, phenobarbital, and phenytoin may decrease the effects of telithromycin.

Restrictions An FDA-approved Medication Guide is available and must be dispensed with every prescription. Copies may be found at: http://www.fda.gov/cder/foi/label/2007/021144s012medg.pdf

Dosage Summary

Oral:

Children <13 years: Dosage not established

Children ≥13 years (unlabeled): 800 mg once daily

Adults: 800 mg once daily

Dosage Forms Excipient information presented when available (limited, particularly for generics); consult specific product labeling.

Tablet:

Ketek®: 300 mg [not available in Canada], 400 mg

Telmisartan (tel mi SAR tan)

Related Information

Angiotensin Agents *on page 1754*

U.S. Brand Names Micardis®

Canadian Brand Names Micardis®

Mexican Brand Names Micardis; Predxal

Pharmacologic Category Angiotensin II Receptor Blocker

Generic Available No

Use Treatment of hypertension; may be used alone or in combination with other antihypertensive agents

Effect on Mental Status May cause dizziness or fatigue, may rarely cause insomnia, anxiety, nervousness, depression, or sedation

Effect on Psychiatric Treatment May decrease lithium clearance, resulting in an increase in serum lithium levels and potential lithium toxicity; monitor serum lithium levels

Pregnancy Risk Factor C (1st trimester); D (2nd and 3rd trimesters)

Pregnancy Considerations Medications which act on the renin-angiotensin system are reported to have the following fetal/neonatal effects: Hypotension, neonatal skull hypoplasia, anuria, renal failure, and death; oligohydramnios is also reported. These effects are reported to occur with exposure during the second and third trimesters. There are no adequate and well-controlled studies in pregnant women. **[U.S. Boxed Warning]: Based on human data, drugs**

that act on the angiotensin system can cause injury and death to the developing fetus when used in the second and third trimesters. Angiotensin receptor blockers should be discontinued as soon as possible once pregnancy is detected.

Lactation Enters breast milk/not recommended

Contraindications Hypersensitivity to telmisartan or any component of the formulation

Warnings/Precautions [U.S. Boxed Warning]: Based on human data, drugs that act on the angiotensin system can cause injury and death to the developing fetus when used in the second and third trimesters. Angiotensin receptor blockers should be discontinued as soon as possible once pregnancy is detected. May cause hyperkalemia; avoid potassium supplementation unless specifically required by healthcare provider. Avoid use or use a smaller dose in patients who are volume depleted; correct depletion first. May be associated with deterioration of renal function and/or increases in serum creatinine, particularly in patients with low renal blood flow (eg, renal artery stenosis, heart failure) whose glomerular filtration rate (GFR) is dependent on efferent arteriolar vasoconstriction by angiotensin II. Use with caution in unstented unilateral/bilateral renal artery stenosis. When unstented bilateral renal artery stenosis is present, use is generally avoided due to the elevated risk of deterioration in renal function unless possible benefits outweigh risks. Use with caution with pre-existing renal insufficiency; significant aortic/mitral stenosis. Use with caution in patients who have biliary obstructive disorders or hepatic dysfunction. Safety and efficacy have not been established in children.

Adverse Reactions May be associated with worsening of renal function in patients dependent on renin-angiotensin-aldosterone system.

1% to 10%:

Cardiovascular: Hypertension (1%), chest pain (1%), peripheral edema (1%)

Central nervous system: Headache (1%), dizziness (1%), pain (1%), fatigue (1%)

Gastrointestinal: Diarrhea (3%), dyspepsia (1%), nausea (1%), abdominal pain (1%)

Genitourinary: Urinary tract infection (1%)

Neuromuscular & skeletal: Back pain (3%), myalgia (1%)

Respiratory: Upper respiratory infection (7%), sinusitis (3%), pharyngitis (1%), cough (2%)

Miscellaneous: Flu-like syndrome (1%)

<1% (Limited to important or life-threatening): Abnormal vision, allergic reaction, anemia, angina, angioedema, angioneurotic edema, atrial fibrillation, bradycardia, creatinine kinase increased, CHF, cramps, depression, dyspnea, edema, eosinophilia, epistaxis, erectile dysfunction, erythema, facial edema, gout, hepatic dysfunction, hyperkalemia, hypersensitivity, hypotension, impotence, increased serum creatinine and BUN, insomnia, MI, migraine, muscle cramps, orthostatic hypotension (more frequent in dialysis patients), paresthesia, pruritus, rhabdomyolysis, rash, renal dysfunction, renal failure, somnolence, syncope, thrombocytopenia, tinnitus, uric acid increased, urticaria, vertigo, weakness

Metabolism/Transport Effects Inhibits CYP2C19 (weak)

Drug Interactions

ACE Inhibitors: Angiotensin II Receptor Blockers may enhance the adverse/toxic effect of ACE Inhibitors. *Risk C: Monitor therapy*

Cardiac Glycosides: Telmisartan may increase the serum concentration of Cardiac Glycosides. *Risk C: Monitor therapy*

Diazoxide: May enhance the hypotensive effect of Antihypertensives. *Risk C: Monitor therapy*

Eplerenone: May enhance the hyperkalemic effect of Angiotensin II Receptor Blockers. *Risk C: Monitor therapy*

Herbs (Hypertensive Properties): May diminish the antihypertensive effect of Antihypertensives. *Risk C: Monitor therapy*

Herbs (Hypotensive Properties): May enhance the hypotensive effect of Antihypertensives. *Risk C: Monitor therapy*

Lithium: Angiotensin II Receptor Blockers may increase the serum concentration of Lithium. Management: Lithium dosage reductions will likely be needed following the addition of an angiotensin II receptor antagonist. *Risk D: Consider therapy modification*

Methylphenidate: May diminish the antihypertensive effect of Antihypertensives. *Risk C: Monitor therapy*

Nonsteroidal Anti-Inflammatory Agents: May diminish the therapeutic effect of Angiotensin II Receptor Blockers. The combination of these two agents may also significantly decrease glomerular filtration and renal function. *Risk C: Monitor therapy*

Potassium Salts: May enhance the hyperkalemic effect of Angiotensin II Receptor Blockers. *Risk C: Monitor therapy*

Potassium-Sparing Diuretics: Angiotensin II Receptor Blockers may enhance the hyperkalemic effect of Potassium-Sparing Diuretics. *Risk C: Monitor therapy*

Prostacyclin Analogues: May enhance the hypotensive effect of Antihypertensives. *Risk C: Monitor therapy*

RiTUXimab: Antihypertensives may enhance the hypotensive effect of RiTUXimab. *Risk D: Consider therapy modification*

Trimethoprim: May enhance the hyperkalemic effect of Angiotensin II Receptor Blockers. *Risk C: Monitor therapy*

Ethanol/Nutrition/Herb Interactions Herb/Nutraceutical: Avoid dong quai if using for hypertension (has estrogenic activity). Avoid ephedra, yohimbe, ginseng (may worsen hypertension). Avoid garlic (may have increased antihypertensive effect).

Mechanism of Action Angiotensin II acts as a vasoconstrictor. In addition to causing direct vasoconstriction, angiotensin II also stimulates the release of aldosterone. Once aldosterone is released, sodium as well as water are reabsorbed. The end result is an elevation in blood pressure. Telmisartan is a nonpeptide AT1 angiotensin II receptor antagonist. This binding prevents angiotensin II from binding to the receptor thereby blocking the vasoconstriction and the aldosterone secreting effects of angiotensin II.

Pharmacodynamics/Kinetics Orally active, not a prodrug

Onset of action: 1-2 hours

Peak effect: 0.5-1 hours

Duration: Up to 24 hours

Protein binding: >99.5%

Metabolism: Hepatic via conjugation to inactive metabolites; not metabolized via CYP

Bioavailability (dose dependent): 42% to 58%

Half-life elimination: Terminal: 24 hours

Excretion: Feces (97%)

Clearance: Total body: 800 mL/minute

Dosage Adults: Oral: Initial: 40 mg once daily; usual maintenance dose range: 20-80 mg/day. Patients with volume depletion should be initiated on the lower dosage with close supervision.

Dosage adjustment in renal impairment: No adjustment required; hemodialysis patients are more susceptible to orthostatic hypotension

Dosage adjustment in hepatic impairment: Supervise patients closely.

Dietary Considerations May be taken without regard to food.

Monitoring Parameters Supine blood pressure, electrolytes, serum creatinine, BUN, urinalysis, symptomatic hypotension, and tachycardia

Dosage Forms Excipient information presented when available (limited, particularly for generics); consult specific product labeling.

Tablet: 20 mg, 40 mg, 80 mg

Telmisartan and Hydrochlorothiazide

(tel mi SAR tan & hye droe klor oh THYE a zide)

U.S. Brand Names Micardis® HCT

Canadian Brand Names Micardis® Plus

Index Terms Hydrochlorothiazide and Telmisartan

Pharmacologic Category Angiotensin II Receptor Blocker; Diuretic, Thiazide

Use Treatment of hypertension; combination product should not be used for initial therapy

Effect on Mental Status May cause dizziness or fatigue; may rarely cause insomnia, anxiety, nervousness, or depression

Effect on Psychiatric Treatment May decrease lithium clearance resulting in an increase in serum lithium levels and potential lithium toxicity; monitor serum lithium levels. May cause photosensitivity; concomitant use with psychotropics may further the risk. Use sunscreen, wear protective clothing and eyewear and avoid direct sunlight.

Dosage Summary

Oral:

Children: Dosage not established

Adults: Initial: Telmisartan 80 mg and hydrochlorothiazide 12.5-25 mg once daily; Maintenance: Telmisartan 80-160 mg and hydrochlorothiazide 12.5-25 mg once daily

Dosage Forms Excipient information presented when available (limited, particularly for generics); consult specific product labeling. [CAN]: Canadian brand name

Tablet:

Micardis® HCT [available in U.S.]:

40/12.5: Telmisartan 40 mg and hydrochlorothiazide 12.5 mg

80/12.5: Telmisartan 80 mg and hydrochlorothiazide 12.5 mg

80/25: Telmisartan 80 mg and hydrochlorothiazide 25 mg

Micardis® Plus [CAN]: 80/25: Telmisartan 80 mg and hydrochlorothiazide 25 mg [Not available in U.S.]

Temazepam (te MAZ e pam)

Medication Safety Issues

Sound-alike/look-alike issues:

Temazepam may be confused with flurazepam, LORazepam

Restoril® may be confused with Vistaril®, Zestril®

Related Information

Benzodiazepines *on page 1774*

CMS: Long-Term Care Facility Thresholds *on page 1815*

Discontinuation of Psychotropic Drugs *on page 1839*

U.S. Brand Names Restoril®

Canadian Brand Names Apo-Temazepam®; CO Temazepam; Dom-Temazepam; Gen-Temazepam; Novo-Temazepam; Nu-Temazepam; PHL-Temazepam; PMS-Temazepam; ratio-Temazepam; Restoril®

Pharmacologic Category Hypnotic, Benzodiazepine

Generic Available Yes

Use Short-term treatment of insomnia

Unlabeled/Investigational Use Treatment of anxiety; adjunct in the treatment of depression; management of panic attacks

Mental Health Comment In 2007, the FDA requested that all manufacturers of sedative-hypnotic drug products revise labeling to include a greater emphasis on the risks of adverse effects. These risks include severe allergic reactions (anaphylaxis, angioedema) and complex sleep-related behaviors, which may include sleep-driving (driving while not fully awake and with no memory of the event), making phone calls, and preparing and eating food while asleep.

There are two subtypes of GABA receptors (GABA-A and GABA-B) and three different benzodiazepine receptors (Bz_1, Bz_2, and Bz_3). Benzodiazepine receptors and effects appear to be linked to the GABA-A receptors. Benzodiazepines do not bind to GABA-B receptors. The role of GABA-B receptors is unclear. Benzodiazepines have no specificity for benzodiazepine receptor subtypes.

Temazepam is a short half-life benzodiazepine. Duration of action after a single dose is determined by redistribution rather than metabolism. Tolerance develops to the sedative, hypnotic, and anticonvulsant effects. It does not develop to the anxiolytic or skeletal muscle relaxing effects. Psychological and physical dependence may occur with prolonged use of benzodiazepines. The onset of withdrawal symptoms is usually seen on the first day without drug and lasts 5-7 days in patients receiving short half-life benzodiazepines, whereas, the onset occurs after 5 days with a duration of 10-14 days after abrupt discontinuance of long half-life benzodiazepines. Risk factors for abuse include personal or family history of substance abuse and personality disorder. Temazepam is slowly absorbed; undergoes phase II metabolism and, therefore, is less likely to be effected in patients with hepatic dysfunction.

Restrictions C-IV

An FDA-approved patient medication guide is available and must be distributed when dispensing an outpatient prescription (new or refill) where this medication is to be used without direct supervision of a healthcare provider. Medication guides are available at http://www.fda.gov/cder/Offices/ODS/medication_guides.htm.

Pregnancy Risk Factor X

Lactation Enters breast milk/not recommended (AAP rates "of concern")

Contraindications Hypersensitivity to temazepam or any component of the formulation (cross-sensitivity with other benzodiazepines may exist); narrow-angle glaucoma (not in product labeling, however, benzodiazepines are contraindicated); pregnancy

Warnings/Precautions As a hypnotic, should be used only after evaluation of potential causes of sleep disturbance. Failure of sleep disturbance to resolve after 7-10 days may indicate psychiatric or medical illness. A worsening of insomnia or the emergence of new abnormalities of thought or behavior may represent unrecognized psychiatric or medical illness and requires immediate and careful evaluation.

Use with caution in elderly or debilitated patients, patients with hepatic disease (including alcoholics), or renal impairment. Use with caution in patients with respiratory disease, or impaired gag reflex. Avoid use inpatients with sleep apnea.

Causes CNS depression (dose-related) resulting in sedation, dizziness, confusion, or ataxia which may impair physical and mental capabilities. Patients must be cautioned about performing tasks which require mental alertness (eg, operating machinery or driving). Use with caution in patients receiving other CNS depressants or psychoactive agents. Postmarketing studies have indicated that the use of hypnotic/sedative agents for sleep has been associated with hypersensitivity reactions including anaphylaxis as well as angioedema. An increased risk for hazardous sleep-related activities such as sleep-driving; cooking and eating food, and making phone calls while asleep have also been noted. Effects with other sedative drugs or ethanol may be potentiated. Benzodiazepines have been associated with falls and traumatic injury and should be used with extreme caution in patients who are at risk of these events (especially the elderly).

Use caution in patients with suicidal risk. Use with caution in patients with a history of drug dependence. Benzodiazepines have been associated with dependence and acute withdrawal symptoms on discontinuation or reduction in dose (may occur after as little as 10 days). Acute withdrawal, including seizures, may be precipitated after administration of flumazenil to patients receiving long-term benzodiazepine therapy.

Benzodiazepines have been associated with anterograde amnesia. Paradoxical reactions, including hyperactive or aggressive behavior, have been reported with benzodiazepines, particularly in adolescent/pediatric or psychiatric patients. Does not have analgesic, antidepressant, or antipsychotic properties.

Adverse Reactions

1% to 10%:

- Central nervous system: Confusion, dizziness, drowsiness, fatigue, anxiety, headache, lethargy, hangover, euphoria, vertigo
- Dermatologic: Rash
- Endocrine & metabolic: Decreased libido
- Gastrointestinal: Diarrhea
- Neuromuscular & skeletal: Dysarthria, weakness
- Ocular: Blurred vision
- Miscellaneous: Diaphoresis

<1% (Limited to important or life-threatening): Amnesia, anaphylaxis, angioedema, ataxia, blood dyscrasias, complex sleep-related behavior (sleep-driving, cooking or eating food, making phone calls), drug dependence, paradoxical reactions, vomiting

Metabolism/Transport Effects Substrate (minor) of CYP2B6, 2C9, 2C19, 3A4

Drug Interactions

Alcohol (Ethyl): CNS Depressants may enhance the CNS depressant effect of Alcohol (Ethyl). *Risk C: Monitor therapy*

Clozapine: Benzodiazepines may enhance the adverse/toxic effect of Clozapine. *Risk D: Consider therapy modification*

CNS Depressants: May enhance the adverse/toxic effect of other CNS Depressants. *Risk C: Monitor therapy*

Phenytoin: Benzodiazepines may increase the serum concentration of Phenytoin. Short-term exposure to benzodiazepines may not present as much risk as chronic therapy. *Risk C: Monitor therapy*

Theophylline Derivatives: May diminish the therapeutic effect of Benzodiazepines. *Risk D: Consider therapy modification*

Ethanol/Nutrition/Herb Interactions

Ethanol: Avoid ethanol (may increase CNS depression).

Food: Serum levels may be increased by grapefruit juice.

Herb/Nutraceutical: St John's wort may decrease temazepam levels. Avoid valerian, St John's wort, kava kava, gotu kola (may increase CNS depression).

Mechanism of Action Binds to stereospecific benzodiazepine receptors on the postsynaptic GABA neuron at several sites within the central nervous system, including the limbic system, reticular formation. Enhancement of the inhibitory effect of GABA on neuronal excitability results by increased neuronal membrane permeability to chloride ions. This shift in chloride ions results in hyperpolarization (a less excitable state) and stabilization.

Pharmacodynamics/Kinetics

Distribution: V_d: 1.4 L/kg

Protein binding: 96%

Metabolism: Hepatic

Half-life elimination: 9.5-12.4 hours

Time to peak, serum: 2-3 hours

Excretion: Urine (80% to 90% as inactive metabolites)

Dosage Oral:

Adults: 15-30 mg at bedtime

Elderly or debilitated patients: 15 mg

Monitoring Parameters Respiratory and cardiovascular status

Reference Range Therapeutic: 26 ng/mL after 24 hours

Additional Information Abrupt discontinuation after sustained use (generally >10 days) may cause withdrawal symptoms.

Dosage Forms Excipient information presented when available (limited, particularly for generics); consult specific product labeling.

Capsule: 15 mg, 22.5 mg, 30 mg

Restoril®: 7.5 mg, 15 mg, 22.5 mg, 30 mg

◆ **Temodar®** *see* Temozolomide *on page 1547*

Temozolomide (te moe ZOE loe mide)

Medication Safety Issues

High alert medication: The Institute for Safe Medication Practices (ISMP) includes this medication among its list of drugs which have a heightened risk of causing significant patient harm when used in error.

U.S. Brand Names Temodar®

Canadian Brand Names Temodal®; Temodar®

Mexican Brand Names Temodal

Index Terms NSC-362856; TMZ

Pharmacologic Category Antineoplastic Agent, Alkylating Agent (Triazene)

Use Treatment of adult patients with refractory anaplastic astrocytoma; newly-diagnosed glioblastoma multiforme

Unlabeled/Investigational Use Metastatic melanoma

Effect on Mental Status Fatigue, dizziness, amnesia, and insomnia are common; may cause somnolence, confusion, anxiety, depression

Effect on Psychiatric Treatment Myelosuppression is common, use caution with clozapine and carbamazepine; nausea is very common, avoid use with SSRIs

Dosage Summary

Oral:

Children: Dosage not established

Adults: Initial: 150 mg/m^2/day for 5 days; Subsequent doses: 100-200 mg/m^2/day for 5 days every 28 days, based upon hematologic tolerance **or** Concomitant phase: 75 mg/m^2/day for 42 days with radiotherapy (60Gy administered in 30 fractions); Maintenance phase: 100-200 mg/m^2/day for 5 days every 28 days, based upon hematologic tolerance (maximum: 6 cycles)

Dosage Forms Excipient information presented when available (limited, particularly for generics); consult specific product labeling.

Capsule:

Temodar®: 5 mg, 20 mg, 100 mg, 140 mg, 180 mg, 250 mg

Temsirolimus (tem sir OH li mus)

Medication Safety Issues

Sound-alike/look-alike issues:

Temsirolimus may be confused with sirolimus, tacrolimus

High alert medication: The Institute for Safe Medication Practices (ISMP) includes this medication among its list of drug classes which have a heightened risk of causing significant patient harm when used in error.

Temsirolimus, for the treatment of advanced renal cell cancer, is a flat dose (25 mg) and is not based on body surface area (BSA).

U.S. Brand Names Torisel®

Canadian Brand Names Torisel®

Index Terms CCI-779; NSC-683864

Pharmacologic Category Antineoplastic Agent, mTOR Kinase Inhibitor

Use Treatment of advanced renal cell cancer (RCC)

Effect on Mental Status Insomnia is common; may produce symptoms of mania or depression

Effect on Psychiatric Treatment Increases in serum glucose are common with temsirolimus and may alter insulin and/or oral hypoglycemic therapy requirements in diabetic patients. Hyperglycemia has also been associated with mental disorders as well as various psychotropic agents (especially atypical antipsychotics). Elevations in cholesterol and triglycerides may also be seen with psychotropics and temsirolimus. Concomitant use of these agents may produce additive effects; monitor metabolic profile. GI side effects are common; concurrent use with SSRIs, lithium, carbamazepine, or valproic acid may produce additive effects. Hematologic side effects are common; concurrent use with clozapine, carbamazepine, or valproic acid may produce additive effects. Temsirolimus is a CYP3A4 substrate; therefore, agents that inhibit its metabolism (nefazodone) may increase toxicity while inducers (eg, carbamazepine, barbiturates, phenytoin) may reduce its efficacy.

Dosage Summary

I.V.:

Children: Dosage not established

Adults: 25 mg weekly

Dosage Forms Excipient information presented when available (limited, particularly for generics); consult specific product labeling.

Injection, solution [concentrate]:

Torisel®: 25 mg/mL [contains dehydrated ethanol, propylene glycol; diluent contains dehydrated ethanol, polyethylene glycol, polysorbate 80]

Tenecteplase (ten EK te plase)

Medication Safety Issues

Sound-alike/look-alike issues:

TNKase® may be confused with t-PA

TNK (occasional abbreviation for TNKase®) is an error-prone abbreviation (mistaken as TPA)

High alert medication: The Institute for Safe Medication Practices (ISMP) includes this medication (I.V.) among its list of drugs which have a heightened risk of causing significant patient harm when used in error.

U.S. Brand Names TNKase®

Canadian Brand Names TNKase®

Mexican Brand Names Metalyse

Pharmacologic Category Thrombolytic Agent

Use Thrombolytic agent used in the management of ST-elevation myocardial infarction (STEMI) for the lysis of thrombi in the coronary vasculature to restore perfusion and reduce mortality.

Recommended criteria for treatment: STEMI: Chest pain ≥20 minutes duration, onset of chest pain within 12 hours of treatment (or within prior 12-24 hours in patients with continuing ischemic symptoms), and S-T segment elevation >0.1 mV in at least two contiguous precordial leads or two adjacent limb leads on ECG or new or presumably new left bundle branch block (LBBB)

Unlabeled/Investigational Use Acute MI - combination regimen of tenecteplase (unlabeled dose), abciximab, and heparin (unlabeled dose)

Effect on Mental Status May cause stroke

Effect on Psychiatric Treatment None reported

Dosage Summary

I.V.:

Children: Dosage not established

Adults <60 kg: 30 mg single dose over 5 seconds

Adults ≥60 to <70 kg: 35 mg single dose over 5 seconds

Adults ≥70 to <80 kg: 40 mg single dose over 5 seconds

Adults ≥80 to <90 kg: 45 mg single dose over 5 seconds

Adults ≥90 kg: 50 mg single dose over 5 seconds

Dosage Forms Excipient information presented when available (limited, particularly for generics); consult specific product labeling.

Injection, powder for reconstitution [recombinant]:

TNKase®: 50 mg

◆ **Tenex®** *see* GuanFACINE *on page 750*

Teniposide (ten i POE side)

Medication Safety Issues

Sound-alike/look-alike issues:

Teniposide may be confused with etoposide

High alert medication: The Institute for Safe Medication Practices (ISMP) includes this medication among its list of drugs which have a heightened risk of causing significant patient harm when used in error.

U.S. Brand Names Vumon®

Canadian Brand Names Vumon®

Mexican Brand Names Vumon

Index Terms EPT; VM-26

Pharmacologic Category Antineoplastic Agent, Miscellaneous

Use Treatment of acute lymphocytic leukemia, small cell lung cancer

Effect on Mental Status None reported

Effect on Psychiatric Treatment Myelosuppression is common; avoid clozapine and carbamazepine

Dosage Forms Excipient information presented when available (limited, particularly for generics); consult specific product labeling.

Injection, solution: 10 mg/mL (5 mL) [contains benzyl alcohol, dehydrated ethanol 42.7%, and polyoxyethylated castor oil]

Tenofovir (te NOE fo veer)

U.S. Brand Names Viread®

Canadian Brand Names Viread®

Mexican Brand Names Viread

Index Terms PMPA; TDF; Tenofovir Disoproxil Fumarate

Pharmacologic Category Antiretroviral Agent, Reverse Transcriptase Inhibitor (Nucleotide)

Use Management of HIV infections in combination with at least two other antiretroviral agents; treatment of chronic hepatitis B virus (HBV)

Effect on Mental Status May cause dizziness and depression

Effect on Psychiatric Treatment Nausea and diarrhea are common; use caution with SSRIs, lithium, and valproic acid. May cause elevation of triglycerides; monitor in patients receiving antipsychotics especially clozapine, olanzapine, and quetiapine.

Dosage Summary

Oral:

Children: Dosage not established

Adults: 300 mg once daily

Dosage Forms Excipient information presented when available (limited, particularly for generics); consult specific product labeling.

Tablet, as disoproxil fumarate: 300 mg [equivalent to 245 mg tenofovir disoproxil]

- ◆ **Tenofovir and Emtricitabine** *see* Emtricitabine and Tenofovir *on page 530*
- ◆ **Tenofovir Disoproxil Fumarate** *see* Tenofovir *on page 1549*
- ◆ **Tenofovir Disoproxil Fumarate, Efavirenz, and Emtricitabine** *see* Efavirenz, Emtricitabine, and Tenofovir *on page 527*
- ◆ **Tenoretic®** *see* Atenolol and Chlorthalidone *on page 150*
- ◆ **Tenormin®** *see* Atenolol *on page 147*

Terazosin (ter AY zoe sin)

Canadian Brand Names Alti-Terazosin; Apo-Terazosin®; Hytrin®; Novo-Terazosin; Nu-Terazosin; PMS-Terazosin

Mexican Brand Names Adecur; Hytrin

Pharmacologic Category $Alpha_1$ Blocker

Generic Available Yes

Use Management of mild to moderate hypertension; alone or in combination with other agents such as diuretics or beta-blockers; benign prostate hyperplasia (BPH)

Unlabeled/Investigational Use Pediatric hypertension

Effect on Mental Status Dizziness is common; may cause drowsiness or nervousness; may rarely cause insomnia or depression

Effect on Psychiatric Treatment None reported

Pregnancy Risk Factor C

Lactation Excretion in breast milk unknown

Contraindications Hypersensitivity to quinazolines (doxazosin, prazosin, terazosin) or any component of the formulation; concurrent use with phosphodiesterase-5 (PDE-5) inhibitors including sildenafil (>25 mg), tadalafil, or vardenafil

Warnings/Precautions Can cause significant orthostatic hypotension and syncope, especially with first dose; anticipate a similar effect if therapy is interrupted for a few days, if dosage is rapidly increased, or if another antihypertensive drug (particularly vasodilators) or a PDE-5 inhibitor is introduced. Discontinue if symptoms of angina occur or worsen. Patients should be cautioned about performing hazardous tasks when starting new therapy or adjusting dosage upward. Prostate cancer should be ruled out before starting for BPH. Use with caution in hepatic impairment. Intraoperative floppy iris syndrome has been observed in cataract surgery patients who were on or were previously treated with $alpha_1$-blockers. Causality has not been established and there appears to be no benefit in discontinuing alpha-blocker therapy prior to surgery. Safety and efficacy in children have not been established.

Adverse Reactions Asthenia, postural hypotension, dizziness, somnolence, nasal congestion/rhinitis, and impotence were the only events noted in clinical trials to occur at a frequency significantly greater than placebo ($p < 0.05$).

>10%:

Central nervous system: Dizziness, headache

Neuromuscular & skeletal: Muscle weakness

1% to 10%:

Cardiovascular: Edema, palpitation, chest pain, peripheral edema (3%), orthostatic hypotension (3% to 4%), tachycardia

Central nervous system: Fatigue, nervousness, drowsiness

Gastrointestinal: Dry mouth

Genitourinary: Urinary incontinence

Ocular: Blurred vision

Respiratory: Dyspnea, nasal congestion

<1% (Limited to important or life-threatening): Allergic reactions, anaphylaxis, atrial fibrillation, priapism, sexual dysfunction, syncope (0.8%), thrombocytopenia

Drug Interactions

Alfuzosin: Alpha1-Blockers may enhance the antihypertensive effect of Alfuzosin. Risk of orthostatic hypotension or syncope may be increased. Alfuzosin may enhance the antihypertensive effect of Alpha1-Blockers. *Risk X: Avoid combination*

Beta-Blockers: May enhance the orthostatic effect of Alpha1-Blockers. The risk associated with ophthalmic products is probably less than systemic products. **Exceptions:** Levobunolol; Metipranolol. *Risk D: Consider therapy modification*

Calcium Channel Blockers: Alpha1-Blockers may enhance the hypotensive effect of Calcium Channel Blockers. *Risk C: Monitor therapy*

Diazoxide: May enhance the hypotensive effect of Antihypertensives. *Risk C: Monitor therapy*

Herbs (Hypertensive Properties): May diminish the antihypertensive effect of Antihypertensives. *Risk C: Monitor therapy*

Herbs (Hypotensive Properties): May enhance the hypotensive effect of Antihypertensives. *Risk C: Monitor therapy*

Methylphenidate: May diminish the antihypertensive effect of Antihypertensives. *Risk C: Monitor therapy*

Phosphodiesterase 5 Inhibitors: May enhance the hypotensive effect of Alpha1-Blockers. *Risk D: Consider therapy modification*

Prostacyclin Analogues: May enhance the hypotensive effect of Antihypertensives. *Risk C: Monitor therapy*

RiTUXimab: Antihypertensives may enhance the hypotensive effect of RiTUXimab. *Risk D: Consider therapy modification*

Tamsulosin: Alpha1-Blockers may enhance the antihypertensive effect of Tamsulosin. Risk of orthostatic hypotension or syncope may be increased. Tamsulosin may enhance the antihypertensive effect of Alpha1-Blockers. *Risk X: Avoid combination*

Ethanol/Nutrition/Herb Interactions Herb/Nutraceutical: Avoid dong quai if using for hypertension (has estrogenic activity). Avoid ephedra, yohimbe, ginseng (may worsen hypertension). Avoid saw palmetto. Avoid garlic (may have increased antihypertensive effect).

Mechanism of Action Alpha$_1$-specific blocking agent with minimal alpha$_2$ effects; this allows peripheral postsynaptic blockade, with the resultant decrease in arterial tone, while preserving the negative feedback loop which is mediated by the peripheral presynaptic alpha$_2$-receptors; terazosin relaxes the smooth muscle of the bladder neck, thus reducing bladder outlet obstruction

Pharmacodynamics/Kinetics

Onset of action: 1-2 hours

Absorption: Rapid

Protein binding: 90% to 95%

Metabolism: Extensively hepatic

Half-life elimination: 9.2-12 hours

Time to peak, serum: ~1 hour

Excretion: Feces (60%); urine (40%)

Dosage Oral:

Hypertension:

Children (unlabeled use): Initial: 1 mg once daily; gradually increase dose as necessary, up to maximum of 20 mg/day

Adults: Initial: 1 mg at bedtime; slowly increase dose to achieve desired blood pressure, up to 20 mg/day; usual dose range (JNC 7): 1-20 mg once daily

Dosage reduction may be needed when adding a diuretic or other antihypertensive agent; if drug is discontinued for greater than several days, consider beginning with initial dose and retitrate as needed; dosage may be given on a twice daily regimen if response is diminished at 24 hours and hypotensive is observed at 2-4 hours following a dose

Benign prostatic hyperplasia: Adults: Initial: 1 mg at bedtime, increasing as needed; most patients require 10 mg day; if no response after 4-6 weeks of 10 mg/day, may increase to 20 mg/day

Dietary Considerations May be taken without regard to meals at the same time each day.

Monitoring Parameters Standing and sitting/supine blood pressure, especially following the initial dose at 2-4 hours following the dose and thereafter at the trough point to ensure adequate control throughout the dosing interval; urinary symptoms

Dosage Forms Excipient information presented when available (limited, particularly for generics); consult specific product labeling.

Capsule: 1 mg, 2 mg, 5 mg, 10 mg

Terbinafine (TER bin a feen)

Medication Safety Issues

Sound-alike/look-alike issues:

Terbinafine may be confused with terbutaline

Lamisil® may be confused with Lamictal®, Lomotil®

International issues:

Lamisil® may be confused with Lemesil® which is a brand name for nimesulide in Greece and Romania

U.S. Brand Names Lamisil AT® [OTC]; Lamisil®

Canadian Brand Names Apo-Terbinafine®; CO Terbinafine; Dom-Terbinafine; Gen-Terbinafine; Lamisil®; Novo-Terbinafine; PMS-Terbinafine

Mexican Brand Names Lamisil

Index Terms Terbinafine Hydrochloride

Pharmacologic Category Antifungal Agent, Oral; Antifungal Agent, Topical

Use Active against most strains of *Trichophyton mentagrophytes*, *Trichophyton rubrum*; may be effective for infections of *Microsporum gypseum* and *M. nanum*, *Trichophyton verrucosum*, *Epidermophyton floccosum*, *Candida albicans*, and *Scopulariopsis brevicaulis*

Oral: Onychomycosis of the toenail or fingernail due to susceptible dermatophytes; treatment of tinea capitis

Topical: Antifungal for the treatment of tinea pedis (athlete's foot), tinea cruris (jock itch), and tinea corporis (ringworm) [OTC/prescription formulations]; tinea versicolor [prescription formulations]

Effect on Mental Status None reported

Effect on Psychiatric Treatment May rarely cause pancytopenia and neutropenia; use caution with clozapine and carbamazepine. May cause GI side effects; concomitant use with SSRIs, carbamazepine, valproic acid, and lithium may produce additive effects. Terbinafine is a potent CYP2D6 inhibitor and may decrease the metabolism of thioridazine and tricyclic antidepressants; combined use with thioridazine should be avoided.

Dosage Summary

Oral granules:

Children <4 years: Dosage not established

Children ≥4 years:

<25 kg: 125 mg once daily for 6 weeks

25-35 kg: 187.5 mg once daily for 6 weeks

>35 kg: 250 mg once daily for 6 weeks

Oral tablet:

Children: Dosage not established

Adults: 250-500 mg daily in 1-2 divided doses

Topical:

Children <12 years: Dosage not established

Children ≥12 years: Apply to affected area once or twice daily

Adults: Apply to affected area once or twice daily

Dosage Forms Excipient information presented when available (limited, particularly for generics); consult specific product labeling.

Cream, topical, as hydrochloride: 1% (12 g, 24 g)

Lamisil AT®: 1% (12 g, 15 g, 24 g, 30 g, 36 g) [contains benzyl alcohol]

Gel, topical:

Lamisil AT®: 1% (6 g, 12 g) [contains benzyl alcohol]

Granules, oral:

Lamisil® 125 mg/packet (42s); 187.5 mg/packet (42s)

Solution, topical, as hydrochloride [spray]:

Lamisil AT®: 1% (30 mL) [contains ethanol]

Tablet, oral: 250 mg

Lamisil®: 250 mg

◆ **Terbinafine Hydrochloride** *see* Terbinafine *on page 1551*

Terbutaline (ter BYOO ta leen)

Medication Safety Issues

Sound-alike/look-alike issues:

Terbutaline may be confused with terbinafine, TOLBUTamide

Canadian Brand Names Bricanyl®

Index Terms Brethaire [DSC]; Bricanyl [DSC]

Pharmacologic Category $Beta_2$-Adrenergic Agonist

Use Bronchodilator in reversible airway obstruction and bronchial asthma

Unlabeled/Investigational Use Tocolytic agent (management of preterm labor)

Effect on Mental Status Restlessness and nervousness are common; may cause dizziness, drowsiness, or insomnia

Effect on Psychiatric Treatment Concurrent use with TCAs or MAO inhibitors may increase toxicity

Dosage Summary

Oral:

Children <12 years (unlabeled use): Initial: 0.05 mg/kg/dose 3 times/day; Maintenance: 0.05-0.15 mg/kg/dose 3-4 times/day (maximum: 5 mg/day)

Children 12-15 years: 2.5 mg every 6 hours 3 times/day (maximum: 7.5 mg/day)

Children >15 years: 2.5-5 mg every 6 hours 3 times/day (maximum: 15 mg/day)

Adults: 2.5-5 mg every 6 hours 3 times/day (maximum: 15 mg/day)

SubQ:

Children <12 years (unlabeled use): 0.005-0.3 mg/kg/dose; may repeat in 15-20 minutes

Children ≥12 years: 0.25 mg/dose; may repeat in 15-30 minutes (maximum: 0.5 mg/4-hour period)

Adults: 0.25 mg/dose; may repeat in 15-30 minutes (maximum: 0.5 mg/4 hour period)

Dosage Forms Excipient information presented when available (limited, particularly for generics); consult specific product labeling. [CAN] = Canadian brand name

Injection, solution, as sulfate: 1 mg/mL (1 mL)

Powder for oral inhalation:

Bricanyl® Turbuhaler [CAN]: 500 mcg/actuation [50 or 200 metered actuations] [not available in U.S.]

Tablet, as sulfate: 2.5 mg, 5 mg

Teriparatide (ter i PAR a tide)

U.S. Brand Names Forteo®
Canadian Brand Names Forteo®
Mexican Brand Names Forteo
Index Terms Parathyroid Hormone (1-34); Recombinant Human Parathyroid Hormone (1-34); rhPTH(1-34)
Pharmacologic Category Parathyroid Hormone Analog
Use Treatment of osteoporosis in postmenopausal women at high risk of fracture; treatment of primary or hypogonadal osteoporosis in men at high risk of fracture
Effect on Mental Status May cause dizziness or depression
Effect on Psychiatric Treatment May cause orthostasis; use caution with psychotropics. May cause GI side effects; use caution with SSRIs.
Restrictions An FDA-approved medication guide must be distributed when dispensing an outpatient prescription (new or refill) where this medication is to be used without direct supervision of a healthcare provider. Medication guides are available at http://www.fda.gov/cder/Offices/ODS/medication_guides.htm.
Dosage Summary
SubQ:
Children: Dosage not established
Adults: 20 mcg once daily
Dosage Forms Excipient information presented when available (limited, particularly for generics); consult specific product labeling.
Injection, solution:
Forteo®: 250 mcg/mL (3 mL) [prefilled syringe, delivers teriparatide 20 mcg/dose]

- **TESPA** *see* Thiotepa *on page 1576*
- **Tessalon®** *see* Benzonatate *on page 180*
- **Testim®** *see* Testosterone *on page 1553*
- **Testopel®** *see* Testosterone *on page 1553*

Testosterone (tes TOS ter one)

Medication Safety Issues
Sound-alike/look-alike issues:
Testosterone may be confused with testolactone
Testoderm® may be confused with Estraderm®

Transdermal patch may contain conducting metal (eg, aluminum); remove patch prior to MRI.
U.S. Brand Names Androderm®; AndroGel®; Delatestryl®; Depo®-Testosterone; First®-Testosterone; First®-Testosterone MC; Striant®; Testim®; Testopel®
Canadian Brand Names Andriol®; Androderm®; AndroGel®; Andropository; Delatestryl®; Depotest® 100; Everone® 200; Virilon® IM
Mexican Brand Names Lowtiyel
Index Terms Testosterone Cypionate; Testosterone Enanthate
Pharmacologic Category Androgen
Use
Injection: Androgen replacement therapy in the treatment of delayed male puberty; male hypogonadism (primary or hypogonadotropic); inoperable metastatic female breast cancer (enanthate only)
Pellet: Androgen replacement therapy in the treatment of delayed male puberty; male hypogonadism (primary or hypogonadotropic)
Topical (buccal system, gel, transdermal system): Male hypogonadism (primary or hypogonadotropic)
Capsule (not available in U.S.): Androgen replacement therapy in the treatment of delayed male puberty; male hypogonadism (primary or hypogonadotropic); replacement therapy in impotence or for male climacteric symptoms due to androgen deficiency
Unlabeled/Investigational Use Androgen deficiency in men with AIDS wasting; postmenopausal women with decreased sexual desire (in combination with estrogen therapy)
Effect on Mental Status May cause anxiety, insomnia, aggressive behavior, or depression
Effect on Psychiatric Treatment May rarely cause neutropenia; use caution with clozapine and carbamazepine

Restrictions C-III

Dosage Summary

Buccal:

Children: Dosage not established

Adults (males): 30 mg every 12 hours

I.M.:

Children: Dosage not established

Adolescents (males): 50-400 mg every 2-4 weeks

Adults: 50-400 mg every 2-4 weeks

SubQ:

Children: Dosage not established

Adolescents (males): 150-450 mg every 3-6 months

Adults (males): 150-450 mg every 3-6 months

Transdermal:

Androderm®:

Children: Dosage not established

Adults (males): Apply 2.5-7.5 mg/day at night time

AndroGel®, Testim®:

Children: Dosage not established

Adults (males): 5-10 g (50-100 mg testosterone) applied once daily in the morning (maximum: 10 g/day)

Dosage Forms Excipient information presented when available (limited, particularly for generics); consult specific product labeling. [CAN] = Canadian brand name

Capsule, gelatin, as undecanoate:

Andriol™ [CAN]: 40 mg (10s) [not available in U.S.]

Gel, topical:

AndroGel®:

1.25 g/actuation (75 g) [1% metered-dose pump; delivers 5 g/4 actuations; provides sixty 1.25 g actuations; contains ethanol 67%; may be chemically synthesized from soy]

2.5 g (30s) [1% unit dose packets; contains ethanol 67%; may be chemically synthesized from soy]

5 g (30s) [1% unit dose packets; contains ethanol; may be chemically synthesized from soy]

Testim®: 5 g (30s) [1% unit-dose tube; contains ethanol 74%; may be chemically synthesized from soy]

Implant, subcutaneous:

Testopel®: 75 mg (10s, 100s)

Injection, in oil, as cypionate: 100 mg/mL (10 mL); 200 mg/mL (1 mL, 10 mL)

Depo®-Testosterone: 100 mg/mL (10 mL); 200 mg/mL (1 mL, 10 mL) [contains benzyl alcohol, benzyl benzoate, and cottonseed oil]

Injection, in oil, as enanthate: 200 mg/mL (5 mL)

Delatestryl®: 200 mg/mL (1 mL, 5 mL) [contains sesame oil]

Kit [for prescription compounding; testosterone 2%]:

First®-Testosterone:

Injection, in oil: Testosterone propionate 100 mg/mL (12 mL) [contains sesame oil and benzyl alcohol]

Ointment: White petrolatum (48 g)

First®-Testosterone MC:

Injection, in oil: Testosterone propionate 100 mg/mL (12 mL) [contains sesame oil and benzyl alcohol]

Cream: Moisturizing cream (48 g)

Mucoadhesive, for buccal application [buccal system]:

Striant®: 30 mg (10s) [may be chemically synthesized from soy]

Transdermal system, topical:

Androderm®: 2.5 mg/day (60s) [contains ethanol]; 5 mg/day (30s) [contains ethanol]

◆ **Testosterone Cypionate** *see* Testosterone *on page 1553*

◆ **Testosterone Enanthate** *see* Testosterone *on page 1553*

◆ **Testred®** *see* MethylTESTOSTERone *on page 1030*

Tetrabenazine (tet ra BEN a zeen)

U.S. Brand Names Xenazine®

Canadian Brand Names Nitoman™

Pharmacologic Category Central Monoamine-Depleting Agent

Use Treatment of chorea associated with Huntington's disease

Canadian labeling: Treatment of hyperkinetic movement disorders, including Huntington's chorea, hemiballismus, senile chorea, Tourette syndrome, and tardive dyskinesia

Restrictions An FDA-approved patient medication guide is available and must be distributed when dispensing an outpatient prescription (new or refill) where this medication is to be used without direct supervision of a healthcare provider.

Pregnancy Risk Factor C

Pregnancy Considerations Adverse events were observed in some animal studies. There are no adequate and well-controlled studies in pregnant women. Avoid use in pregnant women unless the potential benefit justifies the potential risk to the fetus.

Lactation Excretion in breast milk unknown/not recommended

Contraindications

U.S. labeling: Patients who are actively suicidal or with untreated or inadequately treated depression; hepatic impairment; use with or within 14 days of MAO inhibitors; use with or within 20 days of reserpine

Canadian labeling: Hypersensitivity to tetrabenazine or any component of the formulation; history or current episode of clinical depression; use with or within 14 days of MAO inhibitors

Warnings/Precautions **[U.S. Boxed Warning]: May increase risk for depression and suicidal ideation; evaluate immediately if signs and/or symptoms of depression or suicidality are noted. Use with caution in patients with a history of depression; monitor patients closely.** Reduce dose if depression occurs; consider discontinuing if depression/suicidal ideation does not resolve. May induce/exacerbate symptoms of parkinsonism (more common in elderly patients). May cause drowsiness; patients should be warned to use caution when driving or operating machinery, or engaging in other tasks requiring alertness. Due to the possibility of comorbid psychiatric disorders and potential psychiatric adverse effects, patients should be carefully monitored for potential changes in psychiatric status during therapy.

Use has been associated with akathisia; monitor for signs and symptoms of restlessness and agitation. Use has been associated with esophageal dysmotility, dysphagia, and aspiration; use with caution in patients at risk of aspiration pneumonia. Has been shown to prolong the QT interval alone (minimal) and with other drugs with comparable effects on the QT interval (additive). Avoid use in patients with congenital QT prolongation, a history of cardiac arrhythmias, or concomitant drugs known to cause QT prolongation. May cause orthostatic hypotension; monitor patients at risk closely. Has not been studied with concomitant use of neuroleptic drugs (eg, haloperidol, olanzapine); adverse effects may be additive. Use with caution in patients with breast cancer or other prolactin-dependent tumors; elevates prolactin levels. Patients should be tested for the CYP2D6 gene prior to initiating doses >50 mg/day; maximum dosage should not exceed 50 mg/day in poor metabolizers. Safety and efficacy have not been established in children. Should not be used to treat levodopa-induced dyskinesia.

Adverse Reactions Note: Many adverse effects are dose-related and may resolve at lower dosages. Adverse effects reported for adults with chorea associated with Huntington's disease.

>10%:

Central nervous system: Extrapyramidal symptoms (15% to 33%), sedation (31%), somnolence (31%), fatigue (22%), insomnia (22%), akathisia (19%), depression (19%), anxiety (15%)

Gastrointestinal: Nausea (13%)

Neuromuscular & skeletal: Falls (15%)

Respiratory: Upper respiratory tract infection (11%)

1% to 10%:

Central nervous system: Parkinsonism (3% to 10%), irritability (9%), dizziness (4%), headache (4%), obsessive reaction (4%)

Dermatologic: Bruising (6%)

Gastrointestinal: Dysphagia (4% to 10%), vomiting (6%), appetite decreased (4%), diarrhea (2%)

Genitourinary: Dysuria (4%)

Neuromuscular & skeletal: Balance difficulty (9%), bradykinesia (9%), dysarthria (4%), gait disturbance (4%)

Respiratory: Bronchitis (4%), dyspnea (4%)

<1% (Limited to important or life-threatening): Aspiration pneumonia, hyperprolactinemia, orthostatic hypotension, neuroleptic malignant syndrome, QT_c prolongation, restlessness, suicidal ideation, suicide, syncope, transaminases increased

Drug Interactions

Alcohol (Ethyl): CNS Depressants may enhance the CNS depressant effect of Alcohol (Ethyl). *Risk C: Monitor therapy*

Alfuzosin: May enhance the QTc-prolonging effect of QTc-Prolonging Agents. *Risk C: Monitor therapy*

Antipsychotics: Tetrabenazine may enhance the adverse/toxic effect of Antipsychotics. *Risk C: Monitor therapy*

Ciprofloxacin: May enhance the QTc-prolonging effect of QTc-Prolonging Agents. *Risk C: Monitor therapy*

CNS Depressants: May enhance the adverse/toxic effect of other CNS Depressants. *Risk C: Monitor therapy*

CYP2D6 Inhibitors (Moderate): May decrease the metabolism of CYP2D6 Substrates. *Risk C: Monitor therapy*

CYP2D6 Inhibitors (Strong): May increase the serum concentration of Tetrabenazine. Specifically, concentrations of the active alpha- and beta-dihydrotetrabenazine metabolites may be increased. Management: Tetrabenazine dose should be reduced by 50% when starting a strong CYP2D6 inhibitor. Maximum tetrabenazine dose is 50mg/day when used with a strong CYP2D6 inhibitor. *Risk D: Consider therapy modification*

Darunavir: May increase the serum concentration of CYP2D6 Substrates. *Risk C: Monitor therapy*

Gadobutrol: May enhance the QTc-prolonging effect of QTc-Prolonging Agents. *Risk D: Consider therapy modification*

MAO Inhibitors: Tetrabenazine may enhance the adverse/toxic effect of MAO Inhibitors. *Risk X: Avoid combination*

Nilotinib: May enhance the QTc-prolonging effect of QTc-Prolonging Agents. *Risk X: Avoid combination*

QTc-Prolonging Agents: May enhance the QTc-prolonging effect of Tetrabenazine. *Risk X: Avoid combination*

Reserpine: May enhance the adverse/toxic effect of Tetrabenazine. *Risk X: Avoid combination*

Ethanol/Nutrition/Herb Interactions

Ethanol: Avoid ethanol (may increase CNS depression).

Herb/Nutraceutical: Avoid valerian, St John's wort, kava kava, gotu kola (may increase CNS depression).

Stability Store at 25°C (77°F); excursions permitted to 15°C to 30°C (59°F to 86°F).

Mechanism of Action Within basal ganglia, interferes with and depletes monoamine neurotransmitters (including dopamine, serotonin, and norepinephrine) in presynaptic vesicles (likely through actions on vesicle monoamine transporter). Tetrabenazine inhibits presynaptic dopamine release and also blocks CNS dopamine receptors. The effects resemble reserpine but with less peripheral activity and a shorter duration of action. Treatment results in symptomatic improvement of hyperkinetic movement disorders, including Huntington's chorea, hemiballismus, senile chorea, Tic and Hille's de la Tourette syndrome, and tardive dyskinesia.

Pharmacodynamics/Kinetics

Duration of action: 16-24 hours; chorea may recur within 12-18 hours after discontinuation

Protein binding: 82% to 85%; Metabolites: 59% to 68%

Metabolism: Hepatic (rapid and extensive), to alpha and beta hydroxytetrabenazine (HTBZ) via CYP2D6 (primary active moiety)

Bioavailability: Low and erratic (due to extensive first-pass effects); unaffected by food

Half-life elimination: Alpha-HTBZ: 4-8 hours; Beta-HTBZ: 2-4 hours (increased with hepatic impairment)

Time to peak, plasma: Within 1-1.5 hours

Excretion: Urine (75% as metabolites, <10% as alpha and beta HTBZ); feces (7% to 16%)

Dosage Oral: Dose should be individualized; titrate slowly

Chorea associated with Huntington's disease: Adults:

Initial: 12.5 mg once daily, may increase to 12.5 mg twice daily after 1 week

Maintenance: May be increased by 12.5 mg/day at weekly intervals; doses >37.5 mg/day should be divided into 3 doses (maximum single dose 25 mg)

Patients requiring doses >50 mg/day: Genotype for CYP2D6:

Extensive/intermediate metabolizers: Maximum: 100 mg/day; 37.5 mg/dose

Poor metabolizers: Maximum: 50 mg/day; 25 mg/dose

Concomitant use with strong CYP2D6 inhibitors (eg, fluoxetine, paroxetine, quinidine): Dose of tetrabenazine should be reduced by 50% in patients receiving strong CYP2D6 inhibitors, follow dosing for poor CYP2D6

metabolizers. Use caution when adding a CYP2D6 inhibitor to patients already taking tetrabenazine.

Note: If treatment is interrupted for >5 days, retitration is recommended. If treatment is interrupted for <5 days resume at previous maintenance dose.

Canadian labeling: Hyperkinetic movement disorders:

Adults: Initial: 12.5 mg twice daily (may be given 3 times/day); may be increased by 12.5 mg/day every 3-5 days; should be titrated slowly to maximal tolerated and effective dose (dose is individualized)

Usual maximum tolerated dosage: 25 mg 3 times/day; maximum recommended dose: 200 mg/day

Note: If there is no improvement at the maximum tolerated dose after 7 days, improvement is unlikely; discontinuation should be considered.

Elderly and/or debilitated patients: Consider initiation at lower doses; must be titrated slowly to individualize dosage

Dosage adjustment for toxicity: For toxicity/adverse reaction, including akathisia, restlessness, parkinsonism, insomnia, depression, suicidality, anxiety, sedation (intolerable): Suspend upward dosage titration and reduce dose; consider discontinuing if adverse reaction does not resolve (may be discontinued without tapering.

Dosage adjustment in hepatic impairment: Use is contraindicated

Dietary Considerations May be taken with or without food.

Administration May administer with or without food.

Monitoring Parameters Improvement in movement disorder; signs and/or symptoms of depression or suicidal ideation; signs and/or symptoms of NMS; orthostatic blood pressure. Due to the possibility of comorbid psychiatric disorders, and potential psychiatric adverse effects, patients should be carefully monitored for potential changes in psychiatric status during therapy. CYP2D6 genotyping for evaluation of metabolizer status.

Dosage Forms Excipient information presented when available (limited, particularly for generics); consult specific product labeling. [CAN] = Canadian product

Tablet:

Nitoman™ [CAN]: 25 mg [not available in the U.S.]

Xenazine®: 12.5 mg, 25 mg

Tetracaine (TET ra kane)

U.S. Brand Names Pontocaine®; Pontocaine® Niphanoid®

Canadian Brand Names Ametop™; Pontocaine®

Index Terms Amethocaine Hydrochloride; Tetracaine Hydrochloride

Pharmacologic Category Local Anesthetic

Use Spinal anesthesia; local anesthesia in the eye for various diagnostic and examination purposes; topically applied to nose and throat for various diagnostic procedures

Effect on Mental Status May cause dizziness, drowsiness, or nervousness

Effect on Psychiatric Treatment None reported

Dosage Summary

Ophthalmic:

Children: Dosage not established

Adults: Instill 1-2 drops into eye(s)

Subarachnoid injection:

Children: Dosage not established

Adults: 2-15 mg (maximum: 20 mg)

Topical:

Children: Dosage not established

Adults: 0.25 % or 0.5% by direct application or nebulization (maximum: 20 mg total)

Dosage Forms Excipient information presented when available (limited, particularly for generics); consult specific product labeling.

Injection, powder for reconstitution, as hydrochloride [preservative free]:

Pontocaine® Niphanoid®: 20 mg

Injection, solution, as hydrochloride [preservative free]: 1% [10 mg/mL] (2 mL)

Pontocaine®): 1% [10 mg/mL] (2 mL) [contains sodium bisulfite]

Solution, ophthalmic, as hydrochloride: 0.5% [5 mg/mL] (2 mL, 15 mL)

Solution, topical, as hydrochloride (Pontocaine®): 2% [20 mg/mL] (30 mL, 118 mL) [for rhinolaryngology]

◆ **Tetracaine Hydrochloride** *see* Tetracaine *on page 1557*

◆ **Tetracosactide** *see* Cosyntropin *on page 402*

Tetracycline (tet ra SYE kleen)

Medication Safety Issues
Sound-alike/look-alike issues:
Tetracycline may be confused with tetradecyl sulfate
Achromycin may be confused with actinomycin, Adriamycin PFS®

Canadian Brand Names Apo-Tetra®; Nu-Tetra

Mexican Brand Names Acromicina; Ambotetra; Erifor; Quimocyclar; Tetrex

Index Terms Achromycin; TCN; Tetracycline Hydrochloride

Pharmacologic Category Antibiotic, Tetracycline Derivative

Use Treatment of susceptible bacterial infections of both gram-positive and gram-negative organisms; also infections due to *Mycoplasma*, *Chlamydia*, and *Rickettsia*; indicated for acne, exacerbations of chronic bronchitis, and treatment of gonorrhea and syphilis in patients who are allergic to penicillin; as part of a multidrug regimen for *H. pylori* eradication to reduce the risk of duodenal ulcer recurrence

Effect on Mental Status None reported

Effect on Psychiatric Treatment Tetracycline may decrease lithium clearance resulting in an increase in serum lithium levels and potential lithium toxicity although the clinical significance is likely minimal; monitor serum lithium levels

Dosage Summary

Oral:

Children ≤8 years: Dosage not established
Children >8 years: 25-50 mg/kg/day divided every 6 hours
Adults: 250-500 mg 2-4 times/day

Dosage Forms Excipient information presented when available (limited, particularly for generics); consult specific product labeling.
Capsule, as hydrochloride: 250 mg, 500 mg

- ◆ **Tetracycline Hydrochloride** *see* Tetracycline *on page 1558*
- ◆ **Tetracycline, Metronidazole, and Bismuth Subcitrate Potassium** *see* Bismuth, Metronidazole, and Tetracycline *on page 190*
- ◆ **Tetracycline, Metronidazole, and Bismuth Subsalicylate** *see* Bismuth, Metronidazole, and Tetracycline *on page 190*
- ◆ **Tetrahydroaminoacrine** *see* Tacrine *on page 1531*
- ◆ **Tetrahydrocannabinol** *see* Dronabinol *on page 512*

Tetrahydrocannabinol and Cannabidiol
(TET ra hye droe can NAB e nol & can nab e DYE ol)

Canadian Brand Names Sativex®

Index Terms Cannabidiol and Tetrahydrocannabinol; Delta-9-Tetrahydrocannabinol and Cannabinol; GW-1000-02; THC and CBD

Pharmacologic Category Analgesic, Miscellaneous

Generic Available No

Use Adjunctive treatment of neuropathic pain in multiple sclerosis; adjunctive treatment of moderate-to-severe pain in advanced cancer

Effect on Mental Status Dizziness and fatigue are common; may cause mood changes (euphoria, depression), memory impairment, disorientation, dissociation, and impulsivity.

Effect on Psychiatric Treatment Contraindicated in patients with a history of psychotic disorders.

Restrictions Not available in U.S.; CDSA-II

Pregnancy Considerations Cannabinoids have been associated with reproductive toxicity. Animal studies indicate possible effects on fetal development and spermatogenesis. Use in pregnancy is contraindicated. Women of childbearing potential and males who are capable of causing pregnancy should use a reliable form of contraception for the duration of treatment and for 3 months following discontinuation.

Lactation Enters breast milk/contraindicated

Contraindications Hypersensitivity to cannabinoids or any component of the formulation; serious cardiovascular disease (including arrhythmias, severe heart failure, poorly controlled hypertension, and ischemic heart disease); history of psychotic disorders (including schizophrenia); women of childbearing potential who are not using a reliable form of contraception; males intending to start a family; children <18 years of age; pregnancy; breast-feeding

Warnings/Precautions [Canadian Boxed Warnings]: May cause physical and psychological dependence in long-term use; avoid use in patients with a history or risk of drug or alcohol dependency. Prescriptions should

be written for the minimal amount needed between clinic visits. Use may be associated with changes in mood, cognitive performance, memory, impulsivity, and coordination, as well as an altered perception of reality, particularly with respect to an awareness/sensation of time. May impair physical or mental abilities; patients must be cautioned about performing tasks which require mental alertness (eg, operating machinery or driving). **[Canadian Boxed Warnings]: Use with caution in patients with a history of seizures. Concurrent use of ethanol or other CNS active drugs may be additive.** Dosage must be carefully titrated and monitored, with downward adjustment in patients with unacceptable adverse events. Drug discontinuation is recommended, and a period of close observation should be instituted, in patients experiencing a psychotic reaction.

[Canadian Boxed Warning]: May be associated with adverse cardiovascular effects, including tachycardia and alterations in blood pressure (including orthostatic changes).

Use with caution in severe hepatic and renal dysfunction. Use with caution in elderly patients. May be irritating to the buccal mucosa; avoid administration in an area of soreness or inflammation. Use in cancer patients associated with increased risk of urinary retention and infection. Formulation contains ethanol; use may be harmful in patients with alcoholism. Due to accumulation in body fat, cannabinoids may be detectable in the urine and serum for several weeks following drug discontinuation.

Adverse Reactions

>10%:

Central nervous system: Dizziness (up to 32%), somnolence (9% to 15%), fatigue (14%)

Gastrointestinal: Oral application site events (≤20%), nausea (12%)

1% to 10%:

Cardiovascular: Hypotension (2% to 5%), hypertension (2%), flushing (1%), syncope (1%),

Central nervous system: Headache (3%), confusion (1% to 7%), disorientation (5%), impaired balance (3% to 5%), vertigo (4% to 5%), attention disturbance (3% to 5%), memory impairment (1%), dissociation (3%), euphoria (3%), hallucination (up to 3%), insomnia (3%), panic attack (3%), anxiety (2%), lethargy (2%), malaise (2%), amnesia (2%), depression (1% to 2%), paranoia (1%)

Endocrine & metabolic: Thirst (1%)

Gastrointestinal: Xerostomia (8%), diarrhea (5% to 7%), oral discomfort/pain (up to 8%), vomiting (4% to 8%), constipation (4% to 5%), abnormal taste (4%), tooth discoloration (4%), dysgeusia (3% to 5%), oral candidiasis (3%), anorexia (2%), appetite increased (2%), abdominal pain (1%), appetite decreased (1%)

Genitourinary: Urinary retention (5%)

Hepatic: ALT/AST increased (2.6%)

Neuromuscular & skeletal: Weakness (5% to 6%), muscle spasticity (3%), dysarthria (2%), fall (2%), paresthesia (2%)

Ocular: Vision blurred (2%)

Renal: Hematuria (3%)

Respiratory: Pharyngitis (2%), cough (1%), respiratory tract infection (1%), throat irritation (1%)

Miscellaneous: Drunken feeling (5%), sensation of heaviness (1%)

<1% and/or frequency not defined: Auditory hallucination, delusions, suicidal ideation, tachycardia, urinary infection

Metabolism/Transport Effects **Substrate** (minor) of CYP2C9, 2C19, 2D6, 3A4; **Inhibits** (weak) CYP1A2, 2C19, 2D6, 3A4

Drug Interactions

Alcohol (Ethyl): CNS Depressants may enhance the CNS depressant effect of Alcohol (Ethyl). *Risk C: Monitor therapy*

Anticholinergic Agents: May enhance the tachycardic effect of Cannabinoids. *Risk C: Monitor therapy*

CNS Depressants: May enhance the adverse/toxic effect of other CNS Depressants. *Risk C: Monitor therapy*

Cocaine: May enhance the tachycardic effect of Cannabinoids. *Risk C: Monitor therapy*

Sympathomimetics: Cannabinoids may enhance the tachycardic effect of Sympathomimetics. *Risk C: Monitor therapy*

Ethanol/Nutrition/Herb Interactions

Ethanol: Avoid ethanol (may increase CNS depression).

Food: Administration with high-lipid meals may increase absorption.

Stability Prior to first use, store unopened at 2°C to 8°C (36°F to 46°F); do not freeze. After opening, may be stored at room temperature of 15°C to 25°C (59°F to 77°F) for up to 28 days. Avoid heat and direct sunlight.

Mechanism of Action Stimulates cannabinoid receptors CB1 and CB2 in the CNS and dorsal root ganglia as well as other sites in the body. Cannabinoid receptors in the pain pathways of the brain and spinal cord mediate cannabinoid-induced analgesia. Peripheral CB2 receptors modulate immune function through cytokine release.

Pharmacodynamics/Kinetics

Absorption: Rapidly absorbed from the buccal mucosa

Distribution: Widely distributed, particularly to fatty tissues

Protein binding: Extensive

Metabolism: Hepatic, via CYP isoenzymes (2C9, 2C19, 2D6 and 3A4) to THC metabolite 11-hydroxy-tetrahydrocannabinol (11-OH-THC, psycho-active) and CBD metabolite 7-hydroxy-cannabidiol.

Half-life elimination: Initial: 1-2 hours; terminal half-life may require 24-36 hours (or longer) due to redistribution from fatty tissue

Time to peak, plasma: 2-4 hours

Excretion: As metabolites, urine and feces

Dosage Buccal spray: Adults: Neuropathic pain (MS), cancer pain: Initial: One spray every 4 hours to a maximum of 4 sprays on first day

Titration and individualization: Dosage is self-titrated by the patient. In the treatment of MS, the mean daily dosage after titration in clinical trials was 5 sprays per day. The usual maximum dose is 12 sprays per day although some patients may require and tolerate a higher number of sprays per day. In the treatment of cancer pain, the mean daily dosage after titration was 8 sprays per day. Dosage should be adjusted as necessary, based on effect and tolerance. Sprays should be evenly distributed over the course of the day during initial titration. If adverse reactions, including intoxication-type symptoms, are noted the dosage should be suspended until resolution of the symptoms; a dosage reduction or extension of the interval between doses may be used to avoid a recurrence of symptoms. Retitration may be required in the event of adverse reactions and/or worsening of symptoms.

Elderly: Refer to adult dosing. Use with caution and monitor closely.

Dosage adjustment in renal impairment: Use with caution; has not been studied in patients with significant renal dysfunction.

Dosage adjustment in hepatic impairment: Use with caution; has not been studied in patients with significant hepatic dysfunction.

Administration Note: For buccal use only; spray should be directed below the tongue or on the inside of the cheeks (the site should be varied); avoid direction to the pharynx.

Shake vial before use and remove protective cap; replace protective cap following use. Do not apply spray to sore or inflamed mucosa.

Priming: Vial should be held in an upright position and primed prior to the initial use by depression of the actuator 2-3 times until a fine spray appears. Priming should not be required for subsequent uses. Do not spray near an open flame.

Normal use: Hold vial in upright position and spray into mouth; spray should be directed below the tongue or on the inside of the cheeks, avoiding direction to the pharynx. The site should be varied.

Monitoring Parameters Mental status, response to pain; mucosal integrity and inflammation

Dosage Forms Excipient information presented when available (limited, particularly for generics); consult specific product labeling. [CAN] = Canadian brand name

Solution, buccal [spray]:

Sativex® [CAN]: Delta-9 tetrahydrocannabinol 27 mg/mL and cannabidiol 25 mg/mL (5.5 mL) [delivers 100 microliters/spray; 51 metered sprays; contains ethanol 50%, peppermint oil, and propylene glycol] [not available in U.S.]

Tetrahydrozoline (tet ra hye DROZ a leen)

Medication Safety Issues

Sound-alike/look-alike issues:

Visine® may be confused with Visken®

U.S. Brand Names Eye-Sine™ [OTC] [DSC]; Geneye [OTC]; Murine® Tears Plus [OTC]; Opti-Clear [OTC]; Optigene® 3 [OTC] [DSC]; Tyzine®; Tyzine® Pediatric; Visine® Advanced Relief [OTC]; Visine® Original [OTC]

Index Terms Tetrahydrozoline Hydrochloride; Tetryzoline

Pharmacologic Category Adrenergic Agonist Agent; Imidazoline Derivative; Ophthalmic Agent, Vasoconstrictor

Use Symptomatic relief of nasal congestion and conjunctival congestion

Effect on Mental Status None reported

Effect on Psychiatric Treatment MAO inhibitors can cause an exaggerated adrenergic response if taken concurrently or within 21 days of discontinuing MAO inhibitor; beta-blockers can cause hypertensive episodes and increased risk of intracranial hemorrhage

Dosage Summary

Intranasal:

Children <2 years: Dosage not established

Children 2-6 years: Instill 2-3 drops (0.05%) every 4-6 hours as needed (maximum: every 3 hours)

Children >6 years: Instill 2-4 drops (0.1%) **or** 3-4 sprays (0.1%) every 3-4 hours as needed (maximum: every 3 hours)

Adults: Instill 2-4 drops (0.1%) **or** 3-4 sprays (0.1%) every 3-4 hours as needed (maximum: every 3 hours)

Ophthalmic:

Children: Dosage not established

Adults: Instill 1-2 drops in each eye 2-4 times/day

Dosage Forms Excipient information presented when available (limited, particularly for generics); consult specific product labeling. [DSC] = Discontinued product

Solution, intranasal, as hydrochloride [drops]:

Tyzine®: 0.1% (30 mL) [contains benzalkonium chloride]

Tyzine® Pediatric: 0.05% (15 mL) [contains benzalkonium chloride]

Solution, intranasal, as hydrochloride [spray]:

Tyzine®: 0.1% (15 mL) [contains benzalkonium chloride]

Solution, ophthalmic, as hydrochloride: 0.05% (15 mL)

Eye-Sine™ [DSC], Geneye, Optigene® 3 [DSC]: 0.05% (15 mL) [may contain benzalkonium chloride]

Murine® Tears Plus: 0.05% (15 mL) [contains benzalkonium chloride]

Opti-Clear: 0.05% (15 mL)

Visine® Advanced Relief: 0.05% (30 mL) [contains benzalkonium chloride and polyethylene glycol]

Visine® Original: 0.05% (15 mL, 30 mL) [contains benzalkonium chloride; 15 mL size also available with dropper]

- ◆ **Tetrahydrozoline Hydrochloride** *see* Tetrahydrozoline *on page 1560*
- ◆ **2,2,2-tetramine** *see* Trientine *on page 1623*
- ◆ **Tetra Tannate Pediatric** *see* Chlorpheniramine, Ephedrine, Phenylephrine, and Carbetapentane *on page 326*
- ◆ **Tetryzoline** *see* Tetrahydrozoline *on page 1560*
- ◆ **Teveten®** *see* Eprosartan *on page 547*
- ◆ **Teveten® HCT** *see* Eprosartan and Hydrochlorothiazide *on page 549*
- ◆ **Tev-Tropin®** *see* Somatropin *on page 1499*
- ◆ **Texacort®** *see* Hydrocortisone *on page 785*
- ◆ **TG** *see* Thioguanine *on page 1569*
- ◆ **6-TG (error-prone abbreviation)** *see* Thioguanine *on page 1569*
- ◆ **THA** *see* Tacrine *on page 1531*

Thalidomide (tha LI doe mide)

Medication Safety Issues

Sound-alike/look-alike issues:

Thalidomide may be confused with flutamide

High alert medication: The Institute for Safe Medication Practices (ISMP) includes this medication among its list of drugs which have a heightened risk of causing significant patient harm when used in error.

International issues:

Thalomid® may be confused with Thilomide® which is a brand name for lodoxamide in Greece and Turkey

U.S. Brand Names Thalomid®

Canadian Brand Names Thalomid®

Index Terms NSC-66847

Pharmacologic Category Angiogenesis Inhibitor; Immunomodulator, Systemic; Tumor Necrosis Factor (TNF) Blocking Agent

Use Treatment of multiple myeloma; treatment and maintenance of cutaneous manifestations of erythema nodosum leprosum (ENL)

Unlabeled/Investigational Use Treatment of Crohn's disease; graft-versus-host reactions after bone marrow transplantation; AIDS-related aphthous stomatitis; Behçet's syndrome; Waldenström's macroglobulinemia; Langerhans cell histiocytosis; may be effective in rheumatoid arthritis, discoid lupus erythematosus, and erythema multiforme

Effect on Mental Status Sedation is common; may cause dizziness, nervousness, insomnia, agitation, abnormal thinking, amnesia, anxiety, confusion, depression, euphoria, and psychosis

Effect on Psychiatric Treatment May cause leukopenia; use caution with clozapine and carbamazepine; concurrent use with other psychotropics may produce additive sedation

Restrictions Thalidomide is approved for marketing only under a special distribution program. This program, called the "System for Thalidomide Education and Prescribing Safety" (STEPS® 1-888-423-5436), has been approved by the FDA. Prescribers and pharmacists must be registered with the program. No more than a 4-week supply should be dispensed. Blister packs should be dispensed intact (do not repackage capsules). Prescriptions must be filled within 7 days. Subsequent prescriptions may be filled only if fewer than 7 days of therapy remain on the previous prescription. A new prescription is required for further dispensing (a telephone prescription may not be accepted.)

Dosage Summary

Oral:

Children: Dosage not established

Adults:

Cutaneous ENL: Initial: 100-300 mg once daily at bedtime (400 mg/day in severe cases); Maintenance: Continue initial dose until active reaction subsides then taper in 50 mg decrements every 2-4 weeks

Multiple myeloma: 200 mg once daily

Dosage Forms Excipient information presented when available (limited, particularly for generics); consult specific product labeling.

Capsule:

Thalomid®: 50 mg, 100 mg, 200 mg

- ◆ **Thalitone®** *see* Chlorthalidone *on page 340*
- ◆ **Thalomid®** *see* Thalidomide *on page 1561*
- ◆ **THC** *see* Dronabinol *on page 512*
- ◆ **THC and CBD** *see* Tetrahydrocannabinol and Cannabidiol *on page 1558*
- ◆ **Theo-24®** *see* Theophylline *on page 1562*
- ◆ **TheoCap™** *see* Theophylline *on page 1562*
- ◆ **Theochron™** *see* Theophylline *on page 1562*

Theophylline (thee OFF i lin)

Medication Safety Issues

Sound-alike/look-alike issues:

Theolair™ may be confused with Thiola®, Thyrolar®

Related Information

Anticholinergic Effects of Common Psychotropics *on page 1758*

U.S. Brand Names Elixophyllin®; Theo-24®; TheoCap™; Theochron™; Uniphyl®

Canadian Brand Names Apo-Theo LA®; Novo-Theophyl SR; PMS-Theophylline; Pulmophylline; ratio-Theo-Bronc; Theochron® SR; Theolair™; Uniphyl® SRT

Mexican Brand Names Pharmafil

Index Terms Theophylline Anhydrous

Pharmacologic Category Theophylline Derivative

Generic Available Yes: Extended release capsule and tablet, infusion

Use Treatment of symptoms and reversible airway obstruction due to chronic asthma, chronic bronchitis, or COPD

Effect on Mental Status May cause nervousness and restlessness; may rarely cause insomnia and irritability

Effect on Psychiatric Treatment Barbiturates and carbamazepine may decrease serum levels while disulfiram, propranolol, and fluvoxamine may increase theophylline levels

Pregnancy Risk Factor C

Pregnancy Considerations Theophylline crosses the placenta; adverse effects may be seen in the newborn. Theophylline metabolism may change during pregnancy; monitor serum levels.

Lactation Enters breast milk/compatible (AAP rates "compatible")

Contraindications Hypersensitivity to theophylline or any component of the formulation; premixed injection may contain corn-derived dextrose and its use is contraindicated in patients with allergy to corn-related products

Warnings/Precautions If a patient develops signs and symptoms of theophylline toxicity (eg, persistent, repetitive vomiting), a serum theophylline level should be measured and subsequent doses held. Due to potential saturation of theophylline clearance at serum levels in or (in some patients) less than the therapeutic range, dosage adjustment should be made in small increments (maximum: 25%). Due to wider interpatient variability, theophylline serum level measurements must be used to optimize therapy and prevent serious toxicity. Use with caution in patients with peptic ulcer, hyperthyroidism, seizure disorders, and patients with tachyarrhythmias (eg, sinus tachycardia, atrial fibrillation).

Adverse Reactions

Adverse reactions/theophylline serum level: (Adverse effects do not necessarily occur according to serum levels. Arrhythmia and seizure can occur without seeing the other adverse effects).

15-25 mcg/mL: GI upset, diarrhea, nausea/vomiting, abdominal pain, nervousness, headache, insomnia, agitation, dizziness, muscle cramp, tremor

25-35 mcg/mL: Tachycardia, occasional PVC

>35 mcg/mL: Ventricular tachycardia, frequent PVC, seizure

Uncommon at serum theophylline concentrations ≤20 mcg/mL:

1% to 10%:

Cardiovascular: Tachycardia

Central nervous system: Nervousness, restlessness

Gastrointestinal: Nausea, vomiting

<1% (Limited to important or life-threatening): Insomnia, irritability, seizure, tremor

Metabolism/Transport Effects **Substrate** of CYP1A2 (major), 2C9 (minor), 2D6 (minor), 2E1 (major), 3A4 (major); **Inhibits** CYP1A2 (weak)

Drug Interactions

Adenosine: Theophylline Derivatives may diminish the therapeutic effect of Adenosine. *Risk D: Consider therapy modification*

Allopurinol: May increase the serum concentration of Theophylline Derivatives. *Risk C: Monitor therapy*

Aminoglutethimide: May increase the metabolism of Theophylline Derivatives. *Risk C: Monitor therapy*

Barbiturates: May increase the metabolism of Theophylline Derivatives. *Risk C: Monitor therapy*

Benzodiazepines: Theophylline Derivatives may diminish the therapeutic effect of Benzodiazepines. *Risk D: Consider therapy modification*

Beta-Blockers (Beta1 Selective): May diminish the bronchodilatory effect of Theophylline Derivatives. This is true at higher beta-blockers doses where cardioselectivity is lost. *Risk C: Monitor therapy*

Beta-Blockers (Nonselective): May diminish the bronchodilatory effect of Theophylline Derivatives. *Risk D: Consider therapy modification*

Cannabinoids: May enhance the tachycardic effect of Sympathomimetics. *Risk C: Monitor therapy*

CarBAMazepine: May increase the metabolism of Theophylline Derivatives. *Risk C: Monitor therapy*

Cimetidine: May decrease the metabolism of Theophylline Derivatives. *Risk D: Consider therapy modification*

CYP1A2 Inducers (Strong): May increase the metabolism of CYP1A2 Substrates. *Risk C: Monitor therapy*

CYP1A2 Inhibitors (Moderate): May decrease the metabolism of CYP1A2 Substrates. *Risk C: Monitor therapy*

CYP1A2 Inhibitors (Strong): May decrease the metabolism of CYP1A2 Substrates. *Risk D: Consider therapy modification*

CYP2E1 Inhibitors (Moderate): May decrease the metabolism of CYP2E1 Substrates. *Risk C: Monitor therapy*

CYP3A4 Inducers (Strong): May increase the metabolism of CYP3A4 Substrates. *Risk C: Monitor therapy*

CYP3A4 Inhibitors (Moderate): May decrease the metabolism of CYP3A4 Substrates. *Risk C: Monitor therapy*

CYP3A4 Inhibitors (Strong): May decrease the metabolism of CYP3A4 Substrates. *Risk D: Consider therapy modification*

Dasatinib: May increase the serum concentration of CYP3A4 Substrates. *Risk C: Monitor therapy*

Deferasirox: May decrease the serum concentration of CYP3A4 Substrates. *Risk C: Monitor therapy*

Disulfiram: May increase the serum concentration of Theophylline Derivatives. *Risk C: Monitor therapy*

Fluvoxamine: May decrease the metabolism of Theophylline Derivatives. *Risk D: Consider therapy modification*

Herbs (CYP3A4 Inducers): May increase the metabolism of CYP3A4 Substrates. *Risk C: Monitor therapy*

Interferons: May decrease the metabolism of Theophylline Derivatives. *Risk C: Monitor therapy*

Isoniazid: May decrease the metabolism of Theophylline Derivatives. *Risk D: Consider therapy modification*

Lithium: Theophylline Derivatives may increase the excretion of Lithium. *Risk C: Monitor therapy*

Macrolide Antibiotics: May decrease the metabolism of Theophylline Derivatives. **Exceptions:** Azithromycin; Dirithromycin [Off Market]; Spiramycin; Telithromycin. *Risk D: Consider therapy modification*

Mexiletine: May decrease the metabolism of Theophylline Derivatives. *Risk D: Consider therapy modification*

Moricizine: May increase the metabolism of Theophylline Derivatives. *Risk C: Monitor therapy*

Pentoxifylline: May increase the serum concentration of Theophylline Derivatives. *Risk C: Monitor therapy*

Phenytoin: May increase the metabolism of Theophylline Derivatives. Theophylline Derivatives may decrease the serum concentration of Phenytoin. *Risk C: Monitor therapy*

Protease Inhibitors: May decrease the serum concentration of Theophylline Derivatives. **Exceptions:** Amprenavir; Fosamprenavir. *Risk C: Monitor therapy*

Quinolone Antibiotics: May decrease the metabolism of Theophylline Derivatives. Ciprofloxacin and enoxacin are of greatest concern. Theophylline/quinolone therapy might augment the seizure-producing potential of each of the individual agents. **Exceptions:** Gatifloxacin; Gemifloxacin; Levofloxacin; Lomefloxacin; Moxifloxacin; Nalidixic Acid; Sparfloxacin; Trovafloxacin. *Risk D: Consider therapy modification*

Regadenoson: Theophylline may diminish the vasodilatory effect of Regadenoson. *Risk D: Consider therapy modification*

Sympathomimetics: May enhance the adverse/toxic effect of other Sympathomimetics. *Risk C: Monitor therapy*

Tacrine: May decrease the metabolism of Theophylline Derivatives. *Risk C: Monitor therapy*

Thiabendazole: May decrease the metabolism of Theophylline Derivatives. *Risk D: Consider therapy modification*

Thyroid Products: May increase the metabolism of Theophylline Derivatives. *Risk C: Monitor therapy*

Ticlopidine: May decrease the metabolism of Theophylline Derivatives. *Risk C: Monitor therapy*

Zafirlukast: Theophylline Derivatives may decrease the serum concentration of Zafirlukast. *Risk C: Monitor therapy*

Zileuton: May increase the serum concentration of Theophylline. *Risk D: Consider therapy modification*

Ethanol/Nutrition/Herb Interactions Food: Food does not appreciably affect the absorption of liquid, fast-release products, and most sustained release products; however, food may induce a sudden release (dose-dumping) of once-daily sustained release products resulting in an increase in serum drug levels and potential toxicity. Avoid excessive amounts of caffeine. Avoid extremes of dietary protein and carbohydrate intake. Changes in diet may affect the elimination of theophylline; charbroiled foods may increase elimination, reducing half-life by 50%.

Mechanism of Action Causes bronchodilatation, diuresis, CNS and cardiac stimulation, and gastric acid secretion by blocking phosphodiesterase which increases tissue concentrations of cyclic adenine monophosphate (cAMP) which in turn promotes catecholamine stimulation of lipolysis, glycogenolysis, and gluconeogenesis and induces release of epinephrine from adrenal medulla cells

Pharmacodynamics/Kinetics

Absorption: Oral: Dosage form dependent

Distribution: 0.45 L/kg based on ideal body weight

Metabolism: Children >1 year and Adults: Hepatic; involves CYP1A2, 2E1 and 3A4; forms active metabolites (caffeine and 3-methylxanthine)
Half-life elimination: Highly variable and dependent upon age, liver function, cardiac function, lung disease, and smoking history
Time to peak, serum:
Oral: Liquid: 1 hour; Tablet, enteric-coated: 5 hours; Tablet, uncoated: 2 hours
I.V.: Within 30 minutes
Excretion: Urine
Neonates: 50% unchanged
Children >3 months and Adults: 10% unchanged

Dosage Use ideal body weight for obese patients
I.V.: Initial: Maintenance infusion rates:
Children:
6 weeks to 6 months: 0.5 mg/kg/hour
6 months to 1 year: 0.6-0.7 mg/kg/hour

Children >1 year and Adults:
Acute bronchospasm: See table.

Approximate I.V. Theophylline Dosage for Treatment of Acute Bronchospasm

Group	Dosage for Next 12 h[1]	Dosage After 12 h[1]
Infants 6 wk - 6 mo	0.5 mg/kg/h	
Children 6 mo - 1 y	0.6-0.7 mg/kg/h	
Children 1-9 y	0.95 mg/kg/h (1.2 mg/kg/h)	0.79 mg/kg/h (1 mg/kg/h)
Children 9-16 y and young adult smokers	0.79 mg/kg/h (1 mg/kg/h)	0.63 mg/kg/h (0.8 mg/kg/h)
Healthy, nonsmoking adults	0.55 mg/kg/h (0.7 mg/kg/h)	0.39 mg/kg/h (0.5 mg/kg/h)
Older patients and patients with cor pulmonale	0.47 mg/kg/h (0.6 mg/kg/h)	0.24 mg/kg/h (0.3 mg/kg/h)
Patients with congestive heart failure or liver failure	0.39 mg/kg/h (0.5 mg/kg/h)	0.08-0.16 mg/kg/h (0.1-0.2 mg/kg/h)

[1]Equivalent hydrous aminophylline dosage indicated in parentheses.

Approximate I.V. maintenance dosages are based upon continuous infusions; bolus dosing (often used in children <6 months of age) may be determined by multiplying the hourly infusion rate by 24 hours and dividing by the desired number of doses/day. See the following:
Maintenance dose for acute symptoms: See table.

Maintenance Dose for Acute Symptoms

Population Group	Oral Theophylline (mg/kg/day)	I.V. Aminophylline
Premature infant or newborn - 6 wk (for apnea/bradycardia)	4	5 mg/kg/day
6 wk - 6 mo	10	12 mg/kg/day or continuous I.V. infusion[1]
Infants 6 mo - 1 y	12-18	15 mg/kg/day or continuous I.V. infusion[1]
Children 1-9 y	20-24	1 mg/kg/h
Children 9-12 y, and adolescent daily smokers of cigarettes or marijuana, and otherwise healthy adult smokers <50 y	16	0.9 mg/kg/h
Adolescents 12-16 y (nonsmokers)	13	0.7 mg/kg/h
Otherwise healthy nonsmoking adults (including elderly patients)	10 (not to exceed 900 mg/day)	0.5 mg/kg/h
Cardiac decompensation, cor pulmonale, and/or liver dysfunction	5 (not to exceed 400 mg/day)	0.25 mg/kg/h

[1]For continuous I.V. infusion divide total daily dose by 24 = mg/kg/h.

Dosage should be adjusted according to serum level measurements during the first 12- to 24-hour period. See table

Dosage Adjustment After Serum Theophylline Measurement

Serum Theophylline		Guidelines
Within normal limits	10-20 mcg/mL	Maintain dosage if tolerated. Recheck serum theophylline concentration at 6- to 12-month intervals.[1]
Too high	20-25 mcg/mL	Decrease doses by about 10%. Recheck serum theophylline concentration after 3 days and then at 6- to 12-month intervals.[1]
	25-30 mcg/mL	Skip next dose and decrease subsequent doses by about 25%. Recheck serum theophylline.
	>30 mcg/mL	Skip next 2 doses and decrease subsequent doses by 50%. Recheck serum theophylline.
Too low	7.5-10 mcg/mL	Increase dose by about 25%.[2] Recheck serum theophylline concentration after 3 days and then at 6- to 12-month intervals.[1]
	5-7.5 mcg/mL	Increase dose by about 25% to the nearest dose increment[2] and recheck serum theophylline for guidance in further dosage adjustment (another increase will probably be needed, but this provides a safety check).

[1]Finer adjustments in dosage may be needed for some patients.

[2]Dividing the daily dose into 3 doses administered at 8-hour intervals may be indicated if symptoms occur repeatedly at the end of a dosing interval.

From Weinberger M and Hendeles L, "Practical Guide to Using Theophylline," *J Resp Dis*, 1981,2:12-27.

Oral theophylline: Initial dosage recommendation: Loading dose (to achieve a serum level of about 10 mcg/mL; loading doses should be given using a rapidly absorbed oral product **not** a sustained release product):

If no theophylline has been administered in the previous 24 hours: 4-6 mg/kg theophylline

If theophylline has been administered in the previous 24 hours: administer 1/2 loading dose or 2-3 mg/kg theophylline can be given in emergencies when serum levels are not available

On the average, for every 1 mg/kg theophylline given, blood levels will rise 2 mcg/mL

Ideally, defer the loading dose if a serum theophylline concentration can be obtained rapidly. However, if this is not possible, exercise clinical judgment. If the patient is not experiencing theophylline toxicity, this is unlikely to result in dangerous adverse effects.

Oral theophylline dosage for bronchial asthma (by age): See table

Oral Theophylline Dosage for Bronchial Asthma[1]

Age (y)	Initial 3 Days	Second 3 Days	Steady-State Maintenance
<1	0.2 x (age in weeks) + 5		0.3 x (age in weeks) + 8
1-9	16 up to a maximum of 400 mg/24 h	20	22
9-12	16 up to a maximum of 400 mg/24 h	16 up to a maximum of 600 mg/24 h	20 up to a maximum of 800 mg/24 h
12-16	16 up to a maximum of 400 mg/24 h	16 up to a maximum of 600 mg/24 h	18 up to a maximum of 900 mg/24 h
Adults	400 mg/24 h	600 mg/24 h	900 mg/24 h

[1]Dose in mg/kg/24 hours of theophylline.

Increasing dose: The dosage may be increased in approximately 25% increments at 2- to 3-day intervals so long as the drug is tolerated or until the maximum dose is reached

Maintenance dose: In children and healthy adults, a slow-release product can be used; the total daily dose can be divided every 8-12 hours

Dietary Considerations Should be taken with water 1 hour before or 2 hours after meals. Premixed injection may contain corn-derived dextrose and its use is contraindicated in patients with allergy to corn-related products.

Administration Oral: Long-acting preparations should be taken with a full glass of water, swallowed whole, or cut in half if scored. Do **not** crush. Extended release capsule forms may be opened and the contents sprinkled on soft foods; do **not** chew beads.

Additional Information Theophylline salt / theophylline content (percent)
Theophylline anhydrous (eg, most oral solids): 100% theophylline
Theophylline monohydrate (eg, oral solutions): 91% theophylline
Aminophylline (theophylline) (eg, injection): 80% (79% to 86%) theophylline
Oxtriphylline (choline theophylline) (eg, Choledyl®): 64% theophylline

Dosage Forms Excipient information presented when available (limited, particularly for generics); consult specific product labeling. [DSC] = Discontinued product

Capsule, extended release: 100 mg [DSC]; 125 mg [DSC]; 200 mg [DSC]; 300 mg [DSC]
TheoCap™: 125 mg, 200 mg; 300 mg [DSC] [12 hour]
Theo-24®: 100 mg, 200 mg, 300 mg, 400 mg [24 hours]

Elixir:
Elixophyllin®: 80 mg/15 mL (473 mL) [contains alcohol 20%; mixed fruit flavor]

Infusion [premixed in D_5W]: 200 mg (50 mL, 100 mL); 400 mg (100 mL [DSC]; 250 mL, 500 mL); 800 mg (250 mL, 500 mL, 1000 mL)

Tablet, controlled release:
Uniphyl®: 400 mg, 600 mg [24 hours]

Tablet, extended release: 100 mg, 200 mg, 300 mg, 400 mg, 450 mg, 600 mg
Theochron™: 100 mg, 200 mg, 300 mg, 450 mg [12-24 hours]

Theophylline and Guaifenesin (thee OFF i lin & gwye FEN e sin)

U.S. Brand Names Elixophyllin-GG®; Quibron® [DSC]

Index Terms Guaifenesin and Theophylline

Pharmacologic Category Theophylline Derivative

Use Symptomatic treatment of bronchospasm associated with bronchial asthma, chronic bronchitis, and pulmonary emphysema

Effect on Mental Status May cause nervousness, agitation, restlessness, insomnia, or dizziness

Effect on Psychiatric Treatment Barbiturates and carbamazepine may decrease serum levels while disulfiram, propranolol, and fluvoxamine may increase theophylline levels

Dosage Summary

Oral:
Children: Dosage not established
Adults: 16 mg/kg/day **or** 400 mg (theophylline)/day divided every 6-8 hours

Dosage Forms Excipient information presented when available (limited, particularly for generics); consult specific product labeling. [DSC] = Discontinued product

Capsule:
Quibron®: Theophylline 150 mg and guaifenesin 90 mg [DSC]

Liquid:
Elixophyllin-GG®: Theophylline 100 mg and guaifenesin 100 mg per 15 mL (240 mL, 480 mL) [alcohol free, dye free, sugar free; cherry-berry flavor]

◆ **Theophylline Anhydrous** *see* Theophylline *on page 1562*
◆ **Theophylline Ethylenediamine** *see* Aminophylline *on page 88*
◆ **Thermazene®** *see* Silver Sulfadiazine *on page 1485*

Thiabendazole (thye a BEN da zole)

U.S. Brand Names Mintezol®

Index Terms Tiabendazole

Pharmacologic Category Anthelmintic

Use Treatment of strongyloidiasis, cutaneous larva migrans, visceral larva migrans, dracunculiasis, trichinosis, and mixed helminthic infections

Unlabeled/Investigational Use Cutaneous larva migrans (topical application)

Effect on Mental Status May cause drowsiness, dizziness, hallucinations, or delirium

Effect on Psychiatric Treatment May rarely cause leukopenia; use caution with clozapine and carbamazepine

Dosage Summary

Oral:
Children ≤68 kg: 50 mg/kg/day divided every 12 hours (maximum: 3 g/day)
Children >68 kg: 1.5 g every 12 hours (maximum: 3 g/day)
Adults ≤68 kg: 50 mg/kg/day divided every 12 hours (maximum: 3 g/day)
Adults >68 kg: 1.5 g every 12 hours (maximum: 3 g/day)

Topical:

Children: Dosage not established

Adults (unlabeled use): Apply directly to larval tracks 2-6 times/day

Dosage Forms Excipient information presented when available (limited, particularly for generics); consult specific product labeling. [DSC] = Discontinued product

Suspension, oral: 500 mg/5 mL (120 mL) [DSC]

Tablet, chewable: 500 mg [orange flavor]

◆ **Thiamazole** *see* Methimazole *on page 1010*

◆ **Thiamin** *see* Thiamine *on page 1568*

Thiamine (THYE a min)

Medication Safety Issues

Sound-alike/look-alike issues:

Thiamine may be confused with Tenormin®, Thorazine®

International issues:

Doxal® [Brazil] may be confused with Doxil® which is a brand name for doxorubicin in the U.S.

Doxal® [Brazil]: Brand name for doxycycline in Austria; brand name for pyridoxine in Brazil; brand name for doxepin in Finland

Canadian Brand Names Betaxin®

Mexican Brand Names Anerex; Dexabion; Dolo-Neurobion; Dolo-Pangavit; Dolo-Tiaminal; Incremin con Hierro; Neo-Panlacticos; Neurobion; Pagavit; Pharmaton; Suma-B; Tiamidexal; Tiaminal; Tribedoce

Index Terms Aneurine Hydrochloride; Thiamin; Thiamine Hydrochloride; Thiaminium Chloride Hydrochloride; Vitamin B_1

Pharmacologic Category Vitamin, Water Soluble

Generic Available Yes

Use Treatment of thiamine deficiency including beriberi, Wernicke's encephalopathy, Korsakoff's syndrome, neuritis associated with pregnancy, or in alcoholic patients; dietary supplement

Effect on Mental Status Weakness and restlessness have been reported with injection

Effect on Psychiatric Treatment None reported

Pregnancy Risk Factor A/C (dose exceeding RDA recommendation)

Pregnancy Considerations

Thiamine requirements are increased during pregnancy. Severe nausea and vomiting (hyperemesis gravidarum) may lead to thiamine deficiency manifested as Wernicke's encephalopathy.

Lactation Enters breast milk/use caution (AAP rates "compatible")

Contraindications Hypersensitivity to thiamine or any component of the formulation

Warnings/Precautions Use with caution with parenteral route (especially I.V.) of administration. Hypersensitivity reactions have been reported following repeated parenteral doses; consider skin test in individuals with history of allergic reactions. Single vitamin deficiency is rare; evaluate for other deficiencies. Dextrose administration may precipitate acute symptoms of thiamine deficiency; use caution when thiamine status is marginal or suspect. Some parenteral products contain aluminum; use caution in patients with impaired renal function and neonates.

Adverse Reactions Adverse reactions reported with injection. Frequency not defined.

Cardiovascular: Cyanosis

Central nervous system: Restlessness

Dermatologic: Angioneurotic edema, pruritus, urticaria

Gastrointestinal: Hemorrharge into GI tract, nausea, tightness of the throat

Local: Induration and/or tenderness at the injection site (following I.M. administration)

Neuromuscular & skeletal: Weakness

Respiratory: Pulmonary edema

Miscellaneous: Anaphylactic/hypersensitivity reactions (following I.V. administration), diaphoresis, warmth

Drug Interactions

There are no known significant interactions.

Ethanol/Nutrition/Herb Interactions

Ethanol: May decrease thiamine absorption.

Food: High carbohydrate diets may increase thiamine requirement.

Stability Injection: Store at 15°C to 30°C (59°F to 86°F). Protect from light

Mechanism of Action An essential coenzyme in carbohydrate metabolism by combining with adenosine triphosphate to form thiamine pyrophosphate

Pharmacodynamics/Kinetics

Absorption: Oral: Adequate; I.M.: Rapid and complete

Distribution: Highest concentrations found in brain, heart, kidney, liver; crosses the placenta, enters breast milk

Excretion: Urine (as unchanged drug and as pyrimidine after body storage sites become saturated)

Dosage

Adequate Intake:

0-6 months: 0.2 mg/day

7-12 months: 0.3 mg/day

Recommended daily intake:

1-3 years: 0.5 mg

4-8 years: 0.6 mg

9-13 years: 0.9 mg

14-18 years: Female: 1 mg; Male: 1.2 mg

≥19 years: Female: 1.1 mg; Male: 1.2 mg

Pregnancy, lactation: 1.4 mg

Parenteral nutrition supplementation:

Infants: 1.2 mg/day

Adults: 6 mg/day; may be increased to 25-50 mg/day with history of alcohol abuse

Thiamine deficiency (beriberi):

Children: 10-25 mg/dose I.M. or I.V. daily (if critically ill), or 10-50 mg/dose orally every day for 2 weeks, then 5-10 mg/dose orally daily for 1 month

Adults: 5-30 mg/dose I.M. or I.V. 3 times/day (if critically ill); then orally 5-30 mg/day in single or divided doses 3 times/day for 1 month

Alcohol withdrawal syndrome: Adults: 100 mg/day I.M. or I.V. for several days, followed by 50-100 mg/day orally

Wernicke's encephalopathy: Adults: Treatment: Initial: 100 mg I.V., then 50-100 mg/day I.M. or I.V. until consuming a regular, balanced diet. Larger doses may be needed in patients with alcohol abuse.

Dietary Considerations Dietary sources include legumes, pork, beef, whole grains, yeast, and fresh vegetables. A deficiency state can occur in as little as 3 weeks following total dietary absence.

Administration Parenteral form may be administered by I.M. or I.V. injection. Various rates of administration have been reported. Local injection reactions may be minimized by slow administration (~30 minutes) into larger, more proximal veins. Thiamine should be administered prior to parenteral glucose solutions to prevent the precipitation of heart failure.

Reference Range Normal, serum: 1.1-1.6 mg/dL

Test Interactions False-positive for uric acid using the phosphotungstate method and for urobilinogen using the Ehrlich's reagent; large doses may interfere with the spectrophotometric determination of serum theophylline concentration

Dosage Forms Excipient information presented when available (limited, particularly for generics); consult specific product labeling.

Injection, solution, as hydrochloride: 100 mg/mL (2 mL)

Tablet, as hydrochloride: 50 mg, 100 mg, 250 mg, 500 mg

- **Thiamine Hydrochloride** *see* Thiamine *on page 1568*
- **Thiaminium Chloride Hydrochloride** *see* Thiamine *on page 1568*

Thioguanine (thye oh GWAH neen)

Medication Safety Issues

High alert medication: The Institute for Safe Medication Practices (ISMP) includes this medication among its list of drugs which have a heightened risk of causing significant patient harm when used in error.

6-thioguanine and 6-TG are error-prone abbreviations (associated with six-fold overdoses of thioguanine)

U.S. Brand Names Tabloid®

Canadian Brand Names Lanvis®

Index Terms 2-Amino-6-Mercaptopurine; 6-TG (error-prone abbreviation); 6-Thioguanine (error-prone abbreviation); NSC-752; TG; Tioguanine

Pharmacologic Category Antineoplastic Agent, Antimetabolite (Purine Antagonist)

Use Treatment of acute myelogenous (nonlymphocytic) leukemia; treatment of chronic myelogenous leukemia and granulocytic leukemia

Effect on Mental Status None reported

Effect on Psychiatric Treatment Myelosuppression is common; avoid clozapine and carbamazepine

Restrictions The I.V. formulation is not available in U.S.

Dosage Summary

Oral:

Infants: 3.3 mg/kg/day in 2 divided doses for 4 days (combination therapy)

Children <3 years: 3.3 mg/kg/day in 2 divided doses for 4 days (combination therapy)

Children ≥3 years: 2-3 mg/kg/day calculated to nearest 20 mg or 75-200 mg/m^2/day in 1-2 divided doses for 5-7 days or until remission is attained

Adults: 2-3 mg/kg/day calculated to nearest 20 mg or 75-200 mg/m^2/day in 1-2 divided doses for 5-7 days or until remission is attained

Dosage Forms Excipient information presented when available (limited, particularly for generics); consult specific product labeling.

Tablet [scored]:

Tabloid®: 40 mg

◆ **6-Thioguanine (error-prone abbreviation)** *see* Thioguanine *on page 1569*

Thiopental (thye oh PEN tal)

Medication Safety Issues

High alert medication: The Institute for Safe Medication Practices (ISMP) includes this medication among its list of drugs which have a heightened risk of causing significant patient harm when used in error.

U.S. Brand Names Pentothal®

Canadian Brand Names Pentothal®

Index Terms Thiopental Sodium

Pharmacologic Category Anticonvulsant, Barbiturate; Barbiturate; General Anesthetic

Generic Available No

Use Induction of anesthesia; adjunct for intubation in head injury patients; control of convulsive states; treatment of elevated intracranial pressure

Restrictions C-III

Pregnancy Risk Factor C

Contraindications Hypersensitivity to thiopental, barbiturates, or any component of the formulation; status asthmaticus; severe cardiovascular disease; porphyria (variegate or acute intermittent); should not be administered by intra-arterial injection

Warnings/Precautions Laryngospasm or bronchospasms may occur; use with extreme caution in patients with reactive airway diseases (asthma or COPD). Use with caution when the hypnotic may be prolonged or potentiated (excessive premedication, Addison's disease, hepatic or renal dysfunction, myxedema, increased blood urea, severe anemia, or myasthenia gravis). Potential for drug dependency exists, abrupt cessation may precipitate withdrawal, including status epilepticus in epileptic patients. Do not administer to patients in acute pain. Use caution in patients with unstable aneurysms, cardiovascular disease, renal impairment, or hepatic disease. Use caution in elderly, debilitated, or pediatric patients. May cause paradoxical responses, including agitation and hyperactivity, particularly in acute pain and pediatric patients. Effects with other sedative drugs or ethanol may be potentiated. May cause respiratory depression or hypotension. Use with caution in hemodynamically unstable patients (hypotension or shock) or patients with respiratory disease. Repeated dosing or continuous infusions may cause cumulative effects. Extravasation or intra-arterial injection causes necrosis due to pH of 10.6, ensure patient has intravenous access.

Adverse Reactions Frequency not defined.

Cardiovascular: Bradycardia, hypotension, syncope

Central nervous system: Drowsiness, lethargy, CNS excitation or depression, impaired judgment, "hangover" effect, confusion, somnolence, agitation, hyperkinesia, ataxia, nervousness, headache, insomnia, nightmares, hallucinations, anxiety, dizziness, shivering

Dermatologic: Rash, exfoliative dermatitis, Stevens-Johnson syndrome

Gastrointestinal: Nausea, vomiting, constipation

Hematologic: Agranulocytosis, thrombocytopenia, megaloblastic anemia, immune hemolytic anemia (rare)

Local: Pain at injection site, thrombophlebitis with I.V. use

Renal: Oliguria

Respiratory: Laryngospasm, respiratory depression, apnea (especially with rapid I.V. use), hypoventilation, sneezing, cough, bronchospasm

Miscellaneous: Gangrene with inadvertent intra-arterial injection, anaphylaxis, anaphylactic reactions

Drug Interactions

Acetaminophen: Barbiturates may increase the metabolism of Acetaminophen. This may 1) diminish the effect of acetaminophen; and 2) increase the risk of liver damage. *Risk C: Monitor therapy*

Alcohol (Ethyl): CNS Depressants may enhance the CNS depressant effect of Alcohol (Ethyl). *Risk C: Monitor therapy*

Beta-Blockers: Barbiturates may decrease the serum concentration of Beta-Blockers. **Exceptions:** Atenolol; Levobunolol; Metipranolol; Nadolol. *Risk C: Monitor therapy*

Calcium Channel Blockers: Barbiturates may increase the metabolism of Calcium Channel Blockers. **Exceptions:** Clevidipine. *Risk D: Consider therapy modification*

Carbonic Anhydrase Inhibitors: May enhance the adverse/toxic effect of Anticonvulsants (Barbiturate). Specifically, osteomalacia and rickets. **Exceptions:** Brinzolamide; Dorzolamide. *Risk C: Monitor therapy*

Chloramphenicol: May decrease the metabolism of Barbiturates. Barbiturates may increase the metabolism of Chloramphenicol. *Risk D: Consider therapy modification*

CNS Depressants: May enhance the adverse/toxic effect of other CNS Depressants. *Risk C: Monitor therapy*

Contraceptive (Progestins): Barbiturates may diminish the therapeutic effect of Contraceptive (Progestins). Contraceptive failure is possible. *Risk D: Consider therapy modification*

Corticosteroids (Systemic): Barbiturates may increase the metabolism of Corticosteroids (Systemic). *Risk C: Monitor therapy*

CycloSPORINE: Barbiturates may increase the metabolism of CycloSPORINE. *Risk D: Consider therapy modification*

Disopyramide: Barbiturates may increase the metabolism of Disopyramide. *Risk D: Consider therapy modification*

Doxycycline: Barbiturates may decrease the serum concentration of Doxycycline. *Risk D: Consider therapy modification*

Etoposide: Barbiturates may increase the metabolism of Etoposide. *Risk C: Monitor therapy*

Etoposide Phosphate: Barbiturates may decrease the serum concentration of Etoposide Phosphate. Barbiturates may increase the metabolism, via CYP isoenzymes, of etoposide phosphate. *Risk C: Monitor therapy*

Felbamate: May increase the serum concentration of Barbiturates. *Risk C: Monitor therapy*

Ketorolac: May diminish the therapeutic effect of Anticonvulsants. *Risk C: Monitor therapy*

LamoTRIgine: Barbiturates may increase the metabolism of LamoTRIgine. *Risk D: Consider therapy modification*

Mefloquine: May diminish the therapeutic effect of Anticonvulsants. Mefloquine may decrease the serum concentration of Anticonvulsants. Management: Mefloquine is contraindicated in persons with a history of convulsions. If anticonvulsant is being used for another indication monitor response to treatment closely, as concurrent mefloquine may decrease response to treatment. *Risk D: Consider therapy modification*

Meperidine: Barbiturates may enhance the CNS depressant effect of Meperidine. *Risk C: Monitor therapy*

Methadone: Barbiturates may increase the metabolism of Methadone. *Risk D: Consider therapy modification*

Oral Contraceptive (Estrogens): Barbiturates may diminish the therapeutic effect of Oral Contraceptive (Estrogens). Contraceptive failure is possible. *Risk D: Consider therapy modification*

Primidone: May enhance the adverse/toxic effect of Barbiturates. Primidone is converted to phenobarbital, and thus becomes additive with existing barbiturate therapy. *Risk C: Monitor therapy*

Propafenone: Barbiturates may increase the metabolism of Propafenone. *Risk D: Consider therapy modification*

Pyridoxine: May increase the metabolism of Barbiturates. Apparent in high pyridoxine doses (eg, 200 mg/day) *Risk C: Monitor therapy*

QuiNIDine: Barbiturates may increase the metabolism of QuiNIDine. *Risk D: Consider therapy modification*

Rifamycin Derivatives: May increase the metabolism of Barbiturates. *Risk C: Monitor therapy*

Teniposide: Barbiturates may increase the metabolism of Teniposide. *Risk C: Monitor therapy*

Theophylline Derivatives: Barbiturates may increase the metabolism of Theophylline Derivatives. **Exceptions:** Dyphylline. *Risk C: Monitor therapy*

Tricyclic Antidepressants: Barbiturates may increase the metabolism of Tricyclic Antidepressants. *Risk D: Consider therapy modification*

Valproic Acid: May decrease the metabolism of Barbiturates. Barbiturates may decrease the serum concentration of Valproic Acid. *Risk C: Monitor therapy*

Vitamin K Antagonists (eg, warfarin): Barbiturates may increase the metabolism of Vitamin K Antagonists. *Risk D: Consider therapy modification*

Stability Reconstituted solutions remain stable for 3 days at room temperature and 7 days when refrigerated.

Mechanism of Action Short-acting barbiturate with sedative, hypnotic, and anticonvulsant properties. Barbiturates depress the sensory cortex, decrease motor activity, alter cerebellar function, and produce drowsiness, sedation, and hypnosis. In high doses, barbiturates exhibit anticonvulsant activity; barbiturates produce dose-dependent respiratory depression.

Pharmacodynamics/Kinetics

Onset of action: Anesthetic: I.V.: 30-60 seconds

Duration: 5-30 minutes

Distribution: V_d: 1.4 L/kg

Protein binding: 72% to 86%

Metabolism: Hepatic, primarily to inactive metabolites but pentobarbital is also formed

Half-life elimination: 3-11.5 hours; decreased in children

Dosage I.V.:

Induction anesthesia:

Infants: 5-8 mg/kg

Children 1-12 years: 5-6 mg/kg

Adults: 3-5 mg/kg

Maintenance anesthesia:

Children: 1 mg/kg as needed

Adults: 25-100 mg as needed

Increased intracranial pressure: Children and Adults: 1.5-5 mg/kg/dose; repeat as needed to control intracranial pressure

Seizures:

Children: 2-3 mg/kg/dose; repeat as needed

Adults: 75-250 mg/dose; repeat as needed

Dosing adjustment in renal impairment: Cl_{cr} <10 mL/minute: Administer at 75% of normal dose

Note: Accumulation may occur with chronic dosing due to lipid solubility; prolonged recovery may result from redistribution of thiopental from fat stores

Dietary Considerations Sodium content of 1 g (injection): 86.8 mg (3.8 mEq)

Administration Administer slowly over 20-30 seconds. Rapid I.V. injection may cause hypotension or decreased cardiac output; avoid extravasation, necrosis may occur. Check I.V. catheter placement prior to administration.

Monitoring Parameters Respiratory rate, heart rate, blood pressure

Reference Range Therapeutic: Hypnotic: 1-5 mcg/mL (SI: 4.1-20.7 μmol/L); Coma: 30-100 mcg/mL (SI: 124-413 μmol/L); Anesthesia: 7-130 mcg/mL (SI: 29-536 μmol/L); Toxic: >10 mcg/mL (SI: >41 μmol/L)

Additional Information Thiopental switches from linear to nonlinear pharmacokinetics following prolonged continuous infusions.

Dosage Forms Excipient information presented when available (limited, particularly for generics); consult specific product labeling.

Injection, powder for reconstitution, as sodium: 250 mg, 400 mg, 500 mg, 1 g

◆ **Thiopental Sodium** *see* Thiopental *on page 1570*

◆ **Thiophosphoramide** *see* Thiotepa *on page 1576*

Thioridazine (thye oh RID a zeen)

Medication Safety Issues

Sound-alike/look-alike issues:

Thioridazine may be confused with thiothixene, Thorazine®

Mellaril® may be confused with Elavil®, Mebaral®

Related Information

Anticholinergic Effects of Common Psychotropics *on page 1758*

Antipsychotic Agents *on page 1769*

CMS: Long-Term Care Facility Thresholds *on page 1815*

Discontinuation of Psychotropic Drugs *on page 1839*

Liquid Compatibility of Antidepressants, Antipsychotics, and Mood Stabilizers *on page 1788*

Canadian Brand Names Mellaril®
Mexican Brand Names Melleril
Index Terms Thioridazine Hydrochloride
Pharmacologic Category Antipsychotic Agent, Typical, Phenothiazine
Generic Available Yes

Use Management of schizophrenic patients who fail to respond adequately to treatment with other antipsychotic drugs, either because of insufficient effectiveness or the inability to achieve an effective dose due to intolerable adverse effects from those medications

Unlabeled/Investigational Use Behavior problems (children); severe psychoses (children); schizophrenia/psychoses (children); depressive disorders/dementia (children and adults); behavioral symptoms associated with dementia (elderly); psychosis/agitation related to Alzheimer's dementia

Mental Health Comment Thioridazine is a low-potency antipsychotic. Older antipsychotic medications (chlorpromazine, haloperidol), which do not meet specific criteria for "atypical" antipsychotics, are often referred to as typical antipsychotics. They are associated with the troubling side effect, EPS. However, it is commonly believed that in order for a drug to treat psychosis, it must block dopamine is some manner.

Common side effects include sedation and neuroleptic effect (reduced initiative, interest in the environment, and display of emotion or affect). All **typical** antipsychotics are considered to be equally effective if given in equipotent doses. An inverse relationship exists between intrinsic antimuscarinic activity and propensity to cause extrapyramidal side effects. If dystonia or pseudoparkinsonism occurs, antiparkinsonian agents should be considered. If akathisia occurs, beta-blockers (eg, propranolol), benzodiazepines, or antiparkinsonian agents should be considered. Tardive dyskinesia (TD) secondary to typical antipsychotics has an estimated incidence of 3% to 5% per year for the first 5 years of treatment. After this time period, the incidence is estimated to be 2% to 3% per year. Prevalence rates are ~15% to 20%. Female gender and age constitute risk factors for TD. Indeed, prevalence rates have been reported to be as high as 70% in elderly females. No specific treatment exists for TD, however, patients are often initiated on/switched to an atypical antipsychotic because of their lower incidence to cause TD and hopes of suppression.

Typical antipsychotics are usually only indicated for schizophrenia, but are generally effective for mania and psychosis and/or behavioral syndromes secondary to other mental conditions. Nonpsychiatric uses include Tourette's syndrome, Huntington's disease, and occasionally, intractable hiccups, pruritus, nausea, and vomiting.

These drugs are thought to exert their antipsychotic activity by blocking dopamine D_2 receptors in the mesolimbic dopaminergic pathway. Side effects are often related to their ability to antagonize dopamine receptors in the nigrostriatal and tuberoinfundibular pathways.

Thioridazine has a black-box warning for prolongation of QT_c interval.

Coadministration of two or more antipsychotics does not generally improve clinical response and may increase the potential for adverse effects.

In 2008, the FDA issued a warning regarding increased mortality risk with typical **and** atypical antipsychotic drugs when used in elderly patients with dementia-related psychosis.

Pregnancy Risk Factor C

Lactation Excretion in breast milk unknown/not recommended

Contraindications Hypersensitivity to thioridazine or any component of the formulation (cross-reactivity between phenothiazines may occur); severe CNS depression; circulatory collapse; severe hypotension; bone marrow suppression; blood dyscrasias; coma; in combination with other drugs that are known to prolong the QT_c interval; in patients with congenital long QT syndrome or a history of cardiac arrhythmias; concurrent use with medications that inhibit the metabolism of thioridazine (fluoxetine, paroxetine, fluvoxamine, propranolol, pindolol); patients known to have genetic defect leading to reduced levels of activity of CYP2D6

Warnings/Precautions [U.S. Boxed Warning]: Thioridazine has dose-related effects on ventricular repolarization leading to QT_c prolongation, a potentially life-threatening effect. Therefore, it should be reserved for patients with schizophrenia who have failed to respond to adequate levels of other antipsychotic drugs. May cause orthostatic hypotension; use with caution in patients at risk of this effect or those who would tolerate transient hypotensive episodes (cerebrovascular disease, cardiovascular disease, or other medications which may predispose).

Highly sedating, use with caution in disorders where CNS depression is a feature. Use with caution in Parkinson's disease. Use with caution in patients with hemodynamic instability; predisposition to seizures; subcortical brain damage; severe cardiac, hepatic, renal, or respiratory disease. Esophageal dysmotility and aspiration have been associated with antipsychotic use; use with caution in patients at risk of pneumonia (ie, Alzheimer's disease). Caution in breast cancer or other prolactin-dependent tumors (may elevate prolactin levels). May alter temperature regulation or mask toxicity of other drugs due to antiemetic effects. Check blood counts periodically and discontinue at first signs of blood dyscrasias; use is contraindicated in patients with bone marrow suppression.

Elderly patients with dementia-related psychosis treated with antipsychotics are at an increased risk of death compared to placebo. An increased incidence of cerebrovascular adverse events (including fatalities) has been reported in elderly patients with dementia-related psychosis. Thioridazine is not approved for this indication. Phenothiazines may cause anticholinergic effects (confusion, agitation, constipation, xerostomia, blurred vision, urinary retention); therefore, they should be used with caution in patients with decreased gastrointestinal motility, urinary retention, BPH, xerostomia, or visual problems. Conditions which also may be exacerbated by cholinergic blockade include narrow-angle glaucoma (screening is recommended) and worsening of myasthenia gravis. Relative to other neuroleptics, thioridazine has a high potency of cholinergic blockade.

May cause extrapyramidal symptoms (EPS), including pseudoparkinsonism, acute dystonic reactions, akathisia, and tardive dyskinesia (risk of these reactions is low relative to other neuroleptics). Risk of dystonia (and possibly other EPS) may be greater with increased doses, use of conventional antipsychotics, males, and younger patients. Use caution in the elderly. May be associated with neuroleptic malignant syndrome (NMS). Doses exceeding recommended doses may cause pigmentary retinopathy.

Adverse Reactions Frequency not defined.

Cardiovascular: Hypotension, orthostatic hypotension, peripheral edema, ECG changes

Central nervous system: EPS (pseudoparkinsonism, akathisia, dystonias, tardive dyskinesia), dizziness, drowsiness, neuroleptic malignant syndrome (NMS), impairment of temperature regulation, lowering of seizure threshold

Dermatologic: Increased sensitivity to sun, rash, discoloration of skin (blue-gray)

Endocrine & metabolic: Changes in menstrual cycle, libido (changes in), breast pain, galactorrhea, amenorrhea

Gastrointestinal: Constipation, weight gain, nausea, vomiting, stomach pain, xerostomia, diarrhea

Genitourinary: Difficulty in urination, ejaculatory disturbances, urinary retention, priapism

Hematologic: Agranulocytosis, leukopenia

Hepatic: Cholestatic jaundice, hepatotoxicity

Neuromuscular & skeletal: Tremor, seizure

Ocular: Pigmentary retinopathy, blurred vision, cornea and lens changes

Respiratory: Nasal congestion

Metabolism/Transport Effects Substrate of CYP2C19 (minor), 2D6 (major); **Inhibits** CYP1A2 (weak), 2C9 (weak), 2D6 (moderate), 2E1 (weak)

Drug Interactions

Acetylcholinesterase Inhibitors (Central): May enhance the neurotoxic (central) effect of Antipsychotics. Severe extrapyramidal symptoms have occurred in some patients. *Risk C: Monitor therapy*

Alcohol (Ethyl): CNS Depressants may enhance the CNS depressant effect of Alcohol (Ethyl). *Risk C: Monitor therapy*

Alfuzosin: May enhance the QTc-prolonging effect of QTc-Prolonging Agents. *Risk C: Monitor therapy*

Amphetamines: Antipsychotics may diminish the stimulatory effect of Amphetamines. *Risk C: Monitor therapy*

Analgesics (Opioid): Antipsychotic Agents (Phenothiazines) may enhance the hypotensive effect of Analgesics (Opioid). *Risk C: Monitor therapy*

Antacids: May decrease the absorption of Antipsychotic Agents (Phenothiazines). *Risk C: Monitor therapy*

Anticholinergics: May enhance the adverse/toxic effect of other Anticholinergics. **Exceptions:** Paliperidone. *Risk C: Monitor therapy*

Antimalarial Agents: May increase the serum concentration of Antipsychotic Agents (Phenothiazines). *Risk C: Monitor therapy*

Anti-Parkinson's Agents (Dopamine Agonist): Antipsychotics (Typical) may diminish the therapeutic effect of Anti-Parkinson's Agents (Dopamine Agonist). *Risk D: Consider therapy modification*

Beta-Blockers: Antipsychotic Agents (Phenothiazines) may enhance the hypotensive effect of Beta-Blockers. Beta-Blockers may decrease the metabolism of Antipsychotic Agents (Phenothiazines). Antipsychotic Agents (Phenothiazines) may decrease the metabolism of Beta-Blockers. **Exceptions:** Atenolol; Levobunolol; Metipranolol; Nadolol. *Risk C: Monitor therapy*

Ciprofloxacin: May enhance the QTc-prolonging effect of QTc-Prolonging Agents. *Risk C: Monitor therapy*

CNS Depressants: May enhance the adverse/toxic effect of other CNS Depressants. *Risk C: Monitor therapy*

CYP2D6 Inhibitors: May decrease the metabolism of Thioridazine. *Risk X: Avoid combination*

CYP2D6 Substrates: CYP2D6 Inhibitors (Moderate) may decrease the metabolism of CYP2D6 Substrates. **Exceptions:** Tamoxifen. *Risk C: Monitor therapy*

Darunavir: May increase the serum concentration of CYP2D6 Substrates. *Risk C: Monitor therapy*

Fluvoxamine: May increase the serum concentration of Thioridazine. *Risk X: Avoid combination*

Gadobutrol: May enhance the QTc-prolonging effect of QTc-Prolonging Agents. *Risk D: Consider therapy modification*

Lithium formulations: May enhance the neurotoxic effect of Antipsychotics. Lithium formulations may decrease the serum concentration of Antipsychotics. Specifically noted with chlorpromazine. *Risk C: Monitor therapy*

Nilotinib: May enhance the QTc-prolonging effect of QTc-Prolonging Agents. *Risk X: Avoid combination*

Pramlintide: May enhance the anticholinergic effect of Anticholinergics. These effects are specific to the GI tract. *Risk D: Consider therapy modification*

QTc-Prolonging Agents: May enhance the QTc-prolonging effect of Thioridazine. *Risk X: Avoid combination*

Tamoxifen: CYP2D6 Inhibitors (Moderate) may decrease the metabolism of Tamoxifen. Specifically, CYP2D6 inhibitors may decrease the formation of highly potent active metabolites. *Risk D: Consider therapy modification*

Tetrabenazine: May enhance the adverse/toxic effect of Antipsychotics. *Risk C: Monitor therapy*

TraMADol: CYP2D6 Inhibitors (Moderate) may diminish the therapeutic effect of TraMADol. These CYP2D6 inhibitors may prevent the metabolic conversion of tramadol to its active metabolite that accounts for much of its opioid-like effects. *Risk C: Monitor therapy*

Ziprasidone: QTc-Prolonging Agents may enhance the QTc-prolonging effect of Ziprasidone. The risk of a severe arrhythmia may be increased. *Risk X: Avoid combination*

Ethanol/Nutrition/Herb Interactions

Ethanol: Avoid ethanol (may increase CNS depression).

Herb/Nutraceutical: Avoid kava kava, valerian, St John's wort, gotu kola (may increase CNS depression). Avoid dong quai, St John's wort (may also cause photosensitization).

Stability Protect from light.

Mechanism of Action Thioridazine is a piperidine phenothiazine which blocks postsynaptic mesolimbic dopaminergic receptors in the brain; exhibits a strong alpha-adrenergic blocking effect and depresses the release of hypothalamic and hypophyseal hormones

Pharmacodynamics/Kinetics

Duration: 4-5 days

Half-life elimination: 21-25 hours

Time to peak, serum: ~1 hour

Dosage Oral:

Children >2-12 years (unlabeled use): Range: 0.5-3 mg/kg/day in 2-3 divided doses; usual: 1 mg/kg/day; maximum: 3 mg/kg/day

- Behavior problems (unlabeled use): Initial: 10 mg 2-3 times/day, increase gradually
- Severe psychoses (unlabeled use): Initial: 25 mg 2-3 times/day, increase gradually

Children >12 years (unlabeled use) and Adults:

- Schizophrenia/psychoses: Initial: 50-100 mg 3 times/day with gradual increments as needed and tolerated; maximum: 800 mg/day in 2-4 divided doses
- Depressive disorders/dementia (unlabeled use): Initial: 25 mg 3 times/day; maintenance dose: 20-200 mg/day

Elderly: Behavioral symptoms associated with dementia (unlabeled use): Oral: Initial: 10-25 mg 1-2 times/day; increase at 4- to 7-day intervals by 10-25 mg/day; increase dose intervals (once daily, twice daily, etc) as necessary to control response or side effects. Maximum daily dose: 400 mg; gradual increases (titration) may prevent some side effects or decrease their severity.

Hemodialysis: Not dialyzable (0% to 5%)

Administration Do not take antacid within 2 hours of taking drug.

Monitoring Parameters Baseline and periodic ECG; vital signs; serum potassium, lipid profile, fasting blood glucose and Hgb A_{1c}; BMI; mental status, abnormal involuntary movement scale (AIMS); periodic eye exam; do not initiate if QT_c >450 msec

Reference Range Toxic: >1 mg/mL; lethal: 2-8 mg/dL

Test Interactions False-positives for phenylketonuria, urinary amylase, uroporphyrins, urobilinogen

Dosage Forms Excipient information presented when available (limited, particularly for generics); consult specific product labeling. [DSC] = Discontinued product

Tablet, as hydrochloride: 10 mg, 15 mg [DSC], 25 mg, 50 mg, 100 mg, 150 mg [DSC], 200 mg [DSC]

◆ **Thioridazine Hydrochloride** *see* Thioridazine *on page 1572*

◆ **Thiosulfuric Acid Disodium Salt** *see* Sodium Thiosulfate *on page 1497*

Thiotepa (thye oh TEP a)

Medication Safety Issues

High alert medication: The Institute for Safe Medication Practices (ISMP) includes this medication among its list of drugs which have a heightened risk of causing significant patient harm when used in error.

Index Terms TESPA; Thiophosphoramide; Triethylenethiophosphoramide; TSPA

Pharmacologic Category Antineoplastic Agent, Alkylating Agent

Use Treatment of superficial tumors of the bladder; palliative treatment of adenocarcinoma of breast or ovary; lymphomas and sarcomas; controlling intracavitary effusions caused by metastatic tumors; I.T. use: CNS leukemia/lymphoma, CNS metastases

Effect on Mental Status May cause dizziness

Effect on Psychiatric Treatment Myelosuppression is common; avoid clozapine and carbamazepine; barbiturates may increase clearance of thiotepa

Dosage Forms Excipient information presented when available (limited, particularly for generics); consult specific product labeling.

Injection, powder for reconstitution: 15 mg, 30 mg

Thiothixene (thye oh THIKS een)

Medication Safety Issues

Sound-alike/look-alike issues:

Thiothixene may be confused with thioridazine

Navane® may be confused with Norvasc®, Nubain®

Related Information

Anticholinergic Effects of Common Psychotropics *on page 1758*

Antipsychotic Agents *on page 1769*

CMS: Long-Term Care Facility Thresholds *on page 1815*

Discontinuation of Psychotropic Drugs *on page 1839*

Liquid Compatibility of Antidepressants, Antipsychotics, and Mood Stabilizers *on page 1788*

U.S. Brand Names Navane®

Canadian Brand Names Navane®

Index Terms Tiotixene

Pharmacologic Category Antipsychotic Agent, Typical

Generic Available Yes

Use Management of schizophrenia

Unlabeled/Investigational Use Psychotic disorders (children); rapid tranquilization of the agitated patient (children); nonpsychotic patient, dementia behavior (elderly); psychosis/agitation related to Alzheimer's dementia

Mental Health Comment Thiothixene is a high-potency antipsychotic. Older antipsychotic medications (chlorpromazine, haloperidol), which do not meet specific criteria for "atypical" antipsychotics, are often referred to as typical antipsychotics. They are associated with the troubling side effect, EPS. However, it is commonly believed that in order for a drug to treat psychosis, it must block dopamine is some manner.

Common side effects include sedation and neuroleptic effect (reduced initiative, interest in the environment, and display of emotion or affect). All **typical** antipsychotics are considered to be equally effective if given in equipotent doses. An inverse relationship exists between intrinsic antimuscarinic activity and propensity to cause extrapyramidal side effects. If dystonia or pseudoparkinsonism occurs, antiparkinsonian agents should be considered. If akathisia occurs, beta-blockers (eg, propranolol), benzodiazepines, or antiparkinsonian agents should be considered. Tardive dyskinesia (TD) secondary to typical antipsychotics has an estimated incidence of 3% to 5% per year for the first 5 years of treatment. After this time period, the incidence is estimated to be 2% to 3% per year. Prevalence rates are ~15% to 20%. Female gender and age constitute risk factors for TD. Indeed, prevalence rates have been reported to be as high as 70% in elderly females. No specific treatment exists for TD, however, patients are often initiated on/switched to an atypical antipsychotic because of their lower incidence to cause TD and hopes of suppression.

Typical antipsychotics are usually only indicated for schizophrenia, but are generally effective for mania and psychosis and/or behavioral syndromes secondary to other mental conditions. Nonpsychiatric uses include Tourette's syndrome, Huntington's disease, and occasionally, intractable hiccups, pruritus, nausea, and vomiting.

These drugs are thought to exert their antipsychotic activity by blocking dopamine D_2 receptors in the mesolimbic dopaminergic pathway. Side effects are often related to their ability to antagonize dopamine receptors in the nigrostriatal and tuberoinfundibular pathways.

Coadministration of two or more antipsychotics does not generally improve clinical response and may increase the potential for adverse effects.

In 2008, the FDA issued a warning regarding increased mortality risk with typical **and** atypical antipsychotic drugs when used in elderly patients with dementia-related psychosis.

Pregnancy Risk Factor C

Lactation Excretion in breast milk unknown/not recommended

Contraindications Hypersensitivity to thiothixene or any component of the formulation; severe CNS depression; circulatory collapse; blood dyscrasias; coma

Warnings/Precautions **[U.S. Boxed Warning]: Elderly patients with dementia-related psychosis treated with antipsychotics are at an increased risk of death compared to placebo.** An increased incidence of cerebrovascular adverse events (including fatalities) has been reported in elderly patients with dementia-related psychosis. Thiothixene is not approved for this indication.May alter cardiac conduction; life-threatening arrhythmias have occurred with therapeutic doses of antipsychotics. Avoid use in patients with underlying QT prolongation, in those taking medicines that prolong the QT interval, or cause polymorphic ventricular tachycardia; monitor ECG closely for dose-related QT effects. Myelosuppression (eg, leukopenia, agranulocytosis) has been observed with antipsychotic use; check blood counts periodically and discontinue at first signs of blood dyscrasias; use is contraindicated in patients with bone marrow suppression. Antipsychotic use has been associated with esophageal dysmotility and aspiration; use with caution in patients at risk of pneumonia (ie, Alzheimer's disease). May cause extrapyramidal symptoms (EPS), including pseudoparkinsonism, acute dystonic reactions, akathisia, and tardive dyskinesia (risk of these reactions is high relative to other neuroleptics). Risk of dystonia (and possibly other EPS) may be greater with increased doses, use of conventional antispychotics, males, and younger patients. Use may be associated with NMS; monitor for mental status changes, fever, muscle rigidity, and/or autonomic instability (risk may be increased in patients with Parkinson's disease or Lewy body dementia). May cause orthostatic hypotension; use with caution in patients at risk of this effect or in those who would not tolerate transient hypotensive episodes (cerebrovascular disease, cardiovascular disease, hypovolemia, or concurrent medication use which may predispose to hypotension/bradycardia). May be associated with pigmentary retinopathy. May be sedating, use with caution in disorders where CNS depression is a feature; patients must be cautioned about performing tasks which require mental alertness (eg, operating machinery or driving). Impaired core body temperature regulation may occur; caution with strenuous exercise, heat exposure, dehydration, and concomitant medication possessing anticholinergic effects.

May be sedating, use with caution in disorders where CNS depression is a feature; patients must be cautioned about performing tasks which require mental alertness (eg, operating machinery or driving). May cause anticholinergic effects (constipation, xerostomia, blurred vision, urinary retention); use with caution in patients with decreased gastrointestinal motility, paralytic ileus, urinary retention, BPH, xerostomia, or visual problems. Relative to other neuroleptics, thiothixene has a low potency of cholinergic blockade. May mask toxicity of other drugs or conditions (eg, intestinal obstruction, Reye's syndrome, brain tumor) due to antiemetic effects.

Use with caution in patients with severe cardiovascular disease, narrow-angle glaucoma, hepatic impairment, myasthenia gravis, Parkinson's disease, breast cancer or other prolactin-dependent tumors, renal impairment, respiratory disease, or seizure disorder. Safety and efficacy have not been established in children <12 years of age.

Adverse Reactions Frequency not defined.

Cardiovascular: Hypotension, nonspecific ECG changes, syncope, tachycardia

Central nervous system: Agitation, dizziness, drowsiness, extrapyramidal symptoms (akathisia, dystonias, lightheadedness, pseudoparkinsonism, tardive dyskinesia), insomnia restlessness

Dermatologic: Discoloration of skin (blue-gray), photosensitivity, pruritus, rash, urticaria

Endocrine & metabolic: Amenorrhea, breast pain, libido (changes in), changes in menstrual cycle, galactorrhea, gynecomastia, hyper-/hypoglycemia, hyperprolactinemia, lactation

Gastrointestinal: Constipation, nausea, salivation increased, stomach pain, vomiting, weight gain, xerostomia

Genitourinary: Difficulty in urination, ejaculatory disturbances, impotence

Hematologic: Leukocytes, leukopenia

Neuromuscular & skeletal: Tremors

Ocular: Blurred vision, pigmentary retinopathy

Respiratory: Nasal congestion

Miscellaneous: Diaphoresis

Metabolism/Transport Effects **Substrate** of CYP1A2 (major); **Inhibits** CYP2D6 (weak)

Drug Interactions

Acetylcholinesterase Inhibitors (Central): May enhance the neurotoxic (central) effect of Antipsychotics. Severe extrapyramidal symptoms have occurred in some patients. *Risk C: Monitor therapy*

Alcohol (Ethyl): CNS Depressants may enhance the CNS depressant effect of Alcohol (Ethyl). *Risk C: Monitor therapy*

Alfuzosin: May enhance the QTc-prolonging effect of QTc-Prolonging Agents. *Risk C: Monitor therapy*

Amphetamines: Antipsychotics may diminish the stimulatory effect of Amphetamines. *Risk C: Monitor therapy*

Anticholinergics: May enhance the adverse/toxic effect of other Anticholinergics. **Exceptions:** Paliperidone. *Risk C: Monitor therapy*

Anti-Parkinson's Agents (Dopamine Agonist): Antipsychotics (Typical) may diminish the therapeutic effect of Anti-Parkinson's Agents (Dopamine Agonist). *Risk D: Consider therapy modification*

Ciprofloxacin: May enhance the QTc-prolonging effect of QTc-Prolonging Agents. *Risk C: Monitor therapy*

CNS Depressants: May enhance the adverse/toxic effect of other CNS Depressants. *Risk C: Monitor therapy*

CYP1A2 Inducers (Strong): May increase the metabolism of CYP1A2 Substrates. *Risk C: Monitor therapy*

CYP1A2 Inhibitors (Moderate): May decrease the metabolism of CYP1A2 Substrates. *Risk C: Monitor therapy*

CYP1A2 Inhibitors (Strong): May decrease the metabolism of CYP1A2 Substrates. *Risk D: Consider therapy modification*

Gadobutrol: May enhance the QTc-prolonging effect of QTc-Prolonging Agents. *Risk D: Consider therapy modification*

Lithium formulations: May enhance the neurotoxic effect of Antipsychotics. Lithium formulations may decrease the serum concentration of Antipsychotics. Specifically noted with chlorpromazine. *Risk C: Monitor therapy*

Nilotinib: May enhance the QTc-prolonging effect of QTc-Prolonging Agents. *Risk X: Avoid combination*

Pramlintide: May enhance the anticholinergic effect of Anticholinergics. These effects are specific to the GI tract. *Risk D: Consider therapy modification*

QTc-Prolonging Agents: May enhance the adverse/toxic effect of other QTc-Prolonging Agents. Their effects can be additive, causing life-threatening ventricular arrhythmias. *Risk D: Consider therapy modification*

Tetrabenazine: May enhance the adverse/toxic effect of Antipsychotics. *Risk C: Monitor therapy*

Thioridazine: QTc-Prolonging Agents may enhance the QTc-prolonging effect of Thioridazine. *Risk X: Avoid combination*

Ziprasidone: QTc-Prolonging Agents may enhance the QTc-prolonging effect of Ziprasidone. The risk of a severe arrhythmia may be increased. *Risk X: Avoid combination*

Ethanol/Nutrition/Herb Interactions

Ethanol: Avoid ethanol (may increase CNS depression).

Herb/Nutraceutical: Avoid kava kava, valerian, St John's wort, gotu kola (may increase CNS depression).

Mechanism of Action Thiothixene is a thioxanthene antipsychotic which elicits antipsychotic activity by postsynaptic blockade of CNS dopamine receptors resulting in inhibition of dopamine-mediated effects; also has alpha-adrenergic blocking activity

Pharmacodynamics/Kinetics

Metabolism: Extensively hepatic

Half-life elimination: >24 hours with chronic use

Dosage Oral:

Children <12 years (unlabeled use): Schizophrenia/psychoses: 0.25 mg/kg/24 hours in divided doses (dose not well established; use not recommended)

Children >12 years (unlabeled use) and Adults:

Mild-to-moderate psychosis: 2 mg 3 times/day, up to 20-30 mg/day; more severe psychosis: Initial: 5 mg 2 times/day, may increase gradually, if necessary; maximum: 60 mg/day

Rapid tranquilization of the agitated patient (administered every 30-60 minutes): 5-10 mg; average total dose for tranquilization: 15-30 mg

Elderly: Nonpsychotic patient, dementia behavior (unlabeled use): Initial: 1-2 mg 1-2 times/day; increase dose at 4- to 7-day intervals by 1-2 mg/day. Increase dosing intervals (bid, tid, etc) as necessary to control response or side effects; maximum daily dose: 30 mg. Gradual increases in dose may prevent some side effects or decrease their severity.

Hemodialysis: Not dialyzable (0% to 5%)

Child/Adolescent Considerations The use of thiothixene in children <12 years of age is not recommended; safety and efficacy have not been established for this age group.

Monitoring Parameters Vital signs; lipid profile, fasting blood glucose/Hgb A_{1c}; BMI; mental status, abnormal involuntary movement scale (AIMS), extrapyramidal symptoms (EPS)

Test Interactions May cause false-positive pregnancy test

Dosage Forms Excipient information presented when available (limited, particularly for generics); consult specific product labeling. [DSC] = Discontinued product

Capsule: 1 mg, 2 mg, 5 mg, 10 mg

Navane®: 1 mg [DSC], 2 mg, 5 mg, 10 mg, 20 mg

- **Thrive™ [OTC]** *see* Nicotine *on page 1133*
- **Thymocyte Stimulating Factor** *see* Aldesleukin *on page 58*
- **Thymoglobulin®** *see* Antithymocyte Globulin (Rabbit) *on page 126*
- **Thyrel® TRH [DSC]** *see* Protirelin *on page 1363*

Thyroid, Desiccated (THYE roid DES i kay tid)

U.S. Brand Names Armour® Thyroid; Nature-Throid™; Westhroid™

Index Terms Desiccated Thyroid; Thyroid Extract; Thyroid USP

Pharmacologic Category Thyroid Product

Use Replacement or supplemental therapy in hypothyroidism; pituitary TSH suppressants (thyroid nodules, thyroiditis, multinodular goiter, thyroid cancer), thyrotoxicosis, diagnostic suppression tests

Effect on Mental Status May cause nervousness or insomnia

Effect on Psychiatric Treatment Use to augment antidepressants and treat lithium-induced hypothyroidism

Dosage Summary

Oral:

Children 0-6 months: 15-30 mg/day **or** 4.8-6 mg/kg/day

Children 6-12 months: 30-45 mg/day **or** 3.6-4.8 mg/kg/day

Children 1-5 years: 45-60 mg/day **or** 3-3.6 mg/kg/day

Children 6-12 years: 60-90 mg/day **or** 2.4-3 mg/kg/day

Children >12 years: >90 mg/day **or** 1.2-1.8 mg/kg/day

Adults: Initial: 15-30 mg/day; Maintenance: 60-120 mg/day; **Note:** Titration is recommended

Dosage Forms Excipient information presented when available (limited, particularly for generics); consult specific product labeling.

Tablet: 30 mg, 32.5 mg, 60 mg, 65 mg, 120 mg, 130 mg, 180 mg

Armour® Thyroid: 15 mg, 30 mg, 60 mg, 90 mg, 120 mg, 180 mg, 240 mg, 300 mg
Nature-Throid™: 16.25 mg, 32.5 mg, 65 mg, 130 mg, 195 mg
Westhroid™: 32.5 mg, 65 mg, 130 mg

◆ **Thyroid Extract** *see* Thyroid, Desiccated *on page 1579*

◆ **Thyroid USP** *see* Thyroid, Desiccated *on page 1579*

◆ **Thyrolar®** *see* Liotrix *on page 930*

◆ **ThyroSafe™ [OTC]** *see* Potassium Iodide *on page 1317*

◆ **ThyroShield™ [OTC]** *see* Potassium Iodide *on page 1317*

◆ **Thyrotropin Releasing Hormone** *see* Protirelin *on page 1363*

◆ ***L*-Thyroxine Sodium** *see* Levothyroxine *on page 920*

◆ **Tiabendazole** *see* Thiabendazole *on page 1567*

TiaGABine (tye AG a been)

Medication Safety Issues
Sound-alike/look-alike issues:
TiaGABine may be confused with tiZANidine

Related Information
Anticonvulsants By Seizure Type *on page 1759*

U.S. Brand Names Gabitril®

Canadian Brand Names Gabitril®

Index Terms Tiagabine Hydrochloride

Pharmacologic Category Anticonvulsant, Miscellaneous

Generic Available No

Use Adjunctive therapy in adults and children ≥12 years of age in the treatment of partial seizures

Pregnancy Risk Factor C

Lactation Enters breast milk/not recommended

Contraindications Hypersensitivity to tiagabine or any component of the formulation

Warnings/Precautions New-onset seizures and status epilepticus have been associated with tiagabine use when taken for unlabeled indications. Often these seizures have occurred shortly after the initiation of treatment or shortly after a dosage increase. Seizures have also occurred with very low doses or after several months of therapy. In most cases, patients were using concomitant medications (eg, antidepressants, antipsychotics, stimulants, narcotics). In these instances, the discontinuation of tiagabine, followed by an evaluation for an underlying seizure disorder, is suggested. Use for unapproved indications, however, has not been proven to be safe or effective and is not recommended. When tiagabine is used as an adjunct in partial seizures (an FDA-approved indication), it should not be abruptly discontinued because of the possibility of increasing seizure frequency, unless safety concerns require a more rapid withdrawal. Rarely, nonconvulsive status epilepticus has been reported following abrupt discontinuation or dosage reduction.

Use with caution in patients with hepatic impairment. Experience in patients not receiving enzyme-inducing drugs has been limited; caution should be used in treating any patient who is not receiving one of these medications (decreased dose and slower titration may be required). Weakness, sedation, and confusion may occur with tiagabine use. Patients must be cautioned about performing tasks which require mental alertness (eg, operating machinery or driving). Effects with other sedative drugs or ethanol may be potentiated. May cause serious rash, including Stevens-Johnson syndrome. Safety and efficacy have not been established in children <12 years of age.

Adverse Reactions
>10%:
Central nervous system: Concentration decreased, dizziness, nervousness, somnolence
Gastrointestinal: Nausea
Neuromuscular & skeletal: Weakness, tremor

1% to 10%:
Cardiovascular: Chest pain, edema, hypertension, palpitation, peripheral edema, syncope, tachycardia, vasodilation
Central nervous system: Agitation, ataxia, chills, confusion, difficulty with memory, confusion, depersonalization, depression, euphoria, hallucination, hostility, insomnia, malaise, migraine, paranoid reaction, personality disorder, speech disorder
Dermatologic: Alopecia, bruising, dry skin, pruritus, rash

Gastrointestinal: Abdominal pain, diarrhea, gingivitis, increased appetite, mouth ulceration, stomatitis, vomiting, weight gain/loss

Neuromuscular & skeletal: Abnormal gait, arthralgia, dysarthria, hyper-/hypokinesia, hyper-/hypotonia, myasthenia, myalgia, myoclonus, neck pain, paresthesia, reflexes decreased, stupor, twitching, vertigo

Ocular: Abnormal vision, amblyopia, nystagmus

Otic: Ear pain, hearing impairment, otitis media, tinnitus

Respiratory: Bronchitis, cough, dyspnea, epistaxis, pneumonia

Miscellaneous: Allergic reaction, cyst, diaphoresis, flu-like syndrome, lymphadenopathy

<1% (Limited to important or life-threatening): Abortion, abscess, anemia, angina, apnea, asthma, blepharitis, blindness, cellulitis, cerebral ischemia, cholelithiasis, CNS neoplasm, coma, deafness, dehydration, dysphagia, dystonia, electrocardiogram abnormal, encephalopathy, hemorrhage, erythrocytes abnormal, leukopenia, fecal incontinence, herpes simplex/zoster, glossitis, goiter, hematuria, hemoptysis, hepatomegaly, hypercholesteremia, hyper-/hypoglycemia, hyperlipemia, hypokalemia, hyponatremia, hypotension, hypothyroidism, impotence, kidney failure, liver function tests abnormal, MI, neoplasm, peripheral vascular disorder, paralysis, photophobia, psychosis, petechia, photosensitivity, seizure (when used for unlabeled uses), sepsis, spasm, suicide attempt, thrombocytopenia, thrombophlebitis, urinary retention, urinary urgency, urticaria, visual field defect

Metabolism/Transport Effects **Substrate** of 3A4 (major)

Drug Interactions

Alcohol (Ethyl): CNS Depressants may enhance the CNS depressant effect of Alcohol (Ethyl). *Risk C: Monitor therapy*

CNS Depressants: May enhance the adverse/toxic effect of other CNS Depressants. *Risk C: Monitor therapy*

CYP3A4 Inducers (Strong): May increase the metabolism of CYP3A4 Substrates. *Risk C: Monitor therapy*

CYP3A4 Inhibitors (Moderate): May decrease the metabolism of CYP3A4 Substrates. *Risk C: Monitor therapy*

CYP3A4 Inhibitors (Strong): May decrease the metabolism of CYP3A4 Substrates. *Risk D: Consider therapy modification*

Dasatinib: May increase the serum concentration of CYP3A4 Substrates. *Risk C: Monitor therapy*

Deferasirox: May decrease the serum concentration of CYP3A4 Substrates. *Risk C: Monitor therapy*

Herbs (CYP3A4 Inducers): May increase the metabolism of CYP3A4 Substrates. *Risk C: Monitor therapy*

Ketorolac: May diminish the therapeutic effect of Anticonvulsants. *Risk C: Monitor therapy*

Mefloquine: May diminish the therapeutic effect of Anticonvulsants. Mefloquine may decrease the serum concentration of Anticonvulsants. Management: Mefloquine is contraindicated in persons with a history of convulsions. If anticonvulsant is being used for another indication monitor response to treatment closely, as concurrent mefloquine may decrease response to treatment. *Risk D: Consider therapy modification*

Ethanol/Nutrition/Herb Interactions

Ethanol: Avoid ethanol (may increase CNS depression).

Food: Food reduces the rate but not the extent of absorption.

Herb/Nutraceutical: St John's wort may decrease tiagabine levels. Avoid valerian, St John's wort, kava kava, gotu kola (may increase CNS depression).

Mechanism of Action The exact mechanism by which tiagabine exerts antiseizure activity is not definitively known; however, *in vitro* experiments demonstrate that it enhances the activity of gamma aminobutyric acid (GABA), the major neuroinhibitory transmitter in the nervous system; it is thought that binding to the GABA uptake carrier inhibits the uptake of GABA into presynaptic neurons, allowing an increased amount of GABA to be available to postsynaptic neurons; based on *in vitro* studies, tiagabine does not inhibit the uptake of dopamine, norepinephrine, serotonin, glutamate, or choline

Pharmacodynamics/Kinetics

Absorption: Rapid (45 minutes); prolonged with food

Protein binding: 96%, primarily to albumin and α_1-acid glycoprotein

Metabolism: Hepatic via CYP (primarily 3A4)

Bioavailability: Oral: Absolute: 90%

Half-life elimination: 2-5 hours when administered with enzyme inducers; 7-9 hours when administered without enzyme inducers

Time to peak, plasma: 45 minutes

Excretion: Feces (63%); urine (25%); 2% as unchanged drug; primarily as metabolites

Dosage Oral (administer with food):

Patients receiving enzyme-inducing AED regimens:

Children 12-18 years: 4 mg once daily for 1 week; may increase to 8 mg daily in 2 divided doses for 1 week; then may increase by 4-8 mg weekly to response or up to 32 mg daily in 2-4 divided doses

Adults: 4 mg once daily for 1 week; may increase by 4-8 mg weekly to response or up to 56 mg daily in 2-4 divided doses; usual maintenance: 32-56 mg/day

Patients **not** receiving enzyme-inducing AED regimens: The estimated plasma concentrations of tiagabine in patients not taking enzyme-inducing medications is twice that of patients receiving enzyme-inducing AEDs. Lower doses are required; slower titration may be necessary.

Dietary Considerations Take with food.

Monitoring Parameters A reduction in seizure frequency is indicative of therapeutic response to tiagabine in patients with partial seizures; complete blood counts, renal function tests, liver function tests, and routine blood chemistry should be monitored periodically during therapy

Reference Range Maximal plasma level after a 24 mg/dose: 552 ng/mL

Additional Information Animal studies suggest that tiagabine may bind to retina and uvea; however, no treatment-related ophthalmoscopic changes were seen long-term; periodic monitoring may be considered.

Dosage Forms Excipient information presented when available (limited, particularly for generics); consult specific product labeling.

Tablet, as hydrochloride:

Gabitril®: 2 mg, 4 mg, 12 mg, 16 mg

◆ **Tiagabine Hydrochloride** *see* TiaGABine *on page 1580*

◆ **Tiazac®** *see* Diltiazem *on page 473*

Ticarcillin and Clavulanate Potassium

(tye kar SIL in & klav yoo LAN ate poe TASS ee um)

U.S. Brand Names Timentin®

Canadian Brand Names Timentin®

Mexican Brand Names Timentin

Index Terms Ticarcillin and Clavulanic Acid

Pharmacologic Category Antibiotic, Penicillin

Use Treatment of lower respiratory tract, urinary tract, skin and skin structures, bone and joint, gynecologic (endometritis) and intra-abdominal (peritonitis) infections, and septicemia caused by susceptible organisms. Clavulanate expands activity of ticarcillin to include beta-lactamase producing strains of *S. aureus*, *H. influenzae*, *Bacteroides* species, and some other gram-negative bacilli

Effect on Mental Status May cause drowsiness or confusion; penicillins reported to cause apprehension, illusions, hallucinations, depersonalization, agitation, insomnia, and encephalopathy

Effect on Psychiatric Treatment None reported

Dosage Summary

I.V.:

Children <60 kg: 200-300 mg of ticarcillin component/kg/day in divided doses every 4-6 hours

Children ≥60 kg: 3.1 g (ticarcillin 3 g plus clavulanic acid 0.1 g) every 4-6 hours (maximum: 24 g of ticarcillin component/day)

Adults <60 kg: 200-300 mg of ticarcillin component/kg/day in divided doses every 4-6 hours

Adults ≥60 kg: 3.1 g (ticarcillin 3 g plus clavulanic acid 0.1 g) every 4-6 hours (maximum: 24 g of ticarcillin component/day)

Dosage Forms Excipient information presented when available (limited, particularly for generics); consult specific product labeling.

Infusion [premixed, frozen]: Ticarcillin 3 g and clavulanic acid 0.1 g (100 mL) [contains sodium 4.51 mEq and potassium 0.15 mEq per g]

Injection, powder for reconstitution: Ticarcillin 3 g and clavulanic acid 0.1 g (3.1 g, 31 g) [contains sodium 4.51 mEq and potassium 0.15 mEq per g]

◆ **Ticarcillin and Clavulanic Acid** *see* Ticarcillin and Clavulanate Potassium *on page 1582*

◆ **Ticlid® [DSC]** *see* Ticlopidine *on page 1583*

Ticlopidine (tye KLOE pi deen)

U.S. Brand Names Ticlid® [DSC]

Canadian Brand Names Alti-Ticlopidine; Apo-Ticlopidine®; Gen-Ticlopidine; Novo-Ticlopidine; Nu-Ticlopidine; Rhoxal-ticlopidine; Sandoz-Ticlopidine; Ticlid®

Mexican Brand Names Ticlid

Index Terms Ticlopidine Hydrochloride

Pharmacologic Category Antiplatelet Agent

Use Platelet aggregation inhibitor that reduces the risk of thrombotic stroke in patients who have had a stroke or stroke precursors. **Note:** Due to its association with life-threatening hematologic disorders, ticlopidine should be reserved for patients who are intolerant to aspirin, or who have failed aspirin therapy. Adjunctive therapy (with aspirin) following successful coronary stent implantation to reduce the incidence of subacute stent thrombosis.

Unlabeled/Investigational Use Protection of aortocoronary bypass grafts, diabetic microangiopathy, ischemic heart disease, prevention of postoperative DVT, reduction of graft loss following renal transplant

Effect on Mental Status None reported

Effect on Psychiatric Treatment May cause neutropenia; use caution with clozapine and carbamazepine

Dosage Summary

Oral:

Children: Dosage not established

Adults: 250 mg twice daily with food

Dosage Forms Excipient information presented when available (limited, particularly for generics); consult specific product labeling. [DSC] = Discontinued product

Tablet, as hydrochloride: 250 mg

Ticlid®: 250 mg [DSC]

◆ **Ticlopidine Hydrochloride** *see* Ticlopidine *on page 1583*

◆ **Tigan®** *see* Trimethobenzamide *on page 1628*

Tigecycline (tye ge SYE kleen)

U.S. Brand Names Tygacil®

Mexican Brand Names Tygacil

Index Terms GAR-936

Pharmacologic Category Antibiotic, Glycylcycline

Use Treatment of complicated skin and skin structure infections caused by susceptible organisms, including methicillin-resistant *Staphylococcus aureus* and vancomycin-sensitive *Enterococcus faecalis*; treatment of complicated intra-abdominal infections

Effect on Mental Status May cause dizziness or insomnia

Effect on Psychiatric Treatment GI side effects are common; concomitant use with lithium, SSRIs, or valproic acid may produce additive effects

Dosage Summary

I.V.:

Children: Dosage not established

Adults: Initial: 100 mg as a single dose; Maintenance: 50 mg every 12 hours

Dosage Forms Excipient information presented when available (limited, particularly for generics); consult specific product labeling.

Injection, powder for reconstitution:

Tygacil®: 50 mg [contains lactose 100 mg]

◆ **Tikosyn®** *see* Dofetilide *on page 492*

◆ **Tilade® [DSC]** *see* Nedocromil *on page 1115*

◆ **Tilia™ Fe** *see* Ethinyl Estradiol and Norethindrone *on page 597*

Tiludronate (tye LOO droe nate)

Medication Safety Issues

International issues:

Skelid® may be confused with Skaelud® which is a brand name for pyrithione zinc in Denmark

U.S. Brand Names Skelid®

Index Terms Tiludronate Disodium

Pharmacologic Category Bisphosphonate Derivative

Use Treatment of Paget's disease of the bone (osteitis deformans) in patients who have a level of serum alkaline phosphatase (SAP) at least twice the upper limit of normal, or who are symptomatic, or who are at risk for future complications of their disease

Effect on Mental Status May cause dizziness, anxiety, or nervousness

Effect on Psychiatric Treatment None reported

Dosage Summary

Oral:

Children: Dosage not established

Adults: 400 mg once daily for 3 months

Dosage Forms Excipient information presented when available (limited, particularly for generics); consult specific product labeling.

Tablet, tiludronic acid:

Skelid®: 200 mg [equivalent to 240 mg tiludronate disodium]

◆ **Tiludronate Disodium** *see* Tiludronate *on page 1583*

◆ **Time-C [OTC]** *see* Ascorbic Acid *on page 141*

◆ **Time-C-Bio [OTC]** *see* Ascorbic Acid *on page 141*

◆ **Timentin®** *see* Ticarcillin and Clavulanate Potassium *on page 1582*

Timolol (TIM oh lol)

Medication Safety Issues

Sound-alike/look-alike issues:

Timolol may be confused with atenolol, Tylenol®

Timoptic® may be confused with Betoptic® S, Talacen®, Viroptic®

Bottle cap color change:

Timoptic®: Both the 0.25% and 0.5% strengths are now packaged in bottles with yellow caps; previously, the color of the cap on the product corresponded to different strengths.

International issues:

Betimol® may be confused with Betanol® which is a brand name for metipranolol in Monaco

Related Information

Beta-Blockers *on page 1776*

U.S. Brand Names Betimol®; Istalol®; Timolol GFS; Timoptic-XE®; Timoptic®; Timoptic® in OcuDose®

Canadian Brand Names Alti-Timolol; Apo-Timol®; Apo-Timop®; Gen-Timolol; Nu-Timolol; Phoxal-timolol; PMS-Timolol; Sandoz-Timolol; Tim-AK; Timoptic-XE®; Timoptic®

Mexican Brand Names Globitan; Horex; Imot Ofteno; Nyolol; Shemol; Timoptol; Timozzard

Index Terms Timolol Hemihydrate; Timolol Maleate

Pharmacologic Category Beta-Adrenergic Blocker, Nonselective; Ophthalmic Agent, Antiglaucoma

Use

Ophthalmic: Treatment of elevated intraocular pressure such as glaucoma or ocular hypertension

Oral: Treatment of hypertension and angina; to reduce mortality following myocardial infarction; prophylaxis of migraine

Effect on Mental Status May cause dizziness or fatigue; may rarely cause anxiety, depression, or hallucinations

Effect on Psychiatric Treatment Barbiturates and carbamazepine may decrease the effects of beta-blockers

Dosage Summary

Ophthalmic:

Gel-forming solution:

Children: Instill 1 drop (0.25% or 0.5%) once daily

Adults: Instill 1 drop (0.25% or 0.5%) once daily

Solution:

Children: Initial: Instill 1 drop (0.25%) twice daily; Maintenance: Instill 1 drop (0.25% or 0.5%) 1-2 times daily (maximum: 2 drops/day (0.5%)

Adults: Initial: Instill 1 drop (0.25%) twice daily; Maintenance: Instill 1 drop (0.25% or 0.5%) 1-2 times daily (maximum: 2 drops/day (0.5%)

Oral:

Children: Dosage not established

Adults: Initial: 10 mg twice daily; Maintenance: 20-60 mg/day in 2 divided doses (maximum: 60 mg/day)

Dosage Forms Excipient information presented when available (limited, particularly for generics); consult specific product labeling. [DSC] = Discontinued product

Note: Unless otherwise specified, strength expressed as base.

Gel-forming solution, ophthalmic, as maleate:

Timolol GFS: 0.25% (2.5 mL, 5 mL); 0.5% (2.5 mL, 5 mL)

Timoptic-XE®: 0.25% (5 mL); 0.5% (5 mL)

Solution, ophthalmic, as hemihydrate:

Betimol®: 0.25% (5 mL, 10 mL [DSC], 15 mL [DSC]); 0.5% (5 mL, 10 mL, 15 mL) [contains benzalkonium chloride]

Solution, ophthalmic, as maleate: 0.25% (5 mL, 10 mL, 15 mL); 0.5% (5 mL, 10 mL, 15 mL)

Istalol®: 0.5% (10 mL) [contains benzalkonium chloride and potassium sorbate]

Timoptic®: 0.25% (5 mL); 0.5% (5 mL, 10 mL) [contains benzalkonium chloride]

Solution, ophthalmic, as maleate [preservative free]:

Timoptic® in OcuDose®: 0.25% (0.2 mL); 0.5% (0.2 mL)

Tablet, as maleate: 5 mg, 10 mg, 20 mg [strength expressed as salt]

- **Timolol and Dorzolamide** *see* Dorzolamide and Timolol *on page 499*
- **Timolol GFS** *see* Timolol *on page 1584*
- **Timolol Hemihydrate** *see* Timolol *on page 1584*
- **Timolol Maleate** *see* Timolol *on page 1584*
- **Timoptic®** *see* Timolol *on page 1584*
- **Timoptic® in OcuDose®** *see* Timolol *on page 1584*
- **Timoptic-XE®** *see* Timolol *on page 1584*
- **Tinamed® Corn and Callus Remover [OTC]** *see* Salicylic Acid *on page 1454*
- **Tinamed® Wart Remover [OTC]** *see* Salicylic Acid *on page 1454*
- **Tindamax®** *see* Tinidazole *on page 1585*

Tinidazole (tye NI da zole)

U.S. Brand Names Tindamax®

Mexican Brand Names Estovit-T; Fasigyn; Induken

Pharmacologic Category Amebicide; Antibiotic, Miscellaneous; Antiprotozoal, Nitroimidazole

Use Treatment of trichomoniasis caused by *T. vaginalis*; treatment of giardiasis caused by *G. duodenalis* (*G. lamblia*); treatment of intestinal amebiasis and amebic liver abscess caused by *E. histolytica*; treatment of bacterial vaginosis caused by *Bacteroides* spp, *Gardnerella vaginalis*, and *Prevotella* spp in nonpregnant females

Effect on Mental Status May cause fatigue, malaise, ataxia, confusion, depression, giddiness, insomnia, and seizures

Effect on Psychiatric Treatment Bromocriptine, fluvoxamine, and nefazodone may increase levels of tinidazole; barbiturates, carbamazepine, oxcarbazepine, phenytoin, and fosphenytoin may decrease levels of tinidazole; monitor

Dosage Summary

Oral:

Children ≤3 years: Dosage not established

Children >3 years: 50 mg/kg/day (maximum: 2 g/day)

Adults: 1-2 g/day

Dosage Forms Excipient information presented when available (limited, particularly for generics); consult specific product labeling.

Tablet [scored]:

Tindamax®: 250 mg, 500 mg

Tinzaparin (tin ZA pa rin)

Medication Safety Issues

High alert medication: The Institute for Safe Medication Practices (ISMP) includes this medication among its list of drug classes which have a heightened risk of causing significant patient harm when used in error.

2009 National Patient Safety Goals: The Joint Commission on Accreditation of Healthcare Organizations requires healthcare organizations that provide anticoagulant therapy to have a process in place to reduce the risk of anticoagulant-associated patient harm. Patients receiving anticoagulants should receive individualized care through a defined process that includes standardized ordering, dispensing, administration, monitoring and education. This does not apply to routine short-term use of anticoagulants for prevention of venous thromboembolism when the expectation is that the patient's laboratory values will remain within or close to normal values (NPSG.03.05.01).

U.S. Brand Names Innohep®

Canadian Brand Names Innohep®

Index Terms Tinzaparin Sodium

Pharmacologic Category Low Molecular Weight Heparin

Use Treatment of acute symptomatic deep vein thrombosis, with or without pulmonary embolism, in conjunction with warfarin sodium

Effect on Mental Status May cause insomnia, confusion, or dizziness

Effect on Psychiatric Treatment May rarely cause agranulocytosis; use caution with clozapine and carbamazepine

Dosage Summary

SubQ:

Children: Dosage not established

Adults: 175 anti-Xa int. units/kg of body weight once daily

Dosage Forms Excipient information presented when available (limited, particularly for generics); consult specific product labeling.

Injection, solution, as sodium:

Innohep®: 20,000 anti-Xa int. units/mL (2 mL) [contains benzyl alcohol and sodium metabisulfite]

◆ **Tinzaparin Sodium** *see* Tinzaparin *on page 1585*

◆ **Tioguanine** *see* Thioguanine *on page 1569*

◆ **Tiotixene** *see* Thiothixene *on page 1576*

Tipranavir (tip RA na veer)

U.S. Brand Names Aptivus®

Canadian Brand Names Aptivus®

Mexican Brand Names Aptivus

Index Terms PNU-140690E; TPV

Pharmacologic Category Antiretroviral Agent, Protease Inhibitor

Use Treatment of HIV-1 infections in combination with ritonavir and other antiretroviral agents; limited to highly treatment-experienced or multiprotease inhibitor-resistant patients.

Effect on Mental Status May cause fatigue and depression

Effect on Psychiatric Treatment Contraindicated with midazolam, pimozide, and triazolam. May cause hyperlipidemia and hyperglycemia; concurrent use with atypical antipsychotics, valproic acid, and carbamazepine may produce additive effects; monitor. Use caution with disulfiram (capsules contain dehydrated ethanol). Carbamazepine may decrease serum concentration of tipranavir. The effect of methadone may be reduced by tipranavir requiring a dosage adjustment.

Dosage Summary

Oral:

Children <2 years: Dosage not established

Children ≥2 years: 12-14 mg/kg or 290-375 mg/m^2 (maximum: 500 mg/dose) twice daily

Adults: 500 mg twice daily

Dosage Forms Excipient information presented when available (limited, particularly for generics); consult specific product labeling.

Capsule, soft gelatin:

Aptivus®: 250 mg [contains dehydrated ethanol 7% per capsule]

Solution:

Aptivus®: 100 mg/mL (95 mL) [contains vitamin E, propylene glycol; buttermint-butter toffee flavor]

Tirofiban (tye roe FYE ban)

Medication Safety Issues

Sound-alike/look-alike issues:

Aggrastat® may be confused with Aggrenox®, argatroban

High alert medication: The Institute for Safe Medication Practices (ISMP) includes this medication among its list of drugs which have a heightened risk of causing significant patient harm when used in error.

U.S. Brand Names Aggrastat®

Canadian Brand Names Aggrastat®
Mexican Brand Names Agrastat
Index Terms MK383; Tirofiban Hydrochloride
Pharmacologic Category Antiplatelet Agent, Glycoprotein IIb/IIIa Inhibitor
Use In combination with heparin, is indicated for the treatment of acute coronary syndrome, including patients who are to be managed medically and those undergoing PTCA or atherectomy. In this setting, it has been shown to decrease the rate of a combined endpoint of death, new myocardial infarction or refractory ischemia/repeat cardiac procedure.
Effect on Mental Status May cause dizziness
Effect on Psychiatric Treatment Contraindicated in patients with a recent stroke (within 30 days)
Dosage Summary
I.V.:
Children: Dosage not established
Adults: Initial: 0.4 mcg/kg/minute for 30 minutes; Maintenance infusion: 0.1 mcg/kg/minute
Dosage Forms Excipient information presented when available (limited, particularly for generics); consult specific product labeling. [DSC] = Discontinued product
Infusion [premixed in sodium chloride]:
Aggrastat®: 50 mcg/mL (100 mL, 250 mL)
Injection, solution:
Aggrastat®: 250 mcg/mL (50 mL) [DSC]

◆ **Tirofiban Hydrochloride** *see* Tirofiban *on page 1586*
◆ **Tirosint™** *see* Levothyroxine *on page 920*
◆ **Titralac™ [OTC]** *see* Calcium Carbonate *on page 254*

TiZANidine (tye ZAN i deen)

Medication Safety Issues
Sound-alike/look-alike issues:
TiZANidine may be confused with tiaGABine
Zanaflex® capsules and Zanaflex® tablets (or generic tizanidine tablets) are not interchangeable
U.S. Brand Names Zanaflex Capsules™; Zanaflex®
Canadian Brand Names Apo-Tizanidine®; Gen-Tizanidine; Zanaflex®
Mexican Brand Names Sirdalud
Index Terms Sirdalud®
Pharmacologic Category Alpha$_2$-Adrenergic Agonist
Generic Available Yes: Tablet
Use Skeletal muscle relaxant used for treatment of muscle spasticity
Unlabeled/Investigational Use Tension headaches, low back pain, and trigeminal neuralgia
Effect on Mental Status Drowsiness is common; may cause dizziness, anxiety, nervousness, or insomnia; may rarely cause psychosis
Effect on Psychiatric Treatment Concurrent use with psychotropics may produce additive sedation and dry mouth
Pregnancy Risk Factor C
Lactation Excretion in breast milk unknown/not recommended
Contraindications Hypersensitivity to tizanidine or any component of the formulation; concomitant therapy with ciprofloxacin or fluvoxamine (potent CYP1A2 inhibitors)
Warnings/Precautions Significant hypotension (possibly with bradycardia or orthostatic hypotension) and sedation may occur; use caution in patients with cardiac disease or those at risk for severe hypotensive or sedative effects. Avoid concomitant administration with CYP1A2 inhibitors; increased tizanidine levels/effects (severe hypotension and sedation) may occur. These effects may also be increased with concomitant administration with other CNS depressants and/or antihypertensives; use caution. Elderly patients are at risk due to decreased clearance, particulary in elderly patients with renal insufficiency (Cl_{cr} <25 mL/minute) compared to healthy elderly subjects; this may lead to an increased risk of adverse effects and/or a longer duration of effects. Use caution in any patient with renal impairment; reduced initial doses recommended in patient with Cl_{cr} <25 mL/minute. Use with extreme caution or avoid in hepatic impairment due to extensive hepatic metabolism and potential hepatotoxicity; AST/ALT elevations (≥2 times baseline) and rarely hepatic failure have occurred; monitoring recommended.

Use has been associated with visual hallucinations or delusions, generally in first 6 weeks of therapy; use caution in patients with psychiatric disorders. Withdrawal resulting in rebound hypertension, tachycardia, and hypertonia may occur upon discontinuation; doses should be decreased slowly, particularly in patients receiving high doses for prolonged periods. Pharmacokinetics and bioequivalence between capsules and tablets altered by nonfasting vs fasting conditions. Limited data exists for chronic use of single doses >8 mg and multiple doses >24 mg/day. Safety and efficacy have not been established in children.

Adverse Reactions Frequency percentages below reported during multiple-dose studies, unless specified otherwise.

>10%:

Cardiovascular: Hypotension (single-dose study with doses ≥8 mg: 16% to 33%)

Central nervous system: Somnolence (48%), dizziness (16%)

Gastrointestinal: Xerostomia (49%)

Neuromuscular & skeletal: Weakness (41%)

1% to 10%:

Cardiovascular: Bradycardia (single-dose study with doses ≥8 mg: 2% to 10%)

Central nervous system: Nervousness (3%), speech disorder (3%), visual hallucinations/delusions (3%; generally occurring in first 6 weeks of therapy), anxiety (1%), depression (1%), fever (1%)

Dermatologic: Rash (1%), skin ulcer (1%)

Gastrointestinal: Constipation (4%), vomiting (3%), abdominal pain (1%), diarrhea (1%), dyspepsia (1%)

Genitourinary: UTI (10%), urinary frequency (3%)

Hepatic: Liver enzymes increased (3% to 5%)

Neuromuscular & skeletal: Dyskinesia (3%), back pain (1%), myasthenia (1%), paresthesia (1%)

Ocular: Blurred vision (3%)

Respiratory: Pharyngitis (3%), rhinitis (3%)

Miscellaneous: Infection (6%), flu-like syndrome (3%), diaphoresis (1%)

<1%, frequency not defined, and postmarketing experience (limited to important or life-threatening): Adrenal insufficiency, allergic reaction, anemia, angina, arrhythmia, carcinoma, cholelithiasis, deafness, dementia, dyslipidemia, gastrointestinal hemorrhage, glaucoma, heart failure, hepatomegaly, hemiplegia, hepatic failure, hepatitis, hepatoma, hyperglycemia, hypokalemia, hyponatremia, hypoproteinemia, hypothyroidism, jaundice, leukopenia, leukocytosis, MI, optic neuritis, palpitation, postural hypotension, psychotic-like symptoms, pulmonary embolus, respiratory acidosis, retinal hemorrhage, sepsis, suicide attempt, syncope, thrombocythemia, thrombocytopenia, ventricular extrasystoles, ventricular tachycardia

Metabolism/Transport Effects **Substrate** of CYP1A2 (major)

Drug Interactions

Alcohol (Ethyl): CNS Depressants may enhance the CNS depressant effect of Alcohol (Ethyl). *Risk C: Monitor therapy*

Antidepressants (Alpha2-Antagonist): May diminish the hypotensive effect of Alpha2-Agonists. *Risk D: Consider therapy modification*

Beta-Blockers: May enhance the rebound hypertensive effect of Alpha2-Agonists. This effect can occur when the alpha$_2$-agonist is abruptly withdrawn. **Exceptions:** Levobunolol; Metipranolol. *Risk D: Consider therapy modification*

Ciprofloxacin: May decrease the metabolism of TiZANidine. *Risk X: Avoid combination*

CNS Depressants: May enhance the adverse/toxic effect of other CNS Depressants. *Risk C: Monitor therapy*

CYP1A2 Inhibitors (Moderate): May decrease the metabolism of CYP1A2 Substrates. *Risk C: Monitor therapy*

CYP1A2 Inhibitors (Strong): May decrease the metabolism of CYP1A2 Substrates. *Risk D: Consider therapy modification*

Diazoxide: May enhance the hypotensive effect of Antihypertensives. *Risk C: Monitor therapy*

Fluvoxamine: May decrease the metabolism of TiZANidine. *Risk X: Avoid combination*

Herbs (Hypertensive Properties): May diminish the antihypertensive effect of Antihypertensives. *Risk C: Monitor therapy*

Herbs (Hypotensive Properties): May enhance the hypotensive effect of Antihypertensives. *Risk C: Monitor therapy*

Methylphenidate: May diminish the antihypertensive effect of Antihypertensives. *Risk C: Monitor therapy*

Oral Contraceptive (Estrogens): May increase the serum concentration of TiZANidine. *Risk C: Monitor therapy*

Prostacyclin Analogues: May enhance the hypotensive effect of Antihypertensives. *Risk C: Monitor therapy*

RiTUXimab: Antihypertensives may enhance the hypotensive effect of RiTUXimab. *Risk D: Consider therapy modification*

Tricyclic Antidepressants: May diminish the antihypertensive effect of Alpha2-Agonists. *Risk D: Consider therapy modification*

Ethanol/Nutrition/Herb Interactions

Ethanol: Avoid ethanol (may increase CNS depression).

Food: The tablet and capsule dosage forms are not bioequivalent when administered with food. Food increases both the time to peak concentration and the extent of absorption for both the tablet and capsule. However, maximal concentrations of tizanidine achieved when administered with food were increased by 30% for the tablet, but decreased by 20% for the capsule. Under fed conditions, the capsule is approximately 80% bioavailable relative to the tablet.

Herb/Nutraceutical: Avoid valerian, St John's wort, kava kava, gotu kola (may increase CNS depression). Avoid black cohosh, California poppy, coleus, golden seal, hawthorn, mistletoe, periwinkle, quinine, shepherd's purse (may increase hypotensive effects).

Mechanism of Action An alpha$_2$-adrenergic agonist agent which decreases excitatory input to alpha motor neurons; an imidazole derivative chemically-related to clonidine, which acts as a centrally acting muscle relaxant with alpha$_2$-adrenergic agonist properties; acts on the level of the spinal cord

Pharmacodynamics/Kinetics

Duration: 3-6 hours

Absorption: Tablets and capsules are bioequivalent under fasting conditions, but not under nonfasting conditions.

Tablets administered with food: Peak plasma concentration is increased by ~30%; time to peak increased by 25 minutes; extent of absorption increased by ~30%.

Capsules administered with food: Peak plasma concentration decreased by 20%; time to peak increased by 2-3 hours; extent of absorption increased by ~10%.

Capsules opened and sprinkled on applesauce are not bioequivalent to administration of intact capsules under fasting conditions. Peak plasma concentration and AUC are increased by 15% to 20%.

Protein binding: ~30%

Metabolism: Extensively hepatic

Bioavailability: ~40% (extensive first-pass metabolism)

Half-life elimination: 2.5 hours

Time to peak, serum:

Fasting state: Capsule, tablet: 1 hour

Fed state: Capsule: 3-4 hours, Tablet: 1.5 hours

Excretion: Urine (60%); feces (20%)

Dosage

Adults: 2-4 mg 3 times/day

Usual initial dose: 4 mg, may increase by 2-4 mg as needed for satisfactory reduction of muscle tone every 6-8 hours to a maximum of 3 doses in any 24-hour period

Maximum: 36 mg/day

Elderly: No specific dosing guidelines exist; clearance is decreased; dose cautiously

Dosing adjustment in renal impairment: Cl_{cr} <25 mL/minute: Use with caution; clearance reduced >50%. During initial dose titration, use reduced doses. If higher doses necessary, increase dose instead of increasing dosing frequency.

Dosing adjustment in hepatic impairment: Avoid use in hepatic impairment; if used, lowest possible dose should be used initially with close monitoring for adverse effects (eg, hypotension).

Dietary Considerations Administration with food compared to administration in the fasting state results in clinically-significant differences in absorption and other pharmacokinetic parameters. Patients should be consistent and should not switch administration of the tablets or the capsules between the fasting and nonfasting state. In addition, switching between the capsules and the tablets in the fed state will also result in significant differences. Opening capsule contents to sprinkle on applesauce compared to swallowing intact capsules whole will also result in significant absorption differences. Patients should be consistent with regards to administration.

Administration Capsules may be opened and contents sprinkled on food; however, extent of absorption is increased up to 20% relative to administration of the capsule under fasted conditions.

Monitoring Parameters Monitor liver function (aminotransferases) at baseline, 1, 3, 6 months and periodically thereafter; blood pressure; renal function

Dosage Forms Excipient information presented when available (limited, particularly for generics); consult specific product labeling.

Capsule:

Zanaflex Capsules™: 2 mg, 4 mg, 6 mg

Tablet: 2 mg, 4 mg

Zanaflex®: 2 mg [DSC], 4 mg [scored]

- ◆ **TMC-114** *see* Darunavir *on page 420*
- ◆ **TMC125** *see* Etravirine *on page 608*
- ◆ **TMP** *see* Trimethoprim *on page 1629*
- ◆ **TMP-SMZ** *see* Sulfamethoxazole and Trimethoprim *on page 1517*
- ◆ **TMZ** *see* Temozolomide *on page 1547*
- ◆ **TNKase®** *see* Tenecteplase *on page 1548*
- ◆ **TOBI®** *see* Tobramycin *on page 1590*

Tobramycin (toe bra MYE sin)

Medication Safety Issues

Sound-alike/look-alike issues:

Tobramycin may be confused with Trobicin®, vancomycin

AKTob® may be confused with AK-Trol®

Nebcin® may be confused with Inapsine®, Naprosyn®, Nubain®

Tobrex® may be confused with TobraDex®

High alert medication: The Institute for Safe Medication Practices (ISMP) includes this medication (intrathecal administration) among its list of drug classes which have a heightened risk of causing significant patient harm when used in error.

U.S. Brand Names AKTob®; TOBI®; Tobrex®

Canadian Brand Names PMS-Tobramycin; Sandoz-Tobramycin; TOBI®; Tobramycin Injection, USP; Tobrex®

Mexican Brand Names Micitrex; Tobi; Verbram

Index Terms Tobramycin Sulfate

Pharmacologic Category Antibiotic, Aminoglycoside; Antibiotic, Ophthalmic

Use Treatment of documented or suspected infections caused by susceptible gram-negative bacilli including *Pseudomonas aeruginosa*; topically used to treat superficial ophthalmic infections caused by susceptible bacteria. Tobramycin solution for inhalation is indicated for the management of cystic fibrosis patients (>6 years of age) with *Pseudomonas aeruginosa*.

Effect on Mental Status May cause drowsiness

Effect on Psychiatric Treatment None reported

Dosage Summary

I.M.:

Infants: 2.5 mg/kg every 8 hours

Children <5 years: 2.5 mg/kg every 8 hours

Children ≥5 years: 2-3.3 mg/kg every 6-8 hours

Adults: 1-2.5 mg/kg every 8-12 hours (1 mg/kg used for synergy) **or** 4-7 mg/kg/day as a single daily dose

Elderly: 1.5-5 mg/kg/day in 1-2 divided doses

I.V.:

Infants: 2.5 mg/kg every 8 hours

Children <5 years: 2.5 mg/kg every 8 hours

Children ≥5 years: 2-3.3 mg/kg every 6-8 hours

Adults: 1-2.5 mg/kg every 8-12 hours (1 mg/kg/dose used for synergy) **or** 4-7 mg/kg/day as a single daily dose

Elderly: 1.5-5 mg/kg/day in 1-2 divided doses **or** 5-7 mg/kg given every 24, 36, or 48 hours based on Cl_{cr}

Inhalation:

Children <6 years: Dosage not established

Children ≥6 years: 300 mg every 12 hours [TOBI®]

Adults: 300 mg every 12 hours [TOBI®]

Ophthalmic:

Ointment:

Children <2 months: Dosage not established

Children ≥2 months: Apply 2-3 times/day; for severe infections, apply every 3-4 hours
Adults: Apply 2-3 times/day; for severe infections, apply every 3-4 hours
Solution:
Children <2 months: Dosage not established
Children ≥2 months: Instill 1-2 drops every 4 hours
Adults: Instill 1-2 drops every 4 hours

Dosage Forms Excipient information presented when available (limited, particularly for generics); consult specific product labeling.
Infusion [premixed in NS]: 60 mg (50 mL); 80 mg (100 mL)
Injection, powder for reconstitution: 1.2 g
Injection, solution: 10 mg/mL (2 mL, 8 mL); 40 mg/mL (2 mL, 30 mL, 50 mL) [may contain sodium metabisulfite]
Ointment, ophthalmic (Tobrex®): 0.3% (3.5 g)
Solution for nebulization [preservative free] (TOBI®): 60 mg/mL (5 mL)
Solution, ophthalmic (AKTob®, Tobrex®): 0.3% (5 mL) [contains benzalkonium chloride]

◆ **Tobramycin Sulfate** *see* Tobramycin *on page 1590*
◆ **Tobrex®** *see* Tobramycin *on page 1590*

Tocainide (TOE kay nide)

Medication Safety Issues
Sound-alike/look-alike issues:
Tonocard® may be confused with Torecan®

U.S. Brand Names Tonocard® [DSC]

Index Terms Tocainide Hydrochloride

Pharmacologic Category Antiarrhythmic Agent, Class Ib

Use Suppression and prevention of symptomatic life-threatening ventricular arrhythmias

Unlabeled/Investigational Use Trigeminal neuralgia

Effect on Mental Status Dizziness is common; may cause nervousness or confusion

Effect on Psychiatric Treatment May cause agranulocytosis; use caution with clozapine and carbamazepine; barbiturates may decrease the serum levels of tocainide

Dosage Summary
Oral:
Children: Dosage not established
Adults: 1200-2400 mg/day in 3 divided doses (maximum: 2400 mg/day)

Dosage Forms Excipient information presented when available (limited, particularly for generics); consult specific product labeling. [DSC] = Discontinued product
Tablet, as hydrochloride [DSC]: 400 mg, 600 mg

◆ **Tocainide Hydrochloride** *see* Tocainide *on page 1591*
◆ **Tofranil®** *see* Imipramine *on page 812*
◆ **Tofranil-PM®** *see* Imipramine *on page 812*

TOLAZamide (tole AZ a mide)

Medication Safety Issues
Sound-alike/look-alike issues:
TOLAZamide may be confused with tolazoline, TOLBUTamide
Tolinase® may be confused with Orinase®

High alert medication: The Institute for Safe Medication Practices (ISMP) includes this medication among its list of drugs which have a heightened risk of causing significant patient harm when used in error.

Canadian Brand Names Tolinase®

Pharmacologic Category Antidiabetic Agent, Sulfonylurea

Use Adjunct to diet for the management of mild to moderately severe, stable, type 2 diabetes mellitus (noninsulin dependent, NIDDM)

Effect on Mental Status Dizziness is common

Effect on Psychiatric Treatment May cause agranulocytosis; use caution with clozapine and carbamazepine; concurrent use with psychotropics may produce alterations in serum glucose concentrations; monitor glucose; clinical manifestation of hypoglycemia may be blocked by beta-blockers

Dosage Summary

Oral:

Children: Dosage not established

Adults: Initial: 100-250 mg/day with first main meal of day; Maintenance: 100-1000 mg/day in 1-2 (doses >500 mg) divided doses (maximum: 1 g/day); **Note:** Titration is recommended

Dosage Forms Excipient information presented when available (limited, particularly for generics); consult specific product labeling.

Tablet: 250 mg, 500 mg

Tolazoline (tole AZ oh leen)

Medication Safety Issues

Sound-alike/look-alike issues:

Tolazoline may be confused with TOLAZamide

Priscoline® may be confused with Apresoline®

U.S. Brand Names Priscoline® [DSC]

Index Terms Benzazoline Hydrochloride; Tolazoline Hydrochloride

Pharmacologic Category Vasodilator

Use Treatment of persistent pulmonary vasoconstriction and hypertension of the newborn (persistent fetal circulation), peripheral vasospastic disorders

Effect on Mental Status None reported

Effect on Psychiatric Treatment May cause agranulocytosis, caution with clozapine and carbamazepine; use with ethanol may produce "disulfiram reaction"

Dosage Summary

I.M.:

Children: Dosage not established

Adults: 10-50 mg 4 times/day

I.V.:

Neonates: Initial: 1-2 mg/kg over 10-15 minutes; Maintenance: 1-2 mg/kg/hour **or** 0.25 mg/kg/hour (maximum: 6-8 mg/kg/hour)

Children: Dosage not established

Adults: 10-50 mg 4 times/day

SubQ:

Children: Dosage not established

Adults: 10-50 mg 4 times/day

Dosage Forms Excipient information presented when available (limited, particularly for generics); consult specific product labeling. [DSC] = Discontinued product

Injection, solution, as hydrochloride [DSC]: 25 mg/mL (4 mL)

◆ **Tolazoline Hydrochloride** *see* Tolazoline *on page 1592*

TOLBUTamide (tole BYOO ta mide)

Medication Safety Issues

Sound-alike/look-alike issues:

TOLBUTamide may be confused with terbutaline, TOLAZamide

Orinase® may be confused with Orabase®, Ornex®, Tolinase®

High alert medication: The Institute for Safe Medication Practices (ISMP) includes this medication among its list of drugs which have a heightened risk of causing significant patient harm when used in error.

Canadian Brand Names Apo-Tolbutamide®

Mexican Brand Names Artosin; Rastinon

Index Terms Tolbutamide Sodium

Pharmacologic Category Antidiabetic Agent, Sulfonylurea

Use Adjunct to diet for the management of type 2 diabetes mellitus (noninsulin dependent, NIDDM)

Effect on Mental Status Dizziness is common

Effect on Psychiatric Treatment May cause agranulocytosis; use caution with clozapine and carbamazepine; concurrent use with psychotropics may produce alterations in serum glucose concentrations; monitor glucose; clinical manifestation of hypoglycemia may be blocked by beta-blockers

Dosage Summary

Oral:

Children: Dosage not established

Adults: Initial: 1-2 g/day as a single dose or divided doses throughout the day; Maintenance: 0.25-3 g/day as a single dose or divided doses throughout the day

Elderly: Initial: 250 mg 1-3 times/day; Maintenance: 500-2000 mg/day in 1-3 divided doses (maximum: 3 g/day)

Dosage Forms Excipient information presented when available (limited, particularly for generics); consult specific product labeling.
Tablet: 500 mg

◆ **Tolbutamide Sodium** *see* TOLBUTamide *on page 1592*

Tolcapone (TOLE ka pone)

Related Information
Antiparkinsonian Agents *on page 1767*

U.S. Brand Names Tasmar®

Mexican Brand Names Tasmar

Pharmacologic Category Anti-Parkinson's Agent, COMT Inhibitor

Generic Available No

Use Adjunct to levodopa and carbidopa for the treatment of signs and symptoms of idiopathic Parkinson's disease in patients with motor fluctuations not responsive to other therapies

Restrictions A patient signed consent form acknowledging the risks of hepatic injury should be obtained by the treating physician.

Pregnancy Risk Factor C

Pregnancy Considerations Tolcapone may be teratogenic based on animal studies. There are no adequate and well-controlled studies in pregnant women. Use only if benefit outweighs risk.

Lactation Excretion in breast milk unknown/not recommended

Contraindications Hypersensitivity to tolcapone or any component of the formulation; history of liver disease or tolcapone-induced hepatocellular injury; nontraumatic rhabdomyolysis or hyperpyrexia and confusion

Warnings/Precautions **[U.S. Boxed Warning]: Due to reports of fatal liver injury associated with use of this drug, the manufacturer is advising that tolcapone be reserved for patients who are experiencing inadequate symptom control or who are not appropriate candidates for other available treatments.** Patients must provide written consent acknowledging the risks of hepatic injury. Liver disease should be excluded prior to initiation; laboratory monitoring is recommended. Discontinue if signs and/or symptoms of hepatic injury are noted (eg, transaminases >2 times upper limit of normal) or if clinical improvement is not evident after 3 weeks of therapy. Use with caution in patients with pre-existing dyskinesias; exacerbation of pre-existing dyskinesia and severe rhabdomyolysis has been reported. Levodopa dosage reduction may be required, particularly in patients with levodopa dosages >600 mg daily or with moderate-to-severe dyskinesia prior to initiation.

May cause orthostatic hypotension and syncope; Parkinson's disease patients appear to have an impaired capacity to respond to a postural challenge; use with caution in patients at risk of hypotension (such as those receiving antihypertensive drugs) or where transient hypotensive episodes would be poorly tolerated (cardiovascular disease or cerebrovascular disease). Parkinson's patients being treated with dopaminergic agonists ordinarily require careful monitoring for signs and symptoms of postural hypotension, especially during dose escalation, and should be informed of this risk. May cause hallucinations, which may improve with reduction in levodopa therapy. Use with caution in patients with lower gastrointestinal disease or an increased risk of dehydration; tolcapone has been associated with delayed development of diarrhea (onset after 2-12 weeks).

Tolcapone, in conjunction with other drug therapy that alters brain biogenic amine concentrations (eg, MAO inhibitors, SSRIs), has been associated with a syndrome resembling neuroleptic malignant syndrome (hyperpyrexia and confusion - some fatal) on abrupt withdrawal or dosage reduction. Concomitant use of tolcapone and nonselective MAO inhibitors should be avoided. Selegiline is a selective MAO type B inhibitor (when given orally at ≤10 mg/day) and can be taken with tolcapone. Dopaminergic agents from the ergot class have also been associated with fibrotic complications, such as retroperitoneal fibrosis, pulmonary infiltrates or effusion and pleural thickening. It is unknown whether non-ergot, pro-dopaminergic agents like tolcapone confer this risk. Use caution in patients with hepatic impairment or severe renal impairment. Safety and efficacy in pediatric patients have not been established.

Adverse Reactions
>10%:
Cardiovascular: Orthostatic hypotension (17%)

Central nervous system: Sleep disorder (24% to 25%), excessive dreaming (16% to 21%), somnolence (14% to 32%), hallucinations (8% to 24%) dizziness (6% to 13%), headache (10% to 11%), confusion (10% to 11%)
Gastrointestinal: Nausea (28% to 50%), anorexia (19% to 23%), diarrhea (16% to 34%; approximately 3% to 4% severe)
Neuromuscular & skeletal: Dyskinesia (42% to 51%), dystonia (19% to 22%), muscle cramps (17% to 18%)

1% to 10%:
Cardiovascular: Syncope (4% to 5%), chest pain (1% to 3%), hypotension (2%), palpitation
Central nervous system: Fatigue (3% to 7%), loss of balance (2% to 3%), agitation (1%), euphoria (1%), hyperactivity (1%), malaise (1%), panic reaction (1%), irritability (1%), mental deficiency (1%), fever (1%), depression, hypoesthesia, tremor, speech disorder, vertigo, emotional lability, hyperkinesia
Dermatologic: Alopecia (1%), bleeding (1%), tumor (1%), rash
Gastrointestinal: Vomiting (8% to 10%), constipation (6% to 8%), xerostomia (5% to 6%), abdominal pain (5% to 6%), dyspepsia (3% to 4%), flatulence (2% to 4%), tooth disorder
Genitourinary: UTI (5%), hematuria (4% to 5%), urine discoloration (2% to 3%), urination disorder (1% to 2%), uterine tumor (1%), incontinence, impotence
Hepatic: Transaminases increased (1% to 3%; 3 times ULN, usually with first 6 months of therapy)
Neuromuscular & skeletal: Paresthesia (1% to 3%), hyper-/hypokinesia (1% to 3%), arthritis (1% to 2%), neck pain (2%), stiffness (2%), myalgia, rhabdomyolysis
Ocular: Cataract (1%), eye inflammation (1%)
Otic: Tinnitus
Respiratory: Upper respiratory infection (5% to 7%), dyspnea (3%), sinus congestion (1% to 2%), bronchitis, pharyngitis
Miscellaneous: Diaphoresis (4% to 7%), influenza (3% to 4%), burning (1% to 2%), flank pain, injury, infection

<1% (Limited to important or life-threatening): Abnormal stools, abscess, allergic reaction, amnesia, anemia, antisocial reaction, apathy, apnea, arteriosclerosis, arthrosis, asthma, bladder calculus, breast neoplasm, carcinoma, cardiovascular disorder, cellulitis, cerebral ischemia, cerebrovascular accident, chills, cholecystitis, cholelithiasis, choreoathetosis, colitis, cough increased, death, dehydration, delirium, delusions, diabetes mellitus, diplopia, duodenal ulcer, dysphagia, dysuria, ear pain, eczema, edema, encephalopathy, epistaxis, erythema multiforme, esophagitis, extrapyramidal syndrome, eye hemorrhage, eye pain, facial edema, furunculosis, gastroenteritis, gastrointestinal carcinoma, gastrointestinal hemorrhage, glaucoma, hemiplegia, hernia, herpes simplex, herpes zoster, hiccup, hostility, hypercholesteremia, hyperventilation, hypoxia, infection (bacterial), infection (fungal), joint disorder, kidney calculus, lacrimation disorder, laryngitis, leukemia, libido changes, lung edema, manic reaction, meningitis, mouth ulceration, myoclonus, neoplasm, nervousness, neuralgia, neuropathy, nocturia, oliguria, otitis media, ovarian carcinoma, pain, paranoid reaction, parosmia, pericardial effusion, polyuria, prostatic carcinoma, prostatic disorder, pruritus, psychosis, rectal disorder, rhinitis, salivation increased, seborrhea, skin discoloration, skin disorder, stomach atony, surgical procedure, tenosynovitis, thinking abnormal, thirst, thrombocytopenia, thrombosis, tongue disorder, twitching, urinary retention, urinary tract disorder, urticaria, uterine atony, uterine disorder, uterine hemorrhage, vaginitis, viral infection

Metabolism/Transport Effects Inhibits CYP2C9 (weak)

Drug Interactions

Alcohol (Ethyl): CNS Depressants may enhance the CNS depressant effect of Alcohol (Ethyl). *Risk C: Monitor therapy*
CNS Depressants: May enhance the adverse/toxic effect of other CNS Depressants. *Risk C: Monitor therapy*
COMT Substrates: COMT Inhibitors may decrease the metabolism of COMT Substrates. *Risk C: Monitor therapy*
MAO Inhibitors: COMT Inhibitors may enhance the adverse/toxic effect of MAO Inhibitors. *Risk D: Consider therapy modification*

Ethanol/Nutrition/Herb Interactions

Ethanol: Avoid ethanol (may increase CNS depression).
Food: Tolcapone, taken with food within 1 hour before or 2 hours after the dose, decreases bioavailability by 10% to 20%.
Avoid valerian, St John's wort, kava kava, gotu kola (may increase CNS depression).

Stability Store at 20°C to 25°C (68°F to 77°F).

Mechanism of Action Tolcapone is a selective and reversible inhibitor of catechol-o-methyltransferase (COMT). In the presence of a decarboxylase inhibitor (eg, carbidopa), COMT is the major degradation pathway for levodopa. Inhibition of COMT leads to more sustained plasma levels of levodopa and enhanced central dopaminergic activity.

Pharmacodynamics/Kinetics

Absorption: Rapid

Distribution: 9 L

Protein binding: >99.0%

Metabolism: Hepatic, via glucuronidation, to inactive metabolite (>99%)

Bioavailability: 65%

Half-life elimination: 2-3 hours

Time to peak: ~2 hours

Excretion: Urine (60% as metabolites, 0.5% as unchanged drug); feces (40%)

Dosage Note: If clinical improvement is not observed after 3 weeks of therapy (regardless of dose), tolcapone treatment should be discontinued.

Oral: Adults: Initial: 100 mg 3 times/day; may increase as tolerated to 200 mg 3 times/day. **Note:** Levodopa dose may need to be decreased upon initiation of tolcapone (average reduction in clinical trials was 30%). As many as 70% of patients receiving levodopa doses >600 mg daily required levodopa dosage reduction in clinical trials. Patients with moderate-to-severe dyskinesia prior to initiation are also more likely to require dosage reduction.

Dosage adjustment in renal impairment: No adjustment necessary for mild-moderate impairment. Use caution with severe impairment; no safety information available in patients with Cl_{cr}<25 mL/minute.

Dosage adjustment in hepatic impairment: Do not use. Discontinue immediately if signs/symptoms of hepatic impairment develop.

Dietary Considerations May be taken without regard to food.

Administration May be administered with or without food. In clinical studies, the first dose of the day was administered with carbidopa/levodopa, and the subsequent doses were administered 6 hours and 12 hours later.

Monitoring Parameters Blood pressure, symptoms of Parkinson's disease, liver enzymes at baseline and then every 2-4 weeks for the first 6 months of therapy; thereafter, periodic monitoring should be conducted as deemed clinically relevant. If the dose is increased to 200 mg 3 times/day, reinitiate LFT monitoring every 2-4 weeks for 6 months, and then resume periodic monitoring. Discontinue therapy if the ALT or AST exceeds 2 times ULN or if the clinical signs and symptoms suggest the onset of liver failure.

Dosage Forms Excipient information presented when available (limited, particularly for generics); consult specific product labeling.

Tablet:

Tasmar®: 100 mg, 200 mg

◆ **Tolectin** *see* Tolmetin *on page 1595*

Tolmetin (TOLE met in)

Related Information

Nonsteroidal Anti-Inflammatory Agents *on page 1792*

Mexican Brand Names Tolectín

Index Terms Tolectin; Tolmetin Sodium

Pharmacologic Category Nonsteroidal Anti-inflammatory Drug (NSAID), Oral

Use Treatment of rheumatoid arthritis and osteoarthritis, juvenile rheumatoid arthritis

Effect on Mental Status Dizziness is common; may cause nervousness; may rarely cause drowsiness, confusion, insomnia, hallucinations, or depression

Effect on Psychiatric Treatment May rarely cause agranulocytosis; use caution with clozapine and carbamazepine; may decrease lithium clearance resulting in an increase in serum lithium levels and potential lithium toxicity; monitor serum lithium levels

Restrictions An FDA-approved medication guide must be distributed when dispensing an oral outpatient prescription (new or refill) where this medication is to be used without direct supervision of a healthcare provider. Medication guides are available at http://www.fda.gov/cder/Offices/ODS/medication_guides.htm.

Dosage Summary

Oral:

Children <2 years: Dosage not established

Children ≥2 years: Initial: 20 mg/kg/day in 3-4 divided doses; Maintenance: 15-30 mg/kg/day in 3-4 divided doses (maximum 30 mg/kg/day)

Adults: Initial: 400 mg 3 times/day; Maintenance: 600-1800 mg/day in 3 divided doses (maximum: 1.8 g/day)

Dosage Forms Excipient information presented when available (limited, particularly for generics); consult specific product labeling.

Capsule: 400 mg

Tablet: 200 mg, 600 mg

◆ **Tolmetin Sodium** *see* Tolmetin *on page 1595*

Tolterodine (tole TER oh deen)

Medication Safety Issues

Sound-alike/look-alike issues:

Tolterodine may be confused with fesoterodine

Detrol® may be confused with Ditropan®

International issues:

Detrol® may be confused with Desurol® which is a brand name for oxolinic acid in the Czech Republic

U.S. Brand Names Detrol®; Detrol® LA

Canadian Brand Names Detrol®; Detrol® LA; Unidet®

Mexican Brand Names Detrusitol

Index Terms Tolterodine Tartrate

Pharmacologic Category Anticholinergic Agent

Generic Available No

Use Treatment of patients with an overactive bladder with symptoms of urinary frequency, urgency, or urge incontinence

Effect on Mental Status May cause drowsiness, dizziness, hallucinations, or nervousness

Effect on Psychiatric Treatment Fluoxetine and likely paroxetine increase the serum concentration of tolterodine; however, the magnitude of this increase is small (~25%, as reported for fluoxetine) and thus no dosage adjustment is required.

Pregnancy Risk Factor C

Pregnancy Considerations Teratogenic effects were observed in some animal studies. There are no adequate and well-controlled studies in pregnant women. Use during pregnancy only if the potential benefit to the mother outweighs the possible risk to the fetus.

Lactation Excretion in breast milk unknown/not recommended

Contraindications Hypersensitivity to tolterodine or any component of the formulation; urinary retention; gastric retention; uncontrolled narrow-angle glaucoma

Warnings/Precautions May cause drowsiness and/or blurred vision, which may impair physical or mental abilities; patients must be cautioned about performing tasks which require mental alertness (eg, operating machinery or driving). Use with caution in patients with bladder flow obstruction, may increase the risk of urinary retention. Use with caution in patients with gastrointestinal obstructive disorders (ie, pyloric stenosis), may increase the risk of gastric retention. Use with caution in patients with myasthenia gravis and controlled (treated) narrow-angle glaucoma; metabolized in the liver and excreted in the urine and feces, dosage adjustment is required for patients with renal or hepatic impairment. Tolterodine has been associated with QT_c prolongation at high (supratherapeutic) doses. The manufacturer recommends caution in patients with congenital prolonged QT or in patients receiving concurrent therapy with QT_c-prolonging drugs (class Ia or III antiarrhythmics). However, the mean change in QT_c even at supratherapeutic dosages was less than 15 msec. Individuals who are CYP2D6 poor metabolizers or in the presence of inhibitors of CYP2D6 and CYP3A4 may be more likely to exhibit prolongation. Dosage adjustment is recommended in patients receiving CYP3A4 inhibitors (a lower dose of tolterodine is recommended). Safety and efficacy in pediatric patients have not been established.

Adverse Reactions As reported with immediate release tablet, unless otherwise specified

>10%: Gastrointestinal: Dry mouth (35%; extended release capsules 23%)

1% to 10%:

Cardiovascular: Chest pain (2%)

Central nervous system: Headache (7%; extended release capsules 6%), somnolence (3%; extended release capsules 3%), fatigue (4%; extended release capsules 2%), dizziness (5%; extended release capsules 2%), anxiety (extended release capsules 1%)

Dermatologic: Dry skin (1%)

Gastrointestinal: Abdominal pain (5%; extended release capsules 4%), constipation (7%; extended release capsules 6%), dyspepsia (4%; extended release capsules 3%), diarrhea (4%), weight gain (1%)

Genitourinary: Dysuria (2%; extended release capsules 1%)

Neuromuscular & skeletal: Arthralgia (2%)

Ocular: Abnormal vision (2%; extended release capsules 1%), dry eyes (3%; extended release capsules 3%)

Respiratory: Bronchitis (2%), sinusitis (extended release capsules 2%)

Miscellaneous: Flu-like syndrome (3%), infection (1%)

<1% (Limited to important or life-threatening): Anaphylactoid reactions, angioedema, confusion, dementia aggravated, disorientation, hallucinations, memory impairment, palpitation, peripheral edema, QT_c prolongation, tachycardia

Metabolism/Transport Effects Substrate of CYP2C9 (minor), 2C19 (minor), 2D6 (major), 3A4 (major)

Drug Interactions

Acetylcholinesterase Inhibitors (Central): Anticholinergics may diminish the therapeutic effect of Acetylcholinesterase Inhibitors (Central). Acetylcholinesterase Inhibitors (Central) may diminish the therapeutic effect of Anticholinergics. If the anticholinergic action is a side effect of the agent, the result may be beneficial. *Risk C: Monitor therapy*

Anticholinergics: May enhance the adverse/toxic effect of other Anticholinergics. **Exceptions:** Paliperidone. *Risk C: Monitor therapy*

Antifungal Agents (Azole Derivatives, Systemic): May decrease the metabolism of Tolterodine. This is likely only of concern in CYP2D6-deficient patients (ie, "poor metabolizers") *Risk D: Consider therapy modification*

Cannabinoids: Anticholinergic Agents may enhance the tachycardic effect of Cannabinoids. *Risk C: Monitor therapy*

CYP2D6 Inhibitors (Moderate): May decrease the metabolism of CYP2D6 Substrates. *Risk C: Monitor therapy*

CYP2D6 Inhibitors (Strong): May decrease the metabolism of CYP2D6 Substrates. *Risk D: Consider therapy modification*

CYP3A4 Inducers (Strong): May increase the metabolism of CYP3A4 Substrates. *Risk C: Monitor therapy*

CYP3A4 Inhibitors (Moderate): May decrease the metabolism of CYP3A4 Substrates. *Risk C: Monitor therapy*

CYP3A4 Inhibitors (Strong): May decrease the metabolism of CYP3A4 Substrates. *Risk D: Consider therapy modification*

Darunavir: May increase the serum concentration of CYP2D6 Substrates. *Risk C: Monitor therapy*

Dasatinib: May increase the serum concentration of CYP3A4 Substrates. *Risk C: Monitor therapy*

Deferasirox: May decrease the serum concentration of CYP3A4 Substrates. *Risk C: Monitor therapy*

Fluconazole: May decrease the metabolism of Tolterodine. This is likely only of concern in CYP2D6-deficient patients (ie, "poor metabolizers") *Risk C: Monitor therapy*

Herbs (CYP3A4 Inducers): May increase the metabolism of CYP3A4 Substrates. *Risk C: Monitor therapy*

Potassium Chloride: Anticholinergic Agents may enhance the ulcerogenic effect of Potassium Chloride. *Risk D: Consider therapy modification*

Pramlintide: May enhance the anticholinergic effect of Anticholinergics. These effects are specific to the GI tract. *Risk D: Consider therapy modification*

Secretin: Anticholinergic Agents may diminish the stimulatory effect of Secretin. *Risk D: Consider therapy modification*

VinBLAStine: May increase the serum concentration of Tolterodine. Management: Reduce tolterodine dosage to 1 mg twice daily (regular release formulation) or 2 mg daily (extended release formulation) and monitor for increased levels/effects of tolterodine with initiation of vinblastine therapy. *Risk D: Consider therapy modification*

Warfarin: Tolterodine may enhance the anticoagulant effect of Warfarin. *Risk C: Monitor therapy*

Ethanol/Nutrition/Herb Interactions

Food: Increases bioavailability (~53% increase) of tolterodine tablets (dose adjustment not necessary); does not affect the pharmacokinetics of tolterodine extended release capsules. As a CYP3A4 inhibitor, grapefruit juice may increase the serum level and/or toxicity of tolterodine, but unlikely secondary to high oral bioavailability.

Herb/Nutraceutical: St John's wort (*Hypericum*) appears to induce CYP3A enzymes.

Stability Store at 25°C (77°F); excursions permitted to 15°C to 30°C (59°F to 86°F). Protect from light.

Mechanism of Action Tolterodine is a competitive antagonist of muscarinic receptors. In animal models, tolterodine demonstrates selectivity for urinary bladder receptors over salivary receptors. Urinary bladder contraction is mediated by muscarinic receptors. Tolterodine increases residual urine volume and decreases detrusor muscle pressure.

Pharmacodynamics/Kinetics

Absorption: Immediate release tablet: Rapid; ≥77%

Distribution: I.V.: V_d: 113 ± 27 L

Protein binding: >96% (primarily to alpha$_1$-acid glycoprotein)

Metabolism: Extensively hepatic, primarily via CYP2D6 (some metabolites share activity) and 3A4 usually (minor pathway). In patients with a genetic deficiency of CYP2D6, metabolism via 3A4 predominates.

Bioavailability: Immediate release tablet: Increased 53% with food

Half-life elimination:

Immediate release tablet: Extensive metabolizers: ~2 hours; Poor metabolizers: ~10 hours

Extended release capsule: Extensive metabolizers: ~7 hours; Poor metabolizers: ~18 hours

Time to peak: Immediate release tablet: 1-2 hours; Extended release tablet: 2-6 hours

Excretion: Urine (77%); feces (17%); primarily as metabolites (<1% unchanged drug) of which the active 5-hydroxymethyl metabolite accounts for 5% to 14% (<1% in poor metabolizers); as unchanged drug (<1%; <2.5% in poor metabolizers)

Dosage

Oral: Adults: Treatment of overactive bladder:

Immediate release tablet: 2 mg twice daily; the dose may be lowered to 1 mg twice daily based on individual response and tolerability

Dosing adjustment in patients concurrently taking CYP3A4 inhibitors: 1 mg twice daily

Extended release capsule: 4 mg once a day; dose may be lowered to 2 mg daily based on individual response and tolerability

Dosing adjustment in patients concurrently taking CYP3A4 inhibitors: 2 mg daily

Elderly: Safety and efficacy in patients >64 years was found to be similar to that in younger patients; no dosage adjustment is needed based on age

Dosing adjustment in renal impairment: Use with caution (studies conducted in patients with Cl_{cr} 10-30 mL/minute):

Immediate release tablet: 1 mg twice daily

Extended release capsule: 2 mg daily

Dosing adjustment in hepatic impairment:

Immediate release tablet: 1 mg twice daily

Extended release capsule: 2 mg daily

Administration Extended release capsule: Swallow whole; do not crush, chew, or open

Monitoring Parameters Renal function (BUN, creatinine); hepatic function

Dosage Forms Excipient information presented when available (limited, particularly for generics); consult specific product labeling.

Capsule, extended release, as tartrate (Detrol® LA): 2 mg, 4 mg

Tablet, as tartrate (Detrol®): 1 mg, 2 mg

◆ **Tolterodine Tartrate** *see* Tolterodine *on page 1596*

◆ **Tomoxetine** *see* Atomoxetine *on page 151*

◆ **Tonocard® [DSC]** *see* Tocainide *on page 1591*

◆ **Topamax®** *see* Topiramate *on page 1598*

◆ **Topicaine® [OTC]** *see* Lidocaine *on page 924*

Topiramate (toe PYRE a mate)

Medication Safety Issues

Sound-alike/look-alike issues:

Topamax® may be confused with Tegretol®, Tegretol®-XR, Toprol-XL®

Related Information

Anticonvulsants By Seizure Type *on page 1759*

U.S. Brand Names Topamax®

Canadian Brand Names Apo-Topiramate; Co-Topiramate; Dom-Topiramate; Gen-Topiramate; Novo-Topiramate; PHL-Topiramate; PMS-Topiramate; ratio-Topiramate; Sandoz-Topiramate; Topamax®

Mexican Brand Names Topamax

Pharmacologic Category Anticonvulsant, Miscellaneous

Generic Available No

Use Monotherapy or adjunctive therapy for partial onset seizures and primary generalized tonic-clonic seizures; adjunctive treatment of seizures associated with Lennox-Gastaut syndrome; prophylaxis of migraine headache

Unlabeled/Investigational Use Infantile spasms, neuropathic pain, cluster headache

Mental Health Comment Large double-blind studies have failed to differentiate this drug from placebo when used for bipolar disorder.

Pregnancy Risk Factor C

Pregnancy Considerations Topiramate was found to be teratogenic in animal studies; however, there is limited information in pregnant women; use only if benefit to the mother outweighs the risk to the fetus. Based on limited data, topiramate was found to cross the placenta. Postmarketing experience includes reports of hypospadias following *in vitro* exposure to topiramate.

Lactation Enters breast milk/not recommended

Contraindications Hypersensitivity to topiramate or any component of the formulation

Warnings/Precautions Use with caution in patients with hepatic, respiratory, or renal impairment. Topiramate may decrease serum bicarbonate concentrations (up to 67% of patients); treatment-emergent metabolic acidosis is less common. Risk may be increased in patients with a predisposing condition (organ dysfunction, ketogenic diet, or concurrent treatment with other drugs which may cause acidosis). Metabolic acidosis may occur at dosages as low as 50 mg/day. Monitor serum bicarbonate as well as potential complications of chronic acidosis (nephrolithiasis, osteomalacia, and reduced growth rates in children). Kidney stones have been reported in both children and adults; the risk of kidney stones is about 2-4 times that of the untreated population; the risk of this event may be reduced by increasing fluid intake.

Cognitive dysfunction, psychiatric disturbances (mood disorders), and sedation (somnolence or fatigue) may occur with topiramate use; incidence may be related to rapid titration and higher doses. Topiramate may also cause paresthesia, dizziness, and ataxia. Topiramate has been associated with acute myopia and secondary angle-closure glaucoma in adults and children, typically within 1 month of initiation; discontinue in patients with acute onset of decreased visual acuity or ocular pain. Hyperammonemia with or without encephalopathy may occur with concomitant valproate administration; use with caution in patients with inborn errors of metabolism or decreased hepatic mitochondrial activity. Topiramate may be associated (rarely) with severe oligohydrosis and hyperthermia, most frequently in children; use caution and monitor closely during strenuous exercise, during exposure to high environmental temperature, or in patients receiving drugs with anticholinergic activity.

Avoid abrupt withdrawal of topiramate therapy, it should be withdrawn/tapered slowly to minimize the potential of increased seizure frequency. Doses were also gradually withdrawn in migraine prophylaxis studies. Effects with other sedative drugs or ethanol may be potentiated. Safety and efficacy have not been established in children <2 years of age for adjunctive treatment of seizures and <10 years of age for monotherapy treatment of seizures. Safety and efficacy have not been established in children for migraine prophylaxis.

Adverse Reactions Adverse events are reported for placebo-controlled trials of adjunctive therapy in adult and pediatric patients. Unless otherwise noted, the percentages refer to incidence in epilepsy trials. Note: A wide range of dosages were studied; incidence of adverse events was frequently lower in the pediatric population studied.

>10%:

- Central nervous system: Dizziness (4% to 32%), ataxia (6% to 16%), somnolence (15% to 29%), psychomotor slowing (3% to 21%), nervousness (9% to 19%), memory difficulties (2% to 14%), speech problems (2% to 13%), fatigue (9% to 30%), difficulty concentrating (5% to 14%), depression (9% to 13%), confusion (4% to 14%)
- Endocrine & metabolic: Serum bicarbonate decreased (dose-related: 7% to 67%; marked reductions [to <17 mEq/L] 1% to 11%)
- Gastrointestinal: Nausea (6% to 12%; migraine trial: 14%), weight loss (8% to 13%), anorexia (4% to 24%)
- Neuromuscular & skeletal: Paresthesia (1% to 19%; migraine trial: 35% to 51%)

Ocular: Nystagmus (10% to 11%), abnormal vision (<1% to 13%)
Respiratory: Upper respiratory infection (migraine trial: 12% to 13%)
Miscellaneous: Injury (6% to 14%)

1% to 10%:

Cardiovascular: Chest pain (2% to 4%), edema (1% to 2%), bradycardia (1%), pallor (up to 1%), hypertension (1% to 2%)

Central nervous system: Abnormal coordination (4%), hypoesthesia (1% to 2%; migraine trial: 8%), convulsions (1%), depersonalization (1% to 2%), apathy (1% to 3%), cognitive problems (3%), emotional lability (3%), agitation (3%), aggressive reactions (2% to 9%), tremor (3% to 9%), stupor (1% to 2%), mood problems (4% to 9%), anxiety (2% to 10%), insomnia (4% to 8%), neurosis (1%), vertigo (1% to 2%)

Dermatologic: Pruritus (migraine trial: 2% to 4%), skin disorder (1% to 3%), alopecia (2%), dermatitis (up to 2%), hypertrichosis (up to 2%), rash erythematous (up to 2%), eczema (up to 1%), seborrhea (up to 1%), skin discoloration (up to 1%)

Endocrine & metabolic: Hot flashes (1% to 2%); metabolic acidosis (hyperchloremia, nonanion gap), dehydration, breast pain (up to 4%), menstrual irregularities (1% to 2%), hypoglycemia (1%), libido decreased (<1% to 2%)

Gastrointestinal: Dyspepsia (2% to 7%), abdominal pain (5% to 7%), constipation (3% to 5%), xerostomia (2% to 4%), fecal incontinence (1%), gingivitis (1%), diarrhea (2%; migraine trial: 11%), vomiting (1% to 3%), gastroenteritis (1% to 3%), appetite increased (1%), GI disorder (1%), (2% to 4%; migraine trial: 12% to 15%), dysphagia (1%), flatulence (1%), GERD (1%), glossitis (1%), gum hyperplasia (1%), weight increase (1%)

Genitourinary: Impotence, dysuria/incontinence (<1% to 4%), prostatic disorder (2%), UTI (2% to 3%), premature ejaculation (migraine trial: 3%), cystitis (2%)

Hematologic: Leukopenia (1% to 2%), purpura (8%), hematoma (1%), prothrombin time increased (1%), thrombocytopenia (1%)

Neuromuscular & skeletal: Myalgia (2%), weakness (3% to 6%), back pain (1% to 5%), leg pain (2% to 4%), rigors (1%), hypertonia, arthralgia (1% to 7%), gait abnormal (2% to 8%), involuntary muscle contractions (2%; migraine trial: 4%), skeletal pain (1%), hyperkinesia (up to 5%), hyporeflexia (up to 2%)

Ocular: Conjunctivitis (1%), diplopia (2% to 10%), myopia (up to 1%)

Otic: Hearing decreased (1% to 2%), tinnitus (1% to 2%), otitis media (migraine trial: 1% to 2%)

Renal: Nephrolithiasis, renal calculus (1% to 2%), hematuria (<1% to 2%)

Respiratory: Pharyngitis (3% to 6%), sinusitis (4% to 6%; migraine trial: 8% to 10%), epistaxis (1% to 4%), rhinitis (4% to 7%), dyspnea (1% to 2%), pneumonia (5%), coughing (migraine trial: 2% to 3%), bronchitis (migraine trial: 3%)

Miscellaneous: Flu-like syndrome (3% to 7%), allergy (2% to 3%), body odor (up to 1%), fever (migraine trial: 1% to 2%), viral infection (migraine trial: 3% to 4%), infection (<1% to 2%), diaphoresis (≤1%), thirst (2%)

<1% (Limited to important or life-threatening): Accommodation abnormality, anemia, angina, apraxia, AV block, bone marrow depression, deep vein thrombosis, dehydration, delirium, diabetes mellitus, dyskinesia, electrolyte imbalance, encephalopathy (with valproate therapy), eosinophilia, erythema multiforme, euphoria, eye pain, granulocytopenia, hepatic failure, hepatitis, hyperammonemia (with valproate therapy), hyperthermia (severe), hypokalemia, hypotension, liver enzymes increased, lymphadenopathy, lymphopenia, manic reaction, migraine aggravated, neuropathy, oligohydrosis, pancreatitis, pancytopenia, paranoid reaction, pemphigus, photosensitivity, psychosis, pulmonary embolism, rash, renal tubular acidosis, Stevens-Johnson syndrome, suicidal behavior, syncope, syndrome of acute myopia/secondary angle-closure glaucoma, tongue edema, toxic epidermal necrolysis

Metabolism/Transport Effects **Inhibits** CYP2C19 (weak); **Induces** CYP3A4 (weak)

Drug Interactions

Alcohol (Ethyl): CNS Depressants may enhance the CNS depressant effect of Alcohol (Ethyl). *Risk C: Monitor therapy*

CarBAMazepine: May decrease the serum concentration of Topiramate. *Risk D: Consider therapy modification*

CNS Depressants: May enhance the adverse/toxic effect of other CNS Depressants. *Risk C: Monitor therapy*

Ketorolac: May diminish the therapeutic effect of Anticonvulsants. *Risk C: Monitor therapy*

Maraviroc: CYP3A4 Inducers may decrease the serum concentration of Maraviroc. *Risk D: Consider therapy modification*

Mefloquine: May diminish the therapeutic effect of Anticonvulsants. Mefloquine may decrease the serum concentration of Anticonvulsants. Management: Mefloquine is contraindicated in persons with a history of convulsions. If anticonvulsant is being used for another indication monitor response to treatment closely, as concurrent mefloquine may decrease response to treatment. *Risk D: Consider therapy modification*

Oral Contraceptive (Estrogens): Topiramate may decrease the serum concentration of Oral Contraceptive (Estrogens). Contraceptive failure is possible. *Risk D: Consider therapy modification*

Phenytoin: Topiramate may decrease the metabolism of Phenytoin. Phenytoin may increase the metabolism of Topiramate. *Risk C: Monitor therapy*

Valproic Acid: Topiramate may enhance the hepatotoxic effect of Valproic Acid. *Risk C: Monitor therapy*

Ethanol/Nutrition/Herb Interactions

Ethanol: Avoid ethanol (may increase CNS depression).

Food: Ketogenic diet may increase the possibility of acidosis and/or kidney stones.

Herb/Nutraceutical: Avoid evening primrose (seizure threshold decreased).

Stability Store at room temperature of 15°C to 30°C (59°F to 86°F). Protect from moisture.

Mechanism of Action Anticonvulsant activity may be due to a combination of potential mechanisms: Blocks neuronal voltage-dependent sodium channels, enhances GABA(A) activity, antagonizes AMPA/kainate glutamate receptors, and weakly inhibits carbonic anhydrase.

Pharmacodynamics/Kinetics

Absorption: Good, rapid; unaffected by food

Protein binding: 15% to 41% (inversely related to plasma concentrations)

Metabolism: Hepatic via P450 enzymes

Bioavailability: 80%

Half-life elimination: Mean: Adults: Normal renal function: 21 hours; shorter in pediatric patients; clearance is 50% higher in pediatric patients; Elderly: ~24 hours

Time to peak, serum: ~1-4 hours

Excretion: Urine (~70% to 80% as unchanged drug)

Dialyzable: ~30%

Dosage Oral: **Note:** Do not abruptly discontinue therapy; taper dosage gradually to prevent rebound effects. (In clinical trials, adult doses were withdrawn by decreasing in weekly intervals of 50-100 mg/day gradually over 2-8 weeks for seizure treatment, and by decreasing in weekly intervals by 25-50 mg/day for migraine prophylaxis.)

Epilepsy, monotherapy: Children ≥10 years and Adults: Partial onset seizure and primary generalized tonic-clonic seizure: Initial: 25 mg twice daily; may increase weekly by 50 mg/day up to 100 mg twice daily (week 4 dose); thereafter, may further increase weekly by 100 mg/day up to the recommended maximum of 200 mg twice daily.

Epilepsy, adjunctive therapy:

Children 2-16 years:

Partial onset seizure or seizure associated with Lennox-Gastaut syndrome: Initial dose titration should begin at 25 mg (or less, based on a range of 1-3 mg/kg/day) nightly for the first week; dosage may be increased in increments of 1-3 mg/kg/day (administered in 2 divided doses) at 1- or 2-week intervals to a total daily dose of 5-9 mg/kg/day

Primary generalized tonic-clonic seizure: Use initial dose listed above, but use slower initial titration rate; titrate to recommended maintenance dose by the end of 8 weeks

Adolescents ≥17 years and Adults:

Partial onset seizures: Initial: 25-50 mg/day (given in 2 divided doses) for 1 week; increase at weekly intervals by 25-50 mg/day until response; usual maintenance dose: 100-200 mg twice daily. Doses >1600 mg/day have not been studied.

Primary generalized tonic-clonic seizures: Use initial dose as listed above for partial onset seizures, but use slower initial titration rate; titrate upwards to recommended dose by the end of 8 weeks; usual maintenance dose: 200 mg twice daily. Doses >1600 mg/day have not been studied.

Adults:

Migraine prophylaxis: Initial: 25 mg/day (in the evening), titrated at weekly intervals in 25 mg increments, up to the recommended total daily dose of 100 mg/day given in 2 divided doses

Cluster headache (unlabeled use): Initial: 25 mg/day, titrated at weekly intervals in 25 mg increments, up to 200 mg/day

Neuropathic pain (unlabeled use): Initial: 25 mg/day, titrated at weekly intervals in 25-50 mg increments to target dose of 400 mg daily in 2 divided doses. Reported dosage range studied: 25-800 mg/day

Dosing adjustment in renal impairment: Cl_{cr} <70 mL/minute: Administer 50% dose and titrate more slowly

Hemodialysis: Supplemental dose may be needed during hemodialysis

Dosing adjustment in hepatic impairment: Clearance may be reduced

Administration Oral: May be administered without regard to meals

Capsule sprinkles: May be swallowed whole or opened to sprinkle the contents on soft food (drug/food mixture should not be chewed).

Tablet: Because of bitter taste, tablets should not be broken.

Monitoring Parameters Seizure frequency, hydration status; electrolytes (recommended monitoring includes serum bicarbonate at baseline and periodically during treatment), serum creatinine; monitor for symptoms of acute acidosis and complications of long-term acidosis (nephrolithiasis, osteomalacia, and reduced growth rates in children); ammonia level in patients with unexplained lethargy, vomiting, or mental status changes; intraocular pressure, symptoms of secondary angle closure glaucoma

Additional Information May be associated with weight loss in some patients

Dosage Forms Excipient information presented when available (limited, particularly for generics); consult specific product labeling.

Capsule, sprinkle:

Topamax®: 15 mg, 25 mg

Tablet:

Topamax®: 25 mg, 50 mg, 100 mg, 200 mg

◆ **Toposar®** *see* Etoposide *on page 607*

Topotecan (toe poe TEE kan)

Medication Safety Issues

Sound-alike/look-alike issues:

Hycamtin® may be confused with Hycomine®, Mycamine®

High alert medication: The Institute for Safe Medication Practices (ISMP) includes this medication among its list of drugs which have a heightened risk of causing significant patient harm when used in error.

U.S. Brand Names Hycamtin®

Canadian Brand Names Hycamtin®

Index Terms Hycamptamine; NSC-609699; SKF 104864; SKF 104864-A; Topotecan Hydrochloride

Pharmacologic Category Antineoplastic Agent, Camptothecin; Antineoplastic Agent, Natural Source (Plant) Derivative

Use Treatment of ovarian cancer and small cell lung cancer; cervical cancer (in combination with cisplatin)

Unlabeled/Investigational Use Investigational: Treatment of nonsmall cell lung cancer, myelodysplastic syndrome, sarcoma (pediatrics), neuroblastoma (pediatrics), refractory solid tumors (pediatrics)

Effect on Mental Status None reported

Effect on Psychiatric Treatment May cause myelosuppression; use caution with clozapine and carbamazepine

Dosage Summary

Oral:

Children: Dosage not established

Adults: 2.3 mg/m^2/day for 5 days; repeated every 21 days

I.V.:

Children: Dosage not established

Adults: IVPB: 1.5 mg/m^2/day for 5 days; repeated every 21 days **or** 0.75 mg/m^2/day for 3 days every 21 days

Dosage Forms Excipient information presented when available (limited, particularly for generics); consult specific product labeling.

Capsule:

Hycamtin®: 0.25 mg, 1 mg

Injection, powder for reconstitution:

Hycamtin®: 4 mg

◆ **Topotecan Hydrochloride** *see* Topotecan *on page 1602*

◆ **Toprol-XL®** *see* Metoprolol *on page 1036*

Toremifene (tore EM i feen)

U.S. Brand Names Fareston®
Canadian Brand Names Fareston®
Mexican Brand Names Fareston
Index Terms FC1157a; Toremifene Citrate
Pharmacologic Category Antineoplastic Agent, Estrogen Receptor Antagonist; Selective Estrogen Receptor Modulator (SERM)
Use Treatment of postmenopausal metastatic breast cancer (estrogen receptor positive or estrogen receptor status unknown)
Effect on Mental Status Dizziness, anxiety, irritability, insomnia, and depression are common
Effect on Psychiatric Treatment None reported
Dosage Summary
Oral:
Children: Dosage not established
Adults: 60 mg once daily
Dosage Forms Excipient information presented when available (limited, particularly for generics); consult specific product labeling.
Tablet:
Fareston®: 60 mg

◆ **Toremifene Citrate** *see* Toremifene *on page 1603*

◆ **Torisel®** *see* Temsirolimus *on page 1547*

Torsemide (TORE se mide)

Medication Safety Issues
Sound-alike/look-alike issues:
Torsemide may be confused with furosemide
Demadex® may be confused with Denorex®
U.S. Brand Names Demadex®
Pharmacologic Category Diuretic, Loop
Use Management of edema associated with congestive heart failure and hepatic or renal disease; used alone or in combination with antihypertensives in treatment of hypertension; I.V. form is indicated when rapid onset is desired
Effect on Mental Status May cause dizziness
Effect on Psychiatric Treatment May cause agranulocytosis; use caution with clozapine and carbamazepine; may decrease lithium clearance resulting in an increase in serum lithium levels and potential lithium toxicity, however, this is much more common and significant with the thiazide diuretics; monitor serum lithium levels; concurrent use with chloral hydrate may produce hot flashes and hypertension
Dosage Summary
I.V.:
Children: Dosage not established
Adults: 2.5-200 mg once daily; Infusion: 20 mg bolus, then 5-20 mg/hour
Oral:
Children: Dosage not established
Adults: 2.5-200 mg once daily (maximum: 200 mg/day)
Dosage Forms Excipient information presented when available (limited, particularly for generics); consult specific product labeling. [DSC] = Discontinued product
Injection, solution:
Demadex®: 10 mg/mL (2 mL [DSC], 5 mL [DSC])
Tablet: 5 mg, 10 mg, 20 mg, 100 mg
Demadex®: 5 mg, 10 mg, 20 mg, 100 mg [scored]

◆ **Tositumomab I-131** *see* Tositumomab and Iodine I 131 Tositumomab *on page 1603*

Tositumomab and Iodine I 131 Tositumomab

(toe si TYOO mo mab & EYE oh dyne eye one THUR tee one toe si TYOO mo mab)

Medication Safety Issues
High alert medication: The Institute for Safe Medication Practices (ISMP) includes this medication among its list of drugs which have a heightened risk of causing significant patient harm when used in error.
U.S. Brand Names Bexxar®

Index Terms 131 I Anti-B1 Antibody; 131 I-Anti-B1 Monoclonal Antibody; Anti-CD20-Murine Monoclonal Antibody I-131; B1; B1 Antibody; Iodine I 131 Tositumomab and Tositumomab; Tositumomab I-131

Pharmacologic Category Antineoplastic Agent, Monoclonal Antibody; Radiopharmaceutical

Use Treatment of relapsed or refractory CD20 positive, low-grade, follicular, or transformed non-Hodgkin's lymphoma

Effect on Mental Status May cause sedation

Effect on Psychiatric Treatment Hematologic adverse reactions are common; use caution with clozapine, carbamazepine, valproic acid and derivatives, and mirtazapine. Rash is common; consider in differential in patients receiving lamotrigine. GI side effects are common; concurrent use with SSRIs may produce additive effects. May produce hypotension; concurrent use with psychotropic agents may produce additive blood pressure-lowering effects.

Dosage Summary

I.V.:

Tositumomab:

Children: Dosage not established

Adults: Step 1: 450 mg in NS 50 mL over 60 minutes; Step 2: 450 mg in NS 50 mL over 60 minutes

Iodine I-131 tositumomab (Given after tositumomab):

Children: Dosage not established

Adults: Step 1: I-131 5.0 mCi and tositumomab 35 mg in NS 30 mL over 20 minutes; Step 2: I-131 (calculated to deliver 65-75 cGy total body irradiation) and tositumomab 35 mg over 20 minutes

Dosage Forms Excipient information presented when available (limited, particularly for generics); consult specific product labeling.

Note: Not all components are shipped from the same facility. When ordering, ensure that all will arrive on the same day.

Kit [dosimetric package]: Tositumomab 225 mg/16.1 mL [2 vials], tositumomab 35 mg/2.5 mL [1 vial], and iodine I 131 tositumomab 0.1 mg/mL and 0.61mCi/mL (20 mL) [1 vial]

Kit [therapeutic package]: Tositumomab 225 mg/16.1 mL [2 vials], tositumomab 35 mg/2.5 mL [1 vial], and iodine I 131 tositumomab 1.1 mg/mL and 5.6 mCi/mL (20 mL) [1 or 2 vials]

- **Totect™** *see* Dexrazoxane *on page 441*
- **Touro® CC** *see* Guaifenesin, Pseudoephedrine, and Dextromethorphan *on page 748*
- **Touro® CC-LD** *see* Guaifenesin, Pseudoephedrine, and Dextromethorphan *on page 748*
- **Touro® Allergy** *see* Brompheniramine and Pseudoephedrine *on page 206*
- **Touro® DM** *see* Guaifenesin and Dextromethorphan *on page 739*
- **Touro® HC [DSC]** *see* Hydrocodone and Guaifenesin *on page 779*
- **Touro LA®** *see* Guaifenesin and Pseudoephedrine *on page 744*
- **TPV** *see* Tipranavir *on page 1586*
- **tRA** *see* Tretinoin, Oral *on page 1617*

TraMADol (TRA ma dole)

Medication Safety Issues

Sound-alike/look-alike issues:

TraMADol may be confused with Toradol®, Trandate®, traZODone, Voltaren®

Ultram® may be confused with Ultane®, Ultracet®, Voltaren®

International issues:

Theradol® [Netherlands] may be confused with Foradil® which is a brand name for formoterol in the U.S.

Theradol® [Netherlands] may be confused with Terazol® which is a brand name for terconazole in the U.S.

Theradol® [Netherlands] may be confused with Toradol® which is a brand name for ketorolac in the U.S.

U.S. Brand Names Ultram®; Ultram® ER

Canadian Brand Names Ralivia™ ER; Tridural™; Zytram® XL

Mexican Brand Names Durodor Retard; Trexol

Index Terms Tramadol Hydrochloride

Pharmacologic Category Analgesic, Opioid

Generic Available Yes: Excludes extended release tablet

Use Relief of moderate to moderately-severe pain

Effect on Mental Status May cause dizziness, drowsiness, or restlessness

Effect on Psychiatric Treatment Contraindicated with opioid-dependent patients, MAO inhibitors, psychotropics; carbamazepine may decrease the effects of tramadol; concurrent use with MAO inhibitors and TCAs may produce seizures; tramadol has MAO inhibitor activity and should be used cautiously with other antidepressants

Pregnancy Risk Factor C

Pregnancy Considerations Adverse events were observed in animal studies. Tramadol has been shown to cross the human placenta when administered during labor. Postmarketing reports following tramadol use during pregnancy include neonatal seizures, withdrawal syndrome, fetal death, and stillbirth. Not recommended for use during labor and delivery.

Lactation Enters breast milk/not recommended

Contraindications Hypersensitivity to tramadol, opioids, or any component of the formulation; opioid-dependent patients; acute intoxication with alcohol, hypnotics, centrally-acting analgesics, opioids, or psychotropic drugs

Note: Based on Canadian product labeling:

Tramadol is contraindicated during or within 14 days following MAO inhibitor therapy

Extended release formulations (Ralivia™ ER [CAN], Tridural™[CAN], and Zytram® XL [CAN]): Additional contraindications: Severe (Cl_{cr} <30 mL/minute) renal dysfunction, severe (Child-Pugh Class C) hepatic dysfunction

Warnings/Precautions Rare but serious anaphylactoid reactions (including fatalities) often following initial dosing have been reported. Pruritus, hives, bronchospasm, angioedema, toxic epidermal necrolysis (TEN) and Stevens-Johnson syndrome also have been reported with use. Previous anaphylactoid reactions to opioids may increase risks for similar reactions to tramadol. Caution patients to swallow tablets whole. Rapid release and absorption of tramadol from tablets that are broken, crushed, or chewed may lead to a potentially lethal overdose. May cause CNS depression, which may impair physical or mental abilities; patients must be cautioned about performing tasks which require mental alertness (eg, operating machinery or driving). May cause CNS depression and/or respiratory depression, particularly when combined with other CNS depressants. Use with caution and reduce dosage when administered to patients receiving other CNS depressants. An increased risk of seizures may occur in patients receiving serotonin reuptake inhibitors (SSRIs or anorectics), tricyclic antidepressants, other cyclic compounds (including cyclobenzaprine, promethazine), neuroleptics, or drugs which may lower seizure threshold. Patients with a history of seizures, or with a risk of seizures (head trauma, metabolic disorders, CNS infection, or malignancy, or during ethanol/drug withdrawal) are also at increased risk. Avoid use with serotonergic agents such as TCAs, MAO inhibitors (contraindicated in Canadian product labeling), triptans, venlafaxine, trazodone, lithium, sibutramine, meperidine, dextromethorphan, St John's wort, SNRIs and SSRIs; concomitant use has been associated with the development of serotonin syndrome.

Elderly (particularly >75 years of age), debilitated patients and patients with chronic respiratory disorders may be at greater risk of adverse events. Use with caution in patients with increased intracranial pressure or head injury. Avoid use in patients who are suicidal or addiction prone. Use caution in heavy alcohol users. Use caution in treatment of acute abdominal conditions; may mask pain. Use tramadol with caution and reduce dosage in patients with liver disease or renal dysfunction. Tolerance or drug dependence may result from extended use (withdrawal symptoms have been reported); abrupt discontinuation should be avoided. Tapering of dose at the time of discontinuation limits the risk of withdrawal symptoms. Safety and efficacy in pediatric patients have not been established.

Adverse Reactions

>10%:

Cardiovascular: Flushing (8% to 16%)

Central nervous system: Dizziness (16% to 33%), headache (12% to 32%), insomnia (7% to 11%), somnolence (7% to 25%)

Dermatologic: Pruritus (6% to 12%)

Gastrointestinal: Constipation (10% to 46%), nausea (15% to 40%), vomiting (5% to 17%), dyspepsia (1% to 13%)

Neuromuscular & skeletal: Weakness (4% to 12%)

1% to 10%:

Cardiovascular: Chest pain (1% to <5%), postural hypotension (2% to 5%), vasodilation (1% to <5%)

Central nervous system: Anxiety (1% to <5%), confusion (1% to <5%), coordination impaired (1% to <5%), depression (1% to <5%), euphoria (1% to <5%), hypoesthesia (1% to <5%), lethargy (1% to <5%), nervousness (1% to <5%), pain (1% to <5%), pyrexia (1% to <5%), restlessness (1% to <5%), malaise (<1% to <5%)

Dermatologic: Dermatitis (1% to <5%), rash (1% to <5%)

Endocrine & metabolic: Hot flashes (2% to 9%), menopausal symptoms (1% to <5%)

Gastrointestinal: Diarrhea (5% to 10%), xerostomia (5% to 10%), anorexia (1% to <6%), abdominal pain (1% to <5%), appetite decreased (1% to <5%), weight loss (1% to <5%), flatulence (<1% to <5%)

Genitourinary: Urinary tract infection (1% to <5%), urinary frequency (<1% to <5%), urinary retention (<1% to <5%)

Neuromuscular & skeletal: Arthralgia (1% to <5%), back pain (1% to <5%), hypertonia (1% to <5%), rigors (1% to <5%), paresthesia (1% to <5%), tremor (1% to <5%), creatinine phosphokinase increased (1% to <5%)

Ocular: Blurred vision (1% to <5%), miosis (1% to <5%)

Respiratory: Bronchitis (1% to <5%), congestion (nasal/sinus) (1% to <5%), cough (1% to <5%), dyspnea (1% to <5%), nasopharyngitis (1% to <5%), rhinorrhea (1% to <5%), sinusitis (1% to <5%), sneezing (1% to <5%), sore throat (1% to <5%), upper respiratory infection (1% to <5%)

Miscellaneous: Diaphoresis (2% to 9%), flu-like syndrome (1% to < 5%), shivering (<1% to <5%)

<1% (Limited to important or life-threatening): Abnormal ECG, abnormal gait, agitation, allergic reaction, amnesia, anaphylactoid reactions, anaphylaxis, angioedema, appendicitis, ALT/AST increased, bronchospasm, cataracts, cellulitis, cholecystitis, cholelithiasis, clamminess, cognitive dysfunction, concentration difficulty, creatinine increased, deafness, disorientation, dreams abnormal, dysuria, ear infection, edema, gastroenteritis, gastrointestinal bleeding, hallucination, hematuria, hemoglobin decreased, hepatitis, hyperglycemia, hyper-/hypotension, irritability, joint stiffness, libido decreased, liver enzymes increased, liver failure, menstrual disorder, MI, migraine, muscle cramps, muscle spasms, muscle twitching, myalgia, myocardial ischemia, night sweats, palpitation, pancreatitis, peripheral edema, peripheral ischemia, pneumonia, proteinuria, pulmonary edema, pulmonary embolism, sedation, seizure, serotonin syndrome, sleep disorder, speech disorder, Stevens-Johnson syndrome, stomatitis, suicidal tendency, syncope, taste perversion, tachycardia, tinnitus, toxic epidermal necrolysis, urticaria, vertigo, vesicles

A withdrawal syndrome may occur with abrupt discontinuation; includes anxiety, diarrhea, hallucinations (rare), nausea, pain, piloerection, rigors, sweating, and tremor. Uncommon discontinuation symptoms may include severe anxiety, panic attacks, or paresthesia.

Metabolism/Transport Effects Substrate of CYP2D6 (major), 3A4 (major)

Drug Interactions

Alcohol (Ethyl): CNS Depressants may enhance the CNS depressant effect of Alcohol (Ethyl). *Risk C: Monitor therapy*

CNS Depressants: May enhance the adverse/toxic effect of other CNS Depressants. *Risk C: Monitor therapy*

CYP2D6 Inhibitors (Moderate): May diminish the therapeutic effect of TraMADol. These CYP2D6 inhibitors may prevent the metabolic conversion of tramadol to its active metabolite that accounts for much of its opioid-like effects. *Risk C: Monitor therapy*

CYP2D6 Inhibitors (Strong): May diminish the therapeutic effect of TraMADol. These CYP2D6 inhibitors may prevent the metabolic conversion of tramadol to its active metabolite that accounts for much of its opioid-like effects. *Risk C: Monitor therapy*

CYP3A4 Inducers (Strong): May increase the metabolism of CYP3A4 Substrates. *Risk C: Monitor therapy*

CYP3A4 Inhibitors (Moderate): May decrease the metabolism of CYP3A4 Substrates. *Risk C: Monitor therapy*

CYP3A4 Inhibitors (Strong): May decrease the metabolism of CYP3A4 Substrates. *Risk D: Consider therapy modification*

Dasatinib: May increase the serum concentration of CYP3A4 Substrates. *Risk C: Monitor therapy*

Deferasirox: May decrease the serum concentration of CYP3A4 Substrates. *Risk C: Monitor therapy*

Herbs (CYP3A4 Inducers): May increase the metabolism of CYP3A4 Substrates. *Risk C: Monitor therapy*

MAO Inhibitors: TraMADol may enhance the neuroexcitatory and/or seizure-potentiating effect of MAO Inhibitors. *Risk D: Consider therapy modification*

Selective Serotonin Reuptake Inhibitors: May enhance the neuroexcitatory and/or seizure-potentiating effect of TraMADol. TraMADol may enhance the serotonergic effect of Selective Serotonin Reuptake Inhibitors. This may cause serotonin syndrome. *Risk D: Consider therapy modification*

Serotonin Modulators: May enhance the adverse/toxic effect of other Serotonin Modulators. The development of serotonin syndrome may occur. *Risk D: Consider therapy modification*

Sibutramine: May enhance the serotonergic effect of Serotonin Modulators. This may cause serotonin syndrome. *Risk X: Avoid combination*

Tricyclic Antidepressants: May enhance the neuroexcitatory and/or seizure-potentiating effect of TraMADol. *Risk C: Monitor therapy*

Ethanol/Nutrition/Herb Interactions

Ethanol: Avoid ethanol (may increase CNS depression).

Food:

Immediate release: Does not affect the rate or extent of absorption.

Extended release: Reduced C_{max} and AUC and T_{max} occurred 3 hours earlier when taken with a high-fat meal.

Herb/Nutraceutical: Avoid valerian, St John's wort, kava kava, gotu kola (may increase CNS depression).

Stability Store at controlled room temperature of 25°C (77°F).

Mechanism of Action Tramadol and active metabolite (M1) binds to µ-opiate receptors in the CNS causing inhibition of ascending pain pathways, altering the perception of and response to pain; also inhibits the reuptake of norepinephrine and serotonin, which also modifies the ascending pain pathway

Pharmacodynamics/Kinetics

Onset of action: Immediate release: ~1 hour

Duration of action: 9 hours

Absorption: Immediate release formulation: Rapid and complete; Extended release formulation: Delayed

Distribution: V_d: 2.5-3 L/kg

Protein binding, plasma: 20%

Metabolism: Extensively hepatic via demethylation, glucuronidation, and sulfation; has pharmacologically active metabolite formed by CYP2D6 (M1; O-desmethyl tramadol)

Bioavailability: Immediate release: 75%; Extended release: Ultram® ER: 85% to 90% (as compared to immediate release), Zytram® XL, Tridural™: 70%

Half-life elimination: Tramadol: ~6-8 hours; Active metabolite: 7-9 hours; prolonged in elderly, hepatic or renal impairment; Zytram® XL: ~16 hours; Ralivia™ ER, Tridural™: ~5-9 hours

Time to peak: Immediate release: ~2 hours; Extended release: Ultram® ER: ~12 hours, Tridural™: ~4 hours

Excretion: Urine (30% as unchanged drug; 60% as metabolites)

Dosage Moderate-to-severe chronic pain: Oral:

Adults:

Immediate release formulation: 50-100 mg every 4-6 hours (not to exceed 400 mg/day)

For patients not requiring rapid onset of effect, tolerability may be improved by starting dose at 25 mg/day and titrating dose by 25 mg every 3 days, until reaching 25 mg 4 times/day. The total daily dose may then be increased by 50 mg every 3 days as tolerated, to reach dose of 50 mg 4 times/day. After titration, 50-100 mg may be given every 4-6 hours as needed up to a maximum 400 mg/day.

Extended release formulations:

Ultram® ER: Patients not currently on immediate-release: 100 mg once daily; titrate every 5 days (maximum: 300 mg/day); Patients currently on immediate-release: Calculate 24-hour immediate release total and initiate total daily dose (round dose to the next lowest 100 mg increment); titrate (maximum: 300 mg/day)

Ralivia™ ER (Canadian labeling, not available in U.S.): 100 mg once daily; titrate every 5 days as needed based on clinical response and severity of pain (maximum: 300 mg/day)

Tridural™ (Canadian labeling, not available in U.S.): 100 mg once daily; titrate by 100 mg/day every 2 days as needed based on clinical response and severity of pain (maximum: 300 mg/day)

Zytram® XL (Canadian labeling, not available in U.S.): 150 mg once daily; if pain relief is not achieved may titrate by increasing dosage incrementally, with sufficient time to evaluate effect of increased dosage; generally not more often than every 7 days (maximum: 400 mg/day)

Elderly >75 years:

Immediate release: 50 mg every 6 hours (not to exceed 300 mg/day); see dosing adjustments for renal and hepatic impairment.

Extended release formulation: Use with great caution. See adult dosing.

Dosing adjustment in renal impairment:
Immediate release: Cl_{cr} <30 mL/minute: Administer 50-100 mg dose every 12 hours (maximum: 200 mg/day)
Extended release: Should not be used in patients with Cl_{cr} <30 mL/minute
Dosing adjustment in hepatic impairment:
Immediate release: Cirrhosis: Recommended dose: 50 mg every 12 hours
Extended release: Should not be used in patients with severe (Child-Pugh Class C) hepatic dysfunction

Dietary Considerations May be taken with or without food. Extended release formulation: Be consistent; always give with food or always give on an empty stomach.

Administration Extended release tablet: Swallow whole; do not crush, chew, or split

Monitoring Parameters Pain relief, respiratory rate, blood pressure, and pulse; signs of tolerance or abuse

Reference Range 100-300 ng/mL; however, serum level monitoring is not required

Dosage Forms Excipient information presented when available (limited, particularly for generics); consult specific product labeling. [CAN] = Canadian brand name
Tablet, as hydrochloride: 50 mg
Ultram®: 50 mg
Tablet, extended release, as hydrochloride:
Ultram® ER: 100 mg, 200 mg, 300 mg
Ralivia™ ER [CAN]: 100 mg, 200 mg, 300 mg [not available in the U.S.]
Tridural™ [CAN]: 100 mg, 200 mg, 300 mg [not available in the U.S.]
Zytram® XL [CAN]: 150 mg, 200 mg, 300 mg, 400 mg [not available in the U.S.]

◆ **Tramadol Hydrochloride** *see* TraMADol *on page 1604*

◆ **Tramadol Hydrochloride and Acetaminophen** *see* Acetaminophen and Tramadol *on page 38*

◆ **Trandate®** *see* Labetalol *on page 881*

Trandolapril (tran DOE la pril)

Related Information
Angiotensin Agents *on page 1754*

U.S. Brand Names Mavik®

Canadian Brand Names Mavik™

Mexican Brand Names Gopten

Pharmacologic Category Angiotensin-Converting Enzyme (ACE) Inhibitor

Use Treatment of hypertension alone or in combination with other antihypertensive agents; treatment of heart failure or left ventricular dysfunction after myocardial infarction

Unlabeled/Investigational Use As a class, ACE inhibitors are recommended in the treatment of heart failure; to delay the progression of nephropathy and reduce risks of cardiovascular events in hypertensive patients with type 1 or 2 diabetes mellitus

Effect on Mental Status May cause dizziness, drowsiness, nervousness, or insomnia

Effect on Psychiatric Treatment May cause neutropenia; use caution with clozapine and carbamazepine; may decrease lithium clearance resulting in an increase in serum lithium levels and potential lithium toxicity; monitor serum lithium levels; concurrent use with low potency antipsychotics and TCAs may produce additive hypotensive effects

Dosage Summary
Oral:
Children: Dosage not established
Adults: Initial: 1-2 mg once daily; Maintenance: 1-4 mg once daily

Dosage Forms Excipient information presented when available (limited, particularly for generics); consult specific product labeling.
Tablet: 1 mg, 2 mg, 4 mg
Mavik®: 1 mg, 2 mg, 4 mg

Trandolapril and Verapamil (tran DOE la pril & ver AP a mil)

U.S. Brand Names Tarka®

Canadian Brand Names Tarka®

Index Terms Verapamil and Trandolapril

Pharmacologic Category Angiotensin-Converting Enzyme (ACE) Inhibitor; Calcium Channel Blocker

Use Treatment of hypertension; however, not indicated for initial treatment of hypertension

Effect on Mental Status May cause dizziness, drowsiness, nervousness, or insomnia

Effect on Psychiatric Treatment May cause neutropenia; use caution with clozapine and carbamazepine; may decrease lithium clearance resulting in an increase in serum lithium levels and potential lithium toxicity; monitor serum lithium levels; concurrent use with low potency antipsychotics and TCAs may produce additive hypotensive effects; barbiturates may decrease verapamil serum concentrations; verapamil may increase carbamazepine serum concentrations

Dosage Summary

Oral:

Children: Dosage not established

Adults: Trandolapril 1-4 mg and verapamil 180-240 mg once daily

Dosage Forms Excipient information presented when available (limited, particularly for generics); consult specific product labeling.

Tablet, variable release:

1/240: Trandolapril 1 mg [immediate release] and verapamil hydrochloride 240 mg [sustained release]

2/180: Trandolapril 2 mg [immediate release] and verapamil hydrochloride 180 mg [sustained release]

2/240: Trandolapril 2 mg [immediate release] and verapamil hydrochloride 240 mg [sustained release]

4/240: Trandolapril 4 mg [immediate release] and verapamil hydrochloride 240 mg [sustained release]

- ◆ **Transamine Sulphate** *see* Tranylcypromine *on page 1609*
- ◆ **Transderm Scōp®** *see* Scopolamine Derivatives *on page 1463*
- ◆ ***trans*-Retinoic Acid** *see* Tretinoin, Oral *on page 1617*
- ◆ **Trans-Ver-Sal® [OTC]** *see* Salicylic Acid *on page 1454*
- ◆ **Tranxene® SD™** *see* Clorazepate *on page 384*
- ◆ **Tranxene® SD™-Half Strength** *see* Clorazepate *on page 384*
- ◆ **Tranxene T-Tab®** *see* Clorazepate *on page 384*
- ◆ **Tranxene® T-Tab®** *see* Clorazepate *on page 384*

Tranylcypromine (tran il SIP roe meen)

Related Information

Antidepressant Agents *on page 1760*

Tyramine Content of Foods *on page 1848*

U.S. Brand Names Parnate®

Canadian Brand Names Parnate®

Index Terms Transamine Sulphate; Tranylcypromine Sulfate

Pharmacologic Category Antidepressant, Monoamine Oxidase Inhibitor

Generic Available No

Use Treatment of major depressive episode without melancholia

Unlabeled/Investigational Use Post-traumatic stress disorder

Mental Health Comment Not commonly used due to a required low tyramine diet and drug-drug interactions. It is estimated that 20 mg of tranylcypromine = 40 mg of isocarboxazid = 45 mg phenelzine. Phenelzine and isocarboxazid are hydrazine MAO inhibitors and tranylcypromine is a nonhydrazine. These drugs produce irreversible inhibition of MAO inhibitors. The half-life for regeneration is 2-3 days. Therefore, a 2-week period is required when switching from an MAO inhibitor to another antidepressant.

While hypertension and hypertensive crisis are risks associated with MAO inhibitor therapy, orthostatic hypotension may also occur. Orthostasis associated with MAO inhibitor therapy is not related to alpha$_1$-adrenergic receptor blockade. The "false transmitter" concept is used to explain this side effect. This concept states that MAO inhibitors promote gradual accumulation in sympathetic nerve ending of amines lacking direct sympathomimetic activity (octopamine) at the expense of the normal synaptic transmitter, norepinephrine. Since octopamine has little ability to activate either alpha- or beta-adrenergic receptors, a functional impairment of sympathetic neurotransmission occurs.

The MAO inhibitors are usually reserved for patients who do not tolerate or respond to other antidepressants. The brain activity of monoamine oxidase increases with age and even more so in patients with Alzheimer's disease. Therefore, the MAO inhibitors may have an increased role in patients with Alzheimer's disease who are depressed. Phenelzine is less stimulating than tranylcypromine.

Restrictions An FDA-approved medication guide concerning the use of antidepressants in children, adolescents, and young adults must be distributed when dispensing an outpatient prescription (new or refill) where this medication is to be used without direct supervision of a healthcare provider. Medication guides are available at http://www.fda.gov/cder/Offices/ODS/medication_guides.htm. Dispense to parents or guardians of children and adolescents receiving this medication.

Pregnancy Risk Factor C

Lactation Enters breast milk/not recommended

Contraindications Hypersensitivity to tranylcypromine, other MAO inhibitors, dibenzazepine derivatives, or any component of the formulation; cardiovascular disease; cerebrovascular defect; headache history; hepatic disease; hypertension; pheochromocytoma; renal disease; concurrent use of antihistamines, antiparkinson drugs, antihypertensives, bupropion, buspirone, CNS depressants, dexfenfluramine, dextromethorphan, diuretics, ethanol, meperidine, and SSRIs; general anesthesia (discontinue 10 days prior to elective surgery); local vasoconstrictors; spinal anesthesia (hypotension may be exaggerated); sympathomimetics (and related compounds); foods high in tyramine content; supplements containing tyrosine, phenylalanine, tryptophan, or caffeine

Warnings/Precautions **Risk of suicide: [U.S. Boxed Warning]: Antidepressants increase the risk of suicidal thinking and behavior in children, adolescents, and young adults (18-24 years of age) with major depressive disorder (MDD) and other psychiatric disorders;** consider risk prior to prescribing. Short-term studies did not show an increased risk in patients >24 years of age and showed a decreased risk inpatients >65 years. Closely monitor for clinical worsening, suicidality, or unusual changes in behavior such as anxiety, agitation, panic attacks, insomnia, irritability, hostility, impulsivity, akathisia, hypomania, and mania. The patient's family or caregiver should be instructed to closely observe the patient and communicate condition with healthcare provider. Such observation would generally include at least weekly face-to-face contact with patients or their family members or caregivers during the first 4 weeks of treatment, then every other week visits for the next 4 weeks, then at 12 weeks, and as clinically indicated beyond 12 weeks. Additional contact by telephone may be appropriate between face-to-face visits. A medication guide should be dispensed with each prescription. **Tranylcypromine is not FDA approved for treatment of children and adolescents.**

All patients treated with antidepressants should be observed similarly for clinical worsening and suicidality, especially during the initial few months of a course of drug therapy, or at times of dose changes, either increases or decreases. The possibility of a suicide attempt is inherent in major depression and may persist until remission occurs. Worsening depression and severe abrupt suicidality that are not part of the presenting symptoms may require discontinuation or modification of drug therapy. Use caution in high-risk patients during initiation of therapy. Prescriptions should be written for the smallest quantity consistent with good patient care.

Hypertensive crisis may occur with foods/supplements high in tyramine, tryptophan, phenylalanine, or tyrosine content; treatment with phentolamine is recommended for hypertensive crisis. Use with caution in patients who have glaucoma, hyperthyroidism, diabetes or hypotension. May cause orthostatic hypotension (especially at dosages >30 mg/day). Use with caution in patients at risk of seizures, or in patients receiving other drugs which may lower seizure threshold. Discontinue at least 48 hours prior to myelography. May increase the risks associated with electroconvulsive therapy. Consider discontinuing, when possible, prior to elective surgery. Use with caution in patients with renal impairment. Do not use with other MAO inhibitors or antidepressants. Avoid products containing sympathomimetic stimulants or dextromethorphan. Concurrent use with antihypertensive agents may lead to exaggeration of hypotensive effects. May worsen psychosis in some patients or precipitate a shift to mania or hypomania in patients with bipolar disorder. **Tranylcypromine is not FDA approved for the treatment of bipolar depression.**

Elderly patients: Interactions with tyramine or tryptophan-containing foods and orthostasis have limited tranylcypromine's use.

Adverse Reactions Frequency not defined.

Cardiovascular: Edema, orthostatic hypotension, palpitation, tachycardia

Central nervous system: Agitation, akinesia, anxiety, ataxia, chills, confusion, disorientation, dizziness, drowsiness, fatigue, headache, hyper-reflexia, insomnia, mania, memory loss, restlessness, sleep disturbances, twitching

Dermatologic: Alopecia, cystic acne (flare), pruritus, rash, urticaria, scleroderma (localized)

Endocrine & metabolic: Hypernatremia, hypermetabolic syndrome; sexual dysfunction (anorgasmia, ejaculatory disturbances, impotence); SIADH

Gastrointestinal: Abdominal pain, anorexia, constipation, diarrhea, nausea, vomiting, weight gain, xerostomia

Genitourinary: Incontinence, urinary retention

Hematologic: Agranulocytosis, anemia, leukopenia, thrombocytopenia

Hepatic: Hepatitis

Neuromuscular & skeletal: Akinesis, muscle spasm, myoclonus, numbness, paresthesia, tremor, weakness

Ocular: Blurred vision, glaucoma

Otic: Tinnitus

Miscellaneous: Diaphoresis

Metabolism/Transport Effects Inhibits CYP1A2 (moderate), 2A6 (strong), 2C8 (weak), 2C9 (weak), 2C19 (moderate), 2D6 (moderate), 2E1 (weak), 3A4 (weak)

Drug Interactions

Acetylcholinesterase Inhibitors (Central): Anticholinergics may diminish the therapeutic effect of Acetylcholinesterase Inhibitors (Central). Acetylcholinesterase Inhibitors (Central) may diminish the therapeutic effect of Anticholinergics. If the anticholinergic action is a side effect of the agent, the result may be beneficial. *Risk C: Monitor therapy*

Alcohol (Ethyl): CNS Depressants may enhance the CNS depressant effect of Alcohol (Ethyl). *Risk C: Monitor therapy*

Alpha-/Beta-Agonists (Direct-Acting): MAO Inhibitors may enhance the vasopressor effect of Alpha-/Beta-Agonists (Direct-Acting). Primarily with oral administration of phenylephrine. **Exceptions:** Dipivefrin. *Risk D: Consider therapy modification*

Alpha-/Beta-Agonists (Indirect-Acting): MAO Inhibitors may enhance the hypertensive effect of Alpha-/Beta-Agonists (Indirect-Acting). *Risk X: Avoid combination*

Alpha1-Agonists: MAO Inhibitors may enhance the hypertensive effect of Alpha1-Agonists. *Risk X: Avoid combination*

Alpha2-Agonists (Ophthalmic): MAO Inhibitors may enhance the hypertensive effect of Alpha2-Agonists (Ophthalmic). *Risk X: Avoid combination*

Altretamine: May enhance the orthostatic effect of MAO Inhibitors. *Risk C: Monitor therapy*

Amphetamines: MAO Inhibitors may enhance the hypertensive effect of Amphetamines. *Risk X: Avoid combination*

Anilidopiperidine Opioids: May enhance the serotonergic effect of MAO Inhibitors. This could result in serotonin syndrome. Management: Avoid use of fentanyl (and other anilidopiperidine opioids when possible) in patients who have used a monoamine oxidase inhibitor within the past 14 days due to reports of unpredictable but severe adverse effects. *Risk D: Consider therapy modification*

Anticholinergics: May enhance the adverse/toxic effect of other Anticholinergics. **Exceptions:** Paliperidone. *Risk C: Monitor therapy*

Antidepressants (Serotonin/Norepinephrine Reuptake Inhibitor): MAO Inhibitors may enhance the serotonergic effect of Antidepressants (Serotonin/Norepinephrine Reuptake Inhibitor). This may cause serotonin syndrome. *Risk X: Avoid combination*

Atomoxetine: MAO Inhibitors may enhance the neurotoxic (central) effect of Atomoxetine. *Risk X: Avoid combination*

Beta2-Agonists: MAO Inhibitors may enhance the adverse/toxic effect of Beta2-Agonists. *Risk C: Monitor therapy*

BuPROPion: MAO Inhibitors may enhance the neurotoxic (central) effect of BuPROPion. *Risk X: Avoid combination*

BusPIRone: May enhance the adverse/toxic effect of MAO Inhibitors. Elevated blood pressure has been reported. *Risk X: Avoid combination*

CNS Depressants: May enhance the adverse/toxic effect of other CNS Depressants. *Risk C: Monitor therapy*

Codeine: CYP2D6 Inhibitors (Moderate) may diminish the therapeutic effect of Codeine. These CYP2D6 inhibitors may prevent the metabolic conversion of codeine to its active metabolite morphine. *Risk C: Monitor therapy*

COMT Inhibitors: May enhance the adverse/toxic effect of MAO Inhibitors. *Risk D: Consider therapy modification*

Cyclobenzaprine: May enhance the serotonergic effect of MAO Inhibitors. This could result in serotonin syndrome. *Risk X: Avoid combination*

CYP1A2 Substrates: CYP1A2 Inhibitors (Moderate) may decrease the metabolism of CYP1A2 Substrates. *Risk C: Monitor therapy*

CYP2A6 Substrates: CYP2A6 Inhibitors (Strong) may decrease the metabolism of CYP2A6 Substrates. *Risk D: Consider therapy modification*

CYP2C19 Substrates: CYP2C19 Inhibitors (Moderate) may decrease the metabolism of CYP2C19 Substrates. *Risk C: Monitor therapy*

CYP2D6 Substrates: CYP2D6 Inhibitors (Moderate) may decrease the metabolism of CYP2D6 Substrates. **Exceptions:** Tamoxifen. *Risk C: Monitor therapy*

Dexmethylphenidate: MAO Inhibitors may enhance the hypertensive effect of Dexmethylphenidate. *Risk X: Avoid combination*

Dextromethorphan: MAO Inhibitors may enhance the serotonergic effect of Dextromethorphan. This may cause serotonin syndrome. *Risk X: Avoid combination*

Levodopa: May enhance the adverse/toxic effect of MAO Inhibitors. Of particular concern is the development of hypertensive reactions when levodopa is used with nonselective MAOI. *Risk D: Consider therapy modification*

Linezolid: MAO Inhibitors may enhance the adverse/toxic effect of Linezolid. *Risk X: Avoid combination*

Lithium: MAO Inhibitors may enhance the adverse/toxic effect of Lithium. *Risk C: Monitor therapy*

Maprotiline: May enhance the adverse/toxic effect of MAO Inhibitors. *Risk X: Avoid combination*

Meperidine: MAO Inhibitors may enhance the serotonergic effect of Meperidine. This may cause serotonin syndrome. *Risk X: Avoid combination*

Methyldopa: MAO Inhibitors may enhance the adverse/toxic effect of Methyldopa. *Risk X: Avoid combination*

Methylphenidate: MAO Inhibitors may enhance the hypertensive effect of Methylphenidate. *Risk X: Avoid combination*

Mirtazapine: MAO Inhibitors may enhance the neurotoxic (central) effect of Mirtazapine. *Risk X: Avoid combination*

Nebivolol: CYP2D6 Inhibitors (Moderate) may increase the serum concentration of Nebivolol. *Risk C: Monitor therapy*

Pramlintide: May enhance the anticholinergic effect of Anticholinergics. These effects are specific to the GI tract. *Risk D: Consider therapy modification*

Propoxyphene: May enhance the adverse/toxic effect of MAO Inhibitors. Specifically, the risk of serotonin syndrome or other serotonergic adverse events may be increased. *Risk X: Avoid combination*

Rauwolfia Alkaloids: MAO Inhibitors may enhance the adverse/toxic effect of Rauwolfia Alkaloids. Existing MAOI therapy can result in paradoxical effects of added rauwolfia alkaloids (eg, excitation, hypertension). *Risk D: Consider therapy modification*

Selective Serotonin Reuptake Inhibitors: MAO Inhibitors may enhance the serotonergic effect of Selective Serotonin Reuptake Inhibitors. This may cause serotonin syndrome. *Risk X: Avoid combination*

Serotonin 5-HT1D Receptor Agonists: MAO Inhibitors may decrease the metabolism of Serotonin 5-HT1D Receptor Agonists. Management: If MAO inhibitor therapy is required, naratriptan, eletriptan or frovatriptan may be a suitable 5-HT1D agonist to employ. **Exceptions:** Eletriptan; Frovatriptan; Naratriptan. *Risk X: Avoid combination*

Serotonin Modulators: May enhance the adverse/toxic effect of other Serotonin Modulators. The development of serotonin syndrome may occur. *Risk D: Consider therapy modification*

Sibutramine: May enhance the serotonergic effect of Serotonin Modulators. This may cause serotonin syndrome. *Risk X: Avoid combination*

Tamoxifen: CYP2D6 Inhibitors (Moderate) may decrease the metabolism of Tamoxifen. Specifically, CYP2D6 inhibitors may decrease the formation of highly potent active metabolites. *Risk D: Consider therapy modification*

Tetrabenazine: May enhance the adverse/toxic effect of MAO Inhibitors. *Risk X: Avoid combination*

Thioridazine: CYP2D6 Inhibitors may decrease the metabolism of Thioridazine. *Risk X: Avoid combination*

TraMADol: May enhance the neuroexcitatory and/or seizure-potentiating effect of MAO Inhibitors. *Risk D: Consider therapy modification*

Tricyclic Antidepressants: MAO Inhibitors may enhance the serotonergic effect of Tricyclic Antidepressants. This may cause serotonin syndrome. *Risk X: Avoid combination*

Ethanol/Nutrition/Herb Interactions

Ethanol: Avoid ethanol (based on CNS depressant effects and potential tyramine content)

Food: Concurrent ingestion of foods rich in tyramine may cause sudden and severe high blood pressure (hypertensive crisis). Avoid tyramine-containing foods with MAO-Is. Food's freshness is also an important concern; improperly stored or spoiled food can create an environment where tyramine concentrations may increase.

Herb/Nutraceuticals: Avoid valerian, St John's wort, SAMe. Avoid supplements containing caffeine, gingko, yohimbime, ephedra, tyrosine, tryptophan or phenylalanine. Ingestion of large quantities may increase the risk of severe side effects (eg, hypertensive reactions, serotonin syndrome).

Mechanism of Action Tranylcypromine is a nonhydrazine monoamine oxidase inhibitor. It increases endogenous concentrations of epinephrine, norepinephrine, dopamine, and serotonin through inhibition of the enzyme (monoamine oxidase) responsible for the breakdown of these neurotransmitters.

Pharmacodynamics/Kinetics

Onset of action: Therapeutic: 2 days to 3 weeks continued dosing

Half-life elimination: 90-190 minutes

Time to peak, serum: ~2 hours

Excretion: Urine

Dosage Adults: Oral: 10 mg twice daily, increase by 10 mg increments at 1- to 3-week intervals; maximum: 60 mg/day; usual effective dose: 30 mg/day

Dietary Considerations Avoid foods containing tryptophan and caffeine. Avoid tyramine-containing foods/beverages. Some examples include aged or matured cheese, air-dried or cured meats (including sausages and salamis), fava or broad bean pods, tap/draft beers, Marmite concentrate, sauerkraut, soy sauce and other soybean condiments.

Monitoring Parameters Blood pressure, mental status, suicidal ideation (especially at the beginning of therapy or when doses are increased or decreased)

Additional Information Tranylcypromine has a more rapid onset of therapeutic effect than other MAO inhibitors, but causes more severe hypertensive reactions.

Dosage Forms Excipient information presented when available (limited, particularly for generics); consult specific product labeling.

Tablet: 10 mg

◆ **Tranylcypromine Sulfate** *see* Tranylcypromine *on page 1609*

Trastuzumab (tras TU zoo mab)

Medication Safety Issues

High alert medication: The Institute for Safe Medication Practices (ISMP) includes this medication among its list of drug classes which have a heightened risk of causing significant patient harm when used in error.

U.S. Brand Names Herceptin®

Canadian Brand Names Herceptin®

Mexican Brand Names Herceptin

Index Terms NSC-688097

Pharmacologic Category Antineoplastic Agent, Monoclonal Antibody; Monoclonal Antibody

Use Adjuvant treatment of HER-2 overexpressing breast cancer; treatment of HER-2 overexpressing metastatic breast cancer

Effect on Mental Status Insomnia and dizziness are common; may cause depression

Effect on Psychiatric Treatment None reported

Dosage Summary

I.V.:

Children: Dosage not established

Adults: Loading dose: 4 mg/kg; Maintenance: 2 mg/kg once weekly **or** Loading dose: 8 mg/kg; Maintenance: 6 mg/kg every 3 weeks

Dosage Forms Excipient information presented when available (limited, particularly for generics); consult specific product labeling.

Injection, powder for reconstitution:

Herceptin®: 440 mg [packaged with bacteriostatic water for injection; diluent contains benzyl alcohol]

◆ **Trasylol®** *see* Aprotinin *on page 130*

TraZODone (TRAZ oh done)

Medication Safety Issues

Sound-alike/look-alike issues:

Desyrel® may be confused with Demerol®, Delsym®, Zestril®

TraZODone may be confused with traMADol

International issues:

Desyrel® may be confused with Deseril® which is a brand name for methysergide in multiple international markets

Related Information

Anticholinergic Effects of Common Psychotropics *on page 1758*

Antidepressant Agents *on page 1760*

Antidepressant Receptor Profile *on page 1764*

Canadian Brand Names Alti-Trazodone; Apo-Trazodone D®; Apo-Trazodone®; Desyrel®; Gen-Trazodone; Novo-Trazodone; Nu-Trazodone; PMS-Trazodone; ratio-Trazodone; Trazorel®

Index Terms Trazodone Hydrochloride

Pharmacologic Category Antidepressant, Serotonin Reuptake Inhibitor/Antagonist

Generic Available Yes

Use Treatment of depression

Unlabeled/Investigational Use Potential augmenting agent for antidepressants, hypnotic

Restrictions An FDA-approved medication guide concerning the use of antidepressants in children, adolescents, and young adults must be distributed when dispensing an outpatient prescription (new or refill) where this medication is to be used without direct supervision of a healthcare provider. Medication guides are available at http://www.fda.gov/cder/Offices/ODS/medication_guides.htm. Dispense to parents or guardians of children and adolescents receiving this medication.

Pregnancy Risk Factor C

Pregnancy Considerations Trazodone is classified as pregnancy category C due to adverse effects observed in animal studies. When trazodone is taken during pregnancy, an increased risk of major malformations has not been observed in the small number of pregnancies studied. The long-term effects on neurobehavior have not been evaluated.

Women treated for major depression and who are euthymic prior to pregnancy are more likely to experience a relapse when medication is discontinued as compared to pregnant women who continue taking antidepressant medications. Therapy during pregnancy should be individualized; treatment of depression during pregnancy should incorporate the clinical expertise of the mental health clinician, obstetrician, primary healthcare provider, and pediatrician. If treatment during pregnancy is required, consider tapering therapy during the third trimester to prevent potential withdrawal symptoms in the infant. If this is done and the woman is considered to be at risk of relapse from her major depressive disorder, the medication can be restarted following delivery.

Lactation Enters breast milk/use caution (AAP rates "of concern")

Contraindications Hypersensitivity to trazodone or any component of the formulation

Warnings/Precautions [U.S. Boxed Warning]: Antidepressants increase the risk of suicidal thinking and behavior in children, adolescents, and young adults (18-24 years of age) with major depressive disorder (MDD) and other psychiatric disorders; consider risk prior to prescribing. Short-term studies did not show an increased risk in patients >24 years of age and showed a decreased risk in patients ≥65 years. Closely monitor for clinical worsening, suicidality, or unusual changes in behavior; the patient's family or caregiver should be instructed to closely observe the patient and communicate condition with healthcare provider. A medication guide should be dispensed with each prescription. **Trazodone is not FDA approved for use in children.**

The possibility of a suicide attempt is inherent in major depression and may persist until remission occurs. Monitor for worsening of depression or suicidality, especially during initiation of therapy (generally first 1-2 months) or with dose increases or decreases. Use caution in high-risk patients. Worsening depression and severe abrupt suicidality that are not part of the presenting symptoms may require discontinuation or modification of drug therapy. The patient's family or caregiver should be alerted to monitor patients for the emergence of suicidality and associated behaviors (such as agitation, irritability, hostility, impulsivity, and hypomania) and call healthcare provider.

May worsen psychosis in some patients or precipitate a shift to mania or hypomania in patients with bipolar disorder. Patients presenting with depressive symptoms should be screened for bipolar disorder. Monotherapy in patients with bipolar disorder should be avoided. **Trazodone is not FDA approved for the treatment of bipolar depression.**

Priapism, including cases resulting in permanent dysfunction, has occurred with the use of trazodone. Not recommended for use in a patient during the acute recovery phase of MI. Trazodone should be initiated with caution in patients who are receiving concurrent or recent therapy with a MAO inhibitor.

The risks of sedation and/or postural hypotension are high relative to other antidepressants. Trazodone frequently causes sedation, which may result in impaired performance of tasks requiring alertness (eg, operating machinery or driving). Sedative effects may be additive with other CNS depressants and ethanol. Use with caution in patients with a history of cardiovascular disease (including previous MI, stroke, tachycardia, or conduction abnormalities). The risk of conduction abnormalities with this agent is low relative to other antidepressants.

Consider discontinuing, when possible, prior to elective surgery. Therapy should not be abruptly discontinued in patients receiving high doses for prolonged periods. Use caution in patients with a previous seizure disorder or condition predisposing to seizures such as brain damage, alcoholism, or concurrent therapy with other drugs which lower the seizure threshold. Use with caution in patients with hepatic or renal dysfunction and in elderly patients.

Adverse Reactions

>10%:

Central nervous system: Dizziness, headache, sedation

Gastrointestinal: Nausea, xerostomia

Ocular: Blurred vision

1% to 10%:

Cardiovascular: Syncope, hyper-/hypotension, edema

Central nervous system: Confusion, decreased concentration, fatigue, incoordination

Gastrointestinal: Diarrhea, constipation, weight gain/loss

Neuromuscular & skeletal: Tremor, myalgia

Respiratory: Nasal congestion

<1% (Limited to important or life-threatening): Agitation, allergic reactions, alopecia, anxiety, bradycardia, extrapyramidal symptoms, hepatitis, priapism, rash, seizure, speech impairment, tachycardia, urinary retention

Metabolism/Transport Effects Substrate of CYP2D6 (minor), 3A4 (major); **Inhibits** CYP2D6 (moderate), 3A4 (weak)

Drug Interactions

Alcohol (Ethyl): CNS Depressants may enhance the CNS depressant effect of Alcohol (Ethyl). *Risk C: Monitor therapy*

BusPIRone: May enhance the serotonergic effect of Antidepressants (Serotonin Reuptake Inhibitor/Antagonist). This may cause serotonin syndrome. *Risk C: Monitor therapy*

CNS Depressants: May enhance the adverse/toxic effect of other CNS Depressants. *Risk C: Monitor therapy*

Codeine: CYP2D6 Inhibitors (Moderate) may diminish the therapeutic effect of Codeine. These CYP2D6 inhibitors may prevent the metabolic conversion of codeine to its active metabolite morphine. *Risk C: Monitor therapy*

CYP2D6 Substrates: CYP2D6 Inhibitors (Moderate) may decrease the metabolism of CYP2D6 Substrates. **Exceptions:** Tamoxifen. *Risk C: Monitor therapy*

CYP3A4 Inducers (Strong): May increase the metabolism of CYP3A4 Substrates. *Risk C: Monitor therapy*

CYP3A4 Inhibitors (Moderate): May decrease the metabolism of CYP3A4 Substrates. *Risk C: Monitor therapy*

CYP3A4 Inhibitors (Strong): May decrease the metabolism of CYP3A4 Substrates. *Risk D: Consider therapy modification*

Dabigatran Etexilate: P-Glycoprotein Inducers may decrease the serum concentration of Dabigatran Etexilate. *Risk C: Monitor therapy*

Dasatinib: May increase the serum concentration of CYP3A4 Substrates. *Risk C: Monitor therapy*

Deferasirox: May decrease the serum concentration of CYP3A4 Substrates. *Risk C: Monitor therapy*

Herbs (CYP3A4 Inducers): May increase the metabolism of CYP3A4 Substrates. *Risk C: Monitor therapy*

Nebivolol: CYP2D6 Inhibitors (Moderate) may increase the serum concentration of Nebivolol. *Risk C: Monitor therapy*

P-Glycoprotein Substrates: P-Glycoprotein Inducers may decrease the serum concentration of P-Glycoprotein Substrates. P-glycoprotein inducers may also further limit the distribution of p-glycoprotein substrates to specific cells/tissues/organs where p-glycoprotein is present in large amounts (e.g., brain, T-lymphocytes, testes, etc.). *Risk C: Monitor therapy*

Protease Inhibitors: May increase the serum concentration of TraZODone. *Risk D: Consider therapy modification*

Selective Serotonin Reuptake Inhibitors: May enhance the serotonergic effect of Antidepressants (Serotonin Reuptake Inhibitor/Antagonist). This may cause serotonin syndrome. *Risk C: Monitor therapy*

Serotonin Modulators: May enhance the adverse/toxic effect of other Serotonin Modulators. The development of serotonin syndrome may occur. *Risk D: Consider therapy modification*

Sibutramine: May enhance the serotonergic effect of Serotonin Modulators. This may cause serotonin syndrome. *Risk X: Avoid combination*

Tamoxifen: CYP2D6 Inhibitors (Moderate) may decrease the metabolism of Tamoxifen. Specifically, CYP2D6 inhibitors may decrease the formation of highly potent active metabolites. *Risk D: Consider therapy modification*

TraMADol: CYP2D6 Inhibitors (Moderate) may diminish the therapeutic effect of TraMADol. These CYP2D6 inhibitors may prevent the metabolic conversion of tramadol to its active metabolite that accounts for much of its opioid-like effects. *Risk C: Monitor therapy*

Venlafaxine: May enhance the serotonergic effect of TraZODone. This could result in serotonin syndrome. *Risk D: Consider therapy modification*

Ethanol/Nutrition/Herb Interactions

Ethanol: Avoid ethanol (may increase CNS depression).

Food: Time to peak serum levels may be increased if trazodone is taken with food.

Herb/Nutraceutical: Avoid valerian, St John's wort, SAMe, kava kava (may increase risk of serotonin syndrome and/or excessive sedation).

Mechanism of Action Inhibits reuptake of serotonin, causes adrenoreceptor subsensitivity, and induces significant changes in 5-HT presynaptic receptor adrenoreceptors. Trazodone also significantly blocks histamine (H_1) and alpha$_1$-adrenergic receptors.

Pharmacodynamics/Kinetics

Onset of action: Therapeutic (antidepressant): 1-3 weeks; sleep aid: 1-3 hours

Protein binding: 85% to 95%

Metabolism: Hepatic via CYP3A4 to an active metabolite (mCPP)

Half-life elimination: 7-8 hours, two compartment kinetics

Time to peak, serum: 30-100 minutes; delayed with food (up to 2.5 hours)

Excretion: Primarily urine; secondarily feces

Dosage Oral: Therapeutic effects may take up to 6 weeks to occur; therapy is normally maintained for 6-12 months after optimum response is reached to prevent recurrence of depression

Children 6-12 years: Depression (unlabeled use): Initial: 1.5-2 mg/kg/day in divided doses; increase gradually every 3-4 days as needed; maximum: 6 mg/kg/day in 3 divided doses

Adolescents: Depression (unlabeled use): Initial: 25-50 mg/day; increase to 100-150 mg/day in divided doses

Adults:

Depression: Initial: 150 mg/day in 3 divided doses (may increase by 50 mg/day every 3-7 days); maximum: 600 mg/day

Sedation/hypnotic (unlabeled use): 25-50 mg at bedtime (often in combination with daytime SSRIs); may increase up to 200 mg at bedtime

Elderly: 25-50 mg at bedtime with 25-50 mg/day dose increase every 3 days for inpatients and weekly for outpatients, if tolerated; usual dose: 75-150 mg/day

Administration Dosing after meals may decrease lightheadedness and postural hypotension

Monitoring Parameters Suicidal ideation (especially at the beginning of therapy or when doses are increased or decreased)

Reference Range

Plasma levels do not always correlate with clinical effectiveness

Therapeutic: 0.5-2.5 mcg/mL

Potentially toxic: >2.5 mcg/mL

Toxic: >4 mcg/mL

Dosage Forms Excipient information presented when available (limited, particularly for generics); consult specific product labeling.

Tablet, as hydrochloride: 50 mg, 100 mg, 150 mg, 300 mg

◆ **Trazodone Hydrochloride** *see* TraZODone *on page 1614*

◆ **Treanda®** *see* Bendamustine *on page 179*

- **Trecator®** *see* Ethionamide *on page 602*
- **Trelstar® Depot** *see* Triptorelin *on page 1635*
- **Trelstar® LA** *see* Triptorelin *on page 1635*
- **Trental®** *see* Pentoxifylline *on page 1251*
- **Tretinoin and Clindamycin** *see* Clindamycin and Tretinoin *on page 364*
- **Tretinoin and Mequinol** *see* Mequinol and Tretinoin *on page 992*

Tretinoin, Oral (TRET i noyn, oral)

Medication Safety Issues

Sound-alike/look-alike issues:

Tretinoin may be confused with isotretinoin, trientine

High alert medication: The Institute for Safe Medication Practices (ISMP) includes this medication among its list of drugs which have a heightened risk of causing significant patient harm when used in error.

U.S. Brand Names Vesanoid®

Canadian Brand Names Vesanoid®

Mexican Brand Names Vesanoid

Index Terms *trans*-Retinoic Acid; All-*trans*-Retinoic Acid; ATRA; NSC-122758; Ro 5488; tRA

Pharmacologic Category Antineoplastic Agent, Miscellaneous; Retinoic Acid Derivative

Use Induction of remission in patients with acute promyelocytic leukemia (APL), French American British (FAB) classification M3 (including the M3 variant)

Effect on Mental Status Dizziness, anxiety, insomnia, depression, and confusion are common; may cause agitation, hallucinations, or cognitive impairment; may rarely cause mood changes

Effect on Psychiatric Treatment None reported

Dosage Summary

Oral:

Children: Induction: 45 $mg/m^2/day$ in 2-3 divided doses (maximum duration of treatment: 90 days); Maintenance: 45-200 $mg/m^2/day$ in 2-3 divided doses for up to 12 months

Adults: Induction: 45 $mg/m^2/day$ in 2-3 divided doses (maximum duration of treatment: 90 days); Maintenance: 45-200 $mg/m^2/day$ in 2-3 divided doses for up to 12 months

Dosage Forms Excipient information presented when available (limited, particularly for generics); consult specific product labeling.

Capsule: 10 mg

Vesanoid®: 10 mg [contains soybean oil and parabens]

- **Trexall™** *see* Methotrexate *on page 1014*
- **Treximet™** *see* Sumatriptan and Naproxen *on page 1530*
- **TRH** *see* Protirelin *on page 1363*
- **Triall™** *see* Chlorpheniramine, Phenylephrine, and Methscopolamine *on page 329*

Triamcinolone (trye am SIN oh lone)

Medication Safety Issues

Sound-alike/look-alike issues:

Kenalog® may be confused with Ketalar®

Nasacort® may be confused with NasalCrom®

TAC (occasional abbreviation for triamcinolone) is an error-prone abbreviation (mistaken as tetracaine-adrenaline-cocaine)

Related Information

Corticosteroids *on page 1780*

U.S. Brand Names Aristospan®; Azmacort®; Kenalog-10®; Kenalog-40®; Kenalog®; Nasacort® AQ; Tri-Nasal® [DSC]; Triderm®; Triesence™; Trivaris™; Zytopic™

Canadian Brand Names Aristospan®; Kenalog®; Kenalog® in Orabase; Nasacort® AQ; Oracort; Triaderm; Trinasal®

Mexican Brand Names Intralon; Nasacort AQ

Index Terms Triamcinolone Acetonide, Aerosol; Triamcinolone Acetonide, Parenteral; Triamcinolone Diacetate, Oral; Triamcinolone Diacetate, Parenteral; Triamcinolone Hexacetonide; Triamcinolone, Oral

Pharmacologic Category Corticosteroid, Inhalant (Oral); Corticosteroid, Nasal; Corticosteroid, Ophthalmic; Corticosteroid, Systemic; Corticosteroid, Topical

Use

Intra-articular (soft tissue): Acute gouty arthritis, acute/subacute bursitis, acute tenosynovitis, epicondylitis, rheumatoid arthritis, synovitis of osteoarthritis

Intralesional: Alopecia areata, discoid lupus erythematosus, keloids, granuloma annulare lesions (localized hypertrophic, infiltrated, or inflammatory), lichen planus plaques, lichen simplex chronicus plaques, psoriatic plaques, necrobiosis lipoidica diabeticorum, cystic tumors of aponeurosis or tendon (ganglia)

Nasal inhalation: Management of seasonal and perennial allergic rhinitis

Ophthalmic: Intravitreal: treatment of sympathetic ophthalmia, temporal arteritis, uveitis, ocular inflammatory conditions unresponsive to topical corticosteroids

Triesence™: Visualization during vitrectomy

Oral inhalation: Control of bronchial asthma and related bronchospastic conditions

Oral topical: Adjunctive treatment and temporary relief of symptoms associated with oral inflammatory lesions and ulcerative lesions resulting from trauma

Systemic: Adrenocortical insufficiency, dermatologic diseases, endocrine disorders, gastrointestinal diseases, hematologic and neoplastic disorders, nervous system disorders, nephrotic syndrome, rheumatic disorders, allergic states, respiratory diseases, systemic lupus erythematosus (SLE), and other diseases requiring anti-inflammatory or immunosuppressive effects

Topical: Inflammatory dermatoses responsive to steroids

Effect on Mental Status Nervousness and insomnia are common; may cause drowsiness, delirium, euphoria, hallucinations, or mood swings

Effect on Psychiatric Treatment Barbiturates may increase the metabolism of triamcinolone

Dosage Summary

Inhalation:

Nasal inhaler:

Children <6 years: Dosage not established

Children 6-11 years: 220 mcg/day as 2 sprays in each nostril once daily

Children ≥12 years: 220-440 mcg/day as 2-4 sprays in each nostril 1-4 times/day

Adults: 220-440 mcg/day as 2-4 sprays in each nostril 1-4 times/day

Nasal spray:

Children <2 years: Dosage not established

Children 2-5 years: 110 mcg/day as 1 spray in each nostril once daily (maximum: 110 mcg/day)

Children 6-11 years: Initial: 110 mcg/day as 1 spray in each nostril once daily; may increase to 220 mcg/day as 2 sprays in each nostril

Children ≥12 years: 110-220 mcg/day as 1-2 sprays in each nostril once daily

Adults: 110-220 mcg/day as 1-2 sprays in each nostril once daily

Oral:

Children <6 years: Dosage not established

Children 6-12 years: 75-150 mcg 3-4 times/day **or** 150-300 mcg twice daily (maximum dose: 900 mcg/day)

Children >12 years: 150 mcg 3-4 times/day **or** 300 mcg twice daily (maximum dose: 1200 mcg/day)

Adults: 150 mcg 3-4 times/day **or** 300 mcg twice daily (maximum dose: 1200 mcg/day)

I.M.:

Children: Initial: 0.11-1.6 mg/kg/day in 3-4 divided doses

Children 6-12 years: Acetonide: Initial: 40 mg; Range: 2.5-100 mg/day

Children >12 years: Acetonide: Initial: 60 mg; Range: 2.5-100 mg/day

Adults: Acetonide: Initial: 60 mg; Range: 2.5-100 mg/day, may repeat with 20-100 mg when symptoms recur; Multiple sclerosis: 160 mg/day for 1 week, then 64 mg every other day

Intra-articular:

Children: Dosage not established

Adults: Acetonide: 2.5-80 mg; Hexacetonide: 2-20 mg

Intradermal:

Children: Dosage not established

Adults: Acetonide: 1 mg/site

Intralesional:

Children: Dosage not established

Adults: Acetonide: 1-30 mg (usually 1 mg/injection site); Hexacetonide: Up to 0.5 mg/sq inch

Intrasynovial:
Children: Dosage not established
Adults: Acetonide: 5-40 mg

Intravitreal:
Children: Ocular disease: 4 mg as needed; visualization during vitrectomy: 1-4 mg
Adults: Ocular disease: 4 mg as needed; visualization during vitrectomy: 1-4 mg

Tendon Sheath:
Children: Dosage not established
Adults: Acetonide: 2.5-10 mg

Topical:
Children: Dosage not established
Adults: Cream, ointment: Apply thin film to affected areas 2-4 times/day; Oral: Press a small dab (about 1/4 inch) to the lesion until a thin film develops; Spray: Apply to affected area 3-4 times/day

Dosage Forms Excipient information presented when available (limited, particularly for generics); consult specific product labeling. [DSC] = Discontinued product

Aerosol for oral inhalation, as acetonide:
Azmacort®: 75 mcg per actuation (20 g) [contains chlorofluorocarbon; 240 actuations]

Aerosol, topical, as acetonide:
Kenalog®: 0.2 mg/2-second spray (63 g) [contains dehydrated ethanol 10.3%]

Cream, as acetonide: 0.025% (15 g, 80 g, 454 g); 0.1% (15 g, 80 g, 454 g, 2270 g); 0.5% (15 g)
Triderm®: 0.1% (30 g, 85 g)
Zytopic™: 0.1% (85 g)

Injection, suspension, as acetonide:
Kenalog-10®: 10 mg/mL (5 mL) [contains benzyl alcohol, polysorbate 80; not for I.V. or I.M. use]
Kenalog-40®: 40 mg/mL (1 mL, 5 mL, 10 mL) [contains benzyl alcohol, polysorbate 80; not for I.V. or intradermal use]
Triesence™: 40 mg/mL (1 mL) [contains polysorbate 80; not for I.V. use]
Trivaris™: 80 mg/mL (0.1 mL) [preservative free; not for I.V. use; (for intra-articular, intramuscular, intravitreal use)]

Injection, suspension, as hexacetonide:
Aristospan®: 5 mg/mL (5 mL); 20 mg/mL (1 mL, 5 mL) [contains benzyl alcohol, polysorbate 80; not for I.V. use]

Lotion, as acetonide: 0.025% (60 mL); 0.1% (60 mL)

Ointment, topical, as acetonide: 0.025% (15 g, 80 g, 454 g); 0.05% (430 g); 0.1% (15 g, 80 g, 454 g); 0.5% (15 g)

Paste, oral, topical, as acetonide: 0.1% (5 g)

Powder, for prescription compounding, as acetonide [micronized]: Triamcinolone acetonide USP (5 g)

Solution, intranasal, as acetonide [spray]:
Tri-Nasal®: 50 mcg/inhalation (15 mL) [120 actuations] [DSC]

Suspension, intranasal, as acetonide [spray]:
Nasacort® AQ: 55 mcg/inhalation (16.5 g) [120 actuations]

◆ **Triamcinolone Acetonide, Aerosol** *see* Triamcinolone *on page 1617*

◆ **Triamcinolone Acetonide, Parenteral** *see* Triamcinolone *on page 1617*

◆ **Triamcinolone Diacetate, Oral** *see* Triamcinolone *on page 1617*

◆ **Triamcinolone Diacetate, Parenteral** *see* Triamcinolone *on page 1617*

◆ **Triamcinolone Hexacetonide** *see* Triamcinolone *on page 1617*

◆ **Triamcinolone, Oral** *see* Triamcinolone *on page 1617*

◆ **Triaminic® Cold and Allergy [OTC]** *see* Chlorpheniramine and Phenylephrine *on page 323*

◆ **Triaminic® Infant Thin Strips® Decongestant [OTC] [DSC]** *see* Phenylephrine *on page 1273*

◆ **Triaminic® Thin Strips® Cold [OTC]** *see* Phenylephrine *on page 1273*

◆ **Triaminic® Thin Strips™ Cough and Runny Nose [OTC]** *see* DiphenhydrAMINE *on page 481*

◆ **Triaminic® Thin Strips™ Long Acting Cough [OTC]** *see* Dextromethorphan *on page 448*

Triamterene (trye AM ter een)

Medication Safety Issues

Sound-alike/look-alike issues:

Triamterene may be confused with trimipramine

Dyrenium® may be confused with Pyridium®

U.S. Brand Names Dyrenium®

Pharmacologic Category Diuretic, Potassium-Sparing

Use Alone or in combination with other diuretics in treatment of edema and hypertension; decreases potassium excretion caused by kaliuretic diuretics

Effect on Mental Status May cause drowsiness or dizziness

Effect on Psychiatric Treatment Triamterene may increase the side effects of amantadine (dizziness, nausea, dry mouth) necessitating a decrease in dosage; monitor

Dosage Summary

Oral:

Children (unlabeled dose): Initial: 1-2 mg/kg/day in 2 divided doses; maximum: 3-4 mg/kg/day, up to 300 mg/day

Adults: 50-300 mg/day in 1-2 divided doses (maximum: 300 mg/day)

Dosage Forms Excipient information presented when available (limited, particularly for generics); consult specific product labeling.

Capsule: 50 mg, 100 mg [contains benzyl alcohol]

◆ **Triamterene and Hydrochlorothiazide** *see* Hydrochlorothiazide and Triamterene *on page 776*

◆ **Triant-HC™** *see* Phenylephrine, Hydrocodone, and Chlorpheniramine *on page 1277*

Triazolam (trye AY zoe lam)

Medication Safety Issues

Sound-alike/look-alike issues:

Triazolam may be confused with alPRAZolam

Halcion® may be confused with halcinonide, Haldol®

Related Information

Benzodiazepines *on page 1774*

CMS: Long-Term Care Facility Thresholds *on page 1815*

Discontinuation of Psychotropic Drugs *on page 1839*

U.S. Brand Names Halcion®

Canadian Brand Names Apo-Triazo®; Gen-Triazolam; Halcion®

Mexican Brand Names Halcion

Pharmacologic Category Hypnotic, Benzodiazepine

Generic Available Yes

Use Short-term treatment of insomnia

Mental Health Comment In 2007, the FDA requested that all manufacturers of sedative-hypnotic drug products revise labeling to include a greater emphasis on the risks of adverse effects. These risks include severe allergic reactions (anaphylaxis, angioedema) and complex sleep-related behaviors, which may include sleep-driving (driving while not fully awake and with no memory of the event), making phone calls, and preparing and eating food while asleep.

There are two subtypes of GABA receptors (GABA-A and GABA-B) and three different benzodiazepine receptors (Bz_1, Bz_2, and Bz_3). Benzodiazepine receptors and effects appear to be linked to the GABA-A receptors. Benzodiazepines do not bind to GABA-B receptors. The role of GABA-B receptors is unclear. Benzodiazepines have no specificity for benzodiazepine receptor subtypes.

Triazolam is a short half-life benzodiazepine. Duration of action after a single dose is determined by redistribution rather than metabolism. Tolerance develops to the sedative, hypnotic, and anticonvulsant effects. It does not develop to the anxiolytic or skeletal muscle relaxing effects. Psychological and physical dependence may occur with prolonged use of benzodiazepines. The onset of withdrawal symptoms is usually seen on the first day without drug and lasts 5-7 days in patients receiving short half-life benzodiazepines, whereas, the onset occurs after 5 days with a duration of 10-14 days after abrupt discontinuance of long half-life benzodiazepines. Risk factors for abuse include personal or family history of substance abuse and personality disorder.

Restrictions C-IV

An FDA-approved patient medication guide is available and must be distributed when dispensing an outpatient prescription (new or refill) where this medication is to be used without direct supervision of a healthcare provider. Medication guides are available at http://www.fda.gov/cder/Offices/ODS/medication_guides.htm.

Pregnancy Risk Factor X

Pregnancy Considerations Other benzodiazepines are known to cross the placenta and accumulate in the fetus. Teratogenic effects have been reported. Use of triazolam is contraindicated in pregnancy.

Lactation Excretion in breast milk unknown/not recommended

Contraindications Hypersensitivity to triazolam or any component of the formulation (cross-sensitivity with other benzodiazepines may exist); concurrent therapy with itraconazole, ketoconazole, nefazodone, and other moderate/strong CYP3A4 inhibitors; pregnancy

Warnings/Precautions As a hypnotic, should be used only after evaluation of potential causes of sleep disturbance. Failure of sleep disturbance to resolve after 7-10 days may indicate psychiatric or medical illness. A worsening of insomnia or the emergence of new abnormalities of thought or behavior may represent unrecognized psychiatric or medical illness and requires immediate and careful evaluation. Prescription should be written for a maximum of 7-10 days and should not be prescribed in quantities exceeding a 1-month supply. Abrupt discontinuation after sustained use (generally >10 days) may cause withdrawal symptoms.

An increase in daytime anxiety may occur after as few as 10 days of continuous use, which may be related to withdrawal reaction in some patients. Anterograde amnesia may occur at a higher rate with triazolam than with other benzodiazepines. Use with caution in elderly or debilitated patients, patients with hepatic disease (including alcoholics), or renal impairment. Use with caution in patients with respiratory disease or impaired gag reflex. Avoid use in patients with sleep apnea.

Causes CNS depression (dose-related) resulting in sedation, dizziness, confusion, or ataxia which may impair physical and mental capabilities. Patients must be cautioned about performing tasks which require mental alertness (eg, operating machinery or driving). Use with caution in patients receiving other CNS depressants or psychoactive agents. Postmarketing studies have indicated that the use of hypnotic/sedative agents for sleep has been associated with hypersensitivity reactions including anaphylaxis as well as angioedema. An increased risk for hazardous sleep-related activities such as sleep-driving; cooking and eating food, and making phone calls while asleep have also been noted. Effects with other sedative drugs or ethanol may be potentiated. Benzodiazepines have been associated with falls and traumatic injury and should be used with extreme caution in patients who are at risk of these events (especially the elderly).

Use caution with potent CYP3A4 inhibitors, as they may significantly decreased the clearance of triazolam. Use caution in patients with suicidal risk. Use with caution in patients with a history of drug dependence. Benzodiazepines have been associated with dependence and acute withdrawal symptoms on discontinuation or reduction in dose. Acute withdrawal, including seizures, may be precipitated after administration of flumazenil to patients receiving long-term benzodiazepine therapy.

Paradoxical reactions, including hyperactive or aggressive behavior have been reported with benzodiazepines, particularly in adolescent/pediatric or psychiatric patients. Does not have analgesic, antidepressant, or antipsychotic properties.

Adverse Reactions

>10%: Central nervous system: Drowsiness (14%)

1% to 10%:

Central nervous system: Headache (10%), dizziness (8%), nervousness (5%), lightheadedness (5%), ataxia (5%)

Gastrointestinal: Nausea (5%), vomiting (5%)

<1% (Limited to important or life-threatening): Anaphylaxis, angioedema, anterograde amnesia; complex sleep-related behavior (sleep-driving, cooking or eating food, making phone calls); confusion, cramps, depression, dermatitis, dreaming/nightmares, dysesthesia, euphoria, fatigue, memory impairment, pain, paresthesia, tachycardia, visual disturbance, weakness, xerostomia

In addition, the following have been reported in association with triazolam and other benzodiazepines: Chest pain, dysarthria, libido changes; paradoxical reactions (eg, mania, sleep disturbances, hallucination, delusions, aggressiveness, falling, syncope); sedation, slurred speech

Metabolism/Transport Effects Substrate of CYP3A4 (major); **Inhibits** CYP2C8 (weak), 2C9 (weak)

Drug Interactions

Alcohol (Ethyl): CNS Depressants may enhance the CNS depressant effect of Alcohol (Ethyl). *Risk C: Monitor therapy*

Antifungal Agents (Azole Derivatives, Systemic): May decrease the metabolism of Benzodiazepines (metabolized by oxidation). *Risk D: Consider therapy modification*

Aprepitant: May increase the serum concentration of Benzodiazepines (metabolized by oxidation). *Risk C: Monitor therapy*

Calcium Channel Blockers (Nondihydropyridine): May decrease the metabolism of Benzodiazepines (metabolized by oxidation). *Risk D: Consider therapy modification*

CarBAMazepine: May increase the metabolism of Benzodiazepines (metabolized by oxidation). *Risk C: Monitor therapy*

Cimetidine: May decrease the metabolism of Benzodiazepines (metabolized by oxidation). *Risk C: Monitor therapy*

Clozapine: Benzodiazepines may enhance the adverse/toxic effect of Clozapine. *Risk D: Consider therapy modification*

CNS Depressants: May enhance the adverse/toxic effect of other CNS Depressants. *Risk C: Monitor therapy*

CYP3A4 Inducers (Strong): May increase the metabolism of CYP3A4 Substrates. *Risk C: Monitor therapy*

CYP3A4 Inhibitors (Moderate): May decrease the metabolism of CYP3A4 Substrates. *Risk C: Monitor therapy*

CYP3A4 Inhibitors (Strong): May decrease the metabolism of CYP3A4 Substrates. *Risk D: Consider therapy modification*

Dasatinib: May increase the serum concentration of CYP3A4 Substrates. *Risk C: Monitor therapy*

Deferasirox: May decrease the serum concentration of CYP3A4 Substrates. *Risk C: Monitor therapy*

Disulfiram: May decrease the metabolism of Benzodiazepines (metabolized by oxidation). *Risk C: Monitor therapy*

Efavirenz: May increase the serum concentration of Triazolam. *Risk X: Avoid combination*

Fluconazole: May decrease the metabolism of Benzodiazepines (metabolized by oxidation). *Risk D: Consider therapy modification*

Fosaprepitant: May increase the serum concentration of Benzodiazepines (metabolized by oxidation). Specifically, the active metabolite aprepitant is likely responsible for this effect. *Risk C: Monitor therapy*

Grapefruit Juice: May decrease the metabolism of Benzodiazepines (metabolized by oxidation). *Risk D: Consider therapy modification*

Isoniazid: May decrease the metabolism of Benzodiazepines (metabolized by oxidation). *Risk C: Monitor therapy*

Macrolide Antibiotics: May decrease the metabolism of Benzodiazepines (metabolized by oxidation). **Exceptions:** Azithromycin; Dirithromycin [Off Market]; Spiramycin. *Risk D: Consider therapy modification*

Nefazodone: May decrease the metabolism of Benzodiazepines (metabolized by oxidation). *Risk D: Consider therapy modification*

Oral Contraceptive (Estrogens): May decrease the metabolism of Benzodiazepines (metabolized by oxidation). *Risk C: Monitor therapy*

Oral Contraceptive (Progestins): May decrease the metabolism of Benzodiazepines (metabolized by oxidation). *Risk C: Monitor therapy*

Phenytoin: Benzodiazepines may increase the serum concentration of Phenytoin. Short-term exposure to benzodiazepines may not present as much risk as chronic therapy. *Risk C: Monitor therapy*

Protease Inhibitors: May decrease the metabolism of Benzodiazepines (metabolized by oxidation). Management: Amprenavir, atazanavir, darunavir, indinavir, nelfinavir, ritonavir, and tipranavir are contraindicated with midazolam and triazolam according to each protease inhibitor 's prescribing information. *Risk D: Consider therapy modification*

Proton Pump Inhibitors: May increase the serum concentration of Benzodiazepines (metabolized by oxidation). **Exceptions:** Lansoprazole; Pantoprazole; Rabeprazole. *Risk C: Monitor therapy*

Rifamycin Derivatives: May increase the metabolism of Benzodiazepines (metabolized by oxidation). *Risk D: Consider therapy modification*

Selective Serotonin Reuptake Inhibitors: May decrease the metabolism of Benzodiazepines (metabolized by oxidation). **Exceptions:** Citalopram; Escitalopram; PARoxetine; Sertraline. *Risk C: Monitor therapy*

St Johns Wort: May increase the metabolism of Benzodiazepines (metabolized by oxidation). *Risk C: Monitor therapy*

Theophylline Derivatives: May diminish the therapeutic effect of Benzodiazepines. *Risk D: Consider therapy modification*

Ethanol/Nutrition/Herb Interactions

Ethanol: Avoid ethanol (may increase CNS depression).

Food: Food may decrease the rate of absorption. Benzodiazepine serum concentrations may be increased by grapefruit juice; monitor.

Herb/Nutraceutical: St John's wort may decrease levels/effects of benzodiazepines. Avoid valerian, St John's wort, kava kava, gotu kola (may increase CNS depression).

Stability Store at controlled room temperature of 20°C to 25°C (68°F to 77°F).

Mechanism of Action Binds to stereospecific benzodiazepine receptors on the postsynaptic GABA neuron at several sites within the central nervous system, including the limbic system, reticular formation. Enhancement of the inhibitory effect of GABA on neuronal excitability results by increased neuronal membrane permeability to chloride ions. This shift in chloride ions results in hyperpolarization (a less excitable state) and stabilization.

Pharmacodynamics/Kinetics

Onset of action: Hypnotic: 15-30 minutes

Duration: 6-7 hours

Distribution: V_d: 0.8-1.8 L/kg

Protein binding: 89%

Metabolism: Extensively hepatic

Half-life elimination: 1.5-5.5 hours

Excretion: Urine as unchanged drug and metabolites

Dosage Oral (onset of action is rapid, patient should be in bed when taking medication):

Children <18 years: Dosage not established

Adults:

Insomnia (short-term): 0.125-0.25 mg at bedtime (maximum dose: 0.5 mg/day)

Preprocedure sedation (dental): 0.25 mg taken the evening before oral surgery; or 0.25 mg 1 hour before procedure

Elderly: Insomnia (short-term use): Initial: 0.125 mg at bedtime; maximum dose: 0.25 mg/day

Dosing adjustment/comments in hepatic impairment: Reduce dose or avoid use in cirrhosis

Administration May take with food. Tablet may be crushed or swallowed whole. Onset of action is rapid, patient should be in bed when taking medication.

Monitoring Parameters Respiratory and cardiovascular status

Dosage Forms Excipient information presented when available (limited, particularly for generics); consult specific product labeling. [DSC] = Discontinued product

Tablet: 0.125 mg, 0.25 mg

Halcion®: 0.125 mg [DSC], 0.25 mg

- ◆ **Tribavirin** *see* Ribavirin *on page 1417*
- ◆ **Trichloroacetaldehyde Monohydrate** *see* Chloral Hydrate *on page 313*
- ◆ **TriCor®** *see* Fenofibrate *on page 620*
- ◆ **Tricosal** *see* Choline Magnesium Trisalicylate *on page 342*
- ◆ **Triderm®** *see* Triamcinolone *on page 1617*
- ◆ **Trien** *see* Trientine *on page 1623*

Trientine (TRYE en teen)

Medication Safety Issues

Sound-alike/look-alike issues:

Trientine may be confused with Trental®, tretinoin

U.S. Brand Names Syprine®

Canadian Brand Names Syprine®

Index Terms 2,2,2-tetramine; Trien; Trientine Hydrochloride; Triethylene Tetramine Dihydrochloride

Pharmacologic Category Chelating Agent

Use Treatment of Wilson's disease in patients intolerant to penicillamine

Effect on Mental Status May cause drowsiness

Effect on Psychiatric Treatment None reported

Dosage Summary

Oral:

Children <12 years: 20 mg/kg (Roberts, 2003) or 500-750 mg/day in 2-4 divided doses (maximum: 1.5 g/day)

Children ≥12 years: 750-1500 mg/day in 2-4 divided doses (maximum: 2 g/day)

Adults: 750-1500 mg/day in 2-4 divided doses (maximum: 2 g/day)

Dosage Forms Excipient information presented when available (limited, particularly for generics); consult specific product labeling.

Capsule, as hydrochloride: 250 mg

- ◆ **Trientine Hydrochloride** *see* Trientine *on page 1623*
- ◆ **Triesence™** *see* Triamcinolone *on page 1617*
- ◆ **Triethylene Tetramine Dihydrochloride** *see* Trientine *on page 1623*
- ◆ **Triethylenethiophosphoramide** *see* Thiotepa *on page 1576*

Trifluoperazine (trye floo oh PER a zeen)

Medication Safety Issues

Sound-alike/look-alike issues:

Trifluoperazine may be confused with triflupromazine, trihexyphenidyl

Stelazine® may be confused with selegiline

Related Information

Anticholinergic Effects of Common Psychotropics *on page 1758*

Antipsychotic Agents *on page 1769*

CMS: Long-Term Care Facility Thresholds *on page 1815*

Discontinuation of Psychotropic Drugs *on page 1839*

Liquid Compatibility of Antidepressants, Antipsychotics, and Mood Stabilizers *on page 1788*

Canadian Brand Names Apo-Trifluoperazine®; Novo-Trifluzine; PMS-Trifluoperazine; Terfluzine

Mexican Brand Names Flupazine; Stelazine

Index Terms Trifluoperazine Hydrochloride

Pharmacologic Category Antipsychotic Agent, Typical, Phenothiazine

Generic Available Yes

Use Treatment of schizophrenia

Unlabeled/Investigational Use Management of psychotic disorders; behavioral symptoms associated with dementia behavior (elderly); psychosis/agitation related to Alzheimer's dementia

Mental Health Comment Older antipsychotic medications (chlorpromazine, haloperidol), which do not meet specific criteria for "atypical" antipsychotics, are often referred to as typical antipsychotics. They are associated with the troubling side effect, EPS. However, it is commonly believed that in order for a drug to treat psychosis, it must block dopamine is some manner.

Common side effects include sedation and neuroleptic effect (reduced initiative, interest in the environment, and display of emotion or affect). All **typical** antipsychotics are considered to be equally effective if given in equipotent doses. An inverse relationship exists between intrinsic antimuscarinic activity and propensity to cause extrapyramidal side effects. If dystonia or pseudoparkinsonism occurs, antiparkinsonian agents should be considered. If akathisia occurs, beta-blockers (eg, propranolol), benzodiazepines, or antiparkinsonian agents should be considered. Tardive dyskinesia (TD) secondary to typical antipsychotics has an estimated incidence of 3% to 5% per year for the first 5 years of treatment. After this time period, the incidence is estimated to be 2% to 3% per year. Prevalence rates are ~15% to 20%. Female gender and age constitute risk factors for TD. Indeed, prevalence rates have been reported to be as high as 70% in elderly females. No specific treatment exists for TD, however, patients are often initiated on/switched to an atypical antipsychotic because of their lower incidence to cause TD and hopes of suppression.

Typical antipsychotics are usually only indicated for schizophrenia, but are generally effective for mania and psychosis and/or behavioral syndromes secondary to other mental conditions. Nonpsychiatric uses include Tourette's syndrome, Huntington's disease, and occasionally, intractable hiccups, pruritus, nausea, and vomiting.

These drugs are thought to exert their antipsychotic activity by blocking dopamine D_2 receptors in the mesolimbic dopaminergic pathway. Side effects are often related to their ability to antagonize dopamine receptors in the nigrostriatal and tuberoinfundibular pathways.

Coadministration of two or more antipsychotics does not generally improve clinical response and may increase the potential for adverse effects.

In 2008, the FDA issued a warning regarding increased mortality risk with typical **and** atypical antipsychotic drugs when used in elderly patients with dementia-related psychosis.

Pregnancy Risk Factor C

Lactation Enters breast milk/not recommended (AAP rates "of concern")

Contraindications Hypersensitivity to trifluoperazine or any component of the formulation (cross-reactivity between phenothiazines may occur); severe CNS depression; bone marrow suppression; blood dyscrasias; severe hepatic disease; coma

Warnings/Precautions Elderly patients with dementia-related psychosis treated with antipsychotics are at an increased risk of death compared to placebo. An increased incidence of cerebrovascular adverse events (including fatalities) has been reported in elderly patients with dementia-related psychosis. Trifluoperazine is not approved for this indication.

May be sedating, use with caution in disorders where CNS depression is a feature. Use with caution in Parkinson's disease. Caution in patients with hemodynamic instability; predisposition to seizures; subcortical brain damage; hepatic impairment; severe cardiac, renal, or respiratory disease. Esophageal dysmotility and aspiration have been associated with antipsychotic use - use with caution in patients at risk of pneumonia (ie, Alzheimer's disease). Caution in breast cancer or other prolactin-dependent tumors (may elevate prolactin levels). May alter temperature regulation or mask toxicity of other drugs due to antiemetic effects. May alter cardiac conduction - life-threatening arrhythmias have occurred with therapeutic doses of phenothiazines. May cause orthostatic hypotension - use with caution in patients at risk of this effect or those who would tolerate transient hypotensive episodes (cerebrovascular disease, cardiovascular disease or other medications which may predispose). Check blood counts periodically and discontinue at first signs of blood dyscrasias; use is contraindicated in patients with bone marrow suppression. Safety in children <6 years of age has not been established.

Due to anticholinergic effects, should be used with caution in patients with decreased gastrointestinal motility, urinary retention, BPH, xerostomia, visual problems, narrow-angle glaucoma (screening is recommended) and myasthenia gravis. Relative to other antipsychotics, trifluoperazine has a low potency of cholinergic blockade.

May cause extrapyramidal symptoms (EPS), including pseudoparkinsonism, acute dystonic reactions, akathisia, and tardive dyskinesia (risk of these reactions is high relative to other neuroleptics). Risk of dystonia (and possibly other EPS) may be greater with increased doses, use of conventional antipsychotics, males, and younger patients. Use caution in the elderly. May be associated with neuroleptic malignant syndrome (NMS) or pigmentary retinopathy.

Adverse Reactions Frequency not defined.

Cardiovascular: Hypotension, orthostatic hypotension, cardiac arrest

Central nervous system: Extrapyramidal symptoms (pseudoparkinsonism, akathisia, dystonias, tardive dyskinesia), dizziness, headache, neuroleptic malignant syndrome (NMS), impairment of temperature regulation, lowering of seizure threshold

Dermatologic: Increased sensitivity to sun, rash, discoloration of skin (blue-gray), photosensitivity

Endocrine & metabolic: Changes in menstrual cycle, libido (changes in), breast pain, hyperglycemia, hypoglycemia, gynecomastia, lactation, galactorrhea

Gastrointestinal: Constipation, weight gain, nausea, vomiting, stomach pain, xerostomia

Genitourinary: Difficulty in urination, ejaculatory disturbances, urinary retention, priapism

Hematologic: Agranulocytosis, leukopenia, pancytopenia, thrombocytopenic purpura, eosinophilia, hemolytic anemia, aplastic anemia

Hepatic: Cholestatic jaundice, hepatotoxicity

Neuromuscular & skeletal: Tremor

Ocular: Pigmentary retinopathy, cornea and lens changes

Respiratory: Nasal congestion

Metabolism/Transport Effects Substrate of CYP1A2 (major)

Drug Interactions

Acetylcholinesterase Inhibitors (Central): May enhance the neurotoxic (central) effect of Antipsychotics. Severe extrapyramidal symptoms have occurred in some patients. *Risk C: Monitor therapy*

Alcohol (Ethyl): CNS Depressants may enhance the CNS depressant effect of Alcohol (Ethyl). *Risk C: Monitor therapy*

Amphetamines: Antipsychotics may diminish the stimulatory effect of Amphetamines. *Risk C: Monitor therapy*

Analgesics (Opioid): Antipsychotic Agents (Phenothiazines) may enhance the hypotensive effect of Analgesics (Opioid). *Risk C: Monitor therapy*

Antacids: May decrease the absorption of Antipsychotic Agents (Phenothiazines). *Risk C: Monitor therapy*

Anticholinergics: May enhance the adverse/toxic effect of other Anticholinergics. **Exceptions:** Paliperidone. *Risk C: Monitor therapy*

Antimalarial Agents: May increase the serum concentration of Antipsychotic Agents (Phenothiazines). *Risk C: Monitor therapy*

Anti-Parkinson 's Agents (Dopamine Agonist): Antipsychotics (Typical) may diminish the therapeutic effect of Anti-Parkinson 's Agents (Dopamine Agonist). *Risk D: Consider therapy modification*

Beta-Blockers: Antipsychotic Agents (Phenothiazines) may enhance the hypotensive effect of Beta-Blockers. Beta-Blockers may decrease the metabolism of Antipsychotic Agents (Phenothiazines). Antipsychotic Agents (Phenothiazines) may decrease the metabolism of Beta-Blockers. **Exceptions:** Atenolol; Levobunolol; Metipranolol; Nadolol. *Risk C: Monitor therapy*

CNS Depressants: May enhance the adverse/toxic effect of other CNS Depressants. *Risk C: Monitor therapy*

CYP1A2 Inducers (Strong): May increase the metabolism of CYP1A2 Substrates. *Risk C: Monitor therapy*

CYP1A2 Inhibitors (Moderate): May decrease the metabolism of CYP1A2 Substrates. *Risk C: Monitor therapy*

CYP1A2 Inhibitors (Strong): May decrease the metabolism of CYP1A2 Substrates. *Risk D: Consider therapy modification*

Lithium formulations: May enhance the neurotoxic effect of Antipsychotics. Lithium formulations may decrease the serum concentration of Antipsychotics. Specifically noted with chlorpromazine. *Risk C: Monitor therapy*

Pramlintide: May enhance the anticholinergic effect of Anticholinergics. These effects are specific to the GI tract. *Risk D: Consider therapy modification*

Tetrabenazine: May enhance the adverse/toxic effect of Antipsychotics. *Risk C: Monitor therapy*

Ethanol/Nutrition/Herb Interactions

Ethanol: Avoid ethanol (may increase CNS depression).

Herb/Nutraceutical: Avoid kava kava, gotu kola, valerian, St John's wort (may increase CNS depression). Avoid dong quai, St John's wort (may also cause photosensitization).

Mechanism of Action Trifluoperazine is a piperazine phenothiazine antipsychotic which blocks postsynaptic mesolimbic dopaminergic receptors in the brain; exhibits alpha-adrenergic blocking effect and depresses the release of hypothalamic and hypophyseal hormones

Pharmacodynamics/Kinetics

Metabolism: Extensively hepatic

Half-life elimination: >24 hours with chronic use

Dosage Oral:

Children 6-12 years: Schizophrenia/psychoses: Hospitalized or well-supervised patients: Initial: 1 mg 1-2 times/day, gradually increase until symptoms are controlled or adverse effects become troublesome; maximum: 15 mg/day

Adults:

Schizophrenia/psychoses:

Outpatients: 1-2 mg twice daily

Hospitalized or well-supervised patients: Initial: 2-5 mg twice daily with optimum response in the 15-20 mg/day range; do not exceed 40 mg/day

Nonpsychotic anxiety: 1-2 mg twice daily; maximum: 6 mg/day; therapy for anxiety should not exceed 12 weeks; do not exceed 6 mg/day for longer than 12 weeks when treating anxiety; agitation, jitteriness, or insomnia may be confused with original neurotic or psychotic symptoms

Elderly:

Schizophrenia/psychoses:

Refer to adult dosing. Dose selection should start at the low end of the dosage range and titration must be gradual.

Behavioral symptoms associated with dementia behavior (unlabeled use): Initial: 0.5-1 mg 1-2 times/day; increase dose at 4- to 7-day intervals by 0.5-1 mg/day; increase dosing intervals (bid, tid, etc) as necessary to control response or side effects. Maximum daily dose: 40 mg. Gradual increases (titration) may prevent some side effects or decrease their severity.

Hemodialysis: Not dialyzable (0% to 5%)

Dietary Considerations May be taken with food to decrease GI distress.

Monitoring Parameters Vital signs; lipid profile, fasting blood glucose/Hgb A_{1c}; BMI; mental status, abnormal involuntary movement scale (AIMS)

Reference Range Therapeutic response and blood levels have not been established

Test Interactions False-positive for phenylketonuria

Additional Information Do not exceed 6 mg/day for longer than 12 weeks when treating anxiety. Agitation, jitteriness, or insomnia may be confused with original neurotic or psychotic symptoms.

Dosage Forms Excipient information presented when available (limited, particularly for generics); consult specific product labeling.

Tablet: 1 mg, 2 mg, 5 mg, 10 mg

- **Trifluoperazine Hydrochloride** *see* Trifluoperazine *on page 1624*
- **Triglide™** *see* Fenofibrate *on page 620*

Trihexyphenidyl (trye heks ee FEN i dil)

Medication Safety Issues

Sound-alike/look-alike issues:

Trihexyphenidyl may be confused with trifluoperazine

Artane may be confused with Altace®, Anturane®, Aramine®

Related Information

Anticholinergic Effects of Common Psychotropics *on page 1758*

Antiparkinsonian Agents *on page 1767*

Discontinuation of Psychotropic Drugs *on page 1839*

Canadian Brand Names Apo-Trihex®

Mexican Brand Names Hipokinon

Index Terms Artane; Benzhexol Hydrochloride; Trihexyphenidyl Hydrochloride

Pharmacologic Category Anti-Parkinson's Agent, Anticholinergic; Anticholinergic Agent

Generic Available Yes

Use Adjunctive treatment of Parkinson's disease; treatment of drug-induced extrapyramidal symptoms

Mental Health Comment This agent should not be used for an acute dystonic reaction. No injectable dosage form is available. However, oral dosage forms may be utilized to treat akathisia and pseudoparkinsonism. It is considered to be the least sedating antihistamine used to treat drug-induced EPS.

Pregnancy Risk Factor C

Lactation Excretion in breast milk unknown/use caution

Contraindications Hypersensitivity to trihexyphenidyl or any component of the formulation; narrow-angle glaucoma; pyloric or duodenal obstruction; stenosing peptic ulcers; bladder neck obstructions; achalasia; myasthenia gravis

Warnings/Precautions Use with caution in hot weather or during exercise, especially when administered concomitantly with other atropine-like drugs to chronically-ill patients, alcoholics, patients with CNS disease, or persons doing manual labor in a hot environment. Elderly patients require strict dosage regulation. Use with caution in patients with tachycardia, cardiac arrhythmias, hypertension, hypotension, glaucoma, prostatic hyperplasia or any tendency toward urinary retention, liver or kidney disorders, and obstructive disease of the GI or GU tract. May exacerbate mental symptoms when used to treat extrapyramidal symptoms. When given in large doses or to susceptible patients, may cause weakness. Does not improve symptoms of tardive dyskinesias.

Adverse Reactions Frequency not defined.

Cardiovascular: Tachycardia

Central nervous system: Confusion, agitation, euphoria, drowsiness, headache, dizziness, nervousness, delusions, hallucinations, paranoia

Dermatologic: Dry skin, increased sensitivity to light, rash

Gastrointestinal: Constipation, xerostomia, dry throat, ileus, nausea, vomiting, parotitis

Genitourinary: Urinary retention

Neuromuscular & skeletal: Weakness

Ocular: Blurred vision, mydriasis, increase in intraocular pressure, glaucoma, blindness (long-term use in narrow-angle glaucoma)

Respiratory: Dry nose

Miscellaneous: Diaphoresis (decreased)

Drug Interactions

Acetylcholinesterase Inhibitors (Central): Anticholinergics may diminish the therapeutic effect of Acetylcholinesterase Inhibitors (Central). Acetylcholinesterase Inhibitors (Central) may diminish the therapeutic effect of Anticholinergics. If the anticholinergic action is a side effect of the agent, the result may be beneficial. *Risk C: Monitor therapy*

Anticholinergics: May enhance the adverse/toxic effect of other Anticholinergics. **Exceptions:** Paliperidone. *Risk C: Monitor therapy*

Cannabinoids: Anticholinergic Agents may enhance the tachycardic effect of Cannabinoids. *Risk C: Monitor therapy*

Potassium Chloride: Anticholinergic Agents may enhance the ulcerogenic effect of Potassium Chloride. *Risk D: Consider therapy modification*

Pramlintide: May enhance the anticholinergic effect of Anticholinergics. These effects are specific to the GI tract. *Risk D: Consider therapy modification*

Secretin: Anticholinergic Agents may diminish the stimulatory effect of Secretin. *Risk D: Consider therapy modification*

Ethanol/Nutrition/Herb Interactions Ethanol: Avoid ethanol (may increase CNS depression).

Mechanism of Action Exerts a direct inhibitory effect on the parasympathetic nervous system. It also has a relaxing effect on smooth musculature; exerted both directly on the muscle itself and indirectly through parasympathetic nervous system (inhibitory effect)

Pharmacodynamics/Kinetics

Onset of action: Peak effect: ~1 hour

Half-life elimination: 3.3-4.1 hours

Time to peak, serum: 1-1.5 hours

Excretion: Primarily urine

Dosage Adults: Oral: Initial: 1-2 mg/day, increase by 2 mg increments at intervals of 3-5 days; usual dose: 5-15 mg/day in 3-4 divided doses

Administration Tolerated best if given in 3 daily doses and with food. High doses may be divided into 4 doses, at meal times and at bedtime. Patients may be switched to sustained-action capsules when stabilized on conventional dosage forms.

Monitoring Parameters IOP monitoring and gonioscopic evaluations should be performed periodically

Additional Information Incidence and severity of side effects are dose related. Patients may be switched to sustained-action capsules when stabilized on conventional dosage forms.

Dosage Forms Excipient information presented when available (limited, particularly for generics); consult specific product labeling.

Elixir, as hydrochloride: 2 mg/5 mL (480 mL)

Tablet, as hydrochloride: 2 mg, 5 mg

- **Trihexyphenidyl Hydrochloride** *see* Trihexyphenidyl *on page 1627*
- **Tri-Hist** *see* Chlorpheniramine, Pyrilamine, and Phenylephrine *on page 335*
- **Trikof-D® [DSC]** *see* Guaifenesin, Pseudoephedrine, and Dextromethorphan *on page 748*
- **Trileptal®** *see* OXcarbazepine *on page 1195*
- **TriLyte®** *see* Polyethylene Glycol-Electrolyte Solution *on page 1310*

Trimethobenzamide (trye meth oh BEN za mide)

Medication Safety Issues

Sound-alike/look-alike issues:

Tigan® may be confused with Tiazac®, Ticar®, Ticlid®

Trimethobenzamide may be confused with metoclopramide, trimethoprim

U.S. Brand Names Tigan®

Canadian Brand Names Tigan®

Index Terms Trimethobenzamide Hydrochloride

Pharmacologic Category Anticholinergic Agent; Antiemetic

Use Treatment of postoperative nausea and vomiting; treatment of nausea associated with gastroenteritis

Effect on Mental Status Drowsiness is common; may cause dizziness; may rarely cause depression

Effect on Psychiatric Treatment Concurrent use with psychotropics may produce additive sedation

Dosage Summary

I.M.:

Children: Dosage not established

Adults: 200 mg 3-4 times/day **or** 200 mg as a single dose, repeat 1 hour later

Oral:

Children ≤40 kg: Unable to administer recommended dose with available product

Children >40 kg: 300 mg 3-4 times/day

Adults: 300 mg 3-4 times/day

Dosage Forms Excipient information presented when available (limited, particularly for generics); consult specific product labeling.

Capsule, as hydrochloride: 300 mg

Tigan®: 300 mg

Injection, solution, as hydrochloride: 100 mg/mL (2 mL)

Tigan®: 100 mg/mL (20 mL)

Injection, solution, as hydrochloride [preservative free]:

Tigan®: 100 mg/mL (2 mL)

◆ **Trimethobenzamide Hydrochloride** *see* Trimethobenzamide *on page 1628*

Trimethoprim (trye METH oh prim)

Medication Safety Issues

Sound-alike/look-alike issues:

Trimethoprim may be confused with trimethaphan

Proloprim® may be confused with Prolixin®, Protropin®

U.S. Brand Names Primsol®

Canadian Brand Names Apo-Trimethoprim®

Index Terms TMP

Pharmacologic Category Antibiotic, Miscellaneous

Use Treatment of urinary tract infections due to susceptible strains of *E. coli*, *P. mirabilis*, *K. pneumoniae*, *Enterobacter* sp and coagulase-negative *Staphylococcus* including *S. saprophyticus*; acute otitis media in children; acute exacerbations of chronic bronchitis in adults; in combination with other agents for treatment of toxoplasmosis, *Pneumocystis carinii*; treatment of superficial ocular infections involving the conjunctiva and cornea

Effect on Mental Status None reported

Effect on Psychiatric Treatment May cause neutropenia; use caution with clozapine and carbamazepine

Dosage Summary

Oral:

Children ≤2 months: Dosage not established

Children >2 months: 4 mg/kg/day in divided doses every 12 hours

Adults: 100 mg every 12 hours **or** 200 mg every 24 hours; up to 15-20 mg/kg/day may be necessary- see Indication-Specific Dosing

Dosage Forms Excipient information presented when available (limited, particularly for generics); consult specific product labeling.

Solution, oral:

Primsol®: 50 mg (base)/5 mL (473 mL) [dye free, ethanol free; contains propylene glycol, sodium benzoate; bubble gum flavor]

Tablet: 100 mg

◆ **Trimethoprim and Sulfamethoxazole** *see* Sulfamethoxazole and Trimethoprim *on page 1517*

Trimetrexate (tri me TREKS ate)

Medication Safety Issues

High alert medication: The Institute for Safe Medication Practices (ISMP) includes this medication among its list of drugs which have a heightened risk of causing significant patient harm when used in error.

U.S. Brand Names NeuTrexin® [DSC]

Index Terms NSC-352122; Trimetrexate Glucuronate

Pharmacologic Category Antineoplastic Agent, Miscellaneous

Use Alternative therapy for the treatment of moderate-to-severe *Pneumocystis jiroveci* pneumonia (PCP) in immunocompromised patients, including patients with acquired immunodeficiency syndrome (AIDS), who are intolerant of, or are refractory to, sulfamethoxazole/trimethoprim therapy or for whom sulfamethoxazole/trimethoprim and pentamidine are contraindicated

Unlabeled/Investigational Use Treatment of nonsmall cell lung cancer, metastatic colorectal cancer, metastatic head and neck cancer, pancreatic adenocarcinoma, cutaneous T-cell lymphoma

Effect on Mental Status None reported

Effect on Psychiatric Treatment May cause neutropenia; use caution with clozapine and carbamazepine

Dosage Summary

I.V.:

Children: Dosage not established

Adults <50 kg: 1.5 mg/kg/day once daily **or** 45 mg/m^2 once daily with leucovorin

Adults 50-80 kg: 1.2 mg/kg/day once daily **or** 45 mg/m^2 once daily with leucovorin

Adults >80 kg: 1 mg/kg/day once daily **or** 45 mg/m^2 once daily with leucovorin

Dosage Forms Excipient information presented when available (limited, particularly for generics); consult specific product labeling. [DSC] = Discontinued product

Injection, powder for reconstitution [preservative free]:

NeuTrexin®: 25 mg, 200 mg [DSC]

◆ **Trimetrexate Glucuronate** *see* Trimetrexate *on page 1629*

Trimipramine (trye MI pra meen)

Medication Safety Issues

Sound-alike/look-alike issues:

Trimipramine may be confused with triamterene, trimeprazine

Related Information

Antidepressant Agents *on page 1760*
Antidepressant Receptor Profile *on page 1764*
Discontinuation of Psychotropic Drugs *on page 1839*

U.S. Brand Names Surmontil®

Canadian Brand Names Apo-Trimip®; Nu-Trimipramine; Rhotrimine®; Surmontil®

Index Terms Trimipramine Maleate

Pharmacologic Category Antidepressant, Tricyclic (Tertiary Amine)

Generic Available No

Use Treatment of depression

Mental Health Comment Tricyclic antidepressants may be classified as tertiary (amitriptyline, doxepin, clomipramine, imipramine, trimipramine) or secondary amines (nortriptyline, desipramine, protriptyline). The tertiary amines are not recommended to treat depression in the elderly. If a TCA is used in the elderly, it should be a secondary amine. The tertiary amines are commonly used in low dosages for various conditions associated with pain. Toxicity is generally dose dependent. Relatively small overdoses (1-week supply) can be potentially fatal.

Restrictions An FDA-approved medication guide concerning the use of antidepressants in children, adolescents, and young adults must be distributed when dispensing an outpatient prescription (new or refill) where this medication is to be used without direct supervision of a healthcare provider. Medication guides are available at http://www.fda.gov/cder/Offices/ODS/medication_guides.htm. Dispense to parents or guardians of children and adolescents receiving this medication.

Pregnancy Risk Factor C

Lactation Enters breast milk/contraindicated

Contraindications Hypersensitivity to trimipramine, any component of the formulation, or other dibenzodiazepines; use of MAO inhibitors within 14 days; use in a patient during the acute recovery phase of MI

Warnings/Precautions **[U.S. Boxed Warning]: Antidepressants increase the risk of suicidal thinking and behavior in children, adolescents, and young adults (18-24 years of age) with major depressive disorder (MDD) and other psychiatric disorders;** consider risk prior to prescribing. Short-term studies did not show an increased risk in patients >24 years of age and showed a decreased risk in patients ≥65 years. Closely monitor for clinical worsening, suicidality, or unusual changes in behavior; the patient's family or caregiver should be instructed to closely observe the patient and communicate condition with healthcare provider. A medication guide should be dispensed with each prescription. **Trimipramine is not FDA approved for use in children.**

The possibility of a suicide attempt is inherent in major depression and may persist until remission occurs. Monitor for worsening of depression or suicidality, especially during initiation of therapy (generally first 1-2 months) or with dose increases or decreases. Use caution in high-risk patients. Worsening depression and severe abrupt suicidality that are not part of the presenting symptoms may require discontinuation or modification of drug therapy. The patient's family or caregiver should be alerted to monitor patients for the emergence of suicidality and associated behaviors (such as agitation, irritability, hostility, impulsivity, and hypomania) and call healthcare provider.

May worsen psychosis in some patients or precipitate a shift to mania or hypomania in patients with bipolar disorder. Patients presenting with depressive symptoms should be screened for bipolar disorder. Monotherapy in patients with bipolar disorder should be avoided. **Trimipramine is not FDA approved for the treatment of bipolar depression.**

The degree of sedation, anticholinergic effects, orthostasis, and conduction abnormalities are high relative to other antidepressants. Trimipramine often causes drowsiness/sedation, resulting in impaired performance of tasks requiring alertness (eg, operating machinery or driving). Sedative effects may be additive with other CNS depressants and/or ethanol. Use with caution in patients with a history of cardiovascular disease (including previous MI, stroke, tachycardia, or conduction abnormalities). Use with caution in patients with urinary retention, benign prostatic hyperplasia, narrow-angle glaucoma, xerostomia, visual problems, constipation, or a history of bowel obstruction.

May alter glucose control - use with caution in patients with diabetes. Consider discontinuing, when possible, prior to elective surgery. Therapy should not be abruptly discontinued in patients receiving high doses for prolonged periods. May lower seizure threshold - use caution in patients with a previous seizure disorder or condition predisposing to seizures such as brain damage, alcoholism, or concurrent therapy with other drugs which lower the seizure threshold. May increase the risks associated with electroconvulsive therapy. Use with caution in hyperthyroid patients or those receiving thyroid supplementation. Use with caution in patients with hepatic or renal dysfunction and in elderly patients.

Adverse Reactions Frequency not defined.

Cardiovascular: Arrhythmias, hyper-/hypotension, tachycardia, palpitation, heart block, stroke, MI

Central nervous system: Headache, exacerbation of psychosis, confusion, delirium, hallucinations, nervousness, restlessness, delusions, agitation, insomnia, nightmares, anxiety, seizure, drowsiness

Dermatologic: Photosensitivity, rash, petechiae, itching

Endocrine & metabolic: Sexual dysfunction, breast enlargement, galactorrhea, SIADH

Gastrointestinal: Xerostomia, constipation, increased appetite, nausea, unpleasant taste, weight gain, diarrhea, heartburn, vomiting, anorexia, trouble with gums, decreased lower esophageal sphincter tone may cause GE reflux

Genitourinary: Difficult urination, urinary retention, testicular edema

Hematologic: Agranulocytosis, eosinophilia, purpura, thrombocytopenia

Hepatic: Cholestatic jaundice, increased liver enzymes

Neuromuscular & skeletal: Tremors, numbness, tingling, paresthesia, incoordination, ataxia, peripheral neuropathy, extrapyramidal symptoms

Ocular: Blurred vision, eye pain, disturbances in accommodation, mydriasis, increased intraocular pressure

Otic: Tinnitus

Miscellaneous: Allergic reactions

Metabolism/Transport Effects Substrate (major) of CYP2C19, 2D6, 3A4

Drug Interactions

Acetylcholinesterase Inhibitors (Central): Anticholinergics may diminish the therapeutic effect of Acetylcholinesterase Inhibitors (Central). Acetylcholinesterase Inhibitors (Central) may diminish the therapeutic effect of Anticholinergics. If the anticholinergic action is a side effect of the agent, the result may be beneficial. *Risk C: Monitor therapy*

Alcohol (Ethyl): CNS Depressants may enhance the CNS depressant effect of Alcohol (Ethyl). *Risk C: Monitor therapy*

Alfuzosin: May enhance the QTc-prolonging effect of QTc-Prolonging Agents. *Risk C: Monitor therapy*

Alpha-/Beta-Agonists (Direct-Acting): Tricyclic Antidepressants may enhance the vasopressor effect of Alpha-/Beta-Agonists (Direct-Acting). **Exceptions:** Dipivefrin. *Risk D: Consider therapy modification*

Alpha1-Agonists: Tricyclic Antidepressants may enhance the vasopressor effect of Alpha1-Agonists. *Risk D: Consider therapy modification*

Alpha2-Agonists: Tricyclic Antidepressants may diminish the antihypertensive effect of Alpha2-Agonists. **Exceptions:** Apraclonidine; Brimonidine. *Risk D: Consider therapy modification*

Altretamine: May enhance the orthostatic effect of Tricyclic Antidepressants. *Risk C: Monitor therapy*

Amphetamines: Tricyclic Antidepressants may enhance the stimulatory effect of Amphetamines. Tricyclic Antidepressants may also potentiate the cardiovascular effects of Amphetamines. *Risk C: Monitor therapy*

Anticholinergics: May enhance the adverse/toxic effect of other Anticholinergics. **Exceptions:** Paliperidone. *Risk C: Monitor therapy*

Aspirin: Antidepressants (Tricyclic, Tertiary Amine) may enhance the antiplatelet effect of Aspirin. *Risk C: Monitor therapy*

Barbiturates: May increase the metabolism of Tricyclic Antidepressants. *Risk D: Consider therapy modification*

Beta2-Agonists: Tricyclic Antidepressants may enhance the adverse/toxic effect of Beta2-Agonists. *Risk C: Monitor therapy*

BuPROPion: May decrease the metabolism of Tricyclic Antidepressants. *Risk C: Monitor therapy*

CarBAMazepine: May increase the metabolism of Tricyclic Antidepressants. *Risk C: Monitor therapy*

Cimetidine: May decrease the metabolism of Tricyclic Antidepressants. *Risk C: Monitor therapy*

Cinacalcet: May increase the serum concentration of Tricyclic Antidepressants. *Risk C: Monitor therapy*

Ciprofloxacin: May enhance the QTc-prolonging effect of QTc-Prolonging Agents. *Risk C: Monitor therapy*

CNS Depressants: May enhance the adverse/toxic effect of other CNS Depressants. *Risk C: Monitor therapy*

CYP2C19 Inducers (Strong): May increase the metabolism of CYP2C19 Substrates. *Risk C: Monitor therapy*

CYP2C19 Inhibitors (Moderate): May decrease the metabolism of CYP2C19 Substrates. *Risk C: Monitor therapy*

CYP2C19 Inhibitors (Strong): May decrease the metabolism of CYP2C19 Substrates. *Risk D: Consider therapy modification*

CYP2D6 Inhibitors (Moderate): May decrease the metabolism of CYP2D6 Substrates. *Risk C: Monitor therapy*

CYP2D6 Inhibitors (Strong): May decrease the metabolism of CYP2D6 Substrates. *Risk D: Consider therapy modification*

CYP3A4 Inducers (Strong): May increase the metabolism of CYP3A4 Substrates. *Risk C: Monitor therapy*

CYP3A4 Inhibitors (Moderate): May decrease the metabolism of CYP3A4 Substrates. *Risk C: Monitor therapy*

CYP3A4 Inhibitors (Strong): May decrease the metabolism of CYP3A4 Substrates. *Risk D: Consider therapy modification*

Darunavir: May increase the serum concentration of CYP2D6 Substrates. *Risk C: Monitor therapy*

Dasatinib: May increase the serum concentration of CYP3A4 Substrates. *Risk C: Monitor therapy*

Deferasirox: May decrease the serum concentration of CYP3A4 Substrates. *Risk C: Monitor therapy*

Desmopressin: Tricyclic Antidepressants may enhance the adverse/toxic effect of Desmopressin. *Risk C: Monitor therapy*

Dexmethylphenidate: May decrease the metabolism of Tricyclic Antidepressants. *Risk C: Monitor therapy*

DULoxetine: May decrease the metabolism of Tricyclic Antidepressants. *Risk C: Monitor therapy*

Gadobutrol: May enhance the QTc-prolonging effect of QTc-Prolonging Agents. *Risk D: Consider therapy modification*

Lithium: May enhance the neurotoxic effect of Tricyclic Antidepressants. *Risk C: Monitor therapy*

MAO Inhibitors: May enhance the serotonergic effect of Tricyclic Antidepressants. This may cause serotonin syndrome. *Risk X: Avoid combination*

Methylphenidate: May decrease the metabolism of Tricyclic Antidepressants. *Risk C: Monitor therapy*

Nilotinib: May enhance the QTc-prolonging effect of QTc-Prolonging Agents. *Risk X: Avoid combination*

NSAID (COX-2 Inhibitor): Antidepressants (Tricyclic, Tertiary Amine) may enhance the antiplatelet effect of NSAID (COX-2 Inhibitor). *Risk C: Monitor therapy*

NSAID (Nonselective): Antidepressants (Tricyclic, Tertiary Amine) may enhance the antiplatelet effect of NSAID (Nonselective). *Risk C: Monitor therapy*

Pramlintide: May enhance the anticholinergic effect of Anticholinergics. These effects are specific to the GI tract. *Risk D: Consider therapy modification*

Propoxyphene: May enhance the CNS depressant effect of Tricyclic Antidepressants. *Risk C: Monitor therapy*

Protease Inhibitors: May increase the serum concentration of Tricyclic Antidepressants. *Risk C: Monitor therapy*

QTc-Prolonging Agents: May enhance the adverse/toxic effect of other QTc-Prolonging Agents. Their effects can be additive, causing life-threatening ventricular arrhythmias. *Risk D: Consider therapy modification*

QuiNIDine: Tricyclic Antidepressants may enhance the QTc-prolonging effect of QuiNIDine. QuiNIDine may decrease the metabolism of Tricyclic Antidepressants. *Risk D: Consider therapy modification*

Selective Serotonin Reuptake Inhibitors: May decrease the metabolism of Tricyclic Antidepressants. *Risk D: Consider therapy modification*

Serotonin Modulators: May enhance the adverse/toxic effect of other Serotonin Modulators. The development of serotonin syndrome may occur. *Risk D: Consider therapy modification*

Sibutramine: May enhance the serotonergic effect of Serotonin Modulators. This may cause serotonin syndrome. *Risk X: Avoid combination*

St Johns Wort: May increase the metabolism of Tricyclic Antidepressants. The risk of serotonin syndrome may theoretically be increased. *Risk D: Consider therapy modification*

Sulfonylureas: Cyclic Antidepressants may enhance the hypoglycemic effect of Sulfonylureas. *Risk C: Monitor therapy*

Terbinafine: May decrease the metabolism of Tricyclic Antidepressants. *Risk D: Consider therapy modification*

Tetrabenazine: QTc-Prolonging Agents may enhance the QTc-prolonging effect of Tetrabenazine. *Risk X: Avoid combination*

Thioridazine: QTc-Prolonging Agents may enhance the QTc-prolonging effect of Thioridazine. *Risk X: Avoid combination*

TraMADol: Tricyclic Antidepressants may enhance the neuroexcitatory and/or seizure-potentiating effect of TraMADol. *Risk C: Monitor therapy*

Valproic Acid: May increase the serum concentration of Tricyclic Antidepressants. *Risk C: Monitor therapy*

Vitamin K Antagonists (eg, warfarin): Tricyclic Antidepressants may enhance the anticoagulant effect of Vitamin K Antagonists. *Risk C: Monitor therapy*

Ziprasidone: QTc-Prolonging Agents may enhance the QTc-prolonging effect of Ziprasidone. The risk of a severe arrhythmia may be increased. *Risk X: Avoid combination*

Ethanol/Nutrition/Herb Interactions

Ethanol: Avoid ethanol (may increase CNS depression).

Food: Grapefruit juice may inhibit the metabolism of some TCAs and clinical toxicity may result.

Herb/Nutraceutical: Avoid valerian, St John's wort, SAMe, kava kava (may increase risk of serotonin syndrome and/or excessive sedation).

Stability Solutions stable at a pH of 4-5. Turns yellowish or reddish on exposure to light. Slight discoloration does not affect potency; marked discoloration is associated with loss of potency. Capsules stable for 3 years following date of manufacture.

Mechanism of Action Increases the synaptic concentration of serotonin and/or norepinephrine in the central nervous system by inhibition of their reuptake by the presynaptic neuronal membrane

Pharmacodynamics/Kinetics

Distribution: V_d: 17-48 L/kg

Protein binding: 95%; free drug: 3% to 7%

Metabolism: Hepatic; significant first-pass effect

Bioavailability: 18% to 63%

Half-life elimination: 16-40 hours

Excretion: Urine

Dosage Oral:

Adults: 50-150 mg/day as a single bedtime dose up to a maximum of 200 mg/day outpatient and 300 mg/day inpatient

Elderly: Adequate studies have not been done in the elderly. In general, dosing should be cautious, starting at the lower end of dosing range.

Monitoring Parameters Blood pressure and pulse rate prior to and during initial therapy; evaluate mental status, suicidal ideation (especially at the beginning of therapy or when doses are increased or decreased); monitor weight; ECG in older adults

Additional Information May cause alterations in bleeding time.

Dosage Forms Excipient information presented when available (limited, particularly for generics); consult specific product labeling.

Capsule: 25 mg, 50 mg, 100 mg

- ◆ **Trimipramine Maleate** *see* Trimipramine *on page 1630*
- ◆ **Tri-Nasal® [DSC]** *see* Triamcinolone *on page 1617*

- ◆ **TriNessa™** *see* Ethinyl Estradiol and Norgestimate *on page 600*
- ◆ **Tri-Norinyl®** *see* Ethinyl Estradiol and Norethindrone *on page 597*
- ◆ **Trionate® [DSC]** *see* Carbetapentane and Chlorpheniramine *on page 272*
- ◆ **Triostat®** *see* Liothyronine *on page 928*
- ◆ **Triphasil®** *see* Ethinyl Estradiol and Levonorgestrel *on page 595*
- ◆ **Triplex™ AD** *see* Chlorpheniramine, Pyrilamine, and Phenylephrine *on page 335*
- ◆ **Tri-Previfem™** *see* Ethinyl Estradiol and Norgestimate *on page 600*

Triprolidine and Pseudoephedrine

(trye PROE li deen & soo doe e FED rin)

Medication Safety Issues

Sound-alike/look-alike issues:

Aprodine® may be confused with Aphrodyne®

U.S. Brand Names Allerfrim [OTC]; Aprodine® [OTC]; Genac® [OTC]; Silafed® [OTC]; Sudafed® Maximum Strength Sinus Nighttime [OTC] [DSC]; Tri-Sudo® [OTC] [DSC]; Zymine®-D

Canadian Brand Names Actifed®

Mexican Brand Names Actifed

Index Terms Pseudoephedrine and Triprolidine

Pharmacologic Category Alpha/Beta Agonist; Histamine H_1 Antagonist; Histamine H_1 Antagonist, First Generation

Use Temporary relief of nasal congestion, decongest sinus openings, running nose, sneezing, itching of nose or throat and itchy, watery eyes due to common cold, hay fever, or other upper respiratory allergies

Effect on Mental Status Drowsiness, nervousness, and insomnia are common; may cause dizziness; may rarely cause depression, hallucinations, or paradoxical excitement

Effect on Psychiatric Treatment Contraindicated with MAO inhibitors; concurrent use with psychotropics may produce additive sedation

Dosage Summary

Oral:

Children 2-4 years (Zymine®-D): 1.25 mL every 4-6 hours (maximum pseudoephedrine: 60 mg/24 hours)

Children 4-6 years (Zymine®-D): 2.5 mL every 4-6 hours (maximum pseudoephedrine: 60 mg/24 hours)

Children 6-12 years:

Allerfrim, Aprodine®: 5 mL every 4-6 hours (maximum 4 doses/24 hours)

Aprodine® tablet: 1/2 tablet every 4-6 hours (maximum 4 doses/24 hours)

Zymine®-D: 2.5-5 mL every 4-6 hours (maximum pseudoephedrine: 120 mg/24 hours)

Children >12 years:

Allerfrim, Aprodine®: 10 mL every 4-6 hours (maximum 4 doses/24 hours)

Aprodine® tablet: One tablet every 4-6 hours (maximum 4 doses/24 hours)

Zymine®-D: 5-10 mL every 4-6 hours (maximum pseudoephedrine: 240 mg/24 hours)

Adults:

Allerfrim, Aprodine®: 10 mL every 4-6 hours (maximum 4 doses/24 hours)

Aprodine® tablet: One tablet every 4-6 hours (maximum 4 doses/24 hours)

Zymine®-D: 5-10 mL every 4-6 hours (maximum pseudoephedrine: 240 mg/24 hours)

Dosage Forms Excipient information presented when available (limited, particularly for generics); consult specific product labeling. [DSC] = Discontinued product

Liquid:

Zymine®-D: Triprolidine hydrochloride 1.25 mg and pseudoephedrine hydrochloride 45 mg per 5 mL (480 mL)

Syrup: Triprolidine hydrochloride 1.25 mg and pseudoephedrine hydrochloride 30 mg per 5 mL (120 mL) [DSC]

Allerfrim: Triprolidine hydrochloride 1.25 mg and pseudoephedrine hydrochloride 30 mg per 5 mL (120 mL, 480 mL) [contains sodium benzoate]

Aprodine®: Triprolidine hydrochloride 1.25 mg and pseudoephedrine hydrochloride 30 mg per 5 mL (120 mL)

Silafed®: Triprolidine hydrochloride 1.25 mg and pseudoephedrine hydrochloride 30 mg per 5 mL (120 mL, 240 mL)

Tablet:

Allerfrim, Aprodine®, Genac®, Sudafed® Maximum Strength Sinus Nighttime, Tri-Sudo® [DSC]: Triprolidine hydrochloride 2.5 mg and pseudoephedrine hydrochloride 60 mg

◆ **Triprolidine, Codeine, and Pseudoephedrine** *see* Triprolidine, Pseudoephedrine, and Codeine *on page 1635*

Triprolidine, Pseudoephedrine, and Codeine

(trye PROE li deen, soo doe e FED rin, & KOE deen)

Medication Safety Issues
Sound-alike/look-alike issues:
Triacin-C® may be confused with triacetin

Canadian Brand Names CoActifed®; Covan®; ratio-Cotridin

Index Terms Codeine, Pseudoephedrine, and Triprolidine; Codeine, Triprolidine, and Pseudoephedrine; Pseudoephedrine, Codeine, and Triprolidine; Pseudoephedrine, Triprolidine, and Codeine; Triprolidine, Codeine, and Pseudoephedrine

Pharmacologic Category Alpha/Beta Agonist; Analgesic, Opioid; Antitussive; Histamine H_1 Antagonist; Histamine H_1 Antagonist, First Generation

Use Symptomatic relief of upper respiratory symptoms and cough

Effect on Mental Status Drowsiness, nervousness, and insomnia are common; may cause dizziness; may rarely cause depression, hallucinations, or paradoxical excitement

Effect on Psychiatric Treatment May see increased toxicity with MAO inhibitors (hypertensive crisis), sympathomimetics, CNS depressants, ethanol (sedation)

Restrictions C-V (CDSA-I)

Dosage Summary
Oral:
Children <2 years: Dosage not established
Children 2-6 years: 2.5 mL 4 times/day
Children 7-12 years: 5 mL 4 times/day **or** 1/2 tablet 4 times/day
Children >12 years: 10 mL 4 times/day **or** 1 tablet 4 times/day
Adults: 10 mL 4 times/day **or** 1 tablet 4 times/day

Dosage Forms Excipient information presented when available (limited, particularly for generics); consult specific product labeling. [CAN] = Canadian brand name
Syrup:
CoActifed® [CAN], ratio-Cotridin [CAN]: Triprolidine hydrochloride 2 mg, pseudoephedrine hydrochloride 30 mg, and codeine phosphate 10 mg per 5 mL (100 mL, 2000 mL) [not available in U.S.]
CoVan® [CAN]: Triprolidine hydrochloride 2 mg, pseudoephedrine hydrochloride 30 mg, and codeine phosphate 10 mg per 5 mL (500 mL) [not available in U.S.]
Tablet:
CoActifed® [CAN]: Triprolidine hydrochloride 4 mg, pseudoephedrine hydrochloride 60 mg, and codeine phosphate 20 mg (50s) [not available in U.S.]

◆ **TripTone® [OTC]** *see* DimenhyDRINATE *on page 478*

◆ **Triptoraline** *see* Triptorelin *on page 1635*

Triptorelin (trip toe REL in)

U.S. Brand Names Trelstar® Depot; Trelstar® LA

Canadian Brand Names Trelstar® ; Trelstar® Depot; Trelstar® LA

Index Terms AY-25650; CL-118,532; D-Trp(6)-LHRH; Triptoraline; Triptorelin Pamoate; Tryptoreline

Pharmacologic Category Gonadotropin Releasing Hormone Agonist

Use Palliative treatment of advanced prostate cancer as an alternative to orchiectomy or estrogen administration

Unlabeled/Investigational Use Treatment of endometriosis, growth hormone deficiency, hyperandrogenism, *in vitro* fertilization, ovarian carcinoma, pancreatic carcinoma, precocious puberty, uterine leiomyomata

Effect on Mental Status May cause insomnia, fatigue, emotional lability, or dizziness

Effect on Psychiatric Treatment Contraindicated with dopamine antagonists

Dosage Summary
I.M.:
Children: Dosage not established
Adults:
Trelstar® Depot: 3.75 mg once every 28 days
Trelstar ™ LA: 11.25 mg once every 84 days

Dosage Forms Excipient information presented when available (limited, particularly for generics); consult specific product labeling.
Injection, powder for reconstitution:
Trelstar® Depot: 3.75 mg [contains polylactide-co-glycolide; polysorbate 80]
Trelstar® LA: 11.25 mg [contains polylactide-co-glycolide; polysorbate 80]

- **Triptorelin Pamoate** *see* Triptorelin *on page 1635*
- **Trisenox®** *see* Arsenic Trioxide *on page 140*
- **Tri-Sprintec™** *see* Ethinyl Estradiol and Norgestimate *on page 600*
- **Tri-Sudo® [OTC] [DSC]** *see* Triprolidine and Pseudoephedrine *on page 1634*
- **Trital DM** *see* Chlorpheniramine, Phenylephrine, and Dextromethorphan *on page 327*
- **TriTuss®** *see* Guaifenesin, Dextromethorphan, and Phenylephrine *on page 746*
- **TriTuss® ER** *see* Guaifenesin, Dextromethorphan, and Phenylephrine *on page 746*
- **Trivalent Inactivated Influenza Vaccine (TIV)** *see* Influenza Virus Vaccine *on page 820*
- **Trivaris™** *see* Triamcinolone *on page 1617*
- **Tri-Vent™ DM [DSC]** *see* Guaifenesin, Pseudoephedrine, and Dextromethorphan *on page 748*
- **Tri-Vent™ DPC [DSC]** *see* Chlorpheniramine, Phenylephrine, and Dextromethorphan *on page 327*
- **Tri-Vent™ HC [DSC]** *see* Hydrocodone, Carbinoxamine, and Pseudoephedrine *on page 782*
- **Trivora®** *see* Ethinyl Estradiol and Levonorgestrel *on page 595*
- **Trobicin® [DSC]** *see* Spectinomycin *on page 1502*
- **Tronolane® Suppository [OTC]** *see* Phenylephrine *on page 1273*
- **Tropicacyl®** *see* Tropicamide *on page 1636*

Tropicamide (troe PIK a mide)

U.S. Brand Names Mydral™; Mydriacyl®; Tropicacyl®
Canadian Brand Names Diotrope®; Mydriacyl®
Index Terms Bistropamide
Pharmacologic Category Ophthalmic Agent, Mydriatic
Use Short-acting mydriatic used in diagnostic procedures; as well as preoperatively and postoperatively; treatment of some cases of acute iritis, iridocyclitis, and keratitis
Effect on Mental Status May cause drowsiness
Effect on Psychiatric Treatment None reported
Dosage Summary
Ophthalmic:
Children: 0.5%: Instill 1-2 drops 15-20 minutes before exam, may repeat; 1%: Instill 1-2 drops, may repeat in 5 minutes
Adults: 0.5%: Instill 1-2 drops 15-20 minutes before exam, may repeat; 1%: Instill 1-2 drops, may repeat in 5 minutes
Dosage Forms Excipient information presented when available (limited, particularly for generics); consult specific product labeling.
Solution, ophthalmic [drops]: 0.5% (15 mL); 1% (2 mL, 3 mL, 15 mL)
Mydriacyl®: 1% (3 mL, 15 mL) [contains benzalkonium chloride]
Mydral™, Tropicacyl®: 0.5% (15 mL); 1% (15 mL) [contains benzalkonium chloride]

Trospium (TROSE pee um)

U.S. Brand Names Sanctura®; Sanctura® XR
Canadian Brand Names Trosec
Index Terms Trospium Chloride
Pharmacologic Category Anticholinergic Agent
Use Treatment of overactive bladder with symptoms of urgency, incontinence, and urinary frequency
Effect on Mental Status May cause delirium and hallucinations
Effect on Psychiatric Treatment Dry mouth and other anticholinergic effects are common; concurrent use with psychotropics may produce additive effects; use caution in patients with Alzheimer's disease

Dosage Summary

Oral:

Children: Dosage not established

Adults: Immediate release formulation: 20 mg twice daily; Extended release formulation: 60 mg once daily

Elderly ≥75 years: Immediate release formulation: Initial: 20 mg at bedtime; Maintenance: 20 mg once or twice daily

Dosage Forms Excipient information presented when available (limited, particularly for generics); consult specific product labeling.

Capsule, extended release, as chloride:

Sanctura® XR: 60 mg

Tablet, as chloride:

Sanctura®: 20 mg

- ◆ **Trospium Chloride** *see* Trospium *on page 1636*
- ◆ **Trusopt®** *see* Dorzolamide *on page 498*
- ◆ **Truvada®** *see* Emtricitabine and Tenofovir *on page 530*
- ◆ **Tryptoreline** *see* Triptorelin *on page 1635*
- ◆ **TSPA** *see* Thiotepa *on page 1576*
- ◆ **Tucks® Anti-Itch [OTC]** *see* Hydrocortisone *on page 785*
- ◆ **Tums® [OTC]** *see* Calcium Carbonate *on page 254*
- ◆ **Tums® E-X [OTC]** *see* Calcium Carbonate *on page 254*
- ◆ **Tums® Extra Strength Sugar Free [OTC]** *see* Calcium Carbonate *on page 254*
- ◆ **Tums® Smoothies™ [OTC]** *see* Calcium Carbonate *on page 254*
- ◆ **Tums® Ultra [OTC]** *see* Calcium Carbonate *on page 254*
- ◆ **Tur-bi-kal® [OTC]** *see* Phenylephrine *on page 1273*
- ◆ **Tusnel-DM Pediatric®** *see* Guaifenesin, Pseudoephedrine, and Dextromethorphan *on page 748*
- ◆ **Tusnel Liquid®** *see* Guaifenesin, Pseudoephedrine, and Dextromethorphan *on page 748*
- ◆ **Tusnel Pediatric®** *see* Guaifenesin, Pseudoephedrine, and Dextromethorphan *on page 748*
- ◆ **Tussafed® HC [DSC]** *see* Hydrocodone, Phenylephrine, and Guaifenesin *on page 783*
- ◆ **Tussafed® HCG [DSC]** *see* Hydrocodone, Phenylephrine, and Guaifenesin *on page 783*
- ◆ **Tussi-12®** *see* Carbetapentane and Chlorpheniramine *on page 272*
- ◆ **Tussi-12® D** *see* Carbetapentane, Phenylephrine, and Pyrilamine *on page 275*
- ◆ **Tussi-12® DS** *see* Carbetapentane, Phenylephrine, and Pyrilamine *on page 275*
- ◆ **Tussi-12 S™** *see* Carbetapentane and Chlorpheniramine *on page 272*
- ◆ **TussiCaps™** *see* Hydrocodone and Chlorpheniramine *on page 778*
- ◆ **Tussigon®** *see* Hydrocodone and Homatropine *on page 780*
- ◆ **TussiNate™ [DSC]** *see* Hydrocodone, Phenylephrine, and Diphenhydramine *on page 782*
- ◆ **Tussionex®** *see* Hydrocodone and Chlorpheniramine *on page 778*
- ◆ **Tussi-Organidin® DM NR** *see* Guaifenesin and Dextromethorphan *on page 739*
- ◆ **Tussi-Organidin® DM-S NR** *see* Guaifenesin and Dextromethorphan *on page 739*
- ◆ **Tussi-Organidin® NR** *see* Guaifenesin and Codeine *on page 738*
- ◆ **Tussi-Organidin® S-NR** *see* Guaifenesin and Codeine *on page 738*
- ◆ **Tussizone-12 RF™** *see* Carbetapentane and Chlorpheniramine *on page 272*
- ◆ **Tusso-C™** *see* Guaifenesin and Codeine *on page 738*
- ◆ **Tusso-DF® [DSC]** *see* Hydrocodone and Guaifenesin *on page 779*
- ◆ **Tusso™-DMR** *see* Guaifenesin, Dextromethorphan, and Phenylephrine *on page 746*
- ◆ **Tussplex™ DM** *see* Chlorpheniramine, Phenylephrine, and Dextromethorphan *on page 327*
- ◆ **Tustan 12S™** *see* Carbetapentane and Chlorpheniramine *on page 272*
- ◆ **TVP-1012** *see* Rasagiline *on page 1403*
- ◆ **Twelve Resin-K** *see* Cyanocobalamin *on page 404*

- **Twilite® [OTC]** *see* DiphenhydrAMINE *on page 481*
- **Twinject™** *see* EPINEPHrine *on page 543*
- **Tycolene [OTC]** *see* Acetaminophen *on page 30*
- **Tycolene Maximum Strength [OTC]** *see* Acetaminophen *on page 30*
- **Tygacil®** *see* Tigecycline *on page 1583*
- **Tykerb®** *see* Lapatinib *on page 898*
- **Tylenol® [OTC]** *see* Acetaminophen *on page 30*
- **Tylenol® 8 Hour [OTC]** *see* Acetaminophen *on page 30*
- **Tylenol® Allergy Multi-Symptom Nighttime [OTC]** *see* Acetaminophen, Diphenhydramine, and Phenylephrine *on page 44*
- **Tylenol® Arthritis Pain [OTC]** *see* Acetaminophen *on page 30*
- **Tylenol® Children's [OTC]** *see* Acetaminophen *on page 30*
- **Tylenol® Children's with Flavor Creator [OTC]** *see* Acetaminophen *on page 30*
- **Tylenol® Children's Plus Cold Nighttime [OTC] [DSC]** *see* Acetaminophen, Chlorpheniramine, and Pseudoephedrine *on page 40*
- **Tylenol® Cold Day Non-Drowsy [OTC]** *see* Acetaminophen, Dextromethorphan, and Pseudoephedrine *on page 43*
- **Tylenol® Cold Daytime, Children's [OTC]** *see* Acetaminophen and Pseudoephedrine *on page 37*
- **Tylenol® Cold Head Congestion Daytime [OTC]** *see* Acetaminophen, Dextromethorphan, and Phenylephrine *on page 42*
- **Tylenol® Cold, Infants [OTC] [DSC]** *see* Acetaminophen and Pseudoephedrine *on page 37*
- **Tylenol® Cold Multi-Symptom Daytime [OTC]** *see* Acetaminophen, Dextromethorphan, and Phenylephrine *on page 42*
- **Tylenol® Extra Strength [OTC]** *see* Acetaminophen *on page 30*
- **Tylenol® Flu Non-Drowsy Maximum Strength [OTC]** *see* Acetaminophen, Dextromethorphan, and Pseudoephedrine *on page 43*
- **Tylenol® Infants [OTC]** *see* Acetaminophen *on page 30*
- **Tylenol® Junior [OTC]** *see* Acetaminophen *on page 30*
- **Tylenol® Plus Infants Cold & Cough [OTC] [DSC]** *see* Acetaminophen, Dextromethorphan, and Phenylephrine *on page 42*
- **Tylenol® PM [OTC]** *see* Acetaminophen and Diphenhydramine *on page 35*
- **Tylenol® Severe Allergy [OTC]** *see* Acetaminophen and Diphenhydramine *on page 35*
- **Tylenol® Sinus Congestion & Pain Daytime [OTC]** *see* Acetaminophen and Phenylephrine *on page 36*
- **Tylenol® Sinus Daytime [OTC]** *see* Acetaminophen and Pseudoephedrine *on page 37*
- **Tylenol® With Codeine** *see* Acetaminophen and Codeine *on page 34*
- **Tylox®** *see* Oxycodone and Acetaminophen *on page 1205*
- **Tysabri®** *see* Natalizumab *on page 1109*
- **Tyzeka™** *see* Telbivudine *on page 1541*
- **Tyzine®** *see* Tetrahydrozoline *on page 1560*
- **Tyzine® Pediatric** *see* Tetrahydrozoline *on page 1560*
- **506U78** *see* Nelarabine *on page 1120*
- **U-90152S** *see* Delavirdine *on page 424*
- **UCB-P071** *see* Cetirizine *on page 307*
- **UK-88,525** *see* Darifenacin *on page 419*
- **UK-427,857** *see* Maraviroc *on page 971*
- **UK92480** *see* Sildenafil *on page 1482*
- **UK109496** *see* Voriconazole *on page 1678*
- **Ultane®** *see* Sevoflurane *on page 1479*
- **Ultiva®** *see* Remifentanil *on page 1408*
- **Ultracet®** *see* Acetaminophen and Tramadol *on page 38*
- **Ultram®** *see* TraMADol *on page 1604*
- **Ultram® ER** *see* TraMADol *on page 1604*
- **Ultraprin [OTC]** *see* Ibuprofen *on page 803*
- **Unasyn®** *see* Ampicillin and Sulbactam *on page 122*

- ◆ **Unburn®** *see* Lidocaine *on page 924*
- ◆ **Uni-Cof [DSC]** *see* Pseudoephedrine, Dihydrocodeine, and Chlorpheniramine *on page 1371*
- ◆ **Unifed [OTC]** *see* Pseudoephedrine *on page 1367*
- ◆ **Uniphyl®** *see* Theophylline *on page 1562*
- ◆ **Uniretic®** *see* Moexipril and Hydrochlorothiazide *on page 1068*
- ◆ **Unisom® Maximum Strength SleepGels® [OTC]** *see* DiphenhydrAMINE *on page 481*
- ◆ **Unisom® SleepTabs® [OTC]** *see* Doxylamine *on page 510*
- ◆ **Unithroid®** *see* Levothyroxine *on page 920*
- ◆ **Univasc®** *see* Moexipril *on page 1068*
- ◆ **Urecholine®** *see* Bethanechol *on page 186*
- ◆ **Urelle®** *see* Methenamine, Sodium Biphosphate, Phenyl Salicylate, Methylene Blue, and Hyoscyamine *on page 1010*
- ◆ **Urimar-T** *see* Methenamine, Sodium Biphosphate, Phenyl Salicylate, Methylene Blue, and Hyoscyamine *on page 1010*
- ◆ **Urispas®** *see* Flavoxate *on page 633*
- ◆ **Uristat® [OTC] [DSC]** *see* Phenazopyridine *on page 1258*
- ◆ **Uro-Mag® [OTC]** *see* Magnesium Oxide *on page 966*
- ◆ **Uroxatral®** *see* Alfuzosin *on page 65*
- ◆ **Urso 250™** *see* Ursodiol *on page 1639*
- ◆ **Ursodeoxycholic Acid** *see* Ursodiol *on page 1639*

Ursodiol (ur soe DYE ol)

U.S. Brand Names Actigall®; Urso 250™; Urso Forte™

Canadian Brand Names DOM-Ursodiol C; PHL-Ursodiol C; PMS-Ursodiol C; Urso®; Urso® DS

Mexican Brand Names Ursofalk

Index Terms Ursodeoxycholic Acid

Pharmacologic Category Gallstone Dissolution Agent

Use Actigall®: Gallbladder stone dissolution; prevention of gallstones in obese patients experiencing rapid weight loss; Urso®: Primary biliary cirrhosis

Unlabeled/Investigational Use Liver transplantation

Effect on Mental Status May cause drowsiness

Effect on Psychiatric Treatment None reported

Dosage Summary

Oral:

Children: Dosage not established

Adults: 8-15 mg/kg/day in 2-4 divided doses **or** 300 mg twice daily

Dosage Forms Excipient information presented when available (limited, particularly for generics); consult specific product labeling.

Capsule (Actigall®): 300 mg

Tablet:

Urso 250™: 250 mg

Urso Forte™: 500 mg

- ◆ **Urso Forte™** *see* Ursodiol *on page 1639*
- ◆ **Uta®** *see* Methenamine, Sodium Biphosphate, Phenyl Salicylate, Methylene Blue, and Hyoscyamine *on page 1010*
- ◆ **Utira™-C** *see* Methenamine, Sodium Biphosphate, Phenyl Salicylate, Methylene Blue, and Hyoscyamine *on page 1010*
- ◆ **UTI Relief® [OTC]** *see* Phenazopyridine *on page 1258*
- ◆ **Uvadex®** *see* Methoxsalen *on page 1018*

Vaccinia Immune Globulin (Intravenous)

(vax IN ee a i MYUN GLOB yoo lin IN tra VEE nus)

U.S. Brand Names CNJ-016™

Index Terms VIGIV

Pharmacologic Category Immune Globulin

Use Treatment of infectious complications of smallpox (vaccinia virus) vaccination, such as eczema vaccinatum, progressive vaccinia, and severe generalized vaccinia; treatment of vaccinia infections in individuals with concurrent skin conditions or accidental virus exposure to eyes (except vaccinia keratitis), mouth, or other areas where viral infection would pose significant risk

Effect on Mental Status May cause dizziness

Effect on Psychiatric Treatment None reported

Dosage Summary

I.V.:

Cangene:

Children: Dosage not established

Adults: 6000 units/kg, 9000 units/kg may be considered if no response to initial dose

Elderly: Dosage not established

DynPort:

Children: Dosage not established

Adults: 2 mL/kg (100 mg/kg), 200-500 mg/kg may be considered if no response to initial dose

Elderly: Dosage not established

Dosage Forms Excipient information presented when available (limited, particularly for generics); consult specific product labeling.

Injection, solution [preservative free; solvent-detergent treated]:

CNJ-016™ (Cangene product): ≥50,000 units/15 mL (15 mL) [contains maltose 10% and polysorbate 80 0.03%]

DynPort product: 50 mg/mL (50 mL) [contains sucrose 50 mg/mL, human albumin 10 mg/mL, sodium 0.02-0.03 mEq/mL]

- **Vaccinia Vaccine** *see* Smallpox Vaccine *on page 1493*
- **Vagifem®** *see* Estradiol *on page 576*

Valacyclovir (val ay SYE kloe veer)

Medication Safety Issues

Sound-alike/look-alike issues:

Valtrex® may be confused with Valcyte™

Valacyclovir may be confused with valganciclovir, vancomycin

U.S. Brand Names Valtrex®

Canadian Brand Names Valtrex®

Mexican Brand Names Rapivir

Index Terms Valacyclovir Hydrochloride

Pharmacologic Category Antiviral Agent, Oral

Use Treatment of herpes zoster (shingles) in immunocompetent patients; treatment of first-episode and recurrent genital herpes; suppression of recurrent genital herpes and reduction of heterosexual transmission of genital herpes in immunocompetent patients; suppression of genital herpes in HIV-infected individuals; treatment of herpes labialis (cold sores); chickenpox in immunocompetent children

Unlabeled/Investigational Use Prophylaxis of cancer-related HSV, VZV, and CMV infections; treatment of cancer-related HSV, VZV infection

Effect on Mental Status May cause aggression, agitation, confusion, encephalopathy, hallucinations, mania, psychosis

Effect on Psychiatric Treatment Use caution in patients with renal impairment; CNS symptoms have been reported in these patients

Dosage Summary

Oral:

Children <2 years: Dosage not established

Children 2 to <12 years: 20 mg/kg/dose 3 times/day (maximum: 1 g 3 times/day)

Children ≥12 to <18 years: 2 g every 12 hours for 1 day **or** 20 mg/kg/dose 3 times/day (maximum: 1 g 3 times/day)

Adults: 500 mg to 1 g 1-3 times/day **or** 2 g every 12 hours for 1 day

Dosage Forms Excipient information presented when available (limited, particularly for generics); consult specific product labeling.

Caplet:

Valtrex®: 500 mg, 1000 mg

- **Valacyclovir Hydrochloride** *see* Valacyclovir *on page 1640*
- **Valcyte™** *see* Valganciclovir *on page 1642*
- **23-Valent Pneumococcal Polysaccharide Vaccine** *see* Pneumococcal Polysaccharide Vaccine (Polyvalent) *on page 1309*
- ***Valeriana officinalis*** *see* Valerian *(Valeriana officinalis) on page 1641*

Valerian (*Valeriana officinalis*)

Natural Product Category Herb

Synonyms *Valeriana officinalis*; Amantilla; Setwall

Plant Part Root

Dosage and Standardization Oral: 200 mg 1-4 times/day, standardized to contain 0.8% to 1% valerenic acids per dose. Sedative dose: 200-400 mg at bedtime

Reported Uses

Anxiety (Andreatini, 2002; Delsignore, 1980; Kohnen, 1988; Sousa, 1992)

Hyperthyroidism (pharmacologic activity)

Insomnia (sedative/hypnotic) (Balderer, 1985; Dominguez, 2000; Koetter, 2007; Müller, 2006)

Premenstrual syndrome (PMS), menopause; restless motor syndromes and muscle spasms (Houghton, 1988)

Summary Valerian has a long history of use as a sedative and anxiolytic. It is one of the most popular herbal preparations in Europe. It has also been reported that valerian improves sleep quality. It may have benefit for individuals with stress caused by a number of factors and may be useful in premenstrual syndrome (PMS). In addition, it has been used in restless leg syndrome and muscle spasms. When used as a hypnotic, it does not appear to be associated with "hangover" effects, an advantage over many sedative-hypnotic drugs.

Effect on Mental Status May cause sedation

Effect on Psychiatric Treatment Combined use with other psychotropics may produce additive CNS depression

Pharmacology Valerian components include valepotriates, valeric acid, and pungent oils. These have a sedative effect on the central nervous system, and they can induce smooth muscle relaxation in the gastrointestinal tract. Valepotriates and valeric acid are believed to bind to receptor sites which are similar to the benzodiazepines, influencing gamma-aminobutyric acid (GABA) affinity in the CNS.

Theoretical Cautions and Contraindications Based on pharmacologic activities, may cause drowsiness or sedation. Use with caution when driving or operating heavy machinery (German Commission E, 1985). Use caution in individuals taking medications that cause CNS depression, including sedative-hypnotics, antihistamines, antidepressants, and anxiolytics. May increase sleeping time from hypnotic agents (reported with pentobarbital in animal studies) (Hendriks, 1985).

Note: Do not use valerian supplements in children <3 years of age. Use only valepotriate and baldrinal-free in children <12 years of age due to potential mutagenic properties.

General Warnings Use all herbal supplements with extreme caution in children <2 years of age and in pregnancy or lactation. Some herbs are contraindicated in pregnancy or lactation; make sure to observe warnings. Use with caution in individuals on medication and with pre-existing medical conditions. Always review for potential herb-drug interactions (HDIs) and other warnings. Large and prolonged doses may increase the potential for adverse effects. Herbs may cause transient adverse effects such as nausea, vomiting, and GI distress due to a variety of chemical constituents. Use caution in individuals having known allergies to plants.

Theoretical Interactions CNS depressants, sedative-hypnotics (barbiturates), antidepressants, anxiolytics, antihistamines, beta-blockers, antiseizure medications, loperamide, disulfiram, metronidazole, vasopressin, alcohol

References

Andreatini R, Sartori VA, Seabra ML, et al, "Effect of Valepotriates (Valerian Extract) in Generalized Anxiety Disorder: A Randomized Placebo-Controlled Pilot Study," *Phytother Res*, 2002, 16(7):650-4.

Balderer G and Borbely AA, "Effect of Valerian on Human Sleep," *Psvchopharmacology (Berl)*, 1985, 87(4):406-9.

Delsignore R, Orlando S, Costi D, et al, "Placebo Controlled Clinical Trial With Valerian," *Settimana Medica*, 1980, 68(9):437-47.

Dominguez RA, Bravo-Valverde RL, Kaplowitz BR, et al, "Valerian As a Hypnotic for Hispanic Patients," *Cultur Divers Ethni Minor Psychol*, 2000, 6(1):84-92.

Hendriks H, Bos R, Woerdenbag, HJ, et al, "Central Nervous Depressant Activity of Valerenic Acid in the Mouse," *Planta Med*, 1985, (1):28-31.

Houghton PJ, "The Biological Activity of Valerian and Related Plants," *J Ethnopharmacol*, 1988, 22(2):121-42.

Koetter U, Schrader E, Käufeler R, et al, "A Randomized, Double Blind, Placebo-Controlled, Prospective Clinical Study to Demonstrate Clinical Efficacy of a Fixed Valerian Hops Extract Combination (Ze 91019) in Patients Suffering From Non-Organic Sleep Disorder," *Phytother Res*, 2007, 21(9):847-51.

Kohnen R and Oswald WD, "The Effects of Valerian, Propranolol, and Their Combination on Activation, Performance, and Mood of Healthy Volunteers Under Social Stress Conditions," *Pharmacopsychiatry*, 1988, 21(6):447-8.

Müller SF and Klement S, "A Combination of Valerian and Lemon Balm Is Effective in the Treatment of Restlessness and Dyssomnia in Children," *Phytomedicine*, 2006, 13 (6):383-7.

Natural Standard Research Collaboration, Chief Editors: Ulbricht C, Basch E, *Natural Standard Herb and Supplement Reference - Evidence-Based Clinical Reviews*, USA: Elsevier/Mosby, 2005.

Sousa MPd, Pacheco P, and Roldao V, "Double-Blind Comparative Study of the Efficacy and Safety of Valdispert vs Clobazepam," *KlaiChemi Med Research Info*, 1992.

"*Valerianae radix*," German Commission E Monograph, Bundesanzeiger, 1985, No 90.

Valganciclovir (val gan SYE kloh veer)

Medication Safety Issues

Sound-alike/look-alike issues:

Valcyte™ may be confused with Valium®, Valtrex®

Valganciclovir may be confused with valacyclovir

U.S. Brand Names Valcyte™

Canadian Brand Names Valcyte™

Mexican Brand Names Valcyte

Index Terms Valganciclovir Hydrochloride

Pharmacologic Category Antiviral Agent

Use Treatment of cytomegalovirus (CMV) retinitis in patients with acquired immunodeficiency syndrome (AIDS); prevention of CMV disease in high-risk patients (donor CMV positive/recipient CMV negative) undergoing kidney, heart, or kidney/pancreas transplantation

Effect on Mental Status Insomnia is common; may cause confusion and psychosis

Effect on Psychiatric Treatment Gastrointestinal side effects are common; use caution with SSRIs, lithium, and valproic acid. Granulocytopenia is common; use caution with clozapine, carbamazepine, and valproic acid.

Dosage Summary

Oral:

Children: Dosage not established

Adults: 900 mg 1-2 times/day

Dosage Forms Excipient information presented when available (limited, particularly for generics); consult specific product labeling.

Tablet, as hydrochloride: 450 mg [valganciclovir hydrochloride 496.3 mg equivalent to valganciclovir 450 mg]

◆ **Valganciclovir Hydrochloride** *see* Valganciclovir *on page 1642*

◆ **Valium®** *see* Diazepam *on page 451*

◆ **Valorin [OTC]** *see* Acetaminophen *on page 30*

◆ **Valorin Extra [OTC]** *see* Acetaminophen *on page 30*

◆ **Valproate Semisodium** *see* Valproic Acid and Derivatives *on page 1642*

◆ **Valproate Sodium** *see* Valproic Acid and Derivatives *on page 1642*

◆ **Valproic Acid** *see* Valproic Acid and Derivatives *on page 1642*

Valproic Acid and Derivatives (val PROE ik AS id & dah RIV ah tives)

Medication Safety Issues

Sound-alike/look-alike issues:

Depakene® may be confused with Depakote®

Depakote® may be confused with Depakene®, Depakote® ER, Senokot®

Depakote® ER may be confused with Depakote®

Related Information

Adverse Effects of Approved Mood Stabilizers / Anticonvulsants *on page 1751*

Agents Approved for Bipolar Disorder *on page 1752*

Anticonvulsants By Seizure Type *on page 1759*

Clozapine-Induced Side Effects *on page 1818*

Liquid Compatibility of Antidepressants, Antipsychotics, and Mood Stabilizers *on page 1788*

U.S. Brand Names Depacon®; Depakene®; Depakote®; Depakote® ER; Depakote® Sprinkle; Stavzor™

Canadian Brand Names Alti-Divalproex; Apo-Divalproex®; Apo-Valproic®; Depakene®; Dom-Divalproex; Epival® I.V.; Gen-Divalproex; Novo-Divalproex; Nu-Divalproex; PHL-Divalproex; PHL-Valproic Acid; PHL-Valproic Acid E.C.; PMS-Valproic Acid; PMS-Valproic Acid E.C.; ratio-Valproic; ratio-Valproic ECC; Rhoxal-valproic; Sandoz-Valproic

Mexican Brand Names Epival; Vematina

Index Terms 2-Propylpentanoic Acid; 2-Propylvaleric Acid; Dipropylacetic Acid; Divalproex Sodium; DPA; Valproate Semisodium; Valproate Sodium; Valproic Acid

Pharmacologic Category Anticonvulsant, Miscellaneous; Antimanic Agent; Histone Deacetylase Inhibitor

Generic Available Yes: Capsule (excluding delayed release or sprinkle), injection, syrup

Use

Depacon®, Depakene®, Depakote®, Depakote® ER, Depakote® Sprinkle, Stavzor™: Monotherapy and adjunctive therapy in the treatment of patients with complex partial seizures; monotherapy and adjunctive therapy of simple and complex absence seizures; adjunctive therapy in patients with multiple seizure types that include absence seizures

Depakote®, Depakote® ER, Stavzor™: Mania associated with bipolar disorder; migraine prophylaxis

Unlabeled/Investigational Use Status epilepticus

Mental Health Comment Both valproic acid and lithium are considered first-line agents for the management of bipolar disorder. They are useful in patients with mixed and rapid-cycling bipolar disorder. Thrombocytopenia is dose dependent and may be more common in children (Koenig, 2008). Asymptomatic elevations of hepatic transaminases are also dose related and not necessarily associated with hepatic dysfunction. Severe hepatic dysfunction is a rare idiosyncratic reaction; it is not dose related. The majority of cases occur within the first 3 months. The cause is unknown but risk factors include young age (<2 years of age), multiple anticonvulsants, and the presence of a neurologic disease in addition to epilepsy. No hepatic fatalities have been reported in patients >10 years of age who received valproic acid monotherapy.

Valproic acid is one of only a few medications that displays saturation-dependent protein binding pharmacokinetics. Therefore, when large doses are taken, the protein binding sites become saturated. This leads to an increase in unbound drug, which in turn leads to an increase in total clearance with resulting steady-state concentrations less than what might be expected. The response threshold for bipolar disorder appears to be 50 mcg/mL. Serum concentration of the extended release dosage form taken 12 hours after the last dose will result in a 25% increase over the delayed release dosage form. Interpret the levels accordingly.

Use in dementia-related aggression: Valproic acid derivatives have been investigated for over 10 years in the setting of behavioral disturbances in dementia patients. Although a number of earlier investigations suggested that valproate was effective in reducing the severity of symptoms such as aggression and agitation, these studies were commonly limited by small numbers of patients, open-label design, and lack of statistical evaluation (see Pratt and Davis review). More recently, three randomized, controlled trials were reviewed by Sink et al. These studies evaluated the use of both long- and short-acting valproate formulations in a total of 270 nursing home patients presenting with dementia of the Alzheimer's or vascular type. Although each study used a different rating scale for the assessment of neuropsychiatric symptoms, in none of the studies was the primary outcome variable significantly different ($p<0.05$) between valproate treatment and placebo.

In addition, a double-blind, randomized trial conducted by the Alzheimer's Disease Cooperative Study group evaluated the use of divalproex in nursing home patients exhibiting dementia-associated agitation. Patients were randomized to receive divalproex (n=75) or placebo (n=78) for 6 weeks duration. The primary outcome variable was the Brief Psychiatry Rating Scale Agitation factor, with a secondary measure of the Clinical Global Impression of Change. Patients received an average dose of divalproex of 800 mg/day with approximately 88% compliance. There were no differences between treatment groups with respect to safety or tolerability. The results also showed no significant differences between groups in any of the outcome measures.

Taken together, data generated from several randomized, blinded studies do not support the use of valproic acid for the treatment of dementia-related aggression or agitation. Interestingly, there are experimental data both *in vitro* and *in vivo* which suggest a possible role for valproate in slowing the neuronal deterioration process resulting from Alzheimer's pathology. Thus, there are studies ongoing to investigate the potential role that valproic acid may play in slowing disease progression and/or preserving cognitive function.

Koenig S, Gerstner T, Keller A, et al, "High Incidence of Vaproate-Induced Coagulation Disorders in Children Receiving Valproic Acid: A Prospective Study," *Blood Coagul Fibrinolysis*, 2008, 19(5):375-82.

Pratt CE and Davis SM, "Divalproex Sodium Therapy in Elderly With Dementia-Related Agitation," *Ann Pharmacother*, 2002, 36(10):1625-8.

Sink KM, Holden KF, and Yaffe K, "Pharmacological Treatment of neuropsychiatric Symptoms of Dementia: A Review of the Evidence," *JAMA*, 293 (5):596-608.

Tariot PN, Raman R, Jakimovich L, et al, "Divalproex Sodium in Nursing Home Residents With Possible or Probable Alzheimer Disease Complicated by Agitation: A Randomized, Controlled Trial," *Am J Geriatr Psychiatry*, 2005, 13 (11):942-9.

Pregnancy Risk Factor D

Pregnancy Considerations [U.S. Boxed Warning]: May cause teratogenic effects such as neural tube defects (eg, spina bifida). Teratogenic effects have been reported in animals and humans. Valproic acid crosses the placenta. Neural tube, cardiac, facial (characteristic pattern of dysmorphic facial features), skeletal, multiple other defects reported. Epilepsy itself, number of medications, genetic factors, or a combination of these probably influence the teratogenicity of anticonvulsant therapy. Information from the North American Antiepileptic Drug Pregnancy Registry notes a fourfold increase in congenital malformations with exposure to valproic acid monotherapy during the 1st trimester of pregnancy when compared to monotherapy with other antiepileptic drugs (AED). The risk of neural tube defects is ~1% to 2% (general population risk estimated to be 0.14% to 0.2%). The effect of folic acid supplementation to decrease this risk is unknown, however, folic acid supplementation is recommended for all women contemplating pregnancy. An information sheet describing the teratogenic potential is available from the manufacturer.

Nonteratogenic effects have also been reported. Afibrinogenemia leading to fatal hemorrhage and hepatotoxicity have been noted in case reports of infants following *in utero* exposure to valproic acid. Use in women of childbearing potential requires that benefits of use in mother be weighed against the potential risk to fetus, especially when used for conditions not associated with permanent injury or risk of death (eg, migraine). Health professionals and patients are encouraged to contact the North American Antiepileptic Drug Pregnancy registry to monitor outcomes of pregnant women exposed to valproic acid and other AEDs (1-888-233-2334).

Lactation Enters breast milk/not recommended (AAP considers "compatible")

Contraindications Hypersensitivity to valproic acid, derivatives, or any component of the formulation; hepatic disease or significant impairment; urea cycle disorders

Warnings/Precautions

[U.S. Boxed Warning]: Hepatic failure resulting in fatalities has occurred in patients; children <2 years of age are at considerable risk. Other risk factors include organic brain disease, mental retardation with severe seizure disorders, congenital metabolic disorders, and patients on multiple anticonvulsants. Hepatotoxicity has usually been reported within 6 months of therapy initiation. Monitor patients closely for appearance of malaise, weakness, facial edema, anorexia, jaundice, and vomiting; discontinue immediately with signs/ symptom of significant or suspected impairment. Liver function tests should be performed at baseline and at regular intervals after initiation of therapy, especially within the first 6 months. Hepatic dysfunction may progress despite discontinuing treatment. Should only be used as monotherapy in children <2 years of age and patients at high risk for hepatotoxicity. Contraindicated with severe impairment.

[U.S. Boxed Warning]: Cases of life-threatening pancreatitis, occurring at the start of therapy or following years of use, have been reported in adults and children. Some cases have been hemorrhagic with rapid progression of initial symptoms to death. Promptly evaluate symptoms of abdominal pain, nausea, vomiting, and/or anorexia; should generally be discontinued if pancreatitis is diagnosed.

[U.S. Boxed Warning]: May cause teratogenic effects such as neural tube defects (eg, spina bifida). Use in women of childbearing potential requires that benefits of use in mother be weighed against the potential risk to fetus, especially when used for conditions not associated with permanent injury or risk of death (eg, migraine).

May cause severe thrombocytopenia, inhibition of platelet aggregation, and bleeding. Tremors may indicate overdosage; use with caution in patients receiving other anticonvulsants. Hypersensitivity reactions affecting multiple organs have been reported in association with valproic acid use; may include dermatologic and/or hematologic changes (eosinophilia, neutropenia, thrombocytopenia) or symptoms of organ dysfunction.

Hyperammonemia and/or encephalopathy, sometimes fatal, have been reported following the initiation of valproic acid therapy and may be present with normal transaminase levels. Ammonia levels should be measured in patients who develop unexplained lethargy and vomiting, changes in mental status, or in patients who present with hypothermia (unintentional drop in core body temperature to <35°C/95°F). Discontinue therapy if ammonia levels are increased and evaluate for possible urea cycle disorder (UCD); contraindicated in patients with UCD. Evaluation of UCD should be considered for the following patients prior to the start of therapy: History of unexplained encephalopathy or coma; encephalopathy associated with protein load; pregnancy or postpartum encephalopathy; unexplained mental retardation; history of elevated plasma ammonia or glutamine; history of cyclical vomiting and lethargy; episodic extreme irritability, ataxia; low BUN or protein avoidance; family history of UCD or unexplained infant deaths (particularly male); or signs or symptoms of UCD (hyperammonemia, encephalopathy, respiratory alkalosis). Hypothermia has been reported with valproic acid therapy; may or may not be associated with hyperammonemia; may also occur with concomitant topiramate therapy.

In vitro studies have suggested valproic acid stimulates the replication of HIV and CMV viruses under experimental conditions. The clinical consequence of this is unknown, but should be considered when monitoring affected patients.

FDA reports demonstrate a statistically significant increased risk of suicidality; relative risk appears to be higher in patients with epilepsy compared to patients treated for psychiatric or other considerations. Use of Depacon® injection is not recommended for post-traumatic seizure prophylaxis following acute head trauma. Anticonvulsants should not be discontinued abruptly because of the possibility of increasing seizure frequency; valproic acid should be withdrawn gradually to minimize the potential of increased seizure frequency, unless safety concerns require a more rapid withdrawal. Concomitant use with carbapenem antibiotics may reduce valproic acid levels to subtherapeutic levels; monitor levels frequently and consider alternate therapy if levels drop significantly or lack of seizure control occurs. Concomitant use with clonazepam may induce absence status. Patients treated for bipolar disorder should be monitored closely for clinical worsening or suicidality; prescriptions should be written for the smallest quantity consistent with good patient care.

CNS depression may occur with valproic acid use. Patients must be cautioned about performing tasks which require mental alertness (operating machinery or driving). Effects with other sedative drugs or ethanol may be potentiated. Use with caution in the elderly.

Adverse Reactions

>10%:

Central nervous system: Headache (≤31%), somnolence (≤30%), dizziness (12% to 25%), insomnia (>1% to 15%), nervousness (>1% to 11%), pain (1% to 11%)

Dermatologic: Alopecia (>1% to 24%)

Gastrointestinal: Nausea (15% to 48%), vomiting (7% to 27%), diarrhea (7% to 23%), abdominal pain (7% to 23%), dyspepsia (7% to 23%), anorexia (>1% to 12%)

Hematologic: Thrombocytopenia (1% to 24%; dose related)

Neuromuscular & skeletal: Tremor (≤57%), weakness (6% to 27%)

Ocular: Diplopia (>1% to 16%), amblyopia/blurred vision (≤12%)

Miscellaneous: Infection (≤20%), flu-like syndrome (12%)

1% to 10%:

Cardiovascular: Peripheral edema (>1% to 8%), chest pain (>1% to <5%), edema (>1% to <5%), facial edema (>1% to <5%), hypertension (>1% to <5%), hypotension (>1% to <5%), palpitation (>1% to <5%), postural hypotension (>1% to <5%), tachycardia (>1% to <5%), vasodilation(>1% to <5%), arrhythmia

Central nervous system: Ataxia (>1% to 8%), amnesia (>1% to 7%), emotional lability (>1% to 6%), fever (>1% to 6%), abnormal thinking (≤6%), depression (>1% to 5%), abnormal dreams (>1% to <5%), agitation (>1% to <5%), anxiety (>1% to <5%), catatonia (>1% to <5%), chills (>1% to <5%), confusion (>1% to <5%), coordination abnormal (>1% to <5%), hallucination (>1% to <5%), malaise (>1% to <5%), personality disorder (>1% to <5%), speech disorder (>1% to <5%), tardive dyskinesia (>1% to <5%), vertigo (>1% to <5%), euphoria (1%), hypoesthesia (1%)

Dermatologic: Rash (>1% to 6%), bruising (>1% to 5%), discoid lupus erythematosus (>1% to <5%), dry skin (>1% to <5%), furunculosis (>1% to

<5%), petechia (>1% to <5%), pruritus (>1% to <5), seborrhea (>1% to <5%)

Endocrine & metabolic: Amenorrhea (>1% to <5%), dysmenorrhea (>1% to <5%), metrorrhagia (>1% to <5%), hypoproteinemia

Gastrointestinal: Weight gain (4% to 9%), weight loss (6%), appetite increased (≤6%), constipation (>1% to 5%), xerostomia (>1% to 5%), eructation (>1% to <5%), fecal incontinence (>1% to <5%), flatulence (>1% to <5%), gastroenteritis (>1% to <5%), glossitis (>1% to <5%), hematemesis (>1% to <5%), pancreatitis (>1% to <5%), periodontal abscess (>1% to <5%), stomatitis (>1% to <5%), taste perversion (>1% to <5%), dysphagia, gum hemorrhage, mouth ulceration

Genitourinary: Cystitis (>1% to 5%), dysuria (>1% to 5%), urinary frequency (>1% to <5%), urinary incontinence (>1% to <5%), vaginal hemorrhage (>1% to 5%), vaginitis (>1% to <5%)

Hepatic: AST/ALT increased (>1% to <5%)

Local: Injection site pain (3%), injection site reaction (2%), injection site inflammation (1%)

Neuromuscular & skeletal: Back pain (≤8%), abnormal gait (>1% to <5%), arthralgia (>1% to <5%), arthrosis (>1% to <5%), dysarthria (>1% to <5%), hypertonia (>1% to <5%), hypokinesia (>1% to <5%), leg cramps (>1% to <5%), myalgia (>1% to <5%), myasthenia (>1% to <5%), neck pain (>1% to <5%), neck rigidity (>1% to <5%), paresthesia (>1% to <5%), reflex increased (>1% to <5%), twitching (>1% to <5%)

Ocular: Nystagmus (1% to 8%), dry eyes (>1% to 5%), eye pain (>1% to 5%), abnormal vision (>1% to <5%), conjunctivitis (>1% to <5%)

Otic: Tinnitus (1% to 7%), ear pain (>1% to 5%), deafness (>1% to <5%), otitis media (>1% to <5%)

Respiratory: Pharyngitis (2% to 8%), bronchitis (5%), rhinitis (>1% to 5%), dyspnea (1% to 5%), cough (>1% to <5%), epistaxis (>1% to <5%), pneumonia (>1% to <5%), sinusitis (>1% to <5%)

Miscellaneous: Diaphoresis (1%), hiccups

<1% (Limited to important and/or life-threatening): Aggression, agranulocytosis, allergic reaction, anaphylaxis, anemia, aplastic anemia, asterixis, behavioral deterioration, bilirubin increased, bleeding time altered, bone marrow suppression, bone pain, bradycardia, breast enlargement, cutaneous vasculitis, carnitine decreased, cerebral atrophy (reversible), coma (rare), dementia, encephalopathy (rare), enuresis, eosinophilia, erythema multiforme, Fanconi-like syndrome (rare, in children), galactorrhea, hematoma formation, hemorrhage, hepatic failure, hepatotoxicity, hostility, hyperactivity, hyperammonemia, hyperammonemic encephalopathy (in patients with UCD), hyperglycinemia, hypersensitivity reactions (severe, with multiorgan dysfunction), hypofibrinogenemia, hyponatremia, hypothermia, inappropriate ADH secretion, intermittent porphyria, LDH increased, leukopenia, lupus, lymphocytosis, macrocytosis, menstrual irregularities, pancytopenia parkinsonism, parotid gland swelling, photosensitivity, platelet aggregation inhibited, polycystic ovary disease (rare), psychosis, seeing "spots before the eyes," Stevens-Johnson syndrome, suicidal behavior/ideation, thyroid function tests abnormal, toxic epidermal necrolysis (rare), urinary tract infection

Metabolism/Transport Effects For valproic acid: **Substrate** (minor) of CYP2A6, 2B6, 2C9, 2C19, 2E1; **Inhibits** CYP2C9 (weak), 2C19 (weak), 2D6 (weak), 3A4 (weak); **Induces** CYP2A6 (weak)

Drug Interactions

Aminocamptothecin: Valproic Acid may decrease the serum concentration of Aminocamptothecin. *Risk C: Monitor therapy*

Barbiturates: Valproic Acid may decrease the metabolism of Barbiturates. Barbiturates may decrease the serum concentration of Valproic Acid. *Risk C: Monitor therapy*

CarBAMazepine: May increase the metabolism of Valproic Acid. Valproic Acid may decrease the serum concentration of CarBAMazepine. Carbamazepine-Epoxide concentrations might increase, offsetting the decreases in the parent compound. *Risk C: Monitor therapy*

Carbapenems: May decrease the serum concentration of Valproic Acid. *Risk C: Monitor therapy*

ChlorproMAZINE: May increase the serum concentration of Valproic Acid. *Risk C: Monitor therapy*

Ethosuximide: May decrease the serum concentration of Valproic Acid. Valproic Acid may increase the serum concentration of Ethosuximide. *Risk C: Monitor therapy*

Felbamate: May increase the serum concentration of Valproic Acid. *Risk D: Consider therapy modification*

LamoTRIgine: Valproic Acid may enhance the adverse/toxic effect of LamoTRIgine. Valproic Acid may increase the serum concentration of LamoTRIgine. *Risk D: Consider therapy modification*

LORazepam: Valproic Acid may decrease the metabolism of LORazepam. *Risk D: Consider therapy modification*

Methylfolate: May decrease the serum concentration of Valproic Acid. *Risk C: Monitor therapy*

OXcarbazepine: Valproic Acid may decrease the serum concentration of OXcarbazepine. *Risk C: Monitor therapy*

Phenytoin: May increase the metabolism of Valproic Acid. A hepatotoxic metabolite of valproic acid may result. Valproic Acid may decrease the serum concentration of Phenytoin. Continued therapy usually yields a normalization (or slight increase) of serum phenytoin concentrations. Free phenytoin concentrations, however, tend to remain relatively stable (possibly increased with continued therapy). *Risk C: Monitor therapy*

Primidone: Valproic Acid may decrease the metabolism of Primidone. More specifically, the metabolism of phenobarbital, primidone 's primary active metabolite, would be decreased. Primidone may decrease the serum concentration of Valproic Acid. *Risk C: Monitor therapy*

Protease Inhibitors: May decrease the serum concentration of Valproic Acid. *Risk C: Monitor therapy*

Rifampin: May decrease the serum concentration of Valproic Acid. *Risk D: Consider therapy modification*

Risperidone: Valproic Acid may enhance the adverse/toxic effect of Risperidone. Generalized edema has developed. *Risk C: Monitor therapy*

Salicylates: May increase the serum concentration of Valproic Acid. *Risk C: Monitor therapy*

Topiramate: May enhance the hepatotoxic effect of Valproic Acid. *Risk C: Monitor therapy*

Tricyclic Antidepressants: Valproic Acid may increase the serum concentration of Tricyclic Antidepressants. *Risk C: Monitor therapy*

Vorinostat: Valproic Acid may enhance the thrombocytopenic effect of Vorinostat. This may increase the risk of gastrointestinal bleeding. *Risk C: Monitor therapy*

Zidovudine: Valproic Acid may decrease the metabolism of Zidovudine. *Risk C: Monitor therapy*

Ethanol/Nutrition/Herb Interactions

Ethanol: Avoid ethanol (may increase CNS depression).

Food: Food may delay but does not affect the extent of absorption. Valproic acid serum concentrations may be decreased if taken with food. Milk has no effect on absorption.

Herb/Nutraceutical: Avoid evening primrose (seizure threshold decreased).

Stability

Depakote® tablet, Depakene® solution: Store below 30°C (86°F).

Depakote® Sprinkles: Store below 25°C (77°F).

Depakote® ER, Stavzor™: Store at controlled room temperature of 25°C (77°F).

Depakene® capsule: Store at controlled room temperature of 15°C to 25°C (59°F to 77°F).

Depacon®: Store vial at room temperature of 15°C to 30°C (59°F to 86°F). Injection should be diluted in 50 mL of a compatible diluent. Stable in D_5W, NS, and LR for at least 24 hours when stored in glass or PVC.

Mechanism of Action Causes increased availability of gamma-aminobutyric acid (GABA), an inhibitory neurotransmitter, to brain neurons or may enhance the action of GABA or mimic its action at postsynaptic receptor sites

Pharmacodynamics/Kinetics

Distribution: Total valproate: 11 L/1.73 m^2; free valproate 92 L/1.73 m^2

Protein binding (dose dependent): 80% to 90%; decreased in the elderly and with hepatic or renal dysfunction

Metabolism: Extensively hepatic via glucuronide conjugation and mitochondrial beta-oxidation. The relationship between dose and total valproate concentration is nonlinear; concentration does not increase proportionally with the dose, but increases to a lesser extent due to saturable plasma protein binding. The kinetics of unbound drug are linear.

Bioavailability: Depakote® ER: ~90% relative to I.V. dose and ~89% relative to delayed release formulation

Half-life elimination (increased in neonates and with liver disease): Children >2 months: 7-13 hours; Adults: 9-16 hours

Time to peak, serum: Depakote® tablet: ~4 hours; Depakote® ER: 4-17 hours; Stavzor™: 2 hours

Excretion: Urine (30% to 50% as glucuronide conjugate, 3% as unchanged drug)

Dosage

Seizure disorders: **Note:** Administer doses >250 mg/day in divided doses.

Oral:

Simple and complex absence seizures: Children and Adults: Initial: 15 mg/kg/day; increase by 5-10 mg/kg/day at weekly intervals until therapeutic levels are achieved; maximum: 60 mg/kg/day. Larger maintenance doses may be required in younger children.

Complex partial seizures: Children ≥10 years and Adults: Initial: 10-15 mg/kg/day; increase by 5-10 mg/kg/day at weekly intervals until therapeutic levels are achieved; maximum: 60 mg/kg/day. Larger maintenance doses may be required in younger children.

Note: Regular release and delayed release formulations are usually given in 2-4 divided doses/day; extended release formulation (Depakote® ER) is usually given once daily. Conversion to Depakote® ER from a stable dose of Depakote® may require an increase in the total daily dose between 8% and 20% to maintain similar serum concentrations. Depakote® ER is not recommended for use in children <10 years of age.

I.V.: Administer as a 60-minute infusion (≤20 mg/minute) with the same frequency as oral products; switch patient to oral products as soon as possible. Rapid infusions ≤45 mg/kg over 5-10 minutes (1.5-6 mg/kg/minute) were generally well tolerated in a clinical trial.

Rectal (unlabeled): Dilute syrup 1:1 with water for use as a retention enema; loading dose: 17-20 mg/kg one time; maintenance: 10-15 mg/kg/dose every 8 hours

Status epilepticus (unlabeled use): Adults:

Loading dose: I.V.: 15-45 mg/kg administered at ≤6 mg/kg/minute.

Maintenance dose: I.V. infusion: 1-4 mg/kg/hour; titrate dose as needed based upon patient response and evaluation of drug-drug interactions

Mania: Adults: Oral:

Depakote® tablet, Stavzor™: Initial: 750 mg/day in divided doses; dose should be adjusted as rapidly as possible to desired clinical effect; maximum recommended dosage: 60 mg/kg/day

Depakote® ER: Initial: 25 mg/kg/day given once daily; dose should be adjusted as rapidly as possible to desired clinical effect; maximum recommended dose: 60 mg/kg/day.

Migraine prophylaxis:

Children ≥12 years (Stavzor™): 250 mg twice daily; adjust dose based on patient response, up to 1000 mg/day

Children ≥16 years and Adults: Oral:

Depakote® tablet: 250 mg twice daily; adjust dose based on patient response, up to 1000 mg/day

Depakote® ER: 500 mg once daily for 7 days, then increase to 1000 mg once daily; adjust dose based on patient response; usual dosage range 500-1000 mg/day

Elderly: Elimination is decreased in the elderly. Studies of elderly patients with dementia show a high incidence of somnolence. In some patients, this was associated with weight loss. Starting doses should be lower and increases should be slow, with careful monitoring of nutritional intake and dehydration. Safety and efficacy for use in patients >65 years have not been studied for migraine prophylaxis.

Dosing adjustment in renal impairment: A 27% reduction in clearance of unbound valproate is seen in patients with Cl_{cr} <10 mL/minute. Hemodialysis reduces valproate concentrations by 20%, therefore no dose adjustment is needed in patients with renal failure. Protein binding is reduced, monitoring only total valproate concentrations may be misleading.

Dosing adjustment/comments in hepatic impairment: Reduce dose. Clearance is decreased with liver impairment. Hepatic disease is also associated with decreased albumin concentrations and 2- to 2.6-fold increase in the unbound fraction. Free concentrations of valproate may be elevated while total concentrations appear normal. Use is contraindicated in severe impairment.

Dietary Considerations Valproic acid may cause GI upset; take with large amount of water or food to decrease GI upset. May need to split doses to avoid GI upset.

Depakote® Sprinkle capsule contents may be mixed with semisolid food (eg, applesauce or pudding) in patients having difficulty swallowing; particles should be swallowed and not chewed.

Valproate sodium oral solution will generate valproic acid in carbonated beverages and may cause mouth and throat irritation; do not mix valproate sodium oral solution with carbonated beverages.

Administration

Depakote® ER: Swallow whole; do not crush or chew. Patients who need dose adjustments smaller than 500 mg/day for migraine prophylaxis should be changed to Depakote® delayed release tablets.

Depakote® Sprinkle capsules may be swallowed whole or open capsule and sprinkle on small amount (1 teaspoonful) of soft food and use immediately (do not store or chew).

Depacon®: Following dilution to final concentration, administer over 60 minutes at a rate ≤20 mg/minute. Alternatively, single doses up to 45 mg/kg have been administered as a rapid infusion over 5-10 minutes (1.5-6 mg/kg/minute).

Depakene® capsule, Stavzor™: Swallow whole; do not chew.

Monitoring Parameters Liver enzymes (at baseline and during therapy), CBC with platelets (baseline and periodic intervals), PT/PTT (especially prior to surgery), serum ammonia (with symptoms of lethargy, mental status change), serum valproate levels

Reference Range

Therapeutic:

Epilepsy: 50-100 mcg/mL (SI: 350-690 μmol/L)

Mania: 85-125 mcg/mL (SI: 350-860 μmol/L)

Toxic: Some laboratories may report >200 mcg/mL (SI: >1390 μmol/L) as a toxic threshold, although clinical toxicity can occur at lower concentrations. Probability of thrombocytopenia increases with total valproate levels ≥110 mcg/mL in females or ≥135 mcg/mL in males.

Seizure control: May improve at levels >100 mcg/mL (SI: 690 μmol/L), but toxicity may occur at levels of 100-150 mcg/mL (SI: 690-1040 μmol/L)

Mania: Clinical response seen with trough levels between 85-125 mcg/mL; risk of toxicity increases at levels >125 mcg/mL

Test Interactions False-positive result for urine ketones; accuracy of thyroid function tests

Additional Information Extended release tablets have 10% to 20% less fluctuation in serum concentration than delayed release tablets. Extended release tablets are not bioequivalent to delayed release tablets.

Dosage Forms Excipient information presented when available (limited, particularly for generics); consult specific product labeling. **Note:** Strength expressed as valproic acid

Capsule, softgel, as valproic acid: 250 mg

Depakene®: 250 mg

Capsule, softgel, delayed release, as valproic acid:

Stavzor™: 125 mg, 250 mg, 500 mg

Capsule, sprinkles, as divalproex sodium:

Depakote® Sprinkle: 125 mg

Injection, solution, as valproate sodium: 100 mg/mL (5 mL)

Depacon®: 100 mg/mL (5 mL) [contains edetate disodium]

Syrup, as valproic acid: 250 mg/5 mL (5 mL, 10 mL, 480 mL)

Depakene®: 250 mg/5 mL (480 mL)

Tablet, delayed release, as divalproex sodium: 125 mg, 250 mg, 500 mg

Depakote®: 125 mg, 250 mg, 500 mg

Tablet, delayed release, enteric coated, as divalproex sodium: 125 mg, 250 mg, 500 mg

Tablet, extended release, as divalproex sodium:

Depakote® ER: 250 mg, 500 mg

Valrubicin (val ROO bi sin)

Medication Safety Issues

Sound-alike/look-alike issues:

Valstar® may be confused with valsartan

High alert medication: The Institute for Safe Medication Practices (ISMP) includes this medication among its list of drugs which have a heightened risk of causing significant patient harm when used in error.

U.S. Brand Names Valstar® [DSC]

Canadian Brand Names Valstar®; Valtaxin®

Index Terms *N*-trifluoroacetyladriamycin-14-valerate; AD3L

Pharmacologic Category Antineoplastic Agent, Anthracycline

Use Intravesical therapy of BCG-refractory carcinoma *in situ* of the urinary bladder

Effect on Mental Status May cause dizziness or drowsiness

Effect on Psychiatric Treatment None reported

Dosage Summary

Intravesical:

Children: Dosage not established

Adults: 800 mg once weekly

Dosage Forms Excipient information presented when available (limited, particularly for generics); consult specific product labeling. [DSC] = Discontinued product

Injection, solution [DSC]: 40 mg/mL (5 mL) [contains Cremophor® EL 50% (polyoxyethyleneglycol triricinoleate) and dehydrated alcohol 50%]

Valsartan (val SAR tan)

Medication Safety Issues

Sound-alike/look-alike issues:

Valsartan may be confused with losartan, Valstar™

Diovan® may be confused with Darvon®, Dioval®, Zyban®

Related Information

Angiotensin Agents *on page 1754*

U.S. Brand Names Diovan®

Canadian Brand Names Diovan®

Mexican Brand Names Diovan

Pharmacologic Category Angiotensin II Receptor Blocker

Generic Available No

Use Alone or in combination with other antihypertensive agents in the treatment of essential hypertension; reduction of cardiovascular mortality in patients with left ventricular dysfunction postmyocardial infarction; treatment of heart failure (NYHA Class II-IV)

Effect on Mental Status May cause dizziness or drowsiness

Effect on Psychiatric Treatment May rarely cause neutropenia; use caution with clozapine and carbamazepine; barbiturates and carbamazepine may increase the metabolism of valsartan

Pregnancy Risk Factor D

Pregnancy Considerations Medications which act on the renin-angiotensin system are reported to have the following fetal/neonatal effects: Hypotension, neonatal skull hypoplasia, anuria, renal failure, and death; oligohydramnios is also reported. These effects are reported to occur with exposure during the second and third trimesters. **[U.S. Boxed Warning]: Based on human data, drugs that act on the angiotensin system can cause injury and death to the developing fetus when used in the second and third trimesters. Angiotensin receptor blockers should be discontinued as soon as possible once pregnancy is detected.**

Lactation Excretion in breast milk unknown/not recommended

Contraindications

U.S. labeling: There are no contraindications listed in manufacturer's labeling.

Canadian labeling: Hypersensitivity to valsartan or any component of the formulation

Warnings/Precautions [U.S. Boxed Warning]: Based on human data, drugs that act on the angiotensin system can cause injury and death to the developing fetus when used in the second and third trimesters. Angiotensin receptor blockers should be discontinued as soon as possible once pregnancy is detected. May cause hyperkalemia; avoid potassium supplementation unless specifically required by healthcare provider. During the initiation of therapy, hypotension may occur, particularly in patients with heart failure or post-MI patients. Use extreme caution with concurrent administration of potassium-sparing diuretics or potassium supplements, in patients with mild-to-moderate hepatic dysfunction (adjust dose), in those who may be sodium/water depleted (eg, on high-dose diuretics), and in the elderly; correct depletion first.

Use caution with unstented unilateral/bilateral renal artery stenosis. When unstented bilateral renal artery stenosis is present, use is generally avoided due to the elevated risk of deterioration in renal function unless possible benefits outweigh risks. Use with caution with preexisting renal insufficiency; significant aortic/mitral stenosis. May be associated with deterioration of renal function and/or increases in serum creatinine, particularly in patients with low renal blood flow (eg, renal artery stenosis, heart failure) whose glomerular filtration rate (GFR) is dependent on efferent arteriolar vasoconstriction by angiotensin II. Use caution in patients with severe renal impairment or significant hepatic dysfunction. Monitor renal function closely in patients with severe heart failure;

changes in renal function should be anticipated and dosage adjustments of valsartan or concomitant medications may be needed. In Canada, use is not approved in patients <18 years of age.

Adverse Reactions

>10%:

Central nervous system: Dizziness (heart failure trials 17%)

Renal: BUN increased >50% (heart failure trials 17%)

1% to 10%:

Cardiovascular: Hypotension (heart failure trials 7%; MI trial 1%), postural hypotension (heart failure trials 2%), syncope (up to >1%)

Central nervous system: Dizziness (hypertension trial 2% to 8%), fatigue (heart failure trials 3%; hypertension trial 2%), postural dizziness (heart failure trials 2%), headache (heart failure trials >1%), vertigo (up to >1%)

Endocrine & metabolic: Serum potassium increased by >20% (4% to 10%), hyperkalemia (heart failure trials 2%)

Gastrointestinal: Diarrhea (heart failure trials 5%), abdominal pain (2%), nausea (heart failure trials >1%), upper abdominal pain (heart failure trials >1%)

Hematologic: Neutropenia (2%)

Neuromuscular & skeletal: Arthralgia (heart failure trials 3%), back pain (up to 3%)

Ocular: Blurred vision (heart failure trials >1%)

Renal: Creatinine doubled (MI trial 4%), creatinine increased >50% (heart failure trials 4%), renal dysfunction (up to >1%)

Respiratory: Cough (1% to 3%)

Miscellaneous: Viral infection (3%)

All indications: <1% (Limited to important or life-threatening): Allergic reactions, alopecia, anaphylaxis, anemia, angioedema, anorexia, anxiety, chest pain, constipation, dyspepsia, dyspnea, flatulence, hematocrit/hemoglobin decreased, hepatitis, impotence, insomnia, liver function tests increased, microcytic anemia, muscle cramps, myalgia, palpitation, paresthesia, photosensitivity, pruritus, rash, rhabdomyolysis, somnolence, taste disorder, thrombocytopenia, vomiting, weakness, xerostomia

Metabolism/Transport Effects Inhibits CYP2C9 (weak)

Drug Interactions

ACE Inhibitors: Angiotensin II Receptor Blockers may enhance the adverse/toxic effect of ACE Inhibitors. *Risk C: Monitor therapy*

Diazoxide: May enhance the hypotensive effect of Antihypertensives. *Risk C: Monitor therapy*

Eplerenone: May enhance the hyperkalemic effect of Angiotensin II Receptor Blockers. *Risk C: Monitor therapy*

Herbs (Hypertensive Properties): May diminish the antihypertensive effect of Antihypertensives. *Risk C: Monitor therapy*

Herbs (Hypotensive Properties): May enhance the hypotensive effect of Antihypertensives. *Risk C: Monitor therapy*

Lithium: Angiotensin II Receptor Blockers may increase the serum concentration of Lithium. Management: Lithium dosage reductions will likely be needed following the addition of an angiotensin II receptor antagonist. *Risk D: Consider therapy modification*

Methylphenidate: May diminish the antihypertensive effect of Antihypertensives. *Risk C: Monitor therapy*

Nonsteroidal Anti-Inflammatory Agents: May diminish the therapeutic effect of Angiotensin II Receptor Blockers. The combination of these two agents may also significantly decrease glomerular filtration and renal function. *Risk C: Monitor therapy*

Potassium Salts: May enhance the hyperkalemic effect of Angiotensin II Receptor Blockers. *Risk C: Monitor therapy*

Potassium-Sparing Diuretics: Angiotensin II Receptor Blockers may enhance the hyperkalemic effect of Potassium-Sparing Diuretics. *Risk C: Monitor therapy*

Prostacyclin Analogues: May enhance the hypotensive effect of Antihypertensives. *Risk C: Monitor therapy*

RiTUXimab: Antihypertensives may enhance the hypotensive effect of RiTUXimab. *Risk D: Consider therapy modification*

Trimethoprim: May enhance the hyperkalemic effect of Angiotensin II Receptor Blockers. *Risk C: Monitor therapy*

Ethanol/Nutrition/Herb Interactions

Food: Decreases rate and extent of absorption by 50% and 40%, respectively.

Herb/Nutraceutical: Avoid bayberry, blue cohosh, cayenne, ephedra, ginger, ginseng (American), kola, licorice (may worsen hypertension). Avoid black cohosh, California poppy, coleus, golden seal, hawthorn, mistletoe, periwinkle, quinine, shepherd's purse (may have increased antihypertensive effect).

Stability Store at 25°C (77°F); excursions between 15°C to 30°C (59°F to 86°F) permitted. Protect from moisture.

Mechanism of Action Valsartan produces direct antagonism of the angiotensin II (AT2) receptors, unlike the ACE inhibitors. It displaces angiotensin II from the AT1 receptor and produces its blood pressure-lowering effects by antagonizing AT1-induced vasoconstriction, aldosterone release, catecholamine release, arginine vasopressin release, water intake, and hypertrophic responses. This action results in more efficient blockade of the cardiovascular effects of angiotensin II and fewer side effects than the ACE inhibitors.

Pharmacodynamics/Kinetics

Onset of antihypertensive effect: 2 weeks (maximal: 4 weeks)
Distribution: V_d: 17 L (adults)
Protein binding: 95%, primarily albumin
Metabolism: To inactive metabolite
Bioavailability: Tablet: 25% (range 10% to 35%); suspension: ~40% (~1.6 times more than tablet)
Half-life elimination: ~6 hours
Time to peak, serum: 2-4 hours
Excretion: Feces (83%) and urine (13%) as unchanged drug

Dosage Oral:

Hypertension:

Children 6-16 years: Initial: 1.3 mg/kg once daily (maximum: 40 mg/day); dose may be increased to achieve desired effect; doses >2.7 mg/kg (maximum: 160 mg) have not been studied

Adults: Initial: 80 mg or 160 mg once daily (in patients who are not volume depleted); dose may be increased to achieve desired effect; maximum recommended dose: 320 mg/day

Heart failure: Adults: Initial: 40 mg twice daily; titrate dose to 80-160 mg twice daily, as tolerated; maximum daily dose: 320 mg

Left ventricular dysfunction after MI: Adults: Initial: 20 mg twice daily; titrate dose to target of 160 mg twice daily as tolerated; may initiate ≥12 hours following MI

Dosing adjustment in renal impairment:

Children: Use is not recommended if Cl_{cr} <30 mL/minute.

Adults: No dosage adjustment necessary if Cl_{cr} >10 mL/minute.

Dialysis: Not significantly removed

Dosing adjustment in hepatic impairment In mild-to-moderate liver disease no adjustment is needed. Use caution in patients with liver disease. Patients with mild to moderate chronic disease have twice the exposure as healthy volunteers.

Dietary Considerations Avoid salt substitutes which contain potassium. May be taken with or without food.

Administration Administer with or without food.

Monitoring Parameters Baseline and periodic electrolyte panels, renal function, BP; in CHF, serum potassium during dose escalation and periodically thereafter

Additional Information Valsartan may have an advantage over losartan due to minimal metabolism requirements and consequent use in mild-to-moderate hepatic impairment.

Dosage Forms Excipient information presented when available (limited, particularly for generics); consult specific product labeling.

Tablet:

Diovan®: 40 mg, 80 mg, 160 mg, 320 mg

◆ **Valsartan and Amlodipine** *see* Amlodipine and Valsartan *on page 105*

Valsartan and Hydrochlorothiazide

(val SAR tan & hye droe klor oh THYE a zide)

Medication Safety Issues

Sound-alike/look-alike issues:

Diovan® may be confused with Darvon®, Dioval®, Zyban®

U.S. Brand Names Diovan HCT®

Canadian Brand Names Diovan HCT®

Mexican Brand Names CoDiovan

Index Terms Hydrochlorothiazide and Valsartan

Pharmacologic Category Angiotensin II Receptor Blocker; Diuretic, Thiazide

Use Treatment of hypertension

Effect on Mental Status May cause dizziness or drowsiness

Effect on Psychiatric Treatment May rarely cause neutropenia; use caution with clozapine and carbamazepine; barbiturates and carbamazepine may increase the metabolism of valsartan; may decrease lithium clearance resulting in an increase in serum lithium levels and potential lithium toxicity; monitor serum lithium levels

Dosage Summary

Oral:

Children: Dosage not established

Adults: Valsartan 80-160 mg and hydrochlorothiazide 12.5-25 mg once daily (maximum: 25 mg/day [hydrochlorothiazide]; 320 mg/day [valsartan]); **Note:** Titration is recommended

Dosage Forms Excipient information presented when available (limited, particularly for generics); consult specific product labeling.

Tablet:

Diovan HCT® 80 mg/12.5 mg: Valsartan 80 mg and hydrochlorothiazide 12.5 mg

Diovan HCT® 160 mg/12.5 mg: Valsartan 160 mg and hydrochlorothiazide 12.5 mg

Diovan HCT® 160 mg/25 mg: Valsartan 160 mg and hydrochlorothiazide 25 mg

Diovan HCT® 320 mg/12.5 mg: Valsartan 320 mg and hydrochlorothiazide 12.5 mg

Diovan HCT® 320 mg/25 mg: Valsartan 320 mg and hydrochlorothiazide 25 mg

◆ **Valstar® [DSC]** *see* Valrubicin *on page 1649*

◆ **Valtrex®** *see* Valacyclovir *on page 1640*

◆ **Vancocin®** *see* Vancomycin *on page 1653*

Vancomycin (van koe MYE sin)

Medication Safety Issues

Sound-alike/look-alike issues:

I.V. vancomycin may be confused with Invanz®

Vancomycin may be confused with clindamycin, vecuronium

High alert medication: The Institute for Safe Medication Practices (ISMP) includes this medication (intrathecal administration) among its list of drug classes which have a heightened risk of causing significant patient harm when used in error.

U.S. Brand Names Vancocin®

Canadian Brand Names Vancocin®

Mexican Brand Names Vancocin CP

Index Terms Vancomycin Hydrochloride

Pharmacologic Category Antibiotic, Miscellaneous

Use Treatment of patients with infections caused by staphylococcal species and streptococcal species; used orally for staphylococcal enterocolitis or for antibiotic-associated pseudomembranous colitis produced by *C. difficile*

Unlabeled/Investigational Use Bacterial endophthalmitis

Effect on Mental Status None reported

Effect on Psychiatric Treatment May cause neutropenia; use caution with clozapine and carbamazepine

Dosage Summary

I.V.:

Infants >1 month: 40-60 mg/kg/day in divided doses every 6 hours

Children: 40-60 mg/kg/day in divided doses every 6 hours **or** 20 mg/kg 1 hour prior to surgery

Adults: 15-20 mg/kg every 12 hours **or** 30-45 mg/kg/day in divided doses every 8-12 hours **or** 500-750 mg every 6 hours (maximum: 3 g/day) **or** 1 g 1 hour prior to surgery

Intracatheter:

Children: 2 mg/mL in SWIF/NS or D_5W; instill 3-5 mL into catheter port as a flush solution instead of heparin lock

Adults: 2 mg/mL in SWIF/NS or D_5W; instill 3-5 mL into catheter port as a flush solution instead of heparin lock.

Intrathecal:

Children: 5-20 mg/day

Adults: Up to 20 mg/day

Oral:

Children: 40 mg/kg/day in divided doses

Adults: 125 mg 4 times/day

Dosage Forms Excipient information presented when available (limited, particularly for generics); consult specific product labeling.

Capsule (Vancocin®): 125 mg, 250 mg

Infusion [premixed in iso-osmotic dextrose] (Vancocin®): 500 mg (100 mL); 1 g (200 mL)

Injection, powder for reconstitution: 500 mg, 1 g, 5 g, 10 g

- **Vancomycin Hydrochloride** *see* Vancomycin *on page 1653*
- **Vandazole™** *see* MetroNIDAZOLE *on page 1040*
- **Vaniqa™** *see* Eflornithine *on page 527*
- **Vanquish® Extra Strength Pain Reliever [OTC]** *see* Acetaminophen, Aspirin, and Caffeine *on page 39*
- **Vantas™** *see* Histrelin *on page 769*
- **Vantin®** *see* Cefpodoxime *on page 297*
- **Vaprisol®** *see* Conivaptan *on page 400*
- **VAQTA®** *see* Hepatitis A Vaccine *on page 760*

Vardenafil (var DEN a fil)

Medication Safety Issues

Sound-alike/look-alike issues:

Vardenafil may be confused with sildenafil, tadalafil

Levitra® may be confused with Kaletra®, Lexiva®

U.S. Brand Names Levitra®

Canadian Brand Names Levitra®

Mexican Brand Names Levitra

Index Terms Vardenafil Hydrochloride

Pharmacologic Category Phosphodiesterase-5 Enzyme Inhibitor

Generic Available No

Use Treatment of erectile dysfunction (ED)

Effect on Mental Status May cause dizziness; may rarely cause insomnia

Effect on Psychiatric Treatment May cause flu-like syndrome; consider this when evaluating for potential SSRI discontinuation syndrome; the symptoms are similar. Serum concentration of vardenafil may be increased with concurrent use of fluoxetine, fluvoxamine, and nefazodone; monitor.

Pregnancy Risk Factor B

Pregnancy Considerations Teratogenic effects were not observed in animal studies; however, vardenafil is not indicated for use in women. No effects on sperm motility or morphology were observed in healthy males.

Lactation Excretion in breast milk unknown/not indicated for use in women.

Contraindications Hypersensitivity to vardenafil or any component of the formulation; concurrent (regular or intermittent) use of organic nitrates in any form (eg, nitroglycerin, isosorbide dinitrate)

Warnings/Precautions There is a degree of cardiac risk associated with sexual activity; therefore, physicians may wish to consider the patient's cardiovascular status prior to initiating any treatment for erectile dysfunction. Use caution in patients with anatomical deformation of the penis (angulation, cavernosal fibrosis, or Peyronie's disease) and in patients who have conditions which may predispose them to priapism (sickle cell anemia, multiple myeloma, leukemia). Instruct patients to seek immediate medical attention if erection persists >4 hours.

Use is not recommended in patients with hypotension (<90/50 mm Hg); uncontrolled hypertension (>170/100 mm Hg); unstable angina or angina during intercourse; life-threatening arrhythmias, stroke or MI within the last 6 months; cardiac failure or coronary artery disease causing unstable angina. Safety and efficacy have not been studied in these patients. Use caution in patients with left ventricular outflow obstruction (eg, aortic stenosis). Use caution with alpha-blockers, effective CYP3A4 inhibitors, the elderly, or those with hepatic impairment (Child-Pugh class B); dosage adjustment is needed.

Rare cases of nonarteritic ischemic optic neuropathy (NAION) have been reported; risk may be increased with history of vision loss. Other risk factors for NAION include heart disease, diabetes, hypertension, smoking, age >50 years, or history of certain eye problems. Sudden decrease or loss of hearing has been reported rarely; hearing changes may be accompanied by tinnitus and dizziness.

Safety and efficacy have not been studied in patients with the following conditions, therefore, use in these patients is not recommended at this time: Congenital QT prolongation, patients taking medications known to prolong the QT interval (avoid use in patients taking Class Ia or III antiarrhythmics); severe hepatic impairment (Child-Pugh class C); end-stage renal disease requiring dialysis; retinitis pigmentosa or other degenerative retinal disorders. The safety and efficacy of vardenafil with other treatments for erectile dysfunction have not been studied and are not recommended as combination therapy. Concomitant use with all forms of nitrates is contraindicated. If nitrate administration is medically necessary, it is not known when nitrates can be safely administered following the use of vardenafil; the ACC/AHA 2007 guidelines support administration of nitrates only if 24 hours have elapsed. Safety and efficacy have not been established in children. Potential underlying causes of erectile dysfunction should be evaluated prior to treatment.

Adverse Reactions

>10%:

Cardiovascular: Flushing (11%)

Central nervous system: Headache (15%)

2% to 10%:

Central nervous system: Dizziness (2%)

Gastrointestinal: Dyspepsia (4%), nausea (2%)

Neuromuscular & skeletal: CPK increased (2%)

Respiratory: Rhinitis (9%), sinusitis (3%)

Miscellaneous: Flu-like syndrome (3%)

<2% (Limited to important or life-threatening): Abnormal ejaculation, amnesia (transient global), anaphylactic reaction, angina, arthralgia, dyspnea, hearing decreased, hearing loss, hyper-/hypotension, insomnia, liver function tests abnormal, MI, myalgia, nonarteritic ischemic optic neuropathy (NAION), pain, photophobia, photosensitivity, postural hypotension, priapism, pruritus, rash, somnolence, syncope, tachycardia, tinnitus, vertigo, vision abnormal, visual acuity reduced, visual field defects, vision loss (temporary or permanent)

Metabolism/Transport Effects **Substrate** of CYP2C (minor), 3A5 (minor), 3A4 (major)

Drug Interactions

Alpha1-Blockers: Phosphodiesterase 5 Inhibitors may enhance the hypotensive effect of Alpha1-Blockers. **Exceptions:** Dapiprazole [Off Market]. *Risk D: Consider therapy modification*

Antifungal Agents (Azole Derivatives, Systemic): May decrease the metabolism of Phosphodiesterase 5 Inhibitors. *Risk D: Consider therapy modification*

CYP3A4 Inhibitors (Moderate): May decrease the metabolism of CYP3A4 Substrates. *Risk C: Monitor therapy*

CYP3A4 Inhibitors (Strong): May decrease the metabolism of CYP3A4 Substrates. *Risk D: Consider therapy modification*

Dasatinib: May increase the serum concentration of CYP3A4 Substrates. *Risk C: Monitor therapy*

Etravirine: May decrease the serum concentration of Phosphodiesterase 5 Inhibitors. Management: No empiric dosage adjustments are recommended with concomitant therapy; however, dose of the phosphodiesterase inhibitor may need to be altered based on clinical response. *Risk C: Monitor therapy*

Macrolide Antibiotics: May decrease the metabolism of Phosphodiesterase 5 Inhibitors. **Exceptions:** Azithromycin; Dirithromycin [Off Market]; Spiramycin. *Risk D: Consider therapy modification*

Protease Inhibitors: May decrease the metabolism of Phosphodiesterase 5 Inhibitors. Management: Dose restrictions for tadalafil, and/or sildenafil and vardenafil are recommended in combination with ritonavir, atazanavir, indinavir, darunavir and saquinavir. Consult specific prescribing information for detailed recommendations. *Risk D: Consider therapy modification*

Sapropterin: May enhance the hypotensive effect of Phosphodiesterase 5 Inhibitors. *Risk C: Monitor therapy*

Vasodilators (Organic Nitrates): Phosphodiesterase 5 Inhibitors may enhance the vasodilatory effect of Vasodilators (Organic Nitrates). *Risk X: Avoid combination*

Ethanol/Nutrition/Herb Interactions Food: High-fat meals decrease maximum serum concentration 18% to 50%. Serum concentrations/toxicity may be increased with grapefruit juice; avoid concurrent use.

Stability Store at controlled room temperature of 25°C (77°F); excursions permitted to 15°C to 25°C (59°F to 86°F).

Mechanism of Action Does not directly cause penile erections, but affects the response to sexual stimulation. The physiologic mechanism of erection of the penis involves release of nitric oxide (NO) in the corpus cavernosum during sexual stimulation. NO then activates the enzyme guanylate cyclase, which results in increased levels of cyclic guanosine monophosphate (cGMP), producing smooth muscle relaxation and inflow of blood to the corpus cavernosum. Vardenafil enhances the effect of NO by inhibiting phosphodiesterase type 5 (PDE-5), which is responsible for degradation of cGMP in the corpus cavernosum; when sexual stimulation causes local release of NO, inhibition of PDE-5 by vardenafil causes increased levels of cGMP in the corpus cavernosum, resulting in smooth muscle relaxation and inflow of blood to the corpus cavernosum; at recommended doses, it has no effect in the absence of sexual stimulation.

Pharmacodynamics/Kinetics

Onset: ~60 minutes
Absorption: Rapid
Distribution: V_d: 208 L
Protein binding: ~95% (parent drug and metabolite)
Metabolism: Hepatic via CYP3A4 (major), CYP2C and 3A5 (minor); forms metabolite (active)
Bioavailability: ~15%; Elderly (≥65 years): AUC increased by 52%; Hepatic impairment (moderate, Child-Pugh class B): AUC increased by 160%
Half-life elimination: Terminal: Vardenafil and metabolite: 4-5 hours
Time to peak, plasma: 0.5-2 hours
Excretion: Feces (91% to 95% as metabolites); urine (2% to 6%)

Dosage Oral: Adults: Erectile dysfunction: 10 mg 60 minutes prior to sexual activity; dosing range: 5-20 mg; to be given as one single dose and not given more than once daily

Elderly ≥65 years: Initial: 5 mg 60 minutes prior to sexual activity; to be given as one single dose and not given more than once daily

Dosing adjustment with concomitant medications:

Alpha-blocker (dose should be stable at time of vardenafil initiation): Initial vardenafil dose: 5 mg/24 hours; if an alpha-blocker is added to vardenafil therapy, it should be initiated at the smallest possible dose, and titrated carefully.
Atazanavir: Maximum vardenafil dose: 2.5 mg/24 hours
Clarithromycin: Maximum vardenafil dose: 2.5 mg/24 hours
Erythromycin: Maximum vardenafil dose: 5 mg/24 hours
Indinavir: Maximum vardenafil dose: 2.5 mg/24 hours
Itraconazole:
200 mg/day: Maximum vardenafil dose: 5 mg/24 hours
400 mg/day: Maximum vardenafil dose: 2.5 mg/24 hours
Ketoconazole:
200 mg/day: Maximum vardenafil dose: 5 mg/24 hours
400 mg/day: Maximum vardenafil dose: 2.5 mg/24 hours
Ritonavir: Maximum vardenafil dose: 2.5 mg/72 hours
Saquinavir: Maximum vardenafil dose: 2.5 mg/24 hours

Dosage adjustment in renal impairment: Dose adjustment not needed for mild, moderate, or severe impairment; use has not been studied in patients on renal dialysis

Dosage adjustment in hepatic impairment:

Child-Pugh class A: No adjustment required
Child-Pugh class B: Initial: 5 mg 60 minutes prior to sexual activity (maximum dose: 10 mg); to be given as one single dose and not given more than once daily
Child-Pugh class C: Has not been studied; use is not recommended by the manufacturer

Dietary Considerations May take with or without food.

Administration May be administered with or without food, 60 minutes prior to sexual activity.

Monitoring Parameters Monitor for response and adverse reactions.

Dosage Forms Excipient information presented when available (limited, particularly for generics); consult specific product labeling.

Tablet:
Levitra®: 2.5 mg, 5 mg, 10 mg, 20 mg

◆ **Vardenafil Hydrochloride** *see* Vardenafil *on page 1654*

Varenicline (var e NI kleen)

Related Information

Addiction Treatments *on page 1817*

U.S. Brand Names Chantix®

Canadian Brand Names Champix®

Mexican Brand Names Champix

Index Terms Varenicline Tartrate

Pharmacologic Category Partial Nicotine Agonist; Smoking Cessation Aid

Generic Available No

Use Treatment to aid in smoking cessation

Restrictions An FDA-approved medication guide must be distributed when dispensing an outpatient prescription (new or refill) where this medication is to be used without direct supervision of a healthcare provider. Medication guides are available at http://www.fda.gov/cder/Offices/ODS/medication_guides.htm.

Pregnancy Risk Factor C

Pregnancy Considerations Teratogenic effects were not observed in animal studies, however, decreased fertility, decreased fetal weight, and increased auditory startle response were observed in the offspring. There are no adequate or well-controlled studies in pregnant women. Use only if benefit outweighs the potential risk to fetus.

Lactation Excretion in breast milk unknown/not recommended

Contraindications There are no contraindications listed within the manufacturer's labeling.

Warnings/Precautions Dose-dependent nausea may occur; both transient and persistent nausea has been reported. Dosage reduction may be considered for intolerable nausea. Neuropsychiatric symptoms, including suicidal thoughts and erratic/aggressive behavior, have been reported with use and following withdrawal of varenicline. Smoking cessation (with or without treatment) is associated with nicotine withdrawal symptoms and the exacerbation of underlying psychiatric illness; however, behavioral changes were also reported in patients who continued to smoke. Monitor patients for behavioral changes and psychiatric symptoms (eg, agitation, depression, suicidal behavior, suicidal ideation); inform patients to discontinue treatment and contact their healthcare provider immediately if they experience any behavioral and/or mood changes. Patients with pre-existing psychiatric illness (eg, bipolar disorder, major severe depression, schizophrenia) were not studied in clinical trials; safety and efficacy has not been established in these populations. Due to rare neuropsychiatric events, caution is warranted if treatment is initiated; worsening of psychiatric illness has been reported. May cause sedation, which may impair physical or mental abilities; patients must be cautioned about performing tasks which require mental alertness (eg, operating machinery or driving).

Use caution in renal dysfunction; dosage adjustment required. Safety and efficacy of varenicline with other smoking cessation therapies have not been established; increased adverse events when used concurrently with nicotine replacement therapy. The manufacturer does not recommend use in patients <18 years of age.

Adverse Reactions

>10%:

Central nervous system: Insomnia (18% to 19%), headache (15% to 19%), abnormal dreams (9% to 13%)

Gastrointestinal: Nausea (16% to 40%; dose related)

1% to 10%:

Central nervous system: Sleep disorder (≤5%), somnolence (3%), nightmares (1% to 2%), lethargy (1% to 2%), malaise (≤7%)

Dermatologic: Rash (≤3%)

Gastrointestinal: Flatulence (6% to 9%), abdominal pain (≤7%), constipation (5% to 8%), abnormal taste (5% to 8%), xerostomia (≤6%), dyspepsia (5%), vomiting (1% to 5%), appetite increased (3% to 4%), anorexia (≤2%), gastroesophageal reflux (1%)

Respiratory: Dyspnea (≤2%), rhinorrhea (≤1%)

<1% (Limited to important or life-threatening): Acute coronary syndrome, acute renal failure, aggression, agitation, amnesia, anemia, angina, anxiety, arrhythmia, asthma, atrial fibrillation, attention disturbance, behavioral changes, blindness (transient), blurred vision, bradycardia, bradyphrenia, cardiac flutter, cataract, cerebrovascular accident, chest pain, chills, conjunctivitis, coronary artery disease, cor pulmonale, deafness, depression, dermatitis, diabetes mellitus, diarrhea, disorientation, dissociation, dizziness, dysarthria, dysphagia, ECG abnormal, eczema, edema, emotional disorder, enterocolitis, epistaxis, erectile dysfunction, eructation, erythema, esophagitis, euphoria, facial palsy, fever, flu-like syndrome, flushing, gall bladder disorder, gastritis, gastric ulcer, gastrointestinal hemorrhage, gingivitis, hallucinations, hyperhidrosis, hyper-/hypokalemia, hyperlipidemia, hypersensitivity, hyper-/hypotension, hypoglycemia, intestinal obstruction, irritability, leukocytosis, libido decreased, liver function test abnormal, lymphadenopathy, mental impairment, MI, migraine, mood swings, mouth ulceration, muscle enzyme increased, musculoskeletal pain, multiple sclerosis, myositis, nephrolithiasis, night blindness, nocturia, nystagmus,

ocular vascular disorder, osteoporosis, palpitation, pancreatitis, parosmia, peripheral ischemia, photophobia, photosensitivity, pleurisy, polyuria, psoriasis, psychomotor impairment, psychotic disorder, pulmonary embolism, restless leg syndrome, restlessness, seizure, sexual dysfunction, splenomegaly, suicidal behavior, suicidal ideation, suicide, syncope, tachycardia, thinking abnormal, thrombocytopenia, thrombosis, thyroid disorder, tinnitus, transient ischemic attack, tremor, urinary retention, urticaria, ventricular extrasystoles, vertigo, visual field defect, vitreous floaters, weight gain, xerophthalmia

Drug Interactions

There are no known significant interactions.

Stability Store at controlled room temperature of 25°C (77°F).

Mechanism of Action Partial neuronal alpha$_4$ β_2 nicotinic receptor agonist; prevents nicotine stimulation of mesolimbic dopamine system associated with nicotine addiction. Also binds to 5 HT_3 receptor (significance not determined) with moderate affinity. Varenicline stimulates dopamine activity but to a much smaller degree than nicotine does, resulting in decreased craving and withdrawal symptoms.

Pharmacodynamics/Kinetics

Absorption: Well absorbed; unaffected by food
Protein binding: ≤20%
Metabolism: Minimal (<10% of clearance is through metabolism)
Half-life elimination: ~24 hours
Time to peak, plasma: ~3-4 hours
Excretion: Primarily urine (92% as unchanged drug)

Dosage Oral: Adults:

Initial:
Days 1-3: 0.5 mg once daily
Days 4-7: 0.5 mg twice daily
Maintenance (≥ Day 8): 1 mg twice daily

Note: Start 1 week before target quit date. Patients who cannot tolerate adverse events may require temporary reduction in dose. If patient successfully quits smoking during the 12 weeks, may continue for another 12 weeks to help maintain success. If not successful in first 12 weeks, then stop medication and reassess factors contributing to failure.

Dosage adjustment for toxicity: Lower dose for a period of time, then increase again

Dosage adjustment in renal impairment:

Cl_{cr} ≥30 mL/minute: No adjustment required
Cl_{cr} <30 mL/minute: Initial: 0.5 mg once daily; maximum dose: 0.5 mg twice daily
Hemodialysis: Maximum dose: 0.5 mg once daily

Dosage adjustment in hepatic impairment: No adjustment required

Dietary Considerations Should be given with food and a full glass of water to decrease gastric upset.

Administration Administer with food and glass of water.

Monitoring Parameters Monitor for behavioral changes and psychiatric symptoms (eg, agitation, depression, suicidal behavior, suicidal ideation)

Additional Information In all studies, patients received an educational booklet on smoking cessation and received up to 10 minutes of counseling at each weekly visit. Dosing started 1 week before target quit date. Successful cessation of smoking may alter pharmacokinetic properties of other medications (eg, theophylline, warfarin, insulin).

Dosage Forms Excipient information presented when available (limited, particularly for generics); consult specific product labeling.

Tablet:
Chantix®: 0.5 mg, 1 mg

Combination package, oral [dose-pack]:
Chantix®:
Tablet, oral: 0.5 mg (11) [white tablets]
Tablet, oral: 1 mg (42) [light blue tablets]

◆ **Varenicline Tartrate** *see* Varenicline *on page 1656*

◆ **Varicella, Measles, Mumps, and Rubella Vaccine** *see* Measles, Mumps, Rubella, and Varicella Virus Vaccine *on page 972*

◆ **Vaseretic®** *see* Enalapril and Hydrochlorothiazide *on page 536*

Vasopressin (vay soe PRES in)

Medication Safety Issues
Sound-alike/look-alike issues:
Pitressin® may be confused with Pitocin®

Canadian Brand Names Pressyn®; Pressyn® AR

Index Terms 8-Arginine Vasopressin; ADH; Antidiuretic Hormone

Pharmacologic Category Antidiuretic Hormone Analog; Hormone, Posterior Pituitary

Use Treatment of diabetes insipidus; differential diagnosis of diabetes insipidus

Unlabeled/Investigational Use Adjunct in the treatment of GI hemorrhage and esophageal varices; pulseless arrest (ventricular tachycardia [VT]/ ventricular fibrillation [VF], asystole/pulseless electrical activity [PEA]); vasodilatory shock (septic shock)

Effect on Mental Status May cause dizziness

Effect on Psychiatric Treatment May be somewhat useful as a treatment for lithium-induced diabetes insipidus; hydrochlorothiazide and amiloride are more effective, less expensive options

Dosage Summary

Note: Administration and dosage varies by indication.

Endotracheal (unlabeled):
Children: Dosage not established
Adults: 40 units diluted with NS (to a total volume of 10 mL) as a single dose

I.M.:
Children: 2.5-10 units 2-4 times/day as needed
Adults: 5-10 units 2-3 times/day as needed

I.V. (unlabeled):
Children:
Diabetes insipidus: 0.0005 unit/kg/hour as continuous infusion; double dosage as needed every 30 minutes (maximum: 0.01 unit/kg/hour)
GI hemorrhage: I.V. bolus: 0.3 units/kg (maximum: 20 units) may be given; Continuous I.V. infusion: 0.001-0.01 units/kg/minute (maximum: 0.01 unit/ kg/minute)
Adults:
Diabetes insipidus: 0.0005 unit/kg/hour as continuous infusion; double dosage as needed every 30 minutes (maximum: 0.01 unit/kg/hour)
Pulseless arrest: 40 units as a single dose
Variceal hemorrhage: 0.2-0.4 units/minute (maximum 0.8 units/minute)

SubQ:
Children: 2.5-10 units 2-4 times/day as needed
Adults: 5-10 units 2-3 times/day as needed

Dosage Forms Excipient information presented when available (limited, particularly for generics); consult specific product labeling.
Injection, solution: 20 units/mL (0.5 mL, 1 mL, 10 mL)

◆ **Vasotec®** *see* Enalapril *on page 531*
◆ **Vectibix®** *see* Panitumumab *on page 1221*
◆ **Velban** *see* VinBLAStine *on page 1672*
◆ **Velcade®** *see* Bortezomib *on page 192*
◆ **Velivet™** *see* Ethinyl Estradiol and Desogestrel *on page 592*

Venlafaxine (ven la FAX een)

Related Information
Antidepressant Agents *on page 1760*
Antidepressant Receptor Profile *on page 1764*

U.S. Brand Names Effexor XR®; Effexor®

Canadian Brand Names Co-Venlafaxine XR; Effexor® XR; Novo-Venlafaxine XR; PMS-Venlafaxine XR; ratio-Venlafaxine XR

Mexican Brand Names Efexor XR

Pharmacologic Category Antidepressant, Serotonin/Norepinephrine Reuptake Inhibitor

Generic Available Yes: Tablet

Use Treatment of major depressive disorder, generalized anxiety disorder (GAD), social anxiety disorder (social phobia), panic disorder

Unlabeled/Investigational Use Obsessive-compulsive disorder (OCD); hot flashes; neuropathic pain; attention-deficit/hyperactivity disorder (ADHD)

Mental Health Comment Venlafaxine functions like an SSRI in low doses (75 mg/day), a dual mechanism agent in moderate doses (150-225 mg/day) ▶

and affects serotonin, norepinephrine, and dopamine in high doses (375 mg/day). May cause modest dose related increases in systolic blood pressure; monitor blood pressure.

Restrictions An FDA-approved medication guide concerning the use of antidepressants in children, adolescents, and young adults must be distributed when dispensing an outpatient prescription (new or refill) where this medication is to be used without direct supervision of a healthcare provider. Medication guides are available at http://www.fda.gov/cder/Offices/ODS/medication_guides.htm. Dispense to parents or guardians of children and adolescents receiving this medication.

Pregnancy Risk Factor C

Pregnancy Considerations Venlafaxine is classified as pregnancy category C due to adverse effects observed in animal studies. Venlafaxine and its active metabolite ODV cross the human placenta. Neonatal seizures and neonatal abstinence syndrome have been noted in case reports following maternal use of venlafaxine during pregnancy. Nonteratogenic effects in the newborn following SSRI/SNRI exposure late in the third trimester include respiratory distress, cyanosis, apnea, seizures, temperature instability, feeding difficulty, vomiting, hypoglycemia, hyper- or hypotonia, hyper-reflexia, jitteriness, irritability, constant crying, and tremor. The long-term effects on neurobehavior have not been studied.

Due to pregnancy-induced physiologic changes, some pharmacokinetic parameters of venlafaxine may be altered. Women should be monitored for decreased efficacy. Women treated for major depression and who are euthymic prior to pregnancy are more likely to experience a relapse when medication is discontinued as compared to pregnant women who continue taking antidepressant medications. The ACOG recommends that therapy with SSRIs or SNRIs during pregnancy be individualized; treatment of depression during pregnancy should incorporate the clinical expertise of the mental health clinician, obstetrician, primary healthcare provider, and pediatrician. If treatment during pregnancy is required, consider tapering therapy during the third trimester in order to prevent withdrawal symptoms in the infant. If this is done and the woman is considered to be at risk of relapse from her major depressive disorder, the medication can be restarted following delivery, although the dose should be readjusted to that required before pregnancy.

Lactation Enters breast milk/not recommended

Contraindications Hypersensitivity to venlafaxine or any component of the formulation; use of MAO inhibitors within 14 days; should not initiate MAO inhibitor within 7 days of discontinuing venlafaxine

Warnings/Precautions **[U.S. Boxed Warning]: Antidepressants increase the risk of suicidal thinking and behavior in children, adolescents, and young adults (18-24 years of age) with major depressive disorder (MDD) and other psychiatric disorders;** consider risk prior to prescribing. Short-term studies did not show an increased risk in patients >24 years of age and showed a decreased risk in patients ≥65 years. Closely monitor for clinical worsening, suicidality, or unusual changes in behavior; the patient's family or caregiver should be instructed to closely observe the patient and communicate condition with healthcare provider. Reduced growth rate has been observed with venlafaxine therapy in children. A medication guide should be dispensed with each prescription. **Venlafaxine is not FDA approved for use in children.**

The possibility of a suicide attempt is inherent in major depression and may persist until remission occurs. Monitor for worsening of depression or suicidality, especially during initiation of therapy (generally first 1-2 months) or with dose increases or decreases. Use caution in high-risk patients. Worsening depression and severe abrupt suicidality that are not part of the presenting symptoms may require discontinuation or modification of drug therapy. The patient's family or caregiver should be alerted to monitor patients for the emergence of suicidality and associated behaviors (such as agitation, irritability, hostility, impulsivity, and hypomania) and call healthcare provider.

May worsen psychosis in some patients or precipitate a shift to mania or hypomania in patients with bipolar disorder. Patients presenting with depressive symptoms should be screened for bipolar disorder. Monotherapy in patients with bipolar disorder should be avoided. **Venlafaxine is not FDA approved for the treatment of bipolar depression.**

The potential for severe reactions exists when used with MAO inhibitors, SSRIs/SNRIs or triptans (myoclonus, diaphoresis, hyperthermia, NMS features, seizures, and death). May cause sustained increase in blood pressure or tachycardia; dose related and increases are generally modest (12-15 mm Hg diastolic). Control pre-existing hypertension prior to initiation of venlafaxine.

Use caution in patients with recent history of MI, unstable heart disease, or hyperthyroidism; may cause increase in anxiety, nervousness, insomnia; may cause weight loss (use with caution in patients where weight loss is undesirable); may cause increases in serum cholesterol. Use caution with hepatic or renal impairment; dosage adjustments recommended. May cause hyponatremia/SIADH (elderly at increased risk); volume depletion (diuretics may increase risk).

May impair platelet aggregation resulting in increased risk of bleeding events, particularly if used concomitantly with aspirin or NSAIDs. Bleeding related to SSRI or SNRI use has been reported to range from relatively minor bruising and epistaxis to life-threatening hemorrhage. Interstitial lung disease and eosinophilic pneumonia have been rarely reported; may present as progressive dyspnea, cough, and/or chest pain. Prompt evaluation and possible discontinuation of therapy may be necessary. Venlafaxine may increase the risks associated with electroconvulsive therapy. Use cautiously in patients with a history of seizures. The risks of cognitive or motor impairment, as well as the potential for anticholinergic effects are very low. May cause or exacerbate sexual dysfunction.

Abrupt discontinuation or dosage reduction after extended (≥6 weeks) therapy may lead to agitation, dysphoria, nervousness, anxiety, and other symptoms. When discontinuing therapy, dosage should be tapered gradually over at least a 2-week period. If intolerable symptoms occur following a decrease in dosage or upon discontinuation of therapy, then resuming the previous dose with a more gradual taper should be considered. Use caution in patients with increased intraocular pressure or at risk of acute narrow-angle glaucoma.

Adverse Reactions

>10%:

Central nervous system: Headache (25% to 38%), insomnia (15% to 24%), somnolence (12% to 23%), nervousness (6% to 21%), dizziness (11% to 20%)

Gastrointestinal: Nausea (21% to 58%), xerostomia (12% to 22%), anorexia (8% to 20%), constipation (8% to 15%)

Genitourinary: Abnormal ejaculation/orgasm (2% to 19%)

Neuromuscular & skeletal: Weakness (8% to 19%)

Miscellaneous: Diaphoresis (10% to 14%)

1% to 10%:

Cardiovascular: Hypertension (dose related; 3% in patients receiving <100 mg/day, up to 13% in patients receiving >300 mg/day), vasodilation (3% to 4%), palpitation (3%), tachycardia (2%), chest pain (2%), postural hypotension (1%), edema

Central nervous system: Abnormal dreams (3% to 7%), anxiety (5% to 6%), yawning (3% to 5%), agitation (2% to 4%), chills (3%), confusion (2%), abnormal thinking (2%), depersonalization (1%), depression (1% to 3%), fever, migraine, amnesia, hypoesthesia, trismus, vertigo

Dermatologic: Rash (3%), pruritus (1%), bruising

Endocrine & metabolic: Libido decreased (3% to 9%), hypercholesterolemia (5%), triglycerides increased

Gastrointestinal: Diarrhea (6% to 8%), dyspepsia (7%), vomiting (3% to 6%), abdominal pain (6%), flatulence (3% to 4%), taste perversion (2%), weight loss (1% to 4%), appetite increased, weight gain

Genitourinary: Impotence (4% to 10%), urinary frequency (3%), urination impaired (2%), urinary retention (1%), prostatic disorder

Neuromuscular & skeletal: Tremor (4% to 10%), hypertonia (3%), paresthesia (2% to 3%), twitching (1% to 3%), neck pain, arthralgia

Ocular: Abnormal or blurred vision (4% to 6%), mydriasis (2%)

Otic: Tinnitus (2%)

Respiratory: Pharyngitis (7%), sinusitis (2%), cough increased, dyspnea

Miscellaneous: Infection (6%), flu-like syndrome (6%), trauma (2%)

<1% (Limited to important or life-threatening): Agranulocytosis, anaphylaxis, anemia, aplastic anemia, aneurysm, angina pectoris, anuria, appendicitis, arrhythmia (including atrial and ventricular tachycardia, fibrillation, and torsade de pointes), arteritis, asthma, ataxia, atelectasis, atrioventricular block, bacteremia, balance/coordination impaired, basophilia, bigeminy, biliary pain, bilirubinemia, bleeding time increased, bradycardia, bradykinesia, BUN increased, bundle branch block, carcinoma, cardiovascular disorder (mitral valve and circulatory disturbance), cataract, catatonia, cellulitis, cerebral ischemia, cholelithiasis, congestive heart failure, coronary artery disease, creatinine increased, crystalluria, cyanosis, deafness, DVT, dehydration, delusions, dementia, diabetes mellitus, dystonia, ECG abnormalities (including QT prolongation), embolus, eosinophilia, erythema multiforme,

exfoliative dermatitis, extrapyramidal symptoms, extrasystoles, facial paralysis, fasciitis, fatty liver, gastrointestinal ulcer, glaucoma, glycosuria, granuloma, Guillain-Barré syndrome, heart arrest, hematemesis, hematoma, hemorrhage (eye, GI, mucocutaneous, rectal), hepatic necrosis, hepatic failure, hepatitis, homicidal ideation, hostility, hyperacusis, hypercalcinuria, hyperchlorhydria, hyper-/hypoglycemia, hyper-/hypokalemia, hyper-/hypophosphatemia, hyper-/hypothyroidism, hyperuricemia, hypocholesteremia, hyponatremia, hypoproteinemia, hypotension, interstitial lung disease (including eosinophilic pneumonia), intestinal obstruction, jaundice, kidney function abnormal, larynx edema, leukocytosis, leukoderma, leukopenia, liver enzymes increased, loss of consciousness, lymphadenopathy, lymphocytosis, maculopapular rash, menstrual abnormalities, miliaria, moniliasis, multiple myeloma, myasthenia, myocardial infarct, myoclonus, myopathy, neck rigidity, neuroleptic malignant-like syndrome, neuropathy, neutropenia, osteoporosis, pancreatitis, pancytopenia, peripheral vascular disorder, pleurisy, pneumonia, pyelonephritis, pyuria, renal failure, rhabdomyolysis, rheumatoid arthritis, seizure, serotonin syndrome, SIADH, skin atrophy, Stevens-Johnson syndrome, suicidal ideation (reported at a frequency up to 2% in children/adolescents with major depressive disorder), suicide attempt, syncope, tendon rupture, thrombocythemia, thrombocytopenia, tongue edema, toxic epidermal necrolysis, withdrawal syndrome

Metabolism/Transport Effects Substrate of CYP2C9 (minor), 2C19 (minor), 2D6 (major), 3A4 (major); **Inhibits** CYP2B6 (weak), 2D6 (weak), 3A4 (weak)

Drug Interactions

Alcohol (Ethyl): CNS Depressants may enhance the CNS depressant effect of Alcohol (Ethyl). *Risk C: Monitor therapy*

Aspirin: Antidepressants (Serotonin/Norepinephrine Reuptake Inhibitor) may enhance the antiplatelet effect of Aspirin. *Risk C: Monitor therapy*

CNS Depressants: May enhance the adverse/toxic effect of other CNS Depressants. *Risk C: Monitor therapy*

CYP2D6 Inhibitors (Moderate): May decrease the metabolism of CYP2D6 Substrates. *Risk C: Monitor therapy*

CYP2D6 Inhibitors (Strong): May decrease the metabolism of CYP2D6 Substrates. *Risk D: Consider therapy modification*

CYP3A4 Inducers (Strong): May increase the metabolism of CYP3A4 Substrates. *Risk C: Monitor therapy*

CYP3A4 Inhibitors (Moderate): May decrease the metabolism of CYP3A4 Substrates. *Risk C: Monitor therapy*

CYP3A4 Inhibitors (Strong): May decrease the metabolism of CYP3A4 Substrates. *Risk D: Consider therapy modification*

Darunavir: May increase the serum concentration of CYP2D6 Substrates. *Risk C: Monitor therapy*

Dasatinib: May increase the serum concentration of CYP3A4 Substrates. *Risk C: Monitor therapy*

Deferasirox: May decrease the serum concentration of CYP3A4 Substrates. *Risk C: Monitor therapy*

Herbs (CYP3A4 Inducers): May increase the metabolism of CYP3A4 Substrates. *Risk C: Monitor therapy*

Indinavir: Venlafaxine may decrease the serum concentration of Indinavir. *Risk C: Monitor therapy*

MAO Inhibitors: May enhance the serotonergic effect of Antidepressants (Serotonin/Norepinephrine Reuptake Inhibitor). This may cause serotonin syndrome. *Risk X: Avoid combination*

Metoclopramide: May enhance the adverse/toxic effect of Venlafaxine. Specifically, the risk of serotonin syndrome may be increased. *Risk C: Monitor therapy*

NSAID (Nonselective): Antidepressants (Serotonin/Norepinephrine Reuptake Inhibitor) may enhance the antiplatelet effect of NSAID (Nonselective). *Risk C: Monitor therapy*

Serotonin Modulators: May enhance the adverse/toxic effect of other Serotonin Modulators. The development of serotonin syndrome may occur. *Risk D: Consider therapy modification*

Sibutramine: May enhance the serotonergic effect of Serotonin Modulators. This may cause serotonin syndrome. *Risk X: Avoid combination*

TraZODone: Venlafaxine may enhance the serotonergic effect of TraZODone. This could result in serotonin syndrome. *Risk D: Consider therapy modification*

Voriconazole: May enhance the adverse/toxic effect of Venlafaxine. Voriconazole may increase the serum concentration of Venlafaxine. *Risk C: Monitor therapy*

Ethanol/Nutrition/Herb Interactions

Ethanol: Avoid ethanol (may increase CNS effects).

Herb/Nutraceutical: Avoid valerian, St John's wort, SAMe, kava kava, tryptophan (may increase risk of serotonin syndrome and/or excessive sedation).

Stability Store at controlled room temperature of 20°C to 25°C (68°F to 77°F).

Mechanism of Action Venlafaxine and its active metabolite, o-desmethylvenlafaxine (ODV), are potent inhibitors of neuronal serotonin and norepinephrine reuptake and weak inhibitors of dopamine reuptake. Venlafaxine and ODV have no significant activity for muscarinic cholinergic, H_1-histaminergic, or alpha$_2$-adrenergic receptors. Venlafaxine and ODV do not possess MAO-inhibitory activity.

Pharmacodynamics/Kinetics

Absorption: Oral: 92% to 100%; food has no significant effect on the absorption of venlafaxine or formation of the active metabolite O-desmethylvenlafaxine (ODV)

Distribution: At steady state: Venlafaxine 7.5 ± 3.7 L/kg, ODV 5.7 ± 1.8 L/Kg

Protein binding: Bound to human plasma protein: Venlafaxine 27%, ODV 30%

Metabolism: Hepatic via CYP2D6 to active metabolite, O-desmethylvenlafaxine (ODV); other metabolites include N-desmethylvenlafaxine and N,O-didesmethylvenlafaxine

Bioavailability: Absolute: ~45%

Half-life elimination: Venlafaxine: 3-7 hours; ODV: 9-13 hours; Steady-state, plasma: Venlafaxine/ODV: Within 3 days of multiple-dose therapy; prolonged with cirrhosis (Adults: Venlafaxine: ~30%, ODV: ~60%) and with dialysis (Adults: Venlafaxine: ~180%, ODV: ~142%)

Time to peak:

- Immediate release: Venlafaxine: 2 hours, ODV: 3 hours
- Extended release: Venlafaxine: 5.5 hours, ODV: 9 hours

Excretion: Urine (~87%, 5% as unchanged drug, 29% as unconjugated ODV, 26% as conjugated ODV, 27% as minor inactive metabolites) within 48 hours

Clearance at steady state: Venlafaxine: 1.3 ± 0.6 L/hour/kg, ODV: 0.4 ± 0.2 L/hour/kg

- Clearance decreased with:
  - Cirrhosis: Adults: Venlafaxine: ~50%, ODV: ~30%
  - Severe cirrhosis: Adults: Venlafaxine: ~90%
  - Renal impairment (Cl_{cr} 10-70 mL/minute): Adults: Venlafaxine: ~24%
  - Dialysis: Adults: Venlafaxine: ~57%, ODV: ~56%; due to large volume of distribution, a significant amount of drug is not likely to be removed.

Dosage Oral:

Children and Adolescents:

- Attention-deficit/hyperactivity disorder (unlabeled use): Initial: 12.5 mg/day
  - Children <40 kg: Increase by 12.5 mg/week to maximum of 50 mg/day in 2 divided doses
  - Children ≥40 kg: Increase by 25 mg/week to maximum of 75 mg/day in 3 divided doses.
  - Mean dose: 60 mg or 1.4 mg/kg administered in 2-3 divided doses

Adults:

- Depression:
  - Immediate-release tablets: 75 mg/day, administered in 2 or 3 divided doses, taken with food; dose may be increased in 75 mg/day increments at intervals of at least 4 days, up to 225-375 mg/day
  - Extended-release capsules: 75 mg once daily taken with food; for some new patients, it may be desirable to start at 37.5 mg/day for 4-7 days before increasing to 75 mg once daily; dose may be increased by up to 75 mg/day increments every 4 days as tolerated, up to a recommended maximum of 225 mg/day
- Generalized anxiety disorder, social anxiety disorder: Extended-release capsules: 75 mg once daily taken with food; for some new patients, it may be desirable to start at 37.5 mg/day for 4-7 days before increasing to 75 mg once daily; dose may be increased by up to 75 mg/day increments every 4 days as tolerated, up to a maximum of 225 mg/day
- Panic disorder: Extended-release capsules: 37.5 mg once daily for 1 week; may increase to 75 mg daily, with subsequent weekly increases of 75 mg/day up to a maximum of 225 mg/day.
- Obsessive-compulsive disorder (unlabeled use): Titrate to usual dosage range of 150-300 mg/day; however, doses up to 375 mg daily have been used; response may be seen in 4 weeks
- Neuropathic pain (unlabeled use): Dosages evaluated varied considerably based on etiology of chronic pain, but efficacy has been shown for many conditions in the range of 75-225 mg/day; onset of relief may occur in 1-2 weeks, or take up to 6 weeks for full benefit.

Hot flashes (unlabeled use): Doses of 37.5-75 mg/day have demonstrated significant improvement of vasomotor symptoms after 4-8 weeks of treatment; in one study, doses >75 mg/day offered no additional benefit; however, higher doses (225 mg/day) may be beneficial in patients with perimenopausal depression.

Attention-deficit disorder (unlabeled use): Initial: Doses vary between 18.75 to 75 mg/day; may increase after 4 weeks to 150 mg/day; if tolerated, doses up to 225 mg/day have been used

Note: When discontinuing this medication after more than 1 week of treatment, it is generally recommended that the dose be tapered. If venlafaxine is used for 6 weeks or longer, the dose should be tapered over 2 weeks when discontinuing its use.

Elderly: Alzheimer's dementia-related depression:

Immediate-release tablets: Initial: 25 mg/day; may increase at weekly intervals to maximum of 375 mg/day in divided doses

Extended-release capsules: Initial: 37.5 mg/day; may increase at weekly intervals to maximum of 225 mg/day

Dosing adjustment in renal impairment: Cl_{cr} 10-70 mL/minute: Decrease dose by 25%; decrease total daily dose by 50% if dialysis patients; dialysis patients should receive dosing after completion of dialysis

Dosing adjustment in moderate hepatic impairment: Reduce total daily dosage by 50%

Child/Adolescent Considerations Sixteen children and adolescents (mean age: 11.6 years) with attention-deficit/hyperactivity disorder (ADHD) received a mean daily dose of 60 mg (1.4 mg/kg) administered in 2-3 divided doses (Olvera, 1996). Thirty-three children 8-17 years of age with major depression participated in a 6-week trial. For children 8-12 years, doses were initiated at 12.5 mg once daily for 3 days, then increased to 12.5 mg twice daily for 3 days, then increased to 12.5 mg 3 times/day for the rest of the study. Both venlafaxine and placebo patients improved over time, however, no significant differences in symptoms were noted between groups (Mandoki, 1997). Higher initial doses of 37.5 mg/day for 1 week with increases to 75 mg/day for 2-8 weeks are currently being investigated (Weller, 2000). Ten children with autism spectrum disorder were initiated at 12.5 mg/day and adjusted on a flexible basis (mean: 24.4 mg/day; range 6.25-50 mg/day) (Hollander, 2000).

Brent D, Emslie G, Clarke G, et al,"Switching to Another SSRI or to Venlafaxine With or Without Cognitive Behavioral Therapy for Adolescents With SSRI-Resistant Depression: The TORDIA Randomized Controlled Trial," *JAMA*, 2008, 299(8):901-13.

Hollander E, Kaplan A, Cartwright C, et al, "Venlafaxine in Children, Adolescents, and Young Adults With Autism Spectrum Disorders: An Open Retrospective Clinical Report," *J Child Neurol*, 2000, 15(2):132-5.

Mandoki MW, Tapia MR, Tapia MA, et al, "Venlafaxine in the Treatment of Children and Adolescents With Major Depression," *Psychopharmacol Bull*, 1997, 33(1):149-54.

Olvera RL, Pliszka SR, Luh J, et al, "An Open Trial of Venlafaxine in the Treatment of Attention-Deficit/Hyperactivity Disorder in Children and Adolescents," *J Child Adolesc Psychopharmacol*, 1996, 6(4):241-50.

Weller EB, Weller RA, and Davis HP, "Use of Venlafaxine in Children and Adolescents: A Review of Current Literature," *Depression and Anxiety*, 2000, 12(Suppl 1):85-9.

Dietary Considerations Should be taken with food.

Administration Administer with food.

Extended release capsule: Swallow capsule whole; do not crush or chew. Alternatively, contents may be sprinkled on a spoonful of applesauce and swallowed immediately without chewing; followed with a glass of water to ensure complete swallowing of the pellets.

Monitoring Parameters Blood pressure should be regularly monitored, especially in patients with a high baseline blood pressure; may cause mean increase in heart rate of 4-9 beats/minute; cholesterol; mental status for depression, suicidal ideation (especially at the beginning of therapy or when doses are increased or decreased), anxiety, social functioning, mania, panic attacks; height and weight should be monitored in children

Reference Range Peak serum level of 163 ng/mL (325 ng/mL of ODV metabolite) obtained after a 150 mg oral dose

Test Interactions Increased thyroid, uric acid, glucose, potassium, AST, cholesterol (S)

Dosage Forms Excipient information presented when available (limited, particularly for generics); consult specific product labeling.

Capsule, extended release:
Effexor XR®: 37.5 mg, 75 mg, 150 mg
Tablet: 25 mg, 37.5 mg, 50 mg, 75 mg, 100 mg
Effexor®: 25 mg, 37.5 mg, 50 mg, 75 mg, 100 mg

- **Venofer®** *see* Iron Sucrose *on page 858*
- **Ventavis®** *see* Iloprost *on page 810*
- **Ventolin® HFA** *see* Albuterol *on page 54*
- **VePesid® [DSC]** *see* Etoposide *on page 607*
- **Veramyst™** *see* Fluticasone *on page 668*

Verapamil (ver AP a mil)

Medication Safety Issues

Sound-alike/look-alike issues:
Calan® may be confused with Colace®
Covera-HS® may be confused with Provera®
Isoptin® may be confused with Isopto® Tears
Verelan® may be confused with Virilon®, Voltaren®

High alert medication: The Institute for Safe Medication Practices (ISMP) includes this medication (I.V. formulation) among its list of drug classes which have a heightened risk of causing significant patient harm when used in error.

Significant differences exist between oral and I.V. dosing. Use caution when converting from one route of administration to another.

International issues:
Calan®: Brand name for vinpocetine in Japan

Related Information

Calcium Channel Blockers *on page 1778*

U.S. Brand Names Calan®; Calan® SR; Covera-HS®; Isoptin® SR; Verelan®; Verelan® PM

Canadian Brand Names Apo-Verap®; Apo-Verap® SR; Calan®; Chronovera®; Covera-HS®; Covera®; Dom-Verapamil SR; Gen-Verapamil; Gen-Verapamil SR; Isoptin® SR; Med-Verapamil; Novo-Veramil SR; Nu-Verap; PHL-Verapamil; PMS-Verapamil SR; Riva-Verapamil SR; Verapamil Hydrochloride Injection, USP; Verelan SRC

Mexican Brand Names Cronovera; Dilacoran

Index Terms Iproveratril Hydrochloride; Verapamil Hydrochloride

Pharmacologic Category Antiarrhythmic Agent, Class IV; Calcium Channel Blocker

Generic Available Yes

Use Orally for treatment of angina pectoris (vasospastic, chronic stable, unstable) and hypertension; I.V. for supraventricular tachyarrhythmias (PSVT, atrial fibrillation, atrial flutter)

Unlabeled/Investigational Use Migraine; hypertrophic cardiomyopathy; bipolar disorder (manic manifestations)

Effect on Mental Status May cause drowsiness, dizziness, confusion, insomnia, psychotic symptoms, and extrapyramidal symptoms

Effect on Psychiatric Treatment Barbiturates may decrease verapamil serum concentrations; verapamil may increase buspirone, carbamazepine, and midazolam serum concentrations; concurrent use with lithium may cause an increase or decrease in serum lithium concentrations; monitor; verapamil has been used to treat bipolar disorder, mania

Pregnancy Risk Factor C

Pregnancy Considerations Use in pregnancy only when clearly needed and when the benefits outweigh the potential risk to the fetus. Crosses the placenta. One report of suspected heart block when used to control fetal supraventricular tachycardia. May exhibit tocolytic effects.

Lactation Enters breast milk (small amounts)/not recommended

Contraindications Hypersensitivity to verapamil or any component of the formulation; severe left ventricular dysfunction; hypotension (systolic pressure <90 mm Hg) or cardiogenic shock; sick sinus syndrome (except in patients with a functioning artificial pacemaker); second- or third-degree AV block (except in patients with a functioning artificial pacemaker); atrial flutter or fibrillation and an accessory bypass tract (WPW, Lown-Ganong-Levine syndrome)

Warnings/Precautions Increased angina and/or MI has occurred with initiation or dosage titration of calcium channel blockers. The most common side effect is peripheral edema; occurs within 2-3 weeks of starting therapy. Avoid use in heart failure; can exacerbate condition. Symptomatic hypotension with or without syncope can rarely occur; blood pressure must be lowered at a rate appropriate for the patient's clinical condition. Rare increases in liver function tests can be observed. Can cause first-degree AV block or sinus bradycardia. Other conduction abnormalities are rare. Use caution when using verapamil together with a beta-blocker. Avoid use of I.V. verapamil with an I.V. beta-blocker; can result in asystole. Use I.V. with caution in patients with hypertrophic subaortic stenosis (IHSS). Use I.V. with caution in patients with attenuated neuromuscular transmission (Duchenne's muscular dystrophy, myasthenia gravis). Adjust the dose in severe renal dysfunction; may require lower startingdoes in hepatic dysfunction. Verapamil significantly increases digoxin serum concentrations (adjust digoxin's dose). May prolong recovery from nondepolarizing neuromuscular-blocking agents.

Adverse Reactions

>10%: Gastrointestinal: Gingival hyperplasia (up to 19%), constipation (12% up to 42% in clinical trials)

1% to 10%:

Cardiovascular: Bradycardia (1.2 to 1.4%); first-, second-, or third-degree AV block (1.2%); CHF (1.8%); hypotension (2.5% to 3%); peripheral edema (1.9%), symptomatic hypotension (1.5% I.V.); severe tachycardia (1%)

Central nervous system: Dizziness (1.2% to 3.3%), fatigue (1.7%), headache (1.2% to 2.2%)

Dermatologic: Rash (1.2%)

Gastrointestinal: Nausea (0.9% to 2.7%)

Respiratory: Dyspnea (1.4%)

<1% (Limited to important or life-threatening): Alopecia, angina, arthralgia, asystole, atrioventricular dissociation, bronchial/laryngeal spasm, cerebrovascular accident, chest pain, claudication, confusion, diarrhea, dry mouth, ecchymosis, electrical mechanical dissociation (EMD), emotional depression, eosinophilia, equilibrium disorders, erythema multiforme, exanthema, exfoliative dermatitis, galactorrhea/hyperprolactinemia, GI obstruction, gingival hyperplasia, gynecomastia, hair color change, impotence, muscle cramps, MI, myoclonus, paresthesia, Parkinsonian syndrome, psychotic symptoms, purpura (vasculitis), rash, respiratory failure, rotary nystagmus, shakiness, shock, somnolence, Stevens-Johnson syndrome, syncope, urticaria, ventricular fibrillation, vertigo

Metabolism/Transport Effects Substrate of CYP1A2 (minor), 2B6 (minor), 2C9 (minor), 2C18 (minor), 2E1 (minor), 3A4 (major); **Inhibits** CYP1A2 (weak), 2C9 (weak), 2D6 (weak), 3A4 (moderate)

Drug Interactions

Alcohol (Ethyl): Verapamil may increase the serum concentration of Alcohol (Ethyl). *Risk C: Monitor therapy*

Alpha1-Blockers: May enhance the hypotensive effect of Calcium Channel Blockers. *Risk C: Monitor therapy*

Amiodarone: Calcium Channel Blockers (Nondihydropyridine) may enhance the bradycardic effect of Amiodarone. Sinus arrest has been reported. *Risk D: Consider therapy modification*

Anilidopiperidine Opioids: May enhance the bradycardic effect of Calcium Channel Blockers (Nondihydropyridine). Anilidopiperidine Opioids may enhance the hypotensive effect of Calcium Channel Blockers (Nondihydropyridine). *Risk C: Monitor therapy*

Antifungal Agents (Azole Derivatives, Systemic): May decrease the metabolism of Calcium Channel Blockers. *Risk D: Consider therapy modification*

Barbiturates: May increase the metabolism of Calcium Channel Blockers. *Risk D: Consider therapy modification*

Benzodiazepines (metabolized by oxidation): Calcium Channel Blockers (Nondihydropyridine) may decrease the metabolism of Benzodiazepines (metabolized by oxidation). *Risk D: Consider therapy modification*

Beta-Blockers: Calcium Channel Blockers (Nondihydropyridine) may enhance the hypotensive effect of Beta-Blockers. Bradycardia and signs of heart failure have also been reported. Calcium Channel Blockers (Nondihydropyridine) may increase the serum concentration of Beta-Blockers. **Exceptions:** Levobunolol; Metipranolol. *Risk C: Monitor therapy*

BusPIRone: Calcium Channel Blockers (Nondihydropyridine) may decrease the metabolism of BusPIRone. *Risk D: Consider therapy modification*

Calcium Channel Blockers (Dihydropyridine): Calcium Channel Blockers (Nondihydropyridine) may enhance the hypotensive effect of Calcium Channel Blockers (Dihydropyridine). Calcium Channel Blockers (Nondihydropyridine) may decrease the metabolism of Calcium Channel Blockers (Dihydropyridine). **Exceptions:** Clevidipine. *Risk C: Monitor therapy*

Calcium Salts: May diminish the therapeutic effect of Calcium Channel Blockers. *Risk C: Monitor therapy*

CarBAMazepine: Calcium Channel Blockers (Nondihydropyridine) may decrease the metabolism of CarBAMazepine. CarBAMazepine may increase the metabolism of Calcium Channel Blockers (Nondihydropyridine). *Risk D: Consider therapy modification*

Cardiac Glycosides: Calcium Channel Blockers (Nondihydropyridine) may enhance the AV-blocking effect of Cardiac Glycosides. Calcium Channel Blockers (Nondihydropyridine) may decrease the metabolism of Cardiac Glycosides. *Risk D: Consider therapy modification*

Cimetidine: May decrease the metabolism of Calcium Channel Blockers. *Risk D: Consider therapy modification*

Colchicine: Verapamil may enhance the nephrotoxic effect of Colchicine. Colchicine may increase the serum concentration of Verapamil. *Risk C: Monitor therapy*

Corticosteroids (Systemic): Calcium Channel Blockers (Nondihydropyridine) may decrease the metabolism of Corticosteroids (Systemic). *Risk C: Monitor therapy*

CycloSPORINE: Calcium Channel Blockers (Nondihydropyridine) may decrease the metabolism of CycloSPORINE. CycloSPORINE may decrease the metabolism of Calcium Channel Blockers (Nondihydropyridine). *Risk D: Consider therapy modification*

CYP3A4 Inducers (Strong): May increase the metabolism of CYP3A4 Substrates. *Risk C: Monitor therapy*

CYP3A4 Inhibitors (Moderate): May decrease the metabolism of CYP3A4 Substrates. *Risk C: Monitor therapy*

CYP3A4 Inhibitors (Strong): May decrease the metabolism of CYP3A4 Substrates. *Risk D: Consider therapy modification*

CYP3A4 Substrates: CYP3A4 Inhibitors (Moderate) may decrease the metabolism of CYP3A4 Substrates. *Risk C: Monitor therapy*

Dabigatran Etexilate: P-Glycoprotein Inhibitors may increase the serum concentration of Dabigatran Etexilate. *Risk X: Avoid combination*

Dasatinib: May increase the serum concentration of CYP3A4 Substrates. *Risk C: Monitor therapy*

Deferasirox: May decrease the serum concentration of CYP3A4 Substrates. *Risk C: Monitor therapy*

Diazoxide: May enhance the hypotensive effect of Antihypertensives. *Risk C: Monitor therapy*

Dofetilide: Verapamil may increase the serum concentration of Dofetilide. *Risk X: Avoid combination*

Eletriptan: Calcium Channel Blockers (Nondihydropyridine) may decrease the metabolism of Eletriptan. *Risk C: Monitor therapy*

Eplerenone: Calcium Channel Blockers (Nondihydropyridine) may decrease the metabolism of Eplerenone. *Risk C: Monitor therapy*

Fexofenadine: Verapamil may increase the bioavailability of Fexofenadine. *Risk C: Monitor therapy*

Fluconazole: May decrease the metabolism of Calcium Channel Blockers. *Risk C: Monitor therapy*

Grapefruit Juice: May decrease the metabolism of Calcium Channel Blockers. *Risk C: Monitor therapy*

Herbs (CYP3A4 Inducers): May increase the metabolism of CYP3A4 Substrates. *Risk C: Monitor therapy*

Herbs (Hypertensive Properties): May diminish the antihypertensive effect of Antihypertensives. *Risk C: Monitor therapy*

Herbs (Hypotensive Properties): May enhance the hypotensive effect of Antihypertensives. *Risk C: Monitor therapy*

HMG-CoA Reductase Inhibitors: Calcium Channel Blockers (Nondihydropyridine) may decrease the metabolism of HMG-CoA Reductase Inhibitors. **Exceptions:** Fluvastatin; Pravastatin; Rosuvastatin. *Risk D: Consider therapy modification*

Lithium: Calcium Channel Blockers (Nondihydropyridine) may enhance the neurotoxic effect of Lithium. Calcium Channel Blockers (Nondihydropyridine) may increase the serum concentration of Lithium. Decreased or unaltered lithium concentrations have also been reported with this combination. *Risk C: Monitor therapy*

Macrolide Antibiotics: May decrease the metabolism of Calcium Channel Blockers. **Exceptions:** Azithromycin; Dirithromycin [Off Market]; Spiramycin. *Risk D: Consider therapy modification*

Magnesium Salts: Calcium Channel Blockers may enhance the adverse/toxic effect of Magnesium Salts. Magnesium Salts may enhance the hypotensive effect of Calcium Channel Blockers. *Risk C: Monitor therapy*

Maraviroc: CYP3A4 Inhibitors may increase the serum concentration of Maraviroc. *Risk D: Consider therapy modification*

Methylphenidate: May diminish the antihypertensive effect of Antihypertensives. *Risk C: Monitor therapy*

Midodrine: Calcium Channel Blockers (Nondihydropyridine) may enhance the bradycardic effect of Midodrine. *Risk C: Monitor therapy*

Nafcillin: May increase the metabolism of Calcium Channel Blockers. *Risk D: Consider therapy modification*

Neuromuscular-Blocking Agents (Nondepolarizing): Calcium Channel Blockers may enhance the neuromuscular-blocking effect of Neuromuscular-Blocking Agents (Nondepolarizing). *Risk C: Monitor therapy*

Nitroprusside: Calcium Channel Blockers may enhance the hypotensive effect of Nitroprusside. *Risk C: Monitor therapy*

P-Glycoprotein Inducers: May decrease the serum concentration of P-Glycoprotein Substrates. P-glycoprotein inducers may also further limit the distribution of p-glycoprotein substrates to specific cells/tissues/organs where p-glycoprotein is present in large amounts (e.g., brain, T-lymphocytes, testes, etc.). *Risk C: Monitor therapy*

P-Glycoprotein Inhibitors: May increase the serum concentration of P-Glycoprotein Substrates. P-glycoprotein inhibitors may also enhance the distribution of p-glycoprotein substrates to specific cells/tissues/organs where p-glycoprotein is present in large amounts (e.g., brain, T-lymphocytes, testes, etc.). *Risk C: Monitor therapy*

P-Glycoprotein Substrates: P-Glycoprotein Inhibitors may increase the serum concentration of P-Glycoprotein Substrates. P-glycoprotein inhibitors may also enhance the distribution of p-glycoprotein substrates to specific cells/tissues/organs where p-glycoprotein is present in large amounts (e.g., brain, T-lymphocytes, testes, etc.). *Risk C: Monitor therapy*

Phenytoin: Calcium Channel Blockers may decrease the metabolism of Phenytoin. *Risk D: Consider therapy modification*

Pimecrolimus: CYP3A4 Inhibitors (Moderate) may decrease the metabolism of Pimecrolimus. *Risk C: Monitor therapy*

Prostacyclin Analogues: May enhance the hypotensive effect of Antihypertensives. *Risk C: Monitor therapy*

Protease Inhibitors: May decrease the metabolism of Calcium Channel Blockers (Nondihydropyridine). Increased serum concentrations of the calcium channel blocker may increase risk of AV nodal blockade. *Risk D: Consider therapy modification*

QuiNIDine: Calcium Channel Blockers (Nondihydropyridine) may increase the serum concentration of QuiNIDine. *Risk D: Consider therapy modification*

Quinupristin: May decrease the metabolism of Calcium Channel Blockers. *Risk C: Monitor therapy*

Ranolazine: Calcium Channel Blockers (Nondihydropyridine) may decrease the metabolism of Ranolazine. *Risk X: Avoid combination*

Rifamycin Derivatives: May increase the metabolism of Calcium Channel Blockers. This primarily affects oral forms of calcium channel blockers. *Risk D: Consider therapy modification*

Risperidone: Verapamil may increase the serum concentration of Risperidone. *Risk C: Monitor therapy*

RiTUXimab: Antihypertensives may enhance the hypotensive effect of RiTUXimab. *Risk D: Consider therapy modification*

Rivaroxaban: P-Glycoprotein Inhibitors may increase the serum concentration of Rivaroxaban. *Risk X: Avoid combination*

Salicylates: Calcium Channel Blockers (Nondihydropyridine) may enhance the anticoagulant effect of Salicylates. *Risk C: Monitor therapy*

Salmeterol: CYP3A4 Inhibitors (Moderate) may increase the serum concentration of Salmeterol. *Risk C: Monitor therapy*

Tacrolimus: Calcium Channel Blockers (Nondihydropyridine) may decrease the metabolism of Tacrolimus. *Risk C: Monitor therapy*

Topotecan: P-Glycoprotein Inhibitors may increase the serum concentration of Topotecan. *Risk X: Avoid combination*

Ethanol/Nutrition/Herb Interactions

Ethanol: Avoid or limit ethanol (may increase ethanol levels).

Food: Grapefruit juice may increase the serum concentration of verapamil; avoid concurrent use.

Herb/Nutraceutical: St John's wort may decrease levels. Avoid dong quai if using for hypertension (has estrogenic activity). Avoid ephedra, yohimbe, ginseng (may worsen arrhythmia or hypertension). Avoid garlic (may have increased antihypertensive effect).

Stability Store injection at room temperature; do not freeze. Protect from heat. Use only clear solutions. Physically compatible in solutions of pH of 3-6, but may precipitate in solutions having a pH ≥6. Protect I.V. solution from light.

Mechanism of Action Inhibits calcium ion from entering the "slow channels" or select voltage-sensitive areas of vascular smooth muscle and myocardium during depolarization; produces a relaxation of coronary vascular smooth muscle and coronary vasodilation; increases myocardial oxygen delivery in patients with vasospastic angina; slows automaticity and conduction of AV node.

Pharmacodynamics/Kinetics

Onset of action: Peak effect: Oral: Immediate release: 1-2 hours; I.V.: 1-5 minutes

Duration: Oral: Immediate release tablets: 6-8 hours; I.V.: 10-20 minutes

Protein binding: 90%

Metabolism: Hepatic via multiple CYP isoenzymes; extensive first-pass effect

Bioavailability: Oral: 20% to 35%

Half-life elimination: Infants: 4.4-6.9 hours; Adults: Single dose: 2-8 hours, Multiple doses: 4.5-12 hours; prolonged with hepatic cirrhosis

Excretion: Urine (70%, 3% to 4% as unchanged drug); feces (16%)

Dosage

Children: SVT:

I.V.:

<1 year: 0.1-0.2 mg/kg over 2 minutes; repeat every 30 minutes as needed

1-15 years: 0.1-0.3 mg/kg over 2 minutes; maximum: 5 mg/dose, may repeat dose in 15 minutes if adequate response not achieved; maximum for second dose: 10 mg/dose

Oral (dose not well established):

1-5 years: 4-8 mg/kg/day in 3 divided doses **or** 40-80 mg every 8 hours

>5 years: 80 mg every 6-8 hours

Adults:

SVT: I.V.: 2.5-5 mg (over 2 minutes); second dose of 5-10 mg (~0.15 mg/kg) may be given 15-30 minutes after the initial dose if patient tolerates, but does not respond to initial dose; maximum total dose: 20 mg

Angina: Oral: Initial dose: 80-120 mg 3 times/day (elderly or small stature: 40 mg 3 times/day); range: 240-480 mg/day in 3-4 divided doses

Hypertension: Oral:

Immediate release: 80 mg 3 times/day; usual dose range (JNC 7): 80-320 mg/day in 2 divided doses

Sustained release: 240 mg/day; usual dose range (JNC 7): 120-360 mg/day in 1-2 divided doses; 120 mg/day in the elderly or small patients (no evidence of additional benefit in doses >360 mg/day).

Extended release:

Covera-HS®: Usual dose range (JNC 7): 120-360 mg once daily (once-daily dosing is recommended at bedtime)

Verelan® PM: Usual dose range: 200-400 mg once daily at bedtime

Dosing adjustment in renal impairment: Cl_{cr} <10 mL/minute: Administer at 50% to 75% of normal dose.

Dialysis: Not dialyzable (0% to 5%) via hemo- or peritoneal dialysis; supplemental dose is not necessary.

Dosing adjustment/comments in hepatic disease: Reduce dose in cirrhosis, reduce dose to 20% to 50% of normal and monitor ECG.

Dietary Considerations Calan® SR and Isoptin® SR products may be taken with food or milk, other formulations may be administered without regard to meals; sprinkling contents of Verelan® or Verelan® PM capsule onto applesauce does not affect oral absorption.

Administration

Oral: Do not crush or chew sustained or extended release products.

Calan® SR, Isoptin® SR: Administer with food.

Verelan®, Verelan® PM: Capsules may be opened and the contents sprinkled on 1 tablespoonful of applesauce, then swallowed without chewing.

I.V.: Rate of infusion: Over 2 minutes.

Monitoring Parameters Monitor blood pressure closely

Reference Range Therapeutic: 50-200 ng/mL (SI: 100-410 nmol/L) for parent; under normal conditions, norverapamil concentration is the same as parent drug. Toxic: >90 mcg/mL

Dosage Forms Excipient information presented when available (limited, particularly for generics); consult specific product labeling.

Caplet, sustained release, as hydrochloride: 120 mg, 180 mg, 240 mg

Calan® SR: 120 mg

Calan® SR: 180 mg, 240 mg [scored]

Capsule, extended release, oral, as hydrochloride: 120 mg, 180 mg, 240 mg

Capsule, extended release, controlled onset, as hydrochloride: 100 mg, 200 mg, 300 mg

Verelan® PM: 100 mg, 200 mg, 300 mg

Capsule, sustained release, as hydrochloride: 120 mg, 180 mg, 240 mg, 360 mg

Verelan®: 120 mg, 180 mg, 240 mg, 360 mg
Injection, solution, as hydrochloride: 2.5 mg/mL (2 mL, 4 mL)
Tablet, as hydrochloride: 40 mg, 80 mg, 120 mg
Calan®: 40 mg
Calan®: 80 mg, 120 mg [scored]
Tablet, extended release, as hydrochloride: 120 mg, 180 mg, 240 mg
Tablet, extended release, controlled onset, as hydrochloride:
Covera-HS®: 180 mg, 240 mg
Tablet, sustained release, as hydrochloride: 120 mg, 180 mg, 240 mg
Isoptin® SR: 120 mg
Isoptin® SR: 180 mg, 240 mg [scored]

- **Verapamil and Trandolapril** *see* Trandolapril and Verapamil *on page 1608*
- **Verapamil Hydrochloride** *see* Verapamil *on page 1665*
- **Verelan®** *see* Verapamil *on page 1665*
- **Verelan® PM** *see* Verapamil *on page 1665*
- **Vermox® [DSC]** *see* Mebendazole *on page 972*
- **Versed** *see* Midazolam *on page 1046*
- **Versiclear™** *see* Sodium Thiosulfate *on page 1497*
- **Vesanoid®** *see* Tretinoin, Oral *on page 1617*
- **VESIcare®** *see* Solifenacin *on page 1498*
- **VFEND®** *see* Voriconazole *on page 1678*
- **Viadur® [DSC]** *see* Leuprolide *on page 901*
- **Viagra®** *see* Sildenafil *on page 1482*
- **Vibramycin®** *see* Doxycycline *on page 509*
- **Vibra-Tabs®** *see* Doxycycline *on page 509*
- **Vicks® 44® Cough Relief [OTC]** *see* Dextromethorphan *on page 448*
- **Vicks® 44E [OTC]** *see* Guaifenesin and Dextromethorphan *on page 739*
- **Vicks® Casero™ Chest Congestion Relief [OTC]** *see* GuaiFENesin *on page 737*
- **Vicks® DayQuil® Cold/Flu Multi-Symptom Relief [OTC]** *see* Acetaminophen, Dextromethorphan, and Phenylephrine *on page 42*
- **Vicks® Early Defense™ [OTC]** *see* Oxymetazoline *on page 1208*
- **Vicks® Pediatric Formula 44E [OTC]** *see* Guaifenesin and Dextromethorphan *on page 739*
- **Vicks Sinex® 12 Hour [OTC]** *see* Oxymetazoline *on page 1208*
- **Vicks Sinex® 12 Hour Ultrafine Mist [OTC]** *see* Oxymetazoline *on page 1208*
- **Vicks® Sinex® Nasal Spray [OTC]** *see* Phenylephrine *on page 1273*
- **Vicks® Sinex® UltraFine Mist [OTC]** *see* Phenylephrine *on page 1273*
- **Vicks® Vitamin C [OTC]** *see* Ascorbic Acid *on page 141*
- **Vicodin®** *see* Hydrocodone and Acetaminophen *on page 777*
- **Vicodin® ES** *see* Hydrocodone and Acetaminophen *on page 777*
- **Vicodin® HP** *see* Hydrocodone and Acetaminophen *on page 777*
- **Vicoprofen®** *see* Hydrocodone and Ibuprofen *on page 780*
- **Vidaza®** *see* AzaCITIDine *on page 161*
- **Videx®** *see* Didanosine *on page 460*
- **Videx® EC** *see* Didanosine *on page 460*

Vigabatrin (vye GA ba trin)

Related Information
Anticonvulsants By Seizure Type *on page 1759*
Canadian Brand Names Sabril®
Pharmacologic Category Anticonvulsant, Miscellaneous
Generic Available No
Use Active management of partial or secondary generalized seizures not controlled by usual treatments; treatment of infantile spasms
Unlabeled/Investigational Use Spasticity, tardive dyskinesias
Restrictions Not available in U.S.
Pregnancy Risk Factor Not assigned; contraindicated per manufacturer
Pregnancy Considerations There are no adequate and well-controlled studies in pregnant women. Animal studies indicating fetal malformation and neurotoxicity are of concern.

Lactation Excretion in breast milk unknown/contraindicated

Contraindications Hypersensitivity to vigabatrin of any component of the formulation; pregnancy or breast-feeding

Warnings/Precautions May be associated with ophthalmologic toxicities, which may be permanent; baseline and periodic monitoring is required. Patients must be instructed to report changes in vision. Patients must be closely monitored for potential neurotoxicity (observed in animal models but not established in humans). Use caution in patients with a history of psychosis (psychotic/agitated reactions may occur more frequently), depression, or behavioral problems. Use caution in elderly patients and in patients with renal impairment (Cl_{cr} <60 mL/minute). Effects with other sedative drugs or ethanol may be potentiated. May cause an increase in seizure frequency in some patients, use particular caution in patients with myoclonic seizures, which may be more prone to this effect. Do not discontinue abruptly; gradually reduce dose over a 2- to 4-week period.

Adverse Reactions

>10%:

Central nervous system: Fatigue (27%), headache (26%), drowsiness (22%), dizziness (19%), depression (13%), tremor (11%), agitation (11%). **Note:** In pediatric use, hyperactivity (hyperkinesia, agitation, excitation, or restlessness) was reported in 11% of patients.

Endocrine & metabolic: Weight gain (12%)

Ocular: Visual field defects (33%), abnormal vision (11%)

1% to 10%:

Cardiovascular: Chest pain, edema (dependent)

Central nervous system: Abnormal thinking, aggression, amnesia, anxiety, ataxia, concentration impaired, confusion, emotional lability,insomnia, personality disorder, speech disorder, vertigo, nervousness

Dermatologic: Rash (5%, similar to placebo), skin disorder

Endocrine & metabolic: Dysmenorrhea, menstrual disorder

Gastrointestinal: Abdominal pain, appetite increased, constipation, diarrhea, nausea, vomiting

Genitourinary: Urinary tract infection

Hematologic: Purpura

Neuromuscular & skeletal: Abnormal coordination, abnormal gait, arthralgia, arthrosis, back pain, hyporeflexia, paresthesia, weakness

Ocular: Diplopia, eye pain, nystagmus

Otic: Ear pain

Respiratory: Nasal congestion, sinusitis, throat irritation, upper respiratory tract infection

<1% (Limited to important or life-threatening): Bilateral optic disc pallor, optic/retinal atrophy, and rare optic neuritis have been reported (usually in first year of therapy). Additional rare reactions include angioedema, hallucinations, hypersensitivity, hypomania, mania, psychosis, suicidal behavior, stupor, and urticaria.

Drug Interactions

Alcohol (Ethyl): CNS Depressants may enhance the CNS depressant effect of Alcohol (Ethyl). *Risk C: Monitor therapy*

CNS Depressants: May enhance the adverse/toxic effect of other CNS Depressants. *Risk C: Monitor therapy*

Ketorolac: May diminish the therapeutic effect of Anticonvulsants. *Risk C: Monitor therapy*

Mefloquine: May diminish the therapeutic effect of Anticonvulsants. Mefloquine may decrease the serum concentration of Anticonvulsants. Management: Mefloquine is contraindicated in persons with a history of convulsions. If anticonvulsant is being used for another indication monitor response to treatment closely, as concurrent mefloquine may decrease response to treatment. *Risk D: Consider therapy modification*

Phenytoin: Vigabatrin may decrease the serum concentration of Phenytoin. *Risk C: Monitor therapy*

Ethanol/Nutrition/Herb Interactions

Ethanol: Avoid ethanol (may increase CNS depression).

Herb/Nutraceutical: Avoid evening primrose (seizure threshold decreased). Avoid valerian, St John's wort, kava kava, gotu kola (may increase CNS depression).

Stability Store at controlled room temperature of 15°C to 30°C (68°F to 86°F). Protect from moisture.

Mechanism of Action Irreversibly inhibits gamma-aminobutyric acid transaminase (GABA-T), increasing the levels of the inhibitory compound gamma amino butyric acid (GABA) within the brain. Duration of effect is dependent upon rate of GABA-T resynthesis.

Pharmacodynamics/Kinetics

Duration (rate of GABA-T resynthesis dependent): Variable (not strictly correlated to serum concentrations)

Absorption: Rapid

Metabolism: Minimal

Half-life elimination: 5-8 hours; Elderly: Up to 13 hours

Time to peak: 2 hours

Excretion: Urine (70%, as unchanged drug)

Dosage Oral:

Children: **Note:** Administer daily dose in 2 divided doses, especially in the higher dosage ranges:

Adjunctive treatment of seizures: Initial: 40 mg/kg/day; maintenance dosages based on patient weight:

10-15 kg: 0.5-1 g/day

16-30 kg: 1-1.5 g/day

31-50 kg: 1.5-3 g/day

>50 kg: 2-3 g/day

Infantile spasms: 50-100 mg/kg/day, depending on severity of symptoms; higher doses (up to 150 mg/kg/day) have been used in some cases.

Adults: Adjunctive treatment of seizures: Initial: 1 g/day (severe manifestations may require 2 g/day); dose may be given as a single daily dose or divided into 2 equal doses. Increase daily dose by 0.5 g based on response and tolerability. Optimal dose range: 2-3 g/day (maximum dose: 3 g/day).

Elderly: Initiate at low end of dosage range (refer to adult dosing); monitor closely for sedation and confusion

Dosage adjustment in renal impairment: Cl_{cr} <60 mL/minute: Initiate at lower dosage; monitor closely for sedation and confusion

Dietary Considerations May be taken with or without food.

Administration May be administered with or without food.

Sachet: Dissolve powder in 10 mL of water, juice, infant formula, or milk immediately before administration. The appropriate aliquot may be administered using an oral syringe.

Monitoring Parameters Ophthalmologic examination at baseline and periodically during therapy (every 3 months); including mydriatic peripheral fundus examination and visual field perimetry. Observe patient for excessive sedation, especially when instituting or increasing therapy.

Additional Information Not available in U.S.

Dosage Forms Excipient information presented when available (limited, particularly for generics); consult specific product labeling. [CAN] = Canadian brand name

Powder for oral suspension [sachets]:

Sabril® [CAN]: 0.5 g [not available in the U.S.]

Tablet:

Sabril® [CAN]: 500 mg [not available in the U.S.]

◆ **Vigamox™** *see* Moxifloxacin *on page 1084*

◆ **VIGIV** *see* Vaccinia Immune Globulin (Intravenous) *on page 1639*

◆ **Vimpat®** *see* Lacosamide *on page 885*

VinBLAStine (vin BLAS teen)

Medication Safety Issues

Sound-alike/look-alike issues:

VinBLAStine may be confused with vinCRIStine, vinorelbine

High alert medication: The Institute for Safe Medication Practices (ISMP) includes this medication among its list of drug classes which have a heightened risk of causing significant patient harm when used in error.

Note: Must be dispensed in overwrap which bears the statement **"Do not remove covering until the moment of injection. Fatal if given intrathecally. For I.V. use only."** Syringes should be labeled: **"Fatal if given intrathecally. For I.V. use only."**

Mexican Brand Names Lemblastine

Index Terms NSC-49842; Velban; Vinblastine Sulfate; Vincaleukoblastine; VLB

Pharmacologic Category Antineoplastic Agent, Natural Source (Plant) Derivative; Antineoplastic Agent, Vinca Alkaloid

Use Treatment of Hodgkin's and non-Hodgkin's lymphoma; testicular cancer; breast cancer; mycosis fungoides; Kaposi's sarcoma; histiocytosis (Letterer-Siwe disease); choriocarcinoma

Unlabeled/Investigational Use Treatment of bladder cancer, melanoma, nonsmall cell lung cancer (NSCLC), ovarian cancer, prostate cancer, renal cancer, soft tissue sarcoma (desmoid tumors)

Effect on Mental Status May cause depression

Effect on Psychiatric Treatment Bone marrow suppression is common; use caution with clozapine and carbamazepine

Dosage Summary Details concerning dosing in combination regimens should also be consulted.

I.V.:

Children: Initial dose: 3-6.5 mg/m^2; do not administer more frequently than every 7 days

Adults: Initial: 3.7 mg/m^2; adjust dose every 7 days (based on white blood cell response) up to 5.5 mg/m^2 (second dose); 7.4 mg/m^2 (third dose); 9.25 mg/m^2 (fourth dose); and 11.1 mg/m^2 (fifth dose); Usual range: 5.5-7.4 mg/m^2 every 7 days; Maximum dose: 18.5 mg/m^2

Dosage Forms Excipient information presented when available (limited, particularly for generics); consult specific product labeling.

Injection, powder for reconstitution, as sulfate: 10 mg

Injection, solution, as sulfate: 1 mg/mL (10 mL) [contains benzyl alcohol]

◆ **Vinblastine Sulfate** *see* VinBLAStine *on page 1672*

◆ **Vincaleukoblastine** *see* VinBLAStine *on page 1672*

◆ **Vincasar PFS®** *see* VinCRIStine *on page 1673*

VinCRIStine (vin KRIS teen)

Medication Safety Issues

Sound-alike/look-alike issues:

VinCRIStine may be confused with vinBLAStine

Oncovin® may be confused with Ancobon®

High alert medication: The Institute for Safe Medication Practices (ISMP) includes this medication among its list of drugs which have a heightened risk of causing significant patient harm when used in error.

To prevent fatal inadvertent intrathecal injection, it is recommended that all doses be dispensed in a small minibag. If dispensing vincristine in a syringe, vincristine must be packaged in the manufacturer-provided overwrap which bears the statement **"Do not remove covering until the moment of injection. For intravenous use only. Fatal if given intrathecally."**

U.S. Brand Names Vincasar PFS®

Canadian Brand Names Vincasar® PFS®

Mexican Brand Names Citomid RU; Oncovin; Vintec

Index Terms Leurocristine Sulfate; NSC-67574; Oncovin; Vincristine Sulfate

Pharmacologic Category Antineoplastic Agent, Natural Source (Plant) Derivative; Antineoplastic Agent, Vinca Alkaloid

Use Treatment of leukemias, Hodgkin's disease, non-Hodgkin's lymphomas, Wilms' tumor, neuroblastoma, rhabdomyosarcoma

Effect on Mental Status May cause sedation, confusion, depression, or insomnia

Effect on Psychiatric Treatment May cause myelosuppression; use caution with clozapine and carbamazepine

Dosage Summary Note: Doses are often capped at 2 mg; however, this may reduce the efficacy of the therapy and may not be advisable. Refer to individual protocols; orders for single doses >2.5 mg or >5 mg/treatment cycle should be verified with the specific treatment regimen and/or an experienced oncologist prior to dispensing. I.V.:

I.V.:

Children ≤10 kg or BSA <1 m^2: Initial therapy 0.05 mg/kg once weekly then titrate dose

Children >10 kg or BSA ≥1 m^2: 1-2 mg/m^2, may repeat once weekly for 3-6 weeks (maximum: 2 mg/dose)

Adults: 0.4-1.4 mg/m^2, may repeat every week **or** 0.4-0.5 mg/day continuous infusion for 4 days every 4 weeks **or** 0.25-0.5 mg/m^2/day continuous infusion for 5 days every 4 weeks

Dosage Forms Excipient information presented when available (limited, particularly for generics); consult specific product labeling.

Injection, solution, as sulfate [preservative free]:

Vincasar PFS®: 1 mg/mL (1 mL, 2 mL)

◆ **Vincristine Sulfate** *see* VinCRIStine *on page 1673*

Vinorelbine (vi NOR el been)

Medication Safety Issues

Sound-alike/look-alike issues:

Vinorelbine may be confused with vinBLAStine

High alert medication: The Institute for Safe Medication Practices (ISMP) includes this medication among its list of drug classes which have a heightened risk of causing significant patient harm when used in error.

Vinorelbine is intended **for I. V. use only**: Inadvertent intrathecal administration of other vinca alkaloids has resulted in death. Syringes containing vinorelbine should be labeled **"For I.V. use only. Fatal if given intrathecally."**

U.S. Brand Names Navelbine®

Canadian Brand Names Navelbine®; Vinorelbine Injection, USP; Vinorelbine Tartrate for Injection

Mexican Brand Names Navelbine

Index Terms Dihydroxydeoxynorvinkaleukoblastine; Vinorelbine Tartrate

Pharmacologic Category Antineoplastic Agent, Natural Source (Plant) Derivative; Antineoplastic Agent, Vinca Alkaloid

Use Treatment of nonsmall cell lung cancer (NSCLC)

Unlabeled/Investigational Use Treatment of breast cancer, cervical cancer, and ovarian cancer

Effect on Mental Status May cause drowsiness

Effect on Psychiatric Treatment Bone marrow suppression is common; avoid clozapine and carbamazepine

Dosage Summary Note: Details concerning dosing in combination regimens should also be consulted.

I.V.:

Children: Dosage not established

Adults: 30 mg/m^2/dose every 7 days **or** 25-30 mg/m^2/dose every 7 days (in combination with cisplatin)

Dosage Forms Excipient information presented when available (limited, particularly for generics); consult specific product labeling.

Injection, solution [preservative free]: 10 mg/mL (1 mL, 5 mL)

Navelbine®: 10 mg/mL (1 mL, 5 mL)

- **Vinorelbine Tartrate** *see* Vinorelbine *on page 1674*
- **Viosterol** *see* Ergocalciferol *on page 550*
- **Viracept®** *see* Nelfinavir *on page 1120*
- **Viramune®** *see* Nevirapine *on page 1124*
- **Viravan® [DSC]** *see* Phenylephrine and Pyrilamine *on page 1275*
- **Viravan®-DM** *see* Phenylephrine, Pyrilamine, and Dextromethorphan *on page 1278*
- **Virazole®** *see* Ribavirin *on page 1417*
- **Viread®** *see* Tenofovir *on page 1549*
- **Virilon®** *see* MethylTESTOSTERone *on page 1030*
- **Visine-A® [OTC]** *see* Naphazoline and Pheniramine *on page 1102*
- **Visine® Advanced Relief [OTC]** *see* Tetrahydrozoline *on page 1560*
- **Visine® L.R. [OTC]** *see* Oxymetazoline *on page 1208*
- **Visine® Original [OTC]** *see* Tetrahydrozoline *on page 1560*
- **Visipaque™** *see* Iodixanol *on page 850*
- **Vistaril®** *see* HydrOXYzine *on page 797*
- **Vistide®** *see* Cidofovir *on page 344*
- **Vistra 650** *see* Acetaminophen and Phenyltoloxamine *on page 36*
- **Vita-C® [OTC]** *see* Ascorbic Acid *on page 141*
- **Vitamin C** *see* Ascorbic Acid *on page 141*
- **Vitamin D_2** *see* Ergocalciferol *on page 550*
- **Vitamin D_3 and Alendronate** *see* Alendronate and Cholecalciferol *on page 62*
- **Vitamin B_1** *see* Thiamine *on page 1568*
- **Vitamin B_3** *see* Niacin *on page 1124*
- **Vitamin B_6** *see* Pyridoxine *on page 1376*
- **Vitamin B_{12}** *see* Cyanocobalamin *on page 404*
- **Vitamin D3 [OTC]** *see* Cholecalciferol *on page 341*

Vitamin E (VYE ta min ee)

Medication Safety Issues

Sound-alike/look-alike issues:

Aquasol E® may be confused with Anusol®

U.S. Brand Names Alph-E [OTC]; Alph-E-Mixed [OTC]; Aquasol E® [OTC]; Aquavit-E [OTC]; d-Alpha-Gems™ [OTC]; E-Gems Elite® [OTC]; E-Gems Plus® [OTC]; E-Gems® [OTC]; Ester-E™ [OTC]; Gamma E-Gems® [OTC]; Gamma-E Plus [OTC]; High Gamma Vitamin E Complete™ [OTC]; Key-E® Kaps [OTC]; Key-E® [OTC]

Mexican Brand Names Eternal; Ixopolet

Index Terms *d*-Alpha Tocopherol; *dl*-Alpha Tocopherol

Pharmacologic Category Vitamin, Fat Soluble

Generic Available Yes

Use Dietary supplement

Unlabeled/Investigational Use To reduce the risk of bronchopulmonary dysplasia or retrolental fibroplasia in infants exposed to high concentrations of oxygen; prevention and treatment of tardive dyskinesia; prevention and treatment of hemolytic anemia secondary to vitamin E deficiency

Effect on Mental Status May rarely cause drowsiness

Effect on Psychiatric Treatment Used to prevent or treat tardive dyskinesia and Alzheimer's disease

Pregnancy Risk Factor A/C (dose exceeding RDA recommendation)

Lactation Enters breast milk/compatible

Contraindications Hypersensitivity to vitamin E or any component of the formulation

Warnings/Precautions May induce vitamin K deficiency. Necrotizing enterocolitis has been associated with oral administration of large dosages (eg, >200 units/day) of a hyperosmolar vitamin E preparation in low birth weight infants.

Adverse Reactions Frequency not defined.

Central nervous system: Fatigue, headache

Dermatologic: Contact dermatitis with topical preparation

Endocrine & metabolic: Gonadal dysfunction

Gastrointestinal: Diarrhea, intestinal cramps, nausea

Neuromuscular & skeletal: Weakness

Ocular: Blurred vision

Drug Interactions

Vitamin K Antagonists (eg, warfarin): Vitamin E may enhance the anticoagulant effect of Vitamin K Antagonists. *Risk C: Monitor therapy*

Stability Protect from light.

Mechanism of Action Prevents oxidation of vitamin A and C; protects polyunsaturated fatty acids in membranes from attack by free radicals and protects red blood cells against hemolysis

Pharmacodynamics/Kinetics

Absorption: Oral: Depends on presence of bile; reduced in conditions of malabsorption, in low birth weight premature infants, and as dosage increases; water miscible preparations are better absorbed than oil preparations

Distribution: To all body tissues, especially adipose tissue, where it is stored

Metabolism: Hepatic to glucuronides

Excretion: Feces

Dosage Vitamin E may be expressed as alpha-tocopherol equivalents (ATE), which refer to the biologically-active (R) stereoisomer content. Oral:

Recommended daily allowance (RDA):

- Infants (adequate intake; RDA not established):
  - ≤6 months: 4 mg
  - 7-12 months: 6 mg
- Children:
  - 1-3 years: 6 mg; upper limit of intake should not exceed 200 mg/day
  - 4-8 years: 7 mg; upper limit of intake should not exceed 300 mg/day
  - 9-13 years: 11 mg; upper limit of intake should not exceed 600 mg/day
  - 14-18 years: 15 mg; upper limit of intake should not exceed 800 mg/day
- Adults: 15 mg; upper limit of intake should not exceed 1000 mg/day
- Pregnant female:
  - ≤18 years: 15 mg; upper level of intake should not exceed 800 mg/day
  - 19-50 years: 15 mg; upper level of intake should not exceed 1000 mg/day
- Lactating female:
  - ≤18 years: 19 mg; upper level of intake should not exceed 800 mg/day
  - 19-50 years: 19 mg; upper level of intake should not exceed 1000 mg/day

Vitamin E deficiency:
  Children (with malabsorption syndrome): 1 unit/kg/day of water miscible vitamin E (to raise plasma tocopherol concentrations to the normal range within 2 months and to maintain normal plasma concentrations)
  Adults: 60-75 units/day
Prevention of vitamin E deficiency: Adults: 30 units/day
Cystic fibrosis, beta-thalassemia, sickle cell anemia may require higher daily maintenance doses:
  Children:
    Cystic fibrosis: 100-400 units/day
    Beta-thalassemia: 750 units/day
  Adults:
    Sickle cell: 450 units/day
    Tardive dyskinesia (unlabeled use): 1600 units/day

Administration Swallow capsules whole; do not crush or chew.

Monitoring Parameters Plasma tocopherol concentrations (normal range: 6-14 mcg/mL)

Reference Range Therapeutic: 0.8-1.5 mg/dL (SI: 19-35 µmol/L), some method variation

Additional Information The 2R-stereoisomeric forms of α-tocopherol are used to define vitamin E intake and RDA. While international units are no longer recognized, many fortified foods and supplements continue to use this term although USP units are now used by the pharmaceutical industry when labeling vitamin E supplements. Both IUs and USP units are based on the same equivalency. The following can be used to convert international units (IU) of vitamin E (and esters) to milligrams α-tocopherol in order to meet recommended daily intake:

Synthetic (eg, all-racemic α-tocopherol):
dl-α-tocopherol:
  USP: 1.10 IU / mg; 0.91 mg / IU
  Molar: 2.12 µmol / IU
  α-tocopherol: 0.45 mg / IU
dl-α-tocopherol acetate:
  USP: 1 IU / mg; 1 mg / IU
  Molar: 2.12 µmol / IU
  α-tocopherol: 0.45 mg / IU
dl-α-tocopherol succinate:
  USP: 0.89 IU / mg; 1.12 mg / IU
  Molar: 2.12 µmol / IU
  α-tocopherol: 0.45 mg / IU

Natural (eg, RRR-α-tocopherol):
d-α-tocopherol:
  USP: 1.49 IU / mg; 0.67 mg / IU
  Molar: 1.56 µmol / IU
  α-tocopherol: 0.67 mg / IU
d-α-tocopherol acetate:
  USP: 1.36 IU / mg; 0.74mg / IU
  Molar: 1.56 µmol / IU
  α-tocopherol: 0.67 mg / IU
d-α-tocopherol succinate:
  USP: 1.21 IU / mg; 0.83 mg / IU
  Molar: 1.56 µmol / IU
  α-tocopherol: 0.67 mg / IU

Historically, vitamin E supplements have been labeled (incorrectly) as *d*- or *dl*-α-tocopherol. Synthetic vitamin E compounds are racemic mixtures, and may be designated as all-racemic (all rac-α-tocopherol). The natural form contains the only RRR-α-tocopherol. All of these compounds may be present in fortified foods and multivitamins. Not all stereoisomers are capable of performing physiological functions in humans; therefore, cannot be considered to meet vitamin E requirements.

Dosage Forms Excipient information presented when available (limited, particularly for generics); consult specific product labeling.
Capsule: 400 int. units, 1000 int. units
  Key-E® Kaps: 200 int. units, 400 int. units
Capsule, softgel: 200 int. units, 400 int. units, 600 int. units, 1000 int. units
  Alph-E: 200 int. units, 400 int. units
  Alph-E-Mixed: 200 int. units [contains mixed tocopherols]; 400 int. units [contains mixed tocopherols], 1000 int. units [sugar free; contains mixed tocopherols]
  Aqua Gem E®: 200 units, 400 units

d-Alpha-Gems™: 400 int. units [derived from soybean oil]
E-Gems®: 30 int. units, 100 int. units, 200 int. units, 400 int. units, 600 int. units, 800 int. units, 1000 int. units, 1200 int. units [derived from soybean oil]
E-Gems Plus®: 200 int. units, 400 int. units, 800 int. units [contains mixed tocopherols]
E-Gems Elite®: 400 int. units [contains mixed tocopherols]
Ester-E™: 400 int. units
Gamma E-Gems®: 90 int. units [also contains mixed tocopherols]
Gamma-E Plus: 200 int. units [contains soybean oil]
High Gamma Vitamin E Complete™: 200 int. units [contains soybean oil, mixed tocopherols]
Cream: 50 int. units/g (60 g), 100 int. units/g (60 g), 1000 int. units/120 g (120 g), 30,000 int. units/57 g (57 g)
Key-E®: 30 int. units/g (60 g, 120 g, 600 g)
Lip balm (E-Gem® Lip Care): 1000 int. units/tube [contains vitamin A and aloe]
Oil, oral/topical: 100 int. units/0.25 mL (60 mL, 75 mL); 1150 units/0.25 mL (30 mL, 60 mL, 120 mL); 28,000 int. units/30 mL (30 mL)
Alph-E: 28,000 int. units/30 mL (30 mL) [topical]
E-Gems®: 100 units/10 drops (15 mL, 60 mL)
Ointment, topical (Key-E®): 30 units/g (60 g, 120 g, 480 g)
Powder (Key-E®): 700 int. units per 1/4 teaspoon (15 g, 75 g, 1000 g) [derived from soybean oil]
Solution, oral drops: 15 int. units/0.3 mL (30 mL)
Aquasol E®: 15 int. units/0.3 mL (12 mL, 30 mL) [latex free]
Aquavit-E: 15 int. units/0.3 mL (30 mL) [butterscotch flavor]
Suppository, rectal/vaginal (Key-E®): 30 int. units (12s, 24s) [contains coconut oil]
Tablet: 100 int. units, 200 int. units, 400 int. units, 500 int. units
Key-E®: 200 int. units, 400 int. units

◆ **Vitamin K_1** *see* Phytonadione *on page 1289*

Vitamins (Multiple/Injectable) (VYE ta mins, MUL ti pul/in JEK ti bal)

U.S. Brand Names Infuvite® Adult; Infuvite® Pediatric; M.V.I. Adult™; M.V.I. ®-12 ; M.V.I® Pediatric

Pharmacologic Category Vitamin

Use Nutritional supplement in patients receiving parenteral nutrition or requiring intravenous administration

Effect on Mental Status Injectable forms of multivitamins contain aluminum. Aluminum may reach toxic levels with prolonged administration if kidney function is impaired. Aluminum toxicity may manifest as impaired mental function.

Effect on Psychiatric Treatment None reported

Dosage Summary

I.V.:

Children <3 kg: Dosage not established

Children ≥3 kg to 11 years: 5 mL/day (pediatric formulation) added to TPN or ≥100 mL of appropriate solution

Children >11 years: 10 mL/day (adult formulation) added to TPN or ≥500 mL or appropriate solution

Adults: 10 mL/day (adult formulation) added to TPN or ≥500 mL or appropriate solution

Dosage Forms Excipient information presented when available (limited, particularly for generics); consult specific product labeling.

Content varies depending on product used. For more detailed information on ingredients in these and other multivitamins, please refer to package labeling.

◆ **Vitelle™ Irospan® [OTC] [DSC]** *see* Ferrous Sulfate and Ascorbic Acid *on page 628*

◆ **Vitrasert®** *see* Ganciclovir *on page 708*

◆ **Vitussin [DSC]** *see* Hydrocodone and Guaifenesin *on page 779*

◆ **Vivactil®** *see* Protriptyline *on page 1363*

◆ **Vivarin® [OTC]** *see* Caffeine *on page 250*

◆ **Vivelle® [DSC]** *see* Estradiol *on page 576*

◆ **Vivelle-Dot®** *see* Estradiol *on page 576*

◆ **Vivitrol™** *see* Naltrexone *on page 1099*

◆ **VLB** *see* VinBLAStine *on page 1672*

◆ **VM-26** *see* Teniposide *on page 1549*

◆ **Voltaren®** *see* Diclofenac *on page 457*
◆ **Voltaren® Gel** *see* Diclofenac *on page 457*
◆ **Voltaren Ophthalmic®** *see* Diclofenac *on page 457*
◆ **Voltaren®-XR** *see* Diclofenac *on page 457*

Voriconazole (vor i KOE na zole)

U.S. Brand Names VFEND®
Canadian Brand Names VFEND®
Mexican Brand Names VFEND
Index Terms UK109496
Pharmacologic Category Antifungal Agent, Oral; Antifungal Agent, Parenteral
Use Treatment of invasive aspergillosis; treatment of esophageal candidiasis; treatment of candidemia (in non-neutropenic patients); treatment of disseminated *Candida* infections of the skin and viscera; treatment of serious fungal infections caused by *Scedosporium apiospermum* and *Fusarium* spp (including *Fusarium solani*) in patients intolerant of, or refractory to, other therapy
Unlabeled/Investigational Use
Fungal infection prophylaxis in intermediate or high risk neutropenic cancer patients with myelodysplastic syndrome (MDS) or acute myelogenous leukemia (AML), neutropenic allogeneic hematopoietic stem cell recipients, and patients with significant graft-versus-host disease; empiric antifungal therapy (second-line) for persistent neutropenic fever
Effect on Mental Status May cause abnormal dreams, agitation, amnesia, anxiety, confusion, delirium, dementia, depersonalization, depression, dizziness, encephalopathy, euphoria, insomnia, psychosis, somnolence, suicidal ideation
Effect on Psychiatric Treatment Contraindicated with CYP3A4 substrates which may lead to QT_c prolongation (pimozide); coadministration with barbiturates (long acting), carbamazepine, and ergot alkaloids. Blurred vision is common; use caution with anticholinergic agents. Concurrent use with benzodiazepines that are oxidatively metabolized (alprazolam, diazepam, temazepam, triazolam, and midazolam) may result in elevated benzodiazepine serum concentrations and potential risk for toxicity. Buspirone and zolpidem serum concentrations may be increased with concurrent use. St John's wort may decrease voriconazole levels; monitor.
Dosage Summary
I.V.:
Children <12 years: Dosage not established
Children ≥12 years: Initial: 6 mg/kg every 12 hours for 2 doses; Maintenance: 3-4 mg/kg every 12 hours
Adults: Initial: 6 mg/kg every 12 hours for 2 doses; Maintenance: 3-4 mg/kg every 12 hours
Oral:
Children <12 years: Dosage not established
Children ≥12 years: 100-300 mg every 12 hours
Adults: 100-300 mg every 12 hours
Dosage Forms Excipient information presented when available (limited, particularly for generics); consult specific product labeling.
Injection, powder for reconstitution: 200 mg [contains SBECD 3200 mg]
Powder for oral suspension: 200 mg/5 mL (70 mL) [contains sodium benzoate and sucrose; orange flavor]
Tablet: 50 mg, 200 mg [contains lactose]

Vorinostat (vor IN oh stat)

Medication Safety Issues
High alert medication: The Institute for Safe Medication Practices (ISMP) includes this medication among its list of drug classes which have a heightened risk of causing significant patient harm when used in error.
U.S. Brand Names Zolinza™
Index Terms NSC-701852; SAHA; Suberoylanilide Hydroxamic Acid
Pharmacologic Category Antineoplastic Agent, Histone Deacetylase Inhibitor
Use Treatment of progressive, persistent, or recurrent cutaneous T-cell lymphoma (CTCL)
Effect on Mental Status Fatigue is common; may cause dizziness
Effect on Psychiatric Treatment Vorinostat causes dose-related thrombocytopenia; use caution with valproic acid. GI side effects are common; concomitant use with lithium, valproic acid, carbamazepine, and SSRIs may produce additive effects. Hyperglycemia is common; psychotropics may further

alter glucose regulation. Xerostomia is common; concomitant use with psychotropics may produce additive effects.

Dosage Summary

Oral:

Children: Dosage not established

Adults: 400 mg once daily

Dosage Forms Excipient information presented when available (limited, particularly for generics); consult specific product labeling.

Capsule:

Zolinza™: 100 mg

- **VoSpire ER®** *see* Albuterol *on page 54*
- **VP-16** *see* Etoposide *on page 607*
- **VP-16-213** *see* Etoposide *on page 607*
- **V-Tann™ [DSC]** *see* Phenylephrine and Pyrilamine *on page 1275*
- **Vumon®** *see* Teniposide *on page 1549*
- **Vytorin®** *see* Ezetimibe and Simvastatin *on page 611*
- **Vyvanse™** *see* Lisdexamfetamine *on page 931*

Warfarin (WAR far in)

Medication Safety Issues

Sound-alike/look-alike issues:

Coumadin® may be confused with Avandia®, Cardura®, Compazine®, Kemadrin®

Jantoven™ may be confused with Janumet™, Januvia™

High alert medication: The Institute for Safe Medication Practices (ISMP) includes this medication among its list of drugs which have a heightened risk of causing significant patient harm when used in error.

2009 National Patient Safety Goals: The Joint Commission on Accreditation of Healthcare Organizations requires healthcare organizations that provide anticoagulant therapy to have a process in place to reduce the risk of anticoagulant-associated patient harm. Patients receiving anticoagulants should receive individualized care through a defined process that includes standardized ordering, dispensing, administration, monitoring and education. This does not apply to routine short-term use of anticoagulants for prevention of venous thromboembolism when the expectation is that the patient's laboratory values will remain within or close to normal values (NPSG.03.05.01).

Related Information

Anticholinergic Effects of Common Psychotropics *on page 1758*

U.S. Brand Names Coumadin®; Jantoven®

Canadian Brand Names Apo-Warfarin®; Coumadin®; Gen-Warfarin; Novo-Warfarin; Taro-Warfarin

Mexican Brand Names Coumadin

Index Terms Warfarin Sodium

Pharmacologic Category Anticoagulant, Coumarin Derivative; Vitamin K Antagonist

Generic Available Yes: Tablet

Use Prophylaxis and treatment of thromboembolic disorders (eg, venous, pulmonary) and embolic complications arising from atrial fibrillation or cardiac valve replacement; adjunct to reduce risk of systemic embolism (eg, recurrent MI, stroke) after myocardial infarction

Unlabeled/Investigational Use Prevention of recurrent transient ischemic attacks

Effect on Mental Status None reported

Effect on Psychiatric Treatment May cause leukopenia; use caution with clozapine and carbamazepine; barbiturates and carbamazepine may decrease the anticoagulant effect of warfarin; chloral hydrate, alcohol, disulfiram, and SSRIs may enhance the anticoagulant effect

Restrictions An FDA-approved medication guide must be distributed when dispensing an outpatient prescription (new or refill) where this medication is to be used without direct supervision of a healthcare provider. Medication guides are available at http://www.fda.gov/cder/Offices/ODS/medication_guides.htm.

Pregnancy Risk Factor X

Pregnancy Considerations Oral anticoagulants cross the placenta and produce fetal abnormalities. May also cause fatal fetal hemorrhage. Warfarin should not be used during pregnancy because of significant risks. Adjusted-dose heparin can be given safely throughout pregnancy in patients with venous thromboembolism.

Lactation Does not enter breast milk, only metabolites are excreted (AAP rates "compatible")

Contraindications Hypersensitivity to warfarin or any component of the formulation; hemorrhagic tendencies (eg, patients bleeding from the GI, respiratory, or GU tract; aneurysm; cerebrovascular hemorrhage; following spinal puncture and other diagnostic or therapeutic procedures with potential for significant bleeding; history of bleeding diathesis); recent or potential surgery of the eye or CNS; major regional lumbar block anesthesia or surgery resulting in large, open surfaces; blood dyscrasias; severe uncontrolled or malignant hypertension; pericarditis or pericardial effusion; subacute bacterial endocarditis; history of warfarin-induced necrosis; an unreliable, noncompliant patient; alcoholism; patient who has a history of falls or is a significant fall risk; unsupervised senile or psychotic patient; eclampsia/pre-eclampsia, threatened abortion, pregnancy

Warnings/Precautions Use care in the selection of patients appropriate for this treatment. Ensure patient cooperation especially from the alcoholic, illicit drug user, demented, or psychotic patient; ability to comply with routine laboratory monitoring is essential. Use with caution in trauma, acute infection, moderate-severe renal insufficiency, prolonged dietary insufficiencies, moderate-severe hypertension, polycythemia vera, vasculitis, open wound, active TB, any disruption in normal GI flora, history of PUD, anaphylactic disorders, indwelling catheters, severe diabetes, thyroid disease, and menstruating and postpartum women. Use with caution in protein C deficiency. Use with caution in patients with heparin-induced thrombocytopenia and DVT. Warfarin monotherapy is contraindicated in the initial treatment of active HIT. Reduced liver function, regardless of etiology, may impair synthesis of coagulation factors leading to increased warfarin sensitivity.

[U.S. Boxed Warning]: May cause major or fatal bleeding. Risk factors for bleeding include high intensity anticoagulation (INR >4), age (>65 years), variable INRs, history of GI bleeding, hypertension, cerebrovascular disease, serious heart disease, anemia, malignancy, trauma, renal insufficiency, drug-drug interactions, long duration of therapy, or known genetic deficiency in CYP2C9 activity. Patient must be instructed to report bleeding, accidents, or falls. Unrecognized bleeding sites (eg, colon cancer) may be uncovered by anticoagulation. Patient must also report any new or discontinued medications, herbal or alternative products used, or significant changes in smoking or dietary habits. Necrosis or gangrene of the skin and other tissue can occur, usually in conjunction with protein C or S deficiency. "Purple toes syndrome," due to cholesterol microembolization, may rarely occur. Women may be at risk of developing ovarian hemorrhage at the time of ovulation. The elderly may be more sensitive to anticoagulant therapy. Safety and efficacy have not been established in children; monitor closely.

Presence of the CYP2C9*2 or *3 allele and/or polymorphism of the vitamin K oxidoreductase (VKORC1) gene may increase the risk of bleeding. Lower doses may be required in these patients; genetic testing may help determine appropriate dosing.

Adverse Reactions Bleeding is the major adverse effect of warfarin. Hemorrhage may occur at virtually any site. Risk is dependent on multiple variables, including the intensity of anticoagulation and patient susceptibility.

Cardiovascular: Angina, chest pain, edema, hemorrhagic shock, hypotension, pallor, syncope, vasculitis

Central nervous system: Coma, dizziness, fatigue, fever, headache, lethargy, malaise, pain, stroke

Dermatologic: Alopecia, bullous eruptions, dermatitis, rash, pruritus, urticaria

Gastrointestinal: Abdominal cramps, abdominal pain, anorexia, diarrhea, flatulence, gastrointestinal bleeding, mouth ulcers, nausea, taste disturbance, vomiting

Genitourinary: Hematuria, priapism

Hematologic: Agranulocytosis, anemia, leukopenia, retroperitoneal hematoma, unrecognized bleeding sites (eg, colon cancer) may be uncovered by anticoagulation

Hepatic: Cholestatic jaundice, hepatic injury, hepatitis, transaminases increased

Neuromuscular & skeletal: Joint pain, muscle pain, osteoporosis (potential association with long-term use), paralysis, paresthesia, weakness

Respiratory: Dyspnea, tracheobronchial calcification

Miscellaneous: Anaphylactic reaction, cold intolerance, hypersensitivity/allergic reactions, skin necrosis, gangrene, "purple toes" syndrome

Metabolism/Transport Effects Substrate of CYP1A2 (minor), 2C9 (major), 2C19 (minor), 3A4 (minor); **Inhibits** CYP2C9 (moderate), 2C19 (weak)

Drug Interactions

Acetaminophen: May enhance the anticoagulant effect of Vitamin K Antagonists. Most likely with daily acetaminophen doses >1.3 g for >1 week. *Risk C: Monitor therapy*

Allopurinol: May enhance the anticoagulant effect of Vitamin K Antagonists. *Risk D: Consider therapy modification*

Aminoglutethimide: May increase the metabolism of Vitamin K Antagonists. *Risk D: Consider therapy modification*

Amiodarone: May enhance the anticoagulant effect of Vitamin K Antagonists. *Risk D: Consider therapy modification*

Androgens: May enhance the anticoagulant effect of Vitamin K Antagonists. *Risk D: Consider therapy modification*

Anticoagulants: May enhance the anticoagulant effect of other Anticoagulants. *Risk C: Monitor therapy*

Antifungal Agents (Azole Derivatives, Systemic): May decrease the metabolism of Vitamin K Antagonists. *Risk D: Consider therapy modification*

Antineoplastic Agents: May enhance the anticoagulant effect of Vitamin K Antagonists. Antineoplastic Agents may diminish the anticoagulant effect of Vitamin K Antagonists. **Exceptions:** Alitretinoin; Altretamine; Aminoglutethimide; Anastrozole; Asparaginase; AzaCITIDine; Bleomycin; Capecitabine; CARBOplatin; Carmustine; Chlorambucil; CISplatin; Cladribine; Cytarabine; Cytarabine (Liposomal); Dacarbazine; DACTINomycin; DAUNOrubicin Citrate (Liposomal); DAUNOrubicin Hydrochloride; Denileukin Diftitox; Docetaxel; DOXOrubicin (Liposomal); Epirubicin; Estramustine; Etoposide Phosphate; Exemestane; Fludarabine; Goserelin; Hydroxyurea; IDArubicin; Irinotecan; Letrozole; Leuprolide; Lomustine; Mechlorethamine; Megestrol; Mitomycin; Mitoxantrone; Nilutamide; Paclitaxel; Pegaspargase; Pentostatin; Polyestradiol; Porfimer; RiTUXimab; Streptozocin; Tamoxifen; Temozolomide; Teniposide; Thioguanine; Thiotepa; Topotecan; Toremifene; Tretinoin (Oral); Valrubicin; VinBLAStine; Vinorelbine. *Risk C: Monitor therapy*

Antiplatelet Agents: May enhance the anticoagulant effect of Anticoagulants. *Risk C: Monitor therapy*

Antithyroid Agents: May diminish the anticoagulant effect of Vitamin K Antagonists. *Risk D: Consider therapy modification*

Aprepitant: May decrease the serum concentration of Warfarin. *Risk C: Monitor therapy*

Atazanavir: May increase the serum concentration of Warfarin. *Risk C: Monitor therapy*

AzaTHIOprine: May diminish the anticoagulant effect of Vitamin K Antagonists. *Risk C: Monitor therapy*

Barbiturates: May increase the metabolism of Vitamin K Antagonists. *Risk D: Consider therapy modification*

Bile Acid Sequestrants: May decrease the absorption of Vitamin K Antagonists. *Risk C: Monitor therapy*

Bosentan: May increase the metabolism of Vitamin K Antagonists. *Risk C: Monitor therapy*

Capecitabine: May increase the serum concentration of Vitamin K Antagonists. *Risk D: Consider therapy modification*

CarBAMazepine: May decrease the serum concentration of Vitamin K Antagonists. *Risk D: Consider therapy modification*

Cephalosporins: May enhance the anticoagulant effect of Vitamin K Antagonists. **Exceptions:** Cefaclor; Cefadroxil; Cefdinir; Cefepime; Cefixime; Cefonicid; Cefotaxime; Cefpodoxime; Cefprozil; Ceftazidime; Ceftibuten; Ceftizoxime; Ceftobiprole; Cefuroxime; Cephalexin; Cephradine [Off Market]. *Risk C: Monitor therapy*

Cimetidine: May enhance the anticoagulant effect of Vitamin K Antagonists. *Risk D: Consider therapy modification*

Clopidogrel: May enhance the anticoagulant effect of Warfarin. *Risk D: Consider therapy modification*

Coenzyme Q-10: May diminish the anticoagulant effect of Vitamin K Antagonists. *Risk C: Monitor therapy*

Contraceptive (Progestins): May diminish the anticoagulant effect of Vitamin K Antagonists. In contrast, enhanced anticoagulant effects have also been noted with some products. *Risk D: Consider therapy modification*

Corticosteroids (Systemic): May enhance the anticoagulant effect of Warfarin. *Risk C: Monitor therapy*

Cranberry: May enhance the anticoagulant effect of Warfarin. *Risk C: Monitor therapy*

CYP2C9 Inducers (Highly Effective): May increase the metabolism of CYP2C9 Substrates (High risk). *Risk C: Monitor therapy*

CYP2C9 Inhibitors (Moderate): May decrease the metabolism of CYP2C9 Substrates (High risk). *Risk C: Monitor therapy*

CYP2C9 Inhibitors (Strong): May decrease the metabolism of CYP2C9 Substrates (High risk). *Risk D: Consider therapy modification*

CYP2C9 Substrates (High risk): CYP2C9 Inhibitors (Moderate) may decrease the metabolism of CYP2C9 Substrates (High risk). *Risk C: Monitor therapy*

Darunavir: May decrease the serum concentration of Warfarin. *Risk C: Monitor therapy*

Dasatinib: May enhance the anticoagulant effect of Anticoagulants. *Risk C: Monitor therapy*

Dicloxacillin: May diminish the anticoagulant effect of Vitamin K Antagonists. *Risk C: Monitor therapy*

Disulfiram: May increase the serum concentration of Vitamin K Antagonists. *Risk C: Monitor therapy*

Drotrecogin Alfa: Vitamin K Antagonists may enhance the adverse/toxic effect of Drotrecogin Alfa. Bleeding may occur. *Risk D: Consider therapy modification*

Efavirenz: May increase the serum concentration of Vitamin K Antagonists. *Risk C: Monitor therapy*

Etoposide: May enhance the anticoagulant effect of Vitamin K Antagonists. *Risk C: Monitor therapy*

Fenofibrate: May enhance the anticoagulant effect of Warfarin. Fenofibrate may increase the serum concentration of Warfarin. *Risk D: Consider therapy modification*

Fenugreek: May enhance the anticoagulant effect of Vitamin K Antagonists. *Risk D: Consider therapy modification*

Fibric Acid Derivatives: May enhance the anticoagulant effect of Vitamin K Antagonists. *Risk D: Consider therapy modification*

Fluconazole: May decrease the metabolism of Vitamin K Antagonists. *Risk D: Consider therapy modification*

Fluorouracil: May increase the serum concentration of Vitamin K Antagonists. *Risk D: Consider therapy modification*

Fosaprepitant: May decrease the serum concentration of Warfarin. The active metabolite aprepitant is likely responsible for this effect. *Risk C: Monitor therapy*

Gefitinib: May enhance the anticoagulant effect of Vitamin K Antagonists. *Risk C: Monitor therapy*

Ginkgo Biloba: May enhance the anticoagulant effect of Vitamin K Antagonists. *Risk D: Consider therapy modification*

Ginseng (American): May decrease the serum concentration of Warfarin. *Risk C: Monitor therapy*

Glucagon: May enhance the anticoagulant effect of Vitamin K Antagonists. *Risk C: Monitor therapy*

Glutethimide: May increase the metabolism of Vitamin K Antagonists. *Risk D: Consider therapy modification*

Griseofulvin: May increase the metabolism of Vitamin K Antagonists. *Risk C: Monitor therapy*

Herbs (Anticoagulant/Antiplatelet Properties) (eg, Alfalfa, Anise, Bilberry): May enhance the adverse/toxic effect of Anticoagulants. Bleeding may occur. *Risk D: Consider therapy modification*

HMG-CoA Reductase Inhibitors: May enhance the anticoagulant effect of Vitamin K Antagonists. **Exceptions:** Atorvastatin. *Risk C: Monitor therapy*

Ifosfamide: May enhance the anticoagulant effect of Vitamin K Antagonists. *Risk C: Monitor therapy*

Imatinib: May enhance the anticoagulant effect of Warfarin. Imatinib may decrease the metabolism of Warfarin. *Risk D: Consider therapy modification*

Ivermectin: May enhance the anticoagulant effect of Vitamin K Antagonists. *Risk C: Monitor therapy*

Leflunomide: May enhance the anticoagulant effect of Vitamin K Antagonists. *Risk C: Monitor therapy*

Lopinavir: May decrease the serum concentration of Warfarin. *Risk C: Monitor therapy*

Macrolide Antibiotics: May decrease the metabolism of Vitamin K Antagonists. **Exceptions:** Dirithromycin [Off Market]; Spiramycin. *Risk C: Monitor therapy*

Mercaptopurine: May diminish the anticoagulant effect of Vitamin K Antagonists. *Risk C: Monitor therapy*

MetroNIDAZOLE: May decrease the metabolism of Vitamin K Antagonists. *Risk D: Consider therapy modification*

Nafcillin: May diminish the anticoagulant effect of Vitamin K Antagonists. *Risk D: Consider therapy modification*

NSAID (COX-2 Inhibitor): May enhance the anticoagulant effect of Vitamin K Antagonists. *Risk C: Monitor therapy*

NSAID (Nonselective): May enhance the anticoagulant effect of Vitamin K Antagonists. *Risk D: Consider therapy modification*

Omega-3-Acid Ethyl Esters: May enhance the anticoagulant effect of Warfarin. *Risk C: Monitor therapy*

Oral Contraceptive (Estrogens): May diminish the anticoagulant effect of Vitamin K Antagonists. In contrast, enhanced anticoagulant effects have also been noted with some products. *Risk D: Consider therapy modification*

Orlistat: May enhance the anticoagulant effect of Warfarin. *Risk C: Monitor therapy*

Pentosan Polysulfate Sodium: May enhance the anticoagulant effect of Anticoagulants. *Risk C: Monitor therapy*

Phenytoin: May enhance the anticoagulant effect of Vitamin K Antagonists. Vitamin K Antagonists may increase the serum concentration of Phenytoin. *Risk D: Consider therapy modification*

Phytonadione: May diminish the anticoagulant effect of Vitamin K Antagonists. *Risk D: Consider therapy modification*

Propafenone: May increase the serum concentration of Vitamin K Antagonists. *Risk C: Monitor therapy*

Propoxyphene: May decrease the metabolism of Vitamin K Antagonists. *Risk C: Monitor therapy*

Prostacyclin Analogues: May enhance the adverse/toxic effect of Anticoagulants. Specifically, the antiplatelet effects of these agents may lead to an increased risk of bleeding with the combination. *Risk C: Monitor therapy*

Proton Pump Inhibitors: May increase the serum concentration of Warfarin. **Exceptions:** Esomeprazole; Lansoprazole; Pantoprazole; Rabeprazole. *Risk C: Monitor therapy*

QuiNIDine: May enhance the anticoagulant effect of Vitamin K Antagonists. Note that the prothrombin time might be unchanged in the face of increased bleeding. *Risk C: Monitor therapy*

Quinolone Antibiotics: May enhance the anticoagulant effect of Vitamin K Antagonists. *Risk C: Monitor therapy*

Rifamycin Derivatives: May increase the metabolism of Vitamin K Antagonists. *Risk C: Monitor therapy*

Salicylates: May enhance the anticoagulant effect of Vitamin K Antagonists. *Risk D: Consider therapy modification*

Selective Serotonin Reuptake Inhibitors: May enhance the anticoagulant effect of Vitamin K Antagonists. *Risk C: Monitor therapy*

Sitaxsentan: May increase the serum concentration of Warfarin. *Risk D: Consider therapy modification*

Sorafenib: May enhance the anticoagulant effect of Warfarin. Sorafenib may increase the serum concentration of Warfarin. *Risk C: Monitor therapy*

St Johns Wort: May increase the metabolism of Vitamin K Antagonists. *Risk D: Consider therapy modification*

Sulfinpyrazone [Off Market]: May decrease the metabolism of Vitamin K Antagonists. Sulfinpyrazone [Off Market] may decrease the protein binding of Vitamin K Antagonists. *Risk D: Consider therapy modification*

Sulfonamide Derivatives: May enhance the anticoagulant effect of Vitamin K Antagonists. *Risk D: Consider therapy modification*

Tamoxifen: May increase the serum concentration of Vitamin K Antagonists. *Risk X: Avoid combination*

Tetracycline Derivatives: May enhance the anticoagulant effect of Vitamin K Antagonists. *Risk C: Monitor therapy*

Thrombolytic Agents: May enhance the anticoagulant effect of Anticoagulants. *Risk C: Monitor therapy*

Thyroid Products: May enhance the anticoagulant effect of Vitamin K Antagonists. *Risk D: Consider therapy modification*

Tigecycline: May increase the serum concentration of Warfarin. *Risk C: Monitor therapy*

Tolterodine: May enhance the anticoagulant effect of Warfarin. *Risk C: Monitor therapy*

Tricyclic Antidepressants: May enhance the anticoagulant effect of Vitamin K Antagonists. *Risk C: Monitor therapy*

Vitamin A: May enhance the anticoagulant effect of Vitamin K Antagonists. *Risk C: Monitor therapy*

Vitamin E: May enhance the anticoagulant effect of Vitamin K Antagonists. *Risk C: Monitor therapy*

Voriconazole: May increase the serum concentration of Warfarin. *Risk C: Monitor therapy*

Vorinostat: May enhance the anticoagulant effect of Vitamin K Antagonists. *Risk C: Monitor therapy*

Zafirlukast: May decrease the metabolism of Vitamin K Antagonists. *Risk C: Monitor therapy*

Zileuton: May increase the serum concentration of Warfarin. *Risk C: Monitor therapy*

Ethanol/Nutrition/Herb Interactions

Ethanol: Avoid ethanol. Acute ethanol ingestion (binge drinking) decreases the metabolism of warfarin and increases PT/INR. Chronic daily ethanol use increases the metabolism of warfarin and decreases PT/INR.

Food: The anticoagulant effects of warfarin may be decreased if taken with foods rich in vitamin K. Vitamin E may increase warfarin effect. Cranberry juice may increase warfarin effect.

Herb/Nutraceutical: Cranberry, fenugreek, ginkgo biloba, glucosamine, may enhance bleeding or increase warfarin's effect. Ginseng (American), coenzyme Q_{10}, and St John's wort may decrease warfarin levels and effects. Avoid alfalfa, anise, bilberry, bladderwrack, bromelain, cat's claw, celery, chamomile, coleus, cordyceps, dong quai, evening primrose oil, fenugreek, feverfew, garlic, ginger, ginkgo biloba, ginseng (American), ginseng (Panax), ginseng (Siberian), grapeseed, green tea, guggul, horse chestnut seed, horseradish, licorice, omega-3-acids, prickly ash, red clover, reishi, SAMe (s-adenosylmethionine), sweet clover, turmeric, and white willow (all have additional antiplatelet activity).

Stability

Injection: Prior to reconstitution, store at 15°C to 30°C (59°F to 86°F). Following reconstitution with 2.7 mL of sterile water (yields 2 mg/mL solution), stable for 4 hours at 15°C to 30°C (59°F to 86°F). Protect from light.

Tablet: Store at 15°C to 30°C (59°F to 86°F). Protect from light.

Mechanism of Action Hepatic synthesis of coagulation factors II, VII, IX, and X, as well as proteins C and S, requires the presence of vitamin K. These clotting factors are biologically activated by the addition of carboxyl groups to key glutamic acid residues within the proteins' structure. In the process, "active" vitamin K is oxidatively converted to an "inactive" form, which is then subsequently re-activated by vitamin K epoxide reductase complex 1 (VKORC1). Warfarin competitively inhibits the subunit 1 of the multi-unit VKOR complex, thus depleting functional vitamin K reserves and hence reduces synthesis of active clotting factors.

Pharmacodynamics/Kinetics

Onset of action: Anticoagulation: Oral: 24-72 hours

Peak effect: Full therapeutic effect: 5-7 days; INR may increase in 36-72 hours

Duration: 2-5 days

Absorption: Oral: Rapid, complete

Distribution: 0.14 L/kg

Protein binding: 99%

Metabolism: Hepatic, primarily via CYP2C9; minor pathways include CYP2C8, 2C18, 2C19, 1A2, and 3A4

Genomic variants: Approximately 37% reduced clearance of S-warfarin in patients heterozygous for 2C9 (*1/*2 or *1/*3), and ~70% reduced in patients homozygous for reduced function alleles (*2/*2, *2/*3, or *3/*3)

Half-life elimination: 20-60 hours; Mean: 40 hours; highly variable among individuals

Time to peak, plasma: Oral: ~4 hours

Excretion: Urine (92%, primarily as metabolites)

Dosage Note: New labeling identifies genetic factors which may increase patient sensitivity to warfarin. Specifically, genetic variations in the proteins CYP2C9 and VKORC1, responsible for warfarin's primary metabolism and pharmacodynamic activity, respectively, have been identified as predisposing factors associated with decreased dose requirement and increased bleeding risk. A genotyping test is available, and may provide important guidance on initiation of anticoagulant therapy.

Oral:

Infants and Children (unlabeled use): Initial loading dose (if baseline INR is 1-1.3): 0.2 mg/kg (maximum: 10 mg/dose); adjust dose based on INR (reported ranges to maintain INR of 2-3: 0.09-0.33 mg/kg/day). Infants <12 months of age may require doses at or near the high end of this range; consistent anticoagulation may be difficult to maintain in children <5 years of age.

Adults: Initial dosing must be individualized. Consider the patient (hepatic function, cardiac function, age, nutritional status, concurrent therapy, risk of bleeding) in addition to prior dose response (if available) and the clinical situation. Start 2-5 mg daily for 2 days **or** 5-10 mg daily for 1-2 days (Ansell, 2008). Adjust dose according to INR results; usual maintenance dose ranges from 2-10 mg daily (individual patients may require loading and maintenance doses outside these general guidelines).

Note: Lower starting doses may be required for patients with hepatic impairment, poor nutrition, CHF, elderly, high risk of bleeding, or patients who are debilitated, or those with reduced function genomic variants of the catabolic enzymes CYP2C9 (*2 or *3 alleles) or VKORC1 (-1639 polymorphism). Higher initial doses may be reasonable in selected patients (ie, receiving enzyme-inducing agents and with low risk of bleeding).

I.V.: Adults: 2-5 mg/day administered as a slow bolus injection

Dosing adjustment in renal disease: No adjustment required, however, patients with renal failure have an increased risk of bleeding complications. Monitor closely.

Dosing adjustment in hepatic disease: Monitor effect at usual doses; the response to oral anticoagulants may be markedly enhanced in obstructive jaundice (due to reduced vitamin K absorption) and also in hepatitis and cirrhosis (due to decreased production of vitamin K-dependent clotting factors); INR should be closely monitored

Dietary Considerations Foods high in vitamin K (eg, beef liver, pork liver, green tea, and leafy green vegetables) inhibit anticoagulant effect. Do not change dietary habits once stabilized on warfarin therapy. A balanced diet with a consistent intake of vitamin K is essential. Avoid large amounts of alfalfa, asparagus, broccoli, Brussels sprouts, cabbage, cauliflower, green teas, kale, lettuce, spinach, turnip greens, and watercress; decreased efficacy of warfarin. It is recommended that the diet contain a CONSISTENT vitamin K content of 70-140 mcg/day. Check with healthcare provider before changing diet.

Administration

Oral: Administer with or without food. Take at the same time each day.

I.V.: Administer as a slow bolus injection over 1-2 minutes; avoid all I.M. injections

Monitoring Parameters Prothrombin time, hematocrit, INR; consider genotyping of CYP2C9 and VKORC1 prior to initiation of therapy, if available

Reference Range

INR = patient prothrombin time/mean normal prothrombin time

ISI = international sensitivity index

INR should be increased by 2-3.5 times depending upon indication. An INR >4 does not generally add additional therapeutic benefit and is associated with increased risk of bleeding.

Adult INR ranges based upon indication: See table on next page.

Warfarin levels are not used for monitoring degree of anticoagulation. They may be useful if a patient with unexplained coagulopathy is using the drug surreptitiously or if it is unclear whether clinical resistance is due to true drug resistance or lack of drug intake.

Normal prothrombin time (PT): 10.9-12.9 seconds. Healthy premature newborns have prolonged coagulation test screening results (eg, PT, aPTT, TT) which return to normal adult values at approximately 6 months of age. Healthy prematures, however, do not develop spontaneous hemorrhage or thrombotic complications because of a balance between procoagulants and inhibitors.

Additional Information Prospective genotyping is available, and may provide important guidance on initiation of anticoagulant therapy. Commercial testing with PGxPredict™:WARFARIN is now available from PGxHealth™ (Division of Clinical Data, Inc, New Haven, CT). The test genotypes patients for presence of the CYP2C9*2 or *3 alleles and the VKORC1 -1639G>A polymorphism. The results of the test allow patients to be phenotyped as extensive, intermediate, or poor metabolizers (CYP2C9) and as low, intermediate, or high warfarin sensitivity (VKORC1). Ordering information is available at 888-592-7327 or warfarininfo@pgxhealth.com.

Dosage Forms Excipient information presented when available (limited, particularly for generics); consult specific product labeling.

Injection, powder for reconstitution, as sodium:

Coumadin®: 5 mg

Tablet, as sodium: 1 mg, 2 mg, 2.5 mg, 3 mg, 4 mg, 5 mg, 6 mg, 7.5 mg, 10 mg

Coumadin®: 1 mg, 2 mg, 2.5 mg, 3 mg, 4 mg, 5 mg, 6 mg, 7.5 mg [scored]

Coumadin®: 10 mg [scored; dye free]

Jantoven®: 1 mg, 2 mg, 2.5 mg, 3 mg, 4 mg, 5 mg, 6 mg, 7.5 mg [scored]

Jantoven®: 10 mg [scored; dye free]

Adult Target INR Ranges Based Upon Indication

Indication	Targeted INR	Targeted INR Range
Cardiac		
Acute myocardial infarction (high risk)[1]	2.5	2-3[2,3]
Atrial fibrillation or atrial flutter	2.5	2-3
Valvular		
Bileaflet or Medtronic Hall tilting disk mechanical aortic valve in normal sinus rhythm and normal LA size	2.5	2-3
Bileaflet or tilting disk mechanical mitral valve	3	2.5-3.5
Caged ball or caged disk mechanical valve	3	2.5-3.5
Mechanical prosthetic valve with systemic embolism despite adequate anticoagulation	3 or 3.5[4]	2.5-3.5[4] or 3-4[4]
Mechanical valve and risk factors for thromboembolism (eg, AF, MI[5], LA enlargement, hypercoagulable state, low EF) or history of atherosclerotic vascular disease	3	2.5-3.5[6]
Bioprosthetic mitral valve	2.5	2-3[7]
Bioprosthetic mitral or aortic valve with prior history of systemic embolism	2.5	2-3[7]
Bioprosthetic mitral or aortic valve with evidence of LA thrombus at surgery	2.5	2-3[8]
Bioprosthetic mitral or aortic valve with risk factors for thromboembolism (eg, AF, hypercoagulable state or low EF)	2.5	2-3[9]
Prosthetic mitral valve thrombosis (resolved)	4	3.5-4.5[3]
Prosthetic aortic valve thrombosis (resolved)	3.5	3-4[3]
Rheumatic mitral valve disease and normal sinus rhythm (LA diameter >5.5 cm), AF, previous systemic embolism, or LA thrombus	2.5	2-3
Thromboembolism Treatment		
Venous thromboembolism	2.5	2-3[10,11]
Thromboprophylaxis		
Chronic thromboembolic pulmonary hypertension (CTPH)	2.5	2-3
Lupus inhibitor (no other risk factors)	2.5	2-3
Lupus inhibitor and recurrent thromboembolism	3	2.5-3.5
Major trauma patients with impaired mobility undergoing rehabilitation	2.5	2-3
Spinal cord injury (acute) undergoing rehabilitation	2.5	2-3
Total hip or knee replacement (elective) or hip fracture surgery	2.5	2-3[12]
Other Indications		
Cerebral venous sinus thrombosis	2.5	2-3[13]
Ischemic stroke due to AF	2.5	2-3

[1]High-risk includes large anterior MI, significant heart failure, intracardiac thrombus, atrial fibrillation, history of thromboembolism.

[2]Maintain anticoagulation for 3 months.

[3]Combine with aspirin 81 mg/day.

[4]Combine with aspirin 81 mg/day, if not previously receiving, **and/or** if previous target INR was 2.5, then new target INR should be 3 (2.5-3.5). If previous target INR was 3, then new target INR should be 3.5 (3-4).

[5]MI refers to anterior-apical ST-segment elevation myocardial infarction.

[6]Combine with aspirin 81 mg/day unless patient is at high risk of bleeding (eg, history of GI bleed, age >80 years).

[7]Maintain anticoagulation for 3 months after valve insertion then switch to aspirin 81 mg/day if no other indications for warfarin exist or clinically reassess need for warfarin in patients with prior history of systemic embolism.

[8]Maintain anticoagulation with warfarin until thrombus resolution.

[9]If patient has history of atherosclerotic vascular disease, combine with aspirin 81 mg/day unless patient is at high risk of bleeding (eg, history of GI bleed, age >80 years).

[10]Treat for 3 months in patients with VTE due to transient reversible risk factor. Treat for a minimum of 3 months in patients with unprovoked VTE and evaluate for long term therapy. Other risk groups (eg, cancer) may require >3 months of therapy.

[11]In patients with unprovoked VTE who prefer less frequent INR monitoring, low-intensity therapy (INR range: 1.5-1.9) with less frequent monitoring is recommended over stopping treatment.

[12]Continue for at least 10 days and up to 35 days after surgery.

[13]Continue for up to 12 months.

- **Warfarin Sodium** *see* Warfarin *on page 1679*
- **Wart-Off® Maximum Strength [OTC]** *see* Salicylic Acid *on page 1454*
- **4-Way® 12 Hour [OTC]** *see* Oxymetazoline *on page 1208*
- **4 Way® Fast Acting [OTC]** *see* Phenylephrine *on page 1273*
- **4 Way® Menthol [OTC]** *see* Phenylephrine *on page 1273*
- **4 Way® No Drip [OTC]** *see* Phenylephrine *on page 1273*
- **WelChol®** *see* Colesevelam *on page 398*

- **Wellbutrin®** *see* BuPROPion *on page 217*
- **Wellbutrin XL™** *see* BuPROPion *on page 217*
- **Wellbutrin SR®** *see* BuPROPion *on page 217*
- **Westcort®** *see* Hydrocortisone *on page 785*
- **Westhroid™** *see* Thyroid, Desiccated *on page 1579*
- **White Mineral Oil** *see* Mineral Oil *on page 1055*
- **Whitethorn** *see* Hawthorn *(Crataegus oxyacantha) on page 758*
- **Wild Chamomile** *see* Feverfew *(Tanacetum parthenium) on page 628*
- **Wild Quinine** *see* Feverfew *(Tanacetum parthenium) on page 628*
- **WinRho® SDF** *see* Rh_o(D) Immune Globulin *on page 1415*
- **WR-2721** *see* Amifostine *on page 83*
- **WR-139007** *see* Dacarbazine *on page 414*
- **WR-139013** *see* Chlorambucil *on page 315*
- **WR-139021** *see* Carmustine *on page 284*
- **Wycillin [DSC]** *see* Penicillin G Procaine *on page 1241*
- **Xanax®** *see* ALPRAZolam *on page 72*
- **Xanax XR®** *see* ALPRAZolam *on page 72*
- **Xeloda®** *see* Capecitabine *on page 263*
- **Xenazine®** *see* Tetrabenazine *on page 1554*
- **Xenical®** *see* Orlistat *on page 1184*
- **Xifaxan™** *see* Rifaximin *on page 1420*
- **Xilep** *see* Rufinamide *on page 1452*
- **XiraTuss™ [DSC]** *see* Carbetapentane, Phenylephrine, and Chlorpheniramine *on page 274*
- **Xodol® 5/300** *see* Hydrocodone and Acetaminophen *on page 777*
- **Xodol® 7.5/300** *see* Hydrocodone and Acetaminophen *on page 777*
- **Xodol® 10/300** *see* Hydrocodone and Acetaminophen *on page 777*
- **Xolair®** *see* Omalizumab *on page 1174*
- **Xolegel™** *see* Ketoconazole *on page 876*
- **Xopenex®** *see* Levalbuterol *on page 902*
- **Xopenex HFA™** *see* Levalbuterol *on page 902*
- **XPECT™ [OTC]** *see* GuaiFENesin *on page 737*
- **Xpect-HC™ [DSC]** *see* Hydrocodone and Guaifenesin *on page 779*
- **XPECT-PE™ [DSC]** *see* Guaifenesin and Phenylephrine *on page 742*
- **Xylocaine®** *see* Lidocaine *on page 924*
- **Xylocaine® MPF** *see* Lidocaine *on page 924*
- **Xylocaine® Viscous** *see* Lidocaine *on page 924*

Xylometazoline (zye loe met AZ oh leen)

Medication Safety Issues

Sound-alike/look-alike issues:

Otrivin® may be confused with Lotrimin®

U.S. Brand Names Otrivin® Pediatric [OTC] [DSC]; Otrivin® [OTC] [DSC]

Canadian Brand Names Balminil

Index Terms Xylometazoline Hydrochloride

Pharmacologic Category Imidazoline Derivative; Vasoconstrictor, Nasal

Use Symptomatic relief of nasal and nasopharyngeal mucosal congestion

Effect on Mental Status May cause drowsiness or dizziness

Effect on Psychiatric Treatment None reported

Dosage Summary

Nasal:

Children <2 years: Dosage not established

Children 2-12 years: Instill 2-3 drops (0.05%) in each nostril every 8-10 hours

Children >12 years: Instill 2-3 drops or sprays (0.1%) in each nostril every 8-10 hours

Adults: Instill 2-3 drops or sprays (0.1%) in each nostril every 8-10 hours

Dosage Forms Excipient information presented when available (limited, particularly for generics); consult specific product labeling. [DSC] = Discontinued product

Solution, intranasal drops, as hydrochloride:

Otrivin® [DSC]: 0.1% (25 mL)

Otrivin® Pediatric [DSC]: 0.05% (25 mL)

Solution, intranasal spray, as hydrochloride (Otrivin® [DSC]): 0.1% (20 mL)

- **Xylometazoline Hydrochloride** *see* Xylometazoline *on page 1687*
- **Xyrem®** *see* Sodium Oxybate *on page 1495*
- **Xyzal®** *see* Levocetirizine *on page 909*
- **Y-90 Ibritumomab** *see* Ibritumomab *on page 802*
- **Y-90 Zevalin** *see* Ibritumomab *on page 802*
- **Yagona** *see* Kava Kava *(Piper methysticum) on page 874*
- **Yasmin®** *see* Ethinyl Estradiol and Drospirenone *on page 593*
- **Yaz®** *see* Ethinyl Estradiol and Drospirenone *on page 593*
- **YM087** *see* Conivaptan *on page 400*
- **YM905** *see* Solifenacin *on page 1498*
- **YM-08310** *see* Amifostine *on page 83*
- **Yocon®** *see* Yohimbine *on page 1688*
- **Yodoxin®** *see* Iodoquinol *on page 851*

Yohimbine (yo HIM bine)

Medication Safety Issues

Sound-alike/look-alike issues:

Aphrodyne® may be confused with Aprodine®

Yocon® may be confused with Zocor®

U.S. Brand Names Aphrodyne® [DSC]; Yocon®

Canadian Brand Names PMS-Yohimbine; Yocon®

Index Terms Yohimbine Hydrochloride

Pharmacologic Category Miscellaneous Product

Generic Available Yes

Unlabeled/Investigational Use Treatment of SSRI-induced sexual dysfunction; weight loss; impotence; sympathicolytic and mydriatic; may have activity as an aphrodisiac

Effect on Mental Status May cause anxiety, irritability, dizziness, insomnia, mania, panic attacks, and psychosis

Effect on Psychiatric Treatment May cause neutropenia; use caution with clozapine and carbamazepine; antidepressant should not be used with yohimbine; has been used to treat SSRI-induced sexual dysfunction

Contraindications Hypersensitivity to yohimbine or any component of the formulation; renal disease

Warnings/Precautions Do not use in pregnancy; do not use in children; not for use in geriatric, psychiatric, or cardio-renal patients with a history of gastric or duodenal ulcer; generally not for use in females. Should not be used in kidney disease or psychiatric disorders; can cause high blood pressure and anxiety, tachycardia, nausea, or vomiting.

Adverse Reactions Frequency not defined.

Cardiovascular: Tachycardia, hypertension, hypotension (orthostatic), flushing

Central nervous system: Anxiety, mania, hallucinations, irritability, dizziness, psychosis, insomnia, headache, panic attacks

Gastrointestinal: Nausea, vomiting, anorexia, salivation

Neuromuscular & skeletal: Tremors

Miscellaneous: Antidiuretic action, diaphoresis

Metabolism/Transport Effects Substrate of CYP2D6 (minor); **Inhibits** CYP2D6 (weak)

Drug Interactions

There are no known significant interactions.

Mechanism of Action Derived from the bark of the yohimbe tree (*Corynanthe yohimbe*), this indole alkaloid produces a presynaptic alpha$_2$-adrenergic blockade. Peripheral autonomic effect is to increase cholinergic and decrease adrenergic activity; yohimbine exerts a stimulating effect on the mood and a mild antidiuretic effect.

Pharmacodynamics/Kinetics

Duration of action: Usually 3-4 hours, but may last 36 hours

Absorption: 33%

Distribution: V_d: 0.3-3 L/kg

Half-life elimination: 0.6 hour

Dosage Adults: Oral:

Male erectile impotence: 5.4 mg tablet 3 times/day have been used. If side effects occur, reduce to 1/2 tablet (2.7 mg) 3 times/day followed by gradual increases to 1 tablet 3 times/day. Results of therapy >10 weeks are not known.

Orthostatic hypotension: Doses of 12.5 mg/day have been utilized; however, more research is necessary

Additional Information Also a street drug of abuse that can be smoked; has a bitter taste. Dissociative state may resemble phencyclidine intoxication.

Dosage Forms Excipient information presented when available (limited, particularly for generics); consult specific product labeling. [DSC] = Discontinued product

Caplet, oral, as hydrochloride:

Aphrodyne®: 5.4 mg [DSC] [scored]

Tablet, as hydrochloride: 5.4 mg

Yocon®: 5.4 mg

- **Yohimbine Hydrochloride** *see* Yohimbine *on page 1688*
- **Z4942** *see* Ifosfamide *on page 809*
- **Zaditor® [OTC]** *see* Ketotifen *on page 879*

Zafirlukast (za FIR loo kast)

Medication Safety Issues

Sound-alike/look-alike issues:

Accolate® may be confused with Accupril®, Accutane®, Aclovate®

U.S. Brand Names Accolate®

Canadian Brand Names Accolate®

Mexican Brand Names Accolate

Index Terms ICI-204,219

Pharmacologic Category Leukotriene-Receptor Antagonist

Generic Available No

Use Prophylaxis and chronic treatment of asthma in adults and children ≥5 years of age

Effect on Mental Status May cause insomnia, malaise, or dizziness

Effect on Psychiatric Treatment Reports of agranulocytosis in association with zafirlukast; monitor CBC in patients receiving clozapine and carbamazepine

Pregnancy Risk Factor B

Pregnancy Considerations There are no adequate and well-controlled trials in pregnant women. Teratogenic effects not observed in animal studies; fetal defects were observed when administered in maternally toxic doses.

Lactation Enters breast milk/contraindicated

Contraindications Hypersensitivity to zafirlukast or any component of the formulation

Warnings/Precautions Zafirlukast is not FDA approved for use in the reversal of bronchospasm in acute asthma attacks, including status asthmaticus. Therapy with zafirlukast can be continued during acute exacerbations of asthma.

Hepatic adverse events (including hepatitis, hyperbilirubinemia, and hepatic failure) have been reported; female patients may be at greater risk. Discontinue immediately if liver dysfunction is suspected. Periodic testing of liver function may be considered (early detection is generally believed to improve the likelihood of recovery). If hepatic dysfunction is suspected (due to clinical signs/symptoms), liver function tests should be measured immediately. Do not resume or restart if hepatic function studies are consistent with dysfunction. Use caution in patients with alcoholic cirrhosis; clearance is reduced.

Rare cases of eosinophilic vasculitis (Churg-Strauss) have been reported in patients receiving zafirlukast (usually, but not always, associated with reduction in concurrent steroid dosage). No causal relationship established. Monitor for eosinophilic vasculitis, rash, pulmonary symptoms, cardiac symptoms, or neuropathy.

An increased proportion of zafirlukast patients >55 years of age reported infections as compared to placebo-treated patients. These infections were mostly mild or moderate in intensity and predominantly affected the respiratory tract. Infections occurred equally in both sexes, were dose-proportional to total milligrams of zafirlukast exposure, and were associated with coadministration of inhaled corticosteroids. Safety and efficacy have not been established in patients <5 years of age.

Adverse Reactions

>10%: Central nervous system: Headache (13%)

1% to 10%:

Central nervous system: Dizziness (2%), pain (2%), fever (2%)

Gastrointestinal: Nausea (3%), diarrhea (3%), abdominal pain (2%), vomiting (2%), dyspepsia (1%)

Hepatic: ALT increased (2%)

Neuromuscular & skeletal: Back pain (2%), myalgia (2%), weakness (2%)

Miscellaneous: Infection (4%)

<1% (Limited to important or life-threatening): Agranulocytosis, angioedema, arthralgia, behavior/mood changes, bleeding, bruising, edema, eosinophilia (systemic), eosinophilic pneumonia, hepatic failure, hepatitis, hyperbilirubinemia, hypersensitivity reactions, insomnia, malaise, pruritus, rash, suicidality, suicide, urticaria, vasculitis with clinical features of Churg-Strauss syndrome (rare)

Metabolism/Transport Effects Substrate of CYP2C9 (major); **Inhibits** CYP1A2 (weak), 2C8 (weak), 2C9 (moderate), 2C19 (weak), 2D6 (weak), 3A4 (weak)

Drug Interactions

CYP2C9 Inducers (Highly Effective): May increase the metabolism of CYP2C9 Substrates (High risk). *Risk C: Monitor therapy*

CYP2C9 Inhibitors (Moderate): May decrease the metabolism of CYP2C9 Substrates (High risk). *Risk C: Monitor therapy*

CYP2C9 Inhibitors (Strong): May decrease the metabolism of CYP2C9 Substrates (High risk). *Risk D: Consider therapy modification*

CYP2C9 Substrates (High risk): CYP2C9 Inhibitors (Moderate) may decrease the metabolism of CYP2C9 Substrates (High risk). *Risk C: Monitor therapy*

Erythromycin: May decrease the serum concentration of Zafirlukast. *Risk C: Monitor therapy*

Theophylline Derivatives: May decrease the serum concentration of Zafirlukast. **Exceptions:** Dyphylline. *Risk C: Monitor therapy*

Vitamin K Antagonists (eg, warfarin): Zafirlukast may decrease the metabolism of Vitamin K Antagonists. *Risk C: Monitor therapy*

Ethanol/Nutrition/Herb Interactions Food: Decreases bioavailability of zafirlukast by 40%.

Stability Store tablets at controlled room temperature (20°C to 25°C; 68°F to 77°F). Protect from light and moisture; dispense in original airtight container.

Mechanism of Action Zafirlukast is a selectively and competitive leukotriene-receptor antagonist (LTRA) of leukotriene D4 and E4 (LTD4 and LTE4), components of slow-reacting substance of anaphylaxis (SRSA). Cysteinyl leukotriene production and receptor occupation have been correlated with the pathophysiology of asthma, including airway edema, smooth muscle constriction, and altered cellular activity associated with the inflammatory process, which contribute to the signs and symptoms of asthma.

Pharmacodynamics/Kinetics

Protein binding: >99%, primarily to albumin

Metabolism: Extensively hepatic via CYP2C9

Bioavailability: Reduced 40% with food

Half-life elimination: 10 hours

Time to peak, serum: 3 hours

Excretion: Urine (10%); feces

Dosage Oral:

Children <5 years: Safety and effectiveness have not been established

Children 5-11 years: 10 mg twice daily

Children ≥12 years and Adults: 20 mg twice daily

Elderly: The mean dose (mg/kg) normalized AUC and C_{max} increase and plasma clearance decreases with increasing age. In patients >65 years of age, there is a two- to threefold greater C_{max} and AUC compared to younger adults.

Dosing adjustment in renal impairment: Dosage adjustment not required.

Dosing adjustment in hepatic impairment: In patients with hepatic impairment (ie, biopsy-proven cirrhosis), there is a 50% to 60% greater C_{max} and AUC compared to normal subjects.

Dietary Considerations Should be taken on an empty stomach (1 hour before or 2 hours after meals).

Administration Administer at least 1 hour before or 2 hours after a meal.

Monitoring Parameters Monitor for improvements in air flow; monitor closely for sign/symptoms of hepatic injury; periodic monitoring of LFTs may be considered (not proved to prevent serious injury, but early detection may enhance recovery)

Dosage Forms Excipient information presented when available (limited, particularly for generics); consult specific product labeling.

Tablet: 10 mg, 20 mg

Zalcitabine (zal SITE a been)

U.S. Brand Names Hivid® [DSC]
Canadian Brand Names Hivid®
Mexican Brand Names Hivid
Index Terms ddC; Dideoxycytidine
Pharmacologic Category Antiretroviral Agent, Reverse Transcriptase Inhibitor (Nucleoside)
Use In combination with at least two other antiretrovirals in the treatment of patients with HIV infection; it is not recommended that zalcitabine be given in combination with didanosine, stavudine, or lamivudine due to overlapping toxicities, virologic interactions, or lack of clinical data
Effect on Mental Status Drowsiness is common; may cause dizziness
Effect on Psychiatric Treatment May cause granulocytopenia; use caution with clozapine; concurrent use with disulfiram can enhance peripheral neuropathy; avoid combination
Dosage Summary
Oral:
Children <13 years: Dosage not established
Children ≥13 years: 0.75 mg 3 times/day
Adults: 0.75 mg 3 times/day
Dosage Forms Excipient information presented when available (limited, particularly for generics); consult specific product labeling. [DSC] = Discontinued product
Tablet:
Hivid®: 0.375 mg, 0.75 mg [DSC]

Zaleplon (ZAL e plon)

Related Information
CMS: Long-Term Care Facility Thresholds *on page 1815*
Nonbenzodiazepine Anxiolytics and Hypnotics *on page 1791*
U.S. Brand Names Sonata®
Mexican Brand Names Sonata
Pharmacologic Category Hypnotic, Nonbenzodiazepine
Generic Available Yes
Use Short-term (7-10 days) treatment of insomnia (has been demonstrated to be effective for up to 5 weeks in controlled trial)
Mental Health Comment In 2007, the FDA requested that all manufacturers of sedative-hypnotic drug products revise labeling to include a greater emphasis on the risks of adverse effects. These risks include severe allergic reactions (anaphylaxis, angioedema) and complex sleep-related behaviors, which may include sleep-driving (driving while not fully awake and with no memory of the event), making phone calls, and preparing and eating food while asleep. Zaleplon may be associated with a lower potential for abuse compared to benzodiazepines.
Restrictions C-IV

An FDA-approved patient medication guide is available and must be distributed when dispensing an outpatient prescription (new or refill) where this medication is to be used without direct supervision of a healthcare provider. Medication guides are available at http://www.fda.gov/cder/Offices/ODS/medication_guides.htm.
Pregnancy Risk Factor C
Pregnancy Considerations Not recommended for use during pregnancy
Lactation Enters breast milk/not recommended
Contraindications Hypersensitivity to zaleplon or any component of the formulation
Warnings/Precautions Symptomatic treatment of insomnia should be initiated only after careful evaluation of potential causes of sleep disturbance. Failure of sleep disturbance to resolve after 7-10 days may indicate psychiatric and/or medical illness.

Use with caution in patients with depression, particularly if suicidal risk may be present. Use with caution in patients with a history of drug dependence. Abrupt discontinuance may lead to withdrawal symptoms. Hypnotics/sedatives have been associated with abnormal thinking and behavior changes including decreased inhibition, aggression, bizarre behavior, agitation, hallucinations, and depersonalization. These changes may occur unpredictably and may indicate previously unrecognized psychiatric disorders; evaluate appropriately. May impair physical and mental capabilities. Patients must be cautioned about performing tasks which require mental alertness (operating machinery or driving). Amnesia can occur. Use with caution in patients receiving other CNS depressants or psychoactive medications. Effects with other sedative drugs or ethanol may be potentiated. Postmarketing studies have indicated that the use of hypnotic/sedative agents for sleep has been associated with hypersensitivity reactions including anaphylaxis as well as angioedema. An increased risk for hazardous sleep-related activities such as sleep-driving; cooking and eating food, and making phone calls while asleep have also been noted.

Use with caution in the elderly, those with compromised respiratory function, or hepatic impairment (dosage adjustment recommended in mild-to-moderate hepatic impairment; avoid use in severe impairment). Because of the rapid onset of action, zaleplon should be administered immediately prior to bedtime or after the patient has gone to bed and is having difficulty falling asleep. Capsules contain tartrazine (FDC yellow #5); avoid in patients with sensitivity (caution in patients with asthma). Safety and efficacy have not been established in children.

Adverse Reactions

>10 %: Central nervous system: Headache (30% to 42%)

1% to 10%:

Cardiovascular: Chest pain (≥1%), peripheral edema (≤1%)

Central nervous system: Dizziness (7% to 9%), somnolence (5% to 6%), amnesia (2% to 4%), depersonalization (<1% to 2%), hypoesthesia (<1% to 2%), malaise (<1% to 2%), abnormal thinking (≥1%), anxiety (≥1%), depression (≥1%), fever (≥1%), migraine (≥1%), nervousness (≥1%), confusion (≤1%), hallucination (≤1%), vertigo (≤1%)

Dermatologic: Pruritus (≥1%), rash (≥1%), photosensitivity reaction (≤1%)

Endocrine & metabolic: Dysmenorrhea (3% to 4%)

Gastrointestinal: Nausea (6% to 8%), abdominal pain (6%), anorexia (<1% to 2%), constipation (≥1%), dyspepsia (≥1%), taste perversion (≥1%), xerostomia (≥1%), colitis (up to 1%)

Neuromuscular & skeletal: Weakness (5% to 7%), paresthesia (3%), tremor (2%), arthralgia (≥1%), arthritis (≥1%), back pain (≥1%), myalgia (≥1%), hypertonia (1%)

Ocular: Eye pain (3% to 4%), abnormal vision (<1% to 2%), conjunctivitis (≥1%)

Otic: Hyperacusis (1% to 2%), ear pain (≤1%)

Respiratory: Bronchitis (≥1%), epistaxis (≤1%)

Miscellaneous: Parosmia (<1% to 2%)

<1% (Limited to important or life-threatening): Alopecia, ALT increased, anaphylaxis, angioedema, anemia, angina, AST increased, ataxia, bigeminy, bilirubinemia, bleeding gums, bundle branch block, cardiospasm, cerebral ischemia, cholelithiasis, circumoral paresthesia, CNS stimulation; complex sleep-related behavior (sleep-driving, cooking or eating food, making phone calls); cyanosis, delusions, diabetes mellitus, duodenal ulcer, dysarthria, dystonia, dysuria, ecchymosis, eosinophilia, facial paralysis, gastroenteritis, glaucoma, goiter, hematuria, hyper-/hypoglycemia, hyper-/hypotension, hyperuricemia, hypothyroidism, impotence, incontinence, intestinal obstruction, ketosis, lactose intolerance, leukocytosis, lymphocytosis, liver function tests (abnormal), lymphadenopathy, myasthenia, myositis, osteoporosis, palpitation, peptic ulcer, pericardial effusion, photophobia, ptosis, pulmonary embolus, purpura, rash, rectal bleeding, sinus bradycardia, substernal chest pain, syncope, thrombophlebitis, tongue edema, ulcerative stomatitis, urinary retention, ventricular tachycardia, vasodilation, ventricular extrasystoles

Metabolism/Transport Effects Substrate of CYP3A4 (minor)

Drug Interactions

Alcohol (Ethyl): CNS Depressants may enhance the CNS depressant effect of Alcohol (Ethyl). *Risk C: Monitor therapy*

Cimetidine: May decrease the metabolism of Zaleplon. *Risk D: Consider therapy modification*

CNS Depressants: May enhance the adverse/toxic effect of other CNS Depressants. *Risk C: Monitor therapy*

Flumazenil: May diminish the sedative effect of Hypnotics (Nonbenzodiazepine). *Risk C: Monitor therapy*

Rifamycin Derivatives: May increase the metabolism of Zaleplon. *Risk C: Monitor therapy*

Ethanol/Nutrition/Herb Interactions

Ethanol: Avoid ethanol (may increase CNS depression).

Food: High fat meal prolonged absorption; delayed t_{max} by 2 hours, and reduced C_{max} by 35%.

Herb/Nutraceutical: St John's wort may decrease zaleplon levels. Avoid valerian, St John's wort, kava kava, gotu kola (may increase CNS depression).

Stability Store at controlled room temperature of 20°C to 25°C (68°F to 77°F). Protect from light.

Mechanism of Action Zaleplon is unrelated to benzodiazepines, barbiturates, or other hypnotics. However, it interacts with the benzodiazepine GABA receptor complex. Nonclinical studies have shown that it binds selectively to the brain omega-1 receptor situated on the alpha subunit of the GABA-A receptor complex.

Pharmacodynamics/Kinetics

Onset of action: Rapid

Duration: 6-8 hours

Absorption: Rapid and almost complete; high-fat meal delays absorption

Distribution: V_d: ~1.4 L/kg

Protein binding: ~45% to 75%

Metabolism: Extensive, primarily via aldehyde oxidase to form 5-oxo-zaleplon and, to a lesser extent, by CYP3A4 to desethylzaleplon; all metabolites are pharmacologically inactive

Bioavailability: ~30%

Half-life elimination: 1 hour

Time to peak, serum: 1 hour

Excretion: Urine (~70% primarily metabolites, <1% as unchanged drug); feces (~17%)

Clearance: Plasma: Oral: 3 L/hour/kg

Dosage Oral:

Adults: 10 mg at bedtime (range: 5-20 mg); has been used for up to 5 weeks of treatment in controlled trial setting

Elderly: 5 mg at bedtime; recommended maximum: 10 mg/day

Dosage adjustment in renal impairment: No adjustment for mild-to-moderate renal impairment; use in severe renal impairment has not been adequately studied

Dosage adjustment in hepatic impairment: Mild-to-moderate impairment: 5 mg; not recommended for use in patients with severe hepatic impairment

Dietary Considerations Avoid taking with or after a heavy, high-fat meal; reduces absorption.

Administration Immediately before bedtime or when the patient is in bed and cannot fall asleep

Additional Information Prescription quantities should not exceed a 1-month supply.

Dosage Forms Excipient information presented when available (limited, particularly for generics); consult specific product labeling.

Capsule: 5 mg, 10 mg

Sonata®: 5 mg, 10 mg [contains tartrazine]

◆ **Zamicet®** *see* Hydrocodone and Acetaminophen *on page 777*

◆ **Zanaflex®** *see* TiZANidine *on page 1587*

◆ **Zanaflex Capsules™** *see* TiZANidine *on page 1587*

Zanamivir (za NA mi veer)

U.S. Brand Names Relenza®

Canadian Brand Names Relenza®

Mexican Brand Names Relenza

Pharmacologic Category Antiviral Agent; Neuraminidase Inhibitor

Use Treatment of uncomplicated acute illness due to influenza virus A and B in patients who have been symptomatic for no more than 2 days; prophylaxis against influenza virus A and B

The Advisory Committee on Immunization Practices (ACIP) recommends that **treatment** be considered for the following:

- Persons hospitalized with laboratory confirmed influenza (may also have benefit if started >48 hours after onset of illness).
- Persons with laboratory confirmed influenza pneumonia.
- Persons with laboratory confirmed influenza and bacterial infections.
- Persons with laboratory confirmed influenza and who are at higher risk for influenza complications.
- Persons presenting for care within 48 hours of laboratory confirmed influenza onset and who want to decrease duration and/or severity of their symptoms or decrease the risk of transmission to those at high risk for complications.

The ACIP recommends that **prophylaxis** be considered for the following:

- Persons at high risk for influenza infection during the first 2 weeks following vaccination (eg, children <9 years and not previously vaccinated) if the virus is circulating in the community.
- Persons at high risk for influenza infection, but the vaccination is contraindicated.
- Unvaccinated family members or healthcare providers with prolonged exposure to or close contact with high-risk persons, unvaccinated persons, or infants <6 months of age.
- Persons at high risk for influenza infection, their family members and close contacts, and healthcare workers when the circulating strain of influenza is not matched with the vaccine.
- Persons with immune deficiency or those who may not respond to vaccination.
- Unvaccinated staff and persons during response to an outbreak in a closed institutional setting that has patients at high risk for infection (eg, extended care facilities).

Effect on Mental Status May cause dizziness; may rarely cause drowsiness

Effect on Psychiatric Treatment None reported

Dosage Summary

Oral inhalation:

Children ≥5 years: Prophylaxis: 10 mg once daily

Children ≥7 years: Treatment: 10 mg twice daily

Adolescents: Prophylaxis: 10 mg once daily

Adults:

Prophylaxis: 10 mg once daily

Treatment: 10 mg twice daily

Dosage Forms Excipient information presented when available (limited, particularly for generics); consult specific product labeling.

Powder for oral inhalation: 5 mg/blister (20s) [4 blisters per Rotadisk® foil pack, 5 Rotadisk® per package; packaged with Diskhaler® inhalation device; contains lactose]

◆ **Zanosar®** *see* Streptozocin *on page 1510*

◆ **Zantac®** *see* Ranitidine *on page 1399*

◆ **Zantac 75® [OTC]** *see* Ranitidine *on page 1399*

◆ **Zantac 150™ [OTC]** *see* Ranitidine *on page 1399*

◆ **Zantac® EFFERdose®** *see* Ranitidine *on page 1399*

◆ **Zarontin®** *see* Ethosuximide *on page 603*

◆ **Zaroxolyn®** *see* Metolazone *on page 1034*

◆ **Zavesca®** *see* Miglustat *on page 1053*

◆ **Z-chlopenthixol** *see* Zuclopenthixol *on page 1712*

◆ **Z-Cof™ 12DM** *see* Guaifenesin, Pseudoephedrine, and Dextromethorphan *on page 748*

◆ **Z-Cof LA™** *see* Guaifenesin and Dextromethorphan *on page 739*

◆ **ZD1033** *see* Anastrozole *on page 125*

◆ **ZD1839** *see* Gefitinib *on page 709*

◆ **ZDV** *see* Zidovudine *on page 1695*

◆ **Zebeta®** *see* Bisoprolol *on page 190*

◆ **Zebutal™** *see* Butalbital, Acetaminophen, and Caffeine *on page 229*

◆ **Zegerid®** *see* Omeprazole and Sodium Bicarbonate *on page 1179*

◆ **Zelapar™** *see* Selegiline *on page 1466*

◆ **Zeldox** *see* Ziprasidone *on page 1698*

◆ **Zelnorm®** *see* Tegaserod *on page 1541*

◆ **Zemplar®** *see* Paricalcitol *on page 1226*

◆ **Zenapax®** *see* Daclizumab *on page 414*

◆ **Zenchent™** *see* Ethinyl Estradiol and Norethindrone *on page 597*

◆ **Zeneca 182,780** *see* Fulvestrant *on page 698*

◆ **Zerit®** *see* Stavudine *on page 1505*

◆ **ZerLor™** *see* Acetaminophen, Caffeine, and Dihydrocodeine *on page 39*

◆ **Zestoretic®** *see* Lisinopril and Hydrochlorothiazide *on page 938*

◆ **Zestril®** *see* Lisinopril *on page 934*

◆ **Zetia®** *see* Ezetimibe *on page 610*

◆ **Zevalin®** *see* Ibritumomab *on page 802*

- **Zgesic** *see* Acetaminophen and Phenyltoloxamine *on page 36*
- **Ziac®** *see* Bisoprolol and Hydrochlorothiazide *on page 191*
- **Ziagen®** *see* Abacavir *on page 22*
- **Ziana™** *see* Clindamycin and Tretinoin *on page 364*

Ziconotide (zi KOE no tide)

Medication Safety Issues

High alert medication: The Institute for Safe Medication Practices (ISMP) includes this medication among its list of drugs which have a heightened risk of causing significant patient harm when used in error.

U.S. Brand Names Prialt®

Pharmacologic Category Analgesic, Nonopioid; Calcium Channel Blocker, N-Type

Use Management of severe chronic pain in patients requiring intrathecal (I.T.) therapy and who are intolerant or refractory to other therapies

Effect on Mental Status Dizziness and sedation are common. May cause hallucinations, mood changes, cognitive impairment, changes in consciousness, anxiety, nervousness, agitation, abnormal dreams, insomnia, or hostility.

Effect on Psychiatric Treatment Contraindicated in individuals with a history of psychosis. Concomitant use with psychotropic agents may produce additive sedative effects; monitor. GI side effects are common; concomitant use with SSRIs, valproic acid, or lithium may produce additive effects; monitor.

Dosage Summary

I.T.:

Children: Dosage not established

Adults: Initial dose: ≤2.4 mcg/day (0.1 mcg/hour); Maintenance range: 2.4-19.2 mcg/day (0.1-0.8 mcg/hour) (maximum: 19.2 mcg/day (0.8 mcg/hour)); **Note:** Titration is recommended

Dosage Forms Excipient information presented when available (limited, particularly for generics); consult specific product labeling.

Injection, solution, as acetate [preservative free]:

Prialt®: 25 mcg/mL (20 mL); 100 mcg/mL (1 mL, 5 mL)

Zidovudine (zye DOE vyoo deen)

Medication Safety Issues

Sound-alike/look-alike issues:

Azidothymidine may be confused with azaTHIOprine, aztreonam

Retrovir® may be confused with ritonavir

AZT is an error-prone abbreviation (mistaken as azathioprine, aztreonam)

U.S. Brand Names Retrovir®

Canadian Brand Names Apo-Zidovudine®; AZT™; Retrovir®

Mexican Brand Names Retrovir-AZT; Timivudin

Index Terms Azidothymidine; AZT (error-prone abbreviation); Compound S; ZDV

Pharmacologic Category Antiretroviral Agent, Reverse Transcriptase Inhibitor (Nucleoside)

Use Treatment of HIV infection in combination with at least two other antiretroviral agents; prevention of maternal/fetal HIV transmission as monotherapy

Unlabeled/Investigational Use Postexposure prophylaxis for HIV exposure as part of a multidrug regimen

Effect on Mental Status May cause anxiety, confusion, depression, dizziness, drowsiness, insomnia, or mania

Effect on Psychiatric Treatment Granulocytopenia is common; avoid clozapine and carbamazepine. Valproic acid may decrease the clearance of zidovudine. GI side effects are common; concurrent use with SSRIs may produce additive effects.

Dosage Summary

I.V.:

Infants <30 weeks gestation at birth: 1.5 mg/kg/dose every 12 hours; at 4 weeks of age advance to 1.5 mg/kg/dose every 8 hours

Infants ≥30 weeks and <35 weeks gestation at birth: 2 mg/kg/dose every 12 hours; at 2 weeks of age, advance to 1.5 mg/kg/dose every 8 hours

Infants (full term): 1.5 mg/kg/dose every 6 hours

Children 3 months to 12 years: 120 mg/m^2/dose every 6 hours **or** 20 mg/m^2/hour as a continuous infusion

Children >12 years: 1-2 mg/kg/dose every 4 hours around-the-clock **or** 2 mg/kg bolus followed by 1 mg/kg/hour continuous infusion
Adults: 1 mg/kg/dose every 4 hours around-the-clock **or** 2 mg/kg bolus followed by 1 mg/kg/hour continuous infusion

Oral:
Infants <30 weeks gestation at birth: 2 mg/kg/dose every 12 hours; at 4 weeks of age advance to 2 mg/kg/dose every 8 hours
Infants ≥30 weeks and <35 weeks gestation at birth: 2 mg/kg/dose every 12 hours; at 2 weeks of age, advance to 2 mg/kg/dose every 8 hours
Infants (full term): 2 mg/kg/dose every 6 hours
Children 6 weeks to 12 years: 160 mg/m^2/dose every 8 hours (maximum: 200 mg every 8 hours) **or** 240 mg/m^2 every 12 hours (maximum 300 mg twice daily) **or**
4 to <9 kg: 12 mg/kg/dose twice daily **or** 8 mg/kg/dose 3 times a day
≥9 to <30 kg: 9 mg/kg/dose twice daily **or** 6 mg/kg/dose 3 times a day
≥30 kg: 300 mg twice daily **or** 200 mg 3 times a day
Children >12 years: 100 mg 5 times/day **or** 200 mg 3 times/day **or** 300 mg twice daily
Adults: 100 mg 5 times/day **or** 200 mg 3 times/day **or** 300 mg twice daily

Dosage Forms Excipient information presented when available (limited, particularly for generics); consult specific product labeling.
Capsule:
Retrovir®: 100 mg
Injection, solution [preservative free]:
Retrovir®: 10 mg/mL (20 mL)
Syrup:
Retrovir®: 50 mg/5 mL (240 mL) [contains sodium benzoate; strawberry flavor]
Tablet: 300 mg
Retrovir®: 300 mg

Zidovudine and Lamivudine (zye DOE vyoo deen & la MI vyoo deen)

Medication Safety Issues
Sound-alike/look-alike issues:
Combivir® may be confused with Combivent®, Epivir®

AZT is an error-prone abbreviation (mistaken as azaTHIOprine, aztreonam)

U.S. Brand Names Combivir®
Canadian Brand Names Combivir®
Mexican Brand Names Combivir
Index Terms AZT + 3TC (error-prone abbreviation); Lamivudine and Zidovudine
Pharmacologic Category Antiretroviral Agent, Reverse Transcriptase Inhibitor (Nucleoside)
Use Treatment of HIV infection when therapy is warranted based on clinical and/or immunological evidence of disease progression
Effect on Mental Status Dizziness, insomnia, sedation are common; may cause depression. May rarely cause confusion or mania.
Effect on Psychiatric Treatment Leukopenia and granulocytopenia are common; caution with clozapine and carbamazepine. Increased toxicity may result if used concurrently with drugs that inhibit glucuronidation or excretion (lorazepam). Valproic acid increased zidovudine's AUC by 80% and decreased clearance by 38%.

Dosage Summary
Oral:
Children <12 years: Dosage not established
Children ≥12 years: One tablet twice daily
Adults: One tablet twice daily

Dosage Forms Excipient information presented when available (limited, particularly for generics); consult specific product labeling.
Tablet:
Combivir®: Zidovudine 300 mg and lamivudine 150 mg

◆ **Zilactin-L® [OTC]** *see* Lidocaine *on page 924*

Zileuton (zye LOO ton)

U.S. Brand Names Zyflo CR™; Zyflo® [DSC]
Pharmacologic Category 5-Lipoxygenase Inhibitor

Generic Available No

Use Prophylaxis and chronic treatment of asthma in children ≥12 years of age and adults

Effect on Mental Status May cause dizziness, drowsiness, insomnia, or nervousness

Effect on Psychiatric Treatment Concurrent use with propranolol may enhance beta-blocker activity

Pregnancy Risk Factor C

Pregnancy Considerations In developmental studies, reduced body weight and increased skeletal variations were observed in rats. There are no adequate and well-controlled studies in pregnant women.

Lactation Excretion in breast milk unknown/not recommended

Contraindications Hypersensitivity to zileuton or any component of the formulation; active liver disease or transaminase elevations greater than or equal to three times the upper limit of normal (≥3 times ULN)

Warnings/Precautions Not FDA approved for the reversal of bronchospasm in acute asthma attacks, including status asthmaticus; therapy may be continued during acute asthma exacerbations. Hepatic adverse effects have been reported (elevated transaminase levels); females >65 years and patients with pre-existing elevated transaminases may be at greater risk. Serum ALT should be monitored. Discontinue zileuton and follow transaminases until normal if patients develop clinical signs/symptoms of liver dysfunction or with transaminase levels >5 times ULN (use caution with history of liver disease and/or in those patients who consume substantial quantities of ethanol). Safety and efficacy have not been established in children <12 years of age.

Adverse Reactions

>10%: Central nervous system: Headache (23% to 25%)

1% to 10%:

- Central nervous system: Pain (8%)
- Dermatologic: Rash
- Gastrointestinal: Dyspepsia (8%), nausea (6%), abdominal pain (5%), diarrhea, vomiting
- Hematologic: Leukopenia (1% to 3%)
- Hepatic: ALT increased (2% to 3%)
- Neuromuscular & skeletal: Asthenia (4%), myalgia (3%)
- Respiratory: Pharyngitis, sinusitis, upper respiratory tract infection
- Miscellaneous: Hypersensitivity reactions

Frequency not defined:

- Cardiovascular: Chest pain
- Central nervous system: Dizziness, fever, insomnia, malaise, nervousness, somnolence
- Dermatologic: Pruritus
- Gastrointestinal: Constipation, flatulence
- Genitourinary: Urinary tract infection, vaginitis
- Neuromuscular & skeletal: Arthralgia, hypertonia, neck pain/rigidity
- Ocular: Conjunctivitis
- Miscellaneous: Lymphadenopathy

Postmarketing and/or case reports: Behavior/mood changes, hepatitis, hyperbilirubinemia, jaundice, liver failure, suicidality, suicide, urticaria

Metabolism/Transport Effects Substrate (minor) of CYP1A2, 2C9, 3A4; **Inhibits** CYP1A2 (moderate)

Drug Interactions

Propranolol: Zileuton may increase the serum concentration of Propranolol. *Risk C: Monitor therapy*

Theophylline: Zileuton may increase the serum concentration of Theophylline. *Risk D: Consider therapy modification*

Warfarin: Zileuton may increase the serum concentration of Warfarin. *Risk C: Monitor therapy*

Ethanol/Nutrition/Herb Interactions

Ethanol: Avoid ethanol (may increase CNS depression; may increase risk of hepatic toxicity).

Food:

- Zyflo CR™: Improved absorption when administered with food.
- Zyflo®: Absorption not improved when taken with food.

Herb/Nutraceutical: St John's wort may decrease zileuton levels.

Stability Store tablets at 15°C to 30°C (59°F to 86°F). Protect from light.

Mechanism of Action Specific 5-lipoxygenase inhibitor which inhibits leukotriene formation. Leukotrienes augment neutrophil and eosinophil migration, neutrophil and monocyte aggregation, leukocyte adhesion, increased capillary permeability, and smooth muscle contraction (which contribute to inflammation, edema, mucous secretion, and bronchoconstriction in the airway of the asthmatic.)

Pharmacodynamics/Kinetics

Absorption: Rapid
Distribution: 1.2 L/kg
Protein binding: 93%
Metabolism: Hepatic and gastrointestinal; zileuton and N-dehydroxylated metabolite can be metabolized by CYP1A2, 2C9, and 3A4
Bioavailability: Unknown
Half-life elimination: ~3 hours
Time to peak, serum: 1.7 hours
Excretion: Urine (~95% primarily as metabolites); feces (~2%)

Dosage Oral:

Children <12 years: Safety and effectiveness have not been established
Children ≥12 years and Adults:
Zyflo®: 600 mg 4 times/day
Zyflo CR™: 1200 mg twice daily.

Dosing adjustment in renal impairment: Adjustment not required in renal failure or with hemodialysis

Dosing adjustment in hepatic impairment: Contraindicated with hepatic dysfunction

Dietary Considerations Zyflo®: May be taken with or without food; Zyflo CR™: Take with food.

Administration Zyflo®: Administer without regard to meals (eg, with or without food). Zyflo CR™: Do not crush, cut, or chew tablet; administer with food.

Monitoring Parameters Evaluate hepatic transaminases at initiation of, and during therapy. Monitor serum ALT before treatment begins, once-a-month for the first 3 months, every 2-3 months for the remainder of the first year, and periodically thereafter for patients receiving long-term zileuton therapy. If symptoms of liver dysfunction (right upper quadrant pain, nausea, fatigue, lethargy, pruritus, jaundice, or "flu-like" symptoms) develop or transaminase elevations >5 times ULN occur, discontinue therapy and follow transaminase levels until normal.

Dosage Forms Excipient information presented when available (limited, particularly for generics); consult specific product labeling. [DSC] = Discontinued product

Tablet:
Zyflo®: 600 mg [DSC]
Tablet, extended release:
Zyflo CR™: 600 mg

◆ **Zinacef®** *see* Cefuroxime *on page 300*

◆ **Zinecard®** *see* Dexrazoxane *on page 441*

◆ **Zingo™** *see* Lidocaine *on page 924*

Ziprasidone (zi PRAS i done)

Related Information

Agents Approved for Bipolar Disorder *on page 1752*
Antipsychotic Agents *on page 1769*
Antipsychotic Receptor Profile *on page 1772*
Atypical Antipsychotics *on page 1773*
CMS: Long-Term Care Facility Thresholds *on page 1815*
Discontinuation of Psychotropic Drugs *on page 1839*

U.S. Brand Names Geodon®

Canadian Brand Names Zeldox®

Mexican Brand Names Geodon

Index Terms Zeldox; Ziprasidone Hydrochloride; Ziprasidone Mesylate

Pharmacologic Category Antipsychotic Agent, Atypical

Generic Available No

Use Treatment of schizophrenia; treatment of acute manic or mixed episodes associated with bipolar disorder with or without psychosis; acute agitation in patients with schizophrenia

Unlabeled/Investigational Use Tourette's syndrome; psychosis/agitation related to Alzheimer's dementia

Mental Health Comment Ziprasidone is an antipsychotic agent of a class often referred to as atypical. It should be noted that the definition of the term "atypical" is not universally agreed upon. Some prefer to describe antipsychotics based on their pharmacological properties. A common feature of all definitions used to describe "atypical" antipsychotics is the lack of significant acute or subacute

EPS, at dosages generally associated with antipsychotic actions. Other experts have included definitions of atypicality that include a) failure to increase serum prolactin levels; b) superior efficacy for positive, negative, and cognitive symptoms; and c) lack of evidence of tardive dyskinesia or dystonia following chronic administration. Clinically, the dose range for ziprasidone appears to be higher than the approved range (40-160 mg/day); minimum effective dose for most patients is 120 mg/day. Therefore, appropriate dosing with this compound is important. It is also important that this medication be taken with a 500 calorie meal as the bioavailability is increased 100% in the presence of food.

The short-acting I.M. formulation appears to be as efficacious as other available agents for the management of acute agitation; however, comparative trials have not been conducted.

Tardive dyskinesia (TD) secondary to **typical** antipsychotics has an estimated incidence of 3% to 5% per year for the first 5 years of treatment. The incidence of TD associated with the atypical antipsychotics is estimated to be 0.5% to 1%. It is not clear if this estimate represents a risk associated with mental illness or to what extent drug therapy can be implicated. Atypical antipsychotics appear less likely to cause tardive dyskinesia than typical antipsychotics (fluphenazine, haloperidol).

Coadministration of two or more antipsychotics does not generally improve clinical response and may increase the potential for adverse effects.

In 2008, the FDA issued a warning regarding increased mortality risk with typical **and** atypical antipsychotic drugs when used in elderly patients with dementia-related psychosis.

Pregnancy Risk Factor C

Pregnancy Considerations Developmental toxicity demonstrated in animals. There are no adequate and well-controlled studies in pregnant women. Use only if potential benefit justifies risk to the fetus.

Lactation Excretion in breast milk unknown/not recommended

Contraindications Hypersensitivity to ziprasidone or any component of the formulation; history (or current) prolonged QT; congenital long QT syndrome; recent myocardial infarction; history of arrhythmias; uncompensated heart failure; concurrent use of other QT_c-prolonging agents including amiodarone, arsenic trioxide, bretylium, chlorpromazine, cisapride, class la antiarrhythmics (quinidine, procainamide), dofetilide, dolasetron, droperidol, ibutilide, levomethadyl, mefloquine, mesoridazine, pentamidine, pimozide, probucol, some quinolone antibiotics (moxifloxacin), sotalol, tacrolimus, and thioridazine

Warnings/Precautions **[U.S. Boxed Warning]: Elderly patients with dementia-related behavioral disorders treated with atypical antipsychotics are at an increased risk of death compared to placebo.** An increased incidence of cerebrovascular adverse events (including fatalities) has been reported in elderly patients with dementia-related psychosis. Ziprasidone is not approved for this indication.

May result in QT_c prolongation (dose related), which has been associated with the development of malignant ventricular arrhythmias (torsade de pointes) and sudden death. Note contraindications related to this effect. Observed prolongation was greater than with other atypical antipsychotic agents (risperidone, olanzapine, quetiapine), but less than with thioridazine. Avoid hypokalemia, hypomagnesemia. Use caution in patients with bradycardia. Discontinue in patients found to have persistent QT_c intervals >500 msec. Patients with symptoms of dizziness, palpitations, or syncope should receive further cardiac evaluation. May cause orthostatic hypotension.

May cause extrapyramidal symptoms (EPS). Risk of dystonia (and probably other EPS) may be greater with increased doses, use of conventional antipsychotics, males, and younger patients. Impaired core body temperature regulation may occur; caution with strenuous exercise, heat exposure, dehydration, and concomitant medication possessing anticholinergic effects; not reported in premarketing trials of ziprasidone. Antipsychotic use may also be associated with neuroleptic malignant syndrome (NMS). Use with caution in patients at risk of seizures.

Atypical antipsychotics have been associated with development of hyperglycemia. There is limited documentation with ziprasidone and specific risk associated with this agent is not known. Use caution in patients with diabetes or other disorders of glucose regulation; monitor for worsening of glucose control.

Cognitive and/or motor impairment (sedation) is common with ziprasidone. Use with caution in disorders where CNS depression is a feature. Use with caution in Parkinson's disease. Antipsychotic use has been associated with esophageal dysmotility and aspiration; use with caution in patients at risk of pneumonia (ie, Alzheimer's disease). Caution in breast cancer or other prolactin-dependent tumors; elevates prolactin levels. Use caution in renal or hepatic impairment. Ziprasidone has been associated with a fairly high incidence of rash (5%). Significant weight gain has been observed with antipsychotic therapy; incidence varies with product. Monitor waist circumference and BMI. Safety and efficacy have not been established in pediatric patients.

The possibility of a suicide attempt is inherent in psychotic illness or bipolar disorder; use caution in high-risk patients during initiation of therapy. Prescriptions should be written for the smallest quantity consistent with good patient care.

Adverse Reactions Note: Although minor QT_c prolongation (mean: 10 msec at 160 mg/day) may occur more frequently (incidence not specified), clinically-relevant prolongation (>500 msec) was rare (0.06%) and less than placebo (0.23%).

>10%:

Central nervous system: Extrapyramidal symptoms (2% to 31%), somnolence (8% to 31%), headache (3% to 18%), dizziness (3% to 16%)

Gastrointestinal: Nausea (4% to 12%)

1% to 10%:

Cardiovascular: Chest pain (5%), postural hypotension (5%), hypertension (2% to 3%), bradycardia (2%), tachycardia (2%), vasodilation (1%), facial edema, orthostatic hypotension

Central nervous system: Akathisia (2% to 10%), anxiety (2% to 5%), insomnia (3%), agitation (2%), speech disorder (2%), personality disorder (2%), psychosis (1%), akinesia, amnesia, ataxia, chills, confusion, coordination abnormal, delirium, dystonia, fever, hostility, hypothermia, oculogyric crisis, vertigo

Dermatologic: Rash (4%), fungal dermatitis (2%)

Endocrine & metabolic: Dysmenorrhea (2%)

Gastrointestinal: Weight gain (10%), constipation (2% to 9%), dyspepsia (1% to 8%), diarrhea (3% to 5%), vomiting (3% to 5%), salivation increased (4%), xerostomia (1% to 5%), tongue edema (3%), abdominal pain (2%), anorexia (2%), dysphagia (2%), rectal hemorrhage (2%), tooth disorder (1%), buccoglossal syndrome

Genitourinary: Priapism (1%)

Local: Injection site pain (7% to 9%)

Neuromuscular & skeletal: Weakness (2% to 6%), hypoesthesia (2%), myalgia (2%), paresthesia (2%), back pain (1%), cogwheel rigidity (1%), hypertonia (1%), abnormal gait, choreoathetosis, dysarthria, dyskinesia, hyper-/hypokinesia, hypotonia, neuropathy, tremor, twitching

Ocular: Vision abnormal (3% to 6%), diplopia

Respiratory: Infection (8%), rhinitis (1% to 4%), cough (3%), pharyngitis (3%), dyspnea (2%)

Miscellaneous: Diaphoresis (2%), furunculosis (2%), flu-like syndrome (1%), photosensitivity reaction, withdrawal syndrome

<1% (Limited to important or life-threatening): Akinesia, allergic reaction, angina, atrial fibrillation, ataxia, AV block (first degree), bundle branch block, cerebral infarction, cholestatic jaundice, choreoathetosis, delirium, dysarthria, dysphagia, eosinophilia, exfoliative dermatitis, galactorrhea, gout, gynecomastia, hemorrhage, hepatitis, jaundice, myocarditis, neuroleptic malignant syndrome, neuropathy, opisthotonos, photophobia, pneumonia, pulmonary embolism, QT_c prolongation >500 msec (0.06%), seizure (0.4%), sexual dysfunction (male and female), stroke, syncope (0.6%), tardive dyskinesia, tenosynovitis, thrombocytopenia, thyroiditis, torsade de pointes, torticollis, urinary retention

Metabolism/Transport Effects **Substrate** (minor) of CYP1A2, 3A4; **Inhibits** CYP2D6 (weak), 3A4 (weak)

Drug Interactions

Acetylcholinesterase Inhibitors (Central): May enhance the neurotoxic (central) effect of Antipsychotics. Severe extrapyramidal symptoms have occurred in some patients. *Risk C: Monitor therapy*

Alcohol (Ethyl): CNS Depressants may enhance the CNS depressant effect of Alcohol (Ethyl). *Risk C: Monitor therapy*

Alfuzosin: May enhance the QTc-prolonging effect of QTc-Prolonging Agents. *Risk C: Monitor therapy*

Amphetamines: Antipsychotics may diminish the stimulatory effect of Amphetamines. *Risk C: Monitor therapy*

Antifungal Agents (Azole Derivatives, Systemic): May decrease the metabolism of Ziprasidone. *Risk C: Monitor therapy*

Anti-Parkinson's Agents (Dopamine Agonist): Antipsychotics (Atypical) may diminish the therapeutic effect of Anti-Parkinson's Agents (Dopamine Agonist). *Risk D: Consider therapy modification*

CarBAMazepine: May increase the metabolism of Ziprasidone. *Risk C: Monitor therapy*

Ciprofloxacin: May enhance the QTc-prolonging effect of QTc-Prolonging Agents. *Risk C: Monitor therapy*

CNS Depressants: May enhance the adverse/toxic effect of other CNS Depressants. *Risk C: Monitor therapy*

Gadobutrol: May enhance the QTc-prolonging effect of QTc-Prolonging Agents. *Risk D: Consider therapy modification*

Lithium formulations: May enhance the neurotoxic effect of Antipsychotics. Lithium formulations may decrease the serum concentration of Antipsychotics. Specifically noted with chlorpromazine. *Risk C: Monitor therapy*

Nilotinib: May enhance the QTc-prolonging effect of QTc-Prolonging Agents. *Risk X: Avoid combination*

QTc-Prolonging Agents: May enhance the QTc-prolonging effect of Ziprasidone. The risk of a severe arrhythmia may be increased. *Risk X: Avoid combination*

Tetrabenazine: May enhance the adverse/toxic effect of Antipsychotics. *Risk C: Monitor therapy*

Thioridazine: QTc-Prolonging Agents may enhance the QTc-prolonging effect of Thioridazine. *Risk X: Avoid combination*

Ethanol/Nutrition/Herb Interactions

Ethanol: Avoid ethanol (may increase CNS depression).

Food: Administration with food increases serum levels twofold. Grapefruit juice may increase serum concentration of ziprasidone.

Herb/Nutraceutical: St John's wort may decrease serum levels of ziprasidone, due to a potential effect on CYP3A4. This has not been specifically studied. Avoid kava kava, chamomile (may increase CNS depression).

Stability

Capsule: Store at controlled room temperature of 15°C to 30°C (59°F to 86°F).

Vials for injection: Store at controlled room temperature of 15°C to 30°C (59°F to 86°F). Protect from light. Each vial should be reconstituted with 1.2 mL SWI. Shake vigorously. Will form a pale, pink solution containing 20 mg/mL ziprasidone. Following reconstitution, injection may be stored at room temperature up to 24 hours or up to 7 days if refrigerated. Protect from light.

Mechanism of Action Ziprasidone is a benzylisothiazolylpiperazine antipsychotic. The exact mechanism of action is unknown. However, *in vitro* radioligand studies show that ziprasidone has high affinity for D_2, D_3, 5-HT_{2A}, 5-HT_{1A}, 5-HT_{2C}, 5-HT_{1D}, and alpha$_1$-adrenergic; moderate affinity for histamine H_1 receptors; and no appreciable affinity for alpha$_2$-adrenergic receptors, beta-adrenergic, 5-HT_3, 5-HT_4, cholinergic, mu, sigma, or benzodiazepine receptors. Ziprasidone functions as an antagonist at the D_2, 5-HT_{2A}, and 5-HT_{1D} receptors and as an agonist at the 5-HT_{1A} receptor. Ziprasidone moderately inhibits the reuptake of serotonin and norepinephrine.

Pharmacodynamics/Kinetics

Absorption: Well absorbed

Distribution: V_d: 1.5 L/kg

Protein binding: 99%, primarily to albumin and alpha$_1$-acid glycoprotein

Metabolism: Extensively hepatic, primarily via aldehyde oxidase; less than $^1/_3$ of total metabolism via CYP3A4 and CYP1A2 (minor)

Bioavailability: Oral (with food): 60% (up to twofold increase with food); I.M.: 100%

Half-life elimination: Oral: 7 hours; I.M.: 2-5 hours

Time to peak: Oral: 6-8 hours; I.M.: ≤60 minutes

Excretion: Feces (66%) and urine (20%) as metabolites; little as unchanged drug (1% urine, 4% feces)

Clearance: 7.5 mL/minute/kg

Dosage

Children and Adolescents: Tourette's syndrome (unlabeled use): Oral: 5-40 mg/day

Adults:

- Bipolar mania: Oral: Initial: 40 mg twice daily (with food)
  - Adjustment: May increase to 60 or 80 mg twice daily on second day of treatment; average dose 40-80 mg twice daily
- Schizophrenia: Oral: Initial: 20 mg twice daily (with food)
  - Adjustment: Increases (if indicated) should be made no more frequently than every 2 days; ordinarily patients should be observed for improvement over several weeks before adjusting the dose
  - Maintenance: Range 20-100 mg twice daily; however, dosages >80 mg twice daily are generally not recommended

Acute agitation (schizophrenia): I.M.: 10 mg every 2 hours **or** 20 mg every 4 hours; maximum: 40 mg/day; oral therapy should replace I.M. administration as soon as possible

Elderly: No dosage adjustment is recommended; consider initiating at a low end of the dosage range, with slower titration

Dosage adjustment in renal impairment:

Oral: No dosage adjustment is recommended

I.M.: Cyclodextrin, an excipient in the I.M. formulation, is cleared by renal filtration; use with caution.

Ziprasidone is not removed by hemodialysis.

Dosage adjustment in hepatic impairment: No dosage adjustment is recommended

Child/Adolescent Considerations Twenty-eight children 7-17 years of age with Tourette's syndrome and chronic tic disorder were randomly assigned to ziprasidone or placebo for 56 days. Ziprasidone was initiated at 5 mg/day and titrated to a maximum of 40 mg/day (Sallee, 2000).

An open-label trial of ziprasidone in 10 children and adolescents with pervasive developmental disorder showed 50% of patients as "much improved" at the end of the study (McDougle, 2002). Study duration averaged 14 weeks (range: 6-30 weeks) with an initial ziprasidone dosage of 20 mg twice daily, titrated up to an average maintenance of 30 mg twice daily (range: 20-120 mg/day). Sedation was the most common adverse reaction and no cardiovascular events (including QT prolongation) were noted.

McDougle CJ, Kem DL, and Posey DJ, "Case Series: Use of Ziprasidone for Maladaptive Symptoms in Youths With Autism," *J Am Acad Child Adolesc Psychiatry*, 2002, 41(8):921-7.

Sallee FR, Kurlan R, Goetz CG, et al, "Ziprasidone Treatment of Children and Adolescents With Tourette's Syndrome: A Pilot Study," *J Am Acad Child Adolesc Psychiatry*, 2000, 39(3):292-9.

Administration

Oral: Administer with food.

Injection: For I.M. administration only.

Monitoring Parameters Vital signs; serum potassium and magnesium; fasting lipid profile and fasting blood glucose/Hgb A_{1c} (prior to treatment, at 3 months, then annually); BMI, personal/family history of obesity, waist circumference; blood pressure; mental status, abnormal involuntary movement scale (AIMS), extrapyramidal symptoms. Weight should be assessed prior to treatment, at 4 weeks, 8 weeks, 12 weeks, and then at quarterly intervals. Consider titrating to a different antipsychotic agent for a weight gain ≥5% of the initial weight. The value of routine ECG screening or monitoring has not been established.

Test Interactions Increased cholesterol, triglycerides, eosinophils

Additional Information The increased potential to prolong QT_c, as compared to other available antipsychotic agents, should be considered in the evaluation of available alternatives.

Dosage Forms Excipient information presented when available (limited, particularly for generics); consult specific product labeling.

Capsule, as hydrochloride: 20 mg, 40 mg, 60 mg, 80 mg

Injection, powder for reconstitution, as mesylate: 20 mg

◆ **Ziprasidone Hydrochloride** *see* Ziprasidone *on page 1698*

◆ **Ziprasidone Mesylate** *see* Ziprasidone *on page 1698*

◆ **Zithromax®** *see* Azithromycin *on page 163*

◆ **Zithromax® TRI-PAK™** *see* Azithromycin *on page 163*

◆ **Zithromax® Z-PAK®** *see* Azithromycin *on page 163*

◆ **ZM-182,780** *see* Fulvestrant *on page 698*

◆ **Zmax™** *see* Azithromycin *on page 163*

◆ **Zocor®** *see* Simvastatin *on page 1486*

◆ **Zofran®** *see* Ondansetron *on page 1180*

◆ **Zofran® ODT** *see* Ondansetron *on page 1180*

◆ **Zoladex®** *see* Goserelin *on page 735*

◆ **Zoledronate** *see* Zoledronic Acid *on page 1702*

Zoledronic Acid (zoe le DRON ik AS id)

Medication Safety Issues

Sound-alike/look-alike issues:

Zometa® may be confused with Zofran®, Zoladex®

U.S. Brand Names Reclast®; Zometa®
Canadian Brand Names Aclasta®; Zometa®
Mexican Brand Names Zometa
Index Terms CGP-42446; NSC-721517; Zoledronate
Pharmacologic Category Antidote; Bisphosphonate Derivative
Use Treatment of hypercalcemia of malignancy (albumin-corrected serum calcium ≥12 mg/dL), multiple myeloma, bone metastases of solid tumors, Paget's disease of bone; osteoporosis (to reduce the incidence of fractures in postmenopausal women with osteoporosis or to reduce the incidence of new clinical fractures in patients with low-trauma hip fracture)
Unlabeled/Investigational Use Prevention of bone loss associated with aromatase inhibitor therapy in postmenopausal women with breast cancer; prevention of bone loss associated with androgen deprivation therapy in prostate cancer
Effect on Mental Status Insomnia, anxiety, agitation, depression, and dizziness are common; may rarely cause confusion
Effect on Psychiatric Treatment Bisphosphonates have been associated with renal toxicity manifested as deterioration of renal function and potential renal failure. Use caution in patients receiving lithium. GI side effects are common; concomitant use with SSRIs may produce additive effects. May cause neutropenia; use caution with clozapine and carbamazepine.
Dosage Summary
I.V.:
Children: Dosage not established
Adults:
Zometa®: 4 mg as a single dose [hypercalcemia of malignancy] or 4 mg every 3-4 weeks [multiple myeloma or metastatic bone lesions]
Reclast®: 5 mg [Paget's disease] or 5 mg every 12 months [osteoporosis]
Dosage Forms Excipient information presented when available (limited, particularly for generics); consult specific product labeling. [CAN] = Canadian brand name
Infusion, solution [premixed]:
Aclasta® [CAN]: 5 mg (100 mL) [not available in U.S.]
Reclast®: 5 mg (100 mL)
Injection, solution:
Zometa®: 4 mg/5 mL (5 mL) [as monohydrate 4.264 mg]

◆ **Zolinza™** *see* Vorinostat *on page 1678*

Zolmitriptan (zohl mi TRIP tan)

Medication Safety Issues
Sound-alike/look-alike issues:
Zolmitriptan may be confused with SUMAtriptan
Related Information
Antimigraine Drugs: 5-HT_1 Receptor Agonists *on page 1766*
U.S. Brand Names Zomig-ZMT®; Zomig®
Canadian Brand Names Zomig®; Zomig® Nasal Spray; Zomig® Rapimelt
Mexican Brand Names Zomig
Index Terms 311C90
Pharmacologic Category Antimigraine Agent; Serotonin 5-$HT_{1B,\ 1D}$ Receptor Agonist
Generic Available No
Use Acute treatment of migraine with or without aura
Effect on Mental Status Dizziness is common, may cause drowsiness
Effect on Psychiatric Treatment Contraindicated with other serotonin agonists (SSRIs) and MAO inhibitors
Pregnancy Risk Factor C
Pregnancy Considerations There are no adequate and well-controlled studies using sumatriptan in pregnant women. Use only if potential benefit to the mother outweighs the potential risk to the fetus. In animal studies, administration was associated with embryolethality, fetal abnormalities, and pup mortality.
Lactation Excretion in breast milk unknown/use caution
Contraindications Hypersensitivity to zolmitriptan or any component of the formulation; ischemic heart disease or Prinzmetal's angina; signs or symptoms of ischemic heart disease; uncontrolled hypertension; symptomatic Wolff-Parkinson-White syndrome or arrhythmias associated with other cardiac accessory conduction pathway disorders; use with ergotamine derivatives (within 24 hours of); use within 24 hours of another 5-HT_1 agonist; concurrent

administration or within 2 weeks of discontinuing an MAO inhibitor; management of hemiplegic or basilar migraine

Warnings/Precautions Zolmitriptan is indicated only in patient populations with a clear diagnosis of migraine. Not for prophylactic treatment of migraine headaches. Cardiac events (including myocardial infarction, ventricular arrhythmia, cardiac arrest, and death) have been reported with 5-HT_1 agonist administration. Should not be given to patients who have risk factors for CAD without adequate cardiac evaluation. Patients with suspected CAD should have cardiovascular evaluation to rule out CAD before considering zolmitriptan's use; if cardiovascular evaluation negative, first dose would be safest if given in the healthcare provider's office. Periodic evaluation of those without cardiovascular disease, but with continued risk factors, should be done. Significant elevation in blood pressure, including hypertensive crisis, has also been reported. Vasospasm-related reactions have been reported other than coronary artery vasospasm. Peripheral vascular ischemia and colonic ischemia with abdominal pain and bloody diarrhea have occurred. Cerebral/subarachnoid hemorrhage and stroke have been reported with 5-HT_1 agonist administration. Use with caution in patients with hepatic impairment. Zomig-ZMT™ tablets contain phenylalanine. Symptoms of agitation, confusion, hallucinations, hyper-reflexia, myoclonus, shivering, and tachycardia (serotonin syndrome) may occur with concomitant proserotonergic drugs (ie, SSRIs/SNRIs or triptans) or agents which reduce zolmitriptan's metabolism. Concurrent use of serotonin precursors (eg, tryptophan) is not recommended. Safety and efficacy not established in patients <18 years of age.

Adverse Reactions Percentages noted from oral preparations.

1% to 10%:

Cardiovascular: Chest pain (2% to 4%), palpitation (up to 2%)

Central nervous system: Dizziness (6% to 10%), somnolence (5% to 8%), pain (2% to 3%), vertigo (≤2%)

Gastrointestinal: Nausea (4% to 9%), xerostomia (3% to 5%), dyspepsia (1% to 3%), dysphagia (≤2%)

Neuromuscular & skeletal: Paresthesia (5% to 9%), weakness (3% to 9%), warm/cold sensation (5% to 7%), hypoesthesia (1% to 2%), myalgia (1% to 2%), myasthenia (up to 2%)

Miscellaneous: Neck/throat/jaw pain (4% to 10%), diaphoresis (up to 3%), allergic reaction (up to 1%)

<1% (Limited to important or life-threatening): Anaphylactoid reaction, anaphylaxis, angina, apnea, arrhythmia, ataxia, bronchospasm, cerebral ischemia, coronary artery vasospasm, cyanosis, eosinophilia, esophagitis, gastrointestinal infarction/necrosis, hallucinations, headache, hematemesis, hypertension, hypertensive crisis, ischemic colitis, melena, miscarriage, MI, myocardial ischemia, pancreatitis, photosensitivity, QT prolongation, rash, splenic infarction, syncope, tetany, thrombocytopenia, tinnitus, ulcer, urticaria

Events related to other serotonin 5-HT_{1D} receptor agonists: Cardiac arrest, cerebral hemorrhage, peripheral vascular ischemia, stroke, subarachnoid hemorrhage, ventricular fibrillation

Metabolism/Transport Effects Substrate of CYP1A2 (minor)

Drug Interactions

Cimetidine: May increase the serum concentration of Zolmitriptan. *Risk C: Monitor therapy*

Ergot Derivatives: May enhance the vasoconstricting effect of Serotonin 5-HT1D Receptor Agonists. Serotonin 5-HT1D Receptor Agonists may enhance the vasoconstricting effect of Ergot Derivatives. *Risk X: Avoid combination*

MAO Inhibitors: May decrease the metabolism of Serotonin 5-HT1D Receptor Agonists. Management: If MAO inhibitor therapy is required, naratriptan, eletriptan or frovatriptan may be a suitable 5-HT1D agonist to employ. *Risk X: Avoid combination*

Serotonin Modulators: May enhance the adverse/toxic effect of other Serotonin Modulators. The development of serotonin syndrome may occur. *Risk D: Consider therapy modification*

Sibutramine: May enhance the serotonergic effect of Serotonin Modulators. This may cause serotonin syndrome. *Risk X: Avoid combination*

Ethanol/Nutrition/Herb Interactions Ethanol: Limit use (may have additive CNS toxicity).

Stability Store at 20°C to 25°C (68°F to 77°F). Protect from light and moisture.

Mechanism of Action Selective agonist for serotonin (5-HT_{1B} and 5-HT_{1D} receptors) in cranial arteries to cause vasoconstriction and reduce sterile inflammation associated with antidromic neuronal transmission correlating with relief of migraine

Pharmacodynamics/Kinetics

Onset of action: 0.5-1 hour

Absorption: Well absorbed

Distribution: V_d: 7 L/kg

Protein binding: 25%

Metabolism: Converted to an active N-desmethyl metabolite (2-6 times more potent than zolmitriptan)

Bioavailability: 40%

Half-life elimination: 2.8-3.7 hours

Time to peak, serum: Tablet: 1.5 hours; Orally-disintegrating tablet and nasal spray: 3 hours

Excretion: Urine (~60% to 65% total dose); feces (30% to 40%)

Dosage Oral:

Children: Safety and efficacy have not been established

Adults: Migraine:

Tablet: Initial: ≤2.5 mg at the onset of migraine headache; may break 2.5 mg tablet in half

Orally-disintegrating tablet: Initial: 2.5 mg at the onset of migraine headache

Nasal spray: Initial: 1 spray (5 mg) at the onset of migraine headache

Note: Use the lowest possible dose to minimize adverse events. If the headache returns, the dose may be repeated after 2 hours; do not exceed 10 mg within a 24-hour period. Controlled trials have not established the effectiveness of a second dose if the initial one was ineffective.

Elderly: No dosage adjustment needed but elderly patients are more likely to have underlying cardiovascular disease and should have careful evaluation of cardiovascular system before prescribing.

Dosage adjustment in renal impairment: No dosage adjustment recommended. There is a 25% reduction in zolmitriptan's clearance in patients with severe renal impairment (Cl_{cr} 5-25 mL/minute).

Dosage adjustment in hepatic impairment: Administer with caution in patients with liver disease, generally using doses <2.5 mg. Patients with moderate-to-severe hepatic impairment may have decreased clearance of zolmitriptan, and significant elevation in blood pressure was observed in some patients.

Administration Administer as soon as migraine headache starts.

Tablet: May be broken.

Orally-disintegrating tablet: Must be taken whole; do not break, crush or chew. Place on tongue and allow to dissolve. Administration with liquid is not required.

Nasal spray: Blow nose gently prior to use. After removing protective cap, instill device into nostril. Block opposite nostril; breathe in gently through nose while pressing plunger of spray device. One dose (5 mg) is equal to 1 spray in 1 nostril.

Additional Information Not recommended if the patient has risk factors for heart disease (high blood pressure, high cholesterol, obesity, diabetes, smoking, strong family history of heart disease, postmenopausal woman, or a male >40 years of age).

This agent is intended to relieve migraine, but not to prevent or reduce the number of attacks. Use only to treat an actual migraine attack.

Dosage Forms Excipient information presented when available (limited, particularly for generics); consult specific product labeling.

Solution, intranasal [spray]:

Zomig®: 5 mg/0.1 mL (0.1 mL)

Tablet:

Zomig®: 2.5 mg, 5 mg

Tablet, orally disintegrating:

Zomig-ZMT®: 2.5 mg [contains phenylalanine 2.81 mg/tablet; orange flavor]; 5 mg [contains phenylalanine 5.62 mg/tablet; orange flavor]

◆ **Zoloft®** *see* Sertraline *on page 1472*

Zolpidem (zole PI dem)

Medication Safety Issues

Sound-alike/look-alike issues:

Ambien® may be confused with Ambi 10®

Related Information

CMS: Long-Term Care Facility Thresholds *on page 1815*

Nonbenzodiazepine Anxiolytics and Hypnotics *on page 1791*

U.S. Brand Names Ambien CR®; Ambien®

Mexican Brand Names Stilnox

Index Terms Zolpidem Tartrate

Pharmacologic Category Hypnotic, Nonbenzodiazepine

Generic Available Yes: Excludes extended release

Use

Ambien®: Short-term treatment of insomnia (with difficulty of sleep onset)

Ambien CR®: Treatment of insomnia (with difficulty of sleep onset and/or sleep maintenance)

Mental Health Comment In 2007, the FDA requested that all manufacturers of sedative-hypnotic drug products revise labeling to include a greater emphasis on the risks of adverse effects. These risks include severe allergic reactions (anaphylaxis, angioedema) and complex sleep-related behaviors, which may include sleep-driving (driving while not fully awake and with no memory of the event), making phone calls, and preparing and eating food while asleep. Zolpidem may be associated with a lower potential for abuse compared to benzodiazepines.

Restrictions C-IV

An FDA-approved patient medication guide is available and must be distributed when dispensing an outpatient prescription (new or refill) where this medication is to be used without direct supervision of a healthcare provider. The guide provides information about the appropriate use of zolpidem, and discusses concerns relating to "sleep-driving" and other activities of which the patient may have no recollection.

Pregnancy Risk Factor C

Pregnancy Considerations Teratogenic effects were not observed in animal studies. Children born of mothers taking sedative/hypnotics may be at risk for withdrawal; neonatal flaccidity has been reported in infants following maternal use of sedative/hypnotics during pregnancy.

Lactation Enters breast milk/not recommended (AAP rates "compatible")

Contraindications Hypersensitivity to zolpidem or any component of the formulation

Warnings/Precautions Should be used only after evaluation of potential causes of sleep disturbance. Failure of sleep disturbance to resolve after 7-10 days may indicate psychiatric or medical illness. Hypnotics/sedatives have been associated with abnormal thinking and behavior changes including decreased inhibition, aggression, bizarre behavior, agitation, hallucinations, and depersonalization. These changes may occur unpredictably and may indicate previously unrecognized psychiatric disorders; evaluate appropriately. Sedative/hypnotics may produce withdrawal symptoms following abrupt discontinuation. Use with caution in patients with depression; worsening of depression, including suicide or suicidal ideation has been reported with the use of hypnotics. Intentional overdose may be an issue in this population. The minimum dose that will effectively treat the individual patient should be used. Prescriptions should be written for the smallest quantity consistent with good patient care. Causes CNS depression, which may impair physical and mental capabilities. Zolpidem should only be administered when the patient is able to stay in bed a full night (7-8 hours) before being active again. Effects with other sedative drugs or ethanol may be potentiated.

Use caution in patients with myasthenia gravis. Use caution in the elderly; dose adjustment recommended. Closely monitor elderly or debilitated patients for impaired cognitive or motor performance. Avoid use in patients with sleep apnea or a history of sedative-hypnotic abuse. Postmarketing studies have indicated that the use of hypnotic/sedative agents for sleep has been associated with hypersensitivity reactions including anaphylaxis as well as angioedema. An increased risk for hazardous sleep-related activities such as sleep-driving; cooking and eating food, and making phone calls while asleep have also been noted; amnesia may also occur. Discontinue treatment in patients who report a sleep-driving episode.

Use caution with respiratory disease. Use caution with hepatic impairment; dose adjustment required. Because of the rapid onset of action, administer immediately prior to bedtime or after the patient has gone to bed and is having difficulty falling asleep. Safety and efficacy have not been established in pediatric patients.

Adverse Reactions Actual frequency may be dosage form, dose, and/or age dependent

>10%: Central nervous system: Dizziness, headache, somnolence

1% to 10%:

Cardiovascular: Blood pressure increased, chest discomfort/pain, palpitation

Central nervous system: Abnormal dreams, anxiety, apathy, amnesia, ataxia, attention disturbance, body temperature increased, confusion, depersonalization, depression, disinhibition, disorientation, drowsiness, drugged feeling, euphoria, fatigue, fever, hallucinations, hypoesthesia, insomnia, memory disorder, lethargy, lightheadedness, mood swings, sleep disorder, stress

Dermatologic: Rash, urticaria, wrinkling

Endocrine & metabolic: Menorrhagia

Gastrointestinal: Abdominal discomfort, abdominal pain, abdominal tenderness, appetite disorder, constipation, diarrhea, dyspepsia, flatulence, gastroenteritis, gastroesophageal reflux, hiccup, nausea, vomiting, xerostomia

Genitourinary: Urinary tract infection

Neuromuscular & skeletal: Arthralgia, back pain, balance disorder, myalgia, neck pain, paresthesia, psychomotor retardation, tremor, weakness

Ocular: Asthenopia, blurred vision, depth perception altered, diplopia, red eye, visual disturbance

Otic: Labyrinthitis, tinnitus, vertigo

Renal: Dysuria

Respiratory: Pharyngitis, sinusitis, throat irritation, upper respiratory tract infection

Miscellaneous: Allergy, binge eating, flu-like syndrome

<1% (Limited to important or life-threatening): Agitation, anaphylaxis, angioedema, anorexia, arthritis, bronchitis, cerebrovascular disorder, cognition decreased, complex sleep-related behavior (sleep-driving, cooking or eating food, making phone calls), concentrating difficulty, constipation, cough, cystitis, diaphoresis, dysarthria, dysphagia, dyspnea, edema, emotional lability, eye irritation, falling, hepatic function abnormalities, hyperglycemia, hyper-/hypotension, illusion, leg cramps, menstrual disorder, nervousness, pallor, postural hypotension, pruritus, rhinitis, scleritis, somnambulism (sleepwalking), speech disorder, stupor, syncope, tachycardia, taste perversion, thirst, urinary incontinence, vaginitis

Metabolism/Transport Effects Substrate of CYP1A2 (minor), 2C9 (minor), 2C19 (minor), 2D6 (minor), 3A4 (major)

Drug Interactions

Alcohol (Ethyl): CNS Depressants may enhance the CNS depressant effect of Alcohol (Ethyl). *Risk C: Monitor therapy*

Antifungal Agents (Azole Derivatives, Systemic): May decrease the metabolism of Zolpidem. **Exceptions:** Miconazole. *Risk D: Consider therapy modification*

CNS Depressants: May enhance the adverse/toxic effect of other CNS Depressants. *Risk C: Monitor therapy*

CYP3A4 Inducers (Strong): May increase the metabolism of CYP3A4 Substrates. *Risk C: Monitor therapy*

CYP3A4 Inhibitors (Moderate): May decrease the metabolism of CYP3A4 Substrates. *Risk C: Monitor therapy*

CYP3A4 Inhibitors (Strong): May decrease the metabolism of CYP3A4 Substrates. *Risk D: Consider therapy modification*

Dasatinib: May increase the serum concentration of CYP3A4 Substrates. *Risk C: Monitor therapy*

Deferasirox: May decrease the serum concentration of CYP3A4 Substrates. *Risk C: Monitor therapy*

Flumazenil: May diminish the sedative effect of Hypnotics (Nonbenzodiazepine). *Risk C: Monitor therapy*

Herbs (CYP3A4 Inducers): May increase the metabolism of CYP3A4 Substrates. *Risk C: Monitor therapy*

Rifamycin Derivatives: May increase the metabolism of Zolpidem. *Risk C: Monitor therapy*

Ethanol/Nutrition/Herb Interactions

Ethanol: May enhance the adverse/toxic effects of zolpidem; avoid use.

Food: Maximum plasma concentration and bioavailability are decreased with food; time to peak plasma concentration is increased; half-life remains unchanged. Grapefruit juice may decrease the metabolism of zolpidem.

Herb/Nutraceutical: St John's wort may decrease the levels/effects of zolpidem; avoid concomitant use. In addition, concomitant use of valerian, kava kava, and gotu kola should be avoided due to the risk of increased CNS depression.

Stability Store Ambien® at controlled room temperature of 20°C to 25°C (68°F to 77°F). Store Ambien CR® at controlled room temperature of 15°C to 25°C (59°F to 77°F).

Mechanism of Action Zolpidem, an imidazopyridine hypnotic that is structurally dissimilar to benzodiazepines, enhances the activity of the inhibitory neurotransmitter, γ-aminobutyric acid (GABA), via selective agonism at the benzodiazepine-1 (BZ_1) receptor; the result is increased chloride conductance, neuronal hyperpolarization, inhibition of the action potential, and a decrease in neuronal excitability leading to sedative and hypotic effects. Because of its selectivity for the BZ_1 receptor site over the BZ_2 receptor site, zolpidem exhibits minimal anxiolytic, myorelaxant, and anticonvulsant properties (effects largely attributed to agonism at the BZ_2 receptor site).

Pharmacodynamics/Kinetics

Onset of action: 30 minutes

Duration: 6-8 hours

Absorption: Rapid

Distribution: V_d: 0.54 L/kg

Protein binding: ~93%

Metabolism: Hepatic methylation and hydroxylation via CYP3A4 (~60%), CYP2C9 (~22%), CYP1A2 (~14%), CYP2D6 (~3%), and CYP2C19 (~3%) to three inactive metabolites

Bioavailability: 70%

Half-life elimination: ~2.5 hours (range 1.4-4.5 hours); Cirrhosis: Up to 9.9 hours; Elderly: prolonged up to 32%

Time to peak, plasma: 1.6 hours; 2.2 hours with food

Excretion: Urine (48% to 67%, primarily as metabolites); feces (29% to 42%, primarily as metabolites)

Dosage Oral:

Adults:

Ambien®: 10 mg immediately before bedtime; maximum dose: 10 mg

Ambien CR®: 12.5 mg immediately before bedtime

Elderly:

Ambien®: 5 mg immediately before bedtime

Ambien CR®: 6.25 mg immediately before bedtime

Dosing adjustment in renal impairment: Dose adjustment not required; monitor closely

Hemodialysis: Not dialyzable

Dosing adjustment in hepatic impairment:

Ambien®: 5 mg

Ambien CR®: 6.25 mg

Dietary Considerations For faster sleep onset, do not administer with (or immediately after) a meal.

Administration Ingest immediately before bedtime due to rapid onset of action. Ambien CR® tablets should be swallowed whole; do not divide, crush, or chew.

Monitoring Parameters Daytime alertness; respiratory rate; behavior profile

Reference Range 80-150 ng/mL

Additional Information Causes fewer disturbances in sleep stages as compared to benzodiazepines. Time spent in sleep stages 3 and 4 are maintained; zolpidem decreases sleep latency; should not be prescribed in quantities exceeding a 1-month supply.

Dosage Forms Excipient information presented when available (limited, particularly for generics); consult specific product labeling.

Tablet, as tartrate: 5 mg, 10 mg

Ambien®: 5 mg, 10 mg

Tablet, extended release, as tartrate:

Ambien CR®: 6.25 mg, 12.5 mg

- **Zolpidem Tartrate** *see* Zolpidem *on page 1705*
- **Zometa®** *see* Zoledronic Acid *on page 1702*
- **Zomig®** *see* Zolmitriptan *on page 1703*
- **Zomig-ZMT®** *see* Zolmitriptan *on page 1703*
- **Zonalon®** *see* Doxepin *on page 502*
- **Zonegran®** *see* Zonisamide *on page 1708*

Zonisamide (zoe NIS a mide)

Medication Safety Issues

Sound-alike/look-alike issues:

Zonisamide may be confused with lacosamide

Related Information

Anticonvulsants By Seizure Type *on page 1759*

U.S. Brand Names Zonegran®

Canadian Brand Names Zonegran®

Pharmacologic Category Anticonvulsant, Miscellaneous

Generic Available Yes

Use Adjunct treatment of partial seizures in children >16 years of age and adults with epilepsy

Unlabeled/Investigational Use Bipolar disorder

Pregnancy Risk Factor C

Pregnancy Considerations Fetal abnormalities and death have been reported in animals, however, there are no studies in pregnant women. Based on limited case reports, it appears zonisamide crosses the placenta. Use during pregnancy only if the potential benefits outweigh the potential risks.

Lactation Excretion in breast milk unknown/contraindicated

Contraindications Hypersensitivity to zonisamide, sulfonamides, or any component of the formulation

Warnings/Precautions Rare, but potentially fatal sulfonamide reactions have occurred following the use of zonisamide. These reactions include Stevens-Johnson syndrome and toxic epidermal necrolysis, usually appearing within 2-16 weeks of drug initiation. Discontinue zonisamide if rash develops. Chemical similarities are present among sulfonamides, sulfonylureas, carbonic anhydrase inhibitors, thiazides, and loop diuretics (except ethacrynic acid). Use in patients with sulfonamide allergy is specifically contraindicated in product labeling, however, a risk of cross-reaction exists in patients with allergy to any of these compounds; avoid use when previous reaction has been severe.

Decreased sweating (oligohydrosis) and hyperthermia requiring hospitalization have been reported in children. Discontinue zonisamide in patients who develop acute renal failure or a significant sustained increase in creatinine/BUN concentration. Kidney stones have been reported. Use cautiously in patients with renal or hepatic dysfunction. Significant CNS effects include psychiatric symptoms, psychomotor slowing, and fatigue or somnolence. Fatigue and somnolence occur within the first month of treatment, most commonly at doses of 300-500 mg/day. Effects with other sedative drugs or ethanol may be potentiated. Abrupt withdrawal may precipitate seizures; discontinue or reduce doses gradually. Safety and efficacy in children <16 years of age has not been established.

Adverse Reactions Adjunctive therapy: Frequencies noted in patients receiving other anticonvulsants:

>10%:

Central nervous system: Somnolence (17%), dizziness (13%)

Gastrointestinal: Anorexia (13%)

1% to 10%:

Central nervous system: Headache (10%), agitation/irritability (9%), fatigue (8%), tiredness (7%), ataxia (6%), confusion (6%), concentration decreased (6%), memory impairment (6%), depression (6%), insomnia (6%), speech disorders (5%), mental slowing (4%), anxiety (3%), nervousness (2%), schizophrenic/schizophreniform behavior (2%), difficulty in verbal expression (2%), status epilepticus (1%), convulsion (1%), hyperesthesia (1%), incoordination (1%)

Dermatologic: Rash (3%), bruising (2%), pruritus (1%)

Gastrointestinal: Nausea (9%), abdominal pain (6%), diarrhea (5%), dyspepsia (3%), weight loss (3%), constipation (2%), dry mouth (2%), taste perversion (2%), vomiting (1%)

Neuromuscular & skeletal: Paresthesia (4%), abnormal gait (1%), tremor (1%), weakness (1%)

Ocular: Diplopia (6%), nystagmus (4%), amblyopia (1%)

Otic: Tinnitus (1%)

Respiratory: Rhinitis (2%), pharyngitis (1%), increased cough (1%)

Miscellaneous: Flu-like syndrome (4%) accidental injury (1%)

<1% (Limited to important or life threatening symptoms): Agranulocytosis, allergic reaction, alopecia, aplastic anemia, apnea, atrial fibrillation, bladder calculus, cholangitis, cholecystitis, cholestatic jaundice, colitis, deafness, duodenitis, dysarthria, dyskinesia, dyspnea, dystonia, encephalopathy, esophagitis, facial paralysis, gingival hyperplasia, glaucoma, gum hemorrhage, gynecomastia, heart failure, hematemesis, hemoptysis, hirsutism, hyperthermia, impotence, leukopenia, lupus erythematosus, menorrhagia, movement disorder, myoclonus, nephrolithiasis, neuropathy, oculogyric crisis, oligohydrosis, peripheral neuritis, pulmonary embolus, rash, rectal hemorrhage, Stevens-Johnson syndrome, stroke, suicidal behavior/ideation, syncope, thrombocytopenia, toxic epidermal necrolysis, urinary retention, urticaria

Metabolism/Transport Effects Substrate of CYP2C19 (minor), 3A4 (major)

Drug Interactions

Alcohol (Ethyl): CNS Depressants may enhance the CNS depressant effect of Alcohol (Ethyl). *Risk C: Monitor therapy*

CNS Depressants: May enhance the adverse/toxic effect of other CNS Depressants. *Risk C: Monitor therapy*

CYP3A4 Inducers (Strong): May increase the metabolism of CYP3A4 Substrates. *Risk C: Monitor therapy*

CYP3A4 Inhibitors (Moderate): May decrease the metabolism of CYP3A4 Substrates. *Risk C: Monitor therapy*

CYP3A4 Inhibitors (Strong): May decrease the metabolism of CYP3A4 Substrates. *Risk D: Consider therapy modification*

Dasatinib: May increase the serum concentration of CYP3A4 Substrates. *Risk C: Monitor therapy*

Deferasirox: May decrease the serum concentration of CYP3A4 Substrates. *Risk C: Monitor therapy*

Herbs (CYP3A4 Inducers): May increase the metabolism of CYP3A4 Substrates. *Risk C: Monitor therapy*

Ketorolac: May diminish the therapeutic effect of Anticonvulsants. *Risk C: Monitor therapy*

Mefloquine: May diminish the therapeutic effect of Anticonvulsants. Mefloquine may decrease the serum concentration of Anticonvulsants. Management: Mefloquine is contraindicated in persons with a history of convulsions. If anticonvulsant is being used for another indication monitor response to treatment closely, as concurrent mefloquine may decrease response to treatment. *Risk D: Consider therapy modification*

Phenytoin: May increase the metabolism of Zonisamide. *Risk C: Monitor therapy*

Ethanol/Nutrition/Herb Interactions

Ethanol: Avoid ethanol (may increase CNS depression).

Food: Food delays time to maximum concentration, but does not affect bioavailability.

Stability Store at controlled room temperature 25°C (77°F). Protect from moisture and light.

Mechanism of Action The exact mechanism of action is not known. May stabilize neuronal membranes and suppress neuronal hypersynchronization through action at sodium and calcium channels. Does not affect GABA activity.

Pharmacodynamics/Kinetics

Distribution: V_d: 1.45 L/kg

Protein binding: 40%

Metabolism: Hepatic via CYP3A4; forms N-acetyl zonisamide and 2-sulfamoylacetyl phenol (SMAP)

Half-life elimination: 63 hours

Time to peak: 2-6 hours

Excretion: Urine (62%, 35% as unchanged drug, 65% as metabolites); feces (3%)

Dosage Oral:

Children >16 years and Adults:

Adjunctive treatment of partial seizures: Initial: 100 mg/day; dose may be increased to 200 mg/day after 2 weeks. Further dosage increases to 300 mg/day and 400 mg/day can then be made with a minimum of 2 weeks between adjustments, in order to reach steady state at each dosage level. Doses of up to 600 mg/day have been studied, however, there is no evidence of increased response with doses above 400 mg/day.

Mania (unlabeled use): Initial: 100-200 mg/day; maximum: 600 mg/day (Kanba, 1994)

Elderly: Data from clinical trials is insufficient for patients >65 years; begin dosing at the low end of the dosing range.

Dosage adjustment in renal/hepatic impairment: Slower titration and frequent monitoring are indicated in patients with renal or hepatic disease. There is insufficient experience regarding dosing/toxicity in patients with estimated GFR <50 mL/minute. Marked renal impairment (Cl_{cr} <20 mL/minute) was associated with a 35% increase in AUC.

Dietary Considerations May be taken with or without food.

Administration Capsules should be swallowed whole. Dose may be administered once or twice daily. Doses of 300 mg/day and higher are associated with increased side effects. Steady-state levels are reached in 14 days.

Monitoring Parameters Monitor BUN and serum creatinine

Dosage Forms Excipient information presented when available (limited, particularly for generics); consult specific product labeling.

Capsule: 25 mg, 50 mg, 100 mg

Zonegran®: 25 mg, 100 mg

Zopiclone (ZOE pi clone)

Canadian Brand Names Apo-Zopiclone®; CO Zopiclone; Dom-Zopiclone; Gen-Zopiclone; Imovane®; Novo-Zopiclone; Nu-Zopiclone; PMS-Zopiclone; RAN™-Zopiclone; ratio-Zopiclone; Rhovane®; Rhoxal-zopiclone; Riva-Zopiclone; Sandoz-Zopiclone

Mexican Brand Names Imovane

Pharmacologic Category Hypnotic, Nonbenzodiazepine

Generic Available Yes

Use Symptomatic relief of transient and short-term insomnia

Restrictions Not available in U.S.

Pregnancy Risk Factor Not assigned; similar agents rated D

Pregnancy Considerations There is insufficient data on safety in pregnancy; however, benzodiazepines may cause congenital malformations during the 1st trimester and neonatal CNS depression during the last few weeks of pregnancy; it is expected zopiclone may do the same.

Lactation Enters breast milk/not recommended

Contraindications Hypersensitivity to zopiclone or any component of the formulation; patients with severe respiratory impairment (eg, sleep apnea); pregnancy (similar agents)

Warnings/Precautions Causes CNS depression; use with caution in patients who previously manifested paradoxical reactions to ethanol or other sedatives. Symptomatic treatment of insomnia should be initiated only after careful evaluation of potential causes of sleep disturbance. Failure of sleep disturbance to resolve after 7-10 days may indicate psychiatric and/or medical illness; should not be administered for more than 7-10 days consecutively. Use with caution in elderly patients and in patients with hepatic dysfunction, severe pulmonary insufficiency, and depression. Amnesia can occur; do not take unless a full night's sleep and clearance of the drug from the body are possible. Hypnotics/sedatives have been associated with abnormal thinking and behavior changes including decreased inhibition, aggression, bizarre behavior, agitation, hallucinations, and depersonalization. These changes may occur unpredictably and may indicate previously unrecognized psychiatric disorders; evaluate appropriately. Elderly are more susceptible to adverse reactions. May cause dependence; withdrawal symptoms can occur with abrupt discontinuation; the risk of dependence is increased in patients with a history of alcoholism and drug abuse. Use with caution in patients taking strong CYP3A4 inhibitors. Because of the rapid onset of action, administer immediately prior to bedtime or after the patient has gone to bed and is having difficulty falling asleep. Not recommended for use in patients <18 years of age.

Adverse Reactions Frequency not defined.

Cardiovascular: Palpitations

Central nervous system: Agitation, anterograde amnesia, anxiety, asthenia, chills, confusion, depression, dizziness, drowsiness, euphoria, headache, hostility, memory impairment, nervousness, nightmares, somnolence, speech abnormalities

Dermatological: Rash, spots on skin

Endocrine & metabolic: Anorexia; libido decreased; alkaline phosphatase, ALT, and AST increased; appetite increased

Gastrointestinal: Constipation, coated tongue, diarrhea, dry mouth, dyspepsia, halitosis, nausea, taste alteration (bitter taste, common), vomiting

Neuromuscular & skeletal: Coordination impaired, hypotonia, limb heaviness, muscle spasms, paresthesia, tremor

Ocular: Amblyopia

Respiratory: Dyspnea

Miscellaneous: Diaphoresis

Metabolism/Transport Effects Substrate (major) of CYP2C9, 3A4

Drug Interactions

Alcohol (Ethyl): CNS Depressants may enhance the CNS depressant effect of Alcohol (Ethyl). *Risk C: Monitor therapy*

CNS Depressants: May enhance the adverse/toxic effect of other CNS Depressants. *Risk C: Monitor therapy*

CYP2C9 Inducers (Highly Effective): May increase the metabolism of CYP2C9 Substrates (High risk). *Risk C: Monitor therapy*

CYP2C9 Inhibitors (Moderate): May decrease the metabolism of CYP2C9 Substrates (High risk). *Risk C: Monitor therapy*

CYP2C9 Inhibitors (Strong): May decrease the metabolism of CYP2C9 Substrates (High risk). *Risk D: Consider therapy modification*

CYP3A4 Inducers (Strong): May increase the metabolism of CYP3A4 Substrates. *Risk C: Monitor therapy*

CYP3A4 Inhibitors (Moderate): May decrease the metabolism of CYP3A4 Substrates. *Risk C: Monitor therapy*

CYP3A4 Inhibitors (Strong): May decrease the metabolism of CYP3A4 Substrates. *Risk D: Consider therapy modification*

Dasatinib: May increase the serum concentration of CYP3A4 Substrates. *Risk C: Monitor therapy*

Deferasirox: May decrease the serum concentration of CYP3A4 Substrates. *Risk C: Monitor therapy*

Flumazenil: May diminish the sedative effect of Hypnotics (Nonbenzodiazepine). *Risk C: Monitor therapy*

Herbs (CYP3A4 Inducers): May increase the metabolism of CYP3A4 Substrates. *Risk C: Monitor therapy*

Macrolide Antibiotics: May increase the serum concentration of Zopiclone. **Exceptions:** Azithromycin; Dirithromycin [Off Market]; Spiramycin. *Risk D: Consider therapy modification*

Ethanol/Nutrition/Herb Interactions

Ethanol: Avoid ethanol (may increase CNS depression).

Food: Effect/toxicity may be increased by grapefruit juice; avoid concurrent use.

Herb/Nutraceutical: St John's wort may decrease levels. Avoid valerian, St John's wort, kava kava, gotu kola (may increase CNS depression).

Stability Store at room temperature of 15°C to 30°C (59°F to 86°F) in a dry place. Protect from light.

Mechanism of Action Zopiclone is a cyclopyrrolone derivative and has a pharmacological profile similar to benzodiazepines. Zopiclone reduces sleep latency, increases duration of sleep, and decreases the number of nocturnal awakenings.

Pharmacodynamics/Kinetics

Absorption: Elderly: 75% to 94%

Distribution: Rapidly from vascular compartment

Protein binding: ~45%

Metabolism: Extensively hepatic

Half-life elimination: 5 hours; Elderly: 7 hours; Hepatic impairment: 11.9 hours

Time to peak, serum: <2 hours; Hepatic impairment: 3.5 hours

Excretion: Urine (75%); feces (16%)

Dosage Administer just before bedtime: Oral:

Adults: 5-7.5 mg

Patients with chronic respiratory insufficiency: 3.75 mg; may increase up to 7.5 mg with caution in appropriate cases

Elderly: Initial: 3.75 mg; may increase to 5-7.5 mg

Dosage adjustment in hepatic impairment: 3.75 mg; may increase up to 7.5 mg with caution in appropriate cases

Administration Administer just before bedtime.

Monitoring Parameters Monitor for confusion, excessive drowsiness (especially in elderly). Monitor patients with hepatic insufficiency closely.

Additional Information Not available in U.S.

Dosage Forms Excipient information presented when available (limited, particularly for generics); consult specific product labeling. [CAN] = Canadian brand name

Tablet: 5 mg, 7.5 mg [not available in the U.S.]

Apo-Zopiclone® [CAN], Gen-Zopiclone [CAN], Imovane® [CAN], Novo-Zopiclone [CAN], Nu-Zopiclone [CAN], PMS-Zopiclone [CAN], Rhovane® [CAN], Rhoxal-zopiclone [CAN]: 5 mg, 7.5 mg

- ◆ **Zorbtive®** *see* Somatropin *on page 1499*
- ◆ **ZORprin®** *see* Aspirin *on page 143*
- ◆ **Zosyn®** *see* Piperacillin and Tazobactam Sodium *on page 1302*
- ◆ **Zovia®** *see* Ethinyl Estradiol and Ethynodiol Diacetate *on page 594*
- ◆ **Zovirax®** *see* Acyclovir *on page 49*
- ◆ **Ztuss™ Tablet [DSC]** *see* Hydrocodone, Pseudoephedrine, and Guaifenesin *on page 784*
- ◆ **Ztuss™ ZT [DSC]** *see* Hydrocodone and Guaifenesin *on page 779*

Zuclopenthixol (zoo kloe pen THIX ol)

Related Information

Discontinuation of Psychotropic Drugs *on page 1839*

Canadian Brand Names Clopixol-Acuphase®; Clopixol®; Clopixol® Depot

Mexican Brand Names Clopixol; Clopixol Acuphase; Clopixol Depot

Index Terms Z-chlopenthixol; Zuclopenthixol Acetate; Zuclopenthixol Decanoate; Zuclopenthixol Dihydrochloride

Pharmacologic Category Antipsychotic Agent, Typical

Generic Available No

Use Management of schizophrenia; acetate injection is intended for short-term acute treatment; decanoate injection is for long-term management; dihydrochloride tablets may be used in either phase

Unlabeled/Investigational Use Bipolar disorder, psychoses; agitated states

Mental Health Comment Older antipsychotic medications (chlorpromazine, haloperidol), which do not meet specific criteria for "atypical" antipsychotics, are often referred to as typical antipsychotics. They are associated with the troubling side effect, EPS. However, it is commonly believed that in order for a drug to treat psychosis, it must block dopamine is some manner.

Common side effects include sedation and neuroleptic effect (reduced initiative, interest in the environment, and display of emotion or affect). All **typical** antipsychotics are considered to be equally effective if given in equipotent doses. An inverse relationship exists between intrinsic antimuscarinic activity and propensity to cause extrapyramidal side effects. If dystonia or pseudoparkinsonism occurs, antiparkinsonian agents should be considered. If akathisia occurs, beta-blockers (eg, propranolol), benzodiazepines, or antiparkinsonian agents should be considered. Tardive dyskinesia (TD) secondary to typical antipsychotics has an estimated incidence of 3% to 5% per year for the first 5 years of treatment. After this time period, the incidence is estimated to be 2% to 3% per year. Prevalence rates are ~15% to 20%. Female gender and age constitute risk factors for TD. Indeed, prevalence rates have been reported to be as high as 70% in elderly females. No specific treatment exists for TD, however, patients are often initiated on/switched to an atypical antipsychotic because of their lower incidence to cause TD and hopes of suppression.

Typical antipsychotics are usually only indicated for schizophrenia, but are generally effective for mania and psychosis and/or behavioral syndromes secondary to other mental conditions. Nonpsychiatric uses include Tourette's syndrome, Huntington's disease, and occasionally, intractable hiccups, pruritus, nausea, and vomiting.

These drugs are thought to exert their antipsychotic activity by blocking dopamine D_2 receptors in the mesolimbic dopaminergic pathway. Side effects are often related to their ability to antagonize dopamine receptors in the nigrostriatal and tuberoinfundibular pathways.

Coadministration of two or more antipsychotics does not generally improve clinical response and may increase the potential for adverse effects.

In 2008, the FDA issued a warning regarding increased mortality risk with typical **and** atypical antipsychotic drugs when used in elderly patients with dementia-related psychosis.

Restrictions Not available in U.S.

Pregnancy Risk Factor C

Lactation Enters breast milk/not recommended

Contraindications Hypersensitivity to zuclopenthixol, thioxanthenes, or any component of the formulation; acute intoxication (ethanol, barbiturate, or opioid); severe CNS depression; coma; suspected or established subcortical brain damage; circulatory collapse; blood dyscrasias; pheochromocytoma

Warnings/Precautions Elderly patients with dementia-related psychosis treated with antipsychotics are at an increased risk of death compared to placebo. An increased incidence of cerebrovascular adverse events (including fatalities) has been reported in elderly patients with dementia-related psychosis. Zuclopenthixol is not approved for this indication.

May alter cardiac conduction; life-threatening arrhythmias have occurred with therapeutic doses of antipsychotics. Avoid use in patients with underlying QT prolongation, in those taking medicines that prolong the QT interval, or cause polymorphic ventricular tachycardia; monitor ECG closely for dose-related QT effects. Adverse effects of decanoate may be prolonged. Myelosuppression (eg, leukopenia, agranulocytosis) has been observed with antipsychotic use; check blood counts periodically and discontinue at first signs of blood dyscrasias; use is contraindicated in patients with bone marrow suppression. Antipsychotic use has been associated with esophageal dysmotility and aspiration; use with caution in patients at risk of pneumonia (ie, Alzheimer's disease). May cause extrapyramidal symptoms (EPS), including pseudoparkinsonism, acute dystonic reactions, akathisia, and tardive dyskinesia (risk of these reactions is high relative to other neuroleptics). Risk of dystonia (and possibly other EPS) may be greater with increased doses, use of conventional antispychotics, males, and younger patients. Use may be associated with NMS; monitor for mental status changes, fever, muscle rigidity, and/or autonomic instability (risk may be increased in patients with Parkinson's disease or Lewy body dementia). May cause orthostatic hypotension; use with caution in patients at risk of this effect or in those who would not tolerate transient hypotensive episodes (cerebrovascular disease, cardiovascular disease, hypovolemia, or concurrent medication use which may predispose to hypotension/bradycardia). May be associated with pigmentary retinopathy. May be sedating, use with caution in disorders where CNS depression is a feature; patients must be cautioned about performing tasks which require mental alertness (eg, operating machinery or driving). Impaired core body temperature regulation may occur; caution with strenuous exercise, heat exposure, dehydration, and concomitant medication possessing anticholinergic effects.

May be sedating, use with caution in disorders where CNS depression is a feature; patients must be cautioned about performing tasks which require mental alertness (eg, operating machinery or driving). May cause anticholinergic effects (constipation, xerostomia, blurred vision, urinary retention); use with caution in patients with decreased gastrointestinal motility, paralytic ileus, urinary retention, BPH, xerostomia, or visual problems. Relative to other neuroleptics, zuclopenthixol has a low potency of cholinergic blockade. May mask toxicity of other drugs or conditions (eg, intestinal obstruction, Reye's syndrome, brain tumor) due to antiemetic effects.

Use with caution in patients with severe cardiovascular disease, narrow-angle glaucoma, hepatic impairment, myasthenia gravis, Parkinson's disease, breast cancer or other prolactin-dependent tumors, renal impairment, respiratory disease, or seizure disorder. Safety and efficacy have not been established in children.

Adverse Reactions

>10%:

Central nervous system: Somnolence/drowsiness (32%), anxiety/nervousness (17%), insomnia (16%), akathisia (14%), extrapyramidal effects (13%), dizziness (11%)

Gastrointestinal: Xerostomia (15%)

Endocrine & metabolic: Libido decreased (3%), menstrual disorder (2%)

Neuromuscular & skeletal: Hypertonia (19%), tremor (19%), weakness (15%)

1% to 10%:

Central nervous system: Agitation (10%), depression (8%), concentration impaired (8%), headache (5%), vertigo (5%), dystonia (5%), tardive dyskinesia (3%), paresthesia (1%), hallucinations (3%), apathy (3%), confusion (3%), amnesia (3%), abnormal dreams (2%)

Dermatologic: Seborrhea (2%), pruritus (up to 2%)

Gastrointestinal: Constipation (8%), salivation increased (8%), anorexia (4%), vomiting (3%), nausea (2%)

Genitourinary: Micturition disorder (3%)

Neuromuscular & skeletal: Hypokinesia (8%), abnormal gait (2%), myalgia (1%)

Ocular: Abnormal accommodation (6%), abnormal vision (4%)

Miscellaneous: Diaphoresis increased (3%)

<1% (Limited to important or life-threatening): Abdominal pain, agranulocytosis, allergic reaction, anorgasmia, apnea, ataxia, chest pain, corneal deposits, dysphagia, dyspnea, dyskinesia, erectile dysfunction, galactorrhea, glossitis, gynecomastia, hypotension, migraine, oculogyric crisis, neuroleptic malignant syndrome (NMS), paroniria, photosensitivity, purpura, rash, respiratory depression, seizure, speech disorder, tinnitus

Metabolism/Transport Effects Substrate of CYP2D6 (major)

Drug Interactions

Acetylcholinesterase Inhibitors (Central): May enhance the neurotoxic (central) effect of Antipsychotics. Severe extrapyramidal symptoms have occurred in some patients. *Risk C: Monitor therapy*

Alcohol (Ethyl): CNS Depressants may enhance the CNS depressant effect of Alcohol (Ethyl). *Risk C: Monitor therapy*

Alfuzosin: May enhance the QTc-prolonging effect of QTc-Prolonging Agents. *Risk C: Monitor therapy*

Amphetamines: Antipsychotics may diminish the stimulatory effect of Amphetamines. *Risk C: Monitor therapy*

Anticholinergics: May enhance the adverse/toxic effect of other Anticholinergics. **Exceptions:** Paliperidone. *Risk C: Monitor therapy*

Anti-Parkinson's Agents (Dopamine Agonist): Antipsychotics (Typical) may diminish the therapeutic effect of Anti-Parkinson's Agents (Dopamine Agonist). *Risk D: Consider therapy modification*

Ciprofloxacin: May enhance the QTc-prolonging effect of QTc-Prolonging Agents. *Risk C: Monitor therapy*

CNS Depressants: May enhance the adverse/toxic effect of other CNS Depressants. *Risk C: Monitor therapy*

CYP2D6 Inhibitors (Moderate): May decrease the metabolism of CYP2D6 Substrates. *Risk C: Monitor therapy*

CYP2D6 Inhibitors (Strong): May decrease the metabolism of CYP2D6 Substrates. *Risk D: Consider therapy modification*

Darunavir: May increase the serum concentration of CYP2D6 Substrates. *Risk C: Monitor therapy*

Gadobutrol: May enhance the QTc-prolonging effect of QTc-Prolonging Agents. *Risk D: Consider therapy modification*

Lithium formulations: May enhance the neurotoxic effect of Antipsychotics. Lithium formulations may decrease the serum concentration of Antipsychotics. Specifically noted with chlorpromazine. *Risk C: Monitor therapy*

Nilotinib: May enhance the QTc-prolonging effect of QTc-Prolonging Agents. *Risk X: Avoid combination*

Pramlintide: May enhance the anticholinergic effect of Anticholinergics. These effects are specific to the GI tract. *Risk D: Consider therapy modification*

QTc-Prolonging Agents: May enhance the adverse/toxic effect of other QTc-Prolonging Agents. Their effects can be additive, causing life-threatening ventricular arrhythmias. *Risk D: Consider therapy modification*

Tetrabenazine: May enhance the adverse/toxic effect of Antipsychotics. *Risk C: Monitor therapy*

Thioridazine: QTc-Prolonging Agents may enhance the QTc-prolonging effect of Thioridazine. *Risk X: Avoid combination*

Ziprasidone: QTc-Prolonging Agents may enhance the QTc-prolonging effect of Ziprasidone. The risk of a severe arrhythmia may be increased. *Risk X: Avoid combination*

Ethanol/Nutrition/Herb Interactions

Ethanol: Avoid ethanol (may increase CNS depression).

Herb/Nutraceutical: Avoid dong quai, St John's wort (may also cause photosensitization). Avoid kava kava, gotu kola, valerian, St John's wort (may increase CNS depression).

Stability Store at 20°C to 25°C (68°F to 77°F); do not freeze. Protect all dosage forms from light. Acuphase® and depot injections may be mixed together in the same syringe. Clear or slightly yellow solutions may be used. Dispense in amber or opaque vials/bottles.

Mechanism of Action Zuclopenthixol is a thioxanthene antipsychotic with a piperazine side chain; related to fluphenazine, the cis(z)-clopenthixol is the active isomer of this neuroleptic; blocks postsynaptic dopaminergic brain receptors.

Pharmacodynamics/Kinetics

Onset of action: Acetate injection: Sedation within 2 hours

Duration: Acetate injection: 2-3 days; Decanoate injection: 2 weeks

Distribution: V_d: 15-20 L/kg

Metabolism: Hepatic via N-dealkylation

Half-life elimination: Terminal: Oral: 20 hours; Depot: 19 days

Time to peak: Acetate injection: 24-36 hours; Dihydrochloride tablet: 3 hours; Depot: 3-7 days

Dosage Adults:

Oral: Zuclopenthixol dihydrochloride: Initial: 20-30 mg/day in 2-3 divided doses; usual maintenance dose: 20-40 mg/day; maximum daily dose: 100 mg

I.M.:

Zuclopenthixol acetate: 50-150 mg; may be repeated in 2-3 days; no more than 4 injections should be given in the course of treatment; maximum dose during course of treatment: 400 mg (maximum treatment period: 2 weeks)

Transfer of patients from I.M. acetate (Acuphase®) to oral (tablets):

50 mg = 20 mg daily

100 mg = 40 mg daily

150 mg = 60 mg daily

Zuclopenthixol decanoate: 100 mg by deep I.M. injection; additional I.M. doses of 100-200 mg may be given over the following 1-4 weeks; maximum weekly dose: 600 mg; usual maintenance dose: 150-300 mg every 2 weeks

Transfer of patients from oral (tablets) to I.M. decanoate (depot):

≤20 mg daily = 100 mg every 2 weeks

25-40 mg daily = 200 mg every 2 weeks

50-75 mg daily = 300 mg every 2 weeks

>75 mg/day = 400 mg every 2 weeks

Transfer of patients from I.M. acetate (Acuphase®) to I.M. decanoate (depot):

50 mg every 2-3 days = 100 mg every 2 weeks

100 mg every 2-3 days = 200 mg every 2 weeks
150 mg every 2-3 days = 300 mg every 2 weeks

Monitoring Parameters Vital signs; lipid profile, fasting blood glucose/Hgb A_{1c}; BMI; mental status, abnormal involuntary movement scale (AIMS), extrapyramidal symptoms (EPS)

Reference Range Therapeutic z-clopenthixol serum levels are 2-12 ng/mL; ingestion of 2.5 g resulted in a peak blood level of 900 ng/mL

Additional Information Not available in U.S.

Dosage Forms Excipient information presented when available (limited, particularly for generics); consult specific product labeling. [CAN] = Canadian brand name

Injection, as acetate:

Clopixol Acuphase® [CAN]: 50 mg/mL [zuclopenthixol 42.5 mg/mL] (1 mL, 2 mL) [not available in the U.S.]

Injection, as decanoate:

Clopixol® Depot [CAN]: 200 mg/mL [zuclopenthixol 144.4 mg/mL] (10 mL) [not available in the U.S.]

Tablet, as dihydrochloride:

Clopixol® [CAN]: 10 mg, 25 mg, 40 mg [not available in the U.S.]

◆ **Zuclopenthixol Acetate** *see* Zuclopenthixol *on page 1712*
◆ **Zuclopenthixol Decanoate** *see* Zuclopenthixol *on page 1712*
◆ **Zuclopenthixol Dihydrochloride** *see* Zuclopenthixol *on page 1712*
◆ **Zyban®** *see* BuPROPion *on page 217*
◆ **Zydone®** *see* Hydrocodone and Acetaminophen *on page 777*
◆ **Zyflo® [DSC]** *see* Zileuton *on page 1696*
◆ **Zyflo CR™** *see* Zileuton *on page 1696*
◆ **Zyloprim®** *see* Allopurinol *on page 67*
◆ **Zymar®** *see* Gatifloxacin *on page 709*
◆ **Zymine®-D** *see* Triprolidine and Pseudoephedrine *on page 1634*
◆ **Zyprexa®** *see* OLANZapine *on page 1160*
◆ **Zyprexa Zydis** *see* OLANZapine *on page 1160*
◆ **Zyprexa® Zydis®** *see* OLANZapine *on page 1160*
◆ **Zyrtec® [OTC]** *see* Cetirizine *on page 307*
◆ **Zyrtec-D 12 Hour® [DSC]** *see* Cetirizine and Pseudoephedrine *on page 309*
◆ **Zyrtec® Allergy [OTC]** *see* Cetirizine *on page 307*
◆ **Zyrtec®, Children's Allergy [OTC]** *see* Cetirizine *on page 307*
◆ **Zyrtec®, Children's Hives Relief [OTC]** *see* Cetirizine *on page 307*
◆ **Zytopic™** *see* Triamcinolone *on page 1617*
◆ **Zytrec-D® Allergy & Congestion [OTC]** *see* Cetirizine and Pseudoephedrine *on page 309*
◆ **Zyvox®** *see* Linezolid *on page 927*

PSYCHIATRIC SPECIAL TOPICS

TABLE OF CONTENTS

Psychiatric Assessment
Psychiatric Assessment - General Patient.. 1718
Psychiatric Assessment - Rating Scales... 1720

Diagnostic & Statistical Manual of Mental Disorders (DSM-IV)
Diagnostic and Statistical Manual of Mental Disorders (DSM-IV)............... 1729

PSYCHIATRIC ASSESSMENT - GENERAL PATIENT

Evaluation of a patient with a psychiatric disorder is similar to other medical assessments. The evaluation should include a comprehensive medical and psychiatric history including family psychiatric history, medication, allergies, and review of systems. Collateral history from family members is often crucial in furnishing information that the patient may be unable to provide. History of response to previous treatment is essential in cases where pharmacologic therapy is to be initiated. Basic physical evaluations include physical/neurologic exam and laboratory testing including blood chemistries, blood counts, endocrine, hepatic, and other specialized evaluations as indicated. Imaging or lumbar puncture may be indicated in some cases for ruling out neurological or medical diagnoses.

An outline of components of the comprehensive psychiatric assessment is described below.

1. History of present illness: Include patient's age, sex, race, past psychiatric diagnosis, and current presenting problems including duration and history of onset
2. Past psychiatric history: Include previous psychiatric diagnoses, treatments, hospitalizations, and drug therapies
3. Family psychiatric history: Include history of alcoholism, substance abuse, and any suspected psychiatric disorders
4. Past/current medical history: Include all medical/neurologic disorders, treatments, hospitalizations, surgeries, and medications. For women, obtain gynecological history including last menstrual period (rule out pregnancy).
5. Allergies
6. Developmental history: Include birth history, childhood history (including query for childhood abuse), educational level, and significant traumatic events (eg, loss of parent)
7. Social history: Include marital status, employment history, and level of impairment associated with psychiatric disorder
8. Substance abuse history
9. Review of systems
10. Laboratory data as needed; include pregnancy testing for women of childbearing potential
11. Other specialized studies: EEG, MRI, CT, etc as needed
12. Physical exam (unless done recently, should be obtained; required for acute mental status change)
13. Mental status exam: Includes:
    a. General impression: Appearance, state of self care, eye contact, etc
    b. Speech: Note rate, rhythm, coherence
    c. Affect
    d. Cognition: Include gross awareness of person, place, time, concentration, memory, and recall; may require specialized testing if impairment exists
    e. Mood
    f. Risk assessment: Include potential risk of harm to self or others
    g. Perceptual disturbances, such as hallucinations
    h. Thought form: Assess for loosening of associations, formal thought disorder
    i. Thought content: Include delusions/paranoia
    j. Insight: Include determination of patient appreciation of the disorder, its impairing effects, and awareness of risk to self or others
    k. Judgment: In particular judgment based on patient's current status
    l. Psychometric testing as needed
    m. Differential diagnosis and preliminary diagnosis
    n. Treatment plan: Include pharmacotherapy, psychotherapy, additional referrals (eg, marital therapy), nutritional counseling, substance abuse treatment, psychosocial rehabilitation, and other interventions as needed

Most components of the assessment may be done at first patient visit, or shortly thereafter, although some, such as psychometric testing or specialized studies such as EEG, may require more time. Most importantly, the psychiatric diagnosis (and attendant treatments) should not be considered fixed and unchangeable as additional later obtained history may shed insight onto diagnosis (eg, previous "highs" which may clarify a diagnosis of bipolar illness). In acute clinical situations, treatments may be initiated before diagnosis is completely clear, as in the case of the agitated, psychotic patient who is prescribed antipsychotic medication as a full diagnostic assessment is underway.

PSYCHIATRIC ASSESSMENT - RATING SCALES

WHAT RATING SCALES MEASURE

Health assessments measure a variety of components of health. Some are functional measures which focus on the diagnosis, prognosis, and evaluation methods of different illnesses. For example, the measurement of the blood pressure is a health measure that has diagnostic value. Prognostic measures such as Apgar scores or IQ can give us information about expectation of an individual's future health, while some evaluative indices can help to look at the changes that happened with time.

Other health measurements have to do with the topic domains. For example, they are concerned with a particular organ, organ system, or with a disorder. They can be specific, generic, broad spectrum, or classified according to the method used, such as questionnaires or rating scales. In a rating scale, an interviewer, usually a clinician trained in how to use the scale, assesses different aspects of health utilizing an open clinical interview or an interview with different degrees of structure, but finally making the determination depending on his/her clinical experience.

Most of the scales used in psychiatric research are *ordinal* scales in which numbers are used as labels for different categories reflecting an increased order for the item being measured. For instance: 0 = normal, 1 = slight, 2 = mild, 3 = moderate, 4 = severe. This system has the shortcoming of lacking the accuracy of *interval* scales where the unit changes are constant and always represent the same value. In order to achieve consistency with the ordinal scales, it is important to have definitions and/or guidelines for the items/anchoring points in order to assign the proper numerical values and to minimize the personal bias of the rater. Bias in assigning a number could be due to a series of factors. The role of experience in the clinical evaluations is very important. This experience is something that cannot be learned, but is lived, and may be influenced by the professional orientation of the person doing the rating. The next chapter will outline some recommendations on how to execute scales properly, but in general the idea is to provide a number to an observation, statement, affect, symptom, behavior, etc that will permit the statistical manipulation of clinical data in order to assess change.

Other important issues with regard to rating scales and the quality of the measurements are the concepts of *reliability* and *validity*. Reliability is the ability of the scale to convey consistent and reproducible information. Some experts prefer the use of consistency rather than reliability, emphasizing the concept of stability of the measurements across time, patients, and raters.

Validity is the degree to which the scale measures what it is supposed to measure. Most validation studies about a scale start with an assessment of the *content validity*, referring to the clinical appropriateness of the measure and how adequately the questions reflect the aims that were specified in the scope of the measure. These attributes are more subjective than statistical with the clinical credibility of a measure inferred from the comments of experts and/or patients. The statistical attributes are referred to as *criterion validity* which looks at the correlation of the instrument in comparison to a "gold standard." Other concepts associated with the validity of a scale are the *construct validity* and the *factorial validity*. Construct validation begins with a conceptual definition of the topic to be measured and the factorial analysis has to do with the underlying conceptual structure of the instrument and how the items may or may not fall into groupings.

THE PSYCHIATRIC INTERVIEW AND APPLICATION OF RATING SCALES

THE RATING SCALE INTERVIEW

Each scale has its own manual or guideline that explains how to use the scale, the rating system, and other specific information, including definitions of the items and the scale anchoring points. In general, most scales evaluate the patient/patient behavior over a defined period of time, that is usually 7 days prior to the administration of the scale. Most of the information needed to complete rater-administered scales is obtained with a clinical interview which can be structured, semistructured, or nonstructured depending on the preference of the rater and/or the condition of the scale. During the rating process, it is important to rate what is observed or what is reported without taking into consideration psychological, psychodynamic, or any other kinds of explanations. In the case of having difficulties in selecting a severity/grading number (2 vs 3 or 3 vs 4, etc), the rater is advised to select the higher number. It is also advisable that the rater be familiar or have all the information available and necessary to make the appropriate ratings. Inexperienced raters must do ratings under supervision until their "competence" in using a particular scale has been corroborated but, in general, a rater can do a good job if s/he is capable of doing a good interview, is familiar with the scale, and follows the manual.

STEPS TO DOING A GOOD RATING

The following are important points to keep in mind for doing a good scale rating:

1. Have all the information available
2. Be familiar with the scale
3. Perform a good interview
4. Ask all the items
5. Make sure you have established the severity of the symptoms

In several studies, it has been shown that the interview is the main source of error. The reasons are multiple, but in general they have to do with the interviewer not asking about all the items or failing to clarify inconsistencies or completely missing components for the accurate assessment of symptoms severity.

It is important for the interviewer to prepare himself/herself, to prepare the environment, and to prepare the patient in order to eliminate all barriers of communication. It is necessary that the interviewer establish an atmosphere of trust and professionalism, where the patient feels safe and secure to answer all the questions appropriately and accurately.

The interviewer should prepare himself/herself by reviewing all the information available about the patient, and by becoming familiar with the interview and the different items. It is important that s/he be focused and calm. The environment has to be clean, accessible, warm, and conducive to good communication. The patient must be greeted properly and instructed regarding the purpose of the interview with an appropriate introduction to the questions that are going to be asked.

The art of interviewing is knowing which questions to ask and how to ask them. In the case of rating scales, the type of questions are determined by the items composing the scale. It is important to cover all the items and to determine the severity of the symptoms. In many cases, and with the proposed idea of increasing accuracy, the questions are preprepared making the interview semi or structured. In this case, the interviewer has to be careful not to relinquish the control of the interview to the structure of the questioning or to the "leading" quality of preprepared questions. It must be kept in mind that the structured interview is still a clinical activity designed to collect information about the illness of the patient.

The interviewer must ask questions about all items, and once the presence of the symptoms is established, then s/he must ask questions to ascertain the severity of the symptoms. During this process, the interviewer needs to become aware of inconsistencies presented by the patient and must clarify them using appropriate techniques. The repetitive asking of questions to clarify items often gives a mechanical quality to the interviews, which the interviewer should resist, making sure s/he does not interfere with the free associations of the patient and his/her presentation of the different symptoms. It is also important that the interviewer be fully aware of the utilization of time, as the longer the interview, the more difficult it is to keep the attention of the patient.

The interviewer must finish the interview by asking the patient's input at the end, and by summarizing the data obtained in order to make sure that all the questions have been asked, and there are no items being left out. At this time, arrangements for next visits can be made and an outline of what is going to happen next should be presented to the patient and/or family.

It is important to practice interviewing patients with different scales. As we have mentioned, practitioners cannot learn experience from books and/or watching others. They need to interview patients, record these experiences, and be able to discuss their interviews and ratings with colleagues who can give their opinions and comments about the techniques utilized. In addition, scoring can be discussed to reach some sort of consensus, which will help with interrater reliability and homogeneity of the scorings. In summary, if the interviewer is familiar with the scale, uses the manual, and does a good interview, the rating scale scoring will usually accurately reflect the condition of the patient.

SPECIFIC RATING SCALE TYPES

Rating scales may be used for a variety of purposes in differing clinical settings. Some scales are designed to be used as a one-time assessment, while others are meant to be repeated sequentially, so that change over time can be evaluated. Major categories include:

A. Diagnostic Scales

Psychiatric diagnostic scales are assessment tools that identify specific mental disorders. Most of these are lengthy instruments, designed generally as a one-time assessment, often taking 45-90 minutes to administer. Diagnostic scales may be paired with other clinical assessments, or may be done independently. Research studies frequently utilize diagnostic scales to select a homogenous group of research subjects at study initiation. Diagnostic scales are more rarely used in clinical settings, primarily because of the time required for their administration. Diagnostic scales for adults include the Present State Examination (PSE), a diagnostic assessment tool which was developed to standardize diagnostic procedures in international studies of mental illness. The PSE was used in the World Health Organization's (WHO) International Pilot Study of Schizophrenia. The PSE is not used a great deal currently, but has been replaced by other instruments, including the Composite International Diagnostic Interview (CIDI) and the Schedules for Clinical Assessment in Neuropsychiatry (SCAN). Both of these scales were developed using items from the PSE. Both the CIDI and the SCAN were developed by the WHO. Additional information on these scales, including opportunities for training in these instruments, may be obtained on the WHO internet site at www.who.int.

Other commonly used diagnostic scales include the Structured Clinical Interview for Axis I Disorders (SCID), the Schedule for Affective Disorders and Schizophrenia (SADS), and the Diagnostic Interview Schedule (DIS), developed by the National Institute of Mental Health (NIMH).

There are a number of popular instruments to identify and evaluate severity of psychiatric illness in children and adolescents. These include the Schedule for Affective Disorder and Schizophrenia for School-Age children (K-SADS), The National Institute of Mental Health Diagnostic Interview Schedule for Children (NIMH-DISC), and the Child Behavior Checklists (CBCL). Both the K-SADS and the DISC are structured or semistructured interviews which ultimately categorize subjects along DSM diagnostic lines. The CBCL does not furnish a diagnosis, but rather identifies broad groups of symptoms in evaluated subjects.

Because of the length and detail of most diagnostic measures, intensive training is usually required to properly administer these instruments. Clinicians and administrators contemplating the use of diagnostic scales in outcomes studies, must carefully consider the costs and time involved in adequate training versus the potential benefits of using these measures.

B. Symptom-Based Scales

Many rating scales in psychiatry are based on the assessment of a particular symptom or set of symptoms, and are not targeted to a specific psychiatric diagnosis. An example of this is the Brief Psychiatric Rating Scale (BPRS), which evaluates a variety of symptoms including depression, hostility, and uncooperativeness. The BPRS has been used to evaluate individuals with many different psychiatric disorders, including schizophrenia and bipolar disorder.

C. Diagnosis-Specific Scales

There are a smaller number of rating scales in psychiatry designed to be used for specific psychiatric diagnoses. These include the Positive and Negative Syndrome Scale for Schizophrenia (PANSS) and the Calgary Scale for Depression in individuals with schizophrenia who have depressive symptoms. Diagnosis-specific scales exist for many diagnostic categories including depression, anxiety disorders, and cognitive disorders. Some scales, such as the Hamilton Depression Rating Scale (HAM-D), were originally intended as diagnosis-specific scales, but over the years have been used in clinical/research settings as symptom-based scales.

D. Self-Rated vs Rater-Administered Scales

Some rating scales in psychiatry are designed to be self-rated. Advantages to self-rated scales are primarily the ease of administration, with no clinician or professional staff time required for scale administration. Self-rated scales may be useful in evaluating subtle, subjective states. Additionally, self-rated scales can be used in psycho-educational interventions to raise awareness in patient self-identification of illness target symptoms and monitoring of clinical progress. An example is use of the Beck Depression Inventory (BDI), a self-rated depression scale used to identify and monitor mood symptoms in a patient being treated for a major depressive episode.

Disadvantages of self-rated scales primarily center around reliability. This may be more of a problem in disorders where lack of insight is often a key feature of illness, such as may be the case with schizophrenia or bipolar mania. Often, to optimize reliability of outcome determinations, a self-rated scale will be paired with a clinician-rated measure (eg, the Beck Depression Inventory and the Hamilton Rating Scale for Depression being used together).

E. Other Dimensions of Outcome

Other scales in psychiatry are neither symptom- nor disorder-based. This includes the important domain of quality of life. As healthcare has become more consumer-oriented, and as medical technology has advanced, there has been increasing emphasis on the expectation that treatment should lead to not only a reduction in psychopathology, but should also lead to an improved quality of life. There are many instruments that have been developed to evaluate quality of life (QOL). These include the Quality of Life Interview (QOLI) by Lehman, the Quality of Well Being Scale (QWB), and the Sickness Impact Profile (SIP), among others. A disadvantage of many of the currently utilized instruments to evaluate quality of life is their length and complexity. It must be remembered that QOL scales are usually accompanied by at least one measure of illness severity. When designing outcome study plans, the study organizer must take into account the total amount of time which will be required at each assessment interval. The "time to complete scale" portion of the monographs in this book may be helpful in providing this information. However, when clinical data is obtained via a standard clinical interview, it is often possible to rate multiple scales from a single interview.

Another domain of outcome that may be evaluated by rating scales is functional level. Frequently, a functional level scale paired with a symptom severity scale will provide important outcome information. For example, it is not enough to know that the atypical antipsychotic clozapine reduces Brief Psychiatric Rating Scale (BPRS) scores in treatment-refractory schizophrenia. It is also important to identify that the clozapine-related BPRS score reduction is associated with an improvement in patient functional level.

Another increasingly recognized critical factor in clinical outcomes is patient satisfaction and patient perception of care. Many new scales are being developed in this area. Patient perception of care and attitudes towards treatment measures include the Client Satisfaction Questionnaire (CSQ) and the Drug Attitude Inventory (DAI), among others. Patient satisfaction may be helpful in determining how desirable or acceptable treatment or care systems are from the point of view of the patient/consumer. As with all scales, care must be taken in selecting an appropriate sample of individuals to assess using patient satisfaction scales. The sample surveyed should be representative of all patients who use the care system unless it is determined *a priori* that a more select sample is being evaluated. Finally, it must be remembered that patient satisfaction does not necessarily correlate with reduction in symptoms severity.

There are many other domains of clinical outcome including general health status, adverse events, and resource utilization. The best outcome analysis will often evaluate multiple domains of outcome, rather than relying on single dimension, such as symptoms severity. Other important factors of outcome evaluation include sample selection, sample size, and timing of assessment.

F. Self-Rated Scales in Mental Health That Can be Utilized in Clinical Settings

Scale Name	Condition / Situation Assessed	Time Required for Scale Rating
Arizona Sexual Experiences[1]	Sexual functioning	5 minutes
Barratt Impulsiveness Scale[2,3]	Impulsivity	10-15 minutes
Beck Depression Inventory[4,5]	Depression	5-10 minutes
Beck Hopelessness Scale[6]	Negative attitudes about the future/suicidality	5-10 minutes
Beck Scale for Suicide Ideation[7]	Suicide risk	5-10 minutes

Scale Name	Condition / Situation Assessed	Time Required for Scale Rating
Brief Fear of Negative Evaluation Scale[8]	Social phobia	5-10 minutes
Brief Sexual Function Inventory[9]	Sexual functioning in men	5-10 minutes
Burden Interview[10,11]	Caregiver burden	15 minutes
Buss-Durkee Hostility Inventory[12,13]	Anger/hostility	15-20 minutes
CAGE Questionnaire[14-16]	Alcohol abuse	≤5 minutes
Carroll Depression Scale[17]	Depression	20 minutes
Child Behavior Checklist*[,18-20]	Childhood behavior	~15 minutes; may vary by format
Children's Depression Inventory[21]	Childhood depression	Long form: 15 minutes Short form: ≤10 minutes
Conner's Rating Scale*[,22]	Childhood behavior	Long form: 15-20 minutes Short form: 5-10 minutes
Daily Record of Severity of Problems[23]	Premenstrual dysphoric disorder	10-15 minutes
Drug Attitude Inventory[24]	Medication attitudes/ treatment adherence	10-item version: ~10 minutes 30-item version: 15-30 minutes
Eating Attitudes Test[25]	Eating disorder	10 minutes
Eating Disorders Inventory[26,27]	Eating disorder	15-20 minutes
Fagerström Test for Nicotine Dependence[28-30]	Nicotine dependence	<5 minutes
Family Assessment Device[31-33]	Family functioning	15 minutes
Fear Questionnaire[34]	Phobias	10 minutes
Geriatric Depression Scale[35]	Geriatric depression	15-20 minutes
Inventory of Drug-Taking Situations[36]	Alcohol/drug abuse	15-20 minutes
Michigan Alcohol Screening Test[37,38]	Alcohol abuse	15-30 minutes (depending on format)
Mississippi Scale[39,40]	Combat-related post-traumatic stress disorder	10-20 minutes
Mood Disorders Questionnaire[41,42]	Bipolar disorder	5 minutes
Multidimensional Scale of Perceived Social Support[43-45]	Perceived social support	5-10 minutes
Patient Satisfaction Questionnaire[46-49]	Satisfaction with medical care	15 minutes
Post-Traumatic Stress Diagnostic Scale[50,51]	Post-traumatic stress disorder	10-15 minutes
Premenstrual Tension Syndrome Scale*[52,53]	Premenstrual mood symptoms	PMTS-SR: 10 minutes
Psychological General Well Being Schedule[54-57]	Quality of life/inner personal state	10-15 minutes
Revised Children's Manifest Anxiety Scale*[58,59]	Anxiety	15-20 minutes
Reynolds Adolescent Depression Scale[60-62]	Adolescent depression	15 minutes
Rush Sexual Inventory[63]	Sexual function	7-10 minutes
Sheehan Patient-Rated Anxiety Scale[64,65]	Panic disorder	15 minutes
Sleep Disorders Questionnaire[66-68]	Sleep disorders	30 minutes
Social Adjustment Scale*[69-71]	Social functioning	SAS-SR: 15 minutes
State-Trait Anger Expression Inventory[72]	Anger expression	10-15 minutes
Suicide Probability Scale[73]	Suicide risk	15-20 minutes
Symptom Checklist-90-Revised[74,75]	General health status	15-20 minutes
The Client Satisfaction Questionnaire[76-79]	Satisfaction with healthcare services	5-10 minutes
The COOP Charts for Adult Primary Care Practice[80-82]	General health status	5-10 minutes
The Duke Health Profile[83,84]	General health status	<5 minutes

Scale Name	Condition / Situation Assessed	Time Required for Scale Rating
The Nottingham Health Profile[85-87]	Quality of life	10-15 minutes
The Quality of Well Being Scale*[88-92]	Quality of life	7-10 minutes
The Service Satisfaction Scale[93]	Satisfaction with healthcare services	15-20 minutes
The Short Form 36 Health Survey[94-98]	General health status	10 minutes
The Sickness Impact Profile[99-102]	Quality of life	20 minutes
Zung Depression Scale[103-105]	Depression	10 minutes

*Multiple versions exist, including a self-rated version.

[1]McGahuey CA, Gelenberg AJ, Laukes CA, et al, "The Arizona Sexual Experience Scale (ASEX): Reliability and Validity," *J Sex Marital Ther*, 2000, 26(1):25-40.

[2]Barratt ES, "Impulsiveness and Aggression," *Violence and Mental Disorder: Developments in Risk Assessment*, Monahan J and Steadman HJ, eds, Chicago, IL: University of Chicago Press, 1994, 61-79.

[3]Patton JH, Stanford MS, and Barratt ES, "Factor Structure of the Barratt Impulsiveness Scale," *J Clin Psychol*, 1995, 51(6):768-74.

[4]Beck AT and Steer RA, *Manual for the Beck Depression Inventory*, San Antonio: Psychological Corporation, 1993.

[5]Beck AT, Steer RA, and Garbing MG, "Psychometric Properties of the Beck Depression Inventory: Twenty-Five Years of Evaluation," *Clin Psychol Rev*, 1988, 8:77-100.

[6]Beck AT, Weissman A, Lester D, et al, "The Measurement of Pessimism: The Hopelessness Scale," *J Consult Clin Psychol*, 1974, 42(6):861-5.

[7]Beck AT and Steer RA, *Manual for the Beck Scale for Suicide Ideation*, San Antonio, TX: The Psychological Corporation.

[8]Leary MR, "A Brief Version of the Fear of Negative Evaluation Scale," *Personality and Social Psychology*, 1983, 9:371-5.

[9]O'Leary MP, Fowler FJ, Lenderking WR, et al, "A Brief Male Sexual Function Inventory for Urology," *Urology*, 1995, 46(5):697-706.

[10]Zarit SH and Zarit JM, "The Memory and Behavior Problem Checklist and the Burden Interview," (Pennsylvania State University Gerontology Center Reprint Series, No 189, Part 3), College Park, PA: Pennsylvania State University Gerontology Center, 1990.

[11]Zarit SH, Reever KE, and Bach-Peterson J, "Relatives of the Impaired Elderly: Correlates of Feelings of Burden," *Gerontologist*, 1980, 20(6):649-55.

[12]Buss AH and Durkee A, "An Inventory for Assessing Different Kinds of Hostility," *J Consult Psychol*, 1957, 21(4):343-9.

[13]Buss AH and Perry M, "The Aggression Questionnaire," *J Pers Soc Psychol*, 1992, 63 (3):452-9.

[14]Ewing JA and Rouse BA, "Identifying the Hidden Alcoholic," Presented at the 29th International Congress on Alcohol and Drug Dependence, Sydney, Australia, Feb 3, 1970.

[15]Ewing JA, "Detecting Alcoholism: The CAGE Questionnaire," *JAMA*, 1984, 252 (14):1905-7.

[16]Mayfield D, McLeod G, and Hall P, "The CAGE Questionnaire: Validation of a New Alcoholism Screening Instrument," *Am J Psychiatry*, 1974, 131(10):1121-3.

[17]Carroll BJ, Feinberg M, Smouse PE, et al, "The Carroll Rating Scale for Depression. I. Development, Reliability, and Validation," *Br J Psychiatry*, 1981, 138:194-200.

[18]Achenbach TM and Rescorla LA, *Manual for the ASEBA Preschool Forms and Profiles*, Burlington, VT: Department of Psychiatry, 2000.

[19]Achenbach TM, *Integrative Guide for the 1991 CBCL/4-18, YSR, and TRF Profiles*, Burlington, VT: University of Vermont, Department of Psychiatry, 1991.

[20]Achenbach TM, *Manual for the Child Behavior Checklist/4-18 and 1991 Profile*, Burlington, VT: University of Vermont, Department of Psychiatry, 1991.

[21]Kovacs M, "Rating Scales to Assess Depression in School Age Children," *Acta Paedopsychiatrica*, 1981, 46(5-6):305-15.

[22]Conners CK, Sitarenios G, Parker JD, et al, "The Revised Conners' Parent Rating Scale (CPRS-R): Factor Structure, Reliability, and Criterion Validity," *J Abnorm Child Psychol*, 1998, 26(4):257-68.

[23]Endicott J and Harrison W, *Daily Rating of Severity of Problems Form*, Department of Research Assessment and Training, New York, NY: New York State Psychiatric Institute, 1990.

[24]Awad AG, "Subjective Response to Neuroleptics in Schizophrenia," *Schizophr Bull*, 1993, 19(3):609-18.

[25]Garner DM and Garfinkel PE, "The Eating Attitudes Test: An Index of the Symptoms of Anorexia Nervosa," *Psychol Med*, 1979, 9(2):273-9.

[26]Garner DM, *Eating Disorder Inventory-2: Professional Manual*, Odessa, FL: Psychological Assessment Resources, 1991.

[27]Raciti MC and Norcross JC, "The EAT and EDI: Screening, Interrelationships, and Psychometrics," *Int J Eat Disord*, 1987, 6:579-86.

[28]Fagerström KO, "Measuring Degree of Physical Dependence to Tobacco Smoking With Reference to Individualization of Treatment," *Addict Behav*, 1978, 3(3-4):235-41.

[29]Heatherton TF, Kozlowski LT, Frecker RC, et al, "The Fagerström Test for Nicotine Dependence: A Revision of the Fagerström Tolerance Questionnaire," *Br J Addict*, 1991, 86(9):1119-27.

[30]Pomerleau CS, Carton SM, Lutzke ML, et al, "Reliability of the Fagerström Tolerance Questionnaire and the Fagerström Test for Nicotine Dependence," *Addict Behav*, 1994, 19 (1):33-9.

[31]Epstein NB, Baldwin LM, and Bishop DS, "The McMaster Family Assessment Device," *J Marital Fam Ther*, 1983, 9:171-80.
[32]Miller IW, Epstein NB, Bishop DS, et al, "The McMaster Family Assessment Device: Reliability and Validity," *J Marital Fam Ther*, 1985, 11:345-56.
[33]Miller IW, Kabacoff RI, Epstein NB, et al, "The Development of a Clinical Rating Scale for the McMaster Model of Family Functioning," *Fam Process*, 1994, 33(1):53-69.
[34]Marks IM and Mathews AM, "Brief Standard Self-Rating for Phobic Patients," *Behav Res Ther*, 1979, 17(3):263-7.
[35]Yesavage JA, Brink TL, Rose TL, et al, "Development and Validation of a Geriatric Depression Screening Scale: A Preliminary Report," *J Psychiatr Res*, 1982, 17(1):37-49.
[36]Annis HM, Turner NE, and Sklar SM, *Inventory of Drug-Taking Situations User's Guide*, 1997, Toronto, Canada: Addiction Research Foundation.
[37]Selzer ML, "The Michigan Alcoholism Screening Test: The Quest for a New Diagnostic Instrument," *Am J Psychiatry*, 1971, 127(12):1653-8.
[38]Selzer ML, Vinokur A, and van Rooijen L, "A Self-Administered Short Michigan Alcoholism Screening Test (SMAST)," *J Stud Alcohol*, 1975, 36(1):117-26.
[39]Keane TM, Caddell JM, and Taylor KL, "Mississippi Scale for Combat-Related Post-Traumatic Stress Disorder: Three Studies in Reliability and Validity," *J Consult Clin Psychol*, 1988, 56(1):85-90.
[40]Norris FH and Perilla JL, "The Revised Civilian Mississippi Scale for PTSD: Reliability, Validity, and Cross-Language Stability," *J Trauma Stress*, 1996, 9(2):285-98.
[41]Hirschfeld RM, Williams JB, Spitzer RL, et al, "Development and Validation of a Screening Instrument for Bipolar Spectrum Disorder: The Mood Disorder Questionnaire," *Am J Psychiatry*, 2000, 157(11):1873-5.
[42]Mulrow CD, Williams JW Jr, Gerety MB, et al, "Case-Finding Instruments for Depression in Primary Care Settings," *Ann Intern Med*, 1995, 122(12):913-21.
[43]Dahlem NW, Zimet GD, and Walker RR, "The Multidimensional Scale of Perceived Social Support: A Confirmation Study," *J Clin Psychol*, 1991, 47(6):756-61.
[44]Zimet GD, Dahlem NW, Zimet SG, et al, "The Multidimensional Scale of Perceived Social Support," *J Pers Assess*, 1988, 52:31-41.
[45]Zimet GD, Powell SS, Farley GK, et al, "Psychometric Characteristics of the Multidimensional Scale of Perceived Social Support," *J Pers Assess*, 1990, 55(3-4):610-7.
[46]Marshal GN, Hays RD, Sherbourne CD, et al, "The Structure of Patient Satisfaction With Outpatient Medical Care," *Psychol Assess*, 1993, 5:477-83.
[47]Ware JE, Snyder MK, and Wright WR, "Development and Validation of Scales to Measure Patient.Satisfaction With Health Care Services," *Results Regarding Scales Constructed From the Patient Satisfaction Questionnaire and Measures of Other Health Care Perceptions*, Springfield, VA: National Technical Information Service, 1976, Vol 1 of a final report, Pt B, 288-329.
[48]Ware JE, Snyder MK, and Wright WR, "Development and Validation of Scales to Measure Patient Satisfaction With Health Care Services," *Review of Literature, Overview of Methods, and Results Regarding Construction of Scales*, Springfield, VA: National Technical Information Service, 1976, Vol 1 of a final report, Pt A, 288-329.
[49]Ware JE, Snyder MK, Wright WR, et al, "Defining and Measuring Patient Satisfaction With Medical Care," *Eval Program Plann*, 1983, 6(3-4):247-63.
[50]Foa EB, Cahman L, Jaycox L, et al, "The Validation of a Self-Report Measure of Post-Traumatic Stress Disorder: The Post-Traumatic Diagnostic Scale," *Psychol Assess*, 1997, 9:445-51.
[51]Foa EB, *Post-Traumatic Stress Diagnostic Scale: Manual*, Minneapolis, MN: National Computer Systems, 1995.
[52]Steiner M, Haskett RF, and Carroll BJ, "Premenstrual Tension Syndrome: The Development of Research Diagnostic Criteria and New Rating Scales," *Acta Psychiatr Scand*, 1980, 62(2):177-90.
[53]Steiner M, Streiner DL, Steinberg S, et al, "The Measurement of Premenstrual Mood Symptoms," *J Affect Disord*, 1999, 53(3):269-73.
[54]Dupuy HJ, "Self-Representations of General Psychological Well-Being of American Adults," Paper Presented at American Public Health Association Meeting, Los Angeles, October 1978.
[55]Dupuy HJ, "The Psychological General Well-Being Index," *Assessment of Quality of Life in Clinical Trials of Cardiovascular Therapies*, Wenger NK, Mattson ME, Furberg CD, et al, eds, New York, NY: LeJacq, 1984, 170-83.
[56]Himmelfarb S and Murrell SA, "Reliability and Validity of Five Mental Health Scales in Older Persons," *J Gerontol*, 1983, 38(3):333-9.
[57]Stephens T, "Physical Activity and Mental Health in the United States and Canada: Evidence From Four Population Surveys," *Prev Med*, 1988, 17(1):35-47.
[58]Reynolds CR and Richmond BO, "What I Think and Feel: A Revised Measure of Children's Manifest Anxiety," *J Abnorm Child Psychol*, 1978, 6(2):271-80.
[59]Reynolds CR and Richmond BO, "What I Think and Feel: A Revised Measure of Children's Manifest Anxiety," *J Abnorm Child Psychol*, 1997, 25(1):15-20.
[60]Reynolds WM, "A Model for the Screening and Identification of Depressed Children and Adolescents in School Settings," *Professional School Psychology*, 1986, 1:117-29.
[61]Reynolds WM and Mazza JJ, "Reliability and Validity of the Reynolds Adolescent Depression Scale With Young Adolescents," *Journal of School Psychology*, 1998, 36:353-76.
[62]Reynolds WM, *Reynolds Adolescent Depression Scale: Professional Manual*, Odessa, FL: Psychological Assessment Resources, 1987.
[63]Zajecka J, Mitchell S, and Fawcett J, "Treatment-Emergent Changes in Sexual Function With Selective Serotonin Reuptake Inhibitors as Measured With the Rush Sexual Inventory," *Psychopharmacol Bull*, 1997, 33(4):755-60.
[64]Sheehan DV and Harnett-Sheehan K, "Psychometric Assessment of Anxiety Disorders," Ch 8, *Anxiety Psychobiolgoical and Clinical Perspectives*, Sartorius N, Andreoli V, Cassano G, et al, eds, Washington DC: Hemisphere Publishing Corp, 1990, 85-100.

[65]Sheehan DV, "Appendix 2. The Sheehan Patient Rated Anxiety Scale," *J Clin Psychiatry*, 1999, 60(Suppl 18):63-4.

[66]Douglass AB, Bornstein R, Nino-Murcia G, et al, "Creation of the ASDC Sleep Disorders Questionnaire," *Sleep Research*, 1986, 15:117.

[67]Douglass AB, Bornstein R, Nino-Murcia G, et al, "The Sleep Disorders Questionnaire I: Creation and Multivariate Structure of SDQ," *Sleep*, 1994, 17(2):160-7.

[68]Douglass AB, *Sleep Disorders Questionnaire (SDQ) Scoring Manual — Version B*, Ann Arbor, MI: Douglass, 1993.

[69]Edwards DW, Yarvis RM, Mueller DP, et al, "Test-Taking and the Stability of Adjustment Scales: Can We Assess Patient Deterioration?" *Eval Q*, 1978, 2:275-92.

[70]Weissman MM and Bothwell S, "Assessment of Social Adjustment by Patient Self-Report," *Arch Gen Psychiatry*, 1976, 33(9):1111-5.

[71]Weissman MM, Prusoff BA, Thompson WD, et al, "Social Adjustment by Self-Report in a Community Sample and in Psychiatric Outpatients," *J Nerv Ment Dis*, 1978, 166(5):317-26.

[72]Spielberger CD, Johnson EH, Russell SF, et al, "The Experience and Expression of Anger: Construction and Validation of an Anger Expression Scale," *Anger and Hostility in Cardiovascular and Behavioral Disorders*, Chesney MA and Rosenman RH, eds, New York, NY: Hemisphere/McGraw Hill, 1985, 5-30.

[73]Cull JG and Gill WS, "The Suicide Probability Scale," *West Psycholog Serv*, 1982.

[74]Derogatis LR, Lipman RS, and Covi L, "SCL-90: An Outpatient Psychiatric Rating Scale-Preliminary Report," *Psychopharmacol Bull*, 1973, 9(1):13-28.

[75]Derogatis LR, "SCL-90-R, Brief Symptom Inventory: The Matching Clinical Rating Scales in Psychological Testing," *The Use of Psychological Testing for Treatment Planning and Outcome Assessment,* Maruish ME, ed, Hillsdale, NJ: L. Erlbaum Associates, 1994.

[76]Attkisson CC and Greenfield TK, "The Client Satisfaction Questionnaire-8 and the Service Satisfaction Questionnaire-30," *The Use of Psychological Testing for Treatment Planning and Outcome Assessment*, Maruish ME, ed, Hillsdale, NJ: Erlbaum Associates, 1994.

[77]Attkisson CC and Pascoe GC, "Patient Satisfaction in Health and Mental Health Services," *Eval Program Plann*, 1983, 6(Suppl 3 and 4):185-418.

[78]Larsen DL, Attkisson CC, Hargreaves WA, et al, "Assessment of Client/Patient Satisfaction: Development of a General Scale," *Eval Program Plann*, 1979, 2(3):197-207.

[79]Rosenblatt A and Attkisson CC, "Assessing Outcomes for Sufferers of Severe Mental Disorder: A Conceptual Framework and Review," *Eval Program Plann*, 1993, 16:347-63.

[80]Larson CO, Hays RD, and Nelson EC, "Do the Pictures Influence Scores on the Dartmouth COOP Charts?" *Qual Life Res*, 1992, 1(4):247-9.

[81]Meyboom-de Jong B and Smith Rja, "Studies With the Dartmouth COOP Charts in General Practice: Comparison With the Nottingham Health Profile and the General Health Questionnaire," *Functional Status Measurement in Primary Care*, New York, NY: Springer-Verlag, 1990, 132-49.

[82]Nelson E, Wasson J, Kirk J, et al, "Assessment of Function in Routine Clinical Practice: Description of the COOP Chart Method and Preliminary Findings," *J Chronic Dis*, 1987, 40 (Suppl 1):55S-63S.

[83]Beaton DE, Bombardier C, and Hogg-Johnson S, "Choose Your Tool: A Comparison of the Psychometric Properties of Five Generic Health Instruments in Workers With Soft Tissue Injuries," *Qual Life Res*, 1994, 3:50-6.

[84]Parkerson GR Jr, Broadhead WE, and Tse CK, "The Duke Health Profile. A 17-Item Measure of Health and Dysfunction," *Med Care*, 1990, 28(11):1056-72.

[85]Alonso J, Anto JM, and Moreno C, "Spanish Version of the Nottingham Health Profile: Translation and Preliminary Validity," *Am J Public Health*, 1990, 80(6):704-8.

[86]Ebrahim S, Barer D, and Nouri F, "Use of the Nottingham Health Profile With Patients After a Stroke," *J Epidemiol Community Health*, 1986, 40(2):166-9.

[87]Hunt SM, McEwen J, and McKenna SP, "Measuring Health Status: A New Tool for Clinicians and Epidemiologists," *J R Coll Gen Pract*, 1985, 35(273):185-8.

[88]Andresen EM, Rothenberg BM, and Kaplan RM, "Performance of a Self-Administered Mailed Version of the Quality of Well Being (QWB-SA) Questionnaire Among Older Adults," *Medical Care*, 1998, 36(9):1349-60.

[89]Fanshel S and Bush JW, "A Health-Status Index and Its Application to Health-Services Outcomes," *Operations Res*, 1970, 18:1021-65.

[90]Kaplan RI and Atkins CJ, "The Well-Year of Life as a Basis for Patient Decision-Making," *Patient Educ Couns*, 1989, 13(3):281-95.

[91]Kaplan RM and Bush JW, "Health Related Quality of Life Measurement for Evaluation, Research and Policy Analysis," *Health Psychol*, 1982, 1:61-80.

[92]Kaplan RM, Anderson JP, Wu AW, et al, "The Quality of Well-Being Scale: Applications in AIDS, Cystic Fibrosis, and Arthritis," *Med Care*, 1989, 27(Suppl 3):27S-43S.

[93]Greenfield TK and Attkisson CC, "The UCSF Client Satisfaction Scales: II The Service Satisfaction Scale-30," *The Use of Psychological Testing for Treatment Planning and Outcomes Assessment*, 2nd ed, Maruish ME, ed, Mahwah, NJ: Lawrence Erlbaum Associates, 1999, 1347-67.

[94]Hays RD, Wells KB, Sherbourne CD, et al, "Functioning and Well-Being Outcomes of Patients With Depression Compared to Chronic Medical Illnesses," *Arch Gen Psychiat*, 1995, 52(1):11-9.

[95]Medical Outcomes Trust, *How to Score the SF-36 Short Form Health Survey*, Boston, MA: The Medical Outcomes Trust, 1992.

[96]Ware JE Jr and Sherbourne CD, "The MOS 36-Item Short-Form Health Survey (SF-36). I. Conceptual Framework and Item Selection," *Med Care*, 1992, 30(6):473-83.

[97]Ware JE, Kosinski M, and Keller SD, *SF-36 Physical and Mental Health Summary Scores: A User's Manual*, Boston, MA: The Health Institute, New England Medical Center, 1994.

[98]Ware JE, Snow KK, Kosinski M, et al, *SF-36 Health Survey: Manual and Interpretation Guide*, Boston, MA: The Health Institute, New England Medical Center, 1993.

[99]Bergner M, Bobbitt RA, Kressel S, et al, "The Sickness Impact Profile: Conceptual Formulation and Methodology for the Development of a Health Status Measure," *Int J Health Serv*, 1976, 6(3):393-415.

[100]Bergner M, Bobbitt RA, Pollard WE, et al, The Sickness Impact Profile: Validation of a Health Status Measure," *Med Care*, 1976, 14(1):57-67.
[101]Brooks WB, Jordan JS, Divine GW, et al, "The Impact of Psychologic Factors on Measurement of Functional Status: Assessment of the Sickness Impact Profile," *Med Care*, 1990, 28(9):793-804.
[102]Read JL, Quinn RJ, and Hoefer MA, "Measuring Overall Health: An Evaluation of Three Important Approaches," *J Chronic Dis*, 1987, 40(Suppl 1):7S-26S.
[103]Zung WW, "A Self-Rating Depression Scale," *Arch Gen Psychiat*, 1965, 12:63-70.
[104]Zung WW, "Self-Rating Depression Scale (SDS)," *ECDEU Assessment Manual for Psychopharmacology*, Guy W, ed, Washington DC: U.S. Department of Health, Education, and Welfare, 1976, 333-6.
[105]Zung WW, "The Depression Status Inventory: An Adjunct to the Self-Rating Depression Scale," *J Clin Psychol*, 1972, 28(4):539-43.

DIAGNOSTIC AND STATISTICAL MANUAL OF MENTAL DISORDERS (DSM-IV)

AXIS I AND II CATEGORIES AND CODES

An ellipsis (...) is used in the names of certain disorders to indicate that the name of a specific mental disorder or general medical condition should be inserted when recording the name.

An "x" appearing in a diagnostic code indicates that a specific code number is required.

If criteria are currently met, one of the following severity specifiers may be noted after the diagnosis:

- Mild
- Moderate
- Severe

If criteria are no longer met, one of the following specifiers may be noted:

- In partial remission
- In full remission
- Prior history
- NOS = Not otherwise specified

AXIS I: CLINICAL DISORDERS; OTHER CONDITIONS THAT MAY BE A FOCUS OF CLINICAL ATTENTION

Axis I is for reporting all the various disorders or conditions in the Classification except for the Personality Disorders and Mental Retardation (which are reported on Axis II). The major groups of disorders to be reported on Axis I are listed in the box. Also reported on Axis I are Other Conditions That May Be a Focus of Clinical Attention.

AXIS I
Clinical Disorders
Other Conditions That May Be a Focus of Clinical Attention

Disorders Usually First Diagnosed in Infancy, Childhood, or Adolescence (excluding Mental Retardation, which is diagnosed on Axis II)
Delirium, Dementia, and Amnestic and Other Cognitive Disorders
Mental Disorders Due to a General Medical Condition
Substance-Related Disorders
Schizophrenia and Other Psychotic Disorders
Mood Disorders
Anxiety Disorders
Somatoform Disorders
Factitious Disorders
Dissociative Disorders
Sexual and Gender Identity Disorders
Eating Disorders
Sleep Disorders
Impulse-Control Disorders Not Elsewhere Classified
Adjustment Disorders
Other Conditions That May Be a Focus of Clinical Attention

AXIS II: PERSONALITY DISORDERS; MENTAL RETARDATION

Axis II is for reporting Personality Disorders and Mental Retardation. It may also be used for noting prominent maladaptive personality features and defense mechanisms. The listing of Personality Disorders and Mental Retardation on a separate axis ensures that consideration will be given to the possible presence of Personality Disorders and Mental Retardation that might otherwise be overlooked when attention is directed to the usually more florid Axis I disorders. The coding of Personality Disorders on Axis II should not be taken to imply that their pathogenesis or range of appropriate treatment is fundamentally different from that for the disorders coded on Axis I. The disorders to be reported on Axis II are listed in the box.

AXIS II
Personality Disorders
Mental Retardation

Paranoid Personality Disorder
Schizoid Personality Disorder
Schizotypal Personality Disorder
Antisocial Personality Disorder
Borderline Personality Disorder
Histrionic Personality Disorder
Narcissistic Personality Disorder
Avoidant Personality Disorder
Dependent Personality Disorder
Obsessive-Compulsive Personality Disorder
Personality Disorder Not Otherwise Specified
Mental Retardation

DISORDERS USUALLY FIRST DIAGNOSED IN INFANCY, CHILDHOOD, OR ADOLESCENCE

MENTAL RETARDATION

Note: These are coded on Axis II.

317	Mild Mental Retardation
318.0	Moderate Mental Retardation
318.1	Severe Mental Retardation
318.2	Profound Mental Retardation
319	Mental Retardation, Severity Unspecified

LEARNING DISORDERS

315.00	Reading Disorder
315.1	Mathematics Disorder
315.2	Disorder of Written Expression
315.9	Learning Disorder NOS

MOTOR SKILLS DISORDER

315.4	Development Coordination Disorder

COMMUNICATION DISORDERS

315.31	Expressive Language Disorder
315.32	Mixed Receptive-Expressive Language Disorder
315.39	Phonological Disorder
307.0	Stuttering
307.9	Communication Disorder NOS

PERVASIVE DEVELOPMENTAL DISORDERS

299.00	Autistic Disorder
299.80	Rett's Disorder
299.10	Childhood Disintegrative Disorder
299.80	Asperger's Disorder
299.80	Pervasive Developmental Disorder NOS

ATTENTION-DEFICIT AND DISRUPTIVE BEHAVIOR DISORDERS

314.xx	Attention-Deficit/Hyperactivity Disorder
.01	Combined Type
.00	Predominantly Inattentive Type
.01	Predominantly Hyperactive-Impulsive Type
314.9	Attention-Deficit/Hyperactivity Disorder NOS
312.xx	Conduct Disorder

.81	Childhood-Onset Type
.82	Adolescent-Onset Type
.89	Unspecified Onset
313.81	Oppositional Defiant Disorder
312.9	Disruptive Behavior Disorder NOS

FEEDING AND EATING DISORDERS OF INFANCY OR EARLY CHILDHOOD

307.52	Pica
307.53	Rumination Disorder
307.59	Feeding Disorder of Infancy or Early Childhood

TIC DISORDERS

307.23	Tourette's Disorder
307.22	Chronic Motor or Vocal Tic Disorder
307.21	Transient Tic Disorder
	Specify if: Single Episode/Recurrent
307.20	Tic Disorder NOS

ELIMINATION DISORDERS

___.__	Encopresis
787.6	With Constipation and Overflow Incontinence
307.7	Without Constipation and Overflow Incontinence
307.6	Enuresis (Not Due to a General Medical Condition)
	Specify type: Nocturnal Only/Diurnal Only/Nocturnal and Diurnal

OTHER DISORDERS OF INFANCY, CHILDHOOD, OR ADOLESCENCE

309.21	Separation Anxiety Disorder
	Specify if: Early Onset
313.23	Selective Mutism
313.89	Reactive Attachment Disorder of Infancy or Early Childhood
	Specify type: Inhibited Type/Disinhibited Type
307.3	Stereotypic Movement Disorder
	Specify if: With Self-Injurious Behavior
313.9	Disorder of Infancy, Childhood, or Adolescence NOS

DELIRIUM, DEMENTIA, AND AMNESTIC AND OTHER COGNITIVE DISORDERS

DELIRIUM

293.0	Delirium Due to ... [Indicate the General Medical Condition]
___.__	Substance Intoxication Delirium (refer to Substance-Related Disorders for substance-specific codes)
___.__	Substance Withdrawal Delirium (refer to Substance-Related Disorders for substance-specific codes)
___.__	Delirium Due to Multiple Etiologies (code each of the specific etiologies)
780.09	Delirium NOS

DEMENTIA

294.xx	Dementia of the Alzheimer's Type, With Early Onset (also code 331.0 Alzheimer's disease on Axis III)
.10	Without Behavioral Disturbance
.11	With Behavioral Disturbance
294.xx	Dementia of the Alzheimer's Type, With Late Onset (also code 331.0 Alzheimer's disease on Axis III)
.10	Without Behavioral Disturbance
.11	With Behavioral Disturbance
290.xx	Vascular Dementia
.40	Uncomplicated
.41	With Delirium
.42	With Delusions
.43	With Depressed Mood
	Specify if: With Behavioral Disturbance

Code presence or absence of a behavioral disturbance in the fifth digit for Dementia Due to a General Medical Condition:

0 = Without Behavioral Disturbance

1 = With Behavioral Disturbance

294.1x	Dementia Due to HIV Disease (also code 042 HIV on Axis III)
294.1x	Dementia Due to Head Trauma (also code 854.00 head injury on Axis III)
294.1x	Dementia Due to Parkinson's Disease (also code 331.82 Demntia with Lewy bodies on Axis III)
294.1x	Dementia Due to Huntington's Disease (also code 333.4 Huntington's disease on Axis III)
294.1x	Dementia Due to Pick's Disease (also code 331.1 Pick's disease on Axis III)
294.1x	Dementia Due to Creutzfeldt-Jakob Disease (also code 046.1 Creutzfeldt-Jakob disease on Axis III)
294.1x	Dementia Due to ... [Indicate the General Medical Condition not listed above] (also code the general medical condition on Axis III)
___.___	Substance-Induced Persisting Dementia (refer to Substance-Related Disorders for substance-specific codes)
___.___	Dementia Due to Multiple Etiologies (code each of the specific etiologies)
294.8	Dementia NOS

AMNESTIC DISORDERS

294.0	Amnestic Disorder Due to ... [Indicate the General Medical Condition]
	Specify if: Transient/Chronic
___.___	Substance-Induced Persisting Amnestic Disorder (refer to Substance-Related Disorders for substance-specific codes)
294.8	Amnestic Disorder NOS

OTHER COGNITIVE DISORDERS

294.9	Cognitive Disorder NOS

MENTAL DISORDERS DUE TO A GENERAL MEDICAL CONDITION NOT ELSEWHERE CLASSIFIED

293.89	Catatonic Disorder Due to ... [Indicate the General Medical Condition]
310.1	Personality Change Due to ... [Indicate the General Medical Condition]
	Specify type: Labile Type/Disinhibited Type/Aggressive Type/Apathetic Type/Paranoid Type/Other Type/Combined Type/Unspecified Type
293.9	Mental Disorder NOS Due to ... [Indicate the General Medical Condition]

SUBSTANCE-RELATED DISORDERS

The following specifiers apply to Substance Dependence as noted:

[a]With Physiological Dependence/Without Physiological Dependence

[b]Early Full Remission/Early Partial Remission/Sustained Full Remission/ Sustained Partial Remission

[c]In a Controlled Environment

[d]On Agonist Therapy

The following specifiers apply to Substance-Induced Disorders as noted:

[I]With Onset During Intoxication/ [W]With Onset During Withdrawal

ALCOHOL-RELATED DISORDERS

___ **Alcohol Use Disorders**

303.90 Alcohol Dependence[a,b,c]

305.00 Alcohol Abuse

___ **Alcohol-Induced Disorders**

303.00 Alcohol Intoxication

291.81 Alcohol Withdrawal

Specify if: With Perceptual Disturbances

291.0 Alcohol Intoxication Delirium

291.0 Alcohol Withdrawal Delirium

291.2 Alcohol-Induced Persisting Dementia

291.1 Alcohol-Induced Persisting Amnestic Disorder

291.x Alcohol-Induced Psychotic Disorder

.5 With Delusions[I,W]

.3 With Hallucinations[I,W]

291.89 Alcohol-Induced Mood Disorder[I,W]

291.89 Alcohol-Induced Anxiety Disorder[I,W]

291.89 Alcohol-Induced Sexual Dysfunction[I]

291.89 Alcohol-Induced Sleep Disorder[I,W]

291.9 Alcohol-Related Disorder NOS

AMPHETAMINE (or Amphetamine-Like) - RELATED DISORDERS

___ **Amphetamine Use Disorders**

304.40 Amphetamine Dependence[a,b,c]

305.70 Amphetamine Abuse

___ **Amphetamine-Induced Disorders**

292.89 Amphetamine Intoxication

Specify if: With Perceptual Disturbances

292.0 Amphetamine Withdrawal

292.81 Amphetamine Intoxication Delirium

292.xx Amphetamine-Induced Psychotic Disorder

.11 With Delusions[I]

.12 With Hallucinations[I]

292.84 Amphetamine-Induced Mood Disorder[I,W]

292.89 Amphetamine-Induced Anxiety Disorder[I]

292.89 Amphetamine-Induced Sexual Dysfunction[I]

292.89 Amphetamine-Induced Sleep Disorder[I,W]

292.9 Amphetamine-Related Disorder NOS

CAFFEINE-RELATED DISORDERS

___ **Caffeine-Induced Disorders**

305.90 Caffeine Intoxication

292.89 Caffeine-Induced Anxiety Disorder[I]

292.89 Caffeine-Induced Sleep Disorder[I]

292.9 Caffeine-Related Disorder NOS

CANNABIS-RELATED DISORDERS

___ **Cannabis Use Disorders**

304.30 Cannabis Dependence[a,b,c]

305.20 Cannabis Abuse

___ **Cannabis-Induced Disorders**

292.89 Cannabis Intoxication

Specify if: With Perceptual Disturbance

292.81 Cannabis Intoxication Delirium

292.xx Cannabis-Induced Psychotic Disorder

.11 With Delusions[I]

.12 With Hallucinations[I]

292.89 Cannabis-Induced Anxiety Disorder[I]

292.9 Cannabis-Related Disorder NOS

COCAINE-RELATED DISORDERS

___ **Cocaine Use Disorders**

304.20 Cocaine Dependence[a,b,c]

305.60 Cocaine Abuse

___ **Cocaine-Induced Disorders**

292.89 Cocaine Intoxication

Specify if: With Perceptual Disturbances

292.0 Cocaine Withdrawal

292.81 Cocaine Intoxication Delirium

292.xx Cocaine-Induced Psychotic Disorder

.11 With Delusions[I]

.12 With Hallucinations[I]

292.84 Cocaine-Induced Mood Disorder[I,W]

292.89 Cocaine-Induced Anxiety Disorder[I,W]

292.89 Cocaine-Induced Sexual Dysfunction[I]

292.89 Cocaine-Induced Sleep Disorder[I,W]

292.9 Cocaine-Related Disorder NOS

HALLUCINOGEN-RELATED DISORDERS

___ **Hallucinogen Use Disorders**

304.50 Hallucinogen Dependence[b,c]

305.30 Hallucinogen Abuse

___ **Hallucinogen-Induced Disorders**

292.89 Hallucinogen Intoxication

292.89 Hallucinogen Persisting Perception Disorder (Flashbacks)

292.81 Hallucinogen Intoxication Delirium

292.xx Hallucinogen-Induced Psychotic Disorder

.11 With Delusions[I]

.12 With Hallucinations[I]

292.84 Hallucinogen-Induced Mood Disorder[I]
292.89 Hallucinogen-Induced Anxiety Disorder[I]
292.9 Hallucinogen-Related Disorder NOS

INHALANT-RELATED DISORDERS

___ **Inhalant Use Disorders**

304.60 Inhalant Dependence[b,c]
305.90 Inhalant Abuse

___ **Inhalant-Induced Disorders**

292.89 Inhalant Intoxication
292.81 Inhalant Intoxication Delirium
292.82 Inhalant-Induced Persisting Dementia
292.xx Inhalant-Induced Psychotic Disorder
.11 With Delusions[I]
.12 With Hallucinations[I]
292.84 Inhalant-Induced Mood Disorder[I]
292.89 Inhalant-Induced Anxiety Disorder[I]
292.9 Inhalant-Related Disorder NOS

NICOTINE-RELATED DISORDERS

___ **Nicotine Use Disorders**

305.1 Nicotine Dependence[a,b]

___ **Nicotine-Induced Disorders**

292.0 Nicotine Withdrawal
292.9 Nicotine-Related Disorder NOS

OPIOID-RELATED DISORDERS

___ **Opioid Use Disorders**

304.00 Opioid Dependence[a,b,c,d]
305.50 Opioid Abuse

___ **Opioid-Induced Disorders**

292.89 Opioid Intoxication
Specify if: With Perceptual Disturbances
292.0 Opioid Withdrawal
292.81 Opioid Intoxication Delirium
292.xx Opioid-Induced Psychotic Disorder
.11 With Delusions[I]
.12 With Hallucinations[I]
292.84 Opioid-Induced Mood Disorder[I]
292.89 Opioid-Induced Sexual Dysfunction[I]
292.89 Opioid-Induced Sleep Disorder[I,W]
292.9 Opioid-Related Disorder NOS

PHENCYCLIDINE (or Phencyclidine-Like)-RELATED DISORDERS

___ **Phencyclidine Use Disorders**

304.60 Phencyclidine Dependence[b,c]
305.90 Phencyclidine Abuse

___ **Phencyclidine-Induced Disorders**

292.89 Phencyclidine Intoxication
Specify if: With Perceptual Disturbances
292.81 Phencyclidine Intoxication Delirium

292.xx Phencyclidine-Induced Psychotic Disorder
.11 With Delusions[I]
.12 With Hallucinations[I]
292.84 Phencyclidine-Induced Mood Disorder[I]
292.89 Phencyclidine-Induced Anxiety Disorder[I]
292.9 Phencyclidine-Related Disorder NOS

SEDATIVE-, HYPNOTIC-, OR ANXIOLYTIC-RELATED DISORDERS

___ **Sedative, Hypnotic, or Anxiolytic Use Disorders**
304.10 Sedative, Hypnotic, or Anxiolytic Dependence[a,b,c]
305.40 Sedative, Hypnotic, or Anxiolytic Abuse

___ **Sedative-, Hypnotic-, or Anxiolytic-Induced Disorders**
292.89 Sedative, Hypnotic, or Anxiolytic Intoxication
292.0 Sedative, Hypnotic, or Anxiolytic Withdrawal
Specify if: With Perceptual Disturbances
292.81 Sedative, Hypnotic, or Anxiolytic Intoxication Delirium
292.81 Sedative, Hypnotic, or Anxiolytic Withdrawal Delirium
292.82 Sedative-, Hypnotic-, or Anxiolytic-Induced Persisting Dementia
292.83 Sedative-, Hypnotic-, or Anxiolytic-Induced Persisting Amnestic Disorder
292.xx Sedative-, Hypnotic-, or Anxiolytic-Induced Psychotic Disorder
.11 With Delusions[I,W]
.12 With Hallucinations[I,W]
292.84 Sedative-, Hypnotic-, or Anxiolytic-Induced Mood Disorder[I,W]
292.89 Sedative-, Hypnotic-, or Anxiolytic-Induced Anxiety Disorder[W]
292.89 Sedative-, Hypnotic-, or Anxiolytic-Induced Sexual Dysfunction[I]
292.89 Sedative-, Hypnotic-, or Anxiolytic-Induced Sleep Disorder[I,W]
292.9 Sedative-, Hypnotic-, or Anxiolytic-Related Disorder NOS

POLYSUBSTANCE-RELATED DISORDER

304.80 Polysubstance Dependence[a,b,c,d]

OTHER (or Unknown) SUBSTANCE-RELATED DISORDERS

___ **Other (or Unknown) Substance Use Disorders**
304.90 Other (or Unknown) Substance Dependence[a,b,c,d]
305.90 Other (or Unknown) Substance Abuse

___ **Other (or Unknown) Substance-Induced Disorders**
292.89 Other (or Unknown) Substance Intoxication
Specify if: With Perceptual Disturbances
292.0 Other (or Unknown) Substance Withdrawal
Specify if: With Perceptual Disturbances
292.81 Other (or Unknown) Substance-Induced Delirium
292.82 Other (or Unknown) Substance-Induced Persisting Dementia
292.83 Other (or Unknown) Substance-Induced Persisting Amnestic Disorder
292.xx Other (or Unknown) Substance-Induced Psychotic Disorder
.11 With Delusions[I,W]
.12 With Hallucinations[I,W]
292.84 Other (or Unknown) Substance-Induced Mood Disorder[I,W]
292.89 Other (or Unknown) Substance-Induced Anxiety Disorder[I,W]

292.89 Other (or Unknown) Substance-Induced Sexual Dysfunction[I]

292.89 Other (or Unknown) Substance-Induced Sleep Disorder[I,W]

292.9 Other (or Unknown) Substance-Related Disorder NOS

SCHIZOPHRENIA AND OTHER PSYCHOTIC DISORDERS

295.xx Schizophrenia

The following Classification of Longitudinal Course applies to all subtypes of Schizophrenia:

Episodic With Interepisode Residual Symptoms (*specify if:* With Prominent Negative Symptoms)/Episodic With No Interepisode Residual Symptoms

Continuous (*specify if:* With Prominent Negative Symptoms)

Single Episode In Partial Remission (*specify if:* With Prominent Negative Symptoms)/Single Episode In Full Remission

Other or Unspecified Pattern

.30 Paranoid Type

.10 Disorganized Type

.20 Catatonic Type

.90 Undifferentiated Type

.60 Residual Type

295.40 Schizophreniform Disorder

Specify if: Without Good Prognostic Features/With Good Prognostic Features

295.70 Schizoaffective Disorder

Specify type: Bipolar Type/Depressive Type

297.1 Delusional Disorder

Specify type: Erotomanic Type/Grandiose Type/Jealous Type/Persecutory Type/Somatic Type/Mixed Type/Unspecified Type

298.8 Brief Psychotic Disorder

Specify if: With Marked Stressor(s)/Without Marked Stressor(s)/With Postpartum Onset

297.3 Shared Psychotic Disorder

293.xx Psychotic Disorder Due to ... [Indicate the General Medical Condition]

.81 With Delusions

.82 With Hallucinations

___.__ Substance-Induced Psychotic Disorder

(Refer to Substance-Related Disorders for substance-specific codes)

Specify if: With Onset During Intoxication/With Onset During Withdrawal

298.9 Psychotic Disorder NOS

MOOD DISORDERS

Code current state of Major Depressive Disorder or Bipolar I Disorder in fifth digit:

1 = Mild
2 = Moderate
3 = Severe Without Psychotic Features
4 = Severe With Psychotic Features
Specify: Mood-Congruent Psychotic Features/Mood-Incongruent Psychotic Features
5 = In Partial Remission
6 = In Full Remission
0 = Unspecified

The following specifiers apply (for current or most recent episode) to Mood Disorders as noted:

[a]Severity/Psychotic/Remission Specifiers
[b]Chronic
[c]With Catatonic Features
[d]With Melancholic Features
[e]With Atypical Features
[f]With Postpartum Onset

The following specifiers apply to Mood Disorders as noted:

[g]With or Without Full Interepisode Recovery
[h]With Seasonal Pattern
[i]With Rapid Cycling

DEPRESSIVE DISORDERS

296.xx	Major Depressive Disorder
.2x	Single Episode[a,b,c,d,e,f]
.3x	Recurrent[a,b,c,d,e,f,g,h]
300.4	Dysthymic Disorder
	Specify if: Early Onset/Late Onset
	Specify: With Atypical Features
311	Depressive Disorder NOS

BIPOLAR DISORDERS

296.xx	Bipolar I Disorder
.0x	Single Manic Episode[a,c,f]
	Specify if: Mixed
.40	Most Recent Episode Hypomanic[g,h,i]
.4x	Most Recent Episode Manic[a,c,f,g,h,i]
.6x	Most Recent Episode Mixed[a,c,f,g,h,i]
.5x	Most Recent Episode Depressed[a,b,c,d,e,f,g,h,i]
.7	Most Recent Episode Unspecified[g,h,i]
296.89	Bipolar II Disorder[a,b,c,d,e,f,g,h,i]
	Specify (current or most recent episode): Hypomanic/Depressed
301.13	Cyclothymic Disorder
296.80	Bipolar Disorder NOS
293.83	Mood Disorder Due to ... [Indicate the General Medical Condition]
	Specify type: With Depressive Features/With Major Depressive-Like Episode/With Manic Features/With Mixed Features
___.__	Substance-Induced Mood Disorder (refer to Substance-Related Disorders for substance-specific codes)
	Specify type: With Depressive Features/With Manic Features/With Mixed Features
	Specify if: With Onset During Intoxication/With Onset During Withdrawal
296.90	Mood Disorder NOS

ANXIETY DISORDERS

300.01	Panic Disorder Without Agoraphobia
300.21	Panic Disorder With Agoraphobia
300.22	Agoraphobia Without History of Panic Disorder
300.29	Specific Phobia
	Specify type: Animal Type/Natural Environment Type/Blood-Injection-Injury Type/Situational Type/Other Type
300.23	Social Phobia
	Specify if: Generalized
300.3	Obsessive-Compulsive Disorder
	Specify if: With Poor Insight
309.81	Post-traumatic Stress Disorder
	Specify if: Acute/Chronic
	Specify if: With Delayed Onset
308.3	Acute Stress Disorder
300.02	Generalized Anxiety Disorder

293.84 Anxiety Disorder Due to ... [Indicate the General Medical Condition]

Specify if: With Generalized Anxiety/With Panic Attacks/With Obsessive-Compulsive Symptoms

___.___ Substance-Induced Anxiety Disorder (refer to Substance-Related Disorders for substance-specific codes)

Specify if: With Generalized Anxiety/With Panic Attacks/With Obsessive-Compulsive Symptoms/With Phobic Symptoms

Specify if: With Onset During Intoxication/With Onset During Withdrawal

300.00 Anxiety Disorder NOS

SOMATOFORM DISORDERS

300.81 Somatization Disorder

300.82 Undifferentiated Somatoform Disorder

300.11 Conversion Disorder

Specify type: With Motor Symptom or Deficit/With Sensory Symptom or Deficit/With Seizures or Convulsions/With Mixed Presentation

307.xx Pain Disorder

.80 Associated With Psychological Factors

.89 Associated With Both Psychological Factors and a General Medical Condition

Specify if: Acute/Chronic

300.7 Hyperchondriasis

Specify if: With Poor Insight

300.7 Body Dysmorphic Disorder

300.82 Somatoform Disorder NOS

FACTITIOUS DISORDERS

300.xx Factitious Disorder

.16 With Predominantly Psychological Signs and Symptoms

.19 With Predominantly Physical Signs and Symptoms

.19 With Combined Psychological and Physical Signs and Symptoms

300.19 Factitious Disorder NOS

DISSOCIATIVE DISORDERS

300.12 Dissociative Amnesia

300.13 Dissociative Fugue

300.14 Dissociative Identity Disorder

300.6 Depersonalization Disorder

300.15 Dissociative Disorder NOS

SEXUAL AND GENDER IDENTITY DISORDERS

SEXUAL DYSFUNCTION

The following specifiers apply to all primary Sexual Dysfunctions:
Lifelong Type/Acquired Type
Generalized Type/Situational Type
Due to Psychological Factors/Due to Combined Factors

___ **Sexual Desire Disorders**

302.71 Hypoactive Sexual Desire Disorder

302.79 Sexual Aversion Disorder

___ **Sexual Arousal Disorders**

302.72 Female Sexual Arousal Disorder

302.72 Male Erectile Disorder

___ Orgasmic Disorders

302.73 Female Orgasmic Disorder

302.74 Male Orgasmic Disorder

302.75 Premature Ejaculation

___ Sexual Pain Disorders

302.76 Dyspareunia (Not Due to a General Medical Condition)

306.51 Vaginismus (Not Due to a General Medical Condition)

___ Sexual Dysfunction Due to a General Medical Condition

625.8 Female Hypoactive Sexual Desire Disorder Due to ... [Indicate the General Medical Condition]

608.89 Male Hypoactive Sexual Desire Disorder Due to ... [Indicate the General Medical Condition]

607.84 Male Erectile Disorder Due to ... [Indicate the General Medial Condition]

625.0 Female Dyspareunia Due to ... [Indicate the General Medial Condition]

608.89 Male Dyspareunia Due to ... [Indicate the General Medial Condition]

625.8 Other Female Sexual Dysfunction Due to ... [Indicate the General Medial Condition]

608.89 Other Male Sexual Dysfunction Due to ... [Indicate the General Medial Condition]

___.__ Substance-Induced Sexual Dysfunction (refer to Substance-Related Disorders for substance-specific codes)

Specify if: With Impaired Desire/With Impaired Arousal/With Impaired Orgasm/With Sexual Pain

Specify if: With Onset During Intoxication

302.70 Sexual Dysfunction NOS

PARAPHILIAS

302.4 Exhibitionism

302.81 Fetishism

302.89 Frotteurism

302.2 Pedophilia

Specify if: Sexually Attracted to Males/Sexually Attracted to Females/ Sexually Attracted to Both

Specify if: Limited to Incest

Specify type: Exclusive Type/Nonexclusive Type

302.83 Sexual Masochism

302.84 Sexual Sadism

302.3 Transvestic Fetishism

Specify if: With Gender Dysphoria

302.82 Voyeurism

302.9 Paraphilia NOS

GENDER IDENTITY DISORDERS

302.xx Gender Identity Disorder

.6 in Children

.85 in Adolescents or Adults

Specify if: Sexually Attracted to Males/Sexually Attracted to Females/ Sexually Attracted to Both/Sexually Attracted to Neither

302.6 Gender Identity Disorder NOS

302.9 Sexual Disorder NOS

EATING DISORDERS

307.1 Anorexia Nervosa

Specify type: Restricting Type; Binge-Eating/Purging Type

307.51 Bulimia Nervosa

Specify type: Purging Type/Nonpurging Type

307.50 Eating Disorder NOS

SLEEP DISORDERS

PRIMARY SLEEP DISORDERS

___ **Dyssomnias**

307.42	Primary Insomnia
307.44	Primary Hypersomnia
	Specify if: Recurrent
347	Narcolepsy
780.59	Breathing-Related Sleep Disorder
307.45	Circadian Rhythm Sleep Disorder
	Specify type: Delayed Sleep Phase Type/Jet Lag Type/Shift Work Type/ Unspecified Type
307.47	Dyssomnia NOS

___ **Parasomnias**

307.47	Nightmare Disorder
307.46	Sleep Terror Disorder
307.46	Sleepwalking Disorder
307.47	Parasomnia NOS

SLEEP DISORDERS RELATED TO ANOTHER MENTAL DISORDER

307.42	Insomnia Related to ... [Indicate the Axis I or Axis II Disorder]
307.44	Hypersomnia Related to ... [Indicate the Axis I or Axis II Disorder]

OTHER SLEEP DISORDERS

780.xx	Sleep Disorder Due to ... [Indicate the General Medical Condition]
.52	Insomnia Type
.54	Hypersomnia Type
.59	Parasomnia Type
.59	Mixed Type
___.___	Substance-Induced Sleep Disorder (refer to Substance-Related Disorders for substance-specific codes)
	Specify type: Insomnia Type/Hypersomnia Type/Parasomnia Type/Mixed Type
	Specify if: With Onset During Intoxication/With Onset During Withdrawal

IMPULSE-CONTROL DISORDERS NOT ELSEWHERE CLASSIFIED

312.34	Intermittent Explosive Disorder
312.32	Kleptomania
312.33	Pyromania
312.31	Pathological Gambling
312.39	Trichotillomania
312.30	Impulse-Control Disorder NOS

ADJUSTMENT DISORDERS

309.xx	Adjustment Disorder
.0	With Depressed Mood
.24	With Anxiety
.28	With Mixed Anxiety and Depressed Mood
.3	With Disturbance of Conduct
.4	With Mixed Disturbance of Emotions and Conduct
.9	Unspecified
	Specify if: Acute/Chronic

PERSONALITY DISORDERS

Note: These are coded on Axis II.

301.0	Paranoid Personality Disorder
301.20	Schizoid Personality Disorder
301.22	Schizotypal Personality Disorder
301.7	Antisocial Personality Disorder
301.83	Borderline Personality Disorder
301.50	Histrionic Personality Disorder
301.81	Narcissistic Personality Disorder
301.82	Avoidant Personality Disorder
301.6	Dependent Personality Disorder
301.4	Obsessive-Compulsive Personality Disorder
301.9	Personality Disorder NOS

OTHER CONDITIONS THAT MAY BE A FOCUS OF CLINICAL ATTENTION

PSYCHOLOGICAL FACTORS AFFECTING MEDICAL CONDITION

316 ... [Specified Psychological Factor] Affecting
... [Indicate the General Medical Condition]

Choose name based on nature of factors:

Mental Disorder Affecting Medical Condition

Psychological Symptoms Affecting Medical Condition

Personality Traits or Coping Style Affecting Medical Condition

Maladaptive Health Behaviors Affecting Medical Condition

Stress-Related Physiological Response Affecting Medical Condition

Other or Unspecified Psychological Factors Affecting Medical Condition

MEDICATION-INDUCED MOVEMENT DISORDERS

332.1	Neuroleptic-Induced Parkinsonism
333.92	Neuroleptic Malignant Syndrome
333.7	Neuroleptic-Induced Acute Dystonia
333.99	Neuroleptic-Induced Acute Akathisia
333.82	Neuroleptic-Induced Tardive Dyskinesia
333.1	Medication-Induced Postural Tremor
333.90	Medication-Induced Movement Disorder NOS

OTHER MEDICATION-INDUCED DISORDER

995.2	Adverse Effects of Medication NOS

RELATIONAL PROBLEMS

V61.9	Relational Problem Related to a Mental Disorder or General Medical Condition
V61.20	Parent-Child Relational Problem
V61.10	Partner Relational Problem
V61.8	Sibling Relational Problem
V62.81	Relational Problem NOS

PROBLEMS RELATED TO ABUSE OR NEGLECT

V61.21	Physical Abuse of Child (code 995.54 if focus of attention is on victim)
V61.21	Sexual Abuse of Child (code 995.53 if focus of attention is on victim)
V61.21	Neglect of Child (code 995.52 if focus of attention is on victim)
___.__	Physical Abuse of Adult (682)
V61.12	(if by partner)
V62.83	(if by person other than partner) (code 995.81 if focus of attention is on victim)
___.__	Sexual Abuse of Adult (682)
V61.12	(if by partner)
V62.83	(if by person other than partner) (code 995.83 if focus of attention is on victim)

ADDITIONAL CONDITIONS THAT MAY BE A FOCUS OF CLINICAL ATTENTION

V15.81	Noncompliance With Treatment
V65.2	Malingering
V71.01	Adult Antisocial Behavior
V71.02	Child or Adolescent Antisocial Behavior
V62.89	Borderline Intellectual Functioning
	Note: This is coded on Axis II
780.93	Age-Related Cognitive Decline
V62.82	Bereavement
V62.3	Academic Problem
V62.2	Occupational Problem
313.82	Identity Problem
V62.89	Religious or Spiritual Problem
V62.4	Acculturation Problem
V62.89	Phase of Life Problem

ADDITIONAL CODES

300.9	Unspecified Mental Disorder (nonpsychotic)
V71.09	No Diagnosis or Condition on Axis I
799.9	Diagnosis or Condition Deferred on Axis I
V71.09	No Diagnosis on Axis II
799.9	Diagnosis Deferred on Axis II

MULTIAXIAL SYSTEM

Axis I	Clinical Disorders
	Other Conditions That May Be a Focus of Clinical Attention
Axis II	Personality Disorders
	Mental Retardation
Axis III	General Medical Conditions
Axis IV	Psychosocial and Environmental Problems
Axis V	Global Assessment of Functioning

APPENDIX TABLE OF CONTENTS

Abbreviations and Measurements
Body Mass Index (BMI) ... 1746
Body Surface Area of Adults and Children ... 1747
Ideal Body Weight Calculation ... 1748

Assessment of Renal Function
Creatinine Clearance Estimating Methods in Patients With Stable Renal Function ... 1749

Comparative Drug Charts
Adverse Effects of Approved Mood Stabilizers / Anticonvulsants ... 1751
Agents Approved for Bipolar Disorder ... 1752
Angiotensin Agents ... 1754
Anticholinergic Effects of Common Psychotropics ... 1758
Anticonvulsants by Seizure Type ... 1759
Antidepressant Agents ... 1760
Antidepressant Receptor Profile ... 1764
Antimigraine Drugs: 5-HT_1 Receptor Agonists ... 1766
Antiparkinsonian Agents ... 1767
Antipsychotic Agents ... 1769
Antipsychotic Neurological Side Effects ... 1771
Antipsychotic Receptor Profile ... 1772
Atypical Antipsychotics ... 1773
Benzodiazepines ... 1774
Beta-Blockers ... 1776
Calcium Channel Blockers ... 1778
Corticosteroids ... 1780
Hallucinogenic Drugs ... 1783
Laxatives, Classification and Properties ... 1785
Lipid-Lowering Agents ... 1786
Liquid Compatibility of Antidepressants, Antipsychotics, and Mood Stabilizers ... 1788
Narcotic / Opioid Analgesics ... 1789
Nonbenzodiazepine Anxiolytics and Hypnotics ... 1791
Nonsteroidal Anti-Inflammatory Agents ... 1792
Selective Serotonin Reuptake Inhibitors (SSRIs) CYP Profile ... 1793
Selective Serotonin Reuptake Inhibitors (SSRIs) FDA-Approved Indication(s) ... 1794
Selective Serotonin Reuptake Inhibitors (SSRIs) Pharmacokinetics ... 1795
Selective Serotonin Reuptake Inhibitors (SSRIs) Receptor Profile ... 1796
Stimulant Agents Used for ADHD ... 1797

Cytochrome P450 and Drug Interactions
Cytochrome P450 Enzymes: Substrates, Inhibitors, and Inducers ... 1799

Therapy Guidelines
CMS: Long-Term Care Facility Thresholds ... 1815

Therapy Recommendations
Addiction Treatments ... 1817
Clozapine-Induced Side Effects ... 1818
Criteria to Differentiate Pseudo From Idiopathic Parkinsonism ... 1819
Depression ... 1820
Hyperlipidemia Management ... 1821
Hypertension ... 1828

Miscellaneous
Discontinuation of Psychotropic Drugs ... 1839
Drugs of Abuse ... 1840
Laboratory Detection of Drugs ... 1845
Serotonin Syndrome ... 1846
Tyramine Content of Foods ... 1848

BODY MASS INDEX (BMI)

Body Mass Index (BMI), kg/m^2 Height (feet, inches)

Weight (lb)	5'0"	5'3"	5'6"	5'9"	6'0"	6'3"
140	27	25	23	21	19	18
150	29	27	24	22	20	19
160	31	28	26	24	22	20
170	33	30	28	25	23	21
180	35	32	29	27	25	23
190	37	34	31	28	26	24
200	39	36	32	30	27	25
210	41	37	34	31	29	26
220	43	39	36	33	30	28
230	45	41	37	34	31	29
240	47	43	39	36	33	30
250	49	44	40	37	34	31

BODY SURFACE AREA OF ADULTS AND CHILDREN

Calculating Body Surface Area in Children

In a child of average size, find weight and corresponding surface area on the boxed scale to the left; or, use the nomogram to the right. Lay a straightedge on the correct height and weight points for the child, then read the intersecting point on the surface area scale.

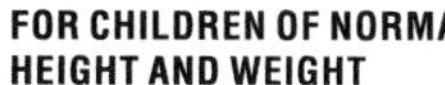

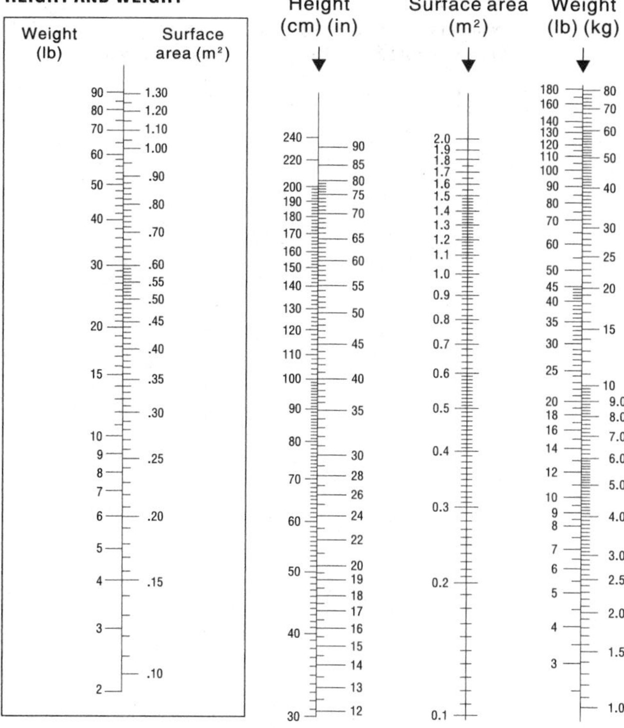

BODY SURFACE AREA FORMULA (Adult and Pediatric)

$$\text{BSA (m}^2) = \sqrt{\frac{\text{Ht (in)} \times \text{Wt (lb)}}{3131}} \quad \text{or, in metric: BSA (m}^2) = \sqrt{\frac{\text{Ht (cm)} \times \text{Wt (kg)}}{3600}}$$

References

Lam TK and Leung DT, "More on Simplified Calculation of Body Surface Area," *N Engl J Med*, 1988, 318(17):1130 (Letter).

Mosteller RD, "Simplified Calculation of Body Surface Area", *N Engl J Med*, 1987, 317(17):1098 (Letter).

IDEAL BODY WEIGHT CALCULATION

Adults (18 years and older) (IBW is in kg)

IBW (male) = 50 + (2.3 x height in inches over 5 feet)

IBW (female) = 45.5 + (2.3 x height in inches over 5 feet)

Children (IBW is in kg; height is in cm)

a. 1-18 years

$$\text{IBW} = \frac{(\text{height}^2 \times 1.65)}{1000}$$

b. 5 feet and taller

IBW (male) = 39 + (2.27 x height in inches over 5 feet)

IBW (female) = 42.2 + (2.27 x height in inches over 5 feet)

CREATININE CLEARANCE ESTIMATING METHODS IN PATIENTS WITH STABLE RENAL FUNCTION

These formulas provide an acceptable estimate of the patient's creatinine clearance **except** in the following instances.

- Patient's serum creatinine is changing rapidly (either increasing or decreasing).
- Patient is markedly emaciated.

In above situations, certain assumptions have to be made.

- In a patient with rapidly rising serum creatinine (ie, >0.5-0.7 mg/dL/day), it is best to assume that the patient's creatinine clearance is probably <10 mL/minute.
- In an emaciated patient, although their actual creatinine clearance is less than their calculated creatinine clearance (because of decreased creatinine production), it is not possible to easily predict how much less.

INFANTS

Estimation of creatinine clearance using serum creatinine and body length (to be used when an adequate timed specimen cannot be obtained). **Note:** This formula may not provide an accurate estimation of creatinine clearance for infants younger than 6 months of age and for patients with severe starvation or muscle wasting.

$$Cl_{cr} = K \times L/S_{cr}$$

where:

Cl_{cr} = creatinine clearance in mL/minute/1.73 m^2
K = constant of proportionality that is age specific

Age	K
Low birth weight ≤1 y	0.33
Full-term ≤1 y	0.45
2-12 y	0.55
13-21 y female	0.55
13-21 y male	0.70

L = length in cm
S_{cr} = serum creatinine concentration in mg/dL

Reference

Schwartz GJ, Brion LP, and Spitzer A, "The Use of Plasma Creatinine Concentration for Estimating Glomerular Filtration Rate in Infants, Children and Adolescents," *Pediatr Clin North Am*, 1987, 34(3):571-90.

CHILDREN (1-18 years)

Method 1: (Traub SL and Johnson CE, *Am J Hosp Pharm*, 1980, 37(2):195-201)

$$Cl_{cr} = 0.48 \times (\text{height}) / S_{cr}$$

where:

Cl_{cr} = creatinine clearance in mL/min/1.73 m^2
S_{cr} = serum creatinine in mg/dL
Height = height in cm

Method 2: Nomogram (Traub SL and Johnson CE, *Am J Hosp Pharm*, 1980, 37 (2):195-201)

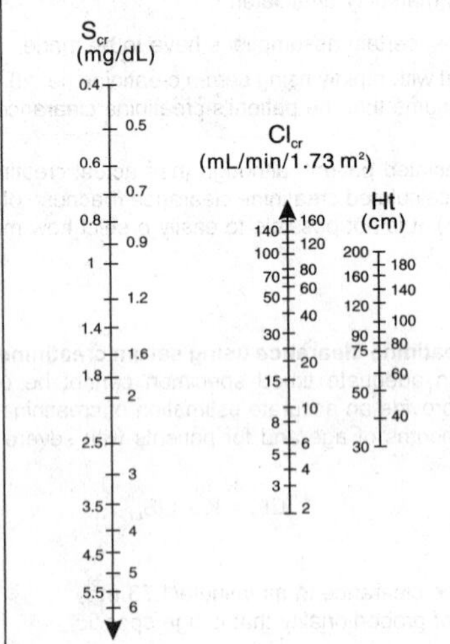

ADULTS (18 years and older)

Method 1: (Cockroft DW and Gault MH, *Nephron*, 1976, 16:31-41)

Estimated creatinine clearance (Cl_{cr}) (mL/min):

Male = (140 – age) x BW (kg) / 72 x S_{cr}
Female = male x 0.85

Note: Use of actual body weight (BW) in obese patients (and possibly patients with ascites) may significantly overestimate creatinine clearance. Some clinicians prefer to use an adjusted ideal body weight (IBW) in such cases [eg, IBW + 0.4(ABW-IBW)], especially when calculating dosages for aminoglycoside antibiotics.

Method 2: (Jelliffe RW, *Ann Intern Med*, 1973, 79:604)

Estimated creatinine clearance (Cl_{cr}) (mL/min/1.73 m^2):

Male = 98 – 0.8 (age – 20) / S_{cr}
Female = male x 0.90

ADVERSE EFFECTS OF APPROVED MOOD STABILIZERS / ANTICONVULSANTS

Drug	Dosage Forms	Somnolence	Weight Gain	Dizziness	Hypothyroidism	Rash	Gastrointestinal Effects	Black Box Warnings
Carbamazepine (Equetro™)	Cap (extended release)	Moderate	Low	High	None	Moderate	Moderate/high	Hematologic
Lamotrigine (Lamictal®)	Tab	Low	Low	High	None	Moderate	Moderate	Dermatologic
Lithium (Eskalith®, Eskalith CR®, Lithobid®)	Cap, syr, tab	Low	Moderate	Low	Moderate	Low	Moderate	Neurotoxicity
Valproic acid and derivatives (Depakote® Delayed Release, Depakote® ER)	Tab (delayed release, extended release)	Moderate	Low/moderate	Low	None	Low	Moderate/high (less with extended-release dosage form)	Hepatic, pancreatitis, teratogen

Ehret MS and Levin GM, "Long-Term Use of Atypical Antipsychotics in Bipolar Disorder," *Pharmacotherapy*, 2006, 26(8):1134-47.

AGENTS APPROVED FOR BIPOLAR DISORDER

Drug	Indication	Dosage Forms	Route of Metabolism/ Excretion	Protein Binding (%)	Bioavailability (%)	Usual Daily Dose	Therapeutic Range	Comments
Mood Stabilizers								
Carbamazepine (Equetro™)	Mania and mixed episodes	Tab, liq	Hepatic/urine	75-90	85	600-1800 mg	N/A	Nausea, headache, dizziness, and sedation common; blood levels >12 mcg/mL associated with toxicity; enzyme inducer
Lamotrigine (Lamictal®)	Maintenance treatment	Tab	Glucuronidation/urine	55	98	100-500 mg	N/A	May have antidepressant and mood-stabilizing effects; dosage adjustment required if receiving valproic acid
Lithium (Eskalith®; Lithane®; Lithobid®; Lithonate®; Lithotabs®)	Mania and maintenance treatment	Tab, cap, liq	None/urine (unchanged)	0	~100	600-1800 mg	0.5-1.5 mEq/L[1]	Nausea, tremor, polydipsia, and polyuria common; may cause hypothyroidism with chronic use
Valproate (Depakote®)	Mania	Tab, cap, liq	Glucuronidation/urine	80-90	95	1-3 g	50-125 mcg/mL[1]	Nausea, sedation, diarrhea, and tremor are common; also indicated for migraine prophylaxis; loading dose: 20 mg/kg PO; monitor LFTs if using combination anticonvulsants
Antipsychotics								
Aripiprazole (Abilify®)	Mania, mixed episodes, and maintenance treatment	Tab, soln	Hepatic	99	87	10-30 mg	N/A	
Chlorpromazine	Mania	Inj, tab	Hepatic	92-97	20	400-600 mg	N/A	Low potency: Sedating

Drug	Indication	Dosage Forms	Route of Metabolism/ Excretion	Protein Binding (%)	Bioavailability (%)	Usual Daily Dose	Therapeutic Range	Comments
Olanzapine (Zyprexa®)	Mania, mixed episodes, and maintenance treatment	Tab, inj, tab (oral-disintegrating)	Glucuronidation	93	57	5-20 mg	N/A	Monotherapy or in combination with lithium or valproate
Quetiapine (Seroquel®)	Mania	Tab	Hepatic	83	9	300-800 mg	N/A	Monotherapy or in combination with lithium or valproate
Risperidone (Risperdal®)	Mania and mixed episodes	Tab, soln, tab (oral-disintegrating)	Hepatic	90	66-70	1-6 mg	N/A	Monotherapy or in combination with lithium or valproate
Ziprasidone (Geodon®)	Mania and mixed episodes	Cap, inj	Hepatic	99	60[2]	80-160 mg	N/A	With or without psychosis
Other								
Olanzapine and Fluoxetine (Symbyax®)	Depression[3]	Cap	Hepatic	93/95	57/?	6-12 mg/ 25-50 mg	N/A	Bipolar depression

N/A = correlation between serum concentration and clinical response have not been established.

[1]Obtain blood level 12 hours after the last dose in the evening.

[2]With food.

[3]Combination treatment in one formulation.

ANGIOTENSIN AGENTS

Comparison of Indications and Adult Dosages

Drug	Hypertension	CHF	Renal Dysfunction	Dialyzable	Strengths (mg)
ACE Inhibitors					
Benazepril (Lotensin®)	10-40 mg/day	Not FDA approved	Cl_{cr} <30 mL/min: 5 mg/day initially Maximum: 40 mg/day	Yes	Tablets 5, 10, 20, 40
Captopril (Capoten®)	25-100 mg/day bid-tid	6.25-100 mg tid Maximum: 450 mg/day	Cl_{cr} 10-50 mL/min: 75% of usual dose Cl_{cr} <10 mL/min: 50% of usual dose	Yes	Tablets 12.5, 25, 50, 100
Enalapril (Vasotec®)	2.5-40 mg/day qd-bid	2.5-20 mg bid Maximum: 20 mg bid	Cl_{cr} 30-80 mL/min: 5 mg/day initially Cl_{cr} <30 mL/min: 2.5 mg/day initially	Yes	Tablets 2.5, 5, 10, 20
Enalaprilat[1]	0.625 mg, 1.25 mg, 2.5 mg q6h Maximum: 5 mg q6h	Not FDA approved	Cl_{cr} <30 mL/min: 0.625 mg q6h	Yes	1.25 mg/mL (1 mL, 2 mL vials)
Fosinopril (Monopril®)	10-40 mg/day	10-40 mg/day	No dosage reduction necessary	Not well dialyzed	Tablets 10, 20, 40
Lisinopril (Prinivil®, Zestril®)	10-40 mg/day Maximum: 40 mg/day	5-40 mg/day	Cl_{cr} 10-30 mL/min: 5 mg/day initially Cl_{cr} <10 mL/min: 2.5 mg/day initially	Yes	Tablets 2.5, 5, 10, 20, 30, 40
Moexipril (Univasc®)	7.5-30 mg/day qd-bid Maximum: 30 mg/day	LV dysfunction (post-MI): 7.5-30 mg/day	Cl_{cr} <40 mL/min: 3.75 mg/day initially Maximum: 15 mg/day	Unknown	Tablets 7.5, 15
Perindopril (Aceon®)	4-8 mg/day	4-8 mg/day Maximum: 16 mg/day	Cl_{cr} 30-60 mL/min: 2 mg/day Cl_{cr} 15-29 mL/min: 2 mg qod Cl_{cr} <15 mL/min: 2 mg on dialysis days	Yes	Tablets 2, 4, 8
Quinapril (Accupril®)	10-40 mg/day qd-bid	5-20 mg bid	Cl_{cr} 30-60 mL/min: 5 mg/day initially Cl_{cr} <10-30 mL/min: 2.5 mg/day initially	Not well dialyzed	Tablets 5, 10, 20, 40
Ramipril (Altace®)	2.5-20 mg/day qd-bid	2.5-10 mg/day	Cl_{cr} <40 mL/min: 25% of normal dose	Unknown	Capsules 1.25, 2.5, 5, 10
Trandolapril (Mavik®)	1-4 mg/day Maximum: 8 mg/day qd-bid	LV dysfunction (post-MI): 1-4 mg/day	Cl_{cr} <30 mL/min: 0.5 mg/day initially	No	Tablets 1, 2, 4

Comparison of Indications and Adult Dosages *continued*

Drug	Hypertension	CHF	Renal Dysfunction	Dialyzable	Strengths (mg)
Angiotensin II Receptor Blockers					
Candesartan (Atacand®)	8-32 mg/day	Target: 32 mg once daily	No dosage adjustment necessary	No	Tablets 4, 8, 16, 32
Eprosartan (Teveten®)	400-800 mg/day qd-bid	Not FDA approved	No dosage adjustment necessary	Unknown	Tablets 400, 600
Irbesartan (Avapro®)	150-300 mg/day	Not FDA approved	No dosage reduction necessary	No	Tablets 75, 150, 300
Losartan (Cozaar®)	25-100 mg qd or bid	Not FDA approved	No dosage adjustment necessary	No	Tablets 25, 50, 100
Olmesartan (Benicar®)	20-40 mg/day	Not FDA approved	No dosage adjustment necessary	Unknown	Tablets 5, 20, 40
Telmisartan (Micardis®)	20-80 mg/day	Not FDA approved	No dosage reduction necessary	No	Tablets 20, 40, 80
Valsartan (Diovan®)	80-320 mg/day	Target: 160 mg bid	Decrease dose only if Cl_{cr} <10 mL/minute	No	Tablets 40, 80, 160, 320
Renin Inhibitors					
Aliskiren (Tekturna®)	150-300 mg once daily	Not FDA approved	No dosage adjustment necessary in mild-to-moderate impairment; not adequately studied in severe impairment	Unknown	Tablets 150, 300

Dosage is based on 70 kg adult with normal hepatic and renal function.

[1]Enalaprilat is the only available ACE inhibitor in a parenteral formulation.

ACE Inhibitors: Comparative Pharmacokinetics

Drug	Prodrug	Absorption (%)	Serum $t_{1/2}$ (h) Normal Renal Function	Serum Protein Binding (%)	Elimination	Onset of BP Lowering Action (h)	Peak BP Lowering Effects (h)	Duration of BP Lowering Effects (h)
Benazepril	Yes	37		~97	Renal (32%), biliary (~12%)	1	2-4	24
Benazeprilat			10-11 (effective)	~95%				
Captopril	No	60-75 (fasting)	1.9 (elimination)	25-30	Renal	0.25-0.5	1-1.5	~6
Enalapril	Yes	55-75	2	50-60	Renal (60%-80%), fecal	1	4-6	12-24
Enalaprilat			11 (effective)					
Fosinopril		36			Renal (~50%), biliary (~50%)	1		24
Fosinoprilat			12 (effective)	>99				
Moexipril	Yes		1	90	Fecal (53%), renal (8%)		1-2	>24
Moexiprilat			2-10	50				
Perindopril	Yes		1.5-3	60	Renal		3-7	
Perindoprilat			3-10 (effective)	10-20				
Quinapril	Yes	>60	0.8	97	Renal (~60%) as metabolite, fecal	1	2-4	24
Quinaprilat			2					
Ramipril	Yes	50-60	1-2	73	Renal (60%), fecal (40%)	1-2	3-6	24
Ramiprilat			13-17 (effective)	56				
Trandolapril	Yes		6	80	Renal (33%), fecal (66%)	1-2	6	≥24
Trandolaprilat			10	65-94				

Angiotensin II Receptor Blockers and Renin Inhibitors: Comparative Pharmacokinetics

	Prodrug	Time to Peak	Bioavailability	Food "Area-Under-the-Curve"	Elimination Half-Life	Elimination Altered in Renal Dysfunction	Precautions in Severe Renal Dysfunction	Elimination Altered in Hepatic Dysfunction	Precautions in Hepatic Dysfunction	Protein Binding
Angiotensin II Receptor Blockers										
Candesartan (Atacand®)	Yes[1]	3-4 h	15%	No effect	9 h	Yes[2]	Yes	No	Yes	>99%
Eprosartan (Teveten®)	No	1-2 h	13%	No effect	5-9 h	No	Yes	No	Yes	98%
Irbesartan (Avapro®)	No	1.5-2 h	60%-80%	No effect	11-15 h	No	Yes	No	No	90%
Losartan (Cozaar®)	Yes[3]	1 h / 3-4 h[3]	33%	9%-10%	1.5-2 h / 6-9 h[3]	No	Yes	Yes	Yes	~99%
Olmesartan (Benicar®)	Yes	1-2 h	26%	No effect	13 h	Yes	Yes	Yes	No	99%
Telmisartan (Micardis®)	No	0.5-1 h	42%-58%	9.6%-20%	24 h	No	Yes	Yes	Yes	>99.5%
Valsartan (Diovan®)	No	2-4 h	25%	9%-40%	6 h	No	Yes	Yes	Yes	95%
Renin Inhibitors										
Aliskiren (Tekturna®)	No	1-3 h	~3%	85% (high-fat meal)	16-32 h	Yes[4]	Yes	No	No	?

[1]Candesartan cilexetil: Active metabolite candesartan.

[2]Dosage adjustments are not necessary.

[3]Losartan: Active metabolite E-3174.

[4]No initial dosage adjustment in mild-to-moderate impairment.

ANTICHOLINERGIC EFFECTS OF COMMON PSYCHOTROPICS

Drug	Atropine Equivalence Factor [1]	Common Daily Dose (mg)	Atropine Equivalent (mg/dose)
Anticholinergics			
Benztropine	0.849	2	1.70
Diphenhydramine	0.011	50	0.55
Trihexyphenidyl	0.828	5	4.14
Neuroleptics			
Chlorpromazine	0.030	500	15.00
Clozapine	0.125	500	62.50
Fluphenazine	0.001	25	0.03
Haloperidol	0.000	20	0.00
Loxapine	0.005	150	0.75
Mesoridazine	0.025	150	3.75
Molindone	0.000	150	0.00
Perphenazine	0.001	32	0.03
Thioridazine	0.104	300	31.20
Thiothixene	0.001	40	0.04
Trifluoperazine	0.003	25	0.08
Antidepressants			
Amitriptyline	0.121	150	18.15
Amoxapine	0.002	150	0.30
Desipramine	0.011	150	1.65
Doxepin	0.026	150	3.90
Fluoxetine	0.001	20	0.02
Imipramine	0.024	150	3.60
Maprotiline	0.004	150	0.60
Nortriptyline	0.015	75	1.13
Trazodone	0.000	100	0.00

[1]Anticholinergic effects of 1 mg of drug in equivalent mg of atropine.

Frequently Prescribed Drugs for the Elderly

Drug [1]	Atropine Equivalent	Common Dose	Anticholinergic Drug Level (ng/mL of atropine equivalents)
Captopril	1.5	75	0.02
Cimetidine	344	400	0.86
Codeine	9.9	90	0.11
Digoxin	0.03	0.125	0.25
Dipyridamole	24.8	225	0.11
Dyazide	2	25/37.5	0.08
Furosemide	8.8	40	0.22
Isosorbide dinitrate	9	60	0.15
Nifedipine	6.6	30	0.22
Prednisolone	11	20	0.55
Ranitidine	33	150	0.22
Theophylline	176	400	0.44
Warfarin	0.6	5	0.12

[1]At a 10^{-8} M concentration.

Adapted from Tune L, Carr S, Hoag E, et al, "Anticholinergic Effects of Drugs Commonly Prescribed for the Elderly: Potential Means for Assessing Risk of Delirium," *Am J Psychiatry*, 1992, 149(10):1393-4.

ANTICONVULSANTS BY SEIZURE TYPE

Antiepileptic Drugs for Children and Adolescents by Seizure Type and Epilepsy Syndrome

Seizure Type or Epilepsy Syndrome	First Line Therapy	Alternatives
Partial seizures (with or without secondary generalization)	Carbamazepine, oxcarbazepine, or phenytoin	**Second choice:** Gabapentin, lamotrigine, topiramate, or valproate **Third choice:** Tiagabine, zonisamide, phenobarbital, or primidone **Consider:** Benzodiazepine, acetazolamide, vigabatrin, or felbamate
Generalized tonic-clonic seizures	Valproate, carbamazepine, or phenytoin	**Second choice:** Topiramate or lamotrigine **Third choice:** Phenobarbital or primidone **Consider:** Zonisamide
Childhood absence epilepsy		
Before 10 years of age	Ethosuximide (only if no convulsive seizures) or valproate	**Second choice:** Lamotrigine **Third choice:** Methsuximide, acetazolamide, benzodiazepine, topiramate, or zonisamide
After 10 years of age	Valproate	**Second choice:** Lamotrigine **Third choice:** Ethosuximide, methsuximide, acetazolamide, benzodiazepine, topiramate, or zonisamide
Juvenile myoclonic epilepsy	Valproate	**Second choice:** Lamotrigine, topiramate, or clonazepam **Third choice:** Phenobarbital, primidone, carbamazepine, or phenytoin **Consider:** Felbamate
Progressive myoclonic epilepsy	Valproate	**Second choice:** Valproate plus clonazepam, or phenobarbital
Lennox-Gastaut and related syndromes	Valproate	**Second choice:** Topiramate, lamotrigine **Third choice:** Ketogenic diet, vagal nerve stimulation, felbamate, benzodiazepine, or phenobarbital **Consider:** Ethosuximide, methsuximide, ACTH or steroids, pyridoxine, vigabatrin, or adjunctive rufinamide
Infantile spasms	ACTH (or steroids), vigabatrin, or valproate	**Second choice:** Topiramate **Third choice:** Lamotrigine, tiagabine, or benzodiazepine **Consider:** Pyridoxine, felbamate, or zonisamide
Benign epilepsy of childhood with centrotemporal spikes	Gabapentin or valproate	**Second choice:** Carbamazepine or phenytoin **Third choice:** Phenobarbital, primidone, or benzodiazepine **Consider:** Lamotrigine or topiramate
Neonatal seizures	Phenobarbital	**Second choice:** Phenytoin **Consider:** Clonazepam, primidone, valproate, or pyridoxine

References

Bourgeois BF, "Antiepileptic Drugs in Pediatric Practice," *Epilepsia*, 1995, 36(Suppl 2):S34-S45.

Bourgeois BF, "New Antiepileptic Drugs in Children: Which Ones for Which Seizures?" *Clin Neuropharmacol*, 2000, 23(3):119-32.

ANTIDEPRESSANT AGENTS

Comparison of Usual Dosage, Mechanism of Action, and Adverse Effects

Drug	Initial Dose	Usual Dosage (mg/d)	Dosage Forms	Adverse Effects						Comments
				ACH	Drowsiness	Orthostatic Hypotension	Conduction Abnormalities	GI Distress	Weight Gain	
Tricyclic Antidepressants and Related Compounds[1]										
Amitriptyline	25-75 mg qhs	100-300	T, I	4+	4+	3+	3+	1	4+	Also used in chronic pain, migraine, and as a hypnotic; contraindicated with cisapride
Amoxapine	50 mg bid	100-400	T	2+	2+	2+	2+	0	2+	May cause extrapyramidal symptom (EPS)
Clomipramine[2] (Anafranil®)	25-75 mg qhs	100-250	C	4+	4+	2+	3+	1+	4+	Approved for OCD
Desipramine (Norpramin®)	25-75 mg qhs	100-300	T	1+	2+	2+	2+	0	1+	Blood levels useful for therapeutic monitoring
Doxepin (Sinequan®, Zonalon®)	25-75 mg qhs	100-300	C, L	3+	4+	2+	2+	0	4+	
Imipramine (Tofranil®, Tofranil-PM®)	25-75 mg qhs	100-300	T, C	3+	3+	4+	3+	1+	4+	Blood levels useful for therapeutic monitoring
Maprotiline	25-75 mg qhs	100-225	T	2+	3+	2+	2+	0	2+	
Nortriptyline (Pamelor®)	25-50 mg qhs	50-150	C, L	2+	2+	1+	2+	0	1+	Blood levels useful for therapeutic monitoring
Protriptyline (Vivactil®)	15 mg qAM	15-60	T	2+	1+	2+	3+	1+	1+	
Trimipramine (Surmontil®)	25-75 mg qhs	100-300	C	4+	4+	3+	3+	0	4+	

Comparison of Usual Dosage, Mechanism of Action, and Adverse Effects *continued*

Drug	Initial Dose	Usual Dosage (mg/d)	Dosage Forms	Adverse Effects						Comments
				ACH	Drowsiness	Orthostatic Hypotension	Conduction Abnormalities	GI Distress	Weight Gain	
Selective Serotonin Reuptake Inhibitors[3]										
Citalopram (Celexa™)	20 mg qAM	20-60	T	0	0	0	0	3+[4]	1+	
Escitalopram (Lexapro™)	10 mg qAM	10-20	T	0	0	0	0	3+	1+	S-enantiomer of citalopram
Fluoxetine (Prozac®, Prozac® Weekly™, Sarafem™)	10-20 mg qAM	20-80	C, L, T	0	0	0	0	3+[4]	1+	CYP2B6 and 2D6 inhibitor
Fluvoxamine[2]	50 mg qhs	100-300	T	0	0	0	0	3+[4]	1+	Contraindicated with pimozide, thioridazine, mesoridazine, CYP1A2, 2B6, 2C19, and 3A4 inhibitors
Paroxetine (Paxil®, Paxil® CR™)	10-20 mg qAM	20-50	T, L	1+	1+	0	0	3+[4]	2+	CYP2B6 and 2D6 inhibitor
Sertraline (Zoloft®)	25-50 mg qAM	50-200	T	0	0	0	0	3+[4]	1+	CYP2B6 and 2C19 inhibitor
Dopamine-Reuptake Blocking Compounds										
Bupropion (Wellbutrin®, Wellbutrin SR®, Wellbutrin XL™, Zyban®)	100 mg bid-tid IR[5] 150 mg qAM-bid SR[6]	300-450[7]	T	0	0	0	1+/0	1+	0	Contraindicated with seizures, bulimia, and anorexia; low incidence of sexual dysfunction IR: A 6-h interval between doses preferred SR: An 8-h interval between doses preferred

Comparison of Usual Dosage, Mechanism of Action, and Adverse Effects *continued*

Drug	Initial Dose	Usual Dosage (mg/d)	Dosage Forms	Adverse Effects						Comments
				ACH	Drowsiness	Orthostatic Hypotension	Conduction Abnormalities	GI Distress	Weight Gain	
Serotonin / Norepinephrine Reuptake Inhibitors[8]										
Duloxetine (Cymbalta®)	40-60 mg/d	40-60	C	1+	1+	0	1+	3+	0	Useful for stress incontinence and chronic pain
Desvenlafaxine (Pristiq™)	50 mg/d	50-100	T/SR	0	1+	1+	0	3+[4]	0	
Venlafaxine (Effexor®, Effexor® XR)	25 mg bid-tid IR 37.5 mg qd XR	75-375	T	1+	1+	0	1+	3+[4]	0	High-dose is useful to treat refractory depression; frequency of hypertension increases with dosage >225 mg/d
5-HT$_2$ Receptor Antagonist Properties										
Nefazodone	100 mg bid	300-600	T	1+	1+	2+	1+	1+	0	Contraindicated with carbamazepine, pimozide, astemizole, cisapride, and terfenadine; caution with triazolam and alprazolam; low incidence of sexual dysfunction
Trazodone (Desyrel®)	50 mg tid	150-600	T	0	4+	3+	1+	1+	2+	
Noradrenergic Antagonist										
Mirtazapine (Remeron®, Remeron® SolTab®)	15 mg qhs	15-45	T	1+	3+	1+	1+	0	3+	Dose >15 mg/d less sedating, low incidence of sexual dysfunction

Comparison of Usual Dosage, Mechanism of Action, and Adverse Effects *continued*

Drug	Initial Dose	Usual Dosage (mg/d)	Dosage Forms	Adverse Effects						Comments
				ACH	Drowsiness	Orthostatic Hypotension	Conduction Abnormalities	GI Distress	Weight Gain	
Monoamine Oxidase Inhibitors										
Isocarboxazid (Marplan®)	10 mg tid	10-30	T	2+	2+	2+	1+	1+	2+	Diet must be low in tyramine; contraindicated with sympathomimetics and other antidepressants
Phenelzine (Nardil®)	15 mg tid	15-90	T	2+	2+	2+	0	1+	3+	
Tranylcypromine (Parnate®)	10 mg bid	10-60	T	2+	1+	2+	1+	1+	2+	
Selegiline (EmSam®)	6 mg/d	6-12	Trans-dermal	2+	1+	2+	0	1+	0	Low tyramine diet not required for 6 mg/d dosage

ACH = anticholinergic effects (dry mouth, blurred vision, urinary retention, constipation); 0 - 4+ = absent or rare - relatively common. T = tablet, L = liquid, I = injectable, C = capsule; IR = immediate release, SR = sustained release.

[1]**Important note:** A 1-week supply taken all at once in a patient receiving the maximum dose can be fatal.

[2]Not approved by FDA for depression. Approved for OCD.

[3]Flat dose response curve, headache, nausea, and sexual dysfunction are common side effects for SSRIs.

[4]Nausea is usually mild and transient.

[5]IR: 100 mg bid, may be increased to 100 mg tid no sooner than 3 days after beginning therapy.

[6]SR: 150 mg qAM, may be increased to 150 mg bid as early as day 4 of dosing.

[7]To minimize seizure risk, do not exceed IR 150 mg/dose or SR 200 mg/dose.

[8]Do not use with sibutramine; relatively safe in overdose.

ANTIDEPRESSANT RECEPTOR PROFILE

Generic Name (Brand Name)	NE-T	5HT-T	DA-T	M_1	H_1	α_1
Amitriptyline	34.5	4.33	3200	**17.9**	1.1	27
Amoxapine	16.1	58.5	4350	1000	25	50
Bupropion (Wellbutrin®; Wellbutrin SR®; Wellbutrin XL™; Zyban®)	52,600	9100	526	40,000	6200	4550
Citalopram (Celexa™)	4000	1.16	28,000	2200	476	1890
Clomipramine (Anafranil®)	37	0.28	2200	**37**	31.2	38.5
Desipramine (Norpramin®)	**0.83**	17.5	3200	196	110	130
Desvenlafaxine (Pristiq™)	3385	40	25,000	No significant activity		
Doxepin (Prudoxin™; Sinequan®; Zonalon®)	29.4	66.7	12,200	83	**0.24**	23.8
Duloxetine (Cymbalta®)[1]	7.5	0.8	240	>1000	2300	8300
Escitalopram (Lexapro™)	7841	1.10	27,410	1242	1973	3870
Fluoxetine (Prozac®; Prozac® Weekly™; Sarafem™)	244	**0.81**	3600	2000	6250	5900
Fluvoxamine	1300	2.22	9100	24,000	>100,000	7700
Imipramine (Tofranil®; Tofranil-PM®)	37	1.41	8300	91	11	90.9
Maprotiline	11.1	5900	1000	560	2.0	90.9
Mirtazapine (Remeron®; Remeron SolTab®)	4760	100,000	100,000	670	**0.14**	500
Nefazodone (Serzone®)	60	200	360	11,000	21.3	25.6
Nortriptyline (Aventyl® HCl; Pamelor®)	4.35	18.5	1140	149	10	58.8
Paroxetine (Paxil®; Paxil CR™)	40	**0.13**	500	108	22,000	>100,000
Protriptyline (Vivactil®)	1.40	19.6	2130	**25**	25	130
Sertraline (Zoloft®)	417	**0.29**	**25**	625	24,000	370

Generic Name (Brand Name)	NE-T	5HT-T	DA-T	M_1	H_1	α_1
Trazodone (Desyrel®)	8300	160	7140	>100,000	345	35.7
Trimipramine (Surmontil®)	2400	1500	10,000	58.8	**0.27**	23.8
Venlafaxine (Effexor®; Effexor® XR)	1060	9.10	9100	>100,000	>100,000	>100,000

Note: These numbers represent inhibitor constants (Ki) in nM. NE-T = norepinephrine transporter; 5HT-T = serotonin transporter; DA-T = dopamine transporter; M_1 = muscarinic$_1$ receptor; H_1 = histamine$_1$ receptor; α_1 = alpha$_1$ receptor.

[1]Bymaster FP, Dreshfield-Ahmad LJ, Threlkeld PG, et al, "Comparative Affinity of Duloxetine and Venlafaxine for Serotonin and Norepinephrine Transporters *in vitro* and *in vivo*, Human Serotonin Receptor Subtypes, and Other Neuronal Receptors," *Neuropsychopharmacology*, 2001, 25(6):871-80.

References

Deecher DC, Beyer CE, Johnston G, et al, "Desvenlafaxine Succinate: A New Serotonin and Norepinephrine Reuptake Inhibitor," *J Pharmacol Exp Ther*, 2006, 318(2):657-65.

Gilman AG, *Goodman and Gilman's The Pharmacological Basis of Therapeutics*, 10th ed, New York, NY: McGraw-Hill, 2001.

ANTIMIGRAINE DRUGS: 5-HT$_1$ RECEPTOR AGONISTS

Pharmacokinetic Differences

Pharmacokinetic Parameter	Almotriptan (Axert™)	Eletriptan (Relpax®)	Frovatriptan (Frova®)	Naratriptan (Amerge®)	Rizatriptan (Maxalt®, Maxalt-MLT®)		Sumatriptan (Imitrex®)			Zolmitriptan (Zomig®, Zomig-ZMT™)	
	Oral (6.25 mg)	Tablets	Oral	Oral	Tablets	Disintegrating Tablets	SubQ (6 mg)	Oral (100 mg)	Nasal (20 mg)	Oral (5 mg)	Oral (10 mg)
Onset	<60 min	<2 h	<2 h	30 min	~30 min	~30 min	10 min	30-60 min	<60 min	0.5-1 h	
Duration	Short	Short	Long	Long	Short	Short	Short	Short	Short	Short	
Time to peak serum concentration (h)	1-3	1.5-2	2-4	2-4	1-1.5	1.6-2.5	5-20	1.5-2.5	1	1.5	2-3.5
Average bioavailability (%)	70	50	20-30	70	45	—	97	15	17	40-46	46-49
Volume of distribution (L)	180-200	138	210-280	170	110-140	110-140	170	170	NA	—	402
Half-life (h)	3-4	4	26	6	2-3	2-3	2	2-2.5[1]	2	2.8-3.4	2.5-3.7
Fraction excreted unchanged in urine (%)	40	—	32	50	14	14	22	3	3	8	8

[1]With extended dosing, the half-life extends to 7 hours.

ANTIPARKINSONIAN AGENTS

Drugs Used for the Treatment of Parkinsonian Symptoms[1]

Drug	Mechanism	Initial Dose	Titration Schedule	Usual Daily Dosage	Recommended Dosing Schedule
Dopaminergic Agents					
Amantadine (Symmetrel®)	NMDA receptor antagonist and inhibits neuronal reuptake of dopamine	100 mg every other day	100 mg/dose every week, up to 300 mg 3 times/d	100-200 mg	Twice daily
Apomorphine (Apokyn™)	D_2 receptors (caudate-putamen)	1-2 mg	Complex; based on tolerance and response to test dose(s)	Variable; <20 mg	Individualized; 3-5 times/d prn
Bromocriptine (Parlodel®)	Moderate affinity for D_2 and D_3 dopamine receptors	1.25 mg twice daily	2.5 mg/d every 2-4 wk	2.5-100 mg	3 times/d
Cabergoline (Dostinex®)[2]	Selective to D_2 dopamine receptors	0.5 mg once daily	0.25-0.5 mg/d every 4 wk	0.5-5 mg	Once daily
Entacapone (Comtan®)	COMT enzyme inhibitor	200 mg 3 times/d	Titrate down the doses of levodopa/carbidopa as required	600-1600 mg	3 times/d; up to 8 times/d
Levodopa/carbidopa (Sinemet® CR)	Converts to dopamine; binds to all CNS dopamine receptors	10-25/100 mg 2-4 times/d	0.5-1 tablet (10 or 25/100 mg) every 1-2 d	50/200 to 200/2000 mg (3-8 tablets)	3 times/d or twice daily (for controlled release)
Levodopa/carbidopa/ entacapone (Stalevo™)	Converts to dopamine; binds to all CNS dopamine receptors; COMT enzyme inhibitor	1 tablet 3-4 times/d (to replace previous dosing with individual agents)	As tolerated based on response and presence of dyskinesias	3-8 tablets per day	3-4 times/d
Pergolide (Permax® [DSC])	Low affinity for D_1 and maximal affinity for D_2 and D_3 dopamine receptors	0.05 mg/night	0.1-0.15 mg/d every 3 d for 12 d, then 0.25 mg/d every 3 d	0.05-5 mg	3 times/d
Pramipexole (Mirapex®)	High affinity for D_2 and D_3 dopamine receptors	0.125 mg 3 times/d	0.125 mg/dose every 5-7 d	1.5-4.5 mg	3 times/d
Rasagiline (Azilect®)	Inhibits MAO-B	0.5-1 mg once daily	≤1 mg daily	0.5-1 mg	Once daily
Ropinirole (Requip®)	High affinity for D_2 and D_3 dopamine receptors	0.25 mg 3 times/d	0.25 mg/dose weekly for 4 wk, then 1.5 mg/d every week up to 9 mg/d; 3 mg/d up to a max of 24 mg/d	0.75-24 mg	3 times/d

Drugs Used for the Treatment of Parkinsonian Symptoms[1] *continued*

Drug	Mechanism	Initial Dose	Titration Schedule	Usual Daily Dosage	Recommended Dosing Schedule
Rotigotine (Neupro® [DSC])	D_1, D_2, D_3 dopamine receptor agonist	2 mg/24 hours transdermal patch	Increase by 2 mg/24 hours weekly; maximum 6 mg/24 hours	2 mg/24 hours, 4 mg/24 hours, or 6 mg/24 hours	Once daily patch
Selegiline (Eldepryl®)	Inhibits MAO-B	5-10 mg twice daily	Titrate down the doses of levodopa/carbidopa as required	5-10 mg	Twice daily
Tolcapone (Tasmar®)	COMT enzyme inhibitor	100 mg 3 times/d	Titrate down the doses of levodopa/carbidopa as required	300-600 mg	3 times/d
Anticholinergic Agents					
Benztropine (Cogentin®)	Blocks cholinergic receptors, also has antihistamine effects	0.5-2 mg/d in 1-4 divided doses	0.5 mg/dose every 5-6 d	2-6 mg	1-2 times/d
Diphenhydramine (Benadryl®)	Blocks cholinergic receptors	12.5-25 mg 3-4 times/d	As tolerated	25-300 mg	3-4 times/d
Procyclidine (Kemadrin®)	Blocks cholinergic receptors	2.5 mg 3 times/d	Gradually as tolerated	7.5-20 mg	3 times/d
Trihexyphenidyl (Artane)	Blocks cholinergic receptors; also some direct effects	1-2 mg/d	2 mg/d at intervals of 3-5 d	5-15 mg	3-4 times/d

[1]The medications listed in the table represent treatment options for both idiopathic Parkinson's disease, as well as Parkinsonian symptoms resulting from other drug therapy.

[2]Cabergoline is not FDA approved for the treatment of Parkinson's disease.

ANTIPSYCHOTIC AGENTS

Antipsychotic Agent	Dosage Forms	I.M./P.O. Potency	Equiv. Dosages (approx) (mg)	Usual Adult Daily Maint. Dose (mg)	Sedation (Incidence)	Extrapyramidal Side Effects	Anticholinergic Side Effects	Orthostatic Hypotension	Comments
Aripiprazole (Abilify™)	Soln, tab		4	10-30	Low	Very low	Very low	Very low	Low weight gain; activating
Chlorpromazine (Thorazine® [DSC])	Conc, inj, supp, syr, tab	4:1	100	200-1000	High	Moderate	Moderate	Moderate / high	
Clozapine (Clozaril®)	Tab		100	75-900	High	Very low	High	High	~1% incidence of agranulocytosis; weekly-biweekly CBC required; potential for weight gain, lipid abnormalities, and diabetes
Fluphenazine (Permitil®, Prolixin®, Prolixin Decanoate®, Prolixin Enanthate®)	Conc, elix, inj, tab	2:1	2	0.5-20	Low	High	Low	Low	
Haloperidol (Haldol®, Haldol® Decanoate)	Conc, inj, tab	2:1	2	0.5-20	Low	High	Low	Low	
Loxapine (Loxitane®, Loxitane® C, Loxitane® I.M.)	Cap, conc, inj		10	25-250	Moderate	Moderate	Low	Low	
Molindone (Moban®)	Conc, tab		15	15-225	Low	Moderate	Low	Low	May cause less weight gain
Olanzapine (Zyprexa®, Zyprexa® Zydis®)	Inj, tab, tab (oral-disintegrating)		4	5-20	Moderate / high	Low	Moderate	Moderate	Potential for weight gain, lipid abnormalities, diabetes
Paliperidone (Invega™)	Tab (extended release)			3-12	Low / moderate	Low	Very low	Moderate	Active metabolite of risperidone

Antipsychotic Agent	Dosage Forms	I.M./P.O. Potency	Equiv. Dosages (approx) (mg)	Usual Adult Daily Maint. Dose (mg)	Sedation (Incidence)	Extrapyramidal Side Effects	Anticholinergic Side Effects	Orthostatic Hypotension	Comments
Perphenazine (Trilafon®)	Conc, inj, tab		10	16-64	Low	Moderate	Low	Low	
Pimozide (Orap™)	Tab		2	1-10	Moderate	High	Moderate	Low	Contraindicated with CYP3A inhibitors
Quetiapine (Seroquel®)	Tab		125	50-800	Moderate / high	Very low	Moderate	Moderate	Moderate weight gain; potential for lipid abnormalities; diabetes
Risperidone (Risperdal®)	Inj, soln, tab, tab (oral-disintegrating)		1	0.5-6	Low / moderate	Low	Very low	Moderate	Low to moderate weight gain; potential for diabetes
Thioridazine (Mellaril®)	Conc, tab		100	200-800	High	Low	High	Moderate / high	May cause irreversible retinitis pigmentosa at doses >800 mg/d; prolongs QTc; use only in treatment of refractory illness
Thiothixene (Navane®)	Cap, conc, powder for inj	4:1	4	5-40	Low	High	Low	Low / moderate	
Trifluoperazine (Stelazine® [DSC])	Conc, inj, tab		5	2-40	Low	High	Low	Low	
Ziprasidone (Geodon®)	Cap, powder for inj	2:1	40	40-160	Low / moderate	Low	Very low	Low / moderate	Low weight gain; contraindicated with QTc-prolonging agents

ANTIPSYCHOTIC NEUROLOGICAL SIDE EFFECTS

Reaction	Features	Period of Maximum Risk	Incidence	Risk Factors	Proposed Mechanism	Treatment
Acute dystonia	Spasm of muscles of tongue, face, neck, back; may mimic seizures; **not** hysteria	1-5 days	2% to 10% ≥40% with risk factors	Young male, use of high potency antipsychotic; history of dystonia	Dopamine/ acetylcholine imbalance	Benztropine or diphenhydramine (I.M., I.V.)
Parkinsonism	Bradykinesia, rigidity, variable tremor, mask-facies, shuffling gait	5-30 days (may persist)	10% to 60%	Use of high potency antipsychotic, high dosage of antipsychotic, female gender, age ≥40 years of age	Dopamine blockade	Antiparkinsonism agents; switch to an atypical antipsychotic
Akathisia	Subjective experience of motor restlessness; may experience anxiety or agitation	5-60 days (commonly persists)	20% to 75%		Unknown	Reduce dose or change drug; low doses of propranolol (30-120 mg/d) antiparkinsonism agents[1] or benzodiazepines
Tardive dyskinesia	Oral-facial dyskinesia; choreoathetosis, sometimes irreversible, rarely progressive	6-24 months (worse on withdrawal)	3% to 5%/year	Female gender, increasing age, duration of exposure to medication, ethnicity, mood disorders, history of extrapyramidal symptoms	Dopamine supersensitivity	Prevention best; use an atypical antipsychotic
"Rabbit" syndrome	Perioral tremor (late parkinsonism variant?); usually reversible	Months or years	Unknown		Unknown	Antiparkinsonism agents; reduce dose of neuroleptic
Neuroleptic malignant syndrome (NMS)	Catatonia, stupor, fever, unstable pulse and blood pressure, myoglobinemia; can be fatal	Weeks	~1% [2]		Unknown	Stop neuroleptic; bromocriptine; dantrolene; general supportive care

Adapted from: Baldessarini RJ, *Chemotherapy in Psychiatry: Principles and Practice*, Cambridge, MA: Harvard University Press, 1985, 70-1.

Note: These side effects may occur with the newer atypical antipsychotics but at a significantly lower rate.

[1]Preferred for patients with akathisia and concurrent parkinsonism

[2]Mortality rate is approximately 10%; patients with myoglobinemia and renal failure have a mortality rate of ~50%

ANTIPSYCHOTIC RECEPTOR PROFILE

Generic Name (Brand Name)	D_1	D_2	D_3	D_4	$5\text{-}HT_{1A}$	$5\text{-}HT_{1D}$	$5\text{-}HT_{2A}$	$5\text{-}HT_{2C}$	α_1/α_2	H_1	M_1	5HT-T	NE-T
Aripiprazole (Abilify®)	265[1]	0.34[1]	0.8[1]	44[1]	1.7[1]		3.4[1]	15[1]	57/-	61[1]	>10,000	98	>10,000
Clozapine (Clozaril®)	85	126	473	35	875	1700	16	16	7/160	6	1.9	3900	390
Haloperidol (Haldol®)	210	0.7	2	3	1100		45	>10,000	6/3800	440	>1500		
Olanzapine (Zyprexa®)	31	11	49	27	>10,000	530	4	23	19/230	7	1.9	>15,000	2000
Paliperidone (Invega™)		2.8			480	19	1.2	48	10/80	3.4	8800		
Quetiapine (Seroquel®)	455	160	340	1600	2800	>5100	295	1500	7/2500	11	120	>18,000	680
Risperidone (Risperdal®)	430	4	10	9	210	170	0.5	25	2/56	20	>10,000	1400	28,000
Ziprasidone (Geodon®)	525	5	7	32	3	2	0.4	1	11/154	50	>1000	53	48

Note: Values represent affinity constants expressed in nanomolar units.

[1]Data with cloned human receptors.

Arnt J and Skarsfeldt T, "Do Novel Antipsychotics Have Similar Pharmacological Characteristics? A Review of the Evidence," *Neuropsychopharmacology*, 1998, 18(2):63-101.

Bymaster FP, Calligaro DO, Falcone JF, et al, "Radioreceptor Binding Profile of the Atypical Antipsychotic Olanzapine," *Neuropsychopharmacology*, 1996, 14(2):87-96.

Gilman AG, *Goodman and Gilman's The Pharmacological Basis of Therapeutics*, 10th ed, New York, NY: McGraw-Hill, 2001.

Richelson E and Souder T, "Binding of Antipsychotic Drugs to Human Brain Receptors Focus on Newer Generation Compounds," *Life Sci*, 2000, 68(1):29-39.

Seeger TF, Seymour PA, Schmidt AW, et al, "Ziprasidone (CP-88, 059): A New Antipsychotic With Combined Dopamine and Serotonin Receptor Antagonist Activity," *J Pharmacol Exp Ther*, 1995, 275(1):101-13.

ATYPICAL ANTIPSYCHOTICS

Drug[1]	DR EPS	PROL	TD[2]	ACH	SZ	OH	LFTs	SED	WT GAIN	NMS	AGRAN	TX REFR	Lipid	DM	QTc
Aripiprazole (Abilify®)	No	No	Uncommon	Very low	Low	Low	Low	Low	Very low	Yes	?	Maybe	Very low	Very low	Low
Clozapine (Clozaril®)	No	No	Uncommon	High	DD	High	Low	High	High	Yes	Yes	Yes	High	High	Low
Olanzapine Zyprexa®, Zyprexa® Zydis®)	Yes	Yes	Uncommon	Moderate	Low	Low/ moderate	Low/ moderate	Moderate	High	Yes	Yes[3]	Maybe	High	High	Low
Paliperidone (Invega™)	Yes	Yes	Uncommon	Very low	Low	Moderate	Low	Low	Low	Yes	?	Maybe	Low	Low	Low
Quetiapine (Seroquel®)	No	No	Uncommon	Moderate	Low	Moderate	Low/ moderate	Moderate	Moderate	Yes	Yes[3]	Maybe	Moderate	Low/ moderate	Low
Risperidone (Risperdal®)	Yes	Yes	Uncommon	Very low	Low	Moderate	Low	Low	Low/ moderate	Yes	Yes[3]	Maybe	Low	Low/ moderate	Low
Ziprasidone (Geodon®)	Yes	Yes	Uncommon	Very low	Low	Low/ moderate	Low	Low	Very low	Yes	Yes[3]	Maybe	Very low	Very low	Moderate[4]

DR EPS = dose related extrapyramidal symptoms; **PROL** = prolactin elevation (may cause amenorrhea, galactorrhea, gynecomastia, impotence); **TD** = tardive dyskinesia; **ACH** = anticholinergic side effects (dry mouth, blurred vision, constipation, urinary hesitancy); **SZ** = seizures; **OH** = orthostatic hypotension (blood pressure drops upon standing); **LFTs** = increased liver function test results; **SED** = sedation; **WT GAIN** = weight gain; **NMS** = neuroleptic malignant syndrome; **AGRAN** = agranulocytosis (without white blood cells to fight infection); **TX REFR** = efficacy in treatment refractory schizophrenia; **Lipid** = lipid abnormalities; cholesterol and/or triglyceride elevations; **DM** = diabetes (based on case reports); **QTc** = QTc prolongation; **DD** = dose dependent

[1]Defined as 1) decrease or no EPS at doses producing antipsychotic effect; 2) minimum or no increase in prolactin; 3) decrease in both positive and negative symptoms of schizophrenia.

[2]Rate of TD ~ 1/5 that seen with conventional antipsychotics.

[3]Case reports.

[4]Dose related within 40-160 mg dosage range.

BENZODIAZEPINES

Agent	FDA-Approved Indication	Dosage Forms	Relative Potency	Peak Blood Levels (oral) (h)	Protein Binding (%)	Volume of Distribution (L/kg)	Major Active Metabolite	Onset	Metabolism	Half-Life (parent) (h)	Half-Life[1] (metabolite) (h)	Elimination	Usual Initial Dose	Adult Oral Dosage Range
Anxiolytic														
Alprazolam (Alprazolam Intensol®, Niravam™; Xanax XR®; Xanax®)	Anxiety, anxiety associated with depression, panic disorder treatment	Sol, tab	0.5	IR: 1-2 XR: 9	80	0.9-1.2	No	Intermediate	Hepatic via CYP3A4	12-15	—	Urine	0.25-0.5 tid	0.75-4 mg/d
Chlordiazepoxide (Librium®)	Anxiety, EtOH withdrawal, adjunct to anesthesia (I.V.)	Cap, powd for inj	10	2-4	90-98	0.3	Yes	Intermediate	Hepatic via CYP3A4	5-30	24-96	Urine	5-25 mg tid-qid	15-100 mg/d
Diazepam (Diastat® Rectal Delivery System, Diazepam Intensol®, Valium®)	Anxiety, EtOH withdrawal, adjunct to anesthesia (I.V.), anxiety/amnesiac during cardioversion (I.V.), anxiety/amnesia in endoscopic procedures, convulsions/status epilepticus (I.V.), adjunct in epilepsy (rectal gel), skeletal muscle spasms	Gel, inj, sol, tab	5	0.5-2	98	1.1	Yes	Rapid	Hepatic via 2C19 and 3A4	20-80	50-100	Urine	2-10 mg bid-qid	4-40 mg/d
Lorazepam (Ativan®) [2]	Anxiety, anxiety associated with depression, adjunct to anesthesia (I.V.), convulsions/status epilepticus (I.V.)	Inj, sol, tab	1	1-6	88-92	1.3	No	Intermediate	Hepatic	10-20	—	Urine and feces (minimal)	0.5-2 mg tid-qid	2-4 mg/d
Oxazepam (Serax®)	Anxiety, anxiety associated with depression, EtOH withdrawal	Cap, tab	15-30	2-4	86-99	0.6-2	No	Slow	Hepatic via glucoronide conjugation	5-20	—	Urine as unchanged (50%) and glucoronide	10-30 mg tid-qid	30-120 mg/d
Sedative / Hypnotic														
Estazolam (ProSom™)	Insomnia	Tab	0.3	2	93	—	No	Slow	Hepatic via CYP3A4	10-24	—	Urine	1 mg qhs	1-2 mg
Flurazepam (Dalmane®)	Insomnia	Cap	5	0.5-2	97	—	Yes	Rapid	Hepatic via CYP3A4	Not significant	40-114	Urine	15 mg qhs	15-60 mg
Quazepam (Doral®)	Insomnia	Tab	5	2	95	5	Yes	Intermediate	Hepatic via CYP3A4	25-41	28-114	Urine	15 mg qhs	7.5-15 mg

Agent	FDA-Approved Indication	Dosage Forms	Relative Potency	Peak Blood Levels (oral) (h)	Protein Binding (%)	Volume of Distribution (L/kg)	Major Active Metabolite	Onset	Metabolism	Half-Life (parent) (h)	Half-Life[1] (metabolite) (h)	Elimination	Usual Initial Dose	Adult Oral Dosage Range
Temazepam (Restoril®)	Insomnia	Cap	5	2-3	96	1.4	No	Slow	Hepatic via CYP2B6, 2C8/9, 2C19, 3A4	10-40	—	Urine as inactive metabolites	15-30 mg qhs	15-30 mg
Triazolam (Halcion®)	Insomnia	Tab	0.1	1	89-94	0.8-1.3	No	Intermediate	Hepatic via CYP3A4	2.3	—	Urine as unchanged drug and metabolites	0.125-0.25 qhs	0.125-0.25 mg
Miscellaneous														
Clonazepam (Klonopin™)	Adjunct in Lennox-Gastuat syndrome, akinetic seizures, myoclonic seizures, adjunct in absence seizures, panic disorder treatment	Tab	0.25-0.5	1-2	86	1.8-4	No	Intermediate	Hepatic via glucoronide and sulfate conjugation	18-50	—	Urine as glucoronide or sulfate conjugate	0.5 mg tid	1.5-20 mg/d
Clorazepate (Tranxene®)	Anxiety, EtOH withdrawal, adjunct in partial seizures	Cap, tab	7.5	1-2	80-95	—	Yes	Rapid	Decarboxylated in acidic stomach prior to absorption and hepatic via CYP3A4	Not significant	50-100	Urine	7.5-15 mg bid-qid	15-60 mg
Midazolam	Adjunct to anesthesia, anxiety/amnesiac during cardioversion, anxiety/amnesia in endoscopic procedures	Inj	NA	0.4-0.7 [3]	95	0.8-6.6	No	Rapid	Hepatic via CYP3A4	2-5 h	—	Urine as glucoronide or feces (2% to 10%)	NA	NA

IR = immediate release; XR = extended release; NA = not available.

Rapid = 15 minutes or less; intermediate = 15-30 minutes; slow = 30-60 minutes.

[1]Significant metabolite.

[2]Reliable bioavailability when given I.M.

[3]I.V. only.

BETA-BLOCKERS

Agent	Adrenergic Receptor Blocking Activity	Lipid Solubility	Protein Bound (%)	Half-Life (h)	Bioavailability (%)	Primary (Secondary) Route of Elimination	Indications	Usual Dosage
Acebutolol (Sectral®)	$beta_1$	Low	15-25	3-4	40 7-fold[1]	Hepatic (renal)	Hypertension, arrhythmias	P.O.: 400-1200 mg/d
Atenolol (Tenormin®)	$beta_1$	Low	<5-10	6-9[2]	50-60 4-fold[1]	Renal (hepatic)	Hypertension, angina pectoris, acute MI	P.O.: 50-200 mg/d I.V.: 5 mg x 2 doses
Betaxolol (Kerlone®)	$beta_1$	Low	50-55	14-22	84-94	Hepatic (renal)	Hypertension	P.O.: 10-20 mg/d
Bisoprolol (Zebeta®)	$beta_1$	Low	26-33	9-12	80	Renal (hepatic)	Hypertension, heart failure	P.O.: 2.5-5 mg
Carteolol (Cartrol®)	$beta_1$ $beta_2$	Low	20-30	6	80-85	Renal	Hypertension	P.O.: 2.5-10 mg/d
Carvedilol (Coreg®)	$beta_1$ $beta_2$ $alpha_1$	ND	98	7-10	25-35	Bile into feces	Hypertension, heart failure (mild to severe)	P.O.: 6.25 mg twice daily
Esmolol (Brevibloc®)	$beta_1$	Low	55	0.15	NA 5-fold[1]	Red blood cell	Supraventricular tachycardia, sinus tachycardia, atrial fibrillation/flutter, hypertension	I.V. infusion: 25-300 mcg/kg/min
Labetalol (Trandate®)	$alpha_1$ $beta_1$ $beta_2$	Moderate	50	5.5-8	18-30 10-fold[1]	Renal (hepatic)	Hypertension	P.O.: 200-2400 mg/d I.V.: 20-80 mg at 10-min intervals up to a maximum of 300 mg **or** continuous infusion of 2 mg/min
Metoprolol (Lopressor®, Toprol-XL®)	$beta_1$	Moderate	10-12	3-7	50 10-fold[1] (Toprol XL®: 77)	Hepatic/renal	Hypertension, angina pectoris, acute MI, heart failure (mild to moderate; XL formulation only)	P.O.: 100-450 mg/d I.V.: Post-MI 15 mg Angina: 15 mg then 2-5 mg/hour Arrhythmias: 0.2 mg/kg

Agent	Adrenergic Receptor Blocking Activity	Lipid Solubility	Protein Bound (%)	Half-Life (h)	Bioavailability (%)	Primary (Secondary) Route of Elimination	Indications	Usual Dosage
Nadolol (Corgard®)	$beta_1$ $beta_2$	Low	25-30	20-24	30 5- to 8-fold[1]	Renal	Hypertension, angina pectoris	P.O.: 40-320 mg/d
Penbutolol (Levatol®)	$beta_1$ $beta_2$	High	80-98	5	~100	Hepatic (renal)	Hypertension	P.O.: 20-80 mg/d
Pindolol	$beta_1$ $beta_2$	Moderate	57	3-4[2]	90 4-fold[1]	Hepatic (renal)	Hypertension	P.O.: 20-60 mg/d
Propranolol (Inderal®, various)	$beta_1$ $beta_2$	High	90	3-5[2]	30 20-fold[1]	Hepatic	Hypertension, angina pectoris, arrhythmias, prophylaxis (post-MI)	P.O.: 40-480 mg/d I.V.: Reflex tachycardia 1-10 mg
Propranolol long-acting (Inderal-LA®)	$beta_1$ $beta_2$	High	90	9-18	20- to 30-fold[1]	Hepatic	Hypertrophic subaortic stenosis, prophylaxis (post-MI)	P.O.: 180-240 mg/d
Sotalol (Betapace®, Betapace AF®, Sorine®)	$beta_1$ $beta_2$	Low	0	12	90-100	Renal	Ventricular arrhythmias/ tachyarrhythmias	P.O. 160-320 mg/d
Timolol (Blocadren®)	$beta_1$ $beta_2$	Low to moderate	<10	4	75 7-fold[1]	Hepatic (renal)	Hypertension, prophylaxis (post-MI)	P.O.: 20-60 mg/d P.O.: 20 mg/d

Dosage is based on 70 kg adult with normal hepatic and renal function.

Note: All $beta_1$-selective agents will inhibit $beta_2$ receptors at higher doses.

[1]Interpatient variations in plasma levels.

[2]Half-life increased to 16-27 hours in creatinine clearance of 15-35 mL/minute and >27 hours in creatinine clearance <15 mL/minute.

CALCIUM CHANNEL BLOCKERS

Comparative Pharmacokinetics

Agent	Bioavailability (%)	Protein Binding (%)	Onset of BP Effect (min)	Duration of BP Effect (h)	Half-Life (h)	Volume of Distribution	Route of Metabolism	Route of Excretion
Dihydropyridines								
Amlodipine (Norvasc®)	64-90	93-98	30-50	24	30-50	21 L/kg	Hepatic; inactive metabolites	Urine; 10% as parent
Clevidipine (Cleviprex™)		>99.5	2-4	5-15 min	1-15 min	0.17 L/kg	Blood and extravascular tissue esterases	Urine(63% to 74%; as metabolites); feces (7% to 22%)
Felodipine (Plendil®)	20	>99	2-5 h	24	11-16	10 L/kg	Hepatic; CYP3A4 substrate (major); inactive metabolites; extensive first pass	Urine (70%; as metabolites); feces 10%
Isradipine (DynaCirc® [DSC]) (immediate release)	15-24	95	20	>12	8	3 L/kg	Hepatic; CYP3A4 substrate (major); inactive metabolites; extensive first pass	Urine as metabolites
Nicardipine (Cardene®) (immediate release)	35	>95	30	≤8	2-4		Hepatic; CYP3A4 substrate (major); saturable first pass	Urine (60%; as metabolites); feces 35%
Nifedipine (Procardia®) (immediate release)	40-77	92-98	Within 20		2-5		Hepatic; CYP3A4 substrate (major); inactive metabolites	Urine as metabolites
Nimodipine (Nimotop®)	13	>95	ND	4-6	1-2		Hepatic; CYP3A4 substrate (major); metabolites inactive or less active than parent; extensive first pass	Urine (50%; as metabolites); feces 32%

Comparative Pharmacokinetics *continued*

Agent	Bioavailability (%)	Protein Binding (%)	Onset of BP Effect (min)	Duration of BP Effect (h)	Half-Life (h)	Volume of Distribution	Route of Metabolism	Route of Excretion
Nisoldipine (Sular®)	5	>99	ND	6-12	7-12		Hepatic; CYP3A4 substrate (major); 1 active metabolite (10% of parent); extensive first pass	Urine as metabolites
Phenylalkylamines								
Verapamil (Calan®) (immediate release)	20-35	90	30	6-8	4.5-12		Hepatic; CYP3A4 substrate (major); 1 active metabolite (20% of parent); extensive first pass	Urine (70%; 3%-4% as unchanged drug); feces 16%
Benzothiazepines								
Diltiazem (Cardizem®) (immediate release)	~40	70-80	30-60	6-8	3-4.5	3-13 L/kg	Hepatic; CYP3A4 substrate (major); 1 major metabolite (20%-50% of parent); extensive first pass	Urine as metabolites

CORTICOSTEROIDS

Corticosteroids, Systemic Equivalencies

Glucocorticoid	Approximate Equivalent Dose (mg)	Routes of Administration	Relative Anti-inflammatory Potency	Relative Mineralocorticoid Potency	Protein Binding (%)	Half-life	
						Plasma (min)	Biologic (h)
Short-Acting							
Cortisone	25	P.O., I.M.	0.8	2	90	30	8-12
Hydrocortisone	20	I.M., I.V.	1	2	90	80-118	8-12
Intermediate-Acting							
Methylprednisolone[1]	4	P.O., I.M., I.V.	5	0	—	78-188	18-36
Prednisolone	5	P.O., I.M., I.V., intra-articular, intradermal, soft tissue injection	4	1	90-95	115-212	18-36
Prednisone	5	P.O.	4	1	70	60	18-36
Triamcinolone[1]	4	P.O., I.M., intra-articular, intradermal, intrasynovial, soft tissue injection	5	0	—	200+	18-36
Long-Acting							
Betamethasone	0.6-0.75	P.O., I.M., intra-articular, intradermal, intrasynovial, soft tissue injection	25	0	64	300+	36-54
Dexamethasone	0.75	P.O., I.M., I.V., intra-articular, intradermal, soft tissue injection	25-30	0	—	110-210	36-54
Mineralocorticoids							
Fludrocortisone	—	P.O.	10	125	42	210+	18-36

[1]May contain propylene glycol as an excipient in injectable forms.

GUIDELINES FOR SELECTION AND USE OF TOPICAL CORTICOSTEROIDS

The quantity prescribed and the frequency of refills should be monitored to reduce the risk of adrenal suppression. In general, short courses of high-potency agents are preferable to prolonged use of low potency. After control is achieved, control should be maintained with a low potency preparation.

1. Low-to-medium potency agents are usually effective for treating thin, acute, inflammatory skin lesions; whereas, high or super-potent agents are often required for treating chronic, hyperkeratotic, or lichenified lesions.
2. Since the stratum corneum is thin on the face and intertriginous areas, low-potency agents are preferred but a higher potency agent may be used for 2 weeks.
3. Because the palms and soles have a thick stratum corneum, high or super-potent agents are frequently required.
4. Low potency agents are preferred for infants and the elderly. Infants have a high body surface area to weight ratio; elderly patients have thin, fragile skin.
5. The vehicle in which the topical corticosteroid is formulated influences the absorption and potency of the drug. Ointment bases are preferred for thick, lichenified lesions; they enhance penetration of the drug. Creams are preferred for acute and subacute dermatoses; they may be used on moist skin areas or intertriginous areas. Solutions, gels, and sprays are preferred for the scalp or for areas where a nonoil-based vehicle is needed.
6. In general, super-potent agents should not be used for longer than 2-3 weeks unless the lesion is limited to a small body area. Medium-to-high potency agents usually cause only rare adverse effects when treatment is limited to 3 months or less, and use on the face and intertriginous areas are avoided. If long-term treatment is needed, intermittent vs continued treatment is recommended.
7. Most preparations are applied once or twice daily. More frequent application may be necessary for the palms or soles because the preparation is easily removed by normal activity and penetration is poor due to a thick stratum corneum. Every-other-day or weekend-only application may be effective for treating some chronic conditions.

Corticosteroids, Topical

	Steroid	Vehicle
	Very High Potency	
0.05%	Betamethasone dipropionate, augmented	Lotion, ointment
0.05%	Clobetasol propionate	Cream, foam, gel, lotion, ointment, shampoo, spray
0.05%	Diflorasone diacetate	Ointment
0.05%	Halobetasol propionate	Cream, ointment
	High Potency	
0.1%	Amcinonide	Cream, ointment, lotion
0.05%	Betamethasone dipropionate, augmented	Cream
0.05%	Betamethasone dipropionate	Cream, ointment
0.1%	Betamethasone valerate	Ointment
0.05%	Desoximetasone	Gel
0.25%	Desoximetasone	Cream, ointment
0.05%	Diflorasone diacetate	Cream, ointment
0.05%	Fluocinonide	Cream, ointment, gel
0.1%	Halcinonide	Cream, ointment
0.5%	Triamcinolone acetonide	Cream
	Intermediate Potency	
0.05%	Betamethasone dipropionate	Lotion
0.1%	Betamethasone valerate	Cream
0.1%	Clocortolone pivalate	Cream
0.05%	Desoximetasone	Cream

Corticosteroids, Topical *continued*

	Steroid	Vehicle
0.025%	Fluocinolone acetonide	Cream, ointment
0.05%	Flurandrenolide	Cream, ointment, lotion, tape
0.005%	Fluticasone propionate	Ointment
0.05%	Fluticasone propionate	Cream
0.1%	Hydrocortisone butyrate[1]	Ointment, solution
0.2%	Hydrocortisone valerate[1]	Cream, ointment
0.1%	Mometasone furoate[1]	Cream, ointment, lotion
0.1%	Prednicarbate	Cream, ointment
0.025%	Triamcinolone acetonide	Cream, ointment, lotion
0.1%	Triamcinolone acetonide	Cream, ointment, lotion
	Low Potency	
0.05%	Alclometasone dipropionate[1]	Cream, ointment
0.05%	Desonide	Cream
0.01%	Fluocinolone acetonide	Cream, solution
0.5%	Hydrocortisone[1]	Cream, ointment, lotion
0.5%	Hydrocortisone acetate[1]	Cream, ointment
1%	Hydrocortisone acetate[1]	Cream, ointment
1%	Hydrocortisone[1]	Cream, ointment, lotion, solution
2.5%	Hydrocortisone[1]	Cream, ointment, lotion

[1]Not fluorinated.

HALLUCINOGENIC DRUGS

Principal Pharmacological Properties of Hallucinogenic Drugs

Drug; Chemical Structure	Duration of Acute Effect (h)	pKa	Route of Metabolism / Excretion	Half-Life	Protein Binding (%)	V_d (L/kg)	Urine Screen Positive for	Duration of Psychotropic Effects	Doses of Abuse	Fatal Dose
Phencyclidine (PCP); arylcyclohexylamine	4-6	8.5	Hepatic/urine	1 h	65	6.2-0.3	2 wk	Up to 1 mo	1-9 mg	1 mg/kg
Cocaine; tropane alkaloid	0.5	5.6	Plasma hydrolysis[1]	48-75 min	9-90	1.2-1.9	4 days (benzoylecgonine)	≤5-7 d	20-200 mg (intranasally)	1-1.2 g
Cannabis; monoterpenoid	0.5-3	10.6	Hepatic hydroxylation	25-57 h	97-99	10	Up to 4 d	≤6 h	5-15 mg THC	
LSD; indole alkylamine	0.7-8	7.8	Hepatic hydroxylation	2.5 h		0.27	5 d	May last for days	100-300 mcg	0.2 mg/kg
Psilocybin; tryptamine	0.5-6						Not detected	12 h	20-100 mushrooms	5-15 mg of psilocybin
Mescaline; phenylalkylamine	4.6	Not known	Hepatic/urine[2]	6 h	None	Not known		12 h	5 mg/kg	20 mg/kg
Morphine; alkaloid/ derivative of opium	4-5	8.05	Glucuronidation/ urine	1.9-3.1 h	35	3.2	48 h	≤6 h	2-20 mg	Variable – dependent on tolerance, nontolerant fatal dose is 120 mg orally or 30 mg parenterally

Principal Pharmacological Properties of Hallucinogenic Drugs *continued*

Drug; Chemical Structure	Duration of Acute Effect (h)	pKa	Route of Metabolism / Excretion	Half-Life	Protein Binding (%)	V_d (L/kg)	Urine Screen Positive for	Duration of Psychotropic Effects	Doses of Abuse	Fatal Dose
Heroin; diacetylmorphine	3.4	7.6	Hepatic[3]	3-20 min	40	25	~40 h	≤6 h	2.2 mg	Variable – dependent on tolerance
Amphetamine; β-(phenylisopropyl)-amine	Variable	9.93	Hepatic[4]	12 h[5]	16-20	3-6	2-4 d	Delusions may remain for months	100-1000 mg/d	Variable – dependent on tolerance

[1]By serum cholinesterase.

[2]60% excreted unchanged.

[3]Converted to morphine.

[4]Converted to phenylacetone.

[5]Urine pH-dependent.

Reprinted with permission from Leikin JB, Krantz AJ, Zell-Kanter M, et al, "Clinical Features and Management of Intoxication Due to Hallucinogenic Drugs," *Med Toxicol Adverse Drug Exp*, 1989, 4(5):328.

LAXATIVES, CLASSIFICATION AND PROPERTIES

Laxative	Onset of Action	Site of Action	Mechanism of Action
Saline			
Magnesium citrate Magnesium hydroxide (Phillips'® Milk of Magnesia)	30 min to 3 h	Small and large intestine	Attract/retain water in intestinal lumen increasing intraluminal pressure; cholecystokinin release
Sodium phosphates (Fleet® Enema)	2-15 min	Colon	
Irritant / Stimulant			
Senna (Senokot®)	6-10 h	Colon	Direct action on intestinal mucosa; stimulate myenteric plexus; alter water and electrolyte secretion
Bisacodyl (Dulcolax®) tablets, suppositories	15 min to 1 h	Colon	
Castor oil	2-6 h	Small intestine	
Bulk-Producing			
Methylcellulose (Citrucel®) Psyllium (Metamucil®)	12-24 h (up to 72 h)	Small and large intestine	Holds water in stool; mechanical distention; malt soup extract reduces fecal pH
Lubricant			
Mineral oil	6-8 h	Colon	Lubricates intestine; retards colonic absorption of fecal water; softens stool
Surfactants / Stool Softener			
Docusate sodium (Colace®) Docusate calcium (Surfak®)	24-72 h	Small and large intestine	Detergent activity; facilitates admixture of fat and water to soften stool
Miscellaneous and Combination Laxatives			
Glycerin suppository	15-30 min	Colon	Local irritation; hyperosmotic action
Lactulose	24-48 h	Colon	Delivers osmotically active molecules to colon
Lubiprostone (Amitiza®)	24-48 h	Apical membrane of the GI epithelium	Activates intestinal chloride channels increasing intestinal fluid
Docusate/senna (Peri-Colace®)	8-12 h	Small and large intestine	Senna – mild irritant; docusate – stool softener
Polyethylene glycol 3350 (GlycoLax™, MiraLax™)	48 h	Small and large intestine	Nonabsorbable solution which acts as an osmotic agent
Sorbitol 70%	24-48 h	Colon	Delivers osmotically active molecules to colon

LIPID-LOWERING AGENTS

Effects on Lipoproteins

Drug	Total Cholesterol (%)	LDLC (%)	HDLC (%)	TG (%)
Bile-acid resins	↓20-25	↓20-35	→	↑5-20
Fibric acid derivatives	↓10	↓10 (↑)	↑10-20	↓40-55
HMG-CoA RI (statins)	↓15-60	↓20-40	↑2-15	↓7-25
Nicotinic acid	↓25	↓20	↑20	↓40
Probucol	↓10-15	↓<10	↓30	→
Ezetimibe	↓12-13	↓16-18	↑1-4	↓5-6

Lipid-Lowering Agents

Drug	Dose / Day	Effect on LDL (%)	Effect on HDL (%)	Effect on TG (%)
HMG-CoA Reductase Inhibitors				
Atorvastatin	10 mg 20 mg 40 mg 80 mg	-39 -43 -50 -60	+6 +9 +6 +5	-19 -26 -29 -37
Fluvastatin	20 mg 40 mg 80 mg	-22 -25 -36	+3 +4 +6	-12 -14 -18
Lovastatin	10 mg 20 mg 40 mg 80 mg	-21 -27 -31 -40	+5 +6 +5 +9.5	-10 -8 -8 -19
Pravastatin	10 mg 20 mg 40 mg 80 mg	-22 -32 -34 -37	+7 +2 +12 +3	-15 -11 -24 -19
Rosuvastatin	5 mg 10 mg 20 mg 40 mg	-45 -52 -55 -63	+13 +14 +8 +10	-35 -10 -23 -28
Simvastatin	5 mg 10 mg 20 mg 40 mg 80 mg	-26 -30 -38 -41 -47	+10 +12 +8 +13 +16	-12 -15 -19 -28 -33
Bile Acid Sequestrants				
Cholestyramine	4-24 g	-15 to -30	+3 to +5	+0 to +20
Colestipol	7-30 g	-15 to -30	+3 to +5	+0 to +20
Colesevelam	6 tablets 7 tablets	-15 -18	+3 +3	+10 +9
Fibric Acid Derivatives				
Fenofibrate	67-200 mg	-20 to -25	+1 to +20	-30 to -50
Gemfibrozil	600 mg twice daily	-5 to -10[1]	+10 to +20	-40 to -60
Niacin	1.5-6 g	-21 to -27	+10 to +35	-10 to -50
2-Azetidinone				
Ezetimibe	10 mg	-18	+1	-8
Omega-3-Acid Ethyl Esters	4 g	+44.5	+9.1	-44.9
Combination Products				
Ezetimibe and fenofibrate	10/160 mg	-20	+19	-44
Ezetimibe and simvastatin	10/10 mg 10/20 mg 10/40 mg 10/80 mg	-45 -52 -55 -60	+8 +10 +6 +6	-23 -24 -23 -31

Lipid-Lowering Agents *continued*

Drug	Dose / Day	Effect on LDL (%)	Effect on HDL (%)	Effect on TG (%)
Niacin and lovastatin	1000/20 mg 1000/40 mg 1500/40 mg 2000/40 mg	-30 -36 -37 -42	+20 +20 +27 +30	-32 -39 -44 -44
Niacin and simvastatin	1000/20 mg 1000/40 mg 2000/20 mg 2000/40 mg	-12 -7 -14 -5	+21 +15 +29 +24	-27 -23 -38 -32

[1]May increase LDL in some patients.

Recommended Liver Function Monitoring for HMG-CoA Reductase Inhibitors

Agent	Initial and After Elevation in Dose	6 Weeks[1]	12 Weeks[1]	Periodically
Atorvastatin (Lipitor®)	x		x	x
Fluvastatin (Lescol®)	x		x	x
Lovastatin (Mevacor®)	x	x	x	x
Pravastatin (Pravachol®)	x			x
Simvastatin (Zocor®)	x			x

[1]After initiation of therapy or any elevation in dose.

LIQUID COMPATIBILITY OF ANTIDEPRESSANTS, ANTIPSYCHOTICS, AND MOOD STABILIZERS

Fruit and Vegetable Juices

Drug	Apple Juice	Grape Juice	Grapefruit Juice	Lemonade	Orange Juice	Pineapple Juice	Prune Juice	Tomato Juice
Aripiprazole								
Carbamazepine*								
Chlorpromazine*	X	X	C		C		U	
Citalopram	C				C			
Doxepin			C		C	C	C	C
Escitalopram	C				C			
Fluoxetine								
Fluphenazine	X		C		C		C	
Haloperidol	C	X	X		C			
Lithium	X	C	C		C		C	
Loxapine			C		C			
PARoxetine								
Risperidone					C			
Sertraline				C	C			
Thioridazine	X	X	C		C		X	
Thiothixene	X		C		C		C	
Trifluoperazine	X	X	C		C		C	
Valproate								

C = compatible; X = incompatible; U = conflicting data; Blank = no data.

*Carbamazepine is not compatible with chlorpromazine.

Other Beverages

Drug	Water	Saline	Milk	Coffee	Tea	Cola	Gingerale	7-Up / Sprite
Aripiprazole								
Carbamazepine*	C	C						
Chlorpromazine*	C	C	C	U	U	U	C	
Citalopram	C							
Doxepin	C		C			X		
Escitalopram	C							
Fluoxetine								
Fluphenazine	C	C	C	X	X	X	X	
Haloperidol	C	X	X	X	X	C		
Lithium	C	C	C	C	C	C	C	
Loxapine				C		C	C	
PARoxetine								
Risperidone	C	C	C	C	X	X		
Sertraline	C						C	C
Thioridazine	C	C	X	X	X	X	C	
Thiothixene	C		C	X	X	X		
Trifluoperazine	C	C	C	U	C	C	C	
Valproate	C	C				X	X	

C = compatible; X = incompatible; U = conflicting data; Blank = no data.

*Carbamazepine is not compatible with chlorpromazine.

NARCOTIC / OPIOID ANALGESICS

Opioid Analgesics – Initial Oral Dosing Commonly Used for Severe Pain

Drug	Equianalgesic Dose (mg)		Initial Oral Dose	
	Oral[1]	Parenteral[2]	Children (mg/kg)	Adults (mg)
Buprenorphine	—	0.4	—	—
Butorphanol	—	2	—	—
Hydromorphone	7.5	1.5	0.06	4-8
Levorphanol	Acute: 4 Chronic: 1	Acute: 2 Chronic: 1	0.04	2-4
Meperidine	300	75	Not recommended	
Methadone	10	5	0.2	5-10
Morphine	30	10	0.3	15-30
Nalbuphine	—	10	—	—
Pentazocine	50	30	—	—
Oxycodone	20	—	0.3	10-20
Oxymorphone	—	1	—	—

From "Principles of Analgesic Use in the Treatment of Acute Pain and Cancer Pain," *Am Pain Soc*, Fifth Ed.

[1]Elderly: Starting dose should be lower for this population group.

[2]Standard parenteral doses for acute pain in adults; can be used to doses for I.V. infusions and repeated small I.V. boluses. Single I.V. boluses, use half the I.M. dose. Children >6 months: I.V. dose = parenteral equianalgesic dose x weight (kg)/100.

Comparative Pharmacology

Drug	Analgesic	Antitussive	Constipation	Respiratory Depression	Sedation	Emesis
Phenanthrenes						
Codeine	+	+++	+	+	+	+
Hydrocodone	++	+++				
Hydromorphone	++	++	+	++	+	+
Levorphanol	++	++		++	++	+
Morphine	++	++	++	++	++	++
Oxycodone	++	+++	++	++	++	++
Oxymorphone	++	+	+++	+++		+++
Phenylpiperidines						
Meperidine	++		+	++	+	
Diphenylheptanes						
Methadone	++	++	+	++	+	+
Propoxyphene	+			+	+	+
Agonist / Antagonist						
Pentazocine	++		+	++	++ or stimulation	++

Adapted from Catalano RB, "The Medical Approach to Management of Pain Caused by Cancer," *Semin Oncol*, 1975, 2(4):379-92.

NONBENZODIAZEPINE ANXIOLYTICS AND HYPNOTICS

Drug	Dosage Forms	Initial Dose	Usual Dosage Range	Onset	Half-Life	Comments
Buspirone (BuSpar®)	Tab	7.5 mg bid	30-60 mg/d	30 min - 1.5 h	2-3 h	Do not use for alcohol or benzodiazepine withdrawal; no sedation or dependence; do not use PRN; use 4 weeks for full therapeutic effect
Chloral hydrate (Aquachloral® Supprettes®, Somnote™)	Cap, rec supp, syr	500 mg - 1 g qhs	500 mg - 2 g/d	30 min	8-11 h	GI irritating; tolerance to hypnotic effect develops rapidly; do not use for alcohol or benzodiazepine withdrawal
Diphenhydramine (Benadryl® Allergy and others)	Sol, cap, tab, cream, lot, syr, elix	25-50 mg qhs	25-200 mg/d	1-3 h	2-8 h	Antihistamine with anticholinergic side effects; max hypnotic dose: 50 mg/d; do not use for alcohol or benzodiazepine withdrawal
Doxylamine (Unisom®, SleepTabs® and others)	Tab	25 mg qhs	25 mg qhs	30 min	10-12 h	Antihistamine with anticholinergic side effects
Eszopiclone (Lunesta™)	Tab	1-2 mg qhs	1-3 mg qhs	30 min	6-9 h	Use caution in patients with depression especially if suicidal
Hydroxyzine (Atarax®, Vistaril®)	Tab, cap, liq, inj, syr	25-100 mg qid	100-600 mg/d	30 min	3-7 h	Antihistamine with anticholinergic side effects; do not use for alcohol or benzodiazepine withdrawal
Propranolol (Inderal®, Inderal® LA, InnoPran XL™, Propranolol Intensol™)	Tab, cap, sol, inj	10 mg tid	80-160 mg/d	1-2 h	4-6 h	Useful for physical manifestations of anxiety (increased heart rate, tremor); second-line agent; do not use for alcohol or benzodiazepine withdrawal
Ramelteon (Rozerem™)	Tab	8 mg qhs	8 mg qhs	30 min	1-3 h	Melatonin receptor agonist; contraindicated with fluvoxamine
Zaleplon (Sonata®)	Cap	5-10 mg qhs	5-20 mg qhs	30 min	1 h	Do not use for alcohol or benzodiazepine withdrawal
Zolpidem (Ambien®)	Tab	10 mg qhs	10 mg qhs	30 min	2.5 h	Do not use for alcohol or benzodiazepine withdrawal

NONSTEROIDAL ANTI-INFLAMMATORY AGENTS

Comparative Dosages and Pharmacokinetics

Drug	Maximum Recommended Daily Dose (mg)	Time to Peak Levels[1] (h)	Half-life (h)
Acetic Acids			
Diclofenac potassium immediate release (Cataflam®)	200	1	1-2
Diclofenac sodium delayed release (Voltaren®)	225	2-3	1-2
Etodolac	1200	1-2	7.3
Indomethacin (Indocin®)	200	1-2	4.5
Indomethacin sustained release (Indocin® SR)	150	2-4	4.5-6
Ketorolac (Toradol®)	I.M.: 120[2] P.O.: 40	0.5-1	3.8-8.6
Sulindac (Clinoril®)	400	2-4	7.8 (16.4)[3]
Tolmetin (Tolectin®)	2000	0.5-1	1-1.5
Fenamates (Anthranilic Acids)			
Meclofenamate	400	0.5-1	2 (3.3)[4]
Mefenamic acid (Ponstel®)	1000	2-4	2-4
Propionic Acids			
Fenoprofen (Nalfon®)	3200	1-2	2-3
Flurbiprofen	300	1.5	5.7
Ibuprofen (various)	3200	1-2	1.8-2.5
Ketoprofen	300	0.5-2	2-4
Naproxen (Naprosyn®)	1500	2-4	12-15
Naproxen sodium (Anaprox®, others)	1375	1-2	12-13
Oxaprozin (Daypro®)	1800	3-5	42-50
Nonacidic Agent			
Nabumetone	2000	3-6	24
Salicylic Acid Derivative			
Diflunisal	1500	2-3	8-12
Salsalate	3000	2-3	7-8
COX-2 Inhibitor			
Celecoxib (Celebrex®)	400	3	11
Oxicam			
Meloxicam (Mobic®)	15	4-5	15-20
Piroxicam (Feldene®)	20	3-5	30-86

Dosage is based on 70 kg adult with normal hepatic and renal function.

[1]Food decreases the rate of absorption and may delay the time to peak levels.

[2]150 mg on the first day.

[3]Half-life of active sulfide metabolite.

[4]Half-life with multiple doses.

SELECTIVE SEROTONIN REUPTAKE INHIBITORS (SSRIS) CYP PROFILE

Generic Name (Brand Name)	1A2	2B6	2C8/9	2C19	2D6	3A4
Citalopram (Celexa®)	Weak	Weak	—	Weak	Weak	—
Escitalopram (Lexapro™)	—	—	—	—	Weak	—
Fluoxetine (Prozac®; Prozac® Weekly™; Sarafem™)	Moderate	Weak	Weak	Moderate	**Strong**	Weak
Fluvoxamine	**Strong**	Weak	Weak	**Strong**	Weak	Weak
Paroxetine (Paxil®; Paxil CR™)	Weak	Moderate	Weak	Weak	**Strong**	Weak
Sertraline (Zoloft®)	Weak	Moderate	Weak	Moderate	Moderate	Moderate

Based on a ratio ([I]/Ki) of the serum concentration [I] of drug achieved under typical dosing conditions and a drug's Ki value (inhibitor constant).

Weak = ratio <0.1.
Moderate = ratio 0.1-0.99.
Strong = ratio ≥1.

SELECTIVE SEROTONIN REUPTAKE INHIBITORS (SSRIS) FDA-APPROVED INDICATION(S)

Generic Name (Brand Name)	Major Depression	Anorexia / Bulimia	Obsessive-Compulsive Disorder) (OCD)	Premenstrual Dysphoric Disorder) (PMDD)	Panic Disorder	Post-traumatic Stress Disorder) (PTSD)	Social Anxiety Disorder	Generalized Anxiety Disorder) (GAD)
Citalopram (Celexa™)	X							X
Escitalopram (Lexapro™)	X							X
Fluoxetine (Prozac®; Prozac® Weekly™; Sarafem™)	X	X	X	X	X			
Fluvoxamine			X					
Paroxetine (Paxil®; Paxil CR™)	X		X	X (Paxil CR™)	X	X	X	X
Sertraline (Zoloft®)	X		X	X	X	X	X	

SELECTIVE SEROTONIN REUPTAKE INHIBITORS (SSRIS) PHARMACOKINETICS

SSRI	Half-Life (h)	Metabolite Half-Life	Peak Plasma Level (h)	% Protein Bound	Bioavailability (%)	Initial Dose
Citalopram (Celexa™)	35	S-desmethyl-citalopram: 59 hours	4	80	80	20 mg qAM
Escitalopram (Lexapro™)	27-32	S-desmethyl-citalopram: 59 hours	5	56	80	10 mg qAM
Fluoxetine (Prozac®, Prozac® Weekly™, Sarafem™)	Initial: 24-72 Chronic: 96-144	Norfluoxetine: 4-16 days	6-8	95	72	10-20 mg qAM
Fluvoxamine	16	N/A	3	80	53	50 mg qhs
Paroxetine (Paxil®, Paxil® CR™)	21	N/A	5	95	>90	10-20 mg qAM
Sertraline (Zoloft®)	26	N-desmethyl-sertraline: 62-104 hours	5-8	98	88	25-50 qAM

SELECTIVE SEROTONIN REUPTAKE INHIBITORS (SSRIS) RECEPTOR PROFILE

Generic Name (Brand Name)	NE-T	5HT-T	DA-T	M_1	H_1	α_1
Citalopram (Celexa™)	4000	1.16	28,000	2200	476	1890
Escitalopram[1] (Lexapro®)	7841	1.10	27,410	1242	1973	3870
Fluoxetine (Prozac®; Prozac® Weekly™; Sarafem™)	244	0.81	3600	2000	6250	5900
Fluvoxamine	1300	2.22	9100	24,000	>100,000	7700
Paroxetine (Paxil®; Paxil CR™)	40	0.13	500	108	22,000	>100,000
Sertraline (Zoloft®)	417	0.29	25	625	24,000	370

Ki (nM; inhibitory constant); NE-T = norepinephrine transporter; 5HT-T = serotonin transporter; DA-T = dopamine transporter; M_1 = muscarinic$_1$ receptor; H_1 = histamine H_1 receptor; α_1 = alpha$_1$ receptor.

[1]Owens MJ, Knight DL, and Nemeroff CB, "Second-Generation SSRIs: Human Monoamine Transporter Binding Profile of Escitalopram and R-Fluoxetine," *Biol Psychiatry*, 2001, 50(5):345-50.

Adapted from Gilman AG, *Goodman and Gilman's The Pharmacological Basis of Therapeutics*, 10th ed, New York, NY: McGraw-Hill, 2001.

STIMULANT AGENTS USED FOR ADHD

Generic Name (Brand Name)	Dosage	Formulations	Comments
Dexmethylphenidate (Focalin™)	2.5 mg bid, increase by 2.5-5 mg at weekly intervals; maximum dose: 20 mg/d	Tablet: 2.5 mg, 5 mg, 10 mg	Doses should be taken at least 4 hours apart; when switching from methylphenidate the starting dose of dexmethylphenidate should be half that of methylphenidate
Dextroamphetamine and Amphetamine (Adderall®)	2.5-5 mg qAM, increase by 2.5-5 mg/wk; maximum dose: 40 mg/d on bid schedule	Tablet: 5 mg, 7.5 mg, 10 mg, 12.5 mg, 15 mg, 20 mg, 30 mg	Also used for narcolepsy; take at least 6 hours before bedtime
Dextroamphetamine and Amphetamine long acting (Adderall XR™)	5-10 mg qAM, increase by 10 mg weekly; maximum dose: 30 mg/d	Capsule: 5 mg, 10 mg, 15 mg, 20 mg, 25 mg, 30 mg	Take dosage before noon; capsule can be opened and sprinkled on applesauce
Dextroamphetamine[1] short acting (Dexedrine®, Dextrostat®)	2.5-5 mg qAM, increase by 2.5-5 mg/wk; maximum dose: 40 mg/d	Tablet: 5 mg, 10 mg	Avoid evening doses; monitor growth; also used for narcolepsy and exogenous obesity
Dextroamphetamine[1] long acting (Dexedrine® Spansules)		Spansules, sustained release: 5 mg, 10 mg, 15 mg	
Lisdexamfetamine (Vyvanse™)	30 mg qAM, increase by 10-20 mg weekly; maximum dose: 70 mg/d	Capsule: 20 mg, 30 mg, 40 mg, 50 mg, 60 mg, 70 mg	
Methamphetamine (Desoxyn®)	2.5-5 mg qd-bid, increase by 5 mg/wk until optimum response is achieved, usually 20-25 mg/d	Tablet: 5 mg	
Methylphenidate extended release (Ritalin® LA)	20 mg qd; may increase by 30 mg weekly; maximum dose: 60 mg/d	Capsule: 20 mg, 30 mg, 40 mg	8 hour duration of action
Methylphenidate short acting (Ritalin®, Methylin™)	2.5-5 mg before breakfast or lunch; increase by 5-10 mg/d at weekly intervals; maximum dose: 90 mg/d	Tablet: 5 mg, 10 mg, 20 mg	
Methylphenidate sustained release (Ritalin SR®)	2.5-5 mg before breakfast or lunch; increase by 5-10 mg/d at weekly intervals; maximum dose: 90 mg/d	Tablet, sustained release: 20 mg	8 hour duration of action

Generic Name (Brand Name)	Dosage	Formulations	Comments
Methylphenidate long acting (Metadate ER®, Methylin™ ER)	2.5-5 mg before breakfast or lunch; increase by 5-10 mg/d at weekly intervals; maximum dose: 90 mg/d	Tablet: 10 mg, 20 mg	8 hour duration of action
Methylphenidate extended release (Metadate CD®)	20 mg qd; may increase by 30 mg weekly; maximum dose: 60 mg/d	Capsule: 10 mg, 20 mg, 30 mg	8 hour duration of action; biphasic peak
Methylphenidate extended release (Concerta™)	18 mg qAM; increase by 18 mg weekly; maximum dose: 54 mg/d	Tablet: 18 mg, 27 mg, 36 mg, 54 mg	12 hour duration of action; take with water, milk, or juice

[1]Available in generic form.

CYTOCHROME P450 ENZYMES: SUBSTRATES, INHIBITORS, AND INDUCERS

INTRODUCTION

Most drugs are eliminated from the body, at least in part, by being chemically altered to less lipid-soluble products (ie, metabolized), and thus are more likely to be excreted via the kidneys or the bile. Phase I metabolism includes drug hydrolysis, oxidation, and reduction, and results in drugs that are more polar in their chemical structure, while Phase II metabolism involves the attachment of an additional molecule onto the drug (or partially metabolized drug) in order to create an inactive and/or more water soluble compound. Phase II processes include (primarily) glucuronidation, sulfation, glutathione conjugation, acetylation, and methylation.

Virtually any of the Phase I and II enzymes can be inhibited by some xenobiotic or drug. Some of the Phase I and II enzymes can be induced. Inhibition of the activity of metabolic enzymes will result in increased concentrations of the substrate (drug), whereas induction of the activity of metabolic enzymes will result in decreased concentrations of the substrate. For example, the well-documented enzyme-inducing effects of PHENobarbital may include a combination of Phase I and II enzymes. Phase II glucuronidation may be increased via induced UDP-glucuronosyltransferase (UGT) activity, whereas Phase I oxidation may be increased via induced cytochrome P450 (CYP) activity. However, for most drugs, the primary route of metabolism (and the primary focus of drug-drug interaction) is Phase I oxidation, and specifically, metabolism.

CYP enzymes may be responsible for the metabolism (at least partial metabolism) of approximately 75% of all drugs, with the CYP3A subfamily responsible for nearly half of this activity. Found throughout plant, animal, and bacterial species, CYP enzymes represent a superfamily of xenobiotic metabolizing proteins. There have been several hundred CYP enzymes identified in nature, each of which has been assigned to a family (1, 2, 3, etc), subfamily (A, B, C, etc), and given a specific enzyme number (1, 2, 3, etc) according to the similarity in amino acid sequence that it shares with other enzymes. Of these many enzymes, only a few are found in humans, and even fewer appear to be involved in the metabolism of xenobiotics (eg, drugs). The key human enzyme subfamilies include CYP1A, CYP2A, CYP2B, CYP2C, CYP2D, CYP2E, and CYP3A.

CYP enzymes are found in the endoplasmic reticulum of cells in a variety of human tissues (eg, skin, kidneys, brain, lungs), but their predominant sites of concentration and activity are the liver and intestine. Though the abundance of CYP enzymes throughout the body is relatively equally distributed among the various subfamilies, the relative contribution to drug metabolism is (in decreasing order of magnitude) CYP3A4 (nearly 50%), CYP2D6 (nearly 25%), CYP2C8/9 (nearly 15%), then CYP1A2, CYP2C19, CYP2A6, and CYP2E1. Owing to their potential for numerous drug-drug interactions, those drugs that are identified in preclinical studies as substrates of CYP3A enzymes are often given a lower priority for continued research and development in favor of drugs that appear to be less affected by (or less likely to affect) this enzyme subfamily.

Each enzyme subfamily possesses unique selectivity toward potential substrates. For example, CYP1A2 preferentially binds medium-sized, planar, lipophilic molecules, while CYP2D6 preferentially binds molecules that possess a basic nitrogen atom. Some CYP subfamilies exhibit polymorphism (ie, multiple allelic variants that manifest differing catalytic properties). The best described polymorphisms involve CYP2C9, CYP2C19, and CYP2D6. Individuals possessing "wild type" gene alleles exhibit normal functioning CYP capacity. Others, however, possess allelic variants that leave the person with a subnormal level of catalytic potential (so called "poor metabolizers"). Poor metabolizers would be more likely to experience toxicity from drugs metabolized by the affected enzymes (or less effects if the enzyme is responsible for converting a prodrug to it's active form as in the case of codeine). The percentage of people classified as poor metabolizers varies by enzyme and population group. As an example, approximately 7% of Caucasians and only about 1% of Orientals appear to be CYP2D6 poor metabolizers.

CYP enzymes can be both inhibited and induced by other drugs, leading to increased or decreased serum concentrations (along with the associated effects), respectively. Induction occurs when a drug causes an increase in the amount of smooth endoplasmic reticulum, secondary to increasing the amount of the affected

CYP enzymes in the tissues. This "revving up" of the CYP enzyme system may take several days to reach peak activity, and likewise, may take several days, even months, to return to normal following discontinuation of the inducing agent.

CYP inhibition occurs via several potential mechanisms. Most commonly, a CYP inhibitor competitively (and reversibly) binds to the active site on the enzyme, thus preventing the substrate from binding to the same site, and preventing the substrate from being metabolized. The affinity of an inhibitor for an enzyme may be expressed by an inhibition constant (Ki) or IC50 (defined as the concentration of the inhibitor required to cause 50% inhibition under a given set of conditions). In addition to reversible competition for an enzyme site, drugs may inhibit enzyme activity by binding to sites on the enzyme other than that to which the substrate would bind, and thereby cause a change in the functionality or physical structure of the enzyme. A drug may also bind to the enzyme in an irreversible (ie, "suicide") fashion. In such a case, it is not the concentration of drug at the enzyme site that is important (constantly binding and releasing), but the number of molecules available for binding (once bound, always bound).

Although an inhibitor or inducer may be known to affect a variety of CYP subfamilies, it may only inhibit one or two in a clinically important fashion. Likewise, although a substrate is known to be at least partially metabolized by a variety of CYP enzymes, only one or two enzymes may contribute significantly enough to its overall metabolism to warrant concern when used with potential inducers or inhibitors. Therefore, when attempting to predict the level of risk of using two drugs that may affect each other via altered CYP function, it is important to identify the relative effectiveness of the inhibiting/inducing drug on the CYP subfamilies that significantly contribute to the metabolism of the substrate. The contribution of a specific CYP pathway to substrate metabolism should be considered not only in light of other known CYP pathways, but also other nonoxidative pathways for substrate metabolism (eg, glucuronidation) and transporter proteins (eg, P-glycoprotein) that may affect the presentation of a substrate to a metabolic pathway.

HOW TO USE THE TABLES

The following CYP SUBSTRATES, INHIBITORS, and INDUCERS tables provide a clinically relevant perspective on drugs that are affected by, or affect, cytochrome P450 (CYP) enzymes. Not all human, drug-metabolizing CYP enzymes are specifically (or separately) included in the tables. Some enzymes have been excluded because they do not appear to significantly contribute to the metabolism of marketed drugs (eg, CYP2C18). In the case of CYP3A4, the industry routinely uses this single enzyme designation to represent all enzymes in the CYP3A subfamily. CYP3A7 is present in fetal livers. It is effectively absent from adult livers. CYP3A4 (adult) and CYP3A7 (fetal) appear to share similar properties in their respective hosts. The impact of CYP3A7 in fetal and neonatal drug interactions has not been investigated.

The **CYP Substrates table** contains a list of drugs reported to be metabolized, at least in part, by one or more CYP enzymes. An enzyme that appears to play a clinically significant (major) role in a drug's metabolism is indicated by "•", and an enzyme whose role appears to be clinically insignificant (minor) is indicated by "○". A clinically significant designation is the result of a two-phase review. The first phase considered the contribution of each CYP enzyme to the overall metabolism of the drug. The enzyme pathway was considered potentially clinically relevant if it was responsible for at least 30% of the metabolism of the drug. If so, the drug was subjected to a second phase. The second phase considered the clinical relevance of a substrate's concentration being increased twofold, or decreased by one-half (such as might be observed if combined with an effective CYP inhibitor or inducer, respectively). If either of these changes was considered to present a clinically significant concern, the CYP pathway for the drug was designated "major." If neither change would appear to present a clinically significant concern, or if the CYP enzyme was responsible for a smaller portion of the overall metabolism (ie, <30%), the pathway was designated "minor."

The **CYP Inhibitors table** contains a list of drugs that are reported to inhibit one or more CYP enzymes. Enzymes that are strongly inhibited by a drug are indicated by "•". Enzymes that are moderately inhibited are indicated by "□". Enzymes that are weakly inhibited are indicated by "○". The designations are the result of a review of published clinical reports, available Ki data, and assessments published by other experts in the field. As it pertains to Ki values set in a ratio with achievable serum drug concentrations ([I]) under normal dosing conditions, the following parameters were employed: [I]/Ki ≥1 = strong; [I]/Ki 0.1-1 = moderate; [I]/Ki <0.1 = weak.

The **CYP Inducers table** contains a list of drugs that are reported to induce one or more CYP enzymes. Enzymes that appear to be effectively induced by a drug are indicated by "•", and enzymes that do not appear to be effectively induced are indicated by "○". The designations are the result of a review of published clinical reports and assessments published by experts in the field.

In general, clinically significant interactions are more likely to occur between substrates and either inhibitors or inducers of the same enzyme(s), all of which have been indicated by "•". However, these assessments possess a degree of subjectivity, at times based on limited indications regarding the significance of CYP effects of particular agents. An attempt has been made to balance a conservative, clinically-sensitive presentation of the data with a desire to avoid the numbing effect of a "beware of everything" approach. Even so, other potential interactions (ie, those involving enzymes indicated by "○") may warrant consideration in some cases. It is important to note that information related to CYP metabolism of drugs is expanding at a rapid pace, and thus, the contents of this table should only be considered to represent a "snapshot" of the information available at the time of publication.

Selected Readings

Bjornsson TD, Callaghan JT, Einolf HJ, et al, "The Conduct of *in vitro* and *in vivo* Drug-Drug Interaction Studies: A PhRMA Perspective," *J Clin Pharmacol*, 2003, 43(5):443-69.

Drug-Drug Interactions, Rodrigues AD, ed, New York, NY: Marcel Dekker, Inc, 2002.

Levy RH, Thummel KE, Trager WF, et al, eds, *Metabolic Drug Interactions*, Philadelphia, PA: Lippincott Williams & Wilkins, 2000.

Michalets EL, "Update: Clinically Significant Cytochrome P-450 Drug Interactions," *Pharmacotherapy*, 1998, 18(1):84-112.

Thummel KE and Wilkinson GR, "*In vitro* and *in vivo* Drug Interactions Involving Human CYP3A," *Annu Rev Pharmacol Toxicol*, 1998, 38:389-430.

Zhang Y and Benet LZ, "The Gut as a Barrier to Drug Absorption: Combined Role of Cytochrome P450 3A and P-Glycoprotein," *Clin Pharmacokinet*, 2001, 40(3):159-68.

Selected Websites

http://www.gentest.com
http://www.imm.ki.se/CYPalleles
http://medicine.iupui.edu/flockhart
http://www.mhc.com/Cytochromes

CYP Substrates

• = major substrate; ○ = minor substrate

Drug	1A2	2A6	2B6	2C8	2C9	2C19	2D6	2E1	3A4
Acenocoumarol	•				•	○			
Acetaminophen	○	○			○		○	○	○
Albendazole	○								○
Alfentanil									•
Alfuzosin									•
Aliskiren									○
Almotriptan							○		○
Alosetron	•				○				○
ALPRAZolam									•
Ambrisentan						•			•
Aminophylline	•							○	○
Amiodarone	○			•		○	○		•
Amitriptyline	○		○		○	○	•		○
AmLODIPine									•
Amoxapine							•		
Amphetamine							•		
Amprenavir					○				•
Anagrelide	○								
Apomorphine	○					○			○
Aprepitant	○					○			•
Arformoterol						○	○		
Argatroban									○
Aripiprazole							•		•
Armodafinil									•
Aspirin					○				
Atazanavir									•

CYP Substrates *continued*

Drug	1A2	2A6	2B6	2C8	2C9	2C19	2D6	2E1	3A4
Atomoxetine						○	●		
Atorvastatin									●
Azelastine	○					○	○		○
Azithromycin									○
Benzphetamine			○						●
Benztropine							○		
Benzydamine	○					○	○		○
Betaxolol	●						●		
Bexarotene									○
Bezafibrate									○
Bisoprolol							○		●
Bortezomib	○				○	●	○		●
Bosentan					●				●
Brinzolamide									○
Bromazepam									●
Bromocriptine									●
Budesonide									●
Bupivacaine	○					○	○		○
Buprenorphine									●
BuPROPion	○	○	●		○		○	○	○
BusPIRone							○		●
Busulfan									●
Caffeine	●				○		○	○	○
Candesartan					○				
Capsaicin								○	
Captopril							●		
CarBAMazepine				○					●
Carisoprodol						●			
Carteolol							○		
Carvedilol	○				●		●	○	○
Celecoxib					●				○
Cetirizine									○
Cevimeline							○		○
ChlordiazePOXIDE									●
Chloroquine							●		●
Chlorpheniramine							○		●
ChlorproMAZINE	○						●		○
ChlorproPAMIDE					○				
Chlorzoxazone	○	○					○	●	○
Ciclesonide							○		●
Cilostazol	○					○	○		●
Cinacalcet	○						○		○
Cisapride	○	○	○		○	○			●
Citalopram						●	○		●
Clarithromycin									●
Clobazam						●			●
ClomiPRAMINE	●					●	●		○
ClonazePAM									●
Clopidogrel	○								○
Clorazepate									●
Clozapine	●	○			○	○	○		○
Cocaine									●
Codeine[1]							●		○
Colchicine									●
Conivaptan									●
Cyclobenzaprine	●						○		○

CYP Substrates *continued*

Drug	1A2	2A6	2B6	2C8	2C9	2C19	2D6	2E1	3A4
Cyclophosphamide[2]		○	●		○	○			●
CycloSPORINE									●
Dacarbazine	●							●	
Dantrolene									●
Dapsone				○	●	○		○	●
Darifenacin							○		●
Darunavir									●
Dasatinib									●
Delavirdine							○		●
Desipramine	○						●		
Desogestrel						●			
Dexamethasone									○
Dexmedetomidine		●							
Dextroamphetamine							●		
Dextromethorphan			○		○	○	●	○	○
Diazepam	○		○		○	●			●
Diclofenac	○		○	○	○	○	○		○
Digoxin									○
Dihydrocodeine[1]							○		
Dihydroergotamine									●
Diltiazem					○		○		●
Disopyramide									●
Disulfiram	○	○	○				○	○	○
Docetaxel									●
Dofetilide									○
Dolasetron					○				○
Domperidone									○
Donepezil							○		○
Dorzolamide					○				○
Doxepin	●						●		●
DOXOrubicin							●		●
Doxycycline									●
Drospirenone									○
DULoxetine	●						●		
Dutasteride									○
Efavirenz			●						●
Eletriptan									●
Enalapril									●
Enflurane								●	
Eplerenone									●
Ergoloid mesylates									●
Ergonovine									●
Ergotamine									●
Erlotinib	○								●
Erythromycin			○						●
Escitalopram						●			●
Esomeprazole						●			●
Estazolam									○
Estradiol	●	○	○		○	○	○	○	●
Estrogens, conjugated A/synthetic	●	○	○		○	○	○	○	●
Estrogens, conjugated equine	●	○	○		○	○	○	○	●
Estrogens, conjugated esterified	●		○		○			○	●
Estropipate	●		○		○			○	●
Eszopiclone								○	●
Ethinyl estradiol					○				●
Ethosuximide									●

CYP Substrates *continued*

Drug	1A2	2A6	2B6	2C8	2C9	2C19	2D6	2E1	3A4
Etonogestrel									○
Etoposide	○							○	•
Exemestane									•
Felbamate								○	•
Felodipine									•
Fenofibrate									○
FentaNYL									•
Fexofenadine									○
Finasteride									○
Flecainide	○						•		
Flunisolide									•
FLUoxetine	○		○		•	○	•	○	○
Fluphenazine							•		
Flurazepam									•
Flurbiprofen					○				
Flutamide	•								•
Fluticasone									•
Fluvastatin				○	•		○		○
Fluvoxamine	•						•		
Formoterol		○			○	○	○		
Fosamprenavir (as amprenavir)					○				•
Fosaprepitant	○					○			•
Fosphenytoin (as phenytoin)					•	•			○
Frovatriptan	○								
Fulvestrant									○
Galantamine							○		○
Gefitinib									•
Gemfibrozil									○
Glimepiride					•				
GlipiZIDE					•				
Granisetron									○
Guanabenz	•								
Haloperidol	○						•		•
Halothane		○	○		○		○	•	○
HYDROcodone[1]							•		
Hydrocortisone									○
Ibuprofen					○	○			
Ifosfamide[3]		•	○	○	○	•			•
Imatinib	○				○	○	○		•
Imipramine	○		○			•	•		○
Imiquimod	○								○
Indinavir							○		•
Indomethacin					○	○			
Irbesartan					○				
Irinotecan			•						•
Isoflurane								•	
Isoniazid								•	
Isosorbide									•
Isosorbide dinitrate									•
Isosorbide mononitrate									•
Isradipine									•
Itraconazole									•
Ivermectin									○
Ixabepilone									•
Ketamine			•		•				•
Ketoconazole									•

CYP Substrates *continued*

Drug	1A2	2A6	2B6	2C8	2C9	2C19	2D6	2E1	3A4
Lansoprazole					○	●			●
Lapatinib				○					●
Letrozole		○							○
Levobupivacaine	○								○
Levonorgestrel									●
Lidocaine	○	○	○		○		●		●
Lomustine							●		
Loperamide			○						
Lopinavir									○
Loratadine							○		○
Losartan					●				●
Lovastatin									●
Lumiracoxib					●				
Maprotiline							●		
Maraviroc									●
MedroxyPROGESTERone									●
Mefenamic acid					○				
Mefloquine									●
Meloxicam					○				○
Meperidine			○			○			○
Mephobarbital			○		○	●			
Mestranol[4]					●				●
Methadone					○	○	○		●
Methamphetamine							●		
Methoxsalen		○							
Methsuximide						●			
Methylergonovine									●
Methylphenidate							●		
MethylPREDNISolone									●
Metoclopramide	○						○		
Metoprolol						○	●		
Mexiletine	●						●		
Micafungin									○
Miconazole									●
Midazolam			○						●
Mifepristone									○
Mirtazapine	●				○		●		●
Moclobemide						●	●		
Modafinil									●
Mometasone									○
Montelukast					●				●
Moricizine									●
Morphine sulfate							○		
Naproxen	○				○				
Nateglinide					●				●
Nebivolol							●		
Nefazodone							●		●
Nelfinavir					○	●	○		●
Nevirapine			○				○		●
NiCARdipine	○				○		○	○	●
Nicotine	○	○	○		○	○	○	○	○
NIFEdipine							○		●
Nilotinib									●
Nilutamide						●			
NiMODipine									●
Nisoldipine									●

CYP Substrates *continued*

Drug	1A2	2A6	2B6	2C8	2C9	2C19	2D6	2E1	3A4
Norelgestromin									○
Norethindrone									●
Norgestrel									●
Nortriptyline	○					○	●		○
OLANZapine	●						○		
Omeprazole		○			○	●	○		●
Ondansetron	○				○		○	○	●
Orphenadrine	○		○				○		○
Oxybutynin									○
OxyCODONE[1]							●		
Paclitaxel				●	●				●
Palonosetron	○						○		○
Pantoprazole					○	●	○		○
Paricalcitol									●
PARoxetine							●		
Pentamidine						●			
Pergolide									●
Perphenazine	○				○	○	●		○
Phencyclidine									●
PHENobarbital					○	●		○	
Phenytoin					●	●			○
Pimecrolimus									○
Pimozide	●								●
Pindolol							●		
Pioglitazone				●					○
Piroxicam					○				
Pravastatin									○
PrednisoLONE									○
PredniSONE									○
Primaquine									●
Procainamide							●		
Progesterone	○	○			○	●	○		●
Proguanil	○					○			○
Promethazine			●				●		
Propafenone	○						●		○
Propofol	○	○	●		●	○	○	○	○
Propranolol	●					○	●		○
Protriptyline							●		
Quazepam									○
QUEtiapine							○		●
QuiNIDine					○			○	●
QuiNINE	○					○			●
Rabeprazole						●			●
Ramelteon	●								○
Ranitidine	○					○	○		
Ranolazine							○		●
Rasagiline	●								
Repaglinide				●					●
Rifabutin									●
Riluzole	●								
Risperidone							●		○
Ritonavir	○		○				●		●
Ropinirole	●								○
Ropivacaine	●		○				○		○
Rosiglitazone				●	○				
Rosuvastatin					○				○

CYP Substrates *continued*

Drug	1A2	2A6	2B6	2C8	2C9	2C19	2D6	2E1	3A4
Salmeterol									●
Saquinavir							○		●
Selegiline	○	○	●	○		○	○		○
Sertraline			○		○	●	●		○
Sevoflurane		○	○					●	○
Sibutramine									●
Sildenafil					○				●
Simvastatin									●
Sirolimus									●
SitaGLIPtin				○					○
Sitaxsentan					○				○
Solifenacin									●
Sorafenib									○
Spiramycin									●
SUFentanil									●
SulfaDIAZINE					●			○	○
Sulfamethoxazole					●				○
Sulfinpyrazone					●				○
SulfiSOXAZOLE					●				
Sunitinib									●
Tacrine	●								
Tacrolimus									●
Tadalafil									●
Tamoxifen		○	○		●		●	○	●
Tamsulosin							●		●
Telithromycin	○								●
Temazepam			○		○	○			○
Temsirolimus									●
Teniposide									●
Terbinafine	○				○	○			○
Testosterone			○		○	○			○
Tetracycline									●
Theophylline	●				○		○	●	●
Thiabendazole	○								
Thioridazine						○	●		
Thiothixene	●								
TiaGABine									●
Ticlopidine									●
Timolol							●		
Tinidazole			○						●
Tiotropium							○		○
Tipranavir									●
TiZANidine	●								
TOLBUTamide					●	○			
Tolcapone					○				
Tolterodine					○	○	●		●
Toremifene	○								●
Torsemide				○	●				
TraMADol[1]							●		○
TraZODone							○		●
Tretinoin		○	○	●	○				
Triazolam									●
Trifluoperazine	●								
Trimethadione					○	○		●	○
Trimethoprim					●				●
Trimipramine						●	●		●

CYP Substrates *continued*

Drug	1A2	2A6	2B6	2C8	2C9	2C19	2D6	2E1	3A4
Valproic acid		○	○		○	○		○	
Vardenafil									•
Venlafaxine					○	○	•		•
Verapamil	○		○		○			○	•
VinBLAStine							○		•
VinCRIStine									•
Vinorelbine							○		•
Voriconazole					•	•			○
Warfarin	○				•	○			○
Yohimbine							○		
Zafirlukast					•				
Zaleplon									○
Zidovudine		○			○	○			○
Zileuton	○				○				○
Ziprasidone	○								○
Zolmitriptan	○								
Zolpidem	○				○	○	○		•
Zonisamide						○			•
Zopiclone					•				•
Zuclopenthixol							•		

[1]This opioid analgesic is bioactivated *in vivo* via CYP2D6. Inhibiting this enzyme would decrease the effects of the analgesic. The active metabolite might also affect, or be affected by, CYP enzymes.

[2]Cyclophosphamide is bioactivated *in vivo* to acrolein via CYP2B6 and 3A4. Inhibiting these enzymes would decrease the effects of cyclophosphamide.

[3]Ifosfamide is bioactivated *in vivo* to acrolein via CYP3A4. Inhibiting this enzyme would decrease the effects of ifosfamide.

[4]Mestranol is bioactivated *in vivo* to ethinyl estradiol via CYP2C8/9.

CYP Inhibitors

• = strong inhibitor; □ = moderate inhibitor; ○ = weak inhibitor

Drug	1A2	2A6	2B6	2C8	2C9	2C19	2D6	2E1	3A4
Acebutolol							○		
Acetaminophen									○
AcetaZOLAMIDE									○
Albendazole	○								
Alosetron	○							○	
Amiodarone	○	□	○		□	○	□		□
Amitriptyline	○				○	○	○	○	
AmLODIPine	□	○	○	○	○		○		○
Amphetamine							○		
Amprenavir						○			•
Anastrozole	○			○	○				○
Apomorphine	○					○			
Aprepitant					○	○			□
Armodafinil						□			
Atazanavir	○			•	○				•
Atorvastatin									○
Azelastine			○		○	○	○		○
Azithromycin									○
Betamethasone									○
Betaxolol							○		
Biperiden							○		
Bortezomib	○				○	□	○		○
Bromazepam								○	
Bromocriptine	○								○
Buprenorphine	○	○				○	○		

CYP Inhibitors *continued*

Drug	1A2	2A6	2B6	2C8	2C9	2C19	2D6	2E1	3A4
BuPROPion							○		
Caffeine	○								□
Candesartan				○	○				
Celecoxib				□			○		
Chloramphenicol					○				○
Chloroquine							□		
Chlorpheniramine							○		
ChlorproMAZINE							●	○	
Chlorzoxazone								○	○
Cholecalciferol					○	○	○		
Cimetidine	□				○	□	□	○	□
Cinacalcet							○		
Ciprofloxacin	●								○
Cisapride							○		○
Citalopram	○		○			○	○		
Clarithromycin	○								●
Clemastine							○		○
ClomiPRAMINE							□		
Clopidogrel					○				
Clotrimazole	○	○	○	○	○	○	○	○	□
Clozapine	○				○	○	□	○	○
Cocaine							●		○
Codeine							○		
Conivaptan									●
Cyclophosphamide									○
CycloSPORINE					○				□
Danazol									○
Darifenacin							□		○
Dasatinib									○
Delavirdine	○				●	●	●		●
Desipramine		□	□				□	○	□
Dexmedetomidine	○				○		●		○
Dextromethorphan							○		
Diazepam						○			○
Diclofenac	□				○			○	○
Dihydroergotamine									○
Diltiazem					○		○		□
Dimethyl sulfoxide					○	○			
DiphenhydrAMINE							□		
Disulfiram	○	○	○		○		○	●	○
Docetaxel									○
Dolasetron							○		
DOXOrubicin			□				○		○
Doxycycline									□
Drospirenone	○				○	○			○
DULoxetine							□		
Econazole								○	
Efavirenz					□	□			□
Entacapone	○	○			○	○	○	○	○
Eprosartan					○				
Ergotamine									○
Erythromycin	○								□
Escitalopram							○		
Esomeprazole						□			
Estradiol	○			○					
Estrogens, conjugated A/synthetic	○								

CYP Inhibitors *continued*

Drug	1A2	2A6	2B6	2C8	2C9	2C19	2D6	2E1	3A4
Estrogens, conjugated equine	○			○					
Ethinyl estradiol	○		○	○		○			○
Ethotoin						○			
Etoposide					○				○
Felbamate						○			
Felodipine				□	○		○		○
Fenofibrate		○		○	○	○			
FentaNYL									○
Fexofenadine							○		
Flavocoxid	○				○	○	○		○
Flecainide							○		
Fluconazole	○				●	●			□
FLUoxetine	□		○		○	□	●		○
Fluphenazine	○				○		○	○	
Flurazepam								○	
Flurbiprofen					●				
Flutamide	○								
Fluvastatin	○			○	□		○		○
Fluvoxamine	●		○		○	●	○		○
Fosamprenavir (as amprenavir)						○			●
Fosaprepitant					○	○			□
Gefitinib						○	○		
Gemfibrozil	□			●	●	●			
GlyBURIDE				○					○
Grapefruit juice									□
Haloperidol							□		□
HydrALAZINE									○
HydrOXYzine							○		
Ibuprofen					●				
Ifosfamide									○
Imatinib					○		□		●
Imipramine	○					○	□	○	
Indinavir					○	○	○		●
Indomethacin					●	○			
Interferon alfa-2a	○								
Interferon alfa-2b	○								
Interferon gamma-1b	○							○	
Irbesartan				□	□		○		○
Isoflurane			○						
Isoniazid	○	□			○	●	□	□	●
Isradipine									○
Itraconazole									●
Ketoconazole	●	□	○	○	●	□	□		●
Ketoprofen					○				
Lansoprazole					○	□	○		○
Leflunomide					○				
Letrozole		●				○			
Lidocaine	●						□		□
Lomustine							○		○
Loratadine				○		□	○		
Losartan	○			□	□	○			○
Lovastatin					○		○		○
Mefenamic acid					●				
Mefloquine							○		○
Meloxicam					○				
Mephobarbital						○			

CYP Inhibitors *continued*

Drug	1A2	2A6	2B6	2C8	2C9	2C19	2D6	2E1	3A4
Mestranol	○		○			○			○
Methadone							□		○
Methimazole	○	○	○		○	○	□	○	○
Methotrimeprazine							○		
Methoxsalen	●	●			○	○	○	○	○
Methsuximide						○			
Methylphenidate							○		
MethylPREDNISolone				○					○
Metoclopramide							○		
Metoprolol							○		
MetroNIDAZOLE					○				□
Metyrapone		○							
Mexiletine	●								
Micafungin									○
Miconazole	□	●	○		●	●	●	□	●
Midazolam				○	○				○
Mifepristone							○		○
Mirtazapine	○								○
Mitoxantrone									○
Moclobemide	○					○	○		
Modafinil	○	○			○	●		○	○
Montelukast				○	○				
Nateglinide					○				
Nefazodone	○		○	○			○		●
Nelfinavir	○		○		○	○	○		●
Nevirapine	○						○		○
NiCARdipine					●	□	□		●
Nicotine		○						○	
NIFEdipine	□				○		○		○
Nilutamide						○			
Nisoldipine	○								○
Nizatidine									○
Norfloxacin	●								□
Nortriptyline							○	○	
Ofloxacin	●								
OLANZapine	○				○	○	○		○
Omeprazole	○				□	●	○		○
Ondansetron	○				○		○		
Orphenadrine	○	○	○		○	○	○	○	○
OXcarbazepine						○			
Oxprenolol							○		
Oxybutynin				○			○		○
Pantoprazole					□				
PARoxetine	○		□		○	○	●		○
Peginterferon alfa-2a	○								
Peginterferon alfa-2b	○								
Pentamidine				○	○	○	○		○
Pentoxifylline	○								
Pergolide							●		○
Perphenazine	○						○		
Phencyclidine									○
Pilocarpine		○						○	○
Pimozide						○	○	○	○
Pindolol							○		
Pioglitazone				□	○	○	□		
Piroxicam					●				

CYP Inhibitors *continued*

Drug	1A2	2A6	2B6	2C8	2C9	2C19	2D6	2E1	3A4
Posaconazole									□
Pravastatin					○		○		○
Praziquantel							○		
PrednisoLONE									○
Primaquine	●						○		○
Probenecid						○			
Progesterone					○	○			○
Promethazine							○		
Propafenone	○						○		
Propofol	□				○	□	○	○	●
Propoxyphene					○		○		○
Propranolol	○						○		
Pyrimethamine					□		□		
QuiNIDine					○		●		●
QuiNINE				□	□		●		○
Quinupristin									○
Rabeprazole				□		□	○		○
Ranitidine	○						○		
Ranolazine							○		○
Risperidone							○		○
Ritonavir				●	○	○	●	○	●
Ropinirole	○						●		
Rosiglitazone				□	○	○	○		
Saquinavir					○	○	○		□
Selegiline	○	○			○	○	○	○	○
Sertraline	○		□	○	○	□	□		□
Sildenafil	○				○	○	○	○	○
Simvastatin				○	○		○		
Sirolimus									○
Sitaxsentan					●	●			□
Sorafenib			□	●	□				
Sulconazole	○	○			○	○	○	○	○
SulfaDIAZINE					●				
Sulfamethoxazole					□				
Sulfinpyrazone					□				
SulfiSOXAZOLE					●				
Tacrine	○								
Tacrolimus									○
Tamoxifen			○	□	○				○
Telithromycin							○		●
Telmisartan						○			
Temsirolimus							○		○
Teniposide					○				○
Tenofovir	○								
Terbinafine							●		
Testosterone									○
Tetracycline									□
Theophylline	○								
Thiabendazole	●								
Thioridazine	○				○		□	○	
Thiotepa			●						
Thiothixene							○		
Ticlopidine	○				○	●	□	○	○
Timolol							○		
Tioconazole	○	○			○	○	○	○	
Tocainide	○								

CYP Inhibitors *continued*

Drug	1A2	2A6	2B6	2C8	2C9	2C19	2D6	2E1	3A4
TOLBUTamide				○	●				
Tolcapone					○				
Topiramate						○			
Torsemide						○			
Tranylcypromine	□	●		○	○	□	□	○	○
TraZODone							□		○
Tretinoin					○				
Triazolam				○	○				
Trimethoprim				□	□				
Triprolidine							○		
Valproic acid					○	○	○		○
Valsartan					○				
Venlafaxine			○				○		○
Verapamil	○				○		○		□
VinBLAStine							○		○
VinCRIStine									○
Vinorelbine							○		○
Voriconazole					○	○			□
Warfarin					□	○			
Yohimbine							○		
Zafirlukast	○			○	□	○	○		○
Zileuton	□								
Ziprasidone							○		○

CYP Inducers

● = effectively induced; ○ = not effectively induced

Drug	1A2	2A6	2B6	2C8	2C9	2C19	2D6	2E1	3A4
Aminoglutethimide	●					●			●
Amobarbital		●							
Aprepitant					○				○
Armodafinil	○								○
Bexarotene									○
Bosentan					●				●
Calcitriol									○
CarBAMazepine	●		●	●	●	●			●
Colchicine				○	○			○	○
Cyclophosphamide			○	○	○				
Dexamethasone		○	○	○	○				●
Dicloxacillin									○
Efavirenz (in liver only)			○						●
Estradiol									○
Estrogens, conjugated A/synthetic									○
Estrogens, conjugated equine									○
Felbamate									○
Fosaprepitant					○				○
Fosphenytoin (as phenytoin)			●	●	●	●			●
Griseofulvin	○			○	○				○
Hydrocortisone									○
Ifosfamide				○	○				
Insulin preparations	○								
Isoniazid (after D/C)								○	
Lansoprazole	○								
MedroxyPROGESTERone									○
Mephobarbital		○							

CYP Inducers *continued*

Drug	1A2	2A6	2B6	2C8	2C9	2C19	2D6	2E1	3A4
Metyrapone									○
Modafinil	○		○						○
Moricizine	○								○
Nafcillin									●
Nevirapine			●						●
Norethindrone						○			
Omeprazole	○								
OXcarbazepine									●
Paclitaxel									○
Pantoprazole	○								○
PENTobarbital		●							●
PHENobarbital	●	●	●	●	●				●
Phenytoin			●	●	●	●			●
Pioglitazone									○
PredniSONE						○			○
Primaquine	○								
Primidone[1]	●		●	●	●				●
Rifabutin									●
Rifampin	●	●	●	●	●	●			●
Rifapentine				●	●				●
Rifaximin									○
Ritonavir (long-term)	○			○	○				○
Secobarbital		●		●	●				
Sulfinpyrazone									○
Terbinafine									○
Topiramate									○
Tretinoin								○	
Valproic acid		○							

[1]Primidone is partially metabolized to PHENobarbital. See PHENobarbital for additional CYP information.

CMS: LONG-TERM CARE FACILITY THRESHOLDS

Select tables from "State Operations Manual: Appendix PP - Guidance to Surveyors for Long Term Care Facilities," available at http://cms.hhs.gov/manuals/Downloads/ som107ap_pp_guidelines_ltcf.pdf

Daily Dose Thresholds for Antipsychotic Medications Used to Manage Behavioral Symptoms Related to Dementing Illnesses

Generic Medication	Dosage (mg)
First Generation	
Chlorpromazine	75
Fluphenazine	4
Haloperidol	2
Loxapine	10
Molindone	10
Perphenazine	8
Pimozide	*
Prochlorperazine	*
Thioridazine	75
Thiothixene	7
Trifluoperazine	8
Second Generation	
Aripiprazole	10
Clozapine	50
Olanzapine	7.5
Quetiapine	150
Risperidone	2
Ziprasidone	*

*Not customarily used for the treatment of behavioral symptoms

Total Daily Dose Thresholds for Anxiolytic Medications

Generic Medication	Dosage (mg)
Alprazolam	0.75
Chlordiazepoxide	20
Clonazepam	1.5
Clorazepate	15
Diazepam	5
Estazolam	0.5
Flurazepam	15
Lorazepam	2
Oxazepam	30
Quazepam	7.5

Daily Dose Thresholds For Sedative-Hypnotic Medications

Generic Medication	Oral Dosage (mg)
Chloral hydrate[1]	500
Diphenhydramine[1]	25
Estazolam	0.5
Eszopiclone	1
Flurazepam[1]	15
Hydroxyzine[1]	50
Lorazepam	1
Oxazepam	15
Quazepam[1]	7.5
Ramelteon	8
Temazepam	15
Triazolam[1]	0.125
Zaleplon	5
Zolpidem IR	5
Zolpidem CR	6.25

IR = immediate release, CR = controlled release

[1]These medications are not considered medications of choice for the management of insomnia, especially in older individuals.

ADDICTION TREATMENTS

Acamprosate (Campral®)	Maintenance of alcohol abstinence: 666 mg 3 times/day; 333 mg 3 times/day in patients with Cl_{cr} 30-50 mL/minute
Buprenorphine (Buprenex®, Subutex®)	Opioid dependence: Induction: 12-16 mg/day Maintenance: 4-24 mg/day Target dose: 16 mg/day
Buprenorphine and Naloxone (Suboxone®)	Opioid dependence: Induction: Not recommended Maintenance: 4-24 mg/day Target dose: 16 mg/day
Bupropion SR (Zyban®)	Smoking cessation: Initiate at 150 mg every morning for 3 days. If tolerated, increase to 150 mg twice daily on day 4 of dosing. Should be an interval of at least 8 hours between successive doses. Target quit date after at least 1 week of treatment. Trial may be up to 12 weeks. Contraindicated in patients with seizures, anorexia, or bulimia.
Clonidine (Catapres®)	Alcohol, nicotine, opioid withdrawal: Initiate 0.1 mg 2-3 times/day
Disulfiram (Antabuse®)	Management of chronic alcoholism: 125-500 mg/day; patients must be free of alcohol for at least 12 hours prior to initiation. Contraindicated with metronidazole and alcohol (including cough syrups).
Methadone (Dolophine®)	Narcotic dependence: 15-60 mg every 6-8 hours; can only be initiated in approved treatment programs
Naltrexone (Depade®, ReVia®, Vivitrol™)	Alcohol dependence: I.M.: 380 mg every 4 weeks Oral: 25 mg; if no withdrawal signs within 1 hour, give another 25 mg; maintenance: 50 mg/day to 100-150 mg 3 time/week Opioid antidote: Oral: 25 mg; if no withdrawal signs within 1 hour, give another 25 mg; maintenance: 50 mg/day to 100-150 mg 3 time/week. Patient should be free of opioid for 7-10 days prior to initiation
Nicotine gum	Smoking cessation: 1-2 pieces/hour; maximum: 30 pieces/day (2 mg/piece). If high tobacco use, give DS (4 mg/piece); maximum: 20/day
Nicotine inhaler	Smoking cessation: 6-16 cartridges/day
Nicotine lozenge	Smoking cessation: One lozenge every 1-2 hours weeks 1-6 One lozenge every 2-4 hours weeks 7-9 One lozenge every 4-8 hours weeks 10-12
Nicotine nasal spray	Smoking cessation: 1 spray in each nostril once or twice per hour; maximum: 80 sprays
Nicotine patches	Smoking cessation: One patch daily for 8 weeks
Varenicline (Chantix™)	Smoking cessation: 0.5 mg/day days 1-3 0.5 mg twice daily days 4-7 1 mg twice daily weeks 2-12

CLOZAPINE-INDUCED SIDE EFFECTS

INCIDENCE AND MANAGEMENT

Effect	Incidence	Management
Sedation & fatigue	35%	Initiate split dosing with long-term goal to administer twice daily with larger portion at bedtime (appears to be dose-dependent). For chronic sedation, consider an empiric trial of methylphenidate 5-20 mg/day.
Sialorrhea	25%	Clozapine may affect the swallowing mechanism; behavioral approach may be best. Consider lowering the dose. Pharmacological management consists of clonidine 0.1-0.9 mg/day (monitor blood pressure) or benztropine 0.5-2 mg/day (monitor for increased anticholinergic side effects).
Weight gain	35%	Diet and exercise best. No pharmacological agent shown to be consistently useful; one study showed the addition of quetiapine to clozapine minimized weight gain; consider lowering dose.
Urinary incontinence	25%	If patient receiving co-pharmacy with typical antipsychotic, consider discontinuing; pharmacological management consists of ephedrine 25-150 mg/d, pseudoephedrine 30-160 mg/d, oxybutynin 5 mg tid, or desmopressin.
Tachycardia	25%	Dose dependent. Beta-blocker; atenolol 50 mg/d or propranolol 10 mg tid (adjust for rate).
Constipation	20%	Discontinue other medications with anticholinergic activity, if possible. May need chronic psyllium and/or docusate.
Seizures	4%	Dose dependent. Valproic acid/valproate; initiate at 250 mg tid or 500 mg bid and titrate to serum level of at least 50 mcg/mL.
Agranulocytosis	0.3% to 1%	Stop drug. Do not rechallenge. Consider filgrastim (G-CSF) or sargramostim (GM-CSF) during acute recovery phase.

CRITERIA TO DIFFERENTIATE PSEUDO FROM IDIOPATHIC PARKINSONISM

Criteria	Pseudoparkinsonism	Idiopathic Parkinson's Disease
Duration of symptoms	Usually transient	Progressive deterioration
Time of onset	Early (<3 months)	Delayed
Age of onset	Any age	Mostly >50 y
Tremor	Less common	During drug free periods
Bilateral signs	Typical	Mid to late stages
Response to anticholinergic agents	Efficacious	Minimal efficacy

DEPRESSION

Medications That May Precipitate Depression

Anti-inflammatory & analgesic agents	Indomethacin, pentazocine, phenacetin, phenylbutazone
Antimicrobial agents	Cycloserine, ethambutol, sulfonamides, select gram-negative antibiotics
Cardiovascular/ antihypertensive agents	Clonidine, digitalis, diuretics, guanethidine, hydralazine, indapamide, methyldopa, prazosin, procainamide, propranolol, reserpine
CNS-agents	Alcohol, amantadine, amphetamine & derivatives (withdrawal), barbiturates, benzodiazepines, chloral hydrate, carbamazepine, cocaine (withdrawal), haloperidol, L-dopa, phenothiazines, succinimide derivatives, levetiracetam
Hormonal agents	ACTH, corticosteroids, estrogen, melatonin, oral contraceptives, progesterone
Miscellaneous	Antineoplastic agents, cimetidine, disulfiram, organic pesticides, physostigmine, mercury

Medical Disorders and Psychiatric Disorders Associated With Depression

Endocrine diseases	Acromegaly, Addison's disease, Cushing's disease, diabetes mellitus, hyperparathyroidism, hypoparathyroidism, hyperthyroidism, hypothyroidism, insulinoma, pheochromocytoma, pituitary dysfunction
Deficiency states	Pellagra, pernicious anemia, severe anemia, Wernicke's encephalopathy
Infections	AIDS, encephalitis, fungal infections, meningitis, neurosyphilis, influenza, mononucleosis, pneumonia, toxoplasmosis, tuberculosis, viral hepatitis
Collagen disorders	Rheumatoid arthritis, systemic lupus erythematosus
Metabolic disorders	Electrolyte imbalance, hypokalemia, hyponatremia, hepatic encephalopathy, Pick's disease, uremia, Wilson's disease
Cardiovascular disease	Cerebral arteriosclerosis, chronic bronchitis, congestive heart failure, emphysema, myocardial infarction, paroxysmal dysrhythmias
Neurologic disorders	Alzheimer's disease, amyotrophic lateral sclerosis, brain tumors, chronic pain syndrome, complex partial seizures, Creutzfeldt-Jakob disease, Huntington's disease, multiple sclerosis, myasthenia gravis, Parkinson's disease, poststroke, sleep apnea, trauma (postconcussion)
Malignant disease	Breast, gastrointestinal, lung, pancreas, prostate
Psychiatric disorders	Alcoholism, anxiety disorders, eating disorders, schizophrenia

HYPERLIPIDEMIA MANAGEMENT

MORTALITY

There is a strong link between serum cholesterol and cardiovascular mortality. This association becomes stronger in patients with established coronary artery disease. Lipid-lowering trials show that reductions in LDL cholesterol are followed by reductions in mortality. In general, each 1% fall in LDL cholesterol confers a 2% reduction in cardiovascular events. The aim of therapy for hyperlipidemia is to decrease cardiovascular morbidity and mortality by lowering cholesterol to a target level using safe and cost-effective treatment modalities. The target LDL cholesterol is determined by the number of patient risk factors (see the following Risk Factors and Goal LDL Cholesterol tables). The goal is achieved through diet, lifestyle modification, and drug therapy. The basis for these recommendations is provided by longitudinal interventional studies, demonstrating that lipid-lowering in patients with prior cardiovascular events (secondary prevention) and in patients with hyperlipidemia but no prior cardiac event (primary prevention) lowers the occurrence of future cardiovascular events, including stroke.

Adult Treatment Panel (ATP) III LDL-C Goals and Cutpoints for Therapeutic Lifestyle Changes (TLC) and Drug Therapy in Different Risk Categories

Risk Category	LDL-C Goal	Initiate TLC	Consider Drug Therapy[1]
High risk: CHD[2] or CHD risk equivalents[3] (10-year risk >20%)	<100 mg/dL (optional goal: <70 mg/dL)[4]	≥100 mg/dL[5]	≥100 mg/dL[6] (<100 mg/dL: Consider drug options)[1]
Moderately high risk: ≥2 risk factors[7] (10-year risk 10% to 20%)[8]	<130 mg/dL[9]	≥130 mg/dL[5]	≥130 mg/dL (100-120 mg/dL: Consider drug options)[10]
Moderate risk: ≥2 risk factors[7] (10-year risk <10%)[8]	<130 mg/dL	≥130 mg/dL	≥160 mg/dL
Lower risk: 0-1 risk factor[11]	<160 mg/dL	≥160 mg/dL	≥190 mg/dL (160-189 mg/dL: LDL-lowering drug optional)

[1]When LDL-lowering drug therapy is employed, it is advised that intensity of therapy be sufficient to achieve at least a 30% to 40% reduction in LDL-C levels.

[2]CHD includes history of myocardial infarction, unstable angina, stable angina, coronary artery procedures (angioplasty or bypass surgery), or evidence of clinically significant myocardial ischemia.

[3]CHD risk equivalents include clinical manifestations of noncoronary forms of atherosclerotic disease (peripheral arterial disease, abdominal aortic aneurysm, and carotid artery disease [transient ischemic attacks or stroke of carotid origin or >50% obstruction of a carotid artery]), diabetes, and 2+ risk factors with 10-year risk for hard CHD >20%.

[4]Very high risk favors the optional LDL-C goal of <70 mg/dL, and in patients with high triglycerides, non-HDL-C <100 mg/dL.

[5]Any person at high risk or moderately high risk who has lifestyle-related risk factors (eg, obesity, physical inactivity, elevated triglyceride, low HDL-C, or metabolic syndrome) is a candidate for therapeutic lifestyle changes to modify these risk factors regardless of LDL-C level.

[6]If baseline LDL-C is <100 mg/dL, institution of an LDL-lowering drug is a therapeutic option on the basis of available clinical trial results. If a high-risk person has high triglycerides or low HDL-C, combining a fibrate or nicotinic acid with an LDL-lowering drug can be considered.

[7]Risk factors include cigarette smoking, hypertension (BP ≥140/90 mm Hg or on antihypertensive medication), low HDL cholesterol (<40 mg/dL), family history of premature CHD (CHD in male first-degree relative <55 years of age; CHD in female first-degree relative <65 years of age), and age (men ≥45 years; women ≥55 years).

[8]Electronic 10-year risk calculators are available at www.nhlbi.nih.gov/guidelines/cholesterol.

[9]Optional LDL-C goal <100 mg/dL.

[10]For moderately high-risk persons, when LDL-C level is 100-129 mg/dL, at baseline or on lifestyle therapy, initiation of an LDL-lowering drug to achieve an LDL-C level <100 mg/dL is a therapeutic option on the basis of available clinical trial results.

[11]Almost all people with zero or 1 risk factor have a 10-year risk <10%, and 10-year risk assessment in people with zero or 1 risk factor thus not necessary.

Major Risk Factors That Modify LDL Goals

Positive risk factors	Male ≥45 years
	Female ≥55 years
	Family history of premature coronary heart disease, defined as CHD in male first-degree relative <55 years; CHD in female first-degree relative <65 years
	Cigarette smoking
	Hypertension (blood pressure ≥140/90 mm Hg) or taking antihypertensive medication
	Low HDL (<40 mg/dL [1.03 mmol/L])
Negative risk factors	High HDL (≥60 mg/dL [1.6 mmol/L])[1]

[1]If HDL is ≥60 mg/dL, may subtract one positive risk factor.

Any person with elevated LDL cholesterol or other form of hyperlipidemia should undergo evaluation to rule out secondary dyslipidemia. Causes of secondary dyslipidemia include diabetes, hypothyroidism, obstructive liver disease, chronic renal failure, and drugs that increase LDL and decrease HDL (progestins, anabolic steroids, corticosteroids).

Elevated Serum Triglyceride Levels

Elevated serum triglyceride levels may be an independent risk factor for coronary heart disease. Factors that contribute to hypertriglyceridemia include obesity, inactivity, cigarette smoking, excess alcohol intake, high carbohydrate diets (>60% of energy intake), type 2 diabetes, chronic renal failure, nephrotic syndrome, certain medications (corticosteroids, estrogens, retinoids, higher doses of beta-blockers), and genetic disorders. Non-HDL cholesterol (total cholesterol minus HDL cholesterol) is a secondary focus for clinicians treating patients with high serum triglyceride levels (≥200 mg/dL). The goal for non-HDL cholesterol in patients with high serum triglyceride levels can be set 30 mg/dL higher than usual LDL cholesterol goals. Patients with serum triglyceride levels <200 mg/dL should aim for the target LDL cholesterol goal.

ATP classification of serum triglyceride levels:

- Normal triglycerides: <150 mg/dL
- Borderline-high: 150-199 mg/dL
- High: 200-499 mg/dL
- Very high: ≥500 mg/dL

NONDRUG THERAPY

Dietary therapy and lifestyle modifications should be individualized for each patient. A total lifestyle change is recommended for all patients. Dietary and lifestyle modifications should be tried for 3 months, if deemed appropriate. Nondrug and drug therapy should be initiated simultaneously in patients with highly elevated cholesterol (see LDL Cholesterol Goals and Cutpoints for Therapeutic Lifestyle Changes and Drug Therapy in Different Risk Categories table). Increasing physical activity and smoking cessation will aid in the treatment of hyperlipidemia and improve cardiovascular health.

Note: Refer to the National Cholesterol Education Program reference for details concerning the calculation of 10-year risk of CHD using Framingham risk scoring. Risk assessment tool is available on-line at http://hin.nhlbi.nih.gov/atpiii/calculator.asp?usertype=prof, last accessed March 14, 2002.

Total Lifestyle Change (TLC) Diet

	Recommended Intake
Total fat	25%-35% of total calories
Saturated fat[1]	<7% of total calories
Polyunsaturated fat	≤10% of total calories
Monounsaturated fat	≤20% of total calories
Carbohydrates[2]	50%-60% of total calories
Fiber	20-30 g/day
Protein	~15% of total calories
Cholesterol	<200 mg/day
Total calories[3]	Balance energy intake and expenditure to maintain desirable body weight/prevent weight gain

[1]*Trans* fatty acids (partially hydrogenated oils) intake should be kept low. These are found in potato chips, other snack foods, margarines and shortenings, and fast-foods.

[2]Complex carbohydrates including grains (especially whole grains, fruits, and vegetables).

[3]Daily energy expenditure should include at least moderate physical activity.

DRUG THERAPY

Drug therapy should be selected based on the patient's lipid profile, concomitant disease states, and the cost of therapy. The following table lists specific advantages and disadvantages for various classes of lipid-lowering medications. The expected reduction in lipids with therapy is listed in the Lipid-Lowering Agents table. Refer to individual drug monographs for detailed information.

Advantages and Disadvantages of Specific Lipid-Lowering Therapies

	Advantages	Disadvantages
Bile acid sequestrants	Good choice for ↑ LDL, especially when combined with a statin (↓ LDL ≤50%); low potential for systemic side effects; good choice for younger patients	May increase triglycerides; higher incidence of adverse effects; moderately expensive; drug interactions; inconvenient dosing
Niacin	Good choice for almost any lipid abnormality; inexpensive; greatest increase in HDL	High incidence of adverse effects; may adversely affect NIDDM and gout; sustained release niacin may decrease the incidence of flushing and circumvent the need for multiple daily dosing; sustained release niacin may not increase HDL cholesterol or decrease triglycerides as well as immediate release niacin
HMG-CoA reductase inhibitors	Produces greatest ↓ in LDL; generally well-tolerated; convenient once-daily dosing; proven decrease in mortality	Expensive
Gemfibrozil	Good choice in patients with ↑ triglycerides where niacin is contraindicated or not well-tolerated; gemfibrozil is well tolerated	Variable effects on LDL
Ezetimibe	Additional cholesterol-lowering effects when combined with HMG-CoA reductase inhibitors	Effects similar to bile acid sequestrants

Lipid-Lowering Agents

Drug	Dose / Day	Effect on LDL (%)	Effect on HDL (%)	Effect on TG (%)
HMG-CoA Reductase Inhibitors				
Atorvastatin	10 mg 20 mg 40 mg 80 mg	-39 -43 -50 -60	+6 +9 +6 +5	-19 -26 -29 -37
Fluvastatin	20 mg 40 mg 80 mg	-22 -25 -36	+3 +4 +6	-12 -14 -18
Lovastatin	10 mg 20 mg 40 mg 80 mg	-21 -27 -31 -40	+5 +6 +5 +9.5	-10 -8 -8 -19
Pravastatin	10 mg 20 mg 40 mg 80 mg	-22 -32 -34 -37	+7 +2 +12 +3	-15 -11 -24 -19
Rosuvastatin	5 mg 10 mg 20 mg 40 mg	-45 -52 -55 -63	+13 +14 +8 +10	-35 -10 -23 -28
Simvastatin	5 mg 10 mg 20 mg 40 mg 80 mg	-26 -30 -38 -41 -47	+10 +12 +8 +13 +16	-12 -15 -19 -28 -33
Bile Acid Sequestrants				
Cholestyramine	4-24 g	-15 to -30	+3 to +5	+0 to +20
Colestipol	7-30 g	-15 to -30	+3 to +5	+0 to +20
Colesevelam	6 tablets 7 tablets	-15 -18	+3 +3	+10 +9
Fibric Acid Derivatives				
Fenofibrate	67-200 mg	-20 to -25	+1 to +20	-30 to -50
Gemfibrozil	600 mg twice daily	-5 to -10[1]	+10 to +20	-40 to -60
Niacin	1.5-6 g	-21 to -27	+10 to +35	-10 to -50
2-Azetidinone				
Ezetimibe	10 mg	-18	+1	-8
Omega-3-Acid Ethyl Esters	4 g	+44.5	+9.1	-44.9
Combination Products				
Ezetimibe and fenofibrate	10/160 mg	-20	+19	-44
Ezetimibe and simvastatin	10/10 mg 10/20 mg 10/40 mg 10/80 mg	-45 -52 -55 -60	+8 +10 +6 +6	-23 -24 -23 -31
Niacin and lovastatin	1000/20 mg 1000/40 mg 1500/40 mg 2000/40 mg	-30 -36 -37 -42	+20 +20 +27 +30	-32 -39 -44 -44
Niacin and simvastatin	1000/20 mg 1000/40 mg 2000/20 mg 2000/40 mg	-12 -7 -14 -5	+21 +15 +29 +24	-27 -23 -38 -32

[1]May increase LDL in some patients.

Recommended Liver Function Monitoring for HMG-CoA Reductase Inhibitors

Agent	Initial and After Elevation in Dose	6 Weeks[1]	12 Weeks[1]	Periodically
Atorvastatin (Lipitor®)	x		x	x
Fluvastatin (Lescol®)	x		x	x
Lovastatin (Mevacor®)	x	x	x	x
Pravastatin (Pravachol®)	x			x
Simvastatin (Zocor®)	x			x

[1]After initiation of therapy or any elevation in dose.

Progression of Drug Therapy in Primary Prevention

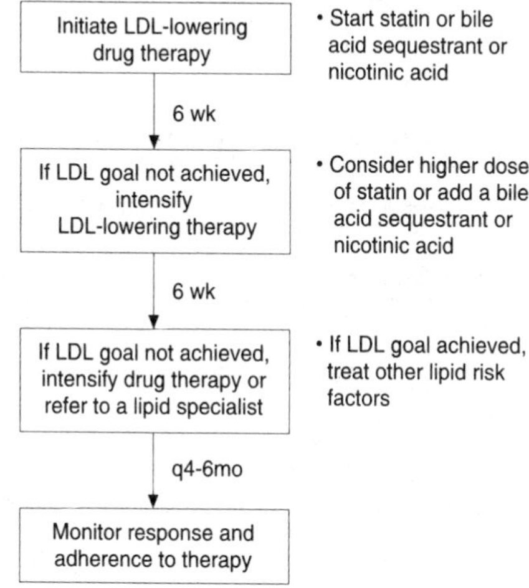

DRUG SELECTION

Lipid Profile	Monotherapy	Combination Therapies
Increased LDL with normal HDL and triglycerides (TG)	Resin Niacin[1] Statin	Resin plus niacin[1] or statin Statin plus niacin[1,2]
Increased LDL and increased TG (200-499 mg/dL)[2]	Intensify LDL-lowering therapy	Statin plus niacin[1,3] Statin plus fibrate[3]
Increased LDL and increased TG (≥500 mg/dL)[2]	Consider combination therapy (niacin,[1] fibrates, statin)	
Increased TG	Niacin[1] Fibrates	Niacin[1] plus fibrates
Increased LDL and low HDL	Niacin[1] Statin	Statin plus niacin[1,2]

[1]Avoid in diabetics.

[2]Emphasize weight reduction and increased physical activity.

[3]Risk of myopathy with combination.

Resins = bile acid sequestrants; statins = HMG-CoA reductase inhibitors; fibrates = fibric acid derivatives (eg, gemfibrozil, fenofibrate).

COMBINATION DRUG THERAPY

If after at least 6 weeks of therapy at the maximum recommended or tolerated dose, the patient's LDL cholesterol is not at target, consider optimizing nondrug measures, prescribing a higher dose of current lipid-lowering drug, or adding another lipid-lowering medication to the current therapy. Successful drug combinations include statin and niacin, statin and bile acid sequestrant, or niacin and bile acid sequestrant. At maximum recommended doses, LDL cholesterol may be decreased by 50% to 60% with combination therapy. This is the same reduction achieved by atorvastatin 40 mg twice daily. If a bile acid sequestrant is used with other lipid-lowering agents, space doses 1 hour before or 4 hours after the bile acid sequestrant administration. Statins combined with either fenofibrate, clofibrate, gemfibrozil, or niacin increase the risk of rhabdomyolysis. In this situation, patient education (muscle pain/weakness) and careful follow-up are warranted.

References

Guidelines

American Diabetes Association, "Standards of Medical Care in Diabetes - 2008," *Diabetes Care*, 2008, 31(Suppl 1):S12-54.

National Cholesterol Education Program, "Third Report of the Expert Panel on Detection, Evaluation, and Treatment of High Blood Cholesterol in Adults (Adult Treatment Panel III)," *JAMA*, 2001, 285(19):2486-97.

Grundy SM, Cleeman JI, Merz CN, et al, "Implications of Recent Clinical Trials for the National Cholesterol Education Program Adult Treatment Panel III Guidelines," *J Am Coll Cardiol*, 2004, 44(3):720-32.

Others

Berthold HK, Sudhop T, and von Bergmann K, "Effect of a Garlic Oil Preparation on Serum Lipoproteins and Cholesterol Metabolism: A Randomized Controlled Trial," *JAMA*, 1998, 279(23):1900-2.

Bertolini S, Bon GB, Campbell LM, et al, "Efficacy and Safety of Atorvastatin Compared to Pravastatin in Patients With Hypercholesterolemia," *Atherosclerosis*, 1997, 130 (1-2):191-7.

Blankenhorn DH, Nessim SA, Johnson RL, et al, "Beneficial Effects of Combined Colestipol-Niacin Therapy on Coronary Atherosclerosis and Venous Bypass Grafts," *JAMA*, 1987, 257(23):3233-40.

Brown G, Albers JJ, Fisher LD, et al, "Regression of Coronary Artery Disease as a Result of Intensive Lipid-Lowering Therapy in Men With High Levels of Apolipoprotein B," *N Engl J Med*, 1990, 323(19):1289-98.

Capuzzi DM, Guyton JR, Morgan JM, et al, "Efficacy and Safety of an Extended-Release Niacin (Niaspan®): A Long-Term Study," *Am J Cardiol*, 1998, 82(12A):74U-81U.

Coronary Drug Project Research Program, "Clofibrate and Niacin in Coronary Heart Disease," *JAMA*, 1975, 231(4):360-81.

Dart A, Jerums G, Nicholson G, et al, "A Multicenter, Double-Blind, One-Year Study Comparing Safety and Efficacy of Atorvastatin Versus Simvastatin in Patients With Hypercholesterolemia," *Am J Cardiol*, 1997, 80(1):39-44.

Davidson MH, Dillon MA, Gordon B, et al, "Colesevelam Hydrochloride (Cholestagel): A New Potent Bile Acid Sequestrant Associated With a Low Incidence of Gastrointestinal Side Effects," *Arch Intern Med*, 1999, 159(16):1893-900.

Davidson M, McKenney J, Stein E, et al, "Comparison of One-Year Efficacy and Safety of Atorvastatin Versus Lovastatin in Primary Hypercholesterolemia," *Am J Cardiol*, 1997, 79 (11):1475-81.

Frick MH, Heinonen OP, Huttunen JK, et al, "Helsinki Heart Study: Primary-Prevention Trial With Gemfibrozil in Middle-Aged Men With Dyslipidemia," *N Engl J Med*, 1987, 317 (20):1237-45.

Garber AM, Browner WS, and Hulley SB, "Clinical Guideline, Part 2: Cholesterol Screening in Asymptomatic Adults, Revisited," *Ann Intern Med*, 1995, 124(5):518-31.

Johannesson M, Jonsson B, Kjekshus J, et al, "Cost-Effectiveness of Simvastatin Treatment to Lower Cholesterol Levels in Patients With Coronary Heart Disease. Scandinavian Simvastatin Survival Study Group," *N Engl N Med*, 1997, 336(5):332-6.

Jones P, Kafonek S, Laurora I, et al, "Comparative Dose Efficacy Study of Atorvastatin Versus Simvastatin, Pravastatin, Lovastatin, and Fluvastatin in Patients With Hypercholesterolemia," *Am J Cardiol*, 1998, 81(5):582-7.

Kasiske BL, Ma JZ, Kalil RS, et al, "Effects of Antihypertensive Therapy on Serum Lipids," *Ann Intern Med*, 1995, 122(2):133-41.

Lipid Research Clinics Program, "The Lipid Research Clinics Coronary Primary Prevention Trial Results: I. Reduction in Incidence of Coronary Heart Disease," *JAMA*, 1984, 251 (3):351-64.

Mauro VF and Tuckerman CE, "Ezetimibe for Management of Hypercholesterolemia," *Ann Pharmacother*, 2003, 37(6):839-48.

Multiple Risk Factor Intervention Trial Research Group, "Multiple Risk Factor Intervention Trial: Risk Factor Changes and Mortality Results," *JAMA*, 1982, 248(12):1465-77.

Pitt B, Waters D, Brown WV, et al, "Aggressive Lipid-Lowering Therapy Compared With Angioplasty in Stable Coronary Artery Disease. Atorvastatin Versus Revascularization Treatment Investigators," *N Engl J Med*, 1999, 341(2):70-6.

Ross SD, Allen IE, Connelly JE, et al, "Clinical Outcomes in Statin Treatment Trials: A Meta-Analysis," *Arch Intern Med*, 1999, 159(15):1793-802.

Sacks FM, Pfeffer MA, Moye LA, et al, "The Effect of Pravastatin on Coronary Events After Myocardial Infarction in Patients With Average Cholesterol Levels," *N Engl J Med*, 1996, 335(14):1001-9.

Scandinavian Simvastatin Survival Study, "Randomized Trial of Cholesterol Lowering in 4444 Patients With Coronary Heart Disease: The Scandinavian Simvastatin Survival Study (4S)," *Lancet*, 1994, 344(8934):1383-9.

Schrott HG, Bittner V, Vittinghoff E, et al, "Adherence to National Cholesterol Education Program Treatment Goals in Postmenopausal Women With Heart Disease. The Heart and Estrogen/Progestin Replacement Study (HERS)," *JAMA*, 1997, 277(16):1281-6.

Shepherd J, Cobbe SM, Ford I, et al, "Prevention of Coronary Heart Disease With Pravastatin in Men With Hypercholesterolemia, The West of Scotland Coronary Prevention Study Group," *N Engl J Med*, 1995, 333(20):1301-7.

Stein EA, Davidson MH, Dobs AS, et al, "Efficacy and Safety of Simvastatin 80 mg/day in Hypercholesterolemic Patients. The Expanded Dose Simvastatin U.S. Study Group," *Am J Cardiol*, 1998, 82(3):311-6.

HYPERTENSION

The optimal blood pressure for adults is <120/80 mm Hg. Consistent systolic pressure ≥140 mm Hg or a diastolic pressure ≥90 mm Hg, in the absence of a secondary cause, defines hypertension. Hypertension affects approximately 25% (50 million people) in the United States. Of those patients on antihypertensive medication, only one in three have their blood pressure controlled (<140/90 mm Hg).

Controlling systolic hypertension has been much more difficult than controlling diastolic hypertension. Educating patients in lifestyle management, cardiovascular risk reduction, and drug therapy aids in improving the morbidity and mortality of patients with hypertension.

The Seventh Report of the Joint National Committee (JNC VII) is an excellent reference and guide for the treatment of hypertension (Chobanian AV, Bakris GL, Black HR, et al, "The Seventh Report of the Joint National Committee on Prevention, Detection, Evaluation, and Treatment of High Blood Pressure: The JNC 7 Report," *JAMA*, 2003, 289(19):2560-71). For adults, hypertension is classified in stages (see following table).

Adult Classification of Blood Pressure

Category	Systolic (mm Hg)		Diastolic (mm Hg)
Normal	<120	and	<80
Prehypertension	120-139	or	80-89
Hypertension			
Stage 1	140-159	or	90-99
Stage 2	≥160	or	≥100

Adapted from Chobanian AV, Bakris GL, Black HR, et al, "The Seventh Report of the Joint National Committee on Prevention, Detection, Evaluation, and Treatment of High Blood Pressure: The JNC 7 Report," *JAMA*, 2003, 289(19):2560-71.

Normal Blood Pressure in Children

Age (y)	Girls' SBP / DBP (mm Hg)		Boys' SBP / DBP (mm Hg)	
	50th Percentile for Height	75th Percentile for Height	50th Percentile for Height	75th Percentile for Height
1	104/58	105/59	102/57	104/58
6	111/73	112/73	114/74	115/75
12	123/80	124/81	123/81	125/82
17	129/84	130/85	136/87	138/88

SBP = systolic blood pressure.

DBP = diastolic blood pressure.

Adapted from the report by the NHBPEP Working Group on Hypertension Control in Children and Adolescents, *Pediatrics*, 1996, 98(4 Pt 1):649-58.

PATIENT ASSESSMENT

- **Cardiovascular Risk Factors:** Hypertension, cigarette smoking, obesity (BMI ≥30), inactive lifestyle, dyslipidemia, diabetes mellitus, microalbuminuria or estimated GFR <60 mL/minute, age (>55 years for men, >65 years for women), family history of premature cardiovascular disease (men <55 years or women >65 years).

  Components of metabolic syndrome include hypertension, obesity, dyslipidemia, diabetes mellitus.
- Identify causes of high BP.
- Assess target-organ damage and CVD.

Target-Organ Disease

Organ System	Manifestation
Cardiac	Clinical, ECG, or radiologic evidence of coronary artery disease; prior MI, angina, post-CABG; left ventricular hypertrophy (LVH); left ventricular dysfunction or cardiac failure, prior coronary revascularization
Cerebrovascular	Transient ischemic attack or stroke
Peripheral vascular	Absence of pulses in extremities (except dorsalis pedis), claudication, aneurysm, peripheral arterial disease
Renal	Serum creatinine ≥130 μmol/L (1.5 mg/dL); proteinuria (≥1+); microalbuminuria, chronic kidney disease
Eye	Hemorrhages or exudates, with or without papilledema; retinopathy

Adapted from Chobanian AV, Bakris GL, Black HR, et al, "The Seventh Report of the Joint National Committee on Prevention, Detection, Evaluation, and Treatment of High Blood Pressure: The JNC 7 Report," *JAMA*, 2003, 289(19):2560-71.

BLOOD PRESSURE MEASUREMENT

At an office visit, patients should be seated quietly for ≥5 minutes in a chair with feet on the floor and arm supported at heart level. At least two measurements should be made. Patients should be given their results and their goal BP.

Ambulatory BP monitoring is useful in evaluating "white coat hypertension" (no end-organ damage), drug resistance, hypotensive symptoms, episodic hypertension, and autonomic dysfunction. Ambulatory BP monitoring correlates better with end-organ damage than office measurements.

Having patients monitor their own BP helps to improve compliance and provides information on response to therapeutic interventions.

Based on these initial assessments, treatment strategies for patients with hypertension are stratified based on their blood pressure and comorbidities (compelling indications).

Management of Blood Pressure

	Management: Based upon highest BP category		
BP Classification	**Lifestyle Modification**	**Initial Therapy Without Compelling Indication**	**Initial Therapy With Compelling Indication[1]**
Normal	Encourage	None	None
Prehypertensive	Yes	None	Treat patients with chronic kidney disease or diabetes to BP goal of <130/80 mm Hg
Hypertension			
Stage 1	Yes	Thiazide-type diuretic for most; consider ACEI, ARB, β-blocker, CCB, or combination	Drugs for the compelling indications; other antihypertensives as needed
Stage 2	Yes	Two drug combos (typically a thiazide-type diuretic and ACEI or ARB or β-blocker or CCB). Use combo cautiously in patients at risk for orthostasis.	Drugs for the compelling indications; other antihypertensives as needed

[1]Compelling Indication: Conditions for which specific classes of antihypertensive drugs have proven beneficial.

Adapted from Chobanian AV, Bakris GL, Black HR, et al, "The Seventh Report of the Joint National Committee on Prevention, Detection, Evaluation, and Treatment of High Blood Pressure: The JNC 7 Report," *JAMA*, 2003, 289(19):2560-71.

ACHIEVING BLOOD PRESSURE CONTROL

Treatment of hypertension should be individualized. Lower blood pressure (goal <130/80 mm Hg) should be achieved in patients with diabetes or chronic renal disease. The following Hypertension Treatment Algorithm may be used to select specific antihypertensives based on compelling indications.

Special consideration for starting combination therapy should be made in each patient.

Starting drug therapy at a low dose and titrating upward if blood pressure is not controlled is recommended.

Most patients with hypertension will require two or more drugs to achieve their BP goals.

Adding a second drug from a different class will help when a single drug at reasonable doses has failed to achieve the goal.

If the untreated BP is >20/10 mm Hg away from the goal, consider initiating therapy with two drugs. Use caution in those at risk for orthostasis (eg, diabetics, geriatrics, and those with autonomic dysfunction).

Low-dose aspirin therapy should be considered when BP is controlled; use in uncontrolled hypertension can increase the risk of hemorrhagic stroke.

Lifestyle modification and risk reduction should always be reviewed and reinforced.

MONITORING THERAPY

Generally, monthly follow-up is recommended until BP control is reached.

More frequent monitoring is required for those patients with Stage 2 hypertension or those with complications.

Serum potassium and serum creatinine should be monitored at least twice yearly.

When BP is at goal and stable, follow-up can be maintained every 3-6 months. Treat other cardiovascular risk factors if present.

Hypertension Treatment Algorithm

Begin or continue lifestyle modifications

↓

Not at goal blood pressure (<140/90 mm Hg or <130/80 mm Hg for patients with diabetes or chronic renal disease)

↓

Initial Drug Choice

Hypertension

Stage I
Thiazide-type diuretic for most. Consider ACEI, ARB, β-blocker, CCB, or combo.

Stage 2
Two-drug combo for most (typically thiazide-type diuretic + ACEI or ARB or β-blocker or CCB)

Compelling Indications

Chronic kidney disease
- ACEI
- ARB

Diabetes mellitus
- ACEI
- ARB
- β-blocker
- CCB
- Diuretic

Heart failure
- ACEI
- Aldosterone blocker
- ARB
- β-blocker
- Diuretic

High coronary risk
- ACEI
- β-blocker
- CCB
- Diuretic

Myocardial infarction
- ACEI
- Aldosterone blocker
- β-blocker

Recurrent stroke prevention
- ACEI
- Diuretic

↓

Not at goal blood pressure

↓ Optimize dosages or add additional drugs until goal BP achieved.

↓ Consider consultation with hypertension specialist.

Additional Considerations for Specific Therapies

Indication	Drug Therapy
Atrial tachyarrhythmias	β-blocker, CCB (non-DHP)
Chronic kidney disease	
Cl_{cr} <60 mL/min or albuminuria	ACEI or ARB
Cl_{cr} <30 mL/min	Increase loop diuretic
Diabetes	Thiazide diuretic, β-blocker, ACEI, ARB, CCB
Nephropathy	ACEI, ARB
Essential tremor	β-blocker (noncardioselective)
Heart failure	
Ventricular dysfunction (asymptomatic)	ACEI, β-blocker
Ventricular dysfunction (symptomatic)	ACEI, β-blocker, ARB, aldosterone blocker, loop diuretic
Hypertensive women who are pregnant	Methyldopa, β-blocker, vasodilator
Ischemic heart disease	
Angina	β-blocker, CCB (long-acting)
Acute coronary syndromes	β-blocker, ACEI
Migraine	β-blocker (noncardioselective), CCB (long-acting, non-DHP)
Osteoporosis	Thiazide diuretic
Perioperative hypertension	β-blocker
Prostatism (BPH)	Alpha-adrenergic blocking agent
Raynaud syndrome	CCB
Thyrotoxicosis	β-blocker

Note: ACEI = angiotensin-converting enzyme inhibitor; ARB = angiotensin receptor blocker; CCB = calcium channel blocker; DHP = dihydropyridine.

May Have Unfavorable Effects on Comorbid Conditions

Condition	Drug Therapy to Avoid
Angioedema	ACEI
Bronchospastic disease	β-blocker
Gout	Thiazide diuretic
Heart block (second or third degree)	β-blocker, CCB (non-DHP)
Hyponatremia	Thiazide diuretic
Potassium >5 mEq/L before treatment	Potassium sparing diuretic, aldosterone antagonist
Pregnancy or those likely to become pregnant	ACEI, ARB

Note: ACEI = angiotensin-converting enzyme inhibitor; ARB = angiotensin receptor blocker; CCB = calcium channel blocker; DHP = dihydropyridine.

HYPERTENSIVE EMERGENCIES AND URGENCIES

General Treatment Principles in the Treatment of Hypertensive Emergencies

Principle	Considerations
Admit the patient to the hospital, preferably in the ICU. Monitor vital signs appropriately.	Establish I.V. access and place patient on a cardiac monitor. Place a femoral intra-arterial line and pulmonary arterial catheter, if indicated, to assess cardiopulmonary function and intravascular volume status.
Perform rapid but thorough history and physical examination.	Determine cause of, or precipitating factors to, hypertensive crisis if possible (remember to obtain a medication history including Rx, OTC, and illicit drugs). Obtain details regarding any prior history of hypertension (severity, duration, treatment), as well as other coexisting illnesses. Assess the extent of hypertensive end organ damage. Determine if a hypertensive urgency or emergency exists.
Determine goal blood pressure based on premorbid level, duration, severity and rapidity of increase of blood pressure, concomitant medical conditions, race, and age.	Acute decreases in blood pressure to normal or subnormal levels during the initial treatment period may reduce perfusion to the brain, heart, and kidneys, and must be avoided except in specific instances (ie, dissecting aortic aneurysm). Gradually establish a normal (or reasonable) blood pressure over the next 1-2 weeks.
Select an appropriate antihypertensive regimen depending on the individual patient and clinical setting.	Initiate a controlled decrease in blood pressure. Avoid concomitant administration of multiple agents that may cause precipitous falls in blood pressure. Select the agent with the best hemodynamic profile based on the primary treatment goal. Avoid diuretics and sodium restriction during the initial treatment period unless there is a clear clinical indication (ie, CHF, pulmonary edema). Avoid sedating antihypertensives in patients with hypertensive encephalopathy, CVA, or other CNS disorders in whom mental status must be monitored. Use caution with direct vasodilating agents that induce reflex tachycardia or increase cardiac output in patients with coronary heart disease, history of angina or myocardial infarction, or dissecting aortic aneurysm. Preferably choose an agent that does not adversely affect glomerular filtration rate or renal blood flow and also agents that have favorable effects on cerebral blood flow and its autoregulation, especially for patients with hypertensive encephalopathy or CVAs. Select the most efficacious agent with the fewest adverse effects based on the underlying cause of the hypertensive crisis and other individual patient factors.
Initiate a chronic antihypertensive regimen after the patient's blood pressure is stabilized	Begin oral antihypertensive therapy once goal blood pressure is achieved before gradually tapering parenteral medications. Select the best oral regimen based on cost, ease of administration, adverse effect profile, and concomitant medical conditions.

Oral Agents Used in the Treatment of Hypertensive Urgencies

Drug	Dose	Onset	Cautions
Captopril[1]	P.O.: 25 mg, repeat as required	15-30 min	Hypotension, renal failure in bilateral renal artery stenosis
Clonidine	P.O.: 0.1-0.2 mg, repeated every hour as needed to a total dose of 0.6 mg	30-60 min	Hypotension, drowsiness, dry mouth
Labetalol	P.O.: 200-400 mg, repeat every 2-3 h	30 min to 2 h	Bronchoconstriction, heart block, orthostatic hypotension

[1]There is no clearly defined clinical advantage in the use of sublingual over oral routes of administration with these agents.

Recommendations for the Use of Intravenous Antihypertensive Drugs in Selected Hypertensive Emergencies

Condition	Agent(s) of Choice	Agent(s) to Avoid or Use With Caution	General Treatment Principles
Hypertensive encephalopathy	Nitroprusside, labetalol	Methyldopa, reserpine	Avoid drugs with CNS-sedating effects.
Acute intracranial or subarachnoid hemorrhage	Nicardipine,[1] nitroprusside	β-blocker	Careful titration with a short-acting agent.

Recommendations for the Use of Intravenous Antihypertensive Drugs in Selected Hypertensive Emergencies *continued*

Condition	Agent(s) of Choice	Agent(s) to Avoid or Use With Caution	General Treatment Principles
Cerebral infarction	Nicardipine,[1] nitroprusside, labetalol	β-blocker, minoxidil	Careful titration with a short-acting agent. Avoid agents that may decrease cerebral blood flow.
Head trauma	Esmolol, labetalol	Methyldopa, reserpine, nitroprusside, nitroglycerin, hydralazine	Avoid drugs with CNS-sedating effects, or those that may increase intracranial pressure.
Acute myocardial infarction, myocardial ischemia	Nitroglycerin, nicardipine[1] (calcium channel blocker), labetalol	Hydralazine, minoxidil	Avoid drugs which cause reflex tachycardia and increased myocardial oxygen consumption.
Acute pulmonary edema	Nitroprusside, nitroglycerin, loop diuretics	β-blocker (labetalol), minoxidil, methyldopa	Avoid drugs which may cause sodium and water retention and edema exacerbation.
Renal dysfunction	Hydralazine, calcium channel blocker	Nitroprusside, ACE inhibitors, β-blocker (labetalol)	Avoid drugs with increased toxicity in renal failure and those that may cause decreased renal blood flow.
Eclampsia	Hydralazine, labetalol, nitroprusside[2]	Diuretics	Avoid drugs that may cause adverse fetal effects, compromise placental circulation, or decrease cardiac output.
Pheochromo- cytoma	Phentolamine, nitroprusside, β-blocker (eg, esmolol) only after alpha blockade (phentolamine)	β-blocker in the absence of alpha blockade, methyldopa, minoxidil	Use drugs of proven efficacy and specificity. Unopposed beta-blockade may exacerbate hypertension.
Dissecting aortic aneurysm	Nitroprusside and beta-blockade	Hydralazine, minoxidil	Avoid drugs which may increase cardiac output.
Postoperative hypertension	Nitroprusside, nicardipine,[1] labetalol, clevidipine		Avoid drugs which may exacerbate postoperative ileus.

[1]The use of nicardipine in these situations is by the recommendation of the author based on a review of the literature.

[2]Reserve nitroprusside for eclamptic patients with life-threatening hypertension unresponsive to other agents due to the potential risk to the fetus (cyanide and thiocyanate metabolites may cross the placenta).

Selected Intravenous Agents for Hypertensive Emergencies

Drug	Dose[1]	Onset of Action	Duration of Action	Adverse Effects[2]	Special Indications
Vasodilators					
Sodium nitroprusside	0.25-10 mcg/kg/min as I.V. infusion[3] (max: 10 min only)	Immediate	1-2 min	Nausea, vomiting, muscle twitching, sweating, thiocyanate and cyanide intoxication	Most hypertensive emergencies; caution with high intracranial pressure or azotemia
Nicardipine hydrochloride	5-15 mg/h I.V.	5-10 min	1-4 h	Tachycardia, headache, flushing, local phlebitis	Most hypertensive emergencies except acute heart failure; caution with coronary ischemia
Clevidipine butyrate	1-21 mg/h I.V.	2-4 min	5-15 min	Atrial fibrillation, nausea, insomnia, fever	Most hypertensive emergencies; caution with lipid disorder
Fenoldopam mesylate	0.1-0.3 mcg/kg/min as I.V. infusion	<5 min	30 min	Tachycardia, headache, nausea, flushing	Most hypertensive emergencies; caution with glaucoma
Nitroglycerin	5-100 mcg/min as I.V. infusion[3]	2-5 min	3-5 min	Headache, vomiting, methemoglobinemia, tolerance with prolonged use	Coronary ischemia
Enalaprilat	1.25-5 mg every 6 hours I.V.	15-30 min	6 h	Precipitous fall in pressure in high-renin states; response variable	Acute left ventricular failure; avoid in acute myocardial infarction
Hydralazine hydrochloride	10-20 mg I.V. 10-50 mg I.M.	10-20 min 20-30 min	3-8 h	Tachycardia, flushing, headache, vomiting, aggravation of angina	Eclampsia

Selected Intravenous Agents for Hypertensive Emergencies *continued*

Drug	Dose[1]	Onset of Action	Duration of Action	Adverse Effects[2]	Special Indications
				Adrenergic Inhibitors	
Labetalol hydrochloride	20-80 mg I.V. bolus every 10 min; 0.5-2 mg/min as I.V. infusion	5-10 min	3-6 h	Vomiting, scalp tingling, burning in throat, dizziness, nausea, heart block, orthostatic hypotension	Most hypertensive emergencies except acute heart failure
Esmolol hydrochloride	250-500 mcg/kg/min for 1 min, then 50-100 mcg/kg/min for 4 min; may repeat	1-2 min	10-20 min	Hypotension, nausea	Aortic dissection, perioperative
Phentolamine	5-15 mg I.V.	1-2 min	3-10 min	Tachycardia, flushing, headache	Catecholamine excess

[1]These doses may vary from those in the *Physicians' Desk Reference* (51st edition).

[2]Hypotension may occur with all agents.

[3]Require special delivery system.

References

Guidelines

"1999 World Health Organization-International Society of Hypertension Guidelines for the Management of Hypertension. Guidelines Subcommittee," *J Hypertens*, 1999, 17 (2):151-83.

Chobanian AV, Bakris GL, Black HR, et al, "The Seventh Report of the Joint National Committee on Prevention, Detection, Evaluation, and Treatment of High Blood Pressure: The JNC 7 Report," *JAMA*, 2003, 289(19):2560-72.

National High Blood Pressure Education Program Working Group on Hypertension Control in Children and Adolescents, "Update on the 1987 Task Force Report on High Blood Pressure in Children and Adolescents: A Working Group Report From the National High Blood Pressure Education Program," *Pediatrics*, 1996, 98(4 Pt 1):649-58.

National High Blood Pressure Education Program Working Group, "1995 Update of the Working Group Reports on Chronic Renal Failure and Renovascular Hypertension," *Arch Intern Med*, 1996, 156(17):1938-47.

"The Sixth Report of the National Committee on Detection, Evaluation, and Treatment of High Blood Pressure (JNC-VI)," *Arch Intern Med*, 1997, 157(21):2413-46.

Others

Appel LJ, Moore TJ, Obarzanek E, et al, "A Clinical Trial of the Effect of Dietary Patterns on Blood Pressure. The DASH Collaborative Research Group," *N Engl J Med*, 1997, 336 (16):1117-24.

Epstein M and Bakris G, "Newer Approaches to Antihypertensive Therapy: Use of Fixed-Dose Combination Therapy," *Arch Intern Med*, 1996, 156(17):1969-78.

Estacio RO and Schrier RW, "Antihypertensive Therapy in Type II Diabetes: Implications of the Appropriate Blood Pressure Control in Diabetes (ABCD) Trial," *Am J Cardiol*, 1998, 82 (9B):9R-14R.

Flack JM, Neaton J, Grimm RJ, et al, "Blood Pressure and Mortality Among Men With Prior Myocardial Infarction. The Multiple Risk Factor Intervention Trial Research Group," *Circulation*, 1995, 92(9):2437-45.

Frishman WH, Bryzinski BS, Coulson LR, et al, "A Multifactorial Trial Design to Assess Combination Therapy in Hypertension: Treatment With Bisoprolol and Hydrochlorothiazide," *Arch Intern Med*, 1994, 154(13):1461-8.

Furberg CD, Psaty BM, and Meyer JV, "Nifedipine: Dose-Related Increase in Mortality in Patients With Coronary Heart Disease," *Circulation*, 1995, 92(5):1326-31.

Glynn RJ, Brock DB, Harris T, et al, "Use of Antihypertensive Drugs and Trends in Blood Pressure in the Elderly," *Arch Intern Med*, 1995, 155:1855-60.

Gradman AH, Cutler NR, Davis PJ, et al, "Combined Enalapril and Felodipine Extended Release (ER) for Systemic Hypertension. The Enalapril-Felodipine ER Factorial Study Group," *Am J Cardiol*, 1997, 79(4):431-5.

Grimm RH Jr, Flack JM, Grandits GA, et al, "Long-Term Effects on Plasma Lipids of Diet and Drugs to Treat Hypertension. The Treatment of Mild Hypertension Study (TOMHS) Research Group," *JAMA*, 1996, 275(20):1549-56.

Grimm RH Jr, Grandits GA, Cutler JA, et al, "Relationships of Quality-of-Life Measures to Long-Term Lifestyle and Drug Treatment in the Treatment of Mild Hypertension Study. The TOMHS Research Group," *Arch Intern Med*, 1997, 157(6):638-48.

Grossman E, Messerli FH, Grodzicki T, et al, "Should a Moratorium Be Placed on Sublingual Nifedipine Capsules Given for Hypertensive Emergencies and Pseudoemergencies?" *JAMA*, 1996, 276(16):1328-31.

Hansson L, Zanchetti A, Carruthers SG, et al, "Effects of Intensive Blood Pressure Lowering and Low-Dose Aspirin in Patients With Hypertension: Principal Results of the Hypertension Optimal Treatment (HOT) Randomized Trial. HOT Study Group," *Lancet*, 1998, 351(9118):1755-62.

Kaplan NM and Gifford RW Jr, "Choice of Initial Therapy for Hypertension," *JAMA*, 1996, 275 (20):1577-80.

Kasiske BL, Ma JZ, Kalil RSN, et al, "Effects of Antihypertensive Therapy in Serum Lipids," *Ann Intern Med*, 1995, 122(2):133-41.

Kostis JB, Davis BR, Cutler J, et al, "Prevention of Heart Failure by Antihypertensive Drug Treatment in Older Persons With Isolated Systolic Hypertension. SHEP Cooperative Research Group," *JAMA*, 1997, 278(3):212-6.

Lazarus JM, Bourgoignie JJ, Buckalew VM, et al, "Achievement and Safety of a Low Blood Pressure Goal in Chronic Renal Disease: The Modification of Diet in Renal Disease Study Group," *Hypertension*, 1997, 29(2):641-50.

Lindheimer MD, "Hypertension in Pregnancy," *Hypertension*, 1993, 22(1):127-37.

Materson BJ, Reda DJ, Cushman WC, et al, "Single-Drug Therapy for Hypertension in Men: A Comparison of Six Antihypertensive Agents With Placebo. The Department of Veterans Affairs Cooperative Study Group on Antihypertensive Agents," *N Engl J Med*, 1993, 328 (13):914-21.

Miller NH, Hill M, Kottke T, et al, "The Multi-Level Compliance Challenge: Recommendations for a Call to Action; A Statement for Healthcare Professionals," *Circulation*, 1997, 95 (4):1085-90.

Neaton JD and Wentworth D, "Serum Cholesterol, Blood Pressure, Cigarette Smoking, and Death From Coronary Heart Disease: Overall Findings and Differences by Age for 316,099 White Men. The Multiple Risk Factor Intervention Trial Research Group," *Arch Intern Med*, 1992, 152(1):56-64.

Neaton JD, Grim RH, Prineas RJ, et al, "Treatment of Mild Hypertension Study. Final Results. Treatment of Mild Hypertension Study Research Group," *JAMA*, 1993, 270 (6):713-24.

Oparil S, Levine JH, Zuschke CA, et al, "Effects of Candesartan Cilexetil in Patients With Severe Systemic Hypertension," *Am J Cardiol*, 1999, 84(3):289-93.

Peacock WF, Varon J, Garrison N, et al, "I.V. Clevidipine for Hypertension: Safety, Efficacy, and Transition to Oral Therapy," *Ann Emerg Med*, 2007, 50(3 Suppl):S8-9.

Perloff D, Grim C, Flack J, et al, "Human Blood Pressure Determination by Sphygmomanometry," *Circulation*, 1993, 88(5 Pt 1):2460-7.

Perry HM Jr, Bingham S, Horney A, et al, "Antihypertensive Efficacy of Treatment Regimens Used in Veterans Administration Hypertension Clinics. Department of Veterans Affairs Cooperative Study Group on Antihypertensive Agents," *Hypertension*, 1998, 31(3):771-9.

Preston RA, Materson BJ, Reda DJ, et al, "Age-Race Subgroup Compared With Renin Profile as Predictors of Blood Pressure Response to Antihypertensive Therapy," *JAMA*, 1998, 280(13):1168-72.

Psaty BM, Smith NL, Siscovick DS, et al, "Health Outcomes Associated With Antihypertensive Therapies Used as First-Line Agents. A Systemic Review and Meta-analysis," *JAMA*, 1997, 277(9):739-45.

Radevski IV, Valtchanova SP, Candy GP, et al, "Comparison of Acebutolol With and Without Hydrochlorothiazide Versus Carvedilol With and Without Hydrochlorothiazide in Black Patients With Mild to Moderate Systemic Hypertension," *Am J Cardiol*, 1999, 84(1):70-5.

Setaro JF and Black HR, "Refractory Hypertension," *N Engl J Med*, 1992, 327(8):543-7.

SHEP Cooperative Research Group, "Prevention of Stroke by Antihypertensive Drug Treatment in Older Persons With Isolated Systolic Hypertension: Final Results of the Systolic Hypertension in the Elderly Program (SHEP)," *JAMA*, 1991, 265(24):3255-64.

Sibai BM, "Treatment of Hypertension in Pregnant Women," *N Engl J Med*, 1996, 335 (4):257-65.

Singla N, Warltier DC, Gandhi SD, et al, "Treatment of Acute Postoperative Hypertension in Cardiac Surgery Patients: An Efficacy Study of Clevidipine Assessing Its Postoperative Antihypertensive Effect in Cardiac Surgery-2 (ESCAPE-2), a Randomized, Double-Blind, Placebo-Controlled Trial," *Anesth Analg*, 2008, 107(1):59-67.

Sowers JR, "Comorbidity of Hypertension and Diabetes: The Fosinopril Versus Amlodipine Cardiovascular Events Trial," *Am J Cardiol*, 1998, 82(9B):15R-19R.

Sternberg H, Rosenthal T, Shamiss A, et al, "Altered Circadian Rhythm of Blood Pressure in Shift Workers," *J Hum Hypertens*, 1995, 9(5):349-53.

"The Hypertension Prevention Trial: Three-Year Effects of Dietary Changes on Blood Pressure. Hypertension Prevention Trial Research Group," *Arch Intern Med*, 1990, 150 (1):153-62.

Trials of Hypertension Prevention Collaborative Research Group, "Effects of Weight Loss and Sodium Reduction Intervention on Blood Pressure and Hypertension Incidence in Overweight People With High-Normal Blood Pressure: The Trials of Hypertension Prevention, Phase II," *Arch Intern Med*, 1997, 157(6):657-67.

Tuomilehto J, Rastenyte D, Birkenhager WH, et al, "Effects of Calcium Channel Blockade in Older Patients With Diabetes and Systolic Hypertension," *N Engl J Med*, 1999, 340 (9):677-84.

Veelken R and Schmieder RE, "Overview of Alpha-1 Adrenoceptor Antagonism and Recent Advances in Hypertensive Therapy," *Am J Hypertens*, 1996, 9(11):139S-49S.

White WB, Black HR, Weber MA, et al, "Comparison of Effects of Controlled Onset Extended Release Verapamil at Bedtime and Nifedipine Gastrointestinal Therapeutic System on Arising on Early Morning Blood Pressure, Heart Rate, and the Heart Rate-Blood Pressure Product," *Am J Cardiol*, 1998, 81(4):424-31.

DISCONTINUATION OF PSYCHOTROPIC DRUGS

Withdrawal Symptoms and Recommendations

Drug	Withdrawal Symptoms	Recommendations
Amantadine	Neuroleptic malignant syndrome, drug-induced catatonia	In Parkinson's disease, dosage should be reduced gradually in order to prevent exacerbation of symptoms
Antipsychotics	Nausea, emesis, anorexia, diarrhea, rhinorrhea, diaphoresis, myalgia, paresthesia, anxiety, agitation, restlessness, insomnia	Reinitiate antipsychotic[1]
Benzodiazepines	Rebound symptoms, tachycardia, insomnia, tremor, seizures, psychosis	Taper dose slowly or switch to benzodiazepine with a long half-life at a high affinity (preferable) for the GABA benzodiazepine receptor site
Benztropine	Nervousness, craving, restlessness, depression, poor concentration, nausea, vomiting, headache, blurred vision, malaise	Dosage should be reduced gradually to prevent sudden increase in adverse symptoms; half-life of benztropine is 24 hours
Biperiden	Anxiety, depression, motor agitation, hallucinations, physical complaints	When discontinuing an antidyskinetic, taper gradually to avoid a rebound of adverse symptoms
Bromocriptine	Recurrence of symptoms, galactorrhea	No definitive information available on dosage reduction; however, when initiating therapy, begin with low dose and increase gradually (2.5 mg every 14-28 days for Parkinson's and 3-7 days for other indications) to prevent development of side effects
Diphenhydramine	Recurrence of insomnia, increased daytime restlessness, irritability, excessive blinking, increased defecation (rebound cholinergic reaction)	No specific recommendations reported
Levodopa	Confusion, fever, seizure activity, hyper-rigidity, profuse diaphoresis, tachycardia, tachypnea, muscle enzyme elevation	Gradually reduce dose to avoid the neuroleptic malignant-like syndrome (NLMLS); after discontinuation, dantrolene and/or bromocriptine have been used in patients with evident NLMLS to decrease fever and avoid a potentially lethal complication
Pergolide [DSC]	Hallucinations, confusion, paranoid ideation, worsening parkinsonism symptoms	No recommendations reported
SSRIs	Dizziness, light-headedness, insomnia, fatigue, anxiety, agitation, nausea, headache, sensory disturbances	Restart SSRI or another antidepressant with a similar pharmacologic profile[2]
TCAs	Malaise, myalgia, anergy, diaphoresis, rhinitis, paresthesia, headache, nausea, vomiting, diarrhea, anorexia, insomnia, irritability, depressed mood	Administer antimuscarinic agents
Trihexyphenidyl	Anxiety, tachycardia, orthostatic hypotension, deterioration of sleep quality, extrapyramidal symptoms, deterioration of psychotic symptomatology, life-threatening respiratory difficulties	Reduce dose gradually to avoid withdrawal symptoms or an increase in psychotic symptoms

[1]Dilsaver SC and Alessi NE, "Antipsychotic Withdrawal Symptoms: Phenomenology and Pathophysiology," *Acta Psychiatr Scand*, 1988, 77(3):241-6.

[2]Zajecka J, Tracy KA, and Mitchell S, "Discontinuation Symptoms After Treatment With Serotonin Reuptake Inhibitors: A Literature Review," *J Clin Psychiatry*, 1997, 58(7):291-7.

DRUGS OF ABUSE

Drugs (Trade or Other Names)	Medical Uses	Physical Dependence	Psychological Dependence	Tolerance	Duration (h)	Usual Method	Possible Effects	Effects of Overdose	Withdrawal Syndrome
Anabolic Steroids									
Testosterone (cypionate, enanthate) (C-III) (Depo®-Testosterone, Delatestryl®)	Hypogonadism	Unknown	Unknown	Unknown	14-28 d	Injected	Virilization, acne, testicular atrophy, gynecomastia, aggressive behavior, edema	Unknown	Possible depression
Nandrolone (decanoate, phenpropionate) (C-III) (Nortestosterone, Durabolin®, Deca-Durabolin®, Deca)	Anemia, breast cancer	Unknown	Unknown	Unknown	30 d	Injected			
Oxymetholone (C-III) (Anadrol®-50)	Anemia	Unknown	Unknown	Unknown	24	Oral			
Cannabis									
Marijuana (C-I) (Pot, Acapulco gold, grass, reefer, sinsemilla, Thai sticks, blunts, mota, yerba, grifa)	None	Unknown	Moderate	Yes	2-4	Smoked, oral	Euphoria, relaxed inhibitions, increased appetite, disorientation	Fatigue, paranoia, possible psychosis	Occasional reports of insomnia, hyperactivity, decreased appetite
Tetrahydrocannabinol (C-I [substance]; C-II [product]) (THC, Marinol®)	Antinauseant, appetite stimulant	Yes	Moderate	Yes	2-4	Smoked, oral			
Hashish and hashish oil (C-I) (Hash, hash oil)	None	Unknown	Moderate	Yes	2-4	Smoked, oral			
Depressants									
Alcohol (beer, wine, liquor)	None	High	High	Yes	1-3	Oral	Impaired memory, slurred speech, drunken behavior, slow onset vitamin deficiency, organ damage	Vomiting, respiratory depression, loss of consciousness, possible death	Trembling, anxiety, insomnia, vitamin deficiency, confusion, hallucinations, convulsions

Drugs (Trade or Other Names)	Medical Uses	Physical Dependence	Psychological Dependence	Tolerance	Duration (h)	Usual Method	Possible Effects	Effects of Overdose	Withdrawal Syndrome
Chloral hydrate (C-IV) (Noctec, Somnos®, Felsules)	Hypnotic	Moderate	Moderate	Yes	5-8	Oral	Slurred speech, disorientation, drunken behavior without odor of alcohol	Shallow respiration, clammy skin, dilated pupils, weak and rapid pulse, coma, possible death	Anxiety, insomnia, tremors, delirium, convulsions, possible death
Barbiturates (C-II, III, IV) (Amytal®, Fiorinal®, Nembutal®, Seconal®, Tuinal®, phenobarbital, pentobarbital)	Anesthetic, anticonvulsant, sedative, hypnotic, veterinary euthanasia agent	High-moderate	High-moderate	Yes	1-16	Oral, injected			
Benzodiazepines (C-IV) (Ativan®, Dalmane®, diazepam, Librium®, Xanax®, Serax®, Valium®, Tranxene®, Verstran, Versed, Halcion®, Paxipam®, Restoril®, rohypnol [roofies; R-2])	Antianxiety, sedative, anticonvulsant, hypnotic	Moderate	Moderate	Yes	1-8	Oral, injected			
Gamma hydroxybutyric acid (C-I [substance]; C-III [product]) (GHB, liquid ecstacy, liquid X, sodium oxybate, Xyrem®)	None in U.S.; anesthetic	Moderate	Moderate	Yes	3-6	Oral			
Hallucinogens									
LSD (C-I) (Acid, microdot sunshine, boomers)	None	None	Unknown	Yes	8-12	Oral	Illusions and hallucinations, altered perception of time and distance	Longer, more intense "trip" episodes, psychosis, possible death	Unknown
MDMA and analogs (C-1) (MDA [love drug], MDEA [Eve], MDMA [ecstacy, XTC, Adam], DOM, DOB, XTC	None	None	Moderate	Yes	4-6	Oral, snorted, smoked	Heightened senses, teeth grinding, and dehydration	Increased body temperature, electrolyte imbalance, cardiac arrest	Muscle aches, drowsiness, depression, acne
Phencyclidine and analogs (C-I, II) (PCE, PCPy, TCP, PCP, hog, loveboat, angel dust, ketamine [Special K])	Anesthetic (ketamine)	Possible	High	Yes	1-12	Oral, smoked, injected, snorted	Illusions and hallucinations, altered perception of time and distance	Longer, more intense "trip" episodes, psychosis, possible death	None
Other hallucinogens (C-I) (DMT, DET, psilocybe mushrooms, psilocin mescaline, peyote cactus, ayahuasca, dextromethorphan [DXM])	None	None	None	Possible	4-8	Oral	Illusions and hallucinations, altered perception of time and distance	Unable to direct movement, feel pain, or remember	Drug seeking behavior not regulated

Drugs (Trade or Other Names)	Medical Uses	Physical Dependence	Psychological Dependence	Tolerance	Duration (h)	Usual Method	Possible Effects	Effects of Overdose	Withdrawal Syndrome
Inhalants									
Amyl and butyl nitrate (pearls, poppers, rush, locker room)	Angina (amyl)	Unknown	Unknown	No	1	Inhaled	Flushing, hypotension, headache	Methemoglobinemia	Agitation
Nitrous oxide (laughing gas, balloons, whippets)	Anesthetic	Unknown	Low	No	0.5	Inhaled	Impaired memory, slurred speech, drunken behavior, slow onset vitamin deficiency, organ damage	Vomiting, respiratory depression, loss of consciousness, possible death	Trembling, anxiety, insomnia, vitamin deficiency, confusion, hallucinations, convulsions
Other inhalants (adhesives, spray paint, hair spray, dry cleaning fluid, spot remover, lighter fluid)	None	Unknown	High	No	0.5-2	Inhaled	Impaired memory, slurred speech, drunken behavior, slow onset vitamin deficiency, organ damage	Vomiting, respiratory depression, loss of consciousness, possible death	Trembling, anxiety, insomnia, vitamin deficiency, confusion, hallucinations, convulsions

Drugs (Trade or Other Names)	Medical Uses	Physical Dependence	Psychological Dependence	Tolerance	Duration (h)	Usual Method	Possible Effects	Effects of Overdose	Withdrawal Syndrome
Narcotics									
Heroin (C-I) (Diacetylmorphine, horse, smack, negra, chiva, black tar)	None in U.S.; analgesic, antitussive	High	High	Yes	3-4	Injected, snorted, smoked	Euphoria, drowsiness, respiratory depression, constricted pupils, nausea	Slow and shallow breathing, clammy skin, convulsions, coma, possible death	Watery eyes, runny nose, yawning, lose of appetite, irritability, tremors, panic, cramps, nausea, chills and sweating
Morphine (C-II) (Duramorph®, MS-Contin®, Roxanol™, Oramorph SR™)	Analgesic	High	High	Yes	3-12	Oral, smoked, injected			
Codeine (C-II [substance]; C-III, V [products]) (Tylenol® w/codeine, Empirin® w/codeine, Robitussin® A-C, Fiorinal® w/codeine, APAP w/ codeine)	Analgesic, antitussive	Moderate	Moderate	Yes	3-4	Oral, injected			
Hydrocodone (C-II [substance]; C-III, V [products]) (Tussionex®, Vicodin®, Hycodan®, Lorcet®)	Analgesic, antitussive	High	High	Yes	3-6	Oral			
Hydromorphone (C-II) (Dilaudid®)	Analgesic	High	High	Yes	3-4	Oral, injected			
Oxycodone (C-II) (Percodan®, Percocet®, Tylox®, Roxicet™, Roxicodone™)	Analgesic	High	High	Yes	3-12	Oral			
Methadone and LAAM (C-I, II) (Dolophine®, methadone, levo-alpha-acetylmethadol, levomethadyl acetate)	Analgesic, treatment of dependence	High	High	Yes	12-72	Oral, injected			
Fentanyl and analogs (C-I, II) (Innovar, Sublimaze®, Alfenta®, Sufenta®, Duragesic®)	Analgesic, adjunct to anesthesia, anesthetic	High	High	Yes	0.1-72	Injected, transdermal patch			
Other narcotics (C-II, III, IV, V) (Percodan®, Percocet®, Tylox®, opium, Darvon®, Talwin®, buprenorphine, meperidine (pethidine), Demerol®)	Analgesic, antidiarrheal	High-low	High-low	Yes	Variable	Oral, injected			

Drugs (Trade or Other Names)	Medical Uses	Physical Dependence	Psychological Dependence	Tolerance	Duration (h)	Usual Method	Possible Effects	Effects of Overdose	Withdrawal Syndrome
Stimulants									
Cocaine (C-II) (Coke, flake, snow, crack, coca, Bianca, perico, nieve, soda)	Local anesthetic	Possible	High	Yes	1-2	Snorted, smoked, injected	Increased alertness, excitation, euphoria, increased pulse rate and blood pressure, insomnia, loss of appetite	Agitation, increased body temperature, hallucinations, convulsions, possible death	Apathy, long periods of sleep, irritability, depression, disorientation
Amphetamine/methamphetamine (C-II) (Adderall®, Desoxyn®, Dexedrine®, ice, crank, crystal, krystal meth, speed)	Attention deficit disorder, narcolepsy, weight control	Possible	High	Yes	2-4	Oral, injected, smoked			
Methylphenidate (C-II) (Concerta®, Focalin™, Metadate®, Ritalin®)	Attention deficit disorder, narcolepsy	Possible	High	Yes	2-4	Oral, injected, smoked, snorted			
Other stimulants (C-III, IV) (Adipex®, Didrex®, Ionamin®, Melfiat®, Tenuate®, Tepanil, Prelu-2®, Preludin)	Weight control	Possible	Moderate	Yes	2-4	Oral			

Adapted from U.S. Department of Justice Drug Enforcement Administration, *Drugs of Abuse*, http://www.usdoj.gov/dea/pubs/abuse/doa-p.pdf, 2005.

LABORATORY DETECTION OF DRUGS

Agent	Time Detectable in Urine[1]
Alcohol	12-24 h
Amobarbital	2-4 d
Amphetamine	2-4 d
Butalbital	2-4 d
Cannabinoids	
Occasional use	2-7 d
Regular use	30 d
Cocaine (benzoylecgonine)	12-72 h
Codeine	2-4 d
Chlordiazepoxide	30 d
Diazepam	30 d
Dilaudid®	2-4 d
Ethanol	12-24 h
Heroin (morphine)	2-4 d
Hydromorphone	2-4 d
Librium®	30 d
Marijuana	
Occasional use	2-7 d
Regular use	30 d
Methamphetamine	2-4 d
Methaqualone	2-4 d
Morphine	2-4 d
Pentobarbital	2-4 d
Phencyclidine (PCP)	
Occasional use	2-7 d
Regular use	30 d
Phenobarbital	30 d
Quaalude®	2-4 d
Secobarbital	2-4 d
Valium®	30 d

[1]The periods of detection for the various abused drugs listed above should be taken as estimates since the actual figures will vary due to metabolism, user, laboratory, and excretion.

Chang JY, "Drug Testing and Interpretation of Results," *Pharmchem Newsletter*, 1989, 17:1.

SEROTONIN SYNDROME

Manifestations of Severe Serotonin Syndrome and Related Clinical Conditions

Condition	Medication History	Time Needed for Condition to Develop	Vital Signs	Pupils	Mucosa	Skin	Bowel Sounds	Neuromuscular Tone	Reflexes	Mental Status
Serotonin syndrome	Proserotonergic drug	<12 hours	Hypertension, tachycardia, tachypnea, hyperthermia (>41.1°C)	Mydriasis	Sialorrhea	Diaphoresis	Hyperactive	Increased, predominantly in lower extremities	Hyper-reflexia, clonus (unless masked by increased muscle tone)	Agitation, coma
Anticholinergic "toxidrome"	Anticholinergic agent	<12 hours	Hypertension (mild), tachycardia, tachypnea, hyperthermia (typically ≤38.8°C)	Mydriasis	Dry	Erythema, hot and dry to touch	Decreased or absent	Normal	Normal	Agitated delirium
Neuroleptic malignant syndrome	Dopamine antagonist	1-3 days	Hypertension, tachycardia, tachypnea, hyperthermia (>41.1°C)	Normal	Sialorrhea	Pallor, diaphoresis	Normal or decreased	"Lead-pipe" rigidity present in all muscle groups	Bradyreflexia	Stupor, alert mutism, coma
Malignant hyperthermia	Inhalational anesthesia	30 minutes to 24 hours after administration of inhalational anesthesia or succinylcholine	Hypertension, tachycardia, tachypnea, hyperthermia (can be as high as 46°C)	Normal	Normal	Mottled appearance, diaphoresis	Decreased	Rigor mortis-like rigidity	Hyporeflexia	Agitation

Reprinted with permission: Boyer EW and Shannon M, "The Serotonin Syndrome," *N Engl J Med,* 2005, 352(11):1112-20.

Management of Serotonin Syndrome

1. Remove precipitating drugs
   a. Serotonergic agents (eg, antidepressants; especially SSRI and MAO Inhibitors)
   b. Be mindful of half-life elimination and active metabolites
2. Supportive care
   a. Intravenous fluids
   b. Correct vital signs
3. Control agitation
   a. Benzodiazepines (diazepam)
   b. Avoid physical restraints
4. 5-HT_{2A} antagonists
   a. Cyproheptadine: 12-32 mg/day (may be crushed and administered via nasogastric tube)
   b. Chlorpromazine: I.M.: 50-100 mg (monitor vitals)
5. Control autonomic instability
   a. Norepinephrine **or**
   b. Phenylephrine **or**
   c. Epinephrine
   d. Nitroprusside or esmolol for hypertension and tachycardia
6. Control hyperthermia
   a. Benzodiazepines
   b. Neuromuscular paralysis with vecuronium (**Note:** Avoid succinylcholine)
   c. Intubation
   d. Do not use antipyretic agents
7. Other
   a. Do not use propranolol, bromocriptine, and dantrolene

TYRAMINE CONTENT OF FOODS

Food[1]	Allowed	Minimize Intake	Not Allowed
Beverages	Decaffeinated beverages (eg, coffee, tea, soda); milk, soy milk, chocolate beverage	Caffeine-containing drinks, clear spirits, wine, bottled/canned beers	**Tap** beer
Breads/cereals	All except those containing cheese	None	Cheese bread and crackers
Dairy products	Cottage cheese, farmers or pot cheese, cream cheese, ricotta cheese, all milk, eggs, ice cream, pudding, yogurt, sour cream, processed cheese, mozzarella	None	All other cheeses (**aged** cheese, American, Camembert, cheddar, Gouda, gruyere, parmesan, provolone, romano, Roquefort, stilton)
Meat, fish, and poultry	All fresh packaged or processed (eg, hot dogs, bologna), or frozen	Pepperoni	**Aged** chicken and beef liver, dried and pickled fish, shrimp paste, summer or dry sausage, dried meats (eg, salami, cacciatore), meat extracts, liverwurst
Starches — potatoes/rice	All	None	Soybean (including paste), tofu
Vegetables	All fresh, frozen, canned, or dried vegetable juices except those not allowed	Chili peppers, Chinese pea pods	Sauerkraut, broad or fava bean pods (not beans)
Fruit	Fresh, frozen, or canned fruits and fruit juices	Avocado, figs	Banana peel, avocado (over-ripened)
Soups	All soups not listed to limit or avoid	None	Soups which contain **aged** cheese, **tap** beer, any made with flavor cubes or meat extract, miso soup, broad or fava bean pods (not beans)
Fats	All except fermented	None	None
Sweets	Sugar, hard candy, honey, molasses, syrups, chocolate candy	None	None
Desserts	Cakes, cookies, gelatin, pastries, sherbets, sorbets, chocolate desserts	None	None
Miscellaneous	Salt, nuts, spices, herbs, flavorings, Worcestershire sauce, Brewer's or Baker's yeast, monosodium glutamate, vitamins with Brewer's yeast	Peanuts	Soy sauce, all aged and fermented products, marmite and other concentrated yeast extracts

[1]Freshness is of primary importance. Food that is spoiled or improperly stored should be avoided.

References:

Shulman KI and Walker SE, "A Reevaluation of Dietary Restrictions for Irreversible Monoamine Oxidase Inhibitors" *Psychiatr Ann*, 2001, 31(6):378-84.

Shulman KI and Walker SE, "Refining the MAOI Diet: Tyramine Content of Pizza and Soy Products," *J Clin Psychiatry*, 1999, 60(3):191-3.

Walker SE, Shulman KI, Tailor SAN, et al, "Tyramine Content of Previously Restricted Foods in Monoamine Oxidase Inhibitor Diets," *J Clin Psychopharmacol*, 1996, 16(5):383-8.

Alphabetical Index

Abacavir ... 22
Abacavir and Lamivudine ... 22
Abacavir Sulfate *See* Abacavir ... 22
Abacavir Sulfate and Lamivudine *See* Abacavir and Lamivudine ... 22
Abatacept ... 22
Abbott-43818 *See* Leuprolide ... 901
ABC *See* Abacavir ... 22
ABCD *See* Amphotericin B Cholesteryl Sulfate Complex ... 119
Abelcet® *See* Amphotericin B, Lipid Complex ... 121
Abenol® (Can) *See* Acetaminophen ... 30
ABI-007 *See* Paclitaxel (Protein Bound) ... 1214
Abilify® *See* Aripiprazole ... 133
Abilify® Discmelt™ *See* Aripiprazole ... 133
ABLC *See* Amphotericin B, Lipid Complex ... 121
Abraxane® *See* Paclitaxel (Protein Bound) ... 1214
ABX-EGF *See* Panitumumab ... 1221
9-AC *See* Aminocamptothecin ... 86
AC 2993 *See* Exenatide ... 609
ACAM2000™ *See* Smallpox Vaccine ... 1493
Acamprosate ... 23
Acamprosate Calcium *See* Acamprosate ... 23
Acarbixin (Mex) *See* Amoxicillin and Clavulanate Potassium ... 115
Acarbose ... 25
ACC (Mex) *See* Acetylcysteine ... 47
Accolate® *See* Zafirlukast ... 1689
AccuHist® *See* Brompheniramine and Pseudoephedrine ... 206
AccuHist® PDX Drops *See* Brompheniramine, Pseudoephedrine, and Dextromethorphan ... 208
AccuNeb® *See* Albuterol ... 54
Accupril® *See* Quinapril ... 1386
Accuretic® *See* Quinapril and Hydrochlorothiazide ... 1386
Accutane® *See* Isotretinoin ... 871
Ac-De (Mex) *See* DACTINomycin ... 415
ACE *See* Captopril ... 264
Acebutolol ... 27
Acebutolol Hydrochloride *See* Acebutolol ... 27
Acenocoumarin *See* Acenocoumarol ... 30
Acenocoumarol ... 30
Aceon® *See* Perindopril Erbumine ... 1254
Acephen™ [OTC] *See* Acetaminophen ... 30
Acerola [OTC] *See* Ascorbic Acid ... 141
Acetadiazol (Mex) *See* AcetaZOLAMIDE ... 46
Acetadote® *See* Acetylcysteine ... 47
Aceta-Gesic [OTC] *See* Acetaminophen and Phenyltoloxamine ... 36
Acetaminophen ... 30
Acetaminophen and Butalbital *See* Butalbital and Acetaminophen ... 236
Acetaminophen and Chlorpheniramine *See* Chlorpheniramine and Acetaminophen ... 322
Acetaminophen and Codeine ... 34
Acetaminophen and Diphenhydramine ... 35
Acetaminophen and Hydrocodone *See* Hydrocodone and Acetaminophen ... 777
Acetaminophen and Oxycodone *See* Oxycodone and Acetaminophen ... 1205
Acetaminophen and Pentazocine *See* Pentazocine and Acetaminophen ... 1245
Acetaminophen and Phenylephrine ... 36
Acetaminophen and Phenyltoloxamine ... 36
Acetaminophen and Propoxyphene *See* Propoxyphene and Acetaminophen ... 1354
Acetaminophen and Pseudoephedrine ... 37
Acetaminophen and Tramadol ... 38
Acetaminophen, Aspirin, and Caffeine ... 39
Acetaminophen, Butalbital, and Caffeine *See* Butalbital, Acetaminophen, and Caffeine ... 229
Acetaminophen, Caffeine, and Dihydrocodeine ... 39
Acetaminophen, Caffeine, Codeine, and Butalbital *See* Butalbital, Acetaminophen, Caffeine, and Codeine ... 232
Acetaminophen, Chlorpheniramine, and Pseudoephedrine ... 40
Acetaminophen, Codeine, and Doxylamine ... 41
Acetaminophen, Dextromethorphan, and Phenylephrine ... 42
Acetaminophen, Dextromethorphan, and Pseudoephedrine ... 43
Acetaminophen, Dichloralphenazone, and Isometheptene *See* Acetaminophen, Isometheptene, and Dichloralphenazone ... 45
Acetaminophen, Diphenhydramine, and Phenylephrine ... 44
Acetaminophen, Isometheptene, and Dichloralphenazone ... 45
Acetaminophen, Phenylephrine, and Diphenhydramine *See* Acetaminophen, Diphenhydramine, and Phenylephrine ... 44
Acetaminophen, Pseudoephedrine, and Chlorpheniramine *See* Acetaminophen, Chlorpheniramine, and Pseudoephedrine ... 40
AcetaZOLAMIDE ... 46
Acetoxymethylprogesterone *See* MedroxyPROGESTERone ... 975
Acetylcholine ... 47
Acetylcholine Chloride *See* Acetylcholine ... 47

Acetylcysteine ... 47
Acetylcysteine Sodium *See* Acetylcysteine ... 47
Acetylcysteine Solution (Can) *See* Acetylcysteine ... 47
Acetylsalicylic Acid *See* Aspirin ... 143
Achromycin *See* Tetracycline ... 1558
Aciclovir *See* Acyclovir ... 49
Acid Mantle (Mex) *See* Calcium Acetate ... 254
Ácido ascórbico (Mex) *See* Ascorbic Acid ... 141
Acid Reducer (Can) *See* Ranitidine ... 1399
Acid Reducer Maximum Strength Non Prescription (Can) *See* Ranitidine ... 1399
Acifur (Mex) *See* Acyclovir ... 49
Acilac (Can) *See* Lactulose ... 886
Acimox (Mex) *See* Amoxicillin ... 112
AcipHex® *See* Rabeprazole ... 1389
Acitfed® Cold & Allergy [OTC] [reformulation] *See* Chlorpheniramine and Phenylephrine 323
Aclasta® (Can) *See* Zoledronic Acid ... 1702
Aclixel (Mex) *See* Paclitaxel ... 1213
Acloral (Mex) *See* Ranitidine ... 1399
Acortiz (Mex) *See* Hydrochlorothiazide ... 773
Acrivastine and Pseudoephedrine ... 48
Acromicina (Mex) *See* Tetracycline ... 1558
ACT *See* DACTINomycin ... 415
Act-D *See* DACTINomycin ... 415
ACTH *See* Corticotropin ... 401
ActHIB® *See* Haemophilus b Conjugate Vaccine ... 753
Actidose-Aqua® [OTC] *See* Charcoal ... 312
Actidose® with Sorbitol [OTC] *See* Charcoal ... 312
Actifed® (Can) *See* Triprolidine and Pseudoephedrine ... 1634
Actifed® Cold and Sinus [OTC] *See* Acetaminophen, Chlorpheniramine, and Pseudoephedrine ... 40
Actigall® *See* Ursodiol ... 1639
Actimmune® *See* Interferon Gamma-1b ... 849
Actinium (Mex) *See* OXcarbazepine ... 1195
Actinomycin *See* DACTINomycin ... 415
Actinomycin D *See* DACTINomycin ... 415
Actinomycin CI *See* DACTINomycin ... 415
Actiq® *See* FentaNYL ... 624
Activated Carbon *See* Charcoal ... 312
Activated Charcoal *See* Charcoal ... 312
Activated Ergosterol *See* Ergocalciferol ... 550
Activella® *See* Estradiol and Norethindrone ... 579
Actonel® *See* Risedronate ... 1424
Actonel® and Calcium *See* Risedronate and Calcium ... 1424
Actoplus Met™ *See* Pioglitazone and Metformin ... 1301
Actos® *See* Pioglitazone ... 1297
Acular® *See* Ketorolac ... 878
Acular LS™ *See* Ketorolac ... 878
Acular® PF *See* Ketorolac ... 878
Acupril (Mex) *See* Quinapril ... 1386
ACV *See* Acyclovir ... 49
Acycloguanosine *See* Acyclovir ... 49
Acyclovir ... 49
Aczone® *See* Dapsone ... 418
AD3L *See* Valrubicin ... 1649
Adalat (Mex) *See* NIFEdipine ... 1136
Adalat® XL® (Can) *See* NIFEdipine ... 1136
Adalat® CC *See* NIFEdipine ... 1136
Adalimumab ... 50
Adalken (Mex) *See* Penicillamine ... 1239
Adamantanamine Hydrochloride *See* Amantadine ... 79
ADD 234037 *See* Lacosamide ... 885
Addaprin [OTC] *See* Ibuprofen ... 803
Adderall® *See* Dextroamphetamine and Amphetamine ... 444
Adderall XR® *See* Dextroamphetamine and Amphetamine ... 444
Adecur (Mex) *See* Terazosin ... 1549
Adefovir ... 51
Adefovir Dipivoxil *See* Adefovir ... 51
Adekon (Mex) *See* Ergocalciferol ... 550
Adel (Mex) *See* Clarithromycin ... 360
Adenocard® *See* Adenosine ... 51
Adenoscan® *See* Adenosine ... 51
Adenosine ... 51
Adenosine Injection, USP (Can) *See* Adenosine ... 51
Aderowest (Mex) *See* Ergocalciferol ... 550
ADH *See* Vasopressin ... 1659
Adinol (Mex) *See* Acetaminophen ... 30
Adipex-P® *See* Phentermine ... 1270

Adiro (Mex) *See* Aspirin ... 143
AdoMet *See* SAMe (S-adenosyl methionine) ... 1460
Adoxa® *See* Doxycycline ... 509
Adrenalin® *See* EPINEPHrine ... 543
Adrenaline *See* EPINEPHrine ... 543
Adrenocorticotropic Hormone *See* Corticotropin ... 401
ADR (error-prone abbreviation) *See* DOXOrubicin ... 507
Adria *See* DOXOrubicin ... 507
Adriamycin® *See* DOXOrubicin ... 507
Adriblastina RD (Mex) *See* DOXOrubicin ... 507
Adrucil® *See* Fluorouracil ... 649
Adsorbent Charcoal *See* Charcoal ... 312
Advagraf™ (Can) *See* Tacrolimus ... 1533
Advair® (Can) *See* Fluticasone and Salmeterol ... 674
Advair Diskus® *See* Fluticasone and Salmeterol ... 674
Advair® HFA *See* Fluticasone and Salmeterol ... 674
Advantan (Mex) *See* MethylPREDNISolone ... 1029
Advicor® *See* Niacin and Lovastatin ... 1127
Advil® (Can) *See* Ibuprofen ... 803
Advil® Children's [OTC] *See* Ibuprofen ... 803
Advil® Cold, Children's [OTC] [DSC] *See* Pseudoephedrine and Ibuprofen ... 1369
Advil® Cold & Sinus (Can) *See* Pseudoephedrine and Ibuprofen ... 1369
Advil® Cold & Sinus [OTC] *See* Pseudoephedrine and Ibuprofen ... 1369
Advil® Infants' [OTC] *See* Ibuprofen ... 803
Advil® Junior [OTC] [DSC] *See* Ibuprofen ... 803
Advil® Migraine [OTC] *See* Ibuprofen ... 803
Advil® [OTC] *See* Ibuprofen ... 803
Aerius® (Can) *See* Desloratadine ... 430
AeroBid® *See* Flunisolide ... 646
AeroBid®-M *See* Flunisolide ... 646
aerohist plus™ *See* Chlorpheniramine, Phenylephrine, and Methscopolamine ... 329
aeroKid™ *See* Chlorpheniramine, Phenylephrine, and Methscopolamine ... 329
Aerosial (Mex) *See* Budesonide ... 210
Afazol Grin (Mex) *See* Naphazoline ... 1101
Afeditab™ CR *See* NIFEdipine ... 1136
Aflamid (Mex) *See* Meloxicam ... 982
Afluria® *See* Influenza Virus Vaccine ... 820
Afrin (Mex) *See* Oxymetazoline ... 1208
Afrinex infantil (Mex) *See* Phenylephrine ... 1273
Afrin® Extra Moisturizing [OTC] *See* Oxymetazoline ... 1208
Afrin® Original [OTC] *See* Oxymetazoline ... 1208
Afrin® Severe Congestion [OTC] *See* Oxymetazoline ... 1208
Afrin® Sinus [OTC] *See* Oxymetazoline ... 1208
Afungil (Mex) *See* Fluconazole ... 635
A.F. Valdecasas (Mex) *See* Folic Acid ... 684
Agalsidase Beta ... 52
Agenerase® (Can) *See* Amprenavir ... 123
Agenerase® [DSC] *See* Amprenavir ... 123
Agglad Ofteno (Mex) *See* Brimonidine ... 199
Aggrastat® *See* Tirofiban ... 1586
Aggrenox® *See* Aspirin and Dipyridamole ... 145
AGN 1135 *See* Rasagiline ... 1403
Agnicin (Mex) *See* Amikacin ... 83
Agrastat (Mex) *See* Tirofiban ... 1586
Agrylin® *See* Anagrelide ... 124
AH-Chew® *See* Chlorpheniramine, Phenylephrine, and Methscopolamine ... 329
AH-Chew™ Ultra *See* Chlorpheniramine, Phenylephrine, and Methscopolamine ... 329
Ahist™ *See* Chlorpheniramine ... 321
A-hydroCort *See* Hydrocortisone ... 785
Airomir (Can) *See* Albuterol ... 54
Akacin (Mex) *See* Amikacin ... 83
AK-Con™ *See* Naphazoline ... 1101
AK-Dilate® *See* Phenylephrine ... 1273
Akne-Mycin® *See* Erythromycin ... 557
Akorazol (Mex) *See* Ketoconazole ... 876
AK-Pentolate™ *See* Cyclopentolate ... 407
Akten™ *See* Lidocaine ... 924
AKTob® *See* Tobramycin ... 1590
Akurza *See* Salicylic Acid ... 1454
Alamag Plus [OTC] *See* Aluminum Hydroxide, Magnesium Hydroxide, and Simethicone ... 78
Alavert™ Allergy and Sinus [OTC] *See* Loratadine and Pseudoephedrine ... 948
Alavert™ Allergy Relief 24-Hour [OTC] *See* Loratadine ... 946
Alavert™ [OTC] *See* Loratadine ... 946
Alaway™ [OTC] *See* Ketotifen ... 879
Albalon® [DSC] *See* Naphazoline ... 1101
Albatrina (Mex) *See* Loratadine ... 946
Albendazole ... 53

Albenza® *See* Albendazole ... 53
Albert® Glyburide (Can) *See* GlyBURIDE ... 730
Albert® Pentoxifylline (Can) *See* Pentoxifylline ... 1251
Albumin-Bound Paclitaxel *See* Paclitaxel (Protein Bound) ... 1214
Albuterol ... 54
Albuterol and Ipratropium *See* Ipratropium and Albuterol ... 854
Albuterol Sulfate *See* Albuterol ... 54
Alcaine® *See* Proparacaine ... 1352
Alcalak [OTC] *See* Calcium Carbonate ... 254
Alcomicin® (Can) *See* Gentamicin ... 714
Aldactazide® *See* Hydrochlorothiazide and Spironolactone ... 776
Aldactazide 25® (Can) *See* Hydrochlorothiazide and Spironolactone ... 776
Aldactazide 50® (Can) *See* Hydrochlorothiazide and Spironolactone ... 776
Aldactone® *See* Spironolactone ... 1503
Aldesleukin ... 58
Aldex™ *See* Guaifenesin and Phenylephrine ... 742
Aldex® AN *See* Doxylamine ... 510
Aldex® CT *See* Diphenhydramine and Phenylephrine ... 485
Aldex®D *See* Phenylephrine and Pyrilamine ... 1275
Aldex® DM *See* Phenylephrine, Pyrilamine, and Dextromethorphan ... 1278
Aldomet (Mex) *See* Methyldopa ... 1021
Aldoril® *See* Methyldopa and Hydrochlorothiazide ... 1021
Aldroxicon I [OTC] *See* Aluminum Hydroxide, Magnesium Hydroxide, and Simethicone ... 78
Aldroxicon II [OTC] *See* Aluminum Hydroxide, Magnesium Hydroxide, and Simethicone ... 78
Alefacept ... 58
Alemtuzumab ... 59
Alendronate ... 59
Alendronate and Cholecalciferol ... 62
Alendronate Sodium *See* Alendronate ... 59
Alendronate Sodium and Cholecalciferol *See* Alendronate and Cholecalciferol ... 62
Aleprozil (Mex) *See* Omeprazole ... 1176
Alepsal (Mex) *See* PHENobarbital ... 1265
Aler-Cap [OTC] *See* DiphenhydrAMINE ... 481
Aler-Dryl [OTC] *See* DiphenhydrAMINE ... 481
Aler-Tab [OTC] *See* DiphenhydrAMINE ... 481
Alertec® (Can) *See* Modafinil ... 1065
Alesse® *See* Ethinyl Estradiol and Levonorgestrel ... 595
Aleval (Mex) *See* Sertraline ... 1472
Aleve®-D Sinus & Cold [OTC] *See* Naproxen and Pseudoephedrine ... 1107
Aleve®-D Sinus & Headache [OTC] *See* Naproxen and Pseudoephedrine ... 1107
Aleve® Cold & Sinus [OTC] [DSC] *See* Naproxen and Pseudoephedrine ... 1107
Aleve® [OTC] *See* Naproxen ... 1102
Aleve® Sinus & Headache [OTC] [DSC] *See* Naproxen and Pseudoephedrine ... 1107
Alfaken (Mex) *See* Lisinopril ... 934
Alfenta® *See* Alfentanil ... 64
Alfentanil ... 64
Alfentanil Hydrochloride *See* Alfentanil ... 64
Alfentanil Injection, USP (Can) *See* Alfentanil ... 64
Alferon® N *See* Interferon Alfa-n3 ... 847
Alfuzosin ... 65
Alfuzosin Hydrochloride *See* Alfuzosin ... 65
Aliclen™ *See* Salicylic Acid ... 1454
Alidol (Mex) *See* Ketorolac ... 878
Alimta® *See* Pemetrexed ... 1238
Alin (Mex) *See* Dexamethasone ... 436
Alinia® *See* Nitazoxanide ... 1146
Aliskiren ... 65
Aliskiren and Hydrochlorothiazide ... 66
Aliskiren Hemifumarate *See* Aliskiren ... 65
Aliskiren Hemifumarate and Hydrochlorothiazide *See* Aliskiren and Hydrochlorothiazide ... 66
Alitretinoin ... 66
Alka-Mints® [OTC] *See* Calcium Carbonate ... 254
Alka-Seltzer Plus® Day Cold [OTC] *See* Acetaminophen, Dextromethorphan, and Phenylephrine ... 42
Alka-Seltzer Plus® Sinus Formula [OTC] *See* Acetaminophen and Phenylephrine ... 36
Alka-Seltzer® P.M. [OTC] *See* Aspirin and Diphenhydramine ... 145
Alkeran® *See* Melphalan ... 983
AllanHist PDX *See* Brompheniramine, Pseudoephedrine, and Dextromethorphan ... 208
AllanTan Pediatric [DSC] *See* Chlorpheniramine and Phenylephrine ... 323
AllanVan-DM *See* Phenylephrine, Pyrilamine, and Dextromethorphan ... 1278
AllanVan-S [DSC] *See* Phenylephrine and Pyrilamine ... 1275
Allegra® *See* Fexofenadine ... 629
Allegra-D® (Can) *See* Fexofenadine and Pseudoephedrine ... 631
Allegra-D® 12 Hour *See* Fexofenadine and Pseudoephedrine ... 631
Allegra-D® 24 Hour *See* Fexofenadine and Pseudoephedrine ... 631
Allegra® ODT *See* Fexofenadine ... 629
Aller-Chlor® [OTC] *See* Chlorpheniramine ... 321

Allerdryl® (Can) *See* DiphenhydrAMINE 481
Allerest® Allergy and Sinus Relief [OTC] *See* Acetaminophen and Pseudoephedrine 37
Allerest® Maximum Strength Allergy and Hay Fever [OTC] *See* Chlorpheniramine and Pseudoephedrine 325
Allerfrim [OTC] *See* Triprolidine and Pseudoephedrine 1634
Allergy Relief [OTC] *See* Loratadine 946
AllerMax® [OTC] *See* DiphenhydrAMINE 481
Allernix (Can) *See* DiphenhydrAMINE 481
AllerTan™ *See* Chlorpheniramine, Pyrilamine, and Phenylephrine 335
AlleRx™-D *See* Pseudoephedrine and Methscopolamine 1370
AlleRx™ Suspension *See* Chlorpheniramine and Phenylephrine 323
Allfen-DM *See* Guaifenesin and Dextromethorphan 739
Allfen Jr *See* GuaiFENesin 737
Alli™ [OTC] *See* Orlistat 1184
Alloprin® (Can) *See* Allopurinol 67
Allopurinol 67
Allopurinol Sodium *See* Allopurinol 67
All-trans-Retinoic Acid *See* Tretinoin, Oral 1617
Almacone Double Strength® [OTC] *See* Aluminum Hydroxide, Magnesium Hydroxide, and Simethicone 78
Almacone® [OTC] *See* Aluminum Hydroxide, Magnesium Hydroxide, and Simethicone 78
Almetec (Mex) *See* Olmesartan 1170
Almotriptan 70
Almotriptan Malate *See* Almotriptan 70
Alocril® *See* Nedocromil 1115
Alomide® *See* Lodoxamide 942
Aloprim™ *See* Allopurinol 67
Alora® *See* Estradiol 576
Alosol (Mex) *See* Polymyxin B 1312
Aloxi® *See* Palonosetron 1218
Alpain *See* Acetaminophen and Phenyltoloxamine 36
Alphadinal (Mex) *See* Naphazoline 1101
Alpha-Galactosidase-A (Recombinant) *See* Agalsidase Beta 52
Alphagan® (Can) *See* Brimonidine 199
Alphagan® P *See* Brimonidine 199
AlphaNine® SD *See* Factor IX 612
Alphapen (Mex) *See* Ampicillin 122
Alph-E-Mixed [OTC] *See* Vitamin E 1675
Alph-E [OTC] *See* Vitamin E 1675
ALPRAZolam 72
Alprazolam Intensol® *See* ALPRAZolam 72
Alprostadil 77
Altace® *See* Ramipril 1395
Altafrin *See* Phenylephrine 1273
Altamisa *See* Feverfew (Tanacetum parthenium) 628
Altarussin DM [OTC] *See* Guaifenesin and Dextromethorphan 739
Altaryl [OTC] *See* DiphenhydrAMINE 481
ALternaGel® [OTC] *See* Aluminum Hydroxide 78
Alti-Alprazolam (Can) *See* ALPRAZolam 72
Alti-Amiodarone (Can) *See* Amiodarone 89
Alti-Amoxi-Clav (Can) *See* Amoxicillin and Clavulanate Potassium 115
Alti-Azathioprine (Can) *See* AzaTHIOprine 162
Alti-Captopril (Can) *See* Captopril 264
Alti-Clindamycin (Can) *See* Clindamycin 363
Alti-Clobazam (Can) *See* Clobazam 364
Alti-Clonazepam (Can) *See* ClonazePAM 373
Alti-Desipramine (Can) *See* Desipramine 426
Alti-Diltiazem CD (Can) *See* Diltiazem 473
Alti-Divalproex (Can) *See* Valproic Acid and Derivatives 1642
Alti-Doxazosin (Can) *See* Doxazosin 500
Alti-Flunisolide (Can) *See* Flunisolide 646
Alti-Flurbiprofen (Can) *See* Flurbiprofen 667
Alti-Fluvoxamine (Can) *See* Fluvoxamine 678
Alti-Ipratropium (Can) *See* Ipratropium 852
Alti-Metformin (Can) *See* MetFORMIN 997
Alti-Minocycline (Can) *See* Minocycline 1056
Alti-MPA (Can) *See* MedroxyPROGESTERone 975
Alti-Nadolol (Can) *See* Nadolol 1090
Alti-Nortriptyline (Can) *See* Nortriptyline 1152
Alti-Ranitidine (Can) *See* Ranitidine 1399
Alti-Salbutamol (Can) *See* Albuterol 54
Alti-Sotalol (Can) *See* Sotalol 1502
Alti-Sulfasalazine (Can) *See* Sulfasalazine 1522
Alti-Terazosin (Can) *See* Terazosin 1549
Alti-Ticlopidine (Can) *See* Ticlopidine 1583
Alti-Timolol (Can) *See* Timolol 1584
Alti-Trazodone (Can) *See* TraZODone 1614

Altoprev® *See* Lovastatin ... 956
Altretamine ... 78
Altruline (Mex) *See* Sertraline ... 1472
Aluminum Hydroxide ... 78
Aluminum Hydroxide, Magnesium Hydroxide, and Simethicone ... 78
Aluminum Sucrose Sulfate, Basic *See* Sucralfate ... 1514
Alupent® *See* Metaproterenol ... 996
Aluprex (Mex) *See* Sertraline ... 1472
Alvesco® *See* Ciclesonide ... 343
Alzam (Mex) *See* ALPRAZolam ... 72
Amantadine ... 79
Amantadine Hydrochloride *See* Amantadine ... 79
Amantilla *See* Valerian (Valeriana officinalis) ... 1641
Amaryl® *See* Glimepiride ... 723
Amatine® (Can) *See* Midodrine ... 1050
Ambenonium ... 82
Ambenonium Chloride *See* Ambenonium ... 82
Ambien® *See* Zolpidem ... 1705
Ambien CR® *See* Zolpidem ... 1705
Ambifed-G *See* Guaifenesin and Pseudoephedrine ... 744
Ambifed-G DM *See* Guaifenesin, Pseudoephedrine, and Dextromethorphan ... 748
AmBisome® *See* Amphotericin B, Liposomal ... 121
Ambotetra (Mex) *See* Tetracycline ... 1558
Amcef (Mex) *See* CefTRIAXone ... 300
Amdry-C *See* Chlorpheniramine, Pseudoephedrine, and Methscopolamine ... 334
Amdry-D *See* Pseudoephedrine and Methscopolamine ... 1370
Amebidal (Mex) *See* MetroNIDAZOLE ... 1040
Amerge® *See* Naratriptan ... 1107
American coneflower *See* Echinacea (Echinacea purpurea, Echinacea angustifolia) ... 523
A-Methapred *See* MethylPREDNISolone ... 1029
Amethocaine Hydrochloride *See* Tetracaine ... 1557
Amethopterin *See* Methotrexate ... 1014
Ametop™ (Can) *See* Tetracaine ... 1557
Amevive® *See* Alefacept ... 58
Amfepramone *See* Diethylpropion ... 460
AMG 073 *See* Cinacalcet ... 345
Amicar® *See* Aminocaproic Acid ... 87
Amicil (Mex) *See* Amoxicillin ... 112
Amidrine [DSC] *See* Acetaminophen, Isometheptene, and Dichloralphenazone ... 45
Amifostine ... 83
A-Migdobis (Mex) *See* Bismuth ... 189
Amigesic® (Can) *See* Salsalate ... 1459
Amigesic® [DSC] *See* Salsalate ... 1459
Amikacin ... 83
Amikacin Sulfate *See* Amikacin ... 83
Amikacin Sulfate Injection, USP (Can) *See* Amikacin ... 83
Amikafur (Mex) *See* Amikacin ... 83
Amikayect (Mex) *See* Amikacin ... 83
Amikin® (Can) *See* Amikacin ... 83
AMILoride ... 84
Amiloride and Hydrochlorothiazide ... 86
Amiloride Hydrochloride *See* AMILoride ... 84
2-Amino-6-Mercaptopurine *See* Thioguanine ... 1569
2-Amino-6-Methoxypurine Arabinoside *See* Nelarabine ... 1120
2-Amino-6-Trifluoromethoxy-benzothiazole *See* Riluzole ... 1421
Aminobenzylpenicillin *See* Ampicillin ... 122
Aminocamptothecin ... 86
9-Aminocamptothecin *See* Aminocamptothecin ... 86
Aminocaproic Acid ... 87
Aminoglutethimide ... 87
Aminophylline ... 88
Aminosalicylate Sodium *See* Aminosalicylic Acid ... 88
Aminosalicylic Acid ... 88
4-Aminosalicylic Acid *See* Aminosalicylic Acid ... 88
5-Aminosalicylic Acid *See* Mesalamine ... 994
Aminoxin [OTC] *See* Pyridoxine ... 1376
Amiodarone ... 89
Amiodarone Hydrochloride *See* Amiodarone ... 89
Amiodarone Hydrochloride for Injection® (Can) *See* Amiodarone ... 89
Amitiza® *See* Lubiprostone ... 963
Amitriptyline ... 90
Amitriptyline and Chlordiazepoxide ... 94
Amitriptyline and Perphenazine ... 98
Amitriptyline Hydrochloride *See* Amitriptyline ... 90
AMJ 9701 *See* Palifermin ... 1214
AmLODIPine ... 100
Amlodipine and Atorvastatin ... 103

Amlodipine and Benazepril 104
Amlodipine and Olmesartan 104
Amlodipine and Valsartan 105
Amlodipine Besylate *See* AmLODIPine 100
Amlodipine Besylate and Olmesartan Medoxomil *See* Amlodipine and Olmesartan 104
Amlodipine Besylate and Valsartan *See* Amlodipine and Valsartan 105
AMN107 *See* Nilotinib 1140
Amnesteem™ *See* Isotretinoin 871
Amobarbital 105
Amobarbital Sodium *See* Amobarbital 105
Amobay (Mex) *See* Amoxicillin 112
Amobay Cl (Mex) *See* Amoxicillin and Clavulanate Potassium 115
Amoclan *See* Amoxicillin and Clavulanate Potassium 115
Amonafide 108
Amonafide Hydrochloride *See* Amonafide 108
Amoxapine 108
Amoxicillin 112
Amoxicillin and Clavulanate Potassium 115
Amoxicillin and Clavulanic Acid *See* Amoxicillin and Clavulanate Potassium 115
Amoxicillin, Lansoprazole, and Clarithromycin *See* Lansoprazole, Amoxicillin, and Clarithromycin 897
Amoxicillin Trihydrate *See* Amoxicillin 112
Amoxiclav (Mex) *See* Amoxicillin and Clavulanate Potassium 115
Amoxiclav-BID (Mex) *See* Amoxicillin and Clavulanate Potassium 115
Amoxifur (Mex) *See* Amoxicillin 112
Amoxil® *See* Amoxicillin 112
Amoxinova (Mex) *See* Amoxicillin 112
Amoxisol (Mex) *See* Amoxicillin 112
Amoxivet (Mex) *See* Amoxicillin 112
Amoxycillin *See* Amoxicillin 112
Amphetamine and Dextroamphetamine *See* Dextroamphetamine and Amphetamine 444
Amphocil (Mex) *See* Amphotericin B (Conventional) 120
Amphocin® [DSC] *See* Amphotericin B (Conventional) 120
Amphojel® (Can) *See* Aluminum Hydroxide 78
Amphotec® *See* Amphotericin B Cholesteryl Sulfate Complex 119
Amphotericin B Cholesteryl Sulfate Complex 119
Amphotericin B Colloidal Dispersion *See* Amphotericin B Cholesteryl Sulfate Complex 119
Amphotericin B (Conventional) 120
Amphotericin B Desoxycholate *See* Amphotericin B (Conventional) 120
Amphotericin B, Lipid Complex 121
Amphotericin B, Liposomal 121
Ampicillin 122
Ampicillin and Sulbactam 122
Ampicillin Sodium *See* Ampicillin 122
Ampicillin Trihydrate *See* Ampicillin 122
Ampi-quim (Mex) *See* Abacavir 22
Amprenavir 123
AMPT *See* Metyrosine 1044
Amrinone Lactate *See* Inamrinone 817
Amrix® *See* Cyclobenzaprine 405
Amsapen (Mex) *See* Ampicillin 122
Amsler (Mex) *See* Azelastine 162
Amyl Nitrite 124
Amylobarbitone *See* Amobarbital 105
Amytal® *See* Amobarbital 105
AN100226 *See* Natalizumab 1109
Anadrol®-50 *See* Oxymetholone 1209
Anafil (Mex) *See* Morphine Sulfate 1077
Anafranil® *See* ClomiPRAMINE 368
Anagrelide 124
Anagrelide Hydrochloride *See* Anagrelide 124
Anakinra 124
Analphen (Mex) *See* Acetaminophen 30
Anandron® (Can) *See* Nilutamide 1140
Anapenil (Mex) *See* Penicillin V Potassium 1242
Anaplex® DM *See* Brompheniramine, Pseudoephedrine, and Dextromethorphan 208
Anaplex® DMX *See* Brompheniramine, Pseudoephedrine, and Dextromethorphan 208
Anaprox® *See* Naproxen 1102
Anaprox® DS *See* Naproxen 1102
Anapsique (Mex) *See* Amitriptyline 90
Anaspaz® *See* Hyoscyamine 799
Anastrozole 125
Ancef *See* CeFAZolin 292
Ancobon® *See* Flucytosine 640
Andehist DM NR *See* Brompheniramine, Pseudoephedrine, and Dextromethorphan 208
Andehist NR Drops [DSC] *See* Carbinoxamine and Pseudoephedrine 280
Andehist NR Syrup *See* Brompheniramine and Pseudoephedrine 206

Andriol® (Can) *See* Testosterone 1553
Androderm® *See* Testosterone 1553
AndroGel® *See* Testosterone 1553
Android® *See* MethylTESTOSTERone 1030
Andropository (Can) *See* Testosterone 1553
Androtin (Mex) *See* Famotidine 613
Androxy™ *See* Fluoxymesterone 657
Anectine® *See* Succinylcholine 1511
Anerex (Mex) *See* Thiamine 1568
Anestacon® *See* Lidocaine 924
Anestafoam™ [OTC] *See* Lidocaine 924
Aneurine Hydrochloride *See* Thiamine 1568
Anexate® (Can) *See* Flumazenil 644
Anextuss *See* Guaifenesin, Dextromethorphan, and Phenylephrine 746
Angeliq® *See* Drospirenone and Estradiol 515
Angiomax® *See* Bivalirudin 191
Angiotrofin (Mex) *See* Diltiazem 473
Angiotrofin Retard (Mex) *See* Diltiazem 473
Anitrim (Mex) *See* Sulfamethoxazole and Trimethoprim 1517
Anolor 300 *See* Butalbital, Acetaminophen, and Caffeine 229
Ansaid® (Can) *See* Flurbiprofen 667
Ansamycin *See* Rifabutin 1418
Antabuse® *See* Disulfiram 489
Antacsal-E (Mex) *See* Aspirin 143
Antadex-H (Mex) *See* Chlorpheniramine 321
Antalgin (Mex) *See* Indomethacin 818
Antara™ *See* Fenofibrate 620
Anti-4 Alpha Integrin *See* Natalizumab 1109
131 I Anti-B1 Antibody *See* Tositumomab and Iodine I 131 Tositumomab 1603
131 I-Anti-B1 Monoclonal Antibody *See* Tositumomab and Iodine I 131 Tositumomab 1603
Anti-CD11a *See* Efalizumab 526
Anti-CD20 Monoclonal Antibody *See* RiTUXimab 1434
Anti-CD20-Murine Monoclonal Antibody I-131 *See* Tositumomab and Iodine I 131 Tositumomab 1603
Antidiuretic Hormone *See* Vasopressin 1659
Antithymocyte Globulin (Equine) 126
Antithymocyte Globulin (Rabbit) 126
Antithymocyte Immunoglobulin *See* Antithymocyte Globulin (Rabbit) 126
Antitumor Necrosis Factor Apha (Human) *See* Adalimumab 50
Anti-VEGF Monoclonal Antibody *See* Bevacizumab 187
Antivert® *See* Meclizine 974
Antizol® *See* Fomepizole 685
Anucort-HC® *See* Hydrocortisone 785
Anu-Med [OTC] *See* Phenylephrine 1273
Anusol-HC® *See* Hydrocortisone 785
Anusol® HC-1 [OTC] *See* Hydrocortisone 785
Anzemet® *See* Dolasetron 493
APAP *See* Acetaminophen 30
APAP and Tramadol *See* Acetaminophen and Tramadol 38
Aphrodyne® [DSC] *See* Yohimbine 1688
Apidra® *See* Insulin Glulisine 829
Aplonidine *See* Apraclonidine 129
Apo-Acebutolol® (Can) *See* Acebutolol 27
Apo-Acetaminophen® (Can) *See* Acetaminophen 30
Apo-Acetazolamide® (Can) *See* AcetaZOLAMIDE 46
Apo-Acyclovir® (Can) *See* Acyclovir 49
Apo-Alendronate® (Can) *See* Alendronate 59
Apo-Allopurinol® (Can) *See* Allopurinol 67
Apo-Alpraz® (Can) *See* ALPRAZolam 72
Apo-Alpraz® TS (Can) *See* ALPRAZolam 72
Apo-Amiloride® (Can) *See* AMILoride 84
Apo-Amilzide® (Can) *See* Amiloride and Hydrochlorothiazide 86
Apo-Amiodarone® (Can) *See* Amiodarone 89
Apo-Amitriptyline® (Can) *See* Amitriptyline 90
Apo-Amoxi® (Can) *See* Amoxicillin 112
Apo-Amoxi-Clav® (Can) *See* Amoxicillin and Clavulanate Potassium 115
Apo-Ampi® (Can) *See* Ampicillin 122
Apo-Atenidone® (Can) *See* Atenolol and Chlorthalidone 150
Apo-Atenol® (Can) *See* Atenolol 147
Apo-Azathioprine® (Can) *See* AzaTHIOprine 162
Apo-Azithromycin® (Can) *See* Azithromycin 163
Apo-Baclofen® (Can) *See* Baclofen 168
Apo-Beclomethasone® (Can) *See* Beclomethasone 171
Apo-Benazepril® (Can) *See* Benazepril 178
Apo-Benztropine® (Can) *See* Benztropine 183
Apo-Bisoprolol® (Can) *See* Bisoprolol 190
Apo-Brimonidine® (Can) *See* Brimonidine 199

Apo-Bromazepam® (Can) *See* Bromazepam 200
Apo-Bromocriptine® (Can) *See* Bromocriptine 202
Apo-Buspirone® (Can) *See* BusPIRone 223
Apo-Butorphanol® (Can) *See* Butorphanol 247
Apo-Cal® (Can) *See* Calcium Carbonate 254
Apo-Calcitonin® (Can) *See* Calcitonin 253
Apo-Capto® (Can) *See* Captopril 264
Apo-Carbamazepine® (Can) *See* CarBAMazepine 265
Apo-Carvedilol® (Can) *See* Carvedilol 286
Apo-Cefaclor® (Can) *See* Cefaclor 291
Apo-Cefadroxil® (Can) *See* Cefadroxil 292
Apo-Cefoxitin® (Can) *See* Cefoxitin 296
Apo-Cefprozil® (Can) *See* Cefprozil 297
Apo-Cefuroxime® (Can) *See* Cefuroxime 300
Apo-Cephalex® (Can) *See* Cephalexin 306
Apo-Cetirizine® (Can) *See* Cetirizine 307
Apo-Chlorax® (Can) *See* Clidinium and Chlordiazepoxide 362
Apo-Chlordiazepoxide® (Can) *See* ChlordiazePOXIDE 316
Apo-Chlorpropamide® (Can) *See* ChlorproPAMIDE 340
Apo-Chlorthalidone® (Can) *See* Chlorthalidone 340
Apo-Cimetidine® (Can) *See* Cimetidine 345
Apo-Ciproflox® (Can) *See* Ciprofloxacin 346
Apo-Citalopram® (Can) *See* Citalopram 354
Apo-Clarithromycin (Can) *See* Clarithromycin 360
Apo-Clindamycin® (Can) *See* Clindamycin 363
Apo-Clobazam® (Can) *See* Clobazam 364
Apo-Clomipramine® (Can) *See* ClomiPRAMINE 368
Apo-Clonazepam® (Can) *See* ClonazePAM 373
Apo-Clonidine® (Can) *See* CloNIDine 377
Apo-Clorazepate® (Can) *See* Clorazepate 384
Apo-Clozapine® (Can) *See* Clozapine 386
Apo-Cromolyn® (Can) *See* Cromolyn 402
Apo-Cyclobenzaprine® (Can) *See* Cyclobenzaprine 405
Apo-Desipramine® (Can) *See* Desipramine 426
Apo-Desmopressin® (Can) *See* Desmopressin 431
Apo-Dexamethasone® (Can) *See* Dexamethasone 436
Apo-Diazepam® (Can) *See* Diazepam 451
Apo-Diclo® (Can) *See* Diclofenac 457
Apo-Diclo Rapide® (Can) *See* Diclofenac 457
Apo-Diclo SR® (Can) *See* Diclofenac 457
Apo-Diflunisal® (Can) *See* Diflunisal 463
Apo-Digoxin® (Can) *See* Digoxin 463
Apo-Diltiaz® (Can) *See* Diltiazem 473
Apo-Diltiaz CD® (Can) *See* Diltiazem 473
Apo-Diltiaz® Injectable (Can) *See* Diltiazem 473
Apo-Diltiaz SR® (Can) *See* Diltiazem 473
Apo-Diltiaz TZ® (Can) *See* Diltiazem 473
Apo-Dimenhydrinate® (Can) *See* DimenhyDRINATE 478
Apo-Dipyridamole FC® (Can) *See* Dipyridamole 488
Apo-Divalproex® (Can) *See* Valproic Acid and Derivatives 1642
Apo-Domperidone® (Can) *See* Domperidone 493
Apo-Doxazosin® (Can) *See* Doxazosin 500
Apo-Doxepin® (Can) *See* Doxepin 502
Apo-Doxy® (Can) *See* Doxycycline 509
Apo-Doxy Tabs® (Can) *See* Doxycycline 509
Apo-Enalapril® (Can) *See* Enalapril 531
Apo-Erythro Base® (Can) *See* Erythromycin 557
Apo-Erythro E-C® (Can) *See* Erythromycin 557
Apo-Erythro-ES® (Can) *See* Erythromycin 557
Apo-Erythro-S® (Can) *See* Erythromycin 557
Apo-Etodolac® (Can) *See* Etodolac 606
Apo-Famciclovir (Can) *See* Famciclovir 613
Apo-Famotidine® (Can) *See* Famotidine 613
Apo-Famotidine® Injectable (Can) *See* Famotidine 613
Apo-Fenofibrate® (Can) *See* Fenofibrate 620
Apo-Feno-Micro® (Can) *See* Fenofibrate 620
Apo-Ferrous Gluconate® (Can) *See* Ferrous Gluconate 627
Apo-Ferrous Sulfate® (Can) *See* Ferrous Sulfate 627
Apo-Flavoxate® (Can) *See* Flavoxate 633
Apo-Flecainide® (Can) *See* Flecainide 633
Apo-Fluconazole® (Can) *See* Fluconazole 635
Apo-Flunisolide® (Can) *See* Flunisolide 646
Apo-Fluoxetine® (Can) *See* FLUoxetine 650
Apo-Fluphenazine® (Can) *See* Fluphenazine 660
Apo-Fluphenazine Decanoate® (Can) *See* Fluphenazine 660
Apo-Flurazepam® (Can) *See* Flurazepam 664
Apo-Flurbiprofen® (Can) *See* Flurbiprofen 667

Apo-Flutamide® (Can) *See* Flutamide 667
Apo-Fluticasone (Can) *See* Fluticasone 668
Apo-Fluvoxamine® (Can) *See* Fluvoxamine 678
Apo-Folic® (Can) *See* Folic Acid 684
Apo-Fosinopril® (Can) *See* Fosinopril 691
Apo-Furosemide® (Can) *See* Furosemide 699
Apo-Gabapentin® (Can) *See* Gabapentin 702
Apo-Gain® (Can) *See* Minoxidil 1057
Apo-Gemfibrozil® (Can) *See* Gemfibrozil 711
Apo-Glimepiride (Can) *See* Glimepiride 723
Apo-Glyburide® (Can) *See* GlyBURIDE 730
Apo-Haloperidol® (Can) *See* Haloperidol 754
Apo-Haloperidol LA® (Can) *See* Haloperidol 754
Apo-Hydralazine® (Can) *See* HydrALAZINE 772
Apo-Hydro® (Can) *See* Hydrochlorothiazide 773
Apo-Hydroxyquine® (Can) *See* Hydroxychloroquine 796
Apo-Hydroxyurea® (Can) *See* Hydroxyurea 796
Apo-Hydroxyzine® (Can) *See* HydrOXYzine 797
Apo-Ibuprofen® (Can) *See* Ibuprofen 803
Apo-Imipramine® (Can) *See* Imipramine 812
Apo-Indapamide® (Can) *See* Indapamide 817
Apo-Indomethacin® (Can) *See* Indomethacin 818
Apo-Ipravent® (Can) *See* Ipratropium 852
Apo-ISDN® (Can) *See* Isosorbide Dinitrate 866
Apo-ISMN® (Can) *See* Isosorbide Mononitrate 869
Apo-K® (Can) *See* Potassium Chloride 1315
Apo-Keto® (Can) *See* Ketoprofen 877
Apo-Ketoconazole® (Can) *See* Ketoconazole 876
Apo-Keto-E® (Can) *See* Ketoprofen 877
Apo-Ketorolac® (Can) *See* Ketorolac 878
Apo-Ketorolac Injectable® (Can) *See* Ketorolac 878
Apo-Keto SR® (Can) *See* Ketoprofen 877
Apokyn® *See* Apomorphine 127
Apo-Labetalol® (Can) *See* Labetalol 881
Apo-Lactulose® (Can) *See* Lactulose 886
Apo-Lamotrigine® (Can) *See* LamoTRIgine 889
Apo-Leflunomide® (Can) *See* Leflunomide 899
Apo-Levetiracetam (Can) *See* Levetiracetam 905
Apo-Levobunolol® (Can) *See* Levobunolol 907
Apo-Levocarb® (Can) *See* Carbidopa and Levodopa 277
Apo-Levocarb® CR (Can) *See* Carbidopa and Levodopa 277
Apo-Lisinopril® (Can) *See* Lisinopril 934
Apo-Lisinopril/Hctz (Can) *See* Lisinopril and Hydrochlorothiazide 938
Apo-Lithium® Carbonate (Can) *See* Lithium 938
Apo-Lithium® Carbonate SR (Can) *See* Lithium 938
Apo-Loperamide® (Can) *See* Loperamide 944
Apo-Loratadine® (Can) *See* Loratadine 946
Apo-Lorazepam® (Can) *See* LORazepam 949
Apo-Lovastatin® (Can) *See* Lovastatin 956
Apo-Loxapine® (Can) *See* Loxapine 960
Apo-Medroxy® (Can) *See* MedroxyPROGESTERone 975
Apo-Mefenamic® (Can) *See* Mefenamic Acid 976
Apo-Mefloquine® (Can) *See* Mefloquine 976
Apo-Megestrol® (Can) *See* Megestrol 977
Apo-Meloxicam® (Can) *See* Meloxicam 982
Apo-Metformin® (Can) *See* MetFORMIN 997
Apo-Methazide® (Can) *See* Methyldopa and Hydrochlorothiazide 1021
Apo-Methazolamide® (Can) *See* Methazolamide 1009
Apo-Methoprazine® (Can) *See* Methotrimeprazine 1015
Apo-Methotrexate® (Can) *See* Methotrexate 1014
Apo-Methyldopa® (Can) *See* Methyldopa 1021
Apo-Methylphenidate® (Can) *See* Methylphenidate 1024
Apo-Methylphenidate® SR (Can) *See* Methylphenidate 1024
Apo-Metoclop® (Can) *See* Metoclopramide 1031
Apo-Metoprolol® (Can) *See* Metoprolol 1036
Apo-Metronidazole® (Can) *See* MetroNIDAZOLE 1040
Apo-Midazolam® (Can) *See* Midazolam 1046
Apo-Midodrine® (Can) *See* Midodrine 1050
Apo-Minocycline® (Can) *See* Minocycline 1056
Apo-Moclobemide® (Can) *See* Moclobemide 1062
Apomorphine 127
Apomorphine Hydrochloride *See* Apomorphine 127
Apomorphine Hydrochloride Hemihydrate *See* Apomorphine 127
Apo-Nabumetone® (Can) *See* Nabumetone 1089
Apo-Nadol® (Can) *See* Nadolol 1090
Apo-Napro-Na® (Can) *See* Naproxen 1102
Apo-Napro-Na DS® (Can) *See* Naproxen 1102

Apo-Naproxen® (Can) *See* Naproxen 1102
Apo-Naproxen EC® (Can) *See* Naproxen 1102
Apo-Naproxen SR® (Can) *See* Naproxen 1102
Apo-Nifed® (Can) *See* NIFEdipine 1136
Apo-Nifed PA® (Can) *See* NIFEdipine 1136
Apo-Nitrofurantoin® (Can) *See* Nitrofurantoin 1147
Apo-Nizatidine® (Can) *See* Nizatidine 1149
Apo-Norflox® (Can) *See* Norfloxacin 1151
Apo-Nortriptyline® (Can) *See* Nortriptyline 1152
Apo-Oflox® (Can) *See* Ofloxacin 1159
Apo-Ofloxacin® (Can) *See* Ofloxacin 1159
Apo-Omeprazole® (Can) *See* Omeprazole 1176
Apo-Ondansetron® (Can) *See* Ondansetron 1180
Apo-Orciprenaline® (Can) *See* Metaproterenol 996
Apo-Oxaprozin® (Can) *See* Oxaprozin 1193
Apo-Oxazepam® (Can) *See* Oxazepam 1193
Apo-Oxybutynin® (Can) *See* Oxybutynin 1199
Apo-Paclitaxel® (Can) *See* Paclitaxel 1213
Apo-Pantoprazole (Can) *See* Pantoprazole 1221
Apo-Paroxetine® (Can) *See* PARoxetine 1226
Apo-Pentoxifylline SR® (Can) *See* Pentoxifylline 1251
Apo-Pen VK® (Can) *See* Penicillin V Potassium 1242
Apo-Perindopril® (Can) *See* Perindopril Erbumine 1254
Apo-Perphenazine® (Can) *See* Perphenazine 1255
Apo-Pimozide® (Can) *See* Pimozide 1290
Apo-Pindol® (Can) *See* Pindolol 1294
Apo-Pioglitazone (Can) *See* Pioglitazone 1297
Apo-Piroxicam® (Can) *See* Piroxicam 1307
Apo-Pramipexole (Can) *See* Pramipexole 1318
Apo-Pravastatin® (Can) *See* Pravastatin 1321
Apo-Prazo® (Can) *See* Prazosin 1325
Apo-Prednisone® (Can) *See* PredniSONE 1327
Apo-Primidone® (Can) *See* Primidone 1336
Apo-Procainamide® (Can) *See* Procainamide 1339
Apo-Prochlorperazine® (Can) *See* Prochlorperazine 1341
Apo-Propafenone® (Can) *See* Propafenone 1351
Apo-Propranolol® (Can) *See* Propranolol 1355
Apo-Quinidine® (Can) *See* QuiNIDine 1387
Apo-Quinine® (Can) *See* QuiNINE 1388
Apo-Ramipril® (Can) *See* Ramipril 1395
Apo-Ranitidine® (Can) *See* Ranitidine 1399
Apo-Risperidone® (Can) *See* Risperidone 1425
Apo-Salvent® (Can) *See* Albuterol 54
Apo-Salvent® CFC Free (Can) *See* Albuterol 54
Apo-Salvent® Respirator Solution (Can) *See* Albuterol 54
Apo-Salvent® Sterules (Can) *See* Albuterol 54
Apo-Selegiline® (Can) *See* Selegiline 1466
Apo-Sertraline® (Can) *See* Sertraline 1472
Apo-Simvastatin® (Can) *See* Simvastatin 1486
Apo-Sotalol® (Can) *See* Sotalol 1502
Apo-Sulfatrim® (Can) *See* Sulfamethoxazole and Trimethoprim 1517
Apo-Sulfatrim® DS (Can) *See* Sulfamethoxazole and Trimethoprim 1517
Apo-Sulfatrim® Pediatric (Can) *See* Sulfamethoxazole and Trimethoprim 1517
Apo-Sulin® (Can) *See* Sulindac 1523
Apo-Sumatriptan® (Can) *See* SUMAtriptan 1527
Apo-Tamox® (Can) *See* Tamoxifen 1537
Apo-Temazepam® (Can) *See* Temazepam 1545
Apo-Terazosin® (Can) *See* Terazosin 1549
Apo-Terbinafine® (Can) *See* Terbinafine 1551
Apo-Tetra® (Can) *See* Tetracycline 1558
Apo-Theo LA® (Can) *See* Theophylline 1562
Apo-Ticlopidine® (Can) *See* Ticlopidine 1583
Apo-Timol® (Can) *See* Timolol 1584
Apo-Timop® (Can) *See* Timolol 1584
Apo-Tizanidine® (Can) *See* TiZANidine 1587
Apo-Tolbutamide® (Can) *See* TOLBUTamide 1592
Apo-Topiramate (Can) *See* Topiramate 1598
Apo-Trazodone® (Can) *See* TraZODone 1614
Apo-Trazodone D® (Can) *See* TraZODone 1614
Apo-Triazide® (Can) *See* Hydrochlorothiazide and Triamterene 776
Apo-Triazo® (Can) *See* Triazolam 1620
Apo-Trifluoperazine® (Can) *See* Trifluoperazine 1624
Apo-Trihex® (Can) *See* Trihexyphenidyl 1627
Apo-Trimethoprim® (Can) *See* Trimethoprim 1629
Apo-Trimip® (Can) *See* Trimipramine 1630
Apo-Valproic® (Can) *See* Valproic Acid and Derivatives 1642
Apo-Verap® (Can) *See* Verapamil 1665

Apo-Verap® SR (Can) *See* Verapamil 1665
Apo-Warfarin® (Can) *See* Warfarin 1679
Apo-Zidovudine® (Can) *See* Zidovudine 1695
Apo-Zopiclone® (Can) *See* Zopiclone 1711
APPG *See* Penicillin G Procaine 1241
Apra Children's [OTC] *See* Acetaminophen 30
Apraclonidine 129
Apraclonidine Hydrochloride *See* Apraclonidine 129
Aprepitant 130
Aprepitant Injection *See* Fosaprepitant 690
Apresazide [DSC] *See* Hydralazine and Hydrochlorothiazide 772
Apresolina (Mex) *See* HydrALAZINE 772
Apresoline® (Can) *See* HydrALAZINE 772
Apresoline [DSC] *See* HydrALAZINE 772
Apri® *See* Ethinyl Estradiol and Desogestrel 592
Aprodine® [OTC] *See* Triprolidine and Pseudoephedrine 1634
Aprotinin 130
Aprovel (Mex) *See* Irbesartan 855
Aptivus® *See* Tipranavir 1586
Aquachloral® Supprettes® [DSC] *See* Chloral Hydrate 313
Aquacort® (Can) *See* Hydrocortisone 785
AquaMEPHYTON® (Can) *See* Phytonadione 1289
Aquanil HC (Mex) *See* Hydrocortisone 785
Aquanil™ HC [OTC] *See* Hydrocortisone 785
Aquasol AD (Mex) *See* Ergocalciferol 550
Aquasol E® [OTC] *See* Vitamin E 1675
Aquatensen® (Can) *See* Methyclothiazide 1020
Aquavit-E [OTC] *See* Vitamin E 1675
Aqueous Procaine Penicillin G *See* Penicillin G Procaine 1241
Ara-C *See* Cytarabine 412
Arabinosylcytosine *See* Cytarabine 412
Aralen® *See* Chloroquine Phosphate 320
Aranelle™ *See* Ethinyl Estradiol and Norethindrone 597
Aranesp® *See* Darbepoetin Alfa 419
Arava® *See* Leflunomide 899
Aredia® *See* Pamidronate 1220
Arformoterol 131
Arformoterol Tartrate *See* Arformoterol 131
8-Arginine Vasopressin *See* Vasopressin 1659
Aricept® *See* Donepezil 495
Aricept® ODT *See* Donepezil 495
Aricept® RDT (Can) *See* Donepezil 495
Arimidex® *See* Anastrozole 125
Aripiprazole 133
Aristospan® *See* Triamcinolone 1617
Armodafinil 138
Armour® Thyroid *See* Thyroid, Desiccated 1579
Aromasin® *See* Exemestane 609
Aropax (Mex) *See* PARoxetine 1226
Arranon® *See* Nelarabine 1120
Arsenic Trioxide 140
Artane *See* Trihexyphenidyl 1627
Artelife (Mex) *See* Pentoxifylline 1251
Arthrotec® *See* Diclofenac and Misoprostol 458
Artosin (Mex) *See* TOLBUTamide 1592
Artrotec (Mex) *See* Diclofenac and Misoprostol 458
Arzobema (Mex) *See* Imipenem and Cilastatin 812
As2O3 *See* Arsenic Trioxide 140
ASA *See* Aspirin 143
5-ASA *See* Mesalamine 994
ASA and Diphenhydramine *See* Aspirin and Diphenhydramine 145
Asacol® *See* Mesalamine 994
Asacol® 800 (Can) *See* Mesalamine 994
Asaphen (Can) *See* Aspirin 143
Asaphen E.C. (Can) *See* Aspirin 143
Asco-Caps [OTC] *See* Ascorbic Acid 141
Ascocid® [OTC] *See* Ascorbic Acid 141
Ascomp® with Codeine *See* Butalbital, Aspirin, Caffeine, and Codeine 242
Ascor L 500® *See* Ascorbic Acid 141
Ascor L NC® *See* Ascorbic Acid 141
Ascorbic Acid 141
Ascorbic Acid and Ferrous Sulfate *See* Ferrous Sulfate and Ascorbic Acid 628
Asco-Tabs [OTC] *See* Ascorbic Acid 141
Ascriptin® Maximum Strength [OTC] *See* Aspirin 143
Ascriptin® [OTC] *See* Aspirin 143
Asendin [DSC] *See* Amoxapine 108
Asian Ginseng *See* Ginseng, Panax (Panax ginseng) 718

Asmanex® Twisthaler® *See* Mometasone 1071
Asotax (Mex) *See* Paclitaxel 1213
Asparaginase 142
Aspart Insulin *See* Insulin Aspart 822
Aspercin [OTC] *See* Aspirin 143
Aspergum® [OTC] *See* Aspirin 143
Aspirin 143
Aspirin, Acetaminophen, and Caffeine *See* Acetaminophen, Aspirin, and Caffeine 39
Aspirina efervescente (Mex) *See* Aspirin 143
Aspirina Junior (Mex) *See* Aspirin 143
Aspirin and Carisoprodol *See* Carisoprodol and Aspirin 284
Aspirin and Diphenhydramine 145
Aspirin and Diphenhydramine Citrate *See* Aspirin and Diphenhydramine 145
Aspirin and Dipyridamole 145
Aspirin and Extended-Release Dipyridamole *See* Aspirin and Dipyridamole 145
Aspirin and Meprobamate *See* Meprobamate and Aspirin 992
Aspirin and Oxycodone *See* Oxycodone and Aspirin 1208
Aspirin and Pravastatin 146
Aspirin, Caffeine and Acetaminophen *See* Acetaminophen, Aspirin, and Caffeine 39
Aspirin, Caffeine, and Butalbital *See* Butalbital, Aspirin, and Caffeine 239
Aspirin, Caffeine, and Propoxyphene *See* Propoxyphene, Aspirin, and Caffeine 1355
Aspirin, Caffeine, Codeine, and Butalbital *See* Butalbital, Aspirin, Caffeine, and Codeine . 242
Aspirin, Carisoprodol, and Codeine *See* Carisoprodol, Aspirin, and Codeine 284
Aspirin Free Anacin® Maximum Strength [OTC] *See* Acetaminophen 30
Aspirin, Orphenadrine, and Caffeine *See* Orphenadrine, Aspirin, and Caffeine 1187
Aspirtab [OTC] *See* Aspirin 143
Assal (Mex) *See* Albuterol 54
Astelin® *See* Azelastine 162
Astin (Mex) *See* Pravastatin 1321
Astramorph/PF™ *See* Morphine Sulfate 1077
Atacand® *See* Candesartan 260
Atacand HCT® *See* Candesartan and Hydrochlorothiazide 262
Atacand® Plus (Can) *See* Candesartan and Hydrochlorothiazide 262
Atarax® (Can) *See* HydrOXYzine 797
Atasol® (Can) *See* Acetaminophen 30
Atazanavir 147
Atazanavir Sulfate *See* Atazanavir 147
Atenolol 147
Atenolol and Chlorthalidone 150
ATG *See* Antithymocyte Globulin (Equine) 126
Atgam® *See* Antithymocyte Globulin (Equine) 126
Athos (Mex) *See* Dextromethorphan 448
Atisuril (Mex) *See* Allopurinol 67
Ativan® *See* LORazepam 949
ATNAA *See* Atropine and Pralidoxime 159
Atoken (Mex) *See* Atenolol 147
Atomoxetine 151
Atomoxetine Hydrochloride *See* Atomoxetine 151
Atorvastatin 153
Atorvastatin Calcium and Amlodipine Besylate *See* Amlodipine and Atorvastatin 103
Atovaquone 157
Atovaquone and Proguanil 157
Atovaquone and Proguanil Hydrochloride *See* Atovaquone and Proguanil 157
ATRA *See* Tretinoin, Oral 1617
Atrexel (Mex) *See* Methotrexate 1014
Atriance™ (Can) *See* Nelarabine 1120
Atripla® *See* Efavirenz, Emtricitabine, and Tenofovir 527
AtroPen® *See* Atropine 158
Atropine 158
Atropine and Difenoxin *See* Difenoxin and Atropine 462
Atropine and Diphenoxylate *See* Diphenoxylate and Atropine 486
Atropine and Pralidoxime 159
Atropine and Pralidoxime Chloride *See* Atropine and Pralidoxime 159
Atropine-Care® *See* Atropine 158
Atropine, Hyoscyamine, Scopolamine, and Phenobarbital *See* Hyoscyamine, Atropine, Scopolamine, and Phenobarbital 800
Atropine Sulfate *See* Atropine 158
Atropine Sulfate and Edrophonium Chloride *See* Edrophonium and Atropine 525
Atrovent® *See* Ipratropium 852
Atrovent® HFA *See* Ipratropium 852
Atuss® HD [DSC] *See* Pseudoephedrine, Hydrocodone, and Chlorpheniramine 1372
Atuss® HX [DSC] *See* Hydrocodone and Guaifenesin 779
Augmentin® *See* Amoxicillin and Clavulanate Potassium 115
Augmentin ES-600® *See* Amoxicillin and Clavulanate Potassium 115
Augmentin XR® *See* Amoxicillin and Clavulanate Potassium 115
Auranofin 160
Aurofox (Mex) *See* CefTRIAXone 300

Aurorex (Mex) *See* Moclobemide 1062
Avage™ *See* Tazarotene 1540
Avalide® *See* Irbesartan and Hydrochlorothiazide 856
Avamys™ (Can) *See* Fluticasone 668
Avandamet® *See* Rosiglitazone and Metformin 1449
Avandaryl™ *See* Rosiglitazone and Glimepiride 1448
Avandia® *See* Rosiglitazone 1444
Avapro® *See* Irbesartan 855
Avapro® HCT *See* Irbesartan and Hydrochlorothiazide 856
Avastin® *See* Bevacizumab 187
Avaxim® (Can) *See* Hepatitis A Vaccine 760
Avaxim®-Pediatric (Can) *See* Hepatitis A Vaccine 760
Avedox-FC (Mex) *See* Albuterol 54
Avelox® *See* Moxifloxacin 1084
Avelox® I.V. *See* Moxifloxacin 1084
Aventyl® (Can) *See* Nortriptyline 1152
Aviane™ *See* Ethinyl Estradiol and Levonorgestrel 595
Avian Influenza Virus Vaccine *See* Influenza Virus Vaccine (H5N1) 821
Aviant (Mex) *See* Desloratadine 430
Avinza® *See* Morphine Sulfate 1077
Aviran (Mex) *See* Indinavir 818
Avistar (Mex) *See* AmLODIPine 100
Avodart® *See* Dutasteride 521
Avonex® *See* Interferon Beta-1a 848
Axed (Mex) *See* Ergocalciferol 550
Axert™ *See* Almotriptan 70
Axid® *See* Nizatidine 1149
Axid® AR [OTC] *See* Nizatidine 1149
Axtar (Mex) *See* CefTRIAXone 300
AY-25650 *See* Triptorelin 1635
Aygestin® *See* Norethindrone 1150
5-Aza-2'-deoxycytidine *See* Decitabine 422
5-AzaC *See* Decitabine 422
AzaCITIDine 161
AZA-CR *See* AzaCITIDine 161
Azactam® *See* Aztreonam 168
Azacytidine *See* AzaCITIDine 161
5-Azacytidine *See* AzaCITIDine 161
Azantac (Mex) *See* Ranitidine 1399
Azasan® *See* AzaTHIOprine 162
AzaSite™ *See* Azithromycin 163
AzaTHIOprine 162
Azathioprine Sodium *See* AzaTHIOprine 162
Azatrilem (Mex) *See* AzaTHIOprine 162
5-AZC *See* AzaCITIDine 161
Azelastine 162
Azelastine Hydrochloride *See* Azelastine 162
Azidothymidine *See* Zidovudine 1695
Azilect® *See* Rasagiline 1403
Azithromycin 163
Azithromycin Dihydrate *See* Azithromycin 163
Azithromycin Hydrogencitrate *See* Azithromycin 163
Azithromycin Monohydrate *See* Azithromycin 163
Azitrocin (Mex) *See* Azithromycin 163
Azitrohexal (Mex) *See* Azithromycin 163
Azmacort® *See* Triamcinolone 1617
Az Ofteno (Mex) *See* Azelastine 162
AZO-Gesic® [OTC] *See* Phenazopyridine 1258
Azo-Max (Mex) *See* Azithromycin 163
Azomyr (Mex) *See* Desloratadine 430
Azopt® *See* Brinzolamide 199
Azor™ *See* Amlodipine and Olmesartan 104
Azoran (Mex) *See* Omeprazole 1176
AZO-Standard® Maximum Strength [OTC] *See* Phenazopyridine 1258
AZO-Standard® [OTC] *See* Phenazopyridine 1258
AZT™ (Can) *See* Zidovudine 1695
AZT + 3TC (error-prone abbreviation) *See* Zidovudine and Lamivudine 1696
AZT (error-prone abbreviation) *See* Zidovudine 1695
Azthreonam *See* Aztreonam 168
Aztreonam 168
Azulfidina (Mex) *See* Sulfasalazine 1522
Azulfidine® *See* Sulfasalazine 1522
Azulfidine® EN-tabs® *See* Sulfasalazine 1522
B1 *See* Tositumomab and Iodine I 131 Tositumomab 1603
B1 Antibody *See* Tositumomab and Iodine I 131 Tositumomab 1603
B2036-PEG *See* Pegvisomant 1237
B 9273 *See* Alefacept 58

BA-16038 *See* Aminoglutethimide ... 87
Babee® Cof Syrup [OTC] *See* Dextromethorphan ... 448
Baclofen ... 168
Bactelan (Mex) *See* Sulfamethoxazole and Trimethoprim ... 1517
Bacteric (Mex) *See* Sulfamethoxazole and Trimethoprim ... 1517
Bactiver (Mex) *See* Sulfamethoxazole and Trimethoprim ... 1517
Bactocin (Mex) *See* Ofloxacin ... 1159
Bactrim™ *See* Sulfamethoxazole and Trimethoprim ... 1517
Bactrim™ DS *See* Sulfamethoxazole and Trimethoprim ... 1517
Bactroban® *See* Mupirocin ... 1085
Bactroban® Nasal *See* Mupirocin ... 1085
Bactropin (Mex) *See* Sulfamethoxazole and Trimethoprim ... 1517
Bagotanilo (Mex) *See* CARBOplatin ... 281
Baking Soda *See* Sodium Bicarbonate ... 1494
BAL *See* Dimercaprol ... 479
Balacet 325™ *See* Propoxyphene and Acetaminophen ... 1354
BAL in Oil® *See* Dimercaprol ... 479
Balminil (Can) *See* Xylometazoline ... 1687
Balminil Decongestant (Can) *See* Pseudoephedrine ... 1367
Balminil DM D (Can) *See* Pseudoephedrine and Dextromethorphan ... 1369
Balminil DM + Decongestant + Expectorant (Can) *See* Guaifenesin, Pseudoephedrine, and Dextromethorphan ... 748
Balminil DM E (Can) *See* Guaifenesin and Dextromethorphan ... 739
Balminil Expectorant (Can) *See* GuaiFENesin ... 737
Balsalazide ... 170
Balsalazide Disodium *See* Balsalazide ... 170
Baltussin *See* Dihydrocodeine, Chlorpheniramine, and Phenylephrine ... 469
Balziva™ *See* Ethinyl Estradiol and Norethindrone ... 597
Band-Aid® Hurt-Free™ Antiseptic Wash [OTC] *See* Lidocaine ... 924
Banophen® Anti-Itch [OTC] *See* DiphenhydrAMINE ... 481
Banophen® [OTC] *See* DiphenhydrAMINE ... 481
Banzel™ *See* Rufinamide ... 1452
Bapex (Mex) *See* Gabapentin ... 702
Baraclude® *See* Entecavir ... 540
Baridium® [OTC] *See* Phenazopyridine ... 1258
Basaljel® (Can) *See* Aluminum Hydroxide ... 78
Basiliximab ... 171
BAY 43-9006 *See* Sorafenib ... 1501
Bayer® Aspirin Extra Strength [OTC] *See* Aspirin ... 143
Bayer® Aspirin Regimen Adult Low Dose [OTC] *See* Aspirin ... 143
Bayer® Aspirin Regimen Children's [OTC] *See* Aspirin ... 143
Bayer® Aspirin Regimen Regular Strength [OTC] *See* Aspirin ... 143
Bayer® Genuine Aspirin [OTC] *See* Aspirin ... 143
Bayer® Plus Extra Strength [OTC] *See* Aspirin ... 143
Bayer® PM [OTC] *See* Aspirin and Diphenhydramine ... 145
Bayer® with Heart Advantage [OTC] *See* Aspirin ... 143
Bayer® Women's Aspirin Plus Calcium [OTC] *See* Aspirin ... 143
BCI-Fluoxetine (Can) *See* FLUoxetine ... 650
BCI-Gabapentin (Can) *See* Gabapentin ... 702
BCI-Metformin (Can) *See* MetFORMIN ... 997
BCI-Ranitidine (Can) *See* Ranitidine ... 1399
BCNU *See* Carmustine ... 284
Bebulin® VH *See* Factor IX Complex (Human) ... 612
Beclazone (Mex) *See* Beclomethasone ... 171
Beclomethasone ... 171
Beclomethasone Dipropionate *See* Beclomethasone ... 171
Beconase (Mex) *See* Beclomethasone ... 171
Beconase® AQ *See* Beclomethasone ... 171
Becotide (Mex) *See* Beclomethasone ... 171
Bedoyecta (Mex) *See* Pyridoxine ... 1376
BeFlex *See* Acetaminophen and Phenyltoloxamine ... 36
Belladonna Alkaloids With Phenobarbital *See* Hyoscyamine, Atropine, Scopolamine, and Phenobarbital ... 800
Belladonna and Opium ... 174
Belladonna, Phenobarbital, and Ergotamine ... 175
Bellamine S [DSC] *See* Belladonna, Phenobarbital, and Ergotamine ... 175
Bellergal® Spacetabs® (Can) *See* Belladonna, Phenobarbital, and Ergotamine ... 175
Benadryl® (Can) *See* DiphenhydrAMINE ... 481
Benadryl-D™ Allergy and Sinus Fastmelt™ [OTC] *See* Diphenhydramine and Pseudoephedrine ... 486
Benadryl-D™ Children's Allergy and Sinus [OTC] *See* Diphenhydramine and Pseudoephedrine ... 486
Benadryl® Allergy and Cold [OTC] *See* Acetaminophen, Diphenhydramine, and Phenylephrine ... 44
Benadryl® Allergy and Sinus Headache [OTC] *See* Acetaminophen, Diphenhydramine, and Phenylephrine ... 44
Benadryl® Allergy [OTC] *See* DiphenhydrAMINE ... 481

Benadryl® Children's Allergy and Cold Fastmelt™ [OTC] *See* Diphenhydramine and Pseudoephedrine 486
Benadryl® Children's Allergy Fastmelt® [OTC] *See* DiphenhydrAMINE 481
Benadryl® Children's Allergy [OTC] *See* DiphenhydrAMINE 481
Benadryl® Children's Dye-Free Allergy [OTC] *See* DiphenhydrAMINE 481
Benadryl® Itch Stopping Extra Strength [OTC] *See* DiphenhydrAMINE 481
Benadryl® Itch Stopping [OTC] *See* DiphenhydrAMINE 481
Benaxima (Mex) *See* Cefotaxime 295
Benaxona (Mex) *See* CefTRIAXone 300
Benazepril 178
Benazepril and Hydrochlorothiazide 179
Benazepril Hydrochloride *See* Benazepril 178
Benazepril Hydrochloride and Amlodipine Besylate *See* Amlodipine and Benazepril 104
Bendamustine 179
Bendamustine Hydrochloride *See* Bendamustine 179
Bendroflumethiazide and Nadolol *See* Nadolol and Bendroflumethiazide 1092
Benecid Valdecasas (Mex) *See* Probenecid 1338
BeneFix® *See* Factor IX 612
Beneflur® (Can) *See* Fludarabine 641
Benemid [DSC] *See* Probenecid 1338
Benicar® *See* Olmesartan 1170
Benicar HCT® *See* Olmesartan and Hydrochlorothiazide 1172
Ben-Tann *See* DiphenhydrAMINE 481
Bentyl® *See* Dicyclomine 459
Bentylol® (Can) *See* Dicyclomine 459
Benuryl™ (Can) *See* Probenecid 1338
Benylin® 3.3 mg-D-E (Can) *See* Guaifenesin, Pseudoephedrine, and Codeine 747
Benylin® D for Infants (Can) *See* Pseudoephedrine 1367
Benylin® DM-D (Can) *See* Pseudoephedrine and Dextromethorphan 1369
Benylin® DM-D-E (Can) *See* Guaifenesin, Pseudoephedrine, and Dextromethorphan 748
Benylin® DM-E (Can) *See* Guaifenesin and Dextromethorphan 739
Benylin® E Extra Strength (Can) *See* GuaiFENesin 737
Benzathine Benzylpenicillin *See* Penicillin G Benzathine 1239
Benzathine Penicillin G *See* Penicillin G Benzathine 1239
Benzazoline Hydrochloride *See* Tolazoline 1592
Benzene Hexachloride *See* Lindane 927
Benzetacil (Mex) *See* Penicillin G Benzathine 1239
Benzhexol Hydrochloride *See* Trihexyphenidyl 1627
Benzisoquinolinedione *See* Amonafide 108
Benzmethyzin *See* Procarbazine 1340
Benzoic Acid, Methenamine, Methylene Blue, Phenyl Salicylate, and Hyoscyamine *See* Methenamine, Phenyl Salicylate, Methylene Blue, Benzoic Acid, and Hyoscyamine 1009
Benzonatate 180
Benzphetamine 181
Benzphetamine Hydrochloride *See* Benzphetamine 181
Benztropine 183
Benztropine Mesylate *See* Benztropine 183
Benzylpenicillin Benzathine *See* Penicillin G Benzathine 1239
Benzylpenicillin Potassium *See* Penicillin G, Parenteral, Aqueous 1241
Benzylpenicillin Sodium *See* Penicillin G, Parenteral, Aqueous 1241
Berinin P (Mex) *See* Factor IX 612
Bestafen (Mex) *See* Ibuprofen 803
9-Beta-D-Ribofuranosyladenine *See* Adenosine 51
Betacaine® (Can) *See* Lidocaine 924
Betaderm (Can) *See* Betamethasone 184
Betaferon (Mex) *See* Interferon Beta-1b 848
Betagan® *See* Levobunolol 907
Beta-HC® *See* Hydrocortisone 785
Betaject™ (Can) *See* Betamethasone 184
Betaloc® (Can) *See* Metoprolol 1036
Betaloc® Durules® (Can) *See* Metoprolol 1036
Betamethasone 184
Betamethasone Dipropionate *See* Betamethasone 184
Betamethasone Dipropionate, Augmented *See* Betamethasone 184
Betamethasone Sodium Phosphate *See* Betamethasone 184
Betamethasone Valerate *See* Betamethasone 184
Betapace® *See* Sotalol 1502
Betapace AF® *See* Sotalol 1502
Beta Sal® [OTC] *See* Salicylic Acid 1454
Betaseron® *See* Interferon Beta-1b 848
Beta-Val® *See* Betamethasone 184
Betaxin® (Can) *See* Thiamine 1568
Betaxolol 186
Betaxolol Hydrochloride *See* Betaxolol 186
Bethanechol 186
Bethanechol Chloride *See* Bethanechol 186

Betimol® *See* Timolol ... 1584
Betnesol® (Can) *See* Betamethasone ... 184
Betnovate® (Can) *See* Betamethasone ... 184
Betoptic® S *See* Betaxolol ... 186
Betsol "Z" (Mex) *See* Sodium Bicarbonate ... 1494
Bevacizumab ... 187
Bexarotene ... 187
Bexxar® *See* Tositumomab and Iodine I 131 Tositumomab ... 1603
BG 9273 *See* Alefacept ... 58
Biaxin® *See* Clarithromycin ... 360
Biaxin® XL *See* Clarithromycin ... 360
Bicalutamide ... 188
Bicillin® L-A *See* Penicillin G Benzathine ... 1239
Bicillin® C-R *See* Penicillin G Benzathine and Penicillin G Procaine ... 1240
Bicillin® C-R 900/300 *See* Penicillin G Benzathine and Penicillin G Procaine ... 1240
Biclin (Mex) *See* Amikacin ... 83
BiCNU® *See* Carmustine ... 284
Biconcor (Mex) *See* Bisoprolol and Hydrochlorothiazide ... 191
BIDA *See* Amonafide ... 108
Bidhist *See* Brompheniramine ... 205
BiDil® *See* Isosorbide Dinitrate and Hydralazine ... 869
Bi-Euglucon M "5" (Mex) *See* Glyburide and Metformin ... 733
Biltricide® *See* Praziquantel ... 1324
Bimxan (Mex) *See* Amoxicillin ... 112
Binarin (Mex) *See* Epirubicin ... 545
Binotal (Mex) *See* Ampicillin ... 122
Bio-Carbamazepine (Can) *See* CarBAMazepine ... 265
Biocilin (Mex) *See* Filgrastim ... 632
Biodaclin (Mex) *See* Clindamycin ... 363
Biodexan Ofteno (Mex) *See* Polymyxin B ... 1312
Biofilen (Mex) *See* Atenolol ... 147
Biofilgran (Mex) *See* Filgrastim ... 632
Biokacin (Mex) *See* Amikacin ... 83
Biomixin (Mex) *See* Doxycycline ... 509
Bioniche Promethazine (Can) *See* Promethazine ... 1347
Bio-Oxazepam (Can) *See* Oxazepam ... 1193
BioQuin® Durules™ (Can) *See* QuiNIDine ... 1387
Biosint (Mex) *See* Cefotaxime ... 295
Biphentin® (Can) *See* Methylphenidate ... 1024
Bird Flu Vaccine *See* Influenza Virus Vaccine (H5N1) ... 821
bis-chloronitrosourea *See* Carmustine ... 284
Bismatrol *See* Bismuth ... 189
Bismatrol Maximum Strength [OTC] *See* Bismuth ... 189
Bismatrol [OTC] *See* Bismuth ... 189
Bismuth ... 189
Bismuth, Metronidazole, and Tetracycline ... 190
Bismuth Subcitrate Potassium, Tetracycline, and Metronidazole *See* Bismuth, Metronidazole, and Tetracycline ... 190
Bismuth Subsalicylate *See* Bismuth ... 189
Bismuth Subsalicylate, Tetracycline, and Metronidazole *See* Bismuth, Metronidazole, and Tetracycline ... 190
Bisoprolol ... 190
Bisoprolol and Hydrochlorothiazide ... 191
Bisoprolol Fumarate *See* Bisoprolol ... 190
Bis-POM PMEA *See* Adefovir ... 51
Bistropamide *See* Tropicamide ... 1636
Bivalirudin ... 191
BL4162A *See* Anagrelide ... 124
Blastocarb RU (Mex) *See* CARBOplatin ... 281
Blastolem RU (Mex) *See* CISplatin ... 354
Blefamide SF (Mex) *See* Sulfacetamide and Prednisolone ... 1516
Blefamide SOP (Mex) *See* Sulfacetamide and Prednisolone ... 1516
Blenoxane® (Can) *See* Bleomycin ... 192
Blenoxane® [DSC] *See* Bleomycin ... 192
Bleo *See* Bleomycin ... 192
Bleolem (Mex) *See* Bleomycin ... 192
Bleomax (Mex) *See* Bleomycin ... 192
Bleomycin ... 192
Bleomycin Injection, USP (Can) *See* Bleomycin ... 192
Bleomycin Sulfate *See* Bleomycin ... 192
Blephamide® *See* Sulfacetamide and Prednisolone ... 1516
BLM *See* Bleomycin ... 192
Blopress (Mex) *See* Candesartan ... 260
Blotex (Mex) *See* Atenolol ... 147
Blugat (Mex) *See* Gabapentin ... 702
BMS-232632 *See* Atazanavir ... 147
BMS 337039 *See* Aripiprazole ... 133

BMS-354825 *See* Dasatinib ... 420
Bonadoxina (Mex) *See* Meclizine ... 974
Bonamine™ (Can) *See* Meclizine ... 974
Bondronat® (Can) *See* Ibandronate ... 801
Bonine® (Can) *See* Meclizine ... 974
Bonine® [OTC] *See* Meclizine ... 974
Boniva® *See* Ibandronate ... 801
Bontril® (Can) *See* Phendimetrazine ... 1259
Bontril PDM® *See* Phendimetrazine ... 1259
Bontril® Slow-Release *See* Phendimetrazine ... 1259
Bonviva (Mex) *See* Ibandronate ... 801
Bortezomib ... 192
B&O Supprettes® [DSC] *See* Belladonna and Opium ... 174
Botox® *See* Botulinum Toxin Type A ... 193
Botox® Cosmetic *See* Botulinum Toxin Type A ... 193
Botulinum Toxin Type A ... 193
Botulinum Toxin Type B ... 197
Brakhor (Mex) *See* Pravastatin ... 1321
Braxan (Mex) *See* Amiodarone ... 89
Bre-A-Col (Mex) *See* Guaifenesin and Dextromethorphan ... 739
Bregamin (Mex) *See* Chlorpheniramine ... 321
Bremagan Flu (Mex) *See* Phenylephrine ... 1273
Brethaire [DSC] *See* Terbutaline ... 1552
Brevibloc® *See* Esmolol ... 569
Brevicon® *See* Ethinyl Estradiol and Norethindrone ... 597
Brevicon® 0.5/35 (Can) *See* Ethinyl Estradiol and Norethindrone ... 597
Brevicon® 1/35 (Can) *See* Ethinyl Estradiol and Norethindrone ... 597
Brevital® (Can) *See* Methohexital ... 1011
Brevital® Sodium *See* Methohexital ... 1011
Bricanyl® (Can) *See* Terbutaline ... 1552
Bricanyl [DSC] *See* Terbutaline ... 1552
Brimonidine ... 199
Brimonidine Tartrate *See* Brimonidine ... 199
Brinzolamide ... 199
Brioschi® [OTC] *See* Sodium Bicarbonate ... 1494
Brispen (Mex) *See* Dicloxacillin ... 459
Bristaxol (Mex) *See* Paclitaxel ... 1213
British Anti-Lewisite *See* Dimercaprol ... 479
BRL 43694 *See* Granisetron ... 736
Brogamax (Mex) *See* Sulfamethoxazole and Trimethoprim ... 1517
Bromaline® DM [OTC] *See* Brompheniramine, Pseudoephedrine, and Dextromethorphan ... 208
Bromaline® [OTC] *See* Brompheniramine and Pseudoephedrine ... 206
Bromatane DX *See* Brompheniramine, Pseudoephedrine, and Dextromethorphan ... 208
Bromazepam ... 200
Brometane DX [DSC] *See* Brompheniramine, Pseudoephedrine, and Dextromethorphan ... 208
Bromfenex® [DSC] *See* Brompheniramine and Pseudoephedrine ... 206
Bromfenex® PD [DSC] *See* Brompheniramine and Pseudoephedrine ... 206
Bromhist DM *See* Brompheniramine, Pseudoephedrine, and Dextromethorphan ... 208
Bromhist-NR *See* Brompheniramine and Pseudoephedrine ... 206
Bromhist PDX *See* Brompheniramine, Pseudoephedrine, and Dextromethorphan ... 208
Bromhist Pediatric *See* Brompheniramine and Pseudoephedrine ... 206
Bromocriptine ... 202
Bromocriptine Mesylate *See* Bromocriptine ... 202
Bromphenex DM *See* Brompheniramine, Pseudoephedrine, and Dextromethorphan ... 208
Brompheniramine ... 205
Brompheniramine and Pseudoephedrine ... 206
Brompheniramine Maleate *See* Brompheniramine ... 205
Brompheniramine Maleate and Pseudoephedrine Hydrochloride *See* Brompheniramine and Pseudoephedrine ... 206
Brompheniramine Maleate and Pseudoephedrine Sulfate *See* Brompheniramine and Pseudoephedrine ... 206
Brompheniramine, Pseudoephedrine, and Dextromethorphan ... 208
Brompheniramine Tannate *See* Brompheniramine ... 205
Bromplex DX *See* Brompheniramine, Pseudoephedrine, and Dextromethorphan ... 208
Brontex® *See* Guaifenesin and Codeine ... 738
Brospina (Mex) *See* Buprenorphine ... 212
Brotapp *See* Brompheniramine and Pseudoephedrine ... 206
Brotapp-DM *See* Brompheniramine, Pseudoephedrine, and Dextromethorphan ... 208
Brovana® *See* Arformoterol ... 131
BroveX™ *See* Brompheniramine ... 205
BroveX™ CT *See* Brompheniramine ... 205
Brovex SR *See* Brompheniramine and Pseudoephedrine ... 206
Brucam (Mex) *See* Piroxicam ... 1307
Brucarcer (Mex) *See* CarBAMazepine ... 265
Brudex (Mex) *See* Dextromethorphan ... 448
Brudifen (Mex) *See* DiphenhydrAMINE ... 481
Brufincol (Mex) *See* Pravastatin ... 1321

Brulin (Mex) *See* Dexamethasone 436
Brupen (Mex) *See* Ampicillin 122
Brurem (Mex) *See* Sulindac 1523
Brusal (Mex) *See* Albuterol 54
Bruzol (Mex) *See* Albendazole 53
B-Tuss™ *See* Phenylephrine, Hydrocodone, and Chlorpheniramine 1277
BTX-A *See* Botulinum Toxin Type A 193
B-type Natriuretic Peptide (Human) *See* Nesiritide 1123
Budeprion XL® *See* BuPROPion 217
Budeprion™ SR *See* BuPROPion 217
Budesonide 210
Buffasal [OTC] *See* Aspirin 143
Buffered Aspirin and Pravastatin Sodium *See* Aspirin and Pravastatin 146
Bufferin® Extra Strength [OTC] *See* Aspirin 143
Bufferin® [OTC] *See* Aspirin 143
Buffinol [OTC] *See* Aspirin 143
Bufigen (Mex) *See* Nalbuphine 1094
Bumetanide 211
Bumex® *See* Bumetanide 211
Bupap *See* Butalbital and Acetaminophen 236
Bupivacaine 211
Bupivacaine Hydrochloride *See* Bupivacaine 211
Buprenex® *See* Buprenorphine 212
Buprenorphine 212
Buprenorphine and Naloxone 215
Buprenorphine Hydrochloride *See* Buprenorphine 212
Buprenorphine Hydrochloride and Naloxone Hydrochloride Dihydrate
See Buprenorphine and Naloxone 215
Buproban™ *See* BuPROPion 217
BuPROPion 217
Burinex® (Can) *See* Bumetanide 211
Burnamycin [OTC] *See* Lidocaine 924
Burn Jel® [OTC] *See* Lidocaine 924
Burn-O-Jel [OTC] *See* Lidocaine 924
Buscopan® (Can) *See* Scopolamine Derivatives 1463
BuSpar® *See* BusPIRone 223
Buspirex (Can) *See* BusPIRone 223
BusPIRone 223
Buspirone Hydrochloride *See* BusPIRone 223
Bustab® (Can) *See* BusPIRone 223
Busulfan 226
Busulfex® *See* Busulfan 226
Butabarbital 226
Butalbital, Acetaminophen, and Caffeine 229
Butalbital, Acetaminophen, Caffeine, and Codeine 232
Butalbital and Acetaminophen 236
Butalbital, Aspirin, and Caffeine 239
Butalbital, Aspirin, Caffeine, and Codeine 242
Butalbital Compound *See* Butalbital, Aspirin, and Caffeine 239
Butalbital Compound and Codeine *See* Butalbital, Aspirin, Caffeine, and Codeine 242
Butifeno (Mex) *See* Ketotifen 879
Butisol Sodium® *See* Butabarbital 226
Butorphanol 247
Butorphanol Tartrate *See* Butorphanol 247
B-Vex *See* Brompheniramine 205
BW-430C *See* LamoTRIgine 889
BW524W91 *See* Emtricitabine 530
Byetta® *See* Exenatide 609
Bystolic™ *See* Nebivolol 1115
C1H *See* Alemtuzumab 59
C2B8 Monoclonal Antibody *See* RiTUXimab 1434
C8-CCK *See* Sincalide 1489
311C90 *See* Zolmitriptan 1703
C225 *See* Cetuximab 310
Cabergoline 248
Caduet® *See* Amlodipine and Atorvastatin 103
Caelyx (Mex) *See* DOXOrubicin 507
Cafcit® *See* Caffeine 250
Cafergor® (Can) *See* Ergotamine and Caffeine 554
Cafergot (Mex) *See* Ergotamine 552
Caffeine 250
Caffeine, Acetaminophen, and Aspirin *See* Acetaminophen, Aspirin, and Caffeine 39
Caffeine, Acetaminophen, Butalbital, and Codeine *See* Butalbital, Acetaminophen, Caffeine, and Codeine 232
Caffeine and Ergotamine *See* Ergotamine and Caffeine 554
Caffeine and Sodium Benzoate *See* Caffeine 250
Caffeine, Aspirin, and Acetaminophen *See* Acetaminophen, Aspirin, and Caffeine 39

Caffeine Citrate *See* Caffeine 250
Caffeine, Dihydrocodeine, and Acetaminophen *See* Acetaminophen, Caffeine, and Dihydrocodeine 39
Caffeine, Orphenadrine, and Aspirin *See* Orphenadrine, Aspirin, and Caffeine 1187
Caffeine, Propoxyphene, and Aspirin *See* Propoxyphene, Aspirin, and Caffeine 1355
Caftar (Mex) *See* Ergotamine 552
Cal-C-Caps [OTC] *See* Calcium Citrate 257
Calan® *See* Verapamil 1665
Calan® SR *See* Verapamil 1665
Calcarb 600 [OTC] *See* Calcium Carbonate 254
Cal-Cee [OTC] *See* Calcium Citrate 257
Calci-Chew® [OTC] *See* Calcium Carbonate 254
Calcimar® (Can) *See* Calcitonin 253
Calci-Mix® [OTC] *See* Calcium Carbonate 254
Calcionate [OTC] *See* Calcium Glubionate 258
Calcite-500 (Can) *See* Calcium Carbonate 254
Calcitonin 253
Calcitonin (Salmon) *See* Calcitonin 253
Cal-Citrate-225 *See* Calcium Citrate 257
Cal-Citrate® 250 [OTC] [DSC] *See* Calcium Citrate 257
Calcium Acetate 254
Calcium Acetylhomotaurinate *See* Acamprosate 23
Calcium and Risedronate *See* Risedronate and Calcium 1424
Calcium Carbonate 254
Calcium Carbonate and Etidronate Disodium *See* Etidronate and Calcium 605
Calcium Carbonate and Magnesium Hydroxide 256
Calcium Carbonate, Magnesium Hydroxide, and Famotidine *See* Famotidine, Calcium Carbonate, and Magnesium Hydroxide 614
Calcium Chloride 256
Calcium Citrate 257
Calcium Glubionate 258
Calcium Gluconate 258
Calcium Lactate 259
Calcival (Mex) *See* Calcium Citrate 257
Caldecort® [OTC] *See* Hydrocortisone 785
Cal-Gest [OTC] *See* Calcium Carbonate 254
Cal-GLU™ *See* Calcium Gluconate 258
Cal-G [OTC] *See* Calcium Gluconate 258
Caliprene (Mex) *See* Pilocarpine 1290
Cal-Mint [OTC] *See* Calcium Carbonate 254
Calmylin with Codeine (Can) *See* Guaifenesin, Pseudoephedrine, and Codeine 747
CaloMist™ *See* Cyanocobalamin 404
Calsan (Mex) *See* Calcium Carbonate 254
Caltine® (Can) *See* Calcitonin 253
Caltrate® (Can) *See* Calcium Carbonate 254
Caltrate® 600 [OTC] *See* Calcium Carbonate 254
Caltrate® Select (Can) *See* Calcium Carbonate 254
Caltrón (Mex) *See* Calcium Carbonate 254
Camila™ *See* Norethindrone 1150
Camomille Grande *See* Feverfew (Tanacetum parthenium) 628
Campath® *See* Alemtuzumab 59
Campath-1H *See* Alemtuzumab 59
Camphorated Tincture of Opium (error-prone synonym) *See* Paregoric 1225
Campral® *See* Acamprosate 23
Camptosar® *See* Irinotecan 856
Camptothecin-11 *See* Irinotecan 856
Canasa® *See* Mesalamine 994
Cancidas® *See* Caspofungin 290
Candesartan 260
Candesartan and Hydrochlorothiazide 262
Candesartan Cilexetil *See* Candesartan 260
Candesartan Cilexetil and Hydrochlorothiazide *See* Candesartan and Hydrochlorothiazide 262
Cannabidiol and Tetrahydrocannabinol *See* Tetrahydrocannabinol and Cannabidiol 1558
Canthacur® (Can) *See* Cantharidin 263
Cantharidin 263
Cantharone® (Can) *See* Cantharidin 263
Cantil® (Can) *See* Mepenzolate 986
Cantil® [DSC] *See* Mepenzolate 986
Capastat® Sulfate *See* Capreomycin 263
Capecitabine 263
Capital® and Codeine *See* Acetaminophen and Codeine 34
Capoten® *See* Captopril 264
Capotena (Mex) *See* Captopril 264
Capozide® *See* Captopril and Hydrochlorothiazide 265
Capreomycin 263
Capreomycin Sulfate *See* Capreomycin 263

Captopril 264
Captopril and Hydrochlorothiazide 265
Captral (Mex) *See* Captopril 264
Carac® *See* Fluorouracil 649
Carafate® *See* Sucralfate 1514
Carapres® (Can) *See* CloNIDine 377
Carbac (Mex) *See* Loracarbef 946
CarBAMazepine 265
Carbaphen 12® *See* Carbetapentane, Phenylephrine, and Chlorpheniramine 274
Carbaphen 12 Ped® *See* Carbetapentane, Phenylephrine, and Chlorpheniramine 274
Carbatrol® *See* CarBAMazepine 265
Carbaxefed RF [DSC] *See* Carbinoxamine and Pseudoephedrine 280
Carbazep (Mex) *See* CarBAMazepine 265
Carbazina (Mex) *See* CarBAMazepine 265
Carbenicillin 272
Carbenicillin Indanyl Sodium *See* Carbenicillin 272
Carbetapentane and Chlorpheniramine 272
Carbetapentane and Phenylephrine 273
Carbetapentane and Pseudoephedrine 273
Carbetapentane, Ephedrine, Phenylephrine, and Chlorpheniramine
See Chlorpheniramine, Ephedrine, Phenylephrine, and Carbetapentane 326
Carbetapentane, Guaifenesin, and Phenylephrine 274
Carbetapentane, Phenylephrine, and Chlorpheniramine 274
Carbetapentane, Phenylephrine, and Pyrilamine 275
Carbetapentane Tannate and Chlorpheniramine Tannate *See* Carbetapentane and Chlorpheniramine 272
Carbetapentane Tannate and Pseudoephedrine Tannate *See* Carbetapentane and Pseudoephedrine 273
Carbetaplex *See* Carbetapentane, Guaifenesin, and Phenylephrine 274
Carbidopa 276
Carbidopa and Levodopa 277
Carbidopa, Levodopa, and Entacapone *See* Levodopa, Carbidopa, and Entacapone 911
Carbinoxamine 280
Carbinoxamine and Pseudoephedrine 280
Carbinoxamine Maleate *See* Carbinoxamine 280
Carbinoxamine, Pseudoephedrine, and Hydrocodone *See* Hydrocodone, Carbinoxamine, and Pseudoephedrine 782
Carbocaine® *See* Mepivacaine 990
Carbofed DM *See* Brompheniramine, Pseudoephedrine, and Dextromethorphan 208
Carbolit (Mex) *See* Lithium 938
Carbolith™ (Can) *See* Lithium 938
Carboplat (Mex) *See* CARBOplatin 281
CARBOplatin 281
Carboprost *See* Carboprost Tromethamine 282
Carboprost Tromethamine 282
Carbotec (Mex) *See* CARBOplatin 281
Carbotural (Mex) *See* Charcoal 312
Carboxine-PSE [DSC] *See* Carbinoxamine and Pseudoephedrine 280
Cardene® *See* NiCARdipine 1128
Cardene® I.V. *See* NiCARdipine 1128
Cardene® SR *See* NiCARdipine 1128
Cardioxane (Mex) *See* Dexrazoxane 441
Cardizem® *See* Diltiazem 473
Cardizem® CD *See* Diltiazem 473
Cardizem® LA *See* Diltiazem 473
Cardizem® SR (Can) *See* Diltiazem 473
Cardura® *See* Doxazosin 500
Cardura-1™ (Can) *See* Doxazosin 500
Cardura-2™ (Can) *See* Doxazosin 500
Cardura-4™ (Can) *See* Doxazosin 500
Cardura® XL *See* Doxazosin 500
Carindacillin *See* Carbenicillin 272
Carisoprodate *See* Carisoprodol 283
Carisoprodol 283
Carisoprodol and Aspirin 284
Carisoprodol, Aspirin, and Codeine 284
Carmustine 284
Carmustinum *See* Carmustine 284
Carnotprim (Mex) *See* Metoclopramide 1031
Carpin (Mex) *See* CarBAMazepine 265
Carteolol 285
Carteolol Hydrochloride *See* Carteolol 285
Cartia XT™ *See* Diltiazem 473
Carvedilol 286
Casodex® *See* Bicalutamide 188
Caspofungin 290
Caspofungin Acetate *See* Caspofungin 290

Cataflam® *See* Diclofenac 457
Catapres® *See* CloNIDine 377
Catapres-TTS® *See* CloNIDine 377
Caverject® *See* Alprostadil 77
Caverject Impulse® *See* Alprostadil 77
CB-1348 *See* Chlorambucil 315
CBDCA *See* CARBOplatin 281
CBZ *See* CarBAMazepine 265
CC-5013 *See* Lenalidomide 899
CCI-779 *See* Temsirolimus 1547
CCNU *See* Lomustine 943
2-CdA *See* Cladribine 360
CDDP *See* CISplatin 354
CDP870 *See* Certolizumab Pegol 307
CDX *See* Bicalutamide 188
CE *See* Estrogens (Conjugated/Equine) 582
Cec (Mex) *See* Cefaclor 291
Ceclor® (Can) *See* Cefaclor 291
Cecon® [OTC] *See* Ascorbic Acid 141
Cedax® *See* Ceftibuten 299
Cedocard®-SR (Can) *See* Isosorbide Dinitrate 866
CEE *See* Estrogens (Conjugated/Equine) 582
CeeNU® *See* Lomustine 943
Cefabiot (Mex) *See* Cefuroxime 300
Cefaclor 291
Cefadroxil 292
Cefadroxil Monohydrate *See* Cefadroxil 292
Cefalver (Mex) *See* Cephalexin 306
Cefaxona (Mex) *See* CefTRIAXone 300
CeFAZolin 292
Cefazolin Sodium *See* CeFAZolin 292
Cefdinir 293
Cefditoren 293
Cefditoren Pivoxil *See* Cefditoren 293
Cefepime 294
Cefepime Hydrochloride *See* Cefepime 294
Cefixime 294
Cefixime Trihydrate *See* Cefixime 294
Cefizox® *See* Ceftizoxime 299
Ceflacid (Mex) *See* Cefaclor 291
Cefotaxime 295
Cefotaxime Sodium *See* Cefotaxime 295
Cefotetan 296
Cefotetan Disodium *See* Cefotetan 296
Cefoxitin 296
Cefoxitin Sodium *See* Cefoxitin 296
Cefpodoxime 297
Cefpodoxime Proxetil *See* Cefpodoxime 297
Cefprozil 297
Cefraden (Mex) *See* CefTRIAXone 300
Ceftazidime 298
Ceftibuten 299
Ceftin® *See* Cefuroxime 300
Ceftizoxime 299
Ceftizoxime Sodium *See* Ceftizoxime 299
Ceftrex (Mex) *See* CefTRIAXone 300
Ceftrianol (Mex) *See* CefTRIAXone 300
CefTRIAXone 300
Ceftriaxone Sodium *See* CefTRIAXone 300
Ceftrilem (Mex) *See* CefTRIAXone 300
Cefuracet (Mex) *See* Cefuroxime 300
Cefuroxime 300
Cefuroxime Axetil *See* Cefuroxime 300
Cefuroxime For Injection (Can) *See* Cefuroxime 300
Cefuroxime Sodium *See* Cefuroxime 300
Cefzil® (Can) *See* Cefprozil 297
Celebrex® *See* Celecoxib 301
Celecoxib 301
Celestone® *See* Betamethasone 184
Celestone® Soluspan® *See* Betamethasone 184
Celexa® *See* Citalopram 354
CellCept® *See* Mycophenolate 1087
Celontin® *See* Methsuximide 1019
Celsentri™ (Can) *See* Maraviroc 971
Celunaf (Mex) *See* Naphazoline 1101
Cemill [OTC] *See* Ascorbic Acid 141
Cenestin® *See* Estrogens (Conjugated A/Synthetic) 581

Cenolate® *See* Ascorbic Acid 141
Centany™ [DSC] *See* Mupirocin 1085
Cephadyn *See* Butalbital and Acetaminophen 236
Cephalexin 306
Cephalexin Monohydrate *See* Cephalexin 306
Ceporex (Mex) *See* Cephalexin 306
Cerebyx® *See* Fosphenytoin 692
Cerezyme® *See* Imiglucerase 811
Ceron *See* Chlorpheniramine and Phenylephrine 323
Ceron-DM *See* Chlorpheniramine, Phenylephrine, and Dextromethorphan 327
Certolizumab Pegol 307
Certuss-D® *See* Guaifenesin, Dextromethorphan, and Phenylephrine 746
Cerubidine® *See* DAUNOrubicin Hydrochloride 421
Cervidil® *See* Dinoprostone 480
C.E.S.® (Can) *See* Estrogens (Conjugated/Equine) 582
Cesamet® *See* Nabilone 1088
Cesia™ *See* Ethinyl Estradiol and Desogestrel 592
Cesol (Mex) *See* Praziquantel 1324
Cetacort® [DSC] *See* Hydrocortisone 785
Cetafen Extra® [OTC] *See* Acetaminophen 30
Cetafen® [OTC] *See* Acetaminophen 30
Cetirizine 307
Cetirizine and Pseudoephedrine 309
Cetirizine Hydrochloride *See* Cetirizine 307
Cetirizine Hydrochloride and Pseudoephedrine Hydrochloride *See* Cetirizine and Pseudoephedrine 309
Cetitev (Mex) *See* Cetirizine 307
Cetoxil (Mex) *See* Cefuroxime 300
Cetuximab 310
Cevalin (Mex) *See* Ascorbic Acid 141
Cevimeline 310
Cevimeline Hydrochloride *See* Cevimeline 310
CFDN *See* Cefdinir 293
CG *See* Chorionic Gonadotropin (Human) 342
C-Gel [OTC] *See* Ascorbic Acid 141
CGP 33101 *See* Rufinamide 1452
CGP-42446 *See* Zoledronic Acid 1702
CGP-57148B *See* Imatinib 810
C-Gram [OTC] *See* Ascorbic Acid 141
CGS-20267 *See* Letrozole 900
Chamomile, German *(Matricaria chamomilla, Matricaria recutita)* 310
Champix® (Can) *See* Varenicline 1656
Chantix® *See* Varenicline 1656
Charcadole® (Can) *See* Charcoal 312
Charcadole®, Aqueous (Can) *See* Charcoal 312
Charcadole® TFS (Can) *See* Charcoal 312
Char-Caps [OTC] *See* Charcoal 312
CharcoAid® G [OTC] *See* Charcoal 312
Charcoal 312
Charcoal Plus® DS [OTC] *See* Charcoal 312
CharcoCaps® [OTC] *See* Charcoal 312
Chemet® *See* Succimer 1511
Cheracol® *See* Guaifenesin and Codeine 738
Cheracol D (Mex) *See* Guaifenesin and Dextromethorphan 739
Cheracol® D [OTC] *See* Guaifenesin and Dextromethorphan 739
Cheracol® Plus [OTC] *See* Guaifenesin and Dextromethorphan 739
Chew-C [OTC] *See* Ascorbic Acid 141
Children's Advil® Cold (Can) *See* Pseudoephedrine and Ibuprofen 1369
Children's Pepto [OTC] *See* Calcium Carbonate 254
Children's Motion Sickness Liquid (Can) *See* DimenhyDRINATE 478
Children's Tylenol® Plus Cold and Allergy [OTC] *See* Acetaminophen, Diphenhydramine, and Phenylephrine 44
Chinese Ephedra *See* Ephedra (Ephedra sinica) 541
Chinese Joint Fir *See* Ephedra (Ephedra sinica) 541
Chirocaine® (Can) *See* Levobupivacaine 908
Chirocaine® [DSC] *See* Levobupivacaine 908
Chloral *See* Chloral Hydrate 313
Chloral Hydrate 313
Chlorambucil 315
Chlorambucilum *See* Chlorambucil 315
Chloraminophene *See* Chlorambucil 315
Chloramphenicol 315
Chlorbutinum *See* Chlorambucil 315
Chlordex GP *See* Dextromethorphan, Chlorpheniramine, Phenylephrine, and Guaifenesin 450
ChlordiazePOXIDE 316
Chlordiazepoxide and Amitriptyline Hydrochloride *See* Amitriptyline and Chlordiazepoxide 94

Chlordiazepoxide and Clidinium *See* Clidinium and Chlordiazepoxide 362
Chlordiazepoxide and Methscopolamine 319
Chlorethazine *See* Mechlorethamine 974
Chlorethazine Mustard *See* Mechlorethamine 974
Chlorex-A *See* Chlorpheniramine, Phenylephrine, and Phenyltoloxamine 331
Chlorex-A 12 [DSC] *See* Chlorpheniramine, Pyrilamine, and Phenylephrine 335
Chlormeprazine *See* Prochlorperazine 1341
Chlor-Mes *See* Chlorpheniramine, Phenylephrine, and Methscopolamine 329
Chlor-Mes-D *See* Chlorpheniramine, Phenylephrine, and Methscopolamine 329
2-Chlorodeoxyadenosine *See* Cladribine 360
Chloromag® *See* Magnesium Chloride 965
Chloromycetin® (Can) *See* Chloramphenicol 315
Chloromycetin® Succinate (Can) *See* Chloramphenicol 315
Chloroquine Phosphate 320
Chlorothiazide 321
Chlorpheniramine 321
Chlorpheniramine, Acetaminophen, and Pseudoephedrine *See* Acetaminophen, Chlorpheniramine, and Pseudoephedrine 40
Chlorpheniramine and Acetaminophen 322
Chlorpheniramine and Carbetapentane *See* Carbetapentane and Chlorpheniramine 272
Chlorpheniramine and Dextromethorphan *See* Dextromethorphan and Chlorpheniramine 449
Chlorpheniramine and Phenylephrine 323
Chlorpheniramine and Pseudoephedrine 325
Chlorpheniramine, Carbetapentane, and Phenylephrine *See* Carbetapentane, Phenylephrine, and Chlorpheniramine 274
Chlorpheniramine, Dextromethorphan, Phenylephrine, and Guaifenesin *See* Dextromethorphan, Chlorpheniramine, Phenylephrine, and Guaifenesin 450
Chlorpheniramine, Ephedrine, Phenylephrine, and Carbetapentane 326
Chlorpheniramine Maleate *See* Chlorpheniramine 321
Chlorpheniramine Maleate and Dextromethorphan Hydrobromide *See* Dextromethorphan and Chlorpheniramine 449
Chlorpheniramine Maleate and Hydrocodone Bitartrate *See* Hydrocodone and Chlorpheniramine 778
Chlorpheniramine Maleate and Phenylephrine Hydrochloride *See* Chlorpheniramine and Phenylephrine 323
Chlorpheniramine Maleate and Pseudoephedrine Hydrochloride *See* Chlorpheniramine and Pseudoephedrine 325
Chlorpheniramine Maleate, Dihydrocodeine Bitartrate, and Phenylephrine Hydrochloride *See* Dihydrocodeine, Chlorpheniramine, and Phenylephrine 469
Chlorpheniramine Maleate, Phenylephrine Hydrochloride, and Guaifenesin *See* Chlorpheniramine, Phenylephrine, and Guaifenesin 329
Chlorpheniramine Maleate, Pseudoephedrine Hydrochloride, and Dextromethorphan Hydrobromide *See* Chlorpheniramine, Pseudoephedrine, and Dextromethorphan 333
Chlorpheniramine, Phenylephrine, and Dextromethorphan 327
Chlorpheniramine, Phenylephrine, and Guaifenesin 329
Chlorpheniramine, Phenylephrine, and Hydrocodone *See* Phenylephrine, Hydrocodone, and Chlorpheniramine 1277
Chlorpheniramine, Phenylephrine, and Methscopolamine 329
Chlorpheniramine, Phenylephrine, and Phenyltoloxamine 331
Chlorpheniramine, Phenylephrine, Codeine, and Potassium Iodide 332
Chlorpheniramine, Pseudoephedrine, and Acetaminophen *See* Acetaminophen, Chlorpheniramine, and Pseudoephedrine 40
Chlorpheniramine, Pseudoephedrine, and Codeine 332
Chlorpheniramine, Pseudoephedrine, and Dextromethorphan 333
Chlorpheniramine, Pseudoephedrine, and Dihydrocodeine *See* Pseudoephedrine, Dihydrocodeine, and Chlorpheniramine 1371
Chlorpheniramine, Pseudoephedrine, and Hydrocodone *See* Pseudoephedrine, Hydrocodone, and Chlorpheniramine 1372
Chlorpheniramine, Pseudoephedrine, and Methscopolamine 334
Chlorpheniramine, Pyrilamine, and Phenylephrine 335
Chlorpheniramine Tannate and Phenylephrine Tannate *See* Chlorpheniramine and Phenylephrine 323
Chlorpheniramine Tannate and Pseudoephedrine Tannate *See* Chlorpheniramine and Pseudoephedrine 325
Chlorpheniramine Tannate, Phenylephrine Tannate, and Guaifenesin *See* Chlorpheniramine, Phenylephrine, and Guaifenesin 329
Chlorpheniramine Tannate, Pseudoephedrine Tannate, and Dextromethorphan Tannate *See* Chlorpheniramine, Pseudoephedrine, and Dextromethorphan 333
Chlorphen [OTC] *See* Chlorpheniramine 321
ChlorproMAZINE 336
Chlorpromazine Hydrochloride *See* ChlorproMAZINE 336
ChlorproPAMIDE 340
Chlor-Tan A 12 [DSC] *See* Chlorpheniramine, Pyrilamine, and Phenylephrine 335
Chlorthalidone 340
Chlorthalidone and Atenolol *See* Atenolol and Chlorthalidone 150
Chlorthalidone and Clonidine *See* Clonidine and Chlorthalidone 380
Chlor-Trimeton® [OTC] *See* Chlorpheniramine 321
Chlor-Tripolon® (Can) *See* Chlorpheniramine 321

Chlor-Tripolon ND® (Can) *See* Loratadine and Pseudoephedrine 948
Chlorzoxazone 341
Cholal modificado (Mex) *See* Magnesium Sulfate 966
Cholecalciferol 341
Cholecalciferol and Alendronate *See* Alendronate and Cholecalciferol 62
Cholestyramine Resin 341
Choline Magnesium Trisalicylate 342
Chooz® [OTC] *See* Calcium Carbonate 254
Choragon (Mex) *See* Chorionic Gonadotropin (Human) 342
Choriogonadotropin Alfa *See* Chorionic Gonadotropin (Recombinant) 343
Choriomon (Mex) *See* Chorionic Gonadotropin (Human) 342
Chorionic Gonadotropin (Human) 342
Chorionic Gonadotropin (Recombinant) 343
Chronovera® (Can) *See* Verapamil 1665
CI-1008 *See* Pregabalin 1332
Cialis® *See* Tadalafil 1534
Ciclesonide 343
Cicloferon (Mex) *See* Acyclovir 49
Ciclonal (Mex) *See* Doxycycline 509
Cidecin *See* DAPTOmycin 418
Cidofovir 344
Cilest (Mex) *See* Ethinyl Estradiol and Norgestimate 600
Cilostazol 344
Ciloxan® *See* Ciprofloxacin 346
Cimetase (Mex) *See* Cimetidine 345
Cimetidine 345
Cimogal (Mex) *See* Ciprofloxacin 346
Cimzia® *See* Certolizumab Pegol 307
Cina (Mex) *See* Levofloxacin 913
Cinacalcet 345
Cinacalcet Hydrochloride *See* Cinacalcet 345
Cipan (Mex) *See* Cetirizine and Pseudoephedrine 309
Cipralex® (Can) *See* Citalopram 354
Cipro® *See* Ciprofloxacin 346
Cipro® XL (Can) *See* Ciprofloxacin 346
Ciprobac (Mex) *See* Ciprofloxacin 346
Ciproflox (Mex) *See* Ciprofloxacin 346
Ciprofloxacin 346
Ciprofloxacin Hydrochloride *See* Ciprofloxacin 346
Ciproton (Mex) *See* Pantoprazole 1221
Ciproxina (Mex) *See* Ciprofloxacin 346
Cipro® XR *See* Ciprofloxacin 346
Cisapride U.S. - Available Via Limited-Access Protocol Only 353
Cisatracurium 353
Cisatracurium Besylate *See* Cisatracurium 353
CISplatin 354
13-cis-Retinoic Acid *See* Isotretinoin 871
Cisticid (Mex) *See* Praziquantel 1324
Citalopram 354
Citalopram Hydrobromide *See* Citalopram 354
Citalopram-ODAN (Can) *See* Citalopram 354
Citomid RU (Mex) *See* VinCRIStine 1673
Citox (Mex) *See* Citalopram 354
Citracal® Kosher [OTC] *See* Calcium Citrate 257
CL-118,532 *See* Triptorelin 1635
CI-719 *See* Gemfibrozil 711
CL-184116 *See* Porfimer 1314
CL-232315 *See* Mitoxantrone 1061
Cladribine 360
Claforan® *See* Cefotaxime 295
Clamoxin (Mex) *See* Amoxicillin and Clavulanate Potassium 115
Claravis™ *See* Isotretinoin 871
Clariflu (Mex) *See* Loratadine and Pseudoephedrine 948
Clarifriol (Mex) *See* Loratadine and Pseudoephedrine 948
Clarinex® *See* Desloratadine 430
Clarinex-D® 12 Hour *See* Desloratadine and Pseudoephedrine 431
Clarinex-D® 24 Hour *See* Desloratadine and Pseudoephedrine 431
Clarithromycin 360
Clarithromycin, Lansoprazole, and Amoxicillin *See* Lansoprazole, Amoxicillin, and Clarithromycin 897
Claritin® (Can) *See* Loratadine 946
Claritin® 24 Hour Allergy [OTC] *See* Loratadine 946
Claritin-D® 12 Hour Allergy & Congestion [OTC] *See* Loratadine and Pseudoephedrine 948
Claritin-D® 24 Hour Allergy & Congestion [OTC] *See* Loratadine and Pseudoephedrine 948
Claritin® Allergic Decongestant (Can) *See* Oxymetazoline 1208
Claritin® Children's Allergy [OTC] *See* Loratadine 946
Claritin® Children's [OTC] *See* Loratadine 946

Claritin® Extra (Can) *See* Loratadine and Pseudoephedrine ... 948
Claritin® Hives Relief [OTC] *See* Loratadine ... 946
Claritin® Kids (Can) *See* Loratadine ... 946
Claritin® Liberator (Can) *See* Loratadine and Pseudoephedrine ... 948
Clarityne (Mex) *See* Loratadine ... 946
Clarus™ (Can) *See* Isotretinoin ... 871
Clavant (Mex) *See* Amoxicillin and Clavulanate Potassium ... 115
Clavipen (Mex) *See* Amoxicillin and Clavulanate Potassium ... 115
Clavucyd (Mex) *See* Amoxicillin and Clavulanate Potassium ... 115
Clavulanic Acid and Amoxicillin *See* Amoxicillin and Clavulanate Potassium ... 115
Clavulin® (Can) *See* Amoxicillin and Clavulanate Potassium ... 115
Clavuser (Mex) *See* Amoxicillin and Clavulanate Potassium ... 115
Clear eyes® for Dry Eyes and ACR Relief [OTC] *See* Naphazoline ... 1101
Clear eyes® for Dry Eyes and Redness Relief [OTC] *See* Naphazoline ... 1101
Clear eyes® Redness Relief [OTC] *See* Naphazoline ... 1101
Clear eyes® Seasonal Relief [OTC] *See* Naphazoline ... 1101
Clemastine ... 361
Clemastine Fumarate *See* Clemastine ... 361
Cleocin® *See* Clindamycin ... 363
Cleocin HCl® *See* Clindamycin ... 363
Cleocin Pediatric® *See* Clindamycin ... 363
Cleocin Phosphate® *See* Clindamycin ... 363
Cleocin T® *See* Clindamycin ... 363
Cleocin® Vaginal Ovule *See* Clindamycin ... 363
Clexane (Mex) *See* Enoxaparin ... 537
Clidets (Mex) *See* Clindamycin ... 363
Clidinium and Chlordiazepoxide ... 362
Climaderm (Mex) *See* Estradiol ... 576
Climara® *See* Estradiol ... 576
Clinamsa (Mex) *See* Clindamycin ... 363
Clindagel® *See* Clindamycin ... 363
ClindaMax® *See* Clindamycin ... 363
Clindamycin ... 363
Clindamycin and Tretinoin ... 364
Clindamycin Hydrochloride *See* Clindamycin ... 363
Clindamycin Injection, USP (Can) *See* Clindamycin ... 363
Clindamycin Palmitate *See* Clindamycin ... 363
Clindamycin Phosphate *See* Clindamycin ... 363
Clindamycin Phosphate and Tretinoin *See* Clindamycin and Tretinoin ... 364
ClindaReach™ *See* Clindamycin ... 363
Clindesse™ *See* Clindamycin ... 363
Clindoxyl® (Can) *See* Clindamycin ... 363
Clinoril® *See* Sulindac ... 1523
Clirbest (Mex) *See* Acyclovir ... 49
Clison (Mex) *See* Sulindac ... 1523
Clobazam ... 364
Clobazam-10 (Can) *See* Clobazam ... 364
Clofarabine ... 367
Clofarex *See* Clofarabine ... 367
Clolar™ *See* Clofarabine ... 367
Clomid® *See* ClomiPHENE ... 368
ClomiPHENE ... 368
Clomiphene Citrate *See* ClomiPHENE ... 368
ClomiPRAMINE ... 368
Clomipramine Hydrochloride *See* ClomiPRAMINE ... 368
Clonapam (Can) *See* ClonazePAM ... 373
Clonapilep (Mex) *See* ClonazePAM ... 373
ClonazePAM ... 373
CloNIDine ... 377
Clonidine and Chlorthalidone ... 380
Clonidine Hydrochloride *See* CloNIDine ... 377
Clopidogrel ... 380
Clopidogrel Bisulfate *See* Clopidogrel ... 380
Clopixol® (Can) *See* Zuclopenthixol ... 1712
Clopixol-Acuphase® (Can) *See* Zuclopenthixol ... 1712
Clopixol® Depot (Can) *See* Zuclopenthixol ... 1712
Clopsine (Mex) *See* Clozapine ... 386
Cloramfeni Ofteno (Mex) *See* Chloramphenicol ... 315
Cloran (Mex) *See* Chloramphenicol ... 315
Clorazepate ... 384
Clorazepate Dipotassium *See* Clorazepate ... 384
Clordil (Mex) *See* Chloramphenicol ... 315
Clorixan (Mex) *See* Acyclovir ... 49
Cloro-Trimeton (Mex) *See* Chlorpheniramine ... 321
Clorpres® *See* Clonidine and Chlorthalidone ... 380
Clostedal (Mex) *See* CarBAMazepine ... 265
Clozapine ... 386

Clozaril® See Clozapine 386
Clozer (Mex) See ClonazePAM 373
Clyvorax (Mex) See Acyclovir 49
CMA-676 See Gemtuzumab Ozogamicin 713
CNJ-016™ See Vaccinia Immune Globulin (Intravenous) 1639
CoActifed® (Can) See Triprolidine, Pseudoephedrine, and Codeine 1635
CO Alendronate (Can) See Alendronate 59
Co-Aprovel (Mex) See Irbesartan and Hydrochlorothiazide 856
CO Azithromycin (Can) See Azithromycin 163
CO Bicalutamide (Can) See Bicalutamide 188
CO Buspirone (Can) See BusPIRone 223
CO Cabergoline (Can) See Cabergoline 248
Cocaine 392
Cocaine Hydrochloride See Cocaine 392
CO Ciprofloxacin (Can) See Ciprofloxacin 346
CO Citalopram (Can) See Citalopram 354
CO Clomipramine (Can) See ClomiPRAMINE 368
CO Clonazepam (Can) See ClonazePAM 373
Codal-DM [OTC] See Phenylephrine, Pyrilamine, and Dextromethorphan 1278
Codeine 394
Codeine, Acetaminophen, Butalbital, and Caffeine See Butalbital, Acetaminophen, Caffeine, and Codeine 232
Codeine and Acetaminophen See Acetaminophen and Codeine 34
Codeine and Butalbital Compound See Butalbital, Aspirin, Caffeine, and Codeine 242
Codeine and Guaifenesin See Guaifenesin and Codeine 738
Codeine and Promethazine See Promethazine and Codeine 1349
Codeine and Pseudoephedrine See Pseudoephedrine and Codeine 1368
Codeine, Aspirin, and Carisoprodol See Carisoprodol, Aspirin, and Codeine 284
Codeine, Butalbital, Aspirin, and Caffeine See Butalbital, Aspirin, Caffeine, and Codeine . 242
Codeine, Chlorpheniramine, and Pseudoephedrine See Chlorpheniramine, Pseudoephedrine, and Codeine 332
Codeine, Chlorpheniramine, Phenylephrine, and Potassium Iodide See Chlorpheniramine, Phenylephrine, Codeine, and Potassium Iodide 332
Codeine Contin® (Can) See Codeine 394
Codeine, Doxylamine, and Acetaminophen See Acetaminophen, Codeine, and Doxylamine 41
Codeine, Guaifenesin, and Pseudoephedrine See Guaifenesin, Pseudoephedrine, and Codeine 747
Codeine Phosphate See Codeine 394
Codeine Phosphate and Pseudoephedrine Hydrochloride See Pseudoephedrine and Codeine 1368
Codeine, Promethazine, and Phenylephrine See Promethazine, Phenylephrine, and Codeine 1350
Codeine, Pseudoephedrine, and Triprolidine See Triprolidine, Pseudoephedrine, and Codeine 1635
Codeine Sulfate See Codeine 394
Codeine, Triprolidine, and Pseudoephedrine See Triprolidine, Pseudoephedrine, and Codeine 1635
Coderit (Mex) See Codeine 394
Codiclear® DH [DSC] See Hydrocodone and Guaifenesin 779
codimal® DM [OTC] See Phenylephrine, Pyrilamine, and Dextromethorphan 1278
CoDiovan (Mex) See Valsartan and Hydrochlorothiazide 1652
Codituss DM [OTC] See Phenylephrine, Pyrilamine, and Dextromethorphan 1278
Coedarone (Mex) See Amiodarone 89
CO Enalapril (Can) See Enalapril 531
Co-Fluconazole (Can) See Fluconazole 635
CO Fluoxetine (Can) See FLUoxetine 650
Cogentin® See Benztropine 183
Co-Gesic® [DSC] See Hydrocodone and Acetaminophen 777
CO Glimepiride (Can) See Glimepiride 723
Cognex® See Tacrine 1531
CO Ipra-Sal (Can) See Ipratropium and Albuterol 854
Col-Alphar (Mex) See Pravastatin 1321
Colazal® See Balsalazide 170
ColBenemid See Colchicine and Probenecid 398
Colchicine 396
Colchicine and Probenecid 398
Colchiquim (Mex) See Colchicine 396
Coldaid (Mex) See Phenylephrine 1273
Coldamine See Chlorpheniramine, Pseudoephedrine, and Methscopolamine 334
Coldcough See Pseudoephedrine, Dihydrocodeine, and Chlorpheniramine 1371
Coldcough HC [DSC] See Pseudoephedrine, Hydrocodone, and Chlorpheniramine 1372
Coldcough PD See Dihydrocodeine, Chlorpheniramine, and Phenylephrine 469
Coldmist DM [DSC] See Guaifenesin, Pseudoephedrine, and Dextromethorphan 748
Colesevelam 398
Colesken (Mex) See Simvastatin 1486
Colestid® See Colestipol 399
Colestipol 399

Colestipol Hydrochloride *See* Colestipol ... 399
CO Levetiracetam (Can) *See* Levetiracetam ... 905
CO Lisinopril (Can) *See* Lisinopril ... 934
Collifrin (Mex) *See* Oxymetazoline ... 1208
Colliprol (Mex) *See* Propranolol ... 1355
Colocort® *See* Hydrocortisone ... 785
CO Lovastatin (Can) *See* Lovastatin ... 956
Colpradin (Mex) *See* Pravastatin ... 1321
Colyte® *See* Polyethylene Glycol-Electrolyte Solution ... 1310
Combantrin™ (Can) *See* Pyrantel Pamoate ... 1373
CombiPatch® *See* Estradiol and Norethindrone ... 579
Combipres® [DSC] *See* Clonidine and Chlorthalidone ... 380
Combivent® *See* Ipratropium and Albuterol ... 854
Combivir® *See* Zidovudine and Lamivudine ... 1696
CO Meloxicam (Can) *See* Meloxicam ... 982
Comhist® [DSC] *See* Chlorpheniramine, Phenylephrine, and Phenyltoloxamine ... 331
CO Mirtazapine (Can) *See* Mirtazapine ... 1058
Commit® [OTC] *See* Nicotine ... 1133
Common Hops *See* Hops (Humulus lupulus) ... 770
Compazine® (Can) *See* Prochlorperazine ... 1341
Compound E *See* Cortisone ... 401
Compound F *See* Hydrocortisone ... 785
Compound S *See* Zidovudine ... 1695
Compound W® One-Step Wart Remover for Feet [OTC] *See* Salicylic Acid ... 1454
Compound W® One-Step Wart Remover for Kids [OTC] *See* Salicylic Acid ... 1454
Compound W® One-Step Wart Remover [OTC] *See* Salicylic Acid ... 1454
Compound W® [OTC] *See* Salicylic Acid ... 1454
Compoz® Nighttime Sleep Aid [OTC] *See* DiphenhydrAMINE ... 481
Compro™ *See* Prochlorperazine ... 1341
Comtan® *See* Entacapone ... 538
Comtrex® Flu Therapy Nighttime [OTC] *See* Acetaminophen, Chlorpheniramine, and Pseudoephedrine ... 40
Comtrex® Sore Throat Maximum Strength [OTC] *See* Acetaminophen ... 30
Comvax® *See* Haemophilus b Conjugate and Hepatitis B Vaccine ... 752
Conal *See* Chlorpheniramine, Pyrilamine, and Phenylephrine ... 335
Conazol (Mex) *See* Ketoconazole ... 876
Concerta® *See* Methylphenidate ... 1024
Concor (Mex) *See* Bisoprolol ... 190
Coneflower *See* Echinacea (Echinacea purpurea, Echinacea angustifolia) ... 523
Congestac® [OTC] *See* Guaifenesin and Pseudoephedrine ... 744
Conivaptan ... 400
Conivaptan Hydrochloride *See* Conivaptan ... 400
Conjugated Estrogen *See* Estrogens (Conjugated/Equine) ... 582
Conjugated Estrogen and Methyltestosterone *See* Estrogens (Esterified) and Methyltestosterone ... 587
CO Norfloxacin (Can) *See* Norfloxacin ... 1151
Constulose *See* Lactulose ... 886
Contac® Cold 12 Hour Relief Non Drowsy (Can) *See* Pseudoephedrine ... 1367
Contac® Cold and Sore Throat, Non Drowsy, Extra Strength (Can) *See* Acetaminophen and Pseudoephedrine ... 37
Contac® Cold-Chest Congestion, Non Drowsy, Regular Strength (Can) *See* Guaifenesin and Pseudoephedrine ... 744
Contac® Cold + Flu Maximum Strength Non-Drowsy [OTC] *See* Acetaminophen and Phenylephrine ... 36
Contac® Complete (Can) *See* Acetaminophen, Dextromethorphan, and Pseudoephedrine ... 43
Contac® Cough, Cold and Flu Day & Night™ (Can) *See* Acetaminophen, Dextromethorphan, and Pseudoephedrine ... 43
Controlip (Mex) *See* Fenofibrate ... 620
CO Paroxetine (Can) *See* PARoxetine ... 1226
Copaxone® *See* Glatiramer Acetate ... 722
COPD *See* Dyphylline and Guaifenesin ... 522
Copegus® *See* Ribavirin ... 1417
CO Pioglitazone (Can) *See* Pioglitazone ... 1297
Copolymer-1 *See* Glatiramer Acetate ... 722
CO Pravastatin (Can) *See* Pravastatin ... 1321
CO Ramipril (Can) *See* Ramipril ... 1395
CO Ranitidine (Can) *See* Ranitidine ... 1399
Cordarone® *See* Amiodarone ... 89
Cordilat (Mex) *See* NIFEdipine ... 1136
Cordron-D NR [DSC] *See* Carbinoxamine and Pseudoephedrine ... 280
Coreg® *See* Carvedilol ... 286
Coreg CR® *See* Carvedilol ... 286
Co-Renitec (Mex) *See* Enalapril and Hydrochlorothiazide ... 536
Corfen DM *See* Chlorpheniramine, Phenylephrine, and Dextromethorphan ... 327
Corgard® *See* Nadolol ... 1090
Coricidin HBP® Chest Congestion and Cough [OTC] *See* Guaifenesin and Dextromethorphan ... 739

Coricidin HBP® Cold and Flu [OTC] *See* Chlorpheniramine and Acetaminophen 322
Coricidin® HBP Cough & Cold [OTC] *See* Dextromethorphan and Chlorpheniramine 449
CO Risperidone (Can) *See* Risperidone 1425
Corlopam® *See* Fenoldopam 623
Coronex® (Can) *See* Isosorbide Dinitrate 866
Corpotasin (Mex) *See* Potassium Chloride 1315
Cortaid® Intensive Therapy [OTC] *See* Hydrocortisone 785
Cortaid® Maximum Strength [OTC] *See* Hydrocortisone 785
Cortaid® Sensitive Skin [OTC] *See* Hydrocortisone 785
Cortamed® (Can) *See* Hydrocortisone 785
Cortef® *See* Hydrocortisone 785
Cortenema® *See* Hydrocortisone 785
Corticool® [OTC] *See* Hydrocortisone 785
Corticotropin 401
Corticotropin, Repository *See* Corticotropin 401
Cortifoam® *See* Hydrocortisone 785
Cortisol *See* Hydrocortisone 785
Cortisone 401
Cortisone Acetate *See* Cortisone 401
Cortisporin Otico (Mex) *See* Polymyxin B 1312
Cortizone®-10 Maximum Strength [OTC] *See* Hydrocortisone 785
Cortizone®-10 Plus Maximum Strength [OTC] *See* Hydrocortisone 785
Cortizone®-10 Quick Shot [OTC] *See* Hydrocortisone 785
Cortrosyn® *See* Cosyntropin 402
Corvert® *See* Ibutilide 808
Corzide® *See* Nadolol and Bendroflumethiazide 1092
CO Sertraline (Can) *See* Sertraline 1472
CO Simvastatin (Can) *See* Simvastatin 1486
Cosmegen® *See* DACTINomycin 415
Cosopt® *See* Dorzolamide and Timolol 499
CO Sotalol (Can) *See* Sotalol 1502
CO Sumatriptan (Can) *See* SUMAtriptan 1527
Cosyntropin 402
CO Temazepam (Can) *See* Temazepam 1545
CO Terbinafine (Can) *See* Terbinafine 1551
Co-Topiramate (Can) *See* Topiramate 1598
Co-Trimoxazole *See* Sulfamethoxazole and Trimethoprim 1517
Coughcold HCM [DSC] *See* Hydrocodone and Pseudoephedrine 781
Coughtuss *See* Phenylephrine, Hydrocodone, and Chlorpheniramine 1277
Coumadin® *See* Warfarin 1679
Covan® (Can) *See* Triprolidine, Pseudoephedrine, and Codeine 1635
Covaryx™ *See* Estrogens (Esterified) and Methyltestosterone 587
Covaryx™ HS *See* Estrogens (Esterified) and Methyltestosterone 587
Co-Venlafaxine XR (Can) *See* Venlafaxine 1659
Covera® (Can) *See* Verapamil 1665
Covera-HS® *See* Verapamil 1665
Coversyl® (Can) *See* Perindopril Erbumine 1254
Co-Vidarabine *See* Pentostatin 1250
Coviracil *See* Emtricitabine 530
Cozaar® *See* Losartan 952
CO Zopiclone (Can) *See* Zopiclone 1711
CP358774 *See* Erlotinib 556
C-Phen *See* Chlorpheniramine and Phenylephrine 323
C-Phen DM *See* Chlorpheniramine, Phenylephrine, and Dextromethorphan 327
CPM *See* Cyclophosphamide 408
CPM-12 *See* Chlorpheniramine 321
CPT-11 *See* Irinotecan 856
CPZ *See* ChlorproMAZINE 336
Crantex HC [DSC] *See* Hydrocodone, Phenylephrine, and Guaifenesin 783
Crantex LA *See* Guaifenesin and Phenylephrine 742
Crataegus oxyacantha *See* Hawthorn (Crataegus oxyacantha) 758
Creomulsion® Cough [OTC] *See* Dextromethorphan 448
Creomulsion® for Children [OTC] *See* Dextromethorphan 448
Creo-Terpin® [OTC] *See* Dextromethorphan 448
Crinone® *See* Progesterone 1345
Crixivan® *See* Indinavir 818
Crolom® *See* Cromolyn 402
Cromoglycic Acid *See* Cromolyn 402
Cromolyn 402
Cromolyn Sodium *See* Cromolyn 402
Cronolevel (Mex) *See* Betamethasone 184
Cronovera (Mex) *See* Verapamil 1665
Cryofaxol (Mex) *See* Cyclophosphamide 408
Cryosid (Mex) *See* Etoposide 607
Cryosolona (Mex) *See* MethylPREDNISolone 1029
Cryostatin (Mex) *See* Octreotide 1158
Cryoxet (Mex) *See* Paclitaxel 1213

Cryselle™ *See* Ethinyl Estradiol and Norgestrel 601
Crystalline Penicillin *See* Penicillin G, Parenteral, Aqueous 1241
Crystapen® (Can) *See* Penicillin G, Parenteral, Aqueous 1241
CsA *See* CycloSPORINE 409
C-Tanna 12 *See* Carbetapentane and Chlorpheniramine 272
C-Tanna 12D *See* Carbetapentane, Phenylephrine, and Pyrilamine 275
C-Time [OTC] *See* Ascorbic Acid 141
CTLA-4Ig *See* Abatacept 22
CTM *See* Chlorpheniramine 321
CTP 30 (Can) *See* Citalopram 354
CTX *See* Cyclophosphamide 408
Cubicin® *See* DAPTOmycin 418
Cuprimine® *See* Penicillamine 1239
Curyken (Mex) *See* Loratadine 946
Cutaclin 1% (Mex) *See* Clindamycin 363
Cutivate® *See* Fluticasone 668
CyA *See* CycloSPORINE 409
Cyanocobalamin 404
Cyclen® (Can) *See* Ethinyl Estradiol and Norgestimate 600
Cyclessa® *See* Ethinyl Estradiol and Desogestrel 592
Cyclizine 405
Cyclizine Hydrochloride *See* Cyclizine 405
Cyclizine Lactate *See* Cyclizine 405
Cyclobenzaprine 405
Cyclobenzaprine Hydrochloride *See* Cyclobenzaprine 405
Cyclogyl® *See* Cyclopentolate 407
Cyclomen® (Can) *See* Danazol 416
Cyclomydril® *See* Cyclopentolate and Phenylephrine 407
Cyclopentolate 407
Cyclopentolate and Phenylephrine 407
Cyclopentolate Hydrochloride *See* Cyclopentolate 407
Cyclophosphamide 408
CycloSERINE 408
Cyclosporin A *See* CycloSPORINE 409
CycloSPORINE 409
Cylate™ *See* Cyclopentolate 407
Cymbalta® *See* DULoxetine 516
Cymevene (Mex) *See* Ganciclovir 708
Cynocuatro (Mex) *See* Levothyroxine 920
Cynomel (Mex) *See* Liothyronine 928
Cyproheptadine 410
Cyproheptadine Hydrochloride *See* Cyproheptadine 410
Cystagon® *See* Cysteamine 412
Cysteamine 412
Cysteamine Bitartrate *See* Cysteamine 412
Cystospaz® *See* Hyoscyamine 799
CYT *See* Cyclophosphamide 408
Cytadren® *See* Aminoglutethimide 87
Cytarabine 412
Cytarabine (Conventional) *See* Cytarabine 412
Cytarabine Hydrochloride *See* Cytarabine 412
Cytarabine (Liposomal) 413
Cytomel® *See* Liothyronine 928
Cytosar® (Can) *See* Cytarabine 412
Cytosar-U *See* Cytarabine 412
Cytosine Arabinosine Hydrochloride *See* Cytarabine 412
Cytostasan *See* Bendamustine 179
Cytovene® *See* Ganciclovir 708
Cytoxan® (Can) *See* Cyclophosphamide 408
Cytoxan® [DSC] *See* Cyclophosphamide 408
Cytuss HC *See* Phenylephrine, Hydrocodone, and Chlorpheniramine 1277
D2E7 *See* Adalimumab 50
D3 *See* Cholecalciferol 341
D3-5™ [OTC] *See* Cholecalciferol 341
D3-50™ [OTC] *See* Cholecalciferol 341
D-3-Mercaptovaline *See* Penicillamine 1239
D-3 [OTC] *See* Cholecalciferol 341
d4T *See* Stavudine 1505
DAB389IL-2 *See* Denileukin Diftitox 425
DAB389 Interleukin-2 *See* Denileukin Diftitox 425
Dabex (Mex) *See* MetFORMIN 997
Dacarbazine 414
Dacex-DM *See* Guaifenesin, Dextromethorphan, and Phenylephrine 746
Daclizumab 414
Dacogen™ *See* Decitabine 422
DACT *See* DACTINomycin 415
DACTINomycin 415

Dalacin® C (Can) *See* Clindamycin ... 363
Dalacin® T (Can) *See* Clindamycin ... 363
Dalacin® Vaginal (Can) *See* Clindamycin ... 363
Dallergy® *See* Chlorpheniramine, Phenylephrine, and Methscopolamine ... 329
Dallergy Drops *See* Chlorpheniramine and Phenylephrine ... 323
Dallergy®-JR *See* Chlorpheniramine and Phenylephrine ... 323
Dalmane® *See* Flurazepam ... 664
d-Alpha-Gems™ [OTC] *See* Vitamin E ... 1675
d-Alpha Tocopherol *See* Vitamin E ... 1675
Danac (Mex) *See* Ondansetron ... 1180
Danaparoid ... 415
Danaparoid Sodium *See* Danaparoid ... 415
Danazol ... 416
Danocrine® (Can) *See* Danazol ... 416
Danocrine® [DSC] *See* Danazol ... 416
Dantrium® *See* Dantrolene ... 416
Dantrolene ... 416
Dantrolene Sodium *See* Dantrolene ... 416
Daonil (Mex) *See* GlyBURIDE ... 730
Dapcin *See* DAPTOmycin ... 418
Dapsoderm-X (Mex) *See* Dapsone ... 418
Dapsone ... 418
DAPTOmycin ... 418
Daranide® *See* Dichlorphenamide ... 457
Daraprim® *See* Pyrimethamine ... 1377
Darbepoetin Alfa ... 419
Darifenacin ... 419
Darifenacin Hydrobromide *See* Darifenacin ... 419
Darunavir ... 420
Darunavir Ethanolate *See* Darunavir ... 420
Darvocet A500® *See* Propoxyphene and Acetaminophen ... 1354
Darvocet-N® 50 *See* Propoxyphene and Acetaminophen ... 1354
Darvocet-N® 100 *See* Propoxyphene and Acetaminophen ... 1354
Darvon® *See* Propoxyphene ... 1353
Darvon® Compound [DSC] *See* Propoxyphene, Aspirin, and Caffeine ... 1355
Darvon-N® *See* Propoxyphene ... 1353
Dasatinib ... 420
Dasav (Mex) *See* Diltiazem ... 473
Daunomycin *See* DAUNOrubicin Hydrochloride ... 421
DAUNOrubicin Citrate (Liposomal) ... 421
DAUNOrubicin Hydrochloride ... 421
DAUNOrubicin Liposomal *See* DAUNOrubicin Citrate (Liposomal) ... 421
DaunoXome® *See* DAUNOrubicin Citrate (Liposomal) ... 421
Daxon (Mex) *See* Nitazoxanide ... 1146
Dayhist® Allergy [OTC] *See* Clemastine ... 361
Daypro® *See* Oxaprozin ... 1193
Daytrana™ *See* Methylphenidate ... 1024
dCF *See* Pentostatin ... 1250
DDAVP® *See* Desmopressin ... 431
DDAVP® Melt (Can) *See* Desmopressin ... 431
ddC *See* Zalcitabine ... 1691
ddI *See* Didanosine ... 460
1-Deamino-8-D-Arginine Vasopressin *See* Desmopressin ... 431
Debequin C (Mex) *See* Guaifenesin and Dextromethorphan ... 739
Decadron (Mex) *See* Dexamethasone ... 436
Decadronal (Mex) *See* Dexamethasone ... 436
Deca-Durabolin® (Can) *See* Nandrolone ... 1101
Dec-Chlorphen *See* Chlorpheniramine and Phenylephrine ... 323
Dec-Chlorphen DM [DSC] *See* Chlorpheniramine, Phenylephrine, and Dextromethorphan ... 327
De-Chlor DM *See* Chlorpheniramine, Phenylephrine, and Dextromethorphan ... 327
De-Chlor DR *See* Chlorpheniramine, Phenylephrine, and Dextromethorphan ... 327
De-Chlor G [DSC] *See* Hydrocodone, Phenylephrine, and Guaifenesin ... 783
De-Chlor HC *See* Phenylephrine, Hydrocodone, and Chlorpheniramine ... 1277
Decitabine ... 422
Declomycin® *See* Demeclocycline ... 424
Deconamine® SR *See* Chlorpheniramine and Pseudoephedrine ... 325
Deconsal® II *See* Guaifenesin and Phenylephrine ... 742
Deconsal® CT *See* Phenylephrine and Pyrilamine ... 1275
Decorex (Mex) *See* Dexamethasone ... 436
Deferasirox ... 423
Deferoxamine ... 423
Deferoxamine Mesylate *See* Deferoxamine ... 423
Deflenol (Mex) *See* GuaiFENesin ... 737
Deflox (Mex) *See* Diclofenac ... 457
Dehistine *See* Chlorpheniramine, Phenylephrine, and Methscopolamine ... 329
Dehydrobenzperidol *See* Droperidol ... 513
Delatestryl® *See* Testosterone ... 1553

Delavirdine 424
Delestrogen® *See* Estradiol 576
Delsym® [OTC] *See* Dextromethorphan 448
Delta-9-tetrahydro-cannabinol *See* Dronabinol 512
Delta-9-Tetrahydrocannabinol and Cannabinol *See* Tetrahydrocannabinol and Cannabidiol 1558
Delta-9 THC *See* Dronabinol 512
Delta-D® [OTC] *See* Cholecalciferol 341
Deltacortisone *See* PredniSONE 1327
Deltadehydrocortisone *See* PredniSONE 1327
Deltahydrocortisone *See* PrednisoLONE 1326
Demadex® *See* Torsemide 1603
Demeclocycline 424
Demeclocycline Hydrochloride *See* Demeclocycline 424
Demerol® *See* Meperidine 986
Demerol HCl (Mex) *See* Meperidine 986
4-Demethoxydaunorubicin *See* IDArubicin 809
Demethylchlortetracycline *See* Demeclocycline 424
Demser® *See* Metyrosine 1044
Demulen® 30 (Can) *See* Ethinyl Estradiol and Ethynodiol Diacetate 594
Denileukin Diftitox 425
Denvar (Mex) *See* Cefixime 294
Deoxycoformycin *See* Pentostatin 1250
2′-Deoxycoformycin *See* Pentostatin 1250
Depacon® *See* Valproic Acid and Derivatives 1642
Depade® *See* Naltrexone 1099
Depakene® *See* Valproic Acid and Derivatives 1642
Depakote® *See* Valproic Acid and Derivatives 1642
Depakote® ER *See* Valproic Acid and Derivatives 1642
Depakote® Sprinkle *See* Valproic Acid and Derivatives 1642
Depen® *See* Penicillamine 1239
Deplin™ *See* Methylfolate 1022
DepoCyt® *See* Cytarabine (Liposomal) 413
DepoDur® *See* Morphine Sulfate 1077
Depo®-Estradiol *See* Estradiol 576
Depofin (Mex) *See* Iodoquinol 851
Depo-Medrol® *See* MethylPREDNISolone 1029
Depo-Prevera® (Can) *See* MedroxyPROGESTERone 975
Depo-Provera® *See* MedroxyPROGESTERone 975
Depo-Provera® Contraceptive *See* MedroxyPROGESTERone 975
depo-subQ provera 104™ *See* MedroxyPROGESTERone 975
Depotest® 100 (Can) *See* Testosterone 1553
Depo®-Testosterone *See* Testosterone 1553
Deprectal (Mex) *See* OXcarbazepine 1195
Deprenyl *See* Selegiline 1466
Dequin (Mex) *See* Guaifenesin and Dextromethorphan 739
Derimeton (Mex) *See* Chlorpheniramine 321
Dermagran® [OTC] *See* Aluminum Hydroxide 78
Dermamycin® [OTC] *See* DiphenhydrAMINE 481
Dermarest Dricort® [OTC] *See* Hydrocortisone 785
Dermarest® Psoriasis Medicated Moisturizer [OTC] *See* Salicylic Acid 1454
Dermarest® Psoriasis Medicated Scalp Treatment [OTC] *See* Salicylic Acid 1454
Dermarest® Psoriasis Medicated Shampoo/Conditioner [OTC] *See* Salicylic Acid 1454
Dermarest® Psoriasis Medicated Skin Treatment [OTC] *See* Salicylic Acid 1454
Dermarest® Psoriasis Overnight Treatment [OTC] *See* Salicylic Acid 1454
Dermarest® Psoriasis Scalp Treatment Mousse [OTC] [DSC] *See* Salicylic Acid 1454
Dermtex® HC [OTC] *See* Hydrocortisone 785
Desferal® *See* Deferoxamine 423
Desferrioxamine *See* Deferoxamine 423
Desiccated Thyroid *See* Thyroid, Desiccated 1579
Desiken (Mex) *See* Ribavirin 1417
Desipramine 426
Desipramine Hydrochloride *See* Desipramine 426
Desloratadine 430
Desloratadine and Pseudoephedrine 431
Desmethylimipramine Hydrochloride *See* Desipramine 426
Desmopressin 431
Desmopressin Acetate *See* Desmopressin 431
Desogen® *See* Ethinyl Estradiol and Desogestrel 592
Desogestrel and Ethinyl Estradiol *See* Ethinyl Estradiol and Desogestrel 592
Desoxyephedrine Hydrochloride *See* Methamphetamine 1006
Desoxyn® *See* Methamphetamine 1006
Desoxyphenobarbital *See* Primidone 1336
Desvenlafaxine 433
Desyrel® (Can) *See* TraZODone 1614
Detemir Insulin *See* Insulin Detemir 825
Detilem (Mex) *See* Dacarbazine 414

Detrol® *See* Tolterodine 1596
Detrol® LA *See* Tolterodine 1596
Detrusitol (Mex) *See* Tolterodine 1596
Detuss [DSC] *See* Pseudoephedrine, Hydrocodone, and Chlorpheniramine 1372
Devil's Shrub *See* Ginseng, Siberian (Eleutherococcus senticosus) 720
Dexabion (Mex) *See* Thiamine 1568
Dexafrin Ofteno (Mex) *See* Dexamethasone 436
Dexamethasone 436
Dexamethasone Intensol™ *See* Dexamethasone 436
Dexamethasone Sodium Phosphate *See* Dexamethasone 436
Dexasone® (Can) *See* Dexamethasone 436
Dexbrompheniramine and Pseudoephedrine 437
Dexchlorpheniramine 437
Dexchlorpheniramine Maleate *See* Dexchlorpheniramine 437
Dexchlorpheniramine Tannate, Pseudoephedrine Tannate, and Dextromethorphan Tannate *See* Chlorpheniramine, Pseudoephedrine, and Dextromethorphan 333
Dexcon-PE *See* Guaifenesin, Dextromethorphan, and Phenylephrine 746
Dexedrine® *See* Dextroamphetamine 441
Dexferrum® *See* Iron Dextran Complex 857
Dexidex (Mex) *See* Nitazoxanide 1146
Dexiron™ (Can) *See* Iron Dextran Complex 857
Dexmedetomidine 438
Dexmedetomidine Hydrochloride *See* Dexmedetomidine 438
Dexmethylphenidate 438
Dexmethylphenidate Hydrochloride *See* Dexmethylphenidate 438
Dexometorfano-Guaifenesina (Mex) *See* Guaifenesin and Dextromethorphan 739
DexPak® 10 Day TaperPak® *See* Dexamethasone 436
DexPak® TaperPak® *See* Dexamethasone 436
Dex PC *See* Chlorpheniramine, Phenylephrine, and Dextromethorphan 327
Dexrazoxane 441
Dexsul (Mex) *See* Polymyxin B 1312
Dextroamphetamine 441
Dextroamphetamine and Amphetamine 444
Dextroamphetamine Sulfate *See* Dextroamphetamine 441
Dextromethorphan 448
Dextromethorphan, Acetaminophen, and Pseudoephedrine *See* Acetaminophen, Dextromethorphan, and Pseudoephedrine 43
Dextromethorphan and Chlorpheniramine 449
Dextromethorphan and Guaifenesin *See* Guaifenesin and Dextromethorphan 739
Dextromethorphan and Promethazine *See* Promethazine and Dextromethorphan 1350
Dextromethorphan and Pseudoephedrine *See* Pseudoephedrine and Dextromethorphan 1369
Dextromethorphan, Chlorpheniramine, and Phenylephrine *See* Chlorpheniramine, Phenylephrine, and Dextromethorphan 327
Dextromethorphan, Chlorpheniramine, and Pseudoephedrine *See* Chlorpheniramine, Pseudoephedrine, and Dextromethorphan 333
Dextromethorphan, Chlorpheniramine, Phenylephrine, and Guaifenesin 450
Dextromethorphan, Guaifenesin, and Pseudoephedrine *See* Guaifenesin, Pseudoephedrine, and Dextromethorphan 748
Dextromethorphan Hydrobromide, Acetaminophen, and Phenylephrine Hydrochloride *See* Acetaminophen, Dextromethorphan, and Phenylephrine 42
Dextromethorphan Hydrobromide and Chlorpheniramine Maleate *See* Dextromethorphan and Chlorpheniramine 449
Dextromethorphan Hydrobromide, Brompheniramine Maleate, and Pseudoephedrine Hydrochloride *See* Brompheniramine, Pseudoephedrine, and Dextromethorphan 208
Dextromethorphan Tannate, Pyrilamine Tannate, and Phenylephrine Tannate *See* Phenylephrine, Pyrilamine, and Dextromethorphan 1278
Dextropropoxyphene *See* Propoxyphene 1353
DextroStat® *See* Dextroamphetamine 441
DFMO *See* Eflornithine 527
DHAD *See* Mitoxantrone 1061
DHAQ *See* Mitoxantrone 1061
DHE *See* Dihydroergotamine 470
D.H.E. 45® *See* Dihydroergotamine 470
DHPG Sodium *See* Ganciclovir 708
DHS™ Sal [OTC] *See* Salicylic Acid 1454
DHT™ [DSC] *See* Dihydrotachysterol 472
DHT™ Intensol™ [DSC] *See* Dihydrotachysterol 472
Diabenese (Mex) *See* ChlorproPAMIDE 340
Diabeta *See* GlyBURIDE 730
Diabetic Tussin C® *See* Guaifenesin and Codeine 738
Diabetic Tussin® Allergy Relief [OTC] *See* Chlorpheniramine 321
Diabetic Tussin® DM Maximum Strength [OTC] *See* Guaifenesin and Dextromethorphan 739
Diabetic Tussin® DM [OTC] *See* Guaifenesin and Dextromethorphan 739
Diabetic Tussin® EX [OTC] *See* GuaiFENesin 737
Diabinese® [DSC] *See* ChlorproPAMIDE 340
Diaβeta® *See* GlyBURIDE 730

Diaminocyclohexane Oxalatoplatinum *See* Oxaliplatin ... 1191
Diaminodiphenylsulfone *See* Dapsone ... 418
Diamode [OTC] *See* Loperamide ... 944
Diamox® (Can) *See* AcetaZOLAMIDE ... 46
Diamox® Sequels® *See* AcetaZOLAMIDE ... 46
Diamsalina (Mex) *See* Dicloxacillin ... 459
Diaperol (Mex) *See* Loperamide ... 944
Diarr-Eze (Can) *See* Loperamide ... 944
Diastabol (Mex) *See* Miglitol ... 1052
Diastat® *See* Diazepam ... 451
Diastat® AcuDial™ *See* Diazepam ... 451
Diastat® Rectal Delivery System (Can) *See* Diazepam ... 451
Diazemuls® (Can) *See* Diazepam ... 451
Diazepam ... 451
Diazepam Intensol® *See* Diazepam ... 451
Diazoxide ... 456
Dibacilina (Mex) *See* Ampicillin ... 122
Dibaprim (Mex) *See* Sulfamethoxazole and Trimethoprim ... 1517
Dibasona (Mex) *See* Dexamethasone ... 436
Dibenzyline® *See* Phenoxybenzamine ... 1270
DIC *See* Dacarbazine ... 414
Dicel™ *See* Chlorpheniramine and Pseudoephedrine ... 325
Dicel™ DM *See* Chlorpheniramine, Pseudoephedrine, and Dextromethorphan ... 333
Dichloralphenazone, Acetaminophen, and Isometheptene *See* Acetaminophen, Isometheptene, and Dichloralphenazone ... 45
Dichloralphenazone, Isometheptene, and Acetaminophen *See* Acetaminophen, Isometheptene, and Dichloralphenazone ... 45
Dichlorphenamide ... 457
Dichysterol *See* Dihydrotachysterol ... 472
Diclectin® (Can) *See* Doxylamine and Pyridoxine ... 511
Diclofenac ... 457
Diclofenac and Misoprostol ... 458
Diclofenac Epolamine *See* Diclofenac ... 457
Diclofenac Potassium *See* Diclofenac ... 457
Diclofenac Sodium *See* Diclofenac ... 457
Diclofenamide *See* Dichlorphenamide ... 457
Dicloxacillin ... 459
Dicloxacillin Sodium *See* Dicloxacillin ... 459
Dicyclomine ... 459
Dicyclomine Hydrochloride *See* Dicyclomine ... 459
Dicycloverine Hydrochloride *See* Dicyclomine ... 459
Didanosine ... 460
Didasten (Mex) *See* Didanosine ... 460
Dideoxycytidine *See* Zalcitabine ... 1691
Dideoxyinosine *See* Didanosine ... 460
Didrex® *See* Benzphetamine ... 181
Didrocal™ (Can) *See* Etidronate and Calcium ... 605
Didronel® *See* Etidronate Disodium ... 605
Diethylpropion ... 460
Diethylpropion Hydrochloride *See* Diethylpropion ... 460
Difenoxin and Atropine ... 462
Difil-G *See* Dyphylline and Guaifenesin ... 522
Difil®-G Forte *See* Dyphylline and Guaifenesin ... 522
Diflucan® *See* Fluconazole ... 635
Diflunisal ... 463
Digezanol (Mex) *See* Albendazole ... 53
Digitek® *See* Digoxin ... 463
Digoxin ... 463
Digoxin CSD (Can) *See* Digoxin ... 463
Dihematoporphyrin Ether *See* Porfimer ... 1314
Dihistine® DH [DSC] *See* Chlorpheniramine, Pseudoephedrine, and Codeine ... 332
Dihydrocodeine, Aspirin, and Caffeine ... 468
Dihydrocodeine Bitartrate, Acetaminophen, and Caffeine *See* Acetaminophen, Caffeine, and Dihydrocodeine ... 39
Dihydrocodeine Bitartrate, Phenylephrine Hydrochloride, and Chlorpheniramine Maleate *See* Phenylephrine, Hydrocodone, and Chlorpheniramine ... 1277
Dihydrocodeine Bitartrate, Pseudoephedrine Hydrochloride, and Chlorpheniramine Maleate *See* Pseudoephedrine, Dihydrocodeine, and Chlorpheniramine ... 1371
Dihydrocodeine, Chlorpheniramine, and Phenylephrine ... 469
Dihydrocodeine Compound *See* Dihydrocodeine, Aspirin, and Caffeine ... 468
Dihydrocodeine, Pseudoephedrine, and Guaifenesin ... 469
DiHydro-CP *See* Pseudoephedrine, Dihydrocodeine, and Chlorpheniramine ... 1371
Dihydroergotamine ... 470
Dihydroergotamine Mesylate *See* Dihydroergotamine ... 470
Dihydroergotoxine *See* Ergoloid Mesylates ... 551
Dihydrogenated Ergot Alkaloids *See* Ergoloid Mesylates ... 551

DiHydro-GP *See* Dihydrocodeine, Pseudoephedrine, and Guaifenesin 469
Dihydrohydroxycodeinone *See* OxyCODONE 1201
Dihydromorphinone *See* HYDROmorphone 791
Dihydrotachysterol 472
Dihydroxyanthracenedione Dihydrochloride *See* Mitoxantrone 1061
Dihydroxydeoxynorvinkaleukoblastine *See* Vinorelbine 1674
Dihydroxypropyl Theophylline *See* Dyphylline 521
Diiodohydroxyquin *See* Iodoquinol 851
Dilacoran (Mex) *See* Verapamil 1665
Dilacor® XR *See* Diltiazem 473
Dilantin® *See* Phenytoin 1280
Dilatrate®-SR *See* Isosorbide Dinitrate 866
Dilatrend (Mex) *See* Carvedilol 286
Dilaudid® *See* HYDROmorphone 791
Dilaudid-HP® *See* HYDROmorphone 791
Dilaudid-HP-Plus® (Can) *See* HYDROmorphone 791
Dilaudid® Sterile Powder (Can) *See* HYDROmorphone 791
Dilaudid-XP® (Can) *See* HYDROmorphone 791
Dilex-G *See* Dyphylline and Guaifenesin 522
Dilor® (Can) *See* Dyphylline 521
Dilor-G® *See* Dyphylline and Guaifenesin 522
Dilt-CD *See* Diltiazem 473
Diltiazem 473
Diltiazem HCl ER® (Can) *See* Diltiazem 473
Diltiazem Hydrochloride *See* Diltiazem 473
Diltiazem Hydrochloride Injection (Can) *See* Diltiazem 473
Dilt-XR *See* Diltiazem 473
Dilucid (Mex) *See* Lovastatin 956
Dimacol (Mex) *See* Guaifenesin and Dextromethorphan 739
Dimaphen [OTC] *See* Brompheniramine and Pseudoephedrine 206
Dimefor (Mex) *See* MetFORMIN 997
Dimegan (Mex) *See* Loratadine 946
Dimegan D (Mex) *See* Loratadine and Pseudoephedrine 948
Dimenhidrinato (Mex) *See* DimenhyDRINATE 478
DimenhyDRINATE 478
Dimercaprol 479
Dimetapp (Mex) *See* Brompheniramine and Pseudoephedrine 206
Dimetapp® Children's Long Acting Cough Plus Cold [OTC] *See* Dextromethorphan and Chlorpheniramine 449
Dimetapp® Children's Nighttime Cold & Congestion [OTC] *See* Diphenhydramine and Phenylephrine 485
Dimetapp® ND Children's [OTC] *See* Loratadine 946
Dimetapp® Toddler's [OTC] *See* Phenylephrine 1273
β,β-Dimethylcysteine *See* Penicillamine 1239
Dimethyl Sulfoxide 480
Dimethyl Sulfoxide Irrigation, USP (Can) *See* Dimethyl Sulfoxide 480
Dimethyl Triazeno Imidazole Carboxamide *See* Dacarbazine 414
Dimicaps (Mex) *See* DimenhyDRINATE 478
Dimodan (Mex) *See* Disopyramide 488
Dimopen (Mex) *See* Amoxicillin 112
Dinate® (Can) *See* DimenhyDRINATE 478
Dinoprostone 480
Diocaine® (Can) *See* Proparacaine 1352
Diocarpine (Can) *See* Pilocarpine 1290
Diochloram® (Can) *See* Chloramphenicol 315
Diodex® (Can) *See* Dexamethasone 436
Diodoquin® (Can) *See* Iodoquinol 851
Diogent® (Can) *See* Gentamicin 714
Diomycin® (Can) *See* Erythromycin 557
Dionephrine® (Can) *See* Phenylephrine 1273
Diopentolate® (Can) *See* Cyclopentolate 407
Diopred® (Can) *See* PrednisoLONE 1326
Dioptic's Atropine Solution (Can) *See* Atropine 158
Dioptimyd® (Can) *See* Sulfacetamide and Prednisolone 1516
Diotame® [OTC] *See* Bismuth 189
Diotrope® (Can) *See* Tropicamide 1636
Diovan® *See* Valsartan 1650
Diovan HCT® *See* Valsartan and Hydrochlorothiazide 1652
Diovol Plus® (Can) *See* Aluminum Hydroxide, Magnesium Hydroxide, and Simethicone 78
Dipentum® *See* Olsalazine 1173
Diphen® AF [OTC] *See* DiphenhydrAMINE 481
Diphenhist [OTC] *See* DiphenhydrAMINE 481
DiphenhydrAMINE 481
Diphenhydramine and Acetaminophen *See* Acetaminophen and Diphenhydramine 35
Diphenhydramine and ASA *See* Aspirin and Diphenhydramine 145
Diphenhydramine and Aspirin *See* Aspirin and Diphenhydramine 145
Diphenhydramine and Phenylephrine 485

Diphenhydramine and Pseudoephedrine ... 486
Diphenhydramine Citrate *See* DiphenhydrAMINE ... 481
Diphenhydramine Citrate and Aspirin *See* Aspirin and Diphenhydramine ... 145
Diphenhydramine Hydrochloride *See* DiphenhydrAMINE ... 481
Diphenhydramine Hydrochloride and Phenylephrine Hydrochloride *See* Diphenhydramine and Phenylephrine ... 485
Diphenhydramine, Hydrocodone, and Phenylephrine *See* Hydrocodone, Phenylephrine, and Diphenhydramine ... 782
Diphenhydramine, Phenylephrine Hydrochloride, and Acetaminophen *See* Acetaminophen, Diphenhydramine, and Phenylephrine ... 44
Diphenhydramine Tannate *See* DiphenhydrAMINE ... 481
Diphenhydramine Tannate and Phenylephrine Tannate *See* Diphenhydramine and Phenylephrine ... 485
Diphen® [OTC] *See* DiphenhydrAMINE ... 481
Diphenoxylate and Atropine ... 486
Diphenylhydantoin *See* Phenytoin ... 1280
Diphtheria and Tetanus Toxoids and Acellular Pertussis Adsorbed, Hepatitis B (Recombinant) and Inactivated Poliovirus Vaccine Combined *See* Diphtheria, Tetanus Toxoids, Acellular Pertussis, Hepatitis B (Recombinant), and Poliovirus (Inactivated) Vaccine ... 487
Diphtheria CRM197 Protein *See* Pneumococcal Conjugate Vaccine, 7-Valent ... 1308
Diphtheria, Tetanus Toxoids, Acellular Pertussis, Hepatitis B (Recombinant), and Poliovirus (Inactivated) Vaccine ... 487
Diphtheria Toxoid Conjugate *See* Haemophilus b Conjugate Vaccine ... 753
Diprivan® *See* Propofol ... 1352
Diprofast (Mex) *See* Betamethasone ... 184
Diprolene® *See* Betamethasone ... 184
Diprolene® AF *See* Betamethasone ... 184
Diprolene® Glycol (Can) *See* Betamethasone ... 184
Dipronova (Mex) *See* Betamethasone ... 184
Dipropylacetic Acid *See* Valproic Acid and Derivatives ... 1642
Diprosone® (Can) *See* Betamethasone ... 184
Diprospan (Mex) *See* Betamethasone ... 184
Dipyridamole ... 488
Dipyridamole and Aspirin *See* Aspirin and Dipyridamole ... 145
Dipyridamole For Injection (Can) *See* Dipyridamole ... 488
Dirpasid (Mex) *See* Metoclopramide ... 1031
Disalicylic Acid *See* Salsalate ... 1459
Dismifen (Mex) *See* Acetaminophen ... 30
Disodium Cromoglycate *See* Cromolyn ... 402
Disodium Thiosulfate Pentahydrate *See* Sodium Thiosulfate ... 1497
d-Isoephedrine Hydrochloride *See* Pseudoephedrine ... 1367
Disopyramide ... 488
Disopyramide Phosphate *See* Disopyramide ... 488
Disulfiram ... 489
Dithioglycerol *See* Dimercaprol ... 479
Ditropan® *See* Oxybutynin ... 1199
Ditropan® XL *See* Oxybutynin ... 1199
Ditterolina (Mex) *See* Dicloxacillin ... 459
Diuril® *See* Chlorothiazide ... 321
Divalproex Sodium *See* Valproic Acid and Derivatives ... 1642
Divigel® *See* Estradiol ... 576
Dixarit® (Can) *See* CloNIDine ... 377
5071-1DL(6) *See* Megestrol ... 977
dl-Alpha Tocopherol *See* Vitamin E ... 1675
D-Mannitol *See* Mannitol ... 968
4-DMDR *See* IDArubicin ... 809
DMSA *See* Succimer ... 1511
DMSO *See* Dimethyl Sulfoxide ... 480
Dobipro (Mex) *See* Beclomethasone ... 171
Docetaxel ... 491
Docusate and Senna ... 491
Dodemina (Mex) *See* Pyridoxine ... 1376
Dofetilide ... 492
Dolac (Mex) *See* Ketorolac ... 878
Dolasetron ... 493
Dolasetron Mesylate *See* Dolasetron ... 493
Dolgic® LQ *See* Butalbital, Acetaminophen, and Caffeine ... 229
Dolgic® Plus *See* Butalbital, Acetaminophen, and Caffeine ... 229
Dolo Bedoyecta (Mex) *See* Pyridoxine ... 1376
Dolobid (Mex) *See* Diflunisal ... 463
Dologesic® *See* Acetaminophen and Phenyltoloxamine ... 36
Dolo-Neurobion (Mex) *See* Thiamine ... 1568
Dolo-Neurobion Retard (Mex) *See* Cyanocobalamin ... 404
Dolo-Pangavit (Mex) *See* Thiamine ... 1568
Dolophine® *See* Methadone ... 1001
Doloral (Can) *See* Morphine Sulfate ... 1077

Dolo-Tiaminal (Mex) *See* Thiamine 1568
Doluvital (Mex) *See* Acetaminophen 30
Dolvifen (Mex) *See* Pyridoxine 1376
Dolviran (Mex) *See* Acetaminophen 30
Dom-Alendronate (Can) *See* Alendronate 59
Dom-Amiodarone (Can) *See* Amiodarone 89
Dom-Anagrelide (Can) *See* Anagrelide 124
Dom-Azithromycin (Can) *See* Azithromycin 163
Dom-Buspirone (Can) *See* BusPIRone 223
Dom-Carbamazepine (Can) *See* CarBAMazepine 265
Dom-Ciprofloxacin (Can) *See* Ciprofloxacin 346
Dom-Citalopram (Can) *See* Citalopram 354
Dom-Clobazam (Can) *See* Clobazam 364
Dom-Diclofenac (Can) *See* Diclofenac 457
Dom-Diclofenac SR (Can) *See* Diclofenac 457
Dom-Divalproex (Can) *See* Valproic Acid and Derivatives 1642
Dom-Domperidone (Can) *See* Domperidone 493
Domer (Mex) *See* Omeprazole 1176
Dom-Fenofibrate Supra (Can) *See* Fenofibrate 620
Dom-Fluconazole (Can) *See* Fluconazole 635
Dom-Fluoxetine (Can) *See* FLUoxetine 650
Dom-Furosemide (Can) *See* Furosemide 699
Domiken (Mex) *See* Doxycycline 509
DOM-Levetiracetam (Can) *See* Levetiracetam 905
Dom-Loperamide (Can) *See* Loperamide 944
Dom-Mefenamic Acid (Can) *See* Mefenamic Acid 976
Dom-Methimazole (Can) *See* Methimazole 1010
Dom-Metoprolol (Can) *See* Metoprolol 1036
Dom-Moclobemide (Can) *See* Moclobemide 1062
Domperidone 493
Domperidone Maleate *See* Domperidone 493
Dom-Propranolol (Can) *See* Propranolol 1355
Dom-Ranitidine (Can) *See* Ranitidine 1399
Dom-Risperidone (Can) *See* Risperidone 1425
Dom-Sertraline (Can) *See* Sertraline 1472
Dom-Simvastatin (Can) *See* Simvastatin 1486
Dom-Sumatriptan (Can) *See* SUMAtriptan 1527
Dom-Temazepam (Can) *See* Temazepam 1545
Dom-Terbinafine (Can) *See* Terbinafine 1551
Dom-Topiramate (Can) *See* Topiramate 1598
DOM-Ursodiol C (Can) *See* Ursodiol 1639
Dom-Verapamil SR (Can) *See* Verapamil 1665
Dom-Zopiclone (Can) *See* Zopiclone 1711
Donatussin *See* Dextromethorphan, Chlorpheniramine, Phenylephrine, and Guaifenesin 450
Donatussin DC [DSC] *See* Hydrocodone, Phenylephrine, and Guaifenesin 783
Donatussin DM [DSC] *See* Chlorpheniramine, Phenylephrine, and Dextromethorphan 327
Donatussin Drops *See* Guaifenesin and Phenylephrine 742
Donepezil 495
Donnatal® *See* Hyoscyamine, Atropine, Scopolamine, and Phenobarbital 800
Donnatal Extentabs® *See* Hyoscyamine, Atropine, Scopolamine, and Phenobarbital 800
DOPamine 498
Dopamine Hydrochloride *See* DOPamine 498
Dopram® *See* Doxapram 499
Doral® *See* Quazepam 1378
Doribax™ *See* Doripenem 498
Doripenem 498
Dormicum (Mex) *See* Midazolam 1046
Doryx® *See* Doxycycline 509
Dorzolamide 498
Dorzolamide and Timolol 499
Dorzolamide Hydrochloride *See* Dorzolamide 498
Dosteril (Mex) *See* Lisinopril 934
Dostinex® (Can) *See* Cabergoline 248
Dostinex® [DSC] *See* Cabergoline 248
Double Tussin DM [OTC] *See* Guaifenesin and Dextromethorphan 739
Doxapram 499
Doxapram Hydrochloride *See* Doxapram 499
Doxazosin 500
Doxazosin Mesylate *See* Doxazosin 500
Doxepin 502
Doxepin Hydrochloride *See* Doxepin 502
Doxercalciferol 507
Doxil® *See* DOXOrubicin (Liposomal) 508
Doxolem (Mex) *See* DOXOrubicin (Liposomal) 508
Doxolem RU (Mex) *See* DOXOrubicin 507
Doxopeg (Mex) *See* DOXOrubicin 507
DOXOrubicin 507

Doxorubicin Hydrochloride *See* DOXOrubicin ... 507
DOXOrubicin Hydrochloride (Liposomal) *See* DOXOrubicin (Liposomal) ... 508
DOXOrubicin (Liposomal) ... 508
Doxotec (Mex) *See* DOXOrubicin ... 507
Doxtie (Mex) *See* DOXOrubicin ... 507
Doxy-100® *See* Doxycycline ... 509
Doxycin (Can) *See* Doxycycline ... 509
Doxycycline ... 509
Doxycycline Calcium *See* Doxycycline ... 509
Doxycycline Hyclate *See* Doxycycline ... 509
Doxycycline Monohydrate *See* Doxycycline ... 509
Doxylamine ... 510
Doxylamine and Pyridoxine ... 511
Doxylamine Succinate *See* Doxylamine ... 510
Doxylamine Succinate and Pyridoxine Hydrochloride *See* Doxylamine and Pyridoxine ... 511
Doxylamine Succinate, Codeine Phosphate, and Acetaminophen *See* Acetaminophen, Codeine, and Doxylamine ... 41
Doxytec (Can) *See* Doxycycline ... 509
DPA *See* Valproic Acid and Derivatives ... 1642
D-Penicillamine *See* Penicillamine ... 1239
DPH *See* Phenytoin ... 1280
D-Phen 1000 *See* Guaifenesin and Phenylephrine ... 742
Drafen (Mex) *See* DiphenhydrAMINE ... 481
Dramamine (Mex) *See* DimenhyDRINATE ... 478
Dramamine® Less Drowsy Formula [OTC] *See* Meclizine ... 974
Dramamine® [OTC] *See* DimenhyDRINATE ... 478
Drenural (Mex) *See* Bumetanide ... 211
Dretinof (Mex) *See* Pilocarpine ... 1290
Dried Smallpox Vaccine *See* Smallpox Vaccine ... 1493
Driken (Mex) *See* Iron Dextran Complex ... 857
Driminate® [OTC] *See* DimenhyDRINATE ... 478
Drinex [OTC] *See* Acetaminophen, Chlorpheniramine, and Pseudoephedrine ... 40
Drisdol® *See* Ergocalciferol ... 550
Dristan™ 12-Hour [OTC] *See* Oxymetazoline ... 1208
Dristan® Long Lasting Nasal (Can) *See* Oxymetazoline ... 1208
Dristan® N.D. (Can) *See* Acetaminophen and Pseudoephedrine ... 37
Dristan® N.D., Extra Strength (Can) *See* Acetaminophen and Pseudoephedrine ... 37
Drixoral® (Can) *See* Dexbrompheniramine and Pseudoephedrine ... 437
Drixoral® Cold & Allergy [OTC] *See* Dexbrompheniramine and Pseudoephedrine ... 437
Drixoral® Nasal (Can) *See* Oxymetazoline ... 1208
Drixoral® ND (Can) *See* Pseudoephedrine ... 1367
Dronabinol ... 512
Droperidol ... 513
Droperidol Injection, USP (Can) *See* Droperidol ... 513
Drospirenone and Estradiol ... 515
Drospirenone and Ethinyl Estradiol *See* Ethinyl Estradiol and Drospirenone ... 593
DroTuss-CP *See* Phenylephrine, Hydrocodone, and Chlorpheniramine ... 1277
Droxia® *See* Hydroxyurea ... 796
Drynalken (Mex) *See* DOPamine ... 498
DSCG *See* Cromolyn ... 402
D-Ser(But)6,Azgly10-LHRH *See* Goserelin ... 735
D-Tann *See* Diphenhydramine and Phenylephrine ... 485
D-Tann HC [DSC] *See* Hydrocodone, Phenylephrine, and Diphenhydramine ... 782
DTaP/IPV/HepB *See* Diphtheria, Tetanus Toxoids, Acellular Pertussis, Hepatitis B (Recombinant), and Poliovirus (Inactivated) Vaccine ... 487
DTIC® (Can) *See* Dacarbazine ... 414
DTO (error-prone abbreviation) *See* Opium Tincture ... 1183
D-Trp(6)-LHRH *See* Triptorelin ... 1635
Duetact™ *See* Pioglitazone and Glimepiride ... 1300
Dull-C® [OTC] *See* Ascorbic Acid ... 141
DULoxetine ... 516
Duloxetine Hydrochloride *See* DULoxetine ... 516
Duodote™ *See* Atropine and Pralidoxime ... 159
Duofilm® (Can) *See* Salicylic Acid ... 1454
Duoforte® 27 (Can) *See* Salicylic Acid ... 1454
Duomax *See* Guaifenesin and Phenylephrine ... 742
DuoNeb® *See* Ipratropium and Albuterol ... 854
DuP 753 *See* Losartan ... 952
Duplat (Mex) *See* Pentoxifylline ... 1251
Durabolin® (Can) *See* Nandrolone ... 1101
Duracef (Mex) *See* Cefadroxil ... 292
Duraclon® *See* CloNIDine ... 377
Duradrin® [DSC] *See* Acetaminophen, Isometheptene, and Dichloralphenazone ... 45
Duradryl® *See* Chlorpheniramine, Phenylephrine, and Methscopolamine ... 329
Duragesic® *See* FentaNYL ... 624
Durahist™ *See* Chlorpheniramine, Pseudoephedrine, and Methscopolamine ... 334
Durahist™ PE *See* Chlorpheniramine, Phenylephrine, and Methscopolamine ... 329

Duralith® (Can) *See* Lithium ... 938
Duramist® Plus [OTC] *See* Oxymetazoline ... 1208
Duramorph® *See* Morphine Sulfate ... 1077
Duraphen™ II DM *See* Guaifenesin, Dextromethorphan, and Phenylephrine ... 746
Duraphen™ DM [DSC] *See* Guaifenesin, Dextromethorphan, and Phenylephrine ... 746
Duraphen™ Forte *See* Guaifenesin, Dextromethorphan, and Phenylephrine ... 746
DuraTan™ Forte *See* Chlorpheniramine, Pseudoephedrine, and Dextromethorphan ... 333
Durater (Mex) *See* Famotidine ... 613
Duration® [OTC] [DSC] *See* Oxymetazoline ... 1208
Duratuss® *See* Guaifenesin and Phenylephrine ... 742
Duratuss® DA *See* Chlorpheniramine and Pseudoephedrine ... 325
Duratuss® DM *See* Guaifenesin and Dextromethorphan ... 739
Duratuss GP® *See* Guaifenesin and Phenylephrine ... 742
Duratuss® HD [DSC] *See* Hydrocodone, Phenylephrine, and Guaifenesin ... 783
Duricef® (Can) *See* Cefadroxil ... 292
Duricef® [DSC] *See* Cefadroxil ... 292
Durodor Retard (Mex) *See* TraMADol ... 1604
Durogesic (Mex) *See* FentaNYL ... 624
Dutasteride ... 521
Duvoid® (Can) *See* Bethanechol ... 186
D-Vi-Sol® (Can) *See* Cholecalciferol ... 341
DW286 *See* Gemifloxacin ... 712
Dyazide® *See* Hydrochlorothiazide and Triamterene ... 776
Dycill® (Can) *See* Dicloxacillin ... 459
Dylix *See* Dyphylline ... 521
Dymaten (Mex) *See* Loratadine ... 946
Dynacin® *See* Minocycline ... 1056
DynaCirc® (Can) *See* Isradipine ... 871
DynaCirc® CR *See* Isradipine ... 871
Dynacirc SRO (Mex) *See* Isradipine ... 871
Dynahist-ER Pediatric® [DSC] *See* Chlorpheniramine and Pseudoephedrine ... 325
Dynatuss-EX *See* Guaifenesin, Dextromethorphan, and Phenylephrine ... 746
Dynex [DSC] *See* Guaifenesin and Pseudoephedrine ... 744
Dyphylline ... 521
Dyphylline and Guaifenesin ... 522
Dyrenium® *See* Triamterene ... 1620
Dytan™ *See* DiphenhydrAMINE ... 481
E2 and DRSP *See* Drospirenone and Estradiol ... 515
E2020 *See* Donepezil ... 495
E 2080 *See* Rufinamide ... 1452
EACA *See* Aminocaproic Acid ... 87
EarSol® HC *See* Hydrocortisone ... 785
Easprin® *See* Aspirin ... 143
Ebixa® (Can) *See* Memantine ... 983
Ecaten (Mex) *See* Captopril ... 264
Echinacea angustifolia *See* Echinacea *(Echinacea purpurea, Echinacea angustifolia)* ... 523
Echinacea *(Echinacea purpurea, Echinacea angustifolia)* ... 523
Echinacea pallida *See* Echinacea *(Echinacea purpurea, Echinacea angustifolia)* ... 523
Echinacea purpurea *See* Echinacea *(Echinacea purpurea, Echinacea angustifolia)* ... 523
EC-Naprosyn® *See* Naproxen ... 1102
E. coli Asparaginase *See* Asparaginase ... 142
Econopred® Plus [DSC] *See* PrednisoLONE ... 1326
Ecotrin (Mex) *See* Aspirin ... 143
Ecotrin® Low Strength [OTC] *See* Aspirin ... 143
Ecotrin® Maximum Strength [OTC] *See* Aspirin ... 143
Ecotrin® [OTC] *See* Aspirin ... 143
Ectaprim (Mex) *See* Sulfamethoxazole and Trimethoprim ... 1517
Ectiva (Mex) *See* Sibutramine ... 1479
Ectosone (Can) *See* Betamethasone ... 184
Ed A-Hist™ *See* Chlorpheniramine and Phenylephrine ... 323
Ed A-Hist DM *See* Chlorpheniramine, Phenylephrine, and Dextromethorphan ... 327
Ed ChlorPed D *See* Chlorpheniramine and Phenylephrine ... 323
Edecam (Mex) *See* Piroxicam ... 1307
Edecrin® *See* Ethacrynic Acid ... 591
Edex® *See* Alprostadil ... 77
Ednapron (Mex) *See* PredniSONE ... 1327
Edrophonium ... 525
Edrophonium and Atropine ... 525
Edrophonium Chloride *See* Edrophonium ... 525
Edrophonium Chloride and Atropine Sulfate *See* Edrophonium and Atropine ... 525
ED-TLC *See* Phenylephrine, Hydrocodone, and Chlorpheniramine ... 1277
ED-Tuss HC *See* Phenylephrine, Hydrocodone, and Chlorpheniramine ... 1277
E.E.M.T. D.S. *See* Estrogens (Esterified) and Methyltestosterone ... 587
E.E.M.T. H.S. *See* Estrogens (Esterified) and Methyltestosterone ... 587
E.E.S.® *See* Erythromycin ... 557
Efalizumab ... 526
Efavirenz ... 526

Efavirenz, Emtricitabine, and Tenofovir ... 527
Efectine (Mex) *See* Loratadine ... 946
Efexor XR (Mex) *See* Venlafaxine ... 1659
Effer-K™ *See* Potassium Bicarbonate and Potassium Citrate ... 1315
Effexor® *See* Venlafaxine ... 1659
Effexor XR® *See* Venlafaxine ... 1659
Efficort Lipo (Mex) *See* Hydrocortisone ... 785
Eflornithine ... 527
Eflornithine Hydrochloride *See* Eflornithine ... 527
Efudex® *See* Fluorouracil ... 649
Efudix (Mex) *See* Fluorouracil ... 649
E-Gems Elite® [OTC] *See* Vitamin E ... 1675
E-Gems® [OTC] *See* Vitamin E ... 1675
E-Gems Plus® [OTC] *See* Vitamin E ... 1675
EHDP *See* Etidronate Disodium ... 605
Elantan (Mex) *See* Isosorbide Mononitrate ... 869
Elavil *See* Amitriptyline ... 90
Eldepryl® *See* Selegiline ... 1466
Electrolyte Lavage Solution *See* Polyethylene Glycol-Electrolyte Solution ... 1310
Elequine (Mex) *See* Levofloxacin ... 913
Elestrin™ *See* Estradiol ... 576
Eletriptan ... 528
Eletriptan Hydrobromide *See* Eletriptan ... 528
Eleutherococcus senticosus *See* Ginseng, Siberian *(Eleutherococcus senticosus)* ... 720
Elica (Mex) *See* Mometasone ... 1071
Eligard® *See* Leuprolide ... 901
Elipten *See* Aminoglutethimide ... 87
Elitek™ *See* Rasburicase ... 1407
Elixophyllin® *See* Theophylline ... 1562
Elixophyllin-GG® *See* Theophylline and Guaifenesin ... 1567
ElixSure® Cough [OTC] *See* Dextromethorphan ... 448
Ellence® *See* Epirubicin ... 545
Elmiron® *See* Pentosan Polysulfate Sodium ... 1250
Elocom® (Can) *See* Mometasone ... 1071
Elocon® *See* Mometasone ... 1071
Elomet (Mex) *See* Mometasone ... 1071
Elovent Twisthaler (Mex) *See* Mometasone ... 1071
Eloxatin® *See* Oxaliplatin ... 1191
Elspar® *See* Asparaginase ... 142
Eltor® (Can) *See* Pseudoephedrine ... 1367
Eltroxin® (Can) *See* Levothyroxine ... 920
Elyzol-S (Mex) *See* MetroNIDAZOLE ... 1040
Emcyt® *See* Estramustine ... 580
Emend® *See* Aprepitant ... 130
Emend® for Injection *See* Fosaprepitant ... 690
Emipastin (Mex) *See* Pravastatin ... 1321
Emo-Cort® (Can) *See* Hydrocortisone ... 785
Emsam® *See* Selegiline ... 1466
Emtricitabine ... 530
Emtricitabine and Tenofovir ... 530
Emtricitabine, Efavirenz, and Tenofovir *See* Efavirenz, Emtricitabine, and Tenofovir ... 527
Emtriva® *See* Emtricitabine ... 530
ENA 713 *See* Rivastigmine ... 1435
Enablex® *See* Darifenacin ... 419
Enalapril ... 531
Enalapril and Felodipine ... 536
Enalapril and Hydrochlorothiazide ... 536
Enalaprilat *See* Enalapril ... 531
Enalapril Maleate *See* Enalapril ... 531
Enalapril Maleate and Felodipine *See* Enalapril and Felodipine ... 536
Enalapril Maleate and Hydrochlorothiazide *See* Enalapril and Hydrochlorothiazide ... 536
Enbrel® *See* Etanercept ... 591
Encort™ *See* Hydrocortisone ... 785
EndaCof-DM *See* Brompheniramine, Pseudoephedrine, and Dextromethorphan ... 208
EndaCof [DSC] *See* Hydrocodone and Guaifenesin ... 779
EndaCof-PD *See* Brompheniramine, Pseudoephedrine, and Dextromethorphan ... 208
EndaCof-XP [DSC] *See* Hydrocodone and Guaifenesin ... 779
Endantadine® (Can) *See* Amantadine ... 79
Endocet® *See* Oxycodone and Acetaminophen ... 1205
Endodan® *See* Oxycodone and Aspirin ... 1208
Endo®-Levodopa/Carbidopa (Can) *See* Carbidopa and Levodopa ... 277
Endometrin® *See* Progesterone ... 1345
Enduron® (Can) *See* Methyclothiazide ... 1020
Enduron® [DSC] *See* Methyclothiazide ... 1020
Enerjets [OTC] *See* Caffeine ... 250
Enfuvirtide ... 537
ENG *See* Etonogestrel ... 606

Engerix-B® *See* Hepatitis B Vaccine ... 764
Eni (Mex) *See* Ciprofloxacin ... 346
Enjuvia™ *See* Estrogens (Conjugated B/Synthetic) ... 581
Enlon® (Can) *See* Edrophonium ... 525
Enlon® [DSC] *See* Edrophonium ... 525
Enlon-Plus™ [DSC] *See* Edrophonium and Atropine ... 525
Enoxaparin ... 537
Enoxaparin Injection (Can) *See* Enoxaparin ... 537
Enoxaparin Sodium *See* Enoxaparin ... 537
Enpresse™ *See* Ethinyl Estradiol and Levonorgestrel ... 595
Entacapone ... 538
Entacapone, Carbidopa, and Levodopa *See* Levodopa, Carbidopa, and Entacapone ... 911
Entacyl® (Can) *See* Piperazine ... 1303
Entecavir ... 540
Enteropride (Mex) *See* Cisapride U.S. - Available Via Limited-Access Protocol Only ... 353
Entex® HC [DSC] *See* Hydrocodone, Pseudoephedrine, and Guaifenesin ... 784
Entex® LA (Can) *See* Guaifenesin and Pseudoephedrine ... 744
Entex® PSE *See* Guaifenesin and Pseudoephedrine ... 744
Entocort® (Can) *See* Budesonide ... 210
Entocort® EC *See* Budesonide ... 210
Entrophen® (Can) *See* Aspirin ... 143
Enulose *See* Lactulose ... 886
Epamin (Mex) *See* Phenytoin ... 1280
Epaq (Mex) *See* MetroNIDAZOLE ... 1040
Eperbel-S [DSC] *See* Belladonna, Phenobarbital, and Ergotamine ... 175
Ephedra (Ephedra sinica) ... 541
Ephedra sinica *See* Ephedra (Ephedra sinica) ... 541
EPHEDrine ... 542
Ephedrine, Chlorpheniramine, Phenylephrine, and Carbetapentane *See* Chlorpheniramine, Ephedrine, Phenylephrine, and Carbetapentane ... 326
Ephedrine Sulfate *See* EPHEDrine ... 542
Epidermal Thymocyte Activating Factor *See* Aldesleukin ... 58
Epilem (Mex) *See* Epirubicin ... 545
EPINEPHrine ... 543
Epinephrine Bitartrate *See* EPINEPHrine ... 543
Epinephrine Hydrochloride *See* EPINEPHrine ... 543
EpiPen® *See* EPINEPHrine ... 543
EpiPen® Jr *See* EPINEPHrine ... 543
Epipodophyllotoxin *See* Etoposide ... 607
Epirubicin ... 545
Epirubicin Hydrochloride *See* Epirubicin ... 545
Epitol® *See* CarBAMazepine ... 265
Epival (Mex) *See* Valproic Acid and Derivatives ... 1642
Epival® I.V. (Can) *See* Valproic Acid and Derivatives ... 1642
Epivir® *See* LamiVUDine ... 888
Epivir-HBV® *See* LamiVUDine ... 888
Eplerenone ... 545
EPO *See* Epoetin Alfa ... 546
Epoetin Alfa ... 546
Epogen® *See* Epoetin Alfa ... 546
Epoprostenol ... 547
Epoprostenol Sodium *See* Epoprostenol ... 547
Eprex® (Can) *See* Epoetin Alfa ... 546
Eprosartan ... 547
Eprosartan and Hydrochlorothiazide ... 549
Eprosartan Mesylate and Hydrochlorothiazide *See* Eprosartan and Hydrochlorothiazide ... 549
Epsilon Aminocaproic Acid *See* Aminocaproic Acid ... 87
Epsom Salts *See* Magnesium Sulfate ... 966
EPT *See* Teniposide ... 1549
Eptifibatide ... 550
Epzicom® *See* Abacavir and Lamivudine ... 22
Equagesic® *See* Meprobamate and Aspirin ... 992
Equanil *See* Meprobamate ... 991
Equetro® *See* CarBAMazepine ... 265
Eranz (Mex) *See* Donepezil ... 495
Erbitux® *See* Cetuximab ... 310
Ergocaf (Mex) *See* Ergotamine ... 552
Ergocalciferol ... 550
Ergoloid Mesylates ... 551
Ergomar® *See* Ergotamine ... 552
Ergometrine Maleate *See* Ergonovine ... 552
Ergonovine ... 552
Ergonovine Maleate *See* Ergonovine ... 552
Ergotamine ... 552
Ergotamine and Caffeine ... 554
Ergotamine Tartrate *See* Ergotamine ... 552

Ergotamine Tartrate and Caffeine *See* Ergotamine and Caffeine 554
Ergotamine Tartrate, Belladonna, and Phenobarbital *See* Belladonna, Phenobarbital, and Ergotamine 175
Ergotrate® *See* Ergonovine 552
Erifor (Mex) *See* Tetracycline 1558
Erispan (Mex) *See* Betamethasone 184
Eritrocap (Mex) *See* Erythromycin 557
Eritropharma-S (Mex) *See* Erythromycin 557
Erlotinib 556
Erlotinib Hydrochloride *See* Erlotinib 556
Errin™ *See* Norethindrone 1150
Ertapenem 557
Ertapenem Sodium *See* Ertapenem 557
Erwinia Asparaginase *See* Asparaginase 142
Eryacnen 4 (Mex) *See* Erythromycin 557
Erybid™ (Can) *See* Erythromycin 557
Eryc® (Can) *See* Erythromycin 557
Eryc® [DSC] *See* Erythromycin 557
Eryderm® [DSC] *See* Erythromycin 557
Erygel® [DSC] *See* Erythromycin 557
EryPed® *See* Erythromycin 557
Ery-Tab® *See* Erythromycin 557
Erythrocin® *See* Erythromycin 557
Erythromycin 557
Erythromycin and Sulfisoxazole 563
Erythromycin Base *See* Erythromycin 557
Erythromycin Ethylsuccinate *See* Erythromycin 557
Erythromycin Lactobionate *See* Erythromycin 557
Erythromycin Stearate *See* Erythromycin 557
Erythropoiesis-Stimulating Agent (ESA) *See* Darbepoetin Alfa 419
Erythropoiesis-Stimulating Protein *See* Darbepoetin Alfa 419
Erythropoietin *See* Epoetin Alfa 546
Erythro-RX *See* Erythromycin 557
Escitalopram 564
Escitalopram Oxalate *See* Escitalopram 564
Esclim® *See* Estradiol 576
Eserine® (Can) *See* Physostigmine 1288
Eserine Salicylate *See* Physostigmine 1288
Esgic® *See* Butalbital, Acetaminophen, and Caffeine 229
Esgic-Plus™ *See* Butalbital, Acetaminophen, and Caffeine 229
Eskalith CR® [DSC] *See* Lithium 938
Eskalith® [DSC] *See* Lithium 938
Eskasole (Mex) *See* Albendazole 53
Esmolol 569
Esmolol Hydrochloride *See* Esmolol 569
Esomeprazole 570
Esomeprazole Magnesium *See* Esomeprazole 570
Esomeprazole Sodium *See* Esomeprazole 570
E.S.P.® *See* Erythromycin and Sulfisoxazole 563
Estalis® (Can) *See* Estradiol and Norethindrone 579
Estalis-Sequi® (Can) *See* Estradiol and Norethindrone 579
Estazolam 574
Ester-E™ [OTC] *See* Vitamin E 1675
Esterified Estrogen and Methyltestosterone *See* Estrogens (Esterified) and Methyltestosterone 587
Esterified Estrogens *See* Estrogens, Esterified 587
Estopein (Mex) *See* Ketorolac 878
Estovit-T (Mex) *See* Tinidazole 1585
Estrace® *See* Estradiol 576
Estraderm® *See* Estradiol 576
Estradiol 576
Estradiol Acetate *See* Estradiol 576
Estradiol and Drospirenone *See* Drospirenone and Estradiol 515
Estradiol and NGM *See* Estradiol and Norgestimate 580
Estradiol and Norethindrone 579
Estradiol and Norgestimate 580
Estradiol Cypionate *See* Estradiol 576
Estradiol Hemihydrate *See* Estradiol 576
Estradiol Transdermal *See* Estradiol 576
Estradiol Valerate *See* Estradiol 576
Estradot® (Can) *See* Estradiol 576
Estramustine 580
Estramustine Phosphate *See* Estramustine 580
Estramustine Phosphate Sodium *See* Estramustine 580
Estrasorb™ *See* Estradiol 576
Estratab® (Can) *See* Estrogens, Esterified 587
Estratest® *See* Estrogens (Esterified) and Methyltestosterone 587

Estratest® H.S. *See* Estrogens (Esterified) and Methyltestosterone 587
Estrepto-Monaxin (Mex) *See* Streptomycin 1510
Estring® *See* Estradiol 576
EstroGel® *See* Estradiol 576
Estrogenic Substances, Conjugated *See* Estrogens (Conjugated/Equine) 582
Estrogens (Conjugated A/Synthetic) 581
Estrogens (Conjugated B/Synthetic) 581
Estrogens (Conjugated/Equine) 582
Estrogens (Conjugated/Equine) and Medroxyprogesterone 583
Estrogens, Esterified 587
Estrogens (Esterified) and Methyltestosterone 587
Estropipate 588
Estrostep® Fe *See* Ethinyl Estradiol and Norethindrone 597
Eszopiclone 589
Etacortilen (Mex) *See* Dexamethasone 436
Etanercept 591
Eternal (Mex) *See* Vitamin E 1675
Ethacrynate Sodium *See* Ethacrynic Acid 591
Ethacrynic Acid 591
Ethambutol 592
Ethambutol Hydrochloride *See* Ethambutol 592
Ethinyl Estradiol and Desogestrel 592
Ethinyl Estradiol and Drospirenone 593
Ethinyl Estradiol and Ethynodiol Diacetate 594
Ethinyl Estradiol and Etonogestrel 594
Ethinyl Estradiol and Levonorgestrel 595
Ethinyl Estradiol and NGM *See* Ethinyl Estradiol and Norgestimate 600
Ethinyl Estradiol and Norelgestromin 597
Ethinyl Estradiol and Norethindrone 597
Ethinyl Estradiol and Norgestimate 600
Ethinyl Estradiol and Norgestrel 601
Ethiofos *See* Amifostine 83
Ethionamide 602
Ethmozine® (Can) *See* Moricizine 1077
Ethmozine® [DSC] *See* Moricizine 1077
Ethosuximide 603
Ethotoin 604
ETH-Oxydose™ *See* OxyCODONE 1201
Ethoxynaphthamido Penicillin Sodium *See* Nafcillin 1093
Ethyl Esters of Omega-3 Fatty Acids *See* Omega-3-Acid Ethyl Esters 1175
Ethylphenylhydantoin *See* Ethotoin 604
Ethynodiol Diacetate and Ethinyl Estradiol *See* Ethinyl Estradiol and Ethynodiol Diacetate 594
Ethyol® *See* Amifostine 83
Etibi® (Can) *See* Ethambutol 592
Etidronate and Calcium 605
Etidronate Disodium 605
Etindrax (Mex) *See* Allopurinol 67
Etodolac 606
Etodolic Acid *See* Etodolac 606
Etonco (Mex) *See* Etoposide 607
Etonogestrel 606
Etonogestrel and Ethinyl Estradiol *See* Ethinyl Estradiol and Etonogestrel 594
Etopophos® *See* Etoposide Phosphate 607
Etopos (Mex) *See* Etoposide 607
Etoposide 607
Etoposide Phosphate 607
Etrafon® (Can) *See* Amitriptyline and Perphenazine 98
Etravirine 608
Eudal®-SR *See* Guaifenesin and Pseudoephedrine 744
Euflex® (Can) *See* Flutamide 667
Euglucon® (Can) *See* GlyBURIDE 730
Eulexin® *See* Flutamide 667
Eun-haeng *See* Ginkgo (Ginkgo biloba) 715
Eutirox (Mex) *See* Levothyroxine 920
Evamist™ *See* Estradiol 576
Everone® 200 (Can) *See* Testosterone 1553
Evista® *See* Raloxifene 1391
Evoclin® *See* Clindamycin 363
Evorel (Mex) *See* Estradiol 576
Evorelconti (Mex) *See* Ethinyl Estradiol and Norethindrone 597
Evoxac® *See* Cevimeline 310
Evra® (Can) *See* Ethinyl Estradiol and Norelgestromin 597
Exacol (Mex) *See* Chloramphenicol 315
Examsa (Mex) *See* Dexamethasone 436
Excedrin® Extra Strength [OTC] *See* Acetaminophen, Aspirin, and Caffeine 39
Excedrin® Migraine [OTC] *See* Acetaminophen, Aspirin, and Caffeine 39

Excedrin® P.M. [OTC] *See* Acetaminophen and Diphenhydramine ... 35
ExeClear [DSC] *See* Hydrocodone and Guaifenesin ... 779
ExeCof *See* Guaifenesin, Dextromethorphan, and Phenylephrine ... 746
ExeCof-XP [DSC] *See* Hydrocodone and Guaifenesin ... 779
ExeFen *See* Guaifenesin and Pseudoephedrine ... 744
ExeFen-DMX *See* Guaifenesin, Pseudoephedrine, and Dextromethorphan ... 748
ExeFen-PD *See* Guaifenesin and Phenylephrine ... 742
Exel (Mex) *See* Meloxicam ... 982
Exelon® *See* Rivastigmine ... 1435
Exemestane ... 609
Exenatide ... 609
Exendin-4 *See* Exenatide ... 609
ExeTuss-DM *See* Guaifenesin, Dextromethorphan, and Phenylephrine ... 746
ExeTuss [DSC] *See* Guaifenesin and Phenylephrine ... 742
ExeTuss-GP *See* Guaifenesin and Phenylephrine ... 742
ExeTuss HC [DSC] *See* Hydrocodone, Phenylephrine, and Guaifenesin ... 783
Exforge® *See* Amlodipine and Valsartan ... 105
Exiadol (Mex) *See* Guaifenesin and Dextromethorphan ... 739
Exjade® *See* Deferasirox ... 423
Extendryl® *See* Chlorpheniramine, Phenylephrine, and Methscopolamine ... 329
Extendryl® GCP *See* Carbetapentane, Guaifenesin, and Phenylephrine ... 274
Extendryl® HC [DSC] *See* Hydrocodone and Guaifenesin ... 779
Extendryl® JR *See* Chlorpheniramine, Phenylephrine, and Methscopolamine ... 329
Extendryl PSE *See* Pseudoephedrine and Methscopolamine ... 1370
Extendryl® SR *See* Chlorpheniramine, Phenylephrine, and Methscopolamine ... 329
Extina® *See* Ketoconazole ... 876
Exubera (Mex) *See* Insulin Inhalation ... 830
Exubera® [DSC] *See* Insulin Inhalation ... 830
EYE001 *See* Pegaptanib ... 1235
Eye-Sine™ [OTC] [DSC] *See* Tetrahydrozoline ... 1560
EZ-Char™ [OTC] *See* Charcoal ... 312
Ezetimibe ... 610
Ezetimibe and Simvastatin ... 611
Ezetrol® (Can) *See* Ezetimibe ... 610
Fabrazyme® *See* Agalsidase Beta ... 52
Facicam (Mex) *See* Piroxicam ... 1307
Facidex (Mex) *See* Famotidine ... 613
Facidmol (Mex) *See* Bismuth ... 189
Factive® *See* Gemifloxacin ... 712
Factor IX ... 612
Factor IX Complex (Human) ... 612
Factor IX Concentrate *See* Factor IX ... 612
Factrel® *See* Gonadorelin ... 734
Famciclovir ... 613
Famotidine ... 613
Famotidine, Calcium Carbonate, and Magnesium Hydroxide ... 614
Famotidine Omega (Can) *See* Famotidine ... 613
Famvir® *See* Famciclovir ... 613
Fansidar® *See* Sulfadoxine and Pyrimethamine ... 1517
Fareston® *See* Toremifene ... 1603
Farmapram (Mex) *See* ALPRAZolam ... 72
Farmorubicin (Mex) *See* Epirubicin ... 545
Farmorubicin RD (Mex) *See* Epirubicin ... 545
Fasiclor (Mex) *See* Cefaclor ... 291
Fasigyn (Mex) *See* Tinidazole ... 1585
Faslodex® *See* Fulvestrant ... 698
Fasturtec® (Can) *See* Rasburicase ... 1407
Father John's® Plus [OTC] *See* Chlorpheniramine, Phenylephrine, and Dextromethorphan ... 327
FazaClo® *See* Clozapine ... 386
5-FC *See* Flucytosine ... 640
FC1157a *See* Toremifene ... 1603
Featherfew *See* Feverfew *(Tanacetum parthenium)* ... 628
Featherfoil *See* Feverfew *(Tanacetum parthenium)* ... 628
Febratic (Mex) *See* Ibuprofen ... 803
Febrifuge Plant *See* Feverfew *(Tanacetum parthenium)* ... 628
Felbamate ... 614
Felbatol® *See* Felbamate ... 614
Feldene® *See* Piroxicam ... 1307
Felodipine ... 617
Felodipine and Enalapril *See* Enalapril and Felodipine ... 536
Femara® *See* Letrozole ... 900
Femcon™ Fe *See* Ethinyl Estradiol and Norethindrone ... 597
femhrt® *See* Ethinyl Estradiol and Norethindrone ... 597
Femiprim (Mex) *See* Ascorbic Acid ... 141
Femiron® [OTC] *See* Ferrous Fumarate ... 626
Fem-Prin® [OTC] *See* Acetaminophen, Aspirin, and Caffeine ... 39

Femring® *See* Estradiol 576
Femtrace® *See* Estradiol 576
Fenesin DM IR *See* Guaifenesin and Dextromethorphan 739
Fenesin IR *See* GuaiFENesin 737
Fenesin PE IR *See* Guaifenesin and Phenylephrine 742
Fenidantoin S (Mex) *See* Phenytoin 1280
Fenitron (Mex) *See* Phenytoin 1280
Fenofibrate 620
Fenoglide™ *See* Fenofibrate 620
Fenoldopam 623
Fenoldopam Mesylate *See* Fenoldopam 623
Fenoprofen 623
Fenoprofen Calcium *See* Fenoprofen 623
Fentanest (Mex) *See* FentaNYL 624
FentaNYL 624
Fentanyl Citrate *See* FentaNYL 624
Fentanyl Citrate Injection, USP (Can) *See* FentaNYL 624
Fentanyl Hydrochloride *See* FentaNYL 624
Fentora® *See* FentaNYL 624
Feosol® [OTC] *See* Ferrous Sulfate 627
Feostat® [OTC] [DSC] *See* Ferrous Fumarate 626
Feraken (Mex) *See* Moclobemide 1062
Feratab® [OTC] *See* Ferrous Sulfate 627
Fer-Gen-Sol [OTC] *See* Ferrous Sulfate 627
Fergon® [OTC] *See* Ferrous Gluconate 627
Fer-In-Sol® (Can) *See* Ferrous Sulfate 627
Fer-In-Sol® [OTC] *See* Ferrous Sulfate 627
Fer-Iron® [OTC] *See* Ferrous Sulfate 627
Fermig (Mex) *See* SUMAtriptan 1527
Ferodan™ (Can) *See* Ferrous Sulfate 627
Fero-Grad 500® [OTC] *See* Ferrous Sulfate and Ascorbic Acid 628
Ferretts [OTC] *See* Ferrous Fumarate 626
Ferrex 150 [OTC] *See* Polysaccharide-Iron Complex 1313
Ferric Gluconate 626
Ferrlecit® *See* Ferric Gluconate 626
Ferro-Sequels® [OTC] *See* Ferrous Fumarate 626
Ferrous Fumarate 626
Ferrous Gluconate 627
Ferrous Sulfate 627
Ferrous Sulfate and Ascorbic Acid 628
Fersivag (Mex) *See* Lisinopril 934
Ferval (Mex) *See* Ferrous Fumarate 626
FeSO4 *See* Ferrous Sulfate 627
FeverALL® [OTC] *See* Acetaminophen 30
Feverfew *(Tanacetum parthenium)* 628
Fexmid™ *See* Cyclobenzaprine 405
Fexofenadine 629
Fexofenadine and Pseudoephedrine 631
Fexofenadine Hydrochloride *See* Fexofenadine 629
Filanc (Mex) *See* Acetaminophen 30
Filatil (Mex) *See* Filgrastim 632
Filgrastim 632
Fioricet® *See* Butalbital, Acetaminophen, and Caffeine 229
Fioricet® with Codeine *See* Butalbital, Acetaminophen, Caffeine, and Codeine 232
Fiorinal® *See* Butalbital, Aspirin, and Caffeine 239
Fiorinal®-C 1/2 (Can) *See* Butalbital, Aspirin, Caffeine, and Codeine 242
Fiorinal®-C 1/4 (Can) *See* Butalbital, Aspirin, Caffeine, and Codeine 242
Fiorinal® with Codeine *See* Butalbital, Aspirin, Caffeine, and Codeine 242
First™-Progesterone VGS *See* Progesterone 1345
First®-Testosterone *See* Testosterone 1553
First®-Testosterone MC *See* Testosterone 1553
Fisalamine *See* Mesalamine 994
Fish Oil *See* Omega-3-Acid Ethyl Esters 1175
Fisopred (Mex) *See* PrednisoLONE 1326
Fixoten (Mex) *See* Pentoxifylline 1251
FK506 *See* Tacrolimus 1533
Flagenase (Mex) *See* MetroNIDAZOLE 1040
Flagyl® *See* MetroNIDAZOLE 1040
Flagyl ER® *See* MetroNIDAZOLE 1040
Flamazine® (Can) *See* Silver Sulfadiazine 1485
Flamicina (Mex) *See* Ampicillin 122
Flankol (Mex) *See* Diclofenac 457
Flavan *See* Flavocoxid 633
Flavit AV (Mex) *See* Phenylephrine 1273
Flavocoxid 633
Flavonoid *See* Flavocoxid 633
Flavoxate 633

Flavoxate Hydrochloride *See* Flavoxate 633
Flebocortid (Mex) *See* Hydrocortisone 785
Flecainide 633
Flecainide Acetate *See* Flecainide 633
Flector® *See* Diclofenac 457
Fleet enema para Adulto (Mex) *See* Mineral Oil 1055
Fleet® Mineral Oil Enema [OTC] *See* Mineral Oil 1055
Flevox (Mex) *See* Levofloxacin 913
Flexeril® *See* Cyclobenzaprine 405
Flexitec (Can) *See* Cyclobenzaprine 405
Flextra 650 *See* Acetaminophen and Phenyltoloxamine 36
Flextra-DS *See* Acetaminophen and Phenyltoloxamine 36
Flixonase (Mex) *See* Fluticasone 668
Flixotide (Mex) *See* Fluticasone 668
Flkeboconadrol (Mex) *See* Hydrocortisone 785
Flolan® *See* Epoprostenol 547
Flomax® *See* Tamsulosin 1537
Flomax® CR (Can) *See* Tamsulosin 1537
Flonase® *See* Fluticasone 668
Flonorm (Mex) *See* Rifaximin 1420
Florazole® ER (Can) *See* MetroNIDAZOLE 1040
Florical® [OTC] *See* Calcium Carbonate 254
Florinef® (Can) *See* Fludrocortisone 641
Florinef® [DSC] *See* Fludrocortisone 641
Flovent® Diskus® *See* Fluticasone 668
Flovent® HFA *See* Fluticasone 668
Floxacin (Mex) *See* Norfloxacin 1151
Floxager (Mex) *See* Ciprofloxacin 346
Floxantina (Mex) *See* Ciprofloxacin 346
Floxil (Mex) *See* Ofloxacin 1159
Floxin® *See* Ofloxacin 1159
Floxin Otic Singles *See* Ofloxacin 1159
Floxstat (Mex) *See* Ofloxacin 1159
Floxuridine 634
Fluanxol® (Can) *See* Flupenthixol 658
Fluarix® *See* Influenza Virus Vaccine 820
Flubenisolone *See* Betamethasone 184
Fluconazole 635
Fluconazole Injection (Can) *See* Fluconazole 635
Fluconazole Omega (Can) *See* Fluconazole 635
Flucoxan (Mex) *See* Fluconazole 635
Flucytosine 640
Fludara® *See* Fludarabine 641
Fludarabine 641
Fludarabine Phosphate *See* Fludarabine 641
Fludrocortisone 641
Fludrocortisone Acetate *See* Fludrocortisone 641
Fluken (Mex) *See* Flutamide 667
FluLaval™ *See* Influenza Virus Vaccine 820
Flulem (Mex) *See* Flutamide 667
Flumadine® *See* Rimantadine 1422
Flumazenil 644
Flumazenil Injection (Can) *See* Flumazenil 644
Flumazenil Injection, USP (Can) *See* Flumazenil 644
Flumedil (Mex) *See* GlipiZIDE 726
FluMist® *See* Influenza Virus Vaccine 820
Flunisolide 646
Fluohydrisone Acetate *See* Fludrocortisone 641
Fluohydrocortisone Acetate *See* Fludrocortisone 641
5-Fluorocytosine *See* Flucytosine 640
Fluorodeoxyuridine *See* Floxuridine 634
9α-Fluorohydrocortisone Acetate *See* Fludrocortisone 641
Fluoroplex® *See* Fluorouracil 649
Fluorouracil 649
5-Fluorouracil *See* Fluorouracil 649
FLUoxetine 650
Fluoxetine and Olanzapine *See* Olanzapine and Fluoxetine 1165
Fluoxetine Hydrochloride *See* FLUoxetine 650
Fluoxymesterone 657
Fluozoid (Mex) *See* Ethosuximide 603
Flupazine (Mex) *See* Trifluoperazine 1624
Flupenthixol 658
Flupenthixol Decanoate *See* Flupenthixol 658
Flupenthixol Dihydrochloride *See* Flupenthixol 658
Fluphenazine 660
Fluphenazine Decanoate *See* Fluphenazine 660
Flurazepam 664

Flurazepam Hydrochloride *See* Flurazepam 664
Flurbiprofen 667
Flurbiprofen Sodium *See* Flurbiprofen 667
5-Flurocytosine *See* Flucytosine 640
Flutamide 667
Fluticasone 668
Fluticasone and Salmeterol 674
Fluticasone Furoate *See* Fluticasone 668
Fluticasone Propionate *See* Fluticasone 668
Fluticasone Propionate and Salmeterol Xinafoate *See* Fluticasone and Salmeterol 674
Fluvastatin 676
Fluviatol NF (Mex) *See* Phenylephrine 1273
Fluviral S/F® (Can) *See* Influenza Virus Vaccine 820
Fluvirin® *See* Influenza Virus Vaccine 820
Fluvoxamine 678
Fluzone® *See* Influenza Virus Vaccine 820
FNI 2B (Mex) *See* Interferon Alfa-2b 844
Focalin® *See* Dexmethylphenidate 438
Focalin® XR *See* Dexmethylphenidate 438
Folacin *See* Folic Acid 684
Folacin-800 [OTC] *See* Folic Acid 684
Folate *See* Folic Acid 684
Folic Acid 684
Folivital (Mex) *See* Folic Acid 684
Fomepizole 685
Fomiken (Mex) *See* Phenytoin 1280
Foradil® (Can) *See* Formoterol 686
Foradil® Aerolizer® *See* Formoterol 686
Forken (Mex) *See* Amiodarone 89
Formoterol 686
Formoterol Fumarate *See* Formoterol 686
Formoterol Fumarate Dihydrate *See* Formoterol 686
Formulation R™ [OTC] *See* Phenylephrine 1273
Formulex® (Can) *See* Dicyclomine 459
Fortamet® *See* MetFORMIN 997
Fortaz® *See* Ceftazidime 298
Forteo® *See* Teriparatide 1553
Fortical® *See* Calcitonin 253
Fortovase (Mex) *See* Saquinavir 1461
Fortum (Mex) *See* Ceftazidime 298
Fosamax® *See* Alendronate 59
Fosamax Plus (Mex) *See* Alendronate and Cholecalciferol 62
Fosamax Plus D™ *See* Alendronate and Cholecalciferol 62
Fosamprenavir 689
Fosamprenavir Calcium *See* Fosamprenavir 689
Fosaprepitant 690
Fosaprepitant Dimeglumine *See* Fosaprepitant 690
Fosavance (Can) *See* Alendronate and Cholecalciferol 62
Foscarnet 690
Foscavir® *See* Foscarnet 690
Fosfomycin 691
Fosfomycin Tromethamine *See* Fosfomycin 691
Fosinopril 691
Fosinopril and Hydrochlorothiazide 692
Fosinopril Sodium *See* Fosinopril 691
Fosphenytoin 692
Fosphenytoin Sodium *See* Fosphenytoin 692
Fosrenol® *See* Lanthanum 898
Fossil Tree *See* Ginkgo (Ginkgo biloba) 715
Fot-Amsa (Mex) *See* Cefotaxime 295
Fotexina (Mex) *See* Cefotaxime 295
Freezone® [OTC] *See* Salicylic Acid 1454
Frisium® (Can) *See* Clobazam 364
Froben® (Can) *See* Flurbiprofen 667
Froben-SR® (Can) *See* Flurbiprofen 667
Frova® *See* Frovatriptan 696
Frovatriptan 696
Frovatriptan Succinate *See* Frovatriptan 696
Frusemide *See* Furosemide 699
FTC *See* Emtricitabine 530
FTC, TDF, and EFV *See* Efavirenz, Emtricitabine, and Tenofovir 527
FU *See* Fluorouracil 649
5-FU *See* Fluorouracil 649
FUDR® *See* Floxuridine 634
5-FUDR *See* Floxuridine 634
Fulcin Forte (Mex) *See* Griseofulvin 736
Fulvestrant 698

Fungizone® (Can) *See* Amphotericin B (Conventional) 120
Fung-O® [OTC] *See* Salicylic Acid 1454
Fungoral (Mex) *See* Ketoconazole 876
Furadantin® *See* Nitrofurantoin 1147
Furadantina (Mex) *See* Nitrofurantoin 1147
Furazosin *See* Prazosin 1325
Furobioxin (Mex) *See* Cefuroxime 300
Furosemide 699
Furosemide Injection, USP (Can) *See* Furosemide 699
Furosemide Special (Can) *See* Furosemide 699
Fuzeon® *See* Enfuvirtide 537
FXT (Can) *See* FLUoxetine 650
Gabantin (Mex) *See* Gabapentin 702
Gabapentin 702
Gabaz (Mex) *See* GlipiZIDE 726
Gabirol (Mex) *See* Rimantadine 1422
Gabitril® *See* TiaGABine 1580
Gadolinium-DTPA *See* Gadopentetate Dimeglumine 705
Gadopentetate Dimeglumine 705
Galantamine 705
Galantamine Hydrobromide *See* Galantamine 705
Galecin (Mex) *See* Clindamycin 363
Galidrin (Mex) *See* Ranitidine 1399
Gallium Nitrate 707
Galsulfase 708
Gamikal (Mex) *See* Amikacin 83
Gamma Benzene Hexachloride *See* Lindane 927
Gamma E-Gems® [OTC] *See* Vitamin E 1675
Gamma-E Plus [OTC] *See* Vitamin E 1675
Gamma Hydroxybutyric Acid *See* Sodium Oxybate 1495
Gammaphos *See* Amifostine 83
Ganciclovir 708
Ganidin NR *See* GuaiFENesin 737
Ganite™ *See* Gallium Nitrate 707
Gani-Tuss DM NR *See* Guaifenesin and Dextromethorphan 739
Gani-Tuss® NR *See* Guaifenesin and Codeine 738
Gantrisin® *See* SulfiSOXAZOLE 1523
Gapridol (Mex) *See* Gabapentin 702
GAR-936 *See* Tigecycline 1583
Garamicina (Mex) *See* Gentamicin 714
Garamsa (Mex) *See* Gentamicin 714
Garamycin® (Can) *See* Gentamicin 714
Gascop (Mex) *See* Albendazole 53
Gastrocrom® *See* Cromolyn 402
Gatifloxacin 709
G-CSF *See* Filgrastim 632
G-CSF (PEG Conjugate) *See* Pegfilgrastim 1236
GCV Sodium *See* Ganciclovir 708
GD-Celecoxib (Can) *See* Celecoxib 301
Gd-DTPA *See* Gadopentetate Dimeglumine 705
GD-Quinapril (Can) *See* Quinapril 1386
Gefitinib 709
Gelusil® (Can) *See* Aluminum Hydroxide, Magnesium Hydroxide, and Simethicone 78
Gelusil® [OTC] *See* Aluminum Hydroxide, Magnesium Hydroxide, and Simethicone 78
Gemcitabine 710
Gemcitabine Hydrochloride *See* Gemcitabine 710
Gemfibrozil 711
Gemifloxacin 712
Gemifloxacin Mesylate *See* Gemifloxacin 712
Gemtuzumab Ozogamicin 713
Gemzar® *See* Gemcitabine 710
Gen-Acebutolol (Can) *See* Acebutolol 27
Genaced™ [OTC] *See* Acetaminophen, Aspirin, and Caffeine 39
Genac® [OTC] *See* Triprolidine and Pseudoephedrine 1634
Genacote™ [OTC] *See* Aspirin 143
Gen-Acyclovir (Can) *See* Acyclovir 49
Genahist® [OTC] *See* DiphenhydrAMINE 481
Gen-Alendronate (Can) *See* Alendronate 59
Gen-Alprazolam (Can) *See* ALPRAZolam 72
Gen-Amilazide (Can) *See* Amiloride and Hydrochlorothiazide 86
Gen-Amiodarone (Can) *See* Amiodarone 89
Gen-Amoxicillin (Can) *See* Amoxicillin 112
Gen-Anagrelide (Can) *See* Anagrelide 124
Genapap™ Children [OTC] *See* Acetaminophen 30
Genapap™ Extra Strength [OTC] *See* Acetaminophen 30
Genapap™ Infant [OTC] *See* Acetaminophen 30
Genapap™ [OTC] *See* Acetaminophen 30

Genapap™ Sinus Maximum Strength [OTC] [DSC] *See* Acetaminophen and Pseudoephedrine 37
Genaphed® [OTC] *See* Pseudoephedrine 1367
Genasal [OTC] *See* Oxymetazoline 1208
Genasec™ [OTC] *See* Acetaminophen and Phenyltoloxamine 36
Gen-Atenolol (Can) *See* Atenolol 147
Genatuss DM® [OTC] *See* Guaifenesin and Dextromethorphan 739
Gen-Azathioprine (Can) *See* AzaTHIOprine 162
Gen-Baclofen (Can) *See* Baclofen 168
Gen-Beclo (Can) *See* Beclomethasone 171
Gen-Bicalutamide (Can) *See* Bicalutamide 188
Gen-Bromazepam (Can) *See* Bromazepam 200
Gen-Budesonide AQ (Can) *See* Budesonide 210
Gen-Buspirone (Can) *See* BusPIRone 223
Gen-Captopril (Can) *See* Captopril 264
Gen-Carbamazepine CR (Can) *See* CarBAMazepine 265
Gen-Cimetidine (Can) *See* Cimetidine 345
Gen-Ciprofloxacin (Can) *See* Ciprofloxacin 346
Gen-Citalopram (Can) *See* Citalopram 354
Gen-Clarithromycin (Can) *See* Clarithromycin 360
Gen-Clindamycin (Can) *See* Clindamycin 363
Gen-Clomipramine (Can) *See* ClomiPRAMINE 368
Gen-Clonazepam (Can) *See* ClonazePAM 373
Gen-Clozapine (Can) *See* Clozapine 386
Gen-Combo Sterinebs (Can) *See* Ipratropium and Albuterol 854
Gen-Cyclobenzaprine (Can) *See* Cyclobenzaprine 405
Gen-Diltiazem (Can) *See* Diltiazem 473
Gen-Diltiazem CD (Can) *See* Diltiazem 473
Gen-Divalproex (Can) *See* Valproic Acid and Derivatives 1642
Gen-Doxazosin (Can) *See* Doxazosin 500
Genebs Extra Strength [OTC] *See* Acetaminophen 30
Genebs [OTC] *See* Acetaminophen 30
Gen-Enalapril (Can) *See* Enalapril 531
Generlac *See* Lactulose 886
Gen-Etidronate (Can) *See* Etidronate Disodium 605
Genexa™ LA [DSC] *See* Guaifenesin and Phenylephrine 742
Geneye [OTC] *See* Tetrahydrozoline 1560
Gen-Famotidine (Can) *See* Famotidine 613
Gen-Fenofibrate Micro (Can) *See* Fenofibrate 620
Gen-Fluconazole (Can) *See* Fluconazole 635
Gen-Fluoxetine (Can) *See* FLUoxetine 650
Gen-Fosinopril (Can) *See* Fosinopril 691
Gen-Gabapentin (Can) *See* Gabapentin 702
Gen-Gemfibrozil (Can) *See* Gemfibrozil 711
Gen-Glybe (Can) *See* GlyBURIDE 730
Gengraf® *See* CycloSPORINE 409
Gen-Hydroxychloroquine (Can) *See* Hydroxychloroquine 796
Gen-Hydroxyurea (Can) *See* Hydroxyurea 796
Gen-Indapamide (Can) *See* Indapamide 817
Gen-Ipratropium (Can) *See* Ipratropium 852
Genkova (Mex) *See* Gentamicin 714
Gen-Lamotrigine (Can) *See* LamoTRIgine 889
Gen-Levothyroxine (Can) *See* Levothyroxine 920
Gen-Lisinopril (Can) *See* Lisinopril 934
Gen-Lisinopril/Hctz (Can) *See* Lisinopril and Hydrochlorothiazide 938
Gen-Lovastatin (Can) *See* Lovastatin 956
Gen-Medroxy (Can) *See* MedroxyPROGESTERone 975
Gen-Meloxicam (Can) *See* Meloxicam 982
Gen-Metformin (Can) *See* MetFORMIN 997
Gen-Metoprolol (Can) *See* Metoprolol 1036
Gen-Minocycline (Can) *See* Minocycline 1056
Gen-Mirtazapine (Can) *See* Mirtazapine 1058
Gen-Nabumetone (Can) *See* Nabumetone 1089
Gen-Naproxen EC (Can) *See* Naproxen 1102
Gen-Nitro (Can) *See* Nitroglycerin 1147
Gen-Nizatidine (Can) *See* Nizatidine 1149
Gen-Nortriptyline (Can) *See* Nortriptyline 1152
Genobiotic-Doxi (Mex) *See* Doxycycline 509
Genoestatina (Mex) *See* Pravastatin 1321
Genoldene (Mex) *See* Piroxicam 1307
Gen-Ondansetron (Can) *See* Ondansetron 1180
Genotropin® *See* Somatropin 1499
Genotropin Miniquick® *See* Somatropin 1499
Genovix (Mex) *See* Acyclovir 49
Gen-Oxybutynin (Can) *See* Oxybutynin 1199
Genozyl (Mex) *See* Allopurinol 67
Gen-Paroxetine (Can) *See* PARoxetine 1226

Gen-Pindolol (Can) *See* Pindolol ... 1294
Gen-Pioglitazone (Can) *See* Pioglitazone ... 1297
Gen-Piroxicam (Can) *See* Piroxicam ... 1307
Genpril® [OTC] [DSC] *See* Ibuprofen ... 803
Gen-Ranidine (Can) *See* Ranitidine ... 1399
Genrex (Mex) *See* Gentamicin ... 714
Gen-Risperidone (Can) *See* Risperidone ... 1425
Gen-Salbutamol (Can) *See* Albuterol ... 54
Gen-Selegiline (Can) *See* Selegiline ... 1466
Gen-Sertraline (Can) *See* Sertraline ... 1472
Gen-Simvastatin (Can) *See* Simvastatin ... 1486
Gen-Sotalol (Can) *See* Sotalol ... 1502
Gen-Sumatriptan (Can) *See* SUMAtriptan ... 1527
Gentak® *See* Gentamicin ... 714
Gentamicin ... 714
Gentamicin Injection, USP (Can) *See* Gentamicin ... 714
Gentamicin Sulfate *See* Gentamicin ... 714
Gentamil (Mex) *See* Gentamicin ... 714
Gen-Tamoxifen (Can) *See* Tamoxifen ... 1537
Gen-Tamsulosin (Can) *See* Tamsulosin ... 1537
Gentasol™ *See* Gentamicin ... 714
Gentazol (Mex) *See* Gentamicin ... 714
Gen-Temazepam (Can) *See* Temazepam ... 1545
Gen-Terbinafine (Can) *See* Terbinafine ... 1551
Gentex HC [DSC] *See* Hydrocodone, Phenylephrine, and Guaifenesin ... 783
Gentex LA [DSC] *See* Guaifenesin and Phenylephrine ... 742
Gentex LQ *See* Carbetapentane, Guaifenesin, and Phenylephrine ... 274
Gen-Ticlopidine (Can) *See* Ticlopidine ... 1583
Gen-Timolol (Can) *See* Timolol ... 1584
Gen-Tizanidine (Can) *See* TiZANidine ... 1587
Gen-Topiramate (Can) *See* Topiramate ... 1598
Gen-Trazodone (Can) *See* TraZODone ... 1614
Gen-Triazolam (Can) *See* Triazolam ... 1620
Gentuss-HC *See* Hydrocodone, Phenylephrine, and Diphenhydramine ... 782
Gen-Verapamil (Can) *See* Verapamil ... 1665
Gen-Verapamil SR (Can) *See* Verapamil ... 1665
Gen-Warfarin (Can) *See* Warfarin ... 1679
Gen-Zopiclone (Can) *See* Zopiclone ... 1711
Geocillin® [DSC] *See* Carbenicillin ... 272
Geodon® *See* Ziprasidone ... 1698
Gepromi (Mex) *See* Progesterone ... 1345
Gervaken (Mex) *See* Clarithromycin ... 360
Geslutin (Mex) *See* Progesterone ... 1345
GF196960 *See* Tadalafil ... 1534
GG *See* GuaiFENesin ... 737
GHB *See* Sodium Oxybate ... 1495
GI87084B *See* Remifentanil ... 1408
Gilphex TR® *See* Guaifenesin and Phenylephrine ... 742
Giltuss® *See* Guaifenesin, Dextromethorphan, and Phenylephrine ... 746
Giltuss HC® [DSC] *See* Hydrocodone, Phenylephrine, and Guaifenesin ... 783
Giltuss Pediatric® *See* Guaifenesin, Dextromethorphan, and Phenylephrine ... 746
Giltuss TR® *See* Guaifenesin, Dextromethorphan, and Phenylephrine ... 746
Gimaclav (Mex) *See* Amoxicillin and Clavulanate Potassium ... 115
Gimalxina (Mex) *See* Amoxicillin ... 112
Ginedisc (Mex) *See* Estradiol ... 576
Ginkgo biloba *See* Ginkgo (Ginkgo biloba) ... 715
Ginkgo (Ginkgo biloba) ... 715
Ginseng, Panax (Panax ginseng) ... 718
Ginseng, Siberian *(Eleutherococcus senticosus)* ... 720
Glargine Insulin *See* Insulin Glargine ... 827
Glatiramer Acetate ... 722
Gleevec® *See* Imatinib ... 810
Gliadel® *See* Carmustine ... 284
Gliadel Wafer® (Can) *See* Carmustine ... 284
Glibenclamide *See* GlyBURIDE ... 730
Glimepiride ... 723
Glimepiride and Pioglitazone *See* Pioglitazone and Glimepiride ... 1300
Glimepiride and Pioglitazone Hydrochloride *See* Pioglitazone and Glimepiride ... 1300
Glimepiride and Rosiglitazone Maleate *See* Rosiglitazone and Glimepiride ... 1448
GlipiZIDE ... 726
Glipizide and Metformin ... 729
Glipizide and Metformin Hydrochloride *See* Glipizide and Metformin ... 729
Glivec (Mex) *See* Imatinib ... 810
Globitan (Mex) *See* Timolol ... 1584
Glubacida (Mex) *See* Polymyxin B ... 1312
Glucal (Mex) *See* GlyBURIDE ... 730
Glucobay™ (Can) *See* Acarbose ... 25

GlucoNorm® (Can) *See* Repaglinide ... 1409
Glucophage® *See* MetFORMIN ... 997
Glucophage® XR *See* MetFORMIN ... 997
Glucotrol® *See* GlipiZIDE ... 726
Glucotrol XL® *See* GlipiZIDE ... 726
Glucovance® *See* Glyburide and Metformin ... 733
Glulisine Insulin *See* Insulin Glulisine ... 829
Glumetza™ *See* MetFORMIN ... 997
Glybenclamide *See* GlyBURIDE ... 730
Glybenzcyclamide *See* GlyBURIDE ... 730
GlyBURIDE ... 730
Glyburide and Metformin ... 733
Glyburide and Metformin Hydrochloride *See* Glyburide and Metformin ... 733
Glycerol Guaiacolate *See* GuaiFENesin ... 737
Glyceryl Trinitrate *See* Nitroglycerin ... 1147
Glycon (Can) *See* MetFORMIN ... 997
Glycopyrrolate ... 734
Glycopyrrolate Injection, USP (Can) *See* Glycopyrrolate ... 734
Glycopyrronium Bromide *See* Glycopyrrolate ... 734
Glydiazinamide *See* GlipiZIDE ... 726
Glynase® PresTab® *See* GlyBURIDE ... 730
Glyset® *See* Miglitol ... 1052
GM-CSF *See* Sargramostim ... 1462
GMD-Azithromycin (Can) *See* Azithromycin ... 163
GMD-Fluconazole (Can) *See* Fluconazole ... 635
GMD-Gemfibrozil (Can) *See* Gemfibrozil ... 711
GMD-Sertraline (Can) *See* Sertraline ... 1472
GnRH *See* Gonadorelin ... 734
GnRH Agonist *See* Histrelin ... 769
Gold Sodium Thiomalate ... 734
GoLYTELY® *See* Polyethylene Glycol-Electrolyte Solution ... 1310
Gonadorelin ... 734
Gonadorelin Acetate *See* Gonadorelin ... 734
Gonadorelin Hydrochloride *See* Gonadorelin ... 734
Gonadotropin Releasing Hormone *See* Gonadorelin ... 734
Good Sense Sleep Aid [OTC] *See* Doxylamine ... 510
Goody's® Extra Strength Headache Powder [OTC] *See* Acetaminophen, Aspirin, and Caffeine ... 39
Goody's® Extra Strength Pain Relief [OTC] *See* Acetaminophen, Aspirin, and Caffeine ... 39
Goody's PM® [OTC] *See* Acetaminophen and Diphenhydramine ... 35
Gopten (Mex) *See* Trandolapril ... 1608
Gordofilm® [OTC] *See* Salicylic Acid ... 1454
Goserelin ... 735
Goserelin Acetate *See* Goserelin ... 735
Gotinal (Mex) *See* Naphazoline ... 1101
GP 47680 *See* OXcarbazepine ... 1195
GR38032R *See* Ondansetron ... 1180
Gralddep (Mex) *See* Loratadine and Pseudoephedrine ... 948
Granisetron ... 736
Granisol™ *See* Granisetron ... 736
Granulocyte Colony Stimulating Factor *See* Filgrastim ... 632
Granulocyte Colony Stimulating Factor (PEG Conjugate) *See* Pegfilgrastim ... 1236
Granulocyte-Macrophage Colony Stimulating Factor *See* Sargramostim ... 1462
Graten (Mex) *See* Morphine Sulfate ... 1077
Gravol® (Can) *See* DimenhyDRINATE ... 478
Grifulvin® V *See* Griseofulvin ... 736
Griseofulvin ... 736
Griseofulvin Microsize *See* Griseofulvin ... 736
Griseofulvin Ultramicrosize *See* Griseofulvin ... 736
Grisovin (Mex) *See* Griseofulvin ... 736
Gris-PEG® *See* Griseofulvin ... 736
Guaicon DM [OTC] *See* Guaifenesin and Dextromethorphan ... 739
Guaicon DMS [OTC] *See* Guaifenesin and Dextromethorphan ... 739
Guaifed® *See* Guaifenesin and Phenylephrine ... 742
Guaifed-PD® *See* Guaifenesin and Phenylephrine ... 742
Guaifen™ DM [DSC] *See* Guaifenesin, Dextromethorphan, and Phenylephrine ... 746
GuaiFENesin ... 737
Guaifenesin AC *See* Guaifenesin and Codeine ... 738
Guaifenesin and Codeine ... 738
Guaifenesin and Dextromethorphan ... 739
Guaifenesin and Dyphylline *See* Dyphylline and Guaifenesin ... 522
Guaifenesin and Hydrocodone *See* Hydrocodone and Guaifenesin ... 779
Guaifenesin and Phenylephrine ... 742
Guaifenesin and Phenylephrine Tannate *See* Guaifenesin and Phenylephrine ... 742
Guaifenesin and Pseudoephedrine ... 744
Guaifenesin and Theophylline *See* Theophylline and Guaifenesin ... 1567

Guaifenesin, Carbetapentane Citrate, and Phenylephrine Hydrochloride *See* Carbetapentane, Guaifenesin, and Phenylephrine 274
Guaifenesin, Chlorpheniramine, Phenylephrine, and Dextromethorphan *See* Dextromethorphan, Chlorpheniramine, Phenylephrine, and Guaifenesin 450
Guaifenesin, Dextromethorphan, and Phenylephrine 746
Guaifenesin, Dextromethorphan Hydrobromide, and Phenylephrine Hydrochloride *See* Guaifenesin, Dextromethorphan, and Phenylephrine 746
Guaifenesin, Dihydrocodeine, and Pseudoephedrine *See* Dihydrocodeine, Pseudoephedrine, and Guaifenesin 469
Guaifenesin, Hydrocodone, and Pseudoephedrine *See* Hydrocodone, Pseudoephedrine, and Guaifenesin 784
Guaifenesin, Hydrocodone Bitartrate, and Phenylephrine Hydrochloride *See* Hydrocodone, Phenylephrine, and Guaifenesin 783
Guaifenesin, Phenylephrine, and Chlorpheniramine *See* Chlorpheniramine, Phenylephrine, and Guaifenesin 329
Guaifenesin, Pseudoephedrine, and Codeine 747
Guaifenesin, Pseudoephedrine, and Dextromethorphan 748
Guaifenesin, Pyrilamine Tannate, and Phenylephrine Tannate *See* Phenylephrine, Pyrilamine, and Guaifenesin 1279
Guaifenex® DM [DSC] *See* Guaifenesin and Dextromethorphan 739
Guaifenex® GP [DSC] *See* Guaifenesin and Pseudoephedrine 744
Guaifenex® PSE [DSC] *See* Guaifenesin and Pseudoephedrine 744
Guaimax-D® *See* Guaifenesin and Pseudoephedrine 744
Guaiphen-D *See* Guaifenesin and Phenylephrine 742
Guaiphen-D 1200 *See* Guaifenesin and Phenylephrine 742
Guaiphen-PD *See* Guaifenesin and Phenylephrine 742
Guaituss AC *See* Guaifenesin and Codeine 738
Guanabenz 750
Guanabenz Acetate *See* Guanabenz 750
GuanFACINE 750
Guanfacine Hydrochloride *See* GuanFACINE 750
Guia-D *See* Guaifenesin and Dextromethorphan 739
Guiaplex™ HC [DSC] *See* Hydrocodone, Phenylephrine, and Guaifenesin 783
Guiatuss DAC *See* Guaifenesin, Pseudoephedrine, and Codeine 747
Guiatuss-DM® [OTC] *See* Guaifenesin and Dextromethorphan 739
Guiatuss™ [OTC] *See* GuaiFENesin 737
GW506U78 *See* Nelarabine 1120
GW-1000-02 *See* Tetrahydrocannabinol and Cannabidiol 1558
GW433908G *See* Fosamprenavir 689
GW572016 *See* Lapatinib 898
Gynodiol® [DSC] *See* Estradiol 576
H5N1 Influenza Vaccine *See* Influenza Virus Vaccine (H5N1) 821
Habitrol® (Can) *See* Nicotine 1133
Haemophilus b Conjugate and Hepatitis B Vaccine 752
Haemophilus b Conjugate Vaccine 753
Haemophilus b (meningococcal protein conjugate) Conjugate Vaccine *See* *Haemophilus* b Conjugate and Hepatitis B Vaccine 752
Haemophilus b Oligosaccharide Conjugate Vaccine *See* *Haemophilus* b Conjugate Vaccine 753
Haemophilus b Polysaccharide Vaccine *See* *Haemophilus* b Conjugate Vaccine 753
Halcion® *See* Triazolam 1620
Haldol® *See* Haloperidol 754
Haldol® Decanoate *See* Haloperidol 754
Halfprin® [OTC] *See* Aspirin 143
Haloperidol 754
Haloperidol Decanoate *See* Haloperidol 754
Haloperidol Injection, USP (Can) *See* Haloperidol 754
Haloperidol-LA (Can) *See* Haloperidol 754
Haloperidol Lactate *See* Haloperidol 754
Haloperidol-LA Omega (Can) *See* Haloperidol 754
Haloperidol Long Acting (Can) *See* Haloperidol 754
Haloperil (Mex) *See* Haloperidol 754
Harkoseride *See* Lacosamide 885
HAVRIX® *See* Hepatitis A Vaccine 760
Havrix 1440 (Mex) *See* Hepatitis A Vaccine 760
Havrix Junior (Mex) *See* Hepatitis A Vaccine 760
Hawthorn (Crataegus oxyacantha) 758
HbCV *See* Haemophilus b Conjugate Vaccine 753
HBIG *See* Hepatitis B Immune Globulin 762
hBNP *See* Nesiritide 1123
hCG *See* Chorionic Gonadotropin (Human) 342
HCTZ (error-prone abbreviation) *See* Hydrochlorothiazide 773
Heavy Mineral Oil *See* Mineral Oil 1055
Hectorol® *See* Doxercalciferol 507
Helidac® *See* Bismuth, Metronidazole, and Tetracycline 190
Hemabate® *See* Carboprost Tromethamine 282
Hematin *See* Hemin 760
Hemin 760

Hemobion (Mex) *See* Ferrous Sulfate ... 627
Hemocyte® [OTC] *See* Ferrous Fumarate ... 626
Hemorrhoidal HC *See* Hydrocortisone ... 785
Hemril®-30 *See* Hydrocortisone ... 785
HepaGam B™ *See* Hepatitis B Immune Globulin ... 762
Hepatitis A Vaccine ... 760
Hepatitis B Immune Globulin ... 762
Hepatitis B Inactivated Virus Vaccine (recombinant DNA) *See* Hepatitis B Vaccine ... 764
Hepatitis B Vaccine ... 764
Hepatitis B Vaccine (Recombinant) *See* *Haemophilus* b Conjugate and Hepatitis B Vaccine ... 752
Hepatron C (Mex) *See* Interferon Alfa-2b and Ribavirin ... 846
Hepsera™ *See* Adefovir ... 51
Heptovir® (Can) *See* LamiVUDine ... 888
Herceptin® *See* Trastuzumab ... 1613
Hercivir (Mex) *See* Acyclovir ... 49
Herklin (Mex) *See* Lindane ... 927
Hexachlorocyclohexane *See* Lindane ... 927
Hexalen® *See* Altretamine ... 78
Hexamethylmelamine *See* Altretamine ... 78
Hexit™ (Can) *See* Lindane ... 927
HEXM *See* Altretamine ... 78
hGH *See* Somatropin ... 1499
Hib Conjugate Vaccine *See* *Haemophilus* b Conjugate Vaccine ... 753
Hib Polysaccharide Conjugate *See* *Haemophilus* b Conjugate Vaccine ... 753
Hidantoína (Mex) *See* Phenytoin ... 1280
Hidramox (Mex) *See* Amoxicillin ... 112
Hidrociclina (Mex) *See* Penicillin G Procaine ... 1241
High Gamma Vitamin E Complete™ [OTC] *See* Vitamin E ... 1675
High-Molecular-Weight Iron Dextran (DexFerrum®) *See* Iron Dextran Complex ... 857
Higroton (Mex) *See* Chlorthalidone ... 340
Hipoden (Mex) *See* Lidocaine ... 924
Hipokinon (Mex) *See* Trihexyphenidyl ... 1627
Hirulog *See* Bivalirudin ... 191
Histacol™ BD *See* Brompheniramine, Pseudoephedrine, and Dextromethorphan ... 208
Histade™ [DSC] *See* Chlorpheniramine and Pseudoephedrine ... 325
Histantil (Can) *See* Promethazine ... 1347
Histatab PH *See* Chlorpheniramine, Phenylephrine, and Methscopolamine ... 329
Hista-Vent® DA [DSC] *See* Chlorpheniramine, Phenylephrine, and Methscopolamine ... 329
Hista-Vent® PSE [DSC] *See* Chlorpheniramine, Pseudoephedrine, and Methscopolamine ... 334
Histex™ *See* Chlorpheniramine and Pseudoephedrine ... 325
Histex® SR *See* Brompheniramine and Pseudoephedrine ... 206
Histinex® HC *See* Phenylephrine, Hydrocodone, and Chlorpheniramine ... 1277
Histrelin ... 769
Histrelin Acetate *See* Histrelin ... 769
Hivid® (Can) *See* Zalcitabine ... 1691
Hivid® [DSC] *See* Zalcitabine ... 1691
HMM *See* Altretamine ... 78
HMR 3647 *See* Telithromycin ... 1542
HN2 *See* Mechlorethamine ... 974
Hold® DM [OTC] *See* Dextromethorphan ... 448
Homatropine ... 769
Homatropine and Hydrocodone *See* Hydrocodone and Homatropine ... 780
Homatropine Hydrobromide *See* Homatropine ... 769
Hops (Humulus lupulus) ... 770
Horex (Mex) *See* Timolol ... 1584
Horse Antihuman Thymocyte Gamma Globulin *See* Antithymocyte Globulin (Equine) ... 126
H.P. Acthar® Gel *See* Corticotropin ... 401
Hp-PAC® (Can) *See* Lansoprazole, Amoxicillin, and Clarithromycin ... 897
HTF919 *See* Tegaserod ... 1541
hu1124 *See* Efalizumab ... 526
Humalog® *See* Insulin Lispro ... 832
Humalog® Mix 25 (Can) *See* Insulin Lispro Protamine and Insulin Lispro ... 834
Humalog® Mix 50/50™ *See* Insulin Lispro Protamine and Insulin Lispro ... 834
Humalog® Mix 75/25™ *See* Insulin Lispro Protamine and Insulin Lispro ... 834
Human Antitumor Necrosis Factor Alpha *See* Adalimumab ... 50
Human Growth Hormone *See* Somatropin ... 1499
Humanized IgG1 Anti-CD52 Monoclonal Antibody *See* Alemtuzumab ... 59
Human LFA-3/IgG(1) Fusion Protein *See* Alefacept ... 58
Humatin® (Can) *See* Paromomycin ... 1226
Humatin® [DSC] *See* Paromomycin ... 1226
Humatrope® *See* Somatropin ... 1499
Humegon® (Can) *See* Chorionic Gonadotropin (Human) ... 342
Humira® *See* Adalimumab ... 50
Humulin® 20/80 (Can) *See* Insulin NPH and Insulin Regular ... 836
Humulin 30 70 (Mex) *See* Insulin NPH and Insulin Regular ... 836
Humulin® 50/50 *See* Insulin NPH and Insulin Regular ... 836

Humulin® 70/30 *See* Insulin NPH and Insulin Regular ... 836
Humulin® N *See* Insulin NPH ... 835
Humulin® R *See* Insulin Regular ... 838
Humulin® R U-500 *See* Insulin Regular ... 838
Humulus lupulus *See* Hops (Humulus lupulus) ... 770
Huperzia serrata *See* HuperzineA (Huperzia serrata) ... 771
HuperzineA (Huperzia serrata) ... 771
HXM *See* Altretamine ... 78
Hyalcrom NF (Mex) *See* Ketotifen ... 879
Hycamptamine *See* Topotecan ... 1602
Hycamtin® *See* Topotecan ... 1602
hycet™ *See* Hydrocodone and Acetaminophen ... 777
Hycodan® [DSC] *See* Hydrocodone and Homatropine ... 780
Hycort™ (Can) *See* Hydrocortisone ... 785
Hycotuss® [DSC] *See* Hydrocodone and Guaifenesin ... 779
Hydeltra T.B.A.® (Can) *See* PrednisoLONE ... 1326
Hydergina (Mex) *See* Ergoloid Mesylates ... 551
Hydergine® (Can) *See* Ergoloid Mesylates ... 551
Hydergine [DSC] *See* Ergoloid Mesylates ... 551
Hyderm (Can) *See* Hydrocortisone ... 785
HydrALAZINE ... 772
Hydralazine and Hydrochlorothiazide ... 772
Hydralazine and Isosorbide Dinitrate *See* Isosorbide Dinitrate and Hydralazine ... 869
Hydralazine Hydrochloride *See* HydrALAZINE ... 772
Hydramine® [OTC] *See* DiphenhydrAMINE ... 481
Hydrated Chloral *See* Chloral Hydrate ... 313
Hydrea® *See* Hydroxyurea ... 796
Hydrisalic™ [OTC] *See* Salicylic Acid ... 1454
Hydrochlorothiazide ... 773
Hydrochlorothiazide and Aliskiren *See* Aliskiren and Hydrochlorothiazide ... 66
Hydrochlorothiazide and Amiloride *See* Amiloride and Hydrochlorothiazide ... 86
Hydrochlorothiazide and Benazepril *See* Benazepril and Hydrochlorothiazide ... 179
Hydrochlorothiazide and Bisoprolol *See* Bisoprolol and Hydrochlorothiazide ... 191
Hydrochlorothiazide and Captopril *See* Captopril and Hydrochlorothiazide ... 265
Hydrochlorothiazide and Enalapril *See* Enalapril and Hydrochlorothiazide ... 536
Hydrochlorothiazide and Eprosartan *See* Eprosartan and Hydrochlorothiazide ... 549
Hydrochlorothiazide and Fosinopril *See* Fosinopril and Hydrochlorothiazide ... 692
Hydrochlorothiazide and Hydralazine *See* Hydralazine and Hydrochlorothiazide ... 772
Hydrochlorothiazide and Irbesartan *See* Irbesartan and Hydrochlorothiazide ... 856
Hydrochlorothiazide and Lisinopril *See* Lisinopril and Hydrochlorothiazide ... 938
Hydrochlorothiazide and Losartan *See* Losartan and Hydrochlorothiazide ... 956
Hydrochlorothiazide and Methyldopa *See* Methyldopa and Hydrochlorothiazide ... 1021
Hydrochlorothiazide and Metoprolol *See* Metoprolol and Hydrochlorothiazide ... 1040
Hydrochlorothiazide and Metoprolol Tartrate *See* Metoprolol and Hydrochlorothiazide ... 1040
Hydrochlorothiazide and Moexipril *See* Moexipril and Hydrochlorothiazide ... 1068
Hydrochlorothiazide and Olmesartan Medoxomil *See* Olmesartan and Hydrochlorothiazide ... 1172
Hydrochlorothiazide and Propranolol *See* Propranolol and Hydrochlorothiazide ... 1361
Hydrochlorothiazide and Quinapril *See* Quinapril and Hydrochlorothiazide ... 1386
Hydrochlorothiazide and Spironolactone ... 776
Hydrochlorothiazide and Telmisartan *See* Telmisartan and Hydrochlorothiazide ... 1544
Hydrochlorothiazide and Triamterene ... 776
Hydrochlorothiazide and Valsartan *See* Valsartan and Hydrochlorothiazide ... 1652
Hydrocodone and Acetaminophen ... 777
Hydrocodone and Chlorpheniramine ... 778
Hydrocodone and Guaifenesin ... 779
Hydrocodone and Homatropine ... 780
Hydrocodone and Ibuprofen ... 780
Hydrocodone and Pseudoephedrine ... 781
Hydrocodone Bitartrate and Ibuprofen *See* Hydrocodone and Ibuprofen ... 780
Hydrocodone Bitartrate, Carbinoxamine Maleate, and Pseudoephedrine Hydrochloride *See* Hydrocodone, Carbinoxamine, and Pseudoephedrine ... 782
Hydrocodone Bitartrate, Phenylephrine Hydrochloride, and Diphenhydramine Hydrochloride *See* Hydrocodone, Phenylephrine, and Diphenhydramine ... 782
Hydrocodone, Carbinoxamine, and Pseudoephedrine ... 782
Hydrocodone, Chlorpheniramine, and Pseudoephedrine *See* Pseudoephedrine, Hydrocodone, and Chlorpheniramine ... 1372
Hydrocodone, Phenylephrine, and Chlorpheniramine *See* Phenylephrine, Hydrocodone, and Chlorpheniramine ... 1277
Hydrocodone, Phenylephrine, and Diphenhydramine ... 782
Hydrocodone, Phenylephrine, and Guaifenesin ... 783
Hydrocodone Polistirex and Chlorpheniramine Polistirex *See* Hydrocodone and Chlorpheniramine ... 778
Hydrocodone, Pseudoephedrine, and Guaifenesin ... 784
Hydrocodone Tannate and Pseudoephedrine Tannate *See* Hydrocodone and Pseudoephedrine ... 781

Hydrocodone Tannate, Phenylephrine Tannate, and Diphenhydramine Tannate *See* Hydrocodone, Phenylephrine, and Diphenhydramine ... 782
Hydrocortisone ... 785
Hydrocortisone Acetate *See* Hydrocortisone ... 785
Hydrocortisone Butyrate *See* Hydrocortisone ... 785
Hydrocortisone Probutate *See* Hydrocortisone ... 785
Hydrocortisone Sodium Succinate *See* Hydrocortisone ... 785
Hydrocortisone Valerate *See* Hydrocortisone ... 785
Hydro DP *See* Hydrocodone, Phenylephrine, and Diphenhydramine ... 782
HydroFed [DSC] *See* Hydrocodone, Phenylephrine, and Guaifenesin ... 783
Hydro-GP [DSC] *See* Hydrocodone, Phenylephrine, and Guaifenesin ... 783
Hydromet® *See* Hydrocodone and Homatropine ... 780
Hydromorph Contin® (Can) *See* HYDROmorphone ... 791
Hydromorph-IR® (Can) *See* HYDROmorphone ... 791
HYDROmorphone ... 791
Hydromorphone HP (Can) *See* HYDROmorphone ... 791
Hydromorphone HP® 10 (Can) *See* HYDROmorphone ... 791
Hydromorphone HP® 20 (Can) *See* HYDROmorphone ... 791
Hydromorphone HP® 50 (Can) *See* HYDROmorphone ... 791
Hydromorphone HP® Forte (Can) *See* HYDROmorphone ... 791
Hydromorphone Hydrochloride *See* HYDROmorphone ... 791
Hydromorphone Hydrochloride Injection, USP (Can) *See* HYDROmorphone ... 791
Hydron CP *See* Phenylephrine, Hydrocodone, and Chlorpheniramine ... 1277
Hydron PSC [DSC] *See* Pseudoephedrine, Hydrocodone, and Chlorpheniramine ... 1372
Hydro-PC II *See* Phenylephrine, Hydrocodone, and Chlorpheniramine ... 1277
Hydro PC II Plus *See* Phenylephrine, Hydrocodone, and Chlorpheniramine ... 1277
Hydro-Rx *See* Hydrocortisone ... 785
Hydro-Tussin™-CBX [DSC] *See* Carbinoxamine and Pseudoephedrine ... 280
Hydro-Tussin™ DHC [DSC] *See* Pseudoephedrine, Dihydrocodeine, and Chlorpheniramine ... 1371
Hydro-Tussin™ DM [DSC] *See* Guaifenesin and Dextromethorphan ... 739
Hydro-Tussin™ EXP [DSC] *See* Dihydrocodeine, Pseudoephedrine, and Guaifenesin ... 469
Hydro-Tussin™ HD [DSC] *See* Hydrocodone, Pseudoephedrine, and Guaifenesin ... 784
Hydro-Tussin™ XP [DSC] *See* Hydrocodone, Pseudoephedrine, and Guaifenesin ... 784
HydroVal® (Can) *See* Hydrocortisone ... 785
4-Hydroxybutyrate *See* Sodium Oxybate ... 1495
Hydroxycarbamide *See* Hydroxyurea ... 796
Hydroxychloroquine ... 796
Hydroxychloroquine Sulfate *See* Hydroxychloroquine ... 796
Hydroxydaunomycin Hydrochloride *See* DOXOrubicin ... 507
1α-Hydroxyergocalciferol *See* Doxercalciferol ... 507
Hydroxyldaunorubicin Hydrochloride *See* DOXOrubicin ... 507
9-hydroxy-risperidone *See* Paliperidone ... 1215
Hydroxyurea ... 796
HydrOXYzine ... 797
Hydroxyzine Hydrochloride *See* HydrOXYzine ... 797
Hydroxyzine Hydrochloride Injection, USP (Can) *See* HydrOXYzine ... 797
Hydroxyzine Pamoate *See* HydrOXYzine ... 797
HydroZone Plus [OTC] *See* Hydrocortisone ... 785
Hyflex-DS® [DSC] *See* Acetaminophen and Phenyltoloxamine ... 36
Hygroton *See* Chlorthalidone ... 340
Hyoscine Butylbromide *See* Scopolamine Derivatives ... 1463
Hyoscine Hydrobromide *See* Scopolamine Derivatives ... 1463
Hyoscyamine ... 799
Hyoscyamine, Atropine, Scopolamine, and Phenobarbital ... 800
Hyoscyamine, Methenamine, Benzoic Acid, Phenyl Salicylate, and Methylene Blue *See* Methenamine, Phenyl Salicylate, Methylene Blue, Benzoic Acid, and Hyoscyamine ... 1009
Hyoscyamine, Methenamine, Sodium Biphosphate, Phenyl Salicylate, and Methylene Blue *See* Methenamine, Sodium Biphosphate, Phenyl Salicylate, Methylene Blue, and Hyoscyamine ... 1010
Hyoscyamine Sulfate *See* Hyoscyamine ... 799
Hyosyne *See* Hyoscyamine ... 799
Hyperforin *See* St John's Wort (Hypericum perforatum) ... 1506
HyperHep B® (Can) *See* Hepatitis B Immune Globulin ... 762
HyperHEP B™ S/D *See* Hepatitis B Immune Globulin ... 762
Hypericum *See* St John's Wort (Hypericum perforatum) ... 1506
Hypericum perforatum *See* St John's Wort (Hypericum perforatum) ... 1506
HyperRHO™ S/D Full Dose *See* Rho(D) Immune Globulin ... 1415
HyperRHO™ S/D Mini Dose *See* Rho(D) Immune Globulin ... 1415
Hyphed [DSC] *See* Pseudoephedrine, Hydrocodone, and Chlorpheniramine ... 1372
Hytakerol® (Can) *See* Dihydrotachysterol ... 472
Hytakerol® [DSC] *See* Dihydrotachysterol ... 472
Hytone® *See* Hydrocortisone ... 785
Hytrin® (Can) *See* Terazosin ... 1549
Hyzaar® *See* Losartan and Hydrochlorothiazide ... 956
Hyzaar® DS (Can) *See* Losartan and Hydrochlorothiazide ... 956

I123 Iobenguane *See* Iobenguane I 123 ... 849
I-123 MIBG *See* Iobenguane I 123 ... 849
Ibandronate ... 801
Ibandronate Sodium *See* Ibandronate ... 801
Ibandronic Acid *See* Ibandronate ... 801
Ibidomide Hydrochloride *See* Labetalol ... 881
Ibritumomab ... 802
Ibritumomab Tiuxetan *See* Ibritumomab ... 802
Ibu® *See* Ibuprofen ... 803
Ibu-200 [OTC] *See* Ibuprofen ... 803
Ibudone™ *See* Hydrocodone and Ibuprofen ... 780
Ibuflam (Mex) *See* Ibuprofen ... 803
Ibuprofen ... 803
Ibuprofen and Hydrocodone *See* Hydrocodone and Ibuprofen ... 780
Ibuprofen and Pseudoephedrine *See* Pseudoephedrine and Ibuprofen ... 1369
Ibuprofen Lysine *See* Ibuprofen ... 803
Ibutilide ... 808
Ibutilide Fumarate *See* Ibutilide ... 808
ICI-182,780 *See* Fulvestrant ... 698
ICI-204,219 *See* Zafirlukast ... 1689
ICI-46474 *See* Tamoxifen ... 1537
ICI-118630 *See* Goserelin ... 735
ICI-176334 *See* Bicalutamide ... 188
ICI-D1033 *See* Anastrozole ... 125
ICL670 *See* Deferasirox ... 423
ICRF-187 *See* Dexrazoxane ... 441
Idamycin® (Can) *See* IDArubicin ... 809
Idamycin PFS® *See* IDArubicin ... 809
IDArubicin ... 809
Idarubicin Hydrochloride *See* IDArubicin ... 809
IDEC-C2B8 *See* RiTUXimab ... 1434
IDEC-Y2B8 *See* Ibritumomab ... 802
IDR *See* IDArubicin ... 809
Ifadex (Mex) *See* Ifosfamide ... 809
Ifa Fonal (Mex) *See* Diazepam ... 451
Ifex® *See* Ifosfamide ... 809
IFLrA *See* Interferon Alfa-2a ... 844
Ifolem (Mex) *See* Ifosfamide ... 809
Ifomida (Mex) *See* Ifosfamide ... 809
Ifosfamide ... 809
IgG4-Kappa Monoclonal Antibody *See* Natalizumab ... 1109
Ignis (Mex) *See* Acyclovir ... 49
IL-1Ra *See* Anakinra ... 124
IL-2 *See* Aldesleukin ... 58
IL-11 *See* Oprelvekin ... 1184
Ileveran (Mex) *See* Enalapril ... 531
Iliadin (Mex) *See* Oxymetazoline ... 1208
Iloprost ... 810
Iloprost Tromethamine *See* Iloprost ... 810
Ilosone (Mex) *See* Erythromycin ... 557
Imatinib ... 810
Imatinib Mesylate *See* Imatinib ... 810
IMC-C225 *See* Cetuximab ... 310
Imdur® *See* Isosorbide Mononitrate ... 869
Imdur 60 (Mex) *See* Isosorbide Mononitrate ... 869
123I-Metaiodobenzylguanidine (MIBG) *See* Iobenguane I 123 ... 849
Imferon *See* Iron Dextran Complex ... 857
IMI 30 *See* IDArubicin ... 809
IMid-3 *See* Lenalidomide ... 899
Imidazole Carboxamide *See* Dacarbazine ... 414
Imidazole Carboxamide Dimethyltriazene *See* Dacarbazine ... 414
Imidex (Mex) *See* Lansoprazole ... 894
Imiglucerase ... 811
Imigran (Mex) *See* SUMAtriptan ... 1527
Iminen (Mex) *See* Imipenem and Cilastatin ... 812
Imipemide *See* Imipenem and Cilastatin ... 812
Imipenem and Cilastatin ... 812
Imipramine ... 812
Imipramine Hydrochloride *See* Imipramine ... 812
Imipramine Pamoate *See* Imipramine ... 812
Imitrex® *See* SUMAtriptan ... 1527
Imitrex® DF (Can) *See* SUMAtriptan ... 1527
Imitrex® Nasal Spray (Can) *See* SUMAtriptan ... 1527
Immunine® VH (Can) *See* Factor IX ... 612
Imodium® (Can) *See* Loperamide ... 944
Imodium® A-D [OTC] *See* Loperamide ... 944
Imodium® Advanced *See* Loperamide and Simethicone ... 944

Imot Ofteno (Mex) *See* Timolol 1584
Imovane® (Can) *See* Zopiclone 1711
Implanon™ *See* Etonogestrel 606
Imuran® *See* AzaTHIOprine 162
In-111 Ibritumomab *See* Ibritumomab 802
In-111 Zevalin *See* Ibritumomab 802
Inamrinone 817
Inapsine® *See* Droperidol 513
Inbumed (Mex) *See* Albuterol 54
Incardel (Mex) *See* Acarbose 25
Increlex™ *See* Mecasermin 973
Incremin con Hierro (Mex) *See* Thiamine 1568
Indaflex (Mex) *See* Indomethacin 818
Indanet (Mex) *See* Indomethacin 818
Indapamide 817
Inderal® *See* Propranolol 1355
Inderalici (Mex) *See* Propranolol 1355
Inderal® LA *See* Propranolol 1355
Inderide® *See* Propranolol and Hydrochlorothiazide 1361
Indilan (Mex) *See* Indinavir 818
Indinavir 818
Indinavir Sulfate *See* Indinavir 818
Indocid (Mex) *See* Indomethacin 818
Indocid® P.D.A. (Can) *See* Indomethacin 818
Indocin® *See* Indomethacin 818
Indocin® I.V. *See* Indomethacin 818
Indofol (Mex) *See* Propofol 1352
Indo-Lemmon (Can) *See* Indomethacin 818
Indometacin *See* Indomethacin 818
Indomethacin 818
Indomethacin Sodium Trihydrate *See* Indomethacin 818
Indotec (Can) *See* Indomethacin 818
Induken (Mex) *See* Tinidazole 1585
Indumir (Mex) *See* DiphenhydrAMINE 481
INF-alpha 2 *See* Interferon Alfa-2b 844
Infantaire [OTC] *See* Acetaminophen 30
INFeD® *See* Iron Dextran Complex 857
Infergen® *See* Interferon Alfacon-1 847
Inflamase® Mild (Can) *See* PrednisoLONE 1326
InFLIXimab 819
Infliximab, Recombinant *See* InFLIXimab 819
Influenza Virus Vaccine 820
Influenza Virus Vaccine (H5N1) 821
Influenza Virus Vaccine (Monovalent) *See* Influenza Virus Vaccine (H5N1) 821
Influenza Virus Vaccine (Purified Surface Antigen) *See* Influenza Virus Vaccine 820
Influenza Virus Vaccine (Split-Virus) *See* Influenza Virus Vaccine 820
Influenza Virus Vaccine (Trivalent, Live) *See* Influenza Virus Vaccine 820
Infufer® (Can) *See* Iron Dextran Complex 857
Infumorph® *See* Morphine Sulfate 1077
Infuvite® Adult *See* Vitamins (Multiple/Injectable) 1677
Infuvite® Pediatric *See* Vitamins (Multiple/Injectable) 1677
INH *See* Isoniazid 862
Inhaled Insulin *See* Insulin Inhalation 830
Inhibitron (Mex) *See* Omeprazole 1176
Inigrin (Mex) *See* Loratadine 946
Inmunef (Mex) *See* Filgrastim 632
Innohep® *See* Tinzaparin 1585
InnoPran XL™ *See* Propranolol 1355
Inprax (Mex) *See* Oxybutynin 1199
Insogen (Mex) *See* ChlorproPAMIDE 340
Inspra™ *See* Eplerenone 545
Inspra IC (Mex) *See* Eplerenone 545
Insulin Aspart 822
Insulin Aspart and Insulin Aspart Protamine *See* Insulin Aspart Protamine and Insulin Aspart 824
Insulin Aspart Protamine and Insulin Aspart 824
Insulin Detemir 825
Insulin Glargine 827
Insulin Glulisine 829
Insulin Inhalation 830
Insulin Lispro 832
Insulin Lispro and Insulin Lispro Protamine *See* Insulin Lispro Protamine and Insulin Lispro 834
Insulin Lispro Protamine and Insulin Lispro 834
Insulin NPH 835
Insulin NPH and Insulin Regular 836
Insulin Regular 838

Insulin Regular and Insulin NPH *See* Insulin NPH and Insulin Regular ... 836
Intal® *See* Cromolyn ... 402
Integrilin® *See* Eptifibatide ... 550
Intelence™ *See* Etravirine ... 608
α-2-interferon *See* Interferon Alfa-2b ... 844
Interferon Alfa-2a ... 844
Interferon Alfa-2a (PEG Conjugate) *See* Peginterferon Alfa-2a ... 1236
Interferon Alfa-2b ... 844
Interferon Alfa-2b and Ribavirin ... 846
Interferon Alfa-2b and Ribavirin Combination Pack *See* Interferon Alfa-2b and Ribavirin ... 846
Interferon Alfa-2b (PEG Conjugate) *See* Peginterferon Alfa-2b ... 1237
Interferon Alfacon-1 ... 847
Interferon Alfa-n3 ... 847
Interferon Alpha-2a *See* Interferon Alfa-2a ... 844
Interferon Alpha-2b *See* Interferon Alfa-2b ... 844
Interferon Beta-1a ... 848
Interferon Beta-1b ... 848
Interferon Gamma-1b ... 849
Interleukin-1 Receptor Antagonist *See* Anakinra ... 124
Interleukin-2 *See* Aldesleukin ... 58
Interleukin-11 *See* Oprelvekin ... 1184
Internol (Mex) *See* Atenolol ... 147
Intralon (Mex) *See* Triamcinolone ... 1617
Intrifiban *See* Eptifibatide ... 550
Intron® A *See* Interferon Alfa-2b ... 844
Intropin *See* DOPamine ... 498
Invanz® *See* Ertapenem ... 557
Invega® *See* Paliperidone ... 1215
Inversine® *See* Mecamylamine ... 973
Invirase® *See* Saquinavir ... 1461
Iobenguane I 123 ... 849
Iobenguane Sulfate I 123 *See* Iobenguane I 123 ... 849
Iodine I 131 Tositumomab and Tositumomab *See* Tositumomab and Iodine I 131 Tositumomab ... 1603
Iodixanol ... 850
Iodoquinol ... 851
Ionamin® *See* Phentermine ... 1270
Ionil® [OTC] *See* Salicylic Acid ... 1454
Ionil Plus® [OTC] *See* Salicylic Acid ... 1454
Iopidine® *See* Apraclonidine ... 129
Iosat™ [OTC] *See* Potassium Iodide ... 1317
Ipecac Syrup ... 851
IPG-Citalopram (Can) *See* Citalopram ... 354
Iplex™ [DSC] *See* Mecasermin ... 973
Ipratropium ... 852
Ipratropium and Albuterol ... 854
Ipratropium Bromide *See* Ipratropium ... 852
I-Prin [OTC] *See* Ibuprofen ... 803
Iproveratril Hydrochloride *See* Verapamil ... 1665
Iqfadina (Mex) *See* Ranitidine ... 1399
Iquix® *See* Levofloxacin ... 913
Irbesartan ... 855
Irbesartan and Hydrochlorothiazide ... 856
Ircon® [OTC] *See* Ferrous Fumarate ... 626
IRESSA® *See* Gefitinib ... 709
Iretron (Mex) *See* Erythromycin ... 557
Irinotecan ... 856
Irinotecan Hydrochloride Trihydrate (Can) *See* Irinotecan ... 856
Irizz. (Mex) *See* ALPRAZolam ... 72
Iron Dextran *See* Iron Dextran Complex ... 857
Iron Dextran Complex ... 857
Iron Fumarate *See* Ferrous Fumarate ... 626
Iron Gluconate *See* Ferrous Gluconate ... 627
Iron-Polysaccharide Complex *See* Polysaccharide-Iron Complex ... 1313
Iron Sucrose ... 858
Iron Sulfate *See* Ferrous Sulfate ... 627
Iron Sulfate and Vitamin C *See* Ferrous Sulfate and Ascorbic Acid ... 628
Irtan (Mex) *See* Nedocromil ... 1115
ISD *See* Isosorbide Dinitrate ... 866
ISDN *See* Isosorbide Dinitrate ... 866
Isentress™ *See* Raltegravir ... 1393
ISMN *See* Isosorbide Mononitrate ... 869
Ismo® *See* Isosorbide Mononitrate ... 869
Isoamyl Nitrite *See* Amyl Nitrite ... 124
Isobamate *See* Carisoprodol ... 283
Isocarboxazid ... 858

Isochron™ *See* Isosorbide Dinitrate ... 866
Isoface (Mex) *See* Isotretinoin ... 871
Isometheptene, Acetaminophen, and Dichloralphenazone *See* Acetaminophen, Isometheptene, and Dichloralphenazone ... 45
Isometheptene, Dichloralphenazone, and Acetaminophen *See* Acetaminophen, Isometheptene, and Dichloralphenazone ... 45
IsonaRif™ *See* Rifampin and Isoniazid ... 1419
Isoniazid ... 862
Isoniazid and Rifampin *See* Rifampin and Isoniazid ... 1419
Isoniazid, Rifampin, and Pyrazinamide *See* Rifampin, Isoniazid, and Pyrazinamide ... 1419
Isonicotinic Acid Hydrazide *See* Isoniazid ... 862
Isonipecaine Hydrochloride *See* Meperidine ... 986
Isophane Insulin *See* Insulin NPH ... 835
Isophane Insulin and Regular Insulin *See* Insulin NPH and Insulin Regular ... 836
Isophosphamide *See* Ifosfamide ... 809
Isoproterenol ... 866
Isoproterenol Hydrochloride *See* Isoproterenol ... 866
Isoptin® SR *See* Verapamil ... 1665
Isopto® Atropine *See* Atropine ... 158
Isopto® Carpine *See* Pilocarpine ... 1290
Isopto® Eserine (Can) *See* Physostigmine ... 1288
Isopto® Homatropine *See* Homatropine ... 769
Isopto® Hyoscine *See* Scopolamine Derivatives ... 1463
Isorbid (Mex) *See* Isosorbide Dinitrate ... 866
Isordil® *See* Isosorbide Dinitrate ... 866
Isosorbide Dinitrate ... 866
Isosorbide Dinitrate and Hydralazine ... 869
Isosorbide Mononitrate ... 869
Isotamine® (Can) *See* Isoniazid ... 862
Isotretinoin ... 871
Isotrex® (Can) *See* Isotretinoin ... 871
Isox (Mex) *See* Itraconazole ... 872
Isradipine ... 871
Istalol® *See* Timolol ... 1584
Isuprel® *See* Isoproterenol ... 866
Itraconazole ... 872
Itranax (Mex) *See* Itraconazole ... 872
Ivermectin ... 873
Ivexterm (Mex) *See* Ivermectin ... 873
IvySoothe® [OTC] *See* Hydrocortisone ... 785
Ixopolet (Mex) *See* Vitamin E ... 1675
JAMP-Citalopram (Can) *See* Citalopram ... 354
Jamp® Travel Tablet (Can) *See* DimenhyDRINATE ... 478
Jantoven® *See* Warfarin ... 1679
Janumet™ *See* Sitagliptin and Metformin ... 1492
Januvia™ *See* SitaGLIPtin ... 1491
Jersin (Mex) *See* Acyclovir ... 49
Jolessa™ *See* Ethinyl Estradiol and Levonorgestrel ... 595
Jolivette™ *See* Norethindrone ... 1150
Junel™ *See* Ethinyl Estradiol and Norethindrone ... 597
Junel™ Fe *See* Ethinyl Estradiol and Norethindrone ... 597
K-10® (Can) *See* Potassium Chloride ... 1315
Kadian® *See* Morphine Sulfate ... 1077
Kaletra® *See* Lopinavir and Ritonavir ... 945
Kanamycin ... 873
Kanamycin Sulfate *See* Kanamycin ... 873
Kantrex® *See* Kanamycin ... 873
Kaon-Cl-10® *See* Potassium Chloride ... 1315
Kao-Paverin® [OTC] *See* Loperamide ... 944
Kaopectate® Extra Strength [OTC] *See* Bismuth ... 189
Kaopectate® [OTC] *See* Bismuth ... 189
Kao-Tin [OTC] *See* Bismuth ... 189
Kapectolin [OTC] *See* Bismuth ... 189
Kariva™ *See* Ethinyl Estradiol and Desogestrel ... 592
Karmikin (Mex) *See* Amikacin ... 83
Kava Kava (Piper methysticum) ... 874
Kawa *See* Kava Kava (Piper methysticum) ... 874
Kay Ciel® [DSC] *See* Potassium Chloride ... 1315
KCl *See* Potassium Chloride ... 1315
K-Dur® (Can) *See* Potassium Chloride ... 1315
Kedrop (Mex) *See* Ketotifen ... 879
Keflex® *See* Cephalexin ... 306
Keftab® (Can) *See* Cephalexin ... 306
Kelefusin (Mex) *See* Potassium Chloride ... 1315
Kelnor™ *See* Ethinyl Estradiol and Ethynodiol Diacetate ... 594
Kemadrin® [DSC] *See* Procyclidine ... 1344
Kemsol® (Can) *See* Dimethyl Sulfoxide ... 480

Kenalog® *See* Triamcinolone ... 1617
Kenalog-10® *See* Triamcinolone ... 1617
Kenalog-40® *See* Triamcinolone ... 1617
Kenalog® in Orabase (Can) *See* Triamcinolone ... 1617
Kenoket (Mex) *See* ClonazePAM ... 373
Kenstatin (Mex) *See* Pravastatin ... 1321
Kentadin (Mex) *See* Pentoxifylline ... 1251
Kenzoflex (Mex) *See* Ciprofloxacin ... 346
Kenzolol (Mex) *See* NiMODipine ... 1141
Keoxifene Hydrochloride *See* Raloxifene ... 1391
Kepivance™ *See* Palifermin ... 1214
Keppra® *See* Levetiracetam ... 905
Keppra XR™ *See* Levetiracetam ... 905
Keralyt® [OTC] *See* Salicylic Acid ... 1454
Keritmon (Mex) *See* Amiodarone ... 89
Kerlone® *See* Betaxolol ... 186
Kerr Insta-Char® [OTC] *See* Charcoal ... 312
Ketalar® *See* Ketamine ... 876
Ketalin (Mex) *See* Ketamine ... 876
Ketamine ... 876
Ketamine Hydrochloride *See* Ketamine ... 876
Ketamine Hydrochloride Injection, USP (Can) *See* Ketamine ... 876
Ketaxal (Mex) *See* Ketotifen ... 879
Ketek® *See* Telithromycin ... 1542
Ketoconazole ... 876
Ketoderm® (Can) *See* Ketoconazole ... 876
3-Keto-desogestrel *See* Etonogestrel ... 606
Ketoprofen ... 877
Ketorolac ... 878
Ketorolac Tromethamine *See* Ketorolac ... 878
Ketorolac Tromethamine Injection, USP (Can) *See* Ketorolac ... 878
Ketotifen ... 879
Ketotifen Fumarate *See* Ketotifen ... 879
Kew *See* Kava Kava (Piper methysticum) ... 874
Kew Tree *See* Ginkgo (Ginkgo biloba) ... 715
Key-E® Kaps [OTC] *See* Vitamin E ... 1675
Key-E® [OTC] *See* Vitamin E ... 1675
KI *See* Potassium Iodide ... 1317
Kiddi Pharmaton (Mex) *See* Cyanocobalamin ... 404
Kidkare Children's Cough and Cold [OTC] *See* Chlorpheniramine, Pseudoephedrine, and Dextromethorphan ... 333
Kidkare Decongestant [OTC] *See* Pseudoephedrine ... 1367
Kidonax (Mex) *See* Nitazoxanide ... 1146
Kidrolase® (Can) *See* Asparaginase ... 142
Kineret® *See* Anakinra ... 124
Kinestase (Mex) *See* Cisapride U.S. - Available Via Limited-Access Protocol Only ... 353
Kinevac® *See* Sincalide ... 1489
Kivexa™ (Can) *See* Abacavir and Lamivudine ... 22
Klamoxyl (Mex) *See* Clindamycin ... 363
Klaricid (Mex) *See* Clarithromycin ... 360
Klarmyn (Mex) *See* Clarithromycin ... 360
Klean-Prep® (Can) *See* Polyethylene Glycol-Electrolyte Solution ... 1310
Klin-Amsa (Mex) *See* Clindamycin ... 363
Klonopin® *See* ClonazePAM ... 373
Klonopin® Wafers *See* ClonazePAM ... 373
K-Lor® *See* Potassium Chloride ... 1315
Klor-Con® *See* Potassium Chloride ... 1315
Klor-Con® 8 *See* Potassium Chloride ... 1315
Klor-Con® 10 *See* Potassium Chloride ... 1315
Klor-Con®/25 *See* Potassium Chloride ... 1315
Klor-Con® M *See* Potassium Chloride ... 1315
Klor-Con®/EF *See* Potassium Bicarbonate and Potassium Citrate ... 1315
K-Lyte® *See* Potassium Bicarbonate and Potassium Citrate ... 1315
K-Lyte®/Cl (Can) *See* Potassium Chloride ... 1315
K-Lyte® DS *See* Potassium Bicarbonate and Potassium Citrate ... 1315
Koffex DM-D (Can) *See* Pseudoephedrine and Dextromethorphan ... 1369
Koffex DM + Decongestant + Expectorant (Can) *See* Guaifenesin, Pseudoephedrine, and Dextromethorphan ... 748
Koffex DM-Expectorant (Can) *See* Guaifenesin and Dextromethorphan ... 739
Koffex Expectorant (Can) *See* GuaiFENesin ... 737
Kolephrin® #1 *See* Guaifenesin and Codeine ... 738
Kolephrin® GG/DM [OTC] *See* Guaifenesin and Dextromethorphan ... 739
Kolephrin® [OTC] *See* Acetaminophen, Chlorpheniramine, and Pseudoephedrine ... 40
Konakion (Can) *See* Phytonadione ... 1289
Konakion MM (Mex) *See* Phytonadione ... 1289
Konaturil (Mex) *See* Ketoconazole ... 876
Kondremul® [OTC] *See* Mineral Oil ... 1055

Koptin (Mex) *See* Azithromycin ... 163
K-Pek II [OTC] *See* Loperamide ... 944
Krenosin (Mex) *See* Adenosine ... 51
Kriadex (Mex) *See* ClonazePAM ... 373
Kristalose® *See* Lactulose ... 886
Krobicin (Mex) *See* Clarithromycin ... 360
K-Tab® *See* Potassium Chloride ... 1315
K-Tan 4 [DSC] *See* Phenylephrine and Pyrilamine ... 1275
K-Tan [DSC] *See* Phenylephrine and Pyrilamine ... 1275
Kuppam (Mex) *See* Pantoprazole ... 1221
Kuric™ *See* Ketoconazole ... 876
Kwelcof® [DSC] *See* Hydrocodone and Guaifenesin ... 779
Kytril® *See* Granisetron ... 736
L-749,345 *See* Ertapenem ... 557
L-758,298 *See* Fosaprepitant ... 690
L-M-X™ 4 [OTC] *See* Lidocaine ... 924
L-M-X™ 5 [OTC] *See* Lidocaine ... 924
L 754030 *See* Aprepitant ... 130
LA 20304a *See* Gemifloxacin ... 712
Labetalol ... 881
Labetalol Hydrochloride *See* Labetalol ... 881
Labetalol Hydrochloride Injection, USP (Can) *See* Labetalol ... 881
Laciken (Mex) *See* Acyclovir ... 49
Lacosamide ... 885
Lactulax (Mex) *See* Lactulose ... 886
Lactulose ... 886
Ladakamycin *See* AzaCITIDine ... 161
Ladogal (Mex) *See* Danazol ... 416
Lagesic™ *See* Acetaminophen and Phenyltoloxamine ... 36
L-All 12 *See* Carbetapentane and Phenylephrine ... 273
L-AmB *See* Amphotericin B, Liposomal ... 121
Lamdra SBK (Mex) *See* LamoTRIgine ... 889
Lamictal® *See* LamoTRIgine ... 889
Lamisil® *See* Terbinafine ... 1551
Lamisil AT® [OTC] *See* Terbinafine ... 1551
LamiVUDine ... 888
Lamivudine and Abacavir *See* Abacavir and Lamivudine ... 22
Lamivudine and Zidovudine *See* Zidovudine and Lamivudine ... 1696
LamoTRIgine ... 889
Landstav (Mex) *See* Stavudine ... 1505
Lanexat (Mex) *See* Flumazenil ... 644
Lanodizol (Mex) *See* Lansoprazole ... 894
Lanoxicaps® (Can) *See* Digoxin ... 463
Lanoxicaps® [DSC] *See* Digoxin ... 463
Lanoxin® *See* Digoxin ... 463
Lansoprazole ... 894
Lansoprazole, Amoxicillin, and Clarithromycin ... 897
Lansoprazole and Naproxen ... 897
Lanthanum ... 898
Lanthanum Carbonate *See* Lanthanum ... 898
Lantus® *See* Insulin Glargine ... 827
Lantus® OptiSet® (Can) *See* Insulin Glargine ... 827
Lanvis® (Can) *See* Thioguanine ... 1569
Lapatinib ... 898
Lapatinib Ditosylate *See* Lapatinib ... 898
Laracit (Mex) *See* Cytarabine ... 412
Largactil® (Can) *See* ChlorproMAZINE ... 336
Lariam® *See* Mefloquine ... 976
Laritol (Mex) *See* Loratadine ... 946
Lartron (Mex) *See* Ondansetron ... 1180
Lasix® *See* Furosemide ... 699
Lasix® Special (Can) *See* Furosemide ... 699
L-asparaginase *See* Asparaginase ... 142
Lauritran (Mex) *See* Erythromycin ... 557
Laxilose (Can) *See* Lactulose ... 886
l-Bunolol Hydrochloride *See* Levobunolol ... 907
LCM *See* Lacosamide ... 885
L-Deoxythymidine *See* Telbivudine ... 1541
L-Deprenyl *See* Selegiline ... 1466
LDP-341 *See* Bortezomib ... 192
Lectopam® (Can) *See* Bromazepam ... 200
Ledertrexate (Mex) *See* Methotrexate ... 1014
Ledoxina (Mex) *See* Cyanocobalamin ... 404
Leena™ *See* Ethinyl Estradiol and Norethindrone ... 597
Leflunomide ... 899
Legatrin PM® [OTC] *See* Acetaminophen and Diphenhydramine ... 35
Lemblastine (Mex) *See* VinBLAStine ... 1672

Leminter (Mex) *See* Pantoprazole 1221
Lenalidomide 899
Lentocaine (Mex) *See* Mepivacaine 990
Lepirudin 900
Lepirudin (rDNA) *See* Lepirudin 900
Leponex (Mex) *See* Clozapine 386
Leptopsique (Mex) *See* Perphenazine 1255
Lertamine (Mex) *See* Loratadine 946
Lertamine D (Mex) *See* Loratadine and Pseudoephedrine 948
Lertus CD (Mex) *See* Codeine 394
Lescol® *See* Fluvastatin 676
Lescol® XL *See* Fluvastatin 676
Lessina™ *See* Ethinyl Estradiol and Levonorgestrel 595
Letrozole 900
Leukeran® *See* Chlorambucil 315
Leukine® *See* Sargramostim 1462
Leuprolide 901
Leuprolide Acetate *See* Leuprolide 901
Leuprorelin Acetate *See* Leuprolide 901
Leurocristine Sulfate *See* VinCRIStine 1673
Leustatin® *See* Cladribine 360
Levalbuterol 902
Levalbuterol Hydrochloride *See* Levalbuterol 902
Levalbuterol Tartrate *See* Levalbuterol 902
Levall™ *See* Carbetapentane, Guaifenesin, and Phenylephrine 274
Levall 5.0 [DSC] *See* Hydrocodone, Phenylephrine, and Guaifenesin 783
Levall G *See* Guaifenesin and Pseudoephedrine 744
Levaquin® *See* Levofloxacin 913
Levarterenol Bitartrate *See* Norepinephrine 1150
Levate® (Can) *See* Amitriptyline 90
Levatol® *See* Penbutolol 1238
Levbid® *See* Hyoscyamine 799
Levemir® *See* Insulin Detemir 825
Levetiracetam 905
Levhexal (Mex) *See* Levothyroxine 920
Levitra® *See* Vardenafil 1654
Levlen® *See* Ethinyl Estradiol and Levonorgestrel 595
Levlite™ *See* Ethinyl Estradiol and Levonorgestrel 595
Levobunolol 907
Levobunolol Hydrochloride *See* Levobunolol 907
Levobupivacaine 908
Levocabastine 909
Levocabastine Hydrochloride *See* Levocabastine 909
Levocetirizine 909
Levocetirizine Dihydrochloride *See* Levocetirizine 909
Levodopa and Carbidopa *See* Carbidopa and Levodopa 277
Levodopa, Carbidopa, and Entacapone 911
Levo-Dromoran® *See* Levorphanol 919
Levofloxacin 913
Levomepromazine *See* Methotrimeprazine 1015
Levonorgestrel 918
Levonorgestrel and Ethinyl Estradiol *See* Ethinyl Estradiol and Levonorgestrel 595
Levophed® *See* Norepinephrine 1150
Levora® *See* Ethinyl Estradiol and Levonorgestrel 595
Levorphanol 919
Levorphanol Tartrate *See* Levorphanol 919
Levorphan Tartrate *See* Levorphanol 919
Levothroid® *See* Levothyroxine 920
Levothyroxine 920
Levothyroxine Sodium (Can) *See* Levothyroxine 920
Levoxyl® *See* Levothyroxine 920
Levsin® *See* Hyoscyamine 799
Levsin®/SL *See* Hyoscyamine 799
Lexapro® *See* Escitalopram 564
Lexiva® *See* Fosamprenavir 689
Lexotan (Mex) *See* Bromazepam 200
Lexxel® (Can) *See* Enalapril and Felodipine 536
Lexxel® [DSC] *See* Enalapril and Felodipine 536
LFA-3/IgG(1) Fusion Protein, Human *See* Alefacept 58
LHRH *See* Gonadorelin 734
LH-RH Agonist *See* Histrelin 769
l-Hyoscyamine Sulfate *See* Hyoscyamine 799
Lialda™ *See* Mesalamine 994
Liberaxim (Mex) *See* HYDROmorphone 791
Libiocid (Mex) *See* Lincomycin 926
Librax® (Can) *See* Clidinium and Chlordiazepoxide 362
Librax® [original formulation] *See* Clidinium and Chlordiazepoxide 362

Librax® [reformulation] [DSC] *See* Chlordiazepoxide and Methscopolamine 319
Librium® *See* ChlordiazePOXIDE 316
LidaMantle® *See* Lidocaine 924
Lidocaine 924
Lidocaine Hydrochloride *See* Lidocaine 924
Lidodan™ (Can) *See* Lidocaine 924
Lidoderm® *See* Lidocaine 924
Lignocaine Hydrochloride *See* Lidocaine 924
Limbitrol® *See* Amitriptyline and Chlordiazepoxide 94
Limbitrol® DS *See* Amitriptyline and Chlordiazepoxide 94
Limbrel™ *See* Flavocoxid 633
Limustin (Mex) *See* Tacrolimus 1533
Lin-Amox (Can) *See* Amoxicillin 112
Lin-Buspirone (Can) *See* BusPIRone 223
Lincocin® *See* Lincomycin 926
Lincomycin 926
Lincomycin Hydrochloride *See* Lincomycin 926
Lindane 927
Linessa® (Can) *See* Ethinyl Estradiol and Desogestrel 592
Linezolid 927
Lin-Fosinopril (Can) *See* Fosinopril 691
Lin-Sotalol (Can) *See* Sotalol 1502
Lioresal® *See* Baclofen 168
Liotec (Can) *See* Baclofen 168
Liothyronine 928
Liothyronine Sodium *See* Liothyronine 928
Liotrix 930
Liperol (Mex) *See* Lovastatin 956
Lipidil EZ® (Can) *See* Fenofibrate 620
Lipidil Micro® (Can) *See* Fenofibrate 620
Lipidil Supra® (Can) *See* Fenofibrate 620
Lipitor® *See* Atorvastatin 153
Lipofen™ *See* Fenofibrate 620
Liposomal DAUNOrubicin *See* DAUNOrubicin Citrate (Liposomal) 421
Liposomal DOXOrubicin *See* DOXOrubicin (Liposomal) 508
Liquadd™ *See* Dextroamphetamine 441
Liquibid-D® *See* Guaifenesin and Phenylephrine 742
Liquid Antidote *See* Charcoal 312
Liqui-Doss® [OTC] [DSC] *See* Mineral Oil 1055
Liquid Paraffin *See* Mineral Oil 1055
Lisdexamfetamine 931
Lisdexamfetamine Dimesylate *See* Lisdexamfetamine 931
Lisdexamphetamine *See* Lisdexamfetamine 931
Lisiken (Mex) *See* Clindamycin 363
Lisinopril 934
Lisinopril and Hydrochlorothiazide 938
Lisobac (Mex) *See* Amikacin 83
Lispro Insulin *See* Insulin Lispro 832
Lithane™ (Can) *See* Lithium 938
Litheum 300 (Mex) *See* Lithium 938
Lithium 938
Lithium Carbonate *See* Lithium 938
Lithium Citrate *See* Lithium 938
Lithobid® *See* Lithium 938
Little Colds® Multi-Symptom Cold Formula
[OTC] [DSC] *See* Acetaminophen, Dextromethorphan, and Phenylephrine 42
Little Fevers™ [OTC] *See* Acetaminophen 30
Little Noses® Decongestant [OTC] *See* Phenylephrine 1273
Live Attenuated Influenza Vaccine (LAIV) *See* Influenza Virus Vaccine 820
Live Smallpox Vaccine *See* Smallpox Vaccine 1493
Livostin® (Can) *See* Levocabastine 909
Livostin® [DSC] *See* Levocabastine 909
L-methylfolate *See* Methylfolate 1022
LNg 20 *See* Levonorgestrel 918
Locoid® *See* Hydrocortisone 785
Locoid Lipocream® *See* Hydrocortisone 785
Lodine (Mex) *See* Etodolac 606
Lodine Retard (Mex) *See* Etodolac 606
Lodosyn® *See* Carbidopa 276
Lodoxamide 942
Lodoxamide Tromethamine *See* Lodoxamide 942
Lodrane® 12D *See* Brompheniramine and Pseudoephedrine 206
Lodrane® 12 Hour *See* Brompheniramine 205
Lodrane® 24 *See* Brompheniramine 205
Lodrane® 24D *See* Brompheniramine and Pseudoephedrine 206
Lodrane® D *See* Brompheniramine and Pseudoephedrine 206
Lodrane® [DSC] *See* Brompheniramine and Pseudoephedrine 206

Lodrane® XR *See* Brompheniramine 205
Loestrin® *See* Ethinyl Estradiol and Norethindrone 597
Loestrin™ 1.5/30 (Can) *See* Ethinyl Estradiol and Norethindrone 597
Loestrin® 24 Fe *See* Ethinyl Estradiol and Norethindrone 597
Loestrin® Fe *See* Ethinyl Estradiol and Norethindrone 597
Lofibra® *See* Fenofibrate 620
LoHist-12 *See* Brompheniramine 205
LoHist 12D *See* Brompheniramine and Pseudoephedrine 206
LoHist-D *See* Chlorpheniramine and Pseudoephedrine 325
LoHist LQ *See* Brompheniramine and Pseudoephedrine 206
LoHist PD *See* Brompheniramine and Pseudoephedrine 206
L-OHP *See* Oxaliplatin 1191
L-Ombrix (Mex) *See* Mebendazole 972
Lomine (Can) *See* Dicyclomine 459
Lomotil® *See* Diphenoxylate and Atropine 486
Lomsin (Mex) *See* Albendazole 53
Lomustine 943
Loniten® (Can) *See* Minoxidil 1057
Lonox® *See* Diphenoxylate and Atropine 486
Lo/Ovral® *See* Ethinyl Estradiol and Norgestrel 601
Loperacap (Can) *See* Loperamide 944
Loperamide 944
Loperamide and Simethicone 944
Loperamide Hydrochloride *See* Loperamide 944
Lopid® *See* Gemfibrozil 711
Lopinavir and Ritonavir 945
Lopremone *See* Protirelin 1363
Lopresor (Mex) *See* Metoprolol 1036
Lopressor® *See* Metoprolol 1036
Lopressor HCT® *See* Metoprolol and Hydrochlorothiazide 1040
Lorabid® (Can) *See* Loracarbef 946
Lorabid® [DSC] *See* Loracarbef 946
Loracarbef 946
Loradamed [OTC] *See* Loratadine 946
Loratadine 946
Loratadine and Pseudoephedrine 948
LORazepam 949
Lorazepam Injection, USP (Can) *See* LORazepam 949
Lorazepam Intensol® *See* LORazepam 949
Lorcet® 10/650 *See* Hydrocodone and Acetaminophen 777
Lorcet® Plus *See* Hydrocodone and Acetaminophen 777
Lorelin (Mex) *See* Leuprolide 901
Loretsin (Mex) *See* Pravastatin 1321
Lorimox (Mex) *See* Loratadine 946
Lornakin (Mex) *See* Cisapride U.S. - Available Via Limited-Access Protocol Only 353
Lortab® *See* Hydrocodone and Acetaminophen 777
Losartan 952
Losartan and Hydrochlorothiazide 956
Losartan Potassium *See* Losartan 952
Losec® (Can) *See* Omeprazole 1176
Losec MUPS® (Can) *See* Omeprazole 1176
Lotan (Mex) *See* Loratadine 946
Lotensin® *See* Benazepril 178
Lotensin® HCT *See* Benazepril and Hydrochlorothiazide 179
Lotrel® *See* Amlodipine and Benazepril 104
Lovastatin 956
Lovastatin and Niacin *See* Niacin and Lovastatin 1127
Lovaza® *See* Omega-3-Acid Ethyl Esters 1175
Lovenox® *See* Enoxaparin 537
Lovenox® HP (Can) *See* Enoxaparin 537
Low-Molecular-Weight Iron Dextran (INFeD®) *See* Iron Dextran Complex 857
Low-Ogestrel® *See* Ethinyl Estradiol and Norgestrel 601
Lowtiyel (Mex) *See* Testosterone 1553
Loxapac® IM (Can) *See* Loxapine 960
Loxapine 960
Loxapine Succinate *See* Loxapine 960
Loxibest (Mex) *See* Meloxicam 982
Loxitane® *See* Loxapine 960
Lozide® (Can) *See* Indapamide 817
Lozol® (Can) *See* Indapamide 817
L-PAM *See* Melphalan 983
LRH *See* Gonadorelin 734
L-Sarcolysin *See* Melphalan 983
LTA® 360 *See* Lidocaine 924
LTG *See* LamoTRIgine 889
Lu-26-054 *See* Escitalopram 564
Lubiprostone 963

Lucrin Depot (Mex) *See* Leuprolide 901
Ludex (Mex) *See* Famotidine 613
Ludiomil (Mex) *See* Maprotiline 968
Luditec (Mex) *See* GlipiZIDE 726
Lufyllin® *See* Dyphylline 521
Lufyllin®-GG *See* Dyphylline and Guaifenesin 522
Lugol's Solution *See* Potassium Iodide and Iodine 1317
Luminal® Sodium *See* PHENobarbital 1265
Lunesta® *See* Eszopiclone 589
LupiCare® Dandruff [OTC] *See* Salicylic Acid 1454
LupiCare® Psoriasis [OTC] *See* Salicylic Acid 1454
LupiCare® Psoriasis Scalp [OTC] [DSC] *See* Salicylic Acid 1454
Lupron® *See* Leuprolide 901
Lupron Depot® *See* Leuprolide 901
Lupron Depot-Ped® *See* Leuprolide 901
Lupulus *See* Hops *(Humulus lupulus)* 770
Lurdex (Mex) *See* Albendazole 53
LuSonal™ *See* Phenylephrine 1273
Luteinizing Hormone Releasing Hormone *See* Gonadorelin 734
Lutera™ *See* Ethinyl Estradiol and Levonorgestrel 595
Lutrepulse™ (Can) *See* Gonadorelin 734
Lutropin Alfa 964
Luveris® *See* Lutropin Alfa 964
Luvox® (Can) *See* Fluvoxamine 678
Luvox® CR *See* Fluvoxamine 678
Luxiq® *See* Betamethasone 184
LY139603 *See* Atomoxetine 151
LY146032 *See* DAPTOmycin 418
LY170053 *See* OLANZapine 1160
LY231514 *See* Pemetrexed 1238
LY248686 *See* DULoxetine 516
LY2148568 *See* Exenatide 609
Lybrel™ *See* Ethinyl Estradiol and Levonorgestrel 595
Lymphocyte Immune Globulin *See* Antithymocyte Globulin (Equine) 126
Lymphocyte Mitogenic Factor *See* Aldesleukin 58
Lyrica® *See* Pregabalin 1332
Lyrinel (Mex) *See* Oxybutynin 1199
Lysodren® *See* Mitotane 1061
Maalox® Max [OTC] *See* Aluminum Hydroxide, Magnesium Hydroxide, and Simethicone 78
Maalox® [OTC] *See* Aluminum Hydroxide, Magnesium Hydroxide, and Simethicone 78
Maalox® Regular Chewable [OTC] *See* Calcium Carbonate 254
Maalox® Total Stomach Relief® [OTC] *See* Bismuth 189
MabCampath® (Can) *See* Alemtuzumab 59
Mabthera (Mex) *See* RiTUXimab 1434
Macrobid® *See* Nitrofurantoin 1147
Macrodantin® *See* Nitrofurantoin 1147
Macrodantina (Mex) *See* Nitrofurantoin 1147
Macrozit (Mex) *See* Azithromycin 163
Macugen® *See* Pegaptanib 1235
Mag 64™ [OTC] *See* Magnesium Chloride 965
Magaldrate and Simethicone 965
Mag-Caps [OTC] *See* Magnesium Oxide 966
Mag Delay® [OTC] *See* Magnesium Chloride 965
MagGel™ [OTC] *See* Magnesium Oxide 966
Magnacet™ *See* Oxycodone and Acetaminophen 1205
Magnesium Chloride 965
Magnesium Hydroxide, Aluminum Hydroxide, and Simethicone *See* Aluminum Hydroxide, Magnesium Hydroxide, and Simethicone 78
Magnesium Hydroxide and Calcium Carbonate *See* Calcium Carbonate and Magnesium Hydroxide 256
Magnesium Hydroxide, Famotidine, and Calcium Carbonate *See* Famotidine, Calcium Carbonate, and Magnesium Hydroxide 614
Magnesium Oxide 966
Magnesium Sulfate 966
Magnevist® *See* Gadopentetate Dimeglumine 705
Mag-Ox® 400 [OTC] *See* Magnesium Oxide 966
Ma Huang *See* Ephedra (Ephedra sinica) 541
Malarone® *See* Atovaquone and Proguanil 157
Malarone® Pediatric (Can) *See* Atovaquone and Proguanil 157
Malival (Mex) *See* Indomethacin 818
Mandrake *See* Podophyllum Resin 1309
Manerix® (Can) *See* Moclobemide 1062
Mannitol 968
Manzida (Mex) *See* Ethambutol 592
Mapap Children's [OTC] *See* Acetaminophen 30
Mapap Extra Strength [OTC] *See* Acetaminophen 30
Mapap Infants [OTC] *See* Acetaminophen 30

Mapap® Multi-Symptom Cold [OTC] *See* Acetaminophen, Dextromethorphan, and Phenylephrine ... 42
Mapap [OTC] *See* Acetaminophen ... 30
Mapap® Sinus Congestion and Pain Daytime [OTC] *See* Acetaminophen and Phenylephrine ... 36
Mapap Sinus Maximum Strength [OTC] *See* Acetaminophen and Pseudoephedrine ... 37
Mapezine® (Can) *See* CarBAMazepine ... 265
Mapluxin (Mex) *See* Digoxin ... 463
Maprotiline ... 968
Maprotiline Hydrochloride *See* Maprotiline ... 968
Maraviroc ... 971
Marcaine® *See* Bupivacaine ... 211
Marcaine® Spinal *See* Bupivacaine ... 211
Marezine® [OTC] *See* Cyclizine ... 405
Margesic® H *See* Hydrocodone and Acetaminophen ... 777
Marinol® *See* Dronabinol ... 512
Mark 1™ *See* Atropine and Pralidoxime ... 159
Marovilina (Mex) *See* Ampicillin ... 122
Marplan® *See* Isocarboxazid ... 858
Marvelon® (Can) *See* Ethinyl Estradiol and Desogestrel ... 592
Matricaria chamomilla *See* Chamomile, German *(Matricaria chamomilla, Matricaria recutita)* ... 310
Matricaria recutita *See* Chamomile, German *(Matricaria chamomilla, Matricaria recutita)* ... 310
Matulane® *See* Procarbazine ... 1340
Mavik® *See* Trandolapril ... 1608
Maxair™ Autohaler™ *See* Pirbuterol ... 1305
Maxalt® *See* Rizatriptan ... 1437
Maxalt-MLT® *See* Rizatriptan ... 1437
Maxalt RPD™ (Can) *See* Rizatriptan ... 1437
Maxef (Mex) *See* Cefepime ... 294
Maxidex® *See* Dexamethasone ... 436
Maxidone® *See* Hydrocodone and Acetaminophen ... 777
Maxifed® *See* Guaifenesin and Pseudoephedrine ... 744
Maxifed DM *See* Guaifenesin, Pseudoephedrine, and Dextromethorphan ... 748
Maxifed DMX *See* Guaifenesin, Pseudoephedrine, and Dextromethorphan ... 748
Maxifed-G® *See* Guaifenesin and Pseudoephedrine ... 744
Maximum D3® *See* Cholecalciferol ... 341
Maxiphen DM *See* Guaifenesin, Dextromethorphan, and Phenylephrine ... 746
Maxipime® *See* Cefepime ... 294
Maxitrol (Mex) *See* Polymyxin B ... 1312
Maxi-Tuss HC® *See* Phenylephrine, Hydrocodone, and Chlorpheniramine ... 1277
Maxi-Tuss HCG [DSC] *See* Hydrocodone and Guaifenesin ... 779
Maxi-Tuss HCX *See* Phenylephrine, Hydrocodone, and Chlorpheniramine ... 1277
Maxzide® *See* Hydrochlorothiazide and Triamterene ... 776
Maxzide®-25 *See* Hydrochlorothiazide and Triamterene ... 776
May Apple *See* Podophyllum Resin ... 1309
Maybush *See* Hawthorn (Crataegus oxyacantha) ... 758
MCV4 *See* Meningococcal Polysaccharide (Groups A / C / Y and W-135) Diphtheria Toxoid Conjugate Vaccine ... 985
MDL 73,147EF *See* Dolasetron ... 493
Measles, Mumps, Rubella, and Varicella Virus Vaccine ... 972
Mebaral® *See* Mephobarbital ... 988
Mebedal (Mex) *See* Mebendazole ... 972
Mebendazol (Mex) *See* Mebendazole ... 972
Mebendazole ... 972
Mebensole (Mex) *See* Mebendazole ... 972
Mecamylamine ... 973
Mecamylamine Hydrochloride *See* Mecamylamine ... 973
Mecasermin ... 973
Mecasermin (rDNA Origin) *See* Mecasermin ... 973
Mecasermin Rinfabate *See* Mecasermin ... 973
Mechlorethamine ... 974
Mechlorethamine Hydrochloride *See* Mechlorethamine ... 974
Meclizine ... 974
Meclizine Hydrochloride *See* Meclizine ... 974
Meclofenamate ... 974
Meclofenamate Sodium *See* Meclofenamate ... 974
Meclomen® (Can) *See* Meclofenamate ... 974
Meclomid (Mex) *See* Metoclopramide ... 1031
Meclozine Hydrochloride *See* Meclizine ... 974
Med-Diltiazem (Can) *See* Diltiazem ... 473
Medent-DM *See* Guaifenesin, Pseudoephedrine, and Dextromethorphan ... 748
Medent LD *See* Guaifenesin and Pseudoephedrine ... 744
Medicinal Carbon *See* Charcoal ... 312
Medicinal Charcoal *See* Charcoal ... 312
Medicone® Suppositories [OTC] *See* Phenylephrine ... 1273
Medigesic® *See* Butalbital, Acetaminophen, and Caffeine ... 229

Medi-Meclizine [OTC] *See* Meclizine ... 974

Medi-Phenyl [OTC] *See* Phenylephrine ... 1273

Mediproxen [OTC] *See* Naproxen ... 1102

Medi-Synal [OTC] *See* Acetaminophen and Pseudoephedrine ... 37

Medrol® *See* MethylPREDNISolone ... 1029

MedroxyPROGESTERone ... 975

Medroxyprogesterone Acetate *See* MedroxyPROGESTERone ... 975

Medroxyprogesterone and Estrogens (Conjugated) *See* Estrogens (Conjugated/Equine) and Medroxyprogesterone ... 583

Medsara (Mex) *See* Cytarabine ... 412

Medsatrexate (Mex) *See* Methotrexate ... 1014

Med-Verapamil (Can) *See* Verapamil ... 1665

Mefenamic-250 (Can) *See* Mefenamic Acid ... 976

Mefenamic Acid ... 976

Mefloquine ... 976

Mefloquine Hydrochloride *See* Mefloquine ... 976

Megace® *See* Megestrol ... 977

Megace® ES *See* Megestrol ... 977

Megace® OS (Can) *See* Megestrol ... 977

Megal (Mex) *See* Guaifenesin and Dextromethorphan ... 739

Megestrol ... 977

Megestrol Acetate *See* Megestrol ... 977

Megestron (Mex) *See* MedroxyPROGESTERone ... 975

Megion (Mex) *See* CefTRIAXone ... 300

Mejoralito Junior (Mex) *See* Acetaminophen ... 30

Mejoralito Pediátrico (Mex) *See* Acetaminophen ... 30

Meladinina (Mex) *See* Methoxsalen ... 1018

Melatonin ... 978

Mellaril® (Can) *See* Thioridazine ... 1572

Melleril (Mex) *See* Thioridazine ... 1572

Melosteral (Mex) *See* Meloxicam ... 982

Meloxicam ... 982

Melphalan ... 983

Memantine ... 983

Memantine Hydrochloride *See* Memantine ... 983

Menactra® *See* Meningococcal Polysaccharide (Groups A / C / Y and W-135) Diphtheria Toxoid Conjugate Vaccine ... 985

Menest® *See* Estrogens, Esterified ... 587

Meningococcal Polysaccharide (Groups A / C / Y and W-135) Diphtheria Toxoid Conjugate Vaccine ... 985

Meningococcal Polysaccharide Vaccine (Groups A / C / Y and W-135) ... 985

Menomune®-A/C/Y/W-135 *See* Meningococcal Polysaccharide Vaccine (Groups A / C / Y and W-135) ... 985

Menostar® *See* Estradiol ... 576

292 MEP® (Can) *See* Meprobamate and Aspirin ... 992

Mepenzolate ... 986

Mepenzolate Bromide *See* Mepenzolate ... 986

Mepergan *See* Meperidine and Promethazine ... 987

Meperidine ... 986

Meperidine and Promethazine ... 987

Meperidine Hydrochloride *See* Meperidine ... 986

Meperitab® *See* Meperidine ... 986

Mephobarbital ... 988

Mephyton® *See* Phytonadione ... 1289

Mepivacaine ... 990

Mepivacaine Hydrochloride *See* Mepivacaine ... 990

Meprobamate ... 991

Meprobamate and Aspirin ... 992

Mepron® *See* Atovaquone ... 157

Mequinol and Tretinoin ... 992

Mercaptopurine ... 993

6-Mercaptopurine (error-prone abbreviation) *See* Mercaptopurine ... 993

Mercapturic Acid *See* Acetylcysteine ... 47

Meridia® *See* Sibutramine ... 1479

Meropenem ... 993

Merrem® (Can) *See* Meropenem ... 993

Merrem® I.V. *See* Meropenem ... 993

Mersyndol® With Codeine (Can) *See* Acetaminophen, Codeine, and Doxylamine ... 41

Mesalamine ... 994

Mesalazine *See* Mesalamine ... 994

Mesasal® (Can) *See* Mesalamine ... 994

Mescryo (Mex) *See* Mesna ... 995

M-Eslon® (Can) *See* Morphine Sulfate ... 1077

Mesna ... 995

Mesnex® *See* Mesna ... 995

Mesnil (Mex) *See* Mesna ... 995

Mesodal (Mex) *See* Mesna ... 995

Mestinon® *See* Pyridostigmine ... 1374
Mestinon®-SR (Can) *See* Pyridostigmine ... 1374
Mestinon® Timespan® *See* Pyridostigmine ... 1374
Mestranol and Norethindrone ... 995
Mestrel (Mex) *See* Megestrol ... 977
Metacortandralone *See* PrednisoLONE ... 1326
Metadate® CD *See* Methylphenidate ... 1024
Metadate® ER *See* Methylphenidate ... 1024
Metadol™ (Can) *See* Methadone ... 1001
Metaglip™ *See* Glipizide and Metformin ... 729
123 Meta-Iodobenzlyguanidine Sulfate *See* Iobenguane I 123 ... 849
Metalyse (Mex) *See* Tenecteplase ... 1548
Metaproterenol ... 996
Metaproterenol Sulfate *See* Metaproterenol ... 996
Metax (Mex) *See* Dexamethasone ... 436
Metaxalone ... 996
MetFORMIN ... 997
Metformin and Glipizide *See* Glipizide and Metformin ... 729
Metformin and Glyburide *See* Glyburide and Metformin ... 733
Metformin and Repaglinide *See* Repaglinide and Metformin ... 1412
Metformin and Rosiglitazone *See* Rosiglitazone and Metformin ... 1449
Metformin and Sitagliptin *See* Sitagliptin and Metformin ... 1492
Metformin Hydrochloride *See* MetFORMIN ... 997
Metformin Hydrochloride and Pioglitazone Hydrochloride *See* Pioglitazone and Metformin ... 1301
Metformin Hydrochloride and Rosiglitazone Maleate *See* Rosiglitazone and Metformin ... 1449
Methadone ... 1001
Methadone Diskets® *See* Methadone ... 1001
Methadone Hydrochloride *See* Methadone ... 1001
Methadone Intensol™ *See* Methadone ... 1001
Methadose® *See* Methadone ... 1001
Methaminodiazepoxide Hydrochloride *See* ChlordiazePOXIDE ... 316
Methamphetamine ... 1006
Methamphetamine Hydrochloride *See* Methamphetamine ... 1006
Methazolamide ... 1009
Methenamine, Phenyl Salicylate, Methylene Blue, Benzoic Acid, and Hyoscyamine ... 1009
Methenamine, Sodium Biphosphate, Phenyl Salicylate, Methylene Blue, and Hyoscyamine ... 1010
Methergin (Mex) *See* Methylergonovine ... 1022
Methergine® *See* Methylergonovine ... 1022
Methimazole ... 1010
Methitest™ *See* MethylTESTOSTERone ... 1030
Methocarbamol ... 1011
Methohexital ... 1011
Methohexital Sodium *See* Methohexital ... 1011
Methotrexate ... 1014
Methotrexate Sodium *See* Methotrexate ... 1014
Methotrimeprazine ... 1015
Methotrimeprazine Hydrochloride *See* Methotrimeprazine ... 1015
Methoxsalen ... 1018
Methoxypsoralen *See* Methoxsalen ... 1018
8-Methoxypsoralen *See* Methoxsalen ... 1018
Methscopolamine ... 1019
Methscopolamine and Pseudoephedrine *See* Pseudoephedrine and Methscopolamine ... 1370
Methscopolamine Bromide *See* Methscopolamine ... 1019
Methscopolamine, Chlorpheniramine, and Pseudoephedrine *See* Chlorpheniramine, Pseudoephedrine, and Methscopolamine ... 334
Methscopolamine Nitrate and Chlordiazepoxide Hydrochloride *See* Chlordiazepoxide and Methscopolamine ... 319
Methscopolamine Nitrate, Chlorpheniramine Maleate, and Phenylephrine Hydrochloride *See* Chlorpheniramine, Phenylephrine, and Methscopolamine ... 329
Methscopolamine, Pseudoephedrine, and Chlorpheniramine *See* Chlorpheniramine, Pseudoephedrine, and Methscopolamine ... 334
Methsuximide ... 1019
Methyclothiazide ... 1020
Methylacetoxyprogesterone *See* MedroxyPROGESTERone ... 975
Methyldopa ... 1021
Methyldopa and Hydrochlorothiazide ... 1021
Methyldopate Hydrochloride *See* Methyldopa ... 1021
Methylene Blue, Methenamine, Benzoic Acid, Phenyl Salicylate, and Hyoscyamine *See* Methenamine, Phenyl Salicylate, Methylene Blue, Benzoic Acid, and Hyoscyamine ... 1009
Methylene Blue, Methenamine, Sodium Biphosphate, Phenyl Salicylate, and Hyoscyamine *See* Methenamine, Sodium Biphosphate, Phenyl Salicylate, Methylene Blue, and Hyoscyamine ... 1010

Methylergometrine Maleate *See* Methylergonovine 1022
Methylergonovine 1022
Methylergonovine Maleate *See* Methylergonovine 1022
Methylfolate 1022
Methylin® *See* Methylphenidate 1024
Methylin® ER *See* Methylphenidate 1024
Methylmorphine *See* Codeine 394
Methylnaltrexone 1023
Methylnaltrexone Bromide *See* Methylnaltrexone 1023
Methylphenidate 1024
Methylphenidate Hydrochloride *See* Methylphenidate 1024
Methylphenobarbital *See* Mephobarbital 988
Methylphenoxy-Benzene Propanamine *See* Atomoxetine 151
Methylphenyl Isoxazolyl Penicillin *See* Oxacillin 1190
Methylphytyl Napthoquinone *See* Phytonadione 1289
MethylPREDNISolone 1029
6-α-Methylprednisolone *See* MethylPREDNISolone 1029
Methylprednisolone Acetate (Can) *See* MethylPREDNISolone 1029
Methylprednisolone Sodium Succinate *See* MethylPREDNISolone 1029
4-Methylpyrazole *See* Fomepizole 685
MethylTESTOSTERone 1030
Meticortelone (Mex) *See* PrednisoLONE 1326
Meticorten (Mex) *See* PredniSONE 1327
Metimyd (Mex) *See* Sulfacetamide and Prednisolone 1516
Metipranolol 1031
Metipranolol Hydrochloride *See* Metipranolol 1031
Metoclopramide 1031
Metoclopramide Hydrochloride Injection (Can) *See* Metoclopramide 1031
Metolazone 1034
Metoprolol 1036
Metoprolol-25 (Can) *See* Metoprolol 1036
Metoprolol and Hydrochlorothiazide 1040
Metoprolol Succinate *See* Metoprolol 1036
Metoprolol Tartrate *See* Metoprolol 1036
Metoprolol Tartrate and Hydrochlorothiazide *See* Metoprolol and Hydrochlorothiazide 1040
Metoprolol Tartrate Injection, USP (Can) *See* Metoprolol 1036
Metoxiprim (Mex) *See* Sulfamethoxazole and Trimethoprim 1517
MetroCream® *See* MetroNIDAZOLE 1040
MetroGel® *See* MetroNIDAZOLE 1040
MetroGel-Vaginal® *See* MetroNIDAZOLE 1040
MetroLotion® *See* MetroNIDAZOLE 1040
MetroNIDAZOLE 1040
Metronidazole, Bismuth Subcitrate Potassium, and Tetracycline *See* Bismuth, Metronidazole, and Tetracycline 190
Metronidazole, Bismuth Subsalicylate, and Tetracycline *See* Bismuth, Metronidazole, and Tetracycline 190
Metronidazole Hydrochloride *See* MetroNIDAZOLE 1040
Metyrosine 1044
Mevacor® *See* Lovastatin 956
Mevinolin *See* Lovastatin 956
Mexiletine 1045
Mexitil® [DSC] *See* Mexiletine 1045
Mezavant® (Can) *See* Mesalamine 994
Mezelol (Mex) *See* Metoprolol 1036
M-FA-142 *See* Amonafide 108
MgSO4 (error-prone abbreviation) *See* Magnesium Sulfate 966
Miacalcic (Mex) *See* Calcitonin 253
Miacalcin® *See* Calcitonin 253
Miacalcin® NS (Can) *See* Calcitonin 253
Mi-Acid™ Double Strength [OTC] *See* Calcium Carbonate and Magnesium Hydroxide 256
Mi-Acid Maximum Strength [OTC] *See* Aluminum Hydroxide, Magnesium Hydroxide, and Simethicone 78
Mi-Acid [OTC] *See* Aluminum Hydroxide, Magnesium Hydroxide, and Simethicone 78
Micafungin 1045
Micafungin Sodium *See* Micafungin 1045
Micardis® *See* Telmisartan 1542
Micardis® HCT *See* Telmisartan and Hydrochlorothiazide 1544
Micardis® Plus (Can) *See* Telmisartan and Hydrochlorothiazide 1544
Miccil (Mex) *See* Bumetanide 211
Micitrex (Mex) *See* Tobramycin 1590
MICRhoGAM® *See* Rho(D) Immune Globulin 1415
Microgestin™ *See* Ethinyl Estradiol and Norethindrone 597
Microgestin™ Fe *See* Ethinyl Estradiol and Norethindrone 597
Microgynon (Mex) *See* Ethinyl Estradiol and Levonorgestrel 595
Microgynon CD (Mex) *See* Ethinyl Estradiol and Levonorgestrel 595
microK® *See* Potassium Chloride 1315

microK® 10 *See* Potassium Chloride ... 1315
Micro-K Extencaps® (Can) *See* Potassium Chloride ... 1315
Micromycin (Mex) *See* Minocycline ... 1056
Micronase® *See* GlyBURIDE ... 730
Micronor® (Can) *See* Norethindrone ... 1150
Microsona (Mex) *See* Hydrocortisone ... 785
Microzide® *See* Hydrochlorothiazide ... 773
Midazolam ... 1046
Midazolam Hydrochloride *See* Midazolam ... 1046
Midazolam Injection (Can) *See* Midazolam ... 1046
Midodrine ... 1050
Midodrine Hydrochloride *See* Midodrine ... 1050
Midol® Cramp and Body Aches [OTC] *See* Ibuprofen ... 803
Midol® Extended Relief *See* Naproxen ... 1102
Midozor (Mex) *See* Midazolam ... 1046
Midrat (Mex) *See* Captopril ... 264
Midrin® *See* Acetaminophen, Isometheptene, and Dichloralphenazone ... 45
Midsummer Daisy *See* Feverfew (Tanacetum parthenium) ... 628
Mifeprex® *See* Mifepristone ... 1051
Mifepristone ... 1051
Miflonide (Mex) *See* Budesonide ... 210
Migergot *See* Ergotamine and Caffeine ... 554
Miglitol ... 1052
Miglustat ... 1053
Migquin [DSC] *See* Acetaminophen, Isometheptene, and Dichloralphenazone ... 45
Migranal® *See* Dihydroergotamine ... 470
Migratine *See* Acetaminophen, Isometheptene, and Dichloralphenazone ... 45
Migrazone® [DSC] *See* Acetaminophen, Isometheptene, and Dichloralphenazone ... 45
Migrin-A [DSC] *See* Acetaminophen, Isometheptene, and Dichloralphenazone ... 45
Mild-C® [OTC] *See* Ascorbic Acid ... 141
Millipred™ *See* PrednisoLONE ... 1326
Milophene® (Can) *See* ClomiPHENE ... 368
Milrinone ... 1055
Milrinone Lactate *See* Milrinone ... 1055
Milrinone Lactate Injection (Can) *See* Milrinone ... 1055
Miltown® [DSC] *See* Meprobamate ... 991
Mineral Oil ... 1055
Minestrin™ 1/20 (Can) *See* Ethinyl Estradiol and Norethindrone ... 597
Minipres (Mex) *See* Prazosin ... 1325
Minipress® *See* Prazosin ... 1325
Minirin® (Can) *See* Desmopressin ... 431
Minitran™ *See* Nitroglycerin ... 1147
Minizide® [DSC] *See* Prazosin and Polythiazide ... 1325
Minocin® (Can) *See* Minocycline ... 1056
Minocin® PAC *See* Minocycline ... 1056
Minocycline ... 1056
Minocycline Hydrochloride *See* Minocycline ... 1056
Minodiab (Mex) *See* GlipiZIDE ... 726
Min-Ovral® (Can) *See* Ethinyl Estradiol and Levonorgestrel ... 595
Minox (Can) *See* Minoxidil ... 1057
Minoxidil ... 1057
Mintab DM *See* Guaifenesin and Dextromethorphan ... 739
Mint-Citalopram (Can) *See* Citalopram ... 354
Mintezol® *See* Thiabendazole ... 1567
Mintox Extra Strength [OTC] *See* Aluminum Hydroxide, Magnesium Hydroxide, and Simethicone ... 78
Mintox Plus [OTC] *See* Aluminum Hydroxide, Magnesium Hydroxide, and Simethicone ... 78
Mintuss DR *See* Chlorpheniramine, Phenylephrine, and Dextromethorphan ... 327
Mintuss G [DSC] *See* Hydrocodone, Phenylephrine, and Guaifenesin ... 783
Mintuss HC *See* Phenylephrine, Hydrocodone, and Chlorpheniramine ... 1277
Mintuss MS *See* Phenylephrine, Hydrocodone, and Chlorpheniramine ... 1277
Miochol®-E *See* Acetylcholine ... 47
Mirapex® *See* Pramipexole ... 1318
Mircette® *See* Ethinyl Estradiol and Desogestrel ... 592
Mirena® *See* Levonorgestrel ... 918
Mirtazapine ... 1058
Misinex (Mex) *See* Gentamicin ... 714
Misoprostol and Diclofenac *See* Diclofenac and Misoprostol ... 458
Mitomycin ... 1061
Mitomycin-X *See* Mitomycin ... 1061
Mitomycin-C *See* Mitomycin ... 1061
Mitotane ... 1061
Mitotie (Mex) *See* Mitomycin ... 1061
Mitoxantrone ... 1061
Mitoxantrone Hydrochloride *See* Mitoxantrone ... 1061
Mitoxantrone Injection® (Can) *See* Mitoxantrone ... 1061
Mitoxgen (Mex) *See* Mitoxantrone ... 1061

Mitozantrone *See* Mitoxantrone 1061
Mitroken (Mex) *See* Ciprofloxacin 346
Mitroxone (Mex) *See* Mitoxantrone 1061
MK383 *See* Tirofiban 1586
MK-0431 *See* SitaGLIPtin 1491
MK462 *See* Rizatriptan 1437
MK 0517 *See* Fosaprepitant 690
MK-0518 *See* Raltegravir 1393
MK594 *See* Losartan 952
MK0826 *See* Ertapenem 557
MK 869 *See* Aprepitant 130
MLN341 *See* Bortezomib 192
MMF *See* Mycophenolate 1087
MMR-V *See* Measles, Mumps, Rubella, and Varicella Virus Vaccine 972
MMRV *See* Measles, Mumps, Rubella, and Varicella Virus Vaccine 972
Moban® *See* Molindone 1069
Mobic® *See* Meloxicam 982
Mobicox® (Can) *See* Meloxicam 982
Moclobemide 1062
Modafinil 1065
Modecate® (Can) *See* Fluphenazine 660
Modecate® Concentrate (Can) *See* Fluphenazine 660
Modicon® *See* Ethinyl Estradiol and Norethindrone 597
Modiodal (Mex) *See* Modafinil 1065
Moduret (Can) *See* Amiloride and Hydrochlorothiazide 86
Moduretic (Mex) *See* Amiloride and Hydrochlorothiazide 86
Moduretic (Combinado con hidroclorotiazida) (Mex) *See* AMILoride 84
Modusik-A Ofteno (Mex) *See* CycloSPORINE 409
Moexipril 1068
Moexipril and Hydrochlorothiazide 1068
Moexipril Hydrochloride *See* Moexipril 1068
Molindone 1069
Molindone Hydrochloride *See* Molindone 1069
Mometasone 1071
Mometasone Furoate *See* Mometasone 1071
Monacolin K *See* Lovastatin 956
Monitan® (Can) *See* Acebutolol 27
Monoclonal Antibody *See* Muromonab-CD3 1086
Monocor® (Can) *See* Bisoprolol 190
Monodox® *See* Doxycycline 509
Monoket® *See* Isosorbide Mononitrate 869
Mono Mack (Mex) *See* Isosorbide Mononitrate 869
MonoNessa™ *See* Ethinyl Estradiol and Norgestimate 600
Mononine® *See* Factor IX 612
Monopril® *See* Fosinopril 691
Monopril-HCT® *See* Fosinopril and Hydrochlorothiazide 692
Montelukast 1074
Montelukast Sodium *See* Montelukast 1074
Monurol® *See* Fosfomycin 691
8-MOP® *See* Methoxsalen 1018
Mopral (Mex) *See* Omeprazole 1176
Moricizine 1077
Moricizine Hydrochloride *See* Moricizine 1077
Morning After Pill *See* Ethinyl Estradiol and Norgestrel 601
Morphine HP® (Can) *See* Morphine Sulfate 1077
Morphine LP® Epidural (Can) *See* Morphine Sulfate 1077
Morphine Sulfate 1077
M.O.S.® 10 (Can) *See* Morphine Sulfate 1077
M.O.S.® 20 (Can) *See* Morphine Sulfate 1077
M.O.S.® 30 (Can) *See* Morphine Sulfate 1077
Mosco® Callus & Corn Remover [OTC] *See* Salicylic Acid 1454
M.O.S.-SR® (Can) *See* Morphine Sulfate 1077
M.O.S.-Sulfate® (Can) *See* Morphine Sulfate 1077
Motilium (Mex) *See* Domperidone 493
Motofen® [DSC] *See* Difenoxin and Atropine 462
Motrin (Mex) *See* Ibuprofen 803
Motrin® (Children's) (Can) *See* Ibuprofen 803
Motrin® Children's [OTC] *See* Ibuprofen 803
Motrin® [DSC] *See* Ibuprofen 803
Motrin® IB (Can) *See* Ibuprofen 803
Motrin® IB [OTC] *See* Ibuprofen 803
Motrin® Infants' [OTC] *See* Ibuprofen 803
Motrin® Junior [OTC] *See* Ibuprofen 803
MoviPrep® *See* Polyethylene Glycol-Electrolyte Solution 1310
Moxifloxacin 1084
Moxifloxacin Hydrochloride *See* Moxifloxacin 1084
Moxlin (Mex) *See* Amoxicillin and Clavulanate Potassium 115

4-MP *See* Fomepizole ... 685
MPA *See* Mycophenolate ... 1087
MPA and Estrogens (Conjugated) *See* Estrogens (Conjugated/Equine) and Medroxyprogesterone ... 583
6-MP (error-prone abbreviation) *See* Mercaptopurine ... 993
MPSV4 *See* Meningococcal Polysaccharide Vaccine (Groups A / C / Y and W-135) ... 985
MS Contin® *See* Morphine Sulfate ... 1077
MS (error-prone abbreviation and should not be used) *See* Morphine Sulfate ... 1077
MS-IR® (Can) *See* Morphine Sulfate ... 1077
MSO4 (error-prone abbreviation and should not be used) *See* Morphine Sulfate ... 1077
MTC *See* Mitomycin ... 1061
MTX (error-prone abbreviation) *See* Methotrexate ... 1014
Mubonet (Mex) *See* Calcium Carbonate ... 254
Mucinex® D Maximum Strength [OTC] *See* Guaifenesin and Pseudoephedrine ... 744
Mucinex®-D [OTC] *See* Guaifenesin and Pseudoephedrine ... 744
Mucinex® Children's Cough [OTC] *See* Guaifenesin and Dextromethorphan ... 739
Mucinex®, Children's Mini-Melts™ [OTC] *See* GuaiFENesin ... 737
Mucinex®, Children's [OTC] *See* GuaiFENesin ... 737
Mucinex® DM Maximum Strength [OTC] *See* Guaifenesin and Dextromethorphan ... 739
Mucinex® DM [OTC] *See* Guaifenesin and Dextromethorphan ... 739
Mucinex® Full force™ [OTC] *See* Oxymetazoline ... 1208
Mucinex®, Junior Mini-Melts™ [OTC] *See* GuaiFENesin ... 737
Mucinex® Maximum Strength [OTC] *See* GuaiFENesin ... 737
Mucinex® moisture smart™ [OTC] *See* Oxymetazoline ... 1208
Mucinex® [OTC] *See* GuaiFENesin ... 737
Mucomyst® (Can) *See* Acetylcysteine ... 47
Multiferon (Mex) *See* Interferon Alfa-2a ... 844
Multitargeted Antifolate *See* Pemetrexed ... 1238
Mumps, Rubella, Varicella, and Measles Vaccine *See* Measles, Mumps, Rubella, and Varicella Virus Vaccine ... 972
Munobal (Mex) *See* Felodipine ... 617
Mupirocin ... 1085
Mupirocin Calcium *See* Mupirocin ... 1085
Murine® Tears Plus [OTC] *See* Tetrahydrozoline ... 1560
Muromonab-CD3 ... 1086
Muse® *See* Alprostadil ... 77
Muse® Pellet (Can) *See* Alprostadil ... 77
Mustargen® *See* Mechlorethamine ... 974
Mustine *See* Mechlorethamine ... 974
Mutamycin® (Can) *See* Mitomycin ... 1061
Mutterkraut *See* Feverfew (Tanacetum parthenium) ... 628
M. V. I. 12 (Mex) *See* Pyridoxine ... 1376
M.V.I. Adult™ *See* Vitamins (Multiple/Injectable) ... 1677
M.V.I.® Pediatric *See* Vitamins (Multiple/Injectable) ... 1677
Myambutol® *See* Ethambutol ... 592
Mycamine® *See* Micafungin ... 1045
Mycobutin® *See* Rifabutin ... 1418
Mycophenolate ... 1087
Mycophenolate Mofetil *See* Mycophenolate ... 1087
Mycophenolate Sodium *See* Mycophenolate ... 1087
Mycophenolic Acid *See* Mycophenolate ... 1087
MyDex *See* Guaifenesin and Phenylephrine ... 742
Mydfrin® *See* Phenylephrine ... 1273
Mydral™ *See* Tropicamide ... 1636
Mydriacyl® *See* Tropicamide ... 1636
Myfortic® *See* Mycophenolate ... 1087
MyHist-DM *See* Phenylephrine, Pyrilamine, and Dextromethorphan ... 1278
MyHist-PD *See* Chlorpheniramine, Pyrilamine, and Phenylephrine ... 335
MyKidz Iron 10™ *See* Ferrous Sulfate ... 627
Mylanta® Children's [OTC] *See* Calcium Carbonate ... 254
Mylanta® Double Strength (Can) *See* Aluminum Hydroxide, Magnesium Hydroxide, and Simethicone ... 78
Mylanta® Extra Strength (Can) *See* Aluminum Hydroxide, Magnesium Hydroxide, and Simethicone ... 78
Mylanta® Gelcaps® [OTC] *See* Calcium Carbonate and Magnesium Hydroxide ... 256
Mylanta® Liquid [OTC] *See* Aluminum Hydroxide, Magnesium Hydroxide, and Simethicone ... 78
Mylanta® Maximum Strength Liquid [OTC] *See* Aluminum Hydroxide, Magnesium Hydroxide, and Simethicone ... 78
Mylanta® Regular Strength (Can) *See* Aluminum Hydroxide, Magnesium Hydroxide, and Simethicone ... 78
Mylanta® Supreme [OTC] *See* Calcium Carbonate and Magnesium Hydroxide ... 256
Mylanta® Ultra [OTC] *See* Calcium Carbonate and Magnesium Hydroxide ... 256
Myleran® *See* Busulfan ... 226
Mylocel™ *See* Hydroxyurea ... 796
Mylotarg® *See* Gemtuzumab Ozogamicin ... 713
Myobloc® *See* Botulinum Toxin Type B ... 197
Myochrysine® *See* Gold Sodium Thiomalate ... 734

Myphetane DX *See* Brompheniramine, Pseudoephedrine, and Dextromethorphan ... 208
myrac™ *See* Minocycline ... 1056
Mysoline® *See* Primidone ... 1336
Mytelase® *See* Ambenonium ... 82
Mytussin® AC *See* Guaifenesin and Codeine ... 738
Mytussin® DAC *See* Guaifenesin, Pseudoephedrine, and Codeine ... 747
N-0923 *See* Rotigotine ... 1449
NAAK *See* Atropine and Pralidoxime ... 159
Nabi-HB® *See* Hepatitis B Immune Globulin ... 762
Nabilone ... 1088
nab-Paclitaxel *See* Paclitaxel (Protein Bound) ... 1214
Nabumetone ... 1089
NAC *See* Acetylcysteine ... 47
N-acetyl-5-methoxytryptamine *See* Melatonin ... 978
N-Acetyl-L-cysteine *See* Acetylcysteine ... 47
N-Acetylcysteine *See* Acetylcysteine ... 47
N-Acetyl-P-Aminophenol *See* Acetaminophen ... 30
Nadolol ... 1090
Nadolol and Bendroflumethiazide ... 1092
Nafacil-S (Mex) *See* Cephalexin ... 306
Nafarelin ... 1093
Nafarelin Acetate *See* Nafarelin ... 1093
Nafcillin ... 1093
Nafcillin Sodium *See* Nafcillin ... 1093
Nafidimide *See* Amonafide ... 108
Nafiset (Mex) *See* Desmopressin ... 431
Naglazyme™ *See* Galsulfase ... 708
NaHCO3 *See* Sodium Bicarbonate ... 1494
Nalbuphine ... 1094
Nalbuphine Hydrochloride *See* Nalbuphine ... 1094
Nalcrom® (Can) *See* Cromolyn ... 402
Nalcryn SP (Mex) *See* Nalbuphine ... 1094
Nalex®-A *See* Chlorpheniramine, Phenylephrine, and Phenyltoloxamine ... 331
Nalex A 12 *See* Chlorpheniramine, Pyrilamine, and Phenylephrine ... 335
Nalfon® *See* Fenoprofen ... 623
Nallpen® (Can) *See* Nafcillin ... 1093
N-allylnoroxymorphine Hydrochloride *See* Naloxone ... 1097
Nalmefene ... 1095
Nalmefene Hydrochloride *See* Nalmefene ... 1095
Naloxone ... 1097
Naloxone and Buprenorphine *See* Buprenorphine and Naloxone ... 215
Naloxone Hydrochloride *See* Naloxone ... 1097
Naloxone Hydrochloride and Pentazocine Hydrochloride *See* Pentazocine ... 1243
Naloxone Hydrochloride Dihydrate and Buprenorphine Hydrochloride *See* Buprenorphine and Naloxone ... 215
Naloxone Hydrochloride Injection® (Can) *See* Naloxone ... 1097
Naltrexone ... 1099
Naltrexone Hydrochloride *See* Naltrexone ... 1099
Namenda™ *See* Memantine ... 983
Nandrolone ... 1101
Nandrolone Decanoate *See* Nandrolone ... 1101
Nandrolone Phenpropionate *See* Nandrolone ... 1101
Naphazoline ... 1101
Naphazoline and Pheniramine ... 1102
Naphazoline Hydrochloride *See* Naphazoline ... 1101
Naphcon-A® (Can) *See* Naphazoline and Pheniramine ... 1102
Naphcon-A® [OTC] *See* Naphazoline and Pheniramine ... 1102
Naphcon Forte® (Can) *See* Naphazoline ... 1101
Naphcon® [OTC] *See* Naphazoline ... 1101
NapraPAC™ *See* Lansoprazole and Naproxen ... 897
Naprelan® *See* Naproxen ... 1102
Naprodil (Mex) *See* Naproxen ... 1102
Naprosyn® *See* Naproxen ... 1102
Naproxen ... 1102
Naproxen and Lansoprazole *See* Lansoprazole and Naproxen ... 897
Naproxen and Pseudoephedrine ... 1107
Naproxen and Sumatriptan *See* Sumatriptan and Naproxen ... 1530
Naproxen Sodium *See* Naproxen ... 1102
Naproxen Sodium and Pseudoephedrine *See* Naproxen and Pseudoephedrine ... 1107
Naproxen Sodium and Sumatriptan *See* Sumatriptan and Naproxen ... 1530
Naproxen Sodium and Sumatriptan Succinate *See* Sumatriptan and Naproxen ... 1530
Naramig (Mex) *See* Naratriptan ... 1107
Naratriptan ... 1107
Naratriptan Hydrochloride *See* Naratriptan ... 1107
Narcan *See* Naloxone ... 1097
Narcanti (Mex) *See* Naloxone ... 1097
Nardil® *See* Phenelzine ... 1261

Nasacort® AQ *See* Triamcinolone ... 1617
NasalCrom® [OTC] *See* Cromolyn ... 402
Nasalide® (Can) *See* Flunisolide ... 646
Nasarel® *See* Flunisolide ... 646
Nasatab® LA *See* Guaifenesin and Pseudoephedrine ... 744
Nascobal® *See* Cyanocobalamin ... 404
Nasex-G *See* Guaifenesin and Phenylephrine ... 742
Nasofed™ *See* Pseudoephedrine ... 1367
Nasonex® *See* Mometasone ... 1071
Nasop12™ *See* Phenylephrine ... 1273
Nastil (Mex) *See* Ketoconazole ... 876
Natalizumab ... 1109
Nateglinide ... 1112
Natele (Mex) *See* Pyridoxine ... 1376
Natrecor® *See* Nesiritide ... 1123
Natriuretic Peptide *See* Nesiritide ... 1123
Natulan® (Can) *See* Procarbazine ... 1340
Nature-Throid™ *See* Thyroid, Desiccated ... 1579
Nauseatol (Can) *See* DimenhyDRINATE ... 478
Navane® *See* Thiothixene ... 1576
Navelbine® *See* Vinorelbine ... 1674
Naxen® (Can) *See* Naproxen ... 1102
Naxen® EC (Can) *See* Naproxen ... 1102
NC-722665 *See* Bicalutamide ... 188
Nebivolol ... 1115
Nebivolol Hydrochloride *See* Nebivolol ... 1115
NebuPent® *See* Pentamidine ... 1242
Necon® 0.5/35 *See* Ethinyl Estradiol and Norethindrone ... 597
Necon® 1/35 *See* Ethinyl Estradiol and Norethindrone ... 597
Necon® 1/50 *See* Mestranol and Norethindrone ... 995
Necon® 7/7/7 *See* Ethinyl Estradiol and Norethindrone ... 597
Necon® 10/11 *See* Ethinyl Estradiol and Norethindrone ... 597
Nedocromil ... 1115
Nedocromil Sodium *See* Nedocromil ... 1115
Nefazodone ... 1116
Nefazodone Hydrochloride *See* Nefazodone ... 1116
Nefryl (Mex) *See* Oxybutynin ... 1199
Nelarabine ... 1120
Nelfinavir ... 1120
Nembutal® *See* PENTobarbital ... 1247
Nembutal® Sodium (Can) *See* PENTobarbital ... 1247
Neoalexil (Mex) *See* Loratadine ... 946
Neobacigrin (Mex) *See* Polymyxin B ... 1312
Neo-Clarosip (Mex) *See* Clarithromycin ... 360
Neo DM *See* Chlorpheniramine, Phenylephrine, and Dextromethorphan ... 327
Neofrin™ *See* Phenylephrine ... 1273
Neolem (Mex) *See* CycloSPORINE ... 409
Neo-Panlacticos (Mex) *See* Thiamine ... 1568
NeoProfen® *See* Ibuprofen ... 803
Neoral® *See* CycloSPORINE ... 409
Neosar *See* Cyclophosphamide ... 408
Neosporin (Mex) *See* Polymyxin B ... 1312
Neostigmine ... 1121
Neostigmine Bromide *See* Neostigmine ... 1121
Neostigmine Methylsulfate *See* Neostigmine ... 1121
Neo-Synephrine® (Can) *See* Phenylephrine ... 1273
Neo-Synephrine® 12 Hour Extra Moisturizing [OTC] *See* Oxymetazoline ... 1208
Neo-Synephrine® 12 Hour [OTC] *See* Oxymetazoline ... 1208
Neo-Synephrine® Extra Strength [OTC] *See* Phenylephrine ... 1273
Neo-Synephrine® Injection *See* Phenylephrine ... 1273
Neo-Synephrine® Mild [OTC] *See* Phenylephrine ... 1273
Neo-Synephrine® Regular Strength [OTC] *See* Phenylephrine ... 1273
Neotrex (Mex) *See* Isotretinoin ... 871
Nephro-Calci® [OTC] *See* Calcium Carbonate ... 254
Nephro-Fer® [OTC] *See* Ferrous Fumarate ... 626
Nerve Agent Antidote Kit *See* Atropine and Pralidoxime ... 159
Nesiritide ... 1123
Neugeron (Mex) *See* CarBAMazepine ... 265
Neulasta® *See* Pegfilgrastim ... 1236
Neuleptil® (Can) *See* Periciazine ... 1252
Neumega® *See* Oprelvekin ... 1184
Neupax (Mex) *See* ALPRAZolam ... 72
Neupogen® *See* Filgrastim ... 632
Neupro® [DSC] *See* Rotigotine ... 1449
Neurobion (Mex) *See* Thiamine ... 1568
Neurolep (Mex) *See* CarBAMazepine ... 265
Neurontin® *See* Gabapentin ... 702

Neut® *See* Sodium Bicarbonate 1494
NeuTrexin® [DSC] *See* Trimetrexate 1629
Neutrogena® Advanced Solutions™ [OTC] *See* Salicylic Acid 1454
Neutrogena® Blackhead Eliminating™ 2-in-1 Foaming Pads [OTC] *See* Salicylic Acid 1454
Neutrogena® Blackhead Eliminating™ Astringent [OTC] [DSC] *See* Salicylic Acid 1454
Neutrogena® Blackhead Eliminating™ Daily Scrub [OTC] *See* Salicylic Acid 1454
Neutrogena® Blackhead Eliminating™ Treatment Mask [OTC] [DSC] *See* Salicylic Acid 1454
Neutrogena® Body Clear® [OTC] *See* Salicylic Acid 1454
Neutrogena® Clear Pore™ Oil-Controlling Astringent [OTC] *See* Salicylic Acid 1454
Neutrogena® Oil-Free Acne Wash 60 Second Mask Scrub [OTC] *See* Salicylic Acid 1454
Neutrogena® Oil-Free Acne Wash Cream Cleanser [OTC] *See* Salicylic Acid 1454
Neutrogena® Oil-Free Acne Wash Foam Cleanser [OTC] *See* Salicylic Acid 1454
Neutrogena® Oil-Free Acne Wash [OTC] *See* Salicylic Acid 1454
Neutrogena® Rapid Clear® Acne Defense [OTC] *See* Salicylic Acid 1454
Neutrogena® Rapid Clear® Acne Eliminating [OTC] *See* Salicylic Acid 1454
Nevirapine 1124
Nexavar® *See* Sorafenib 1501
Nexium® *See* Esomeprazole 570
Nexium IV (Mex) *See* Esomeprazole 570
Nexium-MUPS (Mex) *See* Esomeprazole 570
Nexphen PD *See* Guaifenesin and Phenylephrine 742
NFV *See* Nelfinavir 1120
Niacin 1124
Niacin and Lovastatin 1127
Niacin and Simvastatin 1127
Niacin-Time® *See* Niacin 1124
Niacor® *See* Niacin 1124
Niar (Mex) *See* Selegiline 1466
Niaspan® *See* Niacin 1124
NiCARdipine 1128
Nicardipine Hydrochloride *See* NiCARdipine 1128
Nicoderm® (Can) *See* Nicotine 1133
NicoDerm® CQ® [OTC] *See* Nicotine 1133
Nicorette® (Can) *See* Nicotine 1133
Nicorette® [OTC] *See* Nicotine 1133
Nicorette® Plus (Can) *See* Nicotine 1133
Nicotine 1133
Nicotinell TTS (Mex) *See* Nicotine 1133
Nicotinic Acid *See* Niacin 1124
Nicotrol® (Can) *See* Nicotine 1133
Nicotrol® Inhaler *See* Nicotine 1133
Nicotrol® NS *See* Nicotine 1133
Nicoumalone *See* Acenocoumarol 30
Nidagel™ (Can) *See* MetroNIDAZOLE 1040
Nifar-GB (Mex) *See* NIFEdipine 1136
Nifediac™ CC *See* NIFEdipine 1136
Nifedical™ XL *See* NIFEdipine 1136
Nifedigel (Mex) *See* NIFEdipine 1136
NIFEdipine 1136
Niferex® [OTC] *See* Polysaccharide-Iron Complex 1313
Nifezzard (Mex) *See* NIFEdipine 1136
Niftolid *See* Flutamide 667
Nilandron® *See* Nilutamide 1140
Nilotinib 1140
Nilotinib Hydrochloride Monohydrate *See* Nilotinib 1140
Nilutamide 1140
Nimbex® *See* Cisatracurium 353
NiMODipine 1141
Nimotop® *See* NiMODipine 1141
Ninjin *See* Ginseng, Panax (*Panax ginseng*) 718
Nipent® *See* Pentostatin 1250
Nipresol (Mex) *See* Metoprolol 1036
Niquitin (Mex) *See* Nicotine 1133
Niravam™ *See* ALPRAZolam 72
Nisoldipine 1143
Nistaken (Mex) *See* Propafenone 1351
Nitalapram *See* Citalopram 354
Nitan (Mex) *See* Nitroprusside 1149
Nitazoxanide 1146
Nitisinone 1146
Nitoman™ (Can) *See* Tetrabenazine 1554
Nitradisc (Mex) *See* Nitroglycerin 1147
Nitrek® [DSC] *See* Nitroglycerin 1147

4'-Nitro-3'-Trifluoromethylisobutyrantide *See* Flutamide 667
Nitro-Bid® *See* Nitroglycerin 1147
Nitro-Dur® *See* Nitroglycerin 1147
Nitrofurantoin 1147
Nitrogen Mustard *See* Mechlorethamine 974
Nitroglycerin 1147
Nitroglycerin Injection, USP (Can) *See* Nitroglycerin 1147
Nitroglycerol *See* Nitroglycerin 1147
Nitrol® (Can) *See* Nitroglycerin 1147
Nitrolingual® *See* Nitroglycerin 1147
Nitropress® *See* Nitroprusside 1149
Nitroprusside 1149
Nitroprusside Sodium *See* Nitroprusside 1149
NitroQuick® *See* Nitroglycerin 1147
Nitrostat® *See* Nitroglycerin 1147
NitroTime® *See* Nitroglycerin 1147
Nizatidine 1149
Nizoral® *See* Ketoconazole 876
Nizoral® A-D [OTC] *See* Ketoconazole 876
N-Methylhydrazine *See* Procarbazine 1340
N-methylnaltrexone Bromide *See* Methylnaltrexone 1023
No Doz® Maximum Strength [OTC] *See* Caffeine 250
Nograine (Mex) *See* SUMAtriptan 1527
NoHist *See* Chlorpheniramine and Phenylephrine 323
NoHist-A *See* Chlorpheniramine, Phenylephrine, and Phenyltoloxamine 331
Nolvadex® (Can) *See* Tamoxifen 1537
Nolvadex®-D (Can) *See* Tamoxifen 1537
Nomactril (Mex) *See* Octreotide 1158
Nopatic (Mex) *See* Gabapentin 702
Nora-BE™ *See* Norethindrone 1150
Norace (Mex) *See* Mestranol and Norethindrone 995
Noradrenaline *See* Norepinephrine 1150
Noradrenaline Acid Tartrate *See* Norepinephrine 1150
Norapred (Mex) *See* PredniSONE 1327
Norboral (Mex) *See* GlyBURIDE 730
Norco® *See* Hydrocodone and Acetaminophen 777
Nordeoxyguanosine *See* Ganciclovir 708
Nordet (Mex) *See* Ethinyl Estradiol and Levonorgestrel 595
Nordette® *See* Ethinyl Estradiol and Levonorgestrel 595
Nordinet Infantil (Mex) *See* Acetaminophen 30
Norditropin® *See* Somatropin 1499
Norditropin® NordiFlex® *See* Somatropin 1499
Norel DM™ *See* Chlorpheniramine, Phenylephrine, and Dextromethorphan 327
norel® EX *See* Guaifenesin and Phenylephrine 742
Norelgestromin and Ethinyl Estradiol *See* Ethinyl Estradiol and Norelgestromin 597
Norepinephrine 1150
Norepinephrine Bitartrate *See* Norepinephrine 1150
Norethindrone 1150
Norethindrone Acetate *See* Norethindrone 1150
Norethindrone Acetate and Ethinyl Estradiol *See* Ethinyl Estradiol and Norethindrone 597
Norethindrone and Estradiol *See* Estradiol and Norethindrone 579
Norethindrone and Mestranol *See* Mestranol and Norethindrone 995
Norethisterone *See* Norethindrone 1150
Norfenon (Mex) *See* Propafenone 1351
Norflex™ *See* Orphenadrine 1186
Norfloxacin 1151
Norfloxacine® (Can) *See* Norfloxacin 1151
Norgesic™ (Can) *See* Orphenadrine, Aspirin, and Caffeine 1187
Norgesic™ [DSC] *See* Orphenadrine, Aspirin, and Caffeine 1187
Norgesic™ Forte (Can) *See* Orphenadrine, Aspirin, and Caffeine 1187
Norgesic™ Forte [DSC] *See* Orphenadrine, Aspirin, and Caffeine 1187
Norgestimate and Estradiol *See* Estradiol and Norgestimate 580
Norgestimate and Ethinyl Estradiol *See* Ethinyl Estradiol and Norgestimate 600
Norgestrel and Ethinyl Estradiol *See* Ethinyl Estradiol and Norgestrel 601
Norinyl® 1+35 *See* Ethinyl Estradiol and Norethindrone 597
Norinyl® 1+50 *See* Mestranol and Norethindrone 995
Ñorispez (Mex) *See* Risperidone 1425
Noritate® *See* MetroNIDAZOLE 1040
Norlutate® (Can) *See* Norethindrone 1150
Normodyne® (Can) *See* Labetalol 881
Noroxin® *See* Norfloxacin 1151
Noroxin Oftalmico (Mex) *See* Norfloxacin 1151
Norpace® *See* Disopyramide 488
Norpace® CR *See* Disopyramide 488
Norplant® Implant (Can) *See* Levonorgestrel 918
Norpramin® *See* Desipramine 426
Nor-QD® *See* Norethindrone 1150

Nortemp Children's [OTC] *See* Acetaminophen 30
Nor-Tenz (Mex) *See* Brimonidine 199
Northyx™ *See* Methimazole 1010
Nortrel™ *See* Ethinyl Estradiol and Norethindrone 597
Nortrel™ 7/7/7 *See* Ethinyl Estradiol and Norethindrone 597
Nortriptyline 1152
Nortriptyline Hydrochloride *See* Nortriptyline 1152
Norvas (Mex) *See* AmLODIPine 100
Norvasc® *See* AmLODIPine 100
Norventyl (Can) *See* Nortriptyline 1152
Norvir® *See* Ritonavir 1433
Norvir® SEC (Can) *See* Ritonavir 1433
Nositrol (Mex) *See* Hydrocortisone 785
Novador (Mex) *See* Cefuroxime 300
Novahistex® DM Decongestant (Can) *See* Pseudoephedrine and Dextromethorphan 1369
Novahistex® DM Decongestant Expectorant (Can) *See* Guaifenesin, Pseudoephedrine, and Dextromethorphan 748
Novahistex® Expectorant with Decongestant (Can) *See* Guaifenesin and Pseudoephedrine 744
Novahistine DH *See* Dihydrocodeine, Chlorpheniramine, and Phenylephrine 469
Novahistine® DM Decongestant (Can) *See* Pseudoephedrine and Dextromethorphan 1369
Novahistine® DM Decongestant Expectorant (Can) *See* Guaifenesin, Pseudoephedrine, and Dextromethorphan 748
Novamilor (Can) *See* Amiloride and Hydrochlorothiazide 86
Novamoxin® (Can) *See* Amoxicillin 112
Novantrone® *See* Mitoxantrone 1061
Novaprin (Mex) *See* Danazol 416
Novarel® *See* Chorionic Gonadotropin (Human) 342
Novasen (Can) *See* Aspirin 143
Novaxen (Mex) *See* Naproxen 1102
Noviken LP (Mex) *See* NIFEdipine 1136
Novina (Mex) *See* Pravastatin 1321
Novo-5 ASA (Can) *See* Mesalamine 994
Novo-Acebutolol (Can) *See* Acebutolol 27
Novo-Alendronate (Can) *See* Alendronate 59
Novo-Alprazol (Can) *See* ALPRAZolam 72
Novo-Amiodarone (Can) *See* Amiodarone 89
Novo-Ampicillin (Can) *See* Ampicillin 122
Novo-Atenol (Can) *See* Atenolol 147
Novo-Atenolthalidone (Can) *See* Atenolol and Chlorthalidone 150
Novo-Azathioprine (Can) *See* AzaTHIOprine 162
Novo-Azithromycin (Can) *See* Azithromycin 163
Novo-Bicalutamide (Can) *See* Bicalutamide 188
Novo-Bisoprolol (Can) *See* Bisoprolol 190
Novo-Bromazepam (Can) *See* Bromazepam 200
Novo-Bupropion SR (Can) *See* BuPROPion 217
Novo-Buspirone (Can) *See* BusPIRone 223
Novocain® *See* Procaine 1340
Novo-Captopril (Can) *See* Captopril 264
Novo-Carbamaz (Can) *See* CarBAMazepine 265
Novo-Carvedilol (Can) *See* Carvedilol 286
Novo-Cefaclor (Can) *See* Cefaclor 291
Novo-Cefadroxil (Can) *See* Cefadroxil 292
Novo-Chloroquine (Can) *See* Chloroquine Phosphate 320
Novo-Chlorpromazine (Can) *See* ChlorproMAZINE 336
Novo-Cholamine (Can) *See* Cholestyramine Resin 341
Novo-Cholamine Light (Can) *See* Cholestyramine Resin 341
Novo-Cimetidine (Can) *See* Cimetidine 345
Novo-Ciprofloxacin (Can) *See* Ciprofloxacin 346
Novo-Citalopram (Can) *See* Citalopram 354
Novo-Clavamoxin (Can) *See* Amoxicillin and Clavulanate Potassium 115
Novo-Clindamycin (Can) *See* Clindamycin 363
Novo-Clobazam (Can) *See* Clobazam 364
Novo-Clonazepam (Can) *See* ClonazePAM 373
Novo-Clonidine (Can) *See* CloNIDine 377
Novo-Clopate (Can) *See* Clorazepate 384
Novo-Cycloprine (Can) *See* Cyclobenzaprine 405
Novo-Desmopressin (Can) *See* Desmopressin 431
Novo-Difenac (Can) *See* Diclofenac 457
Novo-Difenac K (Can) *See* Diclofenac 457
Novo-Difenac-SR (Can) *See* Diclofenac 457
Novo-Diflunisal (Can) *See* Diflunisal 463
Novo-Digoxin (Can) *See* Digoxin 463
Novo-Diltazem (Can) *See* Diltiazem 473
Novo-Diltazem-CD (Can) *See* Diltiazem 473
Novo-Diltiazem HCl ER (Can) *See* Diltiazem 473
Novo-Dimenate (Can) *See* DimenhyDRINATE 478

Novo-Dipam (Can) *See* Diazepam ... 451
Novo-Divalproex (Can) *See* Valproic Acid and Derivatives ... 1642
Novo-Domperidone (Can) *See* Domperidone ... 493
Novo-Doxazosin (Can) *See* Doxazosin ... 500
Novo-Doxepin (Can) *See* Doxepin ... 502
Novo-Doxylin (Can) *See* Doxycycline ... 509
Novo-Enalapril (Can) *See* Enalapril ... 531
Novo-Famotidine (Can) *See* Famotidine ... 613
Novo-Fenofibrate (Can) *See* Fenofibrate ... 620
Novo-Fenofibrate-S (Can) *See* Fenofibrate ... 620
Novo-Ferrogluc (Can) *See* Ferrous Gluconate ... 627
Novo-Fluconazole (Can) *See* Fluconazole ... 635
Novo-Fluoxetine (Can) *See* FLUoxetine ... 650
Novo-Flurprofen (Can) *See* Flurbiprofen ... 667
Novo-Flutamide (Can) *See* Flutamide ... 667
Novo-Fluvoxamine (Can) *See* Fluvoxamine ... 678
Novo-Fosinopril (Can) *See* Fosinopril ... 691
Novo-Furantoin (Can) *See* Nitrofurantoin ... 1147
Novo-Gabapentin (Can) *See* Gabapentin ... 702
Novo-Gemfibrozil (Can) *See* Gemfibrozil ... 711
Novo-Gesic (Can) *See* Acetaminophen ... 30
Novo-Glimepiride (Can) *See* Glimepiride ... 723
Novo-Glyburide (Can) *See* GlyBURIDE ... 730
Novo-Hydrazide (Can) *See* Hydrochlorothiazide ... 773
Novo-Hydroxyzin (Can) *See* HydrOXYzine ... 797
Novo-Hylazin (Can) *See* HydrALAZINE ... 772
Novo-Indapamide (Can) *See* Indapamide ... 817
Novo-Ipramide (Can) *See* Ipratropium ... 852
Novo-Keto (Can) *See* Ketoprofen ... 877
Novo-Ketoconazole (Can) *See* Ketoconazole ... 876
Novo-Keto-EC (Can) *See* Ketoprofen ... 877
Novo-Ketorolac (Can) *See* Ketorolac ... 878
Novo-Ketotifen® (Can) *See* Ketotifen ... 879
Novo-Lamotrigine (Can) *See* LamoTRIgine ... 889
Novo-Leflunomide (Can) *See* Leflunomide ... 899
Novo-Levobunolol (Can) *See* Levobunolol ... 907
Novo-Levocarbidopa (Can) *See* Carbidopa and Levodopa ... 277
Novo-Levofloxacin (Can) *See* Levofloxacin ... 913
Novo-Lexin (Can) *See* Cephalexin ... 306
Novolin® 70/30 *See* Insulin NPH and Insulin Regular ... 836
Novolin® ge 30/70 (Can) *See* Insulin NPH and Insulin Regular ... 836
Novolin® ge 40/60 (Can) *See* Insulin NPH and Insulin Regular ... 836
Novolin® ge 50/50 (Can) *See* Insulin NPH and Insulin Regular ... 836
Novolin® ge NPH (Can) *See* Insulin NPH ... 835
Novolin® ge Toronto (Can) *See* Insulin Regular ... 838
Novolin® N *See* Insulin NPH ... 835
Novolin® R *See* Insulin Regular ... 838
Novo-Lisinopril (Can) *See* Lisinopril ... 934
Novo-Lisinopril/Hctz (Can) *See* Lisinopril and Hydrochlorothiazide ... 938
NovoLog® *See* Insulin Aspart ... 822
NovoLog® Mix 70/30 *See* Insulin Aspart Protamine and Insulin Aspart ... 824
Novo-Loperamide (Can) *See* Loperamide ... 944
Novo-Lorazepam (Can) *See* LORazepam ... 949
Novo-Lovastatin (Can) *See* Lovastatin ... 956
Novo-Maprotiline (Can) *See* Maprotiline ... 968
Novo-Medrone (Can) *See* MedroxyPROGESTERone ... 975
Novo-Meloxicam (Can) *See* Meloxicam ... 982
Novo-Meprazine (Can) *See* Methotrimeprazine ... 1015
Novo-Mepro (Can) *See* Meprobamate ... 991
Novo-Metformin (Can) *See* MetFORMIN ... 997
Novo-Methacin (Can) *See* Indomethacin ... 818
Novo-Metoprolol (Can) *See* Metoprolol ... 1036
Novo-Mexiletine (Can) *See* Mexiletine ... 1045
Novo-Minocycline (Can) *See* Minocycline ... 1056
Novo-Mirtazapine (Can) *See* Mirtazapine ... 1058
NovoMix® 30 (Can) *See* Insulin Aspart Protamine and Insulin Aspart ... 824
Novo-Moclobemide (Can) *See* Moclobemide ... 1062
Novo-Morphine SR (Can) *See* Morphine Sulfate ... 1077
Novo-Nabumetone (Can) *See* Nabumetone ... 1089
Novo-Nadolol (Can) *See* Nadolol ... 1090
Novo-Naproc EC (Can) *See* Naproxen ... 1102
Novo-Naprox (Can) *See* Naproxen ... 1102
Novo-Naprox Sodium (Can) *See* Naproxen ... 1102
Novo-Naprox Sodium DS (Can) *See* Naproxen ... 1102
Novo-Naprox SR (Can) *See* Naproxen ... 1102
Novo-Nifedin (Can) *See* NIFEdipine ... 1136
Novo-Nizatidine (Can) *See* Nizatidine ... 1149

Novo-Norfloxacin (Can) *See* Norfloxacin ... 1151
NovoNorm (Mex) *See* Repaglinide ... 1409
Novo-Nortriptyline (Can) *See* Nortriptyline ... 1152
Novo-Ofloxacin (Can) *See* Ofloxacin ... 1159
Novo-Olanzapine (Can) *See* OLANZapine ... 1160
Novo-Ondansetron (Can) *See* Ondansetron ... 1180
Novo-Oxybutynin (Can) *See* Oxybutynin ... 1199
Novo-Paroxetine (Can) *See* PARoxetine ... 1226
Novo-Pen-VK (Can) *See* Penicillin V Potassium ... 1242
Novo-Peridol (Can) *See* Haloperidol ... 754
Novo-Pheniram (Can) *See* Chlorpheniramine ... 321
Novo-Pindol (Can) *See* Pindolol ... 1294
Novo-Pioglitazone (Can) *See* Pioglitazone ... 1297
Novo-Pirocam (Can) *See* Piroxicam ... 1307
Novo-Pramine (Can) *See* Imipramine ... 812
Novo-Pramipexole (Can) *See* Pramipexole ... 1318
Novo-Pranol (Can) *See* Propranolol ... 1355
Novo-Pravastatin (Can) *See* Pravastatin ... 1321
Novo-Prazin (Can) *See* Prazosin ... 1325
Novo-Prednisolone (Can) *See* PrednisoLONE ... 1326
Novo-Prednisone (Can) *See* PredniSONE ... 1327
Novo-Profen (Can) *See* Ibuprofen ... 803
Novo-Propamide (Can) *See* ChlorproPAMIDE ... 340
Novo-Purol (Can) *See* Allopurinol ... 67
Novo-Quinidin (Can) *See* QuiNIDine ... 1387
Novo-Quinine (Can) *See* QuiNINE ... 1388
Novo-Rabeprazole EC (Can) *See* Rabeprazole ... 1389
Novo-Ramipril (Can) *See* Ramipril ... 1395
Novo-Ranidine (Can) *See* Ranitidine ... 1399
NovoRapid® (Can) *See* Insulin Aspart ... 822
Novo-Risperidone (Can) *See* Risperidone ... 1425
Novo-Rythro Estolate (Can) *See* Erythromycin ... 557
Novo-Rythro Ethylsuccinate (Can) *See* Erythromycin ... 557
Novo-Selegiline (Can) *See* Selegiline ... 1466
Novo-Semide (Can) *See* Furosemide ... 699
Novo-Sertraline (Can) *See* Sertraline ... 1472
Novo-Simvastatin (Can) *See* Simvastatin ... 1486
Novo-Sorbide (Can) *See* Isosorbide Dinitrate ... 866
Novo-Sotalol (Can) *See* Sotalol ... 1502
Novo-Soxazole (Can) *See* SulfiSOXAZOLE ... 1523
Novo-Spiroton (Can) *See* Spironolactone ... 1503
Novo-Spirozine (Can) *See* Hydrochlorothiazide and Spironolactone ... 776
Novo-Sucralate (Can) *See* Sucralfate ... 1514
Novo-Sumatriptan (Can) *See* SUMAtriptan ... 1527
Novo-Sundac (Can) *See* Sulindac ... 1523
Novo-Tamoxifen (Can) *See* Tamoxifen ... 1537
Novo-Tamsulosin (Can) *See* Tamsulosin ... 1537
Novo-Temazepam (Can) *See* Temazepam ... 1545
Novo-Terazosin (Can) *See* Terazosin ... 1549
Novo-Terbinafine (Can) *See* Terbinafine ... 1551
Novo-Theophyl SR (Can) *See* Theophylline ... 1562
Novo-Ticlopidine (Can) *See* Ticlopidine ... 1583
Novo-Topiramate (Can) *See* Topiramate ... 1598
Novo-Trazodone (Can) *See* TraZODone ... 1614
Novo-Triamzide (Can) *See* Hydrochlorothiazide and Triamterene ... 776
Novo-Trifluzine (Can) *See* Trifluoperazine ... 1624
Novo-Trimel (Can) *See* Sulfamethoxazole and Trimethoprim ... 1517
Novo-Trimel D.S. (Can) *See* Sulfamethoxazole and Trimethoprim ... 1517
Novo-Triptyn (Can) *See* Amitriptyline ... 90
Novo-Venlafaxine XR (Can) *See* Venlafaxine ... 1659
Novo-Veramil SR (Can) *See* Verapamil ... 1665
Novo-Warfarin (Can) *See* Warfarin ... 1679
Novoxapram® (Can) *See* Oxazepam ... 1193
Novo-Zopiclone (Can) *See* Zopiclone ... 1711
Noxafil® *See* Posaconazole ... 1314
Nozinan® (Can) *See* Methotrimeprazine ... 1015
NPH Insulin *See* Insulin NPH ... 835
NPH Insulin and Regular Insulin *See* Insulin NPH and Insulin Regular ... 836
NRP104 *See* Lisdexamfetamine ... 931
NRS® [OTC] *See* Oxymetazoline ... 1208
NSC-740 *See* Methotrexate ... 1014
NSC-750 *See* Busulfan ... 226
NSC-752 *See* Thioguanine ... 1569
NSC-755 *See* Mercaptopurine ... 993
NSC-762 *See* Mechlorethamine ... 974
NSC-3053 *See* DACTINomycin ... 415
NSC-3088 *See* Chlorambucil ... 315

NSC-8806 *See* Melphalan ... 983
NSC-13875 *See* Altretamine ... 78
NSC-15200 *See* Gallium Nitrate ... 707
NSC-26271 *See* Cyclophosphamide ... 408
NSC-26980 *See* Mitomycin ... 1061
NSC-27640 *See* Floxuridine ... 634
NSC-38721 *See* Mitotane ... 1061
NSC-49842 *See* VinBLAStine ... 1672
NSC-63878 *See* Cytarabine ... 412
NSC-66847 *See* Thalidomide ... 1561
NSC-67574 *See* VinCRIStine ... 1673
NSC-71423 *See* Megestrol ... 977
NSC-77213 *See* Procarbazine ... 1340
NSC-79037 *See* Lomustine ... 943
NSC-82151 *See* DAUNOrubicin Hydrochloride ... 421
NSC-85998 *See* Streptozocin ... 1510
NSC-89199 *See* Estramustine ... 580
NSC-102816 *See* AzaCITIDine ... 161
NSC-105014 *See* Cladribine ... 360
NSC-106977 *(Erwinia) See* Asparaginase ... 142
NSC-109229 *(E. coli) See* Asparaginase ... 142
NSC-109724 *See* Ifosfamide ... 809
NSC-122758 *See* Tretinoin, Oral ... 1617
NSC-123127 *See* DOXOrubicin ... 507
NSC-125066 *See* Bleomycin ... 192
NSC-125973 *See* Paclitaxel ... 1213
NSC-127716 *See* Decitabine ... 422
NSC-147834 *See* Flutamide ... 667
NSC-169780 *See* Dexrazoxane ... 441
NSC-218321 *See* Pentostatin ... 1250
NSC-241240 *See* CARBOplatin ... 281
NSC-256439 *See* IDArubicin ... 809
NSC-256942 *See* Epirubicin ... 545
NSC-266046 *See* Oxaliplatin ... 1191
NSC-301739 *See* Mitoxantrone ... 1061
NSC-308847 *See* Amonafide ... 108
NSC-312887 *See* Fludarabine ... 641
NSC-352122 *See* Trimetrexate ... 1629
NSC-362856 *See* Temozolomide ... 1547
NSC-367982 *See* Interferon Alfa-2a ... 844
NSC-373364 *See* Aldesleukin ... 58
NSC-377523 *See* Interferon Alfa-2b ... 844
NSC-409962 *See* Carmustine ... 284
NSC-603071 *See* Aminocamptothecin ... 86
NSC-606864 *See* Goserelin ... 735
NSC606869 *See* Clofarabine ... 367
NSC-609699 *See* Topotecan ... 1602
NSC-613327 *See* Gemcitabine ... 710
NSC-613795 *See* Sargramostim ... 1462
NSC-614629 *See* Filgrastim ... 632
NSC-616348 *See* Irinotecan ... 856
NSC-628503 *See* Docetaxel ... 491
NSC-644468 *See* Deferoxamine ... 423
NSC-644954 *See* Pegaspargase ... 1235
NSC-671663 *See* Octreotide ... 1158
NSC-673089 *See* Paclitaxel ... 1213
NSC-681239 *See* Bortezomib ... 192
NSC-683864 *See* Temsirolimus ... 1547
NSC-684588 *See* Nilutamide ... 1140
NSC-687451 *See* RiTUXimab ... 1434
NSC-688097 *See* Trastuzumab ... 1613
NSC-697732 *See* DAUNOrubicin Citrate (Liposomal) ... 421
NSC-698037 *See* Pemetrexed ... 1238
NSC-701852 *See* Vorinostat ... 1678
NSC-703813 *See* Lenalidomide ... 899
NSC-704865 *See* Bevacizumab ... 187
NSC-706363 *See* Arsenic Trioxide ... 140
NSC-706725 *See* Raloxifene ... 1391
NSC-712227 *See* DOXOrubicin (Liposomal) ... 508
NSC-712807 *See* Capecitabine ... 263
NSC-714692 *See* Cetuximab ... 310
NSC-714744 *See* Denileukin Diftitox ... 425
NSC-715055 *See* Gefitinib ... 709
NSC-715969 *See* Alemtuzumab ... 59
NSC-716051 *See* Imatinib ... 810
NSC-718781 *See* Erlotinib ... 556
NSC-719344 *See* Anastrozole ... 125

NSC-719345 *See* Letrozole ... 900
NSC-720568 *See* Gemtuzumab Ozogamicin ... 713
NSC-721517 *See* Zoledronic Acid ... 1702
NSC-721631 *See* Rasburicase ... 1407
NSC-722623 *See* Ibandronate ... 801
NSC-722848 *See* Oprelvekin ... 1184
NSC-724223 *See* Epoetin Alfa ... 546
NSC-724577 *See* Anagrelide ... 124
NSC-724772 *See* Sorafenib ... 1501
NSC-725961 *See* Pegfilgrastim ... 1236
NSC-727989 *See* Lapatinib ... 898
NSC-728729 *See* InFLIXimab ... 819
NSC-729969 *See* Darbepoetin Alfa ... 419
NSC-732517 *See* Dasatinib ... 420
NSC-736511 *See* Sunitinib ... 1530
NSC-736631 *See* Paclitaxel (Protein Bound) ... 1214
NSC-742319 *See* Panitumumab ... 1221
NTG *See* Nitroglycerin ... 1147
N-trifluoroacetyladriamycin-14-valerate *See* Valrubicin ... 1649
NTZ *See* Nitazoxanide ... 1146
Nu-Acebutolol (Can) *See* Acebutolol ... 27
Nu-Acyclovir (Can) *See* Acyclovir ... 49
Nu-Alprax (Can) *See* ALPRAZolam ... 72
Nu-Amilzide (Can) *See* Amiloride and Hydrochlorothiazide ... 86
Nu-Amoxi (Can) *See* Amoxicillin ... 112
Nu-Ampi (Can) *See* Ampicillin ... 122
Nu-Atenol (Can) *See* Atenolol ... 147
Nu-Baclo (Can) *See* Baclofen ... 168
Nubain® *See* Nalbuphine ... 1094
Nu-Beclomethasone (Can) *See* Beclomethasone ... 171
Nu-Bromazepam (Can) *See* Bromazepam ... 200
Nu-Buspirone (Can) *See* BusPIRone ... 223
Nu-Capto (Can) *See* Captopril ... 264
Nu-Carbamazepine (Can) *See* CarBAMazepine ... 265
Nu-Cefaclor (Can) *See* Cefaclor ... 291
Nu-Cephalex (Can) *See* Cephalexin ... 306
Nu-Cimet (Can) *See* Cimetidine ... 345
Nu-Clonazepam (Can) *See* ClonazePAM ... 373
Nu-Clonidine (Can) *See* CloNIDine ... 377
Nucofed® *See* Pseudoephedrine and Codeine ... 1368
Nucofed® Expectorant [DSC] *See* Guaifenesin, Pseudoephedrine, and Codeine ... 747
Nucofed® Pediatric Expectorant [DSC] *See* Guaifenesin, Pseudoephedrine, and Codeine ... 747
Nu-Cotrimox (Can) *See* Sulfamethoxazole and Trimethoprim ... 1517
Nu-Cromolyn (Can) *See* Cromolyn ... 402
Nu-Cyclobenzaprine (Can) *See* Cyclobenzaprine ... 405
Nu-Desipramine (Can) *See* Desipramine ... 426
Nu-Diclo (Can) *See* Diclofenac ... 457
Nu-Diclo-SR (Can) *See* Diclofenac ... 457
Nu-Diflunisal (Can) *See* Diflunisal ... 463
Nu-Diltiaz (Can) *See* Diltiazem ... 473
Nu-Diltiaz-CD (Can) *See* Diltiazem ... 473
Nu-Divalproex (Can) *See* Valproic Acid and Derivatives ... 1642
Nu-Domperidone (Can) *See* Domperidone ... 493
Nu-Doxycycline (Can) *See* Doxycycline ... 509
Nu-Erythromycin-S (Can) *See* Erythromycin ... 557
Nu-Famotidine (Can) *See* Famotidine ... 613
Nu-Fenofibrate (Can) *See* Fenofibrate ... 620
Nu-Fluoxetine (Can) *See* FLUoxetine ... 650
Nu-Flurprofen (Can) *See* Flurbiprofen ... 667
Nu-Fluvoxamine (Can) *See* Fluvoxamine ... 678
Nu-Furosemide (Can) *See* Furosemide ... 699
Nu-Gabapentin (Can) *See* Gabapentin ... 702
Nu-Gemfibrozil (Can) *See* Gemfibrozil ... 711
Nu-Glyburide (Can) *See* GlyBURIDE ... 730
Nu-Hydral (Can) *See* HydrALAZINE ... 772
Nu-Ibuprofen (Can) *See* Ibuprofen ... 803
Nu-Indapamide (Can) *See* Indapamide ... 817
Nu-Indo (Can) *See* Indomethacin ... 818
Nu-Ipratropium (Can) *See* Ipratropium ... 852
Nu-Iron® 150 [OTC] *See* Polysaccharide-Iron Complex ... 1313
Nu-Ketoprofen (Can) *See* Ketoprofen ... 877
Nu-Ketoprofen-E (Can) *See* Ketoprofen ... 877
Nu-Ketotifen® (Can) *See* Ketotifen ... 879
NuLev™ [DSC] *See* Hyoscyamine ... 799
Nu-Levocarb (Can) *See* Carbidopa and Levodopa ... 277
Nu-Loraz (Can) *See* LORazepam ... 949

Nu-Lovastatin (Can) *See* Lovastatin ... 956
Nu-Loxapine (Can) *See* Loxapine ... 960
NuLYTELY® *See* Polyethylene Glycol-Electrolyte Solution ... 1310
Numark (Mex) *See* Budesonide ... 210
Nu-Medopa (Can) *See* Methyldopa ... 1021
Nu-Mefenamic (Can) *See* Mefenamic Acid ... 976
Nu-Megestrol (Can) *See* Megestrol ... 977
Nu-Metformin (Can) *See* MetFORMIN ... 997
Nu-Metoclopramide (Can) *See* Metoclopramide ... 1031
Nu-Metop (Can) *See* Metoprolol ... 1036
Nu-Moclobemide (Can) *See* Moclobemide ... 1062
Nu-Naprox (Can) *See* Naproxen ... 1102
Nu-Nifed (Can) *See* NIFEdipine ... 1136
Nu-Nizatidine (Can) *See* Nizatidine ... 1149
Nu-Nortriptyline (Can) *See* Nortriptyline ... 1152
Nu-Oxybutyn (Can) *See* Oxybutynin ... 1199
Nu-Pentoxifylline SR (Can) *See* Pentoxifylline ... 1251
Nu-Pen-VK (Can) *See* Penicillin V Potassium ... 1242
Nupercainal® Hydrocortisone Cream [OTC] *See* Hydrocortisone ... 785
Nu-Pindol (Can) *See* Pindolol ... 1294
Nu-Pirox (Can) *See* Piroxicam ... 1307
Nu-Prazo (Can) *See* Prazosin ... 1325
Nu-Prochlor (Can) *See* Prochlorperazine ... 1341
Nu-Propranolol (Can) *See* Propranolol ... 1355
Nu-Ranit (Can) *See* Ranitidine ... 1399
Nuro-B (Mex) *See* Pyridoxine ... 1376
Nu-Selegiline (Can) *See* Selegiline ... 1466
Nu-Sertraline (Can) *See* Sertraline ... 1472
Nu-Simvastatin (Can) *See* Simvastatin ... 1486
Nu-Sotalol (Can) *See* Sotalol ... 1502
Nu-Sucralate (Can) *See* Sucralfate ... 1514
Nu-Sundac (Can) *See* Sulindac ... 1523
Nu-Temazepam (Can) *See* Temazepam ... 1545
Nu-Terazosin (Can) *See* Terazosin ... 1549
Nu-Tetra (Can) *See* Tetracycline ... 1558
Nu-Ticlopidine (Can) *See* Ticlopidine ... 1583
Nu-Timolol (Can) *See* Timolol ... 1584
Nutracort® *See* Hydrocortisone ... 785
Nutralox® [OTC] *See* Calcium Carbonate ... 254
Nu-Trazodone (Can) *See* TraZODone ... 1614
Nu-Triazide (Can) *See* Hydrochlorothiazide and Triamterene ... 776
Nu-Trimipramine (Can) *See* Trimipramine ... 1630
Nutropin® *See* Somatropin ... 1499
Nutropin AQ® *See* Somatropin ... 1499
Nutropine® (Can) *See* Somatropin ... 1499
NuvaRing® *See* Ethinyl Estradiol and Etonogestrel ... 594
Nu-Verap (Can) *See* Verapamil ... 1665
Nuvigil™ *See* Armodafinil ... 138
Nu-Zopiclone (Can) *See* Zopiclone ... 1711
NVP *See* Nevirapine ... 1124
Nyolol (Mex) *See* Timolol ... 1584
Nytol® (Can) *See* DiphenhydrAMINE ... 481
Nytol® Extra Strength (Can) *See* DiphenhydrAMINE ... 481
Nytol® Quick Caps [OTC] *See* DiphenhydrAMINE ... 481
Nytol® Quick Gels [OTC] *See* DiphenhydrAMINE ... 481
NāSop™ [DSC] *See* Phenylephrine ... 1273
Nōstrilla® [OTC] *See* Oxymetazoline ... 1208
OCBZ *See* OXcarbazepine ... 1195
Occlusal™-HP (Can) *See* Salicylic Acid ... 1454
Occlusal®-HP [OTC] *See* Salicylic Acid ... 1454
Ocella™ *See* Ethinyl Estradiol and Drospirenone ... 593
Octanine F (Mex) *See* Factor IX ... 612
Octex (Mex) *See* Sulfamethoxazole and Trimethoprim ... 1517
Octostim® (Can) *See* Desmopressin ... 431
Octreotide ... 1158
Octreotide Acetate *See* Octreotide ... 1158
Octreotide Acetate Injection (Can) *See* Octreotide ... 1158
Octreotide Acetate Omega (Can) *See* Octreotide ... 1158
Ocufen® *See* Flurbiprofen ... 667
Ocuflox® *See* Ofloxacin ... 1159
OcuNefrin™ [OTC] *See* Phenylephrine ... 1273
Ocupress® Ophthalmic (Can) *See* Carteolol ... 285
O-desmethylvenlafaxine *See* Desvenlafaxine ... 433
ODV *See* Desvenlafaxine ... 433
Oesclim® (Can) *See* Estradiol ... 576
Oestrogel (Mex) *See* Estradiol ... 576
Off-Ezy® Wart Remover [OTC] [DSC] *See* Salicylic Acid ... 1454

Ofloxacin ... 1159
Oftadil (Mex) *See* Chloramphenicol ... 315
Ogastro (Mex) *See* Lansoprazole ... 894
Ogen® *See* Estropipate ... 588
Ogestrel® *See* Ethinyl Estradiol and Norgestrel ... 601
OGMT *See* Metyrosine ... 1044
OGT-918 *See* Miglustat ... 1053
9-OH-risperidone *See* Paliperidone ... 1215
OKT3 *See* Muromonab-CD3 ... 1086
Olan (Mex) *See* Lansoprazole ... 894
OLANZapine ... 1160
Olanzapine and Fluoxetine ... 1165
Olanzapine and Fluoxetine Hydrochloride *See* Olanzapine and Fluoxetine ... 1165
Olexin (Mex) *See* Omeprazole ... 1176
Olipcis (Mex) *See* Oxaliplatin ... 1191
Olmesartan ... 1170
Olmesartan and Amlodipine *See* Amlodipine and Olmesartan ... 104
Olmesartan and Hydrochlorothiazide ... 1172
Olmesartan Medoxomil *See* Olmesartan ... 1170
Olmesartan Medoxomil and Hydrochlorothiazide *See* Olmesartan and Hydrochlorothiazide ... 1172
Olsalazine ... 1173
Olsalazine Sodium *See* Olsalazine ... 1173
Omacor® [DSC] *See* Omega-3-Acid Ethyl Esters ... 1175
Omalizumab ... 1174
Omega-3-Acid Ethyl Esters ... 1175
Omeprazole ... 1176
Omeprazole and Sodium Bicarbonate ... 1179
Omifin (Mex) *See* ClomiPHENE ... 368
Omnaris™ *See* Ciclesonide ... 343
Omnicef® *See* Cefdinir ... 293
Omnicef R (Mex) *See* Cefdinir ... 293
OMNIhist® II L.A. *See* Chlorpheniramine, Phenylephrine, and Methscopolamine ... 329
Omnipen (Mex) *See* Ampicillin ... 122
Omnipred™ *See* PrednisoLONE ... 1326
Omnitrope™ *See* Somatropin ... 1499
Oncaspar® *See* Pegaspargase ... 1235
Oncovin (Mex) *See* VinCRIStine ... 1673
Ondansetron ... 1180
Ondansetron Hydrochloride *See* Ondansetron ... 1180
Ondansetron Injection (Can) *See* Ondansetron ... 1180
Ondansetron-Omega (Can) *See* Ondansetron ... 1180
One Gram C [OTC] *See* Ascorbic Acid ... 141
Onicit (Mex) *See* Palonosetron ... 1218
ONTAK® *See* Denileukin Diftitox ... 425
Onxol® *See* Paclitaxel ... 1213
Opana® *See* Oxymorphone ... 1210
Opana® ER *See* Oxymorphone ... 1210
OPC-13013 *See* Cilostazol ... 344
OPC-14597 *See* Aripiprazole ... 133
OP-CCK *See* Sincalide ... 1489
Opcon-A® [OTC] *See* Naphazoline and Pheniramine ... 1102
Ophthetic® *See* Proparacaine ... 1352
Ophtho-Tate® (Can) *See* PrednisoLONE ... 1326
Opium and Belladonna *See* Belladonna and Opium ... 174
Opium Tincture ... 1183
Opium Tincture, Deodorized *See* Opium Tincture ... 1183
Oprad (Mex) *See* Amikacin ... 83
Oprelvekin ... 1184
Opthavir (Mex) *See* Acyclovir ... 49
Optho-Bunolol® (Can) *See* Levobunolol ... 907
Opti-Clear [OTC] *See* Tetrahydrozoline ... 1560
Opticrom® (Can) *See* Cromolyn ... 402
Optigene® 3 [OTC] [DSC] *See* Tetrahydrozoline ... 1560
OptiPranolol® *See* Metipranolol ... 1031
Optivar® *See* Azelastine ... 162
Optomicin (Mex) *See* Erythromycin ... 557
o,p'-DDD *See* Mitotane ... 1061
Oracea™ *See* Doxycycline ... 509
Oracort (Can) *See* Triamcinolone ... 1617
Oramorph SR® *See* Morphine Sulfate ... 1077
Oranor (Mex) *See* Norfloxacin ... 1151
Oranyl [OTC] *See* Pseudoephedrine ... 1367
Oranyl Plus [OTC] *See* Acetaminophen and Pseudoephedrine ... 37
Orap® *See* Pimozide ... 1290
Orapred® *See* PrednisoLONE ... 1326
Orapred ODT™ *See* PrednisoLONE ... 1326

OraVerse™ *See* Phentolamine 1272
Orciprenaline Sulfate *See* Metaproterenol 996
Orelox (Mex) *See* Cefpodoxime 297
Orencia® *See* Abatacept 22
Orfadin® *See* Nitisinone 1146
Organidin® NR *See* GuaiFENesin 737
Orgaran® (Can) *See* Danaparoid 415
Orlistat 1184
Ornex® Maximum Strength [OTC] *See* Acetaminophen and Pseudoephedrine 37
Ornex® [OTC] *See* Acetaminophen and Pseudoephedrine 37
Orphenace® (Can) *See* Orphenadrine 1186
Orphenadrine 1186
Orphenadrine, Aspirin, and Caffeine 1187
Orphenadrine Citrate *See* Orphenadrine 1186
Orphengesic [DSC] *See* Orphenadrine, Aspirin, and Caffeine 1187
Orphengesic Forte [DSC] *See* Orphenadrine, Aspirin, and Caffeine 1187
Ortho® 0.5/35 (Can) *See* Ethinyl Estradiol and Norethindrone 597
Ortho® 1/35 (Can) *See* Ethinyl Estradiol and Norethindrone 597
Ortho® 7/7/7 (Can) *See* Ethinyl Estradiol and Norethindrone 597
Ortho-Cept® *See* Ethinyl Estradiol and Desogestrel 592
Orthoclone OKT® 3 *See* Muromonab-CD3 1086
Ortho-Cyclen® *See* Ethinyl Estradiol and Norgestimate 600
Ortho-Est® *See* Estropipate 588
Ortho Evra® *See* Ethinyl Estradiol and Norelgestromin 597
Ortho Micronor® *See* Norethindrone 1150
Ortho-Novum (Mex) *See* Norethindrone 1150
Ortho-Novum® 1/50 (Can) *See* Mestranol and Norethindrone 995
Ortho-Novum® 1/50 [DSC] *See* Mestranol and Norethindrone 995
Ortho Prefest *See* Estradiol and Norgestimate 580
Ortho Tri-Cyclen® *See* Ethinyl Estradiol and Norgestimate 600
Ortho Tri-Cyclen® Lo *See* Ethinyl Estradiol and Norgestimate 600
Ortopsique (Mex) *See* Diazepam 451
Oruvail® (Can) *See* Ketoprofen 877
Os-Cal® (Can) *See* Calcium Carbonate 254
Os-Cal® 500 [OTC] [DSC] *See* Calcium Carbonate 254
Oseltamivir 1188
Oseum (Mex) *See* Calcitonin 253
OSI-774 *See* Erlotinib 556
Osmitrol® *See* Mannitol 968
Osteocit® (Can) *See* Calcium Citrate 257
Osteomin (Mex) *See* Calcium Carbonate 254
Ostoforte® (Can) *See* Ergocalciferol 550
Otaxem (Mex) *See* Methotrexate 1014
Otedram (Mex) *See* Bromazepam 200
OTFC (Oral Transmucosal Fentanyl Citrate) *See* FentaNYL 624
Otrivin® [OTC] [DSC] *See* Xylometazoline 1687
Otrivin® Pediatric [OTC] [DSC] *See* Xylometazoline 1687
Otrozol (Mex) *See* MetroNIDAZOLE 1040
Ovcon® *See* Ethinyl Estradiol and Norethindrone 597
Ovelquin (Mex) *See* Levofloxacin 913
Ovidrel® *See* Chorionic Gonadotropin (Recombinant) 343
Ovral® (Can) *See* Ethinyl Estradiol and Norgestrel 601
Oxacillin 1190
Oxacillin Sodium *See* Oxacillin 1190
Oxaliplatin 1191
Oxandrin® *See* Oxandrolone 1191
Oxandrolone 1191
Oxaprozin 1193
Oxazepam 1193
OXcarbazepine 1195
Oxetol (Mex) *See* OXcarbazepine 1195
Oxeze® Turbuhaler® (Can) *See* Formoterol 686
Oxifungol (Mex) *See* Fluconazole 635
Oxilapine Succinate *See* Loxapine 960
Oximetazolina (Mex) *See* Oxymetazoline 1208
Oxis Turbuhaler (Mex) *See* Formoterol 686
Oxpam® (Can) *See* Oxazepam 1193
Oxpentifylline *See* Pentoxifylline 1251
Oxpram® (Can) *See* Oxazepam 1193
Oxsoralen® *See* Methoxsalen 1018
Oxsoralen-Ultra® *See* Methoxsalen 1018
Oxybutynin 1199
Oxybutynin Chloride *See* Oxybutynin 1199
Oxycocet® (Can) *See* Oxycodone and Acetaminophen 1205
Oxycodan® (Can) *See* Oxycodone and Aspirin 1208
OxyCODONE 1201
Oxycodone and Acetaminophen 1205

Oxycodone and Aspirin 1208
Oxycodone Hydrochloride *See* OxyCODONE 1201
OxyContin® *See* OxyCODONE 1201
OxyFast® *See* OxyCODONE 1201
OxyIR® *See* OxyCODONE 1201
Oxylin Liquifilm (Mex) *See* Oxymetazoline 1208
Oxymetazoline 1208
Oxymetazoline Hydrochloride *See* Oxymetazoline 1208
Oxymetholone 1209
Oxymorphone 1210
Oxymorphone Hydrochloride *See* Oxymorphone 1210
Oxytrol® *See* Oxybutynin 1199
Oysco 500 [OTC] *See* Calcium Carbonate 254
Oyst-Cal 500 [OTC] *See* Calcium Carbonate 254
P-V Tussin Tablet [DSC] *See* Hydrocodone and Pseudoephedrine 781
P-071 *See* Cetirizine 307
Pacerone® *See* Amiodarone 89
Paclitaxel 1213
Paclitaxel (Protein Bound) 1214
Pacovanton (Mex) *See* Nitazoxanide 1146
Paferxin (Mex) *See* Cephalexin 306
Pagavit (Mex) *See* Thiamine 1568
Pain Eze [OTC] *See* Acetaminophen 30
Pain-Off [OTC] *See* Acetaminophen, Aspirin, and Caffeine 39
Palafer® (Can) *See* Ferrous Fumarate 626
Palatrin (Mex) *See* Lansoprazole 894
Palgic® *See* Carbinoxamine 280
Palgic®-D [DSC] *See* Carbinoxamine and Pseudoephedrine 280
Palgic®-DS [DSC] *See* Carbinoxamine and Pseudoephedrine 280
Palifermin 1214
Paliperidone 1215
Palivizumab 1218
Palmer's® Skin Success Acne Cleanser [OTC] *See* Salicylic Acid 1454
Palonosetron 1218
Palonosetron Hydrochloride *See* Palonosetron 1218
2-PAM *See* Pralidoxime 1318
Pamelor® *See* Nortriptyline 1152
Pamidronate 1220
Pamidronate Disodium® (Can) *See* Pamidronate 1220
Pamine® *See* Methscopolamine 1019
Pamine® Forte *See* Methscopolamine 1019
p-Aminoclonidine *See* Apraclonidine 129
Pamisol (Mex) *See* Pamidronate 1220
Pamprin® Maximum Strength All Day Relief [OTC] *See* Naproxen 1102
Panax ginseng *See* Ginseng, Panax (Panax ginseng) 718
Pancof® [DSC] *See* Pseudoephedrine, Dihydrocodeine, and Chlorpheniramine 1371
Pancof®-EXP *See* Dihydrocodeine, Pseudoephedrine, and Guaifenesin 469
Pancof-XP [DSC] *See* Hydrocodone and Guaifenesin 779
Pandel® *See* Hydrocortisone 785
Pangavit Pediátrico (Mex) *See* Cyproheptadine 410
Panhematin® *See* Hemin 760
Panitumumab 1221
Panlor® DC *See* Acetaminophen, Caffeine, and Dihydrocodeine 39
Panlor® SS *See* Acetaminophen, Caffeine, and Dihydrocodeine 39
Panretin® *See* Alitretinoin 66
Panto™ I.V. (Can) *See* Pantoprazole 1221
Pantoloc® (Can) *See* Pantoprazole 1221
Pantoloc® M (Can) *See* Pantoprazole 1221
Pantomicina (Mex) *See* Erythromycin 557
Pantoprazole 1221
Pantozol (Mex) *See* Pantoprazole 1221
Papaverine 1225
Papaverine Hydrochloride *See* Papaverine 1225
Para-Aminosalicylate Sodium *See* Aminosalicylic Acid 88
Paracetamol *See* Acetaminophen 30
Parafon Forte® (Can) *See* Chlorzoxazone 341
Parafon Forte® DSC *See* Chlorzoxazone 341
Paramix (Mex) *See* Nitazoxanide 1146
Paraplatin-AQ (Can) *See* CARBOplatin 281
Parathyroid Hormone (1-34) *See* Teriparatide 1553
Para-Time SR® *See* Papaverine 1225
Parcaine™ *See* Proparacaine 1352
Parcopa™ *See* Carbidopa and Levodopa 277
Paregoric 1225
Paricalcitol 1226
Pariet® (Can) *See* Rabeprazole 1389
Pariprazole *See* Rabeprazole 1389

Parlodel® *See* Bromocriptine ... 202
Parlodel® SnapTabs® *See* Bromocriptine ... 202
Parnate® *See* Tranylcypromine ... 1609
Paromomycin ... 1226
Paromomycin Sulfate *See* Paromomycin ... 1226
PARoxetine ... 1226
Paroxetine Hydrochloride *See* PARoxetine ... 1226
Paroxetine Mesylate *See* PARoxetine ... 1226
Parsel (Mex) *See* Dihydroergotamine ... 470
Parvolex® (Can) *See* Acetylcysteine ... 47
PAS *See* Aminosalicylic Acid ... 88
Paser® *See* Aminosalicylic Acid ... 88
Pathocil® (Can) *See* Dicloxacillin ... 459
Pauly (Mex) *See* Pantoprazole ... 1221
Pavabid [DSC] *See* Papaverine ... 1225
Paxil® *See* PARoxetine ... 1226
Paxil CR® *See* PARoxetine ... 1226
Paxosit (Mex) *See* Hydrocortisone ... 785
PCA (error-prone abbreviation) *See* Procainamide ... 1339
PCE® *See* Erythromycin ... 557
P Chlor GG *See* Chlorpheniramine, Phenylephrine, and Guaifenesin ... 329
PCM *See* Chlorpheniramine, Phenylephrine, and Methscopolamine ... 329
PCM Allergy [DSC] *See* Chlorpheniramine, Phenylephrine, and Methscopolamine ... 329
PCV7 *See* Pneumococcal Conjugate Vaccine, 7-Valent ... 1308
PD-Cof *See* Chlorpheniramine, Phenylephrine, and Dextromethorphan ... 327
PD-Hist-D *See* Chlorpheniramine and Phenylephrine ... 323
PediaCare® Infants' Decongestant & Cough [OTC] [DSC] *See* Pseudoephedrine and Dextromethorphan ... 1369
PediaCare® Infants' Long-Acting Cough [OTC] [DSC] *See* Dextromethorphan ... 448
Pediacof® [DSC] *See* Chlorpheniramine, Phenylephrine, Codeine, and Potassium Iodide ... 332
PediaHist DM *See* Brompheniramine, Pseudoephedrine, and Dextromethorphan ... 208
Pediapred® *See* PrednisoLONE ... 1326
Pedia Relief Cough and Cold [OTC] *See* Pseudoephedrine and Dextromethorphan ... 1369
Pedia Relief Infants [OTC] *See* Pseudoephedrine and Dextromethorphan ... 1369
Pedia Relief™ [OTC] *See* Chlorpheniramine, Pseudoephedrine, and Dextromethorphan ... 333
Pediarix® *See* Diphtheria, Tetanus Toxoids, Acellular Pertussis, Hepatitis B (Recombinant), and Poliovirus (Inactivated) Vaccine ... 487
PediaTan™ *See* Chlorpheniramine ... 321
PediaTan™ D *See* Chlorpheniramine and Phenylephrine ... 323
Pediatex™-D [DSC] *See* Carbinoxamine and Pseudoephedrine ... 280
Pediatric Digoxin CSD (Can) *See* Digoxin ... 463
Pediatrix (Can) *See* Acetaminophen ... 30
Pediazole® (Can) *See* Erythromycin and Sulfisoxazole ... 563
PedvaxHIB® *See* Haemophilus b Conjugate Vaccine ... 753
PEG-L-asparaginase *See* Pegaspargase ... 1235
Peganone® *See* Ethotoin ... 604
Pegaptanib ... 1235
Pegaptanib Sodium *See* Pegaptanib ... 1235
Pegaspargase ... 1235
Pegasys® *See* Peginterferon Alfa-2a ... 1236
Pegfilgrastim ... 1236
Peginterferon Alfa-2a ... 1236
Peginterferon Alfa-2b ... 1237
PegIntron™ *See* Peginterferon Alfa-2b ... 1237
PegLyte® (Can) *See* Polyethylene Glycol-Electrolyte Solution ... 1310
Pegtron (Mex) *See* Peginterferon Alfa-2b ... 1237
Pegvisomant ... 1237
Pegylated Interferon Alfa-2a *See* Peginterferon Alfa-2a ... 1236
Pegylated Interferon Alfa-2b *See* Peginterferon Alfa-2b ... 1237
Pegylated Liposomal DOXOrubicin *See* DOXOrubicin (Liposomal) ... 508
PE-Hist DM *See* Chlorpheniramine, Phenylephrine, and Dextromethorphan ... 327
Pemetrexed ... 1238
Pemetrexed Disodium *See* Pemetrexed ... 1238
Penamox (Mex) *See* Amoxicillin ... 112
Penbritin (Mex) *See* Ampicillin ... 122
Penbutolol ... 1238
Penbutolol Sulfate *See* Penbutolol ... 1238
Pendex *See* Guaifenesin and Phenylephrine ... 742
Pendo-5 ASA (Can) *See* Mesalamine ... 994
Pengesod (Mex) *See* Penicillin G, Parenteral, Aqueous ... 1241
Penicillamine ... 1239
Penicillin V Potassium ... 1242
Penicillin G Benzathine ... 1239
Penicillin G Benzathine and Penicillin G Procaine ... 1240
Penicillin G, Parenteral, Aqueous ... 1241
Penicillin G Potassium *See* Penicillin G, Parenteral, Aqueous ... 1241
Penicillin G Procaine ... 1241

Penicillin G Procaine and Benzathine Combined *See* Penicillin G Benzathine and Penicillin G Procaine 1240
Penicillin G Sodium *See* Penicillin G, Parenteral, Aqueous 1241
Pennsaid® (Can) *See* Diclofenac 457
Pentahydrate *See* Sodium Thiosulfate 1497
Pentam-300® *See* Pentamidine 1242
Pentamidine 1242
Pentamidine Isethionate *See* Pentamidine 1242
Pentamidine Isetionate for Injection (Can) *See* Pentamidine 1242
Pentamycetin® (Can) *See* Chloramphenicol 315
Pentasa® *See* Mesalamine 994
Penta-Triamterene HCTZ (Can) *See* Hydrochlorothiazide and Triamterene 776
Pentazocine 1243
Pentazocine and Acetaminophen 1245
Pentazocine Hydrochloride *See* Pentazocine 1243
Pentazocine Hydrochloride and Acetaminophen *See* Pentazocine and Acetaminophen 1245
Pentazocine Hydrochloride and Naloxone Hydrochloride *See* Pentazocine 1243
Pentazocine Lactate *See* Pentazocine 1243
PENTobarbital 1247
Pentobarbital Sodium *See* PENTobarbital 1247
Pentosan Polysulfate Sodium 1250
Pentostatin 1250
Pentothal® *See* Thiopental 1570
Pentoxifylline 1251
Pentoxil® *See* Pentoxifylline 1251
Pentrexyl (Mex) *See* Ampicillin 122
Pen-Vi-K (Mex) *See* Penicillin V Potassium 1242
Pen VK *See* Penicillin V Potassium 1242
Pepcid® *See* Famotidine 613
Pepcid® AC (Can) *See* Famotidine 613
Pepcid® AC Maximum Strength [OTC] *See* Famotidine 613
Pepcid® AC [OTC] *See* Famotidine 613
Pepcid® Complete [OTC] *See* Famotidine, Calcium Carbonate, and Magnesium Hydroxide 614
Pepcidine (Mex) *See* Famotidine 613
Pepcid® I.V. (Can) *See* Famotidine 613
Pepevit (Mex) *See* Niacin 1124
Peptic Relief [OTC] *See* Bismuth 189
Pepto-Bismol® Maximum Strength [OTC] *See* Bismuth 189
Pepto-Bismol® [OTC] *See* Bismuth 189
Pepto Relief [OTC] *See* Bismuth 189
Percocet® *See* Oxycodone and Acetaminophen 1205
Percocet®-Demi (Can) *See* Oxycodone and Acetaminophen 1205
Percodan® *See* Oxycodone and Aspirin 1208
Percogesic® Extra Strength [OTC] *See* Acetaminophen and Diphenhydramine 35
Percogesic® [OTC] *See* Acetaminophen and Phenyltoloxamine 36
Perforomist™ *See* Formoterol 686
Periactin *See* Cyproheptadine 410
Periciazine 1252
Peri-Colace® [OTC] *See* Docusate and Senna 491
Pericyazine *See* Periciazine 1252
Peridane (Mex) *See* Pentoxifylline 1251
Peridol (Can) *See* Haloperidol 754
Perindopril Erbumine 1254
Periostat® *See* Doxycycline 509
Perphenazine 1255
Perphenazine and Amitriptyline Hydrochloride *See* Amitriptyline and Perphenazine 98
Persantin (Mex) *See* Dipyridamole 488
Persantine® *See* Dipyridamole 488
Pesatril (Mex) *See* Lisinopril 934
Pethidine Hydrochloride *See* Meperidine 986
Peucetol (Mex) *See* Pantoprazole 1221
Pexeva® *See* PARoxetine 1226
Pexicam® (Can) *See* Piroxicam 1307
PFA *See* Foscarnet 690
Pfizerpen® *See* Penicillin G, Parenteral, Aqueous 1241
Pfizerpen-AS® (Can) *See* Penicillin G Procaine 1241
PGE1 *See* Alprostadil 77
PGE2 *See* Dinoprostone 480
PGI2 *See* Epoprostenol 547
PGX *See* Epoprostenol 547
Phanasin® Diabetic Choice [OTC] *See* GuaiFENesin 737
Phanasin® [OTC] *See* GuaiFENesin 737
Phanatuss® DM [OTC] *See* Guaifenesin and Dextromethorphan 739
Phanatuss® HC [DSC] *See* Hydrocodone and Guaifenesin 779
Pharmacen-M (Mex) *See* Acetaminophen 30

Pharmafil (Mex) *See* Theophylline 1562
Pharmaton (Mex) *See* Thiamine 1568
Pharmaton Complex (Mex) *See* Ergocalciferol 550
Pharmorubicin® (Can) *See* Epirubicin 545
Phenabid® *See* Chlorpheniramine and Phenylephrine 323
Phenabid DM® *See* Chlorpheniramine, Phenylephrine, and Dextromethorphan 327
Phenadoz™ *See* Promethazine 1347
Phenagesic [OTC] *See* Acetaminophen and Phenyltoloxamine 36
PhenaVent™ D [DSC] *See* Guaifenesin and Phenylephrine 742
PhenaVent™ [DSC] *See* Guaifenesin and Phenylephrine 742
PhenaVent™ LA [DSC] *See* Guaifenesin and Phenylephrine 742
PhenaVent™ Ped [DSC] *See* Guaifenesin and Phenylephrine 742
Phenazo™ (Can) *See* Phenazopyridine 1258
Phenazopyridine 1258
Phenazopyridine Hydrochloride *See* Phenazopyridine 1258
Phencarb GG *See* Carbetapentane, Guaifenesin, and Phenylephrine 274
Phendimetrazine 1259
Phendimetrazine Tartrate *See* Phendimetrazine 1259
Phenelzine 1261
Phenelzine Sulfate *See* Phenelzine 1261
Phenergan® *See* Promethazine 1347
Pheniramine and Naphazoline *See* Naphazoline and Pheniramine 1102
PHENobarbital 1265
Phenobarbital, Belladonna, and Ergotamine Tartrate *See* Belladonna, Phenobarbital, and Ergotamine 175
Phenobarbital, Hyoscyamine, Atropine, and Scopolamine *See* Hyoscyamine, Atropine, Scopolamine, and Phenobarbital 800
Phenobarbital Sodium *See* PHENobarbital 1265
Phenobarbitone *See* PHENobarbital 1265
Phenoxybenzamine 1270
Phenoxybenzamine Hydrochloride *See* Phenoxybenzamine 1270
Phenoxymethyl Penicillin *See* Penicillin V Potassium 1242
Phentermine 1270
Phentermine Hydrochloride *See* Phentermine 1270
Phentolamine 1272
Phentolamine Mesylate *See* Phentolamine 1272
Phenylalanine Mustard *See* Melphalan 983
Phenylazo Diamino Pyridine Hydrochloride *See* Phenazopyridine 1258
Phenylephrine 1273
Phenylephrine CM *See* Chlorpheniramine, Phenylephrine, and Methscopolamine 329
Phenylephrine, Acetaminophen, and Dextromethorphan *See* Acetaminophen, Dextromethorphan, and Phenylephrine 42
Phenylephrine and Chlorpheniramine *See* Chlorpheniramine and Phenylephrine 323
Phenylephrine and Cyclopentolate *See* Cyclopentolate and Phenylephrine 407
Phenylephrine and Diphenhydramine *See* Diphenhydramine and Phenylephrine 485
Phenylephrine and Promethazine *See* Promethazine and Phenylephrine 1350
Phenylephrine and Pyrilamine 1275
Phenylephrine, Chlorpheniramine, and Carbetapentane *See* Carbetapentane, Phenylephrine, and Chlorpheniramine 274
Phenylephrine, Chlorpheniramine, and Dextromethorphan *See* Chlorpheniramine, Phenylephrine, and Dextromethorphan 327
Phenylephrine, Chlorpheniramine, and Dihydrocodeine *See* Dihydrocodeine, Chlorpheniramine, and Phenylephrine 469
Phenylephrine, Chlorpheniramine, and Guaifenesin *See* Chlorpheniramine, Phenylephrine, and Guaifenesin 329
Phenylephrine, Chlorpheniramine, and Phenyltoloxamine *See* Chlorpheniramine, Phenylephrine, and Phenyltoloxamine 331
Phenylephrine, Chlorpheniramine, Codeine, and Potassium Iodide *See* Chlorpheniramine, Phenylephrine, Codeine, and Potassium Iodide 332
Phenylephrine, Dextromethorphan, and Acetaminophen *See* Acetaminophen, Dextromethorphan, and Phenylephrine 42
Phenylephrine, Diphenhydramine, and Hydrocodone *See* Hydrocodone, Phenylephrine, and Diphenhydramine 782
Phenylephrine, Ephedrine, Chlorpheniramine, and Carbetapentane *See* Chlorpheniramine, Ephedrine, Phenylephrine, and Carbetapentane 326
Phenylephrine, Guaifenesin, and Hydrocodone *See* Hydrocodone, Phenylephrine, and Guaifenesin 783
Phenylephrine Hydrochloride *See* Phenylephrine 1273
Phenylephrine Hydrochloride, Acetaminophen, and Diphenhydramine *See* Acetaminophen, Diphenhydramine, and Phenylephrine 44
Phenylephrine Hydrochloride and Acetaminophen *See* Acetaminophen and Phenylephrine 36
Phenylephrine Hydrochloride and Diphenhydramine Hydrochloride *See* Diphenhydramine and Phenylephrine 485
Phenylephrine Hydrochloride and Guaifenesin *See* Guaifenesin and Phenylephrine 742
Phenylephrine Hydrochloride, Carbetapentane Citrate, and Guaifenesin *See* Carbetapentane, Guaifenesin, and Phenylephrine 274

Phenylephrine Hydrochloride, Chlorpheniramine maleate, Dextromethorphan Hydrobromide, and Guaifenesin *See* Dextromethorphan, Chlorpheniramine, Phenylephrine, and Guaifenesin 450
Phenylephrine Hydrochloride, Guaifenesin, and Dextromethorphan Hydrobromide *See* Guaifenesin, Dextromethorphan, and Phenylephrine 746
Phenylephrine Hydrochloride, Hydrocodone Bitartrate, and Chlorpheniramine Maleate *See* Phenylephrine, Hydrocodone, and Chlorpheniramine 1277
Phenylephrine, Hydrocodone, and Chlorpheniramine 1277
Phenylephrine, Promethazine, and Codeine *See* Promethazine, Phenylephrine, and Codeine 1350
Phenylephrine, Pyrilamine, and Dextromethorphan 1278
Phenylephrine, Pyrilamine, and Guaifenesin 1279
Phenylephrine Tannate *See* Phenylephrine 1273
Phenylephrine Tannate and Carbetapentane Tannate *See* Carbetapentane and Phenylephrine 273
Phenylephrine Tannate and Diphenhydramine Tannate *See* Diphenhydramine and Phenylephrine 485
Phenylephrine Tannate, Carbetapentane Tannate, and Pyrilamine Tannate *See* Carbetapentane, Phenylephrine, and Pyrilamine 275
Phenylephrine Tannate, Chlorpheniramine Tannate, and Methscopolamine Nitrate *See* Chlorpheniramine, Phenylephrine, and Methscopolamine 329
Phenylethylmalonylurea *See* PHENobarbital 1265
Phenylgesic [OTC] *See* Acetaminophen and Phenyltoloxamine 36
Phenyl Salicylate, Methenamine, Methylene Blue, Benzoic Acid, and Hyoscyamine *See* Methenamine, Phenyl Salicylate, Methylene Blue, Benzoic Acid, and Hyoscyamine 1009
Phenyl Salicylate, Methenamine, Methylene Blue, Sodium Biphosphate, and Hyoscyamine *See* Methenamine, Sodium Biphosphate, Phenyl Salicylate, Methylene Blue, and Hyoscyamine 1010
Phenyltoloxamine, Chlorpheniramine, and Phenylephrine *See* Chlorpheniramine, Phenylephrine, and Phenyltoloxamine 331
Phenyltoloxamine Citrate and Acetaminophen *See* Acetaminophen and Phenyltoloxamine 36
Phenytek® *See* Phenytoin 1280
Phenytoin 1280
Phenytoin Sodium *See* Phenytoin 1280
Phenytoin Sodium, Extended *See* Phenytoin 1280
Phenytoin Sodium, Prompt *See* Phenytoin 1280
PHL-Alendronate (Can) *See* Alendronate 59
PHL-Alendronate-FC (Can) *See* Alendronate 59
PHL-Amiodarone (Can) *See* Amiodarone 89
PHL-Amoxicillin (Can) *See* Amoxicillin 112
PHL-Anagrelide (Can) *See* Anagrelide 124
PHL-Azithromycin (Can) *See* Azithromycin 163
PHL-Bicalutamide (Can) *See* Bicalutamide 188
PHL-Carbamazepine (Can) *See* CarBAMazepine 265
PHL-Ciprofloxacin (Can) *See* Ciprofloxacin 346
PHL-Citalopram (Can) *See* Citalopram 354
PHL-Divalproex (Can) *See* Valproic Acid and Derivatives 1642
PHL-Domperidone (Can) *See* Domperidone 493
Phlemex *See* Guaifenesin and Dextromethorphan 739
PHL-Fenofibrate Supra (Can) *See* Fenofibrate 620
PHL-Fluconazole (Can) *See* Fluconazole 635
PHL-Fluoxetine (Can) *See* FLUoxetine 650
PHL-Levetiracetam (Can) *See* Levetiracetam 905
PHL-Lorazepam (Can) *See* LORazepam 949
PHL-Methimazole (Can) *See* Methimazole 1010
PHL-Metoprolol (Can) *See* Metoprolol 1036
PHL-Ondansetron (Can) *See* Ondansetron 1180
PHL-Risperidone (Can) *See* Risperidone 1425
PHL-Sertraline (Can) *See* Sertraline 1472
PHL-Simvastatin (Can) *See* Simvastatin 1486
PHL-Sumatriptan (Can) *See* SUMAtriptan 1527
PHL-Temazepam (Can) *See* Temazepam 1545
PHL-Topiramate (Can) *See* Topiramate 1598
PHL-Ursodiol C (Can) *See* Ursodiol 1639
PHL-Valproic Acid (Can) *See* Valproic Acid and Derivatives 1642
PHL-Valproic Acid E.C. (Can) *See* Valproic Acid and Derivatives 1642
PHL-Verapamil (Can) *See* Verapamil 1665
PhosLo® *See* Calcium Acetate 254
Phosphonoformate *See* Foscarnet 690
Phosphonoformic Acid *See* Foscarnet 690
Photoderm Max Bio (Mex) *See* Mannitol 968
Photofrin® *See* Porfimer 1314
Phoxal-timolol (Can) *See* Timolol 1584
Phrenilin® *See* Butalbital and Acetaminophen 236
Phrenilin® Forte *See* Butalbital and Acetaminophen 236

Phrenilin® with Caffeine and Codeine *See* Butalbital, Acetaminophen, Caffeine, and Codeine ... 232
p-Hydroxyampicillin *See* Amoxicillin ... 112
Phyllocontin® (Can) *See* Aminophylline ... 88
Phyllocontin®-350 (Can) *See* Aminophylline ... 88
Phylloquinone *See* Phytonadione ... 1289
Physostigmine ... 1288
Physostigmine Salicylate *See* Physostigmine ... 1288
Physostigmine Sulfate *See* Physostigmine ... 1288
Phytomenadione *See* Phytonadione ... 1289
Phytonadione ... 1289
Pidorubicin *See* Epirubicin ... 545
Pidorubicin Hydrochloride *See* Epirubicin ... 545
Pilocarpine ... 1290
Pilocarpine Hydrochloride *See* Pilocarpine ... 1290
Pilopine HS® *See* Pilocarpine ... 1290
Pimozide ... 1290
Pin-X® [OTC] *See* Pyrantel Pamoate ... 1373
Pindolol ... 1294
Pink Bismuth *See* Bismuth ... 189
Pioglitazone ... 1297
Pioglitazone and Glimepiride ... 1300
Pioglitazone and Metformin ... 1301
Piperacillin ... 1301
Piperacillin and Tazobactam Sodium ... 1302
Piperacillin for Injection, USP (Can) *See* Piperacillin ... 1301
Piperacillin Sodium *See* Piperacillin ... 1301
Piperacillin Sodium and Tazobactam Sodium *See* Piperacillin and Tazobactam Sodium ... 1302
Piperazine ... 1303
Piperazine Citrate *See* Piperazine ... 1303
Piperazine Estrone Sulfate *See* Estropipate ... 588
Piper methysticum *See* Kava Kava (Piper methysticum) ... 874
Piportil® L4 (Can) *See* Pipotiazine ... 1303
Piportil L4 (Mex) *See* Pipotiazine ... 1303
Pipotiazine ... 1303
Pipotiazine Palmitate *See* Pipotiazine ... 1303
Piralgina (Mex) *See* EPHEDrine ... 542
Pirbuterol ... 1305
Pirbuterol Acetate *See* Pirbuterol ... 1305
Pirimir (Mex) *See* Phenazopyridine ... 1258
Pirox (Mex) *See* Piroxicam ... 1307
Piroxicam ... 1307
p-Isobutylhydratropic Acid *See* Ibuprofen ... 803
Pizotifen ... 1307
Pizotifen Malate *See* Pizotifen ... 1307
Pizzard (Mex) *See* Desmopressin ... 431
PK-Merz (Mex) *See* Amantadine ... 79
Plan B™ (Can) *See* Levonorgestrel ... 918
Plan B® [RX/OTC] *See* Levonorgestrel ... 918
Plaquenil® *See* Hydroxychloroquine ... 796
Plasil (Mex) *See* Metoclopramide ... 1031
Plavix® *See* Clopidogrel ... 380
Plegine® (Can) *See* Phendimetrazine ... 1259
Plendil® *See* Felodipine ... 617
Pletal® *See* Cilostazol ... 344
Plexicodim (Mex) *See* OxyCODONE ... 1201
PMPA *See* Tenofovir ... 1549
PMS-Alendronate (Can) *See* Alendronate ... 59
PMS-Alendronate-FC (Can) *See* Alendronate ... 59
PMS-Amantadine (Can) *See* Amantadine ... 79
PMS-Amiodarone (Can) *See* Amiodarone ... 89
PMS-Amitriptyline (Can) *See* Amitriptyline ... 90
PMS-Amoxicillin (Can) *See* Amoxicillin ... 112
PMS-Anagrelide (Can) *See* Anagrelide ... 124
PMS-Atenolol (Can) *See* Atenolol ... 147
PMS-Azithromycin (Can) *See* Azithromycin ... 163
PMS-Baclofen (Can) *See* Baclofen ... 168
PMS-Bethanechol (Can) *See* Bethanechol ... 186
PMS-Bicalutamide (Can) *See* Bicalutamide ... 188
PMS-Bisoprolol (Can) *See* Bisoprolol ... 190
PMS-Brimonidine Tartrate (Can) *See* Brimonidine ... 199
PMS-Bromocriptine (Can) *See* Bromocriptine ... 202
PMS-Buspirone (Can) *See* BusPIRone ... 223
PMS-Butorphanol (Can) *See* Butorphanol ... 247
PMS-Captopril (Can) *See* Captopril ... 264
PMS-Carbamazepine (Can) *See* CarBAMazepine ... 265

PMS-Carvedilol (Can) *See* Carvedilol 286
PMS-Cefaclor (Can) *See* Cefaclor 291
PMS-Chloral Hydrate (Can) *See* Chloral Hydrate 313
PMS-Cholestyramine (Can) *See* Cholestyramine Resin 341
PMS-Cimetidine (Can) *See* Cimetidine 345
PMS-Ciprofloxacin (Can) *See* Ciprofloxacin 346
PMS-Citalopram (Can) *See* Citalopram 354
PMS-Clarithromycin (Can) *See* Clarithromycin 360
PMS-Clindamycin (Can) *See* Clindamycin 363
PMS-Clobazam (Can) *See* Clobazam 364
PMS-Clonazepam (Can) *See* ClonazePAM 373
PMS-Deferoxamine (Can) *See* Deferoxamine 423
PMS-Desipramine (Can) *See* Desipramine 426
PMS-Desmopressin (Can) *See* Desmopressin 431
PMS-Dexamethasone (Can) *See* Dexamethasone 436
PMS-Diclofenac (Can) *See* Diclofenac 457
PMS-Diclofenac SR (Can) *See* Diclofenac 457
PMS-Diphenhydramine (Can) *See* DiphenhydrAMINE 481
PMS-Domperidone (Can) *See* Domperidone 493
PMS-Enalapril (Can) *See* Enalapril 531
PMS-Erythromycin (Can) *See* Erythromycin 557
PMS-Famciclovir (Can) *See* Famciclovir 613
PMS-Fenofibrate Micro (Can) *See* Fenofibrate 620
PMS-Fenofibrate Supra (Can) *See* Fenofibrate 620
PMS-Fluconazole (Can) *See* Fluconazole 635
PMS-Flunisolide (Can) *See* Flunisolide 646
PMS-Fluoxetine (Can) *See* FLUoxetine 650
PMS-Fluphenazine Decanoate (Can) *See* Fluphenazine 660
PMS-Fluvoxamine (Can) *See* Fluvoxamine 678
PMS-Fosinopril (Can) *See* Fosinopril 691
PMS-Furosemide (Can) *See* Furosemide 699
PMS-Gabapentin (Can) *See* Gabapentin 702
PMS-Gemfibrozil (Can) *See* Gemfibrozil 711
PMS-Glimepiride (Can) *See* Glimepiride 723
PMS-Glyburide (Can) *See* GlyBURIDE 730
PMS-Haloperidol LA (Can) *See* Haloperidol 754
PMS-Hydrochlorothiazide (Can) *See* Hydrochlorothiazide 773
PMS-Hydromorphone (Can) *See* HYDROmorphone 791
PMS-Hydroxyzine (Can) *See* HydrOXYzine 797
PMS-Indapamide (Can) *See* Indapamide 817
PMS-Ipratropium (Can) *See* Ipratropium 852
PMS-ISMN (Can) *See* Isosorbide Mononitrate 869
PMS-Isoniazid (Can) *See* Isoniazid 862
PMS-Isosorbide (Can) *See* Isosorbide Dinitrate 866
PMS-Lactulose (Can) *See* Lactulose 886
PMS-Lamotrigine (Can) *See* LamoTRIgine 889
PMS-Levetiracetam (Can) *See* Levetiracetam 905
PMS-Levobunolol (Can) *See* Levobunolol 907
PMS-Lindane (Can) *See* Lindane 927
PMS-Lisinopril (Can) *See* Lisinopril 934
PMS-Lithium Carbonate (Can) *See* Lithium 938
PMS-Lithium Citrate (Can) *See* Lithium 938
PMS-Loperamine (Can) *See* Loperamide 944
PMS-Lorazepam (Can) *See* LORazepam 949
PMS-Lovastatin (Can) *See* Lovastatin 956
PMS-Loxapine (Can) *See* Loxapine 960
PMS-Mefenamic Acid (Can) *See* Mefenamic Acid 976
PMS-Meloxicam (Can) *See* Meloxicam 982
PMS-Metformin (Can) *See* MetFORMIN 997
PMS-Methotrimeprazine (Can) *See* Methotrimeprazine 1015
PMS-Methylphenidate (Can) *See* Methylphenidate 1024
PMS-Metoprolol (Can) *See* Metoprolol 1036
PMS-Minocycline (Can) *See* Minocycline 1056
PMS-Mirtazapine (Can) *See* Mirtazapine 1058
PMS-Moclobemide (Can) *See* Moclobemide 1062
PMS-Mometasone (Can) *See* Mometasone 1071
PMS-Morphine Sulfate SR (Can) *See* Morphine Sulfate 1077
PMS-Naproxen EC (Can) *See* Naproxen 1102
PMS-Nizatidine (Can) *See* Nizatidine 1149
PMS-Norfloxacin (Can) *See* Norfloxacin 1151
PMS-Nortriptyline (Can) *See* Nortriptyline 1152
PMS-Ofloxacin (Can) *See* Ofloxacin 1159
PMS-Ondansetron (Can) *See* Ondansetron 1180
PMS-Oxazepam (Can) *See* Oxazepam 1193
PMS-Oxybutynin (Can) *See* Oxybutynin 1199
PMS-Oxycodone-Acetaminophen (Can) *See* Oxycodone and Acetaminophen 1205
PMS-Pantoprazole (Can) *See* Pantoprazole 1221

PMS-Paroxetine (Can) *See* PARoxetine 1226
PMS-Phenobarbital (Can) *See* PHENobarbital 1265
PMS-Pindolol (Can) *See* Pindolol 1294
PMS-Pioglitazone (Can) *See* Pioglitazone 1297
PMS-Pramipexole (Can) *See* Pramipexole 1318
PMS-Pravastatin (Can) *See* Pravastatin 1321
PMS-Procyclidine (Can) *See* Procyclidine 1344
PMS-Promethazine (Can) *See* Promethazine 1347
PMS-Propafenone (Can) *See* Propafenone 1351
PMS-Propranolol (Can) *See* Propranolol 1355
PMS-Pseudoephedrine (Can) *See* Pseudoephedrine 1367
PMS-Ranitidine (Can) *See* Ranitidine 1399
PMS-Risperidone ODT (Can) *See* Risperidone 1425
PMS-Salbutamol (Can) *See* Albuterol 54
PMS-Sertraline (Can) *See* Sertraline 1472
PMS-Simvastatin (Can) *See* Simvastatin 1486
PMS-Sotalol (Can) *See* Sotalol 1502
PMS-Sucralate (Can) *See* Sucralfate 1514
PMS-Sumatriptan (Can) *See* SUMAtriptan 1527
PMS-Temazepam (Can) *See* Temazepam 1545
PMS-Terazosin (Can) *See* Terazosin 1549
PMS-Terbinafine (Can) *See* Terbinafine 1551
PMS-Theophylline (Can) *See* Theophylline 1562
PMS-Timolol (Can) *See* Timolol 1584
PMS-Tobramycin (Can) *See* Tobramycin 1590
PMS-Topiramate (Can) *See* Topiramate 1598
PMS-Trazodone (Can) *See* TraZODone 1614
PMS-Trifluoperazine (Can) *See* Trifluoperazine 1624
PMS-Ursodiol C (Can) *See* Ursodiol 1639
PMS-Valproic Acid (Can) *See* Valproic Acid and Derivatives 1642
PMS-Valproic Acid E.C. (Can) *See* Valproic Acid and Derivatives 1642
PMS-Venlafaxine XR (Can) *See* Venlafaxine 1659
PMS-Verapamil SR (Can) *See* Verapamil 1665
PMS-Yohimbine (Can) *See* Yohimbine 1688
PMS-Zopiclone (Can) *See* Zopiclone 1711
Pneumo 23™ (Can) *See* Pneumococcal Polysaccharide Vaccine (Polyvalent) 1309
Pneumococcal 7-Valent Conjugate Vaccine *See* Pneumococcal Conjugate Vaccine, 7-Valent 1308
Pneumococcal Conjugate Vaccine, 7-Valent 1308
Pneumococcal Polysaccharide Vaccine (Polyvalent) 1309
Pneumotussin® [DSC] *See* Hydrocodone and Guaifenesin 779
Pneumovax® 23 *See* Pneumococcal Polysaccharide Vaccine (Polyvalent) 1309
PNU-140690E *See* Tipranavir 1586
Podocon-25® *See* Podophyllum Resin 1309
Podofilia No. 2 (Mex) *See* Podophyllum Resin 1309
Podofilm® (Can) *See* Podophyllum Resin 1309
Podophyllin *See* Podophyllum Resin 1309
Podophyllum Resin 1309
Polaramine (Mex) *See* Dexchlorpheniramine 437
Polcotec (Mex) *See* Metoclopramide 1031
Polixin (Mex) *See* Polymyxin B 1312
Polocaine® *See* Mepivacaine 990
Polocaine® Dental *See* Mepivacaine 990
Polocaine® MPF *See* Mepivacaine 990
Poly-B con Vitamina C (Mex) *See* Pyridoxine 1376
Polyethylene Glycol-Electrolyte Solution 1310
Poly-Hist DM *See* Phenylephrine, Pyrilamine, and Dextromethorphan 1278
Poly Hist Forte® *See* Chlorpheniramine, Pyrilamine, and Phenylephrine 335
Poly Hist PD *See* Chlorpheniramine, Pyrilamine, and Phenylephrine 335
Poly-Iron 150 [OTC] *See* Polysaccharide-Iron Complex 1313
Polymox (Mex) *See* Amoxicillin 112
Polymyxin B 1312
Polymyxin B Sulfate *See* Polymyxin B 1312
Poly-Rx *See* Polymyxin B 1312
Polysaccharide-Iron Complex 1313
Polythiazide 1313
Polythiazide and Prazosin *See* Prazosin and Polythiazide 1325
Poly Tussin DM *See* Chlorpheniramine, Phenylephrine, and Dextromethorphan 327
PolyTussin HD *See* Phenylephrine, Hydrocodone, and Chlorpheniramine 1277
Ponstan® (Can) *See* Mefenamic Acid 976
Ponstan-500 (Mex) *See* Mefenamic Acid 976
Ponstel® *See* Mefenamic Acid 976
Pontocaine® *See* Tetracaine 1557
Pontocaine® Niphanoid® *See* Tetracaine 1557
Porfimer 1314
Porfimer Sodium *See* Porfimer 1314
Portia™ *See* Ethinyl Estradiol and Levonorgestrel 595

Posaconazole 1314
Posipen (Mex) *See* Dicloxacillin 459
Postinor-2 (Mex) *See* Levonorgestrel 918
Post Peel Healing Balm [OTC] *See* Hydrocortisone 785
Potassium Bicarbonate and Potassium Citrate 1315
Potassium Bicarbonate and Potassium Citrate (Effervescent) *See* Potassium Bicarbonate and Potassium Citrate 1315
Potassium Chloride 1315
Potassium Iodide 1317
Potassium Iodide and Iodine 1317
Potassium Iodide, Chlorpheniramine, Phenylephrine, and Codeine *See* Chlorpheniramine, Phenylephrine, Codeine, and Potassium Iodide 332
Pota-Vi-Kin (Mex) *See* Penicillin V Potassium 1242
PPS *See* Pentosan Polysulfate Sodium 1250
PPV23 *See* Pneumococcal Polysaccharide Vaccine (Polyvalent) 1309
Pralidoxime 1318
Pralidoxime and Atropine *See* Atropine and Pralidoxime 159
Pralidoxime Chloride *See* Pralidoxime 1318
Pramipexole 1318
Pramlintide 1321
Pramlintide Acetate *See* Pramlintide 1321
PrandiMet™ *See* Repaglinide and Metformin 1412
Prandin® *See* Repaglinide 1409
Pranidol (Mex) *See* Propranolol 1355
Pravachol® *See* Pravastatin 1321
Pravacol (Mex) *See* Pravastatin 1321
PravASA (Can) *See* Aspirin and Pravastatin 146
Pravastatin 1321
Pravastatin and Aspirin *See* Aspirin and Pravastatin 146
Pravastatin Sodium *See* Pravastatin 1321
Pravigard™ PAC [DSC] *See* Aspirin and Pravastatin 146
Praxel (Mex) *See* Paclitaxel 1213
Prazidec (Mex) *See* Omeprazole 1176
Praziquantel 1324
Prazosin 1325
Prazosin and Polythiazide 1325
Prazosin Hydrochloride *See* Prazosin 1325
Precedex™ *See* Dexmedetomidine 438
Precose® *See* Acarbose 25
Pred Forte® *See* PrednisoLONE 1326
Predlitem (Mex) *See* MethylPREDNISolone 1029
Pred Mild® *See* PrednisoLONE 1326
Prednefrin SF (Mex) *See* PrednisoLONE 1326
Pred-NF (Mex) *See* PrednisoLONE 1326
Prednidib (Mex) *See* PredniSONE 1327
PrednisoLONE 1326
Prednisolone Acetate *See* PrednisoLONE 1326
Prednisolone Acetate, Ophthalmic *See* PrednisoLONE 1326
Prednisolone and Sulfacetamide *See* Sulfacetamide and Prednisolone 1516
Prednisolone Sodium Phosphate *See* PrednisoLONE 1326
Prednisolone Sodium Phosphate, Ophthalmic *See* PrednisoLONE 1326
PredniSONE 1327
PredniSONE Intensol™ *See* PredniSONE 1327
Pred Un (Mex) *See* PrednisoLONE 1326
Predxal (Mex) *See* Telmisartan 1542
Prefest™ *See* Estradiol and Norgestimate 580
Pregabalin 1332
Pregnenedione *See* Progesterone 1345
Pregnyl® *See* Chorionic Gonadotropin (Human) 342
Prelar Depot (Mex) *See* Leuprolide 901
Prelone® *See* PrednisoLONE 1326
Premarin® *See* Estrogens (Conjugated/Equine) 582
Premelle (Mex) *See* Estrogens (Conjugated/Equine) and Medroxyprogesterone 583
Premjact® [OTC] *See* Lidocaine 924
Premphase® *See* Estrogens (Conjugated/Equine) and Medroxyprogesterone 583
Premplus® (Can) *See* Estrogens (Conjugated/Equine) and Medroxyprogesterone 583
Prempro™ *See* Estrogens (Conjugated/Equine) and Medroxyprogesterone 583
Preparation H® Hydrocortisone [OTC] *See* Hydrocortisone 785
Preparation H® [OTC] *See* Phenylephrine 1273
Prepidil® *See* Dinoprostone 480
Preservative-Free Cosopt® (Can) *See* Dorzolamide and Timolol 499
Presistin (Mex) *See* Cisapride U.S. - Available Via Limited-Access Protocol Only 353
Pressyn® (Can) *See* Vasopressin 1659
Pressyn® AR (Can) *See* Vasopressin 1659
Pretz-D® [OTC] *See* EPHEDrine 542
Prevacid® *See* Lansoprazole 894
Prevacid® NapraPAC™ *See* Lansoprazole and Naproxen 897

Pseudoephedrine Hydrochloride, Hydrocodone Bitartrate, and Chlorpheniramine Maleate *See* Pseudoephedrine, Hydrocodone, and Chlorpheniramine ... 1372
Pseudoephedrine Hydrochloride, Methscopolamine Nitrate, and Chlorpheniramine Maleate *See* Chlorpheniramine, Pseudoephedrine, and Methscopolamine ... 334
Pseudoephedrine, Hydrocodone, and Carbinoxamine *See* Hydrocodone, Carbinoxamine, and Pseudoephedrine ... 782
Pseudoephedrine, Hydrocodone, and Chlorpheniramine ... 1372
Pseudoephedrine, Hydrocodone, and Guaifenesin *See* Hydrocodone, Pseudoephedrine, and Guaifenesin ... 784
Pseudoephedrine, Methscopolamine, and Chlorpheniramine *See* Chlorpheniramine, Pseudoephedrine, and Methscopolamine ... 334
Pseudoephedrine Sulfate *See* Pseudoephedrine ... 1367
Pseudoephedrine Tannate, Dextromethorphan Tannate, and Brompheniramine Tannate *See* Brompheniramine, Pseudoephedrine, and Dextromethorphan ... 208
Pseudoephedrine, Triprolidine, and Codeine *See* Triprolidine, Pseudoephedrine, and Codeine ... 1635
Pseudofrin (Can) *See* Pseudoephedrine ... 1367
Pseudo GG TR *See* Guaifenesin and Pseudoephedrine ... 744
Pseudo Max *See* Guaifenesin and Pseudoephedrine ... 744
Pseudo Max DMX *See* Guaifenesin, Pseudoephedrine, and Dextromethorphan ... 748
Pseudomonic Acid A *See* Mupirocin ... 1085
Pseudovent™ 400 [DSC] *See* Guaifenesin and Pseudoephedrine ... 744
Pseudovent™ DM [DSC] *See* Guaifenesin, Pseudoephedrine, and Dextromethorphan ... 748
Pseudovent™ [DSC] *See* Guaifenesin and Pseudoephedrine ... 744
Pseudovent™-Ped [DSC] *See* Guaifenesin and Pseudoephedrine ... 744
P&S® [OTC] *See* Salicylic Acid ... 1454
P-Tann D *See* Chlorpheniramine and Phenylephrine ... 323
Pteroylglutamic Acid *See* Folic Acid ... 684
PTU (error-prone abbreviation) *See* Propylthiouracil ... 1361
Pulmicort® (Can) *See* Budesonide ... 210
Pulmicort Flexhaler™ *See* Budesonide ... 210
Pulmicort Respules® *See* Budesonide ... 210
Pulmophylline (Can) *See* Theophylline ... 1562
Puribel 300 (Mex) *See* Allopurinol ... 67
Purinethol® *See* Mercaptopurine ... 993
Purple Coneflower *See* Echinacea (Echinacea purpurea, Echinacea angustifolia) ... 523
Pusarat (Mex) *See* Simvastatin ... 1486
Pylera™ *See* Bismuth, Metronidazole, and Tetracycline ... 190
Pyrantel Pamoate ... 1373
Pyrazinamide ... 1373
Pyrazinamide, Rifampin, and Isoniazid *See* Rifampin, Isoniazid, and Pyrazinamide ... 1419
Pyrazinoic Acid Amide *See* Pyrazinamide ... 1373
Pyri-500 [OTC] *See* Pyridoxine ... 1376
2-Pyridine Aldoxime Methochloride *See* Pralidoxime ... 1318
Pyridium® *See* Phenazopyridine ... 1258
Pyridostigmine ... 1374
Pyridostigmine Bromide *See* Pyridostigmine ... 1374
Pyridoxine ... 1376
Pyridoxine and Doxylamine *See* Doxylamine and Pyridoxine ... 511
Pyridoxine Hydrochloride *See* Pyridoxine ... 1376
Pyrilafen Tannate-12™ *See* Phenylephrine and Pyrilamine ... 1275
Pyrilamine Maleate, Dextromethorphan Hydrobromide, and Phenylephrine Hydrochloride *See* Phenylephrine, Pyrilamine, and Dextromethorphan ... 1278
Pyrilamine, Phenylephrine, and Carbetapentane *See* Carbetapentane, Phenylephrine, and Pyrilamine ... 275
Pyrilamine Tannate and Phenylephrine Tannate *See* Phenylephrine and Pyrilamine ... 1275
Pyrilamine Tannate, Guaifenesin, and Phenylephrine Tannate *See* Phenylephrine, Pyrilamine, and Guaifenesin ... 1279
Pyrimethamine ... 1377
Pyrimethamine and Sulfadoxine *See* Sulfadoxine and Pyrimethamine ... 1517
QDALL® AR *See* Chlorpheniramine ... 321
QDALL® [DSC] *See* Chlorpheniramine and Pseudoephedrine ... 325
Quadrax (Mex) *See* Ibuprofen ... 803
Quadrivalent Meningococcal Conjugate Vaccine *See* Meningococcal Polysaccharide Vaccine (Groups A / C / Y and W-135) ... 985
Quad Tann® *See* Chlorpheniramine, Ephedrine, Phenylephrine, and Carbetapentane ... 326
Quad Tann® Pediatric *See* Chlorpheniramine, Ephedrine, Phenylephrine, and Carbetapentane ... 326
Qualaquin™ *See* QuiNINE ... 1388
Quartuss™ *See* Dextromethorphan, Chlorpheniramine, Phenylephrine, and Guaifenesin ... 450
Quasense™ *See* Ethinyl Estradiol and Levonorgestrel ... 595
Quazepam ... 1378
Quelicin® *See* Succinylcholine ... 1511
Questran® *See* Cholestyramine Resin ... 341
Questran® Light *See* Cholestyramine Resin ... 341
Questran® Light Sugar Free (Can) *See* Cholestyramine Resin ... 341
QUEtiapine ... 1381
Quetiapine Fumarate *See* QUEtiapine ... 1381

Prevacid® SoluTab™ *See* Lansoprazole ... 894
Prevalite® *See* Cholestyramine Resin ... 341
Prevex® B (Can) *See* Betamethasone ... 184
Prevex® HC (Can) *See* Hydrocortisone ... 785
Previfem™ *See* Ethinyl Estradiol and Norgestimate ... 600
Prevnar® *See* Pneumococcal Conjugate Vaccine, 7-Valent ... 1308
Prevpac® *See* Lansoprazole, Amoxicillin, and Clarithromycin ... 897
Prezista® *See* Darunavir ... 420
Prialt® *See* Ziconotide ... 1695
Priftin® *See* Rifapentine ... 1420
Prilosan (Mex) *See* Lansoprazole ... 894
Prilosec® *See* Omeprazole ... 1176
Prilosec OTC™ [OTC] *See* Omeprazole ... 1176
Primaclone *See* Primidone ... 1336
Primacor® *See* Milrinone ... 1055
Primalev™ *See* Oxycodone and Acetaminophen ... 1205
Primaquine ... 1335
Primaquine Phosphate *See* Primaquine ... 1335
Primatene® Mist [OTC] *See* EPINEPHrine ... 543
Primaxin® *See* Imipenem and Cilastatin ... 812
Primaxin® I.V. (Can) *See* Imipenem and Cilastatin ... 812
Primidone ... 1336
Primsol® *See* Trimethoprim ... 1629
Prinac AC (Mex) *See* Folic Acid ... 684
Princol (Mex) *See* Lincomycin ... 926
Prindex (Mex) *See* Carbinoxamine ... 280
Prindex Pediátrico (Mex) *See* Carbinoxamine and Pseudoephedrine ... 280
Prinivil® *See* Lisinopril ... 934
Prinzide® *See* Lisinopril and Hydrochlorothiazide ... 938
Priscoline® [DSC] *See* Tolazoline ... 1592
Pristinamycin *See* Quinupristin and Dalfopristin ... 1388
Pristiq™ *See* Desvenlafaxine ... 433
Privine® [OTC] *See* Naphazoline ... 1101
ProAir™ HFA *See* Albuterol ... 54
Proalid (Mex) *See* Tacrolimus ... 1533
ProAmatine® *See* Midodrine ... 1050
Probenecid ... 1338
Probenecid and Colchicine *See* Colchicine and Probenecid ... 398
Probi RHO (D) (Mex) *See* Rho(D) Immune Globulin ... 1415
Probirina (Mex) *See* Ribavirin ... 1417
Procainamide ... 1339
Procainamide Hydrochloride *See* Procainamide ... 1339
Procainamide Hydrochloride Injection, USP (Can) *See* Procainamide ... 1339
Procaine ... 1340
Procaine Amide Hydrochloride *See* Procainamide ... 1339
Procaine Benzylpenicillin *See* Penicillin G Procaine ... 1241
Procaine Hydrochloride *See* Procaine ... 1340
Procaine Penicillin G *See* Penicillin G Procaine ... 1241
Procanbid® [DSC] *See* Procainamide ... 1339
Procan® SR (Can) *See* Procainamide ... 1339
Procarbazine ... 1340
Procarbazine Hydrochloride *See* Procarbazine ... 1340
Procardia® *See* NIFEdipine ... 1136
Procardia XL® *See* NIFEdipine ... 1136
Procef (Mex) *See* Cefprozil ... 297
Procetofene *See* Fenofibrate ... 620
Prochieve® *See* Progesterone ... 1345
Prochlorperazine ... 1341
Prochlorperazine Edisylate *See* Prochlorperazine ... 1341
Prochlorperazine Maleate *See* Prochlorperazine ... 1341
Proclose (Mex) *See* Octreotide ... 1158
Procrit® *See* Epoetin Alfa ... 546
Proctocort® *See* Hydrocortisone ... 785
ProctoCream® HC *See* Hydrocortisone ... 785
Proctofene *See* Fenofibrate ... 620
Procto-Kit™ *See* Hydrocortisone ... 785
Procto-Pak™ *See* Hydrocortisone ... 785
Proctosert *See* Hydrocortisone ... 785
Proctosol-HC® *See* Hydrocortisone ... 785
Proctozone-HC™ *See* Hydrocortisone ... 785
Procyclidine ... 1344
Procyclidine Hydrochloride *See* Procyclidine ... 1344
Procytox® (Can) *See* Cyclophosphamide ... 408
Prodium® [OTC] *See* Phenazopyridine ... 1258
Pro Doc Limitee Bromazepam (Can) *See* Bromazepam ... 200
Profasi® HP (Can) *See* Chorionic Gonadotropin (Human) ... 342
Profen II DM® *See* Guaifenesin, Pseudoephedrine, and Dextromethorphan ... 748

Profen II® [DSC] *See* Guaifenesin and Pseudoephedrine 744
Profen Forte™ DM *See* Guaifenesin, Pseudoephedrine, and Dextromethorphan 748
Profenid (Mex) *See* Ketoprofen 877
ProFe [OTC] *See* Polysaccharide-Iron Complex 1313
Profercol (Mex) *See* Cisapride U.S. - Available Via Limited-Access Protocol Only 353
Profiben (Mex) *See* Pentoxifylline 1251
Profilnine® SD *See* Factor IX Complex (Human) 612
Proflavanol C™ (Can) *See* Ascorbic Acid 141
Progesterone 1345
Progestin *See* Progesterone 1345
Proglycem® *See* Diazoxide 456
Prograf® *See* Tacrolimus 1533
Proguanil and Atovaquone *See* Atovaquone and Proguanil 157
Proguanil Hydrochloride and Atovaquone *See* Atovaquone and Proguanil 157
Proleukin® *See* Aldesleukin 58
Prolex®-D [DSC] *See* Guaifenesin and Phenylephrine 742
Prolex®-PD [DSC] *See* Guaifenesin and Phenylephrine 742
Promacet *See* Butalbital and Acetaminophen 236
Promecilina (Mex) *See* Ampicillin 122
Promethazine 1347
Promethazine and Codeine 1349
Promethazine and Dextromethorphan 1350
Promethazine and Meperidine *See* Meperidine and Promethazine 987
Promethazine and Phenylephrine 1350
Promethazine Hydrochloride *See* Promethazine 1347
Promethazine, Phenylephrine, and Codeine 1350
Promethegan™ *See* Promethazine 1347
Prometrium® *See* Progesterone 1345
Promiced (Mex) *See* Metoprolol 1036
Pronestyl®-SR (Can) *See* Procainamide 1339
Propaderm® (Can) *See* Beclomethasone 171
Propafenone 1351
Propafenone Hydrochloride *See* Propafenone 1351
Propantheline 1351
Propantheline Bromide *See* Propantheline 1351
Proparacaine 1352
Proparacaine Hydrochloride *See* Proparacaine 1352
Proplex® T [DSC] *See* Factor IX Complex (Human) 612
Propofol 1352
Propoxyphene 1353
Propoxyphene and Acetaminophen 1354
Propoxyphene, Aspirin, and Caffeine 1355
Propoxyphene Hydrochloride *See* Propoxyphene 1353
Propoxyphene Hydrochloride and Acetaminophen *See* Propoxyphene and Acetaminophen 1354
Propoxyphene Hydrochloride, Aspirin, and Caffeine *See* Propoxyphene, Aspirin, and Caffeine 1355
Propoxyphene Napsylate *See* Propoxyphene 1353
Propoxyphene Napsylate and Acetaminophen *See* Propoxyphene and Acetaminophen 1354
Propranolol 1355
Propranolol and Hydrochlorothiazide 1361
Propranolol Hydrochloride *See* Propranolol 1355
Propranolol Hydrochloride Injection, USP (Can) *See* Propranolol 1355
Proprinal® Cold and Sinus [OTC] *See* Pseudoephedrine and Ibuprofen 1369
Proprinal [OTC] *See* Ibuprofen 803
Propulsid® *See* Cisapride U.S. - Available Via Limited-Access Protocol Only 353
2-Propylpentanoic Acid *See* Valproic Acid and Derivatives 1642
Propylthiouracil 1361
Propyl-Thyracil® (Can) *See* Propylthiouracil 1361
2-Propylvaleric Acid *See* Valproic Acid and Derivatives 1642
ProQuad® *See* Measles, Mumps, Rubella, and Varicella Virus Vaccine 972
Proquin® XR *See* Ciprofloxacin 346
Prosed®/DS *See* Methenamine, Phenyl Salicylate, Methylene Blue, Benzoic Acid, and Hyoscyamine 1009
Prosertin (Mex) *See* Sertraline 1472
ProSom® [DSC] *See* Estazolam 574
Prostacyclin *See* Epoprostenol 547
Prostacyclin PGI2 *See* Iloprost 810
Prostaglandin E1 *See* Alprostadil 77
Prostaglandin E2 *See* Dinoprostone 480
Prostaglandin F2 *See* Carboprost Tromethamine 282
Prostigmin® *See* Neostigmine 1121
Prostigmine (Mex) *See* Neostigmine 1121
Prostin E2® *See* Dinoprostone 480
Prostin® VR (Can) *See* Alprostadil 77
Prostin VR Pediatric® *See* Alprostadil 77

Protalgine (Mex) *See* LamoTRIgine 889
Protamine Sulfate 1362
Protein-Bound Paclitaxel *See* Paclitaxel (Protein Bound) 1214
Prothrombin Complex Concentrate *See* Factor IX Complex (Human) 612
Protirelin 1363
Protonix® *See* Pantoprazole 1221
Protopam® *See* Pralidoxime 1318
Protopic® *See* Tacrolimus 1533
Protriptyline 1363
Protriptyline Hydrochloride *See* Protriptyline 1363
Proventil® [DSC] *See* Albuterol 54
Proventil® HFA *See* Albuterol 54
Provera® *See* MedroxyPROGESTERone 975
Provera-Pak (Can) *See* MedroxyPROGESTERone 975
Provigil® *See* Modafinil 1065
Proxymetacaine *See* Proparacaine 1352
Prozac® *See* FLUoxetine 650
Prozac® Weekly™ *See* FLUoxetine 650
Prozolan (Mex) *See* Pantoprazole 1221
PRP-OMP *See* Haemophilus b Conjugate Vaccine 753
PRP-T *See* Haemophilus b Conjugate Vaccine 753
Prudoxin™ *See* Doxepin 502
Prymaccone *See* Primaquine 1335
23PS *See* Pneumococcal Polysaccharide Vaccine (Polyvalent) 1309
PS-341 *See* Bortezomib 192
Pseudacarb™ *See* Carbetapentane and Pseudoephedrine 273
Pseudoephedrine 1367
Pseudoephedrine, Acetaminophen, and Chlorpheniramine *See* Acetaminophen, Chlorpheniramine, and Pseudoephedrine 40
Pseudoephedrine, Acetaminophen, and Dextromethorphan *See* Acetaminophen, Dextromethorphan, and Pseudoephedrine 43
Pseudoephedrine and Acetaminophen *See* Acetaminophen and Pseudoephedrine 37
Pseudoephedrine and Brompheniramine *See* Brompheniramine and Pseudoephedrine 206
Pseudoephedrine and Carbetapentane *See* Carbetapentane and Pseudoephedrine 273
Pseudoephedrine and Carbinoxamine *See* Carbinoxamine and Pseudoephedrine 280
Pseudoephedrine and Chlorpheniramine *See* Chlorpheniramine and Pseudoephedrine 325
Pseudoephedrine and Codeine 1368
Pseudoephedrine and Desloratadine *See* Desloratadine and Pseudoephedrine 431
Pseudoephedrine and Dexbrompheniramine *See* Dexbrompheniramine and Pseudoephedrine 437
Pseudoephedrine and Dextromethorphan 1369
Pseudoephedrine and Diphenhydramine *See* Diphenhydramine and Pseudoephedrine 486
Pseudoephedrine and Fexofenadine *See* Fexofenadine and Pseudoephedrine 631
Pseudoephedrine and Guaifenesin *See* Guaifenesin and Pseudoephedrine 744
Pseudoephedrine and Ibuprofen 1369
Pseudoephedrine and Loratadine *See* Loratadine and Pseudoephedrine 948
Pseudoephedrine and Methscopolamine 1370
Pseudoephedrine and Naproxen *See* Naproxen and Pseudoephedrine 1107
Pseudoephedrine and Triprolidine *See* Triprolidine and Pseudoephedrine 1634
Pseudoephedrine, Chlorpheniramine, and Acetaminophen *See* Acetaminophen, Chlorpheniramine, and Pseudoephedrine 40
Pseudoephedrine, Chlorpheniramine, and Codeine *See* Chlorpheniramine, Pseudoephedrine, and Codeine 332
Pseudoephedrine, Chlorpheniramine, and Dextromethorphan *See* Chlorpheniramine, Pseudoephedrine, and Dextromethorphan 333
Pseudoephedrine, Chlorpheniramine, and Dihydrocodeine *See* Pseudoephedrine, Dihydrocodeine, and Chlorpheniramine 1371
Pseudoephedrine, Codeine, and Triprolidine *See* Triprolidine, Pseudoephedrine, and Codeine 1635
Pseudoephedrine, Dextromethorphan, and Acetaminophen *See* Acetaminophen, Dextromethorphan, and Pseudoephedrine 43
Pseudoephedrine, Dextromethorphan, and Guaifenesin *See* Guaifenesin, Pseudoephedrine, and Dextromethorphan 748
Pseudoephedrine, Dihydrocodeine, and Chlorpheniramine 1371
Pseudoephedrine, Guaifenesin, and Codeine *See* Guaifenesin, Pseudoephedrine, and Codeine 747
Pseudoephedrine Hydrochloride *See* Pseudoephedrine 1367
Pseudoephedrine Hydrochloride and Acrivastine *See* Acrivastine and Pseudoephedrine 48
Pseudoephedrine Hydrochloride and Cetirizine Hydrochloride *See* Cetirizine and Pseudoephedrine 309
Pseudoephedrine Hydrochloride and Codeine Phosphate *See* Pseudoephedrine and Codeine 1368
Pseudoephedrine Hydrochloride and Hydrocodone Bitartrate *See* Hydrocodone and Pseudoephedrine 781
Pseudoephedrine hydrochloride and Methscopolamine Nitrate *See* Pseudoephedrine and Methscopolamine 1370
Pseudoephedrine Hydrochloride, Guaifenesin, and Dihydrocodeine Bitartrate *See* Dihydrocodeine, Pseudoephedrine, and Guaifenesin 469

Quibron® [DSC] *See* Theophylline and Guaifenesin ... 1567
Quimocyclar (Mex) *See* Tetracycline ... 1558
Quinalbarbitone Sodium *See* Secobarbital ... 1464
Quinapril ... 1386
Quinapril and Hydrochlorothiazide ... 1386
Quinapril Hydrochloride *See* Quinapril ... 1386
Quinaretic *See* Quinapril and Hydrochlorothiazide ... 1386
Quinate® (Can) *See* QuiNIDine ... 1387
QuiNIDine ... 1387
Quinidine Gluconate *See* QuiNIDine ... 1387
Quinidine Polygalacturonate *See* QuiNIDine ... 1387
Quinidine Sulfate *See* QuiNIDine ... 1387
QuiNINE ... 1388
Quinine-Odan™ (Can) *See* QuiNINE ... 1388
Quinine Sulfate *See* QuiNINE ... 1388
Quintasa® (Can) *See* Mesalamine ... 994
Quinupristin and Dalfopristin ... 1388
Quirocaine (Mex) *See* Levobupivacaine ... 908
Quixin® *See* Levofloxacin ... 913
QVAR® *See* Beclomethasone ... 171
R 14-15 *See* Erlotinib ... 556
Rabeprazole ... 1389
Racepinephrine *See* EPINEPHrine ... 543
Racovel (Mex) *See* Carbidopa and Levodopa ... 277
Raductil (Mex) *See* Sibutramine ... 1479
R-albuterol *See* Levalbuterol ... 902
Ralivia™ ER (Can) *See* TraMADol ... 1604
Ralix *See* Chlorpheniramine, Phenylephrine, and Methscopolamine ... 329
Raloxifene ... 1391
Raloxifene Hydrochloride *See* Raloxifene ... 1391
Raltegravir ... 1393
Ramelteon ... 1394
Ramipril ... 1395
RAN™-Atenolol (Can) *See* Atenolol ... 147
RAN™-Carvedilol (Can) *See* Carvedilol ... 286
Ran-Cefprozil (Can) *See* Cefprozil ... 297
RAN™-Ciprofloxacin (Can) *See* Ciprofloxacin ... 346
RAN™-Citalopram (Can) *See* Citalopram ... 354
Ranclor (Mex) *See* Cefaclor ... 291
RAN™-Domperidone (Can) *See* Domperidone ... 493
Ranexa® *See* Ranolazine ... 1403
RAN™-Fentanyl Transdermal System (Can) *See* FentaNYL ... 624
RAN-Fosinopril (Can) *See* Fosinopril ... 691
Raniclor™ *See* Cefaclor ... 291
Ranisen (Mex) *See* Ranitidine ... 1399
Ranitidine ... 1399
Ranitidine Hydrochloride *See* Ranitidine ... 1399
Ranitidine Injection, USP (Can) *See* Ranitidine ... 1399
Ran-Levo (Mex) *See* Levofloxacin ... 913
Ran-Lisinopril (Can) *See* Lisinopril ... 934
RAN™-Lovastatin (Can) *See* Lovastatin ... 956
RAN™-Metformin (Can) *See* MetFORMIN ... 997
Ranolazine ... 1403
Ran-Pantoprazole (Can) *See* Pantoprazole ... 1221
Ran-Rabeprazole (Can) *See* Rabeprazole ... 1389
Ran-Risperidone (Can) *See* Risperidone ... 1425
Ranstar (Mex) *See* Stavudine ... 1505
Ran-Tamsulosin (Can) *See* Tamsulosin ... 1537
RAN™-Zopiclone (Can) *See* Zopiclone ... 1711
Rapamune® *See* Sirolimus ... 1490
Raphon [OTC] *See* EPINEPHrine ... 543
Rapivir (Mex) *See* Valacyclovir ... 1640
Raptiva® *See* Efalizumab ... 526
Rasagiline ... 1403
Rasagiline Mesylate *See* Rasagiline ... 1403
Rasburicase ... 1407
Rasilez® (Can) *See* Aliskiren ... 65
Rastinon (Mex) *See* TOLBUTamide ... 1592
rATG *See* Antithymocyte Globulin (Rabbit) ... 126
ratio-Aclavulanate (Can) *See* Amoxicillin and Clavulanate Potassium ... 115
ratio-Acyclovir (Can) *See* Acyclovir ... 49
ratio-Alendronate (Can) *See* Alendronate ... 59
Ratio-Amiodarone (Can) *See* Amiodarone ... 89
Ratio-Amiodarone I.V. (Can) *See* Amiodarone ... 89
ratio-Azithromycin (Can) *See* Azithromycin ... 163
ratio-Bicalutamide (Can) *See* Bicalutamide ... 188
ratio-Brimonidine (Can) *See* Brimonidine ... 199

ratio-Buspirone (Can) *See* BusPIRone ... 223
ratio-Carvedilol (Can) *See* Carvedilol ... 286
ratio-Cefuroxime (Can) *See* Cefuroxime ... 300
ratio-Ciprofloxacin (Can) *See* Ciprofloxacin ... 346
ratio-Citalopram (Can) *See* Citalopram ... 354
ratio-Clarithromycin (Can) *See* Clarithromycin ... 360
ratio-Clindamycin (Can) *See* Clindamycin ... 363
ratio-Clobazam (Can) *See* Clobazam ... 364
ratio-Cotridin (Can) *See* Triprolidine, Pseudoephedrine, and Codeine ... 1635
ratio-Diltiazem CD (Can) *See* Diltiazem ... 473
ratio-Domperidone (Can) *See* Domperidone ... 493
ratio-Emtec (Can) *See* Acetaminophen and Codeine ... 34
ratio-Enalapril (Can) *See* Enalapril ... 531
ratio-Famotidine (Can) *See* Famotidine ... 613
ratio-Fenofibrate MC (Can) *See* Fenofibrate ... 620
ratio-Fentanyl (Can) *See* FentaNYL ... 624
ratio-Fluoxetine (Can) *See* FLUoxetine ... 650
ratio-Fluticasone (Can) *See* Fluticasone ... 668
ratio-Fosinopril (Can) *See* Fosinopril ... 691
ratio-Glimepiride (Can) *See* Glimepiride ... 723
ratio-Glyburide (Can) *See* GlyBURIDE ... 730
ratio-Inspra-Sal (Can) *See* Albuterol ... 54
ratio-Ipra Sal UDV (Can) *See* Ipratropium and Albuterol ... 854
ratio-Ketorolac (Can) *See* Ketorolac ... 878
ratio-Lamotrigine (Can) *See* LamoTRIgine ... 889
ratio-Lenoltec (Can) *See* Acetaminophen and Codeine ... 34
ratio-Lisinopril (Can) *See* Lisinopril ... 934
ratio-Lovastatin (Can) *See* Lovastatin ... 956
ratio-Metformin (Can) *See* MetFORMIN ... 997
ratio-Methotrexate (Can) *See* Methotrexate ... 1014
ratio-Mirtazapine (Can) *See* Mirtazapine ... 1058
ratio-Mometasone (Can) *See* Mometasone ... 1071
Ratio-Morphine (Can) *See* Morphine Sulfate ... 1077
Ratio-Morphine SR (Can) *See* Morphine Sulfate ... 1077
ratio-Omeprazole (Can) *See* Omeprazole ... 1176
ratio-Ondansetron (Can) *See* Ondansetron ... 1180
ratio-Orciprenaline® (Can) *See* Metaproterenol ... 996
ratio-Paroxetine (Can) *See* PARoxetine ... 1226
ratio-Pentoxifylline (Can) *See* Pentoxifylline ... 1251
ratio-Pioglitazone (Can) *See* Pioglitazone ... 1297
ratio-Pravastatin (Can) *See* Pravastatin ... 1321
ratio-Ramipril (Can) *See* Ramipril ... 1395
Ratio-Ranitidine (Can) *See* Ranitidine ... 1399
Ratio-Risperidone (Can) *See* Risperidone ... 1425
ratio-Salbutamol (Can) *See* Albuterol ... 54
ratio-Sertraline (Can) *See* Sertraline ... 1472
ratio-Simvastatin (Can) *See* Simvastatin ... 1486
ratio-Sumatriptan (Can) *See* SUMAtriptan ... 1527
ratio-Tamsulosin (Can) *See* Tamsulosin ... 1537
ratio-Temazepam (Can) *See* Temazepam ... 1545
ratio-Theo-Bronc (Can) *See* Theophylline ... 1562
ratio-Topiramate (Can) *See* Topiramate ... 1598
ratio-Trazodone (Can) *See* TraZODone ... 1614
ratio-Valproic (Can) *See* Valproic Acid and Derivatives ... 1642
ratio-Valproic ECC (Can) *See* Valproic Acid and Derivatives ... 1642
ratio-Venlafaxine XR (Can) *See* Venlafaxine ... 1659
ratio-Zopiclone (Can) *See* Zopiclone ... 1711
Razadyne™ *See* Galantamine ... 705
Razadyne™ ER *See* Galantamine ... 705
Reactine™ (Can) *See* Cetirizine ... 307
Reactine® Allergy and Sinus (Can) *See* Cetirizine and Pseudoephedrine ... 309
ReAzo [OTC] *See* Phenazopyridine ... 1258
Rebetol® *See* Ribavirin ... 1417
Rebetron® *See* Interferon Alfa-2b and Ribavirin ... 846
Rebif® *See* Interferon Beta-1a ... 848
Reclast® *See* Zoledronic Acid ... 1702
Reclipsen™ *See* Ethinyl Estradiol and Desogestrel ... 592
Recofol (Mex) *See* Propofol ... 1352
Recombinant Hirudin *See* Lepirudin ... 900
Recombinant Human Insulin-Like Growth Factor-1 *See* Mecasermin ... 973
Recombinant Human Interleukin-11 *See* Oprelvekin ... 1184
Recombinant Human Luteinizing Hormone *See* Lutropin Alfa ... 964
Recombinant Human Parathyroid Hormone (1-34) *See* Teriparatide ... 1553
Recombinant Interleukin-11 *See* Oprelvekin ... 1184
Recombinant N-Acetylgalactosamine 4-Sulfatase *See* Galsulfase ... 708
Recombinant Urate Oxidase *See* Rasburicase ... 1407
Recombivax HB® *See* Hepatitis B Vaccine ... 764

Rectacaine [OTC] *See* Phenylephrine ... 1273
Redotex (Mex) *See* Atropine ... 158
Reductil (Mex) *See* Sibutramine ... 1479
Reese's® Pinworm Medicine [OTC] *See* Pyrantel Pamoate ... 1373
Refenesen™ 400 [OTC] *See* GuaiFENesin ... 737
Refenesen™ DM [OTC] *See* Guaifenesin and Dextromethorphan ... 739
Refenesen™ [OTC] *See* GuaiFENesin ... 737
Refenesen™ PE [OTC] *See* Guaifenesin and Phenylephrine ... 742
Refenesen Plus [OTC] *See* Guaifenesin and Pseudoephedrine ... 744
Refludan® *See* Lepirudin ... 900
Regad (Mex) *See* Pantoprazole ... 1221
Regaine (Mex) *See* Minoxidil ... 1057
Regitine® (Can) *See* Phentolamine ... 1272
Regitine [DSC] *See* Phentolamine ... 1272
Reglan® *See* Metoclopramide ... 1031
Regonol® *See* Pyridostigmine ... 1374
Regulact (Mex) *See* Lactulose ... 886
Regular Insulin *See* Insulin Regular ... 838
Relacon-DM NR *See* Guaifenesin, Pseudoephedrine, and Dextromethorphan ... 748
Relacon-HC *See* Phenylephrine, Hydrocodone, and Chlorpheniramine ... 1277
Relacum (Mex) *See* Midazolam ... 1046
Relafen® (Can) *See* Nabumetone ... 1089
Relefact® TRH (Can) *See* Protirelin ... 1363
Relenza® *See* Zanamivir ... 1693
Relief® [OTC] [DSC] *See* Phenylephrine ... 1273
Relifex (Mex) *See* Nabumetone ... 1089
Relistor™ *See* Methylnaltrexone ... 1023
Relpax® *See* Eletriptan ... 528
Remeron® *See* Mirtazapine ... 1058
Remeron® RD (Can) *See* Mirtazapine ... 1058
Remeron SolTab® *See* Mirtazapine ... 1058
Remicade® *See* InFLIXimab ... 819
Remifentanil ... 1408
Reminyl® (Can) *See* Galantamine ... 705
Reminyl® [DSC] *See* Galantamine ... 705
Reminyl® ER (Can) *See* Galantamine ... 705
Renedil® (Can) *See* Felodipine ... 617
Renese® *See* Polythiazide ... 1313
Renidac (Mex) *See* Sulindac ... 1523
Repaglinide ... 1409
Repaglinide and Metformin ... 1412
Repaglinide and Metformin Hydrochloride *See* Repaglinide and Metformin ... 1412
Repan® *See* Butalbital, Acetaminophen, and Caffeine ... 229
Replenine-VF (Mex) *See* Factor IX Complex (Human) ... 612
Reprexain® *See* Hydrocodone and Ibuprofen ... 780
Requa® Activated Charcoal [OTC] *See* Charcoal ... 312
Requip® *See* Ropinirole ... 1440
Requip® XL™ *See* Ropinirole ... 1440
Rescon® *See* Chlorpheniramine, Phenylephrine, and Methscopolamine ... 329
Rescon® MX *See* Chlorpheniramine, Phenylephrine, and Methscopolamine ... 329
Rescon DM [OTC] *See* Chlorpheniramine, Pseudoephedrine, and Dextromethorphan ... 333
Rescon GG [OTC] *See* Guaifenesin and Phenylephrine ... 742
Rescon-Jr® *See* Chlorpheniramine and Phenylephrine ... 323
Rescriptor® *See* Delavirdine ... 424
Resectisol® *See* Mannitol ... 968
Reserpine ... 1413
Respa®-1st *See* Guaifenesin and Pseudoephedrine ... 744
Respa-DM® *See* Guaifenesin and Dextromethorphan ... 739
Respahist® *See* Brompheniramine and Pseudoephedrine ... 206
Respaire®-60 SR [DSC] *See* Guaifenesin and Pseudoephedrine ... 744
Respaire®-120 SR [DSC] *See* Guaifenesin and Pseudoephedrine ... 744
Respa® PE [DSC] *See* Guaifenesin and Phenylephrine ... 742
Respi-Tann™ *See* Carbetapentane and Pseudoephedrine ... 273
Restasis® *See* CycloSPORINE ... 409
Restoril® *See* Temazepam ... 1545
Retrovir® *See* Zidovudine ... 1695
Retrovir-AZT (Mex) *See* Zidovudine ... 1695
Reumophan (Mex) *See* Chlorzoxazone ... 341
Reumophan Alka (Mex) *See* Chlorzoxazone ... 341
Reumophan Vit (Mex) *See* Chlorzoxazone ... 341
Revapol (Mex) *See* Mebendazole ... 972
Revatio® *See* Sildenafil ... 1482
Revex® [DSC] *See* Nalmefene ... 1095
ReVia® *See* Naltrexone ... 1099
Revitalose C-1000® (Can) *See* Ascorbic Acid ... 141
Revlimid® *See* Lenalidomide ... 899
Rexivin (Mex) *See* Methocarbamol ... 1011

Reyataz® *See* Atazanavir ... 147
rhASB *See* Galsulfase ... 708
r-hCG *See* Chorionic Gonadotropin (Recombinant) ... 343
Rheumatrex® Dose Pack® *See* Methotrexate ... 1014
r-h α-GAL *See* Agalsidase Beta ... 52
RhIG *See* Rho(D) Immune Globulin ... 1415
rhIGF-1 *See* Mecasermin ... 973
rhIGF-1/rhIGFBP-3 *See* Mecasermin ... 973
rhIL-11 *See* Oprelvekin ... 1184
Rhinacon A *See* Chlorpheniramine, Phenylephrine, and Phenyltoloxamine ... 331
Rhinalar® (Can) *See* Flunisolide ... 646
Rhinall [OTC] *See* Phenylephrine ... 1273
Rhinocort (Mex) *See* Budesonide ... 210
Rhinocort® Aqua® *See* Budesonide ... 210
Rhinocort® Turbuhaler® (Can) *See* Budesonide ... 210
RhinoFlex™ *See* Acetaminophen and Phenyltoloxamine ... 36
RhinoFlex 650 *See* Acetaminophen and Phenyltoloxamine ... 36
r-hLH *See* Lutropin Alfa ... 964
Rho(D) Immune Globulin ... 1415
Rho(D) Immune Globulin (Human) *See* Rho(D) Immune Globulin ... 1415
Rho®-Clonazepam (Can) *See* ClonazePAM ... 373
Rhodacine® (Can) *See* Indomethacin ... 818
Rhodis™ (Can) *See* Ketoprofen ... 877
Rhodis-EC™ (Can) *See* Ketoprofen ... 877
Rhodis SR™ (Can) *See* Ketoprofen ... 877
RhoGAM® *See* Rho(D) Immune Globulin ... 1415
RhoIGIV *See* Rho(D) Immune Globulin ... 1415
RhoIVIM *See* Rho(D) Immune Globulin ... 1415
Rho®-Loperamine (Can) *See* Loperamide ... 944
Rho®-Metformin (Can) *See* MetFORMIN ... 997
Rho®-Nitro (Can) *See* Nitroglycerin ... 1147
Rhophylac® *See* Rho(D) Immune Globulin ... 1415
Rho®-Sotalol (Can) *See* Sotalol ... 1502
Rhotral (Can) *See* Acebutolol ... 27
Rhotrimine® (Can) *See* Trimipramine ... 1630
Rhovane® (Can) *See* Zopiclone ... 1711
Rhoxal-acebutolol (Can) *See* Acebutolol ... 27
Rhoxal-atenolol (Can) *See* Atenolol ... 147
Rhoxal-cyclosporine (Can) *See* CycloSPORINE ... 409
Rhoxal-diltiazem CD (Can) *See* Diltiazem ... 473
Rhoxal-diltiazem SR (Can) *See* Diltiazem ... 473
Rhoxal-diltiazem T (Can) *See* Diltiazem ... 473
Rhoxal-Fluoxetine (Can) *See* FLUoxetine ... 650
Rhoxal-fluvoxamine (Can) *See* Fluvoxamine ... 678
Rhoxal-glimepiride (Can) *See* Glimepiride ... 723
Rhoxal-Loperamide (Can) *See* Loperamide ... 944
Rhoxal-minocycline (Can) *See* Minocycline ... 1056
Rhoxal-mirtazapine (Can) *See* Mirtazapine ... 1058
Rhoxal-mirtazapine FC (Can) *See* Mirtazapine ... 1058
Rhoxal-nabumetone (Can) *See* Nabumetone ... 1089
Rhoxal-orphendrine (Can) *See* Orphenadrine ... 1186
Rhoxal-pamidronate (Can) *See* Pamidronate ... 1220
Rhoxal-paroxetine (Can) *See* PARoxetine ... 1226
Rhoxal-Ranitidine (Can) *See* Ranitidine ... 1399
Rhoxal-salbutamol (Can) *See* Albuterol ... 54
Rhoxal-sertraline (Can) *See* Sertraline ... 1472
Rhoxal-sumatriptan (Can) *See* SUMAtriptan ... 1527
Rhoxal-ticlopidine (Can) *See* Ticlopidine ... 1583
Rhoxal-valproic (Can) *See* Valproic Acid and Derivatives ... 1642
Rhoxal-zopiclone (Can) *See* Zopiclone ... 1711
rhPTH(1-34) *See* Teriparatide ... 1553
rHuEPO-α *See* Epoetin Alfa ... 546
rhuGM-CSF *See* Sargramostim ... 1462
rHu-KGF *See* Palifermin ... 1214
rhuMAb-E25 *See* Omalizumab ... 1174
rHuMAb-EGFr *See* Panitumumab ... 1221
rhuMAb-VEGF *See* Bevacizumab ... 187
RibaPak™ *See* Ribavirin ... 1417
Ribasphere® *See* Ribavirin ... 1417
Ribavirin ... 1417
Ribavirin and Interferon Alfa-2b Combination Pack *See* Interferon Alfa-2b and Ribavirin ... 846
Riclasip (Mex) *See* Amoxicillin and Clavulanate Potassium ... 115
Ridaura® *See* Auranofin ... 160
Ridene (Mex) *See* NiCARdipine ... 1128
Rifabutin ... 1418
Rifadin® *See* Rifampin ... 1418

Rifamate® *See* Rifampin and Isoniazid ... 1419
Rifampicin *See* Rifampin ... 1418
Rifampin ... 1418
Rifampin and Isoniazid ... 1419
Rifampin, Isoniazid, and Pyrazinamide ... 1419
Rifapentine ... 1420
Rifater (Mex) *See* Pyrazinamide ... 1373
Rifaximin ... 1420
Rifinah (Mex) *See* Rifampin and Isoniazid ... 1419
rIFN-A *See* Interferon Alfa-2a ... 844
rIFN beta-1a *See* Interferon Beta-1a ... 848
rIFN beta-1b *See* Interferon Beta-1b ... 848
rIL-11 *See* Oprelvekin ... 1184
Rilutek® *See* Riluzole ... 1421
Riluzole ... 1421
Rimactan (Mex) *See* Rifampin ... 1418
Rimantadine ... 1422
Rimantadine Hydrochloride *See* Rimantadine ... 1422
Rimso-50® *See* Dimethyl Sulfoxide ... 480
Rinate™ Pediatric *See* Chlorpheniramine and Phenylephrine ... 323
Rindal HD Plus *See* Phenylephrine, Hydrocodone, and Chlorpheniramine ... 1277
Rindal HPD [DSC] *See* Hydrocodone, Phenylephrine, and Diphenhydramine ... 782
Rinelon (Mex) *See* Mometasone ... 1071
Riomet® *See* MetFORMIN ... 997
Riopan Plus® Double Strength [OTC] [DSC] *See* Magaldrate and Simethicone ... 965
Riopan Plus® [OTC] [DSC] *See* Magaldrate and Simethicone ... 965
Riphenidate (Can) *See* Methylphenidate ... 1024
Riptam (Mex) *See* Oxaliplatin ... 1191
Risedronate ... 1424
Risedronate and Calcium ... 1424
Risedronate Sodium *See* Risedronate ... 1424
Risedronate Sodium and Calcium Carbonate *See* Risedronate and Calcium ... 1424
Risperdal® *See* Risperidone ... 1425
Risperdal® M-Tab® *See* Risperidone ... 1425
Risperdal® Consta® *See* Risperidone ... 1425
Risperidone ... 1425
Ritalin® *See* Methylphenidate ... 1024
Ritalin® LA *See* Methylphenidate ... 1024
Ritalin-SR® *See* Methylphenidate ... 1024
Ritonavir ... 1433
Ritonavir and Lopinavir *See* Lopinavir and Ritonavir ... 945
Rituxan® *See* RiTUXimab ... 1434
RiTUXimab ... 1434
Riva-Alendronate (Can) *See* Alendronate ... 59
Riva-Atenolol (Can) *See* Atenolol ... 147
Riva-Buspirone (Can) *See* BusPIRone ... 223
Riva-Ciprofloxacin (Can) *See* Ciprofloxacin ... 346
Riva-Citalopram (Can) *See* Citalopram ... 354
Riva-Clindamycin (Can) *See* Clindamycin ... 363
Riva-Diclofenac (Can) *See* Diclofenac ... 457
Riva-Diclofenac-K (Can) *See* Diclofenac ... 457
Riva-Dicyclomine (Can) *See* Dicyclomine ... 459
Riva-Enalapril (Can) *See* Enalapril ... 531
Riva-Famotidine (Can) *See* Famotidine ... 613
Riva-Fluconazole (Can) *See* Fluconazole ... 635
Riva-Fluoxetine (Can) *See* FLUoxetine ... 650
Riva-Fosinopril (Can) *See* Fosinopril ... 691
Riva-Lisinopril (Can) *See* Lisinopril ... 934
Riva-Loperamide (Can) *See* Loperamide ... 944
Riva-Lorazepam (Can) *See* LORazepam ... 949
Riva-Lovastatin (Can) *See* Lovastatin ... 956
Riva-Mirtazapine (Can) *See* Mirtazapine ... 1058
Riva-Naproxen (Can) *See* Naproxen ... 1102
Rivanase AQ (Can) *See* Beclomethasone ... 171
Riva-Norfloxacin (Can) *See* Norfloxacin ... 1151
Riva-Oxazepam (Can) *See* Oxazepam ... 1193
Riva-Oxybutynin (Can) *See* Oxybutynin ... 1199
Riva-Pravastatin (Can) *See* Pravastatin ... 1321
Riva-Ranitidine (Can) *See* Ranitidine ... 1399
Riva-Risperidone (Can) *See* Risperidone ... 1425
Riva-Sertraline (Can) *See* Sertraline ... 1472
Riva-Simvastatin (Can) *See* Simvastatin ... 1486
Riva-Sotalol (Can) *See* Sotalol ... 1502
Rivastigmine ... 1435
Rivastigmine Tartrate *See* Rivastigmine ... 1435
Riva-Sumatriptan (Can) *See* SUMAtriptan ... 1527
Riva-Verapamil SR (Can) *See* Verapamil ... 1665

Riva-Zide (Can) *See* Hydrochlorothiazide and Triamterene ... 776
Riva-Zopiclone (Can) *See* Zopiclone ... 1711
Rivotril® (Can) *See* ClonazePAM ... 373
Rizatriptan ... **1437**
rLFN-α2 *See* Interferon Alfa-2b ... 844
R-modafinil *See* Armodafinil ... 138
Ro 5488 *See* Tretinoin, Oral ... 1617
Roaccutan (Mex) *See* Isotretinoin ... 871
Robafen® AC *See* Guaifenesin and Codeine ... 738
Robafen DM Clear [OTC] *See* Guaifenesin and Dextromethorphan ... 739
Robafen DM [OTC] *See* Guaifenesin and Dextromethorphan ... 739
Robaxin® *See* Methocarbamol ... 1011
Robidrine® (Can) *See* Pseudoephedrine ... 1367
Robinul® *See* Glycopyrrolate ... 734
Robinul® Forte *See* Glycopyrrolate ... 734
Robitussin® (Can) *See* GuaiFENesin ... 737
Robitussin® Childrens Cough & Cold (Can) *See* Pseudoephedrine and Dextromethorphan ... 1369
Robitussin® Children's Cough & Cold Long-Acting [OTC] *See* Dextromethorphan and Chlorpheniramine ... 449
Robitussin® Cold and Cough CF [OTC] *See* Guaifenesin, Dextromethorphan, and Phenylephrine ... 746
Robitussin® Cough and Allergy [OTC] *See* Chlorpheniramine, Phenylephrine, and Dextromethorphan ... 327
Robitussin® Cough and Cold CF [OTC] *See* Guaifenesin, Pseudoephedrine, and Dextromethorphan ... 748
Robitussin® Cough and Cold Infant CF [OTC] *See* Guaifenesin, Pseudoephedrine, and Dextromethorphan ... 748
Robitussin® Cough and Cold Nighttime [OTC] *See* Chlorpheniramine, Phenylephrine, and Dextromethorphan ... 327
Robitussin® Cough and Cold [OTC] *See* Guaifenesin, Pseudoephedrine, and Dextromethorphan ... 748
Robitussin® Cough and Congestion [OTC] *See* Guaifenesin and Dextromethorphan ... 739
Robitussin® Cough & Cold® (Can) *See* Guaifenesin, Pseudoephedrine, and Dextromethorphan ... 748
Robitussin® Cough & Cold Long-Acting [OTC] *See* Dextromethorphan and Chlorpheniramine ... 449
Robitussin® CoughGels™ [OTC] *See* Dextromethorphan ... 448
Robitussin® DM (Can) *See* Guaifenesin and Dextromethorphan ... 739
Robitussin® DM Infant [OTC] [DSC] *See* Guaifenesin and Dextromethorphan ... 739
Robitussin® DM [OTC] *See* Guaifenesin and Dextromethorphan ... 739
Robitussin® Maximum Strength Cough [OTC] *See* Dextromethorphan ... 448
Robitussin® Night Time Cough & Cold [OTC] *See* Diphenhydramine and Phenylephrine ... 485
Robitussin® [OTC] *See* GuaiFENesin ... 737
Robitussin® Pediatric Cold and Cough CF [OTC] *See* Guaifenesin, Dextromethorphan, and Phenylephrine ... 746
Robitussin® Pediatric Cough and Cold Nighttime [OTC] *See* Chlorpheniramine, Phenylephrine, and Dextromethorphan ... 327
Robitussin® Pediatric Cough [OTC] *See* Dextromethorphan ... 448
Robitussin® Sugar Free Cough [OTC] *See* Guaifenesin and Dextromethorphan ... 739
Rocephin® *See* CefTRIAXone ... 300
Rofact™ (Can) *See* Rifampin ... 1418
Roferon®-A (Can) *See* Interferon Alfa-2a ... 844
Roferon®-A [DSC] *See* Interferon Alfa-2a ... 844
Rofucal (Mex) *See* Hydrochlorothiazide ... 773
Rogaine® (Can) *See* Minoxidil ... 1057
Rogaine® Extra Strength for Men [OTC] *See* Minoxidil ... 1057
Rogaine® for Men [OTC] *See* Minoxidil ... 1057
Rogaine® for Women [OTC] *See* Minoxidil ... 1057
Rogitine® (Can) *See* Phentolamine ... 1272
Rolaids® Extra Strength [OTC] *See* Calcium Carbonate and Magnesium Hydroxide ... 256
Rolaids® [OTC] *See* Calcium Carbonate and Magnesium Hydroxide ... 256
Rolaids® Softchews [OTC] *See* Calcium Carbonate ... 254
Rolicytin (Mex) *See* Clarithromycin ... 360
Romazicon® *See* Flumazenil ... 644
Romilar (Mex) *See* Dextromethorphan ... 448
Romilar® AC *See* Guaifenesin and Codeine ... 738
Romycin® *See* Erythromycin ... 557
Rondec® *See* Chlorpheniramine and Phenylephrine ... 323
Rondec®-DM *See* Chlorpheniramine, Phenylephrine, and Dextromethorphan ... 327
Ropinirole ... **1440**
Ropinirole Hydrochloride *See* Ropinirole ... 1440
Roquiferon (Mex) *See* Interferon Alfa-2a ... 844
Rosiglitazone ... **1444**
Rosiglitazone and Glimepiride ... **1448**
Rosiglitazone and Metformin ... **1449**

Rosiglitazone Maleate and Metformin Hydrochloride *See* Rosiglitazone and Metformin ... 1449
Rotigotine ... 1449
Rowasa® *See* Mesalamine ... 994
Roxanol™ *See* Morphine Sulfate ... 1077
Roxicet™ *See* Oxycodone and Acetaminophen ... 1205
Roxicet™ 5/500 *See* Oxycodone and Acetaminophen ... 1205
Roxicodone® *See* OxyCODONE ... 1201
Roychlor® (Can) *See* Potassium Chloride ... 1315
Rozerem™ *See* Ramelteon ... 1394
RP-6976 *See* Docetaxel ... 491
RP-54274 *See* Riluzole ... 1421
RP-59500 *See* Quinupristin and Dalfopristin ... 1388
(R,R)-Formoterol L-Tartrate *See* Arformoterol ... 131
RS-25259 *See* Palonosetron ... 1218
RS-25259-197 *See* Palonosetron ... 1218
R-Tanna *See* Chlorpheniramine and Phenylephrine ... 323
R-Tanna Pediatric *See* Chlorpheniramine and Phenylephrine ... 323
RTCA *See* Ribavirin ... 1417
RU 0211 *See* Lubiprostone ... 963
RU-486 *See* Mifepristone ... 1051
RU-23908 *See* Nilutamide ... 1140
RU-38486 *See* Mifepristone ... 1051
Rubella, Varicella, Measles, and Mumps Vaccine *See* Measles, Mumps, Rubella, and Varicella Virus Vaccine ... 972
Rubex® [DSC] *See* DOXOrubicin ... 507
Rubidexol (Mex) *See* Methadone ... 1001
Rubidomycin Hydrochloride *See* DAUNOrubicin Hydrochloride ... 421
Rubilem (Mex) *See* DAUNOrubicin Hydrochloride ... 421
RUF 331 *See* Rufinamide ... 1452
Rufinamide ... 1452
Ru-Hist Forte *See* Chlorpheniramine, Pyrilamine, and Phenylephrine ... 335
Ru-Tuss DM *See* Guaifenesin, Pseudoephedrine, and Dextromethorphan ... 748
Rutuss Jr *See* Guaifenesin and Pseudoephedrine ... 744
Rylosol (Can) *See* Sotalol ... 1502
Ryna®-12 *See* Phenylephrine and Pyrilamine ... 1275
Ryna-12 S® *See* Phenylephrine and Pyrilamine ... 1275
Ryna-12X® *See* Phenylephrine, Pyrilamine, and Guaifenesin ... 1279
Rynacrom (Mex) *See* Cromolyn ... 402
Rynatan® *See* Chlorpheniramine and Phenylephrine ... 323
Rynatan® Pediatric *See* Chlorpheniramine and Phenylephrine ... 323
Rynatuss® *See* Chlorpheniramine, Ephedrine, Phenylephrine, and Carbetapentane ... 326
Rynesa 12S *See* Phenylephrine and Pyrilamine ... 1275
Ry-T-12 *See* Phenylephrine and Pyrilamine ... 1275
Rythmodan® (Can) *See* Disopyramide ... 488
Rythmodan®-LA (Can) *See* Disopyramide ... 488
Rythmol® *See* Propafenone ... 1351
Rythmol® Gen-Propafenone (Can) *See* Propafenone ... 1351
Rythmol® SR *See* Propafenone ... 1351
S2® [OTC] *See* EPINEPHrine ... 543
S-(+)-3-isobutylgaba *See* Pregabalin ... 1332
6(S)-5-methyltetrahydrofolate *See* Methylfolate ... 1022
6(S)-5-MTHF *See* Methylfolate ... 1022
S-4661 *See* Doripenem ... 498
Sab-Diclofenac (Can) *See* Diclofenac ... 457
SAB-Dimenhydrinate (Can) *See* DimenhyDRINATE ... 478
SAB-Gentamicin (Can) *See* Gentamicin ... 714
Sab-Naproxen (Can) *See* Naproxen ... 1102
Sab-Prenase (Can) *See* PrednisoLONE ... 1326
Sabril® (Can) *See* Vigabatrin ... 1670
S-adenosylmethionine *See* SAMe (S-adenosyl methionine) ... 1460
Safemar (Mex) *See* Lansoprazole ... 894
Safe Tussin® DM [OTC] *See* Guaifenesin and Dextromethorphan ... 739
SAHA *See* Vorinostat ... 1678
Saizen® *See* Somatropin ... 1499
Sal-Acid® [OTC] *See* Salicylic Acid ... 1454
SalAc® [OTC] *See* Salicylic Acid ... 1454
Salactic® [OTC] *See* Salicylic Acid ... 1454
Salagen® *See* Pilocarpine ... 1290
Salazopyrin® (Can) *See* Sulfasalazine ... 1522
Salazopyrin En-Tabs® (Can) *See* Sulfasalazine ... 1522
Salbu-2 (Can) *See* Albuterol ... 54
Salbu-4 (Can) *See* Albuterol ... 54
Salbutalan (Mex) *See* Albuterol ... 54
Salbutamol *See* Albuterol ... 54
Salbutamol and Ipratropium *See* Ipratropium and Albuterol ... 854
Salbutamol Sulphate *See* Albuterol ... 54

Salex® *See* Salicylic Acid ... 1454
Salex™ [DSC] *See* Salicylic Acid ... 1454
Salflex® (Can) *See* Salsalate ... 1459
Salicylazosulfapyridine *See* Sulfasalazine ... 1522
Salicylic Acid ... **1454**
Salicylsalicylic Acid *See* Salsalate ... 1459
Salitop™ *See* Salicylic Acid ... 1454
Salmeterol ... **1457**
Salmeterol and Fluticasone *See* Fluticasone and Salmeterol ... 674
Salmeterol Xinafoate *See* Salmeterol ... 1457
Salofalk® (Can) *See* Mesalamine ... 994
Sal-Plant® [OTC] *See* Salicylic Acid ... 1454
Salsalate ... **1459**
Sal-Tropine™ *See* Atropine ... 158
SAMe *(S-adenosyl methionine)* ... **1460**
Sanctura® *See* Trospium ... 1636
Sanctura® XR *See* Trospium ... 1636
Sancuso® *See* Granisetron ... 736
Sandimmune® *See* CycloSPORINE ... 409
Sandimmune® I.V. (Can) *See* CycloSPORINE ... 409
Sandimmun Neoral (Mex) *See* CycloSPORINE ... 409
Sandomigran® (Can) *See* Pizotifen ... 1307
Sandomigran DS® (Can) *See* Pizotifen ... 1307
Sandostatin® *See* Octreotide ... 1158
Sandostatina (Mex) *See* Octreotide ... 1158
Sandostatin LAR® *See* Octreotide ... 1158
Sandoz-Acebutolol (Can) *See* Acebutolol ... 27
Sandoz Alendronate (Can) *See* Alendronate ... 59
Sandoz-Amiodarone (Can) *See* Amiodarone ... 89
Sandoz-Anagrelide (Can) *See* Anagrelide ... 124
Sandoz-Atenolol (Can) *See* Atenolol ... 147
Sandoz-Azithromycin (Can) *See* Azithromycin ... 163
Sandoz-Betaxolol (Can) *See* Betaxolol ... 186
Sandoz-Bicalutamide (Can) *See* Bicalutamide ... 188
Sandoz-Bisoprolol (Can) *See* Bisoprolol ... 190
Sandoz-Brimonidine (Can) *See* Brimonidine ... 199
Sandoz-Carbamazepine (Can) *See* CarBAMazepine ... 265
Sandoz-Cefprozil (Can) *See* Cefprozil ... 297
Sandoz-Ciprofloxacin (Can) *See* Ciprofloxacin ... 346
Sandoz-Citalopram (Can) *See* Citalopram ... 354
Sandoz-Clonazepam (Can) *See* ClonazePAM ... 373
Sandoz-Cyclosporine (Can) *See* CycloSPORINE ... 409
Sandoz-Diclofenac (Can) *See* Diclofenac ... 457
Sandoz-Diltiazem CD (Can) *See* Diltiazem ... 473
Sandoz-Diltiazem T (Can) *See* Diltiazem ... 473
Sandoz-Enalapril (Can) *See* Enalapril ... 531
Sandoz-Estradiol Derm 50 (Can) *See* Estradiol ... 576
Sandoz-Estradiol Derm 75 (Can) *See* Estradiol ... 576
Sandoz-Estradiol Derm 100 (Can) *See* Estradiol ... 576
Sandoz-Famciclovir (Can) *See* Famciclovir ... 613
Sandoz Fenofibrate S (Can) *See* Fenofibrate ... 620
Sandoz-Fluoxetine (Can) *See* FLUoxetine ... 650
Sandoz-Fluvoxamine (Can) *See* Fluvoxamine ... 678
Sandoz-Glimepiride (Can) *See* Glimepiride ... 723
Sandoz-Glyburide (Can) *See* GlyBURIDE ... 730
Sandoz-Levobunolol (Can) *See* Levobunolol ... 907
Sandoz Lisinopril/Hctz (Can) *See* Lisinopril and Hydrochlorothiazide ... 938
Sandoz-Loperamide (Can) *See* Loperamide ... 944
Sandoz-Lovastatin (Can) *See* Lovastatin ... 956
Sandoz-Metformin FC (Can) *See* MetFORMIN ... 997
Sandoz-Metoprolol (Can) *See* Metoprolol ... 1036
Sandoz-Minocycline (Can) *See* Minocycline ... 1056
Sandoz-Mirtazapine (Can) *See* Mirtazapine ... 1058
Sandoz-Mirtazapine FC (Can) *See* Mirtazapine ... 1058
Sandoz-Nabumetone (Can) *See* Nabumetone ... 1089
Sandoz Omeprazole (Can) *See* Omeprazole ... 1176
Sandoz-Ondansetron (Can) *See* Ondansetron ... 1180
Sandoz-Paroxetine (Can) *See* PARoxetine ... 1226
Sandoz-Pioglitazone (Can) *See* Pioglitazone ... 1297
Sandoz-Pravastatin (Can) *See* Pravastatin ... 1321
Sandoz-Ramipril (Can) *See* Ramipril ... 1395
Sandoz-Ranitidine (Can) *See* Ranitidine ... 1399
Sandoz Risperidone (Can) *See* Risperidone ... 1425
Sandoz-Sertraline (Can) *See* Sertraline ... 1472
Sandoz-Simvastatin (Can) *See* Simvastatin ... 1486
Sandoz-Sumatriptan (Can) *See* SUMAtriptan ... 1527
Sandoz-Tamsulosin (Can) *See* Tamsulosin ... 1537

Sandoz-Ticlopidine (Can) *See* Ticlopidine ... 1583
Sandoz-Timolol (Can) *See* Timolol ... 1584
Sandoz-Tobramycin (Can) *See* Tobramycin ... 1590
Sandoz-Topiramate (Can) *See* Topiramate ... 1598
Sandoz-Valproic (Can) *See* Valproic Acid and Derivatives ... 1642
Sandoz-Zopiclone (Can) *See* Zopiclone ... 1711
Sandrena (Mex) *See* Estradiol ... 576
Sans Acne® (Can) *See* Erythromycin ... 557
Sansacné (Mex) *See* Erythromycin ... 557
Saquinavir ... 1461
Saquinavir Mesylate *See* Saquinavir ... 1461
Sarafem® *See* FLUoxetine ... 650
Sargramostim ... 1462
Sarna® HC (Can) *See* Hydrocortisone ... 785
Sarnol®-HC [OTC] *See* Hydrocortisone ... 785
Sativex® (Can) *See* Tetrahydrocannabinol and Cannabidiol ... 1558
SB-265805 *See* Gemifloxacin ... 712
SC 33428 *See* IDArubicin ... 809
Scandonest® 3% Plain *See* Mepivacaine ... 990
SCH 13521 *See* Flutamide ... 667
SCH 56592 *See* Posaconazole ... 1314
ScheinPharm Ranitidine (Can) *See* Ranitidine ... 1399
S-Citalopram *See* Escitalopram ... 564
Scopace™ *See* Scopolamine Derivatives ... 1463
Scopolamine Base *See* Scopolamine Derivatives ... 1463
Scopolamine Butylbromide *See* Scopolamine Derivatives ... 1463
Scopolamine Derivatives ... 1463
Scopolamine Hydrobromide *See* Scopolamine Derivatives ... 1463
Scopolamine, Hyoscyamine, Atropine, and Phenobarbital *See* Hyoscyamine, Atropine, Scopolamine, and Phenobarbital ... 800
Scot-Tussin DM® Cough Chasers [OTC] [DSC] *See* Dextromethorphan ... 448
Scot-Tussin® DM Maximum Strength [OTC] *See* Dextromethorphan and Chlorpheniramine ... 449
Scot-Tussin® Expectorant [OTC] *See* GuaiFENesin ... 737
Scot-Tussin® Senior [OTC] *See* Guaifenesin and Dextromethorphan ... 739
SD/01 *See* Pegfilgrastim ... 1236
SDX-105 *See* Bendamustine ... 179
SDZ ENA 713 *See* Rivastigmine ... 1435
Seasonale® *See* Ethinyl Estradiol and Levonorgestrel ... 595
Seasonique™ *See* Ethinyl Estradiol and Levonorgestrel ... 595
Sebcur® (Can) *See* Salicylic Acid ... 1454
Sebivo® (Can) *See* Telbivudine ... 1541
Secobarbital ... 1464
Secobarbital Sodium *See* Secobarbital ... 1464
Seconal® *See* Secobarbital ... 1464
Secotex (Mex) *See* Tamsulosin ... 1537
Sectral® *See* Acebutolol ... 27
Sedalito (Mex) *See* Acetaminophen ... 30
Sedapap® *See* Butalbital and Acetaminophen ... 236
Select™ 1/35 (Can) *See* Ethinyl Estradiol and Norethindrone ... 597
Selegiline ... 1466
Selegiline Hydrochloride *See* Selegiline ... 1466
Selfemra™ *See* FLUoxetine ... 650
Seloken-Zok (Mex) *See* Metoprolol ... 1036
Selopres Zok (Mex) *See* Metoprolol and Hydrochlorothiazide ... 1040
Selzentry™ *See* Maraviroc ... 971
Semprex®-D *See* Acrivastine and Pseudoephedrine ... 48
Senna and Docusate *See* Docusate and Senna ... 491
Senna-S *See* Docusate and Senna ... 491
Senokot-S® [OTC] *See* Docusate and Senna ... 491
SenoSol™-SS [OTC] *See* Docusate and Senna ... 491
Sensibit (Mex) *See* Loratadine ... 946
Sensipar® *See* Cinacalcet ... 345
Sensipharma (Mex) *See* Lidocaine ... 924
Sensorcaine® *See* Bupivacaine ... 211
Sensorcaine®-MPF *See* Bupivacaine ... 211
Sensorcaine®-MPF Spinal *See* Bupivacaine ... 211
Sepibest (Mex) *See* CarBAMazepine ... 265
Septilisin (Mex) *See* Polymyxin B ... 1312
Septra® *See* Sulfamethoxazole and Trimethoprim ... 1517
Septra® DS *See* Sulfamethoxazole and Trimethoprim ... 1517
Septra® Injection (Can) *See* Sulfamethoxazole and Trimethoprim ... 1517
Septrin (Mex) *See* Sulfamethoxazole and Trimethoprim ... 1517
Serax® *See* Oxazepam ... 1193
Seretide (Mex) *See* Fluticasone and Salmeterol ... 674
Serevent (Mex) *See* Salmeterol ... 1457
Serevent® Diskhaler® Disk (Can) *See* Salmeterol ... 1457

Serevent® Diskus® *See* Salmeterol ... 1457
Serofene (Mex) *See* ClomiPHENE ... 368
Serolux (Mex) *See* Sertraline ... 1472
Seromycin® *See* CycloSERINE ... 408
Seronex (Mex) *See* Domperidone ... 493
Serophene® *See* ClomiPHENE ... 368
Seropram (Mex) *See* Citalopram ... 354
Seroquel® *See* QUEtiapine ... 1381
Seroquel® XR *See* QUEtiapine ... 1381
Serostim® *See* Somatropin ... 1499
Sertex (Mex) *See* Sertraline ... 1472
Sertraline ... 1472
Sertraline Hydrochloride *See* Sertraline ... 1472
Servamox (Mex) *See* Amoxicillin and Clavulanate Potassium ... 115
Servicef (Mex) *See* Cephalexin ... 306
Serviclor (Mex) *See* Cefaclor ... 291
Servigenta (Mex) *See* Gentamicin ... 714
Servitrim (Mex) *See* Sulfamethoxazole and Trimethoprim ... 1517
Serzone *See* Nefazodone ... 1116
Setwall *See* Valerian (Valeriana officinalis) ... 1641
Sevoflurane ... 1479
Sevorane (Mex) *See* Sevoflurane ... 1479
Sevorane® AF (Can) *See* Sevoflurane ... 1479
Shanzha Rou *See* Hawthorn (Crataegus oxyacantha) ... 758
Shemol (Mex) *See* Timolol ... 1584
Siberian Ginseng *See* Ginseng, Siberian (Eleutherococcus senticosus) ... 720
Sibutramine ... 1479
Sibutramine Hydrochloride Monohydrate *See* Sibutramine ... 1479
Sidevar (Mex) *See* Lovastatin ... 956
Sifrol (Mex) *See* Pramipexole ... 1318
Siladryl® Allergy [OTC] *See* DiphenhydrAMINE ... 481
Silafed® [OTC] *See* Triprolidine and Pseudoephedrine ... 1634
Silapap® Children's [OTC] *See* Acetaminophen ... 30
Silapap® Infants [OTC] *See* Acetaminophen ... 30
Sildec [DSC] *See* Carbinoxamine and Pseudoephedrine ... 280
Sildec PE-DM *See* Chlorpheniramine, Phenylephrine, and Dextromethorphan ... 327
Sildec PE [DSC] *See* Chlorpheniramine and Phenylephrine ... 323
Sildec Syrup *See* Brompheniramine and Pseudoephedrine ... 206
Sildenafil ... 1482
Silexin [OTC] *See* Guaifenesin and Dextromethorphan ... 739
Silfedrine Children's [OTC] *See* Pseudoephedrine ... 1367
Silphen DM® [OTC] *See* Dextromethorphan ... 448
Silphen® [OTC] *See* DiphenhydrAMINE ... 481
Sil-Tex *See* Guaifenesin and Phenylephrine ... 742
Siltussin DAS [OTC] *See* GuaiFENesin ... 737
Siltussin DM DAS [OTC] *See* Guaifenesin and Dextromethorphan ... 739
Siltussin DM [OTC] *See* Guaifenesin and Dextromethorphan ... 739
Siltussin SA [OTC] *See* GuaiFENesin ... 737
Silvadene® *See* Silver Sulfadiazine ... 1485
Silver Apricot *See* Ginkgo *(Ginkgo biloba)* ... 715
Silver Sulfadiazine ... 1485
Simcor® *See* Niacin and Simvastatin ... 1127
Simethicone, Aluminum Hydroxide, and Magnesium Hydroxide *See* Aluminum Hydroxide, Magnesium Hydroxide, and Simethicone ... 78
Simethicone and Loperamide Hydrochloride *See* Loperamide and Simethicone ... 944
Simethicone and Magaldrate *See* Magaldrate and Simethicone ... 965
Simlo (Mex) *See* Simvastatin ... 1486
Simplaqor (Mex) *See* Simvastatin ... 1486
Simply Sleep® (Can) *See* DiphenhydrAMINE ... 481
Simply Sleep® [OTC] *See* DiphenhydrAMINE ... 481
Simuc-DM *See* Guaifenesin and Dextromethorphan ... 739
Simuc [DSC] *See* Guaifenesin and Phenylephrine ... 742
Simulect® *See* Basiliximab ... 171
Simvastatin ... 1486
Simvastatin and Ezetimibe *See* Ezetimibe and Simvastatin ... 611
Simvastatin and Niacin *See* Niacin and Simvastatin ... 1127
Sina-12X *See* Guaifenesin and Phenylephrine ... 742
Sincalide ... 1489
Sincrosa (Mex) *See* Acarbose ... 25
Sinedol (Mex) *See* Acetaminophen ... 30
Sinemet® *See* Carbidopa and Levodopa ... 277
Sinemet® CR *See* Carbidopa and Levodopa ... 277
Sinequan® (Can) *See* Doxepin ... 502
Sinequan® [DSC] *See* Doxepin ... 502
Singloben (Mex) *See* GlipiZIDE ... 726
Singulair® *See* Montelukast ... 1074
Sinogan (Mex) *See* Methotrimeprazine ... 1015

Sinozol (Mex) *See* Itraconazole 872
Sinpebac (Mex) *See* Mupirocin 1085
Sinpet (Mex) *See* Phentermine 1270
Sintrom® (Can) *See* Acenocoumarol 30
Sinufin (Mex) *See* Amoxicillin and Clavulanate Potassium 115
Sinutab® Non Drowsy (Can) *See* Acetaminophen and Pseudoephedrine 37
Sinutab® Non-Drying [OTC] *See* Guaifenesin and Pseudoephedrine 744
Sinutab® Sinus & Allergy (Can) *See* Acetaminophen, Chlorpheniramine, and Pseudoephedrine 40
Sinutab® Sinus Allergy Maximum Strength [OTC] *See* Acetaminophen, Chlorpheniramine, and Pseudoephedrine 40
Sinutab® Sinus [OTC] *See* Acetaminophen and Phenylephrine 36
SINUtuss® DM *See* Guaifenesin, Dextromethorphan, and Phenylephrine 746
SINUvent® PE *See* Guaifenesin and Phenylephrine 742
Sirdalud (Mex) *See* TiZANidine 1587
Sirolimus 1490
Sistopress (Mex) *See* AmLODIPine 100
SitaGLIPtin 1491
Sitagliptin and Metformin 1492
Sitagliptin Phosphate *See* SitaGLIPtin 1491
Sitagliptin Phosphate and Metformin Hydrochloride *See* Sitagliptin and Metformin 1492
Sixol (Mex) *See* Colchicine 396
SJW *See* St John's Wort (Hypericum perforatum) 1506
Skelaxin® *See* Metaxalone 996
Skelid® *See* Tiludronate 1583
SKF 104864 *See* Topotecan 1602
SKF 104864-A *See* Topotecan 1602
Sleep-ettes D [OTC] *See* DiphenhydrAMINE 481
Sleepinal® [OTC] *See* DiphenhydrAMINE 481
Slo-Niacin® [OTC] *See* Niacin 1124
Slo-Pot (Can) *See* Potassium Chloride 1315
Slow FE® [OTC] *See* Ferrous Sulfate 627
Slow-K® (Can) *See* Potassium Chloride 1315
Slow-Mag® [OTC] *See* Magnesium Chloride 965
Smallpox Vaccine 1493
Small Wolf *See* Hops (Humulus lupulus) 770
SMZ-TMP *See* Sulfamethoxazole and Trimethoprim 1517
(+)-(S)-N-Methyl-γ-(1-naphthyloxy)-2-thiophenepropylamine Hydrochloride *See* DULoxetine 516
Sodipen (Mex) *See* Penicillin G, Parenteral, Aqueous 1241
Sodium 2-Mercaptoethane Sulfonate *See* Mesna 995
Sodium 4-Hydroxybutyrate *See* Sodium Oxybate 1495
Sodium L-Triiodothyronine *See* Liothyronine 928
Sodium Acid Carbonate *See* Sodium Bicarbonate 1494
Sodium Aurothiomalate *See* Gold Sodium Thiomalate 734
Sodium Benzoate and Caffeine *See* Caffeine 250
Sodium Bicarbonate 1494
Sodium Biphosphate, Methenamine, Methylene Blue, Phenyl Salicylate, and Hyoscyamine *See* Methenamine, Sodium Biphosphate, Phenyl Salicylate, Methylene Blue, and Hyoscyamine 1010
Sodium Diuril® *See* Chlorothiazide 321
Sodium Etidronate *See* Etidronate Disodium 605
Sodium Ferric Gluconate *See* Ferric Gluconate 626
Sodium Hydrogen Carbonate *See* Sodium Bicarbonate 1494
Sodium Hyposulfate *See* Sodium Thiosulfate 1497
Sodium Nafcillin *See* Nafcillin 1093
Sodium Nitroferricyanide *See* Nitroprusside 1149
Sodium Nitroprusside *See* Nitroprusside 1149
Sodium Oxybate 1495
Sodium PAS *See* Aminosalicylic Acid 88
Sodium Thiosulfate 1497
Sodium Thiosulphate *See* Sodium Thiosulfate 1497
Sojourn™ *See* Sevoflurane 1479
Solage *See* Mequinol and Tretinoin 992
Solagé® *See* Mequinol and Tretinoin 992
Solaraze® *See* Diclofenac 457
Solarcaine® Aloe Extra Burn Relief [OTC] *See* Lidocaine 924
Solciclina (Mex) *See* Amoxicillin 112
Solhidrol (Mex) *See* Hydrocortisone 785
Solia™ *See* Ethinyl Estradiol and Desogestrel 592
Solifenacin 1498
Solifenacin Succinate *See* Solifenacin 1498
Solodyn™ *See* Minocycline 1056
Soltamox™ [DSC] *See* Tamoxifen 1537
Soltrim (Mex) *See* Sulfamethoxazole and Trimethoprim 1517
Solu-Cortef® *See* Hydrocortisone 785
Solu-Medrol® *See* MethylPREDNISolone 1029

Solural (Mex) *See* Calcium Chloride 256
Soluver® (Can) *See* Salicylic Acid 1454
Soluver® Plus (Can) *See* Salicylic Acid 1454
Soma® *See* Carisoprodol 283
Soma® Compound *See* Carisoprodol and Aspirin 284
Soma® Compound w/Codeine [DSC] *See* Carisoprodol, Aspirin, and Codeine 284
Somatrem *See* Somatropin 1499
Somatropin 1499
Somavert® *See* Pegvisomant 1237
Sominex® Maximum Strength [OTC] *See* DiphenhydrAMINE 481
Sominex® [OTC] *See* DiphenhydrAMINE 481
Somnote® *See* Chloral Hydrate 313
Som Pam (Can) *See* Flurazepam 664
Sonata® *See* Zaleplon 1691
Sophipren Ofteno (Mex) *See* PrednisoLONE 1326
Sophivir Ungena (Mex) *See* Acyclovir 49
Sophixin Ofteno (Mex) *See* Ciprofloxacin 346
Sorafenib 1501
Sorafenib Tosylate *See* Sorafenib 1501
Sorifran (Mex) *See* Lansoprazole 894
Sorine® *See* Sotalol 1502
Sotacor® (Can) *See* Sotalol 1502
Sotalol 1502
Sotalol Hydrochloride *See* Sotalol 1502
Sotret® *See* Isotretinoin 871
Sotrexe (Mex) *See* Isotretinoin 871
Spacol [DSC] *See* Hyoscyamine 799
Spacol T/S [DSC] *See* Hyoscyamine 799
Spastrin® [DSC] *See* Belladonna, Phenobarbital, and Ergotamine 175
SPD417 *See* CarBAMazepine 265
Spectinomycin 1502
Spectinomycin Hydrochloride *See* Spectinomycin 1502
Spectracef® *See* Cefditoren 293
SPEF-Pioglitazone (Can) *See* Pioglitazone 1297
SPI 0211 *See* Lubiprostone 963
Spironolactone 1503
Spironolactone and Hydrochlorothiazide *See* Hydrochlorothiazide and Spironolactone 776
SPM 927 *See* Lacosamide 885
Sporanox® *See* Itraconazole 872
SPP100 *See* Aliskiren 65
Spriafil® (Can) *See* Posaconazole 1314
Sprintec™ *See* Ethinyl Estradiol and Norgestimate 600
Sprycel® *See* Dasatinib 420
Sronyx™ *See* Ethinyl Estradiol and Levonorgestrel 595
SSD® *See* Silver Sulfadiazine 1485
SSD® AF *See* Silver Sulfadiazine 1485
SSKI® *See* Potassium Iodide 1317
Stadol® [DSC] *See* Butorphanol 247
Staflex *See* Acetaminophen and Phenyltoloxamine 36
Stagesic™ *See* Hydrocodone and Acetaminophen 777
Stalevo® *See* Levodopa, Carbidopa, and Entacapone 911
Starlix® *See* Nateglinide 1112
Statex® (Can) *See* Morphine Sulfate 1077
Statobex® (Can) *See* Phendimetrazine 1259
Statuss™ DM *See* Chlorpheniramine, Phenylephrine, and Dextromethorphan 327
Stavudine 1505
Stavzor™ *See* Valproic Acid and Derivatives 1642
Stelazine (Mex) *See* Trifluoperazine 1624
Stemetil® (Can) *See* Prochlorperazine 1341
Stenox (Mex) *See* Fluoxymesterone 657
Sterapred® *See* PredniSONE 1327
Sterapred® DS *See* PredniSONE 1327
STI-571 *See* Imatinib 810
Stiemcyn (Mex) *See* Erythromycin 557
Stilnox (Mex) *See* Zolpidem 1705
Stimate® *See* Desmopressin 431
St John's Wort (Hypericum perforatum) 1506
St. Joseph® Adult Aspirin [OTC] *See* Aspirin 143
Stocrin (Mex) *See* Efavirenz 526
Stratasin (Mex) *See* Indomethacin 818
Strattera® *See* Atomoxetine 151
Streptomycin 1510
Streptomycin Sulfate *See* Streptomycin 1510
Streptozocin 1510
Striant® *See* Testosterone 1553
Stridex® Essential Care® [OTC] *See* Salicylic Acid 1454
Stridex® Facewipes To Go® [OTC] *See* Salicylic Acid 1454

Stridex® Maximum Strength [OTC] *See* Salicylic Acid ... 1454
Stridex® Sensitive Skin [OTC] *See* Salicylic Acid ... 1454
Strifon Forte® (Can) *See* Chlorzoxazone ... 341
Stromectol® *See* Ivermectin ... 873
Strong Iodine Solution *See* Potassium Iodide and Iodine ... 1317
SU11248 *See* Sunitinib ... 1530
Suberoylanilide Hydroxamic Acid *See* Vorinostat ... 1678
Sublimaze® *See* FentaNYL ... 624
Suboxone® *See* Buprenorphine and Naloxone ... 215
Subsalicilato de Bismuto (Mex) *See* Bismuth ... 189
Subutex® *See* Buprenorphine ... 212
Succimer ... 1511
Succinylcholine ... 1511
Succinylcholine Chloride *See* Succinylcholine ... 1511
Suclor™ *See* Chlorpheniramine and Pseudoephedrine ... 325
Sucralfate ... 1514
Sudafed (Mex) *See* Pseudoephedrine ... 1367
Sudafed® 12 Hour [OTC] *See* Pseudoephedrine ... 1367
Sudafed® 24 Hour [OTC] *See* Pseudoephedrine ... 1367
Sudafed® Children's Cold & Cough [OTC] *See* Pseudoephedrine and Dextromethorphan ... 1369
Sudafed® Children's [OTC] *See* Pseudoephedrine ... 1367
Sudafed® Cold & Cough Extra Strength (Can) *See* Acetaminophen, Dextromethorphan, and Pseudoephedrine ... 43
Sudafed® Decongestant (Can) *See* Pseudoephedrine ... 1367
Sudafed® Head Cold and Sinus Extra Strength (Can) *See* Acetaminophen and Pseudoephedrine ... 37
Sudafed® Maximum Strength Nasal Decongestant [OTC] *See* Pseudoephedrine ... 1367
Sudafed® Maximum Strength Sinus Nighttime [OTC] [DSC] *See* Triprolidine and Pseudoephedrine ... 1634
Sudafed® Multi-Symptom Sinus and Cold [OTC] *See* Acetaminophen and Pseudoephedrine ... 37
Sudafed PE® Nighttime Cold [OTC] *See* Acetaminophen, Diphenhydramine, and Phenylephrine ... 44
Sudafed PE™ [OTC] *See* Phenylephrine ... 1273
Sudafed PE® Severe Cold [OTC] *See* Acetaminophen, Diphenhydramine, and Phenylephrine ... 44
Sudafed PE® Sinus & Allergy [OTC] *See* Chlorpheniramine and Phenylephrine ... 323
Sudafed PE® Sinus Headache [OTC] *See* Acetaminophen and Phenylephrine ... 36
Sudafed® Sinus Advance (Can) *See* Pseudoephedrine and Ibuprofen ... 1369
Sudafed® Sinus & Allergy [OTC] *See* Chlorpheniramine and Pseudoephedrine ... 325
SudaHist® *See* Chlorpheniramine and Pseudoephedrine ... 325
Sudal® 12 *See* Chlorpheniramine and Pseudoephedrine ... 325
SudaTex-DM *See* Guaifenesin, Pseudoephedrine, and Dextromethorphan ... 748
SudaTex-G *See* Guaifenesin and Pseudoephedrine ... 744
SudoGest Children's [OTC] *See* Pseudoephedrine and Dextromethorphan ... 1369
SudoGest [OTC] *See* Pseudoephedrine ... 1367
Sudo-Tab® [OTC] *See* Pseudoephedrine ... 1367
Sufenta® *See* SUFentanil ... 1516
SUFentanil ... 1516
Sufentanil Citrate *See* SUFentanil ... 1516
Sufentanil Citrate Injection, USP (Can) *See* SUFentanil ... 1516
Sufisal (Mex) *See* Pentoxifylline ... 1251
Suifac (Mex) *See* Omeprazole ... 1176
Sular® *See* Nisoldipine ... 1143
Sulbactam and Ampicillin *See* Ampicillin and Sulbactam ... 122
Sulcrate® (Can) *See* Sucralfate ... 1514
Sulcrate® Suspension Plus (Can) *See* Sucralfate ... 1514
Sulfacetamide and Prednisolone ... 1516
SulfADIAZINE ... 1517
Sulfadoxine and Pyrimethamine ... 1517
Sulfamethoxazole and Trimethoprim ... 1517
Sulfasalazine ... 1522
Sulfatrim® *See* Sulfamethoxazole and Trimethoprim ... 1517
Sulfazine *See* Sulfasalazine ... 1522
Sulfazine EC *See* Sulfasalazine ... 1522
SulfiSOXAZOLE ... 1523
Sulfisoxazole Acetyl *See* SulfiSOXAZOLE ... 1523
Sulfisoxazole and Erythromycin *See* Erythromycin and Sulfisoxazole ... 563
Sulfizole® (Can) *See* SulfiSOXAZOLE ... 1523
Sulfoid Trimetho (Mex) *See* Sulfamethoxazole and Trimethoprim ... 1517
Sulindac ... 1523
Sulphafurazole *See* SulfiSOXAZOLE ... 1523
Suma-B (Mex) *See* Thiamine ... 1568
SUMAtriptan ... 1527
Sumatriptan and Naproxen ... 1530
Sumatriptan Succinate *See* SUMAtriptan ... 1527

Sumatriptan Succinate and Naproxen *See* Sumatriptan and Naproxen ... 1530
Sumatriptan Succinate and Naproxen Sodium *See* Sumatriptan and Naproxen ... 1530
Sumatryx (Can) *See* SUMAtriptan ... 1527
Summer's Eve® SpecialCare™ Medicated Anti-Itch Cream [OTC] [DSC] *See* Hydrocortisone ... 785
Sunicaine (Mex) *See* Lidocaine ... 924
Sunitinib ... 1530
Sunitinib Malate *See* Sunitinib ... 1530
Sunzepam (Mex) *See* Diazepam ... 451
Supeudol® (Can) *See* OxyCODONE ... 1201
Supprelin® LA *See* Histrelin ... 769
Supradol (Mex) *See* Ketorolac ... 878
Suprax® *See* Cefixime ... 294
Supremunn (Mex) *See* CycloSPORINE ... 409
Suretin (Mex) *See* Tazarotene ... 1540
Surmontil® *See* Trimipramine ... 1630
Sustiva® *See* Efavirenz ... 526
Sutent® *See* Sunitinib ... 1530
Su-Tuss DM *See* Guaifenesin and Dextromethorphan ... 739
Su-Tuss®-HD [DSC] *See* Hydrocodone, Pseudoephedrine, and Guaifenesin ... 784
Suxamethonium Chloride *See* Succinylcholine ... 1511
Sydolil (Mex) *See* Ergotamine ... 552
Symax SL *See* Hyoscyamine ... 799
Symax SR *See* Hyoscyamine ... 799
Symbyax (Mex) *See* FLUoxetine ... 650
Symlin® *See* Pramlintide ... 1321
Symmetrel® *See* Amantadine ... 79
SymTan™ [DSC] *See* Hydrocodone and Pseudoephedrine ... 781
Synacthen *See* Cosyntropin ... 402
Synagis® *See* Palivizumab ... 1218
Synalar (Mex) *See* Polymyxin B ... 1312
Synalgos®-DC *See* Dihydrocodeine, Aspirin, and Caffeine ... 468
Synarel® *See* Nafarelin ... 1093
Syn-Diltiazem® (Can) *See* Diltiazem ... 473
Synercid® *See* Quinupristin and Dalfopristin ... 1388
Synphasic® (Can) *See* Ethinyl Estradiol and Norethindrone ... 597
Syntest D.S. [DSC] *See* Estrogens (Esterified) and Methyltestosterone ... 587
Syntest H.S. [DSC] *See* Estrogens (Esterified) and Methyltestosterone ... 587
Syntex (Mex) *See* Polymyxin B ... 1312
Synthroid® *See* Levothyroxine ... 920
Syprine® *See* Trientine ... 1623
Syrup of Ipecac *See* Ipecac Syrup ... 851
Systen (Mex) *See* Estradiol ... 576
T3 Sodium (error-prone abbreviation) *See* Liothyronine ... 928
T3/T4 Liotrix *See* Liotrix ... 930
T4 *See* Levothyroxine ... 920
T-20 *See* Enfuvirtide ... 537
Tabalon 400 (Mex) *See* Ibuprofen ... 803
642® Tablet (Can) *See* Propoxyphene ... 1353
Tabloid® *See* Thioguanine ... 1569
Tacex (Mex) *See* CefTRIAXone ... 300
Tacrine ... 1531
Tacrine Hydrochloride *See* Tacrine ... 1531
Tacrolimus ... 1533
Tadalafil ... 1534
Tadasil (Mex) *See* Cisapride U.S. - Available Via Limited-Access Protocol Only ... 353
Tafenil (Mex) *See* Flutamide ... 667
Tafil (Mex) *See* ALPRAZolam ... 72
Tafirol Flex (Mex) *See* Chlorzoxazone ... 341
Tagal (Mex) *See* Ceftazidime ... 298
Tagamet (Mex) *See* Cimetidine ... 345
Tagamet® HB (Can) *See* Cimetidine ... 345
Tagamet® HB 200 [OTC] *See* Cimetidine ... 345
TAK-375 *See* Ramelteon ... 1394
Talacen® *See* Pentazocine and Acetaminophen ... 1245
Talpramin (Mex) *See* Imipramine ... 812
Talwin® *See* Pentazocine ... 1243
Talwin® Nx *See* Pentazocine ... 1243
Tambocor™ *See* Flecainide ... 633
Tamiflu® *See* Oseltamivir ... 1188
Tamofen® (Can) *See* Tamoxifen ... 1537
Tamoxifen ... 1537
Tamoxifen Citrate *See* Tamoxifen ... 1537
Tamsulosin ... 1537
Tamsulosin Hydrochloride *See* Tamsulosin ... 1537
Tanacetum parthenium *See* Feverfew *(Tanacetum parthenium)* ... 628
TanaCof-XR *See* Brompheniramine ... 205

Tanafed DMX™ *See* Chlorpheniramine, Pseudoephedrine, and Dextromethorphan 333
Tannate-V-DM *See* Phenylephrine, Pyrilamine, and Dextromethorphan 1278
Tannate 12 S *See* Carbetapentane and Chlorpheniramine 272
Tannate PD-DM *See* Chlorpheniramine, Pseudoephedrine, and Dextromethorphan 333
Tannate Pediatric *See* Chlorpheniramine and Phenylephrine 323
Tannic-12 [DSC] *See* Carbetapentane and Chlorpheniramine 272
Tannic-12 S *See* Carbetapentane and Chlorpheniramine 272
Tannihist-12 D [DSC] *See* Carbetapentane, Phenylephrine, and Pyrilamine 275
Tannihist-12 RF [DSC] *See* Carbetapentane and Chlorpheniramine 272
Tanta-Orciprenaline® (Can) *See* Metaproterenol 996
TAP-144 *See* Leuprolide 901
Tapazole® *See* Methimazole 1010
Taporin (Mex) *See* Cefotaxime 295
Tarceva® *See* Erlotinib 556
Targretin® *See* Bexarotene 187
Tarka® *See* Trandolapril and Verapamil 1608
Taro-Carbamazepine Chewable (Can) *See* CarBAMazepine 265
Taro-Ciprofloxacin (Can) *See* Ciprofloxacin 346
Taro-Clindamycin (Can) *See* Clindamycin 363
Taro-Enalapril (Can) *See* Enalapril 531
Taro-Fluconazole (Can) *See* Fluconazole 635
Taro-Mometasone (Can) *See* Mometasone 1071
Taro-Simvastatin (Can) *See* Simvastatin 1486
Taro-Sone® (Can) *See* Betamethasone 184
Taro-Warfarin (Can) *See* Warfarin 1679
Tasedan (Mex) *See* Estazolam 574
Tasigna® *See* Nilotinib 1140
Tasmar® *See* Tolcapone 1593
Tasovak (Mex) *See* Piperacillin and Tazobactam Sodium 1302
Tavanic (Mex) *See* Levofloxacin 913
Tavist® Allergy [OTC] *See* Clemastine 361
Tavist® ND ALLERGY [OTC] *See* Loratadine 946
Tavor (Mex) *See* Oxybutynin 1199
Taxol® *See* Paclitaxel 1213
Taxotere® *See* Docetaxel 491
Tazarotene 1540
Tazicef® *See* Ceftazidime 298
Tazobactam and Piperacillin *See* Piperacillin and Tazobactam Sodium 1302
Tazocin® (Can) *See* Piperacillin and Tazobactam Sodium 1302
Tazorac® *See* Tazarotene 1540
Taztia XT™ *See* Diltiazem 473
Tazun (Mex) *See* ALPRAZolam 72
3TC® (Can) *See* LamiVUDine 888
T-Cell Growth Factor *See* Aldesleukin 58
TCGF *See* Aldesleukin 58
TCN *See* Tetracycline 1558
TDF *See* Tenofovir 1549
Tebegran (Mex) *See* SUMAtriptan 1527
Tebrazid™ (Can) *See* Pyrazinamide 1373
Tebruxim (Mex) *See* Cefotaxime 295
Tecflu (Mex) *See* Fluorouracil 649
Tecnal C 1/2 (Can) *See* Butalbital, Aspirin, Caffeine, and Codeine 242
Tecnal C 1/4 (Can) *See* Butalbital, Aspirin, Caffeine, and Codeine 242
Tecnofen (Mex) *See* Tamoxifen 1537
Tecnoplatin (Mex) *See* CISplatin 354
Tecta (Mex) *See* Pantoprazole 1221
Tegaserod 1541
Tegaserod Maleate *See* Tegaserod 1541
Tegretol® *See* CarBAMazepine 265
Tegretol®-XR *See* CarBAMazepine 265
Tekturna® *See* Aliskiren 65
Tekturna HCT® *See* Aliskiren and Hydrochlorothiazide 66
Telbivudine 1541
Teldrin® HBP [OTC] *See* Chlorpheniramine 321
Telithromycin 1542
Telmisartan 1542
Telmisartan and Hydrochlorothiazide 1544
Telzer (Mex) *See* Fosamprenavir 689
Telzir® (Can) *See* Fosamprenavir 689
Temazepam 1545
Temgesic (Mex) *See* Buprenorphine 212
Temodal® (Can) *See* Temozolomide 1547
Temodar® *See* Temozolomide 1547
Temozolomide 1547
Tempra® (Can) *See* Acetaminophen 30
Temsirolimus 1547
Tenecteplase 1548

Tenex® *See* GuanFACINE ... 750
Teniposide ... 1549
Tenofovir ... 1549
Tenofovir and Emtricitabine *See* Emtricitabine and Tenofovir ... 530
Tenofovir Disoproxil Fumarate *See* Tenofovir ... 1549
Tenofovir Disoproxil Fumarate, Efavirenz, and Emtricitabine *See* Efavirenz, Emtricitabine, and Tenofovir ... 527
Tenolin (Can) *See* Atenolol ... 147
Tenoretic® *See* Atenolol and Chlorthalidone ... 150
Tenormin® *See* Atenolol ... 147
Tensilon® (Can) *See* Edrophonium ... 525
Tenuate® (Can) *See* Diethylpropion ... 460
Tenuate® Dospan® (Can) *See* Diethylpropion ... 460
Tequin (Mex) *See* Gatifloxacin ... 709
Terazosin ... 1549
Terbac (Mex) *See* CefTRIAXone ... 300
Terbinafine ... 1551
Terbinafine Hydrochloride *See* Terbinafine ... 1551
Terbutaline ... 1552
Terfluzine (Can) *See* Trifluoperazine ... 1624
Terican (Mex) *See* Irinotecan ... 856
Teriparatide ... 1553
Terix (Mex) *See* Amphotericin B (Conventional) ... 120
Tesafilm (Mex) *See* Dextromethorphan ... 448
TESPA *See* Thiotepa ... 1576
Tessalon® *See* Benzonatate ... 180
Testim® *See* Testosterone ... 1553
Testopel® *See* Testosterone ... 1553
Testosterone ... 1553
Testosterone Cypionate *See* Testosterone ... 1553
Testosterone Enanthate *See* Testosterone ... 1553
Testred® *See* MethylTESTOSTERone ... 1030
Tetrabenazine ... 1554
Tetracaine ... 1557
Tetracaine Hydrochloride *See* Tetracaine ... 1557
Tetracosactide *See* Cosyntropin ... 402
Tetracycline ... 1558
Tetracycline Hydrochloride *See* Tetracycline ... 1558
Tetracycline, Metronidazole, and Bismuth Subcitrate Potassium *See* Bismuth, Metronidazole, and Tetracycline ... 190
Tetracycline, Metronidazole, and Bismuth Subsalicylate *See* Bismuth, Metronidazole, and Tetracycline ... 190
Tetrahydroaminoacrine *See* Tacrine ... 1531
Tetrahydrocannabinol *See* Dronabinol ... 512
Tetrahydrocannabinol and Cannabidiol ... 1558
Tetrahydrozoline ... 1560
Tetrahydrozoline Hydrochloride *See* Tetrahydrozoline ... 1560
2,2,2-tetramine *See* Trientine ... 1623
Tetra Tannate Pediatric *See* Chlorpheniramine, Ephedrine, Phenylephrine, and Carbetapentane ... 326
Tetrex (Mex) *See* Tetracycline ... 1558
Tetryzoline *See* Tetrahydrozoline ... 1560
Teveten® *See* Eprosartan ... 547
Teveten® HCT *See* Eprosartan and Hydrochlorothiazide ... 549
Teveten® Plus (Can) *See* Eprosartan and Hydrochlorothiazide ... 549
Tev-Tropin® *See* Somatropin ... 1499
Texacort® *See* Hydrocortisone ... 785
Texate (Mex) *See* Methotrexate ... 1014
TG *See* Thioguanine ... 1569
6-TG (error-prone abbreviation) *See* Thioguanine ... 1569
THA *See* Tacrine ... 1531
Thalidomide ... 1561
Thalitone® *See* Chlorthalidone ... 340
Thalomid® *See* Thalidomide ... 1561
THC *See* Dronabinol ... 512
THC and CBD *See* Tetrahydrocannabinol and Cannabidiol ... 1558
Theo-24® *See* Theophylline ... 1562
TheoCap™ *See* Theophylline ... 1562
Theochron™ *See* Theophylline ... 1562
Theochron® SR (Can) *See* Theophylline ... 1562
Theolair™ (Can) *See* Theophylline ... 1562
Theophylline ... 1562
Theophylline and Guaifenesin ... 1567
Theophylline Anhydrous *See* Theophylline ... 1562
Theophylline Ethylenediamine *See* Aminophylline ... 88
Therafilm (Mex) *See* DiphenhydrAMINE ... 481
Theraflu (Mex) *See* Loratadine and Pseudoephedrine ... 948

Thermazene® *See* Silver Sulfadiazine ... 1485
Thiabendazole ... 1567
Thiamazole *See* Methimazole ... 1010
Thiamin *See* Thiamine ... 1568
Thiamine ... 1568
Thiamine Hydrochloride *See* Thiamine ... 1568
Thiaminium Chloride Hydrochloride *See* Thiamine ... 1568
Thioguanine ... 1569
6-Thioguanine (error-prone abbreviation) *See* Thioguanine ... 1569
Thiopental ... 1570
Thiopental Sodium *See* Thiopental ... 1570
Thiophosphoramide *See* Thiotepa ... 1576
Thioridazine ... 1572
Thioridazine Hydrochloride *See* Thioridazine ... 1572
Thiosulfuric Acid Disodium Salt *See* Sodium Thiosulfate ... 1497
Thiotepa ... 1576
Thiothixene ... 1576
Thrive™ [OTC] *See* Nicotine ... 1133
Thymocyte Stimulating Factor *See* Aldesleukin ... 58
Thymoglobulin® *See* Antithymocyte Globulin (Rabbit) ... 126
Thyrel® TRH [DSC] *See* Protirelin ... 1363
Thyroid, Desiccated ... 1579
Thyroid Extract *See* Thyroid, Desiccated ... 1579
Thyroid USP *See* Thyroid, Desiccated ... 1579
Thyrolar® *See* Liotrix ... 930
ThyroSafe™ [OTC] *See* Potassium Iodide ... 1317
ThyroShield™ [OTC] *See* Potassium Iodide ... 1317
Thyrotropin Releasing Hormone *See* Protirelin ... 1363
L-Thyroxine Sodium *See* Levothyroxine ... 920
Tiabendazole *See* Thiabendazole ... 1567
TiaGABine ... 1580
Tiagabine Hydrochloride *See* TiaGABine ... 1580
Tiamidexal (Mex) *See* Thiamine ... 1568
Tiaminal (Mex) *See* Thiamine ... 1568
Tiazac® *See* Diltiazem ... 473
Tiazac® XC (Can) *See* Diltiazem ... 473
Ticarcillin and Clavulanate Potassium ... 1582
Ticarcillin and Clavulanic Acid *See* Ticarcillin and Clavulanate Potassium ... 1582
Ticlid® (Can) *See* Ticlopidine ... 1583
Ticlid® [DSC] *See* Ticlopidine ... 1583
Ticlopidine ... 1583
Ticlopidine Hydrochloride *See* Ticlopidine ... 1583
Tienam (Mex) *See* Imipenem and Cilastatin ... 812
Tigan® *See* Trimethobenzamide ... 1628
Tigecycline ... 1583
Tikosyn® *See* Dofetilide ... 492
Tilade® (Can) *See* Nedocromil ... 1115
Tilade® [DSC] *See* Nedocromil ... 1115
Tilazem (Mex) *See* Diltiazem ... 473
Tilia™ Fe *See* Ethinyl Estradiol and Norethindrone ... 597
Tiludronate ... 1583
Tiludronate Disodium *See* Tiludronate ... 1583
Tim-AK (Can) *See* Timolol ... 1584
Time-C-Bio [OTC] *See* Ascorbic Acid ... 141
Time-C [OTC] *See* Ascorbic Acid ... 141
Timentin® *See* Ticarcillin and Clavulanate Potassium ... 1582
Timexole (Mex) *See* Sulfamethoxazole and Trimethoprim ... 1517
Timivudin (Mex) *See* Zidovudine ... 1695
Timolol ... 1584
Timolol and Dorzolamide *See* Dorzolamide and Timolol ... 499
Timolol GFS *See* Timolol ... 1584
Timolol Hemihydrate *See* Timolol ... 1584
Timolol Maleate *See* Timolol ... 1584
Timoptic® *See* Timolol ... 1584
Timoptic® in OcuDose® *See* Timolol ... 1584
Timoptic-XE® *See* Timolol ... 1584
Timoptol (Mex) *See* Timolol ... 1584
Timozzard (Mex) *See* Timolol ... 1584
Tinamed® Corn and Callus Remover [OTC] *See* Salicylic Acid ... 1454
Tinamed® Wart Remover [OTC] *See* Salicylic Acid ... 1454
Tindamax® *See* Tinidazole ... 1585
Tiniazol (Mex) *See* Ketoconazole ... 876
Tinidazole ... 1585
Tinzaparin ... 1585
Tinzaparin Sodium *See* Tinzaparin ... 1585
Tioguanine *See* Thioguanine ... 1569
Tiotixene *See* Thiothixene ... 1576

Tipranavir ... 1586
Tirofiban ... 1586
Tirofiban Hydrochloride *See* Tirofiban ... 1586
Tiroidine (Mex) *See* Levothyroxine ... 920
Tirosint™ *See* Levothyroxine ... 920
Tirotax (Mex) *See* Cefotaxime ... 295
Tissulest (Mex) *See* Pravastatin ... 1321
Titralac™ [OTC] *See* Calcium Carbonate ... 254
TiZANidine ... 1587
TMC-114 *See* Darunavir ... 420
TMC125 *See* Etravirine ... 608
TMP *See* Trimethoprim ... 1629
TMP-SMZ *See* Sulfamethoxazole and Trimethoprim ... 1517
TMZ *See* Temozolomide ... 1547
TNKase® *See* Tenecteplase ... 1548
TOBI® *See* Tobramycin ... 1590
Tobramycin ... 1590
Tobramycin Injection, USP (Can) *See* Tobramycin ... 1590
Tobramycin Sulfate *See* Tobramycin ... 1590
Tobrex® *See* Tobramycin ... 1590
Tocainide ... 1591
Tocainide Hydrochloride *See* Tocainide ... 1591
Tofranil® *See* Imipramine ... 812
Tofranil-PM® *See* Imipramine ... 812
TOLAZamide ... 1591
Tolazoline ... 1592
Tolazoline Hydrochloride *See* Tolazoline ... 1592
TOLBUTamide ... 1592
Tolbutamide Sodium *See* TOLBUTamide ... 1592
Tolcapone ... 1593
Tolectin *See* Tolmetin ... 1595
Tolectín (Mex) *See* Tolmetin ... 1595
Tolinase® (Can) *See* TOLAZamide ... 1591
Tolmetin ... 1595
Tolmetin Sodium *See* Tolmetin ... 1595
Toloran (Mex) *See* Ketorolac ... 878
Tolterodine ... 1596
Tolterodine Tartrate *See* Tolterodine ... 1596
Tomoxetine *See* Atomoxetine ... 151
Tondex (Mex) *See* Gentamicin ... 714
Tonocard® [DSC] *See* Tocainide ... 1591
Tonopan (Mex) *See* Dihydroergotamine ... 470
Topamax® *See* Topiramate ... 1598
Topicaine® [OTC] *See* Lidocaine ... 924
Topilene® (Can) *See* Betamethasone ... 184
Topiramate ... 1598
Topisone® (Can) *See* Betamethasone ... 184
Toposar® *See* Etoposide ... 607
Topotecan ... 1602
Topotecan Hydrochloride *See* Topotecan ... 1602
Toprol-XL® *See* Metoprolol ... 1036
Toradol® (Can) *See* Ketorolac ... 878
Toradol® IM (Can) *See* Ketorolac ... 878
Toral (Mex) *See* Ketorolac ... 878
Toremifene ... 1603
Toremifene Citrate *See* Toremifene ... 1603
Torisel® *See* Temsirolimus ... 1547
Torkol (Mex) *See* Ketorolac ... 878
Torsemide ... 1603
Tositumomab I-131 *See* Tositumomab and Iodine I 131 Tositumomab ... 1603
Tositumomab and Iodine I 131 Tositumomab ... 1603
Totect™ *See* Dexrazoxane ... 441
Touro® CC *See* Guaifenesin, Pseudoephedrine, and Dextromethorphan ... 748
Touro® CC-LD *See* Guaifenesin, Pseudoephedrine, and Dextromethorphan ... 748
Touro® Allergy *See* Brompheniramine and Pseudoephedrine ... 206
Touro® DM *See* Guaifenesin and Dextromethorphan ... 739
Touro® HC [DSC] *See* Hydrocodone and Guaifenesin ... 779
Touro LA® *See* Guaifenesin and Pseudoephedrine ... 744
TPV *See* Tipranavir ... 1586
tRA *See* Tretinoin, Oral ... 1617
Tradaxin (Mex) *See* Cetirizine ... 307
Tradea (Mex) *See* Methylphenidate ... 1024
Tramacet (Can) *See* Acetaminophen and Tramadol ... 38
TraMADol ... 1604
Tramadol Hydrochloride *See* TraMADol ... 1604
Tramadol Hydrochloride and Acetaminophen *See* Acetaminophen and Tramadol ... 38
Trandate® *See* Labetalol ... 881

Trandolapril ... 1608
Trandolapril and Verapamil ... 1608
Transamine Sulphate *See* Tranylcypromine ... 1609
Transderm-V® (Can) *See* Scopolamine Derivatives ... 1463
Transderm-Nitro® (Can) *See* Nitroglycerin ... 1147
Transderm Scōp® *See* Scopolamine Derivatives ... 1463
Trans-Plantar® (Can) *See* Salicylic Acid ... 1454
trans-Retinoic Acid *See* Tretinoin, Oral ... 1617
Transtec (Mex) *See* Buprenorphine ... 212
Trans-Ver-Sal® (Can) *See* Salicylic Acid ... 1454
Trans-Ver-Sal® [OTC] *See* Salicylic Acid ... 1454
Tranxene (Mex) *See* Clorazepate ... 384
Tranxene® SD™ *See* Clorazepate ... 384
Tranxene® SD™-Half Strength *See* Clorazepate ... 384
Tranxene® T-Tab® *See* Clorazepate ... 384
Tranylcypromine ... 1609
Tranylcypromine Sulfate *See* Tranylcypromine ... 1609
Trastuzumab ... 1613
Trasylol® *See* Aprotinin ... 130
TraZODone ... 1614
Trazodone Hydrochloride *See* TraZODone ... 1614
Trazorel® (Can) *See* TraZODone ... 1614
Treanda® *See* Bendamustine ... 179
Trebanol (Mex) *See* Atenolol ... 147
Trecator® *See* Ethionamide ... 602
Trelstar® (Can) *See* Triptorelin ... 1635
Trelstar® Depot *See* Triptorelin ... 1635
Trelstar® LA *See* Triptorelin ... 1635
Trental® *See* Pentoxifylline ... 1251
Trepina (Mex) *See* CarBAMazepine ... 265
Tretinoin and Clindamycin *See* Clindamycin and Tretinoin ... 364
Tretinoin and Mequinol *See* Mequinol and Tretinoin ... 992
Tretinoin, Oral ... 1617
Trexall™ *See* Methotrexate ... 1014
Trexen (Mex) *See* Clindamycin ... 363
Treximet™ *See* Sumatriptan and Naproxen ... 1530
Trexol (Mex) *See* TraMADol ... 1604
TRH *See* Protirelin ... 1363
Triaderm (Can) *See* Triamcinolone ... 1617
Triaken (Mex) *See* CefTRIAXone ... 300
Triall™ *See* Chlorpheniramine, Phenylephrine, and Methscopolamine ... 329
Triamcinolone ... 1617
Triamcinolone Acetonide, Aerosol *See* Triamcinolone ... 1617
Triamcinolone Acetonide, Parenteral *See* Triamcinolone ... 1617
Triamcinolone Diacetate, Oral *See* Triamcinolone ... 1617
Triamcinolone Diacetate, Parenteral *See* Triamcinolone ... 1617
Triamcinolone Hexacetonide *See* Triamcinolone ... 1617
Triamcinolone, Oral *See* Triamcinolone ... 1617
Triaminic® Cold & Allergy (Can) *See* Chlorpheniramine and Pseudoephedrine ... 325
Triaminic® Cold and Allergy [OTC] *See* Chlorpheniramine and Phenylephrine ... 323
Triaminic® Infant Thin Strips® Decongestant [OTC] [DSC] *See* Phenylephrine ... 1273
Triaminic® Thin Strips® Cold [OTC] *See* Phenylephrine ... 1273
Triaminic® Thin Strips™ Cough and Runny Nose [OTC] *See* DiphenhydrAMINE ... 481
Triaminic® Thin Strips™ Long Acting Cough [OTC] *See* Dextromethorphan ... 448
Triamterene ... 1620
Triamterene and Hydrochlorothiazide *See* Hydrochlorothiazide and Triamterene ... 776
Triant-HC™ *See* Phenylephrine, Hydrocodone, and Chlorpheniramine ... 1277
Triatec-8 (Can) *See* Acetaminophen and Codeine ... 34
Triatec-8 Strong (Can) *See* Acetaminophen and Codeine ... 34
Triatec-30 (Can) *See* Acetaminophen and Codeine ... 34
Triazolam ... 1620
Tribavirin *See* Ribavirin ... 1417
Tribedoce (Mex) *See* Thiamine ... 1568
Tribedoce DX (Mex) *See* Cyanocobalamin ... 404
Tribiot (Mex) *See* Polymyxin B ... 1312
Trichloroacetaldehyde Monohydrate *See* Chloral Hydrate ... 313
TriCor® *See* Fenofibrate ... 620
Tricosal *See* Choline Magnesium Trisalicylate ... 342
Tri-Cyclen® (Can) *See* Ethinyl Estradiol and Norgestimate ... 600
Tri-Cyclen® Lo (Can) *See* Ethinyl Estradiol and Norgestimate ... 600
Triderm® *See* Triamcinolone ... 1617
Tridural™ (Can) *See* TraMADol ... 1604
Trien *See* Trientine ... 1623
Trientine ... 1623
Trientine Hydrochloride *See* Trientine ... 1623
Triesence™ *See* Triamcinolone ... 1617
Triethylene Tetramine Dihydrochloride *See* Trientine ... 1623

Triethylenethiophosphoramide *See* Thiotepa 1576
Trifluoperazine 1624
Trifluoperazine Hydrochloride *See* Trifluoperazine 1624
Triglide™ *See* Fenofibrate 620
Trihexyphenidyl 1627
Trihexyphenidyl Hydrochloride *See* Trihexyphenidyl 1627
Tri-Hist *See* Chlorpheniramine, Pyrilamine, and Phenylephrine 335
Trikacide (Can) *See* MetroNIDAZOLE 1040
Trikof-D® [DSC] *See* Guaifenesin, Pseudoephedrine, and Dextromethorphan 748
Trileptal® *See* OXcarbazepine 1195
TriLyte® *See* Polyethylene Glycol-Electrolyte Solution 1310
Trimethobenzamide 1628
Trimethobenzamide Hydrochloride *See* Trimethobenzamide 1628
Trimethoprim 1629
Trimethoprim and Sulfamethoxazole *See* Sulfamethoxazole and Trimethoprim 1517
Trimetoger (Mex) *See* Sulfamethoxazole and Trimethoprim 1517
Trimetrexate 1629
Trimetrexate Glucuronate *See* Trimetrexate 1629
Trimexazol (Mex) *See* Sulfamethoxazole and Trimethoprim 1517
Trimipramine 1630
Trimipramine Maleate *See* Trimipramine 1630
Trinasal® (Can) *See* Triamcinolone 1617
Tri-Nasal® [DSC] *See* Triamcinolone 1617
Trinergot (Mex) *See* Ergotamine 552
TriNessa™ *See* Ethinyl Estradiol and Norgestimate 600
Trineurovita (Mex) *See* Pyridoxine 1376
Trinipatch® 0.2 (Can) *See* Nitroglycerin 1147
Trinipatch® 0.4 (Can) *See* Nitroglycerin 1147
Trinipatch® 0.6 (Can) *See* Nitroglycerin 1147
Trinordiol (Mex) *See* Ethinyl Estradiol and Levonorgestrel 595
Tri-Norinyl® *See* Ethinyl Estradiol and Norethindrone 597
Trioftín (Mex) *See* Polymyxin B 1312
Trionate® [DSC] *See* Carbetapentane and Chlorpheniramine 272
Triostat® *See* Liothyronine 928
Triox (Mex) *See* CefTRIAXone 300
Triphasil® *See* Ethinyl Estradiol and Levonorgestrel 595
Triplex™ AD *See* Chlorpheniramine, Pyrilamine, and Phenylephrine 335
Tri-Previfem™ *See* Ethinyl Estradiol and Norgestimate 600
Triprolidine and Pseudoephedrine 1634
Triprolidine, Codeine, and Pseudoephedrine *See* Triprolidine, Pseudoephedrine, and Codeine 1635
Triprolidine, Pseudoephedrine, and Codeine 1635
Triptanol (Mex) *See* Amitriptyline 90
TripTone® [OTC] *See* DimenhyDRINATE 478
Triptoraline *See* Triptorelin 1635
Triptorelin 1635
Triptorelin Pamoate *See* Triptorelin 1635
Triquilar® (Can) *See* Ethinyl Estradiol and Levonorgestrel 595
Trisenox® *See* Arsenic Trioxide 140
Tri-Sprintec™ *See* Ethinyl Estradiol and Norgestimate 600
Tri-Sudo® [OTC] [DSC] *See* Triprolidine and Pseudoephedrine 1634
Tritace (Mex) *See* Ramipril 1395
Trital DM *See* Chlorpheniramine, Phenylephrine, and Dextromethorphan 327
TriTuss® *See* Guaifenesin, Dextromethorphan, and Phenylephrine 746
TriTuss® ER *See* Guaifenesin, Dextromethorphan, and Phenylephrine 746
Trivalent Inactivated Influenza Vaccine (TIV) *See* Influenza Virus Vaccine 820
Trivaris™ *See* Triamcinolone 1617
Tri-Vent™ DM [DSC] *See* Guaifenesin, Pseudoephedrine, and Dextromethorphan 748
Tri-Vent™ DPC [DSC] *See* Chlorpheniramine, Phenylephrine, and Dextromethorphan 327
Tri-Vent™ HC [DSC] *See* Hydrocodone, Carbinoxamine, and Pseudoephedrine 782
Trivora® *See* Ethinyl Estradiol and Levonorgestrel 595
Trivorin (Mex) *See* Ribavirin 1417
Trixilem (Mex) *See* Methotrexate 1014
Triyotex (Mex) *See* Liothyronine 928
Trobicin® [DSC] *See* Spectinomycin 1502
Tronolane® Suppository [OTC] *See* Phenylephrine 1273
Tropharma (Mex) *See* Erythromycin 557
Tropicacyl® *See* Tropicamide 1636
Tropicamide 1636
Trosec (Can) *See* Trospium 1636
Trospium 1636
Trospium Chloride *See* Trospium 1636
Trusopt® *See* Dorzolamide 498
Truvada® *See* Emtricitabine and Tenofovir 530
Tryptoreline *See* Triptorelin 1635
TSPA *See* Thiotepa 1576
Tucks® Anti-Itch [OTC] *See* Hydrocortisone 785

Tukol D (Mex) *See* Guaifenesin and Dextromethorphan 739
Tulip (Mex) *See* Simvastatin 1486
Tums (Mex) *See* Calcium Carbonate 254
Tums® E-X [OTC] *See* Calcium Carbonate 254
Tums® Extra Strength Sugar Free [OTC] *See* Calcium Carbonate 254
Tums® [OTC] *See* Calcium Carbonate 254
Tums® Smoothies™ [OTC] *See* Calcium Carbonate 254
Tums® Ultra [OTC] *See* Calcium Carbonate 254
Tur-bi-kal® [OTC] *See* Phenylephrine 1273
Tusitato (Mex) *See* Benzonatate 180
Tusnel-DM Pediatric® *See* Guaifenesin, Pseudoephedrine, and Dextromethorphan 748
Tusnel Liquid® *See* Guaifenesin, Pseudoephedrine, and Dextromethorphan 748
Tusnel Pediatric® *See* Guaifenesin, Pseudoephedrine, and Dextromethorphan 748
Tussafed® HC [DSC] *See* Hydrocodone, Phenylephrine, and Guaifenesin 783
Tussafed® HCG [DSC] *See* Hydrocodone, Phenylephrine, and Guaifenesin 783
Tussi-12® *See* Carbetapentane and Chlorpheniramine 272
Tussi-12® D *See* Carbetapentane, Phenylephrine, and Pyrilamine 275
Tussi-12® DS *See* Carbetapentane, Phenylephrine, and Pyrilamine 275
Tussi-12 S™ *See* Carbetapentane and Chlorpheniramine 272
TussiCaps™ *See* Hydrocodone and Chlorpheniramine 778
Tussigon® *See* Hydrocodone and Homatropine 780
TussiNate™ [DSC] *See* Hydrocodone, Phenylephrine, and Diphenhydramine 782
Tussionex® *See* Hydrocodone and Chlorpheniramine 778
Tussi-Organidin® DM NR *See* Guaifenesin and Dextromethorphan 739
Tussi-Organidin® DM-S NR *See* Guaifenesin and Dextromethorphan 739
Tussi-Organidin® NR *See* Guaifenesin and Codeine 738
Tussi-Organidin® S-NR *See* Guaifenesin and Codeine 738
Tussizone-12 RF™ *See* Carbetapentane and Chlorpheniramine 272
Tusso-C™ *See* Guaifenesin and Codeine 738
Tusso-DF® [DSC] *See* Hydrocodone and Guaifenesin 779
Tusso™-DMR *See* Guaifenesin, Dextromethorphan, and Phenylephrine 746
Tussplex™ DM *See* Chlorpheniramine, Phenylephrine, and Dextromethorphan 327
Tustan 12S™ *See* Carbetapentane and Chlorpheniramine 272
TVP-1012 *See* Rasagiline 1403
Twelve Resin-K *See* Cyanocobalamin 404
Twilite® [OTC] *See* DiphenhydrAMINE 481
Twinject™ *See* EPINEPHrine 543
Tycolene Maximum Strength [OTC] *See* Acetaminophen 30
Tycolene [OTC] *See* Acetaminophen 30
Tygacil® *See* Tigecycline 1583
Tykerb® *See* Lapatinib 898
Tylenol® (Can) *See* Acetaminophen 30
Tylenol® 8 Hour [OTC] *See* Acetaminophen 30
Tylenol® Allergy Multi-Symptom Nighttime [OTC] *See* Acetaminophen, Diphenhydramine, and Phenylephrine 44
Tylenol® Allergy Sinus (Can) *See* Acetaminophen, Chlorpheniramine, and Pseudoephedrine 40
Tylenol® Arthritis Pain [OTC] *See* Acetaminophen 30
Tylenol® Children's [OTC] *See* Acetaminophen 30
Tylenol® Children's with Flavor Creator [OTC] *See* Acetaminophen 30
Tylenol® Children's Plus Cold Nighttime [OTC] [DSC] *See* Acetaminophen, Chlorpheniramine, and Pseudoephedrine 40
Tylenol® Cold Day Non-Drowsy [OTC] *See* Acetaminophen, Dextromethorphan, and Pseudoephedrine 43
Tylenol® Cold Daytime (Can) *See* Acetaminophen, Dextromethorphan, and Pseudoephedrine 43
Tylenol® Cold Daytime, Children's [OTC] *See* Acetaminophen and Pseudoephedrine 37
Tylenol® Cold Head Congestion Daytime [OTC] *See* Acetaminophen, Dextromethorphan, and Phenylephrine 42
Tylenol® Cold, Infants [OTC] [DSC] *See* Acetaminophen and Pseudoephedrine 37
Tylenol® Cold Multi-Symptom Daytime [OTC] *See* Acetaminophen, Dextromethorphan, and Phenylephrine 42
Tylenol® Decongestant (Can) *See* Acetaminophen and Pseudoephedrine 37
Tylenol Elixir with Codeine (Can) *See* Acetaminophen and Codeine 34
Tylenol® Extra Strength [OTC] *See* Acetaminophen 30
Tylenol® Flu Non-Drowsy Maximum Strength [OTC] *See* Acetaminophen, Dextromethorphan, and Pseudoephedrine 43
Tylenol® Infants [OTC] *See* Acetaminophen 30
Tylenol® Junior [OTC] *See* Acetaminophen 30
Tylenol No. 1 (Can) *See* Acetaminophen and Codeine 34
Tylenol No. 1 Forte (Can) *See* Acetaminophen and Codeine 34
Tylenol No. 2 with Codeine (Can) *See* Acetaminophen and Codeine 34
Tylenol No. 3 with Codeine (Can) *See* Acetaminophen and Codeine 34
Tylenol No. 4 with Codeine (Can) *See* Acetaminophen and Codeine 34
Tylenol® [OTC] *See* Acetaminophen 30
Tylenol® Plus Infants Cold & Cough [OTC] [DSC] *See* Acetaminophen, Dextromethorphan, and Phenylephrine 42

Tylenol® PM [OTC] *See* Acetaminophen and Diphenhydramine 35
Tylenol® Severe Allergy [OTC] *See* Acetaminophen and Diphenhydramine 35
Tylenol® Sinus (Can) *See* Acetaminophen and Pseudoephedrine 37
Tylenol® Sinus Congestion & Pain Daytime [OTC] *See* Acetaminophen and Phenylephrine 36
Tylenol® Sinus Daytime [OTC] *See* Acetaminophen and Pseudoephedrine 37
Tylenol® With Codeine *See* Acetaminophen and Codeine 34
Tylex (Mex) *See* Acetaminophen 30
Tylex CD (Mex) *See* Codeine 394
Tylox® *See* Oxycodone and Acetaminophen 1205
Tysabri® *See* Natalizumab 1109
Tyzeka™ *See* Telbivudine 1541
Tyzine® *See* Tetrahydrozoline 1560
Tyzine® Pediatric *See* Tetrahydrozoline 1560
506U78 *See* Nelarabine 1120
U-90152S *See* Delavirdine 424
UCB-P071 *See* Cetirizine 307
UK-88,525 *See* Darifenacin 419
UK-427,857 *See* Maraviroc 971
UK92480 *See* Sildenafil 1482
UK109496 *See* Voriconazole 1678
Ulcidine (Can) *See* Famotidine 613
Uldapril (Mex) *See* Lansoprazole 894
Ulpax (Mex) *See* Lansoprazole 894
Ulsen (Mex) *See* Omeprazole 1176
Ultane® *See* Sevoflurane 1479
Ultiva® *See* Remifentanil 1408
Ultracet® *See* Acetaminophen and Tramadol 38
Ultram® *See* TraMADol 1604
Ultram® ER *See* TraMADol 1604
Ultramop™ (Can) *See* Methoxsalen 1018
Ultraprin [OTC] *See* Ibuprofen 803
Unamol (Mex) *See* Cisapride U.S. - Available Via Limited-Access Protocol Only 353
Unasyn® *See* Ampicillin and Sulbactam 122
Unburn® *See* Lidocaine 924
Unibron (Mex) *See* Albuterol 54
Uniclar (Mex) *See* Mometasone 1071
Uni-Cof [DSC] *See* Pseudoephedrine, Dihydrocodeine, and Chlorpheniramine 1371
Unidet® (Can) *See* Tolterodine 1596
Unifed [OTC] *See* Pseudoephedrine 1367
Unigastrozol (Mex) *See* Pantoprazole 1221
Unipen® (Can) *See* Nafcillin 1093
Uniphyl® *See* Theophylline 1562
Uniphyl® SRT (Can) *See* Theophylline 1562
Uniretic® *See* Moexipril and Hydrochlorothiazide 1068
Unisom®-2 (Can) *See* Doxylamine 510
Unisom® Maximum Strength SleepGels® [OTC] *See* DiphenhydrAMINE 481
Unisom® SleepTabs® [OTC] *See* Doxylamine 510
Unithroid® *See* Levothyroxine 920
Unival (Mex) *See* Sucralfate 1514
Univasc® *See* Moexipril 1068
Unizuric 300 (Mex) *See* Allopurinol 67
Urecholine® *See* Bethanechol 186
Urelle® *See* Methenamine, Sodium Biphosphate, Phenyl Salicylate, Methylene Blue, and Hyoscyamine 1010
Urimar-T *See* Methenamine, Sodium Biphosphate, Phenyl Salicylate, Methylene Blue, and Hyoscyamine 1010
Urispas® *See* Flavoxate 633
Uristat® [OTC] [DSC] *See* Phenazopyridine 1258
Uro-Mag® [OTC] *See* Magnesium Oxide 966
Uromax® (Can) *See* Oxybutynin 1199
Uromitexan (Can) *See* Mesna 995
Uroprot (Mex) *See* Mesna 995
Uroxatral® *See* Alfuzosin 65
Urso® (Can) *See* Ursodiol 1639
Urso 250™ *See* Ursodiol 1639
Ursodeoxycholic Acid *See* Ursodiol 1639
Ursodiol 1639
Urso® DS (Can) *See* Ursodiol 1639
Ursofalk (Mex) *See* Ursodiol 1639
Urso Forte™ *See* Ursodiol 1639
Uta® *See* Methenamine, Sodium Biphosphate, Phenyl Salicylate, Methylene Blue, and Hyoscyamine 1010
Utira™-C *See* Methenamine, Sodium Biphosphate, Phenyl Salicylate, Methylene Blue, and Hyoscyamine 1010
UTI Relief® [OTC] *See* Phenazopyridine 1258
Utradol™ (Can) *See* Etodolac 606

Utrogestan (Mex) *See* Progesterone ... 1345
Uvadex® *See* Methoxsalen ... 1018
Uvega (Mex) *See* Lidocaine ... 924
Vaccinia Immune Globulin (Intravenous) ... 1639
Vaccinia Vaccine *See* Smallpox Vaccine ... 1493
Vagifem® *See* Estradiol ... 576
Valacyclovir ... 1640
Valacyclovir Hydrochloride *See* Valacyclovir ... 1640
Valcyte™ *See* Valganciclovir ... 1642
23-Valent Pneumococcal Polysaccharide Vaccine *See* Pneumococcal Polysacch aride Vaccine (Polyvalent) ... 1309
Valeriana officinalis *See* Valerian *(Valeriana officinalis)* ... 1641
Valerian *(Valeriana officinalis)* ... 1641
Valganciclovir ... 1642
Valganciclovir Hydrochloride *See* Valganciclovir ... 1642
Valifol (Mex) *See* Isoniazid ... 862
Valisone® Scalp Lotion (Can) *See* Betamethasone ... 184
Valium® *See* Diazepam ... 451
Valorin Extra [OTC] *See* Acetaminophen ... 30
Valorin [OTC] *See* Acetaminophen ... 30
Valproate Semisodium *See* Valproic Acid and Derivatives ... 1642
Valproate Sodium *See* Valproic Acid and Derivatives ... 1642
Valproic Acid *See* Valproic Acid and Derivatives ... 1642
Valproic Acid and Derivatives ... 1642
Valrubicin ... 1649
Valsartan ... 1650
Valsartan and Amlodipine *See* Amlodipine and Valsartan ... 105
Valsartan and Hydrochlorothiazide ... 1652
Valstar® (Can) *See* Valrubicin ... 1649
Valstar® [DSC] *See* Valrubicin ... 1649
Valtaxin® (Can) *See* Valrubicin ... 1649
Valtrex® *See* Valacyclovir ... 1640
Vanceril® AEM (Can) *See* Beclomethasone ... 171
Vancocin® *See* Vancomycin ... 1653
Vancocin CP (Mex) *See* Vancomycin ... 1653
Vancomycin ... 1653
Vancomycin Hydrochloride *See* Vancomycin ... 1653
Vandazole™ *See* MetroNIDAZOLE ... 1040
Vaniqa™ *See* Eflornithine ... 527
Vanquish® Extra Strength Pain Reliever [OTC] *See* Acetaminophen, Aspirin, and Caffeine ... 39
Vantas™ *See* Histrelin ... 769
Vantin® *See* Cefpodoxime ... 297
Vantoxyl (Mex) *See* Pentoxifylline ... 1251
Vaprisol® *See* Conivaptan ... 400
VAQTA® *See* Hepatitis A Vaccine ... 760
Vardenafil ... 1654
Vardenafil Hydrochloride *See* Vardenafil ... 1654
Varenicline ... 1656
Varenicline Tartrate *See* Varenicline ... 1656
Varicella, Measles, Mumps, and Rubella Vaccine *See* Measles, Mumps, Rubella, and Varicella Virus Vaccine ... 972
Vaseretic® *See* Enalapril and Hydrochlorothiazide ... 536
Vasocon® (Can) *See* Naphazoline ... 1101
Vasophrinic DH (Can) *See* Pseudoephedrine, Hydrocodone, and Chlorpheniramine ... 1372
Vasopressin ... 1659
Vasotec® *See* Enalapril ... 531
Vasotec® I.V. (Can) *See* Enalapril ... 531
Vaxigrip® (Can) *See* Influenza Virus Vaccine ... 820
Vectibix® *See* Panitumumab ... 1221
Velban *See* VinBLAStine ... 1672
Velcade® *See* Bortezomib ... 192
Velivet™ *See* Ethinyl Estradiol and Desogestrel ... 592
Vematina (Mex) *See* Valproic Acid and Derivatives ... 1642
Venlafaxine ... 1659
Venofer® *See* Iron Sucrose ... 858
Ventavis® *See* Iloprost ... 810
Ventolin® (Can) *See* Albuterol ... 54
Ventolin® Diskus (Can) *See* Albuterol ... 54
Ventolin® HFA *See* Albuterol ... 54
Ventolin® I.V. Infusion (Can) *See* Albuterol ... 54
Ventrodisk (Can) *See* Albuterol ... 54
VePesid® (Can) *See* Etoposide ... 607
VePesid® [DSC] *See* Etoposide ... 607
Veramyst™ *See* Fluticasone ... 668
Verapamil ... 1665
Verapamil and Trandolapril *See* Trandolapril and Verapamil ... 1608

Verapamil Hydrochloride *See* Verapamil 1665
Verapamil Hydrochloride Injection, USP (Can) *See* Verapamil 1665
Verbram (Mex) *See* Tobramycin 1590
Verelan® *See* Verapamil 1665
Verelan® PM *See* Verapamil 1665
Verelan SRC (Can) *See* Verapamil 1665
Vermin-Dazol (Mex) *See* Mebendazole 972
Vermin Plus (Mex) *See* Albendazole 53
Vermox® (Can) *See* Mebendazole 972
Vermox® [DSC] *See* Mebendazole 972
Versed *See* Midazolam 1046
Versiclear™ *See* Sodium Thiosulfate 1497
Vertisal (Mex) *See* MetroNIDAZOLE 1040
Vertizole (Mex) *See* Mebendazole 972
Vesanoid® *See* Tretinoin, Oral 1617
VESIcare® *See* Solifenacin 1498
VFEND® *See* Voriconazole 1678
Viadur® (Can) *See* Leuprolide 901
Viadur® [DSC] *See* Leuprolide 901
Viagra® *See* Sildenafil 1482
Vibramicina (Mex) *See* Doxycycline 509
Vibramycin® *See* Doxycycline 509
Vibra-Tabs® *See* Doxycycline 509
Vicks® 44® Cough Relief [OTC] *See* Dextromethorphan 448
Vicks® 44E [OTC] *See* Guaifenesin and Dextromethorphan 739
Vicks® Casero™ Chest Congestion Relief [OTC] *See* GuaiFENesin 737
Vicks® DayQuil® Cold/Flu Multi-Symptom Relief [OTC] *See* Acetaminophen, Dextromethorphan, and Phenylephrine 42
Vicks® Early Defense™ [OTC] *See* Oxymetazoline 1208
Vicks® Pediatric Formula 44E [OTC] *See* Guaifenesin and Dextromethorphan 739
Vicks Sinex® 12 Hour [OTC] *See* Oxymetazoline 1208
Vicks Sinex® 12 Hour Ultrafine Mist [OTC] *See* Oxymetazoline 1208
Vicks® Sinex® Nasal Spray [OTC] *See* Phenylephrine 1273
Vicks® Sinex® UltraFine Mist [OTC] *See* Phenylephrine 1273
Vicks® Vitamin C [OTC] *See* Ascorbic Acid 141
Vicnite (Mex) *See* DiphenhydrAMINE 481
Vicodin® *See* Hydrocodone and Acetaminophen 777
Vicodin® ES *See* Hydrocodone and Acetaminophen 777
Vicodin® HP *See* Hydrocodone and Acetaminophen 777
Vicoprofen® *See* Hydrocodone and Ibuprofen 780
Victoclir (Mex) *See* Acyclovir 49
Vidaxil (Mex) *See* Digoxin 463
Vidaza® *See* AzaCITIDine 161
Videx® *See* Didanosine 460
Videx® EC *See* Didanosine 460
Vigabatrin 1670
Vigamox™ *See* Moxifloxacin 1084
Vigamoxi (Mex) *See* Moxifloxacin 1084
VIGIV *See* Vaccinia Immune Globulin (Intravenous) 1639
Viken (Mex) *See* Cefotaxime 295
Vilona (Mex) *See* Ribavirin 1417
Vimpat® *See* Lacosamide 885
VinBLAStine 1672
Vinblastine Sulfate *See* VinBLAStine 1672
Vincaleukoblastine *See* VinBLAStine 1672
Vincasar PFS® *See* VinCRIStine 1673
Vincidal (Mex) *See* Loratadine 946
VinCRIStine 1673
Vincristine Sulfate *See* VinCRIStine 1673
Vindacin (Mex) *See* Sulindac 1523
Vinorelbine 1674
Vinorelbine Injection, USP (Can) *See* Vinorelbine 1674
Vinorelbine Tartrate *See* Vinorelbine 1674
Vinorelbine Tartrate for Injection (Can) *See* Vinorelbine 1674
Vintec (Mex) *See* VinCRIStine 1673
Viosterol *See* Ergocalciferol 550
Viracept® *See* Nelfinavir 1120
Viramune® *See* Nevirapine 1124
Viravan®-DM *See* Phenylephrine, Pyrilamine, and Dextromethorphan 1278
Viravan® [DSC] *See* Phenylephrine and Pyrilamine 1275
Virazide (Mex) *See* Ribavirin 1417
Virazole® *See* Ribavirin 1417
Viread® *See* Tenofovir 1549
Virestat (Mex) *See* Acyclovir 49
Virilon® *See* MethylTESTOSTERone 1030
Virilon® IM (Can) *See* Testosterone 1553
Virlix D (Mex) *See* Cetirizine and Pseudoephedrine 309

Visine A. D. (Mex) *See* Oxymetazoline ... 1208
Visine® Advanced Allergy (Can) *See* Naphazoline and Pheniramine ... 1102
Visine® Advanced Relief [OTC] *See* Tetrahydrozoline ... 1560
Visine-A® [OTC] *See* Naphazoline and Pheniramine ... 1102
Visine® L.R. [OTC] *See* Oxymetazoline ... 1208
Visine® Original [OTC] *See* Tetrahydrozoline ... 1560
Visipaque™ *See* Iodixanol ... 850
Visken® (Can) *See* Pindolol ... 1294
Vistaril® *See* HydrOXYzine ... 797
Vistide® *See* Cidofovir ... 344
Vistra 650 *See* Acetaminophen and Phenyltoloxamine ... 36
Vita-C® [OTC] *See* Ascorbic Acid ... 141
Vitalen (Mex) *See* Cyanocobalamin ... 404
Vitamin C *See* Ascorbic Acid ... 141
Vitamin D2 *See* Ergocalciferol ... 550
Vitamin D3 and Alendronate *See* Alendronate and Cholecalciferol ... 62
Vitamin B1 *See* Thiamine ... 1568
Vitamin B3 *See* Niacin ... 1124
Vitamin B6 *See* Pyridoxine ... 1376
Vitamin B12 *See* Cyanocobalamin ... 404
Vitamin D3 [OTC] *See* Cholecalciferol ... 341
Vitamin E ... 1675
Vitamin K1 *See* Phytonadione ... 1289
Vitamins (Multiple/Injectable) ... 1677
Vitelle™ Irospan® [OTC] [DSC] *See* Ferrous Sulfate and Ascorbic Acid ... 628
Vitrasert® *See* Ganciclovir ... 708
Vitussin [DSC] *See* Hydrocodone and Guaifenesin ... 779
Vivactil® *See* Protriptyline ... 1363
Vivarin® [OTC] *See* Caffeine ... 250
Vivelle-Dot® *See* Estradiol ... 576
Vivelle® [DSC] *See* Estradiol ... 576
Vivioptal Junior (Mex) *See* Magnesium Sulfate ... 966
Vivitar (Mex) *See* Spironolactone ... 1503
Vivitrol™ *See* Naltrexone ... 1099
Vivradoxil (Mex) *See* Doxycycline ... 509
VLB *See* VinBLAStine ... 1672
VM-26 *See* Teniposide ... 1549
Voflaxin (Mex) *See* Levofloxacin ... 913
Voltaren® *See* Diclofenac ... 457
Voltaren Forte (Mex) *See* Codeine ... 394
Voltaren® Gel *See* Diclofenac ... 457
Voltaren Ophtha® (Can) *See* Diclofenac ... 457
Voltaren Ophthalmic® *See* Diclofenac ... 457
Voltaren Rapide® (Can) *See* Diclofenac ... 457
Voltaren®-XR *See* Diclofenac ... 457
Vomisin (Mex) *See* DimenhyDRINATE ... 478
Voriconazole ... 1678
Vorinostat ... 1678
VoSpire ER® *See* Albuterol ... 54
VP-16 *See* Etoposide ... 607
VP-16-213 *See* Etoposide ... 607
VP-TEC (Mex) *See* Etoposide ... 607
V-Tann™ [DSC] *See* Phenylephrine and Pyrilamine ... 1275
Vulcasid (Mex) *See* Omeprazole ... 1176
Vuminix (Mex) *See* Fluvoxamine ... 678
Vumon® *See* Teniposide ... 1549
Vytorin® *See* Ezetimibe and Simvastatin ... 611
Vyvanse™ *See* Lisdexamfetamine ... 931
Warfarin ... 1679
Warfarin Sodium *See* Warfarin ... 1679
Wart-Off® Maximum Strength [OTC] *See* Salicylic Acid ... 1454
4-Way® 12 Hour [OTC] *See* Oxymetazoline ... 1208
4 Way® Fast Acting [OTC] *See* Phenylephrine ... 1273
4 Way® Menthol [OTC] *See* Phenylephrine ... 1273
4 Way® No Drip [OTC] *See* Phenylephrine ... 1273
WelChol® *See* Colesevelam ... 398
Wellbutrin® *See* BuPROPion ... 217
Wellbutrin XL™ *See* BuPROPion ... 217
Wellbutrin SR® *See* BuPROPion ... 217
Westcort® *See* Hydrocortisone ... 785
Westenicol (Mex) *See* Chloramphenicol ... 315
Westhroid™ *See* Thyroid, Desiccated ... 1579
White Mineral Oil *See* Mineral Oil ... 1055
Whitethorn *See* Hawthorn *(Crataegus oxyacantha)* ... 758
Wild Chamomile *See* Feverfew *(Tanacetum parthenium)* ... 628
Wild Quinine *See* Feverfew *(Tanacetum parthenium)* ... 628
Winpred™ (Can) *See* PredniSONE ... 1327

WinRho® SDF *See* Rho(D) Immune Globulin 1415
WR-2721 *See* Amifostine 83
WR-139007 *See* Dacarbazine 414
WR-139013 *See* Chlorambucil 315
WR-139021 *See* Carmustine 284
Wycillin® (Can) *See* Penicillin G Procaine 1241
Wycillin [DSC] *See* Penicillin G Procaine 1241
Wytensin® (Can) *See* Guanabenz 750
Xalyn-Or (Mex) *See* Amoxicillin 112
Xanax® *See* ALPRAZolam 72
Xanax TS™ (Can) *See* ALPRAZolam 72
Xanax XR® *See* ALPRAZolam 72
Xatral (Can) *See* Alfuzosin 65
Xatral OD (Mex) *See* Alfuzosin 65
Xedin (Mex) *See* Cefotaxime 295
Xeloda® *See* Capecitabine 263
Xenazine® *See* Tetrabenazine 1554
Xenical® *See* Orlistat 1184
Xifaxan™ *See* Rifaximin 1420
Xilep *See* Rufinamide 1452
Xipen (Mex) *See* Pentoxifylline 1251
XiraTuss™ [DSC] *See* Carbetapentane, Phenylephrine, and Chlorpheniramine 274
XL-Dol Infantil (Mex) *See* Acetaminophen 30
Xodol® 5/300 *See* Hydrocodone and Acetaminophen 777
Xodol® 7.5/300 *See* Hydrocodone and Acetaminophen 777
Xodol® 10/300 *See* Hydrocodone and Acetaminophen 777
Xolair® *See* Omalizumab 1174
Xolegel™ *See* Ketoconazole 876
Xopenex® *See* Levalbuterol 902
Xopenex HFA™ *See* Levalbuterol 902
Xorufec (Mex) *See* Cefuroxime 300
Xpect-HC™ [DSC] *See* Hydrocodone and Guaifenesin 779
XPECT™ [OTC] *See* GuaiFENesin 737
XPECT-PE™ [DSC] *See* Guaifenesin and Phenylephrine 742
Xusal (Mex) *See* Levocetirizine 909
Xylocaina (Mex) *See* Lidocaine 924
Xylocaine® *See* Lidocaine 924
Xylocaine® MPF *See* Lidocaine 924
Xylocaine® Viscous *See* Lidocaine 924
Xylocard® (Can) *See* Lidocaine 924
Xylometazoline 1687
Xylometazoline Hydrochloride *See* Xylometazoline 1687
Xylorane (Mex) *See* Citalopram 354
Xyrem® *See* Sodium Oxybate 1495
Xyzal® *See* Levocetirizine 909
Y-90 Ibritumomab *See* Ibritumomab 802
Y-90 Zevalin *See* Ibritumomab 802
Yagona *See* Kava Kava *(Piper methysticum)* 874
Yasmin® *See* Ethinyl Estradiol and Drospirenone 593
Yaz® *See* Ethinyl Estradiol and Drospirenone 593
Yectamicina (Mex) *See* Gentamicin 714
Yectamid (Mex) *See* Amikacin 83
Yentreve (Mex) *See* DULoxetine 516
YM087 *See* Conivaptan 400
YM905 *See* Solifenacin 1498
YM-08310 *See* Amifostine 83
Yocon® *See* Yohimbine 1688
Yodoxin® *See* Iodoquinol 851
Yohimbine 1688
Yohimbine Hydrochloride *See* Yohimbine 1688
Yuredol (Mex) *See* Cyclobenzaprine 405
Z4942 *See* Ifosfamide 809
Zactos (Mex) *See* Pioglitazone 1297
Zaditen® (Can) *See* Ketotifen 879
Zaditor® (Can) *See* Ketotifen 879
Zaditor® [OTC] *See* Ketotifen 879
Zadolina (Mex) *See* Ceftazidime 298
Zafirlukast 1689
Zalcitabine 1691
Zaldiar (Mex) *See* Acetaminophen and Tramadol 38
Zaleplon 1691
Zamicet® *See* Hydrocodone and Acetaminophen 777
Zanaflex® *See* TiZANidine 1587
Zanaflex Capsules™ *See* TiZANidine 1587
Zanamivir 1693
Zanosar® *See* Streptozocin 1510
Zantac® *See* Ranitidine 1399

Zantac 75® (Can) *See* Ranitidine ... 1399
Zantac 75® [OTC] *See* Ranitidine ... 1399
Zantac 150™ [OTC] *See* Ranitidine ... 1399
Zantac® EFFERdose® *See* Ranitidine ... 1399
Zantac Maximum Strength Non-Prescription (Can) *See* Ranitidine ... 1399
Zarontin® *See* Ethosuximide ... 603
Zaroxolyn® *See* Metolazone ... 1034
Zavesca® *See* Miglustat ... 1053
Z-chlopenthixol *See* Zuclopenthixol ... 1712
Z-Cof™ 12DM *See* Guaifenesin, Pseudoephedrine, and Dextromethorphan ... 748
Z-Cof LA™ *See* Guaifenesin and Dextromethorphan ... 739
ZD1033 *See* Anastrozole ... 125
ZD1839 *See* Gefitinib ... 709
ZDV *See* Zidovudine ... 1695
Zebeta® *See* Bisoprolol ... 190
Zebutal™ *See* Butalbital, Acetaminophen, and Caffeine ... 229
Zegerid® *See* Omeprazole and Sodium Bicarbonate ... 1179
Zeid (Mex) *See* Simvastatin ... 1486
Zelapar™ *See* Selegiline ... 1466
Zeldox® (Can) *See* Ziprasidone ... 1698
Zelmac (Mex) *See* Tegaserod ... 1541
Zelnorm® *See* Tegaserod ... 1541
Zelnorm® [DSC] (Can) *See* Tegaserod ... 1541
Zemplar® *See* Paricalcitol ... 1226
Zenapax® *See* Daclizumab ... 414
Zenchent™ *See* Ethinyl Estradiol and Norethindrone ... 597
Zeneca 182,780 *See* Fulvestrant ... 698
Zentel (Mex) *See* Albendazole ... 53
Zerit® *See* Stavudine ... 1505
ZerLor™ *See* Acetaminophen, Caffeine, and Dihydrocodeine ... 39
Zestoretic® *See* Lisinopril and Hydrochlorothiazide ... 938
Zestril® *See* Lisinopril ... 934
Zetia® *See* Ezetimibe ... 610
Zevalin® *See* Ibritumomab ... 802
Zgesic *See* Acetaminophen and Phenyltoloxamine ... 36
Ziac® *See* Bisoprolol and Hydrochlorothiazide ... 191
Ziagen® *See* Abacavir ... 22
Ziagenavir (Mex) *See* Abacavir ... 22
Ziana™ *See* Clindamycin and Tretinoin ... 364
Zibil (Mex) *See* Albuterol ... 54
Ziconotide ... 1695
Zidovudine ... 1695
Zidovudine and Lamivudine ... 1696
Zient (Mex) *See* Ezetimibe ... 610
Zilactin® (Can) *See* Lidocaine ... 924
Zilactin-L® [OTC] *See* Lidocaine ... 924
Zileuton ... 1696
Zinacef® *See* Cefuroxime ... 300
Zinecard® *See* Dexrazoxane ... 441
Zingo™ *See* Lidocaine ... 924
Zinnat (Mex) *See* Cefuroxime ... 300
Zintrepid (Mex) *See* Ezetimibe and Simvastatin ... 611
Zipra (Mex) *See* Ciprofloxacin ... 346
Ziprasidone ... 1698
Ziprasidone Hydrochloride *See* Ziprasidone ... 1698
Ziprasidone Mesylate *See* Ziprasidone ... 1698
Zirconia (Mex) *See* Acyclovir ... 49
Zithran (Mex) *See* Azithromycin ... 163
Zithromax® *See* Azithromycin ... 163
Zithromax® TRI-PAK™ *See* Azithromycin ... 163
Zithromax® Z-PAK® *See* Azithromycin ... 163
Ziverone (Mex) *See* Acyclovir ... 49
ZM-182,780 *See* Fulvestrant ... 698
Zmax™ *See* Azithromycin ... 163
Zocor® *See* Simvastatin ... 1486
Zofran® *See* Ondansetron ... 1180
Zofran® ODT *See* Ondansetron ... 1180
Zoladex® *See* Goserelin ... 735
Zoladex® LA (Can) *See* Goserelin ... 735
Zoldicam (Mex) *See* Fluconazole ... 635
Zoledronate *See* Zoledronic Acid ... 1702
Zoledronic Acid ... 1702
Zolinza™ *See* Vorinostat ... 1678
Zolmitriptan ... 1703
Zoloft® *See* Sertraline ... 1472
Zolpidem ... 1705
Zolpidem Tartrate *See* Zolpidem ... 1705

Zolpra (Mex) *See* Pantoprazole 1221
Zometa® *See* Zoledronic Acid 1702
Zomig® *See* Zolmitriptan 1703
Zomig® Nasal Spray (Can) *See* Zolmitriptan 1703
Zomig® Rapimelt (Can) *See* Zolmitriptan 1703
Zomig-ZMT® *See* Zolmitriptan 1703
Zomorph® (Can) *See* Morphine Sulfate 1077
Zonalon® *See* Doxepin 502
Zonegran® *See* Zonisamide 1708
Zonisamide 1708
Zopiclone 1711
Zorbtive® *See* Somatropin 1499
Zorced (Mex) *See* Simvastatin 1486
ZORprin® *See* Aspirin 143
Zosyn® *See* Piperacillin and Tazobactam Sodium 1302
Zovia® *See* Ethinyl Estradiol and Ethynodiol Diacetate 594
Zovirax® *See* Acyclovir 49
Ztuss™ Tablet [DSC] *See* Hydrocodone, Pseudoephedrine, and Guaifenesin 784
Ztuss™ ZT [DSC] *See* Hydrocodone and Guaifenesin 779
Zuclopenthixol 1712
Zuclopenthixol Acetate *See* Zuclopenthixol 1712
Zuclopenthixol Decanoate *See* Zuclopenthixol 1712
Zuclopenthixol Dihydrochloride *See* Zuclopenthixol 1712
Zuparex (Mex) *See* Piroxicam 1307
Zurcal (Mex) *See* Pantoprazole 1221
Zyban® *See* BuPROPion 217
Zydone® *See* Hydrocodone and Acetaminophen 777
Zyflo CR™ *See* Zileuton 1696
Zyflo® [DSC] *See* Zileuton 1696
Zyloprim® *See* Allopurinol 67
Zymanta (Mex) *See* ClonazePAM 373
Zymar® *See* Gatifloxacin 709
Zym-Fluconazole (Can) *See* Fluconazole 635
Zymine®-D *See* Triprolidine and Pseudoephedrine 1634
Zyprexa® *See* OLANZapine 1160
Zyprexa® Zydis® *See* OLANZapine 1160
Zyrtec-D (Mex) *See* Cetirizine and Pseudoephedrine 309
Zyrtec-D 12 Hour® [DSC] *See* Cetirizine and Pseudoephedrine 309
Zyrtec® Allergy [OTC] *See* Cetirizine 307
Zyrtec®, Children's Allergy [OTC] *See* Cetirizine 307
Zyrtec®, Children's Hives Relief [OTC] *See* Cetirizine 307
Zyrtec® [OTC] *See* Cetirizine 307
Zytopic™ *See* Triamcinolone 1617
Zytram® XL (Can) *See* TraMADol 1604
Zytrec-D® Allergy & Congestion [OTC] *See* Cetirizine and Pseudoephedrine 309
Zyvox® *See* Linezolid 927
Zyvoxam® (Can) *See* Linezolid 927
Zyxem (Mex) *See* Levocetirizine 909

NOTES

Other Products Offered by Lexi-Comp®

Anesthesiology & Critical Care Drug Handbook *

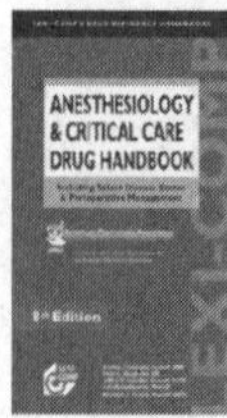

Designed for anesthesiologists, critical care practitioners, and all healthcare professionals involved in the care of surgical or ICU patients.

Includes: Comprehensive drug information to ensure the appropriate clinical management of patients; Intensivist and Anesthesiologist perspective; Over 2000 medications most commonly used in the preoperative and critical care setting; and Special Topics/Issues section with frequently encountered patient conditions

Drug Information Handbook *

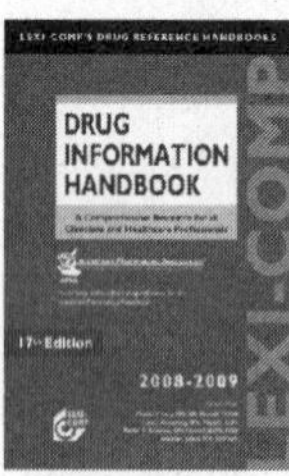

This easy-to-use drug reference is for the pharmacist, physician, or other healthcare professional requiring fast access to comprehensive drug information.

Over 1400 drug monographs are detailed with up to 32 fields of information per monograph. A valuable appendix includes hundreds of charts and reviews of special topics such as guidelines for treatment and therapy recommendations. A pharmacologic category index is also provided.

Drug Information Handbook with International Trade Names Index *

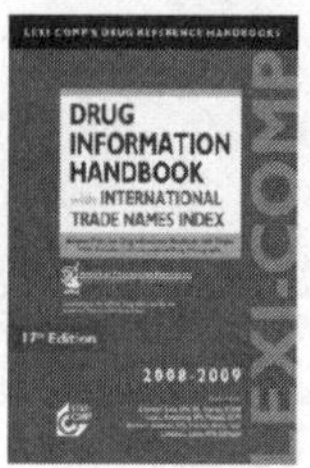

The *Drug Information Handbook with International Trade Names Index* includes the same content of our *Drug Information Handbook*, plus International drug monographs for use worldwide! This easy-to-use drug reference is compiled especially for the pharmacist, physician, or other healthcare professional professional seeking quick access to comprehensive drug information.

Drug Information Handbook for Advanced Practice Nursing

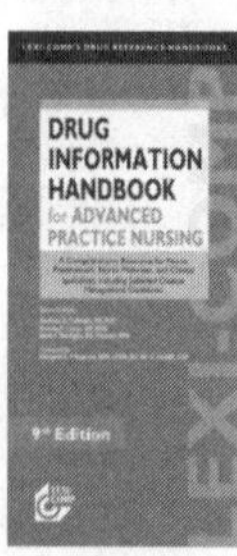

Designed to assist the Advanced Practice Nurse with prescribing, monitoring, and educating patients.

Includes: Over 4800 generic and brand names, cross-referenced by page number; Drug names and important Nursing fields highlighted in RED; Labeled and investigational indications; Adult, Geriatric, and Pediatric dosing; and up to 58 fields of information per monograph, including Patient Education and Physical Assessment.

* Published in cooperation with the American Pharmacists Association® (APhA).

To order, call Customer Service at 1-866-397-3433 or visit www.lexi.com.
Outside of the U.S., call 330-650-6506 or visit www.lexi.com

Other Products Offered by Lexi-Comp®

Drug Information Handbook for Nursing

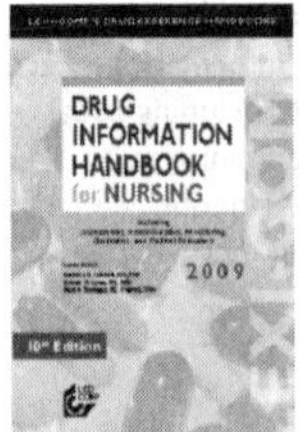

Designed for registered professional nurses and upper-division nursing students requiring dosing, administration, monitoring, and patient education information.

Includes: Over 4800 generic and brand name drugs, cross-referenced by page number; drug names and specific nursing fields highlighted in RED for easy reference, Nursing Actions field includes Physical Assessment and Patient Education guidelines

Drug Information Handbook for Oncology *

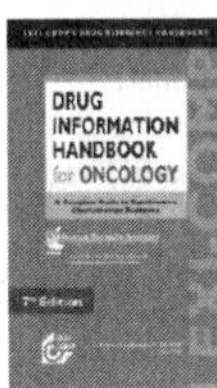

Designed for oncology professionals requiring information on combination chemotherapy regimens and dosing protocols.

Includes: Monographs containing warnings, adverse reaction profiles, drug interactions, dosing for specific indications, vesicant, emetic potential, combination regimens, and more; where applicable, a special Combination Chemotherapy field links to specific oncology monographs; Special Topics such as Cancer Treatment Related Complications, Bone Marrow Transplantation, and Drug Development

Geriatric Dosage Handbook *

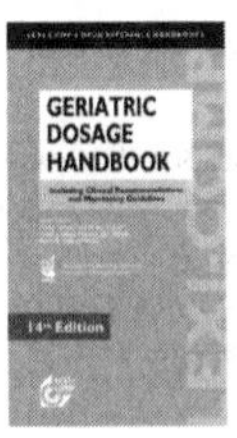

Designed for all healthcare professionals managing geriatric patients.

Includes: Up to 39 fields of information per monograph: complete adult and geriatric dosing and dosing for patients with renal/hepatic impairment; Special Geriatric Considerations; Medication Safety Issues; extensive information on drug interactions

Laboratory Test Handbook

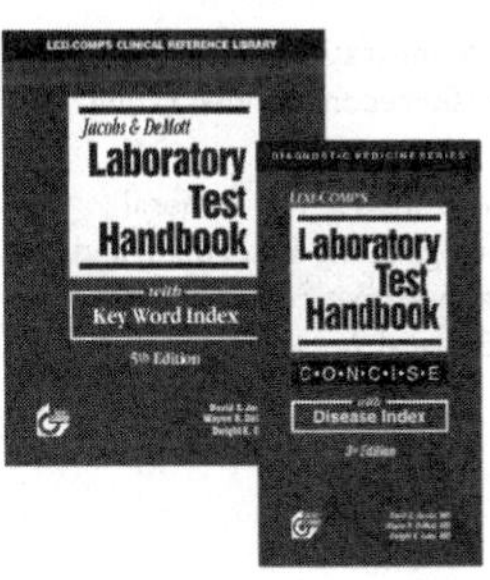

An invaluable source of information for anyone interested in diagnostic laboratory testing. Includes: 960 tests; Up to 25 fields per test; Extensive cross-referencing; Over 12,000 references; and Key Word Index: test result, disease, organ system and syndrome.

Clinicians, nurse practitioners, residents, nurses, and students will appreciate the Concise version of the *Laboratory Test Handbook* for its convenience as a quick reference. This abridged version includes 876 tests.

* Published in cooperation with the American Pharmacists Association® (APhA).

To order, call Customer Service at 1-866-397-3433 or visit www.lexi.com.
Outside of the U.S., call 330-650-6506 or visit www.lexi.com

Other Products Offered by Lexi-Comp®

Pediatric Dosage Handbook *

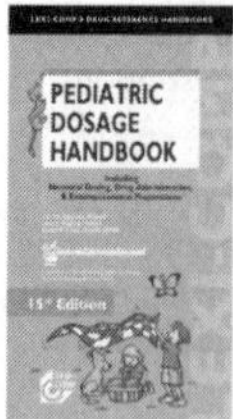

This book is designed for any healthcare professional requiring quick access to comprehensive pediatric drug information. Each monograph contains multiple fields of content, including usual dosage by age group, indication and route of administration. Drug interactions, adverse reactions, extemporaneous preparations, pharmacodynamics/pharma-cokinetics data, and medication safety issue are covered.

Also available:

Manual de Prescripción Pediátrica (Spanish version)

Pediatric Dosage Handbook with International Trade Names Index *

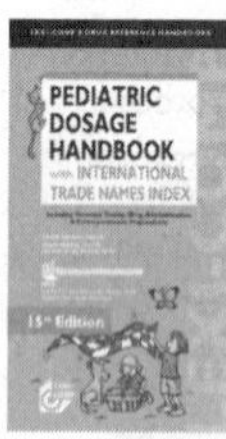

The *Pediatric Dosage Handbook with International Trade Names Index* is the trusted pediatric drug resource for medical professionals worldwide. The International Edition contains all the content of Lexi-Comp's *Pediatric Dosage Handbook*, plus an International Trade Names Index including trade names from 125 countries.

Pharmacogenomics Handbook

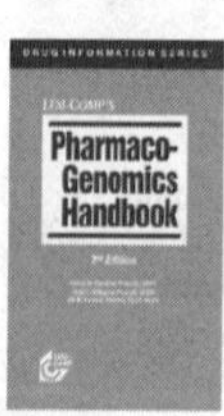

Ideal for any healthcare professional or student wishing to gain insight into the emerging field of pharmacogenomics.

Includes: Information concerning key genetic variations that may influence drug disposition and/or sensitivity; brief introductions to fundamental concepts in genetics and genomics. A foundation for all clinicians who will be called on to integrate rapidly-expanding genomic knowledge into the management of drug therapy.

Rating Scales for Mental Health

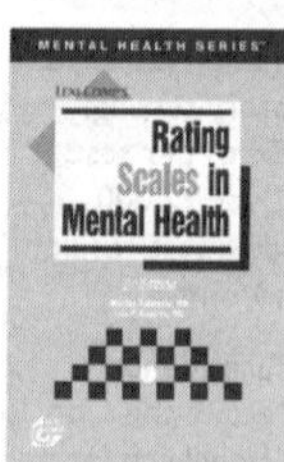

Ideal for clinicians as well as administrators, this book provides an overview of over 100 recommended rating scales for mental assessment.

Includes: Rating scales for conditions such as General Anxiety, Social/Family Functioning, Eating Disorders, and Sleep Disorders; and Monograph format covering such topics as Overview of Scale, General Applications, Psychometric Properties, and References